S0-AWH-704

DRUG INFORMATION HANDBOOK for DENTISTRY

Including Oral Medicine for Medically-Compromised Patients & Specific Oral Conditions

Richard L. Wynn, BSPharm, PhD
Timothy F. Meiller, DDS, PhD
Harold L. Crossley, DDS, PhD

12th Edition

LEXI-COMP

DRUG
INFORMATION
HANDBOOK
for DENTISTRY

Including Oral Medicine for Medically-Compromised Patients & Specific Oral Conditions

Richard L. Wynn, BSPharm, PhD
Professor of Pharmacology
Baltimore College of Dental Surgery
Dental School
University of Maryland Baltimore
Baltimore, Maryland

Timothy F. Meiller, DDS, PhD
Professor
Diagnostic Sciences and Pathology
Baltimore College of Dental Surgery
Professor of Oncology
Greenebaum Cancer Center
University of Maryland Baltimore
Baltimore, Maryland

Harold L. Crossley, DDS, PhD
Professor Emeritus
Baltimore College of Dental Surgery
Dental School
University of Maryland Baltimore
Baltimore, Maryland

LEXI-COMP

NOTICE

This handbook is intended to serve the user as a handy reference and not as a complete drug information resource. It does not include information on every therapeutic agent available. The publication covers a combination of commonly used drugs in dentistry and medicine and is specifically designed to present important aspects of drug data in a more concise format than is typically found in medical literature, exhaustive drug compendia, or product material supplied by manufacturers.

Drug information is constantly evolving because of ongoing research and clinical experience and is often subject to interpretation. While great care has been taken to ensure the accuracy of the information presented, the reader is advised that the authors, editors, reviewers, contributors, and publishers cannot be responsible for the continued currency of the information or for any errors, omissions, or the application of this information, or for any consequences arising therefrom. Therefore, the author(s) and/or the publisher shall have no liability to any person or entity with regard to claims, loss, or damage caused, or alleged to be caused, directly or indirectly, by the use of information contained herein. Because of the dynamic nature of drug information, readers are advised that decisions regarding drug therapy must be based on the independent judgment of the clinician, changing information about a drug (eg, as reflected in the literature and manufacturer's most current product information), and changing medical practices. The editors are not responsible for any inaccuracy of quotation or for any false or misleading implication that may arise due to the text or formulas as used or due to the quotation of revisions no longer official.

The editors, authors, and contributors have written this book in their private capacities. No official support or endorsement by any federal or state agency or pharmaceutical company is intended or inferred.

The publishers have made every effort to trace the copyright holders for borrowed material. If they have inadvertently overlooked any, they will be pleased to make the necessary arrangements at the first opportunity.

If you have any suggestions or questions regarding any information presented in this handbook, please contact our drug information pharmacists at (330) 650-6506.

This manual was produced using the FormuLex™ Program — a complete publishing service of Lexi-Comp, Inc.

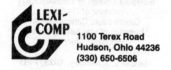

LEXI-COMP

1100 Terex Road
Hudson, Ohio 44236
(330) 650-6506

ISBN 1-59195-145-3

TABLE OF CONTENTS

About the Authors 3

Editorial Advisory Panel 4

Preface to the Twelfth Edition 10

Acknowledgments 11

Description of Sections and Fields 12

Description of Dental Use 15

Controlled Substances 16

FDA Pregnancy Categories 17

FDA Name Differentiation Project – The Use of Tall-Man Letters 18

Prescription Writing 19

Safe Writing Practices 20

ALPHABETICAL LISTING OF DRUGS 21

NATURAL PRODUCTS: HERBAL AND DIETARY SUPPLEMENTS 1609

    Effects on Various Systems 1610

    ALPHABETICAL LISTING OF NATURAL PRODUCTS 1613

ORAL MEDICINE TOPICS

    Part I: Dental Management and Therapeutic Considerations in Medically-Compromised Patients

        Table of Contents 1635

        Cardiovascular Diseases 1636

        Gastrointestinal Disorders 1654

        Respiratory Diseases 1656

        Endocrine Disorders and Pregnancy 1659

        HIV Infection and AIDS 1662

        Rheumatoid Arthritis, Osteoarthritis, and Osteoporosis 1668

        Tuberculosis 1673

        Sexually-Transmitted Diseases 1674

        Systemic Viral Diseases 1675

        Antibiotic Prophylaxis - Preprocedural Guidelines for Dental Patients 1680

    Part II: Dental Management and Therapeutic Considerations in Patients With Specific Oral Conditions and Other Medicine Topics

        Table of Contents 1691

        Oral Pain 1692

        Bacterial Infections 1697

        Periodontal Diseases 1705

        Fungal Infections 1707

        Viral Infections 1709

        Ulcerative and Erosive Disorders 1712

        Dentin Hypersensitivity, High Caries Index, and Xerostomia 1714

        Temporomandibular Dysfunction (TMD) 1724

        Sedation 1727

        Management of Patients Undergoing Cancer Therapy 1728

TABLE OF CONTENTS *(Continued)*

Part III: Sample Prescriptions

Table of Contents 1731
Bacterial Endocarditis (Prevention) 1732
Prosthetic Joint Late Infections (Prevention) 1733
Oral Pain 1734
Bacterial Infections and Periodontal Diseases 1736
Sinus Infection Treatment 1738
Antimicrobial Rinses 1739
Fungal Infections 1740
Viral Infections 1742
Ulcerative and Erosive Disorders 1744
Sedation (Prior to Dental Treatment) 1746

APPENDIX

Abbreviations and Measurements

Abbreviations, Acronyms, and Symbols 1748
Standard Conversions 1752
Apothecary / Metric Equivalents 1752
Pounds / Kilograms Conversion 1753

Pharmacology of Drug Metabolism and Interactions 1754

Infectious Disease Information

Occupational Exposure to Bloodborne Pathogens
(Standard / Universal Precautions) 1770
Immunizations (Vaccines) 1786
Tuberculosis Treatment 1800
Treatment of Sexually Transmitted Infections 1811

Laboratory Values

Normal Blood Values 1814

Over-the-Counter Dental Products

Dentifrice Products 1815
Mouth Pain, Cold Sore, and Canker Sore Products 1828
Oral Rinse Products 1831

Miscellaneous

Top 200 Prescribed Drugs in 2005 1834
Dental Drug Use in Pregnancy and Breast-Feeding 1836
Vasoconstrictor Interactions With Antidepressants 1839

INDEXES

Pharmacologic Category Index 1841
Alphabetical Index 1865

ABOUT THE AUTHORS

Richard L. Wynn, BSPharm, PhD

Richard L. Wynn, PhD, is Professor of Pharmacology at the Baltimore College of Dental Surgery, Dental School, University of Maryland Baltimore. Dr Wynn has served as a dental educator, researcher, and teacher of dental pharmacology and dental hygiene pharmacology for his entire professional career. He holds a BS (pharmacy; registered pharmacist, Maryland), an MS (physiology) and a PhD (pharmacology) from the University of Maryland. Dr Wynn chaired the Department of Pharmacology at the University of Maryland Dental School from 1980 to 1995. Previously, he chaired the Department of Oral Biology at the University of Kentucky College of Dentistry.

Dr Wynn has to his credit over 300 publications including original research articles, textbooks, textbook chapters, monographs, and articles in continuing education journals. He has given over 500 continuing education seminars to dental professionals in the U.S., Canada, and Europe. Dr Wynn has been a consultant to the drug industry for 24 years and his research laboratories have contributed to the development of new analgesics and anesthetics. He is a consultant to the Academy of General Dentistry, the American Dental Association, and a former consultant to the Council on Dental Education, Commission on Accreditation. He is a featured columnist and his drug review articles, entitled *Pharmacology Today*, appear in each issue of *General Dentistry*, a journal published by the Academy. One of his primary interests continues to be keeping dental professionals informed on all aspects of drug use in dental practice.

Timothy F. Meiller, DDS, PhD

Dr Meiller is Professor of Diagnostic Sciences and Pathology at the Baltimore College of Dental Surgery and Professor of Oncology in the Program of Oncology at the Greenebaum Cancer Center, University of Maryland Baltimore. He has held his position in Diagnostic Sciences at the Dental School for 30 years and serves as an attending faculty at the Greenebaum Cancer Center.

Dr Meiller is a Diplomate of the American Board of Oral Medicine and a graduate of Johns Hopkins University and the University of Maryland Dental and Graduate Schools, holding a DDS and a PhD in Immunology/Virology. He has over 200 publications to his credit, maintains an active general dental practice, and is a consultant to the National Institutes of Health. He is currently engaged in ongoing investigations into cellular immune dysfunction in oral diseases associated with AIDS, in cancer patients, and in other medically-compromised patients.

Harold L. Crossley, DDS, PhD

Dr Crossley is Professor Emeritus at the Baltimore College of Dental Surgery, Dental School, University of Maryland Baltimore. A native of Rhode Island, he received a Bachelor of Science degree in Pharmacy from the University of Rhode Island in 1964. He later was awarded the Master of Science (1970) and Doctorate degrees (1972) in the area of Pharmacology. The University of Maryland Dental School in Baltimore awarded Dr Crossley the DDS degree in 1980. He is the Director of Conjoint Sciences and Preclinical Studies at the School of Dentistry and maintains an intramural part-time private dental practice.

Dr Crossley has coauthored a number of articles dealing with law enforcement on both a local and federal level. This liaison with law enforcement agencies keeps him well-acquainted with the "drug culture." He has been appointed to the Governor's Commission on Prescription Drug Abuse and the Maryland State Dental Association's Well-Being Committee. Drawing on this unique background, Dr Crossley has become nationally and internationally recognized as an expert on street drugs and chemical dependency, as well as the clinical pharmacology of dental drugs.

EDITORIAL ADVISORY PANEL

4

Samir Desai, MD
Assistant Professor of Medicine
Department of Medicine
Baylor College of Medicine
Houston, Texas
Staff Physician
Veterans Affairs Medical Center
Houston, Texas

Andrew J. Donnelly, PharmD, MBA
Director of Pharmacy
and
Clinical Professor of Pharmacy Practice
University of Illinois Medical Center at Chicago
Chicago, Illinois

Thom C. Dumsha, DDS
Associate Professor and Chair
Dental School
University of Maryland Baltimore
Baltimore, Maryland

Michael S. Edwards, PharmD, MBA
Assistant Director, Weinberg Pharmacy
Johns Hopkins Hospital
Baltimore, Maryland

Vicki L. Ellingrod, PharmD, BCPP
Associate Professor
University of Iowa
Iowa City, Iowa

Kelley K. Engle, BSPharm
Pharmacotherapy Specialist
Lexi-Comp, Inc
Hudson, Ohio

Margaret A. Fitzgerald, MS, APRN, BC, NP-C, FAANP
President
Fitzgerald Health Education Associates, Inc.
North Andover, Massachusetts
Family Nurse Practitioner
Greater Lawrence Family Health Center
Lawrence, Massachusetts

Matthew A. Fuller, PharmD, BCPS, BCPP, FASHP
Clinical Pharmacy Specialist, Psychiatry
Cleveland Department of Veterans Affairs Medical Center
Brecksville, Ohio
Associate Clinical Professor of Psychiatry
Clinical Instructor of Psychology
Case Western Reserve University
Cleveland, Ohio
Adjunct Associate Professor of Clinical Pharmacy
University of Toledo
Toledo, Ohio

Morton P. Goldman, PharmD
Assistant Director, Pharmacotherapy Services
The Cleveland Clinic Foundation
Cleveland, Ohio

Julie A. Golembiewski, PharmD
Clinical Associate Professor
Colleges of Pharmacy and Medicine
Pharmacotherapist, Anesthesia/Pain
University of Illinois
Chicago, Illinois

Jeffrey P. Gonzales, PharmD
Critical Care Pharmacy Specialist
The Cleveland Clinic Foundation
Cleveland, Ohio

Barbara L. Gracious, MD
Assistant Professor of Psychiatry and Pediatrics
Case Western Reserve University
Director of Child Psychiatry and Training & Education
University Hospitals of Cleveland
Cleveland, Ohio

EDITORIAL ADVISORY PANEL *(Continued)*

Charles Lacy, RPh, PharmD, FCSHP
Vice President, Information Technologies
Professor, Pharmacy Practice
Professor, Business Leadership
University of Southern Nevada
Las Vegas, Nevada

Brenda R. Lance, RN, MSN
Program Development Director
Northcoast HealthCare Management Company
Northcoast Infusion Therapies
Oakwood Village, Ohio

Leonard L. Lance, RPh, BSPharm
Clinical Pharmacist
Lexi-Comp Inc
Hudson, Ohio

Jerrold B. Leikin, MD, FACP, FACEP, FACMT, FAACT
Director, Medical Toxicology
Evanston Northwestern Healthcare-OMEGA
Glenbrook Hospital
Glenview, Illinois
Associate Director
Toxikon Consortium at Cook County Hospital
Chicago, Illinois
Professor of Medicine
Pharmacology and Health Systems Management
Rush Medical College
Chicago, Ilinois
Professor of Medicine
Feinberg School of Medicine
Northwestern University
Chicago, Ilinois

Jeffrey D. Lewis, PharmD
Pharmacotherapy Specialist
Lexi-Comp, Inc
Hudson, Ohio

Jennifer K. Long, PharmD, BCPS
Infectious Diseases Clinical Specialist
The Cleveland Clinic Foundation
Cleveland, Ohio

Laurie S. Mauro, BS, PharmD
Associate Professor of Clinical Pharmacy
Department of Pharmacy Practice
College of Pharmacy
The University of Toledo
Toledo, Ohio

Vincent F. Mauro, BS, PharmD, FCCP
Professor of Clinical Pharmacy
College of Pharmacy
The University of Toledo
Adjunct Professor of Medicine
College of Medicine
Medical University of Ohio at Toledo
Toledo, Ohio

Timothy F. Meiller, DDS, PhD
Professor
Diagnostic Sciences and Pathology
Baltimore College of Dental Surgery
Professor of Oncology
Greenebaum Cancer Center
University of Maryland Baltimore
Baltimore, Maryland

Franklin A. Michota, Jr, MD
Head, Section of Hospital and Preoperative Medicine
Department of General Internal Medicine
The Cleveland Clinic Foundation
Cleveland, Ohio

Michael A. Militello, PharmD, BCPS
Clinical Cardiology Specialist
Department of Pharmacy
The Cleveland Clinic Foundation
Cleveland, Ohio

Elizabeth A. Tomsik, PharmD, BCPS
Pharmacotherapy Specialist
Lexi-Comp, Inc
Hudson, Ohio

Beatrice B. Turkoski, RN, PhD
Associate Professor, Graduate Faculty
Advanced Pharmacology
College of Nursing
Kent State University
Kent, Ohio

David M. Weinstein, PhD
Pharmacotherapy Specialist
Lexi-Comp, Inc.
Hudson, Ohio

Anne Marie Whelan, PharmD
College of Pharmacy
Dalhousie University
Halifax, Nova Scotia

Richard L. Wynn, PhD
Professor of Pharmacology
Baltimore College of Dental Surgery
Dental School
University of Maryland Baltimore
Baltimore, Maryland

PREFACE TO THE TWELFTH EDITION

The *Drug Information Handbook for Dentistry* continues to receive indicators of success and the authors are extremely gratified in this regard. We wish to thank each practitioner and student who has made all of the previous editions so widely accepted in the field of dentistry. In this new 12th edition, we have continued, as always, to respond to all of the comments and creative suggestions that come from our readership each year.

We know that our text remains an excellent companion to oral medicine and medical reference libraries that every clinician has available in their office. We hope that the active general dentist, the specialist, the dental hygienist, and the advanced student of dentistry remain better prepared for patient care while using this new 12th edition.

The authors of the 12th edition of the *Drug Information Handbook for Dentistry* are extremely proud that the book remains as popular and as successful as its readers have affirmed. We are confident that the dental practitioners and dental hygienists who utilize the text have found it to be easy to navigate and their knowledge regarding pharmacotherapeutics and oral medicine questions has been enhanced by its use. The complete cross-referencing of generic and brand names along with the foreign brands, makes the text the complete drug reference guide for dental practice.

The monographs now include over 1,500 drugs and these have been updated in the 12th edition with the fields easier to read and identify for all of the drugs. The drugs most commonly used in dentistry have the added fields regarding specific use considerations in dentistry. Important medical drugs also include dosing and dose formulation information. In addition, the adverse reaction section and the important uses and effects on dental treatment for all drugs have been updated throughout the text. As in each previous edition, the Oral Medicine section has been updated offering a selection of drug possibilities for management of common conditions often seen in the oral cavity. Example prescriptions are now in a stand-alone section for quicker reference. Prescribing information options are outlined and are available for easy cross reference for the dental practitioner.

The alphabetical index at the back of the text guides the reader through the text, as does the alphabetical listing of all drug names (both generic and brand names) throughout the monograph sections. The natural products section, drug synonyms, and U.S., Canadian, and Mexican brand names have all been updated.

Richard L. Wynn

Timothy F. Meiller

Harold L. Crossley

ACKNOWLEDGMENTS

This handbook exists in its present form as a result of the concerted efforts of many individuals, including Jack D. Bolinski, DDS, and Brad F. Bolinski, who recognized the need for a comprehensive dental and medical drug compendium; Robert D. Kerscher, publisher and chief executive officer of Lexi-Comp, Inc; Steven Kerscher, president and chief operating officer; Mark F. Bonfiglio, BS, PharmD, RPh, chief content officer; Stacy S. Robinson, editorial manager; Ginger S. Stein, project manager; David C. Marcus, chief information officer; Leslie Jo Hoppes, pharmacology database manager; Tracey J. Henterly, senior graphic designer; Alexandra Hart, composition specialist; and Brad F. Bolinski, director, dentistry.

Much of the material contained in this book was a result of contributions by pharmacists throughout the United States and Canada. Lexi-Comp has assisted many medical institutions in developing hospital-specific formulary manuals that contain clinical drug information, as well as dosing. Working with these clinical pharmacists, hospital pharmacy and therapeutics committees, and hospital drug information centers, Lexi-Comp has developed an evolutionary drug database that reflects the practice of pharmacy in these major institutions.

Special acknowledgment goes out to all Lexi-Comp staff members for their contributions to this handbook. In addition, the authors wish to thank their families, friends, and colleagues who supported them in their efforts to complete this handbook.

DESCRIPTION OF SECTIONS AND FIELDS

The *Drug Information Handbook for Dentistry, 12th Edition* is organized into six sections: Introductory text; alphabetical listing of drug monographs; natural products; oral medicine topics; appendix; and indexes which include pharmacologic categories and alphabetical listings containing generic product names and synonyms, as well as U.S., Canadian, and Mexican brand names.

INTRODUCTORY TEXT

Helpful guides to understanding the organization and format of the information in this handbook.

DRUG MONOGRAPHS

This alphabetical listing of drugs contains comprehensive monographs for medications commonly prescribed in dentistry and concise monographs for other popular drugs which dental patients may be taking. Monographs may contain the following fields:

Generic Name	U.S. adopted name
Pronunciation	Phonetic pronunciation guide
Related Information	Cross-reference(s) to pertinent information in other sections of this handbook
Related Sample Prescriptions	Cross-reference(s) to sample prescriptions.
U.S. Brand Names	Trade name(s) (manufacturer-specific) found in the United States. The symbol [DSC] appears after trade names that have been recently discontinued.
Canadian Brand Names	Trade name(s) found in Canada
Mexican Brand Names	Trade name(s) found in Mexico
Generic Available	Indicated by a "yes" or "no" if information available
Synonyms	Other names or accepted abbreviations of the generic drug
Pharmacologic Category	Indicates one or more systematic classifications of the drug
Dental Use	Information in the **Dental Use** field indicates when a drug has an established use specific to dentistry and/or oral medicine. In some cases, these uses are considered to be unlabeled, as they are not included in the FDA-approved product labeling. (see Description of Dental Use)
Use	Statements under the **Use** field reflect the approved labeling by the FDA based on accepted clinical evaluation on safety and efficacy of the drug as submitted in the New Drug Application (NDA). The "gold standard" of clinical testing of a new drug requires a randomly-selected cohort of subjects, using a double-blind and placebo controlled protocol and an acceptable method of assessment to test differences between test compound and placebo. It is assumed that by their approval of the labeling, the FDA considers the new drug "safe and effective" for treating a particular condition in a given patient population.
Unlabeled/Investigational Use	Statements under the **Unlabeled/Investigational** use field refer to other conditions, dosages, or routes of administration which are decided by the prescriber, where such uses have not been officially approved by the FDA. Such "off label" use usually occurs in response to published studies supporting a drug's effectiveness in a new use and/or alternative dosing strategy. It is important to note that individual reports do not necessarily indicate in and of themselves that the safety and effectiveness of the drug in question has been established for the new use. If an individual report is one of many studies, the clinician is encouraged to read and critically review all of the studies in order to arrive at a decision on the safety and efficacy for the "off label" use.
Local Anesthetic/Vasoconstrictor Precautions	Specific information to prevent potential drug interactions related to anesthesia
Effects on Dental Treatment	Includes significant side effects of drug therapy which may directly or indirectly affect dental treatment or diagnosis; may also contain suggested management approaches and patient handling or care.
Significant Adverse Effects	Side effects are grouped by percentage of incidence (if known) and/or body system; in the interest of saving space, <1% effects are grouped only by percentage. **Note:** For nondental-specific drugs, this field includes only the most common adverse effects and does not include <1% effects.

Restrictions	The controlled substance classification from the Drug Enforcement Agency (DEA). U.S. schedules are I-V. Schedules vary by country and sometimes state (ie, Massachusetts uses I-VI)
Dental Usual Dosing	The amount of the drug to be typically given or taken during dental treatment for children and adults
Dosage	The amount of the drug to be typically given or taken during therapy for children and adults; also includes any dosing adjustment/comments for renal impairment or hepatic failure
Mechanism of Action	How the drug works in the body to elicit a response
Contraindications	Information pertaining to inappropriate use of the drug
Warnings/Precautions	Precautionary considerations, hazardous conditions related to use of the drug, and disease states or patient populations in which the drug should be cautiously used
Drug Interactions	If a drug has demonstrated involvement with cytochrome P450 enzymes, the initial line of this field will identify the drug as an inhibitor, inducer, or substrate of specific isoenzymes (ie, CYP1A2). Isoenzymes are identified as substrates (minor or major), inhibitors (weak or moderate or strong), and inducers (weak or strong). A summary of this information can also be found in a tabular format within the introductory section. The remainder of the field presents a description of the interaction between the drug listed in the monograph and other drugs or drug classes. May include possible mechanisms and effect of combined therapy. May also include a strategy to manage the patient on combined therapy (ie, quinidine). **Note:** For nondental-specific drugs, the Drug Interactions field is abbreviated and broken down into 3 subcategories: **Cytochrome P450 Effect, Increased Effect/Toxicity, and Decreased Effect**
Ethanol/Nutrition/Herb Interactions	Information regarding potential interactions with food, nutritionals, herbal products, vitamins, or ethanol
Dietary Considerations	Includes information on how the medication should be taken relative to meals or food
Pharmacodynamics/Kinetics	The magnitude of a drug's effect depends on the drug concentration at the site of action. The pharmacodynamics are expressed in terms of onset of action and duration of action. Pharmacokinetics are expressed in terms of absorption, distribution (including appearance in breast milk and crossing of the placenta), protein binding, metabolism, bioavailability, half-life, time to peak serum concentration, and elimination.
Pregnancy Risk Factor	Five categories established by the FDA to indicate the potential of a systemically absorbed drug for causing birth defects
Lactation	Information describing characteristics of using the drug listed in the monograph while breast-feeding (where recommendation of American Academy of Pediatrics differs, notation is made).
Breast-Feeding Considerations	Further information relating to taking the drug while nursing
Dosage Forms	Information with regard to form, strength, and availability of the drug **Note:** For nondental-specific drugs, the information is strung with the forms in all caps and bolded and uses the following abbreviations: AERO = aerosol; CAP = capsule; CONC = concentrate; CRM = cream; CRYST = crystals; ELIX = elixir; GRAN = granules; INF = infusion; INJ = injection; LIQ = liquid; LOZ = lozenge; OINT = ointment; SHAMP = shampoo; SOLN = solution; SUPP = suppository; SUSP = suspension; SYR = syrup; TAB = tablet.
Dental Comment	Pharmacology-related comments and considerations relevant to the dental professional
Selected Readings	Sources and literature where the user may find additional information

DESCRIPTION OF SECTIONS AND FIELDS *(Continued)*

NATURAL PRODUCTS: HERBAL AND DIETARY SUPPLEMENTS

This section is divided into three parts. First, is a brief introduction to popular natural products, followed by an alphabetical listing of herbal and dietary supplements commonly purchased over-the-counter which patients may be taking. Monographs may contain the following:

NATURAL PRODUCT MONOGRAPHS

Name	Common name
Related Information	Cross-reference(s) to related monographs
Synonyms	Other names (scientific or slang) and accepted abbreviations
Use	Information pertaining to appropriate medical indications for the product; some include recommendations from Commission E.
Local Anesthetic/Vasoconstrictor Precautions	Specific information to prevent potential interactions related to anesthesia
Effects on Bleeding	How the product affects bleeding during dental procedures
Warnings/Precautions	Cautions and hazardous conditions related to use

ORAL MEDICINE TOPICS

This section is divided into three major parts and contains text on Oral Medicine topics. In each subsection, the systemic condition or the oral disease state is described briefly, followed by the pharmacologic considerations with which the dentist must be familiar.

Part I: **Dental Management and Therapeutic Considerations in Medically-Compromised Patients:** Focuses on common medical conditions and their associated drug therapies with which the dentist must be familiar. Patient profiles with commonly associated drug regimens are described.

Part II: **Dental Management and Therapeutic Considerations in Patients With Specific Oral Conditions:** Focuses on therapies the dentist may choose to prescribe for patients suffering from oral disease or who are in need of special care. Some overlap between these sections has resulted from systemic conditions that have oral manifestations and vice-versa. Cross-references to the descriptions and the monographs for individual drugs described elsewhere in this handbook allow for easy retrieval of information. Example prescriptions for drugs commonly used in the treatment of each condition are presented so that the clinician can evaluate alternate approaches to treatment. Seldom is there a single drug of choice.

Note: Prescriptions listed represent prototype drugs and popular prescriptions and are examples only. The pharmacologic category index is available for cross-referencing if alternatives or additional drugs are sought.

Part III: **Sample Prescriptions:** Examples provided for prototype drugs and popular prescriptions. Prescriptions included for the following uses: Bacterial endocarditis (prevention), prosthetic joint late infections (prevention), oral pain, bacterial infections and periodontal diseases, sinus infection treatment, antimicrobial rinses, fungal infections, viral infections, ulcerative and erosive disorders, sedation (prior to dental treatment)

APPENDIX

The appendix is broken down into various sections for easy use and offers a compilation of tables and guidelines which can often be helpful when considering patient care. It includes descriptions of most over-the-counter oral care products and dental drug interactions, in addition to, infectious disease information and the top 200 drugs prescribed in 2005.

INDEXES

This section includes a pharmacologic category index with an easy-to-use classification system in alphabetical order and an alphabetical index which provides a quick reference for generic names, synonyms, U.S., Canadian, and Mexican brand names. From this index, the reader can cross-reference to the monographs.

DESCRIPTION OF DENTAL USE

UNLABELED USE AND ROUTES OF ADMINISTRATION IN DENTISTRY AND ORAL MEDICINE

The off-label use of a medication may involve differences in either the intended purpose or the route of administration of a particular medication. In dentistry, there are some situations which are common (clindamycin for endocarditis prophylaxis), and uncommon (application of Kenalog® cream to the oral mucosa) which may be termed "unlabeled use". Depending on the degree of familiarity, the prescription of a drug for an off-label purpose may create concern on the part of healthcare professionals who are less familiar with the dental use of these medications. For example, a pharmacist may note the statement "for external use only" on the label of a tube of topical cream and question whether the drug should be applied to the oral mucosa. Usually, reinforcement of the use of a drug as well as an analysis of the likely systemic exposure/toxicity, can address these concerns.

The dentist who prescribes a drug bears the responsibility for deciding on the purpose of the prescription and the detail of the dosing regimen. These professional decisions are based on information from a variety of sources, including (but not limited to) the official labeling, sound scientific evidence, expert medical judgment, or published literature. In selected situations, these sources may justify the use of a drug in an off-label manner. Accepted professional standards indicate off-label use of a drug must be initiated in good faith, serve the best interest of the patient, and must be undertaken without fraudulent intent. Healthcare providers should recognize that the approved labeling is not intended to limit the practitioners in the exercise of his or her best professional judgment in serving the interest of patients. In addition, the purpose of labeling is not intended to impose liability for off-label use. However, it should be noted that a practitioner may be accountable for the negligent use in a civil action regardless of whether the FDA has approved the use of the drug in question. Based on these assertions, at least one medical organization (the American Academy of Pediatrics) has published in an official policy statement that the practice of medicine may actually require a practitioner to use drugs in an off-label manner in order to provide the most appropriate treatment for a given patient. Off-label use in dentistry and oral medicine is a frequently encountered issue. A discussion of the off-label use of drugs in dentistry appears in the *ADA Guide to Dental Therapeutics*, 3rd Edition, edited by Sebastian G. Ciancio, DDS in cooperation with the ADA Council on Scientific Affairs.

CONTROLLED SUBSTANCES

Schedule I = C-I

The drugs and other substances in this schedule have no legal medical uses except research. They have a **high** potential for abuse. They include selected opiates such as heroin, opium derivatives, and hallucinogens.

Schedule II = C-II

The drugs and other substances in this schedule have legal medical uses and a **high** abuse potential which may lead to severe dependence. They include former "Class A" narcotics, amphetamines, barbiturates, and other drugs.

Schedule III = C-III

The drugs and other substances in this schedule have legal medical uses and a **lesser** degree of abuse potential which may lead to **moderate** dependence. They include former "Class B" narcotics and other drugs.

Schedule IV = C-IV

The drugs and other substances in this schedule have legal medial uses and **low** abuse potential which may lead to **moderate** dependence. They include barbiturates, benzodi-azepines, propoxyphenes, and other drugs.

Schedule V = C-V

The drugs and other substances in this schedule have legal medical uses and **low** abuse potential which may lead to **moderate** dependence. They include narcotic cough preparations, diarrhea preparations, and other drugs.

Note: These are federal classifications. Your individual state may place a substance into a more restricted category. When this occurs, the more restricted category applies. Consult your state law.

FDA PREGNANCY CATEGORIES

Throughout this book there is a field labeled Pregnancy Risk Factor (PRF) and the letter A, B, C, D, or X immediately following which signifies a category. The FDA has established these five categories to indicate the potential of a systemically absorbed drug for causing birth defects. The key differentiation among the categories rests upon the reliability of documentation and the risk:benefit ratio. Pregnancy Category X is particularly notable in that if any data exists that may implicate a drug as a teratogen and the risk:benefit ratio is clearly negative, the drug is contraindicated during pregnancy.

These categories are summarized as follows:

A   Controlled studies in pregnant women fail to demonstrate a risk to the fetus in the first trimester with no evidence of risk in later trimesters. The possibility of fetal harm appears remote.

B   Either animal-reproduction studies have not demonstrated a fetal risk but there are no controlled studies in pregnant women, or animal-reproduction studies have shown an adverse effect (other than a decrease in fertility) that was not confirmed in controlled studies in women in the first trimester and there is no evidence of a risk in later trimesters.

C   Either studies in animals have revealed adverse effects on the fetus (teratogenic or embryocidal effects or other) and there are no controlled studies in women, or studies in women and animals are not available. Drugs should be given only if the potential benefits justify the potential risk to the fetus.

D   There is positive evidence of human fetal risk, but the benefits from use in pregnant women may be acceptable despite the risk (eg, if the drug is needed in a life-threatening situation or for a serious disease for which safer drugs cannot be used or are ineffective).

X   Studies in animals or human beings have demonstrated fetal abnormalities or there is evidence of fetal risk based on human experience, or both, and the risk of the use of the drug in pregnant women clearly outweighs any possible benefit. The drug is contraindicated in women who are or may become pregnant.

FDA NAME DIFFERENTIATION PROJECT: THE USE OF TALL-MAN LETTERS

Confusion between similar drug names is an important cause of medication errors. For years, The Institute For Safe Medication Practices (ISMP), has urged generic manufacturers to use a combination of large and small letters as well as bolding (ie, chlorpro**MA-ZINE** and chlorpro**PAMIDE**) to help distinguish drugs with look-alike names, especially when they share similar strengths. Recently the FDA's Division of Generic Drugs began to issue recommendation letters to manufacturers suggesting this novel way to label their products to help reduce this drug name confusion. Although this project has had marginal success, the method has successfully eliminated problems with products such as diphenhydr**AMINE** and dimenhy**DRINATE**. Hospitals should also follow suit by making similar changes in their own labels, preprinted order forms, computer screens and printouts, and drug storage location labels.

The following is a list of product names and recommended FDA revisions you will find in this book:

Drug Product	Recommended Revision
acetazolamide	aceta**ZOLAMIDE**
acetohexamide	aceto**HEXAMIDE**
bupropion	bu**PROP**ion
buspirone	bus**PIR**one
chlorpromazine	chlorpro**MAZINE**
chlorpropamide	chlorpro**PAMIDE**
clomiphene	clomi**PHENE**
clomipramine	clomi**PRAMINE**
cycloserine	cyclo**SERINE**
cyclosporine	cyclo**SPORINE**
daunorubicin	**DAUNO**rubicin
dimenhydrinate	dimenhy**DRINATE**
diphenhydramine	diphenhydr**AMINE**
dobutamine	**DOBUT**amine
dopamine	**DOP**amine
doxorubicin	**DOXO**rubicin
glipizide	glipi**ZIDE**
glyburide	gly**BURIDE**
hydralazine	hydr**ALAZINE**
hydroxyzine	hydr**OXY**zine
medroxyprogesterone	medroxy**PROGESTER**one
methylprednisolone	methyl**PREDNIS**olone
methyltestosterone	methyl**TESTOSTER**one
nicardipine	ni**CAR**dipine
nifedipine	**NIFE**dipine
prednisolone	predniso**LONE**
prednisone	predni**SONE**
sulfadiazine	sulfa**DIAZINE**
sulfisoxazole	sulfi**SOXAZOLE**
tolazamide	**TOLAZ**amide
tolbutamide	**TOLBUT**amide
vinblastine	vin**BLAS**tine
vincristine	vin**CRIS**tine

Institute for Safe Medication Practices. "New Tall-Man Lettering Will Reduce Mix-Ups Due to Generic Drug Name Confusion," *ISMP Medication Safety Alert*, September 19, 2001. Available at: http://www.ismp.org.

Institute for Safe Medication Practices. "Prescription Mapping, Can Improve Efficiency While Minimizing Errors With Look-Alike Products," *ISMP Medication Safety Alert*, October 6, 1999. Available at: http://www.ismp.org.

U.S. Pharmacopeia, "USP Quality Review: Use Caution-Avoid Confusion," March 2001, No. 76. Available at: http://www.usp.org.

PRESCRIPTION WRITING

Doctor's Name
Address
Phone Number

Patient's Name/Date

Patient's Address/Age

Rx:

Drug Name/Dosage Size

Disp: Number of tablets, capsules, ounces to be dispensed (roman numerals added as precaution for abused drugs)

Sig: Direction on how drug is to be taken

Doctor's signature

State license number

DEA number (if required)

PRESCRIPTION REQUIREMENTS

1. Date
2. Full name and address of patient
3. Name and address of prescriber
4. Signature of prescriber

If Class II drug, Drug Enforcement Agency (DEA) number necessary.

If Class II and Class III narcotic, a triplicate prescription form (in the state of California) is necessary and it must be handwritten by the prescriber.

Please turn to appropriate oral medicine chapters for examples of prescriptions.

SAFE WRITING PRACTICES

Health professionals and their support personnel frequently produce handwritten copies of information they see in print; therefore, such information is subjected to even greater possibilities for error or misinterpretation on the part of others. Thus, particular care must be given to how drug names and strengths are expressed when creating written health-care documents.

The following are a few examples of safe writing rules suggested by the Institute for Safe Medication Practices, Inc.*

1. There should be a space between a number and its units as it is easier to read. There should be no periods after the abbreviations mg or mL.

Correct	Incorrect
10 mg	10mg
100 mg	100mg

2. Never place a decimal and a zero after a whole number (2 mg is correct and 2.0 mg is **incorrect**). If the decimal point is not seen because it falls on a line or because individuals are working from copies where the decimal point is not seen, this causes a tenfold overdose.

3. Just the opposite is true for numbers less than one. Always place a zero before a naked decimal (0.5 mL is correct, .5 mL is **incorrect**).

4. Never abbreviate the word unit. The handwritten U or u, looks like a 0 (zero), and may cause a tenfold overdose error to be made.

5. IU is not a safe abbreviation for international units. The handwritten IU looks like IV. Write out international units or use int. units.

6. Q.D. is not a safe abbreviation for once daily, as when the Q is followed by a sloppy dot, it looks like QID which means four times daily.

7. O.D. is not a safe abbreviation for once daily, as it is properly interpreted as meaning "right eye" and has caused liquid medications such as saturated solution of potassium iodide and Lugol's solution to be administered incorrectly. There is no safe abbreviation for once daily. It must be written out in full.

8. Do not use chemical names such as 6-mercaptopurine or 6-thioguanine, as sixfold overdoses have been given when these were not recognized as chemical names. The proper names of these drugs are mercaptopurine or thioguanine.

9. Do not abbreviate drug names (5FC, 6MP, 5-ASA, MTX, HCTZ, CPZ, PBZ, etc) as they are misinterpreted and cause error.

10. Do not use the apothecary system or symbols.

11. Do not abbreviate microgram as µg; instead use mcg as there is less likelihood of misinterpretation.

12. When writing an outpatient prescription, write a complete prescription. A complete prescription can prevent the prescriber, the pharmacist, and/or the patient from making a mistake and can eliminate the need for further clarification. The legible prescriptions should contain:

   a. patient's full name

   b. for pediatric or geriatric patients: their age (or weight where applicable)

   c. drug name, dosage form and strength; if a drug is new or rarely prescribed, print this information

   d. number or amount to be dispensed

   e. complete instructions for the patient, including the purpose of the medication

   f. when there are recognized contraindications for a prescribed drug, indicate to the pharmacist that you are aware of this fact (ie, when prescribing a potassium salt for a patient receiving an ACE inhibitor, write "K serum leveling being monitored")

*From "Safe Writing" by Davis NM, PharmD and Cohen MR, MS, Lecturers and Consultants for Safe Medication Practices, 1143 Wright Drive, Huntington Valley, PA 19006. Phone: (215) 947-7566.

ALPHABETICAL LISTING OF DRUGS

1370-999-397 *see* Anagrelide *on page 124*

A₁-PI *see* Alpha₁-Proteinase Inhibitor *on page 73*

A200® Lice [OTC] *see* Permethrin *on page 1218*

A-200® Maximum Strength [OTC] *see* Pyrethrins and Piperonyl Butoxide *on page 1315*

A and D® Original [OTC] *see* Vitamin A and Vitamin D *on page 1580*

Abacavir (a BAK a veer)

Related Information
HIV Infection and AIDS *on page 1662*

U.S. Brand Names Ziagen®

Canadian Brand Names Ziagen®

Generic Available No

Synonyms Abacavir Sulfate; ABC

Pharmacologic Category Antiretroviral Agent, Reverse Transcriptase Inhibitor (Nucleoside)

Use Treatment of HIV infections in combination with other antiretroviral agents

Local Anesthetic/Vasoconstrictor Precautions No information available to require special precautions

Effects on Dental Treatment No significant effects or complications reported

Common Adverse Effects Hypersensitivity reactions (which may be fatal) occur in ~5% of patients. Symptoms may include anaphylaxis, fever, rash (including erythema multiforme), fatigue, diarrhea, abdominal pain; respiratory symptoms (eg, pharyngitis, dyspnea, cough, adult respiratory distress syndrome, or respiratory failure); headache, malaise, lethargy, myalgia, myolysis, arthralgia, edema, paresthesia, nausea and vomiting, mouth ulcerations, conjunctivitis, lymphadenopathy, hepatic failure, and renal failure.

Note: Rates of adverse reactions were defined during combination therapy with other antiretrovirals (lamivudine and efavirenz **or** lamivudine and zidovudine). Only reactions which occurred at a higher frequency than in the comparator group are noted. Adverse reaction rates attributable to abacavir alone are not available.

>10%:
  Central nervous system: Headache (7% to 13%), fatigue and malaise (7% to 12%)
  Gastrointestinal: Nausea (7% to 19%, children 9%)
1% to 10%:
  Central nervous system: Depression (6%), dizziness (6%), fever (6%, children 9%), anxiety (5%), abnormal dreams (10%)
  Dermatologic: Rash (5% to 6%, children 7%)
  Gastrointestinal: Diarrhea (7%), vomiting (2% to 10%, children 9%), abdominal pain (6%)
  Hematologic: Thrombocytopenia (1%)
  Hepatic: AST increased (6%)
  Neuromuscular and skeletal: Musculoskeletal pain (5% to 6%)
  Respiratory: Bronchitis (4%), respiratory viral infection (5%)
  Miscellaneous: Hypersensitivity reactions (9%; may include reactions to other components of antiretroviral regimen), infection (EENT 5%)

Restrictions An FDA-approved medication guide is available at http://www.fda.gov/cder/Offices/ODS/labeling.htm; distribute to each patient to whom this medication is dispensed.

Mechanism of Action Nucleoside reverse transcriptase inhibitor. Abacavir is a guanosine analogue which is phosphorylated to carbovir triphosphate which interferes with HIV viral RNA-dependent DNA polymerase resulting in inhibition of viral replication.

Drug Interactions
Increased Effect/Toxicity: Abacavir increases the blood levels of amprenavir. Abacavir may decrease the serum concentration of methadone in some patients. Concomitant use of ribavirin and nucleoside analogues may increase the risk of developing lactic acidosis (includes adefovir, didanosine, lamivudine, stavudine, zalcitabine, zidovudine).

Pharmacodynamics/Kinetics
Absorption: Rapid and extensive absorption

Distribution: V_d: 0.86 L/kg

Protein binding: 50%

Metabolism: Hepatic via alcohol dehydrogenase and glucuronyl transferase to inactive carboxylate and glucuronide metabolites

Bioavailability: 83%

Half-life elimination: 1.5 hours

Time to peak: 0.7-1.7 hours
Excretion: Primarily urine (as metabolites, 1.2% as unchanged drug); feces (16% total dose)
Pregnancy Risk Factor C

Abacavir and Lamivudine (a BAK a veer & la MI vyoo deen)

Related Information
Abacavir *on page 22*
Lamivudine *on page 894*
U.S. Brand Names Epzicom™
Canadian Brand Names Kivexa™
Generic Available No
Synonyms Abacavir Sulfate and Lamivudine; Lamivudine and Abacavir
Pharmacologic Category Antiretroviral Agent, Reverse Transcriptase Inhibitor (Nucleoside)
Use Treatment of HIV infections in combination with other antiretroviral agents
Local Anesthetic/Vasoconstrictor Precautions No information available to require special precautions
Effects on Dental Treatment No significant effects or complications reported
Common Adverse Effects Percentages reported with once daily abacavir, lamivudine, and efavirenz administration. Also see individual agents.
1% to 10%:
Central nervous system: Fatigue/malaise (7%), headache/migraine (7%), insomnia (7%), dizziness/vertigo (6%), pyrexia (5%), abnormal dreams (4%), anxiety (3%)
Dermatologic: Rash (5%)
Gastrointestinal: Nausea (6%), diarrhea (5%), abdominal pain/gastritis (4%)
Miscellaneous: Hypersensitivity (9%)
Restrictions An FDA-approved medication guide is available at www.fda.gov/cder/Offices/ODS/labeling.htm; distribute to each patient to whom this medication is dispensed.
Mechanism of Action Nucleoside reverse transcriptase inhibitor combination.

Abacavir is a guanosine analogue which is phosphorylated to carbovir triphosphate which interferes with HIV viral RNA-dependent DNA polymerase resulting in inhibition of viral replication.

Lamivudine is a cytosine analog. After lamivudine is triphosphorylated, the principle mode of action is inhibition of HIV reverse transcription via viral DNA chain termination; inhibits RNA-dependent DNA polymerase activities of reverse transcriptase.
Drug Interactions
Increased Effect/Toxicity: See individual agents.
Decreased Effect: See individual agents.
Pharmacodynamics/Kinetics See individual agents.
Pregnancy Risk Factor C

Abacavir, Lamivudine, and Zidovudine
(a BAK a veer, la MI vyoo deen, & zye DOE vyoo deen)

Related Information
Abacavir *on page 22*
Lamivudine *on page 894*
Zidovudine *on page 1594*
U.S. Brand Names Trizivir®
Generic Available No
Synonyms Azidothymidine, Abacavir, and Lamivudine; AZT, Abacavir, and Lamivudine; Compound S, Abacavir, and Lamivudine; Lamivudine, Abacavir, and Zidovudine; 3TC, Abacavir, and Zidovudine; ZDV, Abacavir, and Lamivudine; Zidovudine, Abacavir, and Lamivudine
Pharmacologic Category Antiretroviral Agent, Reverse Transcriptase Inhibitor (Nucleoside)
Use Treatment of HIV infection (either alone or in combination with other antiretroviral agents) in patients whose regimen would otherwise contain the components of Trizivir®
Local Anesthetic/Vasoconstrictor Precautions No information available to require special precautions
Effects on Dental Treatment No significant effects or complications reported
Common Adverse Effects Fatal hypersensitivity reactions have occurred in patients taking abacavir (in Trizivir®). If Trizivir® is to be restarted following an
(Continued)

Abacavir, Lamivudine, and Zidovudine *(Continued)*

interruption in therapy, first evaluate the patient for previously unsuspected symptoms of hypersensitivity. Do not restart if hypersensitivity is suspected or if hypersensitivity cannot be ruled out.

The following information is based on CNAAB3003 study data concerning effects noted in patients receiving abacavir, lamivudine, and zidovudine. See individual agents for additional information.

>10%:

Endocrine & metabolic: Triglycerides increased (25%)

Gastrointestinal: Nausea (47%), nausea and vomiting (16%), diarrhea (12%), loss of appetite/anorexia (11%)

1% to 10%:

Central nervous system: Insomnia (7%)

Miscellaneous: Hypersensitivity (5% based on abacavir component)

Other (frequency unknown): GGTP increased, pancreatitis

Restrictions An FDA-approved medication guide is available at www.fda.gov/cder/Offices/ODS/labeling.htm; distribute to each patient to whom this medication is dispensed.

Mechanism of Action The combination of abacavir, lamivudine, and zidovudine is believed to act synergistically to inhibit reverse transcriptase via DNA chain termination after incorporation of the nucleoside analogue as well as to delay the emergence of mutations conferring resistance.

Drug Interactions

Increased Effect/Toxicity: See individual agents.

Decreased Effect: See individual agents.

Pharmacodynamics/Kinetics Bioavailability studies of Trizivir® show no difference in AUC or C_{max} when compared to abacavir, lamivudine, and zidovudine given together as individual agents. See individual agents.

Pregnancy Risk Factor C

Abacavir Sulfate *see* Abacavir *on page 22*

Abacavir Sulfate and Lamivudine *see* Abacavir and Lamivudine *on page 23*

Abarelix *(a ba REL iks)*

U.S. Brand Names Plenaxis™ [DSC]

Generic Available No

Synonyms PPI-149; R-3827

Pharmacologic Category Gonadotropin Releasing Hormone Antagonist

Use Palliative treatment of advanced symptomatic prostate cancer; treatment is limited to men who are not candidates for LHRH therapy, refuse surgical castration, and have one or more of the following complications due to metastases or local encroachment: 1) risk of neurological compromise, 2) ureteral or bladder outlet obstruction, or 3) severe bone pain (persisting despite narcotic analgesia)

Local Anesthetic/Vasoconstrictor Precautions No information available to require special precautions (see Dental Comment)

Effects on Dental Treatment No significant effects or complications reported

Common Adverse Effects

>10%:

Cardiovascular: Hot flushes (79%), peripheral edema (15%)

Central nervous system: Sleep disturbance (44%), pain (31%), dizziness (12%), headache (12%)

Endocrine & metabolic: Breast enlargement (30%), nipple discharge/tenderness (20%)

Gastrointestinal: Constipation (15%), diarrhea (11%)

Neuromuscular & skeletal: Back pain (17%)

Respiratory: Upper respiratory infection (12%)

1% to 10%:

Central nervous system: Fatigue (10%)

Endocrine & metabolic: Serum triglycerides increased (10%)

Gastrointestinal: Nausea (10%)

Genitourinary: Dysuria (10%), micturition frequency (10%), urinary retention (10%), urinary tract infection (10%)

Hepatic: Transaminases increased (2% to 8%)

Miscellaneous: Allergic reactions (urticaria, pruritus, syncope, hypotension): risk increases with prolonged treatment

Restrictions Abarelix is not distributed through retail pharmacies. Prescribing and distribution of abarelix is limited to physicians and hospital pharmacies participating in the Plenaxis™ PLUS program. See Additional Information, or contact Praecis Pharmaceuticals at www.plenaxisplus.com or by calling 1-877-772-3247.

Mechanism of Action Competes with naturally-occurring GnRH for binding on receptors of the pituitary. Suppresses LH and FSH, resulting in decreased testosterone.

Drug Interactions

Increased Effect/Toxicity: When used with other QT_c-prolonging agents, additive QT_c prolongation may occur. Life-threatening ventricular arrhythmias may result; example drugs include class Ia and class III antiarrhythmics, cisapride, selected quinolones, erythromycin, pimozide, mesoridazine, and thioridazine.

Pharmacodynamics/Kinetics

Distribution: V_d: 4040 L ($\pm$ 1607)

Metabolism: Hepatic, via peptide hydrolysis

Half-life elimination: 13 days

Time to peak, serum: 3 days (following I.M. administration)

Excretion: Urine (13% as unchanged drug)

Pregnancy Risk Factor X

Dental Comment

This drug is known to prolong the QT interval. The QT interval is measured as the time and distance between the Q point of the QRS complex and the end of the T wave in the ECG tracing. After adjustment for heart rate, the QT interval is defined as prolonged if it is more than 450 msec in men and 460 msec in women. A long QT syndrome was first described in the 1950s and 60s as a congenital syndrome involving QT interval prolongation and syncope and sudden death. Some of the congenital long QT syndromes were characterized by a peculiar electrocardiographic appearance of the QRS complex involving a premature atria beat followed by a pause, then a subsequent sinus beat showing marked QT prolongation and deformity. This type of cardiac arrhythmia was originally termed "torsade de pointes" (translated from the French as "twisting of the points").

Prolongation of the QT interval is thought to result from delayed ventricular repolarization. The repolarization process within the myocardial cell is due to the efflux of intracellular potassium. The channels associated with this current can be blocked by many drugs, thus, predisposing the electrical propagation cycle to torsade de pointes.

Abarelix is one of the drugs confirmed to prolong the QT interval and is accepted as having a risk of causing torsade de pointes. The risk of drug-induced torsade de pointes is extremely low when a single QT interval prolonging drug is prescribed. In terms of epinephrine, it is not known what effect vasoconstrictors in the local anesthetic regimen will have in patients with a known history of congenital prolonged QT interval or in patients taking any medication that prolongs the QT interval. Until more information is obtained, it is suggested that the clinician consult with the physician prior to the use of a vasoconstrictor in suspected patients, and that the vasoconstrictor (epinephrine, levonordefrin [Neo-Cobefrin®]) be used with caution.

Abatacept (ab a TA sept)

U.S. Brand Names Orencia®

Generic Available No

Synonyms CTLA-4Ig

Pharmacologic Category Antirheumatic, Disease Modifying

Use Treatment of rheumatoid arthritis not responsive to other disease-modifying antirheumatic drugs (DMARD); may be used as monotherapy or in combination with other DMARDs (not in combination with TNF-blocking agents)

Local Anesthetic/Vasoconstrictor Precautions No information available to require special precautions

Effects on Dental Treatment No significant effects or complications reported

Common Adverse Effects Note: Percentages not always reported; COPD patients experienced a higher frequency of COPD-related adverse reactions (COPD exacerbation, cough, dyspnea, pneumonia, rhonchi)

>10%:

Central nervous system: Headache (18%)

Gastrointestinal: Nausea

Respiratory: Nasopharyngitis (12%), upper respiratory tract infection

Miscellaneous: Infection

1% to 10%:

Cardiovascular: Hypertension (7%)

Central nervous system: Dizziness (9%)

Dermatologic: Rash (4%), herpes simplex

Gastrointestinal: Dyspepsia (6%)

Genitourinary: Urinary tract infection (6%)

(Continued)

Abatacept *(Continued)*

Neuromuscular & skeletal: Back pain (7%), limb pain (3%)
Respiratory: Cough (8%), bronchitis, pneumonia, rhinitis, sinusitis
Miscellaneous: Infusion-related reactions (9%), influenza

Mechanism of Action Selective costimulation modulator; inhibits T-cell (T-lymphocyte) activation by binding to CD80 and CD86 on antigen presenting cells (APC), thus blocking the required CD28 interaction between APCs and T cells. Activated T lymphocytes are found in the synovium of rheumatoid arthritis patients.

Drug Interactions

Increased Effect/Toxicity: Abatacept may increase the risk of infections associated with vaccines (live organism). TNF-blocking agents used in combination with abatacept is contraindicated (may increase risk of infections).

Decreased Effect: Abatacept may decrease the efficacy of immune response to live vaccines.

Pharmacodynamics/Kinetics

Distribution: V_{ss}: 0.02-0.13 L/kg

Half-life elimination: 8-25 days

Pregnancy Risk Factor C

Abbott-43818 *see* Leuprolide *on page 906*

ABC *see* Abacavir *on page 22*

ABCD *see* Amphotericin B Cholesteryl Sulfate Complex *on page 112*

Abciximab *(ab SIK si mab)*

Related Information

Cardiovascular Diseases *on page 1636*

U.S. Brand Names ReoPro®

Canadian Brand Names Reopro®

Generic Available No

Synonyms C7E3; 7E3

Pharmacologic Category Antiplatelet Agent, Glycoprotein IIb/IIIa Inhibitor

Use Prevention of acute cardiac ischemic complications in patients at high risk for abrupt closure of the treated coronary vessel and patients at risk of restenosis; an adjunct with heparin to prevent cardiac ischemic complications in patients with unstable angina not responding to conventional therapy when a percutaneous coronary intervention (PCI) is scheduled within 24 hours

Unlabeled/Investigational Use Acute MI — combination regimen of abciximab (full dose), tenecteplase (half dose), and heparin (unlabeled dose)

Local Anesthetic/Vasoconstrictor Precautions No information available to require special precautions

Effects on Dental Treatment Key adverse event(s) related to dental treatment: As with all anticoagulants, bleeding is a potential adverse effect of abciximab during dental surgery; risk is dependent on multiple variables, including the intensity of anticoagulation and patient susceptibility. Medical consult is suggested. It is unlikely that ambulatory patients presenting for dental treatment will be taking intravenous anticoagulant therapy.

Common Adverse Effects As with all drugs which may affect hemostasis, bleeding is associated with abciximab. Hemorrhage may occur at virtually any site. Risk is dependent on multiple variables, including the concurrent use of multiple agents which alter hemostasis and patient susceptibility.

>10%:

Cardiovascular: Hypotension (14%), chest pain (11%)

Gastrointestinal: Nausea (14%)

Hematologic: Minor bleeding (4% to 17%)

Neuromuscular & skeletal: Back pain (18%)

1% to 10%:

Cardiovascular: Bradycardia (5%), peripheral edema (2%)

Central nervous system: Headache (7%)

Gastrointestinal: Vomiting (7%), abdominal pain (3%)

Hematologic: Major bleeding (1% to 14%), thrombocytopenia: <100,000 cells/mm^3 (3% to 6%); <50,000 cells/mm^3 (0.4% to 2%)

Local: Injection site pain (4%)

Mechanism of Action Fab antibody fragment of the chimeric human-murine monoclonal antibody 7E3; this agent binds to platelet IIb/IIIa receptors, resulting in steric hindrance, thus inhibiting platelet aggregation

Drug Interactions

Increased Effect/Toxicity: The risk of bleeding is increased when abciximab is given with heparin, other anticoagulants, thrombolytics, or antiplatelet drugs. However, aspirin and heparin were used concurrently in the majority of patients in the major clinical studies of abciximab. Allergic reactions may be increased in patients who have received diagnostic or therapeutic monoclonal antibodies due to the presence of HACA antibodies. Concomitant use of other glycoprotein IIb/IIIa antagonists is contraindicated.

Pharmacodynamics/Kinetics Half-life elimination: ~30 minutes

Pregnancy Risk Factor C

Abelcet® *see* Amphotericin B (Lipid Complex) *on page 115*

Abilify® *see* Aripiprazole *on page 138*

ABLC *see* Amphotericin B (Lipid Complex) *on page 115*

A/B Otic *see* Antipyrine and Benzocaine *on page 130*

Abraxane™ *see* Paclitaxel (Protein Bound) *on page 1177*

Abreva® [OTC] *see* Docosanol *on page 495*

Absorbable Cotton *see* Cellulose (Oxidized/Regenerated) *on page 300*

Absorbable Gelatin Sponge *see* Gelatin (Absorbable) *on page 728*

9-AC *see* Aminocamptothecin *on page 86*

AC 2993 *see* Exenatide *on page 629*

Acamprosate (a kam PROE sate)

U.S. Brand Names Campral®

Generic Available No

Synonyms Acamprosate Calcium; Calcium Acetylhomotaurinate

Pharmacologic Category GABA Agonist/Glutamate Antagonist

Use Maintenance of alcohol abstinence

Local Anesthetic/Vasoconstrictor Precautions No information available to require special precautions

Effects on Dental Treatment Key adverse event(s) related to dental treatment: Xerostomia and changes in salivation (normal salivary flow resumes upon discontinuation).

Common Adverse Effects

Note: Many adverse effects associated with treatment may be related to alcohol abstinence; reported frequency range may overlap with placebo.

>10%: Gastrointestinal: Diarrhea (10% to 17%)

1% to 10%:

Cardiovascular: Syncope, palpitation, edema (peripheral)

Central nervous system: Insomnia (6% to 9%), anxiety (5% to 8%), depression (4% to 8%), dizziness (3% to 4%), pain (2% to 4%), paresthesia (2% to 3%), headache, somnolence, amnesia, tremor, chills

Dermatologic: Pruritus (3% to 4%), rash

Endocrine and metabolic: Weight gain, libido decreased

Gastrointestinal: Anorexia (2% to 5%), flatulence (1% to 3%), nausea (3% to 4%), abdominal pain, dry mouth (1% to 3%), vomiting, dyspepsia, constipation, appetite increased, taste perversion

Genitourinary: Impotence

Neuromuscular & skeletal: Weakness (5% to 7%), back pain, myalgia, arthralgia

Ocular: Abnormal vision

Respiratory: Rhinitis, dyspnea, pharyngitis, bronchitis

Miscellaneous: Diaphoresis (2% to 3%), suicide attempt

Mechanism of Action Mechanism not fully defined. Structurally similar to gamma-amino butyric acid (GABA), acamprosate appears to increase the activity of the GABA-ergic system, and decreases activity of glutamate within the CNS, including a decrease in activity at N-methyl D-aspartate (NMDA) receptors; may also affect CNS calcium channels. Restores balance to GABA and glutamate activities which appear to be disrupted in alcohol dependence. During therapeutic use, reduces alcohol intake, but does not cause a disulfiram-like reaction following alcohol ingestion.

Drug Interactions

Decreased Effect: No clinically-significant drug-to-drug interactions have been identified.

Pharmacodynamics/Kinetics

Distribution: V_d: 1 L/kg

Protein binding: Negligible

Metabolism: Not metabolized

Bioavailability: 11%

Half-life elimination: 20-33 hours

Excretion: Urine (as unchanged drug)

Pregnancy Risk Factor C

Acamprosate Calcium *see Acamprosate on page 27*

Acarbose (AY car bose)

Related Information
Endocrine Disorders and Pregnancy *on page 1659*
U.S. Brand Names Precose®
Canadian Brand Names Prandase®
Mexican Brand Names Glucobay®
Generic Available No
Pharmacologic Category Antidiabetic Agent, Alpha-Glucosidase Inhibitor
Use
Monotherapy, as indicated as an adjunct to diet to lower blood glucose in patients with type 2 diabetes mellitus (noninsulin dependent, NIDDM) whose hyperglycemia cannot be managed on diet alone

Combination with a sulfonylurea, metformin, or insulin in patients with type 2 diabetes mellitus (noninsulin dependent, NIDDM) when diet plus acarbose do not result in adequate glycemic control. The effect of acarbose to enhance glycemic control is additive to that of other hypoglycemic agents when used in combination.

Local Anesthetic/Vasoconstrictor Precautions No information available to require special precautions

Effects on Dental Treatment No significant effects or complications reported

Common Adverse Effects >10%:
Gastrointestinal: Abdominal pain (21%) and diarrhea (33%) tend to return to pretreatment levels over time, and the frequency and intensity of flatulence (77%) tend to abate with time

Hepatic: Transaminases increased

Mechanism of Action Competitive inhibitor of pancreatic α-amylase and intestinal brush border α-glucosidases, resulting in delayed hydrolysis of ingested complex carbohydrates and disaccharides and absorption of glucose; dose-dependent reduction in postprandial serum insulin and glucose peaks; inhibits the metabolism of sucrose to glucose and fructose

Drug Interactions
Increased Effect/Toxicity: Acarbose may increase the risk of hypoglycemia when used with oral hypoglycemics.

Decreased Effect: The effect of acarbose is antagonized/decreased by thiazide and related diuretics, corticosteroids, phenothiazines, thyroid products, estrogens, oral contraceptives, phenytoin, nicotinic acid, sympathomimetics, calcium channel-blocking drugs, isoniazid, intestinal adsorbents (eg, charcoal), and digestive enzyme preparations (eg, amylase, pancreatin). Acarbose decreases the absorption/serum concentration of digoxin.

Pharmacodynamics/Kinetics
Absorption: <2% as active drug

Metabolism: Exclusively via GI tract, principally by intestinal bacteria and digestive enzymes; 13 metabolites identified

Bioavailability: Low systemic bioavailability of parent compound; acts locally in GI tract

Excretion: Urine (~34%)

Pregnancy Risk Factor B

A-Caro-25® *see Beta-Carotene on page 198*
Accolate® *see Zafirlukast on page 1590*
AccuNeb™ *see Albuterol on page 58*
Accupril® *see Quinapril on page 1322*
Accuretic® *see Quinapril and Hydrochlorothiazide on page 1323*
Accutane® *see Isotretinoin on page 869*
Accuzyme® *see Papain and Urea on page 1186*
ACE *see Captopril on page 257*

Acebutolol (a se BYOO toe lole)

Related Information
Cardiovascular Diseases *on page 1636*
U.S. Brand Names Sectral®
Canadian Brand Names Apo-Acebutolol®; Gen-Acebutolol; Monitan®; Novo-Acebutolol; Nu-Acebutolol; Rhotral; Rhoxal-acebutolol; Sandoz-Acebutolol; Sectral®
Generic Available Yes

Synonyms Acebutolol Hydrochloride

Pharmacologic Category Antiarrhythmic Agent, Class II; Beta Blocker With Intrinsic Sympathomimetic Activity

Use Treatment of hypertension, ventricular arrhythmias, angina

Local Anesthetic/Vasoconstrictor Precautions No information available to require special precautions

Effects on Dental Treatment Acebutolol is a cardioselective beta-blocker. Local anesthetic with vasoconstrictor can be safely used in patients medicated with acebutolol. Nonselective beta-blockers (ie, propranolol, nadolol) enhance the pressor response to epinephrine, resulting in hypertension and bradycardia; this has not been reported for acebutolol. Many nonsteroidal anti-inflammatory drugs, such as ibuprofen and indomethacin, can reduce the hypotensive effect of beta-blockers after 3 or more weeks of therapy with the NSAID. Short-term NSAID use (ie, 3 days) requires no special precautions in patients taking beta-blockers.

Common Adverse Effects

>10%: Central nervous system: Fatigue (11%)

1% to 10%:

Cardiovascular: Chest pain (2%), edema (2%), bradycardia, hypotension, CHF

Central nervous system: Headache (6%), dizziness (6%), insomnia (3%), depression (2%), abnormal dreams (2%), anxiety, hyperesthesia, hypoesthesia, impotence

Dermatologic: Rash (2%), pruritus

Gastrointestinal: Constipation (4%), diarrhea (4%), dyspepsia (4%), nausea (4%), flatulence (3%), vomiting, abdominal pain

Genitourinary: Micturition frequency (3%), dysuria, nocturia, impotence (2%)

Neuromuscular & skeletal: Arthralgia (2%), myalgia (2%), back pain, joint pain

Ocular: Abnormal vision (2%), conjunctivitis, dry eyes, eye pain

Respiratory: Dyspnea (4%), rhinitis (2%), cough (1%), pharyngitis, wheezing

Potential adverse effects (based on experience with other beta-blocking agents) include reversible mental depression, disorientation, catatonia, short-term memory loss, emotional lability, slightly clouded sensorium, laryngospasm, respiratory distress, allergic reactions, erythematous rash, agranulocytosis, purpura, thrombocytopenia, mesenteric artery thrombosis, ischemic colitis, alopecia, Peyronie's disease, claudication

Mechanism of Action Competitively blocks beta$_1$-adrenergic receptors with little or no effect on beta$_2$-receptors except at high doses; exhibits membrane stabilizing and intrinsic sympathomimetic activity

Drug Interactions

Cytochrome P450 Effect: Inhibits CYP2D6 (weak)

Increased Effect/Toxicity: Acebutolol may increase the effects of other drugs which slow AV conduction (digoxin, verapamil, diltiazem), alpha-blockers (prazosin, terazosin), and alpha-adrenergic stimulants (epinephrine, phenylephrine). Acebutolol may mask the tachycardia from hypoglycemia caused by insulin and oral hypoglycemics. In patients receiving concurrent therapy, the risk of hypertensive crisis is increased when either clonidine or the beta-blocker is withdrawn. Reserpine has been shown to enhance the effect of acebutolol. Beta-blockers may increase the action or levels of ethanol, disopyramide, nondepolarizing muscle relaxants, and theophylline although the effects are difficult to predict.

Decreased Effect: Decreased effect of acebutolol with aluminum salts, barbiturates, calcium salts, cholestyramine, colestipol, NSAIDs, penicillins (ampicillin), rifampin, and salicylates due to decreased bioavailability and plasma levels. The effect of sulfonylureas may be decreased by beta-blockers; however, the decreased effect has not been shown with tolbutamide.

Pharmacodynamics/Kinetics

Onset of action: 1-2 hours

Duration: 12-24 hours

Absorption: Oral: 40%

Protein binding: 5% to 15%

Metabolism: Extensive first-pass effect

Half-life elimination: 6-7 hours

Time to peak: 2-4 hours

Excretion: Feces (~55%); urine (35%)

Pregnancy Risk Factor B (manufacturer); D (2nd and 3rd trimesters - expert analysis)

Acebutolol Hydrochloride see Acebutolol on page 28

Acenocoumarin see Acenocoumarol on page 30

Acenocoumarol (a see no KOOM a rol)

Canadian Brand Names Sintrom®
Generic Available No
Synonyms Acenocoumarin; Nicoumalone
Pharmacologic Category Anticoagulant, Coumarin Derivative
Use Prophylaxis and treatment of venous thrombosis, pulmonary embolism, and thromboembolic disorders; atrial fibrillation with risk of embolism; adjunct in the prophylaxis of coronary occlusion and transient ischemic attacks
Local Anesthetic/Vasoconstrictor Precautions No information available to require special precautions
Effects on Dental Treatment Signs of acenocoumarol overdose may first appear as bleeding from gingival tissue; consultation with prescribing physician is advisable prior to surgery to determine temporary dose reduction or withdrawal of medication.
Common Adverse Effects As with all anticoagulants, bleeding is the major adverse effect of acenocoumarol. Hemorrhage may occur at virtually any site. Risk is dependent on multiple variables, including the intensity of anticoagulation and patient susceptibility.

Frequency not defined.
Cardiovascular: Hemorrhagic shock
Central nervous system: Fever, headache, stroke (hemorrhagic)
Dermatologic: Rash, urticaria, skin necrosis
  Skin necrosis/gangrene, due to paradoxical local thrombosis, is a known but rare risk of oral anticoagulant therapy. Its onset is usually within the first few days of therapy and is frequently localized to the limbs, breast, or penis. The risk of this effect is increased in patients with protein C or S deficiency.

Additional adverse reactions associated with warfarin, but likely to also occur with indanediones, include priapism and skin necrosis ("purple toe" syndrome or cutaneous gangrene).
Gastrointestinal: Gastrointestinal bleeding, melena
Genitourinary: Hematuria
Hematologic: Hemorrhage, retroperitoneal hematoma, unrecognized bleeding sites (eg, colon cancer) may be uncovered by anticoagulation. Other hematologic reactions reported with coumarin derivatives include agranulocytosis, red cell aplasia, anemia, thrombocytopenia, eosinophilia.
Hepatic: Hepatitis, hepatotoxicity, hematobilia
Ocular: Ocular hemorrhage
Respiratory: Epistaxis, hemoptysis, pulmonary hemorrhage
Miscellaneous: Hypersensitivity/allergic reactions
Restrictions Not available in U.S.
Dosage Note: Dosage must be individualized. The following information is based on the manufacturer's labeling in Canada. Adults:
Oral: Initial: 8-12 mg on day 1, followed by 4-8 mg on day 2. Subsequent dosage should be based on PT/INR measurements. Usual range of maintenance doses: 1-10 mg/day. Tapering of dosage is recommended prior to discontinuation.
Mechanism of Action Interferes with hepatic synthesis of vitamin K-dependent coagulation factors (II, VII, IX, X)
Contraindications Hypersensitivity to acenocoumarol or any component of the formulation; hemorrhagic tendencies; hemophilia; thrombocytopenia purpura; leukemia; recent or potential surgery of the eye or CNS; major regional lumbar block anesthesia or surgery resulting in large, open surfaces; bleeding from the GI, respiratory, or GU tract; threatened abortion; aneurysm; prolonged dietary insufficiencies (vitamin K deficiency); ascorbic acid deficiency; history of bleeding diathesis; prostatectomy; continuous tube drainage of the small intestine; polyarthritis; diverticulitis; emaciation; malnutrition; cerebrovascular hemorrhage; eclampsia/pre-eclampsia; blood dyscrasias; severe uncontrolled or malignant hypertension; severe hepatic disease; pericarditis or pericardial effusion; subacute bacterial endocarditis; visceral carcinoma; following spinal puncture and other diagnostic or therapeutic procedures with potential for significant bleeding; history of warfarin-induced necrosis; an unreliable, noncompliant patient; alcoholism; patient who has a history of falls or is a significant fall risk; pregnancy
Warnings/Precautions Use care in the selection of patients appropriate for this treatment. Use with caution in trauma, acute infection (antibiotics and fever may alter affects), renal insufficiency, moderate-severe hypertension, polycythemia vera, vasculitis, open wound, active TB, history of PUD, anaphylactic disorders, indwelling catheters, severe diabetes, thyroid disease, and menstruating and postpartum women. Necrosis or gangrene of the skin and other tissues can

occur (rarely) due to early hypercoagulability; risk is increased in patients with protein C deficiency. "Purple toe" syndrome, due to cholesterol microembolization, has been described with coumarin-type anticoagulants. Women may be at risk of developing ovarian hemorrhage at the time of ovulation.

Hemorrhage is the most serious risk of therapy. Patient must be instructed to report bleeding, accidents, or falls. Patient must also report any new or discontinued medications, herbal or alternative products used, significant changes in smoking or dietary habits. Ensure patient cooperation especially from the alcoholic, illicit drug user, demented, or psychotic patient. The elderly may be more sensitive to anticoagulant therapy.

Drug Interactions
Cytochrome P450 Effect: Substrate of CYP1A2 (major), 2C9 (major), 2C19 (minor)

Increased Effect/Toxicity: The following agents may increase the levels and/or effects of acenocoumarol: Acetaminophen, amiodarone, anticoagulants, antiplatelet agents, CYP1A2 inhibitors (example inhibitors include ciprofloxacin, fluvoxamine, ketoconazole, norfloxacin, ofloxacin, and rofecoxib), CYP2C8/9 inhibitors (example inhibitors include delavirdine, fluconazole, gemfibrozil, ketoconazole, nicardipine, pioglitazone, and sulfonamides), miconazole, NSAIDs, salicylates, sulfamethoxazole, sulfinpyrazone, tetracycline antibiotics, and trimethoprim.

Decreased Effect: CYP1A2 and/or 2C9 inducers may decrease the levels/effects of acenocoumarol; example inducers of these enzymes include aminoglutethimide, carbamazepine, phenobarbital, phenytoin, rifampin, rifapentine, and secobarbital.

Ethanol/Nutrition/Herb Interactions
Ethanol: Avoid ethanol. Acute ethanol ingestion (binge drinking) decreases the metabolism of oral anticoagulants and increases PT/INR. Chronic daily ethanol use increases the metabolism of oral anticoagulants and decreases PT/INR.

Food: The anticoagulant effects of acenocoumarol may be decreased if taken with foods rich in vitamin K. Vitamin E may increase anticoagulant effect.

Herb/Nutraceutical: St John's wort may decrease oral anticoagulant levels. Alfalfa contains large amounts of vitamin K as do many enteral products. Coenzyme Q_{10} may decrease response to oral anticoagulants. Avoid cat's claw, dong quai, evening primrose, feverfew, red clover, horse chestnut, garlic, green tea, ginseng, and ginkgo (all have additional antiplatelet activity).

Dietary Considerations Foods high in vitamin K (eg, beef liver, pork liver, green tea, and leafy green vegetables) inhibit anticoagulant effect. Do not change dietary habits once stabilized on acenocoumarol therapy. A balanced diet with a consistent intake of vitamin K is essential. Avoid large amounts of alfalfa, asparagus, broccoli, Brussels sprouts, cabbage, cauliflower, green teas, kale, lettuce, spinach, turnip greens, watercress; these decrease efficacy of oral anticoagulants. It is recommended that the diet contain a CONSISTENT vitamin K content of 70-140 mcg/day. Check with healthcare provider before changing diet. Avoid using multivitamins that contain vitamin K.

Pharmacodynamics/Kinetics
Onset of action: Peak anticoagulant effect: Oral: 36-48 hours
Absorption: Oral: 60%
Protein binding: 99%
Metabolism: Hepatic, via oxidation (possibly by CYP1A2, 2C9, and 2C19) to inactive metabolites
Half-life elimination: 8-11 hours
Time to peak, plasma: 1-3 hours
Excretion: Urine (60%) and feces (29%) as metabolites

Dosage Forms TAB: 1 mg, 4 mg

Aceon® *see* Perindopril Erbumine *on page 1216*
Acephen™ [OTC] *see* Acetaminophen *on page 31*
Acetadote® *see* Acetylcysteine *on page 46*

Acetaminophen (a seet a MIN oh fen)

Related Information
Oral Pain *on page 1692*
Related Sample Prescriptions
Mild/Moderate Oral Pain *on page 1734*
U.S. Brand Names Acephen™ [OTC]; Apra Children's [OTC]; Aspirin Free Anacin® Maximum Strength [OTC]; Cetafen® [OTC]; Cetafen Extra® [OTC]; Comtrex® Sore Throat Maximum Strength [OTC]; ElixSure™ Fever/Pain [OTC] [DSC]; FeverALL® [OTC]; Genapap™ [OTC]; Genapap™ Children [OTC]; Genapap™ Extra Strength [OTC]; Genapap™ Infant [OTC]; Genebs [OTC]; (Continued)

Acetaminophen *(Continued)*

Genebs Extra Strength [OTC]; Infantaire [OTC]; Mapap [OTC]; Mapap Children's [OTC]; Mapap Extra Strength [OTC]; Mapap Infants [OTC]; Nortemp Children's [OTC]; Pain Eze [OTC]; Silapap® Children's [OTC]; Silapap® Infants [OTC]; Tycolene [OTC]; Tycolene Maximum Strength [OTC]; Tylenol® [OTC]; Tylenol® 8 Hour [OTC]; Tylenol® Arthritis Pain [OTC]; Tylenol® Children's [OTC]; Tylenol® Children's with Flavor Creator [OTC]; Tylenol® Extra Strength [OTC]; Tylenol® Infants [OTC]; Tylenol® Junior [OTC]; Valorin [OTC]; Valorin Extra [OTC]

Canadian Brand Names Abenol®; Apo-Acetaminophen®; Atasol®; Novo-Gesic; Pediatrix; Tempra®; Tylenol®

Mexican Brand Names Acetafen®; Andox®; Datril®; Magnidol®; Neodol®; Neodolito®; Sedalito®; Sinedol®; Temperal®; Tempra®; Tylex®

Generic Available Yes: Excludes extended release products

Synonyms APAP; N-Acetyl-P-Aminophenol; Paracetamol

Pharmacologic Category Analgesic, Miscellaneous

Dental Use Treatment of postoperative pain

Use Treatment of mild-to-moderate pain and fever (antipyretic/analgesic); does not have antirheumatic or anti-inflammatory effects

Local Anesthetic/Vasoconstrictor Precautions No information available to require special precautions

Effects on Dental Treatment No significant effects or complications reported (see Dental Comment)

Significant Adverse Effects Frequency not defined.

Dermatologic: Rash

Endocrine & metabolic: May increase chloride, uric acid, glucose; may decrease sodium, bicarbonate, calcium

Hematologic: Anemia, blood dyscrasias (neutropenia, pancytopenia, leukopenia)

Hepatic: Bilirubin increased, alkaline phosphatase increased

Renal: Ammonia increased, nephrotoxicity with chronic overdose, analgesic nephropathy

Miscellaneous: Hypersensitivity reactions (rare)

Dental Usual Dosing Postoperative pain: Oral, rectal:

Children <12 years: 10-15 mg/kg/dose every 4-6 hours as needed; do **not** exceed 5 doses (2.6 g) in 24 hours; alternatively, the following age-based doses may be used

Adults: 325-650 mg every 4-6 hours or 1000 mg 3-4 times/day; do **not** exceed 4 g/day

Dosage Oral, rectal:

Children <12 years: 10-15 mg/kg/dose every 4-6 hours as needed; do **not** exceed 5 doses (2.6 g) in 24 hours; alternatively, the following age-based doses may be used; see table.

Acetaminophen Dosing

Age	Dosage (mg)	Age	Dosage (mg)
0-3 mo	40	4-5 y	240
4-11 mo	80	6-8 y	320
1-2 y	120	9-10 y	400
2-3 y	160	11 y	480

Note: Higher rectal doses have been studied for use in preoperative pain control in children. However, specific guidelines are not available and dosing may be product dependent. The safety and efficacy of alternating acetaminophen and ibuprofen dosing has not been established.

Adults: 325-650 mg every 4-6 hours or 1000 mg 3-4 times/day; do **not** exceed 4 g/day

Dosing interval in renal impairment:

Cl_{cr} 10-50 mL/minute: Administer every 6 hours

Cl_{cr} <10 mL/minute: Administer every 8 hours (metabolites accumulate)

Hemodialysis: Moderately dialyzable (20% to 50%)

Dosing adjustment/comments in hepatic impairment: Use with caution. Limited, low-dose therapy is usually well tolerated in hepatic disease/cirrhosis. However, cases of hepatotoxicity at daily acetaminophen dosages <4 g/day have been reported. Avoid chronic use in hepatic impairment.

Mechanism of Action Inhibits the synthesis of prostaglandins in the central nervous system and peripherally blocks pain impulse generation; produces antipyresis from inhibition of hypothalamic heat-regulating center

Contraindications Hypersensitivity to acetaminophen or any component of the formulation

Warnings/Precautions Limit dose to <4 g/day. May cause severe hepatic toxicity on acute overdose; in addition, chronic daily dosing in adults has resulted in liver damage in some patients. Use with caution in patients with alcoholic liver disease; consuming ≥3 alcoholic drinks/day may increase the risk of liver damage. Use caution in patients with known G6PD deficiency.

OTC labeling: When used for self-medication, patients should be instructed to contact healthcare provider if used for fever lasting >3 days or for pain lasting >10 days in adults or >5 days in children.

Drug Interactions Substrate (minor) of CYP1A2, 2A6, 2C9, 2D6, 2E1, 3A4; **Inhibits** CYP3A4 (weak)

Decreased effect: Barbiturates, carbamazepine, hydantoins, rifampin, sulfinpyrazone may decrease the analgesic effect of acetaminophen. Cholestyramine may decrease acetaminophen absorption (separate dosing by at least 1 hour).

Increased toxicity: Barbiturates, carbamazepine, hydantoins, isoniazid, rifampin, sulfinpyrazone may increase the hepatotoxic potential of acetaminophen. Chronic ethanol abuse increases risk for acetaminophen toxicity; effect of warfarin may be enhanced.

Ethanol/Nutrition/Herb Interactions

Ethanol: Excessive intake of ethanol may increase the risk of acetaminophen-induced hepatotoxicity. Avoid ethanol or limit to <3 drinks/day.

Food: Rate of absorption may be decreased when given with food.

Herb/Nutraceutical: St John's wort may decrease acetaminophen levels.

Dietary Considerations Chewable tablets may contain phenylalanine (amount varies, ranges between 3-12 mg/tablet); consult individual product labeling.

Pharmacodynamics/Kinetics

Onset of action: <1 hour

Duration: 4-6 hours

Absorption: Incomplete; varies by dosage form

Protein binding: 8% to 43% at toxic doses

Metabolism: At normal therapeutic dosages, hepatic to sulfate and glucuronide metabolites, while a small amount is metabolized by CYP to a highly reactive intermediate (acetylimidoquinone) which is conjugated with glutathione and inactivated; at toxic doses (as little as 4 g daily) glutathione conjugation becomes insufficient to meet the metabolic demand causing an increase in acetylimidoquinone concentration, which may cause hepatic cell necrosis

Half-life elimination: Prolonged following toxic doses

Neonates: 2-5 hours

Adults: 1-3 hours (may be increased in elderly; however, this should not affect dosing)

Time to peak, serum: Oral: 10-60 minutes; may be delayed in acute overdoses

Excretion: Urine (2% to 5% unchanged; 55% as glucuronide metabolites; 30% as sulphate metabolites)

Pregnancy Risk Factor B

Lactation Enters breast milk/compatible

Dosage Forms [DSC] = Discontinued product

Caplet: 500 mg

Cetafen Extra® Strength, Genapap™ Extra Strength, Genebs Extra Strength, Mapap Extra Strength, Tycolene Maximum Strength, Tylenol® Extra Strength: 500 mg

Caplet, extended release:

Tylenol® 8 Hour, Tylenol® Arthritis Pain: 650 mg

Capsule: 500 mg

Elixir: 160 mg/5 mL (120 mL, 480 mL, 3780 mL)

Apra Children's: 160 mg/5 mL (120 mL, 480 mL, 3780 mL) [alcohol free; contains benzoic acid; cherry and grape flavors]

Mapap Children's: 160 mg/5 mL (120 mL) [alcohol free; contains benzoic acid and sodium benzoate; cherry flavor]

Gelcap:

Mapap Extra Strength, Tylenol® Extra Strength: 500 mg

Geltab:

Tylenol® Extra Strength: 500 mg

Geltab, extended release:

Tylenol® 8 Hour: 650 mg

Liquid, oral: 500 mg/15 mL (240 mL)

Comtrex® Sore Throat Maximum Strength: 500 mg/15 mL (240 mL) [contains sodium benzoate; honey lemon flavor]

Genapap™ Children: 160 mg/5 mL (120 mL) [contains sodium benzoate; cherry and grape flavors]

(Continued)

Acetaminophen *(Continued)*

Silapap®: 160 mg/5 mL (120 mL, 240 mL, 480 mL) [sugar free; contains sodium benzoate; cherry flavor]

Tylenol® Extra Strength: 500 mg/15 mL (240 mL) [contains sodium benzoate; cherry flavor]

Solution, oral: 160 mg/5 mL (120 mL, 480 mL)

Solution, oral drops: 80 mg/0.8 mL (15 mL) [droppers are marked at 0.4 mL (40 mg) and at 0.8 mL (80 mg)]

Genapap™ Infant: 80 mg/0.8 mL (15 mL) [fruit flavor]

Infantaire: 80 mg/0.8mL (15 mL, 30 mL)

Silapap® Infant's: 80 mg/0.8 mL (15 mL, 30 mL) [contains sodium benzoate; cherry flavor]

Suppository, rectal: 120 mg, 325 mg, 650 mg

Acephen™: 120 mg, 325 mg, 650 mg

FeverALL®: 80 mg, 120 mg, 325 mg, 650 mg

Mapap: 125 mg, 650 mg

Suspension, oral:

Mapap Children's: 160 mg/5 mL (120 mL) [contains sodium benzoate; cherry flavor]

Nortemp Children's: 160 mg/5 mL (120 mL) [alcohol free; contains sodium benzoate; cotton candy flavor]

Tylenol® Children's: 160 mg/5 mL (120 mL, 240 mL) [contains sodium benzoate; bubble gum yum, cherry blast, dye free cherry, grape splash, and very berry strawberry flavors]

Tylenol® Children's with Flavor Creator: 160 mg/5 mL (120 mL) [contains sodium 2 mg/5 mL and sodium benzoate; cherry blast flavor; packaged with apple (4), bubblegum (8), chocolate (4), & strawberry (4) sugar free flavor packets]

Suspension, oral drops:

Mapap Infants: 80 mg/0.8 mL (15 mL, 30 mL) [contains sodium benzoate; cherry flavor]

Tylenol® Infants: 80 mg/0.8 mL (15 mL, 30 mL) [contains sodium benzoate; cherry, dye free cherry, and grape flavors]

Syrup, oral:

ElixSure™ Fever/Pain: 160 mg/5 mL (120 mL) [bubble gum, cherry, and grape flavors] [DSC]

Tablet: 325 mg, 500 mg

Aspirin Free Anacin® Extra Strength, Genapap™ Extra Strength, Genebs Extra Strength, Mapap Extra Strength, Pain Eze, Tylenol® Extra Strength, Valorin Extra: 500 mg

Cetafen®, Genapap™, Genebs, Mapap, Tycolene, Tylenol®, Valorin: 325 mg

Tablet, chewable: 80 mg

Genapap™ Children: 80 mg [contains phenylalanine 6 mg/tablet; fruit and grape flavors]

Mapap Children's: 80 mg [contains phenylalanine 3 mg/tablet; bubble gum, fruit, and grape flavors]

Mapap Junior Strength: 160 mg [contains phenylalanine 12 mg/tablet; grape flavor]

Tylenol® Children's: 80 mg [fruit and grape flavors contain phenylalanine 3 mg/tablet; bubble gum flavor contains phenylalanine 6 mg/tablet] [DSC]

Tylenol® Junior: 160 mg [contains phenylalanine 6 mg/tablet; fruit and grape flavors] [DSC]

Tablet, orally disintegrating: 80 mg, 160 mg

Tylenol® Children's Meltaways: 80 mg [bubble gum, grape, and watermelon flavors]

Tylenol® Junior Meltaways: 160 mg [bubble gum and grape flavors]

Dental Comment Hepatotoxicity caused by acetaminophen is potentiated by chronic ethanol consumption. People who consume ethanol at the same time that they use acetaminophen, even in therapeutic doses, are at risk of developing hepatotoxicity.

A study by Hylek, et al, suggested that the combination of acetaminophen with warfarin (Coumadin®) may cause enhanced anticoagulation. The following recommendations have been made by Hylek, et al, and supported by an editorial in *JAMA* by Bell.

Dose and duration of acetaminophen should be as low as possible, individualized, and monitored.

The study by Hylek reported that for patients who reported taking the equivalent of at least 4 regular strength (325 mg) tablets for longer than a week, the odds of having an INR >6.0 were increased 10-fold above those not taking acetaminophen. Risk decreased with lower intakes of acetaminophen reaching a background level of risk at a dose of 6 or fewer 325 mg tablets per week.

Selected Readings

Ahmad N, Grad HA, Haas DA, et al, "The Efficacy of Nonopioid Analgesics for Postoperative Dental Pain: A Meta-Analysis," *Anesth Prog*, 1997, 44(4):119-26.

Bell WR, "Acetaminophen and Warfarin: Undesirable Synergy," *JAMA*, 1998, 279(9):702-3.

Botting RM, "Mechanism of Action of Acetaminophen: Is There a Cyclooxygenase 3?" *Clin Infect Dis*, 2000, Suppl 5:S202-10.

Chandrasekharan NV, Dai H, Roos KL, et al, "COX-3, a Cyclooxygenase-1 Variant Inhibited by Acetaminophen and Other Analgesic/Antipyretic Drugs: Cloning, Structure, and Expression," *Proc Natl Acad Sci U S A*, 2002, 99(21):13926-31.

Dart RC, Kuffner EK, and Rumack BH, "Treatment of Pain or Fever With Paracetamol (Acetaminophen) in the Alcoholic Patient: A Systematic Review," *Am J Ther*, 2000, 7(2):123-34.

Dionne R, "Additive Analgesia Without Opioid Side Effects," *Compend Contin Educ Dent*, 2000, 21(7):572-4, 576-7.

Dionne RA and Berthold CW, "Therapeutic Uses of Nonsteroidal Anti-inflammatory Drugs in Dentistry," *Crit Rev Oral Biol Med*, 2001, 12(4):315-30.

Graham GG and Scott KF, "Mechanisms of Action of Paracetamol and Related Analgesics," *Inflammopharmacology*, 2003, 11(4):401-13.

Grant JA and Weiler JM, "A Report of a Rare Immediate Reaction After Ingestion of Acetaminophen," *Ann Allergy Asthma Immunol*, 2001, 87(3):227-9.

Hylek EM, Heiman H, Skates SJ, et al, "Acetaminophen and Other Risk Factors for Excessive Warfarin Anticoagulation," *JAMA*, 1998, 279(7):657-62.

Kwan D, Bartle WR, and Walker SE, "The Effects of Acetaminophen on Pharmacokinetics and Pharmacodynamics of Warfarin," *J Clin Pharmacol*, 1999, 39(1):68-75.

Lee WM, "Drug-Induced Hepatotoxicity," *N Engl J Med*, 1995, 333(17):1118-27.

Licht H, Seeff LB, and Zimmerman HJ, "Apparent Potentiation of Acetaminophen Hepatotoxicity by Alcohol," *Ann Intern Med*, 1980, 92(4):511.

McClain CJ, Price S, Barve S, et al, "Acetaminophen Hepatotoxicity: An Update," *Curr Gastroenterol Rep*, 1999, 1(1):42-9.

Nguyen AM, Graham DY, Gage T, et al, "Nonsteroidal Anti-Inflammatory Drug Use in Dentistry: Gastrointestinal Implications," *Gen Dent*, 1999, 47(6):590-6.

Schwab JM, Schluesener HJ, and Laufer S, "COX-3: Just Another COX or the Solitary Elusive Target of Paracetamol?" *Lancet*, 2003, 361(9362):981-2.

Shek KL, Chan LN, and Nutescu E, "Warfarin-Acetaminophen Drug Interaction Revisited," *Pharmacotherapy*, 1999, 19(10):1153-8.

Tanaka E, Yamazaki K, and Misawa S, "Update: The Clinical Importance of Acetaminophen Hepatotoxicity in Nonalcoholic and Alcoholic Subjects," *J Clin Pharm Ther*, 2000, 25(5):325-32.

Wynn RL, "Update on Nonprescription Pain Relievers for Dental Pain," *Gen Dent*, 2004, 52(2):94-8.

Acetaminophen and Chlorpheniramine *see* Chlorpheniramine and Acetaminophen on page 324

Acetaminophen and Codeine (a seet a MIN oh fen & KOE deen)

Related Information

Acetaminophen *on page 31*
Codeine *on page 385*

Related Sample Prescriptions

Moderate/Moderately Severe Oral Pain *on page 1734*

U.S. Brand Names Capital® and Codeine; Tylenol® With Codeine

Canadian Brand Names ratio-Emtec; ratio-Lenoltec; Triatec-8; Triatec-8 Strong; Triatec-30; Tylenol Elixir with Codeine; Tylenol No. 1; Tylenol No. 1 Forte; Tylenol No. 2 with Codeine; Tylenol No. 3 with Codeine; Tylenol No. 4 with Codeine

Generic Available Yes

Synonyms Codeine and Acetaminophen

Pharmacologic Category Analgesic, Narcotic

Dental Use Treatment of postoperative pain

Use Relief of mild-to-moderate pain

Local Anesthetic/Vasoconstrictor Precautions No information available to require special precautions

Effects on Dental Treatment No significant effects or complications reported (see Dental Comment)

Significant Adverse Effects

>10%:
  Central nervous system: Lightheadedness, dizziness, sedation
  Gastrointestinal: Nausea, vomiting
  Respiratory: Dyspnea

1% to 10%:
  Central nervous system: Euphoria, dysphoria
  Dermatologic: Pruritus
  Gastrointestinal: Constipation, abdominal pain
  Miscellaneous: Histamine release

<1% (Limited to important or life-threatening): Antidiuretic hormone release, biliary tract spasm, bradycardia, hypotension, intracranial pressure increased, physical and psychological dependence, respiratory depression, urinary retention

Restrictions C-III; C-V

Note: In countries outside of the U.S., some formulations of Tylenol® with Codeine (eg, Tylenol® No. 3) include caffeine.

(Continued)

Acetaminophen and Codeine *(Continued)*

Dental Usual Dosing Postoperative pain: Adults: Analgesic: Based on codeine (30-60 mg/dose) every 4-6 hours (maximum: 4000 mg/24 hours based on acetaminophen component)

Dosage Doses should be adjusted according to severity of pain and response of the patient. Adult doses ≥60 mg codeine fail to give commensurate relief of pain but merely prolong analgesia and are associated with an appreciably increased incidence of side effects. Oral:

Children: Analgesic:

Codeine: 0.5-1 mg codeine/kg/dose every 4-6 hours

Acetaminophen: 10-15 mg/kg/dose every 4 hours up to a maximum of 2.6 g/24 hours for children <12 years; **alternatively, the following can be used:**

3-6 years: 5 mL 3-4 times/day as needed of elixir

7-12 years: 10 mL 3-4 times/day as needed of elixir

>12 years: 15 mL every 4 hours as needed of elixir

Adults:

Antitussive: Based on codeine (15-30 mg/dose) every 4-6 hours (maximum: 360 mg/24 hours based on codeine component)

Analgesic: Based on codeine (30-60 mg/dose) every 4-6 hours (maximum: 4000 mg/24 hours based on acetaminophen component)

Dosing adjustment in renal impairment: See individual agents.

Dosing adjustment in hepatic impairment: Use with caution. Limited, low-dose therapy is usually well tolerated in hepatic disease/cirrhosis; however, cases of hepatotoxicity at daily acetaminophen dosages <4 g/day have been reported. Avoid chronic use in hepatic impairment.

Mechanism of Action Inhibits the synthesis of prostaglandins in the central nervous system and peripherally blocks pain impulse generation; produces antipyresis from inhibition of hypothalamic heat-regulating center; binds to opiate receptors in the CNS, causing inhibition of ascending pain pathways, altering the perception of and response to pain; causes cough supression by direct central action in the medulla; produces generalized CNS depression. Caffeine (contained in some non-U.S. formulations) is a CNS stimulant; use with acetaminophen and codeine increases the level of analgesia provided by each agent.

Contraindications Hypersensitivity to acetaminophen, codeine, or any component of the formulation; significant respiratory depression (in unmonitored settings); acute or severe bronchial asthma; hypercapnia; paralytic ileus

Warnings/Precautions Use with caution in patients with hypersensitivity reactions to other phenanthrene derivative opioid agonists (morphine, hydrocodone, hydromorphone, levorphanol, oxycodone, oxymorphone); tablets contain metabisulfite which may cause allergic reactions. Tolerance or drug dependence may result from extended use.

Limit total acetaminophen dose to <4 g/day. May cause severe hepatic toxicity on acute overdose; in addition, chronic daily dosing in adults has resulted in liver damage in some patients. Use with caution in patients with alcoholic liver disease; consuming 3 alcoholic drinks/day may increase the risk of liver damage. Use caution in patients with known G6PD deficiency.

This combination should be used with caution in elderly or debilitated patients, hypotension, adrenocortical insufficiency, thyroid disorders, prostatic hyperplasia, urethral stricture, seizure disorder, CNS depression, head injury or increased intracranial pressure. Causes sedation; caution must be used in performing tasks which require alertness (eg, operating machinery or driving). Safety and efficacy in pediatric patients have not been established.

Note: Some non-U.S. formulations (including most Canadian formulations) may contain caffeine as an additional ingredient. Caffeine may cause CNS and cardiovascular stimulation, as well as GI irritation in high doses. Use with caution in patients with a history of peptic ulcer or GERD; avoid in patients with symptomatic cardiac arrhythmias.

Drug Interactions Acetaminophen: **Substrate** (minor) of CYP1A2, 2A6, 2C9, 2D6, 2E1, 3A4; **Inhibits** CYP3A4 (weak)

Increased toxicity: CNS depressants, phenothiazines, tricyclic antidepressants, guanabenz, MAO inhibitors (may also decrease blood pressure); effect of warfarin may be enhanced.

Ethanol/Nutrition/Herb Interactions Ethanol: Excessive intake of ethanol may increase the risk of acetaminophen-induced hepatotoxicity. Avoid ethanol or limit to <3 drinks/day.

Dietary Considerations May be taken with food.

Pharmacodynamics/Kinetics See individual agents.

Pregnancy Risk Factor C

Lactation Enters breast milk/use caution

Dosage Forms [DSC] = Discontinued product; [CAN] = Canadian brand name

Caplet:

ratio-Lenoltec No. 1 [CAN], Tylenol No. 1 [CAN]: Acetaminophen 300 mg, codeine phosphate 8 mg, and caffeine 15 mg [not available in the U.S.]

Tylenol No. 1 Forte [CAN]: Acetaminophen 500 mg, codeine phosphate 8 mg, and caffeine 15 mg [not available in the U.S.]

Elixir, oral [C-V]: Acetaminophen 120 mg and codeine phosphate 12 mg per 5 mL (5 mL, 10 mL, 12.5 mL, 15 mL, 120 mL, 480 mL) [contains alcohol 7%]

Tylenol® with Codeine [DSC]: Acetaminophen 120 mg and codeine phosphate 12 mg per 5 mL (480 mL) [contains alcohol 7%; cherry flavor]

Tylenol Elixir with Codeine [CAN]: Acetaminophen 160 mg and codeine phosphate 8 mg per 5 mL (500 mL) [contains alcohol 7%, sucrose 31%; cherry flavor; not available in the U.S.]

Suspension, oral [C-V] (Capital® and Codeine): Acetaminophen 120 mg and codeine phosphate 12 mg per 5 mL (480 mL) [alcohol free; fruit punch flavor]

Tablet [C-III]: Acetaminophen 300 mg and codeine phosphate 15 mg; acetaminophen 300 mg and codeine phosphate 30 mg; acetaminophen 300 mg and codeine phosphate 60 mg

ratio-Emtec [CAN], Triatec-30 [CAN]: Acetaminophen 300 mg and codeine phosphate 30 mg [not available in the U.S.]

ratio-Lenoltec No. 1 [CAN]: Acetaminophen 300 mg, codeine phosphate 8 mg, and caffeine 15 mg [not available in the U.S.]

ratio-Lenoltec No. 2 [CAN], Tylenol No. 2 with Codeine [CAN]: Acetaminophen 300 mg, codeine phosphate 15 mg, and caffeine 15 mg [not available in the U.S.]

ratio-Lenoltec No. 3 [CAN], Tylenol No. 3 with Codeine [CAN]: Acetaminophen 300 mg, codeine phosphate 30 mg, and caffeine 15 mg [not available in the U.S.]

ratio-Lenoltec No. 4 [CAN], Tylenol No. 4 with Codeine [CAN]: Acetaminophen 300 mg and codeine phosphate 60 mg [not available in the U.S.]

Triatec-8 [CAN]: Acetaminophen 325 mg, codeine phosphate 8 mg, and caffeine 30 mg [not available in the U.S.]

Triatec-8 Strong [CAN]: Acetaminophen 500 mg, codeine phosphate 8 mg, and caffeine 30 mg [not available in the U.S.]

Tylenol® with Codeine No. 3: Acetaminophen 300 mg and codeine phosphate 30 mg [contains sodium metabisulfite]

Tylenol® with Codeine No. 4: Acetaminophen 300 mg and codeine phosphate 60 mg [contains sodium metabisulfite]

Dental Comment Codeine products, as with other narcotic analgesics, are recommended only for acute dosing (ie, 3 days or less). The most common adverse effect you will see in your dental patients from codeine is nausea, followed by sedation and constipation. Codeine has narcotic addiction liability, especially when given long-term. Because of the acetaminophen component, this product should be used with caution in patients with alcoholic liver disease.

A study by Hylek, et al, suggested that the combination of acetaminophen with warfarin (Coumadin®) may cause enhanced anticoagulation. The following recommendations have been made by Hylek, et al, and are supported by an editorial in *JAMA* by Bell.

Dose and duration of acetaminophen should be as low as possible, individualized, and monitored.

The study by Hylek reported that for patients who reported taking the equivalent of at least 4 regular strength (325 mg) tablets for longer than a week, the odds of having an INR >6.0 were increased 10-fold above those not taking acetaminophen. Risk decreased with lower intakes of acetaminophen reaching a background level of risk at a dose of 6 or fewer 325 mg tablets per week.

Selected Readings

Change DJ, Fricke JR, Bird SR, et al, "Rofecoxib Versus Codeine/Acetaminophen in Postoperative Dental Pain: A Double-Blind, Randomized, Placebo- and Active Comparator-Controlled Clinical Trial," *Clin Ther*, 2001, 23(9):1446-55.

Dionne RA, "New Approaches to Preventing and Treating Postoperative Pain," *J Am Dent Assoc*, 1992, 123(6):26-34.

Forbes JA, Butterworth GA, Burchfield WH, et al, "Evaluation of Ketorolac, Aspirin, and an Acetaminophen-Codeine Combination in Postoperative Oral Surgery Pain," *Pharmacotherapy*, 1990, 10(6 Pt 2):77S-93S.

Gobetti JP, "Controlling Dental Pain," *J Am Dent Assoc*, 1992, 123(6):47-52.

Mullican WS and Lacy JR, "Tramadol/Acetaminophen Combination Tablets and Codeine/Acetaminophen Combination Capsules for the Management of Chronic Pain: A Comparative Trial," *Clin Ther*, 2001, 23(9):1429-45.

Wynn RL, "Narcotic Analgesics for Dental Pain: Available Products, Strengths, and Formulations," *Gen Dent*, 2001, 49(2):126-8, 130, 132 passim.

Acetaminophen and Diphenhydramine
(a seet a MIN oh fen & dye fen HYE dra meen)

Related Information
Acetaminophen *on page 31*
DiphenhydrAMINE *on page 483*
U.S. Brand Names Excedrin® P.M. [OTC]; Goody's PM® Powder [OTC]; Legatrin PM® [OTC]; Percogesic® Extra Strength [OTC]; Tylenol® PM [OTC]; Tylenol® Severe Allergy [OTC]
Generic Available Yes: Excludes powder and liquid
Synonyms Diphenhydramine and Acetaminophen
Pharmacologic Category Analgesic, Miscellaneous
Use Aid in the relief of insomnia accompanied by minor pain
Local Anesthetic/Vasoconstrictor Precautions No information available to require special precautions
Effects on Dental Treatment Key adverse event(s) related to dental treatment: Xerostomia (normal salivary flow resumes upon discontinuation).
Common Adverse Effects See individual agents.
Drug Interactions
Cytochrome P450 Effect:
Acetaminophen: **Substrate** (minor) of CYP1A2, 2A6, 2C9, 2D6, 2E1, 3A4; **Inhibits** CYP3A4 (weak)
Diphenhydramine: **Inhibits** CYP2D6 (moderate)
Increased Effect/Toxicity: See individual agents.
Decreased Effect: See individual agents.
Pharmacodynamics/Kinetics See individual agents.

Acetaminophen and Hydrocodone *see* Hydrocodone and Acetaminophen *on page 779*

Acetaminophen and Oxycodone *see* Oxycodone and Acetaminophen *on page 1165*

Acetaminophen and Pentazocine *see* Pentazocine and Acetaminophen *on page 1209*

Acetaminophen and Phenyltoloxamine
(a seet a MIN oh fen & fen il to LOKS a meen)

Related Information
Acetaminophen *on page 31*
U.S. Brand Names Genesec® [OTC]; Percogesic® [OTC]; Phenylgesic® [OTC]
Generic Available Yes
Synonyms Phenyltoloxamine and Acetaminophen
Pharmacologic Category Analgesic, Non-narcotic
Use Relief of mild-to-moderate pain
Local Anesthetic/Vasoconstrictor Precautions No information available to require special precautions
Effects on Dental Treatment No significant effects or complications reported
Drug Interactions
Cytochrome P450 Effect: Acetaminophen: **Substrate** (minor) of CYP1A2, 2A6, 2C9, 2D6, 2E1, 3A4; **Inhibits** CYP3A4 (weak)
Pregnancy Risk Factor B

Acetaminophen and Propoxyphene *see* Propoxyphene and Acetaminophen *on page 1298*

Acetaminophen and Pseudoephedrine
(a seet a MIN oh fen & soo doe e FED rin)

Related Information
Acetaminophen *on page 31*
Pseudoephedrine *on page 1309*
U.S. Brand Names Alka-Seltzer Plus® Cold and Sinus Liqui-Gels [OTC]; Cetafen Cold® [OTC]; Genapap™ Sinus Maximum Strength [OTC]; Mapap Sinus Maximum Strength [OTC]; Medi-Synal [OTC]; Ornex® [OTC]; Ornex® Maximum Strength [OTC]; Sinus-Relief [OTC]; Sinutab® Sinus [OTC]; Sudafed® Sinus and Cold [OTC]; Sudafed® Sinus Headache [OTC]; SudoGest Sinus [OTC]; Tylenol® Cold, Infants [OTC]; Tylenol® Sinus, Children's [OTC]; Tylenol® Sinus Day Non-Drowsy [OTC]
Canadian Brand Names Contac® Cold and Sore Throat, Non Drowsy, Extra Strength; Dristan® N.D.; Dristan® N.D., Extra Strength; Sinutab® Non Drowsy;

Sudafed® Head Cold and Sinus Extra Strength; Tylenol® Decongestant; Tylenol® Sinus

Generic Available Yes

Synonyms Pseudoephedrine and Acetaminophen

Pharmacologic Category Alpha/Beta Agonist; Analgesic, Miscellaneous

Use Relief of mild-to-moderate pain; relief of congestion

Local Anesthetic/Vasoconstrictor Precautions Use with caution since pseudoephedrine is a sympathomimetic amine which could interact with epinephrine to cause a pressor response

Effects on Dental Treatment Key adverse event(s) related to dental treatment: Pseudoephedrine: Xerostomia (normal salivary flow resumes upon discontinuation).

Common Adverse Effects See individual agents.

Drug Interactions

Cytochrome P450 Effect: Acetaminophen: **Substrate** (minor) of CYP1A2, 2A6, 2C9, 2D6, 2E1, 3A4; Inhibits CYP3A4 (weak)

Increased Effect/Toxicity: See individual agents.

Decreased Effect: See individual agents.

Pharmacodynamics/Kinetics See individual agents.

Acetaminophen and Tramadol
(a seet a MIN oh fen & TRA ma dole)

Related Information
Acetaminophen *on page 31*
Tramadol *on page 1514*

Related Sample Prescriptions
Moderate/Moderately Severe Oral Pain *on page 1734*

U.S. Brand Names Ultracet™

Canadian Brand Names Tramacet

Generic Available Yes

Synonyms APAP and Tramadol; Tramadol Hydrochloride and Acetaminophen

Pharmacologic Category Analgesic, Miscellaneous; Analgesic, Non-narcotic

Dental Use Treatment of postoperative pain (≤5 days)

Use Short-term (≤5 days) management of acute pain

Local Anesthetic/Vasoconstrictor Precautions No information available to require special precautions

Effects on Dental Treatment Key adverse event(s) related to dental treatment: Xerostomia and changes in salivation (normal salivary flow resumes upon discontinuation).

Significant Adverse Effects
1% to 10%:
Central nervous system: Somnolence (6%), dizziness (3%), insomnia (2%), anxiety, confusion, euphoria, fatigue, headache, nervousness, tremor
Dermatologic: Pruritus (2%), rash
Endocrine & metabolic: Hot flashes
Gastrointestinal: Constipation (6%), anorexia (3%), diarrhea (3%), nausea (3%), dry mouth (2%), abdominal pain, dyspepsia, flatulence, vomiting
Genitourinary: Prostatic disorder (2%)
Neuromuscular & skeletal: Weakness
Miscellaneous: Diaphoresis increased (4%)
<1% (Limited to important or life-threatening): Allergic reactions, amnesia, anaphylactoid reactions, anaphylaxis, arrhythmia, coma, depersonalization, drug abuse, dysphagia, dyspnea, emotional lability, hallucination, hepatitis, hypertonia, impotence, liver failure, migraine, muscle contractions (involuntary), oliguria, paresthesia, paroniria, pulmonary edema, rigors, seizure, serotonin syndrome, shivering, Stevens-Johnson syndrome, suicidal tendency, stupor, syncope, tinnitus, tongue edema, toxic epidermal necrolysis, urinary retention, urticaria, vertigo
A withdrawal syndrome may occur with abrupt discontinuation; includes anxiety, diarrhea, hallucinations (rare), nausea, pain, piloerection, rigors, sweating, and tremor. Uncommon discontinuation symptoms may include severe anxiety, panic attacks, or paresthesia.

Dental Usual Dosing Acute postoperative pain (≤5 days): Adults: Oral: Two tablets every 4-6 hours as needed for pain relief (maximum: 8 tablets/day); treatment should not exceed 5 days

Dosage Oral: Adults: Acute pain: Two tablets every 4-6 hours as needed for pain relief (maximum: 8 tablets/day); treatment should not exceed 5 days
Dosage adjustment in renal impairment: Cl$_{cr}$ <30 mL/minute: Maximum of 2 tablets every 12 hours; treatment should not exceed 5 days
Dosage adjustment in hepatic impairment: Use is not recommended.
(Continued)

Acetaminophen and Tramadol *(Continued)*

Mechanism of Action

Based on **acetaminophen** component: Inhibits the synthesis of prostaglandins in the central nervous system and peripherally blocks pain impulse generation; produces antipyresis from inhibition of hypothalamic heat-regulating center

Based on **tramadol** component: Binds to μ-opiate receptors in the CNS causing inhibition of ascending pain pathways, altering the perception of and response to pain; also inhibits the reuptake of norepinephrine and serotonin, which also modifies the ascending pain pathway

Contraindications Hypersensitivity to acetaminophen, tramadol, opioids, or any component of the formulation; opioid-dependent patients; acute intoxication with ethanol, hypnotics, narcotics, centrally-acting analgesics, opioids, or psychotropic drugs; hepatic dysfunction

Warnings/Precautions Should be used only with extreme caution in patients receiving MAO inhibitors. Use with caution and reduce dosage when administering to patients receiving other CNS depressants. Seizures may occur when taken within the recommended dosage; risk is increased in patients receiving serotonin reuptake inhibitors (SSRIs or anorectics), tricyclic antidepressants, other cyclic compounds (including cyclobenzaprine, promethazine), neuroleptics, MAO inhibitors, or drugs which may lower seizure threshold. Patients with a history of seizures, or with a risk of seizures (head trauma, metabolic disorders, CNS infection, malignancy, or during alcohol/drug withdrawal) are also at increased risk. Do not use with ethanol or other acetaminophen- or tramadol-containing products.

Limit acetaminophen to <4 g/day. May cause severe hepatic toxicity in acute overdose; in addition, chronic daily dosing in adults has resulted in liver damage in some patients. Use with caution in patients with alcoholic liver disease; consuming ≥3 alcoholic drinks/day may increase the risk of liver damage. Use caution in patients with known G6PD deficiency.

Elderly patients and patients with chronic respiratory disorders may be at greater risk of adverse events. Use with caution in patients with increased intracranial pressure or head injury. Use tramadol with caution and reduce dosage in patients with renal dysfunction. Tolerance or drug dependence may result from extended use (withdrawal symptoms have been reported); abrupt discontinuation should be avoided. Tapering of dose at the time of discontinuation limits the risk of withdrawal symptoms. Safety and efficacy in pediatric patients have not been established.

Drug Interactions

Acetaminophen: **Substrate** (minor) of CYP1A2, 2A6, 2C9, 2D6, 2E1, 3A4; **Inhibits** CYP3A4 (weak)

Tramadol: **Substrate** of CYP2D6 (major), 3A4 (minor)

Amphetamines: May increase the risk of seizures with tramadol.

Anesthetic agents: May increase risk of CNS and respiratory depression; use together with caution and in reduced dosage.

Barbiturates: Barbiturates may increase the hepatotoxic effects of acetaminophen; in addition, acetaminophen levels may be lowered.

Carbamazepine: Carbamazepine decreases half-life of tramadol by 33% to 50%; also have increased risk of seizures; in addition, carbamazepine may increase the hepatotoxic effects and lower serum levels of acetaminophen; concomitant use is not recommended.

CYP2D6 inhibitors: May decrease the effects of tramadol. Example inhibitors include chlorpromazine, delavirdine, fluoxetine, miconazole, paroxetine, pergolide, quinidine, quinine, ritonavir, and ropinirole.

Digoxin: Rare reports of digoxin toxicity with concomitant tramadol use.

Hydantoin anticonvulsants: Phenytoin may increase the hepatotoxic effects of acetaminophen; in addition, acetaminophen levels may be lowered.

MAO inhibitors: May increase the risk of seizures. Use extreme caution.

Naloxone: May increase the risk of seizures (if administered in tramadol overdose).

Neuroleptic agents: May increase the risk of tramadol-associated seizures and may have additive CNS depressant effects.

Narcotics: May increase risk of CNS and respiratory depression; use together with caution and in reduced dosage.

Opioids: May increase the risk of seizures, and may have additive CNS depressant effects. Use together with caution and in reduced dosage.

Phenothiazines: May increase risk of CNS and respiratory depression; use together with caution and in reduced dosage.

Rifampin: Rifampin may increase the clearance of acetaminophen.

Quinidine: May increase the tramadol serum concentrations by inhibiting CYP metabolism.

SSRIs: May increase the risk of seizures with tramadol by inhibiting CYP metabolism (citalopram, fluoxetine, paroxetine, sertraline).

Sulfinpyrazone: Sulfinpyrazone may increase the hepatotoxic effects of acetaminophen; in addition, acetaminophen levels may be lowered.

Tricyclic antidepressants: May increase the risk of seizures.

Warfarin: Acetaminophen and tramadol may lead to an elevation of prothrombin times; monitor.

Ethanol/Nutrition/Herb Interactions

Ethanol: Avoid ethanol (increased liver toxicity with concomitant use).

Food: May delay time to peak plasma levels, however, the extent of absorption is not affected.

Herb/Nutraceutical:

Acetaminophen: Avoid St John's wort (may decrease acetaminophen levels).

Tramadol: Avoid valerian, St John's wort, kava kava, gotu kola (may increase CNS depression).

Dietary Considerations May be taken with or without food. Avoid use of ethanol and ethanol-containing products.

Pharmacodynamics/Kinetics See individual agents.

Pregnancy Risk Factor C

Lactation Tramadol: Enters breast milk/contraindicated

Breast-Feeding Considerations Not recommended for postdelivery analgesia in nursing mothers.

Dosage Forms Tablet: Acetaminophen 325 mg and tramadol hydrochloride 37.5 mg

Selected Readings

Fricke JR Jr, Hewitt DJ, Jordan DM, et al, "A Double-Blind Placebo-Controlled Comparison of Tramadol/Acetaminophen and Tramadol in Patients With Postoperative Dental Pain," *Pain*, 2004, 109(3):250-7.

Fricke JR Jr, Karim R, Jordan D, et al, "A Double-Blind, Single-Dose Comparison of the Analgesic Efficacy of Tramadol/Acetaminophen Combination Tablets, Hydrocodone/Acetaminophen Combination Tablets, and Placebo After Oral Surgery," *Clin Ther*, 2002, 24(6):953-68.

Hiller B and Rosenberg M, "Ultracet: A New Combination Analgesic," *J Mass Dent Soc*, 2003, 52(2):38-40.

Medve RA, Wang J, and Karim R, "Tramadol and Acetaminophen Tablets for Dental Pain," *Anesth Prog*, 2001, 48(3):79-81.

Smith AB, Ravikumar TS, Kamin M, et al, "Combination Tramadol Plus Acetaminophen for Postsurgical Pain," *Am J Surg*, 2004, 187(4):521-7.

Wynn RL, "NSAIDS and Cardiovascular Effects, Celecoxib for Dental Pain, and a New Analgesic - Tramadol with Acetaminophen," *Gen Dent*, 2002, 50(3):218-222.

Acetaminophen, Aspirin, and Caffeine
(a seet a MIN oh fen, AS pir in, & KAF een)

Related Information

Acetaminophen *on page 31*

Aspirin *on page 145*

Caffeine *on page 245*

U.S. Brand Names Excedrin® Extra Strength [OTC]; Excedrin® Migraine [OTC]; Fem-Prin® [OTC]; Genaced™ [OTC]; Goody's® Extra Strength Headache Powder [OTC]; Goody's® Extra Strength Pain Relief [OTC]; Pain-Off [OTC]; Vanquish® Extra Strength Pain Reliever [OTC]

Generic Available Yes

Synonyms Aspirin, Acetaminophen, and Caffeine; Aspirin, Caffeine and Acetaminophen; Caffeine, Acetaminophen, and Aspirin; Caffeine, Aspirin, and Acetaminophen

Pharmacologic Category Analgesic, Miscellaneous

Use Relief of mild-to-moderate pain; mild-to-moderate pain associated with migraine headache

Local Anesthetic/Vasoconstrictor Precautions No information available to require special precautions

Effects on Dental Treatment No significant effects or complications reported

Common Adverse Effects See individual agents.

Drug Interactions

Cytochrome P450 Effect:

Acetaminophen: **Substrate** (minor) of CYP1A2, 2A6, 2C9, 2D6, 2E1, 3A4; **Inhibits** CYP3A4 (weak)

Aspirin: **Substrate** (minor) of CYP2C9

Caffeine: **Substrate** of CYP1A2 (major), 2C9 (minor), 2D6 (minor), 2E1 (minor), 3A4 (minor); **Inhibits** CYP1A2 (weak), 3A4 (moderate)

Increased Effect/Toxicity: See individual agents.

Decreased Effect: See individual agents.

Pharmacodynamics/Kinetics See individual agents.

Pregnancy Risk Factor D

Acetaminophen, Butalbital, and Caffeine see Butalbital, Acetaminophen, and Caffeine on page 239

Acetaminophen, Caffeine, and Dihydrocodeine
(a seet a MIN oh fen, KAF een, & dye hye droe KOE deen)

Related Information
Acetaminophen on page 31
Caffeine on page 245

U.S. Brand Names Panlor® DC; Panlor® SS

Generic Available No

Synonyms Caffeine, Dihydrocodeine, and Acetaminophen; Dihydrocodeine Bitartrate, Acetaminophen, and Caffeine

Pharmacologic Category Analgesic Combination (Narcotic)

Dental Use Relief of moderate to moderately-severe dental pain

Use Relief of moderate to moderately-severe pain

Local Anesthetic/Vasoconstrictor Precautions No information available to require special precautions

Effects on Dental Treatment No significant effects or complications reported

Significant Adverse Effects Frequency not defined. Most common reactions with this combination include:
Central nervous system: Dizziness, drowsiness, lightheadedness, sedation
Dermatologic: Pruritus, skin reactions
Gastrointestinal: Constipation, nausea, vomiting

Restrictions C-III

Dental Usual Dosing Relief of moderate-to-moderately severe dental pain:
Adults: Oral:
Panlor® DC: 2 capsules every 4 hours as needed; adjust dose based on severity of pain (maximum dose: 10 capsules/24 hours)
Panlor® SS: 1 tablet every 4 hours as needed; adjust dose based on severity of pain (maximum dose: 5 tablets/24 hours)

Dosage Oral: Adults: Relief of pain:
Panlor® DC: 2 capsules every 4 hours as needed; adjust dose based on severity of pain (maximum dose: 10 capsules/24 hours)
Panlor® SS: 1 tablet every 4 hours as needed; adjust dose based on severity of pain (maximum dose: 5 tablets/24 hours)

Mechanism of Action
Acetaminophen inhibits the synthesis of prostaglandins in the central nervous system and peripherally blocks pain impulse generation; produces antipyresis from inhibition of hypothalamic heat-regulating center.
Caffeine is a CNS stimulant; use with acetaminophen and dihydrocodeine increases the level of analgesia provided by each agent.
Dihydrocodeine binds to opiate receptors in the CNS, causing inhibition of ascending pain pathways, altering the perception of and response to pain; produces generalized CNS depression.

Contraindications Hypersensitivity to acetaminophen, caffeine, dihydrocodeine, codeine, or any component of the formulation; significant respiratory depression (in unmonitored settings); acute or severe bronchial asthma; hypercapnia; paralytic ileus

Warnings/Precautions Acetaminophen may cause severe hepatotoxicity in acute overdose; limit acetaminophen to <4 g/day; in addition, chronic daily dosing in adults has resulted in liver damage in some patients. Use with caution in patients with alcoholic liver disease; consuming ≥3 alcoholic drinks/day may increase the risk of liver damage. Use caution in patients with known G6PD deficiency. Caffeine may cause CNS and cardiovascular stimulation as well as GI irritation in high doses. Dihydrocodeine should be used with caution in patients with hypersensitivity reactions to other phenanthrene derivative opioid agonists (morphine, hydrocodone, hydromorphone, levorphanol, oxycodone, oxymorphone), respiratory diseases including asthma, emphysema, COPD, or severe hepatic or renal insufficiency. Use caution with MAO inhibitors.

This combination should be used with caution in elderly or debilitated patients, hypotension, adrenocortical insufficiency, thyroid disorders, prostatic hyperplasia, urethral stricture, seizure disorder, CNS depression, head injury or increased intracranial pressure. Causes sedation; caution must be used in performing tasks which require alertness (eg, operating machinery or driving). Safety and efficacy in pediatric patients have not been established.

Drug Interactions
Acetaminophen: **Substrate** (minor) of CYP1A2, 2A6, 2C9, 2D6, 2E1, 3A4; **Inhibits** CYP3A4 (weak)
Caffeine: **Substrate** of CYP1A2 (major), 2C9 (minor), 2D6 (minor), 2E1 (minor), 3A4 (minor); **Inhibits** CYP1A2 (weak), 3A4 (moderate)

Dihydrocodeine: **Substrate** of CYP2D6 (major)

Acetaminophen: See individual agents for associated interactions.

Caffeine:

CYP1A2 inhibitors: May increase the levels/effects of caffeine. Example inhibitors include amiodarone, fluvoxamine, ketoconazole, and rofecoxib.

CYP3A4 substrates: Caffeine may increase the levels/effects of CYP3A4 substrates. Example substrates include benzodiazepines, calcium channel blockers, ergot derivatives, mirtazapine, nateglinide, nefazodone, tacrolimus, and venlafaxine.

Quinolone antibiotics (specifically ciprofloxacin, norfloxacin, ofloxacin): Quinolones may increase the level/effects of caffeine.

Dihydrocodeine:

CYP2D6 inhibitors: May decrease the effects of dihydrocodeine. Example inhibitors include chlorpromazine, delavirdine, fluoxetine, miconazole, paroxetine, pergolide, quinidine, quinine, ritonavir, and ropinirole.

Quinidine: Quinidine may decrease the effects of dihydrocodeine.

Ethanol/Nutrition/Herb Interactions

Ethanol: Excessive intake of ethanol may increase the risk of acetaminophen-induced toxicity. Ethanol may also increase CNS depression.

Pregnancy Risk Factor C

Lactation Enters breast milk/not recommended

Breast-Feeding Considerations Acetaminophen and caffeine are both excreted in breast milk. Specific information for dihydrocodeine is not available; however, similar agents (eg, codeine, morphine) are excreted in breast milk.

Dosage Forms

Capsule (Panlor® DC): Acetaminophen 356.4 mg, caffeine 30 mg, and dihydrocodeine bitartrate 16 mg

Tablet (Panlor® SS): Acetaminophen 712.8 mg, caffeine 60 mg, and dihydrocodeine bitartrate 32 mg

Acetaminophen, Caffeine, Codeine, and Butalbital *see* Butalbital, Acetaminophen, Caffeine, and Codeine *on page 239*

Acetaminophen, Caffeine, Hydrocodone, Chlorpheniramine, and Phenylephrine *see* Hydrocodone, Chlorpheniramine, Phenylephrine, Acetaminophen, and Caffeine *on page 790*

Acetaminophen, Chlorpheniramine, and Pseudoephedrine

(a seet a MIN oh fen, klor fen IR a meen, & soo doe e FED rin)

Related Information

Acetaminophen *on page 31*
Chlorpheniramine *on page 323*
Pseudoephedrine *on page 1309*

U.S. Brand Names Actifed® Cold and Sinus [OTC]; Alka-Seltzer® Plus Cold Liqui-Gels® [OTC]; Comtrex® Flu Therapy Day/Night [OTC]; Comtrex® Flu Therapy Nighttime [OTC]; Comtrex® Maximum Strength Sinus and Nasal Decongestant [OTC] [DSC]; Kolephrin® [OTC]; Sinutab® Sinus Allergy Maximum Strength [OTC]; Thera-Flu® Cold and Sore Throat Night Time [OTC]; Tylenol® Allergy Complete [OTC]; Tylenol® Allergy Sinus [OTC] [DSC]; Tylenol® Children's Plus Cold Nighttime [OTC]

Canadian Brand Names Sinutab® Sinus & Allergy; Tylenol® Allergy Sinus

Generic Available Yes

Synonyms Acetaminophen, Pseudoephedrine, and Chlorpheniramine; Chlorpheniramine, Acetaminophen, and Pseudoephedrine; Chlorpheniramine, Pseudoephedrine, and Acetaminophen; Pseudoephedrine, Acetaminophen, and Chlorpheniramine; Pseudoephedrine, Chlorpheniramine, and Acetaminophen

Pharmacologic Category Analgesic, Miscellaneous; Antihistamine

Use Temporary relief of sinus symptoms

Local Anesthetic/Vasoconstrictor Precautions Use with caution since pseudoephedrine is a sympathomimetic amine which could interact with epinephrine to cause a pressor response

Effects on Dental Treatment Key adverse event(s) related to dental treatment:

Chlorpheniramine: Significant xerostomia with prolonged use (normal salivary flow resumes upon discontinuation).

Pseudoephedrine: Xerostomia (normal salivary flow resumes upon discontinuation).

Common Adverse Effects See individual agents.

(Continued)

Acetaminophen, Chlorpheniramine, and Pseudoephedrine *(Continued)*

Drug Interactions

Cytochrome P450 Effect:

Acetaminophen: **Substrate** (minor) of CYP1A2, 2A6, 2C9, 2D6, 2E1, 3A4; **Inhibits** CYP3A4 (weak)

Chlorpheniramine: **Substrate** of CYP2D6 (minor), 3A4 (major); **Inhibits** CYP2D6 (weak)

Increased Effect/Toxicity: See individual agents.

Decreased Effect: See individual agents.

Pharmacodynamics/Kinetics See individual agents.

Pregnancy Risk Factor B

Acetaminophen, Dextromethorphan, and Pseudoephedrine

(a seet a MIN oh fen, deks troe meth OR fan, & soo doe e FED rin)

Related Information

Acetaminophen *on page 31*

Dextromethorphan *on page 451*

Pseudoephedrine *on page 1309*

U.S. Brand Names Alka-Seltzer® Plus Flu Liqui-Gels® [OTC]; Comtrex® Non-Drowsy Cold and Cough Relief [OTC]; Contac® Severe Cold and Flu/Non-Drowsy [OTC]; Infants' Tylenol® Cold Plus Cough Concentrated Drops [OTC]; Sudafed® Severe Cold [OTC]; Thera-Flu® Severe Cold Non-Drowsy [OTC] [DSC]; Triaminic® Cough and Sore Throat Formula [OTC]; Tylenol® Cold Day Non-Drowsy [OTC]; Tylenol® Flu Non-Drowsy Maximum Strength [OTC]; Vicks® DayQuil® Multi-Symptom Cold and Flu [OTC]

Canadian Brand Names Contac® Complete; Contac® Cough, Cold and Flu Day & Night™; Sudafed® Cold & Cough Extra Strength; Tylenol® Cold Daytime

Generic Available Yes

Synonyms Dextromethorphan, Acetaminophen, and Pseudoephedrine; Pseudoephedrine, Acetaminophen, and Dextromethorphan; Pseudoephedrine, Dextromethorphan, and Acetaminophen

Pharmacologic Category Antihistamine; Antitussive

Use Treatment of mild-to-moderate pain and fever; symptomatic relief of cough and congestion

Local Anesthetic/Vasoconstrictor Precautions Use with caution since pseudoephedrine is a sympathomimetic amine which could interact with epinephrine to cause a pressor response

Effects on Dental Treatment Key adverse event(s) related to dental treatment: Pseudoephedrine: Xerostomia (normal salivary flow resumes upon discontinuation).

Common Adverse Effects See individual agents.

Drug Interactions

Cytochrome P450 Effect:

Acetaminophen: **Substrate** (minor) of CYP1A2, 2A6, 2C9, 2D6, 2E1, 3A4; **Inhibits** CYP3A4 (weak)

Dextromethorphan: **Substrate** of CYP2B6 (minor), 2C9 (minor), 2C19 (minor), 2D6 (major), 2E1 (minor), 3A4 (minor); **Inhibits** CYP2D6 (weak)

Increased Effect/Toxicity: See individual agents.

Decreased Effect: See individual agents.

Pharmacodynamics/Kinetics See individual agents.

Acetaminophen, Dichloralphenazone, and Isometheptene *see* Acetaminophen, Isometheptene, and Dichloralphenazone *on page 44*

Acetaminophen, Isometheptene, and Dichloralphenazone

(a seet a MIN oh fen, eye soe me THEP teen, & dye KLOR al FEN a zone)

Related Information

Acetaminophen *on page 31*

U.S. Brand Names Amidrine; Duradrin®; Midrin®; Migquin; Migratine; Migrazone®; Migrin-A

Generic Available Yes

Synonyms Acetaminophen, Dichloralphenazone, and Isometheptene; Dichloralphenazone, Acetaminophen, and Isometheptene; Dichloralphenazone,

Isometheptene, and Acetaminophen; Isometheptene, Acetaminophen, and Dichloralphenazone; Isometheptene, Dichloralphenazone, and Acetaminophen

Pharmacologic Category Analgesic, Miscellaneous

Use Relief of migraine and tension headache

Local Anesthetic/Vasoconstrictor Precautions No information available to require special precautions

Effects on Dental Treatment No significant effects or complications reported

Common Adverse Effects Frequency not defined.

Central nervous system: Transient dizziness

Dermatological: Rash

Restrictions C-IV

Drug Interactions

Cytochrome P450 Effect: Acetaminophen: **Substrate** (minor) of CYP1A2, 2A6, 2C9, 2D6, 2E1, 3A4; **Inhibits** CYP3A4 (weak)

Increased Effect/Toxicity: See individual agents.

Decreased Effect: See individual agents.

Acetaminophen, Pseudoephedrine, and Chlorpheniramine *see* Acetaminophen, Chlorpheniramine, and Pseudoephedrine *on page 43*

Acetasol® HC *see* Acetic Acid, Propylene Glycol Diacetate, and Hydrocortisone *on page 45*

AcetaZOLAMIDE (a set a ZOLE a mide)

U.S. Brand Names Diamox® Sequels®

Canadian Brand Names Apo-Acetazolamide®; Diamox®

Mexican Brand Names Acetadiazol®

Generic Available Yes: Injection, tablet

Pharmacologic Category Anticonvulsant, Miscellaneous; Carbonic Anhydrase Inhibitor; Diuretic, Carbonic Anhydrase Inhibitor; Ophthalmic Agent, Antiglaucoma

Use Treatment of glaucoma (chronic simple open-angle, secondary glaucoma, preoperatively in acute angle-closure); drug-induced edema or edema due to congestive heart failure (adjunctive therapy); centrencephalic epilepsies (immediate release dosage form); prevention or amelioration of symptoms associated with acute mountain sickness

Unlabeled/Investigational Use Urine alkalinization; respiratory stimulant in COPD; metabolic alkalosis

Local Anesthetic/Vasoconstrictor Precautions No information available to require special precautions

Effects on Dental Treatment Key adverse event(s) related to dental treatment: Metallic taste (resolves upon discontinuation).

Mechanism of Action Reversible inhibition of the enzyme carbonic anhydrase resulting in reduction of hydrogen ion secretion at renal tubule and an increased renal excretion of sodium, potassium, bicarbonate, and water to decrease production of aqueous humor; also inhibits carbonic anhydrase in central nervous system to retard abnormal and excessive discharge from CNS neurons

Pregnancy Risk Factor C

Acetic Acid, Hydrocortisone, and Propylene Glycol Diacetate *see* Acetic Acid, Propylene Glycol Diacetate, and Hydrocortisone *on page 45*

Acetic Acid, Propylene Glycol Diacetate, and Hydrocortisone

(a SEE tik AS id, PRO pa leen GLY kole dye AS e tate, & hye droe KOR ti sone)

Related Information

Hydrocortisone *on page 793*

U.S. Brand Names Acetasol® HC; VoSol® HC

Generic Available Yes

Synonyms Acetic Acid, Hydrocortisone, and Propylene Glycol Diacetate; Hydrocortisone, Acetic Acid, and Propylene Glycol Diacetate; Propylene Glycol Diacetate, Acetic Acid, and Hydrocortisone

Pharmacologic Category Otic Agent, Anti-infective

Use Treatment of superficial infections of the external auditory canal caused by organisms susceptible to the action of the antimicrobial, complicated by swelling

Local Anesthetic/Vasoconstrictor Precautions No information available to require special precautions

Effects on Dental Treatment No significant effects or complications reported

Acetohydroxamic Acid (a SEE toe hye droks am ik AS id)

U.S. Brand Names Lithostat®
Canadian Brand Names Lithostat®
Generic Available No
Synonyms AHA
Pharmacologic Category Urinary Tract Product
Use Adjunctive therapy in chronic urea-splitting urinary infection
Local Anesthetic/Vasoconstrictor Precautions No information available to require special precautions
Effects on Dental Treatment No significant effects or complications reported
Common Adverse Effects Frequency not defined.
Cardiovascular: Deep vein thrombosis (rare), embolism, palpitation, phlebitis
Central nervous system: Anorexia, anxiety, depression, headache, malaise, nervousness, tremor
Dermatologic: Flushing (with ethanol consumption), rash (nonpruritic, macular)
Gastrointestinal: Nausea, vomiting
Hematologic: Hemolytic anemia (15% with laboratory evidence; ~3% severe requiring discontinuation; may be accompanied by GI symptoms or systemic complaints of malaise and/or fatigue); hyperbilirubinemia
Respiratory: Pulmonary embolism (rare)
Mechanism of Action Acetohydroxamic acid inhibits bacterial urease enzymes, decreasing the formation of ammonia in the urine by urea-splitting organisms. A reduction in urinary ammonia may increase the antibacterial activity of some antibiotic agents.
Drug Interactions
Decreased Effect: Acetohydroxamic acid may chelate divalent metals, decreasing the absorption of both agents; avoid concurrent use. Orally-administered iron may be chelated by acetohydroxamic acid, decreasing the absorption of both agents (parenteral iron should be used to treat hypochromic anemia).
Pregnancy Risk Factor X

Acetoxymethylprogesterone see MedroxyPROGESTERone on page 972

Acetylcholine (a se teel KOE leen)

U.S. Brand Names Miochol-E®
Canadian Brand Names Miochol-E®
Generic Available No
Synonyms Acetylcholine Chloride
Pharmacologic Category Cholinergic Agonist; Ophthalmic Agent, Miotic
Use Produces complete miosis in cataract surgery, keratoplasty, iridectomy, and other anterior segment surgery where rapid miosis is required
Local Anesthetic/Vasoconstrictor Precautions No information available to require special precautions
Effects on Dental Treatment No significant effects or complications reported
Mechanism of Action Causes contraction of the sphincter muscles of the iris, resulting in miosis and contraction of the ciliary muscle, leading to accommodation spasm
Pregnancy Risk Factor C

Acetylcholine Chloride see Acetylcholine on page 46

Acetylcysteine (a se teel SIS teen)

U.S. Brand Names Acetadote®
Canadian Brand Names Acetylcysteine Solution; Mucomyst®; Parvolex®
Mexican Brand Names ACC®
Generic Available Yes: Solution for inhalation
Synonyms Acetylcysteine Sodium; Mercapturic Acid; Mucomyst; NAC; N-Acetylcysteine; N-Acetyl-L-cysteine
Pharmacologic Category Antidote; Mucolytic Agent
Use Adjunctive mucolytic therapy in patients with abnormal or viscid mucous secretions in acute and chronic bronchopulmonary diseases; pulmonary complications of surgery and cystic fibrosis; diagnostic bronchial studies; antidote for acute acetaminophen toxicity
Unlabeled/Investigational Use Prevention of radiocontrast-induced renal dysfunction (oral, I.V.); distal intestinal obstruction syndrome (DIOS, previously referred to as meconium ileus equivalent)

Local Anesthetic/Vasoconstrictor Precautions No information available to require special precautions

Effects on Dental Treatment Key adverse event(s) related to dental treatment: Stomatitis, drowsiness, fever, vomiting, nausea, bronchospasm, rhinorrhea, hemoptysis, and dizziness.

Common Adverse Effects

Inhalation: Frequency not defined.
  Central nervous system: Drowsiness, chills, fever
  Gastrointestinal: Vomiting, nausea, stomatitis
  Local: Irritation, stickiness on face following nebulization
  Respiratory: Bronchospasm, rhinorrhea, hemoptysis
  Miscellaneous: Acquired sensitization (rare), clamminess, unpleasant odor during administration

Intravenous:
>10%: Miscellaneous: Anaphylactoid reaction (~17%; reported as severe in 1% or moderate in 10% of patients within 15 minutes of first infusion; severe in 1% or mild to moderate in 6% to 7% of patients after 60-minute infusion)
1% to 10%:
  Cardiovascular: Angioedema (2% to 8%), vasodilation (1% to 6%), hypotension (1% to 4%), tachycardia (1% to 4%), syncope (1% to 3%), chest tightness (1%), flushing (1%)
  Central nervous system: Dysphoria (<1% to 2%)
  Dermatologic: Urticaria (2% to 7%), rash (1% to 5%), facial erythema (≤1%), palmar erythema (≤1%), pruritus (≤1% to 3%), pruritus with rash and vasodilation (2% to 9%)
  Gastrointestinal: Vomiting (<1% to 10%), nausea (1% to 10%), dyspepsia (≤1%)
  Neuromuscular & skeletal: Gait disturbance (<1% to 2%)
  Ocular: Eye pain (<1% to 3%)
  Otic: Ear pain (1%)
  Respiratory: Bronchospasm (1% to 6%), cough (1% to 4%), dyspnea (<1% to 3%), pharyngitis (1%), rhinorrhea (1%), rhonchi (1%), throat tightness (1%)
  Miscellaneous: Diaphoresis (≤1%)

Mechanism of Action Exerts mucolytic action through its free sulfhydryl group which opens up the disulfide bonds in the mucoproteins thus lowering mucous viscosity. The exact mechanism of action in acetaminophen toxicity is unknown; thought to act by providing substrate for conjugation with the toxic metabolite.

Drug Interactions

Decreased Effect: Adsorbed by activated charcoal; clinical significance is minimal, though, once a pure acetaminophen ingestion requiring N-acetylcysteine is established; further charcoal dosing is unnecessary once the appropriate initial charcoal dose is achieved (5-10 g:g acetaminophen)

Pharmacodynamics/Kinetics

Onset of action: Inhalation: 5-10 minutes
Duration: Inhalation: >1 hour
Distribution: 0.47 L/kg
Protein binding, plasma: 83%
Half-life elimination:
  Reduced acetylcysteine: 2 hours
  Total acetylcysteine: Adults: 5.5 hours; Newborns: 11 hours
Time to peak, plasma: Oral: 1-2 hours
Excretion: Urine

Pregnancy Risk Factor B

Acetylcysteine Sodium *see* Acetylcysteine *on page 46*

Acetylsalicylic Acid *see* Aspirin *on page 145*

Achromycin *see* Tetracycline *on page 1467*

Aciclovir *see* Acyclovir *on page 49*

Acidulated Phosphate Fluoride *see* Fluoride *on page 671*

AcipHex® *see* Rabeprazole *on page 1327*

Aclovate® *see* Alclometasone *on page 60*

4-(9-Acridinylamino) Methanesulfon-m-Anisidide *see* Amsacrine *on page 123*

Acridinyl Anisidide *see* Amsacrine *on page 123*

Acrivastine and Pseudoephedrine
  (AK ri vas teen & soo doe e FED rin)

Related Information

Pseudoephedrine *on page 1309*
(Continued)

Acrivastine and Pseudoephedrine *(Continued)*

U.S. Brand Names Semprex®-D

Generic Available No

Synonyms Pseudoephedrine Hydrochloride and Acrivastine

Pharmacologic Category Antihistamine

Use Temporary relief of nasal congestion, decongest sinus openings, running nose, itching of nose or throat, and itchy, watery eyes due to hay fever or other upper respiratory allergies

Local Anesthetic/Vasoconstrictor Precautions Use with caution since pseudoephedrine is a sympathomimetic amine which could interact with epinephrine to cause a pressor response

Effects on Dental Treatment Key adverse event(s) related to dental treatment: Pseudoephedrine: Xerostomia (normal salivary flow resumes upon discontinuation).

Common Adverse Effects

>10%: Central nervous system: Drowsiness, headache

1% to 10%:

Cardiovascular: Tachycardia, palpitation

Central nervous system: Nervousness, dizziness, insomnia, vertigo, light-headedness, fatigue

Gastrointestinal: Nausea, vomiting, xerostomia, diarrhea

Genitourinary: Dysuria

Neuromuscular & skeletal: Weakness

Respiratory: Pharyngitis, cough increased

Miscellaneous: Diaphoresis

Mechanism of Action Refer to Pseudoephedrine; acrivastine is an analogue of triprolidine and it is considered to be relatively less sedating than traditional antihistamines; believed to involve competitive blockade of H_1-receptor sites resulting in the inability of histamine to combine with its receptor sites and exert its usual effects on target cells

Drug Interactions

Increased Effect/Toxicity: Increased risk of hypertensive crisis when acrivastine and pseudoephedrine are given with MAO inhibitors or sympathomimetics. Increased risk of severe CNS depression when given with CNS depressants and ethanol.

Decreased Effect: Decreased effect of guanethidine, reserpine, methyldopa, and beta-blockers when given in conjunction with acrivastine and pseudoephedrine.

Pharmacodynamics/Kinetics

Pseudoephedrine: See Pseudoephedrine.

Acrivastine:

Metabolism: Minimally hepatic

Time to peak: ~1.1 hours

Excretion: Urine (84%); feces (13%)

Pregnancy Risk Factor B

ACT® [OTC] *see* Fluoride *on page 671*

Act-D *see* Dactinomycin *on page 417*

ACTH *see* Corticotropin *on page 395*

ActHIB® *see* Haemophilus b Conjugate Vaccine *on page 534*

Acticin® *see* Permethrin *on page 1218*

Actidose-Aqua® [OTC] *see* Charcoal *on page 311*

Actidose® with Sorbitol [OTC] *see* Charcoal *on page 311*

Actifed® Cold and Allergy [OTC] *see* Triprolidine and Pseudoephedrine *on page 1542*

Actifed® Cold and Sinus [OTC] *see* Acetaminophen, Chlorpheniramine, and Pseudoephedrine *on page 43*

Actigall® *see* Ursodiol *on page 1552*

Actimmune® *see* Interferon Gamma-1b *on page 851*

Actinomycin *see* Dactinomycin *on page 417*

Actinomycin D *see* Dactinomycin *on page 417*

Actinomycin Cl *see* Dactinomycin *on page 417*

Actiq® *see* Fentanyl *on page 644*

Activase® *see* Alteplase *on page 77*

Activated Carbon *see* Charcoal *on page 311*

Activated Charcoal *see* Charcoal *on page 311*

Activated Dimethicone *see* Simethicone *on page 1394*

Activated Ergosterol *see* Ergocalciferol *on page 556*

Activated Methylpolysiloxane *see* Simethicone *on page 1394*

Activated Protein C, Human, Recombinant *see* Drotrecogin Alfa *on page 522*
Activella® *see* Estradiol and Norethindrone *on page 575*
Actonel® *see* Risedronate *on page 1352*
Actonel® and Calcium *see* Risedronate and Calcium *on page 1354*
Actoplus Met™ *see* Pioglitazone and Metformin *on page 1242*
Actos® *see* Pioglitazone *on page 1241*
ACT® Plus [OTC] *see* Fluoride *on page 671*
ACT® x2™ [OTC] *see* Fluoride *on page 671*
Acular® *see* Ketorolac *on page 886*
Acular LS™ *see* Ketorolac *on page 886*
Acular® PF *see* Ketorolac *on page 886*
ACV *see* Acyclovir *on page 49*
Acycloguanosine *see* Acyclovir *on page 49*

Acyclovir (ay SYE kloe veer)

Related Information
Sexually-Transmitted Diseases *on page 1674*
Systemic Viral Diseases *on page 1675*
Valacyclovir *on page 1553*
Viral Infections *on page 1709*
Related Sample Prescriptions
Herpes Simplex (Primary) *on page 1742*
Shingles (Varicella-Zoster Virus) *on page 1742*
U.S. Brand Names Zovirax®
Canadian Brand Names Apo-Acyclovir®; Gen-Acyclovir; Nu-Acyclovir; ratio-Acyclovir; Zovirax®
Mexican Brand Names Acifur®; Cicloferon®; Isavir®; Laciken®; Opthavir®; Zovirax®
Generic Available Yes: Excludes cream, ointment
Synonyms Aciclovir; ACV; Acycloguanosine
Pharmacologic Category Antiviral Agent
Dental Use Treatment of initial and prophylaxis of recurrent mucosal and cutaneous herpes simplex (HSV-1 and HSV-2) infections in immunocompromised patients
Use Treatment of genital herpes simplex virus (HSV), herpes labialis (cold sores), herpes zoster (shingles), HSV encephalitis, neonatal HSV, mucocutaneous HSV in immunocompromised patients, varicella-zoster (chickenpox)
Unlabeled/Investigational Use Prevention of HSV reactivation in HIV-positive patients; prevention of HSV reactivation in hematopoietic stem-cell transplant (HSCT); prevention of HSV reactivation during periods of neutropenia in patients with acute leukemia
Local Anesthetic/Vasoconstrictor Precautions No information available to require special precautions
Effects on Dental Treatment Key adverse event(s) related to dental treatment: Topical (Zovirax® cream): Dry/cracked lips and dry/flaky skin were reported in fewer than 1 in 100 patients in clinical studies.
Significant Adverse Effects
Systemic: Oral:
>10%: Central nervous system: Malaise (12%)
1% to 10%:
Central nervous system: Headache (2%)
Gastrointestinal: Nausea (2% to 5%), vomiting (3%), diarrhea (2% to 3%)
Systemic: Parenteral:
1% to 10%:
Dermatologic: Hives (2%), itching (2%), rash (2%)
Gastrointestinal: Nausea/vomiting (7%)
Hepatic: Liver function tests increased (1% to 2%)
Local: Inflammation at injection site or phlebitis (9%)
Renal: BUN increased (5% to 10%), creatinine increased (5% to 10%), acute renal failure
Topical:
>10%: Dermatologic: Mild pain, burning, or stinging (ointment 30%)
1% to 10%: Dermatologic: Pruritus (ointment 4%), itching
All forms: <1% (Limited to important or life-threatening): Abdominal pain, aggression, agitation, alopecia, anaphylaxis, anemia, angioedema, anorexia, ataxia, coma, confusion, consciousness decreased, delirium, desquamation, diarrhea, disseminated intravascular coagulopathy, dizziness, dry lips, dysarthria, encephalopathy, erythema multiforme, fatigue, fever, gastrointestinal distress, hallucinations, hematuria, hemolysis, hepatitis, hyperbilirubinemia, (Continued)

Acyclovir *(Continued)*

hypotension, insomnia, jaundice, leukocytoclastic vasculitis, leukocytosis, leukopenia, local tissue necrosis (following extravasation), lymphadenopathy, mental depression, myalgia, neutrophilia, paresthesia, peripheral edema, photosensitization, pruritus, psychosis, renal failure, seizure, somnolence, sore throat, Stevens-Johnson syndrome, thrombocytopenia, thrombocytopenic purpura/hemolytic uremic syndrome (TTP/HUS), thrombocytosis, toxic epidermal necrolysis, tremor, urticaria, visual disturbances

Dental Usual Dosing

Herpes labialis (cold sores): Children ≥12 years and Adults: Topical: Cream: Apply 5 times/day for 4 days

Mucocutaneous HSV: Adults:
  Immunocompromised (unlabeled use): Oral: 400 mg 5 times a day for 7-14 days
  Nonlife-threatening, immunocompromised: Topical: Ointment: 1/2" ribbon of ointment for a 4" square surface area every 3 hours (6 times/day) for 7 days

Dosage Note: Obese patients should be dosed using ideal body weight

Genital HSV:

I.V.: Children ≥12 years and Adults (immunocompetent): Initial episode, severe: 5 mg/kg every 8 hours for 5-7 days

Oral:
  Children:
    Initial episode (unlabeled use): 40-80 mg/kg/day divided into 3-4 doses for 5-10 days (maximum: 1 g/day)
    Chronic suppression (unlabeled use; limited data): 80 mg/kg/day in 3 divided doses (maximum: 1 g/day), re-evaluate after 12 months of treatment

  Adults:
    Initial episode: 200 mg every 4 hours while awake (5 times/day) for 10 days (per manufacturer's labeling); 400 mg 3 times/day for 5-10 days has also been reported
    Recurrence: 200 mg every 4 hours while awake (5 times/day) for 5 days (per manufacturer's labeling); begin at earliest signs of disease); 400 mg 3 times/day for 5 days has also been reported
    Chronic suppression: 400 mg twice daily or 200 mg 3-5 times/day, for up to 12 months followed by re-evaluation (per manufacturer's labeling); 400-1200 mg/day in 2-3 divided doses has also been reported

Topical: Adults (immunocompetent): Ointment: Initial episode: 1/2" ribbon of ointment for a 4" square surface area every 3 hours (6 times/day) for 7 days

Herpes labialis (cold sores):
Topical: Children ≥12 years and Adults: Cream: Apply 5 times/day for 4 days

Herpes zoster (shingles):

Oral: Adults (immunocompetent): 800 mg every 4 hours (5 times/day) for 7-10 days

I.V.:
  Children <12 years (immunocompromised): 20 mg/kg/dose every 8 hours for 7 days
  Children ≥12 years and Adults (immunocompromised): 10 mg/kg/dose or 500 mg/m^2/dose every 8 hours for 7 days

HSV encephalitis: I.V.:
  Children 3 months to 12 years: 20 mg/kg/dose every 8 hours for 10 days (per manufacturer's labeling); dosing for 14-21 days also reported
  Children ≥12 years and Adults: 10 mg/kg/dose every 8 hours for 10 days (per manufacturer's labeling); 10-15 mg/kg/dose every 8 hours for 14-21 days also reported

Mucocutaneous HSV:
I.V.:
  Children <12 years (immunocompromised): 10 mg/kg/dose every 8 hours for 7 days
  Children ≥12 years and Adults (immunocompromised): 5 mg/kg/dose every 8 hours for 7 days (per manufacturer's labeling); dosing for up to 14 days also reported

Oral: Adults (immunocompromised, unlabeled use): 400 mg 5 times a day for 7-14 days

Topical: Ointment: Adults (nonlife-threatening, immunocompromised): 1/2" ribbon of ointment for a 4" square surface area every 3 hours (6 times/day) for 7 days

Neonatal HSV: I.V.: Neonate: Birth to 3 months: 10 mg/kg/dose every 8 hours for 10 days (manufacturer's labeling); 15 mg/kg/dose or 20 mg/kg/dose every 8 hours for 14-21 days has also been reported

Varicella-zoster (chickenpox): Begin treatment within the first 24 hours of rash onset:

Oral:

Children ≥2 years and ≤40 kg (immunocompetent): 20 mg/kg/dose (up to 800 mg/dose) 4 times/day for 5 days

Children >40 kg and Adults (immunocompetent): 800 mg/dose 4 times a day for 5 days

I.V.:

Children <1 year (immunocompromised, unlabeled use): 10 mg/kg/dose every 8 hours for 7-10 days

Children ≥1 year and Adults (immunocompromised, unlabeled use): 1500 mg/m^2/day divided every 8 hours or 10 mg/kg/dose every 8 hours for 7-10 days

Prevention of HSV reactivation in HIV-positive patients, for use only when recurrences are frequent or severe (unlabeled use): Oral:

Children: 80 mg/kg/day in 3-4 divided doses

Adults: 200 mg 3 times/day or 400 mg 2 times/day

Prevention of HSV reactivation in HSCT (unlabeled use): Note: Start at the beginning of conditioning therapy and continue until engraftment or until mucositis resolves (~30 days)

Oral: Adults: 200 mg 3 times/day

I.V.:

Children: 250 mg/m^2/dose every 8 hours or 125 mg/m^2/dose every 6 hours

Adults: 250 mg/m^2/dose every 12 hours

Bone marrow transplant recipients (unlabeled use): I.V.: Children and Adults: Allogeneic patients who are HSV and CMV seropositive: 500 mg/m^2/dose (10 mg/kg) every 8 hours; for clinically-symptomatic CMV infection, consider replacing acyclovir with ganciclovir

Dosing adjustment in renal impairment:

Oral:

Cl$_{cr}$ 10-25 mL/minute/1.73 m^2: Normal dosing regimen 800 mg every 4 hours: Administer 800 mg every 8 hours

Cl$_{cr}$ <10 mL/minute/1.73 m^2:

Normal dosing regimen 200 mg every 4 hours, 200 mg every 8 hours, or 400 mg every 12 hours: Administer 200 mg every 12 hours

Normal dosing regimen 800 mg every 4 hours: Administer 800 mg every 12 hours

I.V.:

Cl$_{cr}$ 25-50 mL/minute/1.73 m^2: Administer recommended dose every 12 hours

Cl$_{cr}$ 10-25 mL/minute/1.73 m^2: Administer recommended dose every 24 hours

Cl$_{cr}$ <10 mL/minute/1.73 m^2: Administer 50% of recommended dose every 24 hours

Hemodialysis: Administer dose after dialysis

Peritoneal dialysis: No supplemental dose needed

CAVH: 3.5 mg/kg/day

CVVHD/CVVH: Adjust dose based upon Cl$_{cr}$ 30 mL/minute

Mechanism of Action Acyclovir is converted to acyclovir monophosphate by virus-specific thymidine kinase then further converted to acyclovir triphosphate by other cellular enzymes. Acyclovir triphosphate inhibits DNA synthesis and viral replication by competing with deoxyguanosine triphosphate for viral DNA polymerase and being incorporated into viral DNA.

Contraindications Hypersensitivity to acyclovir, valacyclovir, or any component of the formulation

Warnings/Precautions Use with caution in immunocompromised patients; thrombocytopenic purpura/hemolytic uremic syndrome (TTP/HUS) has been reported. Use caution in the elderly, pre-existing renal disease, or in those receiving other nephrotoxic drugs. Maintain adequate hydration during oral or intravenous therapy. Use I.V. preparation with caution in patients with underlying neurologic abnormalities, serious hepatic or electrolyte abnormalities, or substantial hypoxia.

Safety and efficacy of oral formulations have not been established in pediatric patients <2 years of age.

Chickenpox: Treatment should begin within 24 hours of appearance of rash; oral route not recommended for routine use in otherwise healthy children with varicella, but may be effective in patients at increased risk of moderate to severe infection (>12 years of age, chronic cutaneous or pulmonary disorders, long-term salicylate therapy, corticosteroid therapy).

(Continued)

Acyclovir *(Continued)*

Genital herpes: Physical contact should be avoided when lesions are present; transmission may also occur in the absence of symptoms. Treatment should begin with the first signs or symptoms.

Herpes labialis: For external use only to the lips and face; do not apply to eye or inside the mouth or nose. Treatment should begin with the first signs or symptoms.

Herpes zoster: Acyclovir should be started within 72 hours of appearance of rash to be effective.

Ethanol/Nutrition/Herb Interactions Food: Does not affect absorption of oral acyclovir.

Dietary Considerations May be taken with or without food. Acyclovir 500 mg injection contains sodium ~50 mg (~2 mEq).

Pharmacodynamics/Kinetics

Absorption: Oral: 15% to 30%

Distribution: V_d: 0.8 L/kg (63.6 L): Widely (eg, brain, kidney, lungs, liver, spleen, muscle, uterus, vagina, CSF)

Protein binding: 9% to 33%

Metabolism: Converted by viral enzymes to acyclovir monophosphate, and further converted to diphosphate then triphosphate (active form) by cellular enzymes

Bioavailability: Oral: 10% to 20% with normal renal function (bioavailability decreases with increased dose)

Half-life elimination: Terminal: Neonates: 4 hours; Children 1-12 years: 2-3 hours; Adults: 3 hours

Time to peak, serum: Oral: Within 1.5-2 hours

Excretion: Urine (62% to 90% as unchanged drug and metabolite)

Pregnancy Risk Factor B

Lactation Enters breast milk/use with caution (AAP rates "compatible")

Breast-Feeding Considerations Nursing mothers with herpetic lesions near or on the breast should avoid breast-feeding. Limited data suggest exposure to the nursing infant of ~0.3 mg/kg/day following oral administration of acyclovir to the mother.

Dosage Forms [DSC] = Discontinued product

Capsule: 200 mg
Zovirax®: 200 mg
Cream, topical:
Zovirax®: 5% (2 g)
Injection, powder for reconstitution, as sodium: 500 mg, 1000 mg
Zovirax®: 500 mg [DSC]
Injection, solution, as sodium [preservative free]: 25 mg/mL (20 mL, 40 mL); 50 mg/mL (10 mL, 20 mL)
Ointment, topical:
Zovirax®: 5% (15 g)
Suspension, oral: 200 mg/5 mL (480 mL)
Zovirax®: 200 mg/5 mL (480 mL) [banana flavor]
Tablet: 400 mg, 800 mg
Zovirax®: 400 mg, 800 mg

Aczone™ see Dapsone on page 421
AD3L see Valrubicin on page 1560
Adagen® see Pegademase Bovine on page 1193
Adalat® CC see NIFEdipine on page 1112

Adalimumab *(a da LIM yoo mab)*

Related Information
Rheumatoid Arthritis, Osteoarthritis, and Osteoporosis on page 1668
U.S. Brand Names Humira®
Canadian Brand Names Humira®
Generic Available No
Synonyms Antitumor Necrosis Factor Apha (Human); D2E7; Human Antitumor Necrosis Factor Alpha
Pharmacologic Category Antirheumatic, Disease Modifying; Monoclonal Antibody; Tumor Necrosis Factor (TNF) Blocking Agent
Use Treatment of active rheumatoid and active psoriatic arthritis (moderate to severe). **Note:** May be used alone or in combination with disease-modifying antirheumatic drugs (DMARDs).
Local Anesthetic/Vasoconstrictor Precautions No information available to require special precautions

Effects on Dental Treatment No significant effects or complications reported

Common Adverse Effects

>10%:

Central nervous system: Headache (12%)

Dermatologic: Rash (12%)

Local: Injection site reaction (20%; includes erythema, itching, hemorrhage, pain, swelling)

Respiratory: Upper respiratory tract infection (17%), sinusitis (11%)

5% to 10%:

Cardiovascular: Hypertension (5%)

Endocrine & metabolic: Hyperlipidemia (7%), hypercholesterolemia (6%)

Gastrointestinal: Nausea (9%), abdominal pain (7%)

Genitourinary: Urinary tract infection (8%)

Hepatic: Alkaline phosphatase increased (5%)

Local: Injection-site reaction (8%; other than erythema, itching, hemorrhage, pain, swelling)

Neuromuscular & skeletal: Back pain (6%)

Renal: Hematuria (5%)

Miscellaneous: Accidental injury (10%), flu-like syndrome (7%)

<5%:

Cardiovascular: Arrhythmia, atrial fibrillation, chest pain, CHF, coronary artery disorder, heart arrest, hypertensive encephalopathy, myocardial infarct, palpitation, pericardial effusion, pericarditis, peripheral edema, syncope, tachycardia, thrombosis (leg), vascular disorder

Central nervous system: Confusion, fever, multiple sclerosis, pain in extremity, paresthesia, subdural hematoma, tremor

Dermatologic: Cellulitis

Endocrine & metabolic: Dehydration, menstrual disorder, parathyroid disorder

Gastrointestinal: Diverticulitis, esophagitis, gastroenteritis, gastrointestinal hemorrhage, vomiting

Genitourinary: Cystitis, pelvic pain

Hematologic: Agranulocytosis, granulocytopenia, leukopenia, pancytopenia, polycythemia

Hepatic: Cholecystitis, cholelithiasis, hepatic necrosis

Neuromuscular & skeletal: Arthritis, bone fracture, bone necrosis, joint disorder, muscle cramps, myasthenia, pyogenic arthritis, synovitis, tendon disorder

Ocular: Cataract

Renal: Kidney calculus, paraproteinemia, pyelonephritis

Respiratory: Asthma, bronchospasm, dyspnea, lung function decreased, pleural effusion, pneumonia

Miscellaneous: Adenoma, allergic reactions (1%), carcinoma (including breast, gastrointestinal, skin, urogenital), erysipelas, healing abnormality, herpes zoster, ketosis, lupus erythematosus syndrome, lymphoma, melanoma, postsurgical infection, sepsis, tuberculosis (reactivation of latent infection)

Mechanism of Action Adalimumab is a recombinant monoclonal antibody that binds to human tumor necrosis factor alpha (TNF-alpha), thereby interfering with binding to TNFα receptor sites and subsequent cytokine-driven inflammatory processes. Elevated TNF levels in the synovial fluid are involved in the pathologic pain and joint destruction in immune-mediated arthritis. Adalimumab decreases signs and symptoms of psoriatic and rheumatoid arthritis and inhibits progression of structural damage of rheumatoid arthritis.

Drug Interactions

Increased Effect/Toxicity: Concomitant use with anakinra may increase risk of infections; not recommended.

Decreased Effect: Concomitant use with vaccines (live) has not be studied; currently recommended not to administer live vaccines during adalimumab therapy.

Pharmacodynamics/Kinetics

Distribution: V_d: 4.7-6 L; Synovial fluid concentrations: 31% to 96% of serum

Bioavailability: Absolute: 64%

Half-life elimination: Terminal: ~2 weeks (range 10-20 days)

Time to peak, serum: SubQ: 131 ± 56 hours

Excretion: Clearance increased in the presence of antiadalimumab antibodies; decreased in patients 40 years and older

Pregnancy Risk Factor B

Adamantanamine Hydrochloride see Amantadine on page 81

Adapalene (a DAP a leen)

U.S. Brand Names Differin®
Canadian Brand Names Differin®
Generic Available No
Pharmacologic Category Acne Products
Use Treatment of acne vulgaris
Local Anesthetic/Vasoconstrictor Precautions No information available to require special precautions
Effects on Dental Treatment No significant effects or complications reported
Common Adverse Effects >10%: Dermatologic: Erythema, scaling, dryness, pruritus, burning, pruritus or burning immediately after application
Mechanism of Action Retinoid-like compound which is a modulator of cellular differentiation, keratinization, and inflammatory processes, all of which represent important features in the pathology of acne vulgaris
Pharmacodynamics/Kinetics
Absorption: Topical: Minimal
Excretion: Bile
Pregnancy Risk Factor C

Adderall® *see* Dextroamphetamine and Amphetamine *on page 448*
Adderall XR® *see* Dextroamphetamine and Amphetamine *on page 448*

Adefovir (a DEF o veer)

Related Information
HIV Infection and AIDS *on page 1662*
U.S. Brand Names Hepsera™
Generic Available No
Synonyms Adefovir Dipivoxil
Pharmacologic Category Antiretroviral Agent, Reverse Transcriptase Inhibitor (Nucleoside)
Use Treatment of chronic hepatitis B with evidence of active viral replication (based on persistent elevation of ALT/AST or histologic evidence), including patients with lamivudine-resistant hepatitis B
Local Anesthetic/Vasoconstrictor Precautions No information available to require special precautions
Effects on Dental Treatment No significant effects or complications reported
Common Adverse Effects
>10%: Renal: Hematuria (11% vs 10% in placebo-treated)
1% to 10%:
Central nervous system: Fever, headache
Dermatologic: Rash, pruritus
Gastrointestinal: Dyspepsia (3%), nausea, vomiting, flatulence, diarrhea, abdominal pain
Hepatic: AST/ALT increased, abnormal liver function, hepatic failure
Neuromuscular & skeletal: Weakness
Renal: Serum creatinine increased (4%), renal failure, renal insufficiency
Note: In patients with baseline renal dysfunction, frequency of increased serum creatinine has been observed to be as high as 26% to 37%; the role of adefovir in these changes could not be established.
Respiratory: Cough increased, sinusitis, pharyngitis
Mechanism of Action Acyclic nucleotide reverse transcriptase inhibitor (adenosine analog) which interferes with HBV viral RNA-dependent DNA polymerase resulting in inhibition of viral replication.
Drug Interactions
Increased Effect/Toxicity: Ibuprofen increases the bioavailability of adefovir. Concurrent use of nephrotoxic agents (including aminoglycosides, cyclosporine, NSAIDs, tacrolimus, vancomycin) may increase the risk of nephrotoxicity.
Pharmacodynamics/Kinetics
Distribution: 0.35-0.39 L/kg
Protein binding: ≤4%
Metabolism: Prodrug; rapidly converted to adefovir (active metabolite) in intestine
Bioavailability: 59%
Half-life elimination: 7.5 hours; prolonged in renal impairment
Time to peak: 1.75 hours
Excretion: Urine (45% as active metabolite within 24 hours)
Pregnancy Risk Factor C

Adefovir Dipivoxil *see* Adefovir *on page 54*
Adenocard® *see* Adenosine *on page 55*
Adenoscan® *see* Adenosine *on page 55*

Adenosine (a DEN oh seen)

U.S. Brand Names Adenocard®; Adenoscan®
Canadian Brand Names Adenocard®; Adenoscan®; Adenosine Injection, USP
Generic Available Yes
Synonyms 9-Beta-D-ribofuranosyladenine
Pharmacologic Category Antiarrhythmic Agent, Class IV; Diagnostic Agent
Use
  Adenocard®: Treatment of paroxysmal supraventricular tachycardia (PSVT) including that associated with accessory bypass tracts (Wolff-Parkinson-White syndrome); when clinically advisable, appropriate vagal maneuvers should be attempted prior to adenosine administration; **not effective in atrial flutter, atrial fibrillation, or ventricular tachycardia**
  Adenoscan®: Pharmacologic stress agent used in myocardial perfusion thallium-201 scintigraphy
Unlabeled/Investigational Use
  Adenoscan®: Acute vasodilator testing in pulmonary artery hypertension
Local Anesthetic/Vasoconstrictor Precautions No information available to require special precautions
Effects on Dental Treatment No significant effects or complications reported
Mechanism of Action Slows conduction time through the AV node, interrupting the re-entry pathways through the AV node, restoring normal sinus rhythm
Pregnancy Risk Factor C

ADH *see* Vasopressin *on page 1567*
Adipex-P® *see* Phentermine *on page 1224*
Adoxa™ *see* Doxycycline (Systemic) *on page 514*
Adrenalin® *see* Epinephrine *on page 546*
Adrenaline *see* Epinephrine *on page 546*
Adrenocorticotropic Hormone *see* Corticotropin *on page 395*
ADR (error-prone abbreviation) *see* DOXOrubicin *on page 509*
Adria *see* DOXOrubicin *on page 509*
Adriamycin PFS® *see* DOXOrubicin *on page 509*
Adriamycin RDF® *see* DOXOrubicin *on page 509*
Adrucil® *see* Fluorouracil *on page 674*
Adsorbent Charcoal *see* Charcoal *on page 311*
Advair Diskus® *see* Fluticasone and Salmeterol *on page 690*
Advantage-S™ [OTC] *see* Nonoxynol 9 *on page 1124*
Advate *see* Antihemophilic Factor (Recombinant) *on page 130*
Advicor® *see* Niacin and Lovastatin *on page 1107*
Advil® [OTC] *see* Ibuprofen *on page 808*
Advil® Children's [OTC] *see* Ibuprofen *on page 808*
Advil® Cold, Children's [OTC] *see* Pseudoephedrine and Ibuprofen *on page 1311*
Advil® Cold & Sinus [OTC] *see* Pseudoephedrine and Ibuprofen *on page 1311*
Advil® Infants' [OTC] *see* Ibuprofen *on page 808*
Advil® Junior [OTC] *see* Ibuprofen *on page 808*
Advil® Migraine [OTC] *see* Ibuprofen *on page 808*
AeroBid® *see* Flunisolide *on page 667*
AeroBid®-M *see* Flunisolide *on page 667*
Afeditab™ CR *see* NIFEdipine *on page 1112*
Afrin® Extra Moisturizing [OTC] *see* Oxymetazoline *on page 1172*
Afrin® Original [OTC] *see* Oxymetazoline *on page 1172*
Afrin® Severe Congestion [OTC] *see* Oxymetazoline *on page 1172*
Afrin® Sinus [OTC] *see* Oxymetazoline *on page 1172*
Aftate® Antifungal [OTC] [DSC] *see* Tolnaftate *on page 1506*
AG *see* Aminoglutethimide *on page 87*

Agalsidase Beta (aye GAL si days BAY ta)

U.S. Brand Names Fabrazyme®
Canadian Brand Names Fabrazyme®
Generic Available No
(Continued)

Agalsidase Beta *(Continued)*

Synonyms Alpha-Galactosidase-A (Human, Recombinant); r-h α-GAL

Pharmacologic Category Enzyme

Use Replacement therapy for Fabry disease

Local Anesthetic/Vasoconstrictor Precautions No information available to require special precautions

Effects on Dental Treatment No significant effects or complications reported

Common Adverse Effects Note: The most common and serious adverse reactions are infusion reactions (symptoms may include fever, tachycardia, hypertension, throat tightness, dyspnea, chills, abdominal pain, pruritus, urticaria, vomiting).

>10%:

Cardiovascular: Edema (21%), chest pain (17%), hypotension (14%)

Central nervous system: Fever (48%), headache (45%), anxiety (28%), pain (21%), dizziness (14%), paresthesia (14%)

Dermatologic: Pallor (14%)

Gastrointestinal: Nausea (28%)

Neuromuscular & skeletal: Rigors (52%), skeletal pain (21%)

Respiratory: Rhinitis (38%), pharyngitis (28%)

Miscellaneous: Infusion reactions (alteration of temperature sensation 17%)

1% to 10%:

Cardiovascular: Cardiomegaly (10%), hypertension (10%)

Central nervous system: Depression (10%)

Gastrointestinal: Dyspepsia (10%)

Genitourinary: Testicular pain (7%)

Neuromuscular & skeletal: Arthrosis (10%)

Respiratory: Bronchitis (10%), bronchospasm (7%), laryngitis (7%), sinusitis (7%)

Other reported severe reactions (frequency not established): Arrhythmia, ataxia, bradycardia, cardiac arrest, cardiac output decreased, nephritic syndrome, stroke, vertigo

Mechanism of Action Agalsidase beta is a recombinant form of the enzyme alpha-galactosidase-A, which is required for the hydrolysis of GL-3 and other glycosphingolipids. The compounds may accumulate (over many years) within the tissues of patients with Fabry disease, leading to renal and cardiovascular complications. In clinical trials of limited duration, agalsidase been noted to reduce tissue inclusions of a key sphingolipid (GL-3). It is believed that long-term enzyme replacement may reduce clinical manifestations of renal failure, cardiomyopathy, and stroke. However, the relationship to a reduction in clinical manifestations has not been established.

Pharmacodynamics/Kinetics Half-life elimination: 42-102 minutes (nonlinear)

Pregnancy Risk Factor B

Agenerase® *see* Amprenavir *on page 122*

Aggrastat® *see* Tirofiban *on page 1496*

Aggrenox® *see* Aspirin and Dipyridamole *on page 150*

AgNO₃ *see* Silver Nitrate *on page 1392*

Agrylin® *see* Anagrelide *on page 124*

AGT *see* Aminoglutethimide *on page 87*

AHA *see* Acetohydroxamic Acid *on page 46*

AH-Chew® [DSC] *see* Chlorpheniramine, Phenylephrine, and Methscopolamine *on page 327*

AH-Chew II *see* Chlorpheniramine, Phenylephrine, and Methscopolamine *on page 327*

AH-Chew® D [OTC] [DSC] *see* Phenylephrine *on page 1226*

AHF (Human) *see* Antihemophilic Factor (Human) *on page 129*

AHF (Recombinant) *see* Antihemophilic Factor (Recombinant) *on page 130*

A-hydroCort *see* Hydrocortisone *on page 793*

AICC *see* Anti-inhibitor Coagulant Complex *on page 130*

AK-Con™ *see* Naphazoline *on page 1087*

AK-Dilate® *see* Phenylephrine *on page 1226*

Akineton® *see* Biperiden *on page 208*

Akne-Mycin® *see* Erythromycin *on page 562*

AK-Pentolate® [DSC] *see* Cyclopentolate *on page 402*

AK-Poly-Bac® *see* Bacitracin and Polymyxin B *on page 176*

AK-Pred® *see* PrednisoLONE *on page 1268*

AKTob® *see* Tobramycin *on page 1498*

AK-Tracin® [DSC] *see* Bacitracin *on page 175*

AK-Trol® [DSC] *see* Neomycin, Polymyxin B, and Dexamethasone *on page 1101*

Akwa Tears® [OTC] *see* Artificial Tears *on page 143*

Alamag [OTC] *see* Aluminum Hydroxide and Magnesium Hydroxide *on page 80*

Alamag Plus [OTC] *see* Aluminum Hydroxide, Magnesium Hydroxide, and Simethicone *on page 81*

Alamast® *see* Pemirolast *on page 1199*

Alatrofloxacin Mesylate *see* Trovafloxacin *on page 1546*

Alavert® [OTC] *see* Loratadine *on page 946*

Alavert™ Allergy and Sinus [OTC] *see* Loratadine and Pseudoephedrine *on page 947*

Albalon® *see* Naphazoline *on page 1087*

Albendazole (al BEN da zole)

U.S. Brand Names Albenza®

Mexican Brand Names Bendapar®; Digezanol®; Endoplus®; Eskazole®; Gascop®; Lurdex®; Zentel®

Generic Available No

Pharmacologic Category Anthelmintic

Use Treatment of parenchymal neurocysticercosis caused by *Taenia solium* and cystic hydatid disease of the liver, lung, and peritoneum caused by *Echinococcus granulosus*

Unlabeled/Investigational Use Albendazole has activity against *Ascaris lumbricoides* (roundworm); *Ancylostoma caninum*; *Ancylostoma duodenale* and *Necator americanus* (hookworms); cutaneous larva migrans; *Enterobius vermicularis* (pinworm); *Gnathostoma spinigerum*; *Gongylonema* sp; *Hymenolepis nana* sp (tapeworms); *Mansonella perstans* (filariasis); *Opisthorchis sinensis* and *Opisthorchis viverrini* (liver flukes); *Strongyloides stercoralis* and *Trichuris trichiura* (whipworm); visceral larva migrans (toxocariasis); activity has also been shown against the liver fluke *Clonorchis sinensis*, *Giardia lamblia*, *Cysticercus cellulosae*, and *Echinococcus multilocularis*. Albendazole has also been used for the treatment of intestinal microsporidiosis (*Encephalitozoon intestinalis*), disseminated microsporidiosis (*E. hellem*, *E. cuniculi*, *E. intestinalis*, *Pleistophora* sp, *Trachipleistophora* sp, *Brachiola vesicularum*), and ocular microsporidiosis (*E. hellem*, *E. cuniculi*, *Vittaforma corneae*).

Local Anesthetic/Vasoconstrictor Precautions No information available to require special precautions

Effects on Dental Treatment No significant effects or complications reported

Common Adverse Effects

N = Neurocysticercosis; H = Hydatid disease

>10%:
  Central nervous system: Headache (11% - N; 1% - H)
  Hepatic: LFTs increased (~15% - H; <1% - N)

1% to 10%:
  Central nervous system: Dizziness, vertigo, fever (≤1%), intracranial pressure increased (1% - N), meningeal signs (1% - N)
  Dermatologic: Alopecia (2% - H; <1% - N)
  Gastrointestinal: Abdominal pain (6% - H; 0% - N), nausea/vomiting (3% to 6%)
  Hematologic: Leukopenia (reversible) (<1%)
  Miscellaneous: Allergic reactions (<1%)

Mechanism of Action Active metabolite, albendazole, causes selective degeneration of cytoplasmic microtubules in intestinal and tegmental cells of intestinal helminths and larvae; glycogen is depleted, glucose uptake and cholinesterase secretion are impaired, and desecratory substances accumulate intracellulary. ATP production decreases causing energy depletion, immobilization, and worm death.

Drug Interactions

Cytochrome P450 Effect: Substrate (minor) of CYP1A2, 3A4; **Inhibits** CYP1A2 (weak)

Pharmacodynamics/Kinetics

Absorption: <5%; may increase up to 4-5 times when administered with a fatty meal

Distribution: Well inside hydatid cysts and CSF

Protein binding: 70%

Metabolism: Hepatic; extensive first-pass effect; pathways include rapid sulfoxidation (major), hydrolysis, and oxidation

Half-life elimination: 8-12 hours

Time to peak, serum: 2-2.4 hours

Excretion: Urine (<1% as active metabolite); feces

Pregnancy Risk Factor C

Albenza® *see* Albendazole *on page 57*

Albuterol (al BYOO ter ole)

Related Information
Respiratory Diseases *on page 1656*

U.S. Brand Names AccuNeb™; Proventil®; Proventil® HFA; Ventolin® HFA; VoSpire ER®

Canadian Brand Names Airomir; Alti-Salbutamol; Apo-Salvent®; Gen-Salbutamol; PMS-Salbutamol; ratio-Inspra-Sal; ratio-Salbutamol; Rhoxal-salbutamol; Salbu-2; Salbu-4; Ventolin®; Ventolin® Diskus; Ventolin® HFA; Ventrodisk

Mexican Brand Names Salbulin Autohaler®; Ventolin®; Volmax®

Generic Available Yes: Excludes extended release

Synonyms Albuterol Sulfate; Salbutamol

Pharmacologic Category Beta$_2$-Adrenergic Agonist

Use Bronchodilator in reversible airway obstruction due to asthma or COPD; prevention of exercise-induced bronchospasm

Local Anesthetic/Vasoconstrictor Precautions No information available to require special precautions

Effects on Dental Treatment Key adverse event(s) related to dental treatment: Xerostomia (normal salivary flow resumes upon discontinuation).

Common Adverse Effects Incidence of adverse effects is dependent upon age of patient, dose, and route of administration.

Cardiovascular: Angina, atrial fibrillation, chest discomfort, extrasystoles, flushing, hypertension, palpitation, tachycardia

Central nervous system: CNS stimulation, dizziness, drowsiness, headache, insomnia, irritability, lightheadedness, migraine, nervousness, nightmares, restlessness, sleeplessness, tremor

Dermatologic: Angioedema, erythema multiforme, rash, Stevens-Johnson syndrome, urticaria

Endocrine & metabolic: Hypokalemia, serum glucose increased, serum potassium decreased

Gastrointestinal: Diarrhea, dry mouth, gastroenteritis, nausea, unusual taste, vomiting, tooth discoloration

Genitourinary: Micturition difficulty

Neuromuscular & skeletal: Muscle cramps, weakness

Otic: Otitis media, vertigo

Respiratory: Asthma exacerbation, bronchospasm, cough, epistaxis, laryngitis, oropharyngeal drying/irritation, oropharyngeal edema

Miscellaneous: Allergic reaction, lymphadenopathy

Dosage
Oral:

Children: Bronchospasm (treatment):

2-6 years: 0.1-0.2 mg/kg/dose 3 times/day; maximum dose not to exceed 12 mg/day (divided doses)

6-12 years: 2 mg/dose 3-4 times/day; maximum dose not to exceed 24 mg/day (divided doses)

Extended release: 4 mg every 12 hours; maximum dose not to exceed 24 mg/day (divided doses)

Children >12 years and Adults: Bronchospasm (treatment): 2-4 mg/dose 3-4 times/day; maximum dose not to exceed 32 mg/day (divided doses)

Extended release: 8 mg every 12 hours; maximum dose not to exceed 32 mg/day (divided doses). A 4 mg dose every 12 hours may be sufficient in some patients, such as adults of low body weight.

Elderly: Bronchospasm (treatment): 2 mg 3-4 times/day; maximum: 8 mg 4 times/day

Inhalation: MDI 90 mcg/puff:

Children ≤12 years:

Bronchospasm (acute): 4-8 puffs every 20 minutes for 3 doses, then every 1-4 hours; spacer/holding-chamber device should be used

Exercise-induced bronchospasm (prophylaxis): 1-2 puffs 5 minutes prior to exercise

Children >12 years and Adults:

Bronchospasm (acute): 4-8 puffs every 20 minutes for up to 4 hours, then every 1-4 hours as needed

Exercise-induced bronchospasm (prophylaxis): 2 puffs 5-30 minutes prior to exercise

Children ≥4 years and Adults: Bronchospasm (chronic treatment): 1-2 inhalations every 4-6 hours; maximum: 12 inhalations/day

NIH guidelines: 2 puffs 3-4 times a day as needed; may double dose for mild exacerbations

Nebulization:

Children ≤12 years:

Bronchospasm (treatment): 0.05 mg/kg every 4-6 hours; minimum dose: 1.25 mg, maximum dose: 2.5 mg

2-12 years: AccuNeb™: 0.63 mg or 1.25 mg 3-4 times/day, as needed, delivered over 5-15 minutes

Children >40 kg, patients with more severe asthma, or children 11-12 years: May respond better with a 1.25 mg dose

Bronchospasm (acute): Solution 0.5%: 0.15 mg/kg (minimum dose: 2.5 mg) every 20 minutes for 3 doses, then 0.15-0.3 mg/kg (up to 10 mg) every 1-4 hours as needed; may also use 0.5 mg/kg/hour by continuous infusion. Continuous nebulized albuterol at 0.3 mg/kg/hour has been used safely in the treatment of severe status asthmaticus in children; continuous nebulized doses of 3 mg/kg/hour ± 2.2 mg/kg/hour in children whose mean age was 20.7 months resulted in no cardiac toxicity; the optimal dosage for continuous nebulization remains to be determined.

Note: Use of the 0.5% solution should be used for bronchospasm (acute or treatment) in children <15 kg. AccuNeb™ has not been studied for the treatment of acute bronchospasm; use of the 0.5% concentrated solution may be more appropriate.

Children >12 years and Adults:

Bronchospasm (treatment): 2.5 mg, diluted to a total of 3 mL, 3-4 times/day over 5-15 minutes

NIH guidelines: 1.25-5 mg every 4-8 hours

Bronchospasm (acute) in intensive care patients: 2.5-5 mg every 20 minutes for 3 doses, then 2.5-10 mg every 1-4 hours as needed, **or** 10-15 mg/hour continuously

Hemodialysis: Not removed

Peritoneal dialysis: Significant drug removal is unlikely based on physiochemical characteristics

Mechanism of Action Relaxes bronchial smooth muscle by action on beta$_2$-receptors with little effect on heart rate

Contraindications Hypersensitivity to albuterol, adrenergic amines, or any component of the formulation

Warnings/Precautions Optimize anti-inflammatory treatment before initiating maintenance treatment with albuterol. Do not use as a component of chronic therapy without an anti-inflammatory agent. Only the mildest forms of asthma (Step 1 and/or exercise-induced) would not require concurrent use based upon asthma guidelines. Patient must be instructed to seek medical attention in cases where acute symptoms are not relieved or a previous level of response is diminished. The need to increase frequency of use may indicate deterioration of asthma, and treatment must not be delayed.

Use caution in patients with cardiovascular disease (arrhythmia or hypertension or CHF), convulsive disorders, diabetes, glaucoma, hyperthyroidism, or hypokalemia. Beta agonists may cause elevation in blood pressure, heart rate, and result in CNS stimulation/excitation. Beta$_2$ agonists may increase risk of arrhythmia, increase serum glucose, or decrease serum potassium.

Do not exceed recommended dose; serious adverse events, including fatalities, have been associated with excessive use of inhaled sympathomimetics. Rarely, paradoxical bronchospasm may occur with use of inhaled bronchodilating agents; this should be distinguished from inadequate response. All patients should utilize a spacer device when using a metered-dose inhaler; in addition, face masks should be used in children <4 years of age.

Because of its minimal effect on beta$_1$-receptors and its relatively long duration of action, albuterol is a rational choice in the elderly when an inhaled beta agonist is indicated. Oral use should be avoided in the elderly due to adverse effects. Patient response may vary between inhalers that contain chlorofluorocarbons and those which are chlorofluorocarbon-free.

Drug Interactions

Cytochrome P450 Effect: Substrate of CYP3A4 (major)

Increased Effect/Toxicity: When used with inhaled ipratropium, an increased duration of bronchodilation may occur. Cardiovascular effects are potentiated in patients also receiving MAO inhibitors, tricyclic antidepressants, and sympathomimetic agents (eg, amphetamine, dopamine, dobutamine). Albuterol may increase the risk of malignant arrhythmias with inhaled anesthetics (eg, enflurane, halothane).

Decreased Effect: When used with nonselective beta-adrenergic blockers (eg, propranolol) the effect of albuterol is decreased. Levels/effects of albuterol may be decreased by aminoglutethimide, carbamazepine, nafcillin, nevirapine, phenobarbital, phenytoin, rifamycins, and other CYP3A4 inducers.

(Continued)

Albuterol *(Continued)*

Ethanol/Nutrition/Herb Interactions
Food: Avoid or limit caffeine (may cause CNS stimulation).
Herb/Nutraceutical: Avoid ephedra, yohimbe (may cause CNS stimulation).

Dietary Considerations Oral forms should be administered with water 1 hour before or 2 hours after meals.

Pharmacodynamics/Kinetics
Onset of action: Peak effect:
  Nebulization/oral inhalation: 0.5-2 hours
    CFC-propelled albuterol: 10 minutes
    Ventolin® HFA: 25 minutes
  Oral: 2-3 hours
Duration: Nebulization/oral inhalation: 3-4 hours; Oral: 4-6 hours
Metabolism: Hepatic to an inactive sulfate
Half-life elimination: Inhalation: 3.8 hours; Oral: 3.7-5 hours
Excretion: Urine (30% as unchanged drug)

Pregnancy Risk Factor C

Dosage Forms AERO, for oral inhalation: (Proventil®): 90 mcg/dose (17 g). **AERO, for oral inhalation** [chlorofluorocarbon free]: (Proventil® HFA): 90 mcg/dose (6.7 g); (Ventolin® HFA): 90 mcg/dose (18 g). **SOLN, nebulization:** 0.083% (3 mL); 0.5% (20 mL); (AccuNeb™): 0.63 mg/3 mL (3 mL), 1.25 mg/3 mL (3 mL); (Proventil®): 0.083% (3 mL), 0.5% (20 mL). **SYR:** 2 mg/5 mL (480 mL). **TAB:** 2 mg, 4 mg. **TAB, extended release** (VoSpire®): 4 mg, 8 mg

Albuterol and Ipratropium *see* Ipratropium and Albuterol *on page 857*
Albuterol Sulfate *see* Albuterol *on page 58*
Alcaine® *see* Proparacaine *on page 1296*
Alcalak [OTC] *see* Calcium Carbonate *on page 248*

Alclometasone *(al kloe MET a sone)*

U.S. Brand Names Aclovate®
Generic Available Yes
Synonyms Alclometasone Dipropionate
Pharmacologic Category Corticosteroid, Topical
Dental Use Treatment of inflammation of corticosteroid-responsive dermatosis (low potency topical corticosteroid)
Use Treatment of inflammation of corticosteroid-responsive dermatosis (low potency topical corticosteroid)
Local Anesthetic/Vasoconstrictor Precautions No information available to require special precautions
Effects on Dental Treatment No significant effects or complications reported
Significant Adverse Effects Frequency not defined.
Dermatologic: Acne, allergic dermatitis, hypopigmentation, maceration of the skin, skin atrophy, striae, miliaria, telangiectasia
Endocrine & metabolic: HPA suppression, Cushing's syndrome, growth retardation
Local: Burning, erythema, itching, irritation, dryness, folliculitis, hypertrichosis
Systemic: HPA axis suppression, Cushing's syndrome, hyperglycemia; these reactions occur more frequently with occlusive dressings
Miscellaneous: Secondary infection

Dosage Topical: Apply a thin film to the affected area 2-3 times/day. Therapy should be discontinued when control is achieved; if no improvement is seen, reassessment of diagnosis may be necessary.

Mechanism of Action Stimulates the synthesis of enzymes needed to decrease inflammation, suppress mitotic activity, and cause vasoconstriction

Contraindications Hypersensitivity to alclometasone or any component of the formulation; viral, fungal, or tubercular skin lesions

Warnings/Precautions Adverse systemic effects may occur when used on large areas of the body, denuded areas, for prolonged periods of time, with an occlusive dressing, and/or in infants or small children (not for use in children <1 year of age).

Drug Interactions No data reported
Pregnancy Risk Factor C
Dosage Forms
Cream, as dipropionate: 0.05% (15 g, 45 g, 60 g)
Ointment, as dipropionate: 0.05% (15 g, 45 g, 60 g)

Alclometasone Dipropionate *see* Alclometasone *on page 60*
Aldactazide® *see* Hydrochlorothiazide and Spironolactone *on page 778*
Aldactone® *see* Spironolactone *on page 1413*

Aldara™ *see* Imiquimod *on page 821*

Aldesleukin (al des LOO kin)

U.S. Brand Names Proleukin®
Canadian Brand Names Proleukin®
Mexican Brand Names Proleukin®
Generic Available No
Synonyms Epidermal Thymocyte Activating Factor; ETAF; IL-2; Interleukin-2; Lymphocyte Mitogenic Factor; NSC-373364; T-Cell Growth Factor; TCGF; Thymocyte Stimulating Factor
Pharmacologic Category Biological Response Modulator
Use Treatment of metastatic renal cell cancer, melanoma
Unlabeled/Investigational Use Investigational: Multiple myeloma, HIV infection, and AIDS; may be used in conjunction with lymphokine-activated killer (LAK) cells, tumor-infiltrating lymphocyte (TIL) cells, interleukin-1, and interferons; colorectal cancer; non-Hodgkin's lymphoma
Local Anesthetic/Vasoconstrictor Precautions No information available to require special precautions
Effects on Dental Treatment Key adverse event(s) related to dental treatment: Stomatitis.

Common Adverse Effects
>10%:
  Cardiovascular: Hypotension (85%), dose-limiting, possibly fatal; sinus tachycardia (70%); arrhythmia (22%); edema (47%); angina
  Central nervous system: Mental status changes (transient memory loss, confusion, drowsiness) (73%); dizziness (17%); cognitive changes, fatigue, malaise, somnolence, and disorientation (25%); headaches; insomnia; paranoid delusion
  Dermatologic: Macular erythematous rash (100% of patients on high-dose therapy), pruritus (48%), erythema (41%), rash (26%), exfoliative dermatitis (14%), dry skin (15%)
  Endocrine & metabolic: Fever and chills (89%), electrolyte levels decreased (magnesium, calcium, phosphate, potassium, sodium) (1% to 15%)
  Gastrointestinal: Nausea and vomiting (87%), diarrhea (76%), stomatitis (32%), GI bleeding (13%), weight gain (23%), anorexia (27%)
  Hematologic: Anemia (77%), thrombocytopenia (64%), leukopenia (34%) - may be dose-limiting, coagulation disorders (10%)
  Hepatic: Transient elevations of bilirubin (64%) and enzymes (56%), jaundice (11%)
  Neuromuscular & skeletal: Weakness; rigors - respond to acetaminophen, diphenhydramine, an NSAID, or meperidine
  Renal: Oliguria/anuria (63%, severe in 5% to 6%); proteinuria (12%); renal failure (dose-limiting toxicity) manifested as oliguria noted within 24-48 hours of initiation of therapy; marked fluid retention, azotemia, and increased serum creatinine seen, which may return to baseline within 7 days of discontinuation of therapy; hypophosphatemia
  Respiratory: Congestion (54%), dyspnea (27% to 52%)
  Miscellaneous: Pain (54%), infection (including sepsis and endocarditis) due to neutrophil impairment (23%)
1% to 10%:
  Cardiovascular: Capillary leak syndrome, including peripheral edema, ascites, pulmonary infiltration, and pleural effusion (2% to 4%), may be dose-limiting and potentially fatal; MI (2%)
  Central nervous system: Seizures (1%)
  Endocrine & metabolic: Hypo- and hyperglycemia (2%), electrolyte levels increased (magnesium, calcium, phosphate, potassium, sodium) (1%), hypothyroidism
  Hepatic: Ascites (4%)
  Neuromuscular & skeletal: Arthralgia (6%), myalgia (6%)
  Renal: Hematuria (9%), creatinine increased (5%)
  Respiratory: Pleural effusions, edema (10%)
Mechanism of Action Aldesleukin promotes proliferation, differentiation, and recruitment of T and B cells, natural killer (NK) cells, and thymocytes; causes cytolytic activity in a subset of lymphocytes and subsequent interactions between the immune system and malignant cells; can stimulate lymphokine-activated killer (LAK) cells and tumor-infiltrating lymphocytes (TIL) cells.

Drug Interactions
Increased Effect/Toxicity: Aldesleukin may affect central nervous function; therefore, interactions could occur following concomitant administration of
(Continued)

Aldesleukin *(Continued)*

psychotropic drugs (eg, narcotics, analgesics, antiemetics, sedatives, tran-quilizers).

Concomitant administration of drugs possessing nephrotoxic (eg, aminoglyco-sides, indomethacin), myelotoxic (eg, cytotoxic chemotherapy), cardiotoxic (eg, doxorubicin), or hepatotoxic effects with aldesleukin may increase toxicity in these organ systems.

Beta-blockers and other antihypertensives may potentiate the hypotension seen with aldesleukin.

Decreased Effect: Corticosteroids have been shown to decrease toxicity of aldesleukin, but may reduce the efficacy of the lymphokine.

Pharmacodynamics/Kinetics
Distribution: V_d: 4-7 L; primarily in plasma and then in the lymphocytes
Bioavailability: I.M.: 37%
Half-life elimination: Initial: 6-13 minutes; Terminal: 80-120 minutes

Pregnancy Risk Factor C

Aldex™ *see* Guaifenesin and Phenylephrine *on page 754*

Aldomet *see* Methyldopa *on page 1021*

Aldoril® *see* Methyldopa and Hydrochlorothiazide *on page 1022*

Aldroxicon I [OTC] *see* Aluminum Hydroxide, Magnesium Hydroxide, and Simethi-cone *on page 81*

Aldroxicon II [OTC] *see* Aluminum Hydroxide, Magnesium Hydroxide, and Simethi-cone *on page 81*

Aldurazyme® *see* Laronidase *on page 900*

Alefacept *(a LE fa sept)*

U.S. Brand Names Amevive®
Canadian Brand Names Amevive®
Generic Available No
Synonyms B 9273; BG 9273; Human LFA-3/IgG(1) Fusion Protein; LFA-3/IgG(1) Fusion Protein, Human
Pharmacologic Category Monoclonal Antibody
Use Treatment of moderate to severe chronic plaque psoriasis in adults who are candidates for systemic therapy or phototherapy
Local Anesthetic/Vasoconstrictor Precautions No information available to require special precautions
Effects on Dental Treatment No significant effects or complications reported
Common Adverse Effects
≥10%:
Hematologic: Lymphopenia (up to 10% of patients required temporary discon-tinuation, up to 17% during a second course of therapy)
Local: Injection site reactions (up to 16% of patients; includes pain, inflamma-tion, bleeding, edema, or other reaction)
1% to 10%:
Central nervous system: Chills (6%; primarily during intravenous administra-tion), dizziness (≥2%)
Dermatologic: Pruritus (≥2%)
Gastrointestinal: Nausea (≥2%)
Neuromuscular & skeletal: Myalgia (≥2%)
Respiratory: Pharyngitis (≥2%), cough increased (≥2%)
Miscellaneous: Malignancies (1% vs 0.5% in placebo), antibodies to alefacept (3%; significance unknown), infection (1% requiring hospitalization)
Restrictions Alefacept will be distributed directly to physician offices or to a specialty pharmacy; injections are intended to be administered in the physi-cian's office
Mechanism of Action Binds to CD2, a receptor on the surface of lymphocytes, inhibiting their interaction with leukocyte functional antigen 3 (LFA-3). Interac-tion between CD2 and LFA-3 is important for the activation of T lymphocytes in psoriasis. Activated T lymphocytes secrete a number of inflammatory media-tors, including interferon gamma, which are involved in psoriasis. Since CD2 is primarily expressed on T lymphocytes, treatment results in a reduction in CD4⁺ and CD8⁺ T lymphocytes, with lesser effects on other cell populations (NK and B lymphocytes).
Drug Interactions
Increased Effect/Toxicity: No formal drug interaction studies have been completed.

Decreased Effect: No formal drug interaction studies have been completed.

Pharmacodynamics/Kinetics

Distribution: V_d: 0.094 L/kg

Bioavailability: 63% (following I.M. administration)

Half-life: 270 hours (following I.V. administration)

Excretion: Clearance: 0.25 mL/hour/kg

Pregnancy Risk Factor B

Alemtuzumab (ay lem TU zoo mab)

U.S. Brand Names Campath®

Generic Available No

Synonyms C1H; Campath-1H; DNA-Derived Humanized Monoclonal Antibody; Humanized IgG1 Anti-CD52 Monoclonal Antibody

Pharmacologic Category Antineoplastic Agent, Monoclonal Antibody

Use Treatment of B-cell chronic lymphocytic leukemia (B-CLL)

Unlabeled/Investigational Use Treatment of refractory T-cell prolymphocytic leukemia (T-PLL); rheumatoid arthritis; graft-versus-host disease; multiple myeloma; preconditioning regimen for stem-cell transplantation and renal and liver transplantation; post-transplant rejection (renal)

Local Anesthetic/Vasoconstrictor Precautions No information available to require special precautions

Effects on Dental Treatment Key adverse event(s) related to dental treatment: Stomatitis and mucositis.

Common Adverse Effects

>10%:

Cardiovascular: Hypotension (32%), peripheral edema (13%), hypertension (11%), tachycardia/SVT (11%)

Central nervous system: Fever (85%), fatigue (34%), headache (24%), dysthesias (15%), dizziness (12%)

Dermatologic: Rash (40%), urticaria (30%), pruritus (24%), herpes simplex (11%)

Gastrointestinal: Nausea (54%), vomiting (41%), anorexia (20%), diarrhea (22%), stomatitis/mucositis (14%), abdominal pain (11%)

Hematologic: Neutropenia (85%; grade 3/4: 64%; median duration: 28 days), anemia (80%; grade 3/4: 38%), thrombocytopenia (72%; grade 3/4: 50%; median duration: 21 days)

Neuromuscular & skeletal: Rigors (86%), skeletal muscle pain (24%), weakness (13%), myalgia (11%)

Respiratory: Dyspnea (26%), cough (25%), bronchitis/pneumonitis (21%), pneumonia (16%), pharyngitis (12%)

Miscellaneous: Infection (43% to 66%; incidence is lower if prophylaxis anti-infectives are utilized), diaphoresis (19%), sepsis (15%)

1% to 10%:

Cardiovascular: Chest pain (10%)

Central nervous system: Insomnia (10%), neutropenic fever (10%), malaise (9%), depression (7%), temperature change sensation (5%), somnolence (5%)

Dermatologic: Purpura (8%)

Gastrointestinal: Dyspepsia (10%), constipation (9%)

Hematologic: Pancytopenia/marrow hypoplasia (5% to 6%; grade 3/4: 3%), positive Coombs' test without hemolysis (2%), autoimmune thrombocytopenia (2%), autoimmune hemolytic anemia (1%)

Neuromuscular & skeletal: Back pain (10%), tremor (7%)

Respiratory: Bronchospasm (9%), epistaxis (7%), rhinitis (7%)

Miscellaneous: Moniliasis (8%)

Mechanism of Action Binds to CD52, a nonmodulating antigen present on the surface of B and T lymphocytes, a majority of monocytes, macrophages, NK cells, and a subpopulation of granulocytes. After binding to $CD52^+$ cells, an antibody-dependent lysis occurs.

Drug Interactions

Increased Effect/Toxicity: Monoclonal antibodies may increase the risk for allergic reactions to alemtuzumab due to the presence of HACA antibodies; avoid administration of live vaccines in immunosuppressive therapy.

Pharmacodynamics/Kinetics

Distribution: V_d: 0.18 L/kg

Metabolism: Clearance decreases with repeated dosing (due to loss of CD52 receptors in periphery), resulting in a sevenfold increase in AUC.

Half-life elimination: Initial: 11 hours; 6 days following repeated dosing

Pregnancy Risk Factor C

Alendronate (a LEN droe nate)

Related Information
Rheumatoid Arthritis, Osteoarthritis, and Osteoporosis *on page 1668*

U.S. Brand Names Fosamax®

Canadian Brand Names Apo-Alendronate®; Fosamax®; Novo-Alendronate; ratio-Alendronate

Generic Available No

Synonyms Alendronate Sodium

Pharmacologic Category Bisphosphonate Derivative

Use Treatment and prevention of osteoporosis in postmenopausal females; treatment of osteoporosis in males; Paget's disease of the bone in patients who are symptomatic, at risk for future complications, or with alkaline phosphatase ≥2 times the upper limit of normal; treatment of glucocorticoid-induced osteoporosis in males and females with low bone mineral density who are receiving a daily dosage ≥7.5 mg of prednisone (or equivalent)

Local Anesthetic/Vasoconstrictor Precautions No information available to require special precautions

Effects on Dental Treatment Osteonecrosis of the jaw (ONJ), generally associated with local infection and/or tooth extraction and often with delayed healing, has been reported in patients taking bisphosphonates. Most reported cases of bisphosphonate-associated osteonecrosis have been in cancer patients treated with intravenous bisphosphonates. However, some have occurred in patients with postmenopausal osteoporosis taking oral bisphosphonates. Dental surgery may exacerbate ONJ. For patients requiring dental procedures, there are no data available to suggest whether discontinuation of bisphosphonate treatment reduces the risk of ONJ. See Dental Comment.

Common Adverse Effects Note: Incidence of adverse effects (mostly GI) increases significantly in patients treated for Paget's disease at 40 mg/day.

>10%: Endocrine & metabolic: Hypocalcemia (transient, mild, 18%); hypophosphatemia (transient, mild, 10%)

1% to 10%:
Central nervous system: Headache (up to 3%)
Gastrointestinal: Abdominal pain (1% to 7%), acid reflux (1% to 4%), dyspepsia (1% to 4%), nausea (1% to 4%), flatulence (up to 4%), diarrhea (1% to 3%), gastroesophageal reflux disease (1% to 3%), constipation (up to 3%), esophageal ulcer (up to 2%), abdominal distension (up to 1%), gastritis (up to 1%), vomiting (up to 1%), dysphagia (up to 1%), gastric ulcer (1%), melena (1%)
Neuromuscular & skeletal: Musculoskeletal pain (up to 6%), muscle cramps (up to 1%)

Dosage Oral: Adults: **Note:** Patients treated with glucocorticoids and those with Paget's disease should receive adequate amounts of calcium and vitamin D.

Osteoporosis in postmenopausal females:
Prophylaxis: 5 mg once daily **or** 35 mg once weekly
Treatment: 10 mg once daily **or** 70 mg once weekly

Osteoporosis in males: 10 mg once daily **or** 70 mg once weekly

Osteoporosis secondary to glucocorticoids in males and females: Treatment: 5 mg once daily; a dose of 10 mg once daily should be used in postmenopausal females who are not receiving estrogen.

Paget's disease of bone in males and females: 40 mg once daily for 6 months

Retreatment: Relapses during the 12 months following therapy occurred in 9% of patients who responded to treatment. Specific retreatment data are not available. Following a 6-month post-treatment evaluation period, retreatment with alendronate may be considered in patients who have relapsed based on increases in serum alkaline phosphatase, which should be measured periodically. Retreatment may also be considered in those who failed to normalize their serum alkaline phosphatase.

Elderly: No dosage adjustment is necessary

Dosage adjustment in renal impairment:
Cl_{cr} 35-60 mL/minute: None necessary
Cl_{cr} <35 mL/minute: Alendronate is not recommended due to lack of experience

Dosage adjustment in hepatic impairment: None necessary

Mechanism of Action A bisphosphonate which inhibits bone resorption via actions on osteoclasts or on osteoclast precursors; decreases the rate of bone resorption, leading to an indirect increase in bone mineral density. In Paget's disease, characterized by disordered resorption and formation of bone, inhibition of resorption leads to an indirect decrease in bone formation; but the newly-formed bone has a more normal architecture.

Contraindications Hypersensitivity to alendronate, other bisphosphonates, or any component of the formulation; hypocalcemia; abnormalities of the esophagus which delay esophageal emptying such as stricture or achalasia; inability to stand or sit upright for at least 30 minutes; oral solution should not be used in patients at risk of aspiration

Warnings/Precautions Use caution in patients with renal impairment (not recommended for use in patients with Cl_{cr} <35 mL/minute); hypocalcemia must be corrected before therapy initiation; ensure adequate calcium and vitamin D intake. May cause irritation to upper gastrointestinal mucosa. Esophagitis, esophageal ulcers, esophageal erosions, and esophageal stricture (rare) have been reported; risk increases in patients unable to comply with dosing instructions. Use with caution in patients with dysphagia, esophageal disease, gastritis, duodenitis, or ulcers (may worsen underlying condition).

Bisphosphonate therapy has been associated with osteonecrosis, primarily of the jaw; this has been observed mostly in cancer patients, but also in patients with postmenopausal osteoporosis and other diagnoses. Dental exams and preventative dentistry should be performed prior to placing patients with risk factors on chronic bisphosphonate therapy. Invasive dental procedures should be avoided during treatment.

Infrequent reports of severe (and occasionally debilitating) bone, joint, and/or muscle pain during bisphosphonate treatment; onset of pain ranged from a single day to several months, with relief in most cases upon discontinuation of the drug. Some patients experienced recurrence when rechallenged with same drug or another bisphosphonate.

Safety and efficacy in children have not been established.

Drug Interactions

Increased Effect/Toxicity: Aminoglycosides may lower serum calcium levels with prolonged administration; concomitant use may have an additive hypocalcemic effect. NSAIDs may enhance the gastrointestinal adverse/toxic effects (increased incidence of GI ulcers) of bisphosphonate derivatives. Bisphosphonate derivatives may enhance the hypocalcemic effect of phosphate supplements.

Decreased Effect: The following agents may decrease the absorption of oral bisphosphonate derivatives: Antacids (aluminum, calcium, magnesium), oral calcium salts, oral iron salts, and oral magnesium salts.

Ethanol/Nutrition/Herb Interactions

Ethanol: Avoid ethanol (may increase risk of osteoporosis and gastric irritation).

Food: All food and beverages interfere with absorption. Coadministration with caffeine may reduce alendronate efficacy. Coadministration with dairy products may decrease alendronate absorption. Beverages (especially orange juice and coffee) and food may reduce the absorption of alendronate as much as 60%.

Dietary Considerations Ensure adequate calcium and vitamin D intake; however, wait at least 30 minutes after taking alendronate before taking any supplement. Alendronate must be taken with plain water first thing in the morning and at least 30 minutes before the first food or beverage of the day.

Pharmacodynamics/Kinetics

Distribution: 28 L (exclusive of bone)

Protein binding: ~78%

Metabolism: None

Bioavailability: Fasting: 0.6%; reduced 60% with food or drink

Half-life elimination: Exceeds 10 years

Excretion: Urine; feces (as unabsorbed drug)

Pregnancy Risk Factor C

Dosage Forms SOLN, oral: 70 mg/75 mL. **TAB:** 5 mg, 10 mg, 35 mg, 40 mg, 70 mg

Dental Comment

Novartis Pharmaceuticals Corporation has notified dental health professionals of the risk of osteonecrosis of the jaw (ONJ) and the use of the bisphosphonates, pamidronate, and zoledronic acid. This warning has not been issued for alendronate. There have been reported cases of osteonecrosis of the jaw in association with the use of alendronate to prevent or treat early osteoporosis. Marx has reported 3 cases, Ruggerio 7 cases, and Carter and Gross 1 case. In the three cases reported by Marx, one group was taking 10 mg/day for 6 years and the other two groups were taking 10 mg/day by mouth for 3 years and 2 years respectively.

Previously, Novartis and the Food and Drug Administration (FDA) had notified healthcare providers of a serious adverse event related to the use of bisphosphonates. Osteonecrosis of the jaw has been reported in patients with cancer who were receiving chemotherapy, corticosteroids, and chronic bisphosphonate therapy. The bisphosphonates involved were pamidronate and (Continued)

Alendronate *(Continued)*

zoledronic acid. Dental exams and preventative dentistry should be performed prior to placing patients with risk factors (chemotherapy, corticosteroids, poor oral hygiene) on chronic bisphosphonate therapy. Invasive dental procedures should be avoided during treatment. Product labelings for pamidronate (Aredia®) and zoledronic acid (Zometa®) have been updated. Recently, 63 cases of osteonecrosis associated with the use of bisphosphonates were published (Ruggiero, 2004). In a retrospective review, 56 of the patients received intravenous bisphosphonates for at least one year and 7 patients were on chronic oral therapy. The presenting symptom was a nonhealing extraction socket or an exposed jawbone. These lesions did not show evidence of metastatic disease and required removal of involved bone in most cases.

Bisphosphonates are widely used in the management of metastatic bone disease to treat hypercalcemia associated with malignancies and to treat osteoporosis. In the report by Ruggiero et al, the cluster of patients observed to have necrotic lesions in the jaw shared only one common clinical feature, all received chronic bisphosphonate therapy. The necrosis detected was typical of osteoradionecrosis. It was suggested that because of the trend in the use of chronic bisphosphonate therapy, the observation of an associated risk of osteonecrosis of the jaw should alert practitioners to monitor for this previously unrecognized potential complication.

Selected Readings

Carter GD and Goss AN, "Bisphosphonates and Avascular Necrosis of the Jaws," *Aust Dent J*, 2003, 48(4):268.

Marx RE, Sawatari Y, Fortin M, et al, "Bisphosphonate-Induced Exposed Bone (Osteonecrosis/Osteopetrosis) of the Jaws: Risk Factors, Recognition, Prevention, and Treatment," *J Oral Maxillofac Surg*, 2005, 63(11):1567-75.

Ruggiero SL, Mehrotra B, Rosenberg TJ, et al, "Osteonecrosis of the Jaws Associated With the Use of Bisphosphonates: A Review of 63 Cases," *J Oral Maxillofac Surg*, 2004, 62(5):527-34.

Alendronate and Cholecalciferol
(a LEN droe nate & kole e kal SI fer ole)

U.S. Brand Names Fosamax Plus D™
Canadian Brand Names Fosavance
Generic Available No
Synonyms Alendronate Sodium and Cholecalciferol; Cholecalciferol and Alendronate; Vitamin D_3
Pharmacologic Category Bisphosphonate Derivative; Vitamin D Analog
Use Treatment of osteoporosis in postmenopausal females; increase bone mass in males with osteoporosis
Local Anesthetic/Vasoconstrictor Precautions No information available to require special precautions
Effects on Dental Treatment Osteonecrosis of the jaw (ONJ), generally associated with local infection and/or tooth extraction and often with delayed healing, has been reported in patients taking bisphosphonates. Most reported cases of bisphosphonate-associated osteonecrosis have been in cancer patients treated with intravenous bisphosphonates. However, some have occurred in patients with postmenopausal osteoporosis taking oral bisphosphonates. Dental surgery may exacerbate ONJ. For patients requiring dental procedures, there are no data available to suggest whether discontinuation of bisphosphonate treatment reduces the risk of ONJ. See Dental Comment.
Common Adverse Effects See individual agents.
Mechanism of Action See individual agents.
Drug Interactions
 Increased Effect/Toxicity: See individual agents.
 Decreased Effect: See individual agents.
Pregnancy Risk Factor C
Dental Comment Novartis Pharmaceuticals Corporation has notified dental health professionals of the risk of osteonecrosis of the jaw (ONJ) and the use of the bisphosphonates, pamidronate, and zoledronic acid. This warning has not be issued for alendronate and cholecalciferol combination product.

Previously, Novartis and the Food and Drug Administration (FDA) had notified healthcare providers of a serious adverse event related to the use of bisphosphonates. Osteonecrosis of the jaw has been reported in patients with cancer who were receiving chemotherapy, corticosteroids, and chronic bisphosphonate therapy. The bisphosphonates involved were pamidronate and zoledronic acid. To date, there are no reported associations between alendronate and cholecalciferol and osteonecrosis of the jaw. Dental exams and preventative dentistry should be performed prior to placing patients with risk factors (chemotherapy, corticosteroids, poor oral hygiene) on chronic bisphosphonate therapy. Invasive dental procedures should be avoided during treatment. Product labelings for pamidronate (Aredia®) and zoledronic acid (Zometa®) have been updated. Recently, 63 cases of osteonecrosis associated with the use of bisphosphonates were published (Ruggiero, 2004). In a retrospective review, 56 of the patients received intravenous bisphosphonates for at least 1 year and 7 patients were on chronic oral therapy. The presenting symptom was a nonhealing extraction socket or an exposed jawbone. These lesions did not show evidence of metastatic disease and required removal of involved bone in most cases.

Bisphosphonates are widely used in the management of metastatic bone disease to treat hypercalcemia associated with malignancies and to treat osteoporosis. In the report by Ruggiero et al, the cluster of patients observed to have necrotic lesions in the jaw shared only one common clinical feature, all received chronic bisphosphonate therapy. The necrosis detected was typical of osteoradionecrosis. It was suggested that because of the trend in the use of chronic bisphosphonate therapy, the observation of an associated risk of osteonecrosis of the jaw should alert practitioners to monitor for this previously unrecognized potential complication.

Selected Readings

Ruggiero SL, Mehrotra B, Rosenberg TJ, et al, "Osteonecrosis of the Jaws Associated With the Use of Bisphosphonates: A Review of 63 Cases," *J Oral Maxillofac Surg*, 2004, 62(5):527-34.

Alendronate Sodium *see* Alendronate *on page 64*
Alendronate Sodium and Cholecalciferol *see* Alendronate and Cholecalciferol *on page 66*
Alenic Alka Tablet [OTC] *see* Aluminum Hydroxide and Magnesium Trisilicate *on page 80*
Aler-Cap [OTC] *see* DiphenhydrAMINE *on page 483*
Aler-Dryl [OTC] *see* DiphenhydrAMINE *on page 483*
Aler-Tab [OTC] *see* DiphenhydrAMINE *on page 483*
Alesse® *see* Ethinyl Estradiol and Levonorgestrel *on page 602*
Aleve® [OTC] *see* Naproxen *on page 1089*
Alfenta® *see* Alfentanil *on page 67*

Alfentanil (al FEN ta nil)

U.S. Brand Names Alfenta®
Canadian Brand Names Alfenta®; Alfentanil Injection, USP
Generic Available Yes
Synonyms Alfentanil Hydrochloride
Pharmacologic Category Analgesic, Narcotic
Use Analgesic adjunct given by continuous infusion or in incremental doses in maintenance of anesthesia with barbiturate or N_2O or a primary anesthetic agent for the induction of anesthesia in patients undergoing general surgery in which endotracheal intubation and mechanical ventilation are required

Local Anesthetic/Vasoconstrictor Precautions No information available to require special precautions

Effects on Dental Treatment Key adverse event(s) related to dental treatment: Orthostatic hypotension.
Erythromycin inhibits the liver metabolism of alfentanil resulting in increased sedation and prolonged respiratory depression. Clarithromycin may act similarly.

Common Adverse Effects
>10%:
  Cardiovascular: Bradycardia, peripheral vasodilation
  Central nervous system: Drowsiness, sedation, intracranial pressure increased
  Gastrointestinal: Nausea, vomiting, constipation
  Endocrine & metabolic: Antidiuretic hormone release
  Ocular: Miosis
1% to 10%:
  Cardiovascular: Cardiac arrhythmia, orthostatic hypotension
  Central nervous system: Confusion, CNS depression
  Ocular: Blurred vision

Restrictions C-II
Mechanism of Action Binds with stereospecific receptors at many sites within the CNS, increases pain threshold, alters pain perception, inhibits ascending pain pathways; is an ultra short-acting narcotic
Drug Interactions
  Cytochrome P450 Effect: Substrate of CYP3A4 (major)
  Increased Effect/Toxicity: Dextroamphetamine may enhance the analgesic effect of morphine and other opiate agonists. CNS depressants (eg, benzodiazepines, barbiturates, tricyclic antidepressants), erythromycin, reserpine, beta-blockers may increase the toxic effects of alfentanil. Alfentanil
(Continued)

Alfentanil *(Continued)*

levels/effects may be increased by azole antifungals, clarithromycin, diclofenac, doxycycline, erythromycin, imatinib, isoniazid, nefazodone, nicardipine, propofol, protease inhibitors, quinidine, verapamil, telithromycin, and other inhibitors of CYP3A4.

Pharmacodynamics/Kinetics

Onset of action: Rapid

Duration (dose dependent): 30-60 minutes

Distribution: V_d: Newborns, premature: 1 L/kg; Children: 0.163-0.48 L/kg; Adults: 0.46 L/kg

Half-life elimination: Newborns, premature: 5.33-8.75 hours; Children: 40-60 minutes; Adults: 83-97 minutes

Pregnancy Risk Factor C

Alfentanil Hydrochloride *see* Alfentanil *on page 67*

Alferon® N *see* Interferon Alfa-n3 *on page 848*

Alfuzosin *(al FYOO zoe sin)*

U.S. Brand Names Uroxatral®

Canadian Brand Names Xatral

Generic Available No

Synonyms Alfuzosin Hydrochloride

Pharmacologic Category Alpha$_1$ Blocker

Use Treatment of the functional symptoms of benign prostatic hyperplasia (BPH)

Local Anesthetic/Vasoconstrictor Precautions No information available to require special precautions

Effects on Dental Treatment No significant effects or complications reported

Common Adverse Effects 1% to 10%:

Central nervous system: Dizziness (6%), fatigue (3%), headache (3%), pain (1% to 2%)

Gastrointestinal: Abdominal pain (1% to 2%), constipation (1% to 2%), dyspepsia (1% to 2%), nausea (1% to 2%)

Genitourinary: Impotence (1% to 2%)

Respiratory: Upper respiratory tract infection (3%), bronchitis (1% to 2%), pharyngitis (1% to 2%), sinusitis (1% to 2%)

Mechanism of Action An antagonist of alpha$_1$ adrenoreceptors in the lower urinary tract. Smooth muscle tone is mediated by the sympathetic nervous stimulation of alpha$_1$ adrenoreceptors, which are abundant in the prostate, prostatic capsule, prostatic urethra, and bladder neck. Blockade of these adrenoreceptors can cause smooth muscles in the bladder neck and prostate to relax, resulting in an improvement in urine flow rate and a reduction in symptoms of BPH.

Drug Interactions

Cytochrome P450 Effect: Substrate of CYP3A4 (major)

Increased Effect/Toxicity: Alfuzosin levels/effects may be increased by azole antifungals, clarithromycin, diclofenac, doxycycline, erythromycin, imatinib, isoniazid, nefazodone, nicardipine, propofol, protease inhibitors, quinidine, verapamil, telithromycin, and other CYP3A4 inhibitors. Concurrent use of itraconazole, ketoconazole, or ritonavir is contraindicated.

Decreased Effect: Levels/effects of alfuzosin may be decreased by aminoglutethimide, carbamazepine, nafcillin, nevirapine, phenobarbital, phenytoin, rifamycins, and other CYP3A4 inducers.

Pharmacodynamics/Kinetics

Absorption: Decreased 50% under fasting conditions

Distribution: V_d: 3.2 L/kg

Protein binding: 82% to 90%

Metabolism: Hepatic, primarily via CYP3A4; metabolism includes oxidation, O-demethylation, and N-dealkylation; forms metabolites (inactive)

Bioavailability: 49% following a meal

Half-life elimination: 10 hours

Time to peak, plasma: 8 hours following a meal

Excretion: Feces (69%); urine (24%)

Pregnancy Risk Factor B

Alfuzosin Hydrochloride *see* Alfuzosin *on page 68*

Alglucerase *(al GLOO ser ase)*

U.S. Brand Names Ceredase®

Generic Available No

Synonyms Glucocerebrosidase
Pharmacologic Category Enzyme
Use Replacement therapy for Gaucher's disease (type 1)
Local Anesthetic/Vasoconstrictor Precautions No information available to require special precautions
Effects on Dental Treatment No significant effects or complications reported
Common Adverse Effects Frequency not defined.
  Cardiovascular: Peripheral edema
  Central nervous system: Chills, fatigue, fever, headache, lightheadedness
  Endocrine & metabolic: Hot flashes, menstrual abnormalities
  Gastrointestinal: Abdominal discomfort, diarrhea, nausea, oral ulcerations, vomiting
  Local: Injection site: Abscess, burning, discomfort, pruritus, swelling
  Neuromuscular & skeletal: Backache, weakness
  Miscellaneous: Dysosmia; hypersensitivity reactions (abdominal cramping, angioedema, chest discomfort, flushing, hypotension, nausea, pruritus, respiratory symptoms, urticaria); IgG antibody formation (~13%)
Mechanism of Action Alglucerase is a modified form of glucocerebrosidase; it is prepared from human placental tissue. Glucocerebrosidase is an enzyme deficient in Gaucher's disease. It is needed to catalyze the hydrolysis of glucocerebroside to glucose and ceramide.
Pharmacodynamics/Kinetics Half-life elimination: ~3-11 minutes
Pregnancy Risk Factor C

Alimta® see Pemetrexed on page 1198
Alinia® see Nitazoxanide on page 1117

Alitretinoin (a li TRET i noyn)

U.S. Brand Names Panretin®
Canadian Brand Names Panretin®
Generic Available No
Pharmacologic Category Antineoplastic Agent, Miscellaneous
Use Orphan drug: Topical treatment of cutaneous lesions in AIDS-related Kaposi's sarcoma
Unlabeled/Investigational Use Cutaneous T-cell lymphomas
Local Anesthetic/Vasoconstrictor Precautions No information available to require special precautions
Effects on Dental Treatment No significant effects or complications reported
Common Adverse Effects
  >10%:
    Central nervous system: Pain (0% to 34%)
    Dermatologic: Rash (25% to 77%), pruritus (8% to 11%)
    Neuromuscular & skeletal: Paresthesia (3% to 22%)
  5% to 10%:
    Cardiovascular: Edema (3% to 8%)
    Dermatologic: Exfoliative dermatitis (3% to 9%), skin disorder (0% to 8%)
Mechanism of Action Binds to retinoid receptors to inhibit growth of Kaposi's sarcoma
Drug Interactions
  Increased Effect/Toxicity: Increased toxicity of DEET may occur if products containing this compound are used concurrently with alitretinoin. Due to limited absorption after topical application, interaction with systemic medications is unlikely.
Pharmacodynamics/Kinetics Absorption: Not extensive
Pregnancy Risk Factor D

Alka-Mints® [OTC] see Calcium Carbonate on page 248
Alka-Seltzer Plus® Cold and Cough [OTC] see Chlorpheniramine, Phenylephrine, and Dextromethorphan on page 326
Alka-Seltzer Plus® Cold and Sinus Liqui-Gels [OTC] see Acetaminophen and Pseudoephedrine on page 38
Alka-Seltzer® Plus Cold Liqui-Gels® [OTC] see Acetaminophen, Chlorpheniramine, and Pseudoephedrine on page 43
Alka-Seltzer® Plus Flu Liqui-Gels® [OTC] see Acetaminophen, Dextromethorphan, and Pseudoephedrine on page 44
Alkeran® see Melphalan on page 979
Allbee® C-800 [OTC] see Vitamin B Complex Combinations on page 1581
Allbee® C-800 + Iron [OTC] see Vitamin B Complex Combinations on page 1581
Allbee® with C [OTC] see Vitamin B Complex Combinations on page 1581
Allegra® see Fexofenadine on page 652

Allegra-D® 12 Hour *see* Fexofenadine and Pseudoephedrine *on page 653*
Allegra-D® 24 Hour *see* Fexofenadine and Pseudoephedrine *on page 653*
Aller-Chlor® [OTC] *see* Chlorpheniramine *on page 323*
Allerest® Maximum Strength Allergy and Hay Fever [OTC] *see* Chlorpheniramine and Pseudoephedrine *on page 325*
Allerfrim® [OTC] *see* Triprolidine and Pseudoephedrine *on page 1542*
Allergen® *see* Antipyrine and Benzocaine *on page 130*
AllerMax® [OTC] *see* DiphenhydrAMINE *on page 483*
Allersol® *see* Naphazoline *on page 1087*
Allerx™ *see* Chlorpheniramine and Phenylephrine *on page 324*
Allfen-DM *see* Guaifenesin and Dextromethorphan *on page 754*
Allfen Jr *see* Guaifenesin *on page 752*
Allfen *(reformulation)* *see* Guaifenesin and Potassium Guaiacolsulfonate *on page 755*

Allopurinol (al oh PURE i nole)

U.S. Brand Names Aloprim™; Zyloprim®
Canadian Brand Names Alloprin®; Apo-Allopurinol®; Novo-Purol; Zyloprim®
Mexican Brand Names Atisuril®; Zyloprim®
Generic Available Yes
Synonyms Allopurinol Sodium
Pharmacologic Category Xanthine Oxidase Inhibitor
Use

Oral: Prevention of attack of gouty arthritis and nephropathy; treatment of secondary hyperuricemia which may occur during treatment of tumors or leukemia; prevention of recurrent calcium oxalate calculi

I.V.: Treatment of elevated serum and urinary uric acid levels when oral therapy is not tolerated in patients with leukemia, lymphoma, and solid tumor malignancies who are receiving cancer chemotherapy

Local Anesthetic/Vasoconstrictor Precautions No information available to require special precautions

Effects on Dental Treatment No significant effects or complications reported

Common Adverse Effects

>1%:

Dermatologic: Rash (increased with ampicillin or amoxicillin use, 1.5% per manufacturer, >10% in some reports)

Gastrointestinal: Nausea (1.3%), vomiting (1.2%)

Renal: Renal failure/impairment (1.2%)

Mechanism of Action Allopurinol inhibits xanthine oxidase, the enzyme responsible for the conversion of hypoxanthine to xanthine to uric acid. Allopurinol is metabolized to oxypurinol which is also an inhibitor of xanthine oxidase; allopurinol acts on purine catabolism, reducing the production of uric acid without disrupting the biosynthesis of vital purines.

Drug Interactions

Increased Effect/Toxicity: Allopurinol may increase the effects of azathioprine, chlorpropamide, mercaptopurine, theophylline, and oral anticoagulants. An increased risk of bone marrow suppression may occur when given with myelosuppressive agents (cyclophosphamide, possibly other alkylating agents). Amoxicillin/ampicillin, ACE inhibitors, and thiazide diuretics have been associated with hypersensitivity reactions when combined with allopurinol (rare), and the incidence of rash may be increased with penicillins (ampicillin, amoxicillin). Urinary acidification with large amounts of vitamin C may increase kidney stone formation.

Decreased Effect: Ethanol decreases effectiveness.

Pharmacodynamics/Kinetics

Onset of action: Peak effect: 1-2 weeks

Absorption: Oral: ~80%; Rectal: Poor and erratic

Distribution: V_d: ~1.6 L/kg; V_{ss}: 0.84-0.87 L/kg; enters breast milk

Protein binding: <1%

Metabolism: ~75% to active metabolites, chiefly oxypurinol

Bioavailability: 49% to 53%

Half-life elimination:

Normal renal function: Parent drug: 1-3 hours; Oxypurinol: 18-30 hours

End-stage renal disease: Prolonged

Time to peak, plasma: Oral: 30-120 minutes

Excretion: Urine (76% as oxypurinol, 12% as unchanged drug)

Allopurinol and oxypurinol are dialyzable

Pregnancy Risk Factor C

Allopurinol Sodium *see* Allopurinol *on page 70*

All-*trans*-Retinoic Acid *see* Tretinoin (Oral) *on page 1524*

Almacone® [OTC] *see* Aluminum Hydroxide, Magnesium Hydroxide, and Simethicone *on page 81*

Almacone Double Strength® [OTC] *see* Aluminum Hydroxide, Magnesium Hydroxide, and Simethicone *on page 81*

Almora® [OTC] *see* Magnesium Gluconate *on page 961*

Almotriptan (al moh TRIP tan)

U.S. Brand Names Axert™
Canadian Brand Names Axert™
Generic Available No
Synonyms Almotriptan Malate
Pharmacologic Category Serotonin 5-HT$_{1D}$ Receptor Agonist
Use Acute treatment of migraine with or without aura
Local Anesthetic/Vasoconstrictor Precautions No information available to require special precautions
Effects on Dental Treatment Key adverse effect(s) related to dental treatment: Xerostomia (normal salivary flow resumes upon discontinuation).
Common Adverse Effects 1% to 10%:
  Central nervous system: Headache (>1%), dizziness (>1%), somnolence (>1%)
  Gastrointestinal: Nausea (1% to 2%), xerostomia (1%)
  Neuromuscular & skeletal: Paresthesia (1%)
Dosage Oral: Adults: Migraine: Initial: 6.25-12.5 mg in a single dose; if the headache returns, repeat the dose after 2 hours; no more than 2 doses in 24-hour period
  Note: If the first dose is ineffective, diagnosis needs to be re-evaluated. Safety of treating more than 4 migraines/month has not been established.
  Dosage adjustment in renal impairment: Initial: 6.25 mg in a single dose; maximum daily dose: ≤12.5 mg
  Dosage adjustment in hepatic impairment: Initial: 6.25 mg in a single dose; maximum daily dose: ≤12.5 mg
Mechanism of Action Selective agonist for serotonin (5-HT$_{1B}$, 5-HT$_{1D}$, 5-HT$_{1F}$ receptors) in cranial arteries; causes vasoconstriction and reduce sterile inflammation associated with antidromic neuronal transmission correlating with relief of migraine
Contraindications Hypersensitivity to almotriptan or any component of the formulation; use as prophylactic therapy for migraine; hemiplegic or basilar migraine; cluster headache; known or suspected ischemic heart disease (angina pectoris, MI, documented silent ischemia, coronary artery vasospasm, Prinzmetal's variant angina); peripheral vascular syndromes (including ischemic bowel disease); uncontrolled hypertension; use within 24 hours of another 5-HT$_1$ agonist; use within 24 hours of ergotamine derivative; concurrent administration or within 2 weeks of discontinuing an MAO inhibitor (specifically MAO type A inhibitors)
Warnings/Precautions Almotriptan is indicated only in patients ≥18 years of age with a clear diagnosis of migraine headache. If a patient does not respond to the first dose, the diagnosis of migraine should be reconsidered. Do not give to patients with risk factors for CAD until a cardiovascular evaluation has been performed; if evaluation is satisfactory, the healthcare provider should administer the first dose and cardiovascular status should be periodically re-evaluated. Cardiac events (coronary artery vasospasm, transient ischemia, myocardial infarction, ventricular tachycardia/fibrillation, cardiac arrest, and death), cerebral/subarachnoid hemorrhage, stroke, peripheral vascular ischemia, and colonic ischemia have been reported with 5-HT$_1$ agonist administration. Significant elevation in blood pressure, including hypertensive crisis, has also been reported on rare occasions in patients with and without a history of hypertension. Use with caution in liver or renal dysfunction. Safety and efficacy in pediatric patients have not been established.
Drug Interactions
  Cytochrome P450 Effect: Substrate (minor) of CYP2D6, 3A4
  Increased Effect/Toxicity: Ergot-containing drugs prolong vasospastic reactions; ketoconazole increases almotriptan serum concentration; select serotonin reuptake inhibitors may increase symptoms of hyper-reflexia, weakness, and incoordination; MAO inhibitors may increase toxicity
Dietary Considerations May be taken without regard to meals
Pharmacodynamics/Kinetics
  Absorption: Well absorbed
  Distribution: V$_d$: 180-200 L
  Protein binding: ~35%
  (Continued)

Almotriptan (Continued)

Metabolism: MAO type A oxidative deamination (~27% of dose); via CYP3A4 and 2D6 (~12% of dose) to inactive metabolites

Bioavailability: 70%

Half-life elimination: 3-4 hours

Time to peak: 1-3 hours

Excretion: Urine (40% as unchanged drug); feces (13% unchanged and metabolized)

Pregnancy Risk Factor C

Dosage Forms TAB: 6.25 mg, 12.5 mg

Almotriptan Malate *see* Almotriptan *on page 71*

Alocril® *see* Nedocromil *on page 1095*

Aloe Vesta® 2-n-1 Antifungal [OTC] *see* Miconazole *on page 1039*

Alomide® *see* Lodoxamide *on page 940*

Alophen® [OTC] *see* Bisacodyl *on page 209*

Aloprim™ *see* Allopurinol *on page 70*

Alora® *see* Estradiol *on page 574*

Alosetron (a LOE se tron)

U.S. Brand Names Lotronex®

Mexican Brand Names Lotronex®

Generic Available No

Pharmacologic Category Selective 5-HT₃ Receptor Antagonist

Use Treatment of women with severe diarrhea-predominant irritable bowel syndrome (IBS) who have failed to respond to conventional therapy

Local Anesthetic/Vasoconstrictor Precautions No information available to require special precautions

Effects on Dental Treatment Key adverse event(s) related to dental treatment: Throat and tonsil discomfort and pain.

Common Adverse Effects

>10%: Gastrointestinal: Constipation (dose related) (29%)

1% to 10%: Gastrointestinal: Abdominal discomfort and pain (7%), nausea (6%), gastrointestinal discomfort and pain (6%), abdominal distention (2%), hemorrhoids (2%), regurgitation and reflux (2%)

Restrictions Only physicians enrolled in GlaxoSmithKline's Prescribing Program for Lotronex® may prescribe this medication. Program stickers must be affixed to all prescriptions; no phone, fax, or computerized prescriptions are permitted with this program. An FDA-approved medication guide is available at www.fda.gov/cder/Offices/ODS/labeling.htm; distribute to each patient to whom this medication is dispensed

Mechanism of Action Alosetron is a potent and selective antagonist of a subtype of the serotonin 5-HT₃ receptor. 5-HT₃ receptors are ligand-gated ion channels extensively distributed on enteric neurons in the human gastrointestinal tract, as well as other peripheral and central locations. Activation of these channels affect the regulation of visceral pain, colonic transit, and gastrointestinal secretions. In patients with irritable bowel syndrome, blockade of these channels may reduce pain, abdominal discomfort, urgency, and diarrhea.

Drug Interactions

Cytochrome P450 Effect: Substrate of CYP1A2 (major), 2C9 (minor), 3A4 (minor); Inhibits CYP1A2 (weak), 2E1 (weak)

Increased Effect/Toxicity: CYP1A2 inhibitors may increase the levels/effects of alosetron; example inhibitors include amiodarone, ciprofloxacin, fluvoxamine (contraindicated), ketoconazole, norfloxacin, ofloxacin, and rofecoxib.

Pharmacodynamics/Kinetics

Distribution: V_d: 65-95 L

Protein binding: 82%

Metabolism: Extensive hepatic metabolism. Alosetron is metabolized by CYP2C9, 3A4, and 1A2. Thirteen metabolites have been detected in the urine. Biological activity of these metabolites in unknown.

Bioavailability: Mean: 50% to 60% (range: 30% to >90%); decreased with food (25%)

Half-life elimination: 1.5 hours for alosetron

Time to peak: 1 hour after oral administration

Excretion: Urine (73%) and feces (24%); 7% as unchanged drug (1% feces, 6% urine)

Pregnancy Risk Factor B

Aloxi® *see* Palonosetron *on page 1180*

Alpha₁-Antitrypsin *see* Alpha₁-Proteinase Inhibitor *on page 73*

Alpha₁-PI *see* Alpha₁-Proteinase Inhibitor *on page 73*

Alpha₁-Proteinase Inhibitor, Human *see* Alpha₁-Proteinase Inhibitor *on page 73*

Alpha-Galactosidase-A (Human, Recombinant) *see* Agalsidase Beta *on page 55*

Alphagan® P *see* Brimonidine *on page 220*

Alphanate® *see* Antihemophilic Factor (Human) *on page 129*

AlphaNine® SD *see* Factor IX *on page 632*

Alphaquin HP® *see* Hydroquinone *on page 798*

Alpha₁-Proteinase Inhibitor (al fa won PRO tee in ase in HI bi tor)

U.S. Brand Names Aralast; Prolastin®; Zemaira®
Canadian Brand Names Prolastin®
Generic Available No
Synonyms Alpha₁-Antitrypsin; α₁-PI; Alpha₁-Proteinase Inhibitor, Human; A₁-PI
Pharmacologic Category Antitrypsin Deficiency Agent
Use Replacement therapy in congenital alpha₁-antitrypsin deficiency with clinical emphysema
Local Anesthetic/Vasoconstrictor Precautions No information available to require special precautions
Effects on Dental Treatment Key adverse event(s) related to dental treatment: Pharyngitis.
Common Adverse Effects
  >10%: Hepatic: ALT/AST increased (11%; ~4 times ULN)
  1% to 10%: Respiratory: Pharyngitis (2%)
Mechanism of Action Alpha₁-antitrypsin (AAT) is the principle protease inhibitor in serum. Its major physiologic role is to render proteolytic enzymes (secreted during inflammation) inactive. A decrease in AAT, as seen in congenital AAT deficiency, leads to increased elastic damage in the lung, causing emphysema.
Pharmacodynamics/Kinetics
  Half-life elimination: Metabolic: 5.9 days (Aralast™)
  Time to peak, serum: Threshold levels achieved after 3 weeks
Pregnancy Risk Factor C

Alph-E [OTC] *see* Vitamin E *on page 1581*

Alph-E-Mixed [OTC] *see* Vitamin E *on page 1581*

Alprazolam (al PRAY zoe lam)

Related Information
  Sedation *on page 1727*
  Temporomandibular Dysfunction (TMD) *on page 1724*
Related Sample Prescriptions
  Sedation (Prior to Dental Treatment) *on page 1746*
U.S. Brand Names Alprazolam Intensol®; Niravam™; Xanax®; Xanax XR®
Canadian Brand Names Alti-Alprazolam; Apo-Alpraz®; Gen-Alprazolam; Novo-Alprazol; Nu-Alprax; Xanax®; Xanax TS™
Mexican Brand Names Alzam®; Tafil®
Generic Available Yes: Extended release tablet, immediate release tablet
Pharmacologic Category Benzodiazepine
Dental Use Preoperative sedation
Use Treatment of anxiety disorder (GAD); panic disorder, with or without agoraphobia; anxiety associated with depression
Unlabeled/Investigational Use Anxiety in children
Local Anesthetic/Vasoconstrictor Precautions No information available to require special precautions
Effects on Dental Treatment Key adverse event(s) related to dental treatment: Significant xerostomia and changes in salivation (normal salivary flow resumes upon discontinuation).
Significant Adverse Effects
  >10%:
    Central nervous system: Abnormal coordination, cognitive disorder, depression, drowsiness, fatigue, irritability, lightheadedness, memory impairment, sedation, somnolence
    Gastrointestinal: Appetite increased/decreased, constipation, salivation decreased, weight gain/loss, xerostomia
    Genitourinary: Micturition difficulty
  (Continued)

73

Alprazolam *(Continued)*

Neuromuscular & skeletal: Dysarthria

1% to 10%:

Cardiovascular: Hypotension

Central nervous system: Agitation, attention disturbance, confusion, depersonalization, derealization, disorientation, disinhibition, dizziness, dream abnormalities, fear, hallucinations, hypersomnia, nightmares, seizure, talkativeness

Dermatologic: Dermatitis, pruritus, rash

Endocrine & metabolic: Libido decreased/increased, menstrual disorders

Gastrointestinal: Salivation increased

Genitourinary: Incontinence

Hepatic: Bilirubin increased, jaundice, liver enzymes increased

Neuromuscular & skeletal: Arthralgia, ataxia, myalgia, paresthesia

Ocular: Diplopia

Respiratory: Allergic rhinitis, dyspnea

<1% (Limited to important or life-threatening): Amnesia, falls, galactorrhea, gynecomastia, hepatic failure, hepatitis, hyperprolactinemia, Stevens-Johnson syndrome

Restrictions C-IV

Dental Usual Dosing Preoperative sedation: Adults: Oral: 0.5 mg in evening at bedtime and 0.5 mg 1 hour before procedure

Dosage Oral: **Note:** Treatment >4 months should be re-evaluated to determine the patient's continued need for the drug

Children: Anxiety (unlabeled use): Immediate release: Initial: 0.005 mg/kg/dose or 0.125 mg/dose 3 times/day; increase in increments of 0.125-0.25 mg, up to a maximum of 0.02 mg/kg/dose or 0.06 mg/kg/day (0.375-3 mg/day)

Adults:

Anxiety: Immediate release: Effective doses are 0.5-4 mg/day in divided doses; the manufacturer recommends starting at 0.25-0.5 mg 3 times/day; titrate dose upward; usual maximum: 4 mg/day. Patients requiring doses >4 mg/day should be increased cautiously. Periodic reassessment and consideration of dosage reduction is recommended.

Anxiety associated with depression: Immediate release: Average dose required: 2.5-3 mg/day in divided doses

Ethanol withdrawal (unlabeled use): Immediate release: Usual dose: 2-2.5 mg/day in divided doses

Panic disorder:

Immediate release: Initial: 0.5 mg 3 times/day; dose may be increased every 3-4 days in increments ≤1 mg/day. Mean effective dosage: 5-6 mg/day; many patients obtain relief at 2 mg/day, as much as 10 mg/day may be required

Extended release: 0.5-1 mg once daily; may increase dose every 3-4 days in increments ≤1 mg/day (range: 3-6 mg/day)

Switching from immediate release to extended release: Patients may be switched to extended release tablets by taking the total daily dose of the immediate release tablets and giving it once daily using the extended release preparation.

Preoperative sedation: 0.5 mg in evening at bedtime and 0.5 mg 1 hour before procedure

Dose reduction: Abrupt discontinuation should be avoided. Daily dose may be decreased by 0.5 mg every 3 days, however, some patients may require a slower reduction. If withdrawal symptoms occur, resume previous dose and discontinue on a less rapid schedule.

Elderly: Initial: 0.125-0.25 mg twice daily; increase by 0.125 mg/day as needed. The smallest effective dose should be used. **Note:** Elderly patients may be more sensitive to the effects of alprazolam including ataxia and oversedation. The elderly may also have impaired renal function leading to decreased clearance. Titrate gradually, if needed.

Immediate release: Initial: 0.25 mg 2-3 times/day

Extended release: Initial: 0.5 mg once daily

Dosing adjustment in renal impairment: No guidelines for adjustment; use caution

Dosing adjustment in hepatic impairment: Reduce dose by 50% to 60% or avoid in cirrhosis

Mechanism of Action Binds to stereospecific benzodiazepine receptors on the postsynaptic GABA neuron at several sites within the central nervous system, including the limbic system, reticular formation. Enhancement of the inhibitory effect of GABA on neuronal excitability results by increased neuronal membrane permeability to chloride ions. This shift in chloride ions results in hyperpolarization (a less excitable state) and stabilization.

Contraindications Hypersensitivity to alprazolam or any component of the formulation (cross-sensitivity with other benzodiazepines may exist); narrow-angle glaucoma; concurrent use with ketoconazole or itraconazole; pregnancy

Warnings/Precautions Rebound or withdrawal symptoms, including seizures, may occur 18 hours to 3 days following abrupt discontinuation or large decreases in dose (more common in patients receiving >4 mg/day or prolonged treatment). Dose reductions or tapering must be approached with extreme caution. Breakthrough anxiety may occur at the end of dosing interval. Use with caution in patients receiving concurrent CYP3A4 inhibitors, particularly when these agents are added to therapy. Has weak uricosuric properties, use with caution in renal impairment or predisposition to urate nephropathy. Use with caution in elderly or debilitated patients, patients with hepatic disease (including alcoholics), renal impairment, or obese patients.

Causes CNS depression (dose related) resulting in sedation, dizziness, confusion, or ataxia which may impair physical and mental capabilities. Patients must be cautioned about performing tasks which require mental alertness (eg, operating machinery or driving). Use with caution in patients receiving other CNS depressants or psychoactive agents. Effects with other sedative drugs or ethanol may be potentiated. Benzodiazepines have been associated with falls and traumatic injury and should be used with extreme caution in patients who are at risk of these events (especially the elderly). Use with caution in patients with respiratory disease or impaired gag reflex.

Use caution in patients with depression, particularly if suicidal risk may be present. Episodes of mania or hypomania have occurred in depressed patients treated with alprazolam. May cause physical or psychological dependence - use with caution in patients with a history of drug dependence. Acute withdrawal, including seizures, may be precipitated in patients after administration of flumazenil to patients receiving long-term benzodiazepine therapy.

Benzodiazepines have been associated with anterograde amnesia. Paradoxical reactions, including hyperactive or aggressive behavior, have been reported with benzodiazepines, particularly in adolescent/pediatric or psychiatric patients. Does not have analgesic, antidepressant, or antipsychotic properties.

Benzodiazepines have the potential to cause harm to the fetus, particularly when administered during the first trimester. In addition, withdrawal symptoms may occur in the neonate following *in utero* exposure. Use of alprazolam during pregnancy should be avoided. In addition, symptoms of withdrawal, lethargy, and loss of body weight have been reported in infants exposed to alprazolam and/or benzodiazepines while nursing; use during breast-feeding is not recommended.

Drug Interactions Substrate of CYP3A4 (major)

CNS depressants: Sedative effects and/or respiratory depression may be additive with CNS depressants. Includes ethanol, barbiturates, narcotic analgesics, and other sedative agents; monitor for increased effect.

CYP3A4 inducers: CYP3A4 inducers may decrease the levels/effects of alprazolam. Example inducers include aminoglutethimide, carbamazepine, nafcillin, nevirapine, phenobarbital, phenytoin, and rifamycins.

CYP3A4 inhibitors: May increase the levels/effects of alprazolam. Example inhibitors include azole antifungals, clarithromycin, diclofenac, doxycycline, erythromycin, imatinib, isoniazid, nefazodone, nicardipine, propofol, protease inhibitors, quinidine, telithromycin, and verapamil. Contraindicated with itraconazole and ketoconazole.

Fluoxetine: May increase plasma concentrations/effects of alprazolam.

Oral contraceptives: May increase serum levels/effects of alprazolam.

Theophylline: May partially antagonize some of the effects of benzodiazepines; monitor for decreased response; may require higher doses for sedation.

Tricyclic antidepressants: Plasma concentrations of imipramine and desipramine have been reported to be increased 31% and 20%, respectively, by concomitant administration; monitor.

Ethanol/Nutrition/Herb Interactions

Cigarette smoking: May decrease alprazolam concentrations up to 50%.

Ethanol: Avoid ethanol (may increase CNS depression).

Food: Alprazolam serum concentration is unlikely to be increased by grapefruit juice because of alprazolam's high oral bioavailability. The C_{max} of the extended release formulation is increased by 25% when a high-fat meal is given 2 hours before dosing. T_{max} is decreased 30% when food is given immediately prior to dose. T_{max} is increased by 30% when food is given ≥1 hour after dose.

Herb/Nutraceutical: St John's wort may decrease alprazolam levels. Avoid valerian, St John's wort, kava kava, gotu kola (may increase CNS depression).

(Continued)

75

Alprazolam *(Continued)*

Pharmacodynamics/Kinetics
Distribution: V_d: 0.9-1.2 L/kg; enters breast milk

Protein binding: 80%

Metabolism: Hepatic via CYP3A4; forms two active metabolites (4-hydroxyal-prazolam and α-hydroxyalprazolam)

Bioavailability: 90%

Half-life elimination:

Adults: 11.2 hours (range: 6.3-26.9)

Elderly: 16.3 hours (range: 9-26.9 hours)

Alcoholic liver disease: 19.7 hours (range: 5.8-65.3 hours)

Obesity: 21.8 hours (range: 9.9-40.4 hours)

Time to peak, serum: 1-2 hours

Excretion: Urine (as unchanged drug and metabolites)

Pregnancy Risk Factor D

Lactation Enters breast milk/not recommended (AAP rates "of concern")

Breast-Feeding Considerations Symptoms of withdrawal, lethargy, and loss of body weight have been reported in infants exposed to alprazolam and/or benzodiazepines while nursing. Breast-feeding is not recommended.

Dosage Forms
Solution, oral [concentrate]:

Alprazolam Intensol®: 1 mg/mL (30 mL)

Tablet: 0.25 mg, 0.5 mg, 1 mg, 2 mg

Xanax®: 0.25 mg, 0.5 mg, 1 mg, 2 mg

Tablet, extended release: 0.5 mg, 1 mg, 2 mg, 3 mg

Xanax XR®: 0.5 mg, 1 mg, 2 mg, 3 mg

Tablet, orally disintegrating [scored]:

Niravam™: 0.25 mg, 0.5 mg, 1 mg, 2 mg [orange flavor]

Alprazolam Intensol® *see* Alprazolam *on page 73*

Alprostadil *(al PROS ta dill)*

U.S. Brand Names Caverject®; Caverject Impulse®; Edex®; Muse®; Prostin VR Pediatric®

Canadian Brand Names Caverject®; Muse® Pellet; Prostin VR

Mexican Brand Names Caverject®; Muse®

Generic Available Yes: Solution for injection

Synonyms PGE₁; Prostaglandin E₁

Pharmacologic Category Prostaglandin

Use
Prostin VR Pediatric®: Temporary maintenance of patency of ductus arteriosus in neonates with ductal-dependent congenital heart disease until surgery can be performed. These defects include cyanotic (eg, pulmonary atresia, pulmonary stenosis, tricuspid atresia, Fallot's tetralogy, transposition of the great vessels) and acyanotic (eg, interruption of aortic arch, coarctation of aorta, hypoplastic left ventricle) heart disease.

Caverject®: Treatment of erectile dysfunction of vasculogenic, psychogenic, or neurogenic etiology; adjunct in the diagnosis of erectile dysfunction

Edex®, Muse®: Treatment of erectile dysfunction of vasculogenic, psychogenic, or neurogenic etiology

Unlabeled/Investigational Use Investigational: Treatment of pulmonary hypertension in infants and children with congenital heart defects with left-to-right shunts

Local Anesthetic/Vasoconstrictor Precautions No information available to require special precautions

Effects on Dental Treatment No significant effects or complications reported

Mechanism of Action Causes vasodilation by means of direct effect on vascular and ductus arteriosus smooth muscle; relaxes trabecular smooth muscle by dilation of cavernosal arteries when injected along the penile shaft, allowing blood flow to and entrapment in the lacunar spaces of the penis (ie, corporeal veno-occlusive mechanism)

Pregnancy Risk Factor X/C (Muse®)

Alrex® *see* Loteprednol *on page 953*

Altace® *see* Ramipril *on page 1332*

Altachlore [OTC] *see* Sodium Chloride *on page 1400*

Altafrin *see* Phenylephrine *on page 1226*

Altamist [OTC] *see* Sodium Chloride *on page 1400*

Altarussin DM [OTC] *see* Guaifenesin and Dextromethorphan *on page 754*

Altaryl [OTC] *see* DiphenhydrAMINE *on page 483*

Alteplase (AL te plase)

Related Information
  Cardiovascular Diseases *on page 1636*
U.S. Brand Names Activase®; Cathflo® Activase®
Canadian Brand Names Activase® rt-PA; Cathflo® Activase®
Mexican Brand Names Actilyse®
Generic Available No
Synonyms Alteplase, Recombinant; Alteplase, Tissue Plasminogen Activator, Recombinant; tPA
Pharmacologic Category Thrombolytic Agent
Use Management of acute myocardial infarction for the lysis of thrombi in coronary arteries; management of acute massive pulmonary embolism (PE) in adults

  Acute myocardial infarction (AMI): Chest pain ≥20 minutes, ≤12-24 hours; S-T elevation ≥0.1 mV in at least two ECG leads
  Acute pulmonary embolism (APE): Age ≤75 years: Documented massive pulmonary embolism by pulmonary angiography or echocardiography or high probability lung scan with clinical shock
  Cathflo® Activase®: Restoration of central venous catheter function
Unlabeled/Investigational Use Acute peripheral arterial occlusive disease

Local Anesthetic/Vasoconstrictor Precautions No information available to require special precautions

Effects on Dental Treatment Key adverse event(s) related to dental treatment: As with all drugs which may affect hemostasis, bleeding is the major adverse effect associated with alteplase. Hemorrhage may occur at virtually any site; risk is dependent on multiple variables, including the dosage administered, concurrent use of multiple agents which alter hemostasis, and patient predisposition. Rapid lysis of coronary artery thrombi by thrombolytic agents may be associated with reperfusion-related atrial and/or ventricular arrhythmias.

Common Adverse Effects As with all drugs which may affect hemostasis, bleeding is the major adverse effect associated with alteplase. Hemorrhage may occur at virtually any site. Risk is dependent on multiple variables, including the dosage administered, concurrent use of multiple agents which alter hemostasis, and patient predisposition. Rapid lysis of coronary artery thrombi by thrombolytic agents may be associated with reperfusion-related atrial and/or ventricular arrhythmia. **Note:** Lowest rate of bleeding complications expected with dose used to restore catheter function.

  1% to 10%:
    Cardiovascular: Hypotension
    Central nervous system: Fever
    Dermatologic: Bruising (1%)
    Gastrointestinal: GI hemorrhage (5%), nausea, vomiting
    Genitourinary: GU hemorrhage (4%)
    Hematologic: Bleeding (0.5% major, 7% minor: GUSTO trial)
    Local: Bleeding at catheter puncture site (15.3%, accelerated administration)
  Additional cardiovascular events associated **with use in MI:** AV block, cardiogenic shock, heart failure, cardiac arrest, recurrent ischemia/infarction, myocardial rupture, electromechanical dissociation, pericardial effusion, pericarditis, mitral regurgitation, cardiac tamponade, thromboembolism, pulmonary edema, asystole, ventricular tachycardia, bradycardia, ruptured intracranial AV malformation, seizure, hemorrhagic bursitis, cholesterol crystal embolization
  Additional events associated **with use in pulmonary embolism:** Pulmonary re-embolization, pulmonary edema, pleural effusion, thromboembolism
  Additional events associated **with use in stroke:** Cerebral edema, cerebral herniation, seizure, new ischemic stroke

Mechanism of Action Initiates local fibrinolysis by binding to fibrin in a thrombus (clot) and converts entrapped plasminogen to plasmin

Drug Interactions
  Increased Effect/Toxicity: The potential for hemorrhage with alteplase is increased by oral anticoagulants (warfarin), heparin, low molecular weight heparins, and drugs which affect platelet function (eg, NSAIDs, dipyridamole, ticlopidine, clopidogrel, IIb/IIIa antagonists). Concurrent use with aspirin and heparin may increase the risk of bleeding. However, aspirin and heparin were used concomitantly with alteplase in the majority of patients in clinical studies.
  Decreased Effect: Aminocaproic acid (an antifibrinolytic agent) may decrease the effectiveness of thrombolytic therapy. Nitroglycerin may increase the hepatic clearance of alteplase, potentially reducing lytic activity (limited clinical information).
  (Continued)

Alteplase *(Continued)*

Pharmacodynamics/Kinetics

Duration: >50% present in plasma cleared ~5 minutes after infusion terminated, ~80% cleared within 10 minutes

Excretion: Clearance: Rapidly from circulating plasma (550-650 mL/minute), primarily hepatic; >50% present in plasma is cleared within 5 minutes after the infusion is terminated, ~80% cleared within 10 minutes

Pregnancy Risk Factor C

Alteplase, Recombinant *see Alteplase on page 77*

Alteplase, Tissue Plasminogen Activator, Recombinant *see Alteplase on page 77*

ALternaGel® [OTC] *see Aluminum Hydroxide on page 79*

Altoprev™ *see Lovastatin on page 953*

Altretamine (al TRET a meen)

U.S. Brand Names Hexalen®
Canadian Brand Names Hexalen®
Generic Available No
Synonyms Hexamethylmelamine; HEXM; HMM; HXM; NSC-13875
Pharmacologic Category Antineoplastic Agent, Miscellaneous
Use Palliative treatment of persistent or recurrent ovarian cancer
Local Anesthetic/Vasoconstrictor Precautions No information available to require special precautions
Effects on Dental Treatment No significant effects or complications reported
Common Adverse Effects

>10%:

Central nervous system: Peripheral sensory neuropathy, neurotoxicity (21%; may be progressive and dose-limiting)

Gastrointestinal: Nausea/vomiting (50% to 70%), anorexia (48%), diarrhea (48%)

Hematologic: Anemia, thrombocytopenia (31%), leukopenia (62%), neutropenia

1% to 10%:

Central nervous system: Seizures

Gastrointestinal: Stomach cramps

Hepatic: Alkaline phosphatase increased

Mechanism of Action Although altretamine's clinical antitumor spectrum resembles that of alkylating agents, the drug has demonstrated activity in alkylator-resistant patients. The drug selectively inhibits the incorporation of radioactive thymidine and uridine into DNA and RNA, inhibiting DNA and RNA synthesis; reactive intermediates covalently bind to microsomal proteins and DNA; can spontaneously degrade to demethylated melamines and formaldehyde which are also cytotoxic.

Drug Interactions

Increased Effect/Toxicity: Altretamine may cause severe orthostatic hypotension when administered with MAO inhibitors. Cimetidine may decrease metabolism of altretamine.

Decreased Effect: Phenobarbital may increase metabolism of altretamine which may decrease the effect.

Pharmacodynamics/Kinetics

Absorption: Well absorbed (75% to 89%)

Distribution: Highly concentrated hepatically and renally; low in other organs

Metabolism: Hepatic; rapid and extensive demethylation; active metabolites

Half-life elimination: 13 hours

Time to peak, plasma: 0.5-3 hours

Excretion: Urine (<1% as unchanged drug)

Pregnancy Risk Factor D

Aluminum Chloride (a LOO mi num KLOR ide)

U.S. Brand Names Hemodent™
Generic Available No
Pharmacologic Category Astringent; Hemostatic Agent
Dental Use Hemostatic; gingival retraction; to control bleeding created during a dental procedure
Use Hemostatic
Local Anesthetic/Vasoconstrictor Precautions No information available to require special precautions

Effects on Dental Treatment No significant effects or complications reported

Significant Adverse Effects No data reported

Dental Usual Dosing Control of dental bleeding: Apply retraction cord as directed

Dosage Control of bleeding: Apply retraction cord as directed

Mechanism of Action Precipitates tissue and blood proteins causing a mechanical obstruction to hemorrhage from injured blood vessels

Contraindications No data reported

Warnings/Precautions Since large amounts of astringents may cause tissue irritation and possible damage, only small amounts should be applied.

Drug Interactions No data reported

Dosage Forms
Liquid:
Hemodent™: 21% (10 mL, 20 mL, 40 mL)
Retraction cord [impregnated with 21% solution]:
Hemodent™: Braided cord, thin (7 ft); braided cord medium thin (7 ft); twisted cord #3 (7 ft); twisted cord #9 (7ft)

Aluminum Hydroxide (a LOO mi num hye DROKS ide)

U.S. Brand Names ALternaGel® [OTC]; Dermagran® [OTC]

Canadian Brand Names Amphojel®; Basaljel®

Generic Available Yes: Suspension

Pharmacologic Category Antacid; Antidote; Protectant, Topical

Use Treatment of hyperacidity; hyperphosphatemia; temporary protection of minor cuts, scrapes, and burns

Local Anesthetic/Vasoconstrictor Precautions No information available to require special precautions

Effects on Dental Treatment Key adverse event(s) related to dental treatment: Chalky taste. Aluminum and magnesium ions prevent GI absorption of tetracycline by forming a large ionized chelated molecule with the aluminum ion and tetracyclines in the stomach. Aluminum hydroxide prevents GI absorption of ketoconazole and itraconazole by increasing the pH in the GI tract. Any of these drugs should be administered at least 1 hour before $Al(OH)_3$.

Common Adverse Effects Frequency not defined.
Gastrointestinal: Constipation, stomach cramps, fecal impaction, nausea, vomiting, discoloration of feces (white speckles)
Endocrine & metabolic: Hypophosphatemia, hypomagnesemia

Mechanism of Action Neutralizes hydrochloride in stomach to form $Al (Cl)_3$ salt + H_2O

Drug Interactions
Decreased Effect: Aluminum hydroxide may decrease the absorption of allopurinol, antibiotics (tetracyclines, quinolones, some cephalosporins), bisphosphonate derivatives, corticosteroids, cyclosporine, delavirdine, iron salts, imidazole antifungals, isoniazid, mycophenolate, penicillamine, phosphate supplements, phenytoin, phenothiazines, trientine. Absorption of aluminum hydroxide may be decreased by citric acid derivatives.

Pregnancy Risk Factor C

Aluminum Hydroxide and Magnesium Carbonate
(a LOO mi num hye DROKS ide & mag NEE zhum KAR bun nate)

Related Information
Aluminum Hydroxide *on page 79*

U.S. Brand Names Gaviscon® Extra Strength [OTC]; Gaviscon® Liquid [OTC]

Generic Available Yes

Synonyms Magnesium Carbonate and Aluminum Hydroxide

Pharmacologic Category Antacid

Use Temporary relief of symptoms associated with gastric acidity

Local Anesthetic/Vasoconstrictor Precautions No information available to require special precautions

Effects on Dental Treatment Key adverse event(s) related to dental treatment: Chalky taste. Aluminum and magnesium ions prevent GI absorption of tetracycline by forming a large ionized chelated molecule with the tetracyclines in the stomach. Aluminum hydroxide prevents GI absorption of ketoconazole and itraconazole by increasing the pH in the GI tract. Any of these drugs should be administered at least 1 hour before aluminum hydroxide.

Common Adverse Effects 1% to 10%:
Endocrine & metabolic: Hypermagnesemia, aluminum intoxication (prolonged use and concomitant renal failure), hypophosphatemia
(Continued)

Aluminum Hydroxide and Magnesium Carbonate
(Continued)

Gastrointestinal: Constipation, diarrhea
Neuromuscular & skeletal: Osteomalacia

Drug Interactions
Decreased Effect: Tetracyclines, digoxin, indomethacin, iron salts, isoniazid, allopurinol, benzodiazepines, corticosteroids, penicillamine, phenothiazines, ranitidine, ketoconazole, itraconazole

Aluminum Hydroxide and Magnesium Hydroxide
(a LOO mi num hye DROKS ide & mag NEE zhum hye DROK side)

Related Information
Aluminum Hydroxide *on page 79*
Magnesium Hydroxide *on page 961*

U.S. Brand Names Alamag [OTC]; Rulox [OTC]; Rulox No. 1 [DSC]

Canadian Brand Names Diovol®; Diovol® Ex; Gelusil® Extra Strength; Mylanta™

Generic Available Yes

Synonyms Magnesium Hydroxide and Aluminum Hydroxide

Pharmacologic Category Antacid

Use Antacid, hyperphosphatemia in renal failure

Local Anesthetic/Vasoconstrictor Precautions No information available to require special precautions

Effects on Dental Treatment Key adverse event(s) related to dental treatment: Chalky taste. Aluminum and magnesium ions prevent GI absorption of tetracycline by forming a large ionized chelated molecule with the tetracyclines in the stomach. Aluminum hydroxide prevents GI absorption of ketoconazole and itraconazole by increasing the pH in the GI tract. Any of these drugs should be administered at least 1 hour before aluminum hydroxide.

Common Adverse Effects
>10%: Gastrointestinal: Constipation, chalky taste, stomach cramps, fecal impaction

1% to 10%: Gastrointestinal: Nausea, vomiting, discoloration of feces (white speckles)

Drug Interactions
Decreased Effect: Tetracyclines, digoxin, indomethacin, iron salts, isoniazid, allopurinol, benzodiazepines, corticosteroids, penicillamine, phenothiazines, ranitidine, ketoconazole, itraconazole

Pregnancy Risk Factor C

Aluminum Hydroxide and Magnesium Trisilicate
(a LOO mi num hye DROKS ide & mag NEE zhum trye SIL i kate)

Related Information
Aluminum Hydroxide *on page 79*

U.S. Brand Names Alenic Alka Tablet [OTC]; Gaviscon® Tablet [OTC]; Genaton Tablet [OTC]

Generic Available Yes

Synonyms Magnesium Trisilicate and Aluminum Hydroxide

Pharmacologic Category Antacid

Use Temporary relief of hyperacidity

Local Anesthetic/Vasoconstrictor Precautions No information available to require special precautions

Effects on Dental Treatment Key adverse event(s) related to dental treatment: Chalky taste. Aluminum and magnesium ions prevent GI absorption of tetracycline by forming a large ionized chelated molecule with the tetracyclines in the stomach. Aluminum hydroxide prevents GI absorption of ketoconazole and itraconazole by increasing the pH in the GI tract. Any of these drugs should be administered at least 1 hour before aluminum hydroxide.

Drug Interactions
Decreased Effect: Tetracyclines, digoxin, indomethacin, iron salts, isoniazid, allopurinol, benzodiazepines, corticosteroids, penicillamine, phenothiazines, ranitidine, ketoconazole, itraconazole

Pregnancy Risk Factor C

Aluminum Hydroxide, Magnesium Hydroxide, and Simethicone
(a LOO mi num hye DROKS ide, mag NEE zhum hye DROKS ide, & sye METH i kone)

Related Information
Aluminum Hydroxide *on page 79*
Magnesium Hydroxide *on page 961*
Simethicone *on page 1394*

U.S. Brand Names Alamag Plus [OTC]; Aldroxicon I [OTC]; Aldroxicon II [OTC]; Almacone® [OTC]; Almacone Double Strength® [OTC]; Gelusil® [OTC]; Maalox® [OTC]; Maalox® Max [OTC]; Mi-Acid [OTC]; Mi-Acid Maximum Strength [OTC]; Mintox Extra Strength [OTC]; Mintox Plus [OTC]; Mylanta® Liquid [OTC]; Mylanta® Maximum Strength Liquid [OTC]

Canadian Brand Names Diovol Plus®; Gelusil®; Mylanta® Double Strength; Mylanta® Extra Strength; Mylanta® Regular Strength

Generic Available Yes

Synonyms Magnesium Hydroxide, Aluminum Hydroxide, and Simethicone; Simethicone, Aluminum Hydroxide, and Magnesium Hydroxide

Pharmacologic Category Antacid; Antiflatulent

Use Temporary relief of hyperacidity associated with gas; may also be used for indications associated with other antacids

Local Anesthetic/Vasoconstrictor Precautions No information available to require special precautions

Effects on Dental Treatment Key adverse event(s) related to dental treatment: Chalky taste. Aluminum and magnesium ions prevent GI absorption of tetracycline by forming a large ionized chelated molecule with the tetracyclines in the stomach. Aluminum hydroxide prevents GI absorption of ketoconazole and itraconazole by increasing the pH in the GI tract. Any of these drugs should be administered at least 1 hour before aluminum hydroxide.

Common Adverse Effects
>10%: Gastrointestinal: Chalky taste, stomach cramps, constipation, bowel motility decreased, fecal impaction, hemorrhoids
1% to 10%: Gastrointestinal: Nausea, vomiting, discoloration of feces (white speckles)

Drug Interactions
Decreased Effect: Tetracyclines, digoxin, indomethacin, iron salts, isoniazid, allopurinol, benzodiazepines, corticosteroids, penicillamine, phenothiazines, ranitidine, ketoconazole, itraconazole

Pregnancy Risk Factor C

Aluminum Potassium Sulfate and Epinephrine (Racemic) (Dental) *see* Epinephrine (Racemic) and Aluminum Potassium Sulfate *on page 550*

Aluminum Sucrose Sulfate, Basic *see* Sucralfate *on page 1420*

Aluminum Sulfate and Calcium Acetate
(a LOO mi num SUL fate & KAL see um AS e tate)

Related Information
Calcium Acetate *on page 248*

U.S. Brand Names Domeboro® [OTC]; Gordon Boro-Packs [OTC]; Pedi-Boro® [OTC]

Generic Available No

Synonyms Calcium Acetate and Aluminum Sulfate

Pharmacologic Category Topical Skin Product

Use Astringent wet dressing for relief of inflammatory conditions of the skin; reduce weeping that may occur in dermatitis

Local Anesthetic/Vasoconstrictor Precautions No information available to require special precautions

Effects on Dental Treatment No significant effects or complications reported

Alupent® *see* Metaproterenol *on page 1000*

Amantadine (a MAN ta deen)

Related Information
Respiratory Diseases *on page 1656*
Systemic Viral Diseases *on page 1675*
(Continued)

Amantadine *(Continued)*

U.S. Brand Names Symmetrel®

Canadian Brand Names Endantadine®; PMS-Amantadine; Symmetrel®

Generic Available Yes

Synonyms Adamantanamine Hydrochloride; Amantadine Hydrochloride

Pharmacologic Category Anti-Parkinson's Agent, Dopamine Agonist; Antiviral Agent, Adamantane

Use Prophylaxis and treatment of influenza A viral infection; treatment of parkinsonism; treatment of drug-induced extrapyramidal symptoms

Local Anesthetic/Vasoconstrictor Precautions No information available to require special precautions

Effects on Dental Treatment Key adverse event(s) related to dental treatment: Xerostomia (prolonged use may cause significant xerostomia; normal salivary flow resumes upon discontinuation) and orthostatic hypotension.

Common Adverse Effects 1% to 10%:

Cardiovascular: Orthostatic hypotension, peripheral edema

Central nervous system: Insomnia, depression, anxiety, irritability, dizziness, hallucinations, ataxia, headache, somnolence, nervousness, dream abnormality, agitation, fatigue, confusion

Dermatologic: Livedo reticularis

Gastrointestinal: Nausea, anorexia, constipation, diarrhea, xerostomia

Respiratory: Dry nose

Mechanism of Action As an antiviral, blocks the uncoating of influenza A virus preventing penetration of virus into host; antiparkinsonian activity may be due to its blocking the reuptake of dopamine into presynaptic neurons or by increasing dopamine release from presynaptic fibers

Drug Interactions

Increased Effect/Toxicity: Anticholinergics (benztropine and trihexyphenidyl) may potentiate CNS side effects of amantadine. Hydrochlorothiazide, triamterene, and/or trimethoprim may increase toxicity of amantadine; monitor for altered response.

Pharmacodynamics/Kinetics

Onset of action: Antidyskinetic: Within 48 hours

Absorption: Well absorbed

Distribution: V_d: Normal: 1.5-6.1 L/kg; Renal failure: 5.1 ± 0.2 L/kg; in saliva, tear film, and nasal secretions; in animals, tissue (especially lung) concentrations higher than serum concentrations; crosses blood-brain barrier

Protein binding: Normal renal function: ~67%; Hemodialysis: ~59%

Metabolism: Not appreciable; small amounts of an acetyl metabolite identified

Bioavailability: 86% to 90%

Half-life elimination: Normal renal function: 16 ± 6 hours (9-31 hours); End-stage renal disease: 7-10 days

Excretion: Urine (80% to 90% unchanged) by glomerular filtration and tubular secretion

Total clearance: 2.5-10.5 L/hour

Pregnancy Risk Factor C

Amantadine Hydrochloride *see* Amantadine *on page 81*

Amaryl® *see* Glimepiride *on page 738*

Ambenonium *(am be NOE nee um)*

U.S. Brand Names Mytelase®

Canadian Brand Names Mytelase®

Generic Available No

Synonyms Ambenonium Chloride

Pharmacologic Category Cholinergic Agonist

Use Treatment of myasthenia gravis

Local Anesthetic/Vasoconstrictor Precautions No information available to require special precautions

Effects on Dental Treatment No significant effects or complications reported

Pregnancy Risk Factor C

Ambenonium Chloride *see* Ambenonium *on page 82*

Ambien® *see* Zolpidem *on page 1604*

Ambien CR™ *see* Zolpidem *on page 1604*

Ambifed-G *see* Guaifenesin and Pseudoephedrine *on page 755*

Ambifed-G DM *see* Guaifenesin, Pseudoephedrine, and Dextromethorphan *on page 757*

AmBisome® *see* Amphotericin B (Liposomal) *on page 116*

Amcinonide (am SIN oh nide)

U.S. Brand Names Cyclocort®
Canadian Brand Names Amcort®; Cyclocort®; ratio-Amcinonide
Generic Available Yes
Pharmacologic Category Corticosteroid, Topical
Use Relief of the inflammatory and pruritic manifestations of corticosteroid-responsive dermatoses (high potency corticosteroid)
Local Anesthetic/Vasoconstrictor Precautions No information available to require special precautions
Effects on Dental Treatment No significant effects or complications reported
Common Adverse Effects Frequency not defined.
Dermatologic: Acne, hypopigmentation, allergic dermatitis, maceration of the skin, skin atrophy, striae, miliaria, telangiectasia
Endocrine & metabolic: Cushing's syndrome, growth retardation (long-term use), HPA suppression, hyperglycemia; these reactions occur more frequently with occlusive dressings
Local: Burning, itching, irritation, dryness, folliculitis, hypertrichosis
Miscellaneous: Secondary infection
Mechanism of Action Stimulates the synthesis of enzymes needed to decrease inflammation, suppress mitotic activity, and cause vasoconstriction
Pharmacodynamics/Kinetics
Absorption: Adequate through intact skin; increases with skin inflammation or occlusion
Metabolism: Hepatic
Excretion: Urine and feces
Pregnancy Risk Factor C

Amerge® *see* Naratriptan *on page 1092*
Americaine® [OTC] *see* Benzocaine *on page 190*
Americaine® Hemorrhoidal [OTC] *see* Benzocaine *on page 190*
A-Methapred *see* MethylPREDNISolone *on page 1025*
Amethocaine Hydrochloride *see* Tetracaine *on page 1466*
Amethopterin *see* Methotrexate *on page 1012*
Amevive® *see* Alefacept *on page 62*
Amfepramone *see* Diethylpropion *on page 467*
AMG 073 *see* Cinacalcet *on page 342*
Amibid DM *see* Guaifenesin and Dextromethorphan *on page 754*
Amicar® *see* Aminocaproic Acid *on page 86*
Amidal *see* Guaifenesin and Phenylephrine *on page 754*
Amidate® *see* Etomidate *on page 625*
Amidrine *see* Acetaminophen, Isometheptene, and Dichloralphenazone *on page 44*

Amifostine (am i FOS teen)

U.S. Brand Names Ethyol®
Canadian Brand Names Ethyol®
Mexican Brand Names Ethyol®
Generic Available No
Synonyms Ethiofos; Gammaphos; WR-2721; YM-08310
Pharmacologic Category Adjuvant, Chemoprotective Agent (Cytoprotective); Antidote
Use Reduce the incidence of moderate to severe xerostomia in patients undergoing postoperative radiation treatment for head and neck cancer, where the radiation port includes a substantial portion of the parotid glands; reduce the cumulative renal toxicity associated with repeated administration of cisplatin in patients with advanced ovarian cancer
Local Anesthetic/Vasoconstrictor Precautions No information available to require special precautions
Effects on Dental Treatment No significant effects or complications reported
Common Adverse Effects >10%:
Cardiovascular: Hypotension (15% to 62%; grades 3/4: 3% to 8%; dose dependent)
Gastrointestinal: Nausea/vomiting (53% to 96%; grades 3/4: 8% to 30%; dose dependent)
Mechanism of Action Prodrug that is dephosphorylated by alkaline phosphatase in tissues to a pharmacologically-active free thiol metabolite. The free thiol
(Continued)

Amifostine (Continued)

is available to bind to, and detoxify, reactive metabolites of cisplatin; and can also act as a scavenger of free radicals that may be generated in tissues.

Drug Interactions

Increased Effect/Toxicity: Antihypertensives may potentiate the hypotensive effects of amifostine.

Pharmacodynamics/Kinetics

Distribution: V_d: 3.5 L

Metabolism: Hepatic dephosphorylation to two metabolites (active-free thiol and disulfide)

Half-life elimination: 8-9 minutes

Excretion: Urine

Clearance, plasma: 2.17 L/minute

Pregnancy Risk Factor C

Amigesic® *see* Salsalate *on page 1376*

Amikacin (am i KAY sin)

Related Information

Tuberculosis *on page 1673*

U.S. Brand Names Amikin®

Canadian Brand Names Amikacin Sulfate Injection, USP; Amikin®

Mexican Brand Names Akacin®; Amikafur®; Amikalem®; Amikason's®; Amikayect®; Amikin®; A.M.K.®; Biclin®; Gamikal®; Oprad®; Yectamid®

Generic Available Yes

Synonyms Amikacin Sulfate

Pharmacologic Category Antibiotic, Aminoglycoside

Use Treatment of serious infections due to organisms resistant to gentamicin and tobramycin, including *Pseudomonas*, *Proteus*, *Serratia*, and other gram-negative bacilli (bone infections, respiratory tract infections, endocarditis, and septicemia); documented infection of mycobacterial organisms susceptible to amikacin

Local Anesthetic/Vasoconstrictor Precautions No information available to require special precautions

Effects on Dental Treatment No significant effects or complications reported

Common Adverse Effects 1% to 10%:

Central nervous system: Neurotoxicity

Otic: Ototoxicity (auditory), ototoxicity (vestibular)

Renal: Nephrotoxicity

Mechanism of Action Inhibits protein synthesis in susceptible bacteria by binding to 30S ribosomal subunits

Drug Interactions

Increased Effect/Toxicity: Amikacin may increase or prolong the effect of neuromuscular blocking agents. Concurrent use of amphotericin (or other nephrotoxic drugs) may increase the risk of amikacin-induced nephrotoxicity. The risk of ototoxicity from amikacin may be increased with other ototoxic drugs.

Pharmacodynamics/Kinetics

Absorption:

I.M.: Rapid

Oral: Poorly absorbed

Distribution: Primarily into extracellular fluid (highly hydrophilic); penetrates blood-brain barrier when meninges inflamed; crosses placenta

Relative diffusion of antimicrobial agents from blood into CSF: Good only with inflammation (exceeds usual MICs)

CSF:blood level ratio: Normal meninges: 10% to 20%; Inflamed meninges: 15% to 24%

Half-life elimination (renal function and age dependent):

Infants: Low birth weight (1-3 days): 7-9 hours; Full-term >7 days: 4-5 hours

Children: 1.6-2.5 hours

Adults: Normal renal function: 1.4-2.3 hours; Anuria/end-stage renal disease: 28-86 hours

Time to peak, serum: I.M.: 45-120 minutes

Excretion: Urine (94% to 98%)

Pregnancy Risk Factor D

Amikacin Sulfate *see* Amikacin *on page 84*

Amikin® *see* Amikacin *on page 84*

Amiloride (a MIL oh ride)

Related Information
Cardiovascular Diseases *on page 1636*
U.S. Brand Names Midamor® [DSC]
Canadian Brand Names Apo-Amiloride®
Generic Available Yes
Synonyms Amiloride Hydrochloride
Pharmacologic Category Diuretic, Potassium-Sparing
Use Counteracts potassium loss induced by other diuretics in the treatment of hypertension or edematous conditions including CHF, hepatic cirrhosis, and hypoaldosteronism; usually used in conjunction with more potent diuretics such as thiazides or loop diuretics
Unlabeled/Investigational Use Investigational: Cystic fibrosis; reduction of lithium-induced polyuria
Local Anesthetic/Vasoconstrictor Precautions No information available to require special precautions
Effects on Dental Treatment No significant effects or complications reported
Common Adverse Effects 1% to 10%:
Central nervous system: Headache, fatigue, dizziness
Endocrine & metabolic: Hyperkalemia (up to 10%; risk reduced in patients receiving kaliuretic diuretics), hyperchloremic metabolic acidosis, dehydration, hyponatremia, gynecomastia
Gastrointestinal: Nausea, diarrhea, vomiting, abdominal pain, gas pain, appetite changes, constipation
Genitourinary: Impotence
Neuromuscular & skeletal: Muscle cramps, weakness
Respiratory: Cough, dyspnea
Mechanism of Action Interferes with potassium/sodium exchange (active transport) in the distal tubule, cortical collecting tubule, and collecting duct by inhibiting sodium, potassium-ATPase; decreases calcium excretion; increases magnesium loss
Drug Interactions
Increased Effect/Toxicity: Increased risk of amiloride-associated hyperkalemia with triamterene, spironolactone, ACE inhibitors or angiotensin receptor antagonists, potassium preparations, cyclosporine, tacrolimus, and indomethacin. Amiloride may increase the toxicity of amantadine and lithium by reduction of renal excretion. Quinidine and amiloride together may increase risk of malignant arrhythmias.
Decreased Effect: Decreased effect of amiloride with use of NSAIDs. Amoxicillin's absorption may be reduced with concurrent use.
Pharmacodynamics/Kinetics
Onset of action: 2 hours
Duration: 24 hours
Absorption: ~15% to 25%
Distribution: V_d: 350-380 L
Protein binding: 23%
Metabolism: No active metabolites
Half-life elimination: Normal renal function: 6-9 hours; End-stage renal disease: 8-144 hours
Time to peak, serum: 6-10 hours
Excretion: Urine and feces (equal amounts as unchanged drug)
Pregnancy Risk Factor B

Amiloride and Hydrochlorothiazide
(a MIL oh ride & hye droe klor oh THYE a zide)

Related Information
Amiloride *on page 85*
Hydrochlorothiazide *on page 776*
Canadian Brand Names Apo-Amilzide®; Moduret; Novamilor; Nu-Amilzide
Generic Available Yes
Synonyms Hydrochlorothiazide and Amiloride
Pharmacologic Category Diuretic, Combination
Use Potassium-sparing diuretic; antihypertensive
Local Anesthetic/Vasoconstrictor Precautions No information available to require special precautions
Effects on Dental Treatment No significant effects or complications reported
Common Adverse Effects See individual agents.
(Continued)

Amiloride and Hydrochlorothiazide *(Continued)*

Drug Interactions
Increased Effect/Toxicity: See individual agents.
Decreased Effect: See individual agents.
Pharmacodynamics/Kinetics See individual agents.
Pregnancy Risk Factor B

Amiloride Hydrochloride *see* Amiloride *on page 85*

2-Amino-6-Mercaptopurine *see* Thioguanine *on page 1476*

2-Amino-6-Methoxypurine Arabinoside *see* Nelarabine *on page 1097*

2-Amino-6-Trifluoromethoxy-benzothiazole *see* Riluzole *on page 1350*

Aminobenzylpenicillin *see* Ampicillin *on page 117*

Aminocamptothecin *(a min o camp to THE sin)*

Generic Available No
Synonyms 9-AC; 9-Aminocamptothecin; NSC-603071
Pharmacologic Category Antineoplastic Agent, DNA Binding Agent; Enzyme Inhibitor, Topoisomerase I Inhibitor
Unlabeled/Investigational Use Phase II trials: Relapsed lymphoma, refractory breast cancer, nonsmall cell lung cancer, untreated colorectal carcinoma
Local Anesthetic/Vasoconstrictor Precautions No information available to require special precautions
Effects on Dental Treatment No significant effects or complications reported
Common Adverse Effects Frequency not defined.
Central nervous system: Fatigue
Dermatologic: Alopecia
Gastrointestinal: Nausea, vomiting, diarrhea, mucositis, anorexia
Hematologic: Neutropenia (may be dose limiting), thrombocytopenia (reversible, but may be dose limiting), anemia
Restrictions
Not available in U.S./Investigational
Mechanism of Action Aminocamptothecin binds to topoisomerase I, stabilizing the cleavable DNA-topoisomerase I complex, resulting in arrest of the replication fork and inhibition of DNA synthesis.
Drug Interactions
Decreased Effect: Anticonvulsants may decrease aminocamptothecin levels.
Pharmacodynamics/Kinetics Ratio of lactone to total drug is 8.7 ± 4.7% because of instability of aminocamptothecin lactone in plasma.

Distribution: V_d: 46-92 L
Metabolism: None identified
Half-life elimination: Terminal: 8-17 hours for total aminocamptothecin
Excretion: Urine (32% of total drug delivered)

9-Aminocamptothecin *see* Aminocamptothecin *on page 86*

Aminocaproic Acid *(a mee noe ka PROE ik AS id)*

U.S. Brand Names Amicar®
Generic Available Yes
Synonyms Epsilon Aminocaproic Acid
Pharmacologic Category Hemostatic Agent
Use Treatment of excessive bleeding from fibrinolysis
Unlabeled/Investigational Use Treatment of traumatic hyphema; control bleeding in thrombocytopenia; control oral bleeding in congenital and acquired coagulation disorders
Local Anesthetic/Vasoconstrictor Precautions No information available to require special precautions
Effects on Dental Treatment No significant effects or complications reported (see Dental Comment)
Common Adverse Effects Frequency not defined.
Cardiovascular: Arrhythmia, bradycardia, hypotension, peripheral ischemia, syncope, thrombosis
Central nervous system: Confusion, delirium, dizziness, fatigue, hallucinations, headache, intracranial hypertension, malaise, seizure, stroke
Dermatologic: Rash, pruritus
Gastrointestinal: Abdominal pain, anorexia, cramps, diarrhea, GI irritation, nausea
Genitourinary: Dry ejaculation

Hematologic: Agranulocytosis, bleeding time increased, leukopenia, thrombocytopenia

Neuromuscular & skeletal: CPK increased, myalgia, myositis, myopathy, rhabdomyolysis (rare), weakness

Ophthalmic: Watery eyes, vision decreased

Otic: Tinnitus

Renal: Failure (rare), myoglobinuria (rare)

Respiratory: Dyspnea, nasal congestion, pulmonary embolism

Mechanism of Action Competitively inhibits activation of plasminogen to plasmin, also, a lesser antiplasmin effect

Drug Interactions

Increased Effect/Toxicity: Increased risk of hypercoagulability with oral contraceptives, estrogens. Should not be administered with factor IX complex concentrate or anti-inhibitor complex concentrates due to an increased risk of thrombosis.

Pharmacodynamics/Kinetics

Onset of action: ~1-72 hours

Distribution: Widely through intravascular and extravascular compartments

V_d: Oral: 23 L, I.V.: 30 L

Metabolism: Minimally hepatic

Half-life elimination: 2 hours

Time to peak: Oral: Within 2 hours

Excretion: Urine (65% as unchanged drug, 11% as metabolite)

Pregnancy Risk Factor C

Dental Comment Antifibrinolytic drugs are useful to control bleeding after dental extractions in patients with hemophilia. A clinical trial reported that aminocaproic acid or tranexamic acid reduces both recurrent bleeding and the amount of clotting factor replacement therapy required. In adults, the oral dose was 50-60 mg aminocaproic acid per kg every 4 hours until dental sockets were completely healed.

Extemporaneous solutions incorporating 100 mg aminocaproic acid per 5 mL of oral solution have been used as an oral rinse with some success. Use, however, must be carefully considered since it may not show efficacy in all patients with either drug-induced or hereditary coagulation problems. Studies are ongoing and commercial products may be available in the future.

Amino-Cerv™ *see* Urea *on page 1551*

Aminoglutethimide (a mee noe gloo TETH i mide)

U.S. Brand Names Cytadren®

Generic Available No

Synonyms AG; AGT; BA-16038; Elipten

Pharmacologic Category Antineoplastic Agent, Aromatase Inhibitor; Aromatase Inhibitor; Enzyme Inhibitor; Hormone Antagonist, Anti-Adrenal; Nonsteroidal Aromatase Inhibitor

Use Suppression of adrenal function in selected patients with Cushing's syndrome

Unlabeled/Investigational Use Treatment of breast and prostate cancer (androgen synthesis inhibitor)

Local Anesthetic/Vasoconstrictor Precautions No information available to require special precautions

Effects on Dental Treatment Key adverse event(s) related to dental treatment: Nausea and orthostatic hypotension.

Common Adverse Effects Most adverse effects will diminish in incidence and severity after the first 2-6 weeks

>10%:

Central nervous system: Headache, dizziness, drowsiness, lethargy, clumsiness

Dermatologic: Skin rash

Gastrointestinal: Nausea, anorexia

Hepatic: Cholestatic jaundice

Neuromuscular & skeletal: Myalgia

Renal: Nephrotoxicity

Respiratory: Pulmonary alveolar damage

1% to 10%:

Cardiovascular: Hypotension, tachycardia, orthostasis

Dermatologic: Hirsutism, pruritus

Endocrine & metabolic: Adrenocortical insufficiency

Gastrointestinal: Vomiting

(Continued)

Aminoglutethimide *(Continued)*

Mechanism of Action Blocks the enzymatic conversion of cholesterol to delta-5-pregnenolone, thereby reducing the synthesis of adrenal glucocorticoids, mineralocorticoids, estrogens, aldosterone, and androgens

Drug Interactions

Cytochrome P450 Effect: Induces CYP1A2 (strong), 2C19 (strong), 3A4 (strong)

Decreased Effect: Aminoglutethimide may decrease therapeutic effect of dexamethasone, digitoxin (after 3-8 weeks), warfarin, medroxyprogesterone, megestrol, and tamoxifen. Aminoglutethimide may decrease the levels/effects of aminophylline, benzodiazepines, calcium channel blockers, citalopram, clarithromycin, cyclosporine, diazepam, erythromycin, estrogens, fluvoxamine, methsuximide, mirtazapine, nateglinide, nefazodone, nevirapine, phenytoin, proton pump inhibitors, protease inhibitors, ropinirole, sertraline, tacrolimus, theophylline, venlafaxine, voriconazole, and other drugs metabolized by CYP1A2, 2C19, or 3A4.

Pharmacodynamics/Kinetics

Onset of action: Adrenal suppression: 3-5 days; following withdrawal of therapy, adrenal function returns within 72 hours

Absorption: 90%

Protein binding, plasma: 20% to 25%

Metabolism: Major metabolite is N-acetylaminoglutethimide; induces its own metabolism

Half-life elimination: 7-15 hours; shorter following multiple doses

Excretion: Urine (34% to 50% as unchanged drug, 25% as metabolites)

Pregnancy Risk Factor D

Aminolevulinic Acid *(a MEE noh lev yoo lin ik AS id)*

U.S. Brand Names Levulan® Kerastick®

Canadian Brand Names Levulan®

Generic Available No

Synonyms Aminolevulinic Acid Hydrochloride

Pharmacologic Category Photosensitizing Agent, Topical; Topical Skin Product

Use Treatment of minimally to moderately thick actinic keratoses (grade 1 or 2) of the face or scalp; to be used in conjunction with blue light illumination

Local Anesthetic/Vasoconstrictor Precautions No information available to require special precautions

Effects on Dental Treatment Key adverse event(s) related to dental treatment: Bleeding/hemorrhage.

Common Adverse Effects

Transient stinging, burning, itching, erythema, and edema result from the photosensitizing properties of this agent. Symptoms subside between 1 minute and 24 hours after turning off the blue light illuminator. Severe stinging or burning was reported in at least 50% of patients from at least 1 lesional site treatment.

>10%: Dermatologic: Severe stinging or burning (50%), scaling of the skin/crusted skin (64% to 71%), hyper-/hypopigmentation (22% to 36%), itching (14% to 25%), erosion (2% to 14%)

1% to 10%:

Central nervous system: Dysesthesia (up to 2%)

Dermatologic: Skin ulceration (2% to 4%), vesiculation (4% to 5%), pustular drug eruption (up to 4%), skin disorder (5% to 12%)

Hematologic: Bleeding/hemorrhage (2% to 4%)

Local: Wheal/flare (2% to 7%), local pain (1%), tenderness (1% to 2%), edema (1%), scabbing (up to 2%), ulceration (2% to 4%), excoriation (1%)

Mechanism of Action Aminolevulinic acid is a metabolic precursor of protoporphyrin IX (PpIX), which is a photosensitizer. Photosensitization following application of aminolevulinic acid topical solution occurs through the metabolic conversion to PpIX. When exposed to light of appropriate wavelength and energy, accumulated PpIX produces a photodynamic reaction.

Drug Interactions

Increased Effect/Toxicity: Photosensitizing agents such as griseofulvin, thiazide diuretics, sulfonamides, sulfonylureas, phenothiazines, and tetracyclines theoretically may increase the photosensitizing potential of aminolevulinic acid.

Pharmacodynamics/Kinetics

PpIX:

Peak fluorescence intensity: 11 hours ± 1 hour

Half-life, mean clearance for lesions: 30 ± 10 hours

Pregnancy Risk Factor C

Aminolevulinic Acid Hydrochloride *see* Aminolevulinic Acid *on page 88*

Aminophylline (am in OFF i lin)

Related Information
Respiratory Diseases *on page 1656*
Theophylline *on page 1473*
Canadian Brand Names Phyllocontin®; Phyllocontin®-350
Mexican Brand Names Drafilyn®
Generic Available Yes
Synonyms Theophylline Ethylenediamine
Pharmacologic Category Theophylline Derivative
Use Bronchodilator in reversible airway obstruction due to asthma or COPD; increase diaphragmatic contractility
Local Anesthetic/Vasoconstrictor Precautions No information available to require special precautions
Effects on Dental Treatment Prescribe erythromycin products with caution to patients taking theophylline products. Erythromycin will delay the normal metabolic inactivation of theophyllines leading to increased blood levels; this has resulted in nausea, vomiting, and CNS restlessness.
Common Adverse Effects
Uncommon at serum theophylline concentrations ≤15 mcg/mL
1% to 10%:
Cardiovascular: Tachycardia
Central nervous system: Nervousness, restlessness
Gastrointestinal: Nausea, vomiting
Mechanism of Action Causes bronchodilatation, diuresis, CNS and cardiac stimulation, and gastric acid secretion by blocking phosphodiesterase which increases tissue concentrations of cyclic adenine monophosphate (cAMP) which in turn promote catecholamine stimulation of lipolysis, glycogenolysis, and gluconeogenesis and induce release of epinephrine from adrenal medulla cells
Drug Interactions
Cytochrome P450 Effect: Substrate of CYP1A2 (major), 2E1 (minor), 3A4 (minor)
Increased Effect/Toxicity: Levels/effects of aminophylline may be increased by amiodarone, ciprofloxacin, fluvoxamine, ketoconazole, norfloxacin, ofloxacin, rofecoxib, and other CYP1A2 inhibitors.
Decreased Effect: Levels/effects of aminophylline may be decreased by aminoglutethimide, carbamazepine, phenobarbital, rifampin, and other CYP1A2 inducers.
Pharmacodynamics/Kinetics
Theophylline:
Absorption: Oral: Dosage form dependent
Distribution: 0.45 L/kg based on ideal body weight
Protein binding: 40%, primarily to albumin
Metabolism: Children >1 year and Adults: Hepatic; involves CYP1A2, 2E1, and 3A4; forms active metabolites (caffeine and 3-methylxanthine)
Half-life elimination: Highly variable and dependent upon age, liver function, cardiac function, lung disease, and smoking history
Time to peak, serum:
Oral: Immediate release: 1-2 hours
I.V.: Within 30 minutes
Excretion: Children >3 months and Adults: Urine (10% as unchanged drug)
Pregnancy Risk Factor C

Aminosalicylate Sodium *see* Aminosalicylic Acid *on page 89*

Aminosalicylic Acid (a mee noe sal i SIL ik AS id)

Related Information
Rheumatoid Arthritis, Osteoarthritis, and Osteoporosis *on page 1668*
Tuberculosis *on page 1673*
U.S. Brand Names Paser®
Generic Available No
Synonyms Aminosalicylate Sodium; 4-Aminosalicylic Acid; Para-Aminosalicylate Sodium; PAS; Sodium PAS
Pharmacologic Category Salicylate
Use Adjunctive treatment of tuberculosis used in combination with other anti-tubercular agents
(Continued)

Aminosalicylic Acid *(Continued)*

Unlabeled/Investigational Use Crohn's disease

Local Anesthetic/Vasoconstrictor Precautions No information available to require special precautions

Effects on Dental Treatment NSAID formulations are known to reversibly decrease platelet aggregation via mechanisms different than observed with aspirin. The dentist should be aware of the potential of abnormal coagulation. Caution should also be exercised in the use of NSAIDs in patients already on anticoagulant therapy with drugs such as warfarin (Coumadin®).

Common Adverse Effects Frequency not defined.
  Cardiovascular: Pericarditis, vasculitis
  Central nervous system: Encephalopathy, fever
  Dermatologic: Skin eruptions
  Endocrine & metabolic: Goiter (with or without myxedema), hypoglycemia
  Gastrointestinal: Abdominal pain, diarrhea, nausea, vomiting
  Hematologic: Agranulocytosis, anemia (hemolytic), leukopenia, thrombocytopenia
  Hepatic: Hepatitis, jaundice
  Ocular: Optic neuritis
  Respiratory: Eosinophilic pneumonia

Mechanism of Action Aminosalicylic acid (PAS) is a highly-specific bacteriostatic agent active against *M. tuberculosis*. Structurally related to para-aminobenzoic acid (PABA) and its mechanism of action is thought to be similar to the sulfonamides, a competitive antagonism with PABA; disrupts plate biosynthesis in sensitive organisms.

Drug Interactions
  Decreased Effect: Aminosalicylic acid may decrease serum levels of digoxin and vitamin B_{12}.

Pharmacodynamics/Kinetics
  Absorption: Readily, >90%
  Protein binding: 50% to 60%
  Metabolism: Hepatic (>50%) via acetylation
  Half-life elimination: Reduced with renal impairment
  Time to peak, serum: 6 hours
  Excretion: Urine (>80% as unchanged drug and metabolites)

Pregnancy Risk Factor C

4-Aminosalicylic Acid *see* Aminosalicylic Acid *on page 89*

5-Aminosalicylic Acid *see* Mesalamine *on page 996*

Aminoxin® [OTC] *see* Pyridoxine *on page 1316*

Amiodarone *(a MEE oh da rone)*

Related Information
  Cardiovascular Diseases *on page 1636*
U.S. Brand Names Cordarone®; Pacerone®
Canadian Brand Names Alti-Amiodarone; Amiodarone Hydrochloride for Injection®; Apo-Amiodarone®; Cordarone®; Gen-Amiodarone; Novo-Amiodarone; Rhoxal-amiodarone; Sandoz Amiodarone
Generic Available Yes
Synonyms Amiodarone Hydrochloride
Pharmacologic Category Antiarrhythmic Agent, Class III
Use Management of life-threatening recurrent ventricular fibrillation (VF) or hemodynamically-unstable ventricular tachycardia (VT) refractory to other antiarrhythmic agents or in patients intolerant of other agents used for these conditions

Unlabeled/Investigational Use
  Conversion of atrial fibrillation to normal sinus rhythm; maintenance of normal sinus rhythm
  Prevention of postoperative atrial fibrillation during cardiothoracic surgery
  Paroxysmal supraventricular tachycardia (SVT)
  Control of rapid ventricular rate due to accessory pathway conduction in pre-excited atrial arrhythmias [ACLS guidelines]
  Cardiac arrest with persistent ventricular tachycardia (VT) or ventricular fibrillation (VF) if defibrillation, CPR, and vasopressor administration have failed [ACLS/PALS guidelines]
  Control of hemodynamically-stable VT, polymorphic VT with a normal QT interval, or wide-complex tachycardia of uncertain origin [ACLS/PALS guidelines]

Local Anesthetic/Vasoconstrictor Precautions No information available to require special precautions (see Dental Comment)

Effects on Dental Treatment Key adverse event(s) related to dental treatment: Oral: Abnormal salivation and taste.

Common Adverse Effects In a recent meta-analysis, patients taking lower doses of amiodarone (152-330 mg daily for at least 12 months) were more likely to develop thyroid, neurologic, skin, ocular, and bradycardic abnormalities than those taking placebo (Vorperian, 1997). Pulmonary toxicity was similar in both the low dose amiodarone group and in the placebo group but there was a trend towards increased toxicity in the amiodarone group. Gastrointestinal and hepatic events were seen to a similar extent in both the low dose amiodarone group and placebo group. As the frequency of adverse events varies considerably across studies as a function of route and dose, a consolidation of adverse event rates is provided by Goldschlager, 2000.

Cardiovascular: Hypotension (I.V. 16%, refractory in rare cases)

Central nervous system (3% to 40%): Abnormal gait/ataxia, dizziness, fatigue, headache, malaise, impaired memory, involuntary movement, insomnia, poor coordination, peripheral neuropathy, sleep disturbances, tremor

Dermatologic: Photosensitivity (10% to 75%)

Endocrine & Metabolic: Hypothyroidism (1% to 22%)

Gastrointestinal: Nausea, vomiting, anorexia, and constipation (10% to 33%); AST or ALT level >2x normal (15% to 50%)

Ocular: Corneal microdeposits (>90%; causes visual disturbance in <10%)

1% to 10%:

Cardiovascular: CHF (3%), bradycardia (3% to 5%), AV block (5%), conduction abnormalities, SA node dysfunction (1% to 3%), cardiac arrhythmia, flushing, edema. Additional effects associated with I.V. administration include asystole, cardiac arrest, electromechanical dissociation, ventricular tachycardia, and cardiogenic shock.

Dermatologic: Slate blue skin discoloration (<10%)

Endocrine & metabolic: Hyperthyroidism (<3%), libido decreased

Gastrointestinal: Abdominal pain, abnormal salivation, abnormal taste (oral)

Hematologic: Coagulation abnormalities

Hepatic: Hepatitis and cirrhosis (<3%)

Local: Phlebitis (I.V., with concentrations >3 mg/mL)

Ocular: Visual disturbances (2% to 9%), halo vision (<5% occurring especially at night), optic neuritis (1%)

Respiratory: Pulmonary toxicity has been estimated to occur at a frequency between 2% and 7% of patients (some reports indicate a frequency as high as 17%). Toxicity may present as hypersensitivity pneumonitis; pulmonary fibrosis (cough, fever, malaise); pulmonary inflammation; interstitial pneumonitis; or alveolar pneumonitis. ARDS has been reported in up to 2% of patients receiving amiodarone, and postoperatively in patients receiving oral amiodarone.

Miscellaneous: Abnormal smell (oral)

Restrictions An FDA-approved medication guide is available at www.fda.gov/cder/Offices/ODS/labeling.htm; distribute to each patient to whom this medication is dispensed.

Mechanism of Action Class III antiarrhythmic agent which inhibits adrenergic stimulation (alpha- and beta-blocking properties), affects sodium, potassium, and calcium channels, prolongs the action potential and refractory period in myocardial tissue; decreases AV conduction and sinus node function

Drug Interactions

Cytochrome P450 Effect: Substrate of CYP1A2 (minor), 2C8 (major at low concentration), 2C19 (minor), 2D6 (minor), 3A4 (major); **Inhibits** CYP1A2 (strong), 2A6 (moderate), 2B6 (weak), 2C9 (moderate), 2C19 (weak), 2D6 (moderate), 3A4 (moderate)

Increased Effect/Toxicity: Note: Due to the long half-life of amiodarone, drug interactions may take 1 or more weeks to develop. The effect of drugs which prolong the QT interval, including amitriptyline, azole antifungals, bepridil, cisapride, clarithromycin, disopyramide, erythromycin, gatifloxacin, haloperidol, imipramine, moxifloxacin, quinidine, pimozide, procainamide, sotalol, sparfloxacin, theophylline, and thioridazine may be increased. Cisapride and sparfloxacin are contraindicated. Use of amiodarone with diltiazem, verapamil, digoxin, beta-blockers, and other drugs which delay AV conduction may cause excessive AV block (amiodarone may also decrease the metabolism of some of these agents - see below).

Amiodarone may increase the levels of digoxin (reduce dose by 50% on initiation), flecainide (decrease dose up to 33%), phenothiazines, procainamide (reduce dose), and quinidine. Amiodarone may increase the levels/effects of aminophylline, amphetamines, selected benzodiazepines, selected beta-blockers, calcium channel blockers, cyclosporine, dexmedetomidine, (Continued)

Amiodarone *(Continued)*

dextromethorphan, fluoxetine, fluvoxamine, glimepiride, glipizide, ifosfamide, imatinib, isoniazid, lidocaine, mexiletine, mirtazapine, nateglinide, nefazodone, paroxetine, phenytoin, pioglitazone, risperidone, ritonavir, ropinirole, rosiglitazone, sildenafil (and other PDE-5 inhibitors), sertraline, tacrolimus, telithromycin, theophylline, thioridazine, tricyclic antidepressants, trifluoperazine, venlafaxine, warfarin, and other CYP1A2, 2A6, 2C9, CYP2D6, and/or CYP3A4 substrates. Selected benzodiazepines (midazolam, triazolam), cisapride, ergot alkaloids, selected HMG-CoA reductase inhibitors (lovastatin and simvastatin), mesoridazine, pimozide, and thioridazine are generally contraindicated with strong CYP3A4 inhibitors; example CYP3A4 inhibitors include azole antifungals, clarithromycin, diclofenac, doxycycline, erythromycin, imatinib, isoniazid, nefazodone, nicardipine, propofol, protease inhibitors, quinidine, telithromycin, and verapamil. When used with strong CYP3A4 inhibitors, dosage adjustment/limits are recommended for sildenafil and other PDE-5 inhibitors; consult individual monographs.

The levels/effects of amiodarone may be increased by atazanavir, gemfibrozil, ritonavir, and other CYP2C8 inhibitors.

Concurrent use of fentanyl may lead to bradycardia, sinus arrest, and hypotension. Amiodarone may alter thyroid function and response to thyroid supplements. Amiodarone enhances the myocardial depressant and conduction effects of inhalation anesthetics (monitor).

Decreased Effect: Levels/effects of amiodarone may be decreased by aminoglutethimide, carbamazepine, nafcillin, nevirapine, phenobarbital, phenytoin, rifampin, rifapentine, secobarbital, and other CYP2C8 inducers and CYP3A4 inducers. Amiodarone may decrease the levels/effects of codeine, hydrocodone, oxycodone, tramadol, and other prodrug substrates of CYP2D6. Amiodarone may alter thyroid function and response to thyroid supplements; monitor closely.

Pharmacodynamics/Kinetics

Onset of action: Oral: 2 days to 3 weeks; I.V.: May be more rapid
Peak effect: 1 week to 5 months
Duration after discontinuing therapy: 7-50 days
Note: Mean onset of effect and duration after discontinuation may be shorter in children than adults
Distribution: V_d: 66 L/kg (range: 18-148 L/kg); crosses placenta; enters breast milk in concentrations higher than maternal plasma concentrations
Protein binding: 96%
Metabolism: Hepatic via CYP2C8 and 3A4 to active N-desethylamiodarone metabolite; possible enterohepatic recirculation
Bioavailability: Oral: ~50%
Half-life elimination: Terminal: 40-55 days (range: 26-107 days); shorter in children than adults
Excretion: Feces; urine (<1% as unchanged drug)

Pregnancy Risk Factor D

Dental Comment This drug is known to prolong the QT interval. The QT interval is measured as the time and distance between the Q point of the QRS complex and the end of the T wave in the ECG tracing. After adjustment for heart rate, the QT interval is defined as prolonged if it is more than 450 msec in men and 460 msec in women. A long QT syndrome was first described in the 1950s and 60s as a congenital syndrome involving QT interval prolongation and syncope and sudden death. Some of the congenital long QT syndromes were characterized by a peculiar electrocardiographic appearance of the QRS complex involving a premature atria beat followed by a pause, then a subsequent sinus beat showing marked QT prolongation and deformity. This type of cardiac arrhythmia was originally termed "torsade de pointes" (translated from the French as "twisting of the points").

Prolongation of the QT interval is thought to result from delayed ventricular repolarization. The repolarization process within the myocardial cell is due to the efflux of intracellular potassium. The channels associated with this current can be blocked by many drugs and predispose the electrical propagation cycle to torsade de pointes.

Amiodarone is one of the drugs confirmed to prolong the QT interval and is accepted as having a risk of causing torsade de pointes. The risk of drug-induced torsade de pointes is extremely low when a single QT interval prolonging drug is prescribed. In terms of epinephrine, it is not known what effect vasoconstrictors in the local anesthetic regimen will have in patients with a known history of congenital prolonged QT interval or in patients taking any medication that prolongs the QT interval. Until more information is obtained, it is suggested that the clinician consult with the physician prior to the use of a vasoconstrictor in suspected patients, and that the vasoconstrictor (epinephrine, levonordefrin [Neo-Cobefrin®]) be used with caution.

Amiodarone Hydrochloride *see* Amiodarone *on page 90*

Ami-Tex LA *see* Guaifenesin and Phenylephrine *on page 754*

Ami-Tex PSE *see* Guaifenesin and Pseudoephedrine *on page 755*

Amitiza™ *see* Lubiprostone *on page 957*

Amitone® [OTC] [DSC] *see* Calcium Carbonate *on page 248*

Amitriptyline (a mee TRIP ti leen)

Related Information
Temporomandibular Dysfunction (TMD) *on page 1724*

Canadian Brand Names Apo-Amitriptyline®; Levate®; Novo-Triptyn; PMS-Amitriptyline

Generic Available Yes

Synonyms Amitriptyline Hydrochloride; Elavil

Pharmacologic Category Antidepressant, Tricyclic (Tertiary Amine)

Dental Use Management of chronic neuropathic pain in temporomandibular dysfunction (TMD)

Use Relief of symptoms of depression

Unlabeled/Investigational Use Analgesic for certain chronic and neuropathic pain; prophylaxis against migraine headaches; treatment of depressive disorders in children

Local Anesthetic/Vasoconstrictor Precautions Use with caution; epinephrine and levonordefrin have been shown to have an increased pressor response in combination with TCAs (see Dental Comment)

Effects on Dental Treatment Key adverse event(s) related to dental treatment: Xerostomia and changes in salivation (normal salivary flow resumes upon discontinuation) and orthostatic hypotension. Amitriptyline is the most anticholinergic and sedating of the antidepressants; has pronounced effects on the cardiovascular system. Long-term treatment with TCAs such as amitriptyline increases the risk of caries by reducing salivation and salivary buffer capacity. In a study by Rundergren, et al, pathological alterations were observed in the oral mucosa of 72% of 58 patients; 55% had new carious lesions after taking TCAs for a median of 5¹/₂ years. Current research is investigating the use of the salivary stimulant pilocarpine (Salagen®) to overcome the xerostomia from amitriptyline.

Significant Adverse Effects Anticholinergic effects may be pronounced; moderate to marked sedation can occur (tolerance to these effects usually occurs).

Frequency not defined.

Cardiovascular: Orthostatic hypotension, tachycardia, ECG changes (nonspecific), AV conduction changes, cardiomyopathy (rare), MI, stroke, heart block, arrhythmia, syncope, hypertension, palpitation

Central nervous system: Restlessness, dizziness, insomnia, sedation, fatigue, anxiety, cognitive function impaired, seizure, extrapyramidal symptoms, coma, hallucinations, confusion, disorientation, coordination impaired, ataxia, headache, nightmares, hyperpyrexia

Dermatologic: Allergic rash, urticaria, photosensitivity, alopecia

Endocrine & metabolic: Syndrome of inappropriate ADH secretion

Gastrointestinal: Weight gain, xerostomia, constipation, paralytic ileus, nausea, vomiting, anorexia, stomatitis, peculiar taste, diarrhea, black tongue

Genitourinary: Urinary retention

Hematologic: Bone marrow depression, purpura, eosinophilia

Neuromuscular & skeletal: Numbness, paresthesia, peripheral neuropathy, tremor, weakness

Ocular: Blurred vision, mydriasis, ocular pressure increased

Otic: Tinnitus

Miscellaneous: Diaphoresis, withdrawal reactions (nausea, headache, malaise)

Postmarketing and/or case reports: Neuroleptic malignant syndrome (rare), serotonin syndrome (rare)

Restrictions A medication guide concerning the use of antidepressants in children and teenagers can be found on the FDA website at www.fda.gov/cder/Offices/ODS/labeling.htm. It should be dispensed to parents or guardians of children and teenagers receiving this medication.

Dental Usual Dosing Chronic neuropathic pain in temporomandibular dysfunction (TMD) (unlabeled use): Adults: Oral: Initial: 25 mg at bedtime; may increase as tolerated to 100 mg/day

(Continued)

Amitriptyline *(Continued)*

Dosage

Children:

Chronic pain management (unlabeled use): Oral: Initial: 0.1 mg/kg at bedtime, may advance as tolerated over 2-3 weeks to 0.5-2 mg/kg at bedtime

Depressive disorders (unlabeled use): Oral: Initial doses of 1 mg/kg/day given in 3 divided doses with increases to 1.5 mg/kg/day have been reported in a small number of children (n=9) 9-12 years of age; clinically, doses up to 3 mg/kg/day (5 mg/kg/day if monitored closely) have been proposed

Migraine prophylaxis (unlabeled use): Oral: Initial: 0.25 mg/kg/day, given at bedtime; increase dose by 0.25 mg/kg/day to maximum 1 mg/kg/day. Reported dosing ranges: 0.1-2 mg/kg/day; maximum suggested dose: 10 mg.

Adolescents: Depressive disorders: Oral: Initial: 25-50 mg/day; may administer in divided doses; increase gradually to 100 mg/day in divided doses

Adults:

Depression:

Oral: 50-150 mg/day single dose at bedtime or in divided doses; dose may be gradually increased up to 300 mg/day

Migraine prophylaxis (unlabeled use): Oral: Initial: 10-25 mg at bedtime; usual dose: 150 mg; reported dosing ranges: 10-400 mg/day

Pain management (unlabeled use): Oral: Initial: 25 mg at bedtime; may increase as tolerated to 100 mg/day

Elderly: Depression: Oral: Initial: 10-25 mg at bedtime; dose should be increased in 10-25 mg increments every week if tolerated; dose range: 25-150 mg/day

Dosing interval in hepatic impairment: Use with caution and monitor plasma levels and patient response

Hemodialysis: Nondialyzable

Mechanism of Action Increases the synaptic concentration of serotonin and/or norepinephrine in the central nervous system by inhibition of their reuptake by the presynaptic neuronal membrane

Contraindications Hypersensitivity to amitriptyline or any component of the formulation (cross-sensitivity with other tricyclics may occur); use of MAO inhibitors within past 14 days; acute recovery phase following myocardial infarction; concurrent use of cisapride

Warnings/Precautions Antidepressants increase the risk of suicidal thinking and behavior in children and adolescents with major depressive disorder (MDD) and other depressive disorders; consider risk prior to prescribing. Closely monitor for clinical worsening, suicidality, or unusual changes in behavior; the child's family or caregiver should be instructed to closely observe the patient and communicate condition with healthcare provider. Such observation would generally include at least weekly face-to-face contact with patients or their family members or caregivers during the first 4 weeks of treatment, then every other week visits for the next 4 weeks, then at 12 weeks, and as clinically indicated beyond 12 weeks. Additional contact by telephone may be appropriate between face-to-face visits. Adults treated with antidepressants should be observed similarly for clinical worsening and suicidality, especially during the initial few months of a course of drug therapy, or at times of dose changes, either increases or decreases. A medication guide should be dispensed with each prescription. **Amitriptyline is not FDA-approved for use in children <12 years of age.**

The possibility of a suicide attempt is inherent in major depression and may persist until remission occurs. Monitor for worsening of depression or suicidality, especially during initiation of therapy or with dose increases or decreases. Worsening depression and severe abrupt suicidality that are not part of the presenting symptoms may require discontinuation or modification of drug therapy. Use caution in high-risk patients during initiation of therapy. Prescriptions should be written for the smallest quantity consistent with good patient care. The patient's family or caregiver should be alerted to monitor patients for the emergence of suicidality and associated behaviors such as anxiety, agitation, panic attacks, insomnia, irritability, hostility, impulsivity, akathisia, hypomania, and mania; patients should be instructed to notify their healthcare provider if any of these symptoms or worsening depression occur.

May worsen psychosis in some patients or precipitate a shift to mania or hypomania in patients with bipolar disorder. Monotherapy in patients with bipolar disorder should be avoided. Patients presenting with depressive symptoms should be screened for bipolar disorder. **Amitriptyline is not FDA approved for the treatment of bipolar depression.**

Often causes drowsiness/sedation, resulting in impaired performance of tasks requiring alertness (eg, operating machinery or driving). Sedative effects may be additive with other CNS depressants and/or ethanol. The degree of sedation is very high relative to other antidepressants. May cause hyponatremia/SIADH. May increase the risks associated with electroconvulsive therapy. Consider discontinuing, when possible, prior to elective surgery. Therapy should not be abruptly discontinued in patients receiving high doses for prolonged periods.

May cause orthostatic hypotension; the risk of this problem is very high relative to other antidepressants. Use with caution in patients at risk of hypotension or in patients where transient hypotensive episodes would be poorly tolerated (cardiovascular disease or cerebrovascular disease). The degree of anticholinergic blockade produced by this agent is very high relative to other cyclic antidepressants; use with caution in patients with urinary retention, benign prostatic hyperplasia, narrow-angle glaucoma, xerostomia, visual problems, constipation, or a history of bowel obstruction. May alter glucose control - use with caution in patients with diabetes.

Use with caution in patients with a history of cardiovascular disease (including previous MI, stroke, tachycardia, or conduction abnormalities). The risk of conduction abnormalities with this agent is high relative to other antidepressants. May lower seizure threshold - use caution in patients with a previous seizure disorder or condition predisposing to seizures such as brain damage, alcoholism, or concurrent therapy with other drugs which lower the seizure threshold. Use with caution in hyperthyroid patients or those receiving thyroid supplementation. Use with caution in patients with hepatic or renal dysfunction and in elderly patients.

Drug Interactions Substrate of CYP1A2 (minor), 2B6 (minor), 2C9 (minor), 2C19 (minor), 2D6 (major), 3A4 (minor); **Inhibits** CYP1A2 (weak), 2C9 (weak), 2C19 (weak), 2D6 (weak), 2E1 (weak)

Altretamine: Concurrent use may cause orthostatic hypertension

Amphetamines: TCAs may enhance the effect of amphetamines; monitor for adverse CV effects

Anticholinergics: Combined use with TCAs may produce additive anticholinergic effects

Antihypertensives: Amitriptyline inhibits the antihypertensive response to bethanidine, clonidine, debrisoquin, guanadrel, guanethidine, guanabenz, guanfacine; monitor BP; consider alternate antihypertensive agent

Beta-agonists: When combined with TCAs may predispose patients to cardiac arrhythmias

Bupropion: May increase the levels of tricyclic antidepressants; based on limited information, monitor response

Carbamazepine: Tricyclic antidepressants may increase carbamazepine levels; monitor

Cholestyramine and colestipol: May bind TCAs and reduce their absorption; monitor for altered response

Cisapride: May increase the risk of QT_c prolongation and/or arrhythmia; concurrent use is contraindicated

Clonidine: Abrupt discontinuation of clonidine may cause hypertensive crisis; amitriptyline may enhance the response (also see note on antihypertensives)

CNS depressants: Sedative effects may be additive with TCAs; monitor for increased effect; includes benzodiazepines, barbiturates, antipsychotics, ethanol, and other sedative medications

CYP2D6 inhibitors: May increase the levels/effects of amitriptyline; example inhibitors include chlorpromazine, delavirdine, fluoxetine, miconazole, paroxetine, pergolide, quinidine, quinine, ritonavir, and ropinirole

Epinephrine (and other direct alpha-agonists): Pressor response to I.V. epinephrine, norepinephrine, and phenylephrine may be enhanced in patients receiving TCAs. (**Note:** Effect is unlikely with epinephrine or levonordefrin dosages typically administered as infiltration in combination with local anesthetics.)

Fenfluramine: May increase tricyclic antidepressant levels/effects

Hypoglycemic agents (including insulin): TCAs may enhance the hypoglycemic effects of tolazamide, chlorpropamide, or insulin; monitor for changes in blood glucose levels; reported with chlorpropamide, tolazamide, and insulin

Levodopa: Tricyclic antidepressants may decrease the absorption (bioavailability) of levodopa; rare hypertensive episodes have also been attributed to this combination

Linezolid: Hyperpyrexia, hypertension, tachycardia, confusion, seizures, and **deaths have been reported** with agents which inhibit MAO (serotonin syndrome); this combination should be avoided

Lithium: Concurrent use with a TCA may increase the risk for neurotoxicity

MAO inhibitors: Hyperpyrexia, hypertension, tachycardia, confusion, seizures, and **deaths have been reported** (serotonin syndrome); this combination should be avoided

Methylphenidate: Metabolism of amitriptyline may be decreased
(Continued)

Amitriptyline *(Continued)*

Phenothiazines: Serum concentrations of some TCAs may be increased; in addition, TCAs may increase concentration of phenothiazines; monitor for altered clinical response

QT_c prolonging agents: Concurrent use of tricyclic agents with other drugs which may prolong QT_c interval may increase the risk of potentially fatal arrhythmias; includes type Ia and type III antiarrhythmics agents, selected quinolones (sparfloxacin, gatifloxacin, moxifloxacin, grepafloxacin), cisapride, and other agents

Ritonavir: Combined use of high-dose tricyclic antidepressants with ritonavir may cause serotonin syndrome in HIV-positive patients; monitor

Sucralfate: Absorption of tricyclic antidepressants may be reduced with coadministration

Sympathomimetics, indirect-acting: Tricyclic antidepressants may result in a decreased sensitivity to indirect-acting sympathomimetics; includes dopamine and ephedrine; also see interaction with epinephrine (and direct-acting sympathomimetics)

Tramadol: Tramadol's risk of seizures may be increased with TCAs

Valproic acid: May increase serum concentrations/adverse effects of some tricyclic antidepressants

Warfarin (and other oral anticoagulants): Amitriptyline may increase the anticoagulant effect in patients stabilized on warfarin; monitor INR

Ethanol/Nutrition/Herb Interactions

Ethanol: Avoid ethanol (may increase CNS depression).

Food: Grapefruit juice may inhibit the metabolism of some TCAs and clinical toxicity may result.

Herb/Nutraceutical: St John's wort may decrease amitriptyline levels. Avoid valerian, St John's wort, kava kava, gotu kola (may increase CNS depression).

Pharmacodynamics/Kinetics

Onset of action: Migraine prophylaxis: 6 weeks, higher dosage may be required in heavy smokers because of increased metabolism; Depression: 4-6 weeks, reduce dosage to lowest effective level

Distribution: Crosses placenta; enters breast milk

Metabolism: Hepatic to nortriptyline (active), hydroxy and conjugated derivatives; may be impaired in the elderly

Half-life elimination: Adults: 9-27 hours (average: 15 hours)

Time to peak, serum: ~4 hours

Excretion: Urine (18% as unchanged drug); feces (small amounts)

Pregnancy Risk Factor C

Lactation Enters breast milk/not recommended (AAP rates "of concern")

Breast-Feeding Considerations Generally, it is not recommended to breast-feed if taking antidepressants because of the long half-life, active metabolites, and the potential for side effects in the infant.

Dosage Forms

Tablet, as hydrochloride: 10 mg, 25 mg, 50 mg, 75 mg, 100 mg, 150 mg

Dental Comment This drug is known to prolong the QT interval. The QT interval is measured as the time and distance between the Q point of the QRS complex and the end of the T wave in the ECG tracing. After adjustment for heart rate, the QT interval is defined as prolonged if it is more than 450 msec in men and 460 msec in women. A long QT syndrome was first described in the 1950s and 60s as a congenital syndrome involving QT interval prolongation and syncope and sudden death. Some of the congenital long QT syndromes were characterized by a peculiar electrocardiographic appearance of the QRS complex involving a premature atria beat followed by a pause, then a subsequent sinus beat showing marked QT prolongation and deformity. This type of cardiac arrhythmia was originally termed "torsade de pointes" (translated from the French as "twisting of the points").

Prolongation of the QT interval is thought to result from delayed ventricular repolarization. The repolarization process within the myocardial cell is due to the efflux of intracellular potassium. The channels associated with this current can be blocked by many drugs, thus predisposing the electrical propagation cycle to torsade de pointes.

Amitriptyline is one of the drugs confirmed to prolong the QT interval and is accepted as having a risk of causing torsade de pointes. The risk of drug-induced torsade de pointes is extremely low when a single QT interval prolonging drug is prescribed. In terms of epinephrine, it is not known what effect vasoconstrictors in the local anesthetic regimen will have in patients with a known history of congenital prolonged QT interval or in patients taking any medication that prolongs the QT interval. Until more information is obtained, it is suggested that the clinician consult with the physician prior to the use of a vasoconstrictor in suspected patients, and that the vasoconstrictor (epinephrine, levonordefrin [Neo-Cobefrin®]) be used with caution.

Selected Readings

Boakes AJ, Laurence DR, Teoh PC, et al, "Interactions Between Sympathomimetic Amines and Antidepressant Agents in Man," *Br Med J*, 1973, 1(849):311-5.

Friedlander AH and Mahler ME, "Major Depressive Disorder. Psychopathology, Medical Management, and Dental Implications," *J Am Dent Assoc*, 2001, 132(5):629-38.

Ganzberg S, "Psychoactive Drugs," *ADA Guide to Dental Therapeutics*, 2nd ed, Chicago, IL: ADA Publishing, a Division of ADA Business Enterprises, Inc, 2000, 376-405.

Jastak JT and Yagiela JA, "Vasoconstrictors and Local Anesthesia: A Review and Rationale for Use," *J Am Dent Assoc*, 1983, 107(4):623-30.

Rundegren J, van Dijken J, Mörnstad H, et al, "Oral Conditions in Patients Receiving Long-Term Treatment With Cyclic Antidepressant Drugs," *Swed Dent J*, 1985, 9(2):55-64.

Yagiela JA, "Adverse Drug Interactions in Dental Practice: Interactions Associated With Vasoconstrictors. Part V of a Series," *J Am Dent Assoc*, 1999, 130(5):701-9.

Amitriptyline and Chlordiazepoxide
(a mee TRIP ti leen & klor dye az e POKS ide)

Related Information
Amitriptyline *on page 93*
Chlordiazepoxide *on page 315*

U.S. Brand Names Limbitrol®; Limbitrol® DS

Canadian Brand Names Limbitrol®

Generic Available Yes

Synonyms Chlordiazepoxide and Amitriptyline Hydrochloride

Pharmacologic Category Antidepressant, Tricyclic (Tertiary Amine); Benzodiazepine

Use Treatment of moderate to severe anxiety and/or agitation and depression

Local Anesthetic/Vasoconstrictor Precautions Use with caution; epinephrine and levonordefrin have been shown to have an increased pressor response in combination with TCAs

Effects on Dental Treatment
Amitriptyline: The most anticholinergic and sedating of the antidepressants; pronounced effects on the cardiovascular system; long-term treatment with TCAs such as amitriptyline increases the risk of caries by reducing salivation and salivary buffer capacity. In a study by Rundegren, et al, pathological alterations were observed in the oral mucosa of 72% of 58 patients; 55% had new carious lesions after taking TCAs for a median of 5½ years. Current research is investigating the use of the salivary stimulant pilocarpine (Salagen®) to overcome the xerostomia from amitriptyline.

Chlordiazepoxide: Over 10% of patients will experience xerostomia which disappears with cessation of drug therapy.

Common Adverse Effects See individual agents.

Restrictions C-IV

A medication guide concerning the use of antidepressants in children and teenagers can be found on the FDA website at http://www.fda.gov/cder/Offices/ODS/labeling.htm. It should be dispensed to parents or guardians of children and teenagers receiving this medication.

Mechanism of Action See individual agents.

Drug Interactions
Cytochrome P450 Effect:
Amitriptyline: **Substrate** of CYP1A2 (minor), 2B6 (minor), 2C9 (minor), 2C19 (minor), 2D6 (major), 3A4 (minor); **Inhibits** CYP1A2 (weak), 2C9 (weak), 2C19 (weak), 2D6 (weak), 2E1 (weak)

Chlordiazepoxide: **Substrate** of CYP3A4 (major)

Increased Effect/Toxicity: See individual agents.

Decreased Effect: See individual agents.

Pharmacodynamics/Kinetics See individual agents.

Pregnancy Risk Factor D

Amitriptyline and Perphenazine
(a mee TRIP ti leen & per FEN a zeen)

Related Information
Amitriptyline *on page 93*
Perphenazine *on page 1218*

Canadian Brand Names Etrafon®

Generic Available Yes

Synonyms Perphenazine and Amitriptyline Hydrochloride

Pharmacologic Category Antidepressant, Tricyclic (Tertiary Amine); Antipsychotic Agent, Typical, Phenothiazine

(Continued)

Amitriptyline and Perphenazine *(Continued)*

Use Treatment of patients with moderate to severe anxiety and depression

Unlabeled/Investigational Use Depression with psychotic features

Local Anesthetic/Vasoconstrictor Precautions

Amitriptyline: Use with caution; epinephrine and levonordefrin have been shown to have an increased pressor response in combination with TCAs

Perphenazine: No information available to require special precautions

Effects on Dental Treatment Key adverse event(s) related to dental treatment:

Amitriptyline: Xerostomia (normal salivary flow resumes upon discontinuation). The most anticholinergic and sedating of the antidepressants; pronounced effects on the cardiovascular system; long-term treatment with TCAs, such as amitriptyline, increases the risk of caries by reducing salivation and salivary buffer capacity. In a study by Rundergren, et al, pathological alterations were observed in the oral mucosa of 72% of 58 patients; 55% had new carious lesions after taking TCAs for a median of $5^1/_2$ years. Current research is investigating the use of the salivary stimulant pilocarpine (Salagen®) to overcome the xerostomia from amitriptyline.

Perphenazine: Extrapyramidal symptoms (pseudoparkinsonism, akathisia, dystonias, tardive dyskinesia), dizziness, seizures, headache, drowsiness, paradoxical excitement, restlessness, and hyperactivity.

Tardive dyskinesia: Prevalence rate may be 40% in elderly; development of the syndrome and the irreversible nature are proportional to duration and total cumulative dose over time. Extrapyramidal reactions are more common in elderly with up to 50% developing these reactions after 60 years of age. Drug-induced Parkinson's syndrome occurs often; akathisia is the most common extrapyramidal reaction in elderly.

Increased confusion, memory loss, psychotic behavior, and agitation frequently occur as a consequence of anticholinergic effects. Antipsychotic associated sedation in nonpsychotic patients is extremely unpleasant due to feelings of depersonalization, derealization, and dysphoria.

Common Adverse Effects Frequency not defined.

Based on **amitriptyline** component: Anticholinergic effects may be pronounced; moderate to marked sedation can occur (tolerance to these effects usually occurs).

Cardiovascular: Orthostatic hypotension, tachycardia, ECG changes (nonspecific), AV conduction changes

Central nervous system: Restlessness, dizziness, insomnia, sedation, fatigue, anxiety, cognitive function impaired, seizure, extrapyramidal symptoms

Dermatologic: Allergic rash, urticaria, photosensitivity

Gastrointestinal: Weight gain, xerostomia, constipation

Genitourinary: Urinary retention

Ocular: Blurred vision, mydriasis

Miscellaneous: Diaphoresis

Based on **perphenazine** component:

Cardiovascular: Hyper-/hypotension, orthostatic hypotension, tachycardia, bradycardia, dizziness, cardiac arrest

Central nervous system: Extrapyramidal symptoms (pseudoparkinsonism, akathisia, dystonias, tardive dyskinesia), dizziness, cerebral edema, seizure, headache, drowsiness, paradoxical excitement, restlessness, hyperactivity, insomnia, neuroleptic malignant syndrome (NMS), impairment of temperature regulation

Dermatologic: Sun sensitivity increased, rash, discoloration of skin (blue-gray)

Endocrine & metabolic: Hypoglycemia, hyperglycemia, galactorrhea, lactation, breast enlargement, gynecomastia, menstrual irregularity, amenorrhea, SIADH, libido (changes in)

Gastrointestinal: Constipation, weight gain, vomiting, stomach pain, nausea, xerostomia, salivation, diarrhea, anorexia, ileus

Genitourinary: Difficulty in urination, ejaculatory disturbances, incontinence, polyuria, ejaculating dysfunction, priapism

Hematologic: Agranulocytosis, leukopenia, eosinophilia, hemolytic anemia, thrombocytopenic purpura, pancytopenia

Hepatic: Cholestatic jaundice, hepatotoxicity

Neuromuscular & skeletal: Tremor

Ocular: Pigmentary retinopathy, blurred vision, cornea and lens changes

Respiratory: Nasal congestion

Miscellaneous: Diaphoresis

Restrictions A medication guide concerning the use of antidepressants in children and teenagers can be found on the FDA website at http://www.fda.gov/cder/Offices/ODS/labeling.htm. It should be dispensed to parents or guardians of children and teenagers receiving this medication.

Mechanism of Action

Amitriptyline increases the synaptic concentration of serotonin and/or norepinephrine in the central nervous system by inhibition of their reuptake by the presynaptic neuronal membrane.

Perphenazine is a piperazine phenothiazine antipsychotic which blocks postsynaptic mesolimbic dopaminergic receptors in the brain; exhibits alpha-adrenergic blocking effect and depresses the release of hypothalamic and hypophyseal hormones.

Drug Interactions

Cytochrome P450 Effect:

Amitriptyline: **Substrate** of CYP1A2 (minor), 2B6 (minor), 2C9 (minor), 2C19 (minor), 2D6 (major), 3A4 (minor); **Inhibits** CYP1A2 (weak), 2C9 (weak), 2C19 (weak), 2D6 (weak), 2E1 (weak)

Perphenazine: **Substrate** of CYP1A2 (minor), 2C9 (minor), 2C19 (minor), 2D6 (major), 3A4 (minor); **Inhibits** CYP1A2 (weak), 2D6 (weak)

Increased Effect/Toxicity: See individual agents.

Decreased Effect: See individual agents.

Pharmacodynamics/Kinetics See individual agents.

Pregnancy Risk Factor D

Amitriptyline Hydrochloride *see* Amitriptyline *on page 93*

AMJ 9701 *see* Palifermin *on page 1178*

AmLactin® [OTC] *see* Lactic Acid and Ammonium Hydroxide *on page 893*

Amlexanox (am LEKS an oks)

Related Information

Ulcerative and Erosive Disorders *on page 1712*

Related Sample Prescriptions

Recurrent Aphthous Stomatitis *on page 1744*

U.S. Brand Names Aphthasol®

Generic Available No

Pharmacologic Category Anti-inflammatory, Locally Applied

Dental Use Treatment of aphthous ulcers (ie, canker sores)

Use Treatment of aphthous ulcers (ie, canker sores)

Unlabeled/Investigational Use Allergic disorders

Local Anesthetic/Vasoconstrictor Precautions No information available to require special precautions

Effects on Dental Treatment Key adverse event(s) related to dental treatment: Allergic contact dermatitis and oral irritation. Discontinue therapy if rash or contact mucositis develops (see Dental Comment).

Significant Adverse Effects

1% to 2%:

Dermatologic: Allergic contact dermatitis

Gastrointestinal: Oral irritation

<1% (Limited to important or life-threatening): Contact mucositis

Dosage Topical: Administer (0.5 cm - $^1/_4$") directly on ulcers 4 times/day following oral hygiene, after meals, and at bedtime

Mechanism of Action As a benzopyrano-bipyridine carboxylic acid derivative, amlexanox has anti-inflammatory and antiallergic properties; it inhibits chemical mediatory release of the slow-reacting substance of anaphylaxis (SRS-A) and may have antagonistic effects on interleukin-3

Contraindications Hypersensitivity to amlexanox or any component of the formulation

Warnings/Precautions Discontinue therapy if rash or contact mucositis develops.

Pharmacodynamics/Kinetics

Absorption: Some from swallowed paste

Metabolism: Hydroxylated and conjugated metabolites

Half-life elimination: 3.5 hours

Time to peak, serum: 2 hours

Excretion: Urine (17% as unchanged drug)

Pregnancy Risk Factor B

Lactation Excretion in breast milk unknown/use caution

Dosage Forms Paste: 5% (5 g) [contains benzyl alcohol]

Dental Comment Treatment of canker sores with amlexanox showed a 76% median reduction in ulcer size compared to a 40% reduction with placebo. Greer, et al, reported an overall mean reduction in ulcer size of 1.82 mm² for patients treated with 5% amlexanox versus an average reduction of 0.52 mm² for the control group. Recent studies in over thousands of patients have

(Continued)

Amlexanox *(Continued)*

confirmed that amlexanox accelerates the resolution of pain and healing of aphthous ulcers more significantly than vehicle and no treatment.

Selected Readings

Barrons RW, "Treatment Strategies for Recurrent Oral Aphthous Ulcers," *Am J Health Syst Pharm*, 2001, 58(1):41-50.

Binnie WH, Curro FA, Khandwala A, et al, "Amlexanox Oral Paste: A Novel Treatment That Accelerates the Healing of Aphthous Ulcers," *Compend Contin Educ Dent*, 1997, 18(11):1116-8, 1120-2, 1124.

Eisen D and Lynch DP, "Selecting Topical and Systemic Agents for Recurrent Aphthous Stomatitis," *Cutis*, 2001, 68(3):201-6.

Greer RO Jr, Lindenmuth JE, Juarez T, et al, "A Double-Blind Study of Topically Applied 5% Amlexanox in the Treatment of Aphthous Ulcers," *J Oral Maxillofac Surg*, 1993, 51(3):243-8.

Khandwala A, Van Inwegen RG, and Alfano MC, "5% Amlexanox Oral Paste, A New Treatment for Recurrent Minor Aphthous Ulcers: I. Clinical Demonstration of Acceleration of Healing and Resolution of Pain," *Oral Surg Oral Med Oral Pathol Oral Radiol Endod*, 1997, 83(2):222-30.

Khandwala A, Van Inwegen RG, Charney MR, et al, "5% Amlexanox Oral Paste, A New Treatment for Recurrent Minor Aphthous Ulcers: II. Pharmacokinetics and Demonstration of Clinical Safety," *Oral Surg Oral Med Oral Pathol Oral Radiol Endod*, 1997, 83(2):231-8.

Amlodipine *(am LOE di peen)*

Related Information

Cardiovascular Diseases *on page 1636*

U.S. Brand Names Norvasc®

Canadian Brand Names Norvasc®

Mexican Brand Names Norvas®

Generic Available No

Synonyms Amlodipine Besylate

Pharmacologic Category Calcium Channel Blocker

Use Treatment of hypertension; treatment of symptomatic chronic stable angina, vasospastic (Prinzmetal's) angina (confirmed or suspected); prevention of hospitalization due to angina with documented CAD (limited to patients without heart failure or ejection fraction <40%)

Local Anesthetic/Vasoconstrictor Precautions No information available to require special precautions

Effects on Dental Treatment Fewer reports of gingival hyperplasia with amlodipine than with other CCBs (usually resolves upon discontinuation); consultation with physician is suggested.

Common Adverse Effects

>10%: Cardiovascular: Peripheral edema (2% to 15% dose related)

1% to 10%:

Cardiovascular: Flushing (1% to 3%), palpitation (1% to 4%)

Central nervous system: Headache (7%; similar to placebo 8%), dizziness (1% to 3%), fatigue (4%), somnolence (1% to 2%)

Dermatologic: Rash (1% to 2%), pruritus (1% to 2%)

Endocrine & metabolic: Male sexual dysfunction (1% to 2%)

Gastrointestinal: Nausea (3%), abdominal pain (1% to 2%), dyspepsia (1% to 2%), gingival hyperplasia

Neuromuscular & skeletal: Muscle cramps (1% to 2%), weakness (1% to 2%)

Respiratory: Dyspnea (1% to 2%), pulmonary edema (15% from PRAISE trial, CHF population)

Dosage Oral:

Children 6-17 years: Hypertension: 2.5-5 mg once daily

Adults:

Hypertension: Initial dose: 5 mg once daily; maximum dose: 10 mg once daily. In general, titrate in 2.5 mg increments over 7-14 days. Usual dosage range (JNC 7): 2.5-10 mg once daily.

Angina: Usual dose: 5-10 mg; lower dose suggested in elderly or hepatic impairment; most patients require 10 mg for adequate effect

Elderly: Dosing should start at the lower end of dosing range due to possible increased incidence of hepatic, renal, or cardiac impairment. Elderly patients also show decreased clearance of amlodipine.

Hypertension: 2.5 mg once daily

Angina: 5 mg once daily

Dialysis: Hemodialysis and peritoneal dialysis does not enhance elimination. Supplemental dose is not necessary.

Dosage adjustment in hepatic impairment:

Angina: Administer 5 mg once daily.

Hypertension: Administer 2.5 mg once daily.

Mechanism of Action Inhibits calcium ion from entering the "slow channels" or select voltage-sensitive areas of vascular smooth muscle and myocardium during depolarization, producing a relaxation of coronary vascular smooth muscle and coronary vasodilation; increases myocardial oxygen delivery in patients with vasospastic angina

Contraindications Hypersensitivity to amlodipine or any component of the formulation

Warnings/Precautions Use with caution and titrate dosages for patients with impaired renal or hepatic function; use caution when treating patients with CHF, sick-sinus syndrome, severe left ventricular dysfunction, hypertrophic cardiomyopathy (especially obstructive), concomitant therapy with beta-blockers or digoxin, edema, or increased intracranial pressure with cranial tumors. Do not abruptly withdraw (may cause chest pain); elderly may experience hypotension and constipation more readily.

Drug Interactions

Cytochrome P450 Effect: Substrate of CYP3A4 (major); **Inhibits** CYP1A2 (moderate), 2A6 (weak), 2B6 (weak), 2C8 (weak), 2C9 (weak), 2D6 (weak), 3A4 (weak)

Increased Effect/Toxicity: Amlodipine may increase the levels/effects of aminophylline, fluvoxamine, mexiletine, mirtazapine, ropinirole, theophylline, trifluoperazine and other CYP1A2 substrates. Levels/effects of amlodipine may be increased by azole antifungals, clarithromycin, diclofenac, doxycycline, erythromycin, imatinib, isoniazid, nefazodone, nicardipine, propofol, protease inhibitors, quinidine, telithromycin, verapamil, and other CYP3A4 inhibitors. Cyclosporine levels may be increased by amlodipine. Blood pressure-lowering effects of sildenafil, tadalafil, and vardenafil are additive with amlodipine (use caution).

Decreased Effect: Calcium may reduce the calcium channel blocker's hypotensive effects. Levels/effects of amlodipine may be decreased by aminoglutethimide, carbamazepine, nafcillin, nevirapine, phenobarbital, phenytoin, rifamycins, and other CYP3A4 inducers.

Ethanol/Nutrition/Herb Interactions

Food: Grapefruit juice may modestly increase amlodipine levels.

Herb/Nutraceutical: St John's wort may decrease amlodipine levels. Avoid dong quai if using for hypertension (has estrogenic activity). Avoid ephedra, yohimbe, ginseng (may worsen hypertension). Avoid garlic (may have increased antihypertensive effects).

Dietary Considerations May be taken without regard to meals.

Pharmacodynamics/Kinetics

Onset of action: Antihypertensive: 30-50 minutes

Duration of antihypertensive effect: 24 hours

Absorption: Oral: Well absorbed

Distribution: V_d: 21 L/kg

Protein binding: 93% to 98%

Metabolism: Hepatic (>90%) to inactive metabolite

Bioavailability: 64% to 90%

Half-life elimination: 30-50 hours; increased with hepatic dysfunction

Time to peak, plasma: 6-12 hours

Excretion: Urine (10% as parent, 60% as metabolite)

Pregnancy Risk Factor C

Dosage Forms TAB: 2.5 mg, 5 mg, 10 mg

Selected Readings

Jorgensen MG, "Prevalence of Amlodipine-Related Gingival Hyperplasia," *J Periodontol*, 1997, 68(7):676-8.

Wynn RL, "An Update on Calcium Channel Blocker-Induced Gingival Hyperplasia," *Gen Dent*, 1995, 43(3):218-22.

Wynn RL, "Calcium Channel Blockers and Gingival Hyperplasia," *Gen Dent*, 1991, 39(4):240-3.

Amlodipine and Atorvastatin

(am LOW di peen & a TORE va sta tin)

Related Information

Amlodipine *on page 100*

Atorvastatin *on page 158*

U.S. Brand Names Caduet®

Generic Available No

Synonyms Atorvastatin Calcium and Amlodipine Besylate

Pharmacologic Category Antilipemic Agent, HMG-CoA Reductase Inhibitor; Calcium Channel Blocker

Use For use when treatment with both agents is appropriate:

Amlodipine is used for the treatment of hypertension and angina.

Atorvastatin is used with dietary therapy for the following:

Hyperlipidemias: To reduce elevations in total cholesterol, LDL-C, apolipoprotein B, and triglycerides in patients with primary hypercholesterolemia (elevations of 1 or more components are present in Fredrickson type IIa, IIb,

(Continued)

Amlodipine and Atorvastatin *(Continued)*

III, and IV hyperlipidemias); treatment of homozygous familial hypercholesterolemia

Heterozygous familial hypercholesterolemia (HeFH): In adolescent patients (10-17 years of age, females >1 year postmenarche) with HeFH having LDL-C ≥190 mg/dL **or** LDL-C ≥160 mg/dL with positive family history of premature cardiovascular disease (CVD) or with two or more CVD risk factors in the adolescent patient

Primary prevention of CVD in high-risk patients

Local Anesthetic/Vasoconstrictor Precautions No information available to require special precautions

Effects on Dental Treatment No significant effects or complications reported

Common Adverse Effects See individual agents.

Mechanism of Action

Amlodipine: Inhibits calcium ion from entering the "slow channels" or select voltage-sensitive areas of vascular smooth muscle and myocardium during depolarization, producing a relaxation of coronary vascular smooth muscle and coronary vasodilation; increases myocardial oxygen delivery in patients with vasospastic angina

Atorvastatin: Inhibitor of 3-hydroxy-3-methylglutaryl coenzyme A (HMG-CoA) reductase, the rate limiting enzyme in cholesterol synthesis (reduces the production of mevalonic acid from HMG-CoA); this then results in a compensatory increase in the expression of LDL receptors on hepatocyte membranes and a stimulation of LDL catabolism

Drug Interactions

Cytochrome P450 Effect:

Amlodipine: **Substrate** of CYP3A4 (major); **Inhibits** CYP1A2 (moderate), 2A6 (weak), 2B6 (weak), 2C8 (weak), 2C9 (weak), 2D6 (weak), 3A4 (weak)

Atorvastatin: **Substrate** of CYP3A4 (major); **Inhibits** CYP3A4 (weak)

Pharmacodynamics/Kinetics See individual agents.

Pregnancy Risk Factor X

Amlodipine and Benazepril *(am LOE di peen & ben AY ze pril)*

Related Information

Amlodipine *on page 100*

Benazepril *on page 185*

U.S. Brand Names Lotrel®

Generic Available No

Synonyms Benazepril Hydrochloride and Amlodipine Besylate

Pharmacologic Category Antihypertensive Agent, Combination

Use Treatment of hypertension

Local Anesthetic/Vasoconstrictor Precautions No information available to require special precautions

Effects on Dental Treatment Fewer reports of gingival hyperplasia with amlodipine than with other CCBs (usually resolves upon discontinuation); consultation with physician is suggested.

Common Adverse Effects See individual agents.

Dosage Oral:

Adults: 2.5-10 mg (amlodipine) and 10-40 mg (benazepril) once daily; maximum: Amlodipine: 10 mg/day; benazepril: 40 mg/day

Elderly: Initial dose: 2.5 mg based on amlodipine component

Dosage adjustment in renal impairment: Cl_{cr} ≤30 mL/minute: Use of combination product is not recommended.

Dosage adjustment in hepatic impairment: Initial dose: 2.5 mg based on amlodipine component

Mechanism of Action The mechanism through which benazepril lowers blood pressure is believed to be primarily suppression of the renin-angiotensin-aldosterone system; benazepril has an antihypertensive effect even in patients with low-renin hypertension; amlodipine is a dihydropyridine calcium antagonist that inhibits the transmembrane influx of calcium ions into vascular smooth muscle and cardiac muscle; amlodipine is a peripheral arterial vasodilator that acts directly on vascular smooth muscle to cause a reduction in peripheral vascular resistance and reduction in blood pressure

Contraindications Hypersensitivity to amlodipine, benazepril, other ACE inhibitors, or any component of the formulation; pregnancy (2nd and 3rd trimesters)

Warnings/Precautions Used as a replacement for separate dosing of components or combination therapy when response to single agent is suboptimal. The fixed combination is not indicated for initial treatment of hypertension. See individual agents for additional warnings/precautions.

Drug Interactions
Cytochrome P450 Effect: Amlodipine: **Substrate** of CYP3A4 (major); **Inhibits** CYP1A2 (moderate), 2A6 (weak), 2B6 (weak), 2C8 (weak), 2C9 (weak), 2D6 (weak), 3A4 (weak)
Increased Effect/Toxicity: See individual agents.
Decreased Effect: See individual agents.
Pharmacodynamics/Kinetics See individual agents.
Pregnancy Risk Factor C/D (2nd and 3rd trimesters)
Dosage Forms CAP: (Lotrel® 2.5/10): Amlodipine 2.5 mg and benazepril 10 mg; (Lotrel® 5/10): Amlodipine 5 mg and benazepril 10 mg; (Lotrel® 5/20): Amlodipine 5 mg and benazepril 20 mg; (Lotrel® 5/40): Amlodipine 5 mg and benazepril 40 mg; (Lotrel® 10/20): Amlodipine 10 mg and benazepril 20 mg; (Lotrel® 5/40): Amlodipine 5 mg and benazepril 40 mg

Selected Readings
Wynn RL, "An Update on Calcium Channel Blocker-Induced Gingival Hyperplasia," *Gen Dent*, 1995, 43(3):218-22.
Wynn RL, "Calcium Channel Blockers and Gingival Hyperplasia," *Gen Dent*, 1991, 39(4):240-3.

Amlodipine Besylate *see* Amlodipine *on page 100*
Ammens® Medicated Deodorant [OTC] *see* Zinc Oxide *on page 1597*
Ammonapse *see* Sodium Phenylbutyrate *on page 1403*

Ammonia Spirit (Aromatic)
(a MOE nee ah SPEAR it, air oh MAT ik)

Generic Available Yes
Synonyms Smelling Salts
Pharmacologic Category Respiratory Stimulant
Dental Use Emergency use in syncope
Use Respiratory and circulatory stimulant; treatment of fainting
Local Anesthetic/Vasoconstrictor Precautions No information available to require special precautions
Effects on Dental Treatment No significant effects or complications reported
Significant Adverse Effects 1% to 10%:
Gastrointestinal: Nausea, vomiting
Respiratory: Irritation to nasal mucosa, cough
Dosage Used as "smelling salts" to treat or prevent fainting
Contraindications Hypersensitivity to ammonia or any component of the formulation
Drug Interactions No data reported
Pregnancy Risk Factor C
Dosage Forms Solution for inhalation [ampul]: 1.7% to 2.1% (0.33 mL)

Ammonium Chloride (a MOE nee um KLOR ide)

Generic Available Yes
Pharmacologic Category Electrolyte Supplement, Parenteral
Use Treatment of hypochloremic states or metabolic alkalosis
Local Anesthetic/Vasoconstrictor Precautions No information available to require special precautions
Effects on Dental Treatment No significant effects or complications reported
Common Adverse Effects Frequency not defined.
Central nervous system: Headache, coma, drowsiness, EEG abnormalities, mental confusion, seizure
Dermatologic: Rash
Endocrine & metabolic: Calcium-deficient tetany, hyperchloremia, hypokalemia, metabolic acidosis, potassium and sodium may be decreased
Gastrointestinal: Abdominal pain, gastric irritation, nausea, vomiting
Hepatic: Ammonia may be increased
Local: Pain at site of injection
Neuromuscular & skeletal: Twitching
Respiratory: Hyperventilation
Mechanism of Action Increases acidity by increasing free hydrogen ion concentration
Pharmacodynamics/Kinetics
Metabolism: Hepatic; forms urea and hydrochloric acid
Excretion: Urine
Pregnancy Risk Factor C

Ammonium Lactate *see* Lactic Acid and Ammonium Hydroxide *on page 893*
Amnesteem™ *see* Isotretinoin *on page 869*

Amobarbital (am oh BAR bi tal)

U.S. Brand Names Amytal®
Canadian Brand Names Amytal®
Generic Available No
Synonyms Amobarbital Sodium; Amylobarbitone
Pharmacologic Category Barbiturate
Use Hypnotic in short-term treatment of insomnia; reduce anxiety and provide sedation preoperatively
Unlabeled/Investigational Use Therapeutic or diagnostic "Amytal® Interviewing"; Wada test
Local Anesthetic/Vasoconstrictor Precautions No information available to require special precautions
Effects on Dental Treatment No significant effects or complications reported
Mechanism of Action Interferes with transmission of impulses from the thalamus to the cortex of the brain resulting in an imbalance in central inhibitory and facilitatory mechanisms
Pregnancy Risk Factor D

Amobarbital and Secobarbital
(am oh BAR bi tal & see koe BAR bi tal)

Related Information
Amobarbital *on page 104*
Secobarbital *on page 1381*
U.S. Brand Names Tuinal® [DSC]
Generic Available No
Synonyms Amobarbital Sodium and Secobarbital Sodium; Secobarbital and Amobarbital
Pharmacologic Category Barbiturate
Use Short-term treatment of insomnia
Local Anesthetic/Vasoconstrictor Precautions No information available to require special precautions
Effects on Dental Treatment No significant effects or complications reported
Pregnancy Risk Factor D

Amobarbital Sodium *see* Amobarbital *on page 104*
Amobarbital Sodium and Secobarbital Sodium *see* Amobarbital and Secobarbital *on page 104*

Amonafide (a MON a fide)

Generic Available No
Synonyms Amonafide Hydrochloride; Benzisoquinolinedione; BIDA; M-FA-142; Nafidimide; NSC-308847
Pharmacologic Category Antineoplastic Agent, DNA Binding Agent; Enzyme Inhibitor, Topoisomerase II Inhibitor
Unlabeled/Investigational Use Investigational: Breast, prostate, renal cell, ovarian, pancreatic, and nonsmall cell lung cancers
Local Anesthetic/Vasoconstrictor Precautions No information available to require special precautions
Effects on Dental Treatment No significant effects or complications reported
Common Adverse Effects
>10%:
Gastrointestinal: Nausea and vomiting (mild)
Hematologic: Granulocytopenia, possibly dose-limiting; nadir occurs at days 12-15, recovery by day 21
1% to 10%:
Cardiovascular: Chest pain
Central nervous system: Dizziness, fatigue, headache
Dermatologic: Skin rash, exfoliative dermatitis, alopecia
Local: Inflammatory reactions
Otic: Tinnitus
Neuromuscular & skeletal: Myoclonic jerking, weakness
Mechanism of Action Amonafide acts as a DNA intercalator, stabilizing DNA to thermal denaturation and producing single-strand DNA breaks.

Pharmacodynamics/Kinetics

Distribution: V_d: 370-530 L/m^2

Protein binding: High

Half-life:

Elimination: 3.5-11 hours

Terminal: 3-6 hours

Metabolism: Hepatic, primarily by oxidation and N-acetylation. N-acetylamonafide (active) and amonafide-N'-oxide are the major metabolites. Clearance depends on whether the patient is a fast or slow acetylator. Fast acetylators may experience greater toxicity from the drug.

Excretion: Urine (3% to 22% as unchanged drug)

Amonafide Hydrochloride see Amonafide on page 104

Amoxapine (a MOKS a peen)

Generic Available Yes

Synonyms Asendin [DSC]

Pharmacologic Category Antidepressant, Tricyclic (Secondary Amine)

Use Treatment of depression, psychotic depression, depression accompanied by anxiety or agitation

Local Anesthetic/Vasoconstrictor Precautions Use with caution; epinephrine and levonordefrin have been shown to have an increased pressor response in combination with TCAs

Effects on Dental Treatment Key adverse event(s) related to dental treatment: Xerostomia and changes in salivation (normal salivary flow resumes upon discontinuation). Long-term treatment with TCAs, such as amoxapine, increases the risk of caries by reducing salivation and salivary buffer capacity.

Common Adverse Effects

>10%:

Central nervous system: Drowsiness

Gastrointestinal: Xerostomia, constipation

1% to 10%:

Central nervous system: Dizziness, headache, confusion, nervousness, restlessness, insomnia, ataxia, excitement, anxiety

Dermatologic: Edema, skin rash

Endocrine: Prolactin levels increased

Gastrointestinal: Nausea

Neuromuscular & skeletal: Tremor, weakness

Ocular: Blurred vision

Miscellaneous: Diaphoresis

Restrictions A medication guide concerning the use of antidepressants in children and teenagers can be found on the FDA website at http://www.fda.gov/cder/Offices/ODS/labeling.htm. It should be dispensed to parents or guardians of children and teenagers receiving this medication.

Mechanism of Action Reduces the reuptake of serotonin and norepinephrine. The metabolite, 7-OH-amoxapine has significant dopamine receptor blocking activity similar to haloperidol.

Drug Interactions

Cytochrome P450 Effect: Substrate of CYP2D6 (major)

Increased Effect/Toxicity: Amoxapine increases the effects of amphetamines, anticholinergics, other CNS depressants (sedatives, hypnotics, or ethanol), chlorpropamide, tolazamide, and warfarin. When used with MAO inhibitors, hyperpyrexia, hypertension, tachycardia, confusion, seizures, and **deaths have been reported** (serotonin syndrome). Serotonin syndrome has also been reported with ritonavir (rare). CYP2D6 inhibitors may increase the levels/effects of amoxapine; example inhibitors include chlorpromazine, delavirdine, fluoxetine, miconazole, paroxetine, pergolide, quinidine, quinine, ritonavir, and ropinirole. Use of lithium with a TCA may increase the risk for neurotoxicity. Phenothiazines may increase concentration of some TCAs and TCAs may increase the concentration of phenothiazines. Pressor response to I.V. epinephrine, norepinephrine, and phenylephrine may be enhanced in patients receiving TCAs (**Note:** Effect is unlikely with epinephrine or levonordefrin dosages typically administered as infiltration in combination with local anesthetics). Combined use of beta-agonists or drugs which prolong QT$_c$ (including quinidine, procainamide, disopyramide, cisapride, sparfloxacin, gatifloxacin, moxifloxacin) with TCAs may predispose patients to cardiac arrhythmias.

Decreased Effect: Amoxapine inhibits the antihypertensive effects of bethanidine, clonidine, debrisoquin, guanadrel, guanethidine, guanabenz, or guanfacine. Cholestyramine and colestipol may bind TCAs and reduce their absorption.

(Continued)

Amoxapine (Continued)

Pharmacodynamics/Kinetics

Onset of antidepressant effect: Usually occurs after 1-2 weeks, but may require 4-6 weeks

Absorption: Rapid and well absorbed

Distribution: V_d: 0.9-1.2 L/kg; enters breast milk

Protein binding: 80%

Metabolism: Primarily hepatic

Half-life elimination: Parent drug: 11-16 hours; Active metabolite (8-hydroxy): Adults: 30 hours

Time to peak, serum: 1-2 hours

Excretion: Urine (as unchanged drug and metabolites)

Pregnancy Risk Factor C

Amoxicillin (a moks i SIL in)

Related Information

Antibiotic Prophylaxis *on page 1680*
Bacterial Infections *on page 1697*
Cardiovascular Diseases *on page 1636*
Gastrointestinal Disorders *on page 1654*
Periodontal Diseases *on page 1705*
Sexually-Transmitted Diseases *on page 1674*

Related Sample Prescriptions

Bacterial Endocarditis (Prevention) *on page 1732*
Bacterial Infections and Periodontal Diseases *on page 1736*
Prosthetic Joint Late Infections (Prevention) *on page 1733*

U.S. Brand Names Amoxil®; DisperMox™ [DSC]; Moxilin®; Trimox®

Canadian Brand Names Apo-Amoxi®; Gen-Amoxicillin; Lin-Amox; Novamoxin®; Nu-Amoxi; PMS-Amoxicillin

Generic Available Yes: Excludes tablet for oral suspension

Synonyms Amoxicillin Trihydrate; Amoxycillin; *p*-Hydroxyampicillin

Pharmacologic Category Antibiotic, Penicillin

Dental Use Antibiotic for standard prophylactic regimen for dental patients who are at risk for endocarditis; antibiotic used to treat orofacial infections

Use Treatment of otitis media, sinusitis, and infections caused by susceptible organisms involving the respiratory tract, skin, and urinary tract; prophylaxis of bacterial endocarditis in patients undergoing surgical or dental procedures; as part of a multidrug regimen for *H. pylori* eradication

Unlabeled/Investigational Use Postexposure prophylaxis for anthrax exposure with documented susceptible organisms

Local Anesthetic/Vasoconstrictor Precautions No information available to require special precautions

Effects on Dental Treatment Prolonged use of penicillins may lead to development of oral candidiasis.

Significant Adverse Effects Frequency not defined.

Central nervous system: Hyperactivity, agitation, anxiety, insomnia, confusion, convulsions, behavioral changes, dizziness

Dermatologic: Acute exanthematous pustulosis, erythema maculopapular rash, erythema multiforme, Stevens-Johnson syndrome, exfoliative dermatitis, toxic epidermal necrolysis, hypersensitivity vasculitis, urticaria

Gastrointestinal: Nausea, vomiting, diarrhea, hemorrhagic colitis, pseudomembranous colitis, tooth discoloration (brown, yellow, or gray; rare)

Hematologic: Anemia, hemolytic anemia, thrombocytopenia, thrombocytopenia purpura, eosinophilia, leukopenia, agranulocytosis

Hepatic: AST (SGOT) and ALT (SGPT) increased, cholestatic jaundice, hepatic cholestasis, acute cytolytic hepatitis

Renal: Crystalluria

Dental Usual Dosing Oral:

Children >3 months and <40 kg: Endocarditis (subacute bacterial) prophylaxis: 50 mg/kg 1 hour before procedure

Adults:

Endocarditis prophylaxis: 2 g 1 hour before procedure

Orofacial infection: 250-500 mg every 8 hours or 500-875 mg twice daily

Dosage

Usual dosage range:

Children ≤3 months: Oral: 20-30 mg/kg/day divided every 12 hours

Children >3 months and <40 kg: Oral: 20-50 mg/kg/day in divided doses every 8-12 hours

Adults: Oral: 250-500 mg every 8 hours or 500-875 mg twice daily

Indication-specific dosing:
Children >3 months and <40 kg: Oral:
  Acute otitis media: 80-90 mg/kg/day divided every 12 hours
  Anthrax exposure (CDC guidelines): Note: Postexposure prophylaxis only with documented susceptible organisms: 80 mg/kg/day in divided doses every 8 hours (maximum: 500 mg/dose)
  Ear, nose, throat, genitourinary tract, or skin/skin structure infections:
    Mild to moderate: 25 mg/kg/day in divided doses every 12 hours **or** 20 mg/kg/day in divided doses every 8 hours
    Severe: 45 mg/kg/day in divided doses every 12 hours **or** 40 mg/kg/day in divided doses every 8 hours
  Endocarditis (subacute bacterial) prophylaxis: 50 mg/kg 1 hour before procedure
  Lower respiratory tract infections: 45 mg/kg/day in divided doses every 12 hours **or** 40 mg/kg/day in divided doses every 8 hours
  Lyme disease: 25-50 mg/kg/day divided every 8 hours (maximum: 500 mg)
  Pneumonia:
    4 months to 5 years: 100 mg/kg/day divided every 8 hours
    5-15 years: 100 mg/kg/day divided every 8 hours with clarithromycin, azithromycin, or doxycycline
Adults: Oral:
  Anthrax exposure (CDC guidelines): Note: Postexposure prophylaxis in pregnant or nursing women only with documented susceptible organisms: 500 mg every 8 hours
  Ear, nose, throat, genitourinary tract, or skin/skin structure infections:
    Mild to moderate: 500 mg every 12 hours **or** 250 mg every 8 hours
    Severe: 875 mg every 12 hours **or** 500 mg every 8 hours
  Endocarditis prophylaxis: 2 g 1 hour before procedure
  Helicobacter pylori **eradication:** 1000 mg twice daily; requires combination therapy with at least one other antibiotic and an acid-suppressing agent (proton pump inhibitor or H_2 blocker)
  Lower respiratory tract infections: 875 mg every 12 hours **or** 500 mg every 8 hours
  Lyme disease: 500 mg every 6-8 hours (depending on size of patient) for 21-30 days

Dosing interval in renal impairment: The 875 mg tablet should not be used in patients with Cl_{cr} <30 mL/minute.
  Cl_{cr} 10-30 mL/minute: 250-500 mg every 12 hours
  Cl_{cr} <10 mL/minute: 250-500 mg every 24 hours
Dialysis: Moderately dialyzable (20% to 50%) by hemo- or peritoneal dialysis; approximately 50 mg of amoxicillin per liter of filtrate is removed by continuous arteriovenous or venovenous hemofiltration; dose as per Cl_{cr} <10 mL/minute guidelines

Mechanism of Action Inhibits bacterial cell wall synthesis by binding to one or more of the penicillin-binding proteins (PBPs) which in turn inhibits the final transpeptidation step of peptidoglycan synthesis in bacterial cell walls, thus inhibiting cell wall biosynthesis. Bacteria eventually lyse due to ongoing activity of cell wall autolytic enzymes (autolysins and murein hydrolases) while cell wall assembly is arrested.

Contraindications Hypersensitivity to amoxicillin, penicillin, or any component of the formulation

Warnings/Precautions In patients with renal impairment, doses and/or frequency of administration should be modified in response to the degree of renal impairment; a high percentage of patients with infectious mononucleosis have developed rash during therapy with amoxicillin; a low incidence of cross-allergy with other beta-lactams and cephalosporins exists

Drug Interactions
Allopurinol: Theoretically has an additive potential for amoxicillin rash
Aminoglycosides: May be synergistic against selected organisms
Methotrexate: Penicillins may increase the exposure to methotrexate during concurrent therapy; monitor.
Oral contraceptives: Anecdotal reports suggesting decreased contraceptive efficacy with penicillins have been refuted by more rigorous scientific and clinical data.
Probenecid, disulfiram: May increase levels of penicillins (amoxicillin)
Warfarin: Effects of warfarin may be increased

Dietary Considerations May be taken with food. Amoxil® chewable contains phenylalanine 1.82 mg per 200 mg tablet, phenylalanine 3.64 mg per 400 mg tablet. DisperMox™ contains phenylalanine 5.6 mg in each 200 mg and 400 mg tablet.

Pharmacodynamics/Kinetics
Absorption: Oral: Rapid and nearly complete; food does not interfere
(Continued)

Amoxicillin *(Continued)*

Distribution: Widely to most body fluids and bone; poor penetration into cells, eyes, and across normal meninges

Pleural fluids, lungs, and peritoneal fluid; high urine concentrations are attained; also into synovial fluid, liver, prostate, muscle, and gallbladder; penetrates into middle ear effusions, maxillary sinus secretions, tonsils, sputum, and bronchial secretions; crosses placenta; low concentrations enter breast milk

CSF:blood level ratio: Normal meninges: <1%; Inflamed meninges: 8% to 90%

Protein binding: 17% to 20%

Metabolism: Partially hepatic

Half-life elimination:

Neonates, full-term: 3.7 hours

Infants and Children: 1-2 hours

Adults: Normal renal function: 0.7-1.4 hours

Cl_{cr} <10 mL/minute: 7-21 hours

Time to peak: Capsule: 2 hours; Suspension: 1 hour

Excretion: Urine (80% as unchanged drug); lower in neonates

Pregnancy Risk Factor B

Lactation Enters breast milk/compatible

Dosage Forms [DSC] = Discontinued product

Capsule, as trihydrate: 250 mg, 500 mg

Amoxil®: 500 mg

Moxilin®, Trimox®: 250 mg, 500 mg

Powder for oral suspension, as trihydrate: 125 mg/5 mL (80 mL, 100 mL, 150 mL); 200 mg/5 mL (50 mL, 75 mL, 100 mL); 250 mg/5 mL (80 mL, 100 mL, 150 mL); 400 mg/5 mL (50 mL, 75 mL, 100 mL)

Amoxil®: 200 mg/5 mL (5 mL, 50 mL, 75 mL, 100 mL) [contains sodium benzoate; bubble gum flavor]; 250 mg/5 mL (100 mL, 150 mL) [contains sodium benzoate; bubble gum flavor]; 400 mg/5 mL (5 mL, 50 mL, 75 mL, 100 mL) [contains sodium benzoate; bubble gum flavor]

Moxilin®: 250 mg/5 mL (100 mL, 150 mL)

Trimox®: 125 mg/5 mL (80 mL, 100 mL, 150 mL); 250 mg/5 mL (80 mL, 100 mL, 150 mL) [contains sodium benzoate; raspberry-strawberry flavor]

Powder for oral suspension, as trihydrate [drops] (Amoxil®): 50 mg/mL (30 mL) [bubble gum flavor]

Tablet, as trihydrate (Amoxil®): 500 mg, 875 mg

Tablet, chewable, as trihydrate: 125 mg, 200 mg, 250 mg, 400 mg

Amoxil®: 200 mg [contains phenylalanine 1.82 mg/tablet; cherry banana peppermint flavor]; 400 mg [contains phenylalanine 3.64 mg/tablet; cherry banana peppermint flavor]

Tablet, for oral suspension, as trihydrate (DisperMox™): 200 mg [contains phenylalanine 5.6 mg; strawberry flavor]; 400 mg [contains phenylalanine 5.6 mg; strawberry flavor]; 600 mg [contains phenylalanine 11.23 mg; strawberry flavor] [DSC]

Selected Readings

ADA Division of Legal Affairs, "A Legal Perspective on Antibiotic Prophylaxis," *J Am Dent Assoc,* 2003, 134(9):1260.

American Dental Association; American Academy of Orthopedic Surgeons, "Antibiotic Prophylaxis for Dental Patients With Total Joint Replacements," *J Am Dent Assoc,* 2003, 134(7):895-9.

American Dental Association Council on Scientific Affairs, "Combating Antibiotic Resistance," *J Am Dent Assoc,* 2004, 135(4):484-7.

Dajani AS, Taubert KA, Wilson W, et al, "Prevention of Bacterial Endocarditis. Recommendations by the American Heart Association," *JAMA,* 1997, 277(22):1794-801.

Dajani AS, Taubert KA, Wilson W, et al, "Prevention of Bacterial Endocarditis: Recommendations by the American Heart Association," *J Am Dent Assoc,* 1997, 128(8):1142-51.

Wynn RL, Bergman SA, Meiller TF, et al, "Antibiotics in Treating Oral-Facial Infections of Odontogenic Origin: An Update", *Gen Dent,* 2001, 49(3):238-40, 242, 244 passim.

Amoxicillin and Clavulanate Potassium
(a moks i SIL in & klav yoo LAN ate poe TASS ee um)

Related Information

Amoxicillin *on page 106*

Bacterial Infections *on page 1697*

Related Sample Prescriptions

Bacterial Infections and Periodontal Diseases *on page 1736*

U.S. Brand Names Augmentin®; Augmentin ES-600®; Augmentin XR™

Canadian Brand Names Alti-Amoxi-Clav; Apo-Amoxi-Clav®; Augmentin®; Clavulin®; Novo-Clavamoxin; ratio-Aclavulanate

Generic Available Yes: Excludes extended release

Synonyms Amoxicillin and Clavulanic Acid; Clavulanic Acid and Amoxicillin

Pharmacologic Category Antibiotic, Penicillin

Dental Use Treatment of orofacial infections when beta-lactamase-producing staphylococci and beta-lactamase-producing *Bacteroides* are present

Use Treatment of otitis media, sinusitis, and infections caused by susceptible organisms involving the lower respiratory tract, skin and skin structure, and urinary tract; spectrum same as amoxicillin with additional coverage of beta-lactamase producing *B. catarrhalis*, *H. influenzae*, *N. gonorrhoeae*, and *S. aureus* (not MRSA). The expanded coverage of this combination makes it a useful alternative when amoxicillin resistance is present and patients cannot tolerate alternative treatments.

Local Anesthetic/Vasoconstrictor Precautions No information available to require special precautions

Effects on Dental Treatment Prolonged use of penicillins may lead to development of oral candidiasis (see Dental Comment).

Significant Adverse Effects

>10%: Gastrointestinal: Diarrhea (3% to 34%; incidence varies upon dose and regimen used)

1% to 10%:

Dermatologic: Diaper rash, skin rash, urticaria

Gastrointestinal: Abdominal discomfort, loose stools, nausea, vomiting

Genitourinary: Vaginitis, vaginal mycosis

Miscellaneous: Moniliasis

<1% (Limited to important or life-threatening): Cholestatic jaundice, flatulence, headache, hepatic dysfunction, prothrombin time increased, thrombocytosis

Additional adverse reactions seen with **ampicillin-class antibiotics:** Agitation, agranulocytosis, alkaline phosphatase increased, anaphylaxis, anemia, angioedema, anxiety, behavioral changes, bilirubin increased, black "hairy" tongue, confusion, convulsions, crystalluria, dizziness, enterocolitis, eosinophilia, erythema multiforme, exanthematous pustulosis, exfoliative dermatitis, gastritis, glossitis, hematuria, hemolytic anemia, hemorrhagic colitis, indigestion, insomnia, hyperactivity, interstitial nephritis, leukopenia, mucocutaneous candidiasis, pruritus, pseudomembranous colitis, serum sickness-like reaction, Stevens-Johnson syndrome, stomatitis, transaminases increased, thrombocytopenia, thrombocytopenic purpura, tooth discoloration, toxic epidermal necrolysis

Dental Usual Dosing Orofacial infections: Children >40 kg and Adults: Oral: 250-500 mg every 8 hours or 875 mg every 12 hours

Dosage Note: Dose is based on the amoxicillin component; see "Augmentin® Product-Specific Considerations" table on next page.

Usual dosage range:

Infants <3 months: Oral: 30 mg/kg/day divided every 12 hours using the 125 mg/5 mL suspension

Children ≥3 months and <40 kg: Oral: 20-90 mg/kg/day divided every 8-12 hours

Children >40 kg and Adults: Oral: 250-500 mg every 8 hours or 875 mg every 12 hours

Indication-specific dosing:

Children ≥3 months and <40 kg: Oral:

Lower respiratory tract infections, severe infections, sinusitis: 45 mg/kg/day divided every 12 hours **or** 40 mg/kg/day divided every 8 hours

Mild-to-moderate infections: 25 mg/kg/day divided every 12 hours or 20 mg/kg/day divided every 8 hours

Otitis media (Augmentin® ES-600): 90 mg/kg/day divided every 12 hours for 10 days in children with severe illness and when coverage for β-lactamase-positive *H. influenzae* and *M. catarrhalis* is needed.

Children ≥16 years and Adults: Oral:

Acute bacterial sinusitis: Extended release tablet: Two 1000 mg tablets every 12 hours for 10 days

Bite wounds (animal/human): 875 mg every 12 hours **or** 500 mg every 8 hours

Chronic obstructive pulmonary disease: 875 mg every 12 hours **or** 500 mg every 8 hours

Diabetic foot: Extended release tablet: Two 1000 mg tablets every 12 hours for 7-14 days

Diverticulitis, perirectal abscess: Extended release tablet: Two 1000 mg tablets every 12 hours for 7-10 days

Erysipelas: 875 mg every 12 hours **or** 500 mg every 8 hours

Febrile neutropenia: 875 mg every 12 hours

Pneumonia:

Aspiration: 875 mg every 12 hours

Community-acquired: Extended release tablet: Two 1000 mg tablets every 12 hours for 7-10 days

(Continued)

Amoxicillin and Clavulanate Potassium *(Continued)*

Pyelonephritis (acute, uncomplicated): 875 mg every 12 hours **or** 500 mg every 8 hours

Skin abscess: 875 mg every 12 hours

Dosing interval in renal impairment:

Cl_{cr} <30 mL/minute: Do not use 875 mg tablet or extended release tablets

Cl_{cr} 10-30 mL/minute: 250-500 mg every 12 hours

Cl_{cr} <10 mL/minute: 250-500 every 24 hours

Hemodialysis: Moderately dialyzable (20% to 50%)

250-500 mg every 24 hours; administer dose during and after dialysis. Do not use extended release tablets.

Peritoneal dialysis: Moderately dialyzable (20% to 50%)

Amoxicillin: Administer 250 mg every 12 hours

Clavulanic acid: Dose for Cl_{cr} <10 mL/minute

Continuous arteriovenous or venovenous hemofiltration effects:

Amoxicillin: ~50 mg of amoxicillin/L of filtrate is removed

Clavulanic acid: Dose for Cl_{cr} <10 mL/minute

Augmentin® Product-Specific Considerations

Strength	Form	Consideration
125 mg	CT, S	q8h dosing
	S	For adults having difficulty swallowing tablets, 125 mg/5 mL suspension may be substituted for 500 mg tablet.
200 mg	CT, S	q12h dosing
	CT	Contains phenylalanine
	S	For adults having difficulty swallowing tablets, 200 mg/5 mL suspension may be substituted for 875 mg tablet.
250 mg	CT, S, T	q8h dosing
	CT	Contains phenylalanine
	T	Not for use in patients <40 kg
	CT, T	Tablet and chewable tablet are not interchangeable due to differences in clavulanic acid.
	S	For adults having difficulty swallowing tablets, 250 mg/5 mL suspension may be substituted for 500 mg tablet.
400 mg	CT, S	q12h dosing
	CT	Contains phenylalanine
	S	For adults having difficulty swallowing tablets, 400 mg/5 mL suspension may be substituted for 875 mg tablet.
500 mg	T	q8h or q12h dosing
600 mg	S	q12h dosing
		Contains phenylalanine
		Not for use in adults or children ≥40 kg
		600 mg/5 mL suspension is not equivalent to or interchangeable with 200 mg/5 mL or 400 mg/5 mL due to differences in clavulanic acid.
875 mg	T	q12h dosing; not for use in Cl_{cr} <30 mL/minute
1000 mg	XR	q12h dosing
		Not for use in children <16 years of age
		Not interchangeable with two 500 mg tablets
		Not for use if Cl_{cr} <30 mL/minute or hemodialysis

Legend: CT = chewable tablet, S = suspension, T = tablet, XR = extended release.

Mechanism of Action Clavulanic acid binds and inhibits beta-lactamases that inactivate amoxicillin resulting in amoxicillin having an expanded spectrum of activity. Amoxicillin inhibits bacterial cell wall synthesis by binding to one or more of the penicillin-binding proteins (PBPs) which in turn inhibits the final transpeptidation step of peptidoglycan synthesis in bacterial cell walls, thus inhibiting cell wall biosynthesis. Bacteria eventually lyse due to ongoing activity of cell wall autolytic enzymes (autolysins and murein hydrolases) while cell wall assembly is arrested.

Contraindications Hypersensitivity to amoxicillin, clavulanic acid, penicillin, or any component of the formulation; history of cholestatic jaundice or hepatic dysfunction with amoxicillin/clavulanate potassium therapy; Augmentin XR™: severe renal impairment (Cl_{cr} <30 mL/minute) and hemodialysis patients

Warnings/Precautions Hypersensitivity reactions, including anaphylaxis (some fatal), have been reported. Prolonged use may result in superinfection, including *Pseudomembranous colitis*. In patients with renal impairment, doses and/or frequency of administration should be modified in response to the degree of renal impairment. High percentage of patients with infectious mononucleosis have developed rash during therapy. Incidence of diarrhea is higher than with amoxicillin alone. Use caution in patients with hepatic dysfunction. Hepatic dysfunction, although rare, is more common in elderly and/or males, and occurs more frequently with prolonged treatment, and may occur after therapy is complete. Due to differing content of clavulanic acid, not all formulations are interchangeable. Low incidence of cross-allergy with cephalosporins exists. Some products contain phenylalanine.

Drug Interactions

Allopurinol: Additive potential for amoxicillin rash

Aminoglycosides: May be synergistic against selected organisms

Methotrexate: Penicillins may increase the exposure to methotrexate during concurrent therapy; monitor.

Oral contraceptives: Anecdotal reports suggesting decreased contraceptive efficacy with penicillins have been refuted by more rigorous scientific and clinical data.

Probenecid: May increase levels of penicillins (amoxicillin); concomitant use not recommended.

Warfarin: Effects of warfarin may be increased

Dietary Considerations May be taken with meals or on an empty stomach; take with meals to increase absorption and decrease GI intolerance; may mix with milk, formula, or juice. Extended release tablets should be taken with food. Some products contain phenylalanine; avoid use in phenylketonurics. All dosage forms contain potassium.

Pharmacodynamics/Kinetics Amoxicillin pharmacokinetics are not affected by clavulanic acid.

Amoxicillin: See Amoxicillin.

Clavulanic acid:

Metabolism: Hepatic

Excretion: Urine (30% to 40% as unchanged drug)

Pregnancy Risk Factor B

Lactation Enters breast milk/use caution (AAP rates "compatible")

Breast-Feeding Considerations The AAP considers amoxicillin to be "compatible" with breast-feeding.

Dosage Forms

Powder for oral suspension: 200: Amoxicillin 200 mg and clavulanate potassium 28.5 mg per 5 mL (100 mL) [contains phenylalanine]; 400: Amoxicillin 400 mg and clavulanate potassium 57 mg per 5 mL (100 mL) [contains phenylalanine]; 600: Amoxicillin 600 mg and clavulanic potassium 42.9 mg per 5 mL (75 mL, 125 mL, 200 mL) [contains phenylalanine]

Augmentin®:

125: Amoxicillin 125 mg and clavulanate potassium 31.25 mg per 5 mL (75 mL, 100 mL, 150 mL) [banana flavor]

200: Amoxicillin 200 mg and clavulanate potassium 28.5 mg per 5 mL (50 mL, 75 mL, 100 mL) [contains phenylalanine 7 mg/5 mL; orange-raspberry flavor]

250: Amoxicillin 250 mg and clavulanate potassium 62.5 mg per 5 mL (75 mL, 100 mL, 150 mL) [orange flavor]

400: Amoxicillin 400 mg and clavulanate potassium 57 mg per 5 mL (50 mL, 75 mL, 100 mL) [contains phenylalanine 7 mg/5 mL; orange-raspberry flavor]

Augmentin ES-600®: Amoxicillin 600 mg and clavulanic potassium 42.9 mg per 5 mL (75 mL, 125 mL, 200 mL) [contains phenylalanine 7 mg/5 mL; strawberry cream flavor]

Tablet: 500: Amoxicillin trihydrate 500 mg and clavulanate potassium 125 mg; 875: Amoxicillin trihydrate 875 mg and clavulanate potassium 125 mg

Augmentin®:

250: Amoxicillin trihydrate 250 mg and clavulanate potassium 125 mg

500: Amoxicillin trihydrate 500 mg and clavulanate potassium 125 mg

875: Amoxicillin trihydrate 875 mg and clavulanate potassium 125 mg

Tablet, chewable: 200: Amoxicillin trihydrate 200 mg and clavulanate potassium 28.5 mg [contains phenylalanine]; 400: Amoxicillin trihydrate 400 mg and clavulanate potassium 57 mg [contains phenylalanine]

Augmentin®:

125: Amoxicillin trihydrate 125 mg and clavulanate potassium 31.25 mg [lemon-lime flavor]

200: Amoxicillin trihydrate 200 mg and clavulanate potassium 28.5 mg [contains phenylalanine 2.1 mg/tablet; cherry-banana flavor]

250: Amoxicillin trihydrate 250 mg and clavulanate potassium 62.5 mg [lemon-lime flavor]

400: Amoxicillin trihydrate 400 mg and clavulanate potassium 57 mg [contains phenylalanine 4.2 mg/tablet; cherry-banana flavor]

(Continued)

Amoxicillin and Clavulanate Potassium *(Continued)*

Tablet, extended release (Augmentin XR™): Amoxicillin 1000 mg and clavulanic acid 62.5 mg [contains potassium 29.3 mg (1.27 mEq) and sodium 12.6 mg (0.32 mEq)]

Dental Comment In maxillary sinus, anterior nasal cavity, and deep neck infections, beta-lactamase-producing staphylococci and beta-lactamase-producing *Bacteroides* usually are present. In these situations, antibiotics that resist the beta-lactamase enzyme are indicated. Amoxicillin and clavulanic acid is administered orally for moderate infections. Ampicillin sodium and sulbactam sodium (Unasyn®) is administered parenterally for more severe infections.

Selected Readings

American Dental Association Council on Scientific Affairs, "Combating Antibiotic Resistance," *J Am Dent Assoc*, 2004, 135(4):484-7.

Wynn RL, Bergman SA, Meiller TF, et al, "Antibiotics in Treating Oral-Facial Infections of Odontogenic Origin: An Update," *Gen Dent*, 2001, 49(3):238-40, 242, 244 passim.

Amoxicillin and Clavulanic Acid *see* Amoxicillin and Clavulanate Potassium *on page 108*

Amoxicillin, Lansoprazole, and Clarithromycin *see* Lansoprazole, Amoxicillin, and Clarithromycin *on page 898*

Amoxicillin Trihydrate *see* Amoxicillin *on page 106*

Amoxil® *see* Amoxicillin *on page 106*

Amoxycillin *see* Amoxicillin *on page 106*

Amphadase™ *see* Hyaluronidase *on page 774*

Amphetamine and Dextroamphetamine *see* Dextroamphetamine and Amphetamine *on page 448*

Amphocin® *see* Amphotericin B (Conventional) *on page 113*

Amphotec® *see* Amphotericin B Cholesteryl Sulfate Complex *on page 112*

Amphotericin B Cholesteryl Sulfate Complex
(am foe TER i sin bee kole LES te ril SUL fate KOM plecks)

U.S. Brand Names Amphotec®

Canadian Brand Names Amphotec®

Generic Available No

Synonyms ABCD; Amphotericin B Colloidal Dispersion

Pharmacologic Category Antifungal Agent, Parenteral

Use Treatment of invasive aspergillosis in patients who have failed amphotericin B deoxycholate treatment, or who have renal impairment or experience unacceptable toxicity which precludes treatment with amphotericin B deoxycholate in effective doses.

Unlabeled/Investigational Use Effective in patients with serious *Candida* species infections

Local Anesthetic/Vasoconstrictor Precautions No information available to require special precautions

Effects on Dental Treatment No significant effects or complications reported

Common Adverse Effects

>10%: Central nervous system: Chills, fever

1% to 10%:

Cardiovascular: Hypotension, tachycardia

Central nervous system: Headache

Dermatologic: Rash

Endocrine & metabolic: Hypokalemia, hypomagnesemia

Gastrointestinal: Nausea, diarrhea, abdominal pain

Hematologic: Thrombocytopenia

Hepatic: LFT change

Neuromuscular & skeletal: Rigors

Renal: Creatinine increased

Respiratory: Dyspnea

Note: Amphotericin B colloidal dispersion has an improved therapeutic index compared to conventional amphotericin B, and has been used safely in patients with amphotericin B-related nephrotoxicity; however, continued decline of renal function has occurred in some patients.

Mechanism of Action Binds to ergosterol altering cell membrane permeability in susceptible fungi and causing leakage of cell components with subsequent cell death. Proposed mechanism suggests that amphotericin causes an oxidation-dependent stimulation of macrophages (Lyman, 1992).

Drug Interactions

Increased Effect/Toxicity: Toxic effect with other nephrotoxic drugs (eg, cyclosporine and aminoglycosides) may be additive. Corticosteroids may increase potassium depletion caused by amphotericin. Amphotericin B may predispose patients receiving digitalis glycosides or neuromuscular blocking agents to toxicity secondary to hypokalemia.

Decreased Effect: Pharmacologic antagonism may occur with azole antifungals (eg, ketoconazole, miconazole).

Pharmacodynamics/Kinetics
Distribution: V_d: Total volume increases with higher doses, reflects increasing uptake by tissues (with 4 mg/kg/day = 4 L/kg); predominantly distributed in the liver; concentrations in kidneys and other tissues are lower than observed with conventional amphotericin B
Half-life elimination: 28-29 hours; prolonged with higher doses

Pregnancy Risk Factor B

Amphotericin B Colloidal Dispersion *see* Amphotericin B Cholesteryl Sulfate Complex *on page 112*

Amphotericin B (Conventional)
(am foe TER i sin bee con VEN sha nal)

Related Information
Fungal Infections *on page 1707*
U.S. Brand Names Amphocin®
Canadian Brand Names Fungizone®
Generic Available Yes
Synonyms Amphotericin B Desoxycholate
Pharmacologic Category Antifungal Agent, Parenteral
Use Treatment of severe systemic and central nervous system infections caused by susceptible fungi such as *Candida* species, *Histoplasma capsulatum*, *Cryptococcus neoformans*, *Aspergillus* species, *Blastomyces dermatitidis*, *Torulopsis glabrata*, and *Coccidioides immitis*; fungal peritonitis; irrigant for bladder fungal infections; used in fungal infection in patients with bone marrow transplantation, amebic meningoencephalitis, ocular aspergillosis (intraocular injection), candidal cystitis (bladder irrigation), chemoprophylaxis (low-dose I.V.), immunocompromised patients at risk of aspergillosis (intranasal/nebulized), refractory meningitis (intrathecal), coccidioidal arthritis (intra-articular/I.M.).

Low-dose amphotericin B has been administered after bone marrow transplantation to reduce the risk of invasive fungal disease.

Local Anesthetic/Vasoconstrictor Precautions No information available to require special precautions
Effects on Dental Treatment No significant effects or complications reported
Common Adverse Effects
>10%:
Central nervous system: Fever, chills, headache, malaise, generalized pain
Endocrine & metabolic: Hypokalemia, hypomagnesemia
Gastrointestinal: Anorexia
Hematologic: Anemia
Renal: Nephrotoxicity
1% to 10%:
Cardiovascular: Hypotension, hypertension, flushing
Central nervous system: Delirium, arachnoiditis, pain along lumbar nerves
Gastrointestinal: Nausea, vomiting
Genitourinary: Urinary retention
Hematologic: Leukocytosis
Local: Thrombophlebitis
Neuromuscular & skeletal: Paresthesia (especially with I.T. therapy)
Renal: Renal tubular acidosis, renal failure

Dosage
Premedication: For patients who experience infusion-related immediate reactions, premedicate with the following drugs 30-60 minutes prior to drug administration: NSAID (with or without diphenhydramine) or acetaminophen with diphenhydramine or hydrocortisone 50-100 mg. If the patient experiences rigors during the infusion, meperidine may be administered.
Infants and Children: I.V.:
Test dose: 0.1 mg/kg/dose to a maximum of 1 mg; infuse over 30-60 minutes. Many clinicians believe a test dose is unnecessary.
Maintenance dose: 0.25-1 mg/kg/day given once daily; infuse over 2-6 hours. Once therapy has been established, amphotericin B can be administered on an every-other-day basis at 1-1.5 mg/kg/dose; cumulative dose: 1.5-2 g over 6-10 weeks.
Adults: I.V.:
Test dose: 1 mg infused over 20-30 minutes. Many clinicians believe a test dose is unnecessary.
(Continued)

Amphotericin B (Conventional) *(Continued)*

Maintenance dose: Usual: 0.25-1.5 mg/kg/day; 1-1.5 mg/kg over 4-6 hours every other day may be given once therapy is established; aspergillosis, mucormycosis, rhinocerebral phycomycosis often require 1-1.5 mg/kg/day; do not exceed 1.5 mg/kg/day

Duration of therapy varies with nature of infection: Usual duration is 4-12 weeks or cumulative dose of 1-4 g

Meningitis, coccidioidal or cryptococcal: I.T.:

Children.: 25-100 mcg every 48-72 hours; increase to 500 mcg as tolerated

Adults: Initial: 25-300 mcg every 48-72 hours; increase to 500 mcg to 1 mg as tolerated; maximum total dose: 15 mg has been suggested

Bone marrow transplantation (prophylaxis): Adults: I.V.: Low-dose amphotericin B 0.1-0.25 mg/kg/day has been administered after bone marrow transplantation to reduce the risk of invasive fungal disease.

Bladder irrigation: Candidal cystitis: Irrigate with 50 mcg/mL solution instilled periodically or continuously for 5-10 days or until cultures are clear

Note: Alternative routes of administration and extemporaneous preparations have been used when standard antifungal therapy is not available (eg, inhalation, intraocular injection, subconjunctival application, intracavitary administration into various joints and the pleural space).

Dosing adjustment in renal impairment: If renal dysfunction is due to the drug, the daily total can be decreased by 50% or the dose can be given every other day; I.V. therapy may take several months

Dialysis: Poorly dialyzed; no supplemental dosage necessary when using hemo- or peritoneal dialysis or continuous arteriovenous or venovenous hemodiafiltration effects

Administration in dialysate: Children and Adults: 1-2 mg/L of peritoneal dialysis fluid either with or without low-dose I.V. amphotericin B (a total dose of 2-10 mg/kg given over 7-14 days). Precipitate may form in ionic dialysate solutions.

Mechanism of Action Binds to ergosterol altering cell membrane permeability in susceptible fungi and causing leakage of cell components with subsequent cell death. Proposed mechanism suggests that amphotericin causes an oxidation-dependent stimulation of macrophages (Lyman, 1992).

Contraindications Hypersensitivity to amphotericin or any component of the formulation

Warnings/Precautions Anaphylaxis has been reported with amphotericin B-containing drugs. During the initial dosing, the drug should be administered under close clinical observation. Avoid use with other nephrotoxic drugs; drug-induced renal toxicity usually improves with interrupting therapy, decreasing dosage, or increasing dosing interval. Infusion reactions are most common 1-3 hours after starting the infusion and diminish with continued therapy. Use amphotericin B with caution in patients with decreased renal function.

Drug Interactions

Increased Effect/Toxicity: Use of amphotericin with other nephrotoxic drugs (eg, cyclosporine and aminoglycosides) may result in additive toxicity. Amphotericin may increase the toxicity of flucytosine. Antineoplastic agents may increase the risk of amphotericin-induced nephrotoxicity, bronchospasms, and hypotension. Corticosteroids may increase potassium depletion caused by amphotericin. Amphotericin B may predispose patients receiving digitalis glycosides or neuromuscular-blocking agents to toxicity secondary to hypokalemia.

Decreased Effect: Pharmacologic antagonism may occur with azole antifungal agents (ketoconazole, miconazole).

Pharmacodynamics/Kinetics

Distribution: Minimal amounts enter the aqueous humor, bile, CSF (inflamed or noninflamed meninges), amniotic fluid, pericardial fluid, pleural fluid, and synovial fluid

Protein binding, plasma: 90%

Half-life elimination: Biphasic: Initial: 15-48 hours; Terminal: 15 days

Time to peak: Within 1 hour following a 4- to 6-hour dose

Excretion: Urine (2% to 5% as biologically active form); ~40% eliminated over a 7-day period and may be detected in urine for at least 7 weeks after discontinued use

Pregnancy Risk Factor B

Dosage Forms INJ, powder for reconstitution: 50 mg

Selected Readings

Anderson RP and Clark DA, "Amphotericin B Toxicity Reduced by Administration in Fat Emulsion," *Ann Pharmacother*, 1995, 29(5):496-500.

Arning M, Heer-Sonderhoff A, and Schneider W, "Cardiopulmonary Toxicity After Liposomal Amphotericin B (AmBisome®) in Neutropenic Patients With Acute Leukemia," *Onkologie*, 1994, 17:4.

Arsura EL, Ismail Y, Freedman S, et al, "Amphotericin B-Induced Dilated Cardiomyopathy," *Am J Med*, 1994, 97(6):560-2.

Benson JM and Nahata MC, "Clinical Use of Systemic Antifungal Agents," *Clin Pharm*, 1988, 7(6):424-38.

Benson JM and Nahata MC, "Pharmacokinetics of Amphotericin B in Children," *Antimicrob Agents Chemother*, 1989, 33(11):1989-93.

Bianco JA, Almgren J, Kern DL, et al, "Evidence That Oral Pentoxifylline Reverses Acute Renal Dysfunction in Bone Marrow Transplant Recipients Receiving Amphotericin B and Cyclosporine," *Transplantation*, 1991, 51(4):925-7.

Branch RA, "Prevention of Amphotericin B-Induced Renal Impairment. A Review on the Use of Sodium Supplementation," *Arch Intern Med*, 1988, 148(11):2389-94.

Brent J, Hunt M, Kulig K, et al, "Amphotericin B Overdoses in Infants: Is There a Role for Exchange Transfusion?" *Vet Hum Toxicol*, 1990, 32(2):124-5.

Cruz JM, Peacock JE Jr, Loomer L, et al, "Rapid Intravenous Infusion of Amphotericin B: A Pilot Study," *Am J Med*, 1992, 93:123-30.

Devuyst O, Goffin E, and Van Ypersele de Strihou C, "Recurrent Hemiparesis Under Amphotericin B for *Candida albicans* Peritonitis," *Nephrol Dial Transplant*, 1995, 10(5):699-701.

Edwards JE Jr, Bodey GP, Bowden RA, et al, "International Conference for the Development of a Consensus on the Management and Prevention of Severe Candidal Infections," *Clin Infect Dis*, 1997, 25(1):43-59.

Eggimann P, Francioli P, Bille J, et al, "Fluconazole Prophylaxis Prevents Intra-Abdominal Candidiasis in High-Risk Surgical Patients," *Crit Care Med*, 1999, 27(6):1066-72.

Gales MA and Gales BJ, "Rapid Infusion of Amphotericin B in Dextrose," *Ann Pharmacother*, 1995, 29(5):523-9.

Gallis HA, Drew RH, and Pickard WW, "Amphotericin B: 30 Years of Clinical Experience," *Rev Infect Dis*, 1990, 12(2):308-29.

Goodwin SD, Cleary JD, Walawander CA, et al, "Pretreatment Regimens for Adverse Events Related to Infusion of Amphotericin B," *Clin Infect Dis*, 1995, 20(4):755-61.

Jeffery GM, Beard ME, Ikram RB, et al, "Intranasal Amphotericin B Reduces the Frequency of Invasive Aspergillosis in Neutropenic Patients," *Am J Med*, 1991, 90(6):685-92.

Jones RS, Barman A, Suh B, et al, "Successful Treatment of *Aspergillus vertebral* Osteomyelitis With Amphotericin B Lipid Complex," *Infect Dis Clin Pract*, 1995, 4:237-9.

Kauffman CA and Carver PL, "Antifungal Agents in the 1990s. Current Status and Future Developments," *Drugs*, 1997, 53(4):539-49.

Kintzel PE and Smith GH, "Practical Guidelines for Preparing and Administering Amphotericin B," *Am J Hosp Pharm*, 1992, 49(5):1156-64.

Koren G, Lau A, Klein J, et al, "Pharmacokinetics and Adverse Effects of Amphotericin B in Infants and Children," *J Pediatr*, 1988, 113(3):559-63.

Levy M, Domaratzki J, and Koren G, "Amphotericin-Induced Heart Rate Decrease in Children," *Clin Pediatr (Phila)*, 1995, 34(7):358-64.

Lyman CA and Walsh TJ, "Systemically Administered Antifungal Agents. A Review of Their Clinical Pharmacology and Therapeutic Applications," *Drugs*, 1992, 44(1):9-35.

Patel R, "Antifungal Agents. Part I. Amphotericin B Preparations and Flucytosine," *Mayo Clin Proc*, 1998, 73(12):1205-25.

Rex JH, Bennett JE, Sugar AM, "A Randomized Trial Comparing Fluconazole With Amphotericin B for the Treatment of Candidemia in Patients Without Neutropenia. Candidemia Study Group and the National Institute," *N Engl J Med*, 1994, 331(20):1325-30.

Rex JH, Walsh TJ, Sobel JD, et al, "Practice Guidelines for the Treatment of Candidiasis. Infectious Diseases Society of America," *Clin Infect Dis*, 2000, 30(4):662-78.

Slain D, "Lipid-Based Amphotericin B for the Treatment of Fungal Infections," *Pharmacotherapy*, 1999, 19(3):306-23.

The Ad Hoc Advisory Panel on Peritonitis Management. "Continuous Ambulatory Peritoneal Dialysis (CAPD) Peritonitis Treatment Recommendations: 1989 Update," *Perit Dial Int*, 1989, 9(4):247-56.

Wong-Beringer A, Beringer PM, and Rho JP, "Focus on Amphotericin B Lipid Complex," *Formulary*, 1996, 13(3):169-85.

Amphotericin B Desoxycholate see Amphotericin B (Conventional) on page 113

Amphotericin B (Lipid Complex)
(am foe TER i sin bee LIP id KOM pleks)

U.S. Brand Names Abelcet®

Canadian Brand Names Abelcet®; Amphotec®

Generic Available No

Synonyms ABLC

Pharmacologic Category Antifungal Agent, Parenteral

Use Treatment of aspergillosis or any type of progressive fungal infection in patients who are refractory to or intolerant of conventional amphotericin B therapy

Unlabeled/Investigational Use Effective in patients with serious *Candida* species infections

Local Anesthetic/Vasoconstrictor Precautions No information available to require special precautions

Effects on Dental Treatment No significant effects or complications reported

Common Adverse Effects Nephrotoxicity and infusion-related hyperpyrexia, rigor, and chilling are reduced relative to amphotericin deoxycholate.

>10%:

Central nervous system: Chills, fever

Renal: Serum creatinine increased

Miscellaneous: Multiple organ failure

(Continued)

Amphotericin B (Lipid Complex) *(Continued)*

1% to 10%:
Cardiovascular: Hypotension, cardiac arrest
Central nervous system: Headache, pain
Dermatologic: Rash
Endocrine & metabolic: Bilirubinemia, hypokalemia, acidosis
Gastrointestinal: Nausea, vomiting, diarrhea, gastrointestinal hemorrhage, abdominal pain
Renal: Renal failure
Respiratory: Respiratory failure, dyspnea, pneumonia

Mechanism of Action Binds to ergosterol altering cell membrane permeability in susceptible fungi and causing leakage of cell components with subsequent cell death. Proposed mechanism suggests that amphotericin causes an oxidation-dependent stimulation of macrophages.

Drug Interactions

Increased Effect/Toxicity: See Drug Interactions - Increased Effect/Toxicity in Amphotericin B (Conventional).

Decreased Effect: See Drug Interactions - Decreased Effect in Amphotericin B (Conventional).

Pharmacodynamics/Kinetics

Distribution: V_d: Increases with higher doses; reflects increased uptake by tissues (131 L/kg with 5 mg/kg/day)

Half-life elimination: ~24 hours

Excretion: Clearance: Increases with higher doses (5 mg/kg/day): 400 mL/hour/kg

Pregnancy Risk Factor B

Amphotericin B (Liposomal) *(am foe TER i sin bee lye po SO mal)*

U.S. Brand Names AmBisome®
Canadian Brand Names AmBisome®
Generic Available No
Synonyms L-AmB
Pharmacologic Category Antifungal Agent, Parenteral

Use Empirical therapy for presumed fungal infection in febrile, neutropenic patients; treatment of patients with *Aspergillus* species, *Candida* species, and/or *Cryptococcus* species infections refractory to amphotericin B desoxycholate, or in patients where renal impairment or unacceptable toxicity precludes the use of amphotericin B desoxycholate; treatment of cryptococcal meningitis in HIV-infected patients; treatment of visceral leishmaniasis

Unlabeled/Investigational Use Effective in patients with serious *Candida* species infections

Local Anesthetic/Vasoconstrictor Precautions No information available to require special precautions

Effects on Dental Treatment Key adverse event(s) related to dental treatment: Facial swelling, postural hypotension, mucositis, stomatitis, and ulcerative stomatitis (see Dental Comment).

Common Adverse Effects Percentage of adverse reactions is dependent upon population studied and may vary with respect to premedications and underlying illness. Incidence of decreased renal function and infusion-related events are lower than rates observed with amphotericin B desoxycholate.

>10%:
Cardiovascular: Peripheral edema (15%), edema (12% to 14%), tachycardia (9% to 18%), hypotension (7% to 14%), hypertension (8% to 20%), chest pain (8% to 12%), hypervolemia (8% to 12%)
Central nervous system: Chills (29% to 48%), insomnia (17% to 22%), headache (9% to 20%), anxiety (7% to 14%), pain (14%), confusion (9% to 13%)
Dermatologic: Rash (5% to 25%), pruritus (11%)
Endocrine & metabolic: Hypokalemia (31% to 51%), hypomagnesemia (15% to 50%), hyperglycemia (8% to 23%), hypocalcemia (5% to 18%), hyponatremia (8% to 12%)
Gastrointestinal: Nausea (16% to 40%), vomiting (10% to 32%), diarrhea (11% to 30%), abdominal pain (7% to 20%), constipation (15%), anorexia (10% to 14%)
Hematologic: Anemia (27% to 48%), blood transfusion reaction (9% to 18%), leukopenia (15% to 17%), thrombocytopenia (6% to 13%)
Hepatic: Alkaline phosphatase increased (7% to 22%), BUN increased (7% to 21%), bilirubinemia (9% to 18%), ALT increased (15%), AST increased (13%), liver function tests abnormal (not specified) (4% to 13%)
Local: Phlebitis (9% to 11%)
Neuromuscular & skeletal: Weakness (6% to 13%), back pain (12%)

Renal: Creatinine increased (18% to 40%), hematuria (14%)

Respiratory: Dyspnea (18% to 23%), lung disorder (14% to 18%), cough increased (2% to 18%), epistaxis (8% to 15%), pleural effusion (12%), rhinitis (11%)

Miscellaneous: Sepsis (7% to 14%), infection (11% to 12%)

2% to 10%:

Cardiovascular: Arrhythmia, atrial fibrillation, bradycardia, cardiac arrest, cardiomegaly, facial swelling, flushing, postural hypotension, valvular heart disease, vascular disorder

Central nervous system: Agitation, abnormal thinking, coma, convulsion, depression, dysesthesia, dizziness (7% to 8%), hallucinations, malaise, nervousness, somnolence

Dermatologic: Alopecia, bruising, cellulitis, dry skin, maculopapular rash, petechia, purpura, skin discoloration, skin disorder, skin ulcer, urticaria, vesiculobullous rash

Endocrine & metabolic: Acidosis, fluid overload, hypernatremia (4%), hyperchloremia, hyperkalemia, hypermagnesemia, hyperphosphatemia, hypophosphatemia, hypoproteinemia, lactate dehydrogenase increased, nonprotein nitrogen increased

Gastrointestinal: Constipation, dry mouth, dyspepsia, abdomen enlarged, amylase increased, eructation, fecal incontinence, flatulence, gastrointestinal hemorrhage (10%), hematemesis, hemorrhoids, gum/oral hemorrhage, ileus, mucositis, rectal disorder, stomatitis, ulcerative stomatitis

Genitourinary: Vaginal hemorrhage

Hematologic: Coagulation disorder, hemorrhage, decreased prothrombin, thrombocytopenia

Hepatic: Hepatocellular damage, hepatomegaly, veno-occlusive liver disease

Local: Injection site inflammation

Neuromuscular & skeletal: Arthralgia, bone pain, dystonia, myalgia, neck pain, paresthesia, rigors, tremor

Ocular: Conjunctivitis, dry eyes, eye hemorrhage

Renal: Abnormal renal function, acute kidney failure, dysuria, kidney failure, toxic nephropathy, urinary incontinence

Respiratory: Asthma, atelectasis, cough, dry nose, hemoptysis, hyperventilation, lung edema, pharyngitis, pneumonia, respiratory alkalosis, respiratory insufficiency, respiratory failure, sinusitis, hypoxia (6% to 8%)

Miscellaneous: Allergic reaction, cell-mediated immunological reaction, flu-like syndrome, graft-versus-host disease, herpes simplex, hiccup, procedural complication (8% to 10%), diaphoresis (7%)

Mechanism of Action Binds to ergosterol altering cell membrane permeability in susceptible fungi and causing leakage of cell components with subsequent cell death. Proposed mechanism suggests that amphotericin causes an oxidation-dependent stimulation of macrophages (Lyman, 1992).

Drug Interactions

Increased Effect/Toxicity: Drug interactions have not been studied in a controlled manner; however, drugs that interact with conventional amphotericin B may also interact with amphotericin B liposome for injection. See Drug Interactions - Increased Effect/Toxicity in Amphotericin B (Conventional) monograph.

Pharmacodynamics/Kinetics

Distribution: V_d: 131 L/kg

Half-life elimination: Terminal: 174 hours

Pregnancy Risk Factor B

Dental Comment Amphotericin B, liposomal is a true single bilayer liposomal drug delivery system. Liposomes are closed, spherical vesicles created by mixing specific proportions of amphophilic substances such as phospholipids and cholesterol so that they arrange themselves into multiple concentric bilayer membranes when hydrated in aqueous solutions. Single bilayer liposomes are then formed by microemulsification of multilamellar vesicles using a homogenizer. Amphotericin B, liposomal consists of these unilamellar bilayer liposomes with amphotericin B intercalated within the membrane. Due to the nature and quantity of amphophilic substances used, and the lipophilic moiety in the amphotericin B molecule, the drug is an integral part of the overall structure of the amphotericin B liposomes. Amphotericin B, liposomal contains true liposomes that are <100 nm in diameter.

Ampicillin (am pi SIL in)

Related Information

Antibiotic Prophylaxis on page 1680

Cardiovascular Diseases on page 1636

(Continued)

Ampicillin *(Continued)*

U.S. Brand Names Principen®

Canadian Brand Names Apo-Ampi®; Novo-Ampicillin; Nu-Ampi

Generic Available Yes

Synonyms Aminobenzylpenicillin; Ampicillin Sodium; Ampicillin Trihydrate

Pharmacologic Category Antibiotic, Penicillin

Dental Use I.V. or I.M. administration for the prevention of bacterial endocarditis in patients unable to take oral amoxicillin

Use Treatment of susceptible bacterial infections (nonbeta-lactamase-producing organisms); susceptible bacterial infections caused by streptococci, pneumococci, nonpenicillinase-producing staphylococci, *Listeria*, meningococci; some strains of *H. influenzae*, *Salmonella*, *Shigella*, *E. coli*, *Enterobacter*, and *Klebsiella*

Local Anesthetic/Vasoconstrictor Precautions No information available to require special precautions

Effects on Dental Treatment Key adverse event(s) related to dental treatment: Oral candidiasis.

Significant Adverse Effects Frequency not defined.

Central nervous system: Fever, penicillin encephalopathy, seizure

Dermatologic: Erythema multiforme, exfoliative dermatitis, rash, urticaria

    Note: Appearance of a rash should be carefully evaluated to differentiate (if possible) nonallergic ampicillin rash from hypersensitivity reaction. Incidence is higher in patients with viral infection, *Salmonella* infection, lymphocytic leukemia, or patients that have hyperuricemia.

Gastrointestinal: Black hairy tongue, diarrhea, enterocolitis, glossitis, nausea, pseudomembranous colitis, sore mouth or tongue, stomatitis, vomiting

Hematologic: Agranulocytosis, anemia, hemolytic anemia, eosinophilia, leukopenia, thrombocytopenia purpura

Hepatic: AST increased

Renal: Interstitial nephritis (rare)

Respiratory: Laryngeal stridor

Miscellaneous: Anaphylaxis, serum sickness-like reaction

Dental Usual Dosing Endocarditis prophylaxis: I.M., I.V.: Dental, oral, respiratory tract, or esophageal procedures:

Infants and Children: 50 mg/kg within 30 minutes prior to procedure in patients unable to take oral amoxicillin

Adults: 2 g within 30 minutes prior to procedure in patients unable to take oral amoxicillin

Dosage

Usual dosage range:

Infants and Children:

    Oral: 50-100 mg/kg/day in doses divided every 6 hours (maximum: 2-4 g/day)

    I.M., I.V.: 100-400 mg/kg/day in divided doses every 6 hours (maximum: 12 g/day)

Adults: Oral, I.M., I.V.: 250-500 mg every 6 hours

Indication-specific dosing:

Infants and Children:

    Endocarditis prophylaxis:

      Dental, oral, respiratory tract, or esophageal procedures: I.M., I.V.: 50 mg/kg within 30 minutes prior to procedure in patients unable to take oral amoxicillin

      Genitourinary and gastrointestinal tract (except esophageal) procedures: I.M., I.V.:

        High-risk patients: 50 mg/kg (maximum: 2 g) within 30 minutes prior to procedure, followed by ampicillin 25 mg/kg (or amoxicillin 25 mg/kg orally) 6 hours later; must be used in combination with gentamicin.

        Moderate-risk patients: 50 mg/kg within 30 minutes prior to procedure

    Mild-to-moderate infections:

      Oral: 50-100 mg/kg/day in doses divided every 6 hours (maximum: 2-4 g/day)

      I.M., I.V.: 100-150 mg/kg/day in divided doses every 6 hours (maximum: 2-4 g/day)

    Severe infections, meningitis: I.M., I.V.: 200-400 mg/kg/day in divided doses every 6 hours (maximum: 6-12 g/day)

Adults:

    Actinomycosis: I.V.: 50 mg/kg/day for 4-6 weeks then oral amoxicillin

    Cholangitis (acute): I.V.: 2 g every 4 hours with gentamicin

    Diverticulitis: I.M., I.V.: 2 g every 6 hours with metronidazole

    Endocarditis:

      Infective: I.V.: 12 g/day via continuous infusion or divided every 4 hours

Prophylaxis: Dental, oral, respiratory tract, or esophageal procedures: I.M., I.V.: 2 g within 30 minutes prior to procedure in patients unable to take oral amoxicillin

Genitourinary and gastrointestinal tract (except esophageal) procedures: High-risk patients: I.M., I.V.: 2 g within 30 minutes prior to procedure, followed by ampicillin 1 g (or amoxicillin 1g orally) 6 hours later; must be used in combination with gentamicin.

Moderate-risk patients: I.M., I.V.: 2 g within 30 minutes prior to procedure

Group B strep prophylaxis (intrapartum): I.V.: 2 g initial dose, then 1 g every 4 hours until delivery

***Listeria* infections:** I.V.: 200 mg/kg/day divided every 6 hours

Sepsis/meningitis: I.M., I.V.: 150-250 mg/kg/day divided every 3-4 hours (range: 6-12 g/day)

Urinary tract infections (enterococcus suspected): I.V.: 1-2 g every 6 hours with gentamicin

Dosing interval in renal impairment:

Cl_{cr} >50 mL/minute: Administer every 6 hours

Cl_{cr} 10-50 mL/minute: Administer every 6-12 hours

Cl_{cr} <10 mL/minute: Administer every 12-24 hours

Hemodialysis: Moderately dialyzable (20% to 50%); administer dose after dialysis

Peritoneal dialysis: Moderately dialyzable (20% to 50%)

Administer 250 mg every 12 hours

Continuous arteriovenous or venovenous hemofiltration effects: Dose as for Cl_{cr} 10-50 mL/minute; ~50 mg of ampicillin per liter of filtrate is removed

Mechanism of Action Inhibits bacterial cell wall synthesis by binding to one or more of the penicillin-binding proteins (PBPs) which in turn inhibits the final transpeptidation step of peptidoglycan synthesis in bacterial cell walls, thus inhibiting cell wall biosynthesis. Bacteria eventually lyse due to ongoing activity of cell wall autolytic enzymes (autolysins and murein hydrolases) while cell wall assembly is arrested.

Contraindications Hypersensitivity to ampicillin, any component of the formulation, or other penicillins

Warnings/Precautions Dosage adjustment may be necessary in patients with renal impairment. A low incidence of cross-allergy with other beta-lactams exists. High percentage of patients with infectious mononucleosis have developed rash during therapy with ampicillin. Appearance of a rash should be carefully evaluated to differentiate a nonallergic ampicillin rash from a hypersensitivity reaction. Ampicillin rash occurs in 5% to 10% of children receiving ampicillin and is a generalized dull red, maculopapular rash, generally appearing 3-14 days after the start of therapy. It normally begins on the trunk and spreads over most of the body. It may be most intense at pressure areas, elbows, and knees.

Drug Interactions

Allopurinol: Theoretically has an additive potential for ampicillin/amoxicillin rash

Aminoglycosides: May be synergistic against selected organisms

Methotrexate: Penicillins may increase the exposure to methotrexate during concurrent therapy; monitor.

Oral contraceptives: Anecdotal reports suggesting decreased contraceptive efficacy with penicillins have been refuted by more rigorous scientific and clinical data.

Probenecid, disulfiram: May increase levels of penicillins (ampicillin)

Warfarin: Effects of warfarin may be increased

Ethanol/Nutrition/Herb Interactions Food: Food decreases ampicillin absorption rate; may decrease ampicillin serum concentration.

Dietary Considerations Take on an empty stomach 1 hour before or 2 hours after meals.

Sodium content of 5 mL suspension (250 mg/5 mL): 10 mg (0.4 mEq)

Sodium content of 1 g: 66.7 mg (3 mEq)

Pharmacodynamics/Kinetics

Absorption: Oral: 50%

Distribution: Bile, blister, and tissue fluids; penetration into CSF occurs with inflamed meninges only, good only with inflammation (exceeds usual MICs)

Normal meninges: Nil; Inflamed meninges: 5% to 10%

Protein binding: 15% to 25%

Half-life elimination:

Children and Adults: 1-1.8 hours

Anuria/end-stage renal disease: 7-20 hours

Time to peak: Oral: Within 1-2 hours

Excretion: Urine (~90% as unchanged drug) within 24 hours

Pregnancy Risk Factor B

(Continued)

Ampicillin *(Continued)*

Lactation Enters breast milk/use caution

Dosage Forms

Capsule (Principen®): 250 mg, 500 mg

Injection, powder for reconstitution, as sodium: 125 mg, 250 mg, 500 mg, 1 g, 2 g, 10 g

Powder for oral suspension (Principen®): 125 mg/5 mL (100 mL, 200 mL); 250 mg/5 mL (100 mL, 200 mL)

Selected Readings

ADA Division of Legal Affairs, "A Legal Perspective on Antibiotic Prophylaxis," *J Am Dent Assoc*, 2003, 134(9):1260.

American Dental Association; American Academy of Orthopedic Surgeons, "Antibiotic Prophylaxis for Dental Patients With Total Joint Replacements," *J Am Dent Assoc*, 2003, 134(7):895-9.

American Dental Association Council on Scientific Affairs, "Combating Antibiotic Resistance," *J Am Dent Assoc*, 2004, 135(4):484-7.

Dajani AS, Taubert KA, Wilson W, et al, "Prevention of Bacterial Endocarditis. Recommendations by the American Heart Association," *JAMA*, 1997, 277(22):1794-801.

Dajani AS, Taubert KA, Wilson W, et al, "Prevention of Bacterial Endocarditis: Recommendations by the American Heart Association," *J Am Dent Assoc*, 1997, 128(8):1142-51.

Wynn RL, Bergman SA, Meiller TF, et al, "Antibiotics in Treating Oral-Facial Infections of Odontogenic Origin: An Update", *Gen Dent*, 2001, 49(3):238-40, 242, 244 passim.

Ampicillin and Sulbactam (am pi SIL in & SUL bak tam)

Related Information

Ampicillin *on page 117*

Sexually-Transmitted Diseases *on page 1674*

U.S. Brand Names Unasyn®

Canadian Brand Names Unasyn®

Generic Available Yes

Synonyms Sulbactam and Ampicillin

Pharmacologic Category Antibiotic, Penicillin

Dental Use Parenteral beta-lactamase-resistant antibiotic combination to treat more severe orofacial infections where beta-lactamase-producing staphylococci and beta-lactamase-producing *Bacteroides* are present

Use Treatment of susceptible bacterial infections involved with skin and skin structure, intra-abdominal infections, gynecological infections; spectrum is that of ampicillin plus organisms producing beta-lactamases such as *S. aureus*, *H. influenzae*, *E. coli*, *Klebsiella*, *Acinetobacter*, *Enterobacter*, and anaerobes

Local Anesthetic/Vasoconstrictor Precautions No information available to require special precautions

Effects on Dental Treatment Prolonged use of penicillins may lead to development of oral candidiasis (see Dental Comment).

Significant Adverse Effects Also see Ampicillin.

>10%: Local: Pain at injection site (I.M.)

1% to 10%:

Dermatologic: Rash

Gastrointestinal: Diarrhea

Local: Pain at injection site (I.V.), thrombophlebitis

Miscellaneous: Allergic reaction (may include serum sickness, urticaria, bronchospasm, hypotension, etc)

<1% (Limited to important or life-threatening): Abdominal distension, candidiasis, chest pain, chills, dysuria, edema, epistaxis, erythema, facial swelling, fatigue, flatulence, glossitis, hairy tongue, headache, interstitial nephritis, itching, liver enzymes increased, malaise, mucosal bleeding, nausea, pseudomembranous colitis, seizure, substernal pain, throat tightness, thrombocytopenia, urine retention, vomiting

Dental Usual Dosing Severe orofacial infections: Adults: I.M., I.V.: 1-2 g ampicillin (1.5-3 g Unasyn®) every 6 hours (maximum: 8 g ampicillin/day, 12 g Unasyn®)

Dosage Note: Unasyn® (ampicillin/sulbactam) is a combination product. Dosage recommendations for Unasyn® are based on the ampicillin component.

Usual dosage range:

Children ≥1 year: I.V.: 100-400 mg ampicillin/kg/day divided every 6 hours (maximum: 8 g ampicillin/day, 12 g Unasyn®). **Note:** The American Academy of Pediatrics recommends a dose of up to 300 mg/kg/day for severe infection in infants >1 month of age.

Adults: I.M., I.V.: 1-2 g ampicillin (1.5-3 g Unasyn®) every 6 hours (maximum: 8 g ampicillin/day, 12 g Unasyn®)

Indication-specific dosing:

Children:

Epiglottitis: I.V.: 100-200 mg ampicillin/kg/day divided in 4 doses

Mild-to-moderate infections: I.M., I.V.: 100-200 mg ampicillin/kg/day (150-300 g Unasyn®) divided every 6 hours (maximum: 8 g ampicillin/day, 12 g Unasyn®)

Peritonsillar and retropharyngeal abscess: I.V.: 50 mg ampicillin/kg/dose every 6 hours

Severe infections: I.M., I.V.: 200-400 mg ampicillin/kg/day divided every 6 hours (maximum: 8 g ampicillin/day, 12 g Unasyn®)

Adults: Doses expressed as ampicillin/sulbactam combination:

Amnionitis, cholangitis, diverticulitis, endometritis, endophthalmitis, epididymitis/orchitis, liver abscess, osteomyelitis (diabetic foot), peritonitis: I.V.: 3 g every 6 hours

Endocarditis: I.V.: 3 g every 6 hours with gentamicin or vancomycin for 4-6 weeks

Orbital cellulitis: I.V.: 1.5 g every 6 hours

Parapharyngeal space infections: I.V.: 3 g every 6 hours

Pasteurella multocida (human, canine/feline bites): I.V.: 1.5-3 g every 6 hours

Pelvic inflammatory disease: I.V.: 3 g every 6 hours with doxycycline

Peritonitis (CAPD): Intraperitoneal:
Anuric, intermittent: 3 g every 12 hours
Anuric, continuous: Loading dose: 1.5 g; maintenance dose: 150 mg

Pneumonia:
Aspiration, community-acquired: I.V.: 1.5-3 g every 6 hours
Hospital-acquired: I.V.: 3 g every 6 hours

Urinary tract infections, pyelonephritis: I.V.: 3 g every 6 hours for 14 days

Dosing interval in renal impairment:
Cl_{cr} 15-29 mL/minute: Administer every 12 hours
Cl_{cr} 5-14 mL/minute: Administer every 24 hours

Mechanism of Action The addition of sulbactam, a beta-lactamase inhibitor, to ampicillin extends the spectrum of ampicillin to include some beta-lactamase-producing organisms; inhibits bacterial cell wall synthesis by binding to one or more of the penicillin-binding proteins (PBPs) which in turn inhibits the final transpeptidation step of peptidoglycan synthesis in bacterial cell walls, thus inhibiting cell wall biosynthesis. Bacteria eventually lyse due to ongoing activity of cell wall autolytic enzymes (autolysins and murein hydrolases) while cell wall assembly is arrested.

Contraindications Hypersensitivity to ampicillin, sulbactam, penicillins, or any component of the formulations

Warnings/Precautions Dosage adjustment may be necessary in patients with renal impairment. A low incidence of cross-allergy with other beta-lactams exists. High percentage of patients with infectious mononucleosis have developed rash during therapy with ampicillin. Appearance of a rash should be carefully evaluated to differentiate a nonallergic ampicillin rash from a hypersensitivity reaction. Ampicillin rash occurs in 5% to 10% of children receiving ampicillin and is a generalized dull red, maculopapular rash, generally appearing 3-14 days after the start of therapy. It normally begins on the trunk and spreads over most of the body. It may be most intense at pressure areas, elbows, and knees.

Drug Interactions
Allopurinol: Theoretically has an additive potential for ampicillin/amoxicillin rash
Aminoglycosides: May be synergistic against selected organisms
Methotrexate: Penicillins may increase the exposure to methotrexate during concurrent therapy; monitor.
Oral contraceptives: Anecdotal reports suggesting decreased contraceptive efficacy with penicillins have been refuted by more rigorous scientific and clinical data.
Probenecid, disulfiram: May increase levels of penicillins (ampicillin)
Warfarin: Effects of warfarin may be increased

Dietary Considerations Sodium content of 1.5 g injection: 115 mg (5 mEq)

Pharmacodynamics/Kinetics
Ampicillin: See Ampicillin.
Sulbactam:
Distribution: Bile, blister, and tissue fluids
Protein binding: 38%
Half-life elimination: Normal renal function: 1-1.3 hours
Excretion: Urine (~75% to 85% as unchanged drug) within 8 hours

Pregnancy Risk Factor B

Lactation Enters breast milk/use caution

Dosage Forms Injection, powder for reconstitution (Unasyn®): 1.5 g [ampicillin sodium 1 g and sulbactam sodium 0.5 g]; 3 g [ampicillin sodium 2 g and (Continued)

Ampicillin and Sulbactam *(Continued)*

sulbactam sodium 1 g]; 15 g [ampicillin sodium 10 g and sulbactam sodium 5 g] [bulk package]

Dental Comment In maxillary sinus, anterior nasal cavity, and deep neck infections, beta-lactamase-producing staphylococci and beta-lactamase-producing *Bacteroides* usually are present. In these situations, antibiotics that resist the beta-lactamase enzyme should be administered. Amoxicillin and clavulanic acid is administered orally for moderate infections. Ampicillin sodium and sulbactam sodium (Unasyn®) is administered parenterally for more severe infections.

Ampicillin Sodium *see Ampicillin on page 117*
Ampicillin Trihydrate *see Ampicillin on page 117*

Amprenavir *(am PREN a veer)*

Related Information
HIV Infection and AIDS *on page 1662*
Tuberculosis *on page 1673*
U.S. Brand Names Agenerase®
Canadian Brand Names Agenerase®
Generic Available No
Pharmacologic Category Antiretroviral Agent, Protease Inhibitor
Use Treatment of HIV infections in combination with at least two other antiretroviral agents; oral solution should only be used when capsules or other protease inhibitors are not therapeutic options
Local Anesthetic/Vasoconstrictor Precautions No information available to require special precautions
Effects on Dental Treatment Key adverse event(s) related to dental treatment: Perioral tingling/numbness and taste disorder.
Common Adverse Effects
>10%:
  Central nervous system: Depression/mood disorder (9% to 16%), paresthesia (peripheral 10% to 14%)
  Dermatologic: Rash (20% to 27%)
  Endocrine & metabolic: Hyperglycemia (>160 mg/dL: 37% to 41%), hypertriglyceridemia (>399 mg/dL: 36% to 47%; >750 mg/dL: 8% to 13%)
  Gastrointestinal: Nausea (43% to 74%), vomiting (24% to 34%), diarrhea (39% to 60%), abdominal symptoms
  Miscellaneous: Perioral tingling/numbness (26% to 31%)
1% to 10%:
  Central nervous system: Headache, fatigue
  Dermatologic: Stevens-Johnson syndrome (1% of total, 4% of patients who develop a rash)
  Endocrine & metabolic: Hypercholesterolemia (>260 mg/dL: 4% to 9%), hyperglycemia (>251 mg/dL: 2% to 3%), fat redistribution
  Gastrointestinal: Taste disorders (2% to 10%), amylase increased (3% to 4%)
  Hepatic: AST increased (3% to 5%), ALT increased (4%)
Mechanism of Action Binds to the protease activity site and inhibits the activity of the enzyme. HIV protease is required for the cleavage of viral polyprotein precursors into individual functional proteins found in infectious HIV. Inhibition prevents cleavage of these polyproteins, resulting in the formation of immature, noninfectious viral particles.
Drug Interactions
Cytochrome P450 Effect: **Substrate** of CYP2C9 (minor), 3A4 (major); **Inhibits** CYP2C19 (weak), 3A4 (strong)
Increased Effect/Toxicity: Concurrent use of cisapride, midazolam, pimozide, quinidine, or triazolam is contraindicated. Concurrent use of ergot alkaloids (dihydroergotamine, ergotamine, ergonovine, methylergonovine) with amprenavir is also contraindicated (may cause vasospasm and peripheral ischemia). Concurrent use of oral solution with disulfiram or metronidazole is contraindicated, due to the risk of propylene glycol toxicity.

Serum concentrations of amiodarone, bepridil, lidocaine, quinidine, and other antiarrhythmics may be increased, potentially leading to toxicity; when amprenavir is coadministered with ritonavir, flecainide and propafenone are contraindicated. HMG-CoA reductase inhibitors serum concentrations may be increased by amprenavir, increasing the risk of myopathy/rhabdomyolysis; lovastatin and simvastatin are not recommended; fluvastatin and pravastatin may be safer alternatives.

Amprenavir may increase the levels/effects of selected benzodiazepines (midazolam and triazolam are contraindicated), calcium channel blockers, cyclosporine, mirtazapine, nateglinide, nefazodone, quinidine, sildenafil (and other PDE-5 inhibitors), tacrolimus, venlafaxine, and other CYP3A4 substrates. Amprenavir may increase the levels/effects of trazodone (monitor for signs of hypotension/syncope); reduce dose of trazodone. When used with strong CYP3A4 inhibitors, dosage adjustment/limits are recommended for sildenafil and other PDE-5 inhibitors; refer to individual monographs. Amprenavir may increase the levels/effects of inhaled corticosteroids; monitor for adrenal suppression, Cushing's syndrome; concomitant use of fluticasone with amprenavir/ritonavir is not recommended.

Concurrent therapy with ritonavir may result in increased serum concentrations: dosage adjustment is recommended; avoid concurrent use of amprenavir and ritonavir oral solutions due to metabolic competition between formulation components. Clarithromycin, indinavir, nelfinavir may increase serum concentrations of amprenavir.

Decreased Effect: Serum concentrations of estrogen (oral contraceptives) may be decreased, use alternative (nonhormonal) forms of contraception. Serum concentrations of delavirdine may be decreased; may lead to loss of virologic response and possible resistance to delavirdine; concomitant use is not recommended. Efavirenz and nevirapine may decrease serum concentrations of amprenavir (dosing for combinations not established). Avoid St John's wort (may lead to subtherapeutic concentrations of amprenavir). Effect of amprenavir may be diminished when administered with methadone (consider alternative antiretroviral); in addition, effect of methadone may be reduced (dosage increase may be required). The levels/effects of amprenavir may be decreased by include aminoglutethimide, carbamazepine, nafcillin, nevirapine, phenobarbital, phenytoin, rifamycins, and other CYP3A4 inducers. The administration of antacids and didanosine (buffered formulation) should be separated from amprenavir by 1 hour to limit interaction between formulations.

Pharmacodynamics/Kinetics
Absorption: 63%
Distribution: 430 L
Protein binding: 90%
Metabolism: Hepatic via CYP (primarily CYP3A4)
Bioavailability: Not established; increased sixfold with high-fat meal; oral solution: 86% relative to capsule formulation (14% less bioavailable than capsule)
Half-life elimination: 7.1-10.6 hours
Time to peak: 1-2 hours
Excretion: Feces (75%, ~68% as metabolites); urine (14% as metabolites)

Pregnancy Risk Factor C

AMPT see Metyrosine *on page 1036*

Amrinone Lactate see Inamrinone *on page 827*

AMSA see Amsacrine *on page 123*

Amsacrine (AM sah kreen)

Canadian Brand Names Amsa P-D
Generic Available No
Synonyms 4-(9-Acridinylamino) Methanesulfon-m-Anisidide; Acridinyl Anisidide; AMSA; m-AMSA; NSC-249992
Pharmacologic Category Antineoplastic Agent
Unlabeled/Investigational Use Investigational: Refractory acute lymphocytic and nonlymphocytic leukemias, Hodgkin's disease, and non-Hodgkin's lymphomas; head and neck tumors
Local Anesthetic/Vasoconstrictor Precautions No information available to require special precautions
Effects on Dental Treatment Key adverse event(s) related to dental treatment: Oral ulcerations and stomatitis.
Common Adverse Effects
>10%:
   Cardiovascular: ECG changes (T-wave flattening, S-T wave alterations) consistent with anterolateral ischemia, ventricular fibrillation, ventricular extrasystoles, atrial tachycardia and fibrillation, CHF, cardiac arrest. Patients with hypokalemia, who have received >400 mg/m² of doxorubicin or daunorubicin (or the equivalent), >200 mg/m² of amsacrine within 48 hours, or a total dose of anthracycline + amsacrine >900 mg/m² have an increased risk of cardiac toxicity.
   Dermatologic: Alopecia
   Gastrointestinal: Nausea and vomiting (30%), diarrhea (30%), stomatitis (dose-limiting - 32%), oral ulceration (10%)
   Genitourinary: Orange-red discoloration of the urine
(Continued)

Amsacrine *(Continued)*

Hematologic: Leukopenia (nadir at 10 days); thrombocytopenia (nadir at 12-14 days), with recovery at 21-25 days

Hepatic: Hyperbilirubinemia (30%), liver enzymes increased (10%)

Local: Phlebitis

1% to 10%:

Central nervous system: Headache, dizziness, confusion, convulsions

Hematologic: Anemia

Neuromuscular & skeletal: Paresthesias

Ocular: Blurred vision

Restrictions

Not available in U.S./Investigational

Mechanism of Action Amsacrine has been shown to inhibit DNA synthesis by binding to, and intercalating with, DNA; inhibits topoisomerase II activity.

Pharmacodynamics/Kinetics

Distribution: V_d: 1.67 L/kg; minimal CNS penetration

Protein binding: 96% to 98%

Metabolism: Hepatic, to inactive metabolites (major metabolite is 5′ glutathione conjugate)

Half-life elimination: 1.4-5 hours; Terminal: 5.6-7.8 hours

Excretion: Bile; urine (2% to 10% as unchanged drug)

Amyl Nitrite (AM il NYE trite)

Generic Available Yes

Synonyms Isoamyl Nitrite

Pharmacologic Category Antidote; Vasodilator

Use Coronary vasodilator in angina pectoris; adjunct in treatment of cyanide poisoning; produce changes in the intensity of heart murmurs

Local Anesthetic/Vasoconstrictor Precautions No information available to require special precautions

Effects on Dental Treatment Key adverse event(s) related to dental treatment: Postural hypotension.

Common Adverse Effects 1% to 10%:

Cardiovascular: Postural hypotension; cutaneous flushing of head, neck, and clavicular area; tachycardia

Central nervous system: Headache, restlessness

Gastrointestinal: Nausea, vomiting

Mechanism of Action Relaxes vascular smooth muscle; decreased venous ratios and arterial blood pressure; reduces left ventricular work; decreases myocardial O_2 consumption; in cyanide poisoning, amyl nitrite converts hemoglobin to methemoglobin that binds with cyanide to form cyanate hemoglobin

Drug Interactions

Increased Effect/Toxicity:

Ethanol taken with amyl nitrite may have additive side effects. Avoid concurrent use of sildenafil - severe reactions may result.

Sildenafil: Avoid concurrent use of sildenafil; severe reactions may result.

Pharmacodynamics/Kinetics

Onset of action: Angina: Within 30 seconds

Duration: 3-15 minutes

Pregnancy Risk Factor X

Amylobarbitone *see* Amobarbital *on page 104*

Amytal® *see* Amobarbital *on page 104*

AN100226 *see* Natalizumab *on page 1093*

Anadrol® *see* Oxymetholone *on page 1173*

Anafranil® *see* ClomiPRAMINE *on page 370*

Anagrelide (an AG gre lide)

U.S. Brand Names Agrylin®

Canadian Brand Names Agrylin®; PMS-Anagrelide; Rhoxal-anagrelide; Sandoz-Anagrelide

Generic Available Yes

Synonyms 1370-999-397; Anagrelide Hydrochloride; BL4162A; 6,7-Dichloro-1,5-Dihydroimidazo [2,1b] quinazolin-2(3H)-one Monohydrochloride

Pharmacologic Category Phospholipase A$_2$ Inhibitor

Use Treatment of essential thrombocythemia (ET) and thrombocythemia associated with chronic myelogenous leukemia (CML), polycythemia vera, and other myeloproliferative disorders

Local Anesthetic/Vasoconstrictor Precautions No information available to require special precautions

Effects on Dental Treatment Key adverse event(s) related to dental treatment: Orthostatic hypotension.

Common Adverse Effects

>10%:

Cardiovascular: Palpitations (27%), edema (other than peripheral: 21%)

Central nervous system: Headache (44%), dizziness (15%), pain (15%)

Gastrointestinal: Diarrhea (26%), nausea (17%), abdominal pain (16%)

Neuromuscular & skeletal: Weakness (23%)

Respiratory: Dyspnea (12%)

1% to 10%:

Cardiovascular: Angina, arrhythmias, cardiovascular disease, chest pain (8%), CHF, hypertension, orthostatic hypotension, peripheral edema (9%), syncope, tachycardia (7%), thrombosis, vasodilatation

Central nervous system: Amnesia, chills, confusion, depression, fever (9%), insomnia, malaise (6%), migraine, nervousness, somnolence

Dermatologic: Alopecia, photosensitivity, pruritus (6%), rash (8%), urticaria

Endocrine & skeletal: Dehydration

Gastrointestinal: Anorexia (8%), aphthous stomatitis, constipation, dyspepsia (5%), eructation, flatulence (10%), gastritis, GI distress, GI hemorrhage, melena, vomiting (10%)

Hematologic: Anemia, ecchymosis, hemorrhage, lymphadenoma, thrombocytopenia

Hepatic: Liver enzymes increased

Neuromuscular & skeletal: Arthralgia, back pain (6%), leg cramps, myalgia, paresthesia (6%)

Ocular: Amblyopia, diplopia, tinnitus, visual field abnormality

Renal: Dysuria, hematuria, renal failure

Respiratory: Asthma, bronchitis, cough (6%), epistaxis, pharyngitis (7%), pneumonia, rhinitis, sinusitis

Miscellaneous: Flu-like syndrome

Frequency not defined: Atrial fibrillation, cardiomegaly, cardiomyopathy, cerebrovascular accident, complete heart block, gastric/duodenal ulceration, leukocyte count increased, MI, pancreatitis, pericarditis, pericardial effusion, pleural effusion, pulmonary fibrosis, pulmonary infiltrates, pulmonary hypertension, seizure

Mechanism of Action Anagrelide appears to inhibit cyclic nucleotide phosphodiesterase and the release of arachidonic acid from phospholipase, possibly by inhibiting phospholipase A$_2$. It also causes a dose-related reduction in platelet production, which results from decreased megakaryocyte hypermaturation. The drug disrupts the postmitotic phase of maturation.

Drug Interactions

Cytochrome P450 Effect: Substrate of CYP1A2 (minor)

Increased Effect/Toxicity: Antiplatelet agents may enhance the adverse/toxic effects of drotrecogin alfa. Concurrent use of NSAIDs, salicylates, or treprostinil may enhance the adverse/toxic effects of antiplatelet agents.

Pharmacodynamics/Kinetics

Duration: 6-24 hours

Metabolism: Hepatic

Half-life elimination, plasma: 1.3 hours

Time to peak, serum: 1 hour

Excretion: Urine (<1% as unchanged drug)

Pregnancy Risk Factor C

Anagrelide Hydrochloride *see* Anagrelide *on page 124*

Anakinra (an a KIN ra)

U.S. Brand Names Kineret®

Canadian Brand Names Kineret®

Generic Available No

Synonyms IL-1Ra; Interleukin-1 Receptor Antagonist

Pharmacologic Category Antirheumatic, Disease Modifying; Interleukin-1 Receptor Antagonist

Use Reduction of signs and symptoms of moderately- to severely-active rheumatoid arthritis in adult patients who have failed one or more disease-modifying

(Continued)

Anakinra *(Continued)*

antirheumatic drugs (DMARDs); may be used alone or in combination with DMARDs (other than tumor necrosis factor-blocking agents)

Local Anesthetic/Vasoconstrictor Precautions No information available to require special precautions

Effects on Dental Treatment No significant effects or complications reported

Common Adverse Effects

>10%:

Central nervous system: Headache (12%)

Local: Injection site reaction (majority mild, typically lasting 14-28 days, characterized by erythema, ecchymosis, inflammation, and pain; up to 71%)

Miscellaneous: Infection (39% versus 37% in placebo; serious infection in 3% to 2%)

1% to 10%:

Gastrointestinal: Nausea (8%), diarrhea (7%), abdominal pain (5%)

Hematologic: WBCs decreased (8%)

Respiratory: Sinusitis (7%)

Miscellaneous: Flu-like syndrome (6%)

Mechanism of Action Binds to the interleukin-1 (IL-1) receptor. IL-1 is induced by inflammatory stimuli and mediates a variety of immunological responses, including degradation of cartilage (loss of proteoglycans) and stimulation of bone resorption.

Drug Interactions

Increased Effect/Toxicity: Concurrent use of anakinra and etanercept has been associated with an increased risk of serious infection while American College of Rheumatology (ACR) response rates were not improved, as compared to etanercept alone. Use caution with other drugs known to block or decrease the activity of tumor necrosis factor (TNF); includes infliximab and thalidomide.

Pharmacodynamics/Kinetics

Bioavailability: SubQ: 95%

Half-life elimination: Terminal: 4-6 hours

Time to peak: SubQ: 3-7 hours

Pregnancy Risk Factor B

Ana-Kit® *see* Epinephrine and Chlorpheniramine *on page 549*

Analpram-HC® *see* Pramoxine and Hydrocortisone *on page 1264*

AnaMantle® HC *see* Lidocaine and Hydrocortisone *on page 928*

Anaprox® *see* Naproxen *on page 1089*

Anaprox® DS *see* Naproxen *on page 1089*

Anaspaz® *see* Hyoscyamine *on page 803*

Anastrozole *(an AS troe zole)*

U.S. Brand Names Arimidex®

Canadian Brand Names Arimidex®

Mexican Brand Names Arimidex®

Generic Available No

Synonyms ICI-D1033; ZD1033

Pharmacologic Category Aromatase Inhibitor

Use Treatment of locally-advanced or metastatic breast cancer (ER-positive or hormone receptor unknown) in postmenopausal women; treatment of advanced breast cancer in postmenopausal women with disease progression following tamoxifen therapy; adjuvant treatment of early ER-positive breast cancer in postmenopausal women

Local Anesthetic/Vasoconstrictor Precautions No information available to require special precautions

Effects on Dental Treatment Key adverse event(s) related to dental treatment: Xerostomia (normal salivary flow resumes upon discontinuation).

Common Adverse Effects

>10%:

Cardiovascular: Vasodilatation (25% to 36%), hypertension (5% to 13%)

Central nervous system: Mood disturbance (19%), pain (11% to 17%), headache (10% to 13%), depression (5% to 13%)

Dermatologic: Rash (6% to 11%)

Endocrine & metabolic: Hot flashes (12% to 36%)

Gastrointestinal: Nausea (11% to 19%), vomiting (8% to 13%)

Neuromuscular & skeletal: Weakness (16% to 19%), arthritis (17%), arthralgia (2% to 15%), back pain (10% to 12%), bone pain (6% to 11%), osteoporosis (11%)

Respiratory: Cough increased (8% to 11%), pharyngitis (6% to 14%)

1% to 10%:

Cardiovascular: Peripheral edema (5% to 10%), chest pain (5% to 7%), ischemic cardiovascular disease (4%), venous thromboembolic events (3% to 4%), ischemic cerebrovascular events (2%), angina (2%)

Central nervous system: Insomnia (6% to 10%), dizziness (8%), anxiety (6%), fever (2% to 5%), malaise (2% to 5%), confusion (2% to 5%), nervousness (2% to 5%), somnolence (2% to 5%), lethargy (1%)

Dermatologic: Alopecia (2% to 5%), pruritus (2% to 5%)

Endocrine & metabolic: Hypercholesterolemia (9%), breast pain (2% to 8%)

Gastrointestinal: Constipation (7% to 9%), abdominal pain (7% to 9%), diarrhea (7% to 9%), anorexia (5% to 7%), xerostomia (6%), dyspepsia (7%), weight gain (2% to 9%), weight loss (2% to 5%)

Genitourinary: Urinary tract infection (8%), vulvovaginitis (6%), pelvic pain (5%), vaginal bleeding (1% to 5%), vaginitis (4%), vaginal discharge (4%), vaginal hemorrhage (2% to 4%), leukorrhea (2% to 3%), vaginal dryness (2%)

Hematologic: Anemia (2% to 5%), leukopenia (2% to 5%)

Hepatic: Liver function tests increased (2% to 5%), alkaline phosphatase increased (2% to 5%), gamma GT increased (2% to 5%)

Local: Thrombophlebitis (2% to 5%)

Neuromuscular & skeletal: Fracture (10%), arthrosis (7%), paresthesia (5% to 7%), joint disorder (6%), myalgia (2% to 6%), neck pain (2% to 5%), hypertonia (3%)

Ocular: Cataracts (6%)

Respiratory: Dyspnea (8% to 10%), sinusitis (6%), bronchitis (5%), rhinitis (2% to 5%)

Miscellaneous: Lymph edema (10%), infection (2% to 9%), flu-like syndrome (2% to 7%), diaphoresis (2% to 5%), cyst (5%)

Mechanism of Action Potent and selective nonsteroidal aromatase inhibitor. By inhibiting aromatase, the conversion of androstenedione to estrone, and testosterone to estradiol, is prevented. Anastrozole causes an 85% decrease in estrone sulfate levels.

Drug Interactions

Cytochrome P450 Effect: Inhibits CYP1A2 (weak), 2C8 (weak), 2C9 (weak), 3A4 (weak)

Pharmacodynamics/Kinetics

Onset of estradiol reduction: 24 hours (70% reduction; 80% after 2 weeks therapy)

Duration of estradiol reduction: 6 days

Absorption: Well absorbed (80%); not affected by food

Protein binding, plasma: 40%

Metabolism: Extensively hepatic (85%) via N-dealkylation, hydroxylation, and glucuronidation; primary metabolite inactive

Half-life elimination: 50 hours

Excretion: Feces (~75%); urine (10% as unchanged drug; 60% as metabolites)

Pregnancy Risk Factor D

Anatrast *see* Barium *on page 179*

Anbesol® [OTC] *see* Benzocaine *on page 190*

Anbesol® Baby [OTC] *see* Benzocaine *on page 190*

Anbesol® Cold Sore Therapy [OTC] *see* Benzocaine *on page 190*

Anbesol® Jr. [OTC] *see* Benzocaine *on page 190*

Anbesol® Maximum Strength [OTC] *see* Benzocaine *on page 190*

Ancef® *see* Cefazolin *on page 283*

Ancobon® *see* Flucytosine *on page 662*

Andehist DM NR Drops *see* Carbinoxamine, Pseudoephedrine, and Dextromethorphan *on page 269*

Andehist NR Drops *see* Carbinoxamine and Pseudoephedrine *on page 268*

Andehist NR Syrup *see* Brompheniramine and Pseudoephedrine *on page 223*

Androderm® *see* Testosterone *on page 1462*

AndroGel® *see* Testosterone *on page 1462*

Android® *see* MethylTESTOSTERone *on page 1028*

Anestacon® *see* Lidocaine *on page 920*

Aneurine Hydrochloride *see* Thiamine *on page 1476*

Anexsia® *see* Hydrocodone and Acetaminophen *on page 779*

Anextuss *see* Guaifenesin, Dextromethorphan, and Phenylephrine *on page 756*

Angeliq® *see* Drospirenone and Estradiol *on page 520*

Angiomax® *see* Bivalirudin *on page 213*

Anhydrous Glucose *see* Dextrose *on page 452*

Anidulafungin (ay nid yoo la FUN jin)

U.S. Brand Names Eraxis™
Generic Available No
Synonyms LY303366
Pharmacologic Category Antifungal Agent, Parenteral; Echinocandin
Use Treatment of candidemia and other forms of *Candida* infections (including those of intra-abdominal, peritoneal, and esophageal locus)
Local Anesthetic/Vasoconstrictor Precautions No information available to require special precautions
Effects on Dental Treatment No significant effects or complications reported
Common Adverse Effects 2% to 10%:
Endocrine & metabolic: Hypokalemia (3%)
Gastrointestinal: Diarrhea (3%)
Hepatic: Transaminase increased (<1% to 2%)
Mechanism of Action Noncompetitive inhibitor of 1,3-beta-D-glucan synthase resulting in reduced formation of 1,3-beta-D-glucan, an essential polysaccharide comprising 30% to 60% of *Candida* cell walls (absent in mammalian cells); decreased glucan content leads to osmotic instability and cellular lysis
Pharmacodynamics/Kinetics
Distribution: 30-50 L
Protein binding: 84%
Metabolism: No hepatic metabolism observed; undergoes slow chemical hydrolysis to open-ring peptide-lacking antifungal activity
Half-life elimination: 27 hours
Excretion: Feces (30%, 10% as unchanged drug); urine (<1%)
Pregnancy Risk Factor C

Anolor 300 *see* Butalbital, Acetaminophen, and Caffeine *on page 239*
Ansaid® [DSC] *see* Flurbiprofen *on page 683*
Ansamycin *see* Rifabutin *on page 1345*
Antabuse® *see* Disulfiram *on page 492*
Antagon® *see* Ganirelix *on page 723*
Antara™ *see* Fenofibrate *on page 639*
Antazoline and Naphazoline *see* Naphazoline and Antazoline *on page 1088*

Anthralin (AN thra lin)

U.S. Brand Names Dritho-Scalp®; Psoriatec™
Canadian Brand Names Anthraforte®; Anthranol®; Anthrascalp®; Micanol®
Mexican Brand Names Anthranol®
Generic Available No
Synonyms Dithranol
Pharmacologic Category Antipsoriatic Agent; Keratolytic Agent
Use Treatment of psoriasis (quiescent or chronic psoriasis)
Local Anesthetic/Vasoconstrictor Precautions No information available to require special precautions
Effects on Dental Treatment No significant effects or complications reported
Mechanism of Action Reduction of the mitotic rate and proliferation of epidermal cells in psoriasis by inhibiting synthesis of nucleic protein from inhibition of DNA synthesis to affected areas
Pregnancy Risk Factor C

Anthrax Vaccine (Adsorbed) (AN thraks vak SEEN ad SORBED)

Related Information
Immunizations (Vaccines) *on page 1786*
U.S. Brand Names BioThrax™
Generic Available No
Synonyms AVA
Pharmacologic Category Vaccine
Use Immunization against *Bacillus anthracis*. Recommended for individuals who may come in contact with animal products which come from anthrax endemic areas and may be contaminated with *Bacillus anthracis* spores; recommended for high-risk persons such as veterinarians and other handling potentially infected animals. Routine immunization for the general population is not recommended.

The Department of Defense is implementing an anthrax vaccination program against the biological warfare agent anthrax, which will be administered to all active duty and reserve personnel.

Unlabeled/Investigational Use Postexposure prophylaxis in combination with antibiotics

Local Anesthetic/Vasoconstrictor Precautions No information available to require special precautions

Effects on Dental Treatment No significant effects or complications reported

Common Adverse Effects (Includes pre- and postlicensure data; systemic reactions reported more often in women than in men)

>10%:
  Central nervous system: Malaise (4% to 11%)
  Local: Tenderness (58% to 71%), erythema (12% to 43%), subcutaneous nodule (4% to 39%), induration (8% to 21%), warmth (11% to 19%), local pruritus (7% to 19%)
  Neuromuscular & skeletal: Arm motion limitation (7% to 12%)

1% to 10%:
  Central nervous system: Headache (4% to 7%), fever (<1% to 7%)
  Gastrointestinal: Anorexia (4%), vomiting (4%), nausea (<1% to 4%)
  Local: Mild local reactions (edema/induration <30 mm) (9%), edema (8%)
  Neuromuscular & skeletal: Myalgia (4% to 7%)
  Respiratory: Respiratory difficulty (4%)

Restrictions Not commercially available in the U.S.; presently, all anthrax vaccine lots are owned by the U.S. Department of Defense. The Centers for Disease Control (CDC) does not currently recommend routine vaccination of the general public.

Mechanism of Action Active immunization against *Bacillus anthracis*. The vaccine is prepared from a cell-free filtrate of *B. anthracis*, but no dead or live bacteria.

Drug Interactions

Decreased Effect: Effect of vaccine may be decreased with chemotherapy, corticosteroids (high doses, ≥14 days), immunosuppressant agents, and radiation therapy; consider waiting at least 3 months between discontinuing therapy and administering vaccine.

Pharmacodynamics/Kinetics Duration: Unknown; may be 1-2 years following two inoculations based on animal data

Pregnancy Risk Factor D

Anti-4 Alpha Integrin *see* Natalizumab *on page 1093*

Anti-CD11a *see* Efalizumab *on page 529*

Anti-CD20 Monoclonal Antibody *see* Rituximab *on page 1360*

Antidigoxin Fab Fragments, Ovine *see* Digoxin Immune Fab *on page 474*

Antidiuretic Hormone *see* Vasopressin *on page 1567*

Antihemophilic Factor (Human)
(an tee hee moe FIL ik FAK tor HYU man)

U.S. Brand Names Alphanate®; Hemofil® M; Humate-P®; Koāte®-DVI; Monarc® M; Monoclate-P®

Canadian Brand Names Hemofil® M; Humate-P®

Generic Available Yes

Synonyms AHF (Human); Factor VIII (Human)

Pharmacologic Category Antihemophilic Agent; Blood Product Derivative

Use Management of hemophilia A for patients in whom a deficiency in factor VIII has been demonstrated; can be of significant therapeutic value in patients with acquired factor VIII inhibitors not exceeding 10 Bethesda units/mL

  Humate-P®: In addition, indicated as treatment of spontaneous bleeding in patients with severe von Willebrand disease and in mild and moderate von Willebrand disease where desmopressin is known or suspected to be inadequate

  Orphan status: Alphanate®: Management of von Willebrand disease

Local Anesthetic/Vasoconstrictor Precautions No information available to require special precautions

Effects on Dental Treatment No significant effects or complications reported

Mechanism of Action Protein (factor VIII) in normal plasma which is necessary for clot formation and maintenance of hemostasis; activates factor X in conjunction with activated factor IX; activated factor X converts prothrombin to thrombin, which converts fibrinogen to fibrin, and with factor XIII forms a stable clot

Pharmacodynamics/Kinetics Half-life elimination: Mean: 12-17 hours with hemophilia A; consult specific product labeling

Pregnancy Risk Factor C

Antihemophilic Factor (Recombinant)
(an tee hee moe FIL ik FAK tor ree KOM be nant)

U.S. Brand Names Advate; Helixate® FS; Kogenate® FS; Recombinate™; ReFacto®

Canadian Brand Names Helixate® FS; Kogenate®; Kogenate® FS; Recombinate™; ReFacto®

Generic Available No

Synonyms AHF (Recombinant); Factor VIII (Recombinant); rAHF

Pharmacologic Category Antihemophilic Agent

Use Management of hemophilia A (classic hemophilia) for patients in whom a deficiency in factor VIII has been demonstrated; prevention and control of bleeding episodes; perioperative management of hemophilia A; can be of significant therapeutic value in patients with acquired factor VIII inhibitors ≤10 Bethesda units/mL

Local Anesthetic/Vasoconstrictor Precautions No information available to require special precautions

Effects on Dental Treatment No significant effects or complications reported

Mechanism of Action Factor VIII replacement, necessary for clot formation and maintenance of hemostasis. It activates factor X in conjunction with activated factor IX; activated factor X converts prothrombin to thrombin, which converts fibrinogen to fibrin, and with factor XIII forms a stable clot.

Pharmacodynamics/Kinetics Half-life elimination: Mean: 13-16 hours

Pregnancy Risk Factor C

Anti-inhibitor Coagulant Complex
(an tee-in HI bi tor coe AG yoo lant KOM pleks)

U.S. Brand Names Autoplex® T [DSC]; Feiba VH

Canadian Brand Names Feiba VH Immuno

Generic Available No

Synonyms AICC; Coagulant Complex Inhibitor

Pharmacologic Category Activated Prothrombin Complex Concentrate (aPCC); Antihemophilic Agent; Blood Product Derivative

Use Hemophilia A & B patients with factor VIII inhibitors who are to undergo surgery or those who are bleeding

Local Anesthetic/Vasoconstrictor Precautions No information available to require special precautions

Effects on Dental Treatment No significant effects or complications reported

Common Adverse Effects Frequency not defined.
Cardiovascular: Blood pressure changes, flushing, MI, pulse rate changes
Central nervous system: Headache, lethargy
Dermatologic: Rash, urticaria
Gastrointestinal: Nausea
Hematologic: DIC
Miscellaneous: Allergic reaction, anamnestic response, infusion-related reactions (fever, chills)

Drug Interactions
Increased Effect/Toxicity: Coadministration of aminocaproic acid or tranexamic acid may increase risk of thrombosis.

Pregnancy Risk Factor C

Antipyrine and Benzocaine (an tee PYE reen & BEN zoe kane)

Related Information
Benzocaine *on page 190*

U.S. Brand Names A/B Otic; Allergen®; Aurodex; Auroto

Canadian Brand Names Auralgan®

Generic Available Yes

Synonyms Benzocaine and Antipyrine

Pharmacologic Category Otic Agent, Analgesic; Otic Agent, Cerumenolytic

Use Temporary relief of pain and reduction of swelling associated with acute congestive and serous otitis media, swimmer's ear, otitis externa; facilitates ear wax removal

Local Anesthetic/Vasoconstrictor Precautions No information available to require special precautions

Effects on Dental Treatment No significant effects or complications reported

Pregnancy Risk Factor C

Antiseptic Mouthwash *see* Mouthwash (Antiseptic) *on page 1069*

Antithrombin III (an tee THROM bin three)

U.S. Brand Names Thrombate III®

Canadian Brand Names Thrombate III®

Generic Available No

Synonyms AT-III; Heparin Cofactor I

Pharmacologic Category Anticoagulant; Blood Product Derivative

Use Treatment of hereditary antithrombin III deficiency in connection with surgical procedures, obstetrical procedures, or thromboembolism

Unlabeled/Investigational Use Acquired antithrombin III deficiencies related to disseminated intravascular coagulation (DIC)

Local Anesthetic/Vasoconstrictor Precautions No information available to require special precautions

Effects on Dental Treatment No significant effects or complications reported

Common Adverse Effects 1% to 10%: Central nervous system: Dizziness (2%)

Mechanism of Action Antithrombin III is the primary physiologic inhibitor of *in vivo* coagulation. It is an alpha$_2$-globulin. Its principal actions are the inactivation of thrombin, plasmin, and other active serine proteases of coagulation, including factors IXa, Xa, XIa, and XIIa. The inactivation of proteases is a major step in the normal clotting process. The strong activation of clotting enzymes at the site of every bleeding injury facilitates fibrin formation and maintains normal hemostasis. Thrombosis in the circulation would be caused by active serine proteases if they were not inhibited by antithrombin III after the localized clotting process.

Drug Interactions

Increased Effect/Toxicity: Heparin's anticoagulant effects are potentiated by antithrombin III (half-life of antithrombin III is decreased by heparin). Risk of hemorrhage with antithrombin III may be increased by drotrecogin alfa, thrombolytic agents, oral anticoagulants (warfarin), treprostinil, and drugs which affect platelet function (eg, aspirin, NSAIDs, dipyridamole, ticlopidine, clopidogrel, and IIb/IIIa antagonists).

Pharmacodynamics/Kinetics Half-life elimination: Biologic: 2.5 days (immunologic assay); 3.8 days (functional AT-III assay). Half-life may be decreased following surgery, with hemorrhage, acute thrombosis, and/or during heparin administration.

Pregnancy Risk Factor B

Antithymocyte Globulin (Equine)
(an te THY moe site GLOB yu lin, E kwine)

U.S. Brand Names Atgam®

Canadian Brand Names Atgam®

Generic Available No

Synonyms Antithymocyte Immunoglobulin; ATG; Horse Antihuman Thymocyte Gamma Globulin; Lymphocyte Immune Globulin

Pharmacologic Category Immunosuppressant Agent

Use Prevention and treatment of acute renal allograft rejection; treatment of moderate to severe aplastic anemia in patients not considered suitable candidates for bone marrow transplantation

Unlabeled/Investigational Use Prevention and treatment of other solid organ allograft rejection; prevention of graft-versus-host disease following bone marrow transplantation

Local Anesthetic/Vasoconstrictor Precautions No information available to require special precautions

Effects on Dental Treatment Key adverse event(s) related to dental treatment: Stomatitis.

Common Adverse Effects

>10%:
  Central nervous system: Fever, chills
  Dermatologic: Pruritus, rash, urticaria
  Hematologic: Leukopenia, thrombocytopenia

1% to 10%:
  Cardiovascular: Bradycardia, chest pain, CHF, edema, encephalitis, hyper-/hypotension, myocarditis, tachycardia

(Continued)

Antithymocyte Globulin (Equine) *(Continued)*

Central nervous system: Agitation, headache, lethargy, lightheadedness, listlessness, seizure

Gastrointestinal: Diarrhea, nausea, stomatitis, vomiting

Hepatic: Hepatosplenomegaly, liver function tests abnormal

Local: Pain at injection site, phlebitis, thrombophlebitis, burning soles/palms

Neuromuscular & skeletal: Myalgia, back pain, arthralgia

Ocular: Periorbital edema

Renal: Abnormal renal function tests

Respiratory: Dyspnea, respiratory distress

Miscellaneous: Anaphylaxis, serum sickness, viral infection, night sweats, diaphoresis, lymphadenopathy

Mechanism of Action May involve elimination of antigen-reactive T lymphocytes (killer cells) in peripheral blood or alteration of T-cell function

Pharmacodynamics/Kinetics

Distribution: Poorly into lymphoid tissues; binds to circulating lymphocytes, granulocytes, platelets, bone marrow cells

Half-life elimination, plasma: 1.5-12 days

Excretion: Urine (~1%)

Pregnancy Risk Factor C

Antithymocyte Immunoglobulin *see* Antithymocyte Globulin (Equine) *on page 131*

Antitumor Necrosis Factor Apha (Human) *see* Adalimumab *on page 52*

Anti-VEGF Monoclonal Antibody *see* Bevacizumab *on page 204*

Antivert *see* Meclizine *on page 969*

Antizol *see* Fomepizole *on page 699*

Anucort-HC® *see* Hydrocortisone *on page 793*

Anu-Med [OTC] *see* Phenylephrine *on page 1226*

Anusol-HC® *see* Hydrocortisone *on page 793*

Anusol® HC-1 [OTC] *see* Hydrocortisone *on page 793*

Anusol® Ointment [OTC] *see* Pramoxine *on page 1264*

Anzemet® *see* Dolasetron *on page 498*

APAP *see* Acetaminophen *on page 31*

APAP and Tramadol *see* Acetaminophen and Tramadol *on page 39*

Apatate® [OTC] *see* Vitamin B Complex Combinations *on page 1581*

ApexiCon™ *see* Diflorasone *on page 468*

ApexiCon™ E *see* Diflorasone *on page 468*

Aphedrid™ [OTC] *see* Triprolidine and Pseudoephedrine *on page 1542*

Aphrodyne® *see* Yohimbine *on page 1589*

Aphthasol® *see* Amlexanox *on page 99*

Apidra® *see* Insulin Glulisine *on page 837*

Aplisol® *see* Tuberculin Tests *on page 1548*

Aplonidine *see* Apraclonidine *on page 133*

Apokyn™ *see* Apomorphine *on page 132*

Apomorphine *(a poe MOR feen)*

U.S. Brand Names Apokyn™

Generic Available No

Synonyms Apomorphine Hydrochloride; Apomorphine Hydrochloride Hemihydrate

Pharmacologic Category Anti-Parkinson's Agent, Dopamine Agonist

Use Treatment of hypomobility, "off" episodes with Parkinson's disease

Unlabeled/Investigational Use Treatment of erectile dysfunction

Local Anesthetic/Vasoconstrictor Precautions No information available to require special precautions (see Dental Comment)

Effects on Dental Treatment Key adverse event(s) related to dental treatment: Orthostatic hypotension has been reported in significant numbers of patients.

Common Adverse Effects

>10%:

Cardiovascular: Chest pain/pressure or angina (15%)

Central nervous system: Drowsiness or somnolence (35%), dizziness or orthostatic hypotension (20%)

Gastrointestinal: Nausea and/or vomiting (30%)

Neuromuscular & skeletal: Falls (30%), dyskinesias (24% to 35%)

Respiratory: Yawning (40%), rhinorrhea (20%)

1% to 10%:
    Cardiovascular: Edema (10%), vasodilation (3%), hypotension (2%), syncope (2%), CHF
    Central nervous system: Hallucinations or confusion (10%), anxiety, depression, fatigue, headache, insomnia, pain
    Dermatologic: Bruising
    Endocrine & metabolic: Dehydration
    Gastrointestinal: Constipation, diarrhea
    Local: Injection site reactions
    Neuromuscular & skeletal: Arthralgias, weakness
    Miscellaneous: Diaphoresis increased

Mechanism of Action Stimulates postsynaptic D2-type receptors within the caudate putamen in the brain.

Drug Interactions
    Cytochrome P450 Effect: Substrate (minor) of CYP1A2, 3A4, 2C19; **Inhibits** CYP1A2 (weak), 3A (weak), 2C19 (weak)
    Increased Effect/Toxicity: Antihypertensives, vasodilators, and $5HT_3$ antagonists may increase risk of hypotension. QT_c prolongation may rarely occur with concurrent use of QT_c-prolonging agents. Effects of concomitant levodopa may be increased.
    Decreased Effect: Typical antipsychotics may decrease the efficacy of apomorphine.

Pharmacodynamics/Kinetics
    Onset: SubQ: Rapid
    Distribution: V_d: Mean: 218 L
    Metabolism: Not established; potential routes of metabolism include sulfation, N-demethylation, glucuronidation, and oxidation; catechol-O methyltransferase and nonenzymatic oxidation. CYP isoenzymes do not appear to play a significant role.
    Half-life elimination: Terminal: 40 minutes
    Time to peak, plasma: Improved motor scores: 20 minutes
    Excretion: Urine 93% (as metabolites); feces 16%

Pregnancy Risk Factor C

Dental Comment This drug is known to prolong the QT interval. The QT interval is measured as the time and distance between the Q point of the QRS complex and the end of the T wave in the ECG tracing. After adjustment for heart rate, the QT interval is defined as prolonged if it is more than 450 msec in men and 460 msec in women. A long QT syndrome was first described in the 1950s and 60s as a congenital syndrome involving QT interval prolongation and syncope and sudden death. Some of the congenital long QT syndromes were characterized by a peculiar electrocardiographic appearance of the QRS complex involving a premature atria beat followed by a pause, then a subsequent sinus beat showing marked QT prolongation and deformity. This type of cardiac arrhythmia was originally termed "torsade de pointes" (translated from the French as "twisting of the points").

Prolongation of the QT interval is thought to result from delayed ventricular repolarization. The repolarization process within the myocardial cell is due to the efflux of intracellular potassium. The channels associated with this current can be blocked by many drugs, thus, predisposing the electrical propagation cycle to torsade de pointes.

Apomorphine is one of the drugs confirmed to prolong the QT interval and is accepted as having a risk of causing torsade de pointes. The risk of drug-induced torsade de pointes is extremely low when a single QT interval prolonging drug is prescribed. In terms of epinephrine, it is not known what effect vasoconstrictors in the local anesthetic regimen will have in patients with a known history of congenital prolonged QT interval or in patients taking any medication that prolongs the QT interval. Until more information is obtained, it is suggested that the clinician consult with the physician prior to the use of a vasoconstrictor in suspected patients, and that the vasoconstrictor (epinephrine, levonordefrin [Neo-Cobefrin®]) be used with caution.

Apomorphine Hydrochloride see Apomorphine on page 132
Apomorphine Hydrochloride Hemihydrate see Apomorphine on page 132
APPG see Penicillin G Procaine on page 1204
Apra Children's [OTC] see Acetaminophen on page 31

Apraclonidine (a pra KLOE ni deen)

U.S. Brand Names Iopidine®
Canadian Brand Names Iopidine®
Generic Available No
(Continued)

Apraclonidine (Continued)

Synonyms Aplonidine; Apraclonidine Hydrochloride; p-Aminoclonidine

Pharmacologic Category Alpha$_2$ Agonist, Ophthalmic

Use Prevention and treatment of postsurgical intraocular pressure (IOP) elevation; short-term, adjunctive therapy in patients who require additional reduction of IOP

Local Anesthetic/Vasoconstrictor Precautions No information available to require special precautions

Effects on Dental Treatment Key adverse event(s) related to dental treatment: Xerostomia (normal salivary flow resumes upon discontinuation).

Mechanism of Action Apraclonidine is a potent alpha-adrenergic agent similar to clonidine; relatively selective for alpha$_2$-receptors but does retain some binding to alpha$_1$-receptors; appears to result in reduction of aqueous humor formation; its penetration through the blood-brain barrier is more polar than clonidine which reduces its penetration through the blood-brain barrier and suggests that its pharmacological profile is characterized by peripheral rather than central effects.

Pregnancy Risk Factor C

Apraclonidine Hydrochloride *see Apraclonidine on page 133*

Aprepitant *(ap RE pi tant)*

U.S. Brand Names Emend®

Generic Available No

Synonyms L 754030; MK 869

Pharmacologic Category Antiemetic; Substance P/Neurokinin 1 Receptor Antagonist

Use Prevention of acute and delayed nausea and vomiting associated with moderately- and highly -emetogenic chemotherapy in combination with a corticosteroid and 5-HT$_3$ receptor antagonist

Local Anesthetic/Vasoconstrictor Precautions No information available to require special precautions

Effects on Dental Treatment Key adverse event(s) related to dental treatment: Hiccups.

Common Adverse Effects Note: Adverse reactions reported as part of a combination chemotherapy regimen.

>10%:
    Central nervous system: Fatigue (18% to 22%)
    Dermatologic: Alopecia (24%; placebo 22%)
    Gastrointestinal: Nausea (7% to 13%), constipation (10% to 12%)
    Neuromuscular & skeletal: Weakness (3% to 18%)
    Miscellaneous: Hiccups (11%)

1% to 10%:
    Central nervous system: Dizziness (3% to 7%)
    Endocrine & metabolic: Dehydration (6%), hot flushing (3%)
    Gastrointestinal: Diarrhea (6% to 10%), dyspepsia (8%), abdominal pain (5%), stomatitis (5%), epigastric discomfort (4%), gastritis (4%), mucous membrane disorder (3%), throat pain (3%)
    Hematologic: Neutropenia (3% to 9%), leukopenia (9%), hemoglobin decreased (2% to 5%)
    Hepatic: ALT increased (6%), AST increased (3%)
    Renal: BUN increased (5%), proteinuria (7%), serum creatinine increased (4%)

Mechanism of Action Prevents acute and delayed vomiting by selectively inhibiting the substance P/neurokinin 1 (NK$_1$) receptor.

Drug Interactions

Cytochrome P450 Effect: Substrate of CYP1A2 (minor), 2C19 (minor), 3A4 (major); **Inhibits** CYP2C9 (weak), 2C19 (weak), 3A4 (moderate); **Induces** CYP2C9 (weak), 3A4 (weak)

Increased Effect/Toxicity: Use with cisapride or pimozide is contraindicated. CYP3A4 inhibitors may increase the levels/effects of aprepitant; example inhibitors include azole antifungals, clarithromycin, diclofenac, diltiazem, doxycycline, erythromycin, imatinib, isoniazid, nefazodone, nicardipine, propofol, protease inhibitors, quinidine, telithromycin, and verapamil. Aprepitant may increase the bioavailability of corticosteroids; dose adjustment of dexamethasone and methylprednisolone is needed. Aprepitant may increase the levels/effects of CYP3A4 substrates; example substrates include benzodiazepines, calcium channel blockers, ergot derivatives, mirtazapine, nateglinide, nefazodone, tacrolimus, and venlafaxine.

Decreased Effect: CYP3A4 inducers may decrease the levels/effects of aprepitant; example inducers include aminoglutethimide, carbamazepine, nafcillin, nevirapine, phenobarbital, phenytoin, and rifamycins. Metabolism of warfarin may be induced; monitor INR following the start of each cycle. Efficacy of oral contraceptives may be decreased (plasma levels of ethinyl estradiol and norethindrone decreased with concomitant use).

Pharmacodynamics/Kinetics

Distribution: V_d: 70 L; crosses the blood brain barrier

Protein binding: >95%

Metabolism: Extensively hepatic via CYP3A4 (major); CYP1A2 and CYP2C19 (minor); forms seven metabolites (weakly active)

Bioavailability: 60% to 65%

Half-life elimination: Terminal: 9-13 hours

Time to peak, plasma: 4 hours

Pregnancy Risk Factor B

Apresazide [DSC] *see* Hydralazine and Hydrochlorothiazide *on page 775*

Apresoline [DSC] *see* HydrALAZINE *on page 775*

Apri® *see* Ethinyl Estradiol and Desogestrel *on page 592*

Aprodine® [OTC] *see* Triprolidine and Pseudoephedrine *on page 1542*

Aprotinin (a proe TYE nin)

U.S. Brand Names Trasylol®

Canadian Brand Names Trasylol®

Mexican Brand Names Trasylol®

Generic Available No

Pharmacologic Category Blood Product Derivative; Hemostatic Agent

Use Reduction of blood loss in patients undergoing cardiopulmonary bypass in coronary artery bypass graft surgery

Local Anesthetic/Vasoconstrictor Precautions No information available to require special precautions

Effects on Dental Treatment No significant effects or complications reported

Common Adverse Effects

>10%:

Central nervous system: Fever (15%)

Gastrointestinal: Nausea (11%)

1% to 10%:

Cardiovascular: Atrial flutter (6%), MI (6%; not statistically different from placebo), ventricular extrasystoles (6%), ventricular tachycardia (1% to 5%), heart failure (1% to 5%), arrhythmia (4%), supraventricular arrhythmia (4%), bradycardia (1% to 2%), bundle branch block (1% to 2%), heart block (1% to 2%), hemorrhage (1% to 2%), myocardial ischemia (1% to 2%), pericardia effusion (1% to 2%), shock (<1% to 2%), ventricular fibrillation (1% to 2%), thrombosis (1% to 2%)

Central nervous system: Agitation (1% to 2%), anxiety (1% to 2%), dizziness (1% to 2%), seizure (1% to 2%)

Endocrine & metabolic: Creatinine phosphokinase increase (2%), acidosis (1% to 2%), hyperglycemia (1% to 2%), hypervolemia (1% to 2%), hypokalemia

Gastrointestinal: Diarrhea (3%), dyspepsia (1% to 2%), gastrointestinal hemorrhage (1% to 2%)

Hematologic: Disseminated intravascular coagulation (DIC), leukocytosis (1% to 2%), prothrombin decreased (1% to 2%), thrombocytopenia (1% to 2%)

Hepatic: Liver function tests increased (3%), jaundice (1% to 2%), hepatic failure (1% to 2%)

Neuromuscular & skeletal: Arthralgia (1% to 2%)

Renal: Kidney function abnormality (3%), oliguria (1% to 2%), kidney failure (1%)

Respiratory: Hypoxia (2%), pulmonary hypertension (1% to 2%), pneumonia (1% to 2%), apnea (1% to 2%), cough increased (1% to 2%), lung edema (1% to 2%)

Miscellaneous: Sepsis (1% to 2%), multisystem organ failure (1% to 2%)

Note: In controlled trials, thrombosis has **not** been reported more frequently in the aprotinin versus placebo group. However, thrombosis has been reported in uncontrolled trials, compassionate use trials, and spontaneous postmarketing reports.

Mechanism of Action Bleeding from CABG surgery is thought to result from a systemic inflammatory response induced by the procedure. Contact of blood cells with the cardiopulmonary bypass (CPB) equipment leads to deregulated (Continued)

Aprotinin *(Continued)*

activation of the coagulation and fibrinolysis systems, with concurrent upregulation of proinflammatory cytokines. Aprotinin is a broad spectrum serine protease inhibitor that attenuates the coagulation, fibrinolytic and inflammatory pathways by interfering with the chemical mediators (thrombin, plasmin, kallikrein). Additionally, it protects platelet-expressed glycoproteins from mechanical shear forces. This preserves normal hemostatic activity through protease receptor-independent mechanisms (eg, via ADP, IIb/IIIa), while blocking CPB-induced thrombin-mediated aggregation.

Drug Interactions
Decreased Effect: Aprotinin blocks the fibrinolytic activity of thrombolytic agents (eg, alteplase, streptokinase). The antihypertensive effects of captopril (and other ACE inhibitors) may be blocked.

Pharmacodynamics/Kinetics
Distribution: Extracellular space; renal phagolysosomes
Metabolism: Aprotinin is slowly degraded by lysosomal enzymes.
Half-life elimination: 2.5 hours (plasma); terminal: 10 hours
Excretion: Urine (25% to 40%; <10% as unchanged drug)

Pregnancy Risk Factor B

Aptivus® *see* Tipranavir *on page 1495*

Aquacare® [OTC] *see* Urea *on page 1551*

Aquachloral® Supprettes® *see* Chloral Hydrate *on page 312*

AquaLase™ *see* Balanced Salt Solution *on page 178*

Aquanil™ HC [OTC] *see* Hydrocortisone *on page 793*

Aquaphilic® With Carbamide [OTC] *see* Urea *on page 1551*

AquaSite® [OTC] *see* Artificial Tears *on page 143*

Aquasol A® *see* Vitamin A *on page 1580*

Aquasol E® [OTC] *see* Vitamin E *on page 1581*

Aquavit-E [OTC] *see* Vitamin E *on page 1581*

Aqueous Procaine Penicillin G *see* Penicillin G Procaine *on page 1204*

Ara-C *see* Cytarabine *on page 413*

Arabinosylcytosine *see* Cytarabine *on page 413*

Aralast *see* Alpha₁-Proteinase Inhibitor *on page 73*

Aralen® *see* Chloroquine *on page 320*

Aranelle™ *see* Ethinyl Estradiol and Norethindrone *on page 608*

Aranesp® *see* Darbepoetin Alfa *on page 423*

Arava® *see* Leflunomide *on page 901*

Aredia® *see* Pamidronate *on page 1181*

Arestin™ *see* Minocycline Hydrochloride (Periodontal) *on page 1050*

Argatroban *(ar GA troh ban)*

Related Information
Cardiovascular Diseases *on page 1636*

Generic Available No

Pharmacologic Category Anticoagulant, Thrombin Inhibitor

Use Prophylaxis or treatment of thrombosis in adults with heparin-induced thrombocytopenia; adjunct to percutaneous coronary intervention (PCI) in patients who have or are at risk of thrombosis associated with heparin-induced thrombocytopenia

Local Anesthetic/Vasoconstrictor Precautions No information available to require special precautions

Effects on Dental Treatment Key adverse event(s) related to dental treatment: As with all anticoagulants, bleeding is a potential adverse effect of argatroban during dental surgery; risk is dependent on multiple variables, including the intensity of anticoagulation and patient susceptibility. Medical consult is suggested. It is unlikely that ambulatory patients presenting for dental treatment will be taking intravenous anticoagulant therapy.

Common Adverse Effects As with all anticoagulants, bleeding is the major adverse effect of argatroban. Hemorrhage may occur at virtually any site. Risk is dependent on multiple variables, including the intensity of anticoagulation and patient susceptibility.

>10%:
Cardiovascular: Chest pain (<1% to 15%), hypotension (7% to 11%)
Gastrointestinal: Gastrointestinal bleed (minor, 3% to 14%)
Genitourinary: Genitourinary bleed and hematuria (minor, 2% to 12%)

1% to 10%:
  Cardiovascular: Cardiac arrest (6%), ventricular tachycardia (5%), brady-cardia (5%), myocardial infarction (PCI: 4%), atrial fibrillation (3%), angina (2%), CABG-related bleeding (minor, 2%), myocardial ischemia (2%), cere-brovascular disorder (<1% to 2%), thrombosis (<1% to 2%)
  Central nervous system: Fever (<1% to 7%), headache (5%), pain (5%), intracranial bleeding (1% to 4%)
  Gastrointestinal: Nausea (5% to 7%), diarrhea (6%), vomiting (4% to 6%), abdominal pain (3% to 4%), bleeding (major, <1% to 2%)
  Genitourinary: Urinary tract infection (5%)
  Hematologic: Hemoglobin (<2 g/dL) and hematocrit (minor, 2% to 10%) decreased
  Local: Bleeding at injection or access site (minor, 2% to 5%)
  Neuromuscular & skeletal: Back pain (8%)
  Renal: Abnormal renal function (3%)
  Respiratory: Dyspnea (8% to 10%), cough (3% to 10%), hemoptysis (minor, <1% to 3%), pneumonia (3%)
  Miscellaneous: Sepsis (6%), infection (4%)
Mechanism of Action A direct, highly-selective thrombin inhibitor. Reversibly binds to the active thrombin site of free and clot-associated thrombin. Inhibits fibrin formation; activation of coagulation factors V, VIII, and XIII; protein C; and platelet aggregation.

Drug Interactions
  Cytochrome P450 Effect: Substrate of CYP3A4 (minor)
  Increased Effect/Toxicity: Drugs which affect platelet function (eg, aspirin, NSAIDs, dipyridamole, ticlopidine, clopidogrel), anticoagulants, or thrombolytics may potentiate the risk of hemorrhage. Sufficient time must pass after heparin therapy is discontinued; allow heparin's effect on the aPTT to decrease.
  Concomitant use of argatroban with warfarin increases PT and INR greater than that of warfarin alone. Argatroban is commonly continued during the initiation of warfarin therapy to assure anticoagulation and to protect against possible transient hypercoagulability.

Pharmacodynamics/Kinetics
  Onset of action: Immediate
  Distribution: 174 mL/kg
  Protein binding: Albumin: 20%; α_1-acid glycoprotein: 35%
  Metabolism: Hepatic via hydroxylation and aromatization. Metabolism via CYP3A4/5 to four known metabolites plays a minor role. Unchanged arga-troban is the major plasma component. Plasma concentration of metabolite M1 is 0% to 20% of the parent drug and is three- to fivefold weaker.
  Half-life elimination: 39-51 minutes; Hepatic impairment: ≤181 minutes
  Time to peak: Steady-state: 1-3 hours
  Excretion: Feces (65%); urine (22%); low quantities of metabolites M2-4 in urine
Pregnancy Risk Factor B

Arginine (AR ji neen)

U.S. Brand Names R-Gene®
Generic Available No
Synonyms Arginine Hydrochloride
Pharmacologic Category Diagnostic Agent
Use Pituitary function test (growth hormone)
Unlabeled/Investigational Use Management of severe, uncompensated, metabolic alkalosis (pH ≥7.55) after optimizing therapy with sodium and potas-sium supplements
Local Anesthetic/Vasoconstrictor Precautions No information available to require special precautions
Effects on Dental Treatment No significant effects or complications reported
Mechanism of Action Stimulates pituitary release of growth hormone and prolactin through origins in the hypothalamus; patients with impaired pituitary function have lower or no increase in plasma concentrations of growth hormone after administration of arginine. Arginine hydrochloride has been used for severe metabolic alkalosis due to its high chloride content.
  Arginine hydrochloride has been used investigationally to treat metabolic alka-losis. Arginine contains 475 mEq of hydrogen ions and 475 mEq of chloride ions/L. Arginine is metabolized by the liver to produce hydrogen ions. It may be used in patients with relative hepatic insufficiency because arginine combines with ammonia in the body to produce urea.
Pregnancy Risk Factor B

Arginine Hydrochloride see Arginine on page 137

8-Arginine Vasopressin see Vasopressin on page 1567

Aricept® see Donepezil on page 500

Aricept® ODT see Donepezil on page 500

Arimidex® see Anastrozole on page 126

Aripiprazole (ay ri PIP ray zole)

U.S. Brand Names Abilify®

Generic Available No

Synonyms BMS 337039; OPC-14597

Pharmacologic Category Antipsychotic Agent, Atypical

Use Treatment of schizophrenia; stabilization and maintenance therapy of bipolar disorder (with acute manic or mixed episodes)

Unlabeled/Investigational Use Depression with psychotic features

Local Anesthetic/Vasoconstrictor Precautions No information available to require special precautions

Effects on Dental Treatment Key adverse event(s) related to dental treatment: Extrapyramidal symptoms (similar to placebo) (see Dental Comment).

Common Adverse Effects

>10%:

Central nervous system: Headache (31%), agitation (25%), anxiety (20%), insomnia (20%), extrapyramidal symptoms (6% to 17%), somnolence (12% to 15%, dose related), akathisia (12%), lightheadedness (11%)

Gastrointestinal: Nausea (16%), dyspepsia (15%), constipation (11%), vomiting (11%), weight gain (8% to 30%, highest frequency in patients with BMI <23)

1% to 10%:

Cardiovascular: Edema (peripheral 2%), hypertension (2%), tachycardia, hypotension, bradycardia, chest pain

Central nervous system: Fever, depression, nervousness, mania, confusion, hallucination, hostility, paranoid reaction, suicidal thought, delusion, abnormal dream

Dermatologic: Dry skin, skin ulcer

Endocrine & metabolic: Dehydration

Gastrointestinal: Salivation increased (3%), weight loss

Genitourinary: Urinary incontinence, pelvic pain

Hematologic: Anemia, bruising

Neuromuscular & skeletal: Tremor (4% to 9%), weakness (8%), myalgia (4%), neck pain, neck rigidity, muscle cramp, CPK increased, abnormal gait

Ocular: Blurred vision (3%), conjunctivitis

Respiratory: Rhinitis (4%), pharyngitis (4%), cough (3%), asthma, dyspnea, pneumonia, sinusitis

Miscellaneous: Accidental injury (5%), flu-like syndrome, diaphoresis

Mechanism of Action Aripiprazole is a quinolinone antipsychotic which exhibits high affinity for D_2, D_3, 5-HT_{1A}, and 5-HT_{2A} receptors; moderate affinity for D_4, 5-HT_{2C}, 5-HT_7, alpha, and H_1 receptors. It also possesses moderate affinity for the serotonin reuptake transporter; has no affinity for muscarinic receptors. Aripiprazole functions as a partial agonist at the D_2 and 5-HT_{1A} receptors, and as an antagonist at the 5-HT_{2A} receptor.

Drug Interactions

Cytochrome P450 Effect: Substrate (major) of CYP2D6, 3A4

Increased Effect/Toxicity: CYP2D6 inhibitors may increase the levels/effects of aripiprazole; example inhibitors include chlorpromazine, delavirdine, fluoxetine, miconazole, paroxetine, pergolide, quinidine, quinine, ritonavir, and ropinirole. CYP3A4 inhibitors may increase the levels/effects of aripiprazole; example inhibitors include azole antifungals, clarithromycin, diclofenac, doxycycline, erythromycin, imatinib, isoniazid, nefazodone, nicardipine, propofol, protease inhibitors, quinidine, telithromycin, and verapamil. Manufacturer recommends a 50% reduction in dose during concurrent ketoconazole therapy. Similar reductions in dose may be required with other potent inhibitors. Acetylcholinesterase inhibitors (central) may increase the risk of antipsychotic-related extrapyramidal symptoms.

Decreased Effect: CYP3A4 inducers may decrease the levels/effects of aripiprazole; example inducers include aminoglutethimide, carbamazepine, nafcillin, nevirapine, phenobarbital, phenytoin, and rifamycins. Manufacturer recommends a doubling of the aripiprazole dose when carbamazepine is added. Similar increases may be required with other inducers.

Pharmacodynamics/Kinetics

Onset: Initial: 1-3 weeks

Absorption: Well absorbed

Distribution: V_d: 4.9 L/kg

Protein binding: 99%, primarily to albumin

Metabolism: Hepatic, via CYP2D6, CYP3A4 (dehydro-aripiprazole metabolite has affinity for D_2 receptors similar to the parent drug and represents 40% of the parent drug exposure in plasma)

Bioavailability: 87%

Half-life elimination: Aripiprazole: 75 hours; dehydro-aripiprazole: 94 hours
CYP2D6 poor metabolizers: Aripiprazole: 146 hours

Time to peak, plasma: 3-5 hours
Delayed with high-fat meal: Aripiprazole: 3 hours; dehydro-aripiprazole: 12 hours

Excretion: Feces (55%), urine (25%); primarily as metabolites

Pregnancy Risk Factor C

Dental Comment Aripiprazole works differently from the classic antipsychotics, such as chlorpromazine, in that it does not appear to block central dopaminergic receptors, but rather seems to be a stabilizer of dopamine-serotonin central systems. The risk of extrapyramidal reactions such as pseudoparkinsonism, acute dystonic reactions, akathisia, and tardive dyskinesia are low and the frequencies reported are similar to placebo. Aripiprazole may be associated with neuroleptic malignant syndrome (NMS).

Aristocort® *see* Triamcinolone *on page 1526*

Aristocort® A *see* Triamcinolone *on page 1526*

Aristospan® *see* Triamcinolone *on page 1526*

Arixtra® *see* Fondaparinux *on page 700*

A.R.M® [OTC] *see* Chlorpheniramine and Pseudoephedrine *on page 325*

Armour® Thyroid *see* Thyroid *on page 1482*

Aromasin® *see* Exemestane *on page 628*

Arranon® *see* Nelarabine *on page 1097*

Artane *see* Trihexyphenidyl *on page 1537*

ArthriCare® for Women Extra Moisturizing [OTC] *see* Capsaicin *on page 256*

ArthriCare® for Women Multi-Action [OTC] *see* Capsaicin *on page 256*

ArthriCare® for Women Silky Dry [OTC] *see* Capsaicin *on page 256*

ArthriCare® for Women Ultra Strength [OTC] [DSC] *see* Capsaicin *on page 256*

Arthrotec® *see* Diclofenac and Misoprostol *on page 462*

Articaine and Epinephrine (AR ti kane & ep i NEF rin)

Related Information
Epinephrine *on page 546*
Oral Pain *on page 1692*

U.S. Brand Names Septocaine™; Zorcaine™

Canadian Brand Names Astracaine®; Astracaine® Forte; Septanest® N; Septanest® SP; Ultracaine® D-S; Ultracaine® D-S Forte

Generic Available No

Synonyms Epinephrine and Articaine Hydrochloride

Pharmacologic Category Local Anesthetic

Dental Use Local, infiltrative, or conductive anesthesia in both simple and complex dental and periodontal procedures

Local Anesthetic/Vasoconstrictor Precautions No information available to require special precautions (see Dental Comment)

Effects on Dental Treatment No significant effects or complications reported

Significant Adverse Effects Adverse reactions to Septocaine™ are characteristic of those associated with other amide-type local anesthetics; adverse reactions to this group of drugs may also result from excessive plasma levels which may be due to overdosage, unintentional intravascular injection, or slow metabolic degradation.

≥1% (in controlled trial of 882 patients):
Central nervous system: Headache (4%), paresthesia (1%)
Gastrointestinal: Gingivitis (1%)
Miscellaneous: Pain (body as a whole 13%), facial edema (1%)

<1% (adverse and intercurrent events recorded in 1 or more patients in controlled trials, occurring at an overall rate of <1%, and considered clinically significant): Abdominal pain, accidental injury, arthralgia, asthenia, back pain, constipation, diarrhea, dizziness, dry mouth, dysmenorrhea, dyspepsia, ear pain, ecchymosis, edema, facial paralysis, glossitis, gum hemorrhage, hemorrhage, hyperesthesia, lymphadenopathy, malaise, migraine, mouth ulceration, (Continued)

Articaine and Epinephrine *(Continued)*

myalgia, nausea, neck pain, nervousness, neuropathy, osteomyelitis, pharyngitis, pruritus, rhinitis, salivation increased, skin disorder, somnolence, stomatitis, syncope, tachycardia, taste perversion, thirst, tongue edema, tooth disorder, vomiting

Additional adverse reactions reported with articaine and epinephrine: Arrhythmia, myocardial depression, asthma, convulsions, allergic reactions, injection site reactions, tissue necrosis

Dental Usual Dosing Adults:

Infiltration: Injection volume of 4% solution: 0.5-2.5 mL; total dose: 20-100 mg
Nerve block: Injection volume of 4% solution: 0.5-3.4 mL; total dose: 20-136 mg
Oral surgery: Injection volume of 4% solution: 1-5.1 mL; total dose: 40-204 mg
Note: These dosages are guides only; other dosages may be used; however, do not exceed maximum recommended dose

Special populations: The clinician is reminded that these doses serve only as a guide to the amount of anesthetic required for most routine procedures. The actual volumes to be used depend upon a number of factors, such as type and extent of surgical procedure, depth of anesthesia, degree of muscular relaxation, and condition of the patient. In all cases, the smallest dose that will produce the desired result should be given. Dosages should be reduced for pediatric patients, elderly patients, and patients with cardiac and/or liver disease.

Dosage Summary of recommended volumes and concentrations for various types of anesthetic procedures; dosages (administered by submucosal injection and/or nerve block) apply to normal healthy adults:

Infiltration: Injection volume of 4% solution: 0.5-2.5 mL; total dose: 20-100 mg
Nerve block: Injection volume of 4% solution: 0.5-3.4 mL; total dose: 20-136 mg
Oral surgery: Injection volume of 4% solution: 1-5.1 mL; total dose: 40-204 mg
Note: These dosages are guides only; other dosages may be used; however, do not exceed maximum recommended dose

Special populations: The clinician is reminded that these doses serve only as a guide to the amount of anesthetic required for most routine procedures. The actual volumes to be used depend upon a number of factors, such as type and extent of surgical procedure, depth of anesthesia, degree of muscular relaxation, and condition of the patient. In all cases, the smallest dose that will produce the desired result should be given. Dosages should be reduced for pediatric patients, elderly patients, and patients with cardiac and/or liver disease.

Children <4 years: Safety and efficacy have not been established
Children 4-16 years (dosages in a clinical trial of 61 patients):
Simple procedures: 0.76-5.65 mg/kg (0.9-5.1 mL) was administered safely to 51 patients
Complex procedures: 0.37-7.48 mg/kg (0.7-3.9 mL) was administered safely to 10 patients
Note: Approximately 13% of the pediatric patients required additional injections for complete anesthesia

Geriatric patients (dosages in a clinical trial):
65-75 years:
Simple procedures: 0.43-4.76 mg/kg (0.9-11.9 mL) was administered safely to 35 patients
Complex procedures: 1.05-4.27 mg/kg (1.3-6.8 mL) was administered safely to 19 patients
≥75 years:
Simple procedures: 0.78-4.76 mg/kg (1.3-11.9 mL) was administered safely to 7 patients
Complex procedures: 1.12-2.17 mg/kg (1.3-5.1 mL) was administered safely to 4 patients
Note: Approximately 6% of the patients 65-75 years of age (none of the patients ≥75 years of age) required additional injections for complete anesthesia, compared to 11% of the patients 17-65 years of age who required additional injections.

Maximum recommended dosages:
Children (use in pediatric patients <4 years is not recommended): Not to exceed 7 mg/kg (0.175 mL/kg) **or** 3.2 mg/lb (0.0795 mL/lb) of body weight
Adults (normal, healthy): Submucosal infiltration and/or nerve block: Not to exceed 7 mg/kg (0.175 mL/kg) **or** 3.2 mg/lb (0.0795 mL/lb) of body weight
The following numbers of dental cartridges (1.7 mL) provide the indicated amounts of articaine hydrochloride 4% and epinephrine 1:100,000:
1 cartridge provides 68 mg articaine HCl (4%) and 0.017 mg vasoconstrictor (epinephrine 1:100,000)

2 cartridges provides 136 mg articaine HCl (4%) and 0.034 mg vasoconstrictor (epinephrine 1:100,000)

3 cartridges provides 204 mg articaine HCl (4%) and 0.051 mg vasoconstrictor (epinephrine 1:100,000)

4 cartridges provides 272 mg articaine HCl (4%) and 0.068 mg vasoconstrictor (epinephrine 1:100,000)

5 cartridges provides 340 mg articaine HCl (4%) and 0.085 mg vasoconstrictor (epinephrine 1:100,000)

6 cartridges provides 408 mg articaine HCl (4%) and 0.102 mg vasoconstrictor (epinephrine 1:100,000)

7 cartridges provides 476 mg articaine HCl (4%) and 0.119 mg vasoconstrictor (epinephrine 1:100,000)

8 cartridges provides 544 mg articaine HCl (4%) and 0.136 mg vasoconstrictor (epinephrine 1:100,000)

Mechanism of Action Local anesthetics block the generation and conduction of nerve impulses, presumably by increasing the threshold for electrical excitation in the nerve, by slowing the propagation of the nerve impulse, and by reducing the rate of rise of the action potential. In general, the progression of anesthesia is related to the diameter, myelination, and conduction velocity of the affected nerve fibers. Clinically, the order of loss of nerve function is as follows: 1) pain, 2) temperature, 3) touch, 4) proprioception, and 5) skeletal muscle tone.

Contraindications Hypersensitivity to local anesthetics of the amide type or any component of the formulation

Warnings/Precautions Intravascular injections should be avoided; aspiration should be performed prior to administration; the needle must be repositioned until no return of blood can be elicited by aspiration; however, absence of blood in the syringe does not guarantee that intravascular injection has been avoided. **Accidental intravascular injection may be associated with convulsions, followed by CNS or cardiorespiratory depression and coma, ultimately progressing to respiratory arrest.** Dental practitioners and/or clinicians using local anesthetic agents should be well trained in diagnosis and management of emergencies that may arise from the use of these agents. Resuscitative equipment, oxygen, and other resuscitative drugs should be available for immediate use.

Contains epinephrine, which can cause local tissue necrosis or systemic toxicity, usual precautions for epinephrine administration should be observed. Administration of articaine HCl with epinephrine results in a three- to fivefold increase in plasma epinephrine concentrations compared to baseline; however, in healthy adults, it does not appear to be associated with marked increases in blood pressure or heart rate, except in the case of accidental intravascular injection.

Products may contain sodium metabisulfite, which may cause allergic-type reactions (including anaphylactic symptoms, and life-threatening or less severe asthmatic episodes) in certain susceptible patients. The overall prevalence of the sulfite sensitivity in the general population is unknown, and is seen more frequently in asthmatic than in nonasthmatic persons.

To avoid serious adverse effects and high plasma levels, the lowest dosage resulting in effective anesthesia should be administered. Repeated doses may cause significant increases in blood levels with each repeated dose due to the possibility of accumulation of the drug or its metabolites. Tolerance to elevated blood levels varies with patient status. Reduced dosages, commensurate with age and physical condition, should be given to debilitated patients, elderly patients, acutely-ill patients, and pediatric patients. Use caution in patients with heart block.

Local anesthetic solutions containing a vasoconstrictor should be used cautiously. Patients with peripheral vascular disease or hypertensive vascular disease may exhibit exaggerated vasoconstrictor response, possibly resulting in ischemic injury or necrosis. It should also be used cautiously in patients during or following the administration of a potent general anesthetic agent, since cardiac arrhythmias may occur under these conditions.

Systemic absorption of local anesthetics may produce CNS and cardiovascular effects. Changes in cardiac conduction, excitability, refractoriness, contractility, and peripheral vascular resistance are minimal at blood concentrations produced by therapeutic doses. However, toxic blood concentrations depress cardiac conduction and excitability, which may lead to AV block, ventricular arrhythmias, and cardiac arrest (sometimes resulting in death). In addition, myocardial contractility is depressed and peripheral vasodilation occurs, leading to decreased cardiac output and arterial blood pressure.
(Continued)

Articaine and Epinephrine (Continued)

Careful and constant monitoring of cardiovascular and respiratory (adequacy of ventilation) vital signs and the patient's state of consciousness should be done following each local anesthetic injection; at such times, restlessness, anxiety, tinnitus, dizziness, blurred vision, tremors, depression, or drowsiness may be early warning signs of CNS toxicity.

In vitro studies show that ~5% to 10% of articaine is metabolized by the human liver microsomal P450 isoenzyme system; however, no studies have been performed in patient with liver dysfunction, and caution should be used in patients with severe hepatic disease. Use with caution in patients with impaired cardiovascular function, since they may be less able to compensate for function changes associated with prolonged AV conduction produced by these drugs.

Small doses of local anesthetics injected into dental blocks may produce adverse reactions similar to systemic toxicity seen in unintentional intravascular injections at larger doses. Confusion, convulsions, respiratory depression and/or respiratory arrest, and cardiovascular stimulation or depression have been reported. These reactions may be due to intra-arterial injection of the local anesthetic with retrograde flow to the cerebral circulation. Patients receiving such blocks should be observed constantly with resuscitative equipment and personnel trained in treatment of adverse reactions immediately available. Dosage recommendations should not be exceeded.

Drug Interactions

MAO inhibitors: Administration of local anesthetic solutions containing epinephrine may produce severe, prolonged hypertension.

Phenothiazines, butyrophenones: May reduce or reverse the pressor effects of epinephrine; concurrent use of these agents should be avoided; in situations when concurrent therapy is necessary, careful patient monitoring is essential.

Tricyclic antidepressants: Pressor response to I.V. epinephrine, norepinephrine, and phenylephrine may be enhanced in patients receiving TCAs **(Note:** Effect is unlikely with epinephrine or levonordefrin dosages typically administered as infiltration in combination with local anesthetics).

Pharmacodynamics/Kinetics

Onset of action: 1-6 minutes

Duration: Complete anesthesia: ~1 hour

Metabolism: Hepatic via plasma carboxyesterase to articainic acid (inactive)

Half-life elimination: Articaine: 1.8 hours; Articainic acid: 1.5 hours

Excretion: Urine (primarily as metabolites)

Pregnancy Risk Factor C

Lactation Excretion in breast milk unknown/use caution

Breast-Feeding Considerations It is not known whether articaine is excreted in human milk.

Dosage Forms Injection, solution (Septocaine™, Zorcaine™): Articaine hydrochloride 4% and epinephrine bitartrate 1:100,000 (1.7 mL) [contains sodium metabisulfite]

Additional dosage forms available in Canada: Injection, solution:

Ultracaine DS®: Articaine hydrochloride 4% and epinephrine 1:200,000 (1.7 mL) [contains sodium metabisulfite]

Ultracaine DS Forte®: Articaine hydrochloride 4% and epinephrine 1:100,000 (1.7 mL) [contains sodium metabisulfite]

Dental Comment Septocaine™ (articaine hydrochloride 4% and epinephrine 1:100,000) is the first FDA approval in 30 years of a new local dental anesthetic providing complete pulpal anesthesia for approximately 1 hour. Chemically, articaine contains both an amide linkage and an ester linkage, making it chemically unique in the class of local anesthetics. Since it contains the ester linkage, articaine HCl is rapidly metabolized by plasma carboxyesterase to its primary metabolite, articainic acid, which is an inactive product of this metabolism. According to the manufacturer, *in vitro* studies show that the human liver microsomal P450 isoenzyme system metabolizes approximately 5% to 10% of available articaine with nearly quantitative conversion to articainic acid. The elimination half-life of articaine is about 1.8 hours, and that of articainic acid is about 1.5 hours. Articaine is excreted primarily through urine with 53% to 57% of the administered dose eliminated in the first 24 hours following submucosal administration. Articainic acid is the primary metabolite in urine. A minor metabolite, articainic acid glucuronide, is also excreted in the urine. Articaine constitutes only 2% of the total dose excreted in urine.

Selected Readings

Budenz AW, "Local Anesthetics in Dentistry: Then and Now," *J Calif Dent Assoc*, 2003, 31(5):388-96.

Dower JS Jr, "A Review of Paresthesia in Association With Administration of Local Anesthesia," *Dent Today*, 2003, 22(2):64-9.

Finder RL and Moore PA, "Adverse Drug Reactions to Local Anesthesia," *Dent Clin North Am*, 2002, 46(4):747-57, x.

Haas DA, "An Update on Local Anesthetics in Dentistry," *J Can Dent Assoc*, 2002, 68(9):546-51.

Hawkins JM and Moore PA, "Local Anesthesia: Advances in Agents and Techniques," *Dent Clin North Am*, 2002, 46(4):719-32, ix.

"Injectable Local Anesthetics," *J Am Dent Assoc*, 2003, 134(5):628-9.

Malamed SF, Gagnon S, Leblanc D, "A Comparison Between Articaine HCl and Lidocaine HCl in Pediatric Dental Patients," *Pediatr Dent*, 2000, 22(4):307-11.

Malamed SF, "Allergy and Toxic Reactions to Local Anesthetics," *Dent Today*, 2003, 22(4):114-6, 118-21.

Malamed SF, Gagnon S, Leblanc D, "Articaine Hydrochloride: A Study of the Safety of a New Amide Local Anesthetic," *J Am Dent Assoc*, 2001, 132(2):177-85.

Malamed SF, Gagnon S, Leblanc D, "Efficacy of Articaine: A New Amide Local Anesthetic," *J Am Dent Assoc*, 2000, 131(5):635-42.

Schertzer ER Jr, "Articaine vs lidocaine," *J Am Dent Assoc*, 2000, 131(9):1248, 1250.

Weaver JM, "Articaine, A New Local Anesthetic for American Dentists: Will It Supersede Lidocaine?" *Anesth Prog*, 1999, 46(4):111-2.

Wynn RL, Bergman SA, and Meiller TF, "Paresthesia Associated With Local Anesthetics: A Perspective on Articaine," *Gen Dent*, 2003, 51(6):498-501.

Artificial Tears (ar ti FISH il tears)

U.S. Brand Names Akwa Tears® [OTC]; AquaSite® [OTC]; Bion® Tears [OTC]; HypoTears [OTC]; HypoTears PF [OTC]; Isopto® Tears [OTC]; Liquifilm® Tears [OTC]; Moisture® Eyes [OTC]; Moisture® Eyes PM [OTC]; Murine® Tears [OTC]; Murocel® [OTC]; Nature's Tears® [OTC]; Nu-Tears® [OTC]; Nu-Tears® II [OTC]; OcuCoat® [OTC]; OcuCoat® PF [OTC]; Puralube® Tears [OTC]; Refresh® [OTC]; Refresh Plus® [OTC]; Refresh Tears® [OTC]; Teargen® [OTC]; Teargen® II [OTC]; Tearisol® [OTC]; Tears Again® [OTC]; Tears Naturale® [OTC]; Tears Naturale® Free [OTC]; Tears Naturale® II [OTC]; Tears Plus® [OTC]; Tears Renewed® [OTC]; Ultra Tears® [OTC]; Viva-Drops® [OTC]

Canadian Brand Names Teardrops®

Generic Available Yes

Synonyms Hydroxyethylcellulose; Polyvinyl Alcohol

Pharmacologic Category Ophthalmic Agent, Miscellaneous

Use Ophthalmic lubricant; for relief of dry eyes and eye irritation

Local Anesthetic/Vasoconstrictor Precautions No information available to require special precautions

Effects on Dental Treatment No significant effects or complications reported

Pregnancy Risk Factor C

ASA *see* Aspirin *on page 145*

5-ASA *see* Mesalamine *on page 996*

Asacol® *see* Mesalamine *on page 996*

Ascorbic Acid (a SKOR bik AS id)

U.S. Brand Names C-500-GR™ [OTC]; Cecon® [OTC]; Cevi-Bid® [OTC]; C-Gram [OTC]; Dull-C® [OTC]; Vita-C® [OTC]

Canadian Brand Names Proflavanol C™; Revitalose C-1000®

Mexican Brand Names Cevalin®; Redoxon®

Generic Available Yes

Synonyms Vitamin C

Pharmacologic Category Vitamin, Water Soluble

Use Prevention and treatment of scurvy; acidify the urine

Unlabeled/Investigational Use Investigational: In large doses, to decrease the severity of "colds"; dietary supplementation; a 20-year study was recently completed involving 730 individuals which indicates a possible decreased risk of death by stroke when ascorbic acid at doses ≥45 mg/day was administered

Local Anesthetic/Vasoconstrictor Precautions No information available to require special precautions

Effects on Dental Treatment No significant effects or complications reported

Common Adverse Effects

1% to 10%: Renal: Hyperoxaluria with large doses

Mechanism of Action Not fully understood; necessary for collagen formation and tissue repair; involved in some oxidation-reduction reactions as well as other metabolic pathways, such as synthesis of carnitine, steroids, and catecholamines and conversion of folic acid to folinic acid

Drug Interactions

Increased Effect/Toxicity: Ascorbic acid enhances iron absorption from the GI tract. Concomitant ascorbic acid taken with oral contraceptives may increase contraceptive effect.

Decreased Effect: Ascorbic acid and fluphenazine may decrease fluphenazine levels. Ascorbic acid and warfarin may decrease anticoagulant effect. (Continued)

Ascorbic Acid *(Continued)*

Changes in dose of ascorbic acid when taken with oral contraceptives may reduce the contraceptive effect.

Pharmacodynamics/Kinetics

Absorption: Oral: Readily absorbed; an active process thought to be dose dependent

Distribution: Large

Metabolism: Hepatic via oxidation and sulfation

Excretion: Urine (with high blood levels)

Pregnancy Risk Factor A/C (dose exceeding RDA recommendation)

Ascorbic Acid and Ferrous Sulfate *see* Ferrous Sulfate and Ascorbic Acid *on page 651*

Ascriptin® [OTC] *see* Aspirin *on page 145*

Ascriptin® Extra Strength [OTC] *see* Aspirin *on page 145*

Asendin [DSC] *see* Amoxapine *on page 105*

Asmanex® Twisthaler® *see* Mometasone Furoate *on page 1060*

Asparaginase *(a SPEAR a ji nase)*

U.S. Brand Names Elspar®

Canadian Brand Names Elspar®; Erwinase®; Kidrolase®

Mexican Brand Names Leunase®

Generic Available No

Synonyms *E. coli* Asparaginase; *Erwinia* Asparaginase; L-asparaginase; NSC-106977 (*Erwinia*); NSC-109229 (*E. coli*)

Pharmacologic Category Antineoplastic Agent, Miscellaneous

Use Treatment of acute lymphocytic leukemia, lymphoma

Local Anesthetic/Vasoconstrictor Precautions No information available to require special precautions

Effects on Dental Treatment Key adverse event(s) related to dental treatment: Stomatitis.

Common Adverse Effects Note: Immediate effects: Fever, chills, nausea, and vomiting occur in 50% to 60% of patients.

>10%:

Central nervous system: Fatigue, fever, chills, somnolence, depression, hallucinations, agitation, disorientation, or convulsions (10% to 60%), stupor, confusion, coma (25%)

Endocrine & metabolic: Hyperglycemia (10%)

Gastrointestinal: Nausea, vomiting (50% to 60%), anorexia, abdominal cramps (70%), acute pancreatitis (15%, may be severe in some patients)

Hematologic: Hypofibrinogenemia and depression of clotting factors V and VIII, variable decrease in factors VII and IX, severe protein C deficiency and decrease in antithrombin III (may be dose limiting or fatal)

Hepatic: Transaminases, bilirubin, and alkaline phosphatase increased (transient)

Hypersensitivity: Acute allergic reactions (fever, rash, urticaria, arthralgia, hypotension, angioedema, bronchospasm, anaphylaxis (15% to 35%); may be dose limiting in some patients, may be fatal)

Renal: Azotemia (66%)

1% to 10%:

Endocrine & metabolic: Hyperuricemia

Gastrointestinal: Stomatitis

Mechanism of Action Asparaginase inhibits protein synthesis by hydrolyzing asparagine to aspartic acid and ammonia. Leukemia cells, especially lymphoblasts, require exogenous asparagine; normal cells can synthesize asparagine. Asparaginase is cycle-specific for the G_1 phase.

Drug Interactions

Increased Effect/Toxicity: Increased toxicity has been noticed when asparaginase is administered with vincristine (neuropathy) and prednisone (hyperglycemia). Decreased metabolism when used with cyclophosphamide. Increased hepatotoxicity when used with mercaptopurine.

Decreased Effect: Asparaginase terminates methotrexate action.

Pharmacodynamics/Kinetics

Absorption: I.M.: Produces peak blood levels 50% lower than those from I.V. administration

Distribution: V_d: 4-5 L/kg; 70% to 80% of plasma volume; does not penetrate CSF

Metabolism: Systemically degraded

Half-life elimination: 8-30 hours

Excretion: Urine (trace amounts)
Clearance: Unaffected by age, renal or hepatic function
Pregnancy Risk Factor C

Aspart Insulin *see* Insulin Aspart *on page 835*

Aspercin [OTC] *see* Aspirin *on page 145*

Aspercin Extra [OTC] *see* Aspirin *on page 145*

Aspercreme® [OTC] *see* Triethanolamine Salicylate *on page 1535*

Aspergum® [OTC] *see* Aspirin *on page 145*

Aspirin (AS pir in)

Related Information
Cardiovascular Diseases *on page 1636*
Oral Pain *on page 1692*
Rheumatoid Arthritis, Osteoarthritis, and Osteoporosis *on page 1668*
U.S. Brand Names Ascriptin® [OTC]; Ascriptin® Extra Strength [OTC]; Aspercin [OTC]; Aspercin Extra [OTC]; Aspergum® [OTC]; Bayer® Aspirin [OTC]; Bayer® Aspirin Extra Strength [OTC]; Bayer® Aspirin Regimen Adult Low Strength [OTC]; Bayer® Aspirin Regimen Children's [OTC]; Bayer® Aspirin Regimen Regular Strength [OTC]; Bayer® Extra Strength Arthritis Pain Regimen [OTC]; Bayer® Plus Extra Strength [OTC]; Bayer® Women's Aspirin Plus Calcium [OTC]; Bufferin® [OTC]; Bufferin® Extra Strength [OTC]; Buffinol [OTC]; Buffinol Extra [OTC]; Easprin®; Ecotrin® [OTC]; Ecotrin® Low Strength [OTC]; Ecotrin® Maximum Strength [OTC]; Halfprin® [OTC]; St. Joseph® Adult Aspirin [OTC]; Sureprin 81™ [OTC]; ZORprin®
Canadian Brand Names Asaphen; Asaphen E.C.; Entrophen®; Novasen
Generic Available Yes: Excludes gum
Synonyms Acetylsalicylic Acid; ASA
Pharmacologic Category Salicylate
Dental Use Treatment of postoperative pain
Use Treatment of mild-to-moderate pain, inflammation, and fever; may be used as prophylaxis of myocardial infarction; prophylaxis of stroke and/or transient ischemic episodes; management of rheumatoid arthritis, rheumatic fever, osteoarthritis, and gout (high dose); adjunctive therapy in revascularization procedures (coronary artery bypass graft [CABG], percutaneous transluminal coronary angioplasty [PTCA], carotid endarterectomy), stent implantation
Unlabeled/Investigational Use Low doses have been used in the prevention of pre-eclampsia, complications associated with autoimmune disorders such as lupus or antiphospholipid syndrome
Local Anesthetic/Vasoconstrictor Precautions No information available to require special precautions
Effects on Dental Treatment Key adverse event(s) related to dental treatment: As with all drugs which may affect hemostasis, bleeding is associated with aspirin. Hemorrhage may occur at virtually any site; risk is dependent on multiple variables including dosage, concurrent use of multiple agents which alter hemostasis, and patient susceptibility. Many adverse effects of aspirin are dose related, and are rare at low dosages. Other serious reactions are idiosyncratic, related to allergy or individual sensitivity (see Dental Comment).
Significant Adverse Effects As with all drugs which may affect hemostasis, bleeding is associated with aspirin. Hemorrhage may occur at virtually any site. Risk is dependent on multiple variables including dosage, concurrent use of multiple agents which alter hemostasis, and patient susceptibility. Many adverse effects of aspirin are dose related, and are extremely rare at low dosages. Other serious reactions are idiosyncratic, related to allergy or individual sensitivity. Accurate estimation of frequencies is not possible.

Cardiovascular: Hypotension, tachycardia, dysrhythmias, edema
Central nervous system: Fatigue, insomnia, nervousness, agitation, confusion, dizziness, headache, lethargy, cerebral edema, hyperthermia, coma
Dermatologic: Rash, angioedema, urticaria
Endocrine & metabolic: Acidosis, hyperkalemia, dehydration, hypoglycemia (children), hyperglycemia, hypernatremia (buffered forms)
Gastrointestinal: Nausea, vomiting, dyspepsia, epigastric discomfort, heartburn, stomach pain, gastrointestinal ulceration (6% to 31%), gastric erosions, gastric erythema, duodenal ulcers
Hematologic: Anemia, disseminated intravascular coagulation, prothrombin times prolonged, coagulopathy, thrombocytopenia, hemolytic anemia, bleeding, iron-deficiency anemia
Hepatic: Hepatotoxicity, transaminases increased, hepatitis (reversible)
Neuromuscular & skeletal: Rhabdomyolysis, weakness, acetabular bone destruction (OA)
(Continued)

145

Aspirin *(Continued)*

Otic: Hearing loss, tinnitus

Renal: Interstitial nephritis, papillary necrosis, proteinuria, renal failure (including cases caused by rhabdomyolysis), BUN increased, serum creatinine increased

Respiratory: Asthma, bronchospasm, dyspnea, laryngeal edema, hyperpnea, tachypnea, respiratory alkalosis, noncardiogenic pulmonary edema

Miscellaneous: Anaphylaxis, prolonged pregnancy and labor, stillbirths, low birth weight, peripartum bleeding, Reye's syndrome

Postmarketing and/or case reports: Colonic ulceration, esophageal stricture, esophagitis with esophageal ulcer, esophageal hematoma, oral mucosal ulcers (aspirin-containing chewing gum), coronary artery spasm, conduction defect and atrial fibrillation (toxicity), delirium, ischemic brain infarction, colitis, rectal stenosis (suppository), cholestatic jaundice, periorbital edema, rhinosinusitis

Dental Usual Dosing Postoperative pain:

Analgesic and antipyretic: Oral, rectal:
Children: 10-15 mg/kg/dose every 4-6 hours, up to a total of 4 g/day
Adults: 325-650 mg every 4-6 hours up to 4 g/day

Anti-inflammatory: Oral: Initial:
Children: 60-90 mg/kg/day in divided doses; usual maintenance: 80-100 mg/kg/day divided every 6-8 hours; monitor serum concentrations
Adults: 2.4-3.6 g/day in divided doses; usual maintenance: 3.6-5.4 g/day; monitor serum concentrations

Dosage

Children:

Analgesic and antipyretic: Oral, rectal: 10-15 mg/kg/dose every 4-6 hours, up to a total of 4 g/day

Anti-inflammatory: Oral: Initial: 60-90 mg/kg/day in divided doses; usual maintenance: 80-100 mg/kg/day divided every 6-8 hours; monitor serum concentrations

Antiplatelet effects: Adequate pediatric studies have not been performed; pediatric dosage is derived from adult studies and clinical experience and is not well established; suggested doses have ranged from 3-5 mg/kg/day to 5-10 mg/kg/day given as a single daily dose. Doses are rounded to a convenient amount (eg, $1/2$ of 80 mg tablet).

Mechanical prosthetic heart valves: 6-20 mg/kg/day given as a single daily dose (used in combination with an oral anticoagulant in children who have systemic embolism despite adequate oral anticoagulation therapy (INR 2.5-3.5) and used in combination with low-dose anticoagulation (INR 2-3) and dipyridamole when full-dose oral anticoagulation is contraindicated)

Blalock-Taussig shunts: 3-5 mg/kg/day given as a single daily dose

Kawasaki disease: Oral: 80-100 mg/kg/day divided every 6 hours; monitor serum concentrations; after fever resolves: 3-5 mg/kg/day once daily; in patients without coronary artery abnormalities, give lower dose for at least 6-8 weeks or until ESR and platelet count are normal; in patients with coronary artery abnormalities, low-dose aspirin should be continued indefinitely

Antirheumatic: Oral: 60-100 mg/kg/day in divided doses every 4 hours

Adults:

Analgesic and antipyretic: Oral, rectal: 325-650 mg every 4-6 hours up to 4 g/day

Anti-inflammatory: Oral: Initial: 2.4-3.6 g/day in divided doses; usual maintenance: 3.6-5.4 g/day; monitor serum concentrations

Myocardial infarction prophylaxis: 75-325 mg/day; use of a lower aspirin dosage has been recommended in patients receiving ACE inhibitors

Acute myocardial infarction: 160-325 mg/day (have patient chew tablet if not taking aspirin before presentation)

CABG: 75-325 mg/day starting 6 hours following procedure; if bleeding prevents administration at 6 hours after CABG, initiate as soon as possible

PTCA: Initial: 80-325 mg/day starting 2 hours before procedure; longer pretreatment durations (up to 24 hours) should be considered if lower dosages (80-100 mg) are used

Stent implantation: Oral: 325 mg 2 hours prior to implantation and 160-325 mg daily thereafter

Carotid endarterectomy: 81-325 mg/day preoperatively and daily thereafter

Acute stroke: 160-325 mg/day, initiated within 48 hours (in patients who are not candidates for thrombolytics and are not receiving systemic anticoagulation)

Stroke prevention/TIA: 30-325 mg/day (dosages up to 1300 mg/day in 2-4 divided doses have been used in clinical trials)

Pre-eclampsia prevention (unlabeled use): 60-80 mg/day during gestational weeks 13-26 (patient selection criteria not established)

Dosing adjustment in renal impairment: Cl_{cr} <10 mL/minute: Avoid use.

Hemodialysis: Dialyzable (50% to 100%)

Dosing adjustment in hepatic disease: Avoid use in severe liver disease.

Mechanism of Action Inhibits prostaglandin synthesis, acts on the hypothalamus heat-regulating center to reduce fever, blocks prostaglandin synthetase action which prevents formation of the platelet-aggregating substance thromboxane A_2

Contraindications Hypersensitivity to salicylates, other NSAIDs, or any component of the formulation; asthma; rhinitis; nasal polyps; inherited or acquired bleeding disorders (including factor VII and factor IX deficiency); do not use in children (<16 years of age) for viral infections (chickenpox or flu symptoms), with or without fever, due to a potential association with Reye's syndrome; pregnancy (3rd trimester especially)

Warnings/Precautions Use with caution in patients with platelet and bleeding disorders, renal dysfunction, dehydration, erosive gastritis, or peptic ulcer disease. Heavy ethanol use (>3 drinks/day) can increase bleeding risks. Avoid use in severe renal failure or in severe hepatic failure. Discontinue use if tinnitus or impaired hearing occurs. Caution in mild-to-moderate renal failure (only at high dosages). Patients with sensitivity to tartrazine dyes, nasal polyps, and asthma may have an increased risk of salicylate sensitivity. Surgical patients should avoid ASA if possible, for 1-2 weeks prior to surgery, to reduce the risk of excessive bleeding.

When used for self-medication (OTC labeling): Children and teenagers who have or are recovering from chickenpox or flu-like symptoms should not use this product. Changes in behavior (along with nausea and vomiting) may be an early sign of Reye's syndrome; patients should be instructed to contact their healthcare provider if these occur.

Drug Interactions Substrate of CYP2C9 (minor)

ACE inhibitors: The effects of ACE inhibitors may be blunted by aspirin administration, particularly at higher dosages.

Buspirone increases aspirin's free % *in vitro*.

Carbonic anhydrase inhibitors and corticosteroids have been associated with alteration in salicylate serum concentrations.

Heparin and low molecular weight heparins: Concurrent use may increase the risk of bleeding.

Methotrexate serum levels may be increased; consider discontinuing aspirin 2-3 days before high-dose methotrexate treatment or avoid concurrent use.

NSAIDs may increase the risk of gastrointestinal adverse effects and bleeding. Serum concentrations of some NSAIDs may be decreased by aspirin. Ibuprofen, and possibly other COX-1 inhibitors, may reduce the cardioprotective effects of aspirin. Avoid giving prior to aspirin therapy or on a regular basis in patients with CAD.

Platelet inhibitors (IIb/IIIa antagonists): Risk of bleeding may be increased.

Probenecid effects may be antagonized by aspirin.

Sulfonylureas: The effects of older sulfonylurea agents (tolazamide, tolbutamide) may be potentiated due to displacement from plasma proteins. This effect does not appear to be clinically significant for newer sulfonylurea agents (glyburide, glipizide, glimepiride).

Valproic acid may be displaced from its binding sites which can result in toxicity.

Verapamil may potentiate the prolongation of bleeding time associated with aspirin.

Warfarin and oral anticoagulants may increase the risk of bleeding.

Ethanol/Nutrition/Herb Interactions

Ethanol: Avoid ethanol (may enhance gastric mucosal damage).

Food: Food may decrease the rate but not the extent of oral absorption.

Folic acid: Hyperexcretion of folate; folic acid deficiency may result, leading to macrocytic anemia.

Iron: With chronic aspirin use and at doses of 3-4 g/day, iron-deficiency anemia may result.

Sodium: Hypernatremia resulting from buffered aspirin solutions or sodium salicylate containing high sodium content. Avoid or use with caution in CHF or any condition where hypernatremia would be detrimental.

Benedictine liqueur, prunes, raisins, tea, and gherkins: Potential salicylate accumulation.

Fresh fruits containing vitamin C: Displace drug from binding sites, resulting in increased urinary excretion of aspirin.

Herb/Nutraceutical: Avoid cat's claw, dong quai, evening primrose, feverfew, garlic, ginger, ginkgo, red clover, horse chestnut, green tea, ginseng (all have additional antiplatelet activity). Limit curry powder, paprika, licorice; may

(Continued)

Aspirin *(Continued)*

cause salicylate accumulation. These foods contain 6 mg salicylate/100 g. An ordinarily American diet contains 10-200 mg/day of salicylate.

Dietary Considerations Take with food or large volume of water or milk to minimize GI upset.

Pharmacodynamics/Kinetics

Duration: 4-6 hours

Absorption: Rapid

Distribution: V_d: 10 L; readily into most body fluids and tissues

Metabolism: Hydrolyzed to salicylate (active) by esterases in GI mucosa, red blood cells, synovial fluid, and blood; metabolism of salicylate occurs primarily by hepatic conjugation; metabolic pathways are saturable

Bioavailability: 50% to 75% reaches systemic circulation

Half-life elimination: Parent drug: 15-20 minutes; Salicylates (dose dependent): 3 hours at lower doses (300-600 mg), 5-6 hours (after 1 g), 10 hours with higher doses

Time to peak, serum: ~1-2 hours

Excretion: Urine (75% as salicyluric acid, 10% as salicylic acid)

Pregnancy Risk Factor C/D (full-dose aspirin in 3rd trimester - expert analysis)

Lactation Enters breast milk/use caution

Breast-Feeding Considerations Low amounts of aspirin can be found in breast milk. Milk/plasma ratios ranging from 0.03-0.3 have been reported. Peak levels in breast milk are reported to be at ~9 hours after a dose. Metabolic acidosis was reported in one infant following an aspirin dose of 3.9 g/day in the mother. The AAP states that aspirin should be used with caution while breast-feeding. The WHO considers occasional doses of aspirin to be compatible with breast-feeding, but to avoid long-term therapy and consider monitoring the infant for adverse effects. Other sources suggest avoiding aspirin while breast-feeding due to the theoretical risk of Reye's syndrome.

Dosage Forms

Caplet:

Bayer® Aspirin: 325 mg

Bayer® Aspirin Extra Strength: 500 mg

Bayer® Extra Strength Arthritis Pain Regimen: 500 mg [enteric coated]

Bayer® Women's Aspirin Plus Calcium: 81 mg [contains elemental calcium 300 mg]

Caplet, buffered (Ascriptin® Extra Strength): 500 mg [contains aluminum hydroxide, calcium carbonate, and magnesium hydroxide]

Gelcap (Bayer® Aspirin Extra Strength): 500 mg

Gum (Aspergum®): 227 mg [cherry or orange flavor]

Suppository, rectal: 300 mg, 600 mg

Tablet: 325 mg

Aspercin: 325 mg

Aspercin Extra: 500 mg

Bayer® Aspirin: 325 mg [film coated]

Tablet, buffered: 325 mg

Ascriptin®: 325 mg [contains aluminum hydroxide, calcium carbonate, and magnesium hydroxide]

Bayer® Plus Extra Strength: 500 mg [contains calcium carbonate]

Bufferin®: 325 mg [contains citric acid]

Bufferin® Extra Strength: 500 mg [contains citric acid]

Buffinol: 325 mg [contains magnesium oxide]

Buffinol Extra: 500 mg [contains magnesium oxide]

Tablet, chewable: 81 mg

Bayer® Aspirin Regimen Children's Chewable: 81 mg [cherry, mint or orange flavor]

St. Joseph® Adult Aspirin: 81 mg [orange flavor]

Tablet, controlled release (ZORprin®): 800 mg

Tablet, enteric coated: 81 mg, 325 mg, 500 mg, 650 mg

Bayer® Aspirin Regimen Adult Low Strength, Ecotrin® Low Strength, St. Joseph Adult Aspirin: 81 mg

Bayer® Aspirin Regimen Regular Strength, Ecotrin®: 325 mg

Easprin®: 975 mg

Ecotrin® Maximum Strength: 500 mg

Halfprin®: 81 mg, 162 mg

Sureprin 81™: 81 mg

Dental Comment There is no scientific evidence to warrant discontinuance of aspirin prior to dental surgery. Patients taking one aspirin tablet daily as an antithrombotic and who require dental surgery should be given special consideration in consultation with the physician before removal of the aspirin relative to prevention of postoperative bleeding.

Selected Readings

Daniel NG, Goulet J, Bergeron M, et al, "Antiplatelet Drugs: Is There a Surgical Risk?" *J Can Dent Assoc*, 2002, 68(11):683-7.

Forbes JA, Butterworth GA, Burchfield WH, et al, "Evaluation of Ketorolac, Aspirin, and an Aceta-minophen-Codeine Combination in Postoperative Oral Surgery Pain," *Pharmacotherapy*, 1990, 10(6 Pt 2):77S-93S.

Hurlen M, Erikssen J, Smith P, et al, "Comparison of Bleeding Complications of Warfarin and Warfarin Plus Acetylsalicylic Acid: A Study in 3166 Outpatients," *J Intern Med*, 1994, 236(3):299-304.

Jeske AH, Suchko GD, ADA Council on Scientific Affairs and Division of Science, et al, "Lack of a Scientific Basis for Routine Discontinuation of Oral Anticoagulation Therapy Before Dental Treat-ment," *J Am Dent Assoc*, 2003, 134(11):1492-7.

Little JW, Miller CS, Henry RG, et al, "Antithrombotic Agents: Implications in Dentistry," *Oral Surg Oral Med Oral Pathol Oral Radiol Endod*, 2002, 93(5):544-51.

Schrodi J, Recio L, Fiorellini J, et al, "The Effect of Aspirin on the Periodontal Parameter Bleeding on Probing," *J Periodontol*, 2002, 73(8):871-6.

Scully C and Wolff A, "Oral Surgery in Patients on Anticoagulant Therapy," *Oral Surg Oral Med Oral Pathol Oral Radiol Endod*, 2002, 94(1):57-64.

Aspirin, Acetaminophen, and Caffeine *see* Acetaminophen, Aspirin, and Caffeine *on page 41*

Aspirin and Carisoprodol *see* Carisoprodol and Aspirin *on page 272*

Aspirin and Codeine (AS pir in & KOE deen)

Related Information

Aspirin *on page 145*
Codeine *on page 385*
Oral Pain *on page 1692*

Canadian Brand Names Coryphen® Codeine

Generic Available Yes

Synonyms Codeine Phosphate and Aspirin

Pharmacologic Category Analgesic, Narcotic

Dental Use Treatment of postoperative pain

Use Relief of mild-to-moderate pain

Local Anesthetic/Vasoconstrictor Precautions No information available to require special precautions

Effects on Dental Treatment Key adverse event(s) related to dental treat-ment: Elderly are a high-risk population for adverse effects from nonsteroidal anti-inflammatory agents. As many as 60% of elderly patients with GI complica-tions from NSAIDs can develop peptic ulceration and/or hemorrhage asymp-tomatically. Concomitant disease and drug use contribute to the risk of GI adverse effects. Use lowest effective dose for shortest period possible. Consider renal function decline with age. See Dental Comment.

Significant Adverse Effects Frequency not defined.

Cardiovascular: Palpitations, hypotension, bradycardia, peripheral vasodilation
Central nervous system: CNS depression, intracranial pressure increased
Dermatologic: Pruritus, rash, urticaria
Endocrine & metabolic: Antidiuretic hormone release
Gastrointestinal: Nausea, vomiting, constipation
Hematologic: Occult bleeding
Hepatic: Hepatotoxicity
Respiratory: Respiratory depression, bronchospasm
Ocular: Miosis
Miscellaneous: Physical and psychological dependence, biliary or urinary tract spasm, histamine release, anaphylaxis

Restrictions C-III

Dental Usual Dosing Postoperative pain: Adults: Oral: 1-2 tablets every 4-6 hours as needed for pain

Dosage Oral:

Children:
Aspirin: 10 mg/kg/dose every 4 hours
Codeine: 0.5-1 mg/kg/dose every 4 hours
Adults: 1-2 tablets every 4-6 hours as needed for pain

Dosing adjustment in renal impairment:
Cl_{cr} 10-50 mL/minute: Administer 75% of dose
Cl_{cr} <10 mL/minute: Avoid use

Dosing interval in hepatic disease: Avoid use in severe liver disease

Mechanism of Action Aspirin inhibits prostaglandin synthesis, acts on the hypothalamus heat-regulating center to reduce fever, blocks prostaglandin synthetase action which prevents formation of the platelet-aggregating substance thromboxane A_2; codeine binds to opiate receptors (mu and kappa subtypes) in the CNS causing inhibition of ascending pain pathways, altering the perception of and response to pain

(Continued)

149

Aspirin and Codeine *(Continued)*

Contraindications Hypersensitivity to aspirin, codeine, or any component of the formulation; premature infants or during labor for delivery of a premature infant; pregnancy

Warnings/Precautions Use with caution in patients with impaired renal function, erosive gastritis, or peptic ulcer disease

Enhanced analgesia has been seen in elderly patients on therapeutic doses of narcotics; duration of action may be increased in the elderly; the elderly may be particularly susceptible to the CNS depressant and constipating effects of narcotics

Drug Interactions Aspirin: **Substrate** of CYP2C9 (minor)

Also see individual agents.

Ethanol/Nutrition/Herb Interactions Food: Food decreases rate but not extent of absorption (oral).

Dietary Considerations May be taken with food or milk to minimize GI distress.

Pharmacodynamics/Kinetics See individual agents.

Pregnancy Risk Factor D

Lactation Enters breast milk/use caution

Dosage Forms Tablet:

#3: Aspirin 325 mg and codeine phosphate 30 mg
#4: Aspirin 325 mg and codeine phosphate 60 mg

Dental Comment Codeine products, as with other narcotic analgesics, are recommended only for limited acute dosing (ie, 3 days or less). The most common adverse effect you will see in your dental patients from codeine is nausea, followed by sedation and constipation. Codeine has narcotic addiction liability, especially when given long-term. The aspirin component has anticoagulant effects and can affect bleeding times.

Selected Readings

Dionne RA, "New Approaches to Preventing and Treating Postoperative Pain," *J Am Dent Assoc*, 1992, 123(6):26-34.

Gobetti JP, "Controlling Dental Pain," *J Am Dent Assoc*, 1992, 123(6):47-52.

Aspirin and Dipyridamole *(AS pir in & dye peer ID a mole)*

Related Information

Aspirin *on page 145*
Cardiovascular Diseases *on page 1636*
Dipyridamole *on page 489*

U.S. Brand Names Aggrenox®

Canadian Brand Names Aggrenox®

Generic Available No

Synonyms Aspirin and Extended-Release Dipyridamole; Dipyridamole and Aspirin

Pharmacologic Category Antiplatelet Agent

Use Reduction in the risk of stroke in patients who have had transient ischemia of the brain or completed ischemic stroke due to thrombosis

Local Anesthetic/Vasoconstrictor Precautions No information available to require special precautions

Effects on Dental Treatment No significant effects or complications reported

Common Adverse Effects

>10%:

Central nervous system: Headache (38%)

Gastrointestinal: Dyspepsia, abdominal pain (18%), nausea (16%), diarrhea (13%)

1% to 10%:

Cardiovascular: Cardiac failure (2%), syncope (1%)

Central nervous system: Pain (6%), seizure (2%), fatigue (6%), malaise (2%), amnesia (2%), confusion (1%), somnolence (1%)

Dermatologic: Purpura (1%)

Gastrointestinal: Vomiting (8%), bleeding (4%), rectal bleeding (2%), hemorrhoids (1%), hemorrhage (1%), anorexia (1%)

Hematologic: Anemia (2%)

Neuromuscular & skeletal: Back pain (5%), weakness (2%), arthralgia (6%), arthritis (2%), arthrosis (1%), myalgia (1%)

Respiratory: Cough (2%), upper respiratory tract infection (1%), epistaxis (2%)

Mechanism of Action The antithrombotic action results from additive antiplatelet effects. Dipyridamole inhibits the uptake of adenosine into platelets, endothelial cells, and erythrocytes. Aspirin inhibits platelet aggregation by irreversible inhibition of platelet cyclooxygenase and thus inhibits the generation of thromboxane A_2.

Drug Interactions
　Cytochrome P450 Effect: Aspirin: **Substrate** of CYP2C9 (minor)
　Increased Effect/Toxicity: See individual agents.
　Decreased Effect: See individual agents.
Pharmacodynamics/Kinetics See individual agents.
Pregnancy Risk Factor D

Aspirin and Extended-Release Dipyridamole *see* Aspirin and Dipyridamole *on page 150*

Aspirin and Hydrocodone *see* Hydrocodone and Aspirin *on page 782*

Aspirin and Meprobamate (AS pir in & me proe BA mate)

Related Information
　Aspirin *on page 145*
　Meprobamate *on page 993*
U.S. Brand Names Equagesic®
Canadian Brand Names 292 MEP®
Generic Available No
Synonyms Meprobamate and Aspirin
Pharmacologic Category Antianxiety Agent, Miscellaneous
Use Adjunct to treatment of skeletal muscular disease in patients exhibiting tension and/or anxiety
Local Anesthetic/Vasoconstrictor Precautions No information available to require special precautions
Effects on Dental Treatment Key adverse event(s) related to dental treatment: Elderly are a high-risk population for adverse effects from nonsteroidal anti-inflammatory agents. As many as 60% of elderly patients with GI complications from NSAIDs can develop peptic ulceration and/or hemorrhage asymptomatically. Concomitant disease and drug use contribute to the risk of GI adverse effects. Use lowest effective dose for shortest period possible. Consider renal function decline with age.
Common Adverse Effects See individual agents.
Restrictions C-IV
Drug Interactions
　Cytochrome P450 Effect: Aspirin: **Substrate** of CYP2C9 (minor)
　Increased Effect/Toxicity: See individual agents.
　Decreased Effect: See individual agents.
Pharmacodynamics/Kinetics See individual agents.
Pregnancy Risk Factor D

Aspirin and Oxycodone *see* Oxycodone and Aspirin *on page 1168*

Aspirin and Pravastatin (AS pir in & PRA va stat in)

Related Information
　Aspirin *on page 145*
　Pravastatin *on page 1265*
U.S. Brand Names Pravigard™ PAC [DSC]
Generic Available No
Synonyms Buffered Aspirin and Pravastatin Sodium; Pravastatin and Aspirin
Pharmacologic Category Antilipemic Agent, HMG-CoA Reductase Inhibitor; Salicylate
Use Combination therapy in patients who need treatment with aspirin and pravastatin to reduce the incidence of cardiovascular events, including myocardial infarction, stroke, and death.
Local Anesthetic/Vasoconstrictor Precautions No information available to require special precautions
Effects on Dental Treatment Aspirin: Key adverse event(s) related to dental treatment: As with all drugs which may affect hemostasis, bleeding is associated with aspirin. Hemorrhage may occur at virtually any site; risk is dependent on multiple variables including dosage, concurrent use of multiple agents which alter hemostasis, and patient susceptibility. Many adverse effects of aspirin are dose related, and are rare at low dosages. Other serious reactions are idiosyncratic, related to allergy or individual sensitivity (see Dental Comment).
Common Adverse Effects Clinical studies of this combination product have not been conducted. See individual agents.
(Continued)

Aspirin and Pravastatin *(Continued)*

Mechanism of Action

Aspirin: Inhibits prostaglandin synthesis, acts on the hypothalamus heat-regulating center to reduce fever, blocks prostaglandin synthetase action which prevents formation of the platelet-aggregating substance thromboxane A_2

Pravastatin: Competitive inhibitor of 3-hydroxy-3-methylglutaryl coenzyme A (HMG-CoA) reductase, which is the rate-limiting enzyme involved in *de novo* cholesterol synthesis.

Drug Interactions

Cytochrome P450 Effect:

Aspirin: **Substrate** of CYP2C9 (minor)

Pravastatin: **Substrate** of CYP3A4 (minor); **Inhibits** CYP2C9 (weak), 2D6 (weak), 3A4 (weak)

Increased Effect/Toxicity: See individual agents.

Decreased Effect: See individual agents.

Pharmacodynamics/Kinetics See individual agents.

Pregnancy Risk Factor X

Dental Comment Aspirin: There is no scientific evidence to warrant discontinuance of aspirin prior to dental surgery. Patients taking one aspirin tablet daily as an antithrombotic and who require dental surgery should be given special consideration in consultation with the physician before removal of the aspirin relative to prevention of postoperative bleeding.

Aspirin, Caffeine and Acetaminophen *see* Acetaminophen, Aspirin, and Caffeine *on page 41*

Aspirin, Caffeine, and Butalbital *see* Butalbital, Aspirin, and Caffeine *on page 241*

Aspirin, Caffeine, and Propoxyphene *see* Propoxyphene, Aspirin, and Caffeine *on page 1300*

Aspirin, Caffeine, Codeine, and Butalbital *see* Butalbital, Aspirin, Caffeine, and Codeine *on page 241*

Aspirin, Carisoprodol, and Codeine *see* Carisoprodol, Aspirin, and Codeine *on page 273*

Aspirin Free Anacin® Maximum Strength [OTC] *see* Acetaminophen *on page 31*

Aspirin, Orphenadrine, and Caffeine *see* Orphenadrine, Aspirin, and Caffeine *on page 1152*

Astelin® *see* Azelastine *on page 170*

AsthmaNefrin® *see* Epinephrine (Racemic) *on page 549*

Astramorph/PF™ *see* Morphine Sulfate *on page 1065*

AT-III *see* Antithrombin III *on page 131*

Atacand® *see* Candesartan *on page 252*

Atacand HCT™ *see* Candesartan and Hydrochlorothiazide *on page 254*

Atazanavir *(at a za NA veer)*

U.S. Brand Names Reyataz®

Canadian Brand Names Reyataz®

Generic Available No

Synonyms Atazanavir Sulfate; BMS-232632

Pharmacologic Category Antiretroviral Agent, Protease Inhibitor

Use Treatment of HIV-1 infections in combination with at least two other antiretroviral agents

Note: In patients with prior virologic failure, coadministration with ritonavir is recommended.

Local Anesthetic/Vasoconstrictor Precautions No information available to require special precautions

Effects on Dental Treatment No significant effects or complications reported

Common Adverse Effects Protease inhibitors cause dyslipidemia which includes elevated cholesterol and triglycerides and a redistribution of body fat centrally to cause increased abdominal girth, buffalo hump, facial atrophy, and breast enlargement. These agents also cause hyperglycemia.

>10%:

Dermatologic: Rash (21%; median onset 8 weeks)

Gastrointestinal: Nausea (6% to 14%), amylase increased (14%)

Hepatic: Bilirubin increased (>2.6 times ULN: 35% to 47%)

3% to 10%:

Central nervous system: Depression (4% to 8%), fever (4% to 5%), fatigue (2% to 5%), headache (1% to 6%), peripheral neuropathy (1% to 4%), insomnia (1% to 3%), pain (1% to 3%), dizziness (1% to 2%)

Endocrine & metabolic: Lipodystrophy (1% to 8%)

Gastrointestinal: Abdominal pain (4%), vomiting (3% to 4%), diarrhea (1% to 11%)

Hepatic: Transaminases increased (2% to 9%), jaundice (7% to 8%)

Neuromuscular & skeletal: Myalgia (4%)

Respiratory: Cough increased (3% to 5%)

Mechanism of Action Inhibits the HIV-1 protease; inhibition of the viral protease prevents cleavage of the gag-pol polyprotein resulting in the production of immature, noninfectious virus

Drug Interactions

Cytochrome P450 Effect: Substrate of CYP3A4 (major); **Inhibits** CYP1A2 (weak), 2C8 (strong), 2C9 (weak), 3A4 (strong)

Increased Effect/Toxicity: Serum concentrations of medications significantly metabolized by CYP2C8, CYP3A4, or UGT1A1 may be elevated by atazanavir. Concurrent therapy with cisapride, ergot derivatives (dihydroergotamine, ergonovine, ergotamine, methylergonovine), indinavir, irinotecan, lovastatin, midazolam, pimozide, simvastatin, or triazolam is contraindicated (or not recommended, per manufacturer).

Atazanavir may increase the levels/effects of selected benzodiazepines, calcium channel blockers, cyclosporine, delavirdine, fentanyl, mirtazapine, nateglinide, nefazodone, quinidine, sildenafil (and other PDE-5 inhibitors), tacrolimus, telithromycin, tenofovir, venlafaxine, and other CYP3A4 substrates. When used with strong CYP3A4 inhibitors, dosage adjustment/limits are recommended for sildenafil and other PDE-5 inhibitors; consult individual monographs. Serum concentrations of antiarrhythmics (amiodarone, lidocaine, and quinidine) may be increased; monitor serum concentrations of these agents. Serum concentrations/effects of trazodone may be increased; use caution and reduce trazodone dose.

The levels/effects of atazanavir may be increased by azole antifungals, clarithromycin, delavirdine, diclofenac, doxycycline, erythromycin, imatinib, isoniazid, nefazodone, nicardipine, propofol, protease inhibitors, quinidine, telithromycin, verapamil, and other CYP3A4 inhibitors. Serum concentrations of atazanavir are increased by ritonavir; specific dosing adjustment of atazanavir in combination with ritonavir and efavirenz has been established. Serum concentrations of saquinavir may be increased by atazanavir; dosing recommendations for the combination have not been established. Tenofovir concentrations are increased by atazanavir. Concurrent use of indinavir may increase the risk of hyperbilirubinemia; concomitant administration is not recommended. Serum concentrations of orally inhaled corticosteroids (fluticasone, budesonide) may be increased by atazanavir (with or without ritonavir) resulting in decreased serum cortisol, HPA axis suppression; concurrent use with atazanavir plus ritonavir not recommended.

Atazanavir may increase serum concentrations of clarithromycin, potentially increasing the risk of QT_c prolongation. A 50% reduction in clarithromycin dose or an alternative agent (except in *M. avium* complex infections) should be considered. An increase in rifabutin plasma AUC (>200%) has been observed when coadministered with atazanavir (decrease rifabutin's dose by up to 75%).

Decreased Effect: Concurrent use of proton pump inhibitors may reduce atazanavir absorption; avoid concurrent use. Antacids and buffered formulations (ie, didanosine buffered tablets) may reduce the serum concentrations of atazanavir. Administer atazanavir 2 hours before or 1 hour after these medications. H_2 antagonists may reduce the absorption of atazanavir; avoid concurrent use or administer H_2 antagonist at least 10 hours before or 2 hours after atazanavir. Serum levels/effects of enteric-coated didanosine may be decreased by atazanavir

The levels/effects of atazanavir may be decreased by aminoglutethimide, carbamazepine, nafcillin, nevirapine, phenobarbital, phenytoin, rifamycins, and other CYP3A4 inducers. Rifampin decreases bioavailability of protease inhibitors by ~90%; loss of virologic response and resistance may occur; the two drugs should not be administered together. St John's wort (*Hypericum perforatum*) decreases serum concentrations of protease inhibitors and may lead to treatment failures; concurrent use is contraindicated. Tenofovir may decrease serum concentrations of atazanavir, resulting in a loss of virologic response (specific atazanavir dosing recommendations provided by manufacturer).

(Continued)

Atazanavir *(Continued)*

Pharmacodynamics/Kinetics

Protein binding: 86%

Metabolism: Hepatic, via multiple pathways including CYP3A4; forms two metabolites (inactive)

Half-life elimination: ~7 hours

Time to peak, plasma: 2.5 hours

Excretion: Feces (79%, 20% as unchanged drug); urine (13%, 7% as unchanged drug)

Pregnancy Risk Factor B

Atazanavir Sulfate *see Atazanavir on page 152*

Atenolol *(a TEN oh lole)*

Related Information

Cardiovascular Diseases *on page 1636*

U.S. Brand Names Tenormin®

Canadian Brand Names Apo-Atenol®; Gen-Atenolol; Novo-Atenol; Nu-Atenol; PMS-Atenolol; Rhoxal-atenolol; Riva-Atenolol; Sandoz-Atenolol; Tenolin; Tenormin®

Mexican Brand Names Blokium®; Tenormin®

Generic Available Yes: Tablet

Pharmacologic Category Beta Blocker, Beta₁ Selective

Use Treatment of hypertension, alone or in combination with other agents; management of angina pectoris, postmyocardial infarction patients

Unlabeled/Investigational Use Acute ethanol withdrawal, supraventricular and ventricular arrhythmias, and migraine headache prophylaxis

Local Anesthetic/Vasoconstrictor Precautions No information available to require special precautions

Effects on Dental Treatment Atenolol is a cardioselective beta-blocker. Local anesthetic with vasoconstrictor can be safely used in patients medicated with atenolol. Nonselective beta-blockers (ie, propranolol, nadolol) enhance the pressor response to epinephrine, resulting in hypertension and bradycardia; this has not been reported for atenolol. Many nonsteroidal anti-inflammatory drugs, such as ibuprofen and indomethacin, can reduce the hypotensive effect of beta-blockers after 3 or more weeks of therapy with the NSAID. Short-term NSAID use (ie, 3 days) requires no special precautions in patients taking beta-blockers.

Common Adverse Effects 1% to 10%:

Cardiovascular: Persistent bradycardia, hypotension, chest pain, edema, heart failure, second- or third-degree AV block, Raynaud's phenomenon

Central nervous system: Dizziness, fatigue, insomnia, lethargy, confusion, mental impairment, depression, headache, nightmares

Gastrointestinal: Constipation, diarrhea, nausea

Genitourinary: Impotence

Miscellaneous: Cold extremities

Dosage

Oral:

Children: 0.8-1 mg/kg/dose given daily; range of 0.8-1.5 mg/kg/day; maximum dose: 2 mg/kg/day

Adults:

Hypertension: 25-50 mg once daily, may increase to 100 mg/day. Doses >100 mg are unlikely to produce any further benefit.

Angina pectoris: 50 mg once daily, may increase to 100 mg/day. Some patients may require 200 mg/day.

Postmyocardial infarction: Follow I.V. dose with 100 mg/day or 50 mg twice daily for 6-9 days postmyocardial infarction.

I.V.:

Hypertension: Dosages of 1.25-5 mg every 6-12 hours have been used in short-term management of patients unable to take oral enteral beta-blockers

Postmyocardial infarction: Early treatment: 5 mg slow I.V. over 5 minutes; may repeat in 10 minutes. If both doses are tolerated, may start oral atenolol 50 mg every 12 hours or 100 mg/day for 6-9 days postmyocardial infarction.

Dosing interval for oral atenolol in renal impairment:

Cl_cr 15-35 mL/minute: Administer 50 mg/day maximum.

Cl_cr <15 mL/minute: Administer 50 mg every other day maximum.

Hemodialysis: Moderately dialyzable (20% to 50%) via hemodialysis; administer dose postdialysis or administer 25-50 mg supplemental dose.

Peritoneal dialysis: Elimination is not enhanced; supplemental dose is not necessary.

Mechanism of Action Competitively blocks response to beta-adrenergic stimulation, selectively blocks beta$_1$-receptors with little or no effect on beta$_2$-receptors except at high doses

Contraindications Hypersensitivity to atenolol or any component of the formulation; sinus bradycardia; sinus node dysfunction; heart block greater than first-degree (except in patients with a functioning artificial pacemaker); cardiogenic shock; uncompensated cardiac failure; pulmonary edema; pregnancy

Warnings/Precautions Safety and efficacy in children have not been established. Administer cautiously in compensated heart failure and monitor for a worsening of the condition (efficacy of atenolol in heart failure has not been established). Beta-blocker therapy should not be withdrawn abruptly (particularly in patients with CAD), but gradually tapered to avoid acute tachycardia, hypertension, and/or ischemia. Use caution with concurrent use of beta-blockers and either verapamil or diltiazem; bradycardia or heart block can occur. Avoid concurrent I.V. use of both agents. Beta-blockers should be avoided in patients with bronchospastic disease (asthma) and peripheral vascular disease (may aggravate arterial insufficiency). Atenolol, with B1 selectivity, has been used cautiously in bronchospastic disease with close monitoring. Use cautiously in patients with diabetes - may mask hypoglycemic symptoms. May mask signs of thyrotoxicosis. May cause fetal harm when administered in pregnancy. Use cautiously in the renally impaired (dosage adjustment required). Use care with anesthetic agents which decrease myocardial function. Caution in myasthenia gravis.

Drug Interactions

Increased Effect/Toxicity: Atenolol may increase the effects of other drugs which slow AV conduction (digoxin, verapamil, diltiazem), alpha-blockers (prazosin, terazosin), and alpha-adrenergic stimulants (epinephrine, phenylephrine). Atenolol may mask the tachycardia from hypoglycemia caused by insulin and oral hypoglycemics. In patients receiving concurrent therapy, the risk of hypertensive crisis is increased when either clonidine or the beta-blocker is withdrawn. Reserpine has been shown to enhance the effect of atenolol. Beta-blockers may increase the action or levels of ethanol, disopyramide, nondepolarizing muscle relaxants, and theophylline although the effects are difficult to predict.

Decreased Effect: Decreased effect of atenolol with aluminum salts, barbiturates, calcium salts, cholestyramine, colestipol, NSAIDs, penicillins (ampicillin), rifampin, salicylates, and sulfinpyrazone due to decreased bioavailability and plasma levels. Beta-blockers may decrease the effect of sulfonylureas.

Ethanol/Nutrition/Herb Interactions

Food: Atenolol serum concentrations may be decreased if taken with food.

Herb/Nutraceutical: Avoid dong quai if using for hypertension (has estrogenic activity). Avoid ephedra, yohimbe, ginseng (may worsen hypertension). Avoid garlic (may have increased antihypertensive effect).

Dietary Considerations May be taken without regard to meals.

Pharmacodynamics/Kinetics

Onset of action: Peak effect: Oral: 2-4 hours

Duration: Normal renal function: 12-24 hours

Absorption: Incomplete

Distribution: Low lipophilicity; does not cross blood-brain barrier

Protein binding: 3% to 15%

Metabolism: Limited hepatic

Half-life elimination: Beta:

Neonates: ≤35 hours; Mean: 16 hours

Children: 4.6 hours; children >10 years may have longer half-life (>5 hours) compared to children 5-10 years (<5 hours)

Adults: Normal renal function: 6-9 hours, prolonged with renal impairment; End-stage renal disease: 15-35 hours

Excretion: Feces (50%); urine (40% as unchanged drug)

Pregnancy Risk Factor D

Dosage Forms INJ, solution: 0.5 mg/mL (10 mL). **TAB:** 25 mg, 50 mg, 100 mg

Selected Readings

Foster CA and Aston SJ, "Propranolol-Epinephrine Interaction: A Potential Disaster," *Plast Reconstr Surg*, 1983, 72(1):74-8.

Wong DG, Spence JD, Lamki L, et al, "Effect of Nonsteroidal Anti-inflammatory Drugs on Control of Hypertension of Beta-Blockers and Diuretics," *Lancet*, 1986, 1(8488):997-1001.

Wynn RL, "Dental Nonsteroidal Anti-inflammatory Drugs and Prostaglandin-Based Drug Interactions-Part Two," *Gen Dent*, 1992, 40(2):104, 106, 108.

Wynn RL, "Epinephrine Interactions With Beta-Blockers," *Gen Dent*, 1994, 42(1):16, 18.

Atenolol and Chlorthalidone (a TEN oh lole & klor THAL i done)

Related Information
Atenolol on page 154
Chlorthalidone on page 332
U.S. Brand Names Tenoretic®
Canadian Brand Names Tenoretic®
Generic Available Yes
Synonyms Chlorthalidone and Atenolol
Pharmacologic Category Antihypertensive Agent, Combination
Use Treatment of hypertension with a cardioselective beta-blocker and a diuretic

Local Anesthetic/Vasoconstrictor Precautions No information available to require special precautions

Effects on Dental Treatment Atenolol is a cardioselective beta-blocker. Local anesthetic with vasoconstrictor can be safely used in patients medicated with atenolol. Nonselective beta-blockers (ie, propranolol, nadolol) enhance the pressor response to epinephrine, resulting in hypertension and bradycardia; this has not been reported for atenolol. Many nonsteroidal anti-inflammatory drugs, such as ibuprofen and indomethacin, can reduce the hypotensive effect of beta-blockers after 3 or more weeks of therapy with the NSAID. Short-term NSAID use (ie, 3 days) requires no special precautions in patients taking beta-blockers.

Common Adverse Effects See individual agents.
Drug Interactions
Increased Effect/Toxicity: See individual agents.
Decreased Effect: See individual agents.
Pharmacodynamics/Kinetics See individual agents.
Pregnancy Risk Factor D

ATG see Antithymocyte Globulin (Equine) on page 131
Atgam® see Antithymocyte Globulin (Equine) on page 131
Ativan® see Lorazepam on page 947

Atomoxetine (AT oh mox e teen)

U.S. Brand Names Strattera®
Canadian Brand Names Strattera®
Generic Available No
Synonyms Atomoxetine Hydrochloride; LY139603; Methylphenoxy-Benzene Propanamine; Tomoxetine
Pharmacologic Category Norepinephrine Reuptake Inhibitor, Selective
Use Treatment of attention deficit/hyperactivity disorder (ADHD)
Local Anesthetic/Vasoconstrictor Precautions Use vasoconstrictor with caution. Atomoxetine may increase heart rate or blood pressure in the presence of pressor agents. Pressor agents include the vasoconstrictors epinephrine and levonordefrin (Neo-Cobefrin®)
Effects on Dental Treatment Key adverse event(s) related to dental treatment: Xerostomia (normal salivary flow resumes upon discontinuation).
Common Adverse Effects Percentages as reported in children and adults; some adverse reactions may be increased in "poor metabolizers" (CYP2D6).
>10%:
  Central nervous system: Headache (17% to 27%), insomnia (16%)
  Gastrointestinal: Xerostomia (4% to 21%), abdominal pain (20%), vomiting (15%), appetite decreased (10% to 14%), nausea (12%)
  Respiratory: Cough (11%)
1% to 10%:
  Cardiovascular: Palpitations (4%), diastolic pressure increased (<1% to 5%), systolic blood pressure increased (2% to 9%), orthostatic hypotension (2%), tachycardia (2% to 3%)
  Central nervous system: Fatigue/lethargy (7% to 9%), irritability (8%), somnolence (7%), dizziness (6%), mood swings (5%), abnormal dreams (4%), sleep disturbance (4%), pyrexia (3%), rigors (3%), crying (2%)
  Dermatologic: Dermatitis (2% to 4%)
  Endocrine & metabolic: Dysmenorrhea (7%), libido decreased (6%), menstruation disturbance (2% to 3%), hot flashes (3%), orgasm abnormal (2%)
  Gastrointestinal: Dyspepsia (4% to 6%), diarrhea (4%), flatulence (2%), constipation (3% to 10%), weight loss (2%)
  Genitourinary: Erectile disturbance (7%), ejaculatory disturbance (5%), prostatitis (3%), impotence (3%)
  Neuromuscular & skeletal: Paresthesia (4%), myalgia (3%)

Otic: Ear infection (3%)

Renal: Urinary retention/hesitation (3% to 8%)

Respiratory: Rhinorrhea (4%), sinus headache (3%), sinusitis (6%)

Miscellaneous: Diaphoresis increased (4%), influenza (3%)

Restrictions A medication guide concerning the use of atomoxetine in children and teenagers can be found on the FDA website at http://www.fda.gov/cder/Offices/ODS/labeling.htm. It should be dispensed to parents or guardians of children and teenagers receiving this medication.

Dosage Oral: **Note:** Atomoxetine may be discontinued without the need for tapering dose.

Children and Adolescents ≤70 kg: ADHD: Initial: 0.5 mg/kg/day, increase after minimum of 3 days to ~1.2 mg/kg/day; may administer as either a single daily dose or 2 evenly divided doses in morning and late afternoon/early evening. Maximum daily dose: 1.4 mg/kg or 100 mg, whichever is less.

Dosage adjustment in patients receiving strong CYP2D6 inhibitors (eg, paroxetine, fluoxetine, quinidine): Do not exceed 1.2 mg/kg/day; dose adjustments should occur only after 4 weeks.

Children and Adolescents >70 kg and Adults: ADHD: Initial: 40 mg/day, increased after minimum of 3 days to ~80 mg/day; may administer as either a single daily dose or two evenly divided doses in morning and late afternoon/early evening. May increase to 100 mg in 2-4 additional weeks to achieve optimal response.

Dosage adjustment in patients receiving strong CYP2D6 inhibitors (eg, paroxetine, fluoxetine, quinidine): Do not exceed 80 mg/day; dose adjustments should occur only after 4 weeks.

Elderly: Use has not been evaluated in the elderly

Dosage adjustment in renal impairment: No adjustment needed

Dosage adjustment in hepatic impairment:

Moderate hepatic insufficiency (Child-Pugh class B): All doses should be reduced to 50% of normal

Severe hepatic insufficiency (Child-Pugh class C): All doses should be reduced to 25% of normal

Mechanism of Action Selectively inhibits the reuptake of norepinephrine (Ki 4.5 nM) with little to no activity at the other neuronal reuptake pumps or receptor sites.

Contraindications Hypersensitivity to atomoxetine or any component of the formulation; use with or within 14 days of MAO inhibitors; narrow-angle glaucoma

Warnings/Precautions Use caution with hepatic and renal impairment (dosage adjustments necessary in hepatic impairment). Use may be associated with rare but severe hepatotoxicity; discontinue if signs or symptoms of hepatotoxic reaction (eg, jaundice, pruritus, flu-like symptoms) are noted. May cause increased heart rate or blood pressure; use caution with hypertension or other cardiovascular disease. Use caution in patients who are poor metabolizers of CYP2D6 metabolized drugs ("poor metabolizers"), bioavailability increases. May cause urinary retention/hesitancy; use caution in patients with history of urinary retention or bladder outlet obstruction. Allergic reactions (including angioneurotic edema, urticaria, and rash) may occur. Growth should be monitored during treatment. Height and weight gain may be reduced during the first 9-12 months of treatment, but should recover by 3 years of therapy. Use caution in pediatric patients; may be an increased risk of suicidal ideation. Additional family/caregiver and healthcare provider monitoring suggested during initial months of therapy or at times of dosage changes. Safety and efficacy have not been evaluated in pediatric patients <6 years of age.

Drug Interactions

Cytochrome P450 Effect: Substrate of CYP2C19 (minor), 2D6 (major)

Increased Effect/Toxicity: MAO inhibitors may increase risk of CNS toxicity (combined use is contraindicated). CYP2D6 inhibitors may increase the levels/effects of atomoxetine (dose adjustment may be needed in patients who are extensive metabolizers of CYP2D6); example inhibitors include chlorpromazine, delavirdine, fluoxetine, miconazole, paroxetine, pergolide, quinidine, quinine, ritonavir, and ropinirole. Albuterol may increase risk of cardiovascular toxicity.

Dietary Considerations May be taken with or without food.

Pharmacodynamics/Kinetics

Absorption: Rapid

Distribution: V_d: I.V.: 0.85 L/kg

Protein binding: 98%, primarily albumin

Metabolism: Hepatic, via CYP2D6 and CYP2C19; forms metabolites (4-hydroxyatomoxetine, active, equipotent to atomoxetine; N-desmethylatomoxetine in poor metabolizers, limited activity)

Bioavailability: 63% in extensive metabolizers; 94% in poor metabolizers

(Continued)

Atomoxetine *(Continued)*

Half-life elimination: Atomoxetine: 5 hours (up to 24 hours in poor metabolizers);
Active metabolites: 4-hydroxyatomoxetine: 6-8 hours; N-desmethyl-atomoxetine: 6-8 hours (34-40 hours in poor metabolizers)

Time to peak, plasma: 1-2 hours

Excretion: Urine (80%, as conjugated 4-hydroxy metabolite); feces (17%)

Pregnancy Risk Factor C

Dosage Forms CAP: 10 mg, 18 mg, 25 mg, 40 mg, 60 mg, 80 mg, 100 mg

Atomoxetine Hydrochloride *see* Atomoxetine *on page 156*

Atorvastatin *(a TORE va sta tin)*

Related Information

Cardiovascular Diseases *on page 1636*

U.S. Brand Names Lipitor®

Canadian Brand Names Lipitor®

Mexican Brand Names Lipitor®

Generic Available No

Pharmacologic Category Antilipemic Agent, HMG-CoA Reductase Inhibitor

Use Treatment of dyslipidemias or primary prevention of cardiovascular disease (atherosclerotic) as detailed below:

Primary prevention of cardiovascular disease (high-risk for CVD): To reduce the risk of MI or stroke in patients without evidence of heart disease who have multiple CVD risk factors or type 2 diabetes. Treatment reduces the risk for angina or revascularization procedures in patients with multiple risk factors.

Treatment of dyslipidemias: To reduce elevations in total cholesterol, LDL-C, apolipoprotein B, and triglycerides in patients with elevations of one or more components, and/or to increase HDL-C as present in Fredrickson type IIa, IIb, III, and IV hyperlipidemias; treatment of primary dysbetalipoproteinemia, homozygous familial hypercholesterolemia

Treatment of heterozygous familial hypercholesterolemia (HeFH) in adolescent patients (10-17 years of age, females >1 year postmenarche) having LDL-C ≥190 mg/dL or LDL-C ≥160 mg/dL with positive family history of premature cardiovascular disease (CVD) or with two or more CVD risk factors.

Local Anesthetic/Vasoconstrictor Precautions No information available to require special precautions

Effects on Dental Treatment No significant effects or complications reported

Common Adverse Effects

>10%: Central nervous system: Headache (3% to 17%)

2% to 10%:

Cardiovascular: Chest pain, peripheral edema

Central nervous system: Insomnia, dizziness

Dermatologic: Rash (1% to 4%)

Gastrointestinal: Abdominal pain (up to 4%), constipation (up to 3%), diarrhea (up to 4%), dyspepsia (1% to 3%), flatulence (1% to 3%), nausea

Genitourinary: Urinary tract infection

Hepatic: Transaminases increased (2% to 3% with 80 mg/day dosing)

Neuromuscular & skeletal: Arthralgia (up to 5%), arthritis, back pain (up to 4%), myalgia (up to 6%), weakness (up to 4%)

Respiratory: Sinusitis (up to 6%), pharyngitis (up to 3%), bronchitis, rhinitis

Miscellaneous: Infection (3% to 10%), flu-like syndrome (up to 3%), allergic reaction (up to 3%)

Additional class-related events or case reports (not necessarily reported with atorvastatin therapy): Alkaline phosphatase increased, cataracts, cirrhosis, CPK increased (>10x normal), dermatomyositis, eosinophilia, erectile dysfunction, extraocular muscle movement impaired, fulminant hepatic necrosis, gynecomastia, hemolytic anemia, memory loss, ophthalmoplegia, peripheral nerve palsy, polymyalgia rheumatica, positive ANA, renal failure (secondary to rhabdomyolysis), systemic lupus erythematosus-like syndrome, thyroid dysfunction, tremor, vasculitis, vertigo

Dosage Oral: **Note:** Doses should be individualized according to the baseline LDL-cholesterol levels, the recommended goal of therapy, and patient response; adjustments should be made at intervals of 2-4 weeks

Children 10-17 years (females >1 year postmenarche): HeFH: 10 mg once daily (maximum: 20 mg/day)

Adults:

Hyperlipidemias: Initial: 10-20 mg once daily; patients requiring >45% reduction in LDL-C may be started at 40 mg once daily; range: 10-80 mg once daily

Primary prevention of CVD: 10 mg once daily

Dosing adjustment in renal impairment: No dosage adjustment is necessary.

Dosing adjustment in hepatic impairment: Do not use in active liver disease.

Mechanism of Action Inhibitor of 3-hydroxy-3-methylglutaryl coenzyme A (HMG-CoA) reductase, the rate-limiting enzyme in cholesterol synthesis (reduces the production of mevalonic acid from HMG-CoA); this then results in a compensatory increase in the expression of LDL receptors on hepatocyte membranes and a stimulation of LDL catabolism

Contraindications Hypersensitivity to atorvastatin or any component of the formulation; active liver disease; unexplained persistent elevations of serum transaminases; pregnancy

Warnings/Precautions Secondary causes of hyperlipidemia should be ruled out prior to therapy. May cause hepatic dysfunction. Use with caution in patients who consume large amounts of ethanol or have a history of liver disease. Monitoring is recommended. Rhabdomyolysis with acute renal failure has occurred. Risk is dose related and is increased with concurrent use of lipid-lowering agents which may cause rhabdomyolysis (gemfibrozil, fibric acid derivatives, or niacin at doses ≥1 g/day) or during concurrent use with potent CYP3A4 inhibitors (including amiodarone, clarithromycin, cyclosporine, erythromycin, itraconazole, ketoconazole, nefazodone, grapefruit juice in large quantities, verapamil, or protease inhibitors such as indinavir, nelfinavir, or ritonavir). Weigh the risk versus benefit when combining any of these drugs with atorvastatin. Discontinue in any patient experiencing an acute or serious condition predisposing to renal failure secondary to rhabdomyolysis. Safety and efficacy have not been established in patients <10 years of age or in premenarcheal girls.

Drug Interactions

Cytochrome P450 Effect: Substrate of CYP3A4 (major); **Inhibits** CYP3A4 (weak)

Increased Effect/Toxicity: CYP3A4 inhibitors may increase the levels/effects of atorvastatin; example inhibitors include azole antifungals, clarithromycin, diclofenac, doxycycline, erythromycin, imatinib, isoniazid, nefazodone, nicardipine, propofol, protease inhibitors, quinidine, telithromycin, and verapamil. The risk of myopathy and rhabdomyolysis due to concurrent use of a CYP3A4 inhibitor with atorvastatin is probably less than lovastatin or simvastatin. Cyclosporine, clofibrate, fenofibrate, gemfibrozil, and niacin may also increase the risk of myopathy and rhabdomyolysis. The effect/toxicity of levothyroxine may be increased by atorvastatin. Levels of digoxin and ethinyl estradiol may be increased by atorvastatin.

Decreased Effect: Colestipol, antacids decreased plasma concentrations but effect on LDL-cholesterol was not altered. Cholestyramine may decrease absorption of atorvastatin when administered concurrently.

Ethanol/Nutrition/Herb Interactions

Ethanol: Avoid excessive ethanol consumption (due to potential hepatic effects).

Food: Atorvastatin serum concentrations may be increased by grapefruit juice; avoid concurrent intake of large quantities (>1 quart/day). Red yeast rice contains an estimated 2.4 mg lovastatin per 600 mg rice.

Herb/Nutraceutical: St John's wort may decrease atorvastatin levels.

Dietary Considerations May take with food if desired; may take without regard to time of day. Before initiation of therapy, patients should be placed on a standard cholesterol-lowering diet for 3-6 months and the diet should be continued during drug therapy. Red yeast rice contains an estimated 2.4 mg lovastatin per 600 mg rice.

Pharmacodynamics/Kinetics

Onset of action: Initial changes: 3-5 days; Maximal reduction in plasma cholesterol and triglycerides: 2 weeks

Absorption: Rapid

Distribution: V_d: 318 L

Protein binding: ≥98%

Metabolism: Hepatic; forms active ortho- and parahydroxylated derivates and an inactive beta-oxidation product

Half-life elimination: Parent drug: 14 hours

Time to peak, serum: 1-2 hours

Excretion: Bile; urine (2% as unchanged drug)

Pregnancy Risk Factor X

Dosage Forms TAB: 10 mg, 20 mg, 40 mg, 80 mg

Selected Readings

Siedlik PH, Olson, SC, Yang BB, et al, "Erythromycin Coadministration Increases Plasma Atorvastatin Concentrations," *J Clin Pharmacol*, 1999, 39(5):501-4.

Atorvastatin Calcium and Amlodipine Besylate *see* Amlodipine and Atorvastatin on page 101

Atovaquone (a TOE va kwone)

Related Information
Systemic Viral Diseases *on page 1675*
U.S. Brand Names Mepron®
Canadian Brand Names Mepron®
Generic Available No
Pharmacologic Category Antiprotozoal
Use Acute oral treatment of mild-to-moderate *Pneumocystis carinii* pneumonia (PCP) in patients who are intolerant to co-trimoxazole; prophylaxis of PCP in patients intolerant to co-trimoxazole; treatment/suppression of *Toxoplasma gondii* encephalitis; primary prophylaxis of HIV-infected persons at high risk for developing *Toxoplasma gondii* encephalitis
Local Anesthetic/Vasoconstrictor Precautions No information available to require special precautions
Effects on Dental Treatment Key adverse event(s) related to dental treatment: Oral moniliasis.
Common Adverse Effects Note: Adverse reaction statistics have been compiled from studies including patients with advanced HIV disease; consequently, it is difficult to distinguish reactions attributed to atovaquone from those caused by the underlying disease or a combination thereof.

>10%:
Central nervous system: Headache, fever, insomnia, anxiety
Dermatologic: Rash
Gastrointestinal: Nausea, diarrhea, vomiting
Respiratory: Cough
1% to 10%:
Central nervous system: Dizziness
Dermatologic: Pruritus
Endocrine & metabolic: Hypoglycemia, hyponatremia
Gastrointestinal: Abdominal pain, constipation, anorexia, dyspepsia, amylase increased
Hematologic: Anemia, neutropenia, leukopenia
Hepatic: Liver enzymes increased
Neuromuscular & skeletal: Weakness
Renal: BUN/creatinine increased
Miscellaneous: Oral moniliasis

Mechanism of Action Has not been fully elucidated; may inhibit electron transport in mitochondria inhibiting metabolic enzymes
Drug Interactions
Increased Effect/Toxicity: Possible increased toxicity with other highly protein-bound drugs.
Decreased Effect: Rifamycins (rifampin) used concurrently decrease the steady-state plasma concentrations of atovaquone.
Pharmacodynamics/Kinetics
Absorption: Significantly increased with a high-fat meal
Distribution: 3.5 L/kg
Protein binding: >99%
Metabolism: Undergoes enterohepatic recirculation
Bioavailability: Tablet: 23%; Suspension: 47%
Half-life elimination: 2-3 days
Excretion: Feces (94% as unchanged drug)
Pregnancy Risk Factor C

Atovaquone and Proguanil (a TOE va kwone & pro GWA nil)

Related Information
Atovaquone *on page 160*
U.S. Brand Names Malarone®
Canadian Brand Names Malarone®
Generic Available No
Synonyms Proguanil and Atovaquone
Pharmacologic Category Antimalarial Agent
Use Prevention or treatment of acute, uncomplicated *P. falciparum* malaria
Local Anesthetic/Vasoconstrictor Precautions No information available to require special precautions
Effects on Dental Treatment No significant effects or complications reported

Common Adverse Effects The following adverse reactions were reported in patients being treated for malaria. When used for prophylaxis, reactions are similar to those seen with placebo.

>10%: Gastrointestinal: Abdominal pain (17%), nausea (12%), vomiting (children 10% to 13%, adults 12%)

1% to 10%:
Central nervous system: Headache (10%), dizziness (5%)
Dermatologic: Pruritus (children 6%)
Gastrointestinal: Diarrhea (children 6%, adults 8%), anorexia (5%)
Neuromuscular & skeletal: Weakness (8%)

Mechanism of Action
Atovaquone: Selectively inhibits parasite mitochondrial electron transport.
Proguanil: The metabolite cycloguanil inhibits dihydrofolate reductase, disrupting deoxythymidylate synthesis. Together, atovaquone/cycloguanil affect the erythrocytic and exoerythrocytic stages of development.

Drug Interactions
Cytochrome P450 Effect: Proguanil: **Substrate** (minor) of 1A2, 2C19, 3A4
Decreased Effect: Metoclopramide decreases bioavailability of atovaquone. Rifabutin decreases atovaquone levels by 34%. Rifampin decreases atovaquone levels by 50%. Tetracycline decreases plasma concentrations of atovaquone by 40%.

Pharmacodynamics/Kinetics
Atovaquone: See Atovaquone.
Proguanil:
Absorption: Extensive
Distribution: 42 L/kg
Protein binding: 75%
Metabolism: Hepatic to active metabolites, cycloguanil (via CYP2C19) and 4-chlorophenylbiguanide
Half-life elimination: 12-21 hours
Excretion: Urine (40% to 60%)

Pregnancy Risk Factor C

ATRA see Tretinoin (Oral) on page 1524
Atridox™ see Doxycycline Hyclate (Periodontal) on page 512
AtroPen® see Atropine on page 161

Atropine (A troe peen)

Related Information
Cardiovascular Diseases on page 1636
U.S. Brand Names AtroPen®; Atropine-Care®; Isopto® Atropine; Sal-Tropine™
Canadian Brand Names Dioptic's Atropine Solution; Isopto® Atropine
Mexican Brand Names Tropyn Z®
Generic Available Yes: Excludes tablet
Synonyms Atropine Sulfate
Pharmacologic Category Anticholinergic Agent; Anticholinergic Agent, Ophthalmic; Antidote; Antispasmodic Agent, Gastrointestinal; Ophthalmic Agent, Mydriatic
Dental Use Reduction of salivation and bronchial secretions
Use
Injection: Preoperative medication to inhibit salivation and secretions; treatment of symptomatic sinus bradycardia; AV block (nodal level); ventricular asystole; antidote for organophosphate pesticide poisoning
Ophthalmic: Produce mydriasis and cycloplegia for examination of the retina and optic disc and accurate measurement of refractive errors; uveitis
Oral: Inhibit salivation and secretions
Unlabeled/Investigational Use Pulseless electric activity, asystole, neuromuscular blockade reversal; treatment of nerve agent toxicity (chemical warfare) in combination with pralidoxime
Local Anesthetic/Vasoconstrictor Precautions No information available to require special precautions
Effects on Dental Treatment Key adverse event(s) related to dental treatment: Xerostomia and changes in salivation (normal salivary flow resumes upon discontinuation), dry throat, and nasal dryness.
Significant Adverse Effects Severity and frequency of adverse reactions are dose related and vary greatly; listed reactions are limited to significant and/or life-threatening.

Cardiovascular: Arrhythmia, flushing, hypotension, palpitation, tachycardia
(Continued)

Atropine (Continued)

Central nervous system: Ataxia, coma, delirium, disorientation, dizziness, drowsiness, excitement, fever, hallucinations, headache, insomnia, nervousness

Dermatologic: Anhidrosis, urticaria, rash, scarlatiniform rash

Gastrointestinal: Bloating, constipation, delayed gastric emptying, loss of taste, nausea, paralytic ileus, vomiting, xerostomia

Genitourinary: Urinary hesitancy, urinary retention

Neuromuscular & skeletal: Weakness

Ocular: Angle-closure glaucoma, blurred vision, cycloplegia, dry eyes, mydriasis, ocular tension increased

Respiratory: Dyspnea, laryngospasm, pulmonary edema

Miscellaneous: Anaphylaxis

Restrictions The AtroPen® formulation is available for use primarily by the Department of Defense.

Dental Usual Dosing Inhibit salivation and secretions (preanesthesia): Adults (doses <0.5 mg have been associated with paradoxical bradycardia):

I.M., I.V., SubQ: 0.4-0.6 mg 30-60 minutes preop and repeat every 4-6 hours as needed

Oral: 0.4 mg; may repeat in 4 hours if necessary

Dosage

Neonates, Infants, and Children: Doses <0.1 mg have been associated with paradoxical bradycardia.

Inhibit salivation and secretions (preanesthesia): Oral, I.M., I.V., SubQ:

<5 kg: 0.02 mg/kg/dose 30-60 minutes preop then every 4-6 hours as needed. Use of a minimum dosage of 0.1 mg in neonates <5 kg will result in dosages >0.02 mg/kg. There is no documented minimum dosage in this age group.

>5 kg: 0.01-0.02 mg/kg/dose to a maximum 0.4 mg/dose 30-60 minutes preop; minimum dose: 0.1 mg

Alternate dosing:

3-7 kg (7-16 lb): 0.1 mg

8-11 kg (17-24 lb): 0.15 mg

11-18 kg (24-40 lb): 0.2 mg

18-29 kg (40-65 lb): 0.3 mg

>30 kg (>65 lb): 0.4 mg

Bradycardia: I.V., intratracheal: 0.02 mg/kg, minimum dose 0.1 mg, maximum single dose: 0.5 mg in children and 1 mg in adolescents; may repeat in 5-minute intervals to a maximum total dose of 1 mg in children or 2 mg in adolescents. (**Note:** For intratracheal administration, the dosage must be diluted with normal saline to a total volume of 1-5 mL). When treating bradycardia in neonates, reserve use for those patients unresponsive to improved oxygenation and epinephrine.

Infants and Children: Nerve agent toxicity management (unlabeled use): See **Note** under adult dosing.

Prehospital ("in the field"): I.M.:

Birth to <2 years: Mild-to-moderate symptoms: 0.05 mg/kg; severe symptoms: 0.1 mg/kg

2-10 years: Mild-to-moderate symptoms: 1 mg; severe symptoms: 2 mg

>10 years: Mild-to-moderate symptoms: 2 mg; severe symptoms: 4 mg

Hospital/emergency department: I.M.:

Birth to <2 years: Mild-to-moderate symptoms: 0.05 mg/kg I.M. **or** 0.02 mg/kg I.V.; severe symptoms: 0.1 mg/kg I.M. **or** 0.02 mg/kg I.V.

2-10 years: Mild-to-moderate symptoms: 1 mg; severe symptoms: 2 mg

>10 years: Mild-to-moderate symptoms: 2 mg; severe symptoms: 4 mg

Note: Pralidoxime is a component of the management of nerve agent toxicity; consult Pralidoxime for specific route and dose. For prehospital ("in the field") management, repeat atropine I.M. (children: 0.05-0.1 mg/kg) at 5-10 minute intervals until secretions have diminished and breathing is comfortable or airway resistance has returned to near normal. For hospital management, repeat atropine I.M. (infants 1 mg; all others: 2 mg) at 5-10 minute intervals until secretions have diminished and breathing is comfortable or airway resistance has returned to near normal.

Children: Organophosphate or carbamate poisoning:

I.V.: 0.03-0.05 mg/kg every 10-20 minutes until atropine effect, then every 1-4 hours for at least 24 hours

I.M. (AtroPen®): Mild symptoms: Administer dose listed below as soon as exposure is known or suspected. If severe symptoms develop after first dose, 2 additional doses should be repeated in 10 minutes; do not administer more than 3 doses. Severe symptoms: Immediately administer 3 doses as follows:

<6.8 kg (15 lb): Use of **AtroPen®** formulation not recommended; administer atropine 0.05 mg/kg

6.8-18 kg (15-40 lb): 0.5 mg/dose

18-41 kg (40-90 lb): 1 mg/dose

>41 kg (>90 lb): 2 mg/dose

Adults (doses <0.5 mg have been associated with paradoxical bradycardia):

Asystole or pulseless electrical activity:

I.V.: 1 mg; repeat in 3-5 minutes if asystole persists; total dose of 0.04 mg/kg.

Intratracheal: Administer 2-2.5 times the recommended I.V. dose; dilute in 10 mL NS or distilled water. **Note:** Absorption is greater with distilled water, but causes more adverse effects on PaO_2.

Inhibit salivation and secretions (preanesthesia):

I.M., I.V., SubQ: 0.4-0.6 mg 30-60 minutes preop and repeat every 4-6 hours as needed

Oral: 0.4 mg; may repeat in 4 hours if necessary

Bradycardia: I.V.: 0.5-1 mg every 5 minutes, not to exceed a total of 3 mg or 0.04 mg/kg; may give intratracheally in 10 mL NS (intratracheal dose should be 2-2.5 times the I.V. dose)

Neuromuscular blockade reversal: I.V.: 25-30 mcg/kg 30-60 seconds before neostigmine or 7-10 mcg/kg 30-60 seconds before edrophonium

Organophosphate or carbamate poisoning:

I.V.: 2 mg, followed by 2 mg every 5-60 minutes until adequate atropinization has occurred; initial doses of up to 6 mg may be used in life-threatening cases

I.M. (AtroPen®): Mild symptoms: Administer 2 mg as soon as exposure is known or suspected. If severe symptoms develop after first dose, 2 additional doses should be repeated in 10 minutes; do not administer more than 3 doses. Severe symptoms: Immediately administer three 2 mg doses.

Nerve agent toxicity management (unlabeled use): I.M.: See **Note**. Prehospital ("in the field") or hospital/emergency department: Mild-to-moderate symptoms: 2-4 mg; severe symptoms: 6 mg

Note: Pralidoxime is a component of the management of nerve agent toxicity; consult Pralidoxime for specific route and dose. For prehospital ("in the field") management, repeat atropine I.M. (2 mg) at 5-10 minute intervals until secretions have diminished and breathing is comfortable or airway resistance has returned to near normal. For hospital management, repeat atropine I.M. (2 mg) at 5-10 minute intervals until secretions have diminished and breathing is comfortable or airway resistance has returned to near normal.

Mydriasis, cycloplegia (preprocedure): Ophthalmic (1% solution): Instill 1-2 drops 1 hour before procedure.

Uveitis: Ophthalmic:

1% solution: Instill 1-2 drops 4 times/day

Ointment: Apply a small amount in the conjunctival sac up to 3 times/day; compress the lacrimal sac by digital pressure for 1-3 minutes after instillation

Elderly, frail patients: Nerve agent toxicity management (unlabeled use): I.M.: See **Note** under adult dosing.

Prehospital ("in the field"): Mild-to-moderate symptoms: 1 mg; severe symptoms: 2-4 mg

Hospital/emergency department: Mild-to-moderate symptoms: 1 mg; severe symptoms: 2 mg

Mechanism of Action Blocks the action of acetylcholine at parasympathetic sites in smooth muscle, secretory glands, and the CNS; increases cardiac output, dries secretions, antagonizes histamine and serotonin

Contraindications Hypersensitivity to atropine or any component of the formulation; narrow-angle glaucoma; adhesions between the iris and lens; tachycardia; obstructive GI disease; paralytic ileus; intestinal atony of the elderly or debilitated patient; severe ulcerative colitis; toxic megacolon complicating ulcerative colitis; hepatic disease; obstructive uropathy; renal disease; myasthenia gravis (unless used to treat side effects of acetylcholinesterase inhibitor); asthma; thyrotoxicosis; Mobitz type II block

Warnings/Precautions Heat prostration can occur in the presence of a high environmental temperature. Psychosis can occur in sensitive individuals. The elderly may be sensitive to side effects. Use caution in patients with myocardial ischemia. Use caution in hyperthyroidism, autonomic neuropathy, BPH, CHF, tachyarrhythmias, hypertension, and hiatal hernia associated with reflux esophagitis. Use with caution in children with spastic paralysis.

(Continued)

Atropine *(Continued)*

AtroPen®: There are no absolute contraindications for the use of atropine in organophosphate poisonings, however, use caution in those patients where the use of atropine would be otherwise contraindicated. Formulation for use by trained personnel only.

Drug Interactions

Drugs with anticholinergic activity (including phenothiazines and TCAs) may increase anticholinergic effects when used concurrently.

Sympathomimetic amines may cause tachyarrhythmias; avoid concurrent use.

Pharmacodynamics/Kinetics

Onset of action: I.V.: Rapid

Absorption: Complete

Distribution: Widely throughout the body; crosses placenta; trace amounts enter breast milk; crosses blood-brain barrier

Metabolism: Hepatic

Half-life elimination: 2-3 hours

Excretion: Urine (30% to 50% as unchanged drug and metabolites)

Pregnancy Risk Factor C

Lactation Enters breast milk (trace amounts)/use caution (AAP rates "compatible")

Breast-Feeding Considerations Anticholinergic agents may suppress lactation.

Dosage Forms

Injection, solution, as sulfate: 0.05 mg/mL (5 mL); 0.1 mg/mL (5 mL, 10 mL); 0.4 mg/mL (0.5 mL, 1 mL, 20 mL); 0.5 mg/mL (1 mL); 1 mg/mL (1 mL)

AtroPen® [prefilled autoinjector]: 0.5 mg/0.7 mL (0.7 mL); 1 mg/0.7 mL (0.7 mL); 2 mg/0.7 mL (0.7 mL)

Ointment, ophthalmic, as sulfate: 1% (3.5 g)

Solution, ophthalmic, as sulfate: 1% (5 mL, 15 mL)

Atropine-Care®: 1% (2 mL)

Isopto® Atropine: 1% (5 mL, 15 mL)

Tablet, as sulfate (Sal-Tropine™): 0.4 mg

Atropine and Difenoxin *see* Difenoxin and Atropine *on page 467*

Atropine and Diphenoxylate *see* Diphenoxylate and Atropine *on page 487*

Atropine-Care® *see* Atropine *on page 161*

Atropine, Hyoscyamine, Scopolamine, and Phenobarbital *see* Hyoscyamine, Atropine, Scopolamine, and Phenobarbital *on page 804*

Atropine Sulfate *see* Atropine *on page 161*

Atropine Sulfate and Edrophonium Chloride *see* Edrophonium and Atropine *on page 529*

Atropine Sulfate (Dental Tablets)

(A troe peen SUL fate DEN tal TAB lets)

Related Information

Atropine *on page 161*

Dentin Hypersensitivity, High Caries Index, and Xerostomia *on page 1714*

U.S. Brand Names Sal-Tropine™

Generic Available No

Dental Use Reduction of salivation and bronchial secretions

Use Treatment of GI disorders (eg, peptic ulcer disease, irritable bowel syndrome, hypermotility of colon)

Local Anesthetic/Vasoconstrictor Precautions No information available to require special precautions

Effects on Dental Treatment

Key adverse event(s) related to dental treatment:

Doses <0.1 mg have been associated with paradoxical bradycardia

Children: May produce fever (by inhibiting heat loss by evaporation), scarlitiniform rash

Causes significant xerostomia when used in therapeutic doses (normal salivary flow resumes upon discontinuation):

0.5 mg: Slight dryness of nose and mouth; bradycardia

1 mg: Increased dryness of nose and mouth; thirst; slowing then acceleration of heart rate; mydriasis

2 mg: Significant xerostomia; tachycardia with palpitations; mydriasis; slight blurring of vision; flushing, dry skin

5 mg: Increase in above symptoms plus disturbance of speech; difficulty swallowing; headache; hot, dry skin; restlessness with asthenia

10 mg: Above symptoms to extreme degree plus ataxia, excitement, disorientation, hallucinations, delirium, coma

Dental Usual Dosing Inhibition of salivation and secretions (preanesthesia): Oral:

Neonates, Infants, and Children (no documented minimum dosage):
- 3-7 kg (7-16 lb): 0.1 mg
- 8-11 kg (17-24 lb): 0.15 mg
- 11-18 kg (24-40 lb): 0.2 mg
- 18-29 kg (40-65 lb): 0.3 mg
- >30 kg (>65 lb): 0.4 mg

Adults: 0.4 mg; may repeat in 4 hours, if necessary.

Dosage

Inhibition of salivation and secretions (preanesthesia): Oral:

Neonates, Infants, and Children (no documented minimum dosage):
- 3-7 kg (7-16 lb): 0.1 mg
- 8-11 kg (17-24 lb): 0.15 mg
- 11-18 kg (24-40 lb): 0.2 mg
- 18-29 kg (40-65 lb): 0.3 mg
- >30 kg (>65 lb): 0.4 mg

Adults: 0.4 mg; may repeat in 4 hours, if necessary.

Mechanism of Action Refer to Atropine monograph.

Contraindications Refer to Atropine monograph.

Warnings/Precautions Lower doses (<0.5 mg) may have vagalmimetic effects (ie, increase vagal tone causing paradoxal bradycardia). A total dose of 3 mg (0.04 mg/kg) results in full vagal blockade in humans. Doses of 0.5-1 mg of atropine are mildly stimulating to the CNS. Geriatric patients may be sensitive to side effects; anticholinergic agents are generally not well tolerated in the elderly and their use should be avoided when possible. Larger doses may produce mental disturbances; psychosis can occur in sensitive individuals. Heat prostration can occur in the presence of a high environmental temperature. Use caution in CHF, tachyarrhythmias, hypertension, and hiatal hernia associated with reflux esophagitis. Lower doses (<0.5 mg) may have vagalmimetic effects (ie, increase vagal tone causing paradoxal bradycardia). A total dose of 3 mg (0.04 mg/kg) results in full vagal blockade in humans.

Drug Interactions

Increased Effect: Atropine-induced mouth dryness may be increased if it is given with other drugs that have anticholinergic actions, such as tricyclic antidepressants, antipsychotics, some antihistamines, and antiparkinsonism drugs.

Decreased Effect: May interfere with absorption of other medications.

Breast-Feeding Considerations Although atropine enters breast milk (trace amounts), the AAP rates this drug as "compatible" with breast-feeding; should be used with caution; anticholinergic agents may suppress lactation

Dosage Forms Tablet, as sulfate (Sal-Tropine™): 0.4 mg

Atrovent® *see* Ipratropium *on page 857*

Atrovent® HFA *see* Ipratropium *on page 857*

A/T/S® *see* Erythromycin *on page 562*

Attapulgite (at a PULL gite)

Related Information

Ulcerative and Erosive Disorders *on page 1712*

U.S. Brand Names Children's Kaopectate® [OTC] [DSC]; Diasorb® [OTC]; Kaopectate® Advanced Formula [OTC] [DSC]; Kaopectate® Maximum Strength Caplets [OTC] [DSC]

Canadian Brand Names Kaopectate®

Generic Available Yes

Pharmacologic Category Antidiarrheal

Use Symptomatic treatment of diarrhea

Local Anesthetic/Vasoconstrictor Precautions No information available to require special precautions

Effects on Dental Treatment No significant effects or complications reported

Mechanism of Action Controls diarrhea because of its absorbent action

Pregnancy Risk Factor B

Attenuvax® *see* Measles Virus Vaccine (Live) *on page 967*

Augmentin® *see* Amoxicillin and Clavulanate Potassium *on page 108*

Augmentin ES-600® *see* Amoxicillin and Clavulanate Potassium *on page 108*

Augmentin XR™ *see* Amoxicillin and Clavulanate Potassium *on page 108*

Auranofin (au RANE oh fin)

Related Information
Rheumatoid Arthritis, Osteoarthritis, and Osteoporosis *on page 1668*
U.S. Brand Names Ridaura®
Canadian Brand Names Ridaura®
Generic Available No
Pharmacologic Category Gold Compound
Use Management of active stage of classic or definite rheumatoid arthritis in patients who do not respond to or tolerate other agents; psoriatic arthritis; adjunctive or alternative therapy for pemphigus
Local Anesthetic/Vasoconstrictor Precautions No information available to require special precautions
Effects on Dental Treatment Key adverse event(s) related to dental treatment: Glossitis and stomatitis.
Common Adverse Effects
>10%:
Dermatologic: Itching, rash
Gastrointestinal: Stomatitis
Ocular: Conjunctivitis
Renal: Proteinuria
1% to 10%:
Dermatologic: Urticaria, alopecia
Gastrointestinal: Glossitis
Hematologic: Eosinophilia, leukopenia, thrombocytopenia
Renal: Hematuria
Mechanism of Action The exact mechanism of action of gold is unknown; gold is taken up by macrophages which results in inhibition of phagocytosis and lysosomal membrane stabilization; other actions observed are decreased serum rheumatoid factor and alterations in immunoglobulins. Additionally, complement activation is decreased, prostaglandin synthesis is inhibited, and lysosomal enzyme activity is decreased.
Drug Interactions
Increased Effect/Toxicity: Toxicity of penicillamine, antimalarials, hydroxychloroquine, cytotoxic agents, and immunosuppressants may be increased.
Pharmacodynamics/Kinetics
Onset of action: Delayed; therapeutic response may require as long as 3-4 months
Duration: Prolonged
Absorption: Oral: ~20% gold in dose is absorbed
Protein binding: 60%
Half-life elimination (single or multiple dose dependent): 21-31 days
Time to peak, serum: ~2 hours
Excretion: Urine (60% of absorbed gold); remainder in feces
Pregnancy Risk Factor C

Aurodex *see* Antipyrine and Benzocaine *on page 130*
Aurolate® *see* Gold Sodium Thiomalate *on page 748*
Auroto *see* Antipyrine and Benzocaine *on page 130*
Autoplex® T [DSC] *see* Anti-inhibitor Coagulant Complex *on page 130*
AVA *see* Anthrax Vaccine (Adsorbed) *on page 128*
Avagard™ [OTC] *see* Chlorhexidine Gluconate *on page 316*
Avage™ *see* Tazarotene *on page 1446*
Avalide® *see* Irbesartan and Hydrochlorothiazide *on page 860*
Avandamet™ *see* Rosiglitazone and Metformin *on page 1369*
Avandaryl™ *see* Rosiglitazone and Glimepiride *on page 1369*
Avandia® *see* Rosiglitazone *on page 1367*
Avapro® *see* Irbesartan *on page 858*
Avapro® HCT *see* Irbesartan and Hydrochlorothiazide *on page 860*
Avastin™ *see* Bevacizumab *on page 204*
Avelox® *see* Moxifloxacin *on page 1069*
Avelox® I.V. *see* Moxifloxacin *on page 1069*
Aviane™ *see* Ethinyl Estradiol and Levonorgestrel *on page 602*
Avinza® *see* Morphine Sulfate *on page 1065*
Avita® *see* Tretinoin (Topical) *on page 1525*
Avitene® *see* Collagen Hemostat *on page 392*
Avitene® Flour *see* Collagen Hemostat *on page 392*
Avitene® Ultrafoam *see* Collagen Hemostat *on page 392*
Avitene® UltraWrap™ *see* Collagen Hemostat *on page 392*

Avodart™ *see* Dutasteride *on page 524*

Avonex® *see* Interferon Beta-1a *on page 849*

Axert™ *see* Almotriptan *on page 71*

Axid® *see* Nizatidine *on page 1123*

Axid® AR [OTC] *see* Nizatidine *on page 1123*

AY-25650 *see* Triptorelin *on page 1544*

Aygestin® *see* Norethindrone *on page 1125*

Ayr® Baby Saline [OTC] *see* Sodium Chloride *on page 1400*

Ayr® Saline [OTC] *see* Sodium Chloride *on page 1400*

Ayr® Saline No-Drip [OTC] *see* Sodium Chloride *on page 1400*

Azacitidine (ay za SYE ti deen)

U.S. Brand Names Vidaza™
Generic Available No
Synonyms AZA-CR; 5-Azacytidine; 5-AZC; Ladakamycin; NSC-102816
Pharmacologic Category Antineoplastic Agent, Antimetabolite (Pyrimidine)
Use Treatment of myelodysplastic syndrome (MDS)
Unlabeled/Investigational Use Investigational: Refractory acute lymphocytic and myelogenous leukemia
Local Anesthetic/Vasoconstrictor Precautions No information available to require special precautions
Effects on Dental Treatment Key adverse event(s) related to dental treatment: Mucositis.
Common Adverse Effects Note: Percentages reported are following SubQ administration unless otherwise noted.
>10%:
 Cardiovascular: Hypotension (7%; I.V. 6% to 66% - incidence may be related to dose and rate of infusion), chest pain (16%), pallor (15%), peripheral edema (19%), pitting edema (14%)
 Central nervous system: Pyrexia (52%), fatigue (13% to 36%), headache (22%), dizziness (19%), anxiety (13%), depression (12%), insomnia (11%), malaise (11%), pain (11%)
 Dermatologic: Alopecia (I.V. 20%), bruising (30%), petechiae (24%), erythema (17%), skin lesion (14%), rash (14%)
 Gastrointestinal: Nausea (58% to 85%; more common/more severe with I.V. administration), vomiting (54%; more common/more severe with I.V. administration), mucositis (I.V. 23% to 45%), diarrhea (36%), constipation (34%), anorexia (21%), weight loss (16%), abdominal pain (15%), appetite decreased (13%), abdominal tenderness (12%)
 Hematologic: Anemia (70%), thrombocytopenia (66%), leukopenia (48%), neutropenia (32%), febrile neutropenia (16%)
  Nadir: Day 10-17
  Recovery: Day 28-31
 Hepatic: Hepatic enzymes increased (I.V. 37%)
 Local: Injection site:
  I.V.: Redness, irritation, and induration (80%)
  SubQ: Erythema (35%), pain (23%), bruising (14%)
 Neuromuscular & skeletal: Weakness (49%), rigors (26%), arthralgia (22%), limb pain (20%), back pain (19%), myalgia (16%)
 Respiratory: Cough (30%), dyspnea (5% to 30%), pharyngitis (20%), epistaxis (16%), nasopharyngitis (14%), upper respiratory tract infection (13%), productive cough (11%), pneumonia (11%)
 Miscellaneous: Contusion (19%)
5% to 10%:
 Cardiovascular: Cardiac murmur (10%), tachycardia (9%), peripheral swelling (7%), syncope (6%), chest wall pain (5%), hypoesthesia (5%), postprocedural pain (5%)
 Central nervous system: Lethargy (8%)
 Dermatologic: Cellulitis (8%), urticaria (6%), dry skin (5%), skin nodule (5%)
 Gastrointestinal: Upper abdominal pain (10%), gingival bleeding (9%), oral mucosal petechiae (8%), stomatitis (8%), dyspepsia (7%), hemorrhoids (7%), abdominal distension (6%), loose stools (5%), dysphagia (5%), tongue ulceration (5%)
 Genitourinary: Dysuria (8%), urinary tract infection (8%)
 Hematologic: Hematoma (9%), postprocedural hemorrhage (6%)
 Local: Injection site: Pruritus (7%), granuloma (5%), pigmentation change (5%), swelling (5%)
 Neuromuscular & skeletal: Muscle cramps (6%)
(Continued)

Azacitidine (Continued)

Respiratory: Crackles (10%), rhinorrhea (10%), wheezing (9%), breath sounds decreased (8%), pleural effusion (6%), postnasal drip (6%), rhonchi (6%), nasal congestion (5%), atelectasis (5%), sinusitis (5%)

Miscellaneous: Diaphoresis (10%), lymphadenopathy (9%), herpes simplex (9%), night sweats (9%), transfusion reaction (7%), mouth hemorrhage (5%)

Mechanism of Action Antineoplastic effects may be a result of azacitidine's ability to promote hypomethylation of DNA leading to direct toxicity of abnormal hematopoietic cells in the bone marrow.

Pharmacodynamics/Kinetics

Absorption: SubQ: Rapid and complete

Bioavailability: SubQ: 89%

Distribution: V_d: 76 ± 26 L; does not cross blood-brain barrier

Metabolism: Hepatic; hydrolysis to several metabolites

Half-life elimination: ~4 hours

Time to peak concentration: 30 minutes

Excretion: Urine (50% to 85%); feces (minor)

Pregnancy Risk Factor D

AZA-CR see Azacitidine on page 167

Azactam® see Aztreonam on page 175

5-Azacytidine see Azacitidine on page 167

Azasan® see Azathioprine on page 168

Azathioprine (ay za THYE oh preen)

U.S. Brand Names Azasan®; Imuran®

Canadian Brand Names Alti-Azathioprine; Apo-Azathioprine®; Gen-Azathioprine; Imuran®; Novo-Azathioprine

Mexican Brand Names Azatrilem®; Imuran®

Generic Available Yes

Synonyms Azathioprine Sodium

Pharmacologic Category Immunosuppressant Agent

Dental Use Adjunct with prednisone for managing severe erosive lichen planus, major aphthous stomatitis, erythema multiforme, and benign mucous membrane pemphigoid

Use Adjunctive therapy in prevention of rejection of kidney transplants; active rheumatoid arthritis

Unlabeled/Investigational Use Adjunct in prevention of rejection of solid organ (nonrenal) transplants; maintenance of remission in Crohn's disease

Local Anesthetic/Vasoconstrictor Precautions No information available to require special precautions

Significant Adverse Effects Frequency not defined; dependent upon dose, duration, and concomitant therapy.

Central nervous system: Fever, malaise

Dermatologic: Alopecia, rash

Gastrointestinal: Diarrhea, nausea, pancreatitis, vomiting

Hematologic: Bleeding, leukopenia, macrocytic anemia, pancytopenia, thrombocytopenia

Hepatic: Hepatotoxicity, hepatic veno-occlusive disease, steatorrhea

Neuromuscular & skeletal: Arthralgia, myalgia

Respiratory: Interstitial pneumonitis

Miscellaneous: Hypersensitivity reactions (rare), infection secondary to immunosuppression, neoplasia

Dental Usual Dosing Adjunctive management of severe recurrent aphthous stomatitis (unlabeled use): Adults: Oral: 50 mg once daily in conjunction with prednisone

Dosage I.V. dose is equivalent to oral dose (dosing should be based on ideal body weight):

Children (unlabeled) and Adults:

Renal transplantation: Oral, I.V.: Initial: 3-5 mg/kg/day usually given as a single daily dose, then 1-3 mg/kg/day maintenance

Rheumatoid arthritis: Oral:

Initial: 1 mg/kg/day given once daily or divided twice daily for 6-8 weeks; increase by 0.5 mg/kg every 4 weeks until response or up to 2.5 mg/kg/day; an adequate trial should be a minimum of 12 weeks

Maintenance dose: Reduce dose by 0.5 mg/kg every 4 weeks until lowest effective dose is reached; optimum duration of therapy not specified; may be discontinued abruptly

Adults: Oral: Adjunctive management of severe recurrent aphthous stomatitis (unlabeled use): 50 mg once daily in conjunction with prednisone

Dosing adjustment in renal impairment:
Cl$_{cr}$ 10-50 mL/minute: Administer 75% of normal dose daily
Cl$_{cr}$ <10 mL/minute: Administer 50% of normal dose daily
Hemodialysis: Dialyzable (~45% removed in 8 hours)
Administer dose posthemodialysis: CAPD effects: Unknown; CAVH effects: Unknown

Mechanism of Action Azathioprine is an imidazolyl derivative of mercaptopurine; antagonizes purine metabolism and may inhibit synthesis of DNA, RNA, and proteins; may also interfere with cellular metabolism and inhibit mitosis. The 6-thioguanine nucleotides appear to mediate the majority of azathioprine's immunosuppressive and toxic effects.

Contraindications Hypersensitivity to azathioprine or any component of the formulation; pregnancy

Warnings/Precautions Chronic immunosuppression increases the risk of neoplasia and serious infections. Azathioprine has mutagenic potential to both men and women and with possible hematologic toxicities; hematologic toxicities are dose related and may be more severe with renal transplants undergoing rejection. Gastrointestinal toxicity may occur within the first several weeks of therapy and is reversible. Symptoms may include severe nausea, vomiting, diarrhea, rash, fever, malaise, myalgia, hypotension, and liver enzyme abnormalities. Use with caution in patients with liver disease, renal impairment; monitor hematologic function closely. Patients with genetic deficiency of thiopurine methyltransferase (TPMT) or concurrent therapy with drugs which may inhibit TPMT may be sensitive to myelosuppressive effects.

Drug Interactions
ACE inhibitors: Concomitant therapy may induce anemia and severe leukopenia.
Allopurinol: May increase serum levels of azathioprine's active metabolite (mercaptopurine). Decrease azathioprine dose to $\frac{1}{3}$ to $\frac{1}{4}$ of normal dose.
Aminosalicylates (olsalazine, mesalamine, sulfasalazine): May inhibit TPMT, increasing toxicity/myelosuppression of azathioprine. Use caution.
Warfarin: Effect may be decreased by azathioprine.

Ethanol/Nutrition/Herb Interactions Herb/Nutraceutical: Avoid cat's claw, echinacea (have immunostimulant properties).

Dietary Considerations May be taken with food.

Pharmacodynamics/Kinetics
Distribution: Crosses placenta
Protein binding: ~30%
Metabolism: Hepatic, to 6-mercaptopurine (6-MP), possibly by glutathione S-transferase (GST). Further metabolism of 6-MP (in the liver and GI tract), via three major pathways: Hypoxanthine guanine phosphoribosyltransferase (to 6-thioguanine-nucleotides, or 6-TGN), xanthine oxidase (to 6-thiouric acid), and thiopurine methyltransferase (TPMT), which forms 6-methylmercapotpurine (6-MMP).
Half-life elimination: Parent drug: 12 minutes; mercaptopurine: 0.7-3 hours; End-stage renal disease: Slightly prolonged
Time to peak, plasma: 1-2 hours (including metabolites)
Excretion: Urine (primarily as metabolites)

Pregnancy Risk Factor D
Lactation Enters breast milk/not recommended
Breast-Feeding Considerations Due to risk of immunosuppression, breast-feeding is not recommended.

Dosage Forms
Injection, powder for reconstitution: 100 mg
Tablet [scored]: 50 mg
Azasan®: 75 mg, 100 mg
Imuran®: 50 mg

Azathioprine Sodium see Azathioprine on page 168
5-AZC see Azacitidine on page 167

Azelaic Acid (a zeh LAY ik AS id)

U.S. Brand Names Azelex®; Finacea™
Generic Available No
Pharmacologic Category Topical Skin Product, Acne
Use Topical treatment of inflammatory papules and pustules of mild-to-moderate rosacea; mild-to-moderate inflammatory acne vulgaris
Finacea™: Not FDA-approved for the treatment of acne
Local Anesthetic/Vasoconstrictor Precautions No information available to require special precautions
Effects on Dental Treatment No significant effects or complications reported
(Continued)

Azelaic Acid *(Continued)*

Common Adverse Effects

>5%: Dermatologic: Pruritus (1% to 6%), burning/stinging/itching (1% to 6%)

1% to 5%:

Dermatologic: Acne (<1% to 1%), edema, erythema, rash, peeling, dermatitis, contact dermatitis, irritation, scaling/dry skin/xerosis

Neuromuscular & skeletal: Paresthesia

Mechanism of Action Azelaic acid is a dietary constituent normally found in whole grain cereals; can be formed endogenously. Exact mechanism is not known. *In vitro*, azelaic acid possesses antimicrobial activity against *Propionibacterium acnes* and *Staphylococcus epidermidis*. May decrease microcomedo formation.

Pharmacodynamics/Kinetics

Absorption: Cream: ~3% to 5% penetrates stratum corneum; up to 10% found in epidermis and dermis; 4% systemic

Half-life elimination: Topical: Healthy subjects: 12 hours

Excretion: Urine (as unchanged drug)

Pregnancy Risk Factor B

Azelastine (a ZEL as teen)

U.S. Brand Names Astelin®; Optivar®
Canadian Brand Names Astelin®
Mexican Brand Names Astelin®; Az®
Generic Available No
Synonyms Azelastine Hydrochloride
Pharmacologic Category Antihistamine

Use

Nasal spray: Treatment of the symptoms of seasonal allergic rhinitis such as rhinorrhea, sneezing, and nasal pruritus in children ≥5 years of age and adults; treatment of the symptoms of vasomotor rhinitis in children ≥12 years of age and adults

Ophthalmic: Treatment of itching of the eye associated with seasonal allergic conjunctivitis in children ≥3 years of age and adults

Local Anesthetic/Vasoconstrictor Precautions No information available to require special precautions

Effects on Dental Treatment Key adverse event(s) related to dental treatment: Bitter taste, xerostomia (normal salivary flow resumes upon discontinuation), aphthous stomatitis, glossitis, and burning sensation in throat. Chronic use of antihistamines will inhibit salivary flow, particularly in elderly patients. May contribute to periodontal disease and oral discomfort.

Common Adverse Effects

Nasal spray:

>10%:

Central nervous system: Headache (8% to 15%), somnolence (<1% to 12%)

Gastrointestinal: Bitter taste (8% to 20%)

Respiratory: Cold symptoms/rhinitis (2% to 17%), cough (11%)

2% to 10%:

Central nervous system: Dysesthesia (8%), dizziness (2%), fatigue (2%)

Gastrointestinal: Nausea (3%), weight gain (2%), dry mouth (3%)

Ocular: Conjunctivitis (<2% to 5%)

Respiratory: Asthma (5%), nasal burning (4%), pharyngitis (4%), paroxysmal sneezing (3%), sinusitis (3%), epistaxis (2% to 3%)

<2%:

Cardiovascular: Flushing, hypertension, tachycardia

Central nervous system: Abnormal thinking, anxiety, depersonalization, depression, drowsiness, fever, hypoesthesia, malaise, nervousness, sleep disorder, vertigo

Dermatologic: Contact dermatitis, eczema, furunculosis, hair and follicle infection

Endocrine & metabolic: Amenorrhea, breast pain

Gastrointestinal: Abdominal pain, ALT increased, aphthous stomatitis, appetite increased, constipation, diarrhea, gastroenteritis, glossitis, ulcerative stomatitis, toothache, vomiting

Genitourinary: Albuminuria, hematuria, polyuria

Hepatic: Liver enzymes increased

Neuromuscular & skeletal: Back pain, extremity pain, hyperkinesia, myalgia, rheumatoid arthritis, temporomandibular dislocation

Ocular: Eye pain, watery eyes

Respiratory: Bronchitis, bronchospasm, laryngitis, nasal congestion, nocturnal dyspnea, postnasal drip, sinus hypersecretion, throat burning

Miscellaneous: Allergic reactions, viral infection

<1%, postmarketing, and/or case reports: Anaphylactoid reaction, chest pain, nasal congestion, confusion, diarrhea, dyspnea, facial edema, involuntary muscle contractions, paresthesia, parosmia, pruritus, rash, skin irritation, tolerance, urinary retention, visual abnormalities, xerophthalmia

Ophthalmic:

>10%:
Central nervous system: Headache (15%)
Ocular: Transient burning/stinging (30%)

1% to 10%:
Central nervous system: Fatigue
Genitourinary: Bitter taste (10%)
Ocular: Conjunctivitis, eye pain, blurred vision (temporary)
Respiratory: Asthma, dyspnea, pharyngitis
Miscellaneous: Flu-like syndrome

Mechanism of Action Competes with histamine for H_1-receptor sites on effector cells and inhibits the release of histamine and other mediators involved in the allergic response; when used intranasally, reduces hyper-reactivity of the airways; increases the motility of bronchial epithelial cilia, improving mucociliary transport

Drug Interactions

Cytochrome P450 Effect: Substrate (minor) of CYP1A2, 2C19, 2D6, 3A4; **Inhibits** CYP2B6 (weak), 2C9 (weak), 2C19 (weak), 2D6 (weak), 3A4 (weak)

Increased Effect/Toxicity: Azelastine may increase the CNS effects of ethanol and the arrhythmogenic effects of antipsychotics agents (phenothiazines). Other anticholinergics, cimetidine, CNS depressants and pramlintide may enhance the effects of azelastine.

Decreased Effect: Acetylcholinesterase inhibitors (central) may decreased the effects of azelastine; azelastine may diminish the effects of acetylcholinesterase inhibitors.

Pharmacodynamics/Kinetics
Onset of action: Peak effect: Nasal spray: 3 hours; Ophthalmic solution: 3 minutes
Duration: Nasal spray: 12 hours; Ophthalmic solution: 8 hours
Protein binding: 88%
Metabolism: Hepatic via CYP; active metabolite, desmethylazelastine
Bioavailability: Intranasal: 40%
Half-life elimination: 22 hours
Time to peak, serum: 2-3 hours

Pregnancy Risk Factor C

Azelastine Hydrochloride see Azelastine on page 170

Azelex® see Azelaic Acid on page 169

Azidothymidine see Zidovudine on page 1594

Azidothymidine, Abacavir, and Lamivudine see Abacavir, Lamivudine, and Zidovudine on page 23

Azithromycin (az ith roe MYE sin)

Related Information
Antibiotic Prophylaxis on page 1680
Sexually-Transmitted Diseases on page 1674

Related Sample Prescriptions
Bacterial Endocarditis (Prevention) on page 1732
Bacterial Infections and Periodontal Diseases on page 1736

U.S. Brand Names Zithromax®; Zmax™

Canadian Brand Names Apo-Azithromycin®; GMD-Azithromycin; Novo-Azithromycin; PMS-Azithromycin; ratio-Azithromycin; Sandoz-Azithromycin; Zithromax®

Generic Available Yes: Tablet

Synonyms Azithromycin Dihydrate; Zithromax® TRI-PAK™; Zithromax® Z-PAK®

Pharmacologic Category Antibiotic, Macrolide

Dental Use Alternate antibiotic in the treatment of common orofacial infections caused by aerobic gram-positive cocci and susceptible anaerobes; alternate antibiotic for the prevention of bacterial endocarditis in patients undergoing dental procedures

Use Treatment of acute otitis media due to *H. influenzae*, *M. catarrhalis*, or *S. pneumoniae*; pharyngitis/tonsillitis due to *S. pyogenes*; treatment of mild-to-moderate upper and lower respiratory tract infections, infections of the skin and skin structure, community-acquired pneumonia, pelvic inflammatory disease (PID), sexually-transmitted diseases (urethritis/cervicitis), pharyngitis/
(Continued)

Azithromycin *(Continued)*

tonsillitis (alternative to first-line therapy), and genital ulcer disease (chancroid) due to susceptible strains of *C. trachomatis, M. catarrhalis, H. influenzae, S. aureus, S. pneumoniae, Mycoplasma pneumoniae,* and *C. psittaci;* acute bacterial exacerbations of chronic obstructive pulmonary disease (COPD) due to *H. influenzae, M. catarrhalis,* or *S. pneumoniae;* acute bacterial sinusitis

Unlabeled/Investigational Use Prevention of (or to delay onset of) or treatment of MAC in patients with advanced HIV infection; prophylaxis of bacterial endocarditis in patients who are allergic to penicillin and undergoing surgical or dental procedures; pertussis

Local Anesthetic/Vasoconstrictor Precautions No information available to require special precautions

Effects on Dental Treatment No significant effects or complications reported

Significant Adverse Effects

>10%: Gastrointestinal: Diarrhea (4% to 11%)

1% to 10%:

Central nervous system: Headache

Gastrointestinal: Nausea, abdominal pain, cramping, vomiting (especially with high single-dose regimens)

<1% (Limited to important or life-threatening): Acute renal failure, allergic reaction, aggressive behavior, anaphylaxis, angioedema, arrhythmia (including ventricular tachycardia), cholestatic jaundice, constipation, convulsion, deafness, dehydration, enteritis, erythema multiforme (rare), hearing loss, hepatic necrosis (rare), hepatitis, hypertrophic pyloric stenosis, hypotension, interstitial nephritis, leukopenia, LFTs increased, neutropenia, oral candidiasis, oral moniliasis, palpitations, pancreatitis, paresthesia, pruritus, pseudomembranous colitis, QT_c prolongation (rare), seizure, somnolence, Stevens-Johnson syndrome (rare), syncope, taste perversion, thrombocytopenia, tinnitus, tongue discoloration (rare), torsade de pointes (rare), urticaria, vertigo

Dental Usual Dosing

Prophylaxis for bacterial endocarditis (unlabeled use): Oral:

Children: 15 mg/kg 1 hour before procedure

Adolescents ≥16 years and Adults: 500 mg 1 hour prior to the procedure

Bacterial sinusitis: Oral:

Children ≥6 months: 10 mg/kg once daily for 3 days (maximum: 500 mg/day)

Adolescents ≥16 years and Adults: 500 mg/day for a total of 3 days

Extended release suspension (Zmax™): 2 g as a single dose

Orofacial infections: Adolescents ≥16 years and Adults: Oral: 500 mg/day, then 250 mg days 2-5

Dosage Note: Extended release suspension (Zmax™) is not interchangeable with immediate release formulations. Use should be limited to approved indications. All doses are expressed as immediate release azithromycin unless otherwise specified.

Oral:

Children <6 months: Pertussis (CDC guidelines): 10 mg/kg/day for 5 days

Children ≥6 months:

Community-acquired pneumonia, pertussis (CDC guidelines): 10 mg/kg on day 1 (maximum: 500 mg/day) followed by 5 mg/kg/day once daily on days 2-5 (maximum: 250 mg/day)

Bacterial sinusitis: 10 mg/kg once daily for 3 days (maximum: 500 mg/day)

Otitis media:

1-day regimen: 30 mg/kg as a single dose (maximum dose: 1500 mg)

3-day regimen: 10 mg/kg once daily for 3 days (maximum: 500 mg/day)

5-day regimen: 10 mg/kg on day 1 (maximum: 500 mg/day) followed by 5 mg/kg/day once daily on days 2-5 (maximum: 250 mg/day)

Children ≥2 years: Pharyngitis, tonsillitis: 12 mg/kg/day once daily for 5 days (maximum: 500 mg/day)

Children:

M. avium-infected patients with acquired immunodeficiency syndrome (unlabeled use): 5 mg/kg/day once daily (maximum dose: 250 mg/day) or 20 mg/kg (maximum dose: 1200 mg) once weekly given alone or in combination with rifabutin

Treatment and secondary prevention of disseminated MAC (unlabeled use): 5 mg/kg/day once daily (maximum dose: 250 mg/day) in combination with ethambutol, with or without rifabutin

Prophylaxis for bacterial endocarditis (unlabeled use): 15 mg/kg 1 hour before procedure

Uncomplicated chlamydial urethritis or cervicitis (unlabeled use): Children ≥45 kg: 1 g as a single dose

Adolescents ≥16 years and Adults:

Community-acquired pneumonia: Extended release suspension (Zmax™): 2 g as a single dose

Respiratory tract, skin and soft tissue infections, pertussis (CDC guidelines): 500 mg on day 1 followed by 250 mg/day on days 2-5 (maximum: 500 mg/day)

Alternative regimen: Bacterial exacerbation of COPD: 500 mg/day for a total of 3 days

Bacterial sinusitis: 500 mg/day for a total of 3 days

Extended release suspension (Zmax™): 2 g as a single dose

Orofacial infections: 500 mg/day, then 250 mg days 2-5

Urethritis/cervicitis:

Due to *C. trachomatis*: 1 g as a single dose

Due to *N. gonorrhoeae*: 2 g as a single dose

Chancroid due to *H. ducreyi*: 1 g as a single dose

Prophylaxis of disseminated *M. avium* complex disease in patient with advanced HIV infection (unlabeled use): 1200 mg once weekly (may be combined with rifabutin)

Treatment of disseminated *M. avium* complex disease in patient with advanced HIV infection (unlabeled use): 600 mg daily (in combination with ethambutol 15 mg/kg)

Prophylaxis for bacterial endocarditis (unlabeled use): 500 mg 1 hour prior to the procedure

I.V.: Adults:

Community-acquired pneumonia: 500 mg as a single dose for at least 2 days, follow I.V. therapy by the oral route with a single daily dose of 500 mg to complete a 7-10 day course of therapy

Pelvic inflammatory disease (PID): 500 mg as a single dose for 1-2 days, follow I.V. therapy by the oral route with a single daily dose of 250 mg to complete a 7-day course of therapy

Dosage adjustment in renal impairment: Use caution in patients with Cl_{cr} <10 mL/minute

Dosage adjustment in hepatic impairment: Use with caution due to potential for hepatotoxicity (rare). Specific guidelines for dosing in hepatic impairment have not been established.

Mechanism of Action Inhibits RNA-dependent protein synthesis at the chain elongation step; binds to the 50S ribosomal subunit resulting in blockage of transpeptidation

Contraindications Hypersensitivity to azithromycin, other macrolide antibiotics, or any component of the formulation

Warnings/Precautions Use with caution in patients with hepatic dysfunction; hepatic impairment with or without jaundice has occurred chiefly in older children and adults. It may be accompanied by malaise, nausea, vomiting, abdominal colic, and fever; discontinue use if these occur. May mask or delay symptoms of incubating gonorrhea or syphilis, so appropriate culture and susceptibility tests should be performed prior to initiating azithromycin. Pseudomembranous colitis has been reported with use of macrolide antibiotics; use caution with renal dysfunction. Prolongation of the QT_c interval has been reported with macrolide antibiotics; use caution in patients at risk of prolonged cardiac repolarization. Safety and efficacy have not been established in children <6 months of age with acute otitis media, acute bacterial sinusitis, or community-acquired pneumonia, or in children <2 years of age with pharyngitis/tonsillitis. Suspensions (immediate release and extended release) are not interchangeable.

Drug Interactions Substrate of CYP3A4 (minor); **Inhibits** CYP3A4 (weak)

Cardiac glycosides: Macrolides may increase the serum concentrations of cardiac glycosides; monitor.

Colchicine: Macrolides may increase the adverse/toxic effects of colchicine.

Nelfinavir: May increase azithromycin serum levels; monitor for adverse effects.

Warfarin: Azithromycin and other macrolides may decrease metabolism, via CYP isoenzymes, of warfarin. Monitor for increased effects.

Ethanol/Nutrition/Herb Interactions Food: Rate and extent of GI absorption may be altered depending upon the formulation. Azithromycin suspension, not tablet form, has significantly increased absorption (46%) with food.

Dietary Considerations

Oral suspension, immediate release, may be administered with or without food.

Oral suspension, extended release, should be taken on an empty stomach (at least 1 hour before or 2 hours following a meal).

Tablet may be administered with food to decrease GI effects.

Sodium content:

Injection: 114 mg (4.96 mEq) per vial

(Continued)

Azithromycin *(Continued)*

Oral suspension, immediate release: 3.7 mg per 100 mg/5 mL of constituted suspension; 7.4 mg per 200 mg/5 mL of constituted suspension; 37 mg per 1 g single-dose packet

Oral suspension, extended release: 148 mg per 2 g constituted suspension

Tablet: 0.9 mg/250 mg tablet; 1.8 mg/500 mg tablet; 2.1 mg/600 mg tablet

Pharmacodynamics/Kinetics

Absorption: Rapid

Distribution: Extensive tissue; distributes well into skin, lungs, sputum, tonsils, and cervix; penetration into CSF is poor; I.V.: 33.3 L/kg; Oral: 31.1 L/kg

Protein binding (concentration dependent): 7% to 51%

Metabolism: Hepatic

Bioavailability: 38%, decreased by 17% with extended release suspension; variable effect with food (increased with immediate or delayed release oral suspension, unchanged with tablet)

Half-life elimination: Terminal: Immediate release: 68-72 hours; Extended release: 59 hours

Time to peak, serum: Immediate release: 2-3 hours; Extended release: 5 hours

Excretion: Biliary (major route); urine (6%)

Pregnancy Risk Factor B

Lactation Enters breast milk/use caution

Breast-Feeding Considerations Based on one case report, azithromycin has been shown to accumulate in breast milk.

Dosage Forms Note: Strength expressed as base

Injection, powder for reconstitution, as dihydrate (Zithromax®): 500 mg [contains sodium 114 mg (4.96 mEq) per vial]

Microspheres for oral suspension, extended release, as dihydrate (Zmax™): 2 g [single-dose bottle; contains sodium 148 mg per bottle; cherry and banana flavor]

Powder for oral suspension, immediate release, as dihydrate (Zithromax®): 100 mg/5 mL (15 mL) [contains sodium 3.7 mg/ 5 mL; cherry creme de vanilla and banana flavor]; 200 mg/5 mL (15 mL, 22.5 mL, 30 mL) [contains sodium 7.4 mg/5 mL; cherry creme de vanilla and banana flavor]; 1 g [single-dose packet; contains sodium 37 mg per packet; cherry creme de vanilla and banana flavor]

Tablet, as dihydrate:

Zithromax®: 250 mg [contains sodium 0.9 mg per tablet]; 500 mg [contains sodium 1.8 mg per tablet]; 600 mg [contains sodium 2.1 mg per tablet]

Zithromax® TRI-PAK™ [unit-dose pack]: 500 mg (3s)

Zithromax® Z-PAK® [unit-dose pack]: 250 mg (6s)

Tablet, as monohydrate: 250 mg, 500 mg, 600 mg

Selected Readings

ADA Division of Legal Affairs, "A Legal Perspective on Antibiotic Prophylaxis," *J Am Dent Assoc*, 2003, 134(9):1260.

American Dental Association Council on Scientific Affairs, "Combating Antibiotic Resistance," *J Am Dent Assoc*, 2004, 135(4):484-7.

Cotter CJ and Bierne JC, "Azithromycin for Odontogenic Infection," *J Oral Maxillofac Surg*, 2003, 61(10):1238.

Dajani AS, Taubert KA, Wilson W, et al, "Prevention of Bacterial Endocarditis. Recommendations by the American Heart Association," *JAMA*, 1997, 277(22):1794-801.

Dajani AS, Taubert KA, Wilson W, et al, "Prevention of Bacterial Endocarditis: Recommendations by the American Heart Association," *J Am Dent Assoc*, 1997, 128(8):1142-51.

Moore PA, "Dental Therapeutic Indications for the Newer Long-Acting Macrolide Antibiotics," *J Am Dent Assoc*, 1999, 130(9):1341-3.

Williams JD, Maskell JP, Shain H, et al, "Comparative *In Vitro* Activity of Azithromycin, Macrolides (Erythromycin, Clarithromycin and Spiramycin) and Streptogramin RP 59500 Against Oral Organisms," *J Antimicrob Chemother*, 1992, 30(1):27-37.

Wynn RL, "New Erythromycins," *Gen Dent*, 1996, 44(4):304-7.

Wynn RL, Bergman SA, Meiller TF, et al, "Antibiotics in Treating Oral-Facial Infections of Odontogenic Origin: An Update", *Gen Dent*, 2001, 49(3):238-40, 242, 244 passim.

Azithromycin Dihydrate *see* Azithromycin *on page 171*

Azmacort® *see* Triamcinolone *on page 1526*

AZO-Gesic® [OTC] *see* Phenazopyridine *on page 1220*

Azopt® *see* Brinzolamide *on page 220*

AZO-Standard® [OTC] *see* Phenazopyridine *on page 1220*

AZT + 3TC (error-prone abbreviation) *see* Zidovudine and Lamivudine *on page 1596*

AZT, Abacavir, and Lamivudine *see* Abacavir, Lamivudine, and Zidovudine *on page 23*

AZT (error-prone abbreviation) *see* Zidovudine *on page 1594*

Azthreonam *see* Aztreonam *on page 175*

Aztreonam (AZ tree oh nam)

U.S. Brand Names Azactam®
Canadian Brand Names Azactam®
Generic Available No
Synonyms Azthreonam
Pharmacologic Category Antibiotic, Miscellaneous
Use Treatment of patients with urinary tract infections, lower respiratory tract infections, septicemia, skin/skin structure infections, intra-abdominal infections, and gynecological infections caused by susceptible gram-negative bacilli
Local Anesthetic/Vasoconstrictor Precautions No information available to require special precautions
Effects on Dental Treatment No significant effects or complications reported
Common Adverse Effects As reported in adults: 1% to 10%:
Dermatologic: Rash
Gastrointestinal: Diarrhea, nausea, vomiting
Local: Thrombophlebitis, pain at injection site
Mechanism of Action Inhibits bacterial cell wall synthesis by binding to one or more of the penicillin binding proteins (PBPs) which in turn inhibits the final transpeptidation step of peptidoglycan synthesis in bacterial cell walls, thus inhibiting cell wall biosynthesis. Bacteria eventually lyse due to ongoing activity of cell wall autolytic enzymes (autolysins and murein hydrolases) while cell wall assembly is arrested. Monobactam structure makes cross-allergenicity with beta-lactams unlikely.
Drug Interactions
Decreased Effect: Avoid antibiotics that induce beta-lactamase production (cefoxitin, imipenem).
Pharmacodynamics/Kinetics
Absorption: I.M.: Well absorbed; I.M. and I.V. doses produce comparable serum concentrations
Distribution: Widely to most body fluids and tissues; crosses placenta; enters breast milk
V_d: Children: 0.2-0.29 L/kg; Adults: 0.2 L/kg
Relative diffusion of antimicrobial agents from blood into CSF: Good only with inflammation (exceeds usual MICs)
CSF:blood level ratio: Meninges: Inflamed: 8% to 40%; Normal: ~1%
Protein binding: 56%
Metabolism: Hepatic (minor %)
Half-life elimination:
Children 2 months to 12 years: 1.7 hours
Adults: Normal renal function: 1.7-2.9 hours
End-stage renal disease: 6-8 hours
Time to peak: I.M., I.V. push: Within 60 minutes; I.V. infusion: 1.5 hours
Excretion: Urine (60% to 70% as unchanged drug); feces (~13% to 15%)
Pregnancy Risk Factor B

Azulfidine® see Sulfasalazine on page 1428

Azulfidine® EN-tabs® see Sulfasalazine on page 1428

B-D™ Glucose [OTC] see Dextrose on page 452

B 9273 see Alefacept on page 62

BA-16038 see Aminoglutethimide on page 87

Babee® Cof Syrup [OTC] see Dextromethorphan on page 451

BAC see Benzalkonium Chloride on page 188

Bacid® [OTC] see Lactobacillus on page 535

Baciguent® [OTC] see Bacitracin on page 175

BaciiM® see Bacitracin on page 175

Bacillus Calmette-Guérin (BCG) Live see BCG Vaccine on page 181

Bacitracin (bas i TRAY sin)

U.S. Brand Names AK-Tracin® [DSC]; Baciguent® [OTC]; BaciiM®
Canadian Brand Names Baciguent®; Baciject®
Generic Available Yes
Pharmacologic Category Antibiotic, Miscellaneous; Antibiotic, Ophthalmic; Antibiotic, Topical
Use Treatment of susceptible bacterial infections mainly; has activity against gram-positive bacilli; due to toxicity risks, systemic and irrigant uses of bacitracin should be limited to situations where less toxic alternatives would not be effective
(Continued)

Bacitracin *(Continued)*

Unlabeled/Investigational Use Oral administration: Successful in antibiotic-associated colitis; has been used for enteric eradication of vancomycin-resistant enterococci (VRE)

Local Anesthetic/Vasoconstrictor Precautions No information available to require special precautions

Effects on Dental Treatment No significant effects or complications reported

Common Adverse Effects 1% to 10%:
Cardiovascular: Hypotension, edema of the face/lips, chest tightness
Central nervous system: Pain
Dermatologic: Rash, itching
Gastrointestinal: Anorexia, nausea, vomiting, diarrhea, rectal itching
Hematologic: Blood dyscrasias
Miscellaneous: Diaphoresis

Mechanism of Action Inhibits bacterial cell wall synthesis by preventing transfer of mucopeptides into the growing cell wall

Drug Interactions
Increased Effect/Toxicity: Nephrotoxic drugs, neuromuscular blocking agents, and anesthetics (increased neuromuscular blockade).

Pharmacodynamics/Kinetics
Duration: 6-8 hours
Absorption: Poor from mucous membranes and intact or denuded skin; rapidly following I.M. administration; not absorbed by bladder irrigation, but absorption can occur from peritoneal or mediastinal lavage
Distribution: CSF: Nil even with inflammation
Protein binding, plasma: Minimal
Time to peak, serum: I.M.: 1-2 hours
Excretion: Urine (10% to 40%) within 24 hours

Pregnancy Risk Factor C

Bacitracin and Polymyxin B (bas i TRAY sin & pol i MIKS in bee)

Related Information
Bacitracin *on page 175*
Polymyxin B *on page 1253*

U.S. Brand Names AK-Poly-Bac®; Betadine® First Aid Antibiotics + Moisturizer [OTC]; Polysporin® Ophthalmic; Polysporin® Topical [OTC]

Canadian Brand Names LID-Pack®; Optimyxin®

Generic Available Yes

Synonyms Polymyxin B and Bacitracin

Pharmacologic Category Antibiotic, Ophthalmic; Antibiotic, Topical

Use Treatment of superficial infections caused by susceptible organisms

Local Anesthetic/Vasoconstrictor Precautions No information available to require special precautions

Effects on Dental Treatment No significant effects or complications reported

Common Adverse Effects 1% to 10%: Local: Rash, itching, burning, anaphylactoid reactions, swelling, conjunctival erythema

Mechanism of Action See individual agents.

Pharmacodynamics/Kinetics See individual agents.

Pregnancy Risk Factor C

Bacitracin, Neomycin, and Polymyxin B
(bas i TRAY sin, nee oh MYE sin, & pol i MIKS in bee)

Related Information
Bacitracin *on page 175*
Neomycin *on page 1100*
Polymyxin B *on page 1253*

U.S. Brand Names Neosporin® Neo To Go® [OTC]; Neosporin® Ophthalmic Ointment [DSC]; Neosporin® Topical [OTC]

Canadian Brand Names Neosporin® Ophthalmic Ointment

Generic Available Yes

Synonyms Neomycin, Bacitracin, and Polymyxin B; Polymyxin B, Bacitracin, and Neomycin; Triple Antibiotic

Pharmacologic Category Antibiotic, Ophthalmic; Antibiotic, Topical

Use Helps prevent infection in minor cuts, scrapes, and burns; short-term treatment of superficial external ocular infections caused by susceptible organisms

Local Anesthetic/Vasoconstrictor Precautions No information available to require special precautions

Effects on Dental Treatment No significant effects or complications reported

Common Adverse Effects Frequency not defined.

Dermatologic: Reddening, allergic contact dermatitis

Local: Itching, failure to heal, swelling, irritation

Ophthalmic: Conjunctival edema

Miscellaneous: Anaphylaxis

Mechanism of Action Refer to individual agents, Bacitracin *on page 175*, Neomycin *on page 1100*, and Polymyxin B *on page 1253*.

Pharmacodynamics/Kinetics See individual agents.

Pregnancy Risk Factor C

Bacitracin, Neomycin, Polymyxin B, and Hydrocortisone
(bas i TRAY sin, nee oh MYE sin, pol i MIKS in bee, & hye droe KOR ti sone)

Related Information

Bacitracin *on page 175*

Hydrocortisone *on page 793*

Neomycin *on page 1100*

Polymyxin B *on page 1253*

U.S. Brand Names Cortisporin® Ointment

Canadian Brand Names Cortisporin® Topical Ointment

Generic Available Yes: Ophthalmic ointment

Synonyms Hydrocortisone, Bacitracin, Neomycin, and Polymyxin B; Neomycin, Bacitracin, Polymyxin B, and Hydrocortisone; Polymyxin B, Bacitracin, Neomycin, and Hydrocortisone

Pharmacologic Category Antibiotic, Ophthalmic; Antibiotic, Otic; Antibiotic, Topical; Corticosteroid, Ophthalmic; Corticosteroid, Otic; Corticosteroid, Topical

Use Prevention and treatment of susceptible inflammatory conditions where bacterial infection (or risk of infection) is present

Local Anesthetic/Vasoconstrictor Precautions No information available to require special precautions

Effects on Dental Treatment No significant effects or complications reported

Common Adverse Effects Frequency not defined.

Dermatologic: Rash, generalized itching

Ocular: Irritation

Respiratory: Apnea

Miscellaneous: Secondary infection

Mechanism of Action Refer to individual agents, Bacitracin *on page 175*, Neomycin *on page 1100*, Polymyxin B *on page 1253*, and Hydrocortisone *on page 793*.

Drug Interactions

Cytochrome P450 Effect: Hydrocortisone: **Substrate** of CYP3A4 (minor); **Induces** CYP3A4 (weak)

Pharmacodynamics/Kinetics See individual agents.

Pregnancy Risk Factor C

Bacitracin, Neomycin, Polymyxin B, and Pramoxine
(bas i TRAY sin, nee oh MYE sin, pol i MIKS in bee, & pra MOKS een)

Related Information

Bacitracin *on page 175*

Neomycin *on page 1100*

Polymyxin B *on page 1253*

Pramoxine *on page 1264*

U.S. Brand Names Neosporin® + Pain Ointment [OTC]; Spectrocin Plus™ [OTC]

Generic Available Yes

Synonyms Neomycin, Bacitracin, Polymyxin B, and Pramoxine; Polymyxin B, Neomycin, Bacitracin, and Pramoxine; Pramoxine, Neomycin, Bacitracin, and Polymyxin B

Pharmacologic Category Antibiotic, Topical

Use Prevention and treatment of susceptible superficial topical infections and provide temporary relief of pain or discomfort

Local Anesthetic/Vasoconstrictor Precautions No information available to require special precautions

Effects on Dental Treatment No significant effects or complications reported

Baclofen (BAK loe fen)

U.S. Brand Names Lioresal®
Canadian Brand Names Apo-Baclofen®; Gen-Baclofen; Lioresal®; Liotec; Nu-Baclo; PMS-Baclofen
Generic Available Yes: Tablets only
Pharmacologic Category Skeletal Muscle Relaxant
Use Treatment of reversible spasticity associated with multiple sclerosis or spinal cord lesions
  Orphan drug: Intrathecal: Treatment of intractable spasticity caused by spinal cord injury, multiple sclerosis, and other spinal disease (spinal ischemia or tumor, transverse myelitis, cervical spondylosis, degenerative myelopathy)
Unlabeled/Investigational Use Intractable hiccups, intractable pain relief, bladder spasticity, trigeminal neuralgia, cerebral palsy, Huntington's chorea
Local Anesthetic/Vasoconstrictor Precautions No information available to require special precautions
Effects on Dental Treatment No significant effects or complications reported
Common Adverse Effects
  >10%:
    Central nervous system: Drowsiness, vertigo, psychiatric disturbances, insomnia, slurred speech, ataxia, hypotonia
    Neuromuscular & skeletal: Weakness
  1% to 10%:
    Cardiovascular: Hypotension
    Central nervous system: Fatigue, confusion, headache
    Dermatologic: Rash
    Gastrointestinal: Nausea, constipation
    Genitourinary: Polyuria
Mechanism of Action Inhibits the transmission of both monosynaptic and polysynaptic reflexes at the spinal cord level, possibly by hyperpolarization of primary afferent fiber terminals, with resultant relief of muscle spasticity
Drug Interactions
  Increased Effect/Toxicity: Effects may be additive with CNS depressants.
Pharmacodynamics/Kinetics
  Onset of action: 3-4 days
    Peak effect: 5-10 days
  Absorption (dose dependent): Oral: Rapid
  Protein binding: 30%
  Metabolism: Hepatic (15% of dose)
  Half-life elimination: 3.5 hours
  Time to peak, serum: Oral: Within 2-3 hours
  Excretion: Urine and feces (85% as unchanged drug)
Pregnancy Risk Factor C

BactoShield® CHG [OTC] see Chlorhexidine Gluconate on page 316
Bactrim™ see Sulfamethoxazole and Trimethoprim on page 1425
Bactrim™ DS see Sulfamethoxazole and Trimethoprim on page 1425
Bactroban® see Mupirocin on page 1073
Bactroban® Nasal see Mupirocin on page 1073
Baking Soda see Sodium Bicarbonate on page 1400
BAL see Dimercaprol on page 482
Balacet 325™ see Propoxyphene and Acetaminophen on page 1298

Balanced Salt Solution (BAL anced salt soe LOO shun)

U.S. Brand Names AquaLase™; BSS®; BSS Plus®
Canadian Brand Names BSS®; BSS Plus®; Eye-Stream®
Generic Available Yes
Pharmacologic Category Ophthalmic Agent, Miscellaneous
Use Irrigation solution for ophthalmic surgery:
  AquaLase™, BSS®: Intraocular or extraocular irrigating solution
  BSS® Plus: Intraocular irrigating solution
Local Anesthetic/Vasoconstrictor Precautions No information available to require special precautions
Effects on Dental Treatment No significant effects or complications reported

BAL in Oil® see Dimercaprol on page 482
Balmex® [OTC] see Zinc Oxide on page 1597
Balnetar® [OTC] see Coal Tar on page 383

Balsalazide (bal SAL a zide)

U.S. Brand Names Colazal®
Generic Available No
Synonyms Balsalazide Disodium
Pharmacologic Category 5-Aminosalicylic Acid Derivative; Anti-inflammatory Agent
Use Treatment of mild-to-moderate active ulcerative colitis
Local Anesthetic/Vasoconstrictor Precautions No information available to require special precautions
Effects on Dental Treatment No significant effects or complications reported
Common Adverse Effects 1% to 10%:
  Central nervous system: Headache (8%), insomnia (2%), fatigue (2%), fever (2%), pain (2%), dizziness (1%)
  Gastrointestinal: Abdominal pain (6%), diarrhea (5%), nausea (5%), vomiting (4%), anorexia (2%), dyspepsia (2%), flatulence (2%), rectal bleeding (2%), cramps (1%), constipation (1%), dry mouth (1%), frequent stools (1%)
  Genitourinary: Urinary tract infection (1%)
  Neuromuscular & skeletal: Arthralgia (4%), back pain (2%), myalgia (1%)
  Respiratory: Respiratory infection (4%), cough (2%), pharyngitis (2%), rhinitis (2%), sinusitis (1%)
  Miscellaneous: Flu-like syndrome (1%)
Mechanism of Action Balsalazide is a prodrug, converted by bacterial azoreduction to 5-aminosalicylic acid (active), 4-aminobenzoyl-β-alanine (inert), and their metabolites. 5-aminosalicylic acid may decrease inflammation by blocking the production of arachidonic acid metabolites topically in the colon mucosa.
Drug Interactions
  Decreased Effect: No studies have been conducted. Oral antibiotics may potentially interfere with 5-aminosalicylic acid release in the colon.
Pharmacodynamics/Kinetics
  Onset of action: Delayed; may require several days to weeks
  Absorption: Very low and variable
  Protein binding: ≥99%
  Metabolism: Azoreduced in the colon to 5-aminosalicylic acid (active), 4-aminobenzoyl-β-alanine (inert), and N-acetylated metabolites
  Half-life elimination: Primary effect is topical (colonic mucosa); systemic half-life not determined
  Time to peak: 1-2 hours
  Excretion: Feces (65% as 5-aminosalicylic acid, 4-aminobenzoyl-β-alanine, and N-acetylated metabolites); urine (25% as N-acetylated metabolites); Parent drug: Urine or feces (<1%)
Pregnancy Risk Factor B

Balsalazide Disodium see Balsalazide on page 179

Balsam Peru, Trypsin, and Castor Oil see Trypsin, Balsam Peru, and Castor Oil on page 1547

Baltussin see Dihydrocodeine, Chlorpheniramine, and Phenylephrine on page 476

Bancap HC® see Hydrocodone and Acetaminophen on page 779

Band-Aid® Hurt-Free™ Antiseptic Wash [OTC] see Lidocaine on page 920

Banophen® [OTC] see DiphenhydrAMINE on page 483

Banophen® Anti-Itch [OTC] see DiphenhydrAMINE on page 483

Baraclude™ see Entecavir on page 544

Baricon™ see Barium on page 179

Baridium® [OTC] see Phenazopyridine on page 1220

Barium (BA ree um)

U.S. Brand Names Anatrast; Baricon™; Barobag®; Baro-Cat®; Barosperse®; Bear-E-Yum® CT; Bear-E-Yum® GI; CheeTah®; Digital HD; Enhancer; Entrobar®; EntroEase®; Flo-Coat; HD 85®; HD 200® Plus; Intropaste; Liqui-Coat HD®; Liquid Barosperse®; Medebar® Plus; Medescan; Prepcat; Tomocat®; Tomocat® 1000; Tonopaque
Generic Available No
Synonyms Barium Sulfate
Pharmacologic Category Radiopaque Agents
Use Diagnostic aid for computed tomography or x-ray examinations of the GI tract
  (Continued)

Barium *(Continued)*

Local Anesthetic/Vasoconstrictor Precautions No information available to require special precautions

Effects on Dental Treatment No significant effects or complications reported

Barium Sulfate *see* Barium *on page 179*

Barobag® *see* Barium *on page 179*

Baro-Cat® *see* Barium *on page 179*

Barosperse® *see* Barium *on page 179*

Base Ointment *see* Zinc Oxide *on page 1597*

Basiliximab *(ba si LIK si mab)*

U.S. Brand Names Simulect®
Canadian Brand Names Simulect®
Mexican Brand Names Simulect®
Generic Available No
Pharmacologic Category Monoclonal Antibody
Use Prophylaxis of acute organ rejection in renal transplantation
Local Anesthetic/Vasoconstrictor Precautions No information available to require special precautions

Effects on Dental Treatment Key adverse event(s) related to dental treatment: Facial edema and ulcerative stomatitis. Causes gingival hypertrophy (GH) similar to that caused by cyclosporine; early reports indicate that frequency/incidence of basiliximab-induced GH not as high as cyclosporine-induced GH.

Common Adverse Effects Administration of basiliximab did not appear to increase the incidence or severity of adverse effects in clinical trials. Adverse events were reported in 96% of both the placebo and basiliximab groups.

>10%:
Cardiovascular: Peripheral edema, hypertension, atrial fibrillation
Central nervous system: Fever, headache, insomnia, pain
Dermatologic: Wound complications, acne
Endocrine & metabolic: Hypokalemia, hyperkalemia, hyperglycemia, hyperuricemia, hypophosphatemia, hypercholesterolemia
Gastrointestinal: Constipation, nausea, diarrhea, abdominal pain, vomiting, dyspepsia
Genitourinary: Urinary tract infection
Hematologic: Anemia
Neuromuscular & skeletal: Tremor
Respiratory: Dyspnea, infection (upper respiratory)
Miscellaneous: Viral infection

3% to 10%:
Cardiovascular: Chest pain, cardiac failure, hypotension, arrhythmia, tachycardia, generalized edema, abnormal heart sounds, angina pectoris
Central nervous system: Hypoesthesia, neuropathy, agitation, anxiety, depression, malaise, fatigue, rigors, dizziness
Dermatologic: Cyst, hypertrichosis, pruritus, rash, skin disorder, skin ulceration
Endocrine & metabolic: Dehydration, diabetes mellitus, fluid overload, hypercalcemia, hyperlipidemia, hypoglycemia, hypomagnesemia, acidosis, hypertriglyceridemia, hypocalcemia, hyponatremia
Gastrointestinal: Flatulence, gastroenteritis, GI hemorrhage, gingival hyperplasia, melena, esophagitis, stomatitis, abdomen enlarged, moniliasis, ulcerative stomatitis, weight gain
Genitourinary: Impotence, genital edema, albuminuria, bladder disorder, hematuria, urinary frequency, oliguria, renal function abnormal, renal tubular necrosis, ureteral disorder, urinary retention, dysuria
Hematologic: Hematoma, hemorrhage, purpura, thrombocytopenia, thrombosis, polycythemia, leukopenia
Neuromuscular & skeletal: Arthralgia, arthropathy, cramps, fracture, hernia, myalgia, paresthesia, weakness, back pain, leg pain
Ocular: Cataract, conjunctivitis, abnormal vision
Respiratory: Bronchitis, bronchospasm, pneumonia, pulmonary edema, sinusitis, rhinitis, cough, pharyngitis
Miscellaneous: Accidental trauma, facial edema, sepsis, infection, glucocorticoids increased, herpes infection

Mechanism of Action Chimeric (murine/human) monoclonal antibody which blocks the alpha-chain of the interleukin-2 (IL-2) receptor complex; this receptor is expressed on activated T lymphocytes and is a critical pathway for activating cell-mediated allograft rejection

Drug Interactions
Increased Effect/Toxicity: Basiliximab is an immunoglobulin; specific drug interactions have not been evaluated, but are not anticipated.
Decreased Effect: Basiliximab is an immunoglobulin; specific drug interactions have not been evaluated, but are not anticipated. It is not known if the immune response to vaccines will be impaired during or following basiliximab therapy.

Pharmacodynamics/Kinetics
Duration: Mean: 36 days (determined by IL-2R alpha saturation)
Distribution: Mean: V_d: Children: 5.2 ± 2.8 L; Adults: 8.6 ± 4.1 L
Half-life elimination: Children: 9.4 days; Adults: Mean: 7.2 days
Excretion: Clearance: Children: 20 mL/hour; Adults: Mean: 41 mL/hour

Pregnancy Risk Factor B (manufacturer)

Bausch & Lomb® Computer Eye Drops [OTC] see Glycerin on page 747

BAY 43-9006 see Sorafenib on page 1407

Bayer® Aspirin [OTC] see Aspirin on page 145

Bayer® Aspirin Extra Strength [OTC] see Aspirin on page 145

Bayer® Aspirin Regimen Adult Low Strength [OTC] see Aspirin on page 145

Bayer® Aspirin Regimen Children's [OTC] see Aspirin on page 145

Bayer® Aspirin Regimen Regular Strength [OTC] see Aspirin on page 145

Bayer® Extra Strength Arthritis Pain Regimen [OTC] see Aspirin on page 145

Bayer® Plus Extra Strength [OTC] see Aspirin on page 145

Bayer® Women's Aspirin Plus Calcium [OTC] see Aspirin on page 145

BayGam® see Immune Globulin (Intramuscular) on page 823

BayHep B® see Hepatitis B Immune Globulin on page 768

BayRab® see Rabies Immune Globulin (Human) on page 1328

BayRho-D® Full-Dose see $Rh_o(D)$ Immune Globulin on page 1342

BayRho-D® Mini-Dose see $Rh_o(D)$ Immune Globulin on page 1342

BayTet™ see Tetanus Immune Globulin (Human) on page 1463

Baza® Antifungal [OTC] see Miconazole on page 1039

Baza® Clear [OTC] see Vitamin A and Vitamin D on page 1580

B-Caro-T™ see Beta-Carotene on page 198

BCG, Live see BCG Vaccine on page 181

BCG Vaccine (bee see jee vak SEEN)

Related Information
Immunizations (Vaccines) on page 1786
U.S. Brand Names TheraCys®; TICE® BCG
Canadian Brand Names ImmuCyst®; Oncotice™; Pacis™
Generic Available No
Synonyms Bacillus Calmette-Guérin (BCG) Live; BCG, Live; BCG Vaccine U.S.P. (percutaneous use product)
Pharmacologic Category Biological Response Modulator; Vaccine
Use Immunization against tuberculosis and immunotherapy for cancer; treatment and prophylaxis of carcinoma in situ of the bladder; prophylaxis of primary or recurrent superficial papillary tumors following transurethral resection
Local Anesthetic/Vasoconstrictor Precautions No information available to require special precautions
Effects on Dental Treatment No significant effects or complications reported
Common Adverse Effects All serious adverse reactions must be reported to the U.S. Department of Health and Human Services (DHHS) Vaccine Adverse Event Reporting System (VAERS) 1-800-822-7967.

Adverse reactions associated with **intravesicular administration:**
>10%:
Central nervous system: Malaise (7% to 40%), fever (20% to 38%), chills (34%)
Gastrointestinal: Nausea/vomiting (3% to 16%), anorexia/weight loss (2% to 11%)
Genitourinary: Dysuria (52% to 60%), bladder irritation (50% to 60%), polyuria (40% to 42%), hematuria (26% to 39%), cystitis (6% to 29%), urinary urgency (6% to 18%), urinary tract infection (2% to 18%)
Hematological: Anemia (<1% to 21%)
Miscellaneous: Flu-like syndrome (33%)
1% to 10%:
Central nervous system: Fatigue (7%), headache/dizziness (2%)
Dermatologic: Rash (2%)
(Continued)

BCG Vaccine (Continued)

Gastrointestinal: Diarrhea (6%), abdominal pain (2% to 3%)

Genitourinary: Genital pain (10%), bladder cramps/pain (6%), urinary incontinence (2% to 6%), bladder spasm (5%), nocturia (5%), urinary debris (2%), genital inflammation/abscess (2%)

Hematological: Leukopenia (5%), coagulopathy (3%)

Neuromuscular & skeletal: Arthralgia/myalgia (3% to 7%), cramps/pain (4% to 6%), rigors (3%)

Renal: Renal toxicity (10%)

Respiratory: Pulmonary infection (3%)

Miscellaneous: Infection (3%), allergy (2%)

Adverse reactions associated with **BCG vaccination**: Axillary lymphadenopathy, cervical lymphadenopathy, disseminated BCG infection (BCG osteomyelitis), local reactions (induration, itching, lesions, lymphadenitis, pustule, tenderness, ulceration). Local reactions may persist for up to 3 months; more severe manifestations may occur up to 5 months after vaccination and persist for several weeks.

Mechanism of Action BCG live is an attenuated strain of bacillus Calmette-Guérin (*Mycobacterium bovis*) used as a biological response modifier. BCG live, when used intravesicularly for treatment of bladder carcinoma *in situ*, is thought to cause a local, chronic inflammatory response involving macrophage and leukocyte infiltration of the bladder. By a mechanism not fully understood, this local inflammatory response leads to destruction of superficial tumor cells of the urothelium. BCG is active immunotherapy which stimulates the host's immune mechanism to reject the tumor. Evidence of systemic immune response is also commonly seen, manifested by a positive PPD tuberculin skin test reaction, however, its relationship to clinical efficacy is not well-established.

Drug Interactions

Increased Effect/Toxicity: The following agents may decrease the effectiveness of BCG vaccine: Antimicrobials, immune globulins, immunosuppressants, and other live organism vaccines. Antimicrobials may interfere with the effectiveness of intravesicular BCG.

Decreased Effect: Immunosuppressants may increase the risk of vaccinal infections. BCG vaccination results in a reactive tuberculin skin test.

Pregnancy Risk Factor C

BCG Vaccine U.S.P. *(percutaneous use product)* see BCG Vaccine on page 181

BCNU see Carmustine on page 273

B Complex Combinations see Vitamin B Complex Combinations on page 1581

Bear-E-Yum® CT see Barium on page 179

Bear-E-Yum® GI see Barium on page 179

Bebulin® VH see Factor IX Complex (Human) on page 633

Becaplermin (be KAP ler min)

U.S. Brand Names Regranex®

Canadian Brand Names Regranex®

Generic Available No

Synonyms Recombinant Human Platelet-Derived Growth Factor B; rPDGF-BB

Pharmacologic Category Growth Factor, Platelet-Derived; Topical Skin Product

Use Debridement adjunct for the treatment of diabetic ulcers that occur on the lower limbs and feet

Local Anesthetic/Vasoconstrictor Precautions No information available to require special precautions

Effects on Dental Treatment No significant effects or complications reported

Mechanism of Action Recombinant B-isoform homodimer of human platelet-derived growth factor (rPDGF-BB) which enhances formation of new granulation tissue, induces fibroblast proliferation and differentiation to promote wound healing

Pharmacodynamics/Kinetics

Onset of action: Complete healing: 15% of patients within 8 weeks, 25% at 10 weeks

Absorption: Minimal

Distribution: Binds to PDGF-beta receptors in normal skin and granulation tissue

Pregnancy Risk Factor C

Beclomethasone (be kloe METH a sone)

Related Information
Respiratory Diseases *on page 1656*

U.S. Brand Names Beconase® AQ; QVAR®

Canadian Brand Names Apo-Beclomethasone®; Gen-Beclo; Nu-Beclomethasone; Propaderm®; QVAR®; Rivanase AQ; Vanceril® AEM

Generic Available No

Synonyms Beclomethasone Dipropionate

Pharmacologic Category Corticosteroid, Inhalant (Oral); Corticosteroid, Nasal

Use
Oral inhalation: Maintenance and prophylactic treatment of asthma; includes those who require corticosteroids and those who may benefit from a dose reduction/elimination of systemically-administered corticosteroids. Not for relief of acute bronchospasm.

Nasal aerosol: Symptomatic treatment of seasonal or perennial rhinitis; prevent recurrence of nasal polyps following surgery.

Local Anesthetic/Vasoconstrictor Precautions No information available to require special precautions

Effects on Dental Treatment Key adverse event(s) related to dental treatment: Oral candidiasis, xerostomia (normal salivary flow resumes upon discontinuation), nasal dryness, and dry throat. Localized infections with *Candida albicans* or *Aspergillus niger* occur frequently in the mouth and pharynx with repetitive use of an oral inhaler; may require treatment with appropriate antifungal therapy or discontinuation of inhaler use.

Significant Adverse Effects Frequency not defined.
Central nervous system: Agitation, depression, dizziness, dysphonia, headache, lightheadedness, mental disturbances

Dermatologic: Acneiform lesions, angioedema, atrophy, bruising, pruritus, purpura, striae, rash, urticaria

Endocrine & metabolic: Cushingoid features, growth velocity reduction in children and adolescents, HPA function suppression

Gastrointestinal: Dry/irritated nose, throat and mouth, hoarseness, localized *Candida* or *Aspergillus* infection, loss of smell, loss of taste, nausea, unpleasant smell, unpleasant taste, vomiting, weight gain

Local: Nasal spray: Burning, epistaxis, localized *Candida* infection, nasal septum perforation (rare), nasal stuffiness, nosebleeds, rhinorrhea, sneezing, transient irritation, ulceration of nasal mucosa (rare)

Ocular: Cataracts, glaucoma, intraocular pressure increased

Respiratory: Cough, paradoxical bronchospasm, pharyngitis, sinusitis, wheezing

Miscellaneous: Anaphylactic/anaphylactoid reactions, death (due to adrenal insufficiency, reported during and after transfer from systemic corticosteroids to aerosol in asthmatic patients), immediate and delayed hypersensitivity reactions

Dosage Nasal inhalation and oral inhalation dosage forms are not to be used interchangeably

Inhalation, nasal: Rhinitis, nasal polyps (Beconase® AQ): Children ≥6 years and Adults: 1-2 inhalations each nostril twice daily; total dose 168-336 mcg/day

Inhalation, oral: Asthma (doses should be titrated to the lowest effective dose once asthma is controlled) (QVAR®):

Children 5-11 years: Initial: 40 mcg twice daily; maximum dose: 80 mcg twice daily

Children ≥12 years and Adults:

Patients previously on bronchodilators only: Initial dose 40-80 mcg twice daily; maximum dose: 320 mcg twice day

Patients previously on inhaled corticosteroids: Initial dose 40-160 mcg twice daily; maximum dose: 320 mcg twice daily

NIH Asthma Guidelines (NAEPP, 2002; NIH, 1997): HFA formulation (eg, QVAR®): Administer in divided doses:

Children ≤12 years:
"Low" dose: 80-160 mcg/day
"Medium" dose: 160-320 mcg/day
"High" dose: >320 mcg/day

Children >12 years and Adults:
"Low" dose: 80-240 mcg/day
"Medium" dose: 240-480 mcg/day
"High" dose: >480 mcg/day

Mechanism of Action Controls the rate of protein synthesis; depresses the migration of polymorphonuclear leukocytes, fibroblasts; reverses capillary
(Continued)

Beclomethasone *(Continued)*

permeability and lysosomal stabilization at the cellular level to prevent or control inflammation

Contraindications Hypersensitivity to beclomethasone or any component of the formulation; status asthmaticus

Warnings/Precautions Not to be used in status asthmaticus or for the relief of acute bronchospasm. Safety and efficacy in children <5 years of age have not been established. May cause suppression of hypothalamic-pituitary-adrenal (HPA) axis, particularly in younger children or in patients receiving high doses for prolonged periods. Particular care is required when patients are transferred from systemic corticosteroids to inhaled products due to possible adrenal insufficiency or withdrawal from steroids, including an increase in allergic symptoms. Patients receiving 20 mg per day of prednisone (or equivalent) may be most susceptible. Fatalities have occurred due to adrenal insufficiency in asthmatic patients during and after transfer from systemic corticosteroids to aerosol steroids; aerosol steroids do **not** provide the systemic steroid needed to treat steroid-dependent patients having trauma, surgery, or infections. Withdrawal and discontinuation of the corticosteroid should be done slowly and carefully.

Controlled clinical studies have shown that orally-inhaled and intranasal corticosteroids may cause a reduction in growth velocity in pediatric patients. (In studies of orally-inhaled corticosteroids, the mean reduction in growth velocity was approximately 1 centimeter per year [range 0.3-1.8 cm per year] and appears to be related to dose and duration of exposure.) The growth of pediatric patients receiving inhaled corticosteroids should be monitored routinely (eg, via stadiometry). To minimize the systemic effects of orally-inhaled and intranasal corticosteroids, each patient should be titrated to the lowest effective dose.

May suppress the immune system, patients may be more susceptible to infection. Use with caution in patients with systemic infections or ocular herpes simplex. Avoid exposure to chickenpox and measles. Corticosteroids should be used with caution in patients with diabetes, hypertension, osteoporosis, peptic ulcer, glaucoma, cataracts, or tuberculosis. Use caution in hepatic impairment.

Drug Interactions Salmeterol: The addition of salmeterol has been demonstrated to improve response to inhaled corticosteroids (as compared to increasing steroid dosage).

Pharmacodynamics/Kinetics

Onset of action: Therapeutic effect: 1-4 weeks

Absorption: Readily; quickly hydrolyzed by pulmonary esterases prior to absorption

Distribution: Beclomethasone: 20 L; active metabolite: 424 L

Protein binding: 87%

Metabolism: Hepatic via CYP3A4 to active metabolites

Bioavailability: Of active metabolite, 44% following nasal inhalation (43% from swallowed portion)

Half-life elimination: Initial: 3 hours

Excretion: Feces (60%); urine (12%)

Pregnancy Risk Factor C

Lactation Excretion in breast milk unknown/use caution

Breast-Feeding Considerations Other corticosteroids have been found in breast milk; however, information for beclomethasone is not available. Inhaled corticosteroids are recommended for the treatment of asthma (most information available using budesonide) while breast-feeding.

Dosage Forms

Aerosol for oral inhalation, as dipropionate (QVAR®): 40 mcg/inhalation [100 metered doses] (7.3 g); 80 mcg/inhalation [100 metered doses] (7.3 g)

Suspension, intranasal, aqueous, as dipropionate [spray] (Beconase® AQ): 42 mcg/inhalation [180 metered doses] (25 g)

Beclomethasone Dipropionate *see* Beclomethasone *on page 183*

Beconase® AQ *see* Beclomethasone *on page 183*

Behenyl Alcohol *see* Docosanol *on page 495*

Belladonna Alkaloids With Phenobarbital *see* Hyoscyamine, Atropine, Scopolamine, and Phenobarbital *on page 804*

Belladonna and Opium *(bel a DON a & OH pee um)*

Related Information

Opium Tincture *on page 1149*

U.S. Brand Names B&O Suprettes®

Generic Available Yes

Synonyms Opium and Belladonna

Pharmacologic Category Analgesic Combination (Narcotic); Antispasmodic Agent, Urinary

Use Relief of moderate-to-severe pain associated with rectal or bladder tenesmus that may occur in postoperative states and neoplastic situations; pain associated with ureteral spasms not responsive to non-narcotic analgesics and to space intervals between injections of opiates

Local Anesthetic/Vasoconstrictor Precautions No information available to require special precautions

Effects on Dental Treatment Key adverse event(s) related to dental treatment: Xerostomia and changes in salivation (normal salivary flow resumes upon discontinuation), and dry throat and nose.

Mechanism of Action Anticholinergic alkaloids act primarily by competitive inhibition of the muscarinic actions of acetylcholine on structures innervated by postganglionic cholinergic neurons and on smooth muscle; resulting effects include antisecretory activity on exocrine glands and intestinal mucosa and smooth muscle relaxation. Contains many narcotic alkaloids including morphine; its mechanism for gastric motility inhibition is primarily due to this morphine content. It results in a decrease in digestive secretions, an increase in GI muscle tone, and therefore a reduction in GI propulsion.

Pregnancy Risk Factor C

Belladonna, Phenobarbital, and Ergotamine
(bel a DON a, fee noe BAR bi tal, & er GOT a meen)

Related Information
Ergotamine *on page 558*
Phenobarbital *on page 1221*

U.S. Brand Names Bellamine S; Bel-Tabs

Canadian Brand Names Bellergal® Spacetabs®

Generic Available Yes

Synonyms Ergotamine Tartrate, Belladonna, and Phenobarbital; Phenobarbital, Belladonna, and Ergotamine Tartrate

Pharmacologic Category Ergot Derivative

Use Management and treatment of menopausal disorders, GI disorders, and recurrent throbbing headache

Local Anesthetic/Vasoconstrictor Precautions No information available to require special precautions

Effects on Dental Treatment Key adverse event(s) related to dental treatment: Xerostomia (normal salivary flow resumes upon discontinuation), dry throat, nasal dryness, and difficulty swallowing.

Pregnancy Risk Factor X

Bellamine S *see* Belladonna, Phenobarbital, and Ergotamine *on page 185*

Bel-Tabs *see* Belladonna, Phenobarbital, and Ergotamine *on page 185*

Benadryl® Allergy [OTC] *see* DiphenhydrAMINE *on page 483*

Benadryl® Allergy and Sinus Fastmelt™ [OTC] *see* Diphenhydramine and Pseudoephedrine *on page 487*

Benadryl® Allergy/Sinus [OTC] *see* Diphenhydramine and Pseudoephedrine *on page 487*

Benadryl® Children's Allergy [OTC] *see* DiphenhydrAMINE *on page 483*

Benadryl® Children's Allergy and Cold Fastmelt™ [OTC] *see* Diphenhydramine and Pseudoephedrine *on page 487*

Benadryl® Children's Allergy and Sinus [OTC] *see* Diphenhydramine and Pseudoephedrine *on page 487*

Benadryl® Children's Allergy Fastmelt® [OTC] *see* DiphenhydrAMINE *on page 483*

Benadryl® Dye-Free Allergy [OTC] *see* DiphenhydrAMINE *on page 483*

Benadryl® Injection *see* DiphenhydrAMINE *on page 483*

Benadryl® Itch Stopping [OTC] *see* DiphenhydrAMINE *on page 483*

Benadryl® Itch Stopping Extra Strength [OTC] *see* DiphenhydrAMINE *on page 483*

Benazepril (ben AY ze pril)

Related Information
Cardiovascular Diseases *on page 1636*
(Continued)

Benazepril *(Continued)*

U.S. Brand Names Lotensin®

Canadian Brand Names Apo-Benazepril®; Lotensin®

Mexican Brand Names Lotensin®

Generic Available Yes

Synonyms Benazepril Hydrochloride

Pharmacologic Category Angiotensin-Converting Enzyme (ACE) Inhibitor

Use Treatment of hypertension, either alone or in combination with other antihypertensive agents

Local Anesthetic/Vasoconstrictor Precautions No information available to require special precautions

Effects on Dental Treatment No significant effects or complications reported

Common Adverse Effects 1% to 10%:

Cardiovascular: Postural dizziness (2%)

Central nervous system: Headache (6%), dizziness (4%), fatigue (3%), somnolence (2%)

Endocrine & metabolic: Hyperkalemia (1%), uric acid increased

Gastrointestinal: Nausea (2%)

Renal: Serum creatinine increased (2%), worsening of renal function may occur in patients with bilateral renal artery stenosis or hypovolemia

Respiratory: Cough (1% to 10%)

Eosinophilic pneumonitis, neutropenia, anaphylaxis, renal insufficiency, and renal failure have been reported with other ACE inhibitors. In addition, a syndrome including fever, myalgia, arthralgia, interstitial nephritis, vasculitis, rash, eosinophilia, and elevated ESR has been reported to be associated with ACE inhibitors.

Dosage Oral: Hypertension:

Children ≥6 years: Initial: 0.2 mg/kg/day as monotherapy; dosing range: 0.1-0.6 mg/kg/day (maximum dose: 40 mg/day)

Adults: Initial: 10 mg/day in patients not receiving a diuretic; 20-40 mg/day as a single dose or 2 divided doses; the need for twice-daily dosing should be assessed by monitoring peak (2-6 hours after dosing) and trough responses.

Note: Patients taking diuretics should have them discontinued 2-3 days prior to starting benazepril. If they cannot be discontinued, then initial dose should be 5 mg; restart after blood pressure is stabilized if needed.

Elderly: Oral: Initial: 5-10 mg/day in single or divided doses; usual range: 20-40 mg/day; adjust for renal function; also see **Note** in adult dosing.

Dosing interval in renal impairment: Cl$_{cr}$ <30 mL/minute:

Children: Use is not recommended.

Adults: Administer 5 mg/day initially; maximum daily dose: 40 mg.

Hemodialysis: Moderately dialyzable (20% to 50%); administer dose postdialysis or administer 25% to 35% supplemental dose.

Peritoneal dialysis: Supplemental dose is not necessary.

Mechanism of Action Competitive inhibition of angiotensin I being converted to angiotensin II, a potent vasoconstrictor, through the angiotensin I-converting enzyme (ACE) activity, with resultant lower levels of angiotensin II which causes an increase in plasma renin activity and a reduction in aldosterone secretion

Contraindications Hypersensitivity to benazepril or any component of the formulation; angioedema or serious hypersensitivity related to previous treatment with an ACE inhibitor; bilateral renal artery stenosis; patients with idiopathic or hereditary angioedema; pregnancy (2nd and 3rd trimesters)

Warnings/Precautions Anaphylactic reactions can occur. Angioedema can occur at any time during treatment (especially following first dose). Angioedema can occur at any time during treatment (especially following first dose). It may involve head and neck (potentially affecting the airway) or the intestine (presenting with abdominal pain). Prolonged monitoring may be required especially if tongue, glottis, or larynx are involved as they are associated with airway obstruction. Those with a history of airway surgery in this situation have a higher risk. Careful blood pressure monitoring with first dose (hypotension can occur especially in volume-depleted patients). Dosage adjustment needed in renal impairment. Use with caution in hypovolemia; collagen vascular diseases; valvular stenosis (particularly aortic stenosis); hyperkalemia; or before, during, or immediately after anesthesia. Avoid rapid dosage escalation which may lead to renal insufficiency. Rare toxicities associated with ACE inhibitors include cholestatic jaundice (which may progress to hepatic necrosis) and neutropenia/agranulocytosis with myeloid hyperplasia. Hypersensitivity reactions may be seen during hemodialysis with high-flux dialysis membranes (eg, AN69). Deterioration in renal function can occur with initiation. Use with caution in unilateral renal artery stenosis and pre-existing renal insufficiency.

Drug Interactions

Increased Effect/Toxicity: Potassium supplements, co-trimoxazole (high dose), angiotensin II receptor antagonists (eg, candesartan, losartan, irbesartan), or potassium-sparing diuretics (amiloride, spironolactone, triamterene) may result in elevated serum potassium levels when combined with benazepril. ACE inhibitor effects may be increased by phenothiazines or probenecid (increases levels of captopril). ACE inhibitors may increase serum concentrations/effects of lithium. Diuretics have additive hypotensive effects with ACE inhibitors, and hypovolemia increases the potential for adverse renal effects of ACE inhibitors. In patients with compromised renal function, coadministration with NSAIDs may result in further deterioration of renal function. Allopurinol and ACE inhibitors may cause a higher risk of hypersensitivity reaction when taken concurrently.

Decreased Effect: Aspirin (high dose) may reduce the therapeutic effects of ACE inhibitors; at low dosages this does not appear to be significant. Rifampin may decrease the effect of ACE inhibitors. Antacids may decrease the bioavailability of ACE inhibitors (may be more likely to occur with captopril); separate administration times by 1-2 hours. NSAIDs, specifically indomethacin, may reduce the hypotensive effects of ACE inhibitors.

Ethanol/Nutrition/Herb Interactions Herb/Nutraceutical: Avoid dong quai if using for hypertension (has estrogenic activity). Avoid ephedra, yohimbe, ginseng (may worsen hypertension). Avoid garlic (may have increased antihypertensive effect).

Pharmacodynamics/Kinetics

Reduction in plasma angiotensin-converting enzyme (ACE) activity:
  Onset of action: Peak effect: 1-2 hours after 2-20 mg dose
  Duration: >90% inhibition for 24 hours after 5-20 mg dose
Reduction in blood pressure:
  Peak effect: Single dose: 2-4 hours; Continuous therapy: 2 weeks
Absorption: Rapid (37%); food does not alter significantly; metabolite (benazeprilat) itself unsuitable for oral administration due to poor absorption
Distribution: V_d: ~8.7 L
Metabolism: Rapidly and extensively hepatic to its active metabolite, benazeprilat, via enzymatic hydrolysis; extensive first-pass effect
Half-life elimination: Benazeprilat: Effective: 10-11 hours; Terminal: Children: 5 hours, Adults: 22 hours
Time to peak: Parent drug: 0.5-1 hour
Excretion: Clearance: Nonrenal clearance (ie, biliary, metabolic) appears to contribute to the elimination of benazeprilat (11% to 12%), particularly patients with severe renal impairment; hepatic clearance is the main elimination route of unchanged benazepril
Dialysis: ~6% of metabolite removed within 4 hours of dialysis following 10 mg of benazepril administered 2 hours prior to procedure; parent compound not found in dialysate

Pregnancy Risk Factor C (1st trimester)/D (2nd and 3rd trimesters)

Dosage Forms TAB: 5 mg, 10 mg, 20 mg, 40 mg

Benazepril and Hydrochlorothiazide
(ben AY ze pril & hye droe klor oh THYE a zide)

Related Information
  Benazepril on page 185
  Hydrochlorothiazide on page 776

U.S. Brand Names Lotensin® HCT

Generic Available Yes

Synonyms Hydrochlorothiazide and Benazepril

Pharmacologic Category Antihypertensive Agent, Combination

Use Treatment of hypertension

Local Anesthetic/Vasoconstrictor Precautions No information available to require special precautions

Effects on Dental Treatment No significant effects or complications reported

Common Adverse Effects See individual agents.

Drug Interactions
  Increased Effect/Toxicity: See individual agents.
  Decreased Effect: See individual agents.

Pharmacodynamics/Kinetics See individual agents.

Pregnancy Risk Factor C/D (2nd and 3rd trimesters)

Benazepril Hydrochloride see Benazepril on page 185

Benazepril Hydrochloride and Amlodipine Besylate see Amlodipine and Benazepril on page 102

Bendroflumethiazide and Nadolol *see* Nadolol and Bendroflumethiazide *on page 1080*

BeneFix® *see* Factor IX *on page 632*

Benemid [DSC] *see* Probenecid *on page 1282*

Benicar® *see* Olmesartan *on page 1142*

Benicar HCT® *see* Olmesartan and Hydrochlorothiazide *on page 1143*

Benoquin® *see* Monobenzone *on page 1062*

Bentoquatam (BEN toe kwa tam)

U.S. Brand Names IvyBlock® [OTC]
Generic Available No
Synonyms Quaternium-18 Bentonite
Pharmacologic Category Topical Skin Product
Use Skin protectant for the prevention of allergic contact dermatitis to poison oak, ivy, and sumac

Local Anesthetic/Vasoconstrictor Precautions No information available to require special precautions

Effects on Dental Treatment No significant effects or complications reported

Mechanism of Action An organoclay substance which is capable of absorbing or binding to urushiol, the active principle in poison oak, ivy, and sumac. Bentoquatam serves as a barrier, blocking urushiol skin contact/absorption.

Bentyl® *see* Dicyclomine *on page 464*

Benylin® Adult [OTC] [DSC] *see* Dextromethorphan *on page 451*

Benylin® Expectorant [OTC] [DSC] *see* Guaifenesin and Dextromethorphan *on page 754*

Benylin® Pediatric [OTC] [DSC] *see* Dextromethorphan *on page 451*

Benza® [OTC] *see* Benzalkonium Chloride *on page 188*

Benzac® *see* Benzoyl Peroxide *on page 194*

Benzac® AC *see* Benzoyl Peroxide *on page 194*

Benzac® AC Wash *see* Benzoyl Peroxide *on page 194*

BenzaClin® *see* Clindamycin and Benzoyl Peroxide *on page 364*

Benzac® W *see* Benzoyl Peroxide *on page 194*

Benzac® W Wash *see* Benzoyl Peroxide *on page 194*

Benzagel® *see* Benzoyl Peroxide *on page 194*

Benzagel® Wash [DSC] *see* Benzoyl Peroxide *on page 194*

Benzalkonium Chloride (benz al KOE nee um KLOR ide)

Related Information
Periodontal Diseases *on page 1705*

U.S. Brand Names Benza® [OTC]; HandClens® [OTC]; 3M™ Cavilon™ Skin Cleanser [OTC]; Ony-Clear [OTC] [DSC]; Zephiran® [OTC]
Generic Available Yes
Synonyms BAC
Pharmacologic Category Antibiotic, Topical
Dental Use Surface antiseptic and germicidal preservative
Use Surface antiseptic and germicidal preservative

Local Anesthetic/Vasoconstrictor Precautions No information available to require special precautions

Effects on Dental Treatment No significant effects or complications reported

Significant Adverse Effects 1% to 10%: Hypersensitivity

Dosage Thoroughly rinse anionic detergents and soaps from the skin or other areas prior to use of solutions because they reduce the antibacterial activity of BAC. To protect metal instruments stored in BAC solution, add crushed Anti-Rust Tablets, 4 tablets/quart, to antiseptic solution. Change solution at least once weekly. Not to be used for storage of aluminum or zinc instruments, instruments with lenses fastened by cement, lacquered catheters, or some synthetic rubber goods.

Contraindications Hypersensitivity to benzalkonium or any component of the formulation

Pregnancy Risk Factor C

Dosage Forms [DSC] = Discontinued product
Solution, topical:
Benza®: 1:750 (60 mL, 240 mL, 480 mL, 3840 mL)
HandClens®: 0.13% (120 mL, 480 mL, 800 mL)
Ony-Clear [DSC]: 1% (30 mL)
Zephiran®: 1:750 (240 mL, 3840 mL) [aqueous]
Solution, topical spray (3M™ Cavilon™ Skin Cleanser): 0.11% (240 mL)

Benzalkonium Chloride and Isopropyl Alcohol
(benz al KOE nee um KLOR ide & eye so PRO pil AL koe hol)

Related Information
Benzalkonium Chloride *on page 188*
Viral Infections *on page 1709*

Related Sample Prescriptions
Herpes Simplex (Recurrent) *on page 1742*

U.S. Brand Names Viroxyn® [OTC]

Generic Available No

Synonyms Isopropyl Alcohol Tincture of Benzylkonium Chloride

Pharmacologic Category Antiseptic, Topical

Dental Use Topical: Germicidal for the treatment of cold sores/fever blisters

Local Anesthetic/Vasoconstrictor Precautions No information available to require special precautions

Effects on Dental Treatment No significant effects or complications reported (see Dental Comment)

Significant Adverse Effects Frequency not defined
Ocular: Irritation (following inadvertent contact)
Respiratory: Vapors may cause cough, dyspnea

Dosage Topical: One single application treatment to affected area. Secondary events (new viral load in the initial lesion, which may occur 12-72 hours after initial symptoms) or additional sore presentations will require additional treatment with a new vial. See Dental Comment for application instructions.
Manufacturer states medication should not be used >3 times/day; however, instructions indicate that a single application is generally effective if instructions are followed.

Mechanism of Action Germicidal due to disruption of the viral capsid coat by the quaternary ammonium benzalkonium chloride ingredient.

Contraindications Hypersensitivity to benzalkonium chloride, isopropyl alcohol, or any component of the formulation

Warnings/Precautions For topical use only; ingestion may lead to gastric irritation or distress. Avoid contact with eyes; flush with eye bath if inadvertent contact occurs. Avoid use of anionic cleansers or acidic products for at least 1 hour following application (active ingredient will be neutralized). Avoid the use of soap, toothpaste, cleansers, or drinks containing citric acid (including lemonade and orange juice). Should not be used >3 times/day. Avoid use in pregnant or lactating women. Avoid use in children <2 years of age. Formulation in isopropyl alcohol is flammable; avoid use near sparks, flames, or high temperatures.

Drug Interactions No specific drug interactions have been reported.

Dietary Considerations Avoid citric acid-containing beverages (eg, lemonade or orange juice) for at least 1 hour following application.

Dosage Forms Solution, topical: Benzalkonium 0.13% in isopropyl alcohol [kit includes 3 single-dose applicators]

Dental Comment Use this product according to the following directions from the manufacturer. 1) Prior to treatment, clean area to be treated of all other preparations (ointments, treatments, lipstick). Do not use soap or other cleansers. A dry wipe may be sufficient, or you may use water or alcohol if necessary. 2) Remove cap from vial and replace on the other end over the clear plastic tube. Hold vial between thumb and index finger, applicator end up. Pinch vial in the center at top of cap until the inner ampoule of medication breaks. 3) Hold white applicator down and allow medication to saturate the swab. If necessary, pinch vial gently until a drop of medication just appears. 4) Place the applicator against the area of skin to be treated so that the tip of the applicator is held flat against the skin. The key is to massage medication into the sore and the surrounding area by rubbing. Do not rub so hard that you cause damage to the skin. For best results, the patient should massage drug into the sore by rubbing. The rubbing should proceed for about 10 minutes or until all the drug has been massaged into the sore. The application may sting. This is normal and should subside quickly. For best results, medication must penetrate the subepidermal layers of the skin to site of infection. The ingredients facilitate penetration, but mechanical action is critical. Simply dabbing the drug onto the sore is not likely to give best results. 5) If treating at prodrome (tingling sensation before lesion erupts), a more vigorous rubbing is easily tolerated and gives best results. If the lesion has progressed to vesicle or ulcerated lesion, the patient may prefer to rub less vigorously but for a longer time period. 6) Keep applicator saturated at all times. If necessary, pause and hold vial so as to allow medication to flow into (Continued)

Benzalkonium Chloride and Isopropyl Alcohol
(Continued)

applicator. When finished recap vial. Dispose of immediately. Do not disassemble. Store at room temperature. Flammable; do not expose to high heat or flame. Keep out of reach of children.

Benzalkonium Chloride, Benzocaine, Butyl Aminobenzoate, and Tetracaine Hydrochloride see Benzocaine, Butyl Aminobenzoate, Tetracaine, and Benzalkonium Chloride on page 193

Benzamycin® see Erythromycin and Benzoyl Peroxide on page 567

Benzamycin® Pak see Erythromycin and Benzoyl Peroxide on page 567

Benzashave® see Benzoyl Peroxide on page 194

Benzathine Benzylpenicillin see Penicillin G Benzathine on page 1202

Benzathine Penicillin G see Penicillin G Benzathine on page 1202

Benzazoline Hydrochloride see Tolazoline on page 1501

Benzedrex® [OTC] see Propylhexedrine on page 1305

Benzene Hexachloride see Lindane on page 933

Benzhexol Hydrochloride see Trihexyphenidyl on page 1537

Benziq™ see Benzoyl Peroxide on page 194

Benziq™ LS see Benzoyl Peroxide on page 194

Benzisoquinolinedione see Amonafide on page 104

Benzmethyzin see Procarbazine on page 1284

Benzocaine (BEN zoe kane)

Related Information
Mouth Pain, Cold Sore, and Canker Sore Products on page 1828
Oral Pain on page 1692

Related Sample Prescriptions
Recurrent Aphthous Stomatitis on page 1744

U.S. Brand Names Americaine® [OTC]; Americaine® Hemorrhoidal [OTC]; Anbesol® [OTC]; Anbesol® Baby [OTC]; Anbesol® Cold Sore Therapy [OTC]; Anbesol® Jr. [OTC]; Anbesol® Maximum Strength [OTC]; Benzodent® [OTC]; Cepacol® Sore Throat [OTC]; Chiggerex® [OTC]; Chiggertox® [OTC]; Cylex® [OTC]; Dentapaine [OTC]; Dent's Extra Strength Toothache [OTC]; Dent's Maxi-Strength Toothache [OTC]; Dermoplast® Antibacterial [OTC]; Dermoplast® Pain Relieving [OTC]; Detane® [OTC]; Foille® [OTC]; HDA® Toothache [OTC]; Hurricaine® [OTC]; Ivy-Rid® [OTC]; Kanka® Soft Brush™ [OTC]; Lanacane® [OTC]; Lanacane® Maximum Strength [OTC]; Mycinettes® [OTC]; Orabase® with Benzocaine [OTC]; Orajel® Baby Daytime and Nighttime [OTC]; Orajel® Baby Teething [OTC]; Orajel® Baby Teething Nighttime [OTC]; Orajel® Denture Plus [OTC]; Orajel® Maximum Strength [OTC]; Orajel® Medicated Toothache [OTC]; Orajel® Mouth Sore [OTC]; Orajel® Multi-Action Cold Sore [OTC]; Orajel PM® [OTC]; Orajel® Ultra Mouth Sore [OTC]; Oticaine; Otocaine™; Outgro® [OTC]; Red Cross™ Canker Sore [OTC]; Rid-A-Pain Dental Drops [OTC]; Skeeter Stik [OTC]; Sting-Kill [OTC]; Tanac® [OTC]; Thorets [OTC]; Trocaine® [OTC]; Zilactin®-B [OTC]; Zilactin Toothache and Gum Pain® [OTC]

Canadian Brand Names Anbesol® Baby; Zilactin-B®; Zilactin Baby®

Generic Available Yes: Lozenge, otic drops

Synonyms Ethyl Aminobenzoate

Pharmacologic Category Local Anesthetic

Dental Use Ester-type topical local anesthetic for temporary relief of pain associated with toothache, minor sore throat pain, and canker sore

Use Temporary relief of pain associated with pruritic dermatosis, pruritus, minor burns, acute congestive and serous otitis media, swimmer's ear, otitis externa, bee stings, insect bites; mouth and gum irritations (toothache, minor sore throat pain, canker sores, dentures, orthodontia, teething, mucositis, stomatitis); sunburn; hemorrhoids; anesthetic lubricant for passage of catheters and endoscopic tubes

Local Anesthetic/Vasoconstrictor Precautions No information available to require special precautions

Effects on Dental Treatment No significant effects or complications reported

Significant Adverse Effects Frequency not defined.

Hematologic: Methemoglobinemia

Local: Burning, contact dermatitis, edema, erythema, pruritus, rash, stinging, tenderness, urticaria

Miscellaneous: Hypersensitivity

Dental Usual Dosing Relief of pain (toothache, minor sore throat pain, and canker sore): Children ≥2 years and Adults: Topical (oral): 10% to 20%: Apply thin layer to affected area up to 4 times daily

Dosage Note: These are general dosing guidelines; refer to specific product labeling for dosing instructions.

Children ≥4 months: Topical (oral): Teething pain: 7.5% to 10%: Apply to affected gum area up to 4 times daily

Children ≥2 years and Adults:

Topical:

Bee stings, insect bites, minor burns, sunburn: 5% to 20%: Apply to affected area 3-4 times a day as needed. In cases of bee stings, remove stinger before treatment.

Lubricant for passage of catheters and instruments: 20%: Apply evenly to exterior of instrument prior to use.

Topical (oral): Mouth and gum irritation: 10% to 20%: Apply thin layer to affected area up to 4 times daily

Children ≥5 years and Adults: Oral: Sore throat: Allow one lozenge (10-15 mg) to dissolve slowly in mouth; may repeat every 2 hours as needed

Children ≥12 years and Adults: Rectal: Hemorrhoids: 5% to 20%: Apply externally to affected area up to 6 times daily

Adults: Otic: 20%: Instill 4-5 drops into external auditory canal; may repeat in 1-2 hours if needed

Mechanism of Action Ester local anesthetic blocks both the initiation and conduction of nerve impulses by decreasing the neuronal membrane's permeability to sodium ions, which results in inhibition of depolarization with resultant blockade of conduction

Contraindications Hypersensitivity to benzocaine, other ester-type local anesthetics, or any component of the formulation; secondary bacterial infection of area; ophthalmic use; otic preparations are also contraindicated in the presence of perforated tympanic membrane

Warnings/Precautions Methemoglobinemia has been reported following topical use (rare). When applied as a spray to the mouth or throat, multiple sprays (or sprays of longer than indicated duration) are not recommended. Use caution with breathing problems (asthma, bronchitis, emphysema, in smokers), heart disease, children <6 months of age, and hemoglobin or enzyme abnormalities (glucose-6-phosphodiesterase deficiency, hemoglobin-M disease, NADH-methemoglobin reductase deficiency, pyruvate-kinase deficiency).

When used for self-medication (OTC), notify healthcare provider if condition worsens or does not improve within 7 days, or if swelling, rash, or fever develops. Do not use on open wounds. Avoid contact with the eyes.

Drug Interactions May antagonize actions of sulfonamides

Pharmacodynamics/Kinetics

Absorption: Topical: Poor to intact skin; well absorbed from mucous membranes and traumatized skin

Metabolism: Hepatic (to a lesser extent) and plasma via hydrolysis by cholinesterase

Excretion: Urine (as metabolites)

Pregnancy Risk Factor C

Lactation Excretion in breast milk unknown/use caution

Dosage Forms

Aerosol, oral spray (Hurricaine®): 20% (60 mL) [dye free; cherry flavor]

Aerosol, topical spray:

Americaine®: 20% (60 mL)

Dermoplast® Antibacterial: 20% (83 mL) [contains aloe vera, benzethonium chloride, menthol]

Dermoplast® Pain Relieving: 20% (60 mL, 83 mL) [contains menthol]

Foille®: 5% (92 g) [contains chloroxylenol 0.63% and corn oil]

Ivy-Rid®: 2% (83 mL)

Lanacane® Maximum Strength: 20% (120 mL) [contains alcohol]

Solarcaine®: 20% (120 mL) [contains triclosan 0.13%, alcohol 35%]

Combination package (Orajel® Baby Daytime and Nighttime):

Gel, oral [Daytime Regular Formula]: 7.5% (5.3 g)

Gel, oral [Nighttime Formula]: 10% (5.3 g)

Cream, oral:

Benzodent®: 20% (7.5 g, 30 g)

Orajel PM®: 20% (5.3 g, 7 g)

Cream, topical:

Lanacane®: 6% (30 g, 60 g)

Lanacane® Maximum Strength: 20% (30 g)

Gel, oral:

Anbesol®: 10% (7.5 g) [contains benzyl alcohol; cool mint flavor]

Anbesol® Baby: 7.5% (7.5 g) [contains benzoic acid; grape flavor]

(Continued)

Benzocaine *(Continued)*

Anbesol® Jr.: 10% (7 g) [contains benzyl alcohol; bubble gum flavor]
Anbesol® Maximum Strength: 20% (7.5 g, 10 g) [contains benzyl alcohol]
Dentapaine: 20% (11 g) [contains clove oil]
HDA® Toothache: 6.5% (15 mL) [contains benzyl alcohol]
Hurricaine®: 20% (5 g) [dye free; wild cherry flavor]; (30 g) [dye free; mint, pina colada, watermelon, and wild cherry flavors]
Kanka® Soft Brush™: 20% (2 mL) [packaged in applicator with brush tip]
Orabase® with Benzocaine®: 20% (7 g) [contains ethyl alcohol 48%; mild mint flavor]
Orajel®: 10% (5.3 g, 7 g, 9.4 g)
Orajel® Baby Teething: 7.5% (9.4 g, 11.9 g) [cherry flavor]
Orajel® Baby Teething Nighttime: 10% (5.3 g)
Orajel® Denture Plus: 15% (9 g) [contains menthol 2%, ethyl alcohol 66.7%]
Orajel® Maximum Strength: 20% (5.3 g, 7 g, 9.4 g, 11.9 g)
Orajel® Mouth Sore: 20% (5.3 g, 9.4 g, 11.9 g) [contains benzalkonium chloride 0.02%, zinc chloride 0.1%]
Orajel® Multi-Action Cold Sore: 20% (9.4 g) [contains allantoin 0.5%, camphor 3%, dimethicone 2%]
Orajel® Ultra Mouth Sore: 15% (9.4 g) [contains ethyl alcohol 66.7%, menthol 2%]
Zilactin®-B: 10% (7.5 g)
Gel, topical (Detane®): 7.5% (15 g)
Liquid, oral:
Anbesol®: 10% (9 mL) [cool mint flavor]
Anbesol® Maximum Strength: 20% (9 mL) [contains benzyl alcohol]
Hurricaine®: 20% (30 mL) [pina colada and wild cherry flavors]
Orajel® Baby Teething: 7.5% (13 mL) [very berry flavor]
Orajel® Maximum Strength: 20% (13 mL) [contains ethyl alcohol 44%, tartrazine]
Liquid, oral drop:
Dent's Maxi-Strength Toothache: 20% (3.7 mL) [contains alcohol 74%]
Rid-A-Pain Dental Drops: 6.3% (30 mL) [contains alcohol 70%]
Liquid, topical:
Chiggertox®: 2% (30 mL)
Outgro®: 20% (9 mL)
Skeeter Stik: 5% (14 mL) [contains menthol]
Tanac®: 10% (13 mL) [contains benzalkonium chloride]
Lozenge: 6 mg (18s) [contains menthol]; 15 mg (10s)
Cepacol® Sore Throat: 10 mg (18s) [contains cetylpyridinium, menthol; cherry, citrus, honey lemon, and menthol flavors]
Cepacol® Sore Throat: 10 mg (16s) [sugar free; contains cetylpyridinium, menthol; cherry and menthol flavors]
Cylex®: 15 mg [sugar free; contains cetylpyridinium chloride 5 mg; cherry flavor]
Mycinettes®: 15 mg (12s) [sugar free; contains sodium 9 mg; cherry or regular flavor]
Thorets: 18 mg (500s) [sugar free]
Trocaine®: 10 mg (40s, 400s)
Ointment, oral:
Anbesol® Cold Sore Therapy: 20% (7.1 g) [contains benzyl alcohol, allantoin, aloe, camphor, menthol, vitamin E]
Red Cross™ Canker Sore: 20% (7.5 g) [contains coconut oil]
Ointment, rectal (Americaine® Hemorrhoidal): 20% (30 g)
Ointment, topical:
Chiggerex®: 2% (50 g) [contains aloe vera]
Foille®: 5% (3.5 g, 14 g, 28 g) [contains chloroxylenol 0.1%, benzyl alcohol; corn oil base]
Pads, topical (Sting-Kill): 20% (8s) [contains menthol and tartrazine]
Paste, oral (Orabase® with Benzocaine): 20% (6 g)
Solution, otic drops (Oticaine, Otocaine™): 20% (15 mL)
Swabs, oral:
Hurricaine®: 20% (6s, 100s) [dye free; wild cherry flavor]
Orajel® Baby Teething: 7.5% (12s) [berry flavor]
Orajel® Medicated Mouth Sore, Orajel® Medicated Toothache: 20% (8s, 12s) [contains tartrazine]
Zilactin® Toothache and Gum Pain: 20% (8s) [grape flavor]
Swabs, topical (Sting-Kill): 20% (5s) [contains menthol and tartrazine]
Wax, oral (Dent's Extra Strength Toothache Gum): 20% (1 g)

Benzocaine and Antipyrine *see* Antipyrine and Benzocaine *on page 130*

Benzocaine and Cetylpyridinium Chloride see Cetylpyridinium and Benzocaine on page 309

Benzocaine, Butyl Aminobenzoate, Tetracaine, and Benzalkonium Chloride
(BEN zoe kane, BYOO til a meen oh BENZ oh ate, TET ra kane, & benz al KOE nee um KLOR ide)

Related Information
Benzalkonium Chloride on page 188
Benzocaine on page 190
Tetracaine on page 1466

U.S. Brand Names Cetacaine®

Generic Available No

Synonyms Benzalkonium Chloride, Benzocaine, Butyl Aminobenzoate, and Tetracaine Hydrochloride; Butyl Aminobenzoate, Tetracaine Hydrochloride, Benzocaine, and Benzalkonium Chloride; Tetracaine Hydrochloride, Benzocaine, Butyl Aminobenzoate, and Benzalkonium Chloride

Pharmacologic Category Local Anesthetic

Dental Use Topical anesthetic to control pain or gagging

Use Topical anesthetic to control pain or gagging, pain in surgical or endocscopic procedures; anesthetic for accessible mucous membranes except for the eyes.

Local Anesthetic/Vasoconstrictor Precautions No information available to require special precautions

Effects on Dental Treatment No significant effects or complications reported

Significant Adverse Effects Frequency not defined. Also refer to Benzocaine and Tetracaine monographs.
Local: Contact dermatitis (eg, erythema, pruritus); dehydration of the epithelium; escharotic effect
Miscellaneous: Hypersensitivity reaction

Dental Usual Dosing Control pain or gagging: Adults: Topical: Local anesthetic: Apply to affected area for approximately 1 second

Dosage Apply to affected area for approximately 1 second

Contraindications Hypersensitivity to benzocaine, other ester-type local anesthetics, butyl aminobenzoate, tetracaine, benzalkonium chloride, or any component of the formulation; secondary bacterial infection of area; ophthalmic use; cholinesterase deficiencies; under dentures or cotton rolls; tetracaine in doses >20 mg

Warnings/Precautions Methemoglobinemia has been reported following topical benzocaine use (rare). When applied as a spray to the mouth or throat, multiple sprays or sprays >2 seconds are not recommended. Use caution in breathing problems (asthma, bronchitis, emphysema, in smokers), heart disease, children <4 months of age, and hemoglobin or enzyme abnormalities (glucose-6-phosphodiesterase deficiency, hemoglobin-M disease, NADH-methemoglobin reductase deficiency, pyruvate-kinase deficiency).

Pharmacodynamics/Kinetics
Onset of action: ~30 seconds
Duration: 30-60 minutes

Dosage Forms
Aerosol, topical: Benzocaine 14%, butyl aminobenzoate 2%, tetracaine hydrochloride 2%, and benzalkonium chloride 0.5% (56 g) [also packaged in a kit with various sized cannulas]
Gel, topical: Benzocaine 14%, butyl aminobenzoate 2%, tetracaine hydrochloride 2%, and benzalkonium chloride 0.5% (29 g)
Liquid, topical: Benzocaine 14%, butyl aminobenzoate 2%, tetracaine hydrochloride 2%, and benzalkonium chloride 0.5% (56 mL)

Benzodent® [OTC] see Benzocaine on page 190

Benzoin (BEN zoin)

U.S. Brand Names TinBen® [OTC] [DSC]

Generic Available Yes

Synonyms Gum Benjamin

Pharmacologic Category Antibiotic, Topical; Topical Skin Product

Use Protective application for irritations of the skin; sometimes used in boiling water as steam inhalants for its expectorant and soothing action

Local Anesthetic/Vasoconstrictor Precautions No information available to require special precautions

Effects on Dental Treatment No significant effects or complications reported

Benzonatate (ben ZOE na tate)

Related Information
Management of Patients Undergoing Cancer Therapy *on page 1728*
U.S. Brand Names Tessalon®
Canadian Brand Names Tessalon®
Mexican Brand Names Tesalon®; Tusical®; Tusitato®
Generic Available Yes
Pharmacologic Category Antitussive
Use Symptomatic relief of nonproductive cough
Local Anesthetic/Vasoconstrictor Precautions No information available to require special precautions
Effects on Dental Treatment No significant effects or complications reported
Common Adverse Effects 1% to 10%:
Central nervous system: Sedation, headache, dizziness
Dermatologic: Rash
Gastrointestinal: GI upset
Neuromuscular & skeletal: Chest numbness
Ocular: Burning sensation in eyes
Respiratory: Nasal congestion
Dosage Children >10 years and Adults: Oral: 100 mg 3 times/day or every 4 hours up to 600 mg/day
Mechanism of Action Tetracaine congener with antitussive properties; suppresses cough by topical anesthetic action on the respiratory stretch receptors
Contraindications Hypersensitivity to benzonatate, related compounds (such as tetracaine), or any component of the formulation
Pharmacodynamics/Kinetics
Onset of action: Therapeutic: 15-20 minutes
Duration: 3-8 hours
Pregnancy Risk Factor C
Dosage Forms CAP: 100 mg; (Tessalon®): 100 mg, 200 mg

Benzoyl Peroxide (BEN zoe il peer OKS ide)

U.S. Brand Names Benzac®; Benzac® AC; Benzac® AC Wash; Benzac® W; Benzac® W Wash; Benzagel®; Benzagel® Wash [DSC]; Benzashave®; Benziq™; Benziq™ LS; Brevoxyl®; Brevoxyl® Cleansing; Brevoxyl® Wash; Clearplex [OTC]; Clinac™ BPO; Del Aqua®; Desquam-E™; Desquam-X®; Exact® Acne Medication [OTC]; Fostex® 10% BPO [OTC]; Loroxide® [OTC]; Neutrogena® Acne Mask [OTC]; Neutrogena® On The Spot® Acne Treatment [OTC]; Oxy 10® Balanced Medicated Face Wash [OTC]; Oxy 10® Balance Spot Treatment [OTC]; Palmer's® Skin Success Acne [OTC]; PanOxyl®; PanOxyl®-AQ; PanOxyl® Aqua Gel; PanOxyl® Bar [OTC]; Seba-Gel™; Triaz®; Triaz® Cleanser; Zapzyt® [OTC]; Zoderm®
Canadian Brand Names Acetoxyl®; Benoxyl®; Benzac AC®; Benzac W® Gel; Benzac W® Wash; Desquam-X®; Oxyderm™; PanOxyl®; Solugel®
Mexican Brand Names Benoxyl®; Benzac®; Benzaderm®; Solugel®
Generic Available Yes: Excludes cream, pads, and soap
Pharmacologic Category Topical Skin Product; Topical Skin Product, Acne
Use Adjunctive treatment of mild-to-moderate acne vulgaris and acne rosacea
Local Anesthetic/Vasoconstrictor Precautions No information available to require special precautions
Effects on Dental Treatment No significant effects or complications reported
Common Adverse Effects 1% to 10%: Dermatologic: Irritation, contact dermatitis, dryness, erythema, peeling, stinging
Mechanism of Action Releases free-radical oxygen which oxidizes bacterial proteins in the sebaceous follicles decreasing the number of anaerobic bacteria and decreasing irritating-type free fatty acids
Drug Interactions
Increased Effect/Toxicity: Increased toxicity: Benzoyl peroxide potentiates adverse reactions seen with tretinoin
Pharmacodynamics/Kinetics
Absorption: ~5% via skin; gel more penetrating than cream
Metabolism: Converted to benzoic acid in skin
Pregnancy Risk Factor C

Benzoyl Peroxide and Clindamycin *see* Clindamycin and Benzoyl Peroxide *on page 364*

Benzoyl Peroxide and Erythromycin *see* Erythromycin and Benzoyl Peroxide *on page 567*

Benzoyl Peroxide and Hydrocortisone
(BEN zoe il peer OKS ide & hye droe KOR ti sone)

Related Information
Benzoyl Peroxide *on page 194*
Hydrocortisone *on page 793*
U.S. Brand Names Vanoxide-HC®
Canadian Brand Names Vanoxide-HC®
Generic Available No
Synonyms Hydrocortisone and Benzoyl Peroxide
Pharmacologic Category Topical Skin Product; Topical Skin Product, Acne
Use Treatment of acne vulgaris and oily skin
Local Anesthetic/Vasoconstrictor Precautions No information available to require special precautions
Effects on Dental Treatment No significant effects or complications reported
Common Adverse Effects See individual agents.

Drug Interactions
  Cytochrome P450 Effect: Hydrocortisone: **Substrate** of CYP3A4 (minor); Induces CYP3A4 (weak)
Pharmacodynamics/Kinetics See individual agents.
Pregnancy Risk Factor C

Benzphetamine (benz FET a meen)

U.S. Brand Names Didrex®
Canadian Brand Names Didrex®
Generic Available No
Synonyms Benzphetamine Hydrochloride
Pharmacologic Category Anorexiant
Use Short-term adjunct in exogenous obesity
Local Anesthetic/Vasoconstrictor Precautions Use with caution since amphetamines have actions similar to epinephrine and norepinephrine
Effects on Dental Treatment Key adverse event(s) related to dental treatment: Xerostomia (normal salivary flow resumes upon discontinuation) and metallic taste.
Common Adverse Effects Frequency not defined.
  Cardiovascular: Hypertension, palpitation, tachycardia, chest pain, T-wave changes, arrhythmia, pulmonary hypertension, valvulopathy
  Central nervous system: Euphoria, nervousness, insomnia, restlessness, dizziness, anxiety, headache, agitation, confusion, mental depression, psychosis, CVA, seizure
  Dermatologic: Alopecia, urticaria, skin rash, ecchymosis, erythema
  Endocrine & metabolic: Gynecomastia, libido changes, menstrual irregularities, porphyria
  Gastrointestinal: Nausea, vomiting, abdominal cramps, constipation, xerostomia, metallic taste
  Genitourinary: Impotence
  Hematologic: Bone marrow depression, agranulocytosis, leukopenia
  Neuromuscular & skeletal: Tremor
  Ocular: Blurred vision, mydriasis
Restrictions C-III
Mechanism of Action Noncatechol sympathomimetic amines with pharmacologic actions similar to ephedrine; require breakdown by monoamine oxidase for inactivation; produce central nervous system and respiratory stimulation, a pressor response, mydriasis, bronchodilation, and contraction of the urinary sphincter; thought to have a direct effect on both alpha- and beta-receptor sites in the peripheral system, as well as release stores of norepinephrine in adrenergic nerve terminals; central nervous system action is thought to occur in the cerebral cortex and reticular activating system; anorexigenic effect is probably secondary to the CNS-stimulating effect; the site of action is probably the hypothalamic feeding center.

Drug Interactions
  Cytochrome P450 Effect: Substrate of CYP2B6 (minor), 3A4 (major)
  Increased Effect/Toxicity: Amphetamines may precipitate hypertensive crisis or serotonin syndrome in patients receiving MAO inhibitors (selegiline
  (Continued)

Benzphetamine *(Continued)*

>10 mg/day, isocarboxazid, phenelzine, tranylcypromine, furazolidone). Serotonin syndrome has also been associated with combinations of amphetamines and SSRIs; these combinations should be avoided. TCAs may enhance the effects of amphetamines, potentially leading to hypertensive crisis. Large doses of antacids or urinary alkalinizers increase the half-life and duration of action of amphetamines. May precipitate arrhythmias in patients receiving general anesthetics. Inhibitors of CYP2D6 may increase the effects of amphetamines (includes amiodarone, cimetidine, delavirdine, fluoxetine, paroxetine, propafenone, quinidine, and ritonavir). CYP3A4 inhibitors may increase the levels/effects of benzphetamine; example inhibitors include azole antifungals, clarithromycin, diclofenac, doxycycline, erythromycin, imatinib, isoniazid, nefazodone, nicardipine, propofol, protease inhibitors, quinidine, telithromycin, and verapamil.

Decreased Effect: Amphetamines inhibit the antihypertensive response to guanethidine and guanadrel. Urinary acidifiers decrease the half-life and duration of action of amphetamines. CYP3A4 inducers may decrease the levels/effects of benzphetamine; example inducers include aminoglutethimide, carbamazepine, nafcillin, nevirapine, phenobarbital, phenytoin, and rifamycins.

Pregnancy Risk Factor X

Benzphetamine Hydrochloride *see* Benzphetamine *on page 195*

Benztropine *(BENZ troe peen)*

U.S. Brand Names Cogentin®
Canadian Brand Names Apo-Benztropine®
Generic Available Yes: Tablet
Synonyms Benztropine Mesylate
Pharmacologic Category Anti-Parkinson's Agent, Anticholinergic; Anticholinergic Agent
Use Adjunctive treatment of Parkinson's disease; treatment of drug-induced extrapyramidal symptoms (except tardive dyskinesia)
Local Anesthetic/Vasoconstrictor Precautions No information available to require special precautions
Effects on Dental Treatment Key adverse event(s) related to dental treatment: Xerostomia and changes in salivation (normal salivary flow resumes upon discontinuation), dry throat, and nasal dryness (very prevalent).
Common Adverse Effects Frequency not defined.
Cardiovascular: Tachycardia
Central nervous system: Confusion, disorientation, memory impairment, toxic psychosis, visual hallucinations
Dermatologic: Rash
Endocrine & metabolic: Heat stroke, hyperthermia
Gastrointestinal: Xerostomia, nausea, vomiting, constipation, ileus
Genitourinary: Urinary retention, dysuria
Ocular: Blurred vision, mydriasis
Miscellaneous: Fever
Mechanism of Action Possesses both anticholinergic and antihistaminic effects. *In vitro* anticholinergic activity approximates that of atropine; *in vivo* it is only about half as active as atropine. Animal data suggest its antihistaminic activity and duration of action approach that of pyrilamine maleate. May also inhibit the reuptake and storage of dopamine and thereby, prolong the action of dopamine.
Drug Interactions
Cytochrome P450 Effect: Substrate of CYP2D6 (minor)
Increased Effect/Toxicity: Central and/or peripheral anticholinergic syndrome can occur when benztropine is administered with amantadine, rimantadine, narcotic analgesics, phenothiazines and other antipsychotics (especially with high anticholinergic activity), tricyclic antidepressants, quinidine and some other antiarrhythmics, and antihistamines. Benztropine may increase the absorption of digoxin.
Decreased Effect: May increase gastric degradation of levodopa and decrease the amount of levodopa absorbed by delaying gastric emptying. Therapeutic effects of cholinergic agents (tacrine, donepezil) and neuroleptics may be antagonized.
Pharmacodynamics/Kinetics
Onset of action: Oral: Within 1 hour; Parenteral: Within 15 minutes
Duration: 6-48 hours
Metabolism: Hepatic (N-oxidation, N-dealkylation, and ring hydroxylation)
Bioavailability: 29%
Pregnancy Risk Factor C

Benztropine Mesylate *see* Benztropine *on page 196*

Benzydamine (ben ZID a meen)

Canadian Brand Names Apo-Benzydamine®; Dom-Benzydamine; Novo-Benzydamine; PMS-Benzydamine; ratio-Benzydamine; Sun-Benz®; Tantum®

Mexican Brand Names Lonol®; Vantal®

Generic Available Yes

Synonyms Benzydamine Hydrochloride

Pharmacologic Category Local Anesthetic, Oral

Dental Use Symptomatic treatment of pain associated with acute pharyngitis; treatment of pain associated with radiation-induced oropharyngeal mucositis

Use Symptomatic treatment of pain associated with acute pharyngitis; treatment of pain associated with radiation-induced oropharyngeal mucositis

Local Anesthetic/Vasoconstrictor Precautions No information available to require special precautions

Effects on Dental Treatment Key adverse event(s) related to dental treatment: Numbness, burning/stinging sensation, and xerostomia (normal salivary flow resumes upon discontinuation).

Significant Adverse Effects
Central nervous system: Drowsiness, headache
Gastrointestinal: Nausea and/or vomiting (2%), dry mouth
Local: Numbness (10%), burning/stinging sensation (8%)
Respiratory: Pharyngeal irritation, cough

Restrictions Not available in U.S.

Dental Usual Dosing

Acute pharyngitis: Adults: Oral rinse: Gargle with 15 mL every 1½-3 hours until symptoms resolve. Patient should expel solution from mouth following use; solution should not be swallowed.

Radiation-associated mucositis: Adults: Oral rinse: 15 mL as a gargle or rinse 3-4 times/day; contact between the liquid and the oral mucosa should be maintained for at least 30 seconds, followed by expulsion from the mouth. Clinical studies maintained contact for ~2 minutes, up to 8 times/day. Patient should not swallow the liquid. Begin treatment 1day prior to initiation of radiation therapy and continue daily during treatment. Continue oral rinse treatments after the completion of radiation therapy until desired result/healing is achieved.

Dosage Oral rinse: Adults:
Acute pharyngitis: Gargle with 15 mL of undiluted solution every 1½-3 hours until symptoms resolve. Patient should expel solution from mouth following use; solution should not be swallowed.

Mucositis: 15 mL of undiluted solution as a gargle or rinse 3-4 times/day; contact should be maintained for at least 30 seconds, followed by expulsion from the mouth. Clinical studies maintained contact for ~2 minutes, up to 8 times/day. Patient should not swallow the liquid. Begin treatment 1day prior to initiation of radiation therapy and continue daily during treatment. Continue oral rinse treatments after the completion of radiation therapy until desired result/healing is achieved.

Dosage adjustment in renal impairment: No adjustment required.

Mechanism of Action Local anesthetic and anti-inflammatory, reduces local pain and inflammation. Does not interfere with arachidonic acid metabolism.

Contraindications Hypersensitivity to benzydamine or any component of the formulation

Warnings/Precautions May cause local irritation and/or burning sensation in patients with altered mucosal integrity. Dilution (1:1 in warm water) may attenuate this effect. Use caution in renal impairment. Safety and efficacy have not been established in children ≤5 years of age.

Drug Interactions Substrate (minor) of CYP1A2, 2C19, 2D6, 3A4
No drug interactions established.

Pharmacodynamics/Kinetics
Absorption: Oral rinse may be absorbed, at least in part, through the oral mucosa
Excretion: Urine (primarily as unchanged drug)

Lactation Excretion in breast milk unknown/use caution

Dosage Forms [CAN] = Canadian brand name
Oral rinse: 0.15% (100 mL, 250 mL) [not available in the U.S.]

Benzydamine Hydrochloride *see* Benzydamine *on page 197*

Benzylpenicillin Benzathine *see* Penicillin G Benzathine *on page 1202*

Benzylpenicillin Potassium *see* Penicillin G (Parenteral/Aqueous) *on page 1203*
Benzylpenicillin Sodium *see* Penicillin G (Parenteral/Aqueous) *on page 1203*

Benzylpenicilloyl-polylysine (BEN zil pen i SIL oyl pol i LIE seen)

U.S. Brand Names Pre-Pen® [DSC]
Generic Available No
Synonyms Penicilloyl-polylysine; PPL
Pharmacologic Category Diagnostic Agent
Use Adjunct in assessing the risk of administering penicillin (penicillin or benzyl-penicillin) in adults with a history of clinical penicillin hypersensitivity
Local Anesthetic/Vasoconstrictor Precautions No information available to require special precautions
Effects on Dental Treatment No significant effects or complications reported
Common Adverse Effects Frequency not defined.
  Cardiovascular: Hypotension
  Dermatologic: Angioneurotic edema, pruritus, erythema, urticaria
  Local: Intense local inflammatory response at skin test site, wheal (locally)
  Respiratory: Dyspnea
  Miscellaneous: Systemic allergic reactions occur rarely
Mechanism of Action Elicits IgE antibodies which produce type I accelerate urticarial reactions to penicillins
Drug Interactions
  Decreased Effect: Corticosteroids and other immunosuppressive agents may inhibit the immune response to the skin test.
Pregnancy Risk Factor C

Beractant (ber AKT ant)

U.S. Brand Names Survanta®
Canadian Brand Names Survanta®
Mexican Brand Names Survanta®
Generic Available No
Synonyms Bovine Lung Surfactant; Natural Lung Surfactant
Pharmacologic Category Lung Surfactant
Use Prevention and treatment of respiratory distress syndrome (RDS) in premature infants

Prophylactic therapy: Body weight <1250 g in infants at risk for developing, or with evidence of, surfactant deficiency (administer within 15 minutes of birth)
Rescue therapy: Treatment of infants with RDS confirmed by x-ray and requiring mechanical ventilation (administer as soon as possible - within 8 hours of age)
Local Anesthetic/Vasoconstrictor Precautions No information available to require special precautions
Effects on Dental Treatment No significant effects or complications reported
Common Adverse Effects During the dosing procedure:
  >10%: Cardiovascular: Transient bradycardia
  1% to 10%: Respiratory: Oxygen desaturation
Mechanism of Action Replaces deficient or ineffective endogenous lung surfactant in neonates with respiratory distress syndrome (RDS) or in neonates at risk of developing RDS. Surfactant prevents the alveoli from collapsing during expiration by lowering surface tension between air and alveolar surfaces.
Drug Interactions
  Increased Effect/Toxicity: No data reported
  Decreased Effect: No data reported
Pharmacodynamics/Kinetics Excretion: Clearance: Alveolar clearance is rapid

9-Beta-D-ribofuranosyladenine *see* Adenosine *on page 55*

Beta-Carotene (BAY ta KARE oh teen)

U.S. Brand Names A-Caro-25®; B-Caro-T™; Lumitene™
Generic Available Yes
Pharmacologic Category Vitamin, Fat Soluble
Unlabeled/Investigational Use Prophylaxis and treatment of polymorphous light eruption; prophylaxis against photosensitivity reactions in erythropoietic protoporphyria

Local Anesthetic/Vasoconstrictor Precautions No information available to require special precautions

Effects on Dental Treatment No significant effects or complications reported

Common Adverse Effects >10%: Dermatologic: Carotenodermia (yellowing of palms, hands, or soles of feet, and to a lesser extent the face)

Mechanism of Action The exact mechanism of action in erythropoietic protoporphyria has not as yet been elucidated; although patient must become carotenemic before effects are observed, there appears to be more than a simple internal light screen responsible for the drug's action. A protective effect was achieved when beta-carotene was added to blood samples. The concentrations of solutions used were similar to those achieved in treated patients. Topically applied beta-carotene is considerably less effective than systemic therapy.

Pharmacodynamics/Kinetics

Metabolism: Prior to absorption, converted to vitamin A in the wall of the small intestine, then oxidized to retinoic acid and retinol in the presence of fat and bile acids; small amounts are then stored in the liver; retinol (active) is conjugated with glucuronic acid

Excretion: Urine and feces

Pregnancy Risk Factor C

Betadine® [OTC] see Povidone-Iodine on page 1262

Betadine® First Aid Antibiotics + Moisturizer [OTC] see Bacitracin and Polymyxin B on page 176

Betadine® Ophthalmic see Povidone-Iodine on page 1262

Betagan® see Levobunolol on page 909

Beta-HC® see Hydrocortisone on page 793

Betaine Anhydrous (BAY ta een an HY drus)

U.S. Brand Names Cystadane®
Canadian Brand Names Cystadane®
Generic Available No
Pharmacologic Category Homocystinuria, Treatment Agent
Use Orphan drug: Treatment of homocystinuria to decrease elevated homocysteine blood levels; included within the category of homocystinuria are deficiencies or defects in cystathionine beta-synthase (CBS), 5,10-methylenetetrahydrofolate reductase (MTHFR), and cobalamin cofactor metabolism (CBL).

Local Anesthetic/Vasoconstrictor Precautions No information available to require special precautions

Effects on Dental Treatment No significant effects or complications reported

Common Adverse Effects Minimal; have included nausea, GI distress, and diarrhea

Pregnancy Risk Factor C

BetaMed [OTC] see Pyrithione Zinc on page 1318

Betamethasone (bay ta METH a sone)

Related Information
Respiratory Diseases on page 1656
Related Sample Prescriptions
Recurrent Aphthous Stomatitis on page 1744
U.S. Brand Names Beta-Val®; Celestone®; Celestone® Soluspan®; Diprolene®; Diprolene® AF; Luxiq®; Maxivate®
Canadian Brand Names Betaderm; Betaject™; Betnesol®; Betnovate®; Celestone® Soluspan®; Diprolene® Glycol; Diprosone®; Ectosone; Prevex® B; Taro-Sone®; Topilene®; Topisone®; Valisone® Scalp Lotion
Mexican Brand Names Celestone®
Generic Available Yes: Excludes foam, injection, syrup
Synonyms Betamethasone Dipropionate; Betamethasone Dipropionate, Augmented; Betamethasone Sodium Phosphate; Betamethasone Valerate; Flubenisolone
Pharmacologic Category Corticosteroid, Systemic; Corticosteroid, Topical
Dental Use Treatment of a variety of oral diseases of allergic, inflammatory, or autoimmune origin
Use Inflammatory dermatoses such as seborrheic or atopic dermatitis, neurodermatitis, anogenital pruritus, psoriasis, inflammatory phase of xerosis

Local Anesthetic/Vasoconstrictor Precautions No information available to require special precautions

Effects on Dental Treatment No significant effects or complications reported

(Continued)

Betamethasone *(Continued)*

Significant Adverse Effects

Systemic:

Cardiovascular: Congestive heart failure, edema, hyper-/hypotension

Central nervous system: Dizziness, headache, insomnia, intracranial pressure increased, lightheadedness, nervousness, pseudotumor cerebri, seizure, vertigo

Dermatologic: Ecchymoses, facial erythema, fragile skin, hirsutism, hyper-/hypopigmentation, perioral dermatitis (oral), petechiae, striae, wound healing impaired

Endocrine & metabolic: Amenorrhea, Cushing's syndrome, diabetes mellitus, growth suppression, hyperglycemia, hypokalemia, menstrual irregularities, pituitary-adrenal axis suppression, protein catabolism, sodium retention, water retention

Gastrointestinal: Abdominal distention, appetite increased, hiccups, indigestion, peptic ulcer, pancreatitis, ulcerative esophagitis

Local: Injection site reactions (intra-articular use), sterile abscess

Neuromuscular & skeletal: Arthralgia, muscle atrophy, fractures, muscle weakness, myopathy, osteoporosis, necrosis (femoral and humeral heads)

Ocular: Cataracts, glaucoma, intraocular pressure increased

Miscellaneous: Anaphylactoid reaction, diaphoresis, hypersensitivity, secondary infection

Topical:

Dermatologic: Acneiform eruptions, allergic dermatitis, burning, dry skin, erythema, folliculitis, hypertrichosis, irritation, miliaria, pruritus, skin atrophy, striae, vesiculation

Endocrine and metabolic effects have occasionally been reported with topical use.

Dental Usual Dosing Allergic or inflammatory diseases: Topical: Gel: Apply small quantity with Q-tip to affected area 3-4 times/day

Dosage Base dosage on severity of disease and patient response

Children: Use lowest dose listed as initial dose for adrenocortical insufficiency (physiologic replacement)

I.M.: 0.0175-0.125 mg base/kg/day divided every 6-12 hours **or** 0.5-7.5 mg base/m²/day divided every 6-12 hours

Oral: 0.0175-0.25 mg/kg/day divided every 6-8 hours **or** 0.5-7.5 mg/m²/day divided every 6-8 hours

Topical:

≤12 years: Use is not recommended.

≥13 years: Use minimal amount for shortest period of time to avoid HPA axis suppression

Gel, augmented formulation: Apply once or twice daily; rub in gently. **Note:** Do not exceed 2 weeks of treatment or 50 g/week.

Lotion: Apply a few drops twice daily

Augmented formulation: Apply a few drops once or twice daily; rub in gently. **Note:** Do not exceed 2 weeks of treatment or 50 mL/week.

Cream/ointment: Apply once or twice daily.

Augmented formulation: Apply once or twice daily. **Note:** Do not exceed 2 weeks of treatment or 45 g/week.

Adolescents and Adults:

Oral: 2.4-4.8 mg/day in 2-4 doses; range: 0.6-7.2 mg/day

I.M.: Betamethasone sodium phosphate and betamethasone acetate: 0.6-9 mg/day (generally, ⅓ to ½ of oral dose) divided every 12-24 hours

Adults:

Intrabursal, intra-articular, intradermal: 0.25-2 mL

Intralesional: Rheumatoid arthritis/osteoarthritis:

Very large joints: 1-2 mL

Large joints: 1 mL

Medium joints: 0.5-1 mL

Small joints: 0.25-0.5 mL

Topical:

Foam: Apply to the scalp twice daily, once in the morning and once at night

Gel, augmented formulation: Apply once or twice daily; rub in gently. **Note:** Do not exceed 2 weeks of treatment or 50 g/week.

Lotion: Apply a few drops twice daily

Augmented formulation: Apply a few drops once or twice daily; rub in gently. **Note:** Do not exceed 2 weeks of treatment or 50 mL/week.

Cream/ointment: Apply once or twice daily

Augmented formulation: Apply once or twice daily. **Note:** Do not exceed 2 weeks of treatment or 45 g/week.

Dosing adjustment in hepatic impairment: Adjustments may be necessary in patients with liver failure because betamethasone is extensively metabolized in the liver

Mechanism of Action Controls the rate of protein synthesis; depresses the migration of polymorphonuclear leukocytes, fibroblasts; reverses capillary permeability and lysosomal stabilization at the cellular level to prevent or control inflammation

Contraindications Hypersensitivity to betamethasone, other corticosteroids, or any component of the formulation; systemic fungal infections

Warnings/Precautions Topical use in patients ≤12 years of age is not recommended. May cause suppression of hypothalamic-pituitary-adrenal (HPA) axis, particularly in younger children or in patients receiving high doses for prolonged periods.

Very high potency topical products are not for treatment of rosacea, perioral dermatitis; not for use on face, groin, or axillae; not for use in a diapered area. Avoid concurrent use of other corticosteroids.

May suppress the immune system; patients may be more susceptible to infection. Use with caution in patients with systemic infections or ocular herpes simplex. Avoid exposure to chickenpox and measles.

Use with caution in patients with hypothyroidism, cirrhosis, ulcerative colitis; do not use occlusive dressings on weeping or exudative lesions and general caution with occlusive dressings should be observed; adverse effects may be increased. Discontinue if skin irritation or contact dermatitis should occur; do not use in patients with decreased skin circulation.

Drug Interactions Inhibits CYP3A4 (weak)

Phenytoin, phenobarbital, rifampin increase clearance of betamethasone.

Potassium-depleting diuretics increase potassium loss.

Skin test antigens, immunizations: Betamethasone may decrease response and increase potential infections.

Insulin or oral hypoglycemics: Betamethasone may increase blood glucose.

Ethanol/Nutrition/Herb Interactions

Ethanol: Avoid ethanol (may enhance gastric mucosal irritation).

Food: Betamethasone interferes with calcium absorption.

Herb/Nutraceutical: Avoid cat's claw, echinacea (have immunostimulant properties).

Dietary Considerations May be taken with food to decrease GI distress.

Pharmacodynamics/Kinetics

Protein binding: 64%

Metabolism: Hepatic

Half-life elimination: 6.5 hours

Time to peak, serum: I.V.: 10-36 minutes

Excretion: Urine (<5% as unchanged drug)

Pregnancy Risk Factor C

Lactation Excretion in breast milk unknown/use caution

Breast-Feeding Considerations Systemic corticosteroids are excreted in human milk. The extent of topical absorption is variable. Use with caution while breast-feeding; do not apply to nipples.

Dosage Forms [DSC] = Discontinued product

Note: Potency expressed as betamethasone base.

Cream, topical, as dipropionate: 0.05% (15 g, 45 g)

   Maxivate®: 0.05% (45 g)

Cream, topical, as dipropionate augmented (Diprolene® AF): 0.05% (15 g, 50 g)

Cream, topical, as valerate (Beta-Val®): 0.1% (15 g, 45 g)

Foam, topical, as valerate (Luxiq®): 0.12% (50 g, 100 g, 150 g) [contains alcohol 60.4%]

Gel, topical, as dipropionate augmented: 0.05% (15 g, 50 g)

Injection, suspension (Celestone® Soluspan®): Betamethasone sodium phosphate 3 mg/mL and betamethasone acetate 3 mg/mL [6 mg/mL] (5 mL)

Lotion, topical, as dipropionate (Maxivate®): 0.05% (60 mL)

Lotion, topical, as dipropionate augmented (Diprolene®): 0.05% (30 mL, 60 mL)

Lotion, topical, as valerate (Beta-Val®): 0.1% (60 mL)

Ointment, topical, as dipropionate: 0.05% (15 g, 45 g)

   Maxivate®: 0.05% (45 g)

Ointment, topical, as dipropionate augmented (Diprolene®): 0.05% (15 g, 50 g)

Ointment, topical, as valerate: 0.1% (15 g, 45 g)

Syrup, as base (Celestone®): 0.6 mg/5 mL (118 mL)

Betamethasone and Clotrimazole
(bay ta METH a sone & kloe TRIM a zole)

Related Information
Betamethasone *on page 199*
Clotrimazole *on page 379*

U.S. Brand Names Lotrisone®

Canadian Brand Names Lotriderm®

Generic Available Yes

Synonyms Clotrimazole and Betamethasone

Pharmacologic Category Antifungal Agent, Topical; Corticosteroid, Topical

Dental Use Treatment of a variety of oral diseases of allergic, inflammatory, or autoimmune origin

Use Topical treatment of various dermal fungal infections (including tinea pedis, cruris, and corpora in patients ≥17 years of age)

Local Anesthetic/Vasoconstrictor Precautions No information available to require special precautions

Effects on Dental Treatment No significant effects or complications reported

Significant Adverse Effects Also see individual agents.

1% to 10%:
Dermatologic: Dry skin (2%)
Local: Burning (2%)
Neuromuscular & skeletal: Paresthesia (2%)

<1% (Limited to important or life-threatening): Cushing's syndrome, edema, glycosuria, HPA axis suppression (higher in children), hyperglycemia, rash, secondary infection, stinging. Growth suppression, intracranial hypertension, and striae have also been reported with use in children.

Dental Usual Dosing Allergic or inflammatory diseases: Children ≥17 years and Adults: Topical: Apply to affected area twice daily, morning and evening

Dosage
Children <17 years: Do not use

Children ≥17 years and Adults:

Allergic or inflammatory diseases: Topical: Apply to affected area twice daily, morning and evening

Tinea corporis, tinea cruris: Topical: Massage into affected area twice daily, morning and evening; do not use for longer than 2 weeks; re-evaluate after 1 week if no clinical improvement; do not exceed 45 g cream/week or 45 mL lotion/week

Tinea pedis: Topical: Massage into affected area twice daily, morning and evening; do not use for longer than 4 weeks; re-evaluate after 2 weeks if no clinical improvement; do not exceed 45 g cream/week or 45 mL lotion/week

Elderly: Use with caution; skin atrophy and skin ulceration (rare) have been reported in patients with thinning skin; do not use for diaper dermatitis or under occlusive dressings

Mechanism of Action Betamethasone dipropionate is a corticosteroid. Clotrimazole is an antifungal agent.

Contraindications Hypersensitivity to betamethasone, clotrimazole, other corticosteroids or imidazoles, or any component of the formulation

Warnings/Precautions Systemic absorption of topical corticosteroids may cause hypothalamic-pituitary-adrenal (HPA) axis suppression (reversible); may lead to manifestations of Cushing's syndrome, hyperglycemia, and glucosuria. Risk is increased when used over large surface areas, for prolonged periods of time, or with occlusive dressings. Not for use in patients <17 years of age (striae and growth retardation have been reported with use in infants and children). Do not use for diaper dermatitis.

Drug Interactions
Betamethasone: Inhibits CYP3A4 (weak)

Clotrimazole: Inhibits CYP1A2 (weak), 2A6 (weak), 2B6 (weak), 2C8/9 (weak), 2C19 (weak), 2D6 (weak), 2E1 (weak), 3A4 (moderate)

Also see individual agents.

Pharmacodynamics/Kinetics See individual agents.

Pregnancy Risk Factor C

Lactation Excretion in breast milk unknown/use caution

Breast-Feeding Considerations Betamethasone: Systemic corticosteroids are excreted in human milk. The extent of topical absorption is variable. Use with caution while breast-feeding; do not apply to nipples.

Dosage Forms
Cream: Betamethasone dipropionate 0.05% and clotrimazole 1% (15 g, 45 g) [contains benzyl alcohol]

Lotion: Betamethasone dipropionate 0.05% and clotrimazole 1% (30 mL) [contains benzyl alcohol]

Betamethasone Dipropionate *see* Betamethasone *on page 199*
Betamethasone Dipropionate, Augmented *see* Betamethasone *on page 199*
Betamethasone Sodium Phosphate *see* Betamethasone *on page 199*
Betamethasone Valerate *see* Betamethasone *on page 199*
Betapace® *see* Sotalol *on page 1409*
Betapace AF® *see* Sotalol *on page 1409*
Betasept® [OTC] *see* Chlorhexidine Gluconate *on page 316*
Betaseron® *see* Interferon Beta-1b *on page 850*
Betatar® Gel [OTC] *see* Coal Tar *on page 383*
Beta-Val® *see* Betamethasone *on page 199*

Betaxolol (be TAKS oh lol)

Related Information
Cardiovascular Diseases *on page 1636*
U.S. Brand Names Betoptic® S; Kerlone®
Canadian Brand Names Betoptic® S
Generic Available Yes: Solution, tablet
Synonyms Betaxolol Hydrochloride
Pharmacologic Category Beta Blocker, Beta$_1$ Selective
Use Treatment of chronic open-angle glaucoma and ocular hypertension; management of hypertension
Local Anesthetic/Vasoconstrictor Precautions No information available to require special precautions
Effects on Dental Treatment Betaxolol is a cardioselective beta-blocker. Local anesthetic with vasoconstrictor can be safely used in patients medicated with betaxolol. Nonselective beta-blockers (ie, propranolol, nadolol) enhance the pressor response to epinephrine, resulting in hypertension and bradycardia; this has not been reported for betaxolol. Many nonsteroidal anti-inflammatory drugs, such as ibuprofen and indomethacin, can reduce the hypotensive effect of beta-blockers after 3 or more weeks of therapy with the NSAID. Short-term NSAID use (ie, 3 days) requires no special precautions in patients taking beta-blockers.

Common Adverse Effects
Ophthalmic:
>10%: Ocular: Short-term discomfort (25%)
Frequency not defined: Ocular: Anisocoria, blurred vision, corneal sensitivity decreased, corneal staining, crusty lashes, discharge, dry eyes, edema, erythema, foreign body sensation, inflammation, itching sensation, keratitis, photophobia, tearing, visual acuity decreased

Systemic:
>10%:
Central nervous system: Drowsiness, insomnia
Endocrine & metabolic: Sexual ability decreased
1% to 10%:
Cardiovascular: Bradycardia, palpitation, edema, CHF, peripheral circulation reduced
Central nervous system: Mental depression
Gastrointestinal: Diarrhea or constipation, nausea, vomiting, stomach discomfort
Respiratory: Bronchospasm
Miscellaneous: Cold extremities

Mechanism of Action Competitively blocks beta$_1$-receptors, with little or no effect on beta$_2$-receptors; ophthalmic reduces intraocular pressure by reducing the production of aqueous humor

Drug Interactions
Cytochrome P450 Effect: Substrate (major) of CYP1A2, 2D6; **Inhibits** CYP2D6 (weak)
Increased Effect/Toxicity: Acetylcholinesterase inhibitors, amiodarone, cardiac glycosides, dipyridamole, disopyramide, and SSRIs may enhance the bradycardic effects of beta-blockers. Beta-blockers may enhance the vasopressor effects of alpha-/beta-agonists, the orthostatic effects of alpha$_1$-agonists, and the rebound hypertensive effect of alpha$_2$-agonists after abrupt withdrawal. Aminoquinolones (antimalarial), antipsychotic agents, calcium channel blockers, CYP1A2 inhibitors, 2D6 inhibitors, and propoxyphene may increase the effects of beta-blockers. Beta-blockers may enhance the effects of insulin (hypoglycemia), lidocaine, and sulfonylureas (hypoglycemia).
(Continued)

Betaxolol (Continued)

Decreased Effect: Barbiturates, CYP1A2 inducers, NSAIDs, and rifamycin derivatives may decrease the effects of beta-blockers. Beta₂-agonists may decrease the bradycardic effect of beta-blockers. Beta-blockers may decrease the bronchodilatory effect of theophylline.

Pharmacodynamics/Kinetics

Onset of action: Ophthalmic: 30 minutes; Oral: 1-1.5 hours

Duration: Ophthalmic: ≥12 hours

Absorption: Ophthalmic: Some systemic; Oral: ~100%

Metabolism: Hepatic to multiple metabolites

Protein binding: Oral: 50%

Bioavailability: Oral: 89%

Half-life elimination: Oral: 12-22 hours

Time to peak: Ophthalmic: ~2 hours; Oral: 1.5-6 hours

Excretion: Urine

Pregnancy Risk Factor C (manufacturer); D (2nd and 3rd trimesters - expert analysis)

Betaxolol Hydrochloride *see* Betaxolol *on page 203*

Bethanechol (be THAN e kole)

U.S. Brand Names Urecholine®

Canadian Brand Names Duvoid®; Myotonachol®; PMS-Bethanechol

Generic Available Yes

Synonyms Bethanechol Chloride

Pharmacologic Category Cholinergic Agonist

Use Nonobstructive urinary retention and retention due to neurogenic bladder

Unlabeled/Investigational Use Treatment and prevention of bladder dysfunction caused by phenothiazines; diagnosis of flaccid or atonic neurogenic bladder; gastroesophageal reflux

Local Anesthetic/Vasoconstrictor Precautions No information available to require special precautions

Effects on Dental Treatment This is a cholinergic agent similar to pilocarpine; expect to see salivation and sweating in patients.

Common Adverse Effects Frequency not defined.

Cardiovascular: Hypotension, tachycardia, flushed skin

Central nervous system: Headache, malaise

Gastrointestinal: Abdominal cramps, diarrhea, nausea, vomiting, salivation, eructation

Genitourinary: Urinary urgency

Ocular: Lacrimation, miosis

Respiratory: Asthmatic attacks, bronchial constriction

Miscellaneous: Diaphoresis

Mechanism of Action Stimulates cholinergic receptors in the smooth muscle of the urinary bladder and gastrointestinal tract resulting in increased peristalsis, increased GI and pancreatic secretions, bladder muscle contraction, and increased ureteral peristaltic waves

Drug Interactions

Increased Effect/Toxicity: Bethanechol and ganglionic blockers may cause a critical fall in blood pressure. Cholinergic drugs or anticholinesterase agents may have additive effects with bethanechol.

Decreased Effect: Procainamide, quinidine may decrease the effects of bethanechol. Anticholinergic agents (atropine, antihistamines, TCAs, phenothiazines) may decrease effects.

Pharmacodynamics/Kinetics

Onset of action: 30-90 minutes

Duration: Up to 6 hours

Absorption: Variable

Pregnancy Risk Factor C

Bethanechol Chloride *see* Bethanechol *on page 204*

Betimol® *see* Timolol *on page 1489*

Betoptic® S *see* Betaxolol *on page 203*

Bevacizumab (be vuh SIZ uh mab)

U.S. Brand Names Avastin™

Generic Available No

Synonyms Anti-VEGF Monoclonal Antibody; NSC-704865; rhuMAb-VEGF

Pharmacologic Category Antineoplastic Agent, Monoclonal Antibody; Vascular Endothelial Growth Factor (VEGF) Inhibitor

Use Treatment of metastatic colorectal cancer (in combination with I.V. fluorouracil-based regimen)

Unlabeled/Investigational Use Breast cancer, malignant mesothelioma, prostate cancer, lung cancer (nonsmall cell), renal cell cancer

Investigational: Ovarian cancer (earlier stage)

Local Anesthetic/Vasoconstrictor Precautions No information available to require special precautions

Effects on Dental Treatment No significant effects or complications reported

Common Adverse Effects Percentages reported as part of a combination chemotherapy regimen.

>10%:

Cardiovascular: Hypertension (23% to 34%; grades 3/4: 12%); thromboembolism (18%); hypotension (7% to 15%)

Central nervous system: Pain (61% to 62%); headache (26%); dizziness (19% to 26%)

Dermatologic: Alopecia (6% to 32%), dry skin (7% to 20%), exfoliative dermatitis (3% to 19%), skin discoloration (2% to 16%)

Endocrine & metabolic: Weight loss (15% to 16%), hypokalemia (12% to 16%)

Gastrointestinal: Abdominal pain (50% to 61%); diarrhea (grades 3/4: 34%); vomiting (47% to 52%); anorexia (35% to 43%); constipation (29% to 40%); stomatitis (30% to 32%); gastrointestinal hemorrhage (19% to 24%), dyspepsia (17% to 24%); taste disorder (14% to 21%), flatulence (11% to 19%)

Hematologic: Leukopenia (grades 3/4: 37%), neutropenia (grades 3/4: 21%)

Neuromuscular & skeletal: Weakness (73% to 74%); myalgia (8% to 15%)

Ocular: Tearing increased (6% to 18%)

Renal: Proteinuria (36%)

Respiratory: Upper respiratory infection (40% to 47%), epistaxis (32% to 35%), dyspnea (25% to 26%)

1% to 10%:

Cardiovascular: DVT (6% to 9%; grades 3/4: 9%); arterial thrombosis (4%), syncope (grades 3/4: 3%), intra-abdominal venous thrombosis (grades 3/4: 3%), cardio-/cerebrovascular arterial thrombotic event (2%), CHF (2%)

Central nervous system: Confusion (1% to 6%), abnormal gait (1% to 5%)

Dermatologic: Nail disorder (2% to 8%), skin ulcer (6%)

Gastrointestinal: Xerostomia (4% to 7%), colitis (1% to 6%), gingival bleeding (2%)

Genitourinary: Polyuria/urgency (3% to 6%), vaginal hemorrhage (4%)

Hematologic: Thrombocytopenia (5%)

Hepatic: Bilirubinemia (1% to 6%)

Respiratory: Voice alteration (6% to 9%)

Miscellaneous: Infusion reactions (<3%)

Mechanism of Action Bevacizumab is a recombinant, humanized monoclonal antibody which binds to, and neutralizes, vascular endothelial growth factor (VEGF), preventing its association with endothelial receptors. VEGF binding initiates angiogenesis (endothelial proliferation and the formation of new blood vessels). The inhibition of microvascular growth is believed to retard the growth of all tissues (including metastatic tissue).

Drug Interactions

Increased Effect/Toxicity: Bevacizumab may potentiate the cardiotoxic effects of anthracyclines. Serum concentrations of irinotecan's active metabolite may be increased by bevacizumab; an approximate 33% increase has been observed.

Pharmacodynamics/Kinetics

Distribution: V_d: 46 mL/kg

Half-life elimination: 20 days (range: 11-50 days)

Excretion: Clearance: 2.75-5 mL/kg/day

Pregnancy Risk Factor C

Bexarotene (beks AIR oh teen)

U.S. Brand Names Targretin®

Canadian Brand Names Targretin®

Generic Available No

Pharmacologic Category Antineoplastic Agent, Miscellaneous

Use

Oral: Treatment of cutaneous manifestations of cutaneous T-cell lymphoma in patients who are refractory to at least one prior systemic therapy

(Continued)

Bexarotene *(Continued)*

Topical: Treatment of cutaneous lesions in patients with refractory cutaneous T-cell lymphoma (stage 1A and 1B) or who have not tolerated other therapies

Local Anesthetic/Vasoconstrictor Precautions No information available to require special precautions

Effects on Dental Treatment Key adverse event(s) related to dental treatment: Xerostomia (normal salivary flow resumes upon discontinuation) and gingivitis.

Common Adverse Effects First percentage is at a dose of 300 mg/m^2/day; the second percentage is at a dose >300 mg/m^2/day.

>10%:

Cardiovascular: Peripheral edema (13% to 11%)

Central nervous system: Headache (30% to 42%), chills (10% to 13%)

Dermatologic: Rash (17% to 23%), exfoliative dermatitis (10% to 28%)

Endocrine & metabolic: Hyperlipidemia (about 79% in both dosing ranges), hypercholesteremia (32% to 62%), hypothyroidism (29% to 53%)

Hematologic: Leukopenia (17% to 47%)

Neuromuscular & skeletal: Weakness (20% to 45%)

Miscellaneous: Infection (13% to 23%)

<10%:

Cardiovascular: Hemorrhage, hypertension, angina pectoris, right heart failure, tachycardia, cerebrovascular accident

Central nervous system: Fever (5% to 17%), insomnia (5% to 11%), subdural hematoma, syncope, depression, agitation, ataxia, confusion, dizziness, hyperesthesia

Dermatologic: Dry skin (about 10% for both dosing ranges), alopecia (4% to 11%), skin ulceration, acne, skin nodule, maculopapular rash, serous drainage, vesicular bullous rash, cheilitis

Endocrine & metabolic: Hypoproteinemia, hyperglycemia, weight loss/gain, breast pain

Gastrointestinal: Abdominal pain (11% to 4%), nausea (16% to 8%), diarrhea (7% to 42%), vomiting (4% to 13%), anorexia (2% to 23%), constipation, xerostomia, flatulence, colitis, dyspepsia, gastroenteritis, gingivitis, melena, pancreatitis, serum amylase increased

Genitourinary: Albuminuria, hematuria, urinary incontinence, urinary tract infection, urinary urgency, dysuria, kidney function abnormality

Hematologic: Hypochromic anemia (4% to 13%), anemia (6% to 25%), eosinophilia, thrombocythemia, coagulation time increased, lymphocytosis, thrombocytopenia

Hepatic: LDH increase (7% to 13%), hepatic failure

Neuromuscular & skeletal: Back pain (2% to 11%), arthralgia, myalgia, bone pain, myasthenia, arthrosis, neuropathy

Ocular: Dry eyes, conjunctivitis, blepharitis, corneal lesion, visual field defects, keratitis

Otic: Ear pain, otitis externa

Renal: Creatinine increased

Respiratory: Pharyngitis, rhinitis, dyspnea, pleural effusion, bronchitis, cough increased, lung edema, hemoptysis, hypoxia

Miscellaneous: Flu-like syndrome (4% to 13%), bacterial infection (1% to 13%)

Topical:

Cardiovascular: Edema (10%)

Central nervous system: Headache (14%), weakness (6%), pain (30%)

Dermatologic: Rash (14% to 72%), pruritus (6% to 40%), contact dermatitis (14%), exfoliative dermatitis (6%)

Hematologic: Leukopenia (6%), lymphadenopathy (6%)

Neuromuscular & skeletal: Paresthesia (6%)

Respiratory: Cough (6%), pharyngitis (6%)

Miscellaneous: Diaphoresis (6%), infection (18%)

Mechanism of Action The exact mechanism is unknown. Binds and activates retinoid X receptor subtypes. Once activated, these receptors function as transcription factors that regulate the expression of genes which control cellular differentiation and proliferation. Bexarotene inhibits the growth *in vitro* of some tumor cell lines of hematopoietic and squamous cell origin.

Drug Interactions

Cytochrome P450 Effect: Substrate of CYP3A4 (minor); **Induces** CYP3A4 (weak)

Increased Effect/Toxicity: Bexarotene plasma concentrations may be increased by gemfibrozil. Bexarotene may increase the toxicity of DEET.

Decreased Effect: Bexarotene may decrease the plasma levels of hormonal contraceptives and tamoxifen.

Pharmacodynamics/Kinetics
Absorption: Significantly improved by a fat-containing meal
Protein binding: >99%
Metabolism: Hepatic via CYP3A4 isoenzyme; four metabolites identified; further
metabolized by glucuronidation
Half-life elimination: 7 hours
Time to peak: 2 hours
Excretion: Primarily feces; urine (<1% as unchanged drug and metabolites)
Pregnancy Risk Factor X

BG 9273 see Alefacept on page 62
BI-007 see Paclitaxel (Protein Bound) on page 1177
Biaxin® see Clarithromycin on page 355
Biaxin® XL see Clarithromycin on page 355

Bicalutamide (bye ka LOO ta mide)

U.S. Brand Names Casodex®
Canadian Brand Names Casodex®; CO Bicalutamide; Novo-Bicalutamide;
PMS-Bicalutamide; ratio-Bicalutamide; Sandoz-Bicalutamide
Mexican Brand Names Casodex®
Generic Available No
Synonyms CDX; ICI-176334; NC-722665
Pharmacologic Category Antineoplastic Agent, Antiandrogen
Use In combination therapy with LHRH agonist analogues in treatment of meta-
static prostate cancer
Unlabeled/Investigational Use Monotherapy for locally-advanced prostate
cancer
Local Anesthetic/Vasoconstrictor Precautions No information available to
require special precautions
Effects on Dental Treatment Key adverse event(s) related to dental treat-
ment: Xerostomia (normal salivary flow resumes upon discontinuation).
Common Adverse Effects Adverse reaction percentages reported as part of
combination regimen with an LHRH analogue.
>10%:
Cardiovascular: Peripheral edema (13%)
Central nervous system: Pain (35%)
Endocrine & metabolic: Hot flashes (53%)
Gastrointestinal: Constipation (22%), nausea (15%), diarrhea (12%), abdom-
inal pain (11%)
Genitourinary: Pelvic pain (21%), nocturia (12%), hematuria (12%)
Hematologic: Anemia (11%)
Neuromuscular & skeletal: Back pain (25%), weakness (22%)
Respiratory: Dyspnea (13%)
Miscellaneous: Infection (18%)
≥2% to 10%:
Cardiovascular: Chest pain (8%), hypertension (8%), angina pectoris (2% to
<5%), CHF (2% to <5%), edema (2% to <5%), MI (2% to <5%), coronary
artery disorder (2% to <5%), syncope (2% to <5%)
Central nervous system: Dizziness (10%), headache (7%), insomnia (7%),
anxiety (5%), depression (4%), chills (2% to <5%), confusion (2% to <5%),
fever (2% to <5%), nervousness (2% to <5%), somnolence (2% to <5%)
Dermatologic: Rash (9%), alopecia (2% to <5%), dry skin (2% to <5%),
herpes zoster (2% to <5%), pruritus (2% to <5%), skin carcinoma (2% to
<5%)
Endocrine & metabolic: Gynecomastia (9%), breast pain (6%; up to 39% as
monotherapy), hyperglycemia (6%), dehydration (2% to <5%), gout (2% to
<5%), hypercholesterolemia (2% to <5%), libido decreased (2% to <5%)
Gastrointestinal: Dyspepsia (7%), weight loss (7%), anorexia (6%), flatulence
(6%), vomiting (6%), weight gain (5%), dysphagia (2% to <5%), gastrointestinal carcinoma (2% to <5%), melena (2% to <5%), periodontal abscess (2%
to <5%), rectal hemorrhage (2% to <5%), xerostomia (2% to <5%)
Genitourinary: Urinary tract infection (9%), impotence (7%), polyuria (6%),
urinary retention (5%), urinary impairment (5%), urinary incontinence (4%),
dysuria (2% to <5%), urinary urgency (2% to <5%)
Hepatic: LFTs increased (7%), alkaline phosphatase increased (5%)
Neuromuscular & skeletal: Bone pain (9%), paresthesia (8%), myasthenia
(7%), arthritis (5%), pathological fracture (4%), hypertonia (2% to <5%), leg
cramps (2% to <5%), myalgia (2% to <5%), neck pain (2% to <5%), neurop-
athy (2% to <5%)
Ocular: Cataract (2% to <5%)
Renal: BUN increased, creatinine increased, hydronephrosis
(Continued)

Bicalutamide *(Continued)*

Respiratory: Cough (8%), pharyngitis (8%), bronchitis (6%), pneumonia (4%), rhinitis (4%), asthma (2% to <5%), epistaxis (2% to <5%), sinusitis (2% to <5%)

Miscellaneous: Flu syndrome (7%), diaphoresis (6%), cyst (2% to <5%), hernia (2% to <5%), sepsis (2% to <5%)

Mechanism of Action Pure nonsteroidal antiandrogen that binds to androgen receptors; specifically a competitive inhibitor for the binding of dihydrotestosterone and testosterone; prevents testosterone stimulation of cell growth in prostate cancer

Pharmacodynamics/Kinetics

Absorption: Rapid and complete

Protein binding: 96%

Metabolism: Extensively hepatic; glucuronidation and oxidation of the R (active) enantiomer to inactive metabolites

Half-life elimination: Active enantiomer ~6 days, ~10 days in severe liver disease

Time to peak, plasma: 31 hours

Excretion: Urine (36%, as inactive metabolites); feces (42%, as unchanged drug and inactive metabolites)

Pregnancy Risk Factor X

Bicillin® L-A *see* Penicillin G Benzathine *on page 1202*

Bicillin® C-R *see* Penicillin G Benzathine and Penicillin G Procaine *on page 1203*

Bicillin® C-R 900/300 *see* Penicillin G Benzathine and Penicillin G Procaine *on page 1203*

Bicitra® *see* Sodium Citrate and Citric Acid *on page 1401*

BiCNu® *see* Carmustine *on page 273*

BIDA *see* Amonafide *on page 104*

BiDil® *see* Isosorbide Dinitrate and Hydralazine *on page 867*

Biltricide® *see* Praziquantel *on page 1266*

Bimatoprost *(bi MAT oh prost)*

U.S. Brand Names Lumigan®

Canadian Brand Names Lumigan®

Mexican Brand Names Lumigan®

Generic Available No

Pharmacologic Category Ophthalmic Agent, Antiglaucoma; Prostaglandin, Ophthalmic

Use Reduction of intraocular pressure (IOP) in patients with open-angle glaucoma or ocular hypertension; should be used in patients who are intolerant of other IOP-lowering medications or failed treatment with another IOP-lowering medication

Local Anesthetic/Vasoconstrictor Precautions No information available to require special precautions

Effects on Dental Treatment No significant effects or complications reported

Mechanism of Action As a synthetic analog of prostaglandin with ocular hypotensive activity, bimatoprost decreases intraocular pressure by increasing the outflow of aqueous humor.

Pregnancy Risk Factor C

Biocef® *see* Cephalexin *on page 301*

Biofed [OTC] *see* Pseudoephedrine *on page 1309*

Biolon™ *see* Hyaluronate and Derivatives *on page 773*

Bion® Tears [OTC] *see* Artificial Tears *on page 143*

Bio-Statin® *see* Nystatin *on page 1133*

BioThrax™ *see* Anthrax Vaccine (Adsorbed) *on page 128*

Biperiden *(bye PER i den)*

U.S. Brand Names Akineton®

Canadian Brand Names Akineton®

Mexican Brand Names Akineton®

Generic Available No

Synonyms Biperiden Hydrochloride; Biperiden Lactate

Pharmacologic Category Anti-Parkinson's Agent, Anticholinergic; Anticholinergic Agent

Use Adjunct in the therapy of all forms of Parkinsonism; control of extrapyramidal symptoms secondary to antipsychotics

Local Anesthetic/Vasoconstrictor Precautions No information available to require special precautions

Effects on Dental Treatment Key adverse event(s) related to dental treatment: Xerostomia (normal salivary flow resumes upon discontinuation), nasal dryness, dry throat (very prevalent), and orthostatic hypotension.

Common Adverse Effects Frequency not defined.

Cardiovascular: Orthostatic hypotension, bradycardia

Central nervous system: Drowsiness, euphoria, disorientation, agitation, sleep disorder (decreased REM sleep and increased REM latency)

Gastrointestinal: Constipation, xerostomia

Genitourinary: Urinary retention

Neuromuscular & skeletal: Choreic movements

Ocular: Blurred vision

Mechanism of Action Biperiden is a weak peripheral anticholinergic agent with nicotinolytic activity. The beneficial effects in Parkinson's disease and neuroleptic-induced extrapyramidal symptoms are believed to be due to the inhibition of striatal cholinergic receptors.

Drug Interactions

Cytochrome P450 Effect: Inhibits CYP2D6 (weak)

Increased Effect/Toxicity: Central and/or peripheral anticholinergic syndrome can occur when administered with amantadine (or rimantadine), narcotic analgesics, phenothiazines and other antipsychotics (especially with high anticholinergic activity), tricyclic antidepressants, quinidine and some other antiarrhythmics, and antihistamines. Anticholinergics may increase the bioavailability of atenolol (and possibly other beta-blockers). Anticholinergics may decrease gastric degradation and increase the amount of digoxin or levodopa absorbed by delaying gastric emptying.

Decreased Effect: Anticholinergics may antagonize the therapeutic effect of neuroleptics and cholinergic agents (includes tacrine and donepezil).

Pharmacodynamics/Kinetics

Bioavailability: 29%

Half-life elimination, serum: 18.4-24.3 hours

Time to peak, serum: 1-1.5 hours

Pregnancy Risk Factor C

Biperiden Hydrochloride see Biperiden on page 208
Biperiden Lactate see Biperiden on page 208
Bisac-Evac™ [OTC] see Bisacodyl on page 209

Bisacodyl (bis a KOE dil)

U.S. Brand Names Alophen® [OTC]; Bisac-Evac™ [OTC]; Bisacodyl Uniserts® [OTC]; Correctol® Tablets [OTC]; Doxidan® (reformulation) [OTC]; Dulcolax® [OTC]; Femilax™ [OTC]; Fleet® Bisacodyl Enema [OTC]; Fleet® Stimulant Laxative [OTC]; Gentlax® [OTC] [DSC]; Modane Tablets® [OTC]; Veracolate [OTC]

Canadian Brand Names Apo-Bisacodyl®; Carter's Little Pills®; Dulcolax®; Gentlax®

Mexican Brand Names Dulcolan®

Generic Available Yes: Excludes enema

Pharmacologic Category Laxative, Stimulant

Use Treatment of constipation; colonic evacuation prior to procedures or examination

Local Anesthetic/Vasoconstrictor Precautions No information available to require special precautions

Effects on Dental Treatment No significant effects or complications reported

Mechanism of Action Stimulates peristalsis by directly irritating the smooth muscle of the intestine, possibly the colonic intramural plexus; alters water and electrolyte secretion producing net intestinal fluid accumulation and laxation

Drug Interactions

Decreased Effect: Milk or antacids may decrease the effect of bisacodyl. Bisacodyl may decrease the effect of warfarin.

Pharmacodynamics/Kinetics

Onset of action: Oral: 6-10 hours; Rectal: 0.25-1 hour

Absorption: Oral, rectal: Systemic, <5%

Pregnancy Risk Factor C

Bisacodyl Uniserts® [OTC] see Bisacodyl on page 209
bis-chloronitrosourea see Carmustine on page 273
Bismatrol see Bismuth on page 210

Bismuth (BIZ muth)

Related Information
Gastrointestinal Disorders *on page 1654*

U.S. Brand Names Diotame® [OTC]; Kaopectate® [OTC]; Kaopectate® Extra Strength [OTC]; Kaopectolin *(new formulation)* [OTC]; Maalox® Total Stomach Relief® [OTC]; Pepto-Bismol® [OTC]; Pepto-Bismol® Maximum Strength [OTC]

Generic Available Yes

Synonyms Bismatrol; Bismuth Subgallate; Bismuth Subsalicylate; Pink Bismuth

Pharmacologic Category Antidiarrheal

Use
Subsalicylate formulation: Symptomatic treatment of mild, nonspecific diarrhea; control of traveler's diarrhea (enterotoxigenic *Escherichia coli*); as part of a multidrug regimen for *H. pylori* eradication to reduce the risk of duodenal ulcer recurrence

Subgallate formulation: An aid to reduce fecal odors from a colostomy or ileostomy

Local Anesthetic/Vasoconstrictor Precautions No information available to require special precautions

Effects on Dental Treatment Key adverse event(s) related to dental treatment: Darkening of tongue.

Common Adverse Effects Frequency not defined; subsalicylate formulation:
Central nervous system: Anxiety, confusion, headache, mental depression, slurred speech

Gastrointestinal: Discoloration of the tongue (darkening), grayish black stools, impaction may occur in infants and debilitated patients

Neuromuscular & skeletal: Muscle spasms, weakness

Ocular: Hearing loss, tinnitus

Mechanism of Action Bismuth subsalicylate exhibits both antisecretory and antimicrobial action. This agent may provide some anti-inflammatory action as well. The salicylate moiety provides antisecretory effect and the bismuth exhibits antimicrobial directly against bacterial and viral gastrointestinal pathogens.

Drug Interactions
Increased Effect/Toxicity: Toxicity of aspirin, warfarin, and/or hypoglycemics may be increased.

Decreased Effect: The effects of tetracyclines and uricosurics may be decreased.

Pharmacodynamics/Kinetics
Absorption: Bismuth: <1%; Subsalicylate: >90%

Metabolism: Bismuth subsalicylate is converted to salicylic acid and insoluble bismuth salts in the GI tract.

Half-life elimination: Terminal: Bismuth: Highly variable

Excretion: Bismuth: Urine and feces; Salicylate: Urine

Pregnancy Risk Factor C/D (3rd trimester)

Bismuth Subgallate *see* Bismuth *on page 210*
Bismuth Subsalicylate *see* Bismuth *on page 210*

Bismuth Subsalicylate, Metronidazole, and Tetracycline
(BIZ muth sub sa LIS i late, me troe NI da zole, & tet ra SYE kleen)

Related Information
Bismuth *on page 210*
Metronidazole *on page 1033*
Tetracycline *on page 1467*

U.S. Brand Names Helidac®

Generic Available No

Synonyms Bismuth Subsalicylate, Tetracycline, and Metronidazole; Metronidazole, Bismuth Subsalicylate, and Tetracycline; Tetracycline, Metronidazole, and Bismuth Subsalicylate

Pharmacologic Category Antibiotic, Tetracycline Derivative; Antidiarrheal

Use In combination with an H₂ antagonist, as part of a multidrug regimen for *H. pylori* eradication to reduce the risk of duodenal ulcer recurrence

Local Anesthetic/Vasoconstrictor Precautions No information available to require special precautions

Effects on Dental Treatment Tetracyclines are not recommended for use during pregnancy since they can cause enamel hypoplasia and permanent teeth discoloration; long-term use associated with oral candidiasis.

Common Adverse Effects See individual agents.
>1%:
Central nervous system: Dizziness
Gastrointestinal: Nausea, diarrhea, abdominal pain, vomiting, anal discomfort, anorexia
Neuromuscular & skeletal: Paresthesia
Mechanism of Action Bismuth subsalicylate, metronidazole, and tetracycline individually have demonstrated *in vitro* activity against most susceptible strains of *H. pylori* isolated from patients with duodenal ulcers. Resistance to metronidazole is increasing in the U.S.; an alternative regimen, not containing metronidazole, if *H. pylori* is not eradicated follow therapy.

Drug Interactions
Cytochrome P450 Effect:
Metronidazole: **Inhibits** CYP2C8/9 (weak), 3A4 (moderate)
Tetracycline: **Substrate** of CYP3A4 (major); **Inhibits** CYP3A4 (moderate)
Increased Effect/Toxicity: See individual agents.
Decreased Effect: See individual agents.
Pharmacodynamics/Kinetics See individual agents.
Pregnancy Risk Factor D (tetracycline); B (metronidazole)

Bismuth Subsalicylate, Tetracycline, and Metronidazole *see* Bismuth Subsalicylate, Metronidazole, and Tetracycline *on page 210*

Bisoprolol (bis OH proe lol)

Related Information
Cardiovascular Diseases *on page 1636*
U.S. Brand Names Zebeta®
Canadian Brand Names Monocor®; Zebeta®
Generic Available Yes
Synonyms Bisoprolol Fumarate
Pharmacologic Category Beta Blocker, Beta₁ Selective
Use Treatment of hypertension, alone or in combination with other agents
Unlabeled/Investigational Use Angina pectoris, supraventricular arrhythmias, PVCs, CHF
Local Anesthetic/Vasoconstrictor Precautions No information available to require special precautions
Effects on Dental Treatment Bisoprolol is a cardioselective beta-blocker. Local anesthetic with vasoconstrictor can be safely used in patients medicated with bisoprolol. Nonselective beta-blockers (ie, propranolol, nadolol) enhance the pressor response to epinephrine, resulting in hypertension and bradycardia; this has not been reported for bisoprolol. Many nonsteroidal anti-inflammatory drugs, such as ibuprofen and indomethacin, can reduce the hypotensive effect of beta-blockers after 3 or more weeks of therapy with the NSAID. Short-term NSAID use (ie, 3 days) requires no special precautions in patients taking beta-blockers.

Common Adverse Effects
>10%:
Central nervous system: Drowsiness, insomnia
Endocrine & metabolic: Sexual ability decreased
1% to 10%:
Cardiovascular: Bradycardia, palpitation, edema, CHF, peripheral circulation reduced
Central nervous system: Mental depression
Gastrointestinal: Diarrhea, constipation, nausea, vomiting, stomach discomfort
Ocular: Mild ocular stinging and discomfort, tearing, photophobia, corneal sensitivity decreased, keratitis
Respiratory: Bronchospasm
Miscellaneous: Cold extremities
Mechanism of Action Selective inhibitor of beta₁-adrenergic receptors; competitively blocks beta₁-receptors, with little or no effect on beta₂-receptors at doses <10 mg

Drug Interactions
Cytochrome P450 Effect: Substrate of CYP2D6 (minor), 3A4 (major)
Increased Effect/Toxicity: Bisoprolol may increase the effects of other drugs which slow AV conduction (digoxin, verapamil, diltiazem), alpha-blockers (prazosin, terazosin), and alpha-adrenergic stimulants (epinephrine, phenylephrine). Bisoprolol may mask the tachycardia from hypoglycemia caused by insulin and oral hypoglycemics. In patients receiving concurrent therapy, the risk of hypertensive crisis is increased when either clonidine or the beta-blocker is withdrawn. Reserpine has been shown to
(Continued)

Bisoprolol *(Continued)*

enhance the effect of beta-blockers. Beta-blockers may increase the action or levels of ethanol, disopyramide, nondepolarizing muscle relaxants, and theophylline although the effects are difficult to predict. CYP3A4 inhibitors may increase the levels/effects of bisoprolol; example inhibitors include azole antifungals, clarithromycin, diclofenac, doxycycline, erythromycin, imatinib, isoniazid, nefazodone, nicardipine, propofol, protease inhibitors, quinidine, telithromycin, and verapamil.

Decreased Effect: Decreased effect of bisoprolol with aluminum salts, calcium salts, cholestyramine, colestipol, NSAIDs, penicillins (ampicillin), and salicylates due to decreased bioavailability and plasma levels. The effect of sulfonylureas may be decreased by beta-blockers. CYP3A4 inducers may decrease the levels/effects of bisoprolol; example inducers include aminoglutethimide, carbamazepine, nafcillin, nevirapine, phenobarbital, phenytoin, and rifamycins.

Pharmacodynamics/Kinetics

Onset of action: 1-2 hours

Absorption: Rapid and almost complete

Distribution: Widely; highest concentrations in heart, liver, lungs, and saliva; crosses blood-brain barrier; enters breast milk

Protein binding: 26% to 33%

Metabolism: Extensively hepatic; significant first-pass effect

Half-life elimination: 9-12 hours

Time to peak: 1.7-3 hours

Excretion: Urine (3% to 10% as unchanged drug); feces (<2%)

Pregnancy Risk Factor C (manufacturer); D (2nd and 3rd trimesters - expert analysis)

Bisoprolol and Hydrochlorothiazide

(bis OH proe lol & hye droe klor oh THYE a zide)

Related Information

Bisoprolol *on page 211*

Hydrochlorothiazide *on page 776*

U.S. Brand Names Ziac®

Canadian Brand Names Ziac®

Generic Available Yes

Synonyms Hydrochlorothiazide and Bisoprolol

Pharmacologic Category Antihypertensive Agent, Combination

Use Treatment of hypertension

Local Anesthetic/Vasoconstrictor Precautions No information available to require special precautions

Effects on Dental Treatment Bisoprolol is a cardioselective beta-blocker. Local anesthetic with vasoconstrictor can be safely used in patients medicated with bisoprolol. Nonselective beta-blockers (ie, propranolol, nadolol) enhance the pressor response to epinephrine, resulting in hypertension and bradycardia; this has not been reported for bisoprolol. Many nonsteroidal anti-inflammatory drugs, such as ibuprofen and indomethacin, can reduce the hypotensive effect of beta-blockers after 3 or more weeks of therapy with the NSAID. Short-term NSAID use (ie, 3 days) requires no special precautions in patients taking beta-blockers.

Common Adverse Effects

>10%: Central nervous system: Fatigue

1% to 10%:

Cardiovascular: Chest pain, edema, bradycardia, hypotension

Central nervous system: Headache, dizziness, depression, abnormal dreams, insomnia

Dermatologic: Rash, photosensitivity

Endocrine & metabolic: Hypokalemia, fluid and electrolyte imbalances (hypocalcemia, hypomagnesemia, hyponatremia), hyperglycemia

Gastrointestinal: Constipation, diarrhea, dyspepsia, nausea, flatulence

Genitourinary: Micturition (frequency)

Hematologic: Rarely blood dyscrasias

Neuromuscular & skeletal: Arthralgia, myalgia

Ocular: Abnormal vision

Renal: Prerenal azotemia

Respiratory: Rhinitis, cough, dyspnea

Drug Interactions

Cytochrome P450 Effect: Bisoprolol: **Substrate** of CYP2D6 (minor), 3A4 (major)

Increased Effect/Toxicity: See individual agents.
Decreased Effect: See individual agents.
Pharmacodynamics/Kinetics See individual agents.
Pregnancy Risk Factor C/D (2nd and 3rd trimesters)

Bisoprolol Fumarate *see* Bisoprolol *on page 211*
Bistropamide *see* Tropicamide *on page 1545*

Bivalirudin *(bye VAL i roo din)*

U.S. Brand Names Angiomax®
Canadian Brand Names Angiomax®
Generic Available No
Synonyms Hirulog
Pharmacologic Category Anticoagulant, Thrombin Inhibitor
Use Anticoagulant used in conjunction with aspirin for patients with unstable angina undergoing percutaneous transluminal coronary angioplasty (PTCA) or percutaneous coronary intervention (PCI) with provisional glycoprotein IIb/IIIa inhibitor; anticoagulant used in patients undergoing PCI with (or at risk of) heparin-induced thrombocytopenia (HIT) / thrombosis syndrome (HITTS)
Local Anesthetic/Vasoconstrictor Precautions No information available to require special precautions
Effects on Dental Treatment No significant effects or complications reported
Common Adverse Effects As with all anticoagulants, bleeding is the major adverse effect of bivalirudin. Hemorrhage may occur at virtually any site. Risk is dependent on multiple variables, including the intensity of anticoagulation and patient susceptibility. Additional adverse effects are often related to idiosyncratic reactions, and the frequency is difficult to estimate.

Adverse reactions reported were generally less than those seen with heparin.

>10%:
    Cardiovascular: Hypotension (3% to 12%)
    Central nervous system: Pain (15%), headache (3% to 12%)
    Gastrointestinal: Nausea (3% to 15%)
    Neuromuscular & skeletal: Back pain (9% to 42%)
1% to 10%:
    Cardiovascular: Hypertension (6%), bradycardia (5%), angina (up to 5%)
    Central nervous system: Insomnia (7%), anxiety (6%), fever (5%), nervousness (5%)
    Gastrointestinal: Vomiting (6%), dyspepsia (5%), abdominal pain (5%)
    Genitourinary: Urinary retention (4%)
    Hematologic: Major hemorrhage (2% to 4%, compared to 4% to 9% with heparin); transfusion required (1% to 2%, compared to 2% to 6% with heparin), thrombocytopenia (<1% to 4%)
    Local: Injection site pain (3% to 8%)
    Neuromuscular & skeletal: Pelvic pain (6%)
Mechanism of Action Bivalirudin acts as a specific and reversible direct thrombin inhibitor; it binds to the catalytic and anionic exosite of both circulating and clot-bound thrombin. Catalytic binding site occupation functionally inhibits coagulant effects by preventing thrombin-mediated cleavage of fibrinogen to fibrin monomers, and activation of factors V, VIII, and XIII. Shows linear dose- and concentration-dependent prolongation of ACT, aPTT, PT, and TT.
Drug Interactions
    Increased Effect/Toxicity: Aspirin may increase anticoagulant effect of bivalirudin (**Note:** All clinical trials included coadministration of aspirin). Other anticoagulants may increase the risk of bleeding complications (monitor).Treprostinil may increase risk of bleeding.
Pharmacodynamics/Kinetics
    Onset of action: Immediate
    Duration: Coagulation times return to baseline ~1 hour following discontinuation of infusion
    Distribution: 0.2 L/kg
    Protein binding, plasma: Does not bind other than thrombin
    Half-life elimination: Normal renal function: 25 minutes; Cl$_{cr}$ 10-29 mL/minute: 57 minutes
    Excretion: Urine, proteolytic cleavage
Pregnancy Risk Factor B

BL4162A *see* Anagrelide *on page 124*
Black Draught Tablets [OTC] *see* Senna *on page 1384*
Blenoxane® *see* Bleomycin *on page 214*
Bleo *see* Bleomycin *on page 214*

Bleomycin (blee oh MYE sin)

U.S. Brand Names Blenoxane®
Canadian Brand Names Blenoxane®
Mexican Brand Names Blanoxan®; Bleolem®
Generic Available Yes
Synonyms Bleo; Bleomycin Sulfate; BLM; NSC-125066
Pharmacologic Category Antineoplastic Agent, Antibiotic
Use Treatment of squamous cell carcinomas, melanomas, sarcomas, testicular carcinoma, Hodgkin's lymphoma, and non-Hodgkin's lymphoma
Orphan drug: Sclerosing agent for malignant pleural effusion
Local Anesthetic/Vasoconstrictor Precautions No information available to require special precautions
Effects on Dental Treatment Key adverse event(s) related to dental treatment: Stomatitis.
Common Adverse Effects
>10%:
  Cardiovascular: Raynaud's phenomenon
  Dermatologic: Pain at the tumor site, phlebitis. About 50% of patients develop erythema, induration, hyperkeratosis, and peeling of the skin, particularly on the palmar and plantar surfaces of the hands and feet. Hyperpigmentation (50%), alopecia, nailbed changes may also occur. These effects appear dose related and reversible with discontinuation of the drug.
  Gastrointestinal: Stomatitis and mucositis (30%), anorexia, weight loss
  Respiratory: Tachypnea, rales, acute or chronic interstitial pneumonitis, and pulmonary fibrosis (5% to 10%); hypoxia and death (1%). Symptoms include cough, dyspnea, and bilateral pulmonary infiltrates. The pathogenesis is not certain, but may be due to damage of pulmonary, vascular, or connective tissue. Response to steroid therapy is variable and somewhat controversial.
  Miscellaneous: Acute febrile reactions (25% to 50%); anaphylactoid reactions characterized by hypotension, confusion, fever, chills, and wheezing. Onset may be immediate or delayed for several hours.
1% to 10%:
  Dermatologic: Rash (8%), skin thickening, diffuse scleroderma, onycholysis
  Miscellaneous: Acute anaphylactoid reactions
Mechanism of Action Inhibits synthesis of DNA; binds to DNA leading to single- and double-strand breaks
Drug Interactions
  Increased Effect/Toxicity: Cisplatin may decrease bleomycin elimination.
  Decreased Effect: Bleomycin may decrease plasma levels of digoxin. Concomitant therapy with phenytoin results in decreased phenytoin levels.
Pharmacodynamics/Kinetics
  Absorption: I.M. and intrapleural administration: 30% to 50% of I.V. serum concentrations; intraperitoneal and SubQ routes produce serum concentrations equal to those of I.V.
  Distribution: V_d: 22 L/m^2; highest concentrations in skin, kidney, lung, heart tissues; lowest in testes and GI tract; does not cross blood-brain barrier
  Protein binding: 1%
  Metabolism: Via several tissues including hepatic, GI tract, skin, pulmonary, renal, and serum
  Half-life elimination: Biphasic (renal function dependent):
    Normal renal function: Initial: 1.3 hours; Terminal: 9 hours
    End-stage renal disease: Initial: 2 hours; Terminal: 30 hours
  Time to peak, serum: I.M.: Within 30 minutes
  Excretion: Urine (50% to 70% as active drug)
Pregnancy Risk Factor D

Bleomycin Sulfate *see* Bleomycin *on page 214*
Bleph®-10 *see* Sulfacetamide *on page 1423*
Blephamide® *see* Sulfacetamide and Prednisolone *on page 1424*
Blis-To-Sol® [OTC] *see* Tolnaftate *on page 1506*
BLM *see* Bleomycin *on page 214*
Blocadren® *see* Timolol *on page 1489*
BMS-232632 *see* Atazanavir *on page 152*
BMS 337039 *see* Aripiprazole *on page 138*
Bonine® [OTC] *see* Meclizine *on page 969*
Boniva® *see* Ibandronate *on page 805*
Bontril PDM® *see* Phendimetrazine *on page 1220*
Bontril® Slow-Release *see* Phendimetrazine *on page 1220*

Bortezomib (bore TEZ oh mib)

U.S. Brand Names Velcade®
Canadian Brand Names Velcade®
Generic Available No
Synonyms LDP-341; MLN341; PS-341
Pharmacologic Category Antineoplastic Agent; Proteasome Inhibitor
Use Treatment of multiple myeloma in patients who have had at least one prior therapy
Local Anesthetic/Vasoconstrictor Precautions No information available to require special precautions
Effects on Dental Treatment Key adverse event(s) related to dental treatment: Abnormal taste and stomatitis.
Common Adverse Effects
>10%:
  Cardiovascular: Edema (25%), hypotension (12%)
  Central nervous system: Pyrexia (35% to 36%), psychiatric disturbance (35%), headache (26% to 28%), insomnia (27%), dizziness (14% to 21%, excludes vertigo), anxiety (14%)
  Dermatologic: Rash (18% to 21%), pruritus (11%)
  Endocrine & metabolic: Dehydration (18%)
  Gastrointestinal: Nausea (57% to 64%), diarrhea (51% to 57%), appetite decreased (43%), constipation (42% to 43%), vomiting (35% to 36%), abdominal pain (13% to 16%), abnormal taste (13%), dyspepsia (13%)
  Hematologic: Thrombocytopenia (35% to 43%, Grade 3: 26% to 27%, Grade 4: 3%; Nadir: Day 11), anemia (26% to 32%, Grade 3: 9%), neutropenia (19% to 24%, Grade 3: 13%, Grade 4: 3%)
  Neuromuscular & skeletal: Asthenic conditions (61% to 65%, Grade 3: 12% to 18% - includes fatigue, malaise, weakness), peripheral neuropathy (36% to 37%, Grade 3: 7% to 14%), arthralgia (14% to 26%), limb pain (26%), paresthesia and dysesthesia (23%), bone pain (16%), back pain (14%), muscle cramps (12% to 14%), myalgia (12% to 14%), rigors (11% to 12%)
  Ocular: Blurred vision (11%)
  Respiratory: Dyspnea (20% to 22%), upper respiratory tract infection (18%), cough (17% to 21%), lower respiratory infection (15%), nasopharyngitis (14%)
  Miscellaneous: Herpes zoster (11% to 13%)
1% to 10%: Respiratory: Pneumonia (10%)
Mechanism of Action Bortezomib inhibits proteasomes, enzyme complexes which regulate protein homeostasis within the cell. Specifically, it reversibly inhibits chymotrypsin-like activity at the 26S proteasome, leading to activation of signaling cascades, cell-cycle arrest, and apoptosis.
Drug Interactions
  Cytochrome P450 Effect: Substrate of CYP1A2 (minor), 2C9 (minor), 2C19 (minor), 2D6 (minor), 3A4 (major); **Inhibits** CYP1A2 (weak), 2C9 (weak), 2C19 (moderate), 2D6 (weak), 3A4 (weak)
  Increased Effect/Toxicity: Bortezomib may increase the levels/effects of citalopram, diazepam, methsuximide, phenytoin, propranolol, sertraline, and other CYP2C19 substrates. Levels/effects of bortezomib may be increased by azole antifungals, clarithromycin, diclofenac, doxycycline, erythromycin, imatinib, isoniazid, nefazodone, nicardipine, propofol, protease inhibitors, quinidine, telithromycin, verapamil, and other CYP3A4 inhibitors.
  Decreased Effect: Levels/effects of bortezomib may be decreased by aminoglutethimide, carbamazepine, nafcillin, nevirapine, phenobarbital, phenytoin, rifamycins, and other CYP3A4 inducers.
Pharmacodynamics/Kinetics
  Protein binding: ~83%
  Metabolism: Hepatic via CYP 1A2, 2C9, 2C19, 2D6, 3A4; forms metabolites (inactive)
  Half-life elimination: 9-15 hours
Pregnancy Risk Factor D

Bosentan (boe SEN tan)

U.S. Brand Names Tracleer®
Canadian Brand Names Tracleer®
Generic Available No
(Continued)

Bosentan *(Continued)*

Pharmacologic Category Endothelin Antagonist

Use Treatment of pulmonary artery hypertension (PAH) (WHO Group I) in patients with World Health Organization (WHO) Class III or IV symptoms to improve exercise capacity and decrease the rate of clinical deterioration

Unlabeled/Investigational Use Investigational: Congestive heart failure

Local Anesthetic/Vasoconstrictor Precautions No information available to require special precautions

Effects on Dental Treatment No significant effects or complications reported

Common Adverse Effects

>10%:

Central nervous system: Headache (16% to 22%)

Hematologic: Hemoglobin decreased (≥1 g/dL in up to 57%; typically in first 6 weeks of therapy)

Hepatic: Transaminases increased (>3 times upper limit of normal; up to 11%)

Respiratory: Nasopharyngitis (11%)

1% to 10%:

Cardiovascular: Flushing (7% to 9%), edema (lower limb, 8%; generalized 4%), hypotension (7%), palpitation (5%)

Central nervous system: Fatigue (4%)

Dermatologic: Pruritus (4%)

Gastrointestinal: Dyspepsia (4%)

Hematologic: Anemia (3%)

Hepatic: Abnormal hepatic function (6% to 8%)

Restrictions Bosentan (Tracleer®) is available only through a limited distribution program directly from the manufacturer (Actelion Pharmaceuticals 1-866-228-3546). It will not be available through wholesalers or individual pharmacies. An FDA-approved medication guide is available at www.fda.gov/cder/Offices/ODS/labeling.htm; distribute to each patient to whom this medication is dispensed.

Mechanism of Action Blocks endothelin receptors on vascular endothelium and smooth muscle. Stimulation of these receptors is associated with vasoconstriction. Although bosentan blocks both ET_A and ET_B receptors, the affinity is higher for the A subtype. Improvement in symptoms of pulmonary artery hypertension and a decrease in the rate of clinical deterioration have been demonstrated in clinical trials.

Drug Interactions

Cytochrome P450 Effect: Substrate (major) of CYP2C9, 3A4; **Induces** CYP2C9 (strong), 3A4 (strong)

Increased Effect/Toxicity: An increased risk of serum transaminase elevations was observed during concurrent therapy with glyburide; concurrent use is contraindicated. Cyclosporine increases serum concentrations of bosentan (approximately 3-4 times baseline). Concurrent use of cyclosporine is contraindicated.

CYP2C9 inhibitors may increase the levels/effects of bosentan; example inhibitors include delavirdine, fluconazole, gemfibrozil, ketoconazole, nicardipine, NSAIDs, pioglitazone, and sulfonamides. CYP3A4 inhibitors may increase the levels/effects of bosentan; example inhibitors include azole antifungals, clarithromycin, diclofenac, doxycycline, erythromycin, imatinib, isoniazid, nefazodone, nicardipine, propofol, protease inhibitors, quinidine, telithromycin, and verapamil. Sildenafil may increase the serum concentration of bosentan.

Decreased Effect: Bosentan may enhance the metabolism of cyclosporine, decreasing its serum concentrations by ~50%; effect on sirolimus and/or tacrolimus has not been specifically evaluated, but may be similar. Concurrent use of cyclosporine is contraindicated. CYP2C9 inducers may decrease the levels/effects of bosentan; example inducers include carbamazepine, phenobarbital, phenytoin, rifampin, rifapentine, and secobarbital. Bosentan may decrease the levels/effects of CYP2C9 substrates; example substrates include celecoxib, dapsone, fluoxetine, glimepiride, glipizide, losartan, montelukast, nateglinide, paclitaxel, phenytoin, sulfonamides, trimethoprim, warfarin, and zafirlukast. Bosentan may increase the metabolism, via CYP isoenzymes, of sildenafil.

CYP3A4 inducers may decrease the levels/effects of bosentan; example inducers include aminoglutethimide, carbamazepine, nafcillin, nevirapine, phenobarbital, phenytoin, and rifamycins. Bosentan may enhance the metabolism of methadone resulting in methadone withdrawal. Bosentan may decrease the levels/effects of CYP3A4 substrates; example substrates include benzodiazepines, calcium channel blockers, ergot derivatives, mirtazapine, nateglinide, nefazodone, tacrolimus, and venlafaxine. Bosentan may decrease levels of hormonal contraceptives; additional methods of contraception are recommended.

Pharmacodynamics/Kinetics
Distribution: V_d: 18 L

Protein binding, plasma: >98% primarily to albumin

Metabolism: Hepatic via CYP2C9 and 3A4 to three primary metabolites (one contributing ~10% to 20% pharmacologic activity)

Bioavailability: 50%

Half-life elimination: 5 hours; prolonged with heart failure, possibly in PAH

Time to peak, plasma: 3-5 hours

Excretion: Feces (as metabolites); urine (<3% as unchanged drug)

Pregnancy Risk Factor X

B&O Supprettes® see Belladonna and Opium on page 184

Botox® see Botulinum Toxin Type A on page 217

Botox® Cosmetic see Botulinum Toxin Type A on page 217

Botulinum Toxin Type A (BOT yoo lin num TOKS in type aye)

U.S. Brand Names Botox®; Botox® Cosmetic

Canadian Brand Names Botox®; Botox® Cosmetic

Generic Available No

Synonyms BTX-A

Pharmacologic Category Neuromuscular Blocker Agent, Toxin; Ophthalmic Agent, Toxin

Use Treatment of strabismus and blepharospasm associated with dystonia (including benign essential blepharospasm or VII nerve disorders in patients ≥12 years of age); cervical dystonia (spasmodic torticollis) in patients ≥16 years of age; temporary improvement in the appearance of lines/wrinkles of the face (moderate to severe glabellar lines associated with corrugator and/or procerus muscle activity) in adult patients ≤65 years of age; treatment of severe primary axillary hyperhidrosis in adults not adequately controlled with topical treatments

Orphan drug: Treatment of dynamic muscle contracture in pediatric cerebral palsy patients

Unlabeled/Investigational Use Treatment of oromandibular dystonia, spasmodic dysphonia (laryngeal dystonia) and other dystonias (ie, writer's cramp, focal task-specific dystonias); migraine treatment and prophylaxis

Local Anesthetic/Vasoconstrictor Precautions No information available to require special precautions

Effects on Dental Treatment Key adverse event(s) related to dental treatment: Xerostomia (normal salivary flow resumes upon discontinuation), facial pain, and facial weakness. Affects occur in ~1 week and may last up to several months.

Common Adverse Effects Adverse effects usually occur in 1 week and may last up to several months

>10%:

Central nervous system: Headache (cervical dystonia up to 11%, reduction of glabellar lines up to 13%; can occur with other uses)

Gastrointestinal: Dysphagia (cervical dystonia 19%)

Neuromuscular & skeletal: Neck pain (cervical dystonia 11%)

Ocular: Ptosis (blepharospasm 10% to 40%, strabismus 1% to 38%, reduction of glabellar lines 1% to 5%), vertical deviation (strabismus 17%)

Respiratory: Upper respiratory infection (cervical dystonia 12%)

2% to 10%:

Central nervous system: Anxiety (primary axillary hyperhydrosis), dizziness (cervical dystonia, reduction of glabellar lines), drowsiness (cervical dystonia), fever (cervical dystonia, primary axillary hyperhydrosis), speech disorder (cervical dystonia)

Dermatologic: Nonaxillary sweating (primary axillary hyperhydrosis), pruritus (primary axillary hyperhydrosis)

Gastrointestinal: Xerostomia (cervical dystonia), nausea (cervical dystonia, reduction of glabellar lines)

Local: Injection site reaction

Neuromuscular & skeletal: Back pain (cervical dystonia), facial pain (reduction of glabellar lines), hypertonia (cervical dystonia), weakness (cervical dystonia, reduction of glabellar lines)

Ocular: Dry eyes (blepharospasm 6%), superficial punctate keratitis (blepharospasm 6%)

Respiratory: Cough (cervical dystonia), infection (reduction of glabellar lines, primary axillary hyperhydrosis), pharyngitis (primary axillary hyperhydrosis), rhinitis (cervical dystonia)

(Continued)

Botulinum Toxin Type A *(Continued)*

Miscellaneous: Flu syndrome (cervical dystonia, reduction of glabellar lines, primary axillary hyperhidrosis)

Mechanism of Action Botulinum A toxin is a neurotoxin produced by *Clostridium botulinum*, spore-forming anaerobic bacillus, which appears to affect only the presynaptic membrane of the neuromuscular junction in humans, where it prevents calcium-dependent release of acetylcholine and produces a state of denervation. Muscle inactivation persists until new fibrils grow from the nerve and form junction plates on new areas of the muscle-cell walls.

Drug Interactions

Increased Effect/Toxicity: Aminoglycosides, neuromuscular-blocking agents, and other agents which may block neuromuscular transmission.

Pharmacodynamics/Kinetics

Onset of action (improvement):

Blepharospasm: ~3 days

Cervical dystonia: ~2 weeks

Strabismus: ~1-2 days

Reduction of glabellar lines (Botox® Cosmetic): 1-2 days, increasing in intensity during first week

Duration:

Blepharospasm: ~3 months

Cervical dystonia: <3 months

Strabismus: ~2-6 weeks

Primary axillary hyperhidrosis: 201 days (mean)

Reduction of glabellar lines (Botox® Cosmetic): Up to 3 months

Absorption: Not expected to be present in peripheral blood at recommended doses

Time to peak:

Blepharospasm: 1-2 weeks

Cervical dystonia: ~6 weeks

Strabismus: Within first week

Pregnancy Risk Factor C (manufacturer)

Botulinum Toxin Type B *(BOT yoo lin num TOKS in type bee)*

U.S. Brand Names Myobloc®

Generic Available No

Pharmacologic Category Neuromuscular Blocker Agent, Toxin

Use Treatment of cervical dystonia (spasmodic torticollis)

Unlabeled/Investigational Use Treatment of cervical dystonia in patients who have developed resistance to botulinum toxin type A

Local Anesthetic/Vasoconstrictor Precautions No information available to require special precautions

Effects on Dental Treatment Key adverse event(s) related to dental treatment: Xerostomia (normal salivary flow resumes upon discontinuation), stomatitis, and abnormal taste.

Common Adverse Effects

>10%:

Central nervous system: Headache (10% to 16%), pain (6% to 13%; placebo 10%)

Gastrointestinal: Dysphagia (10% to 25%), xerostomia (3% to 34%)

Local: Injection site pain (12% to 16%)

Neuromuscular & skeletal: Neck pain (up to 17%; placebo: 16%)

Miscellaneous: Infection (13% to 19%; placebo: 15%)

1% to 10%:

Cardiovascular: Chest pain, vasodilation, peripheral edema

Central nervous system: Dizziness (3% to 6%), fever, malaise, migraine, anxiety, tremor, hyperesthesia, somnolence, confusion, vertigo

Dermatologic: Pruritus, bruising

Gastrointestinal: Nausea (3% to 10%; placebo: 5%), dyspepsia (up to 10%; placebo: 5%), vomiting, stomatitis, taste perversion

Genitourinary: Urinary tract infection, cystitis, vaginal moniliasis

Hematologic: Serum neutralizing activity

Neuromuscular & skeletal: Torticollis (up to 8%; placebo: 7%), arthralgia (up to 7%; placebo: 5%), back pain (3% to 7%; placebo: 3%), myasthenia (3% to 6%; placebo: 3%), weakness (up to 6%; placebo: 4%), arthritis

Ocular: Amblyopia, abnormal vision

Otic: Otitis media, tinnitus

Respiratory: Cough (3% to 7%; placebo: 3%), rhinitis (1% to 5%; placebo: 6%), dyspnea, pneumonia

Miscellaneous: Flu-syndrome (6% to 9%), allergic reaction, viral infection, abscess, cyst

Mechanism of Action Botulinum B toxin is a neurotoxin produced by *Clostridium botulinum*, spore-forming anaerobic bacillus. It cleaves synaptic Vesicle Association Membrane Protein (VAMP; synaptobrevin) which is a component of the protein complex responsible for docking and fusion of the synaptic vesicle to the presynaptic membrane. By blocking neurotransmitter release, botulinum B toxin paralyzes the muscle.

Drug Interactions

Increased Effect/Toxicity: Aminoglycosides, neuromuscular-blocking agents, botulinum toxin type A, and other agents which may block neuromuscular transmission

Pharmacodynamics/Kinetics

Duration: 12-16 weeks

Absorption: Not expected to be present in peripheral blood at recommended doses

Pregnancy Risk Factor C (manufacturer)

Boudreaux's® Butt Paste [OTC] *see* Zinc Oxide *on page 1597*
Bovine Lung Surfactant *see* Beractant *on page 198*
Bravelle® *see* Follitropins *on page 698*
Breathe Right® Saline [OTC] *see* Sodium Chloride *on page 1400*
Brethaire [DSC] *see* Terbutaline *on page 1460*
Brethine® *see* Terbutaline *on page 1460*

Bretylium (bre TIL ee um)

Related Information

Cardiovascular Diseases *on page 1636*

Generic Available No

Synonyms Bretylium Tosylate

Pharmacologic Category Antiarrhythmic Agent, Class III

Use Treatment of ventricular tachycardia and fibrillation; treatment of other serious ventricular arrhythmias resistant to lidocaine

Local Anesthetic/Vasoconstrictor Precautions No information available to require special precautions (see Dental Comment)

Effects on Dental Treatment No significant effects or complications reported

Mechanism of Action Class III antiarrhythmic; after an initial release of norepinephrine at the peripheral adrenergic nerve terminals, inhibits further release by postganglionic nerve endings in response to sympathetic nerve stimulation

Pregnancy Risk Factor C

Dental Comment This drug is known to prolong the QT interval. The QT interval is measured as the time and distance between the Q point of the QRS complex and the end of the T wave in the ECG tracing. After adjustment for heart rate, the QT interval is defined as prolonged if it is more than 450 msec in men and 460 msec in women. A long QT syndrome was first described in the 1950s and 60s as a congenital syndrome involving QT interval prolongation and syncope and sudden death. Some of the congenital long QT syndromes were characterized by a peculiar electrocardiographic appearance of the QRS complex involving a premature atria beat followed by a pause, then a subsequent sinus beat showing marked QT prolongation and deformity. This type of cardiac arrhythmia was originally termed "torsade de pointes" (translated from the French as "twisting of the points").

Prolongation of the QT interval is thought to result from delayed ventricular repolarization. The repolarization process within the myocardial cell is due to the efflux of intracellular potassium. The channels associated with this current can be blocked by many drugs, thus predisposing the electrical propagation cycle to torsade de pointes.

Bretylium is one of the drugs confirmed to prolong the QT interval and is accepted as having a risk of causing torsade de pointes. The risk of drug-induced torsade de pointes is extremely low when a single QT interval prolonging drug is prescribed. In terms of epinephrine, it is not known what effect vasoconstrictors in the local anesthetic regimen will have in patients with a known history of congenital prolonged QT interval or in patients taking any medication that prolongs the QT interval. Until more information is obtained, it is suggested that the clinician consult with the physician prior to the use of a vasoconstrictor in suspected patients, and that the vasoconstrictor (epinephrine, levonordefrin [Neo-Cobefrin®]) be used with caution.

Bretylium Tosylate *see* Bretylium *on page 219*
Brevibloc® *see* Esmolol *on page 571*

Brevicon® *see* Ethinyl Estradiol and Norethindrone *on page 608*
Brevital® Sodium *see* Methohexital *on page 1010*
Brevoxyl® *see* Benzoyl Peroxide *on page 194*
Brevoxyl® Cleansing *see* Benzoyl Peroxide *on page 194*
Brevoxyl® Wash *see* Benzoyl Peroxide *on page 194*
Bricanyl [DSC] *see* Terbutaline *on page 1460*

Brimonidine (bri MOE ni deen)

U.S. Brand Names Alphagan® P
Canadian Brand Names Alphagan®; PMS-Brimonidine Tartrate; ratio-Brimonidine
Mexican Brand Names Agglad ofteno®; Alphagan®
Generic Available Yes
Synonyms Brimonidine Tartrate
Pharmacologic Category Alpha₂ Agonist, Ophthalmic; Ophthalmic Agent, Antiglaucoma
Use Lowering of intraocular pressure (IOP) in patients with open-angle glaucoma or ocular hypertension
Local Anesthetic/Vasoconstrictor Precautions No information available to require special precautions
Effects on Dental Treatment Key adverse event(s) related to dental treatment: Xerostomia (normal salivary flow resumes upon discontinuation).
Mechanism of Action Selective agonism for alpha₂-receptors; causes reduction of aqueous humor formation and increased uveoscleral outflow
Pregnancy Risk Factor B

Brimonidine Tartrate *see* Brimonidine *on page 220*

Brinzolamide (brin ZOH la mide)

U.S. Brand Names Azopt®
Canadian Brand Names Azopt®
Generic Available No
Pharmacologic Category Carbonic Anhydrase Inhibitor; Ophthalmic Agent, Antiglaucoma
Use Lowers intraocular pressure in patients with ocular hypertension or open-angle glaucoma
Local Anesthetic/Vasoconstrictor Precautions No information available to require special precautions
Effects on Dental Treatment Key adverse event(s) related to dental treatment: Taste disturbances.
Mechanism of Action Brinzolamide inhibits carbonic anhydrase, leading to decreased aqueous humor secretion. This results in a reduction of intraocular pressure.
Pregnancy Risk Factor C

Brioschi® [OTC] *see* Sodium Bicarbonate *on page 1400*
British Anti-Lewisite *see* Dimercaprol *on page 482*
BRL 43694 *see* Granisetron *on page 751*
Brofed® *see* Brompheniramine and Pseudoephedrine *on page 223*
Bromaline® [OTC] *see* Brompheniramine and Pseudoephedrine *on page 223*
Bromaxefed RF *see* Brompheniramine and Pseudoephedrine *on page 223*

Bromazepam (broe MA ze pam)

Canadian Brand Names Apo-Bromazepam®; Gen-Bromazepam; Lectopam®; Novo-Bromazepam; Nu-Bromazepam
Mexican Brand Names Lexotan®
Generic Available Yes
Pharmacologic Category Benzodiazepine
Use Short-term, symptomatic treatment of anxiety
Local Anesthetic/Vasoconstrictor Precautions No information available to require special precautions
Effects on Dental Treatment Key adverse event(s) related to dental treatment: Xerostomia (normal salivary flow resumes upon discontinuation).
Common Adverse Effects Frequency not defined.
Cardiovascular: Hypotension, palpitation, tachycardia
Central nervous system: Drowsiness, ataxia, dizziness, confusion, depression, euphoria, lethargy, slurred speech, stupor, headache, seizure, anterograde

amnesia. In addition, paradoxical reactions (including excitation, agitation, hallucinations, and psychosis) are known to occur with benzodiazepines.

Dermatologic: Rash, pruritus

Endocrine & metabolic: Hyperglycemia, hypoglycemia

Gastrointestinal: Xerostomia, nausea, vomiting

Genitourinary: Incontinence, libido decreased

Hematologic: Hemoglobin decreased, hematocrit decreased, WBCs increased/decreased

Hepatic: Transaminases increased, alkaline phosphatase increased, bilirubin increased

Neuromuscular & skeletal: Weakness, muscle spasm

Ocular: Blurred vision, depth perception decreased

Restrictions CDSA IV; Not available in U.S.

Mechanism of Action Binds to stereospecific benzodiazepine receptors on the postsynaptic GABA neuron at several sites within the central nervous system, including the limbic system, reticular formation. Enhancement of the inhibitory effect of GABA on neuronal excitability results by increased neuronal membrane permeability to chloride ions. This shift in chloride ions results in hyperpolarization (a less excitable state) and stabilization.

Drug Interactions

　Cytochrome P450 Effect: Substrate of CYP3A4 (major); **Inhibits** CYP2E1 (weak)

　Increased Effect/Toxicity: Benzodiazepines potentiate the CNS depressant effects of narcotic analgesics, barbiturates, phenothiazines, ethanol, antihistamines, MAO inhibitors, sedative-hypnotics, and cyclic antidepressants. CYP3A4 inhibitors may increase the levels/effects of bromazepam; example inhibitors include azole antifungals, clarithromycin, diclofenac, doxycycline, erythromycin, imatinib, isoniazid, nefazodone, nicardipine, propofol, protease inhibitors, quinidine, telithromycin, and verapamil.

　Decreased Effect: CYP3A4 inducers may decrease the levels/effects of bromazepam; example inducers include aminoglutethimide, carbamazepine, nafcillin, nevirapine, phenobarbital, phenytoin, and rifamycins.

Pharmacodynamics/Kinetics

　Protein binding: 70%

　Metabolism: Hepatic

　Bioavailability: 60%

　Half-life elimination: 20 hours

　Excretion: Urine (69%), as metabolites

Pregnancy Risk Factor D (based on other benzodiazepines)

Bromfenac (BROME fen ak)

U.S. Brand Names Xibrom™

Synonyms Bromfenac Sodium

Pharmacologic Category Nonsteroidal Anti-inflammatory Drug (NSAID), Ophthalmic

Use Treatment of postoperative inflammation and reduction in ocular pain following cataract removal

Local Anesthetic/Vasoconstrictor Precautions No information available to require special precautions

Effects on Dental Treatment No significant effects or complications reported

Common Adverse Effects 2% to 7%:

Central nervous system: Headache

Ocular: Abnormal vision, abnormal sensation, conjunctival hyperemia, eye pain, iritis, pruritus

Mechanism of Action Inhibits prostaglandin synthesis by decreasing the activity of the enzyme, cyclooxygenase, which results in decreased formation of prostaglandin precursors.

Drug Interactions

　Increased Effect/Toxicity: Concurrent use of ophthalmic corticosteroids may increase the risk of healing problems.

　Decreased Effect: Bromfenac may decrease the reduction in IOP produced by latanoprost.

Pharmacodynamics/Kinetics

　Absorption: Theoretically, systemic absorption may occur following ophthalmic use (not characterized); anticipated levels are below the limits of assay detection

　Metabolism: Hepatic

　Half-life elimination: 0.5-4 hours (following oral administration)

Pregnancy Risk Factor C/D (3rd trimester)

Bromfenac Sodium see Bromfenac on page 221

Bromfenex® *see* Brompheniramine and Pseudoephedrine *on page 223*

Bromfenex® PD *see* Brompheniramine and Pseudoephedrine *on page 223*

Bromhist-NR *see* Brompheniramine and Pseudoephedrine *on page 223*

Bromhist Pediatric *see* Brompheniramine and Pseudoephedrine *on page 223*

Bromocriptine (broe moe KRIP teen)

U.S. Brand Names Parlodel®

Canadian Brand Names Apo-Bromocriptine®; Parlodel®; PMS-Bromocriptine

Mexican Brand Names Parlodel®; Serocryptin®

Generic Available Yes

Synonyms Bromocriptine Mesylate

Pharmacologic Category Anti-Parkinson's Agent, Dopamine Agonist; Ergot Derivative

Use Treatment of hyperprolactinemia associated with amenorrhea with or without galactorrhea, infertility, or hypogonadism; treatment of prolactin-secreting adenomas; treatment of acromegaly; treatment of Parkinson's disease

Unlabeled/Investigational Use Neuroleptic malignant syndrome

Local Anesthetic/Vasoconstrictor Precautions No information available to require special precautions

Effects on Dental Treatment Key adverse event(s) related to dental treatment: Orthostatic hypotension.

Common Adverse Effects Note: Frequency of adverse effects may vary by dose and/or indication.

>10%:

Cardiovascular: Hypotension (up to 30%)

Central nervous system: Headache, dizziness

Gastrointestinal: Nausea, constipation

1% to 10%:

Cardiovascular: Orthostasis, vasospasm (cold-sensitive), Raynaud's syndrome, syncope

Central nervous system: Fatigue, lightheadedness, drowsiness

Gastrointestinal: Anorexia, vomiting, abdominal cramps, diarrhea, dyspepsia, GI bleeding, xerostomia

Respiratory: Nasal congestion

Withdrawal reactions: Abrupt discontinuation has resulted in rare cases of a withdrawal reaction with symptoms similar to neuroleptic malignant syndrome.

Mechanism of Action Semisynthetic ergot alkaloid derivative and a dopamine receptor agonist which activates postsynaptic dopamine receptors in the tuberoinfundibular (inhibiting pituitary prolactin secretion) and nigrostriatal pathways (enhancing coordinated motor control).

Drug Interactions

Cytochrome P450 Effect: Substrate of CYP3A4 (major); **Inhibits** CYP1A2 (weak), 3A4 (weak)

Increased Effect/Toxicity: Effect/toxiicty of bromocriptine may be increased by alpha agonists/sympathomimetics, antifungals (azole derivatives), macrolide antibiotics, protease inhibitors, and MAO inhibitors. Bromocriptine may increase the effects of sibutramine and other serotonin agonists (serotonin syndrome). CYP3A4 inhibitors may increase the levels/effects of bromocriptine; example inhibitors include azole antifungals, clarithromycin, diclofenac, doxycycline, erythromycin, imatinib, isoniazid, nefazodone, nicardipine, propofol, protease inhibitors, quinidine, telithromycin, and verapamil. Concurrent use of bromocriptine with antihypertensive agents may increase the risk of hypotension. Concurrent use of levodopa may increase the risk of hallucinations (dose-dependant).

Decreased Effect: Effects of bromocriptine may be diminished by antipsychotics, metoclopramide.

Pharmacodynamics/Kinetics

Bioavailability: 28%

Protein binding: 90% to 96%

Metabolism: Primarily hepatic

Half-life elimination: Biphasic: Initial: 6-8 hours; Terminal: 50 hours

Time to peak, serum: 1-2 hours

Excretion: Feces; urine (2% to 6% as unchanged drug)

Pregnancy Risk Factor B

Bromocriptine Mesylate *see* Bromocriptine *on page 222*

Bromodiphenhydramine and Codeine
(brome oh dye fen HYE dra meen & KOE deen)

Related Information
Codeine *on page 385*

Generic Available Yes

Synonyms Codeine and Bromodiphenhydramine

Pharmacologic Category Antihistamine/Antitussive

Use Relief of upper respiratory symptoms and cough associated with allergies or common cold

Local Anesthetic/Vasoconstrictor Precautions No information available to require special precautions

Effects on Dental Treatment Key adverse event(s) related to dental treatment: Bromodiphenhydramine: Xerostomia (normal salivary flow resumes upon discontinuation).

Restrictions C-V

Pregnancy Risk Factor C

Brompheniramine and Pseudoephedrine
(brome fen IR a meen & soo doe e FED rin)

Related Information
Pseudoephedrine *on page 1309*

U.S. Brand Names Andehist NR Syrup; Brofed®; Bromaline® [OTC]; Bromax-efed RF; Bromfenex®; Bromfenex® PD; Bromhist-NR; Bromhist Pediatric; Children's Dimetapp® Elixir Cold & Allergy [OTC]; Histex™ SR; Lodrane®; Lodrane® 12D; Lodrane® LD; Rondec® Syrup [DSC]; Touro™ Allergy

Generic Available Yes: Excludes capsule (sustained release), liquid, tablet (extended release)

Synonyms Brompheniramine Maleate and Pseudoephedrine Hydrochloride; Brompheniramine Maleate and Pseudoephedrine Sulfate; Pseudoephedrine and Brompheniramine

Pharmacologic Category Antihistamine/Decongestant Combination

Use Temporary relief of symptoms of seasonal and perennial allergic rhinitis, and vasomotor rhinitis, including nasal obstruction

Local Anesthetic/Vasoconstrictor Precautions Use with caution since pseudoephedrine is a sympathomimetic amine which could interact with epinephrine to cause a pressor response

Effects on Dental Treatment Key adverse event(s) related to dental treatment:
Brompheniramine: Prolonged use may decrease salivary flow.
Pseudoephedrine: Xerostomia (normal salivary flow resumes upon discontinuation).

Common Adverse Effects Frequency not defined.
Cardiovascular: Arrhythmias, flushing, hypertension, pallor, palpitation, tachycardia
Central nervous system: Convulsions, CNS stimulation, dizziness, excitability (children; rare), giddiness, hallucinations, headache, insomnia, irritability, lassitude, nervousness, sedation
Gastrointestinal: Anorexia, diarrhea, dyspepsia, nausea, vomiting, xerostomia
Neuromuscular skeletal: Tremors, weakness
Ocular: Diplopia
Renal: Dysuria, polyuria, urinary retention (with BPH)
Respiratory: Respiratory difficulty

Mechanism of Action Brompheniramine maleate is an antihistamine with H_1-receptor activity; pseudoephedrine, a sympathomimetic amine and isomer of ephedrine, acts as a decongestant in respiratory tract mucous membranes with less vasoconstrictor action than ephedrine in normotensive individuals.

Pharmacodynamics/Kinetics
See Pseudoephedrine.
Brompheniramine:
Metabolism: Hepatic
Time to peak: Syrup: 5 hours
Excretion: Urine

Pregnancy Risk Factor C

Brompheniramine Maleate and Pseudoephedrine Hydrochloride *see* Brompheniramine and Pseudoephedrine *on page 223*

Brompheniramine Maleate and Pseudoephedrine Sulfate *see* Brompheniramine and Pseudoephedrine *on page 223*

Broncho Saline® [OTC] *see* Sodium Chloride *on page 1400*

Brontex® *see* Guaifenesin and Codeine *on page 753*

BSS® *see* Balanced Salt Solution *on page 178*

BSS Plus® *see* Balanced Salt Solution *on page 178*

BTX-A *see* Botulinum Toxin Type A *on page 217*

B-type Natriuretic Peptide (Human) *see* Nesiritide *on page 1103*

Bubbli-Pred™ [DSC] *see* PrednisoLONE *on page 1268*

Budeprion™ SR *see* BuPROPion *on page 233*

Budesonide (byoo DES oh nide)

U.S. Brand Names Entocort® EC; Pulmicort Respules®; Pulmicort Turbuhaler®; Rhinocort® Aqua®

Canadian Brand Names Entocort®; Gen-Budesonide AQ; Pulmicort®; Rhinocort® Turbuhaler®

Mexican Brand Names Aerosial®; Pulmicort®; Rhinocort®

Generic Available No

Pharmacologic Category Corticosteroid, Inhalant (Oral); Corticosteroid, Nasal; Corticosteroid, Systemic

Use

Intranasal: Children ≥6 years of age and Adults: Management of symptoms of seasonal or perennial rhinitis

Nebulization: Children 12 months to 8 years: Maintenance and prophylactic treatment of asthma

Oral capsule: Treatment of active Crohn's disease (mild to moderate) involving the ileum and/or ascending colon; maintenance of remission (for up to 3 months) of Crohn's disease (mild to moderate) involving the ileum and/or ascending colon

Oral inhalation: Maintenance and prophylactic treatment of asthma; includes patients who require corticosteroids and those who may benefit from systemic dose reduction/elimination

Local Anesthetic/Vasoconstrictor Precautions No information available to require special precautions

Effects on Dental Treatment Key adverse event(s) related to dental treatment: Xerostomia (normal salivary flow resumes upon discontinuation), dry throat, abnormal taste, and herpes simplex. Localized infections with *Candida albicans* or *Aspergillus niger* have occurred frequently in the mouth and pharynx with repetitive use of oral inhaler of corticosteroids. These infections may require treatment with appropriate antifungal therapy or discontinuance of treatment with corticosteroid inhaler.

Common Adverse Effects Reaction severity varies by dose and duration; not all adverse reactions have been reported with each dosage form.

>10%:

Central nervous system: Headache (up to 21%)

Gastrointestinal: Nausea (up to 11%)

Respiratory: Respiratory infection, rhinitis

Miscellaneous: Symptoms of HPA axis suppression and/or hypercorticism may occur in >10% of patients following administration of dosage forms which result in higher systemic exposure (ie, oral capsule), but may be less frequent than rates observed with comparator drugs (prednisolone). These symptoms may be rare (<1%) following administration via methods which result in lower exposures (topical).

1% to 10%:

Cardiovascular: Chest pain, edema, flushing, hypertension, palpitation, syncope, tachycardia

Central nervous system: Dizziness, dysphonia, emotional lability, fatigue, fever, insomnia, migraine, nervousness, pain, vertigo

Dermatologic: Acne, alopecia, bruising, contact dermatitis, eczema, hirsutism, pruritus, pustular rash, rash, striae

Endocrine & metabolic: Adrenal insufficiency, hypokalemia, menstrual disorder

Gastrointestinal: Abdominal pain, anorexia, diarrhea, dry mouth, dyspepsia, flatulence, gastroenteritis, oral candidiasis, taste perversion, vomiting, weight gain

Genitourinary: Dysuria, hematuria, nocturia, pyuria

Hematologic: Cervical lymphadenopathy, leukocytosis, purpura

Hepatic: Alkaline phosphatase increased

Neuromuscular & skeletal: Arthralgia, back pain, fracture, hyperkinesis, hypertonia, myalgia, neck pain, weakness, paresthesia

Ocular: Conjunctivitis, eye infection

Otic: Earache, ear infection, external ear infection

Respiratory: Bronchitis, bronchospasm, cough, epistaxis, nasal irritation, pharyngitis, sinusitis, stridor

Miscellaneous: Abscess, allergic reaction, C-reactive protein increased, erythrocyte sedimentation rate increased, fat distribution (moon face, buffalo hump), flu-like syndrome, herpes simplex, infection, moniliasis, viral infection, voice alteration

Dosage

Nasal inhalation: (Rhinocort® Aqua®): Children ≥6 years and Adults: 64 mcg/day as a single 32 mcg spray in each nostril. Some patients who do not achieve adequate control may benefit from increased dosage. A reduced dosage may be effective after initial control is achieved.

Maximum dose: Children <12 years: 128 mcg/day; Adults: 256 mcg/day

Nebulization: Children 12 months to 8 years: Pulmicort Respules®: Titrate to lowest effective dose once patient is stable; start at 0.25 mg/day or use as follows:

Previous therapy of bronchodilators alone: 0.5 mg/day administered as a single dose or divided twice daily (maximum daily dose: 0.5 mg)

Previous therapy of inhaled corticosteroids: 0.5 mg/day administered as a single dose or divided twice daily (maximum daily dose: 1 mg)

Previous therapy of oral corticosteroids: 1 mg/day administered as a single dose or divided twice daily (maximum daily dose: 1 mg)

Oral inhalation:

Children ≥6 years:

Previous therapy of bronchodilators alone: 200 mcg twice initially which may be increased up to 400 mcg twice daily

Previous therapy of inhaled corticosteroids: 200 mcg twice initially which may be increased up to 400 mcg twice daily

Previous therapy of oral corticosteroids: The highest recommended dose in children is 400 mcg twice daily

Adults:

Previous therapy of bronchodilators alone: 200-400 mcg twice initially which may be increased up to 400 mcg twice daily

Previous therapy of inhaled corticosteroids: 200-400 mcg twice initially which may be increased up to 800 mcg twice daily

Previous therapy of oral corticosteroids: 400-800 mcg twice daily which may be increased up to 800 mcg twice daily

NIH Guidelines (NIH, 1997) (give in divided doses twice daily):

Children:

"Low" dose: 100-200 mcg/day

"Medium" dose: 200-400 mcg/day (1-2 inhalations/day)

"High" dose: >400 mcg/day (>2 inhalation/day)

Adults:

"Low" dose: 200-400 mcg/day (1-2 inhalations/day)

"Medium" dose: 400-600 mcg/day (2-3 inhalations/day)

"High" dose: >600 mcg/day (>3 inhalation/day)

Oral: Adults: Crohn's disease (active): 9 mg once daily in the morning for up to 8 weeks; recurring episodes may be treated with a repeat 8-week course of treatment

Note: Patients receiving CYP3A4 inhibitors should be monitored closely for signs and symptoms of hypercorticism; dosage reduction may be required. If switching from oral prednisolone, prednisolone dosage should be tapered while budesonide (Entocort™ EC) treatment is initiated.

Maintenance of remission: Following treatment of active disease (control of symptoms with CDAI <150), treatment may be continued at a dosage of 6 mg once daily for up to 3 months. If symptom control is maintained for 3 months, tapering of the dosage to complete cessation is recommended. Continued dosing beyond 3 months has not been demonstrated to result in substantial benefit.

Dosage adjustment in hepatic impairment: Monitor closely for signs and symptoms of hypercorticism; dosage reduction may be required.

Mechanism of Action Controls the rate of protein synthesis; depresses the migration of polymorphonuclear leukocytes, fibroblasts; reverses capillary permeability and lysosomal stabilization at the cellular level to prevent or control inflammation

Contraindications Hypersensitivity to budesonide or any component of the formulation

Inhalation: Contraindicated in primary treatment of status asthmaticus, acute episodes of asthma; not for relief of acute bronchospasm

Warnings/Precautions May cause hypercorticism and/or suppression of hypothalamic-pituitary-adrenal (HPA) axis, particularly in younger children or in (Continued)

Budesonide (Continued)

patients receiving high doses for prolonged periods. Particular care is required when patients are transferred from systemic corticosteroids to products with lower systemic bioavailability (ie, inhalation). May lead to possible adrenal insufficiency or withdrawal from steroids, including an increase in allergic symptoms. Patients receiving prolonged therapy ≥20 mg per day of prednisone (or equivalent) may be most susceptible. Aerosol steroids do **not** provide the systemic steroid needed to treat patients having trauma, surgery, or infections.

Controlled clinical studies have shown that orally-inhaled and intranasal corticosteroids may cause a reduction in growth velocity in pediatric patients. (In studies of orally-inhaled corticosteroids, the mean reduction in growth velocity was approximately 1 centimeter per year [range 0.3-1.8 cm per year] and appears to be related to dose and duration of exposure.) To minimize the systemic effects of orally-inhaled and intranasal corticosteroids, each patient should be titrated to the lowest effective dose. Growth should be routinely monitored in pediatric patients.

May suppress the immune system; patients may be more susceptible to infection. Use with caution in patients with systemic infections or ocular herpes simplex. Avoid exposure to chickenpox and measles. Corticosteroids should be used with caution in patients with diabetes, hypertension, osteoporosis, peptic ulcer, glaucoma, cataracts, or tuberculosis. Use caution in hepatic impairment. Enteric-coated capsules should not be crushed or chewed.

Drug Interactions

Cytochrome P450 Effect: Substrate of CYP3A4 (major)

Increased Effect/Toxicity: Cimetidine may decrease the clearance and increase the bioavailability of budesonide, increasing its serum concentrations. In addition, CYP3A4 inhibitors may increase the serum level and/or toxicity of budesonide this effect was shown with ketoconazole, but not erythromycin. Other potential inhibitors include amiodarone, cimetidine, clarithromycin, delavirdine, diltiazem, dirithromycin, disulfiram, fluoxetine, fluvoxamine, grapefruit juice, indinavir, itraconazole, ketoconazole, nefazodone, nevirapine, propoxyphene, quinupristin-dalfopristin, ritonavir, saquinavir, telithromycin, verapamil, zafirlukast, and zileuton. The addition of salmeterol has been demonstrated to improve response to inhaled corticosteroids (as compared to increasing steroid dosage).

Decreased Effect: Theoretically, proton pump inhibitors (omeprazole, pantoprazole) alter gastric pH and may affect the rate of dissolution of enteric-coated capsules. Administration with omeprazole did not alter kinetics of budesonide capsules.

Ethanol/Nutrition/Herb Interactions

Food: Grapefruit juice may double systemic exposure of orally-administered budesonide. Administration of capsules with a high-fat meal delays peak concentration, but does not alter the extent of absorption.

Herb/Nutraceutical: St John's wort may decrease budesonide levels.

Dietary Considerations Avoid grapefruit juice when using oral capsules.

Pharmacodynamics/Kinetics

Onset of action: Respules®: 2-8 days; Rhinocort® Aqua®: ~10 hours; Turbuhaler®: 24 hours

Peak effect: Respules®: 4-6 weeks; Rhinocort® Aqua®: ~2 weeks; Turbuhaler®: 1-2 weeks

Distribution: 2.2-3.9 L/kg

Protein binding: 85% to 90%

Metabolism: Hepatic via CYP3A4 to two metabolites: 16 alpha-hydroxyprednisolone and 6 beta-hydroxybudesonide; minor activity

Bioavailability: Limited by high first-pass effect; Capsule: 9% to 21%; Respules®: 6%; Turbuhaler®: 6% to 13%; Nasal: 34%

Half-life elimination: 2-3.6 hours

Time to peak: Capsule: 0.5-10 hours (variable in Crohn's disease); Respules®: 10-30 minutes; Turbuhaler®: 1-2 hours; Nasal: 1 hour

Excretion: Urine (60%) and feces as metabolites

Pregnancy Risk Factor C/B (Pulmicort Respules® and Turbuhaler®, Rhinocort® Aqua®)

Dosage Forms CAP, enteric coated (Entocort® EC): 3 mg. **POWDER, oral inhalation** (Pulmicort Turbuhaler®): 200 mcg/inhalation (104 g); (additional dosage strengths available in Canada: 100 mcg/inhalation, 400 mcg/inhalation). **SPRAY, intranasal** (Rhinocort® Aqua®): 32 mcg/inhalation (8.6 g). **SUSP, nebulization** (Pulmicort Respules®): 0.25 mg/2 mL (30s), 0.5 mg/2 mL (30s)

Buffered Aspirin and Pravastatin Sodium see Aspirin and Pravastatin on page 151

Bufferin® [OTC] see Aspirin on page 145

Bufferin® Extra Strength [OTC] *see* Aspirin *on page 145*
Buffinol [OTC] *see* Aspirin *on page 145*
Buffinol Extra [OTC] *see* Aspirin *on page 145*

Bumetanide (byoo MET a nide)

Related Information
Cardiovascular Diseases *on page 1636*

U.S. Brand Names Bumex®

Canadian Brand Names Bumex®; Burinex®

Mexican Brand Names Bumedyl®; Drenural®; Miccil®

Generic Available Yes

Pharmacologic Category Diuretic, Loop

Use Management of edema secondary to congestive heart failure or hepatic or renal disease including nephrotic syndrome; may be used alone or in combination with antihypertensives in the treatment of hypertension; can be used in furosemide-allergic patients

Local Anesthetic/Vasoconstrictor Precautions No information available to require special precautions

Effects on Dental Treatment No significant effects or complications reported

Common Adverse Effects
>10%:
  Endocrine & metabolic: Hyperuricemia (18%), hypochloremia (15%), hypokalemia (15%)
  Renal: Azotemia (11%)
1% to 10%:
  Central nervous system: Dizziness (1%)
  Endocrine & metabolic: Hyponatremia (9%); hyperglycemia (7%); variations in phosphorus (5%), CO_2 content (4%), bicarbonate (3%), and calcium (2%)
  Neuromuscular & skeletal: Muscle cramps (1%)
  Otic: Ototoxicity (1%)
  Renal: Serum creatinine increased (7%)

Mechanism of Action Inhibits reabsorption of sodium and chloride in the ascending loop of Henle and proximal renal tubule, interfering with the chloride-binding cotransport system, thus causing increased excretion of water, sodium, chloride, magnesium, phosphate, and calcium; it does not appear to act on the distal tubule

Drug Interactions
Increased Effect/Toxicity: Bumetanide-induced hypokalemia may predispose to digoxin toxicity and may increase the risk of arrhythmia with drugs which may prolong QT interval, including type Ia and type III antiarrhythmic agents, cisapride, and some quinolones (sparfloxacin, gatifloxacin, and moxifloxacin). The risk of toxicity from lithium and salicylates (high dose) may be increased by loop diuretics. Hypotensive effects and/or adverse renal effects of ACE inhibitors and NSAIDs are potentiated by bumetanide-induced hypovolemia. The effects of peripheral adrenergic-blocking drugs or ganglionic blockers may be increased by bumetanide.

Bumetanide may increase the risk of ototoxicity with other ototoxic agents (aminoglycosides, cis-platinum), especially in patients with renal dysfunction. Synergistic diuretic effects occur with thiazide-type diuretics. Diuretics tend to be synergistic with other antihypertensive agents, and hypotension may occur.

Decreased Effect: Glucose tolerance may be decreased by loop diuretics, requiring adjustment of hypoglycemic agents. Cholestyramine or colestipol may reduce bioavailability of bumetanide. Indomethacin (and other NSAIDs) may reduce natriuretic and hypotensive effects of diuretics. Hypokalemia may reduce the efficacy of some antiarrhythmics.

Pharmacodynamics/Kinetics
Onset of action: Oral, I.M.: 0.5-1 hour; I.V.: 2-3 minutes
Duration: 4-6 hours
Distribution: V_d: 13-25 L/kg
Protein binding: 95%
Metabolism: Partially hepatic
Half-life elimination: Neonates: ~6 hours; Infants (1 month): ~2.4 hours; Adults: 1-1.5 hours
Excretion: Primarily urine (as unchanged drug and metabolites)

Pregnancy Risk Factor C (manufacturer); D (expert analysis)

Bumex® *see* Bumetanide *on page 227*
Buphenyl® *see* Sodium Phenylbutyrate *on page 1403*

BUPIVACAINE

Bupivacaine (byoo PIV a kane)

Related Information
Oral Pain *on page 1692*

U.S. Brand Names Marcaine®; Marcaine® Spinal; Sensorcaine®; Sensorcaine®-MPF

Canadian Brand Names Marcaine®; Sensorcaine®

Mexican Brand Names Buvacaina®

Generic Available Yes

Synonyms Bupivacaine Hydrochloride

Pharmacologic Category Local Anesthetic

Dental Use None; not to be confused with bupivacaine and epinephrine dental anesthetic. Refer to Bupivacaine and Epinephrine.

Use Local anesthetic (injectable) for peripheral nerve block, infiltration, sympathetic block, caudal or epidural block, retrobulbar block

Local Anesthetic/Vasoconstrictor Precautions No information available to require special precautions

Effects on Dental Treatment No significant effects or complications reported

Common Adverse Effects Note: Incidence of adverse reactions is difficult to define. Most effects are dose related, and are often due to accelerated absorption from the injection site, unintentional intravascular injection, or slow metabolic degradation. The development of any central nervous system symptoms may be an early indication of more significant toxicity (seizure).

Cardiovascular: Hypotension, bradycardia, palpitation, heart block, ventricular arrhythmia, cardiac arrest

Central nervous system: Restlessness, anxiety, dizziness, seizure (0.1%); rare symptoms (usually associated with unintentional subarachnoid injection during high spinal anesthesia) include persistent anesthesia, paresthesia, paralysis, headache, septic meningitis, and cranial nerve palsies

Gastrointestinal: Nausea, vomiting; rare symptoms (usually associated with unintentional subarachnoid injection during high spinal anesthesia) include fecal incontinence and loss of sphincter control

Genitourinary: Rare symptoms (usually associated with unintentional subarachnoid injection during high spinal anesthesia) include urinary incontinence, loss of perineal sensation, and loss of sexual function

Neuromuscular & skeletal: Weakness

Ocular: Blurred vision, pupillary constriction

Otic: Tinnitus

Respiratory: Apnea, hypoventilation (usually associated with unintentional subarachnoid injection during high spinal anesthesia)

Miscellaneous: Allergic reactions (urticaria, pruritus, angioedema), anaphylactoid reactions

Mechanism of Action Blocks both the initiation and conduction of nerve impulses by decreasing the neuronal membrane's permeability to sodium ions, which results in inhibition of depolarization with resultant blockade of conduction

Drug Interactions

Cytochrome P450 Effect: Substrate (minor) of CYP1A2, 2C19, 2D6, 3A4

Pharmacodynamics/Kinetics

Onset of action: Anesthesia (route and dose dependent): 1-17 minutes

Duration (route and dose dependent): 2-9 hours

Protein binding: ~95%

Metabolism: Hepatic; forms metabolite (PPX)

Half-life elimination (age dependent): Neonates: 8.1 hours; Adults: 1.5-5.5 hours

Excretion: Urine (~6% unchanged)

Pregnancy Risk Factor C

Bupivacaine and Epinephrine (byoo PIV a kane & ep i NEF rin)

Related Information
Bupivacaine *on page 228*
Epinephrine *on page 546*
Oral Pain *on page 1692*

U.S. Brand Names Marcaine® with Epinephrine; Sensorcaine®-MPF with Epinephrine; Sensorcaine® with Epinephrine

Canadian Brand Names Sensorcaine® with Epinephrine

Generic Available Yes

228

Synonyms Epinephrine Bitartrate and Bupivacaine Hydrochloride

Pharmacologic Category Local Anesthetic

Dental Use Local anesthesia

Use Local anesthetic (injectable) for peripheral nerve block, infiltration, sympathetic block, caudal or epidural block, retrobulbar block

Local Anesthetic/Vasoconstrictor Precautions No information available to require special precautions

Effects on Dental Treatment It is common to misinterpret psychogenic responses to local anesthetic injection as an allergic reaction. Intraoral injections are perceived by many patients as a stressful procedure in dentistry. Common symptoms to this stress are diaphoresis, palpitations, and hyperventilation. Patients may exhibit hypersensitivity to bisulfites contained in local anesthetic solution to prevent oxidation of epinephrine. In general, patients reacting to bisulfites have a history of asthma and their airways are hyper-reactive to asthmatic syndrome.

Degree of adverse effects in the CNS and cardiovascular system is directly related to the blood levels of bupivacaine: Bradycardia, hypersensitivity reactions (rare; may be manifest as dermatologic reactions and edema at injection site), asthmatic syndromes.

High blood levels: Anxiety, restlessness, disorientation, confusion, dizziness, tremors, seizures, CNS depression (resulting in somnolence, unconsciousness and possible respiratory arrest), nausea, and vomiting.

Significant Adverse Effects See individual agents.

Dental Usual Dosing Infiltration and nerve block in maxillary and mandibular area: Children >12 years and Adults: 9 mg (1.8 mL) of bupivacaine as a 0.5% solution with epinephrine 1:200,000 per injection site. A second dose may be administered if necessary to produce adequate anesthesia after allowing up to 10 minutes for onset. Up to a maximum of 90 mg of bupivacaine hydrochloride per dental appointment. The effective anesthetic dose varies with procedure, intensity of anesthesia needed, duration of anesthesia required, and physical condition of the patient; always use the lowest effective dose along with careful aspiration.

The following numbers of dental carpules (1.8 mL) provide the indicated amounts of bupivacaine hydrochloride 0.5% and vasoconstrictor (epinephrine 1:200,000). See table.

# of Cartridges (1.8 mL)	mg Bupivacaine (0.5%)	mg Vasoconstrictor (Epinephrine 1:200,000)
1	9	0.009
2	18	0.018
3	27	0.027
4	36	0.036
5	45	0.045
6	54	0.054
7	63	0.063
8	72	0.072
9	81	0.081
10	90	0.090

Note: Adult and children doses of bupivacaine hydrochloride with epinephrine cited from USP Dispensing Information (USP DI), 17th ed, The United States Pharmacopeial Convention, Inc, Rockville, MD, 1997, 134.

Dosage Dose varies with procedure, depth of anesthesia, vascularity of tissues, duration of anesthesia, and condition of patient. Do not use solutions containing preservatives for caudal or epidural block.

Children >12 years and Adults:

Caudal block (preservative free): 15-30 mL of 0.25% or 0.5%

Epidural block (other than caudal block, preservative free): 10-20 mL of 0.25% or 0.5%. Administer in 3-5 mL increments, allowing sufficient time to detect toxic manifestations of inadvertent I.V. or I.T. administration.

Surgical procedures requiring a high degree of muscle relaxation and prolonged effects only: 10-20 mL of 0.75% (**Note:** Not to be used in obstetrical cases)

Local anesthesia: Infiltration: 0.25% infiltrated locally (maximum: 175 mg of bupivacaine)

Peripheral nerve block: 5 mL of 0.25 or 0.5% (maximum: 400 mg/day of bupivacaine)

Retrobulbar anesthesia: 2-4 mL of 0.75%

(Continued)

Bupivacaine and Epinephrine *(Continued)*

Sympathetic nerve block: 20-50 mL of 0.25%

Infiltration and nerve block in maxillary and mandibular area: 9 mg (1.8 mL) of bupivacaine as a 0.5% solution with epinephrine 1:200,000 per injection site. A second dose may be administered if necessary to produce adequate anesthesia after allowing up to 10 minutes for onset. Up to a maximum of 90 mg of bupivacaine hydrochloride per dental appointment. The effective anesthetic dose varies with procedure, intensity of anesthesia needed, duration of anesthesia required, and physical condition of the patient; always use the lowest effective dose along with careful aspiration.

Note: Adult and children doses of bupivacaine hydrochloride with epinephrine cited from USP Dispensing Information (USP DI), 17th ed, The United States Pharmacopeial Convention, Inc, Rockville, MD, 1997, 134.

Mechanism of Action Local anesthetics bind selectively to the intracellular surface of sodium channels to block influx of sodium into the axon. As a result, depolarization necessary for action potential propagation and subsequent nerve function is prevented. The block at the sodium channel is reversible. When drug diffuses away from the axon, sodium channel function is restored and nerve propagation returns.

Epinephrine prolongs the duration of the anesthetic actions of bupivacaine by causing vasoconstriction (alpha adrenergic receptor agonist) of the vasculature surrounding the nerve axons. This prevents the diffusion of bupivacaine away from the nerves resulting in a longer retention in the axon

Contraindications Hypersensitivity to bupivacaine, epinephrine, amide-type local anesthetics, or any component of the formulation

Warnings/Precautions Some commercially available formulations contain sodium metabisulfite, which may cause allergic-type reactions. Do not use solutions containing preservatives for caudal or epidural block. Local anesthetics have been associated with rare occurrences of sudden respiratory arrest. Convulsions due to systemic toxicity leading to cardiac arrest have also been reported, presumably following unintentional intravascular injection. The 0.75% is not recommended for obstetrical anesthesia. A test dose is recommended prior to epidural administration and all reinforcing doses with continuous catheter technique. Use caution with cardiovascular dysfunction, hepatic impairment, or patients with compromised blood supply. Use caution in debilitated, elderly, or acutely ill patients; dose reduction may be required. Not recommended for use in children <12 years of age.

Drug Interactions Bupivacaine: **Substrate** (minor) of CYP1A2, 2C19, 2D6, 3A4 Also see individual agents.

Pharmacodynamics/Kinetics Refer to Bupivacaine; epinephrine reduces the rate of absorption and peak plasma concentration of bupivacaine

Pregnancy Risk Factor C

Lactation Enters breast milk/not recommended

Dosage Forms

Injection, solution [preservative free]: Bupivacaine hydrochloride 0.25% and epinephrine bitartrate 1:200,000 (10 mL, 30 mL); bupivacaine hydrochloride 0.5% and epinephrine bitartrate 1:200,000 (10 mL, 30 mL)

Marcaine® with Epinephrine Preservative Free: Bupivacaine hydrochloride 0.25% and epinephrine bitartrate 1:200,000 (10 mL, 30 mL) [contains sodium metabisulfite]; bupivacaine hydrochloride 0.5% and epinephrine bitartrate 1:200,000 (1.8 mL, 3 mL, 10 mL, 30 mL) [contains sodium metabisulfite]; bupivacaine hydrochloride 0.75% and epinephrine bitartrate 1:200,000 (30 mL) [contains sodium metabisulfite]

Sensorcaine® MPF with Epinephrine: Bupivacaine hydrochloride 0.25% and epinephrine bitartrate 1:200,000 (10 mL, 30 mL) [contains sodium metabisulfite]; bupivacaine hydrochloride 0.5% and epinephrine bitartrate 1:200,000 (10 mL, 30 mL) [contains sodium metabisulfite]

Injection, solution: Bupivacaine hydrochloride 0.25% and epinephrine bitartrate 1:200,000 (50 mL); bupivacaine hydrochloride 0.5% and epinephrine bitartrate 1:200,000 (50 mL)

Marcaine® with Epinephrine, Sensorcaine® with Epinephrine: Bupivacaine hydrochloride 0.25% and epinephrine bitartrate 1:200,000 (50 mL) [contains methylparaben]; bupivacaine hydrochloride 0.5% and epinephrine bitartrate 1:200,000 (50 mL) [contains methylparaben]

Selected Readings

Ayoub ST and Coleman AE, "A Review of Local Anesthetics," *Gen Dent*, 1992, 40(4):285-7, 289-90.

Budenz AW, "Local Anesthetics in Dentistry: Then and Now," *J Calif Dent Assoc*, 2003, 31(5):388-96.

Dower JS Jr, "A Review of Paresthesia in Association With Administration of Local Anesthesia," *Dent Today*, 2003, 22(2):64-9.

Finder RL and Moore PA, "Adverse Drug Reactions to Local Anesthesia," *Dent Clin North Am*, 2002, 46(4):747-57, x.

Haas DA, "An Update on Local Anesthetics in Dentistry," *J Can Dent Assoc*, 2002, 68(9):546-51.

Hawkins JM and Moore PA, "Local Anesthesia: Advances in Agents and Techniques," *Dent Clin North Am*, 2002, 46(4):719-32, ix.

"Injectable Local Anesthetics," *J Am Dent Assoc*, 2003, 134(5):628-9.

Jastak JT and Yagiela JA, "Vasoconstrictors and Local Anesthesia: A Review and Rationale for Use," *J Am Dent Assoc*, 1983, 107(4):623-30.

MacKenzie TA and Young ER, "Local Anesthetic Update," *Anesth Prog*, 1993, 40(2):29-34.

Malamed SF, "Allergy and Toxic Reactions to Local Anesthetics," *Dent Today*, 2003, 22(4):114-6, 118-21.

Wahl MJ, Schmitt MM, Overton DA, et al, "Injection Pain of Bupivacaine With Epinephrine vs. Prilocaine Plain," *J Am Dent Assoc*, 2002, 133(12):1652-6.

Wynn RL, "Epinephrine Interactions With Beta-Blockers," *Gen Dent*, 1994, 42(1):16, 18.

Yagiela JA, "Local Anesthetics," *Anesth Prog*, 1991, 38(4-5):128-41.

Bupivacaine and Lidocaine *see* Lidocaine and Bupivacaine *on page 924*

Bupivacaine Hydrochloride *see* Bupivacaine *on page 228*

Buprenex® *see* Buprenorphine *on page 231*

Buprenorphine (byoo pre NOR feen)

U.S. Brand Names Buprenex®; Subutex®

Canadian Brand Names Buprenex®; Subutex®

Mexican Brand Names Temgesic®

Generic Available Yes: Injection

Synonyms Buprenorphine Hydrochloride

Pharmacologic Category Analgesic, Narcotic

Use
Injection: Management of moderate to severe pain
Tablet: Treatment of opioid dependence

Unlabeled/Investigational Use Injection: Heroin and opioid withdrawal

Local Anesthetic/Vasoconstrictor Precautions No information available to require special precautions

Effects on Dental Treatment No significant effects or complications reported

Common Adverse Effects
Injection:
>10%: Central nervous system: Sedation
1% to 10%:
  Cardiovascular: Hypotension
  Central nervous system: Respiratory depression, dizziness, headache
  Gastrointestinal: Vomiting, nausea
  Ocular: Miosis
  Otic: Vertigo
  Miscellaneous: Diaphoresis

Tablet:
>10%:
  Central nervous system: Headache (30%), pain (24%), insomnia (21% to 25%), Oralety (12%), depression (11%)
  Gastrointestinal: Nausea (10% to 14%), abdominal pain (12%), constipation (8% to 11%)
  Neuromuscular & skeletal: Back pain (14%), weakness (14%)
  Respiratory: Rhinitis (11%)
  Miscellaneous: Withdrawal syndrome (19%; placebo 37%), infection (12% to 20%), diaphoresis (12% to 13%)
(Continued)

Buprenorphine *(Continued)*

1% to 10%:

Central nervous system: Chills (6%), nervousness (6%), somnolence (5%), dizziness (4%), fever (3%)

Gastrointestinal: Vomiting (5% to 8%), diarrhea (5%), dyspepsia (3%)

Ocular: Lacrimation (5%)

Respiratory: Cough (4%), pharyngitis (4%)

Miscellaneous: Flu-like syndrome (6%)

Restrictions Injection: C-V; Tablet: C-III

Prescribing of tablets for opioid dependence is limited to physicians who have met the qualification criteria and have received a DEA number specific to prescribing this product. Tablets will be available through pharmacies and wholesalers which normally provide controlled substances.

Mechanism of Action Buprenorphine exerts its analgesic effect via high affinity binding to μ opiate receptors in the CNS; displays both agonist and antagonist activity

Drug Interactions

Cytochrome P450 Effect: Substrate of CYP3A4 (major); **Inhibits** CYP1A2 (weak), 2A6 (weak), 2C19 (weak), 2D6 (weak)

Increased Effect/Toxicity: Barbiturate anesthetics and other CNS depressants may produce additive respiratory and CNS depression. Respiratory and CV collapse was reported in a patient who received diazepam and buprenorphine. Effects may be additive with other CNS depressants. CYP3A4 inhibitors may increase the levels/effects of buprenorphine; example inhibitors include azole antifungals, clarithromycin, diclofenac, doxycycline, erythromycin, imatinib, isoniazid, nefazodone, nicardipine, propofol, protease inhibitors, quinidine, and verapamil.

Decreased Effect: CYP3A4 inducers may decrease the levels/effects of buprenorphine; example inducers include aminoglutethimide, carbamazepine, nafcillin, nevirapine, phenobarbital, phenytoin, and rifamycins. Naltrexone may antagonize the effect of narcotic analgesics; concurrent use or use within 7-10 days of injection for pain relief is contraindicated.

Pharmacodynamics/Kinetics

Onset of action: Analgesic: 10-30 minutes

Duration: 6-8 hours

Absorption: I.M., SubQ: 30% to 40%

Distribution: V_d: 97-187 L/kg

Protein binding: High

Metabolism: Primarily hepatic; extensive first-pass effect

Half-life elimination: 2.2-3 hours

Excretion: Feces (70%); urine (20% as unchanged drug)

Pregnancy Risk Factor C

Buprenorphine and Naloxone
(byoo pre NOR feen & nal OKS one)

Related Information

Buprenorphine *on page 231*

Naloxone *on page 1084*

U.S. Brand Names Suboxone®

Generic Available No

Synonyms Buprenorphine Hydrochloride and Naloxone Hydrochloride Dihydrate; Naloxone and Buprenorphine; Naloxone Hydrochloride Dihydrate and Buprenorphine Hydrochloride

Pharmacologic Category Analgesic, Narcotic

Use Treatment of opioid dependence

Local Anesthetic/Vasoconstrictor Precautions No information available to require special precautions

Effects on Dental Treatment No significant effects or complications reported

Common Adverse Effects Also see individual agents.

>10%:

Central nervous system: Headache (36%), pain (22%)

Gastrointestinal: Nausea (15%), constipation (12%), abdominal pain (11%)

Miscellaneous: Withdrawal syndrome (25%; placebo 37%), diaphoresis (14%)

1% to 10%:

Cardiovascular: Vasodilation (9%)

Gastrointestinal: Vomiting (7%)

Restrictions C-III; Prescribing of tablets for opioid dependence is limited to physicians who have met the qualification criteria and have received a DEA number specific to prescribing this product. Tablets will be available through pharmacies and wholesalers which normally provide controlled substances.

Mechanism of Action See individual agents.

Drug Interactions
Decreased Effect: See individual agents.

Pharmacodynamics/Kinetics See individual agents.
Absorption: Absorption of the combination product is variable among patients following sublingual use, but variability within each individual patient is low.

Pregnancy Risk Factor C

Buprenorphine Hydrochloride *see* Buprenorphine *on page 231*

Buprenorphine Hydrochloride and Naloxone Hydrochloride Dihydrate *see* Buprenorphine and Naloxone *on page 232*

Buproban™ *see* BuPROPion *on page 233*

BuPROPion (byoo PROE pee on)

U.S. Brand Names Budeprion™ SR; Buproban™; Wellbutrin®; Wellbutrin SR®; Wellbutrin XL™; Zyban®

Canadian Brand Names Novo-Bupropion SR; Wellbutrin®; Wellbutrin XL™; Zyban®

Generic Available Yes: Excludes Wellbutrin XL™

Pharmacologic Category Antidepressant, Dopamine-Reuptake Inhibitor; Smoking Cessation Aid

Use Treatment of depression; adjunct in smoking cessation

Unlabeled/Investigational Use Attention-deficit/hyperactivity disorder (ADHD)

Local Anesthetic/Vasoconstrictor Precautions Part of the mechanism of bupropion is to block reuptake of norepinephrine along with dopamine. Because of the potential for norepinephrine elevation within CNS synapses, it is suggested that vasoconstrictor be administered with caution and to monitor vital signs in dental patients taking antidepressants that affect norepinephrine in this way.

Effects on Dental Treatment Key adverse event(s) related to dental treatment: Abnormal taste, significant xerostomia (normal salivary flow resumes with discontinuation).

Common Adverse Effects Frequencies, when reported, reflect highest incidence reported with sustained release product.
>10%:
Central nervous system: Dizziness (11%), headache (25%), insomnia (16%)
Gastrointestinal: Nausea (18%), xerostomia (24%)
Respiratory: Pharyngitis (11%)
1% to 10%:
Cardiovascular: Arrhythmias, chest pain (4%), flushing, hypertension (may be severe), hypotension, palpitation (5%), syncope, tachycardia
Central nervous system: Agitation (9%), anxiety (6%), confusion, depression, euphoria, hostility, irritability (2%), memory decreased (3%), migraine, nervousness (3%), sleep disturbance, somnolence (3%)
Dermatologic: Pruritus (4%), rash (4%), sweating increased (5%), urticaria (1%)
Endocrine & metabolic: Hot flashes, libido decreased, menstrual complaints
Gastrointestinal: Abdominal pain, anorexia (3%), appetite increased, constipation (5%), diarrhea (7%), dyspepsia, dysphagia (2%), taste perversion (4%), vomiting (2%)
Genitourinary: Urinary frequency (5%)
Neuromuscular & skeletal: Arthralgia (4%), arthritis (2%), myalgia (6%), neck pain, paresthesia (2%), tremor (3%), twitching (2%)
Ocular: Amblyopia (2%), blurred vision
Otic: Auditory disturbance, tinnitus (6%)
Respiratory: Cough increased (2%), sinusitis (1%)
Miscellaneous: Allergic reaction (including anaphylaxis, pruritus, urticaria), infection

Restrictions A medication guide concerning the use of antidepressants in children and teenagers can be found on the FDA website at http://www.fda.gov/cder/Offices/ODS/labeling.htm. It should be dispensed to parents or guardians of children and teenagers receiving this medication.

Dosage Oral:
Children and Adolescents: ADHD (unlabeled use): 1.4-6 mg/kg/day
Adults:
Depression:
Immediate release: 100 mg 3 times/day; begin at 100 mg twice daily; may increase to a maximum dose of 450 mg/day
(Continued)

BuPROPion (Continued)

Sustained release: Initial: 150 mg/day in the morning; may increase to 150 mg twice daily by day 4 if tolerated; target dose: 300 mg/day given as 150 mg twice daily; maximum dose: 400 mg/day given as 200 mg twice daily

Extended release: Initial: 150 mg/day in the morning; may increase as early as day 4 of dosing to 300 mg/day; maximum dose: 450 mg/day

Smoking cessation (Zyban®): Initiate with 150 mg once daily for 3 days; increase to 150 mg twice daily; treatment should continue for 7-12 weeks

Elderly: Depression: 50-100 mg/day, increase by 50-100 mg every 3-4 days as tolerated; there is evidence that the elderly respond at 150 mg/day in divided doses, but some may require a higher dose

Dosing adjustment/comments in renal impairment: Effect of renal disease on bupropion's pharmacokinetics has not been studied; elimination of the major metabolites of bupropion may be affected by reduced renal function. Patients with renal failure should receive a reduced dosage initially and be closely monitored.

Dosing adjustment in hepatic impairment:

Note: The mean AUC increased by ~1.5-fold for hydroxybupropion and ~2.5-fold for erythro/threohydrobupropion; median T_{max} was observed 19 hours later for hydroxybupropion, 31 hours later for erythro/threohydrobupropion; mean half-life for hydroxybupropion increased fivefold, and increased twofold for erythro/threohydrobupropion in patients with severe hepatic cirrhosis compared to healthy volunteers.

Mild-to-moderate hepatic impairment: Use with caution and/or reduced dose/frequency

Severe hepatic cirrhosis: Use with extreme caution; maximum dose:
Wellbutrin®: 75 mg/day
Wellbutrin SR®: 100 mg/day or 150 mg every other day
Wellbutrin XL™: 150 mg every other day
Zyban®: 150 mg every other day

Mechanism of Action Aminoketone antidepressant structurally different from all other marketed antidepressants; like other antidepressants the mechanism of bupropion's activity is not fully understood. Bupropion is a relatively weak inhibitor of the neuronal uptake of serotonin, norepinephrine, and dopamine, and does not inhibit monoamine oxidase. Metabolite inhibits the reuptake of norepinephrine. The primary mechanism of action is thought to be dopaminergic and/or noradrenergic.

Contraindications Hypersensitivity to bupropion or any component of the formulation; seizure disorder; anorexia/bulimia; use of MAO inhibitors within 14 days; patients undergoing abrupt discontinuation of ethanol or sedatives (including benzodiazepines); patients receiving other dosage forms of bupropion

Warnings/Precautions Antidepressants increase the risk of suicidal thinking and behavior in children and adolescents with major depressive disorder (MDD) and other depressive disorders; consider risk prior to prescribing. All patients must be closely monitored for clinical worsening, suicidality, or unusual changes in behavior, especially during the initiation of therapy or following an increase or decrease in dosage. When used in children, the child's family or caregiver should be instructed to closely observe the patient and communicate condition with healthcare provider. A medication guide should be dispensed with each prescription. **Bupropion is not FDA approved for use in children.**

The possibility of a suicide attempt is inherent in major depression and may persist until remission occurs. Use caution in high-risk patients. Worsening depression and severe abrupt suicidality that are not part of the presenting symptoms may require discontinuation or modification of drug therapy. The patient's family or caregiver should be alerted to monitor patients for the emergence of suicidality and associated behaviors (such as agitation, irritability, hostility, impulsivity, and hypomania) and notify the healthcare provider.

May worsen psychosis in some patients or precipitate a shift to mania or hypomania in patients with bipolar disorder. Patients presenting with depressive symptoms should be screened for bipolar disorder. Monotherapy in patients with bipolar disorder should be avoided. **Bupropion is not FDA approved for bipolar depression.**

When using immediate release tablets, seizure risk is increased at total daily dosage >450 mg, individual dosages >150 mg, or by sudden, large increments in dose. Data for the immediate-release formulation of bupropion revealed a seizure incidence of 0.4% in patients treated at doses in the 300-450 mg/day range. The estimated seizure incidence increases almost 10-fold between 450 mg and 600 mg per day. Data for the sustained release dosage form revealed a seizure incidence of 0.1% in patients treated at a dosage range of 100-300 mg/day, and increases to ~0.4% at the maximum recommended dose of 400 mg/day. The risk of seizures is increased in patients with a history of seizures, anorexia/bulimia, head trauma, CNS tumor, severe hepatic cirrhosis, abrupt discontinuation of sedative-hypnotics or ethanol, medications which lower seizure threshold (antipsychotics, antidepressants, theophyllines, systemic steroids), stimulants, or hypoglycemic agents. Discontinue and do not restart in patients experiencing a seizure. May cause CNS stimulation (restlessness, anxiety, insomnia) or anorexia. May increase the risks associated with electro-convulsive therapy. Consider discontinuing, when possible, prior to elective surgery. May cause weight loss; use caution in patients where weight loss is not desirable. The incidence of sexual dysfunction with bupropion is generally lower than with SSRIs.

Use caution in patients with cardiovascular disease, history of hypertension, or coronary artery disease; treatment-emergent hypertension (including some severe cases) has been reported, both with bupropion alone and in combination with nicotine transdermal systems. Use with caution in patients with hepatic or renal dysfunction and in elderly patients. Elderly patients may be at greater risk of accumulation during chronic dosing. May cause motor or cognitive impair-ment in some patients; use with caution if tasks requiring alertness such as operating machinery or driving are undertaken. Arthralgia, myalgia, and fever with rash and other symptoms suggestive of delayed hypersensitivity resem-bling serum sickness reported.

Drug Interactions
Cytochrome P450 Effect: Substrate of CYP1A2 (minor), 2A6 (minor), 2B6 (major), 2C9 (minor), 2D6 (minor), 2E1 (minor), 3A4 (minor); **Inhibits** CYP2D6 (weak)

Increased Effect/Toxicity: Treatment-emergent hypertension may occur in patients treated with bupropion and nicotine patch. Cimetidine may inhibit the metabolism (increase clinical/adverse effects) of bupropion. Toxicity of bupro-pion is enhanced by levodopa and phenelzine (MAO inhibitors). Risk of seizures may be increased with agents that may lower seizure threshold (antipsychotics, antidepressants, theophylline, abrupt discontinuation of benzodiazepines, systemic steroids). Effect of warfarin may be altered by bupropion. Concurrent use with amantadine appears to result in a higher incidence of adverse effects; use caution. CYP2B6 inhibitors may increase the levels/effects of bupropion; example inhibitors include desipramine, parox-etine, and sertraline. Combined use of CYP2B6 inhibitors (orphenadrine, thio-tepa, cyclophosphamide) with bupropion may increase serum concentrations and may result in seizures.

Decreased Effect: CYP2B6 inducers may decrease the levels/effects of bupropion; example inducers include carbamazepine, nevirapine, phenobar-bital, phenytoin, and rifampin. Effect of warfarin may be altered by bupropion.

Ethanol/Nutrition/Herb Interactions
Ethanol: Ethanol (may increase CNS depression).
Herb/Nutraceutical: Avoid valerian, St John's wort, SAMe, gotu kola, kava kava (may increase CNS depression).

Pharmacodynamics/Kinetics
Absorption: Rapid
Distribution: V_d: 19-21 L/kg
Protein binding: 82% to 88%
Metabolism: Extensively hepatic to 3 active metabolites: Hydroxybupropion, erythrohydrobupropion, threohydrobupropion (metabolite activity ranges from $1/5$ to $1/2$ potency of bupropion)
Bioavailability: 5% to 20% in animals
Half-life:
Distribution: 3-4 hours
Elimination: 21 ± 9 hours; Metabolites: Hydroxybupropion: 20 ± 5 hours; Erythrohydrobupropion: 33 ± 10 hours; Threohydrobupropion: 37 ± 13 hours
Time to peak, serum: Bupropion: ~3 hours; bupropion extended release: ~5 hours
Metabolites: Hydroxybupropion, erythrohydrobupropion, threohydrobupro-pion: 6 hours
Excretion: Urine (87%); feces (10%)

Pregnancy Risk Factor B
Dosage Forms TAB (Wellbutrin®): 75 mg, 100 mg. **TAB, extended release:** (Buproban™): 150 mg [equivalent to Zyban®]; (Budeprion™ SR): 100 mg [contains tartrazine; equivalent to Wellbutrin® SR], 150 mg [equivalent to Wellbutrin® SR]; (Wellbutrin XL™): 150 mg, 300 mg. **TAB, sustained release:** 100 mg, 150 mg [equivalent to Wellbutrin® SR], 150 mg [equivalent to Zyban®]; (Wellbutrin® SR): 100 mg, 150 mg, 200 mg; (Zyban®): 150 mg

Selected Readings
Tonstad S and Johnston JA, "Does Bupropion Have Advantages Over Other Medical Therapies in the Cessation of Smoking?" *Expert Opin Pharmacother*, 2004, 5(4):727-34.

Burnamycin [OTC] *see* Lidocaine *on page 920*
Burn Jel [OTC] *see* Lidocaine *on page 920*
Burn-O-Jel [OTC] *see* Lidocaine *on page 920*
BuSpar® *see* BusPIRone *on page 236*

BusPIRone (byoo SPYE rone)

Related Information
Sedation *on page 1727*

U.S. Brand Names BuSpar®

Canadian Brand Names Apo-Buspirone®; BuSpar®; Buspirex; Gen-Buspirone; Lin-Buspirone; Novo-Buspirone; Nu-Buspirone; PMS-Buspirone

Mexican Brand Names Neurosine®

Generic Available Yes

Synonyms Buspirone Hydrochloride

Pharmacologic Category Antianxiety Agent, Miscellaneous

Use Management of generalized anxiety disorder (GAD)

Unlabeled/Investigational Use Management of aggression in mental retardation and secondary mental disorders; major depression; potential augmenting agent for antidepressants; premenstrual syndrome

Local Anesthetic/Vasoconstrictor Precautions No information available to require special precautions

Effects on Dental Treatment Key adverse event(s) related to dental treatment: Xerostomia (normal salivary flow resumes upon discontinuation).

Common Adverse Effects
>10%: Central nervous system: Dizziness
1% to 10%:
Central nervous system: Drowsiness, EPS, serotonin syndrome, confusion, nervousness, lightheadedness, excitement, anger, hostility, headache
Dermatologic: Rash
Gastrointestinal: Diarrhea, nausea
Neuromuscular & skeletal: Muscle weakness, numbness, paresthesia, incoordination, tremor
Ocular: Blurred vision, tunnel vision
Miscellaneous: Diaphoresis, allergic reactions

Dosage Oral:
Generalized anxiety disorder:
Children and Adolescents: Initial: 5 mg daily; increase in increments of 5 mg/day at weekly intervals as needed, to a maximum dose of 60 mg/day divided into 2-3 doses
Adults: 15 mg/day (7.5 mg twice daily); may increase in increments of 5 mg/day every 2-4 days to a maximum of 60 mg/day; target dose for most people is 30 mg/day (15 mg twice daily)
Elderly: Initial: 5 mg twice daily, increase by 5 mg/day every 2-3 days as needed up to 20-30 mg/day; maximum daily dose: 60 mg/day.
Dosing adjustment in renal or hepatic impairment: Buspirone is metabolized by the liver and excreted by the kidneys. Patients with impaired hepatic or renal function demonstrated increased plasma levels and a prolonged half-life of buspirone. Therefore, use in patients with severe hepatic or renal impairment cannot be recommended.

Mechanism of Action The mechanism of action of buspirone is unknown. Buspirone has a high affinity for serotonin 5-HT$_{1A}$ and 5-HT$_2$ receptors, without affecting benzodiazepine-GABA receptors. Buspirone has moderate affinity for dopamine D$_2$ receptors.

Contraindications Hypersensitivity to buspirone or any component of the formulation

Warnings/Precautions Use in hepatic or renal impairment is not recommended; does not prevent or treat withdrawal from benzodiazepines. Low potential for cognitive or motor impairment. Use with MAO inhibitors may result in hypertensive reactions.

Drug Interactions
Cytochrome P450 Effect: Substrate of CYP2D6 (minor), 3A4 (major)
Increased Effect/Toxicity: Concurrent use of buspirone with SSRIs or trazodone may cause serotonin syndrome. Buspirone should not be used concurrently with an MAO inhibitor due to reports of increased blood pressure; theoretically, a selective MAO type B inhibitors (selegiline) has a lower risk of this reaction. Concurrent use of buspirone with nefazodone may increase risk of CNS adverse events; limit buspirone initial dose (eg, 2.5 mg/day). CYP3A4 inhibitors may increase the levels/effects of buspirone; example inhibitors

include azole antifungals, clarithromycin, diclofenac, doxycycline, erythromycin, imatinib, isoniazid, nefazodone, nicardipine, propofol, protease inhibitors, quinidine, telithromycin, and verapamil.

Decreased Effect: CYP3A4 inducers may decrease the levels/effects of buspirone; example inducers include aminoglutethimide, carbamazepine, nafcillin, nevirapine, phenobarbital, phenytoin, and rifamycins.

Ethanol/Nutrition/Herb Interactions

Ethanol: Ethanol (may increase CNS depression).

Food: Food may decrease the absorption of buspirone, but it may also decrease the first-pass metabolism, thereby increasing the bioavailability of buspirone. Grapefruit juice may cause increased buspirone concentrations; avoid concurrent use.

Herb/Nutraceutical: St John's wort may decrease buspirone levels or increase CNS depression. Avoid valerian, gotu kola, kava kava (may increase CNS depression).

Pharmacodynamics/Kinetics

Absorption: Oral: ~100%

Distribution: V_d: 5.3 L/kg

Protein binding: 95%

Metabolism: Hepatic via oxidation; extensive first-pass effect

Bioavailability: ~4%

Half-life elimination: Mean: 2.4 hours (range: 2-11 hours)

Time to peak, serum: Within 0.7-1.5 hours

Excretion: Urine: 65%; feces: 35%; ~1% dose excreted unchanged

Pregnancy Risk Factor B

Dosage Forms TAB: 5 mg, 7.5 mg, 10 mg, 15 mg, 30 mg; (BuSpar®): 5 mg, 10 mg, 15 mg, 30 mg

Buspirone Hydrochloride see BusPIRone on page 236

Busulfan (byoo SUL fan)

U.S. Brand Names Busulfex®; Myleran®

Canadian Brand Names Busulfex®; Myleran®

Mexican Brand Names Myleran®

Generic Available No

Pharmacologic Category Antineoplastic Agent, Alkylating Agent

Use

Oral: Chronic myelogenous leukemia; conditioning regimens for bone marrow transplantation

I.V.: Combination therapy with cyclophosphamide as a conditioning regimen prior to allogeneic hematopoietic progenitor cell transplantation for chronic myelogenous leukemia

Unlabeled/Investigational Use Oral: Bone marrow disorders, such as polycythemia vera and myeloid metaplasia; thrombocytosis

Local Anesthetic/Vasoconstrictor Precautions No information available to require special precautions

Effects on Dental Treatment No significant effects or complications reported

Common Adverse Effects

>10%: Hematologic: Severe pancytopenia, leukopenia, thrombocytopenia, anemia, and bone marrow suppression

Myelosuppressive:

WBC: Moderate

Platelets: Moderate

Onset: 7-10 days

Nadir: 14-21 days

Recovery: 28 days

1% to 10%:

Dermatologic: Hyperpigmentation skin (busulfan tan), urticaria, erythema, alopecia

Endocrine & metabolic: Amenorrhea

Gastrointestinal: Nausea, vomiting, diarrhea; drug has little effect on the GI mucosal lining

Neuromuscular & skeletal: Weakness

Mechanism of Action Reacts with N-7 position of guanosine and interferes with DNA replication and transcription of RNA. Busulfan has a more marked effect on myeloid cells than on lymphoid cells. The drug is also very toxic to hematopoietic stem cells. Busulfan exhibits little immunosuppressive activity. Interferes with the normal function of DNA by alkylation and cross-linking the strands of DNA.

(Continued)

Busulfan (Continued)

Drug Interactions

Cytochrome P450 Effect: Substrate of CYP3A4 (major)

Increased Effect/Toxicity: CYP3A4 inhibitors may increase the levels/effects of busulfan; example inhibitors include azole antifungals, clarithromycin, diclofenac, doxycycline, erythromycin, imatinib, isoniazid, nefazodone, nicardipine, propofol, protease inhibitors, quinidine, telithromycin, and verapamil. Metronidazole may increase busulfan plasma levels. Pulmonary toxicity of other cytotoxic agents may be additive.

Decreased Effect: CYP3A4 inducers may decrease the levels/effects of busulfan; example inducers include aminoglutethimide, carbamazepine, nafcillin, nevirapine, phenobarbital, phenytoin, and rifamycins.

Pharmacodynamics/Kinetics

Duration: 28 days

Absorption: Rapid and complete

Distribution: V_d: ~1 L/kg; into CSF and saliva with levels similar to plasma

Protein binding: ~14%

Metabolism: Extensively hepatic (may increase with multiple doses)

Half-life elimination: After first dose: 3.4 hours; After last dose: 2.3 hours

Time to peak, serum: Oral: Within 4 hours; I.V.: Within 5 minutes

Excretion: Urine (10% to 50% as metabolites) within 24 hours (<2% as unchanged drug)

Pregnancy Risk Factor D

Busulfex® see Busulfan on page 237

Butabarbital (byoo ta BAR bi tal)

U.S. Brand Names Butisol Sodium®
Generic Available No
Pharmacologic Category Barbiturate
Use Sedative; hypnotic
Local Anesthetic/Vasoconstrictor Precautions No information available to require special precautions
Effects on Dental Treatment No significant effects or complications reported

Common Adverse Effects

>10%: Central nervous system: Dizziness, lightheadedness, drowsiness, "hangover" effect

1% to 10%:
Central nervous system: Confusion, mental depression, unusual excitement, nervousness, faint feeling, headache, insomnia, nightmares
Gastrointestinal: Constipation, nausea, vomiting

Restrictions C-III

Mechanism of Action Interferes with transmission of impulses from the thalamus to the cortex of the brain resulting in an imbalance in central inhibitory and facilitatory mechanisms

Drug Interactions

Increased Effect/Toxicity: When butabarbital is combined with other CNS depressants, ethanol, narcotic analgesics, antidepressants, or benzodiazepines, additive respiratory and CNS depression may occur. Barbiturates may enhance the hepatotoxic potential of acetaminophen overdoses. Chloramphenicol, MAO inhibitors, valproic acid, and felbamate may inhibit barbiturate metabolism. Barbiturates may impair the absorption of griseofulvin, and may enhance the nephrotoxic effects of methoxyflurane.

Decreased Effect: Barbiturates, such as butabarbital, are hepatic enzyme inducers, and may increase the metabolism of antipsychotics, some beta-blockers (unlikely with atenolol and nadolol), calcium channel blockers, chloramphenicol, cimetidine, corticosteroids, cyclosporine, disopyramide, doxycycline, ethosuximide, felbamate, furosemide, griseofulvin, lamotrigine, phenytoin, propafenone, quinidine, tacrolimus, TCAs, and theophylline. Barbiturates may increase the metabolism of estrogens and reduce the efficacy of oral contraceptives; an alternative method of contraception should be considered. Barbiturates inhibit the hypoprothrombinemic effects of oral anticoagulants via increased metabolism. Barbiturates may enhance the metabolism of methadone resulting in methadone withdrawal.

Pharmacodynamics/Kinetics

Distribution: V_d: 0.8 L/kg

Protein binding: 26%

Metabolism: Hepatic

Half-life elimination: 1.6 days to 5.8 days

Time to peak, serum: 40-60 minutes

Excretion: Urine (as metabolites)
Pregnancy Risk Factor D

Butalbital, Acetaminophen, and Caffeine
(byoo TAL bi tal, a seet a MIN oh fen, & KAF een)

Related Information
Acetaminophen *on page 31*
Caffeine *on page 245*
U.S. Brand Names Anolor 300; Dolgic® LQ; Dolgic® Plus; Esgic®; Esgic-Plus™; Fioricet®; Medigesic®; Repan®; Zebutal™
Generic Available Yes: Excludes elixir
Synonyms Acetaminophen, Butalbital, and Caffeine
Pharmacologic Category Barbiturate
Use Relief of the symptomatic complex of tension or muscle contraction headache
Local Anesthetic/Vasoconstrictor Precautions No information available to require special precautions
Effects on Dental Treatment No significant effects or complications reported
Common Adverse Effects Note: Specific percentages not reported.
Frequently observed:
Central nervous system: Dizziness, drowsiness, lightheadedness, sedation
Gastrointestinal: Abdominal pain, nausea, vomiting
Respiratory: Dyspnea
Miscellaneous: Intoxicated feeling
Mechanism of Action
Butalbital is a short- to intermediate-acting barbiturate. Barbiturates depress the sensory cortex, decrease motor activity, alter cerebellar function, and produce drowsiness, sedation, hypnosis, and dose-dependent respiratory depression.
Acetaminophen inhibits the synthesis of prostaglandins in the central nervous system and peripherally blocks pain impulse generation; produces antipyresis from inhibition of hypothalamic heat-regulating center
Caffeine increases levels of 3'5' cyclic AMP by inhibiting phosphodiesterase; CNS stimulant which increases medullary respiratory center sensitivity to carbon dioxide, stimulates central inspiratory drive, and improves skeletal muscle contraction (diaphragmatic contractility)
Drug Interactions
Cytochrome P450 Effect:
Acetaminophen: **Substrate** (minor) of CYP1A2, 2A6, 2C9, 2D6, 2E1, 3A4; **Inhibits** CYP3A4 (weak)
Caffeine: **Substrate** of CYP1A2 (major), 2C9 (minor), 2D6 (minor), 2E1 (minor), 3A4 (minor); **Inhibits** CYP1A2 (weak), 3A4 (moderate)
Increased Effect/Toxicity: See Acetaminophen and Caffeine. For butalbital, refer to Phenobarbital.
Pharmacodynamics/Kinetics Also see Acetaminophen and Caffeine.
Absorption: Butalbital: Well absorbed
Protein binding: Butalbital: 45%
Half-life elimination: Butalbital: 35 hours
Excretion: Butalbital: Urine (59% to 88% as unchanged drug and metabolites)
Pregnancy Risk Factor C

Butalbital, Acetaminophen, Caffeine, and Codeine
(byoo TAL bi tal, a seet a MIN oh fen, KAF een, & KOE deen)

Related Information
Acetaminophen *on page 31*
Caffeine *on page 245*
Codeine *on page 385*
U.S. Brand Names Fioricet® with Codeine
Generic Available Yes
Synonyms Acetaminophen, Caffeine, Codeine, and Butalbital; Caffeine, Acetaminophen, Butalbital, and Codeine; Codeine, Acetaminophen, Butalbital, and Caffeine
Pharmacologic Category Analgesic Combination (Narcotic); Barbiturate
Use Relief of symptoms of complex tension (muscle contraction) headache
Local Anesthetic/Vasoconstrictor Precautions No information available to require special precautions
Effects on Dental Treatment Key adverse event(s) related to dental treatment: Xerostomia (normal salivary flow resumes upon discontinuation).
Significant Adverse Effects Frequency not defined.
(Continued)

Butalbital, Acetaminophen, Caffeine, and Codeine
(Continued)

Cardiovascular: Tachycardia, palpitation, hypotension, edema, syncope

Central nervous system: Drowsiness, fatigue, mental confusion, disorientation, nervousness, hallucination, euphoria, depression, seizure, headache, agitation, fainting, excitement, fever

Dermatologic: Rash, erythema, pruritus, urticaria, erythema multiforme, exfoliative dermatitis, toxic epidermal necrolysis

Gastrointestinal: Nausea, xerostomia, constipation, gastrointestinal spasm, heartburn, flatulence

Genitourinary: Urinary retention, diuresis

Neuromuscular & skeletal: Leg pain, weakness, numbness

Otic: Tinnitus

Miscellaneous: Allergic reaction, anaphylaxis

Note: Potential reactions associated with components of Fioricet® with Codeine include agranulocytosis, irritability, nausea, thrombocytopenia, tremor, vomiting

Restrictions C-III

Dosage Oral: Adults: 1-2 capsules every 4 hours. Total daily dosage should not exceed 6 capsules.

Dosing adjustment/comments in hepatic impairment: Use with caution. Limited, low-dose therapy usually well tolerated in hepatic disease/cirrhosis. However, cases of hepatotoxicity at daily acetaminophen dosages <4 g/day have been reported. Avoid chronic use in hepatic impairment.

Mechanism of Action Combination product for the treatment of tension headache. Contains codeine (narcotic analgesic), butalbital (barbiturate), caffeine (CNS stimulant), and acetaminophen (nonopiate, nonsalicylate analgesic).

Contraindications Hypersensitivity to butalbital, codeine, caffeine, acetaminophen, or any component of the formulation; porphyria; known G6PD deficiency; pregnancy (prolonged use or high doses at term)

Warnings/Precautions Limit acetaminophen to <4 g/day. May cause severe hepatic toxicity in acute overdose. In addition, chronic daily dosing in adults has resulted in liver damage in some patients. Use with caution in patients with hypersensitivity reactions to other phenanthrene derivative opioid agonists (eg, morphine, hydrocodone, oxycodone). Use caution with Addison's disease, severe renal or hepatic impairment. Use caution in patients with head injury or other intracranial lesions, acute abdominal conditions, urethral stricture of BPH, or in patients with respiratory diseases. Elderly (not recommended for use) and/or debilitated patients may be more susceptible to CNS depressants, as well as constipating effects of narcotics. Tolerance or drug dependence may result from extended use. Safety and efficacy in pediatric patients have not been established.

Drug Interactions

Acetaminophen: **Substrate** of (minor) CYP1A2, 2A6, 2C9, 2D6, 2E1, 3A4; **Inhibits** CYP3A4 (weak)

Caffeine: **Substrate** of CYP1A2 (major), 2C9 (minor), 2D6 (minor), 2E1 (minor), 3A4 (minor); **Inhibits** CYP1A2 (weak), 3A4 (moderate)

Butalbital: Refer to Phenobarbital.

See also Acetaminophen, Caffeine, and Codeine.

Ethanol/Nutrition/Herb Interactions Ethanol: Avoid ethanol (may increase CNS depression).

Pregnancy Risk Factor C (per manufacturer); D (prolonged use or high doses at term)

Lactation Enters breast milk/not recommended

Breast-Feeding Considerations Codeine, caffeine, barbiturates, and acetaminophen are excreted in breast milk in small amounts. Discontinuation of breast-feeding or discontinuation of the drug should be considered.

Dosage Forms Capsule: Butalbital 50 mg, caffeine 40 mg, acetaminophen 325 mg, and codeine phosphate 30 mg

Selected Readings

Botting RM, "Mechanism of Action of Acetaminophen: Is There a Cyclooxygenase 3?" Clin Infect Dis, 2000, Suppl 5:S202-10.

Dart RC, Kuffner EK, and Rumack BH, "Treatment of Pain or Fever With Paracetamol (Acetaminophen) in the Alcoholic Patient: A Systematic Review," Am J Ther, 2000, 7(2):123-34.

Grant JA and Weiler JM, "A Report of a Rare Immediate Reaction After Ingestion of Acetaminophen," Ann Allergy Asthma Immunol, 2001, 87(3):227-9.

Kwan D, Bartle WR, and Walker SE, "The Effects of Acetaminophen on Pharmacokinetics and Pharmacodynamics of Warfarin," J Clin Pharmacol, 1999, 39(1):68-75.

McClain CJ, Price S, Barve S, et al, "Acetaminophen Hepatotoxicity: An Update," Curr Gastroenterol Rep, 1999, 1(1):42-9.

Shek KL, Chan LN, and Nutescu E, "Warfarin-Acetaminophen Drug Interaction Revisited," Pharmacotherapy, 1999, 19(10):1153-8.

Tanaka E, Yamazaki K, and Misawa S, "Update: The Clinical Importance of Acetaminophen Hepatotoxicity in Nonalcoholic and Alcoholic Subjects," *J Clin Pharm Ther*, 2000, 25(5):325-32.

Butalbital, Aspirin, and Caffeine
(byoo TAL bi tal, AS pir in, & KAF een)

Related Information
Aspirin *on page 145*
Caffeine *on page 245*

U.S. Brand Names Fiorinal®

Canadian Brand Names Fiorinal®

Generic Available Yes

Synonyms Aspirin, Caffeine, and Butalbital; Butalbital Compound

Pharmacologic Category Barbiturate

Use Relief of the symptomatic complex of tension or muscle contraction headache

Local Anesthetic/Vasoconstrictor Precautions No information available to require special precautions

Effects on Dental Treatment No significant effects or complications reported

Common Adverse Effects

>10%:
  Central nervous system: Dizziness, lightheadedness, drowsiness, "hangover" effect
  Gastrointestinal: Heartburn, stomach pain, dyspepsia, epigastric discomfort, nausea

1% to 10%:
  Central nervous system: Confusion, mental depression, unusual excitement, nervousness, faint feeling, headache, insomnia, nightmares, fatigue
  Dermatologic: Skin rash
  Gastrointestinal: Constipation, vomiting, gastrointestinal ulceration
  Hematologic: Hemolytic anemia
  Neuromuscular & skeletal: Weakness
  Respiratory: Troubled breathing
  Miscellaneous: Anaphylactic shock

Restrictions C-III

Drug Interactions

Cytochrome P450 Effect:
  Aspirin: **Substrate** of CYP2C9 (minor)
  Caffeine: **Substrate** of CYP1A2 (major), 2C9 (minor), 2D6 (minor), 2E1 (minor), 3A4 (minor); **Inhibits** CYP1A2 (weak), 3A4 (moderate)

Increased Effect/Toxicity: Enhanced effect/toxicity with oral anticoagulants (warfarin), oral antidiabetic agents, insulin, mercaptopurine, methotrexate, NSAIDs, narcotic analgesics (propoxyphene, meperidine, etc), benzodiazepines, sedative-hypnotics, other CNS depressants. The CNS effects of butalbital may be enhanced by MAO inhibitors.

Decreased Effect: May decrease the effect of uricosuric agents (probenecid and sulfinpyrazone) reducing their effect on gout.

Pregnancy Risk Factor C/D (prolonged use or high doses at term)

Butalbital, Aspirin, Caffeine, and Codeine
(byoo TAL bi tal, AS pir in, KAF een, & KOE deen)

Related Information
Aspirin *on page 145*
Caffeine *on page 245*
Codeine *on page 385*

U.S. Brand Names Fiorinal® With Codeine; Phrenilin® With Caffeine and Codeine

Canadian Brand Names Fiorinal®-C 1/2; Fiorinal®-C 1/4; Tecnal C 1/2; Tecnal C 1/4

Generic Available Yes

Synonyms Aspirin, Caffeine, Codeine, and Butalbital; Butalbital Compound and Codeine; Codeine and Butalbital Compound; Codeine, Butalbital, Aspirin, and Caffeine

Pharmacologic Category Analgesic Combination (Narcotic); Barbiturate

Use Mild-to-moderate pain when sedation is needed

Local Anesthetic/Vasoconstrictor Precautions No information available to require special precautions

Effects on Dental Treatment No significant effects or complications reported

(Continued)

Butalbital, Aspirin, Caffeine, and Codeine *(Continued)*

Common Adverse Effects

>10%:

Central nervous system: Dizziness, lightheadedness, drowsiness

Gastrointestinal: Nausea, heartburn, stomach pain, dyspepsia, epigastric discomfort

1% to 10%:

Central nervous system: Confusion, mental depression, unusual excitement, nervousness, faint feeling, insomnia, nightmares, intoxicated feeling

Dermatologic: Rash

Gastrointestinal: Constipation, GI ulceration

Restrictions C-III

Drug Interactions

Cytochrome P450 Effect:

Aspirin: **Substrate** of CYP2C9 (minor)

Caffeine: **Substrate** of CYP1A2 (major), 2C9 (minor), 2D6 (minor), 2E1 (minor), 3A4 (minor); **Inhibits** CYP1A2 (weak), 3A4 (moderate)

Increased Effect/Toxicity: MAO inhibitors may enhance the CNS effects of butalbital. In patients receiving concomitant corticosteroids during the chronic use of ASA, withdrawal of corticosteroids may result in salicylism. Butalbital compound and codeine may enhance effects of oral anticoagulants. Increased effect with oral antidiabetic agents and insulin, mercaptopurine and methotrexate, NSAIDs, other narcotic analgesics, ethanol, general anesthetics, tranquilizers such as chlordiazepoxide, sedative hypnotics, or other CNS depressants.

Decreased Effect: Aspirin, butalbital, caffeine, and codeine may diminish effects of uricosuric agents such as probenecid and sulfinpyrazone.

Pregnancy Risk Factor C/D (prolonged use or high doses at term)

Butalbital Compound *see* Butalbital, Aspirin, and Caffeine *on page 241*

Butalbital Compound and Codeine *see* Butalbital, Aspirin, Caffeine, and Codeine *on page 241*

Butenafine *(byoo TEN a feen)*

U.S. Brand Names Lotrimin® Ultra™ [OTC]; Mentax®

Generic Available No

Synonyms Butenafine Hydrochloride

Pharmacologic Category Antifungal Agent, Topical

Use Topical treatment of tinea pedis (athlete's foot), tinea cruris (jock itch), tinea corporis (ringworm), and tinea versicolor

Local Anesthetic/Vasoconstrictor Precautions No information available to require special precautions

Effects on Dental Treatment No significant effects or complications reported

Common Adverse Effects >1%: Dermatologic: Burning, stinging, irritation, erythema, pruritus (2%)

Mechanism of Action Butenafine exerts antifungal activity by blocking squalene epoxidation, resulting in inhibition of ergosterol synthesis (antidermatophyte and *Sporothrix schenckii* activity). In higher concentrations, the drug disrupts fungal cell membranes (anticandidal activity).

Pharmacodynamics/Kinetics

Absorption: Minimal systemic

Metabolism: Hepatic via hydroxylation

Half-life elimination: 35 hours

Time to peak, serum: 6 hours

Pregnancy Risk Factor B

Butenafine Hydrochloride *see* Butenafine *on page 242*

Butisol Sodium® *see* Butabarbital *on page 238*

Butoconazole *(byoo toe KOE na zole)*

Related Information

Sexually-Transmitted Diseases *on page 1674*

U.S. Brand Names Gynazole-1®; Mycelex®-3 [OTC]

Canadian Brand Names Femstat® One; Gynazole-1®

Generic Available No

Synonyms Butoconazole Nitrate

Pharmacologic Category Antifungal Agent, Vaginal

Use Local treatment of vulvovaginal candidiasis

Local Anesthetic/Vasoconstrictor Precautions No information available to require special precautions

Effects on Dental Treatment No significant effects or complications reported

Common Adverse Effects Frequency not defined.

Gastrointestinal: Abdominal pain or cramping

Genitourinary: Pelvic pain; vulvar/vaginal burning, itching, soreness, and swelling

Mechanism of Action Increases cell membrane permeability in susceptible fungi (*Candida*)

Pharmacodynamics/Kinetics

Absorption: 2%

Metabolism: Not reported

Time to peak: 12-24 hours

Pregnancy Risk Factor C (use only in 2nd or 3rd trimester)

Butoconazole Nitrate *see* Butoconazole *on page 242*

Butorphanol (byoo TOR fa nole)

U.S. Brand Names Stadol®

Canadian Brand Names Apo-Butorphanol®; PMS-Butorphanol

Generic Available Yes

Synonyms Butorphanol Tartrate

Pharmacologic Category Analgesic, Narcotic

Use

Parenteral: Management of moderate-to-severe pain; preoperative medication; supplement to balanced anesthesia; management of pain during labor

Nasal spray: Management of moderate-to-severe pain, including migraine headache pain

Local Anesthetic/Vasoconstrictor Precautions No information available to require special precautions

Effects on Dental Treatment Key adverse event(s) related to dental treatment: Xerostomia (normal salivary flow resumes upon discontinuation) and unpleasant aftertaste.

Common Adverse Effects

>10%:

Central nervous system: Drowsiness (43%), dizziness (19%), insomnia (Stadol® NS)

Gastrointestinal: Nausea/vomiting (13%)

Respiratory: Nasal congestion (Stadol® NS)

1% to 10%:

Cardiovascular: Vasodilation, palpitation

Central nervous system: Lightheadedness, headache, lethargy, anxiety, confusion, euphoria, somnolence

Dermatologic: Pruritus

Gastrointestinal: Anorexia, constipation, xerostomia, stomach pain, unpleasant aftertaste

Neuromuscular & skeletal: Tremor, paresthesia, weakness

Ocular: Blurred vision

Otic: Ear pain, tinnitus

Respiratory: Bronchitis, cough, dyspnea, epistaxis, nasal irritation, pharyngitis, rhinitis, sinus congestion, sinusitis, upper respiratory infection

Miscellaneous: Diaphoresis increased

Restrictions C-IV

Mechanism of Action Mixed narcotic agonist-antagonist with central analgesic actions; binds to opiate receptors in the CNS, causing inhibition of ascending pain pathways, altering the perception of and response to pain; produces generalized CNS depression

Drug Interactions

Increased Effect/Toxicity: Increased toxicity with CNS depressants, phenothiazines, barbiturates, skeletal muscle relaxants, alfentanil, guanabenz, and MAO inhibitors.

Pharmacodynamics/Kinetics

Onset of action: I.M.: 5-10 minutes; I.V.: <10 minutes; Nasal: Within 15 minutes

Peak effect: I.M.: 0.5-1 hour; I.V.: 4-5 minutes

Duration: I.M., I.V.: 3-4 hours; Nasal: 4-5 hours

Absorption: Rapid and well absorbed

Protein binding: 80%

Metabolism: Hepatic

Bioavailability: Nasal: 60% to 70%

Half-life elimination: 2.5-4 hours

Excretion: Primarily urine

Pregnancy Risk Factor C/D (prolonged use or high doses at term)

Butorphanol Tartrate *see* Butorphanol *on page 243*

Butyl Aminobenzoate, Tetracaine Hydrochloride, Benzocaine, and Benzalkonium Chloride *see* Benzocaine, Butyl Aminobenzoate, Tetracaine, and Benzalkonium Chloride *on page 193*

B Vitamin Combinations *see* Vitamin B Complex Combinations *on page 1581*

BW-430C *see* Lamotrigine *on page 895*

BW524W91 *see* Emtricitabine *on page 536*

Byetta™ *see* Exenatide *on page 629*

C1H *see* Alemtuzumab *on page 63*

C2B8 *see* Rituximab *on page 1360*

C2B8 Monoclonal Antibody *see* Rituximab *on page 1360*

C7E3 *see* Abciximab *on page 26*

C8-CCK *see* Sincalide *on page 1396*

311C90 *see* Zolmitriptan *on page 1603*

C225 *see* Cetuximab *on page 308*

C-500-GR™ [OTC] *see* Ascorbic Acid *on page 143*

Cabergoline (ca BER goe leen)

U.S. Brand Names Dostinex®
Canadian Brand Names Dostinex®
Generic Available Yes
Pharmacologic Category Ergot Derivative
Use Treatment of hyperprolactinemic disorders, either idiopathic or due to pituitary adenomas

Unlabeled/Investigational Use Adjunct for the treatment of Parkinson's disease

Local Anesthetic/Vasoconstrictor Precautions No information available to require special precautions

Effects on Dental Treatment Key adverse event(s) related to dental treatment: Xerostomia (normal salivary flow resumes upon discontinuation), throat irritation, and toothache.

Common Adverse Effects
>10%:
  Central nervous system: Headache (26%), dizziness (17%)
  Gastrointestinal: Nausea (29%)
1% to 10%:
  Body as whole: Asthenia (6%), fatigue (5%), syncope (1%), influenza-like symptoms (1%), malaise (1%), periorbital edema (1%), peripheral edema (1%)
  Cardiovascular: Hot flashes (3%), hypotension (1%), dependent edema (1%), palpitation (1%)
  Central nervous system: Vertigo (4%), depression (3%), somnolence (2%), anxiety (1%), insomnia (1%), concentration impaired (1%), nervousness (1%)
  Dermatologic: Acne (1%), pruritus (1%)
  Endocrine: Breast pain (2%), dysmenorrhea (1%)
  Gastrointestinal: Constipation (7%), abdominal pain (5%), dyspepsia (5%), vomiting (4%), xerostomia (2%), diarrhea (2%), flatulence (2%), throat irritation (1%), toothache (1%), anorexia (1%)
  Neuromuscular & skeletal: Pain (2%), arthralgia (1%), paresthesia (2%)
  Ocular: Abnormal vision (1%)
  Respiratory: Rhinitis (1%)

Mechanism of Action Cabergoline is a long acting dopamine receptor agonist with a high affinity for D_2 receptors; prolactin secretion by the anterior pituitary is predominantly under hypothalamic inhibitory control exerted through the release of dopamine

Drug Interactions
Increased Effect/Toxicity: Cabergoline may increase the effects of sibutramine and other serotonin agonists (serotonin syndrome).
Decreased Effect: Effects of cabergoline may be diminished by antipsychotics, metoclopramide.

Pharmacodynamics/Kinetics
Distribution: Extensive, particularly to the pituitary
Protein binding: 40% to 42%
Metabolism: Extensively hepatic; minimal CYP
Half-life elimination: 63-69 hours

Time to peak: 2-3 hours
Pregnancy Risk Factor B

Ca-DTPA see Diethylene Triamine Penta-Acetic Acid on page 466
Caduet® see Amlodipine and Atorvastatin on page 101
CaEDTA see Edetate Calcium Disodium on page 527
Cafcit® see Caffeine on page 245
Cafergot® see Ergotamine and Caffeine on page 559
Caffedrine® [OTC] see Caffeine on page 245

Caffeine (KAF een)

U.S. Brand Names Cafcit®; Caffedrine® [OTC]; Enerjets [OTC]; Lucidex [OTC]; No Doz® Maximum Strength [OTC]; Vivarin® [OTC]

Generic Available Yes: Caffeine and sodium benzoate injection

Synonyms Caffeine and Sodium Benzoate; Caffeine Citrate; Sodium Benzoate and Caffeine

Pharmacologic Category Stimulant

Use
Caffeine citrate: Treatment of idiopathic apnea of prematurity
Caffeine and sodium benzoate: Treatment of acute respiratory depression (not a preferred agent)
Caffeine [OTC labeling]: Restore mental alertness or wakefulness when experiencing fatigue

Unlabeled/Investigational Use Caffeine and sodium benzoate: Treatment of spinal puncture headache; CNS stimulant; diuretic

Local Anesthetic/Vasoconstrictor Precautions No information available to require special precautions

Effects on Dental Treatment No significant effects or complications reported

Common Adverse Effects Frequency not specified; primarily serum-concentration related.
Cardiovascular: Angina, arrhythmia (ventricular), chest pain, flushing, palpitation, sinus tachycardia, tachycardia (supraventricular), vasodilation
Central nervous system: Agitation, delirium, dizziness, hallucinations, headache, insomnia, irritability, psychosis, restlessness
Dermatologic: Urticaria
Gastrointestinal: Esophageal sphincter tone decreased, gastritis
Neuromuscular & skeletal: Fasciculations
Ocular: Intraocular pressure increased (>180 mg caffeine), miosis
Renal: Diuresis

Mechanism of Action Increases levels of 3'5' cyclic AMP by inhibiting phosphodiesterase; CNS stimulant which increases medullary respiratory center sensitivity to carbon dioxide, stimulates central inspiratory drive, and improves skeletal muscle contraction (diaphragmatic contractility); prevention of apnea may occur by competitive inhibition of adenosine

Drug Interactions
Cytochrome P450 Effect: **Substrate** of CYP1A2 (major), 2C9 (minor), 2D6 (minor), 2E1 (minor), 3A4 (minor); **Inhibits** CYP1A2 (weak), 3A4 (moderate)
Increased Effect/Toxicity: Quinolones (specifically ciprofloxacin, norfloxacin, ofloxacin) and CYP1A2 inhibitors may increase the levels/effects of caffeine; example inhibitors include amiodarone, fluvoxamine, ketoconazole, and rofecoxib
Decreased Effect: Caffeine may diminish the sedative or anxiolytic effects of benzodiazepines. CYP1A2 inducers may decrease the levels/effects of caffeine; example inducers include aminoglutethimide, carbamazepine, phenobarbital, and rifampin.

Pharmacodynamics/Kinetics
Distribution: V_d:
Neonates: 0.8-0.9 L/kg
Children >9 months to Adults: 0.6 L/kg
Protein binding: 17% (children) to 36% (adults)
Metabolism: Hepatic, via demethylation by CYP1A2. Note: In neonates, interconversion between caffeine and theophylline has been reported (caffeine levels are ~25% of measured theophylline after theophylline administration and ~3% to 8% of caffeine would be expected to be converted to theophylline)
Half-life elimination:
Neonates: 72-96 hours (range: 40-230 hours)
Children >9 months and Adults: 5 hours
Time to peak, serum: Oral: Within 30 minutes to 2 hours
(Continued)

Caffeine *(Continued)*

Excretion:

Neonates ≤1 month: 86% excreted unchanged in urine

Infants >1 month and Adults: In urine, as metabolites

Pregnancy Risk Factor C

Caffeine, Acetaminophen, and Aspirin *see* Acetaminophen, Aspirin, and Caffeine *on page 41*

Caffeine, Acetaminophen, Butalbital, and Codeine *see* Butalbital, Acetaminophen, Caffeine, and Codeine *on page 239*

Caffeine and Ergotamine *see* Ergotamine and Caffeine *on page 559*

Caffeine and Sodium Benzoate *see* Caffeine *on page 245*

Caffeine, Aspirin, and Acetaminophen *see* Acetaminophen, Aspirin, and Caffeine *on page 41*

Caffeine Citrate *see* Caffeine *on page 245*

Caffeine, Dihydrocodeine, and Acetaminophen *see* Acetaminophen, Caffeine, and Dihydrocodeine *on page 42*

Caffeine, Hydrocodone, Chlorpheniramine, Phenylephrine, and Acetaminophen *see* Hydrocodone, Chlorpheniramine, Phenylephrine, Acetaminophen, and Caffeine *on page 790*

Caffeine, Orphenadrine, and Aspirin *see* Orphenadrine, Aspirin, and Caffeine *on page 1152*

Caffeine, Propoxyphene, and Aspirin *see* Propoxyphene, Aspirin, and Caffeine *on page 1300*

Caladryl® Clear [OTC] *see* Pramoxine *on page 1264*

CalaMycin® Cool and Clear [OTC] *see* Pramoxine *on page 1264*

Calan® *see* Verapamil *on page 1571*

Calan® SR *see* Verapamil *on page 1571*

Calcarb 600 [OTC] *see* Calcium Carbonate *on page 248*

Calcibind® *see* Cellulose Sodium Phosphate *on page 301*

Calci-Chew® [OTC] *see* Calcium Carbonate *on page 248*

Calciferol™ *see* Ergocalciferol *on page 556*

Calcijex® *see* Calcitriol *on page 247*

Calci-Mix® [OTC] *see* Calcium Carbonate *on page 248*

Calcipotriene *(kal si POE try een)*

U.S. Brand Names Dovonex®

Generic Available No

Pharmacologic Category Topical Skin Product; Vitamin D Analog

Use Treatment of plaque psoriasis

Local Anesthetic/Vasoconstrictor Precautions No information available to require special precautions

Effects on Dental Treatment No significant effects or complications reported

Common Adverse Effects Frequency may vary with site of application.

>10%: Dermatologic: Burning, itching, rash, skin irritation, stinging, tingling

1% to 10%: Dermatologic: Dermatitis, dry skin, erythema, peeling, worsening of psoriasis

Note: Skin atrophy, hypercalciuria, folliculitis, and hypercalcemia are potential adverse effects of calcipotriene.

Mechanism of Action Synthetic vitamin D_3 analog which regulates skin cell production and proliferation

Drug Interactions

Increased Effect/Toxicity: No data reported

Decreased Effect: No data reported

Pharmacodynamics/Kinetics

Onset of action: Improvement begins after 2 weeks; marked improvement seen after 8 weeks

Absorption: When applied to psoriasis plaques: Cream, ointment: ~6%; Solution: <1%

Metabolism: Converted in the skin to inactive metabolites

Pregnancy Risk Factor C

Calcitonin *(kal si TOE nin)*

Related Information

Rheumatoid Arthritis, Osteoarthritis, and Osteoporosis *on page 1668*

U.S. Brand Names Fortical®; Miacalcin®

Canadian Brand Names Apo-Calcitonin®; Calcimar®; Caltine®; Miacalcin® NS

Mexican Brand Names Miacalcic® [salmon]; Oseum® [salmon]; Tonocalcin® [salmon]

Generic Available No

Synonyms Calcitonin (Salmon)

Pharmacologic Category Antidote; Hormone

Use Calcitonin (salmon): Treatment of Paget's disease of bone (osteitis deformans); adjunctive therapy for hypercalcemia; postmenopausal osteoporosis

Local Anesthetic/Vasoconstrictor Precautions No information available to require special precautions

Effects on Dental Treatment No significant effects or complications reported

Common Adverse Effects Unless otherwise noted, frequencies reported are with nasal spray.

>10%: Respiratory: Rhinitis (12%)

1% to 10%:

Cardiovascular: Flushing (nasal spray: <1%; injection: 2% to 5%), angina (1% to 3%), hypertension (1% to 3%)

Central nervous system: Depression (1% to 3%), dizziness (1% to 3%), fatigue (1% to 3%)

Dermatologic: Erythematous rash (1% to 3%)

Gastrointestinal: Abdominal pain (1% to 3%), constipation (1% to 3%), diarrhea (1% to 3%), dyspepsia (1% to 3%), nausea (injection: 10%; nasal spray: 1% to 3%)

Genitourinary: Cystitis (1% to 3%)

Hematologic: Lymphadenopathy (1% to 3%)

Local: Injection site reactions (injection: 10%)

Neuromuscular & skeletal: Back pain (5%), arthrosis (1% to 3%), myalgia (1% to 3%), paresthesia (1% to 3%)

Ocular: Conjunctivitis (1% to 3%), lacrimation abnormality (1% to 3%)

Respiratory: Bronchospasm (1% to 3%), sinusitis (1% to 3%), upper respiratory tract infection (1% to 3%)

Miscellaneous: Flu-like symptoms (1% to 3%), infection (1% to 3%)

Mechanism of Action Peptide sequence similar to human calcitonin; functionally antagonizes the effects of parathyroid hormone. Directly inhibits osteoclastic bone resorption; promotes the renal excretion of calcium, phosphate, sodium, magnesium, and potassium by decreasing tubular reabsorption; increases the jejunal secretion of water, sodium, potassium, and chloride

Pharmacodynamics/Kinetics

Hypercalcemia: I.M. or SubQ:

Onset of action: ~2 hours

Duration: 6-8 hours

Absorption: Nasal: ~3% of I.M. level (range: 0.3% to 31%)

Distribution: Does not cross placenta

Half-life elimination: SubQ: 1.2 hours; Nasal: 43 minutes

Time to peak: Nasal: ~30-40 minutes

Excretion: Urine (as inactive metabolites)

Pregnancy Risk Factor C

Calcitonin (Salmon) *see* Calcitonin *on page 246*

Cal-Citrate® 250 [OTC] *see* Calcium Citrate *on page 250*

Calcitriol (kal si TRYE ole)

U.S. Brand Names Calcijex®; Rocaltrol®

Canadian Brand Names Calcijex®; Rocaltrol®

Mexican Brand Names Altrical®; Rocaltrol®; Tirocal®

Generic Available Yes

Synonyms 1,25 Dihydroxycholecalciferol

Pharmacologic Category Vitamin D Analog

Use Management of hypocalcemia in patients on chronic renal dialysis; management of secondary hyperparathyroidism in moderate-to-severe chronic renal failure; management of hypocalcemia in hypoparathyroidism and pseudohypoparathyroidism

Unlabeled/Investigational Use Decrease severity of psoriatic lesions in psoriatic vulgaris; vitamin D-resistant rickets

Local Anesthetic/Vasoconstrictor Precautions No information available to require special precautions

Effects on Dental Treatment Key adverse event(s) related to dental treatment: Metallic taste and xerostomia (normal salivary flow resumes upon discontinuation).

(Continued)

Calcitriol *(Continued)*

Common Adverse Effects

>10%: Endocrine & metabolic: Hypercalcemia (33%)

Frequency not defined:

Cardiovascular: Cardiac arrhythmia, hyper-/hypotension

Central nervous system: Headache, irritability, seizure (rare), somnolence, psychosis

Dermatologic: Pruritus, erythema multiforme

Endocrine & metabolic: Hypermagnesemia, hyperphosphatemia, polydipsia

Gastrointestinal: Anorexia, constipation, metallic taste, nausea, pancreatitis, vomiting, xerostomia

Hepatic: LFTs increased

Neuromuscular & skeletal: Bone pain, myalgia, dystrophy, soft tissue calcification

Ocular: Conjunctivitis, photophobia

Renal: Polyuria

Mechanism of Action Promotes absorption of calcium in the intestines and retention at the kidneys thereby increasing calcium levels in the serum; decreases excessive serum phosphatase levels, parathyroid hormone levels, and decreases bone resorption; increases renal tubule phosphate resorption

Drug Interactions

Cytochrome P450 Effect: Induces CYP3A4 (weak)

Increased Effect/Toxicity: Risk of hypercalcemia with thiazide diuretics. Risk of hypermagnesemia with magnesium-containing antacids. Risk of digoxin toxicity may be increased (if hypercalcemia occurs).

Decreased Effect: Cholestyramine and colestipol decrease absorption/effect of calcitriol. Thiazide diuretics and corticosteroids may reduce the effect of calcitriol.

Pharmacodynamics/Kinetics

Onset of action: ~2-6 hours

Duration: 3-5 days

Absorption: Oral: Rapid

Protein binding: 99.9%

Metabolism: Primarily to 1,24,25-trihydroxycholecalciferol and 1,24,25-trihydroxy ergocalciferol

Half-life elimination: 3-8 hours

Excretion: Primarily feces; urine (4% to 6%)

Pregnancy Risk Factor C (manufacturer); A/D (dose exceeding RDA recommendation) (expert analysis)

Calcium Acetate *(KAL see um AS e tate)*

Related Information

Rheumatoid Arthritis, Osteoarthritis, and Osteoporosis *on page 1668*

U.S. Brand Names PhosLo®

Generic Available Yes: Solution for injection

Pharmacologic Category Antidote; Calcium Salt; Phosphate Binder

Use

Oral: Control of hyperphosphatemia in end-stage renal failure; does not promote aluminum absorption

I.V.: Calcium supplementation in parenteral nutrition therapy

Local Anesthetic/Vasoconstrictor Precautions No information available to require special precautions

Effects on Dental Treatment No significant effects or complications reported

Mechanism of Action Combines with dietary phosphate to form insoluble calcium phosphate which is excreted in feces

Pregnancy Risk Factor C

Calcium Acetate and Aluminum Sulfate *see* Aluminum Sulfate and Calcium Acetate *on page 81*

Calcium Acetylhomotaurinate *see* Acamprosate *on page 27*

Calcium and Risedronate *see* Risedronate and Calcium *on page 1354*

Calcium Carbonate *(KAL see um KAR bun ate)*

Related Information

Rheumatoid Arthritis, Osteoarthritis, and Osteoporosis *on page 1668*

U.S. Brand Names Alcalak [OTC]; Alka-Mints® [OTC]; Amitone® [OTC] [DSC]; Calcarb 600 [OTC]; Calci-Chew® [OTC]; Calci-Mix® [OTC]; Cal-Gest [OTC]; Cal-Mint [OTC]; Caltrate® 600 [OTC]; Children's Pepto [OTC]; Chooz® [OTC];

Florical® [OTC]; Maalox® Quick Dissolve [OTC]; Mylanta® Children's [OTC]; Nephro-Calci® [OTC]; Nutralox® [OTC]; Os-Cal® 500 [OTC]; Oysco 500 [OTC]; Oyst-Cal 500 [OTC]; Rolaids® Softchews [OTC]; Titralac™ [OTC]; Titralac™ Extra Strength [OTC]; Tums® [OTC]; Tums® E-X [OTC]; Tums® Extra Strength Sugar Free [OTC]; Tums® Smoothies™ [OTC]; Tums® Ultra [OTC]

Canadian Brand Names Apo-Cal®; Calcite-500; Caltrate®; Caltrate® Select; Os-Cal®

Mexican Brand Names Calsan®; Caltrate®; Osteomin®

Generic Available Yes

Pharmacologic Category Antacid; Antidote; Calcium Salt; Electrolyte Supplement, Oral

Use As an antacid; treatment and prevention of calcium deficiency or hyperphosphatemia (eg, osteoporosis, osteomalacia, mild/moderate renal insufficiency, hypoparathyroidism, postmenopausal osteoporosis, rickets); has been used to bind phosphate

Local Anesthetic/Vasoconstrictor Precautions No information available to require special precautions

Effects on Dental Treatment Key adverse event(s) related to dental treatment: Xerostomia (normal salivary flow resumes upon discontinuation).

Mechanism of Action As dietary supplement, used to prevent or treat negative calcium balance; in osteoporosis, it helps to prevent or decrease the rate of bone loss. The calcium in calcium salts moderates nerve and muscle performance and allows normal cardiac function. Also used to treat hyperphosphatemia in patients with advanced renal insufficiency by combining with dietary phosphate to form insoluble calcium phosphate, which is excreted in feces. Calcium salts as antacids neutralize gastric acidity resulting in increased gastric and duodenal bulb pH; they additionally inhibit proteolytic activity of peptic if the pH is increased >4 and increase lower esophageal sphincter tone.

Calcium Carbonate and Etidronate Disodium *see* Etidronate and Calcium *on page 620*

Calcium Carbonate and Magnesium Hydroxide
(KAL see um KAR bun ate & mag NEE zhum hye DROKS ide)

Related Information
Calcium Carbonate *on page 248*
Magnesium Hydroxide *on page 961*

U.S. Brand Names Mi-Acid™ Double Strength [OTC]; Mylanta® Gelcaps® [OTC]; Mylanta® Supreme [OTC]; Mylanta® Ultra [OTC]; Rolaids® [OTC]; Rolaids® Extra Strength [OTC]

Generic Available Yes: Chewable tablet

Synonyms Magnesium Hydroxide and Calcium Carbonate

Pharmacologic Category Antacid

Use Hyperacidity

Local Anesthetic/Vasoconstrictor Precautions No information available to require special precautions

Effects on Dental Treatment No significant effects or complications reported

---

Calcium Carbonate and Simethicone
(KAL see um KAR bun ate & sye METH i kone)

Related Information
Calcium Carbonate *on page 248*
Simethicone *on page 1394*

U.S. Brand Names Gas Ban™ [OTC]; Titralac® Plus [OTC]

Generic Available No

Synonyms Simethicone and Calcium Carbonate

Pharmacologic Category Antacid; Antiflatulent

Use Relief of acid indigestion, heartburn

Local Anesthetic/Vasoconstrictor Precautions No information available to require special precautions

Effects on Dental Treatment Do not give tetracyclines concomitantly.

Pharmacodynamics/Kinetics See individual agents.

Pregnancy Risk Factor C

Calcium Carbonate, Magnesium Hydroxide, and Famotidine *see* Famotidine, Calcium Carbonate, and Magnesium Hydroxide *on page 636*

Calcium Chloride (KAL see um KLOR ide)

Generic Available Yes

Pharmacologic Category Calcium Salt; Electrolyte Supplement, Parenteral

Use Cardiac resuscitation when epinephrine fails to improve myocardial contractions, cardiac disturbances of hyperkalemia, hypocalcemia; emergent treatment of hypocalcemic tetany; treatment of hypermagnesemia

Unlabeled/Investigational Use

Calcium channel blocker overdose

Local Anesthetic/Vasoconstrictor Precautions No information available to require special precautions

Effects on Dental Treatment No significant effects or complications reported

Mechanism of Action Moderates nerve and muscle performance via action potential excitation threshold regulation

Pregnancy Risk Factor C

Calcium Citrate (KAL see um SIT rate)

Related Information

Rheumatoid Arthritis, Osteoarthritis, and Osteoporosis *on page 1668*

U.S. Brand Names Cal-Citrate® 250 [OTC]; Citracal® [OTC]

Canadian Brand Names Osteocit®

Generic Available Yes

Pharmacologic Category Calcium Salt

Use Antacid; treatment and prevention of calcium deficiency or hyperphosphatemia (eg, osteoporosis, osteomalacia, mild/moderate renal insufficiency, hypoparathyroidism, postmenopausal osteoporosis, rickets)

Local Anesthetic/Vasoconstrictor Precautions No information available to require special precautions

Effects on Dental Treatment No significant effects or complications reported

Mechanism of Action Moderates nerve and muscle performance via action potential excitation threshold regulation

Pregnancy Risk Factor C

Calcium Disodium Edetate *see* Edetate Calcium Disodium *on page 527*

Calcium Disodium Versenate® *see* Edetate Calcium Disodium *on page 527*

Calcium EDTA *see* Edetate Calcium Disodium *on page 527*

Calcium Glubionate (KAL see um gloo BYE oh nate)

Related Information

Rheumatoid Arthritis, Osteoarthritis, and Osteoporosis *on page 1668*

Mexican Brand Names Calcium-Sandoz®

Generic Available Yes

Pharmacologic Category Calcium Salt

Use Adjunct in treatment and prevention of postmenopausal osteoporosis; treatment and prevention of calcium depletion or hyperphosphatemia (eg, osteoporosis, osteomalacia, mild-to-moderate renal insufficiency, hypoparathyroidism, rickets)

Local Anesthetic/Vasoconstrictor Precautions No information available to require special precautions

Effects on Dental Treatment No significant effects or complications reported

Mechanism of Action As dietary supplement, used to prevent or treat negative calcium balance; in osteoporosis, it helps to prevent or decrease the rate of bone loss. The calcium in calcium salts moderates nerve and muscle performance and allows normal cardiac function.

Pregnancy Risk Factor C

Calcium Gluconate (KAL see um GLOO koe nate)

Related Information

Rheumatoid Arthritis, Osteoarthritis, and Osteoporosis *on page 1668*

Generic Available Yes

Pharmacologic Category Calcium Salt; Electrolyte Supplement, Oral; Electrolyte Supplement, Parenteral

Use Treatment and prevention of hypocalcemia; treatment of tetany, cardiac disturbances of hyperkalemia, cardiac resuscitation when epinephrine fails to improve myocardial contractions, hypocalcemia; calcium supplementation

Unlabeled/Investigational Use Hydrofluoric acid (HF) burns; calcium channel blocker overdose

Local Anesthetic/Vasoconstrictor Precautions No information available to require special precautions

Effects on Dental Treatment No significant effects or complications reported

Mechanism of Action As dietary supplement, used to prevent or treat negative calcium balance; in osteoporosis, it helps to prevent or decrease the rate of bone loss. The calcium in calcium salts moderates nerve and muscle performance and allows normal cardiac function.

Pregnancy Risk Factor C

Calcium Lactate (KAL see um LAK tate)

Related Information
Rheumatoid Arthritis, Osteoarthritis, and Osteoporosis *on page 1668*
Generic Available Yes
Pharmacologic Category Calcium Salt
Use Adjunct in prevention of postmenopausal osteoporosis; treatment and prevention of calcium depletion

Local Anesthetic/Vasoconstrictor Precautions No information available to require special precautions

Effects on Dental Treatment No significant effects or complications reported

Mechanism of Action As dietary supplement, used to prevent or treat negative calcium balance; in osteoporosis, it helps to prevent or decrease the rate of bone loss. The calcium in calcium salts moderates nerve and muscle performance and allows normal cardiac function.

Pregnancy Risk Factor C

Calcium Leucovorin see Leucovorin on page 905
Calcium Pantothenate see Pantothenic Acid on page 1186

Calcium Phosphate (Tribasic) (KAL see um FOS fate tri BAY sik)

Related Information
Rheumatoid Arthritis, Osteoarthritis, and Osteoporosis *on page 1668*
U.S. Brand Names Posture® [OTC]
Generic Available No
Synonyms Tricalcium Phosphate
Pharmacologic Category Calcium Salt
Use Dietary supplement

Local Anesthetic/Vasoconstrictor Precautions No information available to require special precautions

Effects on Dental Treatment No significant effects or complications reported

Mechanism of Action As dietary supplement, used to prevent or treat negative calcium balance; in osteoporosis, it helps to prevent or decrease the rate of bone loss. The calcium in calcium salts moderates nerve and muscle performance and allows normal cardiac function.

Caldecort® [OTC] see Hydrocortisone on page 793

Calfactant (kaf AKT ant)

U.S. Brand Names Infasurf®
Generic Available No
Pharmacologic Category Lung Surfactant
Use Prevention of respiratory distress syndrome (RDS) in premature infants at high risk for RDS and for the treatment ("rescue") of premature infants who develop RDS

Prophylaxis: Therapy at birth with calfactant is indicated for premature infants <29 weeks of gestational age at significant risk for RDS. Should be administered as soon as possible, preferably within 30 minutes after birth.

Treatment: For infants ≤72 hours of age with RDS (confirmed by clinical and radiologic findings) and requiring endotracheal intubation.

Local Anesthetic/Vasoconstrictor Precautions No information available to require special precautions

Effects on Dental Treatment No significant effects or complications reported

Common Adverse Effects
Cardiovascular: Bradycardia (34%), cyanosis (65%)
Respiratory: Airway obstruction (39%), reflux (21%), requirement for manual ventilation (16%), reintubation (1% to 10%)
(Continued)

Calfactant *(Continued)*

Mechanism of Action Endogenous lung surfactant is essential for effective ventilation because it modifies alveolar surface tension, thereby stabilizing the alveoli. Lung surfactant deficiency is the cause of respiratory distress syndrome (RDS) in premature infants and lung surfactant restores surface activity to the lungs of these infants.

Pharmacodynamics/Kinetics No human studies of absorption, biotransformation, or excretion have been performed

Cal-Gest [OTC] *see* Calcium Carbonate *on page 248*

Callergy Clear [OTC] *see* Pramoxine *on page 1264*

Cal-Mint [OTC] *see* Calcium Carbonate *on page 248*

Caltrate® 600 [OTC] *see* Calcium Carbonate *on page 248*

Camila™ *see* Norethindrone *on page 1125*

Campath® *see* Alemtuzumab *on page 63*

Campath-1H *see* Alemtuzumab *on page 63*

Campho-Phenique® [OTC] *see* Camphor and Phenol *on page 252*

Camphor and Phenol (KAM for & FEE nole)

Related Information
Phenol *on page 1223*
U.S. Brand Names Campho-Phenique® [OTC]
Generic Available Yes: Liquid
Synonyms Phenol and Camphor
Pharmacologic Category Topical Skin Product
Use Relief of pain and itching associated with minor burns, sunburn, minor cuts, insect bites, minor skin irritation; temporary relief of pain from cold sores
Local Anesthetic/Vasoconstrictor Precautions No information available to require special precautions
Effects on Dental Treatment No significant effects or complications reported
Pregnancy Risk Factor C

Camphorated Tincture of Opium (error-prone synonym) *see* Paregoric *on page 1187*

Campral® *see* Acamprosate *on page 27*

Camptosar® *see* Irinotecan *on page 860*

Camptothecin-11 *see* Irinotecan *on page 860*

Canasa™ *see* Mesalamine *on page 996*

Cancidas® *see* Caspofungin *on page 278*

Candesartan (kan de SAR tan)

Related Information
Cardiovascular Diseases *on page 1636*
U.S. Brand Names Atacand®
Canadian Brand Names Atacand®
Generic Available No
Synonyms Candesartan Cilexetil
Pharmacologic Category Angiotensin II Receptor Blocker
Use Alone or in combination with other antihypertensive agents in treating essential hypertension; treatment of heart failure (NYHA class II-IV)
Local Anesthetic/Vasoconstrictor Precautions No information available to require special precautions
Effects on Dental Treatment No significant effects or complications reported
Common Adverse Effects
Cardiovascular: Angina, hypotension (CHF 19%), MI, palpitation, tachycardia
Central nervous system: Dizziness, lightheadedness, drowsiness, headache, vertigo, anxiety, depression, somnolence, fever
Dermatologic: Angioedema, rash
Endocrine & metabolic: Hyperglycemia, hyperkalemia (CHF <1% to 6%), hypertriglyceridemia, hyperuricemia
Gastrointestinal: Dyspepsia, gastroenteritis
Genitourinary: Hematuria
Neuromuscular & skeletal: Back pain, CPK increased, myalgia, paresthesia, weakness
Renal: Serum creatinine increased (up to 13% in patients with CHF with drug discontinuation required in 6%)
Respiratory: Dyspnea, epistaxis, pharyngitis, rhinitis, upper respiratory tract infection
Miscellaneous: Diaphoresis increased

Dosage Adults: Oral:

Hypertension: Usual dose is 4-32 mg once daily; dosage must be individualized. Blood pressure response is dose related over the range of 2-32 mg. The usual recommended starting dose of 16 mg once daily when it is used as monotherapy in patients who are not volume depleted. It can be administered once or twice daily with total daily doses ranging from 8-32 mg. Larger doses do not appear to have a greater effect and there is relatively little experience with such doses.

Congestive heart failure: Initial: 4 mg once daily; double the dose at 2-week intervals, as tolerated; target dose: 32 mg

Note: In selected cases, concurrent therapy with an ACE inhibitor may provide additional benefit.

Elderly: No initial dosage adjustment is necessary for elderly patients (although higher concentrations (C_{max}) and AUC were observed in these populations), for patients with mildly impaired renal function, or for patients with mildly impaired hepatic function.

Dosage adjustment in hepatic impairment: No initial dosage adjustment required in mild hepatic impairment. Consider initiation at lower dosages in moderate hepatic impairment (AUC increased by 145%). No data available concerning dosing in severe hepatic impairment.

Mechanism of Action Candesartan is an angiotensin receptor antagonist. Angiotensin II acts as a vasoconstrictor. In addition to causing direct vasoconstriction, angiotensin II also stimulates the release of aldosterone. Once aldosterone is released, sodium as well as water are reabsorbed. The end result is an elevation in blood pressure. Candesartan binds to the AT1 angiotensin II receptor. This binding prevents angiotensin II from binding to the receptor thereby blocking the vasoconstriction and the aldosterone secreting effects of angiotensin II.

Contraindications Hypersensitivity to candesartan or any component of the formulation; hypersensitivity to other A-II receptor antagonists; bilateral renal artery stenosis; pregnancy (2nd and 3rd trimesters)

Warnings/Precautions Avoid use or use a smaller dose in patients who are volume depleted; correct depletion first. May be associated with deterioration of renal function and/or increases in serum creatinine, particularly in patients dependent on renin-angiotensin-aldosterone system; deterioration may result in oliguria, acute renal failure and progressive azotemia. Small increases in serum creatinine may occur following initiation; consider discontinuation only in patients with progressive and/or significant deterioration in renal function. Use with caution in unilateral renal artery stenosis, hepatic dysfunction, pre-existing renal insufficiency, or significant aortic/mitral stenosis. Use caution when initiating in heart failure; may need to adjust dose, and/or concurrent diuretic therapy, because of candesartan-induced hypotension. Although some properties may be shared between these agents, concurrent therapy with ACE-inhibitor may be rational in selected patients.

Drug Interactions

Cytochrome P450 Effect: Substrate of CYP2C9 (minor); **Inhibits** CYP2C8 (weak), 2C9 (weak)

Increased Effect/Toxicity: The risk of lithium toxicity may be increased by candesartan; monitor lithium levels. Concurrent use with potassium-sparing diuretics (amiloride, spironolactone, triamterene), potassium supplements, or trimethoprim (high-dose) may increase the risk of hyperkalemia.

Ethanol/Nutrition/Herb Interactions

Food: Food reduces the time to maximal concentration and increases the C_{max}.

Herb/Nutraceutical: Avoid dong quai if using for hypertension (has estrogenic activity). Avoid ephedra, yohimbe, ginseng (may worsen hypertension). Avoid garlic (may have increased antihypertensive effect).

Pharmacodynamics/Kinetics

Onset of action: 2-3 hours

Peak effect: 6-8 hours

Duration: >24 hours

Distribution: V_d: 0.13 L/kg

Protein binding: 99%

Metabolism: To candesartan by the intestinal wall cells

Bioavailability: 15%

Half-life elimination (dose dependent): 5-9 hours

Time to peak: 3-4 hours

Excretion: Urine (26%)

Clearance: Total body: 0.37 mL/kg/minute; Renal: 0.19 mL/kg/minute

Pregnancy Risk Factor C/D (2nd and 3rd trimesters)

Dosage Forms TAB: 4 mg, 8 mg, 16 mg, 32 mg

Candesartan and Hydrochlorothiazide
(kan de SAR tan & hye droe klor oh THYE a zide)

Related Information
Candesartan *on page 252*
Cardiovascular Diseases *on page 1636*
Hydrochlorothiazide *on page 776*
U.S. Brand Names Atacand HCT™
Canadian Brand Names Atacand® Plus
Generic Available No
Synonyms Candesartan Cilexetil and Hydrochlorothiazide
Pharmacologic Category Angiotensin II Receptor Blocker Combination; Antihypertensive Agent, Combination; Diuretic, Thiazide
Use Treatment of hypertension; combination product should not be used for initial therapy
Local Anesthetic/Vasoconstrictor Precautions No information available to require special precautions
Effects on Dental Treatment No significant effects or complications reported
Common Adverse Effects Reactions which follow have been reported with the combination product; see individual drug agents for additional adverse reactions that may be expected from each agent.
1% to 10%:
Central nervous system: Dizziness (3%), headache (3%, placebo 5%)
Neuromuscular & skeletal: Back pain (3%)
Respiratory: Upper respiratory tract infection (4%)
Miscellaneous: Flu-like symptoms (2%)
Mechanism of Action
Candesartan: Candesartan is an angiotensin receptor antagonist. Angiotensin II acts as a vasoconstrictor. In addition to causing direct vasoconstriction, angiotensin II also stimulates the release of aldosterone. Once aldosterone is released, sodium as well as water are reabsorbed. The end result is an elevation in blood pressure. Candesartan binds to the AT1 angiotensin II receptor. This binding prevents angiotensin II from binding to the receptor, thereby blocking the vasoconstriction and the aldosterone-secreting effects of angiotensin II.
Hydrochlorothiazide: Inhibits sodium reabsorption in the distal tubules causing increased excretion of sodium and water as well as potassium and hydrogen ions
Drug Interactions
Cytochrome P450 Effect: Candesartan: Substrate of CYP2C9 (minor); Inhibits CYP2C8 (weak), 2C9 (weak)
Increased Effect/Toxicity: See individual agents.
Decreased Effect: See individual agents.
Pharmacodynamics/Kinetics See individual agents.
Pregnancy Risk Factor C/D (2nd and 3rd trimesters)

Candesartan Cilexetil *see* Candesartan *on page 252*

Candesartan Cilexetil and Hydrochlorothiazide *see* Candesartan and Hydrochlorothiazide *on page 254*

Cankaid® [OTC] *see* Carbamide Peroxide *on page 264*

Cannabidiol and Tetrahydrocannabinol *see* Tetrahydrocannabinol and Cannabidiol *on page 1469*

Cantharidin (kan THAR e din)

Canadian Brand Names Canthacur®; Cantharone®
Generic Available No
Pharmacologic Category Keratolytic Agent
Use Removal of ordinary and periungual warts
Local Anesthetic/Vasoconstrictor Precautions No information available to require special precautions
Effects on Dental Treatment No significant effects or complications reported
Common Adverse Effects 1% to 10%:
Cardiovascular: Syncope
Central nervous system: Delirium, ataxia
Dermatologic: Dermal irritation, dermal burns, acantholysis
Gastrointestinal: GI hemorrhage, rectal bleeding, dysphagia

Genitourinary: Priapism
Hepatic: Fatty degeneration
Neuromuscular & skeletal: Hyper-reflexia
Ocular: Conjunctivitis, iritis, keratitis
Renal: Proteinuria, hematuria
Respiratory: Burning of oropharynx
Pregnancy Risk Factor C

Cantil® [DSC] *see* Mepenzolate *on page 983*
Capastat® Sulfate *see* Capreomycin *on page 256*

Capecitabine (ka pe SITE a been)

Related Information
Fluorouracil *on page 674*
U.S. Brand Names Xeloda®
Canadian Brand Names Xeloda®
Mexican Brand Names Xeloda®
Generic Available No
Synonyms NSC-712807
Pharmacologic Category Antineoplastic Agent, Antimetabolite
Use Treatment of metastatic colorectal cancer; adjuvant therapy of Dukes' C colon cancer; treatment of metastatic breast cancer
Local Anesthetic/Vasoconstrictor Precautions No information available to require special precautions
Effects on Dental Treatment Key adverse event(s) related to dental treatment: Stomatitis, abnormal taste, and taste disturbance.
Common Adverse Effects Frequency listed derived from monotherapy trials.
>10%:
Cardiovascular: Edema (9% to 15%)
Central nervous system: Fatigue (16% to 42%), fever (7% to 18%), pain (12%)
Dermatologic: Palmar-plantar erythrodysesthesia (hand-and-foot syndrome) (54% to 60%; grade 3: 11% to 17%; may be dose limiting), dermatitis (27% to 37%)
Gastrointestinal: Diarrhea (47% to 57%; may be dose limiting; grade 3: 12% to 13%; grade 4: 2% to 3%), nausea (34% to 53%), vomiting (15% to 37%), abdominal pain (7% to 35%), stomatitis (22% to 25%), appetite decreased (26%), anorexia (9% to 23%), constipation (9% to 15%)
Hematologic: Lymphopenia (94%; grade 4: 14%), anemia (72% to 80%; grade 4: <1% to 1%), neutropenia (2% to 26%; grade 4: 2%), thrombocytopenia (24%; grade 4: 1%)
Hepatic: Bilirubin increased (22% to 48%; grades 3/4: 11% to 23%)
Neuromuscular & skeletal: Paresthesia (21%)
Ocular: Eye irritation (13% to 15%)
Respiratory: Dyspnea (14%)
5% to 10%:
Cardiovascular: Venous thrombosis (8%), chest pain (6%)
Central nervous system: Headache (5% to 10%), lethargy (10%), dizziness (6% to 8%), insomnia (7% to 8%), mood alteration (5%), depression (5%)
Dermatologic: Nail disorder (7%), rash (7%), skin discoloration (7%), alopecia (6%), erythema (6%)
Endocrine & metabolic: Dehydration (7%)
Gastrointestinal: Motility disorder (10%), oral discomfort (10%), dyspepsia (6% to 8%), upper GI inflammatory disorders (colorectal cancer: 8%), hemorrhage (6%), ileus (6%), taste perversion (colorectal cancer: 6%)
Neuromuscular & skeletal: Back pain (10%), weakness (10%), neuropathy (10%), myalgia (9%), arthralgia (8%), limb pain (6%)
Ocular: Abnormal vision (colorectal cancer: 5%), conjunctivitis (5%)
Respiratory: Cough (7%)
Miscellaneous: Viral infection (colorectal cancer: 5%)
Mechanism of Action Capecitabine is a prodrug of fluorouracil. It undergoes hydrolysis in the liver and tissues to form fluorouracil which is the active moiety. Fluorouracil is a fluorinated pyrimidine antimetabolite that inhibits thymidylate synthetase, blocking the methylation of deoxyuridylic acid to thymidylic acid, interfering with DNA, and to a lesser degree, RNA synthesis. Fluorouracil appears to be phase specific for the G_1 and S phases of the cell cycle.
Drug Interactions
Increased Effect/Toxicity: Phenytoin and warfarin levels or effects may be increased.
Pharmacodynamics/Kinetics
Absorption: Rapid and extensive
(Continued)

Capecitabine *(Continued)*

Protein binding: <60%; ~35% to albumin
Metabolism:
Hepatic: Inactive metabolites: 5'-deoxy-5-fluorocytidine, 5'-deoxy-5-fluorouridine
Tissue: Active metabolite: Fluorouracil
Half-life elimination: 0.5-1 hour
Time to peak: 1.5 hours; Fluorouracil: 2 hours
Excretion: Urine (96%, 57% as α-fluoro-β-alanine); feces (<3%)
Pregnancy Risk Factor D

Capex™ *see Fluocinolone on page 667*

Capital® and Codeine *see Acetaminophen and Codeine on page 35*

Capitrol® [DSC] *see Chloroxine on page 322*

Capoten® *see Captopril on page 257*

Capozide® *see Captopril and Hydrochlorothiazide on page 259*

Capreomycin *(kap ree oh MYE sin)*

Related Information
Tuberculosis *on page 1673*
U.S. Brand Names Capastat® Sulfate
Generic Available No
Synonyms Capreomycin Sulfate
Pharmacologic Category Antibiotic, Miscellaneous; Antitubercular Agent
Use Treatment of tuberculosis in conjunction with at least one other anti-tuberculosis agent
Local Anesthetic/Vasoconstrictor Precautions No information available to require special precautions
Effects on Dental Treatment No significant effects or complications reported
Common Adverse Effects
>10%:
Otic: Ototoxicity [subclinical hearing loss (11%), clinical loss (3%)], tinnitus
Renal: Nephrotoxicity (36%, increased BUN)
1% to 10%: Hematologic: Eosinophilia (dose related, mild)
Mechanism of Action Capreomycin is a cyclic polypeptide antimicrobial. It is administered as a mixture of capreomycin IA and capreomycin IB. The mechanism of action of capreomycin is not well understood. Mycobacterial species that have become resistant to other agents are usually still sensitive to the action of capreomycin. However, significant cross-resistance with viomycin, kanamycin, and neomycin occurs.
Drug Interactions
Increased Effect/Toxicity: May increase effect/duration of nondepolarizing neuromuscular blocking agents. Additive toxicity (nephrotoxicity and ototoxicity), respiratory paralysis may occur with aminoglycosides (eg, streptomycin).
Pharmacodynamics/Kinetics
Half-life elimination: Normal renal function: 4-6 hours
Time to peak, serum: I.M.: ~1 hour
Excretion: Urine (as unchanged drug)
Pregnancy Risk Factor C

Capreomycin Sulfate *see Capreomycin on page 256*

Capsagel® [OTC] *see Capsaicin on page 256*

Capsaicin *(kap SAY sin)*

Related Information
Cayenne *on page 1617*
U.S. Brand Names ArthriCare® for Women Extra Moisturizing [OTC]; ArthriCare® for Women Multi-Action [OTC]; ArthriCare® for Women Silky Dry [OTC]; ArthriCare® for Women Ultra Strength [OTC] [DSC]; Capsagel® [OTC]; Capzasin-HP® [OTC]; Capzasin-P® [OTC]; Zostrix® [OTC]; Zostrix®-HP [OTC]
Canadian Brand Names Zostrix®; Zostrix® H.P.
Generic Available Yes: Cream
Pharmacologic Category Analgesic, Topical; Topical Skin Product
Use Topical treatment of pain associated with postherpetic neuralgia, rheumatoid arthritis, osteoarthritis, diabetic neuropathy; postsurgical pain

Unlabeled/Investigational Use Treatment of pain associated with psoriasis, chronic neuralgias unresponsive to other forms of therapy, and intractable pruritus

Local Anesthetic/Vasoconstrictor Precautions No information available to require special precautions

Effects on Dental Treatment No significant effects or complications reported

Common Adverse Effects Frequency not defined.
  Dermatologic: Itching, stinging sensation, erythema
  Local: Transient burning on application which usually diminishes with repeated use
  Respiratory: Cough

Mechanism of Action Induces release of substance P, the principal chemomediator of pain impulses from the periphery to the CNS, from peripheral sensory neurons; after repeated application, capsaicin depletes the neuron of substance P and prevents reaccumulation

Drug Interactions
  Cytochrome P450 Effect: Substrate of CYP2E1 (minor)

Pharmacodynamics/Kinetics
  Onset of action: 14-28 days
    Peak effect: 4-6 weeks of continuous therapy
  Duration: Several hours

Pregnancy Risk Factor C

Captopril (KAP toe pril)

Related Information
  Cardiovascular Diseases *on page 1636*

U.S. Brand Names Capoten®

Canadian Brand Names Alti-Captopril; Apo-Capto®; Capoten™; Gen-Captopril; Novo-Captopril; Nu-Capto; PMS-Captopril

Mexican Brand Names Capoten®; Captral®; Cardipril®; Cryopril®; Ecaten®; Kenolan®; Lenpryl®; Romir®

Generic Available Yes

Synonyms ACE

Pharmacologic Category Angiotensin-Converting Enzyme (ACE) Inhibitor

Use Management of hypertension; treatment of congestive heart failure, left ventricular dysfunction after myocardial infarction, diabetic nephropathy

Unlabeled/Investigational Use Treatment of hypertensive crisis, rheumatoid arthritis; diagnosis of anatomic renal artery stenosis, hypertension secondary to scleroderma renal crisis; diagnosis of aldosteronism, idiopathic edema, Bartter's syndrome, postmyocardial infarction for prevention of ventricular failure; increase circulation in Raynaud's phenomenon, hypertension secondary to Takayasu's disease

Local Anesthetic/Vasoconstrictor Precautions No information available to require special precautions

Effects on Dental Treatment Key adverse event(s) related to dental treatment: Loss or diminished perception of taste and orthostatic hypotension.

Common Adverse Effects
  1% to 10%:
    Cardiovascular: Hypotension (1% to 3%), tachycardia (1%), chest pain (1%), palpitation (1%)
    Dermatologic: Rash (maculopapular or urticarial) (4% to 7%), pruritus (2%); in patients with rash, a positive ANA and/or eosinophilia has been noted in 7% to 10%.
    Endocrine & metabolic: Hyperkalemia (1% to 11%)
    Hematologic: Neutropenia may occur in up to 4% of patients with renal insufficiency or collagen-vascular disease.
    Renal: Proteinuria (1%), serum creatinine increased, worsening of renal function (may occur in patients with bilateral renal artery stenosis or hypovolemia)
    Respiratory: Cough (<1% to 2%)
    Miscellaneous: Hypersensitivity reactions (rash, pruritus, fever, arthralgia, and eosinophilia) have occurred in 4% to 7% of patients (depending on dose and renal function); dysgeusia - loss of taste or diminished perception (2% to 4%)
  Frequency not defined:
    Cardiovascular: Angioedema, cardiac arrest, cerebrovascular insufficiency, rhythm disturbances, orthostatic hypotension, syncope, flushing, pallor, angina, MI, Raynaud's syndrome, CHF
    Central nervous system: Ataxia, confusion, depression, nervousness, somnolence
  (Continued)

Captopril (Continued)

Dermatologic: Bullous pemphigus, erythema multiforme, Stevens-Johnson syndrome, exfoliative dermatitis

Endocrine & metabolic: Alkaline phosphatase increased, bilirubin increased, gynecomastia

Gastrointestinal: Pancreatitis, glossitis, dyspepsia

Genitourinary: Urinary frequency, impotence

Hematologic: Anemia, thrombocytopenia, pancytopenia, agranulocytosis, anemia

Hepatic: Jaundice, hepatitis, hepatic necrosis (rare), cholestasis, hyponatremia (symptomatic), transaminases increased

Neuromuscular & skeletal: Asthenia, myalgia, myasthenia

Ocular: Blurred vision

Renal: Renal insufficiency, renal failure, nephrotic syndrome, polyuria, oliguria

Respiratory: Bronchospasm, eosinophilic pneumonitis, rhinitis

Miscellaneous: Anaphylactoid reactions

Dosage Note: Dosage must be titrated according to patient's response; use lowest effective dose. Oral:

Infants: Initial: 0.15-0.3 mg/kg/dose; titrate dose upward to maximum of 6 mg/kg/day in 1-4 divided doses; usual required dose: 2.5-6 mg/kg/day

Children: Initial: 0.5 mg/kg/dose; titrate upward to maximum of 6 mg/kg/day in 2-4 divided doses

Older Children: Initial: 6.25-12.5 mg/dose every 12-24 hours; titrate upward to maximum of 6 mg/kg/day

Adolescents: Initial: 12.5-25 mg/dose given every 8-12 hours; increase by 25 mg/dose to maximum of 450 mg/day

Adults:

Acute hypertension (urgency/emergency): 12.5-25 mg, may repeat as needed (may be given sublingually, but no therapeutic advantage demonstrated)

Hypertension:

Initial dose: 12.5-25 mg 2-3 times/day; may increase by 12.5-25 mg/dose at 1- to 2-week intervals up to 50 mg 3 times/day; maximum dose: 150 mg 3 times/day; add diuretic before further dosage increases

Usual dose range (JNC 7): 25-100 mg/day in 2 divided doses

Congestive heart failure:

Initial dose: 6.25-12.5 mg 3 times/day in conjunction with cardiac glycoside and diuretic therapy; initial dose depends upon patient's fluid/electrolyte status

Target dose: 50 mg 3 times/day

LVD after MI: Initial dose: 6.25 mg followed by 12.5 mg 3 times/day; then increase to 25 mg 3 times/day during next several days and then over next several weeks to target dose of 50 mg 3 times/day

Diabetic nephropathy: 25 mg 3 times/day; other antihypertensives often given concurrently

Dosing adjustment in renal impairment:

Cl_{cr} 10-50 mL/minute: Administer at 75% of normal dose.

Cl_{cr} <10 mL/minute: Administer at 50% of normal dose.

Note: Smaller dosages given every 8-12 hours are indicated in patients with renal dysfunction; renal function and leukocyte count should be carefully monitored during therapy.

Hemodialysis: Moderately dialyzable (20% to 50%); administer dose postdialysis or administer 25% to 35% supplemental dose.

Peritoneal dialysis: Supplemental dose is not necessary.

Mechanism of Action Competitive inhibitor of angiotensin-converting enzyme (ACE); prevents conversion of angiotensin I to angiotensin II, a potent vasoconstrictor; results in lower levels of angiotensin II which causes an increase in plasma renin activity and a reduction in aldosterone secretion

Contraindications Hypersensitivity to captopril or any component of the formulation; angioedema related to previous treatment with an ACE inhibitor; idiopathic or hereditary angioedema; bilateral renal artery stenosis; pregnancy (2nd or 3rd trimester)

Warnings/Precautions Anaphylactic reactions can occur. Angioedema can occur at any time during treatment (especially following first dose). It may involve head and neck (potentially affecting the airway) or the intestine (presenting with abdominal pain). Prolonged monitoring may be required especially if tongue, glottis, or larynx are involved as they are associated with airway obstruction. Those with a history of airway surgery in this situation have a higher risk. Careful blood pressure monitoring with first dose (hypotension can occur especially in volume-depleted patients). Use with caution in collagen vascular diseases; valvular stenosis (particularly aortic stenosis); hyperkalemia; or before, during, or immediately after anesthesia. Avoid rapid dosage escalation which may lead to renal insufficiency. Rare toxicities associated with ACE inhibitors include cholestatic jaundice (which may progress to hepatic necrosis) and neutropenia/agranulocytosis with myeloid hyperplasia. If patient has renal impairment, then a baseline WBC with differential and serum creatinine should be evaluated and monitored closely during the first 3 months of therapy. Hypersensitivity reactions may be seen during hemodialysis with high-flux dialysis membranes (eg, AN69). Deterioration in renal function can occur with initiation.

Use with caution and decrease dosage in patients with renal impairment (especially renal artery stenosis), severe CHF, or with coadministered diuretic therapy; experience in children is limited. Severe hypotension may occur in patients who are sodium and/or volume depleted; initiate lower doses and monitor closely when starting therapy in these patients. ACE inhibitors may be preferred agents in elderly patients with CHF and diabetes mellitus (diabetic proteinuria is reduced, minimal CNS effects, and enhanced insulin sensitivity); however, due to decreased renal function, tolerance must be carefully monitored.

Drug Interactions
Cytochrome P450 Effect: Substrate of CYP2D6 (major)
Increased Effect/Toxicity: Potassium supplements, co-trimoxazole (high dose), angiotensin II receptor antagonists (candesartan, losartan, irbesartan, etc), or potassium-sparing diuretics (amiloride, spironolactone, triamterene) may result in elevated serum potassium levels when combined with captopril. CYP2D6 inhibitors may increase the levels/effects of captopril; example inhibitors include chlorpromazine, delavirdine, fluoxetine, miconazole, paroxetine, pergolide, quinidine, quinine, ritonavir, and ropinirole. ACE inhibitor effects may be increased by phenothiazines or probenecid (increases levels of captopril). ACE inhibitors may increase serum concentrations/effects of lithium.

Diuretics have additive hypotensive effects with ACE inhibitors, and hypovolemia increases the potential for adverse renal effects of ACE inhibitors. In patients with compromised renal function, coadministration with NSAIDs may result in further deterioration of renal function. Allopurinol and ACE inhibitors may cause a higher risk of hypersensitivity reaction when taken concurrently.

Decreased Effect: Aspirin (high dose) may reduce the therapeutic effects of ACE inhibitors; at low dosages this does not appear to be significant. Rifampin may decrease the effect of ACE inhibitors. Antacids may decrease the bioavailability of ACE inhibitors (may be more likely to occur with captopril); separate administration times by 1-2 hours. NSAIDs, specifically indomethacin, may reduce the hypotensive effects of ACE inhibitors. More likely to occur in low renin or volume-dependent hypertensive patients.

Ethanol/Nutrition/Herb Interactions
Food: Captopril serum concentrations may be decreased if taken with food. Long-term use of captopril may result in a zinc deficiency which can result in a decrease in taste perception.
Herb/Nutraceutical: Avoid dong quai if using for hypertension (has estrogenic activity). Avoid ephedra, yohimbe, ginseng (may worsen hypertension). Avoid garlic (may have increased antihypertensive effect).
Dietary Considerations Should be taken at least 1 hour before or 2 hours after eating.

Pharmacodynamics/Kinetics
Onset of action: Peak effect: Blood pressure reduction: 1-1.5 hours after dose
Duration: Dose related, may require several weeks of therapy before full hypotensive effect
Absorption: 60% to 75%; reduced 30% to 40% by food
Protein binding: 25% to 30%
Metabolism: 50%
Half-life elimination (renal and cardiac function dependent):
Adults, healthy volunteers: 1.9 hours; Congestive heart failure: 2.06 hours; Anuria: 20-40 hours
Excretion: Urine (95%) within 24 hours
Pregnancy Risk Factor C (1st trimester)/D (2nd and 3rd trimesters)
Dosage Forms TAB: 12.5 mg, 25 mg, 50 mg, 100 mg

Captopril and Hydrochlorothiazide
(KAP toe pril & hye droe klor oh THYE a zide)

Related Information
Captopril on page 257
Cardiovascular Diseases on page 1636
Hydrochlorothiazide on page 776
U.S. Brand Names Capozide®
Canadian Brand Names Capozide®
Generic Available Yes
(Continued)

Captopril and Hydrochlorothiazide *(Continued)*

Synonyms Hydrochlorothiazide and Captopril

Pharmacologic Category Antihypertensive Agent, Combination

Use Management of hypertension and treatment of congestive heart failure

Local Anesthetic/Vasoconstrictor Precautions No information available to require special precautions

Effects on Dental Treatment No significant effects or complications reported

Common Adverse Effects See individual agents.

Mechanism of Action Captopril is a competitive inhibitor of angiotensin-converting enzyme (ACE); prevents conversion of angiotensin I to angiotensin II, a potent vasoconstrictor. This results in lower levels of angiotensin II which causes an increase in plasma renin activity and a reduction in aldosterone secretion. Hydrochlorothiazide inhibits sodium reabsorption in the distal tubules causing increased excretion of sodium and water as well as potassium and hydrogen ions.

Drug Interactions

Cytochrome P450 Effect: Captopril: **Substrate** of CYP2D6 (major)

Increased Effect/Toxicity: See individual agents.

Decreased Effect: See individual agents.

Pharmacodynamics/Kinetics See individual agents.

Pregnancy Risk Factor C/D (2nd and 3rd trimesters)

Capzasin-HP® [OTC] *see* Capsaicin *on page 256*

Capzasin-P® [OTC] *see* Capsaicin *on page 256*

Carac™ *see* Fluorouracil *on page 674*

Carafate® *see* Sucralfate *on page 1420*

Carbachol *(KAR ba kole)*

U.S. Brand Names Carbastat® [DSC]; Isopto® Carbachol; Miostat®

Canadian Brand Names Isopto® Carbachol; Miostat®

Generic Available No

Synonyms Carbacholine; Carbamylcholine Chloride

Pharmacologic Category Cholinergic Agonist; Ophthalmic Agent, Antiglaucoma; Ophthalmic Agent, Miotic

Use Lowers intraocular pressure in the treatment of glaucoma; cause miosis during surgery

Local Anesthetic/Vasoconstrictor Precautions No information available to require special precautions

Effects on Dental Treatment Key adverse event(s) related to dental treatment: Increased salivation.

Mechanism of Action Synthetic direct-acting cholinergic agent that causes miosis by stimulating muscarinic receptors in the eye

Pregnancy Risk Factor C

Carbacholine *see* Carbachol *on page 260*

Carbamazepine *(kar ba MAZ e peen)*

U.S. Brand Names Carbatrol®; Epitol®; Equetro™; Tegretol®; Tegretol®-XR

Canadian Brand Names Apo-Carbamazepine®; Gen-Carbamazepine CR; Novo-Carbamaz; Nu-Carbamazepine; PMS-Carbamazepine; Taro-Carbamazepine Chewable; Tegretol®

Mexican Brand Names Carbazep®; Carbazina®; Clostedal®; Neugeron®; Tegretol®

Generic Available Yes: Excludes capsule (extended release), tablet (extended release)

Synonyms CBZ; SPD417

Pharmacologic Category Anticonvulsant, Miscellaneous

Dental Use Pain relief of trigeminal or glossopharyngeal neuralgia

Use

Carbatrol®, Tegretol®, Tegretol®-XR: Partial seizures with complex symptomatology (psychomotor, temporal lobe), generalized tonic-clonic seizures (grand mal), mixed seizure patterns, trigeminal neuralgia

Equetro™: Acute manic and mixed episodes associated with bipolar 1 disorder

Unlabeled/Investigational Use Treatment of resistant schizophrenia, ethanol withdrawal, restless leg syndrome, psychotic behavior associated with dementia, post-traumatic stress disorders

Local Anesthetic/Vasoconstrictor Precautions No information available to require special precautions

Effects on Dental Treatment Key adverse event(s) related to dental treatment: Oral ulceration.

Significant Adverse Effects Frequency not defined, unless otherwise specified.

Cardiovascular: Arrhythmias, AV block, bradycardia, chest pain (bipolar use), CHF, edema, hyper-/hypotension, lymphadenopathy, syncope, thromboembolism, thrombophlebitis

Central nervous system: Amnesia (bipolar use), anxiety (bipolar use), aseptic meningitis (case report), ataxia (bipolar use 15%), confusion, depression (bipolar use), dizziness (bipolar use 44%), fatigue, headache (bipolar use 22%), sedation, slurred speech, somnolence (bipolar use 32%)

Dermatologic: Alopecia, alterations in skin pigmentation, erythema multiforme, exfoliative dermatitis, photosensitivity reaction, pruritus (bipolar use 8%), purpura, rash, Stevens-Johnson syndrome, toxic epidermal necrolysis, urticaria

Endocrine & metabolic: Chills, fever, hyponatremia, syndrome of inappropriate ADH secretion (SIADH)

Gastrointestinal: Abdominal pain, anorexia, constipation, diarrhea, dyspepsia (bipolar use), gastric distress, nausea (bipolar use 29%), pancreatitis, vomiting (bipolar use 18%), xerostomia (bipolar use)

Genitourinary: Azotemia, impotence, renal failure, urinary frequency, urinary retention

Hematologic: Acute intermittent porphyria, agranulocytosis, aplastic anemia, bone marrow suppression, eosinophilia, leukocytosis, leukopenia, pancytopenia, thrombocytopenia

Hepatic: Abnormal liver function tests, hepatic failure, hepatitis, jaundice

Neuromuscular & skeletal: Back pain, pain (bipolar use 12%), peripheral neuritis, weakness

Ocular: Blurred vision, conjunctivitis, lens opacities, nystagmus

Otic: Hyperacusis, tinnitus

Miscellaneous: Diaphoresis, hypersensitivity (including multiorgan reactions, may include disorders mimicking lymphoma, eosinophilia, hepatosplenomegaly, vasculitis); infection (bipolar use 12%)

Dental Usual Dosing Trigeminal or glossopharyngeal neuralgia: Oral:

Adults: Initial: 100 mg twice daily with food, gradually increasing in increments of 100 mg twice daily as needed

Maintenance: Usual: 400-800 mg daily in 2 divided doses; maximum dose: 1200 mg/day

Elderly: 100 mg 1-2 times daily, increase in increments of 100 mg/day at weekly intervals until therapeutic level is achieved; usual dose: 400-1000 mg/day

Dosage Dosage must be adjusted according to patient's response and serum concentrations. Administer tablets (chewable or conventional) in 2-3 divided doses daily and suspension in 4 divided doses daily. Oral:

Epilepsy:

Children:

<6 years: Initial: 10-20 mg/kg/day divided twice or 3 times daily as tablets or 4 times/day as suspension; increase dose every week until optimal response and therapeutic levels are achieved

Maintenance dose: Divide into 3-4 doses daily (tablets or suspension); maximum recommended dose: 35 mg/kg/day

6-12 years: Initial: 100 mg twice daily (tablets or extended release tablets) or 50 mg of suspension 4 times/day (200 mg/day); increase by up to 100 mg/day at weekly intervals using a twice daily regimen of extended release tablets or 3-4 times daily regimen of other formulations until optimal response and therapeutic levels are achieved

Maintenance: Usual: 400-800 mg/day; maximum recommended dose: 1000 mg/day

Note: Children <12 years who receive ≥400 mg/day of carbamazepine may be converted to extended release capsules (Carbatrol®) using the same total daily dosage divided twice daily

Children >12 years and Adults: Initial: 200 mg twice daily (tablets, extended release tablets, or extended release capsules) or 100 mg of suspension 4 times/day (400 mg daily); increase by up to 200 mg/day at weekly intervals using a twice daily regimen of extended release tablets or capsules, or a 3-4 times/day regimen of other formulations until optimal response and therapeutic levels are achieved; usual dose: 800-1200 mg/day

Maximum recommended doses:

Children 12-15 years: 1000 mg/day

Children >15 years: 1200 mg/day

Adults: 1600 mg/day; however, some patients have required up to 1.6-2.4 g/day

(Continued)

Carbamazepine *(Continued)*

Trigeminal or glossopharyngeal neuralgia: Adults: Initial: 100 mg twice daily with food, gradually increasing in increments of 100 mg twice daily as needed
Maintenance: Usual: 400-800 mg daily in 2 divided doses; maximum dose: 1200 mg/day

Elderly: 100 mg 1-2 times daily, increase in increments of 100 mg/day at weekly intervals until therapeutic level is achieved; usual dose: 400-1000 mg/day

Bipolar disorder (Equetro™): Adults: Initial: 400 mg/day in divided doses, twice daily; may adjust by 200 mg daily increments; maximum dose: 1600 mg/day

Mechanism of Action In addition to anticonvulsant effects, carbamazepine has anticholinergic, antineuralgic, antidiuretic, muscle relaxant, antimanic, antidepressive, and antiarrhythmic properties; may depress activity in the nucleus ventralis of the thalamus or decrease synaptic transmission or decrease summation of temporal stimulation leading to neural discharge by limiting influx of sodium ions across cell membrane or other unknown mechanisms; stimulates the release of ADH and potentiates its action in promoting reabsorption of water; chemically related to tricyclic antidepressants

Contraindications Hypersensitivity to carbamazepine, tricyclic antidepressants, or any component of the formulation; bone marrow depression; with or within 14 days of MAO inhibitor use; pregnancy

Warnings/Precautions Administer carbamazepine with caution to patients with history of cardiac damage, hepatic or renal disease. Potentially fatal blood cell abnormalities have been reported following treatment. Patients with a previous history of adverse hematologic reaction to any drug may be at increased risk. Early detection of hematologic change is important; advise patients of early signs and symptoms including fever, sore throat, mouth ulcers, infections, easy bruising, petechial or purpuric hemorrhage. Prescriptions should be written for the smallest quantity consistent with good patient care. The smallest effective dose is suggested for use in bipolar disorder to reduce the risk for overdose; high-risk patients should be monitored. Actuation of latent psychosis is possible.

Carbamazepine is not effective in absence, myoclonic, or akinetic seizures; exacerbation of certain seizure types have been seen after initiation of carbamazepine therapy in children with mixed seizure disorders. Abrupt discontinuation is not recommended in patients being treated for seizures. Dizziness or drowsiness may occur; caution should be used when performing tasks which require alertness (operating machinery or driving) until the effects are known. Coadministration of carbamazepine and delavirdine may lead to loss of virologic response and possible resistance. Elderly may have increased risk of SIADH-like syndrome. Carbamazepine has mild anticholinergic activity; use with caution in patients with increased intraocular pressure (monitor closely), or sensitivity to anticholinergic effects (urinary retention, constipation). Severe dermatologic reactions, including Lyell and Stevens-Johnson syndromes, although rarely reported, have resulted in fatalities. Drug should be discontinued if there are any signs of hypersensitivity.

Drug Interactions Substrate of CYP2C8 (minor), 3A4 (major); **Induces** CYP1A2 (strong), 2B6 (strong), 2C8 (strong), 2C9 (strong), 2C19 (strong), 3A4 (strong)

Acetaminophen: Carbamazepine may enhance hepatotoxic potential of acetaminophen; risk is greater in acetaminophen overdose.

Antimalarial drugs (chloroquine, mefloquine): Concomitant use with carbamazepine may reduce seizure control by lowering plasma levels; monitor.

Antipsychotics: Carbamazepine may enhance the metabolism (decrease the efficacy) of antipsychotics; monitor for altered response; dose adjustment may be needed.

Barbiturates: May reduce serum concentrations of carbamazepine; monitor.

Benzodiazepines: Serum concentrations and effect of benzodiazepines may be reduced by carbamazepine; monitor for decreased effect.

Calcium channel blockers: Diltiazem and verapamil may increase carbamazepine levels, due to enzyme inhibition (see below); other calcium channel blockers (felodipine) may be decreased by carbamazepine due to enzyme induction.

Chlorpromazine: **Note:** Carbamazepine suspension is incompatible with chlorpromazine solution. Schedule carbamazepine suspension at least 1-2 hours apart from other liquid medicinals.

Corticosteroids: Metabolism may be increased by carbamazepine.

Cyclosporine (and other immunosuppressants): Carbamazepine may enhance the metabolism of immunosuppressants, decreasing its clinical effect; includes both cyclosporine and tacrolimus.

CYP1A2 substrates: Carbamazepine may decrease the levels/effects of CYP1A2 substrates. Example substrates include aminophylline, estrogens, fluvoxamine, mirtazapine, ropinirole, and theophylline.

CYP2B6 substrates: Carbamazepine may decrease the levels/effects of CYP2B6 substrates. Example substrates include bupropion, efavirenz, promethazine, selegiline, and sertraline.

CYP2C8 Substrates: Carbamazepine may decrease the levels/effects of CYP2C8 substrates. Example substrates include amiodarone, paclitaxel, pioglitazone, repaglinide, and rosiglitazone.

CYP2C9 substrates: Carbamazepine may decrease the levels/effects of CYP2C9 substrates. Example substrates include bosentan, celecoxib, dapsone, fluoxetine, glimepiride, glipizide, losartan, montelukast, nateglinide, paclitaxel, phenytoin, sulfonamides, trimethoprim, warfarin, and zafirlukast.

CYP2C19 substrates: Carbamazepine may decrease the levels/effects of CYP2C19 substrates. Example substrates include citalopram, diazepam, methsuximide, phenytoin, propranolol, proton pump inhibitors, sertraline, and voriconazole.

CYP3A4 inducers: CYP3A4 inducers may decrease the levels/effects of carbamazepine. Example inducers include aminoglutethimide, nafcillin, nevirapine, phenobarbital, phenytoin, and rifamycins. Carbamazepine may induce its own metabolism.

CYP3A4 inhibitors: May increase the levels/effects of carbamazepine. Example inhibitors include azole antifungals, clarithromycin, diclofenac, doxycycline, erythromycin, imatinib, isoniazid, nefazodone, nicardipine, propofol, protease inhibitors, quinidine, telithromycin, and verapamil.

CYP3A4 substrates: Carbamazepine may decrease the levels/effects of CYP3A4 substrates. Example substrates include benzodiazepines, calcium channel blockers, clarithromycin, cyclosporine, erythromycin, estrogens, mirtazapine, nateglinide, nefazodone, nevirapine, protease inhibitors, tacrolimus, and venlafaxine.

Danazol: May increase serum concentrations of carbamazepine; monitor.

Delavirdine: May lead to loss of virologic response and possible resistance.

Doxycycline: Carbamazepine may enhance the metabolism of doxycycline, decreasing its clinical effect.

Ethosuximide: Serum levels may be reduced by carbamazepine.

Felbamate: May increase carbamazepine levels and toxicity (increased epoxide metabolite concentrations); carbamazepine may decrease felbamate levels due to enzyme induction.

Immunosuppressants: Carbamazepine may enhance the metabolism of immunosuppressants, decreasing its clinical effect; includes both cyclosporine and tacrolimus.

Isoniazid: May increase the serum concentrations and toxicity of carbamazepine; in addition, carbamazepine may increase the hepatic toxicity of isoniazid (INH).

Isotretinoin: May decrease the effect of carbamazepine.

Lamotrigine: Increases the epoxide metabolite of carbamazepine resulting in toxicity; carbamazepine increases the metabolism of lamotrigine.

Lithium: Neurotoxicity may result in patients receiving concurrent carbamazepine.

Loxapine: May increase concentrations of epoxide metabolite and toxicity of carbamazepine.

Methadone: Carbamazepine may enhance the metabolism of methadone resulting in methadone withdrawal.

Methylphenidate: concurrent use of carbamazepine may reduce the therapeutic effect of methylphenidate; limited documentation; monitor for decreased effect.

Neuromuscular blocking agents, nondepolarizing: Effects may be of shorter duration when administered to patients receiving carbamazepine.

Oral contraceptives: Metabolism may be increased by carbamazepine, resulting in a loss of efficacy.

Phenytoin: Carbamazepine levels may be decreased by phenytoin. Metabolism of phenytoin may be altered by carbamazepine; phenytoin levels may be increased or decreased.

SSRIs: Metabolism may be increased by carbamazepine (due to enzyme induction).

Theophylline: Serum levels may be reduced by carbamazepine.

Thioridazine: **Note:** Carbamazepine suspension is incompatible with thioridazine liquid. Schedule carbamazepine suspension at least 1-2 hours apart from other liquid medicinals.

Thyroid: Serum levels may be reduced by carbamazepine.

Tramadol: Tramadol's risk of seizures may be increased with TCAs (carbamazepine may be associated with similar risk due to chemical similarity to TCAs).
(Continued)

Carbamazepine *(Continued)*

Tricyclic antidepressants: May increase serum concentrations of carbamazepine; carbamazepine may decrease concentrations of tricyclics due to enzyme induction.

Valproic acid: Serum levels may be reduced by carbamazepine; carbamazepine levels may also be altered by valproic acid.

Warfarin: Carbamazepine may inhibit the hypoprothrombinemic effects of oral anticoagulants via increased metabolism; this combination should generally be avoided.

Ethanol/Nutrition/Herb Interactions

Ethanol: Avoid ethanol (may increase CNS depression).

Food: Carbamazepine serum levels may be increased if taken with food. Carbamazepine serum concentration may be increased if taken with grapefruit juice; avoid concurrent use.

Herb/Nutraceutical: Avoid evening primrose (seizure threshold decreased). Avoid valerian, St John's wort, kava kava, gotu kola (may increase CNS depression).

Dietary Considerations Drug may cause GI upset, take with large amount of water or food to decrease GI upset. May need to split doses to avoid GI upset.

Pharmacodynamics/Kinetics

Absorption: Slow

Distribution: V_d: Neonates: 1.5 L/kg; Children: 1.9 L/kg; Adults: 0.59-2 L/kg

Protein binding: Carbamazepine: 75% to 90%, may be decreased in newborns; Epoxide metabolite: 50%

Metabolism: Hepatic via CYP3A4 to active epoxide metabolite; induces hepatic enzymes to increase metabolism

Bioavailability: 85%

Half-life elimination:

Carbamazepine: Initial: 18-55 hours; Multiple doses: Children: 8-14 hours; Adults: 12-17 hours

Epoxide metabolite: Initial: 25-43 hours

Time to peak, serum: Unpredictable:

Immediate release: Suspension: 1.5 hour; tablet: 4-5 hours

Extended release: Carbatrol®, Equetro™: 12-26 hours (single dose), 4-8 hours (multiple doses); Tegretol®-XR: 3-12 hours

Excretion: Urine 72% (1% to 3% as unchanged drug); feces (28%)

Pregnancy Risk Factor D

Lactation Enters breast milk/not recommended (AAP rates "compatible")

Breast-Feeding Considerations Carbamazepine and its metabolites are found in breast milk. The manufacturer does not recommend use while breast-feeding. However, AAP rates this medication "compatible" in breast-feeding.

Dosage Forms

Capsule, extended release (Carbatrol®, Equetro™): 100 mg, 200 mg, 300 mg

Suspension, oral: 100 mg/5 mL (10 mL, 450 mL)

Tegretol®: 100 mg/5 mL (450 mL) [citrus vanilla flavor]

Tablet (Epitol®, Tegretol®): 200 mg

Tablet, chewable (Tegretol®): 100 mg

Tablet, extended release (Tegretol®-XR): 100 mg, 200 mg, 400 mg

Carbamide *see* Urea *on page 1551*

Carbamide Peroxide (KAR ba mide per OKS ide)

Related Information

Oral Rinse Products *on page 1831*

U.S. Brand Names Cankaid® [OTC]; Debrox® [OTC]; Dent's Ear Wax [OTC]; E•R•O [OTC]; Gly-Oxide® [OTC]; Murine® Ear Wax Removal System [OTC]; Orajel® Perioseptic® Spot Treatment [OTC]

Generic Available Yes

Synonyms Urea Peroxide

Pharmacologic Category Anti-inflammatory, Locally Applied; Otic Agent, Cerumenolytic

Dental Use Relief of minor inflammation of gums, oral mucosal surfaces, and lips (including canker sores and dental irritation)

Use Relief of minor inflammation of gums, oral mucosal surfaces, and lips including canker sores and dental irritation; emulsify and disperse ear wax

Local Anesthetic/Vasoconstrictor Precautions No information available to require special precautions

Effects on Dental Treatment No significant effects or complications reported

Significant Adverse Effects Frequency not defined.

Dermatologic: Rash

Local: Irritation, redness

Miscellaneous: Superinfection

Dental Usual Dosing Minor inflammation of gums, oral mucosal surfaces and lips: Children and Adults: Topical: Oral solution (should not be used for >7 days): Apply several drops undiluted on affected area 4 times/day after meals and at bedtime; expectorate after 2-3 minutes **or** place 10 drops onto tongue, mix with saliva, swish for several minutes, expectorate

Dosage Children and Adults:

Oral: Inflammation/dental irritation: Solution (should not be used for >7 days): Oral preparation should not be used in children <2 years of age; apply several drops undiluted on affected area 4 times/day after meals and at bedtime; expectorate after 2-3 minutes **or** place 10 drops onto tongue, mix with saliva, swish for several minutes, expectorate

Otic:

Children <12 years: Tilt head sideways and individualize the dose according to patient size; 3 drops (range: 1-5 drops) twice daily for up to 4 days, tip of applicator should not enter ear canal; keep drops in ear for several minutes by keeping head tilted and placing cotton in ear

Children ≥12 years and Adults: Tilt head sideways and instill 5-10 drops twice daily up to 4 days, tip of applicator should not enter ear canal; keep drops in ear for several minutes by keeping head tilted and placing cotton in ear

Mechanism of Action Carbamide peroxide releases hydrogen peroxide which serves as a source of nascent oxygen upon contact with catalase; deodorant action is probably due to inhibition of odor-causing bacteria; softens impacted cerumen due to its foaming action

Contraindications Hypersensitivity to carbamide peroxide or any component of the formulation; otic preparation should not be used in patients with a perforated tympanic membrane; ear drainage, ear pain, or rash in the ear

Warnings/Precautions

Oral: With prolonged use of oral carbamide peroxide, there is a potential for overgrowth of opportunistic organisms, damage to periodontal tissues, and delayed wound healing; should not be used for longer than 7 days. Not for OTC use in children <2 years of age.

Otic: Do not use if ear drainage or discharge, ear pain, irritation, or rash in ear. Should not be used for longer than 4 days. Not for OTC use in children <12 years of age.

Drug Interactions No data reported

Pharmacodynamics/Kinetics Onset of action: ~24 hours

Pregnancy Risk Factor C

Dosage Forms

Solution, oral: 10% (60 mL)

Cankaid®: 10% (22 mL) [in anhydrous glycerol]

Gly-Oxide®: 10% (15 mL, 60 mL) [contains glycerin]

Orajel® Perioseptic® Spot Treatment: 15% (13.3 mL) [contains anhydrous glycerin]

Solution, otic: 6.5% (15 mL)

Debrox®: 6.5% (15 mL, 30 mL) [contains propylene glycol]

Dent's Ear Wax: 6.5% (3.7 mL) [contains glycerin]

E•R•O: 6.5% (15 mL)

Murine® Ear Wax Removal System: 6.5% (15 mL) [contains alcohol 6.3% and glycerin]

Carbamylcholine Chloride *see* Carbachol *on page 260*

Carbastat® [DSC] *see* Carbachol *on page 260*

Carbatrol® *see* Carbamazepine *on page 260*

Carbaxefed DM RF *see* Carbinoxamine, Pseudoephedrine, and Dextromethorphan *on page 269*

Carbaxefed RF *see* Carbinoxamine and Pseudoephedrine *on page 268*

Carbenicillin (kar ben i SIL in)

U.S. Brand Names Geocillin®

Generic Available No

Synonyms Carbenicillin Indanyl Sodium; Carindacillin

Pharmacologic Category Antibiotic, Penicillin

Use Treatment of serious urinary tract infections and prostatitis caused by susceptible gram-negative aerobic bacilli

Local Anesthetic/Vasoconstrictor Precautions No information available to require special precautions

(Continued)

Carbenicillin *(Continued)*

Effects on Dental Treatment Key adverse event(s) related to dental treatment: Unpleasant taste and glossitis. Prolonged use of penicillins may lead to development of oral candidiasis.

Common Adverse Effects

>10%: Gastrointestinal: Diarrhea

1% to 10%: Gastrointestinal: Nausea, bad taste, vomiting, flatulence, glossitis

Mechanism of Action Inhibits bacterial cell wall synthesis by binding to one or more of the penicillin-binding proteins (PBPs) which in turn inhibits the final transpeptidation step of peptidoglycan synthesis in bacterial cell walls, thus inhibiting cell wall biosynthesis. Bacteria eventually lyse due to ongoing activity of cell wall autolytic enzymes (autolysins and murein hydrolases) while cell wall assembly is arrested.

Drug Interactions

Increased Effect/Toxicity: Increased bleeding effects if taken with high doses of heparin or oral anticoagulants. Aminoglycosides may be synergistic against selected organisms. Penicillins may increase the exposure to methotrexate during concurrent therapy; monitor. Probenecid and disulfiram may increase levels of penicillins (carbenicillin).

Decreased Effect: Decreased effectiveness with tetracyclines. Although anecdotal reports suggest oral contraceptive efficacy could be reduced by penicillins, this has been refuted by more rigorous scientific and clinical data.

Pharmacodynamics/Kinetics

Absorption: 30% to 40%

Distribution: Crosses placenta; small amounts enter breast milk; distributes into bile; low concentrations attained in CSF

Protein binding: ~50%

Half-life elimination: Children: 0.8-1.8 hours; Adults: 1-1.5 hours, prolonged to 10-20 hours with renal insufficiency

Time to peak, serum: Normal renal function: 0.5-2 hours; concentrations are inadequate for treatment of systemic infections

Excretion: Urine (~80% to 99% as unchanged drug)

Pregnancy Risk Factor B

Carbenicillin Indanyl Sodium *see* Carbenicillin *on page 265*

Carbetapentane and Chlorpheniramine
(kar bay ta PEN tane & klor fen IR a meen)

Related Information

Chlorpheniramine *on page 323*

U.S. Brand Names Tannate 12 S; Tannic-12; Tannic-12 S; Tannihist-12 RF; Tussi-12®; Tussi-12 S™; Tussizone-12 RF™

Generic Available Yes

Synonyms Carbetapentane Tannate and Chlorpheniramine Tannate; Chlorpheniramine and Carbetapentane

Pharmacologic Category Antihistamine/Antitussive

Use Symptomatic relief of cough associated with upper respiratory tract conditions, such as the common cold, bronchitis, bronchial asthma

Local Anesthetic/Vasoconstrictor Precautions No information available to require special precautions

Effects on Dental Treatment Key adverse event(s) related to dental treatment: Dry mucous membranes. Chronic use of antihistamines will inhibit salivary flow, particularly in elderly patients; this may contribute to periodontal disease and oral discomfort.

Common Adverse Effects Frequency not defined.

Central nervous system: Drowsiness, excitation (children), sedation

Gastrointestinal: GI motility decreased, dry mucous membranes

Mechanism of Action Carbetapentane is a nonopioid cough suppressant; chlorpheniramine is an H_1-receptor antagonist

Drug Interactions

Increased Effect/Toxicity: Sedative effects of CNS depressants may be potentiated. MAO inhibitors may increase and prolong anticholinergic effects. Avoid use with and within 14 days of treatment with MAO inhibitors.

Pharmacodynamics/Kinetics

Carbetapentane: Data not available

Chlorpheniramine: See individual agents

Pregnancy Risk Factor C

Carbetapentane, Ephedrine, Phenylephrine, and Chlorpheniramine *see* Chlorpheniramine, Ephedrine, Phenylephrine, and Carbetapentane *on page 325*

Carbetapentane, Phenylephrine, and Pyrilamine
(kay bay ta PEN tane, fen il EF rin, & peer II a meen)

Related Information
Phenylephrine *on page 1226*
U.S. Brand Names Tussi-12® D; Tussi-12® DS
Generic Available Yes: Suspension
Synonyms Phenylephrine Tannate, Carbetapentane Tannate, and Pyrilamine Tannate; Pyrilamine, Phenylephrine, and Carbetapentane
Pharmacologic Category Antihistamine; Antihistamine/Decongestant/Antitussive; Antitussive; Decongestant
Use Symptomatic relief of cough associated with respiratory tract conditions such as the common cold, bronchial asthma, acute and chronic bronchitis
Local Anesthetic/Vasoconstrictor Precautions Use with caution since phenylephrine is a sympathomimetic amine which could interact with epinephrine to cause a pressor response
Effects on Dental Treatment Key adverse event(s) related to dental treatment: Tachycardia, palpitations (use vasoconstrictor with caution), and xerostomia (normal salivary flow resumes upon discontinuation).
Mechanism of Action
Carbetapentane is a nonopioid cough suppressant
Phenylephrine hydrochloride is a sympathomimetic agent (primarily alpha), decongestant.
Pyrilamine is an H_1-receptor antagonist.
Pregnancy Risk Factor C

Carbetapentane Tannate and Chlorpheniramine Tannate *see* Carbetapentane and Chlorpheniramine *on page 266*

Carbidopa (kar bi DOE pa)

U.S. Brand Names Lodosyn®
Generic Available No
Pharmacologic Category Anti-Parkinson's Agent, Dopamine Agonist
Use Given with levodopa in the treatment of parkinsonism to enable a lower dosage of levodopa to be used and a more rapid response to be obtained and to decrease side effects; for details of administration and dosage; has no effect without levodopa
Local Anesthetic/Vasoconstrictor Precautions No information available to require special precautions
Effects on Dental Treatment Key adverse event(s) related to dental treatment: Orthostatic hypotension. Dopaminergic therapy in Parkinson's disease includes the use of carbidopa in combination with levodopa. Carbidopa/levodopa combination is associated with orthostatic hypotension. Patients medicated with this drug combination should be carefully assisted from the chair and observed for signs of orthostatic hypotension.
Common Adverse Effects Adverse reactions are associated with concomitant administration with levodopa
>10%: Central nervous system: Anxiety, confusion, nervousness, mental depression
1% to 10%:
Cardiovascular: Orthostatic hypotension, palpitation, cardiac arrhythmia
Central nervous system: Memory loss, insomnia, fatigue, hallucinations, ataxia, dystonic movements
Gastrointestinal: Nausea, vomiting, GI bleeding
Ocular: Blurred vision
Mechanism of Action Carbidopa is a peripheral decarboxylase inhibitor with little or no pharmacological activity when given alone in usual doses. It inhibits the peripheral decarboxylation of levodopa to dopamine; and as it does not cross the blood-brain barrier, unlike levodopa, effective brain concentrations of dopamine are produced with lower doses of levodopa. At the same time, reduced peripheral formation of dopamine reduces peripheral side-effects, notably nausea and vomiting, and cardiac arrhythmias, although the dyskinesias and adverse mental effects associated with levodopa therapy tend to develop earlier.
Pharmacodynamics/Kinetics
Absorption: 40% to 70%
Distribution: Does not cross the blood-brain barrier; in rats, reported to cross placenta and be excreted in milk
Protein binding: 36%
Half-life elimination: 1-2 hours
(Continued)

Carbidopa *(Continued)*

Excretion: Urine (as unchanged drug and metabolites)
Pregnancy Risk Factor C

Carbidopa and Levodopa *see* Levodopa and Carbidopa *on page 911*

Carbidopa, Levodopa, and Entacapone *see* Levodopa, Carbidopa, and Entacapone *on page 912*

Carbihist *see* Carbinoxamine *on page 268*

Carbinoxamine (kar bi NOKS a meen)

U.S. Brand Names Carbihist; Carbinoxamine PD; Carboxine; Histex™ CT; Histex™ I/E; Histex™ PD; Histex™ PD-12; Palgic; Pediatex™; Pediatex™ 12
Generic Available Yes: Liquid
Synonyms Carbinoxamine Maleate; Carbinoxamine Tannate
Pharmacologic Category Antihistamine
Use Seasonal and perennial allergic rhinitis; urticaria

Local Anesthetic/Vasoconstrictor Precautions No information available to require special precautions

Effects on Dental Treatment Key adverse event(s) related to dental treatment: Xerostomia (normal salivary flow resumes upon discontinuation).

Common Adverse Effects Frequency not defined.

Central nervous system: Dizziness, excitability (children), headache, nervousness, sedation

Gastrointestinal: Anorexia, diarrhea, heartburn, nausea, vomiting, xerostomia

Neuromuscular & skeletal: Weakness

Ocular: Diplopia

Renal: Polyuria

Mechanism of Action Carbinoxamine competes with histamine for H_1-receptor sites on effector cells in the gastrointestinal tract, blood vessels, and respiratory tract.

Drug Interactions

Increased Effect/Toxicity: Increased sedation/CNS depression with barbiturates, other CNS depressants, and tricyclic antidepressants. Anticholinergic effects may be increased by MAO inhibitors.

Pharmacodynamics/Kinetics Half-life elimination: 10-20 hours

Pregnancy Risk Factor C

Carbinoxamine and Pseudoephedrine
(kar bi NOKS a meen & soo doe e FED rin)

Related Information

Carbinoxamine *on page 268*

Pseudoephedrine *on page 1309*

U.S. Brand Names Andehist NR Drops; Carbaxefed RF; Carboxine-PSE; Cordron-D NR; Hydro-Tussin™-CBX; Palgic®-D; Palgic®-DS; Pediatex™-D; Rondec® Drops [DSC]; Rondec® Tablets; Rondec-TR®; Sildec
Generic Available Yes
Synonyms Pseudoephedrine and Carbinoxamine
Pharmacologic Category Adrenergic Agonist Agent; Antihistamine, H_1 Blocker; Decongestant
Use Seasonal and perennial allergic rhinitis; vasomotor rhinitis

Local Anesthetic/Vasoconstrictor Precautions Use with caution since pseudoephedrine is a sympathomimetic amine which could interact with epinephrine to cause a pressor response

Effects on Dental Treatment Key adverse event(s) related to dental treatment: Pseudoephedrine: Xerostomia (normal salivary flow resumes upon discontinuation).

Common Adverse Effects Frequency not defined.

Cardiovascular: Arrhythmias, cardiovascular collapse, hypertension, pallor, tachycardia

Central nervous system: Anxiety, convulsions, CNS stimulation, dizziness, excitability (children; rare), fear, hallucinations, headache, insomnia, nervousness, restlessness, sedation

Gastrointestinal: Anorexia, diarrhea, dyspepsia, nausea, vomiting, xerostomia

Neuromuscular skeletal: Tremors, weakness

Ocular: Diplopia

Renal: Dysuria, polyuria, urinary retention (with BPH)

Respiratory: Respiratory difficulty

Mechanism of Action Carbinoxamine competes with histamine for H_1-receptor sites on effector cells in the gastrointestinal tract, blood vessels, and respiratory tract; pseudoephedrine, a sympathomimetic amine and isomer of ephedrine, acts as a decongestant in respiratory tract mucous membranes with less vasoconstrictor action than ephedrine in normotensive individuals

Drug Interactions
Increased Effect/Toxicity: Increased sedation/CNS depression with barbiturates and other CNS depressants. Anticholinergic effects may be increased by MAO inhibitors, tricyclic antidepressants.
Decreased Effect: May decrease effects of antihypertensive agents.

Pregnancy Risk Factor C

Carbinoxamine, Dextromethorphan, and Pseudoephedrine see Carbinoxamine, Pseudoephedrine, and Dextromethorphan on page 269

Carbinoxamine Maleate see Carbinoxamine on page 268

Carbinoxamine PD see Carbinoxamine on page 268

Carbinoxamine, Pseudoephedrine, and Dextromethorphan
(kar bi NOKS a meen, soo doe e FED rin, & deks troe meth OR fan)

Related Information
Carbinoxamine on page 268
Dextromethorphan on page 451
Pseudoephedrine on page 1309
U.S. Brand Names Andehist DM NR Drops; Carbaxefed DM RF; Cordron-DM NR; Decahist-DM; Pediatex™ DM [DSC]; Rondec®-DM Drops [DSC]; Sildec-DM; Tussafed®

Generic Available Yes

Synonyms Carbinoxamine, Dextromethorphan, and Pseudoephedrine; Dextromethorphan, Carbinoxamine, and Pseudoephedrine; Dextromethorphan, Pseudoephedrine, and Carbinoxamine; Pseudoephedrine, Carbinoxamine, and Dextromethorphan; Pseudoephedrine, Dextromethorphan, and Carbinoxamine

Pharmacologic Category Antihistamine/Decongestant/Antitussive

Use Relief of coughs and upper respiratory symptoms, including nasal congestion, associated with allergy or the common cold

Local Anesthetic/Vasoconstrictor Precautions Use with caution since pseudoephedrine is a sympathomimetic amine which could interact with epinephrine to cause a pressor response

Effects on Dental Treatment Key adverse event(s) related to dental treatment: Pseudoephedrine: Xerostomia (normal salivary flow resumes upon discontinuation).

Common Adverse Effects Frequency not defined.
Cardiovascular: Arrhythmias, cardiovascular collapse, hypertension, pallor, tachycardia
Central nervous system: Anxiety, convulsions, CNS stimulation, dizziness, drowsiness, excitability (children; rare), fear, hallucinations, headache, insomnia, nervousness, restlessness, sedation
Gastrointestinal: Anorexia, diarrhea, dyspepsia, GI upset, nausea, vomiting, xerostomia
Neuromuscular skeletal: Tremors, weakness
Ocular: Diplopia
Renal: Dysuria, polyuria, urinary retention (with BPH)
Respiratory: Respiratory difficulty

Mechanism of Action Carbinoxamine competes with histamine for H_1-receptor sites on effector cells in the gastrointestinal tract, blood vessels, and respiratory tract; pseudoephedrine, a sympathomimetic amine and isomer of ephedrine, acts as a decongestant in respiratory tract mucous membranes with less vasoconstrictor action than ephedrine in normotensive individuals; dextromethorphan, a non-narcotic antitussive, increases cough threshold by its activity on the medulla oblongata.

Drug Interactions
Cytochrome P450 Effect: Dextromethorphan: **Substrate** of CYP2B6 (minor), 2C9 (minor), 2C19 (minor), 2D6 (major), 2E1 (minor), 3A4 (minor); **Inhibits** CYP2D6 (weak)

Pregnancy Risk Factor C

Carbinoxamine, Pseudoephedrine, and Hydrocodone see Hydrocodone, Carbinoxamine, and Pseudoephedrine on page 789

Carbinoxamine Tannate see Carbinoxamine on page 268

Carbocaine® see Mepivacaine on page 987

Carbocaine® 2% with Neo-Cobefrin® *see* Mepivacaine and Levonordefrin *on page 991*
Carbolic Acid *see* Phenol *on page 1223*

Carboplatin (KAR boe pla tin)

U.S. Brand Names Paraplatin®
Canadian Brand Names Paraplatin-AQ
Mexican Brand Names Blastocarb®; Carbotec®; Paraplatin®
Generic Available Yes
Synonyms CBDCA
Pharmacologic Category Antineoplastic Agent, Alkylating Agent
Use Treatment of ovarian cancer
Unlabeled/Investigational Use Lung cancer, head and neck cancer, endometrial cancer, esophageal cancer, bladder cancer, breast cancer, cervical cancer, CNS tumors, germ cell tumors, osteogenic sarcoma, and high-dose therapy with stem cell/bone marrow support
Local Anesthetic/Vasoconstrictor Precautions No information available to require special precautions
Effects on Dental Treatment Key adverse event(s) related to dental treatment: Stomatitis.
Common Adverse Effects
>10%:
Dermatologic: Alopecia
Endocrine & metabolic: Hypomagnesemia, hypokalemia, hyponatremia, hypocalcemia; less severe than those seen after cisplatin (usually asymptomatic)
Gastrointestinal: Nausea, vomiting, stomatitis
Hematologic: Myelosuppression (dose related and dose limiting), thrombocytopenia (37% to 80%), leukopenia (27% to 38%)
Nadir: ~21 days following a single dose
Hepatic: Alkaline phosphatase increased, AST increased (usually mild and reversible)
Otic: Hearing loss at high tones (above speech ranges, up to 19%); clinically-important ototoxicity is not usually seen
Renal: BUN and/or creatinine increased
1% to 10%:
Gastrointestinal: Diarrhea, anorexia
Hematologic: Hemorrhagic complications
Local: Pain at injection site
Neuromuscular & skeletal: Peripheral neuropathy (4% to 6%; up to 10% in older and/or previously-treated patients)
Otic: Ototoxicity
Mechanism of Action Carboplatin is an alkylating agent which covalently binds to DNA; possible cross-linking and interference with the function of DNA
Drug Interactions
Increased Effect/Toxicity: Nephrotoxic drugs; aminoglycosides increase risk of ototoxicity. When administered as sequential infusions, observational studies indicate a potential for increased toxicity when platinum derivatives (carboplatin, cisplatin) are administered before taxane derivatives (docetaxel, paclitaxel).
Pharmacodynamics/Kinetics
Distribution: V_d: 16 L/kg; into liver, kidney, skin, and tumor tissue
Protein binding: 0%; platinum is 30% irreversibly bound
Metabolism: Minimally hepatic to aquated and hydroxylated compounds
Half-life elimination: Terminal: 22-40 hours; Cl_{cr} >60 mL/minute: 2.5-5.9 hours
Excretion: Urine (~60% to 90%) within 24 hours
Pregnancy Risk Factor D

Carboprost *see* Carboprost Tromethamine *on page 270*

Carboprost Tromethamine (KAR boe prost tro METH a meen)

U.S. Brand Names Hemabate®
Canadian Brand Names Hemabate®
Generic Available No
Synonyms Carboprost
Pharmacologic Category Abortifacient; Prostaglandin
Use Termination of pregnancy and refractory postpartum uterine bleeding
Unlabeled/Investigational Use Investigational: Hemorrhagic cystitis

Local Anesthetic/Vasoconstrictor Precautions No information available to require special precautions

Effects on Dental Treatment No significant effects or complications reported

Common Adverse Effects
>10%: Gastrointestinal: Nausea (33%)
1% to 10%: Cardiovascular: Flushing (7%)

Mechanism of Action Carboprost tromethamine is a prostaglandin similar to prostaglandin F_2 alpha (dinoprost) except for the addition of a methyl group at the C-15 position. This substitution produces longer duration of activity than dinoprost; carboprost stimulates uterine contractility which usually results in expulsion of the products of conception and is used to induce abortion between 13-20 weeks of pregnancy. Hemostasis at the placentation site is achieved through the myometrial contractions produced by carboprost.

Drug Interactions
Increased Effect/Toxicity: Toxicity may be increased by oxytocic agents.
Pharmacodynamics/Kinetics Excretion: Urine
Pregnancy Risk Factor X

Carbose D see Carboxymethylcellulose on page 271

Carboxine see Carbinoxamine on page 268

Carboxine-PSE see Carbinoxamine and Pseudoephedrine on page 268

Carboxymethylcellulose (kar boks ee meth il SEL yoo lose)

U.S. Brand Names Refresh Liquigel™ [OTC]; Refresh Plus® [OTC]; Refresh Tears® [OTC]; Tears Again® Gel Drops™ [OTC]; Tears Again® Night and Day™ [OTC]; Theratears®
Canadian Brand Names Celluvisc™; Refresh Plus®; Refresh Tears®
Generic Available Yes
Synonyms Carbose D; Carboxymethylcellulose Sodium
Pharmacologic Category Ophthalmic Agent, Miscellaneous
Use Artificial tear substitute
Local Anesthetic/Vasoconstrictor Precautions No information available to require special precautions
Effects on Dental Treatment No significant effects or complications reported

Carboxymethylcellulose Sodium see Carboxymethylcellulose on page 271

Cardene® see NiCARdipine on page 1107

Cardene® I.V. see NiCARdipine on page 1107

Cardene® SR see NiCARdipine on page 1107

Cardizem® see Diltiazem on page 479

Cardizem® CD see Diltiazem on page 479

Cardizem® LA see Diltiazem on page 479

Cardizem® SR [DSC] see Diltiazem on page 479

Cardura® see Doxazosin on page 503

Cardura® XL see Doxazosin on page 503

Carimune™ NF see Immune Globulin (Intravenous) on page 824

Carindacillin see Carbenicillin on page 265

Carisoprodate see Carisoprodol on page 271

Carisoprodol (kar eye soe PROE dole)

U.S. Brand Names Soma®
Canadian Brand Names Soma®
Generic Available Yes
Synonyms Carisoprodate; Isobamate
Pharmacologic Category Skeletal Muscle Relaxant
Dental Use Treatment of muscle spasms and pain associated with acute temporomandibular joint (TMJ) pain
Use Skeletal muscle relaxant
Local Anesthetic/Vasoconstrictor Precautions No information available to require special precautions
Effects on Dental Treatment No significant effects or complications reported
Significant Adverse Effects
>10%: Central nervous system: Drowsiness
1% to 10%:
Cardiovascular: Tachycardia, tightness in chest, flushing of face, syncope
Central nervous system: Mental depression, allergic fever, dizziness, lightheadedness, headache, paradoxical CNS stimulation
Dermatologic: Angioedema, dermatitis (allergic)
(Continued)

Carisoprodol *(Continued)*

Gastrointestinal: Nausea, vomiting, stomach cramps
Neuromuscular & skeletal: Trembling
Ocular: Burning eyes
Respiratory: Dyspnea
Miscellaneous: Hiccups

<1% (Limited to important or life-threatening): Aplastic anemia, clumsiness, eosinophilia, erythema multiforme, leukopenia, rash, urticaria

Dental Usual Dosing Treatment of muscle spasms and pain associated with acute TMJ pain: Adults: Oral: 350 mg 3-4 times/day; take last dose at bedtime; compound: 1-2 tablets 4 times/day

Dosage Oral: Adults: 350 mg 3-4 times/day; take last dose at bedtime; compound: 1-2 tablets 4 times/day

Mechanism of Action Precise mechanism is not yet clear, but many effects have been ascribed to its central depressant actions

Contraindications Hypersensitivity to carisoprodol, meprobamate, or any component of the formulation; acute intermittent porphyria

Warnings/Precautions May cause CNS depression, which may impair physical or mental abilities. Effects with other sedative drugs or ethanol may be potentiated. Use with caution in patients with hepatic/renal dysfunction. Tolerance or drug dependence may result from extended use.

Drug Interactions Substrate of CYP2C19 (major)Increased toxicity: Ethanol, CNS depressants, phenothiazines

CYP2C19 inhibitors: May increase the levels/effects of carisoprodol. Example inhibitors include delavirdine, fluconazole, fluvoxamine, gemfibrozil, isoniazid, omeprazole, and ticlopidine.

Ethanol/Nutrition/Herb Interactions Ethanol: Avoid ethanol (may increase CNS depression).

Pharmacodynamics/Kinetics
Onset of action: ~30 minutes
Duration: 4-6 hours
Distribution: Crosses placenta; high concentrations enter breast milk
Metabolism: Hepatic
Half-life elimination: 8 hours
Excretion: Urine

Pregnancy Risk Factor C

Lactation Enters breast milk (high concentrations)/not recommended

Dosage Forms Tablet: 350 mg

Carisoprodol and Aspirin *(kar eye soe PROE dole & AS pir in)*

Related Information
Aspirin *on page 145*
Carisoprodol *on page 271*

U.S. Brand Names Soma® Compound

Generic Available Yes

Synonyms Aspirin and Carisoprodol

Pharmacologic Category Skeletal Muscle Relaxant

Dental Use Treatment of muscle spasms and pain associated with acute temporomandibular joint pain (TMJ)

Use Skeletal muscle relaxant

Local Anesthetic/Vasoconstrictor Precautions No information available to require special precautions

Effects on Dental Treatment Key adverse event(s) related to dental treatment: Elderly are a high-risk population for adverse effects from nonsteroidal anti-inflammatory agents. As many as 60% of elderly patients with GI complications from NSAIDs can develop peptic ulceration and/or hemorrhage asymptomatically. Concomitant disease and drug use contribute to the risk of GI adverse effects. Use lowest effective dose for shortest period possible. Consider renal function decline with age.

Dental Usual Dosing Treatment of muscle spasms and pain associated with acute TMJ pain: Adults: Oral: 1-2 tablets 4 times/day

Dosage Oral: Adults: 1-2 tablets 4 times/day

Drug Interactions
Carisoprodol: **Substrate** of CYP2C19 (major)
Aspirin: **Substrate** of CYP2C9 (minor)
Also see individual agents.

Ethanol/Nutrition/Herb Interactions Ethanol: Avoid ethanol (may increase CNS depression).

Pharmacodynamics/Kinetics See individual agents.

Pregnancy Risk Factor C/D (full-dose aspirin in 3rd trimester)
Lactation Enters breast milk/contraindicated
Dosage Forms Tablet: Carisoprodol 200 mg and aspirin 325 mg

Carisoprodol, Aspirin, and Codeine
(kar eye soe PROE dole, AS pir in, and KOE deen)

Related Information
Aspirin *on page 145*
Carisoprodol *on page 271*
Codeine *on page 385*
U.S. Brand Names Soma® Compound w/Codeine
Generic Available Yes
Synonyms Aspirin, Carisoprodol, and Codeine; Codeine, Aspirin, and Carisoprodol
Pharmacologic Category Skeletal Muscle Relaxant
Dental Use Treatment of muscle spasms and pain associated with acute temporomandibular joint pain (TMJ)
Use Skeletal muscle relaxant
Local Anesthetic/Vasoconstrictor Precautions No information available to require special precautions
Effects on Dental Treatment Key adverse event(s) related to dental treatment: Elderly are a high-risk population for adverse effects from nonsteroidal anti-inflammatory agents. As many as 60% of elderly patients with GI complications from NSAIDs can develop peptic ulceration and/or hemorrhage asymptomatically. Concomitant disease and drug use contribute to the risk of GI adverse effects. Use lowest effective dose for shortest period possible. Consider renal function decline with age.
Restrictions C-III
Dental Usual Dosing Treatment of muscle spasms and pain associated with acute TMJ pain: Adults: Oral: 1 or 2 tablets 4 times/day
Dosage Oral: Adults: 1 or 2 tablets 4 times/day
Drug Interactions
Carisoprodol: **Substrate** of CYP2C19 (major)
Aspirin: **Substrate** of CYP2C9 (minor)
Also see individual agents.
Ethanol/Nutrition/Herb Interactions Ethanol: Avoid ethanol (may increase CNS depression).
Pharmacodynamics/Kinetics See individual agents.
Pregnancy Risk Factor C/D (full-dose aspirin in 3rd trimester)
Lactation Enters breast milk/contraindicated
Dosage Forms Tablet: Carisoprodol 200 mg, aspirin 325 mg, and codeine phosphate 16 mg

Carmol® 10 [OTC] *see Urea on page 1551*
Carmol® 20 [OTC] *see Urea on page 1551*
Carmol® 40 *see Urea on page 1551*
Carmol® Deep Cleaning *see Urea on page 1551*
Carmol-HC® *see Urea and Hydrocortisone on page 1551*
Carmol® Scalp *see Sulfacetamide on page 1423*

Carmustine (kar MUS teen)

U.S. Brand Names BiCNu®; Gliadel®
Canadian Brand Names BiCNu®; Gliadel Wafer®
Mexican Brand Names BiCNu®
Generic Available No
Synonyms BCNU; bis-chloronitrosourea; Carmustinum; NSC-409962; WR-139021
Pharmacologic Category Antineoplastic Agent; Antineoplastic Agent, Alkylating Agent (Nitrosourea); Antineoplastic Agent, DNA Adduct-Forming Agent; Antineoplastic Agent, DNA Binding Agent
Use
Injection: Treatment of brain tumors (glioblastoma, brainstem glioma, medulloblastoma, astrocytoma, ependymoma, and metastatic brain tumors), multiple myeloma, Hodgkin's disease, non-Hodgkin's lymphomas, melanoma, lung cancer, colon cancer
Wafer (implant): Adjunct to surgery in patients with recurrent glioblastoma multiforme; adjunct to surgery and radiation in patients with high-grade malignant glioma
(Continued)

Carmustine *(Continued)*

Local Anesthetic/Vasoconstrictor Precautions No information available to require special precautions

Effects on Dental Treatment Key adverse event(s) related to dental treatment: Stomatitis.

Common Adverse Effects

>10%:

Cardiovascular: Hypotension (with high dose therapy, due to the alcohol content of the diluent)

Central nervous system: Dizziness, ataxia; Wafers: Seizures (54%) postoperatively

Dermatologic: Hyperpigmentation of skin (with skin contact)

Gastrointestinal: Severe nausea and vomiting, usually begins within 2-4 hours of drug administration and lasts for 4-6 hours; dose related. Patients should receive a prophylactic antiemetic regimen.

Hematologic: Myelosuppression - cumulative, dose related, delayed, thrombocytopenia is usually more common and more severe than leukopenia

Onset (days): 7-14

Nadir (days): 21-35

Recovery (days): 42-56

Hepatic: Reversible increases in bilirubin, alkaline phosphatase, and SGOT occur in 20% to 25% of patients

Local: Pain and burning at injection site; phlebitis

Ocular: Ocular toxicities (transient conjunctival flushing and blurred vision), retinal hemorrhages

Respiratory: Interstitial fibrosis occurs in up to 50% of patients receiving a cumulative dose >1400 mg/m^2, or bone marrow transplantation doses; may be delayed up to 3 years; rare in patients receiving lower doses. A history of lung disease or concomitant bleomycin therapy may increase the risk of this reaction. Patients with forced vital capacity (FVC) or carbon monoxide diffusing capacity of the lungs (DLCO) <70% of predicted are at higher risk.

1% to 10%:

Central nervous system: Wafers: Amnesia, aphasia, ataxia, cerebral edema, confusion, convulsion, depression, diplopia, dizziness, headache, hemiplegia, hydrocephalus, insomnia, meningitis, somnolence, stupor

Dermatologic: Facial flushing, probably due to the alcohol diluent; alopecia

Gastrointestinal: Anorexia, constipation, diarrhea, stomatitis

Hematologic: Anemia

Mechanism of Action Interferes with the normal function of DNA by alkylation and cross-linking the strands of DNA, and by possible protein modification

Drug Interactions

Increased Effect/Toxicity: Carmustine given in combination with cimetidine is reported to cause bone marrow depression. Carmustine given in combination with etoposide is reported to cause severe hepatic dysfunction with hyperbilirubinemia, ascites, and thrombocytopenia. Diluent for infusion contains alcohol; avoid concurrent use of medications that inhibit aldehyde dehydrogenase-2 or cause disulfiram-like reactions.

Pharmacodynamics/Kinetics

Distribution: Readily crosses blood-brain barrier producing CSF levels equal to 15% to 70% of blood plasma levels; enters breast milk; highly lipid soluble

Metabolism: Rapidly hepatic

Half-life elimination: Biphasic: Initial: 1.4 minutes; Secondary: 20 minutes (active metabolites: plasma half-life of 67 hours)

Excretion: Urine (~60% to 70%) within 96 hours; lungs (6% to 10% as CO_2)

Pregnancy Risk Factor D

Carmustinum *see* Carmustine *on page 273*

Carnitor® *see* Levocarnitine *on page 910*

Carrington Antifungal [OTC] *see* Miconazole *on page 1039*

Carteolol *(KAR tee oh lole)*

Related Information

Cardiovascular Diseases *on page 1636*

U.S. Brand Names Cartrol®; Ocupress® [DSC]

Canadian Brand Names Cartrol® Oral; Ocupress® Ophthalmic

Generic Available Yes: Ophthalmic solution

Synonyms Carteolol Hydrochloride

Pharmacologic Category Beta Blocker With Intrinsic Sympathomimetic Activity; Ophthalmic Agent, Antiglaucoma

Use Management of hypertension; treatment of chronic open-angle glaucoma and intraocular hypertension

Local Anesthetic/Vasoconstrictor Precautions No information available to require special precautions

Effects on Dental Treatment Carteolol is a nonselective beta-blocker and may enhance the pressor response to epinephrine, resulting in hypertension and bradycardia. Many nonsteroidal anti-inflammatory drugs, such as ibuprofen and indomethacin, can reduce the hypotensive effect of beta-blockers after 3 or more weeks of therapy with the NSAID. Short-term NSAID use (ie, 3 days) requires no special precautions in patients taking beta-blockers.

Common Adverse Effects
Ophthalmic:
>10%: Ocular: Conjunctival hyperemia
1% to 10%: Ocular: Anisocoria, corneal punctate keratitis, corneal sensitivity decreased, corneal staining, eye pain, vision disturbances
Systemic:
>10%:
 Central nervous system: Drowsiness, insomnia
 Endocrine & metabolic: Sexual ability decreased
1% to 10%:
 Cardiovascular: Bradycardia, palpitation, edema, CHF, peripheral circulation reduced
 Central nervous system: Mental depression
 Gastrointestinal: Constipation, diarrhea, nausea, vomiting, stomach discomfort
 Respiratory: Bronchospasm
 Miscellaneous: Cold extremities

Mechanism of Action Blocks both beta$_1$- and beta$_2$-receptors and has mild intrinsic sympathomimetic activity; has negative inotropic and chronotropic effects and can significantly slow AV nodal conduction

Drug Interactions
Cytochrome P450 Effect: Substrate of CYP2D6 (minor)
Increased Effect/Toxicity: Carteolol may increase the effects of other drugs which slow AV conduction (digoxin, verapamil, diltiazem), alpha-blockers (prazosin, terazosin), and alpha-adrenergic stimulants (epinephrine, phenylephrine). Carteolol may mask the tachycardia from hypoglycemia caused by insulin and oral hypoglycemics. In patients receiving concurrent therapy, the risk of hypertensive crisis is increased when either clonidine or the beta-blocker is withdrawn. Reserpine has been shown to enhance the effect of beta-blockers. Beta-blockers may increase the action or levels of ethanol, disopyramide, nondepolarizing muscle relaxants, and theophylline although the effects are difficult to predict.
Decreased Effect: Decreased effect of beta-blockers with aluminum salts, barbiturates, calcium salts, cholestyramine, colestipol, NSAIDs, penicillins (ampicillin), rifampin, salicylates, and sulfinpyrazone due to decreased bioavailability and plasma levels. Beta-blockers may decrease the effect of sulfonylureas (possibly hyperglycemia). Nonselective beta-blockers blunt the effect of beta-2 adrenergic agonists (albuterol).

Pharmacodynamics/Kinetics
Onset of action: Oral: 1-1.5 hours
 Peak effect: 2 hours
Duration: 12 hours
Absorption: Oral: 80%
Protein binding: 23% to 30%
Metabolism: 30% to 50%
Half-life elimination: 6 hours
Excretion: Urine (as metabolites)
Pregnancy Risk Factor C (manufacturer); D (2nd and 3rd trimesters - expert analysis)

Carteolol Hydrochloride see Carteolol *on page 274*

Cartia XT™ see Diltiazem *on page 479*

Cartrol® see Carteolol *on page 274*

Carvedilol (KAR ve dil ole)

Related Information
Cardiovascular Diseases *on page 1636*
U.S. Brand Names Coreg®
Canadian Brand Names Apo-Carvedilol®; Coreg®; Novo-Carvedilol; PMS-Carvedilol; ratio-Carvedilol
(Continued)

Carvedilol *(Continued)*

Mexican Brand Names Dilatrend®

Generic Available No

Pharmacologic Category Beta Blocker With Alpha-Blocking Activity

Use Mild-to-severe heart failure of ischemic or cardiomyopathic origin (usually in addition to standardized therapy); left ventricular dysfunction following myocardial infarction (MI); management of hypertension

Unlabeled/Investigational Use Angina pectoris

Local Anesthetic/Vasoconstrictor Precautions Use with caution, epinephrine has interacted with noncardioselective beta-blockers to result in initial hypertensive episode followed by bradycardia

Effects on Dental Treatment Key adverse event(s) related to dental treatment: Postural hypotension and periodontitis. Noncardioselective beta-blockers enhance the pressor response to epinephrine, resulting in hypertension and bradycardia. Many nonsteroidal anti-inflammatory drugs, such as ibuprofen and indomethacin, can reduce the hypotensive effect of beta-blockers after 3 or more weeks of therapy with the NSAID. Short-term NSAID use (ie, 3 days) requires no special precautions in patients taking beta-blockers.

Common Adverse Effects Note: Frequency ranges include data from hypertension and heart failure trials. Higher rates of adverse reactions have generally been noted in patients with CHF. However, the frequency of adverse effects associated with placebo is also increased in this population. Events occurring at a frequency > placebo in clinical trials.

>10%:

Cardiovascular: Hypotension (9% to 20%)

Central nervous system: Dizziness (6% to 32%), fatigue (4% to 24%)

Endocrine & metabolic: Hyperglycemia (5% to 12%), weight gain (10% to 12%)

Gastrointestinal: Diarrhea (2% to 12%)

Neuromuscular & skeletal: Weakness (11%)

1% to 10%:

Cardiovascular: Bradycardia (2% to 10%), hypertension (3%), AV block (3%), angina (2% to 6%), postural hypotension (2%), syncope (3% to 8%), dependent edema (4%), palpitation, peripheral edema (1% to 7%), generalized edema (5% to 6%)

Central nervous system: Headache (5% to 8%), fever (3%), paresthesia (2%), somnolence (2%), insomnia (2%), malaise, hypoesthesia, vertigo

Endocrine & metabolic: Alkaline phosphatase increased, gout (6%), hypercholesterolemia (4%), dehydration (2%), hyperkalemia (3%), hypervolemia (2%), hypertriglyceridemia (1%), hyperuricemia, hypoglycemia, hyponatremia

Gastrointestinal: Nausea (4% to 9%), vomiting (6%), melena, periodontitis

Genitourinary: Hematuria (3%), impotence

Hematologic: Thrombocytopenia (1% to 2%), prothrombin decreased, purpura

Hepatic: Transaminases increased

Neuromuscular & skeletal: Back pain (2% to 7%), arthralgia (6%), myalgia (3%), muscle cramps

Ocular: Blurred vision (3% to 5%), lacrimation

Renal: BUN increased (6%), renal function abnormal, albuminuria, glycosuria, creatinine increased (3%), kidney failure

Respiratory: Rhinitis (2%), cough increased (5%)

Miscellaneous: Injury (3% to 6%), allergy, sudden death

Dosage Oral: Adults: Reduce dosage if heart rate drops to <55 beats/minute.

Hypertension: 6.25 mg twice daily; if tolerated, dose should be maintained for 1-2 weeks, then increased to 12.5 mg twice daily. Dosage may be increased to a maximum of 25 mg twice daily after 1-2 weeks. Maximum dose: 50 mg/day.

Congestive heart failure: 3.125 mg twice daily for 2 weeks; if this dose is tolerated, may increase to 6.25 mg twice daily. Double the dose every 2 weeks to the highest dose tolerated by patient. (Prior to initiating therapy, other heart failure medications should be stabilized and fluid retention minimized.)

Maximum recommended dose:

Mild-to-moderate heart failure:

<85 kg: 25 mg twice daily

>85 kg: 50 mg twice daily

Severe heart failure: 25 mg twice daily

Left ventricular dysfunction following MI: Initial 3.125-6.25 mg twice daily; increase dosage incrementally (ie, from 6.25-12.5 mg twice daily) at intervals of 3-10 days, based on tolerance, to a target dose of 25 mg twice daily.

Note: Should be initiated only after patient is hemodynamically stable and fluid retention has been minimized.

Angina pectoris (unlabeled use): 25-50 mg twice daily

Dosing adjustment in renal impairment: None necessary

Dosing adjustment in hepatic impairment: Use is contraindicated in severe liver dysfunction.

Mechanism of Action As a racemic mixture, carvedilol has nonselective beta-adrenoreceptor and alpha-adrenergic blocking activity. No intrinsic sympathomimetic activity has been documented. Associated effects in hypertensive patients include reduction of cardiac output, exercise- or beta agonist-induced tachycardia, reduction of reflex orthostatic tachycardia, vasodilation, decreased peripheral vascular resistance (especially in standing position), decreased renal vascular resistance, reduced plasma renin activity, and increased levels of atrial natriuretic peptide. In CHF, associated effects include decreased pulmonary capillary wedge pressure, decreased pulmonary artery pressure, decreased heart rate, decreased systemic vascular resistance, increased stroke volume index, and decreased right arterial pressure (RAP).

Contraindications Hypersensitivity to carvedilol or any component of the formulation; patients with decompensated cardiac failure requiring intravenous inotropic therapy; bronchial asthma or related bronchospastic conditions; second- or third-degree AV block, sick sinus syndrome, and severe bradycardia (except in patients with a functioning artificial pacemaker); cardiogenic shock; severe hepatic impairment; pregnancy (2nd and 3rd trimesters)

Warnings/Precautions Initiate cautiously and monitor for possible deterioration in patient status (including symptoms of CHF). Adjustment of other medications (ACE inhibitors and/or diuretics) may be required. In severe chronic heart failure, trial patients were excluded if they had cardiac-related rales, ascites, or a serum creatinine >2.8 mg/dL. Congestive heart failure patients may experience a worsening of renal function; risks include ischemic disease, diffuse vascular disease, underlying renal dysfunction; systolic BP <100 mm Hg. Patients should be advised to avoid driving or other hazardous tasks during initiation of therapy due to the risk of syncope. Avoid abrupt discontinuation (may exacerbate underlying condition), particularly in patients with coronary artery disease; dose should be tapered over 1-2 weeks with close monitoring.

Manufacturer recommends discontinuation of therapy if liver injury occurs (confirmed by laboratory testing). Use caution in patients with PVD (can aggravate arterial insufficiency). Use caution with concurrent use of verapamil or diltiazem; bradycardia or heart block can occur. Use caution in patients with bronchospastic disease. Use cautiously in diabetics because it can mask prominent hypoglycemic symptoms. May mask signs of thyrotoxicosis. Use care with anesthetic agents that decrease myocardial function. Safety and efficacy in children <18 years of age have not been established.

Drug Interactions

Cytochrome P450 Effect: Substrate of CYP1A2 (minor), 2C9 (major), 2D6 (major), 2E1 (minor), 3A4 (minor)

Increased Effect/Toxicity: CYP2C9 Inhibitors may increase the levels/ effects of carvedilol; example inhibitors include delavirdine, fluconazole, gemfibrozil, ketoconazole, nicardipine, NSAIDs, sulfonamides and tolbutamide. CYP2D6 inhibitors may increase the levels/effects of carvedilol; example inhibitors include chlorpromazine, delavirdine, fluoxetine, miconazole, paroxetine, pergolide, quinidine, quinine, ritonavir, and ropinirole. Cimetidine increase the serum levels and effects of carvedilol. Carvedilol may increase the effects of other drugs which slow AV conduction (digoxin, verapamil, diltiazem) and alpha-blockers (prazosin, terazosin). Carvedilol may mask the tachycardia from hypoglycemia caused by insulin and oral hypoglycemics. SSRIs may decrease the metabolism of carvedilol.

Decreased Effect: CYP2C9 inducers may decrease the levels/effects of carvedilol; example inducers include carbamazepine, phenobarbital, phenytoin, rifampin, rifapentine, and secobarbital. Decreased antihypertensive effect of beta-blockers has occurred with concurrent NSAID or salicylate use. Beta-blockers may alter the effect of sulfonylureas. Disopyramide may exacerbate heart failure or enhance bradycardic effect of beta-blockers. Beta-blockers may counteract desired effects of beta-agonists.

Ethanol/Nutrition/Herb Interactions Herb/Nutraceutical: Avoid dong quai if using for hypertension (has estrogenic activity). Avoid ephedra, yohimbe, ginseng (may worsen hypertension). Avoid garlic (may have increased antihypertensive effect).

Dietary Considerations Should be taken with food to minimize the risk of orthostatic hypotension.

Pharmacodynamics/Kinetics

Onset of action: 1-2 hours

Peak antihypertensive effect: ~1-2 hours

(Continued)

Carvedilol *(Continued)*

Absorption: Rapid; food decreases rate but not extent of absorption; administration with food minimizes risks of orthostatic hypotension

Distribution: V_d: 115 L

Protein binding: >98%, primarily to albumin

Metabolism: Extensively hepatic, via **CYP2C9, 2D6**, 3A4, and 2C19 (2% excreted unchanged); three active metabolites (4-hydroxyphenyl metabolite is 13 times more potent than parent drug for beta-blockade); first-pass effect; plasma concentrations in the elderly and those with cirrhotic liver disease are 50% and 4-7 times higher, respectively

Bioavailability: 25% to 35%

Half-life elimination: 7-10 hours

Excretion: Primarily feces

Pregnancy Risk Factor C (manufacturer); D (2nd and 3rd trimesters - expert analysis)

Dosage Forms TAB: 3.125 mg, 6.25 mg, 12.5 mg, 25 mg

Selected Readings

Foster CA and Aston SJ, "Propranolol-Epinephrine Interaction: A Potential Disaster," *Plast Reconstr Surg*, 1983, 72(1):74-8.

Wong DG, Spence JD, Lamki L, et al, "Effect of Nonsteroidal Anti-inflammatory Drugs on Control of Hypertension of Beta-Blockers and Diuretics," *Lancet*, 1986, 1(8488):997-1001.

Wynn RL, "Dental Nonsteroidal Anti-inflammatory Drugs and Prostaglandin-Based Drug Interactions, Part Two," *Gen Dent*, 1992, 40(2):104, 106, 108.

Wynn RL, "Epinephrine Interactions With Beta-Blockers," *Gen Dent*, 1994, 42(1):16, 18.

Casanthranol and Docusate *see* Docusate and Casanthranol *on page 496*

Casodex® *see* Bicalutamide *on page 207*

Caspofungin *(kas poe FUN jin)*

U.S. Brand Names Cancidas®

Canadian Brand Names Cancidas®

Mexican Brand Names Cancidas®

Generic Available No

Synonyms Caspofungin Acetate

Pharmacologic Category Antifungal Agent, Parenteral; Echinocandin

Use Treatment of invasive *Aspergillus* infections in patients who are refractory or intolerant of other therapy; treatment of candidemia and other *Candida* infections (intra-abdominal abscesses, esophageal, peritonitis, pleural space); empirical treatment for presumed fungal infections in febrile neutropenic patient

Local Anesthetic/Vasoconstrictor Precautions No information available to require special precautions

Effects on Dental Treatment No significant effects or complications reported

Common Adverse Effects

>10%:

Central nervous system: Headache (up to 11%), fever (3% to 26%), chills (up to 14%)

Endocrine & metabolic: Hypokalemia (4% to 11%)

Hematologic: Hemoglobin decreased (1% to 12%)

Hepatic: Serum alkaline phosphatase increased (3% to 11%), transaminases increased (up to 13%)

Local: Infusion site reactions (2% to 12%), phlebitis/thrombophlebitis (up to 16%)

1% to 10%:

Cardiovascular: Flushing (2% to 3%), facial edema (up to 3%), hypertension (1% to 2%), tachycardia (1% to 2%), hypotension (1%)

Central nervous system: Dizziness (2%), pain (1% to 5%), insomnia (1%)

Dermatologic: Rash (<1% to 6%), pruritus (1% to 3%), erythema (1% to 2%)

Gastrointestinal: Nausea (2% to 6%), vomiting (1% to 4%), abdominal pain (1% to 4%), diarrhea (1% to 4%), anorexia (1%)

Hematologic: Eosinophils increased (3%), neutrophils decreased (2% to 3%), WBC decreased (5% to 6%), anemia (up to 4%), platelet count decreased (2% to 3%)

Hepatic: Bilirubin increased (3%)

Local: Induration (up to 3%)

Neuromuscular & skeletal: Myalgia (up to 3%), paresthesia (1% to 3%), tremor (≤2%)

Renal: Nephrotoxicity (8%)*, proteinuria (5%), hematuria (2%), serum creatinine increased (<1% to 4%), urinary WBCs increased (up to 8%), urinary RBCs increased (1% to 4%), blood urea nitrogen increased (1%)

*Nephrotoxicity defined as serum creatinine ≥2x baseline value or ≥1 mg/dL in patients with serum creatinine above ULN range (patients with Cl_{cr} <30 mL/minute were excluded)

Miscellaneous: Flu-like syndrome (3%), diaphoresis (up to 3%)

Mechanism of Action Inhibits synthesis of β(1,3)-D-glucan, an essential component of the cell wall of susceptible fungi. Highest activity in regions of active cell growth. Mammalian cells do not require β(1,3)-D-glucan, limiting potential toxicity.

Drug Interactions

Increased Effect/Toxicity: Concurrent administration of cyclosporine may increase caspofungin concentrations; hepatic serum transaminases may be observed.

Decreased Effect: Caspofungin may decrease blood concentrations of tacrolimus. Dosage adjustment of caspofungin to 70 mg is required for patients on rifampin.

Pharmacodynamics/Kinetics

Protein binding: 97% to albumin

Metabolism: Slowly, via hydrolysis and *N*-acetylation as well as by spontaneous degradation, with subsequent metabolism to component amino acids. Overall metabolism is extensive.

Half-life elimination: Beta (distribution): 9-11 hours; Terminal: 40-50 hours

Excretion: Urine (41% as metabolites, 1% to 9% unchanged) and feces (35% as metabolites)

Pregnancy Risk Factor C

Caspofungin Acetate *see* Caspofungin *on page 278*

Castellani Paint Modified [OTC] *see* Phenol *on page 1223*

Castor Oil (KAS tor oyl)

U.S. Brand Names Emulsoil® [OTC] [DSC]; Purge® [OTC]

Generic Available Yes: Oil

Synonyms Oleum Ricini

Pharmacologic Category Laxative, Miscellaneous

Use Preparation for rectal or bowel examination or surgery; rarely used to relieve constipation; also applied to skin as emollient and protectant

Local Anesthetic/Vasoconstrictor Precautions No information available to require special precautions

Effects on Dental Treatment No significant effects or complications reported

Mechanism of Action Acts primarily in the small intestine; hydrolyzed to ricinoleic acid which reduces net absorption of fluid and electrolytes and stimulates peristalsis

Pregnancy Risk Factor X

Castor Oil, Trypsin, and Balsam Peru *see* Trypsin, Balsam Peru, and Castor Oil *on page 1547*

Cataflam® *see* Diclofenac *on page 459*

Catapres® *see* Clonidine *on page 373*

Catapres-TTS® *see* Clonidine *on page 373*

Cathflo® Activase® *see* Alteplase *on page 77*

Caverject® *see* Alprostadil *on page 76*

Caverject Impulse® *see* Alprostadil *on page 76*

CaviRinse™ *see* Fluoride *on page 671*

CB-1348 *see* Chlorambucil *on page 313*

CBDCA *see* Carboplatin *on page 270*

CBZ *see* Carbamazepine *on page 260*

CC-5013 *see* Lenalidomide *on page 903*

CCNU *see* Lomustine *on page 941*

2-CdA *see* Cladribine *on page 354*

CDDP *see* Cisplatin *on page 350*

CDX *see* Bicalutamide *on page 207*

Cecon® [OTC] *see* Ascorbic Acid *on page 143*

Cedax® *see* Ceftibuten *on page 292*

CEE *see* Estrogens (Conjugated/Equine) *on page 580*

CeeNU® *see* Lomustine *on page 941*

Cefaclor (SEF a klor)

U.S. Brand Names Raniclor™

Canadian Brand Names Apo-Cefaclor®; Ceclor®; Novo-Cefaclor; Nu-Cefaclor; PMS-Cefaclor

(Continued)

Cefaclor *(Continued)*

Mexican Brand Names Ceclor®

Generic Available Yes: Excludes chewable tablet

Pharmacologic Category Antibiotic, Cephalosporin (Second Generation)

Dental Use Alternative antibiotic for treatment of orofacial infections in patients allergic to penicillins; susceptible bacteria including aerobic gram-positive bacteria and anaerobes

Use Treatment of susceptible bacterial infections including otitis media, lower respiratory tract infections, acute exacerbations of chronic bronchitis, pharyngitis and tonsillitis, urinary tract infections, skin and skin structure infections

Local Anesthetic/Vasoconstrictor Precautions No information available to require special precautions

Effects on Dental Treatment No significant effects or complications reported (see Dental Comment)

Significant Adverse Effects

1% to 10%:

Dermatologic: Rash (maculopapular, erythematous, or morbilliform) (1% to 2%)

Gastrointestinal: Diarrhea (3%)

Genitourinary: Vaginitis (2%)

Hematologic: Eosinophilia (2%)

Hepatic: Transaminases increased (3%)

Miscellaneous: Moniliasis (2%)

<1% (Limited to important or life-threatening): Agitation, agranulocytosis, anaphylaxis, angioedema, aplastic anemia, arthralgia, cholestatic jaundice, CNS irritability, confusion, dizziness, hallucinations, hemolytic anemia, hepatitis, hyperactivity, insomnia, interstitial nephritis, nausea, nervousness, neutropenia, paresthesia, PT prolonged, pruritus, pseudomembranous colitis, seizure, serum-sickness, somnolence, Stevens-Johnson syndrome, thrombocytopenia, toxic epidermal necrolysis, urticaria, vomiting

Reactions reported with other cephalosporins include abdominal pain, cholestasis, fever, hemorrhage, renal dysfunction, superinfection, toxic nephropathy

Dental Usual Dosing Orofacial infections: Adults: Oral: Dosing range: 250-500 mg every 8 hours

Dosage

Usual dosage range:

Children >1 month: Oral: 20-40 mg/kg/day divided every 8-12 hours (maximum dose: 1 g/day)

Adults: Oral: 250-500 mg every 8 hours

Indication-specific dosing:

Children: Oral:

Otitis media: 40 mg/kg/day divided every 12 hours

Pharyngitis: 20 mg/kg/day divided every 12 hours

Dosing adjustment in renal impairment:

Cl_{cr} 10-50 mL/minute: Administer 50% to 100% of dose

Cl_{cr} <10 mL/minute: Administer 50% of dose

Hemodialysis: Moderately dialyzable (20% to 50%)

Mechanism of Action Inhibits bacterial cell wall synthesis by binding to one or more of the penicillin-binding proteins (PBPs) which in turn inhibits the final transpeptidation step of peptidoglycan synthesis in bacterial cell walls, thus inhibiting cell wall biosynthesis. Bacteria eventually lyse due to ongoing activity of cell wall autolytic enzymes (autolysins and murein hydrolases) while cell wall assembly is arrested.

Contraindications Hypersensitivity to cefaclor, any component of the formulation, or other cephalosporins

Warnings/Precautions Modify dosage in patients with severe renal impairment. Prolonged use may result in superinfection. Use with caution in patients with a history of penicillin allergy, especially IgE-mediated reactions (eg, anaphylaxis, urticaria). Beta-lactamase-negative, ampicillin-resistant (BLNAR) strains of *H. influenzae* should be considered resistant to cefaclor. Extended release tablets are not approved for use in children <16 years of age.

Drug Interactions

Aminoglycosides: May be additive to nephrotoxicity.

Furosemide: May be additive to nephrotoxicity.

Probenecid: May decrease cephalosporin elimination.

Ethanol/Nutrition/Herb Interactions

Food: Cefaclor serum levels may be decreased slightly if taken with food. The bioavailability of cefaclor extended release tablets is decreased 23% and the maximum concentration is decreased 67% when taken on an empty stomach.

Dietary Considerations Capsule, chewable tablet, and suspension may be taken with or without food. Raniclor™ contains phenylalanine 2.8 mg/cefaclor 125 mg.

Pharmacodynamics/Kinetics

Absorption: Well absorbed, acid stable

Distribution: Widely throughout the body and reaches therapeutic concentration in most tissues and body fluids, including synovial, pericardial, pleural, peritoneal fluids; bile, sputum, and urine; bone, myocardium, gallbladder, skin and soft tissue; crosses placenta; enters breast milk

Protein binding: 25%

Metabolism: Partially hepatic

Half-life elimination: 0.5-1 hour; prolonged with renal impairment

Time to peak: Capsule: 60 minutes; Suspension: 45 minutes

Excretion: Urine (80% as unchanged drug)

Pregnancy Risk Factor B

Lactation Enters breast milk/use caution

Breast-Feeding Considerations Theoretically, drug absorbed by nursing infant may change bowel flora or affect fever work-up result. Small amounts can be detected in breast milk (trace amounts after 1 hour, increasing to 0.16 mcg/mL at 5 hours). **Note:** As a class, cephalosporins are used to treat bacterial infections in infants.

Dosage Forms

Capsule: 250 mg, 500 mg

Powder for oral suspension: 125 mg/5 mL (75 mL, 150 mL); 187 mg/5 mL (50 mL, 100 mL); 250 mg/5 mL (75 mL, 150 mL); 375 mg/5 mL (50 mL, 100 mL)

Tablet, chewable (Raniclor™): 125 mg [contains phenylalanine 2.8 mg; fruity flavor], 187 mg [contains phenylalanine 4.2 mg; fruity flavor]

Dental Comment Patients allergic to penicillins can use a cephalosporin; the incidence of cross-reactivity between penicillins and cephalosporins is 1% when the allergic reaction to penicillin is delayed. Cefaclor is effective against anaerobic bacteria, but the sensitivity of alpha-hemolytic *Streptococcus* varies; approximately 10% of strains are resistant. Nearly 70% are intermediately sensitive. If the patient has a history of immediate reaction to penicillin, the incidence of cross-reactivity is 20%; cephalosporins are contraindicated in these patients.

Cefadroxil (sef a DROKS il)

Related Information

Antibiotic Prophylaxis *on page 1680*

U.S. Brand Names Duricef®

Canadian Brand Names Apo-Cefadroxil®; Duricef®; Novo-Cefadroxil

Mexican Brand Names Cefamox®; Duracef®

Generic Available Yes

Synonyms Cefadroxil Monohydrate

Pharmacologic Category Antibiotic, Cephalosporin (First Generation)

Dental Use Alternative antibiotic for prevention of bacterial endocarditis. Individuals allergic to amoxicillin (penicillins) may receive cefadroxil provided they have not had an immediate, local, or systemic IgE-mediated anaphylactic allergic reaction to penicillin.

Use Treatment of susceptible bacterial infections, including those caused by group A beta-hemolytic *Streptococcus*; prophylaxis against bacterial endocarditis in patients who are allergic to penicillin and undergoing surgical or dental procedures

Local Anesthetic/Vasoconstrictor Precautions No information available to require special precautions

Effects on Dental Treatment No significant effects or complications reported

Significant Adverse Effects

1% to 10%: Gastrointestinal: Diarrhea

<1% (Limited to important or life-threatening): Abdominal pain, agranulocytosis, anaphylaxis, angioedema, arthralgia, cholestasis, dyspepsia, erythema multiforme, fever, nausea, neutropenia, pruritus, pseudomembranous colitis, rash (maculopapular and erythematous), serum sickness, Stevens-Johnson syndrome, thrombocytopenia, transaminases increased, urticaria, vaginitis, vomiting

Reactions reported with other cephalosporins include abdominal pain, aplastic anemia, BUN increased, creatinine increased, eosinophilia, hemolytic anemia, hemorrhage, pancytopenia, prothrombin time prolonged, renal dysfunction, seizure, superinfection, toxic epidermal necrolysis, toxic nephropathy

(Continued)

281

Cefadroxil *(Continued)*

Dental Usual Dosing Prophylaxis against bacterial endocarditis: Oral:
Children: 50 mg/kg 1 hour prior to the procedure
Adults: 2 g 1 hour prior to the procedure

Dosage
Usual dosage range: Oral:
Children: 30 mg/kg/day divided twice daily up to a maximum of 2 g/day
Adults: 1-2 g/day in 2 divided doses

Indication-specific dosing:
Prophylaxis against bacterial endocarditis:
Children: Oral: 50 mg/kg 1 hour prior to the procedure
Adults: Oral: 2 g 1 hour prior to the procedure

Dosing interval in renal impairment:
Cl_{cr} 10-25 mL/minute: Administer every 24 hours
Cl_{cr} <10 mL/minute: Administer every 36 hours

Mechanism of Action Inhibits bacterial cell wall synthesis by binding to one or more of the penicillin-binding proteins (PBPs) which in turn inhibits the final transpeptidation step of peptidoglycan synthesis in bacterial cell walls, thus inhibiting cell wall biosynthesis. Bacteria eventually lyse due to ongoing activity of cell wall autolytic enzymes (autolysins and murein hydrolases) while cell wall assembly is arrested.

Contraindications Hypersensitivity to cefadroxil, any component of the formulation, or other cephalosporins

Warnings/Precautions Modify dosage in patients with severe renal impairment. Prolonged use may result in superinfection. Use with caution in patients with a history of penicillin allergy, especially IgE-mediated reactions (eg, anaphylaxis, angioedema, urticaria). May cause antibiotic-associated colitis or colitis secondary to *C. difficile*.

Drug Interactions
Increased effect: Probenecid may decrease cephalosporin elimination.
Increased toxicity: Furosemide, aminoglycosides may be a possible additive to nephrotoxicity.

Ethanol/Nutrition/Herb Interactions Food: Concomitant administration with food, infant formula, or cow's milk does **not** significantly affect absorption.

Pharmacodynamics/Kinetics
Absorption: Rapid and well absorbed
Distribution: Widely throughout the body and reaches therapeutic concentrations in most tissues and body fluids, including synovial, pericardial, pleural, and peritoneal fluids; bile, sputum, and urine; bone, myocardium, gallbladder, skin and soft tissue; crosses placenta; enters breast milk
Protein binding: 20%
Half-life elimination: 1-2 hours; Renal failure: 20-24 hours
Time to peak, serum: 70-90 minutes
Excretion: Urine (>90% as unchanged drug)

Pregnancy Risk Factor B

Lactation Enters breast milk (small amounts)/use caution (AAP rates "compatible")

Breast-Feeding Considerations Theoretically, drug absorbed by nursing infant may change bowel flora or affect fever work-up result. **Note:** As a class, cephalosporins are used to treat infections in infants.

Dosage Forms
Capsule, as monohydrate: 500 mg
Duricef®: 500 mg
Powder for oral suspension, as monohydrate: 250 mg/5 mL (50 mL, 100 mL); 500 mg/5 mL (75 mL, 100 mL)
Duricef®: 250 mg/5 mL (50 mL, 100 mL); 500 mg/5 mL (75 mL, 100 mL) [contains sodium benzoate; orange-pineapple flavor]
Tablet, as monohydrate: 1 g
Duricef®: 1 g

Selected Readings

ADA Division of Legal Affairs, "A Legal Perspective on Antibiotic Prophylaxis," *J Am Dent Assoc*, 2003, 134(9):1260.

"Advisory Statement. Antibiotic Prophylaxis for Dental Patients With Total Joint Replacements. American Dental Association; American Academy of Orthopedic Surgeons," *J Am Dent Assoc*, 1997, 128(7):1004-8.

American Dental Association Council on Scientific Affairs, "Combating Antibiotic Resistance," *J Am Dent Assoc*, 2004, 135(4):484-7.

Dajani AS, Taubert KA, Wilson W, et al, "Prevention of Bacterial Endocarditis. Recommendations by the American Heart Association," *JAMA*, 1997, 277(22):1794-801.

Dajani AS, Taubert KA, Wilson W, et al, "Prevention of Bacterial Endocarditis: Recommendations by the American Heart Association," *J Am Dent Assoc*, 1997, 128(8):1142-51.

Donowitz GR and Mandell GL, "Drug Therapy. Beta-Lactam Antibiotics (1)," *N Engl J Med*, 1988, 318(7):419-26.

Donowitz GR and Mandell GL, "Drug Therapy. Beta-Lactam Antibiotics (2)," *N Engl J Med*, 1988, 318(8):490-500.

Gustaferro CA and Steckelberg JM, "Cephalosporin Antimicrobial Agents and Related Compounds," *Mayo Clin Proc*, 1991, 66(10):1064-73.

Cefadroxil Monohydrate *see* Cefadroxil *on page 281*

Cefazolin (sef A zoe lin)

Related Information
Antibiotic Prophylaxis *on page 1680*

U.S. Brand Names Ancef®

Generic Available Yes

Synonyms Cefazolin Sodium

Pharmacologic Category Antibiotic, Cephalosporin (First Generation)

Dental Use
Alternative antibiotic for prevention of bacterial endocarditis when parenteral administration is needed. Individuals allergic to amoxicillin (penicillins) may receive cefazolin provided they have not had an immediate, local, or systemic IgE-mediated anaphylactic allergic reaction to penicillin. Alternate antibiotic for premedication in patients not allergic to penicillin who may be at potential increased risk of hematogenous total joint infection when parenteral administration is needed.

Use
Treatment of respiratory tract, skin and skin structure, genital, urinary tract, biliary tract, bone and joint infections, and septicemia due to susceptible gram-positive cocci (except enterococcus); some gram-negative bacilli including *E. coli*, *Proteus*, and *Klebsiella* may be susceptible; perioperative prophylaxis

Unlabeled/Investigational Use
Prophylaxis against bacterial endocarditis

Local Anesthetic/Vasoconstrictor Precautions
No information available to require special precautions

Effects on Dental Treatment
No significant effects or complications reported

Significant Adverse Effects
Frequency not defined.

Central nervous system: Fever, seizure

Dermatologic: Rash, pruritus, Stevens-Johnson syndrome

Gastrointestinal: Diarrhea, nausea, vomiting, abdominal cramps, anorexia, pseudomembranous colitis, oral candidiasis

Genitourinary: Vaginitis

Hepatic: Transaminases increased, hepatitis

Hematologic: Eosinophilia, neutropenia, leukopenia, thrombocytopenia, thrombocytosis

Local: Pain at injection site, phlebitis

Renal: BUN increased, serum creatinine increased, renal failure

Miscellaneous: Anaphylaxis

Reactions reported with other cephalosporins include toxic epidermal necrolysis, abdominal pain, cholestasis, superinfection, toxic nephropathy, aplastic anemia, hemolytic anemia, hemorrhage, prothrombin time prolonged, pancytopenia

Dental Usual Dosing
Prophylaxis against bacterial endocarditis: I.M., I.V.:

Infants and Children: 25 mg/kg 30 minutes before procedure; maximum dose: 1 g

Adults: 1 g 30 minutes before procedure

Dosage
Usual dosage range: I.M., I.V.:

Children >1 month: 25-100 mg/kg/day divided every 6-8 hours; maximum: 6 g/day

Adults: 250 mg to 2 g every 6-12 (usually 8) hours, depending on severity of infection; maximum dose: 12 g/day

Indication-specific dosing:

Prophylaxis against bacterial endocarditis (unlabeled use):

Infants and Children: 25 mg/kg 30 minutes before procedure; maximum dose: 1 g

Adults: 1 g 30 minutes before procedure

Mild-to-moderate infections: Adults: 500 mg to 1 g every 6-8 hours

Mild infection with gram-positive cocci: Adults: 250-500 mg every 8 hours

Perioperative prophylaxis: Adults: 1 g given 30 minutes prior to surgery (repeat with 500 mg to 1 g during prolonged surgery); followed by 500 mg to 1 g every 6-9 hours for 24 hours postop

Pneumococcal pneumonia: Adults: 500 mg every 12 hours

Severe infection: Adults: 1-2 g every 6 hours

Prophylaxis against bacterial endocarditis (unlabeled use): Adults: 1 g 30 minutes before procedure

UTI (uncomplicated): Adults: 1 g every 12 hours

(Continued)

Cefazolin (Continued)

Dosing adjustment in renal impairment:
Cl_{cr} 10-30 mL/minute: Administer every 12 hours
Cl_{cr} <10 mL/minute: Administer every 24 hours
Hemodialysis: Moderately dialyzable (20% to 50%); administer dose postdialysis or administer supplemental dose of 0.5-1 g after dialysis
Peritoneal dialysis: Administer 0.5 g every 12 hours
Continuous arteriovenous or venovenous hemofiltration: Dose as for Cl_{cr} 10-30 mL/minute; removes 30 mg of cefazolin per liter of filtrate per day

Mechanism of Action Inhibits bacterial cell wall synthesis by binding to one or more of the penicillin-binding proteins (PBPs) which in turn inhibits the final transpeptidation step of peptidoglycan synthesis in bacterial cell walls, thus inhibiting cell wall biosynthesis. Bacteria eventually lyse due to ongoing activity of cell wall autolytic enzymes (autolysins and murein hydrolases) while cell wall assembly is arrested.

Contraindications Hypersensitivity to cefazolin sodium, any component of the formulation, or other cephalosporins

Warnings/Precautions Modify dosage in patients with severe renal impairment. Prolonged use may result in superinfection. Use with caution in patients with a history of penicillin allergy, especially IgE-mediated reactions (eg, anaphylaxis, angioedema, urticaria). May cause antibiotic-associated colitis or colitis secondary to *C. difficile*.

Drug Interactions
Aminoglycosides: Aminoglycosides increase nephrotoxic potential.
Probenecid: High-dose probenecid decreases clearance.
Warfarin: Cefazolin may increase the hypothrombinemic response to warfarin (due to alteration of GI microbial flora).

Dietary Considerations Sodium content of 1 g: 48 mg (2 mEq)

Pharmacodynamics/Kinetics
Distribution: Widely into most body tissues and fluids including gallbladder, liver, kidneys, bone, sputum, bile, pleural, and synovial; CSF penetration is poor; crosses placenta; enters breast milk
Protein binding: 74% to 86%
Metabolism: Minimally hepatic
Half-life elimination: 90-150 minutes; prolonged with renal impairment
Time to peak, serum: I.M.: 0.5-2 hours
Excretion: Urine (80% to 100% as unchanged drug)

Pregnancy Risk Factor B

Lactation Enters breast milk (small amounts)/use caution (AAP rates "compatible")

Breast-Feeding Considerations Theoretically, drug absorbed by nursing infant may change bowel flora or affect fever work-up result. **Note:** As a class, cephalosporins are used to treat infections in infants.

Dosage Forms [DSC] = Discontinued product
Infusion [premixed in D_5W]: 500 mg (50 mL); 1 g (50 mL)
Injection, powder for reconstitution: 500 mg, 1 g, 10 g, 20 g
Ancef®: 1 g; 10 g [DSC]

Selected Readings

ADA Division of Legal Affairs, "A Legal Perspective on Antibiotic Prophylaxis," *J Am Dent Assoc*, 2003, 134(9):1260.

"Advisory Statement. Antibiotic Prophylaxis for Dental Patients With Total Joint Replacements. American Dental Association; American Academy of Orthopedic Surgeons," *J Am Dent Assoc*, 1997, 128(7):1004-8.

American Dental Association; American Academy of Orthopedic Surgeons, "Antibiotic Prophylaxis for Dental Patients With Total Joint Replacements," *J Am Dent Assoc*, 2003, 134(7):895-9.

American Dental Association Council on Scientific Affairs, "Combating Antibiotic Resistance," *J Am Dent Assoc*, 2004, 135(4):484-7.

Dajani AS, Taubert KA, Wilson W, et al, "Prevention of Bacterial Endocarditis. Recommendations by the American Heart Association," *JAMA*, 1997, 277(22):1794-801.

Dajani AS, Taubert KA, Wilson W, et al, "Prevention of Bacterial Endocarditis: Recommendations by the American Heart Association," *J Am Dent Assoc*, 1997, 128(8):1142-51.

Donowitz GR and Mandell GL, "Drug Therapy. Beta-Lactam Antibiotics (1)," *N Engl J Med*, 1988, 318(7):419-26.

Donowitz GR and Mandell GL, "Drug Therapy. Beta-Lactam Antibiotics (2)," *N Engl J Med*, 1988, 318(8):490-500.

Gustaferro CA and Steckelberg JM, "Cephalosporin Antimicrobial Agents and Related Compounds," *Mayo Clin Proc*, 1991, 66(10):1064-73.

Cefazolin Sodium *see* Cefazolin *on page 283*

Cefdinir (SEF di ner)

U.S. Brand Names Omnicef®
Canadian Brand Names Omnicef®
Generic Available No

Synonyms CFDN

Pharmacologic Category Antibiotic, Cephalosporin (Third Generation)

Use Treatment of community-acquired pneumonia, acute exacerbations of chronic bronchitis, acute bacterial otitis media, acute maxillary sinusitis, pharyngitis/tonsillitis, and uncomplicated skin and skin structure infections.

Local Anesthetic/Vasoconstrictor Precautions No information available to require special precautions

Effects on Dental Treatment No significant effects or complications reported

Common Adverse Effects

>10%: Gastrointestinal: Diarrhea (8% to 15%)

1% to 10%:

Central nervous system: Headache (2%)

Dermatologic: Rash (≤3%)

Gastrointestinal: Nausea (≤3%), abdominal pain (≤1%), vomiting (≤1%)

Genitourinary: Vaginal moniliasis (≤4%), urine leukocytes increased (2%), urine protein increased (1% to 2%), vaginitis (≤1%)

Hematologic: Eosinophils increased (1%)

Hepatic: Alkaline phosphatase increased (≤1%), platelets increased (1%)

Renal: Microhematuria (1%)

Miscellaneous: Lymphocytes increased (≤2%), GGT increased (1%), lactate dehydrogenase increased (≤1%), bicarbonate decreased (≤1%), lymphocytes decreased (≤1%), PMN changes (≤1%)

Reactions reported with other cephalosporins include dizziness, fever, encephalopathy, asterixis, neuromuscular excitability, seizure, aplastic anemia, interstitial nephritis, toxic nephropathy, angioedema, hemorrhage, PT prolonged, and superinfection

Mechanism of Action Inhibits bacterial cell wall synthesis by binding to one or more of the penicillin-binding proteins (PBPs) which in turn inhibits the final transpeptidation step of peptidoglycan synthesis in bacterial cell walls, thus inhibiting cell wall biosynthesis. Bacteria eventually lyse due to ongoing activity of cell wall autolytic enzymes (autolysins and murein hydrolases) while cell wall assembly is arrested.

Drug Interactions

Increased Effect/Toxicity: Probenecid may increase the effects of cefdinir by decreasing renal elimination (peak plasma levels of cefdinir are increased by 54% and half-life is prolonged by 50%).

Decreased Effect: Coadministration with iron or antacids reduces the rate and extent of cefdinir absorption.

Pharmacodynamics/Kinetics

Distribution: V_d:

Children 6 months to 12 years: 0.29-1.05 L/kg

Adults: 0.06-0.64 L/kg

Protein binding: 60% to 70%

Metabolism: Minimally hepatic

Bioavailability: Capsule: 16% to 21%; suspension 25%

Half-life elimination: 100 minutes

Excretion: Primarily urine

Pregnancy Risk Factor B

Cefditoren (sef de TOR en)

U.S. Brand Names Spectracef™

Generic Available No

Synonyms Cefditoren Pivoxil

Pharmacologic Category Antibiotic, Cephalosporin

Dental Use Bactericidal antibiotic for infections due to susceptible organisms

Use Treatment of acute bacterial exacerbation of chronic bronchitis or community-acquired pneumonia (due to susceptible organisms including *Haemophilus influenzae*, *Haemophilus parainfluenzae*, *Streptococcus pneumoniae*-penicillin susceptible only, *Moraxella catarrhalis*); pharyngitis or tonsillitis (*Streptococcus pyogenes*); and uncomplicated skin and skin-structure infections (*Staphylococcus aureus* - not MRSA, *Streptococcus pyogenes*)

Local Anesthetic/Vasoconstrictor Precautions No information available to require special precautions

Effects on Dental Treatment No significant effects or complications reported

Significant Adverse Effects

>10%: Gastrointestinal: Diarrhea (11% to 15%)

1% to 10%:

Central nervous system: Headache (2% to 3%)

Endocrine & metabolic: Glucose increased (1% to 2%)

(Continued)

Cefditoren *(Continued)*

Gastrointestinal: Nausea (4% to 6%), abdominal pain (2%), dyspepsia (1% to 2%), vomiting (1%)

Genitourinary: Vaginal moniliasis (3% to 6%)

Hematologic: Hematocrit decreased (2%)

Renal: Hematuria (3%), urinary white blood cells increased (2%)

<1% (Limited to important or life-threatening): Acute renal failure, albumin decreased, allergic reaction, arthralgia, asthma, BUN increased, calcium decreased, eosinophilic pneumonia, coagulation time increased, erythema multiforme, fungal infection, hyperglycemia, interstitial pneumonia, leukopenia, leukorrhea, positive direct Coombs' test, potassium increased, pseudomembranous colitis, rash, sodium decreased, Stevens-Johnson syndrome, thrombocythemia, thrombocytopenia, toxic epidermal necrolysis, white blood cells increased/decreased

Additional adverse effects seen with cephalosporin antibiotics: Anaphylaxis, aplastic anemia, cholestasis, hemorrhage, hemolytic anemia, renal dysfunction, reversible hyperactivity, serum sickness-like reaction, toxic nephropathy

Dental Usual Dosing Dental infections (unlabeled use): Children ≥12 years and Adults: Oral: 400 mg twice daily for 10 days

Dosage

Usual dosage range:

Children ≥12 years and Adults: Oral: 200-400 mg twice daily

Indication-specific dosing:

Children ≥12 years and Adults: Oral:

Acute bacterial exacerbation of chronic bronchitis: 400 mg twice daily for 10 days

Dental infections (unlabeled use): 400 mg twice daily for 10 days

Community-acquired pneumonia: 400 mg twice daily for 14 days

Pharyngitis, tonsillitis, uncomplicated skin and skin structure infections: 200 mg twice daily for 10 days

Dosage adjustment in renal impairment:

Cl_{cr} 30-49 mL/minute/1.73 m^2: Maximum dose: 200 mg twice daily

Cl_{cr} <30 mL/minute/1.73 m^2: Maximum dose: 200 mg once daily

End-stage renal disease: Appropriate dosing not established

Dosage adjustment in hepatic impairment:

Mild-to-moderate impairment: Adjustment not required

Severe impairment (Child-Pugh Class C): Specific guidelines not available

Mechanism of Action Inhibits bacterial cell wall synthesis by binding to one or more of the penicillin binding proteins (PBPs) which in turn inhibits the final transpeptidation step of peptidoglycan synthesis in bacterial cell walls, thus inhibiting cell wall biosynthesis. Bacteria eventually lyse due to ongoing activity of cell wall autolytic enzymes (autolysins and murein hydrolases) while cell wall assembly is arrested.

Contraindications Hypersensitivity to cefditoren, any component of the formulation, other cephalosporins, or milk protein; carnitine deficiency

Warnings/Precautions Use with caution in patients with a history of penicillin allergy, especially IgE-mediated reactions (eg, anaphylaxis, urticaria). May cause antibiotic-associated colitis or colitis secondary to *C. difficile*. Prolonged use may result in superinfection. Caution in individuals with seizure disorders. Use caution in patients with renal or hepatic impairment; modify dosage in patients with severe renal impairment. Cefditoren causes renal excretion of carnitine; do not use in patients with carnitine deficiency; not for long-term therapy due to the possible development of carnitine deficiency over time. May prolong prothrombin time; use with caution in patients with a history of bleeding disorder. Cefditoren tablets contain sodium caseinate, which may cause hypersensitivity reactions in patients with milk protein hypersensitivity; this does not affect patients with lactose intolerance. Safety and efficacy have not been established in children <12 years of age.

Drug Interactions

Probenecid: Serum concentration of cefditoren may be increased.

Warfarin: Prothrombin time may be prolonged by cefditoren; monitor.

Ethanol/Nutrition/Herb Interactions Food: Moderate- to high-fat meals increase bioavailability and maximum plasma concentration.

Dietary Considerations Cefditoren should be taken with meals. Plasma carnitine levels are decreased during therapy (39% with 200 mg dosing, 63% with 400 mg dosing); normal concentrations return within 7-10 days after treatment is discontinued.

Pharmacodynamics/Kinetics

Distribution: 9.3 ± 1.6 L

Protein binding: 88% (*in vitro*), primarily to albumin

Metabolism: Cefditoren pivoxil is hydrolyzed to cefditoren (active) and pivalate

Bioavailability: ~14% to 16%, increased by moderate to high-fat meal

Half-life elimination: 1.6 ± 0.4 hours
Time to peak: 1.5-3 hours
Excretion: Urine (as cefditoren and pivaloylcarnitine)
Pregnancy Risk Factor B
Lactation Excretion in breast milk unknown/use caution
Dosage Forms Tablet, as pivoxil: 200 mg [equivalent to cefditoren; contains sodium caseinate]

Cefditoren Pivoxil see Cefditoren on page 285

Cefepime (SEF e pim)

U.S. Brand Names Maxipime®
Canadian Brand Names Maxipime®
Mexican Brand Names Maxipime®
Generic Available No
Synonyms Cefepime Hydrochloride
Pharmacologic Category Antibiotic, Cephalosporin (Fourth Generation)
Use Treatment of uncomplicated and complicated urinary tract infections, including pyelonephritis caused by typical urinary tract pathogens; monotherapy for febrile neutropenia; uncomplicated skin and skin structure infections caused by *Streptococcus pyogenes*; moderate-to-severe pneumonia caused by pneumococcus, *Pseudomonas aeruginosa*, and other gram-negative organisms; complicated intra-abdominal infections (in combination with metronidazole). Also active against methicillin-susceptible staphylococci, *Enterobacter* sp, and many other gram-negative bacilli.

Children 2 months to 16 years: Empiric therapy of febrile neutropenia patients, uncomplicated skin/soft tissue infections, pneumonia, and uncomplicated/complicated urinary tract infections.

Local Anesthetic/Vasoconstrictor Precautions No information available to require special precautions
Effects on Dental Treatment No significant effects or complications reported
Common Adverse Effects
>10%: Hematologic: Positive Coombs' test without hemolysis
1% to 10%:
Central nervous system: Fever (1%), headache (1%)
Dermatologic: Rash, pruritus
Gastrointestinal: Diarrhea, nausea, vomiting
Local: Erythema at injection site, pain
Reactions reported with other cephalosporins include aplastic anemia, erythema multiforme, hemolytic anemia, hemorrhage, pancytopenia, PT prolonged, renal dysfunction, Stevens-Johnson syndrome, superinfection, toxic epidermal necrolysis, toxic nephropathy, vaginitis
Mechanism of Action Inhibits bacterial cell wall synthesis by binding to one or more of the penicillin-binding proteins (PBPs) which in turn inhibits the final transpeptidation step of peptidoglycan synthesis in bacterial cell walls, thus inhibiting cell wall biosynthesis. Bacteria eventually lyse due to ongoing activity of cell wall autolytic enzymes (autolysis and murein hydrolases) while cell wall assembly is arrested.
Drug Interactions
Increased Effect/Toxicity: High-dose probenecid decreases clearance and increases effect of cefepime. Aminoglycosides increase nephrotoxic potential when taken with cefepime.
Pharmacodynamics/Kinetics
Absorption: I.M.: Rapid and complete
Distribution: V_d: Adults: 14-20 L; penetrates into inflammatory fluid at concentrations ~80% of serum levels and into bronchial mucosa at levels ~60% of those reached in the plasma; crosses blood-brain barrier
Protein binding, plasma: 16% to 19%
Metabolism: Minimally hepatic
Half-life elimination: 2 hours
Time to peak: 0.5-1.5 hours
Excretion: Urine (85% as unchanged drug)
Pregnancy Risk Factor B

Cefepime Hydrochloride see Cefepime on page 287

Cefixime (sef IKS eem)

Related Information
Sexually-Transmitted Diseases on page 1674
(Continued)

Cefixime *(Continued)*

U.S. Brand Names Suprax®
Canadian Brand Names Suprax®
Mexican Brand Names Denvar®
Generic Available No
Pharmacologic Category Antibiotic, Cephalosporin (Third Generation)
Use Treatment of urinary tract infections, otitis media, respiratory infections due to susceptible organisms including *S. pneumoniae* and *S. pyogenes, H. influenzae*, and many Enterobacteriaceae; uncomplicated cervical/urethral gonorrhea due to *N. gonorrhoeae*

Local Anesthetic/Vasoconstrictor Precautions No information available to require special precautions

Effects on Dental Treatment No significant effects or complications reported

Common Adverse Effects
>10%: Gastrointestinal: Diarrhea (16%)
2% to 10%: Gastrointestinal: Abdominal pain, nausea, dyspepsia, flatulence, loose stools

Reactions reported with other cephalosporins include interstitial nephritis, aplastic anemia, hemolytic anemia, hemorrhage, pancytopenia, agranulocytosis, colitis, superinfection

Mechanism of Action Inhibits bacterial cell wall synthesis by binding to one or more of the penicillin binding proteins (PBPs); which in turn inhibits the final transpeptidation step of peptidoglycan synthesis in bacterial cell walls, thus inhibiting cell wall biosynthesis. Bacteria eventually lyse due to ongoing activity of cell wall autolytic enzymes (autolysins and murein hydrolases) while cell wall assembly is arrested.

Drug Interactions
Increased Effect/Toxicity: Aminoglycosides and furosemide may be possible additives to nephrotoxicity. Probenecid increases cefixime concentration. Cefixime may increase carbamazepine. Cefixime may increase prothrombin time when administered with warfarin.

Pharmacodynamics/Kinetics
Absorption: 40% to 50%
Distribution: Widely throughout the body and reaches therapeutic concentration in most tissues and body fluids, including synovial, pericardial, pleural, peritoneal; bile, sputum, and urine; bone, myocardium, gallbladder, and skin and soft tissue
Protein binding: 65%
Half-life elimination: Normal renal function: 3-4 hours; Renal failure: Up to 11.5 hours
Time to peak, serum: 2-6 hours; delayed with food
Excretion: Urine (50% of absorbed dose as active drug); feces (10%)
Pregnancy Risk Factor B

Cefizox® *see* Ceftizoxime *on page 293*
Cefotan® [DSC] *see* Cefotetan *on page 289*

Cefotaxime *(sef oh TAKS eem)*

Related Information
Sexually-Transmitted Diseases *on page 1674*
U.S. Brand Names Claforan®
Canadian Brand Names Claforan®
Mexican Brand Names Benaxima®; Biosint®; Cefradil®; Claforan®; Fotexina®; Taporin®; Viken®
Generic Available Yes: Powder
Synonyms Cefotaxime Sodium
Pharmacologic Category Antibiotic, Cephalosporin (Third Generation)
Use Treatment of susceptible infection in respiratory tract, skin and skin structure, bone and joint, urinary tract, gynecologic as well as septicemia, and documented or suspected meningitis. Active against most gram-negative bacilli (not *Pseudomonas*) and gram-positive cocci (not enterococcus). Active against many penicillin-resistant pneumococci.

Local Anesthetic/Vasoconstrictor Precautions No information available to require special precautions

Effects on Dental Treatment No significant effects or complications reported

Common Adverse Effects
1% to 10%:
Dermatologic: Rash, pruritus
Gastrointestinal: Diarrhea, nausea, vomiting, colitis
Local: Pain at injection site

Reactions reported with other cephalosporins include agranulocytosis, aplastic anemia, cholestasis, hemolytic anemia, hemorrhage, nephropathy, pancytopenia, renal dysfunction, seizure, superinfection.

Mechanism of Action Inhibits bacterial cell wall synthesis by binding to one or more of the penicillin-binding proteins (PBPs) which in turn inhibits the final transpeptidation step of peptidoglycan synthesis in bacterial cell walls, thus inhibiting cell wall biosynthesis. Bacteria eventually lyse due to ongoing activity of cell wall autolytic enzymes (autolysins and murein hydrolases) while cell wall assembly is arrested.

Drug Interactions

Increased Effect/Toxicity: Probenecid may decrease cephalosporin elimination resulting in increased levels. Furosemide, aminoglycosides in combination with cefotaxime may result in additive nephrotoxicity.

Pharmacodynamics/Kinetics

Distribution: Widely to body tissues and fluids including aqueous humor, ascitic and prostatic fluids, bone; penetrates CSF best when meninges are inflamed; crosses placenta; enters breast milk

Metabolism: Partially hepatic to active metabolite, desacetylcefotaxime

Half-life elimination:

Cefotaxime: Premature neonates <1 week: 5-6 hours; Full-term neonates <1 week: 2-3.4 hours; Adults: 1-1.5 hours; prolonged with renal and/or hepatic impairment

Desacetylcefotaxime: 1.5-1.9 hours; prolonged with renal impairment

Time to peak, serum: I.M.: Within 30 minutes

Excretion: Urine (as unchanged drug and metabolites)

Pregnancy Risk Factor B

Cefotaxime Sodium see Cefotaxime on page 288

Cefotetan (SEF oh tee tan)

Related Information

Sexually-Transmitted Diseases on page 1674

U.S. Brand Names Cefotan® [DSC]

Canadian Brand Names Cefotan®

Generic Available No

Synonyms Cefotetan Disodium

Pharmacologic Category Antibiotic, Cephalosporin (Second Generation)

Use Surgical prophylaxis; intra-abdominal infections and other mixed infections; respiratory tract, skin and skin structure, bone and joint, urinary tract and gynecologic as well as septicemia; active against gram-negative enteric bacilli including *E. coli*, *Klebsiella*, and *Proteus*; less active against staphylococci and streptococci than first generation cephalosporins, but active against anaerobes including *Bacteroides fragilis*

Local Anesthetic/Vasoconstrictor Precautions No information available to require special precautions

Effects on Dental Treatment No significant effects or complications reported

Common Adverse Effects

1% to 10%:

Gastrointestinal: Diarrhea (1%)

Hepatic: Transaminases increased (1%)

Miscellaneous: Hypersensitivity reactions (1%)

Reactions reported with other cephalosporins include seizure, Stevens-Johnson syndrome, toxic epidermal necrolysis, renal dysfunction, toxic nephropathy, cholestasis, aplastic anemia, hemolytic anemia, hemorrhage, pancytopenia, agranulocytosis, colitis, superinfection

Mechanism of Action Inhibits bacterial cell wall synthesis by binding to one or more of the penicillin-binding proteins (PBPs) which in turn inhibits the final transpeptidation step of peptidoglycan synthesis in bacterial cell walls, thus inhibiting cell wall biosynthesis. Bacteria eventually lyse due to ongoing activity of cell wall autolytic enzymes (autolysins and murein hydrolases) while cell wall assembly is arrested.

Drug Interactions

Increased Effect/Toxicity: Disulfiram-like reaction may occur if ethanol is consumed by a patient taking cefotetan. Probenecid may increase cefotetan plasma levels. Cefotetan may increase risk of bleeding in patients receiving warfarin.

Pharmacodynamics/Kinetics

Distribution: Widely to body tissues and fluids including bile, sputum, prostatic, peritoneal; low concentrations enter CSF; crosses placenta; enters breast milk

Protein binding: 76% to 90%

(Continued)

Cefotetan *(Continued)*

Half-life elimination: 3-5 hours
Time to peak, serum: I.M.: 1.5-3 hours
Excretion: Primarily urine (as unchanged drug); feces (20%)
Pregnancy Risk Factor B

Cefotetan Disodium *see* Cefotetan *on page 289*

Cefoxitin *(se FOKS i tin)*

Related Information
Sexually-Transmitted Diseases *on page 1674*
U.S. Brand Names Mefoxin®
Generic Available Yes: Powder for injection
Synonyms Cefoxitin Sodium
Pharmacologic Category Antibiotic, Cephalosporin (Second Generation)
Use Less active against staphylococci and streptococci than first generation cephalosporins, but active against anaerobes including *Bacteroides fragilis*; active against gram-negative enteric bacilli including *E. coli*, *Klebsiella*, and *Proteus*; used predominantly for respiratory tract, skin and skin structure, bone and joint, urinary tract and gynecologic as well as septicemia; surgical prophylaxis; intra-abdominal infections and other mixed infections; indicated for bacterial *Eikenella corrodens* infections
Local Anesthetic/Vasoconstrictor Precautions No information available to require special precautions
Effects on Dental Treatment No significant effects or complications reported
Common Adverse Effects
1% to 10%: Gastrointestinal: Diarrhea
Reactions reported with other cephalosporins include Agranulocytosis, aplastic anemia, cholestasis, colitis, erythema multiforme, hemolytic anemia, hemorrhage, pancytopenia, renal dysfunction, serum-sickness reactions, seizure, Stevens-Johnson syndrome, superinfection, toxic nephropathy, vaginitis
Mechanism of Action Inhibits bacterial cell wall synthesis by binding to one or more of the penicillin-binding proteins (PBPs) which in turn inhibits the final transpeptidation step of peptidoglycan synthesis in bacterial cell walls, thus inhibiting cell wall biosynthesis. Bacteria eventually lyse due to ongoing activity of cell wall autolytic enzymes (autolysins and murein hydrolases) while cell wall assembly is arrested.
Drug Interactions
Increased Effect/Toxicity: Probenecid may decrease cephalosporin elimination. Furosemide, aminoglycosides in combination with cefoxitin may result in additive nephrotoxicity.
Pharmacodynamics/Kinetics
Distribution: Widely to body tissues and fluids including pleural, synovial, ascitic, bile; poorly penetrates into CSF even with inflammation of the meninges; crosses placenta; small amounts enter breast milk
Protein binding: 65% to 79%
Half-life elimination: 45-60 minutes; significantly prolonged with renal impairment
Time to peak, serum: I.M.: 20-30 minutes
Excretion: Urine (85% as unchanged drug)
Pregnancy Risk Factor B

Cefoxitin Sodium *see* Cefoxitin *on page 290*

Cefpodoxime *(sef pode OKS eem)*

U.S. Brand Names Vantin®
Canadian Brand Names Vantin®
Mexican Brand Names Orelox®
Generic Available Yes: Tablet
Synonyms Cefpodoxime Proxetil
Pharmacologic Category Antibiotic, Cephalosporin (Third Generation)
Use Treatment of susceptible acute, community-acquired pneumonia caused by *S. pneumoniae* or nonbeta-lactamase producing *H. influenzae*; acute uncomplicated gonorrhea caused by *N. gonorrhoeae*; uncomplicated skin and skin structure infections caused by *S. aureus* or *S. pyogenes*; acute otitis media caused by *S. pneumoniae*, *H. influenzae*, or *M. catarrhalis*; pharyngitis or tonsillitis; and uncomplicated urinary tract infections caused by *E. coli*, *Klebsiella*, and *Proteus*
Local Anesthetic/Vasoconstrictor Precautions No information available to require special precautions

Effects on Dental Treatment No significant effects or complications reported

Common Adverse Effects

>10%:
   Dermatologic: Diaper rash (12%)
   Gastrointestinal: Diarrhea in infants and toddlers (15%)

1% to 10%:
   Central nervous system: Headache (1%)
   Dermatologic: Rash (1%)
   Gastrointestinal: Diarrhea (7%), nausea (4%), abdominal pain (2%), vomiting (1% to 2%)
   Genitourinary: Vaginal infection (3%)

Reactions reported with other cephalosporins include seizure, Stevens-Johnson syndrome, toxic epidermal necrolysis, erythema multiforme, urticaria, serum-sickness reactions, renal dysfunction, interstitial nephritis toxic nephropathy, cholestasis, aplastic anemia, hemolytic anemia, hemorrhage, pancytopenia, agranulocytosis, colitis, vaginitis, superinfection

Mechanism of Action Inhibits bacterial cell wall synthesis by binding to one or more of the penicillin-binding proteins (PBPs) which in turn inhibits the final transpeptidation step of peptidoglycan synthesis in bacterial cell walls, thus inhibiting cell wall biosynthesis. Bacteria eventually lyse due to ongoing activity of cell wall autolytic enzymes (autolysins and murein hydrolases) while cell wall assembly is arrested.

Drug Interactions
   Increased Effect/Toxicity: Probenecid may decrease cephalosporin elimination. Furosemide, aminoglycosides in combination with cefpodoxime may result in additive nephrotoxicity.
   Decreased Effect: Antacids and H_2-receptor antagonists reduce absorption and serum concentration of cefpodoxime.

Pharmacodynamics/Kinetics
   Absorption: Rapid and well absorbed (50%), acid stable; enhanced in the presence of food or low gastric pH
   Distribution: Good tissue penetration, including lung and tonsils; penetrates into pleural fluid
   Protein binding: 18% to 23%
   Metabolism: De-esterified in GI tract to active metabolite, cefpodoxime
   Half-life elimination: 2.2 hours; prolonged with renal impairment
   Time to peak: Within 1 hour
   Excretion: Urine (80% as unchanged drug) in 24 hours

Pregnancy Risk Factor B

Cefpodoxime Proxetil *see* Cefpodoxime *on page 290*

Cefprozil (sef PROE zil)

U.S. Brand Names Cefzil®
Canadian Brand Names Cefzil®
Mexican Brand Names Procef®
Generic Available Yes
Pharmacologic Category Antibiotic, Cephalosporin (Second Generation)
Use Treatment of otitis media and infections involving the respiratory tract and skin and skin structure; active against methicillin-sensitive staphylococci, many streptococci, and various gram-negative bacilli including *E. coli*, some *Klebsiella*, *P. mirabilis*, *H. influenzae*, and *Moraxella*.

Local Anesthetic/Vasoconstrictor Precautions No information available to require special precautions

Effects on Dental Treatment No significant effects or complications reported

Common Adverse Effects

1% to 10%:
   Central nervous system: Dizziness (1%)
   Dermatologic: Diaper rash (2%)
   Gastrointestinal: Diarrhea (3%), nausea (4%), vomiting (1%), abdominal pain (1%)
   Genitourinary: Vaginitis, genital pruritus (2%)
   Hepatic: Transaminases increased (2%)
   Miscellaneous: Superinfection

Reactions reported with other cephalosporins include seizure, toxic epidermal necrolysis, renal dysfunction, interstitial nephritis, toxic nephropathy, aplastic anemia, hemolytic anemia, hemorrhage, pancytopenia, agranulocytosis, colitis, vaginitis, superinfection

Mechanism of Action Inhibits bacterial cell wall synthesis by binding to one or more of the penicillin-binding proteins (PBPs) which in turn inhibits the final transpeptidation step of peptidoglycan synthesis in bacterial cell walls, thus

(Continued)

Cefprozil (Continued)

inhibiting cell wall biosynthesis. Bacteria eventually lyse due to ongoing activity of cell wall autolytic enzymes (autolysins and murein hydrolases) while cell wall assembly is arrested.

Drug Interactions

Increased Effect/Toxicity: Probenecid may decrease cephalosporin elimination. Furosemide, aminoglycosides in combination with cefprozil may result in additive nephrotoxicity.

Pharmacodynamics/Kinetics

Absorption: Well absorbed (94%)

Distribution: Low amounts enter breast milk

Protein binding: 35% to 45%

Half-life elimination: Normal renal function: 1.3 hours

Time to peak, serum: Fasting: 1.5 hours

Excretion: Urine (61% as unchanged drug)

Pregnancy Risk Factor B

Ceftazidime (SEF tay zi deem)

U.S. Brand Names Ceptaz® [DSC]; Fortaz®; Tazicef®

Canadian Brand Names Fortaz®

Mexican Brand Names Fortum®; Izadima®; Tagal®; Taxifur®

Generic Available No

Pharmacologic Category Antibiotic, Cephalosporin (Third Generation)

Use Treatment of documented susceptible *Pseudomonas aeruginosa* infection and infections due to other susceptible aerobic gram-negative organisms; empiric therapy of a febrile, granulocytopenic patient

Local Anesthetic/Vasoconstrictor Precautions No information available to require special precautions

Effects on Dental Treatment No significant effects or complications reported

Common Adverse Effects

1% to 10%:

Gastrointestinal: Diarrhea (1%)

Local: Pain at injection site (1%)

Miscellaneous: Hypersensitivity reactions (2%)

Reactions reported with other cephalosporins include seizure, urticaria, serum-sickness reactions, renal dysfunction, interstitial nephritis, toxic nephropathy, elevated BUN, elevated creatinine, cholestasis, aplastic anemia, hemolytic anemia, pancytopenia, agranulocytosis, colitis, prolonged PT, hemorrhage, superinfection

Mechanism of Action Inhibits bacterial cell wall synthesis by binding to one or more of the penicillin-binding proteins (PBPs) which in turn inhibits the final transpeptidation step of peptidoglycan synthesis in bacterial cell walls, thus inhibiting cell wall biosynthesis. Bacteria eventually lyse due to ongoing activity of cell wall autolytic enzymes (autolysins and murein hydrolases) while cell wall assembly is arrested.

Drug Interactions

Increased Effect/Toxicity: Probenecid may decrease cephalosporin elimination. Aminoglycosides: *in vitro* studies indicate additive or synergistic effect against some strains of Enterobacteriaceae and *Pseudomonas aeruginosa*. Furosemide, aminoglycosides in combination with ceftazidime may result in additive nephrotoxicity.

Pharmacodynamics/Kinetics

Distribution: Widely throughout the body including bone, bile, skin, CSF (higher concentrations achieved when meninges are inflamed), endometrium, heart, pleural and lymphatic fluids

Protein binding: 17%

Half-life elimination: 1-2 hours, prolonged with renal impairment; Neonates <23 days: 2.2-4.7 hours

Time to peak, serum: I.M.: ~1 hour

Excretion: Urine (80% to 90% as unchanged drug)

Pregnancy Risk Factor B

Ceftibuten (sef TYE byoo ten)

Related Information

Bacterial Infections *on page 1697*

U.S. Brand Names Cedax®

Mexican Brand Names Cedax®

Generic Available No

Pharmacologic Category Antibiotic, Cephalosporin (Third Generation)

Use Oral cephalosporin for treatment of bronchitis, otitis media, and pharyngitis/tonsillitis due to *H. influenzae* and *M. catarrhalis*, both beta-lactamase-producing and nonproducing strains, as well as *S. pneumoniae* (weak) and *S. pyogenes*

Local Anesthetic/Vasoconstrictor Precautions No information available to require special precautions

Effects on Dental Treatment No significant effects or complications reported

Common Adverse Effects

1% to 10%:

Central nervous system: Headache (3%), dizziness (1%)

Gastrointestinal: Nausea (4%), diarrhea (3%), dyspepsia (2%), vomiting (1%), abdominal pain (1%)

Hematologic: Increased eosinophils (3%), decreased hemoglobin (2%), thrombocytosis

Hepatic: Increased ALT (1%), increased bilirubin (1%)

Renal: Increased BUN (4%)

Reactions reported with other cephalosporins include anaphylaxis, fever, paresthesia, pruritus, Stevens-Johnson syndrome, toxic epidermal necrolysis, erythema multiforme, angioedema, pseudomembranous colitis, hemolytic anemia, candidiasis, vaginitis, encephalopathy, asterixis, neuromuscular excitability, seizure, serum-sickness reactions, renal dysfunction, interstitial nephritis, toxic nephropathy, cholestasis, aplastic anemia, hemolytic anemia, pancytopenia, agranulocytosis, colitis, prolonged PT, hemorrhage, superinfection

Dosage

Usual dosage range:

Children <12 years: Oral: 9 mg/kg/day for 10 days (maximum dose: 400 mg/day)

Children ≥12 years and Adults: Oral: 400 mg once daily for 10 days (maximum dose: 400 mg/day)

Dosage adjustment in renal impairment:

Cl_{cr} 30-49 mL/minute: Administer 4.5 mg/kg or 200 mg every 24 hours

Cl_{cr} <29 mL/minute: Administer 2.25 mg/kg or 100 mg every 24 hours

Mechanism of Action Inhibits bacterial cell wall synthesis by binding to one or more of the penicillin-binding proteins (PBPs) which in turn inhibits the final transpeptidation step of peptidoglycan synthesis in bacterial cell walls, thus inhibiting cell wall biosynthesis. Bacteria eventually lyse due to ongoing activity of cell wall autolytic enzymes (autolysins and murein hydrolases) while cell wall assembly is arrested.

Contraindications Hypersensitivity to ceftibuten, any component of the formulation, or other cephalosporins

Warnings/Precautions Modify dosage in patients with severe renal impairment, prolonged use may result in superinfection; use with caution in patients with a history of penicillin allergy, especially IgE-mediated reactions (eg, anaphylaxis, urticaria). May cause antibiotic-associated colitis or colitis secondary to *C. difficile*.

Drug Interactions

Increased Effect/Toxicity: High-dose probenecid decreases clearance. Aminoglycosides in combination with ceftibuten may increase nephrotoxic potential.

Dietary Considerations

Capsule: Take without regard to food.

Suspension: Take 2 hours before or 1 hour after meals; contains 1 g of sucrose per 5 mL

Pharmacodynamics/Kinetics

Absorption: Rapid; food decreases peak concentrations, delays T_{max}, and lowers AUC

Distribution: V_d: Children: 0.5 L/kg; Adults: 0.21 L/kg

Half-life elimination: 2 hours

Time to peak: 2-3 hours

Excretion: Urine

Pregnancy Risk Factor B

Dosage Forms CAP: 400 mg. **POWDER, oral suspension:** 90 mg/5 mL (30 mL, 60 mL, 120 mL)

Ceftin® *see* Cefuroxime *on page 295*

Ceftizoxime (sef ti ZOKS eem)

Related Information

Sexually-Transmitted Diseases *on page 1674*

(Continued)

Ceftizoxime *(Continued)*

U.S. Brand Names Cefizox®
Canadian Brand Names Cefizox®
Generic Available No
Synonyms Ceftizoxime Sodium
Pharmacologic Category Antibiotic, Cephalosporin (Third Generation)
Use Treatment of susceptible bacterial infection, mainly respiratory tract, skin and skin structure, bone and joint, urinary tract and gynecologic, as well as septicemia; active against many gram-negative bacilli (not *Pseudomonas*), some gram-positive cocci (not *Enterococcus*), and some anaerobes

Local Anesthetic/Vasoconstrictor Precautions No information available to require special precautions
Effects on Dental Treatment No significant effects or complications reported
Common Adverse Effects
1% to 10%:
Central nervous system: Fever
Dermatologic: Rash, pruritus
Hematologic: Eosinophilia, thrombocytosis
Hepatic: Alkaline phosphatase increased, transaminases increased
Local: Pain, burning at injection site

Other reactions reported with cephalosporins include Stevens-Johnson syndrome, toxic epidermal necrolysis, erythema multiforme, pseudomembranous colitis, angioedema, hemolytic anemia, candidiasis, encephalopathy, asterixis, neuromuscular excitability, seizure, serum-sickness reactions, renal dysfunction, interstitial nephritis, toxic nephropathy, cholestasis, aplastic anemia, hemolytic anemia, pancytopenia, agranulocytosis, colitis, prolonged PT, hemorrhage, superinfection

Mechanism of Action Inhibits bacterial cell wall synthesis by binding to one or more of the penicillin-binding proteins (PBPs) which in turn inhibits the final transpeptidation step of peptidoglycan synthesis in bacterial cell walls, thus inhibiting cell wall biosynthesis. Bacteria eventually lyse due to ongoing activity of cell wall autolytic enzymes (autolysins and murein hydrolases) while cell wall assembly is arrested.

Drug Interactions
Increased Effect/Toxicity: Probenecid may decrease cephalosporin elimination. Furosemide, aminoglycosides in combination with ceftizoxime may result in additive nephrotoxicity.

Pharmacodynamics/Kinetics
Distribution: V_d: 0.35-0.5 L/kg; widely into most body tissues and fluids including gallbladder, liver, kidneys, bone, sputum, bile, pleural and synovial fluids; has good CSF penetration; crosses placenta; small amounts enter breast milk
Protein binding: 30%
Half-life elimination: 1.6 hours; Cl_{cr} <10 mL/minute: 25 hours
Time to peak, serum: I.M.: 0.5-1 hour
Excretion: Urine (as unchanged drug)
Pregnancy Risk Factor B

Ceftizoxime Sodium see Ceftizoxime *on page 293*

Ceftriaxone *(sef trye AKS one)*

Related Information
Sexually-Transmitted Diseases *on page 1674*
U.S. Brand Names Rocephin®
Canadian Brand Names Rocephin®
Mexican Brand Names Amcef®; Benaxona®; Cefaxona®; Ceftrex®; Rocephin®; Tacex®; Terbac®; Triaken®
Generic Available Yes
Synonyms Ceftriaxone Sodium
Pharmacologic Category Antibiotic, Cephalosporin (Third Generation)
Use Treatment of lower respiratory tract infections, acute bacterial otitis media, skin and skin structure infections, bone and joint infections, intra-abdominal and urinary tract infections, pelvic inflammatory disease (PID), uncomplicated gonorrhea, bacterial septicemia, and meningitis; used in surgical prophylaxis
Unlabeled/Investigational Use Treatment of chancroid, epididymitis, complicated gonococcal infections; sexually-transmitted diseases (STD); periorbital or buccal cellulitis; salmonellosis or shigellosis; atypical community-acquired pneumonia; Lyme disease; used in chemoprophylaxis for high-risk contacts and persons with invasive meningococcal disease; sexual assault
Local Anesthetic/Vasoconstrictor Precautions No information available to require special precautions

Effects on Dental Treatment No significant effects or complications reported

Common Adverse Effects

1% to 10%:

Dermatologic: Rash (2%)

Gastrointestinal: Diarrhea (3%)

Hematologic: Eosinophilia (6%), thrombocytosis (5%), leukopenia (2%)

Hepatic: Transaminases increased (3.1% to 3.3%)

Local: Pain, induration at injection site (I.V. 1%); warmth, tightness, induration (5% to 17%) following I.M. injection

Renal: Increased BUN (1%)

Mechanism of Action Inhibits bacterial cell wall synthesis by binding to one or more of the penicillin-binding proteins (PBPs) which in turn inhibits the final transpeptidation step of peptidoglycan synthesis in bacterial cell walls, thus inhibiting cell wall biosynthesis. Bacteria eventually lyse due to ongoing activity of cell wall autolytic enzymes (autolysins and murein hydrolases) while cell wall assembly is arrested.

Drug Interactions

Increased Effect/Toxicity: Cephalosporins may increase the anticoagulant effect of coumarin derivatives (eg, dicumarol, warfarin).

Decreased Effect: Uricosuric agents (eg, probenecid, sulfinpyrazone) may decrease the excretion of cephalosporin; monitor for toxic effects.

Pharmacodynamics/Kinetics

Absorption: I.M.: Well absorbed

Distribution: Widely throughout the body including gallbladder, lungs, bone, bile, CSF (higher concentrations achieved when meninges are inflamed); crosses placenta; enters amniotic fluid and breast milk

Protein binding: 85% to 95%

Half-life elimination: Normal renal and hepatic function: 5-9 hours

Time to peak, serum: I.M.: 1-2 hours

Excretion: Urine (33% to 65% as unchanged drug); feces

Pregnancy Risk Factor B

Ceftriaxone Sodium see Ceftriaxone on page 294

Cefuroxime (se fyoor OKS eem)

U.S. Brand Names Ceftin®; Zinacef®

Canadian Brand Names Apo-Cefuroxime®; Ceftin®; ratio-Cefuroxime; Zinacef®

Mexican Brand Names Cefuracet®; Cetoxil®; Froxal®; Zinnat®

Generic Available Yes

Synonyms Cefuroxime Axetil; Cefuroxime Sodium

Pharmacologic Category Antibiotic, Cephalosporin (Second Generation)

Use Treatment of infections caused by staphylococci, group B streptococci, *H. influenzae* (type A and B), *E. coli*, *Enterobacter*, *Salmonella*, and *Klebsiella*; treatment of susceptible infections of the lower respiratory tract, otitis media, urinary tract, skin and soft tissue, bone and joint, sepsis and gonorrhea

Local Anesthetic/Vasoconstrictor Precautions No information available to require special precautions

Effects on Dental Treatment No significant effects or complications reported

Common Adverse Effects

1% to 10%:

Endocrine & metabolic: Alkaline phosphatase increased (2%)

Hematologic: Eosinophilia (7%), decreased hemoglobin and hematocrit (10%)

Hepatic: Transaminases increased (4%)

Local: Thrombophlebitis (2%)

Reactions reported with other cephalosporins include agranulocytosis, aplastic anemia, asterixis, encephalopathy, hemorrhage, neuromuscular excitability, serum-sickness reactions, superinfection, toxic nephropathy

Mechanism of Action Inhibits bacterial cell wall synthesis by binding to one or more of the penicillin-binding proteins (PBPs) which in turn inhibits the final transpeptidation step of peptidoglycan synthesis in bacterial cell walls, thus inhibiting cell wall biosynthesis. Bacteria eventually lyse due to ongoing activity of cell wall autolytic enzymes (autolysins and murein hydrolases) while cell wall assembly is arrested.

Drug Interactions

Increased Effect/Toxicity: High-dose probenecid decreases clearance. Aminoglycosides in combination with cefuroxime may result in additive nephrotoxicity.

Pharmacodynamics/Kinetics

Absorption: Oral (cefuroxime axetil): Increases with food

(Continued)

Cefuroxime *(Continued)*

Distribution: Widely to body tissues and fluids; crosses blood-brain barrier; therapeutic concentrations achieved in CSF even when meninges are not inflamed; crosses placenta; enters breast milk

Protein binding: 33% to 50%

Bioavailability: Tablet: Fasting: 37%; Following food: 52%

Half-life elimination: Adults: 1-2 hours; prolonged with renal impairment

Time to peak, serum: I.M.: ~15-60 minutes; I.V.: 2-3 minutes

Excretion: Urine (66% to 100% as unchanged drug)

Pregnancy Risk Factor B

Cefuroxime Axetil *see* Cefuroxime *on page 295*

Cefuroxime Sodium *see* Cefuroxime *on page 295*

Cefzil® *see* Cefprozil *on page 291*

Celebrex® *see* Celecoxib *on page 296*

Celecoxib *(se le KOKS ib)*

Related Information
Rheumatoid Arthritis, Osteoarthritis, and Osteoporosis *on page 1668*

U.S. Brand Names Celebrex®

Canadian Brand Names Celebrex®

Generic Available No

Pharmacologic Category Nonsteroidal Anti-inflammatory Drug (NSAID), COX-2 Selective

Dental Use Management of acute dental pain

Use Relief of the signs and symptoms of osteoarthritis, ankylosing spondylitis, and rheumatoid arthritis; management of acute pain; treatment of primary dysmenorrhea; decreasing intestinal polyps in familial adenomatous polyposis (FAP). **Note:** The Notice of Compliance for the use of celecoxib in FAP has been suspended by Health Canada.

Local Anesthetic/Vasoconstrictor Precautions No information available to require special precautions

Effects on Dental Treatment Key adverse event(s) related to dental treatment: Stomatitis, abnormal taste, xerostomia (normal salivary flow resumes upon discontinuation), and tooth disorder. Nonselective NSAIDs are known to reversibly decrease platelet aggregation via mechanisms different than observed with aspirin. According to the manufacturer, celecoxib, at single doses up to 800 mg and multiple doses of 600 mg twice daily, had no effect on platelet aggregation or bleeding time. Comparative NSAIDs (naproxen 500 mg twice daily, ibuprofen 800 mg three times daily, or diclofenac 75 mg twice daily) significantly reduced platelet aggregation and prolonged the bleeding times. See Dental Comment.

Significant Adverse Effects

>10%: Central nervous system: Headache (15.8%)

2% to 10%:

Cardiovascular: Peripheral edema (2.1%)

Central nervous system: Insomnia (2.3%), dizziness (2%)

Dermatologic: Skin rash (2.2%)

Gastrointestinal: Dyspepsia (8.8%), diarrhea (5.6%), abdominal pain (4.1%), nausea (3.5%), flatulence (2.2%)

Neuromuscular & skeletal: Back pain (2.8%)

Respiratory: Upper respiratory tract infection (8.1%), sinusitis (5%), pharyngitis (2.3%), rhinitis (2%)

Miscellaneous: Accidental injury (2.9%)

<2%, postmarketing, and/or case reports (limited to important or life-threatening): Acute renal failure, agranulocytosis, albuminuria, allergic reactions, alopecia, anaphylactoid reactions, angioedema, aplastic anemia, arthralgia, aseptic meningitis, ataxia, bronchospasm, cerebrovascular accident, CHF, colitis, conjunctivitis, cystitis, deafness, diabetes mellitus, dyspnea, dysuria, ecchymosis, erythema multiforme, esophageal perforation, esophagitis, exfoliative dermatitis, flu-like syndrome, gangrene, gastroenteritis, gastroesophageal reflux, gastrointestinal bleeding, glaucoma, hematuria, hepatic failure, hepatitis, hypertension, hypoglycemia, hypokalemia, hyponatremia, interstitial nephritis, intestinal perforation, intracranial hemorrhage (fatal in association with warfarin), jaundice, leukopenia, melena, migraine, myalgia, MI, neuralgia, neuropathy, pancreatitis, pancytopenia, paresthesia, photosensitivity, prostate disorder, pulmonary embolism, rash, renal calculi, sepsis, Stevens-Johnson syndrome, stomatitis, sudden death, syncope, thrombophlebitis, tinnitus, toxic epidermal necrolysis, urticaria, vaginal bleeding, vaginitis, vasculitis, ventricular fibrillation, vertigo, vomiting

Restrictions A medication guide should be dispensed with each prescription. A template for the required MedGuide can be found on the FDA website at http://www.fda.gov/medwatch/SAFETY/2005/safety05.htm#NSAID

Dental Usual Dosing Acute dental pain: Adults: Oral: 400 mg, followed by an additional 200 mg if needed on day 1; maintenance dose: 200 mg twice daily as needed

Dosage Adults: Oral:

Acute pain or primary dysmenorrhea: Initial dose: 400 mg, followed by an additional 200 mg if needed on day 1; maintenance dose: 200 mg twice daily as needed

Ankylosing spondylitis: 200 mg/day as a single dose or in divided doses twice daily; if no effect after 6 weeks, may increase to 400 mg/day. If no response following 6 weeks of treatment with 400 mg/day, consider discontinuation and alternative treatment.

Familial adenomatous polyposis: 400 mg twice daily

Osteoarthritis: 200 mg/day as a single dose or in divided dose twice daily

Rheumatoid arthritis: 100-200 mg twice daily

Elderly: No specific adjustment is recommended. However, the AUC in elderly patients may be increased by 50% as compared to younger subjects. Use the lowest recommended dose in patients weighing <50 kg.

Dosing adjustment in renal impairment: No specific dosage adjustment is recommended; not recommended in patients with advanced renal disease

Dosing adjustment in hepatic impairment: Reduced dosage is recommended (AUC may be increased by 40% to 180%); decrease dose by 50% in patients with moderate hepatic impairment (Child-Pugh class B)

Mechanism of Action Inhibits prostaglandin synthesis by decreasing the activity of the enzyme, cyclooxygenase-2 (COX-2), which results in decreased formation of prostaglandin precursors. Celecoxib does not inhibit cyclooxygenase-1 (COX-1) at therapeutic concentrations.

Contraindications Hypersensitivity to celecoxib, sulfonamides, aspirin, other NSAIDs, or any component of the formulation; perioperative pain in the setting of coronary artery bypass surgery (CABG); pregnancy (3rd trimester)

Warnings/Precautions NSAIDs are associated with an increased risk of adverse cardiovascular events, including MI, and new onset or worsening of pre-existing hypertension. Risk may be increased with duration of use or pre-existing cardiovascular risk factors or disease. Carefully evaluate individual cardiovascular risk profiles prior to prescribing. Use caution with fluid retention, CHF, cerebrovascular disease, ischemic heart disease, or hypertension.

NSAIDs may increase risk of gastrointestinal irritation, ulceration, bleeding, and perforation. These events may occur at any time during therapy and without warning. Use caution with a history of GI disease (bleeding or ulcers), concurrent therapy with aspirin, anticoagulants and/or corticosteroids, smoking, use of alcohol, the elderly or debilitated patients.

Use the lowest effective dose for the shortest duration of time, consistent with individual patient goals, to reduce risk of cardiovascular or GI adverse events. Alternate therapies should be considered for patients at high risk.

NSAIDs may cause serious skin adverse events including exfoliative dermatitis, Stevens-Johnson syndrome (SJS), and toxic epidermal necrolysis (TEN). Anaphylactoid reactions may occur, even without prior exposure; patients with "aspirin triad" (bronchial asthma, aspirin intolerance, rhinitis) may be at increased risk. Do not use in patients who experience bronchospasm, asthma, rhinitis, or urticaria with NSAID or aspirin therapy.

Use with caution in patients with dehydration, decreased renal or hepatic function. Use of NSAIDs can compromise existing renal function, especially when Cl_{cr} <30 mL/minute. Not recommended for use in severe renal or hepatic impairment.

Anaphylactoid reactions may occur, even with no prior exposure to celecoxib. Use caution in patients with known or suspected deficiency of cytochrome P450 isoenzyme 2C9. Safety and efficacy have not been established in patients <18 years of age.

Drug Interactions Substrate of CYP2C9 (major), 3A4 (minor); **Inhibits** CYP2C8 (moderate), 2D6 (weak)

ACE inhibitors: Antihypertensive effect may be diminished by celecoxib.

Aminoglycosides: Celecoxib may decrease excretion; monitor levels.

Aspirin: Low-dose aspirin may be used with celecoxib, however, monitor for GI complications.

Beta-blockers: Antihypertensive effect may be diminished by celecoxib.

Bile acid sequestrants: May decrease absorption of NSAIDs.

(Continued)

Celecoxib *(Continued)*

CYP2C8 Substrates: Celecoxib may increase the levels/effects of CYP2C8 substrates. Example substrates include amiodarone, paclitaxel, pioglitazone, repaglinide, and rosiglitazone.

Cyclosporine: NSAIDs may increase levels/nephrotoxicity of cyclosporine.

Fluconazole: Fluconazole increases celecoxib concentrations twofold. Lowest dose of celecoxib should be used.

Hydralazine: Antihypertensive effect may be diminished by celecoxib.

Lithium: Plasma levels of lithium are increased by ~17% when used with celecoxib. Monitor lithium levels closely when treatment with celecoxib is started or withdrawn.

Loop diuretics (bumetanide, furosemide, torsemide): Natriuretic effect of furosemide and other loop diuretics may be decreased by celecoxib.

Methotrexate: Severe bone marrow suppression, aplastic anemia, and GI toxicity have been reported with concomitant NSAID therapy. Selective COX-2 inhibitors appear to have a lower risk of this toxicity, however, caution is warranted.

Thiazide diuretics: Natriuretic effects of thiazide diuretics may be decreased by celecoxib.

Vancomycin: Celecoxib may decrease excretion; monitor levels.

Warfarin: Bleeding events (including rare intracranial hemorrhage in association with increased prothrombin time) have been reported with concomitant use. Monitor closely, especially in the elderly.

Ethanol/Nutrition/Herb Interactions

Ethanol: Avoid ethanol (increased GI irritation).

Food: Peak concentrations are delayed and AUC is increased by 10% to 20% when taken with a high-fat meal.

Dietary Considerations
Lower doses (200 mg twice daily) may be taken without regard to meals. Larger doses should be taken with food to improve absorption.

Pharmacodynamics/Kinetics

Distribution: V_d (apparent): 400 L

Protein binding: 97% to albumin

Metabolism: Hepatic via CYP2C9; forms inactive metabolites

Bioavailability: Absolute: Unknown

Half-life elimination: 11 hours (fasted)

Time to peak: 3 hours

Excretion: Urine (27% as metabolites, <3% as unchanged drug); feces (57%)

Pregnancy Risk Factor C/D (3rd trimester)

Lactation
Enters breast milk/not recommended (contraindicated in Canadian labeling)

Breast-Feeding Considerations
Based on limited data, celecoxib has been found to be excreted in milk; a decision should be made whether to discontinue nursing or discontinue the drug, taking into account the importance of the drug to the mother.

Dosage Forms
Capsule: 100 mg, 200 mg, 400 mg

Dental Comment The Food and Drug Administration (FDA) has announced product labeling changes for all NSAIDs, including COX-2 selective and over-the-counter (OTC) medications. These changes are the result of the Arthritis and Drug Safety and Risk Management Advisory Committee meeting held in February, 2005.

The FDA has asked that all labels be revised to include information related to the potential for increased risk of cardiovascular (CV) events and gastrointestinal (GI) bleeding associated with their use. In addition, prescription nonselective NSAIDs are being asked to add a contraindication for use in patients who have recently undergone coronary artery bypass graft (CABG) surgery and a boxed warning concerning the CV and GI events. Medication guides will be required for all prescription products. Manufacturers of OTC products are being asked to include a warning about potential skin reactions, which is already included in prescription labeling. The FDA will be working with manufacturers to conduct long-term clinical trials to assess the safety of these agents.

Pfizer, Inc, the manufacturer of celecoxib (Celebrex®) has reported an increased risk of cardiovascular events in one clinical trial during an interim analysis. The increased risk was observed in a trial evaluating celecoxib in patients at risk of colon cancer, prompting the National Cancer Institute to end the study. Other similar clinical studies (which were subjected to analysis by data monitoring committees) are continuing, since an interim analysis of these trials did not reveal an increased risk of cardiovascular events. Further analysis of risk factors related to cardiovascular risk appear warranted. A notice posted by the Food and Drug Administration (FDA) states that the agency "will obtain all available data on these and other ongoing Celebrex® trials as soon as possible and will determine the appropriate regulatory action."

The FDA further notes that these new findings for celecoxib are similar to results with other drugs in this class. Increased cardiovascular risk noted in a study of rofecoxib (Vioxx®) led to a voluntary withdrawal of the product by Merck. In addition, another drug in this class, valdecoxib (Bextra®) demonstrated an increased risk for cardiovascular events in patients following cardiovascular surgery. Valdecoxib (Bextra®) was withdrawn from the market in May 2005.

In their statement, the FDA encourages physicians to consider this developing information in risk-to-benefit evaluations as they consider the use of celecoxib in individual patients. In addition, the FDA advises an evaluation of alternative therapy. If physicians determine that continued use is appropriate for individual patients, the lowest effective dose of celecoxib should be prescribed. Pfizer has not announced a decision to withdraw celecoxib from the market as of December 20, 2004.

The association between selective COX-2 inhibitors and increased cardiovascular risk has been noted previously and prompted by publication of a meta-analysis entitled "Risk of Cardiovascular Events Associated With Selective COX-2 Inhibitors" in the August 22, 2001, edition of the *Journal of the American Medical Association (JAMA).* The researchers reanalyzed four previously published trials, assessing cardiovascular events in patients receiving either celecoxib or rofecoxib. They found an association between the use of COX-2 inhibitors and cardiovascular events (including MI and ischemic stroke). The annualized MI rate was found to be significantly higher in patients receiving celecoxib or rofecoxib than in the control (placebo) group from a recent meta-analysis of primary prevention trials. Although cause and effect cannot be established (these trials were originally designed to assess GI effects, not cardiovascular ones), the authors believe the available data raise a cautionary flag concerning the risk of cardiovascular events with the use of COX-2 inhibitors. The manufacturers of these agents, as well as other healthcare professionals, dispute the methods and validity of the study's conclusions. To date, the FDA has not required any change in the labeling of these agents. Further study is required before any potential risk may be defined.

Cross-reactivity, including bronchospasm, between aspirin and other NSAIDs has been reported in aspirin-sensitive patients. The manufacturer suggests that celecoxib should not be administered to patients with this type of aspirin sensitivity and should be used with caution in patients with pre-existing asthma.

The manufacturer studied the effect of celecoxib on the anticoagulant effect of warfarin and found no alteration of anticoagulant effect, as determined by prothrombin time, in patients taking 2 mg to 5 mg daily. However, the manufacturer has issued a caution when using celecoxib with warfarin since those patients are at increased risk of bleeding complications.

Selected Readings

Dionne R, "COX-2 Inhibitors: Better Than Ibuprofen for Dental Pain?" *Compend Contin Educ Dent,* 1999, 20(6):518-20, 522-4.

Doyle G, Jayawardena S, Ashraf E, et al, "Efficacy and Tolerability of Nonprescription Ibuprofen Versus Celecoxib for Dental Pain," *J Clin Pharmacol,* 2002, 42(8):912-9.

Everts B, Wahrborg P, and Hedner T, "COX-2 Specific Inhibitors - The Emergence of a New Class of Analgesic and Anti-inflammatory Drugs," *Clin Rheumatol,* 2000, 19(5):331-43.

Geis GS, et al, "Efficacy and Safety of Celecoxib, A Specific COX-2 Inhibitor, in Patients With Rheumatoid Arthritis," *Arthritis Rheum,* 1998, 41(9 Suppl):316:1699.

Jeske AH, "COX-2 Inhibitors and Dental Pain Control," *J Gt Houst Dent Soc,* 1999, 71(4):39-40.

Jeske AH, "Selecting New Drugs for Pain Control: Evidence-Based Decisions or Clinical Impressions?" *J Am Dent Assoc,* 2002, 133(8):1052-6.

Jouzeau JY, Terlain B, Abid A, et al, "Cyclo-oxygenase Isoenzymes. How Recent Findings Affect Thinking About Nonsteroidal Anti-inflammatory Drugs," *Drugs,* 1997, 53(4):563-82.

Kaplan-Machlis B and Klostermeyer BS, "The Cyclo-oxygenase-2 Inhibitors: Safety and Effectiveness," *Ann Pharmacother,* 1999, 33(9):979-88.

Karim A, et al, "Celecoxib, A Specific COX-2 Inhibitor, Lacks Significant Drug-Drug Interactions With Methotrexate or Warfarin," *Arthritis Rheum,* 1998, 41(9 Suppl):315:1698.

Kellstein D, Ott D, Jayawardene S, et al, "Analgesic Efficacy of a Single Dose of Lumiracoxib Compared With Rofecoxib, Celecoxib and Placebo in the Treatment of Post-Operative Dental Pain," *Int J Clin Pract,* 2004, 58(3):244-50.

Kurumbail RG, Stevens AM, Gierse JK, et al, "Structural Basis for Selective Inhibition of Cyclo-oxygenase-2 By Anti-inflammatory Agents," *Nature,* 1996, 384(6610):644-8.

Lane NE, "Pain Management in Osteoarthritis: The Role of COX-2 Inhibitors," *J Rheumatol,* 1997, 24(Suppl 49):20-4.

Lipsky PE and Isakson PC, "Outcome of Specific COX-2 Inhibition in Rheumatoid Arthritis," *J Rheumatol,* 1997, 24(Suppl 49):9-14.

Malmstrom K, Daniels S, Kotey P, et al, "Comparison of Rofecoxib and Celecoxib, Two Cyclooxygenase-2 Inhibitors, in Postoperative Dental Pain: A Randomized Placebo- and Active-Comparator-Controlled Clinical Trial," *Clin Ther,* 1999, 21(10):1653-63.

McAdam BF, Catella-Lawson F, Mardini IA, et al, "Systemic Biosynthesis of Prostacyclin by Cyclo-oxygenase (COX)-2: The Human Pharmacology of a Selective Inhibitor of COX-2," *Proc Natl Acad Sci U S A,* 1999, 96(1):272-7.

(Continued)

Celecoxib *(Continued)*

Mengle-Gaw L, et al, "A Study of the Platelet Effects of SC-58635, A Novel COX-2 Selective Inhibitor," *Arthritis Rheum*, 1998, 41(9 Suppl):93-374.

Moore PA and Hersh EV, "Celecoxib and Rofecoxib. The Role of COX-2 Inhibitors in Dental Practice," *J Am Dent Assoc*, 2001, 132(4):451-6.

Needleman P and Isakson PC, "The Discovery and Function of COX-2," *J Rheumatol*, 1997, 24(S49):6-8.

Simon LS, et al, "Preliminary Study of the Safety and Efficacy of SC-58635, A Novel Cyclo-oxygenase 2 Inhibitor: Efficacy and Safety in Two Placebo-Controlled Trials in Osteoarthritis and Rheumatoid Arthritis, and Studies of Gastrointestinal and Platelet Effects," *Arthritis Rheum*, 1998, 41:1591-1602.

Whelton A, Maurath CJ, Verburg KM, et al, "Renal Safety and Tolerability of Celecoxib, a Novel Cyclo-oxygenase-2 Inhibitor," *Am J Ther*, 2000, 7(3):159-75.

Wynn RL, "The New COX-2 Inhibitors: Celecoxib and Rofecoxib," *Home Health Care Consultant*, 2001, 8(10):24-31.

Wynn RL, "The New COX-2 Inhibitors: Rofecoxib (Vioxx®) and Celecoxib (Celebrex™)," *Gen Dent*, 2000, 48(1):16-20.

Wynn RL, "NSAIDS and Cardiovascular Effects, Celecoxib for Dental Pain, and a New Analgesic - Tramadol With Acetaminophen," *Gen Dent*, 2002, 50(3):218-22.

Celestone® *see* Betamethasone *on page 199*

Celestone® Soluspan® *see* Betamethasone *on page 199*

Celexa® *see* Citalopram *on page 351*

CellCept® *see* Mycophenolate *on page 1075*

Cellugel® *see* Hydroxypropyl Methylcellulose *on page 800*

Cellulose (Oxidized/Regenerated)

(SEL yoo lose, OKS i dyzed re JEN er aye ted)

U.S. Brand Names Surgicel®; Surgicel® Fibrillar; Surgicel® NuKnit

Generic Available No

Synonyms Absorbable Cotton; Oxidized Regenerated Cellulose

Pharmacologic Category Hemostatic Agent

Dental Use To control bleeding created during a dental procedure

Use Hemostatic; temporary packing for the control of capillary, venous, or small arterial hemorrhage

Local Anesthetic/Vasoconstrictor Precautions No information available to require special precautions

Effects on Dental Treatment No significant effects or complications reported

Significant Adverse Effects Frequency not defined.

Central nervous system: Headache

Respiratory: Nasal burning or stinging, sneezing (rhinological procedures)

Miscellaneous: Encapsulation of fluid, foreign body reactions (with or without) infection

Postmarketing and/or case reports: Numbness, pain, paralysis

Dental Usual Dosing Control bleeding created during a dental procedure: Topical: Minimal amounts of the fabric strip are laid on the bleeding site or held firmly against the tissues until hemostasis occurs; remove excess material

Dosage Minimal amounts of the fabric strip are laid on the bleeding site or held firmly against the tissues until hemostasis occurs; remove excess material

Mechanism of Action Cellulose, oxidized regenerated is saturated with blood at the bleeding site and swells into a brownish or black gelatinous mass which aids in the formation of a clot. When used in small amounts, it is absorbed from the sites of implantation with little or no tissue reaction. In addition to providing hemostasis, oxidized regenerated cellulose also has been shown *in vitro* to have bactericidal properties.

Contraindications Hypersensitivity to any component of the formulation; implantation into bone defects; hemorrhage from large arteries; nonhemorrhagic oozing; use as an adhesion product

Warnings/Precautions Pain, numbness, or paralysis have been reported if used near a bony or neural space and left inside patient; use minimum amount necessary to achieve hemostasis. Remove as much of agent as possible after hemostasis is achieved. Do not leave in a contaminated or infected space. Always remove completely following hemostasis if applied in proximity to foramina in bone, areas of bony confine, the spinal cord or optic nerve and chasm; product may swell and exert unwanted pressure. The material should not be moistened before insertion since the hemostatic effect is greater when applied dry. The material should not be impregnated with anti-infective agents. Its hemostatic effect is not enhanced by the addition of thrombin.

Drug Interactions No data reported

Pharmacodynamics/Kinetics Absorption: 7-14 days

Pregnancy Risk Factor No data reported

Dosage Forms
Fabric, fibrous (Surgicel® Fibrillar):
  1" x 2" (10s)
  2" x 4" (10s)
  4" x 4" (10s)
Fabric, knitted (Surgicel® NuKnit):
  1" x 1" (24s)
  1" x 3½" (10s)
  3" x 4" (24s)
  6" x 9" (10s)
Fabric, sheer weave (Surgicel®):
  ½" x 2" (24s)
  2" x 3" (24s)
  2" x 14" (24s)
  4" x 8" (24s)

Cellulose Sodium Phosphate
(sel yoo lose SOW dee um FOS fate)

U.S. Brand Names Calcibind®
Canadian Brand Names Calcibind®
Generic Available No
Synonyms CSP; Sodium Cellulose Phosphate
Pharmacologic Category Urinary Tract Product
Use Adjunct to dietary restriction to reduce renal calculi formation in absorptive hypercalciuria type I
Local Anesthetic/Vasoconstrictor Precautions No information available to require special precautions
Effects on Dental Treatment No significant effects or complications reported
Pregnancy Risk Factor C

Celontin® see Methsuximide on page 1019
Cenestin® see Estrogens (Conjugated A/Synthetic) on page 578
Centany™ see Mupirocin on page 1073
Centrum® [OTC] see Vitamins (Multiple/Oral) on page 1582
Centrum® Performance™ [OTC] see Vitamins (Multiple/Oral) on page 1582
Centrum® Silver® [OTC] see Vitamins (Multiple/Oral) on page 1582
Cepacol® Antibacterial Mouthwash [OTC] see Cetylpyridinium on page 309
Cepacol® Antibacterial Mouthwash Gold [OTC] see Cetylpyridinium on page 309
Cepacol® Sore Throat [OTC] see Benzocaine on page 190
Cepastat® [OTC] see Phenol on page 1223
Cepastat® Extra Strength [OTC] see Phenol on page 1223

Cephalexin (sef a LEKS in)

Related Information
Antibiotic Prophylaxis on page 1680
Bacterial Infections on page 1697
Related Sample Prescriptions
Bacterial Endocarditis (Prevention) on page 1732
Bacterial Infections and Periodontal Diseases on page 1736
Prosthetic Joint Late Infections (Prevention) on page 1733
U.S. Brand Names Biocef®; Keflex®; Panixine DisperDose™ [DSC]
Canadian Brand Names Apo-Cephalex®; Keftab®; Novo-Lexin; Nu-Cephalex
Generic Available Yes: Excludes tablet for oral suspension
Synonyms Cephalexin Monohydrate
Pharmacologic Category Antibiotic, Cephalosporin (First Generation)
Dental Use Prophylaxis in total joint replacement patients undergoing dental procedures which produce bacteremia; alternative antibiotic for prevention of bacterial endocarditis
  Note: Individuals allergic to amoxicillin (penicillins) may receive cephalexin provided they have not had an immediate, local, or systemic IgE-mediated anaphylactic allergic reaction to penicillin.
Use Treatment of susceptible bacterial infections including respiratory tract infections, otitis media, skin and skin structure infections, bone infections, and genitourinary tract infections, including acute prostatitis; alternative therapy for acute bacterial endocarditis prophylaxis
Local Anesthetic/Vasoconstrictor Precautions No information available to require special precautions
(Continued)

Cephalexin *(Continued)*

Effects on Dental Treatment No significant effects or complications reported (see Dental Comment)

Significant Adverse Effects Frequency not defined.

Central nervous system: Agitation, confusion, dizziness, fatigue, hallucinations, headache

Dermatologic: Angioedema, erythema multiforme (rare), rash, Stevens-Johnson syndrome (rare), toxic epidermal necrolysis (rare), urticaria

Gastrointestinal: Abdominal pain, diarrhea, dyspepsia, gastritis, nausea (rare), pseudomembranous colitis, vomiting (rare)

Genitourinary: Genital pruritus, genital moniliasis, vaginitis, vaginal discharge

Hematologic: Eosinophilia, neutropenia, thrombocytopenia

Hepatic: AST/ALT increased, cholestatic jaundice (rare), transient hepatitis (rare)

Neuromuscular & skeletal: Arthralgia, arthritis, joint disorder

Renal: Interstitial nephritis (rare)

Miscellaneous: Allergic reactions

Dental Usual Dosing Prophylaxis of bacterial endocarditis (dental, oral, respiratory tract, or esophageal procedures): Oral:

Children >1 year: 50 mg/kg 1 hour prior to procedure (maximum: 2 g)

Children >15 years and Adults: 2 g 1 hour prior to procedure

Dosage

Usual dosage range:

Children >1 year: Oral: 25-100 mg/kg/day every 6-8 hours (maximum: 4 g/day)

Adults: Oral: 250-1000 mg every 6 hours; maximum: 4 g/day

Indication-specific dosing:

Children >1 year: Oral:

Furunculosis: 25-50 mg/kg/day in 4 divided doses

Impetigo: 25 mg/kg/day in 4 divided doses

Otitis media: 75-100 mg/kg/day in 4 divided doses

Prophylaxis of bacterial endocarditis (dental, oral, respiratory tract, or esophageal procedures): 50 mg/kg 1 hour prior to procedure (maximum: 2 g)

Severe infections: 50-100 mg/kg/day in divided doses every 6-8 hours

Skin abscess: 50 mg/kg/day in 4 divided doses (maximum: 4 g)

Streptococcal pharyngitis, skin and skin structure infections: 25-50 mg/kg/day divided every 12 hours

Children >15 years and Adults: Oral:

Cellulitis and mastitis: 500 mg every 6 hours

Furunculosis/skin abscess: 250 mg 4 times/day

Prophylaxis of bacterial endocarditis (dental, oral, respiratory tract, or esophageal procedures): 2 g 1 hour prior to procedure

Streptococcal pharyngitis, skin and skin structure infections: 500 mg every 12 hours

Uncomplicated cystitis: 500 mg every 12 hours for 7-14 days

Dosing adjustment in renal impairment: Adults: Cl_{cr} <10 mL/minute: 250-500 mg every 12 hours

Hemodialysis: Moderately dialyzable (20% to 50%)

Mechanism of Action Inhibits bacterial cell wall synthesis by binding to one or more of the penicillin-binding proteins (PBPs) which in turn inhibits the final transpeptidation step of peptidoglycan synthesis in bacterial cell walls, thus inhibiting cell wall biosynthesis. Bacteria eventually lyse due to ongoing activity of cell wall autolytic enzymes (autolysins and murein hydrolases) while cell wall assembly is arrested.

Contraindications Hypersensitivity to cephalexin, any component of the formulation, or other cephalosporins

Warnings/Precautions Modify dosage in patients with severe renal impairment; prolonged use may result in superinfection. Use with caution in patients with a history of penicillin allergy, especially IgE-mediated reactions (eg, anaphylaxis, urticaria). May cause antibiotic-associated colitis or colitis secondary to *C. difficile*.

Drug Interactions

Aminoglycosides: Increase nephrotoxic potential.

Probenecid: High-dose probenecid decreases clearance of cephalexin.

Ethanol/Nutrition/Herb Interactions Food: Peak antibiotic serum concentration is lowered and delayed, but total drug absorbed is not affected. Cephalexin serum levels may be decreased if taken with food.

Dietary Considerations Take without regard to food. If GI distress, take with food. Panixine DisperDose™ contains phenylalanine 2.8 mg/cephalexin 125 mg.

Pharmacodynamics/Kinetics

Absorption: Delayed in young children

Distribution: Widely into most body tissues and fluids, including gallbladder, liver, kidneys, bone, sputum, bile, and pleural and synovial fluids; CSF penetration is poor; crosses placenta; enters breast milk

Protein binding: 6% to 15%

Half-life elimination: Adults: 0.5-1.2 hours; prolonged with renal impairment

Time to peak, serum: ~1 hour

Excretion: Urine (80% to 100% as unchanged drug) within 8 hours

Pregnancy Risk Factor B

Lactation Enters breast milk (small amounts)/use caution

Breast-Feeding Considerations Theoretically, drug absorbed by nursing infant may change bowel flora or affect fever work-up result. Cephalexin levels can be detected in breast milk, reaching a maximum concentration 4 hours after a single oral dose and gradually decreasing by 8 hours after administration. **Note:** As a class, cephalosporins are used to treat bacterial infections in infants.

Dosage Forms [DSC] = Discontinued product

Capsule: 250 mg, 500 mg

Biocef®: 500 mg

Keflex®: 250 mg, 500 mg

Powder for oral suspension: 125 mg/5 mL (100 mL, 200 mL); 250 mg/5 mL (100 mL, 200 mL)

Biocef®: 125 mg/5 mL (100 mL); 250 mg/5 mL (100 mL)

Keflex®: 125 mg/5 mL (100 mL, 200 mL); 250 mg/5 mL (100 mL, 200 mL)

Tablet, for oral suspension (Panixine DisperDose™): 125 mg [contains phenylalanine 2.8 mg; peppermint flavor], 250 mg [contains phenylalanine 5.6 mg; peppermint flavor] [DSC]

Dental Comment Cephalexin is effective against anaerobic bacteria, but the sensitivity of alpha-hemolytic *Streptococcus* vary; approximately 10% of strains are resistant. Nearly 70% are intermediately sensitive. Patients allergic to penicillins can use a cephalosporin; the incidence of cross-reactivity between penicillins and cephalosporins is 1% when the allergic reaction to penicillin is delayed. If the patient has a history of immediate reaction to penicillin, the incidence of cross-reactivity is 20%; cephalosporins are contraindicated in these patients.

Selected Readings

ADA Division of Legal Affairs, "A Legal Perspective on Antibiotic Prophylaxis," *J Am Dent Assoc*, 2003, 134(9):1260.

"Advisory Statement. Antibiotic Prophylaxis for Dental Patients With Total Joint Replacements. American Dental Association; American Academy of Orthopedic Surgeons," *J Am Dent Assoc*, 1997, 128(7):1004-8.

American Dental Association; American Academy of Orthopedic Surgeons, "Antibiotic Prophylaxis for Dental Patients With Total Joint Replacements," *J Am Dent Assoc*, 2003, 134(7):895-9.

American Dental Association Council on Scientific Affairs, "Combating Antibiotic Resistance," *J Am Dent Assoc*, 2004, 135(4):484-7.

Dajani AS, Taubert KA, Wilson W, et al, "Prevention of Bacterial Endocarditis. Recommendations by the American Heart Association," *JAMA*, 1997, 277(22):1794-801.

Dajani AS, Taubert KA, Wilson W, et al, "Prevention of Bacterial Endocarditis: Recommendations by the American Heart Association," *J Am Dent Assoc*, 1997, 128(8):1142-51.

Saxon A, Beall GN, Rohr AS, et al, "Immediate Hypersensitivity Reactions to Beta-Lactam Antibiotics," *Ann Intern Med*, 1987, 107(2):204-15.

Wynn RL, Bergman SA, Meiller TF, et al, "Antibiotics in Treating Oral-Facial Infections of Odontogenic Origin: An Update," *Gen Dent*, 2001, 49(3):238-40, 242, 244 passim.

Cephalexin Monohydrate *see* Cephalexin *on page 301*

Cephalothin (sef A loe thin)

Generic Available Yes

Synonyms Cephalothin Sodium

Pharmacologic Category Antibiotic, Cephalosporin (First Generation)

Use Treatment of infections when caused by susceptible strains in respiratory, genitourinary, gastrointestinal, skin and soft tissue, bone and joint infections; septicemia; treatment of susceptible gram-positive bacilli and cocci (never enterococcus); some gram-negative bacilli including *E. coli*, *Proteus*, and *Klebsiella* may be susceptible

Local Anesthetic/Vasoconstrictor Precautions No information available to require special precautions

Effects on Dental Treatment No significant effects or complications reported

Common Adverse Effects Frequency not defined.

Dermatologic: Maculopapular and erythematous rash

Gastrointestinal: Diarrhea, nausea, vomiting, dyspepsia, pseudomembranous colitis

Local: Bleeding, pain and induration at injection site

(Continued)

Cephalothin *(Continued)*

Reactions reported with other cephalosporins include anaphylaxis, erythema multiforme, toxic epidermal necrolysis, Stevens-Johnson syndrome, dizziness, fever, headache, CNS irritability, seizure, hemoglobin decreased, neutropenia, leukopenia, agranulocytosis, pancytopenia, aplastic anemia, hemolytic anemia, interstitial nephritis, toxic nephropathy, vaginitis, angioedema, cholestasis, hemorrhage, prolonged PT, serum-sickness reactions, superinfection

Mechanism of Action Inhibits bacterial cell wall synthesis by binding to one or more of the penicillin-binding proteins (PBPs) which in turn inhibits the final transpeptidation step of peptidoglycan synthesis in bacterial cell walls, thus inhibiting cell wall biosynthesis. Bacteria eventually lyse due to ongoing activity of cell wall autolytic enzymes (autolysins and murein hydrolases) while cell wall assembly is arrested.

Drug Interactions

Increased Effect/Toxicity: Probenecid may decrease cephalosporin elimination. Aminoglycosides may increase nephrotoxic potential.

Pharmacodynamics/Kinetics

Distribution: Does not penetrate CSF unless meninges are inflamed; crosses placenta; small amounts enter breast milk

Protein binding: 65% to 80%

Metabolism: Partially hepatic and renal via deacetylation

Half-life elimination: 30-60 minutes

Excretion: Urine (50% to 75% as unchanged drug)

Pregnancy Risk Factor B

Cephalothin Sodium *see* Cephalothin *on page 303*

Cephradine *(SEF ra deen)*

Related Information

Antibiotic Prophylaxis *on page 1680*

U.S. Brand Names Velosef®

Generic Available No

Pharmacologic Category Antibiotic, Cephalosporin (First Generation)

Dental Use Prophylaxis in total joint replacement patients undergoing dental procedures which produce bacteremia

Use Treatment of infections when caused by susceptible strains in respiratory, genitourinary, gastrointestinal, skin and soft tissue, bone and joint infections; treatment of susceptible gram-positive bacilli and cocci (never enterococcus); some gram-negative bacilli including *E. coli*, *Proteus*, and *Klebsiella* may be susceptible

Local Anesthetic/Vasoconstrictor Precautions No information available to require special precautions

Effects on Dental Treatment No significant effects or complications reported

Significant Adverse Effects Frequency not defined.

Central nervous system: Dizziness

Dermatologic: Rash, pruritus

Gastrointestinal: Diarrhea, nausea, vomiting, pseudomembranous colitis

Hematologic: Leukopenia, neutropenia, eosinophilia

Neuromuscular & skeletal: Joint pain

Renal: BUN increased, creatinine increased

Reactions reported with other cephalosporins include anaphylaxis, erythema multiforme, toxic epidermal necrolysis, Stevens-Johnson syndrome, fever, headache, encephalopathy, asterixis, neuromuscular excitability, seizure, agranulocytosis, pancytopenia, aplastic anemia, hemolytic anemia, interstitial nephritis, toxic nephropathy, vaginitis, angioedema, cholestasis, hemorrhage, prolonged PT, serum-sickness reactions, superinfection

Dental Usual Dosing Prophylaxis in total joint replacement patients undergoing dental procedures which produce bacteremia: Adults: Oral: 2 g 1 hour prior to procedure

Dosage

Usual dosage range:

Children ≥9 months: Oral: 25-100 mg/kg/day in divided doses every 6 or 12 hours (maximum: 4 g/day)

Adults: Oral: 250-500 mg every 6-12 hours

Indication-specific dosing:

Children ≥9 months: Oral:

Otitis media: 75-100 mg/kg/day in divided doses every 6 or 12 hours (maximum: 4 g/day)

Dosing adjustment in renal impairment: Adults:
Cl$_{cr}$ 10-50 mL/minute: 250 mg every 6 hours
Cl$_{cr}$ <10 mL/minute: 125 mg every 6 hours

Mechanism of Action Inhibits bacterial cell wall synthesis by binding to one or more of the penicillin-binding proteins (PBPs) which in turn inhibits the final transpeptidation step of peptidoglycan synthesis in bacterial cell walls, thus inhibiting cell wall biosynthesis. Bacteria eventually lyse due to ongoing activity of cell wall autolytic enzymes (autolysins and murein hydrolases) while cell wall assembly is arrested.

Contraindications Hypersensitivity to cephradine, any component of the formulation, or cephalosporins

Warnings/Precautions Use caution with renal impairment; dose adjustment required. Prolonged use may result in superinfection; use with caution in patients with a history of penicillin allergy, especially IgE-mediated reactions (eg, anaphylaxis, urticaria). May cause antibiotic-associated colitis or colitis secondary to *C. difficile*.

Drug Interactions
Increased effect: High-dose probenecid decreases clearance.
Increased toxicity: Aminoglycosides may increase nephrotoxic potential.

Ethanol/Nutrition/Herb Interactions Food: Food delays cephradine absorption but does not decrease extent.

Dietary Considerations May administer with food to decrease GI distress.

Pharmacodynamics/Kinetics
Absorption: Well absorbed
Distribution: Widely into most body tissues and fluids including gallbladder, liver, kidneys, bone, sputum, bile, and pleural and synovial fluids; CSF penetration is poor; crosses placenta; enters breast milk
Protein binding: 18% to 20%
Half-life elimination: 1-2 hours; prolonged with renal impairment
Time to peak, serum: 1-2 hours
Excretion: Urine (~80% to 90% as unchanged drug) within 6 hours

Pregnancy Risk Factor B

Lactation Enters breast milk/use caution

Breast-Feeding Considerations Theoretically, drug absorbed by nursing infant may change bowel flora or affect fever work-up result. **Note:** As a class, cephalosporins are used to treat infections in infants.

Dosage Forms [DSC] = Discontinued product
Capsule: 250 mg, 500 mg [DSC]
Powder for oral suspension: 250 mg/5 mL (100 mL) [fruit flavor]

Selected Readings
ADA Division of Legal Affairs, "A Legal Perspective on Antibiotic Prophylaxis," *J Am Dent Assoc*, 2003, 134(9):1260.
"Advisory Statement. Antibiotic Prophylaxis for Dental Patients With Total Joint Replacements. American Dental Association; American Academy of Orthopedic Surgeons," *J Am Dent Assoc*, 1997, 128(7):1004-8.
American Dental Association; American Academy of Orthopedic Surgeons, "Antibiotic Prophylaxis for Dental Patients With Total Joint Replacements," *J Am Dent Assoc*, 2003, 134(7):895-9.
American Dental Association Council on Scientific Affairs, "Combating Antibiotic Resistance," *J Am Dent Assoc*, 2004, 135(4):484-7.
Donowitz GR and Mandell GL, "Drug Therapy. Beta-Lactam Antibiotics (1)," *N Engl J Med*, 1988, 318(7):419-26.
Donowitz GR and Mandell GL, "Drug Therapy. Beta-Lactam Antibiotics (2)," *N Engl J Med*, 1988, 318(8):490-500.
Gustaferro CA and Steckelberg JM, "Cephalosporin Antimicrobial Agents and Related Compounds," *Mayo Clin Proc*, 1991, 66(10):1064-73.

Ceptaz® [DSC] *see* Ceftazidime *on page 292*
Cerebyx® *see* Fosphenytoin *on page 710*
Ceredase® *see* Alglucerase *on page 68*
Cerezyme® *see* Imiglucerase *on page 819*
Cerovel™ *see* Urea *on page 1551*
Certuss-D® *see* Guaifenesin, Dextromethorphan, and Phenylephrine *on page 756*
Cerubidine® *see* DAUNOrubicin Hydrochloride *on page 426*
Cerumenex® [DSC] *see* Triethanolamine Polypeptide Oleate-Condensate *on page 1535*
Cervidil® *see* Dinoprostone *on page 482*
C.E.S. *see* Estrogens (Conjugated/Equine) *on page 580*
Cesia™ *see* Ethinyl Estradiol and Desogestrel *on page 592*
Cetacaine® *see* Benzocaine, Butyl Aminobenzoate, Tetracaine, and Benzalkonium Chloride *on page 193*
Cetacort® *see* Hydrocortisone *on page 793*
Cetafen® [OTC] *see* Acetaminophen *on page 31*
Cetafen Cold® [OTC] *see* Acetaminophen and Pseudoephedrine *on page 38*
Cetafen Extra® [OTC] *see* Acetaminophen *on page 31*

Ceta-Plus® *see* Hydrocodone and Acetaminophen *on page 779*

Cetirizine (se TI ra zeen)

U.S. Brand Names Zyrtec®
Canadian Brand Names Apo-Cetirizine®; Reactine™
Mexican Brand Names Virlix®; Zyrtec®
Generic Available No
Synonyms Cetirizine Hydrochloride; P-071; UCB-P071
Pharmacologic Category Antihistamine
Use Perennial and seasonal allergic rhinitis and other allergic symptoms including urticaria; chronic idiopathic urticaria
Local Anesthetic/Vasoconstrictor Precautions No information available to require special precautions
Effects on Dental Treatment Key adverse event(s) related to dental treatment: Xerostomia and increased salivation (normal salivary flow resumes upon discontinuation), stomatitis, loss of taste, abnormal taste, tongue discoloration, and ulcerative stomatitis.
Common Adverse Effects
>10%: Central nervous system: Headache (children 11% to 14%, placebo 12%), somnolence (adults 14%, children 2% to 4%)
2% to 10%:
Central nervous system: Insomnia (children 9%, adults <2%), fatigue (adults 6%), malaise (4%), dizziness (adults 2%)
Gastrointestinal: Abdominal pain (children 4% to 6%), dry mouth (adults 5%), diarrhea (children 2% to 3%), nausea (children 2% to 3%, placebo 2%), vomiting (children 2% to 3%)
Respiratory: Epistaxis (children 2% to 4%, placebo 3%), pharyngitis (children 3% to 6%, placebo 3%), bronchospasm (children 2% to 3%, placebo 2%)
Dosage Oral:
Children:
6-12 months: Chronic urticaria, perennial allergic rhinitis: 2.5 mg once daily
12 months to <2 years: Chronic urticaria, perennial allergic rhinitis: 2.5 mg once daily; may increase to 2.5 mg every 12 hours if needed
2-5 years: Chronic urticaria, perennial or seasonal allergic rhinitis: Initial: 2.5 mg once daily; may be increased to 2.5 mg every 12 hours **or** 5 mg once daily
Children ≥6 years and Adults: Chronic urticaria, perennial or seasonal allergic rhinitis: 5-10 mg once daily, depending upon symptom severity
Elderly: Initial: 5 mg once daily; may increase to 10 mg/day. **Note:** Manufacturer recommends 5 mg/day in patients ≥77 years of age.
Dosage adjustment in renal/hepatic impairment:
Children <6 years: Cetirizine use not recommended
Children 6-11 years: <2.5 mg once daily
Children ≥12 and Adults:
Cl_{cr} 11-31 mL/minute, hemodialysis, or hepatic impairment: Administer 5 mg once daily
Cl_{cr} <11 mL/minute, not on dialysis: Cetirizine use not recommended
Mechanism of Action Competes with histamine for H_1-receptor sites on effector cells in the gastrointestinal tract, blood vessels, and respiratory tract
Contraindications Hypersensitivity to cetirizine, hydroxyzine, or any component of the formulation
Warnings/Precautions Cetirizine should be used cautiously in patients with hepatic or renal dysfunction, the elderly and in nursing mothers. May cause drowsiness; use caution performing tasks which require alertness (eg, operating machinery or driving). Safety and efficacy in pediatric patients <6 months of age have not been established.
Drug Interactions
Cytochrome P450 Effect: Substrate of CYP3A4 (minor)
Increased Effect/Toxicity: Increased toxicity with CNS depressants and anticholinergics.
Ethanol/Nutrition/Herb Interactions Ethanol: Avoid ethanol (may increase CNS depression).
Dietary Considerations May be taken with or without food.
Pharmacodynamics/Kinetics
Onset of action: 15-30 minutes
Absorption: Rapid
Protein binding, plasma: Mean: 93%
Metabolism: Limited hepatic
Half-life elimination: 8 hours
Time to peak, serum: 1 hour

Excretion: Urine (70%); feces (10%)
Pregnancy Risk Factor B
Dosage Forms SYR: 5 mg/5 mL (120 mL, 480 mL). **TAB:** 5 mg, 10 mg. **TAB, chewable:** 5 mg, 10 mg

---

Cetirizine and Pseudoephedrine
(se TI ra zeen & soo doe e FED rin)

Related Information
Cetirizine on page 306
Pseudoephedrine on page 1309
U.S. Brand Names Zyrtec-D 12 Hour™
Canadian Brand Names Reactine® Allergy and Sinus
Generic Available No
Synonyms Cetirizine Hydrochloride and Pseudoephedrine Hydrochloride; Pseudoephedrine Hydrochloride and Cetirizine Hydrochloride
Pharmacologic Category Antihistamine/Decongestant Combination
Use Treatment of symptoms of seasonal or perennial allergic rhinitis
Local Anesthetic/Vasoconstrictor Precautions Use with caution since pseudoephedrine is a sympathomimetic amine which could interact with epinephrine to cause a pressor response
Effects on Dental Treatment Key adverse event(s) related to dental treatment: Pseudoephedrine: Xerostomia (normal salivary flow resumes upon discontinuation).
Common Adverse Effects Percentages reported with combination product. Additional adverse effects reported; refer to individual agents.
1% to 10%:
Central nervous system: Insomnia (4%), fatigue (2%), somnolence (2%), dizziness (1%)
Gastrointestinal: Xerostomia (4%)
Respiratory: Pharyngitis (2%), epistaxis (1%)
Mechanism of Action Cetirizine is an antihistamine; exhibits selective inhibition of H_1 receptors. Pseudoephedrine is a sympathomimetic and exerts a decongestant action on nasal mucosa.
Drug Interactions
Cytochrome P450 Effect: Cetirizine: **Substrate** of CYP3A4 (minor)
Increased Effect/Toxicity: See individual agents.
Decreased Effect: See individual agents.
Pharmacodynamics/Kinetics
Zyrtec-D 12 Hour™:
Half-life elimination: Cetirizine: 7.9 hours; Pseudoephedrine: 6 hours
Time to peak: Cetirizine: 2.2 hours; Pseudoephedrine: 4.4 hours
Excretion: Urine (70%); feces (10%)
See individual agents.
Pregnancy Risk Factor C

Cetirizine Hydrochloride see Cetirizine on page 306
Cetirizine Hydrochloride and Pseudoephedrine Hydrochloride see Cetirizine and Pseudoephedrine on page 307

Cetrorelix (set roe REL iks)

U.S. Brand Names Cetrotide®
Canadian Brand Names Cetrotide®
Generic Available No
Synonyms Cetrorelix Acetate
Pharmacologic Category Gonadotropin Releasing Hormone Antagonist
Use Inhibits premature luteinizing hormone (LH) surges in women undergoing controlled ovarian stimulation
Local Anesthetic/Vasoconstrictor Precautions No information available to require special precautions
Effects on Dental Treatment No significant effects or complications reported
Common Adverse Effects
1% to 10%:
Central nervous system: Headache (1%)
Endocrine & metabolic: Ovarian hyperstimulation syndrome, WHO grade II or III (4%)
Gastrointestinal: Nausea (1%)
Hepatic: ALT, AST, GGT, and alkaline phosphatase increased (1% to 2%)
(Continued)

Cetrorelix *(Continued)*

Mechanism of Action Competes with naturally-occurring GnRH for binding on receptors of the pituitary. This delays luteinizing hormone surge, preventing ovulation until the follicles are of adequate size.

Drug Interactions

Increased Effect/Toxicity: No formal studies have been performed.

Decreased Effect: No formal studies have been performed.

Pharmacodynamics/Kinetics

Onset of action: 0.25 mg dose: 2 hours; 3 mg dose: 1 hour

Duration: 3 mg dose (single dose): 4 days

Absorption: Rapid

Protein binding: 86%

Metabolism: Transformed by peptidases; cetrorelix and peptides (1-9), (1-7), (1-6), and (1-4) are found in the bile; peptide (1-4) is the predominant metabolite

Bioavailability: 85%

Half-life elimination: 0.25 mg dose: 5 hours; 0.25 mg multiple doses: 20.6 hours; 3 mg dose: 62.8 hours

Time to peak: 0.25 mg dose: 1 hour; 3 mg dose: 1.5 hours

Excretion: Feces (5% to 10% as unchanged drug and metabolites); urine (2% to 4% as unchanged drug); within 24 hours

Pregnancy Risk Factor X

Cetrorelix Acetate *see* Cetrorelix *on page 307*

Cetrotide® *see* Cetrorelix *on page 307*

Cetuximab *(se TUK see mab)*

U.S. Brand Names Erbitux®

Canadian Brand Names Erbitux®

Generic Available No

Synonyms C225; IMC-C225; NSC-714692

Pharmacologic Category Antineoplastic Agent, Monoclonal Antibody; Epidermal Growth Factor Receptor (EGFR) Inhibitor

Use Treatment of metastatic colorectal cancer; treatment of squamous cell cancer of the head and neck

Unlabeled/Investigational Use Breast cancer, tumors overexpressing EGFR

Local Anesthetic/Vasoconstrictor Precautions No information available to require special precautions

Effects on Dental Treatment No significant effects or complications reported

Common Adverse Effects Except where noted, percentages reported for cetuximab monotherapy.

>10%:

Central nervous system: Malaise (48%), pain (17% to 28%), fever (5% to 27%), headache (26%)

Dermatologic: Acneform rash (76% to 90%; grades 3/4: 1% to 8%), nail disorder (16%), pruritus (11%)

Endocrine & metabolic: Hypomagnesemia (50%; grades 3/4: 10% to 15%)

Gastrointestinal: Nausea (mild to moderate 29%), weight loss (7% to 27%), constipation (26%), abdominal pain (26%), diarrhea (25%), vomiting (25%), anorexia (23%)

Neuromuscular & skeletal: Weakness (45% to 48%)

Respiratory: Dyspnea (17%), cough (11%)

Miscellaneous: Infusion reaction (19% to 21%; grades 3/4: 2% to 4%; 90% with first infusion), infection (14%)

1% to 10%:

Cardiovascular: Peripheral edema (10%), cardiopulmonary arrest (2%; with radiation therapy)

Central nervous system: Insomnia (10%), depression (7%)

Dermatologic: Alopecia (4%), skin disorder (4%)

Endocrine & metabolic: Dehydration (2% to 10%)

Gastrointestinal: Stomatitis (10%), dyspepsia (6%)

Hematologic: Anemia (9%)

Hepatic: Alkaline phosphatase increased (5% to 10%), transaminases increased (5% to 10%)

Neuromuscular & skeletal: Back pain (10%)

Ocular: Conjunctivitis (7%)

Renal: Kidney failure (2%)

Respiratory: Pulmonary embolus (1%)

Miscellaneous: Sepsis (3%)

Mechanism of Action Recombinant human/mouse chimeric monoclonal antibody which binds specifically to the epidermal growth factor receptor (EGFR, HER1, c-ErbB-1) and competitively inhibits the binding of epidermal growth factor (EGF) and other ligands. Binding to the EGFR blocks phosphorylation and activation of receptor-associated kinases, resulting in inhibition of cell growth, induction of apoptosis, and decreased matrix metalloproteinase and vascular endothelial growth factor production.

Drug Interactions
Increased Effect/Toxicity: Interactions have not been evaluated in clinical trials.

Pharmacodynamics/Kinetics
Distribution: V_d: ~2-3 L/m^2
Half-life elimination: 112 hours (range: 63-230 hours)

Pregnancy Risk Factor C

Cetylpyridinium (SEE til peer i DI nee um)

U.S. Brand Names Cepacol® Antibacterial Mouthwash [OTC]; Cepacol® Antibacterial Mouthwash Gold [OTC]; DiabetAid Gingivitis Mouth Rinse [OTC]
Generic Available No
Synonyms Cetylpyridinium Chloride; CPC
Pharmacologic Category Antiseptic, Oral Mouthwash
Dental Use Antiseptic to aid in the prevention and reduction of plaque and gingivitis, and to freshen breath
Use Antiseptic to aid in the prevention and reduction of plaque and gingivitis, and to freshen breath
Local Anesthetic/Vasoconstrictor Precautions No information available to require special precautions
Effects on Dental Treatment Key adverse event(s) related to dental treatment: Tooth and tongue staining and oral irritation.
Significant Adverse Effects Frequency not defined: Gastrointestinal: Tooth and tongue staining, oral irritation
Dental Usual Dosing Prevention and reduction of plaque and gingivitis, and to freshen breath: Children ≥6 years and Adults: Oral (OTC labeling): Rinse or gargle as directed; may be used before or after brushing (2-3 times/day)
Dosage Children ≥6 years and Adults: Oral (OTC labeling): Rinse or gargle to freshen mouth; may be used before or after brushing
Contraindications Hypersensitivity to cetylpyridinium or any component of the formulation
Warnings/Precautions Not labeled for OTC use in children <6 years of age.
Pregnancy Risk Factor C
Dosage Forms Liquid, as chloride, oral [mouthwash/gargle]:
Cepacol® Antibacterial Mouthwash Gold: 0.05% (120 mL, 360 mL, 720 mL, 960 mL) [contains alcohol 14% and tartrazine; original flavor]
Cepacol® Antibacterial Mouthwash: 0.05% (120 mL, 360 mL, 720 mL, 960 mL) [contains alcohol 14% and tartrazine; mint flavor]
DiabetAid Gingivitis Mouth Rinse: 0.1% (480 mL) [sugar free]

Cetylpyridinium and Benzocaine
(SEE til peer i DI nee um & BEN zoe kane)

Related Information
Benzocaine on page 190
Cetylpyridinium on page 309
Canadian Brand Names Cepacol®; Kank-A®
Synonyms Benzocaine and Cetylpyridinium Chloride; Cetylpyridinium Chloride and Benzocaine
Pharmacologic Category Local Anesthetic
Dental Use Antiseptic/anesthetic for oral cavity
Use Symptomatic relief of sore throat
Local Anesthetic/Vasoconstrictor Precautions No information available to require special precautions
Effects on Dental Treatment No significant effects or complications reported
Restrictions Not available in U.S.
Dosage Antiseptic/anesthetic: Oral: Dissolve in mouth as needed for sore throat
Drug Interactions See individual agents.
Pregnancy Risk Factor C

Cetylpyridinium Chloride see Cetylpyridinium on page 309

Cetylpyridinium Chloride and Benzocaine *see* Cetylpyridinium and Benzocaine *on page 309*

Cevi-Bid® [OTC] *see* Ascorbic Acid *on page 143*

Cevimeline (se vi ME leen)

Related Information
Management of Patients Undergoing Cancer Therapy *on page 1728*

U.S. Brand Names Evoxac®

Canadian Brand Names Evoxac®

Generic Available No

Synonyms Cevimeline Hydrochloride

Pharmacologic Category Cholinergic Agonist

Dental Use Treatment of symptoms of dry mouth in patients with Sjögren's syndrome

Use Treatment of symptoms of dry mouth in patients with Sjögren's syndrome

Local Anesthetic/Vasoconstrictor Precautions No information available to require special precautions

Effects on Dental Treatment Key adverse event(s) related to dental treatment: Excessive salivation, salivary gland pain, xerostomia (normal salivary flow resumes upon discontinuation), ulcerative stomatitis, and tooth disorder.

Significant Adverse Effects

>10%:
Central nervous system: Headache (14%; placebo 20%)
Gastrointestinal: Nausea (14%), diarrhea (10%)
Respiratory: Rhinitis (11%), sinusitis (12%), upper respiratory infection (11%)
Miscellaneous: Diaphoresis increased (19%)

1% to 10%:
Cardiovascular: Peripheral edema, chest pain, edema, palpitation
Central nervous system: Dizziness (4%), fatigue (3%), pain (3%), insomnia (2%), anxiety (1%), fever, depression, migraine, hypoesthesia, vertigo
Dermatologic: Rash (4%; placebo 6%), pruritus, skin disorder, erythematous rash
Endocrine & metabolic: Hot flashes (2%)
Gastrointestinal: Dyspepsia (8%; placebo 9%), abdominal pain (8%), vomiting (5%), excessive salivation (2%), constipation, salivary gland pain, dry mouth, sialoadenitis, gastroesophageal reflux, flatulence, ulcerative stomatitis, eructation, amylase increased, anorexia, tooth disorder
Genitourinary: Urinary tract infection (6%), vaginitis, cystitis
Hematologic: Anemia
Local: Abscess
Neuromuscular & skeletal: Back pain (5%), arthralgia (4%), skeletal pain (3%), rigors (1%), hypertonia, tremor, myalgia, hyporeflexia, leg cramps
Ocular: Conjunctivitis (4%), abnormal vision, eye pain, eye abnormality, xerophthalmia
Otic: Earache, otitis media
Respiratory: Coughing (6%), bronchitis (4%), pneumonia, epistaxis
Miscellaneous: Flu-like syndrome, infection, fungal infection, allergy, hiccups

<1% (Limited to important or life-threatening): Aggravated multiple sclerosis, aggressive behavior, alopecia, angina, anterior chamber hemorrhage, aphasia, apnea, arrhythmia, arthropathy, avascular necrosis (femoral head), bronchospasm, bullous eruption, bundle branch block, cholecystitis, cholelithiasis, cholinergic syndrome, coma, deafness, delirium, dementia, depersonalization, dyskinesia, eosinophilia, esophageal stricture, esophagitis, fall, gastric ulcer, gastrointestinal hemorrhage, gingival hyperplasia, glaucoma, granulocytopenia, hallucination, hematuria, hypothyroidism, ileus, impotence, intestinal obstruction, leukopenia, lymphocytosis, manic reaction, MI, neuropathy, paralysis, paranoia, paresthesia, peptic ulcer, pericarditis, peripheral ischemia, photosensitivity reaction, pleural effusion, pulmonary embolism, pulmonary fibrosis, renal calculus, seizure, sepsis, somnolence, syncope, systemic lupus erythematosus, tenosynovitis, thrombocytopenia, thrombocytopenic purpura, thrombophlebitis, T-wave inversion, urinary retention, vasculitis

Dental Usual Dosing Dry mouth (in Sjögren's syndrome): Adults: Oral: 30 mg 3 times/day

Dosage Adults: Oral: 30 mg 3 times/day

Dosage adjustment in renal/hepatic impairment: Not studied; no specific dosage adjustment is recommended

Elderly: No specific dosage adjustment is recommended; however, use caution when initiating due to potential for increased sensitivity

Mechanism of Action Binds to muscarinic (cholinergic) receptors, causing an increase in secretion of exocrine glands (including salivary glands)

Contraindications Hypersensitivity to cevimeline or any component of the formulation; uncontrolled asthma; narrow-angle glaucoma; acute iritis; other conditions where miosis is undesirable

Warnings/Precautions May alter cardiac conduction and/or heart rate; use caution in patients with significant cardiovascular disease, including angina, myocardial infarction, or conduction disturbances. Cevimeline has the potential to increase bronchial smooth muscle tone, airway resistance, and bronchial secretions; use with caution in patients with controlled asthma, COPD, or chronic bronchitis. May cause decreased visual acuity (particularly at night and in patients with central lens changes) and impaired depth perception. Patients should be cautioned about driving at night or performing hazardous activities in reduced lighting. May cause a variety of parasympathomimetic effects, which may be particularly dangerous in elderly patients; excessive sweating may lead to dehydration in some patients.

Use with caution in patients with a history of biliary stones or nephrolithiasis; cevimeline may induce smooth muscle spasms, precipitating cholangitis, cholecystitis, biliary obstruction, renal colic, or ureteral reflux in susceptible patients. Patients with a known or suspected deficiency of CYP2D6 may be at higher risk of adverse effects. Safety and efficacy has not been established in pediatric patients.

Drug Interactions Substrate (minor) of CYP2D6, CYP3A4

Increased effect: The effects of other cholinergic agents may be increased during concurrent administration with cevimeline. Concurrent use of cevimeline and beta-blockers may increase the potential for conduction disturbances.

Decreased effect: Anticholinergic agents (atropine, TCAs, phenothiazines) may antagonize the effects of cevimeline.

Dietary Considerations Take with or without food.

Pharmacodynamics/Kinetics

Distribution: V_d: 6 L/kg

Protein binding: <20%

Metabolism: Hepatic via CYP2D6 and CYP3A4

Half-life elimination: 5 hours

Time to peak: 1.5-2 hours

Excretion: Urine (as metabolites and unchanged drug)

Pregnancy Risk Factor C

Lactation Excretion in breast milk unknown/not recommended

Dosage Forms Capsule, as hydrochloride: 30 mg

Cevimeline Hydrochloride *see* Cevimeline *on page 310*

CFDN *see* Cefdinir *on page 284*

CG *see* Chorionic Gonadotropin (Human) *on page 336*

CGP-42446 *see* Zoledronic Acid *on page 1600*

CGP-57148B *see* Imatinib *on page 817*

C-Gram [OTC] *see* Ascorbic Acid *on page 143*

CGS-20267 *see* Letrozole *on page 904*

Char-Caps [OTC] *see* Charcoal *on page 311*

CharcoAid G® [OTC] [DSC] *see* Charcoal *on page 311*

Charcoal (CHAR kole)

U.S. Brand Names Actidose-Aqua® [OTC]; Actidose® with Sorbitol [OTC]; Char-Caps [OTC]; CharcoAid G® [OTC] [DSC]; Charcoal Plus® DS [OTC]; Charcocaps® [OTC]; EZ-Char™ [OTC]; Kerr Insta-Char® [OTC]

Canadian Brand Names Charcadole®; Charcadole®, Aqueous; Charcadole® TFS

Generic Available Yes

Synonyms Activated Carbon; Activated Charcoal; Adsorbent Charcoal; Liquid Antidote; Medicinal Carbon; Medicinal Charcoal

Pharmacologic Category Antidote

Use Emergency treatment in poisoning by drugs and chemicals; aids the elimination of certain drugs and improves decontamination of excessive ingestions of sustained-release products or in the presence of bezoars; repetitive doses have proven useful to enhance the elimination of certain drugs (eg, theophylline, phenobarbital, and aspirin); repetitive doses for gastric dialysis in uremia to adsorb various waste products; dietary supplement (digestive aid)

Local Anesthetic/Vasoconstrictor Precautions No information available to require special precautions

Effects on Dental Treatment No significant effects or complications reported (Continued)

Charcoal *(Continued)*

Mechanism of Action Adsorbs toxic substances or irritants, thus inhibiting GI absorption; adsorbs intestinal gas; the addition of sorbitol results in hyperosmotic laxative action causing catharsis

Pregnancy Risk Factor C

Charcoal Plus® DS [OTC] *see Charcoal on page 311*

Charcocaps® [OTC] *see Charcoal on page 311*

CheeTah® *see Barium on page 179*

Cheracol® *see Guaifenesin and Codeine on page 753*

Cheracol® D [OTC] *see Guaifenesin and Dextromethorphan on page 754*

Cheracol® Plus [OTC] *see Guaifenesin and Dextromethorphan on page 754*

Cheratussin AC *see Guaifenesin and Codeine on page 753*

CHG *see Chlorhexidine Gluconate on page 316*

Chiggerex® [OTC] *see Benzocaine on page 190*

Chiggertox® [OTC] *see Benzocaine on page 190*

Children's Dimetapp® Elixir Cold & Allergy [OTC] *see Brompheniramine and Pseudoephedrine on page 223*

Children's Kaopectate® [OTC] [DSC] *see Attapulgite on page 165*

Children's Pepto [OTC] *see Calcium Carbonate on page 248*

Chirocaine® [DSC] *see Levobupivacaine on page 909*

Chloral *see Chloral Hydrate on page 312*

Chloral Hydrate *(KLOR al HYE drate)*

U.S. Brand Names Aquachloral® Supprettes®; Somnote™

Canadian Brand Names PMS-Chloral Hydrate

Generic Available Yes: Syrup

Synonyms Chloral; Hydrated Chloral; Trichloroacetaldehyde Monohydrate

Pharmacologic Category Hypnotic, Nonbenzodiazepine

Dental Use Short-term sedative/hypnotic for dental procedures

Use Short-term sedative and hypnotic (<2 weeks); sedative/hypnotic for diagnostic procedures; sedative prior to EEG evaluations

Local Anesthetic/Vasoconstrictor Precautions No information available to require special precautions

Effects on Dental Treatment No significant effects or complications reported

Significant Adverse Effects Frequency not defined.

Central nervous system: Ataxia, disorientation, sedation, excitement (paradoxical), dizziness, fever, headache, confusion, lightheadedness, nightmares, hallucinations, drowsiness, "hangover" effect

Dermatologic: Rash, urticaria

Gastrointestinal: Gastric irritation, nausea, vomiting, diarrhea, flatulence

Hematologic: Leukopenia, eosinophilia, acute intermittent porphyria

Miscellaneous: Physical and psychological dependence may occur with prolonged use of large doses

Restrictions C-IV

Dental Usual Dosing

Conscious sedation: Children: Oral: 50-75 mg/kg/dose 30-60 minutes prior to procedure; may repeat 30 minutes after initial dose if needed, to a total maximum dose of 120 mg/kg or 1 g total

Hypnotic: Adults: Oral, rectal: 500-1000 mg at bedtime or 30 minutes prior to procedure, not to exceed 2 g/24 hours

Sedation, anxiety: Oral, rectal:

Children: 5-15 mg/kg/dose every 8 hours (maximum: 500 mg/dose)

Adults: 250 mg 3 times/day

Dosage

Children:

Sedation or anxiety: Oral, rectal: 5-15 mg/kg/dose every 8 hours (maximum: 500 mg/dose)

Prior to EEG: Oral, rectal: 20-25 mg/kg/dose, 30-60 minutes prior to EEG; may repeat in 30 minutes to maximum of 100 mg/kg or 2 g total

Hypnotic: Oral, rectal: 20-40 mg/kg/dose up to a maximum of 50 mg/kg/24 hours or 1 g/dose or 2 g/24 hours

Conscious sedation: Oral: 50-75 mg/kg/dose 30-60 minutes prior to procedure; may repeat 30 minutes after initial dose if needed, to a total maximum dose of 120 mg/kg or 1 g total

Adults: Oral, rectal:

Sedation, anxiety: 250 mg 3 times/day

Hypnotic: 500-1000 mg at bedtime or 30 minutes prior to procedure, not to exceed 2 g/24 hours

Discontinuation: Withdraw gradually over 2 weeks if patient has been maintained on high doses for prolonged period of time. Do not stop drug abruptly; sudden withdrawal may result in delirium.

Dosing adjustment/comments in renal impairment: Cl$_{cr}$ <50 mL/minute: Avoid use

Hemodialysis: Dialyzable (50% to 100%); supplemental dose is not necessary

Dosing adjustment/comments in hepatic impairment: Avoid use in patients with severe hepatic impairment

Mechanism of Action Central nervous system depressant effects are due to its active metabolite trichloroethanol, mechanism unknown

Contraindications Hypersensitivity to chloral hydrate or any component of the formulation; hepatic or renal impairment; gastritis or ulcers; severe cardiac disease

Warnings/Precautions Use with caution in patients with porphyria. Use with caution in neonates. Drug may accumulate with repeated use; prolonged use in neonates associated with hyperbilirubinemia. Tolerance to hypnotic effect develops, therefore, not recommended for use >2 weeks. Taper dosage to avoid withdrawal with prolonged use. Trichloroethanol (TCE), a metabolite of chloral hydrate, is a carcinogen in mice; there is no data in humans. Chloral hydrate is considered a second line hypnotic agent in the elderly. Recent interpretive guidelines from the Centers for Medicare and Medicaid Services (CMS) discourage the use of chloral hydrate in residents of long-term care facilities.

Drug Interactions

CNS depressants: Sedative effects and/or respiratory depression with chloral hydrate may be additive with other CNS depressants; monitor for increased effect; includes ethanol, sedatives, antidepressants, narcotic analgesics, and benzodiazepines.

Furosemide: Diaphoresis, flushing, and hypertension have occurred in patients who received I.V. furosemide within 24 hours after administration of chloral hydrate; consider using a benzodiazepine.

Phenytoin: Half-life may be decreased by chloral hydrate; limited documentation (small, single-dose study); monitor.

Warfarin: Effect of oral anticoagulants may be increased by chloral hydrate; monitor INR; warfarin dosage may require adjustment. Chloral hydrate's metabolite may displace warfarin from its protein binding sites resulting in an increase in the hypoprothrombinemic response to warfarin.

Ethanol/Nutrition/Herb Interactions

Ethanol: Avoid ethanol (may increase CNS depression).

Herb/Nutraceutical: Avoid valerian, St John's wort, kava kava, gotu kola (may increase CNS depression).

Pharmacodynamics/Kinetics

Onset of action: Peak effect: 0.5-1 hour

Duration: 4-8 hours

Absorption: Oral, rectal: Well absorbed

Distribution: Crosses placenta; negligible amounts enter breast milk

Metabolism: Rapidly hepatic to trichloroethanol (active metabolite); variable amounts hepatically and renally to trichloroacetic acid (inactive)

Half-life elimination: Active metabolite: 8-11 hours

Excretion: Urine (as metabolites); feces (small amounts)

Pregnancy Risk Factor C

Lactation Enters breast milk/compatible

Dosage Forms

Capsule (Somnote™): 500 mg

Suppository, rectal (Aquachloral® Supprettes®): 325 mg [contains tartrazine], 650 mg

Syrup: 500 mg/5 mL (480 mL) [contains sodium benzoate]

Chlorambucil (klor AM byoo sil)

U.S. Brand Names Leukeran®

Canadian Brand Names Leukeran®

Mexican Brand Names Leukeran®

Generic Available No

Synonyms CB-1348; Chlorambucilum; Chloraminophene; Chlorbutinum; NSC-3088; WR-139013

Pharmacologic Category Antineoplastic Agent, Alkylating Agent

Use Management of chronic lymphocytic leukemia, Hodgkin's and non-Hodgkin's lymphoma; breast and ovarian carcinoma; Waldenström's macroglobulinemia, testicular carcinoma, thrombocythemia, choriocarcinoma

Local Anesthetic/Vasoconstrictor Precautions No information available to require special precautions

(Continued)

Chlorambucil (Continued)

Effects on Dental Treatment Key adverse event(s) related to dental treatment: Stomatitis.

Common Adverse Effects Frequency not defined.

Central nervous system: Agitation, ataxia, confusion, focal/generalized seizures (rare), hallucinations

Dermatologic: Angioneurotic edema, erythema multiforme (rare), skin hypersensitivity, Stevens-Johnson syndrome (rare), toxic epidermal necrolysis (rare), urticaria

Endocrine & metabolic: Amenorrhea, azoospermia, chromosomal damage, infertility, sterility

Gastrointestinal: Hepatotoxicity, jaundice, diarrhea (infrequent), nausea (infrequent), stomatitis (infrequent), vomiting (infrequent)

Genitourinary: Sterile cystitis

Hematologic: Myelosuppression (common), leukemia, lymphopenia, neutropenia, secondary malignancies

Hepatic: Hepatotoxicity, jaundice

Neuromuscular & skeletal: Flaccid paresis, muscular twitching, myoclonia, neuropathy (peripheral), tremor

Respiratory: Interstitial pneumonia, pulmonary fibrosis, SIADH (rare)

Miscellaneous: Fever, secondary malignancies

Mechanism of Action Interferes with DNA replication and RNA transcription by alkylation and cross-linking the strands of DNA

Drug Interactions

Decreased Effect: Patients may experience impaired immune response to vaccines; possible infection after administration of live vaccines in patients receiving immunosuppressants.

Pharmacodynamics/Kinetics

Absorption: Rapid and complete

Distribution: V_d: 0.14-0.24 L/kg

Protein binding: ~99%

Metabolism: Hepatic; active metabolite, phenylacetic acid mustard

Bioavailability: Reduced 10% to 20% with food

Half-life elimination: ~1.5 hours; Phenylacetic acid mustard: 2.5 hours

Time to peak, plasma: Within 1 hour; Phenylacetic acid mustard: 1.2-2.6 hours

Excretion: Urine (15% to 60% primarily as metabolites, <1% as unchanged drug or phenylacetic acid mustard: 2.5 hours)

Pregnancy Risk Factor D

Chlorambucilum *see* Chlorambucil *on page 313*

Chloraminophene *see* Chlorambucil *on page 313*

Chloramphenicol (klor am FEN i kole)

U.S. Brand Names Chloromycetin® Sodium Succinate

Canadian Brand Names Chloromycetin®; Diochloram®; Pentamycetin®

Generic Available Yes

Pharmacologic Category Antibiotic, Miscellaneous

Use Treatment of serious infections due to organisms resistant to other less toxic antibiotics or when its penetrability into the site of infection is clinically superior to other antibiotics to which the organism is sensitive; useful in infections caused by *Bacteroides, H. influenzae, Neisseria meningitidis, Salmonella,* and *Rickettsia*; active against many vancomycin-resistant enterococci

Local Anesthetic/Vasoconstrictor Precautions No information available to require special precautions

Effects on Dental Treatment No significant effects or complications reported

Common Adverse Effects

Three (3) major toxicities associated with chloramphenicol include:

Aplastic anemia, an idiosyncratic reaction which can occur with any route of administration; usually occurs 3 weeks to 12 months after initial exposure to chloramphenicol.

Bone marrow suppression is thought to be dose related with serum concentrations >25 mcg/mL and reversible once chloramphenicol is discontinued; anemia and neutropenia may occur during the first week of therapy.

Gray syndrome is characterized by circulatory collapse, cyanosis, acidosis, abdominal distention, myocardial depression, coma, and death. Reaction appears to be associated with serum levels ≥50 mcg/mL. May result from drug accumulation in patients with impaired hepatic or renal function.

Additional adverse reactions, frequency not defined:

Central nervous system: Confusion, delirium, depression, fever, headache

Dermatologic: Angioedema, rash, urticaria

Gastrointestinal: Diarrhea, enterocolitis, glossitis, nausea, stomatitis, vomiting
Hematologic: Granulocytopenia, hypoplastic anemia, pancytopenia, thrombo-
cytopenia
Ocular: Optic neuritis
Miscellaneous: Anaphylaxis, hypersensitivity reactions

Mechanism of Action Reversibly binds to 50S ribosomal subunits of susceptible organisms preventing amino acids from being transferred to growing
peptide chains thus inhibiting protein synthesis

Drug Interactions
Cytochrome P450 Effect: Inhibits CYP2C9 (weak), 3A4 (weak)
Increased Effect/Toxicity: Chloramphenicol increases serum concentra-
tions of chlorpropamide, phenytoin, and oral anticoagulants.
Decreased Effect: Phenobarbital and rifampin may decrease serum concen-
trations of chloramphenicol.

Pharmacodynamics/Kinetics
Distribution: To most tissues and body fluids; readily crosses placenta; enters
breast milk
CSF:blood level ratio: Normal meninges: 66%; Inflamed meninges: >66%
Protein binding: 60%
Metabolism: Extensively hepatic (90%) to inactive metabolites, principally by
glucuronidation; chloramphenicol sodium succinate is hydrolyzed by ester-
ases to active base
Half-life elimination:
Normal renal function: 1.6-3.3 hours
End-stage renal disease: 3-7 hours
Cirrhosis: 10-12 hours
Excretion: Urine (5% to 15%)
Pregnancy Risk Factor C

ChloraPrep® [OTC] see Chlorhexidine Gluconate on page 316
Chloraseptic® Gargle [OTC] see Phenol on page 1223
Chloraseptic® Mouth Pain [OTC] see Phenol on page 1223
Chloraseptic® Rinse [OTC] see Phenol on page 1223
Chloraseptic® Spray [OTC] see Phenol on page 1223
Chloraseptic® Spray for Kids [OTC] see Phenol on page 1223
Chlorbutinum see Chlorambucil on page 313

Chlordiazepoxide (klor dye az e POKS ide)

U.S. Brand Names Librium®
Canadian Brand Names Apo-Chlordiazepoxide®
Generic Available Yes: Capsule
Synonyms Methaminodiazepoxide Hydrochloride
Pharmacologic Category Benzodiazepine
Use Management of anxiety disorder or for the short-term relief of symptoms of
anxiety; withdrawal symptoms of acute alcoholism; preoperative apprehension
and anxiety
Local Anesthetic/Vasoconstrictor Precautions No information available to
require special precautions
Effects on Dental Treatment Key adverse event(s) related to dental treat-
ment: Xerostomia (normal salivary flow resumes upon discontinuation).
Common Adverse Effects
>10%:
Central nervous system: Drowsiness, fatigue, ataxia, lightheadedness,
memory impairment, dysarthria, irritability
Dermatologic: Rash
Endocrine & metabolic: Libido decreased, menstrual disorders
Gastrointestinal: Xerostomia, salivation decreased, appetite increased or
decreased, weight gain/loss
Genitourinary: Micturition difficulties
1% to 10%:
Cardiovascular: Hypotension
Central nervous system: Confusion, dizziness, disinhibition, akathisia
Dermatologic: Dermatitis
Endocrine & metabolic: Libido increased
Gastrointestinal: Salivation increased
Genitourinary: Sexual dysfunction, incontinence
Neuromuscular & skeletal: Rigidity, tremor, muscle cramps
Otic: Tinnitus
Respiratory: Nasal congestion
Restrictions C-IV
(Continued)

Chlordiazepoxide *(Continued)*

Mechanism of Action Binds to stereospecific benzodiazepine receptors on the postsynaptic GABA neuron at several sites within the central nervous system, including the limbic system, reticular formation. Enhancement of the inhibitory effect of GABA on neuronal excitability results by increased neuronal membrane permeability to chloride ions. This shift in chloride ions results in hyperpolarization (a less excitable state) and stabilization.

Drug Interactions

Cytochrome P450 Effect: Substrate of CYP3A4 (major)

Increased Effect/Toxicity: Chlordiazepoxide potentiates the CNS depressant effects of narcotic analgesics, barbiturates, phenothiazines, ethanol, antihistamines, MAO inhibitors, sedative-hypnotics, and cyclic antidepressants. CYP3A4 inhibitors may increase the levels/effects of chlordiazepoxide; example inhibitors include azole antifungals, clarithromycin, diclofenac, doxycycline, erythromycin, imatinib, isoniazid, nefazodone, nicardipine, propofol, protease inhibitors, quinidine, telithromycin, and verapamil.

Decreased Effect: CYP3A4 inducers may decrease the levels/effects of chlordiazepoxide; example inducers include aminoglutethimide, carbamazepine, nafcillin, nevirapine, phenobarbital, phenytoin, and rifamycins.

Pharmacodynamics/Kinetics

Distribution: V_d: 3.3 L/kg; crosses placenta; enters breast milk

Protein binding: 90% to 98%

Metabolism: Extensively hepatic to desmethyldiazepam (active and long-acting)

Half-life elimination: 6.6-25 hours; End-stage renal disease: 5-30 hours; Cirrhosis: 30-63 hours

Time to peak, serum: Oral: Within 2 hours; I.M.: Results in lower peak plasma levels than oral

Excretion: Urine (minimal as unchanged drug)

Pregnancy Risk Factor D

Chlordiazepoxide and Amitriptyline Hydrochloride *see* Amitriptyline and Chlordiazepoxide *on page 97*

Chlordiazepoxide and Clidinium *see* Clidinium and Chlordiazepoxide *on page 360*

Chlordiazepoxide and Methscopolamine

(klor dye az e POKS ide & meth skoe POL a meen)

U.S. Brand Names Librax® *[reformulation]* [DSC]

Generic Available No

Synonyms Methscopolamine Nitrate and Chlordiazepoxide Hydrochloride

Pharmacologic Category Anticholinergic Agent; Benzodiazepine

Use Adjunctive treatment of peptic ulcer; treatment of irritable bowel syndrome, acute enterocolitis

Local Anesthetic/Vasoconstrictor Precautions No information available to require special precautions

Effects on Dental Treatment Key adverse event(s) related to dental treatment: Xerostomia and changes in salivation (normal salivary flow resumes upon discontinuation).

Common Adverse Effects See individual agents.

Restrictions C-IV

Mechanism of Action Chlordiazepoxide binds to stereospecific benzodiazepine (BZD) binding sites on GABA (A) receptor complexes at several sites within the central nervous system, including the limbic system and reticular formation. BZDs enhance GABA-mediated chloride influx through GABA receptor channels, causing membrane hyperpolarization. The net neuroinhibitory effects result in the observed sedative, hypnotic, anxiolytic, and muscle relaxant properties.

Methscopolamine is a peripheral anticholinergic agent with limited ability to cross the blood-brain barrier and provides a peripheral blockade of muscarinic receptors. This agent reduces the volume and the total acid content of gastric secretions, inhibits salivation, and reduces gastrointestinal motility.

Pharmacodynamics/Kinetics See individual agents.

Pregnancy Risk Factor C

Chlorhexidine Gluconate (klor HEKS i deen GLOO koe nate)

Related Information

Bacterial Infections *on page 1697*

Dentin Hypersensitivity, High Caries Index, and Xerostomia *on page 1714*

Management of Patients Undergoing Cancer Therapy *on page 1728*

Periodontal Diseases *on page 1705*
Ulcerative and Erosive Disorders *on page 1712*

Related Sample Prescriptions
Antimicrobial Oral Rinse *on page 1739*

U.S. Brand Names Avagard™ [OTC]; BactoShield® CHG [OTC]; Betasept® [OTC]; ChloraPrep® [OTC]; Dyna-Hex® [OTC]; Hibiclens® [OTC]; Hibistat® [OTC]; Operand® Chlorhexidine Gluconate [OTC]; Peridex®; PerioChip®; Perio-Gard®

Canadian Brand Names Apo-Chlorhexadine®; Hibidil® 1:2000; ORO-Clense

Generic Available Yes: Oral liquid

Synonyms CHG; 3M™ Avagard™ [OTC]

Pharmacologic Category Antibiotic, Oral Rinse; Antibiotic, Topical

Dental Use
Antibacterial dental rinse; chlorhexidine is active against gram-positive and gram-negative organisms, facultative anaerobes, aerobes, and yeast

Chip, for periodontal pocket insertion: Indicated as an adjunct to scaling and root planing procedures for reduction of pocket depth in patients with adult periodontitis; may be used as part of a periodontal maintenance program

Use Skin cleanser for surgical scrub, cleanser for skin wounds, preoperative skin preparation, germicidal hand rinse, and as antibacterial dental rinse. Chlorhexidine is active against gram-positive and gram-negative organisms, facultative anaerobes, aerobes, and yeast.

Orphan drug: Peridex®: Oral mucositis with cytoreductive therapy when used for patients undergoing bone marrow transplant

Local Anesthetic/Vasoconstrictor Precautions No information available to require special precautions

Effects on Dental Treatment Key adverse event(s) related to dental treatment: Increased tartar on teeth, altered taste perception, staining of oral surfaces (mucosa, teeth, dorsum of tongue), and oral/tongue irritation. Staining may be visible as soon as 1 week after therapy begins and is more pronounced when there is a heavy accumulation of unremoved plaque and when teeth fillings have rough surfaces. Stain does not have a clinically adverse effect but because removal may not be possible, patient with frontal restoration should be advised of the potential permanency of the stain.

Significant Adverse Effects
Oral:
>10%: Increase of tartar on teeth, changes in taste. Staining of oral surfaces (mucosa, teeth, dorsum of tongue) may be visible as soon as 1 week after therapy begins and is more pronounced when there is a heavy accumulation of unremoved plaque and when teeth fillings have rough surfaces. Stain does not have a clinically adverse effect but because removal may not be possible, patient with frontal restoration should be advised of the potential permanency of the stain.

1% to 10%: Gastrointestinal: Tongue irritation, oral irritation

<1% (Limited to important or life-threatening): Dyspnea, facial edema, nasal congestion

Topical: Skin erythema and roughness, dryness, sensitization, allergic reactions

Dental Usual Dosing Adults:
Oral rinse (Peridex®, PerioGard®):
Floss and brush teeth, completely rinse toothpaste from mouth and swish 15 mL (one capful) undiluted oral rinse around in mouth for 30 seconds, then expectorate. Caution patient not to swallow the medicine and instruct not to eat for 2-3 hours after treatment. (Cap on bottle measures 15 mL.)

Treatment of gingivitis: Oral prophylaxis: Swish for 30 seconds with 15 mL chlorhexidine, then expectorate; repeat twice daily (morning and evening). Patient should have a re-evaluation followed by a dental prophylaxis every 6 months.

Periodontal chip: One chip is inserted into a periodontal pocket with a probing pocket depth ≥5 mm. Up to 8 chips may be inserted in a single visit. Treatment is recommended every 3 months in pockets with a remaining depth ≥5 mm. If dislodgment occurs 7 days or more after placement, the subject is considered to have had the full course of treatment. If dislodgment occurs within 48 hours, a new chip should be inserted. The chip biodegrades completely and does not need to be removed. Patients should avoid dental floss at the site of PerioChip® insertion for 10 days after placement because flossing might dislodge the chip.

Insertion of periodontal chip: Pocket should be isolated and surrounding area dried prior to chip insertion. The chip should be grasped using forceps with the rounded edges away from the forceps. The chip should be inserted into the periodontal pocket to its maximum depth. It may be maneuvered into position using the tips of the forceps or a flat instrument.

(Continued)

Chlorhexidine Gluconate *(Continued)*

Dosage Adults:

Oral rinse (Peridex®, PerioGard®):

Floss and brush teeth, completely rinse toothpaste from mouth and swish 15 mL (one capful) undiluted oral rinse around in mouth for 30 seconds, then expectorate. Caution patient not to swallow the medicine and instruct not to eat for 2-3 hours after treatment. (Cap on bottle measures 15 mL.)

Treatment of gingivitis: Oral prophylaxis: Swish for 30 seconds with 15 mL chlorhexidine, then expectorate; repeat twice daily (morning and evening). Patient should have a re-evaluation followed by a dental prophylaxis every 6 months.

Periodontal chip: One chip is inserted into a periodontal pocket with a probing pocket depth ≥5 mm. Up to 8 chips may be inserted in a single visit. Treatment is recommended every 3 months in pockets with a remaining depth ≥5 mm. If dislodgment occurs 7 days or more after placement, the subject is considered to have had the full course of treatment. If dislodgment occurs within 48 hours, a new chip should be inserted. The chip biodegrades completely and does not need to be removed. Patients should avoid dental floss at the site of PerioChip® insertion for 10 days after placement because flossing might dislodge the chip.

Insertion of periodontal chip: Pocket should be isolated and surrounding area dried prior to chip insertion. The chip should be grasped using forceps with the rounded edges away from the forceps. The chip should be inserted into the periodontal pocket to its maximum depth. It may be maneuvered into position using the tips of the forceps or a flat instrument.

Cleanser:

Surgical scrub: Scrub 3 minutes and rinse thoroughly, wash for an additional 3 minutes

Hand sanitizer (Avagard™): Dispense 1 pumpful in palm of one hand; dip fingertips of opposite hand into solution and work it under nails. Spread remainder evenly over hand and just above elbow, covering all surfaces. Repeat on other hand. Dispense another pumpful in each hand and reapply to each hand up to the wrist. Allow to dry before gloving.

Hand wash: Wash for 15 seconds and rinse

Hand rinse: Rub 15 seconds and rinse

Mechanism of Action The bactericidal effect of chlorhexidine is a result of the binding of this cationic molecule to negatively charged bacterial cell walls and extramicrobial complexes. At low concentrations, this causes an alteration of bacterial cell osmotic equilibrium and leakage of potassium and phosphorous resulting in a bacteriostatic effect. At high concentrations of chlorhexidine, the cytoplasmic contents of the bacterial cell precipitate and result in cell death.

Contraindications Hypersensitivity to chlorhexidine gluconate or any component of the formulation

Warnings/Precautions

Oral: Staining of oral surfaces (mucosa, teeth, tooth restorations, dorsum of tongue) may occur; may be visible as soon as 1 week after therapy begins and is more pronounced when there is a heavy accumulation of unremoved plaque and when teeth fillings have rough surfaces. Stain does not have a clinically adverse effect, but because removal may not be possible, patient with frontal restoration should be advised of the potential permanency of the stain.

Topical: For topical use only. Keep out of eyes and ears. May stain fabric. There have been case reports of anaphylaxis following chlorhexidine disinfection. Not for preoperative preparation of face or head; avoid contact with meninges.

Drug Interactions No data reported

Pharmacodynamics/Kinetics

Topical hand sanitizer (Avagard™): Duration of antimicrobial protection: 6 hours

Oral rinse (Peridex®, PerioGard®):

Absorption: ~30% retained in the oral cavity following rinsing and slowly released into oral fluids; poorly absorbed

Time to peak, plasma: Oral rinse: Detectable levels not present after 12 hours

Excretion: Feces (~90%); urine (<1%)

Pregnancy Risk Factor B

Dosage Forms

Chip, for periodontal pocket insertion (PerioChip®): 2.5 mg

Liquid, topical [surgical scrub]:

Avagard™: 1% (500 mL) [contains ethyl alcohol and moisturizers]

BactoShield® CHG: 2% (120 mL, 480 mL, 750 mL, 1000 mL, 3800 mL); 4% (120 mL, 480 mL, 750 mL, 1000 mL, 3800 mL) [contains isopropyl alcohol]

Betasept®: 4% (120 mL, 240 mL, 480 mL, 960 mL, 3840 mL) [contains isopropyl alcohol]

ChloraPrep®: 2% (0.67 mL, 1.5 mL, 3 mL, 10.5 mL) [contains isopropyl alcohol 70%; prefilled applicator]

Dyna-Hex®: 2% (120 mL, 960 mL, 3840 mL); 4% (120 mL, 960 mL, 3840 mL)

Hibiclens®: 4% (15 mL, 120 mL, 240 mL, 480 mL, 960 mL, 3840 mL) [contains isopropyl alcohol]

Operand® Chlorhexidine Gluconate: 2% (120 mL); 4% (120 mL, 240 mL, 480 mL, 960 mL, 3840 mL) [contains isopropyl alcohol]

Liquid, oral rinse: 0.12% (480 mL)

Peridex®: 0.12% (480 mL) [contains alcohol 11.6%]

PerioGard®: 0.12% (480 mL) [contains alcohol 11.6%; mint flavor]

Pad [prep pad] (Hibistat®): 0.5% (50s) [contains isopropyl alcohol]

Sponge/Brush (BactoShield® CHG): 4% per sponge/brush [contains isopropyl alcohol]

Selected Readings

al-Tannir MA and Goodman HS, "A Review of Chlorhexidine and Its Use in Special Populations," *Spec Care Dentist*, 1994, 14(3):116-22.

Ercan E, Ozekinci T, Atakul F, et al, "Antibacterial Activity of 2% Chlorhexidine Gluconate and 5.25% Sodium Hypochlorite in Infected Root Canal: In Vivo Study," *J Endod*, 2004, 30(2):84-7.

Ferretti GA, Brown AT, Raybould TP, et al, "Oral Antimicrobial Agents - Chlorhexidine," *NCI Monogr*, 1990, 9:51-5.

Greenstein G, Berman C, and Jaffin R, "Chlorhexidine. An Adjunct to Periodontal Therapy," *J Periodontol*, 1986, 57(6):370-7.

Johnson BT, "Uses of Chlorhexidine in Dentistry," *Gen Dent*, 1995, 43(2):126-32, 134-40.

Noiri Y, Okami Y, Narimatsu M, et al, "Effects of Chlorhexidine, Minocycline, and Metronidazole on Porphyromonas Gingivalis Strain 381 in Biofilms," *J Periodontol*, 2003, 74(11):1647-51.

Reddy MS, Jeffcoat MK, Geurs NC, et al, "Efficacy of Controlled-Release Subgingival Chlorhexidine to Enhance Periodontal Regeneration," *J Periodontol*, 2003, 74(4):411-9.

Soskolne WA, Proskin HM, and Stabholz A, "Probing Depth Changes Following 2 Years of Periodontal Maintenance Therapy Including Adjunctive Controlled Release of Chlorhexidine," *J Periodontol*, 2003, 74(4):420-7.

Yusof ZA, "Chlorhexidine Mouthwash: A Review of Its Pharmacological Activity, Clinical Effects, Uses and Abuses," *Dent J Malays*, 1988, 10(1):9-16.

Chlormeprazine *see* Prochlorperazine *on page 1285*

Chlor-Mes-D *see* Chlorpheniramine, Phenylephrine, and Methscopolamine *on page 327*

2-Chlorodeoxyadenosine *see* Cladribine *on page 354*

Chloroethane *see* Ethyl Chloride *on page 620*

Chloromag® *see* Magnesium Chloride *on page 960*

Chloromycetin® Sodium Succinate *see* Chloramphenicol *on page 314*

Chlorophyll (KLOR oh fil)

U.S. Brand Names Nullo® [OTC]

Generic Available No

Synonyms Chlorophyllin

Pharmacologic Category Gastrointestinal Agent, Miscellaneous

Use Control fecal odors in colostomy or ileostomy

Local Anesthetic/Vasoconstrictor Precautions No information available to require special precautions

Effects on Dental Treatment No significant effects or complications reported

Common Adverse Effects Frequency not defined: Gastrointestinal: Diarrhea, green stools, abdominal cramping

Chlorophyllin *see* Chlorophyll *on page 319*

Chlorophyllin Copper Complex Sodium, Papain, and Urea *see* Chlorophyllin, Papain, and Urea *on page 319*

Chlorophyllin, Papain, and Urea
(KLOR oh fil in, pa PAY in, & yoor EE a)

U.S. Brand Names Panafil®; Ziox™

Generic Available Yes: Ointment

Synonyms Chlorophyllin Copper Complex Sodium, Papain, and Urea; Papain, Urea, and Chlorophyllin; Urea, Chlorophyllin, and Papain

Pharmacologic Category Enzyme, Topical Debridement

Use Treatment of acute and chronic lesions, such as varicose, diabetic decubitus ulcers, burns, postoperative wounds, pilonidal cyst wounds, carbuncles, and miscellaneous traumatic or infected wounds

Local Anesthetic/Vasoconstrictor Precautions No information available to require special precautions

Effects on Dental Treatment No significant effects or complications reported

Common Adverse Effects Local: Burning sensation, skin irritation

(Continued)

Chlorophyllin, Papain, and Urea (Continued)

Mechanism of Action
Papain: Potent digestant of nonviable protein matter; harmless to viable tissue. Requires activation to exert its function.

Urea: Exposes papain activators (sulfhydryl groups) and denatures nonviable protein matter making it more susceptible to enzymatic digestion.

Chlorophyllin copper complex sodium: Inhibits the hemagglutinating and inflammatory properties of protein degradation products in the wound; the resulting healthy granulation, decreased local inflammation, and decreased wound odor promotes wound healing.

Drug Interactions
Decreased Effect: Heavy metals, hydrogen peroxide

Chloroprocaine (klor oh PROE kane)

Related Information
Oral Pain *on page 1692*

U.S. Brand Names Nesacaine®; Nesacaine®-MPF

Canadian Brand Names Nesacaine®-CE

Generic Available Yes

Synonyms Chloroprocaine Hydrochloride

Pharmacologic Category Local Anesthetic

Use Infiltration anesthesia and peripheral and epidural anesthesia

Local Anesthetic/Vasoconstrictor Precautions No information available to require special precautions

Effects on Dental Treatment No significant effects or complications reported

Common Adverse Effects Frequency not defined.
Cardiovascular: Bradycardia, cardiac arrest, hypotension, ventricular arrhythmia

Central nervous system: Anxiety, dizziness, restlessness, tinnitus, unconsciousness

Dermatologic: Angioneurotic edema, erythema, pruritus, urticaria

Ocular: Blurred vision

Respiratory: Respiratory arrest

Miscellaneous: Allergic reactions, anaphylactoid reactions

Mechanism of Action Chloroprocaine HCl is benzoic acid, 4-amino-2-chloro-2-(diethylamino) ethyl ester monohydrochloride. Chloroprocaine is an ester-type local anesthetic, which stabilizes the neuronal membranes and prevents initiation and transmission of nerve impulses thereby affecting local anesthetic actions. Local anesthetics including chloroprocaine, reversibly prevent generation and conduction of electrical impulses in neurons by decreasing the transient increase in permeability to sodium. The differential sensitivity generally depends on the size of the fiber; small fibers are more sensitive than larger fibers and require a longer period for recovery. Sensory pain fibers are usually blocked first, followed by fibers that transmit sensations of temperature, touch, and deep pressure. High concentrations block sympathetic somatic sensory and somatic motor fibers. The spread of anesthesia depends upon the distribution of the solution. This is primarily dependent on the volume of drug injected.

Drug Interactions
Decreased Effect: The para-aminobenzoic acid metabolite of chloroprocaine may decrease the efficacy of sulfonamide antibiotics.

Pharmacodynamics/Kinetics
Onset of action: 6-12 minutes

Duration: 30-60 minutes

Distribution: V_d: Depends upon route of administration; high concentrations found in highly perfused organs such as liver, lungs, heart, and brain

Metabolism: Plasma cholinesterases

Excretion: Urine

Pregnancy Risk Factor C

Chloroprocaine Hydrochloride *see* Chloroprocaine *on page 320*

Chloroquine (KLOR oh kwin)

U.S. Brand Names Aralen®

Canadian Brand Names Aralen®; Novo-Chloroquine

Generic Available Yes

Synonyms Chloroquine Phosphate

Pharmacologic Category Aminoquinoline (Antimalarial)

Use Suppression or chemoprophylaxis of malaria; treatment of uncomplicated or mild-to-moderate malaria; extraintestinal amebiasis

Unlabeled/Investigational Use Rheumatoid arthritis; discoid lupus erythematosus

Local Anesthetic/Vasoconstrictor Precautions No information available to require special precautions

Effects on Dental Treatment Key adverse event(s) related to dental treatment: Stomatitis.

Common Adverse Effects Frequency not defined.

Cardiovascular: Hypotension (rare), ECG changes (rare; including T-wave inversion), cardiomyopathy

Central nervous system: Fatigue, personality changes, headache, psychosis, seizure, delirium, depression

Dermatologic: Pruritus, hair bleaching, pleomorphic skin eruptions, alopecia, lichen planus eruptions, alopecia, mucosal pigmentary changes (blue-black), photosensitivity

Gastrointestinal: Nausea, diarrhea, vomiting, anorexia, stomatitis, abdominal cramps

Hematologic: Aplastic anemia, agranulocytosis (reversible), neutropenia, thrombocytopenia

Neuromuscular & skeletal: Rare cases of myopathy, neuromyopathy, proximal muscle atrophy, and depression of deep tendon reflexes have been reported

Ocular: Retinopathy (including irreversible changes in some patients long-term or high-dose therapy), blurred vision

Otic: Nerve deafness, tinnitus, reduced hearing (risk increased in patients with pre-existing auditory damage)

Mechanism of Action Binds to and inhibits DNA and RNA polymerase; interferes with metabolism and hemoglobin utilization by parasites; inhibits prostaglandin effects; chloroquine concentrates within parasite acid vesicles and raises internal pH resulting in inhibition of parasite growth; may involve aggregates of ferriprotoporphyrin IX acting as chloroquine receptors causing membrane damage; may also interfere with nucleoprotein synthesis

Drug Interactions

Cytochrome P450 Effect: Substrate (major) of CYP2D6, 3A4; **Inhibits** CYP2D6 (moderate)

Increased Effect/Toxicity: Chloroquine may increase the levels/effects of dextromethorphan, fluoxetine, lidocaine, mirtazapine, nefazodone, paroxetine, risperidone, ritonavir, thioridazine, tricyclic antidepressants, venlafaxine, and other CYP2D6 substrates. Chloroquine may increase the levels/effects of cyclosporine. The levels/effects of chloroquine may be increased by azole antifungals, chlorpromazine, cimetidine, clarithromycin, delavirdine, diclofenac, doxycycline, erythromycin, fluoxetine, imatinib, isoniazid, miconazole, nefazodone, nicardipine, paroxetine, pergolide, propofol, protease inhibitors, quinidine, quinine, ritonavir, ropinirole, telithromycin, verapamil, and other CYP2D6 or 3A4 inhibitors.

Decreased Effect: Chloroquine levels may be decreased by antacids or kaolin. Chloroquine may decrease ampicillin and/or praziquantel levels. Chloroquine may decrease the levels/effects of CYP2D6 prodrug substrates; example prodrug substrates include codeine, hydrocodone, oxycodone, and tramadol. The levels/effects of chloroquine may be decreased by aminoglutethimide, carbamazepine, nafcillin, nevirapine, phenobarbital, phenytoin, rifamycins, and other CYP3A4 inducers.

Pharmacodynamics/Kinetics

Duration: Small amounts may be present in urine months following discontinuation of therapy

Absorption: Oral: Rapid (~89%)

Distribution: Widely in body tissues (eg, eyes, heart, kidneys, liver, lungs) where retention prolonged; crosses placenta; enters breast milk

Metabolism: Partially hepatic

Half-life elimination: 3-5 days

Time to peak, serum: 1-2 hours

Excretion: Urine (~70% as unchanged drug); acidification of urine increases elimination

Pregnancy Risk Factor C

Chloroquine Phosphate see Chloroquine on page 320

Chlorothiazide (klor oh THYE a zide)

Related Information
Cardiovascular Diseases *on page 1636*
U.S. Brand Names Diuril®
Canadian Brand Names Diuril®
Generic Available Yes: Tablet
Pharmacologic Category Diuretic, Thiazide
Use Management of mild-to-moderate hypertension; adjunctive treatment of edema

Local Anesthetic/Vasoconstrictor Precautions No information available to require special precautions

Effects on Dental Treatment Key adverse event(s) related to dental treatment: Orthostatic hypotension.

Common Adverse Effects Frequency not defined.
Cardiovascular: Hypotension, orthostatic hypotension, necrotizing angiitis
Central nervous system: Dizziness, headache, restlessness, vertigo
Dermatologic: Alopecia, erythema multiforme, exfoliative dermatitis, photosensitivity, Stevens-Johnson syndrome, toxic epidermal necrolysis
Endocrine & metabolic: Cholesterol increased, hypokalemia, hypomagnesemia, triglycerides increased
Gastrointestinal: Abdominal cramping, anorexia, constipation, diarrhea, gastric irritation, nausea, pancreatitis, sialadenitis, vomiting
Genitourinary: Impotence
Hematologic: Agranulocytosis, aplastic anemia, hemolytic anemia, leukopenia, thrombocytopenia
Hepatic: Jaundice
Neuromuscular & skeletal: Muscle spasm, paresthesia, weakness
Ocular: Blurred vision, xanthopsia
Renal: Azotemia, hematuria, interstitial nephritis, renal failure, renal dysfunction
Respiratory: Pneumonitis, pulmonary edema, respiratory distress
Miscellaneous: Anaphylactic reactions, systemic lupus erythematosus

Mechanism of Action Inhibits sodium reabsorption in the distal tubules causing increased excretion of sodium and water as well as potassium and hydrogen ions, magnesium, phosphate, calcium

Drug Interactions
Increased Effect/Toxicity: Increased effect of chlorothiazide with furosemide and other loop diuretics. Increased hypotension and/or renal adverse effects of ACE inhibitors may result in aggressively diuresed patients. Beta-blockers increase hyperglycemic effects of thiazides in Type 2 diabetes mellitus. Cyclosporine and thiazides can increase the risk of gout or renal toxicity. Digoxin toxicity can be exacerbated if a thiazide induces hypokalemia or hypomagnesemia. Lithium toxicity can occur with thiazides due to reduced renal excretion of lithium. Thiazides may prolong the duration of action with neuromuscular-blocking agents. Corticosteroids may increase electrolyte-depletion effects of chlorothiazide.
Decreased Effect: Effects of oral hypoglycemics may be decreased. Decreased absorption of chlorothiazide with cholestyramine and colestipol. NSAIDs can decrease the efficacy of thiazides, reducing the diuretic and antihypertensive effects.

Pharmacodynamics/Kinetics
Onset of action: Diuresis: Oral: 2 hours; I.V.: 15 minutes
Duration of diuretic action: Oral: 6-12 hours; I.V.: ~2 hours
Absorption: Oral: Poor
Half-life elimination: 1-2 hours
Time to peak, serum: Oral: ~4 hours; I.V.: 30 minutes
Excretion: Urine (as unchanged drug)
Pregnancy Risk Factor C (manufacturer); D (expert analysis)

Chloroxine (klor OKS een)

U.S. Brand Names Capitrol® [DSC]
Canadian Brand Names Capitrol®
Generic Available No
Pharmacologic Category Topical Skin Product
Use Treatment of dandruff or seborrheic dermatitis of the scalp
Local Anesthetic/Vasoconstrictor Precautions No information available to require special precautions
Effects on Dental Treatment No significant effects or complications reported
Pregnancy Risk Factor C

Chlorphen [OTC] *see* Chlorpheniramine *on page 323*

Chlorpheniramine (klor fen IR a meen)

Related Information
Bacterial Infections *on page 1697*
Related Sample Prescriptions
Sinus Infection Treatment *on page 1738*
U.S. Brand Names Aller-Chlor® [OTC]; Chlorphen [OTC]; Chlor-Trimeton® [OTC]; Diabetic Tussin® Allergy Relief [OTC]; Teldrin® HBP [OTC]
Canadian Brand Names Chlor-Tripolon®; Novo-Pheniram
Generic Available Yes
Synonyms Chlorpheniramine Maleate; CTM
Pharmacologic Category Antihistamine
Dental Use Treatment of histamine-induced allergic symptoms
Use Perennial and seasonal allergic rhinitis and other allergic symptoms including urticaria
Local Anesthetic/Vasoconstrictor Precautions No information available to require special precautions
Effects on Dental Treatment Key adverse event(s) related to dental treatment: Xerostomia (normal salivary flow resumes upon discontinuation). Chronic use of antihistamines will inhibit salivary flow, particularly in elderly patients; this may contribute to periodontal disease and oral discomfort.
Significant Adverse Effects
>10%:
Central nervous system: Slight to moderate drowsiness
Respiratory: Thickening of bronchial secretions
1% to 10%:
Central nervous system: Headache, excitability, fatigue, nervousness, dizziness
Gastrointestinal: Nausea, xerostomia, diarrhea, abdominal pain, appetite increase, weight gain
Genitourinary: Urinary retention
Neuromuscular & skeletal: Arthralgia, weakness
Ocular: Diplopia
Renal: Polyuria
Respiratory: Pharyngitis
Dosage
Children: Oral: 0.35 mg/kg/day in divided doses every 4-6 hours
2-6 years: 1 mg every 4-6 hours, not to exceed 6 mg in 24 hours
6-12 years: 2 mg every 4-6 hours, not to exceed 12 mg/day or sustained release 8 mg at bedtime
Children >12 years and Adults: Oral: 4 mg every 4-6 hours, not to exceed 24 mg/day or sustained release 8-12 mg every 8-12 hours, not to exceed 24 mg/day
Elderly: Oral: 4 mg once or twice daily. **Note:** Duration of action may be 36 hours or more when serum concentrations are low.
Hemodialysis: Supplemental dose is not necessary
Mechanism of Action Competes with histamine for H_1-receptor sites on effector cells in the gastrointestinal tract, blood vessels, and respiratory tract
Contraindications Hypersensitivity to chlorpheniramine maleate or any component of the formulation; narrow-angle glaucoma; bladder neck obstruction; symptomatic prostate hypertrophy; during acute asthmatic attacks; stenosing peptic ulcer; pyloroduodenal obstruction. Avoid use in premature and term newborns due to possible association with SIDS.
Warnings/Precautions Causes sedation, caution must be used in performing tasks which require alertness (eg, operating machinery or driving). Sedative effects of CNS depressants or ethanol are potentiated. Use with caution in patients with angle-closure glaucoma, pyloroduodenal obstruction (including stenotic peptic ulcer), urinary tract obstruction (including bladder neck obstruction and symptomatic prostatic hyperplasia), hyperthyroidism, increased intraocular pressure, and cardiovascular disease (including hypertension and tachycardia). High sedative and anticholinergic properties, therefore may not be considered the antihistamine of choice for prolonged use in the elderly. May cause paradoxical excitation in pediatric patients, and can result in hallucinations, coma, and death in overdose.
Drug Interactions Substrate of CYP2D6 (minor), 3A4 (major); **Inhibits** CYP2D6 (weak)
Increased toxicity (CNS depression): CNS depressants, MAO inhibitors, tricyclic antidepressants, phenothiazines
(Continued)

Chlorpheniramine *(Continued)*

CYP3A4 inhibitors: May increase the levels/effects of chlorpheniramine. Example inhibitors include azole antifungals, clarithromycin, diclofenac, doxycycline, erythromycin, imatinib, isoniazid, nefazodone, nicardipine, propofol, protease inhibitors, quinidine, telithromycin, and verapamil.

Ethanol/Nutrition/Herb Interactions Ethanol: Avoid ethanol (may increase CNS depression).

Dietary Considerations May be taken with food or water.

Pharmacodynamics/Kinetics Half-life elimination, serum: 20-24 hours

Pregnancy Risk Factor B

Dosage Forms

Syrup, as maleate:

Aller-Chlor®: 2 mg/5 mL (120 mL) [contains alcohol 5%]

Diabetic Tussin® Allergy Relief: 2 mg/5 mL (120 mL) [alcohol free, dye free, sugar free]

Tablet, as maleate (Aller-Chlor®, Chlor-Trimeton®, Chlorphen, Teldrin® HBP): 4 mg

Tablet, extended release, as maleate (Chlor-Trimeton®): 12 mg

Chlorpheniramine, Acetaminophen, and Pseudoephedrine *see* Acetaminophen, Chlorpheniramine, and Pseudoephedrine *on page 43*

Chlorpheniramine and Acetaminophen

(klor fen IR a meen & a seet a MIN oh fen)

Related Information

Acetaminophen *on page 31*
Chlorpheniramine *on page 323*

U.S. Brand Names Coricidin HBP® Cold and Flu [OTC]

Generic Available No

Synonyms Acetaminophen and Chlorpheniramine

Pharmacologic Category Antihistamine/Analgesic

Use Symptomatic relief of congestion, headache, aches and pains of colds and flu

Local Anesthetic/Vasoconstrictor Precautions No information available to require special precautions

Effects on Dental Treatment Key adverse event(s) related to dental treatment: Chronic use of antihistamines will inhibit salivary flow, particularly in elderly patients; this may contribute to periodontal disease and oral discomfort.

Common Adverse Effects See individual agents.

Drug Interactions

Cytochrome P450 Effect:

Acetaminophen: **Substrate** (minor) of CYP1A2, 2A6, 2C9, 2D6, 2E1, 3A4; **Inhibits** CYP3A4 (weak)

Chlorpheniramine: **Substrate** of CYP2D6 (minor), 3A4 (major); **Inhibits** CYP2D6 (weak)

Pharmacodynamics/Kinetics See individual agents.

Chlorpheniramine and Carbetapentane *see* Carbetapentane and Chlorpheniramine *on page 266*

Chlorpheniramine and Phenylephrine

(klor fen IR a meen & fen il EF rin)

Related Information

Chlorpheniramine *on page 323*
Phenylephrine *on page 1226*

U.S. Brand Names Allerx™; Dallergy-JR®; Ed A-Hist®; Rescon-Jr; Rondec® *[reformulation]*; R-Tanna; Rynatan®; Rynatan® Pediatric Suspension

Generic Available Yes: Tannate formulations

Synonyms Chlorpheniramine Maleate and Phenylephrine Hydrochloride; Chlorpheniramine Tannate and Phenylephrine Tannate; Phenylephrine and Chlorpheniramine

Pharmacologic Category Antihistamine/Decongestant Combination

Use Temporary relief of upper respiratory conditions such as nasal congestion, runny nose, and sneezing due to the common cold, hay fever, or allergic or vasomotor rhinitis

Local Anesthetic/Vasoconstrictor Precautions Use with caution since phenylephrine is a sympathomimetic amine which could interact with epinephrine to cause a pressor response

Effects on Dental Treatment Key adverse event(s) related to dental treatment:

Chlorpheniramine: Prolonged use will cause significant xerostomia (normal salivary flow resumes upon discontinuation).

Phenylephrine: Up to 10% of patients could experience tachycardia, palpitations, and xerostomia (prolonged use worsens); use vasoconstrictor with caution.

Common Adverse Effects See individual agents.

Drug Interactions

Cytochrome P450 Effect: Chlorpheniramine: **Substrate** of CYP2D6 (minor), 3A4 (major); **Inhibits** CYP2D6 (weak)

Increased Effect/Toxicity: See individual agents.

Decreased Effect: See individual agents.

Pharmacodynamics/Kinetics See individual agents.

Pregnancy Risk Factor C

Chlorpheniramine and Pseudoephedrine
(klor fen IR a meen & soo doe e FED rin)

Related Information
Chlorpheniramine on page 323
Pseudoephedrine on page 1309

U.S. Brand Names Allerest® Maximum Strength Allergy and Hay Fever [OTC]; A.R.M® [OTC]; Chlor-Trimeton® Allergy D [OTC]; C-Phed Tannate; Deconamine®; Deconamine® SR; Histade™; Histex™; Kronofed-A®; Kronofed-A®-Jr; LoHist-D; PediaCare® Cold and Allergy [OTC]; Sudafed® Sinus & Allergy [OTC]; Sudal® 12; Triaminic® Cold and Allergy [OTC]

Canadian Brand Names Triaminic® Cold & Allergy

Generic Available Yes: Tablet, extended release capsule, suspension

Synonyms Chlorpheniramine Maleate and Pseudoephedrine Hydrochloride; Chlorpheniramine Tannate and Pseudoephedrine Tannate; Pseudoephedrine and Chlorpheniramine

Pharmacologic Category Alpha/Beta Agonist; Antihistamine

Use Relief of nasal congestion associated with the common cold, hay fever, and other allergies, sinusitis, eustachian tube blockage, and vasomotor and allergic rhinitis

Local Anesthetic/Vasoconstrictor Precautions Use with caution since pseudoephedrine is a sympathomimetic amine which could interact with epinephrine to cause a pressor response

Effects on Dental Treatment Key adverse event(s) related to dental treatment:

Chlorpheniramine: Prolonged use will cause significant xerostomia (normal salivary flow resumes upon discontinuation).

Pseudoephedrine: Xerostomia (prolonged use worsens; normal salivary flow resumes upon discontinuation).

Common Adverse Effects See individual agents.

Mechanism of Action

Chlorpheniramine competes with histamine for H_1-receptor sites on effector cells in the gastrointestinal tract, blood vessels, and respiratory tract.

Pseudoephedrine is a sympathomimetic amine and isomer of ephedrine; acts as a decongestant in respiratory tract mucous membranes with less vasoconstrictor action than ephedrine in normotensive individuals.

Drug Interactions

Cytochrome P450 Effect: Chlorpheniramine: **Substrate** of CYP2D6 (minor), 3A4 (major); **Inhibits** CYP2D6 (weak)

Increased Effect/Toxicity: See individual agents.

Decreased Effect: See individual agents.

Pharmacodynamics/Kinetics See individual agents.

Pregnancy Risk Factor C

Chlorpheniramine, Ephedrine, Phenylephrine, and Carbetapentane
(klor fen IR a meen, e FED rin, fen il EF rin, & kar bay ta PEN tane)

Related Information
Chlorpheniramine on page 323
Ephedrine on page 545
Phenylephrine on page 1226
(Continued)

Chlorpheniramine, Ephedrine, Phenylephrine, and Carbetapentane *(Continued)*

U.S. Brand Names Rynatuss®; Rynatuss® Pediatric [DSC]; Tetra Tannate Pediatric

Generic Available Yes: Suspension

Synonyms Carbetapentane, Ephedrine, Phenylephrine, and Chlorpheniramine; Ephedrine, Chlorpheniramine, Phenylephrine, and Carbetapentane; Phenylephrine, Ephedrine, Chlorpheniramine, and Carbetapentane

Pharmacologic Category Antihistamine/Decongestant/Antitussive

Use Symptomatic relief of cough with a decongestant and an antihistamine

Local Anesthetic/Vasoconstrictor Precautions

Ephedrine: Use vasoconstrictor with caution since ephedrine may enhance cardiostimulation and vasopressor effects of sympathomimetics

Phenylephrine: Use with caution since phenylephrine is a sympathomimetic amine which could interact with epinephrine to cause a pressor response

Effects on Dental Treatment Key adverse event(s) related to dental treatment:

Chlorpheniramine: Prolonged use will cause significant xerostomia (normal salivary flow resumes upon discontinuation).

Ephedrine: No significant effects or complications reported.

Phenylephrine: Up to 10% of patients could experience tachycardia, palpitations, and xerostomia; use vasoconstrictor with caution.

Drug Interactions

Cytochrome P450 Effect: Chlorpheniramine: **Substrate** of CYP2D6 (minor), 3A4 (major); **Inhibits** CYP2D6 (weak)

Increased Effect/Toxicity: See individual agents.

Decreased Effect: See individual agents.

Pregnancy Risk Factor C

Chlorpheniramine, Hydrocodone, Phenylephrine, Acetaminophen, and Caffeine *see* Hydrocodone, Chlorpheniramine, Phenylephrine, Acetaminophen, and Caffeine *on page 790*

Chlorpheniramine Maleate *see* Chlorpheniramine *on page 323*

Chlorpheniramine Maleate and Hydrocodone Bitartrate *see* Hydrocodone and Chlorpheniramine *on page 784*

Chlorpheniramine Maleate and Phenylephrine Hydrochloride *see* Chlorpheniramine and Phenylephrine *on page 324*

Chlorpheniramine Maleate and Pseudoephedrine Hydrochloride *see* Chlorpheniramine and Pseudoephedrine *on page 325*

Chlorpheniramine Maleate, Dihydrocodeine Bitartrate, and Phenylephrine Hydrochloride *see* Dihydrocodeine, Chlorpheniramine, and Phenylephrine *on page 476*

Chlorpheniramine, Phenylephrine, and Dextromethorphan

(klor fen IR a meen, fen il EF rin, & deks troe meth OR fan)

Related Information

Chlorpheniramine *on page 323*
Dextromethorphan *on page 451*
Phenylephrine *on page 1226*

U.S. Brand Names Alka-Seltzer Plus® Cold and Cough [OTC]; Coldtuss DR; Corfen DM; De-Chlor DM; De-Chlor DR; Dex PC; Phenabid DM®; Rondec®-DM *[reformulation]*; Tri-Vent™ DPC

Generic Available Yes: Excludes drops, effervescent tablet, timed release tablet

Synonyms Dextromethorphan, Chlorpheniramine, and Phenylephrine; Phenylephrine, Chlorpheniramine, and Dextromethorphan

Pharmacologic Category Antihistamine/Decongestant/Antitussive

Use Temporary relief of cough and upper respiratory symptoms associated with allergies or the common cold

Local Anesthetic/Vasoconstrictor Precautions

Chlorpheniramine, Dextromethorphan: No information available to require special precautions

Phenylephrine: Use with caution since phenylephrine is a sympathomimetic amine which could interact with epinephrine to cause a pressor response

Effects on Dental Treatment Key adverse event(s) related to dental treatment:

Chlorpheniramine: Prolonged use will cause significant xerostomia (normal salivary flow resumes upon discontinuation).

Dextromethorphan: No significant effects or complications reported

Phenylephrine: Up to 10% of patients could experience tachycardia, palpitations, and xerostomia (prolonged use worsens); use vasoconstrictor with caution.

Common Adverse Effects See individual agents.

Drug Interactions

Cytochrome P450 Effect:

Chlorpheniramine: **Substrate** of CYP2D6 (minor), 3A4 (major); **Inhibits** CYP2D6 (weak)

Dextromethorphan: **Substrate** of CYP2B6 (minor), 2C9 (minor), 2C19 (minor), 2D6 (major), 2E1 (minor), 3A4 (minor); **Inhibits** CYP2D6 (weak)

Increased Effect/Toxicity: See individual agents.

Decreased Effect: See individual agents.

Pharmacodynamics/Kinetics See individual agents.

Pregnancy Risk Factor C

Chlorpheniramine, Phenylephrine, and Methscopolamine
(klor fen IR a meen, fen il EF rin, & meth skoe POL a meen)

Related Information

Chlorpheniramine *on page 323*
Methscopolamine *on page 1019*
Phenylephrine *on page 1226*

U.S. Brand Names AH-Chew® [DSC]; AH-Chew II; Chlor-Mes-D; Dallergy®; Dehistine; Drize®-R; Extendryl; Extendryl JR; Extendryl SR; Hista-Vent® DA; PCM; PCM Allergy

Generic Available Yes

Synonyms Methscopolamine, Chlorpheniramine, and Phenylephrine; Phenylephrine, Chlorpheniramine, and Methscopolamine

Pharmacologic Category Antihistamine/Decongestant/Anticholinergic

Use Treatment of upper respiratory symptoms such as respiratory congestion, allergic rhinitis, vasomotor rhinitis, sinusitis, and allergic skin reactions of urticaria and angioedema

Local Anesthetic/Vasoconstrictor Precautions Use with caution since phenylephrine is a sympathomimetic amine which could interact with epinephrine to cause a pressor response

Effects on Dental Treatment Key adverse event(s) related to dental treatment:

Chlorpheniramine: Significant xerostomia with prolonged use (normal salivary flow resumes upon discontinuation).

Methscopolamine: Anticholinergic side effects can cause a reduction of saliva production or secretion contributes to discomfort and dental disease (ie, caries, oral candidiasis and periodontal disease).

Phenylephrine: Tachycardia, palpitations, and xerostomia; use vasoconstrictor with caution.

Common Adverse Effects Frequency not defined.

Cardiovascular: Arrhythmias, bradycardia, cardiovascular collapse, flushing, hypotension, pallor, palpitation, tachycardia

Central nervous system: Anxiety, convulsions, CNS depression, dizziness, drowsiness, excitability, fear, giddiness, hallucinations, headache, insomnia, irritability, lassitude, restlessness, tenseness, tremor

Gastrointestinal: Constipation, dysphagia, gastric irritation, nausea, xerostomia

Genitourinary: Dysuria, urinary retention

Neuromuscular & skeletal: Weakness

Ocular: Blurred vision, mydriasis

Respiratory: Dry nose, dry throat, respiratory difficulty

Mechanism of Action

Chlorpheniramine maleate: Antihistamine

Phenylephrine hydrochloride: Sympathomimetic agent (primarily alpha), decongestant

Methscopolamine nitrate: Derivative of scopolamine, antisecretory effects

Drug Interactions

Cytochrome P450 Effect: Chlorpheniramine: **Substrate** of CYP2D6 (minor), 3A4 (major); **Inhibits** CYP2D6 (weak)

Increased Effect/Toxicity: Increased effects/toxicity seen with concomitant use of antihistamines, beta-adrenergic blockers, CNS depressants, and MAO inhibitors

Decreased Effect: Decreased effects of antihypertensive agents seen with concomitant use

(Continued)

Chlorpheniramine, Phenylephrine, and Methscopolamine *(Continued)*

Pharmacodynamics/Kinetics See individual agents.
Pregnancy Risk Factor C

Chlorpheniramine, Phenylephrine, and Phenyltoloxamine

(klor fen IR a meen, fen il EF rin, & fen il tole LOKS a meen)

Related Information
Chlorpheniramine *on page 323*
Phenylephrine *on page 1226*

U.S. Brand Names Comhist®; Nalex®-A

Generic Available Yes: Liquid, prolonged release tablet

Synonyms Phenylephrine, Chlorpheniramine, and Phenyltoloxamine; Phenyltoloxamine, Chlorpheniramine, and Phenylephrine

Pharmacologic Category Antihistamine/Decongestant Combination

Use Symptomatic relief of rhinitis and nasal congestion due to colds or allergy

Local Anesthetic/Vasoconstrictor Precautions Use with caution since phenylephrine is a sympathomimetic amine which could interact with epinephrine to cause a pressor response

Effects on Dental Treatment Key adverse event(s) related to dental treatment:

Chlorpheniramine: Prolonged use will cause significant xerostomia (normal salivary flow resumes upon discontinuation).

Phenylephrine: Up to 10% of patients could experience tachycardia, palpitations, and xerostomia; use vasoconstrictor with caution.

Common Adverse Effects Frequency not defined.

Cardiovascular: Hypotension, palpitation

Central nervous system: Headache, dizziness, sedation, excitation (children), nervousness, seizure

Dermatologic: Urticaria, drug rash

Gastrointestinal: Dry mouth, anorexia, nausea, vomiting, diarrhea, constipation, GI upset

Genitourinary: Urinary frequency, urinary retention

Hematologic: Agranulocytosis, leukopenia, thrombocytopenia

Ocular: Blurred vision

Respiratory: Dry nose/throat, thickening of bronchial secretions, wheezing, stuffy nose, tightness of chest

Drug Interactions

Cytochrome P450 Effect: Chlorpheniramine: **Substrate** of CYP2D6 (minor), 3A4 (major); **Inhibits** CYP2D6 (weak)

Increased Effect/Toxicity: See individual agents.

Decreased Effect: See individual agents.

Pregnancy Risk Factor C

Chlorpheniramine, Phenylephrine, Codeine, and Potassium Iodide

(klor fen IR a meen, fen il EF rin, KOE deen, & poe TASS ee um EYE oh dide)

Related Information
Chlorpheniramine *on page 323*
Codeine *on page 385*
Phenylephrine *on page 1226*
Potassium Iodide *on page 1260*

U.S. Brand Names Pediacof® [DSC]

Generic Available No

Synonyms Codeine, Chlorpheniramine, Phenylephrine, and Potassium Iodide; Phenylephrine, Chlorpheniramine, Codeine, and Potassium Iodide; Potassium Iodide, Chlorpheniramine, Phenylephrine, and Codeine

Pharmacologic Category Antihistamine/Decongestant/Antitussive/Expectorant

Use Symptomatic relief of rhinitis, nasal congestion and cough due to colds or allergy

Local Anesthetic/Vasoconstrictor Precautions Use with caution since phenylephrine is a sympathomimetic amine which could interact with epinephrine to cause a pressor response

Effects on Dental Treatment Key adverse event(s) related to dental treatment:
Chlorpheniramine: Prolonged use will cause significant xerostomia (normal salivary flow resumes upon discontinuation).
Phenylephrine: Up to 10% of patients could experience tachycardia, palpitations, and xerostomia (prolonged use worsens); use vasoconstrictor with caution.

Restrictions C-V

Drug Interactions
Cytochrome P450 Effect: Chlorpheniramine: **Substrate** of CYP2D6 (minor), 3A4 (major); **Inhibits** CYP2D6 (weak)
Increased Effect/Toxicity: See individual agents.
Decreased Effect: See individual agents.

Chlorpheniramine, Pseudoephedrine, and Acetaminophen *see* Acetaminophen, Chlorpheniramine, and Pseudoephedrine *on page 43*

Chlorpheniramine, Pseudoephedrine, and Codeine
(klor fen IR a meen, soo doe e FED rin, & KOE deen)

Related Information
Chlorpheniramine *on page 323*
Codeine *on page 385*
Pseudoephedrine *on page 1309*

U.S. Brand Names Dihistine® DH

Generic Available Yes

Synonyms Codeine, Chlorpheniramine, and Pseudoephedrine; Pseudoephedrine, Chlorpheniramine, and Codeine

Pharmacologic Category Antihistamine/Decongestant/Antitussive

Use Temporary relief of cough associated with minor throat or bronchial irritation or nasal congestion due to common cold, allergic rhinitis, or sinusitis

Local Anesthetic/Vasoconstrictor Precautions Use with caution since pseudoephedrine is a sympathomimetic amine which could interact with epinephrine to cause a pressor response

Effects on Dental Treatment Key adverse event(s) related to dental treatment:
Chlorpheniramine: Significant xerostomia with prolonged use (normal salivary flow resumes upon discontinuation).
Pseudoephedrine: Xerostomia (normal salivary flow resumes upon discontinuation).

Common Adverse Effects See individual agents.

Restrictions C-V

Drug Interactions
Cytochrome P450 Effect: Chlorpheniramine: **Substrate** of CYP2D6 (minor), 3A4 (major); **Inhibits** CYP2D6 (weak)
Increased Effect/Toxicity: See individual agents.
Decreased Effect: See individual agents.
Pharmacodynamics/Kinetics See individual agents.
Pregnancy Risk Factor C

Chlorpheniramine, Pseudoephedrine, and Dihydrocodeine *see* Pseudoephedrine, Dihydrocodeine, and Chlorpheniramine *on page 1312*

Chlorpheniramine Tannate and Phenylephrine Tannate *see* Chlorpheniramine and Phenylephrine *on page 324*

Chlorpheniramine Tannate and Pseudoephedrine Tannate *see* Chlorpheniramine and Pseudoephedrine *on page 325*

ChlorproMAZINE (klor PROE ma zeen)

Canadian Brand Names Apo-Chlorpromazine®; Largactil®; Novo-Chlorpromazine

Mexican Brand Names Largactil®

Generic Available Yes

Synonyms Chlorpromazine Hydrochloride; CPZ

Pharmacologic Category Antipsychotic Agent, Typical, Phenothiazine

Use Control of mania; treatment of schizophrenia; control of nausea and vomiting; relief of restlessness and apprehension before surgery; acute intermittent porphyria; adjunct in the treatment of tetanus; intractable hiccups; combativeness and/or explosive hyperexcitable behavior in children 1-12 years of age and in short-term treatment of hyperactive children

Unlabeled/Investigational Use Management of psychotic disorders
(Continued)

ChlorproMAZINE *(Continued)*

Local Anesthetic/Vasoconstrictor Precautions Most pharmacology textbooks state that in presence of phenothiazines, systemic doses of epinephrine paradoxically decrease the blood pressure. This is the so called "epinephrine reversal" phenomenon. This has never been observed when epinephrine is given by infiltration as part of the anesthesia procedure. See Dental Comment.

Effects on Dental Treatment Key adverse event(s) related to dental treatment:

Significant hypotension may occur, especially when the drug is administered parenterally. Orthostatic hypotension is due to alpha-receptor blockade; elderly are at greater risk.

Tardive dyskinesia: Prevalence rate may be 40% in elderly; development of the syndrome and the irreversible nature are proportional to duration and total cumulative dose over time. Extrapyramidal reactions are more common in elderly with up to 50% developing these reactions after 60 years of age. Drug-induced Parkinson's syndrome occurs often; akathisia is the most common extrapyramidal reaction in elderly.

Increased confusion, memory loss, psychotic behavior, and agitation frequently occur as a consequence of anticholinergic effects. Antipsychotic-associated sedation in nonpsychotic patients is extremely unpleasant due to feelings of depersonalization, derealization, and dysphoria.

Common Adverse Effects Frequency not defined.

Cardiovascular: Postural hypotension, tachycardia, dizziness, nonspecific QT changes

Central nervous system: Drowsiness, dystonias, akathisia, pseudoparkinsonism, tardive dyskinesia, neuroleptic malignant syndrome, seizure

Dermatologic: Photosensitivity, dermatitis, skin pigmentation (slate gray)

Endocrine & metabolic: Lactation, breast engorgement, false-positive pregnancy test, amenorrhea, gynecomastia, hyper- or hypoglycemia

Gastrointestinal: Xerostomia, constipation, nausea

Genitourinary: Urinary retention, ejaculatory disorder, impotence

Hematologic: Agranulocytosis, eosinophilia, leukopenia, hemolytic anemia, aplastic anemia, thrombocytopenic purpura

Hepatic: Jaundice

Ocular: Blurred vision, corneal and lenticular changes, epithelial keratopathy, pigmentary retinopathy

Mechanism of Action Chlorpromazine is an aliphatic phenothiazine antipsychotic which blocks postsynaptic mesolimbic dopaminergic receptors in the brain; exhibits a strong alpha-adrenergic blocking effect and depresses the release of hypothalamic and hypophyseal hormones; believed to depress the reticular activating system, thus affecting basal metabolism, body temperature, wakefulness, vasomotor tone, and emesis

Drug Interactions

Cytochrome P450 Effect: Substrate of CYP1A2 (minor), 2D6 (major), 3A4 (minor); Inhibits CYP2D6 (strong), 2E1 (weak)

Increased Effect/Toxicity: The levels/effects of chlorpromazine may be increased by delavirdine, fluoxetine, miconazole, paroxetine, pergolide, quinidine, quinine, ritonavir, ropinirole, and other CYP2D6 inhibitors. Effects on CNS depression may be additive when chlorpromazine is combined with CNS depressants (narcotic analgesics, ethanol, barbiturates, cyclic antidepressants, antihistamines, or sedative-hypnotics). Chlorpromazine may increase the levels/effects of amphetamines, selected beta-blockers, dextromethorphan, fluoxetine, lidocaine, mirtazapine, nefazodone, paroxetine, risperidone, ritonavir, thioridazine, tricyclic antidepressants, and venlafaxine and other CYP2D6 substrates. Chlorpromazine may increase the effects/toxicity of anticholinergics, antihypertensives, lithium (rare neurotoxicity), trazodone, or valproic acid. Concurrent use with TCA may produce increased toxicity or altered therapeutic response. Chloroquine and propranolol may increase chlorpromazine concentrations. Hypotension may occur when chlorpromazine is combined with epinephrine. May increase the risk of arrhythmia when combined with antiarrhythmics, cisapride, pimozide, sparfloxacin, or other drugs which prolong QT interval. Metoclopramide may increase risk of extrapyramidal symptoms (EPS). Acetylcholinesterase inhibitors (central) may increase the risk of antipsychotic-related EPS.

Decreased Effect: Chlorpromazine may decrease the levels/effects of CYP2D6 prodrug substrates; example prodrug substrates include codeine, hydrocodone, oxycodone, and tramadol. Phenothiazines inhibit the ability of bromocriptine to lower serum prolactin concentrations. Benztropine (and other anticholinergics) may inhibit the therapeutic response to chlorpromazine and excess anticholinergic effects may occur. Antihypertensive effects of guanethidine and guanadrel may be inhibited by chlorpromazine. Chlorpromazine may inhibit the antiparkinsonian effect of levodopa. Chlorpromazine and possibly other low potency antipsychotics may reverse the pressor effects of epinephrine.

Pharmacodynamics/Kinetics

Onset of action: I.M.: 15 minutes; Oral: 30-60 minutes

Absorption: Rapid

Distribution: V_d: 20 L/kg; crosses the placenta; enters breast milk

Protein binding: 92% to 97%

Metabolism: Extensively hepatic to active and inactive metabolites

Bioavailability: 20%

Half-life, biphasic: Initial: 2 hours; Terminal: 30 hours

Excretion: Urine (<1% as unchanged drug) within 24 hours

Pregnancy Risk Factor C

Dental Comment

This drug is known to prolong the QT interval. The QT interval is measured as the time and distance between the Q point of the QRS complex and the end of the T wave in the ECG tracing. After adjustment for heart rate, the QT interval is defined as prolonged if it is more than 450 msec in men and 460 msec in women. A long QT syndrome was first described in the 1950s and 60s as a congenital syndrome involving QT interval prolongation and syncope and sudden death. Some of the congenital long QT syndromes were characterized by a peculiar electrocardiographic appearance of the QRS complex involving a premature atria beat followed by a pause, then a subsequent sinus beat showing marked QT prolongation and deformity. This type of cardiac arrhythmia was originally termed "torsade de pointes" (translated from the French as "twisting of the points").

Prolongation of the QT interval is thought to result from delayed ventricular repolarization. The repolarization process within the myocardial cell is due to the efflux of intracellular potassium. The channels associated with this current can be blocked by many drugs, thus, predisposing the electrical propagation cycle to torsade de pointes.

Chlorpromazine is one of the drugs confirmed to prolong the QT interval and is accepted as having a risk of causing torsade de pointes. The risk of drug-induced torsade de pointes is extremely low when a single QT interval prolonging drug is prescribed. In terms of epinephrine, it is not known what effect vasoconstrictors in the local anesthetic regimen will have in patients with a known history of congenital prolonged QT interval or in patients taking any medication that prolongs the QT interval. Until more information is obtained, it is suggested that the clinician consult with the physician prior to the use of a vasoconstrictor in suspected patients, and that the vasoconstrictor (epinephrine, levonordefrin [Neo-Cobefrin®]) be used with caution.

Chlorpromazine Hydrochloride *see* ChlorproMAZINE *on page 329*

ChlorproPAMIDE (klor PROE pa mide)

Related Information

Endocrine Disorders and Pregnancy *on page 1659*

U.S. Brand Names Diabinese®

Canadian Brand Names Apo-Chlorpropamide®; Novo-Propamide

Mexican Brand Names Diabinese®; Insogen®

Generic Available Yes

Pharmacologic Category Antidiabetic Agent, Sulfonylurea

Use Management of blood sugar in type 2 diabetes mellitus (noninsulin dependent, NIDDM)

Unlabeled/Investigational Use Neurogenic diabetes insipidus

Local Anesthetic/Vasoconstrictor Precautions No information available to require special precautions

Effects on Dental Treatment Chlorpropamide-dependent diabetics (noninsulin dependent, Type 2) should be appointed for dental treatment in morning in order to minimize chance of stress-induced hypoglycemia.

Common Adverse Effects

>10%:

Central nervous system: Headache, dizziness

Gastrointestinal: Anorexia, constipation, heartburn, epigastric fullness, nausea, vomiting, diarrhea

1% to 10%: Dermatologic: Skin rash, urticaria, photosensitivity

Mechanism of Action Stimulates insulin release from the pancreatic beta cells; reduces glucose output from the liver; insulin sensitivity is increased at peripheral target sites

(Continued)

ChlorproPAMIDE (Continued)

Drug Interactions
Cytochrome P450 Effect: Substrate of CYP2C8/9 (minor)

Increased Effect/Toxicity: A possible interaction between chlorpropamide and fluoroquinolone antibiotics has been reported resulting in a potentiation of hypoglycemic action of chlorpropamide. Toxic potential is increased when given concomitantly with other highly protein bound drugs (ie, phenylbutazone, oral anticoagulants, hydantoins, salicylates, NSAIDs, beta-blockers, sulfonamides) - increase hypoglycemic effect. Ethanol may be associated with disulfiram reactions. Phenylbutazone may increase hypoglycemic effects. Possible interactions between chlorpropamide and coumarin derivatives have been reported that may either potentiate or weaken the effects of coumarin derivatives.

Decreased Effect: Certain drugs tend to produce hyperglycemia and may lead to loss of control (ie, thiazides and other diuretics, corticosteroids, phenothiazines, thyroid products, estrogens, oral contraceptives, phenytoin, nicotinic acid, sympathomimetics, calcium channel blocking drugs, and isoniazid). Possible interactions between chlorpropamide and coumarin derivatives have been reported that may either potentiate or weaken the effects of coumarin derivatives.

Pharmacodynamics/Kinetics
Onset of action: Peak effect: ~6-8 hours
Distribution: V_d: 0.13-0.23 L/kg; enters breast milk
Protein binding: 60% to 90%
Metabolism: Extensively hepatic (~80%)
Half-life elimination: 30-42 hours; prolonged in elderly or with renal impairment
  End-stage renal disease: 50-200 hours
Time to peak, serum: 3-4 hours
Excretion: Urine (10% to 30% as unchanged drug)

Pregnancy Risk Factor C

Chlorthalidone (klor THAL i done)

Related Information
Cardiovascular Diseases *on page 1636*

U.S. Brand Names Thalitone®
Canadian Brand Names Apo-Chlorthalidone®
Generic Available Yes
Synonyms Hygroton
Pharmacologic Category Diuretic, Thiazide
Use Management of mild-to-moderate hypertension when used alone or in combination with other agents; treatment of edema associated with congestive heart failure or nephrotic syndrome. Recent studies have found chlorthalidone effective in the treatment of isolated systolic hypertension in the elderly.

Local Anesthetic/Vasoconstrictor Precautions No information available to require special precautions
Effects on Dental Treatment No significant effects or complications reported

Common Adverse Effects 1% to 10%:
Dermatologic: Photosensitivity
Endocrine & metabolic: Hypokalemia
Gastrointestinal: Anorexia, epigastric distress

Mechanism of Action Sulfonamide-derived diuretic that inhibits sodium and chloride reabsorption in the cortical-diluting segment of the ascending loop of Henle

Drug Interactions
Increased Effect/Toxicity: Increased effect of chlorthalidone with furosemide and other loop diuretics. Increased hypotension and/or renal adverse effects of ACE inhibitors may result in aggressively diuresed patients. Beta-blockers increase hyperglycemic effects of thiazides in Type 2 diabetes mellitus. Cyclosporine and thiazides can increase the risk of gout or renal toxicity. Digoxin toxicity can be exacerbated if a thiazide induces hypokalemia or hypomagnesemia. Lithium toxicity can occur with thiazides due to reduced renal excretion of lithium. Thiazides may prolong the duration of action with neuromuscular blocking agents.

Decreased Effect: Effects of oral hypoglycemics may be decreased. Decreased absorption of chlorthalidone with cholestyramine and colestipol. NSAIDs can decrease the efficacy of chlorthalidone, reducing the diuretic and antihypertensive effects.

Pharmacodynamics/Kinetics
Onset of action: Peak effect: 2-6 hours

Duration: 24-72 hours
Absorption: 65%
Distribution: Crosses placenta; enters breast milk
Metabolism: Hepatic
Half-life elimination: 35-55 hours; may be prolonged with renal impairment; Anuria: 81 hours
Excretion: Urine (~50% to 65% as unchanged drug)
Pregnancy Risk Factor B (manufacturer); D (expert analysis)

Chlorthalidone and Atenolol *see* Atenolol and Chlorthalidone *on page 156*

Chlorthalidone and Clonidine *see* Clonidine and Chlorthalidone *on page 376*

Chlor-Trimeton® [OTC] *see* Chlorpheniramine *on page 323*

Chlor-Trimeton® Allergy D [OTC] *see* Chlorpheniramine and Pseudoephedrine *on page 325*

Chlorzoxazone (klor ZOKS a zone)

Related Information
Temporomandibular Dysfunction (TMD) *on page 1724*
U.S. Brand Names Parafon Forte® DSC
Canadian Brand Names Parafon Forte®; Strifon Forte®
Generic Available Yes
Pharmacologic Category Skeletal Muscle Relaxant
Dental Use Treatment of muscle spasm and pain associated with acute temporomandibular joint pain (TMJ)
Use Symptomatic treatment of muscle spasm and pain associated with acute musculoskeletal conditions
Local Anesthetic/Vasoconstrictor Precautions No information available to require special precautions
Effects on Dental Treatment No significant effects or complications reported
Significant Adverse Effects Frequency not defined.
Central nervous system: Dizziness, drowsiness, lightheadedness, paradoxical stimulation, malaise
Dermatologic: Rash, petechiae, ecchymoses (rare), angioneurotic edema
Gastrointestinal: Nausea, vomiting, stomach cramps
Genitourinary: Urine discoloration
Hepatic: Liver dysfunction
Miscellaneous: Anaphylaxis (very rare)
Dental Usual Dosing Treatment of muscle spasm and pain associated with acute TMJ pain: Oral:
Children: 20 mg/kg/day or 600 mg/m^2/day in 3-4 divided doses
Adults: 250-500 mg 3-4 times/day up to 750 mg 3-4 times/day
Dosage Oral:
Children: 20 mg/kg/day or 600 mg/m^2/day in 3-4 divided doses
Adults: 250-500 mg 3-4 times/day up to 750 mg 3-4 times/day
Mechanism of Action Acts on the spinal cord and subcortical levels by depressing polysynaptic reflexes
Contraindications Hypersensitivity to chlorzoxazone or any component of the formulation; impaired liver function
Drug Interactions Substrate of CYP1A2 (minor), 2A6 (minor), 2D6 (minor), 2E1 (major), 3A4 (minor); **Inhibits** CYP2E1 (weak), 3A4 (weak)
CNS depressants: Effects may be increased by chlorzoxazone.
CYP2E1 inhibitors: May increase the levels/effects of chlorzoxazone. Example inhibitors include disulfiram, isoniazid, and miconazole.
Disulfiram: May increase chlorzoxazone concentration; monitor.
Isoniazid: May increase chlorzoxazone concentration; monitor.
Ethanol/Nutrition/Herb Interactions Ethanol: Avoid ethanol (may increase CNS depression).
Pharmacodynamics/Kinetics
Onset of action: ~1 hour
Duration: 6-12 hours
Absorption: Readily absorbed
Metabolism: Extensively hepatic via glucuronidation
Excretion: Urine (as conjugates)
Pregnancy Risk Factor C
Lactation Excretion in breast milk unknown/not recommended
Dosage Forms
Caplet (Parafon Forte® DSC): 500 mg
Tablet: 250 mg, 500 mg

Cholecalciferol (kole e kal SI fer ole)

U.S. Brand Names Delta-D®
Canadian Brand Names D-Vi-Sol®
Generic Available Yes
Synonyms D_3
Pharmacologic Category Vitamin D Analog
Use Dietary supplement, treatment of vitamin D deficiency, or prophylaxis of deficiency
Local Anesthetic/Vasoconstrictor Precautions No information available to require special precautions
Effects on Dental Treatment Key adverse event(s) related to dental treatment: Metallic taste and xerostomia (normal salivary flow resumes upon discontinuation).
Common Adverse Effects Frequency not defined.
Cardiovascular: Arrhythmia, hyper-/hypotension, cardiac arrhythmia
Central nervous system: Irritability, headache, somnolence, overt psychosis (rare)
Dermatologic: Pruritus
Endocrine & metabolic: Polydipsia
Gastrointestinal: Nausea, vomiting, anorexia, pancreatitis, metallic taste, dry mouth, constipation, weight loss
Genitourinary: Albuminuria, polyuria
Hepatic: Increased liver function test
Neuromuscular & skeletal: Bone pain, myalgia, weakness, muscle pain
Ocular: Conjunctivitis, photophobia
Renal: Azotemia, nephrocalcinosis
Drug Interactions
Cytochrome P450 Effect: Inhibits CYP2C9 (weak), 2C19 (weak), 2D6 (weak)
Pharmacodynamics/Kinetics
Distribution: Primarily hepatic
Protein binding: Extensively to vitamin D-binding protein
Metabolism: Primary liver and kidney hydroxylation; glucuronidation (minimal)
Half-life elimination: 14 hours
Time to peak, plasma: 11 hours
Excretion: As metabolites, urine (2.4%) and feces (4.9%)
Pregnancy Risk Factor C

Cholecalciferol and Alendronate *see* Alendronate and Cholecalciferol *on page 66*

Cholestyramine Resin (koe LES teer a meen REZ in)

Related Information
Cardiovascular Diseases *on page 1636*
U.S. Brand Names Prevalite®; Questran®; Questran® Light
Canadian Brand Names Novo-Cholamine; Novo-Cholamine Light; PMS-Cholestyramine; Questran®; Questran® Light Sugar Free
Generic Available Yes
Pharmacologic Category Antilipemic Agent, Bile Acid Sequestrant
Use Adjunct in the management of primary hypercholesterolemia; pruritus associated with elevated levels of bile acids; diarrhea associated with excess fecal bile acids; binding toxicologic agents; pseudomembranous colitis
Local Anesthetic/Vasoconstrictor Precautions No information available to require special precautions
Effects on Dental Treatment No significant effects or complications reported
Common Adverse Effects
>10%: Gastrointestinal: Constipation, heartburn, nausea, vomiting, stomach pain
1% to 10%:
Central nervous system: Headache
Gastrointestinal: Belching, bloating, diarrhea
Mechanism of Action Forms a nonabsorbable complex with bile acids in the intestine, releasing chloride ions in the process; inhibits enterohepatic reuptake of intestinal bile salts and thereby increases the fecal loss of bile salt-bound low density lipoprotein cholesterol

Drug Interactions
Decreased Effect:

Cholestyramine can reduce the absorption of numerous medications when used concurrently. Give other medications 1 hour before or 4-6 hours after giving cholestyramine. Medications which may be affected include HMG-CoA reductase inhibitors, thiazide diuretics, propranolol (and potentially other beta-blockers), corticosteroids, thyroid hormones, digoxin, valproic acid, NSAIDs, loop diuretics, sulfonylureas, troglitazone (and potentially other agents in this class).

Warfarin and other oral anticoagulants: Hypoprothrombinemic effects may be reduced by cholestyramine. Separate administration times (as detailed above) and monitor INR closely when initiating or discontinuing.

Pharmacodynamics/Kinetics
Onset of action: Peak effect: 21 days
Absorption: None
Excretion: Feces (as insoluble complex with bile acids)

Pregnancy Risk Factor C

Choline Magnesium Trisalicylate
(KOE leen mag NEE zhum trye sa LIS i late)

Related Information
Rheumatoid Arthritis, Osteoarthritis, and Osteoporosis *on page 1668*
Temporomandibular Dysfunction (TMD) *on page 1724*

U.S. Brand Names Trilisate® [DSC]

Generic Available Yes

Synonyms Tricosal

Pharmacologic Category Salicylate

Use Management of osteoarthritis, rheumatoid arthritis, and other arthritis; acute painful shoulder

Local Anesthetic/Vasoconstrictor Precautions No information available to require special precautions

Effects on Dental Treatment NSAID formulations are known to reversibly decrease platelet aggregation via mechanisms different than observed with aspirin. The dentist should be aware of the potential of abnormal coagulation. Caution should also be exercised in the use of NSAIDs in patients already on anticoagulant therapy with drugs such as warfarin (Coumadin®).

Common Adverse Effects
<20%:
Gastrointestinal: Nausea, vomiting, diarrhea, heartburn, dyspepsia, epigastric pain, constipation
Otic: Tinnitus

<2%:
Central nervous system: Headache, lightheadedness, dizziness, drowsiness, lethargy
Otic: Hearing impairment

Dosage Oral (based on total salicylate content):
Children <37 kg: 50 mg/kg/day given in 2 divided doses; 2250 mg/day for heavier children
Adults: 500 mg to 1.5 g 2-3 times/day **or** 3 g at bedtime; usual maintenance dose: 1-4.5 g/day
Elderly: 750 mg 3 times/day
Dosing adjustment/comments in renal impairment: Avoid use in severe renal impairment

Mechanism of Action Inhibits prostaglandin synthesis; acts on the hypothalamus heat-regulating center to reduce fever; blocks the generation of pain impulses

Contraindications Hypersensitivity to salicylates, other nonacetylated salicylates, other NSAIDs, or any component of the formulation; bleeding disorders; pregnancy (3rd trimester)

Warnings/Precautions Salicylate salts may not inhibit platelet aggregation and, therefore, should not be substituted for aspirin in the prophylaxis of thrombosis. Use with caution in patients with impaired renal function, dehydration, erosive gastritis, asthma, or peptic ulcer. Discontinue use 1 week prior to surgical procedures. Children and teenagers who have or are recovering from chickenpox or flu-like symptoms should not use this product. Changes in behavior (along with nausea and vomiting) may be an early sign of Reye's syndrome; patients should be instructed to contact their healthcare provider if these occur.
(Continued)

Choline Magnesium Trisalicylate *(Continued)*

Elderly are a high-risk population for adverse effects from NSAIDs. As many as 60% of elderly can develop peptic ulceration and/or hemorrhage asymptomatically. Use lowest effective dose for shortest period possible. Tinnitus or impaired hearing may indicate toxicity. Tinnitus may be a difficult and unreliable indication of toxicity due to age-related hearing loss or eighth cranial nerve damage. CNS adverse effects may be observed in the elderly at lower doses than younger adults.

Drug Interactions

Increased Effect/Toxicity: Choline magnesium trisalicylate may increase the hypoprothrombinemic effect of warfarin.

Decreased Effect: Antacids may decrease choline magnesium trisalicylate absorption/salicylate concentrations.

Ethanol/Nutrition/Herb Interactions

Ethanol: Avoid ethanol (may enhance gastric mucosal irritation).

Food: May decrease the rate but not the extent of oral absorption.

Herb/Nutraceutical: Avoid cat's claw, dong quai, evening primrose, feverfew, garlic, ginger, ginkgo, red clover, horse chestnut, green tea, ginseng (all have additional antiplatelet activity). Limit curry powder, paprika, licorice, Benedictine liqueur, prunes, raisins, tea, and gherkins; may cause salicylate accumulation. These foods contain 6 mg salicylate/100 g.

Dietary Considerations Take with food or large volume of water or milk to minimize GI upset. Liquid may be mixed with fruit juice just before drinking. Hypermagnesemia resulting from magnesium salicylate; avoid or use with caution in renal insufficiency.

Pharmacodynamics/Kinetics

Onset of action: Peak effect: ~2 hours

Absorption: Stomach and small intestines

Distribution: Readily into most body fluids and tissues; crosses placenta; enters breast milk

Half-life elimination (dose dependent): Low dose: 2-3 hours; High dose: 30 hours

Time to peak, serum: ~2 hours

Pregnancy Risk Factor C/D (3rd trimester)

Dosage Forms LIQ: 500 mg/5 mL (240 mL). **TAB:** 500 mg, 750 mg, 1000 mg

Cholografin® Meglumine *see* Iodipamide Meglumine *on page 853*

Chondroitin Sulfate and Sodium Hyaluronate
(kon DROY tin SUL fate & SOW de um hye al yoor ON ate)

Related Information

Chondroitin Sulfate *on page 1618*

U.S. Brand Names Viscoat®

Generic Available No

Synonyms Sodium Hyaluronate and Chondroitin Sulfate

Pharmacologic Category Ophthalmic Agent, Viscoelastic

Use Surgical aid in anterior segment procedures; protects corneal endothelium and coats intraocular lens thus protecting it

Local Anesthetic/Vasoconstrictor Precautions No information available to require special precautions

Effects on Dental Treatment No significant effects or complications reported

Mechanism of Action Functions as a tissue lubricant and is thought to play an important role in modulating the interactions between adjacent tissues

Pregnancy Risk Factor C

Chooz® [OTC] *see* Calcium Carbonate *on page 248*

Choriogonadotropin Alfa *see* Chorionic Gonadotropin (Recombinant) *on page 337*

Chorionic Gonadotropin (Human)
(kor ee ON ik goe NAD oh troe pin, HYU man)

Related Information

Chorionic Gonadotropin (Recombinant) *on page 337*

U.S. Brand Names Novarel™; Pregnyl®

Canadian Brand Names Humegon®; Pregnyl®; Profasi® HP

Generic Available Yes

Synonyms CG; hCG

Pharmacologic Category Ovulation Stimulator

Use Induces ovulation and pregnancy in anovulatory, infertile females; treatment of hypogonadotropic hypogonadism, prepubertal cryptorchidism; spermatogenesis induction with follitropin alfa or follitropin beta

Local Anesthetic/Vasoconstrictor Precautions No information available to require special precautions

Effects on Dental Treatment No significant effects or complications reported

Common Adverse Effects

1% to 10%:
Central nervous system: Mental depression, fatigue
Endocrine & metabolic: Pelvic pain, ovarian cysts, breast enlargement, precocious puberty
Local: Pain at the injection site
Neuromuscular & skeletal: Premature closure of epiphyses

Mechanism of Action Stimulates production of gonadal steroid hormones by causing production of androgen by the testes; as a substitute for luteinizing hormone (LH) to stimulate ovulation

Drug Interactions

Increased Effect/Toxicity: No data reported

Decreased Effect: No data reported

Pharmacodynamics/Kinetics

Half-life elimination: Biphasic: Initial: 11 hours; Terminal: 23 hours
Excretion: Urine (as unchanged drug) within 3-4 days

Pregnancy Risk Factor C

Chorionic Gonadotropin (Recombinant)
(kor ee ON ik goe NAD oh troe pin ree KOM be nant)

Related Information

Chorionic Gonadotropin (Human) *on page 336*

U.S. Brand Names Ovidrel®

Canadian Brand Names Ovidrel®

Generic Available No

Synonyms Choriogonadotropin Alfa; r-hCG

Pharmacologic Category Gonadotropin; Ovulation Stimulator

Use As part of an assisted reproductive technology (ART) program, induces ovulation in infertile females who have been pretreated with follicle stimulating hormones (FSH); induces ovulation and pregnancy in infertile females when the cause of infertility is functional

Local Anesthetic/Vasoconstrictor Precautions No information available to require special precautions

Effects on Dental Treatment No significant effects or complications reported

Common Adverse Effects

2% to 10%:
Endocrine & metabolic: Ovarian cyst (3%), ovarian hyperstimulation (<2% to 3%)
Gastrointestinal: Abdominal pain (3% to 4%), nausea (3%), vomiting (3%)
Local: Injection site: Pain (8%), bruising (3% to 5%), reaction (<2% to 3%), inflammation (<2% to 2%)
Miscellaneous: Postoperative pain (5%)

<2%:
Cardiovascular: Cardiac arrhythmia, heart murmur
Central nervous system: Dizziness, emotional lability, fever, headache, insomnia, malaise
Dermatologic: Pruritus, rash
Endocrine & metabolic: Breast pain, hot flashes, hyperglycemia, intermenstrual bleeding, vaginal hemorrhage
Gastrointestinal: Abdominal enlargement, diarrhea, flatulence
Genitourinary: Cervical carcinoma, cervical lesion, dysuria, genital herpes, genital moniliasis, leukorrhea, urinary incontinence, urinary tract infection, vaginitis
Hematologic: Leukocytosis
Neuromuscular & skeletal: Back pain, paresthesia
Renal: Albuminuria
Respiratory: Cough, pharyngitis, upper respiratory tract infection
Miscellaneous: Ectopic pregnancy, hiccups

In addition, the following have been reported with menotropin therapy: Adnexal torsion, hemoperitoneum, mild-to-moderate ovarian enlargement, pulmonary and vascular complications. Ovarian neoplasms have also been reported (rare) (Continued)

Chorionic Gonadotropin (Recombinant) *(Continued)*

with multiple drug regimens used for ovarian induction (relationship not established).

Mechanism of Action Luteinizing hormone analogue produced by recombinant DNA techniques; stimulates rupture of the ovarian follicle once follicular development has occurred.

Drug Interactions

Increased Effect/Toxicity: Specific drug interaction studies have not been conducted.

Decreased Effect: Specific drug interaction studies have not been conducted.

Pharmacodynamics/Kinetics

Distribution: V_d: 5.9 ± 1 L

Bioavailability: 40%

Half-life elimination: Initial: 4 hours; Terminal: 29 hours

Time to peak: 12-24 hours

Excretion: Urine (10% of dose)

Pregnancy Risk Factor X

Chromium see Trace Metals on page 1513
CI-1008 see Pregabalin on page 1274
Cialis® see Tadalafil on page 1441

Ciclopirox (sye kloe PEER oks)

Related Information

Fungal Infections *on page 1707*

U.S. Brand Names Loprox®; Penlac®

Canadian Brand Names Loprox®; Penlac®; Stieprox®

Mexican Brand Names Loprox®

Generic Available Yes: Cream, topical suspension

Synonyms Ciclopirox Olamine

Pharmacologic Category Antifungal Agent, Topical

Use

Cream/suspension: Treatment of tinea pedis (athlete's foot), tinea cruris (jock itch), tinea corporis (ringworm), cutaneous candidiasis, and tinea versicolor (pityriasis)

Gel: Treatment of tinea pedis (athlete's foot), tinea corporis (ringworm); seborrheic dermatitis of the scalp

Lacquer (solution): Topical treatment of mild-to-moderate onychomycosis of the fingernails and toenails due to *Trichophyton rubrum* (not involving the lunula) and the immediately-adjacent skin

Shampoo: Treatment of seborrheic dermatitis of the scalp

Local Anesthetic/Vasoconstrictor Precautions No information available to require special precautions

Effects on Dental Treatment No significant effects or complications reported

Common Adverse Effects

>10%: Local: Burning sensation (gel: 34%; ≤1% with other forms)

1% to 10%:

Central nervous system: Headache

Dermatologic: Erythema, nail disorder, pruritus, rash

Local: Irritation, redness, or pain

Mechanism of Action Inhibiting transport of essential elements in the fungal cell disrupting the synthesis of DNA, RNA, and protein

Drug Interactions

Increased Effect/Toxicity: No data reported

Decreased Effect: No data reported

Pharmacodynamics/Kinetics

Absorption: Cream, solution: <2% through intact skin; increased with gel; <5% with lacquer

Distribution: Scalp application: To epidermis, corium (dermis), including hair, hair follicles, and sebaceous glands

Protein binding: 94% to 98%

Half-life elimination: Biologic: 1.7 hours (solution); elimination: 5.5 hours (gel)

Excretion: Urine (gel: 3% to 10%); feces (small amounts)

Pregnancy Risk Factor B

Ciclopirox Olamine see Ciclopirox on page 338
Cidecin see Daptomycin on page 423

Cidofovir (si DOF o veer)

Related Information
Systemic Viral Diseases *on page 1675*
U.S. Brand Names Vistide®
Generic Available No
Pharmacologic Category Antiviral Agent
Use Treatment of cytomegalovirus (CMV) retinitis in patients with acquired immunodeficiency syndrome (AIDS). **Note:** Should be administered with probenecid.
Local Anesthetic/Vasoconstrictor Precautions No information available to require special precautions
Effects on Dental Treatment Key adverse event(s) related to dental treatment: Stomatitis and abnormal taste.

Common Adverse Effects
>10%:
Central nervous system: Chills, fever, headache, pain
Dermatologic: Alopecia, rash
Gastrointestinal: Nausea, vomiting, diarrhea, anorexia
Hematologic: Anemia, neutropenia
Neuromuscular & skeletal: Weakness
Ocular: Intraocular pressure decreased, iritis, ocular hypotony, uveitis
Renal: Creatinine increased, proteinuria, renal toxicity
Respiratory: Cough, dyspnea
Miscellaneous: Infection, oral moniliasis, serum bicarbonate decreased
1% to 10%:
Renal: Fanconi syndrome
Respiratory: Pneumonia

Frequency not defined (limited to important or life-threatening reactions):
Cardiovascular: Cardiomyopathy, cardiovascular disorder, CHF, edema, postural hypotension, shock, syncope, tachycardia
Central nervous system: Agitation, amnesia, anxiety, confusion, convulsion, dizziness, hallucinations, insomnia, malaise, vertigo
Dermatologic: Photosensitivity reaction, skin discoloration, urticaria
Endocrine & metabolic: Adrenal cortex insufficiency
Gastrointestinal: Abdominal pain, aphthous stomatitis, colitis, constipation, dysphagia, fecal incontinence, gastritis, GI hemorrhage, gingivitis, melena, proctitis, splenomegaly, stomatitis, tongue discoloration
Genitourinary: Urinary incontinence
Hematologic: Hypochromic anemia, leukocytosis, leukopenia, lymphadenopathy, lymphoma-like reaction, pancytopenia, thrombocytopenia, thrombocytopenic purpura
Hepatic: Hepatomegaly, hepatosplenomegaly, jaundice, liver function tests abnormal, liver damage, liver necrosis
Local: Injection site reaction
Neuromuscular & skeletal: Tremor
Ocular: Amblyopia, blindness, cataract, conjunctivitis, corneal lesion, diplopia, vision abnormal
Otic: Hearing loss
Miscellaneous: Allergic reaction, sepsis

Mechanism of Action Cidofovir is converted to cidofovir diphosphate which is the active intracellular metabolite; cidofovir diphosphate suppresses CMV replication by selective inhibition of viral DNA synthesis. Incorporation of cidofovir into growing viral DNA chain results in reductions in the rate of viral DNA synthesis.

Drug Interactions
Increased Effect/Toxicity: Drugs with nephrotoxic potential (eg, amphotericin B, aminoglycosides, foscarnet, and I.V. pentamidine) should not be used with or within 7 days of cidofovir therapy. Due to concomitant probenecid administration, temporarily discontinue or decrease zidovudine dose by 50% on the day of cidofovir administration only.

Pharmacodynamics/Kinetics The following pharmacokinetic data is based on a combination of cidofovir administered with probenecid:
Distribution: V_d: 0.54 L/kg; does not cross significantly into CSF
Protein binding: <6%
Metabolism: Minimal; phosphorylation occurs intracellularly
Half-life elimination, plasma: ~2.6 hours
Excretion: Urine
Pregnancy Risk Factor C

Cilazapril (sye LAY za pril)

Canadian Brand Names Inhibace®; Novo-Cilazapril
Mexican Brand Names Inibace®
Synonyms Cilazapril Monohydrate
Pharmacologic Category Angiotensin-Converting Enzyme (ACE) Inhibitor
Use Management of hypertension; treatment of congestive heart failure
Local Anesthetic/Vasoconstrictor Precautions No information available to require special precautions
Effects on Dental Treatment Key adverse event(s) related to dental treatment: Orthostatic hypotension.
Common Adverse Effects 1% to 10%
Cardiovascular: Palpitation (up to 1%), hypotension (symptomatic, up to 1% in CHF patients), orthostatic hypotension (2%)
Central nervous system: Headache (3% to 5%), dizziness (3% to 8%), fatigue (2% to 3%)
Gastrointestinal: Nausea (1% to 3%)
Neuromuscular & skeletal: Weakness (0.3% to 2%)
Renal: Serum creatinine increased
Respiratory: Cough (2% in hypertension, up to 7.5% in CHF patients)
Restrictions Not available in U.S.
Mechanism of Action Competitive inhibitor of angiotensin-converting enzyme (ACE); prevents conversion of angiotensin I to angiotensin II, a potent vasoconstrictor; results in lower levels of angiotensin II which causes an increase in plasma renin activity and a reduction in aldosterone secretion.
Drug Interactions
Increased Effect/Toxicity: Potassium supplements, sulfamethoxazole/trimethoprim (high dose), angiotensin II receptor antagonists (eg, candesartan, losartan, irbesartan), or potassium-sparing diuretics (amiloride, spironolactone, triamterene) may result in elevated serum potassium levels when combined with cilazapril. ACE inhibitor effects may be increased by phenothiazines or probenecid (increases levels of other ACE inhibitors). ACE inhibitors may increase serum concentrations/effects of lithium.

Diuretics have additive hypotensive effects with ACE inhibitors, and hypovolemia increases the potential for adverse renal effects of ACE inhibitors. In patients with compromised renal function, coadministration with nonsteroidal anti-inflammatory drugs may result in further deterioration of renal function. Allopurinol and ACE inhibitors may cause a higher risk of hypersensitivity reaction when taken concurrently.
Decreased Effect: Aspirin (high dose) may reduce the therapeutic effects of ACE inhibitors; at low dosages this does not appear to be significant. Rifampin may decrease the effect of ACE inhibitors. Antacids may decrease the bioavailability of ACE inhibitors (may be more likely to occur with captopril); separate administration times by 1-2 hours. NSAIDs, specifically indomethacin, may reduce the hypotensive effects of ACE inhibitors. More likely to occur in low renin or volume-dependent hypertensive patients.
Pharmacodynamics/Kinetics
Onset of action: Antihypertensive: ~1 hour
Duration: Therapeutic effect: 24 hours
Absorption: Rapid
Metabolism: To active form (cilazaprilat)
Bioavailability: 57%
Half-life elimination: Cilazaprilat: Terminal: 36-49 hours
Time to peak: 3-7 hours
Excretion: In urine (91%)
Pregnancy Risk Factor Not assigned; C/D (2nd and 3rd trimesters) based on other ACE inhibitors

Cilazapril Monohydrate see Cilazapril on page 340

Cilostazol (sil OH sta zol)

U.S. Brand Names Pletal®
Canadian Brand Names Pletal®
Generic Available Yes
Synonyms OPC-13013
Pharmacologic Category Antiplatelet Agent; Phosphodiesterase Enzyme Inhibitor
Use Symptomatic management of peripheral vascular disease, primarily intermittent claudication

Unlabeled/Investigational Use Treatment of acute coronary syndromes and for graft patency improvement in percutaneous coronary interventions with or without stenting

Local Anesthetic/Vasoconstrictor Precautions No information available to require special precautions

Effects on Dental Treatment Key adverse event(s) related to dental treatment: Postural hypotension and tongue edema (per manufacturer). If a patient is to undergo elective surgery and an antiplatelet effect is not desired, a medical consult is suggested to consider reduction or discontinuation of cilostazol dose prior to surgery.

Common Adverse Effects

>10%:
Central nervous system: Headache (27% to 34%)
Gastrointestinal: Abnormal stools (12% to 15%), diarrhea (12% to 19%)
Respiratory: Rhinitis (7% to 12%)
Miscellaneous: Infection (10% to 14%)

2% to 10%:
Cardiovascular: Peripheral edema (7% to 9%), palpitation (5% to 10%), tachycardia (4%)
Central nervous system: Dizziness (9% to 10%), vertigo (up to 3%)
Gastrointestinal: Dyspepsia (6%), nausea (6% to 7%), abdominal pain (4% to 5%), flatulence (2% to 3%)
Neuromuscular & skeletal: Back pain (6% to 7%), myalgia (2% to 3%)
Respiratory: Pharyngitis (7% to 10%), cough (3% to 4%)

Mechanism of Action Cilostazol and its metabolites are inhibitors of phosphodiesterase III. As a result, cyclic AMP is increased leading to reversible inhibition of platelet aggregation and vasodilation. Other effects of phosphodiesterase III inhibition include increased cardiac contractility, accelerated AV nodal conduction, increased ventricular automaticity, heart rate, and coronary blood flow.

Drug Interactions

Cytochrome P450 Effect: Substrate of CYP1A2 (minor), 2C19 (minor), 2D6 (minor), 3A4 (major)

Increased Effect/Toxicity: Cilostazol serum concentrations may be increased by antifungal agents (midazole), macrolide antibiotics, and omeprazole. Increased concentrations of cilostazol may be anticipated during concurrent therapy with other inhibitors of CYP3A4 (eg, clarithromycin, diclofenac, doxycycline, erythromycin, imatinib, isoniazid, nefazodone, nicardipine, propofol, protease inhibitors, quinidine, telithromycin, and verapamil) or inhibitors of CYP2C19 (eg, delavirdine, fluconazole, fluvoxamine, gemfibrozil, isoniazid, omeprazole, and ticlopidine). Aspirin-induced inhibition of platelet aggregation is potentiated by concurrent cilostazol. Concurrent use of drotrecogin alfa, NSAIDs, or treprostinil may cause increased bleeding.

Pharmacodynamics/Kinetics

Onset of action: 2-4 weeks; may require up to 12 weeks
Protein binding: 97% to 98%
Metabolism: Hepatic via CYP3A4 (primarily), 1A2, 2C19, and 2D6; at least one metabolite has significant activity
Half-life elimination: 11-13 hours
Excretion: Urine (74%) and feces (20%) as metabolites

Pregnancy Risk Factor C

Ciloxan® *see* Ciprofloxacin *on page 343*

Cimetidine (sye MET i deen)

Related Information
Gastrointestinal Disorders *on page 1654*

U.S. Brand Names Tagamet®; Tagamet® HB 200 [OTC]

Canadian Brand Names Apo-Cimetidine®; Gen-Cimetidine; Novo-Cimetidine; Nu-Cimet; PMS-Cimetidine; Tagamet® HB

Mexican Brand Names Cimetase®; Tagamet®

Generic Available Yes

Pharmacologic Category Histamine H_2 Antagonist

Use Short-term treatment of active duodenal ulcers and benign gastric ulcers; long-term prophylaxis of duodenal ulcer; gastric hypersecretory states; gastroesophageal reflux; prevention of upper GI bleeding in critically-ill patients; labeled for OTC use for prevention or relief of heartburn, acid indigestion, or sour stomach

Unlabeled/Investigational Use Part of a multidrug regimen for *H. pylori* eradication to reduce the risk of duodenal ulcer recurrence
(Continued)

Cimetidine *(Continued)*

No information available to require special precautions

No significant effects or complications reported

Common Adverse Effects 1% to 10%:

Central nervous system: Headache (2% to 4%), dizziness (1%), somnolence (1%), agitation

Endocrine & metabolic: Gynecomastia (<1% to 4%)

Gastrointestinal: Diarrhea (1%), nausea, vomiting

Adverse reactions reported with H_2 antagonists: Alopecia, AV heart block, bradycardia, erythema multiforme, exfoliative dermatitis, Stevens-Johnson syndrome, toxic epidermal necrolysis

Mechanism of Action Competitive inhibition of histamine at H_2 receptors of the gastric parietal cells resulting in reduced gastric acid secretion, gastric volume and hydrogen ion concentration reduced

Drug Interactions

Cytochrome P450 Effect: Inhibits CYP1A2 (moderate), 2C9 (weak), 2C19 (moderate), 2D6 (moderate), 2E1 (weak), 3A4 (moderate)

Increased Effect/Toxicity: Cimetidine may increase the levels/effects of aminophylline, amphetamines, selected beta-blockers, selected benzodiazepines, calcium channel blockers, cyclosporine, dextromethorphan, dofetilide, ergot derivatives, lidocaine, meperidine, metformin, methsuximide, metronidazole, mexiletine, mirtazapine, moricizine, nateglinide, nefazodone, paroxetine (and other SSRIs), phenytoin, procainamide, propafenone, propranolol, quinidine, quinolone antibiotics, risperidone, ritonavir, ropinirole, sildenafil (and other PDE-5 inhibitors), sulfonylureas, tacrine, tacrolimus, theophylline, thioridazine, triamterene, tricyclic antidepressants, trifluoperazine, venlafaxine, and other CYP1A2, 2C19, or 2D6 substrates.

Cimetidine increases warfarin's effect in a dose-related manner. Cimetidine increases carmustine's myelotoxicity; avoid concurrent use.

Decreased Effect: Cimetidine may decrease the levels/effects of CYP2D6 prodrug substrates (eg, codeine, hydrocodone, oxycodone, and tramadol). Ketoconazole, fluconazole, itraconazole (especially capsule) decrease serum concentration; avoid concurrent use with H_2 antagonists. Absorption of delavirdine and atazanavir may be decreased; avoid concurrent use of delavirdine with H_2 antagonists.

Pharmacodynamics/Kinetics

Onset of action: 1 hour

Duration: 4-8 hours

Absorption: Rapid

Distribution: Crosses placenta; enters breast milk

Protein binding: 20%

Metabolism: Partially hepatic

Bioavailability: 60% to 70%

Half-life elimination: Neonates: 3.6 hours; Children: 1.4 hours; Adults: Normal renal function: 2 hours

Time to peak, serum: Oral: 1-2 hours

Excretion: Primarily urine (48% as unchanged drug); feces (some)

Pregnancy Risk Factor B

Cinacalcet *(sin a KAL cet)*

U.S. Brand Names Sensipar™

Generic Available No

Synonyms AMG 073; Cinacalcet Hydrochloride

Pharmacologic Category Calcimimetic

Use Treatment of secondary hyperparathyroidism in dialysis patients; treatment of hypercalcemia in patients with parathyroid carcinoma

Unlabeled/Investigational Use Primary hyperparathyroidism

No information available to require special precautions

No significant effects or complications reported

Common Adverse Effects

>10%:

Endocrine & metabolic: Hypocalcemia

Gastrointestinal: Nausea (31%), vomiting (27%), diarrhea (21%)

Neuromuscular & skeletal: Myalgia (15%)

1% to 10%:

Cardiovascular: Hypertension (7%)

Central nervous system: Dizziness (10%), seizure (1%)

Endocrine & metabolic: Testosterone decreased
Gastrointestinal: Anorexia (6%)
Neuromuscular & skeletal: Weakness (7%), chest pain (6%)

Mechanism of Action Increases the sensitivity of the calcium-sensing receptor on the parathyroid gland.

Drug Interactions
Cytochrome P450 Effect: Substrate of CYP1A2, 2D6, 3A4; **Inhibits** CYP2D6
Increased Effect/Toxicity: Cinacalcet increases levels of amitriptyline and nortriptyline. Ketoconazole may increase cinacalcet levels.

Pharmacodynamics/Kinetics
Distribution: V_d: 1000 L
Protein binding: 93% to 97%
Metabolism: Hepatic via CYP3A4, 2D6, 1A2; forms inactive metabolites
Half-life elimination: Terminal: 30-40 hours
Time to peak, plasma: Nadir in iPTH levels: 2-6 hours postdose
Excretion: Urine 80% (as metabolites); feces 15%

Pregnancy Risk Factor C

Cinacalcet Hydrochloride *see* Cinacalcet *on page 342*
Cipro® *see* Ciprofloxacin *on page 343*
Ciprodex® *see* Ciprofloxacin and Dexamethasone *on page 348*

Ciprofloxacin (sip roe FLOKS a sin)

Related Information
Sexually-Transmitted Diseases *on page 1674*
Tuberculosis *on page 1673*
U.S. Brand Names Ciloxan®; Cipro®; Cipro® XR; Proquin® XR
Canadian Brand Names Apo-Ciproflox®; Ciloxan®; Cipro®; Cipro® XL; CO Ciprofloxacin; Gen-Ciprofloxacin; Novo-Ciprofloxacin; PMS-Ciprofloxacin; ratio-Ciprofloxacin; Rhoxal-ciprofloxacin
Mexican Brand Names Cimogal®; Ciprobiotic®; Ciproflox®; Ciprofur®; Ciproxina®; Eni®; Kenzoflex®; Microgran®; Mitroken®; Nivoflox®; Novoquin®; Opthaflox®; Quinoflox®; Sophixin®; Suiflox®; Zipra®
Generic Available Yes: Suspension, tablet
Synonyms Ciprofloxacin Hydrochloride
Pharmacologic Category Antibiotic, Ophthalmic; Antibiotic, Quinolone
Dental Use Useful as a single agent or in combination with metronidazole in the treatment of periodontitis associated with the presence of *Actinobacillus actinomycetemcomitans* (AA), as well as enteric rods/pseudomonads
Use
Children: Complicated urinary tract infections and pyelonephritis due to *E. coli*. **Note:** Although effective, ciprofloxacin is not the drug of first choice in children.
Children and adults: To reduce incidence or progression of disease following exposure to aerolized *Bacillus anthracis*. Ophthalmologically, for superficial ocular infections (corneal ulcers, conjunctivitis) due to susceptible strains
Adults: Treatment of the following infections when caused by susceptible bacteria: Urinary tract infections; acute uncomplicated cystitis in females; chronic bacterial prostatitis; lower respiratory tract infections (including acute exacerbations of chronic bronchitis); acute sinusitis; skin and skin structure infections; bone and joint infections; complicated intra-abdominal infections (in combination with metronidazole); infectious diarrhea; typhoid fever due to *Salmonella typhi* (eradication of chronic typhoid carrier state has not been proven); uncomplicated cervical and urethra gonorrhea (due to *N. gonorrhoeae*); nosocomial pneumonia; empirical therapy for febrile neutropenic patients (in combination with piperacillin)
Unlabeled/Investigational Use Acute pulmonary exacerbations in cystic fibrosis (children); cutaneous/gastrointestinal/oropharyngeal anthrax (treatment, children and adults); disseminated gonococcal infection (adults); chancroid (adults); prophylaxis to *Neisseria meningitidis* following close contact with an infected person
Local Anesthetic/Vasoconstrictor Precautions No information available to require special precautions
Effects on Dental Treatment No significant effects or complications reported
Significant Adverse Effects
1% to 10%:
Central nervous system: Neurologic events (children 2%, includes dizziness, insomnia, nervousness, somnolence); fever (children 2%); headache (I.V. administration); restlessness (I.V. administration)
(Continued)

Ciprofloxacin *(Continued)*

Dermatologic: Rash (children 2%, adults 1%)

Gastrointestinal: Nausea (children/adults 3%); diarrhea (children 5%, adults 2%); vomiting (children 5%, adults 1%); abdominal pain (children 3%, adults <1%); dyspepsia (children 3%)

Hepatic: ALT/AST increased (adults 1%)

Local: Injection site reactions (I.V. administration)

Respiratory: Rhinitis (children 3%)

<1% (Limited to important or life-threatening): Abnormal gait, acute renal failure, agitation, agranulocytosis, albuminuria, allergic reactions, anaphylactic shock, anaphylaxis, anemia, angina pectoris, angioedema, anorexia, anosmia, arthralgia, ataxia, atrial flutter, bone marrow depression (life-threatening), breast pain, bronchospasm, candidiasis, canduria, cardiopulmonary arrest, cerebral thrombosis, chills, cholestatic jaundice, chromatopsia, confusion, constipation, crystalluria (particularly in alkaline urine), cylindruria, delirium, depersonalization, depression, dizziness, drowsiness, dyspepsia (adults), dysphagia, dyspnea, edema, eosinophilia, erythema multiforme, erythema nodosum, exfoliative dermatitis, fever (adults), fixed eruption, flatulence, gastrointestinal bleeding, hallucinations, headache (oral), hematuria, hemolytic anemia, hepatic failure, hepatic necrosis, hyperesthesia, hyperglycemia, hyperpigmentation, hyper-/hypotension, hypertonia, insomnia, interstitial nephritis, intestinal perforation, irritability, jaundice, joint pain, laryngeal edema, lightheadedness, lymphadenopathy, malaise, manic reaction, methemoglobinemia, MI, migraine, moniliasis, myalgia, myasthenia gravis, myoclonus, nephritis, nightmares, nystagmus, orthostatic hypotension, palpitation, pancreatitis, pancytopenia (life-threatening or fatal), paranoia, paresthesia, peripheral neuropathy, petechia, photosensitivity, prolongation of PT/INR, pseudomembranous colitis, psychosis, pulmonary edema, renal calculi, seizure; serum cholesterol, glucose, triglycerides increased; serum sickness-like reactions, Stevens-Johnson syndrome, syncope, tachycardia, taste loss, tendon rupture, tendonitis, thrombophlebitis, tinnitus, torsade de pointes, toxic epidermal necrolysis (Lyell's syndrome), tremor, twitching, urethral bleeding, vaginal candidiasis, vaginitis, vasculitis, ventricular ectopy, visual disturbance, weakness

Dental Usual Dosing Treatment of periodontitis: Adults: Oral: 500 mg every 12 hours for 10 days

Dosage Note: Extended release tablets and immediate release formulations are not interchangeable. Unless otherwise specified, oral dosing reflects the use of immediate release formulations.

Usual dosage ranges:

Children (see Warnings/Precautions):

Oral: 20-30 mg/kg/day in 2 divided doses; maximum dose: 1.5 g/day

I.V.: 20-30 mg/kg/day divided every 12 hours; maximum dose: 800 mg/day

Adults:

Oral: 250-750 mg every 12 hours

I.V.: 200-400 mg every 12 hours

Indication-specific dosing:

Children:

Anthrax:

Inhalational (postexposure prophylaxis):

Oral: 15 mg/kg/dose every 12 hours for 60 days; maximum: 500 mg/dose

I.V.: 10 mg/kg/dose every 12 hours for 60 days; do **not** exceed 400 mg/dose (800 mg/day)

Cutaneous (treatment, CDC guidelines): Oral: 10-15 mg/kg every 12 hours for 60 days (maximum: 1 g/day); amoxicillin 80 mg/kg/day divided every 8 hours is an option for completion of treatment after clinical improvement. **Note:** In the presence of systemic involvement, extensive edema, lesions on head/neck, refer to I.V. dosing for treatment of inhalational/gastrointestinal/oropharyngeal anthrax.

Inhalational/gastrointestinal/oropharyngeal (treatment, CDC guidelines): I.V.: Initial: 10-15 mg/kg every 12 hours for 60 days (maximum: 500 mg/dose); switch to oral therapy when clinically appropriate; refer to adult dosing for notes on combined therapy and duration

Bacterial conjunctivitis: See adult dosing

Corneal ulcer: See adult dosing

Cystic fibrosis (unlabeled use):

Oral: 40 mg/kg/day divided every 12 hours administered following 1 week of I.V. therapy has been reported in a clinical trial; total duration of therapy: 10-21 days

I.V.: 30 mg/kg/day divided every 8 hours for 1 week, followed by oral therapy, has been reported in a clinical trial

Urinary tract infection (complicated) or pyelonephritis:
  Oral: 20-30 mg/kg/day in 2 divided doses (every 12 hours) for 10-21 days; maximum: 1.5 g/day
  I.V.: 6-10 mg/kg every 8 hours for 10-21 days (maximum: 400 mg/dose)
Adults:
Anthrax:
  Inhalational (postexposure prophylaxis):
    Oral: 500 mg every 12 hours for 60 days
    I.V.: 400 mg every 12 hours for 60 days
  Cutaneous (treatment, CDC guidelines): Oral: Immediate release formulation: 500 mg every 12 hours for 60 days. **Note:** In the presence of systemic involvement, extensive edema, lesions on head/neck, refer to I.V. dosing for treatment of inhalational/gastrointestinal/oropharyngeal anthrax
  Inhalational/gastrointestinal/oropharyngeal (treatment, CDC guidelines): I.V.: 400 mg every 12 hours. **Note:** Initial treatment should include two or more agents predicted to be effective (per CDC recommendations). Agents suggested for use in conjunction with ciprofloxacin or doxycycline include rifampin, vancomycin, imipenem, penicillin, ampicillin, chloramphenicol, clindamycin, and clarithromycin. May switch to oral antimicrobial therapy when clinically appropriate. Continue combined therapy for 60 days.
Bacterial conjunctivitis:
  Ophthalmic solution: Instill 1-2 drops in eye(s) every 2 hours while awake for 2 days and 1-2 drops every 4 hours while awake for the next 5 days
  Ophthalmic ointment: Apply a ½" ribbon into the conjunctival sac 3 times/day for the first 2 days, followed by a ½" ribbon applied twice daily for the next 5 days
Bone/joint infections:
  Oral: 500-750 mg twice daily for 4-6 weeks, depending on severity and susceptibility
  I.V.: Mild to moderate: 400 mg every 12 hours for 4-6 weeks; Severe/complicated: 400 mg every 8 hours for 4-6 weeks
Chancroid (CDC guidelines): Oral: 500 mg twice daily for 3 days
Corneal ulcer: Ophthalmic solution: Instill 2 drops into affected eye every 15 minutes for the first 6 hours, then 2 drops into the affected eye every 30 minutes for the remainder of the first day. On day 2, instill 2 drops into the affected eye hourly. On days 3-14, instill 2 drops into affected eye every 4 hours. Treatment may continue after day 14 if re-epithelialization has not occurred.
Febrile neutropenia (with piperacillin): I.V.: 400 mg every 8 hours for 7-14 days
Gonococcal infections:
  Urethral/cervical gonococcal infections: Oral: 250-500 mg as a single dose (CDC recommends concomitant doxycycline or azithromycin due to developing resistance; avoid use in Asian or Western Pacific travelers)
  Disseminated gonococcal infection (CDC guidelines): Oral: 500 mg twice daily to complete 7 days of therapy (initial treatment with ceftriaxone 1 g I.M./I.V. daily for 24-48 hours after improvement begins)
Infectious diarrhea: Oral:
  Salmonella: 500 mg twice daily for 5-7 days
  Shigella: 500 mg twice daily for 3 days
  Traveler's diarrhea: Mild: 750 mg for one dose; Severe: 500 mg twice daily for 3 days
  Vibrio cholerae: 1 g for one dose
Intra-abdominal (in combination with metronidazole):
  Oral: 500 mg every 12 hours for 7-14 days
  I.V.: 400 mg every 12 hours for 7-14 days
Lower respiratory tract, skin/skin structure infections:
  Oral: 500-750 mg twice daily for 7-14 days depending on severity and susceptibility
  I.V.: Mild to moderate: 400 mg every 12 hours for 7-14 days; Severe/complicated: 400 mg every 8 hours for 7-14 days
Nosocomial pneumonia: I.V.: 400 mg every 8 hours for 10-14 days
Prostatitis (chronic, bacterial):
  Oral: 500 mg every 12 hours for 28 days
  I.V.: 400 mg every 12 hours for 28 days
Sinusitis (acute):
  Oral: 500 mg every 12 hours for 10 days
  I.V.: 400 mg every 12 hours for 10 days
Typhoid fever: Oral: 500 mg every 12 hours for 10 days
(Continued)

Ciprofloxacin *(Continued)*

Urinary tract infection:

Acute uncomplicated: Oral: Immediate release formulation: 250 mg every 12 hours for 3 days; Extended release formulation (Cipro® XR, Proquin® XR): 500 mg every 24 hours for 3 days

Acute uncomplicated pyelonephritis: Oral: Extended release formulation (Cipro® XR): 1000 mg every 24 hours for 7-14 days

Mild to moderate:

Oral: Immediate release formulation: 250 mg every 12 hours for 7-14 days

I.V.: 200 mg every 12 hours for 7-14 days

Severe/complicated:

Oral:

Immediate release formulation: 500 mg every 12 hours for 7-14 days

Extended release formulation (Cipro® XR): 1000 mg every 24 hours for 7-14 days

I.V.: 400 mg every 12 hours for 7-14 days

Elderly: No adjustment needed in patients with normal renal function

Dosing adjustment in renal impairment: Adults:

Cl_{cr} 30-50 mL/minute: Oral: 250-500 mg every 12 hours

Cl_{cr} <30 mL/minute: Acute uncomplicated pyelonephritis or complicated UTI: Oral: Extended release formulation: 500 mg every 24 hours

Cl_{cr} 5-29 mL/minute:

Oral: 250-500 mg every 18 hours

I.V.: 200-400 mg every 18-24 hours

Dialysis: Only small amounts of ciprofloxacin are removed by hemo- or peritoneal dialysis (<10%); usual dose: Oral: 250-500 mg every 24 hours following dialysis

Continuous arteriovenous or venovenous hemodiafiltration effects: Administer 200-400 mg I.V. every 12 hours

Mechanism of Action Inhibits DNA-gyrase in susceptible organisms; inhibits relaxation of supercoiled DNA and promotes breakage of double-stranded DNA

Contraindications Hypersensitivity to ciprofloxacin, any component of the formulation, or other quinolones; concurrent administration of tizanidine

Warnings/Precautions CNS stimulation may occur (tremor, restlessness, confusion, and very rarely hallucinations or seizures). Use with caution in patients with known or suspected CNS disorder. Prolonged use may result in superinfection. Tendon inflammation and/or rupture have been reported with ciprofloxacin and other quinolone antibiotics. Risk may be increased with concurrent corticosteroids, particularly in the elderly. Discontinue at first sign of tendon inflammation or pain. Adverse effects, including those related to joints and/or surrounding tissues, are increased in pediatric patients and therefore, ciprofloxacin should not be considered as drug of choice in children (exception is anthrax treatment). Rare cases of peripheral neuropathy may occur.

Severe hypersensitivity reactions, including anaphylaxis, have occurred with quinolone therapy. Quinolones may exacerbate myasthenia gravis, use with caution (rare, potentially life-threatening weakness of respiratory muscles may occur). Use caution in renal impairment. Avoid excessive sunlight; may cause moderate-to-severe phototoxicity reactions.

Ciprofloxacin is a potent inhibitor of CYP1A2. Coadministration of drugs which depend on this pathway may lead to substantial increases in serum concentrations and adverse effects.

Drug Interactions Inhibits CYP1A2 (strong), 3A4 (weak)

Caffeine: Ciprofloxacin may decrease the metabolism of caffeine.

Corticosteroids: Concurrent use may increase the risk of tendon rupture, particularly in elderly patients (overall incidence rare).

CYP1A2 substrates: Ciprofloxacin may increase the levels/effects of CYP1A2 substrates. Example substrates include aminophylline, fluvoxamine, mexiletine, mirtazapine, ropinirole, tizanidine, and trifluoperazine.

Foscarnet: Concomitant use with ciprofloxacin has been associated with an increased risk of seizures.

Glyburide: Quinolones may increase the effect of glyburide; monitor.

Metal cations (aluminum, calcium, iron, magnesium, and zinc) bind quinolones in the gastrointestinal tract and inhibit absorption. Concurrent administration of most antacids, oral electrolyte supplements, quinapril, sucralfate, some didanosine formulations (chewable/buffered tablets and pediatric powder for oral suspension), and other highly-buffered oral drugs, should be avoided. Ciprofloxacin should be administered 2 hours before or 6 hours after these agents.

Methotrexate: Ciprofloxacin may decrease renal secretion of methotrexate; monitor.

Pentoxifylline: Monitor for headache during concomitant therapy.

Phenytoin: Ciprofloxacin may decrease phenytoin levels; monitor.

Probenecid: May decrease renal secretion of quinolones.

Ropivacaine: Ciprofloxacin may decrease the metabolism of ropivacaine.

Sevelamer: May decrease absorption of oral ciprofloxacin.

Theophylline: Serum levels may be increased by ciprofloxacin; in addition, CNS stimulation/seizures may occur at lower theophylline serum levels due to additive CNS effects.

Tizanidine: Ciprofloxacin may increase serum levels of tizanidine. Concurrent administration is contraindicated.

Warfarin: The hypoprothrombinemic effect of warfarin may be enhanced by ciprofloxacin; monitor INR.

Ethanol/Nutrition/Herb Interactions

Food: Food decreases rate, but not extent, of absorption. Ciprofloxacin serum levels may be decreased if taken with dairy products or calcium-fortified juices. Ciprofloxacin may increase serum caffeine levels if taken with caffeine. Enteral feedings may decrease plasma concentrations of ciprofloxacin probably by >30% inhibition of absorption. Ciprofloxacin should not be administered with enteral feedings. The feeding would need to be discontinued for 1-2 hours prior to and after ciprofloxacin administration. Nasogastric administration produces a greater loss of ciprofloxacin bioavailability than does nasoduodenal administration.

Herb/Nutraceutical: Avoid dong quai, St John's wort (may also cause photosensitization).

Dietary Considerations

Food: Drug may cause GI upset; take without regard to meals (manufacturer prefers that immediate release tablet is taken 2 hours after meals). Extended release tablet may be taken with meals that contain dairy products (calcium content <800 mg), but not with dairy products alone.

Dairy products, calcium-fortified juices, oral multivitamins, and mineral supplements: Absorption of ciprofloxacin is decreased by divalent and trivalent cations. The manufacturer states that the usual dietary intake of calcium (including meals which include dairy products) has not been shown to interfere with ciprofloxacin absorption. Immediate release ciprofloxacin and Cipro® XR may be taken 2 hours before or 6 hours after, and Proquin® XR may be taken 4 hours before or 6 hours after, any of these products.

Caffeine: Patients consuming regular large quantities of caffeinated beverages may need to restrict caffeine intake if excessive cardiac or CNS stimulation occurs.

Pharmacodynamics/Kinetics

Absorption: Oral: Immediate release tablet: Rapid (~50% to 85%)

Distribution: V_d: 2.1-2.7 L/kg; tissue concentrations often exceed serum concentrations especially in kidneys, gallbladder, liver, lungs, gynecological tissue, and prostatic tissue; CSF concentrations: 10% of serum concentrations (noninflamed meninges), 14% to 37% (inflamed meninges); crosses placenta; enters breast milk

Protein binding: 20% to 40%

Metabolism: Partially hepatic; forms 4 metabolites (limited activity)

Half-life elimination: Children: 2.5 hours; Adults: Normal renal function: 3-5 hours

Time to peak: Oral:

Immediate release tablet: 0.5-2 hours

Extended release tablet: Cipro® XR: 1-2.5 hours, Proquin® XR: 3.5-8.7 hours

Excretion: Urine (30% to 50% as unchanged drug); feces (15% to 43%)

Pregnancy Risk Factor C

Lactation Enters breast milk/not recommended (AAP rates "compatible")

Breast-Feeding Considerations Ciprofloxacin is excreted in breast milk; however, the exposure to the infant is considered small and one source suggests that the decision to breast-feed be independent of the need for the antibiotic in the mother. Another source recommends the mother wait 48 hours after the last dose of ciprofloxacin to continue nursing. The manufacturer recommends to discontinue nursing or to discontinue ciprofloxacin.

Dosage Forms [DSC] = Discontinued product

Infusion [premixed in D_5W] (Cipro®): 200 mg (100 mL); 400 mg (200 mL) [latex free]

Injection, solution (Cipro®): 10 mg/mL (20 mL, 40 mL, 120 mL [DSC])

Microcapsules for oral suspension (Cipro®): 250 mg/5 mL (100 mL); 500 mg/5 mL (100 mL) [strawberry flavor]

Ointment, ophthalmic, as hydrochloride (Ciloxan®): 3.33 mg/g [0.3% base] (3.5 g)

Solution, ophthalmic, as hydrochloride (Ciloxan®): 3.5 mg/mL [0.3% base] (2.5 mL, 5 mL, 10 mL) [contains benzalkonium chloride]

(Continued)

Ciprofloxacin *(Continued)*

Tablet: 250 mg, 500 mg, 750 mg

Cipro®: 100 mg, 250 mg, 500 mg, 750 mg

Tablet, extended release:

Cipro® XR: 500 mg [equivalent to ciprofloxacin hydrochloride 287.5 mg and ciprofloxacin base 212.6 mg]; 1000 mg [equivalent to ciprofloxacin hydrochloride 574.9 mg and ciprofloxacin base 425.2 mg]

Proquin® XR: 500 mg

Tablet, extended release [dose pack]:

Proquin® XR: 500 mg (3s)

Selected Readings

Rams TE and Slots J, "Antibiotics in Periodontal Therapy: An Update," *Compendium*, 1992, 13(12):1130, 1132, 1134.

Wynn RL, Bergman SA, Meiller TF, et al, "Antibiotics in Treating Oral-Facial Infections of Odontogenic Origin: An Update," *Gen Dent*, 2001, 49(3):238-40, 242, 244 passim.

Ciprofloxacin and Dexamethasone

(sip roe FLOKS a sin & deks a METH a sone)

Related Information

Ciprofloxacin *on page 343*

Dexamethasone *on page 439*

U.S. Brand Names Ciprodex®

Canadian Brand Names Ciprodex®

Generic Available No

Synonyms Ciprofloxacin Hydrochloride and Dexamethasone; Dexamethasone and Ciprofloxacin

Pharmacologic Category Antibiotic/Corticosteroid, Otic

Use Treatment of acute otitis media in pediatric patients with tympanostomy tubes or acute otitis externa in children and adults

Local Anesthetic/Vasoconstrictor Precautions No information available to require special precautions

Effects on Dental Treatment No significant effects or complications reported

Mechanism of Action Ciprofloxacin is a quinolone antibiotic; dexamethasone is a corticosteroid used to decrease inflammation accompanying bacterial infections

Pregnancy Risk Factor C

Ciprofloxacin and Hydrocortisone

(sip roe FLOKS a sin & hye droe KOR ti sone)

Related Information

Ciprofloxacin *on page 343*

Hydrocortisone *on page 793*

U.S. Brand Names Cipro® HC

Canadian Brand Names Cipro® HC

Generic Available No

Synonyms Ciprofloxacin Hydrochloride and Hydrocortisone; Hydrocortisone and Ciprofloxacin

Pharmacologic Category Antibiotic/Corticosteroid, Otic

Use Treatment of acute otitis externa, sometimes known as "swimmer's ear"

Local Anesthetic/Vasoconstrictor Precautions No information available to require special precautions

Effects on Dental Treatment No significant effects or complications reported

Ciprofloxacin Hydrochloride *see* Ciprofloxacin *on page 343*

Ciprofloxacin Hydrochloride and Dexamethasone *see* Ciprofloxacin and Dexamethasone *on page 348*

Ciprofloxacin Hydrochloride and Hydrocortisone *see* Ciprofloxacin and Hydrocortisone *on page 348*

Cipro® HC *see* Ciprofloxacin and Hydrocortisone *on page 348*

Cipro® XR *see* Ciprofloxacin *on page 343*

Cisapride (SIS a pride)

U.S. Brand Names Propulsid®

Mexican Brand Names Enteropride®; Kinestase®; Prepulsid®; Unamol®

Generic Available No

Pharmacologic Category Gastrointestinal Agent, Prokinetic

Use Treatment of nocturnal symptoms of gastroesophageal reflux disease (GERD); has demonstrated effectiveness for gastroparesis, refractory constipation, and nonulcer dyspepsia

Local Anesthetic/Vasoconstrictor Precautions No information available to require special precautions (see Dental Comment)

Effects on Dental Treatment Key adverse event(s) related to dental treatment: Xerostomia (normal salivary flow resumes upon discontinuation).

Common Adverse Effects

>5%:

Central nervous system: Headache

Dermatologic: Rash

Gastrointestinal: Diarrhea, GI cramping, dyspepsia, flatulence, nausea, xerostomia

Respiratory: Rhinitis

<5%:

Cardiovascular: Tachycardia

Central nervous system: Extrapyramidal effects, somnolence, fatigue, seizure, insomnia, anxiety

Hematologic: Thrombocytopenia, increased LFTs, pancytopenia, leukopenia, granulocytopenia, aplastic anemia

Respiratory: Sinusitis, cough, upper respiratory tract infection, increased incidence of viral infection

Restrictions In U.S., available via limited-access protocol only (1-800-JANSSEN).

Mechanism of Action Enhances the release of acetylcholine at the myenteric plexus. *In vitro* studies have shown cisapride to have serotonin-4 receptor agonistic properties which may increase gastrointestinal motility and cardiac rate; increases lower esophageal sphincter pressure and lower esophageal peristalsis; accelerates gastric emptying of both liquids and solids.

Drug Interactions

Cytochrome P450 Effect: Substrate of CYP1A2 (minor), 2A6 (minor), 2B6 (minor), 2C9 (minor), 2C19 (minor), 3A4 (major); **Inhibits** CYP2D6 (weak), 3A4 (weak)

Increased Effect/Toxicity: Cisapride may increase blood levels of warfarin, diazepam, cimetidine, ranitidine, and CNS depressants. The risk of cisapride-induced malignant arrhythmias may be increased by azole antifungals (fluconazole, itraconazole, ketoconazole, miconazole), antiarrhythmics (Class Ia; quinidine, procainamide, and Class III; amiodarone, sotalol), bepridil, cimetidine, maprotiline, macrolide antibiotics (erythromycin, clarithromycin, troleandomycin), molindone, nefazodone, protease inhibitors (amprenavir, atazanavir, indinavir, nelfinavir, ritonavir), phenothiazines (eg, prochlorperazine, promethazine), sertindole, tricyclic antidepressants (eg amitriptyline), and some quinolone antibiotics (sparfloxacin, gatifloxacin, moxifloxacin). Other strong inhibitors of CYP3A4 (including diclofenac, doxycycline, imatinib, isoniazid, nefazodone, nicardipine, propofol, telithromycin, and verapamil) should be avoided. Cardiovascular disease or electrolyte imbalances (potentially due to diuretic therapy) increase the risk of malignant arrhythmias.

Decreased Effect: Cisapride may decrease the effect of atropine and digoxin.

Pharmacodynamics/Kinetics

Onset of action: 0.5-1 hour

Protein binding: 97.5% to 98%

Metabolism: Extensively hepatic to norcisapride

Bioavailability: 35% to 40%

Half-life elimination: 6-12 hours

Excretion: Urine and feces (<10%)

Pregnancy Risk Factor C

Dental Comment

This drug is known to prolong the QT interval. The QT interval is measured as the time and distance between the Q point of the QRS complex and the end of the T wave in the ECG tracing. After adjustment for heart rate, the QT interval is defined as prolonged if it is more than 450 msec in men and 460 msec in women. A long QT syndrome was first described in the 1950s and 60s as a congenital syndrome involving QT interval prolongation and syncope and sudden death. Some of the congenital long QT syndromes were characterized by a peculiar electrocardiographic appearance of the QRS complex involving a premature atria beat followed by a pause, then a subsequent sinus beat showing marked QT prolongation and deformity. This type of cardiac arrhythmia was originally termed "torsade de pointes" (translated from the French as "twisting of the points").

(Continued)

Cisapride *(Continued)*

Prolongation of the QT interval is thought to result from delayed ventricular repolarization. The repolarization process within the myocardial cell is due to the efflux of intracellular potassium. The channels associated with this current can be blocked by many drugs, thus, predisposing the electrical propagation cycle to torsade de pointes.

Cisapride is one of the drugs confirmed to prolong the QT interval and is accepted as having a risk of causing torsade de pointes. The risk of drug-induced torsade de pointes is extremely low when a single QT interval prolonging drug is prescribed. In terms of epinephrine, it is not known what effect vasoconstrictors in the local anesthetic regimen will have in patients with a known history of congenital prolonged QT interval or in patients taking any medication that prolongs the QT interval. Until more information is obtained, it is suggested that the clinician consult with the physician prior to the use of a vasoconstrictor in suspected patients, and that the vasoconstrictor (epinephrine, levonordefrin [Neo-Cobefrin®]) be used with caution.

Cisplatin (SIS pla tin)

U.S. Brand Names Platinol®-AQ [DSC]
Mexican Brand Names Blastolem®; Platinol®; Tecnoplatin®
Generic Available Yes
Synonyms CDDP
Pharmacologic Category Antineoplastic Agent, Alkylating Agent
Use Treatment of bladder, testicular, and ovarian cancer
Unlabeled/Investigational Use Treatment of head and neck, breast, gastric, lung, esophageal, cervical, prostate and small cell lung cancer; Hodgkin's and non-Hodgkin's lymphoma; neuroblastoma; sarcomas; myeloma, melanoma, mesothelioma, and osteosarcoma
Local Anesthetic/Vasoconstrictor Precautions No information available to require special precautions
Effects on Dental Treatment No significant effects or complications reported
Common Adverse Effects
>10%:
  Central nervous system: Neurotoxicity: Peripheral neuropathy is dose- and duration-dependent.
  Dermatologic: Mild alopecia
  Gastrointestinal: Nausea and vomiting (76% to 100%)
  Hematologic: Myelosuppression (25% to 30%; mild with moderate doses, mild to moderate with high-dose therapy)
    WBC: Mild
    Platelets: Mild
    Onset: 10 days
    Nadir: 14-23 days
    Recovery: 21-39 days
  Hepatic: Liver enzymes increased
  Renal: Nephrotoxicity (acute renal failure and chronic renal insufficiency)
  Otic: Ototoxicity (10% to 30%; manifested as high frequency hearing loss; ototoxicity is especially pronounced in children)
1% to 10%:
  Gastrointestinal: Diarrhea
  Local: Tissue irritation
Mechanism of Action Inhibits DNA synthesis by the formation of DNA cross-links; denatures the double helix; covalently binds to DNA bases and disrupts DNA function; may also bind to proteins; the *cis*-isomer is 14 times more cytotoxic than the *trans*-isomer; both forms cross-link DNA but cis-platinum is less easily recognized by cell enzymes and, therefore, not repaired. Cisplatin can also bind two adjacent guanines on the same strand of DNA producing intrastrand cross-linking and breakage.
Drug Interactions
  Increased Effect/Toxicity: Cisplatin and ethacrynic acid have resulted in severe ototoxicity in animals. Delayed bleomycin elimination with decreased glomerular filtration rate. When administered as sequential infusions, observational studies indicate a potential for increased toxicity when platinum derivatives (carboplatin, cisplatin) are administered before taxane derivatives (docetaxel, paclitaxel).
  Decreased Effect: Sodium thiosulfate and amifostine theoretically inactivate drug systemically; have been used clinically to reduce systemic toxicity with administration of cisplatin.

Pharmacodynamics/Kinetics

Distribution: I.V.: Rapidly into tissue; high concentrations in kidneys, liver, ovaries, uterus, and lungs

Protein binding: >90%

Metabolism: Nonenzymatic; inactivated (in both cell and bloodstream) by sulfhydryl groups; covalently binds to glutathione and thiosulfate

Half-life elimination: Initial: 20-30 minutes; Beta: 60 minutes; Terminal: ~24 hours; Secondary half-life: 44-73 hours

Excretion: Urine (>90%); feces (10%)

Pregnancy Risk Factor D

13-*cis*-Retinoic Acid *see* Isotretinoin *on page 869*

Citalopram (sye TAL oh pram)

Related Information
Escitalopram *on page 568*

U.S. Brand Names Celexa®

Canadian Brand Names Apo-Citalopram®; Celexa®; CO Citalopram; Dom-Citalopram; Gen-Citalopram; Novo-Citalopram; PHL-Citalopram; PMS-Citalopram; ratio-Citalopram; Rhoxal-citalopram

Mexican Brand Names Seropram®

Generic Available Yes

Synonyms Citalopram Hydrobromide; Nitalapram

Pharmacologic Category Antidepressant, Selective Serotonin Reuptake Inhibitor

Use Treatment of depression

Unlabeled/Investigational Use Treatment of dementia, smoking cessation, ethanol abuse, obsessive-compulsive disorder (OCD) in children, diabetic neuropathy

Local Anesthetic/Vasoconstrictor Precautions Although caution should be used in patients taking tricyclic antidepressants, no interactions have been reported with vasoconstrictors and citalopram, a nontricyclic antidepressant which acts to increase serotonin; no precautions appear to be needed

Effects on Dental Treatment Key adverse event(s) related to dental treatment: Xerostomia (normal salivary flow resumes upon discontinuation). Premarketing trials reported abnormal taste. See Dental Comment.

Common Adverse Effects

>10%:
Central nervous system: Somnolence, insomnia
Gastrointestinal: Nausea, xerostomia
Miscellaneous: Diaphoresis

<10%:
Central nervous system: Anxiety, anorexia, agitation, yawning
Dermatologic: Rash, pruritus
Endocrine & metabolic: Sexual dysfunction
Gastrointestinal: Diarrhea, dyspepsia, vomiting, abdominal pain, weight gain
Neuromuscular & skeletal: Tremor, arthralgia, myalgia
Respiratory: Cough, rhinitis, sinusitis

Restrictions A medication guide concerning the use of antidepressants in children and teenagers can be found on the FDA website at http://www.fda.gov/cder/Offices/ODS/labeling.htm. It should be dispensed to parents or guardians of children and teenagers receiving this medication.

Dosage Oral:
Children and Adolescents: OCD (unlabeled use): 10-40 mg/day
Adults: Depression: Initial: 20 mg/day, generally with an increase to 40 mg/day; doses of more than 40 mg are not usually necessary. Should a dose increase be necessary, it should occur in 20 mg increments at intervals of no less than 1 week. Maximum dose: 60 mg/day; reduce dosage in elderly or those with hepatic impairment.

Mechanism of Action A bicyclic phthalane derivative, citalopram selectively inhibits serotonin reuptake in the presynaptic neurons

Contraindications Hypersensitivity to citalopram or any component of the formulation; hypersensitivity or other adverse sequelae during therapy with other SSRIs; concomitant use with MAO inhibitors or within 2 weeks of discontinuing MAO inhibitors

Warnings/Precautions Antidepressants increase the risk of suicidal thinking and behavior in children and adolescents with major depressive disorder (MDD) and other depressive disorders; consider risk prior to prescribing. All patients must be closely monitored for clinical worsening, suicidality, or unusual changes in behavior, especially during the initiation of therapy or following an increase or decrease in dosage. When used in children, the child's family or caregiver
(Continued)

Citalopram *(Continued)*

should be instructed to closely observe the patient and communicate condition with healthcare provider. A medication guide should be dispensed with each prescription. **Citalopram is not FDA approved for use in children.**

The possibility of a suicide attempt is inherent in major depression and may persist until remission occurs. Use caution in high-risk patients. Worsening depression and severe abrupt suicidality that are not part of the presenting symptoms may require discontinuation or modification of drug therapy. The patient's family or caregiver should be alerted to monitor patients for the emergence of suicidality and associated behaviors (such as agitation, irritability, hostility, impulsivity, and hypomania) and call healthcare provider.

May worsen psychosis in some patients or precipitate a shift to mania or hypomania in patients with bipolar disorder. Patients presenting with depressive symptoms should be screened for bipolar disorder. Monotherapy in patients with bipolar disorder should be avoided. **Citalopram is not FDA approved for the treatment of bipolar depression.**

The potential for severe reaction exists when used with MAO inhibitors; serotonin syndrome (hyperthermia, muscular rigidity, mental status changes/agitation, autonomic instability) may occur. May increase the risks associated with electroconvulsive therapy. Has a low potential to impair cognitive or motor performance; caution operating hazardous machinery or driving.

Use with caution in patients with hepatic or renal dysfunction, in elderly patients, concomitant CNS depressants, and pregnancy (high doses of citalopram have been associated with teratogenicity in animals). Use caution with concomitant use of NSAIDs, ASA, or other drugs that affect coagulation; the risk of bleeding is potentiated. May cause hyponatremia/SIADH. May cause or exacerbate sexual dysfunction. Upon discontinuation of citalopram therapy, gradually taper dose. If intolerable symptoms occur following a decrease in dosage or upon discontinuation of therapy, then resuming the previous dose with a more gradual taper should be considered.

Drug Interactions

Cytochrome P450 Effect: Substrate of CYP2C19 (major), 2D6 (minor), 3A4 (major); **Inhibits** CYP1A2 (weak), 2B6 (weak), 2C19 (weak), 2D6 (weak)

Increased Effect/Toxicity: Citalopram should not be used with nonselective MAO inhibitors (phenelzine, isocarboxazid) or other drugs with MAO inhibition (linezolid); fatal reactions have been reported. Wait 5 weeks after stopping citalopram before starting a nonselective MAO inhibitor and 2 weeks after stopping an MAO inhibitor before starting citalopram. Concurrent selegiline has been associated with mania, hypertension, or serotonin syndrome (risk may be reduced relative to nonselective MAO inhibitors).

CYP2C19 inhibitors may increase the levels/effects of citalopram; example inhibitors include delavirdine, fluconazole, fluvoxamine, gemfibrozil, isoniazid, omeprazole, and ticlopidine. CYP3A4 inhibitors may increase the levels/effects of citalopram; example inhibitors include azole antifungals, clarithromycin, diclofenac, doxycycline, erythromycin, imatinib, isoniazid, nefazodone, nicardipine, propofol, protease inhibitors, quinidine, telithromycin, and verapamil.

Combined use of SSRIs and amphetamines, buspirone, meperidine, nefazodone, serotonin agonists (such as sumatriptan), sibutramine, other SSRIs, sympathomimetics, ritonavir, tramadol, and venlafaxine may increase the risk of serotonin syndrome. Risk of hyponatremia may increase with concurrent use of loop diuretics (bumetanide, furosemide, torsemide). Citalopram may increase the hypoprothrombinemic response to warfarin. Concomitant use of citalopram and NSAIDs, aspirin, or other drugs affecting coagulation has been associated with an increased risk of bleeding; monitor.

Combined use of sumatriptan (and other serotonin agonists) may result in toxicity; weakness, hyper-reflexia, and incoordination have been observed with sumatriptan and SSRIs. In addition, concurrent use may theoretically increase the risk of serotonin syndrome; includes sumatriptan, naratriptan, rizatriptan, and zolmitriptan.

Decreased Effect: CYP2C19 inducers may decrease the levels/effects of citalopram; example inducers include aminoglutethimide, carbamazepine, phenytoin, and rifampin. Cyproheptadine may inhibit the effects of serotonin reuptake inhibitors. CYP3A4 inducers may decrease the levels/effects of citalopram; example inducers include aminoglutethimide, carbamazepine, nafcillin, nevirapine, phenobarbital, phenytoin, and rifamycins.

Ethanol/Nutrition/Herb Interactions

Ethanol: Avoid ethanol (may increase CNS depression).

Herb/Nutraceutical: Avoid valerian, St John's wort, SAMe, kava kava, and gotu kola (may increase CNS depression).

Dietary Considerations May be taken without regard to food.

Pharmacodynamics/Kinetics

Distribution: V_d: 12 L/kg

Protein binding, plasma: ~80%

Metabolism: Extensively hepatic, including CYP, to N-demethylated, N-oxide, and deaminated metabolites

Bioavailability: 80%

Half-life elimination: 24-48 hours; average 35 hours (doubled with hepatic impairment)

Time to peak, serum: 1-6 hours, average within 4 hours

Excretion: Urine (10% as unchanged drug)

Note: Clearance was decreased, while AUC and half-life were significantly increased in elderly patients and in patients with hepatic impairment. Mild-to-moderate renal impairment may reduce clearance (17%) and prolong half-life of citalopram. No pharmacokinetic information is available concerning patients with severe renal impairment.

Pregnancy Risk Factor C

Dosage Forms SOLN, oral: 10 mg/5 mL (240 mL). **TAB:** 10 mg, 20 mg, 40 mg

Dental Comment Problems with SSRI-induced bruxism have been reported and may preclude their use; clinicians attempting to evaluate any patient with bruxism or involuntary muscle movement, who is simultaneously being treated with an SSRI drug, should be aware of the potential association.

Citalopram Hydrobromide *see* Citalopram *on page 351*

Citanest® Forte Dental *see* Prilocaine and Epinephrine *on page 1278*

Citanest® Plain *see* Prilocaine *on page 1277*

Citracal® [OTC] *see* Calcium Citrate *on page 250*

Citrate of Magnesia *see* Magnesium Citrate *on page 960*

Citric Acid and d-gluconic Acid Irrigant *see* Citric Acid, Magnesium Carbonate, and Glucono-Delta-Lactone *on page 353*

Citric Acid and Potassium Citrate *see* Potassium Citrate and Citric Acid *on page 1259*

Citric Acid Bladder Mixture *see* Citric Acid, Magnesium Carbonate, and Glucono-Delta-Lactone *on page 353*

Citric Acid, Magnesium Carbonate, and Glucono-Delta-Lactone

(SI trik AS id, mag NEE see um KAR bo nate, and GLOO kon o DEL ta LAK tone)

U.S. Brand Names Renacidin®

Generic Available No

Synonyms Citric Acid and d-gluconic Acid Irrigant; Citric Acid Bladder Mixture; Citric Acid, Magnesium Hydroxycarbonate, D-Gluconic Acid, Magnesium Acid Citrate, and Calcium Carbonate; Hemiacidrin

Pharmacologic Category Urinary Tract Product

Use Prevention of formation of calcifications of indwelling urinary tract catheters; treatment of renal and bladder calculi of the apatite or struvite type

Local Anesthetic/Vasoconstrictor Precautions No information available to require special precautions

Effects on Dental Treatment No significant effects or complications reported

Common Adverse Effects

>10%:

Central nervous system: Fever (20% to 40%)

Genitourinary: Urothelial ulceration with or without edema (13%)

Miscellaneous: Transient flank pain

1% to 10%:

Endocrine & metabolic: Hypermagnesemia, hyperphosphatemia

Genitourinary: Urinary tract infection, dysuria, hematuria, bladder irritability

Neuromuscular & skeletal: Back pain

Renal: Creatinine increased

Mechanism of Action Magnesium from the irrigating solution is exchanged for calcium in the stone matrix. The magnesium stones are soluble and are able to dissolve in the acidic pH of the solution.

Pregnancy Risk Factor C

Citric Acid, Magnesium Hydroxycarbonate, D-Gluconic Acid, Magnesium Acid Citrate, and Calcium Carbonate *see* Citric Acid, Magnesium Carbonate, and Glucono-Delta-Lactone *on page 353*

Citric Acid, Sodium Citrate, and Potassium Citrate
(SIT rik AS id, SOW dee um SIT rate, & poe TASS ee um SIT rate)

Related Information
Potassium Citrate *on page 1259*
U.S. Brand Names Cytra-3; Polycitra®; Polycitra®-LC
Generic Available Yes
Synonyms Potassium Citrate, Citric Acid, and Sodium Citrate; Sodium Citrate, Citric Acid, and Potassium Citrate
Pharmacologic Category Alkalinizing Agent, Oral
Use Conditions where long-term maintenance of an alkaline urine is desirable as in control and dissolution of uric acid and cystine calculi of the urinary tract
Local Anesthetic/Vasoconstrictor Precautions No information available to require special precautions
Effects on Dental Treatment No significant effects or complications reported
Common Adverse Effects Frequency not defined.
Cardiovascular: Cardiac abnormalities
Endocrine & metabolic: Metabolic alkalosis, calcium levels, hyperkalemia, hypernatremia
Gastrointestinal: Diarrhea
Neuromuscular & skeletal: Tetany
Drug Interactions
Increased Effect/Toxicity: Increased toxicity/levels of amphetamines, ephedrine, pseudoephedrine, flecainide, quinidine, and quinine due to urinary alkalinization.
Decreased Effect: Decreased effect/levels of lithium, chlorpropamide, and salicylates due to urinary alkalinization.
Pregnancy Risk Factor Not established

Citrovorum Factor *see Leucovorin on page 905*
Citrucel® [OTC] *see Methylcellulose on page 1021*
CL-118,532 *see Triptorelin on page 1544*
CI-719 *see Gemfibrozil on page 730*
CL-825 *see Pentostatin on page 1211*
CL-184116 *see Porfimer on page 1256*

Cladribine (KLA dri been)

U.S. Brand Names Leustatin®
Canadian Brand Names Leustatin®
Generic Available Yes
Synonyms 2-CdA; 2-Chlorodeoxyadenosine
Pharmacologic Category Adjuvant, Radiosensitizing Agent; Antineoplastic Agent, Antimetabolite; Antineoplastic Agent, Antimetabolite (Purine Antagonist)
Use Treatment of hairy cell leukemia, chronic lymphocytic leukemia (CLL), chronic myelogenous leukemia (CML)
Unlabeled/Investigational Use Non-Hodgkin's lymphomas, progressive multiple sclerosis
Local Anesthetic/Vasoconstrictor Precautions No information available to require special precautions
Effects on Dental Treatment No significant effects or complications reported
Common Adverse Effects
>10%:
Allergic: Fever (70%), chills (18%), skin reactions (erythema, itching) at the catheter site (18%)
Central nervous system: Fatigue (17%), headache (13%)
Dermatologic: Rash
Hematologic: Myelosuppression, common, dose limiting; leukopenia (70%); anemia (37%); thrombocytopenia (12%)
Nadir: 5-10 days
Recovery: 4-8 weeks
1% to 10%:
Cardiovascular: Edema, tachycardia
Central nervous system: Dizziness; pains; chills; malaise; severe infection, possibly related to thrombocytopenia
Dermatologic: Pruritus, erythema
Gastrointestinal: Nausea, mild to moderate, usually not seen at doses <0.3 mg/kg/day; constipation; abdominal pain
Neuromuscular & skeletal: Myalgia, arthralgia, weakness
Renal: Renal failure at high (>0.3 mg/kg/day) doses

Miscellaneous: Diaphoresis, delayed herpes zoster infection, tumor lysis syndrome

Mechanism of Action A purine nucleoside analogue; prodrug which is activated via phosphorylation by deoxycytidine kinase to a 5'-triphosphate derivative. This active form incorporates into DNA to result in the breakage of DNA strand and shutdown of DNA synthesis. This also results in a depletion of nicotinamide adenine dinucleotide and adenosine triphosphate (ATP). Cladribine is cell-cycle nonspecific.

Pharmacodynamics/Kinetics
Absorption: Oral: 55%; SubQ: 100%; Rectal: 20%
Distribution: V_d: 4.52 ± 2.82 L/kg
Protein binding, plasma: 20%
Metabolism: Hepatic; 5'-triphosphate moiety-active
Half-life elimination: Biphasic: Alpha: 25 minutes; Beta: 6.7 hours; Terminal, mean: Normal renal function: 5.4 hours
Excretion: Urine (21% to 44%)
  Clearance: Estimated systemic: 640 mL/hour/kg

Pregnancy Risk Factor D

Claforan® *see* Cefotaxime *on page 288*

Claravis™ *see* Isotretinoin *on page 869*

Clarinex® *see* Desloratadine *on page 435*

Clarinex-D® 12 Hour *see* Desloratadine and Pseudoephedrine *on page 436*

Clarinex-D® 24 Hour *see* Desloratadine and Pseudoephedrine *on page 436*

Claripel™ *see* Hydroquinone *on page 798*

Clarithromycin (kla RITH roe mye sin)

Related Information
Antibiotic Prophylaxis *on page 1680*
Bacterial Infections *on page 1697*
Gastrointestinal Disorders *on page 1654*
Respiratory Diseases *on page 1656*
U.S. Brand Names Biaxin®; Biaxin® XL
Canadian Brand Names Biaxin®; Biaxin® XL; ratio-Clarithromycin
Mexican Brand Names Adel®; Klaricid®; Mabicrol®
Generic Available Yes: Tablet
Pharmacologic Category Antibiotic, Macrolide
Dental Use Alternate antibiotic in the treatment of common orofacial infections caused by aerobic gram-positive cocci and susceptible anaerobes alternate antibiotic for the prevention of bacterial endocarditis in patients undergoing dental procedures

Use
Children:
  Pharyngitis/tonsillitis, acute maxillary sinusitis, uncomplicated skin/skin structure infections, and mycobacterial infections
  Acute otitis media (*H. influenzae, M. catarrhalis,* or *S. pneumoniae*)
  Prevention of disseminated mycobacterial infections due to MAC disease in patients with advanced HIV infection
Adults:
  Pharyngitis/tonsillitis due to susceptible *S. pyogenes*
  Acute maxillary sinusitis and acute exacerbation of chronic bronchitis due to susceptible *H. influenzae, M. catarrhalis,* or *S. pneumoniae*
  Community-acquired pneumonia due to susceptible *H. influenzae, H. parainfluenzae, Mycoplasma pneumoniae, S. pneumoniae,* or *Chlamydia pneumoniae* (TWAR)
  Uncomplicated skin/skin structure infections due to susceptible *S. aureus, S. pyogenes*
  Disseminated mycobacterial infections due to *M. avium* or *M. intracellulare*
  Prevention of disseminated mycobacterial infections due to *M. avium* complex (MAC) disease (eg, patients with advanced HIV infection)
  Duodenal ulcer disease due to *H. pylori* in regimens with other drugs including amoxicillin and lansoprazole or omeprazole, ranitidine bismuth citrate, bismuth subsalicylate, tetracycline, and/or an H_2 antagonist
  Alternate antibiotic for prophylaxis of bacterial endocarditis in patients who are allergic to penicillin and undergoing surgical or dental procedures

Unlabeled/Investigational Use Pertussis
Local Anesthetic/Vasoconstrictor Precautions No information available to require special precautions (see Dental Comment)
Effects on Dental Treatment Key adverse event(s) related to dental treatment: Abnormal taste.
(Continued)

Clarithromycin *(Continued)*

Significant Adverse Effects

1% to 10%:

Central nervous system: Headache (adults and children 2%)

Dermatologic: Rash (children 3%)

Gastrointestinal: Abnormal taste (adults 3% to 7%), diarrhea (adults 3% to 6%; children 6%), vomiting (children 6%), nausea (adults 3%), heartburn (adults 2%), abdominal pain (adults 2%; children 3%), dyspepsia 2%

Hepatic: Prothrombin time increased (1%)

Renal: BUN increased (4%)

<1% (Limited to important or life-threatening): *Clostridium difficile* colitis, alkaline phosphatase increased, anaphylaxis, anorexia, anxiety, behavioral changes, bilirubin increased, confusion, disorientation, dizziness, dyspnea, glossitis, hallucinations, hearing loss (reversible), hepatic dysfunction, hepatic failure, hepatitis, hypoglycemia, insomnia, interstitial nephritis, jaundice, leukopenia, manic behavior, neuromuscular blockade (case reports), neutropenia, nightmares, oral moniliasis, pancreatitis, psychosis, QT prolongation, seizure, serum creatinine increased, smell alteration, Stevens-Johnson syndrome, stomatitis, thrombocytopenia, tinnitus, tongue discoloration, tooth discoloration, torsade de pointes, toxic epidermal necrolysis, transaminases increased, tremor, urticaria, ventricular tachycardia, ventricular arrhythmia, vertigo

Dental Usual Dosing Prophylaxis of bacterial endocarditis: Oral:

Children ≥6 months: 15 mg/kg 1 hour before procedure (maximum dose: 500 mg)

Adults: 500 mg 1 hour prior to procedure

Dosage Oral:

Children ≥1 months: Pertussis (CDC guidelines): 15 mg/kg/day divided every 12 hours for 7 days; maximum: 1 g/day

Children ≥6 months:

Community-acquired pneumonia, sinusitis, bronchitis, skin infections: 15 mg/kg/day divided every 12 hours for 10 days

Mycobacterial infection (prevention and treatment): 7.5 mg/kg twice daily, up to 500 mg twice daily. **Note:** Safety of clarithromycin for MAC not studied in children <20 months.

Prophylaxis of bacterial endocarditis: 15 mg/kg 1 hour before procedure (maximum dose: 500 mg)

Adults:

Usual dose: 250-500 mg every 12 hours **or** 1000 mg (two 500 mg extended release tablets) once daily for 7-14 days

Upper respiratory tract: 250-500 mg every 12 hours for 10-14 days

Pharyngitis/tonsillitis: 250 mg every 12 hours for 10 days

Acute maxillary sinusitis: 500 mg every 12 hours **or** 1000 mg (two 500 mg extended release tablets) once daily for 14 days

Lower respiratory tract: 250-500 mg every 12 hours for 7-14 days

Acute exacerbation of chronic bronchitis due to:

M. catarrhalis and *S. pneumoniae*: 250 mg every 12 hours for 7-14 days or 1000 mg (two 500 mg extended release tablets) once daily for 7 days

H. influenzae: 500 mg every 12 hours for 7-14 days or 1000 mg (two 500 mg extended release tablets) once daily for 7 days

H. parainfluenzae: 500 mg every 12 hours for 7 days or 1000 mg (two 500 mg extended release tablets) for 7 days

Pneumonia due to:

C. pneumoniae, M. pneumoniae, and *S. pneumoniae*: 250 mg every 12 hours for 7-14 days **or** 1000 mg (two 500 mg extended release tablets) once daily for 7 days

H. influenzae: 250 mg every 12 hours for 7 days **or** 1000 mg (two 500 mg extended release tablets) once daily for 7 days

Mycobacterial infection (prevention and treatment): 500 mg twice daily (use with other antimycobacterial drugs, eg, ethambutol, clofazimine, or rifampin)

Pertussis (CDC guidelines): 500 mg twice daily for 7 days

Prophylaxis of bacterial endocarditis: 500 mg 1 hour prior to procedure

Uncomplicated skin and skin structure: 250 mg every 12 hours for 7-14 days

Helicobacter pylori: Dual or triple combination regimen with bismuth subsalicylate, tetracycline, clarithromycin, and an H$_2$-receptor; or combination of omeprazole and clarithromycin: 500 mg every 8-12 hours for 10-14 days

Elderly: Pharmacokinetics are similar to those in younger adults; may have age-related reductions in renal function; monitor and adjust dose if necessary

Dosing adjustment in renal impairment:

Cl$_{cr}$ <30 mL/minute: Half the normal dose or double the dosing interval

In combination with ritonavir:

Cl$_{cr}$ 30-60 mL/minute: Decrease clarithromycin dose by 50%

Cl$_{cr}$ <30 mL/minute: Decrease clarithromycin dose by 75%

Dosing adjustment in hepatic impairment: No dosing adjustment is needed as long as renal function is normal

Mechanism of Action Exerts its antibacterial action by binding to 50S ribosomal subunit resulting in inhibition of protein synthesis. The 14-OH metabolite of clarithromycin is twice as active as the parent compound against certain organisms.

Contraindications Hypersensitivity to clarithromycin, erythromycin, or any macrolide antibiotic; use with ergot derivatives, pimozide, cisapride; combination with ranitidine bismuth citrate should not be used in patients with history of acute porphyria or Cl$_{cr}$ <25 mL/minute

Warnings/Precautions Dosage adjustment required with severe renal impairment, decreased dosage or prolonged dosing interval may be appropriate; antibiotic-associated colitis has been reported with use of clarithromycin. Macrolides (including clarithromycin) have been associated with rare QT prolongation and ventricular arrhythmias, including torsade de pointes. The extended release formulation consists of drug within a nondeformable matrix; following drug release/absorption, the matrix/shell is expelled in the stool. The use of nondeformable products in patients with known stricture/narrowing of the GI tract has been associated with symptoms of obstruction. Safety and efficacy in children <6 months of age have not been established.

Drug Interactions Substrate of CYP3A4 (major); **Inhibits** CYP1A2 (weak), 3A4 (strong)

Alfentanil (and possibly other narcotic analgesics): Serum levels may be increased by clarithromycin; monitor for increased effect.

Benzodiazepines (those metabolized by CYP3A4, including alprazolam, midazolam, triazolam): Serum levels may be increased by clarithromycin; somnolence and confusion have been reported.

Bromocriptine: Serum levels may be increased by clarithromycin; monitor for increased effect.

Buspirone: Serum levels may be increased by clarithromycin; monitor.

Calcium channel blockers (felodipine, verapamil, and potentially others metabolized by CYP3A4): Serum levels may be increased by clarithromycin; monitor.

Carbamazepine: Serum levels may be increased by clarithromycin; monitor.

Cilostazol: Serum levels may be increased by clarithromycin; monitor.

Cisapride: Serum levels may be increased by clarithromycin; serious arrhythmias have occurred; concurrent use contraindicated.

Clopidogrel: Therapeutic effect may be decreased by clarithromycin; monitor.

Clozapine: Serum levels may be increased by clarithromycin; monitor.

Colchicine: Serum levels/toxicity may be increased by clarithromycin; monitor. Avoid use, if possible.

Cyclosporine: Serum levels may be increased by clarithromycin; monitor serum levels.

CYP3A4 inducers: CYP3A4 inducers may decrease the levels/effects of clarithromycin. Example inducers include aminoglutethimide, carbamazepine, nafcillin, nevirapine, phenobarbital, phenytoin, and rifamycins.

CYP3A4 inhibitors: May increase the levels/effects of clarithromycin. Example inhibitors include azole antifungals, diclofenac, doxycycline, erythromycin, imatinib, isoniazid, nefazodone, nicardipine, propofol, protease inhibitors, quinidine, telithromycin, and verapamil.

CYP3A4 substrates: Clarithromycin may increase the levels/effects of CYP3A4 substrates. Example substrates include benzodiazepines, calcium channel blockers, mirtazapine, nateglinide, nefazodone, tacrolimus, and venlafaxine. Selected benzodiazepines (midazolam and triazolam), cisapride, ergot alkaloids, selected HMG-CoA reductase inhibitors (lovastatin and simvastatin), and pimozide are generally contraindicated with strong CYP3A4 inhibitors.

Delavirdine: Serum levels may be increased by clarithromycin; monitor.

Digoxin: Serum levels may be increased by clarithromycin; digoxin toxicity and potentially fatal arrhythmias have been reported; monitor digoxin levels.

Disopyramide: Serum levels may be increased by clarithromycin; in addition, QT$_c$ prolongation and risk of malignant arrhythmia may be increased; avoid combination.

Ergot alkaloids: Concurrent use may lead to acute ergot toxicity (severe peripheral vasospasm and dysesthesia).

Fluconazole: Increases clarithromycin levels and AUC by ~25%

HMG-CoA reductase inhibitors (atorvastatin, lovastatin, and simvastatin); Clarithromycin may increase serum levels of "statins" metabolized by CYP3A4, increasing the risk of myopathy/rhabdomyolysis (does not include fluvastatin and pravastatin). Switch to pravastatin/fluvastatin or suspend treatment during course of clarithromycin therapy.

Methylprednisolone: Serum levels may be increased by clarithromycin; monitor. (Continued)

Clarithromycin (Continued)

Phenytoin: Serum levels may be increased by clarithromycin; other evidence suggested phenytoin levels may be decreased in some patients; monitor.

Pimozide: Serum levels may be increased, leading to malignant arrhythmias; concomitant use is contraindicated.

Protease inhibitors (amprenavir, nelfinavir, and ritonavir): May increase serum levels of clarithromycin.

QT_c-prolonging agents: Concomitant use may increase the risk of malignant arrhythmias.

Quinidine: Serum levels may be increased by clarithromycin; in addition, the risk of QT_c prolongation and malignant arrhythmias may be increased during concurrent use.

Quinolone antibiotics (sparfloxacin, gatifloxacin, or moxifloxacin): Concurrent use may increase the risk of malignant arrhythmias.

Rifabutin: Serum levels may be increased by clarithromycin; monitor.

Sildenafil, tadalafil, vardenafil: Serum levels may be increased by clarithromycin. Do not exceed single sildenafil doses of 25 mg in 48 hours, a single tadalafil dose of 10 mg in 72 hours, or a single vardenafil dose of 2.5 mg in 24 hours.

Tacrolimus: Serum levels may be increased by clarithromycin; monitor serum concentration.

Theophylline: Serum levels may be increased by clarithromycin; monitor.

Thioridazine: Risk of QT_c prolongation and malignant arrhythmias may be increased.

Valproic acid (and derivatives): Serum levels may be increased by clarithromycin; monitor.

Vinblastine (and vincristine): Serum levels may be increased by clarithromycin.

Warfarin: Effects may be potentiated; monitor INR closely and adjust warfarin dose as needed or choose another antibiotic

Zidovudine: Peak levels (but not AUC) of zidovudine may be increased; other studies suggest levels may be decreased.

Zopiclone: Serum levels may be increased by clarithromycin; monitor.

Ethanol/Nutrition/Herb Interactions

Food: Delays absorption; total absorption remains unchanged.

Herb/Nutraceutical: St John's wort may decrease clarithromycin levels.

Dietary Considerations May be taken with or without meals; may be taken with Biaxin® XL should be taken with food.

Pharmacodynamics/Kinetics

Absorption: Highly stable in presence of gastric acid (unlike erythromycin); food delays but does not affect extent of absorption

Distribution: Widely into most body tissues except CNS

Metabolism: Partially hepatic via CYP3A4; converted to 14-OH clarithromycin (active metabolite)

Bioavailability: 50%

Half-life elimination: Clarithromycin: 3-7 hours; 14-OH-clarithromycin: 5-9 hours

Time to peak: 2-4 hours

Excretion: Primarily urine

Clearance: Approximates normal GFR

Pregnancy Risk Factor C

Lactation Excretion in breast milk unknown/use caution

Breast-Feeding Considerations Erythromycins may be taken while breast-feeding. Use caution.

Dosage Forms

Granules for oral suspension (Biaxin®): 125 mg/5 mL (50 mL, 100 mL); 250 mg/5 mL (50 mL, 100 mL) [fruit punch flavor]

Tablet (Biaxin®): 250 mg, 500 mg

Tablet, extended release (Biaxin® XL): 500 mg

Dental Comment

The FDA issued a special alert in December 2005 stating that short-term therapy with clarithromycin in patients with stable coronary artery disease may cause significantly higher cardiovascular mortality. The use of 500 mg clarithromycin daily for 14 days in patients with the above condition resulted in significantly higher all-cause mortality compared to patients taking placebo. This information is provided to the dental practitioner on the possible association between short-term use of clarithromycin for infections and increases in mortality in patients with a history of stable coronary artery disease.

This drug is known to prolong the QT interval. The QT interval is measured as the time and distance between the Q point of the QRS complex and the end of the T wave in the ECG tracing. After adjustment for heart rate, the QT interval is defined as prolonged if it is more than 450 msec in men and 460 msec in women. A long QT syndrome was first described in the 1950s and 60s as a congenital syndrome involving QT interval prolongation and syncope and sudden death. Some of the congenital long QT syndromes were characterized by a peculiar electrocardiographic appearance of the QRS complex involving a premature atria beat followed by a pause, then a subsequent sinus beat showing marked QT prolongation and deformity. This type of cardiac arrhythmia was originally termed "torsade de pointes" (translated from the French as "twisting of the points").

Prolongation of the QT interval is thought to result from delayed ventricular repolarization. The repolarization process within the myocardial cell is due to the efflux of intracellular potassium. The channels associated with this current can be blocked by many drugs, thus, predisposing the electrical propagation cycle to torsade de pointes.

Clarithromycin is one of the drugs confirmed to prolong the QT interval and is accepted as having a risk of causing torsade de pointes. The risk of drug-induced torsade de pointes is extremely low when a single QT interval prolonging drug is prescribed. In terms of epinephrine, it is not known what effect vasoconstrictors in the local anesthetic regimen will have in patients with a known history of congenital prolonged QT interval or in patients taking any medication that prolongs the QT interval. Until more information is obtained, it is suggested that the clinician consult with the physician prior to the use of a vasoconstrictor in suspected patients, and that the vasoconstrictor (epinephrine, levonordefrin [Neo-Cobefrin®]) be used with caution.

Selected Readings

ADA Division of Legal Affairs, "A Legal Perspective on Antibiotic Prophylaxis," *J Am Dent Assoc*, 2003, 134(9):1260.

American Dental Association Council on Scientific Affairs, "Combating Antibiotic Resistance," *J Am Dent Assoc*, 2004, 135(4):484-7.

Amsden GW, "Erythromycin, Clarithromycin, and Azithromycin: Are the Differences Real?" *Clin Ther*, 1996, 18(1):56-72.

Dajani AS, Taubert KA, Wilson W, et al, "Prevention of Bacterial Endocarditis. Recommendations by the American Heart Association," *JAMA*, 1997, 277(22):1794-801.

Dajani AS, Taubert KA, Wilson W, et al, "Prevention of Bacterial Endocarditis. Recommendations by the American Heart Association," *J Am Dent Assoc*, 1997, 128(8):1142-51.

Moore PA, "Dental Therapeutic Indications for the Newer Long-Acting Macrolide Antibiotics," *J Am Dent Assoc*, 1999, 130(9):1341-3.

"Pimozide (Orap) Contraindicated With Clarithromycin (Biaxin®) and Other Macrolide Antibiotics," *FDA Medical Bulletin*, October 1996, 26 (3).

Wynn RL, "New Erythromycins," *Gen Dent*, 1996, 44(4):304-7.

Wynn RL, Bergman SA, Meiller TF, et al, "Antibiotics in Treating Oral-Facial Infections of Odontogenic Origin: An Update," *Gen Dent*, 2001, 49(3):238-40, 242, 244 passim.

Clarithromycin, Lansoprazole, and Amoxicillin *see* Lansoprazole, Amoxicillin, and Clarithromycin *on page 898*

Claritin® 24 Hour Allergy [OTC] *see* Loratadine *on page 946*

Claritin-D® 12-Hour [OTC] *see* Loratadine and Pseudoephedrine *on page 947*

Claritin-D® 24-Hour [OTC] *see* Loratadine and Pseudoephedrine *on page 947*

Claritin® Hives Relief [OTC] *see* Loratadine *on page 946*

Clavulanic Acid and Amoxicillin *see* Amoxicillin and Clavulanate Potassium *on page 108*

Clear Eyes® ACR [OTC] *see* Naphazoline *on page 1087*

Clear Eyes® Extra Relief [OTC] *see* Naphazoline *on page 1087*

Clearplex [OTC] *see* Benzoyl Peroxide *on page 194*

Clemastine (KLEM as teen)

U.S. Brand Names Dayhist® Allergy [OTC]; Tavist® Allergy [OTC]
Mexican Brand Names Tavist®
Generic Available Yes
Synonyms Clemastine Fumarate
Pharmacologic Category Antihistamine
Use Perennial and seasonal allergic rhinitis and other allergic symptoms including urticaria
Local Anesthetic/Vasoconstrictor Precautions No information available to require special precautions
Effects on Dental Treatment Key adverse event(s) related to dental treatment: Xerostomia (normal salivary flow resumes upon discontinuation).
Common Adverse Effects Frequency not defined.
Cardiovascular: Palpitations, hypotension, tachycardia
Central nervous system: Dyscoordination, sedation, somnolence slight to moderate, sleepiness, confusion, restlessness, nervousness, insomnia, irritability, fatigue, headache, dizziness increased
Dermatologic: Rash, photosensitivity
Gastrointestinal: Diarrhea, nausea, xerostomia, epigastric distress, vomiting, constipation
(Continued)

Clemastine *(Continued)*

Genitourinary: Urinary frequency, difficult urination, urinary retention
Hematologic: Hemolytic anemia, thrombocytopenia, agranulocytosis
Ocular: Blurred vision
Otic: Tinnitus
Respiratory: Thickening of bronchial secretions
Miscellaneous: Anaphylaxis

Mechanism of Action Competes with histamine for H_1-receptor sites on effector cells in the gastrointestinal tract, blood vessels, and respiratory tract

Drug Interactions

Cytochrome P450 Effect: Inhibits CYP2D6 (weak), 3A4 (weak)

Increased Effect/Toxicity: CNS depressants may increase the degree of sedation and respiratory depression with antihistamines. May increase the absorption of digoxin. Central and/or peripheral anticholinergic syndrome can occur when administered with amantadine, rimantadine, narcotic analgesics, phenothiazines and other antipsychotics (especially with high anticholinergic activity), tricyclic antidepressants, quinidine, disopyramide, procainamide, and antihistamines.

Decreased Effect: May increase gastric degradation of levodopa and decrease the amount of levodopa absorbed by delaying gastric emptying. Therapeutic effects of cholinergic agents (tacrine, donepezil) and neuroleptics may be antagonized.

Pharmacodynamics/Kinetics

Onset of action: Peak effect: Therapeutic: 5-7 hours
Duration: 8-16 hours
Absorption: Almost complete
Metabolism: Hepatic
Excretion: Urine

Pregnancy Risk Factor B

Clemastine Fumarate *see* Clemastine *on page 359*

Cleocin® *see* Clindamycin *on page 361*

Cleocin HCl® *see* Clindamycin *on page 361*

Cleocin Pediatric® *see* Clindamycin *on page 361*

Cleocin Phosphate® *see* Clindamycin *on page 361*

Cleocin T® *see* Clindamycin *on page 361*

Clidinium and Chlordiazepoxide

(kli DI nee um & klor dye az e POKS ide)

Related Information

Chlordiazepoxide *on page 315*

U.S. Brand Names Librax® *[original formulation]*
Canadian Brand Names Apo-Chlorax®; Librax®
Generic Available Yes
Synonyms Chlordiazepoxide and Clidinium
Pharmacologic Category Antispasmodic Agent, Gastrointestinal; Benzodiazepine

Use Adjunct treatment of peptic ulcer; treatment of irritable bowel syndrome

Local Anesthetic/Vasoconstrictor Precautions No information available to require special precautions

Effects on Dental Treatment Key adverse event(s) related to dental treatment: Xerostomia and changes in salivation (normal salivary flow resumes upon discontinuation).

Common Adverse Effects 1% to 10%:

Central nervous system: Drowsiness, ataxia, confusion, anticholinergic side effects

Gastrointestinal: Dry mouth, constipation, nausea

Drug Interactions

Cytochrome P450 Effect: Chlordiazepoxide: **Substrate** of CYP3A4 (major)

Increased Effect/Toxicity: Additive effects may result from concomitant benzodiazepine and/or anticholinergic therapy. CYP3A4 inhibitors may increase the levels/effects of chlordiazepoxide; example inhibitors include azole antifungals, clarithromycin, diclofenac, doxycycline, erythromycin, imatinib, isoniazid, nefazodone, nicardipine, propofol, protease inhibitors, quinidine, telithromycin, and verapamil.

Decreased Effect: CYP3A4 inducers may decrease the levels/effects of chlordiazepoxide. Example inducers include aminoglutethimide, carbamazepine, nafcillin, nevirapine, phenobarbital, phenytoin, and rifamycins.

Pregnancy Risk Factor D

Climara® see Estradiol on page 574
Clinac™ BPO see Benzoyl Peroxide on page 194
Clindagel® see Clindamycin on page 361
ClindaMax™ see Clindamycin on page 361

Clindamycin (klin da MYE sin)

Related Information
Antibiotic Prophylaxis on page 1680
Bacterial Infections on page 1697
Cardiovascular Diseases on page 1636
Periodontal Diseases on page 1705
Sexually-Transmitted Diseases on page 1674

Related Sample Prescriptions
Bacterial Endocarditis (Prevention) on page 1732
Bacterial Infections and Periodontal Diseases on page 1736
Prosthetic Joint Late Infections (Prevention) on page 1733

U.S. Brand Names Cleocin®; Cleocin HCl®; Cleocin Pediatric®; Cleocin Phosphate®; Cleocin T®; Clindagel®; ClindaMax™; Clindesse™; Clindets®; Evoclin™

Canadian Brand Names Alti-Clindamycin; Apo-Clindamycin®; Clindoxyl®; Dalacin® C; Dalacin® T; Dalacin® Vaginal; Novo-Clindamycin

Mexican Brand Names Clindazyn®; Cutaclin®; Dalacin C®; Dalacin T®; Dalacin V®; Galecin®; Klyndaken®

Generic Available Yes: Excludes foam, vaginal suppositories, vaginal cream

Synonyms Clindamycin Hydrochloride; Clindamycin Palmitate; Clindamycin Phosphate

Pharmacologic Category Antibiotic, Lincosamide

Dental Use Alternate antibiotic, when amoxicillin cannot be used, for the standard regimen for prevention of bacterial endocarditis in patients undergoing dental procedures; alternate antibiotic in the treatment of common orofacial infections caused by aerobic gram-positive cocci and susceptible anaerobes; alternate antibiotic for prophylaxis for dental patients with total joint replacement

Use Treatment against aerobic and anaerobic streptococci (except enterococci), most staphylococci, *Bacteroides* sp and *Actinomyces*; bacterial vaginosis (vaginal cream, vaginal suppository); pelvic inflammatory disease (I.V.); topically in treatment of severe acne; vaginally for *Gardnerella vaginalis*

Unlabeled/Investigational Use May be useful in PCP; alternate treatment for toxoplasmosis

Local Anesthetic/Vasoconstrictor Precautions No information available to require special precautions

Effects on Dental Treatment No significant effects or complications reported (see Dental Comment)

Significant Adverse Effects
Systemic:
>10%: Gastrointestinal: Diarrhea, abdominal pain
1% to 10%:
  Cardiovascular: Hypotension
  Dermatologic: Urticaria, rash, Stevens-Johnson syndrome
  Gastrointestinal: Pseudomembranous colitis, nausea, vomiting
  Local: Thrombophlebitis, sterile abscess at I.M. injection site
  Miscellaneous: Fungal overgrowth, hypersensitivity
<1% (Limited to important or life-threatening): Granulocytopenia, neutropenia, polyarthritis, renal dysfunction (rare), thrombocytopenia

Topical:
>10%: Dermatologic: Dryness, burning, itching, scaliness, erythema, or peeling of skin (lotion, solution); oiliness (gel, lotion)
1% to 10%: Central nervous system: Headache
<1% (Limited to important or life-threatening): Pseudomembranous colitis, nausea, vomiting, diarrhea (severe), abdominal pain, folliculitis, hypersensitivity reactions

Vaginal:
>10%: Genitourinary: Fungal vaginosis, vaginitis or vulvovaginal pruritus (from *Candida albicans*)
1% to 10%:
  Central nervous system: Back pain, headache
  Gastrointestinal: Constipation, diarrhea
  Genitourinary: Urinary tract infection
  Respiratory: Nasopharyngitis
  Miscellaneous: Fungal infection
<1% (Limited to important or life-threatening): Atrophic vaginitis, bladder infection, bladder spasm, cervical dysplasia, diarrhea, dizziness, epistaxis, (Continued)

Clindamycin *(Continued)*

erythema, fever, hypersensitivity, hyperthyroidism, local edema, menstrual disorder, nausea, pain, palpable lymph node, pruritus, pyelonephritis, pyrexia, rash, sciatica, stomach cramps, upper respiratory urticaria, uterine cervical disorder, uterine spasm, vaginal burning, vertigo, vomiting, vulvar erythema, vulvar laceration, wheezing

Dental Usual Dosing

Orofacial infection: Adults: Oral: 150-450 mg/dose every 6-8 hours; maximum dose: 1.8 g/day

Prevention of bacterial endocarditis (unlabeled use): Oral:

Children: 20 mg/kg 1 hour before procedure with no follow-up dose needed

Adults: 600 mg 1 hour before procedure with no follow-up dose needed

Dosage

Usual dosage ranges:

Infants and Children:

Oral: 8-20 mg/kg/day as hydrochloride; 8-25 mg/kg/day as palmitate in 3-4 divided doses (minimum dose of palmitate: 37.5 mg 3 times/day)

I.M., I.V.:

<1 month: 15-20 mg/kg/day

>1 month: 20-40 mg/kg/day in 3-4 divided doses

Adults:

Oral: 150-450 mg/dose every 6-8 hours; maximum dose: 1.8 g/day

I.M., I.V.: 1.2-1.8 g/day in 2-4 divided doses; maximum dose: 4.8 g/day

Indication-specific dosing:

Children:

Anthrax: I.V.: 7.5 mg/kg every 6 hours

Babesiosis: Oral: 20-40 mg/kg/day divided every 8 hours for 7 days plus quinine

Orofacial infections: 8-25 mg/kg in 3-4 equally divided doses

Prevention of bacterial endocarditis (unlabeled use):

Oral: 20 mg/kg 1 hour before procedure with no follow-up dose needed

I.V.: 20 mg/kg within 30 minutes before procedure

Children ≥12 years and Adults:

Acne vulgaris: Topical:

Gel, pledget, lotion, solution: Apply a thin film twice daily

Foam (Evoclin™): Apply once daily

Adults:

Amnionitis: I.V.: 450-900 mg every 8 hours

Anthrax: I.V.: 900 mg every 8 hours with ciprofloxacin or doxycycline

Babesiosis:

Oral: 600 mg 3 times/day for 7 days with quinine

I.V.: 1.2 g twice daily

Bacterial vaginosis: Intravaginal:

Suppositories: Insert one ovule (100 mg clindamycin) daily into vagina at bedtime for 3 days

Cream:

Cleocin®: One full applicator inserted intravaginally once daily before bedtime for 3 or 7 consecutive days in nonpregnant patients or for 7 consecutive days in pregnant patients

Clindesse™: One full applicator inserted intravaginally as a single dose at anytime during the day in nonpregnant patients

Bite wounds (canine): Oral: 300 mg 4 times/day with a fluoroquinolone

Gangrenous myositis: I.V.: 900 mg every 8 hours with penicillin G

Group B streptococcus (neonatal prophylaxis): I.V.: 900 mg every 8 hours until delivery

Orofacial/parapharyngeal space infections:

Oral: 150-450 mg every 6 hours for 7 days, maximum 1.8 g/day

I.V.: 600-900 mg every 8 hours

Pelvic inflammatory disease: I.V.: 900 mg every 8 hours with gentamicin 2 mg/kg, then 1.5 mg/kg every 8 hours; continue after discharge with doxy-cycline 100 mg twice daily to complete 14 days of total therapy

Pneumocystis jiroveci pneumonia (unlabeled use):

Oral: 300-450 mg 4 times/day with primaquine

I.M., I.V.: 1200-2400 mg/day with pyrimethamine or 600 mg 4 times/day with primaquine

Prevention of bacterial endocarditis (unlabeled use):

Oral: 600 mg 1 hour before procedure with no follow-up dose needed

I.V.: 600 mg within 30 minutes before procedure

Toxic shock syndrome: I.V.: 900 mg every 8 hours with penicillin G or ceftriaxone

Toxoplasmosis (unlabeled use): Oral, I.V.: 600 mg every 6 hours with pyrimethamine and folinic acid

Dosing adjustment in hepatic impairment: Adjustment recommended in patients with severe hepatic disease

Mechanism of Action Reversibly binds to 50S ribosomal subunits preventing peptide bond formation thus inhibiting bacterial protein synthesis; bacteriostatic or bactericidal depending on drug concentration, infection site, and organism

Contraindications Hypersensitivity to clindamycin or any component of the formulation; previous pseudomembranous colitis; regional enteritis, ulcerative colitis

Warnings/Precautions Dosage adjustment may be necessary in patients with severe hepatic dysfunction; can cause severe and possibly fatal colitis; discontinue drug if significant diarrhea, abdominal cramps, or passage of blood and mucus occurs. Vaginal products may weaken latex or rubber condoms, or contraceptive diaphragms. Barrier contraceptives are not recommended concurrently or for 3-5 days (depending on the product) following treatment. Some dosage forms contain benzyl alcohol or tartrazine. Use caution in atopic patients.

Drug Interactions Increased duration of neuromuscular blockade from tubocurarine, pancuronium

Ethanol/Nutrition/Herb Interactions
Food: Peak concentrations may be delayed with food.
Herb/Nutraceutical: St John's wort may decrease clindamycin levels.

Dietary Considerations May be taken with food.

Pharmacodynamics/Kinetics
Absorption: Topical: ~10%; Oral: Rapid (90%)
Distribution: High concentrations in bone and urine; no significant levels in CSF, even with inflamed meninges; crosses placenta; enters breast milk
Metabolism: Hepatic
Bioavailability: Topical: <1%
Half-life elimination: Neonates: Premature: 8.7 hours; Full-term: 3.6 hours; Adults: 1.6-5.3 hours (average: 2-3 hours)
Time to peak, serum: Oral: Within 60 minutes; I.M.: 1-3 hours
Excretion: Urine (10%) and feces (~4%) as active drug and metabolites

Pregnancy Risk Factor B

Lactation Enters breast milk/compatible

Dosage Forms Note: Strength is expressed as base
Capsule, as hydrochloride: 150 mg, 300 mg
   Cleocin HCl®: 75 mg [contains tartrazine], 150 mg [contains tartrazine], 300 mg
Cream, vaginal, as phosphate:
   Cleocin®: 2% (40 g) [contains benzyl alcohol and mineral oil; packaged with 7 disposable applicators]
   Clindesse™: 2% (5 g) [contains mineral oil; prefilled single disposable applicator]
Foam, topical, as phosphate (Evoclin™): 1% (50 g, 100 g) [contains ethanol 58%]
Gel, topical, as phosphate: 1% [10 mg/g] (30 g, 60 g)
   Cleocin T®: 1% [10 mg/g] (30 g, 60 g)
   Clindagel®: 1% [10 mg/g] (40 mL, 75 mL)
   ClindaMax™: 1% (30 g, 60 g)
Granules for oral solution, as palmitate (Cleocin Pediatric®): 75 mg/5 mL (100 mL) [cherry flavor]
Infusion, as phosphate [premixed in D₅W] (Cleocin Phosphate®): 300 mg (50 mL); 600 mg (50 mL); 900 mg (50 mL)
Injection, solution, as phosphate (Cleocin Phosphate®): 150 mg/mL (2 mL, 4 mL, 6 mL, 60 mL) [contains benzyl alcohol and disodium edetate 0.5 mg]
Lotion, as phosphate (Cleocin T®, ClindaMax™): 1% [10 mg/mL] (60 mL)
Pledgets, topical: 1% (60s) [contains alcohol]
   Cleocin T®: 1% (60s) [contains isopropyl alcohol 50%]
   Clindets®: 1% (69s) [contains isopropyl alcohol 52%]
Solution, topical, as phosphate (Cleocin T®): 1% [10 mg/mL] (30 mL, 60 mL) [contains isopropyl alcohol 50%]
Suppository (ovule), vaginal, as phosphate (Cleocin®): 100 mg (3s) [contains oleaginous base; single reusable applicator]

Dental Comment Clindamycin has not been shown to interfere with oral contraceptive activity; however, it reduces GI microflora, thus, oral contraceptive users should be advised to use additional methods of birth control. About 1% of clindamycin users develop pseudomembranous colitis. Symptoms may occur 2-9 days after initiation of therapy; however, it has never occurred with the 1-dose regimen of clindamycin used to prevent bacterial endocarditis.

Selected Readings
ADA Division of Legal Affairs, "A Legal Perspective on Antibiotic Prophylaxis," *J Am Dent Assoc*, 2003, 134(9):1260.

(Continued)

Clindamycin *(Continued)*

"Advisory Statement. Antibiotic Prophylaxis for Dental Patients With Total Joint Replacements. American Dental Association; American Academy of Orthopedic Surgeons," *J Am Dent Assoc*, 1997, 128(7):1004-8.

American Dental Association; American Academy of Orthopedic Surgeons, "Antibiotic Prophylaxis for Dental Patients With Total Joint Replacements," *J Am Dent Assoc*, 2003, 134(7):895-9.

American Dental Association Council on Scientific Affairs, "Combating Antibiotic Resistance," *J Am Dent Assoc*, 2004, 135(4):484-7.

Dajani AS, Taubert KA, Wilson W, et al, "Prevention of Bacterial Endocarditis. Recommendations by the American Heart Association," *JAMA*, 1997, 277(22):1794-801.

Dajani AS, Taubert KA, Wilson W, et al, "Prevention of Bacterial Endocarditis. Recommendations by the American Heart Association," *J Am Dent Assoc*, 1997, 128(8):1142-51.

Sandor GK, Low DE, Judd PL, et al, "Antimicrobial Treatment Options in the Management of Odontogenic Infections," *J Can Dent Assoc*, 1998, 64(7):508-14.

Wynn RL, "Clindamycin: An Often Forgotten But Important Antibiotic," *AGD Impact*, 1994, 22:10.

Wynn RL and Bergman SA, "Antibiotics and Their Use in the Treatment of Orofacial Infections, Part I," *Gen Dent*, 1994, 42(5):398, 400, 402.

Wynn RL and Bergman SA, "Antibiotics and Their Use in the Treatment of Orofacial Infections, Part II," *Gen Dent*, 1994, 42(6):498-502.

Wynn RL, Bergman SA, Meiller TF, et al, "Antibiotics in Treating Oral-Facial Infections of Odontogenic Origin: An Update," *Gen Dent*, 2001, 49(3):238-40, 242, 244 passim.

Clindamycin and Benzoyl Peroxide

(klin da MYE sin & BEN zoe il peer OKS ide)

Related Information

Benzoyl Peroxide *on page 194*

Clindamycin *on page 361*

U.S. Brand Names BenzaClin®; Duac™

Canadian Brand Names BenzaClin®

Generic Available No

Synonyms Benzoyl Peroxide and Clindamycin; Clindamycin Phosphate and Benzoyl Peroxide

Pharmacologic Category Topical Skin Product; Topical Skin Product, Acne

Use Topical treatment of acne vulgaris

Local Anesthetic/Vasoconstrictor Precautions No information available to require special precautions

Effects on Dental Treatment No significant effects or complications reported

Common Adverse Effects

>10%: Dermatologic: Peeling (2% to 17%), dry skin (1% to 15%)

1% to 10%: Dermatologic: Pruritus (2%), erythema (1% to 5%), sunburn (1%), burning (<1% to 5%)

Mechanism of Action Clindamycin and benzoyl peroxide have activity against *Propionibacterium acnes in vitro*. This organism has been associated with acne vulgaris. Benzoyl peroxide releases free-radical oxygen which oxidizes bacterial proteins in the sebaceous follicles decreasing the number of anaerobic bacteria and decreasing irritating-type free fatty acids. Clindamycin reversibly binds to 50S ribosomal subunits preventing peptide bond formation thus inhibiting bacterial protein synthesis; bacteriostatic or bactericidal depending on drug concentration, infection site, and organism.

Drug Interactions

Increased Effect/Toxicity: Tretinoin may cause increased adverse events with concurrent use.

Decreased Effect: Erythromycin may antagonize clindamycin's effects.

Pharmacodynamics/Kinetics See individual agents.

Pregnancy Risk Factor C

Clindamycin Hydrochloride *see* Clindamycin *on page 361*

Clindamycin Palmitate *see* Clindamycin *on page 361*

Clindamycin Phosphate *see* Clindamycin *on page 361*

Clindamycin Phosphate and Benzoyl Peroxide *see* Clindamycin and Benzoyl Peroxide *on page 364*

Clindesse™ *see* Clindamycin *on page 361*

Clindets® *see* Clindamycin *on page 361*

Clinoril® *see* Sulindac *on page 1430*

Clobazam (KLOE ba zam)

Canadian Brand Names Alti-Clobazam; Apo-Clobazam®; Clobazam-10; Dom-Clobazam; Frisium®; Novo-Clobazam; PMS-Clobazam; ratio-Clobazam

Mexican Brand Names Frisium®

Generic Available Yes

Pharmacologic Category Benzodiazepine

Use Adjunctive treatment of epilepsy

Unlabeled/Investigational Use Monotherapy for epilepsy or intermittent seizures

Local Anesthetic/Vasoconstrictor Precautions No information available to require special precautions

Effects on Dental Treatment Key adverse event(s) related to dental treatment: Xerostomia (normal salivary flow resumes upon discontinuation). Paradoxical reactions (including excitation, agitation, hallucinations, and psychosis) are known to occur with benzodiazepines.

Common Adverse Effects

Central nervous system: Drowsiness (17%), ataxia (4%), dizziness (2%), behavior disorder (1%), confusion, depression, lethargy, slurred speech, tremor, anterograde amnesia. In addition, paradoxical reactions (including excitation, agitation, hallucinations, and psychosis) are known to occur with benzodiazepines.

Dermatologic: Rash, pruritus, urticaria

Gastrointestinal: Weight gain (2%); dose related: Xerostomia, constipation, nausea

Hematologic: Decreased WBCs and other hematologic abnormalities have been rarely associated with benzodiazepines

Neuromuscular & skeletal: Muscle spasm

Ocular: Blurred vision (1%)

Restrictions Not available in U.S.

Mechanism of Action Clobazam is a 1,5 benzodiazepine which binds to stereospecific benzodiazepine receptors on the postsynaptic GABA neuron at several sites within the central nervous system, including the limbic system, reticular formation. Enhancement of the inhibitory effect of GABA on neuronal excitability results by increased neuronal membrane permeability to chloride ions. This shift in chloride ions results in hyperpolarization (a less excitable state) and stabilization.

Drug Interactions

Cytochrome P450 Effect: Substrate (major) of CYP2C19 and 3A4

Increased Effect/Toxicity: Benzodiazepines potentiate the CNS depressant effects of narcotic analgesics, barbiturates, phenothiazines, ethanol, antihistamines, MAO inhibitors, sedative-hypnotics, and cyclic antidepressants. CYP2C19 inhibitors may increase the levels/effects of clobazam; example inhibitors include delavirdine, fluconazole, fluvoxamine, gemfibrozil, isoniazid, omeprazole, and ticlopidine. CYP3A4 inhibitors may increase the levels/effects of clobazam; example inhibitors include azole antifungals, clarithromycin, diclofenac, doxycycline, erythromycin, imatinib, isoniazid, nefazodone, nicardipine, propofol, protease inhibitors, quinidine, telithromycin, and verapamil.

Decreased Effect: CYP3A4 inducers may decrease the levels/effects of clobazam; example inducers include aminoglutethimide, carbamazepine, nafcillin, nevirapine, phenobarbital, phenytoin, and rifamycins.

Pharmacodynamics/Kinetics

Absorption: Rapid

Protein binding: 85% to 91%

Metabolism: Hepatic via N-dealkylation (likely via CYP) to active metabolite (N-desmethyl), and glucuronidation

Bioavailability: 87%

Half-life elimination: 18 hours; N-desmethyl (active): 42 hours

Time to peak: 15 minutes to 4 hours

Excretion: Urine (90%), as metabolites

Pregnancy Risk Factor Not assigned; similar agents rated D. Contraindicated in 1st trimester (per manufacturer).

Clobetasol (kloe BAY ta sol)

Related Information

Ulcerative and Erosive Disorders *on page 1712*

Related Sample Prescriptions

Erosive Lichen Planus and Major Aphthae *on page 1745*

Recurrent Aphthous Stomatitis *on page 1744*

U.S. Brand Names Clobevate®; Clobex®; Cormax®; Embeline™; Embeline™ E; Olux®; Temovate®; Temovate E®

Canadian Brand Names Clobex®; Dermovate®; Gen-Clobetasol; Novo-Clobetasol

Generic Available Yes: Excludes foam, lotion, shampoo, spray

(Continued)

Clobetasol *(Continued)*

Synonyms Clobetasol Propionate

Pharmacologic Category Corticosteroid, Topical

Dental Use Short-term relief of oral mucosal inflammation

Use Short-term relief of inflammation of moderate-to-severe corticosteroid-responsive dermatoses (very high potency topical corticosteroid)

Local Anesthetic/Vasoconstrictor Precautions No information available to require special precautions

Effects on Dental Treatment No significant effects or complications reported

Significant Adverse Effects Frequency not defined; may depend upon formulation used, length of application, surface area covered, and the use of occlusive dressings.

Endocrine & metabolic: Adrenal suppression, Cushing's syndrome, hyperglycemia

Local: Application site: Burning, cracking/fissuring of the skin, dryness, erythema, folliculitis, irritation, numbness, pruritus, skin atrophy, stinging, telangiectasia

Renal: Glucosuria

Effects reported with other high-potency topical steroids: Acneiform eruptions, allergic contact dermatitis, hypertrichosis, hypopigmentation, maceration of the skin, miliaria, perioral dermatitis, secondary infection

Dental Usual Dosing Oral mucosal inflammation: Children ≥12 years and Adults: Cream: Apply twice daily for up to 2 weeks (maximum dose: 50 g/week); discontinue application when control is achieved; if no improvement is seen, reassessment of diagnosis may be necessary

Dosage Topical: Discontinue when control achieved; if improvement not seen within 2 weeks, reassessment of diagnosis may be necessary.

Children <12 years: Use is not recommended

Children ≥12 years and Adults:

Oral mucosal inflammation, dental (unlabeled use): Cream: Apply twice daily for up to 2 weeks (maximum dose: 50 g/week); discontinue application when control is achieved; if no improvement is seen, reassessment of diagnosis may be necessary

Steroid-responsive dermatoses:

Cream, emollient cream, gel, ointment: Apply twice daily for up to 2 weeks (maximum dose: 50 g/week)

Foam, solution: Apply to affected scalp twice daily for up to 2 weeks (maximum dose: 50 g/week or 50 mL/week)

Mild-to-moderate plaque-type psoriasis of nonscalp areas: Foam: Apply to affected area twice daily for up to 2 weeks (maximum dose: 50 g/week); do not apply to face or intertriginous areas

Children ≥16 years and Adults: Moderate-to-severe plaque-type psoriasis: Emollient cream, lotion: Apply twice daily for up to 2 weeks, has been used for up to 4 weeks when application is <10% of body surface area; use with caution (maximum dose: 50 g/week)

Children ≥18 years and Adults:

Moderate-to-severe plaque-type psoriasis: Spray: Apply by spraying directly onto affected area twice daily; should be gently rubbed into skin. Should be used for not longer than 4 weeks; treatment beyond 2 weeks should be limited to localized lesions which have not improved sufficiently. Total dose should not exceed 50 g/week or 59 mL/week.

Scalp psoriasis: Shampoo: Apply thin film to dry scalp once daily; leave in place for 15 minutes, then add water, lather; rinse thoroughly

Steroid-responsive dermatoses: Lotion: Apply twice daily for up to 2 weeks (maximum dose: 50 g/week)

Mechanism of Action Stimulates the synthesis of enzymes needed to decrease inflammation, suppress mitotic activity, and cause vasoconstriction

Contraindications Hypersensitivity to clobetasol or any component of the formulation; viral, fungal, or tubercular skin lesions

Warnings/Precautions Clobetasol propionate has been shown to suppress the HPA axis; risk may be decreased by treating small surface areas for <2 continuous weeks. Monitor for HPA axis suppression when large surface areas must be covered or if occlusive dressings are used. Not to be used with occlusive dressings unless directed by healthcare provider. Use of any product in children <12 years of age is not recommended. Selected products approved for use in adolescents.

Drug Interactions No data reported

Pharmacodynamics/Kinetics

Absorption: Percutaneous absorption is variable and dependent upon many factors including vehicle used, integrity of epidermis, dose, and use of occlusive dressings

Metabolism: Hepatic

Excretion: Urine and feces

Pregnancy Risk Factor C

Lactation Excretion in breast milk unknown/use caution

Breast-Feeding Considerations It is not known if topical application will result in detectable quantities in breast milk.

Dosage Forms [DSC] = Discontinued product

Cream, as propionate: 0.05% (15 g, 30 g, 45 g, 60 g)

  Cormax®: 0.05% (15 g [DSC], 30 g, 45 g, 60 g [DSC])

  Embeline™, Temovate®: 0.05% (15 g, 30 g, 45 g, 60 g)

Cream, as propionate [in emollient base]: 0.05% (15 g, 30 g, 60 g)

  Embeline™ E: 0.05% (15 g, 30 g, 60 g)

  Temovate E®: 0.05% (15 g [DSC], 30 g, 60 g)

Foam, topical, as propionate [for scalp application] (Olux®): 0.05% (50 g, 100 g) [contains ethanol 60%]

Gel, as propionate: 0.05% (15 g, 30 g, 60 g)

  Clobevate®, Embeline™: 0.05% (15 g, 30 g, 60 g)

  Temovate®: 0.05% (15 g [DSC], 30 g, 60 g)

Lotion, as propionate (Clobex®): 0.05% (30 mL, 59 mL)

Ointment, as propionate: 0.05% (15 g, 30 g, 45 g, 60 g)

  Cormax®: 0.05% (15 g, 45 g)

  Embeline™: 0.05% (15 g, 30 g, 45 g, 60 g)

  Temovate®: 0.05% (15 g, 30 g, 45 g [DSC], 60 g)

Shampoo, as propionate:

  Clobex®: 0.05% (120 mL) [contains alcohol]

Solution, topical, as propionate [for scalp application]: 0.05% (25 mL, 50 mL)

  Cormax®, Embeline™, Temovate®: 0.05% (25 mL, 50 mL) [contains isopropyl alcohol 40%]

Spray, topical, as propionate (Clobex®): 0.05% (60 mL) [contains alcohol]

Clobetasol Propionate *see* Clobetasol *on page 365*

Clobevate® *see* Clobetasol *on page 365*

Clobex® *see* Clobetasol *on page 365*

Clocortolone (kloe KOR toe lone)

U.S. Brand Names Cloderm®

Canadian Brand Names Cloderm®

Generic Available No

Synonyms Clocortolone Pivalate

Pharmacologic Category Corticosteroid, Topical

Use Inflammation of corticosteroid-responsive dermatoses (intermediate-potency topical corticosteroid)

Local Anesthetic/Vasoconstrictor Precautions No information available to require special precautions

Effects on Dental Treatment No significant effects or complications reported

Common Adverse Effects

1% to 10%:

  Dermatologic: Itching, erythema

  Local: Burning, dryness, irritation, papular rash

Mechanism of Action Stimulates the synthesis of enzymes needed to decrease inflammation, suppress mitotic activity, and cause vasoconstriction

Drug Interactions

Increased Effect/Toxicity: No data reported

Decreased Effect: No data reported

Pharmacodynamics/Kinetics

Absorption: Percutaneous absorption is variable and dependent upon many factors including vehicle used, integrity of epidermis, dose, and use of occlusive dressings; small amounts enter circulatory system via skin

Metabolism: Hepatic

Excretion: Urine and feces

Pregnancy Risk Factor C

Clocortolone Pivalate *see* Clocortolone *on page 367*

Cloderm® *see* Clocortolone *on page 367*

Clofarabine (klo FARE a been)

U.S. Brand Names Clolar™

Generic Available No

(Continued)

Clofarabine *(Continued)*

Synonyms Clofarex; NSC606869

Pharmacologic Category Antineoplastic Agent, Antimetabolite (Purine Antagonist)

Use Treatment of relapsed or refractory acute lymphoblastic leukemia

Unlabeled/Investigational Use Adults: Relapsed and refractory acute myeloid leukemia (AML), chronic myeloid leukemia (CML) in blast phase, acute lymphocytic leukemia (ALL), myelodysplastic syndrome

Local Anesthetic/Vasoconstrictor Precautions No information available to require special precautions

Effects on Dental Treatment Key adverse event(s) related to dental treatment: Mucosal inflammation and gingival bleeding.

Common Adverse Effects

>10%:

Cardiovascular: Pericardial effusion (35%), tachycardia (34%), hypotension (29%), left ventricular systolic dysfunction (27%), edema (20%), flushing (18%), hypertension (11%)

Central nervous system: Headache (46%), pyrexia (41%), fatigue (36%) anxiety (22%), pain (19%), dizziness (16%), depression (11%), irritability (11%), lethargy (1%)

Dermatologic: Pruritus (47%), dermatitis (41%), petechiae (29%), erythema (18%), palmar-plantar erythrodysesthesia syndrome (13%), oral candidiasis (13%), cellulitis (11%)

Gastrointestinal: Vomiting (83%), nausea (75%), diarrhea (53%), abdominal pain (36%), anorexia (30%), constipation (21%), mucosal inflammation (18%), gingival bleeding (15%), sore throat (14%), appetite decreased (11%)

Genitourinary: Hematuria (17%)

Hematologic: Febrile neutropenia (57%)

Hepatic: ALT increased (44%), AST increased (38%), bilirubin increased (15%), hepatomegaly (15%), jaundice (15%)

Neuromuscular & skeletal: Rigors (38%), pain in limb (29%), myalgia (14%), back pain (13%), arthralgia (11%)

Respiratory: Epistaxis (31%), cough (19%), respiratory distress (14%), dyspnea (13%)

Miscellaneous: Infection (85%), injection site pain (14%), staphylococcal infection (13%), herpes simplex (11%)

1% to 10%:

Central nervous system: Somnolence (10%)

Gastrointestinal: Weight gain (10%)

Genitourinary: Creatinine increased (6%)

Neuromuscular & skeletal: Tremor (10%)

Respiratory: Pleural effusion (10%), pneumonia (10%), systemic inflammatory response syndrome (SIRS)/capillary leak syndrome

Miscellaneous: Transfusion reaction (10%), bacteremia (10%)

Mechanism of Action Clofarabine, a purine (deoxyadenosine) nucleoside analog, is metabolized to clofarabine 5'-triphosphate. Clofarabine 5'-triphosphate decreases cell replication and repair as well as causing cell death. To decrease cell replication and repair, clofarabine 5'-triphosphate competes with deoxyadenosine triphosphate for the enzymes ribonucleotide reductase and DNA polymerase. Cell replication is decreased when clofarabine 5'-triphosphate inhibits ribonucleotide reductase from reacting with deoxyadenosine triphosphate to produce deoxynucleotide triphosphate which is needed for DNA synthesis. Cell replication is also decreased when clofarabine 5'-triphosphate competes with DNA polymerase for incorporation into the DNA chain; when done during the repair process, cell repair is affected. To cause cell death, clofarabine 5'-triphosphate alters the mitochondrial membrane by releasing proteins, an inducing factor and cytochrome C.

Drug Interactions

Increased Effect/Toxicity: None known

Decreased Effect: None known

Pharmacodynamics/Kinetics

Distribution: V_d: 172 L/m²

Protein binding: 47%

Metabolism: Intracellulary by deoxycytidine kinase and mono- and diphosphokinases to active metabolite clofarabine 5'-triphosphate

Half-life elimination: ~5.2 hours

Excretion: Urine (49% to 60% unchanged)

Pregnancy Risk Factor D

Clofarex *see* Clofarabine *on page 367*

Clofazimine (kloe FA zi meen)

Related Information
  Tuberculosis *on page 1673*
U.S. Brand Names Lamprene® [DSC]
Canadian Brand Names Lamprene®
Generic Available No
Synonyms Clofazimine Palmitate
Pharmacologic Category Leprostatic Agent
Use Treatment of lepromatous leprosy including dapsone-resistant leprosy and lepromatous leprosy with erythema nodosum leprosum; multibacillary leprosy
Unlabeled/Investigational Use Investigational: Multidrug-resistant tuberculosis
Local Anesthetic/Vasoconstrictor Precautions No information available to require special precautions
Effects on Dental Treatment No significant effects or complications reported
Common Adverse Effects
  >10%:
    Dermatologic: Dry skin
    Gastrointestinal: Abdominal pain, nausea, vomiting, diarrhea
    Miscellaneous: Pink to brownish-black discoloration of the skin
  1% to 10%:
    Dermatologic: Rash, pruritus
    Endocrine & metabolic: Blood sugar elevated
    Gastrointestinal: Fecal discoloration
    Genitourinary: Discoloration of urine
    Ocular: Discoloration of conjunctiva; irritation, burning, and itching of the eyes
    Miscellaneous: Discoloration of sputum, sweat
Restrictions Clofazimine is no longer available through most U.S. pharmacies. Requests for clofazimine to treat leprosy should be directed to the National Hansen's Disease Program (a division of the U.S. Department of Health and Human Services), which holds the IND for this indication. The Administrative Officer may be contacted at 225-578-9861 (phone) or 225-578-9856 (fax). Requests for clofazimine to treat MDRTB must be directed to the Division of Special Pathogen and Immunologic Drug Products (HFD-590) at 301-827-2127 (phone). These requests will be distributed by single-patient INDs administered by the FDA. A physician must register as an investigator for this indication.
Mechanism of Action Binds preferentially to mycobacterial DNA to inhibit mycobacterial growth; also has some anti-inflammatory activity through an unknown mechanism
Drug Interactions
  Cytochrome P450 Effect: Inhibits CYP3A4 (weak)
  Decreased Effect: Combined use may decrease effect with dapsone (unconfirmed).
Pharmacodynamics/Kinetics
  Absorption: Variable (45% to 62%)
  Distribution: Highly lipophilic; deposited primarily in fatty tissue and cells of the reticuloendothelial system; taken up by macrophages throughout the body; distributed to breast milk, mesenteric lymph nodes, adrenal glands, subcutaneous fat, liver, bile, gallbladder, spleen, small intestine, muscles, bones, and skin; does not appear to cross blood-brain barrier; remains in tissues for prolonged periods
  Metabolism: Partially hepatic to two metabolites
  Half-life elimination: Terminal: 8 days; Tissue: 70 days
  Time to peak, serum: Chronic therapy: 1-6 hours
  Excretion: Primarily feces; urine (negligible amounts as unchanged drug); sputum, saliva, and sweat (small amounts)
Pregnancy Risk Factor C

Clofazimine Palmitate *see* Clofazimine *on page 369*
Clolar™ *see* Clofarabine *on page 367*
Clomid® *see* ClomiPHENE *on page 369*

ClomiPHENE (KLOE mi feen)

U.S. Brand Names Clomid®; Serophene®
Canadian Brand Names Clomid®; Milophene®; Serophene®
Generic Available Yes
  (Continued)

ClomiPHENE *(Continued)*

Synonyms Clomiphene Citrate

Pharmacologic Category Ovulation Stimulator

Use Treatment of ovulatory failure in patients desiring pregnancy

Unlabeled/Investigational Use Male infertility

Local Anesthetic/Vasoconstrictor Precautions No information available to require special precautions

Effects on Dental Treatment No significant effects or complications reported

Common Adverse Effects

>10%: Endocrine & metabolic: Hot flashes, ovarian enlargement

1% to 10%:

Cardiovascular: Thromboembolism

Central nervous system: Mental depression, headache

Endocrine & metabolic: Breast enlargement (males), breast discomfort (females), abnormal menstrual flow

Gastrointestinal: Distention, bloating, nausea, vomiting

Hepatic: Hepatotoxicity

Ocular: Blurring of vision, diplopia, floaters, after-images, phosphenes, photophobia

Mechanism of Action Induces ovulation by stimulating the release of pituitary gonadotropins

Drug Interactions

Decreased Effect: Decreased response when used with danazol. Decreased estradiol response when used with clomiphene.

Pharmacodynamics/Kinetics

Metabolism: Undergoes enterohepatic recirculation

Half-life elimination: 5-7 days

Excretion: Primarily feces; urine (small amounts)

Pregnancy Risk Factor X

Clomiphene Citrate *see* ClomiPHENE *on page 369*

ClomiPRAMINE *(kloe MI pra meen)*

U.S. Brand Names Anafranil®

Canadian Brand Names Anafranil®; Apo-Clomipramine®; CO Clomipramine; Gen-Clomipramine

Mexican Brand Names Anafranil®

Generic Available Yes

Synonyms Clomipramine Hydrochloride

Pharmacologic Category Antidepressant, Tricyclic (Tertiary Amine)

Use Treatment of obsessive-compulsive disorder (OCD)

Unlabeled/Investigational Use Depression, panic attacks, chronic pain

Local Anesthetic/Vasoconstrictor Precautions Use with caution; epinephrine and levonordefrin have been shown to have an increased pressor response in combination with TCAs

Effects on Dental Treatment Key adverse event(s) related to dental treatment: Xerostomia and changes in salivation (normal salivary flow resumes upon discontinuation). Long-term treatment with TCAs, such as clomipramine, increases the risk of caries by reducing salivation and salivary buffer capacity.

Common Adverse Effects

>10%:

Central nervous system: Dizziness, drowsiness, headache, insomnia, nervousness

Endocrine & metabolic: Libido changes

Gastrointestinal: Xerostomia, constipation, appetite increased, nausea, weight gain, dyspepsia, anorexia, abdominal pain

Neuromuscular & skeletal: Fatigue, tremor, myoclonus

Miscellaneous: Diaphoresis increased

1% to 10%:

Cardiovascular: Hypotension, palpitation, tachycardia

Central nervous system: Confusion, hypertonia, sleep disorder, yawning, speech disorder, abnormal dreaming, paresthesia, memory impairment, anxiety, twitching, coordination impaired, agitation, migraine, depersonalization, emotional lability, flushing, fever

Dermatologic: Rash, pruritus, dermatitis

Gastrointestinal: Diarrhea, vomiting

Genitourinary: Difficult urination

Ocular: Blurred vision, eye pain

Restrictions A medication guide concerning the use of antidepressants in children and teenagers can be found on the FDA website at http://www.fda.gov/

cder/Offices/ODS/labeling.htm. It should be dispensed to parents or guardians of children and teenagers receiving this medication.

Mechanism of Action Clomipramine appears to affect serotonin uptake while its active metabolite, desmethylclomipramine, affects norepinephrine uptake

Drug Interactions

Cytochrome P450 Effect: Substrate of CYP1A2 (major), 2C19 (major), 2D6 (major), 3A4 (minor); **Inhibits** CYP2D6 (moderate)

Increased Effect/Toxicity: The levels/effects of clomipramine may be increased by amiodarone, chlorpromazine, ciprofloxacin, delavirdine, fluconazole, fluoxetine, fluvoxamine, gemfibrozil, isoniazid, ketoconazole, miconazole, norfloxacin, ofloxacin, omeprazole, paroxetine, pergolide, quinidine, quinine, ritonavir, rofecoxib, ropinirole, ticlopidine, and other CYP1A2, 2C19, or 2D6 inhibitors. Clomipramine may increase the levels/effects of amphetamines, selected beta-blockers, dextromethorphan, fluoxetine, lidocaine, mirtazapine, nefazodone, paroxetine, risperidone, ritonavir, thioridazine, tricyclic antidepressants, venlafaxine, and other CYP2D6 substrates.

Clomipramine increases the effects of amphetamines, anticholinergics, lithium, other CNS depressants (sedatives, hypnotics, ethanol), chlorpropamide, tolazamide, phenothiazines, and warfarin. When used with MAO inhibitors or other serotonergic drugs, serotonin syndrome may occur. Serotonin syndrome has also been reported with ritonavir (rare). Pressor response to I.V. epinephrine, norepinephrine, and phenylephrine may be enhanced in patients receiving TCAs. (**Note:** Effect is unlikely with epinephrine or levonordefrin dosages typically administered as infiltration in combination with local anesthetics.) Combined use of beta-agonists or drugs which prolong QT_c (including quinidine, procainamide, disopyramide, cisapride, sparfloxacin, gatifloxacin, moxifloxacin) with TCAs may predispose patients to cardiac arrhythmias.

Decreased Effect: The levels/effects of clomipramine may be decreased by aminoglutethimide, carbamazepine, phenobarbital, phenytoin, rifampin, and other CYP1A2 or 2C19 inducers. Clomipramine may decrease the levels/effects of CYP2D6 prodrug substrates (eg, codeine, hydrocodone, oxycodone, tramadol). Clomipramine inhibits the antihypertensive response to bethanidine, clonidine, debrisoquin, guanadrel, guanethidine, guanabenz, and guanfacine. Cholestyramine and colestipol may decrease the absorption of clomipramine.

Pharmacodynamics/Kinetics

Absorption: Rapid

Metabolism: Hepatic to desmethylclomipramine (active); extensive first-pass effect

Half-life elimination: 20-30 hours

Pregnancy Risk Factor C

Clomipramine Hydrochloride *see* ClomiPRAMINE *on page 370*

Clonazepam (kloe NA ze pam)

U.S. Brand Names Klonopin®

Canadian Brand Names Alti-Clonazepam; Apo-Clonazepam®; Clonapam; Gen-Clonazepam; Klonopin®; Novo-Clonazepam; Nu-Clonazepam; PMS-Clonazepam; Rho®-Clonazepam; Rivotril®; Sandoz-Clonazepam

Mexican Brand Names Kenoket®; Rivotril®

Generic Available Yes

Pharmacologic Category Benzodiazepine

Dental Use Burning mouth syndrome

Use Alone or as an adjunct in the treatment of petit mal variant (Lennox-Gastaut), akinetic, and myoclonic seizures; petit mal (absence) seizures unresponsive to succimides; panic disorder with or without agoraphobia

Unlabeled/Investigational Use Restless legs syndrome; neuralgia; multifocal tic disorder; parkinsonian dysarthria; bipolar disorder; adjunct therapy for schizophrenia

Local Anesthetic/Vasoconstrictor Precautions No information available to require special precautions

Effects on Dental Treatment Key adverse event(s) related to dental treatment: Xerostomia and changes in salivation (normal salivary flow resumes upon discontinuation).

Significant Adverse Effects Reactions reported in patients with seizure and/or panic disorder. Frequency not defined.

Cardiovascular: Edema (ankle or facial), palpitation

Central nervous system: Amnesia, ataxia (seizure disorder ~30%; panic disorder 5%), behavior problems (seizure disorder ~25%), coma, confusion, (Continued)

Clonazepam *(Continued)*

depression, dizziness, drowsiness (seizure disorder ~50%), emotional lability, fatigue, fever, hallucinations, headache, hypotonia, hysteria, insomnia, intellectual ability reduced, memory disturbance, nervousness; paradoxical reactions (including aggressive behavior, agitation, anxiety, excitability, hostility, irritability, nervousness, nightmares, sleep disturbance, vivid dreams); psychosis, slurred speech, somnolence (panic disorder 37%), suicidal attempt, vertigo

Dermatologic: Hair loss, hirsutism, skin rash

Endocrine & metabolic: Dysmenorrhea, libido increased/decreased

Gastrointestinal: Abdominal pain, anorexia, appetite increased/decreased, coated tongue, constipation, dehydration, diarrhea, gastritis, gum soreness, nausea, weight changes (loss/gain), xerostomia

Genitourinary: Colpitis, dysuria, ejaculation delayed, enuresis, impotence, micturition frequency, nocturia, urinary retention, urinary tract infection

Hematologic: Anemia, eosinophilia, leukopenia, thrombocytopenia

Hepatic: Alkaline phosphatase increased (transient), hepatomegaly, transaminases increased (transient)

Neuromuscular & skeletal: Choreiform movements, coordination abnormal, dysarthria, muscle pain, muscle weakness, myalgia, tremor

Ocular: Blurred vision, eye movements abnormal, diplopia, nystagmus

Respiratory: Chest congestion, cough, bronchitis, hypersecretions, pharyngitis, respiratory depression, respiratory tract infection, rhinitis, rhinorrhea, shortness of breath, sinusitis

Miscellaneous: Allergic reaction, aphonia, dysdiadochokinesis, encopresis, "glassy-eyed" appearance, hemiparesis, lymphadenopathy

Restrictions C-IV

Dental Usual Dosing Burning mouth syndrome: Adults: Oral: 0.25-3 mg/day in 2 divided doses, in morning and evening

Dosage Oral:

Children <10 years or 30 kg: Seizure disorders:

Initial daily dose: 0.01-0.03 mg/kg/day (maximum: 0.05 mg/kg/day) given in 2-3 divided doses; increase by no more than 0.5 mg every third day until seizures are controlled or adverse effects seen

Usual maintenance dose: 0.1-0.2 mg/kg/day divided 3 times/day, not to exceed 0.2 mg/kg/day

Adults:

Burning mouth syndrome (dental use): 0.25-3 mg/day in 2 divided doses, in morning and evening

Seizure disorders:

Initial daily dose not to exceed 1.5 mg given in 3 divided doses; may increase by 0.5-1 mg every third day until seizures are controlled or adverse effects seen (maximum: 20 mg/day)

Usual maintenance dose: 0.05-0.2 mg/kg; do not exceed 20 mg/day

Panic disorder: 0.25 mg twice daily; increase in increments of 0.125-0.25 mg twice daily every 3 days; target dose: 1 mg/day (maximum: 4 mg/day)

Discontinuation of treatment: To discontinue, treatment should be withdrawn gradually. Decrease dose by 0.125 mg twice daily every 3 days until medication is completely withdrawn.

Elderly: Initiate with low doses and observe closely

Hemodialysis: Supplemental dose is not necessary

Mechanism of Action The exact mechanism is unknown, but believed to be related to its ability to enhance the activity of GABA; suppresses the spike-and-wave discharge in absence seizures by depressing nerve transmission in the motor cortex

Contraindications Hypersensitivity to clonazepam or any component of the formulation (cross-sensitivity with other benzodiazepines may exist); significant liver disease; narrow-angle glaucoma; pregnancy

Warnings/Precautions Use with caution in elderly or debilitated patients, patients with hepatic disease (including alcoholics), or renal impairment. Use with caution in patients with respiratory disease or impaired gag reflex or ability to protect the airway from secretions (salivation may be increased). Worsening of seizures may occur when added to patients with multiple seizure types. Concurrent use with valproic acid may result in absence status. Monitoring of CBC and liver function tests has been recommended during prolonged therapy.

Causes CNS depression (dose related) resulting in sedation, dizziness, confusion, or ataxia which may impair physical and mental capabilities. Patients must be cautioned about performing tasks which require mental alertness (eg, operating machinery or driving). Use with caution in patients receiving other CNS depressants or psychoactive agents. Effects with other sedative drugs or ethanol may be potentiated. Benzodiazepines have been associated with falls and traumatic injury and should be used with extreme caution in patients who are at risk of these events (especially the elderly).

Use caution in patients with depression, particularly if suicidal risk may be present. Use with caution in patients with a history of drug dependence. Benzodiazepines have been associated with dependence and acute withdrawal symptoms, including seizures, on discontinuation or reduction in dose. Acute withdrawal, including seizures, may be precipitated in patients after administration of flumazenil to patients receiving long-term benzodiazepine therapy.

Benzodiazepines have been associated with anterograde amnesia. Paradoxical reactions, including hyperactive or aggressive behavior, have been reported with benzodiazepines, particularly in adolescent/pediatric or psychiatric patients. Does not have analgesic, antidepressant, or antipsychotic properties.

Drug Interactions Substrate of CYP3A4 (major)

CNS depressants: Sedative effects and/or respiratory depression may be additive with CNS depressants; includes ethanol, barbiturates, narcotic analgesics, and other sedative agents; monitor for increased effect.

CYP3A4 inducers: CYP3A4 inducers may decrease the levels/effects of clonazepam. Example inducers include aminoglutethimide, carbamazepine, nafcillin, nevirapine, phenobarbital, phenytoin, and rifamycins.

CYP3A4 inhibitors: May increase the levels/effects of clonazepam. Example inhibitors include azole antifungals, clarithromycin, diclofenac, doxycycline, erythromycin, imatinib, isoniazid, nefazodone, nicardipine, propofol, protease inhibitors, quinidine, telithromycin, and verapamil.

Disulfiram: Disulfiram may inhibit the metabolism of clonazepam; monitor for increased benzodiazepine effect.

Levodopa: Therapeutic effects may be diminished in some patients following the addition of a benzodiazepine; limited/inconsistent data.

Oral contraceptives: May decrease the clearance of some benzodiazepines (those which undergo oxidative metabolism); monitor for increased benzodiazepine effect.

Theophylline: May partially antagonize some of the effects of benzodiazepines; monitor for decreased response; may require higher doses for sedation.

Valproic acid: The combined use of clonazepam and valproic acid has been associated with absence seizures.

Ethanol/Nutrition/Herb Interactions

Ethanol: Avoid ethanol (may increase CNS depression).

Food: Clonazepam serum concentration is unlikely to be increased by grapefruit juice because of clonazepam's high oral bioavailability.

Herb/Nutraceutical: St John's wort may decrease clonazepam levels. Avoid valerian, St John's wort, kava kava, gotu kola (may increase CNS depression).

Pharmacodynamics/Kinetics

Onset of action: 20-60 minutes

Duration: Infants and young children: 6-8 hours; Adults: ≤12 hours

Absorption: Well absorbed

Distribution: Adults: V_d: 1.5-4.4 L/kg

Protein binding: 85%

Metabolism: Extensively hepatic via glucuronide and sulfate conjugation

Half-life elimination: Children: 22-33 hours; Adults: 19-50 hours

Time to peak, serum: 1-3 hours; Steady-state: 5-7 days

Excretion: Urine (<2% as unchanged drug); metabolites excreted as glucuronide or sulfate conjugates

Pregnancy Risk Factor D

Lactation Enters breast milk/not recommended

Breast-Feeding Considerations Clonazepam enters breast milk; clinical effects on the infant include CNS depression, respiratory depression reported (no recommendation from the AAP).

Dosage Forms

Tablet: 0.5 mg, 1 mg, 2 mg

Tablet, orally disintegrating [wafer]: 0.125 mg, 0.25 mg, 0.5 mg, 1 mg, 2 mg

---

Clonidine (KLON i deen)

Related Information

Cardiovascular Diseases on page 1636

U.S. Brand Names Catapres®; Catapres-TTS®; Duraclon™

Canadian Brand Names Apo-Clonidine®; Carapres®; Dixarit®; Novo-Clonidine; Nu-Clonidine

Generic Available Yes: Tablet

(Continued)

Clonidine *(Continued)*

Synonyms Clonidine Hydrochloride

Pharmacologic Category Alpha$_2$-Adrenergic Agonist

Use Management of mild-to-moderate hypertension; either used alone or in combination with other antihypertensives

Orphan drug: Duraclon™: For continuous epidural administration as adjunctive therapy with intraspinal opiates for treatment of cancer pain in patients tolerant to or unresponsive to intraspinal opiates

Unlabeled/Investigational Use Heroin or nicotine withdrawal; severe pain; dysmenorrhea; vasomotor symptoms associated with menopause; ethanol dependence; prophylaxis of migraines; glaucoma; diabetes-associated diarrhea; impulse control disorder, attention-deficit/hyperactivity disorder (ADHD), clozapine-induced sialorrhea

Local Anesthetic/Vasoconstrictor Precautions No information available to require special precautions

Effects on Dental Treatment Key adverse event(s) related to dental treatment: Significant xerostomia (normal salivary flow resumes upon discontinuation), orthostatic hypotension, and abnormal taste.

Common Adverse Effects Incidence of adverse events is not always reported.

>10%:
>
> Central nervous system: Drowsiness (35% oral, 12% transdermal), dizziness (16% oral, 2% transdermal)
>
> Dermatologic: Transient localized skin reactions characterized by pruritus, and erythema (15% to 50% transdermal)
>
> Gastrointestinal: Dry mouth (40% oral, 25% transdermal)

1% to 10%:

> Cardiovascular: Orthostatic hypotension (3% oral)
>
> Central nervous system: Headache (1% oral, 5% transdermal), sedation (3% transdermal), fatigue (6% transdermal), lethargy (3% transdermal), insomnia (2% transdermal), nervousness (3% oral, 1% transdermal), mental depression (1% oral)
>
> Dermatologic: Rash (1% oral), allergic contact sensitivity (5% transdermal), localized vesiculation (7%), hyperpigmentation (5% at application site), edema (3%), excoriation (3%), burning (3%), throbbing, blanching (1%), papules (1%), and generalized macular rash (1%) has occurred in patients receiving transdermal clonidine.
>
> Endocrine & metabolic: Sodium and water retention, sexual dysfunction (3% oral, 2% transdermal), impotence (3% oral, 2% transdermal), weakness (10% transdermal)
>
> Gastrointestinal: Nausea (5% oral, 1% transdermal), vomiting (5% oral), anorexia and malaise (1% oral), constipation (10% oral, 1% transdermal), dry throat (2% transdermal), taste disturbance (1% transdermal), weight gain (1% oral)
>
> Genitourinary: Nocturia (1% oral)
>
> Hepatic: Liver function test (mild abnormalities, 1% oral)
>
> Miscellaneous: Withdrawal syndrome (1% oral)

Dosage

Children:

> Oral:
>
>> Hypertension: Initial: 5-10 mcg/kg/day in divided doses every 8-12 hours; increase gradually at 5- to 7-day intervals to 25 mcg/kg/day in divided doses every 6 hours; maximum: 0.9 mg/day
>>
>> Clonidine tolerance test (test of growth hormone release from pituitary): 0.15 mg/m^2 or 4 mcg/kg as single dose
>>
>> ADHD (unlabeled use): Initial: 0.05 mg/day; increase every 3-7 days by 0.05 mg/day to 3-5 mcg/kg/day given in divided doses 3-4 times/day (maximum dose: 0.3-0.4 mg/day)
>
> Epidural infusion: Pain management: Reserved for patients with severe intractable pain, unresponsive to other analgesics or epidural or spinal opiates: Initial: 0.5 mcg/kg/hour; adjust with caution, based on clinical effect

Adults:

> Oral:
>
>> Acute hypertension (urgency): Initial 0.1-0.2 mg; may be followed by additional doses of 0.1 mg every hour, if necessary, to a maximum total dose of 0.6 mg.
>>
>>> Unlabeled route of administration: Sublingual clonidine 0.1-0.2 mg twice daily may be effective in patients unable to take oral medication
>>
>> Hypertension: Initial dose: 0.1 mg twice daily (maximum recommended dose: 2.4 mg/day); usual dose range (JNC 7): 0.1-0.8 mg/day in 2 divided doses
>>
>> Nicotine withdrawal symptoms: 0.1 mg twice daily to maximum of 0.4 mg/day for 3-4 weeks

Transdermal: Hypertension: Apply once every 7 days; for initial therapy start with 0.1 mg and increase by 0.1 mg at 1- to 2-week intervals (dosages >0.6 mg do not improve efficacy); usual dose range (JNC 7): 0.1-0.3 mg once weekly

Note: If transitioning from oral to transdermal therapy, overlap oral regimen for 1-2 days; transdermal route takes 2-3 days to achieve therapeutic effects.

Epidural infusion: Pain management: Starting dose: 30 mcg/hour; titrate as required for relief of pain or presence of side effects; minimal experience with doses >40 mcg/hour; should be considered an adjunct to intraspinal opiate therapy

Elderly: Initial: 0.1 mg once daily at bedtime, increase gradually as needed

Dosing adjustment in renal impairment: Cl_{cr} <10 mL/minute: Administer 50% to 75% of normal dose initially

Dialysis: Not dialyzable (0% to 5%) via hemo- or peritoneal dialysis; supplemental dose not necessary

Mechanism of Action Stimulates alpha$_2$-adrenoceptors in the brain stem, thus activating an inhibitory neuron, resulting in reduced sympathetic outflow from the CNS, producing a decrease in peripheral resistance, renal vascular resistance, heart rate, and blood pressure; epidural clonidine may produce pain relief at spinal presynaptic and postjunctional alpha$_2$-adrenoceptors by preventing pain signal transmission; pain relief occurs only for the body regions innervated by the spinal segments where analgesic concentrations of clonidine exist

Contraindications Hypersensitivity to clonidine hydrochloride or any component of the formulation

Warnings/Precautions Gradual withdrawal is needed (over 1 week for oral, 2-4 days with epidural) if drug needs to be stopped. Patients should be instructed about abrupt discontinuation (causes rapid increase in BP and symptoms of sympathetic overactivity). In patients on both a beta-blocker and clonidine where withdrawal of clonidine is necessary, withdraw the beta-blocker first and several days before clonidine. Then slowly decrease clonidine.

Use with caution in patients with severe coronary insufficiency; conduction disturbances; recent MI, CVA, or chronic renal insufficiency. Caution in sinus node dysfunction. Discontinue within 4 hours of surgery then restart as soon as possible after. Clonidine injection should be administered via a continuous epidural infusion device. Epidural clonidine is not recommended for perioperative, obstetrical, or postpartum pain. It is not recommended for use in patients with severe cardiovascular disease or hemodynamic instability. In all cases, the epidural may lead to cardiovascular instability (hypotension, bradycardia). Transdermal patch may contain conducting metal (eg, aluminum); remove patch prior to MRI. Due to the potential for altered electrical conductivity, remove transdermal patch before cardioversion or defibrillation. Clonidine cause significant CNS depression and xerostomia. Caution in patients with pre-existing CNS disease or depression. Elderly may be at greater risk for CNS depressive effects, favoring other agents in this population.

Drug Interactions

Increased Effect/Toxicity: Concurrent use with antipsychotics (especially low potency), narcotic analgesics, or nitroprusside may produce additive hypotensive effects. Clonidine may decrease the symptoms of hypoglycemia with oral hypoglycemic agents or insulin. Alcohol, barbiturates, and other CNS depressants may have additive CNS effects when combined with clonidine. Epidural clonidine may prolong the sensory and motor blockade of local anesthetics. Clonidine may increase cyclosporine (and perhaps tacrolimus) serum concentrations. Beta-blockers may potentiate bradycardia in patients receiving clonidine and may increase the rebound hypertension of withdrawal. Tricyclic antidepressants may also enhance the hypertensive response associated with abrupt clonidine withdrawal.

Decreased Effect: Tricyclic antidepressants (TCAs) antagonize the hypotensive effects of clonidine.

Ethanol/Nutrition/Herb Interactions

Ethanol: Avoid ethanol (may increase CNS depression).

Herb/Nutraceutical: Avoid dong quai if using for hypertension (has estrogenic activity). Avoid ephedra, yohimbe, ginseng (may worsen hypertension). Avoid valerian, St John's wort, kava kava, gotu kola (may increase CNS depression).

Dietary Considerations Hypertensive patients may need to decrease sodium and calories in diet.

Pharmacodynamics/Kinetics

Onset of action: Oral: 0.5-1 hour; Transdermal: Initial application: 2-3 days

Duration: 6-10 hours

Distribution: V_d: Adults: 2.1 L/kg; highly lipid soluble; distributes readily into extravascular sites

(Continued)

Clonidine *(Continued)*

Protein binding: 20% to 40%

Metabolism: Extensively hepatic to inactive metabolites; undergoes enterohepatic recirculation

Bioavailability: 75% to 95%

Half-life elimination: Adults: Normal renal function: 6-20 hours; Renal impairment: 18-41 hours

Time to peak: 2-4 hours

Excretion: Urine (65%, 32% as unchanged drug); feces (22%)

Pregnancy Risk Factor C

Dosage Forms INJ, epidural solution [preservative free] (Duraclon™): 100 mcg/mL (10 mL); 500 mcg/mL (10 mL). **PATCH, transdermal** [once-weekly patch]: (Catapres-TTS®-1): 0.1 mg/24 hours (4s); (Catapres-TTS®-2): 0.2 mg/24 hours (4s); (Catapres-TTS®-3): 0.3 mg/24 hours (4s). **TAB** (Catapres®): 0.1 mg, 0.2 mg, 0.3 mg

---

Clonidine and Chlorthalidone (KLON i deen & klor THAL i done)

Related Information
Chlorthalidone *on page 332*
Clonidine *on page 373*

U.S. Brand Names Clorpres®; Combipres® [DSC]

Generic Available No

Synonyms Chlorthalidone and Clonidine

Pharmacologic Category Antihypertensive Agent, Combination

Use Management of mild-to-moderate hypertension

Local Anesthetic/Vasoconstrictor Precautions No information available to require special precautions

Effects on Dental Treatment No significant effects or complications reported

Common Adverse Effects See individual agents.

Drug Interactions
Increased Effect/Toxicity: See individual agents.
Decreased Effect: See individual agents.

Pharmacodynamics/Kinetics See individual agents.

Pregnancy Risk Factor C

Clonidine Hydrochloride *see* Clonidine *on page 373*

Clopidogrel (kloh PID oh grel)

Related Information
Cardiovascular Diseases *on page 1636*

U.S. Brand Names Plavix®

Canadian Brand Names Plavix®

Generic Available No

Synonyms Clopidogrel Bisulfate

Pharmacologic Category Antiplatelet Agent

Use Reduce atherosclerotic events (myocardial infarction, stroke, vascular deaths) in patients with atherosclerosis documented by recent myocardial infarction (MI), recent stroke, or established peripheral arterial disease; acute coronary syndrome (unstable angina or non-Q-wave MI) managed medically or through PCI (with or without stent)

Unlabeled/Investigational Use In aspirin-allergic patients, prevention of coronary artery bypass graft closure (saphenous vein)

Local Anesthetic/Vasoconstrictor Precautions No information available to require special precautions

Effects on Dental Treatment If a patient is to undergo elective surgery and an antiplatelet effect is not desired, clopidogrel should be discontinued 7 days prior to surgery only upon approval via a medical consult with prescribing physician. As with all drugs which may affect hemostasis, bleeding is associated with clopidogrel. Hemorrhage may occur at virtually any site; risk is dependent on multiple variables, including the concurrent use of multiple agents which alter hemostasis and patient susceptibility. See Dental Comment.

Common Adverse Effects As with all drugs which may affect hemostasis, bleeding is associated with clopidogrel. Hemorrhage may occur at virtually any site. Risk is dependent on multiple variables, including the concurrent use of multiple agents which alter hemostasis and patient susceptibility.

>10%: Gastrointestinal: The overall incidence of gastrointestinal events (including abdominal pain, vomiting, dyspepsia, gastritis and constipation) has been documented to be 27% compared to 30% in patients receiving aspirin.

3% to 10%:
Cardiovascular: Chest pain (8%), edema (4%), hypertension (4%)
Central nervous system: Headache (3% to 8%), dizziness (2% to 6%), depression (4%), fatigue (3%), general pain (6%)
Dermatologic: Rash (4%), pruritus (3%)
Endocrine & metabolic: Hypercholesterolemia (4%)
Gastrointestinal: Abdominal pain (2% to 6%), dyspepsia (2% to 5%), diarrhea (2% to 5%), nausea (3%)
Genitourinary: Urinary tract infection (3%)
Hematologic: Bleeding (major 4%; minor 5%), purpura (5%), epistaxis (3%)
Hepatic: Liver function test abnormalities (<3%; discontinued in 0.11%)
Neuromuscular & skeletal: Arthralgia (6%), back pain (6%)
Respiratory: Dyspnea (5%), rhinitis (4%), bronchitis (4%), cough (3%), upper respiratory infection (9%)
Miscellaneous: Flu-like syndrome (8%)
1% to 3%:
Cardiovascular: Atrial fibrillation, cardiac failure, palpitation, syncope
Central nervous system: Fever, insomnia, vertigo, anxiety
Dermatologic: Eczema
Endocrine & metabolic: Gout, hyperuricemia
Gastrointestinal: Constipation, GI hemorrhage, vomiting
Genitourinary: Cystitis
Hematologic: Hematoma, anemia
Neuromuscular & skeletal: Arthritis, leg cramps, neuralgia, paresthesia, weakness
Ocular: Cataract, conjunctivitis

Dosage Oral: Adults:
Recent MI, recent stroke, or established arterial disease: 75 mg once daily
Acute coronary syndrome: Initial: 300 mg loading dose, followed by 75 mg once daily (in combination with aspirin 75-325 mg once daily). **Note:** A loading dose of 600 mg has been used in some investigations; limited research exists comparing the two doses.
Prevention of coronary artery bypass graft closure (saphenous vein): Aspirin-allergic patients (unlabeled use): Loading dose: 300 mg 6 hours following procedure; maintenance: 50-100 mg/day
Dosing adjustment in renal impairment and elderly: None necessary

Mechanism of Action Blocks the ADP receptors, which prevent fibrinogen binding at that site and thereby reduce the possibility of platelet adhesion and aggregation

Contraindications Hypersensitivity to clopidogrel or any component of the formulation; active pathological bleeding such as PUD or intracranial hemorrhage; coagulation disorders

Warnings/Precautions Use with caution in patients who may be at risk of increased bleeding, including patients with peptic ulcer disease, trauma, or surgery. Consider discontinuing 5 days before elective surgery. Use caution in concurrent treatment with other antiplatelet drugs; bleeding risk is increased. Use with caution in patients with severe liver disease (experience is limited). Cases of thrombotic thrombocytopenic purpura (usually occurring within the first 2 weeks of therapy) have been reported; urgent referral to a hematologist is required.

Drug Interactions
Cytochrome P450 Effect: Substrate (minor) of CYP1A2, 3A4; **Inhibits** CYP2C9 (weak)
Increased Effect/Toxicity: At high concentrations, clopidogrel may interfere with the metabolism of amiodarone, cisapride, cyclosporine, diltiazem, fluvastatin, irbesartan, losartan, oral hypoglycemics, paclitaxel, phenytoin, quinidine, sildenafil, tamoxifen, torsemide, verapamil, and some NSAIDs which may result in toxicity. Clopidogrel and naproxen resulted in an increase of GI occult blood loss. Anticoagulants (warfarin, thrombolytics, drotrecogin alfa) or other antiplatelet agents may increase the risk of bleeding. Rifampin may increase the effects of clopidogrel (monitor).
Decreased Effect: Atorvastatin may attenuate the effects of clopidogrel; monitor. CYP3A4-inhibiting macrolide antibiotics may attenuate the effects of clopidogrel (including clarithromycin, erythromycin, and troleandomycin); monitor.

Ethanol/Nutrition/Herb Interactions Herb/Nutraceutical: Avoid cat's claw, dong quai, evening primrose, feverfew, garlic, ginger, ginkgo, red clover, horse chestnut, green tea, ginseng (all have additional antiplatelet activity).

Dietary Considerations May be taken without regard to meals.

Pharmacodynamics/Kinetics
Onset of action: Inhibition of platelet aggregation detected: 2 hours after 300 mg administered; after second day of treatment with 50-100 mg/day
(Continued)

Clopidogrel *(Continued)*

Peak effect: 50-100 mg/day: Bleeding time: 5-6 days; Platelet function: 3-7 days

Absorption: Well absorbed

Metabolism: Extensively hepatic via hydrolysis; biotransformation primarily to carboxyl acid derivative (inactive). The active metabolite that inhibits platelet aggregation has not been isolated.

Half-life elimination: ~8 hours

Time to peak, serum: ~1 hour

Excretion: Urine

Pregnancy Risk Factor B

Dosage Forms TAB, film coated: 75 mg

Dental Comment There is no scientific evidence to warrant the discontinuance of clopidogrel prior to dental surgery. Patients taking one clopidogrel tablet daily as an antithrombotic and who require dental surgery should be given special consideration in consultation with physician.

Selected Readings

Daniel NG, Goulet J, Bergeron M, et al, "Antiplatelet Drugs: Is There a Surgical Risk?" *J Can Dent Assoc*, 2002, 68(11):683-7.

Jeske AH, Suchko GD, ADA Council on Scientific Affairs and Division of Science, et al, "Lack of a Scientific Basis for Routine Discontinuation of Oral Anticoagulation Therapy Before Dental Treatment," *J Am Dent Assoc*, 2003, 134(11):1492-7.

Little JW, Miller CS, Henry RG, et al, "Antithrombotic Agents: Implications in Dentistry," *Oral Surg Oral Med Oral Pathol Oral Radiol Endod*, 2002, 93(5):544-51.

Scully C and Wolff A, "Oral Surgery in Patients on Anticoagulant Therapy," *Oral Surg Oral Med Oral Pathol Oral Radiol Endod*, 2002, 94(1):57-64.

Wynn RL, "Clopidogrel (Plavix): Dental Considerations of an Antiplatelet Drug," *Gen Dent*, 2001, 49(6):564-8.

Clopidogrel Bisulfate *see Clopidogrel on page 376*

Clorazepate *(klor AZ e pate)*

U.S. Brand Names Tranxene® SD™; Tranxene® SD™-Half Strength; Tranxene® T-Tab®

Canadian Brand Names Apo-Clorazepate®; Novo-Clopate

Mexican Brand Names Tranxene®

Generic Available Yes

Synonyms Clorazepate Dipotassium; Tranxene T-Tab®

Pharmacologic Category Benzodiazepine

Use Treatment of generalized anxiety disorder; management of ethanol withdrawal; adjunct anticonvulsant in management of partial seizures

Local Anesthetic/Vasoconstrictor Precautions No information available to require special precautions

Effects on Dental Treatment Key adverse event(s) related to dental treatment: Xerostomia (normal salivary flow resumes upon discontinuation). Many patients will experience drowsiness; orthostatic hypotension is possible. It is suggested that narcotic analgesics not be given for pain control to patients taking clorazepate due to enhanced sedation.

Common Adverse Effects Frequency not defined.

Cardiovascular: Hypotension

Central nervous system: Drowsiness, fatigue, ataxia, lightheadedness, memory impairment, insomnia, anxiety, headache, depression, slurred speech, confusion, nervousness, dizziness, irritability

Dermatologic: Rash

Endocrine & metabolic: Libido decreased

Gastrointestinal: Xerostomia, constipation, diarrhea, nausea, salivation decreased, vomiting, appetite increased or decreased

Neuromuscular & skeletal: Dysarthria, tremor

Ocular: Blurred vision, diplopia

Restrictions C-IV

Mechanism of Action Binds to stereospecific benzodiazepine receptors on the postsynaptic GABA neuron at several sites within the central nervous system, including the limbic system, reticular formation. Enhancement of the inhibitory effect of GABA on neuronal excitability results by increased neuronal membrane permeability to chloride ions. This shift in chloride ions results in hyperpolarization (a less excitable state) and stabilization.

Drug Interactions

Cytochrome P450 Effect: Substrate of CYP3A4 (major)

Increased Effect/Toxicity: Clorazepate potentiates the CNS depressant effects of narcotic analgesics, barbiturates, phenothiazines, ethanol, antihistamines, MAO inhibitors, sedative-hypnotics, and cyclic antidepressants. CYP3A4 inhibitors may increase the levels/effects of clorazepate; example inhibitors include azole antifungals, clarithromycin, diclofenac, doxycycline, erythromycin, imatinib, isoniazid, nefazodone, nicardipine, propofol, protease inhibitors, quinidine, telithromycin, and verapamil.

Decreased Effect: CYP3A4 inducers may decrease the levels/effects of clorazepate; example inducers include aminoglutethimide, carbamazepine, nafcillin, nevirapine, phenobarbital, phenytoin, and rifamycins.

Pharmacodynamics/Kinetics

Onset of action: 1-2 hours

Duration: Variable, 8-24 hours

Distribution: Crosses placenta; appears in urine

Metabolism: Rapidly decarboxylated to desmethyldiazepam (active) in acidic stomach prior to absorption; hepatically to oxazepam (active)

Half-life elimination: Adults: Desmethyldiazepam: 48-96 hours; Oxazepam: 6-8 hours

Time to peak, serum: ~1 hour

Excretion: Primarily urine

Pregnancy Risk Factor D

Clorazepate Dipotassium *see* Clorazepate *on page 378*

Clorpactin® WCS-90 [OTC] *see* Oxychlorosene *on page 1163*

Clorpres® *see* Clonidine and Chlorthalidone *on page 376*

Clotrimazole (kloe TRIM a zole)

Related Information

Fungal Infections *on page 1707*

Sexually-Transmitted Diseases *on page 1674*

Related Sample Prescriptions

Topical Fungal Infections *on page 1740*

U.S. Brand Names Cruex® Cream [OTC]; Gyne-Lotrimin® 3 [OTC]; Lotrimin® AF Athlete's Foot Cream [OTC]; Lotrimin® AF Athlete's Foot Solution [OTC]; Lotrimin® AF Jock Itch Cream [OTC]; Mycelex®; Mycelex®-7 [OTC]; Mycelex® Twin Pack [OTC]

Canadian Brand Names Canesten® Topical; Canesten® Vaginal; Clotrimaderm; Trivagizole-3®

Mexican Brand Names Altenal®; Candimon®; Lotrimin®

Generic Available Yes: Cream, solution, troche

Pharmacologic Category Antifungal Agent, Oral Nonabsorbed; Antifungal Agent, Topical; Antifungal Agent, Vaginal

Dental Use Treatment of susceptible fungal infections, including oropharyngeal candidiasis; limited data suggests that the use of clotrimazole troches may be effective for prophylaxis against oropharyngeal candidiasis in neutropenic patients

Use Treatment of susceptible fungal infections, including oropharyngeal candidiasis, dermatophytoses, superficial mycoses, and cutaneous candidiasis, as well as vulvovaginal candidiasis; limited data suggest that clotrimazole troches may be effective for prophylaxis against oropharyngeal candidiasis in neutropenic patients

Local Anesthetic/Vasoconstrictor Precautions No information available to require special precautions

Effects on Dental Treatment No significant effects or complications reported

Significant Adverse Effects

Oral:

>10%: Hepatic: Abnormal liver function tests

1% to 10%:

Gastrointestinal: Nausea and vomiting may occur in patients on clotrimazole troches

Local: Mild burning, irritation, stinging to skin or vaginal area

Vaginal:

1% to 10%: Genitourinary: Vulvar/vaginal burning

<1% (Limited to important or life-threatening): Burning or itching of penis of sexual partner; polyuria; vulvar itching, soreness, edema, or discharge

Dental Usual Dosing

Oropharyngeal candidiasis: Children >3 years and Adults: Oral:

Prophylaxis: 10 mg troche dissolved 3 times/day for the duration of chemotherapy or until steroids are reduced to maintenance levels

Treatment: 10 mg troche dissolved slowly 5 times/day for 14 consecutive days

Cutaneous candidiasis: Children >3 years and Adults: Topical (cream, solution): Apply twice daily; if no improvement occurs after 4 weeks of therapy, re-evaluate diagnosis.

(Continued)

Clotrimazole *(Continued)*

Dosage

Children >3 years and Adults:

Oral:

Prophylaxis: 10 mg troche dissolved 3 times/day for the duration of chemotherapy or until steroids are reduced to maintenance levels

Treatment: 10 mg troche dissolved slowly 5 times/day for 14 consecutive
days

Topical (cream, solution): Apply twice daily; if no improvement occurs after 4
weeks of therapy, re-evaluate diagnosis

Children >12 years and Adults:

Vaginal:

Cream:

1%: Insert 1 applicatorful vaginal cream daily (preferably at bedtime) for 7
consecutive days

2%: Insert 1 applicatorful vaginal cream daily (preferably at bedtime) for 3
consecutive days

Tablet: Insert 100 mg/day for 7 days or 500 mg single dose

Topical (cream, solution): Apply to affected area twice daily (morning and
evening) for 7 consecutive days

Mechanism of Action Binds to phospholipids in the fungal cell membrane
altering cell wall permeability resulting in loss of essential intracellular elements

Contraindications Hypersensitivity to clotrimazole or any component of the
formulation

Warnings/Precautions Clotrimazole should not be used for treatment of
systemic fungal infection. Safety and effectiveness of clotrimazole lozenges
(troches) in children <3 years of age have not been established. When using
topical formulation, avoid contact with eyes.

Drug Interactions Inhibits CYP1A2 (weak), 2A6 (weak), 2B6 (weak), 2C8
(weak), 2C9 (weak), 2C19 (weak), 2D6 (weak), 2E1 (weak), 3A4 (moderate)

CYP3A4 substrates: Clotrimazole may increase the levels/effects of CYP3A4
substrates. Example substrates include benzodiazepines, calcium channel
blockers, cyclosporine, mirtazapine, nateglinide, nefazodone, sildenafil (and
other PDE-5 inhibitors), tacrolimus, and venlafaxine. Selected benzodiazepines (midazolam and triazolam), cisapride, ergot alkaloids, selected
HMG-CoA reductase inhibitors (lovastatin and simvastatin), and pimozide are
generally contraindicated with strong CYP3A4 inhibitors.

Pharmacodynamics/Kinetics

Absorption: Topical: Negligible through intact skin

Time to peak, serum:

Oral topical (troche): Salivary levels occur within 3 hours following 30 minutes
of dissolution time

Vaginal cream: High vaginal levels: 8-24 hours

Vaginal tablet: High vaginal levels: 1-2 days

Excretion: Feces (as metabolites)

Pregnancy Risk Factor B (topical); C (troches)

Lactation Excretion in breast milk unknown

Dosage Forms

Combination pack (Mycelex®-7): Vaginal tablet 100 mg (7s) and vaginal cream
1% (7 g)

Cream, topical: 1% (15 g, 30 g, 45 g)

Cruex®: 1% (15 g)

Lotrimin® AF Athlete's Foot: 1% (12 g, 24 g)

Lotrimin® AF Jock Itch: 1% (12 g)

Cream, vaginal: 2% (21 g)

Mycelex®-7: 1% (45 g)

Solution, topical: 1% (10 mL, 30 mL)

Lotrimin® AF Athlete's Foot: 1% (10 mL)

Tablet, vaginal (Gyne-Lotrimin® 3): 200 mg (3s)

Troche (Mycelex®): 10 mg

Clotrimazole and Betamethasone *see* Betamethasone and Clotrimazole *on
page 202*

Cloxacillin *(kloks a SIL in)*

Canadian Brand Names Apo-Cloxi®; Novo-Cloxin; Nu-Cloxi; Riva-Cloxacillin

Generic Available Yes

Synonyms Cloxacillin Sodium

Pharmacologic Category Antibiotic, Penicillin

Dental Use Treatment of susceptible orofacial infections (notably penicillinase-producing staphylococci)

Use Treatment of susceptible bacterial infections, notably penicillinase-producing staphylococci causing respiratory tract, skin and skin structure, bone and joint, urinary tract infections

Local Anesthetic/Vasoconstrictor Precautions No information available to require special precautions

Effects on Dental Treatment Key adverse event(s) related to dental treatment: Prolonged use of penicillins may lead to development of oral candidiasis.

Significant Adverse Effects

1% to 10%: Gastrointestinal: Nausea, diarrhea, abdominal pain

<1% (Limited to important or life-threatening): Agranulocytosis, anemia, BUN increased, creatinine increased, eosinophilia, fever, hematuria, hemolytic anemia, hepatotoxicity, hypersensitivity, interstitial nephritis, leukopenia, neutropenia, PT prolonged, pseudomembranous colitis, rash (maculopapular to exfoliative), seizure with extremely high doses and/or renal failure, serum sickness-like reactions, thrombocytopenia, transient elevated LFTs, vaginitis, vomiting

Restrictions Not available in U.S.

Dental Usual Dosing Susceptible orofacial infections: Children >20 kg and Adults: Oral: 250-500 mg every 6 hours

Dosage

Usual dosage range:

Children >1 month and <20 kg: Oral: 50-100 mg/kg/day in divided doses every 6 hours; (maximum: 4 g/day)

Children >20 kg and Adults: Oral: 250-500 mg every 6 hours

Hemodialysis: Not dialyzable (0% to 5%)

Mechanism of Action Inhibits bacterial cell wall synthesis by binding to one or more of the penicillin-binding proteins (PBPs) which in turn inhibits the final transpeptidation step of peptidoglycan synthesis in bacterial cell walls, thus inhibiting cell wall biosynthesis. Bacteria eventually lyse due to ongoing activity of cell wall autolytic enzymes (autolysins and murein hydrolases) while cell wall assembly is arrested.

Contraindications Hypersensitivity to cloxacillin, any component of the formulation, or penicillins

Warnings/Precautions Monitor PT if patient is concurrently on warfarin. Elimination of drug is slow in renally impaired. Use with caution in patients allergic to cephalosporins due to a low incidence of cross-hypersensitivity.

Drug Interactions

Methotrexate: Penicillins may increase the exposure to methotrexate during concurrent therapy; monitor.

Oral contraceptives: Anecdotal reports suggesting decreased contraceptive efficacy with penicillins have been refuted by more rigorous scientific and clinical data.

Probenecid, disulfiram: May increase levels of penicillins (cloxacillin).

Warfarin: Effects of warfarin may be increased.

Dietary Considerations Should be taken 1 hour before or 2 hours after meals with water.

Sodium content of 250 mg capsule: 13.8 mg (0.6 mEq)

Sodium content of suspension 5 mL of 125 mg/5 mL: 11 mg (0.48 mEq)

Pharmacodynamics/Kinetics

Absorption: Oral: ~50%

Distribution: Widely to most body fluids and bone; penetration into cells, into eye, and across normal meninges is poor; crosses placenta; enters breast milk; inflammation increases amount that crosses blood-brain barrier

Protein binding: 90% to 98%

Metabolism: Extensively hepatic to active and inactive metabolites

Half-life elimination: 0.5-1.5 hours; prolonged with renal impairment and in neonates

Time to peak, serum: 0.5-2 hours

Excretion: Urine and feces

Pregnancy Risk Factor B

Lactation Excretion in breast milk unknown

Breast-Feeding Considerations No data reported; however, other penicillins may be taken while breast-feeding.

Dosage Forms

Capsule, as sodium: 250 mg, 500 mg

Powder for oral suspension, as sodium: 125 mg/5 mL (100 mL, 200 mL)

Cloxacillin Sodium see Cloxacillin on page 380

Clozapine (KLOE za peen)

U.S. Brand Names Clozaril®; FazaClo®
Canadian Brand Names Apo-Clozapine®; Clozaril®; Gen-Clozapine
Generic Available Yes
Pharmacologic Category Antipsychotic Agent, Atypical
Use Treatment-refractory schizophrenia; to reduce risk of recurrent suicidal behavior in schizophrenia or schizoaffective disorder
Unlabeled/Investigational Use Schizoaffective disorder, bipolar disorder, childhood psychosis, severe obsessive-compulsive disorder
Local Anesthetic/Vasoconstrictor Precautions Most pharmacology textbooks state that in presence of phenothiazines, systemic doses of epinephrine paradoxically decrease the blood pressure. This is the so called "epinephrine reversal" phenomenon. This has never been observed when epinephrine is given by infiltration as part of the local anesthesia procedure.
Effects on Dental Treatment Key adverse event(s) related to dental treatment: Sialorrhea and xerostomia (normal salivary flow resumes upon discontinuation). Many patients may experience orthostatic hypotension with clozapine; precautions should be taken; do not use atropine-like drugs for xerostomia in patients taking clozapine due to significant potentiation.
Common Adverse Effects
>10%:
  Cardiovascular: Tachycardia (25%)
  Central nervous system: Drowsiness (39% to 46%), dizziness (19% to 27%), insomnia (2% to 20%)
  Gastrointestinal: Constipation (14% to 25%), weight gain (4% to 31%), sialorrhea (31% to 48%), nausea/vomiting (3% to 17%)
1% to 10%:
  Cardiovascular: Angina (1%), ECG changes (1%), hypertension (4%), hypotension (9%), syncope (6%)
  Central nervous system: Akathisia (3%), seizure (3%), headache (7%), nightmares (4%), akinesia (4%), confusion (3%), myoclonic jerks (1%), restlessness (4%), agitation (4%), lethargy (1%), ataxia (1%), slurred speech (1%), depression (1%), anxiety (1%)
  Dermatologic: Rash (2%)
  Gastrointestinal: Abdominal discomfort/heartburn (4% to 14%), anorexia (1%), diarrhea (2%), xerostomia (6%), throat discomfort (1%)
  Genitourinary: Urinary abnormalities (eg, abnormal ejaculation, retention, urgency, incontinence; 1% to 2%)
  Hematologic: Eosinophilia (1%), leukopenia, leukocytosis, agranulocytosis (1%)
  Hepatic: Liver function tests abnormal (1%)
  Neuromuscular & skeletal: Tremor (6%), hypokinesia (4%), rigidity (3%), hyperkinesia (1%), weakness (1%), pain (1%), spasm (1%)
  Ocular: Visual disturbances (5%)
  Respiratory: Dyspnea (1%), nasal congestion (1%)
  Miscellaneous: Diaphoresis increased, fever, tongue numbness (1%)
Restrictions Patient-specific registration is required to dispense clozapine. Monitoring systems for individual clozapine manufacturers are independent. If a patient is switched from one brand/manufacturer of clozapine to another, the patient must be entered into a new registry (must be completed by the prescriber and delivered to the dispensing pharmacy). Healthcare providers, including pharmacists dispensing clozapine, should verify the patient's hematological status and qualification to receive clozapine with all existing registries. The manufacturer of Clozaril® requests that healthcare providers submit all WBC/ANC values following discontinuation of therapy to the Clozaril National Registry for all nonrechallengable patients until WBC is ≥3500/mm^3 and ANC is ≥2000/mm^3.
Mechanism of Action Clozapine (dibenzodiazepine antipsychotic) exhibits weak antagonism of D_1, D_2, D_3, and D_5 dopamine receptor subtypes, but shows high affinity for D_4; in addition, it blocks the serotonin ($5HT_2$), alpha-adrenergic, histamine H_1, and cholinergic receptors
Drug Interactions
  Cytochrome P450 Effect: Substrate of CYP1A2 (major), 2A6 (minor), 2C9 (minor), 2C19 (minor), 2D6 (minor), 3A4 (minor); **Inhibits** CYP1A2 (weak), 2C9 (weak), 2C19 (weak), 2D6 (moderate), 2E1 (weak), 3A4 (weak)
  Increased Effect/Toxicity: May potentiate anticholinergic and hypotensive effects of other drugs. Benzodiazepines in combination with clozapine may produce respiratory depression and hypotension, especially during the first few weeks of therapy. May potentiate effect/toxicity of risperidone. Clozapine serum concentrations may be increased by inhibitors of CYP1A2; example

inhibitors include amiodarone, ciprofloxacin, fluvoxamine, ketoconazole, norfloxacin, ofloxacin, and rofecoxib. Clozapine may increase the levels/ effects of amphetamines, selected beta-blockers, substrates; example substrates include dextromethorphan, fluoxetine, lidocaine, mirtazapine, nefazodone, paroxetine, risperidone, ritonavir, thioridazine, tricyclic antidepressants, venlafaxine, and other CYP2D6 substrates. Sedative effects may be additive with other CNS depressants (eg, ethanol, barbiturates, benzodiazepines, narcotic analgesics, and other sedatives). Metoclopramide may increase risk of extrapyramidal symptoms (EPS). Acetylcholinesterase inhibitors (central) may increase the risk of antipsychotic-related EPS. Citalopram may increase the levels/effects of clozapine. Omeprazole may alter the concentrations/effects of clozapine.

Decreased Effect: Clozapine may decrease the levels/effects of CYP2D6 prodrug substrates; example prodrug substrates include codeine, hydrocodone, oxycodone, and tramadol. The levels/effects of clozapine may be decreased by carbamazepine, phenobarbital, primidone, rifampin, and other CYP1A2 inducers. Cigarette smoking (nicotine) may enhance the metabolism of clozapine. Clozapine may reverse the pressor effect of epinephrine (avoid in treatment of drug-induced hypotension). Omeprazole may alter the concentrations/effects of clozapine.

Pharmacodynamics/Kinetics

Protein binding: 97% to serum proteins

Metabolism: Extensively hepatic; forms metabolites with limited or no activity

Bioavailability: 12% to 81% (not affected by food)

Half-life elimination: Steady state: 12 hours (range: 4-66 hours)

Time to peak: 2.5 hours (range: 1-6 hours)

Excretion: Urine (~50%) and feces (30%) with trace amounts of unchanged drug

Pregnancy Risk Factor B

Clozaril® see Clozapine on page 382

CMA-676 see Gemtuzumab Ozogamicin on page 732

CNJ-016™ see Vaccinia Immune Globulin (Intravenous) on page 1553

Coagulant Complex Inhibitor see Anti-inhibitor Coagulant Complex on page 130

Coagulation Factor VIIa see Factor VIIa (Recombinant) on page 632

Coal Tar (KOLE tar)

U.S. Brand Names Balnetar® [OTC]; Betatar® Gel [OTC]; Cutar® [OTC]; Denorex® Original Therapeutic Strength [OTC]; DHS™ Tar [OTC]; DHS™ Targel [OTC]; Doak® Tar [OTC]; Exorex®; Fototar® [OTC]; Ionil T® [OTC]; Ionil T® Plus [OTC]; MG 217® [OTC]; MG 217® Medicated Tar [OTC]; Neutrogena® T/Gel [OTC]; Neutrogena® T/Gel Extra Strength [OTC]; Neutrogena® T/Gel Stubborn Itch Control [OTC]; Oxipor® VHC [OTC]; Polytar® [OTC]; PsoriGel® [OTC] [DSC]; Reme-T™ [OTC]; Tera-Gel™ [OTC]; Zetar® [OTC]

Canadian Brand Names Balnetar®; Estar®; Targel®

Generic Available No

Synonyms Crude Coal Tar; LCD; Pix Carbonis

Pharmacologic Category Topical Skin Product

Use Topically for controlling dandruff, seborrheic dermatitis, or psoriasis

Local Anesthetic/Vasoconstrictor Precautions No information available to require special precautions

Effects on Dental Treatment No significant effects or complications reported

Pregnancy Risk Factor C

Coal Tar and Salicylic Acid (KOLE tar & sal i SIL ik AS id)

Related Information

Coal Tar on page 383

Salicylic Acid on page 1374

U.S. Brand Names Tarsum® [OTC]; X-Seb T® Pearl [OTC]; X-Seb T® Plus [OTC]

Canadian Brand Names Sebcur/T®

Generic Available Yes

Synonyms Salicylic Acid and Coal Tar

Pharmacologic Category Topical Skin Product

Use Seborrheal dermatitis, dandruff, psoriasis

Local Anesthetic/Vasoconstrictor Precautions No information available to require special precautions

Effects on Dental Treatment No significant effects or complications reported

Pregnancy Risk Factor C

Cocaine (koe KANE)

Generic Available Yes

Synonyms Cocaine Hydrochloride

Pharmacologic Category Local Anesthetic

Use Topical anesthesia for mucous membranes

Local Anesthetic/Vasoconstrictor Precautions Although plain local anesthetic is not contraindicated, vasoconstrictor is absolutely contraindicated in any patient under the influence of or within 2 hours of cocaine use

Effects on Dental Treatment Key adverse event(s) related to dental treatment: Loss of taste perception. See Dental Comment.

Common Adverse Effects

>10%:

Central nervous system: CNS stimulation

Gastrointestinal: Loss of taste perception

Respiratory: Rhinitis, nasal congestion

Miscellaneous: Loss of smell

1% to 10%:

Cardiovascular: Heart rate (decreased) with low doses, tachycardia with moderate doses, hypertension, cardiomyopathy, cardiac arrhythmia, myocarditis, QRS prolongation, Raynaud's phenomenon, cerebral vasculitis, thrombosis, fibrillation (atrial), flutter (atrial), sinus bradycardia, CHF, pulmonary hypertension, sinus tachycardia, tachycardia (supraventricular), arrhythmia (ventricular), vasoconstriction

Central nervous system: Fever, nervousness, restlessness, euphoria, excitation, headache, psychosis, hallucinations, agitation, seizure, slurred speech, hyperthermia, dystonic reactions, cerebral vascular accident, vasculitis, clonic-tonic reactions, paranoia, sympathetic storm

Dermatologic: Skin infarction, pruritus, madarosis

Gastrointestinal: Nausea, anorexia, colonic ischemia, spontaneous bowel perforation

Genitourinary: Priapism, uterine rupture

Hematologic: Thrombocytopenia

Neuromuscular & skeletal: Chorea (extrapyramidal), paresthesia, tremor, fasciculations

Ocular: Mydriasis (peak effect at 45 minutes; may last up to 12 hours), sloughing of the corneal epithelium, ulceration of the cornea, iritis, mydriasis, chemosis

Renal: Myoglobinuria, necrotizing vasculitis

Respiratory: Tachypnea, nasal mucosa damage (when snorting), hyposmia, bronchiolitis obliterans organizing pneumonia

Miscellaneous: "Washed-out" syndrome

Restrictions C-II

Mechanism of Action Ester local anesthetic blocks both the initiation and conduction of nerve impulses by decreasing the neuronal membrane's permeability to sodium ions, which results in inhibition of depolarization with resultant blockade of conduction; interferes with the uptake of norepinephrine by adrenergic nerve terminals producing vasoconstriction

Drug Interactions

Cytochrome P450 Effect: Substrate of CYP3A4 (major); **Inhibits** CYP2D6 (strong), 3A4 (weak)

Increased Effect/Toxicity: Cocaine may increase the levels/effects of CYP2D6 substrates (eg, amphetamines, selected beta-blockers, dextromethorphan, fluoxetine, lidocaine, mirtazapine, nefazodone, paroxetine, risperidone, ritonavir, thioridazine, tricyclic antidepressants, venlafaxine). Increased toxicity with MAO inhibitors. Use with epinephrine may cause extreme hypertension and/or cardiac arrhythmias. CYP3A4 inhibitors may increase the levels/effects of cocaine (eg, azole antifungals, clarithromycin, diclofenac, doxycycline, erythromycin, imatinib, isoniazid, nefazodone, nicardipine, propofol, protease inhibitors, quinidine, telithromycin, verapamil).

Pharmacodynamics/Kinetics Following topical administration to mucosa:

Onset of action: ~1 minute

Peak effect: ~5 minutes

Duration (dose dependent): ≥30 minutes; cocaine metabolites may appear in urine of neonates up to 5 days after birth due to maternal cocaine use shortly before birth

Absorption: Well absorbed through mucous membranes; limited by drug-induced vasoconstriction; enhanced by inflammation

Distribution: Enters breast milk

Metabolism: Hepatic; major metabolites are ecgonine methyl ester and benzoyl ecgonine

Half-life elimination: 75 minutes

Excretion: Primarily urine (<10% as unchanged drug and metabolites)

Pregnancy Risk Factor C/X (nonmedicinal use)

Dental Comment The cocaine user, regardless of how the cocaine was administered, presents a potential life-threatening situation in the dental operatory. A patient under the influence of cocaine could be compared to a car going 100 mph. Blood pressure is elevated, heart rate is likely increased, and the use of a local anesthetic with epinephrine may result in a medical emergency. Such patients can be identified by their jitteriness, irritability, talkativeness, tremors, and short, abrupt speech patterns. These same signs and symptoms may also be seen in a normal dental patient with preoperative dental anxiety; therefore, the dentist must be particularly alert in order to identify the potential cocaine abuser. If cocaine use is suspected, the patient should never be given a local anesthetic with vasoconstrictor, for fear of exacerbating the cocaine-induced sympathetic response. Life-threatening episodes of cardiac arrhythmias and hypertensive crises have been reported when local anesthetic with vasoconstrictor was administered to a patient under the influence of cocaine. No local anesthetic, used by any dentist, can interfere with, nor test positive by cocaine in any urine testing screen. Therefore, the dentist does not need to be concerned with any false drug-use accusations associated with dental anesthesia.

Cocaine Hydrochloride see Cocaine on page 384

Codeine (KOE deen)

Related Information

Oral Pain on page 1692

Canadian Brand Names Codeine Contin®

Generic Available Yes

Synonyms Codeine Phosphate; Codeine Sulfate; Methylmorphine

Pharmacologic Category Analgesic, Narcotic; Antitussive

Dental Use Treatment of postoperative pain

Use Treatment of mild-to-moderate pain; antitussive in lower doses; dextromethorphan has equivalent antitussive activity but has much lower toxicity in accidental overdose

Local Anesthetic/Vasoconstrictor Precautions No information available to require special precautions

Effects on Dental Treatment No significant effects or complications reported (see Dental Comment)

Significant Adverse Effects

>10%:

Central nervous system: Drowsiness

Gastrointestinal: Constipation

1% to 10%:

Cardiovascular: Tachycardia or bradycardia, hypotension

Central nervous system: Dizziness, lightheadedness, false feeling of well being, malaise, headache, restlessness, paradoxical CNS stimulation, confusion

Dermatologic: Rash, urticaria

Gastrointestinal: Dry mouth, anorexia, nausea, vomiting

Hepatic: Transaminases increased

Genitourinary: Decreased urination, ureteral spasm

Local: Burning at injection site

Neuromuscular & skeletal: Weakness

Ocular: Blurred vision

Respiratory: Dyspnea

Miscellaneous: Physical and psychological dependence, histamine release

<1% (Limited to important or life-threatening): Convulsions, hallucinations, insomnia, mental depression, nightmares

Restrictions C-II

Dental Usual Dosing Postoperative pain: Adults: Oral: 30 mg every 4-6 hours as needed; patients with prior opiate exposure may require higher initial doses. Usual range: 15-120 mg every 4-6 hours as needed

Dosage Note: These are guidelines and do not represent the maximum doses that may be required in all patients. Doses should be titrated to pain relief/prevention. Doses >1.5 mg/kg body weight are not recommended.

(Continued)

Codeine *(Continued)*

Analgesic:

Children: Oral, I.M., SubQ: 0.5-1 mg/kg/dose every 4-6 hours as needed; maximum: 60 mg/dose

Adults:

Oral: 30 mg every 4-6 hours as needed; patients with prior opiate exposure may require higher initial doses. Usual range: 15-120 mg every 4-6 hours as needed

Oral, controlled release formulation (Codeine Contin®, not available in U.S.): 50-300 mg every 12 hours. **Note:** A patient's codeine requirement should be established using prompt release formulations; conversion to long acting products may be considered when chronic, continuous treatment is required. Higher dosages should be reserved for use only in opioid-tolerant patients.

I.M., SubQ: 30 mg every 4-6 hours as needed; patients with prior opiate exposure may require higher initial doses. Usual range: 15-120 mg every 4-6 hours as needed; more frequent dosing may be needed

Antitussive: Oral (for nonproductive cough):

Children: 1-1.5 mg/kg/day in divided doses every 4-6 hours as needed; Alternative dose according to age:

2-6 years: 2.5-5 mg every 4-6 hours as needed; maximum: 30 mg/day

6-12 years: 5-10 mg every 4-6 hours as needed; maximum: 60 mg/day

Adults: 10-20 mg/dose every 4-6 hours as needed; maximum: 120 mg/day

Dosing adjustment in renal impairment:

Cl_{cr} 10-50 mL/minute: Administer 75% of dose

Cl_{cr} <10 mL/minute: Administer 50% of dose

Dosing adjustment in hepatic impairment: Probably necessary in hepatic insufficiency

Mechanism of Action Binds to opiate receptors in the CNS, causing inhibition of ascending pain pathways, altering the perception of and response to pain; causes cough supression by direct central action in the medulla; produces generalized CNS depression

Contraindications Hypersensitivity to codeine or any component of the formulation; pregnancy (prolonged use or high doses at term)

Warnings/Precautions An opioid-containing analgesic regimen should be tailored to each patient's needs and based upon the type of pain being treated (acute versus chronic), the route of administration, degree of tolerance for opioids (naive versus chronic user), age, weight, and medical condition. The optimal analgesic dose varies widely among patients. Doses should be titrated to pain relief/prevention.

Use with caution in patients with hypersensitivity reactions to other phenanthrene derivative opioid agonists (morphine, hydrocodone, hydromorphone, levorphanol, oxycodone, oxymorphone); respiratory diseases including asthma, emphysema, COPD, or severe liver or renal insufficiency; some preparations contain sulfites which may cause allergic reactions; tolerance or drug dependence may result from extended use

Not recommended for use for cough control in patients with a productive cough; not recommended as an antitussive for children <2 years of age; the elderly may be particularly susceptible to the CNS depressant and confusion as well as constipating effects of narcotics

Not approved for I.V. administration (although this route has been used clinically). If given intravenously, must be given slowly and the patient should be lying down. Rapid intravenous administration of narcotics may increase the incidence of serious adverse effects, in part due to limited opportunity to assess response prior to administration of the full dose. Access to respiratory support should be immediately available

Drug Interactions Substrate of CYP2D6 (major), 3A4 (minor); **Inhibits** CYP2D6 (weak)

CYP2D6 inhibitors: May decrease the effects of codeine. Example inhibitors include chlorpromazine, delavirdine, fluoxetine, miconazole, paroxetine, pergolide, quinidine, quinine, ritonavir, and ropinirole.

Decreased effect with cigarette smoking

Increased toxicity: CNS depressants, phenothiazines, TCAs, other narcotic analgesics, guanabenz, MAO inhibitors, neuromuscular blockers

Ethanol/Nutrition/Herb Interactions

Ethanol: Avoid or limit ethanol (may increase CNS depression).

Herb/Nutraceutical: St John's wort may decrease codeine levels. Avoid valerian, St John's wort, kava kava, gotu kola (may increase CNS depression).

Pharmacodynamics/Kinetics

Onset of action: Oral: 0.5-1 hour; I.M.: 10-30 minutes

Peak effect: Oral: 1-1.5 hours; I.M.: 0.5-1 hour

Duration: 4-6 hours

Absorption: Oral: Adequate

Distribution: Crosses placenta; enters breast milk

Protein binding: 7%

Metabolism: Hepatic to morphine (active)

Half-life elimination: 2.5-3.5 hours

Excretion: Urine (3% to 16% as unchanged drug, norcodeine, and free and conjugated morphine)

Pregnancy Risk Factor C/D (prolonged use or high doses at term)

Lactation Enters breast milk/use caution (AAP rates "compatible")

Dosage Forms [CAN] = Canadian brand name

Injection, as phosphate: 15 mg/mL (2 mL); 30 mg/mL (2 mL) [contains sodium metabisulfite]

Solution, oral, as phosphate: 15 mg/5 mL (5 mL, 500 mL) [strawberry flavor]

Tablet, as phosphate: 30 mg, 60 mg

Tablet, as sulfate: 15 mg, 30 mg, 60 mg

Tablet, controlled release (Codeine Contin®) [CAN]: 50 mg, 100 mg, 150 mg, 200 mg [not available in U.S.]

Dental Comment It is recommended that codeine not be used as the sole entity for analgesia because of moderate efficacy along with relatively high incidence of nausea, sedation, and constipation. In addition, codeine has some narcotic addiction liability. Codeine in combination with acetaminophen or aspirin is recommended. Maximum effective analgesic dose of codeine is 60 mg (1 grain). Beyond 60 mg increases respiratory depression only. Sodium thiosulfate is an effective chemical antidote for codeine poisoning.

Selected Readings

Desjardins PJ, Cooper SA, Gallegos TL, et al, "The Relative Analgesic Efficacy of Propiram Fumarate, Codeine, Aspirin, and Placebo in Postimpaction Dental Pain," *J Clin Pharmacol*, 1984, 24(1):35-42.

Forbes JA, Keller CK, Smith JW, et al, "Analgesic Effect of Naproxen Sodium, Codeine, a Naproxen-Codeine Combination and Aspirin on the Postoperative Pain of Oral Surgery," *Pharmacotherapy*, 1986, 6(5):211-8.

Codeine, Acetaminophen, Butalbital, and Caffeine see Butalbital, Acetaminophen, Caffeine, and Codeine on page 239

Codeine and Acetaminophen see Acetaminophen and Codeine on page 35

Codeine and Bromodiphenhydramine see Bromodiphenhydramine and Codeine on page 223

Codeine and Butalbital Compound see Butalbital, Aspirin, Caffeine, and Codeine on page 241

Codeine and Guaifenesin see Guaifenesin and Codeine on page 753

Codeine and Promethazine see Promethazine and Codeine on page 1291

Codeine, Aspirin, and Carisoprodol see Carisoprodol, Aspirin, and Codeine on page 273

Codeine, Butalbital, Aspirin, and Caffeine see Butalbital, Aspirin, Caffeine, and Codeine on page 241

Codeine, Chlorpheniramine, and Pseudoephedrine see Chlorpheniramine, Pseudoephedrine, and Codeine on page 329

Codeine, Chlorpheniramine, Phenylephrine, and Potassium Iodide see Chlorpheniramine, Phenylephrine, Codeine, and Potassium Iodide on page 328

Codeine, Guaifenesin, and Pseudoephedrine see Guaifenesin, Pseudoephedrine, and Codeine on page 756

Codeine Phosphate see Codeine on page 385

Codeine Phosphate and Aspirin see Aspirin and Codeine on page 149

Codeine, Promethazine, and Phenylephrine see Promethazine, Phenylephrine, and Codeine on page 1293

Codeine, Pseudoephedrine, and Triprolidine see Triprolidine, Pseudoephedrine, and Codeine on page 1543

Codeine Sulfate see Codeine on page 385

Codeine, Triprolidine, and Pseudoephedrine see Triprolidine, Pseudoephedrine, and Codeine on page 1543

Codiclear® DH see Hydrocodone and Guaifenesin on page 785

Cod Liver Oil see Vitamin A and Vitamin D on page 1580

Cogentin® see Benztropine on page 196

Co-Gesic® see Hydrocodone and Acetaminophen on page 779

Cognex® see Tacrine on page 1436

Colace® [OTC] see Docusate on page 496

Colace® Adult/Children Suppositories [OTC] see Glycerin on page 747

Colace® Infant/Children Suppositories [OTC] see Glycerin on page 747

Colazal® see Balsalazide on page 179

ColBenemid see Colchicine and Probenecid on page 388

Colchicine (KOL chi seen)

Mexican Brand Names Colchiquim®

Generic Available Yes

Pharmacologic Category Colchicine

Use Treatment of acute gouty arthritis attacks and prevention of recurrences of such attacks

Unlabeled/Investigational Use Primary biliary cirrhosis; management of familial Mediterranean fever; pericarditis

Local Anesthetic/Vasoconstrictor Precautions No information available to require special precautions

Effects on Dental Treatment No significant effects or complications reported

Common Adverse Effects

>10%: Gastrointestinal: Nausea, vomiting, diarrhea, abdominal pain

1% to 10%:

Dermatologic: Alopecia

Gastrointestinal: Anorexia

Mechanism of Action Decreases leukocyte motility, decreases phagocytosis in joints and lactic acid production, thereby reducing the deposition of urate crystals that perpetuates the inflammatory response

Drug Interactions

Cytochrome P450 Effect: Substrate of CYP3A4 (major); **Induces** CYP2C8 (weak), 2C9 (weak), 2E1 (weak), 3A4 (weak)

Increased Effect/Toxicity: Concurrent use of cyclosporine with colchicine may increase toxicity of colchicine. CYP3A4 inhibitors may increase the levels/effects of colchicine (example inhibitors include azole antifungals, diclofenac, doxycycline, imatinib, isoniazid, nefazodone, nicardipine, propofol, protease inhibitors, quinidine, and verapamil. Macrolide antibiotics (clarithromycin, erythromycin, troleandomycin) and telithromycin may decrease the metabolism of colchicine resulting in severe colchicine toxicity; avoid, if possible. Verapamil may increase colchicine toxicity (especially nephrotoxicity).

Pharmacodynamics/Kinetics

Onset of action: Oral: Pain relief: ~12 hours if adequately dosed

Distribution: Concentrates in leukocytes, kidney, spleen, and liver; does not distribute in heart, skeletal muscle, and brain

Protein binding: 10% to 31%

Metabolism: Partially hepatic via deacetylation

Half-life elimination: 12-30 minutes; End-stage renal disease: 45 minutes

Time to peak, serum: Oral: 0.5-2 hours, declining for the next 2 hours before increasing again due to enterohepatic recycling

Excretion: Primarily feces; urine (10% to 20%)

Pregnancy Risk Factor C (oral); D (parenteral)

Colchicine and Probenecid (KOL chi seen & proe BEN e sid)

Related Information

Colchicine on page 388

Probenecid on page 1282

Generic Available Yes

Synonyms ColBenemid; Probenecid and Colchicine

Pharmacologic Category Anti-inflammatory Agent; Antigout Agent; Uricosuric Agent

Use Treatment of chronic gouty arthritis when complicated by frequent, recurrent acute attacks of gout

Local Anesthetic/Vasoconstrictor Precautions No information available to require special precautions

Effects on Dental Treatment No significant effects or complications reported

Common Adverse Effects 1% to 10%:

Cardiovascular: Flushing

Central nervous system: Headache, dizziness

Dermatologic: Rash, alopecia

Gastrointestinal: Anorexia, nausea, vomiting, diarrhea, abdominal pain

Hematologic: Anemia, leukopenia, aplastic anemia, agranulocytosis

Hepatic: Hepatic necrosis, hepatotoxicity

Neuromuscular & skeletal: Peripheral neuritis, myopathy

Renal: Nephrotic syndrome, uric acid stones, polyuria

Miscellaneous: Hypersensitivity reactions

Drug Interactions
 Cytochrome P450 Effect:
  Colchicine: **Substrate** of CYP3A4 (major); **Induces** CYP2C8 (weak), 2C9 (weak), 2E1 (weak), 3A4 (weak)
  Probenecid: **Inhibits** CYP2C19 (weak)
Pharmacodynamics/Kinetics See individual agents.
Pregnancy Risk Factor C

Coldcough PD *see* Dihydrocodeine, Chlorpheniramine, and Phenylephrine *on page 476*

Coldtuss DR *see* Chlorpheniramine, Phenylephrine, and Dextromethorphan *on page 326*

Colesevelam (koh le SEV a lam)

Related Information
  Cardiovascular Diseases *on page 1636*
U.S. Brand Names WelChol®
Canadian Brand Names WelChol®
Generic Available No
Pharmacologic Category Antilipemic Agent, Bile Acid Sequestrant
Use Adjunctive therapy to diet and exercise in the management of elevated LDL in primary hypercholesterolemia (Fredrickson type IIa) when used alone or in combination with an HMG-CoA reductase inhibitor
Local Anesthetic/Vasoconstrictor Precautions No information available to require special precautions
Effects on Dental Treatment No significant effects or complications reported
Common Adverse Effects
  >10%: Gastrointestinal: Constipation (11%)
  2% to 10%:
   Gastrointestinal: Dyspepsia (8%)
   Neuromuscular & skeletal: Weakness (4%), myalgia (2%)
   Respiratory: Pharyngitis (3%)
  Incidence less than or equal to placebo: Infection, headache, pain, back pain, abdominal pain, flu syndrome, flatulence, diarrhea, nausea, sinusitis, rhinitis, cough
Dosage Adult: Oral:
  Monotherapy: 3 tablets twice daily with meals or 6 tablets once daily with a meal; maximum dose: 7 tablets/day
  Combination therapy with an HMG-CoA reductase inhibitor: 4-6 tablets daily; maximum dose: 6 tablets/day
  Dosage adjustment in renal impairment: No recommendations made
  Dosage adjustment in hepatic impairment: No recommendations made
  Elderly: No recommendations made
Mechanism of Action Colesevelam binds bile acids including glycocholic acid in the intestine, impeding their reabsorption. Increases the fecal loss of bile salt-bound LDL-C
Contraindications Hypersensitivity to colesevelam or any component of the formulation; bowel obstruction
Warnings/Precautions Use caution in treating patients with serum triglyceride levels >300 mg/dL (excluded from trials). Safety and efficacy has not been established in pediatric patients. Use caution in dysphagia, swallowing disorders, severe GI motility disorders, major GI tract surgery, pregnancy, nursing mothers, and in patients susceptible to fat-soluble vitamin deficiencies (vitamins A,D,E and K). Minimal effects are seen on HDL-C and triglyceride levels. Secondary causes of hypercholesterolemia should be excluded before initiation.
Drug Interactions
  Increased Effect/Toxicity: Refer to Decreased Effect.
  Decreased Effect: Sustained-release verapamil AUC and C_{max} were reduced. Clinical significance unknown.
   Digoxin, lovastatin, metoprolol, quinidine, valproic acid, or warfarin absorption was not significantly affected with concurrent administration.
   Clinical effects of atorvastatin, lovastatin, and simvastatin were not changed by concurrent administration.
Dietary Considerations Should be taken with meal(s). Follow dietary guidelines.
Pharmacodynamics/Kinetics
  Onset of action: Peak effect: Therapeutic: ~2 weeks
  Absorption: Insignificant
  Excretion: Urine (0.05%) after 1 month of chronic dosing
Pregnancy Risk Factor B
(Continued)

Colesevelam *(Continued)*

Dosage Forms TAB, film coated: 625 mg

Selected Readings

Davidson MH, Dillon MA, Gordon B, et al, "Colesevelam Hydrochloride (Cholestagel): A New, Potent Bile Acid Sequestrant Associated With a Low Incidence of Gastrointestinal Side Effects," *Arch Intern Med*, 1999, 159(16):1893-900.

"Executive Summary of The Third Report of The National Cholesterol Education Program (NCEP) Expert Panel on Detection, Evaluation, And Treatment of High Blood Cholesterol In Adults (Adult Treatment Panel III)," *JAMA*, 2001, 285(19):2486-97.

Steinmetz KL, "Colesevelam Hydrochloride," *Am J Health Syst Pharm*, 2002, 59:932-9.

Colestid® *see* Colestipol *on page 390*

Colestipol *(koe LES ti pole)*

Related Information

Cardiovascular Diseases *on page 1636*

U.S. Brand Names Colestid®

Canadian Brand Names Colestid®

Generic Available No

Synonyms Colestipol Hydrochloride

Pharmacologic Category Antilipemic Agent, Bile Acid Sequestrant

Use Adjunct in management of primary hypercholesterolemia; regression of arteriosclerosis; relief of pruritus associated with elevated levels of bile acids; possibly used to decrease plasma half-life of digoxin in toxicity

Local Anesthetic/Vasoconstrictor Precautions No information available to require special precautions

Effects on Dental Treatment No significant effects or complications reported

Common Adverse Effects

>10%: Gastrointestinal: Constipation

1% to 10%:

Central nervous system: Headache, dizziness, anxiety, vertigo, drowsiness, fatigue

Gastrointestinal: Abdominal pain and distention, belching, flatulence, nausea, vomiting, diarrhea

Mechanism of Action Binds with bile acids to form an insoluble complex that is eliminated in feces; it thereby increases the fecal loss of bile acid-bound low density lipoprotein cholesterol

Drug Interactions

Decreased Effect: Colestipol can reduce the absorption of numerous medications when used concurrently. Give other medications 1 hour before or 4 hours after giving colestipol. Medications which may be affected include HMG-CoA reductase inhibitors, thiazide diuretics, propranolol (and potentially other beta-blockers), corticosteroids, thyroid hormones, digoxin, valproic acid, NSAIDs, loop diuretics, sulfonylureas, troglitazone (and potentially other agents in this class - pioglitazone and rosiglitazone).

Warfarin and other oral anticoagulants: Absorption is reduced by cholestyramine and may also be reduced by colestipol. Separate administration times (as detailed above).

Pharmacodynamics/Kinetics

Absorption: None

Excretion: Feces

Pregnancy Risk Factor C

Colestipol Hydrochloride *see* Colestipol *on page 390*

Colgate Total® *see* Triclosan and Fluoride *on page 1534*

Colistimethate *(koe lis ti METH ate)*

U.S. Brand Names Coly-Mycin® M

Canadian Brand Names Coly-Mycin® M

Generic Available Yes

Synonyms Colistimethate Sodium

Pharmacologic Category Antibiotic, Miscellaneous

Use Treatment of infections due to sensitive strains of certain gram-negative bacilli which are resistant to other antibacterials or in patients allergic to other antibacterials

Unlabeled/Investigational Use Used as inhalation in the prevention of *Pseudomonas aeruginosa* respiratory tract infections in immunocompromised patients, and used as inhalation adjunct agent for the treatment of *P. aeruginosa* infections in patients with cystic fibrosis and other seriously ill or chronically ill patients

Local Anesthetic/Vasoconstrictor Precautions No information available to require special precautions

Effects on Dental Treatment No significant effects or complications reported

Common Adverse Effects 1% to 10%:
Central nervous system: Vertigo, slurring of speech
Dermatologic: Urticaria
Gastrointestinal: GI upset
Respiratory: Respiratory arrest
Renal: Nephrotoxicity

Mechanism of Action Hydrolyzed to colistin, which acts as a cationic detergent which damages the bacterial cytoplasmic membrane causing leaking of intracellular substances and cell death

Drug Interactions
Increased Effect/Toxicity: Other nephrotoxic drugs, neuromuscular blocking agents.

Pharmacodynamics/Kinetics
Distribution: Widely, except for CNS, synovial, pleural, and pericardial fluids
Half-life elimination: 1.5-8 hours; Anuria: ≤2-3 days
Time to peak: ~2 hours
Excretion: Primarily urine (as unchanged drug)

Pregnancy Risk Factor C

Colistimethate Sodium see Colistimethate on page 390

CollaCote® see Collagen (Absorbable) on page 391

Collagen see Collagen Hemostat on page 392

Collagen (Absorbable) (KOL la jen, ab SORB able)

U.S. Brand Names CollaCote®; CollaPlug®; CollaTape®
Generic Available Yes
Pharmacologic Category Hemostatic Agent
Dental Use Control of bleeding created during dental surgery
Use Hemostatic
Local Anesthetic/Vasoconstrictor Precautions No information available to require special precautions
Effects on Dental Treatment No significant effects or complications reported
Significant Adverse Effects No data reported
Dental Usual Dosing Control of bleeding: Children and Adults: Topical: A sufficiently large dressing should be selected so as to completely cover the oral wound
Dosage Children and Adults: A sufficiently large dressing should be selected so as to completely cover the oral wound
Mechanism of Action The highly porous sponge structure absorbs blood and wound exudate. The collagen component causes aggregation of platelets which bind to collagen fibrils. The aggregated platelets degranulate, releasing coagulation factors that promote the formation of fibrin.
Contraindications No data reported
Warnings/Precautions Should not be used on infected or contaminated wounds
Drug Interactions No data reported
Lactation Compatible
Dosage Forms Wound dressing:
$^3/_8$" x $^3/_4$"
$^3/_4$" x 1 $^1/_2$"
1" x 3"

Collagen Absorbable Hemostat see Collagen Hemostat on page 392

Collagenase (KOL la je nase)

U.S. Brand Names Santyl®
Generic Available No
Pharmacologic Category Enzyme, Topical Debridement
Use Promotes debridement of necrotic tissue in dermal ulcers and severe burns
Orphan drug: Injection: Treatment of Peyronie's disease; treatment of Dupytren's disease
Local Anesthetic/Vasoconstrictor Precautions No information available to require special precautions
Effects on Dental Treatment No significant effects or complications reported
Common Adverse Effects Frequency not defined.
Local: Irritation, Pain and burning may occur at site of application
(Continued)

Collagenase (Continued)

Mechanism of Action Collagenase is an enzyme derived from the fermentation of *Clostridium histolyticum* and differs from other proteolytic enzymes in that its enzymatic action has a high specificity for native and denatured collagen. Collagenase will not attack collagen in healthy tissue or newly formed granulation tissue. In addition, it does not act on fat, fibrin, keratin, or muscle.

Drug Interactions

Decreased Effect: Enzymatic activity is inhibited by detergents, benzalkonium chloride, hexachlorophene, nitrofurazone, tincture of iodine, and heavy metal ions (silver and mercury).

Pregnancy Risk Factor C

Collagen Hemostat (KOL la jen HEE moe stat)

U.S. Brand Names Avitene®; Avitene® Flour; Avitene® Ultrafoam; Avitene® UltraWrap™; EndoAvitene®; Helistat®; Helitene®; Instat™; Instat™ MCH; SyringeAvitene™

Generic Available No

Synonyms Collagen; Collagen Absorbable Hemostat; MCH; Microfibrillar Collagen Hemostat

Pharmacologic Category Hemostatic Agent

Dental Use Adjunct to hemostasis when control of bleeding by ligature is ineffective or impractical

Use Adjunct to hemostasis when control of bleeding by ligature is ineffective or impractical

Local Anesthetic/Vasoconstrictor Precautions No information available to require special precautions

Effects on Dental Treatment No significant effects or complications reported

Significant Adverse Effects Frequency not defined.

Miscellaneous: Adhesion formation, allergic reaction, edema, foreign body reaction, hematoma, inflammation, potentiation of infection

Postmarketing and/or case reports: Numbness, pain, paralysis, subgaleal seroma; alveolalgia and transient laryngospasm with dental use

Dental Usual Dosing Hemostasis: Adults: Topical: Apply dry directly to source of bleeding; remove excess material after ~10-15 minutes

Dosage Apply dry directly to source of bleeding; remove excess material after ~10-15 minutes

Mechanism of Action Collagen hemostat is an absorbable topical hemostatic agent prepared from purified bovine corium collagen and shredded into fibrils. Physically, microfibrillar collagen hemostat yields a large surface area. Chemically, it is collagen with hydrochloric acid noncovalently bound to some of the available amino groups in the collagen molecules. When in contact with a bleeding surface, collagen hemostat attracts platelets which adhere to its fibrils and undergo the release phenomenon. This triggers aggregation of the platelets into thrombi in the interstices of the fibrous mass, initiating the formation of a physiologic platelet plug.

Contraindications Hypersensitivity to any component of the formulation; products of bovine origin; closure of skin incisions, contaminated wounds; application to bone surfaces to which prosthetic materials are attached with methylmethacrylate adhesives

Warnings/Precautions Pain, numbness, or paralysis have been reported if used near a bony or neural space and left inside patient; use minimum amount necessary to achieve hemostasis. Remove as much of agent as possible after hemostasis is achieved. Do not leave in a contaminated or infected space. Fragments of MCH may pass through filters of blood scavenging systems; avoid reintroduction of blood from operative sites treated with MCH. Not intended to treat systemic coagulation disorders. Not for use when origin of bleeding is unknown.

Drug Interactions No data reported

Pharmacodynamics/Kinetics

Onset: Hemostasis: 2-5 minutes

Absorption: ≥8 weeks

Dosage Forms

Pad (Instat™) [bovine derived]: 1 inch x 2 inch (24s); 3 inch x 4 inch (24s)

Powder:

Avitene® Flour [microfibrillar product, bovine derived]: 0.5 g, 1 g, 5 g

Helitene® [bovine derived]: 0.5 g, 1 g

Instat™ MCH [microfibrillar product, bovine derived]: 0.5 g, 1 g

SyringeAvitene™ [microfibrillar product, bovine derived, prefilled syringe]: 1 g

Sheet:
  Avitene® [microfibrillar product, bovine derived, nonwoven web]: 35 mm x 35 mm (1s); 70 mm x 35 mm (6s, 12s); 70 mm x 70 mm (6s, 12s)
  EndoAvitene® [microfibrillar product, bovine derived, preloaded applicator]: 5 mm diameter (6s); 10 mm diameter (6s)
Sponge:
  Avitene® Ultrafoam [microfibrillar product, bovine derived]: 2 cm x 6.25 cm x 7 mm (12s); 8 cm x 6.25 cm x 1 cm (6s); 8 cm x 12.5 cm x 1 cm (6s); 8 cm x 12.5 cm x 3 mm (6s)
  Avitene® UltraWrap™ [microfibrillar product, bovine derived]: 8 cm x 12.5 cm (6s)
  Helistat® [bovine derived]: 0.5 inch x 1 inch x 7 mm (18s) [packaged as 3 strips of 6 sponges]; 3 inch x 4 inch x 5 inch (10s)

CollaPlug® see Collagen (Absorbable) on page 391
CollaTape® see Collagen (Absorbable) on page 391
Colocort® see Hydrocortisone on page 793
Coly-Mycin® M see Colistimethate on page 390
Colyte® see Polyethylene Glycol-Electrolyte Solution on page 1253
CombiPatch® see Estradiol and Norethindrone on page 575
Combipres® [DSC] see Clonidine and Chlorthalidone on page 376
Combivent® see Ipratropium and Albuterol on page 857
Combivir® see Zidovudine and Lamivudine on page 1596
Combunox™ see Oxycodone and Ibuprofen on page 1170
Comhist® see Chlorpheniramine, Phenylephrine, and Phenyltoloxamine on page 328
Commit™ [OTC] see Nicotine on page 1109
Compazine see Prochlorperazine on page 1285
Compound E see Cortisone on page 395
Compound F see Hydrocortisone on page 793
Compound S see Zidovudine on page 1594
Compound S, Abacavir, and Lamivudine see Abacavir, Lamivudine, and Zidovudine on page 23
Compound W® [OTC] see Salicylic Acid on page 1374
Compound W® One Step Wart Remover [OTC] see Salicylic Acid on page 1374
Compoz® Nighttime Sleep Aid [OTC] see DiphenhydrAMINE on page 483
Compro™ see Prochlorperazine on page 1285
Comtan® see Entacapone on page 543
Comtrex® Flu Therapy Day/Night [OTC] see Acetaminophen, Chlorpheniramine, and Pseudoephedrine on page 43
Comtrex® Flu Therapy Nighttime [OTC] see Acetaminophen, Chlorpheniramine, and Pseudoephedrine on page 43
Comtrex® Maximum Strength Sinus and Nasal Decongestant [OTC] [DSC] see Acetaminophen, Chlorpheniramine, and Pseudoephedrine on page 43
Comtrex® Non-Drowsy Cold and Cough Relief [OTC] see Acetaminophen, Dextromethorphan, and Pseudoephedrine on page 44
Comtrex® Sore Throat Maximum Strength [OTC] see Acetaminophen on page 31
Conceptrol® [OTC] see Nonoxynol 9 on page 1124
Concerta® see Methylphenidate on page 1023
Condylox® see Podofilox on page 1251
Congestac® [OTC] see Guaifenesin and Pseudoephedrine on page 755

Conivaptan (koe NYE vap tan)

U.S. Brand Names Vaprisol®
Generic Available No
Synonyms Conivaptan Hydrochloride; YM087
Pharmacologic Category Vasopressin Antagonist
Use Treatment of euvolemic hyponatremia in hospitalized patients
Local Anesthetic/Vasoconstrictor Precautions No information available to require special precautions
Effects on Dental Treatment Key adverse event(s) related to dental treatment: Dry mouth, oral candidiasis.
Common Adverse Effects
  >10%:
    Central nervous system: Headache (12%)
(Continued)

Conivaptan *(Continued)*

Local: Injection site reactions including pain, erythema, phlebitis, swelling (53%)

1% to 10%:

Cardiovascular: Hypertension (6%), phlebitis (5%), atrial fibrillation (3%), hypotension (3%; orthostatic 6%)

Central nervous system: Fever (4%), confusion (4%), insomnia (3%), pain (2%)

Dermatologic: Erythema (3%)

Endocrine & metabolic: Hypokalemia (10%), hyper-/hypoglycemia (3%), hypomagnesemia (2%), hyponatremia (3%)

Gastrointestinal: Vomiting (7%), diarrhea (6%), constipation (5%), dry mouth (4%), nausea (4%), dehydration (2%), oral candidiasis (2%)

Genitourinary: Urinary tract infection (3%)

Hematologic: Anemia (4%)

Renal: Polyuria (5% to 6%), hematuria (2%)

Respiratory: Pneumonia (3%)

Miscellaneous: Thirst (10%)

Mechanism of Action Conivaptan is an arginine vasopressin (AVP) receptor antagonist with affinity for AVP receptor subtypes V_{1A} and V_2. The antidiuretic action of AVP is mediated through activation of the V_2 receptor, which functions to regulate water and electrolyte balance at the level of the collecting ducts in the kidney. Serum levels of AVP are commonly elevated in euvolemic or hypervolemic hyponatremia, which results in the dilution of serum sodium and the relative hyponatremic state. Antagonism of the V_2 receptor by conivaptan promotes the excretion of free water (without loss of serum electrolytes) resulting in net fluid loss, increased urine output, decreased urine osmolality, and subsequent restoration of normal serum sodium levels.

Drug Interactions

Cytochrome P450 Effect: Substrate of CYP3A4 (major); **Inhibits** CYP3A4 (strong)

Increased Effect/Toxicity: Conivaptan may increase the levels/effects of CYP3A4 substrates (eg, benzodiazepines, calcium channel blockers, clarithromycin, cyclosporine, erythromycin, estrogens, mirtazapine, nateglinide, nefazodone, nevirapine, protease inhibitors, tacrolimus, and venlafaxine) and digoxin. CYP3A4 inhibitors may increase the levels/effects of conivaptan; example inhibitors include ketoconazole, itraconazole, ritonavir, indinavir, and clarithromycin. Concurrent use of conivaptan and strong CYP3A4 inhibitors is contraindicated.

Decreased Effect: CYP3A4 inducers may decrease the levels/effects of conivaptan; example inducers include aminoglutethimide, carbamazepine, nafcillin, nevirapine, phenobarbital, phenytoin, and rifamycins.

Pharmacodynamics/Kinetics

Protein binding: 99%

Metabolism: Hepatic via CYP3A4 to four minimally-active metabolites

Half-life elimination: 6.7-8.6 hours

Excretion: Feces (83%); urine (12%)

Pregnancy Risk Factor C

Conivaptan Hydrochloride *see* Conivaptan *on page 393*

Conjugated Estrogen and Methyltestosterone *see* Estrogens (Esterified) and Methyltestosterone *on page 585*

Conray® *see* Iothalamate Meglumine *on page 855*

Conray® 30 *see* Iothalamate Meglumine *on page 855*

Conray® 43 *see* Iothalamate Meglumine *on page 855*

Conray® 400 *see* Iothalamate Sodium *on page 855*

Constulose® *see* Lactulose *on page 893*

Contac® Severe Cold and Flu/Non-Drowsy [OTC] *see* Acetaminophen, Dextromethorphan, and Pseudoephedrine *on page 44*

Contact® Cold [OTC] *see* Pseudoephedrine *on page 1309*

ControlRx® *see* Fluoride *on page 671*

Copaxone® *see* Glatiramer Acetate *on page 736*

Copegus® *see* Ribavirin *on page 1343*

Copolymer-1 *see* Glatiramer Acetate *on page 736*

Copper *see* Trace Metals *on page 1513*

Cordarone® *see* Amiodarone *on page 90*

Cordran® *see* Flurandrenolide *on page 681*

Cordran® SP *see* Flurandrenolide *on page 681*

Cordron-D NR *see* Carbinoxamine and Pseudoephedrine *on page 268*

Cordron-DM NR see Carbinoxamine, Pseudoephedrine, and Dextromethorphan on page 269

Coreg® see Carvedilol on page 275

Corfen DM see Chlorpheniramine, Phenylephrine, and Dextromethorphan on page 326

Corgard® see Nadolol on page 1079

Coricidin HBP® Chest Congestion and Cough [OTC] see Guaifenesin and Dextromethorphan on page 754

Coricidin HBP® Cold and Flu [OTC] see Chlorpheniramine and Acetaminophen on page 324

Corlopam® see Fenoldopam on page 641

Cormax® see Clobetasol on page 365

Correctol® Tablets [OTC] see Bisacodyl on page 209

Cortaid® Intensive Therapy [OTC] see Hydrocortisone on page 793

Cortaid® Maximum Strength [OTC] see Hydrocortisone on page 793

Cortaid® Sensitive Skin [OTC] see Hydrocortisone on page 793

Cortef® see Hydrocortisone on page 793

Corticool® [OTC] see Hydrocortisone on page 793

Corticotropin (kor ti koe TROE pin)

U.S. Brand Names H.P. Acthar® Gel
Generic Available No
Synonyms ACTH; Adrenocorticotropic Hormone; Corticotropin, Repository
Pharmacologic Category Corticosteroid, Systemic
Use Acute exacerbations of multiple sclerosis; diagnostic aid in adrenocortical insufficiency, severe muscle weakness in myasthenia gravis
Cosyntropin is preferred over corticotropin for diagnostic test of adrenocortical insufficiency (cosyntropin is less allergenic and test is shorter in duration)
Local Anesthetic/Vasoconstrictor Precautions No information available to require special precautions
Effects on Dental Treatment No significant effects or complications reported
Common Adverse Effects Frequency not defined.
Central nervous system: Insomnia, nervousness
Dermatologic: Hirsutism
Endocrine & metabolic: Diabetes mellitus
Gastrointestinal: Increased appetite, indigestion
Neuromuscular & skeletal: Arthralgia
Ocular: Cataracts
Respiratory: Epistaxis
Mechanism of Action Stimulates the adrenal cortex to secrete adrenal steroids (including hydrocortisone, cortisone), androgenic substances, and a small amount of aldosterone
Pregnancy Risk Factor C

Corticotropin, Repository see Corticotropin on page 395

Cortifoam® see Hydrocortisone on page 793

Cortisol see Hydrocortisone on page 793

Cortisone (KOR ti sone)

Related Information
Respiratory Diseases on page 1656
Triamcinolone on page 1526
Generic Available Yes
Synonyms Compound E; Cortisone Acetate
Pharmacologic Category Corticosteroid, Systemic
Use Management of adrenocortical insufficiency
Local Anesthetic/Vasoconstrictor Precautions No information available to require special precautions
Effects on Dental Treatment A compromised immune response may occur if patient has been taking systemic cortisone. The need for corticosteroid coverage in these patients should be considered before any dental treatment; consult with physician.
Common Adverse Effects
>10%:
Central nervous system: Insomnia, nervousness
Gastrointestinal: Increased appetite, indigestion
1% to 10%:
Dermatologic: Hirsutism
(Continued)

Cortisone *(Continued)*

Endocrine & metabolic: Diabetes mellitus
Neuromuscular & skeletal: Arthralgia
Ocular: Cataracts, glaucoma
Respiratory: Epistaxis

Mechanism of Action Decreases inflammation by suppression of migration of polymorphonuclear leukocytes and reversal of increased capillary permeability

Drug Interactions

Increased Effect/Toxicity: Estrogens may increase cortisone effects. Cortisone may increase ulcerogenic potential of NSAIDs, and may increase potassium deletion due to diuretics.

Decreased Effect: Enzyme inducers (barbiturates, phenytoin, rifampin) may decrease cortisone effects. Effect of live virus vaccines may be decreased. Anticholinesterase agents may decrease effect of cortisone.

Cortisone may decrease effects of warfarin and salicylates.

Pharmacodynamics/Kinetics

Onset of action: Peak effect: Oral: ~2 hours; I.M.: 20-48 hours
Duration: 30-36 hours
Absorption: Slow
Distribution: Muscles, liver, skin, intestines, and kidneys; crosses placenta; enters breast milk
Metabolism: Hepatic to inactive metabolites
Half-life elimination: 0.5-2 hours; End-stage renal disease: 3.5 hours
Excretion: Urine and feces

Pregnancy Risk Factor D

Cortisone Acetate see Cortisone on page 395

Cortisporin® Cream see Neomycin, Polymyxin B, and Hydrocortisone on page 1101

Cortisporin® Ointment see Bacitracin, Neomycin, Polymyxin B, and Hydrocortisone on page 177

Cortisporin® Ophthalmic see Neomycin, Polymyxin B, and Hydrocortisone on page 1101

Cortisporin® Otic see Neomycin, Polymyxin B, and Hydrocortisone on page 1101

Cortizone®-10 Maximum Strength [OTC] see Hydrocortisone on page 793

Cortizone®-10 Plus Maximum Strength [OTC] see Hydrocortisone on page 793

Cortizone®-10 Quick Shot [OTC] see Hydrocortisone on page 793

Cortrosyn® see Cosyntropin on page 396

Corvert® see Ibutilide on page 813

Corzide® see Nadolol and Bendroflumethiazide on page 1080

Cosmegen® see Dactinomycin on page 417

Cosopt® see Dorzolamide and Timolol on page 501

Cosyntropin *(koe sin TROE pin)*

U.S. Brand Names Cortrosyn®
Canadian Brand Names Cortrosyn®
Generic Available No
Synonyms Synacthen; Tetracosactide
Pharmacologic Category Diagnostic Agent
Use Diagnostic test to differentiate primary adrenal from secondary (pituitary) adrenocortical insufficiency
Local Anesthetic/Vasoconstrictor Precautions No information available to require special precautions
Effects on Dental Treatment No significant effects or complications reported
Common Adverse Effects Frequency not defined.
Cardiovascular: Bradycardia, hypertension, peripheral edema, tachycardia
Dermatologic: Rash
Local: Whealing with redness at the injection site
Miscellaneous: Anaphylaxis, hypersensitivity reaction
Mechanism of Action Stimulates the adrenal cortex to secrete adrenal steroids (including hydrocortisone, cortisone), androgenic substances, and a small amount of aldosterone
Pharmacodynamics/Kinetics Time to peak, serum: I.M., IVP: ~1 hour; plasma cortisol levels rise in healthy individuals within 5 minutes
Pregnancy Risk Factor C

Co-Trimoxazole see Sulfamethoxazole and Trimethoprim on page 1425

Coumadin® see Warfarin on page 1585

Covera-HS® *see* Verapamil *on page 1571*

Co-Vidarabine *see* Pentostatin *on page 1211*

Coviracil *see* Emtricitabine *on page 536*

Cozaar® *see* Losartan *on page 950*

CP-99,219-27 *see* Trovafloxacin *on page 1546*

CP358774 *see* Erlotinib *on page 560*

CPC *see* Cetylpyridinium *on page 309*

C-Phed Tannate *see* Chlorpheniramine and Pseudoephedrine *on page 325*

CPM *see* Cyclophosphamide *on page 403*

CPT-11 *see* Irinotecan *on page 860*

CPZ *see* ChlorproMAZINE *on page 329*

Crantex ER *see* Guaifenesin and Phenylephrine *on page 754*

Crantex HC *see* Hydrocodone, Phenylephrine, and Guaifenesin *on page 791*

Crantex LA *see* Guaifenesin and Phenylephrine *on page 754*

Creomulsion® Cough [OTC] *see* Dextromethorphan *on page 451*

Creomulsion® for Children [OTC] *see* Dextromethorphan *on page 451*

Creon® *see* Pancrelipase *on page 1183*

Creo-Terpin® [OTC] *see* Dextromethorphan *on page 451*

Crestor® *see* Rosuvastatin *on page 1370*

Cresylate® *see* m-Cresyl Acetate *on page 966*

Crinone® *see* Progesterone *on page 1289*

Critic-Aid Skin Care® [OTC] *see* Zinc Oxide *on page 1597*

Crixivan® *see* Indinavir *on page 829*

Crolom® *see* Cromolyn *on page 397*

Cromoglycic Acid *see* Cromolyn *on page 397*

Cromolyn (KROE moe lin)

Related Information
Respiratory Diseases *on page 1656*

U.S. Brand Names Crolom®; Gastrocrom®; Intal®; NasalCrom® [OTC]; Opticrom®

Canadian Brand Names Apo-Cromolyn®; Intal®; Nalcrom®; Nu-Cromolyn; Opticrom®

Generic Available Yes: Excludes aerosol, oral solution

Synonyms Cromoglycic Acid; Cromolyn Sodium; Disodium Cromoglycate; DSCG

Pharmacologic Category Mast Cell Stabilizer

Use
Inhalation: May be used as an adjunct in the prophylaxis of allergic disorders, including asthma; prevention of exercise-induced bronchospasm
Nasal: Prevention and treatment of seasonal and perennial allergic rhinitis
Oral: Systemic mastocytosis
Ophthalmic: Treatment of vernal keratoconjunctivitis, vernal conjunctivitis, and vernal keratitis

Unlabeled/Investigational Use Oral: Food allergy, treatment of inflammatory bowel disease

Local Anesthetic/Vasoconstrictor Precautions No information available to require special precautions

Effects on Dental Treatment Key adverse event(s) related to dental treatment:
Inhalation: Unpleasant taste.
Intranasal: Xerostomia (normal salivary flow resumes upon discontinuation).
Systemic: Glossitis, stomatitis, and unpleasant taste.

Common Adverse Effects
Inhalation: >10%: Gastrointestinal: Unpleasant taste in mouth
Nasal:
>10%: Respiratory: Increase in sneezing, burning, stinging, or irritation inside of nose
1% to 10%:
Central nervous system: Headache
Gastrointestinal: Unpleasant taste
Respiratory: Hoarseness, cough, postnasal drip
<1% (Limited to important or life-threatening): Anaphylactic reactions, epistaxis
Ophthalmic: Frequency not defined:
Ocular: Conjunctival injection, dryness around the eye, edema, eye irritation, immediate hypersensitivity reactions, itchy eyes, puffy eyes, styes, rash, watery eyes
Respiratory: Dyspnea
(Continued)

Cromolyn (Continued)

Systemic: Frequency not defined:

Cardiovascular: Angioedema, chest pain, edema, flushing, palpitation, premature ventricular contractions, tachycardia

Central nervous system: Anxiety, behavior changes, convulsions, depression, dizziness, fatigue, hallucinations, headache, irritability, insomnia, lethargy, migraine, nervousness, hypoesthesia, postprandial lightheadedness, psychosis

Dermatologic: Erythema, photosensitivity, pruritus, purpura, rash, urticaria

Gastrointestinal: Abdominal pain, constipation, diarrhea, dyspepsia, dysphagia, esophagospasm, flatulence, glossitis, nausea, stomatitis, unpleasant taste, vomiting

Genitourinary: Dysuria, urinary frequency

Hematologic: Neutropenia, pancytopenia, polycythemia

Hepatic: Liver function test abnormal

Local: Burning

Neuromuscular & skeletal: Arthralgia, leg stiffness, leg weakness, myalgia, paresthesia

Otic: Tinnitus

Respiratory: Dyspnea, pharyngitis

Miscellaneous: Lupus erythematosus

Mechanism of Action Prevents the mast cell release of histamine, leukotrienes and slow-reacting substance of anaphylaxis by inhibiting degranulation after contact with antigens

Pharmacodynamics/Kinetics

Onset: Response to treatment:

Nasal spray: May occur at 1-2 weeks

Ophthalmic: May be seen within a few days; treatment for up to 6 weeks is often required

Oral: May occur within 2-6 weeks

Absorption:

Inhalation: ~8% reaches lungs upon inhalation; well absorbed

Oral: <1% of dose absorbed

Half-life elimination: 80-90 minutes

Time to peak, serum: Inhalation: ~15 minutes

Excretion: Urine and feces (equal amounts as unchanged drug); exhaled gases (small amounts)

Pregnancy Risk Factor B

Cromolyn Sodium *see* Cromolyn *on page 397*

Crosseal™ *see* Fibrin Sealant Kit *on page 653*

Crotamiton (kroe TAM i tonn)

U.S. Brand Names Eurax®

Mexican Brand Names Eurax®

Generic Available No

Pharmacologic Category Scabicidal Agent

Use Treatment of scabies (*Sarcoptes scabiei*) and symptomatic treatment of pruritus

Local Anesthetic/Vasoconstrictor Precautions No information available to require special precautions

Effects on Dental Treatment No significant effects or complications reported

Common Adverse Effects Frequency not defined. Topical:

Dermatologic: Pruritus, contact dermatitis, rash

Local: Local irritation

Miscellaneous: Allergic sensitivity reactions, warm sensation

Mechanism of Action Crotamiton has scabicidal activity against *Sarcoptes scabiei*; mechanism of action unknown

Pregnancy Risk Factor C

Crude Coal Tar *see* Coal Tar *on page 383*

Cruex® Cream [OTC] *see* Clotrimazole *on page 379*

Cryselle™ *see* Ethinyl Estradiol and Norgestrel *on page 616*

Crystalline Penicillin *see* Penicillin G (Parenteral/Aqueous) *on page 1203*

Crystal Violet *see* Gentian Violet *on page 735*

Crystodigin *see* Digitoxin *on page 471*

CsA *see* CycloSPORINE *on page 406*

CSP *see* Cellulose Sodium Phosphate *on page 301*

CTLA-4Ig *see* Abatacept *on page 25*

CTM *see* Chlorpheniramine *on page 323*

CTX *see* Cyclophosphamide *on page 403*

Cubicin® *see* Daptomycin *on page 423*

Culturelle® [OTC] *see* Lactobacillus *on page 535*

Cuprimine® *see* Penicillamine *on page 1201*

Curasore® [OTC] *see* Pramoxine *on page 1264*

Curosurf® *see* Poractant Alfa *on page 1255*

Cutar® [OTC] *see* Coal Tar *on page 383*

Cutivate® *see* Fluticasone *on page 686*

CyA *see* CycloSPORINE *on page 406*

Cyanocobalamin (sye an oh koe BAL a min)

U.S. Brand Names Nascobal®; Twelve Resin-K
Generic Available Yes
Synonyms Vitamin B_{12}
Pharmacologic Category Vitamin, Water Soluble
Use Treatment of pernicious anemia; vitamin B_{12} deficiency due to malabsorption diseases, inadequaste secretion of intrinisic factor, and inadequate utilization of B_{12} (eg, during neoplastic treatment); increased B_{12} requirements due to pregnancy, thyrotoxicosis, hemorrhage, malignancy, liver or kidney disease
Local Anesthetic/Vasoconstrictor Precautions No information available to require special precautions
Effects on Dental Treatment No significant effects or complications reported
Significant Adverse Effects
>10%:
    Cardiovascular: Peripheral vascular disease
    Central nervous system: Headache (2% to 11%)
1% to 10%:
    Central nervous system: Anxiety, dizziness, pain, nervousness, hypoesthesia
    Dermatologic: Itching
    Gastrointestinal: Sore throat, nausea and vomiting, dyspepsia, diarrhea
    Neuromuscular & skeletal: Weakness (1% to 4%), back pain, arthritis, myalgia, paresthesia, abnormal gait, incoordination
    Respiratory: Dyspnea, rhinitis
    Miscellaneous: Infection
Frequency not defined: Peripheral vascular thrombosis, urticaria, anaphylaxis, CHF, pulmonary edema, polycythemia vera, transient exanthema
Dosage
Recommended daily allowance (RDA):
    Children: 0.9-2.4 mcg/day
    Adults: 2.4 mcg/day
        Pregnancy: 2.6 mcg/day
        Lactation: 2.8 mcg/day
Vitamin B_{12} deficiency:
    Intranasal: 500 mcg in one nostril once weekly
    Oral: 250 mcg/day
    I.M., deep SubQ:
        Children (dosage not well established): 0.2 mcg/kg for 2 days, followed by 1000 mcg/day for 2-7 days, followed by 100 mcg/week for one month; for malabsorptive causes of B_{12} deficiency, monthly maintenance doses of 100 mcg have been recommended **or** as an alternative 100 mcg/day for 10-15 days, then once or twice weekly for several months
        Adults: Initial: 30 mcg/day for 5-10 days; maintenance: 100-200 mcg/month
Pernicious anemia: I.M., deep SubQ (administer concomitantly with folic acid if needed, 1 mg/day for 1 month):
    Children: 30-50 mcg/day for 2 or more weeks (to a total dose of 1000-5000 mcg), then follow with 100 mcg/month as maintenance dosage
    Adults: 100 mcg/day for 6-7 days; if improvement, administer same dose on alternate days for 7 doses, then every 3-4 days for 2-3 weeks; once hematologic values have returned to normal, maintenance dosage: 100 mcg/month. **Note:** Alternative dosing of 1000 mcg/day for 5 days (followed by 500-1000 mcg/month) has been used.
Hematologic remission (without evidence of nervous system involvement):
    Intranasal gel: 500 mcg in one nostril once weekly
    Oral: 1000-2000 mcg/day
    I.M., SubQ: 100-1000 mcg/month
Schilling test: I.M.: 1000 mcg
Mechanism of Action Coenzyme for various metabolic functions, including fat and carbohydrate metabolism and protein synthesis, used in cell replication and hematopoiesis
(Continued)

Cyanocobalamin *(Continued)*

Contraindications Hypersensitivity to cyanocobalamin or any component of the formulation, cobalt; hereditary optic nerve atrophy (Leber's disease)

Warnings/Precautions I.M. route used to treat pernicious anemia; vitamin B_{12} deficiency for >3 months results in irreversible degenerative CNS lesions; treatment of vitamin B_{12} megaloblastic anemia may result in severe hypokalemia, sometimes fatal, due to intracellular potassium shift upon anemia resolution. B_{12} deficiency masks signs of polycythemia vera; vegetarian diets may result in B_{12} deficiency; pernicious anemia occurs more often in gastric carcinoma than in general population. Patients with Leber's disease may suffer rapid optic atrophy when treated with vitamin B_{12}; an intradermal test dose of parenteral B_{12} is recommended prior to administration of intranasal product in patients suspected of cyanocobalamin sensitivity; do not use folic acid as substitute for vitamin B_{12} in preventing anemia, as progression of spinal cord degeneration may occur; some parenteral products contain aluminum: use caution in neonates and patients with renal impairment.

Drug Interactions Neomycin, colchicine, anticonvulsants, and metformin may decrease oral absorption of B_{12}, chloramphenicol may decrease B_{12} effects

Ethanol/Nutrition/Herb Interactions Ethanol: Heavy consumption may impair vitamin B_{12} absorption.

Dietary Considerations Vegetarian diets may result in vitamin B_{12} deficiency; use intranasal product at least 1 hour before or after ingestion of hot foods or liquids due to increased nasal secretions

Pharmacodynamics/Kinetics

Absorption: Oral: Variable from the terminal ileum; requires the presence of calcium and gastric "intrinsic factor" to transfer the compound across the intestinal mucosa

Distribution: Principally stored in the liver and bone marrow, also stored in the kidneys and adrenals

Protein binding: To transcobalamin II

Metabolism: Converted in tissues to active coenzymes, methylcobalamin and deoxyadenosylcobalamin

Bioavailability: Intranasal:

Gel: 8.9% (relative to I.M.)

Solution: 6.1% (relative to I.M.)

Pregnancy Risk Factor A/C (dose exceeding RDA recommendation); C (intranasal)

Lactation Enters breast milk/compatible

Dosage Forms [DSC] = Discontinued product

Gel, intranasal (Nascobal®): 500 mcg/0.1 mL (2.3 mL) [contains benzalkonium chloride; delivers 8 doses] [DSC]

Injection, solution: 1000 mcg/mL (1 mL, 10 mL, 30 mL) [may contain benzyl alcohol and/or aluminum]

Lozenge [OTC]: 100 mcg, 250 mcg, 500 mcg

Solution, intranasal spray (Nascobal®): 500 mcg/0.1 mL actuation (2.3 mL) [contains benzalkonium chloride; delivers 8 doses]

Tablet [OTC]: 50 mcg, 100 mcg, 250 mcg, 500 mcg, 1000 mcg, 5000 mcg

Twelve Resin-K: 1000 mcg [may be used as oral, sublingual, or buccal]

Tablet, extended release [OTC]: 1500 mcg

Tablet, sublingual [OTC]: 2500 mcg

Cyanocobalamin, Folic Acid, and Pyridoxine *see* Folic Acid, Cyanocobalamin, and Pyridoxine *on page 697*

Cyclessa® *see* Ethinyl Estradiol and Desogestrel *on page 592*

Cyclizine *(SYE kli zeen)*

U.S. Brand Names Marezine® [OTC]

Generic Available No

Synonyms Cyclizine Hydrochloride; Cyclizine Lactate

Pharmacologic Category Antihistamine

Use Prevention and treatment of nausea, vomiting, and vertigo associated with motion sickness; control of postoperative nausea and vomiting

Local Anesthetic/Vasoconstrictor Precautions No information available to require special precautions

Effects on Dental Treatment Key adverse event(s) related to dental treatment: Xerostomia (normal salivary flow resumes upon discontinuation).

Common Adverse Effects

>10%:

Central nervous system: Drowsiness

Gastrointestinal: Xerostomia

1% to 10%:
Central nervous system: Headache
Dermatologic: Dermatitis
Gastrointestinal: Nausea
Genitourinary: Urinary retention
Ocular: Diplopia
Renal: Polyuria

Mechanism of Action Cyclizine is a piperazine derivative with properties of histamines. The precise mechanism of action in inhibiting the symptoms of motion sickness is not known. It may have effects directly on the labyrinthine apparatus and central actions on the labyrinthine apparatus and on the chemoreceptor trigger zone. Cyclizine exerts a central anticholinergic action.

Drug Interactions
Increased Effect/Toxicity: Increased effect/toxicity with CNS depressants, alcohol.

Pregnancy Risk Factor B

Cyclizine Hydrochloride *see* Cyclizine *on page 400*
Cyclizine Lactate *see* Cyclizine *on page 400*

Cyclobenzaprine (sye kloe BEN za preen)

Related Information
Temporomandibular Dysfunction (TMD) *on page 1724*
U.S. Brand Names Flexeril®
Canadian Brand Names Apo-Cyclobenzaprine®; Flexeril®; Flexitec; Gen-Cyclobenzaprine; Novo-Cycloprine; Nu-Cyclobenzaprine
Generic Available Yes
Synonyms Cyclobenzaprine Hydrochloride
Pharmacologic Category Skeletal Muscle Relaxant
Dental Use Treatment of muscle spasm associated with acute temporomandibular joint pain (TMJ)
Use Treatment of muscle spasm associated with acute painful musculoskeletal conditions
Local Anesthetic/Vasoconstrictor Precautions No information available to require special precautions
Effects on Dental Treatment Key adverse event(s) related to dental treatment: Xerostomia and changes in salivation (normal salivary flow resumes upon discontinuation).
Significant Adverse Effects
>10%:
Central nervous system: Drowsiness (29% to 39%), dizziness (1% to 11%)
Gastrointestinal: Xerostomia (21% to 32%)
1% to 10%:
Central nervous system: Fatigue (1% to 6%), confusion (1% to 3%), headache (1% to 3%), irritability (1% to 3%), mental acuity decreased (1% to 3%), nervousness (1% to 3%)
Gastrointestinal: Abdominal pain (1% to 3%), constipation (1% to 3%), diarrhea (1% to 3%), dyspepsia (1% to 3%), nausea (1% to 3%)
Neuromuscular & skeletal: Muscle weakness (1% to 3%)
Ocular: Blurred vision (1% to 3%)
Respiratory: Pharyngitis (1% to 3%)
<1% (Limited to important or life-threatening): Ageusia, agitation, anaphylaxis, angioedema, anorexia, arrhythmia, cholestasis, diplopia, facial edema, gastritis, hallucinations, hepatitis (rare), hypertonia, hypotension, insomnia, jaundice, liver function tests abnormal, malaise, palpitation, paresthesia, pruritus, psychosis, rash, seizure, tachycardia, thinking abnormal, tinnitus, tongue edema, tremor, urinary frequency, urinary retention, urticaria, vertigo, vomiting
Dental Usual Dosing Treatment of muscle spasm associated with acute TMJ pain (**Note:** Do not use longer than 2-3 weeks): Oral:
Adults: Initial: 5 mg 3 times/day; may increase to 10 mg 3 times/day if needed
Elderly: 5 mg 3 times/day; plasma concentration and incidence of adverse effects are increased in the elderly; dose should be titrated slowly
Dosage Oral: **Note:** Do not use longer than 2-3 weeks
Adults: Initial: 5 mg 3 times/day; may increase to 10 mg 3 times/day if needed
Elderly: 5 mg 3 times/day; plasma concentration and incidence of adverse effects are increased in the elderly; dose should be titrated slowly
Dosage adjustment in hepatic impairment:
Mild: 5 mg 3 times/day; use with caution and titrate slowly
Moderate to severe: Use not recommended
(Continued)

Cyclobenzaprine *(Continued)*

Mechanism of Action Centrally-acting skeletal muscle relaxant pharmacologically related to tricyclic antidepressants; reduces tonic somatic motor activity influencing both alpha and gamma motor neurons

Contraindications Hypersensitivity to cyclobenzaprine or any component of the formulation; do not use concomitantly or within 14 days of MAO inhibitors; hyperthyroidism; congestive heart failure; arrhythmias; acute recovery phase of MI

Warnings/Precautions Cyclobenzaprine shares the toxic potentials of the tricyclic antidepressants and the usual precautions of tricyclic antidepressant therapy should be observed; use with caution in patients with urinary hesitancy, angle-closure glaucoma, hepatic impairment, or in the elderly. Do not use concomitantly or within 14 days after MAO inhibitors; combination may cause hypertensive crisis, severe convulsions. Safety and efficacy have not been established in patients <15 years of age.

Drug Interactions Substrate of CYP1A2 (major), 2D6 (minor), 3A4 (minor)

Anticholinergics: Because of cyclobenzaprine's anticholinergic action, use with caution in patients receiving these agents.

CNS depressants: Effects may be enhanced by cyclobenzaprine.

CYP1A2 inhibitors: May increase the levels/effects of cyclobenzaprine. Example inhibitors include amiodarone, ciprofloxacin, fluvoxamine, ketoconazole, norfloxacin, ofloxacin, and rofecoxib.

Guanethidine: Antihypertensive effect of guanethidine may be decreased; effect seen with tricyclic antidepressants.

MAO inhibitors: Do not use concomitantly or within 14 days after MAO inhibitors.

Tramadol: May increase risk of seizure; effect seen with tricyclic antidepressants and tramadol.

Ethanol/Nutrition/Herb Interactions

Ethanol: Avoid ethanol (may increase CNS depression).

Herb/Nutraceutical: Avoid valerian, kava kava, gotu kola (may increase CNS depression).

Pharmacodynamics/Kinetics

Onset of action: ~1 hour

Duration: 12-24 hours

Absorption: Complete

Metabolism: Hepatic via CYP3A4, 1A2, and 2D6; may undergo enterohepatic recirculation

Bioavailability: 33% to 55%

Half-life elimination: 18 hours (range: 8-37 hours)

Time to peak, serum: 3-8 hours

Excretion: Urine (as inactive metabolites); feces (as unchanged drug)

Pregnancy Risk Factor B

Lactation Excretion in breast milk unknown/not recommended

Dosage Forms

Tablet, as hydrochloride: 5 mg, 10 mg

Flexeril®: 5 mg, 10 mg

Cyclobenzaprine Hydrochloride *see* Cyclobenzaprine *on page 401*

Cyclocort® *see* Amcinonide *on page 83*

Cyclogyl® *see* Cyclopentolate *on page 402*

Cyclomydril® *see* Cyclopentolate and Phenylephrine *on page 403*

Cyclopentolate *(sye kloe PEN toe late)*

U.S. Brand Names AK-Pentolate® [DSC]; Cyclogyl®; Cylate®

Canadian Brand Names Cyclogyl®; Diopentolate®

Generic Available Yes

Synonyms Cyclopentolate Hydrochloride

Pharmacologic Category Anticholinergic Agent, Ophthalmic

Use Diagnostic procedures requiring mydriasis and cycloplegia

Local Anesthetic/Vasoconstrictor Precautions No information available to require special precautions

Effects on Dental Treatment No significant effects or complications reported

Mechanism of Action Prevents the muscle of the ciliary body and the sphincter muscle of the iris from responding to cholinergic stimulation, causing mydriasis and cycloplegia

Pregnancy Risk Factor C

Cyclopentolate and Phenylephrine (sye kloe PEN toe late & fen il EF rin)

Related Information
Cyclopentolate *on page 402*
Phenylephrine *on page 1226*

U.S. Brand Names Cyclomydril®

Generic Available No

Synonyms Phenylephrine and Cyclopentolate

Pharmacologic Category Ophthalmic Agent, Antiglaucoma

Use Induce mydriasis greater than that produced with cyclopentolate HCl alone

Local Anesthetic/Vasoconstrictor Precautions No information available to require special precautions

Effects on Dental Treatment No significant effects or complications reported

Pregnancy Risk Factor C

Cyclopentolate Hydrochloride *see* Cyclopentolate *on page 402*

Cyclophosphamide (sye kloe FOS fa mide)

U.S. Brand Names Cytoxan®

Canadian Brand Names Cytoxan®; Procytox®

Mexican Brand Names Genoxal®; Ledoxina®

Generic Available Yes: Tablet

Synonyms CPM; CTX; CYT; NSC-26271

Pharmacologic Category Antineoplastic Agent, Alkylating Agent

Dental Use Treatment of Wegener's granulomatosis, systemic lupus erythematosus

Use

Oncologic: Treatment of Hodgkin's and non-Hodgkin's lymphoma, Burkitt's lymphoma, chronic lymphocytic leukemia (CLL), chronic myelocytic leukemia (CML), acute myelocytic leukemia (AML), acute lymphocytic leukemia (ALL), mycosis fungoides, multiple myeloma, neuroblastoma, retinoblastoma, rhabdomyosarcoma, Ewing's sarcoma; breast, testicular, endometrial, ovarian, and lung cancers, and in conditioning regimens for bone marrow transplantation

Nononcologic: Prophylaxis of rejection for kidney, heart, liver, and bone marrow transplants, severe rheumatoid disorders, nephrotic syndrome, Wegener's granulomatosis, idiopathic pulmonary hemosideroses, myasthenia gravis, multiple sclerosis, systemic lupus erythematosus, lupus nephritis, autoimmune hemolytic anemia, idiopathic thrombocytic purpura (ITP), macroglobulinemia, and antibody-induced pure red cell aplasia

Local Anesthetic/Vasoconstrictor Precautions No information available to require special precautions

Effects on Dental Treatment Key adverse event(s) related to dental treatment: Mucositis and stomatitis.

Significant Adverse Effects

>10%:
Dermatologic: Alopecia (40% to 60%) but hair will usually regrow although it may be a different color and/or texture. Hair loss usually begins 3-6 weeks after the start of therapy.

Endocrine & metabolic: Fertility: May cause sterility; interferes with oogenesis and spermatogenesis; may be irreversible in some patients; gonadal suppression (amenorrhea)

Gastrointestinal: Nausea and vomiting, usually beginning 6-10 hours after administration; anorexia, diarrhea, mucositis, and stomatitis are also seen

Genitourinary: Severe, potentially fatal acute hemorrhagic cystitis (7% to 40%)

Hematologic: Thrombocytopenia and anemia are less common than leukopenia
Onset: 7 days
Nadir: 10-14 days
Recovery: 21 days

1% to 10%:
Cardiovascular: Facial flushing
Central nervous system: Headache
Dermatologic: Skin rash
Renal: SIADH may occur, usually with doses >50 mg/kg (or 1 g/m^2); renal tubular necrosis, which usually resolves with discontinuation of the drug, is also reported

(Continued)

403

Cyclophosphamide *(Continued)*

Respiratory: Nasal congestion occurs when I.V. doses are administered too rapidly; patients experience runny eyes, rhinorrhea, sinus congestion, and sneezing during or immediately after the infusion.

<1% (Limited to important or life-threatening): High-dose therapy may cause cardiac dysfunction manifested as CHF; cardiac necrosis or hemorrhagic myocarditis has occurred rarely, but may be fatal. Cyclophosphamide may also potentiate the cardiac toxicity of anthracyclines. Other adverse reactions include anaphylactic reactions, darkening of skin/fingernails, dizziness, hemorrhagic colitis, hemorrhagic ureteritis, hepatotoxicity, hyperuricemia, hypokalemia, jaundice, neutrophilic eccrine hidradenitis, radiation recall, renal tubular necrosis, secondary malignancy (eg, bladder carcinoma), Stevens-Johnson syndrome, toxic epidermal necrolysis; interstitial pneumonitis and pulmonary fibrosis are occasionally seen with high doses

BMT:

Cardiovascular: Heart failure, cardiac necrosis, pericardial tamponade

Endocrine & metabolic: Hyponatremia

Hematologic: Methemoglobinemia

Gastrointestinal: Severe nausea and vomiting

Miscellaneous: Hemorrhagic cystitis, secondary malignancy

Dosage Refer to individual protocols

Children:

SLE: I.V.: 500-750 mg/m^2 every month; maximum dose: 1 g/m^2

JRA/vasculitis: I.V.: 10 mg/kg every 2 weeks

Children and Adults:

Oral: 50-100 mg/m^2/day as continuous therapy or 400-1000 mg/m^2 in divided doses over 4-5 days as intermittent therapy

I.V.:

Single doses: 400-1800 mg/m^2 (30-50 mg/kg) per treatment course (1-5 days) which can be repeated at 2-4 week intervals

Continuous daily doses: 60-120 mg/m^2 (1-2.5 mg/kg) per day

Autologous BMT: IVPB: 50 mg/kg/dose x 4 days or 60 mg/kg/dose for 2 days; total dose is usually divided over 2-4 days

Nephrotic syndrome: Oral: 2-3 mg/kg/day every day for up to 12 weeks when corticosteroids are unsuccessful

Dosing adjustment in renal impairment: A large fraction of cyclophosphamide is eliminated by hepatic metabolism

Some authors recommend no dose adjustment unless severe renal insufficiency (Cl$_{cr}$ <20 mL/minute)

Cl$_{cr}$ >10 mL/minute: Administer 100% of normal dose

Cl$_{cr}$ <10 mL/minute: Administer 75% of normal dose

Hemodialysis: Moderately dialyzable (20% to 50%); administer dose posthemodialysis

CAPD effects: Unknown

CAVH effects: Unknown

Dosing adjustment in hepatic impairment: The pharmacokinetics of cyclophosphamide are not significantly altered in the presence of hepatic insufficiency. No dosage adjustments are recommended.

Mechanism of Action Cyclophosphamide is an alkylating agent that prevents cell division by cross-linking DNA strands and decreasing DNA synthesis. It is a cell cycle phase nonspecific agent. Cyclophosphamide also possesses potent immunosuppressive activity. Cyclophosphamide is a prodrug that must be metabolized to active metabolites in the liver.

Contraindications Hypersensitivity to cyclophosphamide or any component of the formulation; pregnancy

Warnings/Precautions Hazardous agent - use appropriate precautions for handling and disposal. Dosage adjustment needed for renal or hepatic failure.

Drug Interactions Substrate of CYP2A6 (minor), 2B6 (major), 2C9 (minor), 2C19 (minor), 3A4 (major); **Inhibits** CYP3A4 (weak); **Induces** CYP2B6 (weak), 2C8 (weak), 2C9 (weak)

Allopurinol may cause increase in bone marrow depression and may result in significant elevations of cyclophosphamide cytotoxic metabolites.

Anesthetic agents: Cyclophosphamide reduces serum pseudocholinesterase concentrations and may prolong the neuromuscular blocking activity of succinylcholine; use with caution with halothane, nitrous oxide, and succinylcholine.

Chloramphenicol results in prolonged cyclophosphamide half-life to increase toxicity.

CYP2B6 inducers: May increase the levels/effects of acrolein (the active metabolite of cyclophosphamide). Example inducers include carbamazepine, nevirapine, phenobarbital, phenytoin, and rifampin.

CYP2B6 inhibitors: May decrease the levels/effects of acrolein (the active metabolite of cyclophosphamide). Example inhibitors include desipramine, paroxetine, and sertraline.

CYP3A4 inducers: CYP3A4 inducers may increase the levels/effects of acrolein (the active metabolite of cyclophosphamide). Example inducers include aminoglutethimide, carbamazepine, nafcillin, nevirapine, phenobarbital, phenytoin, and rifamycins.

CYP3A4 inhibitors: May decrease the levels/effects of acrolein (the active metabolite of cyclophosphamide). Example inhibitors include azole antifungals, ciprofloxacin, clarithromycin, diclofenac, doxycycline, erythromycin, imatinib, isoniazid, nefazodone, nicardipine, propofol, protease inhibitors, quinidine, and verapamil.

Digoxin: Cyclophosphamide may decrease digoxin serum levels.

Doxorubicin: Cyclophosphamide may enhance cardiac toxicity of anthracyclines.

Tetrahydrocannabinol results in enhanced immunosuppression in animal studies.

Thiazide diuretics: Leukopenia may be prolonged.

Ethanol/Nutrition/Herb Interactions Herb/Nutraceutical: Avoid black cohosh, dong quai in estrogen-dependent tumors.

Dietary Considerations Tablets should be administered during or after meals.

Pharmacodynamics/Kinetics

Absorption: Oral: Well absorbed

Distribution: V_d: 0.48-0.71 L/kg; crosses placenta; crosses into CSF (not in high enough concentrations to treat meningeal leukemia)

Protein binding: 10% to 56%

Metabolism: Hepatic to active metabolites acrolein, 4-aldophosphamide, 4-hydroperoxycyclophosphamide, and nor-nitrogen mustard

Bioavailability: >75%

Half-life elimination: 4-8 hours

Time to peak, serum: Oral: ~1 hour

Excretion: Urine (<30% as unchanged drug, 85% to 90% as metabolites)

Pregnancy Risk Factor D

Lactation Enters breast milk/contraindicated

Dosage Forms

Injection, powder for reconstitution (Cytoxan®): 500 mg, 1 g, 2 g [contains mannitol 75 mg per cyclophosphamide 100 mg]

Tablet (Cytoxan®): 25 mg, 50 mg

CycloSERINE (sye kloe SER een)

Related Information

Tuberculosis *on page 1673*

U.S. Brand Names Seromycin®

Generic Available No

Pharmacologic Category Antibiotic, Miscellaneous; Antitubercular Agent

Use Adjunctive treatment in pulmonary or extrapulmonary tuberculosis

Unlabeled/Investigational Use Treatment of Gaucher's disease

Local Anesthetic/Vasoconstrictor Precautions No information available to require special precautions

Effects on Dental Treatment No significant effects or complications reported

Common Adverse Effects Frequency not defined.

Cardiovascular: Cardiac arrhythmia

Central nervous system: Drowsiness, headache, dizziness, vertigo, seizure, confusion, psychosis, paresis, coma

Dermatologic: Rash

Endocrine & metabolic: Vitamin B_{12} deficiency

Hematologic: Folate deficiency

Hepatic: Liver enzymes increased

Neuromuscular & skeletal: Tremor

Mechanism of Action Inhibits bacterial cell wall synthesis by competing with amino acid (D-alanine) for incorporation into the bacterial cell wall; bacteriostatic or bactericidal

Drug Interactions

Increased Effect/Toxicity: Alcohol, isoniazid, and ethionamide increase toxicity of cycloserine. Cycloserine inhibits the hepatic metabolism of phenytoin and may increase risk of epileptic seizures.

Pharmacodynamics/Kinetics

Absorption: ~70% to 90%

(Continued)

CycloSERINE (Continued)

Distribution: Widely to most body fluids and tissues including CSF, breast milk, bile, sputum, lymph tissue, lungs, and ascitic, pleural, and synovial fluids; crosses placenta

Half-life elimination: Normal renal function: 10 hours

Metabolism: Hepatic

Time to peak, serum: 3-4 hours

Excretion: Urine (60% to 70% as unchanged drug) within 72 hours; feces (small amounts); remainder metabolized

Pregnancy Risk Factor C

Cyclosporin A see CycloSPORINE on page 406

CycloSPORINE (SYE kloe spor een)

U.S. Brand Names Gengraf®; Neoral®; Restasis®; Sandimmune®

Canadian Brand Names Apo-Cyclosporine®; Neoral®; Rhoxal-cyclosporine; Sandimmune® I.V.; Sandoz-Cyclosporine

Generic Available Yes

Synonyms CsA; CyA; Cyclosporin A

Pharmacologic Category Immunosuppressant Agent

Dental Use Used as an immunosuppressive agent

Use Prophylaxis of organ rejection in kidney, liver, and heart transplants, has been used with azathioprine and/or corticosteroids; severe, active rheumatoid arthritis (RA) not responsive to methotrexate alone; severe, recalcitrant plaque psoriasis in nonimmunocompromised adults unresponsive to or unable to tolerate other systemic therapy

Ophthalmic emulsion (Restasis®): Increase tear production when suppressed tear production is presumed to be due to keratoconjunctivitis sicca-associated ocular inflammation (in patients not already using topical anti-inflammatory drugs or punctal plugs)

Unlabeled/Investigational Use Short-term, high-dose cyclosporine as a modulator of multidrug resistance in cancer treatment; allogenic bone marrow transplants for prevention and treatment of graft-versus-host disease; also used in some cases of severe autoimmune disease (eg, SLE, myasthenia gravis) that are resistant to corticosteroids and other therapy; focal segmental glomerulosclerosis

Local Anesthetic/Vasoconstrictor Precautions No information available to require special precautions

Effects on Dental Treatment Key adverse event(s) related to dental treatment: Gingival hypertrophy, mouth sores, swallowing difficulty, gingivitis, gum hyperplasia, xerostomia (normal salivary flow resumes upon discontinuation), abnormal taste, tongue disorder, tooth disorder, gum hyperplasia, and gingival bleeding.

Significant Adverse Effects Adverse reactions reported with systemic use, including rheumatoid arthritis, psoriasis, and transplantation (kidney, liver, and heart). Percentages noted include the highest frequency regardless of indication/dosage. Frequencies may vary for specific conditions or formulation.

>10%:

Cardiovascular: Hypertension (8% to 53%), edema (5% to 14%)

Central nervous system: Headache (2% to 25%)

Dermatologic: Hirsutism (21% to 45%), hypertrichosis (5% to 19%)

Endocrine & metabolic: Triglycerides increased (15%), female reproductive disorder (9% to 11%)

Gastrointestinal: Nausea (23%), diarrhea (3% to 13%), gum hyperplasia (2% to 16%), abdominal discomfort (<1% to 15%), dyspepsia (2% to 12%)

Neuromuscular & skeletal: Tremor (7% to 55%), paresthesia (1% to 11%), leg cramps/muscle contractions (2% to 12%)

Renal: Renal dysfunction/nephropathy (10% to 38%), creatinine increased (16% to ≥50%)

Respiratory: Upper respiratory infection (1% to 14%)

Miscellaneous: Infection (3% to 25%)

1% to 10%:

Cardiovascular: Chest pain (4% to 6%), arrhythmia (2% to 5%), abnormal heart sounds, cardiac failure, flushes (<1% to 5%), MI, peripheral ischemia

Central nervous system: Dizziness (8%), pain (6%), convulsions (1% to 5%), insomnia (4%), psychiatric events (4% to 5%), pain (3% to 4%), depression (1% to 6%), migraine (2% to 3%), anxiety, confusion, fever, hypoesthesia, emotional lability, impaired concentration, insomnia, lethargy, malaise, nervousness, paranoia, somnolence, vertigo

Dermatologic: Hypertrichosis (5% to 7%), purpura (3% to 4%), acne (1% to 6%), brittle fingernails, hair breaking, abnormal pigmentation, angioedema, cellulitis, dermatitis, dry skin, eczema, folliculitis, keratosis, pruritus, rash, skin disorder, skin malignancies, urticaria

Endocrine & metabolic: Gynecomastia (<1% to 4%), menstrual disorder (1% to 3%), breast fibroadenosis, breast pain, hyper-/hypoglycemia, diabetes mellitus, goiter, hot flashes, hyperkalemia, hyperuricemia, libido increased/decreased

Gastrointestinal: Vomiting (2% to 10%), flatulence (5%), gingivitis (up to 4%), cramps (up to 4%), anorexia, constipation, dry mouth, dysphagia, enanthema, eructation, esophagitis, gastric ulcer, gastritis, gastroenteritis, gastrointestinal bleeding (upper), gingival bleeding, glossitis, mouth sores, peptic ulcer, pancreatitis, swallowing difficulty, salivary gland enlargement, taste perversion, tongue disorder, tooth disorder, weight loss/gain

Genitourinary: Leukorrhea (1%), abnormal urine, micturition increased, micturition urgency, nocturia, polyuria, pyelonephritis, urinary incontinence, uterine hemorrhage

Hematologic: Leukopenia (<1% to 6%), anemia, bleeding disorder, clotting disorder, platelet disorder, red blood cell disorder, thrombocytopenia

Hepatic: Hepatotoxicity (<1% to 7%), hyperbilirubinemia

Neuromuscular & skeletal: Arthralgia (1% to 6%), bone fracture, joint dislocation, joint pain, muscle pain, myalgia, neuropathy, stiffness, synovial cyst, tendon disorder, tingling, weakness

Ocular: Abnormal vision, cataract, conjunctivitis, eye pain, visual disturbance

Otic: Deafness, hearing loss, tinnitus, vestibular disorder

Renal: BUN increased, hematuria, renal abscess

Respiratory: Sinusitis (<1% to 7%), bronchospasm (up to 5%), cough (3% to 5%), pharyngitis (3% to 5%), dyspnea (1% to 5%), rhinitis (up to 5%), abnormal chest sounds, epistaxis, respiratory infection, pneumonia (up to 1%)

Miscellaneous: Flu-like symptoms (8% to 10%), lymphoma (<1% to 6% reported in transplant), abscess, allergic reactions, bacterial infection, carcinoma, diaphoresis increased, fungal infection, herpes simplex, herpes zoster, hiccups, lymphadenopathy, moniliasis, night sweats, tonsillitis, viral infection

Postmarketing and/or case reports (any indication): Anaphylaxis/anaphylactoid reaction (possibly associated with Cremophor® EL vehicle in injection formulation), benign intracranial hypertension, cholesterol increased, death (due to renal deterioration), encephalopathy, gout, hyperbilirubinemia, hyperkalemia, hypomagnesemia (mild), impaired consciousness, neurotoxicity, papilloedema, pulmonary edema (noncardiogenic), uric acid increased

Ophthalmic emulsion (Restasis®):
>10%: Ocular: Burning (17%)

1% to 10%: Ocular: Hyperemia (conjunctival 5%), eye pain, pruritus, stinging

Dental Usual Dosing Note: Neoral®/Genraf® and Sandimmune® are not bioequivalent and cannot be used interchangeably.

Autoimmune diseases: Adults: 1-3 mg/kg/day

Dosage Neoral®/Genraf® and Sandimmune® are not bioequivalent and cannot be used interchangeably.

Children: Transplant: Refer to adult dosing; children may require, and are able to tolerate, larger doses than adults.

Adults:

Newly-transplanted patients: Adjunct therapy with corticosteroids is recommended. Initial dose should be given 4-12 hours prior to transplant or may be given postoperatively; adjust initial dose to achieve desired plasma concentration

Oral: Dose is dependent upon type of transplant and formulation:

Cyclosporine (modified):

Renal: 9 ± 3 mg/kg/day, divided twice daily

Liver: 8 ± 4 mg/kg/day, divided twice daily

Heart: 7 ± 3 mg/kg/day, divided twice daily

Cyclosporine (non-modified): Initial dose: 15 mg/kg/day as a single dose (range 14-18 mg/kg); lower doses of 10-14 mg/kg/day have been used for renal transplants. Continue initial dose daily for 1-2 weeks; taper by 5% per week to a maintenance dose of 5-10 mg/kg/day; some renal transplant patients may be dosed as low as 3 mg/kg/day

Note: When using the non-modified formulation, cyclosporine levels may increase in liver transplant patients when the T-tube is closed; dose may need decreased

I.V.: Cyclosporine (non-modified): Manufacturer's labeling: Initial dose: 5-6 mg/kg/day as a single dose (⅓ the oral dose), infused over 2-6 hours; use

(Continued)

CycloSPORINE *(Continued)*

should be limited to patients unable to take capsules or oral solution; patients should be switched to an oral dosage form as soon as possible

Note: Many transplant centers administer cyclosporine as 'divided dose' infusions (in 2-3 doses/day) or as a continuous (24-hour) infusion; dosages range from 3-7.5 mg/kg/day. Specific institutional protocols should be consulted.

Conversion to cyclosporine (modified) from cyclosporine (non-modified): Start with daily dose previously used and adjust to obtain preconversion cyclosporine trough concentration. Plasma concentrations should be monitored every 4-7 days and dose adjusted as necessary, until desired trough level is obtained. When transferring patients with previously poor absorption of cyclosporine (non-modified), monitor trough levels at least twice weekly (especially if initial dose exceeds 10 mg/kg/day); high plasma levels are likely to occur.

Rheumatoid arthritis: Oral: Cyclosporine (modified): Initial dose: 2.5 mg/kg/day, divided twice daily; salicylates, NSAIDs, and oral glucocorticoids may be continued (refer to Drug Interactions); dose may be increased by 0.5-0.75 mg/kg/day if insufficient response is seen after 8 weeks of treatment; additional dosage increases may be made again at 12 weeks (maximum dose: 4 mg/kg/day). Discontinue if no benefit is seen by 16 weeks of therapy.

Note: Increase the frequency of blood pressure monitoring after each alteration in dosage of cyclosporine. Cyclosporine dosage should be decreased by 25% to 50% in patients with no history of hypertension who develop sustained hypertension during therapy and, if hypertension persists, treatment with cyclosporine should be discontinued.

Psoriasis: Oral: Cyclosporine (modified): Initial dose: 2.5 mg/kg/day, divided twice daily; dose may be increased by 0.5 mg/kg/day if insufficient response is seen after 4 weeks of treatment. Additional dosage increases may be made every 2 weeks if needed (maximum dose: 4 mg/kg/day). Discontinue if no benefit is seen by 6 weeks of therapy. Once patients are adequately controlled, the dose should be decreased to the lowest effective dose. Doses lower than 2.5 mg/kg/day may be effective. Treatment longer than 1 year is not recommended.

Note: Increase the frequency of blood pressure monitoring after each alteration in dosage of cyclosporine. Cyclosporine dosage should be decreased by 25% to 50% in patients with no history of hypertension who develop sustained hypertension during therapy and, if hypertension persists, treatment with cyclosporine should be discontinued.

Focal segmental glomerulosclerosis (unlabeled use): Initial: 3 mg/kg/day divided every 12 hours

Autoimmune diseases (unlabeled use): 1-3 mg/kg/day

Keratoconjunctivitis sicca: Ophthalmic: Children ≥16 years and Adults: Instill 1 drop in each eye every 12 hours

Dosage adjustment in renal impairment: For severe psoriasis:

Serum creatinine levels ≥25% above pretreatment levels: Take another sample within 2 weeks; if the level remains ≥25% above pretreatment levels, decrease dosage of cyclosporine (modified) by 25% to 50%. If two dosage adjustments do not reverse the increase in serum creatinine levels, treatment should be discontinued.

Serum creatinine levels ≥50% above pretreatment levels: Decrease cyclosporine dosage by 25% to 50%. If two dosage adjustments do not reverse the increase in serum creatinine levels, treatment should be discontinued.

Hemodialysis: Supplemental dose is not necessary.

Peritoneal dialysis: Supplemental dose is not necessary.

Dosage adjustment in hepatic impairment: Probably necessary; monitor levels closely

Mechanism of Action Inhibition of production and release of interleukin II and inhibits interleukin II-induced activation of resting T-lymphocytes.

Contraindications Hypersensitivity to cyclosporine or any component of the formulation. Rheumatoid arthritis and psoriasis: Abnormal renal function, uncontrolled hypertension, malignancies. Concomitant treatment with PUVA or UVB therapy, methotrexate, other immunosuppressive agents, coal tar, or radiation therapy are also contraindications for use in patients with psoriasis. Ophthalmic emulsion is contraindicated in patients with active ocular infections.

Warnings/Precautions Use caution with other potentially nephrotoxic drugs (eg, acyclovir, aminoglycoside antibiotics, amphotericin B, ciprofloxacin). Increased risk of lymphomas, other malignancies, infection. May cause hypertension. Use caution when changing dosage forms; products are not equally interchangeable. Cyclosporine (modified) refers to the capsule dosage formulation of cyclosporine in an aqueous dispersion (previously referred to as "microemulsion"). Cyclosporine (modified) has increased bioavailability as compared to cyclosporine (non-modified) and cannot be used interchangeably without close monitoring. Monitor cyclosporine concentrations closely following the addition, modification, or deletion of other medications; live, attenuated vaccines may be less effective; use should be avoided.

Transplant patients: To be used initially with corticosteroids. May cause significant hyperkalemia and hyperuricemia. May cause seizures, particularly if used with high-dose corticosteroids. Encephalopathy has been reported, predisposing factors include hypertension, hypomagnesemia, hypocholesterolemia, high-dose corticosteroids, high cyclosporine serum concentration, and graft-versus-host disease; may be more common in patients with liver transplant. Make dose adjustments based on cyclosporine blood concentrations. Adjustment of dose should only be made under the direct supervision of an experienced physician. Anaphylaxis has been reported with I.V. use; reserve for patients who cannot take oral form.

Psoriasis: Patients should avoid excessive sun exposure; safety and efficacy in children <18 years of age have not been established. Risk of skin cancer may be increased with a history of PUVA and possibly methotrexate or other immunosuppressants, UVB, coal tar, or radiation.

Rheumatoid arthritis: Safety and efficacy for use in juvenile rheumatoid arthritis have not been established. If receiving other immunosuppressive agents, radiation or UV therapy, concurrent use of cyclosporine is not recommended.

Ophthalmic emulsion: Safety and efficacy have not been established in patients <16 years of age.

Products may contain corn oil, castor oil, ethanol, or propylene glycol; injection also contains Cremophor® EL (polyoxyethylated castor oil), which has been associated with rare anaphylactic reactions.

Drug Interactions Substrate of CYP3A4 (major); **Inhibits** CYP2C9 (weak), 3A4 (moderate)

ACE inhibitors: May enhance nephrotoxic effects of cyclosporine.

Allopurinol: Increases cyclosporine concentrations by inhibiting cyclosporine metabolism.

Amiodarone: May increase cyclosporine concentrations by inhibiting cyclosporine metabolism.

Antibiotics: Concomitant use may potentiate renal dysfunction (seen with ciprofloxacin, gentamicin, tobramycin, vancomycin, trimethoprim and sulfamethoxazole); increased cyclosporine concentrations by inhibiting cyclosporine metabolism (seen with azithromycin, clarithromycin, erythromycin, and norfloxacin, quinupristin/dalfopristin); may decrease cyclosporine concentrations by inducing cyclosporine metabolism (seen with nafcillin, and rifampin); may decrease immunosuppressant effects (seen with ciprofloxacin); CNS disturbances, seizures (seen with imipenem).

Anticonvulsants: May decrease cyclosporine concentrations by inducing cyclosporine metabolism (seen with carbamazepine, phenobarbital, and phenytoin)

Antineoplastics: Concomitant use may potentiate renal dysfunction (seen with melphalan)

Antifungals: Concomitant use may potentiate renal dysfunction (seen with amphotericin B, ketoconazole); increase cyclosporine concentrations by inhibiting cyclosporine metabolism (seen with fluconazole, itraconazole, and ketoconazole)

Bosentan: Cyclosporine may increase the serum concentration of bosentan. Bosentan may decrease the serum concentration of cyclosporine. Concurrent use is contraindicated..

Bromocriptine: Increases cyclosporine concentrations by inhibiting cyclosporine metabolism

Calcium channel blockers (diltiazem, nicardipine, verapamil): Increase cyclosporine concentrations by inhibiting cyclosporine metabolism. Nifedipine has been reported to increase the risk of gingival hyperplasia.

Colchicine: May potentiate renal dysfunction; colchicine may increase cyclosporine concentrations by inhibiting metabolism. Cyclosporine may decrease the clearance of colchicine.

Corticosteroids: Systemic corticosteroids may increase the serum concentration of cyclosporine (reported with methylprednisolone). Cyclosporine may increase the serum concentration of systemic corticosteroids. Convulsions have been reported with high-dose methylprednisolone.

CYP3A4 inducers: CYP3A4 inducers may decrease the levels/effects of cyclosporine. Example inducers include aminoglutethimide, carbamazepine, nafcillin, nevirapine, phenobarbital, phenytoin, and rifamycins.

CYP3A4 inhibitors: May increase the levels/effects of cyclosporine. Example inhibitors include azole antifungals, clarithromycin, diclofenac, doxycycline, (Continued)

CycloSPORINE *(Continued)*

erythromycin, imatinib, isoniazid, nefazodone, nicardipine, propofol, protease inhibitors, quinidine, telithromycin, and verapamil.

CYP3A4 substrates: Cyclosporine may increase the levels/effects of CYP3A4 substrates. Example substrates include benzodiazepines, calcium channel blockers, cyclosporine, mirtazapine, nateglinide, nefazodone, sildenafil (and other PDE-5 inhibitors), tacrolimus, and venlafaxine. Selected benzodiazepines (midazolam and triazolam), cisapride, ergot alkaloids, selected HMG-CoA reductase inhibitors (lovastatin and simvastatin), and pimozide are generally contraindicated with strong CYP3A4 inhibitors.

Danazol: Increases cyclosporine concentrations by inhibiting cyclosporine metabolism

Digoxin: Decreased clearance and decreased volume of distribution of digoxin; severe digitalis toxicity has been observed.

Fibric acid derivatives: May increase the risk of renal dysfunction and may alter cyclosporine concentrations; monitor.

H$_2$ blockers: Concomitant use may potentiate renal dysfunction (seen with cimetidine, ranitidine).

HMG-CoA reductase inhibitors: Cyclosporine may increase levels/effects of HMG-CoA reductase inhibitors, resulting in myalgias, rhabdomyolysis, acute renal failure; dosage adjustments of HMG-CoA reductase inhibitors are recommended.

Imatinib: May increase cyclosporine serum concentrations by inhibiting cyclosporine metabolism.

Immunosuppressives: Concomitant use may potentiate renal dysfunction (seen with tacrolimus, muromonab-CD3).

Metoclopramide: Increases cyclosporine concentrations by inhibiting cyclosporine metabolism.

Methotrexate: Cyclosporine increases plasma levels of methotrexate and decreases plasma levels of its metabolite; monitor closely for signs of toxicity.

Minoxidil: Concomitant use may lead to severe hypertrichosis.

NSAIDs: Concomitant use may potentiate renal dysfunction, especially in dehydrated patients (seen with diclofenac, naproxen, sulindac). In addition, diclofenac plasma levels are doubled when given with cyclosporine; the lowest possible dose of diclofenac should be used. Monitor serum creatinine.

Octreotide: May decrease cyclosporine concentrations by inducing cyclosporine metabolism.

Oral contraceptives (hormonal): May increase serum levels of cyclosporine; monitor for signs of toxicity.

Orlistat: May decrease absorption of cyclosporine; avoid concomitant use.

Protease inhibitors: Formal interaction studies have not been done; protease inhibitors are known to induce CYP3A4; use caution when using cyclosporine with indinavir, nelfinavir, ritonavir, or saquinavir.

Rifabutin: Formal interaction studies have not been done; rifabutin is known to increase the metabolism of medications via CYP3A4.

Sirolimus: Cyclosporine may increase serum levels/effects; monitor. Concurrent therapy may increase the risk of HUS/TTP/TMA. Administer sirolimus 4 hours after cyclosporine to minimize the increase in sirolimus blood levels.

Sulfinpyrazone: May decrease cyclosporine levels by inducing cyclosporine metabolism; monitor.

Ticlopidine: May decrease cyclosporine concentrations by inducing cyclosporine metabolism.

Vaccines: Vaccination may be less effective; avoid use of live vaccines during therapy.

Voriconazole: Cyclosporine serum concentrations may be increased; monitor serum concentrations and renal function. Decrease cyclosporine dosage by 50% when initiating voriconazole.

Ethanol/Nutrition/Herb Interactions

Food: Grapefruit juice increases absorption; unsupervised use should be avoided.

Herb/Nutraceutical: Avoid St John's wort; as an enzyme inducer, it may increase the metabolism of and decrease plasma levels of cyclosporine; organ rejection and graft loss have been reported. Avoid cat's claw, echinacea (have immunostimulant properties).

Dietary Considerations Administer this medication consistently with relation to time of day and meals. Avoid grapefruit juice.

Pharmacodynamics/Kinetics

Absorption:

Ophthalmic emulsion: Serum concentrations not detectable.

Oral:

Cyclosporine (non-modified): Erratic and incomplete; dependent on presence of food, bile acids, and GI motility; larger oral doses are needed in pediatrics due to shorter bowel length and limited intestinal absorption

Cyclosporine (modified): Erratic and incomplete; increased absorption, up to 30% when compared to cyclosporine (non-modified); less dependent on food, bile acids, or GI motility when compared to cyclosporine (non-modified)

Distribution: Widely in tissues and body fluids including the liver, pancreas, and lungs; crosses placenta; enters breast milk

V_{dss}: 4-6 L/kg in renal, liver, and marrow transplant recipients (slightly lower values in cardiac transplant patients; children <10 years have higher values)

Protein binding: 90% to 98% to lipoproteins

Metabolism: Extensively hepatic via CYP3A4; forms at least 25 metabolites; extensive first-pass effect following oral administration

Bioavailability: Oral:

Cyclosporine (non-modified): Dependent on patient population and transplant type (<10% in adult liver transplant patients and as high as 89% in renal transplant patients; bioavailability of Sandimmune® capsules and oral solution are equivalent; bioavailability of oral solution is ~30% of the I.V. solution

Children: 28% (range: 17% to 42%); gut dysfunction common in BMT patients and oral bioavailability is further reduced

Cyclosporine (modified): Bioavailability of Neoral® capsules and oral solution are equivalent:

Children: 43% (range: 30% to 68%)

Adults: 23% greater than with cyclosporine (non-modified) in renal transplant patients; 50% greater in liver transplant patients

Half-life elimination: Oral: May be prolonged in patients with hepatic impairment and shorter in pediatric patients due to the higher metabolism rate

Cyclosporine (non-modified): Biphasic: Alpha: 1.4 hours; Terminal: 19 hours (range: 10-27 hours)

Cyclosporine (modified): Biphasic: Terminal: 8.4 hours (range: 5-18 hours)

Time to peak, serum: Oral:

Cyclosporine (non-modified): 2-6 hours; some patients have a second peak at 5-6 hours

Cyclosporine (modified): Renal transplant: 1.5-2 hours

Excretion: Primarily feces; urine (6%, 0.1% as unchanged drug and metabolites)

Pregnancy Risk Factor C

Lactation Enters breast milk/not recommended

Breast-Feeding Considerations The AAP does not recommend breast-feeding during therapy due to possible immune suppression in the infant as well as the unknown effects on growth or association with carcinogenesis.

Dosage Forms

Capsule, soft gel, modified: 25 mg, 100 mg [contains castor oil, ethanol]

Gengraf®: 25 mg, 100 mg [contains ethanol, castor oil, propylene glycol]

Neoral®: 25 mg, 100 mg [contains dehydrated ethanol, corn oil, castor oil, propylene glycol]

Capsule, soft gel, non-modified (Sandimmune®): 25 mg, 100 mg [contains dehydrated ethanol, corn oil]

Emulsion, ophthalmic [preservative free, single-use vial] (Restasis®): 0.05% (0.4 mL) [contains glycerin, castor oil, polysorbate 80, carbomer 1342; 32 vials/box]

Injection, solution, non-modified (Sandimmune®): 50 mg/mL (5 mL) [contains Cremophor® EL (polyoxyethylated castor oil), ethanol]

Solution, oral, modified:

Gengraf®: 100 mg/mL (50 mL) [contains castor oil, propylene glycol]

Neoral®: 100 mg/mL (50 mL) [contains dehydrated ethanol, corn oil, castor oil, propylene glycol]

Solution, oral, non-modified (Sandimmune®): 100 mg/mL (50 mL) [contains olive oil, ethanol]

Selected Readings

Ferrari SL, Goffin E, Mourad M, et al, "The Interaction Between Clarithromycin and Cyclosporine in Kidney Transplant Recipients," *Transplantation*, 1994, 58(6):725-7.

Harnett JD, Parfrey PS, Paul MD, et al, "Erythromycin-Cyclosporine Interaction in Renal Transplant Recipients," *Transplantation*, 1987, 43(2):316-8.

Cyklokapron® *see* Tranexamic Acid *on page 1518*

Cylate® *see* Cyclopentolate *on page 402*

Cylert® [DSC] *see* Pemoline *on page 1199*

Cylex® [OTC] *see* Benzocaine *on page 190*

Cymbalta® *see* Duloxetine *on page 523*

Cyproheptadine (si proe HEP ta deen)

Mexican Brand Names Viternum®
Generic Available Yes
Synonyms Cyproheptadine Hydrochloride; Periactin
Pharmacologic Category Antihistamine
Use Perennial and seasonal allergic rhinitis and other allergic symptoms including urticaria
Unlabeled/Investigational Use Appetite stimulation, blepharospasm, cluster headaches, migraine headaches, Nelson's syndrome, pruritus, schizophrenia, spinal cord damage associated spasticity, and tardive dyskinesia
Local Anesthetic/Vasoconstrictor Precautions No information available to require special precautions
Effects on Dental Treatment Key adverse event(s) related to dental treatment: Xerostomia (normal salivary flow resumes upon discontinuation).
Common Adverse Effects
>10%:
  Central nervous system: Slight to moderate drowsiness
  Respiratory: Thickening of bronchial secretions
1% to 10%:
  Central nervous system: Headache, fatigue, nervousness, dizziness
  Gastrointestinal: Appetite stimulation, nausea, diarrhea, abdominal pain, xerostomia
  Neuromuscular & skeletal: Arthralgia
  Respiratory: Pharyngitis
Mechanism of Action A potent antihistamine and serotonin antagonist, competes with histamine for H_1-receptor sites on effector cells in the gastrointestinal tract, blood vessels, and respiratory tract
Drug Interactions
Increased Effect/Toxicity: Cyproheptadine may potentiate the effect of CNS depressants. MAO inhibitors may cause hallucinations when taken with cyproheptadine.
Pharmacodynamics/Kinetics
Absorption: Completely
Metabolism: Almost completely hepatic
Excretion: Urine (>50% primarily as metabolites); feces (~25%)
Pregnancy Risk Factor B

Cyproheptadine Hydrochloride see Cyproheptadine on page 412
Cystadane® see Betaine Anhydrous on page 199
Cystagon® see Cysteamine on page 412

Cysteamine (sis TEE a meen)

U.S. Brand Names Cystagon®
Generic Available No
Synonyms Cysteamine Bitartrate
Pharmacologic Category Anticystine Agent; Urinary Tract Product
Use Orphan drug: Treatment of nephropathic cystinosis
Local Anesthetic/Vasoconstrictor Precautions No information available to require special precautions
Effects on Dental Treatment No significant effects or complications reported
Mechanism of Action Reacts with cystine in the lysosome to convert it to cysteine and to a cysteine-cysteamine mixed disulfide, both of which can then exit the lysosome in patients with cystinosis, an inherited defect of lysosomal transport
Pregnancy Risk Factor C

Cysteamine Bitartrate see Cysteamine on page 412

Cysteine (SIS te een)

Generic Available Yes
Synonyms Cysteine Hydrochloride
Pharmacologic Category Nutritional Supplement
Use Supplement to crystalline amino acid solutions, in particular the specialized pediatric formulas (eg, Aminosyn® PF, TrophAmine®) to meet the intravenous amino acid nutritional requirements of infants receiving parenteral nutrition (PN)
Local Anesthetic/Vasoconstrictor Precautions No information available to require special precautions

Effects on Dental Treatment No significant effects or complications reported

Mechanism of Action Cysteine is a sulfur-containing amino acid synthesized from methionine via the transulfuration pathway. It is a precursor of the tripeptide glutathione and also of taurine. Newborn infants have a relative deficiency of the enzyme necessary to affect this conversion. Cysteine may be considered an essential amino acid in infants.

Cysteine Hydrochloride *see* Cysteine *on page 412*

Cysto-Conray® II *see* Iothalamate Meglumine *on page 855*

Cystografin® *see* Diatrizoate Meglumine *on page 453*

Cystografin® Dilute *see* Diatrizoate Meglumine *on page 453*

Cystospaz® *see* Hyoscyamine *on page 803*

Cystospaz-M® [DSC] *see* Hyoscyamine *on page 803*

CYT *see* Cyclophosphamide *on page 403*

Cytadren® *see* Aminoglutethimide *on page 87*

Cytarabine (sye TARE a been)

U.S. Brand Names Cytosar-U®

Canadian Brand Names Cytosar®

Mexican Brand Names Laracit®

Generic Available Yes

Synonyms Arabinosylcytosine; Ara-C; Cytarabine Hydrochloride; Cytosine Arabinosine Hydrochloride; NSC-63878

Pharmacologic Category Antineoplastic Agent, Antimetabolite; Antineoplastic Agent, Antimetabolite (Purine Antagonist)

Use Treatment of acute myelogenous leukemia; lymphoma, meningeal leukemia, and meningeal lymphoma; has little use in the treatment of solid tumors

Local Anesthetic/Vasoconstrictor Precautions No information available to require special precautions

Effects on Dental Treatment Key adverse event(s) related to dental treatment: Mucositis.

Common Adverse Effects

>10%:

Central nervous system: Fever (>80%)

Dermatologic: Alopecia

Gastrointestinal: Nausea, vomiting, diarrhea, and mucositis which subside quickly after discontinuing the drug; GI effects may be more pronounced with divided I.V. bolus doses than with continuous infusion

Hematologic: Myelosuppression; neutropenia and thrombocytopenia are severe, anemia may also occur

Onset: 4-7 days

Nadir: 14-18 days

Recovery: 21-28 days

Hepatic: Hepatic dysfunction, mild jaundice, transaminases increased (acute)

Ocular: Tearing, ocular pain, foreign body sensation, photophobia, and blurred vision may occur with high-dose therapy; ophthalmic corticosteroids or 0.9% NaCl usually prevents or relieves the condition

1% to 10%:

Cardiovascular: Thrombophlebitis, cardiomegaly

Central nervous system: Dizziness, headache, somnolence, confusion, malaise; a severe cerebellar toxicity occurs in about 8% of patients receiving a high dose (>36-48 g/m^2/cycle); it is irreversible or fatal in about 1%

Dermatologic: Skin freckling, itching, cellulitis at injection site; rash, pain, erythema, and skin sloughing of the palmar and plantar surfaces may occur with high-dose therapy. Prophylactic topical steroids and/or skin moisturizers may be useful.

Genitourinary: Urinary retention

Neuromuscular & skeletal: Myalgia, bone pain

Respiratory: Syndrome of sudden respiratory distress, including tachypnea, hypoxemia, interstitial and alveolar infiltrates progressing to pulmonary edema, pneumonia

Mechanism of Action Inhibition of DNA synthesis. Cytosine gains entry into cells by a carrier process, and then must be converted to its active compound, aracytidine triphosphate. Cytosine is a purine analog and is incorporated into DNA; however, the primary action is inhibition of DNA polymerase resulting in decreased DNA synthesis and repair. The degree of cytotoxicity correlates linearly with incorporation into DNA; therefore, incorporation into the DNA is responsible for drug activity and toxicity. Cytarabine is specific for the S phase of the cell cycle.

(Continued)

Cytarabine *(Continued)*

Drug Interactions

Increased Effect/Toxicity: Alkylating agents and radiation and purine analogs when coadministered with cytarabine may result in increased toxic effects. Methotrexate, when administered prior to cytarabine, may enhance the efficacy and toxicity of cytarabine; some combination treatment regimens (eg, hyper-CVAD) have been designed to take advantage of this interaction.

Decreased Effect: Decreased effect of gentamicin, flucytosine. Decreased digoxin oral tablet absorption.

Pharmacodynamics/Kinetics

Distribution: V_d: Total body water; widely and rapidly since it enters the cells readily; crosses blood-brain barrier with CSF levels of 40% to 50% of plasma level

Metabolism: Primarily hepatic; aracytidine triphosphate is the active moiety; about 86% to 96% of dose is metabolized to inactive uracil arabinoside

Half-life elimination: Initial: 7-20 minutes; Terminal: 0.5-2.6 hours

Excretion: Urine (~80% as metabolites) within 24-36 hours

Pregnancy Risk Factor D

Cytarabine Hydrochloride *see* Cytarabine *on page 413*

Cytarabine (Liposomal) *(sye TARE a been lip po SOE mal)*

U.S. Brand Names DepoCyt™

Canadian Brand Names DepoCyt™

Generic Available No

Pharmacologic Category Antineoplastic Agent, Antimetabolite

Use Treatment of neoplastic (lymphomatous) meningitis

Local Anesthetic/Vasoconstrictor Precautions No information available to require special precautions

Effects on Dental Treatment No significant effects or complications reported

Common Adverse Effects

>10%:

Central nervous system: Headache (28%), confusion (14%), somnolence (12%), fever (11%), pain (11%); chemical arachnoiditis is commonly observed, and may include neck pain, neck rigidity, headache, fever, nausea, vomiting, and back pain; may occur in up to 100% of cycles without dexamethasone prophylaxis; incidence is reduced to 33% when dexamethasone is used concurrently

Gastrointestinal: Vomiting (12%), nausea (11%)

1% to 10%:

Cardiovascular: Peripheral edema (7%)

Gastrointestinal: Constipation (7%)

Genitourinary: Incontinence (3%)

Hematologic: Neutropenia (9%), thrombocytopenia (8%), anemia (1%)

Neuromuscular & skeletal: Back pain (7%), weakness (19%), abnormal gait (4%)

Mechanism of Action This is a sustained-release formulation of the active ingredient cytarabine, which acts through inhibition of DNA synthesis; cell cycle-specific for the S phase of cell division; cytosine gains entry into cells by a carrier process, and then must be converted to its active compound; cytosine acts as an analog and is incorporated into DNA; however, the primary action is inhibition of DNA polymerase resulting in decreased DNA synthesis and repair; degree of its cytotoxicity correlates linearly with its incorporation into DNA; therefore, incorporation into the DNA is responsible for drug activity and toxicity

Drug Interactions

Increased Effect/Toxicity: No formal studies of interactions with other medications have been conducted. The limited systemic exposure minimizes the potential for interaction between liposomal cytarabine and other medications.

Decreased Effect: No formal studies of interactions with other medications have been conducted. The limited systemic exposure minimizes the potential for interaction between liposomal cytarabine and other medications.

Pharmacodynamics/Kinetics

Absorption: Systemic exposure following intrathecal administration is negligible since transfer rate from CSF to plasma is slow

Metabolism: In plasma to ara-U (inactive)

Half-life elimination, CSF: 100-263 hours

Time to peak, CSF: Intrathecal: ~5 hours

Excretion: Primarily urine (as metabolites - ara-U)

Pregnancy Risk Factor D

Cytomel® see Liothyronine on page 934
Cytosar-U® see Cytarabine on page 413
Cytosine Arabinosine Hydrochloride see Cytarabine on page 413
Cytotec® see Misoprostol on page 1053
Cytovene® see Ganciclovir on page 722
Cytoxan® see Cyclophosphamide on page 403
Cytra-2 see Sodium Citrate and Citric Acid on page 1401
Cytra-3 see Citric Acid, Sodium Citrate, and Potassium Citrate on page 354
Cytra-K see Potassium Citrate and Citric Acid on page 1259
Cepacol® Dual Action Maximum Strength [OTC] see Dyclonine on page 525
D2E7 see Adalimumab on page 52
D₃ see Cholecalciferol on page 334
D-3-Mercaptovaline see Penicillamine on page 1201
d4T see Stavudine on page 1416
D₅W see Dextrose on page 452
D₁₀W see Dextrose on page 452
D₂₅W see Dextrose on page 452
D₃₀W see Dextrose on page 452
D₄₀W see Dextrose on page 452
D₅₀W see Dextrose on page 452
D₆₀W see Dextrose on page 452
D₇₀W see Dextrose on page 452
DAB₃₈₉IL-2 see Denileukin Diftitox on page 432

Dacarbazine (da KAR ba zeen)

U.S. Brand Names DTIC-Dome®
Canadian Brand Names DTIC®
Generic Available Yes
Synonyms DIC; Dimethyl Triazeno Imidazole Carboxamide; DTIC; Imidazole Carboxamide; Imidazole Carboxamide Dimethyltriazene; WR-139007
Pharmacologic Category Antineoplastic Agent, Alkylating Agent (Triazene)
Use Treatment of malignant melanoma, Hodgkin's disease, soft-tissue sarcomas, fibrosarcomas, rhabdomyosarcoma, islet cell carcinoma, medullary carcinoma of the thyroid, and neuroblastoma
Local Anesthetic/Vasoconstrictor Precautions No information available to require special precautions
Effects on Dental Treatment Key adverse event(s) related to dental treatment: Metallic taste.
Common Adverse Effects
>10%:
   Gastrointestinal: Nausea and vomiting (>90%), can be severe and dose-limiting; nausea and vomiting decrease on successive days when dacarbazine is given daily for 5 days; diarrhea
   Hematologic: Myelosuppression, leukopenia, thrombocytopenia - dose-limiting
   Onset: 5-7 days
   Nadir: 7-10 days
   Recovery: 21-28 days
   Local: Pain on infusion, may be minimized by administration through a central line, or by administration as a short infusion (eg, 1-2 hours as opposed to bolus injection)
1% to 10%:
   Dermatologic: Alopecia, rash, photosensitivity
   Gastrointestinal: Anorexia, metallic taste
   Miscellaneous: Flu-like syndrome (fever, myalgia, malaise)
Mechanism of Action Alkylating agent which appears to form methyl-carbonium ions that attack nucleophilic groups in DNA; cross-links strands of DNA resulting in the inhibition of DNA, RNA, and protein synthesis, the exact mechanism of action is still unclear.
Drug Interactions
   Cytochrome P450 Effect: Substrate (major) of CYP1A2, 2E1
   Increased Effect/Toxicity: CYP1A2 inhibitors may increase the levels/effects of dacarbazine; example inhibitors include amiodarone, ciprofloxacin, fluvoxamine, ketoconazole, norfloxacin, ofloxacin, and rofecoxib. CYP2E1 inhibitors may increase the levels/effects of dacarbazine; example inhibitors include disulfiram, isoniazid, and miconazole.
   Decreased Effect: CYP1A2 inducers may decrease the levels/effects of dacarbazine; example inducers include aminoglutethimide, carbamazepine, (Continued)

Dacarbazine *(Continued)*

phenobarbital, and rifampin. Patients may experience impaired immune response to vaccines; possible infection after administration of live vaccines in patients receiving immunosuppressants.

Pharmacodynamics/Kinetics

Onset of action: I.V.: 18-24 days

Distribution: V_d: 0.6 L/kg, exceeding total body water; suggesting binding to some tissue (probably liver)

Protein binding: 5%

Metabolism: Extensively hepatic; hepatobiliary excretion is probably of some importance; metabolites may also have an antineoplastic effect

Half-life elimination: Biphasic: Initial: 20-40 minutes; Terminal: 5 hours

Excretion: Urine (~30% to 50% as unchanged drug)

Pregnancy Risk Factor C

Dacex-DM *see* Guaifenesin, Dextromethorphan, and Phenylephrine *on page 756*

Daclizumab *(dac KLYE zue mab)*

U.S. Brand Names Zenapax®

Canadian Brand Names Zenapax®

Generic Available No

Pharmacologic Category Immunosuppressant Agent

Use Part of an immunosuppressive regimen (including cyclosporine and corticosteroids) for the prophylaxis of acute organ rejection in patients receiving renal transplant

Unlabeled/Investigational Use Graft-versus-host disease; prevention of organ rejection after heart transplant

Local Anesthetic/Vasoconstrictor Precautions No information available to require special precautions

Effects on Dental Treatment No significant effects or complications reported

Common Adverse Effects Although reported adverse events are frequent, when daclizumab is compared with placebo the incidence of adverse effects is similar between the two groups. Many of the adverse effects reported during clinical trial use of daclizumab may be related to the patient population, transplant procedure, and concurrent transplant medications. Diarrhea, fever, postoperative pain, pruritus, respiratory tract infection, urinary tract infection, and vomiting occurred more often in children than adults.

≥5%:

Cardiovascular: Chest pain, edema, hyper-/hypotension, tachycardia, thrombosis

Central nervous system: Dizziness, fatigue, fever, headache, insomnia, pain, post-traumatic pain, tremor

Dermatologic: Acne, cellulitis, wound healing impaired

Gastrointestinal: Abdominal distention, abdominal pain, constipation, diarrhea, dyspepsia, epigastric pain, nausea, pyrosis, vomiting

Genitourinary: Dysuria

Hematologic: Bleeding

Neuromuscular & skeletal: Back pain, musculoskeletal pain

Renal: Oliguria, renal tubular necrosis

Respiratory: Cough, dyspnea, pulmonary edema,

Miscellaneous: Lymphocele, wound infection

≥2% to <5%:

Central nervous system: Anxiety, depression, shivering

Dermatologic: Hirsutism, pruritus, rash

Endocrine & metabolic: Dehydration, diabetes mellitus, fluid overload

Gastrointestinal: Flatulence, gastritis, hemorrhoids

Genitourinary: Urinary retention, urinary tract bleeding

Local: Application site reaction

Neuromuscular & skeletal: Arthralgia, leg cramps, myalgia, weakness

Ocular: Vision blurred

Renal: Hydronephrosis, renal damage, renal insufficiency

Respiratory: Atelectasis, congestion, hypoxia, pharyngitis, pleural effusion, rales, rhinitis

Miscellaneous: Night sweats, prickly sensation, diaphoresis

Mechanism of Action Daclizumab is a chimeric (90% human, 10% murine) monoclonal IgG antibody produced by recombinant DNA technology. Daclizumab inhibits immune reactions by binding and blocking the alpha-chain of the interleukin-2 receptor (CD25) located on the surface of activated lymphocytes.

Drug Interactions

Increased Effect/Toxicity: The combined use of daclizumab, cyclosporine, mycophenolate mofetil, and corticosteroids has been associated with an increased mortality in a population of cardiac transplant recipients, particularly in patients who received antilymphocyte globulin and in patients with severe infections.

Pharmacodynamics/Kinetics

Distribution: V_d:

Adults: Central compartment: 0.031 L/kg; Peripheral compartment: 0.043 L/kg

Children: Central compartment: 0.067 L/kg; Peripheral compartment: 0.047 L/kg

Half-life elimination (estimated): Adults: Terminal: 20 days; Children: 13 days

Pregnancy Risk Factor C

DACT see Dactinomycin on page 417

Dactinomycin (dak ti noe MYE sin)

U.S. Brand Names Cosmegen®

Canadian Brand Names Cosmegen®

Generic Available No

Synonyms ACT; Act-D; Actinomycin; Actinomycin Cl; Actinomycin D; DACT; NSC-3053

Pharmacologic Category Antineoplastic Agent, Antibiotic

Use Treatment of testicular tumors, melanoma, choriocarcinoma, Wilms' tumor, neuroblastoma, retinoblastoma, rhabdomyosarcoma, uterine sarcomas, Ewing's sarcoma, Kaposi's sarcoma, sarcoma botryoides, and soft tissue sarcoma

Local Anesthetic/Vasoconstrictor Precautions No information available to require special precautions

Effects on Dental Treatment Key adverse event(s) related to dental treatment: Stomatitis and mucositis.

Common Adverse Effects Frequency not defined.

Central nervous system: Fatigue, fever, lethargy, malaise

Dermatologic: Acne, alopecia (reversible), cheilitis; increased pigmentation, sloughing, or erythema of previously irradiated skin; skin eruptions

Endocrine & metabolic: Growth retardation, hypocalcemia

Gastrointestinal: Abdominal pain, anorexia, diarrhea, dysphagia, esophagitis, GI ulceration, mucositis, nausea, pharyngitis, proctitis, stomatitis, vomiting

Hematologic: Agranulocytosis, anemia, leukopenia, pancytopenia, reticulocytopenia, thrombocytopenia, myelosuppression (onset: 7 days, nadir: 14-21 days, recovery: 21-28 days)

Hepatic: Ascites, hepatic failure, hepatitis, hepatomegaly, hepatotoxicity, liver function test abnormality, veno-occlusive disease

Local: Tissue necrosis, pain, and ulceration (following extravasation)

Neuromuscular & skeletal: Myalgia

Renal: Renal function abnormality

Respiratory: Pneumonitis

Miscellaneous: Anaphylactoid reaction, infection

Mechanism of Action Binds to the guanine portion of DNA intercalating between guanine and cytosine base pairs inhibiting DNA and RNA synthesis and protein synthesis

Drug Interactions

Increased Effect/Toxicity: Dactinomycin potentiates the effects of radiation therapy. Avoid administration of live vaccines in immunosuppressive therapy.

Pharmacodynamics/Kinetics

Distribution: High concentrations found in bone marrow and tumor cells, submaxillary gland, liver, and kidney; crosses placenta; poor CSF penetration

Metabolism: Hepatic, minimal

Half-life elimination: 36 hours

Time to peak, serum: I.V.: 2-5 minutes

Excretion: Bile (50%); feces (14%); urine (~10% as unchanged drug)

Pregnancy Risk Factor D

DAD see Mitoxantrone on page 1055

Dakin's Solution see Sodium Hypochlorite Solution on page 1402

Dallergy® see Chlorpheniramine, Phenylephrine, and Methscopolamine on page 327

Dallergy-JR® see Chlorpheniramine and Phenylephrine on page 324

Dalmane® see Flurazepam on page 681

d-Alpha-Gems™ [OTC] see Vitamin E on page 1581

d-Alpha Tocopherol see Vitamin E on page 1581

Dalteparin (dal TE pa rin)

Related Information
Cardiovascular Diseases *on page 1636*
U.S. Brand Names Fragmin®
Canadian Brand Names Fragmin®
Generic Available No
Pharmacologic Category Low Molecular Weight Heparin
Use Prevention of deep vein thrombosis which may lead to pulmonary embolism, in patients requiring abdominal surgery who are at risk for thromboembolism complications (eg, patients >40 years of age, obesity, patients with malignancy, history of deep vein thrombosis or pulmonary embolism, and surgical procedures requiring general anesthesia and lasting >30 minutes); prevention of DVT in patients undergoing hip-replacement surgery; patients immobile during an acute illness; acute treatment of unstable angina or non-Q-wave myocardial infarction; prevention of ischemic complications in patients on concurrent aspirin therapy
Unlabeled/Investigational Use Active treatment of deep vein thrombosis
Local Anesthetic/Vasoconstrictor Precautions No information available to require special precautions
Effects on Dental Treatment No significant effects or complications reported
Common Adverse Effects 1% to 10%:
Hematologic: Bleeding (3% to 5%), wound hematoma (0.1% to 3%)
Local: Pain at injection site (up to 12%), injection site hematoma (0.2% to 7%)
Mechanism of Action Low molecular weight heparin analog with a molecular weight of 4000-6000 daltons; the commercial product contains 3% to 15% heparin with a molecular weight <3000 daltons, 65% to 78% with a molecular weight of 3000-8000 daltons and 14% to 26% with a molecular weight >8000 daltons; while dalteparin has been shown to inhibit both factor Xa and factor IIa (thrombin), the antithrombotic effect of dalteparin is characterized by a higher ratio of antifactor Xa to antifactor IIa activity (ratio = 4)
Drug Interactions
Increased Effect/Toxicity: The risk of bleeding with dalteparin may be increased by drugs which affect platelet function (eg, aspirin, NSAIDs, dipyridamole, ticlopidine, clopidogrel), oral anticoagulants, and thrombolytic agents. Although the risk of bleeding may be increased during concurrent warfarin therapy, dalteparin is commonly continued during the initiation of warfarin therapy to assure anticoagulation and to protect against possible transient hypercoagulability.
Pharmacodynamics/Kinetics
Onset of action: 1-2 hours
Duration: >12 hours
Half-life elimination (route dependent): 2-5 hours
Time to peak, serum: 4 hours
Pregnancy Risk Factor B

Damason-P® *see* Hydrocodone and Aspirin *on page 782*

Danaparoid (da NAP a roid)

Canadian Brand Names Organ®
Generic Available No
Synonyms Danaparoid Sodium
Pharmacologic Category Anticoagulant
Use Prevention of postoperative deep vein thrombosis following elective hip replacement surgery
Unlabeled/Investigational Use Systemic anticoagulation for patients with heparin-induced thrombocytopenia: factor Xa inhibition is used to monitor degree of anticoagulation if necessary
Local Anesthetic/Vasoconstrictor Precautions No information available to require special precautions
Effects on Dental Treatment Key adverse event(s) related to dental treatment: As with all anticoagulants, bleeding is the major adverse effect of danaparoid. Hemorrhage may occur at virtually any site; risk is dependent on multiple variables.
Common Adverse Effects As with all anticoagulants, bleeding is the major adverse effect of danaparoid. Hemorrhage may occur at virtually any site. Risk is dependent on multiple variables.
>10%:
Central nervous system: Fever (22%)

Gastrointestinal: Nausea (4% to 14%), constipation (4% to 11%)

1% to 10%:

Cardiovascular: Peripheral edema (3%), edema (3%)

Central nervous system: Insomnia (3%), headache (3%), asthenia (2%), dizziness (2%), pain (9%)

Dermatologic: Rash (2% to 5%), pruritus (4%)

Gastrointestinal: Vomiting (3%)

Genitourinary: Urinary tract infection (3% to 4%), urinary retention (2%)

Hematologic: Anemia (2%)

Local: Injection site pain (8% to 14%), injection site hematoma (5%)

Neuromuscular & skeletal: Joint disorder (3%)

Miscellaneous: Infection (2%)

Restrictions Not available in U.S.

Mechanism of Action Prevents fibrin formation in coagulation pathway via thrombin generation inhibition by anti-Xa and anti-IIa effects.

Drug Interactions

Increased Effect/Toxicity: The risk of hemorrhage associated with danaparoid may be increased with thrombolytic agents, oral anticoagulants (warfarin) and drugs which affect platelet function (eg, aspirin, NSAIDs, dipyridamole, ticlopidine, clopidogrel).

Pharmacodynamics/Kinetics

Onset of action: Peak effect: SubQ: Maximum antifactor Xa and antithrombin (antifactor IIa) activities occur in 2-5 hours

Half-life elimination, plasma: Mean: Terminal: ~24 hours

Excretion: Primarily urine

Pregnancy Risk Factor B

Danaparoid Sodium *see* Danaparoid *on page 418*

Danazol (DA na zole)

U.S. Brand Names Danocrine® [DSC]

Canadian Brand Names Cyclomen®; Danocrine®

Mexican Brand Names Ladogal®; Norciden®

Generic Available Yes

Pharmacologic Category Androgen

Use Treatment of endometriosis, fibrocystic breast disease, and hereditary angioedema

Local Anesthetic/Vasoconstrictor Precautions No information available to require special precautions

Effects on Dental Treatment No significant effects or complications reported

Common Adverse Effects Frequency not defined.

Cardiovascular: Benign intracranial hypertension (rare), edema, flushing, hypertension

Central nervous system: Anxiety (rare), chills (rare), convulsions (rare), depression, dizziness, emotional lability, fainting, fever (rare), Guillain-Barré syndrome, headache, nervousness, sleep disorders, tremor

Dermatologic: Acne, hair loss, mild hirsutism, maculopapular rash, papular rash, petechial rash, pruritus, purpuric rash, seborrhea, Stevens-Johnson syndrome (rare), photosensitivity (rare), urticaria, vesicular rash

Endocrine & metabolic: Amenorrhea (which may continue post therapy), breast size reduction, clitoris hypertrophy, glucose intolerance, HDL decreased, LDL increased, libido changes, nipple discharge, menstrual disturbances (spotting, altered timing of cycle), semen abnormalities (changes in volume, viscosity, sperm count/motility), spermatogenesis reduction

Gastrointestinal: Appetite changes (rare), bleeding gums (rare), constipation, gastroenteritis, nausea, pancreatitis (rare), vomiting, weight gain

Genitourinary: Vaginal dryness, vaginal irritation, pelvic pain

Hematologic: Eosinophilia, erythrocytosis (reversible), leukocytosis, leukopenia, platelet count increased, polycythemia, RBC increased, thrombocytopenia

Hepatic: Cholestatic jaundice, hepatic adenoma, jaundice, liver enzymes (elevated), malignant tumors (after prolonged use), peliosis hepatis

Neuromuscular & skeletal: Back pain, carpal tunnel syndrome (rare), extremity pain, joint lockup, joint pain, joint swelling, muscle cramps, neck pain, paresthesia, spasms, weakness

Ocular: Cataracts (rare), visual disturbances

Renal: Hematuria

Respiratory: Nasal congestion (rare)

Miscellaneous: Voice change (hoarseness, sore throat, instability, deepening of pitch), diaphoresis

Mechanism of Action Suppresses pituitary output of follicle-stimulating hormone and luteinizing hormone that causes regression and atrophy of normal

(Continued)

Danazol *(Continued)*

and ectopic endometrial tissue; decreases rate of growth of abnormal breast tissue; reduces attacks associated with hereditary angioedema by increasing levels of C4 component of complement

Drug Interactions

Cytochrome P450 Effect: Inhibits CYP3A4 (weak)

Increased Effect/Toxicity: Danazol may increase serum levels of carbamazepine, cyclosporine, tacrolimus, and warfarin leading to toxicity; dosage adjustment may be needed; monitor. Concomitant use of danazol and HMG-CoA reductase inhibitors may lead to severe myopathy or rhabdomyolysis. Danazol may enhance the glucose-lowering effect of hypoglycemic agents.

Decreased Effect: Danazol may decrease effectiveness of hormonal contraceptives. Nonhormonal birth control methods are recommended.

Pharmacodynamics/Kinetics

Onset of action: Therapeutic: ~4 weeks

Metabolism: Extensively hepatic, primarily to 2-hydroxymethylethisterone

Half-life elimination: 4.5 hours (variable)

Time to peak, serum: Within 2 hours

Excretion: Urine

Pregnancy Risk Factor X

Danocrine® [DSC] see Danazol on page 419

Dantrium® see Dantrolene on page 420

Dantrolene *(DAN troe leen)*

U.S. Brand Names Dantrium®

Canadian Brand Names Dantrium®

Generic Available No

Synonyms Dantrolene Sodium

Pharmacologic Category Skeletal Muscle Relaxant

Use Treatment of spasticity associated with spinal cord injury, stroke, cerebral palsy, or multiple sclerosis; treatment of malignant hyperthermia

Unlabeled/Investigational Use Neuroleptic malignant syndrome (NMS)

Local Anesthetic/Vasoconstrictor Precautions No information available to require special precautions

Effects on Dental Treatment No significant effects or complications reported

Common Adverse Effects

>10%:

Central nervous system: Drowsiness, dizziness, lightheadedness, fatigue

Dermatologic: Rash

Gastrointestinal: Diarrhea (mild), nausea, vomiting

Neuromuscular & skeletal: Muscle weakness

1% to 10%:

Cardiovascular: Pleural effusion with pericarditis

Central nervous system: Chills, fever, headache, insomnia, nervousness, mental depression

Gastrointestinal: Diarrhea (severe), constipation, anorexia, stomach cramps

Ocular: Blurred vision

Respiratory: Respiratory depression

Mechanism of Action Acts directly on skeletal muscle by interfering with release of calcium ion from the sarcoplasmic reticulum; prevents or reduces the increase in myoplasmic calcium ion concentration that activates the acute catabolic processes associated with malignant hyperthermia

Drug Interactions

Cytochrome P450 Effect: Substrate of CYP3A4 (major)

Increased Effect/Toxicity: Increased toxicity with estrogens (hepatotoxicity), CNS depressants (sedation), MAO inhibitors, phenothiazines, clindamycin (increased neuromuscular blockade), verapamil (hyperkalemia and cardiac depression), warfarin, clofibrate, and tolbutamide. CYP3A4 inhibitors may increase the levels/effects of dantrolene; example inhibitors include azole antifungals, clarithromycin, diclofenac, doxycycline, erythromycin, imatinib, isoniazid, nefazodone, nicardipine, propofol, protease inhibitors, quinidine, telithromycin, and verapamil.

Decreased Effect: CYP3A4 inducers may decrease the levels/effects of dantrolene; example inducers include aminoglutethimide, carbamazepine, nafcillin, nevirapine, phenobarbital, phenytoin, and rifamycins.

Pharmacodynamics/Kinetics

Absorption: Oral: Slow and incomplete

Metabolism: Hepatic

Half-life elimination: 8.7 hours
Excretion: Feces (45% to 50%); urine (25% as unchanged drug and metabo-lites)
Pregnancy Risk Factor C

Dantrolene Sodium *see Dantrolene on page 420*
Dapcin *see Daptomycin on page 423*

Dapiprazole (DA pi pray zole)

U.S. Brand Names Rēv-Eyes™
Generic Available No
Synonyms Dapiprazole Hydrochloride
Pharmacologic Category Alpha$_1$ Blocker, Ophthalmic
Use Reverse dilation due to drugs (adrenergic or parasympathomimetic) after eye exams
Local Anesthetic/Vasoconstrictor Precautions No information available to require special precautions
Effects on Dental Treatment No significant effects or complications reported
Mechanism of Action Dapiprazole is a selective alpha-adrenergic blocking agent, exerting effects primarily on alpha$_1$-adrenoreceptors. It induces miosis via relaxation of the smooth dilator (radial) muscle of the iris, which causes pupillary constriction. It is devoid of cholinergic effects. Dapiprazole also partially reverses the cycloplegia induced with parasympatholytic agents such as tropicamide. Although the drug has no significant effect on the ciliary muscle *per se*, it may increase accommodative amplitude, therefore relieving the symp-toms of paralysis of accommodation.
Pregnancy Risk Factor B

Dapiprazole Hydrochloride *see Dapiprazole on page 421*

Dapsone (DAP sone)

Related Information
HIV Infection and AIDS *on page 1662*
U.S. Brand Names Aczone™
Generic Available Yes: Tablet
Synonyms Diaminodiphenylsulfone
Pharmacologic Category Antibiotic, Miscellaneous
Dental Use Used in lupus and in selected ulcerative conditions in consult with patient's physician
Use Treatment of leprosy and dermatitis herpetiformis (infections caused by *Mycobacterium leprae*); treatment of acne vulgaris
Unlabeled/Investigational Use Prophylaxis of toxoplasmosis in severely-immunocompromised patients; alternative agent for *Pneumocystis carinii* pneumonia prophylaxis (monotherapy) and treatment (in combination with trimethoprim)
Local Anesthetic/Vasoconstrictor Precautions No information available to require special precautions
Effects on Dental Treatment No significant effects or complications reported
Significant Adverse Effects
>10%: Hematologic: Hemolysis (dose-related; seen in patients with and without G6PD deficiency), hemoglobin decrease (1-2 g/dL- almost all patients), reticulocyte increase (2% to 12%), methemoglobinemia, red cell life span shortened

Frequency not defined.
Cardiovascular: Tachycardia
Central nervous system: Fever, headache, insomnia, psychosis, tonic-clonic movement (topical), vertigo
Dermatologic: Bullous and exfoliative dermatitis, erythema nodosum, exfolia-tive dermatitis (oral), morbilliform and scarlatiniform reactions, phototoxicity (oral), Stevens-Johnson syndrome, toxic epidural necrolysis, urticaria
Endocrine & metabolic: Hypoalbuminemia (without proteinuria), male infertility
Gastrointestinal: Abdominal pain (oral, topical), nausea, pancreatitis (oral, topical), vomiting
Hematologic: Agranulocytosis, anemia, leukopenia, pure red cell aplasia (case report)
Hepatic: Cholestatic jaundice, hepatitis
Neuromuscular & skeletal: Drug-induced lupus erythematosus, lower motor neuron toxicity (prolonged therapy), peripheral neuropathy (rare, nonleprosy patients)
(Continued)

Dapsone *(Continued)*

Ocular: Blurred vision

Otic: Tinnitus

Renal: Albuminuria, nephrotic syndrome, renal papillary necrosis

Respiratory: Interstitial pneumonitis, pharyngitis (topical), pulmonary eosinophilia

Miscellaneous: Infectious mononucleosis-like syndrome (rash, fever, lymphadenopathy, hepatic dysfunction)

Dosage Oral:

Leprosy:

Children: 1-2 mg/kg/24 hours, up to a maximum of 100 mg/day

Adults: 50-100 mg/day for 3-10 years

Dermatitis herpetiformis: Adults: Start at 50 mg/day, increase to 300 mg/day, or higher to achieve full control, reduce dosage to minimum level as soon as possible

Pneumocystis carinii pneumonia (unlabeled use):

Prophylaxis:

Children >1 month: 2 mg/kg/day once daily (maximum dose: 100 mg/day) or 4 mg/kg/dose once weekly (maximum dose: 200 mg)

Adults: 100 mg/day

Treatment: Adults: 100 mg/day in combination with trimethoprim (15-20 mg/kg/day) for 21 days

Topical: Acne vulgaris: Children ≥12 years and Adults: Apply pea-sized amount twice daily

Dosing in renal impairment: No specific guidelines are available

Mechanism of Action Competitive antagonist of para-aminobenzoic acid (PABA) and prevents normal bacterial utilization of PABA for the synthesis of folic acid

Contraindications Hypersensitivity to dapsone or any component of the formulation

Warnings/Precautions Use with caution in patients with severe anemia, G6PD, methemoglobin reductase or hemoglobin M deficiency; hypersensitivity to other sulfonamides; aplastic anemia, agranulocytosis and other severe blood dyscrasias have resulted in death; monitor carefully; treat severe anemia prior to therapy; serious dermatologic reactions (including toxic epidermal necrolysis) are rare but potential occurrences; sulfone reactions may also occur as potentially fatal hypersensitivity reactions; these, but not leprosy reactional states, require drug discontinuation; dapsone is carcinogenic in small animals. Safety and efficacy of topical dapsone has not been adequately evaluated in patient with G6PD deficiency or in patients <12 years of age.

Drug Interactions Substrate of CYP2C8 (minor), 2C9 (major), 2C19 (minor), 2E1 (minor), 3A4 (major)

CYP2C9 Inducers may decrease the levels/effects of dapsone. Example inducers include carbamazepine, phenobarbital, phenytoin, rifampin, rifapentine, and secobarbital.

CYP2C9 Inhibitors may increase the levels/effects of dapsone. Example inhibitors include delavirdine, fluconazole, gemfibrozil, ketoconazole, nicardipine, NSAIDs, sulfonamides and tolbutamide.

CYP3A4 inducers: May decrease the levels/effects of dapsone. Example inducers include aminoglutethimide, carbamazepine, efavirenz, fosphenytoin, nafcillin, nevirapine, oxcarbazine, phenobarbital, phenytoin, primidone, and rifamycins.

CYP3A4 inhibitors: May increase the levels/effects of dapsone. Example inhibitors include azole antifungals, clarithromycin, diclofenac, doxycycline, erythromycin, imatinib, isoniazid, nefazodone, nicardipine, propofol, protease inhibitors, quinidine, telithromycin, and verapamil.

Didanosine: May decrease absorption of dapsone. Didanosine enteric coated capsules should not affect dapsone. Avoid other forms of didanosine.

Folic acid antagonists: May increase the risk of hematologic reactions of dapsone.

Probenecid: Decreases dapsone excretion.

Rifamycin derivatives: Increase metabolism of dapsone.

Trimethoprim: May increase toxic effects of both drugs.

Ethanol/Nutrition/Herb Interactions Herb/Nutraceutical: St John's wort may decrease dapsone levels.

Dietary Considerations Do not administer with antacids, alkaline foods, or drugs.

Pharmacodynamics/Kinetics

Absorption:

Oral: Well absorbed

Topical: ~1% of the absorption of 100 mg tablet

Distribution: V_d: 1.5 L/kg; throughout total body water and present in all tissues, especially liver and kidney
Metabolism: Hepatic; forms metabolite
Half-life elimination: 30 hours (range: 10-50 hours)
Excretion: Urine (~85%)
Pregnancy Risk Factor C
Lactation Enters breast milk/not recommended (AAP rates "compatible")
Dosage Forms
Gel, topical (Aczone™): 5% (30 g)
Tablet: 25 mg, 100 mg

Daptomycin (DAP toe mye sin)

U.S. Brand Names Cubicin®
Generic Available No
Synonyms Cidecin; Dapcin; LY146032
Pharmacologic Category Antibiotic, Cyclic Lipopeptide
Use Treatment of complicated skin and skin structure infections caused by susceptible aerobic Gram-positive organisms
Unlabeled/Investigational Use Treatment of bacteremia, endocarditis, and other severe infections caused by MRSA or VRE
Local Anesthetic/Vasoconstrictor Precautions No information available to require special precautions
Effects on Dental Treatment No significant effects or complications reported
Common Adverse Effects 1% to 10%:
Cardiovascular: Hypotension (2%), hypertension (1%)
Central nervous system: Headache (5%), insomnia (5%), dizziness (2%), fever (2%)
Dermatologic: Rash (4%), pruritus (3%)
Gastrointestinal: Constipation (6%), nausea (6%), diarrhea (5%), vomiting (3%), dyspepsia (1%)
Genitourinary: Urinary tract infection (2%)
Hematologic: Anemia (2%)
Hepatic: Transaminases increased (3%)
Local: Injection site reaction (6%)
Neuromuscular & skeletal: CPK increased (3%), limb pain (2%), arthralgia (1%)
Renal: Renal failure (2%)
Respiratory: Dyspnea (2%)
Miscellaneous: Infection (fungal, 3%)
Mechanism of Action Daptomycin binds to components of the cell membrane of susceptible organisms and causes rapid depolarization, inhibiting intracellular synthesis of DNA, RNA, and protein. Daptomycin is bactericidal in a concentration-dependent manner.
Drug Interactions
Increased Effect/Toxicity: No clinically-significant interactions have been identified.
Pharmacodynamics/Kinetics
Distribution: 0.09 L/kg
Protein binding: 92%
Half-life elimination: 8-9 hours (up to 28 hours in renal impairment)
Excretion: Urine (78%; primarily as unchanged drug); feces (6%)
Pregnancy Risk Factor B

Daranide® *see Dichlorphenamide on page 459*
Daraprim® *see Pyrimethamine on page 1317*

Darbepoetin Alfa (dar be POE e tin AL fa)

U.S. Brand Names Aranesp®
Canadian Brand Names Aranesp®
Generic Available No
Synonyms Erythropoiesis Stimulating Protein
Pharmacologic Category Colony Stimulating Factor; Growth Factor; Recombinant Human Erythropoietin
Use Treatment of anemia associated with chronic renal failure (CRF), including patients on dialysis (ESRD) and patients not on dialysis; anemia associated with chemotherapy for nonmyeloid malignancies
Local Anesthetic/Vasoconstrictor Precautions No information available to require special precautions
Effects on Dental Treatment No significant effects or complications reported
(Continued)

Darbepoetin Alfa *(Continued)*

Common Adverse Effects Note: Frequency of adverse events cited in patients with CRF or cancer and may be, in part, a reflection of population in which the drug is used and/or associated with dialysis procedures.

>10%:
  Cardiovascular: Hypertension (4% to 23%), hypotension (22%), edema (21%), peripheral edema (11%)
  Central nervous system: Fatigue (9% to 33%), fever (4% to 19%), headache (12% to 16%), dizziness (8% to 14%)
  Gastrointestinal: Diarrhea (16% to 22%), constipation (5% to 18%), vomiting (2% to 15%), nausea (14%), abdominal pain (12%)
  Neuromuscular & skeletal: Myalgia (8% to 21%), arthralgia (11% to 13%)
  Respiratory: Upper respiratory infection (14%), dyspnea (2% to 12%)
  Miscellaneous: Infection (27%)

1% to 10%:
  Cardiovascular: Arrhythmia (10%), angina/chest pain (6% to 8%), fluid overload (6%), CHF (6%), thrombosis (6%), MI (2%)
  Central nervous system: Seizure (≤1%), stroke (1%), TIA (1%)
  Dermatologic: Pruritus (8%), rash (7%)
  Endocrine & metabolic: Dehydration (3% to 5%)
  Local: Vascular access thrombosis (8%), injection site pain (7%), vascular access hemorrhage (6%), vascular access infection (6%)
  Neuromuscular & skeletal: Limb pain (10%), back pain (8%), weakness (5%)
  Respiratory: Cough (10%), bronchitis (6%), pneumonia (3%), pulmonary embolism (1%)
  Miscellaneous: Death (7%), flu-like symptoms (6%)

Postmarketing and/or case reports: Deep vein thrombosis, pure red cell aplasia, severe anemia (with or without other cytopenias), thromboembolism, thrombophlebitis

Mechanism of Action Induces erythropoiesis by stimulating the division and differentiation of committed erythroid progenitor cells; induces the release of reticulocytes from the bone marrow into the bloodstream, where they mature to erythrocytes. There is a dose response relationship with this effect. This results in an increase in reticulocyte counts followed by a rise in hematocrit and hemoglobin levels. When administered SubQ or I.V., darbepoetin's half-life is ~3 times that of epoetin alfa concentrations.

Pharmacodynamics/Kinetics
Onset of action: Increased hemoglobin levels not generally observed until 2-6 weeks after initiating treatment
Absorption: SubQ: Slow
Distribution: V_d: 0.06 L/kg
Bioavailability: CRF: SubQ: ~37% (range: 30% to 50%)
Half-life elimination: CRF: Terminal: I.V.: 21 hours, SubQ: 49 hours; cancer: SubQ: 74 hours
  Note: Half-life is ~3 times as long as epoetin alfa
Time to peak: SubQ: CRF: 34 hours (range: 24-72 hours); Cancer: 90 hours (range: 71-123 hours)

Pregnancy Risk Factor C

Darifenacin *(dar i FEN a sin)*

U.S. Brand Names Enablex®
Generic Available No
Synonyms Darifenacin Hydrobromide; UK-88,525
Pharmacologic Category Anticholinergic Agent
Use Management of symptoms of bladder overactivity (urge incontinence, urgency, and frequency)
Local Anesthetic/Vasoconstrictor Precautions No information available to require special precautions
Effects on Dental Treatment Key adverse event(s) related to dental treatment: Xerostomia (normal salivary flow resumes upon discontinuation). Prolonged xerostomia may contribute to discomfort and dental disease (eg, caries, periodontal disease, and oral candidiasis).
Common Adverse Effects
>10%: Gastrointestinal: Xerostomia (19% to 35%), constipation (15% to 21%)
1% to 10%:
  Cardiovascular: Hypertension, peripheral edema
  Central nervous system: Headache (7%), dizziness (1% to 2%)
  Dermatological: Dry skin, pruritis, rash
  Gastrointestinal: Dyspepsia (3% to 8%), abdominal pain (2% to 4%), nausea (2% to 4%), diarrhea (1% to 2%), vomiting, weight gain

Genitourinary: Urinary tract infection (4% to 5%), urinary retention, urinary tract disorder, vaginitis

Neuromuscular & skeletal: Weakness (2% to 3%), arthralgia, back pain

Ocular: Dry eyes (2%), abnormal vision

Respiratory: Bronchitis, pharyngitis, rhinitis, sinusitis

Miscellaneous: Flu-like syndrome (<1% to 3%), accidental injury (<1% to 3%)

Mechanism of Action Selective antagonist of the M3 muscarinic (cholinergic) receptor subtype. Blockade of the receptor limits bladder contractions, reducing the symptoms of bladder irritability/overactivity (urge incontinence, urgency and frequency).

Drug Interactions

Cytochrome P450 Effect: Substrate of CYP2D6 (minor), CYP3A4 (major); **Inhibits** CYP2D6 (moderate), 3A4 (weak)

Increased Effect/Toxicity: Adverse anticholinergic effects may be additive with other anticholinergic agents (includes tricyclic antidepressants, antihistamines, and phenothiazines). Coadministration with pramlintide may result an additive reduction in gut motility. Darifenacin may increase the levels/effects of CYP2D6 substrates; example substrates include amphetamines, selected beta-blockers, dextromethorphan, fluoxetine, lidocaine, mirtazapine, nefazodone, paroxetine, risperidone, ritonavir, thioridazine, tricyclic antidepressants, and venlafaxine. CYP3A4 inhibitors may increase the levels/effects of darifenacin; example inhibitors include azole antifungals, clarithromycin, diclofenac, doxycycline, erythromycin, imatinib, isoniazid, nefazodone, nicardipine, propofol, protease inhibitors, quinidine, telithromycin, and verapamil.

Decreased Effect: Darifenacin may decrease the levels/effects of CYP2D6 prodrug substrates; example prodrug substrates include codeine, hydrocodone, oxycodone, and tramadol. CYP3A4 inducers may decrease the levels/effects of darifenacin; example inducers include aminoglutethimide, carbamazepine, nafcillin, nevirapine, phenobarbital, phenytoin, and rifamycins. Concomitant use with acetylcholinesterase inhibitors may reduce the therapeutic efficacy of darifenacin.

Pharmacodynamics/Kinetics

Distribution: V_{dss}: 163 L

Protein binding: 98%

Metabolism: Hepatic, via CYP3A4 (major) and CYP2D6 (minor)

Bioavailability: 15% to 19%

Half-life elimination: 13-19 hours

Time to peak, plasma: 7 hours

Excretion: As metabolites (inactive); urine (60%), feces (40%)

Pregnancy Risk Factor C

Darifenacin Hydrobromide *see* Darifenacin *on page 424*

Darvocet A500™ *see* Propoxyphene and Acetaminophen *on page 1298*

Darvocet-N® 50 *see* Propoxyphene and Acetaminophen *on page 1298*

Darvocet-N® 100 *see* Propoxyphene and Acetaminophen *on page 1298*

Darvon® *see* Propoxyphene *on page 1297*

Darvon® Compound [DSC] *see* Propoxyphene, Aspirin, and Caffeine *on page 1300*

Darvon-N® *see* Propoxyphene *on page 1297*

Daunomycin *see* DAUNOrubicin Hydrochloride *on page 426*

DAUNOrubicin Citrate (Liposomal)
(daw noe ROO bi sin SI trate lip po SOE mal)

U.S. Brand Names DaunoXome®

Generic Available No

Pharmacologic Category Antineoplastic Agent, Anthracycline

Use First-line cytotoxic therapy for advanced HIV-associated Kaposi's sarcoma

Local Anesthetic/Vasoconstrictor Precautions No information available to require special precautions

Effects on Dental Treatment Key adverse event(s) related to dental treatment: Stomatitis.

Common Adverse Effects

>10%:

Central nervous system: Fatigue (51%), headache (28%), neuropathy (13%)

Hematologic: Myelosuppression, neutropenia (51%), thrombocytopenia, anemia

Onset: 7 days

Nadir: 14 days

Recovery: 21 days

(Continued)

DAUNOrubicin Citrate (Liposomal) *(Continued)*

Gastrointestinal: Abdominal pain, vomiting, anorexia (23%); diarrhea (38%); nausea (55%)

Respiratory: Cough (28%), dyspnea (26%), rhinitis

Miscellaneous: Allergic reactions (24%)

1% to 10%:

Cardiovascular: CHF (incidence unknown), hypertension, palpitation, syncope, tachycardia, chest pain, edema

Dermatologic: Alopecia (8%), pruritus (7%)

Endocrine & metabolic: Hot flashes

Gastrointestinal: Constipation (7%), stomatitis (10%)

Neuromuscular & skeletal: Arthralgia (7%), myalgia (7%)

Ocular: Conjunctivitis, eye pain (5%)

Respiratory: Sinusitis

Mechanism of Action Liposomes have been shown to penetrate solid tumors more effectively, possibly because of their small size and longer circulation time. Once in tissues, daunorubicin is released. Daunorubicin inhibits DNA and RNA synthesis by intercalation between DNA base pairs and by steric obstruction; and intercalates at points of local uncoiling of the double helix. Although the exact mechanism is unclear, it appears that direct binding to DNA (intercalation) and inhibition of DNA repair (topoisomerase II inhibition) result in blockade of DNA and RNA synthesis and fragmentation of DNA.

Drug Interactions

Decreased Effect: Patients may experience impaired immune response to vaccines; possible infection after administration of live vaccines in patients receiving immunosuppressants.

Pharmacodynamics/Kinetics

Distribution: V_d: 3-6.4 L

Metabolism: Similar to daunorubicin, but metabolite plasma levels are low

Half-life elimination: Distribution: 4.4 hours; Terminal: 3-5 hours

Excretion: Primarily feces; some urine

Clearance, plasma: 17.3 mL/minute

Pregnancy Risk Factor D

DAUNOrubicin Hydrochloride

(daw noe ROO bi sin hye droe KLOR ide)

U.S. Brand Names Cerubidine®

Canadian Brand Names Cerubidine®

Mexican Brand Names Rubilem®

Generic Available Yes

Synonyms Daunomycin; DNR; NSC-82151; Rubidomycin Hydrochloride

Pharmacologic Category Antineoplastic Agent, Anthracycline

Use Treatment of acute lymphocytic (ALL) and nonlymphocytic (ANLL) leukemias

Local Anesthetic/Vasoconstrictor Precautions No information available to require special precautions

Effects on Dental Treatment Key adverse event(s) related to dental treatment: Stomatitis and discoloration of saliva.

Common Adverse Effects

>10%:

Cardiovascular: Transient ECG abnormalities (supraventricular tachycardia, S-T wave changes, atrial or ventricular extrasystoles); generally asymptomatic and self-limiting. CHF, dose related, may be delayed for 7-8 years after treatment. Cumulative dose, radiation therapy, age, and use of cyclophosphamide all increase the risk. Recommended maximum cumulative doses:

No risk factors: 550-600 mg/m^2

Concurrent radiation: 450 mg/m^2

Regardless of cumulative dose, if the left ventricular ejection fraction is <30% to 40%, the drug is usually not given

Dermatologic: Alopecia, radiation recall

Gastrointestinal: Mild nausea or vomiting, stomatitis

Genitourinary: Discoloration of urine (red)

Hematologic: Myelosuppression, primarily leukopenia; thrombocytopenia and anemia

Onset: 7 days

Nadir: 10-14 days

Recovery: 21-28 days

1% to 10%:

Dermatologic: Skin "flare" at injection site; discoloration of saliva, sweat, or tears

Endocrine & metabolic: Hyperuricemia

Gastrointestinal: GI ulceration, diarrhea

Mechanism of Action Inhibition of DNA and RNA synthesis by intercalation between DNA base pairs and by steric obstruction. Daunomycin intercalates at points of local uncoiling of the double helix. Although the exact mechanism is unclear, it appears that direct binding to DNA (intercalation) and inhibition of DNA repair (topoisomerase II inhibition) result in blockade of DNA and RNA synthesis and fragmentation of DNA.

Drug Interactions

Decreased Effect: Patients may experience impaired immune response to vaccines; possible infection after administration of live vaccines in patients receiving immunosuppressants.

Pharmacodynamics/Kinetics

Distribution: Many body tissues, particularly the liver, kidneys, lung, spleen, and heart; not into CNS; crosses placenta; V_d: 40 L/kg

Metabolism: Primarily hepatic to daunorubicinol (active), then to inactive aglycones, conjugated sulfates, and glucuronides

Half-life elimination: Distribution: 2 minutes; Elimination: 14-20 hours; Terminal: 18.5 hours; Daunorubicinol plasma half-life: 24-48 hours

Excretion: Feces (40%); urine (~25% as unchanged drug and metabolites)

Pregnancy Risk Factor D

DaunoXome® *see* DAUNOrubicin Citrate (Liposomal) *on page 425*

DAVA *see* Vindesine *on page 1577*

1-Day™ [OTC] *see* Tioconazole *on page 1493*

Dayhist® Allergy [OTC] *see* Clemastine *on page 359*

Daypro® *see* Oxaprozin *on page 1155*

Daytrana™ *see* Methylphenidate *on page 1023*

dCF *see* Pentostatin *on page 1211*

DDAVP® *see* Desmopressin *on page 437*

ddC *see* Zalcitabine *on page 1590*

ddI *see* Didanosine *on page 465*

Deacetyl Vinblastine Carboxamide *see* Vindesine *on page 1577*

1-Deamino-8-D-Arginine Vasopressin *see* Desmopressin *on page 437*

Debacterol® *see* Sulfonated Phenolics in Aqueous Solution *on page 1429*

Debrox® [OTC] *see* Carbamide Peroxide *on page 264*

Decadron® *see* Dexamethasone *on page 439*

Decadron® Phosphate [DSC] *see* Dexamethasone *on page 439*

Decahist-DM *see* Carbinoxamine, Pseudoephedrine, and Dextromethorphan *on page 269*

Decapinol® *see* Delmopinol *on page 430*

De-Chlor DM *see* Chlorpheniramine, Phenylephrine, and Dextromethorphan *on page 326*

De-Chlor DR *see* Chlorpheniramine, Phenylephrine, and Dextromethorphan *on page 326*

De-Chlor G *see* Hydrocodone, Phenylephrine, and Guaifenesin *on page 791*

Declomycin® *see* Demeclocycline *on page 431*

Deconamine® *see* Chlorpheniramine and Pseudoephedrine *on page 325*

Deconamine® SR *see* Chlorpheniramine and Pseudoephedrine *on page 325*

Deconsal® II *see* Guaifenesin and Phenylephrine *on page 754*

Deep Sea [OTC] *see* Sodium Chloride *on page 1400*

Deferasirox (de FER a sir ox)

U.S. Brand Names Exjade®

Generic Available No

Synonyms ICL670

Pharmacologic Category Antidote; Chelating Agent

Use Treatment of chronic iron overload due to blood transfusions

Local Anesthetic/Vasoconstrictor Precautions No information available to require special precautions

Effects on Dental Treatment No significant effects or complications reported

Common Adverse Effects

>10%:

Central nervous system: Fever (19%), headache (16%)

Gastrointestinal: Abdominal pain (8% to 14%), diarrhea (12%), nausea (11%)

Renal: Serum creatinine increased (2% to 38%), proteinuria (19%)

Respiratory: Cough (14%), nasopharyngitis (13%), pharyngolaryngeal pain (11%)

Miscellaneous: Influenza (11%)

(Continued)

Deferasirox (Continued)

1% to 10%:
Central nervous system: Fatigue (6%)
Dermatologic: Rash (8%), urticaria (4%)
Gastrointestinal: Vomiting (10%)
Hepatic: ALT increased (6% to 8%), transaminitis (4%)
Neuromuscular & skeletal: Arthralgia (7%), back pain (6%)
Otic: Ear infection (5%)
Respiratory: Respiratory tract infection (10%), bronchitis (9%), pharyngitis (8%), acute tonsillitis (6%), rhinitis (6%)

Mechanism of Action Selectively binds iron, forming a complex which is excreted primarily through the feces.

Drug Interactions
Decreased Effect: Aluminum-containing antacids may decrease absorption of deferasirox.

Pharmacodynamics/Kinetics
Distribution: Adults: 14 L
Protein binding: 99% to serum albumin
Metabolism: Hepatic via glucuronidation by UGT1A1 and UGT1A3; minor oxidation by CYP450; undergoes enterohepatic recirculation
Bioavailability: 70%
Half-life elimination: 8-16 hours
Time to peak, plasma: 1-4 hours
Excretion: Feces (84%), urine (6% to 8%)

Pregnancy Risk Factor B

Deferoxamine (de fer OKS a meen)

U.S. Brand Names Desferal®
Canadian Brand Names Desferal®; PMS-Deferoxamine
Generic Available Yes
Synonyms Deferoxamine Mesylate
Pharmacologic Category Antidote
Use Acute iron intoxication or when clinical signs of significant iron toxicity exist; chronic iron overload secondary to multiple transfusions
Unlabeled/Investigational Use Removal of corneal rust rings following surgical removal of foreign bodies; diagnosis or treatment of aluminum induced toxicity associated with chronic kidney disease (CKD)
Local Anesthetic/Vasoconstrictor Precautions No information available to require special precautions
Effects on Dental Treatment No significant effects or complications reported
Common Adverse Effects Frequency not defined.
Cardiovascular: Flushing, hypotension, tachycardia, shock, edema
Central nervous system: Fever, dizziness, neuropathy, seizure, exacerbation of aluminum-related encephalopathy (dialysis), headache
Dermatologic: Angioedema, rash, urticaria
Endocrine & metabolic: Growth retardation (children), hypocalcemia
Gastrointestinal: Abdominal discomfort, abdominal pain, diarrhea, nausea, vomiting
Genitourinary: Dysuria
Hematologic: Thrombocytopenia, leukopenia
Local: Injection site: Burning, crust, edema, erythema, eschar, induration, infiltration, irritation, pain, pruritus, swelling, vesicles
Neuromuscular & skeletal: Arthralgia, leg cramps, myalgia, paresthesias
Ocular: Acuity decreased, blurred vision, dichromatopsia, visual loss, scotoma, visual field defects, optic neuritis, cataracts, retinal pigmentary abnormalities, night blindness
Otic: Hearing loss, tinnitus
Renal: Renal impairment, urine discoloration (vin-rose color)
Respiratory: Acute respiratory distress syndrome, asthma
Miscellaneous: Anaphylaxis, hypersensitivity reaction, infections (*Yersinia*, mucormycosis)
Mechanism of Action Complexes with trivalent ions (ferric ions) to form ferrioxamine, which are removed by the kidneys
Drug Interactions
Increased Effect/Toxicity: May cause loss of consciousness or coma when administered with prochlorperazine. Concomitant treatment with vitamin C (>500 mg/day) has been associated with cardiac impairment.
Pharmacodynamics/Kinetics
Absorption: I.M.: Erratic

Metabolism: Hepatic; binds with iron to form ferrioxamine
Half-life elimination: Parent drug: 6.1 hours; Ferrioxamine: 5.8 hours
Excretion: Urine (as unchanged drug and ferrioxamine)
Pregnancy Risk Factor C

Deferoxamine Mesylate *see* Deferoxamine *on page 428*

Dehistine *see* Chlorpheniramine, Phenylephrine, and Methscopolamine *on page 327*

Dehydrobenzperidol *see* Droperidol *on page 519*

Del Aqua® *see* Benzoyl Peroxide *on page 194*

Delatestryl® *see* Testosterone *on page 1462*

Delavirdine (de la VIR deen)

Related Information
HIV Infection and AIDS *on page 1662*
Tuberculosis *on page 1673*
U.S. Brand Names Rescriptor®
Canadian Brand Names Rescriptor®
Generic Available No
Synonyms U-90152S
Pharmacologic Category Antiretroviral Agent, Reverse Transcriptase Inhibitor (Non-nucleoside)
Use Treatment of HIV-1 infection in combination with at least two additional antiretroviral agents
Local Anesthetic/Vasoconstrictor Precautions No information available to require special precautions
Effects on Dental Treatment No significant effects or complications reported
Common Adverse Effects
>10%: Dermatologic: Rash (3.2% required discontinuation)
1% to 10%:
Central nervous system: Headache, fatigue
Dermatologic: Pruritus
Gastrointestinal: Nausea, diarrhea, vomiting
Metabolic: Increased ALT (SGPT), increased AST (SGOT)
Mechanism of Action Delavirdine binds directly to reverse transcriptase, blocking RNA-dependent and DNA-dependent DNA polymerase activities
Drug Interactions
Cytochrome P450 Effect: Substrate of CYP2D6 (minor), 3A4 (major); **Inhibits** CYP1A2 (weak), 2C9 (strong), 2C19 (strong), 2D6 (strong), 3A4 (strong)
Increased Effect/Toxicity: Delavirdine has been reported to increase the serum concentrations of amprenavir, indinavir, nelfinavir, ritonavir, and saquinavir. Dose reduction of indinavir and saquinavir should be considered. Plasma concentrations of delavirdine may be increased by fluoxetine and ketoconazole. Clarithromycin and methadone serum concentrations may be increased by delavirdine.
Delavirdine may increase the levels/effects of CYP2C9, 2C19, or 2D6 substrates. Example substrates include amiodarone, amphetamines, selected beta-blockers, bosentan, citalopram, dapsone, dextromethorphan, diazepam, fluoxetine, glimepiride, glipizide, lidocaine, methsuximide, nateglinide, nefazodone, paroxetine, phenytoin, pioglitazone, propranolol, risperidone, ritonavir, rosiglitazone, sertraline, thioridazine, tricyclic antidepressants, venlafaxine, and warfarin.
Delavirdine may increase the levels/effects of CYP3A4 substrates. Example substrates include benzodiazepines, calcium channel blockers, cisapride, cyclosporine, mirtazapine, nateglinide, nefazodone, sildenafil (and other PDE-5 inhibitors), tacrolimus, and venlafaxine. Concomitant use with alprazolam, cisapride, ergot alkaloids, midazolam, pimozide, or triazolam is contraindicated. Use with lovastatin or simvastatin is not recommended.
Decreased Effect: Antacids, histamine-2 receptor antagonists, or proton pump inhibitors (omeprazole, lansoprazole) may reduce the absorption of delavirdine. Separate administration of didanosine buffered tablets or antacids and delavirdine by 1 hour. Concomitant use with histamine-2 receptor antagonists, omeprazole, or lansoprazole is not recommended.
Decreased delavirdine concentrations may occur when used with amprenavir and nelfinavir. Delavirdine decreases plasma concentrations of didanosine and didanosine may decrease plasma concentrations of delavirdine. Separate administration of didanosine buffered tablets and delavirdine by 1 hour.
Delavirdine may decrease the levels/effects of CYP2D6 prodrug substrates. Example prodrug substrates include codeine, hydrocodone, oxycodone,
(Continued)

Delavirdine *(Continued)*

and tramadol. CYP3A4 inducers may decrease the levels/effects of delavirdine. Example inducers include aminoglutethimide, carbamazepine, nafcillin, nevirapine, phenobarbital, phenytoin, and rifamycins. Carbamazepine, phenobarbital, phenytoin and rifamycins should not be coadministered with delavirdine. Dexamethasone may decrease the plasma concentrations of delavirdine.

Pharmacodynamics/Kinetics
Absorption: Rapid
Distribution: Low concentration in saliva and semen; CSF 0.4% concurrent plasma concentration
Protein binding: ~98%, primarily albumin
Metabolism: Hepatic via CYP3A4 and 2D6 (**Note:** May reduce CYP3A activity and inhibit its own metabolism.)
Bioavailability: 85%
Half-life elimination: 2-11 hours
Time to peak, plasma: 1 hour
Excretion: Urine (51%, <5% as unchanged drug); feces (44%); nonlinear kinetics exhibited

Pregnancy Risk Factor C

Delestrogen® *see Estradiol on page 574*

Delfen® [OTC] *see Nonoxynol 9 on page 1124*

Delmopinol (del MOE pi nol)

U.S. Brand Names Decapinol®
Generic Available No
Synonyms Delmopinol Hydrochloride
Pharmacologic Category Antibacterial, Oral Rinse
Dental Use Treatment of gingivitis; used to decrease the adhesion of oral plaque
Local Anesthetic/Vasoconstrictor Precautions No information available to require special precautions
Effects on Dental Treatment No significant effects or complications reported
Significant Adverse Effects
Local: Anesthetic effect (transient, local), taste alteration, dry mouth, dental calculus increased
Restrictions
Decapinol® is regulated as a medical device in both the U.S. and in Europe.

Preliminary monograph: At the time of publication, it is not possible to determine when this product will be available in the U.S. market.

Additional detail concerning FDA approval may be found at: www.fda.gov/bbs/topics/news/2005/NEW01174.html
Dental Usual Dosing Treatment of gingivitis; used to decrease the adhesion of oral plaque: Adults: Oral: Rinse mouth with 10 mL for 1 minute twice daily (after brushing and flossing)
Mechanism of Action Reduces adhesion of plaque-causing bacteria, reducing the formation of new plaque and promoting the removal of deposits with normal mechanical disruption (brushing and flossing). Ultimately causes a reduction in both plaque and gingivitis. Decapinol® is regulated as a medical device because the primary mode of action is to serve as a physical barrier without chemical activity.
Contraindications Hypersensitivity to delmopinol or any component of the formulation
Warnings/Precautions Not for ingestion, patients should be instructed not to swallow solution. May cause transient anesthetic effects, dry mouth, or changes in taste following use. Light staining may occur, which may be removed by brushing the teeth. Patients should be instructed to avoid eating or drinking for 30 minutes following use. Should be used as an adjunct to normal mechanical hygiene. Avoid use in pregnant women (lack of data). Not recommended for use in children <12 years of age. **Note:** Preliminary monograph: A decision to market this product within the U.S. is pending. At the time of publication, it is not possible to determine when this product will be available in the U.S. market.
Drug Interactions Delmopinol does not interact with toothpaste.
Pregnancy Risk Factor The manufacturer does not recommend use in pregnant women.
Lactation Excretion unknown/not recommended
Dosage Forms Liquid, oral rinse: 0.2%

Selected Readings

Hase JC, Attstrom R, Edwardsson S, et al, "6-Month Use of 0.2% Delmopinol Hydrochloride in Comparison With 0.2% Chlorhexidine Digluconate and Placebo (I). Effect on Plaque Formation and Gingivitis," *J Clin Periodontol*, 1998, 25(9):746-53.

Klinge B, Matsson L, Attstrom R, et al, "Effect of Local Application of Delmopinol Hydrochloride on Developing and Early Established Supragingival Plaque in Humans," *J Clin Periodontol*, 1996, 23(6):543-7.

Lang NP, Hase JC, Grassi M, et al, "Plaque Formation and Gingivitis After Supervised Mouthrinsing With 0.2% Delmopinol Hydrochloride, 0.2% Chlorhexidine Digluconate and Placebo for 6 Months," *Oral Dis*, 1998, 4(2):105-13.

◆ **Delmopinol Hydrochloride** *see* Delmopinol *on page 430*

◆ **Delsym® [OTC]** *see* Dextromethorphan *on page 451*

◆ **Delta-9-tetrahydro-cannabinol** *see* Dronabinol *on page 518*

◆ **Delta-9-Tetrahydrocannabinol and Cannabinol** *see* Tetrahydrocannabinol and Cannabidiol *on page 1469*

◆ **Delta-9 THC** *see* Dronabinol *on page 518*

◆ **Delta-D®** *see* Cholecalciferol *on page 334*

◆ **Deltacortisone** *see* PredniSONE *on page 1271*

◆ **Deltadehydrocortisone** *see* PredniSONE *on page 1271*

◆ **Deltahydrocortisone** *see* PrednisoLONE *on page 1268*

◆ **Demadex®** *see* Torsemide *on page 1512*

Demeclocycline *(dem e kloe SYE kleen)*

U.S. Brand Names Declomycin®
Canadian Brand Names Declomycin®
Generic Available Yes
Synonyms Demeclocycline Hydrochloride; Demethylchlortetracycline
Pharmacologic Category Antibiotic, Tetracycline Derivative
Use Treatment of susceptible bacterial infections (acne, gonorrhea, pertussis and urinary tract infections) caused by both gram-negative and gram-positive organisms
Unlabeled/Investigational Use Treatment of chronic syndrome of inappropriate secretion of antidiuretic hormone (SIADH)
Local Anesthetic/Vasoconstrictor Precautions No information available to require special precautions
Effects on Dental Treatment Tetracyclines are not recommended for use during pregnancy or in children ≤8 years of age since they have been reported to cause enamel hypoplasia and permanent teeth discoloration. Tetracyclines should only be used in these patients if other agents are contraindicated or alternative antimicrobials will not eradicate the organism. Long-term use associated with oral candidiasis.
Common Adverse Effects Frequency not defined.
Cardiovascular: Pericarditis
Central nervous system: Bulging fontanels (infants), dizziness, headache, pseudotumor cerebri (adults)
Dermatologic: Angioneurotic edema, erythema multiforme, erythematous rash, maculopapular rash, photosensitivity, pigmentation of skin, Stevens-Johnson syndrome (rare), urticaria
Endocrine & metabolic: Discoloration of thyroid gland (brown/black), nephrogenic diabetes insipidus
Gastrointestinal: Anorexia, diarrhea, dysphagia, enterocolitis, esophageal ulcerations, glossitis, nausea, pancreatitis, vomiting
Genitourinary: Balanitis
Hematologic: Eosinophilia, neutropenia, hemolytic anemia, thrombocytopenia
Hepatic: Hepatitis (rare), hepatotoxicity (rare), liver enzymes increased, liver failure (rare)
Neuromuscular & skeletal: Myasthenic syndrome, polyarthralgia, tooth discoloration (children <8 years, rarely in adults)
Ocular: Visual disturbances
Otic: Tinnitus
Renal: Acute renal failure
Respiratory: Pulmonary infiltrates
Miscellaneous: Anaphylaxis, anaphylactoid purpura, lupus-like syndrome, systemic lupus erythematosus exacerbation
Mechanism of Action Inhibits protein synthesis by binding with the 30S and possibly the 50S ribosomal subunit(s) of susceptible bacteria; may also cause alterations in the cytoplasmic membrane; inhibits the action of ADH in patients with chronic SIADH
Drug Interactions
Increased Effect/Toxicity: Methoxyflurane anesthesia may cause fatal nephrotoxicity; retinoic acid derivatives may increase adverse and toxic *(Continued)*

Demeclocycline *(Continued)*

effects; warfarin may result in increased anticoagulation; methotrexate levels may be increased

Decreased Effect: Antacid preparations containing calcium, magnesium, aluminum bismuth, or sodium bicarbonate may decrease tetracycline absorption; bile acid sequestrants, quinapril (magnesium-containing formulation), iron, or zinc may also decrease absorption; penicillin decrease therapeutic effect of tetracyclines. Although anecdotal reports suggest oral contraceptive efficacy could be reduced by tetracyclines, this has been refuted by more rigorous scientific and clinical data.

Pharmacodynamics/Kinetics

Onset of action: SIADH: Several days

Absorption: ~50% to 80%; reduced by food and dairy products

Protein binding: 41% to 50%

Metabolism: Hepatic (small amounts) to inactive metabolites; undergoes enterohepatic recirculation

Half-life elimination: 10-17 hours

Time to peak, serum: 3-6 hours

Excretion: Urine (42% to 50% as unchanged drug)

Pregnancy Risk Factor D

Demeclocycline Hydrochloride *see* Demeclocycline *on page 431*

Demerol® *see* Meperidine *on page 983*

4-Demethoxydaunorubicin *see* Idarubicin *on page 814*

Demethylchlortetracycline *see* Demeclocycline *on page 431*

Demser® *see* Metyrosine *on page 1036*

Demulen® *see* Ethinyl Estradiol and Ethynodiol Diacetate *on page 597*

Denavir® *see* Penciclovir *on page 1200*

Denileukin Diftitox *(de ni LOO kin DIF ti toks)*

U.S. Brand Names ONTAK®

Generic Available No

Synonyms DAB$_{389}$IL-2; NSC-714744

Pharmacologic Category Antineoplastic Agent, Miscellaneous

Use Treatment of persistent or recurrent cutaneous T-cell lymphoma whose malignant cells express the CD25 component of the IL-2 receptor

Local Anesthetic/Vasoconstrictor Precautions No information available to require special precautions

Effects on Dental Treatment No significant effects or complications reported

Common Adverse Effects

The following list of symptoms reported during treatment includes all levels of severity:

>10%:

Cardiovascular: Edema (47%; grade 3 and 4, 15%), hypotension (36%), chest pain (24%), vasodilation (22%), tachycardia (12%)

Central nervous system: Fever/chills (81%; grade 3 and 4, 22%), headache (26%), pain (48%; grade 3 and 4, 13%), dizziness (22%), nervousness (11%)

Dermatologic: Rash (34%; grade 3 and 4, 13%), pruritus (20%)

Endocrine & metabolic: Hypoalbuminemia (83%; grade 3 and 4, 14%), hypocalcemia (17%), weight loss (14%)

Gastrointestinal: Nausea/vomiting (64%; grade 3 and 4, 14%), anorexia (36%), diarrhea (29%)

Hematologic: Lymphocyte count decreased (34%), anemia (18%)

Hepatic: Transaminases increased (61%; grade 3 and 4, 15%)

Neuromuscular & skeletal: Weakness (66%; grade 3 and 4, 22%), myalgia (17%), paresthesia (13%)

Respiratory: Dyspnea (29%; grade 3 and 4, 14%), cough increased (26%), pharyngitis (17%), rhinitis (13%)

Miscellaneous: Flu-like syndrome (91%; beginning several hours to days following infusion), hypersensitivity (69%; reactions are variable, but may include hypotension, back pain, dyspnea, vasodilation, rash, chest pain, tachycardia, dysphagia, syncope, or anaphylaxis), infection (48%; grade 3 and 4, 24%), vascular leak syndrome (27%; characterized by hypotension, edema, or hypoalbuminemia; the syndrome usually developed within the first 2 weeks of infusion; 6% of patients who developed this syndrome required hospitalization; the symptoms may persist or even worsen despite cessation of denileukin diftitox)

1% to 10%:
    Cardiovascular: Thrombotic events (7%), hypertension (6%), arrhythmia (6%), MI (1%)
    Central nervous system: Insomnia (9%), confusion (8%)
    Endocrine & metabolic: Dehydration (9%), hypokalemia (6%), hyperthyroidism (<5%), hypothyroidism (<5%)
    Gastrointestinal: Constipation (9%), dyspepsia (7%), dysphagia (6%), oral ulcer (<5%), pancreatitis (<5%)
    Hematologic: Thrombocytopenia (8%), leukopenia (6%)
    Local: Injection site reaction (8%), anaphylaxis (1%)
    Neuromuscular & skeletal: Arthralgia (8%)
    Renal: Hematuria (10%), albuminuria (10%), pyuria (10%), creatinine increased (7%), acute renal insufficiency (<5%)
    Respiratory: Lung disorder (8%)
    Miscellaneous: Anaphylaxis (1%), diaphoresis decreased (10%)
    Postmarketing and/or case reports: Toxic epidermal necrolysis, visual loss

Mechanism of Action Denileukin diftitox is a fusion protein (a combination of amino acid sequences from diphtheria toxin and interleukin-2) which selectively delivers the cytotoxic activity of diphtheria toxin to targeted cells. It interacts with the high-affinity IL-2 receptor on the surface of malignant cells to inhibit intracellular protein synthesis, rapidly leading to cell death.

Pharmacodynamics/Kinetics
    Distribution: V_d: 0.06-0.08 L/kg
    Metabolism: Hepatic via proteolytic degradation (animal studies)
    Half-life elimination: Distribution: 2-5 minutes; Terminal: 70-80 minutes

Pregnancy Risk Factor C

Denorex® Original Therapeutic Strength [OTC] *see* Coal Tar *on page 383*

Denta 5000 Plus *see* Fluoride *on page 671*

DentaGel *see* Fluoride *on page 671*

Dentapaine [OTC] *see* Benzocaine *on page 190*

DentiPatch® *see* Lidocaine (Transoral) *on page 931*

Dent's Ear Wax [OTC] *see* Carbamide Peroxide *on page 264*

Dent's Extra Strength Toothache [OTC] *see* Benzocaine *on page 190*

Dent's Maxi-Strength Toothache [OTC] *see* Benzocaine *on page 190*

Deoxycoformycin *see* Pentostatin *on page 1211*

2'-Deoxycoformycin *see* Pentostatin *on page 1211*

Depacon® *see* Valproic Acid and Derivatives *on page 1556*

Depade® *see* Naltrexone *on page 1086*

Depakene® *see* Valproic Acid and Derivatives *on page 1556*

Depakote® Delayed Release *see* Valproic Acid and Derivatives *on page 1556*

Depakote® ER *see* Valproic Acid and Derivatives *on page 1556*

Depakote® Sprinkle® *see* Valproic Acid and Derivatives *on page 1556*

Depen® *see* Penicillamine *on page 1201*

DepoCyt™ *see* Cytarabine (Liposomal) *on page 414*

DepoDur™ *see* Morphine Sulfate *on page 1065*

Depo®-Estradiol *see* Estradiol *on page 574*

Depo-Medrol® *see* MethylPREDNISolone *on page 1025*

Depo-Provera® *see* MedroxyPROGESTERone *on page 972*

Depo-Provera® Contraceptive *see* MedroxyPROGESTERone *on page 972*

depo-subQ provera 104™ *see* MedroxyPROGESTERone *on page 972*

Depo®-Testosterone *see* Testosterone *on page 1462*

Deprenyl *see* Selegiline *on page 1382*

DermaFungal [OTC] *see* Miconazole *on page 1039*

Dermagran® [OTC] *see* Aluminum Hydroxide *on page 79*

Dermagran® AF [OTC] *see* Miconazole *on page 1039*

Dermamycin® [OTC] *see* DiphenhydrAMINE *on page 483*

Dermarest Dricort® [OTC] *see* Hydrocortisone *on page 793*

Dermarest® Insect Bite [OTC] *see* DiphenhydrAMINE *on page 483*

Dermarest® Plus [OTC] *see* DiphenhydrAMINE *on page 483*

Dermarest® Skin Correction Cream Plus [OTC] *see* Hydroquinone *on page 798*

Derma-Smoothe/FS® *see* Fluocinolone *on page 667*

Dermatop® *see* Prednicarbate *on page 1268*

Dermazene® *see* Iodoquinol and Hydrocortisone *on page 853*

DermaZinc™ [OTC] *see* Pyrithione Zinc *on page 1318*

Dermoplast® Antibacterial [OTC] *see* Benzocaine *on page 190*

Dermoplast® Pain Relieving [OTC] *see* Benzocaine *on page 190*

Dermtex® HC [OTC] *see* Hydrocortisone *on page 793*

Desacetyl Vinblastine Amide Sulfate *see* Vindesine *on page 1577*

Desferal® *see* Deferoxamine *on page 428*

Desiccated Thyroid *see* Thyroid *on page 1482*

Desipramine (des IP ra meen)

U.S. Brand Names Norpramin®

Canadian Brand Names Alti-Desipramine; Apo-Desipramine®; Norpramin®; Nu-Desipramine; PMS-Desipramine

Generic Available Yes

Synonyms Desipramine Hydrochloride; Desmethylimipramine Hydrochloride

Pharmacologic Category Antidepressant, Tricyclic (Secondary Amine)

Use Treatment of depression

Unlabeled/Investigational Use Analgesic adjunct in chronic pain; peripheral neuropathies; substance-related disorders (eg, cocaine withdrawal); attention-deficit/hyperactivity disorder (ADHD); depression in children ≤12 years of age

Local Anesthetic/Vasoconstrictor Precautions Use with caution; epinephrine and levonordefrin have been shown to have an increased pressor response in combination with TCAs

Effects on Dental Treatment Key adverse event(s) related to dental treatment: Xerostomia and changes in salivation (normal salivary flow resumes upon discontinuation), and unpleasant taste. Long-term treatment with TCAs increases the risk of caries by reducing salivation and salivary buffer capacity.

Common Adverse Effects Frequency not defined.

Cardiovascular: Arrhythmias, edema, flushing, heart block, hyper-/hypotension, MI, palpitation, stroke, tachycardia

Central nervous system: Agitation, anxiety, ataxia, confusion, delirium, disorientation, dizziness, drowsiness, drug fever, exacerbation of psychosis, extrapyramidal symptoms, fatigue, hallucinations, headache, hypomania, incoordination, insomnia, nervousness, parkinsonian syndrome, restlessness, seizure

Dermatologic: Alopecia, itching, petechiae, photosensitivity, skin rash, urticaria

Endocrine & metabolic: Breast enlargement, galactorrhea, hyper-/hypoglycemia, impotence, libido changes, SIADH

Gastrointestinal: Abdominal cramps, anorexia, black tongue, constipation, decreased lower esophageal sphincter tone may cause GE reflux, diarrhea, heartburn, nausea, paralytic ileus, stomatitis, unpleasant taste, vomiting, weight gain/loss, xerostomia

Genitourinary: Difficult urination, polyuria, sexual dysfunction, testicular edema, urinary retention

Hematologic: Agranulocytosis, eosinophilia, purpura, thrombocytopenia

Hepatic: Cholestatic jaundice, hepatitis, liver enzymes increased

Neuromuscular & skeletal: Fine muscle tremor, numbness, paresthesia of extremities, peripheral neuropathy, tingling, weakness

Ocular: Blurred vision, disturbances of accommodation, intraocular pressure increased, mydriasis

Otic: Tinnitus

Miscellaneous: Allergic reaction, diaphoresis (excessive)

Restrictions A medication guide concerning the use of antidepressants in children and teenagers can be found on the FDA website at http://www.fda.gov/cder/Offices/ODS/labeling.htm. It should be dispensed to parents or guardians of children and teenagers receiving this medication.

Mechanism of Action Traditionally believed to increase the synaptic concentration of norepinephrine (and to a lesser extent, serotonin) in the central nervous system by inhibition of its reuptake by the presynaptic neuronal membrane. However, additional receptor effects have been found including desensitization of adenyl cyclase, down regulation of beta-adrenergic receptors, and down regulation of serotonin receptors.

Drug Interactions

Cytochrome P450 Effect: Substrate of CYP1A2 (minor), 2D6 (major); Inhibits CYP2A6 (moderate), 2B6 (moderate), 2D6 (moderate), 2E1 (weak), 3A4 (moderate)

Increased Effect/Toxicity: Desipramine increases the effects of amphetamines, anticholinergics, other CNS depressants (sedatives, hypnotics, or ethanol), chlorpropamide, tolazamide, and warfarin. When used with MAO inhibitors, or other serotonin modulators (eg, SSRIs), enhanced serotonergic effects, including serotonin syndrome may occur. Concurrent use with sibutramine is contraindicated. Serotonin syndrome has also been reported with ritonavir (rare). The levels/effects of desipramine may be increased by chlor-promazine, delavirdine, fluoxetine, miconazole, paroxetine, pergolide, quini-dine, quinine, ritonavir, ropinirole, and other CYP2D6 inhibitors.

Cimetidine, grapefruit juice, indinavir, methylphenidate, diltiazem, and verap-amil may increase the serum concentration of TCAs. Use of lithium with a TCA may increase the risk for neurotoxicity. Phenothiazines may increase concentration of some TCAs and TCAs may increase concentration of pheno-thiazines. Pressor response to I.V. epinephrine, norepinephrine, and phenyl-ephrine may be enhanced in patients receiving TCAs (**Note:** Effect is unlikely with epinephrine or levonordefrin dosages typically administered as infiltration in combination with local anesthetics). Combined use of beta-agonists or drugs which prolong QT_c (including quinidine, procainamide, disopyramide, cisapride, sparfloxacin, gatifloxacin, moxifloxacin) with TCAs may predispose patients to cardiac arrhythmias.

Desipramine may increase the levels/effects of selected benzodiazepines, bupropion, calcium channel blockers, cisapride, dexmedetomidine, dextro-methorphan, ergot derivatives, ifosfamide, fluoxetine, selected HMG-CoA reductase inhibitors, lidocaine, mesoridazine, mirtazapine, nateglinide, nefazodone, paroxetine, pimozide, promethazine, propofol, quinidine, risper-idone, ritonavir, selegiline, sertraline, sildenafil (and other PDE-5 inhibitors), tacrolimus, thioridazine, tricyclic antidepressants, venlafaxine, and other CYP2A6, 2B6, 2D6, or 3A4 substrates.

Decreased Effect: Desipramine may decrease the levels/effects of CYP2D6 prodrug substrates (eg, codeine, hydrocodone, oxycodone, tramadol). Desi-pramine's serum levels/effect may be decreased by carbamazepine, chole-styramine, colestipol, phenobarbital, and rifampin. Desipramine may inhibit the antihypertensive effect of clonidine, guanadrel, or methyldopa.

Pharmacodynamics/Kinetics
Onset of action: 1-3 weeks; Maximum antidepressant effect: >2 weeks
Absorption: Well absorbed
Metabolism: Hepatic
Half-life elimination: Adults: 7-60 hours
Time to peak, plasma: 4-6 hours
Excretion: Urine (70%)

Pregnancy Risk Factor C

Desipramine Hydrochloride *see* Desipramine *on page 434*
Desitin® [OTC] *see* Zinc Oxide *on page 1597*
Desitin® Creamy [OTC] *see* Zinc Oxide *on page 1597*

Desloratadine (des lor AT a deen)

U.S. Brand Names Clarinex®
Canadian Brand Names Aerius®
Generic Available No
Pharmacologic Category Antihistamine, Nonsedating
Use Relief of nasal and non-nasal symptoms of seasonal allergic rhinitis (SAR) and perennial allergic rhinitis (PAR); treatment of chronic idiopathic urticaria (CIU)

Local Anesthetic/Vasoconstrictor Precautions No information available to require special precautions

Effects on Dental Treatment Key adverse event(s) related to dental treat-ment: Xerostomia (normal salivary flow resumes upon discontinuation).

Common Adverse Effects
>10%: Central nervous system: Headache (14%)
1% to 10%:
Central nervous system: Fatigue (2% to 5%), somnolence (2%), dizziness (4%)
Endocrine & metabolic: Dysmenorrhea (2%)
Gastrointestinal: Xerostomia (3%), nausea (5%), dyspepsia (3%)
Neuromuscular & skeletal: Myalgia (2% to 3%)
Respiratory: Pharyngitis (3% to 4%)

Dosage Oral:
Children:
6-11 months: 1 mg once daily
12 months to 5 years: 1.25 mg once daily
6-11 years: 2.5 mg once daily
Children ≥12 years and Adults: 5 mg once daily
Dosage adjustment in renal/hepatic impairment:
Children: Not established
Adults: 5 mg every other day
(Continued)

Desloratadine (Continued)

Mechanism of Action Desloratadine, a major metabolite of loratadine, is a long-acting tricyclic antihistamine with selective peripheral histamine H_1 receptor antagonistic activity and additional anti-inflammatory properties.

Contraindications Hypersensitivity to desloratadine, loratadine, or any component of the formulation

Warnings/Precautions Dose should be adjusted in patients with liver or renal impairment. Use with caution in patients known to be slow metabolizers of desloratadine (incidence of side effects may be increased). RediTabs® contain phenylalanine. Safety and efficacy have not been established for children <6 months of age.

Drug Interactions

Increased Effect/Toxicity: With concurrent use of desloratadine and erythromycin or ketoconazole, the C_{max} and AUC of desloratadine and its metabolite are increased; however, no clinically-significant changes in the safety profile of desloratadine were observed in clinical studies.

Ethanol/Nutrition/Herb Interactions Food: Does not affect bioavailability.

Dietary Considerations May be taken with or without food. Orally-disintegrating tablets contain phenylalanine.

Pharmacodynamics/Kinetics

Protein binding: Desloratadine: 82% to 87%; 3-hydroxydesloratadine: 85% to 89%

Metabolism: Hepatic to active metabolite, 3-hydroxydesloratadine (specific enzymes not identified); undergoes glucuronidation. Decreased in slow metabolizers of desloratadine. Not expected to affect or be affected by medications metabolized by CYP with normal doses.

Half-life elimination: 27 hours

Time to peak: 3 hours

Excretion: Urine and feces (as metabolites)

Pregnancy Risk Factor C

Dosage Forms SYR (Clarinex®): 0.5 mg/mL (120 mL, 480 mL). **TAB** (Clarinex®): 5 mg. **TAB, orally-disintegrating** (Clarinex® RediTabs®): 2.5 mg, 5 mg

---

Desloratadine and Pseudoephedrine
(des lor AT a deen & soo doe e FED rin)

U.S. Brand Names Clarinex-D® 12 Hour; Clarinex-D® 24 Hour

Generic Available No

Synonyms Pseudoephedrine and Desloratadine

Pharmacologic Category Antihistamine/Decongestant Combination, Nonsedating

Use Relief of symptoms of seasonal allergic rhinitis, in children ≥12 years of age and adults

Local Anesthetic/Vasoconstrictor Precautions No information available to require special precautions

Effects on Dental Treatment Key adverse event(s) related to dental treatment: Pseudoephedrine: Xerostomia (normal salivary flow resumes upon discontinuation).

Common Adverse Effects See also individual agents. Percentages as reported with the combination products:

1% to 10%:

Central nervous system: Insomnia (5% to 10%), headache (6% to 8%), fatigue (3% to 4%), somnolence (3%), dizziness (2% to 3%), hyperactivity (2%), nervousness (2%)

Gastrointestinal: Xerostomia (8%), anorexia (2%), nausea (2%)

Respiratory: Pharyngitis (3%)

Miscellaneous: Infection (2%)

Mechanism of Action

Desloratadine, a major metabolite of loratadine, is a long-acting tricyclic antihistamine with selective peripheral histamine H_1 receptor antagonistic activity and additional anti-inflammatory properties.

Pseudoephedrine directly stimulates alpha-adrenergic receptors of respiratory mucosa causing vasoconstriction; directly stimulates beta-adrenergic receptors causing bronchial relaxation, increased heart rate and contractility.

Drug Interactions

Increased Effect/Toxicity: See individual agents.

Decreased Effect: See individual agents.

Pharmacodynamics/Kinetics Also see individual agents.

Onset: Antihistaminic activity: 1 hour

Time to peak, plasma: Desloratadine: 4-7 hours; pseudoephedrine: 6-9 hours
Pregnancy Risk Factor C

Desmethylimipramine Hydrochloride see Desipramine on page 434

Desmopressin (des moe PRES in)

U.S. Brand Names DDAVP®; Stimate™
Canadian Brand Names Apo-Desmopressin®; DDAVP®; Minirin®; Octostim®
Mexican Brand Names Minirin®
Generic Available Yes
Synonyms 1-Deamino-8-D-Arginine Vasopressin; Desmopressin Acetate
Pharmacologic Category Antihemophilic Agent; Hemostatic Agent; Vasopressin Analog, Synthetic
Use
Injection: Treatment of diabetes insipidus; control of bleeding in hemophilia A, and mild-to-moderate classic von Willebrand disease (type I)
Tablet, nasal solution: Treatment of diabetes insipidus; primary nocturnal enuresis
Local Anesthetic/Vasoconstrictor Precautions No information available to require special precautions
Effects on Dental Treatment No significant effects or complications reported
Common Adverse Effects Frequency not defined (may be dose or route related).
Cardiovascular: Acute cerebrovascular thrombosis, acute MI, blood pressure increased/decreased, chest pain, edema, facial flushing, palpitation
Central nervous system: Agitation, chills, coma, dizziness, headache, insomnia, somnolence
Dermatologic: Rash
Endocrine & metabolic: Hyponatremia, water intoxication
Gastrointestinal: Abdominal cramps, dyspepsia, nausea, sore throat, vomiting
Genitourinary: Balanitis, vulval pain
Local: Injection: Burning pain, erythema, and swelling at the injection site
Ocular: Conjunctivitis, eye edema, lacrimation disorder
Respiratory: Cough, epistaxis, nasal congestion, rhinitis
Miscellaneous: Allergic reactions (rare), anaphylaxis (rare)
Mechanism of Action Enhances reabsorption of water in the kidneys by increasing cellular permeability of the collecting ducts; possibly causes smooth muscle constriction with resultant vasoconstriction; raises plasma levels of von Willebrand factor and factor VIII
Drug Interactions
Increased Effect/Toxicity: Chlorpropamide, fludrocortisone may increase ADH response.
Decreased Effect: Demeclocycline and lithium may decrease ADH response.
Pharmacodynamics/Kinetics
Intranasal administration:
Onset of increased factor VIII activity: 30 minutes (dose related)
Peak effect 1.5 hours
Bioavailability: 3.2%
I.V. infusion:
Onset of increased factor VIII activity: 30 minutes (dose related)
Peak effect: 1.5-2 hours
Half-life elimination: Terminal: 3 hours (up to 9 hours in renal dysfunction)
Excretion: Urine
Oral tablet:
Onset of action: ADH: ~1 hour
Peak effect: 4-7 hours
Bioavailability: 5% compared to intranasal; 0.16% compared to I.V.
Half-life elimination: 1.5-2.5 hours
Pregnancy Risk Factor B

Desmopressin Acetate see Desmopressin on page 437

Desogen® see Ethinyl Estradiol and Desogestrel on page 592

Desogestrel and Ethinyl Estradiol see Ethinyl Estradiol and Desogestrel on page 592

Desonide (DES oh nide)

U.S. Brand Names DesOwen®; LoKara™; Tridesilon®
Canadian Brand Names Desocort®; PMS-Desonide
Mexican Brand Names Desowen®
Generic Available Yes
(Continued)

Desonide *(Continued)*

Pharmacologic Category Corticosteroid, Topical

Use Adjunctive therapy for inflammation in acute and chronic corticosteroid responsive dermatosis (low potency corticosteroid)

Local Anesthetic/Vasoconstrictor Precautions No information available to require special precautions

Effects on Dental Treatment No significant effects or complications reported

Mechanism of Action Stimulates the synthesis of enzymes needed to decrease inflammation, suppress mitotic activity, and cause vasoconstriction

Pharmacodynamics/Kinetics
Onset of action: ~7 days
Absorption: Extensive from scalp, face, axilla, and scrotum; adequate through epidermis on appendages; may be increased with occlusion or addition of penetrants (eg, urea, DMSO)
Metabolism: Hepatic
Excretion: Primarily urine

Pregnancy Risk Factor C

DesOwen® *see* Desonide *on page 437*

Desoximetasone *(des oks i MET a sone)*

U.S. Brand Names Topicort®; Topicort®-LP
Canadian Brand Names Taro-Desoximetasone; Topicort®
Generic Available Yes
Pharmacologic Category Corticosteroid, Topical
Dental Use Short-term relief of inflammation of moderate to severe corticosteroid-responsive dermatosis (intermediate- to high-potency topical corticosteroid)
Use Relieves inflammation and pruritic symptoms of corticosteroid-responsive dermatosis (intermediate- to high-potency topical corticosteroid)
Local Anesthetic/Vasoconstrictor Precautions No information available to require special precautions
Effects on Dental Treatment No significant effects or complications reported
Significant Adverse Effects <1% (Limited to important or life-threatening): Acneiform eruptions, allergic contact dermatitis, burning, dry skin, erythema, folliculitis, folliculopustular lesions, hypertrichosis, hypopigmentation, itching; local burning, irritation, miliaria; perioral dermatitis, secondary infection, skin atrophy, skin maceration, striae, vesiculation
Dosage Desoximetasone is a potent fluorinated topical corticosteroid. Therapy should be discontinued when control is achieved; if no improvement is seen, reassessment of diagnosis may be necessary.

Cream, gel: Children and Adults: Apply a thin film to affected area twice daily
Ointment: Children ≥10 years and Adults: Apply a thin film to affected area twice daily
Mechanism of Action Stimulates the synthesis of enzymes needed to decrease inflammation, suppress mitotic activity, and cause vasoconstriction
Contraindications Hypersensitivity to desoximetasone or any component of the formulation; topical fungal infections; tuberculosis of skin herpes simplex
Warnings/Precautions Use with caution in patients with impaired circulation; skin infections. Systemic absorption of topical corticosteroids has been shown to suppress the HPA axis. Monitor for HPA axis suppression when used over large areas, prolonged use, or with occlusive dressings. Absorption may be greater in pediatric patients. Use should be limited to the least effective amount. Chronic use of corticosteroids in children may interfere with growth and development. Safety and efficacy of desoximetasone ointment have not been established in children <10 years of age.
Drug Interactions No data reported
Pharmacodynamics/Kinetics
Absorption: May be increased with occlusion, inflammation, or vary with site of application
Ointment: Systemic absorption with occlusion: 7%
Metabolism: Hepatic
Half-life elimination: Emollient cream: 15-17 hours
Excretion: Urine, feces
Pregnancy Risk Factor C
Lactation Excretion in breast milk unknown/use caution
Dosage Forms
Cream, topical: 0.25% (15 g, 60 g); 0.05% (15 g, 60 g)
Topicort®: 0.25% (15 g, 60 g)
Topicort®-LP: 0.05% (15 g, 60 g)

Gel, topical (Topicort®): 0.05% (15 g, 60 g) [contains alcohol 20%]
Ointment, topical (Topicort®): 0.25% (15 g, 60 g)

Desoxyephedrine Hydrochloride see Methamphetamine on page 1005

Desoxyn® see Methamphetamine on page 1005

Desoxyphenobarbital see Primidone on page 1281

Desquam-X® see Benzoyl Peroxide on page 194

Desquam-E™ see Benzoyl Peroxide on page 194

Desyrel® see Trazodone on page 1521

Detane® [OTC] see Benzocaine on page 190

Detemir Insulin see Insulin Detemir on page 836

Detrol® see Tolterodine on page 1506

Detrol® LA see Tolterodine on page 1506

Dex4® Glucose [OTC] see Dextrose on page 452

Dexalone® [OTC] see Dextromethorphan on page 451

Dexamethasone (deks a METH a sone)

Related Information
Respiratory Diseases on page 1656
Ulcerative and Erosive Disorders on page 1712
Related Sample Prescriptions
Erosive Lichen Planus and Major Aphthae on page 1745
Recurrent Aphthous Stomatitis on page 1744
U.S. Brand Names Decadron®; Decadron® Phosphate [DSC]; Dexamethasone Intensol®; DexPak® TaperPak®; Maxidex®
Canadian Brand Names Apo-Dexamethasone®; Dexasone®; Diodex®; Maxidex®; PMS-Dexamethasone
Mexican Brand Names Adrecort®; Alin®; Alin Depot®; Decadron®; Decadronal®; Decadron®; Dexagrin®; Dibasona®; Indarzona®
Generic Available Yes
Synonyms Dexamethasone Sodium Phosphate
Pharmacologic Category Anti-inflammatory Agent; Anti-inflammatory Agent, Ophthalmic; Antiemetic; Corticosteroid, Ophthalmic; Corticosteroid, Systemic; Corticosteroid, Topical
Dental Use Treatment of a variety of oral diseases of allergic, inflammatory or autoimmune origin
Use Systemically and locally for chronic swelling; allergic, hematologic, neoplastic, and autoimmune diseases; may be used in management of cerebral edema, septic shock, as a diagnostic agent, antiemetic
Unlabeled/Investigational Use General indicator consistent with depression; diagnosis of Cushing's syndrome
Local Anesthetic/Vasoconstrictor Precautions No information available to require special precautions
Effects on Dental Treatment No significant effects or complications reported
Significant Adverse Effects Frequency not defined.
Cardiovascular: Edema, hypertension, arrhythmia, cardiomyopathy, myocardial rupture (post-MI), syncope, thromboembolism, thrombophlebitis, vasculitis
Central nervous system: Insomnia, nervousness, vertigo, seizure, psychosis, pseudotumor cerebri (usually following discontinuation), headache, mood swings, delirium, hallucinations, euphoria
Dermatologic: Hirsutism, acne, skin atrophy, bruising, hyperpigmentation, pruritus (generalized), perianal pruritus (following I.V. injection), urticaria
Endocrine & metabolic: Diabetes mellitus, adrenal suppression, hyperlipidemia, Cushing's syndrome, pituitary-adrenal axis suppression, growth suppression, glucose intolerance, gynecomastia, hypokalemia, alkalosis, amenorrhea, sodium and water retention, hyperglycemia, hypercalciuria, weight gain
Gastrointestinal: Appetite increased, indigestion, peptic ulcer, nausea, vomiting, abdominal distention, ulcerative esophagitis, pancreatitis, intestinal perforation
Genitourinary: Altered (increased or decreased) spermatogenesis
Hematologic: Transient leukocytosis
Hepatic: Transaminases increased, hepatomegaly
Neuromuscular & skeletal: Arthralgia, muscle weakness, osteoporosis, fractures, myopathy (particularly in conjunction with neuromuscular disease or neuromuscular blocking agents), tendon rupture, vertebral compression fractures, neuropathy, neuritis, parasthesia
Ocular: Cataracts, glaucoma, exophthalmos, intraocular pressure increased
Miscellaneous: Infections, anaphylactoid reaction, anaphylaxis, angioedema, avascular necrosis, secondary malignancy, Kaposi's sarcoma, intractable hiccups, impaired wound healing, abnormal fat deposition, moon face
(Continued)

Dexamethasone *(Continued)*

Topical: <1%: Itching, dryness, folliculitis, hypertrichosis, acneiform eruptions, hypopigmentation, perioral dermatitis, allergic contact dermatitis, skin maceration, skin atrophy, striae, miliaria, local burning, irritation. secondary infection

Dental Usual Dosing Anti-inflammatory: Adults: Topical: Apply 1-4 times/day. Therapy should be discontinued when control is achieved; if no improvement is seen, reassessment of diagnosis may be necessary.

Dosage

Children:

Antiemetic (prior to chemotherapy): I.V. (should be given as sodium phosphate): 5-20 mg given 15-30 minutes before treatment

Anti-inflammatory immunosuppressant: Oral, I.M., I.V. (injections should be given as sodium phosphate): 0.08-0.3 mg/kg/day **or** 2.5-10 mg/m^2/day in divided doses every 6-12 hours

Extubation or airway edema: Oral, I.M., I.V. (injections should be given as sodium phosphate): 0.5-2 mg/kg/day in divided doses every 6 hours beginning 24 hours prior to extubation and continuing for 4-6 doses afterwards

Cerebral edema: I.V. (should be given as sodium phosphate): Loading dose: 1-2 mg/kg/dose as a single dose; maintenance: 1-1.5 mg/kg/day (maximum: 16 mg/day) in divided doses every 4-6 hours for 5 days then taper for 5 days, then discontinue

Bacterial meningitis in infants and children >2 months: I.V. (should be given as sodium phosphate): 0.6 mg/kg/day in 4 divided doses every 6 hours for the first 4 days of antibiotic treatment; start dexamethasone at the time of the first dose of antibiotic

Physiologic replacement: Oral, I.M., I.V.: 0.03-0.15 mg/kg/day **or** 0.6-0.75 mg/m^2/day in divided doses every 6-12 hours

Adults:

Antiemetic:

Prophylaxis: Oral, I.V.: 10-20 mg 15-30 minutes before treatment on each treatment day

Continuous infusion regimen: Oral or I.V.: 10 mg every 12 hours on each treatment day

Mildly emetogenic therapy: Oral, I.M., I.V.: 4 mg every 4-6 hours

Delayed nausea/vomiting: Oral: 4-10 mg 1-2 times/day for 2-4 days **or**

8 mg every 12 hours for 2 days; then

4 mg every 12 hours for 2 days **or**

20 mg 1 hour before chemotherapy; then

10 mg 12 hours after chemotherapy; then

8 mg every 12 hours for 4 doses; then

4 mg every 12 hours for 4 doses

Anti-inflammatory:

Oral, I.M., I.V. (injections should be given as sodium phosphate): 0.75-9 mg/day in divided doses every 6-12 hours

Intra-articular, intralesional, or soft tissue (as sodium phosphate): 0.4-6 mg/day

Ophthalmic:

Ointment: Apply thin coating into conjunctival sac 3-4 times/day; gradually taper dose to discontinue

Suspension: Instill 2 drops into conjunctival sac every hour during the day and every other hour during the night; gradually reduce dose to every 3-4 hours, then to 3-4 times/day

Topical: Apply 1-4 times/day. Therapy should be discontinued when control is achieved; if no improvement is seen, reassessment of diagnosis may be necessary.

Chemotherapy: Oral, I.V.: 40 mg every day for 4 days, repeated every 4 weeks (VAD regimen)

Cerebral edema: I.V. 10 mg stat, 4 mg I.M./I.V. (should be given as sodium phosphate) every 6 hours until response is maximized, then switch to oral regimen, then taper off if appropriate; dosage may be reduced after 24 days and gradually discontinued over 5-7 days

Dexamethasone suppression test (depression indicator) (unlabeled use): Oral: 1 mg at 11 PM, draw blood at 8 AM the following day for plasma cortisol determination

Cushing's syndrome, diagnostic: Oral: 1 mg at 11 PM, draw blood at 8 AM; greater accuracy for Cushing's syndrome may be achieved by the following:

Dexamethasone 0.5 mg by mouth every 6 hours for 48 hours (with 24-hour urine collection for 17-hydroxycorticosteroid excretion)

Differentiation of Cushing's syndrome due to ACTH excess from Cushing's due to other causes: Oral: Dexamethasone 2 mg every 6 hours for 48 hours (with 24-hour urine collection for 17-hydroxycorticosteroid excretion)

Multiple sclerosis (acute exacerbation): 30 mg/day for 1 week, followed by 4-12 mg/day for 1 month

Physiological replacement: Oral, I.M., I.V. (should be given as sodium phosphate): 0.03-0.15 mg/kg/day **or** 0.6-0.75 mg/m^2/day in divided doses every 6-12 hours

Treatment of shock:

Addisonian crisis/shock (ie, adrenal insufficiency/responsive to steroid therapy): I.V. (given as sodium phosphate): 4-10 mg as a single dose, which may be repeated if necessary

Unresponsive shock (ie, unresponsive to steroid therapy): I.V. (given as sodium phosphate): 1-6 mg/kg as a single I.V. dose or up to 40 mg initially followed by repeat doses every 2-6 hours while shock persists

Hemodialysis: Supplemental dose is not necessary

Peritoneal dialysis: Supplemental dose is not necessary

Mechanism of Action Decreases inflammation by suppression of neutrophil migration, decreased production of inflammatory mediators, and reversal of increased capillary permeability; suppresses normal immune response. Dexamethasone's mechanism of antiemetic activity is unknown.

Contraindications Hypersensitivity to dexamethasone or any component of the formulation; active untreated infections; ophthalmic use in viral, fungal, or tuberculosis diseases of the eye

Warnings/Precautions Use with caution in patients with hypothyroidism, cirrhosis, hypertension, CHF, ulcerative colitis, or thromboembolic disorders. Corticosteroids should be used with caution in patients with diabetes, osteoporosis, peptic ulcer, glaucoma, cataracts, or tuberculosis. Use caution following acute MI (corticosteroids have been associated with myocardial rupture). Use caution in hepatic impairment. Because of the risk of adverse effects, systemic corticosteroids should be used cautiously in the elderly in the smallest possible effective dose for the shortest duration.

May cause suppression of hypothalamic-pituitary-adrenal (HPA) axis, particularly in younger children or in patients receiving high doses for prolonged periods. Symptoms of adrenocortical insufficiency in suppressed patients may result from rapid discontinuation/withdrawal; deficits in HPA response may persist for months following discontinuation and require supplementation during metabolic stress. Patients receiving 20 mg/day of prednisone (or equivalent) may be most susceptible. Particular care is required when patients are transferred from systemic corticosteroids to inhaled products due to possible adrenal insufficiency or exacerbation of underlying disease, including an increase in allergic symptoms. Fatalities have occurred due to adrenal insufficiency in asthmatic patients during and after transfer from systemic corticosteroids to aerosol steroids; aerosol steroids do **not** provide the systemic steroid needed to treat patients having trauma, surgery, or infections. Dexamethasone does not provide adequate mineralocorticoid activity in adrenal insufficiency (may be employed as a single dose while cortisol assays are performed).

Controlled clinical studies have shown that orally-inhaled and intranasal corticosteroids may cause a reduction in growth velocity in pediatric patients. (In studies of orally-inhaled corticosteroids, the mean reduction in growth velocity was ~1 cm per year [range 0.3-1.8 cm per year] and appears to be related to dose and duration of exposure). The growth of pediatric patients receiving inhaled corticosteroids, should be monitored routinely (eg, via stadiometry). To minimize the systemic effects of orally-inhaled and intranasal corticosteroids, each patient should be titrated to the lowest effective dose.

May suppress the immune system; patients may be more susceptible to infection. Use with caution in patients with systemic infections or ocular herpes simplex. Avoid exposure to chickenpox and measles.

Drug Interactions Substrate of CYP3A4 (minor); **Induces** CYP2A6 (weak), 2B6 (weak), 2C8 (weak), 2C9 (weak), 3A4 (weak)

Aminoglutethimide: May reduce the serum levels/effects of dexamethasone; likely via induction of microsomal isoenzymes.

Antacids: May increase the absorption of corticosteroids; separate administration by 2 hours.

Anticholinesterases: Concurrent use may lead to severe weakness in patients with myasthenia gravis.

Aprepitant: May increase the serum levels of corticosteroids; monitor.

Azole antifungals: May increase the serum levels of corticosteroids; monitor.

Bile acid sequestrants: May reduce the absorption of corticosteroids; separate administration by 2 hours.

Calcium channel blockers (nondihydropyridine): May increase the serum levels of corticosteroids; monitor.

Cyclosporine: Corticosteroids may increase the serum levels of cyclosporine. In addition, cyclosporine may increase levels of corticosteroids

(Continued)

Dexamethasone *(Continued)*

Estrogens: May increase the serum levels of corticosteroids; monitor.

Fluoroquinolones: Concurrent use may increase the risk of tendon rupture, particularly in elderly patients (overall incidence rare).

Isoniazid: Serum concentrations may be decreased by corticosteroids.

Neuromuscular-blocking agents: Concurrent use with corticosteroids may increase the risk of myopathy.

Nonsteroidal anti-inflammatory drugs (NSAIDs): Concurrent use with corticosteroids may lead to an increased incidence of gastrointestinal adverse effects; use caution.

Phenytoin: Dexamethasone may decrease serum levels/effects of phenytoin; monitor.

Salicylates: Salicylates may increase the gastrointestinal adverse effects of corticosteroids.

Thalidomide: Concurrent use with corticosteroids may increase the risk of selected adverse effects (toxic epidermal necrolysis and DVT); use caution

Vaccines, toxoids: Corticosteroids may suppress the response to vaccinations. The use of live vaccines is contraindicated in immunosuppressed patients. In patients receiving high doses of systemic corticosteroids for ≥14 days, wait at least 1 month between discontinuing steroid therapy and administering immunization.

Warfarin: Corticosteroids may lead to a reduction in warfarin effect; monitor.

Ethanol/Nutrition/Herb Interactions

Ethanol: Avoid ethanol (may enhance gastric mucosal irritation).

Food: Dexamethasone interferes with calcium absorption. Limit caffeine.

Herb/Nutraceutical: Avoid cat's claw, echinacea (have immunostimulant properties).

Dietary Considerations May be taken with meals to decrease GI upset. May need diet with increased potassium, pyridoxine, vitamin C, vitamin D, folate, calcium, and phosphorus.

Pharmacodynamics/Kinetics

Onset of action: Acetate: Prompt

Duration of metabolic effect: 72 hours; acetate is a long-acting repository preparation

Metabolism: Hepatic

Half-life elimination: Normal renal function: 1.8-3.5 hours; Biological half-life: 36-54 hours

Time to peak, serum: Oral: 1-2 hours; I.M.: ~8 hours

Excretion: Urine and feces

Pregnancy Risk Factor C

Lactation Excretion in breast milk unknown

Dosage Forms [DSC] = Discontinued product

Elixir, as base: 0.5 mg/5 mL (240 mL) [contains alcohol 5%; raspberry flavor]

Injection, solution, as sodium phosphate: 4 mg/mL (1 mL, 5 mL, 10 mL, 25 mL, 30 mL); 10 mg/mL (1 mL, 10 mL)

Decadron® Phosphate: 4 mg/mL (5 mL, 25 mL); 24 mg/mL (5 mL) [contains sodium bisulfite] [DSC]

Ointment, ophthalmic, as sodium phosphate: 0.05% (3.5 g)

Solution, ophthalmic, as sodium phosphate: 0.1% (5 mL)

Solution, oral: 0.5 mg/5 mL (500 mL) [cherry flavor]

Solution, oral concentrate (Dexamethasone Intensol®): 1 mg/mL (30 mL) [contains alcohol 30%]

Suspension, ophthalmic (Maxidex®): 0.1% (5 mL, 15 mL)

Tablet: 0.25 mg, 0.5 mg, 0.75 mg, 1 mg, 1.5 mg, 2 mg, 4 mg, 6 mg [some 0.5 mg tablets may contain tartrazine]

Decadron®: 0.5 mg, 0.75 mg, 4 mg

DexPak® TaperPak®: 1.5 mg [51 tablets on taper dose card]

Dexamethasone and Ciprofloxacin *see* Ciprofloxacin and Dexamethasone *on page 348*

Dexamethasone and Tobramycin *see* Tobramycin and Dexamethasone *on page 1499*

Dexamethasone Intensol® *see* Dexamethasone *on page 439*

Dexamethasone, Neomycin, and Polymyxin B *see* Neomycin, Polymyxin B, and Dexamethasone *on page 1101*

Dexamethasone Sodium Phosphate *see* Dexamethasone *on page 439*

Dexbrompheniramine and Pseudoephedrine

(deks brom fen EER a meen & soo doe e FED rin)

Related Information

Pseudoephedrine *on page 1309*

U.S. Brand Names Drixoral® Cold & Allergy [OTC]

Canadian Brand Names Drixoral®

Generic Available Yes

Synonyms Pseudoephedrine and Dexbrompheniramine

Pharmacologic Category Antihistamine/Decongestant Combination

Use Relief of symptoms of upper respiratory mucosal congestion in seasonal and perennial nasal allergies, acute rhinitis, rhinosinusitis and eustachian tube blockage

Local Anesthetic/Vasoconstrictor Precautions Use with caution since pseudoephedrine is a sympathomimetic amine which could interact with epinephrine to cause a pressor response

Effects on Dental Treatment Key adverse event(s) related to dental treatment: Pseudoephedrine: Xerostomia (normal salivary flow resumes upon discontinuation).

Pregnancy Risk Factor B

Dexchlorpheniramine (deks klor fen EER a meen)

Generic Available Yes

Synonyms Dexchlorpheniramine Maleate

Pharmacologic Category Antihistamine

Use Perennial and seasonal allergic rhinitis and other allergic symptoms including urticaria

Local Anesthetic/Vasoconstrictor Precautions No information available to require special precautions

Effects on Dental Treatment Key adverse event(s) related to dental treatment: Significant xerostomia (normal salivary flow resumes upon discontinuation).

Common Adverse Effects

>10%:

Central nervous system: Slight to moderate drowsiness

Respiratory: Thickening of bronchial secretions

1% to 10%:

Central nervous system: Headache, fatigue, nervousness, dizziness

Gastrointestinal: Appetite increase, weight gain, nausea, diarrhea, abdominal pain, xerostomia

Neuromuscular & skeletal: Arthralgia

Respiratory: Pharyngitis

Mechanism of Action Competes with histamine for H_1-receptor sites on effector cells in the gastrointestinal tract, blood vessels, and respiratory tract. Dexchlorpheniramine is the predominant active isomer of chlorpheniramine and is approximately twice as active as the racemic compound.

Drug Interactions

Increased Effect/Toxicity: CNS depressants may increase the degree of sedation and respiratory depression with antihistamines. May increase the absorption of digoxin. Central and/or peripheral anticholinergic syndrome can occur when administered with amantadine, rimantadine, narcotic analgesics, phenothiazines and other antipsychotics (especially with high anticholinergic activity), tricyclic antidepressants, quinidine, disopyramide, procainamide, and antihistamines.

Decreased Effect: May increase gastric degradation of levodopa and decrease the amount of levodopa absorbed by delaying gastric emptying. Therapeutic effects of cholinergic agents (tacrine, donepezil) and neuroleptics may be antagonized.

Pharmacodynamics/Kinetics

Onset of action: ~1 hour

Duration: 3-6 hours

Absorption: Well absorbed

Metabolism: Hepatic

Pregnancy Risk Factor B

Dexchlorpheniramine and Pseudoephedrine
(deks klor fen EER a meen & soo doe e FED rin)

U.S. Brand Names Duotan PD; Tanafed DP™

Generic Available Yes

Synonyms Pseudoephedrine Tannate and Dexchlorpheniramine Tannate

Pharmacologic Category Alpha/Beta Agonist; Antihistamine

Use Relief of nasal congestion associated with the common cold, hay fever, and other allergies, sinusitis, and vasomotor and allergic rhinitis

(Continued)

Dexchlorpheniramine and Pseudoephedrine
(Continued)

Local Anesthetic/Vasoconstrictor Precautions No information available to require special precautions

Effects on Dental Treatment Key adverse event(s) related to dental treatment: Significant xerostomia (normal salivary flow resumes upon discontinuation).

Common Adverse Effects See individual monographs for dexchlorpheniramine and pseudoephedrine.

Mechanism of Action
Chlorpheniramine competes with histamine for H_1-receptor sites on effector cells in the gastrointestinal tract, blood vessels, and respiratory tract. Dexchlorpheniramine is the predominant active isomer of chlorpheniramine and is approximately twice as active as the racemic compound.

Pseudoephedrine is a sympathomimetic amine and isomer of ephedrine; acts as a decongestant in respiratory tract mucous membranes with less vasoconstrictor action than ephedrine in normotensive individuals.

Drug Interactions
Cytochrome P450 Effect: See individual monographs for dexchlorpheniramine and pseudoephedrine.

Increased Effect/Toxicity: See individual monographs for dexchlorpheniramine and pseudoephedrine.

Decreased Effect: See individual monographs for chlorpheniramine and pseudoephedrine.

Pregnancy Risk Factor C

Dexchlorpheniramine Maleate see Dexchlorpheniramine on page 443

Dexcon-DM see Guaifenesin, Dextromethorphan, and Phenylephrine on page 756

Dexcon-PE see Guaifenesin, Dextromethorphan, and Phenylephrine on page 756

Dexedrine® see Dextroamphetamine on page 447

Dexferrum® see Iron Dextran Complex on page 862

Dexmedetomidine (deks MED e toe mi deen)

U.S. Brand Names Precedex™
Canadian Brand Names Precedex™
Generic Available No
Synonyms Dexmedetomidine Hydrochloride
Pharmacologic Category Alpha$_2$-Adrenergic Agonist; Sedative
Use Sedation of initially intubated and mechanically ventilated patients during treatment in an intensive care setting; duration of infusion should not exceed 24 hours

Unlabeled/Investigational Use Unlabeled uses include premedication prior to anesthesia induction with thiopental; relief of pain and reduction of opioid dose following laparoscopic tubal ligation; as an adjunct anesthetic in ophthalmic surgery; treatment of shivering; premedication to attenuate the cardiostimulatory and postanesthetic delirium of ketamine

Local Anesthetic/Vasoconstrictor Precautions No information available to require special precautions

Effects on Dental Treatment Key adverse event(s) related to dental treatment: Xerostomia and changes in salivation (normal salivary flow resumes upon discontinuation).

Common Adverse Effects
>10%:
  Cardiovascular: Hypotension (30%)
  Gastrointestinal: Nausea (11%)
1% to 10%:
  Cardiovascular: Bradycardia (8%), atrial fibrillation (7%)
  Central nervous system: Pain (3%)
  Hematologic: Anemia (3%), leukocytosis (2%)
  Renal: Oliguria (2%)
  Respiratory: Hypoxia (6%), pulmonary edema (2%), pleural effusion (3%)
  Miscellaneous: Infection (2%), thirst (2%)

Mechanism of Action Selective alpha$_2$-adrenoceptor agonist with sedative properties; alpha$_1$ activity was observed at high doses or after rapid infusions

Drug Interactions
Cytochrome P450 Effect: Substrate of CYP2A6 (major); Inhibits CYP1A2 (weak), 2C9 (weak), 2D6 (strong), 3A4 (weak)

Increased Effect/Toxicity: The levels/effects of dexmedetomidine may be increased by isoniazid, methoxsalen, miconazole, and other CYP2A6 inhibitors. Dexmedetomidine may increase the levels/effects of amphetamines, selected beta-blockers, dextromethorphan, fluoxetine, lidocaine, mirtazapine, nefazodone, paroxetine, risperidone, ritonavir, thioridazine, tricyclic antidepressants, venlafaxine, and other CYP2D6 substrates. Hypotension and/or bradycardia may be increased by vasodilators and heart rate-lowering agents.

Decreased Effect: Dexmedetomidine may decrease the levels/effects of CYP2D6 prodrug substrates; example prodrug substrates include codeine, hydrocodone, oxycodone, and tramadol.

Pharmacodynamics/Kinetics
Onset of action: Rapid
Distribution: V_{ss}: Approximately 118 L; rapid
Protein binding: 94%
Metabolism: Hepatic via glucuronidation and CYP2A6
Half-life elimination: 6 minutes; Terminal: 2 hours
Excretion: Urine (95%); feces (4%)

Pregnancy Risk Factor C

Dexmedetomidine Hydrochloride *see* Dexmedetomidine *on page 444*

Dexmethylphenidate (dex meth il FEN i date)

U.S. Brand Names Focalin™; Focalin™ XR
Generic Available No
Synonyms Dexmethylphenidate Hydrochloride
Pharmacologic Category Central Nervous System Stimulant
Use Treatment of attention-deficit/hyperactivity disorder (ADHD)
Local Anesthetic/Vasoconstrictor Precautions No information available to require special precautions
Effects on Dental Treatment No significant effects or complications reported
Common Adverse Effects
>10%:
  Central nervous system: Headache (25% to 26%), feeling jittery (12%)
  Gastrointestinal: Appetite decreased (30%), abdominal pain (15%)
1% to 10%:
  Cardiovascular: Tachycardia (3%)
  Central nervous system: Dizziness (6%), anxiety (5% to 6%), fever (5%)
  Gastrointestinal: Nausea (9%), dyspepsia (5% to 8%), xerostomia (7%), anorexia (6%), pharyngolaryngeal pain (4%)

Also refer to Methylphenidate monograph for adverse effects seen with methylphenidate.

Restrictions C-II
Mechanism of Action Dexmethylphenidate is the more active, *d-threo*-enantiomer, of racemic methylphenidate. It is a CNS stimulant; blocks the reuptake of norepinephrine and dopamine, and increases their release into the extraneuronal space.

Drug Interactions
Increased Effect/Toxicity: Methylphenidate may cause hypertensive effects when used in combination with MAO inhibitors or drugs with MAO-inhibiting activity (linezolid). Risk may be less with selegiline (MAO type B selective at low doses); it is best to avoid this combination. NMS has been reported in a patient receiving methylphenidate and venlafaxine. Methylphenidate may increase levels of phenytoin and TCAs. Increased toxicity with clonidine, sibutramine, or other sympathomimetics.

Decreased Effect: Effectiveness of antihypertensive agents may be decreased. Carbamazepine may decrease the effect of methylphenidate.

Pharmacodynamics/Kinetics
Duration of action: Capsule: 12 hours
Absorption: Tablet: Rapid; Capsule: Bimodal
Distribution: V_d: 1.54-3.76 L/kg
Metabolism: Via de-esterification to inactive metabolite, *d*-α-phenyl-piperidine acetate (*d*-ritalinic acid)
Bioavailability: 22% to 25%
Half-life elimination: 2-4.5 hours
Time to peak: Fasting:
  Tablet: 1-1.5 hours
  Capsule: First peak: 1.5 hours (range: 1-4 hours); Second peak: 6.5 hours (range: 4.5-7 hours)
Excretion: Urine (90%, primarily as inactive metabolite)

Pregnancy Risk Factor C

Dexmethylphenidate Hydrochloride *see* Dexmethylphenidate *on page 445*
DexPak® TaperPak® *see* Dexamethasone *on page 439*

Dexpanthenol (deks PAN the nole)

U.S. Brand Names Panthoderm® [OTC]
Generic Available Yes: Injection
Synonyms Pantothenyl Alcohol
Pharmacologic Category Gastrointestinal Agent, Stimulant; Topical Skin Product
Use Prophylactic use to minimize paralytic ileus; treatment of postoperative distention; topical to relieve itching and to aid healing of minor dermatoses
Local Anesthetic/Vasoconstrictor Precautions No information available to require special precautions
Effects on Dental Treatment No significant effects or complications reported
Common Adverse Effects Frequency not defined.
 Cardiovascular: Slight drop in blood pressure
 Central nervous system: Agitation
 Dermatologic: Dermatitis, irritation, itching, urticaria
 Gastrointestinal: Diarrhea, hyperperistalsis, vomiting
 Neuromuscular & skeletal: Paresthesia
 Respiratory: Dyspnea
 Miscellaneous: Allergic reactions
Mechanism of Action A pantothenic acid B vitamin analog that is converted to coenzyme A internally; coenzyme A is essential to normal fatty acid synthesis, amino acid synthesis and acetylation of choline in the production of the neuro-transmitter, acetylcholine
Drug Interactions
 Increased Effect/Toxicity: Increased/prolonged effect when dexpanthenol injection is given with succinylcholine; do not give dexpanthenol within 1 hour of succinylcholine.
Pregnancy Risk Factor C

Dex PC *see* Chlorpheniramine, Phenylephrine, and Dextromethorphan *on page 326*

Dexrazoxane (deks ray ZOKS ane)

U.S. Brand Names Zinecard®
Canadian Brand Names Zinecard®
Generic Available No
Synonyms ICRF-187
Pharmacologic Category Cardioprotectant
Use Reduction of the incidence and severity of cardiomyopathy associated with doxorubicin administration in women with metastatic breast cancer who have received a cumulative doxorubicin dose of 300 mg/m^2 and who would benefit from continuing therapy with doxorubicin. It is not recommended for use with the initiation of doxorubicin therapy.
Local Anesthetic/Vasoconstrictor Precautions No information available to require special precautions
Effects on Dental Treatment No significant effects or complications reported
Common Adverse Effects Adverse reactions listed are those which were greater in the dexrazoxane arm in a trial comparison of dexrazoxane plus fluorouracil, doxorubicin, and cyclophosphamide (FAC) to FAC alone. (Most adverse reactions are thought to be attributed to FAC except for myelosuppression (increased) and pain at injection site).
 Central nervous system: Fatigue/malaise, fever
 Dermatologic: Alopecia, extravasation, streaking/erythema
 Endocrine & metabolic: Serum amylase increased, serum calcium decreased, serum triglycerides increased
 Hematologic: Hemorrhage, granulocytopenia, leukopenia, myelosuppression, thrombocytopenia
 Hepatic: AST/ALT increased, bilirubin increased
 Local: Pain at injection site, phlebitis
 Neuromuscular & skeletal: Neurotoxicity
 Miscellaneous: Infection, sepsis
Mechanism of Action Derivative of EDTA; potent intracellular chelating agent. The mechanism of cardioprotectant activity is not fully understood. Appears to be converted intracellularly to a ring-opened chelating agent that interferes with iron-mediated oxygen free radical generation thought to be responsible, in part, for anthracycline-induced cardiomyopathy.

Pharmacodynamics/Kinetics
Distribution: V_d: 22-22.4 L/m^2
Protein binding: None
Half-life elimination: 2.1-2.5 hours
Excretion: Urine (42%)
Clearance, renal: 3.35 L/hour/m^2; Plasma: 6.25-7.88 L/hour/m^2
Pregnancy Risk Factor C

Dextran (DEKS tran)

Related Information
Dextran 1 on page 447
U.S. Brand Names Gentran®; LMD®
Canadian Brand Names Gentran®
Mexican Brand Names Rheomacrodex®
Generic Available Yes
Synonyms Dextran 40; Dextran 70; Dextran, High Molecular Weight; Dextran, Low Molecular Weight
Pharmacologic Category Plasma Volume Expander
Use Blood volume expander used in treatment of shock or impending shock when blood or blood products are not available; dextran 40 is also used as a priming fluid in cardiopulmonary bypass and for prophylaxis of venous thrombosis and pulmonary embolism in surgical procedures associated with a high risk of thromboembolic complications
Local Anesthetic/Vasoconstrictor Precautions No information available to require special precautions
Effects on Dental Treatment No significant effects or complications reported
Mechanism of Action Produces plasma volume expansion by virtue of its highly colloidal starch structure, similar to albumin
Drug Interactions
Increased Effect/Toxicity: Dextran may enhance the anticoagulant effect of abciximab; avoid concurrent use.
Pharmacodynamics/Kinetics
Onset of action: Minutes to 1 hour (depending upon the molecular weight polysaccharide administered)
Excretion: Urine (~75%) within 24 hours
Pregnancy Risk Factor C

Dextran 1 (DEKS tran won)

Related Information
Dextran on page 447
U.S. Brand Names Promit®
Generic Available No
Pharmacologic Category Plasma Volume Expander
Use Prophylaxis of serious anaphylactic reactions to I.V. infusion of dextran
Local Anesthetic/Vasoconstrictor Precautions No information available to require special precautions
Effects on Dental Treatment No significant effects or complications reported
Mechanism of Action Binds to dextran-reactive immunoglobulin without bridge formation and no formation of large immune complexes
Pregnancy Risk Factor C

Dextran 40 see Dextran on page 447
Dextran 70 see Dextran on page 447
Dextran, High Molecular Weight see Dextran on page 447
Dextran, Low Molecular Weight see Dextran on page 447

Dextroamphetamine (deks troe am FET a meen)

U.S. Brand Names Dexedrine®; Dextrostat®
Canadian Brand Names Dexedrine®
Generic Available Yes
Synonyms Dextroamphetamine Sulfate
Pharmacologic Category Stimulant
Use Narcolepsy; attention-deficit/hyperactivity disorder (ADHD)
Unlabeled/Investigational Use Exogenous obesity; depression; abnormal behavioral syndrome in children (minimal brain dysfunction)
Local Anesthetic/Vasoconstrictor Precautions Use vasoconstrictor with caution in patients taking dextroamphetamine. Amphetamines enhance the
(Continued)

Dextroamphetamine *(Continued)*

sympathomimetic response of epinephrine and norepinephrine leading to potential hypertension and cardiotoxicity.

Effects on Dental Treatment Key adverse event(s) related to dental treatment: Xerostomia (normal salivary flow resumes upon discontinuation). Up to 10% of patients taking dextroamphetamines may present with hypertension. Monitor blood pressure prior to using local anesthetic with vasoconstrictors.

Common Adverse Effects Frequency not defined.

Cardiovascular: Palpitations, tachycardia, hypertension, cardiomyopathy

Central nervous system: Overstimulation, euphoria, dyskinesia, dysphoria, exacerbation of motor and phonic tics, restlessness, insomnia, dizziness, headache, psychosis, Tourette's syndrome

Dermatologic: Rash, urticaria

Endocrine & metabolic: Changes in libido

Gastrointestinal: Diarrhea, constipation, anorexia, weight loss, xerostomia, unpleasant taste

Genitourinary: Impotence

Neuromuscular & skeletal: Tremor

Restrictions C-II

Mechanism of Action Blocks reuptake of dopamine and norepinephrine from the synapse, thus increases the amount of circulating dopamine and norepinephrine in cerebral cortex to reticular activating system; inhibits the action of monoamine oxidase and causes catecholamines to be released. Peripheral actions include elevated blood pressure, weak bronchodilator, and respiratory stimulant action.

Drug Interactions

Cytochrome P450 Effect: Substrate of CYP2D6 (major)

Increased Effect/Toxicity: CYP2D6 inhibitors may increase the levels/ effects of dextroamphetamine; example inhibitors include chlorpromazine, delavirdine, fluoxetine, miconazole, paroxetine, pergolide, quinidine, quinine, ritonavir, and ropinirole. Dextroamphetamine may precipitate hypertensive crisis or serotonin syndrome in patients receiving MAO inhibitors (selegiline >10 mg/day, isocarboxazid, phenelzine, tranylcypromine, furazolidone). Serotonin syndrome has also been associated with combinations of amphetamines and SSRIs; these combinations should be avoided. TCAs may enhance the effects of amphetamines. Large doses of antacids or urinary alkalinizers increase the half-life and duration of action of amphetamines. May precipitate arrhythmias in patients receiving general anesthetics.

Decreased Effect: Amphetamines inhibit the antihypertensive response to guanethidine and guanadrel. Urinary acidifiers decrease the half-life and duration of action of amphetamines.

Pharmacodynamics/Kinetics

Onset of action: 1-1.5 hours

Distribution: V_d: Adults: 3.5-4.6 L/kg; distributes into CNS; mean CSF concentrations are 80% of plasma; enters breast milk

Metabolism: Hepatic via CYP monooxygenase and glucuronidation

Half-life elimination: Adults: 10-13 hours

Time to peak, serum: T_{max}: Immediate release: 3 hours; sustained release: 8 hours

Excretion: Urine (as unchanged drug and inactive metabolites)

Pregnancy Risk Factor C

Dextroamphetamine and Amphetamine

(deks troe am FET a meen & am FET a meen)

Related Information

Dextroamphetamine *on page 447*

U.S. Brand Names Adderall®; Adderall XR®

Canadian Brand Names Adderall XR®

Generic Available Yes: Tablet

Synonyms Amphetamine and Dextroamphetamine

Pharmacologic Category Stimulant

Use Attention-deficit/hyperactivity disorder (ADHD); narcolepsy

Local Anesthetic/Vasoconstrictor Precautions Use vasoconstrictor with caution in patients taking dextroamphetamine. Amphetamines enhance the sympathomimetic response of epinephrine and norepinephrine leading to potential hypertension and cardiotoxicity.

Effects on Dental Treatment Key adverse event(s) related to dental treatment: Up to 10% of patients taking dextroamphetamines may present with hypertension. Monitor blood pressure prior to using local anesthetic with vasoconstrictors.

Common Adverse Effects

As reported with Adderall XR®:

>10%:

Central nervous system: Insomnia (12% to 27%), headache (up to 26% in adults)

Gastrointestinal: Appetite decreased (22% to 36%), abdominal pain (11% to 14%), dry mouth (2% to 35%), weight loss (4% to 11%)

1% to 10%:

Cardiovascular: Palpitation (2% to 4%), tachycardia (up to 6% in adults)

Central nervous system: Emotional lability (2% to 9%), agitation (up to 8% in adults), anxiety (8%), dizziness (2% to 7%), nervousness (6%), fever (5%), somnolence (2% to 4%)

Dermatologic: Photosensitization (2% to 4%)

Endocrine & metabolic: Dysmenorrhea (2% to 4%), impotence (2% to 4%), libido decreased (2% to 4%)

Gastrointestinal: Nausea (2% to 8%), vomiting (2% to 7%), diarrhea (2% to 6%), constipation (2% to 4%), dyspepsia (2% to 4%)

Neuromuscular & skeletal: Twitching (2% to 4%), weakness (2% to 6%)

Respiratory: Dyspnea (2% to 4%)

Miscellaneous: Diaphoresis (2% to 4%), infection (2% to 4%), speech disorder (2% to 4%)

<1% (Limited to important or life-threatening): MI, seizure, stroke, sudden death

Adverse reactions reported with other amphetamines include: Cardiomyopathy, dyskinesia, dysphoria, euphoria, exacerbation of motor and phonic tics, exacerbation of Tourette's syndrome, headache, hypertension, overstimulation, palpitation, psychosis, rash, restlessness, tachycardia, tremor, urticaria

Restrictions C-II

Dosage Oral: Note: Use lowest effective individualized dose; administer first dose as soon as awake

ADHD:

Children: <3 years: Not recommended

Children: 3-5 years (Adderall®): Initial 2.5 mg/day given every morning; increase daily dose in 2.5 mg increments at weekly intervals until optimal response is obtained (maximum dose: 40 mg/day given in 1-3 divided doses); use intervals of 4-6 hours between additional doses

Children: ≥6 years:

Adderall®: Initial: 5 mg 1-2 times/day; increase daily dose in 5 mg increments at weekly intervals until optimal response is obtained (usual maximum dose: 40 mg/day given in 1-3 divided doses); use intervals of 4-6 hours between additional doses

Adderall XR®: 5-10 mg once daily in the morning; if needed, may increase daily dose in 5-10 mg increments at weekly intervals (maximum dose: 30 mg/day)

Adolescents 13-17 years (Adderall XR®): 10 mg once daily in the morning; maybe increased to 20 mg/day after 1 week if symptoms are not controlled; higher doses (up to 60 mg)/day have been evaluated; however, there is not adequate evidence that higher doses afforded additional benefit.

Adults: Adderall XR®: Initial: 20 mg once daily in the morning; higher doses (up to 60 mg once daily) have been evaluated; however, there is not adequate evidence that higher doses afforded additional benefit

Narcolepsy (Adderall®):

Children: 6-12 years: Initial: 5 mg/day; increase daily dose in 5 mg at weekly intervals until optimal response is obtained (maximum dose: 60 mg/day given in 1-3 divided doses)

Children >12 years and Adults: Initial: 10 mg/day; increase daily dose in 10 mg increments at weekly intervals until optimal response is obtained (maximum dose: 60 mg/day given in 1-3 divided doses)

Mechanism of Action Blocks reuptake of dopamine and norepinephrine from the synapse, thus increases the amount of circulating dopamine and norepinephrine in cerebral cortex to reticular activating system; inhibits the action of monoamine oxidase and causes catecholamines to be released. Peripheral actions include elevation of blood pressure, weak bronchodilation, and respiratory stimulation.

Contraindications Hypersensitivity to dextroamphetamine, amphetamine, or any component of the formulation; advanced arteriosclerosis; symptomatic cardiovascular disease; moderate to severe hypertension; hyperthyroidism; hypersensitivity or idiosyncrasy to the sympathomimetic amines; glaucoma; agitated states; patients with a history of drug abuse; with or within 14 days following MAO inhibitor (hypertensive crisis)

(Continued)

Dextroamphetamine and Amphetamine *(Continued)*

Warnings/Precautions Amphetamine has a high abuse potential; prolonged use may lead to dependency. Avoid use in patients with structural cardiac abnormalities; has been associated with sudden death. Use caution in patients with hypertension (including mildly hypertensive patients); sustained increases in blood pressure may require dosage reduction or antihypertensive therapy. Amphetamines may impair the ability to engage in potentially hazardous activities. In psychotic children, amphetamines may exacerbate symptoms of behavior disturbance and thought disorder. Stimulants may unmask tics in individuals with coexisting Tourette's syndrome. Appetite suppresson may occur; monitor weight during therapy, particularly in children. Not recommended for children <3 years of age. Avoid abrupt discontinuation.

Drug Interactions
Cytochrome P450 Effect:
Dextroamphetamine: **Substrate** of CYP2D6 (major)

Amphetamine: **Substrate** of CYP2D6 (major); **Inhibits** CYP2D6 (weak)

Increased Effect/Toxicity: CYP2D6 inhibitors may increase the levels/effects of amphetamine and dextroamphetamine; example inhibitors include chlorpromazine, delavirdine, fluoxetine, miconazole, paroxetine, pergolide, quinidine, quinine, ritonavir, and ropinirole. Dextroamphetamine and amphetamine may precipitate hypertensive crisis or serotonin syndrome in patients receiving MAO inhibitors (selegiline >10 mg/day, isocarboxazid, phenelzine, tranylcypromine, furazolidone). Serotonin syndrome has also been associated with combinations of amphetamines and SSRIs; these combinations should be avoided. TCAs may enhance the effects of amphetamines, potentially leading to hypertensive crisis. Large doses of antacids or urinary alkalinizers increase the half-life and duration of action of amphetamines. May precipitate arrhythmias in patients receiving general anesthetics.

Decreased Effect: Amphetamines inhibit the antihypertensive response to guanethidine and guanadrel. Urinary acidifiers decrease the half-life and duration of action of amphetamines. Efficacy of amphetamines may be decreased by antipsychotics.

Ethanol/Nutrition/Herb Interactions
Ethanol: Avoid ethanol (may increase CNS depression).

Food: Dextroamphetamine serum levels may be altered if taken with acidic food, juices, or vitamin C. Avoid caffeine.

Herb/Nutraceutical: Avoid ephedra (may cause hypertension or arrhythmias).

Pharmacodynamics/Kinetics
Onset: 30-60 minutes

Duration: 4-6 hours

Absorption: Well-absorbed

Distribution: V_d: Adults: 3.5-4.6 L/kg; concentrates in breast milk (avoid breast-feeding); distributes into CNS, mean CSF concentrations are 80% of plasma

Half-life elimination:

Children 6-12 years: d-amphetamine: 9 hours; l-amphetamine: 11 hours

Adolescents 13-17 years: d-amphetamine: 11 hours; l-amphetamine: 13-14 hours

Adults: d-amphetamine: 10 hours; l-amphetamine: 13 hours

Metabolism: Hepatic via cytochrome P450 monooxygenase and glucuronidation

Time to peak: T_{max}: Adderall®: 3 hours; Adderall XR®: 7 hours

Excretion: Urine (highly dependent on urinary pH); 70% of a single dose is eliminated within 24 hours; excreted as unchanged amphetamine (30%, may range from ~1% in alkaline urine to ~75% in acidic urine), benzoic acid, hydroxyamphetamine, hippuric acid, norephedrine, and *p*-hydroxynorephedrine

Pregnancy Risk Factor C

Dosage Forms CAP, extended release (Adderall XR®): 5 mg [dextroamphetamine sulfate 1.25 mg, dextroamphetamine saccharate 1.25 mg, amphetamine aspartate monohydrate 1.25 mg, amphetamine sulfate 1.25 mg]; 10 mg [dextroamphetamine sulfate 2.5 mg, dextroamphetamine saccharate 2.5 mg, amphetamine aspartate monohydrate 2.5 mg, amphetamine sulfate 2.5 mg]; 15 mg [dextroamphetamine sulfate 3.75 mg, dextroamphetamine saccharate 3.75 mg, amphetamine aspartate monohydrate 3.75 mg, amphetamine sulfate 3.75 mg]; 20 mg [dextroamphetamine sulfate 5 mg, dextroamphetamine saccharate 5 mg, amphetamine aspartate monohydrate 5 mg, amphetamine sulfate 5 mg]; 25 mg [dextroamphetamine sulfate 6.25 mg, dextroamphetamine saccharate 6.25 mg, amphetamine aspartate monohydrate 6.25 mg, amphetamine sulfate 6.25 mg]; 30 mg [dextroamphetamine sulfate 7.5 mg, dextroamphetamine saccharate 7.5 mg, amphetamine aspartate monohydrate 7.5 mg, amphetamine sulfate 7.5 mg]. **TAB** (Adderall®): 5 mg [dextroamphetamine sulfate 1.25 mg, dextroamphetamine saccharate 1.25 mg, amphetamine aspartate 1.25 mg, amphetamine sulfate 1.25 mg]; 7.5 mg [dextroamphetamine 1.875 mg, dextroamphetamine saccharate 1.875 mg, amphetamine aspartate 1.875 mg, amphetamine sulfate 1.875 mg]; 10 mg [dextroamphetamine sulfate 2.5 mg, dextroamphetamine saccharate 2.5 mg, amphetamine aspartate 2.5 mg, amphetamine sulfate 2.5 mg]; 12.5 mg [dextroamphetamine sulfate 3.125 mg, dextroamphetamine saccharate 3.125 mg, amphetamine aspartate 3.125 mg, amphetamine sulfate 3.125 mg]; 15 mg [dextroamphetamine sulfate 3.75 mg, dextroamphetamine saccharate 3.75 mg, amphetamine aspartate 3.75 mg, amphetamine sulfate 3.75 mg]; 20 mg [dextroamphetamine sulfate 5 mg, dextroamphetamine saccharate 5 mg, amphetamine aspartate 5 mg, amphetamine sulfate 5 mg]; 30 mg [dextroamphetamine sulfate 7.5 mg, dextroamphetamine saccharate 7.5 mg, amphetamine aspartate 7.5 mg, amphetamine sulfate 7.5 mg]

Dextroamphetamine Sulfate *see Dextroamphetamine on page 447*

Dextromethorphan (deks troe meth OR fan)

U.S. Brand Names Babee® Cof Syrup [OTC]; Benylin® Adult [OTC] [DSC]; Benylin® Pediatric [OTC] [DSC]; Creomulsion® Cough [OTC]; Creomulsion® for Children [OTC]; Creo-Terpin® [OTC]; Delsym® [OTC]; Dexalone® [OTC]; Elix-Sure™ Cough [OTC]; Hold® DM [OTC]; PediaCare® Children's Medicated Freezer Pops Long Acting Cough [OTC]; PediaCare® Infants' Long-Acting Cough [OTC]; Robitussin® CoughGels™ [OTC]; Robitussin® Honey Cough [OTC]; Robitussin® Maximum Strength Cough [OTC]; Robitussin® Pediatric Cough [OTC]; Scot-Tussin DM® Cough Chasers [OTC]; Silphen DM® [OTC]; Simply Cough® [OTC]; Triaminic® Thin Strips™ Long Acting Cough [OTC]; Vicks® 44® Cough Relief [OTC]

Mexican Brand Names Athos®; Bekidiba Dex®; Neopulmonier®; Romilar®

Generic Available Yes: Excludes strip, liquid freezer pop

Pharmacologic Category Antitussive

Use Symptomatic relief of coughs caused by minor viral upper respiratory tract infections or inhaled irritants; most effective for a chronic nonproductive cough

Unlabeled/Investigational Use *N*-methyl-D-aspartate (NMDA) antagonist in cerebral injury

Local Anesthetic/Vasoconstrictor Precautions No information available to require special precautions

Effects on Dental Treatment No significant effects or complications reported

Mechanism of Action Chemical relative of morphine lacking narcotic properties except in overdose; controls cough by depressing the medullary cough center

Drug Interactions

Cytochrome P450 Effect: Substrate of CYP2B6 (minor), 2C9 (minor), 2C19 (minor), 2D6 (major), 2E1 (minor), 3A4 (minor); Inhibits CYP2D6 (weak)

Increased Effect/Toxicity: CYP2D6 inhibitors may increase the levels/effects of dextromethorphan; example inhibitors include chlorpromazine, delavirdine, fluoxetine, miconazole, paroxetine, pergolide, quinidine, quinine, ritonavir, and ropinirole. Dextromethorphan may increase effect/toxicity of MAO inhibitors.

Pharmacodynamics/Kinetics

Onset of action: Antitussive: 15-30 minutes

Duration: ≤6 hours

Pregnancy Risk Factor C

Dextromethorphan, Acetaminophen, and Pseudoephedrine *see Acetaminophen, Dextromethorphan, and Pseudoephedrine on page 44*

Dextromethorphan and Guaifenesin *see Guaifenesin and Dextromethorphan on page 754*

Dextromethorphan and Promethazine *see Promethazine and Dextromethorphan on page 1292*

Dextromethorphan and Pseudoephedrine *see Pseudoephedrine and Dextromethorphan on page 1311*

Dextromethorphan, Carbinoxamine, and Pseudoephedrine *see Carbinoxamine, Pseudoephedrine, and Dextromethorphan on page 269*

Dextromethorphan, Chlorpheniramine, and Phenylephrine *see Chlorpheniramine, Phenylephrine, and Dextromethorphan on page 326*

Dextromethorphan, Guaifenesin, and Pseudoephedrine *see Guaifenesin, Pseudoephedrine, and Dextromethorphan on page 757*

Dextromethorphan, Pseudoephedrine, and Carbinoxamine *see Carbinoxamine, Pseudoephedrine, and Dextromethorphan on page 269*

Dextropropoxyphene *see Propoxyphene on page 1297*

Dextrose (DEKS trose)

U.S. Brand Names B-D™ Glucose [OTC]; Dex4® Glucose [OTC]; Enfamil® Glucose; Glutol™ [OTC]; Glutose™ [OTC]; Insta-Glucose® [OTC]; Similac® Glucose

Generic Available Yes

Synonyms Anhydrous Glucose; Dextrose Monohydrate; D_5W; $D_{10}W$; $D_{25}W$; $D_{30}W$; $D_{40}W$; $D_{50}W$; $D_{60}W$; $D_{70}W$; Glucose; Glucose Monohydrate; Glycosum

Pharmacologic Category Antidote, Hypoglycemia; Intravenous Nutritional Therapy

Use

Oral: Treatment of hypoglycemia

5% and 10% solutions: Peripheral infusion to provide calories and fluid replacement

25% (hypertonic) solution: Treatment of acute symptomatic episodes of hypoglycemia in infants and children to restore depressed blood glucose levels; adjunctive treatment of hyperkalemia when combined with insulin

50% (hypertonic) solution: Treatment of insulin-induced hypoglycemia (hyperinsulinemia or insulin shock) and adjunctive treatment of hyperkalemia in adolescents and adults

≥10% solutions: Infusion after admixture with amino acids for nutritional support

Local Anesthetic/Vasoconstrictor Precautions No information available to require special precautions

Effects on Dental Treatment No significant effects or complications reported

Common Adverse Effects Frequency not defined. **Note:** Most adverse effects are associated with excessive dosage or rate of infusion.

Cardiovascular: Venous thrombosis, phlebitis, hypovolemia, hypervolemia, dehydration, edema

Central nervous system: Fever, mental confusion, unconsciousness, hyperosmolar syndrome

Endocrine & metabolic: Hyperglycemia, hypokalemia, acidosis, hypophosphatemia, hypomagnesemia

Genitourinary: Polyuria, glycosuria, ketonuria

Gastrointestinal: Polydipsia, nausea, diarrhea (oral)

Local: Pain, vein irritation, tissue necrosis

Respiratory: Tachypnea, pulmonary edema

Mechanism of Action Dextrose, a monosaccharide, is a source of calories and fluid for patients unable to obtain an adequate oral intake; may decrease body protein and nitrogen losses; promotes glycogen deposition in the liver. When used in the treatment of hyperkalemia (combined with insulin), dextrose stimulates the uptake of potassium by cells, especially in muscle tissue, lowering serum potassium.

Pharmacodynamics/Kinetics

Onset of action: Treatment of hypoglycemia: Oral: 10 minutes

Maximum effect: Treatment of hyperkalemia: I.V.: 30 minutes

Absorption: Rapidly from the small intestine by an active mechanism

Metabolism: Metabolized to carbon dioxide and water

Time to peak, serum: Oral: 40 minutes

Pregnancy Risk Factor C/A (oral)

Dextrose and Tetracaine see Tetracaine and Dextrose on page 1467

Dextrose, Levulose and Phosphoric Acid see Fructose, Dextrose, and Phosphoric Acid on page 713

Dextrose Monohydrate see Dextrose on page 452

Dextrostat® see Dextroamphetamine on page 447

DFMO see Eflornithine on page 532

DHAD see Mitoxantrone on page 1055

DHAQ see Mitoxantrone on page 1055

DHE see Dihydroergotamine on page 477

D.H.E. 45® see Dihydroergotamine on page 477

DHPG Sodium see Ganciclovir on page 722

DHS™ Sal [OTC] see Salicylic Acid on page 1374

DHS™ Tar [OTC] see Coal Tar on page 383

DHS™ Targel [OTC] see Coal Tar on page 383

DHS™ Zinc [OTC] see Pyrithione Zinc on page 1318

DHT™ [DSC] see Dihydrotachysterol on page 478

DHT™ Intensol™ [DSC] see Dihydrotachysterol on page 478

Diabeta see GlyBURIDE on page 744

DiabetAid™ Antifungal Foot Bath [OTC] see Miconazole on page 1039

DiabetAid Gingivitis Mouth Rinse [OTC] *see* Cetylpyridinium *on page 309*

Diabetic Tussin C® *see* Guaifenesin and Codeine *on page 753*

Diabetic Tussin® Allergy Relief [OTC] *see* Chlorpheniramine *on page 323*

Diabetic Tussin® DM [OTC] *see* Guaifenesin and Dextromethorphan *on page 754*

Diabetic Tussin® DM Maximum Strength [OTC] *see* Guaifenesin and Dextromethorphan *on page 754*

Diabetic Tussin® EX [OTC] *see* Guaifenesin *on page 752*

Diabinese® *see* ChlorproPAMIDE *on page 331*

Diaβeta® *see* GlyBURIDE *on page 744*

Diaminocyclohexane Oxalatoplatinum *see* Oxaliplatin *on page 1154*

Diaminodiphenylsulfone *see* Dapsone *on page 421*

Diamode [OTC] *see* Loperamide *on page 942*

Diamox® Sequels® *see* AcetaZOLAMIDE *on page 45*

Diasorb® [OTC] *see* Attapulgite *on page 165*

Diastat® *see* Diazepam *on page 454*

Diastat® AcuDial™ *see* Diazepam *on page 454*

Diatrizoate Meglumine (dye a tri ZOE ate MEG loo meen)

U.S. Brand Names Cystografin®; Cystografin® Dilute; Hypaque-Cysto™; Hypaque™ Meglumine; Reno-30®; Reno-60®; Reno-Dip®

Generic Available No

Pharmacologic Category Iodinated Contrast Media; Radiological/Contrast Media, Ionic

Use
Solution for instillation: Retrograde cystourethrography; retrograde or ascending pyelography

Solution for injection: Arthrography, cerebral angiography, direct cholangiography, discography, drip infusion pyelography, excretory urography, peripheral arteriography, splenoportography, venography; contrast enhancement of computed tomographic head imaging

Local Anesthetic/Vasoconstrictor Precautions No information available to require special precautions

Effects on Dental Treatment No significant effects or complications reported

Pregnancy Risk Factor C

Diatrizoate Meglumine and Diatrizoate Sodium
(dye a tri ZOE ate MEG loo meen & dye a tri ZOE ate SOW dee um)

U.S. Brand Names Gastrografin®; Hypaque™-76; MD-76®R; MD-Gastroview®; RenoCal-76®; Renografin®-60

Generic Available No

Synonyms Diatrizoate Sodium and Diatrizoate Meglumine

Pharmacologic Category Iodinated Contrast Media; Radiological/Contrast Media, Ionic

Use
Oral/rectal: Examination of GI tract; adjunct to contrast enhancement in computed tomography of the torso

Injection: Angiocardiography, aortography, central venography, cerebral angiography, cholangiography, digital arteriography, excretory urography, nephrotomography, peripheral angiography, peripheral arteriography, renal arteriography, renal venography, splenoportography, visceral arteriography; contrast enhancement of computed tomographic imaging

Local Anesthetic/Vasoconstrictor Precautions No information available to require special precautions

Effects on Dental Treatment No significant effects or complications reported

Pregnancy Risk Factor B/C (manufacturer dependent)

Diatrizoate Meglumine and Iodipamide Meglumine
(dye a tri ZOE ate MEG loo meen & eye oh DI pa mide MEG loo meen)

U.S. Brand Names Sinografin®

Generic Available No

Synonyms Iodipamide Meglumine and Diatrizoate Meglumine

Pharmacologic Category Iodinated Contrast Media; Radiological/Contrast Media, Ionic

Use Hysterosalpingography

(Continued)

453

Diatrizoate Meglumine and Iodipamide Meglumine
(Continued)

Local Anesthetic/Vasoconstrictor Precautions No information available to require special precautions

Effects on Dental Treatment No significant effects or complications reported

---

Diatrizoate Sodium (dye a tri ZOE ate SOW dee um)

U.S. Brand Names Hypaque™ Sodium

Generic Available No

Pharmacologic Category Iodinated Contrast Media; Radiological/Contrast Media, Ionic

Use

Powder: Radiographic examination of GI tract

Solution for injection: Aortography, cerebral angiography, direct cholangiography, excretory urography, hysterosalpingography, intraosseous venography, peripheral angiography, splenoportography; contrast enhancement of computed tomographic head imaging

Local Anesthetic/Vasoconstrictor Precautions No information available to require special precautions

Effects on Dental Treatment No significant effects or complications reported

Pregnancy Risk Factor C

Diatrizoate Sodium and Diatrizoate Meglumine see Diatrizoate Meglumine and Diatrizoate Sodium on page 453

Diatx™ see Vitamin B Complex Combinations on page 1581

DiatxFe™ see Vitamin B Complex Combinations on page 1581

Diazepam (dye AZ e pam)

Related Information

Sedation on page 1727

Temporomandibular Dysfunction (TMD) on page 1724

Related Sample Prescriptions

Sedation (Prior to Dental Treatment) on page 1746

U.S. Brand Names Diastat®; Diastat® AcuDial™; Diazepam Intensol®; Valium®

Canadian Brand Names Apo-Diazepam®; Diastat®; Diazemuls®; Novo-Dipam; Valium®

Mexican Brand Names Alboral®; Ortopsique®; Pacitran®; Valium®

Generic Available Yes: Injection, tablet, solution only

Pharmacologic Category Benzodiazepine

Dental Use Oral medication for preoperative dental anxiety; sedative component in I.V. conscious sedation in oral surgery patients; skeletal muscle relaxant

Use Management of anxiety disorders, ethanol withdrawal symptoms; skeletal muscle relaxant; treatment of convulsive disorders

Orphan drug: Viscous solution for rectal administration: Management of selected, refractory epilepsy patients on stable regimens of antiepileptic drugs (AEDs) requiring intermittent use of diazepam to control episodes of increased seizure activity

Unlabeled/Investigational Use Panic disorders; preoperative sedation, light anesthesia, amnesia

Local Anesthetic/Vasoconstrictor Precautions No information available to require special precautions

Effects on Dental Treatment Key adverse event(s) related to dental treatment: Xerostomia and changes in salivation (normal salivary flow resumes upon discontinuation).

Significant Adverse Effects Frequency not defined. Adverse reactions may vary by route of administration.

Cardiovascular: Hypotension, vasodilatation

Central nervous system: Agitation, amnesia, anxiety, ataxia, confusion, depression, dizziness, drowsiness, emotional lability, euphoria, fatigue, headache, incoordination, insomnia, memory impairment, paradoxical excitement or rage, seizure, slurred speech, somnolence, vertigo

Dermatologic: Rash

Endocrine & metabolic: Changes in libido

Gastrointestinal: Changes in salivation, constipation, diarrhea, nausea

Genitourinary: Incontinence, urinary retention

Hepatic: Jaundice

Local: Phlebitis, pain with injection

Neuromuscular & skeletal: Dysarthria, tremor, weakness

Ocular: Blurred vision, diplopia
Respiratory: Apnea, asthma, decrease in respiratory rate

Restrictions C-IV

Dental Usual Dosing

Anxiety/sedation/skeletal muscle relaxant: Adults:
Oral: 2-10 mg 2-4 times/day
I.M., I.V.: 2-10 mg, may repeat in 3-4 hours if needed

Anxiety: Elderly: Oral: Initial: 1-2 mg 1-2 times/day; increase gradually as needed, rarely need to use >10 mg/day (watch for hypotension and excessive sedation)

Skeletal muscle relaxant: Elderly: Oral: Initial: 2-5 mg 2-4 times/day

Dosage Oral absorption is more reliable than I.M.

Children:
Conscious sedation for procedures: Oral: 0.2-0.3 mg/kg (maximum: 10 mg) 45-60 minutes prior to procedure

Sedation/muscle relaxant/anxiety:
Oral: 0.12-0.8 mg/kg/day in divided doses every 6-8 hours
I.M., I.V.: 0.04-0.3 mg/kg/dose every 2-4 hours to a maximum of 0.6 mg/kg within an 8-hour period if needed

Status epilepticus:
Infants 30 days to 5 years: I.V.: 0.05-0.3 mg/kg/dose given over 2-3 minutes, every 15-30 minutes to a maximum total dose of 5 mg; repeat in 2-4 hours as needed **or** 0.2-0.5 mg/dose every 2-5 minutes to a maximum total dose of 5 mg

>5 years: I.V.: 0.05-0.3 mg/kg/dose given over 2-3 minutes every 15-30 minutes to a maximum total dose of 10 mg; repeat in 2-4 hours as needed **or** 1 mg/dose given over 2-3 minutes, every 2-5 minutes to a maximum total dose of 10 mg

Rectal: 0.5 mg/kg, then 0.25 mg/kg in 10 minutes if needed

Anticonvulsant (acute treatment): Rectal gel:
Infants <6 months: Not recommended
Children <2 years: Safety and efficacy have not been studied
Children 2-5 years: 0.5 mg/kg
Children 6-11 years: 0.3 mg/kg
Children ≥12 years: 0.2 mg/kg

Note: Dosage should be rounded upward to the next available dose, 2.5, 5, 10, 12.5, 15, 17.5, and 20 mg/dose; dose may be repeated in 4-12 hours if needed; do not use for more than 5 episodes per month or more than one episode every 5 days

Adolescents: Conscious sedation for procedures:
Oral: 10 mg
I.V.: 5 mg, may repeat with ½ dose if needed

Adults:
Anticonvulsant (acute treatment): Rectal gel: 0.2 mg/kg
Note: Dosage should be rounded upward to the next available dose, 2.5, 5, 10, 12.5, 15, 17.5, and 20 mg/dose; dose may be repeated in 4-12 hours if needed; do not use for more than 5 episodes per month or more than one episode every 5 days.

Anxiety/sedation/skeletal muscle relaxant:
Oral: 2-10 mg 2-4 times/day
I.M., I.V.: 2-10 mg, may repeat in 3-4 hours if needed

Sedation in the ICU patient: I.V.: 0.03-0.1 mg/kg every 30 minutes to 6 hours

Status epilepticus: I.V.: 5-10 mg every 10-20 minutes, up to 30 mg in an 8-hour period; may repeat in 2-4 hours if necessary

Rapid tranquilization of agitated patient (administer every 30-60 minutes):
Oral: 5-10 mg; average total dose for tranquilization: 20-60 mg

Elderly:
Anticonvulsant: Rectal gel: Due to the increased half-life in elderly and debilitated patients, consider reducing dose.
Anxiety: Oral: Initial: 1-2 mg 1-2 times/day; increase gradually as needed, rarely need to use >10 mg/day (watch for hypotension and excessive sedation)
Skeletal muscle relaxant: Oral: Initial: 2-5 mg 2-4 times/day

Hemodialysis: Not dialyzable (0% to 5%); supplemental dose is not necessary

Dosing adjustment in hepatic impairment: Reduce dose by 50% in cirrhosis and avoid in severe/acute liver disease

Mechanism of Action Binds to stereospecific benzodiazepine receptors on the postsynaptic GABA neuron at several sites within the central nervous system, including the limbic system, reticular formation. Enhancement of the inhibitory effect of GABA on neuronal excitability results by increased neuronal membrane permeability to chloride ions. This shift in chloride ions results in hyperpolarization (a less excitable state) and stabilization.
(Continued)

Diazepam *(Continued)*

Contraindications Hypersensitivity to diazepam or any component of the formulation (cross-sensitivity with other benzodiazepines may exist); narrow-angle glaucoma; not for use in children <6 months of age (oral, rectal gel) or <30 days of age (parenteral); pregnancy

Warnings/Precautions Diazepam has been associated with increasing the frequency of grand mal seizures. Withdrawal has also been associated with an increase in the seizure frequency. Use with caution with drugs which may decrease diazepam metabolism. Use with caution in elderly or debilitated patients, patients with hepatic disease (including alcoholics), or renal impairment. Active metabolites with extended half-lives may lead to delayed accumulation and adverse effects. Use with caution in patients with respiratory disease or impaired gag reflex.

Acute hypotension, muscle weakness, apnea, and cardiac arrest have occurred with parenteral administration. Acute effects may be more prevalent in patients receiving concurrent barbiturates, narcotics, or ethanol. Appropriate resuscitative equipment and qualified personnel should be available during administration and monitoring. Avoid use of the injection in patients with shock, coma, or acute ethanol intoxication. Intra-arterial injection or extravasation of the parenteral formulation should be avoided. Parenteral formulation contains propylene glycol, which has been associated with toxicity when administered in high dosages. Administration of rectal gel should only be performed by individuals trained to recognize characteristic seizure activity for which the product is indicated, and capable of monitoring response to determine need for additional medical intervention.

Causes CNS depression (dose-related) resulting in sedation, dizziness, confusion, or ataxia which may impair physical and mental capabilities. Patients must be cautioned about performing tasks which require mental alertness (eg, operating machinery or driving). Use with caution in patients receiving other CNS depressants or psychoactive agents. Effects with other sedative drugs or ethanol may be potentiated. The dosage of narcotics should be reduced by approximately 1/3 when diazepam is added. Benzodiazepines have been associated with falls and traumatic injury and should be used with extreme caution in patients who are at risk of these events (especially the elderly).

Use caution in patients with depression, particularly if suicidal risk may be present. Use with caution in patients with a history of drug dependence. Benzodiazepines have been associated with dependence and acute withdrawal symptoms on discontinuation or reduction in dose. Acute withdrawal, including seizures, may be precipitated in patients after administration of flumazenil to patients receiving long-term benzodiazepine therapy.

Diazepam has been associated with anterograde amnesia. Paradoxical reactions, including hyperactive or aggressive behavior, have been reported with benzodiazepines, particularly in adolescent/pediatric or psychiatric patients. Does not have analgesic, antidepressant, or antipsychotic properties.

Drug Interactions Substrate of CYP1A2 (minor), 2B6 (minor), 2C9 (minor), 2C19 (major), 3A4 (major); **Inhibits** CYP2C19 (weak), 3A4 (weak)

CNS depressants: Sedative effects and/or respiratory depression may be additive with CNS depressants; includes ethanol, barbiturates, narcotic analgesics, and other sedative agents; monitor for increased effect

CYP2C19 inducers: May decrease the levels/effects of diazepam. Example inducers include aminoglutethimide, carbamazepine, phenytoin, and rifampin.

CYP2C19 inhibitors: May increase the levels/effects of diazepam. Example inhibitors include delavirdine, fluconazole, fluvoxamine, gemfibrozil, isoniazid, omeprazole, and ticlopidine.

CYP3A4 inducers: CYP3A4 inducers may decrease the levels/effects of diazepam. Example inducers include aminoglutethimide, carbamazepine, nafcillin, nevirapine, phenobarbital, phenytoin, and rifamycins.

CYP3A4 inhibitors: May increase the levels/effects of diazepam. Example inhibitors include azole antifungals, clarithromycin, diclofenac, doxycycline, erythromycin, imatinib, isoniazid, nefazodone, nicardipine, propofol, protease inhibitors, quinidine, telithromycin, and verapamil.

Levodopa: Therapeutic effects may be diminished in some patients following the addition of a benzodiazepine; limited/inconsistent data

Oral contraceptives: May decrease the clearance of some benzodiazepines (those which undergo oxidative metabolism); monitor for increased benzodiazepine effect

Theophylline: May partially antagonize some of the effects of benzodiazepines; monitor for decreased response; may require higher doses for sedation

Ethanol/Nutrition/Herb Interactions

Ethanol: Avoid ethanol (may increase CNS depression).

Food: Diazepam serum levels may be increased if taken with food. Diazepam effect/toxicity may be increased by grapefruit juice; avoid concurrent use.

Herb/Nutraceutical: St John's wort may decrease diazepam levels. Avoid valerian, St John's wort, kava kava, gotu kola (may increase CNS depression).

Pharmacodynamics/Kinetics

I.V.: Status epilepticus:
Onset of action: Almost immediate
Duration: 20-30 minutes
Absorption: Oral: 85% to 100%, more reliable than I.M.
Protein binding: 98%
Metabolism: Hepatic
Half-life elimination: Parent drug: Adults: 20-50 hours; increased half-life in neonates, elderly, and those with severe hepatic disorders; Active major metabolite (desmethyldiazepam): 50-100 hours; may be prolonged in neonates

Pregnancy Risk Factor D

Lactation Enters breast milk/contraindicated (AAP rates "of concern")

Breast-Feeding Considerations Clinical effects on the infant include sedation; AAP reports that USE MAY BE OF CONCERN.

Dosage Forms

Gel, rectal:
Diastat®: Pediatric rectal tip [4.4 cm]: 5 mg/mL (2.5 mg, 5 mg) [contains ethyl alcohol 10%, sodium benzoate, benzyl alcohol 1.5%; twin pack]
Diastat® AcuDial™ delivery system:
10 mg: Pediatric/adult rectal tip [4.4 cm]: 5 mg/mL (delivers set doses of 5 mg, 7.5 mg, and 10 mg) [contains ethyl alcohol 10%, sodium benzoate, benzyl alcohol 1.5%; twin pack]
20 mg: Adult rectal tip [6 cm]: 5 mg/mL (delivers set doses of 10 mg, 12.5 mg, 15 mg, 17.5 mg, and 20 mg) [contains ethyl alcohol 10%, sodium benzoate, benzyl alcohol 1.5%; twin pack]
Injection, solution: 5 mg/mL (2 mL, 10 mL) [may contain benzyl alcohol, sodium benzoate, benzoic acid]
Solution, oral: 5 mg/5 mL (5 mL, 500 mL) [wintergreen-spice flavor]
Solution, oral concentrate (Diazepam Intensol®): 5 mg/mL (30 mL)
Tablet (Valium®): 2 mg, 5 mg, 10 mg

Diazepam Intensol® *see* Diazepam *on page 454*

Diazoxide (dye az OKS ide)

U.S. Brand Names Hyperstat®; Proglycem®
Canadian Brand Names Proglycem®
Mexican Brand Names Sefulken®
Generic Available No
Pharmacologic Category Antihypertensive; Antihypoglycemic Agent

Use

Oral: Hypoglycemia related to islet cell adenoma, carcinoma, hyperplasia, or adenomatosis, nesidioblastosis, leucine sensitivity, or extrapancreatic malignancy
I.V.: Severe hypertension

Local Anesthetic/Vasoconstrictor Precautions No information available to require special precautions

Effects on Dental Treatment No significant effects or complications reported

Common Adverse Effects 1% to 10%:
Cardiovascular: Hypotension
Central nervous system: Dizziness
Gastrointestinal: Nausea, vomiting
Neuromuscular & skeletal: Weakness

Mechanism of Action Inhibits insulin release from the pancreas; produces direct smooth muscle relaxation of the peripheral arterioles which results in decrease in blood pressure and reflex increase in heart rate and cardiac output

Drug Interactions

Increased Effect/Toxicity: Diuretics and hypotensive agents may potentiate diazoxide adverse effects. Diazoxide may decrease warfarin protein binding.

Decreased Effect: Diazoxide may increase phenytoin metabolism or free fraction.

Pharmacodynamics/Kinetics

Onset of action: Hyperglycemic: Oral: ~1 hour
Peak effect: Hypotensive: I.V.: ~5 minutes
Duration: Hyperglycemic: Oral: Normal renal function: 8 hours; Hypotensive: I.V.: Usually 3-12 hours
Protein binding: 90%
(Continued)

Diazoxide *(Continued)*

Half-life elimination: Children: 9-24 hours; Adults: 20-36 hours; End-stage renal disease: >30 hours

Excretion: Urine (50% as unchanged drug)

Pregnancy Risk Factor C

Dibenzyline® *see* Phenoxybenzamine *on page 1224*

Dibucaine (DYE byoo kane)

U.S. Brand Names Nupercainal® [OTC]
Generic Available Yes
Pharmacologic Category Local Anesthetic
Dental Use Amide derivative local anesthetic for minor skin conditions
Use Fast, temporary relief of pain and itching due to hemorrhoids, minor burns
Local Anesthetic/Vasoconstrictor Precautions No information available to require special precautions
Effects on Dental Treatment No significant effects or complications reported
Significant Adverse Effects 1% to 10%:
Dermatologic: Angioedema, contact dermatitis
Local: Burning
Dental Usual Dosing Local pain (local anesthetic): Children and Adults: Topical: Apply gently to the affected areas; no more than 30 g for adults or 7.5 g for children should be used in any 24-hour period
Dosage Children and Adults: Topical: Apply gently to the affected areas; no more than 30 g for adults or 7.5 g for children should be used in any 24-hour period
Mechanism of Action Local anesthetics bind selectively to the intracellular surface of sodium channels to block influx of sodium into the axon. As a result, depolarization necessary for action potential propagation and subsequent nerve function is prevented. The block at the sodium channel is reversible. When drug diffuses away from the axon, sodium channel function is restored and nerve propagation returns.
Contraindications Hypersensitivity to amide-type anesthetics, ophthalmic use
Drug Interactions No data reported
Pharmacodynamics/Kinetics
Onset of action: ~15 minutes
Duration: 2-4 hours
Absorption: Poor through intact skin; well absorbed through mucous membranes and excoriated skin
Pregnancy Risk Factor C
Breast-Feeding Considerations No data reported; however, topical administration is probably compatible.
Dosage Forms
Ointment: 1% (30 g, 454 g)
Nupercainal®: 1% (30 g, 60g) [contains sodium bisulfite]

DIC *see* Dacarbazine *on page 415*

Dichloralphenazone, Acetaminophen, and Isometheptene *see* Acetaminophen, Isometheptene, and Dichloralphenazone *on page 44*

Dichloralphenazone, Isometheptene, and Acetaminophen *see* Acetaminophen, Isometheptene, and Dichloralphenazone *on page 44*

6,7-Dichloro-1,5-Dihydroimidazo [2,1b] quinazolin-2(3H)-one Monohydrochloride *see* Anagrelide *on page 124*

Dichlorodifluoromethane and Trichloromonofluoromethane (dye klor oh dye flor oh METH ane & tri klor oh mon oh flor oh METH ane)

Related Information
Temporomandibular Dysfunction (TMD) *on page 1724*
U.S. Brand Names Fluori-Methane®
Generic Available No
Synonyms Trichloromonofluoromethane and Dichlorodifluoromethane
Pharmacologic Category Analgesic, Topical
Dental Use Topical application in the management of myofascial pain, restricted motion, and muscle spasm
Use Management of pain associated with injections
Local Anesthetic/Vasoconstrictor Precautions No information available to require special precautions

Effects on Dental Treatment No significant effects or complications reported

Significant Adverse Effects No data reported

Dosage Invert bottle over treatment area approximately 12" away from site of application; open dispenseal spring valve completely, allowing liquid to flow in a stream from the bottle. The rate of spraying is approximately 10 cm/second and should be continued until entire muscle has been covered.

Contraindications Hypersensitivity to dichlorofluoromethane and/or trichloro-monofluoromethane, or any component of the formulation; patients having vascular impairment of the extremities

Warnings/Precautions For external use only; care should be taken to minimize inhalation of vapors, especially with application to head and neck; avoid contact with eyes; should not be applied to the point of frost formation

Drug Interactions No data reported

Pharmacodynamics/Kinetics No data reported

Dosage Forms Aerosol, topical: Dichlorodifluoromethane 15% and trichloro-monofluoromethane 85% (103 mL) [contains chlorofluorocarbons]

Dichlorotetrafluoroethane and Ethyl Chloride *see* Ethyl Chloride and Dichlorotet-rafluoroethane *on page 620*

Dichlorphenamide (dye klor FEN a mide)

U.S. Brand Names Daranide®

Canadian Brand Names Daranide®

Generic Available No

Synonyms Diclofenamide

Pharmacologic Category Carbonic Anhydrase Inhibitor; Diuretic, Carbonic Anhydrase Inhibitor; Ophthalmic Agent, Antiglaucoma

Use Adjunct in treatment of open-angle glaucoma and perioperative treatment for angle-closure glaucoma

Local Anesthetic/Vasoconstrictor Precautions No information available to require special precautions

Effects on Dental Treatment Key adverse event(s) related to dental treatment: Metallic taste.

Pregnancy Risk Factor C

Dichysterol *see* Dihydrotachysterol *on page 478*

Diclofenac (dye KLOE fen ak)

Related Information
Rheumatoid Arthritis, Osteoarthritis, and Osteoporosis *on page 1668*
Temporomandibular Dysfunction (TMD) *on page 1724*

U.S. Brand Names Cataflam®; Solaraze®; Voltaren®; Voltaren Ophthalmic®; Voltaren®-XR

Canadian Brand Names Apo-Diclo®; Apo-Diclo Rapide®; Apo-Diclo SR®; Cataflam®; Novo-Difenac; Novo-Difenac K; Novo-Difenac-SR; Nu-Diclo; Nu-Diclo-SR; Pennsaid®; PMS-Diclofenac; PMS-Diclofenac SR; Riva-Diclofenac; Riva-Diclofenac-K; Voltaren®; Voltaren Ophtha®; Voltaren Rapide®

Generic Available Yes: Excludes gel, ophthalmic solution

Synonyms Diclofenac Potassium; Diclofenac Sodium

Pharmacologic Category Nonsteroidal Anti-inflammatory Drug (NSAID); Nonsteroidal Anti-inflammatory Drug (NSAID), Ophthalmic; Nonsteroidal Anti-inflammatory Drug (NSAID), Oral

Dental Use Immediate-release tablets: Acute treatment of mild to moderate pain

Use
Immediate release: Ankylosing spondylitis; primary dysmenorrhea; acute and chronic treatment of rheumatoid arthritis, osteoarthritis

Delayed-release tablets: Acute and chronic treatment of rheumatoid arthritis, osteoarthritis, ankylosing spondylitis

Extended-release tablets: Chronic treatment of osteoarthritis, rheumatoid arthritis

Ophthalmic solution: Postoperative inflammation following cataract extraction; temporary relief of pain and photophobia in patients undergoing corneal refractive surgery

Topical gel: Actinic keratosis (AK) in conjunction with sun avoidance

Unlabeled/Investigational Use Juvenile rheumatoid arthritis

Local Anesthetic/Vasoconstrictor Precautions No information available to require special precautions

(Continued)

Diclofenac *(Continued)*

Effects on Dental Treatment NSAID formulations are known to reversibly decrease platelet aggregation via mechanisms different than observed with aspirin. The dentist should be aware of the potential of abnormal coagulation. Caution should also be exercised in the use of NSAIDs in patients already on anticoagulant therapy with drugs such as warfarin (Coumadin®).

Significant Adverse Effects

>10%:

Local: Application site reactions (gel): Pruritus (31% to 52%), rash (35% to 46%), contact dermatitis (19% to 33%), dry skin (25% to 27%), pain (15% to 26%), exfoliation (6% to 24%), paresthesia (8% to 20%)

Ocular: Ophthalmic drops (incidence may be dependent upon indication): Lacrimation (30%), keratitis (28%), elevated IOP (15%), transient burning/stinging (15%)

1% to 10%:

Central nervous system: Headache (7%), dizziness (3%)

Dermatologic: Pruritus (1% to 3%), rash (1% to 3%)

Endocrine & metabolic: Fluid retention (1% to 3%)

Gastrointestinal: Abdominal cramps (3% to 9%), abdominal pain (3% to 9%), constipation (3% to 9%), diarrhea (3% to 9%), flatulence (3% to 9%), indigestion (3% to 9%), nausea (3% to 9%), abdominal distention (1% to 3%), peptic ulcer/GI bleed (0.6% to 2%)

Hepatic: Increased ALT/AST (2%)

Local: Application site reactions (gel): Edema (4%)

Ocular: Ophthalmic drops: Abnormal vision, acute elevated IOP, blurred vision, conjunctivitis, corneal deposits, corneal edema, corneal opacity, corneal lesions, discharge, eyelid swelling, injection, iritis, irritation, itching, lacrimation disorder, ocular allergy

Otic: Tinnitus (1% to 3%)

<1% (Limited to important or life-threatening): Oral dosage forms: Acute renal failure, agranulocytosis, allergic purpura, alopecia, anaphylactoid reactions, anaphylaxis, angioedema, aplastic anemia, aseptic meningitis, asthma, bullous eruption, cirrhosis, CHF, eosinophilia, erythema multiforme major, GI hemorrhage, hearing loss, hemolytic anemia, hepatic necrosis, hepatitis, hepatorenal syndrome, interstitial nephritis, jaundice, laryngeal edema, leukopenia, nephrotic syndrome, pancreatitis, papillary necrosis, photosensitivity, purpura, Stevens-Johnson syndrome, swelling of lips and tongue, thrombocytopenia, urticaria, visual changes, vomiting

Restrictions A medication guide should be dispensed with each prescription. A template for the required MedGuide can be found on the FDA website at http://www.fda.gov/medwatch/SAFETY/2005/safety05.htm#NSAID

Dental Usual Dosing Pain: Adults: Oral: Starting dose: 50 mg 3 times/day; maximum dose: 150 mg/day

Dosage Adults:

Oral:

Analgesia/primary dysmenorrhea: Starting dose: 50 mg 3 times/day; maximum dose: 150 mg/day

Rheumatoid arthritis: 150-200 mg/day in 2-4 divided doses (100 mg/day of sustained release product)

Osteoarthritis: 100-150 mg/day in 2-3 divided doses (100-200 mg/day of sustained release product)

Ankylosing spondylitis: 100-125 mg/day in 4-5 divided doses

Ophthalmic:

Cataract surgery: Instill 1 drop into affected eye 4 times/day beginning 24 hours after cataract surgery and continuing for 2 weeks

Corneal refractive surgery: Instill 1-2 drops into affected eye within the hour prior to surgery, within 15 minutes following surgery, and then continue for 4 times/day, up to 3 days

Topical: Apply gel to lesion area twice daily for 60-90 days

Dosage adjustment in renal impairment: Not recommended in patients with advanced renal disease

Dosage adjustment in hepatic impairment: No specific dosing recommendations

Elderly: No specific dosing recommendations; elderly may demonstrate adverse effects at lower doses than younger adults, and >60% may develop asymptomatic peptic ulceration with or without hemorrhage; monitor renal function

Mechanism of Action Inhibits prostaglandin synthesis by decreasing the activity of the enzyme, cyclooxygenase, which results in decreased formation of prostaglandin precursors. Mechanism of action for the treatment of AK has not been established.

Contraindications Hypersensitivity to diclofenac, aspirin, other NSAIDs, or any component of the formulation; perioperative pain in the setting of coronary artery bypass surgery (CABG); pregnancy (3rd trimester)

Warnings/Precautions NSAIDs are associated with an increased risk of adverse cardiovascular events, including MI, stroke, and new onset or worsening of pre-existing hypertension. Risk may be increased with duration of use or pre-existing cardiovascular risk factors or disease. Carefully evaluate individual cardiovascular risk profiles prior to prescribing. Use caution with fluid retention, CHF, or hypertension.

Use of NSAIDs can compromise existing renal function. Renal toxicity can occur in patient with impaired renal function, dehydration, heart failure, liver dysfunction, those taking diuretics and ACEI, and the elderly. Rehydrate patient before starting therapy. Monitor renal function closely. Not recommended for use in patients with advanced renal disease.

NSAIDs may increase risk of gastrointestinal irritation, ulceration, bleeding, and perforation. These events may occur at any time during therapy and without warning. Use caution with a history of GI disease (bleeding or ulcers), concurrent therapy with aspirin, anticoagulants and/or corticosteroids, smoking, use of alcohol, the elderly or debilitated patients.

Use the lowest effective dose for the shortest duration of time, consistent with individual patient goals, to reduce risk of cardiovascular or GI adverse events. Alternate therapies should be considered for patients at high risk.

NSAIDs may cause serious skin adverse events including exfoliative dermatitis, Stevens-Johnson syndrome (SJS), and toxic epidermal necrolysis (TEN). Anaphylactoid reactions may occur, even without prior exposure; patients with 'aspirin triad' (bronchial asthma, aspirin intolerance, rhinitis) may be at increased risk. Do not use in patients who experience bronchospasm, asthma, rhinitis, or urticaria with NSAID or aspirin therapy.

Use with caution in patients with decreased hepatic function. Closely monitor patients with any abnormal LFT. Severe hepatic reactions (eg, fulminant hepatitis, liver failure) have occurred with NSAID use, rarely; discontinue if signs or symptoms of liver disease develop, or if systemic manifestations occur.

The elderly are at increased risk for adverse effects (especially peptic ulceration, CNS effects, renal toxicity) from NSAIDs even at low doses.

Withhold for at least 4-6 half-lives prior to surgical or dental procedures.

Topical gel should not be applied to the eyes, open wounds, infected areas, or to exfoliative dermatitis. Monitor patients for 1 year following application of ophthalmic drops for corneal refractive procedures. Patients using ophthalmic drops should not wear soft contact lenses. Ophthalmic drops may slow/delay healing or prolong bleeding time following surgery.

Drug Interactions Substrate (minor) of CYP1A2, 2B6, 2C8, 2C9, 2C19, 2D6, 3A4; **Inhibits** CYP1A2 (moderate), 2C9 (weak), 2E1 (weak), 3A4 (strong)

ACE inhibitors: Antihypertensive effects may be decreased by concurrent therapy with NSAIDs; monitor blood pressure

Angiotensin II antagonists: Antihypertensive effects may be decreased by concurrent therapy with NSAIDs; monitor blood pressure

Anticoagulants (warfarin, heparin, LMWHs) in combination with NSAIDs can cause increased risk of bleeding.

Antiplatelet drugs (ticlopidine, clopidogrel, aspirin, abciximab, dipyridamole, eptifibatide, tirofiban) can cause an increased risk of bleeding.

Beta-blockers: NSAIDs may decrease the antihypertensive effect of beta-blockers. Monitor.

Cholestyramine (and other bile acid sequestrants): May decrease the absorption of NSAIDs. Separate by at least 2 hours.

Corticosteroids may increase the risk of GI ulceration; avoid concurrent use.

Cyclosporine: NSAIDs may increase serum creatinine, potassium, blood pressure, and cyclosporine levels; monitor cyclosporine levels and renal function carefully.

CYP1A2 substrates: Diclofenac may increase the levels/effects of CYP1A2 substrates. Example substrates include aminophylline, fluvoxamine, mexiletine, mirtazapine, ropinirole, theophylline, and trifluoperazine.

CYP3A4 substrates: Diclofenac may increase the levels/effects of CYP3A4 substrates. Example substrates include benzodiazepines, calcium channel blockers, mirtazapine, nateglinide, nefazodone, tacrolimus, and venlafaxine. Selected benzodiazepines (midazolam and triazolam), cisapride, ergot alkaloids, selected HMG-CoA reductase inhibitors (lovastatin and simvastatin), and pimozide are generally contraindicated with strong CYP3A4 inhibitors.

Gentamicin and amikacin serum concentrations are increased by indomethacin in premature infants. Results may apply to other aminoglycosides and NSAIDs.

(Continued)

Diclofenac *(Continued)*

Hydralazine's antihypertensive effect is decreased; avoid concurrent use.

Lithium levels can be increased; avoid concurrent use if possible or monitor lithium levels and adjust dose. Sulindac may have the least effect. When NSAID is stopped, lithium will need adjustment again.

Loop diuretics efficacy (diuretic and antihypertensive effect) is reduced. Indomethacin reduces this efficacy, however, it may be anticipated with any NSAID.

Methotrexate: Severe bone marrow suppression, aplastic anemia, and GI toxicity have been reported with concomitant NSAID therapy. Avoid use during moderate or high-dose methotrexate (increased and prolonged methotrexate levels). NSAID use during low-dose treatment of rheumatoid arthritis has not been fully evaluated; extreme caution is warranted.

Thiazides antihypertensive effects are decreased; avoid concurrent use.

Verapamil plasma concentration is decreased by diclofenac; avoid concurrent use.

Warfarin's INRs may be increased by piroxicam. Other NSAIDs may have the same effect depending on dose and duration. Monitor INR closely. Use the lowest dose of NSAIDs possible and for the briefest duration.

Ethanol/Nutrition/Herb Interactions

Ethanol: Avoid ethanol (may enhance gastric mucosal irritation).

Herb/Nutraceutical: Avoid alfalfa, anise, bilberry, bladderwrack, bromelain, cat's claw, celery, coleus, cordyceps, dong quai, evening primrose, feverfew, fenugreek, garlic, ginger, ginkgo biloboa, red clover, horse chestnut, grapeseed, green tea, ginseng, guggul, horse chestnut seed, horseradish, licorice, prickly ash, red clover, reishi, SAMe, sweet clover, turmeric, white willow (all have additional antiplatelet activity).

Dietary Considerations May be taken with food to decrease GI distress.

Diclofenac potassium = Cataflam®; potassium content: 5.8 mg (0.15 mEq) per 50 mg tablet

Pharmacodynamics/Kinetics

Onset of action: Cataflam® is more rapid than sodium salt (Voltaren®) because it dissolves in the stomach instead of the duodenum

Absorption: Topical gel: 10%

Protein binding: 99% to albumin

Metabolism: Hepatic to several metabolites

Half-life elimination: 2 hours

Time to peak, serum: Cataflam®: ~1 hour; Voltaren®: ~2 hours

Excretion: Urine (65%); feces (35%)

Pregnancy Risk Factor B (topical); C (oral)/D (3rd trimester)

Lactation Excretion in breast milk unknown/not recommended

Dosage Forms [DSC] = Discontinued product

Gel, as sodium:

Solaraze®: 30 mg/g (50 g)

Solution, ophthalmic, as sodium:

Voltaren Ophthalmic®: 0.1% (2.5 mL, 5 mL)

Tablet, as potassium: 50 mg

Cataflam®: 50 mg

Tablet, delayed release, enteric coated, as sodium: 50 mg, 75 mg

Voltaren®: 25 mg [DSC], 50 mg [DSC], 75 mg

Tablet, extended release, as sodium: 100 mg

Voltaren®-XR: 100 mg

Selected Readings

Kubitzek F, Ziegler G, Gold MS, et al, "Analgesic Efficacy of Low-Dose Diclofenac Versus Paracetamol and Placebo in Postoperative Dental Pain," *J Orofac Pain*, 2003, 17(3):237-44.

Diclofenac and Misoprostol

(dye KLOE fen ak & mye soe PROST ole)

Related Information

Diclofenac *on page 459*

Misoprostol *on page 1053*

Rheumatoid Arthritis, Osteoarthritis, and Osteoporosis *on page 1668*

U.S. Brand Names Arthrotec®

Canadian Brand Names Arthrotec®

Generic Available No

Synonyms Misoprostol and Diclofenac

Pharmacologic Category Nonsteroidal Anti-inflammatory Drug (NSAID), Oral; Prostaglandin

Use The diclofenac component is indicated for the treatment of osteoarthritis and rheumatoid arthritis; the misoprostol component is indicated for the prophylaxis of NSAID-induced gastric and duodenal ulceration

Local Anesthetic/Vasoconstrictor Precautions No information available to require special precautions

Effects on Dental Treatment No significant effects or complications reported

Common Adverse Effects Also see individual agents.

>10%: Gastrointestinal: Abdominal pain (21%), diarrhea (19%), nausea (11%), dyspepsia (14%)

1% to 10%:
Endocrine & metabolic: Transaminases increased
Gastrointestinal: Flatulence (9%)
Hematologic: Anemia
Miscellaneous: Anaphylactic reactions

Restrictions
A medication guide should be dispensed with each prescription. A template for the required MedGuide can be found on the FDA website at http://www.fda.gov/medwatch/SAFETY/2005/safety05.htm#NSAID

Mechanism of Action See individual agents.

Drug Interactions
Cytochrome P450 Effect: Diclofenac: **Substrate** (minor) of CYP1A2, 2B6, 2C8, 2C9, 2C19, 2D6, 3A4; **Inhibits** CYP1A2 (moderate), 2C9 (weak), 2E1 (weak), 3A4 (strong)

Increased Effect/Toxicity: Aspirin (shared toxicity), digoxin (elevated digoxin levels), warfarin (synergistic bleeding potential), methotrexate (increased methotrexate levels), cyclosporine (increased nephrotoxicity), lithium (increased lithium levels). Diclofenac may increase the levels/effects of CYP3A4 substrates (eg, benzodiazepines, calcium channel blockers, mirtazapine, nateglinide, nefazodone, tacrolimus, and venlafaxine). Selected benzodiazepines (midazolam and triazolam), cisapride, ergot alkaloids, selected HMG-CoA reductase inhibitors (lovastatin and simvastatin), and pimozide are generally contraindicated with strong CYP3A4 inhibitors.

Decreased Effect: Aspirin (displaces diclofenac from binding sites), antihypertensive agents (decreased blood pressure control), antacids (may decrease absorption). Antihypertensive effects of ACE inhibitors, angiotensin antagonists, beta blockers, hydralazine, and thiazides may be decreased by concurrent therapy with NSAIDs. Cholestyramine (and other bile acid sequestrants) may decrease the absorption of NSAIDs; separate by at least 2 hours.

Pharmacodynamics/Kinetics See individual agents.

Pregnancy Risk Factor X

Diclofenac Potassium see Diclofenac on page 459

Diclofenac Sodium see Diclofenac on page 459

Diclofenamide see Dichlorphenamide on page 459

Dicloxacillin (dye kloks a SIL in)

Related Information
Bacterial Infections on page 1697
Canadian Brand Names Dycill®; Pathocil®
Generic Available Yes
Synonyms Dicloxacillin Sodium
Pharmacologic Category Antibiotic, Penicillin
Dental Use Treatment of susceptible orofacial infections (notably penicillinase-producing staphylococci)
Use Treatment of systemic infections such as pneumonia, skin and soft tissue infections, and osteomyelitis caused by penicillinase-producing staphylococci

Local Anesthetic/Vasoconstrictor Precautions No information available to require special precautions

Effects on Dental Treatment Key adverse event(s) related to dental treatment: Prolonged use of penicillins may lead to development of oral candidiasis.

Significant Adverse Effects
1% to 10%: Gastrointestinal: Nausea, diarrhea, abdominal pain
<1% (Limited to important or life-threatening): Agranulocytosis, eosinophilia, hemolytic anemia, hepatotoxicity, hypersensitivity, interstitial nephritis, leukopenia, neutropenia, prolonged PT, pseudomembranous colitis, rash (maculopapular to exfoliative), seizure with extremely high doses and/or renal failure, serum sickness-like reactions, thrombocytopenia, vaginitis, vomiting

Dental Usual Dosing Susceptible orofacial infections: Children >40 kg and Adults: 125-250 mg every 6 hours

(Continued)

Dicloxacillin (Continued)

Dosage
Usual dosage range:
Newborns: Use not recommended
Children <40 kg: Oral: 12.5-100 mg/kg/day divided every 6 hours
Children >40 kg: Oral: 125-250 mg every 6 hours
Adults: Oral: 125-1000 mg every 6 hours

Indication-specific dosing:
Children: Oral:
Furunculosis: 25-50 mg/kg/day divided every 6 hours
Osteomyelitis: 50-100 mg/kg/day in divided doses every 6 hours
Adults: Oral:
Erysipelas, furunculosis, impetigo, mastitis, otitis externa, septic bursitis, skin abscess: 500 mg every 6 hours
Prosthetic joint (long-term suppression therapy): 250 mg twice daily
***Staphylococcus aureus*, methicillin susceptible infection if no I.V. access:** 500-1000 mg every 6-8 hours

Dosage adjustment in renal impairment: Not necessary
Hemodialysis: Not dialyzable (0% to 5%); supplemental dosage not necessary
Peritoneal dialysis: Supplemental dosage not necessary
Continuous arteriovenous or venovenous hemofiltration: Supplemental dosage not necessary

Mechanism of Action Inhibits bacterial cell wall synthesis by binding to one or more of the penicillin binding proteins (PBPs) which in turn inhibits the final transpeptidation step of peptidoglycan synthesis in bacterial cell walls, thus inhibiting cell wall biosynthesis. Bacteria eventually lyse due to ongoing activity of cell wall autolytic enzymes (autolysins and murein hydrolases) while cell wall assembly is arrested.

Contraindications Hypersensitivity to dicloxacillin, penicillin, or any component of the formulation

Warnings/Precautions Monitor PT if patient concurrently on warfarin; elimination of drug is slow in neonates; use with caution in patients allergic to cephalosporins

Drug Interactions Induces CYP3A4 (weak)
Methotrexate: Penicillins may increase the exposure to methotrexate during concurrent therapy; monitor.
Oral contraceptives: Anecdotal reports suggesting decreased contraceptive efficacy with penicillins have been refuted by more rigorous scientific and clinical data.
Probenecid, disulfiram: May increase levels of penicillins (dicloxacillin)
Warfarin: Concurrent use may decrease effect of warfarin

Ethanol/Nutrition/Herb Interactions Food: Decreases drug absorption rate; decreases drug serum concentration.

Dietary Considerations Administer on an empty stomach 1 hour before or 2 hours after meals. Sodium content of 250 mg capsule: 13 mg (0.6 mEq)

Pharmacodynamics/Kinetics
Absorption: 35% to 76%; rate and extent reduced by food
Distribution: Throughout body with highest concentrations in kidney and liver; CSF penetration is low; crosses placenta; enters breast milk
Protein binding: 96%
Half-life elimination: 0.6-0.8 hour; slightly prolonged with renal impairment
Time to peak, serum: 0.5-2 hours
Excretion: Feces; urine (56% to 70% as unchanged drug); prolonged in neonates

Pregnancy Risk Factor B

Lactation Excretion in breast milk unknown (probably similar to penicillin G)

Breast-Feeding Considerations No data reported; however, other penicillins may be taken while breast-feeding.

Dosage Forms Capsule: 250 mg, 500 mg

Dicloxacillin Sodium *see* Dicloxacillin *on page 463*

Dicyclomine (dye SYE kloe meen)

U.S. Brand Names Bentyl®
Canadian Brand Names Bentylol®; Formulex®; Lomine; Riva-Dicyclomine
Generic Available Yes: Excludes syrup
Synonyms Dicyclomine Hydrochloride; Dicycloverine Hydrochloride
Pharmacologic Category Anticholinergic Agent
Use Treatment of functional disturbances of GI motility such as irritable bowel syndrome
Unlabeled/Investigational Use Urinary incontinence

Local Anesthetic/Vasoconstrictor Precautions No information available to require special precautions

Effects on Dental Treatment Key adverse event(s) related to dental treatment: Xerostomia and changes in salivation (normal salivary flow resumes upon discontinuation).

Common Adverse Effects Adverse reactions are included here that have been reported for pharmacologically similar drugs with anticholinergic/antispasmodic action; frequency not defined.

Cardiovascular: Syncope, tachycardia, palpitation

Central nervous system: Dizziness, lightheadedness, tingling, headache, drowsiness, nervousness, numbness, mental confusion and/or excitement, dyskinesia, lethargy, speech disturbance, insomnia

Dermatologic: Rash, urticaria, itching, and other dermal manifestations; severe allergic reaction or drug idiosyncrasies including anaphylaxis

Endocrine & metabolic: Suppression of lactation

Gastrointestinal: Xerostomia, nausea, vomiting, constipation, bloated feeling, abdominal pain, taste loss, anorexia

Genitourinary: Urinary hesitancy, urinary retention, impotence

Neuromuscular & skeletal: Weakness

Ocular: Blurred vision, diplopia, mydriasis, cycloplegia, increased ocular tension

Respiratory: Dyspnea, apnea, asphyxia, nasal stuffiness or congestion, sneezing, throat congestion

Miscellaneous: Decreased diaphoresis

Mechanism of Action Blocks the action of acetylcholine at parasympathetic sites in smooth muscle, secretory glands and the CNS

Drug Interactions

Increased Effect/Toxicity: Dicyclomine taken with anticholinergics, amantadine, narcotic analgesics, Type I antiarrhythmics, antihistamines, phenothiazines, tricyclic antidepressants may result in increased toxicity.

Decreased Effect: Decreased effect with phenothiazines, anti-Parkinson's drugs, haloperidol, sustained release dosage forms, and with antacids.

Pharmacodynamics/Kinetics

Onset of action: 1-2 hours

Duration: ≤4 hours

Absorption: Oral: Well absorbed

Metabolism: Extensive

Half-life elimination: Initial: 1.8 hours; Terminal: 9-10 hours

Excretion: Urine (small amounts as unchanged drug)

Pregnancy Risk Factor B

Dicyclomine Hydrochloride *see* Dicyclomine *on page 464*

Dicycloverine Hydrochloride *see* Dicyclomine *on page 464*

Di-Dak-Sol *see* Sodium Hypochlorite Solution *on page 1402*

Didanosine (dye DAN oh seen)

Related Information

HIV Infection and AIDS *on page 1662*

U.S. Brand Names Videx®; Videx® EC

Canadian Brand Names Videx®; Videx® EC

Generic Available Yes: Delayed release capsule

Synonyms ddI; Dideoxyinosine

Pharmacologic Category Antiretroviral Agent, Reverse Transcriptase Inhibitor (Nucleoside)

Use Treatment of HIV infection; always to be used in combination with at least two other antiretroviral agents

Local Anesthetic/Vasoconstrictor Precautions No information available to require special precautions

Effects on Dental Treatment Key adverse event(s) related to dental treatment: Xerostomia (normal salivary flow resumes upon discontinuation).

Common Adverse Effects As reported in monotherapy studies; risk of toxicity may increase when combined with other agents.

>10%:

Gastrointestinal: Increased amylase (15% to 17%), abdominal pain (7% to 13%), diarrhea (19% to 28%)

Neuromuscular & skeletal: Peripheral neuropathy (17% to 20%)

1% to 10%:

Dermatologic: Rash, pruritus

Endocrine & metabolic: Increased uric acid

Gastrointestinal: Pancreatitis; patients >65 years of age had a higher frequency of pancreatitis than younger patients

(Continued)

Didanosine (Continued)

Hepatic: Increased SGOT, increased SGPT, increased alkaline phosphatase

Mechanism of Action Didanosine, a purine nucleoside (adenosine) analog and the deamination product of dideoxyadenosine (ddA), inhibits HIV replication *in vitro* in both T cells and monocytes. Didanosine is converted within the cell to the mono-, di-, and triphosphates of ddA. These ddA triphosphates act as substrate and inhibitor of HIV reverse transcriptase substrate and inhibitor of HIV reverse transcriptase thereby blocking viral DNA synthesis and suppressing HIV replication.

Drug Interactions

Increased Effect/Toxicity: Concomitant administration of other drugs which have the potential to cause peripheral neuropathy or pancreatitis may increase the risk of these toxicities Allopurinol may increase didanosine concentration; avoid concurrent use. Concomitant use of antacids with buffered tablet or pediatric didanosine solution may potentiate adverse effects of aluminum- or magnesium-containing antacids. Ganciclovir may increase didanosine concentration; monitor. Hydroxyurea may precipitate didanosine-induced pancreatitis if added to therapy; concomitant use is not recommended. Coadministration with ribavirin or tenofovir may increase exposure to didanosine and/or its active metabolite increasing the risk or severity of didanosine toxicities, including pancreatitis, lactic acidosis, and peripheral neuropathy; monitor closely and suspend therapy if signs or symptoms of toxicity are noted. Additionally, concomitant tenofovir administration has been associated with hyperglycemia, decreased CD4 cell counts, and reduced virologic response.

Decreased Effect: Didanosine buffered tablets and pediatric oral solution may decrease absorption of quinolones or tetracyclines (administer 2 hours prior to didanosine buffered formulations). Didanosine should be held during PCP treatment with pentamidine. Didanosine may decrease levels of indinavir. Drugs whose absorption depends on the level of acidity in the stomach such as ketoconazole, itraconazole, and dapsone should be administered at least 2 hours prior to the buffered formulations of didanosine (not affected by delayed release capsules). Methadone may decrease didanosine concentrations.

Pharmacodynamics/Kinetics

Absorption: Subject to degradation by acidic pH of stomach; some formulations are buffered to resist acidic pH; ≤50% reduction in peak plasma concentration is observed in presence of food. Delayed release capsules contain enteric-coated beadlets which dissolve in the small intestine.

Distribution: V_d: Children: 35.6 L/m^2; Adults: 1.08 L/kg

Protein binding: <5%

Metabolism: Has not been evaluated in humans; studies conducted in dogs show extensive metabolism with allantoin, hypoxanthine, xanthine, and uric acid being the major metabolites found in urine

Bioavailability: 42%

Half-life elimination:

Children and Adolescents: 0.8 hour

Adults: Normal renal function: 1.5 hours; active metabolite, ddATP, has an intracellular half-life >12 hours *in vitro*; Renal impairment: 2.5-5 hours

Time to peak: Buffered tablets: 0.67 hours; Delayed release capsules: 2 hours

Excretion: Urine (~55% as unchanged drug)

Clearance: Total body: Averages 800 mL/minute

Pregnancy Risk Factor B

Dideoxycytidine see Zalcitabine on page 1590

Dideoxyinosine see Didanosine on page 465

Didrex® see Benzphetamine on page 195

Didronel® see Etidronate Disodium on page 621

Diethylene Triamine Penta-Acetic Acid
(dye ETH i leen TRYE a meen PEN ta a SEE tik AS id)

Generic Available No

Synonyms Ca-DTPA; Diethylenetriamine Pentaacetic Acid; DTPA; Pentetate Calcium Trisodium; Pentetate Zinc Trisodium; Trisodium Calcium Diethylenetriaminepentaacetate (Ca-DTPA); Zinc Diethylenetriaminepentaacetate (Zn-DTPA); Zn-DTPA

Pharmacologic Category Antidote

Use Treatment of known or suspected internal contamination with plutonium, americium, or curium

Local Anesthetic/Vasoconstrictor Precautions No information available to require special precautions

Effects on Dental Treatment Key adverse event(s) related to dental treatment: Metallic taste.

Mechanism of Action Ca-DTPA and Zn-DTPA form chelates with metal ions. The radioactive chelates are then excreted in the urine. Treatment is most effective when radiocontaminants are in circulation or interstitial fluids. Radiocontaminants eventually sequester in liver and bone, therefore, effectiveness of treatment decreases with time after exposure.

Pregnancy Risk Factor C (Ca-DTPA)/B (Zn-DTPA)

Diethylpropion (dye eth il PROE pee on)

U.S. Brand Names Tenuate®; Tenuate® Dospan®
Canadian Brand Names Tenuate®; Tenuate® Dospan®
Mexican Brand Names Ifa Norex®; Neobes®
Generic Available Yes
Synonyms Amfepramone; Diethylpropion Hydrochloride
Pharmacologic Category Anorexiant
Use Short-term adjunct in a regimen of weight reduction based on exercise, behavioral modification, and caloric reduction in the management of exogenous obesity for patients with an initial body mass index ≥30 kg/m² or ≥27 kg/m² in the presence of other risk factors (diabetes, hypertension)
Unlabeled/Investigational Use Migraine

Local Anesthetic/Vasoconstrictor Precautions Use vasoconstrictor with caution in patients taking diethylpropion. Amphetamine-like drugs such as diethylpropion enhance the sympathomimetic response of epinephrine and norepinephrine leading to potential hypertension and cardiotoxicity.

Effects on Dental Treatment Key adverse event(s) related to dental treatment: Xerostomia and changes in salivation (normal salivary flow resumes upon discontinuation), and metallic taste (the use of local anesthetic without vasoconstrictor is recommended in these patients).

Mechanism of Action Diethylpropion is used as an anorexiant agent possessing pharmacological and chemical properties similar to those of amphetamines. The mechanism of action of diethylpropion in reducing appetite appears to be secondary to CNS effects, specifically stimulation of the hypothalamus to release catecholamines into the central nervous system; anorexiant effects are mediated via norepinephrine and dopamine metabolism. An increase in physical activity and metabolic effects (inhibition of lipogenesis and enhancement of lipolysis) may also contribute to weight loss.

Pregnancy Risk Factor B

Diethylpropion Hydrochloride see Diethylpropion on page 467

Difenoxin and Atropine (dye fen OKS in & A troe peen)

Related Information
Atropine on page 161
U.S. Brand Names Motofen®
Generic Available No
Synonyms Atropine and Difenoxin
Pharmacologic Category Antidiarrheal
Use Treatment of diarrhea

Local Anesthetic/Vasoconstrictor Precautions No information available to require special precautions

Effects on Dental Treatment Key adverse event(s) related to dental treatment: Xerostomia (normal salivary flow resumes upon discontinuation).

Common Adverse Effects 1% to 10%:
Central nervous system: Dizziness, drowsiness, lightheadedness, headache
Gastrointestinal: Nausea, vomiting, xerostomia, epigastric distress

Restrictions C-IV

Drug Interactions
Increased Effect/Toxicity: Concurrent use with MAO inhibitors may precipitate hypertensive crisis. May potentiate action of barbiturates, tranquilizers, narcotics, and alcohol. Difenoxin has the potential to prolong biological half-life of drugs for which the rate of elimination is dependent on the microsomal drug metabolizing enzyme system.

Pharmacodynamics/Kinetics
Absorption: Rapid and well absorbed
Metabolism: To inactive hydroxylated metabolite
Time to peak, plasma: Within 40-60 minutes
(Continued)

Difenoxin and Atropine *(Continued)*

Excretion: Urine and feces (primarily as conjugates)
Pregnancy Risk Factor C

Differin® *see Adapalene on page 54*

Diflorasone *(dye FLOR a sone)*

U.S. Brand Names ApexiCon™; ApexiCon™ E; Florone®; Psorcon® e™
Canadian Brand Names Florone®; Psorcon®
Generic Available Yes
Synonyms Diflorasone Diacetate
Pharmacologic Category Corticosteroid, Topical
Use Relieves inflammation and pruritic symptoms of corticosteroid-responsive dermatosis (high to very high potency topical corticosteroid)

Maxiflor®: High potency topical corticosteroid
Psorcon®: Very high potency topical corticosteroid

Local Anesthetic/Vasoconstrictor Precautions No information available to require special precautions
Effects on Dental Treatment No significant effects or complications reported
Mechanism of Action Decreases inflammation by suppression of migration of polymorphonuclear leukocytes and reversal of increased capillary permeability
Pharmacodynamics/Kinetics
Absorption: Negligible, around 1% reaches dermal layers or systemic circulation; occlusive dressings increase absorption percutaneously
Metabolism: Primarily hepatic
Pregnancy Risk Factor C

Diflorasone Diacetate *see Diflorasone on page 468*
Diflucan® *see Fluconazole on page 659*

Diflunisal *(dye FLOO ni sal)*

Related Information
Oral Pain *on page 1692*
Rheumatoid Arthritis, Osteoarthritis, and Osteoporosis *on page 1668*
Temporomandibular Dysfunction (TMD) *on page 1724*
Related Sample Prescriptions
Mild/Moderate Oral Pain *on page 1734*
U.S. Brand Names Dolobid® [DSC]
Canadian Brand Names Apo-Diflunisal®; Novo-Diflunisal; Nu-Diflunisal
Generic Available Yes
Pharmacologic Category Nonsteroidal Anti-inflammatory Drug (NSAID), Oral
Dental Use Treatment of postoperative pain
Use Management of inflammatory disorders usually including rheumatoid arthritis and osteoarthritis; can be used as an analgesic for treatment of mild to moderate pain
Local Anesthetic/Vasoconstrictor Precautions No information available to require special precautions
Effects on Dental Treatment NSAID formulations are known to reversibly decrease platelet aggregation via mechanisms different than observed with aspirin. The dentist should be aware of the potential of abnormal coagulation. Caution should also be exercised in the use of NSAIDs in patients already on anticoagulant therapy with drugs such as warfarin (Coumadin®). See Dental Comment.
Significant Adverse Effects
1% to 10%:
Central nervous system: Headache (3% to 9%), dizziness (1% to 3%), insomnia (1% to 3%), somnolence (1% to 3%), fatigue (1% to 3%)
Dermatologic: Rash (3% to 9%)
Gastrointestinal: Nausea (3% to 9%), dyspepsia (3% to 9%), GI pain (3% to 9%), diarrhea (3% to 9%), constipation (1% to 3%), flatulence (1% to 3%), vomiting (1% to 3%), GI ulceration
Otic: Tinnitus (1% to 3%)
<1% (Limited to important or life-threatening): Acute anaphylactic reaction, agranulocytosis, allergic reactions, angioedema, anorexia, blurred vision, bronchospasm, confusion, chest pain, cholestasis, cystitis, depression, diaphoresis, disorientation, dry mucous membranes, dyspnea, dysuria, edema, eructation, erythema multiforme, esophagitis, exfoliative dermatitis, flushing, gastritis, GI bleeding, GI perforation, hallucinations, hearing

decreased, hearing loss, hematuria, hemolytic anemia, hepatitis, hypersensitivity syndrome, hypersensitivity vasculitis, interstitial nephritis, itching, jaundice, mental depression, muscle cramps, necrotizing fasciitis, nephrotic syndrome, nervousness, palpitations, paresthesia, peptic ulcer, peripheral neuropathy, photosensitivity, proteinuria, pruritus, renal impairment, renal failure, seizure, Stevens-Johnson syndrome, stomatitis, syncope, tachycardia, thrombocytopenia, toxic epidermal necrolysis, trembling, urticaria, vasculitis, vertigo, weakness, wheezing

Restrictions A medication guide should be dispensed with each prescription. A template for the required MedGuide can be found on the FDA website at http://www.fda.gov/medwatch/SAFETY/2005/safety05.htm#NSAID

Dental Usual Dosing Mild-to-moderate pain: Adults: Oral: Initial: 500-1000 mg followed by 250-500 mg every 8-12 hours; maximum daily dose: 1.5 g

Dosage Adults: Oral:

Mild-to-moderate pain: Initial: 500-1000 mg followed by 250-500 mg every 8-12 hours; maximum daily dose: 1.5 g

Arthritis: 500-1000 mg/day in 2 divided doses; maximum daily dose: 1.5 g

Dosing adjustment in renal impairment: Use with caution; Cl_{cr} <50 mL/minute: Administer 50% of normal dose (Aronoff, 1998)

Hemodialysis: No supplement required

CAPD: No supplement require

CAVH: Dose for GFR 10-50

Mechanism of Action Inhibits prostaglandin synthesis by decreasing the activity of the enzyme, cyclooxygenase, which results in decreased formation of prostaglandin precursors

Contraindications Hypersensitivity to diflunisal, aspirin, other NSAIDs, or any component of the formulation; perioperative pain in the setting of coronary artery bypass surgery (CABG); pregnancy (3rd trimester)

Warnings/Precautions NSAIDs are associated with an increased risk of adverse cardiovascular events, including MI, stroke, and new onset or worsening of pre-existing hypertension. Risk may be increased with duration of use or pre-existing cardiovascular risk-factors or disease. Carefully evaluate individual cardiovascular risk profiles prior to prescribing. Use caution with fluid retention, CHF, or hypertension.

NSAIDs may increase risk of gastrointestinal irritation, ulceration, bleeding, and perforation. These events may occur at any time during therapy and without warning. Use caution with a history of GI disease (bleeding or ulcers), concurrent therapy with aspirin, anticoagulants and/or corticosteroids, smoking, use of alcohol, the elderly or debilitated patients.

Use of NSAIDs can compromise existing renal function. Renal toxicity can occur in patient with impaired renal function, dehydration, heart failure, liver dysfunction, those taking diuretics and ACEI and the elderly. Rehydrate patient before starting therapy. Monitor renal function closely. Diflunisal is not recommended for patients with advanced renal disease.

Use the lowest effective dose for the shortest duration of time, consistent with individual patient goals, to reduce risk of cardiovascular or GI adverse events. Alternate therapies should be considered for patients at high risk.

NSAIDs may cause serious skin adverse events including exfoliative dermatitis, Stevens-Johnson syndrome (SJS), and toxic epidermal necrolysis (TEN). Anaphylactoid reactions may occur, even without prior exposure; patients with "aspirin triad" (bronchial asthma, aspirin intolerance, rhinitis) may be at increased risk. Do not use in patients who experience bronchospasm, asthma, rhinitis, or urticaria with NSAID or aspirin therapy.

A hypersensitivity syndrome has been reported; monitor for constitutional symptoms and cutaneous findings; other organ dysfunction may be involved.

Use with caution in patients with decreased hepatic function. Closely monitor patients with any abnormal LFT. Severe hepatic reactions (eg, fulminant hepatitis, liver failure) have occurred with NSAID use, rarely; discontinue if signs or symptoms of liver disease develop, or if systemic manifestations occur.

Diflunisal is a derivative of acetylsalicylic acid and therefore may be associated with Reye's syndrome. Withhold for at least 4-6 half-lives prior to surgical or dental procedures. Safety and efficacy have not been established in children <12 years of age.

Drug Interactions

ACE inhibitors: Antihypertensive effects may be decreased by concurrent therapy with NSAIDs; monitor blood pressure.

Aminoglycosides: NSAIDs may decrease the excretion of aminoglycosides.

Angiotensin II antagonists: Antihypertensive effects may be decreased by concurrent therapy with NSAIDs; monitor blood pressure.

(Continued)

Diflunisal *(Continued)*

Anticoagulants (warfarin, heparin, LMWHs) in combination with NSAIDs can cause increased risk of bleeding.

Antiplatelet agents (ticlopidine, clopidogrel, aspirin, abciximab, dipyridamole, eptifibatide, tirofiban) can cause an increased risk of bleeding.

Beta-blockers: NSAIDs may diminish the antihypertensive effects of beta blockers.

Bisphosphonates: NSAIDs may increase the risk of gastrointestinal ulceration.

Cholestyramine (and other bile acid sequestrants): May decrease the absorption of NSAIDs. Separate by at least 2 hours.

Corticosteroids may increase the risk of GI ulceration; avoid concurrent use.

Cyclosporine: NSAIDs may increase serum creatinine, potassium, blood pressure, and cyclosporine levels; monitor cyclosporine levels and renal function carefully.

Hydralazine's antihypertensive effect is decreased; avoid concurrent use.

Lithium levels can be increased; avoid concurrent use if possible or monitor lithium levels and adjust dose.

Sulindac may have the least effect. When NSAID is stopped, lithium will need adjustment again.

Loop diuretics efficacy (diuretic and antihypertensive effect) is reduced. Indomethacin reduces this efficacy, however, it may be anticipated with any NSAID.

Methotrexate: Severe bone marrow suppression, aplastic anemia, and GI toxicity have been reported with concomitant NSAID therapy. Avoid use during moderate or high-dose methotrexate (increased and prolonged methotrexate levels). NSAID use during low-dose treatment of rheumatoid arthritis has not been fully evaluated; extreme caution is warranted.

Pemetrexed: NSAIDs may decrease the excretion of pemetrexed. Patients with Cl_{cr} 45-79 mL/minute should avoid long acting NSAIDs for 5 days before and 2 days after pemetrexed treatment.

Thiazides antihypertensive effects are decreased; avoid concurrent use.

Treprostinil: May enhance the risk of bleeding with concurrent use.

Vancomycin: NSAIDs may decrease the excretion of vancomycin.

Ethanol/Nutrition/Herb Interactions

Ethanol: Avoid ethanol (may enhance gastric mucosal irritation).

Herb/Nutraceutical: Avoid alfalfa, anise, bilberry, bladderwrack, bromelain, cat's claw, celery, coleus, cordyceps, dong quai, evening primrose, feverfew, fenugreek, garlic, ginger, ginkgo biloboa, red clover, horse chestnut, grapeseed, green tea, ginseng, guggul, horse chestnut seed, horseradish, licorice, prickly ash, red clover, reishi, SAMe, sweet clover, turmeric, white willow (all have additional antiplatelet activity).

Dietary Considerations Should be taken with food to decrease GI distress.

Pharmacodynamics/Kinetics

Onset of action: Analgesic: ~1 hour; maximal effect: 2-3 hours

Duration: 8-12 hours

Absorption: Well absorbed

Protein binding: >99%

Distribution: Enters breast milk

Metabolism: Extensively hepatic; metabolic pathways are saturable

Half-life elimination: 8-12 hours; prolonged with renal impairment

Time to peak, serum: 2-3 hours

Excretion: Urine (~3% as unchanged drug, 90% as glucuronide conjugates) within 72-96 hours

Pregnancy Risk Factor C (1st and 2nd trimesters)/D (3rd trimester)

Lactation Enters breast milk/not recommended

Dosage Forms

Tablet: 500 mg

Dolobid®: 250 mg, 500 mg [DSC]

Dental Comment The advantage of diflunisal as a pain reliever is its 12-hour duration of effect. In many cases, this long effect will ensure a full night sleep during the postoperative pain period.

Selected Readings

Ahmad N, Grad HA, Haas DA, et al, "The Efficacy of Nonopioid Analgesics for Postoperative Dental Pain: A Meta-Analysis," *Anesth Prog*, 1997, 44(4):119-26.

Brooks PM and Day RO, "Nonsteroidal Anti-inflammatory Drugs - Differences and Similarities," *N Engl J Med*, 1991, 324(24):1716-25.

Dionne R, "Additive Analgesia Without Opioid Side Effects," *Compend Contin Educ Dent*, 2000, 21(7):572-4, 576-7.

Dionne RA, "New Approaches to Preventing and Treating Postoperative Pain," *J Am Dent Assoc*, 1992, 123(6):26-34.

Dionne RA and Berthold CW, "Therapeutic Uses of Nonsteroidal Anti-inflammatory Drugs in Dentistry," *Crit Rev Oral Biol Med*, 2001, 12(4):315-30.

Forbes JA, Calderazzo JP, Bowser MW, et al, "A 12-Hour Evaluation of the Analgesic Efficacy of Diflunisal, Aspirin, and Placebo in Postoperative Dental Pain," *J Clin Pharmacol*, 1982, 22(2-3):89-96.

Gobetti JP, "Controlling Dental Pain," *J Am Dent Assoc*, 1992, 123(6):47-52.

Nguyen AM, Graham DY, Gage T, et al, "Nonsteroidal Anti-inflammatory Drug Use in Dentistry: Gastrointestinal Implications," *Gen Dent*, 1999, 47(6):590-6.

Selcuk E, Gomel M, Bellibas SE, et al, "Comparison of the Analgesic Effects of Diflunisal and Paracetamol in the Treatment of Postoperative Dental Pain," *Int J Clin Pharmacol Res*, 1996, 16(2-3):57-65.

Digibind® see Digoxin Immune Fab *on page 474*

DigiFab™ see Digoxin Immune Fab *on page 474*

Digital HD see Barium *on page 179*

Digitek® see Digoxin *on page 471*

Digitoxin (di ji TOKS in)

Related Information
Cardiovascular Diseases *on page 1636*
Digoxin *on page 471*
Digoxin Immune Fab *on page 474*

Generic Available No

Synonyms Crystodigin

Pharmacologic Category Antiarrhythmic Agent, Class IV

Use Treatment of congestive heart failure, atrial fibrillation, atrial flutter, paroxysmal atrial tachycardia, and cardiogenic shock

Local Anesthetic/Vasoconstrictor Precautions Use vasoconstrictor with caution due to risk of cardiac arrhythmias with digitoxin.

Effects on Dental Treatment Sensitive gag reflex may cause difficulty in taking a dental impression.

Common Adverse Effects 1% to 10%: Gastrointestinal: Anorexia, nausea, vomiting

Restrictions Not available in U.S.

Mechanism of Action Digitalis binds to and inhibits magnesium and adenosine triphosphate dependent sodium and potassium ATPase thereby increasing the influx of calcium ions, from extracellular to intracellular cytoplasm due to the inhibition of sodium and potassium ion movement across the myocardial membranes; this increase in calcium ions results in a potentiation of the activity of the contractile heart muscle fibers and an increase in the force of myocardial contraction (positive inotropic effect); digitalis may also increase intracellular entry of calcium via slow calcium channel influx; stimulates release and blocks reuptake of norepinephrine; decreases conduction through the SA and AV nodes

Drug Interactions
Cytochrome P450 Effect: Substrate of CYP3A4 (major)

Increased Effect/Toxicity: CYP3A4 inhibitors may increase the levels/effects of digitoxin; example inhibitors include azole antifungals, clarithromycin, diclofenac, doxycycline, erythromycin, imatinib, isoniazid, nefazodone, nicardipine, propofol, protease inhibitors, quinidine, telithromycin, and verapamil.

Decreased Effect: CYP3A4 inducers may decrease the levels/effects of digitoxin (eg, aminoglutethimide, carbamazepine, nafcillin, nevirapine, phenobarbital, phenytoin, and rifamycins).

Pharmacodynamics/Kinetics
Absorption: 90% to 100%
Distribution: V_d: 7 L/kg
Protein binding: 90% to 97%
Metabolism: Hepatic (50% to 70%)
Half-life elimination: 7-8 days
Time to peak: 8-12 hours
Excretion: Urine and feces (30% to 50% as unchanged drug)

Pregnancy Risk Factor C

Digoxin (di JOKS in)

Related Information
Cardiovascular Diseases *on page 1636*
Digitoxin *on page 471*
Digoxin Immune Fab *on page 474*

U.S. Brand Names Digitek®; Lanoxicaps®; Lanoxin®

Canadian Brand Names Digoxin CSD; Lanoxicaps®; Lanoxin®; Novo-Digoxin; Pediatric Digoxin CSD
(Continued)

Digoxin *(Continued)*

Mexican Brand Names Lanoxin®; Mapluxin®

Generic Available Yes: Excludes capsule

Pharmacologic Category Antiarrhythmic Agent, Class IV; Cardiac Glycoside

Use Treatment of congestive heart failure and to slow the ventricular rate in tachyarrhythmias such as atrial fibrillation, atrial flutter, and supraventricular tachycardia (paroxysmal atrial tachycardia); cardiogenic shock

Local Anesthetic/Vasoconstrictor Precautions Use vasoconstrictor with caution due to risk of cardiac arrhythmias with digoxin

Effects on Dental Treatment Sensitive gag reflex may cause difficulty in taking a dental impression.

Common Adverse Effects Incidence of reactions are not always reported.

Cardiovascular: Heart block; first-, second- (Wenckebach), or third-degree heart block; asystole; atrial tachycardia with block; AV dissociation; accelerated junctional rhythm; ventricular tachycardia or ventricular fibrillation; PR prolongation; ST segment depression

Central nervous system: Visual disturbances (blurred or yellow vision), headache (3%), dizziness (5%), apathy, confusion, mental disturbances (4%), anxiety, depression, delirium, hallucinations, fever

Dermatologic: Maculopapular rash (2%), erythematous, scarlatiniform, papular, vesicular or bullous rash, urticaria, pruritus, facial, angioneurotic or laryngeal edema, shedding of fingernails or toenails, alopecia

Gastrointestinal: Nausea (3%), vomiting (2%), diarrhea (3%), abdominal pain

Neuromuscular & skeletal: Weakness

Children are more likely to experience cardiac arrhythmia as a sign of excessive dosing. The most common are conduction disturbances or tachyarrhythmia (atrial tachycardia with or without block) and junctional tachycardia. Ventricular tachyarrhythmia are less common. In infants, sinus bradycardia may be a sign of digoxin toxicity. Any arrhythmia seen in a child on digoxin should be considered as digoxin toxicity. The gastrointestinal and central nervous system symptoms are not frequently seen in children.

Dosage When changing from oral (tablets or liquid) or I.M. to I.V. therapy, dosage should be reduced by 20% to 25%. Refer to the following: See table.

Dosage Recommendations for Digoxin

Age	Total Digitalizing Dose[2] (mcg/kg[1])		Daily Maintenance Dose[3] (mcg/kg[1])	
	P.O.	I.V. or I.M.	P.O.	I.V. or I.M.
Preterm infant[1]	20-30	15-25	5-7.5	4-6
Full-term infant[1]	25-35	20-30	6-10	5-8
1 mo - 2 y[1]	35-60	30-50	10-15	7.5-12
2-5 y[1]	30-40	25-35	7.5-10	6-9
5-10 y[1]	20-35	15-30	5-10	4-8
>10 y[1]	10-15	8-12	2.5-5	2-3
Adults	0.75-1.5 mg	0.5-1 mg	0.125-0.5 mg	0.1-0.4 mg

[1]Based on lean body weight and normal renal function for age. Decrease dose in patients with ↓ renal function; digitalizing dose often not recommended in infants and children.

[2]Give one-half of the total digitalizing dose (TDD) in the initial dose, then give one-quarter of the TDD in each of two subsequent doses at 8- to 12-hour intervals. Obtain ECG 6 hours after each dose to assess potential toxicity.

[3]Divided every 12 hours in infants and children <10 years of age. Given once daily to children >10 years of age and adults.

Dosing adjustment/interval in renal impairment:

Cl_{cr} 10-50 mL/minute: Administer 25% to 75% of dose or every 36 hours

Cl_{cr} <10 mL/minute: Administer 10% to 25% of dose or every 48 hours

Reduce loading dose by 50% in ESRD

Hemodialysis: Not dialyzable (0% to 5%)

Mechanism of Action

Congestive heart failure: Inhibition of the sodium/potassium ATPase pump which acts to increase the intracellular sodium-calcium exchange to increase intracellular calcium leading to increased contractility

Supraventricular arrhythmias: Direct suppression of the AV node conduction to increase effective refractory period and decrease conduction velocity - positive inotropic effect, enhanced vagal tone, and decreased ventricular rate to fast atrial arrhythmias. Atrial fibrillation may decrease sensitivity and increase tolerance to higher serum digoxin concentrations.

Contraindications Hypersensitivity to digoxin or any component of the formulation; hypersensitivity to cardiac glycosides (another may be tried); history of toxicity; ventricular tachycardia or fibrillation; idiopathic hypertrophic subaortic stenosis; constrictive pericarditis; amyloid disease; second- or third-degree heart block (except in patients with a functioning artificial pacemaker); Wolff-Parkinson-White syndrome and atrial fibrillation concurrently

Warnings/Precautions Use with caution in patients with hypoxia, myxedema, hypothyroidism, acute myocarditis; patients with incomplete AV block (Stokes-Adams attack) may progress to complete block with digitalis drug administration; use with caution in patients with acute myocardial infarction, severe pulmonary disease, advanced heart failure, idiopathic hypertrophic subaortic stenosis, Wolff-Parkinson-White syndrome, sick-sinus syndrome (bradyarrhythmias), amyloid heart disease, and constrictive cardiomyopathies; adjust dose with renal impairment and when verapamil, quinidine or amiodarone are added to a patient on digoxin; elderly and neonates may develop exaggerated serum/tissue concentrations due to age-related alterations in clearance and pharmacodynamic differences; exercise will reduce serum concentrations of digoxin due to increased skeletal muscle uptake; recent studies indicate photopsia, chromatopsia and decreased visual acuity may occur even with therapeutic serum drug levels; reduce or hold dose 1-2 days before elective electrical cardioversion

Drug Interactions

Cytochrome P450 Effect: Substrate of CYP3A4 (minor)

Increased Effect/Toxicity: Beta-blocking agents (propranolol), verapamil, and diltiazem may have additive effects on heart rate. Carvedilol has additive effects on heart rate and inhibits the metabolism of digoxin. Digoxin levels may be increased by amiodarone (reduce digoxin dose 50%), bepridil, cyclosporine, diltiazem, indomethacin, itraconazole, some macrolides (erythromycin, clarithromycin), methimazole, nitrendipine, propafenone, propylthiouracil, quinidine (reduce digoxin dose 33% to 50% on initiation), tetracyclines, and verapamil. Moricizine may increase the toxicity of digoxin (mechanism undefined). Spironolactone may interfere with some digoxin assays, but may also increase blood levels directly. Succinylcholine administration to patients on digoxin has been associated with an increased risk of arrhythmias. Rare cases of acute digoxin toxicity have been associated with parenteral calcium (bolus) administration. The following medications have been associated with increased digoxin blood levels which appear to be of limited clinical significance: Famciclovir, flecainide, ibuprofen, fluoxetine, nefazodone, cimetidine, famotidine, ranitidine, omeprazole, trimethoprim.

Decreased Effect: Amiloride and spironolactone may reduce the inotropic response to digoxin. Cholestyramine, colestipol, kaolin-pectin, and metoclopramide may reduce digoxin absorption. Levothyroxine (and other thyroid supplements) may decrease digoxin blood levels. Penicillamine has been associated with reductions in digoxin blood levels The following reported interactions appear to be of limited clinical significance: Aminoglutethimide, aminosalicylic acid, aluminum-containing antacids, sucralfate, sulfasalazine, neomycin, ticlopidine.

Ethanol/Nutrition/Herb Interactions

Food: Digoxin peak serum levels may be decreased if taken with food. Meals containing increased fiber (bran) or foods high in pectin may decrease oral absorption of digoxin.

Herb/Nutraceutical: Avoid ephedra (risk of cardiac stimulation). Avoid natural licorice (causes sodium and water retention and increases potassium loss).

Dietary Considerations Maintain adequate amounts of potassium in diet to decrease risk of hypokalemia (hypokalemia may increase risk of digoxin toxicity).

Pharmacodynamics/Kinetics

Onset of action: Oral: 1-2 hours; I.V.: 5-30 minutes

Peak effect: Oral: 2-8 hours; I.V.: 1-4 hours

Duration: Adults: 3-4 days both forms

Absorption: By passive nonsaturable diffusion in the upper small intestine; food may delay, but does not affect extent of absorption

Distribution:

Normal renal function: 6-7 L/kg

V_d: Extensive to peripheral tissues, with a distinct distribution phase which lasts 6-8 hours; concentrates in heart, liver, kidney, skeletal muscle, and intestines. Heart/serum concentration is 70:1. Pharmacologic effects are delayed and do not correlate well with serum concentrations during distribution phase.

Hyperthyroidism: Increased V_d

Hyperkalemia, hyponatremia: Decreased digoxin distribution to heart and muscle

Hypokalemia: Increased digoxin distribution to heart and muscles

Concomitant quinidine therapy: Decreased V_d

Chronic renal failure: 4-6 L/kg

(Continued)

Digoxin (Continued)

Decreased sodium/potassium ATPase activity - decreased tissue binding
Neonates, full-term: 7.5-10 L/kg
Children: 16 L/kg
Adults: 7 L/kg, decreased with renal disease
Protein binding: 30%; in uremic patients, digoxin is displaced from plasma protein binding sites
Metabolism: Via sequential sugar hydrolysis in the stomach or by reduction of lactone ring by intestinal bacteria (in ~10% of population, gut bacteria may metabolize up to 40% of digoxin dose); metabolites may contribute to therapeutic and toxic effects of digoxin; metabolism is reduced with CHF
Bioavailability: Oral (formulation dependent): Elixir: 75% to 85%; Tablet: 70% to 80%
Half-life elimination (age, renal and cardiac function dependent):
Neonates: Premature: 61-170 hours; Full-term: 35-45 hours
Infants: 18-25 hours
Children: 35 hours
Adults: 38-48 hours
Adults, anephric: 4-6 days
Half-life elimination: Parent drug: 38 hours; Metabolites: Digoxigenin: 4 hours; Monodigitoxoside: 3-12 hours
Time to peak, serum: Oral: ~1 hour
Excretion: Urine (50% to 70% as unchanged drug)
Pregnancy Risk Factor C
Dosage Forms CAP (Lanoxicaps®): 100 mcg, 200 mcg. **ELIX:** 50 mcg/mL (2.5 mL, 5 mL, 60 mL). **INJ:** 250 mcg/mL (1 mL, 2 mL); (Lanoxin®): 250 mcg/mL (2 mL). **INJ, pediatric:** 100 mcg/mL (1 mL). **TAB:** 125 mcg, 250 mcg; (Digitek®, Lanoxin®): 125 mcg, 250 mcg

---

Digoxin Immune Fab (di JOKS in i MYUN fab)

Related Information
Digitoxin on page 471
Digoxin on page 471
U.S. Brand Names Digibind®; DigiFab™
Canadian Brand Names Digibind®
Generic Available No
Synonyms Antidigoxin Fab Fragments, Ovine
Pharmacologic Category Antidote
Use Treatment of life-threatening or potentially life-threatening digoxin intoxication, including:

- acute digoxin ingestion (ie, >10 mg in adults or >4 mg in children)
- chronic ingestions leading to steady-state digoxin concentrations >6 ng/mL in adults or >4 ng/mL in children
- manifestations of digoxin toxicity due to overdose (life-threatening ventricular arrhythmias, progressive bradycardia, second- or third-degree heart block not responsive to atropine, serum potassium >5 mEq/L in adults or >6 mEq in children)

Local Anesthetic/Vasoconstrictor Precautions No information available to require special precautions
Effects on Dental Treatment No significant effects or complications reported
Common Adverse Effects Frequency not defined.
Cardiovascular: Effects (due to withdrawal of digitalis) include exacerbation of low cardiac output states and CHF, rapid ventricular response in patients with atrial fibrillation; postural hypotension
Endocrine & metabolic: Hypokalemia
Local: Phlebitis
Miscellaneous: Allergic reactions, serum sickness
Mechanism of Action Digoxin immune antigen-binding fragments (Fab) are specific antibodies for the treatment of digitalis intoxication in carefully selected patients; binds with molecules of digoxin or digitoxin and then is excreted by the kidneys and removed from the body
Drug Interactions
Increased Effect/Toxicity: Digoxin: Following administration of digoxin immune Fab, serum digoxin levels are markedly increased due to bound complexes (may be clinically misleading, since bound complex cannot interact with receptors).
Pharmacodynamics/Kinetics
Onset of action: I.V.: Improvement in 2-30 minutes for toxicity
Half-life elimination: 15-20 hours; prolonged with renal impairment
Excretion: Urine; undetectable amounts within 5-7 days
Pregnancy Risk Factor C

Dihematoporphyrin Ether *see* Porfimer *on page 1256*

Dihistine® DH *see* Chlorpheniramine, Pseudoephedrine, and Codeine *on page 329*

Dihydrocodeine, Aspirin, and Caffeine
(dye hye droe KOE deen, AS pir in, & KAF een)

Related Information
Aspirin *on page 145*
Caffeine *on page 245*
Oral Pain *on page 1692*
U.S. Brand Names Synalgos®-DC
Generic Available No
Synonyms Dihydrocodeine Compound
Pharmacologic Category Analgesic, Narcotic
Dental Use Management of postoperative pain
Use Management of mild to moderate pain that requires relaxation
Local Anesthetic/Vasoconstrictor Precautions No information available to require special precautions
Effects on Dental Treatment Key adverse event(s) related to dental treatment: Dihydrocodeine: nausea, followed by sedation and constipation. Elderly are a high-risk population for adverse effects from nonsteroidal anti-inflammatory agents. As many as 60% of elderly patients with GI complications from NSAIDs can develop peptic ulceration and/or hemorrhage asymptomatically. Concomitant disease and drug use contribute to the risk of GI adverse effects. Use lowest effective dose for shortest period possible. Consider renal function decline with age.

Significant Adverse Effects
>10%:
Central nervous system: Lightheadedness, dizziness, drowsiness, sedation
Dermatologic: Pruritus, skin reactions
Gastrointestinal: Nausea, vomiting, constipation

1% to 10%:
Cardiovascular: Hypotension, palpitation, bradycardia, peripheral vasodilation
Central nervous system: Increased intracranial pressure
Endocrine & metabolic: Antidiuretic hormone release
Gastrointestinal: Biliary tract spasm
Genitourinary: Urinary tract spasm
Ocular: Miosis
Respiratory: Respiratory depression
Miscellaneous: Histamine release, physical and psychological dependence with prolonged use

Restrictions C-III
Dental Usual Dosing Management of postoperative pain: Oral:
Adults: 1-2 capsules every 4-6 hours as needed for pain
Elderly: Initial dosing should be cautious (low end of adult dosing range)

Dosage
Adults: Oral: 1-2 capsules every 4-6 hours as needed for pain
Elderly: Initial dosing should be cautious (low end of adult dosing range)

Mechanism of Action Binds to opiate receptors in the CNS, causing inhibition of ascending pain pathways, altering the perception of and response to pain; causes cough suppression by direct central action in the medulla; produces generalized CNS depression

Contraindications Hypersensitivity to dihydrocodeine or any component of the formulation; pregnancy (prolonged use or high doses at term)

Warnings/Precautions Use with caution in patients with hypersensitivity reactions to other phenanthrene derivative opioid agonists (morphine, hydrocodone, hydromorphone, levorphanol, oxycodone, oxymorphone); respiratory diseases including asthma, emphysema, COPD, or severe liver or renal insufficiency; some preparations contain sulfites which may cause allergic reactions; dextromethorphan has equivalent antitussive activity but has much lower toxicity in accidental overdose; tolerance of drug dependence may result from extended use

Drug Interactions Substrate of CYP2D6 (major) based on dihydrocodeine CYP2D6 inhibitors: May decrease the effects of dihydrocodeine. Example inhibitors include chlorpromazine, delavirdine, fluoxetine, miconazole, paroxetine, pergolide, quinidine, quinine, ritonavir, and ropinirole.
MAO inhibitors may increase adverse symptoms

Ethanol/Nutrition/Herb Interactions Ethanol: Avoid ethanol (may increase CNS depression).

(Continued)

Dihydrocodeine, Aspirin, and Caffeine *(Continued)*

Pharmacodynamics/Kinetics
Onset of action: 10-30 minutes
Duration: 4-6 hours
Metabolism: Hepatic
Half-life elimination, serum: 3.8 hours
Time to peak, serum: 30-60 minutes

Pregnancy Risk Factor B/D (prolonged use or high doses at term)

Lactation Excretion in breast milk unknown/use caution

Breast-Feeding Considerations
Acetaminophen: May be taken while breast-feeding.
Aspirin: Use cautiously due to potential adverse effects in nursing infants.
Dihydrocodeine: No data reported.

Dosage Forms Capsule: Dihydrocodeine bitartrate 16 mg, aspirin 356.4 mg, and caffeine 30 mg

Dihydrocodeine Bitartrate, Acetaminophen, and Caffeine *see* Acetaminophen, Caffeine, and Dihydrocodeine *on page 42*

Dihydrocodeine Bitartrate, Pseudoephedrine Hydrochloride, and Chlorpheniramine Maleate *see* Pseudoephedrine, Dihydrocodeine, and Chlorpheniramine *on page 1312*

Dihydrocodeine, Chlorpheniramine, and Phenylephrine (dye hye droe KOE, klor fen IR a meen, & fen il EF rin)

Related Information
Chlorpheniramine *on page 323*
Codeine *on page 385*
Phenylephrine *on page 1226*

U.S. Brand Names Baltussin; Coldcough PD; Pancof®-PD

Generic Available Yes

Synonyms Chlorpheniramine Maleate, Dihydrocodeine Bitartrate, and Phenylephrine Hydrochloride; Phenylephrine, Chlorpheniramine, and Dihydrocodeine

Pharmacologic Category Antihistamine; Antihistamine/Decongestant/Antitussive; Antitussive; Decongestant

Use Symptomatic relief of cough and congestion associated with the upper respiratory tract

Local Anesthetic/Vasoconstrictor Precautions No information available to require special precautions

Effects on Dental Treatment Key adverse event(s) related to dental treatment:
Chlorpheniramine: Prolonged use will cause significant xerostomia (normal salivary flow resumes upon discontinuation).
Phenylephrine: Up to 10% of patients could experience tachycardia, palpitations, and xerostomia; use vasoconstrictor with caution.

Common Adverse Effects Refer to individual monographs for codeine, chlorpheniramine, and phenylephrine

Restrictions C-III/C-V

Mechanism of Action
Dihydrocodeine: Binds to opiate receptors in the CNS; suppresses cough in medullary center; produces generalized CNS depression
Chlorpheniramine: Competes with histamine for H_1-receptor sites on effector cells in the gastrointestinal tract, blood vessels, and respiratory tract
Phenylephrine: Potent, direct-acting alpha-adrenergic stimulator with weak beta-adrenergic activity; causes vasoconstriction of the arterioles of the nasal mucosa and conjunctiva

Drug Interactions
Increased Effect/Toxicity: Refer to individual monographs for codeine, chlorpheniramine, and phenylephrine

Pregnancy Risk Factor C

Dihydrocodeine Compound *see* Dihydrocodeine, Aspirin, and Caffeine *on page 475*

Dihydrocodeine, Pseudoephedrine, and Guaifenesin (dye hye droe KOE, soo doe e FED rin, & gwye FEN e sin)

Related Information
Codeine *on page 385*
Guaifenesin *on page 752*
Pseudoephedrine *on page 1309*

U.S. Brand Names DiHydro-GP; Hydro-Tussin™ EXP; Pancof®-EXP

Generic Available Yes

Synonyms Guaifenesin, Dihydrocodeine, and Pseudoephedrine; Pseudoephedrine Hydrochloride, Guaifenesin, and Dihydrocodeine Bitartrate

Pharmacologic Category Antitussive/Decongestant/Expectorant

Use Temporary relief of cough and congestion associated with upper respiratory tract infections and allergies

Local Anesthetic/Vasoconstrictor Precautions Use with caution since pseudoephedrine is a sympathomimetic amine which could interact with epinephrine to cause a pressor response

Effects on Dental Treatment No significant effects or complications reported

Common Adverse Effects Refer to individual monographs for Codeine, Pseudoephedrine, and Guaifenesin.

Mechanism of Action

Dihydrocodeine is an antitussive and analgesic chemically related to codeine. Codeine binds to opiate receptors in the CNS, causing inhibition of ascending pain pathways, altering the perception of and response to pain; causes cough supression by direct central action in the medulla; produces generalized CNS depression.

Pseudoephedrine directly stimulates alpha-adrenergic receptors of respiratory mucosa causing vasoconstriction; directly stimulates beta-adrenergic receptors causing bronchial relaxation, increased heart rate and contractility.

Guaifenesin is thought to act as an expectorant by irritating the gastric mucosa and stimulating respiratory tract secretions, thereby increasing respiratory fluid volumes and decreasing phlegm viscosity.

Drug Interactions

Increased Effect/Toxicity: Refer to individual monographs for Codeine, Pseudoephedrine, and Guaifenesin.

Pregnancy Risk Factor C

DiHydro-CP see Pseudoephedrine, Dihydrocodeine, and Chlorpheniramine on page 1312

Dihydroergotamine (dye hye droe er GOT a meen)

U.S. Brand Names D.H.E. 45®; Migranal®

Canadian Brand Names Migranal®

Generic Available Yes: Injection

Synonyms DHE; Dihydroergotamine Mesylate

Pharmacologic Category Ergot Derivative

Use Treatment of migraine headache with or without aura; injection also indicated for treatment of cluster headaches

Unlabeled/Investigational Use Adjunct for DVT prophylaxis for hip surgery, for orthostatic hypotension, xerostomia secondary to antidepressant use, and pelvic congestion with pain

Local Anesthetic/Vasoconstrictor Precautions No information available to require special precautions

Effects on Dental Treatment Key adverse event(s) related to dental treatment: Rhinitis and abnormal taste.

Common Adverse Effects

>10%: Nasal spray: Respiratory: Rhinitis (26%)

1% to 10%: Nasal spray:

Central nervous system: Dizziness (4%), somnolence (3%)

Endocrine & metabolic: Hot flashes (1%)

Gastrointestinal: Nausea (10%), taste disturbance (8%), vomiting (4%), diarrhea (2%)

Local: Application site reaction (6%)

Neuromuscular & skeletal: Weakness (1%), stiffness (1%)

Respiratory: Pharyngitis (3%)

Mechanism of Action Ergot alkaloid alpha-adrenergic blocker directly stimulates vascular smooth muscle to vasoconstrict peripheral and cerebral vessels; also has effects on serotonin receptors

Drug Interactions

Cytochrome P450 Effect: Substrate of CYP3A4 (major); **Inhibits** CYP3A4 (weak)

Increased Effect/Toxicity: CYP3A4 inhibitors may increase the levels/effects of dihydroergotamine; example inhibitors include azole antifungals, clarithromycin, diclofenac, doxycycline, erythromycin, imatinib, isoniazid, nefazodone, nicardipine, propofol, protease inhibitors, quinidine, telithromycin, and verapamil. Ergot alkaloids are contraindicated with potent CYP3A4 inhibitors. Dihydroergotamine may increase the effects of 5-HT$_1$

(Continued)

Dihydroergotamine *(Continued)*

agonists (eg, sumatriptan), MAO inhibitors, sibutramine, and other serotonin agonists (serotonin syndrome). Severe vasoconstriction may occur when peripheral vasoconstrictors or beta-blockers are used in patients receiving ergot alkaloids; concurrent use is contraindicated.

Decreased Effect: Effects of dihydroergotamine may be diminished by antipsychotics, metoclopramide. Antianginal effects of nitrates may be reduced by ergot alkaloids.

Pharmacodynamics/Kinetics

Onset of action: 15-30 minutes
Duration: 3-4 hours
Distribution: V_d: 14.5 L/kg
Protein binding: 93%
Metabolism: Extensively hepatic
Half-life elimination: 1.3-3.9 hours
Time to peak, serum: I.M.: 15-30 minutes
Excretion: Primarily feces; urine (10% mostly as metabolites)

Pregnancy Risk Factor X

Dihydroergotamine Mesylate *see* Dihydroergotamine *on page 477*
Dihydroergotoxine *see* Ergoloid Mesylates *on page 557*
Dihydrogenated Ergot Alkaloids *see* Ergoloid Mesylates *on page 557*
DiHydro-GP *see* Dihydrocodeine, Pseudoephedrine, and Guaifenesin *on page 476*
Dihydrohydroxycodeinone *see* Oxycodone *on page 1163*
Dihydromorphinone *see* Hydromorphone *on page 797*

Dihydrotachysterol *(dye hye droe tak ISS ter ole)*

U.S. Brand Names DHT™ [DSC]; DHT™ Intensol™ [DSC]; Hytakerol® [DSC]
Canadian Brand Names Hytakerol®
Generic Available No
Synonyms Dichysterol
Pharmacologic Category Vitamin D Analog
Use Treatment of hypocalcemia associated with hypoparathyroidism; prophylaxis of hypocalcemic tetany following thyroid surgery
Local Anesthetic/Vasoconstrictor Precautions No information available to require special precautions
Effects on Dental Treatment No significant effects or complications reported
Common Adverse Effects >10%:
Endocrine & metabolic: Hypercalcemia
Renal: Elevated serum creatinine, hypercalciuria
Mechanism of Action Synthetic analogue of vitamin D with a faster onset of action; stimulates calcium and phosphate absorption from the small intestine, promotes secretion of calcium from bone to blood; promotes renal tubule resorption of phosphate

Drug Interactions

Increased Effect/Toxicity: Thiazide diuretics may increase calcium levels.
Decreased Effect: Decreased effect/levels of vitamin D if taken with cholestyramine, colestipol, or mineral oil. Phenytoin and phenobarbital may inhibit activation leading to decreased effectiveness.

Pharmacodynamics/Kinetics

Onset of action: Peak effect: Calcium: 2-4 weeks
Duration: ≤9 weeks
Absorption: Well absorbed
Distribution: Stored in liver, fat, skin, muscle, and bone
Excretion: Feces

Pregnancy Risk Factor A/D (dose exceeding RDA recommendation)

Dihydroxyanthracenedione Dihydrochloride *see* Mitoxantrone *on page 1055*
1,25 Dihydroxycholecalciferol *see* Calcitriol *on page 247*
Dihydroxydeoxynorvinkaleukoblastine *see* Vinorelbine *on page 1578*
Dihydroxypropyl Theophylline *see* Dyphylline *on page 526*
Diiodohydroxyquin *see* Iodoquinol *on page 853*
Dilacor® XR *see* Diltiazem *on page 479*
Dilantin® *see* Phenytoin *on page 1228*
Dilatrate®-SR *see* Isosorbide Dinitrate *on page 866*
Dilaudid® *see* Hydromorphone *on page 797*
Dilaudid-HP® *see* Hydromorphone *on page 797*
Dilor® *see* Dyphylline *on page 526*

Diltia XT® *see* Diltiazem *on page 479*

Diltiazem (dil TYE a zem)

Related Information

Cardiovascular Diseases *on page 1636*

U.S. Brand Names Cardizem®; Cardizem® CD; Cardizem® LA; Cardizem® SR [DSC]; Cartia XT™; Dilacor® XR; Diltia XT®; Taztia XT™; Tiazac®

Canadian Brand Names Alti-Diltiazem CD; Apo-Diltiaz®; Apo-Diltiaz CD®; Apo-Diltiaz SR®; Cardizem®; Cardizem® CD; Cardizem® SR; Gen-Diltiazem; Gen-Diltiazem CD; Med-Diltiazem; Novo-Diltiazem; Novo-Diltiazem-CD; Nu-Diltiaz; Nu-Diltiaz-CD; ratio-Diltiazem CD; Rhoxal-diltiazem CD; Rhoxal-diltiazem SR; Sandoz-Diltiazem CD; Sandoz-Diltiazem T; Syn-Diltiazem®; Tiazac®; Tiazac® XC

Mexican Brand Names Angiotrofin®; Tilazem®

Generic Available Yes

Synonyms Diltiazem Hydrochloride

Pharmacologic Category Calcium Channel Blocker

Use

Oral: Essential hypertension; chronic stable angina or angina from coronary artery spasm

Injection: Atrial fibrillation or atrial flutter; paroxysmal supraventricular tachycardia (PSVT)

Unlabeled/Investigational Use Investigational: Therapy of Duchenne muscular dystrophy

Local Anesthetic/Vasoconstrictor Precautions No information available to require special precautions

Effects on Dental Treatment Key adverse event(s) related to dental treatment: Diltiazem has been reported to cause >10% incidence of gingival hyperplasia; usually disappears with discontinuation (consultation with physician is suggested).

Common Adverse Effects Note: Frequencies represent ranges for various dosage forms. Patients with impaired ventricular function and/or conduction abnormalities may have higher incidence of adverse reactions.

>10%:

Cardiovascular: Edema (2% to 15%)

Central nervous system: Headache (5% to 12%)

2% to 10%:

Cardiovascular: AV block (first degree 2% to 8%), edema (lower limb 2% to 8%), pain (6%), bradycardia (2% to 6%), hypotension (<2% to 4%), vasodilation (2% to 3%), extrasystoles (2%), flushing (1% to 2%), palpitation (1% to 2%)

Central nervous system: Dizziness (3% to 10%), nervousness (2%)

Dermatologic: Rash (1% to 4%)

Endocrine & metabolic: Gout (1% to 2%)

Gastrointestinal: Dyspepsia (1% to 6%), constipation (<2% to 4%), vomiting (2%), diarrhea (1% to 2%)

Local: Injection site reactions: Burning, itching (4%)

Neuromuscular & skeletal: Weakness (1% to 4%), myalgia (2%)

Respiratory: Rhinitis (<2% to 10%), pharyngitis (2% to 6%), dyspnea (1% to 6%), bronchitis (1% to 4%), sinus congestion (1% to 2%)

Dosage Adults:

Oral:

Angina:

Capsule, extended release (Cardizem® CD, Cartia XT™, Dilacor® XR, Diltia XT®, Tiazac®): Initial: 120-180 mg once daily (maximum dose: 480 mg/day)

Tablet, extended release (Cardizem® LA): 180 mg once daily; may increase at 7- to 14-day intervals (maximum recommended dose: 360 mg/day)

Tablet, immediate release (Cardizem®): Usual starting dose: 30 mg 4 times/day; usual range: 180-360 mg/day

Hypertension:

Capsule, extended release (Cardizem® CD, Cartia XT™, Dilacor® XR, Diltia XT®, Tiazac®): Initial: 180-240 mg once daily; dose adjustment may be made after 14 days; usual dose range (JNC 7): 180-420 mg/day; Tiazac®: usual dose range: 120-540 mg/day

Capsule, sustained release (Cardizem® SR): Initial: 60-120 mg twice daily; dose adjustment may be made after 14 days; usual range: 240-360 mg/day

(Continued)

Diltiazem *(Continued)*

Tablet, extended release (Cardizem® LA): Initial: 180-240 mg once daily; dose adjustment may be made after 14 days; usual dose range (JNC 7): 120-540 mg/day

Note: Elderly: Patients ≥60 years may respond to a lower initial dose (ie, 120 mg once daily using extended release capsule)

I.V.: Atrial fibrillation, atrial flutter, PSVT:

Initial bolus dose: 0.25 mg/kg actual body weight over 2 minutes (average adult dose: 20 mg)

Repeat bolus dose (may be administered after 15 minutes if the response is inadequate.): 0.35 mg/kg actual body weight over 2 minutes (average adult dose: 25 mg)

Continuous infusion (requires an infusion pump; infusions >24 hours or infusion rates >15 mg/hour are not recommended.): Initial infusion rate of 10 mg/hour; rate may be increased in 5 mg/hour increments up to 15 mg/hour as needed; some patients may respond to an initial rate of 5 mg/hour.

If diltiazem injection is administered by continuous infusion for >24 hours, the possibility of decreased diltiazem clearance, prolonged elimination half-life, and increased diltiazem and/or diltiazem metabolite plasma concentrations should be considered.

Conversion from I.V. diltiazem to oral diltiazem: Start oral approximately 3 hours after bolus dose.

Oral dose (mg/day) is approximately equal to [rate (mg/hour) x 3 + 3] x 10.

3 mg/hour = 120 mg/day
5 mg/hour = 180 mg/day
7 mg/hour = 240 mg/day
11 mg/hour = 360 mg/day

Dosing comments in renal/hepatic impairment: Use with caution as extensively metabolized by the liver and excreted in the kidneys and bile.

Dialysis: Not removed by hemo- or peritoneal dialysis; supplemental dose is not necessary.

Mechanism of Action Inhibits calcium ion from entering the "slow channels" or select voltage-sensitive areas of vascular smooth muscle and myocardium during depolarization, producing a relaxation of coronary vascular smooth muscle and coronary vasodilation; increases myocardial oxygen delivery in patients with vasospastic angina

Contraindications Hypersensitivity to diltiazem or any component of the formulation; sick sinus syndrome; second- or third-degree AV block (except in patients with a functioning artificial pacemaker); hypotension (systolic <90 mm Hg); acute MI and pulmonary congestion

Warnings/Precautions Use with caution and titrate dosages for patients with hypotension or patients taking antihypertensives, impaired renal or hepatic function, or when treating patients with CHF. Use caution with concomitant therapy with beta-blockers or digoxin. Monitor LFTs during therapy since these enzymes may rarely be increased and symptoms of hepatic injury may occur; usually reverses with drug discontinuation; avoid abrupt withdrawal of calcium blockers since rebound angina is theoretically possible.

Drug Interactions

Cytochrome P450 Effect: Substrate of CYP2C9 (minor), 2D6 (minor), 3A4 (major); **Inhibits** CYP2C9 (weak), 2D6 (weak), 3A4 (moderate)

Increased Effect/Toxicity: Diltiazem effects may be additive with amiodarone, beta-blockers, or digoxin, which may lead to bradycardia, other conduction delays, and decreased cardiac output. The levels/effects of diltiazem may be increased by azole antifungals, clarithromycin, diclofenac, doxycycline, erythromycin, imatinib, isoniazid, nefazodone, nicardipine, propofol, protease inhibitors, quinidine, telithromycin, verapamil, and other CYP3A4 inhibitors.

Diltiazem may increase the levels/effects of selected benzodiazepines, calcium channel blockers, cisapride, cyclosporine, ergot alkaloids, selected HMG-CoA reductase inhibitors, mesoridazine, mirtazapine, nateglinide, nefazodone, pimozide, quinidine, sildenafil (and other PDE-5 inhibitors), tacrolimus, thioridazine, venlafaxine, and other CYP3A4 substrates. Blood pressure-lowering effects may be additive with sildenafil, tadalafil, and vardenafil (use caution).

Decreased Effect: Levels/effects of diltiazem may be decreased by aminoglutethimide, carbamazepine, nafcillin, nevirapine, phenobarbital, phenytoin, rifamycins, and other CYP3A4 inducers.

Ethanol/Nutrition/Herb Interactions

Ethanol: Avoid ethanol (may increase risk of hypotension or vasodilation).

Food: Diltiazem serum levels may be elevated if taken with food. Serum concentrations were not altered by grapefruit juice in small clinical trials.

Herb/Nutraceutical: St John's wort may decrease diltiazem levels. Avoid dong quai if using for hypertension (has estrogenic activity). Avoid ephedra (may worsen arrhythmia or hypertension). Avoid yohimbe, ginseng (may worsen hypertension). Avoid garlic (may have increased antihypertensive effect).

Pharmacodynamics/Kinetics

Onset of action: Oral: Immediate release tablet: 30-60 minutes

Absorption: 70% to 80%

Distribution: V_d: 3-13 L/kg; enters breast milk

Protein binding: 70% to 80%

Metabolism: Hepatic; extensive first-pass effect; following single I.V. injection, plasma concentrations of N-monodesmethyldiltiazem and desacetyldiltiazem are typically undetectable; however, these metabolites accumulate to detectable concentrations following 24-hour constant rate infusion. N-monodesmethyldiltiazem appears to have 20% of the potency of diltiazem; desacetyldiltiazem is about 25% to 50% as potent as the parent compound.

Bioavailability: Oral: ~40%

Half-life elimination: Immediate release tablet: 3-4.5 hours, may be prolonged with renal impairment

Time to peak, serum: Immediate release tablet: 2-4 hours

Excretion: Urine and feces (primarily as metabolites)

Pregnancy Risk Factor C

Dosage Forms CAP, extended release [once-daily dosing]: 120 mg, 180 mg, 240 mg, 300 mg; (Cardizem® CD, Taztia XT™): 120 mg, 180 mg, 240 mg, 300 mg, 360 mg; (Cartia XT™): 120 mg, 180 mg, 240 mg, 300 mg; (Dilacor® XR, Diltia XT®): 120 mg, 180 mg, 240 mg; (Tiazac®): 120 mg, 180 mg, 240 mg, 300 mg, 360 mg, 420 mg. **CAP, sustained release** [twice-daily dosing]: 60 mg, 90 mg, 120 mg. **INJ, solution:** 5 mg/mL (5 mL, 10 mL, 25 mL). **INJ, powder for reconstitution** (Cardizem®): 25 mg, 100 mg. **TAB** (Cardizem®): 30 mg, 60 mg, 90 mg, 120 mg **TAB, extended release** (Cardizem® LA): 120 mg, 180 mg, 240 mg, 300 mg, 360 mg, 420 mg

Diltiazem Hydrochloride *see* Diltiazem *on page 479*

DimenhyDRINATE (dye men HYE dri nate)

U.S. Brand Names Dramamine® [OTC]; TripTone® [OTC]

Canadian Brand Names Apo-Dimenhydrinate®; Children's Motion Sickness Liquid; Dinate®; Gravol®; Jamp® Travel Tablet; Nauseatol; Novo-Dimenate; SAB-Dimenhydrinate

Mexican Brand Names Dramamine®; Vomisin®

Generic Available Yes

Pharmacologic Category Antihistamine

Use Treatment and prevention of nausea, vertigo, and vomiting associated with motion sickness

Dosage forms available in Canada (not available in the U.S.), including parenteral formulations and suppositories, are also approved for the treatment of postoperative nausea and vomiting and treatment of radiation sickness.

Unlabeled/Investigational Use Treatment of Meniere's disease

Local Anesthetic/Vasoconstrictor Precautions No information available to require special precautions

Effects on Dental Treatment Key adverse event(s) related to dental treatment: Significant xerostomia (normal salivary flow resumes upon discontinuation).

Common Adverse Effects

>10%:

Central nervous system: Slight to moderate drowsiness

Respiratory: Thickening of bronchial secretions

1% to 10%:

Central nervous system: Headache, fatigue, nervousness, dizziness

Gastrointestinal: Appetite increase, weight gain, nausea, diarrhea, abdominal pain, xerostomia

Neuromuscular & skeletal: Arthralgia

Respiratory: Pharyngitis

Mechanism of Action Competes with histamine for H_1-receptor sites on effector cells in the gastrointestinal tract, blood vessels, and respiratory tract; blocks chemoreceptor trigger zone, diminishes vestibular stimulation, and depresses labyrinthine function through its central anticholinergic activity

(Continued)

DimenhyDRINATE *(Continued)*

Drug Interactions

Increased Effect/Toxicity: CNS depressants may increase the degree of sedation and respiratory depression with antihistamines. May increase the absorption of digoxin. Central and/or peripheral anticholinergic syndrome can occur when administered with amantadine, rimantadine, narcotic analgesics, phenothiazines and other antipsychotics (especially with high anticholinergic activity), tricyclic antidepressants, quinidine, disopyramide, procainamide, and antihistamines.

Decreased Effect: May increase gastric degradation of levodopa and decrease the amount of levodopa absorbed by delaying gastric emptying. Therapeutic effects of cholinergic agents (tacrine, donepezil) and neuroleptics may be antagonized.

Pharmacodynamics/Kinetics

Onset of action: Oral: ~15-30 minutes

Absorption: Oral: Well absorbed

Pregnancy Risk Factor B

Dimercaprol *(dye mer KAP role)*

U.S. Brand Names BAL in Oil®

Generic Available No

Synonyms BAL; British Anti-Lewisite; Dithioglycerol

Pharmacologic Category Antidote

Use Antidote to gold, arsenic (except arsine), and mercury poisoning (except nonalkyl mercury); adjunct to edetate calcium disodium in lead poisoning; possibly effective for antimony, bismuth, chromium, copper, nickel, tungsten, or zinc

Local Anesthetic/Vasoconstrictor Precautions No information available to require special precautions

Effects on Dental Treatment No significant effects or complications reported

Common Adverse Effects

>10%:

Cardiovascular: Hypertension, tachycardia (dose related)

Central nervous system: Headache

1% to 10%: Gastrointestinal: Nausea, vomiting

Mechanism of Action Sulfhydryl group combines with ions of various heavy metals to form relatively stable, nontoxic, soluble chelates which are excreted in urine

Drug Interactions

Increased Effect/Toxicity: Toxic complexes with iron, cadmium, selenium, or uranium.

Pharmacodynamics/Kinetics

Distribution: To all tissues including the brain

Metabolism: Rapidly hepatic to inactive metabolites

Time to peak, serum: 0.5-1 hour

Excretion: Urine

Pregnancy Risk Factor C

Dimetapp® 12-Hour Non-Drowsy Extentabs® [OTC] *see* Pseudoephedrine *on page 1309*

Dimetapp® Cold and Congestion [OTC] *see* Guaifenesin, Pseudoephedrine, and Dextromethorphan *on page 757*

Dimetapp® Decongestant Infant [OTC] *see* Pseudoephedrine *on page 1309*

Dimetapp® Infant Decongestant Plus Cough [OTC] *see* Pseudoephedrine and Dextromethorphan *on page 1311*

β,β-Dimethylcysteine *see* Penicillamine *on page 1201*

Dimethyl Triazeno Imidazole Carboxamide *see* Dacarbazine *on page 415*

Dinoprostone *(dye noe PROST one)*

U.S. Brand Names Cervidil®; Prepidil®; Prostin E₂®

Canadian Brand Names Cervidil®; Prepidil®; Prostin E₂®

Mexican Brand Names Prepidil®; Propess®

Generic Available No

Synonyms PGE₂; Prostaglandin E₂

Pharmacologic Category Abortifacient; Prostaglandin

Use

Gel: Promote cervical ripening prior to labor induction; usage for gel include any patient undergoing induction of labor with an unripe cervix, most commonly for pre-eclampsia, eclampsia, postdates, diabetes, intrauterine growth retardation, and chronic hypertension

Suppositories: Terminate pregnancy from 12th through 28th week of gestation; evacuate uterus in cases of missed abortion or intrauterine fetal death; manage benign hydatidiform mole

Vaginal insert: Initiation and/or cervical ripening in patients at or near term in whom there is a medical or obstetrical indication for the induction of labor

Local Anesthetic/Vasoconstrictor Precautions No information available to require special precautions

Effects on Dental Treatment No significant effects or complications reported

Common Adverse Effects

>10%:

Central nervous system: Headache

Gastrointestinal: Vomiting, diarrhea, nausea

1% to 10%:

Cardiovascular: Bradycardia

Central nervous system: Fever

Neuromuscular & skeletal: Back pain

Mechanism of Action A synthetic prostaglandin E_2 abortifacient that stimulates uterine contractions similar to those seen during natural labor

Drug Interactions

Increased Effect/Toxicity: Dinoprostone may increase the effect of oxytocin; wait 6-12 hours after dinoprostone administration before initiating oxytocin.

Pharmacodynamics/Kinetics

Onset of action (uterine contractions): Within 10 minutes

Duration: Up to 2-3 hours

Absorption: Vaginal: Slow

Metabolism: In many tissues including renal, pulmonary, and splenic systems

Excretion: Primarily urine; feces (small amounts)

Pregnancy Risk Factor C

Diocto® [OTC] *see* Docusate *on page 496*

Diocto C® [DSC] [OTC] *see* Docusate and Casanthranol *on page 496*

Dioctyl Calcium Sulfosuccinate *see* Docusate *on page 496*

Dioctyl Sodium Sulfosuccinate *see* Docusate *on page 496*

Diotame® [OTC] *see* Bismuth *on page 210*

Diovan® *see* Valsartan *on page 1561*

Diovan HCT® *see* Valsartan and Hydrochlorothiazide *on page 1562*

Dipentum® *see* Olsalazine *on page 1144*

Diphen® [OTC] *see* DiphenhydrAMINE *on page 483*

Diphen® AF [OTC] *see* DiphenhydrAMINE *on page 483*

Diphenhist [OTC] *see* DiphenhydrAMINE *on page 483*

DiphenhydrAMINE (dye fen HYE dra meen)

Related Information

Management of Patients Undergoing Cancer Therapy *on page 1728*

Ulcerative and Erosive Disorders *on page 1712*

Viral Infections *on page 1709*

Related Sample Prescriptions

Recurrent Aphthous Stomatitis *on page 1744*

U.S. Brand Names Aler-Cap [OTC]; Aler-Dryl [OTC]; Aler-Tab [OTC]; AllerMax® [OTC]; Altaryl [OTC]; Banophen® [OTC]; Banophen® Anti-Itch [OTC]; Benadryl® Allergy [OTC]; Benadryl® Children's Allergy [OTC]; Benadryl® Children's Allergy Fastmelt® [OTC]; Benadryl® Dye-Free Allergy [OTC]; Benadryl® Injection; Benadryl® Itch Stopping [OTC]; Benadryl® Itch Stopping Extra Strength [OTC]; Compoz® Nighttime Sleep Aid [OTC]; Dermamycin® [OTC]; Dermarest® Insect Bite [OTC]; Dermarest® Plus [OTC]; Diphen® [OTC]; Diphen® AF [OTC]; Diphenhist [OTC]; Dytan™; Genahist® [OTC]; Hydramine® [OTC]; Nytol® Quick Caps [OTC]; Nytol® Quick Gels [OTC]; Q-Dryl [OTC]; Quenalin [OTC]; Siladryl® Allergy [OTC]; Siladryl® DAS [OTC]; Silphen® [OTC]; Simply Sleep® [OTC]; Sleep-ettes D [OTC]; Sleepinal® [OTC]; Sominex® [OTC]; Sominex® Maximum Strength [OTC]; Triaminic® Thin Strips™ Cough and Runny Nose [OTC]; Twilite® [OTC]; Unisom® Maximum Strength SleepGels® [OTC]

Canadian Brand Names Allerdryl®; Allernix; Benadryl®; Nytol®; Nytol® Extra Strength; PMS-Diphenhydramine; Simply Sleep®

Mexican Brand Names Tzoali®

Generic Available Yes: Excludes chewable tablet, orally-disintegrating tablet, suspension, stick, strip

Synonyms Diphenhydramine Citrate; Diphenhydramine Hydrochloride; Diphenhydramine Tannate

(Continued)

483

DiphenhydrAMINE *(Continued)*

Pharmacologic Category Antihistamine

Dental Use Symptomatic relief of nasal mucosal congestion

Use Symptomatic relief of allergic symptoms caused by histamine release which include nasal allergies and allergic dermatosis; can be used for mild nighttime sedation; prevention of motion sickness and as an antitussive; has antinauseant and topical anesthetic properties; treatment of antipsychotic-induced extrapyramidal symptoms

Local Anesthetic/Vasoconstrictor Precautions No information available to require special precautions

Effects on Dental Treatment Key adverse event(s) related to dental treatment: Xerostomia (normal salivary flow resumes upon discontinuation) and dry mucous membranes. Chronic use of antihistamines will inhibit salivary flow, particularly in elderly patients; may contribute to periodontal disease and oral discomfort. See Dental Comment.

Significant Adverse Effects Frequency not defined.

Cardiovascular: Hypotension, palpitation, tachycardia

Central nervous system: Sedation, sleepiness, dizziness, disturbed coordination, headache, fatigue, nervousness, paradoxical excitement, insomnia, euphoria, confusion

Dermatologic: Photosensitivity, rash, angioedema, urticaria

Gastrointestinal: Nausea, vomiting, diarrhea, abdominal pain, xerostomia, appetite increase, weight gain, dry mucous membranes, anorexia

Genitourinary: Urinary retention, urinary frequency, difficult urination

Hematologic: Hemolytic anemia, thrombocytopenia, agranulocytosis

Neuromuscular & skeletal: Tremor, paresthesia

Ocular: Blurred vision

Respiratory: Thickening of bronchial secretions

Dental Usual Dosing Symptomatic relief of nasal mucosal congestion: Adults: Oral: 25-50 mg every 6-8 hours

Dosage

Children:

Oral, I.M., I.V.:

Treatment of moderate to severe allergic reactions: 5 mg/kg/day or 150 mg/m^2/day in divided doses every 6-8 hours, not to exceed 300 mg/day

Minor allergic rhinitis or motion sickness:

2 to <6 years: 6.25 mg every 4-6 hours; maximum: 37.5 mg/day

6 to <12 years: 12.5-25 mg every 4-6 hours; maximum: 150 mg/day

≥12 years: 25-50 mg every 4-6 hours; maximum: 300 mg/day

Night-time sleep aid: 30 minutes before bedtime:

2 to <12 years: 1 mg/kg/dose; maximum: 50 mg/dose

≥12 years: 50 mg

Oral: Antitussive:

2 to <6 years: 6.25 mg every 4 hours; maximum 37.5 mg/day

6 to <12 years: 12.5 mg every 4 hours; maximum 75 mg/day

≥12 years: 25 mg every 4 hours; maximum 150 mg/day

I.M., I.V.: Treatment of dystonic reactions: 0.5-1 mg/kg/dose

Adults:

Oral: 25-50 mg every 6-8 hours

Minor allergic rhinitis or motion sickness: 25-50 mg every 4-6 hours; maximum: 300 mg/day

Moderate to severe allergic reactions: 25-50 mg every 4 hours, not to exceed 400 mg/day

Nighttime sleep aid: 50 mg at bedtime

I.M., I.V.: 10-50 mg in a single dose every 2-4 hours, not to exceed 400 mg/day

Dystonic reaction: 50 mg in a single dose; may repeat in 20-30 minutes if necessary

Topical: For external application, not longer than 7 days

Mechanism of Action Competes with histamine for H$_1$-receptor sites on effector cells in the gastrointestinal tract, blood vessels, and respiratory tract; anticholinergic and sedative effects are also seen

Contraindications Hypersensitivity to diphenhydramine or any component of the formulation; acute asthma; not for use in neonates

Warnings/Precautions Causes sedation, caution must be used in performing tasks which require alertness (eg, operating machinery or driving). Sedative effects of CNS depressants or ethanol are potentiated. Use with caution in patients with angle-closure glaucoma, pyloroduodenal obstruction (including stenotic peptic ulcer), urinary tract obstruction (including bladder neck obstruction and symptomatic prostatic hyperplasia), hyperthyroidism, increased intraocular pressure, and cardiovascular disease (including hypertension and tachycardia). Diphenhydramine has high sedative and anticholinergic properties, so it may not be considered the antihistamine of choice for prolonged use in the elderly. May cause paradoxical excitation in pediatric patients, and can result in hallucinations, coma, and death in overdose. Some preparations contain sodium bisulfite; syrup formulations may contain alcohol. Some preparations contain soy protein; patients with soy protein or peanut allergies should avoid.

Drug Interactions Inhibits CYP2D6 (moderate)

Amantadine, rimantadine: Central and/or peripheral anticholinergic syndrome can occur when administered with amantadine or rimantadine

Anticholinergic agents: Central and/or peripheral anticholinergic syndrome can occur when administered with narcotic analgesics, phenothiazines and other antipsychotics (especially with high anticholinergic activity), tricyclic antidepressants, quinidine and some other antiarrhythmics, and antihistamines

Atenolol: Drugs with high anticholinergic activity may increase the bioavailability of atenolol (and possibly other beta-blockers); monitor for increased effect

Cholinergic agents: Drugs with high anticholinergic activity may antagonize the therapeutic effect of cholinergic agents; includes donepezil, rivastigmine, and tacrine

CNS depressants: Sedative effects may be additive with CNS depressants; includes ethanol, benzodiazepines, barbiturates, narcotic analgesics, and other sedative agents; monitor for increased effect

CYP2D6 substrates: Diphenhydramine may increase the levels/effects of CYP2D6 substrates. Example substrates include amphetamines, selected beta-blockers, dextromethorphan, fluoxetine, lidocaine, mirtazapine, nefazodone, paroxetine, risperidone, ritonavir, thioridazine, tricyclic antidepressants, and venlafaxine.

CYP2D6 prodrug substrates: Diphenhydramine may decrease the levels/effects of CYP2D6 prodrug substrates. Example prodrug substrates include codeine, hydrocodone, oxycodone, and tramadol.

Digoxin: Drugs with high anticholinergic activity may decrease gastric degradation and increase the amount of digoxin absorbed by delaying gastric emptying

Ethanol: Syrup should not be given to patients taking drugs that can cause disulfiram reactions (ie, metronidazole, chlorpropamide) due to high alcohol content

Levodopa: Drugs with high anticholinergic activity may increase gastric degradation and decrease the amount of levodopa absorbed by delaying gastric emptying

Neuroleptics: Drugs with high anticholinergic activity may antagonize the therapeutic effects of neuroleptics

Ethanol/Nutrition/Herb Interactions

Ethanol: Avoid ethanol (may increase CNS depression).

Herb/Nutraceutical: Avoid valerian, St John's wort, kava kava, gotu kola (may increase CNS depression).

Dietary Considerations Tablet:

Chewable, as hydrochloride: Contains phenylalanine 4.2 mg per 12.5 mg tablet

Chewable, as tannate: Contains phenylalanine 1.5 mg per 25 mg tablet

Orally-disintegrating, as citrate: Contains phenylalanine 4.5 mg per 19 mg [equivalent to diphenhydramine hydrochloride 12.5 mg] tablet; contains soy protein isolate (contraindicated in patients with soy protein allergies; use caution in peanut allergic individuals, ~10% are estimated to also have soy protein allergies)

Pharmacodynamics/Kinetics

Onset of action: Maximum sedative effect: 1-3 hours

Duration: 4-7 hours

Protein binding: 78%

Metabolism: Extensively hepatic; smaller degrees in pulmonary and renal systems; significant first-pass effect

Bioavailability: Oral: 40% to 60%

Half-life elimination: 2-8 hours; Elderly: 13.5 hours

Time to peak, serum: 2-4 hours

Excretion: Urine (as unchanged drug)

Pregnancy Risk Factor B

Lactation Enters breast milk/contraindicated

Breast-Feeding Considerations Infants may be more sensitive to the effects of antihistamines.

Dosage Forms

Caplet, as hydrochloride: 25 mg, 50 mg

Aler-Dryl, AllerMax®, Compoz® Nighttime Sleep Aid, Sleep-ettes D, Sominex® Maximum Strength, Twilite®: 50 mg

Simply Sleep®, Nytol® Quick Caps: 25 mg

(Continued)

DiphenhydrAMINE *(Continued)*

Capsule, as hydrochloride: 25 mg, 50 mg
Aler-Cap, Banophen®, Benadryl® Allergy, Diphen®, Diphenhist, Genahist®, Q-Dryl: 25 mg
Sleepinal®: 50 mg
Capsule, softgel, as hydrochloride: 50 mg
Benadryl® Dye-Free Allergy: 25 mg [dye-free]
Compoz® Nighttime Sleep Aid, Nytol® Quick Gels, Sleepinal®, Unisom® Maximum Strength SleepGels®: 50 mg
Captab, as hydrochloride (Diphenhist®): 25 mg
Cream, as hydrochloride: 2% (30 g) [contains zinc acetate 0.1%]
Banophen® Anti-Itch: 2% (30 g) [contains zinc acetate 0.1%]
Benadryl® Itch Stopping: 1% (30 g) [contains zinc acetate 0.1%]
Benadryl® Itch Stopping Extra Strength: 2% (30 g) [contains zinc acetate 0.1%]
Diphenhist®: 2% (30 g) [contains zinc acetate 0.1%]
Elixir, as hydrochloride:
Altaryl: 12.5 mg/5 mL (120 mL, 480 mL, 3840 mL) [cherry flavor]
Banophen®: 12.5 mg/5 mL (120 mL)
Diphen AF: 12.5 mg/5 mL (120 mL, 240 mL, 480 mL) [alcohol free; cherry flavor]
Q-Dryl: 12.5 mg/5 mL (480 mL) [alcohol free]
Gel, topical, as hydrochloride:
Benadryl® Itch Stopping Extra Strength: 2% (120 mL)
Dermarest® Plus: 2% (28 g, 42 g) [contains menthol 1%]
Injection, solution, as hydrochloride: 50 mg/mL (1 mL)
Benadryl®: 50 mg/mL (1 mL, 10 mL)
Liquid, as hydrochloride:
AllerMax®: 12.5 mg/5 mL (120 mL)
Benadryl® Allergy: 12.5 mg/5 mL (120 mL, 240 mL) [alcohol free; contains sodium benzoate; cherry flavor]
Benadryl® Dye-Free Allergy: 12.5 mg/5 mL (120 mL) [alcohol free, dye free, sugar free; contains sodium benzoate; bubble gum flavor]
Genahist®: 12.5 mg/5 mL (120 mL) [alcohol free, sugar free; contains sodium benzoate; cherry flavor]
Hydramine®: 12.5 mg/5 mL (120 mL, 480 mL) [alcohol free]
Q-Dryl: 12.5 mg/5 mL (120 mL) [alcohol free; cherry flavor]
Quenalin: 12.5 mg/5 mL (120 mL) [fruit flavor]
Siladryl® Allergy: 12.5 mg/5 mL (120 mL, 240 mL, 480 mL) [alcohol free, sugar free; black cherry flavor]
Siladryl® DAS: 12.5 mg/5 mL (120 mL) [alcohol free, dye free, sugar free; black cherry flavor]
Liquid, topical, as hydrochloride [stick] (Benadryl® Itch Stopping Extra Strength): 2% (14 mL) [contains zinc acetate 0.1% and alcohol]
Solution, oral, as hydrochloride:
Banophen®: 12.5 mg/5mL (480 mL) [sugar free]
Diphenhist: 12.5 mg/5 mL (120 mL, 480 mL) [alcohol free; contains sodium benzoate]
Solution, topical, as hydrochloride [spray]:
Benadryl® Itch Stopping Extra Strength: 2% (60 mL) [contains zinc acetate 0.1% and alcohol]
Dermamycin®, Dermarest® Insect Bite: 2% (60 mL) [contains menthol 1%]
Strips, oral, as hydrochloride (Triaminic® Thin Strips™ Cough and Runny Nose): 12. 5 mg (16s) [grape flavor]
Suspension, as tannate (Dytan™): 25 mg/5 mL (120 mL) [strawberry flavor]
Syrup, as hydrochloride (Silphen® Cough): 12.5 mg/5 mL (120 mL, 240 mL, 480 mL) [contains alcohol; 5%; strawberry flavor]
Tablet, as hydrochloride: 25 mg, 50 mg
Aler-Tab, Benadryl® Allergy, Genahist®, Sleepinal®, Sominex®: 25 mg
Tablet, chewable, as hydrochloride (Benadryl® Children's Allergy): 12.5 mg [contains phenylalanine 4.2 mg/tablet; grape flavor]
Tablet, chewable, as tannate (Dytan™): 25 mg [contains phenylalanine; strawberry flavor]
Tablet, orally disintegrating, as citrate (Benadryl® Children's Allergy Fastmelt®): 19 mg [equivalent to diphenhydramine hydrochloride 12.5 mg; contains phenylalanine 4.5 mg/tablet and soy protein isolate; cherry flavor]
Dental Comment 25-50 mg of diphenhydramine orally every 4-6 hours can be used to treat mild dermatologic manifestations of allergic reactions to penicillin and other antibiotics. Diphenhydramine is not recommended as local anesthetic for either infiltration route or nerve block since the vehicle has caused local necrosis upon injection. A 50:50 mixture of diphenhydramine liquid (12.5

mg/5mL) in Kaopectate® or Maalox® is used as a local application for recurrent aphthous ulcers; swish 1 tablespoonful for 2 minutes 4 times/day.

Diphenhydramine and Acetaminophen *see* Acetaminophen and Diphenhydramine on page 38

Diphenhydramine and Pseudoephedrine
(dye fen HYE dra meen & soo doe e FED rin)

Related Information
DiphenhydrAMINE on page 483
Pseudoephedrine on page 1309

U.S. Brand Names Benadryl® Allergy and Sinus Fastmelt™ [OTC]; Benadryl® Allergy/Sinus [OTC]; Benadryl® Children's Allergy and Cold Fastmelt™ [OTC]; Benadryl® Children's Allergy and Sinus [OTC]

Generic Available No

Synonyms Pseudoephedrine and Diphenhydramine

Pharmacologic Category Antihistamine/Decongestant Combination

Use Relief of symptoms of upper respiratory mucosal congestion in seasonal and perennial nasal allergies, acute rhinitis, rhinosinusitis, and eustachian tube blockage

Local Anesthetic/Vasoconstrictor Precautions Use with caution since pseudoephedrine is a sympathomimetic amine which could interact with epinephrine to cause a pressor response

Effects on Dental Treatment Key adverse event(s) related to dental treatment: Pseudoephedrine: Xerostomia (normal salivary flow resumes upon discontinuation). Chronic use of antihistamines will inhibit salivary flow, particularly in elderly patients; this may contribute to periodontal disease and oral discomfort.

Common Adverse Effects See individual agents.

Drug Interactions
Cytochrome P450 Effect: Diphenhydramine: **Inhibits** CYP2D6 (moderate)
Increased Effect/Toxicity: See individual agents.
Decreased Effect: See individual agents.

Diphenhydramine Citrate *see* DiphenhydrAMINE on page 483

Diphenhydramine Hydrochloride *see* DiphenhydrAMINE on page 483

Diphenhydramine, Hydrocodone, and Phenylephrine *see* Hydrocodone, Phenylephrine, and Diphenhydramine on page 791

Diphenhydramine Tannate *see* DiphenhydrAMINE on page 483

Diphenoxylate and Atropine (dye fen OKS i late & A troe peen)

Related Information
Atropine on page 161

U.S. Brand Names Lomotil®; Lonox®

Canadian Brand Names Lomotil®

Generic Available Yes

Synonyms Atropine and Diphenoxylate

Pharmacologic Category Antidiarrheal

Use Treatment of diarrhea

Local Anesthetic/Vasoconstrictor Precautions No information available to require special precautions

Effects on Dental Treatment Key adverse event(s) related to dental treatment: Significant xerostomia (normal salivary flow resumes upon discontinuation).

Common Adverse Effects 1% to 10%:
Central nervous system: Nervousness, restlessness, dizziness, drowsiness, headache, mental depression
Gastrointestinal: Paralytic ileus, xerostomia
Genitourinary: Urinary retention and dysuria
Ocular: Blurred vision
Respiratory: Respiratory depression

Restrictions C-V

Mechanism of Action Diphenoxylate inhibits excessive GI motility and GI propulsion; commercial preparations contain a subtherapeutic amount of atropine to discourage abuse

Drug Interactions
Increased Effect/Toxicity: MAO inhibitors (hypertensive crisis), CNS depressants when taken with diphenoxylate may result in increased adverse
(Continued)

Diphenoxylate and Atropine *(Continued)*

effects, antimuscarinics (paralytic ileus). May prolong half-life of drugs metabolized in liver.

Pharmacodynamics/Kinetics

Atropine: See Atropine monograph.

Diphenoxylate:

Onset of action: Antidiarrheal: 45-60 minutes

Peak effect: Antidiarrheal: ~2 hours

Duration: Antidiarrheal: 3-4 hours

Absorption: Well absorbed

Metabolism: Extensively hepatic to diphenoxylic acid (active)

Half-life elimination: 2.5 hours

Time to peak, serum: 2 hours

Excretion: Primarily feces (as metabolites); urine (~14%, <1% as unchanged drug)

Pregnancy Risk Factor C

Diphenylhydantoin *see Phenytoin on page 1228*

Diphtheria and Tetanus Toxoids and Acellular Pertussis Adsorbed, Hepatitis B (Recombinant) and Inactivated Poliovirus Vaccine Combined *see* Diphtheria, Tetanus Toxoids, Acellular Pertussis, Hepatitis B (Recombinant), and Poliovirus (Inactivated) Vaccine *on page 488*

Diphtheria CRM$_{197}$ Protein *see Pneumococcal Conjugate Vaccine (7-Valent) on page 1250*

Diphtheria CRM$_{197}$ Protein Conjugate *see Haemophilus b Conjugate Vaccine on page 534*

Diphtheria, Tetanus Toxoids, Acellular Pertussis, Hepatitis B (Recombinant), and Poliovirus (Inactivated) Vaccine

(dif THEER ee a, TET a nus TOKS oyds, ay CEL yoo lar per TUS sis, hep a TYE tis bee ree KOM be nant, & POE lee oh VYE rus vak SEEN, in ak ti VAY ted vak SEEN)

Related Information

Hepatitis B Vaccine *on page 769*

Immunizations (Vaccines) *on page 1786*

Poliovirus Vaccine (Inactivated) *on page 1252*

Tetanus Toxoid (Adsorbed) *on page 1464*

Tetanus Toxoid (Fluid) *on page 1464*

U.S. Brand Names Pediarix™

Canadian Brand Names Pediarix™

Generic Available No

Synonyms Diphtheria and Tetanus Toxoids and Acellular Pertussis Adsorbed, Hepatitis B (Recombinant) and Inactivated Poliovirus Vaccine Combined

Pharmacologic Category Vaccine

Use Combination vaccine for the active immunization against diphtheria, tetanus, pertussis, hepatitis B virus (all known subtypes), and poliomyelitis (caused by poliovirus types 1, 2, and 3)

Local Anesthetic/Vasoconstrictor Precautions No information available to require special precautions

Effects on Dental Treatment No significant effects or complications reported

Common Adverse Effects All serious adverse reactions must be reported to the U.S. Department of Health and Human Services (DHHS) Vaccine Adverse Event Reporting System (VAERS) 1-800-822-7967.

As reported in a U.S. lot Consistency Study:

>10%:

Central nervous system:

Sleeping increased (28% to 47%, grade 3: <1% to 2%)

Restlessness (28% to 30%, grade 3: ≤1%)

Fever ≥100.4°F (26% to 31%); >103.1°F (<1%); incidence of fever is higher than reported with separately administered vaccines

Gastrointestinal: Appetite decreased (19% to 22%, grade 3: <1%)

Local: Injection site:

Redness (25% to 36%, >20 mm: ≤1%)

Pain (23% to 30%, grade 3: ≤1%)

Swelling (15% to 22%; >20 mm: 1%)

Miscellaneous: Fussiness (57% to 64%; grade 3: 2% to 3%)

Refer to individual product monographs for additional adverse reactions, including postmarketing and case reports.

Mechanism of Action Promotes active immunity to diphtheria, tetanus, pertussis, hepatitis B and poliovirus (types 1, 2 and 3) by inducing production of specific antibodies and antitoxins.

Drug Interactions

Decreased Effect: Immunosuppressant medications or therapies (antimetabolites, alkylating agents, cytotoxic drugs, corticosteroids, irradiation) may decrease vaccine effectiveness, consider deferring vaccination for 3 months after immunosuppressant therapy is discontinued.

Pharmacodynamics/Kinetics Onset of action: Immune response observed to all components 1 month following the 3-dose series

Pregnancy Risk Factor C

Diphtheria Toxoid Conjugate *see Haemophilus* b Conjugate Vaccine *on page 534*

Dipivalyl Epinephrine *see* Dipivefrin *on page 489*

Dipivefrin (dye PI ve frin)

U.S. Brand Names Propine®
Canadian Brand Names Ophtho-Dipivefrin™; PMS-Dipivefrin; Propine®
Generic Available Yes
Synonyms Dipivalyl Epinephrine; Dipivefrin Hydrochloride; DPE
Pharmacologic Category Alpha/Beta Agonist; Ophthalmic Agent, Antiglaucoma; Ophthalmic Agent, Vasoconstrictor
Use Reduces elevated intraocular pressure in chronic open-angle glaucoma; also used to treat ocular hypertension, low tension, and secondary glaucomas

Local Anesthetic/Vasoconstrictor Precautions No information available to require special precautions

Effects on Dental Treatment No significant effects or complications reported

Mechanism of Action Dipivefrin is a prodrug of epinephrine which is the active agent that stimulates alpha- and/or beta-adrenergic receptors increasing aqueous humor outflow

Pregnancy Risk Factor B

Dipivefrin Hydrochloride *see* Dipivefrin *on page 489*

Diprivan® *see* Propofol *on page 1296*

Diprolene® *see* Betamethasone *on page 199*

Diprolene® AF *see* Betamethasone *on page 199*

Dipropylacetic Acid *see* Valproic Acid and Derivatives *on page 1556*

Dipyridamole (dye peer ID a mole)

U.S. Brand Names Persantine®
Canadian Brand Names Apo-Dipyridamole FC®; Persantine®
Generic Available Yes
Pharmacologic Category Antiplatelet Agent; Vasodilator
Use

Oral: Used with warfarin to decrease thrombosis in patients after artificial heart valve replacement

I.V.: Diagnostic agent in CAD

Unlabeled/Investigational Use Treatment of proteinuria in pediatric renal disease

Local Anesthetic/Vasoconstrictor Precautions No information available to require special precautions

Effects on Dental Treatment No significant effects or complications reported

Common Adverse Effects

Oral:

>10%: Dizziness (14%)

1% to 10%:

Central nervous system: Headache (2%)

Dermatologic: Rash (2%)

Gastrointestinal: Abdominal distress (6%)

Frequency not defined: Diarrhea, vomiting, flushing, pruritus, angina pectoris, liver dysfunction

I.V.:

>10%:

Cardiovascular: Exacerbation of angina pectoris (20%)

Central nervous system: Dizziness (12%), headache (12%)

(Continued)

Dipyridamole *(Continued)*

1% to 10%:
Cardiovascular: Hypotension (5%), hypertension (2%), blood pressure lability (2%), ECG abnormalities (ST-T changes, extrasystoles; 5% to 8%), pain (3%), tachycardia (3%)
Central nervous system: Flushing (3%), fatigue (1%)
Gastrointestinal: Nausea (5%)
Neuromuscular & skeletal: Paresthesia (1%)
Respiratory: Dyspnea (3%)

Mechanism of Action Inhibits the activity of adenosine deaminase and phosphodiesterase, which causes an accumulation of adenosine, adenine nucleotides, and cyclic AMP; these mediators then inhibit platelet aggregation and may cause vasodilation; may also stimulate release of prostacyclin or PGD_2; causes coronary vasodilation

Drug Interactions

Increased Effect/Toxicity: Adenosine blood levels and pharmacologic effects are increased with dipyridamole; consider reduced doses of adenosine.

Decreased Effect: Decreased vasodilation from I.V. dipyridamole when given to patients taking theophylline. Theophylline may reduce the pharmacologic effects of dipyridamole (hold theophylline preparations for 36-48 hours before dipyridamole facilitated stress test). Dipyridamole may counteract effect of cholinesterase inhibitor and may aggravate myasthenia gravis.

Pharmacodynamics/Kinetics
Absorption: Readily, but variable
Distribution: Adults: V_d: 2-3 L/kg
Protein binding: 91% to 99%
Metabolism: Hepatic
Half-life elimination: Terminal: 10-12 hours
Time to peak, serum: 2-2.5 hours
Excretion: Feces (as glucuronide conjugates and unchanged drug)

Pregnancy Risk Factor B

Dipyridamole and Aspirin *see* Aspirin and Dipyridamole *on page 150*

Dirithromycin *(dye RITH roe mye sin)*

U.S. Brand Names Dynabac® [DSC]
Generic Available No
Pharmacologic Category Antibiotic, Macrolide
Use Treatment of mild to moderate upper and lower respiratory tract infections due to *Moraxella catarrhalis*, *Streptococcus pneumoniae*, *Legionella pneumophila*, *H. influenzae*, or *S. pyogenes*, ie, acute exacerbation of chronic bronchitis, secondary bacterial infection of acute bronchitis, community-acquired pneumonia, pharyngitis/tonsillitis, and uncomplicated infections of the skin and skin structure due to *Staphylococcus aureus*

Local Anesthetic/Vasoconstrictor Precautions No information available to require special precautions
Effects on Dental Treatment No significant effects or complications reported
Common Adverse Effects 1% to 10%:
Central nervous system: Headache, dizziness, vertigo, insomnia
Dermatologic: Rash, pruritus, urticaria
Endocrine & metabolic: Hyperkalemia
Gastrointestinal: Abdominal pain, nausea, diarrhea, vomiting, dyspepsia, flatulence
Hematologic: Thrombocytosis, eosinophilia, segmented neutrophils
Neuromuscular & skeletal: Weakness, pain, increased CPK
Respiratory: Increased cough, dyspnea

Mechanism of Action After being converted during intestinal absorption to its active form, erythromycylamine, dirithromycin inhibits protein synthesis by binding to the 50S ribosomal subunits of susceptible microorganisms

Drug Interactions

Cytochrome P450 Effect: Substrate of CYP3A4 (minor)
Increased Effect/Toxicity: Absorption of dirithromycin is slightly enhanced with concomitant antacids and H_2 antagonists. Dirithromycin may, like erythromycin, increase the effect of alfentanil, anticoagulants, bromocriptine, carbamazepine, cyclosporine, digoxin, disopyramide, ergots, methylprednisolone, cisapride, and triazolam.

Note: Interactions with nonsedating antihistamines (eg, astemizole) or theophylline are not known to occur; however, caution is advised with coadministration.

Pharmacodynamics/Kinetics
Absorption: Rapid
Distribution: V_d: 800 L; rapidly and widely (higher levels in tissues than plasma)
Protein binding: 14% to 30%
Metabolism: Hydrolyzed to erythromycylamine
Bioavailability: 10%
Half-life elimination: 8 hours (range: 2-36 hours)
Time to peak: 4 hours
Excretion: Feces (81% to 97%)

Pregnancy Risk Factor C

Disalicylic Acid see Salsalate on page 1376
Disodium Cromoglycate see Cromolyn on page 397
Disodium Thiosulfate Pentahydrate see Sodium Thiosulfate on page 1404
d-Isoephedrine Hydrochloride see Pseudoephedrine on page 1309

Disopyramide (dye soe PEER a mide)

Related Information
Cardiovascular Diseases on page 1636
U.S. Brand Names Norpace®; Norpace® CR
Canadian Brand Names Norpace®; Rythmodan®; Rythmodan®-LA
Generic Available Yes
Synonyms Disopyramide Phosphate
Pharmacologic Category Antiarrhythmic Agent, Class Ia
Use Suppression and prevention of unifocal and multifocal atrial and premature, ventricular premature complexes, coupled ventricular tachycardia; effective in the conversion of atrial fibrillation, atrial flutter, and paroxysmal atrial tachycardia to normal sinus rhythm and prevention of the recurrence of these arrhythmias after conversion by other methods
Unlabeled/Investigational Use Hypertrophic obstructive cardiomyopathy (HOCM)
Local Anesthetic/Vasoconstrictor Precautions No information available to require special precautions (see Dental Comment)
Effects on Dental Treatment Key adverse event(s) related to dental treatment: Xerostomia (normal salivary flow resumes upon discontinuation).
Common Adverse Effects The most common adverse effects are related to cholinergic blockade. The most serious adverse effects of disopyramide are hypotension and CHF.

>10%:
Gastrointestinal: Xerostomia (32%), constipation (11%)
Genitourinary: Urinary hesitancy (14% to 23%)

1% to 10%:
Cardiovascular: CHF, hypotension, cardiac conduction disturbance, edema, syncope, chest pain
Central nervous system: Fatigue, headache, malaise, dizziness, nervousness
Dermatologic: Rash, generalized dermatoses, pruritus
Endocrine & metabolic: Hypokalemia, elevated cholesterol, elevated triglycerides
Gastrointestinal: Dry throat, nausea, abdominal distension, flatulence, abdominal bloating, anorexia, diarrhea, vomiting, weight gain
Genitourinary: Urinary retention, urinary frequency, urinary urgency, impotence (1% to 3%)
Neuromuscular & skeletal: Muscle weakness, muscular pain
Ocular: Blurred vision, dry eyes
Respiratory: Dyspnea

Mechanism of Action Class Ia antiarrhythmic: Decreases myocardial excitability and conduction velocity; reduces disparity in refractory between normal and infarcted myocardium; possesses anticholinergic, peripheral vasoconstrictive, and negative inotropic effects

Drug Interactions
Cytochrome P450 Effect: Substrate of CYP3A4 (major)
Increased Effect/Toxicity: Disopyramide may increase the effects/toxicity of anticholinergics, beta-blockers, flecainide, procainamide, quinidine, or propafenone. Digoxin and quinidine serum concentrations may be increased by disopyramide.

CYP3A4 inhibitors may increase the levels/effects of disopyramide. Example inhibitors include azole antifungals, clarithromycin, diclofenac, doxycycline, erythromycin, imatinib, isoniazid, nefazodone, nicardipine, propofol, protease inhibitors, quinidine, telithromycin, and verapamil.
(Continued)

Disopyramide *(Continued)*

Disopyramide effect/toxicity may be additive with drugs which may prolong the QT interval - amiodarone, amitriptyline, bepridil, cisapride (use is contraindicated), disopyramide, erythromycin, haloperidol, imipramine, pimozide, quinidine, sotalol, and thioridazine. In addition concurrent use with sparfloxacin, gatifloxacin, and moxifloxacin may result in additional prolongation of the QT interval; concurrent use is contraindicated.

Decreased Effect: CYP3A4 inducers may decrease the levels/effects of disopyramide; example inducers include aminoglutethimide, carbamazepine, nafcillin, nevirapine, phenobarbital, phenytoin, and rifamycins.

Pharmacodynamics/Kinetics

Onset of action: 0.5-3.5 hours

Duration: 1.5-8.5 hours

Absorption: 60% to 83%

Protein binding (concentration dependent): 20% to 60%

Metabolism: Hepatic to inactive metabolites

Half-life elimination: Adults: 4-10 hours; prolonged with hepatic or renal impairment

Excretion: Urine (40% to 60% as unchanged drug); feces (10% to 15%)

Pregnancy Risk Factor C

Dental Comment

This drug is known to prolong the QT interval. The QT interval is measured as the time and distance between the Q point of the QRS complex and the end of the T wave in the ECG tracing. After adjustment for heart rate, the QT interval is defined as prolonged if it is more than 450 msec in men and 460 msec in women. A long QT syndrome was first described in the 1950s and 60s as a congenital syndrome involving QT interval prolongation and syncope and sudden death. Some of the congenital long QT syndromes were characterized by a peculiar electrocardiographic appearance of the QRS complex involving a premature atria beat followed by a pause, then a subsequent sinus beat showing marked QT prolongation and deformity. This type of cardiac arrhythmia was originally termed "torsade de pointes" (translated from the French as "twisting of the points").

Prolongation of the QT interval is thought to result from delayed ventricular repolarization. The repolarization process within the myocardial cell is due to the efflux of intracellular potassium. The channels associated with this current can be blocked by many drugs and predisposes the electrical propagation cycle to torsade de pointes.

Disopyramide is one of the drugs confirmed to prolong the QT interval and is accepted as having a risk of causing torsade de pointes. The risk of drug-induced torsade de pointes is extremely low when a single QT interval prolonging drug is prescribed. In terms of epinephrine, it is not known what effect vasoconstrictors in the local anesthetic regimen will have in patients with a known history of congenital prolonged QT interval or in patients taking any medication that prolongs the QT interval. Until more information is obtained, it is suggested that the clinician consult with the physician prior to the use of a vasoconstrictor in suspected patients, and that the vasoconstrictor (epinephrine, levonordefrin [Neo-Cobefrin®]) be used with caution.

Disopyramide Phosphate *see* Disopyramide *on page 491*
DisperMox™ [DSC] *see* Amoxicillin *on page 106*

Disulfiram *(dye SUL fi ram)*

U.S. Brand Names Antabuse®
Generic Available No
Pharmacologic Category Aldehyde Dehydrogenase Inhibitor
Use Management of chronic alcoholism
Local Anesthetic/Vasoconstrictor Precautions No information available to require special precautions
Effects on Dental Treatment No significant effects or complications reported
Common Adverse Effects Frequency not defined.
Central nervous system: Drowsiness, headache, fatigue, psychosis
Dermatologic: Rash, acneiform eruptions, allergic dermatitis
Gastrointestinal: Metallic or garlic-like aftertaste
Genitourinary: Impotence
Hepatic: Hepatitis (cholestatic and fulminant), hepatic failure (multiple case reports)
Neuromuscular & skeletal: Peripheral neuritis, polyneuritis, peripheral neuropathy
Ocular: Optic neuritis

Mechanism of Action Disulfiram is a thiuram derivative which interferes with aldehyde dehydrogenase. When taken concomitantly with alcohol, there is an increase in serum acetaldehyde levels. High acetaldehyde causes uncomfortable symptoms including flushing, nausea, thirst, palpitations, chest pain, vertigo, and hypotension. This reaction is the basis for disulfiram use in postwithdrawal long-term care of alcoholism.

Drug Interactions
Cytochrome P450 Effect: Substrate (minor) of CYP1A2, 2A6, 2B6, 2D6, 2E1, 3A4; **Inhibits** CYP1A2 (weak), 2A6 (weak), 2B6 (weak), 2C9 (weak), 2D6 (weak), 2E1 (strong), 3A4 (weak)

Increased Effect/Toxicity: Disulfiram results in severe ethanol intolerance (disulfiram reaction) secondary to disulfiram's ability to inhibit aldehyde dehydrogenase; this combination should be avoided. Combined use with isoniazid, metronidazole, or MAO inhibitors may result in adverse CNS effects; this combination should be avoided. Some pharmaceutic dosage forms include ethanol, including elixirs and intravenous trimethoprim-sulfamethoxazole (contains 10% ethanol as a solubilizing agent); these may inadvertently provoke a disulfiram reaction. Disulfiram may increase the levels/effects of inhalational anesthetics, trimethadione, and other CYP2E1 substrates. Disulfiram may increase serum concentrations of benzodiazepines that undergo oxidative metabolism (all but oxazepam, lorazepam, temazepam). Disulfiram increases phenytoin and theophylline serum concentrations; toxicity may occur. Disulfiram inhibits the metabolism of warfarin resulting in an increased hypoprothrombinemic response.

Pharmacodynamics/Kinetics
Onset of action: Full effect: 12 hours
Duration: ~1-2 weeks after last dose
Absorption: Rapid
Metabolism: To diethylthiocarbamate
Excretion: Feces and exhaled gases (as metabolites)

Pregnancy Risk Factor C

Dithioglycerol see Dimercaprol on page 482

Dithranol see Anthralin on page 128

Ditropan® see Oxybutynin on page 1162

Ditropan® XL see Oxybutynin on page 1162

Diuril® see Chlorothiazide on page 322

Divalproex Sodium see Valproic Acid and Derivatives on page 1556

5071-1DL(6) see Megestrol on page 976

dl-Alpha Tocopherol see Vitamin E on page 1581

4-DMDR see Idarubicin on page 814

DNA-Derived Humanized Monoclonal Antibody see Alemtuzumab on page 63

DNase see Dornase Alfa on page 501

DNR see DAUNOrubicin Hydrochloride on page 426

Doak® Tar [OTC] see Coal Tar on page 383

Doan's® [OTC] see Magnesium Salicylate on page 962

Doan's® Extra Strength [OTC] see Magnesium Salicylate on page 962

DOBUTamine (doe BYOO ta meen)

Related Information
Cardiovascular Diseases on page 1636
Canadian Brand Names Dobutrex®
Mexican Brand Names Dobuject®; Dobutrex®; Oxiken®
Generic Available Yes
Synonyms Dobutamine Hydrochloride
Pharmacologic Category Adrenergic Agonist Agent
Use Short-term management of patients with cardiac decompensation
Unlabeled/Investigational Use Positive inotropic agent for use in myocardial dysfunction of sepsis
Local Anesthetic/Vasoconstrictor Precautions No information available to require special precautions
Effects on Dental Treatment No significant effects or complications reported
Common Adverse Effects Incidence of adverse events is not always reported.
Cardiovascular: Increased heart rate, increased blood pressure, increased ventricular ectopic activity, hypotension, premature ventricular beats (5%, dose related), anginal pain (1% to 3%), nonspecific chest pain (1% to 3%), palpitation (1% to 3%)
Central nervous system: Fever (1% to 3%), headache (1% to 3%), paresthesia
(Continued)

DOBUTamine *(Continued)*

Endocrine & metabolic: Slight decrease in serum potassium

Gastrointestinal: Nausea (1% to 3%)

Hematologic: Thrombocytopenia (isolated cases)

Local: Phlebitis, local inflammatory changes and pain from infiltration, cutaneous necrosis (isolated cases)

Neuromuscular & skeletal: Mild leg cramps

Respiratory: Dyspnea (1% to 3%)

Mechanism of Action Stimulates beta$_1$-adrenergic receptors, causing increased contractility and heart rate, with little effect on beta$_2$- or alpha-receptors

Drug Interactions

Increased Effect/Toxicity: General anesthetics (eg, halothane or cyclopropane) and usual doses of dobutamine have resulted in ventricular arrhythmias in animals. Bretylium and may potentiate dobutamine's effects. Beta-blockers (nonselective ones) may increase hypertensive effect; avoid concurrent use. Cocaine may cause malignant arrhythmias. Guanethidine, MAO inhibitors, methyldopa, reserpine, and tricyclic antidepressants can increase the pressor response to sympathomimetics.

Decreased Effect: Beta-adrenergic blockers may decrease effect of dobutamine and increase risk of severe hypotension.

Pharmacodynamics/Kinetics

Onset of action: I.V.: 1-10 minutes

Peak effect: 10-20 minutes

Metabolism: In tissues and hepatically to inactive metabolites

Half-life elimination: 2 minutes

Excretion: Urine (as metabolites)

Pregnancy Risk Factor B

Dobutamine Hydrochloride *see* DOBUTamine *on page 493*

Docetaxel *(doe se TAKS el)*

U.S. Brand Names Taxotere®

Canadian Brand Names Taxotere®

Generic Available No

Synonyms NSC-628503; RP-6976

Pharmacologic Category Antineoplastic Agent, Natural Source (Plant) Derivative

Use Second-line treatment of locally-advanced or metastatic breast cancer; adjuvant treatment of operable node-positive breast cancer (in combination with doxorubicin and cyclophosphamide); treatment of locally-advanced or metastatic nonsmall cell lung cancer (NSCLC) (single agent for failure of platinum based regimen; in combination with cisplatin in treatment of patients who have not previously received chemotherapy for unresected NSCLC); treatment of hormone refractory, metastatic prostate cancer; treatment (in combination with cisplatin and fluorouracil) for chemo-naïve advanced gastric adenocarcinoma

Unlabeled/Investigational Use Investigational: Treatment of pancreatic, head and neck, and ovarian cancers, soft tissue sarcoma, and melanoma

Local Anesthetic/Vasoconstrictor Precautions No information available to require special precautions

Effects on Dental Treatment Key adverse event(s) related to dental treatment: Mucositis, stomatitis, and taste perversion.

Common Adverse Effects Percentages reported for docetaxel monotherapy; frequency may vary depending on diagnosis, dose, liver function, prior treatment, and premedication. The incidence of adverse events was usually higher in patients with elevated liver function tests.

>10%:

Cardiovascular: Fluid retention (13% to 60%; dose dependent)

Central nervous system: Neurosensory events (20% to 58%; including neuropathy), fever (31% to 35%), neuromotor events (16%)

Dermatologic: Alopecia (74% to 76%), cutaneous events (20% to 48%), nail disorder (11% to 41%)

Gastrointestinal: Stomatitis (19% to 53%; severe 1% to 8%), diarrhea (23% to 43%; severe: 5% to 6%), nausea (34% to 42%), vomiting (22% to 23%)

Hematologic: Neutropenia (84% to 99%; grade 4: 75% to 86%; onset: 4-7 days, nadir: 5-9 days, recovery: 21 days; dose dependent), leukopenia (84% to 99%; grade 4: 32% to 44%), anemia (8% to 94%; dose dependent), thrombocytopenia (8% to 14%; grade 4: 1%; dose dependent), febrile neutropenia (6% to 12%; dose dependent)

Hepatic: Transaminases increased (4% to 19%)

Neuromuscular and skeletal: Weakness (53% to 66%; severe 13% to 18%), myalgia (3% to 23%)

Respiratory: Pulmonary events (41%)

Miscellaneous: Infection (1% to 33%; dose dependent), hypersensitivity (1% to 21%; with premedication 15%)

1% to 10%:

Cardiovascular: Hypotension (3%)

Dermatologic: Rash/erythema (2%)

Gastrointestinal: Taste perversion (6%)

Hepatic: Bilirubin increased (9%), alkaline phosphatase increased (4% to 7%)

Local: Infusion-site reactions (4%, including hyperpigmentation, inflammation, redness, dryness, phlebitis, extravasation, swelling of the vein)

Neuromuscular and skeletal: Arthralgia (3% to 9%)

Ocular: Epiphora associated with canalicular stenosis (up to 77% with weekly administration; up to 1% with every-3-week administration)

Mechanism of Action Docetaxel promotes the assembly of microtubules from tubulin dimers, and inhibits the depolymerization of tubulin which stabilizes microtubules in the cell. This results in inhibition of DNA, RNA, and protein synthesis. Most activity occurs during the M phase of the cell cycle.

Drug Interactions

Cytochrome P450 Effect: Substrate of CYP3A4 (major); **Inhibits** CYP3A4 (weak)

Increased Effect/Toxicity: CYP3A4 inhibitors may increase the levels/ effects of docetaxel; example inhibitors include azole antifungals, clarithromycin, diclofenac, doxycycline, erythromycin, imatinib, isoniazid, nefazodone, nicardipine, propofol, protease inhibitors, quinidine, telithromycin, and verapamil. When administered as sequential infusions, observational studies indicate a potential for increased toxicity when platinum derivatives (carboplatin, cisplatin) are administered before taxane derivatives (docetaxel, paclitaxel).

Decreased Effect: CYP3A4 inducers may decrease the levels/effects of docetaxel; example inducers include aminoglutethimide, carbamazepine, nafcillin, nevirapine, phenobarbital, phenytoin, and rifamycins.

Pharmacodynamics/Kinetics Exhibits linear pharmacokinetics at the recommended dosage range

Distribution: Extensive extravascular distribution and/or tissue binding; V_d: 80-90 L/m^2, V_{dss}: 113 L (mean steady state)

Protein binding: >94%, primarily to alpha$_1$-acid glycoprotein, albumin, and lipoproteins

Metabolism: Hepatic; oxidation via CYP3A4 to metabolites

Half-life elimination: Terminal: 11 hours

Excretion: Feces (75%); urine (6%); ~80% within 48 hours

Clearance: Total body: Mean: 21 L/hour/m^2

Pregnancy Risk Factor D

Docosanol (doe KOE san ole)

Related Sample Prescriptions

Herpes Simplex (Recurrent) *on page 1742*

U.S. Brand Names Abreva® [OTC]

Generic Available No

Synonyms Behenyl Alcohol; *n*-Docosanol

Pharmacologic Category Antiviral Agent, Topical

Dental Use Treatment of herpes simplex of the face or lips

Use Treatment of herpes simplex of the face or lips

Local Anesthetic/Vasoconstrictor Precautions No information available to require special precautions

Effects on Dental Treatment No significant effects or complications reported (see Dental Comment)

Significant Adverse Effects Limited information; headache reported (frequency similar to placebo)

Dental Usual Dosing Herpes simplex (face/lips): Children ≥12 years and Adults: Topical: Apply 5 times/day to affected area of face or lips. Start at first sign of cold sore or fever blister and continue until healed.

Dosage Children ≥12 years and Adults: Topical: Apply 5 times/day to affected area of face or lips. Start at first sign of cold sore or fever blister and continue until healed.

Mechanism of Action Prevents viral entry and replication at the cellular level

Contraindications Hypersensitivity to docosanol or any component of the formulation

(Continued)

Docosanol *(Continued)*

Warnings/Precautions For external use only. Do not apply to inside of mouth or around eyes. Not for use in children <12 years of age.

Dosage Forms Cream: 10% (2 g)

Dental Comment Wash hands before and after applying cream. Begin treatment at first tingle of cold sore or fever blister. Rub into area gently, but completely. Do not apply directly to inside of mouth or around eyes. Contact healthcare provider if sore gets worse or does not heal within 10 days. Do not share this product with others, may spread infection. Notify healthcare professional if pregnant or breast-feeding.

Docusate *(DOK yoo sate)*

U.S. Brand Names Colace® [OTC]; Diocto® [OTC]; Docusoft-S™ [OTC]; DOK™ [OTC]; DOS® [OTC]; D-S-S® [OTC]; Dulcolax® Stool Softener [OTC]; Enemeez® [OTC]; Fleet® Sof-Lax® [OTC]; Genasoft® [OTC]; Phillips'® Stool Softener Laxative [OTC]; Silace [OTC]; Surfak® [OTC]

Canadian Brand Names Apo-Docusate-Calcium®; Apo-Docusate-Sodium®; Colace®; Colax-C®; Novo-Docusate Calcium; Novo-Docusate Sodium; PMS-Docusate Calcium; PMS-Docusate Sodium; Regulex®; Selax®; Soflax™

Generic Available Yes: Excludes gelcap

Synonyms Dioctyl Calcium Sulfosuccinate; Dioctyl Sodium Sulfosuccinate; Docusate Calcium; Docusate Potassium; Docusate Sodium; DOSS; DSS

Pharmacologic Category Stool Softener

Use Stool softener in patients who should avoid straining during defecation and constipation associated with hard, dry stools; prophylaxis for straining (Valsalva) following myocardial infarction. A safe agent to be used in elderly; some evidence that doses <200 mg are ineffective; stool softeners are unnecessary if stool is well hydrated or "mushy" and soft; shown to be ineffective used long-term.

Unlabeled/Investigational Use Ceruminolytic

Local Anesthetic/Vasoconstrictor Precautions No information available to require special precautions

Effects on Dental Treatment Key adverse event(s) related to dental treatment: Throat irritation.

Common Adverse Effects 1% to 10%:
Gastrointestinal: Intestinal obstruction, diarrhea, abdominal cramping
Miscellaneous: Throat irritation

Mechanism of Action Reduces surface tension of the oil-water interface of the stool resulting in enhanced incorporation of water and fat allowing for stool softening

Pharmacodynamics/Kinetics
Onset of action: 12-72 hours
Excretion: Feces

Pregnancy Risk Factor C

Docusate and Casanthranol *(DOK yoo sate & ka SAN thra nole)*

Related Information
Docusate *on page 496*

U.S. Brand Names Diocto C® [DSC] [OTC]; Docusoft Plus™ [DSC] [OTC]; Doxidan® [DSC] [OTC]; Fleet® Sof-Lax® Overnight [DSC] [OTC]; Genasoft® Plus [DSC] [OTC]; Peri-Colace® [DSC] [OTC]

Generic Available No

Synonyms Casanthranol and Docusate; DSS With Casanthranol

Pharmacologic Category Laxative/Stool Softener

Use Treatment of constipation generally associated with dry, hard stools and decreased intestinal motility

Local Anesthetic/Vasoconstrictor Precautions No information available to require special precautions

Effects on Dental Treatment Key adverse event(s) related to dental treatment: Throat irritation.

Common Adverse Effects 1% to 10%:
Dermatologic: Rash
Gastrointestinal: Intestinal obstruction, diarrhea, abdominal cramping, throat irritation

Pregnancy Risk Factor C

Docusate Calcium *see* Docusate *on page 496*
Docusate Potassium *see* Docusate *on page 496*

Docusate Sodium *see* Docusate *on page 496*

Docusoft Plus™ [DSC] [OTC] *see* Docusate and Casanthranol *on page 496*

Docusoft-S™ [OTC] *see* Docusate *on page 496*

Dofetilide (doe FET il ide)

Related Information
Cardiovascular Diseases *on page 1636*

U.S. Brand Names Tikosyn™

Canadian Brand Names Tikosyn™

Generic Available No

Pharmacologic Category Antiarrhythmic Agent, Class III

Use Maintenance of normal sinus rhythm in patients with chronic atrial fibrillation/atrial flutter of longer than 1-week duration who have been converted to normal sinus rhythm; conversion of atrial fibrillation and atrial flutter to normal sinus rhythm

Local Anesthetic/Vasoconstrictor Precautions No information available to require special precautions (see Dental Comment)

Effects on Dental Treatment No significant effects or complications reported

Common Adverse Effects

Supraventricular arrhythmia patients (incidence > placebo)

>10%: Central nervous system: Headache (11%)

2% to 10%:
Central nervous system: Dizziness (8%), insomnia (4%)
Cardiovascular: Ventricular tachycardia (2.6% to 3.7%), chest pain (10%), torsade de pointes (3.3% in CHF patients and 0.9% in patients with a recent MI; up to 10.5% in patients receiving doses in excess of those recommended). Torsade de pointes occurs most frequently within the first 3 days of therapy.
Dermatologic: Rash (3%)
Gastrointestinal: Nausea (5%), diarrhea (3%), abdominal pain (3%)
Neuromuscular & skeletal: Back pain (3%)
Respiratory: Dyspnea (6%), respiratory tract infection (7%)
Miscellaneous: Flu syndrome (4%)

<2%:
Central nervous system: CVA, facial paralysis, flaccid paralysis, migraine, paralysis
Cardiovascular: AV block (0.4% to 1.5%), ventricular fibrillation (0% to 0.4%), bundle branch block, heart block, edema, heart arrest, myocardial infarct, sudden death, syncope
Dermatologic: Angioedema
Gastrointestinal: Liver damage
Neuromuscular & skeletal: Paresthesia
Respiratory: Cough

>2% (incidence ≤ placebo): Anxiety, pain, angina, atrial fibrillation, hypertension, palpitation, supraventricular tachycardia, peripheral edema, urinary tract infection, weakness, arthralgia, diaphoresis

Mechanism of Action Vaughan Williams Class III antiarrhythmic activity. Blockade of the cardiac ion channel carrying the rapid component of the delayed rectifier potassium current. Dofetilide has no effect on sodium channels, adrenergic alpha-receptors, or adrenergic beta-receptors. It increases the monophasic action potential duration due to delayed repolarization. The increase in the QT interval is a function of prolongation of both effective and functional refractory periods in the His-Purkinje system and the ventricles. Changes in cardiac conduction velocity and sinus node function have not been observed in patients with or without structural heart disease. PR and QRS width remain the same in patients with pre-existing heart block and or sick sinus syndrome.

Drug Interactions
Cytochrome P450 Effect: Substrate of CYP3A4 (minor)

Increased Effect/Toxicity: Dofetilide concentrations are increased by cimetidine, verapamil, hydrochlorothiazide, ketoconazole, and trimethoprim (concurrent use of these agents is contraindicated). Dofetilide levels may also be increased by renal cationic transport inhibitors (including triamterene, metformin, amiloride, and megestrol). Diuretics and other drugs which may deplete potassium and/or magnesium (aminoglycoside antibiotics, amphotericin, cyclosporine) may increase dofetilide's toxicity (torsade de pointes); concurrent use of hydrochlorothiazide is contraindicated. Use of QT_c-prolonging agents (including bepridil, cisapride, clarithromycin, erythromycin, tricyclic antidepressants, phenothiazines, sparfloxacin, gatifloxacin, (Continued)

Dofetilide *(Continued)*

moxifloxacin) is contraindicated. Itraconazole may decrease the metabolism of dofetilide (concurrent use is contraindicated).

Pharmacodynamics/Kinetics

Absorption: >90%

Distribution: V_d: 3 L/kg

Protein binding: 60% to 70%

Metabolism: Hepatic via CYP3A4, but low affinity for it; metabolites formed by N-dealkylation and N-oxidation

Bioavailability: >90%

Half-life elimination: 10 hours

Time to peak: Fasting: 2-3 hours

Excretion: Urine (80%, 80% as unchanged drug, 20% as inactive or minimally active metabolites); renal elimination consists of glomerular filtration and active tubular secretion via cationic transport system

Pregnancy Risk Factor C

Dental Comment

This drug is known to prolong the QT interval. The QT interval is measured as the time and distance between the Q point of the QRS complex and the end of the T wave in the ECG tracing. After adjustment for heart rate, the QT interval is defined as prolonged if it is more than 450 msec in men and 460 msec in women. A long QT syndrome was first described in the 1950s and 60s as a congenital syndrome involving QT interval prolongation and syncope and sudden death. Some of the congenital long QT syndromes were characterized by a peculiar electrocardiographic appearance of the QRS complex involving a premature atria beat followed by a pause, then a subsequent sinus beat showing marked QT prolongation and deformity. This type of cardiac arrhythmia was originally termed "torsade de pointes" (translated from the French as "twisting of the points").

Prolongation of the QT interval is thought to result from delayed ventricular repolarization. The repolarization process within the myocardial cell is due to the efflux of intracellular potassium. The channels associated with this current can be blocked by many drugs and predisposes the electrical propagation cycle to torsade de pointes.

Dofetilide is one of the drugs confirmed to prolong the QT interval and is accepted as having a risk of causing torsade de pointes. The risk of drug-induced torsade de pointes is extremely low when a single QT interval prolonging drug is prescribed. In terms of epinephrine, it is not known what effect vasoconstrictors in the local anesthetic regimen will have in patients with a known history of congenital prolonged QT interval or in patients taking any medication that prolongs the QT interval. Until more information is obtained, it is suggested that the clinician consult the physician prior to the use of a vasoconstrictor in suspected patients, and that the vasoconstrictor (epinephrine, levonordefrin [Neo-Cobefrin®]) be used with caution.

Dofus [OTC] *see Lactobacillus on page 535*

DOK™ [OTC] *see Docusate on page 496*

Dolasetron *(dol A se tron)*

U.S. Brand Names Anzemet®

Canadian Brand Names Anzemet®

Mexican Brand Names Anzemet®

Generic Available No

Synonyms Dolasetron Mesylate; MDL 73,147EF

Pharmacologic Category Antiemetic; Selective 5-HT$_3$ Receptor Antagonist

Use Prevention of nausea and vomiting associated with emetogenic cancer chemotherapy; prevention of postoperative nausea and vomiting; treatment of postoperative nausea and vomiting (injectable form only)

Not recommended for treatment of existing chemotherapy-induced emesis (CIE).

Local Anesthetic/Vasoconstrictor Precautions No information available to require special precautions (see Dental Comment)

Effects on Dental Treatment Key adverse event(s) related to dental treatment: Taste alterations.

Common Adverse Effects Adverse events may vary according to indication

>10%:

Central nervous system: Headache (7% to 24%)

Gastrointestinal: Diarrhea (2% to 12%)

1% to 10%:
Cardiovascular: Bradycardia (5%), hypotension (5%), hypertension (2% to 3%), tachycardia (2% to 3%)
Central nervous system: Dizziness (1% to 6%), fatigue (3% to 6%), fever (3% to 5%), chills/shivering (1% to 2%), sedation (2%)
Dermatological: Pruritus (3% to 4%)
Gastrointestinal: Dyspepsia (2% to 3%), abdominal pain (3%)
Hepatic: Abnormal hepatic function (4%)
Neuromuscular & skeletal: Pain (3%)
Renal: Oliguria (1% to 3%), urinary retention (2%)

Mechanism of Action Selective serotonin receptor (5-HT$_3$) antagonist, blocking serotonin both peripherally (primary site of action) and centrally at the chemoreceptor trigger zone

Drug Interactions

Cytochrome P450 Effect: **Substrate** (minor) of CYP2C9, 3A4; **Inhibits** CYP2D6 (weak)

Increased Effect/Toxicity: Due to reports of profound hypotension during concomitant therapy with ondansetron, the manufacturer of apomorphine contraindicates its use with all 5-HT$_3$ antagonists. Use caution with QT$_c$-prolonging agents (includes but may not be limited to amitriptyline, bepridil, disopyramide, erythromycin, haloperidol, imipramine, quinidine, pimozide, procainamide, sotalol, and thioridazine); effect/toxicity of dolasetron and other QT$_c$-prolonging agents may be increased

Decreased Effect: Blood levels of active metabolite are decreased during coadministration of rifampin.

Pharmacodynamics/Kinetics

Absorption: Rapid and complete

Distribution: 5.8 L/kg

Protein binding: Hydrodolasetron: 69% to 77% (50% bound to alpha$_1$-acid glycoprotein)

Metabolism: Hepatic; reduction by carbonyl reductase to hydrodolasetron (active metabolite); further metabolized by CYP3A and flavin monooxygenase

Bioavailability: 75%

Half-life elimination: Dolasetron: 10 minutes; hydrodolasetron: Adults: 6-8 hours; Children: 4-6 hours

Time to peak, plasma: I.V.: 0.6 hours; Oral: 1 hour

Excretion: Urine ~67% (53% to 61% as active metabolite hydrodolasetron); feces ~33%

Pregnancy Risk Factor B

Dental Comment

This drug is known to prolong the QT interval. The QT interval is measured as the time and distance between the Q point of the QRS complex and the end of the T wave in the ECG tracing. After adjustment for heart rate, the QT interval is defined as prolonged if it is more than 450 msec in men and 460 msec in women. A long QT syndrome was first described in the 1950s and 60s as a congenital syndrome involving QT interval prolongation and syncope and sudden death. Some of the congenital long QT syndromes were characterized by a peculiar electrocardiographic appearance of the QRS complex involving a premature atria beat followed by a pause, then a subsequent sinus beat showing marked QT prolongation and deformity. This type of cardiac arrhythmia was originally termed "torsade de pointes" (translated from the French as "twisting of the points").

Prolongation of the QT interval is thought to result from delayed ventricular repolarization. The repolarization process within the myocardial cell is due to the efflux of intracellular potassium. The channels associated with this current can be blocked by many drugs and predisposes the electrical propagation cycle to torsade de pointes.

Dolasetron is one of the drugs confirmed to prolong the QT interval and is accepted as having a risk of causing torsade de pointes. The risk of drug-induced torsade de pointes is extremely low when a single QT interval prolonging drug is prescribed. In terms of epinephrine, it is not known what effect vasoconstrictors in the local anesthetic regimen will have in patients with a known history of congenital prolonged QT interval or in patients taking any medication that prolongs the QT interval. Until more information is obtained, it is suggested that the clinician consult with the physician prior to the use of a vasoconstrictor in suspected patients, and that the vasoconstrictor (epinephrine, levonordefrin [Neo-Cobefrin®]) be used with caution.

Dolasetron Mesylate *see* Dolasetron *on page 498*

Dolgic® LQ *see* Butalbital, Acetaminophen, and Caffeine *on page 239*

Dolgic® Plus *see* Butalbital, Acetaminophen, and Caffeine *on page 239*

Dolobid® [DSC] *see* Diflunisal *on page 468*

Dolophine® *see* Methadone *on page 1004*

Domeboro® [OTC] *see* Aluminum Sulfate and Calcium Acetate *on page 81*

Dome Paste Bandage *see* Zinc Gelatin *on page 1597*

Donepezil (doh NEP e zil)

U.S. Brand Names Aricept®; Aricept® ODT

Canadian Brand Names Aricept®

Mexican Brand Names Eranz®

Generic Available No

Synonyms E2020

Pharmacologic Category Acetylcholinesterase Inhibitor (Central)

Use Treatment of mild to moderate dementia of the Alzheimer's type

Unlabeled/Investigational Use Attention-deficit/hyperactivity disorder (ADHD), behavioral syndromes in dementia

Local Anesthetic/Vasoconstrictor Precautions No information available to require special precautions

Effects on Dental Treatment No significant effects or complications reported

Common Adverse Effects

>10%:

Central nervous system: Insomnia (6% to 14%)

Gastrointestinal: Nausea (5% to 19%), diarrhea (8% to 15%)

1% to 10%:

Cardiovascular: Syncope (2%), chest pain, hyper-/hypotension, atrial fibrillation, hot flashes

Central nervous system: Abnormal dreams (3%), depression (3%), dizziness (8%), fatigue (3% to 8%), headache (10%), somnolence

Dermatologic: Bruising (4%), pruritus, urticaria

Endocrine & metabolic: Dehydration

Gastrointestinal: Anorexia (3% to 7%), vomiting (3% to 8%), weight loss (3%), fecal incontinence, GI bleeding, bloating, epigastric pain, toothache

Genitourinary: Frequent urination (2%), urinary incontinence, nocturia

Neuromuscular & skeletal: Muscle cramps (3% to 8%), arthritis (2%), body pain, bone fracture

Ocular: Blurred vision, cataract, eye irritation

Respiratory: Influenza, dyspnea, bronchitis

Miscellaneous: Diaphoresis

Mechanism of Action Alzheimer's disease is characterized by cholinergic deficiency in the cortex and basal forebrain, which contributes to cognitive deficits. Donepezil reversibly and noncompetitively inhibits centrally-active acetylcholinesterase, the enzyme responsible for hydrolysis of acetylcholine. This appears to result in increased concentrations of acetylcholine available for synaptic transmission in the central nervous system.

Drug Interactions

Cytochrome P450 Effect: Substrate (minor) of CYP2D6, 3A4

Increased Effect/Toxicity: A synergistic effect may be seen with concurrent administration of succinylcholine or cholinergic agonists (bethanechol).

Decreased Effect: Anticholinergic agents (benztropine) may inhibit the effects of donepezil. Acetylcholinesterase inhibitors (central) may increase the risk of antipsychotic-related extrapyramidal symptoms.

Pharmacodynamics/Kinetics

Absorption: Well absorbed

Protein binding: 96%, primarily to albumin (75%) and α_1-acid glycoprotein (21%)

Metabolism: Extensively to four major metabolites (two are active) via CYP2D6 and 3A4; undergoes glucuronidation

Bioavailability: 100%

Half-life elimination: 70 hours; time to steady-state: 15 days

Time to peak, plasma: 3-4 hours

Excretion: Urine 57% (17% as unchanged drug); feces 15%

Pregnancy Risk Factor C

Donnatal® *see* Hyoscyamine, Atropine, Scopolamine, and Phenobarbital *on page 804*

Donnatal Extentabs® *see* Hyoscyamine, Atropine, Scopolamine, and Phenobarbital *on page 804*

Dopram® *see* Doxapram *on page 502*

Doral® *see* Quazepam *on page 1318*

Dornase Alfa (DOOR nase AL fa)

U.S. Brand Names Pulmozyme®
Canadian Brand Names Pulmozyme™
Mexican Brand Names Pulmozyme®
Generic Available No
Synonyms DNase; Recombinant Human Deoxyribonuclease
Pharmacologic Category Enzyme
Use Management of cystic fibrosis patients to reduce the frequency of respiratory infections that require parenteral antibiotics, and to improve pulmonary function
Unlabeled/Investigational Use Treatment of chronic bronchitis
Local Anesthetic/Vasoconstrictor Precautions No information available to require special precautions
Effects on Dental Treatment Key adverse event(s) related to dental treatment: Pharyngitis.
Common Adverse Effects
>10%:
    Respiratory: Pharyngitis
    Miscellaneous: Voice alteration
1% to 10%:
    Cardiovascular: Chest pain
    Dermatologic: Rash
    Ocular: Conjunctivitis
    Respiratory: Laryngitis, cough, dyspnea, hemoptysis, rhinitis, hoarse throat, wheezing
Mechanism of Action The hallmark of cystic fibrosis lung disease is the presence of abundant, purulent airway secretions composed primarily of highly polymerized DNA. The principal source of this DNA is the nuclei of degenerating neutrophils, which is present in large concentrations in infected lung secretions. The presence of this DNA produces a viscous mucous that may contribute to the decreased mucociliary transport and persistent infections that are commonly seen in this population. Dornase alfa is a deoxyribonuclease (DNA) enzyme produced by recombinant gene technology. Dornase selectively cleaves DNA, thus reducing mucous viscosity and as a result, airflow in the lung is improved and the risk of bacterial infection may be decreased.
Pharmacodynamics/Kinetics
Onset of action: Nebulization: Enzyme levels are measured in sputum in ~15 minutes
Duration: Rapidly declines
Pregnancy Risk Factor B

Doryx® see Doxycycline (Systemic) on page 514

Dorzolamide (dor ZOLE a mide)

U.S. Brand Names Trusopt®
Canadian Brand Names Trusopt®
Generic Available No
Synonyms Dorzolamide Hydrochloride
Pharmacologic Category Carbonic Anhydrase Inhibitor; Ophthalmic Agent, Antiglaucoma
Use Lowers intraocular pressure in patients with ocular hypertension or open-angle glaucoma
Local Anesthetic/Vasoconstrictor Precautions No information available to require special precautions
Effects on Dental Treatment No significant effects or complications reported
Mechanism of Action Reversible inhibition of the enzyme carbonic anhydrase resulting in reduction of hydrogen ion secretion at renal tubule and an increased renal excretion of sodium, potassium, bicarbonate, and water to decrease production of aqueous humor; also inhibits carbonic anhydrase in central nervous system to retard abnormal and excessive discharge from CNS neurons
Pregnancy Risk Factor C

Dorzolamide and Timolol (dor ZOLE a mide & TYE moe lole)

Related Information
Dorzolamide on page 501
Timolol on page 1489
(Continued)

Dorzolamide and Timolol *(Continued)*

U.S. Brand Names Cosopt®

Canadian Brand Names Cosopt®

Generic Available No

Synonyms Timolol and Dorzolamide

Pharmacologic Category Beta-Adrenergic Blocker; Carbonic Anhydrase Inhibitor

Use Reduction of intraocular pressure in patients with ocular hypertension or open-angle glaucoma

Local Anesthetic/Vasoconstrictor Precautions No information available to require special precautions

Effects on Dental Treatment No significant effects or complications reported

Common Adverse Effects Percentages as reported with combination product. Also see individual agents.

>5%:

Gastrointestinal: Taste perversion (≤30%)

Ocular: Burning/stinging (≤30%), conjunctival hyperemia (5% to 15%), blurred vision (5% to 15%), superficial punctuate keratitis (5% to 15%), itching (5% to 15%)

1% to 5%:

Cardiovascular: Hypertension

Central nervous system: Dizziness, headache

Gastrointestinal: Abdominal pain, dyspepsia, nausea

Genitourinary: UTI

Neuromuscular & skeletal: Back pain

Ocular: Blepharitis, cloudy vision, conjunctival discharge, conjunctival edema, conjunctival follicles, conjunctivitis, corneal erosion, corneal staining, cortical lens opacity, dryness, eye debris, eye/eyelid discharge, eye/eyelid pain, eye debris, eye/eyelid discharge, eye/eyelid pain, tearing, eyelid edema, eyelid erythema, foreign body sensation, glaucomatous cupping, lens nucleus discoloration, lens opacity, post-capsular cataract, tearing, visual field defect, vitreous detachment

Respiratory: Bronchitis, cough, sinusitis, URTI

Miscellaneous: Flu

Drug Interactions

Cytochrome P450 Effect:

Dorzolamide: **Substrate** (minor) of CYP2C8/9, 3A4

Timolol: **Substrate** of CYP2D6 (major); **Inhibits** CYP2D6 (weak)

Increased Effect/Toxicity: See individual agents.

Decreased Effect: See individual agents.

Pharmacodynamics/Kinetics See individual agents.

Pregnancy Risk Factor C

Dorzolamide Hydrochloride see Dorzolamide on page 501

DOS® [OTC] see Docusate on page 496

DOSS see Docusate on page 496

Dostinex® see Cabergoline on page 244

Dovonex® see Calcipotriene on page 246

Doxapram *(DOKS a pram)*

U.S. Brand Names Dopram®

Generic Available Yes

Synonyms Doxapram Hydrochloride

Pharmacologic Category Respiratory Stimulant; Stimulant

Use Respiratory and CNS stimulant for respiratory depression secondary to anesthesia, drug-induced CNS depression; acute hypercapnia secondary to COPD

Local Anesthetic/Vasoconstrictor Precautions No information available to require special precautions

Effects on Dental Treatment No significant effects or complications reported

Common Adverse Effects Frequency not defined.

Cardiovascular: Arrhythmia, blood pressure increased, chest pain, chest tightness, flushing, heart rate changes, T waves lowered, ventricular tachycardia, ventricular fibrillation

Central nervous system: Apprehension, Babinski turns positive, disorientation, dizziness, hallucinations, headache, hyperactivity, pyrexia, seizure

Dermatologic: Burning sensation, pruritus

Gastrointestinal: Defecation urge, diarrhea, nausea, vomiting

Genitourinary: Spontaneous voiding, urinary retention

Hematologic: Hematocrit decreased, hemoglobin decreased, hemolysis, red blood cell count decreased

Local: Phlebitis

Neuromuscular & skeletal: Clonus, deep tendon reflexes increase, fasciculations, involuntary muscle movement, muscle spasm, paresthesia

Ocular: Pupillary dilatation

Renal: Albuminuria, BUN increased

Respiratory: Bronchospasm, cough, dyspnea, hiccups, hyperventilation, laryngospasm, rebound hypoventilation, tachypnea

Miscellaneous: Diaphoresis

Mechanism of Action Stimulates respiration through action on respiratory center in medulla or indirectly on peripheral carotid chemoreceptors

Drug Interactions

Increased Effect/Toxicity: Increased blood pressure with sympathomimetics, MAO inhibitors. Halothane, cyclopropane, and enflurane may sensitize the myocardium to catecholamine and epinephrine which is released at the initiation of doxapram, hence, separate discontinuation of anesthetics and start of doxapram until the volatile agent has been excreted.

Pharmacodynamics/Kinetics

Onset of action: Respiratory stimulation: I.V.: 20-40 seconds

Peak effect: 1-2 minutes

Duration: 5-12 minutes

Half-life elimination, serum: Adults: Mean: 3.4 hours

Pregnancy Risk Factor B

Doxapram Hydrochloride *see* Doxapram *on page 502*

Doxazosin (doks AY zoe sin)

Related Information

Cardiovascular Diseases *on page 1636*

U.S. Brand Names Cardura®; Cardura® XL

Canadian Brand Names Alti-Doxazosin; Apo-Doxazosin®; Cardura-1™; Cardura-2™; Cardura-4™; Gen-Doxazosin; Novo-Doxazosin

Mexican Brand Names Cardura®

Generic Available Yes: Immediate release tablet

Synonyms Doxazosin Mesylate

Pharmacologic Category Alpha₁ Blocker

Use Treatment of hypertension alone or in conjunction with diuretics, ACE inhibitors, or calcium antagonists; treatment of urinary outflow obstruction and/or obstructive and irritative symptoms associated with benign prostatic hyperplasia (BPH), particularly useful in patients with troublesome symptoms who are unable or unwilling to undergo invasive procedures, but who require rapid symptomatic relief; can be used in combination with finasteride

Local Anesthetic/Vasoconstrictor Precautions No information available to require special precautions

Effects on Dental Treatment Key adverse event(s) related to dental treatment: Xerostomia (normal salivary flow resumes upon discontinuation) and orthostatic hypotension.

Common Adverse Effects Note: Type and frequency of adverse reactions reflect combined data from trials with immediate release and extended release products.

>10%: Central nervous system: Dizziness (5% to 19%), headache (5% to 14%)

1% to 10%:

Cardiovascular: Orthostatic hypotension (dose related; 0.3% up to 2%), edema (3% to 4%), hypotension (2%), palpitation (1% to 2%), chest pain (1% to 2%), arrhythmia (1%), syncope (1%), flushing (1%)

Central nervous system: Fatigue (8% to 12%), somnolence (1% to 5%), nervousness (2%), pain (2%), vertigo (2% to 4%), insomnia (1%), anxiety (1%), paresthesia (1%), movement disorder (1%), ataxia (1%), hypertonia (1%), depression (1%)

Dermatologic: Rash (1%), pruritus (1%)

Endocrine & metabolic: Sexual dysfunction (2%)

Gastrointestinal: Abdominal pain (2%), diarrhea (2%), dyspepsia (1% to 2%), nausea (1% to 3%), xerostomia (1% to 2%), constipation (1%), flatulence (1%)

Genitourinary: Urinary tract infection (1%), impotence (1%), polyuria (2%), incontinence (1%)

Neuromuscular & skeletal: Back pain (2% to 3%), weakness (1% to 7%), arthritis (1%), muscle weakness (1%), myalgia (≤1%), muscle cramps (1%)

Ocular: Abnormal vision (1% to 2%), conjunctivitis (1%)

Otic: Tinnitus (1%)

(Continued)

Doxazosin *(Continued)*

Respiratory: Respiratory tract infection (5%), rhinitis (3%), dyspnea (1% to 3%), respiratory disorder (1%), epistaxis (1%)

Miscellaneous: Diaphoresis increased (1%), flu-like syndrome (1%)

Dosage Oral: Adults:

Immediate release: 1 mg once daily in morning or evening; may be increased to 2 mg once daily. Thereafter titrate upwards, if needed, over several weeks, balancing therapeutic benefit with doxazosin-induced postural hypotension. In the elderly, initiate at 0.5 mg once daily

Hypertension: Maximum dose: 16 mg/day

BPH: Goal: 4-8 mg/day; maximum dose: 8 mg/day

Extended release: BPH: 4 mg once daily with breakfast; titrate based on response and tolerability every 3-4 weeks to maximum recommended dose of 8 mg/day

Reinitiation of therapy: If therapy is discontinued for several days, restart at 4 mg dose and titrate as before.

Conversion to extended release from immediate release: Initiate with 4 mg once daily; omit final evening dose of immediate release prior to starting morning dosing with extended release product.

Dosing adjustment in hepatic impairment: Use with caution in mild-to-moderate hepatic dysfunction. Do not use with severe impairment.

Mechanism of Action

Hypertension: Competitively inhibits postsynaptic alpha1-adrenergic receptors which results in vasodilation of veins and arterioles and a decrease in total peripheral resistance and blood pressure; ~50% as potent on a weight by weight basis as prazosin.

BPH: Competitively inhibits postsynaptic alpha$_1$-adrenergic receptors in prostatic stromal and bladder neck tissues. This reduces the sympathetic tone-induced urethral stricture causing BPH symptoms.

Contraindications Hypersensitivity to quinazolines (prazosin, terazosin), doxazosin, or any component of the formulation

Warnings/Precautions Can cause significant orthostatic hypotension and syncope, especially with first dose; anticipate a similar effect if therapy is interrupted for a few days, if dosage is rapidly increased, or if another antihypertensive drug (particularly vasodilators) or a PDE5 inhibitor is introduced. Patients should be cautioned about performing hazardous tasks when starting new therapy or adjusting dosage upward. Prostate cancer should be ruled out before starting for BPH. Use with caution in mild to moderate hepatic impairment; not recommended in severe dysfunction. Intraoperative floppy iris syndrome has been observed in cataract surgery patients who were on or were previously treated with alpha1 blockers. Causality has not been established and there appears to be no benefit in discontinuing alpha blocker therapy prior to surgery. Safety and efficacy in children have not been established.

The extended release formulation consists of drug within a nondeformable matrix; following drug release/absorption, the matrix/shell is expelled in the stool. The use of nondeformable products in patients with known stricture/narrowing of the GI tract has been associated with symptoms of obstruction. Use caution in patients with increased GI retention (eg, chronic constipation) as doxazosin exposure may be increased.

Drug Interactions

Increased Effect/Toxicity: Increased hypotensive effect with beta-blockers, diuretics, ACE inhibitors, calcium channel blockers, other antihypertensive medications, sildenafil (use with extreme caution at a dose ≤25 mg), tadalafil, and vardenafil.

Ethanol/Nutrition/Herb Interactions Herb/Nutraceutical: Avoid dong quai if using for hypertension (has estrogenic activity). Avoid ephedra, yohimbe, ginseng (may worsen hypertension). Avoid saw palmetto when used for BPH (due to limited experience with this combination). Avoid garlic (may have increased antihypertensive effect).

Dietary Considerations Cardura® XL: Take with morning meal.

Pharmacodynamics/Kinetics Not significantly affected by increased age

Duration: >24 hours

Protein binding: Extended release: 98%

Metabolism: Extensively hepatic to active metabolites; primarily via CYP3A4; secondary pathways involve CYP2D6 and 2C19

Bioavailability: Extended release relative to immediate release: 54% to 59%

Half-life elimination: 15-22 hours

Time to peak, serum: Immediate release: 2-3 hours; extended release: 8-9 hours

Excretion: Feces (63% primarily as metabolites); urine (9%)

Pregnancy Risk Factor C

Dosage Forms TAB: 1 mg, 2 mg, 4 mg, 8 mg

Doxazosin Mesylate *see* Doxazosin *on page 503*

Doxepin (DOKS e pin)

U.S. Brand Names Prudoxin™; Sinequan® [DSC]; Zonalon®
Canadian Brand Names Apo-Doxepin®; Novo-Doxepin; Sinequan®; Zonalon®
Generic Available Yes: Capsule, solution
Synonyms Doxepin Hydrochloride
Pharmacologic Category Antidepressant, Tricyclic (Tertiary Amine); Topical Skin Product
Dental Use Cream: Treatment of burning mouth syndrome and neuropathic pain
Use

Oral: Depression
Topical: Short-term (<8 days) management of moderate pruritus in adults with atopic dermatitis or lichen simplex chronicus

Unlabeled/Investigational Use Analgesic for certain chronic and neuropathic pain; anxiety

Local Anesthetic/Vasoconstrictor Precautions Use with caution; epinephrine and levonordefrin have been shown to have an increased pressor response in combination with TCAs

Effects on Dental Treatment Key adverse event(s) related to dental treatment: Xerostomia and changes in salivation (normal salivary flow resumes upon discontinuation).

Oral: Aphthous stomatitis, unpleasant taste, trouble with gums.
Topical: Taste alteration

Long-term treatment with TCAs increases the risk of caries by reducing salivation and salivary buffer capacity.

Significant Adverse Effects

Oral: Frequency not defined.
Cardiovascular: Hyper-/hypotension, tachycardia
Central nervous system: Drowsiness, dizziness, headache, disorientation, ataxia, confusion, seizure
Dermatologic: Alopecia, photosensitivity, rash, pruritus
Endocrine & metabolic: Breast enlargement, galactorrhea, SIADH, increase or decrease in blood sugar, increased or decreased libido
Gastrointestinal: Xerostomia, constipation, vomiting, indigestion, anorexia, aphthous stomatitis, nausea, unpleasant taste, weight gain, diarrhea, trouble with gums, decreased lower esophageal sphincter tone may cause GE reflux
Genitourinary: Urinary retention, testicular edema
Hematologic: Agranulocytosis, leukopenia, eosinophilia, thrombocytopenia, purpura
Neuromuscular & skeletal: Weakness, tremor, numbness, paresthesia, extrapyramidal symptoms, tardive dyskinesia
Ocular: Blurred vision
Otic: Tinnitus
Miscellaneous: Diaphoresis (excessive), allergic reactions

Topical:
>10%:
Central nervous system: Drowsiness (22%)
Dermatologic: Stinging/burning (23%)
1% to 10%:
Cardiovascular: Edema: (1%)
Central nervous system: Dizziness (2%), emotional changes (2%)
Gastrointestinal: Xerostomia (10%), taste alteration (2%)
<1% (Limited to important or life-threatening): Contact dermatitis, tongue numbness, anxiety

Restrictions A medication guide concerning the use of antidepressants in children and teenagers can be found on the FDA website at http://www.fda.gov/cder/Offices/ODS/labeling.htm. It should be dispensed to parents or guardians of children and teenagers receiving this medication.

Dental Usual Dosing Treatment of burning mouth syndrome and neuropathic pain: Adults: Oral: Topical: Cream: Apply 3-4 times daily

Dosage

Oral: Topical: Burning mouth syndrome (dental use): Cream: Apply 3-4 times daily
Oral (entire daily dose may be given at bedtime):
Depression or anxiety:
Children (unlabeled use): 1-3 mg/kg/day in single or divided doses

(Continued)

505

Doxepin *(Continued)*

Adolescents: Initial: 25-50 mg/day in single or divided doses; gradually increase to 100 mg/day

Adults: Initial: 25-150 mg/day at bedtime or in 2-3 divided doses; may gradually increase up to 300 mg/day; single dose should not exceed 150 mg; select patients may respond to 25-50 mg/day

Elderly: Use a lower dose and adjust gradually

Chronic urticaria, angioedema, nocturnal pruritus: Adults and Elderly: 10-30 mg/day

Dosing adjustment in hepatic impairment: Use a lower dose and adjust gradually

Topical: Pruritus: Adults and Elderly: Apply a thin film 4 times/day with at least 3- to 4-hour interval between applications; not recommended for use >8 days. **Note:** Low-dose (25-50 mg) oral administration has also been used to treat pruritus, but systemic effects are increased.

Mechanism of Action Increases the synaptic concentration of serotonin and norepinephrine in the central nervous system by inhibition of their reuptake by the presynaptic neuronal membrane

Contraindications Hypersensitivity to doxepin, drugs from similar chemical class, or any component of the formulation; narrow-angle glaucoma; urinary retention; use of MAO inhibitors within 14 days; use in a patient during acute recovery phase of MI

Warnings/Precautions Antidepressants increase the risk of suicidal thinking and behavior in children and adolescents with major depressive disorder (MDD) and other depressive disorders; consider risk prior to prescribing. Closely monitor for clinical worsening, suicidality, or unusual changes in behavior; the child's family or caregiver should be instructed to closely observe the patient and communicate condition with healthcare provider. Such observation would generally include at least weekly face-to-face contact with patients or their family members or caregivers during the first 4 weeks of treatment, then every other week visits for the next 4 weeks, then at 12 weeks, and as clinically indicated beyond 12 weeks. Additional contact by telephone may be appropriate between face-to-face visits. Adults treated with antidepressants should be observed similarly for clinical worsening and suicidality, especially during the initial few months of a course of drug therapy, or at times of dose changes, either increases or decreases. A medication guide should be dispensed with each prescription. **Doxepin is approved for treatment of depression in adolescents.**

The possibility of a suicide attempt is inherent in major depression and may persist until remission occurs. Monitor for worsening of depression or suicidality, especially during initiation of therapy or with dose increases or decreases. Worsening depression and severe abrupt suicidality that are not part of the presenting symptoms may require discontinuation or modification of drug therapy. Use caution in high-risk patients during initiation of therapy. Prescriptions should be written for the smallest quantity consistent with good patient care. The patient's family or caregiver should be alerted to monitor patients for the emergence of suicidality and associated behaviors such as anxiety, agitation, panic attacks, insomnia, irritability, hostility, impulsivity, akathisia, hypomania, and mania; patients should be instructed to notify their healthcare provider if any of these symptoms or worsening depression occur.

May worsen psychosis in some patients or precipitate a shift to mania or hypomania in patients with bipolar disorder. Monotherapy in patients with bipolar disorder should be avoided. Patients presenting with depressive symptoms should be screened for bipolar disorder. **Doxepin is not FDA approved for the treatment of bipolar depression.**

Often causes sedation, which may result in impaired performance of tasks requiring alertness (eg, operating machinery or driving). Sedative effects may be additive with other CNS depressants and/or ethanol. The degree of sedation is very high relative to other antidepressants. May increase the risks associated with electroconvulsive therapy. Consider discontinuing, when possible, prior to elective surgery. Therapy should not be abruptly discontinued in patients receiving high doses for prolonged periods.

May cause orthostatic hypotension (risk is moderate relative to other antidepressants) - use with caution in patients at risk of hypotension or in patients where transient hypotensive episodes would be poorly tolerated (cardiovascular disease or cerebrovascular disease). The degree of anticholinergic blockade produced by this agent is high relative to other cyclic antidepressants - use caution in patients with benign prostatic hyperplasia, xerostomia, visual problems, constipation, or history of bowel obstruction.

Use with caution in patients with a history of cardiovascular disease (including previous MI, stroke, tachycardia, or conduction abnormalities). The risk conduction abnormalities with this agent is moderate relative to other antidepressants. Use caution in patients with a previous seizure disorder or condition predisposing to seizures such as brain damage, alcoholism, or concurrent therapy with other drugs which lower the seizure threshold. Use with caution in hyperthyroid patients or those receiving thyroid supplementation. Use with caution in patients with hepatic or renal dysfunction and in elderly patients. Cream formulation is for external use only (not for ophthalmic, vaginal, or oral use). Do not use occlusive dressings. Use for >8 days may increase risk of contact sensitization. Doxepin is significantly absorbed following topical administration; plasma levels may be similar to those achieved with oral administration.

Drug Interactions Substrate (major) of CYP1A2, 2D6, 3A4

Altretamine: Concurrent use may cause orthostatic hypertension

Amphetamines: TCAs may enhance the effect of amphetamines; monitor for adverse CV effects

Anticholinergics: Combined use with TCAs may produce additive anticholinergic effects

Antihypertensives: TCAs may inhibit the antihypertensive response to bethanidine, clonidine, debrisoquin, guanadrel, guanethidine, guanabenz, guanfacine; monitor BP; consider alternate antihypertensive agent

Beta-agonists (nonselective): When combined with TCAs may predispose patients to cardiac arrhythmias

Bupropion: May increase the levels of tricyclic antidepressants; based on limited information; monitor response

Carbamazepine: Tricyclic antidepressants may increase carbamazepine levels; monitor

Cholestyramine and colestipol: May bind TCAs and reduce their absorption; monitor for altered response

Clonidine: Abrupt discontinuation of clonidine may cause hypertensive crisis, amitriptyline may enhance the response

CNS depressants: Sedative effects may be additive with TCAs; monitor for increased effect; includes benzodiazepines, barbiturates, antipsychotics, ethanol and other sedative medications

CYP1A2 inducers: May decrease the levels/effects of doxepin. Example inducers include aminoglutethimide, carbamazepine, phenobarbital, and rifampin.

CYP1A2 inhibitors: May increase the levels/effects of doxepin. Example inhibitors include amiodarone, ciprofloxacin, fluvoxamine, ketoconazole, norfloxacin, ofloxacin, and rofecoxib.

CYP2D6 inhibitors: May increase the levels/effects of doxepin. Example inhibitors include chlorpromazine, delavirdine, fluoxetine, miconazole, paroxetine, pergolide, quinidine, quinine, ritonavir, and ropinirole.

CYP3A4 inducers: CYP3A4 inducers may decrease the levels/effects of doxepin. Example inducers include aminoglutethimide, carbamazepine, nafcillin, nevirapine, phenobarbital, phenytoin, and rifamycins.

CYP3A4 inhibitors: May increase the levels/effects of doxepin. Example inhibitors include azole antifungals, clarithromycin, diclofenac, doxycycline, erythromycin, imatinib, isoniazid, nefazodone, nicardipine, propofol, protease inhibitors, quinidine, telithromycin, and verapamil.

Epinephrine (and other direct alpha-agonists): Pressor response to I.V. epinephrine, norepinephrine, and phenylephrine may be enhanced in patients receiving TCAs (**Note:** Effect is unlikely with epinephrine or levonordefrin dosages typically administered as infiltration in combination with local anesthetics)

Fenfluramine: May increase tricyclic antidepressant levels/effects

Hypoglycemic agents (including insulin): TCAs may enhance the hypoglycemic effects of tolazamide, chlorpropamide, or insulin; monitor for changes in blood glucose levels; reported with chlorpropamide, tolazamide, and insulin

Levodopa: Tricyclic antidepressants may decrease the absorption (bioavailability) of levodopa; rare hypertensive episodes have also been attributed to this combination

Linezolid: Hyperpyrexia, hypertension, tachycardia, confusion, seizures, and **deaths have been reported** with agents which inhibit MAO (serotonin syndrome); this combination should be avoided

Lithium: Concurrent use with a TCA may increase the risk for neurotoxicity

MAO inhibitors: Hyperpyrexia, hypertension, tachycardia, confusion, seizures, and **deaths have been reported** (serotonin syndrome); this combination is contraindicated

Methylphenidate: Metabolism of TCAs may be decreased

Phenothiazines: Serum concentrations of some TCAs may be increased; in addition, TCAs may increase concentration of phenothiazines; monitor for altered clinical response

(Continued)

Doxepin *(Continued)*

QT$_c$-prolonging agents: Concurrent use of tricyclic agents with other drugs which may prolong QT$_c$ interval may increase the risk of potentially fatal arrhythmias; includes type Ia and type III antiarrhythmics agents, selected quinolones (sparfloxacin, gatifloxacin, moxifloxacin, grepafloxacin), cisapride, and other agents

Ritonavir: Combined use of high-dose tricyclic antidepressants with ritonavir may cause serotonin syndrome in HIV-positive patients; monitor

Sucralfate: Absorption of tricyclic antidepressants may be reduced with coadministration

Sympathomimetics, indirect-acting: Tricyclic antidepressants may result in a decreased sensitivity to indirect-acting sympathomimetics; includes dopamine and ephedrine; also see interaction with epinephrine (and direct-acting sympathomimetics)

Tramadol: Tramadol's risk of seizures may be increased with TCAs

Valproic acid: May increase serum concentrations/adverse effects of some tricyclic antidepressants

Warfarin (and other oral anticoagulants): TCAs may increase the anticoagulant effect in patients stabilized on warfarin; monitor INR

Ethanol/Nutrition/Herb Interactions

Ethanol: Avoid ethanol (may increase CNS depression).

Food: Grapefruit juice may inhibit the metabolism of some TCAs and clinical toxicity may result.

Herb/Nutraceutical: Avoid valerian, St John's wort, SAMe, kava kava (may increase risk of serotonin syndrome and/or excessive sedation).

Pharmacodynamics/Kinetics

Onset of action: Peak effect: Antidepressant: Usually >2 weeks; Anxiolytic: may occur sooner

Absorption: Following topical application, plasma levels may be similar to those achieved with oral administration

Distribution: Crosses placenta; enters breast milk

Protein binding: 80% to 85%

Metabolism: Hepatic; metabolites include desmethyldoxepin (active)

Half-life elimination: Adults: 6-8 hours

Excretion: Urine

Pregnancy Risk Factor B (cream); C (all other forms)

Lactation Enters breast milk/not recommended (AAP rates "of concern")

Breast-Feeding Considerations Generally, it is not recommended to breast-feed if taking antidepressants because of the long half-life, active metabolites, and the potential for side effects in the infant.

Dosage Forms [DSC] = Discontinued product

Capsule, as hydrochloride: 10 mg, 25 mg, 50 mg, 75 mg, 100 mg, 150 mg

Sinequan®: 10 mg, 25 mg, 50 mg, 75 mg, 100 mg, 150 mg [DSC]

Cream, as hydrochloride:

Prudoxin™: 5% (45 g) [contains benzyl alcohol]

Zonalon®: 5% (30 g, 45 g) [contains benzyl alcohol]

Solution, oral concentrate, as hydrochloride (Sinequan®): 10 mg/mL (120 mL)

Sinequan®: 10 mg/mL (120 mL) [DSC]

Selected Readings

Friedlander AH and Mahler ME, "Major Depressive Disorder. Psychopathology, Medical Management, and Dental Implications," *J Am Dent Assoc,* 2001, 132(5):629-38.

Ganzberg S, "Psychoactive Drugs," *ADA Guide to Dental Therapeutics,* 2nd ed, Chicago, IL: ADA Publishing, a Division of ADA Business Enterprises, Inc, 2000, 376-405.

Jastak JT and Yagiela JA, "Vasoconstrictors and Local Anesthesia: A Review and Rationale for Use," *J Am Dent Assoc,* 1983, 107(4):623-30.

Rundegren J, van Dijken J, Mörnstad H, et al, "Oral Conditions in Patients Receiving Long-Term Treatment With Cyclic Antidepressant Drugs," *Swed Dent J,* 1985, 9(2):55-64.

Yagiela JA, "Adverse Drug Interactions in Dental Practice: Interactions Associated With Vasoconstrictors. Part V of a Series," *J Am Dent Assoc,* 1999, 130(5):701-9.

Doxepin Hydrochloride *see* Doxepin *on page 505*

Doxercalciferol *(doks er kal si fe FEER ole)*

U.S. Brand Names Hectorol®

Canadian Brand Names Hectorol®

Generic Available No

Synonyms 1α-Hydroxyergocalciferol

Pharmacologic Category Vitamin D Analog

Use Treatment of secondary hyperparathyroidism in patients with chronic kidney disease

Local Anesthetic/Vasoconstrictor Precautions No information available to require special precautions

Effects on Dental Treatment No significant effects or complications reported

Common Adverse Effects
Note: As reported in dialysis patients.

>10%:
 Cardiovascular: Edema (34%)
 Central nervous system: Headache (28%), malaise (28%), dizziness (12%)
 Gastrointestinal: Nausea/vomiting (24%)
 Respiratory: Dyspnea (12%)

1% to 10%:
 Cardiovascular: Bradycardia (7%)
 Central nervous system: Sleep disorder (3%)
 Dermatologic: Pruritus (8%)
 Gastrointestinal: Anorexia (5%), constipation (3%), dyspepsia (5%), weight gain (5%)
 Neuromuscular & skeletal: Arthralgia (5%)
 Miscellaneous: Abscess (3%)

Mechanism of Action Doxercalciferol is metabolized to the active form of vitamin D. The active form of vitamin D controls the intestinal absorption of dietary calcium, the tubular reabsorption of calcium by the kidneys, and in conjunction with PTH, the mobilization of calcium from the skeleton.

Drug Interactions
 Increased Effect/Toxicity: Doxercalciferol toxicity may be increased by concurrent use of other vitamin D supplements or magnesium-containing antacids and supplements.
 Decreased Effect: Absorption of doxercalciferol is reduced with mineral oil and cholestyramine.

Pharmacodynamics/Kinetics
 Metabolism: Hepatic via CYP27
 Half-life elimination: Active metabolite: 32-37 hours; up to 96 hours

Pregnancy Risk Factor B

Doxidan® [DSC] [OTC] see Docusate and Casanthranol on page 496
Doxidan® (reformulation) [OTC] see Bisacodyl on page 209
Doxil® see DOXOrubicin (Liposomal) on page 511

DOXOrubicin (doks oh ROO bi sin)

Related Information
 DOXOrubicin (Liposomal) on page 511
U.S. Brand Names Adriamycin PFS®; Adriamycin RDF®; Rubex®
Canadian Brand Names Adriamycin®
Mexican Brand Names Adriblastina®; Adriblastina RD®; Caelyx®; Doxolem®; Doxotec®
Generic Available Yes
Synonyms ADR (error-prone abbreviation); Adria; Doxorubicin Hydrochloride; Hydroxydaunomycin Hydrochloride; Hydroxyldaunorubicin Hydrochloride; NSC-123127
Pharmacologic Category Antineoplastic Agent, Anthracycline
Use Treatment of leukemias, lymphomas, multiple myeloma, osseous and nonosseous sarcomas, mesotheliomas, germ cell tumors of the ovary or testis, and carcinomas of the head and neck, thyroid, lung, breast, stomach, pancreas, liver, ovary, bladder, prostate, uterus, and neuroblastoma
Local Anesthetic/Vasoconstrictor Precautions No information available to require special precautions
Effects on Dental Treatment Key adverse event(s) related to dental treatment: Stomatitis.
Common Adverse Effects
>10%:
 Dermatologic: Alopecia, radiation recall
 Gastrointestinal: Nausea, vomiting, stomatitis, GI ulceration, anorexia, diarrhea
 Genitourinary: Discoloration of urine, mild dysuria, urinary frequency, hematuria, bladder spasms, cystitis following bladder instillation
 Hematologic: Myelosuppression, primarily leukopenia (75%); thrombocytopenia and anemia
 Onset: 7 days
 Nadir: 10-14 days
 Recovery: 21-28 days

(Continued)

DOXOrubicin *(Continued)*

1% to 10%:

Cardiovascular: Transient ECG abnormalities (supraventricular tachycardia, S-T wave changes, atrial or ventricular extrasystoles); generally asymptomatic and self-limiting. CHF, dose related, may be delayed for 7-8 years after treatment. Cumulative dose, mediastinal/pericardial radiation therapy, cardiovascular disease, age, and use of cyclophosphamide (or other cardiotoxic agents) all increase the risk.

Recommended maximum cumulative doses:

No risk factors: 550 mg/m^2

Concurrent radiation: 450 mg/m^2

Note: Regardless of cumulative dose, if the left ventricular ejection fraction is <30% to 40%, the drug is usually not given.

Dermatologic: Skin "flare" at injection site; discoloration of saliva, sweat, or tears

Endocrine & metabolic: Hyperuricemia

Mechanism of Action Inhibition of DNA and RNA synthesis by intercalation between DNA base pairs by inhibition of topoisomerase II and by steric obstruction. Doxorubicin intercalates at points of local uncoiling of the double helix. Although the exact mechanism is unclear, it appears that direct binding to DNA (intercalation) and inhibition of DNA repair (topoisomerase II inhibition) result in blockade of DNA and RNA synthesis and fragmentation of DNA. Doxorubicin is also a powerful iron chelator; the iron-doxorubicin complex can bind DNA and cell membranes and produce free radicals that immediately cleave the DNA and cell membranes.

Drug Interactions

Cytochrome P450 Effect: Substrate (major) of CYP2D6, 3A4; **Inhibits** CYP2B6 (moderate), 2D6 (weak), 3A4 (weak)

Increased Effect/Toxicity: Allopurinol may enhance the antitumor activity of doxorubicin (animal data only). Cyclosporine may increase doxorubicin levels, enhancing hematologic toxicity or may induce coma or seizures. Cyclophosphamide enhances the cardiac toxicity of doxorubicin by producing additional myocardial cell damage. Mercaptopurine increases doxorubicin toxicities. Streptozocin greatly enhances leukopenia and thrombocytopenia. Verapamil alters the cellular distribution of doxorubicin and may result in increased cell toxicity by inhibition of the P-glycoprotein pump. Paclitaxel reduces doxorubicin clearance and increases toxicity if administered prior to doxorubicin. High doses of progesterone enhance toxicity (neutropenia and thrombocytopenia).

Doxorubicin may increase the levels/effects of bupropion, promethazine, propofol, selegiline, sertraline, and other CYP2B6 substrates. The levels/effects of doxorubicin may be increased by azole antifungals, chlorpromazine, clarithromycin, delavirdine, diclofenac, doxycycline, erythromycin, fluoxetine, imatinib, isoniazid, miconazole, nefazodone, nicardipine, paroxetine, pergolide, propofol, protease inhibitors, quinidine, quinine, ritonavir, ropinirole, telithromycin, verapamil and other inhibitors of CYP2D6 or 3A4. Based on mouse studies, cardiotoxicity may be enhanced by verapamil. Concurrent therapy with actinomycin-D may result in recall pneumonitis following radiation.

Decreased Effect: The levels/effects of doxorubicin may be decreased by aminoglutethimide, carbamazepine, nafcillin, nevirapine, phenobarbital, phenytoin, rifamycins, and other CYP3A4 inducers. Doxorubicin may decrease plasma levels and effectiveness of digoxin. Doxorubicin may decrease the antiviral activity of zidovudine.

Pharmacodynamics/Kinetics

Absorption: Oral: Poor (<50%)

Distribution: V_d: 25 L/kg; to many body tissues, particularly liver, spleen, kidney, lung, heart; does not distribute into the CNS; crosses placenta

Protein binding, plasma: 70%

Metabolism: Primarily hepatic to doxorubicinol (active), then to inactive aglycones, conjugated sulfates, and glucuronides

Half-life elimination:

Distribution: 10 minutes

Elimination: Doxorubicin: 1-3 hours; Metabolites: 3-3.5 hours

Terminal: 17-30 hours

Male: 54 hours; Female: 35 hours

Excretion: Feces (~40% to 50% as unchanged drug); urine (~3% to 10% as metabolites, 1% doxorubicinol, <1% Adriamycin aglycones, and unchanged drug)

Clearance: Male: 113 L/hour; Female: 44 L/hour

Pregnancy Risk Factor D

Doxorubicin Hydrochloride *see* DOXOrubicin *on page 509*
Doxorubicin Hydrochloride (Liposomal) *see* DOXOrubicin (Liposomal) *on page 511*

DOXOrubicin (Liposomal) (doks oh ROO bi sin lip pah SOW mal)

Related Information
DOXOrubicin *on page 509*

U.S. Brand Names Doxil®

Canadian Brand Names Caelyx®

Generic Available No

Synonyms Doxorubicin Hydrochloride (Liposomal)

Pharmacologic Category Antineoplastic Agent, Anthracycline

Use Treatment of AIDS-related Kaposi's sarcoma, breast cancer, ovarian cancer, solid tumors

Local Anesthetic/Vasoconstrictor Precautions No information available to require special precautions

Effects on Dental Treatment Key adverse event(s) related to dental treatment: Mucositis.

Common Adverse Effects
>10%:
  Cardiovascular: Peripheral edema (up to 11%)
  Central nervous system: Fever (8% to 12%), headache (up to 11%), pain (up to 21%)
  Dermatologic: Alopecia (9% to 19%); palmar-plantar erythrodysesthesia/hand-foot syndrome (up to 51% in ovarian cancer, 4% in Kaposi's sarcoma), rash (up to 29% in ovarian cancer, up to 5% in Kaposi's sarcoma)
  Gastrointestinal: Stomatitis (5% to 41%), vomiting (8% to 33%), nausea (18% to 46%), mucositis (up to 14%), constipation (up to 30%), anorexia (up to 20%), diarrhea (5% to 21%), dyspepsia (up to 12%), intestinal obstruction (up to 11%)
  Hematologic: Myelosuppression, neutropenia (12% to 62%), leukopenia (36%), thrombocytopenia (13% to 65%), anemia (6% to 74%)
    Onset: 7 days
    Nadir: 10-14 days
    Recovery: 21-28 days
  Neuromuscular & skeletal: Weakness (7% to 40%), back pain (up to 12%)
  Respiratory: Pharyngitis (up to 16%), dyspnea (up to 15%)
1% to 10%:
  Cardiovascular: Cardiac arrest, chest pain, edema, hypotension, pallor, tachycardia, vasodilation
  Central nervous system: Agitation, anxiety, chills, confusion, depression, dizziness, emotional lability, insomnia, somnolence, vertigo
  Dermatologic: Acne, dry skin (6%), dermatitis, furunculosis, herpes simplex/zoster, maculopapular rash, pruritus, rash, skin discoloration, vesiculobullous rash
  Endocrine & metabolic: Dehydration, hyperbilirubinemia, hyperglycemia, hypocalcemia, hypokalemia, hyponatremia
  Gastrointestinal: Abdomen enlarged, ascites, cachexia, dyspepsia, dysphagia, esophagitis, flatulence, gingivitis, glossitis, ileus, mouth ulceration, rectal bleeding, taste perversion, weight loss, xerostomia
  Genitourinary: Cystitis, dysuria, leukorrhea, pelvic pain, polyuria, urinary incontinence, urinary tract infection, urinary urgency, vaginal bleeding
  Hematologic: Ecchymosis, hemolysis, prothrombin time increased
  Hepatic: ALT increased
  Local: Thrombophlebitis
  Neuromuscular & skeletal: Arthralgia, hypertonia, myalgia, neuralgia, neuritis (peripheral), neuropathy, paresthesia (up to 10%), pathological fracture,
  Ocular: Conjunctivitis, dry eyes, retinitis
  Otic: Ear pain
  Renal: Albuminuria, hematuria
  Respiratory: Apnea, cough increased (up to 10%), epistaxis, pleural effusion, pneumonia, rhinitis, sinusitis
  Miscellaneous: Allergic reaction; infusion-related reactions (bronchospasm, chest tightness, chills, dyspnea, facial edema, flushing, headache, hypotension, pruritus); moniliasis, diaphoresis

Mechanism of Action Doxorubicin inhibits DNA and RNA synthesis by intercalating between DNA base pairs causing steric obstruction and inhibits topoisomerase-II at the point of DNA cleavage. Doxorubicin is also a powerful iron chelator. The iron-doxorubicin complex can bind DNA and cell membranes, producing free hydroxyl (OH) radicals that cleave DNA and cell membranes. Active throughout entire cell cycle.

(Continued)

DOXOrubicin (Liposomal) (Continued)

Drug Interactions

Cytochrome P450 Effect: Substrate (major) of CYP2D6, 3A4; **Inhibits** CYP2B6 (moderate), 2D6 (weak), 3A4 (weak)

Increased Effect/Toxicity: Allopurinol may enhance the antitumor activity of doxorubicin (animal data only). Cyclosporine may increase doxorubicin levels, enhancing hematologic toxicity or may induce coma or seizures. Cyclophosphamide enhances the cardiac toxicity of doxorubicin by producing additional myocardial cell damage. Mercaptopurine increases doxorubicin toxicities. Streptozocin greatly enhances leukopenia and thrombocytopenia. Verapamil alters the cellular distribution of doxorubicin and may result in increased cell toxicity by inhibition of the P-glycoprotein pump. Paclitaxel reduces doxorubicin clearance and increases toxicity if administered prior to doxorubicin. High doses of progesterone enhance toxicity (neutropenia and thrombocytopenia).

Doxorubicin may increase the levels/effects of bupropion, promethazine, propofol, selegiline, sertraline, and other CYP2B6 substrates. The levels/effects of doxorubicin may be increased by azole antifungals, chlorpromazine, clarithromycin, delavirdine, diclofenac, doxycycline, erythromycin, fluoxetine, imatinib, isoniazid, miconazole, nefazodone, nicardipine, paroxetine, pergolide, propofol, protease inhibitors, quinidine, quinine, ritonavir, ropinirole, telithromycin, verapamil and other inhibitors of CYP2D6 or 3A4. Based on mouse studies, cardiotoxicity may be enhanced by verapamil. Concurrent therapy with actinomycin-D may result in recall pneumonitis following radiation.

Decreased Effect: The levels/effects of doxorubicin may be decreased by aminoglutethimide, carbamazepine, nafcillin, nevirapine, phenobarbital, phenytoin, rifamycins, and other CYP3A4 inducers. Doxorubicin may decrease plasma levels and effectiveness of digoxin. Doxorubicin may decrease the antiviral activity of zidovudine.

Pharmacodynamics/Kinetics

Distribution: V_{dss}: 2.8 L/m^2

Protein binding, plasma: Unknown; nonliposomal doxorubicin 70%

Half-life elimination: Terminal: Distribution: 4.7-5.2 hours, Elimination: 44-55 hours

Metabolism: Hepatic and in plasma to doxorubicinol and the sulfate and glucuronide conjugates of 4-demethyl,7-deoxyaglycones

Excretion: Urine (5% as doxorubicin or doxorubicinol)

Clearance: Mean: 0.041 L/hour/m^2

Pregnancy Risk Factor D

Doxy-100® see Doxycycline (Systemic) on page 514

Doxycycline Calcium see Doxycycline (Systemic) on page 514

Doxycycline Hyclate see Doxycycline (Systemic) on page 514

Doxycycline Hyclate (Periodontal)

(doks i SYE kleen HI klayt pair ee oh DON tol)

Related Information

Doxycycline (Systemic) on page 514

U.S. Brand Names Atridox™

Canadian Brand Names Atridox™

Generic Available No

Pharmacologic Category Antibiotic, Tetracycline Derivative

Dental Use Treatment of chronic adult periodontitis for gain in clinical attachment, reduction in probing depth, and reduction in bleeding upon probing

Use Used exclusively in dental applications

Local Anesthetic/Vasoconstrictor Precautions No information available to require special precautions

Effects on Dental Treatment Key adverse event(s) related to dental treatment: Discoloration of teeth (in children), gum discomfort, toothache, periodontal abscess, tooth sensitivity, broken tooth, tooth mobility, endodontic abscess, and jaw pain

Mechanical oral hygiene procedures (ie, tooth brushing, flossing) should be avoided in any treated area for 7 days.

Effects reported in clinical trials were similar in incidence between doxycycline-containing product and vehicle alone; comparable to standard therapies including scaling and root planing or oral hygiene. Although there is no known relationship between doxycycline and hypertension, unspecified essential hypertension was noted in 1.6% of the doxycycline gel group, as compared to

0.2% in the vehicle group (allergic reactions to the vehicle were also reported in two patients).

Significant Adverse Effects Systemic: Gastrointestinal: Diarrhea (3%)

Dental Usual Dosing Oral, subgingival: Dose depends on size, shape and number of pockets treated. Application may be repeated four months after initial treatment. The delivery system consists of 2 separate syringes in a single pouch. Syringe A contains 450 mg of a bioabsorbable polymer gel; syringe B contains doxycycline hyclate 50 mg. To prepare for instillation, couple syringe A to syringe B. Inject contents of syringe A (purple stripe) into syringe B, then push contents back into syringe A. Repeat this mixing cycle at a rate of one cycle per second for 100 cycles. If syringes are stored prior to use (a maximum of 3 days), repeat mixing cycle 10 times before use. After appropriate mixing, contents should be in syringe A. Holding syringes vertically, with syringe A at the bottom, pull back on the syringe A plunger, allowing contents to flow down barrel for several seconds. Uncouple syringes and attach enclosed blunt cannula to syringe A. Local anesthesia is not required for placement. Cannula tip may be bent to resemble periodontal probe and used to explore pocket. Express product from syringe until pocket is filled. To separate tip from formulation, turn tip towards the tooth and press against tooth surface to achieve separation. An appropriate dental instrument may be used to pack gel into the pocket. Pockets may be covered with either Coe-pak™ or Octyldent™ dental adhesive.

Dosage Oral, subgingival: Dose depends on size, shape and number of pockets treated. Application may be repeated four months after initial treatment. The delivery system consists of 2 separate syringes in a single pouch. Syringe A contains 450 mg of a bioabsorbable polymer gel; syringe B contains doxycycline hyclate 50 mg. To prepare for instillation, couple syringe A to syringe B. Inject contents of syringe A (purple stripe) into syringe B, then push contents back into syringe A. Repeat this mixing cycle at a rate of one cycle per second for 100 cycles. If syringes are stored prior to use (a maximum of 3 days), repeat mixing cycle 10 times before use. After appropriate mixing, contents should be in syringe A. Holding syringes vertically, with syringe A at the bottom, pull back on the syringe A plunger, allowing contents to flow down barrel for several seconds. Uncouple syringes and attach enclosed blunt cannula to syringe A. Local anesthesia is not required for placement. Cannula tip may be bent to resemble periodontal probe and used to explore pocket. Express product from syringe until pocket is filled. To separate tip from formulation, turn tip towards the tooth and press against tooth surface to achieve separation. An appropriate dental instrument may be used to pack gel into the pocket. Pockets may be covered with either Coe-pak™ or Octyldent™ dental adhesive.

Mechanism of Action Inhibits protein synthesis by binding with the 30S and possibly the 50S ribosomal subunit(s) of susceptible bacteria; may also cause alterations in the cytoplasmic membrane

Doxycycline inhibits collagenase *in vitro* and has been shown to inhibit collagenase in the gingival crevicular fluid in adults with periodontitis

Contraindications Hypersensitivity to doxycycline, tetracycline or any component of the formulation; children <8 years of age; severe hepatic dysfunction; pregnancy

Warnings/Precautions Do not use during pregnancy; use of tetracyclines during tooth development may cause permanent discoloration of the teeth and enamel hypoplasia. Prolonged use may result in superinfection, including oral or vaginal candidiasis. Photosensitivity may occur; avoid prolonged exposure to sunlight or tanning equipment. Atridox™ has not been evaluated or tested in immunocompromised patients, those with oral candidiasis, or conditions characterized by severe periodontal defects with little remaining periodontium. May result in overgrowth of nonsusceptible organisms, including fungi. Effects of treatment >6 months have not been evaluated; has not been evaluated for use in regeneration of alveolar bone.

Drug Interactions Iron and bismuth subsalicylate may decrease doxycycline bioavailability; barbiturates, phenytoin, and carbamazepine decrease doxycycline's half-life; increased effect of warfarin. Concurrent use of tetracycline and Penthrane® has been reported to result in fatal renal toxicity.

Dietary Considerations May be taken with food, milk, or water.

Pharmacodynamics/Kinetics Systemic absorption from dental subgingival gel may occur, but is limited by the slow rate of dissolution from this formulation over 7 days.

Pregnancy Risk Factor D

Breast-Feeding Considerations Tetracyclines enter breast milk and breast-feeding is not recommended. Use of tetracyclines during tooth development may cause permanent discoloration of the teeth and enamel hypoplasia. Tetracyclines also form a complex in bone-forming tissue, leading to a decreased fibula growth rate when given to premature infants.

(Continued)

Doxycycline Hyclate (Periodontal) *(Continued)*

Dosage Forms Gel, subgingival (Atridox™): 50 mg in each 500 mg of blended formulation [2-syringe system includes doxycycline syringe (50 mg) and delivery system syringe (450 mg) with a blunt cannula]

Doxycycline Monohydrate see Doxycycline (Systemic) on page 514

Doxycycline (Subantimicrobial)
(doks i SYE kleen, sub an tee mye KROE bee ul)

Related Information
Doxycycline (Systemic) *on page 514*

U.S. Brand Names Periostat®

Generic Available No

Pharmacologic Category Antibiotic, Tetracycline Derivative

Dental Use Treatment of periodontitis associated with presence of *Actinobacillus actinomycetemcomitans* (AA). Periostat® is indicated for use as an adjunct to scaling and root planing to promote attachment level gain and to reduce pocket depth in adult periodontitis (systemic levels are subinhibitory against bacteria)

Local Anesthetic/Vasoconstrictor Precautions No information available to require special precautions

Effects on Dental Treatment No significant effects or complications reported

Dental Usual Dosing Adjunctive treatment for periodontitis: Adults: Oral: 20 mg twice daily at least 1 hour before or 2 hours after morning and evening meals for up to 9 months

Dosage Adults: **Adjunctive treatment for periodontitis:** Oral: 20 mg twice daily at least 1 hour before or 2 hours after morning and evening meals for up to 9 months

Mechanism of Action Has been shown to inhibit collagenase activity *in vitro*; has been noted to reduce elevated collagenase activity in the gingival crevicular fluid of patients with periodontal disease; systemic levels do not reach inhibitory concentrations against bacteria

Contraindications Hypersensitivity to doxycycline, tetracycline or any component of the formulation; children <8 years of age; pregnancy

Warnings/Precautions Do not use during pregnancy; use of tetracyclines during tooth development may cause permanent discoloration of the teeth and enamel hypoplasia. Prolonged use may result in superinfection, including oral or vaginal candidiasis. Photosensitivity may occur; avoid prolonged exposure to sunlight or tanning equipment. Effectiveness has not been established in patients with coexisting oral candidiasis; use with caution in patients with a history or predisposition to oral candidiasis.

Breast-Feeding Considerations Tetracyclines enter breast milk and breast-feeding is not recommended. Use of tetracyclines during tooth development may cause permanent discoloration of the teeth and enamel hypoplasia. Tetracyclines also form a complex in bone-forming tissue, leading to a decreased fibula growth rate when given to premature infants.

Dosage Forms Tablet (Periostat®): 20 mg

Selected Readings

Lee HM, Ciancio SG, Tuter G, et al, "Subantimicrobial Dose Doxycycline Efficacy as a Matrix Metalloproteinase Inhibitor in Chronic Periodontitis Patients is Enhanced When Combined With a Non-Steroidal Anti-inflammatory Drug," *J Periodontol*, 2004, 75(3):453-63.

Doxycycline (Systemic) (doks i SYE kleen sis TEM ik)

Related Information
Periodontal Diseases *on page 1705*
Sexually-Transmitted Diseases *on page 1674*

U.S. Brand Names Adoxa™; Doryx®; Doxy-100®; Monodox®; Vibramycin®; Vibra-Tabs®

Canadian Brand Names Apo-Doxy®; Apo-Doxy Tabs®; Doxycin; Doxytec; Novo-Doxylin; Nu-Doxycycline; Vibra-Tabs®

Mexican Brand Names Vibramicina®

Generic Available Yes: Excludes powder for oral solution, syrup

Synonyms Doxycycline Calcium; Doxycycline Hyclate; Doxycycline Monohydrate

Pharmacologic Category Antibiotic, Tetracycline Derivative

Dental Use See Dental Use in Doxycycline Hyclate (Periodontal) *on page 512* and Doxycycline (Subantimicrobial) *on page 514.*

Use Principally in the treatment of infections caused by susceptible *Rickettsia*, *Chlamydia*, and *Mycoplasma*; alternative to mefloquine for malaria prophylaxis;

treatment for syphilis, uncomplicated *Neisseria gonorrhoeae, Listeria, Actinomyces israelii,* and *Clostridium* infections in penicillin-allergic patients; for community-acquired pneumonia and other common infections due to susceptible organisms; anthrax due to *Bacillus anthracis,* including inhalational anthrax (postexposure); treatment of infections caused by uncommon susceptible gram-negative and gram-positive organisms including *Borrelia recurrentis, Ureaplasma urealyticum, Haemophilus ducreyi, Yersinia pestis, Francisella tularensis, Vibrio cholerae, Campylobacter fetus, Brucella* spp, *Bartonella bacilliformis,* and *Calymmatobacterium granulomatis*

Unlabeled/Investigational Use Sclerosing agent for pleural effusion injection; treatment of vancomycin-resistant enterococci (VRE)

Local Anesthetic/Vasoconstrictor Precautions No information available to require special precautions

Effects on Dental Treatment Key adverse event(s) related to dental treatment: Glossitis and tooth discoloration (children). Opportunistic "superinfection" with *Candida albicans;* tetracyclines are not recommended for use during pregnancy or in children ≤8 years of age since they have been reported to cause enamel hypoplasia and permanent teeth discoloration. The use of tetracyclines should only be used in these patients if other agents are contraindicated or alternative antimicrobials will not eradicate the organism.

Significant Adverse Effects Frequency not defined:

Cardiovascular: Intracranial hypertension, pericarditis

Dermatologic: Angioneurotic edema, exfoliative dermatitis (rare), photosensitivity, rash, urticaria

Endocrine & metabolic: Brown/black discoloration of thyroid gland (no dysfunction reported)

Gastrointestinal: Anorexia, diarrhea, enterocolitis, inflammatory lesions in anogenital region

Hematologic: Eosinophilia, hemolytic anemia, neutropenia, thrombocytopenia

Renal: Increased BUN

Miscellaneous: Anaphylactoid purpura, bulging fontanels (infants), SLE exacerbation

Dosage

Children:

Anthrax: Doxycycline should be used in children if antibiotic susceptibility testing, exhaustion of drug supplies, or allergic reaction preclude use of penicillin or ciprofloxacin. For treatment, the consensus recommendation does not include a loading dose for doxycycline.

Inhalational (postexposure prophylaxis) (*MMWR,* 2001, 50:889-893): Oral, I.V. (use oral route when possible):

≤8 years: 2.2 mg/kg every 12 hours for 60 days

>8 years and ≤45 kg: 2.2 mg/kg every 12 hours for 60 days

>8 years and >45 kg: 100 mg every 12 hours for 60 days

Cutaneous (treatment): Oral: See dosing for "Inhalational (postexposure prophylaxis)"

Note: In the presence of systemic involvement, extensive edema, and/or lesions on head/neck, doxycycline should initially be administered I.V.

Inhalational/GI/oropharyngeal (treatment): I.V.: Refer to dosing for inhalational anthrax (postexposure prophylaxis). Switch to oral therapy when clinically appropriate; refer to "Note" on combined therapy and duration under Adult dosing.

Note: If liquid doxycycline is unavailable for the treatment of anthrax, emergency doses may be prepared for children using the tablets: Crush one 100 mg tablet and grind into a fine powder. Mix with 4 teaspoons of food or drink (lowfat milk, chocolate milk, chocolate pudding, or apple juice). Appropriate dose may be taken from this mixture. Mixture may be stored for up to 24 hours. Dairy mixtures should be refrigerated; apple juice may be stored at room temperature.

U.S. Food and Drug Administration, Center for Drug Evaluation and Research, "How to Prepare Emergency Dosages of Doxycycline at Home for Infants and Children," April 25, 2003, viewable at http://www.fda.gov/cder/drug/infopage/penG_doxy/doxycyclinePeds.htm, last accessed May 8, 2003.

Children ≥8 years (<45 kg): **Susceptible infections:** Oral, I.V.: 2-5 mg/kg/day in 1-2 divided doses, not to exceed 200 mg/day

Children >8 years (>45 kg) and Adults: **Susceptible infections:** Oral, I.V.: 100-200 mg/day in 1-2 divided doses

Acute gonococcal infection (PID) in combination with another antibiotic: 100 mg every 12 hours until improved, followed by 100 mg orally twice daily to complete 14 days

Community-acquired pneumonia: 100 mg twice daily

Lyme disease: Oral: 100 mg twice daily for 14-21 days

(Continued)

Doxycycline (Systemic) *(Continued)*

Early syphilis: 200 mg/day in divided doses for 14 days

Late syphilis: 200 mg/day in divided doses for 28 days

Uncomplicated chlamydial infections: 100 mg twice daily for ≥7 days

Endometritis, salpingitis, parametritis, or peritonitis: 100 mg I.V. twice daily with cefoxitin 2 g every 6 hours for 4 days and for ≥48 hours after patient improves; then continue with oral therapy 100 mg twice daily to complete a 10- to 14-day course of therapy

Sclerosing agent for pleural effusion injection (unlabeled use): 500 mg as a single dose in 30-50 mL of NS or SWI

Adults:

Anthrax:

Inhalational (postexposure prophylaxis): Oral, I.V. (use oral route when possible): 100 mg every 12 hours for 60 days (*MMWR*, 2001, 50:889-93); **Note:** Preliminary recommendation, FDA review and update is anticipated.

Cutaneous (treatment): Oral: 100 mg every 12 hours for 60 days. **Note:** In the presence of systemic involvement, extensive edema, lesions on head/neck, refer to I.V. dosing for treatment of inhalational/GI/oropharyngeal anthrax

Inhalational/GI/oropharyngeal (treatment): I.V.: Initial: 100 mg every 12 hours; switch to oral therapy when clinically appropriate; some recommend initial loading dose of 200 mg, followed by 100 mg every 8-12 hours (*JAMA*, 1997, 278:399-411). **Note:** Initial treatment should include two or more agents predicted to be effective (per CDC recommendations). Agents suggested for use in conjunction with doxycycline or ciprofloxacin include rifampin, vancomycin, imipenem, penicillin, ampicillin, chloramphenicol, clindamycin, and clarithromycin. May switch to oral antimicrobial therapy when clinically appropriate. Continue combined therapy for 60 days

Dialysis: Not dialyzable; 0% to 5% by hemo- and peritoneal methods or by continuous arteriovenous or venovenous hemofiltration. Supplemental dosage unnecessary.

Mechanism of Action Inhibits protein synthesis by binding with the 30S and possibly the 50S ribosomal subunit(s) of susceptible bacteria; may also cause alterations in the cytoplasmic membrane

Doxycycline inhibits collagenase *in vitro* and has been shown to inhibit collagenase in the gingival crevicular fluid in adults with periodontitis

Contraindications Hypersensitivity to doxycycline, tetracycline or any component of the formulation; children <8 years of age, except in treatment of anthrax (including inhalational anthrax postexposure prophylaxis); severe hepatic dysfunction; pregnancy

Warnings/Precautions Do not use during pregnancy; use of tetracyclines during tooth development may cause permanent discoloration of the teeth and enamel hypoplasia. Prolonged use may result in superinfection, including oral or vaginal candidiasis. Photosensitivity reaction may occur with this drug; avoid prolonged exposure to sunlight or tanning equipment. Avoid in children ≤8 years of age.

Drug Interactions Substrate of CYP3A4 (major); **Inhibits** CYP3A4 (strong)

Antacids (containing aluminum, calcium, or magnesium): Decreased absorption of tetracyclines

Anticoagulants: Tetracyclines may decrease plasma thrombin activity; monitor

Barbiturates: Decreased half-life of doxycycline

Carbamazepine: Decreased half-life of doxycycline

CYP3A4 inducers: CYP3A4 inducers may decrease the levels/effects of doxycycline. Example inducers include aminoglutethimide, carbamazepine, nafcillin, nevirapine, phenobarbital, phenytoin, and rifamycins.

CYP3A4 substrates: Doxycycline may increase the levels/effects of CYP3A4 substrates. Example substrates include benzodiazepines, calcium channel blockers, mirtazapine, nateglinide, nefazodone, tacrolimus, and venlafaxine. Selected benzodiazepines (midazolam and triazolam), cisapride, ergot alkaloids, selected HMG-CoA reductase inhibitors (lovastatin and simvastatin), and pimozide are generally contraindicated with strong CYP3A4 inhibitors.

Iron-containing products: Decreased absorption of tetracyclines

Methoxyflurane: Concomitant use may cause fatal renal toxicity.

Oral contraceptives: Anecdotal reports suggesting decreased contraceptive efficacy with tetracyclines have been refuted by more rigorous scientific and clinical data.

Phenytoin: Decreased half-life of doxycycline

Ethanol/Nutrition/Herb Interactions

Ethanol: Avoid or limit use (<3 drinks/day); chronic ingestion may decrease serum concentration.

Food: Administer with food or milk due to GI intolerance; may decrease absorption up to 20%. Of currently available tetracyclines, doxycycline has the least affinity for calcium; may decrease absorption of amino acids, calcium, iron, magnesium, and zinc. Administration with calcium or iron may decrease doxycycline absorption. Boiled milk, buttermilk, or yogurt may reduce diarrhea.

Crushed tablets may be mixed with 4 teaspoons of food or drink (lowfat milk, chocolate milk, chocolate pudding, or apple juice) for emergency pediatric dosing if liquid unavailable for treatment of anthrax (see Dosage).

Herb/Nutraceutical: Avoid dong quai; may cause additional photosensitization. Avoid St John's wort; may decrease serum concentration and cause additional photosensitization.

Dietary Considerations

Take with food if gastric irritation occurs. While administration with food may decrease GI absorption of doxycycline by up to 20%, administration on an empty stomach is not recommended due to GI intolerance. Of currently available tetracyclines, doxycycline has the least affinity for calcium.

Doryx® 75 mg and 100 mg tablets contain sodium 4.5 mg and 6 mg, respectively.

Pharmacodynamics/Kinetics

Absorption: Oral: Almost complete; reduced by food or milk by 20%

Distribution: Widely into body tissues and fluids including synovial, pleural, prostatic, seminal fluids, and bronchial secretions; saliva, aqueous humor, and CSF penetration is poor; readily crosses placenta; enters breast milk

Protein binding: 90%

Metabolism: Not hepatic; partially inactivated in GI tract by chelate formation

Half-life elimination: 12-15 hours (usually increases to 22-24 hours with multiple doses); End-stage renal disease: 18-25 hours

Time to peak, serum: 1.5-4 hours

Excretion: Feces (30%); urine (23%)

Pregnancy Risk Factor D

Lactation Enters breast milk/not recommended

Breast-Feeding Considerations Tetracyclines enter breast milk and breast-feeding is not recommended. Use of tetracyclines during tooth development may cause permanent discoloration of the teeth and enamel hypoplasia. Tetracyclines also form a complex in bone-forming tissue, leading to a decreased fibula growth rate when given to premature infants.

Dosage Forms

Capsule, as hyclate: 50 mg, 100 mg
    Vibramycin®: 100 mg
Capsule, as monohydrate (Monodox®): 50 mg, 100 mg
Capsule, coated pellets, as hyclate (Doryx®): 75 mg, 100 mg
Injection, powder for reconstitution, as hyclate (Doxy-100®): 100 mg
Powder for oral suspension, as monohydrate (Vibramycin®): 25 mg/5 mL (60 mL) [raspberry flavor]
Syrup, as calcium (Vibramycin®): 50 mg/5 mL (480 mL) [contains sodium metabisulfite; raspberry-apple flavor]
Tablet, as hyclate: 100 mg
    Vibra-Tabs®: 100 mg
Tablet, as monohydrate (Adoxa™): 50 mg, 75 mg, 100 mg

Doxylamine (dox IL a meen)

U.S. Brand Names Good Sense Sleep Aid [OTC]; Unisom® SleepTabs® [OTC]

Canadian Brand Names Unisom®-2

Generic Available Yes

Synonyms Doxylamine Succinate

Pharmacologic Category Antihistamine

Use Treatment of short-term insomnia

Local Anesthetic/Vasoconstrictor Precautions No information available to require special precautions

Effects on Dental Treatment Key adverse event(s) related to dental treatment: Dry mucous membranes and significant xerostomia (normal salivary flow resumes upon discontinuation).

Common Adverse Effects Frequency not defined.

Cardiovascular: Palpitations, tachycardia

Central nervous system: Dizziness, disorientation, drowsiness, headache, paradoxical CNS stimulation, vertigo

(Continued)

Doxylamine *(Continued)*

Gastrointestinal: Anorexia, dry mucous membranes, diarrhea, constipation, epigastric pain, xerostomia

Genitourinary: Dysuria, urinary retention

Ocular: Blurred vision, diplopia

Mechanism of Action Doxylamine competes with histamine for H_1-receptor sites on effector cells; blocks chemoreceptor trigger zone, diminishes vestibular stimulation, and depresses labyrinthine function through its central anticholinergic activity.

Drug Interactions

Increased Effect/Toxicity: Enhances sedative effects of other CNS depressants, may potentiate anticholinergic effects of narcotic analgesics, phenothiazines (and other antipsychotics with high anticholinergic activity), tricyclic antidepressants, quinidine and some other antiarrhythmics, and antihistamines.

Decreased Effect: Theoretically, may decrease the effect of cholinergic agents (donepezil, rivastigmine, and tacrine).

Pharmacodynamics/Kinetics

Absorption: Well absorbed

Distribution: V_d: 2.5 L/kg

Metabolism: Via multiple metabolic pathways including N-demethylation, oxidation, hydroxylation, N-acetylation to metabolites including nordoxylamine, dinordoxylamine

Half-life elimination: 10-12 hours

Excretion: Urine (primarily as metabolites)

Pregnancy Risk Factor B

Doxylamine Succinate *see* Doxylamine *on page 517*

DPA *see* Valproic Acid and Derivatives *on page 1556*

DPE *see* Dipivefrin *on page 489*

D-Penicillamine *see* Penicillamine *on page 1201*

DPH *see* Phenytoin *on page 1228*

DPM™ [OTC] *see* Urea *on page 1551*

Dramamine® [OTC] *see* DimenhyDRINATE *on page 481*

Dramamine® Less Drowsy Formula [OTC] *see* Meclizine *on page 969*

Drisdol® *see* Ergocalciferol *on page 556*

Dristan® Sinus [OTC] *see* Pseudoephedrine and Ibuprofen *on page 1311*

Dritho-Scalp® *see* Anthralin *on page 128*

Drituss DM *see* Guaifenesin and Dextromethorphan *on page 754*

Drixoral® Cold & Allergy [OTC] *see* Dexbrompheniramine and Pseudoephedrine *on page 442*

Drize®-R *see* Chlorpheniramine, Phenylephrine, and Methscopolamine *on page 327*

Dronabinol *(droe NAB i nol)*

U.S. Brand Names Marinol®

Canadian Brand Names Marinol®

Generic Available No

Synonyms Delta-9-tetrahydro-cannabinol; Delta-9 THC; Tetrahydrocannabinol; THC

Pharmacologic Category Antiemetic; Appetite Stimulant

Use Chemotherapy-associated nausea and vomiting refractory to other antiemetic; AIDS-related anorexia

Unlabeled/Investigational Use

Cancer-related anorexia

Local Anesthetic/Vasoconstrictor Precautions No information available to require special precautions

Effects on Dental Treatment Key adverse event(s) related to dental treatment: Xerostomia (normal salivary flow resumes upon discontinuation) and orthostatic hypotension.

Common Adverse Effects

>10%:

Central nervous system: Drowsiness (48%), sedation (53%), confusion (30%), dizziness (21%), detachment, anxiety, difficulty concentrating, mood change

Gastrointestinal: Appetite increased (when used as an antiemetic), xerostomia (38% to 50%)

1% to 10%:

Cardiovascular: Orthostatic hypotension, tachycardia

Central nervous system: Ataxia (4%), depression (7%), headache, vertigo, hallucinations (5%), memory lapse (4%)

Neuromuscular & skeletal: Paresthesia, weakness

Restrictions C-III

Mechanism of Action Unknown, may inhibit endorphins in the emetic center, suppress prostaglandin synthesis, and/or inhibit medullary activity through an unspecified cortical action

Drug Interactions

Increased Effect/Toxicity: Sedative effects may be additive with CNS depressants (includes barbiturates, narcotic analgesics, and other sedative agents).

Pharmacodynamics/Kinetics

Onset of action: Within 1 hour

Peak effect: 2-4 hours

Duration: 24 hours (appetite stimulation)

Absorption: Oral: 90% to 95%; 10% to 20% of dose gets into systemic circulation

Distribution: V_d: 10 L/kg; dronabinol is highly lipophilic and distributes to adipose tissue

Protein binding: 97% to 99%

Metabolism: Hepatic to at least 50 metabolites, some of which are active; 11-hydroxy-delta-9-tetrahydrocannabinol (11-OH-THC) is the major metabolite; extensive first-pass effect

Half-life elimination: Dronabinol: 25-36 hours (terminal); Dronabinol metabolites: 44-59 hours

Time to peak, serum: 0.5-4 hours

Excretion: Feces (50% as unconjugated metabolites, 5% as unchanged drug); urine (10% to 15% as acid metabolites and conjugates)

Pregnancy Risk Factor C

Droperidol (droe PER i dole)

U.S. Brand Names Inapsine®

Mexican Brand Names Dehydrobenzperidol®

Generic Available Yes

Synonyms Dehydrobenzperidol

Pharmacologic Category Antiemetic; Antipsychotic Agent, Typical

Use Antiemetic in surgical and diagnostic procedures; preoperative medication in patients when other treatments are ineffective or inappropriate

Local Anesthetic/Vasoconstrictor Precautions Manufacturer's information states that droperidol may block vasopressor activity of epinephrine. This has not been observed during use of epinephrine as a vasoconstrictor in local anesthesia. See Dental Comment.

Effects on Dental Treatment Key adverse event(s) related to dental treatment: Orthostatic hypotension.

Common Adverse Effects

>10%:

Cardiovascular: QT_c prolongation (dose dependent)

Central nervous system: Restlessness, anxiety, extrapyramidal symptoms, dystonic reactions, pseudoparkinsonian signs and symptoms, tardive dyskinesia, seizure, altered central temperature regulation, sedation, drowsiness

Endocrine & metabolic: Swelling of breasts

Gastrointestinal: Weight gain, constipation

1% to 10%:

Cardiovascular: Hypotension (especially orthostatic), tachycardia, abnormal T waves with prolonged ventricular repolarization, hypertension

Central nervous system: Hallucinations, persistent tardive dyskinesia, akathisia

Gastrointestinal: Nausea, vomiting

Genitourinary: Dysuria

Mechanism of Action Droperidol is a butyrophenone antipsychotic; antiemetic effect is a result of blockade of dopamine stimulation of the chemoreceptor trigger zone. Other effects include alpha-adrenergic blockade, peripheral vascular dilation, and reduction of the pressor effect of epinephrine resulting in hypotension and decreased peripheral vascular resistance; may also reduce pulmonary artery pressure

Drug Interactions

Increased Effect/Toxicity: Droperidol in combination with certain forms of conduction anesthesia may produce peripheral vasodilitation and hypotension. Droperidol and CNS depressants will likely have additive CNS effects. Droperidol and cyclobenzaprine may have an additive effect on prolonging the

(Continued)

Droperidol *(Continued)*

QT interval. Use caution with other agents known to prolong QT interval (Class I or Class III antiarrhythmics, some quinolone antibiotics, cisapride, some phenothiazines, pimozide, tricyclic antidepressants). Potassium- or magnesium-depleting agents (diuretics, aminoglycosides, amphotericin B, cyclosporine) may increase risk of arrhythmias. Metoclopramide may increase risk of extrapyramidal symptoms (EPS). Acetylcholinesterase inhibitors (central) may increase the risk of antipsychotic-related EPS.

Pharmacodynamics/Kinetics

Onset of action: Peak effect: Parenteral: ~30 minutes

Duration: Parenteral: 2-4 hours, may extend to 12 hours

Absorption: I.M.: Rapid

Distribution: Crosses blood-brain barrier and placenta

V_d: Children: ~0.25-0.9 L/kg; Adults: ~2 L/kg

Protein binding: Extensive

Metabolism: Hepatic, to *p*-fluorophenylacetic acid, benzimidazolone, *p*-hydroxypiperidine

Half-life elimination: Adults: 2.3 hours

Excretion: Urine (75%, <1% as unchanged drug); feces (22%, 11% to 50% as unchanged drug)

Pregnancy Risk Factor C

Dental Comment

This drug is known to prolong the QT interval. The QT interval is measured as the time and distance between the Q point of the QRS complex and the end of the T wave in the ECG tracing. After adjustment for heart rate, the QT interval is defined as prolonged if it is more than 450 msec in men and 460 msec in women. A long QT syndrome was first described in the 1950s and 60s as a congenital syndrome involving QT interval prolongation and syncope and sudden death. Some of the congenital long QT syndromes were characterized by a peculiar electrocardiographic appearance of the QRS complex involving a premature atria beat followed by a pause, then a subsequent sinus beat showing marked QT prolongation and deformity. This type of cardiac arrhythmia was originally termed "torsade de pointes" (translated from the French as "twisting of the points").

Prolongation of the QT interval is thought to result from delayed ventricular repolarization. The repolarization process within the myocardial cell is due to the efflux of intracellular potassium. The channels associated with this current can be blocked by many drugs and predisposes the electrical propagation cycle to torsade de pointes.

Droperidol is one of the drugs confirmed to prolong the QT interval and is accepted as having a risk of causing torsade de pointes. The risk of drug-induced torsade de pointes is extremely low when a single QT interval prolonging drug is prescribed. In terms of epinephrine, it is not known what effect vasoconstrictors in the local anesthetic regimen will have in patients with a known history of congenital prolonged QT interval or in patients taking any medication that prolongs the QT interval. Until more information is obtained, it is suggested that the clinician consult with the physician prior to the use of a vasoconstrictor in suspected patients, and that the vasoconstrictor (epinephrine, levonordefrin [Neo-Cobefrin®]) be used with caution.

Drospirenone and Estradiol *(droh SPYE re none & es tra DYE ole)*

U.S. Brand Names Angeliq®

Canadian Brand Names Angeliq®

Generic Available No

Synonyms E2 and DRSP; Estradiol and Drospirenone

Pharmacologic Category Estrogen and Progestin Combination

Use Treatment of moderate-to-severe vasomotor symptoms associated with menopause; treatment of vulvar and vaginal atrophy associated with menopause

Local Anesthetic/Vasoconstrictor Precautions No information available to require special precautions

Effects on Dental Treatment When prescribing antibiotics, patient must be warned to use additional methods of birth control if on oral contraceptives.

Common Adverse Effects

>10%:

Endocrine & metabolic: Breast pain (19%)

Gastrointestinal: Abdominal pain (11%)

Respiratory: Upper respiratory tract infection (19%)

1% to 10%:
Cardiovascular: Peripheral edema (2%)
Central nervous system: Headache (10%), pain (8%)
Gastrointestinal: Abdomen enlarged (7%)
Genitourinary: Vaginal hemorrhage (9%), endometrial disorder (2%), leukorrhea (1%)
Neuromuscular & skeletal: Back pain (7%)
Respiratory: Flu-like syndrome (7%), sinusitis (5%)
Additional adverse effects reported with estrogens and/or progestins: Abdominal cramps, acne, abnormal uterine bleeding, aggravation of porphyria, amenorrhea, anaphylactoid reactions, anaphylaxis, antifactor Xa decreased, antithrombin III decreased, appetite changes, bloating, breast enlargement, breast tenderness, cerebral embolism, cerebral thrombosis, chloasma, cholestatic jaundice, cholecystitis, cholelithiasis, chorea, contact lens intolerance, cystitis-like syndrome, decreased carbohydrate tolerance, depression, dementia, dizziness, dysmenorrhea; factors VII, VIII, IX, X, XII, VII-X complex, and II-VII-X complex increased; endometrial hyperplasia, erythema multiforme, erythema nodosum, galactorrhea, hemorrhagic eruption, fatigue, fibrinogen increased, impaired glucose tolerance, HDL-cholesterol increased, hirsutism, hypertension, increase in size of uterine leiomyomata, gallbladder disease, insomnia, LDL-cholesterol decreased, libido changes, loss of scalp hair, melasma, migraine, mood disturbances, nausea, nervousness, optic neuritis, pancreatitis, platelet aggregability and platelet count increased, premenstrual-like syndrome, PT and PTT accelerated, pulmonary embolism, pyrexia, retinal thrombosis, somnolence, steepening of corneal curvature, stroke, thrombophlebitis, thyroid-binding globulin increased, total thyroid hormone (T$_4$) increased, triglycerides increased, urticaria, vaginal candidiasis, vomiting, weight gain/loss

Mechanism of Action

Drospirenone is a synthetic progestin and spironolactone analog with antimineralocorticoid and antiandrogenic activity. Counteracts estrogen effects causing endometrial thinning.

Estrogens are responsible for the development and maintenance of the female reproductive system and secondary sexual characteristics. Estradiol is the principal intracellular human estrogen and is more potent than estrone and estriol at the receptor level; it is the primary estrogen secreted prior to menopause. Following menopause, estrone and estrone sulfate are more highly produced. Estrogens modulate the pituitary secretion of gonadotropins, luteinizing hormone, and follicle-stimulating hormone through a negative feedback system; estrogen replacement reduces elevated levels of these hormones in postmenopausal women.

Drug Interactions

Cytochrome P450 Effect:

Drospirenone: **Substrate** of CYP3A4 (minor); **Inhibits** CYP1A2 (weak), 2C9 (weak), 2C19 (weak), 3A4 (weak)

Estradiol: **Substrate** of CYP1A2 (major), 2A6 (minor), 2B6 (minor), 2C9 (minor), 2C19 (minor), 2D6 (minor), 2E1 (minor), 3A4 (major); **Inhibits** CYP1A2 (weak), 2C8 (weak); **Induces** CYP3A4 (weak)

Increased Effect/Toxicity: Potential for hyperkalemia with concomitant use of ACE inhibitors, aldosterone, angiotensin II receptor antagonists, heparin, NSAIDs (when taken daily, long term), and potassium-sparing diuretics; monitor serum potassium during first cycle. Potential for hyperkalemia with concomitant use of aldosterone antagonists; monitor serum potassium during first cycle. Aminoglutethimide may increase CYP metabolism of progestins. Oral contraceptives may increase or decrease the effects of coumarin derivatives.

Decreased Effect: Pregnancy has been reported following concomitant use of antibiotics (ampicillin, griseofulvin, tetracycline), however, pharmacokinetic studies have not shown consistent effects with these antibiotics on plasma concentrations of synthetic steroids. Oral contraceptives may increase or decrease the effects of coumarin derivatives. Anticonvulsants (carbamazepine, felbamate, phenobarbital, phenytoin, topiramate) increase the metabolism of ethinyl estradiol and/or some progestins, leading to possible decrease in contraceptive effectiveness. Phenylbutazones may decrease contraceptive effectiveness and increase menstrual irregularities.

Pharmacodynamics/Kinetics

Distribution: Drospirenone: 4.2 L/kg
Protein binding:
Drospirenone: 97%; does not bind to sex hormone binding globulin or corticosteroid binding globulin
Estradiol: 37% bound to sex hormone binding globulin; 61% bound to albumin
Metabolism: Hepatic
(Continued)

Drospirenone and Estradiol *(Continued)*

Drospirenone forms two metabolites (inactive)
Estradiol: Converted to estrone and estriol; also undergoes enterohepatic recirculation; estrone sulfite is the main metabolite in postmenopausal women
Bioavailability: Drospirenone: 76% to 85%
Time to peak, plasma: Drospirenone: 1 hour; Estradiol: 6-8 hours

Drospirenone and Ethinyl Estradiol *see* Ethinyl Estradiol and Drospirenone *on page 595*

Drotrecogin Alfa *(dro TRE coe jin AL fa)*

U.S. Brand Names Xigris®
Canadian Brand Names Xigris®
Generic Available No
Synonyms Activated Protein C, Human, Recombinant; Drotrecogin Alfa, Activated; Protein C (Activated), Human, Recombinant
Pharmacologic Category Protein C (Activated)
Use Reduction of mortality from severe sepsis (associated with organ dysfunction) in adults at high risk of death (eg, APACHE II score ≥25)
Unlabeled/Investigational Use Purpura fulminans
Local Anesthetic/Vasoconstrictor Precautions No information available to require special precautions
Effects on Dental Treatment Key adverse event(s) related to dental treatment: As with all drugs which may affect hemostasis, bleeding is the major adverse effect associated with drotrecogin alfa. Hemorrhage may occur at virtually any site; risk is dependent on multiple variables, including the dosage administered, concurrent use of multiple agents which alter hemostasis, and patient predisposition.
Common Adverse Effects As with all drugs which may affect hemostasis, bleeding is the major adverse effect associated with drotrecogin alfa. Hemorrhage may occur at virtually any site. Risk is dependent on multiple variables, including the dosage administered, concurrent use of multiple agents which alter hemostasis, and patient predisposition.

>10%:
Dermatologic: Bruising
Gastrointestinal: Gastrointestinal bleeding
1% to 10%: Hematologic: Bleeding (serious 2.4% during infusion vs 3.5% during 28-day study period; individual events listed as <1%)

Mechanism of Action Inhibits factors Va and VIIIa, limiting thrombotic effects. Additional *in vitro* data suggest inhibition of plasminogen activator inhibitor-1 (PAF-1) resulting in profibrinolytic activity, inhibition of macrophage production of tumor necrosis factor, blocking of leukocyte adhesion, and limitation of thrombin-induced inflammatory responses. Relative contribution of effects on the reduction of mortality from sepsis is not completely understood.

Drug Interactions
Increased Effect/Toxicity: Concurrent use of antiplatelet agents, including aspirin (>650 mg/day, recent use within 7 days), cilostazol, clopidogrel, dipyridamole, ticlopidine, NSAIDs, or glycoprotein IIb/IIIa antagonists (recent use within 7 days) may increase risk of bleeding. Concurrent use of low molecular weight heparins or heparin at therapeutic rates of infusion may increase the risk of bleeding. However, the use of low-dose prophylactic heparin does not appear to affect safety. Recent use of thrombolytic agents (within 3 days) may increase the risk of bleeding. Recent use of warfarin (within 7 days or elevation of INR ≥3) may increase the risk of bleeding. Other drugs which interfere with coagulation may increase risk of bleeding (including antithrombin III, danaparoid, direct thrombin inhibitors)

Pharmacodynamics/Kinetics
Duration: Plasma nondetectable within 2 hours of discontinuation
Metabolism: Inactivated by endogenous plasma protease inhibitors; mean clearance: 40 L/hour; increased with severe sepsis (~50%)
Half-life elimination: 1.6 hours
Pregnancy Risk Factor C

Drotrecogin Alfa, Activated *see* Drotrecogin Alfa *on page 522*
Droxia® *see* Hydroxyurea *on page 800*
Dr. Scholl's® Callus Remover [OTC] *see* Salicylic Acid *on page 1374*
Dr. Scholl's® Clear Away [OTC] *see* Salicylic Acid *on page 1374*
DSCG *see* Cromolyn *on page 397*
D-Ser(Bu^t)^6,Azgly^{10}-LHRH *see* Goserelin *on page 750*

D-S-S® [OTC] *see* Docusate *on page 496*

DSS With Casanthranol *see* Docusate and Casanthranol *on page 496*

DTIC *see* Dacarbazine *on page 415*

DTIC-Dome® *see* Dacarbazine *on page 415*

DTO (error-prone abbreviation) *see* Opium Tincture *on page 1149*

DTPA *see* Diethylene Triamine Penta-Acetic Acid *on page 466*

D-Trp(6)-LHRH *see* Triptorelin *on page 1544*

Duac™ *see* Clindamycin and Benzoyl Peroxide *on page 364*

Dulcolax® [OTC] *see* Bisacodyl *on page 209*

Dulcolax® Milk of Magnesia [OTC] *see* Magnesium Hydroxide *on page 961*

Dulcolax® Stool Softener [OTC] *see* Docusate *on page 496*

Dull-C® [OTC] *see* Ascorbic Acid *on page 143*

Duloxetine (doo LOX e teen)

U.S. Brand Names Cymbalta®

Generic Available No

Synonyms Duloxetine Hydrochloride; LY248686; (+)-(S)-N-Methyl-γ-(1-naphthyloxy)-2-thiophenepropylamine Hydrochloride

Pharmacologic Category Antidepressant, Serotonin/Norepinephrine Reuptake Inhibitor

Use Treatment of major depressive disorder; management of pain associated with diabetic neuropathy

Unlabeled/Investigational Use Treatment of stress incontinence; management of chronic pain syndromes; management of fibromyalgia

Local Anesthetic/Vasoconstrictor Precautions Although duloxetine is not a tricyclic antidepressant, it does block norepinephrine reuptake within the CNS synapses as part of its mechanism. It has been suggested that vasoconstrictors be administered with caution and to monitor vital signs in dental patients taking antidepressants that affect norepinephrine in this way.

Effects on Dental Treatment Key adverse event(s) related to dental treatment: Xerostomia and changes in salivation (normal salivary flow resumes upon discontinuation).

Common Adverse Effects

>10%:
  Central nervous system: Somnolence (7% to 15%), dizziness (6% to 14%), headache (13%), insomnia (8% to 11%)
  Gastrointestinal: Nausea (14% to 22%), xerostomia (5% to 15%), diarrhea (8% to 13%), constipation (5% to 11%)

1% to 10%:
  Cardiovascular: Palpitations (1%)
  Central nervous system: Fatigue (2% to 10%), anxiety (3%), fever (1% to 2%), hypoesthesia (1%), irritability (1%), lethargy (1%), nervousness (1%), nightmares (1%), restlessness (1%), sleep disorder (1%), vertigo (1%), yawning (1%)
  Dermatologic: Hyperhydrosis (6%), pruritus (1%), rash (1%)
  Endocrine & metabolic: Libido decreased (3% to 6%), orgasm abnormality (3% to 4%), hot flushes (2%), anorgasmia (1%), hypoglycemia (1%)
  Gastrointestinal: Appetite decreased (3% to 8%), vomiting (5% to 6%), dyspepsia (4%), loose stools (2% to 3%), weight loss (1% to 2%), gastritis (1%)
  Genitourinary: Erectile dysfunction (1% to 4%), ejaculation delayed (3%), ejaculatory dysfunction (3%), pollakiuria (1% to 3%), dysuria (1%), urinary symptoms (hesitancy, obstructive symptoms; 1%)
  Hepatic: Transaminases increased: Occasionally associated with hyperbilirubinemia and/or increased alkaline phosphatase (1%)
  Neuromuscular & skeletal: Muscle cramp (4% to 5%), weakness (2% to 4%), myalgia (1% to 3%), tremor (1% to 3%), muscle tightness (1%), muscle twitching (1%), rigors (1%)
  Ocular: Blurred vision (4%)
  Respiratory: Nasopharyngitis (7% to 9%), cough (3% to 6%), pharyngolaryngeal pain (1% to 3%)
  Miscellaneous: Diaphoresis increased (6%), night sweats (1%)

Restrictions A medication guide concerning the use of antidepressants in children and teenagers can be found on the FDA website at http://www.fda.gov/cder/Offices/ODS/labeling.htm. It should be dispensed to parents or guardians of children and teenagers receiving this medication.

Mechanism of Action Duloxetine is a potent inhibitor of neuronal serotonin and norepinephrine reuptake and a weak inhibitor of dopamine reuptake. Duloxetine has no significant activity for muscarinic cholinergic, H_1-histaminergic, or

(Continued)

Duloxetine *(Continued)*

alpha$_2$-adrenergic receptors. Duloxetine does not possess MAO-inhibitory activity.

Drug Interactions

Cytochrome P450 Effect: Substrate (major) of CYP1A2, 2D6; **inhibits** CYP2D6 (moderate)

Increased Effect/Toxicity: Hyperpyrexia, hypertension, tachycardia, confusion, seizures, and deaths have been reported with MAO inhibitors (serotonin syndrome); this combination is contraindicated. Avoid use of linezolid (due to MAO activity). Duloxetine may increase serum concentrations of thioridazine, which has been associated with the development of malignant ventricular arrhythmias. Serum levels/effects of tricyclic antidepressants may be increased by duloxetine.

Concurrent use of duloxetine with buspirone, meperidine, moclobemide, nefazodone, SSRIs, sibutramine, tramadol and trazodone and venlafaxine may cause serotonin syndrome; avoid concurrent use. Concurrent use of selegiline with SSRIs has been reported to cause serotonin syndrome (less than with nonselective MAO inhibitors). Concurrent use of sumatriptan and similar drugs (serotonin agonists) may result in weakness, hyper-reflexia, and incoordination.

CYP1A2 and CYP2D6 inhibitors may increase the levels/effects of duloxetine. Example inhibitors include amiodarone, chlorpromazine, ciprofloxacin, delavirdine, fluvoxamine, fluoxetine, ketoconazole, miconazole, norfloxacin, ofloxacin, paroxetine, pergolide, quinidine, quinine, rofecoxib, ritonavir, and ropinirole.

Decreased Effect: CYP1A2 inducers may decrease the levels/effects of duloxetine. Example inducers include aminoglutethimide, carbamazepine, phenobarbital, and rifampin.

Pharmacodynamics/Kinetics

Absorption: Well absorbed, 2-hour delay in absorption after ingestion

Distribution: 1640 L

Protein binding: >90%

Metabolism: Hepatic, via CYP1A2 and CYP2D6; forms multiple metabolites (inactive)

Half-life elimination: 12 hours (range 8-17 hours)

Time to peak: 6 hours

Excretion: As metabolites; urine (70%), feces (20%)

Pregnancy Risk Factor C

Duloxetine Hydrochloride *see* Duloxetine *on page 523*

Duocaine™ *see* Lidocaine and Bupivacaine *on page 924*

DuoFilm® [OTC] *see* Salicylic Acid *on page 1374*

DuoNeb™ *see* Ipratropium and Albuterol *on page 857*

DuoPlant® [DSC] [OTC] *see* Salicylic Acid *on page 1374*

Duotan PD *see* Dexchlorpheniramine and Pseudoephedrine *on page 443*

DuP 753 *see* Losartan *on page 950*

Duraclon™ *see* Clonidine *on page 373*

Duradrin® *see* Acetaminophen, Isometheptene, and Dichloralphenazone *on page 44*

Duragesic® *see* Fentanyl *on page 644*

Duramist® Plus [OTC] *see* Oxymetazoline *on page 1172*

Duramorph® *see* Morphine Sulfate *on page 1065*

Duraphen™ II DM *see* Guaifenesin, Dextromethorphan, and Phenylephrine *on page 756*

Duraphen™ DM *see* Guaifenesin, Dextromethorphan, and Phenylephrine *on page 756*

Duraphen™ Forte *see* Guaifenesin, Dextromethorphan, and Phenylephrine *on page 756*

Duration® [OTC] *see* Oxymetazoline *on page 1172*

Duratuss® DM *see* Guaifenesin and Dextromethorphan *on page 754*

Duricef® *see* Cefadroxil *on page 281*

Dutasteride *(doo TAS teer ide)*

U.S. Brand Names Avodart™

Canadian Brand Names Avodart™

Generic Available No

Pharmacologic Category 5 Alpha-Reductase Inhibitor

Use Treatment of symptomatic benign prostatic hyperplasia (BPH)

Unlabeled/Investigational Use Treatment of male patterned baldness

Local Anesthetic/Vasoconstrictor Precautions No information available to require special precautions

Effects on Dental Treatment No significant effects or complications reported

Common Adverse Effects

>10%: Endocrine & metabolic: Serum testosterone increased, thyroid-stimulating hormone increased

1% to 10%: Endocrine & metabolic: Impotence (1% to 5%), libido decreased (1% to 3%), ejaculation disorders (1%), gynecomastia (including breast tenderness, breast enlargement) (1%)

Note: Frequency of adverse events (except gynecomastia) tends to decrease with continued use (>6 months).

Mechanism of Action Dutasteride is a 4-azo analog of testosterone and is a competitive, selective inhibitor of both reproductive tissues (type 2) and skin and hepatic (type 1) 5α-reductase. This results in inhibition of the conversion of testosterone to dihydrotestosterone and markedly suppresses serum dihydrotestosterone levels.

Drug Interactions

Cytochrome P450 Effect: Substrate of CYP3A4 (minor)

Increased Effect/Toxicity: Calcium channel blockers, nondihydropyridine (diltiazem, verapamil) increase dutasteride levels with concurrent use.

Pharmacodynamics/Kinetics

Absorption: Via skin when handling capsules

Distribution: ~12% of serum concentrations partitioned into semen

Protein binding: 99% to albumin; ~97% to α_1-acid glycoprotein; >96% to semen protein

Metabolism: Hepatic via CYP3A4 isoenzyme; forms metabolites: 6-hydroxydutasteride has activity similar to parent compound, 4'-hydroxydutasteride and 1,2-dihydrodutasteride are much less potent than parent *in vitro*

Bioavailability: 60% (range: 40% to 94%)

Half-life elimination: Terminal: ~5 weeks

Time to peak: 2-3 hours

Excretion: Feces (40% as metabolites, 5% as unchanged drug); urine (<1% as unchanged drug); 55% of dose unaccounted for

Pregnancy Risk Factor X

DVA see Vindesine on page 1577

DW286 see Gemifloxacin on page 731

Dyazide® see Hydrochlorothiazide and Triamterene on page 778

Dyclonine (DYE kloe neen)

U.S. Brand Names Cēpacol® Dual Action Maximum Strength [OTC]; Sucrets® [OTC]

Generic Available No

Synonyms Dyclonine Hydrochloride

Pharmacologic Category Local Anesthetic, Oral

Use Temporary relief of pain associated with oral mucosa

Local Anesthetic/Vasoconstrictor Precautions No information available to require special precautions

Effects on Dental Treatment No significant effects or complications reported

Common Adverse Effects The following were reported with the previously available 0.5% and 1% topical solutions; effects are similar to other local anesthetic agents and are generally dose related; frequency not defined:

Cardiovascular: Bradycardia, hypotension

Central nervous system: Apprehension, confusion, convulsion, dizziness, drowsiness, euphoria, lightheadedness, nervousness

Gastrointestinal: Vomiting

Neuromuscular & skeletal: Numbness, tremor, twitching

Ocular: Blurred vision, double vision

Otic: Tinnitus

Respiratory: Respiratory depression

Miscellaneous: Allergic reactions, cold/heat sensation

Pharmacodynamics/Kinetics

Onset of action: Local anesthetic: 2-10 minutes

Duration: ~30 minutes

Absorption: Systemic absorption increased in presence of severely traumatized mucosa

Dyclonine Hydrochloride see Dyclonine on page 525

Dygase see Pancrelipase on page 1183

Dynabac® [DSC] see Dirithromycin on page 490

Dynacin® *see* Minocycline *on page 1049*

DynaCirc® [DSC] *see* Isradipine *on page 871*

DynaCirc® CR *see* Isradipine *on page 871*

Dyna-Hex® [OTC] *see* Chlorhexidine Gluconate *on page 316*

Dynex *see* Guaifenesin and Pseudoephedrine *on page 755*

Dyphylline (DYE fi lin)

U.S. Brand Names Dilor®; Lufyllin®
Canadian Brand Names Dilor®; Lufyllin®
Generic Available No
Synonyms Dihydroxypropyl Theophylline
Pharmacologic Category Theophylline Derivative
Use Bronchodilator in reversible airway obstruction due to asthma or COPD
Local Anesthetic/Vasoconstrictor Precautions No information available to require special precautions
Effects on Dental Treatment Do not prescribe any erythromycin product to patients taking theophylline products. Erythromycin will delay the normal metabolic inactivation of theophyllines leading to increased blood levels; this has resulted in nausea, vomiting and CNS restlessness.
Pregnancy Risk Factor C

Dyrenium® *see* Triamterene *on page 1531*

Dytan™ *see* DiphenhydrAMINE *on page 483*

E2 and DRSP *see* Drospirenone and Estradiol *on page 520*

7E3 *see* Abciximab *on page 26*

E2020 *see* Donepezil *on page 500*

EarSol® HC *see* Hydrocortisone *on page 793*

Easprin® *see* Aspirin *on page 145*

Echothiophate Iodide (ek oh THYE oh fate EYE oh dide)

U.S. Brand Names Phospholine Iodide®
Generic Available No
Synonyms Ecostigmine Iodide
Pharmacologic Category Ophthalmic Agent, Antiglaucoma; Ophthalmic Agent, Miotic
Use Used as miotic in treatment of open-angle glaucoma; may be useful in specific case of narrow-angle glaucoma; accommodative esotropia
Local Anesthetic/Vasoconstrictor Precautions No information available to require special precautions
Effects on Dental Treatment No significant effects or complications reported
Mechanism of Action Produces miosis and changes in accommodation by inhibiting cholinesterase, thereby preventing the breakdown of acetylcholine; acetylcholine is, therefore, allowed to continuously stimulate the iris and ciliary muscles of the eye
Pregnancy Risk Factor C

EC-Naprosyn® *see* Naproxen *on page 1089*

E. coli Asparaginase *see* Asparaginase *on page 144*

Econazole (e KONE a zole)

U.S. Brand Names Spectazole®
Canadian Brand Names Ecostatin®; Spectazole™
Mexican Brand Names Micostyl®; Pevaryl Lipogel®
Generic Available Yes
Synonyms Econazole Nitrate
Pharmacologic Category Antifungal Agent, Topical
Use Topical treatment of tinea pedis (athlete's foot), tinea cruris (jock itch), tinea corporis (ringworm), tinea versicolor, and cutaneous candidiasis
Local Anesthetic/Vasoconstrictor Precautions No information available to require special precautions
Effects on Dental Treatment No significant effects or complications reported
Common Adverse Effects 1% to 10%: Genitourinary: Vulvar/vaginal burning
Mechanism of Action Alters fungal cell wall membrane permeability; may interfere with RNA and protein synthesis, and lipid metabolism

Drug Interactions
Cytochrome P450 Effect: Inhibits CYP2E1 (weak)
Pharmacodynamics/Kinetics
Absorption: <10%
Metabolism: Hepatic to more than 20 metabolites
Excretion: Urine; feces (<1%)
Pregnancy Risk Factor C

Econazole Nitrate *see* Econazole *on page 526*
Econopred® Plus *see* PrednisoLONE *on page 1268*
Ecostigmine Iodide *see* Echothiophate Iodide *on page 526*
Ecotrin® [OTC] *see* Aspirin *on page 145*
Ecotrin® Low Strength [OTC] *see* Aspirin *on page 145*
Ecotrin® Maximum Strength [OTC] *see* Aspirin *on page 145*
Ed A-Hist® *see* Chlorpheniramine and Phenylephrine *on page 324*
Edathamil Disodium *see* Edetate Disodium *on page 527*
Edecrin® *see* Ethacrynic Acid *on page 590*

Edetate Calcium Disodium
(ED e tate KAL see um dye SOW dee um)

U.S. Brand Names Calcium Disodium Versenate®
Generic Available No
Synonyms CaEDTA; Calcium Disodium Edetate; Calcium EDTA; EDTA (Calcium Disodium)
Pharmacologic Category Chelating Agent
Use Treatment of symptomatic acute and chronic lead poisoning or for symptomatic patients with high blood lead levels; used as an aid in the diagnosis of lead poisoning; possibly useful in poisoning by zinc, manganese, and certain heavy radioisotopes
Local Anesthetic/Vasoconstrictor Precautions No information available to require special precautions
Effects on Dental Treatment No significant effects or complications reported
Common Adverse Effects Frequency not defined.
Cardiovascular: Arrhythmias, ECG changes, hypotension
Central nervous system: Chills, fever, headache
Dermatologic: Cheilosis, skin lesions
Endocrine & metabolic: Hypercalcemia
Gastrointestinal: Anorexia, GI upset, nausea, vomiting
Hematologic: Anemia, bone marrow suppression (transient)
Hepatic: Liver function test increased (mild)
Local: Thrombophlebitis following I.V. infusion (when concentration >5 mg/mL), pain at injection site following I.M. injection
Neuromuscular & skeletal: Arthralgia, numbness, tremor, paresthesia
Ocular: Lacrimation
Renal: Renal tubular necrosis, microscopic hematuria, proteinuria
Respiratory: Nasal congestion, sneezing
Miscellaneous: Zinc deficiency
Mechanism of Action Calcium is displaced by divalent and trivalent heavy metals, forming a nonionizing soluble complex that is excreted in urine
Drug Interactions
Decreased Effect: Do not use simultaneously with zinc insulin preparations; do not mix in the same syringe with dimercaprol.
Pharmacodynamics/Kinetics
Onset of action: Chelation of lead: I.V.: 1 hour
Absorption: I.M., SubQ: Well absorbed
Distribution: Into extracellular fluid; minimal CSF penetration
Half-life elimination, plasma: I.M.: 1.5 hours; I.V.: 20 minutes
Excretion: Urine (as metal chelates or unchanged drug); decreased GFR decreases elimination
Pregnancy Risk Factor B

Edetate Disodium (ED e tate dye SOW dee um)

U.S. Brand Names Endrate®
Generic Available Yes
Synonyms Edathamil Disodium; EDTA (Disodium); Na2EDTA; Sodium Edetate
Pharmacologic Category Chelating Agent
Use Emergency treatment of hypercalcemia; control digitalis-induced cardiac dysrhythmias (ventricular arrhythmias)
(Continued)

Edetate Disodium *(Continued)*

Local Anesthetic/Vasoconstrictor Precautions No information available to require special precautions

Effects on Dental Treatment No significant effects or complications reported

Common Adverse Effects Rapid I.V. administration or excessive doses may cause a sudden drop in serum calcium concentration which may lead to hypocalcemic tetany, seizure, arrhythmia, and death from respiratory arrest. Do **not** exceed recommended dosage and rate of administration.

1% to 10%: Gastrointestinal: Nausea, vomiting, abdominal cramps, diarrhea

Mechanism of Action Chelates with divalent or trivalent metals to form a soluble complex that is then eliminated in urine

Drug Interactions

Increased Effect/Toxicity: Increased effect of insulin (edetate disodium may decrease blood glucose concentrations and reduce insulin requirements in diabetic patients treated with insulin).

Pharmacodynamics/Kinetics

Metabolism: None

Half-life elimination: 20-60 minutes

Time to peak: I.V.: 24-48 hours

Excretion: Following chelation: Urine (95%); chelates within 24-48 hours

Pregnancy Risk Factor C

Edex® *see Alprostadil on page 76*

Edrophonium *(ed roe FOE nee um)*

U.S. Brand Names Enlon®; Reversol®

Canadian Brand Names Enlon®

Generic Available No

Synonyms Edrophonium Chloride

Pharmacologic Category Antidote; Cholinergic Agonist; Diagnostic Agent

Use Diagnosis of myasthenia gravis; differentiation of cholinergic crises from myasthenia crises; reversal of nondepolarizing neuromuscular blockers; adjunct treatment of respiratory depression caused by curare overdose

Local Anesthetic/Vasoconstrictor Precautions No information available to require special precautions

Effects on Dental Treatment No significant effects or complications reported

Common Adverse Effects Frequency not defined.

Cardiovascular: Arrhythmias (especially bradycardia), hypotension, decreased carbon monoxide, tachycardia, AV block, nodal rhythm, nonspecific ECG changes, cardiac arrest, syncope, flushing

Central nervous system: Convulsions, dysarthria, dysphonia, dizziness, loss of consciousness, drowsiness, headache

Dermatologic: Skin rash, thrombophlebitis (I.V.), urticaria

Gastrointestinal: Hyperperistalsis, nausea, vomiting, salivation, diarrhea, stomach cramps, dysphagia, flatulence

Genitourinary: Urinary urgency

Neuromuscular & skeletal: Weakness, fasciculations, muscle cramps, spasms, arthralgia

Ocular: Small pupils, lacrimation

Respiratory: Increased bronchial secretions, laryngospasm, bronchiolar constriction; respiratory muscle paralysis, dyspnea, respiratory depression, respiratory arrest, bronchospasm

Miscellaneous: Diaphoresis (increased), anaphylaxis, allergic reactions

Mechanism of Action Inhibits destruction of acetylcholine by acetylcholinesterase. This facilitates transmission of impulses across myoneural junction and results in increased cholinergic responses such as miosis, increased tonus of intestinal and skeletal muscles, bronchial and ureteral constriction, bradycardia, and increased salivary and sweat gland secretions.

Drug Interactions

Increased Effect/Toxicity: Digoxin may enhance bradycardia potential of edrophonium. Effects of succinylcholine, decamethonium, nondepolarizing muscle relaxants (eg, pancuronium, vecuronium) are prolonged by edrophonium. I.V. acetazolamide, neostigmine, physostigmine, and acute muscle weakness may increase the effects of edrophonium.

Decreased Effect: Atropine, nondepolarizing muscle relaxants, procainamide, and quinidine may antagonize the effects of edrophonium.

Pharmacodynamics/Kinetics

Onset of action: I.M.: 2-10 minutes; I.V.: 30-60 seconds

Duration: I.M.: 5-30 minutes; I.V.: 10 minutes

Distribution: V_d: Adults: 1.1 L/kg

Half-life elimination: Adults:1.2-2.4 hours; Anephric patients: 2.4-4.4 hours
Excretion: Adults: Primarily urine (67%)
Pregnancy Risk Factor C

Edrophonium and Atropine (ed roe FOE nee um & A troe peen)

Related Information
  Atropine *on page 161*
U.S. Brand Names Enlon-Plus™
Generic Available No
Synonyms Atropine Sulfate and Edrophonium Chloride; Edrophonium Chloride and Atropine Sulfate
Pharmacologic Category Anticholinergic Agent; Antidote; Cholinergic Agonist
Use Reversal of nondepolarizing neuromuscular blockers; adjunct treatment of respiratory depression caused by curare overdose
Local Anesthetic/Vasoconstrictor Precautions Bradyarrhythmias, tachycardia, and premature ventricular contractions have been reported; use vasoconstrictor with caution
Effects on Dental Treatment No significant effects or complications reported
Common Adverse Effects Also see individual agents.
  >10%: Cardiovascular: Bradycardia, junctional rhythm, tachycardia
  1% to 10%: Cardiovascular: Atrial premature contractions (3% to 10%), first-degree AV block (3% to 10%), P-wave changes (3% to 10%), second-degree AV block (3% to 10%), third-degree AV block (1% to 3%), premature ventricular contractions (1% to 3%)
Mechanism of Action
  Edrophonium: Inhibits destruction of acetylcholine by acetylcholinesterase. This facilitates transmission of impulses across myoneural junction and results in increased cholinergic response.
  Atropine: Minimizes or prevents the muscarinic cholinergic effects caused by edrophonium (eg, bradycardia, bronchocontriction, and increased secretions).
Drug Interactions
  Increased Effect/Toxicity: Concurrent use with narcotic analgesics (without an inhaled anesthetic), beta blockers, or nondepolarizing-neuromuscular blockers without vagolytic activity may result in increased bradyarrhythmias. Concurrent use with other anticholinergics may increase incidence of anticholinergic adverse events.
Pharmacodynamics/Kinetics See individual agents.
  Onset of action: Edrophonium: Antagonism of nondepolarizing muscle relaxants: 3 minutes; Atropine: Heart rate: Immediate
  Duration: Edrophonium: Antagonism of nondepolarizing muscle relaxants: 70 minutes; Atropine: Heart rate: 170 minutes
  Protein binding: Atropine: 14%
  Half-life elimination: Edrophonium: Adults: 1.2-2.4 hours; Anephric patients: 2.4-4.4 hours
  Time to peak, plasma: Edrophonium: Antagonism of nondepolarizing muscle relaxants: 1.2 minutes; Atropine: Heart rate: 2-16 minutes
  Excretion: Edrophonium: Primarily urine (67%)
Pregnancy Risk Factor C

Edrophonium Chloride *see* Edrophonium *on page 528*

Edrophonium Chloride and Atropine Sulfate *see* Edrophonium and Atropine *on page 529*

EDTA (Calcium Disodium) *see* Edetate Calcium Disodium *on page 527*

EDTA (Disodium) *see* Edetate Disodium *on page 527*

E.E.S.® *see* Erythromycin *on page 562*

Efalizumab (e fa li ZOO mab)

U.S. Brand Names Raptiva®
Generic Available No
Synonyms Anti-CD11a; hu1124
Pharmacologic Category Immunosuppressant Agent; Monoclonal Antibody
Use Treatment of chronic moderate-to-severe plaque psoriasis in patients who are candidates for systemic therapy or phototherapy
Local Anesthetic/Vasoconstrictor Precautions No information available to require special precautions
Effects on Dental Treatment No significant effects or complications reported
(Continued)

Efalizumab *(Continued)*

Common Adverse Effects

>10%:

Central nervous system: Headache (32%), chills (13%)

Gastrointestinal: Nausea (11%)

Hematologic: Lymphocytosis (40%), leukocytosis (26%)

Miscellaneous: First-dose reaction (29%, described as chills, fever, headache, myalgia, and nausea occurring within 2 days of the first injection; percent reported in patients receiving a 1 mg/kg dose; severity decreased with 0.7 mg/kg dose); infection (29%, serious infection <1%)

1% to 10%:

Cardiovascular: Peripheral edema (1% to 2%)

Central nervous system: Pain (1% to 2%), fever (7%)

Dermatologic: Acne (4%), psoriasis (1% to 2%), urticaria (1%)

Hepatic: Alkaline phosphatase elevated (4%)

Neuromuscular & skeletal: Myalgia (8%), back pain (4%), arthralgia (1% to 2%), weakness (1% to 2%)

Miscellaneous: Antibodies to efalizumab (6%); hypersensitivity reaction, including asthma, dyspnea, angioedema, urticaria, or maculopapular rash (8%); flu-like syndrome (7%)

Mechanism of Action Efalizumab is a recombinant monoclonal antibody which binds to CD11a, a subunit of leukocyte function antigen-1 (LFA-1) found on leukocytes. By binding to CD11a, efalizumab blocks multiple T-cell mediated responses involved in the pathogenesis of psoriatic plaques.

Drug Interactions

Increased Effect/Toxicity: Concurrent use of immunosuppressants may increase risk of infection.

Decreased Effect: Note: Formal drug interaction studies have not been conducted. Acellular, live, and live-attenuated vaccines should not be administered during therapy.

Pharmacodynamics/Kinetics

Onset: Reduction of CD11a expression and free CD11a-binding sites seen 1-2 days after the first dose; time to steady state serum concentration: 4 weeks

Response to therapy (75% reduction from baseline of PASI score): Observed after 12 weeks

Duration: CD11a expression was ~74% of baseline at 5-13 weeks after discontinuing dose; free CD11a binding sites were at ~86% of baseline at 8-13 weeks following discontinuation; response to therapy (75% reduction from baseline PASI score) continued 1-2 months after discontinuation

Bioavailability: SubQ: 50%

Excretion: Time to eliminate (at steady state): 25 days (range: 13-35 days)

Pregnancy Risk Factor C

Efavirenz *(e FAV e renz)*

Related Information

HIV Infection and AIDS *on page 1662*
Tuberculosis *on page 1673*

U.S. Brand Names Sustiva®

Canadian Brand Names Sustiva®

Generic Available No

Pharmacologic Category Antiretroviral Agent, Reverse Transcriptase Inhibitor (Non-nucleoside)

Use Treatment of HIV-1 infections in combination with at least two other antiretroviral agents

Local Anesthetic/Vasoconstrictor Precautions No information available to require special precautions

Effects on Dental Treatment Key adverse event(s) related to dental treatment: Xerostomia (normal salivary flow resumes upon discontinuation) and abnormal taste.

Common Adverse Effects

>10%:

Central nervous system: Dizziness* (2% to 28%), depression (1% to 16%), insomnia (6% to 16%), anxiety (1% to 11%), pain* (1% to 13%)

Dermatologic: Rash* (NCI grade 1: 9% to 11%, NCI grade 2: 15% to 32%, NCI grade 3 or 4: <1%); 26% experienced new rash vs 17% in control groups; up to 46% of pediatric patients experience rash (median onset: 8 days)

Endocrine & metabolic: HDL increased (25% to 35%), total cholesterol increased (20% to 40%)

Gastrointestinal: Diarrhea* (3% to 14%), nausea* (2% to 12%)

1% to 10%:

Central nervous system: Impaired concentration (2% to 8%), headache* (2% to 7%), somnolence (2% to 7%), fatigue (2% to 7%), abnormal dreams (1% to 6%), nervousness (2% to 6%), severe depression (2%), hallucinations (1%)

Dermatologic: Pruritus (1% to 9%)

Gastrointestinal: Vomiting* (6% to 7%), dyspepsia (3%), abdominal pain (1% to 3%), anorexia (1% to 2%)

Miscellaneous: Diaphoresis increased (1% to 2%)

*Adverse effect reported in ≥10% of patients 3-16 years of age

Mechanism of Action As a non-nucleoside reverse transcriptase inhibitor, efavirenz has activity against HIV-1 by binding to reverse transcriptase. It consequently blocks the RNA-dependent and DNA-dependent DNA polymerase activities including HIV-1 replication. It does not require intracellular phosphorylation for antiviral activity.

Drug Interactions

Cytochrome P450 Effect: Substrate (major) of CYP2B6, 3A4; **Inhibits** CYP2C9 (moderate), 2C19 (moderate), 3A4 (moderate); **Induces** CYP2B6 (weak), 3A4 (strong)

Increased Effect/Toxicity: Coadministration with medications metabolized by these enzymes may lead to increased concentration-related effects. Cisapride, midazolam, triazolam, and ergot alkaloids may result in life-threatening toxicities; concurrent use is contraindicated. May increase (or decrease) effect of warfarin. Efavirenz may increase the levels/effects of CYP2C9 substrates; example substrates include bosentan, dapsone, fluoxetine, glimepiride, glipizide, losartan, montelukast, nateglinide, paclitaxel, phenytoin, warfarin, and zafirlukast. CYP2C19 substrates: Efavirenz may increase the levels/effects of CYP2C19 substrates; example substrates include citalopram, diazepam, methsuximide, phenytoin, propranolol, and sertraline. Efavirenz may alter the levels/effects of CYP3A4 substrates; example substrates include benzodiazepines, calcium channel blockers, ergot derivatives, mirtazapine, nateglinide, nefazodone, tacrolimus, and venlafaxine.

Decreased Effect: CYP2B6 inducers may decrease the levels/effects of efavirenz; example inducers include carbamazepine, nevirapine, phenobarbital, phenytoin, and rifampin. St John's wort may decrease serum concentrations of efavirenz. Concentrations of atazanavir, indinavir, and/or lopinavir may be reduced; dosage adjustments required. Concentrations of saquinavir may be decreased (use as sole protease inhibitor is not recommended). Serum concentrations of methadone may be decreased; monitor for withdrawal. May decrease (or increase) effect of warfarin. Serum concentrations of sertraline may be decreased by efavirenz. CYP3A4 inducers may decrease the levels/effects of efavirenz; example inducers include aminoglutethimide, carbamazepine, nafcillin, nevirapine, phenobarbital, phenytoin, and rifamycins. Voriconazole serum levels may be reduced by efavirenz (concurrent use is contraindicated).

Efavirenz may increase the levels/effects of CYP2C8/9 substrates; example substrates include fluoxetine, glimepiride, glipizide, nateglinide, phenytoin, pioglitazone, rosiglitazone, sertraline, and warfarin. Efavirenz may increase the levels/effects of CYP2C19 substrates; example substrates include citalopram, diazepam, methsuximide, phenytoin, propranolol, and sertraline. Efavirenz may alter the levels/effects of CYP3A4 substrates; example substrates include benzodiazepines, calcium channel blockers, ergot derivatives, mirtazapine, nateglinide, nefazodone, tacrolimus, and venlafaxine.

Pharmacodynamics/Kinetics

Absorption: Increased by fatty meals

Distribution: CSF concentrations exceed free fraction in serum

Protein binding: >99%, primarily to albumin

Metabolism: Hepatic via CYP3A4 and 2B6; may induce its own metabolism

Half-life elimination: Single dose: 52-76 hours; Multiple doses: 40-55 hours

Time to peak: 3-8 hours

Excretion: Feces (16% to 41% primarily as unchanged drug); urine (14% to 34% as metabolites)

Pregnancy Risk Factor D

Effer-K™ see Potassium Bicarbonate and Potassium Citrate on page 1258

Effexor® see Venlafaxine on page 1568

Effexor® XR see Venlafaxine on page 1568

Eflone® [DSC] see Fluorometholone on page 674

Eflornithine (ee FLOR ni theen)

U.S. Brand Names Vaniqa™
Generic Available No
Synonyms DFMO; Eflornithine Hydrochloride
Pharmacologic Category Antiprotozoal; Topical Skin Product
Use Cream: Females ≥12 years: Reduce unwanted hair from face and adjacent areas under the chin

Orphan status: Injection: Treatment of meningoencephalitic stage of *Trypanosoma brucei gambiense* infection (sleeping sickness)

Local Anesthetic/Vasoconstrictor Precautions No information available to require special precautions

Effects on Dental Treatment No significant effects or complications reported

Common Adverse Effects
Injection:
>10%: Hematologic (reversible): Anemia (55%), leukopenia (37%), thrombocytopenia (14%)
1% to 10%:
Central nervous system: Seizures (may be due to the disease) (8%), dizziness
Dermatologic: Alopecia
Gastrointestinal: Vomiting, diarrhea
Hematologic: Eosinophilia
Otic: Hearing impairment
Topical:
>10%: Dermatologic: Acne (11% to 21%), pseudofolliculitis barbae (5% to 15%)
1% to 10%:
Central nervous system: Headache (4% to 5%), dizziness (1%), vertigo (0.3% to 1%)
Dermatologic: Pruritus (3% to 4%), burning skin (2% to 4%), tingling skin (1% to 4%), dry skin (2% to 3%), rash (1% to 3%), facial edema (0.3% to 3%), alopecia (1% to 2%), skin irritation (1% to 2%), erythema (0% to 2%), ingrown hair (0.3% to 2%), folliculitis (0% to 1%)
Gastrointestinal: Dyspepsia (2%), anorexia (0.7% to 2%)

Mechanism of Action Eflornithine exerts antitumor and antiprotozoal effects through specific, irreversible ("suicide") inhibition of the enzyme ornithine decarboxylase (ODC). ODC is the rate-limiting enzyme in the biosynthesis of putrescine, spermine, and spermidine, the major polyamines in nucleated cells. Polyamines are necessary for the synthesis of DNA, RNA, and proteins and are, therefore, necessary for cell growth and differentiation. Although many microorganisms and higher plants are able to produce polyamines from alternate biochemical pathways, all mammalian cells depend on ornithine decarboxylase to produce polyamines. Eflornithine inhibits ODC and rapidly depletes animal cells of putrescine and spermidine; the concentration of spermine remains the same or may even increase. Rapidly dividing cells appear to be most susceptible to the effects of eflornithine. Topically, the inhibition of ODC in the skin leads to a decreased rate of hair growth.

Drug Interactions
Increased Effect/Toxicity: Cream: Possible interactions with other topical products have not been studied.
Decreased Effect: Cream: Possible interactions with other topical products have not been studied.

Pharmacodynamics/Kinetics
Absorption: Topical: <1%
Half-life elimination: I.V.: 3-3.5 hours; Topical: 8 hours
Excretion: Primarily urine (as unchanged drug)

Pregnancy Risk Factor C

Eflornithine Hydrochloride *see* Eflornithine *on page 532*
Efudex® *see* Fluorouracil *on page 674*
E-Gems® [OTC] *see* Vitamin E *on page 1581*
E-Gems Elite® [OTC] *see* Vitamin E *on page 1581*
E-Gems Plus® [OTC] *see* Vitamin E *on page 1581*
EHDP *see* Etidronate Disodium *on page 621*
Elavil *see* Amitriptyline *on page 93*
Eldepryl® *see* Selegiline *on page 1382*
Eldisine Lilly 99094 *see* Vindesine *on page 1577*
Eldopaque® [OTC] *see* Hydroquinone *on page 798*
Eldopaque Forte® *see* Hydroquinone *on page 798*

Eldoquin® [OTC] *see* Hydroquinone *on page 798*

Eldoquin Forte® *see* Hydroquinone *on page 798*

Electrolyte Lavage Solution *see* Polyethylene Glycol-Electrolyte Solution *on page 1253*

Elestat™ *see* Epinastine *on page 546*

Eletriptan (el e TRIP tan)

U.S. Brand Names Relpax®
Canadian Brand Names Relpax®
Mexican Brand Names Relpax®
Generic Available No
Synonyms Eletriptan Hydrobromide
Pharmacologic Category Serotonin 5-HT$_{1B, 1D}$ Receptor Agonist
Use Acute treatment of migraine, with or without aura
Local Anesthetic/Vasoconstrictor Precautions No information available to require special precautions
Effects on Dental Treatment Key adverse event(s) related to dental treatment: Xerostomia (normal salivary flow resumes upon discontinuation).
Common Adverse Effects 1% to 10%:
  Cardiovascular: Chest pain/tightness (1% to 4%; placebo 1%), palpitation
  Central nervous system: Dizziness (3% to 7%; placebo 3%), somnolence (3% to 7%; placebo 4%), headache (3% to 4%; placebo 3%), chills, pain, vertigo
  Gastrointestinal: Nausea (4% to 8%; placebo 5%), xerostomia (2% to 4%; placebo 2%), dysphagia (1% to 2%), abdominal pain/discomfort (1% to 2%; placebo 1%), dyspepsia (1% to 2%; placebo 1%)
  Neuromuscular & skeletal: Weakness (4% to 10%), paresthesia (3% to 4%), back pain, hypertonia, hypoesthesia
  Respiratory: Pharyngitis
  Miscellaneous: Diaphoresis
Mechanism of Action Selective agonist for serotonin (5-HT$_{1B}$, 5-HT$_{1D}$, 5-HT$_{1F}$ receptors) in cranial arteries; causes vasoconstriction and reduce sterile inflammation associated with antidromic neuronal transmission correlating with relief of migraine
Drug Interactions
  Cytochrome P450 Effect: Substrate of CYP3A4 (major)
  Increased Effect/Toxicity: CYP3A4 inhibitors increase serum concentration and half-life of eletriptan; do not use eletriptan within 72 hours of potent CYP3A4 inhibitors (eg, azole antifungals, clarithromycin, diclofenac, doxycycline, erythromycin, imatinib, isoniazid, nefazodone, nicardipine, propofol, protease inhibitors, quinidine, telithromycin, verapamil). Ergot-containing drugs prolong vasospastic reactions; do not use within 24 hours of eletriptan.
Pharmacodynamics/Kinetics
  Absorption: Well absorbed
  Distribution: V$_d$: 138 L
  Protein binding: ~85%
  Metabolism: Hepatic via CYP3A4; forms one metabolite (active)
  Bioavailability: ~50%, increased with high-fat meal
  Half-life elimination: 4 hours (Elderly: 4.4-5.7 hours); Metabolite: ~13 hours
  Time to peak, plasma: 1.5-2 hours
Pregnancy Risk Factor C

Eletriptan Hydrobromide *see* Eletriptan *on page 533*

Elidel® *see* Pimecrolimus *on page 1237*

Eligard® *see* Leuprolide *on page 906*

Elimite® *see* Permethrin *on page 1218*

Elipten *see* Aminoglutethimide *on page 87*

Elitek™ *see* Rasburicase *on page 1337*

Elixophyllin® *see* Theophylline *on page 1473*

Elixophyllin-GG® *see* Theophylline and Guaifenesin *on page 1475*

ElixSure™ Congestion [OTC] *see* Pseudoephedrine *on page 1309*

ElixSure™ Cough [OTC] *see* Dextromethorphan *on page 451*

ElixSure™ Fever/Pain [OTC] [DSC] *see* Acetaminophen *on page 31*

ElixSure™ IB [OTC] *see* Ibuprofen *on page 808*

Ellence® *see* Epirubicin *on page 550*

Elmiron® *see* Pentosan Polysulfate Sodium *on page 1211*

Elocon® *see* Mometasone Furoate *on page 1060*

Eloxatin™ *see* Oxaliplatin *on page 1154*

Elspar® *see* Asparaginase *on page 144*

Emadine® *see* Emedastine *on page 534*
Embeline™ *see* Clobetasol *on page 365*
Embeline™ E *see* Clobetasol *on page 365*
Emcyt® *see* Estramustine *on page 578*

Emedastine (em e DAS teen)

U.S. Brand Names Emadine®
Synonyms Emedastine Difumarate
Pharmacologic Category Antihistamine, H₁ Blocker, Ophthalmic
Use Treatment of allergic conjunctivitis
Local Anesthetic/Vasoconstrictor Precautions No information available to require special precautions
Effects on Dental Treatment No significant effects or complications reported
Mechanism of Action Selective histamine H₁-receptor antagonist for topical ophthalmic use
Pregnancy Risk Factor B

Emedastine Difumarate *see* Emedastine *on page 534*
Emend® *see* Aprepitant *on page 134*
Emetrol® [OTC] *see* Fructose, Dextrose, and Phosphoric Acid *on page 713*
Emko® [OTC] [DSC] *see* Nonoxynol 9 *on page 1124*
EMLA® *see* Lidocaine and Prilocaine *on page 928*

Haemophilus b Conjugate Vaccine
(he MOF fi lus bee KON joo gate vak SEEN)

Related Information
Immunizations (Vaccines) *on page 1786*
U.S. Brand Names ActHIB®; HibTITER®; PedvaxHIB®
Canadian Brand Names ActHIB®; PedvaxHIB®
Generic Available No
Synonyms Diphtheria CRM₁₉₇ Protein Conjugate; Diphtheria Toxoid Conjugate; *Haemophilus* b Oligosaccharide Conjugate Vaccine; *Haemophilus* b Polysaccharide Vaccine; HbCV; HbOC; Hib Polysaccharide Conjugate; PRP-OMP; PRP-T
Pharmacologic Category Vaccine
Use Routine immunization of children 2 months to 5 years of age against invasive disease caused by *H. influenzae*

Unimmunized children ≥5 years of age with a chronic illness known to be associated with increased risk of *Haemophilus influenzae* type b disease, specifically, persons with anatomic or functional asplenia or sickle cell anemia or those who have undergone splenectomy, should receive *Haemophilus influenzae* type b (Hib) vaccine.

Haemophilus b conjugate vaccines are not indicated for prevention of bronchitis or other infections due to *H. influenzae* in adults; adults with specific dysfunction or certain complement deficiencies who are at especially high risk of *H. influenzae* type b infection (HIV-infected adults); patients with Hodgkin's disease (vaccinated at least 2 weeks before the initiation of chemotherapy or 3 months after the end of chemotherapy)

Local Anesthetic/Vasoconstrictor Precautions No information available to require special precautions
Effects on Dental Treatment No significant effects or complications reported
Common Adverse Effects All serious adverse reactions must be reported to the U.S. Department of Health and Human Services (DHHS) Vaccine Adverse Event Reporting System (VAERS) 1-800-822-7967. Frequency not defined:

Central nervous system: Crying (unusual, high pitched, prolonged); fever, irritability, pain, sleepiness
Dermatologic: Rash
Gastrointestinal: Anorexia, diarrhea, vomiting
Local: Injection site: Erythema, induration, pain, soreness, swelling
Otic: Otitis media
Respiratory: Upper respiratory tract infection
Mechanism of Action Stimulates production of anticapsular antibodies and provides active immunity to *Haemophilus influenzae*

Drug Interactions

Decreased Effect: The effect of the vaccine may be decreased with immuno-suppressive agents; consider deferring vaccination for 3 months after immunosuppressant therapy is discontinued.

Pharmacodynamics/Kinetics Seroconversion following one dose of Hib vaccine for children 18 months or 24 months of age or older is 75% to 90% respectively.

Onset of action: Serum antibody response: 1-2 weeks

Duration: Immunity: 1.5 years

Pregnancy Risk Factor C

Lactobacillus (lak toe ba SIL us)

Related Information
Bifidobacterium bifidum / Lactobacillus acidophilus on page 1615
Ulcerative and Erosive Disorders *on page 1712*

U.S. Brand Names Bacid® [OTC]; Culturelle® [OTC]; Dofus [OTC]; Flora-Q™ [OTC]; Kala® [OTC]; Lactinex™ [OTC]; Lacto-Bifidus [OTC]; Lacto-Key [OTC]; Lacto-Pectin [OTC]; Lacto-TriBlend [OTC]; Megadophilus® [OTC]; MoreDophilus® [OTC]; Superdophilus® [OTC]

Canadian Brand Names Bacid®; Fermalac

Generic Available Yes

Synonyms *Lactobacillus acidophilus*; *Lactobacillus bifidus*; *Lactobacillus bulgaricus*; *Lactobacillus casei*; *Lactobacillus paracasei*; *Lactobacillus reuteri*; *Lactobacillus rhamnosus* GG

Pharmacologic Category Dietary Supplement; Probiotic

Dental Use Treatment of uncomplicated diarrhea, particularly that caused by antibiotic therapy; re-establish normal physiologic and bacterial flora of the intestinal tract

Use Promote normal bacterial flora of the intestinal tract

Local Anesthetic/Vasoconstrictor Precautions No information available to require special precautions

Effects on Dental Treatment No significant effects or complications reported

Significant Adverse Effects Gastrointestinal: Flatulence

Dosage
Dietary supplement: Oral: Dosing varies by manufacturer; consult product labeling

Children (Culturelle®): 1 capsule daily

Adults:
Bacid®: 2 caplets/day
Culturelle®: 1 capsule daily; may increase to twice daily
Flora-Q™: 1 capsule/day
Lacto-Key 100 or 600: 1-2 capsules/day
Lactinex™: 1 packet or 4 tablets 3-4 times/day

Mechanism of Action Helps re-establish normal intestinal flora; suppresses the growth of potentially pathogenic microorganisms by producing lactic acid which favors the establishment of an aciduric flora.

Contraindications Hypersensitivity to any component of the formulation

Warnings/Precautions *Lactobacillus* species have been studied for various gastrointestinal disorders including diarrhea, inflammatory bowel disease, gastrointestinal infection. Effectiveness may be dependant upon actual species used; studies are ongoing. Currently, there are no FDA-approved disease-prevention or therapeutic indications for these products.

Drug Interactions No data reported

Dietary Considerations
Products may contain whey, evaporated milk, soy peptone casein and/or beef extract; consult individual product labeling. Lactinex™ contains sodium 5.6 mg/4 tablets

Pharmacodynamics/Kinetics
Absorption: Oral: None
Distribution: Local, primarily colon
Excretion: Feces

Dosage Forms
Capsule:
Culturelle®: *L. rhamnosus* GG 10 billion colony-forming units [contains casein and whey]
Dofus: *L. acidophilus* and *L. bifidus* 10:1 ratio [beet root powder base]
Flora-Q™: *L. acidophilus* and *L. paracasei* ≥8 billion colony-forming units [also contains *Bifidobacterium* and *S. thermophilus*]

(Continued)

Lactobacillus (Continued)

Lacto-Key:
    100: *L. acidophilus* 1 billion colony-forming units [milk, soy, and yeast free; rice derived]
    600: *L. acidophilus* 6 billion colony-forming units [milk, soy, and yeast free; rice derived]

Lacto-Bifidus:
    100: *L. bifidus* 1 billion colony-forming units [milk, soy, and yeast free; rice derived]
    600: *L. bifidus* 6 billion colony-forming units [milk, soy, and yeast free; rice derived]

Lacto-Pectin: *L. acidophilus* and *L. casei* ≥5 billion colony-forming units [also contains *Bifidobacterium lactis* and citrus pectin cellulose complex]

Lacto-TriBlend:
    100: *L. acidophilus*, *L. bifidus*, and *L. bulgaricus* 1 billion colony-forming units [milk, soy and yeast free; rice derived]
    600: *L. acidophilus*, *L. bifidus*, and *L. bulgaricus* 6 billion colony-forming units [milk, soy and yeast free; rice derived]

Megadophilus®, Superdophilus®: *L. acidophilus* 2 billion units [available in dairy based or dairy free formulations]

Capsule, softgel: *L. acidophilus* 100 active units

Caplet (Bacid®): *L. acidophilus* 80% and *L. bulgaricus* 10% [also contains *Bifidobacterium biffidum* 5% and *S. thermophilus* 5%]

Granules (Lactinex™): *L. acidophilus* and *L. bulgaricus* 100 million live cells per 1 g packet (12s) [contains whey, evaporated milk, soy peptone, lactose, and beef extract]

Powder:
    Lacto-TriBlend: *L. acidophilus*, *L. bifidus*, and *L. bulgaricus* 10 billion colony-forming units per ¼ teaspoon (60 g) [milk, soy, and yeast free; rice derived]

    Megadophilus®, Superdophilus®: *L. acidophilus* 2 billion units per half-teaspoon (49 g, 70 g, 84 g, 126 g) [available in dairy based or dairy free (garbanzo bean) formulations]

    MoreDophilus®: *L. acidophilus* 12.4 billion units per teaspoon (30 g, 120 g) [dairy free, yeast free; soy and carrot derived]

Tablet:
    Kala®: *L. acidophilus* 200 million units [dairy free, yeast free; soy based]
    Lactinex™: *L. acidophilus* and *L. bulgaricus* 1 million live cells [contains whey, evaporated milk, soy peptone, lactose, and beef extract; contains sodium 5.6 mg/4 tablets]

Tablet, chewable: *L. reuteri* 100 million organisms

Wafer: *L. acidophilus* 90 mg and *L. bifidus* 25 mg (100s) [provides 1 billion organisms/wafer at time of manufacture; milk free]

Emsam® *see* Selegiline *on page 1382*

Emtricitabine (em trye SYE ta been)

U.S. Brand Names Emtriva®
Generic Available No
Synonyms BW524W91; Coviracil; FTC
Pharmacologic Category Antiretroviral Agent, Reverse Transcriptase Inhibitor (Nucleoside)
Use Treatment of HIV infection in combination with at least two other antiretroviral agents
Unlabeled/Investigational Use Hepatitis B (with HIV coinfection)
Local Anesthetic/Vasoconstrictor Precautions No information available to require special precautions
Effects on Dental Treatment No significant effects or complications reported
Common Adverse Effects Clinical trials were conducted in patients receiving other antiretroviral agents, and it is not possible to correlate frequency of adverse events with emtricitabine alone. The range of frequencies of adverse events is generally comparable to comparator groups, with the exception of hyperpigmentation, which occurred more frequently in patients receiving emtricitabine. Unless otherwise noted, percentages are as reported in adults.
>10%:
    Central nervous system: Dizziness (4% to 25%), headache (13% to 22%), fever (children 18%), insomnia (7% to 16%), abnormal dreams (2% to 11%)

536

Dermatologic: Hyperpigmentation (adults 2% to 4%; children 32%; primarily of palms and/or soles but may include tongue, arms, lip and nails; generally mild and nonprogressive without associated local reactions such as pruritus or rash); rash (17% to 30%; includes pruritus, maculopapular rash, vesiculobullous rash, pustular rash, and allergic reaction)

Gastrointestinal: Diarrhea (adults 23%; children 20%), vomiting (adults 9%; children 23%), nausea (13% to 18%), abdominal pain (8% to 14%), gastroenteritis (children 11%)

Neuromuscular & skeletal: Weakness (12% to 16%), CPK increased (11% to 12%)

Otic: Otitis media (children 23%)

Respiratory: Cough (adults 14%; children 28%), rhinitis (adults 12% to 18%; children 20%), pneumonia (children 15%)

Miscellaneous: Infection (children 44%)

1% to 10%:
Central nervous system: Depression (6% to 9%), neuropathy/neuritis (4%)

Endocrine & metabolic: Serum triglycerides increased (9% to 10%), disordered glucose homeostasis (2% to 3%), serum amylase increased (adults 2% to 5%; children 9%), serum lipase increased (≤1%)

Gastrointestinal: Dyspepsia (4% to 8%)

Hematologic: Anemia (children: 7%)

Hepatic: Transaminases increased (2% to 6%), bilirubin increased (1%)

Neuromuscular & skeletal: Myalgia (4% to 6%), paresthesia (5% to 6%), arthralgia (3% to 5%)

Mechanism of Action Nucleoside reverse transcriptase inhibitor; emtricitabine is a cytosine analogue which is phosphorylated intracellularly to emtricitabine 5'-triphosphate which interferes with HIV viral RNA dependent DNA polymerase resulting in inhibition of viral replication.

Drug Interactions
Increased Effect/Toxicity: Concomitant use of ribavirin and nucleoside analogues may increase the risk of developing lactic acidosis.

Pharmacodynamics/Kinetics
Absorption: Rapid, extensive
Protein binding: <4%
Metabolism: Limited, via oxidation and conjugation (not via CYP isoenzymes)
Bioavailability: Capsule: 93%; solution: 75%
Half-life elimination: Normal renal function: Adults: 10 hours; children: 5-18 hours
Time to peak, plasma: 1-2 hours
Excretion: Urine (86% primarily as unchanged drug, 13% as metabolites); feces (14%)

Pregnancy Risk Factor B

Emtricitabine and Tenofovir
(em trye SYE ta been & te NOE fo veer)

Related Information
Emtricitabine *on page 536*
Tenofovir *on page 1457*

U.S. Brand Names Truvada®

Canadian Brand Names Truvada®

Generic Available No

Synonyms Tenofovir and Emtricitabine

Pharmacologic Category Antiretroviral Agent, Reverse Transcriptase Inhibitor (Nucleoside); Antiretroviral Agent, Reverse Transcriptase Inhibitor (Nucleotide)

Use Treatment of HIV infection in combination with other antiretroviral agents

Local Anesthetic/Vasoconstrictor Precautions No information available to require special precautions

Effects on Dental Treatment No significant effects or complications reported

Common Adverse Effects The adverse reaction profile of combination therapy has not been established. See individual agents.

Mechanism of Action Nucleoside and nucleotide reverse transcriptase inhibitor combination; emtricitabine is a cytosine analogue while tenofovir disoproxil fumarate (TDF) is an analog of adenosine 5'-monophosphate. Each drug interferes with HIV viral RNA dependent DNA polymerase resulting in inhibition of viral replication.

Drug Interactions
Increased Effect/Toxicity: Refer to individual agents.

Pharmacodynamics/Kinetics Refer to individual monographs.

Pregnancy Risk Factor B

Emtriva® *see* Emtricitabine *on page 536*
Emulsoil® [OTC] [DSC] *see* Castor Oil *on page 279*
ENA 713 *see* Rivastigmine *on page 1361*
Enablex® *see* Darifenacin *on page 424*

Enalapril (e NAL a pril)

Related Information
Cardiovascular Diseases *on page 1636*
U.S. Brand Names Vasotec®
Canadian Brand Names Vasotec®
Mexican Brand Names Enaladil®; Feliberal®; Glioten®; Kenopril®; Norpril®; Palane®; Pulsol®; Renitec®
Generic Available Yes
Synonyms Enalaprilat; Enalapril Maleate
Pharmacologic Category Angiotensin-Converting Enzyme (ACE) Inhibitor
Use Management of mild to severe hypertension; treatment of congestive heart failure, left ventricular dysfunction after myocardial infarction
Unlabeled/Investigational Use
Unlabeled: Hypertensive crisis, diabetic nephropathy, rheumatoid arthritis, diagnosis of anatomic renal artery stenosis, hypertension secondary to scleroderma renal crisis, diagnosis of aldosteronism, idiopathic edema, Bartter's syndrome, postmyocardial infarction for prevention of ventricular failure
Investigational: Severe congestive heart failure in infants, neonatal hypertension, acute pulmonary edema
Local Anesthetic/Vasoconstrictor Precautions No information available to require special precautions
Effects on Dental Treatment Key adverse event(s) related to dental treatment: Abnormal taste and orthostatic hypotension.
Common Adverse Effects Note: Frequency ranges include data from hypertension and heart failure trials. Higher rates of adverse reactions have generally been noted in patients with CHF. However, the frequency of adverse effects associated with placebo is also increased in this population.

1% to 10%:
Cardiovascular: Hypotension (0.9% to 7%), chest pain (2%), syncope (0.5% to 2%), orthostasis (2%), orthostatic hypotension (2%)
Central nervous system: Headache (2% to 5%), dizziness (4% to 8%), fatigue (2% to 3%)
Dermatologic: Rash (2%)
Gastrointestinal: Abnormal taste, abdominal pain, vomiting, nausea, diarrhea, anorexia, constipation
Neuromuscular & skeletal: Weakness
Renal: Increased serum creatinine (0.2% to 20%), worsening of renal function (in patients with bilateral renal artery stenosis or hypovolemia)
Respiratory (1% to 2%): Bronchitis, cough, dyspnea

Dosage Use lower listed initial dose in patients with hyponatremia, hypovolemia, severe congestive heart failure, decreased renal function, or in those receiving diuretics.
Oral: **Enalapril:** Children 1 month to 16 years: Hypertension: Initial: 0.08 mg/kg (up to 5 mg) once daily; adjust dosage based on patient response; doses >0.58 mg/kg (40 mg) have not been evaluated in pediatric patients
Investigational: Congestive heart failure: Initial oral doses of **enalapril:** 0.1 mg/kg/day increasing as needed over 2 weeks to 0.5 mg/kg/day have been used in infants
Investigational: Neonatal hypertension: I.V. doses of **enalaprilat:** 5-10 mcg/kg/dose administered every 8-24 hours have been used; monitor patients carefully; select patients may require higher doses
Adults:
Oral: **Enalapril:**
Hypertension: 2.5-5 mg/day then increase as required, usually at 1- to 2-week intervals; usual dose range (JNC 7): 2.5-40 mg/day in 1-2 divided doses. **Note:** Initiate with 2.5 mg if patient is taking a diuretic which cannot be discontinued. May add a diuretic if blood pressure cannot be controlled with enalapril alone.
Heart failure: Initial: 2.5 mg once or twice daily (usual range: 5-40 mg/day in 2 divided doses). Titrate slowly at 1- to 2-week intervals. Target dose: 10-20 mg twice daily (ACC/AHA 2005 Heart Failure Guidelines)
Asymptomatic left ventricular dysfunction: 2.5 mg twice daily, titrated as tolerated to 20 mg/day

I.V.: Enalaprilat:

Hypertension: 1.25 mg/dose, given over 5 minutes every 6 hours; doses as high as 5 mg/dose every 6 hours have been tolerated for up to 36 hours. **Note:** If patients are concomitantly receiving diuretic therapy, begin with 0.625 mg I.V. over 5 minutes; if the effect is not adequate after 1 hour, repeat the dose and administer 1.25 mg at 6-hour intervals thereafter; if adequate, administer 0.625 mg I.V. every 6 hours.

Heart failure: Avoid I.V. administration in patients with unstable heart failure or those suffering acute myocardial infarction.

Conversion from I.V. to oral therapy if not concurrently on diuretics: 5 mg once daily; subsequent titration as needed; if concurrently receiving diuretics and responding to 0.625 mg I.V. every 6 hours, initiate with 2.5 mg/day.

Dosing adjustment in renal impairment:

Oral: Enalapril:

Cl_{cr} 30-80 mL/minute: Administer 5 mg/day titrated upwards to maximum of 40 mg.

Cl_{cr} <30 mL/minute: Administer 2.5 mg day; titrated upward until blood pressure is controlled.

For heart failure patients with sodium <130 mEq/L or serum creatinine >1.6 mg/dL, initiate dosage with 2.5 mg/day, increasing to twice daily as needed. Increase further in increments of 2.5 mg/dose at >4-day intervals to a maximum daily dose of 40 mg.

I.V.: Enalaprilat:

Cl_{cr} >30 mL/minute: Initiate with 1.25 mg every 6 hours and increase dose based on response.

Cl_{cr} <30 mL/minute: Initiate with 0.625 mg every 6 hours and increase dose based on response.

Hemodialysis: Moderately dialyzable (20% to 50%); administer dose postdialysis (eg, 0.625 mg I.V. every 6 hours) or administer 20% to 25% supplemental dose following dialysis; Clearance: 62 mL/minute.

Peritoneal dialysis: Supplemental dose is not necessary, although some removal of drug occurs.

Dosing adjustment in hepatic impairment: Hydrolysis of enalapril to enalaprilat may be delayed and/or impaired in patients with severe hepatic impairment, but the pharmacodynamic effects of the drug do not appear to be significantly altered; no dosage adjustment.

Mechanism of Action Competitive inhibitor of angiotensin-converting enzyme (ACE); prevents conversion of angiotensin I to angiotensin II, a potent vasoconstrictor; results in lower levels of angiotensin II which causes an increase in plasma renin activity and a reduction in aldosterone secretion

Contraindications Hypersensitivity to enalapril or enalaprilat; angioedema related to previous treatment with an ACE inhibitor; patients with idiopathic or hereditary angioedema; bilateral renal artery stenosis; pregnancy (2nd and 3rd trimesters)

Warnings/Precautions Anaphylactic reactions can occur. Angioedema can occur at any time during treatment (especially following first dose). It may involve head and neck (potentially affecting the airway) or the intestine (presenting with abdominal pain). Prolonged monitoring may be required especially if tongue, glottis, or larynx are involved as they are associated with airway obstruction. Those with a history of airway surgery in this situation have a higher risk. Careful blood pressure monitoring with first dose (hypotension can occur especially in volume-depleted patients). Dosage adjustment needed in renal impairment. Use with caution in hypovolemia; collagen vascular diseases; valvular stenosis (particularly aortic stenosis); hyperkalemia; or before, during, or immediately after anesthesia. Avoid rapid dosage escalation which may lead to renal insufficiency.

Rare toxicities associated with ACE inhibitors include cholestatic jaundice (which may progress to hepatic necrosis) and neutropenia/agranulocytosis with myeloid hyperplasia. Hypersensitivity reactions may be seen during hemodialysis with high-flux dialysis membranes (eg, AN69). Hyperkalemia may rarely occur. If patient has renal impairment then a baseline WBC with differential and serum creatinine should be evaluated and monitored closely during the first 3 months of therapy. Use with caution in unilateral renal artery stenosis and pre-existing renal insufficiency. Experience in children is limited.

Drug Interactions

Cytochrome P450 Effect: Substrate of CYP3A4 (major)

Increased Effect/Toxicity: Potassium supplements, co-trimoxazole (high dose), angiotensin II receptor antagonists (eg, candesartan, losartan, irbesartan), or potassium-sparing diuretics (amiloride, spironolactone, triamterene) may result in elevated serum potassium levels when combined with enalapril. ACE inhibitor effects may be increased by phenothiazines or (Continued)

Enalapril *(Continued)*

probenecid (increases levels of captopril). ACE inhibitors may increase serum concentrations/effects of lithium.

Diuretics have additive hypotensive effects with ACE inhibitors, and hypovolemia increases the potential for adverse renal effects of ACE inhibitors. In patients with compromised renal function, coadministration with NSAIDs may result in further deterioration of renal function. Allopurinol and ACE inhibitors may cause a higher risk of hypersensitivity reaction when taken concurrently.

Decreased Effect: Aspirin (high dose) may reduce the therapeutic effects of ACE inhibitors; at low dosages this does not appear to be significant. Antacids may decrease the bioavailability of ACE inhibitors (may be more likely to occur with captopril); separate administration times by 1-2 hours. NSAIDs may reduce the hypotensive effects of ACE inhibitors. More likely to occur in low renin or volume-dependent hypertensive patients. CYP3A4 inducers may decrease the levels/effects of enalapril; example inducers include aminoglutethimide, carbamazepine, nafcillin, nevirapine, phenobarbital, phenytoin, and rifamycins.

Ethanol/Nutrition/Herb Interactions Herb/Nutraceutical: St John's wort may decrease enalapril levels. Avoid dong quai if using for hypertension (has estrogenic activity). Avoid ephedra, yohimbe, ginseng (may worsen hypertension). Avoid natural licorice (causes sodium and water retention and increases potassium loss). Avoid garlic (may have increased antihypertensive effect).

Dietary Considerations Limit salt substitutes or potassium-rich diet.

Pharmacodynamics/Kinetics

Onset of action: Oral: ~1 hour

Duration: Oral: 12-24 hours

Absorption: Oral: 55% to 75%

Protein binding: 50% to 60%

Metabolism: Prodrug, undergoes hepatic biotransformation to enalaprilat

Half-life elimination:

Enalapril: Adults: Healthy: 2 hours; Congestive heart failure: 3.4-5.8 hours

Enalaprilat: Infants 6 weeks to 8 months old: 6-10 hours; Adults: 35-38 hours

Time to peak, serum: Oral: Enalapril: 0.5-1.5 hours; Enalaprilat (active): 3-4.5 hours

Excretion: Urine (60% to 80%); some feces

Pregnancy Risk Factor C (1st trimester)/D (2nd and 3rd trimesters)

Dosage Forms INJ, solution, as enalaprilat 1.25 mg/mL (1 mL, 2 mL). **TAB,** as maleate (Vasotec®): 2.5 mg, 5 mg, 10 mg, 20 mg

Enalapril and Felodipine *(e NAL a pril & fe LOE di peen)*

Related Information

Enalapril *on page 538*

Felodipine *on page 638*

U.S. Brand Names Lexxel®

Canadian Brand Names Lexxel®

Generic Available No

Synonyms Felodipine and Enalapril

Pharmacologic Category Antihypertensive Agent, Combination

Use Treatment of hypertension, however, not indicated for initial treatment of hypertension; replacement therapy in patients receiving separate dosage forms (for patient convenience); when monotherapy with one component fails to achieve desired antihypertensive effect, or when dose-limiting adverse effects limit upward titration of monotherapy

Local Anesthetic/Vasoconstrictor Precautions No information available to require special precautions

Effects on Dental Treatment Key adverse event(s) related to dental treatment: Gingival hyperplasia (fewer reports with felodipine than with other CCBs); resolves upon discontinuation (consultation with physician is suggested).

Common Adverse Effects See individual agents.

Mechanism of Action See individual agents.

Drug Interactions

Cytochrome P450 Effect:

Enalapril: **Substrate** of CYP3A4 (major)

Felodipine: **Substrate** of CYP3A4 (major); **Inhibits** CYP2C8 (moderate), 2C9 (weak), 2D6 (weak), 3A4 (weak)

Increased Effect/Toxicity: See individual agents.

Decreased Effect: See individual agents.

Pharmacodynamics/Kinetics See individual agents.

Pregnancy Risk Factor C/D (2nd and 3rd trimesters)

Enalapril and Hydrochlorothiazide
(e NAL a pril & hye droe klor oh THYE a zide)

Related Information
  Cardiovascular Diseases *on page 1636*
  Enalapril *on page 538*
  Hydrochlorothiazide *on page 776*
U.S. Brand Names Vaseretic®
Canadian Brand Names Vaseretic®
Generic Available Yes
Synonyms Hydrochlorothiazide and Enalapril
Pharmacologic Category Antihypertensive Agent, Combination
Use Treatment of hypertension
Local Anesthetic/Vasoconstrictor Precautions No information available to require special precautions
Effects on Dental Treatment No significant effects or complications reported
Common Adverse Effects See individual agents.
Drug Interactions
  Cytochrome P450 Effect: Enalapril: **Substrate** of CYP3A4 (major)
Pharmacodynamics/Kinetics See individual agents.
Pregnancy Risk Factor C/D (2nd and 3rd trimesters)

Enalaprilat *see* Enalapril *on page 538*

Enalapril Maleate *see* Enalapril *on page 538*

Enbrel® *see* Etanercept *on page 588*

Encare® [OTC] *see* Nonoxynol 9 *on page 1124*

Encort™ *see* Hydrocortisone *on page 793*

Endal® *see* Guaifenesin and Phenylephrine *on page 754*

Endal® HD *see* Hydrocodone, Phenylephrine, and Diphenhydramine *on page 791*

EndoAvitene® *see* Collagen Hemostat *on page 392*

Endocet® *see* Oxycodone and Acetaminophen *on page 1165*

Endodan® [DSC] *see* Oxycodone and Aspirin *on page 1168*

Endrate® *see* Edetate Disodium *on page 527*

Enduron® [DSC] *see* Methyclothiazide *on page 1020*

Enemeez® [OTC] *see* Docusate *on page 496*

Enerjets [OTC] *see* Caffeine *on page 245*

Enfamil® Glucose *see* Dextrose *on page 452*

Enfuvirtide (en FYOO vir tide)

U.S. Brand Names Fuzeon™
Canadian Brand Names Fuzeon™
Generic Available No
Synonyms T-20
Pharmacologic Category Antiretroviral Agent, Fusion Protein Inhibitor
Use Treatment of HIV-1 infection in combination with other antiretroviral agents in treatment-experienced patients with evidence of HIV-1 replication despite ongoing antiretroviral therapy
Local Anesthetic/Vasoconstrictor Precautions No information available to require special precautions
Effects on Dental Treatment Key adverse event(s) related to dental treatment: Taste disturbance.
Common Adverse Effects
  >10%:
    Central nervous system: Insomnia (11%)
    Local: Injection site reactions (98%; may include pain, erythema, induration, pruritus, ecchymosis, nodule or cyst formation)
  1% to 10%:
    Central nervous system: Depression (9%), anxiety (6%)
    Dermatologic: Pruritus (5%)
    Endocrine & metabolic: Weight loss (7%), anorexia (3%)
    Gastrointestinal: Triglycerides increased (9%), appetite decreased (6%), constipation (4%), abdominal pain (3%), pancreatitis (2%), taste disturbance (2%), serum amylase increased (6%)
    Hematologic: Eosinophilia (8%), anemia (2%)
    Hepatic: Transaminases increased (4%)
    Local: Injection site infection (1%)
    Neuromuscular & skeletal: Neuropathy (9%), weakness (6%), myalgia (5%)
    Ocular: Conjunctivitis (2%)
(Continued)

Enfuvirtide *(Continued)*

Respiratory: Cough (7%), pneumonia (4.7 events per 100 patient years vs 0.61 events per 100 patient years in control group), sinusitis (6%)

Miscellaneous: Infections (4% to 6%), flu-like symptoms (2%), lymphadenopathy (2%)

Mechanism of Action Binds to the first heptad-repeat (HR1) in the gp41 subunit of the viral envelope glycoprotein. Inhibits the fusion of HIV-1 virus with CD4 cells by blocking the conformational change in gp41 required for membrane fusion and entry into CD4 cells

Drug Interactions

Increased Effect/Toxicity: No significant interactions identified.

Decreased Effect: No significant interactions identified.

Pharmacodynamics/Kinetics

Distribution: V_d: 5.5 L

Protein binding: 92%

Metabolism: Proteolytic hydrolysis (CYP isoenzymes do not appear to contribute to metabolism); clearance: 24.8 mL/hour/kg

Half-life elimination: 3.8 hours

Time to peak: 8 hours

Pregnancy Risk Factor B

Engerix-B® *see* Hepatitis B Vaccine *on page 769*

Engerix-B® and Havrix® *see* Hepatitis A Inactivated and Hepatitis B (Recombinant) Vaccine *on page 766*

Enhanced-potency Inactivated Poliovirus Vaccine *see* Poliovirus Vaccine (Inactivated) *on page 1252*

Enhancer *see* Barium *on page 179*

Enlon® *see* Edrophonium *on page 528*

Enlon-Plus™ *see* Edrophonium and Atropine *on page 529*

Enoxaparin *(ee noks a PA rin)*

Related Information

Cardiovascular Diseases *on page 1636*

U.S. Brand Names Lovenox®

Canadian Brand Names Lovenox®; Lovenox® HP

Mexican Brand Names Clexane®

Generic Available No

Synonyms Enoxaparin Sodium

Pharmacologic Category Low Molecular Weight Heparin

Use

DVT Treatment (acute): Inpatient treatment (patients with and without pulmonary embolism) and outpatient treatment (patients without pulmonary embolism)

DVT prophylaxis: Following hip or knee replacement surgery, abdominal surgery, or in medical patients with severely-restricted mobility during acute illness in patients at risk of thromboembolic complications

Note: High-risk patients include those with one or more of the following risk factors: >40 years of age, obesity, general anesthesia lasting >30 minutes, malignancy, history of deep vein thrombosis or pulmonary embolism

Unstable angina and non-Q-wave myocardial infarction (to prevent ischemic complications)

Unlabeled/Investigational Use Prophylaxis and treatment of thromboembolism in children

Local Anesthetic/Vasoconstrictor Precautions No information available to require special precautions

Effects on Dental Treatment Key adverse event(s) related to dental treatment: As with all anticoagulants, bleeding is the major adverse effect of enoxaparin. Hemorrhage may occur at virtually any site; risk is dependent on multiple variables. At the recommended doses, single injections of enoxaparin do not significantly influence platelet aggregation or affect global clotting time (ie, PT or aPTT).

Common Adverse Effects As with all anticoagulants, bleeding is the major adverse effect of enoxaparin. Hemorrhage may occur at virtually any site. Risk is dependent on multiple variables. At the recommended doses, single injections of enoxaparin do not significantly influence platelet aggregation or affect global clotting time (ie, PT or aPTT).

1% to 10%:

Central nervous system: Fever (5% to 8%), confusion, pain

Dermatologic: Erythema, bruising

Gastrointestinal: Nausea (3%), diarrhea

Hematologic: Hemorrhage (5% to 13%), thrombocytopenia (2%), hypochromic anemia (2%)

Hepatic: Increased ALT/AST

Local: Injection site hematoma (9%), local reactions (irritation, pain, ecchymosis, erythema)

Thrombocytopenia with thrombosis: Cases of heparin-induced thrombocytopenia (some complicated by organ infarction, limb ischemia, or death) have been reported.

Mechanism of Action Standard heparin consists of components with molecular weights ranging from 4000-30,000 daltons with a mean of 16,000 daltons. Heparin acts as an anticoagulant by enhancing the inhibition rate of clotting proteases by antithrombin III impairing normal hemostasis and inhibition of factor Xa. Low molecular weight heparins have a small effect on the activated partial thromboplastin time and strongly inhibit factor Xa. Enoxaparin is derived from porcine heparin that undergoes benzylation followed by alkaline depolymerization. The average molecular weight of enoxaparin is 4500 daltons which is distributed as (≤20%) 2000 daltons (≥68%) 2000-8000 daltons, and (≤15%) >8000 daltons. Enoxaparin has a higher ratio of antifactor Xa to antifactor IIa activity than unfractionated heparin.

Drug Interactions

Increased Effect/Toxicity: Risk of bleeding with enoxaparin may be increased with thrombolytic agents, oral anticoagulants (warfarin), drugs which affect platelet function (eg, aspirin, NSAIDs, dipyridamole, ticlopidine, clopidogrel, and IIb/IIIa antagonists). Although the risk of bleeding may be increased during concurrent therapy with warfarin, enoxaparin is commonly continued during the initiation of warfarin therapy to assure anticoagulation and to protect against possible transient hypercoagulability. Some cephalosporins and penicillins may block platelet aggregation, theoretically increasing the risk of bleeding.

Pharmacodynamics/Kinetics

Onset of action: Peak effect: SubQ: Antifactor Xa and antithrombin (antifactor IIa): 3-5 hours

Duration: 40 mg dose: Antifactor Xa activity: ~12 hours

Metabolism: Hepatic, to lower molecular weight fragments (little activity)

Protein binding: Does not bind to heparin binding proteins

Half-life elimination, plasma: 2-4 times longer than standard heparin, independent of dose; based on anti-Xa activity: 4.5-7 hours

Excretion: Urine (40% of dose; 10% as active fragments)

Pregnancy Risk Factor B

Enoxaparin Sodium *see* Enoxaparin *on page 542*

Enpresse™ *see* Ethinyl Estradiol and Levonorgestrel *on page 602*

Entacapone (en TA ka pone)

U.S. Brand Names Comtan®

Canadian Brand Names Comtan®

Generic Available No

Pharmacologic Category Anti-Parkinson's Agent, COMT Inhibitor

Use Adjunct to levodopa/carbidopa therapy in patients with idiopathic Parkinson's disease who experience "wearing-off" symptoms at the end of a dosing interval

Local Anesthetic/Vasoconstrictor Precautions No information available to require special precautions

Effects on Dental Treatment Key adverse event(s) related to dental treatment: Orthostatic hypotension and abnormal taste. Dopaminergic therapy in Parkinson's disease (ie, treatment with levodopa) is associated with orthostatic hypotension. Entacapone enhances levodopa bioavailability and may increase the occurrence of hypotension/syncope in the dental patient. The patient should be carefully assisted from the chair and observed for signs of orthostatic hypotension.

Common Adverse Effects

>10%:

Gastrointestinal: Nausea (14%)

Neuromuscular & skeletal: Dyskinesia (25%), placebo (15%)

1% to 10%:

Cardiovascular: Orthostatic hypotension (4%), syncope (1%)

Central nervous system: Dizziness (8%), fatigue (6%), hallucinations (4%), anxiety (2%), somnolence (2%), agitation (1%)

Dermatologic: Purpura (2%)

(Continued)

Entacapone (Continued)

Gastrointestinal: Diarrhea (10%), abdominal pain (8%), constipation (6%), vomiting (4%), dry mouth (3%), dyspepsia (2%), flatulence (2%), gastritis (1%), taste perversion (1%)

Genitourinary: Brown-orange urine discoloration (10%)

Neuromuscular & skeletal: Hyperkinesia (10%), hypokinesia (9%), back pain (4%), weakness (2%)

Respiratory: Dyspnea (3%)

Miscellaneous: Diaphoresis increased (2%), bacterial infection (1%)

Mechanism of Action Entacapone is a reversible and selective inhibitor of catechol-O-methyltransferase (COMT). When entacapone is taken with levodopa, the pharmacokinetics are altered, resulting in more sustained levodopa serum levels compared to levodopa taken alone. The resulting levels of levodopa provide for increased concentrations available for absorption across the blood-brain barrier, thereby providing for increased CNS levels of dopamine, the active metabolite of levodopa.

Drug Interactions

Cytochrome P450 Effect: Inhibits CYP1A2 (weak), 2A6 (weak), 2C9 (weak), 2C19 (weak), 2D6 (weak), 2E1 (weak), 3A4 (weak)

Increased Effect/Toxicity: Entacapone may decrease the metabolism and increase the side effects of COMT substrates (eg, apomorphine, bitolterol, dobutamine, dopamine, epinephrine, norepinephrine, isoproterenol, isoetharine, and methyldopa). Effects on mental status may be additive with other CNS depressants; includes barbiturates, benzodiazepines, TCAs, antipsychotics, ethanol, narcotic analgesics, and other sedative-hypnotics. Concurrent use of nonselective MAO inhibitors with entacapone may increase the risk of cardiovascular side effects; selective MAO inhibitors (eg, selegiline) appear to pose limited risk.

Pharmacodynamics/Kinetics

Onset of action: Rapid

Peak effect: 1 hour

Absorption: Rapid

Distribution: I.V.: V_{dss}: 20 L

Protein binding: 98%, primarily to albumin

Metabolism: Isomerization to the cis-isomer, followed by direct glucuronidation of the parent and cis-isomer

Bioavailability: 35%

Half-life elimination: B phase: 0.4-0.7 hours; Y phase: 2.4 hours

Time to peak, serum: 1 hour

Excretion: Feces (90%); urine (10%)

Pregnancy Risk Factor C

Entacapone, Carbidopa, and Levodopa see Levodopa, Carbidopa, and Entacapone on page 912

Entecavir (en TE ka veer)

U.S. Brand Names Baraclude™

Generic Available No

Pharmacologic Category Antiretroviral Agent, Reverse Transcriptase Inhibitor (Nucleoside)

Use Treatment of chronic hepatitis B infection in adults with evidence of active viral replication and either evidence of persistent transaminase elevations or histologically-active disease

Local Anesthetic/Vasoconstrictor Precautions No information available to require special precautions

Effects on Dental Treatment No significant effects or complications reported

Common Adverse Effects

>10%: Hepatic: Alanine aminotransferase increased (2% to 12%)

1% to 10%:

Central nervous system: Headache (2% to 4%), fatigue (1% to 3%)

Endocrine & metabolic: Hyperglycemia (2%)

Gastrointestinal: Lipase increased (7% to 8%), amylase increased (2% to 3%), diarrhea (≤1%), dyspepsia (≤1%)

Hepatic: Aspartate aminotransferase increased (5%), bilirubin increased (2% to 3%)

Renal: Hematuria (9%), glycosuria (4%), creatinine increased (1% to 2%),

Mechanism of Action Entecavir is intracellularly phosphorylated to guanosine triphosphate which competes with natural substrates to effectively inhibit hepatitis B viral polymerase; enzyme inhibition blocks reverse transcriptase activity thereby reducing viral DNA synthesis.

Pharmacodynamics/Kinetics
Distribution: Extensive (V_d in excess of body water)
Protein binding: 13%
Metabolism: Minor hepatic glucuronide/sulfate conjugation
Half-life elimination: Terminal: 5-6 days; accumulation: 24 hours
Time to peak, plasma: 0.5-1.5 hours
Excretion: Urine (60% to 70% as unchanged drug)

Pregnancy Risk Factor C

Enterex® Glutapak-10® [OTC] see Glutamine on page 743

Entertainer's Secret® [OTC] see Saliva Substitute on page 1374

Entex® see Guaifenesin and Phenylephrine on page 754

Entex® ER see Guaifenesin and Phenylephrine on page 754

Entex® LA see Guaifenesin and Phenylephrine on page 754

Entex® PSE see Guaifenesin and Pseudoephedrine on page 755

Entocort® EC see Budesonide on page 224

Entrobar® see Barium on page 179

EntroEase® see Barium on page 179

Entsol® [OTC] see Sodium Chloride on page 1400

Enulose® see Lactulose on page 893

Enzone® see Pramoxine and Hydrocortisone on page 1264

Ephedrine (e FED rin)

U.S. Brand Names Pretz-D® [OTC]
Generic Available Yes
Synonyms Ephedrine Sulfate
Pharmacologic Category Alpha/Beta Agonist
Use Treatment of bronchial asthma, nasal congestion, acute bronchospasm, idiopathic orthostatic hypotension, hypotension induced by spinal anesthesia
Local Anesthetic/Vasoconstrictor Precautions Use vasoconstrictor with caution since ephedrine may enhance cardiostimulation and vasopressor effects of sympathomimetics such as epinephrine
Effects on Dental Treatment Key adverse event(s) related to dental treatment: Xerostomia (normal salivary flow resumes upon discontinuation).
Common Adverse Effects Frequency not defined.
Cardiovascular: Hypertension, tachycardia, palpitation, elevation or depression of blood pressure, unusual pallor, chest pain, arrhythmia
Central nervous system: CNS stimulating effects, nervousness, anxiety, apprehension, fear, tension, agitation, excitation, restlessness, irritability, insomnia, hyperactivity, dizziness, headache
Gastrointestinal: Xerostomia, nausea, anorexia, GI upset, vomiting
Genitourinary: Painful urination
Neuromuscular & skeletal: Trembling, tremor (more common in the elderly), weakness
Respiratory: Dyspnea
Miscellaneous: Diaphoresis (increased)
Mechanism of Action Releases tissue stores of epinephrine and thereby produces an alpha- and beta-adrenergic stimulation; longer-acting and less potent than epinephrine
Drug Interactions
Increased Effect/Toxicity: Increased (toxic) cardiac stimulation with other sympathomimetic agents, theophylline, cardiac glycosides, or general anesthetics. Increased blood pressure with atropine or MAO inhibitors.
Decreased Effect: Alpha- and beta-adrenergic blocking agents decrease ephedrine vasopressor effects.
Pharmacodynamics/Kinetics
Onset of action: Oral: Bronchodilation: 0.25-1 hour
Duration: Oral: 3-6 hours
Distribution: Crosses placenta; enters breast milk
Metabolism: Minimally hepatic
Half-life elimination: 2.5-3.6 hours
Excretion: Urine (60% to 77% as unchanged drug) within 24 hours
Pregnancy Risk Factor C

Ephedrine, Chlorpheniramine, Phenylephrine, and Carbetapentane see Chlorpheniramine, Ephedrine, Phenylephrine, and Carbetapentane on page 325

Ephedrine Sulfate see Ephedrine on page 545

Epidermal Thymocyte Activating Factor see Aldesleukin on page 61

Epifoam® see Pramoxine and Hydrocortisone on page 1264

Epinastine (ep i NAS teen)

U.S. Brand Names Elestat™
Mexican Brand Names Flurinol®
Generic Available No
Synonyms Epinastine Hydrochloride
Pharmacologic Category Antihistamine, H_1 Blocker, Ophthalmic
Use Treatment of allergic conjunctivitis
Local Anesthetic/Vasoconstrictor Precautions No information available to require special precautions
Effects on Dental Treatment No significant effects or complications reported
Mechanism of Action Selective H_1-receptor antagonist; inhibits release of histamine from the mast cell
Pregnancy Risk Factor C

Epinastine Hydrochloride see Epinastine on page 546

Epinephrine (ep i NEF rin)

Related Information
Respiratory Diseases on page 1656
U.S. Brand Names Adrenalin®; EpiPen®; EpiPen® Jr; Primatene® Mist [OTC]; Raphon [OTC]; S2® [OTC]; Twinject™
Canadian Brand Names Adrenalin®; EpiPen®; EpiPen® Jr
Generic Available Yes: Solution for injection
Synonyms Adrenaline; Epinephrine Bitartrate; Epinephrine Hydrochloride; Racepinephrine
Pharmacologic Category Alpha/Beta Agonist; Antidote
Dental Use Emergency drug for treatment of anaphylactic reactions; used as vasoconstrictor to prolong local anesthesia
Use Treatment of bronchospasms, bronchial asthma, nasal congestion, viral croup, anaphylactic reactions, cardiac arrest; added to local anesthetics to decrease systemic absorption of local anesthetics and increase duration of action; decrease superficial hemorrhage
Unlabeled/Investigational Use ACLS guidelines: Ventricular fibrillation (VF) or pulseless ventricular tachycardia (VT) unresponsive to initial defibrillatory shocks; pulseless electrical activity, asystole, hypotension unresponsive to volume resuscitation; symptomatic bradycardia or hypotension unresponsive to atropine or pacing; inotropic support
Local Anesthetic/Vasoconstrictor Precautions No information available to require special precautions
Effects on Dental Treatment No effects or complications reported
Significant Adverse Effects Frequency not defined.
Cardiovascular: Angina, cardiac arrhythmia, chest pain, flushing, hypertension, increased myocardial oxygen consumption, pallor, palpitation, sudden death, tachycardia (parenteral), vasoconstriction, ventricular ectopy
Central nervous system: Anxiety, dizziness, headache, insomnia, lightheadedness, nervousness, restlessness
Gastrointestinal: Dry throat, nausea, vomiting, xerostomia
Genitourinary: Acute urinary retention in patients with bladder outflow obstruction
Neuromuscular & skeletal: Trembling, weakness
Ocular: Allergic lid reaction, burning, eye pain, ocular irritation, precipitation of or exacerbation of narrow-angle glaucoma, transient stinging
Renal: Decreased renal and splanchnic blood flow
Respiratory: Dyspnea, wheezing
Miscellaneous: Diaphoresis (increased)
Dental Usual Dosing Hypersensitivity reaction:
Infants and Children:
SubQ, I.V.: 0.01 mg/kg every 20 minutes; larger doses or continuous infusion may be needed for some anaphylactic reactions
SubQ, I.M.:
15-30 kg: Twinject™: 0.15 mg (for self-administration following severe allergic reactions to insect stings, food, etc)
>30 kg: Refer to Adults dosing
I.M.:
<30 kg: Epipen® Jr: 0.15 mg (for self-administration following severe allergic reactions to insect stings, food, etc)
>30 kg: Refer to Adults dosing

Adults:
I.M., SubQ: 0.3-0.5 mg (1:1000) every 15-20 minutes if condition requires (I.M route is preferred)
>30 kg: Twinject™: 0.3 mg (for self-administration following severe allergic reactions to insect stings, food, etc)
I.M.: >30 kg: Epipen®: 0.3 mg (for self-administration following severe allergic reactions to insect stings, food, etc)
I.V.: 0.1 mg (1:10,000) over 5 minutes. May infuse at 1-4 mcg/minute to prevent the need to repeat injections frequently.

Dosage
Neonates: Cardiac arrest: I.V.: 0.01-0.03 mg/kg (0.1-0.3 mL/kg of **1:10,000** solution) every 3-5 minutes as needed. Although I.V. route is preferred, may consider administration of doses up to 0.1 mg/kg through the endotracheal tube until I.V. access established; dilute intratracheal doses to 1-2 mL with normal saline.

Infants and Children:
Asystole/pulseless arrest, bradycardia, VT/VF (after failed defibrillations):
I.V., I.O.: 0.01 mg/kg (0.1 mL/kg of **1:10,000** solution) every 3-5 minutes as needed (maximum: 1 mg)
Intratracheal: 0.1 mg/kg (0.1 mL/kg of **1:1000** solution) every 3-5 minutes (maximum: 10 mg)
Continuous I.V. infusion: 0.1-1 mcg/kg/; doses <0.3 mcg/kg/minute generally produce β-adrenergic effects and higher doses generally produce α-adrenergic vasoconstriction; titrate dosage to desired effect
Bronchodilator: SubQ: 0.01 mg/kg (0.01 mL/kg of **1:1000**) (single doses not to exceed 0.5 mg) every 20 minutes for 3 doses
Nebulization: 1-3 inhalations up to every 3 hours using solution prepared with 10 drops of 1:100
Children <4 years: S2® (racepinephrine, OTC labeling): Croup: 0.05 mL/kg (max 0.5 mL/dose); dilute in NS 3 mL. Administer over ~15 minutes; do not administer more frequently than every 2 hours.
Inhalation: Children ≥4 years: Primatene® Mist: Refer to Adults dosing.
Decongestant: Children ≥6 years: Refer to Adults dosing
Hypersensitivity reaction:
SubQ, I.V.: 0.01 mg/kg every 20 minutes; larger doses or continuous infusion may be needed for some anaphylactic reactions
SubQ, I.M.:
15-30 kg: Twinject™: 0.15 mg (for self-administration following severe allergic reactions to insect stings, food, etc)
>30 kg: Refer to Adults dosing
I.M.:
<30 kg: Epipen® Jr: 0.15 mg (for self-administration following severe allergic reactions to insect stings, food, etc)
>30 kg: Refer to Adults dosing

Adults:
Asystole/pulseless arrest, bradycardia, VT/VF:
I.V., I.O.: 1 mg every 3-5 minutes; if this approach fails, higher doses of epinephrine (up to 0.2 mg/kg) may be indicated for treatment of specific problems (eg, beta-blocker or calcium channel blocker overdose)
Intratracheal: Administer 2-2.5 mg for VF or pulseless VT if I.V./I.O. access is delayed or cannot be established; dilute in 5-10 mL NS or distilled water. **Note:** Absorption is greater with distilled water, but causes more adverse effects on PaO₂.
Bradycardia (symptomatic) or hypotension (not responsive to atropine or pacing): I.V. infusion: 2-10 mcg/minute; titrate to desired effect
Bronchodilator:
SubQ: 0.3-0.5 mg **(1:1000)** every 20 minutes for 3 doses
Nebulization: 1-3 inhalations up to every 3 hours using solution prepared with 10 drops of the **1:100** product
S2® (racepinephrine, OTC labeling): 0.5 mL (~10 drops). Dose may be repeated not more frequently than very 3-4 hours if needed. Solution should be diluted if using jet nebulizer.
Inhalation: Primatene® Mist (OTC labeling): One inhalation, wait at least 1 minute; if relieved, may use once more. Do not use again for at least 3 hours.
Decongestant: Intranasal: Apply 1:1000 locally as drops or spray or with sterile swab
Hypersensitivity reaction:
I.M., SubQ: 0.3-0.5 mg (1:1000) every 15-20 minutes if condition requires (I.M route is preferred)
>30 kg: Twinject™: 0.3 mg (for self-administration following severe allergic reactions to insect stings, food, etc)

(Continued)

Epinephrine *(Continued)*

I.M.: >30 kg: Epipen®: 0.3 mg (for self-administration following severe allergic reactions to insect stings, food, etc)

I.V.: 0.1 mg (1:10,000) over 5 minutes. May infuse at 1-4 mcg/minute to prevent the need to repeat injections frequently.

Mechanism of Action Stimulates alpha-, beta₁-, and beta₂-adrenergic receptors resulting in relaxation of smooth muscle of the bronchial tree, cardiac stimulation, and dilation of skeletal muscle vasculature; small doses can cause vasodilation via beta₂-vascular receptors; large doses may produce constriction of skeletal and vascular smooth muscle

Contraindications Hypersensitivity to epinephrine or any component of the formulation; cardiac arrhythmias; angle-closure glaucoma

Warnings/Precautions Use with caution in elderly patients, patients with diabetes mellitus, cardiovascular diseases (angina, tachycardia, myocardial infarction), thyroid disease, or cerebral arteriosclerosis, Parkinson's; some products contain sulfites as preservatives. Rapid I.V. infusion may cause death from cerebrovascular hemorrhage or cardiac arrhythmias. Oral inhalation of epinephrine is **not** the preferred route of administration. Avoid topical application where reduced perfusion could lead to ischemic tissue damage (eg, penis, ears, digits).

Drug Interactions Increased toxicity: Increased cardiac irritability if administered concurrently with halogenated inhalational anesthetics, beta-blocking agents, alpha-blocking agents

Ethanol/Nutrition/Herb Interactions Herb/Nutraceutical: Avoid ephedra, yohimbe (may cause CNS stimulation).

Pharmacodynamics/Kinetics

Onset of action: Bronchodilation: SubQ: ~5-10 minutes; Inhalation: ~1 minute

Distribution: Crosses placenta

Metabolism: Taken up into the adrenergic neuron and metabolized by monoamine oxidase and catechol-o-methyltransferase; circulating drug hepatically metabolized

Excretion: Urine (as inactive metabolites, metanephrine, and sulfate and hydroxy derivatives of mandelic acid, small amounts as unchanged drug)

Pregnancy Risk Factor C

Lactation Excretion in breast milk unknown

Dosage Forms

Aerosol for oral inhalation:

Primatene® Mist: 0.22 mg/inhalation (15 mL, 22.5 mL) [contains CFCs]

Injection, solution [prefilled auto injector]:

EpiPen®: 0.3 mg/0.3 mL [1:1000] (2 mL) [contains sodium metabisulfite; available as single unit or in double-unit pack with training unit]

EpiPen® Jr: 0.15 mg/0.3 mL [1:2000] (2 mL) [contains sodium metabisulfite; available as single unit or in double-unit pack with training unit]

Twinject™: 0.15 mg/0.15 mL [1:1000] (1.1 mL) [contains sodium bisulfite; two 0.15 mg doses per injector]; 0.3 mg/0.3 mL [1:1000] (1.1 mL) [contains sodium bisulfite; two 0.3 mg doses per injector]

Injection, solution, as hydrochloride: 0.1 mg/mL [1:10,000] (10 mL); 1 mg/mL [1:1000] (1 mL) [products may contain sodium metabisulfite]

Adrenalin®: 1 mg/mL [1:1000] (1 mL, 30 mL) [contains sodium bisulfite]

Solution for oral inhalation, as hydrochloride:

Adrenalin®: 1% [10 mg/mL, 1:100] (7.5 mL) [contains sodium bisulfite]

Solution for oral inhalation [racepinephrine]:

S2®: 2.25% (0.5 mL, 15 mL) [as d-epinephrine 1.125% and l-epinephrine 1.125%; contains metabisulfites]

Solution, topical [racepinephrine]:

Raphon: 2.25% (15 mL) [as d-epinephrine 1.125% and l-epinephrine 1.125%; contains metabisulfites]

Selected Readings

"2005 American Heart Association Guidelines for Cardiopulmonary Resuscitation and Emergency Cardiovascular Care," *Circulation*, 2005, 112(24 Suppl): 1-211.

Cydulka R, Davison R, Grammer L, et al, "The Use of Epinephrine in the Treatment of Older Adult Asthmatics," *Ann Emerg Med*, 1988, 17(4):322-6.

Davis C and Wax P, "Subcutaneous Epinephrine O.D. in a Child Resulting in Dysrhythmias and Myocardial Ischemia," *Vet Hum Toxicol*, 1994, 36:367.

Illi A, Sundberg S, Ojala-Karlsson P, et al, "The Effect of Entacapone on the Disposition and Hemodynamic Effects of Intravenous Isoproterenol and Epinephrine," *Clin Pharmacol Ther*, 1995, 58(2):221-7.

Klein JS, Rich MR, and Yuninger JW, "Myocardial Ischemia Without Coronary Artery Disease After Epinephrine Overdose for Insect Sting Reaction," *J Allergy Clin Immunol*, 1995, 95(2):371.

Kuracheck SC and Rockoff MA, "Inadvertent Intravenous Administration of Racemic Epinephrine," *JAMA*, 1984, 253(10):1441-2.

Murphy FT, Manow TJ, Knutson SW, et al, "Epinephrine-Induced Lactic Acidosis in the Setting of Status Asthmaticus," *South Med J*, 1995, 88(5):577-9.

National Asthma Education and Prevention Program, "Expert Panel Report 2: Guidelines for the Diagnosis and Management of Asthma," Bethesda, MD, National Institutes of Health, 1997. NIH publication 97-4051.

Nicholson KE and Rogers JE, "Cocaine and Adrenaline Paste: A Fatal Combination?" *BMJ*, 1995, 311(6999):250-1.

Riou B, Barriot P, Rimailho A, et al, "Treatment of Severe Chloroquine Poisoning," *N Engl J Med*, 1988, 318(1):1-6.

Scalzo A, Keith G, and Thompson M, "Fatal Outcome After Massive Epinephrine Overdose by Intravenous Injection of an OTC Asthma Inhaler," *Clin Toxicol*, 1995, 33(5):501-2.

Stiell IG, Hebert PC, Wells GA, et al, "Vasopressin Versus Epinephrine for Inhospital Cardiac Arrest: A Randomised Controlled Trial," *Lancet*, 2001, 358(9276):105-9.

Waisman Y, Klein BL, Boenning DA, et al, "Prospective Randomized Double-Blind Study Comparing L-Epinephrine and Racemic Epinephrine Aerosols in the Treatment of Laryngotracheitis (Croup)," *Pediatrics*, 1992, 89(2):302-6.

Wenzel V, Krismer AC, Arntz HR, et al, "A Comparison of Vasopressin and Epinephrine for Out-of-Hospital Cardiopulmonary Resuscitation. European Resuscitation Council Vasopressor during Cardiopulmonary Resuscitation Study Group," *N Engl J Med*, 2004, 350(2):105-13.

Epinephrine and Articaine Hydrochloride *see* Articaine and Epinephrine *on page 139*

Epinephrine and Chlorpheniramine
(ep i NEF rin & klor fen IR a meen)

Related Information
Chlorpheniramine *on page 323*
Epinephrine *on page 546*
U.S. Brand Names Ana-Kit®
Generic Available No
Synonyms Insect Sting Kit
Pharmacologic Category Antidote
Use Anaphylaxis emergency treatment of insect bites or stings by the sensitive patient that may occur within minutes of insect sting or exposure to an allergic substance
Local Anesthetic/Vasoconstrictor Precautions No information available to require special precautions
Effects on Dental Treatment No significant effects or complications reported
Drug Interactions
Cytochrome P450 Effect: Chlorpheniramine: **Substrate** of CYP2D6 (minor), 3A4 (major); **Inhibits** CYP2D6 (weak)

Epinephrine and Lidocaine *see* Lidocaine and Epinephrine *on page 924*

Epinephrine and Prilocaine (Dental) *see* Prilocaine and Epinephrine *on page 1278*

Epinephrine Bitartrate *see* Epinephrine *on page 546*

Epinephrine Bitartrate and Bupivacaine Hydrochloride *see* Bupivacaine and Epinephrine *on page 228*

Epinephrine Hydrochloride *see* Epinephrine *on page 546*

Epinephrine (Racemic) (ep i NEF rin, ra SEE mik)

U.S. Brand Names AsthmaNefrin®; microNefrin®; S-2®
Generic Available Yes
Pharmacologic Category Alpha/Beta Agonist; Vasoconstrictor
Dental Use Emergency drug for treatment of bronchoconstriction
Use Emergency drug for treatment of bronchoconstriction
Local Anesthetic/Vasoconstrictor Precautions No information available to require special precautions
Effects on Dental Treatment No significant effects or complications reported
Significant Adverse Effects Refer to Epinephrine monograph
Dental Usual Dosing Bronchoconstriction: Oral Inhalation: 1-3 inhalations (via nebulization); use minimum number of inhalations necessary to achieve response
Dosage Bronchoconstriction: Oral Inhalation: 1-3 inhalations (via nebulization); use minimum number of inhalations necessary to achieve response
Contraindications Hypersensitivity to epinephrine or any component of the formulation; cardiac arrhythmias; angle-closure glaucoma
Warnings/Precautions Use with caution in elderly patients, patients with diabetes mellitus, cardiovascular diseases (angina, tachycardia, myocardial infarction), thyroid disease, or cerebral arteriosclerosis, Parkinson's; some products contain sulfites as preservatives. Rapid I.V. infusion may cause death from cerebrovascular hemorrhage or cardiac arrhythmias. Oral inhalation of (Continued)

Epinephrine (Racemic) *(Continued)*

epinephrine is **not** the preferred route of administration. Avoid topical application where reduced perfusion could lead to ischemic tissue damage (eg, penis, ears, digits).

Drug Interactions Refer to Epinephrine monograph

Pharmacodynamics/Kinetics Onset of action: Bronchodilation: Inhalation: ~1 minute

Dosage Forms Solution for oral inhalation (AsthmaNefrin®, microNefrin®, S-2®): Racepinephrine 2.25% [epinephrine base 1.125%] (7.5 mL, 15 mL, 30 mL)

Epinephrine (Racemic) and Aluminum Potassium Sulfate

(ep i NEF rin, ra SEE mik and a LOO mi num poe TASS ee um SUL fate)

Related Information
Epinephrine *on page 546*

U.S. Brand Names Van R Gingibraid®

Generic Available No

Synonyms Aluminum Potassium Sulfate and Epinephrine (Racemic) (Dental)

Pharmacologic Category Adrenergic Agonist Agent; Alpha/Beta Agonist; Astringent; Vasoconstrictor

Dental Use Gingival retraction

Local Anesthetic/Vasoconstrictor Precautions No information available to require special precautions

Effects on Dental Treatment Key adverse event(s) related to dental treatment: Tissue retraction around base of the tooth (therapeutic effect).

Significant Adverse Effects No data reported

Dental Usual Dosing Gingival retraction: Adults: Pass the impregnated yarn around the neck of the tooth and place into gingival sulcus; normal tissue moisture, water, or gingival retraction solutions activate impregnated yarn. Limit use to one quadrant of the mouth at a time; recommended use is for 3-8 minutes in the mouth.

Mechanism of Action Epinephrine stimulates alpha$_1$ adrenergic receptors to cause vasoconstriction in blood vessels in gingiva; aluminum potassium sulfate, precipitates tissue and blood proteins

Contraindications Hypersensitivity to epinephrine or any component of the formulation; cardiovascular disease, hyperthyroidism, or diabetes; do not apply to areas of heavy or deep bleeding or over exposed bone

Warnings/Precautions Caution should be exercised whenever using gingival retraction cords with epinephrine since it delivers vasoconstrictor doses of racemic epinephrine to patients; the general medical history should be thoroughly evaluated before using in any patient

Drug Interactions No data reported

Pharmacodynamics/Kinetics No data reported

Dosage Forms Yarn, saturated in solution of 8% racemic epinephrine and 7% aluminum potassium sulfate:
Type "0e": 0.20 ± 0.10 mg epinephrine/inch
Type "1e": 0.40 ± 0.20 mg epinephrine/inch
Type "2e": 0.60 ± 0.20 mg epinephrine/inch

EpiPen® *see* Epinephrine *on page 546*

EpiPen® Jr *see* Epinephrine *on page 546*

Epipodophyllotoxin *see* Etoposide *on page 626*

EpiQuin™ Micro *see* Hydroquinone *on page 798*

Epirubicin (ep i ROO bi sin)

U.S. Brand Names Ellence®

Canadian Brand Names Ellence®; Pharmorubicin®

Mexican Brand Names Epilem®; Farmorubicin®

Generic Available No

Synonyms Pidorubicin; Pidorubicin Hydrochloride

Pharmacologic Category Antineoplastic Agent, Anthracycline

Use Adjuvant therapy for primary breast cancer

Local Anesthetic/Vasoconstrictor Precautions No information available to require special precautions

Effects on Dental Treatment Key adverse event(s) related to dental treatment: Mucositis.

Common Adverse Effects

>10%:
Central nervous system: Lethargy (1% to 46%)
Dermatologic: Alopecia (69% to 95%)
Endocrine & metabolic: Amenorrhea (69% to 72%), hot flashes (5% to 39%)
Gastrointestinal: Nausea, vomiting (83% to 92%), mucositis (9% to 59%), diarrhea (7% to 25%)
Hematologic: Leukopenia (49% to 80%; Grade 3 and 4: 1.5% to 58.6%), neutropenia (54% to 80%), anemia (13% to 72%), thrombocytopenia (5% to 49%)
Local: Injection site reactions (3% to 20%)
Ocular: Conjunctivitis (1% to 15%)
Miscellaneous: Infection (15% to 21%)

1% to 10%:
Cardiovascular: CHF (0.4% to 1.5%), decreased LVEF (asymptomatic) (1.4% to 2.1%); recommended maximum cumulative dose: 900 mg/m^2
Central nervous system: Fever (1% to 5%)
Dermatologic: Rash (1% to 9%), skin changes (0.7% to 5%)
Gastrointestinal: Anorexia (2% to 3%)
Other reactions (percentage not specified): Acute lymphoid leukemia, acute myelogenous leukemia (0.3% at 3 years, 0.5% at 5 years, 0.6% at 8 years), anaphylaxis, hypersensitivity, photosensitivity reaction, premature menopause in women, pulmonary embolism, radiation recall, skin and nail hyperpigmentation, thromboembolic phenomena, thrombophlebitis, transaminases increased, urticaria

Mechanism of Action Epirubicin is an anthracycline antibiotic. Epirubicin is known to inhibit DNA and RNA synthesis by steric obstruction after intercalating between DNA base pairs; active throughout entire cell cycle. Intercalation triggers DNA cleavage by topoisomerase II, resulting in cytocidal activity. Epirubicin also inhibits DNA helicase, and generates cytotoxic free radicals.

Drug Interactions

Increased Effect/Toxicity: Cimetidine increased the blood levels of epirubicin (AUC increased by 50%).

Pharmacodynamics/Kinetics

Distribution: V$_{ss}$ 21-27 L/kg
Protein binding: 77% to albumin
Metabolism: Extensively via hepatic and extrahepatic (including RBCs) routes
Half-life elimination: Triphasic; Mean terminal: 33 hours
Excretion: Feces; urine (lesser extent)

Pregnancy Risk Factor D

Epitol® see Carbamazepine on page 260
Epivir® see Lamivudine on page 894
Epivir-HBV® see Lamivudine on page 894

Eplerenone (e PLER en one)

U.S. Brand Names Inspra™
Generic Available No
Pharmacologic Category Diuretic, Potassium-Sparing; Selective Aldosterone Blocker
Use Treatment of hypertension (may be used alone or in combination with other antihypertensive agents); treatment of CHF following acute MI
Local Anesthetic/Vasoconstrictor Precautions No information available to require special precautions
Effects on Dental Treatment No significant effects or complications reported

Common Adverse Effects

>10%: Endocrine & metabolic: Hypertriglyceridemia (1% to 15%, dose related)
1% to 10%:
Central nervous system: Dizziness (3%), fatigue (2%)
Endocrine & metabolic: Breast pain (males <1% to 1%), serum creatinine increased (6% in CHF), gynecomastia (males <1% to 1%), hyponatremia (2%, dose related), hypercholesterolemia (<1% to 1%); hyperkalemia (mild-to-moderate hypertension <1%; left ventricular dysfunction ~6% had serum potassium ≥6 mEq/L)
Gastrointestinal: Diarrhea (2%), abdominal pain (1%)
Genitourinary: Abnormal vaginal bleeding (<1% to 2%)
Renal: Albuminuria (1%)
Respiratory: Cough (2%)
Miscellaneous: Flu-like syndrome (2%)

Mechanism of Action Aldosterone increases blood pressure primarily by inducing sodium reabsorption. Eplerenone reduces blood pressure by blocking
(Continued)

Eplerenone *(Continued)*

aldosterone binding at mineralocorticoid receptors found in the kidney, heart, blood vessels and brain.

Drug Interactions

Cytochrome P450 Effect: Substrate of CYP3A4 (major)

Increased Effect/Toxicity: ACE inhibitors, angiotensin II receptor antagonists, NSAIDs, potassium supplements, and potassium-sparing diuretics increase the risk of hyperkalemia; concomitant use with potassium supplements and potassium-sparing diuretics is contraindicated; monitor potassium levels with ACE inhibitors and angiotensin II receptor antagonists. Potent CYP3A4 inhibitors (eg, itraconazole, ketoconazole) lead to fivefold increase in eplerenone; concurrent use is contraindicated. Less potent CYP3A4 inhibitors (eg, erythromycin, fluconazole, saquinavir, verapamil) lead to approximately twofold increase in eplerenone; starting dose should be decreased to 25 mg/day. Although interaction studies have not been conducted, monitoring of lithium levels is recommended.

Decreased Effect: NSAIDs may decrease the antihypertensive effects of eplerenone. CYP3A4 inducers may decrease the levels/effects of eplerenone; example inducers include aminoglutethimide, carbamazepine, nafcillin, nevirapine, phenobarbital, phenytoin, and rifamycins.

Pharmacodynamics/Kinetics

Distribution: V_d: 43-90 L

Protein binding: ~50%; primarily to alpha$_1$-acid glycoproteins

Metabolism: Primarily hepatic via CYP3A4; metabolites inactive

Half-life elimination: 4-6 hours

Time to peak, plasma: 1.5 hours; may take up to 4 weeks for full therapeutic effect

Excretion: Urine (67%; <5% as unchanged drug), feces (32%)

Pregnancy Risk Factor B

EPO see Epoetin Alfa on page 552

Epoetin Alfa *(e POE e tin AL fa)*

U.S. Brand Names Epogen®; Procrit®

Canadian Brand Names Eprex®

Mexican Brand Names Epomax®; Eprex®

Generic Available No

Synonyms EPO; Erythropoietin; rHuEPO-α

Pharmacologic Category Colony Stimulating Factor

Use Treatment of anemia related to HIV therapy, chronic renal failure, antineoplastic therapy; reduction of allogeneic blood transfusion for elective, noncardiac, nonvascular surgery

Unlabeled/Investigational Use Anemia associated with rheumatic disease; hypogenerative anemia of Rh hemolytic disease; sickle cell anemia; acute renal failure; Gaucher's disease; Castleman's disease; paroxysmal nocturnal hemoglobinuria; anemia of critical illness (limited documentation); anemia of prematurity

Local Anesthetic/Vasoconstrictor Precautions No information available to require special precautions

Effects on Dental Treatment No significant effects or complications reported

Common Adverse Effects Note: Adverse drug reaction incidences vary based on condition being treated and dose administered.

>10%:

Cardiovascular: Edema, hypertension

Central nervous system: Fever, headache, insomnia

Dermatologic: Pruritus, rash

Gastrointestinal: Dyspepsia, nausea, vomiting

Local: Injection site reaction

Neuromuscular & skeletal: Arthralgia, paresthesia, weakness

Respiratory: Congestion, cough, dyspnea, upper respiratory infection

1% to 10%:

Cardiovascular: Chest pain

Central nervous system: Fatigue, seizure

Gastrointestinal: Diarrhea

Hematologic: Clotted access, deep vein thrombosis

Mechanism of Action Induces erythropoiesis by stimulating the division and differentiation of committed erythroid progenitor cells; induces the release of reticulocytes from the bone marrow into the bloodstream, where they mature to erythrocytes. There is a dose response relationship with this effect. This results in an increase in reticulocyte counts followed by a rise in hematocrit and hemoglobin levels.

Pharmacodynamics/Kinetics
Onset of action: Several days
  Peak effect: 2-3 weeks
Distribution: V_d: 9 L; rapid in the plasma compartment; concentrated in liver, kidneys, and bone marrow
Metabolism: Some degradation does occur
Bioavailability: SubQ: ~21% to 31%; intraperitoneal epoetin: 3% (a few patients)
Half-life elimination: Circulating: Chronic renal failure: 4-13 hours; Healthy volunteers: 20% shorter
Time to peak, serum: SubQ: Chronic renal failure: 5-24 hours
Excretion: Feces (majority); urine (small amounts, 10% unchanged in normal volunteers)

Pregnancy Risk Factor C

Epogen® see Epoetin Alfa on page 552

Epoprostenol (e poe PROST en ole)

U.S. Brand Names Flolan®
Canadian Brand Names Flolan®
Generic Available No
Synonyms Epoprostenol Sodium; PGI₂; PGX; Prostacyclin
Pharmacologic Category Prostaglandin
Use Treatment of idiopathic pulmonary arterial hypertension [IPAH]; pulmonary hypertension associated with the scleroderma spectrum of disease [SSD] in NYHA Class III and Class IV patients who do not respond adequately to conventional therapy
Local Anesthetic/Vasoconstrictor Precautions No information available to require special precautions
Effects on Dental Treatment No significant effects or complications reported
Common Adverse Effects
  Note: Adverse events reported during dose initiation and escalation include flushing (58%), headache (49%), nausea/vomiting (32%), hypotension (16%), anxiety/nervousness/agitation (11%), chest pain (11%); abdominal pain, back pain, bradycardia, diaphoresis, dizziness, dyspepsia, dyspnea, hypoesthesia/paresthesia, musculoskeletal pain, and tachycardia are also reported. The following adverse events have been reported during chronic administration for IPAH. Although some may be related to the underlying disease state, anxiety, diarrhea, flu-like symptoms, flushing, headache, jaw pain, nausea, nervousness, and vomiting are clearly contributed to epoprostenol.
  >10%:
    Cardiovascular: Chest pain (67%), palpitation (63%), flushing (42%), tachycardia (35%), arrhythmia (27%), hemorrhage (19%), bradycardia (15%)
    Central nervous system: Dizziness (83%), headache (83%), chills/fever/sepsis/flu-like symptoms (25%), anxiety/nervousness/tremor (21%)
    Gastrointestinal: Nausea/vomiting (67%), diarrhea (37%)
    Genitourinary: Weight loss (27%)
    Local: Injection-site reactions: Infection (21%), pain (13%)
    Neuromuscular & skeletal: Weakness (87%), jaw pain (54%), myalgia (44%), musculoskeletal pain (35%; predominantly involving legs and feet), hypoesthesia/hyperparesthesia/paresthesia (12%)
    Respiratory: Dyspnea (90%)
  1% to 10%:
    Cardiovascular: Supraventricular tachycardia (8%), cerebrovascular accident (4%)
    Central nervous system: Convulsion (4%)
    Dermatologic: Rash (10%; conventional therapy 13%), pruritus (4%)
    Endocrine & metabolic: Hypokalemia (6%)
    Gastrointestinal: Constipation (6%), weight gain (6%)
    Neuromuscular & skeletal: Arthralgia (6%)
    Ocular: Amblyopia (8%), vision abnormality (4%)
    Respiratory: Epistaxis (4%), pleural effusion (4%)
Restrictions Orders for epoprostenol are distributed by two sources in the United States. Information on orders or reimbursement assistance may be obtained from either Accredo Health, Inc (1-800-935-6526) or TheraCom, Inc (1-877-356-5264).
Mechanism of Action Epoprostenol is also known as prostacyclin and PGI₂. It is a strong vasodilator of all vascular beds. In addition, it is a potent endogenous inhibitor of platelet aggregation. The reduction in platelet aggregation results
(Continued)

Epoprostenol *(Continued)*

from epoprostenol's activation of intracellular adenylate cyclase and the resultant increase in cyclic adenosine monophosphate concentrations within the platelets. Additionally, it is capable of decreasing thrombogenesis and platelet clumping in the lungs by inhibiting platelet aggregation.

Drug Interactions

Increased Effect/Toxicity: The hypotensive effects of epoprostenol may be exacerbated by other vasodilators, diuretics, or by using acetate in dialysis fluids. Patients treated with anticoagulants (heparins, warfarin, thrombin inhibitors) or antiplatelet agents (ticlopidine, clopidogrel, IIb/IIIa antagonists, aspirin) and epoprostenol should be monitored for increased bleeding risk.

Pharmacodynamics/Kinetics

Metabolism: Rapidly hydrolyzed; subject to some enzymatic degradation; forms one active metabolite and 13 inactive metabolites

Half-life elimination: 6 minutes

Excretion: Urine (84%); feces (4%)

Pregnancy Risk Factor B

Epoprostenol Sodium *see* Epoprostenol *on page 553*

Eprosartan *(ep roe SAR tan)*

Related Information

Cardiovascular Diseases *on page 1636*

U.S. Brand Names Teveten®

Canadian Brand Names Teveten®

Generic Available No

Pharmacologic Category Angiotensin II Receptor Blocker

Use Treatment of hypertension; may be used alone or in combination with other antihypertensives

Local Anesthetic/Vasoconstrictor Precautions No information available to require special precautions

Effects on Dental Treatment No significant effects or complications reported

Common Adverse Effects 1% to 10%:

Central nervous system: Fatigue (2%), depression (1%)

Endocrine & metabolic: Hypertriglyceridemia (1%)

Gastrointestinal: Abdominal pain (2%)

Genitourinary: Urinary tract infection (1%)

Respiratory: Upper respiratory tract infection (8%), rhinitis (4%), pharyngitis (4%), cough (4%)

Miscellaneous: Viral infection (2%), injury (2%)

Dosage Adults: Oral: Dosage must be individualized; can administer once or twice daily with total daily doses of 400-800 mg. Usual starting dose is 600 mg once daily as monotherapy in patients who are euvolemic. Limited clinical experience with doses >800 mg.

Dosage adjustment in renal impairment: No starting dosage adjustment is necessary; however, carefully monitor the patient

Dosage adjustment in hepatic impairment: No starting dosage adjustment is necessary; however, carefully monitor the patient

Elderly: No starting dosage adjustment is necessary; however, carefully monitor the patient

Mechanism of Action Angiotensin II is formed from angiotensin I in a reaction catalyzed by angiotensin-converting enzyme (ACE, kininase II). Angiotensin II is the principal pressor agent of the renin-angiotensin system, with effects that include vasoconstriction, stimulation of synthesis and release of aldosterone, cardiac stimulation, and renal reabsorption of sodium. Eprosartan blocks the vasoconstrictor and aldosterone-secreting effects of angiotensin II by selectively blocking the binding of angiotensin II to the AT1 receptor in many tissues, such as vascular smooth muscle and the adrenal gland. Its action is therefore independent of the pathways for angiotensin II synthesis. Blockade of the renin-angiotensin system with ACE inhibitors, which inhibit the biosynthesis of angiotensin II from angiotensin I, is widely used in the treatment of hypertension. ACE inhibitors also inhibit the degradation of bradykinin, a reaction also catalyzed by ACE. Because eprosartan does not inhibit ACE (kininase II), it does not affect the response to bradykinin. Whether this difference has clinical relevance is not yet known. Eprosartan does not bind to or block other hormone receptors or ion channels known to be important in cardiovascular regulation.

Contraindications Hypersensitivity to eprosartan or any component of the formulation; sensitivity to other A-II receptor antagonists; bilateral renal artery stenosis; pregnancy (2nd and 3rd trimesters)

Warnings/Precautions Avoid use or use a smaller dose in patients who are volume depleted; correct depletion first. Deterioration in renal function can occur with initiation. Use with caution in unilateral renal artery stenosis and pre-existing renal insufficiency; significant aortic/mitral stenosis. Safety and efficacy not established in pediatric patients.

Drug Interactions
Cytochrome P450 Effect: Inhibits CYP2C9 (weak)
Increased Effect/Toxicity: Eprosartan may increase risk of lithium toxicity. May increase risk of hyperkalemia with potassium-sparing diuretics (eg, amiloride, potassium, spironolactone, triamterene), potassium supplements, or high doses of trimethoprim.
Ethanol/Nutrition/Herb Interactions Herb/Nutraceutical: Avoid dong quai if using for hypertension (has estrogenic activity). Avoid ephedra, yohimbe, ginseng (may worsen hypertension). Avoid garlic (may have increased antihypertensive effect).

Pharmacodynamics/Kinetics
Protein binding: 98%
Metabolism: Minimally hepatic
Bioavailability: 300 mg dose: 13%
Half-life elimination: Terminal: 5-9 hours
Time to peak, serum: Fasting: 1-2 hours
Excretion: Feces (90%); urine (7%, mostly as unchanged drug)
Clearance: 7.9 L/hour
Pregnancy Risk Factor C (1st trimester); D (2nd and 3rd trimesters)
Dosage Forms TAB: 400 mg, 600 mg

Eprosartan and Hydrochlorothiazide
(ep roe SAR tan & hye droe klor oh THYE a zide)

Related Information
Eprosartan *on page 554*
Hydrochlorothiazide *on page 776*
U.S. Brand Names Teveten® HCT
Canadian Brand Names Teveten® HCT; Teveten® Plus
Generic Available No
Synonyms Eprosartan Mesylate and Hydrochlorothiazide; Hydrochlorothiazide and Eprosartan
Pharmacologic Category Angiotensin II Receptor Blocker Combination; Antihypertensive Agent, Combination; Diuretic, Thiazide
Use Treatment of hypertension (not indicated for initial treatment)
Local Anesthetic/Vasoconstrictor Precautions No information available to require special precautions
Effects on Dental Treatment No significant effects or complications reported
Common Adverse Effects Percentages reported with combination product; other reactions have been reported (see individual agents for additional information)
1% to 10%:
Central nervous system: Dizziness (4%), headache (3%), fatigue (2%)
Hematologic: Neutrophil count decreased (1%)
Neuromuscular & skeletal: Back pain (3%)
Renal: BUN elevated (1%)
Mechanism of Action Hydrochlorothiazide inhibits sodium reabsorption in the distal tubules causing increased excretion of sodium and water as well as potassium and hydrogen ions. **Eprosartan** blocks the vasoconstrictor and aldosterone-secreting effects of angiotensin II by selectively blocking the binding of angiotensin II to the AT1 receptor in many tissues, such as vascular smooth muscle and the adrenal gland.

Drug Interactions
Increased Effect/Toxicity: See individual agents.
Decreased Effect: See individual agents.
Pharmacodynamics/Kinetics See individual agents.
Pregnancy Risk Factor C/D (2nd and 3rd trimesters)

Eprosartan Mesylate and Hydrochlorothiazide *see* Eprosartan and Hydrochlorothiazide *on page 555*
Epsilon Aminocaproic Acid *see* Aminocaproic Acid *on page 86*
Epsom Salts *see* Magnesium Sulfate *on page 963*
EPT *see* Teniposide *on page 1456*
Eptacog Alfa (Activated) *see* Factor VIIa (Recombinant) *on page 632*

Eptifibatide (ep TIF i ba tide)

Related Information
Cardiovascular Diseases *on page 1636*
U.S. Brand Names Integrilin®
Canadian Brand Names Integrilin®
Generic Available No
Synonyms Intrifiban
Pharmacologic Category Antiplatelet Agent, Glycoprotein IIb/IIIa Inhibitor
Use Treatment of patients with acute coronary syndrome (unstable angina/non-Q wave myocardial infarction [UA/NQMI]), including patients who are to be managed medically and those undergoing percutaneous coronary intervention (PCI including angioplasty, intracoronary stenting)
Local Anesthetic/Vasoconstrictor Precautions No information available to require special precautions
Effects on Dental Treatment Key adverse event(s) related to dental treatment: Bleeding; patients weighing <70 kg may have an increased risk of major bleeding.
Common Adverse Effects Bleeding is the major drug-related adverse effect. Access site is often primary source of bleeding complications. Incidence of bleeding is also related to heparin intensity. Patients weighing <70 kg may have an increased risk of major bleeding.

>10%: Hematologic: Bleeding (major: 1% to 11%; minor: 3% to 14%; transfusion required: 2% to 13%)
1% to 10%:
Cardiovascular: Hypotension (up to 7%)
Hematologic: Thrombocytopenia (1% to 3%)
Local: Injection site reaction

Mechanism of Action Eptifibatide is a cyclic heptapeptide which blocks the platelet glycoprotein IIb/IIIa receptor, the binding site for fibrinogen, von Willebrand factor, and other ligands. Inhibition of binding at this final common receptor reversibly blocks platelet aggregation and prevents thrombosis.
Drug Interactions
Increased Effect/Toxicity: Eptifibatide effect may be increased by other drugs which affect hemostasis include thrombolytics, oral anticoagulants, NSAIDs, dipyridamole, heparin, low molecular weight heparins, ticlopidine, and clopidogrel. Avoid concomitant use of other IIb/IIIa inhibitors. Cephalosporins which contain the MTT side chain may theoretically increase the risk of hemorrhage. Use with aspirin and heparin may increase bleeding over aspirin and heparin alone. However, aspirin and heparin were used concurrently in the majority of patients in the major clinical studies of eptifibatide. Antiplatelet agents (eg, eptifibatide) may enhance the adverse/toxic effect of drotrecogin alfa; bleeding may occur.
Pharmacodynamics/Kinetics
Onset of action: Within 1 hour
Duration: Platelet function restored ~4 hours following discontinuation
Protein binding: ~25%
Half-life elimination: 2.5 hours
Excretion: Primarily urine (as eptifibatide and metabolites); significant renal impairment may alter disposition of this compound
Clearance: Total body: 55-58 mL/kg/hour; Renal: ~50% of total in healthy subjects
Pregnancy Risk Factor B

Epzicom™ *see* Abacavir and Lamivudine *on page 23*
Equagesic® *see* Aspirin and Meprobamate *on page 151*
Equalactin® [OTC] *see* Polycarbophil *on page 1252*
Equalizer Gas Relief [OTC] *see* Simethicone *on page 1394*
Equanil *see* Meprobamate *on page 993*
Equetro™ *see* Carbamazepine *on page 260*
Eraxis™ *see* Anidulafungin *on page 128*
Erbitux® *see* Cetuximab *on page 308*

Ergocalciferol (er goe kal SIF e role)

U.S. Brand Names Calciferol™; Drisdol®
Canadian Brand Names Drisdol®; Ostoforte®
Generic Available Yes: Capsule

Synonyms Activated Ergosterol; Viosterol; Vitamin D_2

Pharmacologic Category Vitamin D Analog

Use Treatment of refractory rickets, hypophosphatemia, hypoparathyroidism; dietary supplement

Local Anesthetic/Vasoconstrictor Precautions No information available to require special precautions

Effects on Dental Treatment Key adverse event(s) related to dental treatment: Metallic taste and xerostomia (normal salivary flow resumes upon discontinuation).

Common Adverse Effects Generally well tolerated

Frequency not defined: Cardiac arrhythmia, hypertension (late), irritability, headache, psychosis (rare), somnolence, hyperthermia (late), pruritus, decreased libido (late), hypercholesterolemia, mild acidosis (late), polydipsia (late), nausea, vomiting, anorexia, pancreatitis, metallic taste, weight loss (rare), xerostomia, constipation, polyuria (late), increased BUN (late), increased LFTs (late), bone pain, myalgia, weakness, conjunctivitis, photophobia (late), vascular/nephrocalcinosis (rare)

Mechanism of Action Stimulates calcium and phosphate absorption from the small intestine, promotes secretion of calcium from bone to blood; promotes renal tubule phosphate resorption

Drug Interactions

Increased Effect/Toxicity: Thiazide diuretics may increase vitamin D effects. Cardiac glycosides may increase toxicity.

Decreased Effect: Cholestyramine, colestipol, mineral oil may decrease oral absorption.

Pharmacodynamics/Kinetics

Onset of action: Peak effect: ~1 month following daily doses

Absorption: Readily; requires bile

Metabolism: Inactive until hydroxylated hepatically and renally to calcifediol and then to calcitriol (most active form)

Pregnancy Risk Factor A/C (dose exceeding RDA recommendation)

Ergoloid Mesylates (ER goe loid MES i lates)

Canadian Brand Names Hydergine®

Generic Available Yes

Synonyms Dihydroergotoxine; Dihydrogenated Ergot Alkaloids; Hydergine [DSC]

Pharmacologic Category Ergot Derivative

Use Treatment of cerebrovascular insufficiency in primary progressive dementia, Alzheimer's dementia, and senile onset

Local Anesthetic/Vasoconstrictor Precautions No information available to require special precautions

Effects on Dental Treatment Key adverse event(s) related to dental treatment: Orthostatic hypotension.

Common Adverse Effects Adverse effects are minimal; most common include transient nausea, gastrointestinal disturbances and sublingual irritation with SL tablets; other common side effects include:

Cardiovascular: Orthostatic hypotension, bradycardia

Dermatologic: Skin rash, flushing

Ocular: Blurred vision

Respiratory: Nasal congestion

Mechanism of Action Ergoloid mesylates do not have the vasoconstrictor effects of the natural ergot alkaloids; exact mechanism in dementia is unknown; originally classed as peripheral and cerebral vasodilator, now considered a "metabolic enhancer"; there is no specific evidence which clearly establishes the mechanism by which ergoloid mesylate preparations produce mental effects, nor is there conclusive evidence that the drug particularly affects cerebral arteriosclerosis or cerebrovascular insufficiency

Drug Interactions

Cytochrome P450 Effect: Substrate of CYP3A4 (major)

Increased Effect/Toxicity: CYP3A4 inhibitors may increase the levels/effects of ergoloid mesylates; example inhibitors include azole antifungals, clarithromycin, diclofenac, doxycycline, erythromycin, imatinib, isoniazid, nefazodone, nicardipine, propofol, protease inhibitors, quinidine, telithromycin, and verapamil. Ergot alkaloids are contraindicated with potent CYP3A4 inhibitors. Ergoloid mesylates may increase the effects of 5-HT$_1$ agonists (eg, sumatriptan), MAO inhibitors, sibutramine, and other serotonin agonists (serotonin syndrome). Severe vasoconstriction may occur when
(Continued)

Ergoloid Mesylates (Continued)

peripheral vasoconstrictors or beta-blockers are used in patients receiving ergot alkaloids; concurrent use is contraindicated.

Decreased Effect: Effects of ergoloid mesylates may be diminished by antipsychotics, metoclopramide. Antianginal effects of nitrates may be reduced by ergot alkaloids.

Pharmacodynamics/Kinetics

Absorption: Rapid yet incomplete

Half-life elimination, serum: 3.5 hours

Time to peak, serum: ~1 hour

Pregnancy Risk Factor C

Ergomar® see Ergotamine on page 558

Ergometrine Maleate see Ergonovine on page 558

Ergonovine (er goe NOE veen)

Generic Available No

Synonyms Ergometrine Maleate; Ergonovine Maleate

Pharmacologic Category Ergot Derivative

Use Prevention and treatment of postpartum and postabortion hemorrhage caused by uterine atony or subinvolution

Unlabeled/Investigational Use Migraine headaches, diagnostically to identify Prinzmetal's angina

Local Anesthetic/Vasoconstrictor Precautions No information available to require special precautions

Effects on Dental Treatment No significant effects or complications reported

Common Adverse Effects 1% to 10%: Gastrointestinal: Nausea, vomiting

Mechanism of Action Ergot alkaloid alpha-adrenergic agonist directly stimulates vascular smooth muscle to vasoconstrict peripheral and cerebral vessels; may also have antagonist effects on serotonin

Drug Interactions

Cytochrome P450 Effect: Substrate of CYP3A4 (major)

Increased Effect/Toxicity: CYP3A4 inhibitors may increase the levels/ effects of ergonovine; example inhibitors include azole antifungals, clarithromycin, diclofenac, doxycycline, erythromycin, imatinib, isoniazid, nefazodone, nicardipine, propofol, protease inhibitors, quinidine, telithromycin, troleandomycin, and verapamil. Ergot alkaloids are contraindicated with potent CYP3A4 inhibitors. Ergonovine may increase the effects of 5-HT$_1$ agonists (eg, sumatriptan), MAO inhibitors, sibutramine, and other serotonin agonists (serotonin syndrome). Severe vasoconstriction may occur when peripheral vasoconstrictors or beta-blockers are used in patients receiving ergot alkaloids; concurrent use is contraindicated.

Decreased Effect: Effects of ergonovine may be diminished by antipsychotics, metoclopramide. Antianginal effects of nitrates may be reduced by ergot alkaloids.

Pharmacodynamics/Kinetics

Onset of action: I.M.: ~2-5 minutes

Duration: I.M.: Uterine effect: 3 hours; I.V.: ~45 minutes

Metabolism: Hepatic

Excretion: Primarily feces; urine

Pregnancy Risk Factor X

Ergonovine Maleate see Ergonovine on page 558

Ergotamine (er GOT a meen)

U.S. Brand Names Ergomar®

Generic Available No

Synonyms Ergotamine Tartrate

Pharmacologic Category Ergot Derivative

Use Abort or prevent vascular headaches, such as migraine, migraine variants, or so-called "histaminic cephalalgia"

Local Anesthetic/Vasoconstrictor Precautions No information available to require special precautions

Effects on Dental Treatment Key adverse event(s) related to dental treatment: Xerostomia and changes in salivation (normal salivary flow resumes upon discontinuation).

Common Adverse Effects Frequency not defined.

Cardiovascular: Absence of pulse, bradycardia, cardiac valvular fibrosis, cyanosis, edema, ECG changes, gangrene, hypertension, ischemia, precordial distress and pain, tachycardia, vasospasm

Central nervous system: Vertigo

Dermatologic: Itching

Gastrointestinal: Nausea, vomiting

Genitourinary: Retroperitoneal fibrosis

Neuromuscular & skeletal: Muscle pain, numbness, paresthesia, weakness

Respiratory: Pleuropulmonary fibrosis

Miscellaneous: Cold extremities

Mechanism of Action Has partial agonist and/or antagonist activity against tryptaminergic, dopaminergic and alpha-adrenergic receptors depending upon their site; is a highly active uterine stimulant; it causes constriction of peripheral and cranial blood vessels and produces depression of central vasomotor centers

Drug Interactions

Cytochrome P450 Effect: Substrate of CYP3A4 (major); Inhibits CYP3A4 (weak)

Increased Effect/Toxicity: CYP3A4 inhibitors may increase the levels/effects of ergotamine; example inhibitors include azole antifungals, clarithromycin, diclofenac, doxycycline, erythromycin, imatinib, isoniazid, nefazodone, nicardipine, propofol, protease inhibitors, quinidine, telithromycin, troleandomycin, and verapamil. Ergot alkaloids are contraindicated with strong CYP3A4 inhibitors. Ergotamine may increase the effects of 5-HT$_1$ agonists (eg, sumatriptan), MAO inhibitors, sibutramine, and other serotonin agonists (serotonin syndrome). Severe vasoconstriction may occur when peripheral vasoconstrictors or beta-blockers are used in patients receiving ergot alkaloids; concurrent use is contraindicated.

Decreased Effect: Effects of ergotamine may be diminished by antipsychotics, metoclopramide. Antianginal effects of nitrates may be reduced by ergot alkaloids.

Pharmacodynamics/Kinetics

Absorption: Oral: Erratic; enhanced by caffeine coadministration

Metabolism: Extensively hepatic

Time to peak, serum: 0.5-3 hours

Half-life elimination: 2 hours

Excretion: Feces (90% as metabolites)

Pregnancy Risk Factor X

Ergotamine and Caffeine (er GOT a meen & KAF een)

Related Information

Caffeine *on page 245*

Ergotamine *on page 558*

U.S. Brand Names Cafergot®; Wigraine®

Canadian Brand Names Cafergor®

Generic Available No

Synonyms Caffeine and Ergotamine; Ergotamine Tartrate and Caffeine

Pharmacologic Category Ergot Derivative; Stimulant

Use Abort or prevent vascular headaches, such as migraine, migraine variants, or so-called "histaminic cephalalgia"

Local Anesthetic/Vasoconstrictor Precautions No information available to require special precautions

Effects on Dental Treatment No significant effects or complications reported

Common Adverse Effects Frequency not defined.

Cardiovascular: Absence of pulse, bradycardia, cardiac valvular fibrosis, cyanosis, edema, ECG changes, gangrene, hypertension, ischemia, precordial distress and pain, tachycardia, vasospasm

Central nervous system: Vertigo

Dermatologic: Itching

Gastrointestinal: Anal or rectal ulcer (with overuse of suppository), nausea, vomiting

Genitourinary: Retroperitoneal fibrosis

Neuromuscular & skeletal: Muscle pain, numbness, paresthesia, weakness

Respiratory: Pleuropulmonary fibrosis

Miscellaneous: Cold extremities

Mechanism of Action Has partial agonist and/or antagonist activity against tryptaminergic, dopaminergic and alpha-adrenergic receptors depending upon their site; is a highly active uterine stimulant; it causes constriction of peripheral and cranial blood vessels and produces depression of central vasomotor centers

(Continued)

Ergotamine and Caffeine *(Continued)*

Drug Interactions

Cytochrome P450 Effect:

Ergotamine: **Substrate** of CYP3A4 (major); **Inhibits** CYP3A4 (weak)

Caffeine: **Substrate** of CYP1A2 (major), 2C9 (minor), 2D6 (minor), 2E1 (minor), 3A4 (minor); **Inhibits** CYP1A2 (weak), 3A4 (moderate)

Increased Effect/Toxicity: See Ergotamine monograph for related interactions. CYP1A2 inhibitors may increase the levels/effects of caffeine; example inhibitors include amiodarone, fluvoxamine, ketoconazole, and rofecoxib. CYP3A4 inhibitors may increase the levels/effects of ergotamine; example inhibitors include azole antifungals, ciprofloxacin, clarithromycin, diclofenac, doxycycline, erythromycin, imatinib, isoniazid, nefazodone, nicardipine, propofol, protease inhibitors, quinidine, and verapamil. Caffeine may increase the levels/effects of CYP3A4 substrates; example substrates include benzodiazepines, calcium channel blockers, ergot derivatives, mirtazapine, nateglinide, nefazodone, tacrolimus, and venlafaxine. Caffeine levels may be increased by selected quinolone antibiotics (ciprofloxacin, norfloxacin, ofloxacin).

Decreased Effect: See Ergotamine monograph for related interactions.

Pharmacodynamics/Kinetics

Absorption: Ergotamine: Oral, rectal: Erratic; enhanced by caffeine coadministration

Metabolism: Extensively hepatic

Time to peak, serum: Ergotamine: 0.5-3 hours

Half-life elimination: 2 hours

Excretion: Feces (90% as metabolites)

Pregnancy Risk Factor X

Ergotamine Tartrate *see* Ergotamine *on page 558*

Ergotamine Tartrate and Caffeine *see* Ergotamine and Caffeine *on page 559*

Ergotamine Tartrate, Belladonna, and Phenobarbital *see* Belladonna, Phenobarbital, and Ergotamine *on page 185*

Erlotinib *(er LOE tye nib)*

U.S. Brand Names Tarceva™

Generic Available No

Synonyms CP358774; Erlotinib Hydrochloride; NSC-718781; OSI-774; R 14-15

Pharmacologic Category Antineoplastic Agent, Tyrosine Kinase Inhibitor; Epidermal Growth Factor Receptor (EGFR) Inhibitor

Use Treatment of refractory advanced or metastatic nonsmall-cell lung cancer (NSCLC); pancreatic cancer (first-line therapy in combination with gemcitabine)

Unlabeled/Investigational Use Treatment of advanced or metastatic breast cancer, colorectal cancer, head and neck tumors, ovarian cancer, and renal cell cancer

Local Anesthetic/Vasoconstrictor Precautions No information available to require special precautions

Effects on Dental Treatment Key adverse event(s) related to dental treatment: Stomatitis.

Common Adverse Effects Percentages as reported with monotherapy; frequency of adverse event with combination chemotherapy (gemcitabine) noted where applicable

>10%:

Cardiovascular: Edema (37% combination)

Central nervous system: Fatigue (14% to 55%; 73% combination), pyrexia (36% combination), anxiety (21%), headache (17%), depression (16%; 19% combination), dizziness (15% combination), insomnia (12%; 15% combination)

Dermatologic: Acneiform rash (50% to 88%; grade 3/4: 9%), pruritus (13% to 55%), dry skin (12% to 35%), erythema (18%), alopecia (14% combination)

Gastrointestinal: Diarrhea (30% to 56%; grade 3/4: 6%), anorexia (23% to 52%), nausea (11% to 33%; 60% combination), vomiting (23%; 42% combination), mucositis (17% to 18%), glossodynia (18%), stomatitis (17%; 22% combination), xerostomia (17%), pain (14%), flatulence (13% combination); constipation (12%; 31% combination), dyspepsia (12%; 17% combination), dysphagia (12%), weight loss (12%; 39% combination), abnormal taste (11%), abdominal pain (11%; 46% combination)

Hepatic: ALT increased (4%; combination grade 2: 31%, grade 3: 13%, grade 4: <1%), AST increased (combination grade 2: 24%, grade 3: 10%, grade 4 <1%), hyperbilirubinemia (20%; combination grade 2: 17%, grade 3: 10%, grade 4: <1%)

Neuromuscular & skeletal: Bone pain (25% combination), myalgia (21% combination), arthralgia (14%), neuropathy (13% combination), rigors (12% combination), paresthesia (11%)

Ocular: Conjunctivitis (12%; <1% combination), keratoconjunctivitis sicca (12%)

Respiratory: Dyspnea (21% to 41%), cough (16% to 33%)

Miscellaneous: Infection (24%; 39% combination)

1% to 10%:

Cardiovascular (reported with combination chemotherapy): Deep venous thrombosis (4%), arrhythmia, cerebrovascular accidents (including cerebral hemorrhage), MI, myocardial ischemia, syncope

Gastrointestinal (reported with combination chemotherapy): Ileus, pancreatitis

Hematologic (reported with combination chemotherapy): Hemolytic anemia, microangiopathic hemolytic anemia with thrombocytopenia

Ocular: Keratitis (6%; <1% combination)

Renal (reported with combination chemotherapy): Renal insufficiency

Respiratory: Pneumonitis (6%)

Mechanism of Action The mechanism of erlotinib's antitumor action is not fully characterized. The drug is known to inhibit overall epidermal growth factor receptor (HER1/EGFR)- tyrosine kinase. Active competitive inhibition of adenosine triphosphate inhibits downstream signal transduction of ligand dependent HER1/EGFR activation.

Drug Interactions

Cytochrome P450 Effect: Substrate of CYP1A2 (minor), 3A4 (major)

Increased Effect/Toxicity: Ketoconazole and CYP3A4 inhibitors may increase erlotinib levels/effects; example inhibitors include azole antifungals, clarithromycin, diclofenac, doxycycline, erythromycin, imatinib, isoniazid, nefazodone, nicardipine, propofol, protease inhibitors, quinidine, telithromycin, and verapamil.

Decreased Effect: Rifamycins and CYP3A4 inducers may decrease erlotinib levels/effects; example inducers include aminoglutethimide, carbamazepine, nafcillin, nevirapine, phenobarbital, and phenytoin.

Pharmacodynamics/Kinetics

Absorption: Oral: 60% on an empty stomach; ~100% on a full stomach

Distribution: 94-232 L

Protein binding: 92% to 95%, albumin and α_1-acid glycoprotein

Metabolism: Hepatic, CYP3A4 (major), CYP1A1 (minor), CYP1A2 (minor), and CYP1C (minor)

Bioavailability: 100% when given with food; 60% without food

Half-life elimination: 24-36 hours

Time to peak, plasma: 1-7 hours

Excretion: Primarily as metabolites: Feces (83%); urine (8%)

Pregnancy Risk Factor D

Erlotinib Hydrochloride *see* Erlotinib *on page 560*

Errin™ *see* Norethindrone *on page 1125*

Ertaczo™ *see* Sertaconazole *on page 1385*

Ertapenem (er ta PEN em)

U.S. Brand Names Invanz®
Canadian Brand Names Invanz®
Generic Available No
Synonyms Ertapenem Sodium; L-749,345; MK0826
Pharmacologic Category Antibiotic, Carbapenem
Use Treatment of the following moderate-severe infections: Complicated intra-abdominal infections, complicated skin and skin structure infections (including diabetic foot infections without osteomyelitis), complicated UTI (including pyelonephritis), acute pelvic infections, and community-acquired pneumonia. Antibacterial coverage includes aerobic gram-positive organisms, aerobic gram-negative organisms, anaerobic organisms.

Note: Methicillin-resistant *Staphylococcus*, *Enterococcus* spp, penicillin-resistant strains of *Streptococcus pneumoniae*, beta-lactamase-positive strains of *Haemophilus influenzae* are **resistant** to ertapenem, as are most *Pseudomonas aeruginosa*.

Local Anesthetic/Vasoconstrictor Precautions No information available to require special precautions

Effects on Dental Treatment Key adverse event(s) related to dental treatment: Oral candidiasis.

(Continued)

Ertapenem *(Continued)*

Common Adverse Effects Note: Percentages reported in adults.

1% to 10%:

Cardiovascular: Swelling/edema (3%), chest pain (1%), hypertension (0.7% to ≤2%), hypotension (1% to 2%), tachycardia (1% to 2%)

Central nervous system: Headache (6% to 7%), altered mental status (ie, agitation, confusion, disorientation, decreased mental acuity, changed mental status, somnolence, stupor) (3% to 5%), fever (2% to 5%), insomnia (3%), dizziness (2%), fatigue (1%), anxiety (0.8% to ≤1%)

Dermatologic: Rash (2% to 3%), pruritus (1% to 2%), erythema (1% to 2%)

Gastrointestinal: Diarrhea (9% to 10%), nausea (6% to 9%), abdominal pain (4%), vomiting (4%), constipation (3% to 4%), acid regurgitation (1% to 2%), dyspepsia (1%), oral candidiasis (0.1% to ≤1%)

Genitourinary: Vaginitis (1% to 3%)

Hematologic: Platelet count increased (4% to 7%), eosinophils increased (1% to 2%)

Hepatic: Hepatic enzyme elevations (7% to 9%), alkaline phosphatase increase (4% to 7%)

Local: Infused vein complications (5% to 7%), phlebitis/thrombophlebitis (2%), extravasation (0.7% to ≤2%)

Neuromuscular & skeletal: Leg pain (0.4% to 1%)

Respiratory: Dyspnea (1% to 3%), cough (1% to 2%), pharyngitis (0.7% to ≤1%), rales/rhonchi (0.5% to ≤1%), respiratory distress (0.2% to ≤1%)

Mechanism of Action Inhibits bacterial cell wall synthesis by binding to one or more of the penicillin binding proteins; which in turn inhibits the final transpeptidation step of peptidoglycan synthesis in bacterial cell walls, thus inhibiting cell wall biosynthesis. Bacteria eventually lyse due to ongoing activity of cell wall autolytic enzymes (autolysins and murein hydrolases) while cell wall assembly is arrested.

Drug Interactions

Increased Effect/Toxicity: Probenecid may increase serum concentrations of ertapenem; use caution.

Decreased Effect: Ertapenem may decrease valproic acid serum concentrations to subtherapeutic levels; monitor.

Pharmacodynamics/Kinetics

Absorption: I.M.: Almost complete

Distribution: V$_{dss}$:

Children 3 months to 12 years: 0.2 L/kg

Children 13-17 years: 0.16 L/kg

Adults: 0.12 L/kg

Protein binding (concentration dependent): 85% at 300 mcg/mL, 95% at <100 mcg/mL

Metabolism: Hydrolysis to inactive metabolite

Bioavailability: I.M.: 90%

Half-life elimination:

Children 3 months to 12 years: 2.5 hours

Children ≥13 years and Adults: 4 hours

Time to peak: I.M.: 2.3 hours

Excretion: Urine (80% as unchanged drug and metabolite); feces (10%)

Pregnancy Risk Factor B

Ertapenem Sodium *see* Ertapenem *on page 561*

Erwinia Asparaginase *see* Asparaginase *on page 144*

Eryc® *see* Erythromycin *on page 562*

Eryderm® *see* Erythromycin *on page 562*

Erygel® *see* Erythromycin *on page 562*

EryPed® *see* Erythromycin *on page 562*

Ery-Tab® *see* Erythromycin *on page 562*

Erythrocin® *see* Erythromycin *on page 562*

Erythromycin *(er ith roe MYE sin)*

Related Information

Bacterial Infections *on page 1697*

Cardiovascular Diseases *on page 1636*

Respiratory Diseases *on page 1656*

Sexually-Transmitted Diseases *on page 1674*

Viral Infections *on page 1709*

Related Sample Prescriptions

Bacterial Infections and Periodontal Diseases *on page 1736*

U.S. Brand Names Akne-Mycin®; A/T/S®; E.E.S.®; Eryc®; Eryderm®; Erygel®; EryPed®; Ery-Tab®; Erythrocin®; PCE®; Romycin®; Staticin® [DSC]; Theramycin Z®; T-Stat® [DSC]

Canadian Brand Names Apo-Erythro Base®; Apo-Erythro E-C®; Apo-Erythro-ES®; Apo-Erythro-S®; Diomycin®; EES®; Erybid™; Eryc®; Novo-Rythro Estolate; Novo-Rythro Ethylsuccinate; Nu-Erythromycin-S; PCE®; PMS-Erythromycin; Sans Acne®

Mexican Brand Names Eryacnen®; Eryderm®; Ilosone®; Latotryd®; Lauricin®; Lauritran®; Optomicin®; Pantomicina®; Procephal®; Sans-Acne®; Stiemycin®

Generic Available Yes

Synonyms Erythromycin Base; Erythromycin Estolate; Erythromycin Ethylsuccinate; Erythromycin Glucceptate; Erythromycin Lactobionate; Erythromycin Stearate

Pharmacologic Category Antibiotic, Macrolide; Antibiotic, Ophthalmic; Antibiotic, Topical; Topical Skin Product; Topical Skin Product, Acne

Dental Use Systemic: Alternative to penicillin VK for treatment of orofacial infections

Use
Systemic: Treatment of susceptible bacterial infections including *S. pyogenes*, some *S. pneumoniae*, some *S. aureus*, *M. pneumoniae*, *Legionella pneumophila*, diphtheria, pertussis, chancroid, *Chlamydia*, erythrasma, *N. gonorrhoeae*, *E. histolytica*, syphilis and nongonococcal urethritis, and *Campylobacter* gastroenteritis; used in conjunction with neomycin for decontaminating the bowel
Ophthalmic: Treatment of superficial eye infections involving the conjunctiva or cornea; neonatal ophthalmia
Topical: Treatment of acne vulgaris

Unlabeled/Investigational Use Systemic: Treatment of gastroparesis

Local Anesthetic/Vasoconstrictor Precautions No information available to require special precautions (see Dental Comment)

Effects on Dental Treatment Key adverse event(s) related to dental treatment: Oral candidiasis.

Significant Adverse Effects
Systemic:
Cardiovascular: Ventricular arrhythmia, QT_c prolongation, torsade de pointes (rare), ventricular tachycardia (rare)
Central nervous system: Headache (8%), pain (2%), fever, seizure
Dermatitis: Rash (3%), pruritus (1%)
Gastrointestinal: Abdominal pain (8%), cramping, nausea (8%), oral candidiasis, vomiting (3%), diarrhea (7%), dyspepsia (2%), flatulence (2%), anorexia, pseudomembranous colitis, hypertrophic pyloric stenosis (including cases in infants or IHPS), pancreatitis
Hematologic: Eosinophilia (1%)
Hepatic: Cholestatic jaundice (most common with estolate), increased liver function tests (2%)
Local: Phlebitis at the injection site, thrombophlebitis
Neuromuscular & skeletal: Weakness (2%)
Respiratory: Dyspnea (1%), cough (3%)
Miscellaneous: Hypersensitivity reactions, allergic reactions
Topical: 1% to 10%: Dermatologic: Erythema, desquamation, dryness, pruritus

Dental Usual Dosing Treatment of orofacial infections: Adults: Oral:
Base: 250-500 mg every 6-12 hours
Ethylsuccinate: 400-800 mg every 6-12 hours

Dosage
Neonates: Ophthalmic: Prophylaxis of neonatal gonococcal or chlamydial conjunctivitis: 0.5-1 cm ribbon of ointment should be instilled into each conjunctival sac
Infants and Children:
Usual dosage range:
Oral: (**Note:** Due to differences in absorption, 400 mg erythromycin ethylsuccinate produces the same serum levels as 250 mg erythromycin base, sterate or estolate):
Base: 30-50 mg/kg/day in 2-4 divided doses; do not exceed 2 g/day
Estolate: 30-50 mg/kg/day in 2-4 divided doses; do not exceed 2 g/day
Ethylsuccinate: 30-50 mg/kg/day in 2-4 divided doses; do not exceed 3.2 g/day
Stearate: 30-50 mg/kg/day in 2-4 divided doses; do not exceed 2 g/day
I.V.: Lactobionate: 15-50 mg/kg/day divided every 6 hours, not to exceed 4 g/day
Indication-specific dosing: Oral:
Acne vulgaris (unlabeled use): Adolescents: 250-1500 mg/day in 2 divided doses; therapy may be continued for 4-6 weeks at lowest possible dose
(Continued)

Erythromycin *(Continued)*

Pharyngitis: 40 mg/kg/day in 2 doses; maximum: 1600 mg/day; short-course therapy for 5 days may be considered

Pertussis (CDC guidelines): 40-50 mg/kg/day in 4 divided doses for 14 days; maximum 2 g/day (not preferred agent for infants <1 month)

Preop bowel preparation: 20 mg/kg erythromycin base at 1, 2, and 11 PM on the day before surgery combined with mechanical cleansing of the large intestine and oral neomycin

Children and Adults:

Ophthalmic: Instill ½" (1.25 cm) 2-6 times/day depending on the severity of the infection

Topical: Apply over the affected area twice daily after the skin has been thoroughly washed and patted dry

Adults:

Usual dosage range:

Oral:

Base: 250-500 mg every 6-12 hours

Ethylsuccinate: 400-800 mg every 6-12 hours

I.V. (lactobionate): 15-20 mg/kg/day divided every 6 hours or 500 mg to 1 g every 6 hours, or given as a continuous infusion over 24 hours (maximum: 4 g/24 hours)

Indication-specific dosing:

Cervicitis: Oral: 500 mg 4 times/day for 7 days

Chancroid (unlabeled use; not a preferred agent): Oral: 500 mg 4 times/day for 7 days

Community-acquired pneumonia, bronchitis: Oral, I.V.: 500-1000 mg 4 times/day for 10-14 days. If *Legionella* is suspected/confirmed, 750-1000 mg 4 times/day for 21 days or more may be recommended. **Note:** Other macrolides and/or fluoroquinolones may be preferred and better tolerated.

Lymphogranuloma venereum: Oral: 500 mg 4 times/day for 21 days

Nongonococcal urethritis (recurrent): Oral: CDC Guidelines for the Treatment of Sexually Transmitted Diseases recommendation: Metronidazole (2 g as a single dose) plus 7 days of erythromycin base (500 mg 4 times/day) or erythromycin ethylsuccinate (800 mg 4 times/day)

Pertussis (CDC guidelines): Oral: 500 mg every 6 hours for 14 days

Preop bowel preparation (unlabeled use): Oral: 1 g erythromycin base at 1, 2, and 11 PM on the day before surgery combined with mechanical cleansing of the large intestine and oral neomycin

Gastrointestinal prokinetic (unlabeled use): Oral: Erythromycin has been used as a prokinetic agent to improve gastric emptying time and intestinal motility. In adults, 200 mg was infused I.V. initially followed by 250 mg orally 3 times/day 30 minutes before meals. Lower dosages have been used in some trials.

Dosage adjustment in renal impairment: Dialysis: Slightly dialyzable (5% to 20%); no supplemental dosage necessary in hemo- or peritoneal dialysis or in continuous arteriovenous or venovenous hemofiltration

Mechanism of Action Inhibits RNA-dependent protein synthesis at the chain elongation step; binds to the 50S ribosomal subunit resulting in blockage of transpeptidation

Contraindications Hypersensitivity to erythromycin or any component of the formulation

Systemic: Pre-existing liver disease (erythromycin estolate); concomitant use with ergot derivatives, pimozide, or cisapride

Warnings/Precautions Systemic: Use caution with hepatic impairment with or without jaundice has occurred, it may be accompanied by malaise, nausea, vomiting, abdominal colic, and fever; discontinue use if these occur; avoid using erythromycin lactobionate in neonates since formulations may contain benzyl alcohol which is associated with toxicity in neonates; observe for superinfections. Use in infants has been associated with infantile hypertrophic pyloric stenosis (IHPS). Macrolides have been associated with rare QT prolongation and ventricular arrhythmias, including torsade de pointes. Elderly may be at increased risk of adverse events, including hearing loss and/or torsade de pointes when dosage ≥4 g/day, particularly if concurrent renal/hepatic impairment.

Drug Interactions Substrate of CYP2B6 (minor), 3A4 (major); **Inhibits** CYP1A2 (weak), 3A4 (moderate)

Alfentanil (and possibly other narcotic analgesics): Serum levels may be increased by erythromycin; monitor for increased effect.

Antipsychotic agents (particularly mesoridazine and thioridazine): Risk of QT_c prolongation and malignant arrhythmias may be increased.

Benzodiazepines (those metabolized by CYP3A4, including alprazolam and triazolam): Serum levels may be increased by erythromycin; somnolence and confusion have been reported.

Bromocriptine: Serum levels may be increased by erythromycin; monitor for increased effect.

Buspirone: Serum levels may be increased by erythromycin; monitor.

Calcium channel blockers (felodipine, verapamil, and potentially others metabolized by CYP3A4): Serum levels may be increased by erythromycin; monitor.

Carbamazepine: Serum levels may be increased by erythromycin; monitor.

Cilostazol: Serum levels may be increased by erythromycin.

Cisapride: Serum levels may be increased by erythromycin; serious arrhythmias have occurred; concurrent use contraindicated.

Clindamycin (and lincomycin): Use with erythromycin may result in pharmacologic antagonism; manufacturer recommends avoiding this combination.

Clozapine: Serum levels may be increased by erythromycin; monitor.

Colchicine: serum levels/toxicity may be increased by erythromycin; monitor. Avoid use, if possible.

Cyclosporine: Serum levels may be increased by erythromycin; monitor serum levels.

CYP3A4 inducers: CYP3A4 inducers may decrease the levels/effects of erythromycin. Example inducers include aminoglutethimide, carbamazepine, nafcillin, nevirapine, phenobarbital, phenytoin, and rifamycins.

CYP3A4 inhibitors: May increase the levels/effects of erythromycin. Example inhibitors include azole antifungals, clarithromycin, diclofenac, doxycycline, imatinib, isoniazid, nefazodone, nicardipine, propofol, protease inhibitors, quinidine, telithromycin, and verapamil.

CYP3A4 substrates: Erythromycin may increase the levels/effects of CYP3A4 substrates. Example substrates include benzodiazepines, calcium channel blockers, cyclosporine, mirtazapine, nateglinide, nefazodone, sildenafil (and other PDE-5 inhibitors), tacrolimus, and venlafaxine. Selected benzodiazepines (midazolam and triazolam), cisapride, ergot alkaloids, selected HMG-CoA reductase inhibitors (lovastatin and simvastatin), and pimozide are generally contraindicated with strong CYP3A4 inhibitors.

Delavirdine: Serum levels of erythromycin may be increased; also, serum levels of delavirdine may increased by erythromycin (low risk); monitor.

Digoxin: Serum levels may be increased by erythromycin; monitor digoxin levels.

Disopyramide: Serum levels may be increased by erythromycin; in addition, QT_c prolongation and risk of malignant arrhythmia may be increased; avoid combination.

Ergot alkaloids: Concurrent use may lead to acute ergot toxicity (severe peripheral vasospasm and dysesthesia).

HMG-CoA reductase inhibitors (atorvastatin, lovastatin, and simvastatin); Erythromycin may increase serum levels of "statins" metabolized by CYP3A4, increasing the risk of myopathy/rhabdomyolysis (does not include fluvastatin and pravastatin). Switch to pravastatin/fluvastatin or suspend treatment during course of erythromycin therapy.

Loratadine: Serum levels may be increased by erythromycin; monitor.

Methylprednisolone: Serum levels may be increased by erythromycin; monitor.

Neuromuscular-blocking agents: May be potentiated by erythromycin (case reports).

Phenytoin: Serum levels may be increased by erythromycin; other evidence suggested phenytoin levels may be decreased in some patients; monitor.

Pimozide: Serum levels may be increased, leading to malignant arrhythmias; concomitant use is contraindicated.

Protease inhibitors (amprenavir, nelfinavir, and ritonavir): May increase serum levels of erythromycin.

QT_c-prolonging agents: Concomitant use may increase the risk of malignant arrhythmias.

Quinidine: Serum levels may be increased by erythromycin; in addition, the risk of QT_c prolongation and malignant arrhythmias may be increased during concurrent use.

Quinolone antibiotics (sparfloxacin, gatifloxacin, and moxifloxacin): Concurrent use may increase the risk of malignant arrhythmias.

Rifabutin: Serum levels may be increased by erythromycin; monitor.

Sildenafil, tadalafil, vardenafil: Serum concentration may be substantially increased by erythromycin. Do not exceed single sildenafil doses of 25 mg in 48 hours, a single tadalafil dose of 10 mg in 72 hours, or a single vardenafil dose of 2.5 mg in 24 hours.

Tacrolimus: Serum levels may be increased by erythromycin; monitor serum concentration.

Theophylline: Serum levels may be increased by erythromycin; monitor.

(Continued)

Erythromycin *(Continued)*

Valproic acid (and derivatives): Serum levels may be increased by erythromycin; monitor.

Vinblastine (and vincristine): Serum levels may be increased by erythromycin.

Warfarin: Effects may be potentiated; monitor INR closely and adjust warfarin dose as needed or choose another antibiotic.

Zafirlukast: Serum levels may be decreased by erythromycin; monitor.

Zopiclone: Serum levels may be increased by erythromycin; monitor.

Ethanol/Nutrition/Herb Interactions

Ethanol: Avoid ethanol (may decrease absorption of erythromycin or enhance ethanol effects).

Food: Increased drug absorption with meals; erythromycin serum levels may be altered if taken with food.

Herb/Nutraceutical: St John's wort may decrease erythromycin levels.

Dietary Considerations Systemic: Drug may cause GI upset; may take with food.

Pharmacodynamics/Kinetics

Absorption: Oral: Variable but better with salt forms than with base form; 18% to 45%; ethylsuccinate may be better absorbed with food

Distribution: Crosses placenta; enters breast milk

Relative diffusion from blood into CSF: Minimal even with inflammation

CSF:blood level ratio: Normal meninges: 1% to 12%; Inflamed meninges: 7% to 25%

Protein binding: 75% to 90%

Metabolism: Hepatic via demethylation

Half-life elimination: Peak: 1.5-2 hours; End-stage renal disease: 5-6 hours

Time to peak, serum: Base: 4 hours; Ethylsuccinate: 0.5-2.5 hours; delayed with food due to differences in absorption

Excretion: Primarily feces; urine (2% to 15% as unchanged drug)

Pregnancy Risk Factor B

Lactation Enters breast milk/use caution (AAP considers "compatible")

Dosage Forms [DSC] = Discontinued product; [CAN] = Canadian brand name

Capsule, delayed release, enteric-coated pellets, as base (Eryc®): 250 mg

Gel, topical: 2% (30 g, 60 g)

A/T/S®: 2% (30 g) [contains alcohol 92%]

Erygel®: 2% (30 g, 60 g) [contains alcohol 92%]

Granules for oral suspension, as ethylsuccinate (E.E.S.®): 200 mg/5 mL (100 mL, 200 mL) [cherry flavor]

Injection, powder for reconstitution, as lactobionate (Erythrocin®): 500 mg, 1 g

Ointment, ophthalmic: 0.5% [5 mg/g] (1 g, 3.5 g)

Romycin®: 0.5% [5 mg/g] (3.5 g)

Ointment, topical (Akne-Mycin®): 2% (25 g)

Powder for oral suspension, as ethylsuccinate (EryPed®): 200 mg/5 mL (100 mL, 200 mL) [fruit flavor]; 400 mg/5 mL (100 mL, 200 mL) [banana flavor]

Powder for oral suspension, as ethylsuccinate [drops] (EryPed®): 100 mg/2.5 mL (50 mL) [fruit flavor]

Solution, topical: 2% (60 mL)

A/T/S®: 2% (60 mL) [contains alcohol 66%]

Eryderm®, T-Stat® [DSC], Theramycin Z®: 2% (60 mL) [contain alcohol]

Sans Acne® [CAN]: 2% (60 mL) [contains ethyl alcohol 44%; not available in U.S.]

Staticin®: 1.5% (60 mL) [DSC]

Suspension, oral, as estolate: 125 mg/5 mL (480 mL); 250 mg/5 mL (480 mL)

Suspension, oral, as ethylsuccinate: 200 mg/5 mL (480 mL); 400 mg/5 mL (480 mL)

E.E.S.®: 200 mg/5 mL (100 mL, 480 mL) [fruit flavor]; 400 mg/5 mL (100 mL, 480 mL) [orange flavor]

Swab (T-Stat® [DSC]): 2% (60s)

Tablet, chewable, as ethylsuccinate (EryPed®): 200 mg [fruit flavor] [DSC]

Tablet, delayed release, enteric coated, as base (Ery-Tab®): 250 mg, 333 mg, 500 mg

Tablet, as base: 250 mg, 500 mg

Tablet, as ethylsuccinate (E.E.S.®): 400 mg

Tablet, as stearate: 250 mg

Erythrocin®: 250 mg, 500 mg

Tablet [polymer-coated particles], as base (PCE®): 333 mg, 500 mg

Dental Comment

This drug is known to prolong the QT interval. The QT interval is measured as the time and distance between the Q point of the QRS complex and the end of the T wave in the ECG tracing. After adjustment for heart rate, the QT interval is defined as prolonged if it is more than 450 msec in men and 460 msec in women. A long QT syndrome was first described in the 1950s and 60s as a congenital syndrome involving QT interval prolongation and syncope and sudden death. Some of the congenital long QT syndromes were characterized by a peculiar electrocardiographic appearance of the QRS complex involving a premature atria beat followed by a pause, then a subsequent sinus beat showing marked QT prolongation and deformity. This type of cardiac arrhythmia was originally termed "torsade de pointes" (translated from the French as "twisting of the points").

Prolongation of the QT interval is thought to result from delayed ventricular repolarization. The repolarization process within the myocardial cell is due to the efflux of intracellular potassium. The channels associated with this current can be blocked by many drugs and predisposes the electrical propagation cycle to torsade de pointes.

Erythromycin is one of the drugs confirmed to prolong the QT interval and is accepted as having a risk of causing torsade de pointes. The risk of drug-induced torsade de pointes is extremely low when a single QT interval prolonging drug is prescribed. In terms of epinephrine, it is not known what effect vasoconstrictors in the local anesthetic regimen will have in patients with a known history of congenital prolonged QT interval or in patients taking any medication that prolongs the QT interval. Until more information is obtained, it is suggested that the clinician consult with the physician prior to the use of a vasoconstrictor in suspected patients, and that the vasoconstrictor (epinephrine, levonordefrin [Neo-Cobefrin®]) be used with caution.

Many patients cannot tolerate erythromycin because of abdominal pain and nausea; the mechanism of this adverse effect appears to be the motilin agonistic properties of erythromycin in the GI tract. For these patients, clindamycin is indicated as the alternative antibiotic for treatment of orofacial infections.

HMG-CoA reductase inhibitors, also known as the statins, effectively decrease the hepatic cholesterol biosynthesis resulting in the reduction of blood LDL-cholesterol concentrations. The AUC of atorvastatin (Lipitor®) was increased 33% by erythromycin administration. Combination of erythromycin and lovastatin (Mevacor®) has been associated with rhabdomyolysis (Ayanian, et al). The mechanism of erythromycin is inhibiting the CYP3A4 metabolism of atorvastatin, lovastatin, and cerivastatin. Simvastatin (Zocor®) would likely be affected in a similar manner by the coadministration of erythromycin. Clarithromycin (Biaxin®) may exert a similar effect as erythromycin on atorvastatin, lovastatin, cerivastatin, and simvastatin. Erythromycin 3 times/day had no effect on pravastatin (Pravachol®) plasma concentrations (Bottorff, et al).

Selected Readings

American Dental Association Council on Scientific Affairs, "Combating Antibiotic Resistance," *J Am Dent Assoc*, 2004, 135(4):484-7.

Ayanian JZ, Fuchs CS, and Stone RM, "Lovastatin and Rhabdomyolysis," *Ann Intern Med*, 1988, 109(8):682-3.

"Pimozide (Orap) Contraindicated With Clarithromycin (Biaxin®) and Other Macrolide Antibiotics," *FDA Medical Bulletin*, October 1996, 26(3).

Wynn RL and Bergman SA, "Antibiotics and Their Use in the Treatment of Orofacial Infections, Part I," *Gen Dent*, 1994, 42(5):398, 400, 402.

Wynn RL and Bergman SA, "Antibiotics and Their Use in the Treatment of Orofacial Infections, Part II," *Gen Dent*, 1994, 42(6):498-502.

Wynn RL, "Current Concepts of the Erythromycins," *Gen Dent*, 1991, 39(6):408,10-1.

Erythromycin and Benzoyl Peroxide
(er ith roe MYE sin & BEN zoe il per OKS ide)

Related Information
Benzoyl Peroxide *on page 194*
Erythromycin *on page 562*

U.S. Brand Names Benzamycin®; Benzamycin® Pak

Generic Available No

Synonyms Benzoyl Peroxide and Erythromycin

Pharmacologic Category Topical Skin Product; Topical Skin Product, Acne

Use Topical control of acne vulgaris

Local Anesthetic/Vasoconstrictor Precautions No information available to require special precautions

Effects on Dental Treatment No significant effects or complications reported

Drug Interactions
Cytochrome P450 Effect: Erythromycin: **Substrate** of CYP2B6 (minor), 3A4 (major); **Inhibits** CYP1A2 (weak), 3A4 (moderate)

Pharmacodynamics/Kinetics See individual agents.

Pregnancy Risk Factor C

Erythromycin and Sulfisoxazole (er ith roe MYE sin & sul fi SOKS a zole)

Related Information
Erythromycin *on page 562*
SulfiSOXAZOLE *on page 1429*

U.S. Brand Names Pediazole®

Canadian Brand Names Pediazole®

Generic Available Yes

Synonyms Sulfisoxazole and Erythromycin

Pharmacologic Category Antibiotic, Macrolide; Antibiotic, Macrolide Combination; Antibiotic, Sulfonamide Derivative

Use Treatment of susceptible bacterial infections of the upper and lower respiratory tract, otitis media in children caused by susceptible strains of *Haemophilus influenzae*, and many other infections in patients allergic to penicillin

Local Anesthetic/Vasoconstrictor Precautions No information available to require special precautions

Effects on Dental Treatment No significant effects or complications reported

Common Adverse Effects Frequency not defined.
Cardiovascular: Ventricular arrhythmia,
Central nervous system: Headache, fever
Dermatologic: Rash, Stevens-Johnson syndrome, toxic epidermal necrolysis
Gastrointestinal: Abdominal pain, cramping, nausea, vomiting, oral candidiasis, hypertrophic pyloric stenosis, diarrhea, pseudomembranous colitis
Hematologic: Agranulocytosis, aplastic anemia, eosinophilia
Hepatic: Hepatic necrosis, cholestatic jaundice
Local: Phlebitis at the injection site, thrombophlebitis
Renal: Toxic nephrosis, crystalluria
Miscellaneous: Hypersensitivity reactions

Mechanism of Action Erythromycin inhibits bacterial protein synthesis; sulfisoxazole competitively inhibits bacterial synthesis of folic acid from para-aminobenzoic acid

Drug Interactions
Cytochrome P450 Effect:
Erythromycin: **Substrate** of CYP2B6 (minor), 3A4 (major); **Inhibits** CYP1A2 (weak), 3A4 (moderate)
Sulfisoxazole: **Substrate** of CYP2C8/9 (major); **Inhibits** CYP2C8/9 (strong)
Increased Effect/Toxicity: See individual agents.
Decreased Effect: See individual agents.

Pharmacodynamics/Kinetics See individual agents.

Pregnancy Risk Factor C

Erythromycin Base *see* Erythromycin *on page 562*
Erythromycin Estolate *see* Erythromycin *on page 562*
Erythromycin Ethylsuccinate *see* Erythromycin *on page 562*
Erythromycin Gluceptate *see* Erythromycin *on page 562*
Erythromycin Lactobionate *see* Erythromycin *on page 562*
Erythromycin Stearate *see* Erythromycin *on page 562*
Erythropoiesis Stimulating Protein *see* Darbepoetin Alfa *on page 423*
Erythropoietin *see* Epoetin Alfa *on page 552*

Escitalopram (es sye TAL oh pram)

Related Information
Citalopram *on page 351*

U.S. Brand Names Lexapro®

Canadian Brand Names Cipralex®

Generic Available No

Synonyms Escitalopram Oxalate; Lu-26-054; S-Citalopram

Pharmacologic Category Antidepressant, Selective Serotonin Reuptake Inhibitor

Use Treatment of major depressive disorder; generalized anxiety disorders (GAD)

Local Anesthetic/Vasoconstrictor Precautions Although caution should be used in patients taking tricyclic antidepressants, no interactions have been reported with vasoconstrictors and escitalopram, a nontricyclic antidepressant which acts to increase serotonin; no precautions appear to be needed

Effects on Dental Treatment Key adverse event(s) related to dental treatment: Xerostomia (normal salivary flow resumes upon discontinuation) and toothache.

Common Adverse Effects

>10%:

Central nervous system: Headache (24%), somnolence (6% to 13%), insomnia (9% to 12%)

Gastrointestinal: Nausea (15%)

Genitourinary: Ejaculation disorder (9% to 14%)

1% to 10%:

Cardiovascular: Chest pain, hypertension, palpitation

Central nervous system: Dizziness (5%), fatigue (5% to 8%), dreaming abnormal, concentration impaired, fever, irritability, lethargy, lightheadedness, migraine, vertigo, yawning

Dermatologic: Rash

Endocrine & metabolic: Libido decreased (3% to 7%), anorgasmia (2% to 6%), hot flashes, menstrual cramps, menstrual disorder

Gastrointestinal: Diarrhea (8%), xerostomia (6% to 9%), appetite decreased (3%), constipation (3% to 5%), indigestion (3%), abdominal pain (2%), abdominal cramps, appetite increased, flatulence, gastroenteritis, gastroesophageal reflux, heartburn, toothache, vomiting, weight gain/loss

Genitourinary: Impotence (3%), urinary tract infection, urinary frequency

Neuromuscular & skeletal: Arthralgia, limb pain, muscle cramp, myalgia, neck/shoulder pain, paresthesia, tremor

Ocular: Blurred vision

Otic: Earache, tinnitus

Respiratory: Rhinitis (5%), sinusitis (3%), bronchitis, cough, nasal or sinus congestion, sinus headache

Miscellaneous: Diaphoresis (4% to 5%), flu-like syndrome (5%), allergy

Restrictions A medication guide concerning the use of antidepressants in children and teenagers can be found on the FDA website at http://www.fda.gov/cder/Offices/ODS/labeling.htm. It should be dispensed to parents or guardians of children and teenagers receiving this medication.

Dosage Oral:

Adults: Depression, GAD: Initial: 10 mg/day; dose may be increased to 20 mg/day after at least 1 week

Elderly: 10 mg/day; bioavailability and half-life are increased by 50% in the elderly

Dosage adjustment in renal impairment:

Mild to moderate impairment: No dosage adjustment needed

Severe impairment: Cl_{cr} <20 mL/minute: Use caution

Dosage adjustment in hepatic impairment: 10 mg/day

Mechanism of Action Escitalopram is the S-enantiomer of the racemic derivative citalopram, which selectively inhibits the reuptake of serotonin with little to no effect on norepinephrine or dopamine reuptake. It has no or very low affinity for 5-HT$_{1-7}$, alpha- and beta-adrenergic, D$_{1-5}$, H$_{1-3}$, M$_{1-5}$, and benzodiazepine receptors. Escitalopram does not bind or has low affinity for Na$^+$, K$^+$, Cl$^-$, and Ca^{++} ion channels.

Contraindications Hypersensitivity to escitalopram, citalopram, or any component of the formulation; concomitant use or within 2 weeks of MAO inhibitors

Warnings/Precautions Antidepressants increase the risk of suicidal thinking and behavior in children and adolescents with major depressive disorder (MDD) and other depressive disorders; consider risk prior to prescribing. All patients must be closely monitored for clinical worsening, suicidality, or unusual changes in behavior, especially during the initiation of therapy or following an increase or decrease in dosage. When used in children, the child's family or caregiver should be instructed to closely observe the patient and communicate condition with healthcare provider. A medication guide should be dispensed with each prescription. Escitalopram is not FDA approved for use in children

The possibility of a suicide attempt is inherent in major depression and may persist until remission occurs. Use caution in high-risk patients. Worsening depression and severe abrupt suicidality that are not part of the presenting symptoms may require discontinuation or modification of drug therapy. The patient's family or caregiver should be alerted to monitor patients for the emergence of suicidality and associated behaviors (such as agitation, irritability, hostility, impulsivity, and hypomania) and call healthcare provider.

May worsen psychosis in some patients or precipitate a shift to mania or hypomania in patients with bipolar disorder. Patients presenting with depressive symptoms should be screened for bipolar disorder. Monotherapy in patients with bipolar disorder should be avoided. Escitalopram is not FDA approved for the treatment of bipolar depression.

(Continued)

Escitalopram *(Continued)*

The potential for a severe reaction exists when used with MAO inhibitors; serotonin syndrome (hyperthermia, muscular rigidity, mental status changes/ agitation, autonomic instability) may occur. May increase the risks associated with electroconvulsive therapy. Has a low potential to impair cognitive or motor performance; caution operating hazardous machinery or driving.

Use caution with a previous seizure disorder or condition predisposing to seizures such as brain damage, alcoholism, or concurrent therapy with other drugs which lower the seizure threshold. May cause hyponatremia/SIADH. May cause or exacerbate sexual dysfunction. Use caution with renal or liver impairment; concomitant CNS depressants; pregnancy (high doses of citalopram has been associated with teratogenicity in animals). Use caution with concomitant use of NSAIDs, ASA, or other drugs that affect coagulation; the risk of bleeding is potentiated.

Upon discontinuation of escitalopram therapy, gradually taper dose. If intolerable symptoms occur following a decrease in dosage or upon discontinuation of therapy, then resuming the previous dose with a more gradual taper should be considered.

Drug Interactions

Cytochrome P450 Effect: Substrate (major) of CYP2C19, 3A4; **Inhibits** CYP2D6 (weak)

Increased Effect/Toxicity: Escitalopram should not be used with nonselective MAO inhibitors (phenelzine, isocarboxazid) or other drugs with MAO inhibition (linezolid); fatal reactions have been reported. Wait 5 weeks after stopping escitalopram before starting a nonselective MAO inhibitor and 2 weeks after stopping an MAO inhibitor before starting escitalopram. Concurrent selegiline has been associated with mania, hypertension, or serotonin syndrome (risk may be reduced relative to nonselective MAO inhibitors).

CYP2C19 inhibitors may increase the levels/effects of imipramine; example inhibitors include delavirdine, fluconazole, fluvoxamine, gemfibrozil, isoniazid, omeprazole, and ticlopidine. CYP3A4 inhibitors may increase the levels/ effects of escitalopram; example inhibitors include azole antifungals, clarithromycin, diclofenac, doxycycline, erythromycin, imatinib, isoniazid, nefazodone, nicardipine, propofol, protease inhibitors, quinidine, telithromycin, and verapamil.

Combined use of SSRIs and buspirone, meperidine, moclobemide, nefazodone, other SSRIs, tramadol, trazodone, and venlafaxine may increase the risk of serotonin syndrome. Escitalopram increases serum levels/effects of CYP2D6 substrates (tricyclic antidepressants). Escitalopram may increase desipramine levels.

Combined use of sumatriptan (and other serotonin agonists) may result in toxicity; weakness, hyper-reflexia, and incoordination have been observed with sumatriptan and SSRIs. In addition, concurrent use may theoretically increase the risk of serotonin syndrome; includes sumatriptan, naratriptan, rizatriptan, and zolmitriptan.

Concomitant use of escitalopram and NSAIDs, aspirin, or other drugs affecting coagulation has been associated with an increased risk of bleeding; monitor.

Decreased Effect: CYP2C19 inducers may decrease the levels/effects of imipramine; example inducers include aminoglutethimide, carbamazepine, phenytoin, and rifampin. CYP3A4 inducers may decrease the levels/effects of escitalopram; example inducers include aminoglutethimide, carbamazepine, nafcillin, nevirapine, phenobarbital, phenytoin, and rifamycins.

Ethanol/Nutrition/Herb Interactions

Ethanol: Avoid ethanol (may increase CNS depression).

Herb/Nutraceutical: Avoid valerian, St John's wort, SAMe, kava kava, and gotu kola (may increase CNS depression).

Dietary Considerations May be taken with or without food.

Pharmacodynamics/Kinetics

Protein binding: 56% to plasma proteins

Metabolism: Hepatic via CYP2C19 and 3A4 to an active metabolite, S-desmethylcitalopram (S-DCT; 1/7 the activity); S-DCT is metabolized to S-didesmethylcitalopram (S-DDCT; active; 1/27 the activity) via CYP2D6

Half-life elimination: Escitalopram: 27-32 hours; S-desmethylcitalopram: 59 hours

Time to peak: Escitalopram: 5 ± 1.5 hours; S-desmethylcitalopram: 14 hours

Excretion: Urine (Escitalopram: 8%; S-DCT: 10%)

Clearance: Total body: 37-40 L/hour; Renal: Escitalopram: 2.7 L/hour; S-desmethylcitalopram: 6.9 L/hour

Pregnancy Risk Factor C
Dosage Forms SOLN, oral: 1 mg/mL (240 mL). **TAB:** 5 mg, 10 mg, 20 mg;
(Cipralex® [CAN]): 10 mg, 20 mg

Escitalopram Oxalate *see* Escitalopram *on page 568*
Esclim® *see* Estradiol *on page 574*
Eserine Salicylate *see* Physostigmine *on page 1232*
Esgic® *see* Butalbital, Acetaminophen, and Caffeine *on page 239*
Esgic-Plus™ *see* Butalbital, Acetaminophen, and Caffeine *on page 239*
Eskalith® [DSC] *see* Lithium *on page 939*
Eskalith CR® *see* Lithium *on page 939*

Esmolol (ES moe lol)

U.S. Brand Names Brevibloc®
Canadian Brand Names Brevibloc®
Mexican Brand Names Brevibloc®
Generic Available Yes: Excludes infusion
Synonyms Esmolol Hydrochloride
Pharmacologic Category Antiarrhythmic Agent, Class II; Beta Blocker, Beta$_1$ Selective
Use Treatment of supraventricular tachycardia (SVT) and atrial fibrillation/flutter (control ventricular rate); treatment of tachycardia and/or hypertension (especially intraoperative or postoperative); treatment of noncompensatory sinus tachycardia
Unlabeled/Investigational Use In children, for SVT and postoperative hypertension
Local Anesthetic/Vasoconstrictor Precautions No information available to require special precautions
Effects on Dental Treatment Esmolol is a cardioselective beta-blocker. Local anesthetic with vasoconstrictor can be safely used in patients medicated with esmolol. Nonselective beta-blockers (ie, propranolol, nadolol) enhance the pressor response to epinephrine, resulting in hypertension and bradycardia; this has not been reported for esmolol. Many nonsteroidal anti-inflammatory drugs, such as ibuprofen and indomethacin, can reduce the hypotensive effect of beta-blockers after 3 or more weeks of therapy with the NSAID. Short-term NSAID use (ie, 3 days) requires no special precautions in patients taking beta-blockers.
Common Adverse Effects
>10%:
  Cardiovascular: Asymptomatic hypotension (dose-related: 25% to 38%), symptomatic hypotension (dose-related: 12%)
  Miscellaneous: Diaphoresis (10%)
1% to 10%:
  Cardiovascular: Peripheral ischemia (1%)
  Central nervous system: Dizziness (3%), somnolence (3%), confusion (2%), headache (2%), agitation (2%), fatigue (1%)
  Gastrointestinal: Nausea (7%), vomiting (1%)
  Local: Pain on injection (8%), infusion site reaction
Mechanism of Action Class II antiarrhythmic: Competitively blocks response to beta$_1$-adrenergic stimulation with little or no effect of beta$_2$-receptors except at high doses, no intrinsic sympathomimetic activity, no membrane stabilizing activity
Drug Interactions
  Increased Effect/Toxicity: Anticholinesterase inhibitors, amiodarone, cardiac glycosides dipyridamole (I.V.) increase bradycardia; beta blockers increase alpha$_1$ blockers orthostasis, alpha/beta agonists (direct acting) vasopressor effects, alpha$_2$ agonists rebound hypertension when withdrawn. Beta-blockers may enhance the hypoglycemia and mask most symptoms of hypoglycemia in patients on insulin or sulfonylureas. Calcium channel blockers increase hypotension
  Decreased Effect: Alpha$_2$ agonists decrease the effectiveness of beta blockers (beta$_1$ selective). NSAIDs may diminish the antihypertensive effects of beta blockers.
Pharmacodynamics/Kinetics
  Onset of action: Beta-blockade: I.V.: 2-10 minutes (quickest when loading doses are administered)
  Duration of hemodynamic effects: 10-30 minutes; prolonged following higher cumulative doses, extended duration of use
  Protein binding: 55%
  Metabolism: In blood by red blood cell esterases
  (Continued)

Esmolol *(Continued)*

Half-life elimination: Adults: 9 minutes; elimination of metabolite decreases with end stage renal disease

Excretion: Urine (~69% as metabolites, 2% unchanged drug)

Pregnancy Risk Factor C (manufacturer); D (2nd and 3rd trimesters - expert analysis)

Esmolol Hydrochloride *see* Esmolol *on page 571*

Esomeprazole (es oh ME pray zol)

Related Information
Omeprazole *on page 1145*
U.S. Brand Names Nexium®
Canadian Brand Names Nexium®
Generic Available No
Synonyms Esomeprazole Magnesium
Pharmacologic Category Proton Pump Inhibitor; Substituted Benzimidazole
Use

Oral: Short-term (4-8 weeks) treatment of erosive esophagitis; maintaining symptom resolution and healing of erosive esophagitis; treatment of symptomatic gastroesophageal reflux disease (GERD); as part of a multidrug regimen for *Helicobacter pylori* eradication in patients with duodenal ulcer disease (active or history of within the past 5 years); prevention of gastric ulcers in patients at risk (age ≥60 years and/or history of gastric ulcer) associated with continuous NSAID therapy

I.V.: Short-term (≤10 weeks) treatment of gastroesophageal reflux disease (GERD) when oral therapy is not possible or appropriate

Local Anesthetic/Vasoconstrictor Precautions No information available to require special precautions

Effects on Dental Treatment Key adverse event(s) related to dental treatment: Xerostomia (normal salivary flow resumes upon discontinuation).

Common Adverse Effects Unless otherwise specified, percentages represent adverse reactions identified in clinical trials evaluating the intravenous formulation.

>10%: Central nervous system: Headache (I.V. 11%; oral 4% to 8%)

1% to 10%:

Central nervous system: Dizziness (3%)

Dermatologic: Pruritus (≤1%)

Gastrointestinal: Flatulence (10%), nausea (2% to 6%), abdominal pain (6%; oral 3% to 4%), diarrhea (4%), xerostomia (2% to 4%), dyspepsia (<1% to 6%), constipation (3%)

Local: Injection site reaction (2%)

Respiratory: Sinusitis (≤2%), respiratory infection (1%)

Dosage Note: Delayed-release capsules should be swallowed whole and taken at least 1 hour before eating

Adolescents 12-17 years: Oral: GERD: 20-40 mg once daily for up to 8 weeks

Adults:

Oral:

Erosive esophagitis (healing): Initial: 20-40 mg once daily for 4-8 weeks; if incomplete healing, may continue for an additional 4-8 weeks; maintenance: 20 mg once daily

Symptomatic GERD: 20 mg once daily for 4 weeks; may continue an additional 4 weeks if symptoms persist

Helicobacter pylori eradication: 40 mg once daily for 10 days; requires combination therapy

Prevention of NSAID-induced gastric ulcers: 20-40 mg once daily for up to 6 months

I.V.: GERD: 20 mg or 40 mg once daily for ≤10 days; change to oral therapy as soon as appropriate

Elderly: No dosage adjustment needed

Dosage adjustment in renal impairment: No dosage adjustment needed
Dosage adjustment in hepatic impairment:

Mild-to-moderate hepatic impairment (Child-Pugh Class A or B): No dosage adjustment needed

Severe hepatic impairment (Child-Pugh Class C): Dose should not exceed 20 mg/day

Mechanism of Action Proton pump inhibitor suppresses gastric acid secretion by inhibition of the H^+/K^+-ATPase in the gastric parietal cell

Contraindications Hypersensitivity to esomeprazole, substituted benzimidazoles (ie, lansoprazole, omeprazole, pantoprazole, rabeprazole), or any component of the formulation

Warnings/Precautions Relief of symptoms does not preclude the presence of a gastric malignancy. Atrophic gastritis (by biopsy) has been noted with long-term omeprazole therapy; this may also occur with esomeprazole. No reports of enterochromaffin-like (ECL) cell carcinoids, dysplasia, or neoplasia has occurred. No reports of enterochromaffin-like (ECL) cell carcinoids, dysplasia, or neoplasia has occurred. Safety and efficacy in children <12 years of age have not been established.

Drug Interactions

Cytochrome P450 Effect: Substrate of CYP2C19 (major), 3A4 (minor); Inhibits CYP2C19 (moderate)

Increased Effect/Toxicity: Esomeprazole and omeprazole may increase the levels of carbamazepine, HMG CoA reductase inhibitors, and CYP2C19 substrates, including benzodiazepines metabolized by oxidation (eg, diazepam, midazolam, triazolam).

Decreased Effect: CYP2C19 inducers may decrease the levels/effects of esomeprazole; example inducers include aminoglutethimide, carbamazepine, phenytoin, and rifampin. Proton pump inhibitors may decrease the absorption of atazanavir, indinavir, iron salts, itraconazole, and ketoconazole.

Ethanol/Nutrition/Herb Interactions Food: Absorption is decreased by 43% to 53% when taken with food.

Dietary Considerations Take at least 1 hour before meals; best if taken before breakfast. The contents of the capsule may be mixed in applesauce or water; pellets also remain intact when exposed to orange juice, apple juice, and yogurt.

Pharmacodynamics/Kinetics

Distribution: V_{dss}: 16 L

Protein binding: 97%

Metabolism: Hepatic via CYP2C19 and 3A4 enzymes to hydroxy, desmethyl, and sulfone metabolites (all inactive)

Bioavailability: 90% with repeat dosing

Half-life elimination: 1-1.5 hours

Time to peak: 1.5 hours

Excretion: Urine (80%); feces (20%)

Pregnancy Risk Factor B

Dosage Forms CAP, delayed release: 20 mg, 40 mg **INJ, powder for reconstitution:** 20 mg, 40 mg

Esomeprazole Magnesium *see* Esomeprazole *on page 572*

Esoterica® Regular [OTC] *see* Hydroquinone *on page 798*

Especol® [OTC] *see* Fructose, Dextrose, and Phosphoric Acid *on page 713*

Estazolam (es TA zoe lam)

U.S. Brand Names ProSom®

Mexican Brand Names Tasedan®

Generic Available Yes

Pharmacologic Category Benzodiazepine

Use Short-term management of insomnia

Local Anesthetic/Vasoconstrictor Precautions No information available to require special precautions

Effects on Dental Treatment Key adverse event(s) related to dental treatment: Significant xerostomia (normal salivary flow resumes upon discontinuation).

Common Adverse Effects

>10%:

Central nervous system: Somnolence

Neuromuscular & skeletal: Weakness

1% to 10%:

Cardiovascular: Flushing, palpitation

Central nervous system: Anxiety, confusion, dizziness, hypokinesia, abnormal coordination, hangover effect, agitation, amnesia, apathy, emotional lability, euphoria, hostility, seizure, sleep disorder, stupor, twitch

Dermatologic: Dermatitis, pruritus, rash, urticaria

Gastrointestinal: Xerostomia, constipation, decreased appetite, flatulence, gastritis, increased appetite, perverse taste

Genitourinary: Frequent urination, menstrual cramps, urinary hesitancy, urinary frequency, vaginal discharge/itching

Neuromuscular & skeletal: Paresthesia

Ocular: Photophobia, eye pain, eye swelling

Respiratory: Cough, dyspnea, asthma, rhinitis, sinusitis

(Continued)

Estazolam (Continued)

Miscellaneous: Diaphoresis

Restrictions C-IV

Mechanism of Action Binds to stereospecific benzodiazepine receptors on the postsynaptic GABA neuron at several sites within the central nervous system, including the limbic system, reticular formation. Enhancement of the inhibitory effect of GABA on neuronal excitability results by increased neuronal membrane permeability to chloride ions. This shift in chloride ions results in hyperpolarization (a less excitable state) and stabilization.

Drug Interactions

Cytochrome P450 Effect: Substrate of CYP3A4 (minor)

Increased Effect/Toxicity: Sedative effects and/or respiratory depression may be additive with CNS depressants; includes ethanol, barbiturates, narcotic analgesics, and other sedative agents; monitor for increased effect. Levodopa therapeutic effects may be diminished in some patients following the addition of a benzodiazepine; limited/inconsistent data. Oral contraceptives may decrease the clearance of some benzodiazepines (those which undergo oxidative metabolism); monitor for increased benzodiazepine effect. Theophylline may partially antagonize some of the effects of benzodiazepines; monitor for decreased response; may require higher doses for sedation. Concurrent use with itraconazole or ketoconazole is contraindicated (per manufacturer); however, estazolam is a minor CYP3A4 substrate and an effect has not been documented in clinical studies.

Pharmacodynamics/Kinetics

Onset of action: ~1 hour

Duration: Variable

Metabolism: Extensively hepatic

Half-life elimination: 10-24 hours (no significant changes in elderly)

Time to peak, serum: 0.5-1.6 hours

Excretion: Urine (<5% as unchanged drug)

Pregnancy Risk Factor X

Ester-E™ [OTC] see Vitamin E on page 1581

Esterified Estrogen and Methyltestosterone see Estrogens (Esterified) and Methyltestosterone on page 585

Esterified Estrogens see Estrogens (Esterified) on page 584

Estrace® see Estradiol on page 574

Estraderm® see Estradiol on page 574

Estradiol (es tra DYE ole)

Related Information

Endocrine Disorders and Pregnancy on page 1659

Rheumatoid Arthritis, Osteoarthritis, and Osteoporosis on page 1668

U.S. Brand Names Alora®; Climara®; Delestrogen®; Depo®-Estradiol; Esclim®; Estrace®; Estraderm®; Estrasorb™; Estring®; EstroGel®; Femring™; Femtrace®; Gynodiol®; Menostar™; Vagifem®; Vivelle®; Vivelle-Dot®

Canadian Brand Names Climara®; Depo®-Estradiol; Estrace®; Estraderm®; Estradot®; Estring®; EstroGel®; Oesclim®; Sandoz-Estradiol Derm 50; Sandoz-Estradiol Derm 75; Sandoz-Estradiol Derm 100; Vagifem®

Mexican Brand Names Benzo-Ginestryl®; Climaderm®; Estraderm MTX®; Estraderm TTS®; Fem7®; Ginedisc®; Primogyn®; System®

Generic Available Yes: Oral tablet, patch

Synonyms Estradiol Acetate; Estradiol Cypionate; Estradiol Hemihydrate; Estradiol Transdermal; Estradiol Valerate

Pharmacologic Category Estrogen Derivative

Use Treatment of moderate-to-severe vasomotor symptoms associated with menopause; treatment of vulvar and vaginal atrophy; hypoestrogenism (due to hypogonadism, castration, or primary ovarian failure); prostatic cancer (palliation), breast cancer (palliation), osteoporosis (prophylaxis); abnormal uterine bleeding due to hormonal imbalance; postmenopausal urogenital symptoms of the lower urinary tract (urinary urgency, dysuria)

Local Anesthetic/Vasoconstrictor Precautions No information available to require special precautions

Effects on Dental Treatment No significant effects or complications reported

Common Adverse Effects Frequency not defined.

Cardiovascular: Edema, hypertension, MI, venous thromboembolism

Central nervous system: Anxiety, dizziness, epilepsy exacerbation, headache, irritability, mental depression, migraine, mood disturbances, nervousness

Dermatologic: Chloasma, erythema multiforme, erythema nodosum, hemorrhagic eruption, hirsutism, loss of scalp hair, melasma, rash, pruritus

Endocrine & metabolic: Breast enlargement, breast tenderness, libido (changes in), increased thyroid-binding globulin, increased total thyroid hormone (T_4), increased serum triglycerides/phospholipids, increased HDL-cholesterol, decreased LDL-cholesterol, impaired glucose tolerance, hypercalcemia

Gastrointestinal: Abdominal cramps, abdominal pain, bloating, cholecystitis, cholelithiasis, diarrhea, flatulence, gallbladder disease, nausea, pancreatitis, vomiting, weight gain/loss

Genitourinary: Alterations in frequency and flow of menses, changes in cervical secretions, endometrial cancer, increased size of uterine leiomyomata, Pap smear suspicious, vaginal candidiasis

Vaginal: Trauma from applicator insertion may occur in women with severely atrophic vaginal mucosa

Hematologic: Aggravation of porphyria, antithrombin III and antifactor Xa decreased, levels of fibrinogen increased, platelet aggregability increased and platelet count; increased prothrombin and factors VII, VIII, IX, X

Hepatic: Cholestatic jaundice

Local: Transdermal patches: Burning, erythema, irritation, thrombophlebitis

Neuromuscular & skeletal: Chorea, back pain

Ocular: Intolerance to contact lenses, steeping of corneal curvature

Respiratory: Pulmonary thromboembolism

Miscellaneous: Anaphylactoid/anaphylactic reactions, carbohydrate intolerance

Mechanism of Action Estrogens are responsible for the development and maintenance of the female reproductive system and secondary sexual characteristics. Estradiol is the principle intracellular human estrogen and is more potent than estrone and estriol at the receptor level; it is the primary estrogen secreted prior to menopause. Following menopause, estrone and estrone sulfate are more highly produced. Estrogens modulate the pituitary secretion of gonadotropins, luteinizing hormone, and follicle-stimulating hormone through a negative feedback system; estrogen replacement reduces elevated levels of these hormones in postmenopausal women.

Drug Interactions

Cytochrome P450 Effect: Substrate of CYP1A2 (major), 2A6 (minor), 2B6 (minor), 2C9 (minor), 2C19 (minor), 2D6 (minor), 2E1 (minor), 3A4 (major); **Inhibits** CYP1A2 (weak), 2C8 (weak); **Induces** CYP3A4 (weak)

Increased Effect/Toxicity: Estradiol with hydrocortisone increases corticosteroid toxic potential. Anticoagulants and estradiol increase the potential for thromboembolic events.

Decreased Effect: CYP1A2 inducers may decrease the levels/effects of estradiol; example inducers include aminoglutethimide, carbamazepine, phenobarbital, and rifampin. CYP3A4 inducers may decrease the levels/effects of estradiol; example inducers include aminoglutethimide, carbamazepine, nafcillin, nevirapine, phenobarbital, phenytoin, and rifamycins.

Pharmacodynamics/Kinetics

Absorption: Oral, topical: Well absorbed

Distribution: Crosses placenta; enters breast milk

Protein binding: 37% to sex hormone-binding globulin; 61% to albumin

Metabolism: Hepatic via oxidation and conjugation in GI tract; hydroxylated via CYP3A4 to metabolites; first-pass effect; enterohepatic recirculation; reversibly converted to estrone and estriol

Excretion: Primarily urine (as metabolites estrone and estriol); feces (small amounts)

Pregnancy Risk Factor X

Estradiol Acetate *see* Estradiol *on page 574*

Estradiol and Drospirenone *see* Drospirenone and Estradiol *on page 520*

Estradiol and NGM *see* Estradiol and Norgestimate *on page 576*

Estradiol and Norethindrone (es tra DYE ole & nor eth IN drone)

Related Information
Estradiol *on page 574*
Norethindrone *on page 1125*

U.S. Brand Names Activella®; CombiPatch®

Canadian Brand Names Estalis®; Estalis-Sequi®

Generic Available No

Synonyms Norethindrone and Estradiol

Pharmacologic Category Estrogen and Progestin Combination

Use Women with an intact uterus:

Tablet: Treatment of moderate-to-severe vasomotor symptoms associated with menopause; treatment of vulvar and vaginal atrophy; prophylaxis for postmenopausal osteoporosis

(Continued)

Estradiol and Norethindrone *(Continued)*

Transdermal patch: Treatment of moderate-to-severe vasomotor symptoms associated with menopause; treatment of vulvar and vaginal atrophy; treatment of hypoestrogenism due to hypogonadism, castration, or primary ovarian failure

Local Anesthetic/Vasoconstrictor Precautions No information available to require special precautions

Effects on Dental Treatment No significant effects or complications reported

Common Adverse Effects Frequency not defined.

Cardiovascular: Altered blood pressure, cardiovascular accident, edema, venous thromboembolism

Central nervous system: Dizziness, fatigue, headache, insomnia, mental depression, migraine, nervousness

Dermatologic: Chloasma, erythema multiforme, erythema nodosum, hemorrhagic eruption, hirsutism, itching, loss of scalp hair, melasma, pruritus, skin rash

Endocrine & metabolic: Breast enlargement, breast tenderness, breast pain, libido (changes in)

Gastrointestinal: Abdominal pain, bloating, changes in appetite, flatulence, gallbladder disease, nausea, pancreatitis, vomiting, weight gain/loss

Genitourinary: Alterations in frequency and flow of menses, changes in cervical secretions, cystitis-like syndrome, increased size of uterine leiomyomata, premenstrual-like syndrome, vaginal candidiasis, vaginitis

Hematologic: Aggravation of porphyria

Hepatic: Cholestatic jaundice

Local: Application site reaction (transdermal patch)

Neuromuscular & skeletal: Arthralgia, back pain, chorea, myalgia, weakness

Ocular: Intolerance to contact lenses, steeping of corneal curvature

Respiratory: Pharyngitis, pulmonary thromboembolism, rhinitis

Miscellaneous: Allergic reactions, carbohydrate intolerance, flu-like syndrome

Drug Interactions

Cytochrome P450 Effect:

Estradiol: **Substrate** of CYP1A2 (major), 2A6 (minor), 2B6 (minor), 2C9 (minor), 2C19 (minor), 2D6 (minor), 2E1 (minor), 3A4 (major); **Inhibits** CYP1A2 (weak), 2C8 (weak); **Induces** CYP3A4 (weak)

Norethindrone: **Substrate** of CYP3A4 (major); **Induces** CYP2C19 (weak)

Pharmacodynamics/Kinetics

Activella®:

Bioavailability: Estradiol: 50%; Norethindrone: 100%

Half-life elimination: Estradiol: 12-14 hours; Norethindrone: 8-11 hours

Time to peak: Estradiol: 5-8 hours

See individual agents.

Pregnancy Risk Factor X

Estradiol and Norgestimate *(es tra DYE ole & nor JES ti mate)*

Related Information

Estradiol *on page 574*

U.S. Brand Names Prefest™

Generic Available No

Synonyms Estradiol and NGM; Norgestimate and Estradiol; Ortho Prefest

Pharmacologic Category Estrogen and Progestin Combination

Use Women with an intact uterus: Treatment of moderate to severe vasomotor symptoms associated with menopause; treatment of atrophic vaginitis; prevention of osteoporosis

Local Anesthetic/Vasoconstrictor Precautions No information available to require special precautions

Effects on Dental Treatment No significant effects or complications reported

Common Adverse Effects

>10%:

Central nervous system: Headache (23%)

Endocrine & metabolic: Breast pain (16%)

Gastrointestinal: Abdominal pain (12%)

Neuromuscular & skeletal: Back pain (12%)

Respiratory: Upper respiratory tract infection (21%)

Miscellaneous: Flu-like symptoms (11%)

1% to 10%:

Central nervous system: Fatigue (6%), pain (6%), depression (5%), dizziness (5%)

Endocrine & metabolic: Vaginal bleeding (9%), dysmenorrhea (8%), vaginitis (7%)

Gastrointestinal: Nausea (6%), flatulence (5%)
Neuromuscular & skeletal: Arthralgia (9%), myalgia (5%)
Respiratory: Sinusitis (8%), pharyngitis (7%), cough (5%)
Miscellaneous: Viral infection (6%)

Additional adverse effects associated with **estrogens and progestins**; frequency not defined:

Cardiovascular: Edema, hypertension, MI, stroke, venous thrombosis
Central nervous system: Anxiety, epilepsy exacerbation, insomnia, irritability, migraine, mood disturbances, nervousness, pyrexia, somnolence
Dermatologic: Acne, chloasma, erythema multiforme, erythema nodosum, hemorrhagic eruptions, hirsutism, itching, melasma, pruritus, rash, scalp hair loss, urticaria
Endocrine & metabolic: Amenorrhea, breast cancer, breast discharge, breast enlargement, Breast tenderness, carbohydrate tolerance decreased, endometrial cancer, endometrial hyperplasia, fibrocystic breast changes, galactorrhea, hypocalcemia, libido changes, ovarian cancer, triglycerides increased
Gastrointestinal: Abdominal cramps, appetite changes, bloating, gallbladder disease, pancreatitis, vomiting, weight gain/loss
Genitourinary: Abnormal withdrawal bleeding/flow, breakthrough bleeding, cervical secretion changes, cystitis syndrome, uterine leiomyomata size increased, vaginal candidiasis, vaginal bleeding/spotting
Hematologic: Anemia, porphyria
Hepatic: Cholestatic jaundice
Local: Thrombophlebitis
Neuromuscular & skeletal: Chorea
Ocular: Contact lens intolerance, corneal curvature steepening, neuro-ocular lesions
Respiratory: Asthma exacerbation, pulmonary embolism
Miscellaneous: Anaphylaxis

Mechanism of Action Estrogens are responsible for the development and maintenance of the female reproductive system and secondary sexual characteristics. Estradiol is the principle intracellular human estrogen and is more potent than estrone and estriol at the receptor level; it is the primary estrogen secreted prior to menopause. Following menopause, estrone and estrone sulfate are more highly produced. Estrogens modulate the pituitary secretion of gonadotropins, luteinizing hormone, and follicle-stimulating hormone through a negative feedback system; estrogen replacement reduces elevated levels of these hormones in postmenopausal women.

Progestins inhibit gonadotropin production which then prevents follicular maturation and ovulation. In women with adequate estrogen, progestins transform a proliferative endometrium into a secretory endometrium; when administered with estradiol, reduces the incidence of endometrial hyperplasia and risk of adenocarcinoma.

Drug Interactions
Cytochrome P450 Effect:
Estradiol: **Substrate** of CYP1A2 (major), 2A6 (minor), 2B6 (minor), 2C9 (minor), 2C19 (minor), 2D6 (minor), 2E1 (minor), 3A4 (major); **Inhibits** CYP1A2 (weak), 2C8 (weak); **Induces** CYP3A4 (weak)
Increased Effect/Toxicity: Acetaminophen and ascorbic acid may increase plasma levels of estrogen component. Atorvastatin and indinavir increase plasma levels of estrogen/progestin combinations. Estrogen/progestin combinations increase the plasma levels of alprazolam, chlordiazepoxide, cyclosporine, diazepam, prednisolone, selegiline, theophylline, tricyclic antidepressants. Estrogen/progestin combinations may increase (or decrease) the effects of coumarin derivatives.
Decreased Effect: Estrogen/progestin combinations may decrease plasma levels of acetaminophen, clofibric acid, lorazepam, morphine, oxazepam, salicylic acid, temazepam. Estrogen/progestin levels decreased by aminoglutethimide, amprenavir, anticonvulsants, griseofulvin, lopinavir, nelfinavir, nevirapine, rifampin, and ritonavir. Estrogen/progestin combinations may decrease (or increase) the effects of coumarin derivatives.

Pharmacodynamics/Kinetics
Estradiol: See Estradiol monograph.
Norgestimate:
Protein binding: 17-deacetylnorgestimate: 99%
Metabolism: Forms 17-deacetylnorgestimate (major active metabolite) and other metabolites; first-pass effect
Half-life elimination: 17-deacetylnorgestimate: 37 hours
Excretion: Norgestimate metabolites: Urine and feces
Pregnancy Risk Factor X

Estradiol Cypionate see Estradiol on page 574

Estradiol Hemihydrate see Estradiol on page 574

Estradiol Transdermal see Estradiol on page 574

Estradiol Valerate see Estradiol on page 574

Estramustine (es tra MUS teen)

U.S. Brand Names Emcyt®
Canadian Brand Names Emcyt®
Generic Available No
Synonyms Estramustine Phosphate Sodium; NSC-89199
Pharmacologic Category Antineoplastic Agent, Alkylating Agent; Antineoplastic Agent, Hormone; Antineoplastic Agent, Hormone (Estrogen/Nitrogen Mustard)
Use Palliative treatment of prostatic carcinoma (progressive or metastatic)
Local Anesthetic/Vasoconstrictor Precautions No information available to require special precautions
Effects on Dental Treatment No significant effects or complications reported
Common Adverse Effects
>10%:
Cardiovascular: Impaired arterial circulation; ischemic heart disease; venous thromboembolism; cardiac decompensation (58%), about 50% of complications occur within the first 2 months of therapy, 85% occur within the first year; edema
Endocrine & metabolic: Sodium and water retention, gynecomastia, breast tenderness, libido decreased
Gastrointestinal: Nausea, vomiting, may be dose-limiting
Hematologic: Thrombocytopenia
Local: Thrombophlebitis (nearly 100% with I.V. administration)
Respiratory: Dyspnea
1% to 10%:
Cardiovascular: Myocardial infarction
Central nervous system: Insomnia, lethargy
Gastrointestinal: Diarrhea, anorexia, flatulence
Hematologic: Leukopenia
Hepatic: Serum transaminases increased, jaundice
Neuromuscular & skeletal: Leg cramps
Respiratory: Pulmonary embolism
Mechanism of Action Mechanism is not completely clear. It appears to bind to microtubule proteins, preventing normal tubulin function. The antitumor effect may be due solely to an estrogenic effect. Estramustine causes a marked decrease in plasma testosterone and an increase in estrogen levels.
Drug Interactions
Decreased Effect: Milk products and calcium-rich foods/drugs may impair the oral absorption of estramustine phosphate sodium.
Pharmacodynamics/Kinetics
Absorption: Oral: 75%
Metabolism:
GI tract: Initial dephosphorylation
Hepatic: Oxidation and hydrolysis; metabolites include estramustine, estrone, estradiol, nitrogen mustard
Half-life elimination: Terminal: 20-24 hours
Time to peak, serum: 2-3 hours
Excretion: Feces (2.9% to 4.8% as unchanged drug)
Pregnancy Risk Factor C

Estramustine Phosphate Sodium see Estramustine on page 578

Estrasorb™ see Estradiol on page 574

Estratest® see Estrogens (Esterified) and Methyltestosterone on page 585

Estratest® H.S. see Estrogens (Esterified) and Methyltestosterone on page 585

Estring® see Estradiol on page 574

EstroGel® see Estradiol on page 574

Estrogenic Substances, Conjugated see Estrogens (Conjugated/Equine) on page 580

Estrogens (Conjugated A/Synthetic)
(ES troe jenz, KON joo gate ed, aye, sin THET ik)

Related Information
Endocrine Disorders and Pregnancy on page 1659

U.S. Brand Names Cenestin®

Generic Available No

Pharmacologic Category Estrogen Derivative

Use Treatment of moderate-to-severe vasomotor symptoms of menopause; treatment of vulvar and vaginal atrophy

Local Anesthetic/Vasoconstrictor Precautions No information available to require special precautions

Effects on Dental Treatment No significant effects or complications reported

Common Adverse Effects

>10%:

Central nervous system: Headache (11% to 68%), dizziness (11%), pain (11%)

Endocrine & metabolic: Breast pain (29%), endometrial thickening (19%), metrorrhagia (14%)

Gastrointestinal: Abdominal pain (9% to 28%), nausea (9% to 18%)

Neuromuscular & skeletal: Paresthesia (8% to 33%), back pain (14%)

Respiratory: Upper respiratory tract infection (13%)

Miscellaneous: Infection (2% to 14%)

1% to 10%:

Central nervous system: Anxiety (6%), fever (1%)

Gastrointestinal: Dyspepsia (10%), vomiting (7%), constipation (6%), diarrhea (6%), weight gain (6%)

Genitourinary: Vaginitis (8%)

Neuromuscular & skeletal: Leg cramps (10%), hypertonia (6%)

Respiratory: Rhinitis (6% to 8%), cough (6%)

In addition, the following have been reported with estrogen and/or progestin therapy:

Cardiovascular: Edema, hypertension, MI, stroke, venous thromboembolism

Central nervous system: Epilepsy exacerbation, irritability, mental depression, migraine, mood disturbances, nervousness

Dermatologic: Angioedema, chloasma, erythema multiforme, erythema nodosum, hemorrhagic eruption, hirsutism, loss of scalp hair, melasma, pruritus, rash, urticaria

Endocrine & metabolic: Breast cancer, breast enlargement, breast tenderness, HDL-cholesterol increased, hyper-/hypocalcemia, impaired glucose tolerance, LDL-cholesterol decreased, libido (changes in), serum triglycerides/phospholipids increased, thyroid-binding globulin increased, total thyroid hormone (T_4) increased

Gastrointestinal: Abdominal cramps, bloating, cholecystitis, cholelithiasis, gallbladder disease, pancreatitis, weight gain/loss

Genitourinary: Alterations in frequency and flow of menses, changes in cervical secretions, endometrial cancer, endometrial hyperplasia, increased size of uterine leiomyomata, vaginal candidiasis

Hematologic: Aggravation of porphyria, antithrombin III and antifactor Xa decreased, fibrinogen levels increased, platelet aggregability and platelet count increased; prothrombin and factors VII, VIII, IX, X increased

Hepatic: Cholestatic jaundice, hepatic hemangiomas enlarged

Neuromuscular & skeletal: Arthralgias, chorea, leg cramps

Local: Thrombophlebitis

Ocular: Intolerance to contact lenses, retinal vascular thrombosis, steeping of corneal curvature

Respiratory: Asthma exacerbation, pulmonary thromboembolism

Miscellaneous: Anaphylactoid/anaphylactic reactions, carbohydrate intolerance

Mechanism of Action Conjugated A/synthetic estrogens contain a mixture of 9 synthetic estrogen substances, including sodium estrone sulfate, sodium equilin sulfate, sodium 17 alpha-dihydroequilin, sodium 17 alpha-estradiol and sodium 17 beta-dihydroequilin. Estrogens are responsible for the development and maintenance of the female reproductive system and secondary sexual characteristics. Estradiol is the principle intracellular human estrogen and is more potent than estrone and estriol at the receptor level; it is the primary estrogen secreted prior to menopause. Following menopause, estrone and estrone sulfate are more highly produced. Estrogens modulate the pituitary secretion of gonadotropins, luteinizing hormone, and follicle-stimulating hormone through a negative feedback system; estrogen replacement reduces elevated levels of these hormones in postmenopausal women.

Drug Interactions

Cytochrome P450 Effect: Based on estradiol and estrone: **Substrate** of CYP1A2 (major), 2A6 (minor), 2B6 (minor), 2C9 (minor), 2C19 (minor), 2D6 (minor), 2E1 (minor), 3A4 (major); **Inhibits** CYP1A2 (weak); **Induces** CYP3A4 (weak)

(Continued)

Estrogens (Conjugated A/Synthetic) *(Continued)*

Increased Effect/Toxicity: Anticoagulants increase the potential for thromboembolic events. Estrogens may enhance the effects of hydrocortisone and prednisone. Estrogen derivatives may enhance the hepatotoxic effect of cyclosporine. Estrogen derivatives may increase the serum concentration of cyclosporine.

Decreased Effect: CYP1A2 inducers may decrease the levels/effects of estrogens; example inducers include aminoglutethimide, carbamazepine, phenobarbital, and rifampin. CYP3A4 inducers may decrease the levels/effects of estrogen; example inducers include aminoglutethimide, carbamazepine, nafcillin, nevirapine, phenobarbital, phenytoin, and rifamycins. Estrogen derivatives may diminish the therapeutic effect of thyroid products.

Pharmacodynamics/Kinetics

Absorption: Well absorbed over a period of several hours

Protein-binding: Sex hormone-binding globulin (SHBG) and albumin

Metabolism: Hepatic via CYP3A4; estradiol is converted to estrone and estriol; also undergoes enterohepatic recirculation; estrone sulfate is the main metabolite in postmenopausal women

Excretion: Urine (primarily estriol, also as estradiol, estrone, and conjugates)

Estrogens (Conjugated/Equine)
(ES troe jenz KON joo gate ed, EE kwine)

Related Information

Endocrine Disorders and Pregnancy *on page 1659*

U.S. Brand Names Premarin®

Canadian Brand Names Cenestin; C.E.S.®; Premarin®

Generic Available No

Synonyms CEE; C.E.S.; Estrogenic Substances, Conjugated

Pharmacologic Category Estrogen Derivative

Use Treatment of moderate to severe vasomotor symptoms associated with menopause; treatment of vulvar and vaginal atrophy; hypoestrogenism (due to hypogonadism, castration, or primary ovarian failure); prostatic cancer (palliation); breast cancer (palliation); osteoporosis (prophylaxis, postmenopausal women at significant risk only); abnormal uterine bleeding

Unlabeled/Investigational Use Uremic bleeding

Local Anesthetic/Vasoconstrictor Precautions No information available to require special precautions

Effects on Dental Treatment No significant effects or complications reported

Common Adverse Effects

Note: Percentages reported in postmenopausal women.

>10%:

Central nervous system: Headache (26% to 32%; placebo 28%)

Endocrine & metabolic: Breast pain (7% to 12%; placebo 9%)

Gastrointestinal: Abdominal pain (15% to 17%)

Genitourinary: Vaginal hemorrhage (2% to 14%)

Neuromuscular & skeletal: Back pain (13% to 14%)

1% to 10%:

Central nervous system: Nervousness (2% to 5%)

Endocrine & metabolic: Leukorrhea (4% to 7%)

Gastrointestinal: Flatulence (6% to 7%)

Genitourinary: Vaginitis (5% to 7%), vaginal moniliasis (5% to 6%)

Neuromuscular & skeletal: Weakness (7% to 8%), leg cramps (3% to 7%)

In addition, the following have been reported with estrogen and/or progestin therapy:

Cardiovascular: Edema, hypertension, MI, stroke, venous thromboembolism

Central nervous system: Dizziness, epilepsy exacerbation, headache, irritability, mental depression, migraine, mood disturbances, nervousness

Dermatologic: Angioedema, chloasma, erythema multiforme, erythema nodosum, hemorrhagic eruption, hirsutism, loss of scalp hair, melasma, pruritus, rash, urticaria

Endocrine & metabolic: Breast cancer, breast enlargement, breast tenderness, libido (changes in), increased thyroid-binding globulin, increased total thyroid hormone (T_4), increased serum triglycerides/phospholipids, increased HDL-cholesterol, decreased LDL-cholesterol, impaired glucose tolerance, hypercalcemia, hypocalcemia

Gastrointestinal: Abdominal cramps, bloating, cholecystitis, cholelithiasis, gallbladder disease, nausea, pancreatitis, vomiting, weight gain/loss

Genitourinary: Alterations in frequency and flow of menses, changes in cervical secretions, endometrial cancer, endometrial hyperplasia, increased size of uterine leiomyomata, vaginal candidiasis

Hematologic: Aggravation of porphyria, decreased antithrombin III and antifactor Xa, increased levels of fibrinogen, increased platelet aggregability and platelet count; increased prothrombin and factors VII, VIII, IX, X

Hepatic: Cholestatic jaundice, hepatic hemangiomas enlarged

Neuromuscular & skeletal: Arthralgias, chorea, leg cramps

Local: Thrombophlebitis

Ocular: Intolerance to contact lenses, retinal vascular thrombosis, steeping of corneal curvature

Respiratory: Asthma exacerbation, pulmonary thromboembolism

Miscellaneous: Anaphylactoid/anaphylactic reactions, carbohydrate intolerance

Dosage Adults:

Male: Androgen-dependent prostate cancer palliation: Oral: 1.25-2.5 mg 3 times/day

Female:

Prevention of postmenopausal osteoporosis: Oral: Initial: 0.3 mg/day cyclically* or daily, depending on medical assessment of patient. Dose may be adjusted based on bone mineral density and clinical response. The lowest effective dose should be used.

Moderate to severe vasomotor symptoms associated with menopause: Oral: Initial: 0.3 mg/day, cyclically* or daily, depending on medical assessment of patient. The lowest dose that will control symptoms should be used. Medication should be discontinued as soon as possible.

Vulvar and vaginal atrophy:

Oral: Initial: 0.3 mg/day; the lowest dose that will control symptoms should be used. May be given cyclically* or daily, depending on medical assessment of patient. Medication should be discontinued as soon as possible.

Vaginal cream: Intravaginal: ½ to 2 g/day given cyclically*

Abnormal uterine bleeding:

Acute/heavy bleeding:

Oral (unlabeled route): 1.25 mg, may repeat every 4 hours for 24 hours, followed by 1.25 mg once daily for 7-10 days

I.M., I.V.: 25 mg, may repeat in 6-12 hours if needed

Note: Treatment should be followed by a low-dose oral contraceptive; medroxyprogesterone acetate along with or following estrogen therapy can also be given

Nonacute/lesser bleeding: Oral (unlabeled route): 1.25 mg once daily for 7-10 days

Female hypogonadism: Oral: 0.3-0.625 mg/day given cyclically*; dose may be titrated in 6- to 12-month intervals; progestin treatment should be added to maintain bone mineral density once skeletal maturity is achieved.

Female castration, primary ovarian failure: Oral: 1.25 mg/day given cyclically*; adjust according to severity of symptoms and patient response. For maintenance, adjust to the lowest effective dose.

*Cyclic administration: Either 3 weeks on, 1 week off **or** 25 days on, 5 days off

Male and Female:

Breast cancer palliation, metastatic disease in selected patients: Oral: 10 mg 3 times/day for at least 3 months

Uremic bleeding (unlabeled use): I.V.: 0.6 mg/kg/day for 5 days

Elderly: Refer to Adults dosing; a higher incidence of stroke and invasive breast cancer was observed in women >75 years in a WHI substudy.

Mechanism of Action Conjugated estrogens contain a mixture of estrone sulfate, equilin sulfate, 17 alpha-dihydroequilin, 17 alpha-estradiol and 17 beta-dihydroequilin. Estrogens are responsible for the development and maintenance of the female reproductive system and secondary sexual characteristics. Estradiol is the principle intracellular human estrogen and is more potent than estrone and estriol at the receptor level; it is the primary estrogen secreted prior to menopause. Following menopause, estrone and estrone sulfate are more highly produced. Estrogens modulate the pituitary secretion of gonadotropins, luteinizing hormone, and follicle-stimulating hormone through a negative feedback system; estrogen replacement reduces elevated levels of these hormones in postmenopausal women.

Contraindications Hypersensitivity to estrogens or any component of the formulation; undiagnosed abnormal vaginal bleeding; history of or current thrombophlebitis or venous thromboembolic disorders (including DVT, PE); active or recent (within 1 year) arterial thromboembolic disease (eg, stroke, MI); carcinoma of the breast (except in appropriately selected patients being treated (Continued)

Estrogens (Conjugated/Equine) *(Continued)*

for metastatic disease); estrogen-dependent tumor; hepatic dysfunction or disease; pregnancy

Warnings/Precautions

Cardiovascular-related considerations: Estrogens with or without progestin should not be used to prevent coronary heart disease. Use caution with cardiovascular disease or dysfunction. May increase the risks of hypertension, myocardial infarction (MI), stroke, pulmonary emboli (PE), and deep vein thrombosis; incidence of these effects was shown to be significantly increased in postmenopausal women using conjugated equine estrogens (CEE) in combination with medroxyprogesterone acetate (MPA). Nonfatal MI, PE, and thrombophlebitis have also been reported in males taking high doses of CEE (eg, for prostate cancer). Estrogen compounds are generally associated with lipid effects such as increased HDL-cholesterol and decreased LDL-cholesterol. Triglycerides may also be increased; use with caution in patients with familial defects of lipoprotein metabolism. Whenever possible, estrogens should be discontinued at least 4 weeks prior to and for 2 weeks following elective surgery associated with an increased risk of thromboembolism or during periods of prolonged immobilization.

Neurological considerations: The risk of dementia may be increased in postmenopausal women; increased incidence was observed in women ≥65 years of age taking CEE alone or in combination with MPA.

Cancer-related considerations: Unopposed estrogens may increase the risk of endometrial carcinoma in postmenopausal women. Estrogens may exacerbate endometriosis. Malignant transformation of residual endometrial implants has been reported post-hysterectomy with estrogen only therapy. Consider adding a progestin in women with residual endometriosis post-hysterectomy. Estrogens may increase the risk of breast cancer. An increased risk of invasive breast cancer was observed in postmenopausal women using CEE in combination with MPA; a smaller increase in risk was seen with estrogen therapy alone in observational studies. An increase in abnormal mammograms has also been reported with estrogen and progestin therapy. Estrogen use may lead to severe hypercalcemia in patients with breast cancer and bone metastases; discontinue estrogen if hypercalcemia occurs.

Estrogens may cause retinal vascular thrombosis; discontinue permanently if papilledema or retinal vascular lesions are observed on examination. Use with caution in patients with diseases which may be exacerbated by fluid retention, including asthma, epilepsy, migraine, diabetes or renal dysfunction. Use with caution in patients with a history of severe hypocalcemia, SLE, hepatic hemangiomas, porphyria, endometriosis, and gallbladder disease. Use caution with history of cholestatic jaundice associated with past estrogen use or pregnancy. Safety and efficacy in pediatric patients have not been established. Prior to puberty, estrogens may cause premature closure of the epiphyses, premature breast development in girls or gynecomastia in boys. Vaginal bleeding and vaginal cornification may also be induced in girls.

Before prescribing estrogen therapy to postmenopausal women, the risks and benefits must be weighed for each patient. Women should be informed of these risks and benefits, as well as possible effects of progestin when added to estrogen therapy. Estrogens with or without progestin should be used for shortest duration possible consistent with treatment goals. Conduct periodic risk:benefit assessments.

When used solely for prevention of osteoporosis in women at significant risk, nonestrogen treatment options should be considered. When used solely for the treatment of vulvar and vaginal atrophy, topical vaginal products should be considered. Use caution applying topical products to severely atrophic vaginal mucosa.

Drug Interactions

Cytochrome P450 Effect:

Based on estradiol and estrone: **Substrate** of CYP1A2 (major), 2A6 (minor), 2B6 (minor), 2C9 (minor), 2C19 (minor), 2D6 (minor), 2E1 (minor), 3A4 (major); Inhibits CYP1A2 (weak), 2C8 (weak); Induces CYP3A4 (weak)

Increased Effect/Toxicity: Hydrocortisone taken with estrogen may cause corticosteroid-induced toxicity. Increased potential for thromboembolic events with anticoagulants.

Decreased Effect: CYP1A2 inducers may decrease the levels/effects of estrogens; example inducers include aminoglutethimide, carbamazepine, phenobarbital, and rifampin. CYP3A4 inducers may decrease the levels/effects of estrogens; example inducers include aminoglutethimide, carbamazepine, nafcillin, nevirapine, phenobarbital, phenytoin, and rifamycins.

Ethanol/Nutrition/Herb Interactions

Ethanol: Avoid ethanol (routine use increases estrogen level and risk of breast cancer). Ethanol may also increase the risk of osteoporosis.

Food: Folic acid absorption may be decreased.

Herb/Nutraceutical: St John's wort may decrease levels. Avoid black cohosh, dong quai (has estrogenic activity). Avoid red clover, saw palmetto, ginseng (due to potential hormonal effects).

Dietary Considerations Ensure adequate calcium and vitamin D intake when used for the prevention of osteoporosis. Powder for reconstitution for injection (25 mg) contains lactose 200 mg.

Pharmacodynamics/Kinetics

Absorption: Well absorbed

Metabolism: Hepatic via CYP3A4; estradiol is converted to estrone and estriol; also undergoes enterohepatic recirculation; estrone sulfite is the main metabolite in postmenopausal women

Excretion: Urine (primarily estriol, also as estradiol, estrone, and conjugates

Pregnancy Risk Factor X

Dosage Forms CRM, vaginal: 0.625 mg/g (42.5 g). **INJ, powder for reconstitution:** 25 mg. **TAB:** 0.3 mg, 0.45 mg, 0.625 mg, 0.9 mg, 1.25 mg

---

Estrogens (Conjugated/Equine) and Medroxyprogesterone

(ES troe jenz KON joo gate ed/EE kwine & me DROKS ee proe JES te rone)

Related Information

Endocrine Disorders and Pregnancy on page 1659
Estrogens (Conjugated/Equine) on page 580
MedroxyPROGESTERone on page 972

U.S. Brand Names Premphase®; Prempro™

Canadian Brand Names Premphase®; Premplus®; Prempro™

Generic Available No

Synonyms Medroxyprogesterone and Estrogens (Conjugated); MPA and Estrogens (Conjugated)

Pharmacologic Category Estrogen and Progestin Combination

Use Women with an intact uterus: Treatment of moderate to severe vasomotor symptoms associated with menopause; treatment of atrophic vaginitis; osteoporosis (prophylaxis)

Local Anesthetic/Vasoconstrictor Precautions No information available to require special precautions

Effects on Dental Treatment No significant effects or complications reported

Common Adverse Effects

>10%:
  Central nervous system: Headache (28% to 37%), pain (11% to 13%), depression (6% to 11%)
  Endocrine & metabolic: Breast pain (32% to 38%), dysmenorrhea (8% to 13%)
  Gastrointestinal: Abdominal pain (16% to 23%), nausea (9% to 11%)
  Neuromuscular & skeletal: Back pain (13% to 16%)
  Respiratory: Pharyngitis (11% to 13%)
  Miscellaneous: Infection (16% to 18%), flu-like syndrome (10% to 13%)

1% to 10%:
  Cardiovascular: Peripheral edema (3% to 4%)
  Central nervous system: Dizziness (3% to 5%)
  Dermatologic: Pruritus (5% to 10%), rash (4% to 6%)
  Endocrine & metabolic: Leukorrhea (5% to 9%)
  Gastrointestinal: Flatulence (8% to 9%), diarrhea (5% to 6%), dyspepsia (5% to 6%)
  Genitourinary: Vaginitis (5% to 7%), cervical changes (4% to 5%), vaginal hemorrhage (1% to 3%)
  Neuromuscular & skeletal: Weakness (6% to 10%), arthralgia (7% to 9%), leg cramps (3% to 5%), hypertonia (3% to 4%)
  Respiratory: Sinusitis (7% to 8%), rhinitis (6% to 8%)

Additional adverse effects reported with conjugated estrogens and/or progestins: Abdominal cramps, acne, abnormal uterine bleeding, aggravation of porphyria, amenorrhea, anaphylactoid reactions, anaphylaxis, antifactor Xa decreased, antithrombin III decreased, appetite changes, bloating, breast enlargement, breast tenderness, cerebral embolism, cerebral thrombosis, chloasma, cholestatic jaundice, cholecystitis, cholelithiasis, chorea, contact lens intolerance, cystitis-like syndrome, decreased carbohydrate tolerance, dizziness; factors VII, VIII, IX, X, XII, VII-X complex, and II-VII-X complex increased; endometrial hyperplasia, erythema multiforme, erythema

(Continued)

Estrogens (Conjugated/Equine) and Medroxyprogesterone *(Continued)*

nodosum, galactorrhea, hemorrhagic eruption, fatigue, fibrinogen increased, impaired glucose tolerance, HDL-cholesterol increased, hirsutism, hypertension, increase in size of uterine leiomyomata, gallbladder disease, insomnia, LDL-cholesterol decreased, libido changes, loss of scalp hair, melasma, migraine, nervousness, optic neuritis, pancreatitis, platelet aggregability and platelet count increased, premenstrual like syndrome, PT and PTT accelerated, pulmonary embolism, pyrexia, retinal thrombosis, somnolence, steepening of corneal curvature, thrombophlebitis, thyroid-binding globulin increased, total thyroid hormone (T_4) increased, triglycerides increased, urticaria, vaginal candidiasis, vomiting, weight gain/loss

Mechanism of Action

Conjugated estrogens contain a mixture of estrone sulfate, equilin sulfate, 17 alpha-dihydroequilin, 17 alpha-estradiol, and 17 beta-dihydroequilin. Estrogens are responsible for the development and maintenance of the female reproductive system and secondary sexual characteristics. Estradiol is the principle intracellular human estrogen and is more potent than estrone and estriol at the receptor level; it is the primary estrogen secreted prior to menopause. Following menopause, estrone and estrone sulfate are more highly produced. Estrogens modulate the pituitary secretion of gonadotropins, luteinizing hormone, and follicle-stimulating hormone through a negative feedback system; estrogen replacement reduces elevated levels of these hormones in postmenopausal women.

MPA inhibits gonadotropin production which then prevents follicular maturation and ovulation. In women with adequate estrogen, MPA transforms a proliferative endometrium into a secretory endometrium; when administered with conjugated estrogens, reduces the incidence of endometrial hyperplasia and risk of adenocarcinoma.

Drug Interactions

Cytochrome P450 Effect:

Based on estradiol and estrone: **Substrate** of CYP1A2 (major), 2A6 (minor), 2B6 (minor), 2C9 (minor), 2C19 (minor), 2D6 (minor), 2E1 (minor), 3A4 (major); **Inhibits** CYP1A2 (weak), 2C8 (weak); **Induces** CYP3A4 (weak)

Medroxyprogesterone: **Substrate** of CYP3A4 (major); **Induces** CYP3A4 (weak)

Increased Effect/Toxicity: Hydrocortisone taken with estrogen may cause corticosteroid-induced toxicity. Increased potential for thromboembolic events with anticoagulants.

Decreased Effect:

Conjugated estrogens:

Anticonvulsants which are enzyme inducers (barbiturates, carbamazepine, phenobarbital, phenytoin, primidone) may potentially decrease estrogen levels.

Rifampin, nelfinavir, and ritonavir decrease estradiol serum concentrations

MPA: Aminoglutethimide: May decrease effects by increasing hepatic metabolism

Pharmacodynamics/Kinetics See individual agents.

Pregnancy Risk Factor X

Estrogens (Esterified) (ES troe jenz, es TER i fied)

Related Information

Endocrine Disorders and Pregnancy *on page 1659*

U.S. Brand Names Menest®

Canadian Brand Names Estratab®; Menest®

Generic Available No

Synonyms Esterified Estrogens

Pharmacologic Category Estrogen Derivative

Use Treatment of moderate to severe vasomotor symptoms associated with menopause; treatment of vulvar and vaginal atrophy; hypoestrogenism (due to hypogonadism, castration, or primary ovarian failure); prostatic cancer (palliation); breast cancer (palliation); osteoporosis (prophylaxis, in women at significant risk only)

Local Anesthetic/Vasoconstrictor Precautions No information available to require special precautions

Effects on Dental Treatment No significant effects or complications reported

Common Adverse Effects Frequency not defined.

Cardiovascular: Edema, hypertension, venous thromboembolism

Central nervous system: Dizziness, headache, mental depression, migraine

Dermatologic: Chloasma, erythema multiforme, erythema nodosum, hemorrhagic eruption, hirsutism, loss of scalp hair, melasma

Endocrine & metabolic: Breast enlargement, breast tenderness, libido (changes in), increased thyroid-binding globulin, increased total thyroid hormone (T_4), increased serum triglycerides/phospholipids, increased HDL-cholesterol, decreased LDL-cholesterol, impaired glucose tolerance, hypercalcemia

Gastrointestinal: Abdominal cramps, bloating, cholecystitis, cholelithiasis, gallbladder disease, nausea, pancreatitis, vomiting, weight gain/loss

Genitourinary: Alterations in frequency and flow of menses, changes in cervical secretions, endometrial cancer, increased size of uterine leiomyomata, vaginal candidiasis

Hematologic: Aggravation of porphyria, decreased antithrombin III and antifactor Xa, increased levels of fibrinogen, increased platelet aggregability and platelet count; increased prothrombin and factors VII, VIII, IX, X

Hepatic: Cholestatic jaundice

Neuromuscular & skeletal: Chorea

Ocular: Intolerance to contact lenses, steeping of corneal curvature

Respiratory: Pulmonary thromboembolism

Miscellaneous: Carbohydrate intolerance

Mechanism of Action Esterified estrogens contain a mixture of estrogenic substances; the principle component is estrone. Preparations contain 75% to 85% sodium estrone sulfate and 6% to 15% sodium equilin sulfate such that the total is not <90%. Estrogens are responsible for the development and maintenance of the female reproductive system and secondary sexual characteristics. Estradiol is the principle intracellular human estrogen and is more potent than estrone and estriol at the receptor level; it is the primary estrogen secreted prior to menopause. In males and following menopause in females, estrone and estrone sulfate are more highly produced. Estrogens modulate the pituitary secretion of gonadotropins, luteinizing hormone, and follicle-stimulating hormone through a negative feedback system; estrogen replacement reduces elevated levels of these hormones.

Drug Interactions

Cytochrome P450 Effect: Based on estrone: **Substrate** of CYP1A2 (major), 2B6 (minor), 2C9 (minor), 2E1 (minor), 3A4 (major)

Increased Effect/Toxicity: Hydrocortisone taken with estrogen may cause corticosteroid-induced toxicity. Increased potential for thromboembolic events with anticoagulants.

Decreased Effect: CYP1A2 inducers may decrease the levels/effects of estrogens; example inducers include aminoglutethimide, carbamazepine, phenobarbital, and rifampin. CYP3A4 inducers may decrease the levels/effects of estrogens; example inducers include aminoglutethimide, carbamazepine, nafcillin, nevirapine, phenobarbital, phenytoin, and rifamycins.

Pharmacodynamics/Kinetics

Absorption: Readily

Metabolism: Rapidly hepatic to estrone sulfate, conjugated and unconjugated metabolites; first-pass effect

Excretion: Urine (as unchanged drug and as glucuronide and sulfate conjugates)

Pregnancy Risk Factor X

Estrogens (Esterified) and Methyltestosterone
(ES troe jenz es TER i fied & meth il tes TOS te rone)

Related Information

Endocrine Disorders and Pregnancy *on page 1659*

Estrogens (Esterified) *on page 584*

MethylTESTOSTERone *on page 1028*

U.S. Brand Names Estratest®; Estratest® H.S.; Syntest D.S.; Syntest H.S.

Canadian Brand Names Estratest®

Generic Available Yes

Synonyms Conjugated Estrogen and Methyltestosterone; Esterified Estrogen and Methyltestosterone

Pharmacologic Category Estrogen and Progestin Combination

Use Vasomotor symptoms of menopause

Local Anesthetic/Vasoconstrictor Precautions No information available to require special precautions

Effects on Dental Treatment No significant effects or complications reported

Common Adverse Effects 1% to 10%:

Cardiovascular: Increase in blood pressure, edema, thromboembolic disorder

Central nervous system: Depression, headache

Dermatologic: Chloasma, melasma

(Continued)

Estrogens (Esterified) and Methyltestosterone
(Continued)

Endocrine & metabolic: Breast tenderness, change in menstrual flow, hypercalcemia

Gastrointestinal: Nausea, vomiting

Hepatic: Cholestatic jaundice

Mechanism of Action

Conjugated estrogens: Activate estrogen receptors (DNA protein complex) located in estrogen-responsive tissues. Once activated, regulate transcription of certain genes leading to observed effects.

Testosterone: Increases synthesis of DNA, RNA, and various proteins in target tissues

Drug Interactions

Cytochrome P450 Effect: Based on estrone: **Substrate** of CYP1A2 (major), 2B6 (minor), 2C9 (minor), 2E1 (minor), 3A4 (major)

Pharmacodynamics/Kinetics See individual agents.

Pregnancy Risk Factor X

Estropipate (ES troe pih pate)

Related Information

Endocrine Disorders and Pregnancy *on page 1659*

U.S. Brand Names Ogen®; Ortho-Est®

Canadian Brand Names Ogen®

Mexican Brand Names Ogen®

Generic Available Yes

Synonyms Ortho Est; Piperazine Estrone Sulfate

Pharmacologic Category Estrogen Derivative

Use Treatment of moderate to severe vasomotor symptoms associated with menopause; treatment of vulvar and vaginal atrophy; hypoestrogenism (due to hypogonadism, castration, or primary ovarian failure); osteoporosis (prophylaxis, in women at significant risk only)

Local Anesthetic/Vasoconstrictor Precautions No information available to require special precautions

Effects on Dental Treatment No significant effects or complications reported

Common Adverse Effects Frequency not defined.

Cardiovascular: Edema, hypertension, venous thromboembolism

Central nervous system: Dizziness, headache, mental depression, migraine

Dermatologic: Chloasma, erythema multiforme, erythema nodosum, hemorrhagic eruption, hirsutism, loss of scalp hair, melasma

Endocrine & metabolic: Breast enlargement, breast tenderness, libido (changes in), increased thyroid-binding globulin, increased total thyroid hormone (T_4), increased serum triglycerides/phospholipids, increased HDL-cholesterol, decreased LDL-cholesterol, impaired glucose tolerance, hypercalcemia

Gastrointestinal: Abdominal cramps, bloating, cholecystitis, cholelithiasis, gallbladder disease, nausea, pancreatitis, vomiting, weight gain/loss

Genitourinary: Alterations in frequency and flow of menses, changes in cervical secretions, endometrial cancer, increased size of uterine leiomyomata, vaginal candidiasis

Hematologic: Aggravation of porphyria, decreased antithrombin III and antifactor Xa, increased levels of fibrinogen, increased platelet aggregability and platelet count; increased prothrombin and factors VII, VIII, IX, X

Hepatic: Cholestatic jaundice

Neuromuscular & skeletal: Chorea

Ocular: Intolerance to contact lenses, steeping of corneal curvature

Respiratory: Pulmonary thromboembolism

Miscellaneous: Carbohydrate intolerance

Mechanism of Action Estrogens are responsible for the development and maintenance of the female reproductive system and secondary sexual characteristics. Estradiol is the principle intracellular human estrogen and is more potent than estrone and estriol at the receptor level; it is the primary estrogen secreted prior to menopause. In males and following menopause in females, estrone and estrone sulfate are more highly produced. Estrogens modulate the pituitary secretion of gonadotropins, luteinizing hormone, and follicle-stimulating hormone through a negative feedback system; estrogen replacement reduces elevated levels of these hormones. Estropipate is prepared from purified crystalline estrone that has been solubilized as the sulfate and stabilized with piperazine.

Drug Interactions

Cytochrome P450 Effect: Based on estrone: **Substrate** of CYP1A2 (major), 2B6 (minor), 2C9 (minor), 2E1 (minor), 3A4 (major)

Increased Effect/Toxicity: Hydrocortisone taken with estrogen may cause corticosteroid-induced toxicity. Increased potential for thromboembolic events with anticoagulants.

Decreased Effect: CYP1A2 inducers may decrease the levels/effects of estrogens; example inducers include aminoglutethimide, carbamazepine, phenobarbital, and rifampin. CYP3A4 inducers may decrease the levels/effects of estrogens; example inducers include aminoglutethimide, carbamazepine, nafcillin, nevirapine, phenobarbital, phenytoin, and rifamycins.

Pharmacodynamics/Kinetics

Absorption: Well absorbed

Metabolism: Hepatic and in target tissues; first-pass effect

Pregnancy Risk Factor X

Estrostep® Fe see Ethinyl Estradiol and Norethindrone on page 608

Eszopiclone (es zoe PIK lone)

U.S. Brand Names Lunesta™

Generic Available No

Pharmacologic Category Hypnotic, Nonbenzodiazepine

Dental Use Not established at this time

Use Treatment of insomnia

Local Anesthetic/Vasoconstrictor Precautions No information available to require special precautions

Effects on Dental Treatment Key adverse event(s) related to dental treatment: Unpleasant taste and xerostomia (normal salivary flow resumes upon discontinuation).

Common Adverse Effects

>10%:
Central nervous system: Headache (15% to 21%)
Gastrointestinal: Unpleasant taste (8% to 34%)

1% to 10%:
Cardiovascular: Chest pain, peripheral edema
Central nervous system: Somnolence (8% to 10%), dizziness (5% to 7%), hallucinations (1% to 3%), anxiety (1% to 3%), nervousness (up to 5%), confusion (up to 3%), depression (1% to 4%), abnormal dreams (1% to 3%), migraine
Dermatologic: Rash (3% to 4%), pruritus (1% to 4%)
Endocrine & metabolic: Libido decreased (up to 3%), dysmenorrhea (up to 3%), gynecomastia (males up to 3%)
Gastrointestinal: Xerostomia (3% to 7%), dyspepsia (5% to 6%), nausea (5%), diarrhea (2% to 4%), vomiting (up to 3%)
Genitourinary: Urinary tract infection (up to 3%)
Neuromuscular & skeletal: Neuralgia (up to 3%)
Miscellaneous: Infection (5% to 10%), viral infection (3%)

Restrictions C-IV

Dosage Oral:

Adults: Insomnia: Initial: 2 mg before bedtime (maximum dose: 3 mg)
Concurrent use with strong CYP3A4 inhibitor: 1 mg before bedtime; if needed, dose may be increased to 2 mg

Elderly:
Difficulty falling asleep: Initial: 1 mg before bedtime; maximum dose: 2 mg
Difficulty staying asleep: 2 mg before bedtime
Dosage adjustment in renal impairment: None required
Dosage adjustment in hepatic impairment:
Mild-to-moderate: Use with caution; dosage adjustment unnecessary
Severe: Maximum dose: 2 mg

Mechanism of Action May interact with GABA-receptor complexes at binding domains located close to or allosterically coupled to benzodiazepine receptors.

Contraindications Hypersensitivity to eszopiclone or any component of the formulation

Warnings/Precautions Symptomatic treatment of insomnia should be initiated only after careful evaluation of potential causes of sleep disturbance. Tolerance did not develop over 6 months of use. Use with caution in patients with depression or a history of drug dependence. Abrupt discontinuance may lead to withdrawal symptoms. Use with caution in patients receiving other CNS depressants or psychoactive medications. May impair physical and mental capabilities. Use caution in patients with respiratory compromise, hepatic (Continued)

Eszopiclone *(Continued)*

dysfunction, or those taking strong CYP3A4 inhibitors. Safety and efficacy in children have not been established.

Drug Interactions

Cytochrome P450 Effect: Substrate of CYP2E1 (minor), 3A4 (major)

Increased Effect/Toxicity: CYP3A4 inhibitors may increase the levels/effects of eszopiclone; example inhibitors include azole antifungals, clarithromycin, diclofenac, doxycycline, erythromycin, imatinib, isoniazid, nefazodone, nicardipine, propofol, protease inhibitors, quinidine, telithromycin, and verapamil. Concurrent use with olanzapine may lead to decreased psychomotor function.

Decreased Effect: CYP3A4 inducers may decrease the levels/effects of eszopiclone; example inducers include aminoglutethimide, carbamazepine, nafcillin, nevirapine, phenobarbital, phenytoin, and rifamycins.

Ethanol/Nutrition/Herb Interactions

Ethanol: Use caution with concurrent use. Effects are additive and may decrease psychomotor function.

Food: Onset of action may be reduced if taken with or immediately after a heavy meal.

Herb/Nutraceutical: Avoid valerian, St John's wort, kava kava, gotu kola (may increase CNS depression).

Dietary Considerations Avoid taking after a heavy meal; may delay onset.

Pharmacodynamics/Kinetics

Absorption: Rapid; high-fat/heavy meal may delay absorption

Protein binding: 52% to 59%

Metabolism: Hepatic via oxidation and demethylation (CYP2E1, 3A4); 2 primary metabolites; one with activity less than parent.

Half-life elimination: 6 hours; Elderly (≥65 years): ~9 hours

Time to peak, plasma: 1 hour

Excretion: Urine (75%, primarily as metabolites; <10% as parent drug)

Pregnancy Risk Factor C

Dosage Forms TAB: 1 mg, 2 mg, 3 mg

Selected Readings

Krystal AD, Walsh JK, Laska E, et al, "Sustained Efficacy of Eszopiclone Over 6 Months of Nightly Treatment: Results of a Randomized, Double-Blind, Placebo-Controlled Study in Adults With Chronic Insomnia," *Sleep*, 2003, 26(7):793-9.

ETAF see Aldesleukin on page 61

Etanercept *(et a NER sept)*

Related Information

Rheumatoid Arthritis, Osteoarthritis, and Osteoporosis on page 1668

U.S. Brand Names Enbrel®

Canadian Brand Names Enbrel®

Generic Available No

Pharmacologic Category Antirheumatic, Disease Modifying; Tumor Necrosis Factor (TNF) Blocking Agent

Use Treatment of moderately- to severely-active rheumatoid arthritis, moderately- to severely-active polyarticular juvenile arthritis (in patients with inadequate response to at least one disease-modifying antirheumatic drug), psoriatic arthritis, active ankylosing spondylitis (AS); moderate-to-severe chronic plaque psoriasis

Local Anesthetic/Vasoconstrictor Precautions No information available to require special precautions

Effects on Dental Treatment No significant effects or complications reported

Common Adverse Effects

>10%:

Central nervous system: Headache (17%)

Local: Injection site reaction (14% to 37%)

Respiratory: Respiratory tract infection (upper, 29%; other than upper, 38%), rhinitis (12%)

Miscellaneous: Infection (35%), positive ANA (11%), positive antidouble-stranded DNA antibodies (15% by RIA, 3% by *Crithidia luciliae* assay)

≥3% to 10%:

Central nervous system: Dizziness (7%)

Dermatologic: Rash (5%)

Gastrointestinal: Abdominal pain (5%), dyspepsia (4%), nausea (9%), vomiting (3%)

Neuromuscular & skeletal: Weakness (5%)

Respiratory: Pharyngitis (7%), respiratory disorder (5%), sinusitis (3%), cough (6%)
Pediatric patients (JRA): The percentages of patients reporting abdominal pain (17%) and vomiting (13%) were higher than in adult RA. Two patients developed varicella infection associated with aseptic meningitis which resolved without complications (see Warnings/Precautions).

Dosage SubQ:
Children 4-17 years: Juvenile rheumatoid arthritis:
Once-weekly dosing: 0.8 mg/kg (maximum: 50 mg/dose) once weekly
Twice-weekly dosing: 0.4 mg/kg (maximum: 25 mg/dose) twice weekly (individual doses should be separated by 72-96 hours)
Adults:
Rheumatoid arthritis, psoriatic arthritis, ankylosing spondylitis:
Once-weekly dosing: 50 mg once weekly
Twice weekly dosing: 25 mg given twice weekly (individual doses should be separated by 72-96 hours)
Note: If the physician determines that it is appropriate, patients may self-inject after proper training in injection technique.
Plaque psoriasis:
Initial: 50 mg twice weekly, 3-4 days apart (starting doses of 25 or 50 mg once weekly have also been used successfully); maintain initial dose for 3 months
Maintenance dose: 50 mg weekly
Elderly: Although greater sensitivity of some elderly patients cannot be ruled out, no overall differences in safety or effectiveness were observed.

Mechanism of Action Etanercept is a recombinant DNA-derived protein composed of tumor necrosis factor receptor (TNFR) linked to the Fc portion of human IgG1. Etanercept binds tumor necrosis factor (TNF) and blocks its interaction with cell surface receptors. TNF plays an important role in the inflammatory processes and the resulting joint pathology of rheumatoid arthritis (RA), polyarticular-course juvenile arthritis (JRA), ankylosing spondylitis (AS), and plaque psoriasis.

Contraindications Hypersensitivity to etanercept or any component of the formulation; patients with sepsis (mortality may be increased); active infections (including chronic or local infection)

Warnings/Precautions Etanercept may affect defenses against infections and malignancies. Safety and efficacy in patients with immunosuppression or chronic infections have not been evaluated. Rare reactivation of hepatitis B has occurred in chronic virus carriers; evaluate prior to initiation and during treatment. Discontinue administration if patient develops a serious infection. Do not start drug in patients with an active infection. Use caution in patients predisposed to infection, such as poorly-controlled diabetes.

Impact on the development and course of malignancies is not fully defined. As compared to the general population, an increased risk of lymphoma has been noted in clinical trials; however, rheumatoid arthritis has been previously associated with an increased rate of lymphoma. Etanercept is not recommended for use in patients with Wegener's granulomatosis who are receiving immunosuppressive therapy. Treatment may result in the formation of autoimmune antibodies; cases of autoimmune disease have not been described. Non-neutralizing antibodies to etanercept may also be formed. Rarely, a reversible lupus-like syndrome has occurred. The safety of etanercept has not been studied in children <4 years of age.

Use caution in patients with pre-existing or recent-onset demyelinating CNS disorders. Use caution in patients with CHF; has been associated with worsening and new-onset CHF. Use caution in patients with a history of significant hematologic abnormalities; has been associated with pancytopenia and aplastic anemia (rare). Discontinue if significant hematologic abnormalities are confirmed.

Patients should be brought up to date with all immunizations before initiating therapy. Live vaccines should not be given concurrently. Patients with a significant exposure to varicella virus should temporarily discontinue etanercept. Treatment with varicella zoster immune globulin should be considered.

Drug Interactions
Increased Effect/Toxicity: Specific drug interaction studies have not been conducted with etanercept. An increased rate of serious infections has been noted with concurrent anakinra therapy, without additional improvement in American College of Rheumatology (ACR) response criteria. Cyclophosphamide may increase the risk of noncutaneous solid malignancy when used with etanercept (concurrent therapy is not recommended).
Decreased Effect: Specific drug interaction studies have not been conducted with etanercept. Live vaccines should not be given during therapy.
(Continued)

Etanercept (Continued)

Pharmacodynamics/Kinetics
Onset of action: ~2-3 weeks
Half-life elimination: 115 hours (range: 98-300 hours)
Time to peak: 72 hours (range: 48-96 hours)
Excretion: Clearance: Children: 45.9 mL/hour/m^2; Adults: 89 mL/hour (52 mL/hour/m^2)

Pregnancy Risk Factor B

Dosage Forms INJ, powder for reconstitution: 25 mg. INJ, solution: 50 mg/mL (0.98 mL)

Ethacrynate Sodium see Ethacrynic Acid on page 590

Ethacrynic Acid (eth a KRIN ik AS id)

Related Information
Cardiovascular Diseases on page 1636

U.S. Brand Names Edecrin®

Canadian Brand Names Edecrin®

Generic Available No

Synonyms Ethacrynate Sodium

Pharmacologic Category Diuretic, Loop

Use Management of edema associated with congestive heart failure; hepatic cirrhosis or renal disease; short-term management of ascites due to malignancy, idiopathic edema, and lymphedema

Local Anesthetic/Vasoconstrictor Precautions No information available to require special precautions

Effects on Dental Treatment No significant effects or complications reported

Common Adverse Effects Frequency not defined.
Central nervous system: Headache, fatigue, apprehension, confusion, fever, chills, encephalopathy (patients with pre-existing liver disease); vertigo
Dermatologic: Skin rash, Henoch-Schönlein purpura (in patient with rheumatic heart disease)
Endocrine & metabolic: Hyponatremia, hyperglycemia, variations in phosphorus, CO_2 content, bicarbonate, and calcium; reversible hyperuricemia, gout, hyperglycemia, hypoglycemia (occurred in two uremic patients who received doses above those recommended)
Gastrointestinal: Anorexia, malaise, abdominal discomfort or pain, dysphagia, nausea, vomiting, diarrhea, gastrointestinal bleeding, acute pancreatitis (rare)
Genitourinary: Hematuria
Hepatic: Jaundice, abnormal liver function tests
Hematology: Agranulocytosis, severe neutropenia, thrombocytopenia
Local: Thrombophlebitis (with intravenous use), local irritation and pain,
Ocular: Blurred vision
Otic: Tinnitus, temporary or permanent deafness
Renal: Serum creatinine increased

Mechanism of Action Inhibits reabsorption of sodium and chloride in the ascending loop of Henle and distal renal tubule, interfering with the chloride-binding cotransport system, thus causing increased excretion of water, sodium, chloride, magnesium, and calcium

Drug Interactions
Increased Effect/Toxicity: Ethacrynic acid-induced hypokalemia may predispose to digoxin toxicity and may increase the risk of arrhythmia with drugs which may prolong QT interval, including type Ia and type III antiarrhythmic agents, cisapride, and some quinolones (sparfloxacin, gatifloxacin, and moxifloxacin). The risk of toxicity from lithium and salicylates (high dose) may be increased by loop diuretics. Hypotensive effects and/or adverse renal effects of ACE inhibitors and NSAIDs are potentiated by ethacrynic acid-induced hypovolemia. The effects of peripheral adrenergic-blocking drugs or ganglionic blockers may be increased by ethacrynic acid.

Ethacrynic acid may increase the risk of ototoxicity with other ototoxic agents (aminoglycosides, cis-platinum), especially in patients with renal dysfunction. Synergistic diuretic effects occur with thiazide-type diuretics. Diuretics tend to be synergistic with other antihypertensive agents, and hypotension may occur. Nephrotoxicity has been associated with concomitant use of cephaloridine or cephalexin.

Decreased Effect: Probenecid decreases diuretic effects of ethacrynic acid. Glucose tolerance may be decreased by loop diuretics, requiring adjustment of hypoglycemic agents. Cholestyramine or colestipol may reduce bioavailability of ethacrynic acid. Indomethacin (and other NSAIDs) may reduce natriuretic and hypotensive effects of diuretics.

Pharmacodynamics/Kinetics
Onset of action: Diuresis: Oral: ~30 minutes; I.V.: 5 minutes
Peak effect: Oral: 2 hours; I.V.: 30 minutes
Duration: Oral: 12 hours; I.V.: 2 hours
Absorption: Oral: Rapid
Protein binding: >90%
Metabolism: Hepatic (35% to 40%) to active cysteine conjugate
Half-life elimination: Normal renal function: 2-4 hours
Excretion: Feces and urine (30% to 60% as unchanged drug)
Pregnancy Risk Factor B

Ethambutol (e THAM byoo tole)

Related Information
Tuberculosis *on page 1673*
U.S. Brand Names Myambutol®
Canadian Brand Names Etibi®
Generic Available Yes
Synonyms Ethambutol Hydrochloride
Pharmacologic Category Antitubercular Agent
Use Treatment of tuberculosis and other mycobacterial diseases in conjunction with other antituberculosis agents
Local Anesthetic/Vasoconstrictor Precautions No information available to require special precautions
Effects on Dental Treatment No significant effects or complications reported
Common Adverse Effects Frequency not defined.
Cardiovascular: Myocarditis, pericarditis
Central nervous system: Headache, confusion, disorientation, malaise, mental confusion, fever, dizziness, hallucinations
Dermatologic: Rash, pruritus, dermatitis, exfoliative dermatitis
Endocrine & metabolic: Acute gout or hyperuricemia
Gastrointestinal: Abdominal pain, anorexia, nausea, vomiting
Hematologic: Leukopenia, thrombocytopenia, eosinophilia, neutropenia, lymphadenopathy
Hepatic: Abnormal LFTs, hepatotoxicity (possibly related to concurrent therapy), hepatitis
Neuromuscular & skeletal: Peripheral neuritis, arthralgia
Ocular: Optic neuritis; symptoms may include decreased acuity, scotoma, color blindness, or visual defects (usually reversible with discontinuation, irreversible blindness has been described)
Renal: Nephritis
Respiratory: Infiltrates (with or without eosinophilia), pneumonitis
Miscellaneous: Anaphylaxis, anaphylactoid reaction; hypersensitivity syndrome (rash, eosinophilia, and organ-specific inflammation)
Mechanism of Action Suppresses mycobacteria multiplication by interfering with RNA synthesis
Drug Interactions
Decreased Effect: Decreased absorption with aluminum hydroxide. Avoid concurrent administration of aluminum-containing antacids for at least 4 hours following ethambutol.
Pharmacodynamics/Kinetics
Absorption: ~80%
Distribution: Widely throughout body; concentrated in kidneys, lungs, saliva, and red blood cells
Relative diffusion from blood into CSF: Adequate with or without inflammation (exceeds usual MICs)
CSF:blood level ratio: Normal meninges: 0%; Inflamed meninges: 25%
Protein binding: 20% to 30%
Metabolism: Hepatic (20%) to inactive metabolite
Half-life elimination: 2.5-3.6 hours; End-stage renal disease: 7-15 hours
Time to peak, serum: 2-4 hours
Excretion: Urine (~50%) and feces (20%) as unchanged drug
Pregnancy Risk Factor C

Ethambutol Hydrochloride *see Ethambutol on page 591*
Ethamolin® *see Ethanolamine Oleate on page 591*

Ethanolamine Oleate (ETH a nol a meen OH lee ate)

U.S. Brand Names Ethamolin®
Generic Available No
(Continued)

Ethanolamine Oleate *(Continued)*

Synonyms Monoethanolamine

Pharmacologic Category Sclerosing Agent

Use Orphan drug: Sclerosing agent used for bleeding esophageal varices

Local Anesthetic/Vasoconstrictor Precautions No information available to require special precautions

Effects on Dental Treatment No significant effects or complications reported

Common Adverse Effects 1% to 10%:
Central nervous system: Pyrexia (1.8%)
Gastrointestinal: Esophageal ulcer (2%), esophageal stricture (1.3%)
Respiratory: Pleural effusion (2%), pneumonia (1.2%)
Miscellaneous: Retrosternal pain (1.6%)

Mechanism of Action Derived from oleic acid and similar in physical properties to sodium morrhuate; however, the exact mechanism of the hemostatic effect used in endoscopic injection sclerotherapy is not known. Intravenously injected ethanolamine oleate produces a sterile inflammatory response resulting in fibrosis and occlusion of the vein; a dose-related extravascular inflammatory reaction occurs when the drug diffuses through the venous wall. Autopsy results indicate that variceal obliteration occurs secondary to mural necrosis and fibrosis. Thrombosis appears to be a transient reaction.

Pregnancy Risk Factor C

EtheDent™ *see* Fluoride *on page 671*

Ethezyme™ *see* Papain and Urea *on page 1186*

Ethezyme™ 830 *see* Papain and Urea *on page 1186*

Ethinyl Estradiol and Desogestrel
(ETH in il es tra DYE ole & des oh JES trel)

U.S. Brand Names Apri®; Cesia™; Cyclessa®; Desogen®; Kariva™; Mircette®; Ortho-Cept®; Reclipsen™; Solia™; Velivet™

Canadian Brand Names Marvelon®; Ortho-Cept®

Generic Available Yes

Synonyms Desogestrel and Ethinyl Estradiol; Ortho Cept

Pharmacologic Category Contraceptive; Estrogen and Progestin Combination

Use Prevention of pregnancy

Unlabeled/Investigational Use Treatment of hypermenorrhea (menorrhagia); pain associated with endometriosis; dysmenorrhea; dysfunctional uterine bleeding

Local Anesthetic/Vasoconstrictor Precautions No information available to require special precautions

Effects on Dental Treatment When prescribing antibiotics, patient must be warned to use additional methods of birth control if on oral contraceptives.

Common Adverse Effects Frequency not defined.
Cardiovascular: Arterial thromboembolism, cerebral hemorrhage, cerebral thrombosis, edema, hypertension, mesenteric thrombosis, MI
Central nervous system: Depression, dizziness, headache, migraine, nervousness, premenstrual syndrome, stroke
Dermatologic: Acne, erythema multiforme, erythema nodosum, hirsutism, loss of scalp hair, melasma (may persist), rash (allergic)
Endocrine & metabolic: Amenorrhea, breakthrough bleeding, breast enlargement, breast secretion, breast tenderness, carbohydrate intolerance, lactation decreased (postpartum), glucose tolerance decreased, libido changes, menstrual flow changes, sex hormone-binding globulins (SHBG) increased, spotting, temporary infertility (following discontinuation), thyroid-binding globulin increased, triglycerides increased
Gastrointestinal: Abdominal cramps, appetite changes, bloating, cholestasis, colitis, gallbladder disease, jaundice, nausea, vomiting, weight gain/loss
Genitourinary: Cervical erosion changes, cervical secretion changes, cystitis-like syndrome, vaginal candidiasis, vaginitis
Hematologic: Antithrombin III decreased, folate levels decreased, hemolytic uremic syndrome, norepinephrine induced platelet aggregability increased, porphyria, prothrombin increased; factors VII, VIII, IX, and X
Hepatic: Benign liver tumors, Budd-Chiari syndrome, cholestatic jaundice, hepatic adenomas
Local: Thrombophlebitis
Ocular: Cataracts, change in corneal curvature (steepening), contact lens intolerance, optic neuritis, retinal thrombosis
Renal: Impaired renal function
Respiratory: Pulmonary thromboembolism

Miscellaneous: Hemorrhagic eruption

Dosage Oral: Adults: Female: Contraception:

Schedule 1 (Sunday starter): Dose begins on first Sunday after onset of menstruation; if the menstrual period starts on Sunday, take first tablet that very same day. **With a Sunday start, an additional method of contraception should be used until after the first 7 days of consecutive administration.**

For 21-tablet package: Dosage is 1 tablet daily for 21 consecutive days, followed by 7 days off of the medication; a new course begins on the 8th day after the last tablet is taken.

For 28-tablet package: Dosage is 1 tablet daily without interruption.

Schedule 2 (Day 1 starter): Dose starts on first day of menstrual cycle taking 1 tablet daily.

For 21-tablet package: Dosage is 1 tablet daily for 21 consecutive days, followed by 7 days off of the medication; a new course begins on the 8th day after the last tablet is taken.

For 28-tablet package: Dosage is 1 tablet daily without interruption.

If all doses have been taken on schedule and one menstrual period is missed, continue dosing cycle. If two consecutive menstrual periods are missed, pregnancy test is required before new dosing cycle is started.

Missed doses **monophasic formulations** (refer to package insert for complete information):

One dose missed: Take as soon as remembered or take 2 tablets next day

Two consecutive doses missed in the first 2 weeks: Take 2 tablets as soon as remembered or 2 tablets next 2 days. **An additional method of contraception should be used for 7 days after missed dose.**

Two consecutive doses missed in week 3 or three consecutive doses missed at any time:

Schedule 1 (Sunday starter): Continue to take 1 tablet daily until Sunday, then discard the rest of the pack, and a new pack is started that same day.

Schedule 2 (Day 1 starter): Current pack should be discarded, and a new pack started that same day. **An additional method of contraception should be used for 7 days after missed dose.**

Missed doses **biphasic/triphasic formulations** (refer to package insert for complete information):

One dose missed: Take as soon as remembered or take 2 tablets next day.

Two consecutive doses missed in week 1 or week 2 of the pack: Take 2 tablets as soon as remembered and 2 tablets the next day. Resume taking 1 tablet daily until the pack is empty. **An additional method of contraception should be used for 7 days after a missed dose.**

Two consecutive doses missed in week 3 of the pack; **an additional method of contraception must be used for 7 days after a missed dose:**

Schedule 1 (Sunday starter): Take 1 tablet every day until Sunday. Discard the remaining pack and start a new pack of pills on the same day.

Schedule 2 (Day 1 starter): Discard the remaining pack and start a new pack the same day.

Three or more consecutive doses missed; **an additional method of contraception must be used for 7 days after a missed dose:**

Schedule 1 (Sunday starter): Take 1 tablet every day until Sunday; on Sunday, discard the pack and start a new pack.

Schedule 2 (Day 1 starter): Discard the remaining pack and begin new pack of tablets starting on the same day.

Dosage adjustment in renal impairment: Specific guidelines not available; use with caution and monitor blood pressure closely. Consider other forms of contraception.

Dosage adjustment in hepatic impairment: Contraindicated in patients with hepatic impairment

Mechanism of Action Combination hormonal contraceptives inhibit ovulation via a negative feedback mechanism on the hypothalamus, which alters the normal pattern of gonadotropin secretion of a follicle-stimulating hormone (FSH) and luteinizing hormone by the anterior pituitary. The follicular phase FSH and midcycle surge of gonadotropins are inhibited. In addition, combination hormonal contraceptives produce alterations in the genital tract, including changes in the cervical mucus, rendering it unfavorable for sperm penetration even if ovulation occurs. Changes in the endometrium may also occur, producing an unfavorable environment for nidation. Combination hormonal contraceptive drugs may alter the tubal transport of the ova through the fallopian tubes. Progestational agents may also alter sperm fertility.

Contraindications Hypersensitivity to ethinyl estradiol, etonogestrel, desogestrel, or any component of the formulation; history of or current thrombophlebitis or venous thromboembolic disorders (including DVT, PE); active or recent (within 1 year) arterial thromboembolic disease (eg, stroke, MI); cerebral (Continued)

Ethinyl Estradiol and Desogestrel *(Continued)*

vascular disease, coronary artery disease, valvular heart disease with complications, severe hypertension; diabetes mellitus with vascular involvement; severe headache with focal neurological symptoms; known or suspected breast carcinoma, endometrial cancer, estrogen-dependent neoplasms, undiagnosed abnormal genital bleeding; hepatic dysfunction or tumor, cholestatic jaundice of pregnancy, jaundice with prior combination hormonal contraceptive use; major surgery with prolonged immobilization; heavy smoking (≥15 cigarettes/day) in patients >35 years of age; pregnancy

Warnings/Precautions Combination hormonal contraceptives do not protect against HIV infection or other sexually-transmitted diseases. The risk of cardiovascular side effects increases in women who smoke cigarettes, especially those who are >35 years of age; women who use combination hormonal contraceptives should be strongly advised not to smoke. Combination hormonal contraceptives may lead to increased risk of myocardial infarction, use with caution in patients with risk factors for coronary artery disease. May increase the risk of thromboembolism. Whenever possible, combination hormonal contraceptives should be discontinued at least 4 weeks prior to and for 2 weeks following elective surgery associated with an increased risk of thromboembolism or during periods of prolonged immobilization. Combination hormonal contraceptives may have a dose-related risk of vascular disease, hypertension, and gallbladder disease. Women with hypertension or renal disease should be encouraged to use another form of contraception. The use of combination hormonal contraceptives has been associated with a slight increase in frequency of breast cancer, however, studies are not consistent. Combination hormonal contraceptives may cause glucose intolerance. Retinal thrombosis has been reported (rarely). Use caution in conditions that may be aggravated by fluid retention, depression, or history of migraine. Not for use prior to menarche.

The minimum dosage combination of estrogen/progestin that will effectively treat the individual patient should be used. New patients should be started on products containing ≤0.035 mg of estrogen per tablet.

Drug Interactions
Cytochrome P450 Effect:
Ethinyl estradiol: **Substrate** of CYP2C9 (minor), 3A4 (major), 3A5-7 (minor); **Inhibits** CYP1A2 (weak), 2B6 (weak), 2C8 (weak), 2C19 (weak), 3A4 (weak)

Desogestrel: **Substrate** of CYP2C19 (major)

Increased Effect/Toxicity: Acetaminophen, ascorbic acid, and repaglinide may increase plasma levels of estrogen component. Atorvastatin and indinavir increase plasma levels of combination hormonal contraceptives. Combination hormonal contraceptives increase the plasma levels of alprazolam, chlordiazepoxide, cyclosporine, diazepam, prednisolone, selegiline, theophylline, tricyclic antidepressants. Combination hormonal contraceptives may increase (or decrease) the effects of coumarin derivatives.

Decreased Effect: CYP2C19 inducers may decrease the levels/effects of desogestrel; example inducers include aminoglutethimide, carbamazepine, phenytoin, and rifampin. CYP3A4 inducers may decrease the levels/effects of ethinyl estradiol; example inducers include aminoglutethimide, carbamazepine, nafcillin, phenobarbital, phenytoin, and rifamycins. Combination hormonal contraceptives may decrease plasma levels of acetaminophen, clofibric acid, lorazepam, morphine, oxazepam, salicylic acid, temazepam. Contraceptive effect decreased by acitretin, amprenavir, griseofulvin, lopinavir, nelfinavir, nevirapine, penicillins (effect not consistent), ritonavir, tetracyclines (effect not consistent), troglitazone. Combination hormonal contraceptives may decrease (or increase) the effects of coumarin derivatives.

Ethanol/Nutrition/Herb Interactions
Food: CNS effects of caffeine may be enhanced if combination hormonal contraceptives are used concurrently with caffeine. Grapefruit juice increases ethinyl estradiol concentrations and would be expected to increase progesterone serum levels as well; clinical implications are unclear.

Herb/Nutraceutical: St John's wort may decrease the effectiveness of combination hormonal contraceptives by inducing hepatic enzymes. Avoid dong quai and black cohosh (have estrogen activity). Avoid saw palmetto, red clover, ginseng.

Dietary Considerations Should be taken at same time each day.
Pharmacodynamics/Kinetics
Desogestrel:
Absorption: Rapid and complete

Protein binding: Etonogestrel (active metabolite): 98%, primarily to sex hormone-binding globulin

Metabolism: Hepatic via CYP2C9 to active metabolite etonogestrel (3-keto-desogestrel); etonogestrel metabolized via CYP3A4

Half-life elimination: 37.1 hours

Excretion: Urine and feces (as metabolites)

Pregnancy Risk Factor X

Dosage Forms TAB, low-dose (Kariva™, Mircette®): Day 1-21: Ethinyl estradiol 0.02 mg and desogestrel 0.15 mg, Day 22-23: Inactive, Day 24-28: Ethinyl estradiol 0.01 mg (28s). **TAB, monophasic:** (Apri® 28): Ethinyl estradiol 0.03 mg and desogestrel 0.15 mg (28s); (Desogen®, Reclipsen™, Solia™): Ethinyl estradiol 0.03 mg and desogestrel 0.15 mg (28s); (Ortho-Cept® 28): Ethinyl estradiol 0.03 mg and desogestrel 0.15 mg (28s). **TAB, triphasic** (Cesia™, Cyclessa®): Day 1-7: Ethinyl estradiol 0.025 mg and desogestrel 0.1 mg, Day 8-14: Ethinyl estradiol 0.025 mg and desogestrel 0.125 mg, Day 14-21: Ethinyl estradiol 0.025 mg and desogestrel 0.15 mg, Day 21-28: Inactive (28s); (Velivet™): Day 1-7: Ethinyl estradiol 0.025 mg and desogestrel 0.1 mg, Day 8-14: Ethinyl estradiol 0.025 mg and desogestrel 0.125 mg, Day 14-21: Ethinyl estradiol 0.025 mg and desogestrel 0.15 mg, Day 21-28: Inactive (28s)

Ethinyl Estradiol and Drospirenone
(ETH in il es tra DYE ole & droh SPYE re none)

U.S. Brand Names Yasmin®; Yaz

Canadian Brand Names Yasmin®

Generic Available No

Synonyms Drospirenone and Ethinyl Estradiol

Pharmacologic Category Contraceptive; Estrogen and Progestin Combination

Use Prevention of pregnancy

Unlabeled/Investigational Use Treatment of hypermenorrhea (menorrhagia); pain associated with endometriosis; dysmenorrhea; dysfunctional uterine bleeding

Local Anesthetic/Vasoconstrictor Precautions No information available to require special precautions

Effects on Dental Treatment When prescribing antibiotics, patient must be warned to use additional methods of birth control if on oral contraceptives

Common Adverse Effects

>1%:

Central nervous system: Depression, dizziness, emotional lability, fever, headache, migraine, nervousness

Dermatologic: Acne, pruritus, rash

Endocrine & metabolic: Amenorrhea, breast pain, dysmenorrhea, intermenstrual bleeding, menstrual irregularities

Gastrointestinal: Abdominal pain, diarrhea, dyspepsia, gastroenteritis, nausea, vomiting, weight gain

Genitourinary: Cystitis, leukorrhea, papanicolaou smear suspicious, pelvic pain, UTI, vaginal moniliasis, vaginitis

Neuromuscular & skeletal: Back pain, extremity pain, weakness

Respiratory: Bronchitis, cough, pharyngitis, rhinitis, sinusitis, upper respiratory infection

Miscellaneous: Allergic reaction, flu-like syndrome, infection

Adverse reactions reported with other oral contraceptives: Appetite changes, antithrombin III decreased, arterial thromboembolism, benign liver tumors, breast changes, Budd-Chiari syndrome, carbohydrate intolerance, cataracts, cerebral hemorrhage, cerebral thrombosis, cervical changes, change in corneal curvature (steepening), cholestatic jaundice, colitis, contact lens intolerance, decreased lactation (postpartum), deep vein thrombosis, diplopia, edema, erythema multiforme, erythema nodosum; factors VII, VIII, IX, X increased; folate serum concentrations decreased, gallbladder disease, glucose intolerance, hemorrhagic eruption, hemolytic uremic syndrome, hepatic adenomas, hirsutism, hypercalcemia, hypertension, hyperglycemia, libido changes, melasma, mesenteric thrombosis, MI, papilledema, platelet aggregability increased, porphyria, premenstrual syndrome, proptosis, prothrombin increased, pulmonary thromboembolism, renal function impairment, retinal thrombosis, sex hormone-binding globulin increased, thrombophlebitis, thyroid-binding globulin increased, total thyroid hormone (T_4) increased, triglycerides/phospholipids increased, vaginal candidiasis, weight changes

Dosage Oral: Adults: Female: Contraception: Dosage is 1 tablet daily for 28 consecutive days. Dose should be taken at the same time each day, either after the evening meal or at bedtime. Dosing may be started on the first day of menstrual period (Day 1 starter) or on the first Sunday after the onset of the menstrual period (Sunday starter).

(Continued)

Ethinyl Estradiol and Drospirenone *(Continued)*

Day 1 starter: Dose starts on first day of menstrual cycle taking 1 tablet daily.

Sunday starter: Dose begins on first Sunday after onset of menstruation; if the menstrual period starts on Sunday, take first tablet that very same day. **With a Sunday start, an additional method of contraception should be used until after the first 7 days of consecutive administration.**

If all doses have been taken on schedule and one menstrual period is missed, continue dosing cycle. If two consecutive menstrual periods are missed, pregnancy test is required before new dosing cycle is started.

If doses have been missed during the first 3 weeks and the menstrual period is missed, pregnancy should be ruled out prior to continuing treatment.

Missed doses (monophasic formulations) (refer to package insert for complete information):

One dose missed: Take as soon as remembered or take 2 tablets next day

Two consecutive doses missed in the first 2 weeks: Take 2 tablets as soon as remembered or 2 tablets next 2 days. **An additional method of contraception should be used for 7 days after missed dose.**

Two consecutive doses missed in week 3 or three consecutive doses missed at any time: **An additional method of contraception must be used for 7 days after a missed dose.**

Day 1 starter: Current pack should be discarded, and a new pack should be started that same day.

Sunday starter: Continue dose of 1 tablet daily until Sunday, then discard the rest of the pack, and a new pack should be started that same day.

Any number of doses missed in week 4: Continue taking one pill each day until pack is empty; no back-up method of contraception is needed

Dosage adjustment in renal impairment: Contraindicated in patients with renal dysfunction (Cl_{cr} ≤50 mL/minute)

Dosage adjustment in hepatic impairment: Contraindicated in patients with hepatic dysfunction

Mechanism of Action Combination oral contraceptives inhibit ovulation via a negative feedback mechanism on the hypothalamus, which alters the normal pattern of gonadotropin secretion of a follicle-stimulating hormone (FSH) and luteinizing hormone by the anterior pituitary. The follicular phase FSH and midcycle surge of gonadotropins are inhibited. In addition, oral contraceptives produce alterations in the genital tract, including changes in the cervical mucus, rendering it unfavorable for sperm penetration even if ovulation occurs. Changes in the endometrium may also occur, producing an unfavorable environment for nidation. Oral contraceptive drugs may alter the tubal transport of the ova through the fallopian tubes. Progestational agents may also alter sperm fertility. Drospirenone is a spironolactone analogue with antimineralocorticoid and antiandrogenic activity.

Contraindications Hypersensitivity to ethinyl estradiol, drospirenone, or to any component of the formulation; history of or current thrombophlebitis or venous thromboembolic disorders (including DVT, PE); active or recent (within 1 year) arterial thromboembolic disease (eg, stroke, MI); cerebral vascular disease, coronary artery disease, severe hypertension; diabetes with vascular involvement; headache with focal neurological symptoms; known or suspected breast carcinoma, endometrial cancer, estrogen-dependent neoplasms, undiagnosed abnormal genital bleeding; renal insufficiency, hepatic dysfunction or tumor, adrenal insufficiency, cholestatic jaundice of pregnancy, jaundice with prior oral contraceptive use; heavy smoking (≥15 cigarettes/day) in patients >35 years of age; pregnancy

Warnings/Precautions Oral contraceptives do not protect against HIV infection or other sexually-transmitted diseases. The risk of cardiovascular side effects increases in women who smoke cigarettes, especially those who are >35 years of age; women who use oral contraceptives should be strongly advised not to smoke. Oral contraceptives may lead to increased risk of myocardial infarction, use with caution in patients with risk factors for coronary artery disease. May increase the risk of thromboembolism. Whenever possible, combination hormonal contraceptives should be discontinued at least 4 weeks prior to and for 2 weeks following elective surgery associated with an increased risk of thromboembolism or during periods of prolonged immobilization. Oral contraceptives may cause glucose intolerance. Retinal thrombosis has been reported (rarely) with oral contraceptive use. Use with caution in patients with conditions that may be aggravated by fluid retention, depression, or patients with history of migraine. Not for use prior to menarche.

Drospirenone has antimineralocorticoid activity that may lead to hyperkalemia in patients with renal insufficiency, hepatic dysfunction, or adrenal insufficiency. Use caution with medications that may increase serum potassium.

Drug Interactions
  Cytochrome P450 Effect:
    Ethinyl estradiol: **Substrate** of CYP2C9 (minor), 3A4 (major), 3A5-7 (minor); **Inhibits** CYP1A2 (weak), 2B6 (weak), 2C8 (weak), 2C19 (weak), 3A4 (weak)
    Drospirenone: **Substrate** of CYP3A4 (minor); **Inhibits** CYP1A2 (weak), 2C9 (weak), 2C19 (weak), 3A4 (weak)
  Increased Effect/Toxicity: ACE inhibitors, aldosterone antagonists, angiotensin II receptor antagonists, heparin, NSAIDs (when taken daily, long term), and potassium-sparing diuretics increase risk of hyperkalemia with concomitant use. Acetaminophen, ascorbic acid, and atorvastatin may increase plasma concentrations of oral contraceptives. Ethinyl estradiol may increase plasma concentrations of cyclosporine, prednisolone, selegiline, and theophylline. Oral contraceptives may increase (or decrease) the effects of coumarin derivatives.
  Decreased Effect: Acitretin may diminish the therapeutic effect of progestins; contraceptive failure is possible. Oral contraceptives may decrease the plasma concentration of acetaminophen, clofibric acid, lamotrigine, morphine, salicylic acid, and temazepam. Aminoglutethimide, anticonvulsants (carbamazepine, felbamate, oxcarbazepine, phenobarbital, phenytoin, topiramate), aprepitant, phenylbutazone, rifampin, and ritonavir may increase metabolism leading to decreased effect of oral contraceptives. Griseofulvin may diminish the therapeutic effect of contraceptive (progestins). Oral contraceptives may decrease (or increase) the effects of coumarin derivatives. Modafinil and topiramate may decrease the serum concentration of oral contraceptive (estrogens).

Ethanol/Nutrition/Herb Interactions
  Food: CNS effects of caffeine may be enhanced if oral contraceptives are used concurrently with caffeine. Grapefruit juice increases ethinyl estradiol concentrations; clinical implications are unclear.
  Herb/Nutraceutical: St John's wort may decrease the effectiveness of oral contraceptives by inducing hepatic enzymes; may also result in breakthrough bleeding.

Pharmacodynamics/Kinetics
  Distribution: Drospirenone: 4 L/kg; Ethinyl estradiol: 4-5 L/kg
  Protein binding: Drospirenone: Serum proteins (excluding sex hormone-binding globulin and corticosteroid-binding globulin): 97%; Ethinyl estradiol: ~98%
  Metabolism: Drospirenone: To inactive metabolites, minor metabolism hepatically via CYP3A4; Ethinyl estradiol: Hepatic via CYP3A4; forms metabolites
  Bioavailability: Drospirenone: 76%
  Half-life elimination: Drospirenone: 30 hours; Ethinyl estradiol: ~ 24 hours
  Time to peak: Drospirenone: 1-3 hours
  Excretion: Drospirenone, ethinyl estradiol: Urine and feces

Pregnancy Risk Factor X
Dosage Forms TAB: Ethinyl estradiol 0.03 mg and drospirenone 3 mg (28s)

Ethinyl Estradiol and Ethynodiol Diacetate
  (ETH in il es tra DYE ole & e thye noe DYE ole dye AS e tate)

U.S. Brand Names Demulen®; Kelnor™; Zovia™
Canadian Brand Names Demulen® 30
Generic Available Yes
Synonyms Ethynodiol Diacetate and Ethinyl Estradiol
Pharmacologic Category Contraceptive; Estrogen and Progestin Combination
Use Prevention of pregnancy
Unlabeled/Investigational Use Treatment of hypermenorrhea (menorrhagia); pain associated with endometriosis; dysmenorrhea; dysfunctional uterine bleeding
Local Anesthetic/Vasoconstrictor Precautions No information available to require special precautions
Effects on Dental Treatment When prescribing antibiotics, patient must be warned to use additional methods of birth control if on oral contraceptives
Common Adverse Effects Frequency not defined.
  Cardiovascular: Arterial thromboembolism, cerebral hemorrhage, cerebral thrombosis, edema, hypertension, mesenteric thrombosis, MI
  Central nervous system: Depression, dizziness, headache, migraine, nervousness, premenstrual syndrome, stroke
  Dermatologic: Acne, erythema multiforme, erythema nodosum, hirsutism, loss of scalp hair, melasma (may persist), rash (allergic)
(Continued)

Ethinyl Estradiol and Ethynodiol Diacetate *(Continued)*

Endocrine & metabolic: Amenorrhea, breakthrough bleeding, breast enlargement, breast secretion, breast tenderness, carbohydrate intolerance, lactation decreased (postpartum), glucose tolerance decreased, libido changes, menstrual flow changes, sex hormone-binding globulins (SHBG) increased, spotting, temporary infertility (following discontinuation), thyroid-binding globulin increased, triglycerides increased

Gastrointestinal: Abdominal cramps, appetite changes, bloating, cholestasis, colitis, gallbladder disease, jaundice, nausea, vomiting, weight gain/loss

Genitourinary: Cervical erosion changes, cervical secretion changes, cystitis-like syndrome, vaginal candidiasis, vaginitis

Hematologic: Antithrombin III decreased, folate levels decreased, hemolytic uremic syndrome, norepinephrine induced platelet aggregability increased, porphyria, prothrombin increased; factors VII, VIII, IX, and X increased

Hepatic: Benign liver tumors, Budd-Chiari syndrome, cholestatic jaundice, hepatic adenomas

Local: Thrombophlebitis

Ocular: Cataracts, change in corneal curvature (steepening), contact lens intolerance, optic neuritis, retinal thrombosis

Renal: Impaired renal function

Respiratory: Pulmonary thromboembolism

Miscellaneous: Hemorrhagic eruption

Dosage Oral: Adults: Female: Contraception:

Schedule 1 (Sunday starter): Dose begins on first Sunday after onset of menstruation; if the menstrual period starts on Sunday, take first tablet that very same day. **With a Sunday start, an additional method of contraception should be used until after the first 7 days of consecutive administration.**

For 21-tablet package: 1 tablet/day for 21 consecutive days, followed by 7 days off of the medication; a new course begins on the 8th day after the last tablet is taken.

For 28-tablet package: 1 tablet/day without interruption.

Schedule 2 (Day 1 starter): Dose starts on first day of menstrual cycle taking 1 tablet daily.

For 21-tablet package: 1 tablet/day for 21 consecutive days, followed by 7 days off of the medication; a new course begins on the 8th day after the last tablet is taken.

For 28-tablet package: 1 tablet/day without interruption.

If all doses have been taken on schedule and one menstrual period is missed, continue dosing cycle. If two consecutive menstrual periods are missed, pregnancy test is required before new dosing cycle is started.

Missed doses **monophasic formulations** (refer to package insert for complete information):

One dose missed: Take as soon as remembered or take 2 tablets next day

Two consecutive doses missed in the first 2 weeks: Take 2 tablets as soon as remembered or 2 tablets next 2 days. **An additional method of contraception should be used for 7 days after missed dose.**

Two consecutive doses missed in week 3 or three consecutive doses missed at any time: **An additional method of contraception should be used for 7 days after missed dose:**

Schedule 1 (Sunday starter): Continue dose of 1 tablet daily until Sunday, then discard the rest of the pack, and a new pack should be started that same day.

Schedule 2 (Day 1 starter): Current package should be discarded, and a new pack should be started that same day.

Dosage adjustment in renal impairment: Specific guidelines not available; use with caution and monitor blood pressure closely. Consider other forms of contraception.

Dosage adjustment in hepatic impairment: Contraindicated in patients with hepatic impairment

Mechanism of Action Combination hormonal contraceptives inhibit ovulation via a negative feedback mechanism on the hypothalamus, which alters the normal pattern of gonadotropin secretion of a follicle-stimulating hormone (FSH) and luteinizing hormone by the anterior pituitary. The follicular phase FSH and midcycle surge of gonadotropins are inhibited. In addition, combination hormonal contraceptives produce alterations in the genital tract, including changes in the cervical mucus, rendering it unfavorable for sperm penetration even if ovulation occurs. Changes in the endometrium may also occur, producing an unfavorable environment for nidation. Combination hormonal contraceptive drugs may alter the tubal transport of the ova through the fallopian tubes. Progestational agents may also alter sperm fertility.

Contraindications Hypersensitivity to ethinyl estradiol, ethynodiol diacetate, or any component of the formulation; history of or current thrombophlebitis or venous thromboembolic disorders (including DVT, PE); active or recent (within 1 year) arterial thromboembolic disease (eg, stroke, MI); cerebral vascular disease, coronary artery disease, valvular heart disease with complications, severe hypertension; diabetes mellitus with vascular involvement; severe headache with focal neurological symptoms; known or suspected breast carcinoma, endometrial cancer, estrogen-dependent neoplasms, undiagnosed abnormal genital bleeding; hepatic dysfunction or tumor, cholestatic jaundice of pregnancy, jaundice with prior combination hormonal contraceptive use; major surgery with prolonged immobilization; heavy smoking (≥15 cigarettes/day) in patients >35 years of age; pregnancy

Warnings/Precautions Combination hormonal contraceptives do not protect against HIV infection or other sexually-transmitted diseases. The risk of cardiovascular side effects increases in women who smoke cigarettes, especially those who are >35 years of age; women who use combination hormonal contraceptives should be strongly advised not to smoke. Combination hormonal contraceptives may lead to increased risk of myocardial infarction, use with caution in patients with risk factors for coronary artery disease. May increase the risk of thromboembolism. Whenever possible, combination hormonal contraceptives should be discontinued at least 4 weeks prior to and for 2 weeks following elective surgery associated with an increased risk of thromboembolism or during periods of prolonged immobilization. Combination hormonal contraceptives may have a dose-related risk of vascular disease, hypertension, and gallbladder disease. Women with hypertension or renal disease should be encouraged to use a nonhormonal form of contraception. The use of combination hormonal contraceptives has been associated with a slight increase in frequency of breast cancer, however, studies are not consistent. Combination hormonal contraceptives may cause glucose intolerance. Retinal thrombosis has been reported (rarely). Use caution with conditions that may be aggravated by fluid retention, depression, or history of migraine. Not for use prior to menarche.

The minimum dosage combination of estrogen/progestin that will effectively treat the individual patient should be used. New patients should be started on products containing ≤0.035 mg of estrogen per tablet.

Drug Interactions

Cytochrome P450 Effect: Ethinyl estradiol: **Substrate** of CYP2C9 (minor), 3A4 (major), 3A5-7 (minor); **Inhibits** CYP1A2 (weak), 2B6 (weak), 2C8 (weak), 2C19 (weak), 3A4 (weak)

Increased Effect/Toxicity: Acetaminophen and ascorbic acid may increase plasma levels of estrogen component. Atorvastatin and indinavir increase plasma levels of combination hormonal contraceptives. Combination hormonal contraceptives increase the plasma levels of alprazolam, chlordiazepoxide, cyclosporine, diazepam, prednisolone, selegiline, theophylline, tricyclic antidepressants. Combination hormonal contraceptives may increase (or decrease) the effects of coumarin derivatives.

Decreased Effect: CYP3A4 inducers may decrease the levels/effects of ethinyl estradiol; example inducers include aminoglutethimide, carbamazepine, nafcillin, nevirapine, phenobarbital, phenytoin, and rifamycins. Combination hormonal contraceptives may decrease plasma levels of acetaminophen, clofibric acid, lorazepam, morphine, oxazepam, salicylic acid, temazepam. Contraceptive effect decreased by acitretin, aminoglutethimide, amprenavir, anticonvulsants, griseofulvin, lopinavir, nelfinavir, penicillins (effect not consistent), rifampin, ritonavir, tetracyclines (effect not consistent). Combination hormonal contraceptives may decrease (or increase) the effects of coumarin derivatives.

Ethanol/Nutrition/Herb Interactions

Food: CNS effects of caffeine may be enhanced if combination hormonal contraceptives are used concurrently with caffeine. Grapefruit juice increases ethinyl estradiol concentrations and would be expected to increase progesterone serum levels as well; clinical implications are unclear.

Herb/Nutraceutical: St John's wort may decrease the effectiveness of combination hormonal contraceptives by inducing hepatic enzymes. Avoid dong quai and black cohosh (have estrogen activity). Avoid saw palmetto, red clover, ginseng.

Dietary Considerations Should be taken with food at same time each day.

Pharmacodynamics/Kinetics

Ethynodiol diacetate (converted to norethindrone)

Metabolism: Hepatic conjugation

Half-life elimination: Terminal: 5-14 hours

See Norethindrone monograph.

Pregnancy Risk Factor X

(Continued)

Ethinyl Estradiol and Ethynodiol Diacetate *(Continued)*

Dosage Forms TAB, monophasic: (Demulen® 1/35-28, Kelnor™ 1/35, Zovia™ 1/35-28): Ethinyl estradiol 0.035 mg and ethynodiol 1 mg (28s)

Ethinyl Estradiol and Etonogestrel
(ETH in il es tra DYE ole & et oh noe JES trel)

U.S. Brand Names NuvaRing®
Canadian Brand Names NuvaRing®
Generic Available No
Synonyms Etonogestrel and Ethinyl Estradiol
Pharmacologic Category Contraceptive; Estrogen and Progestin Combination
Use Prevention of pregnancy
Unlabeled/Investigational Use Treatment of hypermenorrhea (menorrhagia); pain associated with endometriosis; dysmenorrhea; dysfunctional uterine bleeding
Local Anesthetic/Vasoconstrictor Precautions No information available to require special precautions
Effects on Dental Treatment When prescribing antibiotics, patient must be warned to use additional methods of birth control if on oral contraceptives.
Common Adverse Effects Adverse reactions associated with oral combination hormonal contraceptive agents are also likely to appear with vaginally-administered products (frequency difficult to anticipate). Refer to oral contraceptive monographs for additional information.
5% to 14%:
  Central nervous system: Headache
  Gastrointestinal: Nausea, weight gain
  Genitourinary: Leukorrhea, vaginitis
  Respiratory: Sinusitis, upper respiratory tract infection
Frequency not defined:
  Central nervous system: Emotional lability
  Genitourinary: Bleeding irregularities, coital problems, device expulsion, foreign body sensation, toxic shock syndrome (in some cases associated with tampon use), vaginal discomfort
Dosage Vaginal: Adults: Female: Contraception: One ring, inserted vaginally and left in place for 3 consecutive weeks, then removed for 1 week. A new ring is inserted 7 days after the last was removed (even if bleeding is not complete) and should be inserted at approximately the same time of day the ring was removed the previous week.
Initial treatment should begin as follows (pregnancy should always be ruled out first):
  No hormonal contraceptive use in the past month: Using the first day of menstruation as "Day 1," insert the ring on or prior to "Day 5," even if bleeding is not complete. **An additional form of contraception should be used for the following 7 days.***
  Switching from combination oral contraceptive: Ring can be inserted on any day within 7 days after the last **active** tablet in the cycle was taken and no later than the first day a new cycle of tablets would begin. Additional forms of contraception are not needed.
  Switching from progestin-only contraceptive: **An additional form of contraception should be used for the following 7 days with any of the following.***
    If previously using a progestin-only mini-pill, insert the ring on any day of the month; do not skip days between the last pill and insertion of the ring.
    If previously using an implant, insert the ring on the same day of implant removal.
    If previously using a progestin-containing IUD, insert the ring on day of IUD removal.
    If previously using a progestin injection, insert the ring on the day the next injection would be given.
  Following complete 1st trimester abortion: Insert ring within the first five days of abortion. If not inserted within five days, follow instructions for "No hormonal contraceptive use within the past month" and instruct patient to use a nonhormonal contraceptive in the interim.
  Following delivery or 2nd trimester abortion: Insert ring 4 weeks postpartum (in women who are not breast-feeding) or following 2nd trimester abortion. **An additional form of contraception should be used for the following 7 days.***
  If the ring is accidentally removed from the vagina at anytime during the 3-week period of use, it may be rinsed with cool or lukewarm water (not hot) and

reinserted as soon as possible. If the ring is not reinserted within three hours, contraceptive effectiveness will be decreased. **An additional form of contraception should be used until the ring has been in place for 7 consecutive days.***

If the ring has been removed for longer than 1 week, pregnancy must be ruled out prior to restarting therapy. **An additional form of contraception should be used for the following 7 days.***

If the ring has been left in place for >3 weeks, a new ring should be inserted following a 1-week (ring-free) interval. Pregnancy must be ruled out prior to insertion and **an additional form of contraception should be used for the following 7 days.***

Disconnected ring: In the event the ring disconnects at the weld joint, discard and replace with a new ring.

*Note: Diaphragms may interfere with proper ring placement, and therefore, are not recommended for use as an additional form of contraception.

Dosage adjustment in renal impairment: Specific guidelines not available; use with caution and monitor blood pressure closely. Consider other forms of contraception.

Dosage adjustment in hepatic impairment: Contraindicated in patients with hepatic impairment

Mechanism of Action Combination hormonal contraceptives inhibit ovulation via a negative feedback mechanism on the hypothalamus, which alters the normal pattern of gonadotropin secretion of a follicle-stimulating hormone (FSH) and luteinizing hormone by the anterior pituitary. The follicular phase FSH and midcycle surge of gonadotropins are inhibited. In addition, combination hormonal contraceptives produce alterations in the genital tract, including changes in the cervical mucus, rendering it unfavorable for sperm penetration even if ovulation occurs. Changes in the endometrium may also occur, producing an unfavorable environment for nidation. Combination hormonal contraceptive drugs may alter the tubal transport of the ova through the fallopian tubes. Progestational agents may also alter sperm fertility.

Contraindications Hypersensitivity to ethinyl estradiol, etonogestrel, or any component of the formulation; history of or current thrombophlebitis or venous thromboembolic disorders (including DVT, PE); active or recent (within 1 year) arterial thromboembolic disease (eg, stroke, MI); major surgery with prolonged immobilization, cerebral vascular disease, coronary artery disease, valvular heart disease with complications, severe hypertension; diabetes mellitus with vascular involvement; severe headache with focal neurological symptoms; known or suspected breast carcinoma, endometrial cancer, estrogen-dependent neoplasms, undiagnosed abnormal genital bleeding; hepatic dysfunction or tumor, cholestatic jaundice of pregnancy, jaundice with prior combination hormonal contraceptive use; heavy smoking (≥15 cigarettes/day) in patients >35 years of age; conditions which make the vagina susceptible to irritation or ulceration; pregnancy

Warnings/Precautions Combination hormonal contraceptive agents do not protect against HIV infection or other sexually-transmitted diseases. The risk of cardiovascular side effects increases in women who smoke cigarettes, especially those who are >35 years of age; women who use combination hormonal contraceptives should be strongly advised not to smoke. May lead to increased risk of myocardial infarction, use with caution in patients with risk factors for coronary artery disease. May increase the risk of thromboembolism. Whenever possible, combination hormonal contraceptives should be discontinued at least 4 weeks prior to and for 2 weeks following elective surgery associated with an increased risk of thromboembolism or during periods of prolonged immobilization. May have a dose-related risk of vascular disease, hypertension, and gallbladder disease. Women with hypertension or renal disease should be encouraged to use another form of contraception. May cause glucose intolerance. Retinal thrombosis has been reported (rarely). Use caution with conditions that may be aggravated by fluid retention, depression, or history of migraine. Not for use prior to menarche.

Vaginally-administered combination hormonal contraceptive agents may have a similar adverse effects associated with oral contraceptive products. In order to reduce some of the possible risks, the minimum dosage combination of estrogen/progestin that will effectively treat the individual patient should be used.

Drug Interactions
Cytochrome P450 Effect:
Ethinyl estradiol: **Substrate** of CYP2C9 (minor), 3A4 (major), 3A5-7 (minor); **Inhibits** CYP1A2 (weak), 2B6 (weak), 2C8 (weak), 2C19 (weak), 3A4 (weak)

Etonogestrel: **Substrate** of CYP3A4 (minor)

(Continued)

Ethinyl Estradiol and Etonogestrel *(Continued)*

Increased Effect/Toxicity: Acetaminophen and ascorbic acid may increase plasma levels of estrogen component. Atorvastatin and indinavir increase plasma levels of combination hormonal contraceptives. Combination hormonal contraceptives increase the plasma levels of alprazolam, chlordiazepoxide, cyclosporine, diazepam, prednisolone, selegiline, theophylline, tricyclic antidepressants. Combination hormonal contraceptives may increase (or decrease) the effects of coumarin derivatives.

Decreased Effect: Combination hormonal contraceptives may decrease plasma levels of acetaminophen, clofibric acid, lorazepam, morphine, oxazepam, salicylic acid, temazepam. Contraceptive effect decreased by acitretin, aminoglutethimide, amprenavir, anticonvulsants, griseofulvin, lopinavir, nelfinavir, nevirapine, penicillins (effect not consistent), rifampin, ritonavir, tetracyclines (effect not consistent). Combination hormonal contraceptives may decrease (or increase) the effects of coumarin derivatives.

Ethanol/Nutrition/Herb Interactions

Food: CNS effects of caffeine may be enhanced if combination hormonal contraceptives are used concurrently with caffeine. Grapefruit juice increases ethinyl estradiol concentrations and would be expected to increase progesterone serum levels as well; clinical implications are unclear.

Herb/Nutraceutical: St John's wort may decrease the effectiveness of combination hormonal contraceptives by inducing hepatic enzymes. Avoid dong quai and black cohosh (have estrogen activity). Avoid saw palmetto, red clover, ginseng.

Pharmacodynamics/Kinetics

Duration: Serum levels (contraceptive effectiveness) decrease after 3 weeks of continuous use

Absorption: Ethinyl estradiol and etonogestrel: Rapid
Tampons do not interfere with absorption.

Protein binding:
Ethinyl estradiol: 98%, primarily to albumin
Etonogestrel: 32% to sex hormone-binding globulin (SHBG) and 66% to albumin; SHBG capacity is affected by plasma ethinyl estradiol levels

Metabolism:
Ethinyl estradiol: Hepatic via CYP3A4; forms metabolites (weak estrogenic activity)
Etonogestrel: Hepatic via CYP3A4; forms metabolites (activity not known)

Bioavailability: Ethinyl estradiol: ~56% Etonogestrel: 100%

Half-life elimination: Ethinyl estradiol: 45 hours; Etonogestrel: 29 hours

Excretion: Ethinyl estradiol and etonogestrel: Urine, bile, and feces

Pregnancy Risk Factor X

Dosage Forms RING, vaginal [3-week duration]: Ethinyl estradiol 0.015 mg/day and etonogestrel 0.12 mg/day (1s) [3-week duration]

Ethinyl Estradiol and Levonorgestrel

(ETH in il es tra DYE ole & LEE voe nor jes trel)

Related Information

Levonorgestrel *on page 916*

U.S. Brand Names Alesse®; Aviane™; Enpresse™; Lessina™; Levlen®; Levlite™; Levora®; Lutera™; Nordette®; Portia™; PREVEN®; Seasonale®; Tri-Levlen®; Triphasil®; Trivora®

Canadian Brand Names Alesse®; Min-Ovral®; Triphasil®; Triquilar®

Generic Available Yes

Synonyms Levonorgestrel and Ethinyl Estradiol

Pharmacologic Category Contraceptive; Estrogen and Progestin Combination

Use Prevention of pregnancy; postcoital contraception

Unlabeled/Investigational Use Treatment of hypermenorrhea (menorrhagia); pain associated with endometriosis; dysmenorrhea; dysfunctional uterine bleeding

Local Anesthetic/Vasoconstrictor Precautions No information available to require special precautions

Effects on Dental Treatment When prescribing antibiotics, patient must be warned to use additional methods of birth control if on oral contraceptives.

Common Adverse Effects Frequency not defined.

Cardiovascular: Arterial thromboembolism, cerebral hemorrhage, cerebral thrombosis, edema, hypertension, mesenteric thrombosis, MI

Central nervous system: Depression, dizziness, headache, migraine, nervousness, premenstrual syndrome, stroke

Dermatologic: Acne, erythema multiforme, erythema nodosum, hirsutism, loss of scalp hair, melasma (may persist), rash (allergic)

Endocrine & metabolic: Amenorrhea, breakthrough bleeding, breast enlargement, breast secretion, breast tenderness, carbohydrate intolerance, lactation decreased (postpartum), glucose tolerance decreased, libido changes, menstrual flow changes, sex hormone-binding globulins (SHBG) increased, spotting, temporary infertility (following discontinuation), thyroid-binding globulin increased, triglycerides increased

Gastrointestinal: Abdominal cramps, appetite changes, bloating, cholestasis, colitis, gallbladder disease, jaundice, nausea, vomiting, weight gain/loss

Genitourinary: Cervical erosion changes, cervical secretion changes, cystitis-like syndrome, vaginal candidiasis, vaginitis

Hematologic: Antithrombin III decreased, folate levels decreased, hemolytic uremic syndrome, norepinephrine induced platelet aggregability increased, porphyria, prothrombin increased; factors VII, VIII, IX, and X increased

Hepatic: Benign liver tumors, Budd-Chiari syndrome, cholestatic jaundice, hepatic adenomas

Local: Thrombophlebitis

Ocular: Cataracts, change in corneal curvature (steepening), contact lens intolerance, optic neuritis, retinal thrombosis

Renal: Impaired renal function

Respiratory: Pulmonary thromboembolism

Miscellaneous: Hemorrhagic eruption

Dosage Oral: Adults: Female:

Contraception, 28-day cycle:

Schedule 1 (Sunday starter): Dose begins on first Sunday after onset of menstruation; if the menstrual period starts on Sunday, take first tablet that very same day. With a Sunday start, an additional method of contraception should be used until after the first 7 days of consecutive administration:

For 21-tablet package: 1 tablet/day for 21 consecutive days, followed by 7 days off of the medication; a new course begins on the 8th day after the last tablet is taken

For 28-tablet package: 1 tablet/day without interruption

Schedule 2 (Day 1 starter): Dose starts on first day of menstrual cycle taking 1 tablet/day:

For 21-tablet package: 1 tablet/day for 21 consecutive days, followed by 7 days off of the medication; a new course begins on the 8th day after the last tablet is taken

For 28-tablet package: 1 tablet/day without interruption

If all doses have been taken on schedule and one menstrual period is missed, continue dosing cycle. If two consecutive menstrual periods are missed, pregnancy test is required before new dosing cycle is started.

Missed doses **monophasic formulations** (refer to package insert for complete information):

One dose missed: Take as soon as remembered or take 2 tablets next day

Two consecutive doses missed in the first 2 weeks: Take 2 tablets as soon as remembered or 2 tablets next 2 days. An additional method of contraception should be used for 7 days after missed dose.

Two consecutive doses missed in week 3 or three consecutive doses missed at any time: An additional method of contraception must be used for 7 days after a missed dose:

Schedule 1 (Sunday starter): Continue dose of 1 tablet daily until Sunday, then discard the rest of the pack, and a new pack should be started that same day.

Schedule 2 (Day 1 starter): Current pack should be discarded, and a new pack should be started that same day.

Missed doses **biphasic/triphasic formulations** (refer to package insert for complete information):

One dose missed: Take as soon as remembered or take 2 tablets next day.

Two consecutive doses missed in week 1 or week 2 of the pack: Take 2 tablets as soon as remembered and 2 tablets the next day. Resume taking 1 tablet daily until the pack is empty. An additional method of contraception should be used for 7 days after a missed dose.

Two consecutive doses missed in week 3 of the pack: An additional method of contraception must be used for 7 days after a missed dose.

Schedule 1 (Sunday starter): Take 1 tablet every day until Sunday. Discard the remaining pack and start a new pack of pills on the same day.

Schedule 2 (Day 1 starter): Discard the remaining pack and start a new pack the same day.

Three or more consecutive doses missed: An additional method of contraception must be used for 7 days after a missed dose.

(Continued)

Ethinyl Estradiol and Levonorgestrel *(Continued)*

Schedule 1 (Sunday starter): Take 1 tablet every day until Sunday; on Sunday, discard the pack and start a new pack.

Schedule 2 (Day 1 starter): Discard the remaining pack and begin new pack of tablets starting on the same day.

Contraception, 91-day cycle (Seasonale®): One active tablet/day for 84 consecutive days, followed by 1 inactive tablet/day for 7 days; if all doses have been taken on schedule and one menstrual period is missed, pregnancy should be ruled out prior to continuing therapy.

Missed doses:

One dose missed: Take as soon as remembered or take 2 tablets the next day

Two consecutive doses missed: Take 2 tablets as soon as remembered or 2 tablets the next 2 days. An additional nonhormonal method of contraception should be used for 7 consecutive days after the missed dose.

Three or more consecutive doses missed: Do not take the missed doses; continue taking 1 tablet/day until pack is complete. Bleeding may occur during the following week. An additional nonhormonal method of contraception should be used for 7 consecutive days after the missed dose.

Emergency contraception (PREVEN®): Initial: 2 tablets as soon as possible (but within 72 hours of unprotected intercourse), followed by a second dose of 2 tablets 12 hours later. Repeat dose or use antiemetic if vomiting occurs within 1 hour of dose.

Dosage adjustment in renal impairment: Specific guidelines not available; use with caution and monitor blood pressure closely. Consider other forms of contraception.

Dosage adjustment in hepatic impairment: Contraindicated in patients with hepatic impairment

Mechanism of Action Combination hormonal contraceptives inhibit ovulation via a negative feedback mechanism on the hypothalamus, which alters the normal pattern of gonadotropin secretion of a follicle-stimulating hormone (FSH) and luteinizing hormone by the anterior pituitary. The follicular phase FSH and midcycle surge of gonadotropins are inhibited. In addition, combination hormonal contraceptives produce alterations in the genital tract, including changes in the cervical mucus, rendering it unfavorable for sperm penetration even if ovulation occurs. Changes in the endometrium may also occur, producing an unfavorable environment for nidation. Combination hormonal contraceptive drugs may alter the tubal transport of the ova through the fallopian tubes. Progestational agents may also alter sperm fertility.

Contraindications Hypersensitivity to ethinyl estradiol, levonorgestrel, or any component of the formulation; history of or current thrombophlebitis or venous thromboembolic disorders (including DVT, PE); active or recent (within 1 year) arterial thromboembolic disease (eg, stroke, MI); cerebral vascular disease, coronary artery disease, valvular heart disease with complications, severe hypertension; diabetes mellitus with vascular involvement; severe headache with focal neurological symptoms; known or suspected breast carcinoma, endometrial cancer, estrogen-dependent neoplasms, undiagnosed abnormal genital bleeding; hepatic dysfunction or tumor, cholestatic jaundice of pregnancy, jaundice with prior combination hormonal contraceptive use; major surgery with prolonged immobilization; heavy smoking (≥15 cigarettes/day) in patients >35 years of age; pregnancy

Warnings/Precautions Combination hormonal contraceptives do not protect against HIV infection or other sexually-transmitted diseases. The risk of cardiovascular side effects increases in women who smoke cigarettes, especially those who are >35 years of age; women who use combination hormonal contraceptives should be strongly advised not to smoke. Combination hormonal contraceptives may lead to increased risk of myocardial infarction, use with caution in patients with risk factors for coronary artery disease. May increase the risk of thromboembolism. Whenever possible, combination hormonal contraceptives should be discontinued at least 4 weeks prior to and for 2 weeks following elective surgery associated with an increased risk of thromboembolism or during periods of prolonged immobilization. Combination hormonal contraceptives may have a dose-related risk of vascular disease, hypertension, and gallbladder disease. Women with hypertension or renal disease should be encouraged to use another form of contraception. The use of combination hormonal contraceptives has been associated with a slight increase in frequency of breast cancer, however, studies are not consistent. Combination hormonal contraceptives may cause glucose intolerance. Retinal thrombosis has been reported (rarely). Use caution with conditions that may be aggravated by fluid retention, depression, or history of migraine. Not for use prior to menarche.

The minimum dosage combination of estrogen/progestin that will effectively treat the individual patient should be used. New patients should be started on products containing ≤0.035 mg of estrogen per tablet.

Drug Interactions

Cytochrome P450 Effect:

Ethinyl estradiol: **Substrate** of CYP2C9 (minor), 3A4 (major), 3A5-7 (minor); **Inhibits** CYP1A2 (weak), 2B6 (weak), 2C8 (weak), 2C19 (weak), 3A4 (weak)

Levonorgestrel: **Substrate** of CYP3A4 (major)

Increased Effect/Toxicity: Acetaminophen and ascorbic acid may increase plasma levels of estrogen component. Atorvastatin and indinavir increase plasma levels of combination hormonal contraceptives. Combination hormonal contraceptives increase the plasma levels of alprazolam, chlordiazepoxide, cyclosporine, diazepam, prednisolone, selegiline, theophylline, tricyclic antidepressants. Combination hormonal contraceptives may increase (or decrease) the effects of coumarin derivatives.

Decreased Effect: CYP3A4 inducers may decrease the levels/effects of ethinyl estradiol and/or levonorgestrel; example inducers include aminoglutethimide, carbamazepine, nafcillin, nevirapine, phenobarbital, phenytoin, and rifamycins. Combination hormonal contraceptives may decrease plasma levels of acetaminophen, clofibric acid, lorazepam, morphine, oxazepam, salicylic acid, temazepam. Contraceptive effect decreased by acitretin, aminoglutethimide, amprenavir, anticonvulsants, griseofulvin, lopinavir, nelfinavir, penicillins (effect not consistent), rifampin, ritonavir, tetracyclines (effect not consistent). Combination hormonal contraceptives may decrease (or increase) the effects of coumarin derivatives.

Ethanol/Nutrition/Herb Interactions

Food: CNS effects of caffeine may be enhanced if combination hormonal contraceptives are used concurrently with caffeine. Grapefruit juice increases ethinyl estradiol concentrations and would be expected to increase progesterone serum levels as well; clinical implications are unclear.

Herb/Nutraceutical: St John's wort may decrease the effectiveness of combination hormonal contraceptives by inducing hepatic enzymes. Avoid dong quai and black cohosh (have estrogen activity). Avoid saw palmetto, red clover, ginseng.

Dietary Considerations Should be taken at the same time each day.

Pharmacodynamics/Kinetics See individual agents.

Pregnancy Risk Factor X

Dosage Forms KIT [4 tablets and a pregnancy test] (PREVEN®): Ethinyl estradiol 0.05 mg and levonorgestrel 0.25 mg (4s). **TAB** (PREVEN®): Ethinyl estradiol 0.05 mg and levonorgestrel 0.25 mg (4s). **TAB, low-dose:** (Alesse®, Lessina™, Levlite™. Lutera™): Ethinyl estradiol 0.02 mg and levonorgestrel 0.1 mg (28s); (Aviane™ 28): Ethinyl estradiol 0.02 mg and levonorgestrel 0.1 mg. **TAB, monophasic:** (Nordette®): Ethinyl estradiol 0.03 mg and levonorgestrel 0.15 mg (21s, 28s); (Seasonale®): Ethinyl estradiol 0.03 mg and levonorgestrel 0.15 mg (91s). **TAB, triphasic:** (Enpresse™): Day 1-6: Ethinyl estradiol 0.03 mg and levonorgestrel 0.05, Day 7-11: Ethinyl estradiol 0.04 mg and levonorgestrel 0.075, Day 12-21: Ethinyl estradiol 0.03 mg and levonorgestrel 0.125; (Tri-Levlen® 28, Triphasil® 28): Day 1-6: Ethinyl estradiol 0.03 mg and levonorgestrel 0.05 mg, Day 7-11: Ethinyl estradiol 0.04 mg and levonorgestrel 0.075 mg, Day 12-21: Ethinyl estradiol 0.03 mg and levonorgestrel 0.125 mg, Day 22-28: Inactive (28s); (Trivora® 28): Day 1-6: Ethinyl estradiol 0.03 mg and levonorgestrel 0.05 mg, Day 7-11: Ethinyl estradiol 0.04 mg and levonorgestrel 0.075 mg, Day 12-21: Ethinyl estradiol 0.03 mg and levonorgestrel 0.125 mg, Day 22-28: Inactive (28s)

Ethinyl Estradiol and NGM *see* Ethinyl Estradiol and Norgestimate *on page 613*

Ethinyl Estradiol and Norelgestromin
(ETH in il es tra DYE ole & nor el JES troe min)

U.S. Brand Names Ortho Evra®

Canadian Brand Names Evra®

Synonyms Norelgestromin and Ethinyl Estradiol; Ortho-Evra

Pharmacologic Category Contraceptive; Estrogen and Progestin Combination

Use Prevention of pregnancy

Local Anesthetic/Vasoconstrictor Precautions No information available to require special precautions

Effects on Dental Treatment When prescribing antibiotics, patient must be warned to use additional methods of birth control if on oral contraceptives.

(Continued)

Ethinyl Estradiol and Norelgestromin *(Continued)*

Common Adverse Effects The following reactions have been reported with the contraceptive patch. Adverse reactions associated with oral combination hormonal contraceptive agents are also likely to appear with the topical contraceptive patch (frequency difficult to anticipate). Refer to individual **oral** contraceptive monographs for additional information.

9% to 22%: Abdominal pain, application site reaction, breast symptoms, headache, menstrual cramps, nausea, upper respiratory infection

Dosage Topical: Adults: Female:

Contraception: Apply one patch each week for 3 weeks (21 total days); followed by one week that is patch-free. Each patch should be applied on the same day each week ("patch change day") and only one patch should be worn at a time. No more than 7 days should pass during the patch-free interval.

Schedule 1 (Sunday starter): Dose begins on first Sunday after onset of menstruation; if the menstrual period starts on Sunday, apply one patch that very same day. **With a Sunday start, an additional method of contraception (nonhormonal) should be used until after the first 7 days of consecutive administration.** Each patch change will then occur on Sunday.

Schedule 2 (Day 1 starter): Dose starts on first day of menstrual cycle, applying one patch during the first 24 hours of menstrual cycle. No back-up method of contraception is needed as long as the patch is applied on the first day of cycle. Each patch change will then occur on that same day of the week.

Additional dosing considerations:

No bleeding during patch-free week/missed menstrual period: If patch has been applied as directed, continue treatment on usual "patch change day". If used correctly, no bleeding during patch-free week does not necessarily indicate pregnancy. However, if no withdrawal bleeding occurs for 2 consecutive cycles, pregnancy should be ruled out. If patch has not been applied as directed, and one menstrual period is missed, pregnancy should be ruled out prior to continuing treatment.

If a patch becomes partially or completely detached for <24 hours: Try to reapply to same place, or replace with a new patch immediately. Do not reapply if patch is no longer sticky, if it is sticking to itself or another surface, or if it has material sticking to it.

If a patch becomes partially or completely detached for >24 hours (or time period is unknown): Apply a new patch and use this day of the week as the new "patch change day" from this point on. **An additional method of contraception (nonhormonal) should be used until after the first 7 days of consecutive administration.**

Switching from oral contraceptives: Apply first patch on the first day of withdrawal bleeding. If there is no bleeding within 5 days of taking the last active tablet, pregnancy must first be ruled out. If patch is applied later than the first day of bleeding, **an additional method of contraception (nonhormonal) should be used until after the first 7 days of consecutive administration**

Use after childbirth: Therapy should not be started <4 weeks after childbirth. Pregnancy should be ruled out prior to treatment if menstrual periods have not restarted. **An additional method of contraception (nonhormonal) should be used until after the first 7 days of consecutive administration.**

Use after abortion or miscarriage: Therapy may be started immediately if abortion/miscarriage occur within the first trimester. If therapy is not started within 5 days, follow instructions for first time use. If abortion/miscarriage occur during the second trimester, therapy should not be started for at least 4 weeks. Follow directions for use after childbirth.

Dosage adjustment in renal impairment: Specific guidelines not available; use with caution and monitor blood pressure closely. Consider other forms of contraception.

Dosage adjustment in hepatic impairment: Contraindicated in patients with hepatic impairment

Mechanism of Action Combination hormonal contraceptives inhibit ovulation via a negative feedback mechanism on the hypothalamus, which alters the normal pattern of gonadotropin secretion of a follicle-stimulating hormone (FSH) and luteinizing hormone by the anterior pituitary. The follicular phase FSH and midcycle surge of gonadotropins are inhibited. In addition, combination hormonal contraceptives produce alterations in the genital tract, including changes in the cervical mucus, rendering it unfavorable for sperm penetration even if ovulation occurs. Changes in the endometrium may also occur, producing an unfavorable environment for nidation. Combination hormonal contraceptive drugs may alter the tubal transport of the ova through the fallopian tubes. Progestational agents may also alter sperm fertility.

Contraindications Hypersensitivity to ethinyl estradiol, norelgestromin, or any component of the formulation; history of or current thrombophlebitis or venous thromboembolic disorders (including DVT, PE); active or recent (within 1 year) arterial thromboembolic disease (eg, stroke, MI); cerebral vascular disease, coronary artery disease, valvular heart disease with complications, severe hypertension; diabetes mellitus with vascular involvement; severe headache with focal neurological symptoms; known or suspected breast carcinoma, endometrial cancer, estrogen-dependent neoplasms, undiagnosed abnormal genital bleeding; hepatic dysfunction or tumor, cholestatic jaundice of pregnancy, jaundice with prior combination hormonal contraceptive use; major surgery with prolonged immobilization; heavy smoking (≥15 cigarettes/day) in patients >35 years of age; pregnancy

Warnings/Precautions Combination hormonal contraceptives do not protect against HIV infection or other sexually-transmitted diseases. The risk of cardiovascular side effects increases in women who smoke cigarettes, especially those who are >35 years of age; women who use combination hormonal contraceptives should be strongly advised not to smoke. Combination hormonal contraceptives may lead to increased risk of myocardial infarction, use with caution in patients with risk factors for coronary artery disease. May increase the risk of thromboembolism. Whenever possible, combination hormonal contraceptives should be discontinued at least 4 weeks prior to and for 2 weeks following elective surgery associated with an increased risk of thromboembolism or during periods of prolonged immobilization. Combination hormonal contraceptives may have a dose-related risk of vascular disease, hypertension, and gallbladder disease. Women with hypertension or renal disease should be encouraged to use a nonhormonal form of contraception. The use of combination hormonal contraceptives has been associated with a slight increase in frequency of breast cancer, however, studies are not consistent. Combination hormonal contraceptives may cause glucose intolerance. Retinal thrombosis has been reported (rarely). Use caution with conditions that may be aggravated by fluid retention, depression, or history of migraine. Not for use prior to menarche.

The combination hormonal contraceptive patch may have adverse effects similar to those associated with oral contraceptive products. The topical patch may be less effective in patients weighing ≥90 kg (198 lb) and an increased incidence of pregnancy has been reported in this population; consider another form of contraception. Transdermal patch may contain conducting metal (eg, aluminum); remove patch prior to MRI. The amount of ethinyl estradiol absorbed from the patch results in greater exposure than achieved if administered orally. The increased estrogen exposure from the topical patch should be balanced against the potential for pregnancy if compliance using an oral contraceptive tablet is poor; the difference in risk of serious adverse effects between the two dosage forms is not known. Variability in actual estrogen exposure may be greater in women using the topical patch when compared to women using the oral tablet. The minimum dosage combination of estrogen/progestin that will effectively treat the individual patient should be used.

Drug Interactions
  Cytochrome P450 Effect:
    Ethinyl estradiol: **Substrate** of CYP2C9 (minor), 3A4 (major), 3A5-7 (minor); **Inhibits** CYP1A2 (weak), 2B6 (weak), 2C8 (weak), 2C19 (weak), 3A4 (weak)

    Norelgestromin: **Substrate** of CYP3A4 (minor)

  Increased Effect/Toxicity: Acetaminophen and ascorbic acid may increase plasma levels of estrogen component. Atorvastatin and indinavir increase plasma levels of combination hormonal contraceptives. Combination hormonal contraceptives increase the plasma levels of alprazolam, chlordiazepoxide, cyclosporine, diazepam, prednisolone, selegiline, theophylline, tricyclic antidepressants. Combination hormonal contraceptives may increase (or decrease) the effects of coumarin derivatives.

  Decreased Effect: CYP3A4 inducers may decrease the levels/effects of ethinyl estradiol; example inducers include aminoglutethimide, carbamazepine, nafcillin, nevirapine, phenobarbital, phenytoin, and rifamycins. Combination hormonal contraceptives may decrease plasma levels of acetaminophen, clofibric acid, lorazepam, morphine, oxazepam, salicylic acid, temazepam. Contraceptive effect decreased by acitretin, aminoglutethimide, amprenavir, anticonvulsants, griseofulvin, lopinavir, nelfinavir, penicillins (effect not consistent), rifampin, ritonavir, tetracyclines (effect not consistent), troglitazone. Combination hormonal contraceptives may decrease (or increase) the effects of coumarin derivatives.

Ethanol/Nutrition/Herb Interactions
  Food: CNS effects of caffeine may be enhanced if combination hormonal contraceptives are used concurrently with caffeine. Grapefruit juice increases
(Continued)

Ethinyl Estradiol and Norelgestromin *(Continued)*

ethinyl estradiol concentrations and would be expected to increase progesterone serum levels as well; clinical implications are unclear.

Herb/Nutraceutical: St John's wort may decrease the effectiveness of combination hormonal contraceptives by inducing hepatic enzymes. Avoid dong quai and black cohosh (have estrogen activity). Avoid saw palmetto, red clover, ginseng.

Pharmacodynamics/Kinetics

Ortho Evra®:

Absorption: Topical: Equivalent when applied to abdomen, buttock, upper outer arm, and upper torso

Ethinyl estradiol and norelgestromin: Rapid; reaches plateau by ~48 hours. Absorption of ethinyl estradiol may be increased with heat exposure due to sauna, whirlpool, or treadmill.

The amount of ethinyl estradiol absorbed is 20 mcg/day and results in greater exposure than produced by oral ethinyl estradiol 20 mcg. In contrast, peak levels of ethinyl estradiol are higher in women taking oral tablets.

Protein binding: Norelgestromin: >97% to albumin

Metabolism: Topical:

Ethinyl estradiol: First-pass effect avoided; forms metabolites

Norelgestromin: Hepatic to norgestrel and others; first-pass effect avoided

Bioavailability: Ethinyl estradiol: ~60% greater using the topical patch when compared to oral tablets.

Half-life elimination: Topical:

Ethinyl estradiol: 17 hours

Norelgestromin: 28 hours

Excretion: Ethinyl estradiol and norelgestromin: Urine and feces

Pregnancy Risk Factor X

Dosage Forms PATCH, transdermal: Ethinyl estradiol 0.75 mg and norelgestromin 6 mg (1s, 3s)

Canadian Formulation: **PATCH, transdermal:** Ethinyl estradiol 0.6 mg and norelgestromin 6 mg (1s, 3s).**Note:** The formulation available in Canada differs from the U.S. product in both composition and the manufacturing process (although delivery rates appear similar).

Ethinyl Estradiol and Norethindrone

(ETH in il es tra DYE ole & nor eth IN drone)

Related Information

Norethindrone *on page 1125*

U.S. Brand Names Aranelle™; Brevicon®; Estrostep® Fe; femhrt®; Junel™; Junel™ Fe; Leena™; Loestrin®; Loestrin® 24 Fe; Loestrin® Fe; Microgestin™; Microgestin™ Fe; Modicon®; Necon® 0.5/35; Necon® 1/35; Necon® 7/7/7; Necon® 10/11; Norinyl® 1+35; Nortrel™; Nortrel™ 7/7/7; Ortho-Novum®; Ovcon®; Tri-Norinyl®

Canadian Brand Names Brevicon® 0.5/35; Brevicon® 1/35; FemHRT®; Loestrin™ 1.5/30; Minestrin™ 1/20; Ortho® 0.5/35; Ortho® 1/35; Ortho® 7/7/7; Select™ 1/35; Synphasic®

Generic Available Yes

Synonyms Norethindrone Acetate and Ethinyl Estradiol; Ortho Novum

Pharmacologic Category Contraceptive; Estrogen and Progestin Combination

Use Prevention of pregnancy; treatment of acne; moderate to severe vasomotor symptoms associated with menopause; prevention of osteoporosis (in women at significant risk only)

Unlabeled/Investigational Use Treatment of hypermenorrhea (menorrhagia); pain associated with endometriosis, dysmenorrhea; dysfunctional uterine bleeding

Local Anesthetic/Vasoconstrictor Precautions No information available to require special precautions

Effects on Dental Treatment When prescribing antibiotics, patient must be warned to use additional methods of birth control if on oral contraceptives.

Common Adverse Effects As reported with oral contraceptive agents. Frequency not defined.

Cardiovascular: Arterial thromboembolism, cerebral hemorrhage, cerebral thrombosis, edema, hypertension, mesenteric thrombosis, MI

Central nervous system: Depression, dizziness, headache, migraine, nervousness, premenstrual syndrome, stroke

Dermatologic: Acne, erythema multiforme, erythema nodosum, hirsutism, loss of scalp hair, melasma (may persist), rash (allergic)

Endocrine & metabolic: Amenorrhea, breakthrough bleeding, breast enlargement, breast secretion, breast tenderness, carbohydrate intolerance, lactation decreased (postpartum), glucose tolerance decreased, libido changes, menstrual flow changes, sex hormone-binding globulins (SHBG) increased, spotting, temporary infertility (following discontinuation), thyroid-binding globulin increased, triglycerides increased

Gastrointestinal: Abdominal cramps, appetite changes, bloating, cholestasis, colitis, gallbladder disease, jaundice, nausea, vomiting, weight gain/loss

Genitourinary: Cervical erosion changes, cervical secretion changes, cystitis-like syndrome, vaginal candidiasis, vaginitis

Hematologic: Antithrombin III decreased, folate levels decreased, hemolytic uremic syndrome, norepinephrine induced platelet aggregability increased, porphyria, prothrombin increased; factors VII, VIII, IX, and X

Hepatic: Benign liver tumors, Budd-Chiari syndrome, cholestatic jaundice, hepatic adenomas

Local: Thrombophlebitis

Ocular: Cataracts, change in corneal curvature (steepening), contact lens intolerance, optic neuritis, retinal thrombosis

Renal: Impaired renal function

Respiratory: Pulmonary thromboembolism

Miscellaneous: Hemorrhagic eruption

Dosage Oral:

Adolescents ≥15 years and Adults: Female: Acne: Estrostep®: Refer to dosing for contraception

Adults: Female:

Moderate-to-severe vasomotor symptoms associated with menopause: Initial: femhrt® 0.5/2.5: 1 tablet daily; patient should be re-evaluated at 3- to 6-month intervals to determine if treatment is still necessary; patient should be maintained at the lowest effective dose

Prevention of osteoporosis: Initial: femhrt® 0.5/2.5: 1 tablet daily; patient should be maintained on the lowest effective dose

Contraception:

Schedule 1 (Sunday starter): Dose begins on first Sunday after onset of menstruation; if the menstrual period starts on Sunday, take first tablet that very same day. With a Sunday start, an additional method of contraception should be used until after the first 7 days of consecutive administration.

For 21-tablet package: Dosage is 1 tablet daily for 21 consecutive days, followed by 7 days off of the medication; a new course begins on the 8th day after the last tablet is taken.

For 28-tablet package: Dosage is 1 tablet daily without interruption.

Schedule 2 (Day 1 starter): Dose starts on first day of menstrual cycle taking 1 tablet daily.

For 21-tablet package: Dosage is 1 tablet daily for 21 consecutive days, followed by 7 days off of the medication; a new course begins on the 8th day after the last tablet is taken.

For 28-tablet package: Dosage is 1 tablet daily without interruption.

If all doses have been taken on schedule and one menstrual period is missed, continue dosing cycle. If two consecutive menstrual periods are missed, pregnancy test is required before new dosing cycle is started.

Missed doses **monophasic formulations** (refer to package insert for complete information):

One dose missed: Take as soon as remembered or take 2 tablets next day

Two consecutive doses missed in the first 2 weeks: Take 2 tablets as soon as remembered or 2 tablets next 2 days. An additional method of contraception should be used for 7 days after missed dose.

Two consecutive doses missed in week 3 or three consecutive doses missed at any time: An additional method of contraception must be used for 7 days after a missed dose.

Schedule 1 (Sunday starter): Continue dose of 1 tablet daily until Sunday, then discard the rest of the pack, and a new pack should be started that same day.

Schedule 2 (Day 1 starter): Current pack should be discarded, and a new pack should be started that same day.

Missed doses **biphasic/triphasic formulations** (refer to package insert for complete information):

One dose missed: Take as soon as remembered or take 2 tablets next day.

Two consecutive doses missed in week 1 or week 2 of the pack: Take 2 tablets as soon as remembered and 2 tablets the next day. Resume taking 1 tablet daily until the pack is empty. An additional method of contraception should be used for 7 days after a missed dose.

(Continued)

Ethinyl Estradiol and Norethindrone *(Continued)*

Two consecutive doses missed in week 3 of the pack: An additional method of contraception must be used for 7 days after a missed dose.

Schedule 1 (Sunday Starter): Take 1 tablet every day until Sunday. Discard the remaining pack and start a new pack of pills on the same day.

Schedule 2 (Day 1 starter): Discard the remaining pack and start a new pack the same day.

Three or more consecutive doses missed: An additional method of contraception must be used for 7 days after a missed dose.

Schedule 1 (Sunday Starter): Take 1 tablet every day until Sunday; on Sunday, discard the pack and start a new pack.

Schedule 2 (Day 1 Starter): Discard the remaining pack and begin new pack of tablets starting on the same day.

Dosage adjustment in renal impairment: Specific guidelines not available; use with caution and monitor blood pressure closely. Consider other forms of contraception.

Dosage adjustment in hepatic impairment: Contraindicated in patients with hepatic impairment.

Mechanism of Action Combination oral contraceptives inhibit ovulation via a negative feedback mechanism on the hypothalamus, which alters the normal pattern of gonadotropin secretion of a follicle-stimulating hormone (FSH) and luteinizing hormone by the anterior pituitary. The follicular phase FSH and midcycle surge of gonadotropins are inhibited. In addition, combination hormonal contraceptives produce alterations in the genital tract, including changes in the cervical mucus, rendering it unfavorable for sperm penetration even if ovulation occurs. Changes in the endometrium may also occur, producing an unfavorable environment for nidation. Combination hormonal contraceptive drugs may alter the tubal transport of the ova through the fallopian tubes. Progestational agents may also alter sperm fertility.

In postmenopausal women, exogenous estrogen is used to replace decreased endogenous production. The addition of progestin reduces the incidence of endometrial hyperplasia and risk of endometrial cancer in women with an intact uterus.

Contraindications Hypersensitivity to ethinyl estradiol, norethindrone, norethindrone acetate, or any component of the formulation; history of or current thrombophlebitis or venous thromboembolic disorders (including DVT, PE); active or recent (within 1 year) arterial thromboembolic disease (eg, stroke, MI); cerebral vascular disease, coronary artery disease, severe hypertension; diabetes mellitus with vascular involvement; severe headache with focal neurological symptoms; known or suspected breast carcinoma, endometrial cancer, estrogen-dependent neoplasms, undiagnosed abnormal genital bleeding; hepatic dysfunction or tumor, cholestatic jaundice of pregnancy, jaundice with prior combination hormonal contraceptive use; major surgery with prolonged immobilization; heavy smoking (≥15 cigarettes/day) in patients >35 years of age; pregnancy

Warnings/Precautions

Cardiovascular-related considerations: Use caution with cardiovascular disease or dysfunction. Combination estrogen/progestin therapy has been associated with an increased risk of cardiovascular disease, which may be dose related. May increase the risks of hypertension, myocardial infarction (MI), stroke, pulmonary emboli (PE), and deep vein thrombosis; incidence of these effects was shown to be significantly increased in postmenopausal women using conjugated equine estrogens (CEE) in combination with medroxyprogesterone acetate (MPA). Nonfatal MI, PE, and thrombophlebitis have also been reported in males taking high doses of CEE (eg, for prostate cancer). An increased risk of MI has been noted with use of combination hormonal contraceptives, primarily in women with underlying risk factors. The risk of cardiovascular events increases in women who smoke cigarettes, especially those who are >35 years of age; women who use combination hormonal contraceptives should be strongly advised not to smoke. Women with hypertension or renal disease should be encouraged to use another form of contraception. Estrogen compounds are generally associated with lipid effects such as increased HDL-cholesterol and decreased LDL-cholesterol. Triglycerides may also be increased; use with caution in patients with familial defects of lipoprotein metabolism. Estrogens with or without progestin should not be used to prevent coronary heart disease in postmenopausal women. Whenever possible, combination hormonal contraceptives should be discontinued at least 4 weeks prior to and for 2 weeks following elective surgery associated with an increased risk of thromboembolism or during periods of prolonged immobilization.

Cancer-related considerations: Estrogens may increase the risk of breast cancer. The use of combination hormonal contraceptives has been associated with a slight increase in frequency of breast cancer, however studies are not consistent. An increased risk of invasive breast cancer was observed in post-menopausal women using CEE in combination with MPA; a smaller increase in risk was seen with estrogen therapy alone in observational studies. An increase in abnormal mammograms has also been reported with estrogen and progestin therapy in postmenopausal women. Unopposed estrogens may increase the risk of endometrial carcinoma in postmenopausal women. Estrogens may exacerbate endometriosis. Malignant transformation of residual endometrial implants has been reported post-hysterectomy with estrogen only therapy. Consider adding a progestin in women with residual endometriosis post-hysterectomy. Estrogen use may lead to severe hypercalcemia in postmenopausal patients with breast cancer and bone metastases; discontinue estrogen if hypercalcemia occurs.

Use with caution in patients with diseases which may be exacerbated by fluid retention, including asthma, epilepsy, migraine, or diabetes. Use with caution in patients with a history of severe hypocalcemia, SLE, hepatic hemangiomas, porphyria, endometriosis, and gallbladder disease. Use caution with history of cholestatic jaundice associated with past estrogen use or pregnancy.

Estrogens may cause retinal vascular thrombosis. Discontinue pending examination in cases of sudden partial or complete vision loss, sudden onset of proptosis, diplopia, or migraine; discontinue permanently if papilledema or retinal vascular lesions are observed on examination.

Combination hormonal contraceptives do not protect against HIV infection or other sexually-transmitted diseases. The minimum dosage combination of estrogen/progestin that will effectively treat the individual patient should be used. New patients should be started on products containing ≤0.035 mg of estrogen per tablet. When used for acne, use only in females ≥15 years, who also desire combination hormonal contraceptive therapy, are unresponsive to topical treatments, and have no contraindications to combination hormonal contraceptive use. Not for use prior to menarche.

The risk of dementia may be increased in postmenopausal women; increased incidence was observed in women ≥65 years of age taking CEE alone or in combination with MPA. Before prescribing estrogen therapy to postmenopausal women, the risks and benefits must be weighed for each patient. Women should be informed of these risks and benefits, as well as possible effects of progestin when added to estrogen therapy. Estrogens with or without progestin should be used for shortest duration possible consistent with treatment goals. Conduct periodic risk:benefit assessments. When used solely for prevention of osteoporosis in women at significant risk, nonestrogen treatment options should be considered.

Drug Interactions

Cytochrome P450 Effect:

Ethinyl estradiol: **Substrate** of CYP2C9 (minor), 3A4 (major), 3A5-7 (minor); **Inhibits** CYP1A2 (weak), 2B6 (weak), 2C8 (weak), 2C19 (weak), 3A4 (weak)

Norethindrone: **Substrate** of CYP3A4 (major); Induces CYP2C19 (weak)

Increased Effect/Toxicity: Acetaminophen and ascorbic acid may increase plasma levels of estrogen component. Atorvastatin and indinavir increase plasma levels of combination hormonal contraceptives. Combination hormonal contraceptives increase the plasma levels of alprazolam, chlordiazepoxide, cyclosporine, diazepam, prednisolone, selegiline, theophylline, tricyclic antidepressants. Combination hormonal contraceptives may increase (or decrease) the effects of coumarin derivatives.

Decreased Effect: CYP3A4 inducers may decrease the levels/effects of ethinyl estradiol and norethindrone; example inducers include aminoglutethimide, carbamazepine, nafcillin, nevirapine, phenobarbital, phenytoin, and rifamycins. Combination hormonal contraceptives may decrease plasma levels of acetaminophen, clofibric acid, lorazepam, morphine, oxazepam, salicylic acid, temazepam. Contraceptive effect decreased by acitretin, aminoglutethimide, amprenavir, anticonvulsants, griseofulvin, lopinavir, nelfinavir, penicillins (effect not consistent), rifampin, ritonavir, tetracyclines (effect not consistent), troglitazone. Oral contraceptives may decrease (or increase) the effects of coumarin derivatives.

Ethanol/Nutrition/Herb Interactions

Ethanol: Routine use increases estrogen level and risk of breast cancer; avoid ethanol. Ethanol may also increase the risk of osteoporosis.

Food: CNS effects of caffeine may be enhanced if combination hormonal contraceptives are used concurrently with caffeine. Grapefruit juice increases

(Continued)

Ethinyl Estradiol and Norethindrone *(Continued)*

ethinyl estradiol concentrations and would be expected to increase progesterone serum levels as well; clinical implications are unclear. Norethindrone absorption is increased by 27% following administration with food.

Herb/Nutraceutical: St John's wort may decrease the effectiveness of combination hormonal contraceptives by inducing hepatic enzymes. Avoid dong quai and black cohosh (have estrogen activity). Avoid saw palmetto, red clover, ginseng.

Dietary Considerations Should be taken at same time each day. May be taken with or without food. Ensure adequate calcium and vitamin D intake when used for the prevention of osteoporosis.

Pharmacodynamics/Kinetics

Norethindrone: See individual monograph.

Ethinyl estradiol:

Absorption: Rapid

Bioavailability: 43% to 55%

Distribution: V_d: 2-4 L/kg

Protein binding: >95% to albumin

Metabolism: Hepatic via oxidation and conjugation in GI tract; hydroxylated via CYP3A4 to metabolites; first-pass effect; enterohepatic recirculation; reversibly converted to estrone and estriol

Half-life elimination: 19-24 hours

Excretion: Urine (as estradiol, estrone, and estriol); feces

Pregnancy Risk Factor X

Dosage Forms TAB (femhrt® 1/5): Ethinyl estradiol 5 mcg and norethindrone 1 mg; (femhrt® 0.5/2.5): Ethinyl estradiol 2.5 mcg and norethindrone 1 mg. **TAB, monophasic** (Brevicon®): Ethinyl estradiol 0.035 mg and norethindrone 0.5 mg (28s); (Junel™ 21 1/20, Loestrin® 21 1/20, Microgestin™ 1/20): Ethinyl estradiol 0.02 mg and norethindrone 1 mg (21s); (Junel™ 21 1.5/30, Loestrin® 21 1.5/30, Microgestin™ 1.5/30): Ethinyl estradiol 0.03 mg and norethindrone 1.5 mg (21s); (Junel™ Fe 1/20, Loestrin® 24 Fe, Loestrin® Fe 1/20, Microgestin™ Fe 1/20): Ethinyl estradiol 0.02 mg and norethindrone 1 mg and ferrous fumarate 75 mg (28s); (Junel™ Fe 1.5/30, Loestrin® Fe 1.5/30, Microgestin™ Fe 1.5/30): Ethinyl estradiol 0.03 mg and norethindrone 1.5 mg and ferrous fumarate 75 mg (28s); (Modicon® 28): Ethinyl estradiol 0.035 mg and norethindrone 0.5 mg (28s); (Necon® 0.5/35-28): Ethinyl estradiol 0.035 mg and norethindrone 0.5 mg (28s); (Necon® 1/35-28): Ethinyl estradiol 0.035 mg and norethindrone 1 mg (28s); (Norinyl® 1+35): Ethinyl estradiol 0.035 mg and norethindrone 1 mg (28s); (Nortrel™ 0.5/35 mg): Ethinyl estradiol 0.035 mg and norethindrone 0.5 mg (21s); Ethinyl estradiol 0.035 mg and norethindrone 0.5 mg (28s); (Nortrel™ 1/35 mg): Ethinyl estradiol 0.035 mg and norethindrone 1 mg (21s); Ethinyl estradiol 0.035 mg and norethindrone 1 mg (28s); (Ortho-Novum® 1/35 28): Ethinyl estradiol 0.035 mg and norethindrone 1 mg (28s); (Ovcon® 35 21-day): Ethinyl estradiol 0.035 mg and norethindrone 0.4 mg (21s); (Ovcon® 35 28-day): Ethinyl estradiol 0.035 mg and norethindrone 0.4 mg (28s); (Ovcon® 50): Ethinyl estradiol 0.05 mg and norethindrone 1 mg (28s). **TAB, biphasic** (Necon® 10/11-28): Day 1-10: Ethinyl estradiol 0.035 mg and norethindrone 0.5 mg, Day 11-21: Ethinyl estradiol 0.035 mg and norethindrone 1 mg, Day 22-28: Inactive (28s); (Ortho-Novum® 10/11-28): Day 1-10: Ethinyl estradiol 0.035 mg and norethindrone 0.5 mg, Day 11-21: Ethinyl estradiol 0.035 mg and norethindrone 1 mg, Day 22-28: Inactive (28s). **TAB, triphasic:** (Aranelle™, Tri-Norinyl® 28): Day 1-7: Ethinyl estradiol 0.035 mg and norethindrone 0.5 mg, Day 8-16: Ethinyl estradiol 0.035 mg and norethindrone 1 mg, Day 17-21: Ethinyl estradiol 0.035 mg and norethindrone 0.5 mg, Day 22-28: Inactive (28s); (Estrostep® Fe): Day 1-5: Ethinyl estradiol 0.02 mg and norethindrone acetate 1 mg, Day 6-12: Ethinyl estradiol 0.03 mg and norethindrone acetate 1 mg, Day 13-21: Ethinyl estradiol 0.035 mg and norethindrone acetate 1 mg, Day 22-28: Ferrous fumarate 75 mg (28s); (Leena™): Day 1-7: Ethinyl estradiol 0.035 mg and norethindrone 0.5 mg, Day 1-7: Ethinyl estradiol 0.035 mg and norethindrone 0.5 mg, Day 8-16: Ethinyl estradiol 0.035 mg and norethindrone 1 mg, Day 17-21: Ethinyl estradiol 0.035 mg and norethindrone 0.5 mg, Day 22-28: Inactive; (Necon® 7/7/7, Ortho-Novum® 7/7/7 28): Day 1-7: Ethinyl estradiol 0.035 mg and norethindrone 0.5 mg, Day 8-14: Ethinyl estradiol 0.035 mg and norethindrone 0.75 mg, Day 15-21: Ethinyl estradiol 0.035 mg and norethindrone 1 mg, Day 22-28: Inactive (28s); (Nortrel™ 7/7/7 28): Day 1-7: Ethinyl estradiol 0.035 mg and norethindrone 0.5 mg; Day 8-14: Ethinyl estradiol 0.035 mg and norethindrone 0.75 mg; Day 15-21: Ethinyl estradiol 0.035 mg and norethindrone 1 mg; Day 22-28: Inactive (28s); (Ortho-Novum® 7/7/7 28): Day 1-7: Ethinyl estradiol 0.035 mg and norethindrone 0.5 mg, Day 8-14: Ethinyl estradiol 0.035 mg and norethindrone 0.75 mg, Day 15-21: Ethinyl estradiol 0.035 mg and norethindrone 5 mg, Day 22-28: Inactive (28s)

Ethinyl Estradiol and Norgestimate
(ETH in il es tra DYE ole & nor JES ti mate)

U.S. Brand Names MonoNessa™; Ortho-Cyclen®; Ortho Tri-Cyclen®; Ortho Tri-Cyclen® Lo; Previfem™; Sprintec™; TriNessa™; Tri-Previfem™; Tri-Sprintec™

Canadian Brand Names Cyclen®; Tri-Cyclen®; Tri-Cyclen® Lo

Generic Available Yes

Synonyms Ethinyl Estradiol and NGM; Norgestimate and Ethinyl Estradiol; Ortho Tri Cyclen; Ortho Tri Cyclen

Pharmacologic Category Contraceptive; Estrogen and Progestin Combination

Use Prevention of pregnancy; treatment of acne

Unlabeled/Investigational Use Treatment of hypermenorrhea (menorrhagia); pain associated with endometriosis; dysmenorrhea; dysfunctional uterine bleeding

Local Anesthetic/Vasoconstrictor Precautions No information available to require special precautions

Effects on Dental Treatment When prescribing antibiotics, patient must be warned to use additional methods of birth control if on oral contraceptives.

Common Adverse Effects Frequency not defined.

Cardiovascular: Arterial thromboembolism, cerebral hemorrhage, cerebral thrombosis, edema, hypertension, mesenteric thrombosis, MI

Central nervous system: Depression, dizziness, headache, migraine, nervousness, premenstrual syndrome, stroke

Dermatologic: Acne, erythema multiforme, erythema nodosum, hirsutism, loss of scalp hair, melasma (may persist), rash (allergic)

Endocrine & metabolic: Amenorrhea, breakthrough bleeding, breast enlargement, breast secretion, breast tenderness, carbohydrate intolerance, lactation decreased (postpartum), glucose tolerance decreased, libido changes, menstrual flow changes, sex hormone-binding globulins (SHBG) increased, spotting, temporary infertility (following discontinuation), thyroid-binding globulin increased, triglycerides increased

Gastrointestinal: Abdominal cramps, appetite changes, bloating, cholestasis, colitis, gallbladder disease, jaundice, nausea, vomiting, weight gain/loss

Genitourinary: Cervical erosion changes, cervical secretion changes, cystitis-like syndrome, vaginal candidiasis, vaginitis

Hematologic: Antithrombin III decreased, folate levels decreased, hemolytic uremic syndrome, norepinephrine induced platelet aggregability increased, porphyria, prothrombin increased; factors VII, VIII, IX, and X increased

Hepatic: Benign liver tumors, Budd-Chiari syndrome, cholestatic jaundice, hepatic adenomas

Local: Thrombophlebitis

Ocular: Cataracts, change in corneal curvature (steepening), contact lens intolerance, optic neuritis, retinal thrombosis

Renal: Impaired renal function

Respiratory: Pulmonary thromboembolism

Miscellaneous: Hemorrhagic eruption

Dosage Oral:

Children ≥15 years and Adults: Female: Acne (Ortho Tri-Cyclen®): Refer to dosing for contraception

Adults: Female:

Contraception:

Schedule 1 (Sunday starter): Dose begins on first Sunday after onset of menstruation; if the menstrual period starts on Sunday, take first tablet that very same day. **With a Sunday start, an additional method of contraception should be used until after the first 7 days of consecutive administration.**

For 21-tablet package: Dosage is 1 tablet daily for 21 consecutive days, followed by 7 days off of the medication; a new course begins on the 8th day after the last tablet is taken.

For 28-tablet package: Dosage is 1 tablet daily without interruption.

Schedule 2 (Day 1 starter): Dose starts on first day of menstrual cycle taking 1 tablet daily.

For 21-tablet package: Dosage is 1 tablet daily for 21 consecutive days, followed by 7 days off of the medication; a new course begins on the 8th day after the last tablet is taken.

For 28-tablet package: Dosage is 1 tablet daily without interruption.

If all doses have been taken on schedule and one menstrual period is missed, continue dosing cycle. If two consecutive menstrual periods are missed, pregnancy test is required before new dosing cycle is started.

(Continued)

Ethinyl Estradiol and Norgestimate (Continued)

Missed doses **monophasic formulations** (refer to package insert for complete information):

One dose missed: Take as soon as remembered or take 2 tablets next day

Two consecutive doses missed in the first 2 weeks: Take 2 tablets as soon as remembered or 2 tablets next 2 days. **An additional method of contraception should be used for 7 days after missed dose.**

Two consecutive doses missed in week 3 or three consecutive doses missed at any time: **An additional method of contraception must be used for 7 days after a missed dose:**

Schedule 1 (Sunday starter): Continue dose of 1 tablet daily until Sunday, then discard the rest of the pack, and a new pack should be started that same day.

Schedule 2 (Day 1 starter): Current pack should be discarded, and a new pack should be started that same day.

Missed doses **biphasic/triphasic formulations** (refer to package insert for complete information):

One dose missed: Take as soon as remembered or take 2 tablets next day.

Two consecutive doses missed in week 1 or week 2 of the pack: Take 2 tablets as soon as remembered and 2 tablets the next day. Resume taking 1 tablet daily until the pack is empty. **An additional method of contraception must be used for 7 days after a missed dose.**

Two consecutive doses missed in week 3 of the pack. **An additional method of contraception must be used for 7 days after a missed dose.**

Schedule 1 (Sunday starter): Take 1 tablet every day until Sunday. Discard the remaining pack and start a new pack of pills on the same day.

Schedule 2 (Day 1 starter): Discard the remaining pack and start a new pack the same day.

Three or more consecutive doses missed. **An additional method of contraception must be used for 7 days after a missed dose.**

Schedule 1 (Sunday starter): Take 1 tablet every day until Sunday; on Sunday, discard the pack and start a new pack.

Schedule 2 (Day 1 starter): Discard the remaining pack and begin new pack of tablets starting on the same day.

Dosage adjustment in renal impairment: Specific guidelines not available; use with caution and monitor blood pressure closely. Consider other forms of contraception.

Dosage adjustment in hepatic impairment: Contraindicated in patients with hepatic impairment.

Mechanism of Action Combination hormonal contraceptives inhibit ovulation via a negative feedback mechanism on the hypothalamus, which alters the normal pattern of gonadotropin secretion of a follicle-stimulating hormone (FSH) and luteinizing hormone by the anterior pituitary. The follicular phase FSH and midcycle surge of gonadotropins are inhibited. In addition, combination hormonal contraceptives produce alterations in the genital tract, including changes in the cervical mucus, rendering it unfavorable for sperm penetration even if ovulation occurs. Changes in the endometrium may also occur, producing an unfavorable environment for nidation. Combination hormonal contraceptive drugs may alter the tubal transport of the ova through the fallopian tubes. Progestational agents may also alter sperm fertility.

Contraindications Hypersensitivity to ethinyl estradiol, norgestimate, or any component of the formulation; history of or current thrombophlebitis or venous thromboembolic disorders (including DVT, PE); active or recent (within 1 year) arterial thromboembolic disease (eg, stroke, MI); cerebral vascular disease, coronary artery disease, valvular heart disease with complications, severe hypertension; severe headache with focal neurological symptoms; known or suspected breast carcinoma, endometrial cancer, estrogen-dependent neoplasms, undiagnosed abnormal genital bleeding; hepatic dysfunction or tumor, cholestatic jaundice of pregnancy, jaundice with prior combination hormonal contraceptive use; heavy smoking (≥15 cigarettes/day) in patients >35 years of age; pregnancy

Warnings/Precautions Combination hormonal contraceptives do not protect against HIV infection or other sexually-transmitted diseases. The risk of cardiovascular side effects increases in women who smoke cigarettes, especially those who are >35 years of age; women who use combination hormonal contraceptives should be strongly advised not to smoke. Combination hormonal contraceptives may lead to increased risk of myocardial infarction, use with caution in patients with risk factors for coronary artery disease. May increase the risk of thromboembolism. Whenever possible, combination hormonal contraceptives should be discontinued at least 4 weeks prior to and for 2 weeks following elective surgery associated with an increased risk of thromboembolism or during periods of prolonged immobilization. Combination hormonal contraceptives may have a dose-related risk of vascular disease, hypertension, and gallbladder disease. Women with hypertension or renal disease should be encouraged to use a nonhormonal form of contraception. The use of combination hormonal contraceptives has been associated with a slight increase in frequency of breast cancer, however, studies are not consistent. Combination hormonal contraceptives may cause glucose intolerance. Retinal thrombosis has been reported (rarely). Use caution with conditions that may be aggravated by fluid retention, depression, or history of migraine. Not for use prior to menarche.

The minimum dosage combination of estrogen/progestin that will effectively treat the individual patient should be used. New patients should be started on products containing ≤0.035 mg of estrogen per tablet.

Acne: For use only in females ≥15 years, who also desire combination hormonal contraceptive therapy, are unresponsive to topical treatments, and have no contraindications to combination hormonal contraceptive use.

Drug Interactions
Cytochrome P450 Effect: Ethinyl estradiol: **Substrate** of CYP2C9 (minor), 3A4 (major), 3A5-7 (minor); **Inhibits** CYP1A2 (weak), 2B6 (weak), 2C8 (weak), 2C19 (weak), 3A4 (weak)

Increased Effect/Toxicity: Acetaminophen and ascorbic acid may increase plasma levels of estrogen component. Atorvastatin and indinavir increase plasma levels of combination hormonal contraceptives. Combination hormonal contraceptives increase the plasma levels of alprazolam, chlordiazepoxide, cyclosporine, diazepam, prednisolone, selegiline, theophylline, tricyclic antidepressants. Combination hormonal contraceptives may increase (or decrease) the effects of coumarin derivatives.

Decreased Effect: CYP3A4 inducers may decrease the levels/effects of ethinyl estradiol; example inducers include aminoglutethimide, carbamazepine, nafcillin, nevirapine, phenobarbital, phenytoin, and rifamycins. Combination hormonal contraceptives may decrease plasma levels of acetaminophen, clofibric acid, lorazepam, morphine, oxazepam, salicylic acid, temazepam. Contraceptive effect decreased by acitretin, aminoglutethimide, amprenavir, anticonvulsants, griseofulvin, lopinavir, nelfinavir, nevirapine, penicillins (effect not consistent), rifampin, ritonavir, tetracyclines (effect not consistent). Combination hormonal contraceptives may decrease (or increase) the effects of coumarin derivatives.

Ethanol/Nutrition/Herb Interactions
Food: CNS effects of caffeine may be enhanced if combination hormonal contraceptives are used concurrently with caffeine. Grapefruit juice increases ethinyl estradiol concentrations and would be expected to increase progesterone serum levels as well; clinical implications are unclear.

Herb/Nutraceutical: St John's wort may decrease the effectiveness of combination hormonal contraceptives by inducing hepatic enzymes. Avoid dong quai and black cohosh (have estrogen activity). Avoid saw palmetto, red clover, ginseng.

Dietary Considerations Should be taken at same time each day.

Pharmacodynamics/Kinetics
Norgestimate:
Absorption: Well absorbed

Protein binding: To albumin and sex hormone-binding globulin (SHBG); SHBG capacity is affected by plasma ethinyl estradiol levels

Metabolism: Hepatic; forms 17-deacetylnorgestimate (major active metabolite) and other metabolites

Half-life elimination: 17-deacetylnorgestimate: 12-30 hours

Excretion: Urine and feces

Pregnancy Risk Factor X

Dosage Forms TAB, monophasic (MonoNessa™, Ortho-Cyclen®, Previfem™, Sprintec™): Ethinyl estradiol 0.035 mg and norgestimate 0.25 mg (28s). **TAB, triphasic** (Ortho Tri-Cyclen®, Tri-Previfem™, TriNessa™, Tri-Sprintec™): Day 1-7: Ethinyl estradiol 0.035 mg and norgestimate 0.18 mg, Day 8-14: Ethinyl estradiol 0.035 mg and norgestimate 0.215 mg, Day 15-21: Ethinyl estradiol 0.035 mg and norgestimate 0.25 mg, Day 22-28: Inactive (28s); (Ortho Tri-Cyclen® Lo): Day 1-7: Ethinyl estradiol 0.025 mg and norgestimate 0.18 mg, Day 8-14: Ethinyl estradiol 0.025 mg and norgestimate 0.215 mg, Day 15-21: Ethinyl estradiol 0.025 and norgestimate 0.25 mg, Day 22-28: Inactive (28s)

Ethinyl Estradiol and Norgestrel
(ETH in il es tra DYE ole & nor JES trel)

Related Information
Norgestrel *on page 1127*

U.S. Brand Names Crysselle™; Lo/Ovral®; Low-Ogestrel®; Ogestrel®

Canadian Brand Names Ovral®

Generic Available Yes

Synonyms Morning After Pill; Norgestrel and Ethinyl Estradiol

Pharmacologic Category Contraceptive; Estrogen and Progestin Combination

Use Prevention of pregnancy; postcoital contraceptive or "morning after" pill

Unlabeled/Investigational Use Treatment of hypermenorrhea (menorrhagia); pain associated with endometriosis; dysmenorrhea; dysfunctional uterine bleeding

Local Anesthetic/Vasoconstrictor Precautions No information available to require special precautions

Effects on Dental Treatment When prescribing antibiotics, patient must be warned to use additional methods of birth control if on oral contraceptives.

Common Adverse Effects Frequency not defined.

Cardiovascular: Arterial thromboembolism, cerebral hemorrhage, cerebral thrombosis, edema, hypertension, mesenteric thrombosis, MI

Central nervous system: Depression, dizziness, headache, migraine, nervousness, premenstrual syndrome, stroke

Dermatologic: Acne, erythema multiforme, erythema nodosum, hirsutism, loss of scalp hair, melasma (may persist), rash (allergic)

Endocrine & metabolic: Amenorrhea, breakthrough bleeding, breast enlargement, breast secretion, breast tenderness, carbohydrate intolerance, lactation decreased (postpartum), glucose tolerance decreased, libido changes, menstrual flow changes, sex hormone-binding globulins (SHBG) increased, spotting, temporary infertility (following discontinuation), thyroid-binding globulin increased, triglycerides increased

Gastrointestinal: Abdominal cramps, appetite changes, bloating, cholestasis, colitis, gallbladder disease, jaundice, nausea, vomiting, weight gain/loss

Genitourinary: Cervical erosion changes, cervical secretion changes, cystitis-like syndrome, vaginal candidiasis, vaginitis

Hematologic: Antithrombin III decreased, folate levels decreased, hemolytic uremic syndrome, norepinephrine induced platelet aggregability increased, porphyria, prothrombin increased; factors VII, VIII, IX, and X

Hepatic: Benign liver tumors, Budd-Chiari syndrome, cholestatic jaundice, hepatic adenomas

Local: Thrombophlebitis

Ocular: Cataracts, change in corneal curvature (steepening), contact lens intolerance, optic neuritis, retinal thrombosis

Renal: Impaired renal function

Respiratory: Pulmonary thromboembolism

Miscellaneous: Hemorrhagic eruption

Dosage Oral: Adults: Female:

Contraception:

Schedule 1 (Sunday starter): Dose begins on first Sunday after onset of menstruation; if the menstrual period starts on Sunday, take first tablet that very same day. **With a Sunday start, an additional method of contraception should be used until after the first 7 days of consecutive administration.**

For 21-tablet package: Dosage is 1 tablet daily for 21 consecutive days, followed by 7 days off of the medication; a new course begins on the 8th day after the last tablet is taken.

For 28-tablet package: Dosage is 1 tablet daily without interruption.

Schedule 2 (Day 1 starter): Dose starts on first day of menstrual cycle taking 1 tablet daily.

For 21-tablet package: Dosage is 1 tablet daily for 21 consecutive days, followed by 7 days off of the medication; a new course begins on the 8th day after the last tablet is taken.

For 28-tablet package: Dosage is 1 tablet daily without interruption.

If all doses have been taken on schedule and one menstrual period is missed, continue dosing cycle. If two consecutive menstrual periods are missed, pregnancy test is required before new dosing cycle is started.

Missed doses **monophasic formulations** (refer to package insert for complete information):

One dose missed: Take as soon as remembered or take 2 tablets next day

Two consecutive doses missed in the first 2 weeks: Take 2 tablets as soon as remembered or 2 tablets next 2 days. **An additional method of contraception should be used for 7 days after missed dose.**

Two consecutive doses missed in week 3 or three consecutive doses missed at any time:

Schedule 1 (Sunday starter): Continue to take 1 tablet daily until Sunday, then discard the rest of the pack, and a new pack is started that same day.

Schedule 2 (Day 1 starter): Current pack should be discarded, and a new pack started that same day. **An additional method of contraception should be used for 7 days after missed dose.**

Postcoital contraception:

Ethinyl estradiol 0.03 mg and norgestrel 0.3 mg formulation: 4 tablets within 72 hours of unprotected intercourse and 4 tablets 12 hours after first dose

Ethinyl estradiol 0.05 mg and norgestrel 0.5 mg formulation: 2 tablets within 72 hours of unprotected intercourse and 2 tablets 12 hours after first dose

Dosage adjustment in renal impairment: Specific guidelines not available; use with caution and monitor blood pressure closely. Consider other forms of contraception.

Dosage adjustment in hepatic impairment: Contraindicated in patients with hepatic impairment.

Mechanism of Action Combination hormonal contraceptives inhibit ovulation via a negative feedback mechanism on the hypothalamus, which alters the normal pattern of gonadotropin secretion of a follicle-stimulating hormone (FSH) and luteinizing hormone by the anterior pituitary. The follicular phase FSH and midcycle surge of gonadotropins are inhibited. In addition, combination hormonal contraceptives produce alterations in the genital tract, including changes in the cervical mucus, rendering it unfavorable for sperm penetration even if ovulation occurs. Changes in the endometrium may also occur, producing an unfavorable environment for nidation. Combination hormonal contraceptive drugs may alter the tubal transport of the ova through the fallopian tubes. Progestational agents may also alter sperm fertility.

Contraindications Hypersensitivity to ethinyl estradiol, norgestrel, or any component of the formulation; history of or current thrombophlebitis or venous thromboembolic disorders (including DVT, PE); active or recent (within 1 year) arterial thromboembolic disease (eg, stroke, MI); cerebral vascular disease, coronary artery disease, valvular heart disease with complications, severe hypertension; diabetes mellitus with vascular involvement; severe headache with focal neurological symptoms; known or suspected breast carcinoma, endometrial cancer, estrogen-dependent neoplasms, undiagnosed abnormal genital bleeding; hepatic dysfunction or tumor, cholestatic jaundice of pregnancy, jaundice with prior combination hormonal contraceptive use; major surgery with prolonged immobilization; heavy smoking (≥15 cigarettes/day) in patients >35 years of age; pregnancy

Warnings/Precautions Combination hormonal contraceptives do not protect against HIV infection or other sexually-transmitted diseases. The risk of cardiovascular side effects increases in women who smoke cigarettes, especially those who are >35 years of age; women who use combination hormonal contraceptives should be strongly advised not to smoke. Combination hormonal contraceptives may lead to increased risk of myocardial infarction, use with caution in patients with risk factors for coronary artery disease. May increase the risk of thromboembolism. Whenever possible, combination hormonal contraceptives should be discontinued at least 4 weeks prior to and for 2 weeks following elective surgery associated with an increased risk of thromboembolism or during periods of prolonged immobilization. Combination hormonal contraceptives may have a dose-related risk of vascular disease, hypertension, and gallbladder disease. Women with hypertension or renal disease should be encouraged to use another form of contraception. The use of combination hormonal contraceptives has been associated with a slight increase in frequency of breast cancer, however, studies are not consistent. Combination hormonal contraceptives may cause glucose intolerance. Retinal thrombosis has been reported (rarely). Use caution with conditions that may be aggravated by fluid retention, depression, or history of migraine. Not for use prior to menarche.

The minimum dosage combination of estrogen/progestin that will effectively treat the individual patient should be used. New patients should be started on products containing ≤0.035 mg of estrogen per tablet.

Drug Interactions

Cytochrome P450 Effect:

Ethinyl estradiol: **Substrate** of CYP2C9 (minor), 3A4 (major), 3A5-7 (minor); **Inhibits** CYP1A2 (weak), 2B6 (weak), 2C8 (weak), 2C19 (weak), 3A4 (weak)

(Continued)

Ethinyl Estradiol and Norgestrel *(Continued)*

Norgestrel: **Substrate** of CYP3A4 (major)

Increased Effect/Toxicity: Acetaminophen and ascorbic acid may increase plasma levels of estrogen component. Atorvastatin and indinavir increase plasma levels of combination hormonal contraceptives. Combination hormonal contraceptives increase the plasma levels of alprazolam, chlordiazepoxide, cyclosporine, diazepam, prednisolone, selegiline, theophylline, tricyclic antidepressants. Combination hormonal contraceptives may increase (or decrease) the effects of coumarin derivatives.

Decreased Effect: CYP3A4 inducers may decrease the levels/effects of norgestrel; example inducers include aminoglutethimide, carbamazepine, nafcillin, nevirapine, phenobarbital, phenytoin, and rifamycins. Combination hormonal contraceptives may decrease plasma levels of acetaminophen, clofibric acid, lorazepam, morphine, oxazepam, salicylic acid, temazepam. Contraceptive effect decreased by acitretin, aminoglutethimide, amprenavir, anticonvulsants, griseofulvin, lopinavir, nelfinavir, nevirapine, penicillins (effect not consistent), rifampin, ritonavir, tetracyclines (effect not consistent). Combination hormonal contraceptives may decrease (or increase) the effects of coumarin derivatives.

Ethanol/Nutrition/Herb Interactions

Food: CNS effects of caffeine may be enhanced if combination hormonal contraceptives are used concurrently with caffeine. Grapefruit juice increases ethinyl estradiol concentrations and would be expected to increase progesterone serum levels as well; clinical implications are unclear.

Herb/Nutraceutical: St John's wort may decrease the effectiveness of combination hormonal contraceptives by inducing hepatic enzymes. Avoid dong quai and black cohosh (have estrogen activity). Avoid saw palmetto, red clover, ginseng.

Dietary Considerations Should be taken at same time each day.

Pharmacodynamics/Kinetics See individual agents.

Pregnancy Risk Factor X

Dosage Forms TAB, monophasic: (Cryselle™): Ethinyl estradiol 0.03 mg and norgestrel 0.3 mg (28s); (Low-Ogestrel® 28): Ethinyl estradiol 0.03 mg and norgestrel 0.3 mg (28s); (Lo/Ovral® 28): Ethinyl estradiol 0.03 mg and norgestrel 0.3 mg (28s); (Orgestrel® 28): Ethinyl estradiol 0.05 mg and norgestrel 0.5 mg (28s)

Ethiofos *see* Amifostine *on page 83*

Ethionamide *(e thye on AM ide)*

Related Information

Tuberculosis *on page 1673*

U.S. Brand Names Trecator®

Canadian Brand Names Trecator®

Generic Available No

Pharmacologic Category Antitubercular Agent

Use Treatment of tuberculosis and other mycobacterial diseases, in conjunction with other antituberculosis agents, when first-line agents have failed or resistance has been demonstrated

Local Anesthetic/Vasoconstrictor Precautions No information available to require special precautions

Effects on Dental Treatment Key adverse event(s) related to dental treatment: Postural hypotension, metallic taste, and stomatitis.

Common Adverse Effects Frequency not defined.

Cardiovascular: Postural hypotension

Central nervous system: Depression, dizziness, drowsiness, headache, psychiatric disturbances, restlessness, seizure

Dermatologic: Acne, alopecia, photosensitivity, purpura, rash

Endocrine & metabolic: Gynecomastia, hypoglycemia, hypothyroidism or goiter, pellagra-like syndrome

Gastrointestinal: Abdominal pain, anorexia, diarrhea, excessive salivation, metallic taste, nausea, stomatitis, vomiting, weight loss

Genitourinary: Impotence

Hematologic: Thrombocytopenia

Hepatic: Hepatitis, jaundice, liver function tests increased

Neuromuscular & skeletal: Peripheral neuritis, weakness (common)

Ocular: Blurred vision, diplopia, optic neuritis

Respiratory: Olfactory disturbances

Miscellaneous: Hypersensitivity reaction

Mechanism of Action Inhibits peptide synthesis

Pharmacodynamics/Kinetics
Absorption: Rapid, complete
Distribution: Crosses placenta; V_d: 93.5 L
Protein binding: ~30%
Metabolism: Extensively hepatic to active and inactive metabolites
Bioavailability: 80%
Half-life elimination: 2-3 hours
Time to peak, serum: 1 hour
Excretion: Urine (<1% as unchanged drug; as active and inactive metabolites)
Pregnancy Risk Factor C

Ethmozine® *see* Moricizine *on page 1064*

Ethosuximide (eth oh SUKS i mide)

U.S. Brand Names Zarontin®
Canadian Brand Names Zarontin®
Generic Available Yes
Pharmacologic Category Anticonvulsant, Succinimide
Use Management of absence (petit mal) seizures
Local Anesthetic/Vasoconstrictor Precautions No information available to require special precautions
Effects on Dental Treatment No significant effects or complications reported
Common Adverse Effects Frequency not defined.
Central nervous system: Ataxia, drowsiness, sedation, dizziness, lethargy, euphoria, headache, irritability, hyperactivity, fatigue, night terrors, disturbance in sleep, inability to concentrate, aggressiveness, mental depression (with cases of overt suicidal intentions), paranoid psychosis
Dermatologic: Stevens-Johnson syndrome, SLE, rash, hirsutism
Endocrine & metabolic: Increased libido
Gastrointestinal: Weight loss, gastric upset, cramps, epigastric pain, diarrhea, nausea, vomiting, anorexia, abdominal pain, gum hypertrophy, tongue swelling
Genitourinary: Vaginal bleeding, microscopic hematuria
Hematologic: Leukopenia, agranulocytosis, pancytopenia, eosinophilia
Ocular: Myopia
Miscellaneous: Hiccups
Mechanism of Action Increases the seizure threshold and suppresses paroxysmal spike-and-wave pattern in absence seizures; depresses nerve transmission in the motor cortex
Drug Interactions
Cytochrome P450 Effect: Substrate of CYP3A4 (major)
Increased Effect/Toxicity: Ethosuximide may elevate phenytoin levels. Valproic acid has been reported to both increase and decrease ethosuximide levels. CYP3A4 inhibitors may increase the levels/effects of ethosuximide; example inhibitors include azole antifungals, clarithromycin, diclofenac, doxycycline, erythromycin, imatinib, isoniazid, nefazodone, nicardipine, propofol, protease inhibitors, quinidine, telithromycin, and verapamil.
Decreased Effect: CYP3A4 inducers may decrease the levels/effects of ethosuximide; example inducers include aminoglutethimide, carbamazepine, nafcillin, nevirapine, phenobarbital, phenytoin, and rifamycins.
Pharmacodynamics/Kinetics
Distribution: Adults: V_d: 0.62-0.72 L/kg
Metabolism: Hepatic (~80% to 3 inactive metabolites)
Half-life elimination, serum: Children: 30 hours; Adults: 50-60 hours
Time to peak, serum: Capsule: ~2-4 hours; Syrup: <2-4 hours
Excretion: Urine, slowly (50% as metabolites, 10% to 20% as unchanged drug); feces (small amounts)
Pregnancy Risk Factor C

Ethotoin (ETH oh toyn)

U.S. Brand Names Peganone®
Canadian Brand Names Peganone®
Generic Available No
Synonyms Ethylphenylhydantoin
Pharmacologic Category Anticonvulsant, Hydantoin
Use Generalized tonic-clonic or complex-partial seizures
Local Anesthetic/Vasoconstrictor Precautions No information available to require special precautions
Effects on Dental Treatment No significant effects or complications reported
(Continued)

Ethotoin *(Continued)*

Common Adverse Effects Frequency not defined.

Cardiovascular: Arrhythmias, ataxia, cardiovascular collapse, venous irritation and pain

Central nervous system: Psychiatric changes, slurred speech, trembling, dizziness, drowsiness, headache, insomnia

Dermatologic: Skin rash, Stevens-Johnson syndrome

Gastrointestinal: Constipation, nausea, vomiting, gingival hyperplasia, anorexia, weight loss

Hematologic: Leukopenia, blood dyscrasias

Hepatic: Hepatitis

Local: Thrombophlebitis

Neuromuscular & skeletal: Paresthesia, peripheral neuropathy

Renal: Serum creatinine increased

Ocular: Nystagmus

Miscellaneous: Lymphadenopathy, SLE-like syndrome

Drug Interactions

Cytochrome P450 Effect: Inhibits CYP2C19 (weak)

Pregnancy Risk Factor D

Ethoxynaphthamido Penicillin Sodium *see* Nafcillin *on page 1082*

Ethyl Aminobenzoate *see* Benzocaine *on page 190*

Ethyl Chloride *(ETH il KLOR ide)*

U.S. Brand Names Gebauer's Ethyl Chloride®

Generic Available No

Synonyms Chloroethane

Pharmacologic Category Local Anesthetic

Use Local anesthetic in minor operative procedures and to relieve pain caused by insect stings and burns, and irritation caused by myofascial and visceral pain syndromes

Local Anesthetic/Vasoconstrictor Precautions No information available to require special precautions

Effects on Dental Treatment Key adverse event(s) related to dental treatment: Mucous membrane irritation. See Dental Comment.

Common Adverse Effects 1% to 10%: Mucous membrane irritation, freezing may alter skin pigment

Pregnancy Risk Factor C

Dental Comment Spray for a few seconds to the point of frost formation when the tissue becomes white; avoid prolonged spraying of skin beyond this point

---

Ethyl Chloride and Dichlorotetrafluoroethane

(ETH il KLOR ide & dye klor oh te tra floo or oh ETH ane)

Related Information

Ethyl Chloride *on page 620*

U.S. Brand Names Fluro-Ethyl®

Generic Available No

Synonyms Dichlorotetrafluoroethane and Ethyl Chloride

Pharmacologic Category Local Anesthetic

Use Topical refrigerant anesthetic to control pain associated with minor surgical procedures, dermabrasion, injections, contusions, and minor strains

Local Anesthetic/Vasoconstrictor Precautions No information available to require special precautions

Effects on Dental Treatment No significant effects or complications reported

Pregnancy Risk Factor C

Ethylphenylhydantoin *see* Ethotoin *on page 619*

Ethynodiol Diacetate and Ethinyl Estradiol *see* Ethinyl Estradiol and Ethynodiol Diacetate *on page 597*

Ethyol® *see* Amifostine *on page 83*

Etidronate and Calcium *(e ti DROE nate & KAL see um)*

Related Information

Calcium Carbonate *on page 248*

Etidronate Disodium *on page 621*

Canadian Brand Names Didrocal™

Synonyms Calcium Carbonate and Etidronate Disodium

Pharmacologic Category Bisphosphonate Derivative; Calcium Salt

Use Treatment and prevention of postmenopausal osteoporosis; prevention of corticosteroid-induced osteoporosis

Local Anesthetic/Vasoconstrictor Precautions No information available to require special precautions

Effects on Dental Treatment Osteonecrosis of the jaw (ONJ), generally associated with local infection and/or tooth extraction and often with delayed healing, has been reported in patients taking bisphosphonates. Most reported cases of bisphosphonate-associated osteonecrosis have been in cancer patients treated with intravenous bisphosphonates. However, some have occurred in patients with postmenopausal osteoporosis taking oral bisphosphonates. Dental surgery may exacerbate ONJ. For patients requiring dental procedures, there are no data available to suggest whether discontinuation of bisphosphonate treatment reduces the risk of ONJ. See Dental Comment.

Common Adverse Effects >10%:

Central nervous system: Dizziness (16%), headache (13%)

Gastrointestinal: Diarrhea (37%), nausea (18%), flatulence (17%), constipation (13%), dyspepsia (12%), vomiting (11%)

Restrictions Not available in U.S.

Mechanism of Action See individual agents.

Drug Interactions

Decreased Effect: See individual agents. **Note:** Since etidronate and calcium carbonate are administered sequentially, there is no interaction between the two components. Concurrent administration may result in reduced absorption of etidronate.

Pharmacodynamics/Kinetics See individual agents.

Pregnancy Risk Factor C (based on U.S. labeling)

Dental Comment

Novartis Pharmaceuticals Corporation has notified dental health professionals of the risk of osteonecrosis of the jaw (ONJ) and the use of the bisphosphonates, pamidronate, and zoledronic acid. This warning has not be issued for etidronate disodium.

Previously, Novartis and the Food and Drug Administration (FDA) had notified healthcare providers of a serious adverse event related to the use of bisphosphonates. Osteonecrosis of the jaw has been reported in patients with cancer who were receiving chemotherapy, corticosteroids, and chronic bisphosphonate therapy. The bisphosphonates involved were pamidronate and zoledronic acid. To date, there are no reported associations between etidronate disodium and osteonecrosis of the jaw. Dental exams and preventative dentistry should be performed prior to placing patients with risk factors (chemotherapy, corticosteroids, poor oral hygiene) on chronic bisphosphonate therapy. Invasive dental procedures should be avoided during treatment. Product labelings for pamidronate (Aredia®) and zoledronic acid (Zometa®) have been updated. Recently, 63 cases of osteonecrosis associated with the use of bisphosphonates were published (Ruggiero, 2004). In a retrospective review, 56 of the patients received intravenous bisphosphonates for at least one year and 7 patients were on chronic oral therapy. The presenting symptom was a nonhealing extraction socket or an exposed jawbone. These lesions did not show evidence of metastatic disease and required removal of involved bone in most cases.

Bisphosphonates are widely used in the management of metastatic bone disease to treat hypercalcemia associated with malignancies and to treat osteoporosis. In the report by Ruggiero et al, the cluster of patients observed to have necrotic lesions in the jaw shared only one common clinical feature, all received chronic bisphosphonate therapy. The necrosis detected was typical of osteoradionecrosis. It was suggested that because of the trend in the use of chronic bisphosphonate therapy, the observation of an associated risk of osteonecrosis of the jaw should alert practitioners to monitor for this previously unrecognized potential complication.

Selected Readings

Ruggiero SL, Mehrotra B, Rosenberg TJ, et al, "Osteonecrosis of the Jaws Associated With the Use of Bisphosphonates: A Review of 63 Cases," *J Oral Maxillofac Surg*, 2004, 62(5):527-34.

Etidronate Disodium (e ti DROE nate dye SOW dee um)

Related Information

Rheumatoid Arthritis, Osteoarthritis, and Osteoporosis *on page 1668*

U.S. Brand Names Didronel®

Canadian Brand Names Apo-Etidronate®; Didronel®; Gen-Etidronate

(Continued)

Etidronate Disodium *(Continued)*

Generic Available No

Synonyms EHDP; Sodium Etidronate

Pharmacologic Category Bisphosphonate Derivative

Use Symptomatic treatment of Paget's disease; prevention and treatment of heterotopic ossification due to spinal cord injury or after total hip replacement

Local Anesthetic/Vasoconstrictor Precautions No information available to require special precautions

Effects on Dental Treatment Key adverse event(s) related to dental treatment: Abnormal taste.

Osteonecrosis of the jaw (ONJ), generally associated with local infection and/or tooth extraction and often with delayed healing, has been reported in patients taking bisphosphonates. Most reported cases of bisphosphonate-associated osteonecrosis have been in cancer patients treated with intravenous bisphosphonates. However, some have occurred in patients with postmenopausal osteoporosis taking oral bisphosphonates. Dental surgery may exacerbate ONJ. For patients requiring dental procedures, there are no data available to suggest whether discontinuation of bisphosphonate treatment reduces the risk of ONJ. See Dental Comment.

Common Adverse Effects Frequency not defined.

Gastrointestinal: Diarrhea, nausea

Neuromuscular & skeletal: Bone pain

Mechanism of Action Decreases bone resorption by inhibiting osteocystic osteolysis; decreases mineral release and matrix or collagen breakdown in bone

Drug Interactions

Increased Effect/Toxicity: Aminoglycosides may lower serum calcium levels with prolonged administration; concomitant use may have an additive hypocalcemic effect. NSAIDs may enhance the gastrointestinal adverse/toxic effects (increased incidence of GI ulcers) of bisphosphonate derivatives. Bisphosphonate derivatives may enhance the hypocalcemic effect of phosphate supplements.

Decreased Effect: The following agents may decrease the absorption of oral bisphosphonate derivatives: Antacids (aluminum, calcium, magnesium), oral calcium salts, oral iron salts, and oral magnesium salts

Pharmacodynamics/Kinetics

Onset of action: 1-3 months

Duration: Can persist for 12 months without continuous therapy

Absorption: ~3%

Metabolism: None

Half-life elimination: 1-6 hours

Excretion: Primarily urine (as unchanged drug); feces (as unabsorbed drug)

Pregnancy Risk Factor C

Dental Comment

Novartis Pharmaceuticals Corporation has notified dental health professionals of the risk of osteonecrosis of the jaw (ONJ) and the use of the bisphosphonates, pamidronate, and zoledronic acid. This warning has not been issued for etidronate disodium.

Previously, Novartis and the Food and Drug Administration (FDA) had notified healthcare providers of a serious adverse event related to the use of bisphosphonates. Osteonecrosis of the jaw has been reported in patients with cancer who were receiving chemotherapy, corticosteroids, and chronic bisphosphonate therapy. The bisphosphonates involved were pamidronate and zoledronic acid. To date, there are no reported associations between etidronate disodium and osteonecrosis of the jaw. Dental exams and preventative dentistry should be performed prior to placing patients with risk factors (chemotherapy, corticosteroids, poor oral hygiene) on chronic bisphosphonate therapy. Invasive dental procedures should be avoided during treatment. Product labelings for pamidronate (Aredia®) and zoledronic acid (Zometa®) have been updated. Recently, 63 cases of osteonecrosis associated with the use of bisphosphonates were published (Ruggiero, 2004). In a retrospective review, 56 of the patients received intravenous bisphosphonates for at least one year and 7 patients were on chronic oral therapy. The presenting symptom was a nonhealing extraction socket or an exposed jawbone. These lesions did not show evidence of metastatic disease and required removal of involved bone in most cases.

Bisphosphonates are widely used in the management of metastatic bone disease to treat hypercalcemia associated with malignancies and to treat osteoporosis. In the report by Ruggiero et al, the cluster of patients observed to have necrotic lesions in the jaw shared only one common clinical feature, all received chronic bisphosphonate therapy. The necrosis detected was typical of osteoradionecrosis. It was suggested that because of the trend in the use of chronic bisphosphonate therapy, the observation of an associated risk of osteonecrosis of the jaw should alert practitioners to monitor for this previously unrecognized potential complication.

Selected Readings

Ruggiero SL, Mehrotra B, Rosenberg TJ, et al, "Osteonecrosis of the Jaws Associated With the Use of Bisphosphonates: A Review of 63 Cases," *J Oral Maxillofac Surg*, 2004, 62(5):527-34.

Etodolac (ee toe DOE lak)

Related Information

Rheumatoid Arthritis, Osteoarthritis, and Osteoporosis *on page 1668*
Temporomandibular Dysfunction (TMD) *on page 1724*

U.S. Brand Names Lodine® [DSC]; Lodine® XL [DSC]

Canadian Brand Names Apo-Etodolac®; Lodine®; Utradol™

Generic Available Yes

Synonyms Etodolic Acid

Pharmacologic Category Nonsteroidal Anti-inflammatory Drug (NSAID), Oral

Dental Use Management of postoperative pain

Use Acute and long-term use in the management of signs and symptoms of osteoarthritis; rheumatoid arthritis and juvenile rheumatoid arthritis; management of acute pain

Local Anesthetic/Vasoconstrictor Precautions No information available to require special precautions

Effects on Dental Treatment NSAID formulations are known to reversibly decrease platelet aggregation via mechanisms different than observed with aspirin. The dentist should be aware of the potential of abnormal coagulation. Caution should also be exercised in the use of NSAIDs in patients already on anticoagulant therapy with drugs such as warfarin (Coumadin®).

Significant Adverse Effects

1% to 10%:
Central nervous system: Dizziness (3% to 9 %), chills/fever (1% to 3%), depression (1% to 3%), nervousness (1% to 3%)
Dermatologic: Rash (1% to 3%), pruritus (1% to 3%)
Gastrointestinal: Abdominal cramps (3% to 9%), nausea (3% to 9%), vomiting (1% to 3%), dyspepsia (10%), diarrhea (3% to 9%), constipation (1% to 3%), flatulence (3% to 9%), melena (1% to 3%), gastritis (1% to 3%)
Genitourinary: Dysuria (1% to 3%)
Neuromuscular & skeletal: Weakness (3% to 9%)
Ocular: Blurred vision (1% to 3%)
Otic: Tinnitus (1% to 3%)
Renal: Polyuria (1% to 3%)

<1% (Limited to important or life-threatening): Agranulocytosis, allergic reaction, allergic/necrotizing vasculitis, alopecia, anaphylactic/anaphylactoid reactions, anemia, angioedema, anorexia, arrhythmia, aseptic meningitis, asthma, bleeding time increased, CHF, confusion, conjunctivitis, CVA, cystitis, duodenitis, dyspnea, ecchymosis, edema, erythema multiforme, esophagitis (+/- stricture or cardiospasm), exfoliative dermatitis, GI ulceration, hallucinations, headache, hearing decreased, hematemesis, hematuria, hepatic failure, hepatitis, hyperglycemia (in controlled diabetics), hyperpigmentation, hypertension, infection, insomnia, interstitial nephritis, irregular uterine bleeding, jaundice, LFTs increased, leukopenia, MI, palpitations, pancreatitis, pancytopenia, paresthesia, peptic ulcer (+/- bleeding/perforation), peripheral neuropathy, photophobia, photosensitivity, pulmonary infiltration (eosinophilia), rectal bleeding, renal calculus, renal failure, renal insufficiency, shock, Stevens-Johnson syndrome, syncope, thrombocytopenia, toxic epidermal necrolysis, ulcerative stomatitis, urticaria, vesiculobullous rash, renal papillary necrosis, visual disturbances

Restrictions A medication guide should be dispensed with each prescription. A template for the required MedGuide can be found on the FDA website at http://www.fda.gov/medwatch/SAFETY/2005/safety05.htm#NSAID

Dental Usual Dosing Acute pain: Adults: Oral: 200-400 mg every 6-8 hours, as needed, not to exceed total daily doses of 1000 mg

Dosage Note: For chronic conditions, response is usually observed within 2 weeks.
Children 6-16 years: Oral: Juvenile rheumatoid arthritis (Lodine® XL):
20-30 kg: 400 mg once daily
31-45 kg: 600 mg once daily
46-60 kg: 800 mg once daily
>60 kg: 1000 mg once daily
Adults: Oral:
Acute pain: 200-400 mg every 6-8 hours, as needed, not to exceed total daily doses of 1000 mg
Rheumatoid arthritis, osteoarthritis: 400 mg 2 times/day **or** 300 mg 2-3 times/day **or** 500 mg 2 times/day (doses >1000 mg/day have not been evaluated)
(Continued)

Etodolac *(Continued)*

Lodine® XL: 400-1000 mg once daily

Elderly: Refer to adult dosing; in patients ≥65 years, no dosage adjustment required based on pharmacokinetics. The elderly are more sensitive to antiprostaglandin effects and may need dosage adjustments.

Dosage adjustment in renal impairment:

Mild to moderate: No adjustment required

Severe: Use not recommended; use with caution

Hemodialysis: Not removed

Dosage adjustment in hepatic impairment: No adjustment required.

Mechanism of Action Inhibits prostaglandin synthesis by decreasing the activity of the enzyme, cyclooxygenase, which results in decreased formation of prostaglandin precursors

Contraindications Hypersensitivity to etodolac, aspirin, other NSAIDs, or any component of the formulation; perioperative pain in the setting of coronary artery bypass surgery (CABG); pregnancy

Warnings/Precautions NSAIDs are associated with an increased risk of adverse cardiovascular events, including MI, stroke, and new onset or worsening of pre-existing hypertension. Risk may be increased with duration of use or pre-existing cardiovascular risk-factors or disease. Carefully evaluate individual cardiovascular risk profiles prior to prescribing. Use caution with fluid retention, CHF, or hypertension.

NSAIDs may increase risk of gastrointestinal irritation, ulceration, bleeding, and perforation. These events may occur at any time during therapy and without warning. Use caution with a history of GI disease (bleeding or ulcers), concurrent therapy with aspirin, anticoagulants and/or corticosteroids, smoking, use of alcohol, the elderly or debilitated patients.

Use of NSAIDs can compromise existing renal function. Renal toxicity can occur in patient with impaired renal function, dehydration, heart failure, liver dysfunction, those taking diuretics and ACE inhibitors and the elderly. Rehydrate patient before starting therapy. Monitor renal function closely. Etodolac is not recommended for patients with advanced renal disease.

Use the lowest effective dose for the shortest duration of time, consistent with individual patient goals, to reduce risk of cardiovascular or GI adverse events. Alternate therapies should be considered for patients at high risk.

NSAIDs may cause serious skin adverse events including exfoliative dermatitis, Stevens-Johnson syndrome (SJS), and toxic epidermal necrolysis (TEN). Anaphylactoid reactions may occur, even without prior exposure; patients with "aspirin triad" (bronchial asthma, aspirin intolerance, rhinitis) may be at increased risk. Do not use in patients who experience bronchospasm, asthma, rhinitis, or urticaria with NSAID or aspirin therapy.

Use with caution in patients with decreased hepatic function. Closely monitor patients with any abnormal LFT. Severe hepatic reactions (eg, fulminant hepatitis, liver failure) have occurred with NSAID use, rarely; discontinue if signs or symptoms of liver disease develop, or if systemic manifestations occur. The elderly are at increased risk for adverse effects (especially peptic ulceration, CNS effects, renal toxicity) from NSAIDs even at low doses.

Withhold for at least 4-6 half-lives prior to surgical or dental procedures.

Use of extended release product consisting of a nondeformable matrix should be avoided in patients with stricture/narrowing of the GI tract; symptoms of obstruction have been associated with nondeformable products.

Drug Interactions

ACE inhibitors: Antihypertensive effects may be decreased by concurrent therapy with NSAIDs; monitor blood pressure.

Aminoglycosides: NSAIDs may decrease the excretion of aminoglycosides.

Angiotensin II antagonists: Antihypertensive effects may be decreased by concurrent therapy with NSAIDs; monitor blood pressure.

Anticoagulants (warfarin, heparin, LMWHs) in combination with NSAIDs can cause increased risk of bleeding.

Antiplatelet agents (ticlopidine, clopidogrel, aspirin, abciximab, dipyridamole, eptifibatide, tirofiban) can cause an increased risk of bleeding.

Beta-blockers: NSAIDs may diminish the antihypertensive effects of beta-blockers.

Bisphosphonates: NSAIDs may increase the risk of gastrointestinal ulceration.

Cholestyramine and colestipol reduce the bioavailability of some NSAIDs; separate administration times.

Corticosteroids may increase the risk of GI ulceration; avoid concurrent use.

Cyclosporine: NSAIDs may increase serum creatinine, potassium, blood pressure, and cyclosporine levels; monitor cyclosporine levels and renal function carefully.

Hydralazine's antihypertensive effect is decreased; avoid concurrent use.

Lithium levels can be increased; avoid concurrent use if possible or monitor lithium levels and adjust dose. Sulindac may have the least effect. When NSAID is stopped, lithium will need adjustment again.

Loop diuretics efficacy (diuretic and antihypertensive effect) is reduced. Indomethacin reduces this efficacy, however, it may be anticipated with any NSAID.

Methotrexate: Severe bone marrow suppression, aplastic anemia, and GI toxicity have been reported with concomitant NSAID therapy. Avoid use during moderate or high-dose methotrexate (increased and prolonged methotrexate levels). NSAID use during low-dose treatment of rheumatoid arthritis has not been fully evaluated; extreme caution is warranted.

Pemetrexed: NSAIDs may decrease the excretion of pemetrexed. Patients with Cl_{cr} 45-79 mL/minute should avoid short acting NSAIDs for 2 days before and 2 days after pemetrexed treatment.

Thiazides antihypertensive effects are decreased; avoid concurrent use.

Treprostinil: May enhance the risk of bleeding with concurrent use.

Vancomycin: NSAIDs may decrease the excretion of vancomycin. Avoid concurrent use.

Verapamil plasma concentration is decreased by some NSAIDs; avoid concurrent use.

Ethanol/Nutrition/Herb Interactions

Ethanol: Avoid ethanol (may enhance gastric mucosal irritation).

Food: Etodolac peak serum levels may be decreased if taken with food.

Herb/Nutraceutical: Avoid alfalfa, anise, bilberry, bladderwrack, bromelain, cat's claw, celery, coleus, cordyceps, dong quai, evening primrose, feverfew, fenugreek, garlic, ginger, ginkgo biloba, red clover, horse chestnut, grapeseed, green tea, ginseng, guggul, horse chestnut seed, horseradish, licorice, prickly ash, red clover, reishi, SAMe, sweet clover, turmeric, white willow (all have additional antiplatelet activity)

Dietary Considerations May be taken with food to decrease GI distress.

Pharmacodynamics/Kinetics

Onset of action: Analgesic: 2-4 hours; Maximum anti-inflammatory effect: A few days

Absorption: ≥80%

Distribution: V_d:

Immediate release: Adults:0.4 L/kg

Extended release: Adults: 0.57 L/kg; Children (6-16 years): 0 .08 L/kg

Protein binding: ≥99%, primarily albumin

Metabolism: Hepatic

Half-life elimination: Terminal: Adults: 5-8 hours

Extended release: Children (6-16 years): 12 hours

Time to peak, serum:

Immediate release: Adults: 1-2 hours

Extended release: Extended release: 5-7 hours, increased 1.4-3.8 hours with food

Excretion: Urine 73% (1% unchanged); feces 16%

Pregnancy Risk Factor C/D (3rd trimester)

Lactation Excretion in breast milk unknown/not recommended

Dosage Forms [DSC] = Discontinued product

Capsule: 200 mg, 300 mg

Lodine®: 200 mg, 300 mg [DSC]

Tablet: 400 mg, 500 mg

Tablet, extended release (Lodine® XL): 400 mg, 500 mg [DSC]

Selected Readings

Brooks PM and Day RO, "Nonsteroidal Anti-inflammatory Drugs - Differences and Similarities," *N Engl J Med*, 1991, 324(24):1716-25.

Tucker PW, Smith JR, and Adams DF, "A Comparison of 2 Analgesic Regimens for the Control of Postoperative Periodontal Discomfort," *J Periodontol*, 1996, 67(2):125-9.

Etodolic Acid see Etodolac on page 623

Etomidate (e TOM i date)

U.S. Brand Names Amidate®

Canadian Brand Names Amidate®

Generic Available Yes

Pharmacologic Category General Anesthetic

Use Induction and maintenance of general anesthesia

Unlabeled/Investigational Use Sedation for diagnosis of seizure foci

(Continued)

Etomidate (Continued)

Local Anesthetic/Vasoconstrictor Precautions No information available to require special precautions

Effects on Dental Treatment Key adverse event(s) related to dental treatment: Hiccups.

Common Adverse Effects

>10%:

Endocrine & metabolic: Adrenal suppression

Gastrointestinal: Nausea, vomiting on emergence from anesthesia

Local: Pain at injection site (30% to 80%)

Neuromuscular & skeletal: Myoclonus (33%), transient skeletal movements, uncontrolled eye movements

1% to 10%: Hiccups

Mechanism of Action Ultrashort-acting nonbarbiturate hypnotic (benzylimidazole) used for the induction of anesthesia; chemically, it is a carboxylated imidazole which produces a rapid induction of anesthesia with minimal cardiovascular effects; produces EEG burst suppression at high doses

Drug Interactions

Increased Effect/Toxicity: Fentanyl decreases etomidate elimination. Verapamil may increase the anesthetic and respiratory depressant effects of etomidate.

Pharmacodynamics/Kinetics

Onset of action: 30-60 seconds

Peak effect: 1 minute

Duration: 3-5 minutes; terminated by redistribution

Distribution: V_d: 2-4.5 L/kg

Protein binding: 76%;

Metabolism: Hepatic and plasma esterases

Half-life elimination: Terminal: 2.6 hours

Pregnancy Risk Factor C

Etonogestrel and Ethinyl Estradiol see Ethinyl Estradiol and Etonogestrel on page 600

Etopophos® see Etoposide Phosphate on page 627

Etoposide (e toe POE side)

U.S. Brand Names Toposar®; VePesid®

Canadian Brand Names VePesid®

Mexican Brand Names Etopos®; Lastet®; VePesid®; Vp-Tec®

Generic Available Yes

Synonyms Epipodophyllotoxin; VP-16; VP-16-213

Pharmacologic Category Antineoplastic Agent, Podophyllotoxin Derivative

Use Treatment of refractory testicular tumors; treatment of small cell lung cancer

Unlabeled/Investigational Use Treatment of lymphomas, acute nonlymphocytic leukemia (ANLL); lung, bladder, and prostate carcinoma; hepatoma, rhabdomyosarcoma, uterine carcinoma, neuroblastoma, mycosis fungoides, Kaposi's sarcoma, histiocytosis, gestational trophoblastic disease, Ewing's sarcoma, Wilms' tumor, brain tumors

Local Anesthetic/Vasoconstrictor Precautions No information available to require special precautions

Effects on Dental Treatment Key adverse event(s) related to dental treatment: Mucositis (especially at high doses).

Common Adverse Effects

>10%:

Dermatologic: Alopecia (8% to 66%)

Endocrine & metabolic: Ovarian failure (38%), amenorrhea

Gastrointestinal: Nausea/vomiting (31% to 43%), anorexia (10% to 13%), diarrhea (1% to 13%), mucositis/esophagitis (with high doses)

Hematologic: Leukopenia (60% to 91%; grade 4: 3% to 17%; onset: 5-7 days; nadir: 7-14 days; recovery: 21-28 days), thrombocytopenia (22% to 41%; grades 3/4: 1% to 20%; nadir 9-16 days), anemia (up to 33%)

1% to 10%:

Cardiovascular: Hypotension (1% to 2%; due to rapid infusion)

Gastrointestinal: Stomatitis (1% to 6%), abdominal pain (up to 2%)

Hepatic: Hepatic toxicity (up to 3%)

Neuromuscular & skeletal: Peripheral neuropathy (1% to 2%)

Miscellaneous: Anaphylactic-like reaction (I.V. infusion: 1% to 2%; including chills, fever, tachycardia, bronchospasm, dyspnea)

Mechanism of Action Etoposide has been shown to delay transit of cells through the S phase and arrest cells in late S or early G_2 phase. The drug may inhibit mitochondrial transport at the NADH dehydrogenase level or inhibit uptake of nucleosides into HeLa cells. It is a topoisomerase II inhibitor and appears to cause DNA strand breaks. Etoposide does not inhibit microtubular assembly.

Drug Interactions

Cytochrome P450 Effect: Substrate of CYP1A2 (minor), 2E1 (minor), 3A4 (major); Inhibits CYP2C9 (weak), 3A4 (weak)

Increased Effect/Toxicity: Cyclosporine may increase the levels of etoposide; consider reducing the dose of etoposide by 50%. Etoposide may increase the effects/toxicity of warfarin. CYP3A4 inhibitors may increase the levels/effects of etoposide; example inhibitors include azole antifungals, clarithromycin, diclofenac, doxycycline, erythromycin, imatinib, isoniazid, nefazodone, nicardipine, propofol, protease inhibitors, quinidine, telithromycin, and verapamil.

Decreased Effect: Barbiturates and phenytoin may decrease the levels/effects of etoposide; monitor. CYP3A4 inducers may decrease the levels/effects of etoposide; example inducers include aminoglutethimide, carbamazepine, nafcillin, nevirapine, phenobarbital, phenytoin, and rifamycins.

Pharmacodynamics/Kinetics

Absorption: Oral: 25% to 75%; significant inter- and intrapatient variation

Distribution: Average V_d: 7-17 L/m^2; poor penetration across the blood-brain barrier; CSF concentrations <10% of plasma concentrations

Protein binding: 94% to 97%

Metabolism: Hepatic to hydroxy acid and cislactone metabolites

Bioavailability: Oral: ~50% (range 25% to 75%)

Half-life elimination: Terminal: 4-11 hours; Children: Normal renal/hepatic function: 6-8 hours

Time to peak, serum: Oral: 1-1.5 hours

Excretion:

Children: Urine (≤55% as unchanged drug)

Adults: Urine (42% to 67%; 8% to 35% as unchanged drug) within 24 hours; feces (up to 44%)

Pregnancy Risk Factor D

Etoposide Phosphate (e toe POE side FOS fate)

Related Information

Etoposide on page 626

U.S. Brand Names Etopophos®

Generic Available No

Pharmacologic Category Antineoplastic Agent, Podophyllotoxin Derivative

Use Treatment of refractory testicular tumors; treatment of small cell lung cancer

Local Anesthetic/Vasoconstrictor Precautions No information available to require special precautions

Effects on Dental Treatment Key adverse event(s) related to dental treatment: Mucositis (especially at high doses) and stomatitis.

Common Adverse Effects Note: Also see adverse reactions for **etoposide**. Since etoposide phosphate is converted to etoposide, adverse reactions experienced with etoposide would also be expected with etoposide phosphate.

>10%:

Central nervous system: Chills/fever (24%)

Dermatologic: Alopecia (33% to 44%)

Gastrointestinal: Nausea/vomiting (37%), anorexia (16%), mucositis (11%)

Hematologic: Leukopenia (91%; grade 4: 17%), neutropenia (88%; grade 4: 37%), anemia (72%; grades 3/4: 19%), thrombocytopenia (23%; grade 4: 9%)

Neuromuscular and skeletal: Weakness/malaise (39%)

1% to 10%:

Cardiovascular: Hypotension (5%), hypertension (3%), facial flushing (2%)

Central nervous system: Dizziness (5%)

Dermatologic: Skin rash (3%)

Gastrointestinal: Constipation (8%), abdominal pain (7%), diarrhea (6%), taste perversion (6%)

Local: Extravasation/phlebitis (5%)

Miscellaneous: Anaphylactic-type reactions (3%; including chills, diaphoresis, fever, rigor, tachycardia, bronchospasm, dyspnea, pruritus)

Mechanism of Action Etoposide phosphate is converted *in vivo* to the active moiety, etoposide, by dephosphorylation. Etoposide inhibits mitotic activity; inhibits cells from entering prophase; inhibits DNA synthesis. Initially thought to be mitotic inhibitors similar to podophyllotoxin, but actually have no effect on microtubule assembly. However, later shown to induce DNA strand breakage (Continued)

Etoposide Phosphate *(Continued)*

and inhibition of topoisomerase II (an enzyme which breaks and repairs DNA); etoposide acts in late S or early G2 phases.

Drug Interactions

Cytochrome P450 Effect: **Substrate** of CYP1A2 (minor), 2E1 (minor), 3A4 (major); **Inhibits** CYP2C9 (weak), 3A4 (weak)

Increased Effect/Toxicity: Cyclosporine may increase the levels of etoposide; consider reducing the dose of etoposide by 50%. Etoposide may increase the effects/toxicity of warfarin. CYP3A4 inhibitors may increase the levels/effects of etoposide; example inhibitors include azole antifungals, clarithromycin, diclofenac, doxycycline, erythromycin, imatinib, isoniazid, nefazodone, nicardipine, propofol, protease inhibitors, quinidine, telithromycin, and verapamil.

Decreased Effect: Barbiturates and phenytoin may decrease the levels/effects of etoposide; monitor. CYP3A4 inducers may decrease the levels/effects of etoposide; example inducers include aminoglutethimide, carbamazepine, nafcillin, nevirapine, phenobarbital, phenytoin, and rifamycins.

Pharmacodynamics/Kinetics

Distribution: Average V_d: 7-17 L/m^2; poor penetration across blood-brain barrier; concentrations in CSF being <10% that of plasma

Protein binding: 94% to 97%

Metabolism:

Etoposide phosphate: Rapidly and completely converted to etoposide in plasma

Etoposide: Hepatic to hydroxy acid and cislactone metabolites

Half-life elimination: Terminal: 4-11 hours; Children: Normal renal/hepatic function: 6-8 hours

Excretion: Urine (as unchanged drug and metabolites); feces (2% to 16%)

Children: I.V.: Urine (≤55% as unchanged drug)

Pregnancy Risk Factor D

Eudal®-SR *see* Guaifenesin and Pseudoephedrine *on page 755*

Euflexxa™ *see* Hyaluronate and Derivatives *on page 773*

Eulexin® *see* Flutamide *on page 686*

Eurax® *see* Crotamiton *on page 398*

Evac-U-Gen [OTC] *see* Senna *on page 1384*

Evista® *see* Raloxifene *on page 1329*

Evoclin™ *see* Clindamycin *on page 361*

Evoxac® *see* Cevimeline *on page 310*

Exact® Acne Medication [OTC] *see* Benzoyl Peroxide *on page 194*

Excedrin® Extra Strength [OTC] *see* Acetaminophen, Aspirin, and Caffeine *on page 41*

Excedrin® Migraine [OTC] *see* Acetaminophen, Aspirin, and Caffeine *on page 41*

Excedrin® P.M. [OTC] *see* Acetaminophen and Diphenhydramine *on page 38*

Exelderm® *see* Sulconazole *on page 1422*

Exelon® *see* Rivastigmine *on page 1361*

Exemestane *(ex e MES tane)*

U.S. Brand Names Aromasin®

Canadian Brand Names Aromasin®

Generic Available No

Pharmacologic Category Antineoplastic Agent, Aromatase Inactivator

Use Treatment of advanced breast cancer in postmenopausal women whose disease has progressed following tamoxifen therapy; adjuvant treatment of postmenopausal estrogen receptor-positive early breast cancer following 2-3 years of tamoxifen (for a total of 5 years of adjuvant therapy)

Local Anesthetic/Vasoconstrictor Precautions No information available to require special precautions

Effects on Dental Treatment No significant effects or complications reported

Common Adverse Effects

>10%:

Cardiovasucular: Hypertension (5% to 15%)

Central nervous system: Fatigue (8% to 22%), insomnia (11% to 14%), pain (13%), headache (7% to 13%), depression (6% to 13%)

Dermatological: Hyperhidrosis (4% to 18%), alopecia (15%)

Endocrine & metabolic: Hot flashes (13% to 21%)

Gastrointestinal: Nausea (9% to 18%), abdominal pain (6% to 11%)

Hepatic: Alkaline phosphatase increased (14% to 15%)

Neuromuscular & skeletal: Arthralgia (15% to 29%)

1% to 10%:

Cardiovascular: Edema (6% to 7%); cardiac ischemic events (2%: MI, angina, myocardial ischemia); chest pain

Central nervous system: Dizziness (8% to 10%), anxiety (4% to 10%), fever (5%), confusion, hypoesthesia

Dermatologic: Dermatitis (8%), itching, rash

Endocrine & metabolic: Weight gain (8%)

Gastrointestinal: Diarrhea (4% to 10%), vomiting (7%), anorexia (6%), constipation (5%), appetite increased (3%), dyspepsia

Genitourinary: Urinary tract infection

Hepatic: Bilirubin increased (5% to 7%)

Neuromuscular & skeletal: Back pain (9%), limb pain (9%), osteoarthritis (6%), weakness (6%), osteoporosis (5%), pathological fracture (4%), paresthesia (3%), carpal tunnel syndrome (2%), cramps (2%)

Ocular: Visual disturbances (5%)

Renal: Creatinine increased (6%)

Respiratory: Dyspnea (10%), cough (6%), bronchitis, pharyngitis, rhinitis, sinusitis, upper respiratory infection

Miscellaneous: Influenza-like symptoms (6%), diaphoresis (6%), lymphedema, infection

A dose-dependent decrease in sex hormone-binding globulin has been observed with daily doses of 25 mg or more. Serum luteinizing hormone and follicle-stimulating hormone levels have increased with this medicine.

Mechanism of Action Exemestane is an irreversible, steroidal aromatase inactivator. It prevents conversion of androgens to estrogens by tying up the enzyme aromatase. In breast cancers where growth is estrogen-dependent, this medicine will lower circulating estrogens.

Drug Interactions

Cytochrome P450 Effect: Substrate of CYP3A4 (major)

Decreased Effect: CYP3A4 inducers may decrease the levels/effects of exemestane; example inducers include aminoglutethimide, carbamazepine, efavirenz, fosphenytoin, nafcillin, nevirapine, oxcarbazepine, pentobarbital, phenobarbital, phenytoin, primidone, rifabutin, rifampin, and rifapentine; adjustment required with potent inducers.

Pharmacodynamics/Kinetics

Absorption: Rapid and moderate (~42%) following oral administration; absorption increases ~40% following high-fat meal

Distribution: Extensive

Protein binding: 90%, primarily to albumin and α_1-acid glycoprotein

Metabolism: Extensively hepatic; oxidation (CYP3A4) of methylene group, reduction of 17-keto group with formation of many secondary metabolites; metabolites are inactive

Half-life elimination: 24 hours

Time to peak: Women with breast cancer: 1.2 hours

Excretion: Urine (<1% as unchanged drug, 39% to 45% as metabolites); feces (36% to 48%)

Pregnancy Risk Factor D

Exenatide (ex EN a tide)

U.S. Brand Names Byetta™

Generic Available No

Synonyms AC002993; Exendin-4; LY2148568

Pharmacologic Category Antidiabetic Agent, Incretin Mimetic

Use Management (adjunctive) of type 2 diabetes mellitus (noninsulin dependent, NIDDM)

Local Anesthetic/Vasoconstrictor Precautions No information available to require special precautions

Effects on Dental Treatment No significant effects or complications reported

Common Adverse Effects

>10%:

Endocrine & metabolic: Hypoglycemia (with concurrent sulfonylurea therapy 14% to 36%; frequency similar to placebo with metformin therapy)

Gastrointestinal: Nausea (44%), vomiting (13%), diarrhea (13%)

Miscellaneous: Anti-exenatide antibodies (low titers 38%, high titers 6%)

1% to 10%:

Central nervous system: Dizziness (9%), headache (9%)

Endocrine & metabolic: Appetite decreased

Gastrointestinal: Dyspepsia (6%), GERD

Neuromuscular & skeletal: Weakness

(Continued)

Exenatide *(Continued)*

Miscellaneous: Feeling jittery (9%), diaphoresis increased

Mechanism of Action Exenatide is an analog of the hormone incretin (glucagon-like peptide 1 or GLP-1) which increases insulin secretion, increases B-cell growth/replication, slows gastric emptying, and may decrease food intake. When added to sulfonylureas and/or metformin, it results in additional lowering of hemoglobin A_{1c} by approximately 0.5% to 1%.

Drug Interactions

Decreased Effect: Note: Due to its effects on gastric emptying, exenatide may reduce the rate and extent of absorption of orally-administered drugs. Should be used with caution in patients receiving medications which require rapid absorption from the gastrointestinal tract. Administration of medications 1 hour prior to the use of exenatide has been recommended by the manufacturer when optimal drug absorption and peak levels are important to the overall therapeutic effect (such as with antibiotics and/or oral contraceptives).

Pharmacodynamics/Kinetics

Distribution: V_d: 28.3 L

Metabolism: Minimal systemic metabolism; proteolytic degradation may occur following glomerular filtration

Half-life elimination: 2.4 hours

Time to peak, plasma: SubQ: 2.1 hours

Excretion: Urine (majority of dose)

Pregnancy Risk Factor C

Exendin-4 see Exenatide on page 629

Exjade® see Deferasirox on page 427

ex-lax® [OTC] see Senna on page 1384

ex-lax® Maximum Strength [OTC] see Senna on page 1384

Exorex® see Coal Tar on page 383

Extendryl see Chlorpheniramine, Phenylephrine, and Methscopolamine on page 327

Extendryl JR see Chlorpheniramine, Phenylephrine, and Methscopolamine on page 327

Extendryl SR see Chlorpheniramine, Phenylephrine, and Methscopolamine on page 327

Extraneal® see Icodextrin on page 814

Exubera® see Insulin Inhalation on page 837

EYE001 see Pegaptanib on page 1193

Eye-Sine™ [OTC] see Tetrahydrozoline on page 1470

EZ-Char™ [OTC] see Charcoal on page 311

Ezetimibe *(ez ET i mibe)*

U.S. Brand Names Zetia™

Canadian Brand Names Ezetrol®

Generic Available No

Pharmacologic Category Antilipemic Agent, 2-Azetidinone

Use Use in combination with dietary therapy for the treatment of primary hypercholesterolemia (as monotherapy or in combination with HMG-CoA reductase inhibitors); homozygous sitosterolemia; homozygous familial hypercholesterolemia (in combination with atorvastatin or simvastatin)

Local Anesthetic/Vasoconstrictor Precautions No information available to require special precautions

Effects on Dental Treatment No significant effects or complications reported

Common Adverse Effects 1% to 10%:

Cardiovascular: Chest pain (3%), dizziness (3%), fatigue (2%)

Central nervous system: Headache (8%)

Gastrointestinal: Diarrhea (3% to 4%), abdominal pain (3%)

Neuromuscular & skeletal: Arthralgia (4%)

Respiratory: Sinusitis (4% to 5%), pharyngitis (2% to 3%), placebo 2%)

Dosage Oral:

Hyperlipidemias: Children ≥10 years and Adults: 10 mg/day

Sitosterolemia: Adults: 10 mg/day

Elderly: Refer to Adults dosing

Dosage adjustment in renal impairment: Bioavailability increased with severe impairment; no dosing adjustment recommended

Dosage adjustment in hepatic impairment: Bioavailability increased with hepatic impairment

Mild impairment (Child-Pugh score 5-6): No dosing adjustment necessary

Moderate to severe impairment (Child-Pugh score 7-15): Use of ezetimibe not recommended

Mechanism of Action Inhibits absorption of cholesterol at the brush border of the small intestine, leading to a decreased delivery of cholesterol to the liver, reduction of hepatic cholesterol stores and an increased clearance of cholesterol from the blood; decreases total C, LDL-cholesterol (LDL-C), ApoB, and triglycerides (TG) while increasing HDL-cholesterol (HDL-C).

Contraindications Hypersensitivity to ezetimibe or any component of the formulation

Warnings/Precautions Secondary causes of hyperlipidemia should be ruled out prior to therapy. Use caution with renal or mild hepatic impairment; not recommended for use with moderate or severe hepatic impairment. Safety and efficacy have not been established in patients <10 years of age.

Drug Interactions

Increased Effect/Toxicity: Cyclosporine may increase plasma levels of ezetimibe. Fibric acid derivatives may increase bioavailability of ezetimibe (safety and efficacy of concomitant use not established). Ezetimibe may increase serum levels of cyclosporine.

Decreased Effect: Bile acid sequestrants may decrease ezetimibe bioavailability; administer ezetimibe ≥2 hours before or ≥4 hours after bile acid sequestrants.

Dietary Considerations May be taken without regard to meals. Before initiation of therapy, patients should be placed on a standard cholesterol-lowering diet for 6 weeks and the diet should be continued during drug therapy.

Pharmacodynamics/Kinetics

Protein binding: >90% to plasma proteins

Metabolism: Undergoes conjugation in the small intestine and liver; forms metabolite (active); may undergo enterohepatic recycling

Bioavailability: Variable

Half-life: 22 hours (ezetimibe and metabolite)

Time to peak, plasma: 4-12 hours

Excretion: Feces (78%, 69% as ezetimibe); urine (11%, 9% as metabolite)

Pregnancy Risk Factor C

Dosage Forms TAB: 10 mg

Ezetimibe and Simvastatin (ez ET i mibe & SIM va stat in)

Related Information

Ezetimibe *on page 630*
Simvastatin *on page 1394*

U.S. Brand Names Vytorin™

Generic Available No

Pharmacologic Category Antilipemic Agent, 2-Azetidinone; Antilipemic Agent, HMG-CoA Reductase Inhibitor

Use Used in combination with dietary modification for the treatment of primary hypercholesterolemia and homozygous familial hypercholesterolemia

Local Anesthetic/Vasoconstrictor Precautions No information available to require special precautions

Effects on Dental Treatment No significant effects or complications reported

Common Adverse Effects Percentages below refer to combination Vytorin™. Also see individual agents.

1% to 10%:

Central nervous system: Headache (7%)

Neuromuscular & skeletal: Myalgia (4%), pain in extremity (2%)

Respiratory: Upper respiratory infection (4%)

Miscellaneous: Influenza (3%)

Mechanism of Action

Ezetimibe: Inhibits absorption of cholesterol at the brush border of the small intestine, leading to a decreased delivery of cholesterol to the liver.

Simvastatin: A methylated derivative of lovastatin that acts by competitively inhibiting 3-hydroxy-3-methylglutaryl-coenzyme A (HMG-CoA) reductase, the enzyme that catalyzes the rate-limiting step in cholesterol biosynthesis.

Drug Interactions

Cytochrome P450 Effect: Simvastatin: **Substrate** of CYP3A4 (major); **Inhibits** CYP2C8/9 (weak), 2D6 (weak)

Increased Effect/Toxicity: See individual agents.

Pharmacodynamics/Kinetics See individual agents.

Bioavailability: Vytorin™ is equivalent to coadministered ezetimibe and simvastatin.

Pregnancy Risk Factor X

E•R•O [OTC] *see* Carbamide Peroxide *on page 264*

F₃T *see* Trifluridine *on page 1536*

Fabrazyme® *see* Agalsidase Beta *on page 55*

Factive® *see* Gemifloxacin *on page 731*

Factor VIIa (Recombinant) (FAK ter SEV en ree KOM be nant)

U.S. Brand Names NovoSeven®
Canadian Brand Names Niastase®
Generic Available No
Synonyms Coagulation Factor VIIa; Eptacog Alfa (Activated); rFVIIa
Pharmacologic Category Antihemophilic Agent; Blood Product Derivative
Use Treatment of bleeding episodes and prevention of bleeding in surgical interventions in patients with hemophilia A or B with inhibitors to factor VIII or factor IX and in patients with congenital factor VII deficiency
Local Anesthetic/Vasoconstrictor Precautions No information available to require special precautions
Effects on Dental Treatment No significant effects or complications reported
Common Adverse Effects 1% to 10%:
Cardiovascular: Hypertension
Central nervous system: Fever
Hematologic: Hemorrhage, decreased plasma fibrinogen
Neuromuscular & skeletal: Hemarthrosis
Mechanism of Action Recombinant factor VIIa, a vitamin K-dependent glycoprotein, promotes hemostasis by activating the extrinsic pathway of the coagulation cascade. It replaces deficient activated coagulation factor VII, which complexes with tissue factor and may activate coagulation factor X to Xa and factor IX to IXa. When complexed with other factors, coagulation factor Xa converts prothrombin to thrombin, a key step in the formation of a fibrin-platelet hemostatic plug.
Pharmacodynamics/Kinetics
Distribution: V_d: 103 mL/kg (78-139)
Half-life elimination: 2.3 hours (1.7-2.7)
Excretion: Clearance: 33 mL/kg/hour (27-49)
Pregnancy Risk Factor C

Factor VIII (Human) *see* Antihemophilic Factor (Human) *on page 129*

Factor VIII (Recombinant) *see* Antihemophilic Factor (Recombinant) *on page 130*

Factor IX (FAK ter nyne)

U.S. Brand Names AlphaNine® SD; BeneFix®; Mononine®
Canadian Brand Names BeneFix®; Immunine® VH; Mononine®
Generic Available No
Pharmacologic Category Antihemophilic Agent; Blood Product Derivative
Use Control bleeding in patients with factor IX deficiency (hemophilia B or Christmas disease)
Local Anesthetic/Vasoconstrictor Precautions No information available to require special precautions
Effects on Dental Treatment No significant effects or complications reported
Common Adverse Effects Frequency not defined.
Cardiovascular: Angioedema, cyanosis, flushing, hypotension, tightness in chest, tightness in neck, (thrombosis following high dosages because of presence of activated clotting factors)
Central nervous system: Fever, headache, chills, somnolence, dizziness, drowsiness, lightheadedness
Dermatologic: Urticaria, rash
Gastrointestinal: Nausea, vomiting, abnormal taste
Hematologic: Disseminated intravascular coagulation (DIC)
Local: Injection site discomfort
Neuromuscular & skeletal: Tingling
Respiratory: Dyspnea, laryngeal edema, allergic rhinitis
Miscellaneous: Transient fever (following rapid administration), anaphylaxis, burning sensation in jaw/skull
Mechanism of Action Replaces deficient clotting factor IX; concentrate of factor IX; hemophilia B, or Christmas disease, is an X-linked inherited disorder of blood coagulation characterized by insufficient or abnormal synthesis of the clotting protein factor IX. Factor IX is a vitamin K-dependent coagulation factor which is synthesized in the liver. Factor IX is activated by factor XIa in the intrinsic coagulation pathway. Activated factor IX (IXa), in combination with factor VII:C activates factor X to Xa, resulting ultimately in the conversion of prothrombin to thrombin and the formation of a fibrin clot. The infusion of

exogenous factor IX to replace the deficiency present in hemophilia B temporarily restores hemostasis.

Drug Interactions
  Increased Effect/Toxicity: Do not coadminister with aminocaproic acid; may increase risk for thrombosis.
Pharmacodynamics/Kinetics Half-life elimination: IX component: 23-31 hours
Pregnancy Risk Factor C

Factor IX Complex (Human) (FAK ter nyne KOM pleks HYU man)

U.S. Brand Names Bebulin® VH; Profilnine® SD; Proplex® T
Generic Available No
Synonyms Prothrombin Complex Concentrate
Pharmacologic Category Antihemophilic Agent; Blood Product Derivative
Use
  Control bleeding in patients with factor IX deficiency (hemophilia B or Christmas disease) **Note:** Factor IX concentrate containing **only** factor IX is also available and preferable for this indication.
  Prevention/control of bleeding in hemophilia A patients with inhibitors to factor VIII
  Prevention/control of bleeding in patients with factor VII deficiency
  Emergency correction of the coagulopathy of warfarin excess in critical situations.
Local Anesthetic/Vasoconstrictor Precautions No information available to require special precautions
Effects on Dental Treatment No significant effects or complications reported
Common Adverse Effects 1% to 10%:
  Central nervous system: Fever, headache, chills
  Neuromuscular & skeletal: Tingling
  Miscellaneous: Following rapid administration: Transient fever
Mechanism of Action Replaces deficient clotting factor including factor X; hemophilia B, or Christmas disease, is an X-linked recessively inherited disorder of blood coagulation characterized by insufficient or abnormal synthesis of the clotting protein factor IX. Factor IX is a vitamin K-dependent coagulation factor which is synthesized in the liver. Factor IX is activated by factor XIa in the intrinsic coagulation pathway. Activated factor IX (IXa), in combination with factor VII:C activates factor X to Xa, resulting ultimately in the conversion of prothrombin to thrombin and the formation of a fibrin clot. The infusion of exogenous factor IX to replace the deficiency present in hemophilia B temporarily restores hemostasis.
Drug Interactions
  Increased Effect/Toxicity: Do not coadminister with aminocaproic acid; may increase risk for thrombosis.
Pharmacodynamics/Kinetics
  Half-life elimination:
  VII component: Initial: 4-6 hours; Terminal: 22.5 hours
  IX component: 24 hours
Pregnancy Risk Factor C

Factrel® see Gonadorelin on page 749

Famciclovir (fam SYE kloe veer)

Related Information
  Sexually-Transmitted Diseases on page 1674
  Systemic Viral Diseases on page 1675
Related Sample Prescriptions
  Herpes Simplex (Recurrent) on page 1742
  Shingles (Varicella-Zoster Virus) on page 1742
U.S. Brand Names Famvir®
Canadian Brand Names Famvir®
Generic Available No
Pharmacologic Category Antiviral Agent
Dental Use Management of acute herpes zoster (shingles); treatment of recurrent herpes labialis in immunocompetent patients
Use Management of acute herpes zoster (shingles); treatment and suppression of recurrent episodes of genital herpes in immunocompetent patients; treatment of recurrent mucocutaneous/genital herpes simplex in HIV-infected patients
  (Continued)

Famciclovir *(Continued)*

Local Anesthetic/Vasoconstrictor Precautions No information available to require special precautions

Effects on Dental Treatment No significant effects or complications reported

Significant Adverse Effects

>10%:
- Central nervous system: Headache (17% to 39%)
- Gastrointestinal: Nausea (7% to 13%)

1% to 10%:
- Central nervous system: Fatigue (4% to 6%), migraine (1% to 3%)
- Dermatologic: Pruritus (1% to 4%), rash (<1% to 3%)
- Endocrine and metabolic: Dysmenorrhea (up to 8%)
- Gastrointestinal: Diarrhea (5% to 9%), flatulence (2% to 5%), vomiting (1% to 5%), abdominal pain (1% to 8%)
- Hematologic: Neutropenia (3%), leukopenia (1%)
- Hepatic: Transaminases increased (2% to 3%), bilirubin increased (2%)
- Neuromuscular & skeletal: Paresthesia (1% to 3%)

Postmarketing and/or case reports: Confusion, delirium, disorientation, dizziness, erythema multiforme, hallucinations, jaundice, somnolence, thrombocytopenia, urticaria

Dosage Adults: Oral:

Acute herpes zoster: 500 mg every 8 hours for 7 days (**Note:** Initiate therapy within 72 hours of rash onset.)

Recurrent genital herpes simplex in immunocompetent patients:
- Initial: 125 mg twice daily for 5 days (**Note:** initiate therapy within 6 hours of symptoms/lesions.)
- Suppressive therapy: 250 mg twice daily for up to 1 year

Recurrent mucocutaneous/genital herpes simplex in HIV patients: 500 mg twice daily for 7 days

Dosing interval in renal impairment:

Herpes zoster:
- Cl_{cr} 40-59 mL/minute: Administer 500 mg every 12 hours
- Cl_{cr} 20-39 mL/minute: Administer 500 mg every 24 hours
- Cl_{cr} <20 mL/minute: Administer 250 mg every 24 hours
- Hemodialysis: Administer 250 mg after each dialysis session.

Recurrent genital herpes:
- Cl_{cr} 20-39 mL/minute: Administer 125 mg every 24 hours
- Cl_{cr} <20 mL/minute: Administer 125 mg every 24 hours
- Hemodialysis: Administer 125 mg after each dialysis session.

Suppression of recurrent genital herpes:
- Cl_{cr} 20-39 mL/minute: Administer 125 mg every 12 hours
- Cl_{cr} <20 mL/minute: Administer 125 mg every 24 hours
- Hemodialysis: Administer 125 mg after each dialysis session.

Recurrent orolabial or genital herpes in HIV-infected patients:
- Cl_{cr} 20-39 mL/minute: Administer 500 mg every 24 hours
- Cl_{cr} <20 mL/minute: Administer 250 mg every 24 hours
- Hemodialysis: Administer 250 mg after each dialysis session.

Mechanism of Action Famciclovir undergoes rapid biotransformation to the active compound, penciclovir, which is phosphorylated by viral thymidine kinase in HSV-1, HSV-2, and VZV-infected cells to a monophosphate form; this is then converted to penciclovir triphosphate and competes with deoxyguanosine triphosphate to inhibit HSV-2 polymerase (eg, herpes viral DNA synthesis/replication is selectively inhibited)

Contraindications Hypersensitivity to famciclovir, penciclovir, or any component of the formulation

Warnings/Precautions Has not been established for use in initial episodes of genital herpes, patients with ophthalmic or disseminated zoster, or in immunocompromised patients with herpes zoster; dosage adjustment is required in patients with renal insufficiency and in patients with noncompensated hepatic disease. Tablets contain lactose; do not use with galactose intolerance, severe lactase deficiency, or glucose-galactose malabsorption syndromes. Safety and efficacy have not been established in children <18 years of age.

Ethanol/Nutrition/Herb Interactions Food: Rate of absorption and/or conversion to penciclovir and peak concentration are reduced with food, but bioavailability is not affected.

Dietary Considerations May be taken with food or on an empty stomach.

Pharmacodynamics/Kinetics

Absorption: Food decreases maximum peak concentration and delays time to peak; AUC remains the same

Distribution: V_{dss}: 0.91-1.25 L/kg

Protein binding: ≤20%

Metabolism: Rapidly deacetylated and oxidized to penciclovir; not via CYP

Bioavailability: 69% to 85%

Half-life elimination: Penciclovir: 2-3 hours (10, 20, and 7 hours in HSV-1, HSV-2, and VZV-infected cells, respectively); prolonged with renal impairment

Time to peak: 0.9 hours; C_{max} and T_{max} are decreased and prolonged with noncompensated hepatic impairment

Excretion: Urine (94% mostly as penciclovir)

Pregnancy Risk Factor B

Lactation Excretion in breast milk unknown/use caution

Breast-Feeding Considerations There is no specific data describing the excretion of famciclovir in breast milk. Breast feeding should be avoided if herpes lesions are on breast in order to avoid transmission to infant.

Dosage Forms Tablet: 125 mg, 250 mg, 500 mg [contains lactose]

Famotidine (fa MOE ti deen)

Related Information
Gastrointestinal Disorders on page 1654

U.S. Brand Names Fluxid™; Pepcid®; Pepcid® AC [OTC]

Canadian Brand Names Apo-Famotidine®; Famotidine Omega; Gen-Famotidine; Novo-Famotidine; Nu-Famotidine; Pepcid®; Pepcid® AC; Pepcid® I.V.; ratio-Famotidine; Riva-Famotidine

Mexican Brand Names Durater®; Famoxal®; Farmotex®; Pepcidine®; Sigafam®

Generic Available Yes: Injection, tablet

Pharmacologic Category Histamine H_2 Antagonist

Use Therapy and treatment of duodenal ulcer, gastric ulcer, control gastric pH in critically-ill patients, symptomatic relief in gastritis, gastroesophageal reflux, active benign ulcer, and pathological hypersecretory conditions

OTC labeling: Relief of heartburn, acid indigestion, and sour stomach

Unlabeled/Investigational Use Part of a multidrug regimen for *H. pylori* eradication to reduce the risk of duodenal ulcer recurrence

Local Anesthetic/Vasoconstrictor Precautions No information available to require special precautions

Effects on Dental Treatment No significant effects or complications reported

Common Adverse Effects
Note: Agitation and vomiting have been reported in up to 14% of pediatric patients <1 year of age.

1% to 10%:

Central nervous system: Dizziness (1%), headache (5%)

Gastrointestinal: Constipation (1%), diarrhea (2%)

Dosage
Children: Treatment duration and dose should be individualized

Peptic ulcer: 1-16 years:

Oral: 0.5 mg/kg/day at bedtime or divided twice daily (maximum dose: 40 mg/day); doses of up to 1 mg/kg/day have been used in clinical studies

I.V.: 0.25 mg/kg every 12 hours (maximum dose: 40 mg/day); doses of up to 0.5 mg/kg have been used in clinical studies

GERD: Oral:

<3 months: 0.5 mg/kg once daily

3-12 months: 0.5 mg/kg twice daily

1-16 years: 1 mg/kg/day divided twice daily (maximum dose: 40 mg twice daily); doses of up to 2 mg/kg/day have been used in clinical studies

Children ≥12 years and Adults: Heartburn, indigestion, sour stomach: OTC labeling: Oral: 10-20 mg every 12 hours; dose may be taken 15-60 minutes before eating foods known to cause heartburn

Adults:

Duodenal ulcer: Oral: Acute therapy: 40 mg/day at bedtime for 4-8 weeks; maintenance therapy: 20 mg/day at bedtime

Helicobacter pylori eradication (unlabeled use): 40 mg once daily; requires combination therapy with antibiotics

Gastric ulcer: Oral: Acute therapy: 40 mg/day at bedtime

Hypersecretory conditions: Oral: Initial: 20 mg every 6 hours, may increase in increments up to 160 mg every 6 hours

GERD: Oral: 20 mg twice daily for 6 weeks

Esophagitis and accompanying symptoms due to GERD: Oral: 20 mg or 40 mg twice daily for up to 12 weeks

Patients unable to take oral medication: I.V.: 20 mg every 12 hours

Dosing adjustment in renal impairment: Cl_{cr} <50 mL/minute: Manufacturer recommendation: Administer 50% of dose or increase the dosing interval to every 36-48 hours (to limit potential CNS adverse effects).

(Continued)

Famotidine *(Continued)*

Mechanism of Action Competitive inhibition of histamine at H_2 receptors of the gastric parietal cells, which inhibits gastric acid secretion

Contraindications Hypersensitivity to famotidine, other H_2 antagonists, or any component of the formulation

Warnings/Precautions Modify dose in patients with renal impairment; chewable tablets contain phenylalanine; multidose vials contain benzyl alcohol

OTC labeling: When used for self-medication, patients should be instructed not to use if they have difficulty swallowing, have vomiting with blood, or bloody or black stools. Not for use with other acid reducers.

Drug Interactions

Decreased Effect: Decreased serum levels of ketoconazole and itraconazole (reduced absorption).

Ethanol/Nutrition/Herb Interactions

Ethanol: Avoid ethanol (may cause gastric mucosal irritation).

Food: Famotidine bioavailability may be increased if taken with food.

Dietary Considerations Phenylalanine content: Pepcid® AC chewable: Each 10 mg tablet contains phenylalanine 1.4 mg

Pharmacodynamics/Kinetics

Onset of action: GI: Oral: Within 1-3 hour

Duration: 10-12 hours

Protein binding: 15% to 20%

Bioavailability: Oral: 40% to 50%

Half-life elimination:

Injection, oral suspension, tablet: 2.5-3.5 hours; prolonged with renal impairment; Oliguria: 20 hours

Orally-disintegrating tablet: 2.5-5 hours

Time to peak, serum: Oral: ~1-3 hours

Excretion: Urine (as unchanged drug)

Pregnancy Risk Factor B

Dosage Forms GELCAP (Pepcid® AC): 10 mg. INF [premixed in NS] (Pepcid®): 20 mg (50 mL). INJ, solution 10 mg/mL (4 mL, 20 mL, 50 mL); (Pepcid®): 10 mg/mL (20 mL). INJ, solution [preservative free] (Pepcid®): 10 mg/mL (2 mL). POWDER, oral suspension (Pepcid®): 40 mg/5 mL (50 mL). TAB: 10 mg [OTC], 20 mg, 40 mg; (Pepcid®): 20 mg, 40 mg; (Pepcid® AC): 10 mg, 20 mg. TAB, chewable (Pepcid® AC): 10 mg. TAB, orally-disintegrating (Fluxid™): 20 mg, 40 mg

---

Famotidine, Calcium Carbonate, and Magnesium Hydroxide

(fa MOE ti deen, KAL see um KAR bun ate, & mag NEE zhum hye DROKS ide)

Related Information

Calcium Carbonate *on page 248*

Famotidine *on page 635*

Magnesium Hydroxide *on page 961*

U.S. Brand Names Pepcid® Complete [OTC]

Canadian Brand Names Pepcid® Complete [OTC]

Generic Available No

Synonyms Calcium Carbonate, Magnesium Hydroxide, and Famotidine; Magnesium Hydroxide, Famotidine, and Calcium Carbonate

Pharmacologic Category Antacid; Histamine H_2 Antagonist

Use Relief of heartburn due to acid indigestion

Local Anesthetic/Vasoconstrictor Precautions No information available to require special precautions

Effects on Dental Treatment No significant effects or complications reported

Common Adverse Effects See individual agents.

Mechanism of Action

Famotidine: H_2 antagonist

Calcium carbonate: Antacid

Magnesium hydroxide: Antacid

Drug Interactions

Increased Effect/Toxicity: See individual agents.

Decreased Effect: See individual agents.

Pharmacodynamics/Kinetics See individual agents.

Famvir® *see* Famciclovir *on page 633*

Fansidar® *see* Sulfadoxine and Pyrimethamine *on page 1424*

Fareston® *see* Toremifene *on page 1512*

Faslodex® *see* Fulvestrant *on page 713*

Fat Emulsion (fat e MUL shun)

U.S. Brand Names Intralipid®; Liposyn® III
Canadian Brand Names Intralipid®
Generic Available No
Synonyms Intravenous Fat Emulsion
Pharmacologic Category Caloric Agent
Use Source of calories and essential fatty acids for patients requiring parenteral nutrition of extended duration
Local Anesthetic/Vasoconstrictor Precautions No information available to require special precautions
Effects on Dental Treatment No significant effects or complications reported
Common Adverse Effects Frequency not defined.
  Cardiovascular: Cyanosis, flushing, chest pain
  Central nervous system: Headache, dizziness
  Endocrine & metabolic: Hyperlipemia, hypertriglyceridemia
  Gastrointestinal: Nausea, vomiting, diarrhea
  Hematologic: Hypercoagulability, thrombocytopenia in neonates (rare)
  Hepatic: Hepatomegaly, pancreatitis
  Local: Thrombophlebitis
  Respiratory: Dyspnea
  Miscellaneous: Sepsis, diaphoresis, brown pigment deposition in the reticuloendothelial system (significance unknown)
Mechanism of Action Essential for normal structure and function of cell membranes
Pharmacodynamics/Kinetics
  Metabolism: Undergoes lipolysis to free fatty acids which are utilized by reticuloendothelial cells
  Half-life elimination: 0.5-1 hour
Pregnancy Risk Factor C

FazaClo® *see* Clozapine *on page 382*
5-FC *see* Flucytosine *on page 662*
FC1157a *see* Toremifene *on page 1512*
Feiba VH *see* Anti-inhibitor Coagulant Complex *on page 130*

Felbamate (FEL ba mate)

U.S. Brand Names Felbatol®
Generic Available No
Pharmacologic Category Anticonvulsant, Miscellaneous
Use Not as a first-line antiepileptic treatment; only in those patients who respond inadequately to alternative treatments and whose epilepsy is so severe that a substantial risk of aplastic anemia and/or liver failure is deemed acceptable in light of the benefits conferred by its use. Patient must be fully advised of risk and provide signed written informed consent. Felbamate can be used as either monotherapy or adjunctive therapy in the treatment of partial seizures (with and without generalization) and in adults with epilepsy.
  Orphan drug: Adjunctive therapy in the treatment of partial and generalized seizures associated with Lennox-Gastaut syndrome in children
Local Anesthetic/Vasoconstrictor Precautions No information available to require special precautions
Effects on Dental Treatment Key adverse event(s) related to dental treatment: Xerostomia (normal salivary flow resumes upon discontinuation) and abnormal taste.
Common Adverse Effects
  >10%:
    Central nervous system: Somnolence, headache, fatigue, dizziness
    Gastrointestinal: Nausea, anorexia, vomiting, constipation
  1% to 10%:
    Cardiovascular: Chest pain, palpitation, tachycardia
    Central nervous system: Depression or behavior changes, nervousness, anxiety, ataxia, stupor, malaise, agitation, psychological disturbances, aggressive reaction
    Dermatologic: Skin rash, acne, pruritus
    Gastrointestinal: Xerostomia, diarrhea, abdominal pain, weight gain, taste perversion
    Neuromuscular & skeletal: Tremor, abnormal gait, paresthesia, myalgia
    Ocular: Diplopia, abnormal vision
  (Continued)

Felbamate (Continued)

Respiratory: Sinusitis, pharyngitis
Miscellaneous: ALT increase

Restrictions A patient "informed consent" form should be completed and signed by the patient and physician. Copies are available from Wallace Pharmaceuticals by calling 609-655-6147.

Mechanism of Action Mechanism of action is unknown but has properties in common with other marketed anticonvulsants; has weak inhibitory effects on GABA-receptor binding, benzodiazepine receptor binding, and is devoid of activity at the MK-801 receptor binding site of the NMDA receptor-ionophore complex.

Drug Interactions

Cytochrome P450 Effect: Substrate of CYP2E1 (minor), 3A4 (major); **Inhibits** CYP2C19 (weak); **Induces** CYP3A4 (weak)

Increased Effect/Toxicity: Felbamate increases serum phenytoin, phenobarbital, and valproic acid concentrations which may result in toxicity; consider decreasing phenytoin or phenobarbital dosage by 25%. A decrease in valproic acid dosage may also be necessary. CYP3A4 inhibitors may increase the levels/effects of felbamate; example inhibitors include azole antifungals, clarithromycin, diclofenac, doxycycline, erythromycin, imatinib, isoniazid, nefazodone, nicardipine, propofol, protease inhibitors, quinidine, telithromycin, and verapamil.

Decreased Effect: Felbamate may decrease carbamazepine levels and increase levels of the active metabolite of carbamazepine (10,11-epoxide) resulting in carbamazepine toxicity; monitor for signs of carbamazepine toxicity (dizziness, ataxia, nystagmus, drowsiness). CYP3A4 inducers may decrease the levels/effects of felbamate; example inducers include aminoglutethimide, carbamazepine, nafcillin, nevirapine, phenobarbital, phenytoin, and rifamycins.

Pharmacodynamics/Kinetics

Absorption: Rapid and almost complete; food has no effect upon the tablet's absorption

Distribution: V_d: 0.7-1 L/kg

Protein binding: 22% to 25%, primarily to albumin

Half-life elimination: 20-23 hours (average); prolonged in renal dysfunction

Time to peak, serum: ~3 hours

Excretion: Urine (40% to 50% as unchanged drug, 40% as inactive metabolites)

Pregnancy Risk Factor C

Felbatol® see Felbamate on page 637
Feldene® see Piroxicam on page 1248

Felodipine (fe LOE di peen)

Related Information

Cardiovascular Diseases on page 1636

U.S. Brand Names Plendil®

Canadian Brand Names Plendil®; Renedil®

Mexican Brand Names Munobal®; Plendil®

Generic Available No

Pharmacologic Category Calcium Channel Blocker

Use Treatment of hypertension

Local Anesthetic/Vasoconstrictor Precautions No information available to require special precautions

Effects on Dental Treatment Key adverse event(s) related to dental treatment: Gingival hyperplasia (fewer reports than other CCBs, resolves upon discontinuation, consultation with physician is suggested).

Common Adverse Effects

>10%: Central nervous system: Headache (11% to 15%)

2% to 10%: Cardiovascular: Peripheral edema (2% to 17%), tachycardia (0.4% to 2.5%), flushing (4% to 7%)

Mechanism of Action Inhibits calcium ions from entering the "slow channels" or select voltage-sensitive areas of vascular smooth muscle and myocardium during depolarization, producing a relaxation of coronary vascular smooth muscle and coronary vasodilation; increases myocardial oxygen delivery in patients with vasospastic angina

Drug Interactions

Cytochrome P450 Effect: Substrate of CYP3A4 (major); **Inhibits** CYP2C8 (moderate), 2C9 (weak), 2D6 (weak), 3A4 (weak)

Increased Effect/Toxicity: Felodipine may increase the levels/effects of CYP2C8 substrates; example substrates include amiodarone, paclitaxel, pioglitazone, repaglinide, and rosiglitazone. CYP3A4 inhibitors may increase the levels/effects of felodipine; example inhibitors include azole antifungals, clarithromycin, diclofenac, doxycycline, erythromycin, imatinib, isoniazid, nefazodone, nicardipine, propofol, protease inhibitors, quinidine, telithromycin, and verapamil. Beta-blockers may have increased pharmacokinetic or pharmacodynamic interactions with felodipine. Cyclosporine increases felodipine's serum concentration. Blood pressure-lowering effects may be additive with sildenafil, tadalafil, and vardenafil (use caution). Felodipine may increase tacrolimus serum levels (monitor).

Decreased Effect: Felodipine may decrease pharmacologic actions of theophylline. Calcium may reduce the calcium channel blocker's effects, particularly hypotension. Felodipine may decrease pharmacologic actions of theophylline. CYP3A4 inducers may decrease the levels/effects of felodipine; example inducers include aminoglutethimide, carbamazepine, nafcillin, nevirapine, phenobarbital, phenytoin, and rifamycins.

Pharmacodynamics/Kinetics
Onset of action: Antihypertensive: 2-5 hours
Duration of antihypertensive effect: 24 hours
Absorption: 100%; Absolute: 20% due to first-pass effect
Protein binding: >99%
Metabolism: Hepatic; CYP3A4 substrate (major); extensive first-pass effect
Half-life elimination: Immediate release: 11-16 hours
Excretion: Urine (70% as metabolites); feces 10%

Pregnancy Risk Factor C

Felodipine and Enalapril see Enalapril and Felodipine on page 540

Femara® see Letrozole on page 904

femhrt® see Ethinyl Estradiol and Norethindrone on page 608

Femilax™ [OTC] see Bisacodyl on page 209

Femiron® [OTC] see Ferrous Fumarate on page 650

Fem-Prin® [OTC] see Acetaminophen, Aspirin, and Caffeine on page 41

Femring® see Estradiol on page 574

Femtrace® see Estradiol on page 574

Fenofibrate (fen oh FYE brate)

Related Information
Cardiovascular Diseases on page 1636
U.S. Brand Names Antara™; Lipofen™; Lofibra™; TriCor®; Triglide™
Canadian Brand Names Apo-Fenofibrate®; Apo-Feno-Micro®; Gen-Fenofibrate Micro; Lipidil EZ®; Lipidil Micro®; Lipidil Supra®; Novo-Fenofibrate; Nu-Fenofibrate; PMS-Fenofibrate Micro; ratio-Fenofibrate MC; TriCor®
Mexican Brand Names Controlip®; Lipidil®
Generic Available No
Synonyms Procetofene; Proctofene
Pharmacologic Category Antilipemic Agent, Fibric Acid
Use Adjunct to dietary therapy for the treatment of adults with elevations of serum triglyceride levels (types IV and V hyperlipidemia); adjunct to dietary therapy for the reduction of low density lipoprotein cholesterol (LDL-C), total cholesterol (total-C), triglycerides, and apolipoprotein B (apo B) in adult patients with primary hypercholesterolemia or mixed dyslipidemia (Fredrickson types IIa and IIb)

Local Anesthetic/Vasoconstrictor Precautions No information available to require special precautions

Effects on Dental Treatment No significant effects or complications reported

Common Adverse Effects
>10%: Hepatic: ALT/AST increased (3% to 13%)
1% to 10%:
 Gastrointestinal: Abdominal pain (5%), constipation (2%)
 Neuromuscular & skeletal: Back pain (3%)
 Respiratory: Respiratory disorder (6%), rhinitis (2%)

Frequency not defined:
 Cardiovascular: Angina pectoris, arrhythmia, atrial fibrillation, cardiovascular disorder, chest pain, coronary artery disorder, edema, electrocardiogram abnormality, extrasystoles, hyper-/hypotension, MI, palpitation, peripheral edema, peripheral vascular disorder, phlebitis, tachycardia, varicose veins, vasodilatation
 Central nervous system: Anxiety, depression, dizziness, fever, headache, insomnia, malaise, nervousness, neuralgia, pain, somnolence, vertigo
(Continued)

Fenofibrate *(Continued)*

Dermatologic: Acne, alopecia, bruising, contact dermatitis, eczema, fungal dermatitis, maculopapular rash, nail disorder, photosensitivity reaction, pruritus, skin ulcer, Stevens-Johnson syndrome, toxic epidermal necrolysis, urticaria

Endocrine & metabolic: Diabetes mellitus, gout, gynecomastia, hypoglycemia, hyperuricemia, libido decreased

Gastrointestinal: Anorexia, appetite increased, colitis, diarrhea, dry mouth, duodenal ulcer, dyspepsia, eructation, esophagitis, flatulence, gastroenteritis, gastritis, gastrointestinal disorder, nausea, peptic ulcer, rectal disorder, rectal hemorrhage, tooth disorder, vomiting, weight gain/loss

Genitourinary: Cystitis, dysuria, prostatic disorder, libido decreased, pregnancy (unintended), urinary frequency, urolithiasis, vaginal moniliasis

Hematologic: Agranulocytosis, anemia, eosinophilia, leukopenia, lymphadenopathy, thrombocytopenia

Hepatic: Cholelithiasis, cholecystitis, creatine phosphokinase increased, fatty liver deposits, liver function tests abnormal

Neuromuscular & skeletal: Arthralgia, arthritis, arthrosis, bursitis, hypertonia, joint disorder, leg cramps, muscle pain, myalgia, myasthenia, myopathy, myositis, paresthesia, rhabdomyolysis, tenderness, tenosynovitis, weakness

Ocular: Abnormal vision, amblyopia, cataract, conjunctivitis, eye disorder, refraction disorder

Otic: Ear pain, otitis media

Renal: Creatinine increased, kidney function abnormality

Respiratory: Asthma, bronchitis, cough increased, dyspnea, laryngitis, pharyngitis, pneumonia, sinusitis

Miscellaneous: Allergic reaction, cyst, diaphoresis, hernia, herpes simplex, herpes zoster, hypersensitivity reaction, infection

Dosage Oral:

Adults:

Hypertriglyceridemia: Initial:
Antara™: 43-130 mg/day
Lipofen™: 50-150 mg/day; maximum dose: 150 mg/day
Lofibra™: 67 mg/day with meals, up to 200 mg/day
TriCor®: 48 mg/day, up to 145 mg/day
Triglide™: 50-160 mg/day

Hypercholesterolemia or mixed hyperlipidemia:
Antara™: 130 mg/day
Lipofen™: 150 mg/day
Lofibra™: 200 mg/day with meals
TriCor®: 145 mg/day
Triglide™: 160 mg/day

Elderly: Initial:
Antara™: 43 mg/day
Lipofen™: 50 mg/day
Lofibra™: 67 mg/day
TriCor®: 48 mg/day
Triglide™: 50 mg/day

Dosage adjustment/interval in renal impairment: Monitor renal function and lipid panel before adjusting. Decrease dose or increase dosing interval for patients with renal failure: Initial:
Antara™: 43 mg/day
Lipofen™: 50 mg/day
Lofibra™: 67 mg/day
TriCor®: 48 mg/day
Triglide™: 50 mg/day

Mechanism of Action Fenofibric acid is believed to increase VLDL catabolism by enhancing the synthesis of lipoprotein lipase; as a result of a decrease in VLDL levels, total plasma triglycerides are reduced by 30% to 60%; modest increase in HDL occurs in some hypertriglyceridemic patients

Contraindications Hypersensitivity to fenofibrate or any component of the formulation; hepatic or severe renal dysfunction including primary biliary cirrhosis and unexplained persistent liver function abnormalities; pre-existing gallbladder disease

Warnings/Precautions Hepatic transaminases can become significantly elevated (dose-related); hepatocellular, chronic active, and cholestatic hepatitis have been reported. Regular monitoring of liver function tests is required. May cause cholelithiasis. Use caution with warfarin; adjustments in warfarin therapy may be required. Use caution with HMG-CoA reductase inhibitors (may lead to myopathy, rhabdomyolysis). Therapy should be withdrawn if an adequate response is not obtained after 2 months of therapy at the maximal daily dose.

May cause mild to moderate decreases in hemoglobin, hematocrit and WBC upon initiation of therapy which usually stabilizes with long-term therapy. Rare hypersensitivity reactions may occur. Dose adjustment is required for renal impairment and elderly patients. Safety and efficacy in children have not been established.

Drug Interactions

Cytochrome P450 Effect: Substrate of CYP3A4 (minor); **Inhibits** CYP2A6 (weak), 2C8 (moderate), 2C9 (moderate), 2C19 weak

Increased Effect/Toxicity: Fenofibrate may increase the effects of sulfonylureas and warfarin. Concurrent use of fenofibrate with HMG-CoA reductase inhibitors may increase the risk of myopathy and rhabdomyolysis. Ezetimibe's serum concentration may be increased with concurrent use. Fenofibrate may increase the levels/effects of CYP2C8 substrates (example substrates include amiodarone, paclitaxel, pioglitazone, repaglinide, and rosiglitazone). Fenofibrate may increase the levels/effects of CYP2C9 substrates (example substrates include bosentan, dapsone, fluoxetine, glimepiride, glipizide, losartan, montelukast, nateglinide, paclitaxel, phenytoin, warfarin, and zafirlukast).

Decreased Effect: Bile acid sequestrants may decrease absorption of fenofibrate (separate administration).

Dietary Considerations

Lofibra™: Take with meals.

Antara™, Lipofen™, TriCor®, Triglide™: May be taken with or without food.

Pharmacodynamics/Kinetics

Absorption: Increased when taken with meals

Distribution: Widely to most tissues

Protein binding: >99%

Metabolism: Tissue and plasma via esterases to active form, fenofibric acid; undergoes inactivation by glucuronidation hepatically or renally

Half-life elimination: Fenofibric acid: Mean: 20 hours (range: 10-35 hours)

Time to peak: 3-8 hours

Excretion: Urine (60% as metabolites); feces (25%); hemodialysis has no effect on removal of fenofibric acid from plasma

Pregnancy Risk Factor C

Dosage Forms CAP (Lipofen™): 50 mg, 100 mg, 150 mg. **CAP [micronized]:** (Antara™): 43 mg, 87 mg, 130 mg; (Lofibra™): 67 mg, 134 mg, 200 mg. **TAB** (TriCor®): 48 mg, 145 mg; (Triglide™): 50 mg, 160 mg

---

Fenoldopam (fe NOL doe pam)

U.S. Brand Names Corlopam®

Canadian Brand Names Corlopam®

Generic Available Yes

Synonyms Fenoldopam Mesylate

Pharmacologic Category Dopamine Agonist

Use Treatment of severe hypertension (up to 48 hours in adults), including in patients with renal compromise; short-term (up to 4 hours) blood pressure reduction in pediatric patients

Local Anesthetic/Vasoconstrictor Precautions No information available to require special precautions

Effects on Dental Treatment Key adverse event(s) related to dental treatment: Xerostomia and changes in salivation (normal salivary flow resumes upon discontinuation).

Common Adverse Effects Frequency not always defined.

Cardiovascular: Angina, asymptomatic T wave flattening on ECG, chest pain, edema, facial flushing (>5%), fibrillation (atrial), flutter (atrial), hypotension (>5%), tachycardia

Central nervous system: Dizziness, headache (>5%)

Endocrine & metabolic: Hypokalemia

Gastrointestinal: Abdominal pain/fullness, diarrhea, nausea (>5%), vomiting, xerostomia

Local: Injection site reactions

Ocular: Intraocular pressure (increased), blurred vision

Hepatic: Increases in portal pressure in cirrhotic patients

Mechanism of Action A selective postsynaptic dopamine agonist (D_1-receptors) which exerts hypotensive effects by decreasing peripheral vasculature resistance with increased renal blood flow, diuresis, and natriuresis; 6 times as potent as dopamine in producing renal vasodilitation; has minimal adrenergic effects

(Continued)

Fenoldopam *(Continued)*

Drug Interactions
Increased Effect/Toxicity: Concurrent acetaminophen may increase fenoldopam levels (30% to 70%). Beta-blockers increase the risk of hypotension; avoid concurrent use. If used concurrently with beta-blockers, close monitoring is recommended.

Pharmacodynamics/Kinetics
Onset of action: I.V.: 10 minutes

Duration: I.V.: 1 hour

Distribution: V_d: 0.6 L/kg

Half-life elimination: I.V.: Children: 3-5 minutes; Adults: ~5 minutes

Metabolism: Hepatic via methylation, glucuronidation, and sulfation; the 8-sulfate metabolite may have some activity; extensive first-pass effect

Excretion: Urine (90%); feces (10%)

Pregnancy Risk Factor B

Fenoldopam Mesylate *see* Fenoldopam *on page 641*

Fenoprofen *(fen oh PROE fen)*

Related Information
Rheumatoid Arthritis, Osteoarthritis, and Osteoporosis *on page 1668*
Temporomandibular Dysfunction (TMD) *on page 1724*

U.S. Brand Names Nalfon®

Canadian Brand Names Nalfon®

Generic Available Yes: Tablet

Synonyms Fenoprofen Calcium

Pharmacologic Category Nonsteroidal Anti-inflammatory Drug (NSAID), Oral

Use Symptomatic treatment of acute and chronic rheumatoid arthritis and osteo-arthritis; relief of mild to moderate pain

Local Anesthetic/Vasoconstrictor Precautions No information available to require special precautions

Effects on Dental Treatment NSAID formulations are known to reversibly decrease platelet aggregation via mechanisms different than observed with aspirin. The dentist should be aware of the potential of abnormal coagulation. Caution should also be exercised in the use of NSAIDs in patients already on anticoagulant therapy with drugs such as warfarin (Coumadin®).

Common Adverse Effects
>10%:
Central nervous system: Dizziness (7% to 15%), somnolence (9% to 15%)

Gastrointestinal: Abdominal cramps (2% to 4%), heartburn, indigestion, nausea (8% to 14%), dyspepsia (10% to 14%), flatulence (14%), anorexia (14%), constipation (7% to 14%), occult blood in stool (14%), vomiting (3% to 14%), diarrhea (2% to 14%)

1% to 10%:
Central nervous system: Headache (9%)

Dermatologic: Itching

Endocrine & metabolic: Fluid retention

Restrictions A medication guide should be dispensed with each prescription. A template for the required MedGuide can be found on the FDA website at http://www.fda.gov/medwatch/SAFETY/2005/safety05.htm#NSAID

Dosage Adults: Oral:
Rheumatoid arthritis: 300-600 mg 3-4 times/day up to 3.2 g/day

Mild to moderate pain: 200 mg every 4-6 hours as needed

Dosage adjustment in renal impairment: Not recommended in patients with advanced renal disease

Mechanism of Action Inhibits prostaglandin synthesis by decreasing the activity of the enzyme, cyclooxygenase, which results in decreased formation of prostaglandin precursors

Contraindications Hypersensitivity to fenoprofen, aspirin, or other NSAIDs, or any component of the formulation; perioperative pain in the setting of coronary artery bypass surgery (CABG); significant renal dysfunction; pregnancy (3rd trimester)

Warnings/Precautions NSAIDs are associated with an increased risk of adverse cardiovascular events, including MI, stroke, and new onset or worsening of pre-existing hypertension. Risk may be increased with duration of use or pre-existing cardiovascular risk-factors or disease. Carefully evaluate individual cardiovascular risk profiles prior to prescribing. Use caution with fluid retention, CHF, or hypertension.

Use of NSAIDs can compromise existing renal function. Renal toxicity can occur in patient with impaired renal function, dehydration, heart failure, liver dysfunction, those taking diuretics and ACEI, and the elderly. Rehydrate patient before starting therapy. Monitor renal function closely. Not recommended for use in patients with advanced renal disease.

NSAIDs may increase risk of gastrointestinal irritation, ulceration, bleeding, and perforation. These events may occur at any time during therapy and without warning. Use caution with a history of GI disease (bleeding or ulcers), concurrent therapy with aspirin, anticoagulants and/or corticosteroids, smoking, use of alcohol, the elderly or debilitated patients.

Use the lowest effective dose for the shortest duration of time, consistent with individual patient goals, to reduce risk of cardiovascular or GI adverse events. Alternate therapies should be considered for patients at high risk.

NSAIDs may cause serious skin adverse events including exfoliative dermatitis, Stevens-Johnson syndrome (SJS), and toxic epidermal necrolysis (TEN). Anaphylactoid reactions may occur, even without prior exposure; patients with "aspirin triad" (bronchial asthma, aspirin intolerance, rhinitis) may be at increased risk. Do not use in patients who experience bronchospasm, asthma, rhinitis, or urticaria with NSAID or aspirin therapy.

Use with caution in patients with decreased hepatic function. Closely monitor patients with any abnormal LFT. Severe hepatic reactions (eg, fulminant hepatitis, liver failure) have occurred with NSAID use, rarely; discontinue if signs or symptoms of liver disease develop, or if systemic manifestations occur.

The elderly are at increased risk for adverse effects (especially peptic ulceration, CNS effects, renal toxicity) from NSAIDs even at low doses.

Withhold for at least 4-6 half-lives prior to surgical or dental procedures. Safety and efficacy have not been established in children <18 years of age.

Drug Interactions

Increased Effect/Toxicity: Increased effect/toxicity of phenytoin, sulfonamides, sulfonylureas, salicylates, and oral anticoagulants. Serum concentration/toxicity of methotrexate may be increased.

Decreased Effect: Decreased effect with phenobarbital. Thiazide efficacy (diuretic and antihypertensive effect) may be reduced (indomethacin may reduce this efficacy and it may be anticipated with any NSAID). NSAIDs may decrease the antihypertensive effect of ACE inhibitors, angiotensin antagonists, beta-blockers, or hydralazine. Cholestyramine (and other bile acid sequestrants) may decrease the absorption of NSAIDs; separate by at least 2 hours.

Ethanol/Nutrition/Herb Interactions

Ethanol: Avoid ethanol (may enhance gastric mucosal irritation).

Food: Fenoprofen peak serum levels may be decreased if taken with food.

Herb/Nutraceutical: Avoid alfalfa, anise, bilberry, bladderwrack, bromelain, cat's claw, celery, coleus, cordyceps, dong quai, evening primrose, feverfew, fenugreek, garlic, ginger, ginkgo biloboa, red clover, horse chestnut, grapeseed, green tea, ginseng, guggul, horse chestnut seed, horseradish, licorice, prickly ash, red clover, reishi, SAMe, sweet clover, turmeric, white willow (all have additional antiplatelet activity).

Dietary Considerations May be taken with food to decrease GI distress.

Pharmacodynamics/Kinetics

Onset of action: A few days

Absorption: Rapid, 80%

Distribution: Does not cross the placenta

Protein binding: 99%

Metabolism: Extensively hepatic

Half-life elimination: 2.5-3 hours

Time to peak, serum: ~2 hours

Excretion: Urine (2% to 5% as unchanged drug); feces (small amounts)

Pregnancy Risk Factor C/D (3rd trimester)

Dosage Forms CAP (Nalfon®): 200 mg, 300 mg. **TAB:** 600 mg

Fenoprofen Calcium *see* Fenoprofen *on page 642*

Fenoterol (fen oh TER ole)

Canadian Brand Names Berotec®
Mexican Brand Names Partusisten®
Synonyms Fenoterol Hydrobromide
Pharmacologic Category Beta$_2$-Adrenergic Agonist
Use Treatment and prevention of symptoms of reversible obstructive pulmonary disease (including asthma and acute bronchospasm), chronic bronchitis, emphysema
Local Anesthetic/Vasoconstrictor Precautions No information available to require special precautions
Effects on Dental Treatment No significant effects or complications reported
Common Adverse Effects Note: Frequency of most effects may be dose related, approximate frequencies noted below. In the treatment of acute bronchospasm (high-dose nebulization), symptoms of headache (up to 12%), tremor (32%), and tachycardia (up to 21%) are frequently noted.

>10%: Endocrine & metabolic: Serum glucose increased, serum potassium decreased

1% to 10%:
Cardiovascular: Palpitations, tachycardia
Central nervous system: Headache, dizziness, nervousness
Neuromuscular & skeletal: Tremor, muscle cramps
Respiratory: Pharyngeal irritation, cough

Restrictions Not available in U.S.
Mechanism of Action Relaxes bronchial smooth muscle by action on beta$_2$ receptors with little effect on heart rate.
Drug Interactions
Increased Effect/Toxicity: When used with inhaled ipratropium, an increased duration of bronchodilation may occur. Cardiovascular effects are potentiated in patients also receiving MAO inhibitors, tricyclic antidepressants, and sympathomimetic agents (eg, amphetamine, dopamine, dobutamine). Fenoterol may increase the risk of malignant arrhythmias with inhaled anesthetics (eg, enflurane, halothane). Concurrent use with diuretics may increase the risk of hypokalemia.
Decreased Effect: When used with nonselective beta-adrenergic blockers (eg, propranolol), the effect of fenoterol is decreased.
Pharmacodynamics/Kinetics
Onset of action: 5 minutes
Peak effect: 30-60 minutes
Duration: 3-4 hours (up to 6-8 hours)
Pregnancy Risk Factor Not available; similar agents rated C

Fenoterol Hydrobromide *see* Fenoterol *on page 644*

Fentanyl (FEN ta nil)

U.S. Brand Names Actiq®; Duragesic®; Sublimaze®
Canadian Brand Names Actiq®; Duragesic®
Generic Available Yes: Excludes lozenge
Synonyms Fentanyl Citrate
Pharmacologic Category Analgesic, Narcotic; General Anesthetic
Dental Use Adjunct in preoperative intravenous conscious sedation in patients undergoing dental surgery
Use
Injection: Sedation, relief of pain, preoperative medication, adjunct to general or regional anesthesia
Transdermal: Management of moderate-to-severe chronic pain
Transmucosal (Actiq®): Management of breakthrough cancer pain
Local Anesthetic/Vasoconstrictor Precautions No information available to require special precautions
Effects on Dental Treatment Key adverse event(s) related to dental treatment: Xerostomia, changes in salivation (normal salivary flow resumes upon discontinuation), and orthostatic hypotension. Actiq® may contribute to dental carries due to sugar content of oral lozenge; advise patients to maintain good oral hygiene. See Dental Comment.
Significant Adverse Effects
>10%:
Cardiovascular: Hypotension, bradycardia
Central nervous system: CNS depression, confusion, drowsiness, sedation
Gastrointestinal: Nausea, vomiting, constipation, xerostomia

Neuromuscular & skeletal: Chest wall rigidity (high dose I.V.), weakness
Ocular: Miosis
Respiratory: Respiratory depression
Miscellaneous: Diaphoresis
1% to 10%:
Cardiovascular: Cardiac arrhythmia, edema, orthostatic hypotension, hypertension, syncope
Central nervous system: Abnormal dreams, abnormal thinking, agitation, amnesia, dizziness, euphoria, fatigue, fever, hallucinations, headache, insomnia, nervousness, paranoid reaction
Dermatologic: Erythema, papules, pruritus, rash
Gastrointestinal: Abdominal pain, anorexia, biliary tract spasm, diarrhea, dyspepsia, flatulence
Local: Application site reaction
Neuromuscular & skeletal: Abnormal coordination, abnormal gait, back pain, paresthesia, rigors, tremor
Respiratory: Apnea, bronchitis, dyspnea, hemoptysis, pharyngitis, rhinitis, sinusitis, upper respiratory infection
Miscellaneous: Hiccups, flu-like syndrome, speech disorder
<1% (Limited to important or life-threatening): Abdominal distention, ADH release, amblyopia, anorgasmia, aphasia, bladder pain, blurred vision, bradycardia, bronchospasm, circulatory depression, CNS excitation or delirium, cold/clammy skin, convulsions, dental caries (Actiq®), depersonalization, dysesthesia, ejaculatory difficulty, exfoliative dermatitis, gum line erosion (Actiq®), hyper-/hypotonia, hostility, laryngospasm, libido decreased, oliguria, paradoxical dizziness, physical and psychological dependence with prolonged use, polyuria, pustules, stertorous breathing, stupor, tachycardia, tooth loss (Actiq®), urinary tract spasm, urticaria, vertigo, weight loss

Restrictions C-II
Dental Usual Dosing Surgery: Adults:
Premedication: I.M., slow I.V.: 25-100 mcg/dose 30-60 minutes prior to surgery
Adjunct to regional anesthesia: Slow I.V.: 25-100 mcg/dose over 1-2 minutes.
Note: An I.V. should be in place with regional anesthesia so the I.M. route is rarely used but still maintained as an option in the package labeling.
Dosage Note: These are guidelines and do not represent the maximum doses that may be required in all patients. Doses should be titrated to pain relief/prevention. Monitor vital signs routinely. Single I.M. doses have a duration of 1-2 hours, single I.V. doses last 0.5-1 hour.
Sedation for minor procedures/analgesia:
Children 1-12 years:
Sedation for minor procedures/analgesia: I.M., I.V.: 1-2 mcg/kg/dose; may repeat at 30- to 60-minute intervals. **Note:** Children 18-36 months of age may require 2-3 mcg/kg/dose
Continuous sedation/analgesia: Initial I.V. bolus: 1-2 mcg/kg; then 1-3 mcg/kg/hour to a maximum dose of 5 mcg/kg/hour
Children >12 years and Adults: I.V.: 25-50 mcg; may repeat every 3-5 minutes to desired effect or adverse event; maximum dose of 500 mcg/4 hours; higher doses are used for major procedures

Surgery: Adults:
Premedication: I.M., slow I.V.: 25-100 mcg/dose 30-60 minutes prior to surgery
Adjunct to regional anesthesia: Slow I.V.: 25-100 mcg/dose over 1-2 minutes. **Note:** An I.V. should be in place with regional anesthesia so the I.M. route is rarely used but still maintained as an option in the package labeling.
Adjunct to general anesthesia: Slow I.V.:
Low dose: 0.5-2 mcg/kg/dose depending on the indication. For example, 0.5 mcg/kg will provide analgesia or reduce the amount of propofol needed for laryngeal mask airway insertion with minimal respiratory depression. However, to blunt the hemodynamic response to intubation 2 mcg/kg is often necessary.
Moderate dose: Initial: 2-15 mcg/kg/dose; Maintenance (bolus or infusion): 1-2 mcg/kg/hour. Discontinuing fentanyl infusion 30-60 minutes prior to the end of surgery will usually allow adequate ventilation upon emergence from anesthesia. For "fast-tracking" and early extubation following major surgery, total fentanyl doses are limited to 10-15 mcg/kg.
High dose: **Note:** High-dose (20-50 mcg/kg/dose) fentanyl is rarely used, but is still maintained in the package labeling.

Acute pain management: Adults:
Severe: I.M, I.V.: 50-100 mcg/dose every 1-2 hours as needed; patients with prior opiate exposure may tolerate higher initial doses
Patient-controlled analgesia (PCA): I.V.: Usual concentration: 10 mcg/mL
(Continued)

Fentanyl *(Continued)*

Demand dose: Usual: 10 mcg; range: 10-50 mcg

Lockout interval: 5-8 minutes

Mechanically-ventilated patients (based on 70 kg patient): Slow I.V.: 0.35-1.5 mcg/kg every 30-60 minutes as needed; infusion: 0.7-10 mcg/kg/hour

Breakthrough cancer pain:

Adults: Transmucosal: Actiq® dosing should be individually titrated to provide adequate analgesia with minimal side effects. For patients who are tolerant to and currently receiving opioid therapy for persistent cancer pain. Initial starting dose: 200 mcg; the second dose may be started 15 minutes after completion of the first dose. Consumption should be limited to 4 units/day or less. Patients needing more than 4 units/day should have the dose of their long-term opioid re-evaluated.

Elderly >65 years: Transmucosal: Actiq®: Dose should be reduced to 2.5-5 mcg/kg

Chronic pain management: Children ≥2 years and Adults (opioid-tolerant patients): Transdermal:

Initial: To convert patients from oral or parenteral opioids to transdermal formulation, a 24-hour analgesic requirement should be calculated (based on prior opiate use). Using the tables, the appropriate initial dose can be determined. The initial fentanyl dosage may be approximated from the 24-hour morphine dosage and titrated to minimize adverse effects and provide analgesia. With the initial application, the absorption of transdermal fentanyl requires several hours to reach plateau; therefore transdermal fentanyl is inappropriate for management of acute pain. Change patch every 72 hours.

Conversion from continuous infusion of fentanyl: In patients who have adequate pain relief with a fentanyl infusion, fentanyl may be converted to transdermal dosing at a rate equivalent to the intravenous rate. A two-step taper of the infusion to be completed over 12 hours has been recommended (Kornick, 2001) after the patch is applied. The infusion is decreased to 50% of the original rate six hours after the application of the first patch, and subsequently discontinued twelve hours after application.

Titration: Short-acting agents may be required until analgesic efficacy is established and/or as supplements for "breakthrough" pain. The amount of supplemental doses should be closely monitored. Appropriate dosage increases may be based on daily supplemental dosage using the ratio of 45 mg/24 hours of oral morphine to a 12.5 mcg/hour increase in fentanyl dosage.

Frequency of adjustment: The dosage should not be titrated more frequently than every 3 days after the initial dose or every 6 days thereafter. Patients should wear a consistent fentanyl dosage through two applications (6 days) before dosage increase based on supplemental opiate dosages can be estimated.

Frequency of application: The majority of patients may be controlled on every 72-hour administration; however, a small number of patients require every 48-hour administration.

Recommended Initial Duragesic® Dose Based Upon Daily Oral Morphine Dose[1]

Oral 24-Hour Morphine (mg/d)	Duragesic® Dose (mcg/h)
60-134[2]	25
135-224[2]	50
225-314	75
315-404	100
405-494	125
495-584	150
585-674	175
675-764	200
765-854	225
855-944	250
945-1034	275
1035-1124	300

[1] The table should NOT be used to convert from transdermal fentanyl to other opioid analgesics. Rather, following removal of the patch, titrate the dose of the new opioid until adequate analgesia is achieved.

[2] Pediatric patients initiating therapy on a 25 mcg/hour Duragesic® system should be opioid-tolerant and receiving at least 60 mg oral morphine equivalents per day.

Dose conversion guidelines for transdermal fentanyl[1] (see tables below and on previous page).

Dosing Conversion Guidelines [1,2]

Current Analgesic	Daily Dosage (mg/day)			
Morphine (I.M./I.V.)	10-22	23-37	38-52	53-67
Oxycodone (oral)	30-67	67.5-112	112.5-157	157.5-202
Oxycodone (I.M./I.V.)	15-33	33.1-56	56.1-78	78.1-101
Codeine (oral)	150-447	448-747	748-1047	1048-1347
Hydromorphone (oral)	8-17	17.1-28	28.1-39	39.1-51
Hydromorphone (I.V.)	1.5-3.4	3.5-5.6	5.7-7.9	8-10
Meperidine (I.M.)	75-165	166-278	279-390	391-503
Methadone (oral)	20-44	45-74	75-104	105-134
Methadone (I.M.)	10-22	23-37	38-52	53-67
Fentanyl transdermal recommended dose (mcg/h)	25 mcg/h	50 mcg/h	75 mcg/h	100 mcg/h

[1] The table should NOT be used to convert from transdermal fentanyl to other opioid analgesics. Rather, following removal of the patch, titrate the dose of the new opioid until adequate analgesia is achieved.

[2] Duragesic® product insert, Janssen Pharmaceutica, Feb 2005.

Opioid Analgesics Initial Oral Dosing Commonly Used for Severe Pain

Drug	Equianalgesic Dose (mg)		Initial Oral Dose	
	Oral[1]	Parenteral[2]	Children (mg/kg)	Adults (mg)
Buprenorphine	—	0.4	—	—
Butorphanol	—	2	—	—
Hydromorphone	7.5	1.5	0.06	4-8
Levorphanol	4 (acute) 1 (chronic)	2 (acute) 1 (chronic)	0.04	2-4
Meperidine	300	75	Not Recommended	
Methadone	10	5	0.2	0.2
Morphine	30	10	0.3	15-30
Nalbuphine	—	10	—	—
Pentazocine	50	30	—	—
Oxycodone	20	—	0.3	10-20
Oxymorphone	1	—	—	—

From "Principles of Analgesic Use in the Treatment of Acute Pain and Cancer Pain," *Am Pain Soc*, Fifth Ed.

[1] Elderly: Starting dose should be lower for this population group

[2] Standard parenteral doses for acute pain in adults; can be used to doses for I.V. infusions and repeated small I.V. boluses. Single I.V. boluses, use half the I.M. dose. Children >6 months: I.V. dose = parenteral equianalgesic dose x weight (kg)/100

Dosing adjustment in hepatic impairment: Actiq®: Although fentanyl kinetics may be altered in hepatic disease, Actiq® can be used successfully in the management of breakthrough cancer pain. Doses should be titrated to reach clinical effect with careful monitoring of patients with severe hepatic disease.

Mechanism of Action Binds with stereospecific receptors at many sites within the CNS, increases pain threshold, alters pain reception, inhibits ascending pain pathways
(Continued)

Fentanyl *(Continued)*

Contraindications Hypersensitivity to fentanyl or any component of the formulation; increased intracranial pressure; severe respiratory disease or depression including acute asthma (unless patient is mechanically ventilated); paralytic ileus; severe liver or renal insufficiency; pregnancy (prolonged use or high doses near term)

Transmucosal lozenges (Actiq®) or transdermal patches must not be used in patients who are not opioid tolerant. Patients are considered opioid-tolerant if they are taking at least 60 mg morphine/day, 30 mg oral oxycodone/day, 8 mg oral hydromorphone/day, 25 mcg transdermal fentanyl/hour, or an equivalent dose of another opioid for ≥1 week. Transdermal patches are not for use in acute pain, mild pain, intermittent pain, or postoperative pain management.

Warnings/Precautions An opioid-containing analgesic regimen should be tailored to each patient's needs and based upon the type of pain being treated (acute versus chronic), the route of administration, degree of tolerance for opioids (naive versus chronic user), age, weight, and medical condition. The optimal analgesic dose varies widely among patients. Doses should be titrated to pain relief/prevention. When using with other CNS depressants, reduce dose of one or both agents. Fentanyl shares the toxic potentials of opiate agonists, and precautions of opiate agonist therapy should be observed; use with caution in patients with bradycardia; rapid I.V. infusion may result in skeletal muscle and chest wall rigidity leading to respiratory distress and/or apnea, bronchoconstriction, laryngospasm; inject slowly over 3-5 minutes. Tolerance or drug dependence may result from extended use. Use caution in patients with a history of drug dependence or abuse. The elderly may be particularly susceptible to the CNS depressant and constipating effects of narcotics. Use extreme caution in patients with COPD or other chronic respiratory conditions.

Actiq® should be used only for the care of cancer patients and is intended for use by specialists who are knowledgeable in treating cancer pain. For patients who have received transmucosal product within 6-12 hours, it is recommended that if other narcotics are required, they should be used at starting doses ¼ to ⅓ those usually recommended. Actiq® preparations contain an amount of medication that can be fatal to children. Keep all units out of the reach of children and discard any open units properly. Patients and caregivers should be counseled on the dangers to children including the risk of exposure to partially-consumed units.

Topical patches: Serious or life-threatening hypoventilation may occur, even in opioid-tolerant patients. Serum fentanyl concentrations may increase approximately one-third for patients with a body temperature of 40°C secondary to a temperature-dependent increase in fentanyl release from the system and increased skin permeability. Avoid exposure of application site to direct external heat sources. Patients who experience adverse reactions should be monitored for at least 24 hours after removal of the patch. Transdermal patch may contain conducting metal (eg, aluminum); remove patch prior to MRI. Safety and efficacy of transdermal system have been limited to children ≥2 years of age who are opioid tolerant.

Drug Interactions Substrate of CYP3A4 (major); **Inhibits** CYP3A4 (weak)
CNS depressants: Increased sedation with CNS depressants, phenothiazines
CYP3A4 inhibitors: May increase the levels/effects of fentanyl. Potentially fatal respiratory depression may occur when a potent inhibitor is used in a patient receiving chronic fentanyl (eg, transdermal). Example inhibitors include azole antifungals, clarithromycin, diclofenac, doxycycline, erythromycin, imatinib, isoniazid, nefazodone, nicardipine, propofol, protease inhibitors, quinidine, telithromycin, and verapamil.
MAO inhibitors: Not recommended to use Actiq® within 14 days. Severe and unpredictable potentiation by MAO inhibitors has been reported with opioid analgesics.

Ethanol/Nutrition/Herb Interactions
Ethanol: Avoid ethanol (may increase CNS depression).
Food: Glucose may cause hyperglycemia.
Herb/Nutraceutical: St John's wort may decrease fentanyl levels. Avoid valerian, St John's wort, kava kava, gotu kola (may increase CNS depression).

Dietary Considerations Actiq® contains 2 g sugar per unit.

Pharmacodynamics/Kinetics
Onset of action: Analgesic: I.M.: 7-15 minutes; I.V.: Almost immediate; Transmucosal: 5-15 minutes
Peak effect: Transmucosal: Analgesic: 20-30 minutes
Duration: I.M.: 1-2 hours; I.V.: 0.5-1 hour; Transmucosal: Related to blood level; respiratory depressant effect may last longer than analgesic effect
Absorption: Transmucosal: Rapid, ~25% from the buccal mucosa; 75% swallowed with saliva and slowly absorbed from GI tract

Distribution: Highly lipophilic, redistributes into muscle and fat

Metabolism: Hepatic, primarily via CYP3A4

Bioavailability: Transmucosal: ~50% (range: 36% to 71%)

Half-life elimination: 2-4 hours; Transmucosal: 6.6 hours (range: 5-15 hours); Transdermal: 17 hours (half-life is influenced by absorption rate)

Time to peak: Transdermal: 24-72 hours

Excretion: Urine (primarily as metabolites, 10% as unchanged drug)

Pregnancy Risk Factor C/D (prolonged use or high doses at term)

Lactation Enters breast milk/not recommended (AAP rates "compatible")

Breast-Feeding Considerations Fentanyl is excreted in low concentrations into breast milk. Breast-feeding is considered acceptable following single doses to the mother; however, no information is available when used long-term.

Dosage Forms

Infusion [premixed in NS]: 0.05 mg (10 mL); 1 mg (100 mL); 1.25 mg (250 mL); 2 mg (100 mL); 2.5 mg (250 mL)

Injection, solution, as citrate [preservative free]: 0.05 mg/mL (2 mL, 5 mL, 10 mL, 20 mL, 30 mL, 50 mL)

Sublimaze®: 0.05 mg/mL (2 mL, 5 mL, 10 mL, 20 mL)

Lozenge, oral transmucosal, as citrate:

Actiq®: 200 mcg, 400 mcg, 600 mcg, 800 mcg, 1200 mcg, 1600 mcg [mounted on a plastic radiopaque handle; raspberry flavor]

Transdermal system: 25 mcg/hour [6.25 cm^2] (5s); 50 mcg/hour [12.5 cm^2] (5s); 75 mcg/hour [18.75 cm^2]; 100 mcg/hour [25 cm^2] (5s)

Duragesic®: 12 [delivers 12.5 mcg/hour; 5 cm^2; contains alcohol 0.1 mL/10 cm^2] (5s); 25 [delivers 25 mcg/hour; 10 cm^2; contains alcohol 0.1 mL/10 cm^2] (5s); 50 [delivers 50 mcg/hour; 20 cm^2; contains alcohol 0.1 mL/10 cm^2] (5s); 75 [delivers 75 mcg/hour; 30 cm^2; contains alcohol 0.1 mL/10 cm^2]; 100 [delivers 100 mcg/hour; 40 cm^2; contains alcohol 0.1 mL/10 cm^2] (5s)

Dental Comment Transdermal fentanyl should not be used as a pain reliever in dentistry due to danger of hypoventilation

Selected Readings

Dionne RA, Yagiela JA, Moore PA, et al, "Comparing Efficacy and Safety of Four Intravenous Sedation Regimens in Dental Outpatients," *Am Dent Assoc*, 2001, 132(6):740-51.

Fentanyl Citrate *see* Fentanyl *on page 644*

Feosol® [OTC] *see* Ferrous Sulfate *on page 651*

Feostat® [OTC] [DSC] *see* Ferrous Fumarate *on page 650*

Feratab® [OTC] *see* Ferrous Sulfate *on page 651*

Fer-Gen-Sol [OTC] *see* Ferrous Sulfate *on page 651*

Fergon® [OTC] *see* Ferrous Gluconate *on page 651*

Feridex I.V.® *see* Ferumoxides *on page 652*

Fer-In-Sol® [OTC] *see* Ferrous Sulfate *on page 651*

Fer-Iron® [OTC] *see* Ferrous Sulfate *on page 651*

Fero-Grad 500® [OTC] *see* Ferrous Sulfate and Ascorbic Acid *on page 651*

Ferretts [OTC] *see* Ferrous Fumarate *on page 650*

Ferrex 150 [OTC] *see* Polysaccharide-Iron Complex *on page 1254*

Ferric (III) Hexacyanoferrate (II) *see* Ferric Hexacyanoferrate *on page 650*

Ferric Gluconate (FER ik GLOO koe nate)

U.S. Brand Names Ferrlecit®

Canadian Brand Names Ferrlecit®

Generic Available No

Synonyms Sodium Ferric Gluconate

Pharmacologic Category Iron Salt

Use Repletion of total body iron content in patients with iron-deficiency anemia who are undergoing hemodialysis in conjunction with erythropoietin therapy

Local Anesthetic/Vasoconstrictor Precautions No information available to require special precautions

Effects on Dental Treatment Key adverse event(s) related to dental treatment: Xerostomia (normal salivary flow resumes upon discontinuation). Do not prescribe tetracyclines simultaneously with iron since GI tract absorption of both tetracycline and iron may be inhibited.

Common Adverse Effects Major adverse reactions include hypotension and hypersensitivity reactions. Hypersensitivity reactions have included pruritus, chest pain, hypotension, nausea, abdominal pain, flank pain, fatigue and rash.

Cardiovascular: Hypotension (serious hypotension in 1%), chest pain, hypertension, syncope, tachycardia, angina, MI, pulmonary edema, hypovolemia, peripheral edema

(Continued)

Ferric Gluconate *(Continued)*

Central nervous system: Headache, fatigue, fever, malaise, dizziness, paresthesia, insomnia, agitation, somnolence, pain

Dermatologic: Pruritus, rash

Endocrine & metabolic: Hyperkalemia, hypoglycemia, hypokalemia

Gastrointestinal: Abdominal pain, nausea, vomiting, diarrhea, rectal disorder, dyspepsia, flatulence, melena, epigastric pain

Genitourinary: Urinary tract infection

Hematologic: Anemia, abnormal erythrocytes, lymphadenopathy

Local: Injection site reactions, pain

Neuromuscular & skeletal: Weakness, back pain, leg cramps, myalgia, arthralgia, paresthesia, groin pain

Ocular: Blurred vision, conjunctivitis

Respiratory: Dyspnea, cough, rhinitis, upper respiratory infection, pneumonia

Miscellaneous: Hypersensitivity reactions, infection, rigors, chills, flu-like syndrome, sepsis, carcinoma, diaphoresis increased

Mechanism of Action Supplies a source to elemental iron necessary to the function of hemoglobin, myoglobin and specific enzyme systems; allows transport of oxygen via hemoglobin

Drug Interactions

Decreased Effect: Chloramphenicol may decrease effect of ferric gluconate injection; ferric gluconate injection may decrease the absorption of oral iron

Pharmacodynamics/Kinetics Half-life elimination: Bound: 1 hour

Pregnancy Risk Factor B

Ferric Hexacyanoferrate *(FER ik hex a SYE an oh fer ate)*

U.S. Brand Names Radiogardase™

Generic Available No

Synonyms Ferric (III) Hexacyanoferrate (II); Insoluble Prussian Blue; Prussian Blue

Pharmacologic Category Antidote

Use Treatment of known or suspected internal contamination with radioactive cesium and/or radioactive or nonradioactive thallium

Local Anesthetic/Vasoconstrictor Precautions No information available to require special precautions

Effects on Dental Treatment No significant effects or complications reported

Common Adverse Effects

>10%: Gastrointestinal: Constipation (24%)

1% to 10%: Endocrine & metabolic: Hypokalemia (7%)

Frequency not defined: Gastrointestinal: Gastric distress, fecal discoloration (blue)

Mechanism of Action Binds to cesium and thallium isotopes in the gastrointestinal tract following their ingestion or excretion in the bile; reduces their gastrointestinal reabsorption (enterohepatic circulation)

Pharmacodynamics/Kinetics

Absorption: Ferric hexacyanoferrate: Oral: None

Half-life elimination:

Cesium-137: Effective: Adults: 80 days, decreased by 69% with ferric hexacyanoferrate; adolescents: 62 days, decreased by 46% with ferric hexacyanoferrate; children: 42 days, decreased by 43% with ferric hexacyanoferrate

Nonradioactive thallium: Biological: 8-10 days; with ferric hexacyanoferrate: 3 days

Excretion:

Cesium-137: Without ferric hexacyanoferrate: Urine (~80%), feces (~20%)

Thallium: Without ferric hexacyanoferrate: Fecal to urine excretion ration: 2:1

Ferric hexacyanoferrate: Feces (99%, unchanged)

Pregnancy Risk Factor C

Ferrlecit® see Ferric Gluconate on page 649

Ferro-Sequels® [OTC] see Ferrous Fumarate on page 650

Ferrous Fumarate *(FER us FYOO ma rate)*

U.S. Brand Names Femiron® [OTC]; Feostat® [OTC] [DSC]; Ferretts [OTC]; Ferro-Sequels® [OTC]; Hemocyte® [OTC]; Ircon® [OTC]; Nephro-Fer® [OTC]

Canadian Brand Names Palafer®

Mexican Brand Names Ferval®

Generic Available Yes: Tablet

Synonyms Iron Fumarate
Pharmacologic Category Iron Salt
Use Prevention and treatment of iron-deficiency anemias
Local Anesthetic/Vasoconstrictor Precautions No information available to require special precautions
Effects on Dental Treatment Key adverse event(s) related to dental treatment: Staining of teeth. Do not prescribe tetracyclines simultaneously with iron since GI tract absorption of both tetracycline and iron may be inhibited.
Mechanism of Action Replaces iron found in hemoglobin, myoglobin, and enzymes; allows the transportation of oxygen via hemoglobin
Pregnancy Risk Factor A

Ferrous Gluconate (FER us GLOO koe nate)

U.S. Brand Names Fergon® [OTC]
Canadian Brand Names Apo-Ferrous Gluconate®; Novo-Ferrogluc
Generic Available Yes
Synonyms Iron Gluconate
Pharmacologic Category Iron Salt
Use Prevention and treatment of iron-deficiency anemias
Local Anesthetic/Vasoconstrictor Precautions No information available to require special precautions
Effects on Dental Treatment Key adverse event(s) related to dental treatment: Staining of teeth. Do not prescribe tetracyclines simultaneously with iron since GI tract absorption of both tetracycline and iron may be inhibited.
Mechanism of Action Replaces iron found in hemoglobin, myoglobin, and enzymes; allows the transportation of oxygen via hemoglobin
Pregnancy Risk Factor A

Ferrous Sulfate (FER us SUL fate)

U.S. Brand Names Feosol® [OTC]; Feratab® [OTC]; Fer-Gen-Sol [OTC]; Fer-In-Sol® [OTC]; Fer-Iron® [OTC]; Slow FE® [OTC]
Canadian Brand Names Apo-Ferrous Sulfate®; Fer-In-Sol®; Ferodan™
Mexican Brand Names Hemobion®
Generic Available Yes
Synonyms FeSO$_4$; Iron Sulfate
Pharmacologic Category Iron Salt
Use Prevention and treatment of iron-deficiency anemias
Local Anesthetic/Vasoconstrictor Precautions No information available to require special precautions
Effects on Dental Treatment Do not prescribe tetracyclines simultaneously with iron since GI tract absorption of both tetracycline and iron may be inhibited. Liquid preparations may temporarily stain the teeth.
Mechanism of Action Replaces iron, found in hemoglobin, myoglobin, and other enzymes; allows the transportation of oxygen via hemoglobin
Pregnancy Risk Factor A

Ferrous Sulfate and Ascorbic Acid
(FER us SUL fate & a SKOR bik AS id)

Related Information
Ascorbic Acid *on page 143*
Ferrous Sulfate *on page 651*
U.S. Brand Names Fero-Grad 500® [OTC]; Vitelle™ Irospan® [OTC] [DSC]
Generic Available No
Synonyms Ascorbic Acid and Ferrous Sulfate; Iron Sulfate and Vitamin C
Pharmacologic Category Iron Salt; Vitamin
Use Treatment of iron deficiency in nonpregnant adults; treatment and prevention of iron deficiency in pregnant adults
Local Anesthetic/Vasoconstrictor Precautions No information available to require special precautions
Effects on Dental Treatment Do not prescribe tetracyclines simultaneously with iron since GI tract absorption of both tetracycline and iron may be inhibited. Liquid preparations may temporarily stain the teeth.
Common Adverse Effects Based on **ferrous sulfate** component:
>10%: Gastrointestinal: GI irritation, epigastric pain, nausea, dark stools, vomiting, stomach cramping, constipation
(Continued)

Ferrous Sulfate and Ascorbic Acid (Continued)

1% to 10%:
Gastrointestinal: Heartburn, diarrhea
Genitourinary: Discoloration of urine
Miscellaneous: Liquid preparations may temporarily stain the teeth

Drug Interactions

Increased Effect/Toxicity: Concurrent administration of ≥200 mg vitamin C per 30 mg elemental iron increases absorption of oral iron.

Decreased Effect: Absorption of oral preparation of iron and tetracyclines are decreased when both of these drugs are given together. Absorption of quinolones may be decreased due to formation of a ferric ion-quinolone complex when given concurrently. Concurrent administration of antacids and H_2 blockers (cimetidine) may decrease iron absorption. Iron may decrease absorption of levodopa, methyldopa, penicillamine when given at the same time. Response to iron therapy may be delayed by chloramphenicol.

Pharmacodynamics/Kinetics See individual agents.

Ferumoxides (fer yoo MOX ides)

U.S. Brand Names Feridex I.V.®
Generic Available No
Pharmacologic Category Radiological/Contrast Media, Nonionic
Use For I.V. administration as an adjunct to MRI (in adult patients) to enhance the T2 weighted images used in the detection and evaluation of lesions of the liver
Local Anesthetic/Vasoconstrictor Precautions No information available to require special precautions
Effects on Dental Treatment No significant effects or complications reported
Pregnancy Risk Factor C

FeSO₄ see Ferrous Sulfate on page 651
Fe-Tinic™ 150 [OTC] [DSC] see Polysaccharide-Iron Complex on page 1254
FeverALL® [OTC] see Acetaminophen on page 31

Fexofenadine (feks oh FEN a deen)

U.S. Brand Names Allegra®
Canadian Brand Names Allegra®
Mexican Brand Names Allegra®
Generic Available Yes
Synonyms Fexofenadine Hydrochloride
Pharmacologic Category Antihistamine, Nonsedating
Use Relief of symptoms associated with seasonal allergic rhinitis; treatment of chronic idiopathic urticaria
Local Anesthetic/Vasoconstrictor Precautions No information available to require special precautions
Effects on Dental Treatment No significant effects or complications reported
Common Adverse Effects
>10%: Central nervous system: Headache (5% to 11%)
1% to 10%:
Central nervous system: Fever (2%), dizziness (2%), pain (2%), drowsiness (1%), fatigue (1%)
Endocrine & metabolic: Dysmenorrhea (2%)
Gastrointestinal: Nausea (2%), dyspepsia (1% to 5%)
Neuromuscular & skeletal: Back pain (2% to 3%), myalgia (3%)
Otic: Otitis media (2%)
Respiratory: Cough (4%), upper respiratory tract infection (2% to 4%), nasopharyngitis (2%)
Miscellaneous: Viral infection (3%)
Dosage Oral: Chronic idiopathic urticaria, seasonal allergic rhinitis:
Children 6-11 years: 30 mg twice daily
Children ≥12 years and Adults: 60 mg twice daily **or** 180 mg once daily
Dosing adjustment in renal impairment: Cl$_{cr}$ <80 mL/minute:
Children 6-11 years: Initial: 30 mg once daily
Children ≥12 years and Adults: Initial: 60 mg once daily
Mechanism of Action Fexofenadine is an active metabolite of terfenadine and like terfenadine it competes with histamine for H_1-receptor sites on effector cells in the gastrointestinal tract, blood vessels and respiratory tract; it appears that fexofenadine does not cross the blood brain barrier to any appreciable degree, resulting in a reduced potential for sedation

Contraindications Hypersensitivity to fexofenadine or any component of the formulation

Warnings/Precautions Safety and efficacy in children <6 years of age have not been established.

Drug Interactions
  Cytochrome P450 Effect: Substrate of CYP3A4 (minor); **Inhibits** CYP2D6 (weak)
  Increased Effect/Toxicity: Erythromycin and ketoconazole increased the levels of fexofenadine; however, no increase in adverse events or QT$_c$ intervals was noted. The effect of other macrolide agents or azoles has not been investigated.
  Decreased Effect: Aluminum- and magnesium-containing antacids decrease plasma levels of fexofenadine; separate administration is recommended.

Ethanol/Nutrition/Herb Interactions
  Ethanol: Avoid ethanol (although limited with fexofenadine, may increase risk of sedation).
  Food: Fruit juice (apple, grapefruit, orange, pineapple) may decrease bioavailability of fexofenadine by ~36%.
  Herb/Nutraceutical: St John's wort may decrease fexofenadine levels.

Pharmacodynamics/Kinetics
  Onset of action: 60 minutes
  Duration: Antihistaminic effect: ≥12 hours
  Protein binding: 60% to 70%, primarily albumin and alpha$_1$-acid glycoprotein
  Metabolism: Minimal (~5%)
  Half-life elimination: 14.4 hours
  Time to peak, serum: ~2.6 hours
  Excretion: Feces (~80%) and urine (~11%) as unchanged drug

Pregnancy Risk Factor C

Dosage Forms TAB: 30 mg, 60 mg, 180 mg

Fexofenadine and Pseudoephedrine
(feks oh FEN a deen & soo doe e FED rin)

Related Information
  Fexofenadine *on page 652*
  Pseudoephedrine *on page 1309*

U.S. Brand Names Allegra-D® 12 Hour; Allegra-D® 24 Hour

Canadian Brand Names Allegra-D®

Generic Available No

Synonyms Pseudoephedrine and Fexofenadine

Pharmacologic Category Antihistamine/Decongestant Combination

Use Relief of symptoms associated with seasonal allergic rhinitis in adults and children ≥12 years of age

Local Anesthetic/Vasoconstrictor Precautions Use with caution since pseudoephedrine is a sympathomimetic amine which could interact with epinephrine to cause a pressor response

Effects on Dental Treatment Key adverse event(s) related to dental treatment: Pseudoephedrine: Xerostomia (normal salivary flow resumes upon discontinuation).

Common Adverse Effects See individual agents.

Drug Interactions
  Cytochrome P450 Effect: Fexofenadine: **Substrate** of CYP3A4 (minor); **Inhibits** CYP2D6 (weak)

Pharmacodynamics/Kinetics See individual agents.

Pregnancy Risk Factor C

Fexofenadine Hydrochloride *see Fexofenadine on page 652*

Fiberall® *see Psyllium on page 1313*

FiberCon® [OTC] *see Polycarbophil on page 1252*

FiberEase™ [OTC] *see Methylcellulose on page 1021*

Fiber-Lax® [OTC] *see Polycarbophil on page 1252*

Fibrin Sealant Kit (FI brin SEEL ent kit)

U.S. Brand Names Crosseal™; Tisseel® VH

Canadian Brand Names Tisseel® VH

Generic Available No

(Continued)

Fibrin Sealant Kit *(Continued)*

Synonyms FS

Pharmacologic Category Hemostatic Agent

Use

Crosseal™: Adjunct to hemostasis in liver surgery

Tisseel® VH: Adjunct to hemostasis in cardiopulmonary bypass surgery and splenic injury (due to blunt or penetrating trauma to the abdomen) when the control of bleeding by conventional surgical techniques is ineffective or impractical; adjunctive sealant for closure of colostomies; hemostatic agent in heparinized patients undergoing cardiopulmonary bypass

Local Anesthetic/Vasoconstrictor Precautions No information available to require special precautions

Effects on Dental Treatment No significant effects or complications reported

Mechanism of Action Formation of a biodegradable adhesive is done by duplicating the last step of the coagulation cascade, the formation of fibrin from fibrinogen. Fibrinogen is the main component of the sealant solution. The solution also contains thrombin, which transforms fibrinogen from the sealer protein solution into fibrin, and fibrinolysis inhibitor (aprotinin), which prevents the premature degradation of fibrin. When mixed as directed, a viscous solution forms that sets into an elastic coagulum.

Drug Interactions

Decreased Effect: Decreased effect (Tisseel® VH): Local concentrations/applications of alcohol, heavy-metal ions, iodine; oxycellulose preparations

Pharmacodynamics/Kinetics Onset of action:

Crosseal™: Time to hemostasis: 5.3 minutes

Tisseel® VH: Time to hemostasis: 5 minutes (65% of patients); Final prepared sealant: 70% strength: ~10 minutes; Full strength: ~2 hours

Pregnancy Risk Factor C

Fibro-XL [OTC] *see* Psyllium *on page 1313*

Fibro-Lax [OTC] *see* Psyllium *on page 1313*

Filgrastim *(fil GRA stim)*

U.S. Brand Names Neupogen®

Canadian Brand Names Neupogen®

Mexican Brand Names Neupogen®

Generic Available No

Synonyms G-CSF; Granulocyte Colony Stimulating Factor

Pharmacologic Category Colony Stimulating Factor

Use Stimulation of granulocyte production in chemotherapy-induced neutropenia (nonmyeloid malignancies, acute myeloid leukemia, and bone marrow transplantation); severe chronic neutropenia (SCN); patients undergoing peripheral blood progenitor cell (PBPC) collection

Local Anesthetic/Vasoconstrictor Precautions No information available to require special precautions

Effects on Dental Treatment Key adverse event(s) related to dental treatment: Mucositis.

Comparative Effects — Filgrastim vs Sargramostim

Proliferation/Differentiation	Filgrastim	Sargramostim
Neutrophils	Yes	Yes
Eosinophils	No	Yes
Macrophages	No	Yes
Neutrophil migration	Enhanced	Inhibited

Common Adverse Effects

>10%:

Central nervous system: Fever (12%)

Dermatologic: Petechiae (17%), rash (12%)

Gastrointestinal: Splenomegaly (≤33% of patients with cyclic neutropenia/congenital agranulocytosis receiving filgrastim for ≥14 days; rare in other patients)

Hepatic: Alkaline phosphatase increased (21%)

Neuromuscular & skeletal: Bone pain (22% to 33%), commonly in the lower back, posterior iliac crest, and sternum

Respiratory: Epistaxis (9% to 15%)

1% to 10%:

Cardiovascular: Hyper-/hypotension (4%), S-T segment depression (3%), myocardial infarction/arrhythmias (3%)

Central nervous system: Headache (7%)
Gastrointestinal: Nausea (10%), vomiting (7%), peritonitis (2%)
Hematologic: Leukocytosis (2%)

Mechanism of Action Stimulates the production, maturation, and activation of neutrophils; filgrastim activates neutrophils to increase both their migration and cytotoxicity. See table on previous page.

Pharmacodynamics/Kinetics

Onset of action: ~24 hours; plateaus in 3-5 days

Duration: ANC decreases by 50% within 2 days after discontinuing filgrastim; white counts return to the normal range in 4-7 days; peak plasma levels can be maintained for up to 12 hours

Absorption: SubQ: 100%

Distribution: V_d: 150 mL/kg; no evidence of drug accumulation over a 11- to 20-day period

Metabolism: Systemically degraded

Half-life elimination: 1.8-3.5 hours

Time to peak, serum: SubQ: 2-6 hours

Pregnancy Risk Factor C

Finacea™ see Azelaic Acid on page 169

Finasteride (fi NAS teer ide)

U.S. Brand Names Propecia®; Proscar®
Canadian Brand Names Propecia®; Proscar®
Mexican Brand Names Propeshia®; Proscar®
Generic Available No
Pharmacologic Category 5 Alpha-Reductase Inhibitor
Use

Propecia®: Treatment of male pattern hair loss in **men only**. Safety and efficacy were demonstrated in men between 18-41 years of age.

Proscar®: Treatment of symptomatic benign prostatic hyperplasia (BPH); can be used in combination with an alpha blocker, doxazosin

Unlabeled/Investigational Use Adjuvant monotherapy after radical prostatectomy in the treatment of prostatic cancer; female hirsutism

Local Anesthetic/Vasoconstrictor Precautions No information available to require special precautions

Effects on Dental Treatment No significant effects or complications reported

Common Adverse Effects Note: "Combination therapy" refers to finasteride and doxazosin.

>10%:
Endocrine & metabolic: Impotence (19%; combination therapy 23%), libido decreased (10%; combination therapy 12%)
Genitourinary: Neuromuscular & skeletal: Weakness (5%; combination therapy 17%)

1% to 10%:
Cardiovascular: Postural hypotension (9%; combination therapy 18%), edema (1%, combination therapy 3%)
Central nervous system: Dizziness (7%; combination therapy 23%), somnolence (2%; combination therapy 3%)
Genitourinary: Ejaculation disturbances (7%; combination therapy 14%), decreased volume of ejaculate
Endocrine & metabolic: Gynecomastia (2%)
Respiratory: Dyspnea (1%; combination therapy 2%), rhinitis (1%; combination therapy 2%)

Mechanism of Action Finasteride is a competitive inhibitor of both tissue and hepatic 5-alpha reductase. This results in inhibition of the conversion of testosterone to dihydrotestosterone and markedly suppresses serum dihydrotestosterone levels

Drug Interactions
Cytochrome P450 Effect: Substrate of CYP3A4 (minor)

Pharmacodynamics/Kinetics

Onset of action: 3-6 months of ongoing therapy

Duration:
After a single oral dose as small as 0.5 mg: 65% depression of plasma dihydrotestosterone levels persists 5-7 days
After 6 months of treatment with 5 mg/day: Circulating dihydrotestosterone levels are reduced to castrate levels without significant effects on circulating testosterone; levels return to normal within 14 days of discontinuation of treatment

Distribution: V_{dss}: 76 L

Protein binding: 90%

(Continued)

Finasteride *(Continued)*

Metabolism: Hepatic via CYP3A4; two active metabolites (<20% activity of finasteride)

Bioavailability: Mean: 63%

Half-life elimination, serum: Elderly: 8 hours; Adults: 6 hours (3-16)

Time to peak, serum: 2-6 hours

Excretion: Feces (57%) and urine (39%) as metabolites

Pregnancy Risk Factor X

Fioricet® *see* Butalbital, Acetaminophen, and Caffeine *on page 239*

Fioricet® with Codeine *see* Butalbital, Acetaminophen, Caffeine, and Codeine *on page 239*

Fiorinal® *see* Butalbital, Aspirin, and Caffeine *on page 241*

Fiorinal® With Codeine *see* Butalbital, Aspirin, Caffeine, and Codeine *on page 241*

First® Testosterone *see* Testosterone *on page 1462*

First® Testosterone MC *see* Testosterone *on page 1462*

Fisalamine *see* Mesalamine *on page 996*

FK506 *see* Tacrolimus *on page 1437*

Flagyl® *see* Metronidazole *on page 1033*

Flagyl ER® *see* Metronidazole *on page 1033*

Flagyl® I.V. RTU™ *see* Metronidazole *on page 1033*

Flarex® *see* Fluorometholone *on page 674*

Flavan *see* Flavocoxid *on page 656*

Flavocoxid *(fla vo KOKS id)*

U.S. Brand Names Limbrel™

Synonyms Flavan; Flavonoid

Pharmacologic Category Anti-inflammatory Agent

Use Clinical dietary management of osteoarthritis, including associated inflammation

Local Anesthetic/Vasoconstrictor Precautions No information available to require special precautions

Effects on Dental Treatment No significant effects or complications reported

Common Adverse Effects

≥2%:

Cardiovascular: Hypertension, varicose veins

Dermatologic: Psoriasis

Gastrointestinal: Occult stools (statistically similar to placebo)

Neuromuscular & skeletal: Fluid on the knee

Mechanism of Action Exerts anti-inflammatory properties through nonspecific inhibition of cyclooxygenase (COX) and lipoxygenase (5-LOX) pathways; may also possess general analgesic and antioxidant/anticytokine properties

Drug Interactions

Cytochrome P450 Effect: Inhibits CYP1A2 (weak), 2C9 (weak), 2C19 (weak), 2D6 (weak), 3A4 (weak)

Increased Effect/Toxicity:

Concomitant use with NSAIDs may increase the risk of gastrointestinal bleeding.

Pharmacodynamics/Kinetics

Onset of action: 1-2 hours

Metabolism: Primarily via glucuronidation and sulfation

Flavonoid *see* Flavocoxid *on page 656*

Flavoxate *(fla VOKS ate)*

U.S. Brand Names Urispas®

Canadian Brand Names Apo-Flavoxate®; Urispas®

Mexican Brand Names Bladuril®

Generic Available Yes

Synonyms Flavoxate Hydrochloride

Pharmacologic Category Antispasmodic Agent, Urinary

Use Antispasmodic to provide symptomatic relief of dysuria, nocturia, suprapubic pain, urgency, and incontinence due to detrusor instability and hyper-reflexia in elderly with cystitis, urethritis, urethrocystitis, urethrotrigonitis, and prostatitis

Local Anesthetic/Vasoconstrictor Precautions No information available to require special precautions

Effects on Dental Treatment Key adverse event(s) related to dental treatment: Xerostomia and changes in salivation (normal salivary flow resumes upon discontinuation), and dry throat.

Common Adverse Effects Frequency not defined.

Cardiovascular: Tachycardia, palpitation

Central nervous system: Drowsiness, confusion (especially in the elderly), nervousness, fatigue, vertigo, headache, hyperpyrexia

Dermatologic: Rash, urticaria

Gastrointestinal: Constipation, nausea, vomiting, xerostomia, dry throat

Genitourinary: Dysuria

Hematologic: Leukopenia

Ocular: Increased intraocular pressure, blurred vision

Mechanism of Action Synthetic antispasmotic with similar actions to that of propantheline; it exerts a direct relaxant effect on smooth muscles via phosphodiesterase inhibition, providing relief to a variety of smooth muscle spasms; it is especially useful for the treatment of bladder spasticity, whereby it produces an increase in urinary capacity

Pharmacodynamics/Kinetics

Onset of action: 55-60 minutes

Metabolism: To methyl; flavone carboxylic acid active

Excretion: Urine (10% to 30%) within 6 hours

Pregnancy Risk Factor B

Flavoxate Hydrochloride *see* Flavoxate *on page 656*

Flecainide (fle KAY nide)

Related Information

Cardiovascular Diseases *on page 1636*

U.S. Brand Names Tambocor™

Canadian Brand Names Apo-Flecainide®; Tambocor™

Mexican Brand Names Tambocor™

Generic Available Yes

Synonyms Flecainide Acetate

Pharmacologic Category Antiarrhythmic Agent, Class Ic

Use Prevention and suppression of documented life-threatening ventricular arrhythmias (eg, sustained ventricular tachycardia); controlling symptomatic, disabling supraventricular tachycardias in patients without structural heart disease in whom other agents fail

Local Anesthetic/Vasoconstrictor Precautions No information available to require special precautions (see Dental Comment)

Effects on Dental Treatment No significant effects or complications reported

Common Adverse Effects

>10%:

Central nervous system: Dizziness (19% to 30%)

Ocular: Visual disturbances (16%)

Respiratory: Dyspnea (~10%)

1% to 10%:

Cardiovascular: Palpitations (6%), chest pain (5%), edema (3.5%), tachycardia (1% to 3%), proarrhythmic (4% to 12%), sinus node dysfunction (1.2%)

Central nervous system: Headache (4% to 10%), fatigue (8%), nervousness (5%) additional symptoms occurring at a frequency between 1% and 3%: fever, malaise, hypoesthesia, paresis, ataxia, vertigo, syncope, somnolence, tinnitus, anxiety, insomnia, depression

Dermatologic: Rash (1% to 3%)

Gastrointestinal: Nausea (9%), constipation (1%), abdominal pain (3%), anorexia (1% to 3%), diarrhea (0.7% to 3%)

Neuromuscular & skeletal: Tremor (5%), weakness (5%), paresthesia (1%)

Ocular: Diplopia (1% to 3%), blurred vision

Mechanism of Action Class Ic antiarrhythmic; slows conduction in cardiac tissue by altering transport of ions across cell membranes; causes slight prolongation of refractory periods; decreases the rate of rise of the action potential without affecting its duration; increases electrical stimulation threshold of ventricle, His-Purkinje system; possesses local anesthetic and moderate negative inotropic effects

Drug Interactions

Cytochrome P450 Effect: Substrate of CYP1A2 (minor), 2D6 (major); Inhibits CYP2D6 (weak)

Increased Effect/Toxicity: CYP2D6 inhibitors may increase the levels/effects of flecainide; example inhibitors include chlorpromazine, delavirdine, fluoxetine, miconazole, paroxetine, pergolide, quinidine, quinine, ritonavir, and (Continued)

Flecainide *(Continued)*

ropinirole. Flecainide concentrations may be increased by amiodarone (reduce flecainide 25% to 33%), and propranolol. Beta-adrenergic blockers, disopyramide, verapamil may enhance flecainide's negative inotropic effects. Alkalinizing agents (ie, high-dose antacids, cimetidine, carbonic anhydrase inhibitors, sodium bicarbonate) may decrease flecainide clearance, potentially increasing toxicity. Propranolol blood levels are increased by flecainide.

Decreased Effect: Smoking and acid urine increase flecainide clearance.

Pharmacodynamics/Kinetics

Absorption: Oral: Rapid

Distribution: Adults: V_d: 5-13.4 L/kg

Protein binding: Alpha$_1$ glycoprotein: 40% to 50%

Metabolism: Hepatic

Bioavailability: 85% to 90%

Half-life elimination: Infants: 11-12 hours; Children: 8 hours; Adults: 7-22 hours, increased with congestive heart failure or renal dysfunction; End-stage renal disease: 19-26 hours

Time to peak, serum: ~1.5-3 hours

Excretion: Urine (80% to 90%, 10% to 50% as unchanged drug and metabolites)

Pregnancy Risk Factor C

Dental Comment

This drug is known to prolong the QT interval. The QT interval is measured as the time and distance between the Q point of the QRS complex and the end of the T wave in the ECG tracing. After adjustment for heart rate, the QT interval is defined as prolonged if it is more than 450 msec in men and 460 msec in women. A long QT syndrome was first described in the 1950s and 60s as a congenital syndrome involving QT interval prolongation and syncope and sudden death. Some of the congenital long QT syndromes were characterized by a peculiar electrocardiographic appearance of the QRS complex involving a premature atria beat followed by a pause, then a subsequent sinus beat showing marked QT prolongation and deformity. This type of cardiac arrhythmia was originally termed "torsade de pointes" (translated from the French as "twisting of the points").

Prolongation of the QT interval is thought to result from delayed ventricular repolarization. The repolarization process within the myocardial cell is due to the efflux of intracellular potassium. The channels associated with this current can be blocked by many drugs and predisposes the electrical propagation cycle to torsade de pointes.

Flecainide is one of the drugs confirmed to prolong the QT interval and is accepted as having a risk of causing torsade de pointes. The risk of drug-induced torsade de pointes is extremely low when a single QT interval prolonging drug is prescribed. In terms of epinephrine, it is not known what effect vasoconstrictors in the local anesthetic regimen will have in patients with a known history of congenital prolonged QT interval or in patients taking any medication that prolongs the QT interval. Until more information is obtained, it is suggested that the clinician consult with the physician prior to the use of a vasoconstrictor in suspected patients, and that the vasoconstrictor (epinephrine, levonordefrin [Neo-Cobefrin®]) be used with caution.

Flecainide Acetate *see* Flecainide *on page 657*

Fleet® Accu-Prep® [OTC] *see* Sodium Phosphates *on page 1403*

Fleet® Babylax® [OTC] *see* Glycerin *on page 747*

Fleet® Bisacodyl Enema [OTC] *see* Bisacodyl *on page 209*

Fleet® Enema [OTC] *see* Sodium Phosphates *on page 1403*

Fleet® Glycerin Suppositories [OTC] *see* Glycerin *on page 747*

Fleet® Glycerin Suppositories Maximum Strength [OTC] *see* Glycerin *on page 747*

Fleet® Liquid Glycerin Suppositories [OTC] *see* Glycerin *on page 747*

Fleet® Phospho-Soda® [OTC] *see* Sodium Phosphates *on page 1403*

Fleet® Sof-Lax® [OTC] *see* Docusate *on page 496*

Fleet® Sof-Lax® Overnight [DSC] [OTC] *see* Docusate and Casanthranol *on page 496*

Fleet® Stimulant Laxative [OTC] *see* Bisacodyl *on page 209*

Fletcher's® Castoria® [OTC] *see* Senna *on page 1384*

Flexeril® *see* Cyclobenzaprine *on page 401*

Flex-Power [OTC] *see* Triethanolamine Salicylate *on page 1535*

Flo-Coat *see* Barium *on page 179*

Flolan® *see* Epoprostenol *on page 553*

Flomax® *see* Tamsulosin *on page 1445*

Flonase® see Fluticasone on page 686

Flora-Q™ [OTC] see Lactobacillus on page 535

Florical® [OTC] see Calcium Carbonate on page 248

Florinef® see Fludrocortisone on page 664

Florone® see Diflorasone on page 468

Flovent® HFA see Fluticasone on page 686

Floxin® see Ofloxacin on page 1137

Floxin Otic Singles see Ofloxacin on page 1137

Floxuridine (floks YOOR i deen)

U.S. Brand Names FUDR®
Canadian Brand Names FUDR®
Generic Available Yes
Synonyms Fluorodeoxyuridine; FUDR; 5-FUDR; NSC-27640
Pharmacologic Category Antineoplastic Agent, Antimetabolite (Pyrimidine Antagonist)
Use Management of hepatic metastases of colorectal and gastric cancers
Local Anesthetic/Vasoconstrictor Precautions No information available to require special precautions
Effects on Dental Treatment Key adverse event(s) related to dental treatment: Stomatitis.
Common Adverse Effects
>10%:
  Gastrointestinal: Stomatitis, diarrhea; may be dose-limiting
  Hematologic: Myelosuppression, may be dose-limiting; leukopenia, thrombocytopenia, anemia
    Onset: 4-7 days
    Nadir: 5-9 days
    Recovery: 21 days
1% to 10%:
  Dermatologic: Alopecia, photosensitivity, hyperpigmentation of the skin, localized erythema, dermatitis
  Gastrointestinal: Anorexia
  Hepatic: Biliary sclerosis, cholecystitis, jaundice
Mechanism of Action Mechanism of action and pharmacokinetics are very similar to fluorouracil; floxuridine is the deoxyribonucleotide of fluorouracil. Floxuridine is a fluorinated pyrimidine antagonist which inhibits DNA and RNA synthesis and methylation of deoxyuridylic acid to thymidylic acid.
Drug Interactions
  Increased Effect/Toxicity: Any form of therapy which adds to the stress of the patient, interferes with nutrition, or depresses bone marrow function will increase the toxicity of floxuridine. Pentostatin and floxuridine administered together has resulted in fatal pulmonary toxicity.
  Decreased Effect: Patients may experience impaired immune response to vaccines; possible infection after administration of live vaccines in patients receiving immunosuppressants.
Pharmacodynamics/Kinetics
  Metabolism: Hepatic; Active metabolites: Floxuridine monophosphate (FUDR-MP) and fluorouracil; Inactive metabolites: Urea, CO_2, α-fluoro-β-alanine, α-fluoro-β-guanidopropionic acid, α-fluoro-β-ureidopropionic acid, and dihydrofluorouracil
  Excretion: Urine: Fluorouracil, urea, α-fluoro-β-alanine, α-fluoro-β-guanidopropionic acid, α-fluoro-β-ureidopropionic acid, and dihydrofluorouracil; exhaled gases (CO_2)
Pregnancy Risk Factor D

Fluarix™ see Influenza Virus Vaccine on page 833

Flubenisolone see Betamethasone on page 199

Flucaine® see Proparacaine and Fluorescein on page 1296

Fluconazole (floo KOE na zole)

Related Information
  Fungal Infections on page 1707
  Sexually-Transmitted Diseases on page 1674
Related Sample Prescriptions
  Systemic Fungal Infections on page 1740
(Continued)

Fluconazole *(Continued)*

U.S. Brand Names Diflucan®

Canadian Brand Names Apo-Fluconazole®; Diflucan®; Fluconazole Omega; Gen-Fluconazole; Novo-Fluconazole

Mexican Brand Names Afungil®; Diflucan®; Neofomiral®; Oxifungol®; Zonal®

Generic Available Yes

Pharmacologic Category Antifungal Agent, Oral; Antifungal Agent, Parenteral

Dental Use Treatment of susceptible fungal infections in the oral cavity including candidiasis, oral thrush, and chronic mucocutaneous candidiasis treatment of esophageal and oropharyngeal candidiasis caused by *Candida* species; treatment of severe, chronic mucocutaneous candidiasis caused by *Candida* species

Use Treatment of candidiasis (vaginal, oropharyngeal, esophageal, urinary tract infections, peritonitis, pneumonia, and systemic infections); cryptococcal meningitis; antifungal prophylaxis in allogeneic bone marrow transplant recipients

Local Anesthetic/Vasoconstrictor Precautions No information available to require special precautions

Effects on Dental Treatment Key adverse event(s) related to dental treatment: Abnormal taste.

Significant Adverse Effects Frequency not always defined.

Cardiovascular: Angioedema, pallor, QT prolongation, torsade de pointes

Central nervous system: Headache (2% to 13%), seizure, dizziness

Dermatologic: Rash (2%), alopecia, toxic epidermal necrolysis, Stevens-Johnson syndrome

Endocrine & metabolic: Hypercholesterolemia, hypertriglyceridemia, hypokalemia

Gastrointestinal: Nausea (4% to 7%), vomiting (2%), abdominal pain (2% to 6%), diarrhea (2% to 3%), taste perversion, dyspepsia

Hematologic: Agranulocytosis, leukopenia, neutropenia, thrombocytopenia

Hepatic: Hepatic failure (rare), hepatitis, cholestasis, jaundice, increased ALT/AST, increased alkaline phosphatase

Respiratory: Dyspnea

Miscellaneous: Anaphylactic reactions (rare)

Dental Usual Dosing Candidiasis: Adults:

Usual dosage range: 200-400 mg/day; duration and dosage depends on severity of infection

Oropharyngeal (long-term suppression): 200 mg/day; chronic therapy is recommended in immunocompromised patients with history of oropharyngeal candidiasis (OPC)

Dosage The daily dose of fluconazole is the same for oral and I.V. administration

Usual dosage ranges:

Neonates: First 2 weeks of life, especially premature neonates: Same dose as older children every 72 hours

Children: Loading dose: 6-12 mg/kg; maintenance: 3-12 mg/kg/day; duration and dosage depends on severity of infection

Adults: 200-400 mg/day; duration and dosage depends on severity of infection

Indication-specific dosing:

Children:

Candidiasis:

Oropharyngeal: Loading dose: 6 mg/kg; maintenance: 3 mg/kg/day for 2 weeks

Esophageal: Loading dose: 6 mg/kg; maintenance: 3-12 mg/kg/day for 21 days and at least 2 weeks following resolution of symptoms

Systemic infection: 6 mg/kg every 12 hours for 28 days

Meningitis, cryptococcal: Loading dose: 12 mg/kg; maintenance: 6-12 mg/kg/day for 10-12 weeks following negative CSF culture; relapse suppression: 6 mg/kg/day

Adults:

Candidiasis:

Candidemia, primary therapy, non-neutropenic: 400-800 mg/day for 14 days after last positive blood culture and resolution of signs/symptoms

Alternate therapy: 800 mg/day with amphotericin B for 4-7 days followed by 800 mg/day for 14 days after last positive blood culture and resolution of signs/symptoms

Candidemia, secondary, neutropenic: 6-12 mg/kg/day for 14 days after last positive blood culture and resolution of signs/symptoms

Chronic, disseminated: 6 mg/kg/day for 3-6 months

Oropharyngeal (long-term suppression): 200 mg/day; chronic therapy is recommended in immunocompromised patients with history of oropharyngeal candidiasis (OPC)

Osteomyelitis: 6 mg/kg/day for 6-12 months

Esophageal: 200 mg on day 1, then 100-200 mg/day for 2-3 weeks after clinical improvement

Prophylaxis in bone marrow transplant: 400 mg/day; begin 3 days before onset of neutropenia and continue for 7 days after neutrophils >1000 cells/mm^3

Urinary: 200 mg/day for 1-2 weeks

Vaginal: 150 mg as a single dose

Coccidiomycosis: 400 mg/day; doses of 800-1000 mg/day have been used for meningeal disease; usual duration of therapy ranges from 3-6 months for primary uncomplicated infections and up to 1 year for pulmonary (chronic and diffuse) infection

Endocarditis, prosthetic valve, early: 6-12 mg/kg/day for 6 weeks after valve replacement

Endophthalmitis: 6-12 mg/kg/day or 400-800 mg/day for 6-12 weeks after surgical intervention. **Note:** *C. krusei* and *C. galbrata* infection acquired exogenously should be treated with voriconazole.

Meningitis, cryptococcal: 400-800 mg/day for 10-12 weeks or with flucytosine 100-150 mg/day for 6 weeks; maintenance: 200-400 mg/day

Pneumonia, cryptococcal (mild-to-moderate): 200-400 mg/day for 6-12 months (life-long in HIV-positive patients)

Dosing adjustment/interval in renal impairment:
No adjustment for vaginal candidiasis single-dose therapy
For multiple dosing, administer usual load then adjust daily doses
Cl$_{cr}$ ≤50 mL/minute (no dialysis): Administer 50% of recommended dose or administer every 48 hours.
Hemodialysis: 50% is removed by hemodialysis; administer 100% of daily dose (according to indication) after each dialysis treatment.
Continuous arteriovenous or venovenous hemofiltration: Dose as for Cl$_{cr}$ 10-50 mL/minute.

Mechanism of Action Interferes with cytochrome P450 activity, decreasing ergosterol synthesis (principal sterol in fungal cell membrane) and inhibiting cell membrane formation

Contraindications Hypersensitivity to fluconazole, other azoles, or any component of the formulation; concomitant administration with cisapride

Warnings/Precautions Should be used with caution in patients with renal and hepatic dysfunction or previous hepatotoxicity from other azole derivatives. Patients who develop abnormal liver function tests during fluconazole therapy should be monitored closely and discontinued if symptoms consistent with liver disease develop. Use caution in patients at risk of proarrhythmias.

Drug Interactions Inhibits CYP1A2 (weak), 2C9 (strong), 2C19 (strong), 3A4 (moderate)

Benzodiazepines (metabolized by oxidation, eg, alprazolam, triazolam, midazolam, diazepam) serum concentrations are increased by fluconazole which may cause increased CNS sedation. Consider a benzodiazepine not metabolized by CYP3A4 or another antifungal.

Caffeine's metabolism is decreased; monitor for tachycardia, nervousness, and anxiety.

Calcium channel blockers may have increased serum concentrations; consider another agent instead of a calcium channel blocker, another antifungal, or reduce the dose of the calcium channel blocker. Monitor blood pressure.

Cisapride's serum concentration is increased which may lead to malignant arrhythmias; concurrent use is contraindicated.

Cyclosporine's serum concentration is increased; monitor cyclosporine's serum concentration and renal function.

CYP2C9 Substrates: Fluconazole may increase the levels/effects of CYP2C9 substrates. Example substrates include bosentan, dapsone, fluoxetine, glimepiride, glipizide, losartan, montelukast, nateglinide, paclitaxel, phenytoin, warfarin, and zafirlukast.

CYP2C19 substrates: Fluconazole may increase the levels/effects of CYP2C19 substrates. Example substrates include citalopram, diazepam, methsuximide, phenytoin, propranolol, and sertraline.

CYP3A4 substrates: Fluconazole may increase the levels/effects of CYP3A4 substrates. Example substrates include benzodiazepines, calcium channel blockers, cyclosporine, mirtazapine, nateglinide, nefazodone, sildenafil (and other PDE-5 inhibitors), tacrolimus, and venlafaxine. Selected benzodiazepines (midazolam and triazolam), cisapride, ergot alkaloids, selected HMG-CoA reductase inhibitors (lovastatin and simvastatin), and pimozide are generally contraindicated with strong CYP3A4 inhibitors.

(Continued)

Fluconazole *(Continued)*

HMG-CoA reductase inhibitors (except pravastatin and fluvastatin) have increased serum concentrations; switch to pravastatin/fluvastatin or monitor for development of myopathy.

Losartan's active metabolite is reduced in concentration; consider another anti-hypertensive agent unaffected by the azole antifungals, another antifungal, or monitor blood pressure closely.

Phenytoin's serum concentration is increased; monitor phenytoin levels and adjust dose as needed.

Rifampin decreases fluconazole's serum concentration; monitor infection status.

Tacrolimus's serum concentration is increased; monitor tacrolimus's serum concentration and renal function.

Warfarin's effects are increased; monitor INR and adjust warfarin's dose as needed.

Dietary Considerations Take with or without regard to food.

Pharmacodynamics/Kinetics

Distribution: Widely throughout body with good penetration into CSF, eye, peri-toneal fluid, sputum, skin, and urine

Relative diffusion blood into CSF: Adequate with or without inflammation (exceeds usual MICs)

CSF:blood level ratio: Normal meninges: 70% to 80%; Inflamed meninges: >70% to 80%

Protein binding, plasma: 11% to 12%

Bioavailability: Oral: >90%

Half-life elimination: Normal renal function: ~30 hours

Time to peak, serum: Oral: 1-2 hours

Excretion: Urine (80% as unchanged drug)

Pregnancy Risk Factor C

Lactation Enters breast/not recommended (AAP rates "compatible")

Breast-Feeding Considerations Fluconazole is found in breast milk at concentration similar to plasma.

Dosage Forms

Infusion [premixed in sodium chloride]: 2 mg/mL (100 mL, 200 mL)

Diflucan® [premixed in sodium chloride or dextrose] 2 mg/mL (100 mL, 200 mL)

Powder for oral suspension (Diflucan®): 10 mg/mL (35 mL); 40 mg/mL (35 mL) [contains sodium benzoate; orange flavor]

Tablet (Diflucan®): 50 mg, 100 mg, 150 mg, 200 mg

Flucytosine *(floo SYE toe seen)*

U.S. Brand Names Ancobon®

Canadian Brand Names Ancobon®

Generic Available No

Synonyms 5-FC; 5-Fluorocytosine; 5-Flurocytosine

Pharmacologic Category Antifungal Agent, Oral

Use Adjunctive treatment of susceptible fungal infections (usually *Candida* or *Cryptococcus*); synergy with amphotericin B for certain fungal infections (*Cryptococcus* spp., *Candida* spp.)

Local Anesthetic/Vasoconstrictor Precautions No information available to require special precautions

Effects on Dental Treatment No significant effects or complications reported

Common Adverse Effects Frequency not defined.

Cardiovascular: Cardiac arrest, myocardial toxicity, ventricular dysfunction, chest pain

Central nervous system: Confusion, headache, hallucinations, dizziness, drowsiness, psychosis, parkinsonism, ataxia, sedation, pyrexia, seizure, fatigue

Dermatologic: Rash, photosensitivity, pruritus, urticaria, Lyell's syndrome

Endocrine & metabolic: Temporary growth failure, hypoglycemia, hypokalemia

Gastrointestinal: Nausea, vomiting, diarrhea, abdominal pain, loss of appetite, dry mouth, hemorrhage, ulcerative colitis

Hematologic: Bone marrow suppression, anemia, leukopenia, thrombocyto-penia, agranulocytosis, aplastic anemia, eosinophilia, pancytopenia

Hepatic: Liver enzymes increased, hepatitis, jaundice, azotemia, bilirubin increased

Neuromuscular & skeletal: Peripheral neuropathy, paresthesia, weakness

Otic: Hearing loss

Renal: BUN and serum creatinine increased, renal failure, azotemia, crystalluria

Respiratory: Respiratory arrest, dyspnea

Miscellaneous: Anaphylaxis, allergic reaction

Mechanism of Action Penetrates fungal cells and is converted to fluorouracil which competes with uracil interfering with fungal RNA and protein synthesis

Drug Interactions

Increased Effect/Toxicity: Increased effect with amphotericin B. Amphotericin B-induced renal dysfunction may predispose patient to flucytosine accumulation and myelosuppression.

Decreased Effect: Cytarabine may inactivate flucytosine activity.

Pharmacodynamics/Kinetics

Absorption: 75% to 90%

Distribution: Into CSF, aqueous humor, joints, peritoneal fluid, and bronchial secretions; V_d: 0.6 L/kg

Protein binding: 2% to 4%

Metabolism: Minimally hepatic; deaminated, possibly via gut bacteria, to 5-fluorouracil

Half-life elimination:

Normal renal function: 2-5 hours

Anuria: 85 hours (range: 30-250)

End stage renal disease: 75-200 hours

Time to peak, serum: ~2-6 hours

Excretion: Urine (>90% as unchanged drug)

Pregnancy Risk Factor C

Fludara® *see* Fludarabine *on page 663*

Fludarabine (floo DARE a been)

U.S. Brand Names Fludara®
Canadian Brand Names Fludara®
Mexican Brand Names Fludara®
Generic Available Yes
Synonyms Fludarabine Phosphate
Pharmacologic Category Antineoplastic Agent, Antimetabolite (Purine Antagonist)

Use

I.V.: Treatment of chronic lymphocytic leukemia (CLL) (including refractory CLL); non-Hodgkin's lymphoma in adults

Oral (formulation not available in U.S.): Approved in Canada for treatment of CLL

Unlabeled/Investigational Use Treatment of non-Hodgkin's lymphoma and acute leukemias in pediatric patients; reduced-intensity conditioning regimens prior to allogeneic hematopoietic stem cell transplantation (generally administered in combination with busulfan and antithymocyte globulin or lymphocyte immune globulin, or in combination with melphalan and alemtuzumab)

Local Anesthetic/Vasoconstrictor Precautions No information available to require special precautions

Effects on Dental Treatment Key adverse event(s) related to dental treatment: Stomatitis.

Common Adverse Effects

>10%:

Cardiovascular: Edema

Central nervous system: Fatigue, somnolence (30%), chills, fever, pain

Dermatologic: Rash

Hematologic: Myelosuppression, common, dose-limiting toxicity, primarily leukopenia and thrombocytopenia

Nadir: 10-14 days

Recovery: 5-7 weeks

Neuromuscular & skeletal: Paresthesia, myalgia, weakness

Respiratory: Pneumonia

1% to 10%:

Cardiovascular: CHF

Central nervous system: Malaise, headache

Dermatologic: Alopecia

Endocrine & metabolic: Hyperglycemia, tumor lysis syndrome

Gastrointestinal: Anorexia, stomatitis (1.5%), diarrhea (1.8%), mild nausea/vomiting (3% to 10%)

Hematologic: Eosinophilia, hemolytic anemia, may be dose-limiting, possibly fatal in some patients

Mechanism of Action Fludarabine inhibits DNA synthesis by inhibition of DNA polymerase and ribonucleotide reductase.

(Continued)

Fludarabine *(Continued)*

Drug Interactions
Increased Effect/Toxicity: Combined use with pentostatin may lead to severe, even fatal, pulmonary toxicity.

Pharmacodynamics/Kinetics
Distribution: V_d: 38-96 L/m^2; widely with extensive tissue binding

Metabolism: I.V.: Fludarabine phosphate is rapidly dephosphorylated to 2-fluoro-vidarabine, which subsequently enters tumor cells and is phosphorylated to the active triphosphate derivative; rapidly dephosphorylated in the serum

Bioavailability: 75%

Half-life elimination: 2-fluoro-vidarabine: 9 hours

Excretion: Urine (60%, 23% as 2-fluoro-vidarabine) within 24 hours

Pregnancy Risk Factor D

Fludarabine Phosphate *see* Fludarabine *on page 663*

Fludrocortisone *(floo droe KOR ti sone)*

U.S. Brand Names Florinef®

Canadian Brand Names Florinef®

Generic Available Yes

Synonyms 9α-Fluorohydrocortisone Acetate; Fludrocortisone Acetate; Fluohydrisone Acetate; Fluohydrocortisone Acetate

Pharmacologic Category Corticosteroid, Systemic

Use Partial replacement therapy for primary and secondary adrenocortical insufficiency in Addison's disease; treatment of salt-losing adrenogenital syndrome

Local Anesthetic/Vasoconstrictor Precautions No information available to require special precautions

Effects on Dental Treatment No significant effects or complications reported

Significant Adverse Effects Frequency not defined.

Cardiovascular: Hypertension, edema, CHF

Central nervous system: Convulsions, headache, dizziness

Dermatologic: Acne, rash, bruising

Endocrine & metabolic: Hypokalemic alkalosis, suppression of growth, hyperglycemia, HPA suppression

Gastrointestinal: Peptic ulcer

Neuromuscular & skeletal: Muscle weakness

Ocular: Cataracts

Miscellaneous: Diaphoresis, anaphylaxis (generalized)

Dosage Oral:

Infants and Children: 0.05-0.1 mg/day

Adults: 0.1-0.2 mg/day with ranges of 0.1 mg 3 times/week to 0.2 mg/day

Addison's disease: Initial: 0.1 mg/day; if transient hypertension develops, reduce the dose to 0.05 mg/day. Preferred administration with cortisone (10-37.5 mg/day) or hydrocortisone (10-30 mg/day).

Salt-losing adrenogenital syndrome: 0.1-0.2 mg/day

Mechanism of Action Promotes increased reabsorption of sodium and loss of potassium from renal distal tubules

Contraindications Hypersensitivity to fludrocortisone or any component of the formulation; systemic fungal infections

Warnings/Precautions Taper dose gradually when therapy is discontinued; use with caution with Addison's disease, sodium retention and potassium loss

Drug Interactions Decreased effect:

Anticholinesterases effects are antagonized

Decreased corticosteroid effects by rifampin, barbiturates, and hydantoins

Decreased salicylate levels

Dietary Considerations Systemic use of mineralocorticoids/corticosteroids may require a diet with increased potassium, vitamins A, B$_6$, C, D, folate, calcium, zinc, and phosphorus, and decreased sodium. With fludrocortisone, a decrease in dietary sodium is often not required as the increased retention of sodium is usually the desired therapeutic effect.

Pharmacodynamics/Kinetics

Absorption: Rapid and complete

Protein binding: 42%

Metabolism: Hepatic

Half-life elimination, plasma: 30-35 minutes; Biological: 18-36 hours

Time to peak, serum: ~1.7 hours

Pregnancy Risk Factor C

Lactation Excretion in breast milk unknown

Dosage Forms Tablet, as acetate: 0.1 mg

Fludrocortisone Acetate *see* Fludrocortisone *on page 664*
Flumadine® *see* Rimantadine *on page 1351*

Flumazenil (FLOO may ze nil)

U.S. Brand Names Romazicon®
Canadian Brand Names Anexate®; Romazicon®
Mexican Brand Names Anexate®; Lanexat®
Generic Available Yes
Pharmacologic Category Antidote
Use Benzodiazepine antagonist; reverses sedative effects of benzodiazepines used in conscious sedation and general anesthesia; treatment of benzodiazepine overdose
Local Anesthetic/Vasoconstrictor Precautions No information available to require special precautions
Effects on Dental Treatment Key adverse event(s) related to dental treatment: Xerostomia (normal salivary flow resumes upon discontinuation).
Common Adverse Effects
>10%: Gastrointestinal: Vomiting, nausea
1% to 10%:
Cardiovascular: Palpitations
Central nervous system: Headache, anxiety, nervousness, insomnia, abnormal crying, euphoria, depression, agitation, dizziness, emotional lability, ataxia, depersonalization, increased tears, dysphoria, paranoia, fatigue, vertigo
Endocrine & metabolic: Hot flashes
Gastrointestinal: Xerostomia
Local: Pain at injection site
Neuromuscular & skeletal: Tremor, weakness, paresthesia
Ocular: Abnormal vision, blurred vision
Respiratory: Dyspnea, hyperventilation
Miscellaneous: Diaphoresis
Dosage
Children and Adults: I.V.: See table.

Flumazenil

Pediatric Dosage (further studies needed)	
Pediatric dosage for **reversal of conscious sedation and general anesthesia:**	
Initial dose	0.01 mg/kg over 15 seconds (maximum: 0.2 mg)
Repeat doses (maximum: 4 doses)	0.005-0.01 mg/kg (maximum: 0.2 mg) repeated at 1-minute intervals
Maximum total cumulative dose	1 mg or 0.05 mg/kg (whichever is lower)
Adult Dosage	
Adult dosage for **reversal of conscious sedation and general anesthesia:**	
Initial dose	0.2 mg intravenously over 15 seconds
Repeat doses	If desired level of consciousness is not obtained, 0.2 mg may be repeated at 1-minute intervals.
Maximum total cumulative dose	1 mg (usual dose: 0.6-1 mg) **In the event of resedation:** Repeat doses may be given at 20-minute intervals with maximum of 1 mg/dose and 3 mg/hour.
Adult dosage for **suspected benzodiazepine overdose:**	
Initial dose	0.2 mg intravenously over 30 seconds; if the desired level of consciousness is not obtained, 0.3 mg can be given over 30 seconds
Repeat doses	0.5 mg over 30 seconds repeated at 1-minute intervals
Maximum total cumulative dose	3 mg (usual dose 1-3 mg) Patients with a partial response at 3 mg may require additional titration up to a total dose of 5 mg. If a patient has not responded 5 minutes after cumulative dose of 5 mg, the major cause of sedation is not likely due to benzodiazepines. **In the event of resedation:** May repeat doses at 20-minute intervals with maximum of 1 mg/dose and 3 mg/hour.

Resedation: Repeated doses may be given at 20-minute intervals as needed; repeat treatment doses of 1 mg (at a rate of 0.5 mg/minute) should be given at any time and no more than 3 mg should be given in any hour. After intoxication with high doses of benzodiazepines, the duration of a single dose of flumazenil is not expected to exceed 1 hour; if desired, the period of wakefulness may be prolonged with repeated low intravenous doses of flumazenil, or
(Continued)

Flumazenil *(Continued)*

by an infusion of 0.1-0.4 mg/hour. Most patients with benzodiazepine overdose will respond to a cumulative dose of 1-3 mg and doses >3 mg do not reliably produce additional effects. Rarely, patients with a partial response at 3 mg may require additional titration up to a total dose of 5 mg. **If a patient has not responded 5 minutes after receiving a cumulative dose of 5 mg, the major cause of sedation is not likely to be due to benzodiazepines.**

Elderly: No differences in safety or efficacy have been reported. However, increased sensitivity may occur in some elderly patients.

Dosing in renal impairment: Not significantly affected by renal failure (Cl_{cr} <10 mL/minute) or hemodialysis beginning 1 hour after drug administration

Dosing in hepatic impairment: Initial dose of flumazenil used for initial reversal of benzodiazepine effects is not changed; however, subsequent doses in liver disease patients should be reduced in size or frequency

Mechanism of Action Competitively inhibits the activity at the benzodiazepine recognition site on the GABA/benzodiazepine receptor complex. Flumazenil does not antagonize the CNS effect of drugs affecting GABA-ergic neurons by means other than the benzodiazepine receptor (ethanol, barbiturates, general anesthetics) and does not reverse the effects of opioids

Contraindications Hypersensitivity to flumazenil, benzodiazepines, or any component of the formulation; patients given benzodiazepines for control of potentially life-threatening conditions (eg, control of intracranial pressure or status epilepticus); patients who are showing signs of serious cyclic-antidepressant overdosage

Warnings/Precautions Benzodiazepine reversal may result in seizures in some patients. Patients who may develop seizures include patients on benzodiazepines for long-term sedation, tricyclic antidepressant overdose patients, concurrent major sedative-hypnotic drug withdrawal, recent therapy with repeated doses of parenteral benzodiazepines, myoclonic jerking or seizure activity prior to flumazenil administration. Flumazenil does not reverse respiratory depression/hypoventilation or cardiac depression. Resedation occurs more frequently in patients where a large single dose or cumulative dose of a benzodiazepine is administered along with a neuromuscular blocking agent and multiple anesthetic agents. Flumazenil should be used with caution in the intensive care unit because of increased risk of unrecognized benzodiazepine dependence in such settings. Should not be used to diagnose benzodiazepine-induced sedation. Reverse neuromuscular blockade before considering use. Flumazenil does not antagonize the CNS effects of other GABA agonists (such as ethanol, barbiturates, or general anesthetics); nor does it reverse narcotics. Use with caution in patients with a history of panic disorder; may provoke panic attacks. Use caution in drug and ethanol-dependent patients; these patients may also be dependent on benzodiazepines. Not recommended for treatment of benzodiazepine dependence. Use with caution in head injury patients. Use caution in patients with mixed drug overdoses; toxic effects of other drugs taken may emerge once benzodiazepine effects are reversed. Flumazenil does not consistently reverse amnesia; patient may not recall verbal instructions after procedure. Use caution in severe hepatic dysfunction and in patients relying on a benzodiazepine for seizure control. Safety and efficacy have not been established in children >1 year of age.

Drug Interactions

Increased Effect/Toxicity: Flumazenil reverses the effects of these nonbenzodiazepine hypnotics (zaleplon, zolpidem, zopiclone).

Pharmacodynamics/Kinetics

Onset of action: 1-3 minutes; 80% response within 3 minutes

Peak effect: 6-10 minutes

Duration: Resedation: ~1 hour; duration related to dose given and benzodiazepine plasma concentrations; reversal effects of flumazenil may wear off before effects of benzodiazepine

Distribution: Initial V_d: 0.5 L/kg; V_{dss} 0.77-1.6 L/kg

Protein binding: 40% to 50%

Metabolism: Hepatic; dependent upon hepatic blood flow

Half-life elimination: Adults: Alpha: 7-15 minutes; Terminal: 41-79 minutes

Excretion: Feces; urine (0.2% as unchanged drug)

Pregnancy Risk Factor C

Dosage Forms INJ, solution: 0.1 mg/mL (5 mL, 10 mL)

fluMist® *see* Influenza Virus Vaccine *on page 833*

Flunisolide (floo NISS oh lide)

Related Information
Respiratory Diseases *on page 1656*

U.S. Brand Names AeroBid®; AeroBid®-M; Nasarel®

Canadian Brand Names Alti-Flunisolide; Apo-Flunisolide®; Nasalide®; Rhinalar®

Generic Available Yes: Nasal spray

Pharmacologic Category Corticosteroid, Inhalant (Oral); Corticosteroid, Nasal

Use Steroid-dependent asthma; nasal solution is used for seasonal or perennial rhinitis

Local Anesthetic/Vasoconstrictor Precautions No information available to require special precautions

Effects on Dental Treatment Key adverse event(s) related to dental treatment: *Candida* infections of the nose or pharynx, atrophic rhinitis, sore throat, bitter taste, palpitations, dizziness, headache, nervousness, GI irritation, sneezing, coughing, upper respiratory tract infection, bronchitis, nasal congestion, nasal dryness and burning, increased susceptibility to infections, xerostomia (normal salivary flow resumes upon discontinuation), dry throat, loss of taste, epistaxis, and diaphoresis.

Common Adverse Effects
>10%:
- Cardiovascular: Pounding heartbeat
- Central nervous system: Dizziness, headache, nervousness
- Dermatologic: Itching, rash
- Endocrine & metabolic: Adrenal suppression, menstrual problems
- Gastrointestinal: GI irritation, anorexia, sore throat, bitter taste
- Local: Nasal burning, *Candida* infection of the nose or pharynx, atrophic rhinitis
- Respiratory: Sneezing, cough, upper respiratory tract infection, bronchitis, nasal congestion, nasal dryness
- Miscellaneous: Increased susceptibility to infection

1% to 10%:
- Central nervous system: Insomnia, psychic changes
- Dermatologic: Acne, urticaria
- Gastrointestinal: Increase in appetite, xerostomia, dry throat, loss of taste perception
- Ocular: Cataracts
- Respiratory: Epistaxis
- Miscellaneous: Diaphoresis, loss of smell

Mechanism of Action Decreases inflammation by suppression of migration of polymorphonuclear leukocytes and reversal of increased capillary permeability; does not depress hypothalamus

Drug Interactions
Increased Effect/Toxicity: Expected interactions similar to other corticosteroids
Salmeterol: The addition of salmeterol has been demonstrated to improve response to inhaled corticosteroids (as compared to increasing steroid dosage).

Pharmacodynamics/Kinetics
Absorption: Nasal inhalation: ~50%
Metabolism: Rapidly hepatic to active metabolites
Bioavailability: 40% to 50%
Half-life elimination: 1.8 hours
Excretion: Urine and feces (equal amounts)

Pregnancy Risk Factor C

Fluocinolone (floo oh SIN oh lone)

U.S. Brand Names Capex™; Derma-Smoothe/FS®; Retisert™; Synalar®

Canadian Brand Names Capex™; Derma-Smoothe/FS®; Synalar®

Mexican Brand Names Synalar®

Generic Available Yes: Excludes ocular implant, oil, shampoo

Synonyms Fluocinolone Acetonide

Pharmacologic Category Corticosteroid, Ophthalmic; Corticosteroid, Topical

Dental Use Relief of inflammatory and pruritic manifestations (low, medium, high potency topical corticosteroid)
(Continued)

Fluocinolone *(Continued)*

Use Relief of susceptible inflammatory dermatosis [low, medium, high potency topical corticosteroid]; psoriasis of the scalp; atopic dermatitis in children ≥2 years of age

Ocular implant (Retisert™): Treatment of chronic, noninfectious uveitis affecting the posterior segment of the eye.

Local Anesthetic/Vasoconstrictor Precautions No information available to require special precautions

Effects on Dental Treatment No significant effects or complications reported

Significant Adverse Effects Topical: Frequency not defined.

Dermatologic: Acneiform eruptions, allergic contact dermatitis, burning, dryness, folliculitis, irritation, itching, hypertrichosis, hypopigmentation, miliaria, perioral dermatitis, skin atrophy, striae

Endocrine & metabolic: Cushing's syndrome, HPA axis suppression

Miscellaneous: Secondary infection

Ocular implant:

>50%: Ocular: Cataract, intraocular pressure increased, eye pain; procedural complications (eg, cataract fragments, implant migration, wound complications)

10% to 35%:

Central nervous system: Dizziness (5% to 15%), headache (31%), pain (5% to 15%), pyrexia (5% to 15%)

Dermatologic: Rash (5% to 15%)

Gastrointestinal (5% to 15%): Nausea, vomiting

Neuromuscular & skeletal (5% to 15%): Arthralgia, back pain, limb pain

Ocular: Blurred vision, conjunctival hemorrhage, conjunctival hyperemia, dry eye, eye irritation/inflammation, eyelid edema, glaucoma, hypotony, maculopathy, pruritus, ptosis, tearing, visual acuity decrease, vitreous floaters, vitreous hemorrhage

Respiratory (5% to 15%): Cough, influenza, nasopharyngitis, sinusitis, upper respiratory infection

5% to 9%: Ocular: Blepharitis, choroidal detachment, conjunctival edema/chemosis, corneal edema, eye discharge, eye swelling, macular edema, photophobia, photopsia, retinal hemorrhage, visual disturbance, vitreous opacitites

Frequency not specified: Miscellaneous: Secondary infection (bacterial, viral, or fungal)

Dental Usual Dosing Inflammatory and pruritic manifestations: Adults: Topical: Apply to oral lesion 4 times/day, after meals and at bedtime

Dosage

Children ≥2 years: Topical: Atopic dermatitis (Derma-Smoothe/FS®): Moisten skin; apply to affected area twice daily; do not use for longer than 4 weeks

Children and Adults: Topical: Corticosteroid-responsive dermatoses: Cream, ointment, solution: Apply a thin layer to affected area 2-4 times/day; may use occlusive dressings to manage psoriasis or recalcitrant conditions

Adults:

Topical:

Atopic dermatitis (Derma-Smoothe/FS®): Apply thin film to affected area 3 times/day

Inflammatory and pruritic manifestations (dental use): Apply to oral lesion 4 times/day, after meals and at bedtime

Scalp psoriasis (Derma-Smoothe/FS®): Massage thoroughly into wet or dampened hair/scalp; cover with shower cap. Leave on overnight (or for at least 4 hours). Remove by washing hair with shampoo and rinsing thoroughly.

Seborrheic dermatitis of the scalp (Capex™): Apply no more than 1 ounce to scalp once daily; work into lather and allow to remain on scalp for ~5 minutes. Remove from hair and scalp by rinsing thoroughly with water.

Ocular implant: Chronic uveitis: One silicone-encased tablet (0.59 mg) surgically implanted into the posterior segment of the eye is designed to release 0.6 mcg/day, decreasing over 30 days to a steady-state release rate of 0.3-0.4 mcg/day for 30 months. Recurrence of uveitis denotes depletion of tablet, requiring reimplantation.

Mechanism of Action A synthetic corticosteroid which differs structurally from triamcinolone acetonide in the presence of an additional fluorine atom in the 6-alpha position on the steroid nucleus. The mechanism of action for all topical corticosteroids is not well defined, however, is believed to be a combination of anti-inflammatory, antipruritic, and vasoconstrictive properties.

Contraindications Hypersensitivity to fluocinolone or any component of the formulation; TB of skin, herpes (including varicella)

Ocular implant: Additional contraindications include ocular infections of viral or fungal origin

Warnings/Precautions Adverse systemic effects may occur when used on large areas of the body, denuded areas, for prolonged periods of time, with an occlusive dressing, and/or in infants or small children. Infants and small children may be more susceptible to adrenal axis suppression from topical corticosteroid therapy. Derma-Smoothe/FS® contains peanut oil; use caution in peanut-sensitive children.

Ocular implant: May cause transient decrease in visual acuity of 1-4 weeks duration; caution with use in glaucoma patients; routine monitoring of IOP recommended. May require IOP-lowering treatments within 2 years postimplantation. Prolonged use of ocular corticosteroids may increase risk of secondary infection, cataract formation, optic nerve damage, and/or glaucoma. Recommend unilateral implantation only to minimize risk of postoperative infections developing in both eyes. Safety and efficacy have not been established in children <12 years of age.

Drug Interactions No data reported

Pharmacodynamics/Kinetics

Absorption:

Topical: Dependent on strength of preparation, amount applied, nature of skin at application site, vehicle, and use of occlusive dressing; increased in areas of skin damage, inflammation, or occlusion

Ocular implant: Systemic absorption is negligible

Duration: Ocular implant: Releases fluocinolone acetonide at a rate of 0.6 mcg/day, decreasing over 30 days to a steady-state release rate of 0.3-0.4 mcg/day for 30 months

Distribution:

Topical: Throughout local skin; absorbed drug is distributed rapidly into muscle, liver, skin, intestines, and kidneys

Ocular implant: Aqueous and vitreous humor

Metabolism: Primarily in skin; small amount absorbed into systemic circulation is primarily hepatic to inactive compounds

Excretion: Urine (primarily as glucuronide and sulfate, also as unconjugated products); feces (small amounts)

Pregnancy Risk Factor C

Lactation Excretion in breast milk unknown/use caution

Breast-Feeding Considerations Systemic corticosteroids are excreted in human milk. It is not known if sufficient quantities of fluocinolone are absorbed following topical or ocular administration to produce detectable amounts in breast milk. Hypertension in the nursing infant has been reported following corticosteroid ointment applied to the nipples. Use with caution.

Dosage Forms

Cream, as acetonide: 0.01% (15 g, 60 g); 0.025% (15 g, 60 g)

Synalar®: 0.025% (15 g, 60 g)

Oil, as acetonide:

Derma-Smoothe/FS® [eczema oil]: 0.01% (120 mL) [contains peanut oil]

Derma-Smoothe/FS® [scalp oil]: 0.01% (120 mL) [contains peanut oil; packaged with shower caps]

Ointment, as acetonide (Synalar®): 0.025% (15 g, 60 g)

Shampoo, as acetonide (Capex™): 0.01% (120 mL)

Solution, as acetonide: 0.01% (60 mL)

Synalar®: 0.01% (20 mL, 60 mL)

Tablet, ocular implant, as acetonide (Retisert™): 0.59 mg [enclosed in silicone elastomer]

Fluocinolone Acetonide *see Fluocinolone on page 667*

Fluocinolone, Hydroquinone, and Tretinoin
(floo oh SIN oh lone, HYE droe kwin one, & TRET i noyn)

Related Information

Fluocinolone *on page 667*

Hydroquinone *on page 798*

U.S. Brand Names Tri-Luma™

Generic Available No

Synonyms Hydroquinone, Fluocinolone Acetonide, and Tretinoin; Tretinoin, Fluocinolone Acetonide, and Hydroquinone

Pharmacologic Category Corticosteroid, Topical; Depigmenting Agent; Retinoic Acid Derivative

Use Short-term treatment of moderate to severe melasma of the face

Local Anesthetic/Vasoconstrictor Precautions No information available to require special precautions

(Continued)

Fluocinolone, Hydroquinone, and Tretinoin *(Continued)*

Effects on Dental Treatment Key adverse event(s) related to dental treatment: Xerostomia (normal salivary flow resumes upon discontinuation).

Common Adverse Effects
>10%:
  Dermatologic: Erythema (41%), desquamation (38%), burning (18%), dry skin (14%), pruritus (11%)
1% to 10%:
  Cardiovascular: Telangiectasia (3%)
  Central nervous system: Paresthesia (3%), hyperesthesia (2%)
  Dermatologic: Acne (5%), pigmentation change (2%), irritation (2%), papules (1%), rash (1%), rosacea (1%), vesicles (1%)
  Gastrointestinal: Xerostomia (1%)

Mechanism of Action Not clearly defined. Hydroquinone may interrupt melanin synthesis (tyrosine-tyrosinase pathway); reduces hyperpigmentation.

Drug Interactions
  Cytochrome P450 Effect: Tretinoin: **Substrate** (minor) of CYP2A6, 2B6, 2C8/9; **Inhibits** CYP2C8/9 (weak); **Induces** CYP2E1 (weak)
  Increased Effect/Toxicity: Avoid soaps/cosmetic preparations which are medicated, abrasive, irritating, or any product with strong drying effects (including alcohol, astringent, benzoyl peroxide, resorcinol, salicylic acid, sulfur). Drugs with photosensitizing effects should also be avoided (includes tetracyclines, thiazides, fluoroquinolones, phenothiazines, sulfonamides).

Pharmacodynamics/Kinetics
  Absorption: Minimal
  Metabolism: Hepatic for the small amount absorbed
  Excretion: Urine and feces
Pregnancy Risk Factor C

Fluocinonide *(floo oh SIN oh nide)*

Related Information
  Ulcerative and Erosive Disorders *on page 1712*
Related Sample Prescriptions
  Mild Lichen Planus *on page 1745*
  Recurrent Aphthous Stomatitis *on page 1744*
U.S. Brand Names Lidex®; Lidex-E®; Vanos™
Canadian Brand Names Lidemol®; Lidex®; Lyderm®; Tiamol®; Topsyn®
Mexican Brand Names Topsyn®
Generic Available Yes
Pharmacologic Category Corticosteroid, Topical
Dental Use Relief of inflammatory and pruritic manifestations (high potency topical corticosteroid)
Use Anti-inflammatory, antipruritic; treatment of plaque-type psoriasis (up to 10% of body surface area) [high-potency topical corticosteroid]
Local Anesthetic/Vasoconstrictor Precautions No information available to require special precautions
Effects on Dental Treatment No significant effects or complications reported
Significant Adverse Effects Frequency not defined.
  Cardiovascular: Intracranial hypertension
  Dermatologic: Acne, allergic dermatitis, contact dermatitis, dry skin, folliculitis, hypertrichosis, hypopigmentation, maceration of the skin, miliaria, perioral dermatitis, pruritus, skin atrophy, striae, telangiectasia
  Endocrine & metabolic: Cushing's syndrome, growth retardation, HPA suppression, hyperglycemia
  Local: Burning, irritation
  Renal: Glycosuria
  Miscellaneous: Secondary infection
Dental Usual Dosing Pruritus and inflammation: Children and Adults: Topical (0.5% cream): Apply thin layer to affected area 2-4 times/day depending on the severity of the condition. Therapy should be discontinued when control is achieved; if no improvement is seen, reassessment of diagnosis may be necessary.
Dosage
  Children and Adults: Pruritus and inflammation: Topical (0.5% cream): Apply thin layer to affected area 2-4 times/day depending on the severity of the condition. Therapy should be discontinued when control is achieved; if no improvement is seen, reassessment of diagnosis may be necessary.
  Children ≥12 years and Adults: Plaque-type psoriasis (Vanos™): Topical (0.1% cream): Apply a thin layer once or twice daily to affected areas (limited to

<10% of body surface area). **Note:** Not recommended for use >2 consecutive weeks or >60 g/week total exposure. Discontinue when control is achieved.

Mechanism of Action Fluorinated topical corticosteroid considered to be of high potency. The mechanism of action for all topical corticosteroids is not well defined, however, is felt to be a combination of three important properties: anti-inflammatory activity, immunosuppressive properties, and antiproliferative actions.

Contraindications Hypersensitivity to fluocinonide or any component of the formulation; viral, fungal, or tubercular skin lesions; herpes simplex

Warnings/Precautions Adverse systemic effects may occur when used on large areas of the body, denuded areas, for prolonged periods of time, with an occlusive dressing, and/or in infants or small children. Pediatric patients may be more susceptible to HPA axis suppression. Lower-strength cream (0.05%) may be used cautiously on face or opposing skin surfaces that may rub or touch (eg, skin folds of the groin, axilla, and breasts); higher-strength (0.1%) should not be used on the face, groin, or axillae. Use of the 0.1% cream for >2 weeks or in patients <12 years of age is not recommended.

Drug Interactions No data reported. Concomitant use with other corticosteroids (by any route) may increase the risk of HPA axis suppression.

Pharmacodynamics/Kinetics

Absorption: Dependent on strength of product, amount applied, and nature of skin at application site; ranges from ~1% in areas of thick stratum corneum (palms, soles, elbows, etc) to 36% in areas of thin stratum corneum (face, eyelids, etc); increased in areas of skin damage, inflammation, or occlusion

Distribution: Throughout local skin; absorbed drug into muscle, liver, skin, intestines, and kidneys

Metabolism: Primarily in skin; small amount absorbed into systemic circulation is primarily hepatic to inactive compounds

Excretion: Urine (primarily as glucuronide and sulfate, also as unconjugated products); feces (small amounts as metabolites)

Pregnancy Risk Factor C

Dosage Forms

Cream, anhydrous, emollient (Lidex®): 0.05% (15 g, 30 g, 60 g)
Cream, aqueous, emollient (Lidex-E®): 0.05% (15 g, 30 g, 60 g)
Cream (Vanos™): 0.1% (30 g, 60 g)
Gel (Lidex®): 0.05% (15 g, 30 g, 60 g)
Ointment (Lidex®): 0.05% (15 g, 30 g, 60 g)
Solution (Lidex®): 0.05% (60 mL) [contains alcohol 35%]

Fluohydrisone Acetate see Fludrocortisone on page 664

Fluohydrocortisone Acetate see Fludrocortisone on page 664

Fluoracaine® see Proparacaine and Fluorescein on page 1296

Fluor-A-Day see Fluoride on page 671

Fluorescein and Proparacaine see Proparacaine and Fluorescein on page 1296

Fluoride (FLOR ide)

Related Information

Dentin Hypersensitivity, High Caries Index, and Xerostomia on page 1714
Management of Patients Undergoing Cancer Therapy on page 1728

U.S. Brand Names ACT® [OTC]; ACT® Plus [OTC]; ACT® x2™ [OTC]; CaviRinse™; ControlRx®; Denta 5000 Plus; DentaGel; EtheDent™; Fluor-A-Day; Fluorigard® [OTC]; Fluorinse®; Flura-Drops®; Gel-Kam® [OTC]; Gel-Kam® Rinse; Just for Kids™ [OTC]; Lozi-Flur™; Luride®; Luride® Lozi-Tab®; Neutra-Care®; NeutraGard® [OTC]; NeutraGard® Advanced; NeutraGard® Plus; Omnii Gel™ [OTC]; Pediaflor® [DSC]; PerioMed™; Pharmaflur®; Pharmaflur® 1.1; Phos-Flur®; Phos-Flur® Rinse [OTC]; PreviDent®; PreviDent® 5000 Plus™; StanGard®; StanGard® Perio; Stop®; Thera-Flur-N®

Canadian Brand Names Fluor-A-Day; Fluotic®

Mexican Brand Names Audifluor®

Generic Available Yes: Excludes lozenge, gel drops

Synonyms Acidulated Phosphate Fluoride; Sodium Fluoride; Stannous Fluoride

Pharmacologic Category Nutritional Supplement

Dental Use Prevention of dental caries

Use Prevention of dental caries

Local Anesthetic/Vasoconstrictor Precautions No information available to require special precautions

Effects on Dental Treatment Key adverse event(s) related to dental treatment: Products containing stannous fluoride may stain teeth. See Dental Comment.

(Continued)

Fluoride *(Continued)*

Significant Adverse Effects <1% (Limited to important or life-threatening): Discoloration of teeth, rash, nausea, vomiting

Dosage Oral:

The recommended daily dose of oral fluoride supplement (mg), based on fluoride ion content (ppm) in drinking water (2.2 mg of sodium fluoride is equivalent to 1 mg of fluoride ion): See table.

Fluoride Ion

Fluoride Content of Drinking Water	Daily Dose, Oral (mg)
<0.3 ppm	
Birth - 6 mo	None
6 mo - 3 y	0.25
3-6 y	0.5
6-16 y	1
0.3-0.6 ppm	
Birth - 6 mo	None
6 mo - 3 y	None
3-6 y	0.25
6-16 y	0.5

Adapted from Recommended Dosage Schedule of The American Dental Association, The American Academy of Pediatric Dentistry, and The American Academy of Pediatrics.

Cream: Children ≥6 years and Adults: Brush teeth with cream once daily regardless of fluoride content of drinking water

Dental rinse or gel:

Children 6-12 years: 5-10 mL rinse or apply to teeth and spit daily after brushing

Adults: 10 mL rinse or apply to teeth and spit daily after brushing

PreviDent® rinse: Children >6 years and Adults: Once weekly, rinse 10 mL vigorously around and between teeth for 1 minute, then spit; this should be done preferably at bedtime, after thoroughly brushing teeth; for maximum benefit, do not eat, drink, or rinse mouth for at least 30 minutes after treatment; do not swallow

Fluorinse®: Children >6 years and Adults: Once weekly, vigorously swish 5-10 mL in mouth for 1 minute, then spit

Lozenge (Lozi-Flur™): Adults: One lozenge daily regardless of fluoride content of drinking water

Mechanism of Action Promotes remineralization of decalcified enamel; inhibits the cariogenic microbial process in dental plaque; increases tooth resistance to acid dissolution

Contraindications Hypersensitivity to fluoride, tartrazine, or any component of the formulation; when fluoride content of drinking water exceeds 0.7 ppm; low sodium or sodium-free diets; do not use 1 mg tablets in children <3 years of age or when drinking water fluoride content is ≥0.3 ppm; do not use 1 mg/5 mL rinse (as supplement) in children <6 years of age

Warnings/Precautions Prolonged ingestion with excessive doses may result in dental fluorosis and osseous changes; do **not** exceed recommended dosage; some products contain tartrazine

Drug Interactions Decreased effect/absorption with magnesium-, aluminum-, and calcium-containing products

Dietary Considerations Do not administer with milk; do **not** allow eating or drinking for 30 minutes after use.

Pharmacodynamics/Kinetics

Absorption: Oral: Rapid and complete; sodium fluoride; other soluble fluoride salts; calcium, iron, or magnesium may delay absorption

Distribution: 50% of fluoride is deposited in teeth and bone after ingestion; topical application works superficially on enamel and plaque; crosses placenta; enters breast milk

Excretion: Urine and feces

Pregnancy Risk Factor C

Dosage Forms [DSC] = Discontinued product

Cream, oral, as sodium [toothpaste]: 1.1% (51 g) [fluoride 2.5 mg/dose]

Denta 5000 Plus: 1.1% (51g) [fluoride 2.5 mg/dose; spearmint flavor]

EtheDent™: 1.1% (51g) [fluoride 2.5 mg/dose]

Gel-drops, as sodium fluoride (Thera-Flur-N®): 1.1% (24 mL) [fluoride 0.5%; neutral pH; no artificial color or flavor]

Gel, topical, as acidulated phosphate fluoride (Phos-Flur®): 1.1% (60 g) [fluoride 0.5%; cherry and mint flavors]

Gel, topical, as sodium fluoride: 1.1% (56 g) [fluoride 2 mg/dose]

DentaGel, EtheDent™: 1.1% (56 g) [fluoride 2 mg/dose; fresh mint flavor]

NeutraCare®: 1.1% (60 g) [neutral pH; grape and mint flavors]

NeutraGard® Advanced: 1.1% (60 g) [cinnamon and mint flavors]

PreviDent®: 1.1% (60 g) [fluoride 2 mg/dose; berry, cherry, and mint flavors]

Gel, topical, as stannous fluoride:

Gel-Kam®: 0.4% (129 g) [bubble gum, cinnamon, fruit/berry, and mint flavors]

Just for Kids™: 0.4% (122 g) [bubble gum, fruit punch, and grapey grape flavors]

Omnii Gel™: 0.4% (122 g) [cinnamon, grape, natural, mint, and raspberry flavors]

StanGard®: 0.4% (122 g) [bubble gum, cherry, mint, and raspberry flavors]

Stop®: 0.4% (120 g) [bubble gum, cinnamon, grape, and mint flavors]

Lozenge, as sodium (Lozi-Flur™): 2.21 mg [fluoride 1 mg; cherry flavor]

Paste, oral, as sodium [toothpaste] (ControlRx®): 1.1% (56 g) [vanilla mint flavor]

Solution, oral drops, as sodium: 1.1 mg/mL (50 mL) [fluoride 0.5 mg/mL]

Flura-Drops®: 0.55 mg/drop (24 mL) [fluoride 0.25 mg/drop; dye free, sugar free]

Luride®: 1.1 mg/mL (50 mL) [fluoride 0.5 mg/mL; sugar free]

Pediaflor®: 1.1 mg/mL (50 mL) [fluoride 0.5 mg/mL; contains alcohol <0.5%; sugar free; cherry flavor] [DSC]

Solution, oral rinse, as sodium:

ACT®: 0.05% (530 mL) [fluoride 0.02%; bubble gum, cinnamon (contains tartrazine), and mint flavors]

ACT® Plus: 0.05% (530 mL) [fluoride 0.02%; alcohol free; icy cool mint flavor]

ACT® x2™: 0.5% (530 mL) [fluoride 0.02%; contains alcohol 11%; icy cool mint and spearmint flavors]

CaviRinse™: 0.2% (240 mL) [mint flavor]

Fluorigard®: 0.05% (480 mL) [alcohol free, sugar free; contains sodium benzoate and tartrazine; mint flavor]

Fluorinse®: 0.2% (480 mL) [alcohol free; cinnamon and mint flavors]

NeutraGard®: 0.05% (480 mL) [neutral pH; mint and tropical blast flavors]

NeutraGard® Plus: 0.2% (480 mL) [neutral pH; mint and tropical blast flavors]

Phos-Flur®: 0.44% (500 mL) [bubble gum, cherry, grape, and mint flavors]

PreviDent®: 0.2% (250 mL) [contains alcohol; mint flavor]

Solution, oral rinse concentrate, as stannous fluoride:

Gel-Kam®: 0.63% (300 mL) [fluoride 0.1%/dose; cinnamon and mint flavors]

PerioMed™: 0.63% (284 mL) [fluoride 7 mg/30 mL; alcohol free; cinnamon, mint and tropical fruit flavors]

StanGard® Perio: 0.63% (284 mL) [mint flavor]

Tablet, chewable, as sodium: 0.5 mg [fluoride 0.25 mg]; 1.1 mg [fluoride 0.5 mg]; 2.2 mg [fluoride 1 mg]

EtheDent™:

0.55 mg [fluoride 0.25 mg; sugar free; contains aspartame; vanilla flavor]

1.1 mg [fluoride 0.5 mg; sugar free; contains aspartame; grape flavor]

2.2 mg [fluoride 1 mg; sugar free; contains aspartame; cherry flavor]

Fluor-A-Day:

0.56 mg [fluoride 0.25 mg; raspberry flavor]

1.1 mg [fluoride 0.5 mg; raspberry flavor]

2.21 mg [fluoride 1 mg; raspberry flavor]

Luride® Lozi-Tab®:

0.55 mg [fluoride 0.25 mg; sugar free; vanilla flavor]

1.1 mg [fluoride 0.5 mg; sugar free; grape flavor]

2.2 mg [fluoride 1 mg; sugar free; cherry flavor]

Pharmaflur®: 2.2 mg [fluoride 1 mg; dye free, sugar free; cherry flavor]

Pharmaflur® 1.1: 1.1 mg [fluoride 0.5 mg; dye free, sugar free; grape flavor]

Dental Comment Neutral pH fluoride preparations are preferred in patients with oral mucositis to reduce tissue irritation; long-term use of acidulated fluorides has been associated with enamel demineralization and damage to porcelain crowns

Selected Readings

Wynn RC, "Fluoride: After 50 Years, a Clearer Picture of Its Mechanism," *Gen Dent*, 2002, 50(2):118-22, 124, 126.

Fluoride and Triclosan (Dental) *see* Triclosan and Fluoride *on page* 1534

Fluorigard® [OTC] *see* Fluoride *on page* 671

Fluori-Methane® *see* Dichlorodifluoromethane and Trichloromonofluoromethane *on page* 458

Fluorinse® *see* Fluoride *on page 671*

5-Fluorocytosine *see* Flucytosine *on page 662*

Fluorodeoxyuridine *see* Floxuridine *on page 659*

9α-Fluorohydrocortisone Acetate *see* Fludrocortisone *on page 664*

Fluorometholone (flure oh METH oh lone)

U.S. Brand Names Eflone® [DSC]; Flarex®; Fluor-Op® [DSC]; FML®; FML® Forte

Canadian Brand Names Flarex®; FML®; FML Forte®; PMS-Fluorometholone

Generic Available Yes: Suspension (as base)

Pharmacologic Category Corticosteroid, Ophthalmic

Use Treatment of steroid-responsive inflammatory conditions of the eye

Local Anesthetic/Vasoconstrictor Precautions No information available to require special precautions

Effects on Dental Treatment No significant effects or complications reported

Mechanism of Action Decreases inflammation by suppression of migration of polymorphonuclear leukocytes and reversal of increased capillary permeability

Pregnancy Risk Factor C

Fluorometholone and Sulfacetamide *see* Sulfacetamide and Fluorometholone *on page 1423*

Fluor-Op® [DSC] *see* Fluorometholone *on page 674*

Fluoroplex® *see* Fluorouracil *on page 674*

Fluorouracil (flure oh YOOR a sil)

Related Information
Capecitabine *on page 255*

U.S. Brand Names Adrucil®; Carac™; Efudex®; Fluoroplex®

Canadian Brand Names Efudex®

Generic Available Yes: Injection, topical solution

Synonyms 5-Fluorouracil; FU; 5-FU

Pharmacologic Category Antineoplastic Agent, Antimetabolite (Pyrimidine Antagonist)

Use Treatment of carcinomas of the breast, colon, head and neck, pancreas, rectum, or stomach; topically for the management of actinic or solar keratoses and superficial basal cell carcinomas

Local Anesthetic/Vasoconstrictor Precautions No information available to require special precautions

Effects on Dental Treatment Key adverse event(s) related to dental treatment: Stomatitis.

Common Adverse Effects Toxicity depends on route and duration of treatment

I.V.:
Cardiovascular: Angina, myocardial ischemia, nail changes

Central nervous system: Acute cerebellar syndrome, confusion, disorientation, euphoria, headache, nystagmus

Dermatologic: Alopecia, dermatitis, dry skin, fissuring, palmar-plantar erythrodysesthesia syndrome, pruritic maculopapular rash, photosensitivity, vein pigmentations

Gastrointestinal: Anorexia, bleeding, diarrhea, esophagopharyngitis, nausea, sloughing, stomatitis, ulceration, vomiting

Hematologic: Agranulocytosis, anemia, leukopenia, pancytopenia, thrombocytopenia

Myelosuppression:
  Onset: 7-10 days
  Nadir: 9-14 days
  Recovery: 21-28 days

Local: Thrombophlebitis

Ocular: Lacrimation, lacrimal duct stenosis, photophobia, visual changes

Respiratory: Epistaxis

Miscellaneous: Anaphylaxis, generalized allergic reactions, loss of nails

Topical: Note: Systemic toxicity normally associated with parenteral administration (including neutropenia, neurotoxicity, and gastrointestinal toxicity) has been associated with topical use particularly in patients with a genetic deficiency of dihydropyrimidine dehydrogenase (DPD).

Central nervous system: Headache, insomnia, irritability

Dermatologic: Alopecia, photosensitivity, pruritus, rash, scarring, telangiectasia

Gastrointestinal: Medicinal taste, stomatitis

Hematologic: Leukocytosis, thrombocytopenia

Local: Application site reactions: Allergic contact dermatitis, burning, crusting, dryness, edema, erosion, erythema, hyperpigmentation, irritation, pain, soreness, ulceration

Ocular: Eye irritation (burning, watering, sensitivity, stinging, itching)

Miscellaneous: Birth defects, herpes simplex, miscarriage

Mechanism of Action A pyrimidine antimetabolite that interferes with DNA synthesis by blocking the methylation of deoxyuridylic acid; fluorouracil inhibits thymidylate synthetase (TS), or is incorporated into RNA. The reduced folate cofactor is required for tight binding to occur between the 5-FdUMP and TS.

Drug Interactions

Increased Effect/Toxicity: Fluorouracil may increase effects of warfarin.

Pharmacodynamics/Kinetics

Duration: ~3 weeks

Distribution: V_d: ~22% of total body water; penetrates extracellular fluid, CSF, and third space fluids (eg, pleural effusions and ascitic fluid)

Metabolism: Hepatic (90%); via a dehydrogenase enzyme; FU must be metabolized to be active

Bioavailability: <75%, erratic and unpredependable

Half-life elimination: Biphasic: Initial: 6-20 minutes; two metabolites, FdUMP and FUTP, have prolonged half-lives depending on the type of tissue

Excretion: Lung (large amounts as CO_2); urine (5% as unchanged drug) in 6 hours

Pregnancy Risk Factor D (injection); X (topical)

5-Fluorouracil *see* Fluorouracil *on page 674*

Fluoxetine (floo OKS e teen)

U.S. Brand Names Prozac®; Prozac® Weekly™; Sarafem®

Canadian Brand Names Alti-Fluoxetine; Apo-Fluoxetine®; CO Fluoxetine; FXT; Gen-Fluoxetine; Novo-Fluoxetine; Nu-Fluoxetine; PMS-Fluoxetine; Prozac®; Rhoxal-fluoxetine; Sandoz-Fluoxetine

Mexican Brand Names Fluoxac®; Prozac®; Siqual®

Generic Available Yes: Excludes delayed release capsule

Synonyms Fluoxetine Hydrochloride

Pharmacologic Category Antidepressant, Selective Serotonin Reuptake Inhibitor

Use Treatment of major depressive disorder (MDD); treatment of binge-eating and vomiting in patients with moderate-to-severe bulimia nervosa; obsessive-compulsive disorder (OCD); premenstrual dysphoric disorder (PMDD); panic disorder with or without agoraphobia

Unlabeled/Investigational Use Selective mutism

Local Anesthetic/Vasoconstrictor Precautions Although caution should be used in patients taking tricyclic antidepressants, no interactions have been reported with vasoconstrictors and fluoxetine, a nontricyclic antidepressant which acts to increase serotonin; no precautions appear to be needed (see Dental Comment)

Effects on Dental Treatment Key adverse event(s) related to dental treatment: Xerostomia (normal salivary flow resumes upon discontinuation) and taste perversion. Problems with SSRI-induced bruxism have been reported and may preclude their use; clinicians attempting to evaluate any patient with bruxism or involuntary muscle movement, who is simultaneously being treated with an SSRI drug, should be aware of this potential association.

Common Adverse Effects Percentages listed for adverse effects as reported in placebo-controlled trials and were generally similar in adults and children; actual frequency may be dependent upon diagnosis and in some cases the range presented may be lower than or equal to placebo for a particular disorder.

>10%:

Central nervous system: Insomnia (10% to 33%), headache (21%), anxiety (6% to 15%), nervousness (8% to 14%), somnolence (5% to 17%)

Endocrine & metabolic: Libido decreased (1% to 11%)

Gastrointestinal: Nausea (12% to 29%), diarrhea (8% to 18%), anorexia (4% to 11%), xerostomia (4% to 12%)

Neuromuscular & skeletal: Weakness (7% to 21%), tremor (3% to 13%)

Respiratory: Pharyngitis (3% to 11%), yawn (<1% to 11%)

1% to 10%:

Cardiovascular: Vasodilation (1% to 5%), fever (2%), chest pain, hemorrhage, hypertension, palpitation

(Continued)

Fluoxetine *(Continued)*

Central nervous system: Dizziness (9%), dream abnormality (1% to 5%), thinking abnormality (2%), agitation, amnesia, chills, confusion, emotional lability, sleep disorder

Dermatologic: Rash (2% to 6%), pruritus (4%)

Endocrine & metabolic: Ejaculation abnormal (<1% to 7%), impotence (<1% to 7%)

Gastrointestinal: Dyspepsia (6% to 10%), constipation (5%), flatulence (3%), vomiting (3%), weight loss (2%), appetite increased, taste perversion, weight gain

Genitourinary: Urinary frequency

Ocular: Vision abnormal (2%)

Otic: Ear pain, tinnitus

Respiratory: Sinusitis (1% to 6%)

Miscellaneous: Flu-like syndrome (3% to 10%), diaphoresis (2% to 8%)

Restrictions A medication guide concerning the use of antidepressants in children and teenagers can be found on the FDA website at http://www.fda.gov/cder/Offices/ODS/labeling.htm. It should be dispensed to parents or guardians of children and teenagers receiving this medication.

Dosage Oral: **Note:** Upon discontinuation of fluoxetine therapy, gradually taper dose. If intolerable symptoms occur following a dose reduction, consider resuming the previously prescribed dose and/or decrease dose at a more gradual rate.

Children:

Depression: 8-18 years: 10-20 mg/day; lower-weight children can be started at 10 mg/day, may increase to 20 mg/day after 1 week if needed

OCD: 7-18 years: Initial: 10 mg/day; in adolescents and higher-weight children, dose may be increased to 20 mg/day after 2 weeks. Range: 10-60 mg/day

Selective mutism (unlabeled use):

<5 years: No dosing information available

5-18 years: Initial: 5-10 mg/day; titrate upwards as needed (usual maximum dose: 60 mg/day)

Adults: 20 mg/day in the morning; may increase after several weeks by 20 mg/day increments; maximum: 80 mg/day; doses >20 mg may be given once daily or divided twice daily. **Note:** Lower doses of 5-10 mg/day have been used for initial treatment.

Usual dosage range:

Bulimia nervosa: 60-80 mg/day

Depression: 20-40 mg/day; patients maintained on Prozac® 20 mg/day may be changed to Prozac® Weekly™ 90 mg/week, starting dose 7 days after the last 20 mg/day dose

OCD: 40-80 mg/day

Panic disorder: Initial: 10 mg/day; after 1 week, increase to 20 mg/day; may increase after several weeks; doses >60 mg/day have not been evaluated

PMDD (Sarafem™): 20 mg/day continuously, **or** 20 mg/day starting 14 days prior to menstruation and through first full day of menses (repeat with each cycle)

Elderly: Depression: Some patients may require an initial dose of 10 mg/day with dosage increases of 10 and 20 mg every several weeks as tolerated; should not be taken at night unless patient experiences sedation

Dosing adjustment in renal impairment:

Single dose studies: Pharmacokinetics of fluoxetine and norfluoxetine were similar among subjects with all levels of impaired renal function, including anephric patients on chronic hemodialysis

Chronic administration: Additional accumulation of fluoxetine or norfluoxetine may occur in patients with severely impaired renal function

Hemodialysis: Not removed by hemodialysis; use of lower dose or less frequent dosing is not usually necessary.

Dosing adjustment in hepatic impairment: Elimination half-life of fluoxetine is prolonged in patients with hepatic impairment; a lower or less frequent dose of fluoxetine should be used in these patients

Cirrhosis patients: Administer a lower dose or less frequent dosing interval

Compensated cirrhosis without ascites: Administer 50% of normal dose

Mechanism of Action Inhibits CNS neuron serotonin reuptake; minimal or no effect on reuptake of norepinephrine or dopamine; does not significantly bind to alpha-adrenergic, histamine, or cholinergic receptors

Contraindications Hypersensitivity to fluoxetine or any component of the formulation; patients currently receiving MAO inhibitors, pimozide, or thioridazine

Note: MAO inhibitor therapy must be stopped for 14 days before fluoxetine is initiated. Treatment with MAO inhibitors, thioridazine, or mesoridazine should not be initiated until 5 weeks after the discontinuation of fluoxetine.

Warnings/Precautions Antidepressants increase the risk of suicidal thinking and behavior in children and adolescents with major depressive disorder (MDD) and other depressive disorders; consider risk prior to prescribing. All patients must be closely monitored for clinical worsening, suicidality, or unusual changes in behavior, especially during the initiation of therapy or following an increase or decrease in dosage. When used in children, the child's family or caregiver should be instructed to closely observe the patient and communicate condition with healthcare provider. A medication guide should be dispensed with each prescription. **Fluoxetine is FDA approved for the treatment of OCD in children ≥7 years of age and MDD in children ≥8 years of age.**

The possibility of a suicide attempt is inherent in major depression and may persist until remission occurs. Use caution in high-risk patients. Worsening depression and severe abrupt suicidality that are not part of the presenting symptoms may require discontinuation or modification of drug therapy. The patient's family or caregiver should be alerted to monitor patients for the emergence of suicidality and associated behaviors (such as agitation, irritability, hostility, impulsivity, and hypomania) and call healthcare provider.

May worsen psychosis in some patients or precipitate a shift to mania or hypomania in patients with bipolar disorder. Patients presenting with depressive symptoms should be screened for bipolar disorder. Monotherapy in patients with bipolar disorder should be avoided. **Fluoxetine is not FDA approved for the treatment of bipolar depression.** May cause insomnia, anxiety, nervousness or anorexia. Use with caution in patients where weight loss is undesirable. May impair cognitive or motor performance; caution operating hazardous machinery or driving.

The potential for severe reactions exists when used with MAO inhibitors; serotonin syndrome (hyperthermia, muscular rigidity, mental status changes/agitation, autonomic instability) may occur. Fluoxetine may elevate plasma levels of thioridazine and increase the risk of QT_c interval prolongation. This may lead to serious ventricular arrhythmias such as torsade de pointes-type arrhythmias and sudden death. Fluoxetine use has been associated with occurrences of significant rash and allergic events, including vasculitis, lupus-like syndrome, laryngospasm, anaphylactoid reactions, and pulmonary inflammatory disease. Discontinue if underlying cause of rash cannot be identified.

Use caution in patients with a previous seizure disorder or condition predisposing to seizures such as brain damage, alcoholism, or concurrent therapy with other drugs which lower the seizure threshold. Use with caution in patients with hepatic or renal dysfunction and in elderly patients. May cause hyponatremia/SIADH. May increase the risks associated with electroconvulsive treatment. Use with caution in patients at risk of bleeding or receiving concurrent anticoagulant therapy - may cause impairment in platelet function. Use caution with history of MI or unstable hearst disease; use in these patients is limited. May alter glycemic control in patients with diabetes. Due to the long half-life of fluoxetine and its metabolites, the effects and interactions noted may persist for prolonged periods following discontinuation. May cause or exacerbate sexual dysfunction. Discontinuation symptoms (eg, dysphoric mood, irritability, agitation, confusion, anxiety, insomnia, hypomania) may occur upon abrupt discontinuation. Taper dose when discontinuing therapy.

Drug Interactions

Cytochrome P450 Effect: Substrate of CYP1A2 (minor), 2B6 (minor), 2C9 (major), 2C19 (minor), 2D6 (major), 2E1 (minor), 3A4 (minor); **Inhibits** CYP1A2 (moderate), 2B6 (weak), 2C9 (weak), 2C19 (moderate), 2D6 (strong), 3A4 (weak)

Increased Effect/Toxicity: Fluoxetine should not be used with nonselective MAO inhibitors (phenelzine, isocarboxazid) or other drugs with MAO inhibition (linezolid); fatal reactions have been reported. Wait 5 weeks after stopping fluoxetine before starting a nonselective MAO inhibitor and 2 weeks after stopping an MAO inhibitor before starting fluoxetine. Concurrent selegiline has been associated with mania, hypertension, or serotonin syndrome (risk may be reduced relative to nonselective MAO inhibitors).

Due to potential QT_c interval prolongation, concomitant use of pimozide is contraindicated. Fluoxetine may inhibit the metabolism of thioridazine, resulting in increased plasma levels and increasing the risk of QT_c interval prolongation. This may lead to serious ventricular arrhythmias, such as torsade de pointes-type arrhythmias and sudden death. Do not use together. Wait at least 5 weeks after discontinuing fluoxetine prior to starting thioridazine.

(Continued)

Fluoxetine *(Continued)*

Fluoxetine may increase the levels/effects of aminophylline, amphetamines, selected beta-blockers, citalopram, dextromethorphan, diazepam, fluvoxamine, lidocaine, mexiletine, methsuximide, mirtazapine, nefazodone, paroxetine, phenytoin, propranolol, risperidone, ritonavir, ropinirole, sertraline, theophylline, thioridazine, tricyclic antidepressants, trifluoperazine, venlafaxine, and other substrates of CYP1A2, 2C19, or 2D6.

Combined use of SSRIs and amphetamines, buspirone, meperidine, nefazodone, serotonin agonists (such as sumatriptan), sibutramine, other SSRIs, sympathomimetics, ritonavir, tramadol, and venlafaxine may increase the risk of serotonin syndrome. Combined use of sumatriptan (and other serotonin agonists) may result in toxicity; weakness, hyper-reflexia, and incoordination have been observed with sumatriptan and SSRIs. In addition, concurrent use may theoretically increase the risk of serotonin syndrome.

Concurrent lithium may increase risk of neurotoxicity, and lithium levels may be increased. Risk of hyponatremia may increase with concurrent use of loop diuretics (bumetanide, furosemide, torsemide). Fluoxetine may increase the hypoprothrombinemic response to warfarin. Concomitant use of fluoxetine and NSAIDs, aspirin, or other drugs affecting coagulation has been associated with an increased risk of bleeding; monitor.

The levels/effects of fluoxetine may be increased by chlorpromazine, delavirdine, fluconazole, gemfibrozil, ketoconazole, miconazole, nicardipine, NSAIDs, paroxetine, pergolide, quinidine, quinine, ritonavir, sulfonamides, ropinirole, tolbutamide, and other CYP2C9 or 2D6 inhibitors.

Decreased Effect: The levels/effects of fluoxetine may be decreased by carbamazepine, phenobarbital, phenytoin, rifampin, rifapentine, secobarbital and other CYP2C9 inducers. Fluoxetine may decrease the levels/effects of CYP2D6 prodrug substrates (eg, codeine, hydrocodone, oxycodone, tramadol). Cyproheptadine may inhibit the effects of serotonin reuptake inhibitors. Lithium levels may be decreased by fluoxetine (in addition to reports of increased lithium levels).

Ethanol/Nutrition/Herb Interactions

Ethanol: Avoid ethanol (may increase CNS depression). Depressed patients should avoid/limit intake.

Herb/Nutraceutical: Avoid valerian, St John's wort, kava kava, gotu kola (may increase CNS depression).

Dietary Considerations May be taken with or without food.

Pharmacodynamics/Kinetics

Absorption: Well absorbed; delayed 1-2 hours with weekly formulation

Protein binding: 95%

Metabolism: Hepatic to norfluoxetine (activity equal to fluoxetine)

Half-life elimination: Adults:

Parent drug: 1-3 days (acute), 4-6 days (chronic), 7.6 days (cirrhosis)

Metabolite (norfluoxetine): 9.3 days (range: 4-16 days), 12 days (cirrhosis)

Time to peak: 6-8 hours

Excretion: Urine (10% as norfluoxetine, 2.5% to 5% as fluoxetine)

Note: Weekly formulation results in greater fluctuations between peak and trough concentrations of fluoxetine and norfluoxetine compared to once-daily dosing (24% daily/164% weekly; 17% daily/43% weekly, respectively). Trough concentrations are 76% lower for fluoxetine and 47% lower for norfluoxetine than the concentrations maintained by 20 mg once-daily dosing. Steady-state fluoxetine concentrations are ~50% lower following the once-weekly regimen compared to 20 mg once daily. Average steady-state concentrations of once-daily dosing were highest in children ages 6 to <13 (fluoxetine 171 ng/mL; norfluoxetine 195 ng/mL), followed by adolescents ages 13 to <18 (fluoxetine 86 ng/mL; norfluoxetine 113 ng/mL); concentrations were considered to be within the ranges reported in adults (fluoxetine 91-302 ng/mL; norfluoxetine 72-258 ng/mL).

Pregnancy Risk Factor C

Dosage Forms CAP: 10 mg, 20 mg, 40 mg; (Prozac®): 10 mg, 20 mg, 40 mg; (Sarafem®): 10 mg, 20 mg. **CAP, delayed release** (Prozac® Weekly™): 90 mg. **SOLN, oral** (Prozac®): 20 mg/5 mL (120 mL). **TAB:** 10 mg, 20 mg

Dental Comment

This drug is known to prolong the QT interval. The QT interval is measured as the time and distance between the Q point of the QRS complex and the end of the T wave in the ECG tracing. After adjustment for heart rate, the QT interval is defined as prolonged if it is more than 450 msec in men and 460 msec in women. A long QT syndrome was first described in the 1950s and 60s as a congenital syndrome involving QT interval prolongation and syncope and sudden death. Some of the congenital long QT syndromes were characterized by a peculiar electrocardiographic appearance of the QRS complex involving a premature atria beat followed by a pause, then a subsequent sinus beat showing marked QT prolongation and deformity. This type of cardiac arrhythmia was originally termed "torsade de pointes" (translated from the French as "twisting of the points").

Prolongation of the QT interval is thought to result from delayed ventricular repolarization. The repolarization process within the myocardial cell is due to the efflux of intracellular potassium. The channels associated with this current can be blocked by many drugs and predisposes the electrical propagation cycle to torsade de pointes.

Fluoxetine is one of the drugs confirmed to prolong the QT interval and is accepted as having a risk of causing torsade de pointes. The risk of drug-induced torsade de pointes is extremely low when a single QT interval prolonging drug is prescribed. In terms of epinephrine, it is not known what effect vasoconstrictors in the local anesthetic regimen will have in patients with a known history of congenital prolonged QT interval or in patients taking any medication that prolongs the QT interval. Until more information is obtained, it is suggested that the clinician consult with the physician prior to the use of a vasoconstrictor in suspected patients, and that the vasoconstrictor (epinephrine, levonordefrin [Neo-Cobefrin®]) be used with caution.

Selected Readings

Friedlander AH and Mahler ME, "Major Depressive Disorder. Psychopathology, Medical Management, and Dental Implications," *J Am Dent Assoc*, 2001, 132(5):629-38.

Gerber PE and Lynd LD, "Selective Serotonin Reuptake Inhibitor-induced Movement Disorders," *Ann Pharmacother*, 1998, 32(6):692-8.

Wynn RL, "New Antidepressant Medications," *Gen Dent*, 1997, 45(1):24-8.

Fluoxetine and Olanzapine *see* Olanzapine and Fluoxetine *on page 1141*

Fluoxetine Hydrochloride *see* Fluoxetine *on page 675*

Fluoxymesterone (floo oks i MES te rone)

U.S. Brand Names Halotestin®
Mexican Brand Names Stenox®
Generic Available Yes
Pharmacologic Category Androgen
Use Replacement of endogenous testicular hormone; in females, palliative treatment of breast cancer
Unlabeled/Investigational Use Stimulation of erythropoiesis, angioneurotic edema
Local Anesthetic/Vasoconstrictor Precautions No information available to require special precautions
Effects on Dental Treatment No significant effects or complications reported
Common Adverse Effects
>10%:
  Male: Priapism
  Female: Menstrual problems (amenorrhea), virilism, breast soreness
  Cardiovascular: Edema
  Dermatologic: Acne
1% to 10%:
  Male: Prostatic carcinoma, hirsutism (increase in pubic hair growth), impotence, testicular atrophy
  Cardiovascular: Edema
  Gastrointestinal: GI irritation, nausea, vomiting
  Genitourinary: Prostatic hyperplasia
  Hepatic: Hepatic dysfunction
Restrictions C-III
Mechanism of Action Synthetic androgenic anabolic hormone responsible for the normal growth and development of male sex hormones and development of male sex organs and maintenance of secondary sex characteristics; synthetic testosterone derivative with significant androgen activity; stimulates RNA polymerase activity resulting in an increase in protein production; increases bone development; halogenated derivative of testosterone with up to 5 times the activity of methyltestosterone
Drug Interactions
  Increased Effect/Toxicity: Fluoxymesterone may suppress clotting factors II, V, VII, and X; therefore, bleeding may occur in patients on anticoagulant therapy May elevate cyclosporine serum levels. May enhance hypoglycemic effect of insulin therapy; may decrease blood glucose concentrations and insulin requirements in patients with diabetes. Lithium may potentiate EPS and other CNS effect. May potentiate the effects of narcotics including respiratory depression
  (Continued)

Fluoxymesterone *(Continued)*

Decreased Effect: May decrease barbiturate levels and fluphenazine effectiveness.

Pharmacodynamics/Kinetics

Absorption: Rapid

Protein binding: 98%

Metabolism: Hepatic; enterohepatic recirculation

Half-life elimination: 10-100 minutes

Excretion: Urine (90%)

Pregnancy Risk Factor X

Fluphenazine *(floo FEN a zeen)*

U.S. Brand Names Prolixin® [DSC]; Prolixin Decanoate®

Canadian Brand Names Apo-Fluphenazine®; Apo-Fluphenazine Decanoate®; Modecate®; PMS-Fluphenazine Decanoate

Generic Available Yes: Injection, tablet

Synonyms Fluphenazine Decanoate

Pharmacologic Category Antipsychotic Agent, Typical, Phenothiazine

Use Management of manifestations of psychotic disorders and schizophrenia; depot formulation may offer improved outcome in individuals with psychosis who are nonadherent with oral antipsychotics

Unlabeled/Investigational Use Pervasive developmental disorder

Local Anesthetic/Vasoconstrictor Precautions Most pharmacology textbooks state that in presence of phenothiazines, systemic doses of epinephrine paradoxically decrease the blood pressure. This is the so called "epinephrine reversal" phenomenon. This has never been observed when epinephrine is given by infiltration as part of the anesthesia procedure.

Effects on Dental Treatment Key adverse event(s) related to dental treatment: Xerostomia and increased salivation (normal salivary flow resumes upon discontinuation). Orthostatic hypotension and nasal congestion are possible and since the drug is a dopamine antagonist, extrapyramidal symptoms of the TMJ are a possibility.

Common Adverse Effects Frequency not defined.

Cardiovascular: Hyper-/hypotension, tachycardia, fluctuations in blood pressure, arrhythmia, edema

Central nervous system: Parkinsonian symptoms, akathisia, dystonias, tardive dyskinesia, dizziness, hyper-reflexia, headache, cerebral edema, drowsiness, lethargy, restlessness, excitement, bizarre dreams, EEG changes, depression, seizure, NMS, altered central temperature regulation

Dermatologic: Dermatitis, eczema, erythema, itching, photosensitivity, rash, seborrhea, skin pigmentation, urticaria

Endocrine & metabolic: Changes in menstrual cycle, breast pain, amenorrhea, galactorrhea, gynecomastia, libido (changes in), elevated prolactin, SIADH

Gastrointestinal: Weight gain, loss of appetite, salivation, xerostomia, constipation, paralytic ileus, laryngeal edema

Genitourinary: Ejaculatory disturbances, impotence, polyuria, bladder paralysis, enuresis

Hematologic: Agranulocytosis, leukopenia, thrombocytopenia, nonthrombocytopenic purpura, eosinophilia, pancytopenia

Hepatic: Cholestatic jaundice, hepatotoxicity

Neuromuscular & skeletal: Trembling of fingers, SLE, facial hemispasm

Ocular: Pigmentary retinopathy, cornea and lens changes, blurred vision, glaucoma

Respiratory: Nasal congestion, asthma

Mechanism of Action Fluphenazine is a piperazine phenothiazine antipsychotic which blocks postsynaptic mesolimbic dopaminergic D_1 and D_2 receptors in the brain; depresses the release of hypothalamic and hypophyseal hormones; believed to depress the reticular activating system thus affecting basal metabolism, body temperature, wakefulness, vasomotor tone, and emesis

Drug Interactions

Cytochrome P450 Effect: Substrate of CYP2D6 (major); **Inhibits** CYP1A2 (weak), 2C9 (weak), 2D6 (weak), 2E1 (weak)

Increased Effect/Toxicity: CYP2D6 inhibitors may increase the levels/effects of fluphenazine; example inhibitors include chlorpromazine, delavirdine, fluoxetine, miconazole, paroxetine, pergolide, quinidine, quinine, ritonavir, and ropinirole. Effects on CNS depression may be additive when fluphenazine is combined with CNS depressants (narcotic analgesics, ethanol, barbiturates, cyclic antidepressants, antihistamines, sedative-hypnotics). Fluphenazine may increase the effects/toxicity of anticholinergics, antihypertensives, lithium (rare neurotoxicity), trazodone, or valproic acid. Concurrent use with TCA may produce increased toxicity or altered therapeutic response. Chloroquine and propranolol may increase chlorpromazine concentrations. Hypotension may occur when fluphenazine is combined with epinephrine. May increase the risk of arrhythmia when combined with antiarrhythmics, cisapride, pimozide, sparfloxacin, or other drugs which prolong QT interval. Metoclopramide may increase risk of extrapyramidal symptoms (EPS). Acetylcholinesterase inhibitors (central) may increase the risk of antipsychotic-related EPS.

Decreased Effect: Phenothiazines inhibit the activity of guanethidine, guanadrel, levodopa, and bromocriptine. Barbiturates and cigarette smoking may enhance the hepatic metabolism of fluphenazine. Fluphenazine and possibly other low potency antipsychotics may reverse the pressor effects of epinephrine.

Pharmacodynamics/Kinetics
Onset of action: I.M., SubQ (derivative dependent): Hydrochloride salt: ~1 hour
Peak effect: Neuroleptic: Decanoate: 48-96 hours
Duration: Hydrochloride salt: 6-8 hours; Decanoate: 24-72 hours
Absorption: Oral: Erratic and variable
Distribution: Crosses placenta; enters breast milk
Protein binding: 91% and 99%
Metabolism: Hepatic
Half-life elimination (derivative dependent): Hydrochloride: 33 hours; Decanoate: 163-232 hours
Excretion: Urine (as metabolites)

Pregnancy Risk Factor C

Fluphenazine Decanoate see Fluphenazine on page 680
Flura-Drops® see Fluoride on page 671

Flurandrenolide (flure an DREN oh lide)

U.S. Brand Names Cordran®; Cordran® SP
Canadian Brand Names Cordran®
Generic Available No
Synonyms Flurandrenolone
Pharmacologic Category Corticosteroid, Topical
Use Inflammation of corticosteroid-responsive dermatoses [medium potency topical corticosteroid]
Local Anesthetic/Vasoconstrictor Precautions No information available to require special precautions
Effects on Dental Treatment No significant effects or complications reported
Common Adverse Effects Frequency not defined.
Cardiovascular: Intracranial hypertension
Dermatologic: Itching, dry skin, folliculitis, hypertrichosis, acneiform eruptions, hyperpigmentation, perioral dermatitis, allergic contact dermatitis, skin atrophy, striae, miliaria, acne, maceration of the skin
Endocrine & metabolic: Cushing's syndrome, growth retardation, HPA suppression
Local: Burning, irritation
Miscellaneous: Secondary infection
Mechanism of Action Decreases inflammation by suppression of migration of polymorphonuclear leukocytes and reversal of increased capillary permeability
Pharmacodynamics/Kinetics
Absorption: Adequate with intact skin; repeated applications lead to depot effects on skin, potentially resulting in enhanced percutaneous absorption
Metabolism: Hepatic
Excretion: Urine; feces (small amounts)
Pregnancy Risk Factor C

Flurandrenolone see Flurandrenolide on page 681

Flurazepam (flure AZ e pam)

U.S. Brand Names Dalmane®
Canadian Brand Names Apo-Flurazepam®
Generic Available Yes
Synonyms Flurazepam Hydrochloride
Pharmacologic Category Hypnotic, Benzodiazepine
Use Short-term treatment of insomnia
Local Anesthetic/Vasoconstrictor Precautions No information available to require special precautions
(Continued)

Flurazepam *(Continued)*

Effects on Dental Treatment Key adverse event(s) related to dental treatment: Xerostomia and changes in salivation (normal salivary flow resumes upon discontinuation), and bitter taste.

Common Adverse Effects Frequency not defined.

Cardiovascular: Palpitations, chest pain

Central nervous system: Drowsiness, ataxia, lightheadedness, memory impairment, depression, headache, hangover effect, confusion, nervousness, dizziness, falling, apprehension, irritability, euphoria, slurred speech, restlessness, hallucinations, paradoxical reactions, talkativeness

Dermatologic: Rash, pruritus

Gastrointestinal: Xerostomia, constipation, increased/excessive salivation, heartburn, upset stomach, nausea, vomiting, diarrhea, increased or decreased appetite, bitter taste, weight gain/loss

Hematologic: Granulocytopenia

Hepatic: Elevated AST/ALT, total bilirubin, alkaline phosphatase, cholestatic jaundice

Neuromuscular & skeletal: Dysarthria, body/joint pain, reflex slowing, weakness

Ocular: Blurred vision, burning eyes, difficulty focusing

Otic: Tinnitus

Respiratory: Apnea, dyspnea

Miscellaneous: Diaphoresis, drug dependence

Restrictions C-IV

Dosage Oral:

Children: Insomnia:

≤15 years: Dose not established

>15 years: 15 mg at bedtime

Adults: Insomnia: 15-30 mg at bedtime

Elderly: Insomnia: Oral: 15 mg at bedtime; avoid use if possible

Mechanism of Action Binds to stereospecific benzodiazepine receptors on the postsynaptic GABA neuron at several sites within the central nervous system, including the limbic system, reticular formation. Enhancement of the inhibitory effect of GABA on neuronal excitability results by increased neuronal membrane permeability to chloride ions. This shift in chloride ions results in hyperpolarization (a less excitable state) and stabilization.

Contraindications Hypersensitivity to flurazepam or any component of the formulation (cross-sensitivity with other benzodiazepines may exist); narrow-angle glaucoma; pregnancy

Warnings/Precautions Use with caution in patients receiving other CNS depressants, patients with low albumin, hepatic dysfunction, and in the elderly; do not use in pregnant women; may cause drug dependency; safety and efficacy have not been established in children <15 years of age

Drug Interactions

Cytochrome P450 Effect: **Substrate** of CYP3A4 (major); **Inhibits** CYP2E1 (weak)

Increased Effect/Toxicity: CYP3A4 inhibitors may increase the levels/effects of flurazepam; example inhibitors include azole antifungals, clarithromycin, diclofenac, doxycycline, erythromycin, imatinib, isoniazid, nefazodone, nicardipine, propofol, protease inhibitors, quinidine, telithromycin, and verapamil. Serum levels and response to flurazepam may be increased by cimetidine, clozapine, CNS depressants, diltiazem, disulfiram, digoxin, ethanol, fluconazole, fluoxetine, fluvoxamine, grapefruit juice, labetalol, levodopa, loxapine, metoprolol, metronidazole, nelfinavir, omeprazole, and valproic acid.

Decreased Effect: CYP3A4 inducers may decrease the levels/effects of flurazepam; example inducers include aminoglutethimide, carbamazepine, nafcillin, nevirapine, phenobarbital, phenytoin, and rifamycins.

Ethanol/Nutrition/Herb Interactions

Ethanol: Avoid ethanol (may increase CNS depression).

Food: Serum levels and response to flurazepam may be increased by grapefruit juice, but unlikely because of flurazepam's high oral bioavailability.

Herb/Nutraceutical: Avoid valerian, St John's wort, kava kava, gotu kola (may increase CNS depression).

Pharmacodynamics/Kinetics

Onset of action: Hypnotic: 15-20 minutes

Peak effect: 3-6 hours

Duration: 7-8 hours

Metabolism: Hepatic to N-desalkylflurazepam (active)

Half-life elimination: Desalkylflurazepam:

Adults: Single dose: 74-90 hours; Multiple doses: 111-113 hours

Elderly (61-85 years): Single dose: 120-160 hours; Multiple doses: 126-158 hours

Pregnancy Risk Factor X
Dosage Forms CAP: 15 mg, 30 mg

Flurazepam Hydrochloride *see* Flurazepam *on page 681*

Flurbiprofen (flure BI proe fen)

Related Information
  Rheumatoid Arthritis, Osteoarthritis, and Osteoporosis *on page 1668*
  Temporomandibular Dysfunction (TMD) *on page 1724*
U.S. Brand Names Ansaid® [DSC]; Ocufen®
Canadian Brand Names Alti-Flurbiprofen; Ansaid®; Apo-Flurbiprofen®;
  Froben®; Froben-SR®; Novo-Flurprofen; Nu-Flurprofen; Ocufen®
Generic Available Yes
Synonyms Flurbiprofen Sodium
Pharmacologic Category Nonsteroidal Anti-inflammatory Drug (NSAID),
  Ophthalmic; Nonsteroidal Anti-inflammatory Drug (NSAID), Oral
Dental Use Oral: Management of postoperative pain
Use
  Oral: Treatment of rheumatoid arthritis and osteoarthritis
  Ophthalmic: Inhibition of intraoperative miosis
Local Anesthetic/Vasoconstrictor Precautions No information available to
require special precautions
Effects on Dental Treatment NSAID formulations are known to reversibly
decrease platelet aggregation via mechanisms different than observed with
aspirin. The dentist should be aware of the potential of abnormal coagulation.
Caution should also be exercised in the use of NSAIDs in patients already on
anticoagulant therapy with drugs such as warfarin (Coumadin®).
Significant Adverse Effects
  Ophthalmic: Frequency not defined: Ocular: Slowing of corneal wound healing,
  mild ocular stinging, itching and burning, ocular irritation, fibrosis, miosis,
  mydriasis, bleeding tendency increased
  Oral:
  >1%:
    Cardiovascular: Edema
    Central nervous system: Amnesia, anxiety, depression, dizziness, headache,
      insomnia, malaise, nervousness, somnolence
    Dermatologic: Rash
    Gastrointestinal: Abdominal pain, constipation, diarrhea, dyspepsia, flatu-
      lence, GI bleeding, nausea, vomiting, weight changes
    Hepatic: Liver enzymes elevated
    Neuromuscular & skeletal: Reflexes increased, tremor, vertigo, weakness
    Ocular: Vision changes
    Otic: Tinnitus
    Respiratory: Rhinitis
  <1% (Limited to important or life-threatening): Anaphylactic reaction, anemia,
    angioedema, asthma, bruising, cerebrovascular ischemia, CHF, confusion,
    eczema, eosinophilia, epistaxis, exfoliative dermatitis, fever, gastric/peptic
    ulcer, hematocrit decreased, hematuria, hemoglobin decreased, hepatitis,
    hypertension, hyperuricemia, interstitial nephritis, jaundice, leukopenia,
    paresthesia, parosmia, photosensitivity, pruritus, purpura, renal failure,
    stomatitis, thrombocytopenia, toxic epidermal necrolysis, urticaria, vasodila-
    tion
Restrictions A medication guide should be dispensed with each prescription. A
template for the required MedGuide can be found on the FDA website at: http://
www.fda.gov/medwatch/SAFETY/2005/safety05.htm#NSAID
Dental Usual Dosing Management of postoperative pain: Adults: Oral: 100 mg
every 12 hours
Dosage
  Oral:
    Rheumatoid arthritis and osteoarthritis: 200-300 mg/day in 2-, 3-, or 4 divided
      doses; do not administer more than 100 mg for any single dose; maximum:
      300 mg/day
    Dental: Management of postoperative pain: 100 mg every 12 hours
  Ophthalmic: Instill 1 drop every 30 minutes, beginning 2 hours prior to surgery
    (total of 4 drops in each affected eye)
  Dosage adjustment in renal impairment: Not recommended in patients with
  advanced renal disease
Mechanism of Action Inhibits prostaglandin synthesis by decreasing the
activity of the enzyme, cyclooxygenase, which results in decreased formation of
prostaglandin precursors
(Continued)

Flurbiprofen *(Continued)*

Contraindications Hypersensitivity to flurbiprofen, aspirin, other NSAIDs, or any component of the formulation; perioperative pain in the setting of coronary artery bypass surgery (CABG); dendritic keratitis; pregnancy (3rd trimester)

Warnings/Precautions NSAIDs are associated with an increased risk of adverse cardiovascular events, including MI, stroke, and new onset or worsening of pre-existing hypertension. Risk may be increased with duration of use or pre-existing cardiovascular risk-factors or disease. Carefully evaluate individual cardiovascular risk profiles prior to prescribing. Use caution with fluid retention, CHF, or hypertension.

Use of NSAIDs can compromise existing renal function. Renal toxicity can occur in patient with impaired renal function, dehydration, heart failure, liver dysfunction, those taking diuretics and ACEI, and the elderly. Rehydrate patient before starting therapy. Monitor renal function closely. Not recommended for use in patients with advanced renal disease.

NSAIDs may increase risk of gastrointestinal irritation, ulceration, bleeding, and perforation. These events may occur at any time during therapy and without warning. Use caution with a history of GI disease (bleeding or ulcers), concurrent therapy with aspirin, anticoagulants and/or corticosteroids, smoking, use of alcohol, the elderly or debilitated patients.

Use the lowest effective dose for the shortest duration of time, consistent with individual patient goals, to reduce risk of cardiovascular or GI adverse events. Alternate therapies should be considered for patients at high risk.

NSAIDs may cause serious skin adverse events including exfoliative dermatitis, Stevens-Johnson syndrome (SJS), and toxic epidermal necrolysis (TEN). Anaphylactoid reactions may occur, even without prior exposure; patients with "aspirin triad" (bronchial asthma, aspirin intolerance, rhinitis) may be at increased risk. Do not use in patients who experience bronchospasm, asthma, rhinitis, or urticaria with NSAID or aspirin therapy.

Use with caution in patients with decreased hepatic function. Closely monitor patients with any abnormal LFT. Severe hepatic reactions (eg, fulminant hepatitis, liver failure) have occurred with NSAID use, rarely; discontinue if signs or symptoms of liver disease develop, or if systemic manifestations occur.

The elderly are at increased risk for adverse effects (especially peptic ulceration, CNS effects, renal toxicity) from NSAIDs even at low doses.

Withhold for at least 4-6 half-lives prior to surgical or dental procedures. Safety and efficacy have not been established in children <18 years of age.

Drug Interactions Substrate of CYP2C9 (minor); **Inhibits** CYP2C9 (strong)

ACE inhibitors: Antihypertensive effects may be decreased by concurrent therapy with NSAIDs; monitor blood pressure.

Angiotensin II antagonists: Antihypertensive effects may be decreased by concurrent therapy with NSAIDs; monitor blood pressure.

Anticoagulants (warfarin, heparin, LMWHs) in combination with NSAIDs can cause increased risk of bleeding.

Antiplatelet drugs (ticlopidine, clopidogrel, aspirin, abciximab, dipyridamole, eptifibatide, tirofiban) can cause an increased risk of bleeding.

Beta-blockers: NSAIDs may decrease the antihypertensive effect of beta-blockers. Monitor.

Cholestyramine (and other bile acid sequestrants): May decrease the absorption of NSAIDs. Separate by at least 2 hours.

Corticosteroids may increase the risk of GI ulceration; avoid concurrent use.

Cyclosporine: NSAIDs may increase serum creatinine, potassium, blood pressure, and cyclosporine levels; monitor cyclosporine levels and renal function carefully.

CYP2C9 Substrates: Flurbiprofen may increase the levels/effects of CYP2C9 substrates. Example substrates include bosentan, dapsone, fluoxetine, glimepiride, glipizide, losartan, montelukast, nateglinide, paclitaxel, phenytoin, warfarin, and zafirlukast.

Gentamicin and amikacin serum concentrations are increased by indomethacin in premature infants. Results may apply to other aminoglycosides and NSAIDs.

Hydralazine's antihypertensive effect is decreased; avoid concurrent use.

Lithium levels can be increased; avoid concurrent use if possible or monitor lithium levels and adjust dose. Sulindac may have the least effect. When NSAID is stopped, lithium will need adjustment again.

Loop diuretics efficacy (diuretic and antihypertensive effect) is reduced. Indomethacin reduces this efficacy, however, it may be anticipated with any NSAID.

Methotrexate: Severe bone marrow suppression, aplastic anemia, and GI toxicity have been reported with concomitant NSAID therapy. Avoid use during moderate or high-dose methotrexate (increased and prolonged methotrexate levels). NSAID use during low-dose treatment of rheumatoid arthritis has not been fully evaluated; extreme caution is warranted.

Thiazides antihypertensive effects are decreased; avoid concurrent use.

Warfarin's INRs may be increased by piroxicam. Other NSAIDs may have the same effect depending on dose and duration. Monitor INR closely. Use the lowest dose of NSAIDs possible and for the briefest duration.

Verapamil plasma concentration is decreased by some NSAIDs; avoid concurrent use.

Ethanol/Nutrition/Herb Interactions

Ethanol: Avoid ethanol (may enhance gastric mucosal irritation).

Food: Food may decrease the rate but not the extent of absorption.

Herb/Nutraceutical: Avoid alfalfa, anise, bilberry, bladderwrack, bromelain, cat's claw, celery, coleus, cordyceps, dong quai, evening primrose, feverfew, fenugreek, garlic, ginger, ginkgo biloboa, red clover, horse chestnut, grapeseed, green tea, ginseng, guggul, horse chestnut seed, horseradish, licorice, prickly ash, red clover, reishi, SAMe, sweet clover, turmeric, white willow (all have additional antiplatelet activity).

Dietary Considerations Tablet may be taken with food, milk, or antacid to decrease GI effects.

Pharmacodynamics/Kinetics

Onset of action: ~1-2 hours

Distribution: V_d: 0.12 L/kg

Protein binding: 99%, primarily albumin

Metabolism: Hepatic via CYP2C9; forms metabolites such as 4-hydroxy-flurbiprofen (inactive)

Half-life elimination: 5.7 hours

Time to peak: 1.5 hours

Excretion: Urine (primarily as metabolites)

Pregnancy Risk Factor C/D (3rd trimester)

Lactation Enters breast milk/not recommended

Dosage Forms [DSC] = Discontinued product

Solution, ophthalmic, as sodium (Ocufen®): 0.03% (2.5 mL) [contains thimerosal]

Tablet: 50 mg, 100 mg

Ansaid®: 50 mg, 100 mg [DSC]

Selected Readings

Ahmad N, Grad HA, Haas DA, et al, "The Efficacy of Nonopioid Analgesics for Postoperative Dental Pain: A Meta-Analysis," *Anesth Prog*, 1997, 44(4):119-26.

Bragger U, Muhle T, Fourmousis I, et al, "Effect of the NSAID Flurbiprofen on Remodeling After Periodontal Surgery," *J Periodontal Res*, 1997, 32(7):575-82.

Cooper SA and Kupperman A, "The Analgesic Efficacy of Flurbiprofen Compared to Acetaminophen With Codeine," *J Clin Dent*, 1991, 2(3):70-4.

Dionne R, "Additive Analgesia Without Opioid Side Effects," *Compend Contin Educ Dent*, 2000, 21(7):572-4, 576-7.

Dionne RA, "Suppression of Dental Pain by the Preoperative Administration of Flurbiprofen," *Am J Med*, 1986, 80(3A):41-9.

Dionne RA and Berthold CW, "Therapeutic Uses of Nonsteroidal Anti-inflammatory Drugs in Dentistry," *Crit Rev Oral Biol Med*, 2001, 12(4):315-30.

Dionne RA, Snyder J, and Hargreaves KM, "Analgesic Efficacy of Flurbiprofen in Comparison With Acetaminophen, Acetaminophen Plus Codeine, and Placebo After Impacted Third Molar Removal," *J Oral Maxillofac Surg*, 1994, 52(9):919-24.

Doroschak AM, Bowles WR, and Hargreaves KM, "Evaluation of the Combination of Flurbiprofen and Tramadol for Management of Endodontic Pain," *J Endod*, 1999, 25(10):660-3.

Forbes JA, Yorio CC, Selinger LR, et al, "An Evaluation of Flurbiprofen, Aspirin, and Placebo in Postoperative Oral Surgery Pain," *Pharmacotherapy*, 1989, 9(2):66-73.

Gallardo F and Rossi E, "Analgesic Efficacy of Flurbiprofen as Compared to Acetaminophen and Placebo After Periodontal Surgery," *J Periodontol*, 1990, 61(4):224-7.

Jeffcoat MK, Reddy MS, Haigh S, et al, "A Comparison of Topical Ketorolac, Systemic Flurbiprofen, and Placebo for the Inhibition of Bone Loss in Adult Periodontitis," *J Periodontol*, 1995, 66(5):329-38.

Jeffcoat MK, Reddy MS, Wang IC, et al, "The Effect of Systemic Flurbiprofen on Bone Supporting Dental Implants," *J Am Dent Assoc*, 1995, 126(3):305-11.

Malmberg AB and Yaksh TL, "Antinociception Produced by Spinal Delivery of the S and R Enantiomers of Flurbiprofen in the Formalin Test," *Eur J Pharmacol*, 1994, 256(2):205-9.

Nguyen AM, Graham DY, Gage T, et al, "Nonsteroidal Anti-inflammatory Drug Use in Dentistry: Gastrointestinal Implications," *Gen Dent*, 1999, 47(6):590-6.

Flurbiprofen Sodium *see* Flurbiprofen *on page 683*

5-Flurocytosine *see* Flucytosine *on page 662*

Fluro-Ethyl® *see* Ethyl Chloride and Dichlorotetrafluoroethane *on page 620*

Flutamide (FLOO ta mide)

U.S. Brand Names Eulexin®
Canadian Brand Names Apo-Flutamide®; Euflex®; Eulexin®; Novo-Flutamide
Mexican Brand Names Eulexin®; Fluken®; Flulem®
Generic Available Yes
Synonyms Niftolid; NSC-147834; 4'-Nitro-3'-Trifluoromethylisobutyrantide; SCH 13521
Pharmacologic Category Antineoplastic Agent, Antiandrogen
Use Treatment of metastatic prostatic carcinoma in combination therapy with LHRH agonist analogues
Unlabeled/Investigational Use Female hirsutism
Local Anesthetic/Vasoconstrictor Precautions No information available to require special precautions
Effects on Dental Treatment No significant effects or complications reported
Common Adverse Effects
>10%:
Endocrine & metabolic: Gynecomastia, hot flashes, breast tenderness, galactorrhea (9% to 42%); impotence; decreased libido; tumor flare
Gastrointestinal: Nausea, vomiting (11% to 12%)
Hepatic: Increased AST (SGOT) and LDH levels, transient, mild
1% to 10%:
Cardiovascular: Hypertension (1%), edema
Central nervous system: Drowsiness, confusion, depression, anxiety, nervousness, headache, dizziness, insomnia
Dermatologic: Pruritus, ecchymosis, photosensitivity, herpes zoster
Gastrointestinal: Anorexia, increased appetite, constipation, indigestion, upset stomach (4% to 6%); diarrhea
Hematologic: Anemia (6%), leukopenia (3%), thrombocytopenia (1%)
Neuromuscular & skeletal: Weakness (1%)
Mechanism of Action Nonsteroidal antiandrogen that inhibits androgen uptake or inhibits binding of androgen in target tissues
Drug Interactions
Cytochrome P450 Effect: Substrate (major) of CYP1A2, 3A4; **Inhibits** CYP1A2 (weak)
Increased Effect/Toxicity: CYP1A2 inhibitors may increase the levels/effects of flutamide; example inhibitors include amiodarone, ciprofloxacin, fluvoxamine, ketoconazole, lomefloxacin, ofloxacin, and rofecoxib. CYP3A4 inhibitors may increase the levels/effects of flutamide; example inhibitors include azole antifungals, clarithromycin, diclofenac, doxycycline, erythromycin, imatinib, isoniazid, nefazodone, nicardipine, propofol, protease inhibitors, quinidine, telithromycin, and verapamil. Warfarin effects may be increased.
Decreased Effect: CYP1A2 inducers may decrease the levels/effects of flutamide; example inducers include aminoglutethimide, carbamazepine, phenobarbital, and rifampin. CYP3A4 inducers may decrease the levels/effects of flutamide; example inducers include aminoglutethimide, carbamazepine, nafcillin, nevirapine, phenobarbital, phenytoin, and rifamycins.
Pharmacodynamics/Kinetics
Absorption: Oral: Rapid and complete
Protein binding: Parent drug: 94% to 96%; 2-hydroxyflutamide: 92% to 94%
Metabolism: Extensively hepatic to more than 10 metabolites, primarily 2-hydroxyflutamide (active)
Half-life elimination: 5-6 hours (2-hydroxyflutamide)
Excretion: Primarily urine (as metabolites)
Pregnancy Risk Factor D

Fluticasone (floo TIK a sone)

Related Information
Respiratory Diseases *on page 1656*
U.S. Brand Names Cutivate®; Flonase®; Flovent® HFA
Canadian Brand Names Cutivate™; Flonase®; Flovent® Diskus®; Flovent® HFA
Mexican Brand Names Cutivate®; Flixonase®; Flixotide®
Generic Available Yes: Cream, nasal spray, ointment
Synonyms Fluticasone Propionate
Pharmacologic Category Corticosteroid, Inhalant (Oral); Corticosteroid, Nasal; Corticosteroid, Topical; Corticosteroid, Topical (Medium Potency)

Use

Inhalation: Maintenance treatment of asthma as prophylactic therapy. It is also indicated for patients requiring oral corticosteroid therapy for asthma to assist in total discontinuation or reduction of total oral dose

Intranasal: Management of seasonal and perennial allergic rhinitis and nonallergic rhinitis

Topical: Relief of inflammation and pruritus associated with corticosteroid-responsive dermatoses; atopic dermatitis

Local Anesthetic/Vasoconstrictor Precautions No information available to require special precautions

Effects on Dental Treatment Localized infections with *Candida albicans* or *Aspergillus niger* have occurred frequently in the mouth and pharynx with repetitive use of oral inhaler of corticosteroids. These infections may require treatment with appropriate antifungal therapy or discontinuation of treatment with corticosteroid inhaler.

Common Adverse Effects

Oral inhalation:

>10%:

Central nervous system: Headache (5% to 11%)

Respiratory: Upper respiratory tract infection (16% to 18%)

3% to 10%:

Respiratory: Throat irritation (8% to 10%), sinusitis/sinus infection (4% to 7%), cough (4% to 6%), bronchitis (2% to 6%), hoarseness/dysphonia (2% to 6%), upper respiratory tract inflammation (2% to 5%)

Miscellaneous: Candidiasis (2% to 5%)

1% to 3%:

Cardiovascular: Chest symptoms

Central nervous system: Dizziness, fever, migraine, pain

Gastrointestinal: Diarrhea, dyspepsia, gastrointestinal infection (viral), gastrointestinal discomfort/pain, hyposalivation

Genitourinary: Urinary tract infection

Neuromuscular & skeletal: Musculoskeletal pain, muscle pain, muscle stiffness/tightness/rigidity

Respiratory: Rhinitis, pharyngitis/throat infection, rhinorrhea/postnasal drip, nasal sinus disorder, laryngitis

Miscellaneous: Viral infection, injuries (including muscle, soft tissue)

Postmarketing and/or case reports: Aggression, agitation, anaphylactic reaction, angioedema, aphonia, asthma exacerbation, bronchospasm (immediate and delayed), cataracts, chest tightness, Churg-Strauss syndrome, contusion, Cushingoid features, cutaneous hypersensitivity, depression, dyspnea, ecchymoses, facial edema, growth velocity reduction in children/adolescents, HPA axis suppression, hyperglycemia, hypersensitivity reactions (immediate and delayed), oropharyngeal edema, osteoporosis, paradoxical bronchospasm, pneumonia, pruritus, rash, restlessness, throat soreness, urticaria, vasculitis, weight gain, wheeze

Nasal inhalation:

>10%: Central nervous system: Headache (7% to 16%)

1% to 10%:

Central nervous system: Dizziness (1% to 3%), fever (1% to 3%)

Gastrointestinal: Nausea/vomiting (3% to 5%), abdominal pain (1% to 3%), diarrhea (1% to 3%)

Respiratory: Pharyngitis (6% to 8%), epistaxis (6% to 7%), asthma symptoms (3% to 7%), cough (4%), blood in nasal mucous (1% to 3%), runny nose (1% to 3%), bronchitis (1% to 3%)

Miscellaneous: Aches and pains (1% to 3%), flu-like symptoms (1% to 3%)

<1% and postmarketing reports: Alteration or loss of sense of taste and/or smell, anaphylaxis/anaphylactoid reactions, angioedema, blurred vision, bronchospasm, cataracts, conjunctivitis, dry/irritated eyes, dry throat, dyspnea, edema (face and tongue), glaucoma, hoarseness, hypersensitivity reactions, increased intraocular pressure, nasal septal perforation (rare), nasal ulcer, pruritus, skin rash, sore throat, throat irritation, urticaria, voice changes, wheezing

Topical: 1% to 10%:

Dermatologic: Dry skin (7%), skin burning/stinging (2% to 5%), pruritus (3%), skin irritation (3%), viral skin infection (1% to 3%), exacerbation of eczema (2%)

Neuromuscular & skeletal: Numbness of fingers (1%)

Reported with other topical corticosteroids (in decreasing order of occurrence): Irritation, folliculitis, acneiform eruptions, hypopigmentation, perioral dermatitis, allergic contact dermatitis, secondary infection, skin atrophy, striae, miliaria, pustular psoriasis from chronic plaque psoriasis

(Continued)

Fluticasone *(Continued)*

Dosage

Children:

Asthma: Inhalation, oral:

Flovent® HFA:

Children 4-11 years: 88 mcg twice daily

Children ≥12 years: Refer to Adults dosing.

Note: NIH Asthma Guidelines (administer in divided doses twice daily):

"Low" dose: 88-176 mcg/day

"Medium" dose: 176-440 mcg/day

"High" dose: >440 mcg/day

Flovent® Diskus® [CAN]:

Children 4-16 years: Usual starting dose: 50-100 mcg twice daily; may increase to 200 mcg twice daily in patients not adequately controlled; titrate to the lowest effective dose once asthma stability is achieved

Children ≥16 years: Refer to Adults dosing.

Corticosteroid-responsive dermatoses: Topical: Children ≥3 months: Cream: Apply sparingly to affected area twice daily. If no improvement is seen within 2 weeks, reassessment of diagnosis may be necessary. **Note:** Safety and efficacy of treatment >4 weeks duration have not been established.

Atopic dermatitis: Topical:

Children ≥3 months: Cream: Apply sparingly to affected area 1-2 times/day. If no improvement is seen within 2 weeks, reassessment of diagnosis may be necessary.

Children ≥1 year: Lotion: Apply sparingly to affected area once daily

Note: Safety and efficacy of treatment >4 weeks duration have not been established.

Rhinitis: Intranasal: Children ≥4 years and Adolescents: Initial: 1 spray (50 mcg/spray) per nostril once daily; patients not adequately responding or patients with more severe symptoms may use 2 sprays (100 mcg) per nostril. Depending on response, dosage may be reduced to 100 mcg daily. Total daily dosage should not exceed 2 sprays in each nostril (200 mcg)/day. Dosing should be at regular intervals.

Adults:

Asthma: Inhalation, oral: **Note:** Titrate to the lowest effective dose once asthma stability is achieved

Flovent® HFA: Manufacturers labeling: Dosing based on previous therapy

Bronchodilator alone: Recommended starting dose: 88 mcg twice daily; highest recommended dose: 440 mcg twice daily

Inhaled corticosteroids: Recommended starting dose: 88-220 mcg twice daily; highest recommended dose: 440 mcg twice daily; a higher starting dose may be considered in patients previously requiring higher doses of inhaled corticosteroids

Oral corticosteroids: Recommended starting dose:

Flovent® HFA: 440 mcg twice daily

Highest recommended dose: 880 mcg twice daily; starting dose is patient dependent. In patients on chronic oral corticosteroids therapy, reduce prednisone dose no faster than 2.5-5 mg/day on a weekly basis; begin taper after 1 week of fluticasone therapy

NIH Asthma Guidelines (administer in divided doses twice daily).

"Low" dose: 88-264 mcg/day

"Medium" dose: 264-660 mcg/day

"High" dose: >660 mcg/day

Flovent® Diskus® [CAN]:

Mild asthma: 100-250 mcg twice daily

Moderate asthma: 250-500 mcg twice daily

Severe asthma: 500 mcg twice daily; may increase to 1000 mcg twice daily in very severe patients requiring high doses of corticosteroids

Corticosteroid-responsive dermatoses: Topical: Cream, lotion, ointment: Apply sparingly to affected area twice daily. If no improvement is seen within 2 weeks, reassessment of diagnosis may be necessary.

Atopic dermatitis: Topical: Cream, lotion: Apply sparingly to affected area once or twice daily. If no improvement is seen within 2 weeks, reassessment of diagnosis may be necessary

Rhinitis: Intranasal: Initial: 2 sprays (50 mcg/spray) per nostril once daily; may also be divided into 100 mcg twice a day. After the first few days, dosage may be reduced to 1 spray per nostril once daily for maintenance therapy. Dosing should be at regular intervals.

Elderly: No differences in safety have been observed in the elderly when compared to younger patients. Based on current data, no dosage adjustment is needed based on age.

Dosage adjustment in hepatic impairment: Fluticasone is primarily cleared in the liver. Fluticasone plasma levels may be increased in patients with hepatic impairment, use with caution; monitor.

Mechanism of Action Fluticasone belongs to a new group of corticosteroids which utilizes a fluorocarbothioate ester linkage at the 17 carbon position; extremely potent vasoconstrictive and anti-inflammatory activity; has a weak HPA inhibitory potency when applied topically, which gives the drug a high therapeutic index. The effectiveness of inhaled fluticasone is due to its direct local effect. The mechanism of action for all topical corticosteroids is believed to be a combination of three important properties: anti-inflammatory activity, immunosuppressive properties, and antiproliferative actions.

Contraindications Hypersensitivity to fluticasone or any component of the formulation; primary treatment of status asthmaticus or acute bronchospasm
Topical: Do not use if infection is present at treatment site, in the presence of skin atrophy, or for the treatment of rosacea or perioral dermatitis

Warnings/Precautions May cause hypercorticism or suppression of hypothalamic-pituitary-adrenal (HPA) axis, particularly in younger children or in patients receiving high doses for prolonged periods. HPA axis suppression may lead to adrenal crisis. Fluticasone may cause less HPA axis suppression than therapeutically equivalent oral doses of prednisone. Particular care is required when patients are transferred from systemic corticosteroids to inhaled products due to possible adrenal insufficiency or withdrawal from steroids, including an increase in allergic symptoms. Patients receiving 20 mg per day of prednisone (or equivalent) may be most susceptible. Concurrent use of ritonavir (and potentially other strong inhibitors of CYP3A4) may increase fluticasone levels and effects on HPA suppression.

Controlled clinical studies have shown that orally-inhaled and intranasal corticosteroids may cause a reduction in growth velocity in pediatric patients. (In studies of orally-inhaled corticosteroids, the mean reduction in growth velocity was approximately 1 centimeter per year [range 0.3-1.8 cm per year] and appears to be related to dose and duration of exposure.) To minimize the systemic effects of orally-inhaled and intranasal corticosteroids, each patient should be titrated to the lowest effective dose.

May suppress the immune system, patients may be more susceptible to infection. Use with caution, if at all, in patients with systemic infections, active or quiescent tuberculosis infection, or ocular herpes simplex. Avoid exposure to chickenpox and measles.

Supplemental steroids (oral or parenteral) may be needed during stress or severe asthma attacks. Rare cases of vasculitis (Churg-Strauss syndrome) or other eosinophilic conditions can occur.

Inhalation: Not to be used in status asthmaticus or for the relief of acute bronchospasm. Flovent® Diskus® [CAN] contain lactose; very rare anaphylactic reactions have been reported in patients with severe milk protein allergy.

Topical: May also cause suppression of HPA axis, especially when used on large areas of the body, denuded areas, for prolonged periods of time or with an occlusive dressing. Pediatric patients may be more susceptible to systemic toxicity.

Drug Interactions
Cytochrome P450 Effect: Substrate of CYP3A4 (major)
Increased Effect/Toxicity: CYP3A4 inhibitors: May increase the levels/effects of fluticasone; example inhibitors include azole antifungals, clarithromycin, diclofenac, doxycycline, erythromycin, imatinib, isoniazid, nefazodone, nicardipine, propofol, protease inhibitors, quinidine, telithromycin, and verapamil. Ritonavir may increase serum levels (due to CYP3A4 inhibition) and the potential for steroid-related adverse effects (eg, Cushing syndrome, adrenal suppression).
The addition of salmeterol has been demonstrated to improve response to inhaled corticosteroids (as compared to increasing steroid dosage).

Ethanol/Nutrition/Herb Interactions Herb/Nutraceutical: In theory, St John's wort may decrease serum levels of fluticasone by inducing CYP3A4 isoenzymes.

Dietary Considerations Flovent® Diskus® [CAN] contains lactose; very rare anaphylactic reactions have been reported with Flovent® Rotadisk® in patients with severe milk protein allergy.

Pharmacodynamics/Kinetics
Onset: Flovent® HFA: Maximal benefit may take 1-2 weeks or longer
Absorption:
Topical cream: 5% (increased with inflammation)
Oral inhalation: Absorbed systemically (DISKUS®: ~18%) primarily via lungs, minimal GI absorption (<1%) due to presystemic metabolism
(Continued)

Fluticasone *(Continued)*

Distribution: 4.2 L/kg

Protein binding: 91%

Metabolism: Hepatic via CYP3A4 to 17β-carboxylic acid (negligible activity)

Bioavailability: Nasal: ≤2%; Oral inhalation: (~18% to 21%)

Excretion: Feces (as parent drug and metabolites); urine (<5% as metabolites)

Pregnancy Risk Factor C

Dosage Forms AERO, oral inhalation [CFC free] (Flovent® HFA): 44 mcg/ inhalation (10.6 g); 110 mcg/inhalation (12 g); 220 mcg/inhalation (12 g). **CRM** (Cutivate®): 0.05% (15 g, 30 g, 60 g). **LOT** (Cutivate®): 0.05% (60 mL)**OINT** (Cutivate®): 0.005% (15 g, 30 g, 60 g). **POWDER, for oral inhalation, as propionate** [prefilled blister pack]: (Flovent® Diskus®) [CAN; not available in the United States]: 50 mcg (28s, 60s); 100 mcg (28s, 60s); 250 mcg (28s, 60s); 500 mcg (28s, 60s). **SUSP, intranasal spray** (Flonase®): 50 mcg/inhalation (16 g)

Fluticasone and Salmeterol *(floo TIK a sone & sal ME te role)*

Related Information

Fluticasone *on page 686*

Salmeterol *on page 1375*

U.S. Brand Names Advair Diskus®

Canadian Brand Names Advair Diskus®

Generic Available No

Synonyms Salmeterol and Fluticasone

Pharmacologic Category Beta₂-Adrenergic Agonist; Corticosteroid, Inhalant (Oral)

Use Maintenance treatment of asthma in children ≥4 years and adults; maintenance treatment of COPD associated with chronic bronchitis

Local Anesthetic/Vasoconstrictor Precautions No information available to require special precautions

Effects on Dental Treatment Localized infections with *Candida albicans* or *Aspergillus niger* have occurred frequently in the mouth and pharynx with repetitive use of oral inhaler of corticosteroids. These infections may require treatment with appropriate antifungal therapy or discontinuance of treatment with corticosteroid inhaler.

Common Adverse Effects Percentages reported in patients with asthma

>10%:

Central nervous system: Headache (12% to 13%)

Respiratory: Upper respiratory tract infection (21% to 27%), pharyngitis (10% to 13%)

>3% to 10%:

Gastrointestinal: Nausea/vomiting (4% to 6%), diarrhea (2% to 4%), pain/ discomfort (1% to 4%), oral candidiasis (1% to 4%)

Neuromuscular & skeletal: Musculoskeletal pain (2% to 4%)

Respiratory: Bronchitis (2% to 8%), upper respiratory tract inflammation (6% to 7%), cough (3% to 6%), sinusitis (4% to 5%), hoarseness/dysphonia (2% to 5%), viral respiratory tract infection (4%), epistaxis (4%)

1% to 3%:

Cardiovascular: Chest symptoms, fluid retention, palpitation, syncope

Central nervous system: Compressed nerve syndromes, hypnagogic effects, pain, sleep disorders, tremor

Dermatologic: Hives, skin flakiness/ichthyosis, urticaria, viral skin infection

Endocrine & metabolic: Hypothyroidism

Gastrointestinal: Appendicitis, constipation, dental discomfort/pain, gastrointestinal disorder, gastrointestinal infection, gastrointestinal signs and symptoms (nonspecified), oral discomfort/pain, oral erythema/rash, oral ulcerations, unusual taste, viral GI infection (0% to 3%)

Hematologic: Contusions/hematomas, lymphatic signs and symptoms (nonspecified)

Hepatic: Abnormal liver function tests

Neuromuscular & skeletal: Arthralgia, articular rheumatism, bone/cartilage disorders, fractures, muscle injuries, muscle stiffness, tightness/rigidity

Ocular: Conjunctivitis, eye redness, keratitis, xerophthalmia

Otic: Ear signs and symptoms (nonspecified)

Respiratory: Blood in nasal mucosa, congestion, ear/nose/throat infection, laryngitis, lower respiratory tract infection, lower respiratory signs and symptoms (nonspecified), nasal irritation, nasal signs and symptoms (nonspecified), nasal sinus disorders, pneumonia, rhinitis, rhinorrhea/post nasal drip, sneezing, wheezing

Miscellaneous: Allergies/allergic reactions, bacterial infection, burns, candidiasis (0% to 3%), diaphoresis, sweat/sebum disorders, viral infection, wounds and lacerations

Restrictions An FDA-approved medication guide is available at http://www.fda.gov/cder/Offices/ODS/labeling.htm; distribute to each patient to whom this medication is dispensed.

Dosage Oral inhalation: **Note:** Do not use to transfer patients from systemic corticosteroid therapy.

COPD: Adults: Fluticasone 250 mcg/salmeterol 50 mcg twice daily, 12 hours apart. **Note:** This is the maximum dose.

Asthma:
Children 4-11 years: Fluticasone 100 mcg/salmeterol 50 mcg twice daily, 12 hours apart. **Note:** This is the maximum dose.

Children ≥12 and Adults: One inhalation twice daily, morning and evening, 12 hours apart

Note: Advair Diskus® is available in 3 strengths of fluticasone, initial dose prescribed should be based upon previous dose of inhaled-steroid asthma therapy. Dose should be increased after 2 weeks if adequate response is not achieved. Patients should be titrated to lowest effective dose once stable. (Because each strength contains salmeterol 50 mcg/inhalation, dose adjustments must be made by changing inhaler strength. No more than 1 inhalation of any strength should be taken more than twice daily). Maximum dose: Fluticasone 500 mcg/salmeterol 50 mcg, 1 inhalation twice daily.

Patients not currently on inhaled corticosteroids: Fluticasone 100 mcg/salmeterol 50 mcg **or** fluticasone 250 mcg/salmeterol 50 mcg

Patients currently using inhaled beclomethasone dipropionate:
≤160 mcg/day: Fluticasone 100 mcg/salmeterol 50 mcg
320 mcg/day: Fluticasone 250 mcg/salmeterol 50 mcg
650 mcg/day: Fluticasone 500 mcg/salmeterol 50 mcg

Patients currently using inhaled budesonide:
≤400 mcg/day: Fluticasone 100 mcg/salmeterol 50 mcg
800-1200 mcg/day: Fluticasone 250 mcg/salmeterol 50 mcg
1600 mcg/day: Fluticasone 500 mcg/salmeterol 50 mcg

Patients currently using inhaled flunisolide:
≤1000 mcg/day: Fluticasone 100 mcg/salmeterol 50 mcg
1250-2000 mcg/day: Fluticasone 250 mcg/salmeterol 50 mcg

Patients currently using inhaled fluticasone propionate aerosol:
≤176 mcg/day: Fluticasone 100 mcg/salmeterol 50 mcg
440 mcg/day: Fluticasone 250 mcg/salmeterol 50 mcg
660-880 mcg/day: Fluticasone 500 mcg/salmeterol 50 mcg

Patients currently using inhaled fluticasone propionate powder:
≤200 mcg/day: Fluticasone 100 mcg/salmeterol 50 mcg
500 mcg/day: Fluticasone 250 mcg/salmeterol 50 mcg
1000 mcg/day: Fluticasone 500 mcg/salmeterol 50 mcg

Patients currently using inhaled mometasone furoate powder:
220 mcg/day: Fluticasone 100 mcg/salmeterol 50 mcg
440 mcg/day: Fluticasone 250 mcg/salmeterol 50 mcg
880 mcg/day: Fluticasone 500 mcg/salmeterol 50 mcg

Patients currently using inhaled triamcinolone acetonide:
≤1000 mcg/day: Fluticasone 100 mcg/salmeterol 50 mcg
1100-1600 mcg/day: Fluticasone 250 mcg/salmeterol 50 mcg

Elderly: No differences in safety or effectiveness have been seen in studies of patients ≥65 years of age. However, increased sensitivity may be seen in the elderly. Use with caution in patients with concomitant cardiovascular disease.

Dosage adjustment in renal impairment: Specific guidelines are not available

Dosage adjustment in hepatic impairment: Fluticasone is cleared by hepatic metabolism. No dosing adjustment suggested. Use with caution in patients with impaired liver function.

Mechanism of Action Combination of fluticasone (corticosteroid) and salmeterol (long-acting beta$_2$ agonist) designed to improve pulmonary function and control over what is produced by either agent when used alone. Because fluticasone and salmeterol act locally in the lung, plasma levels do not predict therapeutic effect.

Fluticasone: The mechanism of action for all topical corticosteroids is believed to be a combination of three important properties: Anti-inflammatory activity, immunosuppressive properties, and antiproliferative actions. Fluticasone has extremely potent vasoconstrictive and anti-inflammatory activity.

Salmeterol: Relaxes bronchial smooth muscle by selective action on beta$_2$-receptors with little effect on heart rate

Contraindications Hypersensitivity to fluticasone, salmeterol, or any component of the formulation; status asthmaticus; acute episodes of asthma

(Continued)

Fluticasone and Salmeterol *(Continued)*
Warnings/Precautions
Asthma treatment: Long-acting beta$_2$ agonists may increase the risk of asthma-related deaths. In a large, randomized clinical trial (SMART, 2006), salmeterol was associated with an increase in asthma-related deaths (when added to usual asthma therapy); risk may be greater in African-American patients versus Caucasians. Should only be used as adjuvant therapy in patients not adequately controlled on inhaled corticosteroids or whose disease requires two maintenance therapies. Salmeterol is not meant to relieve acute asthmatic symptoms, should not be initiated in patients with significantly worsening or acutely deteriorating asthma, and is not a substitute for inhaled or oral corticosteroids. Short-acting beta$_2$ agonist should be used for acute symptoms and symptoms occurring between treatments. Corticosteroids should not be stopped or reduced when salmeterol is initiated. During the initiation of salmeterol watch for signs of worsening asthma.

Concurrent diseases: Use caution in patients with cardiovascular disease (eg, arrhythmia, hypertension, or CHF), seizure disorders, diabetes, glaucoma, hyperthyroidism, hepatic impairment, or hypokalemia. Beta agonists may cause elevation in blood pressure, heart rate, CNS stimulation/excitation, increase risk of arrhythmia, increase serum glucose, decrease serum potassium.

Adverse events: Salmeterol should not be used more than twice daily; do not exceed recommended dose; do not use with other long-acting beta$_2$ agonists; serious adverse events, have been associated with excessive use of inhaled sympathomimetics. Rarely, paradoxical bronchospasm may occur with use of inhaled bronchodilating agents; this should be distinguished from inadequate response. Powder for oral inhalation contains lactose; very rare anaphylactic reactions have been reported in patients with severe milk protein allergy. Immediate hypersensitivity reactions (urticaria, angioedema, rash, bronchospasm) have been reported. Rare cases of vasculitis (Churg-Strauss syndrome) have been reported with fluticasone use. Glaucoma, increased intraocular pressure, and cataracts have occurred with fluticasone inhalation; consider routine eye exams in chronic users. Local yeast infections (eg, oral pharyngeal candidiasis) may occur.

Adrenal suppression: Fluticasone may cause hypercorticism or suppression of hypothalamic-pituitary-adrenal (HPA) axis, particularly in younger children or in patients receiving high doses for prolonged periods. Withdrawal and discontinuation of a corticosteroid should be done slowly and carefully. Particular care is required when patients are transferred from systemic corticosteroids to inhaled products. Concurrent use of ritonavir (and potentially other strong inhibitors of CYP3A4) may increase fluticasone levels and effects on HPA suppression. Fatalities have occurred due to adrenal insufficiency in asthmatic patients during and after transfer from systemic corticosteroids to aerosol steroids; aerosol steroids do not provide the systemic steroid needed to treat patients having trauma, surgery, or infections. Do not use this product to transfer patients from oral corticosteroid therapy.

Immune system: Fluticasone may suppress the immune system; use with caution in patients with systemic infections or ocular herpes simplex. Patient should avoid exposure to chickenpox and measles.

Growth: Controlled clinical studies have shown that orally-inhaled and intranasal corticosteroids like fluticasone may cause a reduction in growth velocity in pediatric patients; related to dose and duration. Long-term use may affect bone mineral density in adults. To minimize the systemic effects of orally-inhaled and intranasal corticosteroids, each patient should be titrated to the lowest effective dose.

Safety and efficacy have not been established in children <4 years of age.
Drug Interactions
Cytochrome P450 Effect: Fluticasone: **Substrate** of CYP3A4 (major); Salmeterol: **Substrate** of CYP3A4 (major);

Increased Effect/Toxicity: CYP3A4 inhibitors may increase the levels/effects of fluticasone and salmeterol; example inhibitors include amprenavir, atazanavir, clarithromycin, delavirdine, diclofenac, fosamprenavir, imatinib, indinavir, isoniazid, itraconazole, ketoconazole, miconazole, nefazodone, nelfinavir, nicardipine, propofol, quinidine, ritonavir, and telithromycin. Atomoxetine may enhance the tachycardia effect of beta$_2$agonists. Protease inhibitors may decrease the metabolism, via CYP isoenzymes, of corticosteroids (orally inhaled); examples include amprenavir, atazanavir, fosamprenavir, indinavir, lopinavir, nelfinavir, ritonavir, and saquinavir; **exception** is tipranavir. Sympathomimetics may enhance the adverse/toxic effect of salmeterol. Antifungal agents (imidazole) may decrease the metabolism, via CYP isoenzymes, of corticosteroids (orally inhaled).

Decreased Effect: Beta$_2$-agonists may diminish the bradycardia effect of beta-blockers (beta$_1$ selective). Beta-blockers (nonselective) may diminish the bronchodilator effect of beta$_2$-agonists.

Dietary Considerations Powder for oral inhalation contains lactose; very rare anaphylactic reactions have been reported in patients with severe milk protein allergy.

Pharmacodynamics/Kinetics

Advair Diskus®:
Onset of action: 30-60 minutes
Peak effect: ≥1 week for full effect
Duration: 12 hours
See individual agents.

Pregnancy Risk Factor C

Dosage Forms POWDER, oral inhalation: 100/50: Fluticasone 100 mcg and salmeterol 50 mcg (28s, 60s); 250/50: Fluticasone 250 mcg and salmeterol 50 mcg (28s, 60s); 500/50: Fluticasone 500 mcg and salmeterol 50 mcg (28s, 60s)

Fluticasone Propionate *see* Fluticasone *on page 686*

Fluvastatin (FLOO va sta tin)

Related Information
Cardiovascular Diseases *on page 1636*

U.S. Brand Names Lescol®; Lescol® XL

Canadian Brand Names Lescol®

Mexican Brand Names Canef®; Lescol®

Generic Available No

Pharmacologic Category Antilipemic Agent, HMG-CoA Reductase Inhibitor

Use To be used as a component of multiple risk factor intervention in patients at risk for atherosclerosis vascular disease due to hypercholesterolemia

Adjunct to dietary therapy to reduce elevated total cholesterol (total-C), LDL-C, triglyceride, and apolipoprotein B (apo-B) levels and to increase HDL-C in primary hypercholesterolemia and mixed dyslipidemia (Fredrickson types IIa and IIb); to slow the progression of coronary atherosclerosis in patients with coronary heart disease; reduce risk of coronary revascularization procedures in patients with coronary heart disease

Local Anesthetic/Vasoconstrictor Precautions No information available to require special precautions

Effects on Dental Treatment No significant effects or complications reported

Common Adverse Effects As reported with fluvastatin capsules; in general, adverse reactions reported with fluvastatin extended release tablet were similar, but the incidence was less.

1% to 10%:
Central nervous system: Headache (9%), fatigue (3%), insomnia (3%)
Gastrointestinal: Dyspepsia (8%), diarrhea (5%), abdominal pain (5%), nausea (3%)
Genitourinary: Urinary tract infection (2%)
Neuromuscular & skeletal: Myalgia (5%)
Respiratory: Sinusitis (3%), bronchitis (2%)

Mechanism of Action Acts by competitively inhibiting 3-hydroxyl-3-methylglutaryl-coenzyme A (HMG-CoA) reductase, the enzyme that catalyzes the reduction of HMG-CoA to mevalonate; this is an early rate-limiting step in cholesterol biosynthesis. HDL is increased while total, LDL and VLDL cholesterols, apolipoprotein B, and plasma triglycerides are decreased.

Drug Interactions

Cytochrome P450 Effect: Substrate of CYP2C9 (major), 2C8 (minor), 2D6 (minor), 3A4 (minor); **Inhibits** CYP1A2 (weak), 2C8 (weak), 2C9 (moderate), 2D6 (weak), 3A4 (weak)

Increased Effect/Toxicity: Fibric acid derivatives may increase the risk of myopathy and rhabdomyolysis. Fluvastatin levels/effects may be increased by omeprazole, phenytoin, fluconazole, NSAIDs, sulfonamides, or other CYP2C9 inhibitors. The anticoagulant effect of warfarin may be increased by fluvastatin. Cholestyramine effect may be additive with fluvastatin if administration times are separated. Fluvastatin may increase the levels/effects of fluoxetine, glimepiride, glipizide, and other CYP2C9 substrates.

Decreased Effect: Administration of cholestyramine at the same time with fluvastatin reduces absorption and clinical effect of fluvastatin. Separate administration times by at least 4 hours. Rifampin and rifabutin may decrease fluvastatin blood levels.

(Continued)

Fluvastatin (Continued)

Pharmacodynamics/Kinetics

Onset: Peak effect: Maximal LDL-C reductions achieved within 4 weeks

Distribution: V_d: 0.35 L/kg

Protein binding: >98%

Metabolism: To inactive and active metabolites (oxidative metabolism via CYP2C9 [75%], 2C8 [~5%], and 3A4 [~20%] isoenzymes); active forms do not circulate systemically; extensive (saturable) first-pass hepatic extraction

Bioavailability: Absolute: Capsule: 24%; Extended release tablet: 29%

Half-life elimination: Capsule: <3 hours; Extended release tablet: 9 hours

Time to peak: Capsule: 1 hour; Extended release tablet: 3 hours

Excretion: Feces (90%): urine (5%)

Pregnancy Risk Factor X

Fluvirin® see Influenza Virus Vaccine on page 833

Fluvoxamine (floo VOKS a meen)

Canadian Brand Names Alti-Fluvoxamine; Apo-Fluvoxamine®; Luvox®; Novo-Fluvoxamine; Nu-Fluvoxamine; PMS-Fluvoxamine; Rhoxal-fluvoxamine

Mexican Brand Names Luvox®

Generic Available Yes

Synonyms Luvox

Pharmacologic Category Antidepressant, Selective Serotonin Reuptake Inhibitor

Use Treatment of obsessive-compulsive disorder (OCD) in children ≥8 years of age and adults

Unlabeled/Investigational Use Treatment of major depression; panic disorder; anxiety disorders in children

Local Anesthetic/Vasoconstrictor Precautions Although caution should be used in patients taking tricyclic antidepressants, no interactions have been reported with vasoconstrictors and fluvoxamine, a nontricyclic antidepressant which acts to increase serotonin; no precautions appear to be needed

Effects on Dental Treatment Key adverse event(s) related to dental treatment: Xerostomia (normal salivary flow resumes upon discontinuation) and abnormal taste. Problems with SSRI-induced bruxism have been reported and may preclude their use; clinicians attempting to evaluate any patient with bruxism or involuntary muscle movement, who is simultaneously being treated with an SSRI drug, should be aware of the potential association. See Dental Comment.

Common Adverse Effects

>10%:

Central nervous system: Headache (22%), somnolence (22%), insomnia (21%), nervousness (12%), dizziness (11%)

Gastrointestinal: Nausea (40%), diarrhea (11%), xerostomia (14%)

Neuromuscular & skeletal: Weakness (14%)

1% to 10%:

Cardiovascular: Palpitations

Central nervous system: Somnolence, mania, hypomania, vertigo, abnormal thinking, agitation, anxiety, malaise, amnesia, yawning, hypertonia, CNS stimulation, depression

Endocrine & metabolic: Decreased libido

Gastrointestinal: Abdominal pain, vomiting, dyspepsia, constipation, abnormal taste, anorexia, flatulence, weight gain

Genitourinary: Delayed ejaculation, impotence, anorgasmia, urinary frequency, urinary retention

Neuromuscular & skeletal: Tremors

Ocular: Blurred vision

Respiratory: Dyspnea

Miscellaneous: Diaphoresis

Restrictions A medication guide concerning the use of antidepressants in children and teenagers can be found on the FDA website at http://www.fda.gov/cder/Offices/ODS/labeling.htm. It should be dispensed to parents or guardians of children and teenagers receiving this medication.

Dosage Oral: **Note:** When total daily dose exceeds 50 mg, the dose should be given in 2 divided doses:

Children 8-17 years: Initial: 25 mg at bedtime; adjust in 25 mg increments at 4- to 7-day intervals, as tolerated, to maximum therapeutic benefit: Range: 50-200 mg/day

Maximum: Children: 8-11 years: 200 mg/day, adolescents: 300 mg/day; lower doses may be effective in female versus male patients

Adults: Initial: 50 mg at bedtime; adjust in 50 mg increments at 4- to 7-day intervals; usual dose range: 100-300 mg/day; divide total daily dose into 2 doses; administer larger portion at bedtime

Elderly: Reduce dose, titrate slowly

Dosage adjustment in hepatic impairment: Reduce dose, titrate slowly

Mechanism of Action Inhibits CNS neuron serotonin uptake; minimal or no effect on reuptake of norepinephrine or dopamine; does not significantly bind to alpha-adrenergic, histamine or cholinergic receptors

Contraindications Hypersensitivity to fluvoxamine or any component of the formulation; concurrent use with alosetron, pimozide, thioridazine, tizanidine, mesoridazine, or cisapride; use of MAO inhibitors within 14 days

Warnings/Precautions Antidepressants increase the risk of suicidal thinking and behavior in children and adolescents with major depressive disorder (MDD) and other depressive disorders; consider risk prior to prescribing. All patients must be closely monitored for clinical worsening, suicidality, or unusual changes in behavior, especially during the initiation of therapy or following an increase or decrease in dosage. When used in children, the child's family or caregiver should be instructed to closely observe the patient and communicate condition with healthcare provider. A medication guide should be dispensed with each prescription. **Fluvoxamine is FDA approved for the treatment of OCD in children ≥8 years of age.**

The possibility of a suicide attempt is inherent in major depression and may persist until remission occurs. Use caution in high-risk patients. Worsening depression and severe abrupt suicidality that are not part of the presenting symptoms may require discontinuation or modification of drug therapy. The patient's family or caregiver should be alerted to monitor patients for the emergence of suicidality and associated behaviors (such as agitation, irritability, hostility, impulsivity, and hypomania) and call healthcare provider.

May worsen psychosis in some patients or precipitate a shift to mania or hypomania in patients with bipolar disorder. Patients presenting with depressive symptoms should be screened for bipolar disorder. Monotherapy in patients with bipolar disorder should be avoided. **Fluvoxamine is not FDA approved for the treatment of bipolar depression.**

The potential for severe reaction exits when used with MAO inhibitors - serotonin syndrome (hyperthermia, muscular rigidity, mental status changes/agitation, autonomic instability) may occur. Fluvoxamine has a low potential to impair cognitive or motor performance; caution operating hazardous machinery or driving. Use caution in patients with a previous seizure disorder or condition predisposing to seizures such as brain damage, alcoholism, or concurrent therapy with other drugs which lower the seizure threshold.

May increase the risks associated with electroconvulsive therapy. Use with caution in patients with hepatic or renal dysfunction and in elderly patients. May cause hyponatremia/SIADH. Use with caution in patients with renal insufficiency or other concurrent illness (cardiovascular disease). Use with caution in patients at risk of bleeding or receiving concurrent anticoagulant therapy, although not consistently noted, fluvoxamine may cause impairment in platelet function. May cause or exacerbate sexual dysfunction.

Drug Interactions

Cytochrome P450 Effect: Substrate (major) of CYP1A2, 2D6; **Inhibits** CYP1A2 (strong), 2B6 (weak), 2C9 (weak), 2C19 (strong), 2D6 (weak), 3A4 (weak)

Increased Effect/Toxicity: Fluvoxamine should not be used with nonselective MAO inhibitors (phenelzine, isocarboxazid) and drugs with MAO inhibitor properties (linezolid); fatal reactions have been reported. Wait 5 weeks after stopping fluvoxamine before starting a nonselective MAO inhibitor and 2 weeks after stopping an MAO inhibitor before starting fluvoxamine. Concurrent selegiline has been associated with mania, hypertension, or serotonin syndrome (risk may be reduced relative to nonselective MAO inhibitors).

Fluvoxamine may inhibit the metabolism of thioridazine or mesoridazine, resulting in increased plasma levels and increasing the risk of QT_c interval prolongation. This may lead to serious ventricular arrhythmias, such as torsade de pointes-type arrhythmias and sudden death. Do not use together. Wait at least 5 weeks after discontinuing fluvoxamine prior to starting thioridazine. Fluvoxamine may increase the levels/effects of aminophylline, citalopram, diazepam, mexiletine, mirtazapine, methsuximide, phenytoin, propranolol, ropinirole, sertraline, theophylline, trifluoperazine and other substrates of CYP1A2 or 2C19. Fluvoxamine may increase the concentrations of alosetron and tizanidine; concurrent use is not recommended.

The levels/effects of fluvoxamine may be increased by amiodarone, amphetamines, selected beta-blockers, chlorpromazine, ciprofloxacin, delavirdine, (Continued)

Fluvoxamine *(Continued)*

fluoxetine, ketoconazole, miconazole, norfloxacin, ofloxacin, paroxetine, pergolide, quinidine, quinine, ritonavir, rofecoxib, ropinirole, and other CYP1A2 or 2D6 inhibitors.

Combined use of SSRIs and amphetamines, buspirone, meperidine, nefazodone, serotonin agonists (such as sumatriptan), sibutramine, other SSRIs, sympathomimetics, ritonavir, tramadol, and venlafaxine may increase the risk of serotonin syndrome. Combined use of sumatriptan (and other serotonin agonists) may result in toxicity; weakness, hyper-reflexia, and inco-ordination have been observed with sumatriptan and SSRIs. In addition, concurrent use may theoretically increase the risk of serotonin syndrome; includes sumatriptan, naratriptan, rizatriptan, and zolmitriptan.

Concurrent lithium may increase risk of nephrotoxicity. Risk of hyponatremia may increase with concurrent use of loop diuretics (bumetanide, furosemide, torsemide). Fluvoxamine may increase the hypoprothrombinemic response to warfarin. Concomitant use of fluvoxamine and NSAIDs, aspirin, or other drugs affecting coagulation has been associated with an increased risk of bleeding; monitor.

Decreased Effect: The levels/effects of fluvoxamine may be decreased by aminoglutethimide, carbamazepine, phenobarbital, rifampin, and other CYP1A2 inducers. Cyproheptadine, a serotonin antagonist, may inhibit the effects of serotonin reuptake inhibitors (fluvoxamine); monitor for altered anti-depressant response.

Ethanol/Nutrition/Herb Interactions

Ethanol: Avoid ethanol. Depressed patients should avoid/limit intake.

Food: The bioavailability of melatonin has been reported to be increased by fluvoxamine.

Herb/Nutraceutical: Avoid valerian, St John's wort, SAMe, kava kava (may increase risk of serotonin syndrome and/or excessive sedation).

Pharmacodynamics/Kinetics

Absorption: Steady-state plasma concentrations have been noted to be 2-3 times higher in children than those in adolescents; female children demonstrated a significantly higher AUC than males

Distribution: V_d: ~25 L/kg

Protein binding: ~80%, primarily to albumin

Metabolism: Hepatic

Bioavailability: 53%; not significantly affected by food

Half-life elimination: ~15 hours

Time to peak, plasma: 3-8 hours

Excretion: Urine

Pregnancy Risk Factor C

Dosage Forms TAB: 25 mg, 50 mg, 100 mg

Dental Comment Problems with SSRI-induced bruxism have been reported and may preclude their use; clinicians attempting to evaluate any patient with bruxism or involuntary muscle movement, who is simultaneously being treated with an SSRI drug, should be aware of the potential association.

Selected Readings

Friedlander AH and Mahler ME, "Major Depressive Disorder. Psychopathology, Medical Management, and Dental Implications," *J Am Dent Assoc*, 2001, 132(5):629-38.

Gerber PE and Lynd LD, "Selective Serotonin Reuptake Inhibitor-induced Movement Disorders," *Ann Pharmacother*, 1998, 32(6):692-8.

Wynn RL, "New Antidepressant Medications," *Gen Dent*, 1997, 45(1):24-8.

Fluxid™ *see* Famotidine *on page 635*

Fluzone® *see* Influenza Virus Vaccine *on page 833*

FML® *see* Fluorometholone *on page 674*

FML® Forte *see* Fluorometholone *on page 674*

FML-S® *see* Sulfacetamide and Fluorometholone *on page 1423*

Focalin™ *see* Dexmethylphenidate *on page 445*

Focalin™ XR *see* Dexmethylphenidate *on page 445*

Foille® [OTC] *see* Benzocaine *on page 190*

Folacin *see* Folic Acid *on page 697*

Folacin, Vitamin B$_{12}$, and Vitamin B$_6$ *see* Folic Acid, Cyanocobalamin, and Pyridoxine *on page 697*

Folate *see* Folic Acid *on page 697*

Folbee *see* Folic Acid, Cyanocobalamin, and Pyridoxine *on page 697*

Folgard® [OTC] *see* Folic Acid, Cyanocobalamin, and Pyridoxine *on page 697*

Folgard RX 2.2® [DSC] *see* Folic Acid, Cyanocobalamin, and Pyridoxine *on page 697*

Folic Acid (FOE lik AS id)

Canadian Brand Names Apo-Folic®
Mexican Brand Names AF Valdecasas®
Generic Available Yes
Synonyms Folacin; Folate; Pteroylglutamic Acid
Pharmacologic Category Vitamin, Water Soluble
Use Treatment of megaloblastic and macrocytic anemias due to folate deficiency; dietary supplement to prevent neural tube defects
Local Anesthetic/Vasoconstrictor Precautions No information available to require special precautions
Effects on Dental Treatment No significant effects or complications reported
Significant Adverse Effects Frequency not defined.
  Allergic reaction, bronchospasm, flushing (slight), malaise (general), pruritus, rash
Dosage
  Oral, I.M., I.V., SubQ: Anemia:
    Infants: 0.1 mg/day
    Children <4 years: Up to 0.3 mg/day
    Children >4 years and Adults: 0.4 mg/day
    Pregnant and lactating women: 0.8 mg/day
  Oral:
    RDA: Expressed as dietary folate equivalents:
      Children:
        1-3 years: 150 mcg/day
        4-8 years: 200 mcg/day
        9-13 years: 300 mcg/day
      Children ≥14 years and Adults: 400 mcg/day
      Elderly: Vitamin B_{12} deficiency must be ruled out before initiating folate therapy due to frequency of combined nutritional deficiencies: RDA requirements (1999): 400 mcg/day (0.4 mg) minimum
    Prevention of neural tube defects:
      Females of childbearing potential: 400 mcg/day
      Females at high risk or with family history of neural tube defects: 4 mg/day
Mechanism of Action Folic acid is necessary for formation of a number of coenzymes in many metabolic systems, particularly for purine and pyrimidine synthesis; required for nucleoprotein synthesis and maintenance in erythropoiesis; stimulates WBC and platelet production in folate deficiency anemia
Contraindications Hypersensitivity to folic acid or any component of the formulation
Warnings/Precautions Not appropriate for monotherapy with pernicious, aplastic, or normocytic anemias when anemia is present with vitamin D deficiency. Doses >0.1 mg/day may obscure pernicious anemia with continuing irreversible nerve damage progression. Resistance to treatment may occur with depressed hematopoiesis, alcoholism, deficiencies of other vitamins. Injection contains benzyl alcohol (1.5%) as preservative (use care in administration to neonates).
Drug Interactions
  Phenytoin: Folic acid may decrease phenytoin concentrations
  Raltitrexed: Folic acid may diminish the therapeutic effect of raltitrexed
Dietary Considerations As of January 1998, the FDA has required manufacturers of enriched flour, bread, corn meal, pasta, rice and other grain products to add folic acid to their products. The intent is to help decrease the risk of neural tube defects by increasing folic acid intake. Other foods which contain folic acid include dark green leafy vegetables, citrus fruits and juices, and lentils.
Pharmacodynamics/Kinetics
  Onset of effect: Peak effect: Oral: 0.5-1 hour
  Absorption: Proximal part of small intestine
Pregnancy Risk Factor A
Lactation Enters breast milk/compatible
Dosage Forms
  Injection, solution, as sodium folate: 5 mg/mL (10 mL) [contains benzyl alcohol]
  Tablet: 0.4 mg, 0.8 mg, 1 mg

Folic Acid, Cyanocobalamin, and Pyridoxine
(FOE lik AS id, sye an oh koe BAL a min, & peer i DOKS een)

Related Information
  Cyanocobalamin *on page 399*
  Folic Acid *on page 697*
  (Continued)

Folic Acid, Cyanocobalamin, and Pyridoxine
(Continued)

Pyridoxine *on page 1316*

U.S. Brand Names Folbee; Folgard® [OTC]; Folgard RX 2.2® [DSC]; Foltx®; Tricardio B

Generic Available Yes

Synonyms Cyanocobalamin, Folic Acid, and Pyridoxine; Folacin, Vitamin B$_{12}$, and Vitamin B$_6$; Pyridoxine, Folic Acid, and Cyanocobalamin

Pharmacologic Category Vitamin

Use Nutritional supplement in end-stage renal failure, dialysis, hyperhomocysteinemia, homocystinuria, malabsorption syndromes, dietary deficiencies

Local Anesthetic/Vasoconstrictor Precautions No information available to require special precautions

Effects on Dental Treatment No significant effects or complications reported

Common Adverse Effects See individual agents.

Folinic Acid *see Leucovorin on page 905*

Follistim® AQ *see Follitropins on page 698*

Follitropin Alfa *see Follitropins on page 698*

Follitropin Alpha *see Follitropins on page 698*

Follitropin Beta *see Follitropins on page 698*

Follitropins (foe li TRO pins)

U.S. Brand Names Bravelle®; Follistim® AQ; Gonal-f®; Gonal-f® RFF

Canadian Brand Names Gonal-f®; Puregon®

Mexican Brand Names Follitrin®; Gonal-f®; Puregon®[biosyn.]

Generic Available No

Synonyms Follitropin Alfa; Follitropin Alpha; Follitropin Beta; Recombinant Human Follicle Stimulating Hormone; rFSH-alpha; rFSH-beta; rhFSH-alpha; rhFSH-beta; Urofollitropin

Pharmacologic Category Gonadotropin; Ovulation Stimulator

Use

Urofollitropin (Bravelle®): Ovulation induction in patients who previously received pituitary suppression; Assisted Reproductive Technologies (ART)

Follitropin alfa:

Gonal-f®: Ovulation induction in patients in whom the cause of infertility is functional and not caused by primary ovarian failure; ART; spermatogenesis induction

Gonal-f® RFF: Ovulation induction in patients in whom the cause of infertility is functional and not caused by primary ovarian failure; ART

Follitropin beta (Follistim® AQ): Ovulation induction in patients in whom the cause of infertility is functional and not caused by primary ovarian failure; ART

Local Anesthetic/Vasoconstrictor Precautions No information available to require special precautions

Effects on Dental Treatment No significant effects or complications reported

Common Adverse Effects Actual frequency varies by specific product, route of administration and indication.

Adverse reactions reported in females:

Cardiovascular: Hypertension, hypotension, palpitation, tachycardia

Central nervous system: Depression, dizziness, emotional lability, fatigue, febrile reaction, fever, headache, nervousness, pain, somnolence

Dermatologic: Acne, dry skin, erythema, exfoliative dermatitis, hair loss, hives, rash

Endocrine & metabolic: Adnexal torsion, breast pain, breast tenderness, hot flashes, OHSS, ovarian cyst, ovarian pain

Gastrointestinal: Abdomen enlarged, abdominal cramps, abdominal pain, constipation, diarrhea, dehydration, flatulence, nausea, weight gain

Genitourinary: Leukorrhea, ovarian enlargement, pelvic pain, uterine spasms, vaginal hemorrhage, vaginal spotting

Local: Injection site reaction

Neuromuscular & skeletal: Back pain, neck pain

Respiratory: Acute respiratory distress syndrome, anaphylactic reaction, atelectasis, dyspnea, hypersensitivity, sinusitis, tachypnea, upper respiratory tract infection

Miscellaneous: Flu-like syndrome, hemoperitoneum

Adverse reactions reported in males: Acne, breast pain, fatigue, gynecomastia, hemoptysis, injection site reaction, lymphadenopathy, pain, pilonidal cyst infection, varicocele

Mechanism of Action Urofollitropin is a preparation of highly purified follicle-stimulating hormone (FSH) extracted from the urine of postmenopausal women. Follitropin alfa and follitropin beta are human FSH preparations of recombinant DNA origin. Follitropins stimulate ovarian follicular growth in women who do not have primary ovarian failure, and stimulate spermatogenesis in men with hypogonadotrophic hypogonadism. FSH is required for normal follicular growth, maturation, gonadal steroid production, and spermatogenesis.

Pharmacodynamics/Kinetics

Onset of action: Peak effect:
   Spermatogenesis, median: 6.8-12.4 months (range 2.7-15.7 months)
   Follicle development: Within cycle

Absorption:
   Follitropin alfa: I.M., SubQ.: Absorption rate is slower than the elimination rate
   Follitropin beta: SubQ: 78%

Distribution: Mean V_d: Follitropin alfa: 10 L; Follitropin beta: 8 L

Bioavailability: Ranges from ~66% to 82% depending on agent

Half-life elimination:
   Follitropin alfa:
     I.M.:50 hours, 24 hours following multiple doses
     SubQ: 24 hours
   Follitropin beta: SubQ: 33.4 hours
   Urofollitropin:
     I.M.: 37 hours, 15 hours following multiple doses
     SubQ: 32 hours, 21 hours following multiple doses

Time to peak:
   Follitropin alfa: SubQ: 16 hours; I.M.: 25 hours
   Follitropin beta: SubQ: 13 hours
   Urofollitropin: Single dose: SubQ: 20 hours, I.M.: 17 hours; Multiple doses: I.M., SubQ: 10 hours

Excretion: Clearance: Follitropin alfa: I.V.: 0.6 L/hour

Pregnancy Risk Factor X

Foltx® *see* Folic Acid, Cyanocobalamin, and Pyridoxine *on page 697*

Fomepizole (foe ME pi zole)

U.S. Brand Names Antizol®

Generic Available No

Synonyms 4-Methylpyrazole; 4-MP

Pharmacologic Category Antidote

Use Orphan drug: Treatment of methanol or ethylene glycol poisoning alone or in combination with hemodialysis

Unlabeled/Investigational Use Known or suspected propylene glycol toxicity

Local Anesthetic/Vasoconstrictor Precautions No information available to require special precautions

Effects on Dental Treatment Key adverse event(s) related to dental treatment: Bad/metallic taste.

Common Adverse Effects

>10%:
   Central nervous system: Headache (14%)
   Gastrointestinal: Nausea (11%)

1% to 10% (≤3% unless otherwise noted):
   Cardiovascular: Bradycardia, facial flush, hypotension, phlebosclerosis, shock, tachycardia
   Central nervous system: Dizziness (6%), increased drowsiness (6%), agitation, anxiety, lightheadedness, seizure, vertigo
   Dermatologic: Rash
   Gastrointestinal: Bad/metallic taste (6%), abdominal pain, decreased appetite, diarrhea, heartburn, vomiting
   Hematologic: Anemia, disseminated intravascular coagulation, eosinophilia, lymphangitis
   Hepatic: Increased liver function tests
   Local: Application site reaction, inflammation at the injection site, pain during injection, phlebitis
   Neuromuscular & skeletal: Backache
   Ocular: Nystagmus, transient blurred vision, visual disturbances
   Renal: Anuria
   Respiratory: Abnormal smell, hiccups, pharyngitis
   Miscellaneous: Multiorgan failure, speech disturbances

Mechanism of Action Fomepizole competitively inhibits alcohol dehydrogenase, an enzyme which catalyzes the metabolism of ethanol, ethylene glycol, *(Continued)*

Fomepizole *(Continued)*

and methanol to their toxic metabolites. Ethylene glycol is metabolized to glyco-aldehyde, then oxidized to glycolate, glyoxylate, and oxalate. Glycolate and oxalate are responsible for metabolic acidosis and renal damage. Methanol is metabolized to formaldehyde, then oxidized to formic acid. Formic acid is responsible for metabolic acidosis and visual disturbances.

Pharmacodynamics/Kinetics
Onset of effect: Peak effect: Maximum: 1.5-2 hours
Absorption: Oral: Readily absorbed
Distribution: V_d: 0.6-1.02 L/kg; rapidly into total body water
Protein binding: Negligible
Metabolism: Hepatic to 4-carboxypyrazole (80% to 85% of dose), 4-hydrox-ymethylpyrazole, and their N-glucuronide conjugates; following multiple doses, induces its own metabolism via CYP oxidases after 30-40 hours
Half-life elimination: Has not been calculated; varies with dose
Excretion: Urine (1% to 3.5% as unchanged drug and metabolites)

Pregnancy Risk Factor C

Fomivirsen *(foe MI vir sen)*

Related Information
Systemic Viral Diseases *on page 1675*
U.S. Brand Names Vitravene™ [DSC]
Canadian Brand Names Vitravene™
Generic Available No
Synonyms Fomivirsen Sodium
Pharmacologic Category Antiviral Agent, Ophthalmic
Use Local treatment of cytomegalovirus (CMV) retinitis in patients with acquired immunodeficiency syndrome who are intolerant or insufficiently responsive to other treatments for CMV retinitis or when other treatments for CMV retinitis are contraindicated
Local Anesthetic/Vasoconstrictor Precautions No information available to require special precautions
Effects on Dental Treatment No significant effects or complications reported
Mechanism of Action Inhibits synthesis of viral protein by binding to mRNA which blocks replication of cytomegalovirus through an antisense mechanism

Fomivirsen Sodium *see* Fomivirsen *on page 700*

Fondaparinux *(fon da PARE i nuks)*

U.S. Brand Names Arixtra®
Canadian Brand Names Arixtra®
Generic Available No
Synonyms Fondaparinux Sodium
Pharmacologic Category Factor Xa Inhibitor
Use Prophylaxis of deep vein thrombosis (DVT) in patients undergoing surgery for hip replacement, knee replacement, hip fracture (including extended prophylaxis following hip fracture surgery), or abdominal surgery (in patients at risk for thromboembolic complications); treatment of acute pulmonary embolism (PE); treatment of acute DVT without PE
Local Anesthetic/Vasoconstrictor Precautions No information available to require special precautions
Effects on Dental Treatment Key adverse event(s) related to dental treatment: Hemorrhage may occur at any site; risk increased in renal dysfunction, patients >75 years and/or <50 kg; major bleeding increased as high as 5% in patients receiving initial dose <6 hours postsurgery.
Common Adverse Effects As with all anticoagulants, bleeding is the major adverse effect. Hemorrhage may occur at any site. Risk appears increased by a number of factors including renal dysfunction, age (>75 years), and weight (<50 kg).
>10%:
Central nervous system: Fever (4% to 14%)
Gastrointestinal: Nausea (11%)
Hematologic: Anemia (20%)
1% to 10%:
Cardiovascular: Edema (9%), hypotension (4%), confusion (3%)
Central nervous system: Insomnia (5%), dizziness (4%), headache (2% to 5%), pain (2%)
Dermatologic: Rash (8%), purpura (4%), bullous eruption (3%)

Endocrine & metabolic: Hypokalemia (1% to 4%)

Gastrointestinal: Constipation (5% to 9%), nausea (3%), vomiting (6%), diarrhea (3%), dyspepsia (2%)

Genitourinary: Urinary tract infection (4%), urinary retention (3%)

Hematologic: Moderate thrombocytopenia (50,000-100,000/mm^3: 3%), major bleeding (1% to 3%), minor bleeding (2% to 4%), hematoma (3%); risk of major bleeding increased as high as 5% in patients receiving initial dose <6 hours following surgery

Hepatic: SGOT increased (2%), SGPT increased (3%)

Local: Injection site reaction (bleeding, rash, pruritus)

Miscellaneous: Wound drainage increased (5%)

Mechanism of Action Fondaparinux is a synthetic pentasaccharide that causes an antithrombin III-mediated selective inhibition of factor Xa. Neutralization of factor Xa interrupts the blood coagulation cascade and inhibits thrombin formation and thrombus development.

Drug Interactions

Increased Effect/Toxicity: Anticoagulants, antiplatelet agents, drotrecogin alfa, NSAIDs, salicylates, and thrombolytic agents may enhance the anticoagulant effect and/or increase the risk of bleeding.

Pharmacodynamics/Kinetics

Absorption: Rapid and complete

Distribution: V_d: 7-11 L; mainly in blood

Protein binding: ≥94% to antithrombin III

Bioavailability: 100%

Half-life elimination: 17-21 hours; prolonged with worsening renal impairment

Time to peak: 2-3 hours

Excretion: Urine (as unchanged drug); decreased clearance in patients <50 kg

Pregnancy Risk Factor B

Fondaparinux Sodium see Fondaparinux on page 700

Foradil® Aerolizer™ see Formoterol on page 701

Formoterol (for MOH te rol)

U.S. Brand Names Foradil® Aerolizer™

Canadian Brand Names Foradil®; Oxeze® Turbuhaler®

Generic Available No

Synonyms Formoterol Fumarate

Pharmacologic Category Beta$_2$-Adrenergic Agonist

Use Maintenance treatment of asthma and prevention of bronchospasm in patients ≥5 years of age with reversible obstructive airway disease, including patients with symptoms of nocturnal asthma, who require regular treatment with inhaled, short-acting beta$_2$ agonists; maintenance treatment of bronchoconstriction in patients with COPD; prevention of exercise-induced bronchospasm in patients ≥5 years of age

Note: Oxeze® is also approved in Canada for acute relief of symptoms ("on demand" treatment) in patients ≥6 years of age.

Local Anesthetic/Vasoconstrictor Precautions No information available to require special precautions

Effects on Dental Treatment Key adverse event(s) related to dental treatment: Xerostomia (normal salivary flow resumes upon discontinuation).

Common Adverse Effects Children are more likely to have infection, inflammation, abdominal pain, nausea, and dyspepsia.

>10%:

Endocrine & metabolic: Serum glucose increased, serum potassium decreased

Miscellaneous: Viral infection (17%)

1% to 10%:

Cardiovascular: Chest pain (2%)

Central nervous system: Tremor (2%), dizziness (2%), insomnia (2%), dysphonia (1%)

Dermatologic: Rash (1%)

Respiratory: Bronchitis (5%), infection (3%), dyspnea (2%), tonsillitis (1%)

Mechanism of Action Relaxes bronchial smooth muscle by selective action on beta$_2$ receptors with little effect on heart rate. Formoterol has a long-acting effect.

Drug Interactions

Cytochrome P450 Effect: Substrate (minor) of CYP2A6, 2C9, 2C19, 2D6

Increased Effect/Toxicity: Adrenergic agonists, antidepressants (tricyclic), beta-blockers, corticosteroids, diuretics, drugs that prolong QT$_c$ interval, MAO inhibitors, theophylline derivatives

(Continued)

Formoterol (Continued)

Pharmacodynamics/Kinetics

Onset: Within 3 minutes

Peak effect: 80% of peak effect within 15 minutes

Duration: Improvement in FEV_1 observed for 12 hours in most patients

Absorption: Rapidly into plasma

Protein binding: 61% to 64% *in vitro* at higher concentrations than achieved with usual dosing

Metabolism: Hepatic via direct glucuronidation and O-demethylation; CYP2D6, CYP2C8/9, CYP2C19, CYP2A6 involved in O-demethylation

Half-life elimination: ~10-14 hours

Time to peak: Maximum improvement in FEV_1 in 1-3 hours

Excretion:

Children 5-12 years: Urine (7% to 9% as direct glucuronide metabolites, 6% as unchanged drug)

Adults: Urine (15% to 18% as direct glucuronide metabolites, 10% as unchanged drug)

Pregnancy Risk Factor C

Formoterol Fumarate *see* Formoterol *on page 701*

Formula EM [OTC] *see* Fructose, Dextrose, and Phosphoric Acid *on page 713*

Formulation R™ [OTC] *see* Phenylephrine *on page 1226*

5-Formyl Tetrahydrofolate *see* Leucovorin *on page 905*

Fortamet™ *see* Metformin *on page 1001*

Fortaz® *see* Ceftazidime *on page 292*

Forteo™ *see* Teriparatide *on page 1461*

Fortical® *see* Calcitonin *on page 246*

Fortovase® [DSC] *see* Saquinavir *on page 1377*

Fosamax® *see* Alendronate *on page 64*

Fosamax Plus D™ *see* Alendronate and Cholecalciferol *on page 66*

Fosamprenavir (FOS am pren a veer)

Related Information

HIV Infection and AIDS *on page 1662*

U.S. Brand Names Lexiva™

Canadian Brand Names Telzir®

Generic Available No

Synonyms Fosamprenavir Calcium; GW433908G

Pharmacologic Category Antiretroviral Agent, Protease Inhibitor

Use Treatment of HIV infections in combination with at least two other antiretroviral agents

Local Anesthetic/Vasoconstrictor Precautions No information available to require special precautions

Effects on Dental Treatment No significant effects or complications reported

Common Adverse Effects

>10%:

Central nervous system: Headache (19% to 21%), fatigue (10% to 18%)

Dermatologic: Rash (17% to 35%; moderate to severe reactions 3% to 8%)

Gastrointestinal: Nausea (37% to 39%), diarrhea (34% to 52%), vomiting (16% to 20%), abdominal pain (5% to 11%)

1% to 10%:

Central nervous system: Depression (8%), fatigue, headache, paresthesia

Dermatologic: Pruritus (3% to 8%)

Endocrine & metabolic: Hypertriglyceridemia (0% to 11%), serum lipase increased (6% to 8%), hyperglycemia (<1% to 2%)

Hematologic: Neutropenia (3%)

Hepatic: Transaminases increased (4% to 8%)

Miscellaneous: Perioral tingling/numbness (2% to 10%)

Mechanism of Action Fosamprenavir is rapidly and almost completely converted to amprenavir *in vivo*. Amprenavir binds to the protease activity site and inhibits the activity of the enzyme. HIV protease is required for the cleavage of viral polyprotein precursors into individual functional proteins found in infectious HIV. Inhibition prevents cleavage of these polyproteins, resulting in the formation of immature, noninfectious viral particles.

Drug Interactions

Cytochrome P450 Effect: As amprenavir: Substrate of CYP2C9 (minor), 3A4 (major); Inhibits CYP2C19 (weak), 3A4 (strong)

Increased Effect/Toxicity: Concurrent use of cisapride, midazolam, pimozide, quinidine, or triazolam is contraindicated. Concurrent use of ergot alkaloids (dihydroergotamine, ergotamine, ergonovine, methylergonovine) with amprenavir is also contraindicated (may cause vasospasm and peripheral ischemia). Concurrent use of oral solution with disulfiram or metronidazole is contraindicated, due to the risk of propylene glycol toxicity.

Serum concentrations of orally-inhaled corticosteroids, trazodone, and some antiarrhythmics (eg, amiodarone, bepridil, lidocaine, and quinidine) may be increased, potentially leading to toxicity; when amprenavir is coadministered with ritonavir, flecainide and propafenone are contraindicated. HMG-CoA reductase inhibitors serum concentrations may be increased by amprenavir, increasing the risk of myopathy/rhabdomyolysis; lovastatin and simvastatin are not recommended; fluvastatin and pravastatin may be safer alternatives.

Amprenavir may increase the levels/effects of selected benzodiazepines (midazolam and triazolam are contraindicated), calcium channel blockers, cyclosporine, mirtazapine, nateglinide, nefazodone, quinidine, sildenafil (and other PDE-5 inhibitors), tacrolimus, venlafaxine, and other CYP3A4 substrates. When used with strong CYP3A4 inhibitors, dosage adjustment/limits are recommended for sildenafil and other PDE-5 inhibitors; refer to individual monographs.

Concurrent therapy with ritonavir may result in increased serum concentrations: dosage adjustment is recommended. Clarithromycin, indinavir, nelfinavir may increase serum concentrations of amprenavir.

Decreased Effect: CYP3A4 inducers may decrease the levels/effects of amprenavir; example inducers include aminoglutethimide, carbamazepine, nafcillin, nevirapine, phenobarbital, phenytoin, and rifamycins. The administration of didanosine (buffered formulation) should be separated from amprenavir by 1 hour to limit interaction between formulations. Serum concentrations of estrogen (oral contraceptives) may be decreased, use alternative (nonhormonal) forms of contraception. Dexamethasone may decrease the therapeutic effect of amprenavir. Serum concentrations of delavirdine may be decreased; may lead to loss of virologic response and possible resistance to delavirdine; concomitant use is not recommended. Efavirenz and nevirapine may decrease serum concentrations of amprenavir (dosing for combinations not established). Avoid St John's wort (may lead to subtherapeutic concentrations of amprenavir). Effect of amprenavir may be diminished when administered with methadone (consider alternative antiretroviral); in addition, effect of methadone may be reduced (dosage increase may be required). Ranitidine may impair absorption of fosamprenavir, leading to reduced serum levels of amprenavir; separate doses.

Pharmacodynamics/Kinetics

Absorption: 63%

Bioavailability: Not established; food does not have a significant effect on absorption

Protein-binding: 90%

Half-Life elimination: 7.7 hours

Time to peak, plasma: 1.5-4 hours

Metabolism: Fosamprenavir is rapidly and almost completely converted to amprenavir by cellular phosphatases; amprenavir is hepatically metabolized via CYP isoenzymes (primarily CYP3A4)

Excretion: Feces (75%); urine (14% as metabolites; <1% as unchanged drug)

Pregnancy Risk Factor C

Fosamprenavir Calcium see Fosamprenavir on page 702

Foscarnet (fos KAR net)

Related Information

Systemic Viral Diseases on page 1675

U.S. Brand Names Foscavir®

Canadian Brand Names Foscavir®

Generic Available No

Synonyms PFA; Phosphonoformate; Phosphonoformic Acid

Pharmacologic Category Antiviral Agent

Dental Use Treatment of herpes virus infections suspected to be caused by acyclovir (HSV, VZV) or ganciclovir (CMV) resistant strains (this occurs almost exclusively in persons with advanced AIDS who have received prolonged treatment for herpes infection)

Use

Treatment of herpes virus infections suspected to be caused by acyclovir-resistant (HSV, VZV) or ganciclovir-resistant (CMV) strains; this

(Continued)

Foscarnet *(Continued)*

occurs almost exclusively in immunocompromised persons (eg, with advanced AIDS) who have received prolonged treatment for a herpes virus infection

Treatment of CMV retinitis in persons with AIDS

Unlabeled/Investigational Use Other CMV infections in persons unable to tolerate ganciclovir; may be given in combination with ganciclovir in patients who relapse after monotherapy with either drug

Local Anesthetic/Vasoconstrictor Precautions No information available to require special precautions (see Dental Comment)

Effects on Dental Treatment No significant effects or complications reported

Significant Adverse Effects

>10%:

Central nervous system: Fever, headache, seizure

Endocrine & metabolic: Electrolyte disorders (hyper- or hypocalcemia; hyper- or hypomagnesemia, hyper- or hypophosphatemia, or hypokalemia)

Gastrointestinal: Nausea, diarrhea, vomiting

Hematologic: Anemia

Renal: Nephrotoxicity (abnormal renal function, decreased creatinine clearance)

1% to 10%:

Central nervous system: Seizures (in up to 10% of HIV patients), fatigue, malaise, dizziness, hypoesthesia, depression, confusion, anxiety

Dermatologic: Rash

Gastrointestinal: Anorexia

Hematologic: Granulocytopenia, leukopenia

Local: Injection site pain

Neuromuscular & skeletal: Paresthesia, involuntary muscle contractions, rigors, neuropathy (peripheral), weakness

Ocular: Vision abnormalities

Respiratory: Coughing, dyspnea

Miscellaneous: Sepsis, diaphoresis (increased)

<1% (Limited to important or life-threatening): Arrhythmias, ascites, bradycardia, cardiac failure, cerebral edema, cholecystitis, cholelithiasis, hepatitis, hepatosplenomegaly, leg edema, peripheral edema, substernal chest pain, syncope, vocal cord paralysis

Dental Usual Dosing Herpes simplex infections (acyclovir-resistant): Induction: I.V.: 40 mg/kg/dose every 8-12 hours for 14-21 days

Dosage

CMV retinitis: I.V.:

Induction treatment: 60 mg/kg/dose every 8 hours **or** 100 mg/kg every 12 hours for 14-21 days

Maintenance therapy: 90-120 mg/kg/day as a single infusion

Herpes simplex infections (acyclovir-resistant): Induction: I.V.: 40 mg/kg/dose every 8-12 hours for 14-21 days

Dosage adjustment in renal impairment:

Induction and maintenance dosing schedules based on creatinine clearance (mL/minute/kg): See tables below and on next page.

Maintenance Dosing of Foscarnet in Patients With Abnormal Renal Function

Cl$_{cr}$ (mL/min/kg)	CMV Equivalent to 90 mg/kg q24h	CMV Equivalent to 120 mg/kg q24h
<0.4	Not recommended	Not recommended
≥0.4-0.5	50 mg/kg every 48 hours	65 mg/kg every 48 hours
>0.5-0.6	60 mg/kg every 48 hours	80 mg/kg every 48 hours
>0.6-0.8	80 mg/kg every 48 hours	105 mg/kg every 48 hours
>0.8-1.0	50 mg/kg every 24 hours	65 mg/kg every 24 hours
>1.0-1.4	70 mg/kg every 24 hours	90 mg/kg every 24 hours
>1.4	90 mg/kg every 24 hours	120 mg/kg every 24 hours

Hemodialysis:

Foscarnet is highly removed by hemodialysis (30% in 4 hours HD)

Doses of 50 mg/kg/dose posthemodialysis have been found to produce similar serum concentrations as doses of 90 mg/kg twice daily in patients with normal renal function

Doses of 60-90 mg/kg/dose loading dose (posthemodialysis) followed by 45 mg/kg/dose posthemodialysis (3 times/week) with the monitoring of weekly plasma concentrations to maintain peak plasma concentrations in the range of 400-800 µMolar has been recommended by some clinicians

Continuous arteriovenous or venovenous hemodiafiltration effects: Dose as for Cl_{cr} 10-50 mL/minute

Induction Dosing of Foscarnet in Patients With Abnormal Renal Function

Cl_{cr} (mL/min/kg)	HSV	HSV	CMV	CMV
	Equivalent to 40 mg/kg q12h	Equivalent to 40 mg/kg q8h	Equivalent to 60 mg/kg q8h	Equivalent to 90 mg/kg q12h
<0.4	Not recommended	Not recommended	Not recommended	Not recommended
≥0.4-0.5	20 mg/kg every 24 hours	35 mg/kg every 24 hours	50 mg/kg every 24 hours	50 mg/kg every 24 hours
>0.5-0.6	25 mg/kg every 24 hours	40 mg/kg every 24 hours	60 mg/kg every 24 hours	60 mg/kg every 24 hours
>0.6-0.8	35 mg/kg every 24 hours	25 mg/kg every 12 hours	40 mg/kg every 12 hours	80 mg/kg every 24 hours
>0.8-1.0	20 mg/kg every 12 hours	35 mg/kg every 12 hours	50 mg/kg every 12 hours	50 mg/kg every 12 hours
>1.0-1.4	30 mg/kg every 12 hours	30 mg/kg every 8 hours	45 mg/kg every 8 hours	70 mg/kg every 12 hours
>1.4	40 mg/kg every 12 hours	40 mg/kg every 8 hours	60 mg/kg every 8 hours	90 mg/kg every 12 hours

Mechanism of Action Pyrophosphate analogue which acts as a noncompetitive inhibitor of many viral RNA and DNA polymerases as well as HIV reverse transcriptase. Similar to ganciclovir, foscarnet is a virostatic agent. Foscarnet does not require activation by thymidine kinase.

Contraindications Hypersensitivity to foscarnet or any component of the formulation; Cl_{cr} <0.4 mL/minute/kg during therapy

Warnings/Precautions Hazardous agent — use appropriate precautions for handling and disposal. Renal impairment occurs to some degree in the majority of patients treated with foscarnet; renal impairment may occur at any time and is usually reversible within 1 week following dose adjustment or discontinuation of therapy, however, several patients have died with renal failure within 4 weeks of stopping foscarnet; therefore, renal function should be closely monitored. Foscarnet is deposited in teeth and bone of young, growing animals; it has adversely affected tooth enamel development in rats; safety and effectiveness in children have not been studied. Imbalance of serum electrolytes or minerals occurs in 6% to 18% of patients (hypocalcemia, low ionized calcium, hypo- or hyperphosphatemia, hypomagnesemia or hypokalemia).

Patients with a low ionized calcium may experience perioral tingling, numbness, paresthesias, tetany, and seizures. Seizures have been experienced by up to 10% of AIDS patients. Risk factors for seizures include a low baseline absolute neutrophil count (ANC), impaired baseline renal function and low total serum calcium. Some patients who have experienced seizures have died, while others have been able to continue or resume foscarnet treatment after their mineral or electrolyte abnormality has been corrected, their underlying disease state treated, or their dose decreased. Foscarnet has been shown to be mutagenic in vitro and in mice at very high doses. Information on the use of foscarnet is lacking in the elderly; dose adjustments and proper monitoring must be performed because of the decreased renal function common in older patients.

Drug Interactions
Ciprofloxacin: Concurrent use with ciprofloxacin increases seizure potential.
Cyclosporine: Acute renal failure (reversible) has been reported with cyclosporine due most likely to toxic synergistic effect.
Nephrotoxic drugs (amphotericin B, I.V. pentamidine, aminoglycosides, etc): Should be avoided, if possible, to minimize additive renal risk with foscarnet.
Pentamidine: Increases hypocalcemia.
Ritonavir, saquinavir: Increased risk of renal impairment has been associated with concurrent use with foscarnet.

Pharmacodynamics/Kinetics
Distribution: Up to 28% of cumulative I.V. dose may be deposited in bone
Metabolism: Biotransformation does not occur
Half-life elimination: ~3 hours
Excretion: Urine (≤28% as unchanged drug)

Pregnancy Risk Factor C

Lactation Excretion in breast milk unknown/contraindicated

Breast-Feeding Considerations The CDC recommends **not** to breast-feed if diagnosed with HIV to avoid postnatal transmission of the virus.

Dosage Forms [DSC] = Discontinued product
Injection, solution: 24 mg/mL (250 mL [DSC], 500 mL)
(Continued)

Foscarnet (Continued)

Dental Comment This drug is known to prolong the QT interval. The QT interval is measured as the time and distance between the Q point of the QRS complex and the end of the T wave in the ECG tracing. After adjustment for heart rate, the QT interval is defined as prolonged if it is more than 450 msec in men and 460 msec in women. A long QT syndrome was first described in the 1950s and 60s as a congenital syndrome involving QT interval prolongation and syncope and sudden death. Some of the congenital long QT syndromes were characterized by a peculiar electrocardiographic appearance of the QRS complex involving a premature atria beat followed by a pause, then a subsequent sinus beat showing marked QT prolongation and deformity. This type of cardiac arrhythmia was originally termed "torsade de pointes" (translated from the French as "twisting of the points").

Prolongation of the QT interval is thought to result from delayed ventricular repolarization. The repolarization process within the myocardial cell is due to the efflux of intracellular potassium. The channels associated with this current can be blocked by many drugs and predisposes the electrical propagation cycle to torsade de pointes.

Foscarnet is one of the drugs confirmed to prolong the QT interval and is accepted as having a risk of causing torsade de pointes. The risk of drug-induced torsade de pointes is extremely low when a single QT interval prolonging drug is prescribed. In terms of epinephrine, it is not known what effect vasoconstrictors in the local anesthetic regimen will have in patients with a known history of congenital prolonged QT interval or in patients taking any medication that prolongs the QT interval. Until more information is obtained, it is suggested that the clinician consult with the physician prior to the use of a vasoconstrictor in suspected patients, and that the vasoconstrictor (epinephrine, levonordefrin [Neo-Cobefrin®]) be used with caution.

Selected Readings

Chilukuri S and Rosen T, "Management of Acyclovir-Resistant Herpes Simplex Virus," *Dermatol Clin*, 2003, 21(2):311-20.

Foscavir® *see* Foscarnet *on page 703*

Fosfomycin (fos foe MYE sin)

U.S. Brand Names Monurol™
Canadian Brand Names Monurol™
Mexican Brand Names Fosfocil®; Monurol™
Generic Available No
Synonyms Fosfomycin Tromethamine
Pharmacologic Category Antibiotic, Miscellaneous
Use Single oral dose in the treatment of uncomplicated urinary tract infections in women due to susceptible strains of *E. coli* and *Enterococcus*; may have an advantage over other agents since it maintains high concentration in the urine for up to 48 hours
Unlabeled/Investigational Use Multiple doses have been investigated for complicated urinary tract infections in men
Local Anesthetic/Vasoconstrictor Precautions No information available to require special precautions
Effects on Dental Treatment No significant effects or complications reported
Common Adverse Effects
1% to 10%:
   Central nervous system: Headache (47%), dizziness (1%)
   Dermatologic: Rash (1%)
   Gastrointestinal: Diarrhea (2% to 10%), nausea (4%), epigastric discomfort (1%), abdominal pain
   Genitourinary: Vaginitis
   Neuromuscular & skeletal: Weakness (1%)
Mechanism of Action As a phosphoric acid derivative, fosfomycin inhibits bacterial wall synthesis (bactericidal) by inactivating the enzyme, pyruvyl transferase, which is critical in the synthesis of cell walls by bacteria; the tromethamine salt is preferable to the calcium salt due to its superior absorption
Drug Interactions
   Decreased Effect: Antacids or calcium salts may cause precipitate formation and decrease fosfomycin absorption. Increased gastrointestinal motility due to metoclopramide may lower fosfomycin tromethamine serum concentrations and urinary excretion. This drug interaction possibly could be extrapolated to other medications which increase gastrointestinal motility.
Pharmacodynamics/Kinetics
   Absorption: Well absorbed

Distribution: V_d: 2 L/kg; high concentrations in urine; well into other tissues; crosses maximally into CSF with inflamed meninges

Protein binding: <3%

Bioavailability: 34% to 58%

Half-life elimination: 4-8 hours; Cl_{cr} <10 mL/minute: 50 hours

Time to peak, serum: 2 hours

Excretion: Urine (as unchanged drug); high urinary levels (100 mcg/mL) persist for >48 hours

Pregnancy Risk Factor B

Fosfomycin Tromethamine see Fosfomycin on page 706

Fosinopril (foe SIN oh pril)

Related Information
Cardiovascular Diseases on page 1636

U.S. Brand Names Monopril®

Canadian Brand Names Apo-Fosinopril®; Monopril®; Novo-Fosinopril; ratio-Fosinopril

Generic Available Yes

Synonyms Fosinopril Sodium

Pharmacologic Category Angiotensin-Converting Enzyme (ACE) Inhibitor

Use Treatment of hypertension, either alone or in combination with other antihypertensive agents; treatment of congestive heart failure, left ventricular dysfunction after myocardial infarction

Local Anesthetic/Vasoconstrictor Precautions No information available to require special precautions

Effects on Dental Treatment Key adverse event(s) related to dental treatment: Orthostatic hypotension.

Common Adverse Effects Note: Frequency ranges include data from hypertension and heart failure trials. Higher rates of adverse reactions have generally been noted in patients with CHF. However, the frequency of adverse effects associated with placebo is also increased in this population.

>10%: Central nervous system: Dizziness (2% to 12%)

1% to 10%:
Cardiovascular: Orthostatic hypotension (1% to 2%), palpitation (1%)
Central nervous system: Dizziness (1% to 2%; up to 12% in CHF patients), headache (3%), fatigue (1% to 2%)
Endocrine & metabolic: Hyperkalemia (2.6%)
Gastrointestinal: Diarrhea (2%), nausea/vomiting (1.2% to 2.2%)
Hepatic: Transaminases increased
Neuromuscular & skeletal: Musculoskeletal pain (<1% to 3%), noncardiac chest pain (<1% to 2%), weakness (1%)
Renal: Increased serum creatinine, worsening of renal function (in patients with bilateral renal artery stenosis or hypovolemia)
Respiratory: Cough (2% to 10%)
Miscellaneous: Upper respiratory infection (2%)

>1% but ≤ frequency in patients receiving placebo: Sexual dysfunction, fever, flu-like syndrome, dyspnea, rash, headache, insomnia

Other events reported with ACE inhibitors: Neutropenia, agranulocytosis, eosinophilic pneumonitis, cardiac arrest, pancytopenia, hemolytic anemia, anemia, aplastic anemia, thrombocytopenia, acute renal failure, hepatic failure, jaundice, symptomatic hyponatremia, bullous pemphigus, exfoliative dermatitis, Stevens-Johnson syndrome. In addition, a syndrome which may include fever, myalgia, arthralgia, interstitial nephritis, vasculitis, rash, eosinophilia and positive ANA, and elevated ESR has been reported for other ACE inhibitors.

Dosage Oral:
Children >50 kg: Hypertension: Initial: 5-10 mg once daily
Adults:
Hypertension: Initial: 10 mg/day; most patients are maintained on 20-40 mg/day. May need to divide the dose into two if trough effect is inadequate; discontinue the diuretic, if possible 2-3 days before initiation of therapy; resume diuretic therapy carefully, if needed.
Heart failure: Initial: 10 mg/day (5 mg if renal dysfunction present) and increase, as needed, to a maximum of 40 mg once daily over several weeks; usual dose: 20-40 mg/day. If hypotension, orthostasis, or azotemia occur during titration, consider decreasing concomitant diuretic dose, if any.
Dosing adjustment/comments in renal impairment: None needed since hepatobiliary elimination compensates adequately diminished renal elimination.
Hemodialysis: Moderately dialyzable (20% to 50%)
(Continued)

Fosinopril (Continued)

Mechanism of Action Competitive inhibitor of angiotensin-converting enzyme (ACE); prevents conversion of angiotensin I to angiotensin II, a potent vasoconstrictor; results in lower levels of angiotensin II which causes an increase in plasma renin activity and a reduction in aldosterone secretion; a CNS mechanism may also be involved in hypotensive effect as angiotensin II increases adrenergic outflow from CNS; vasoactive kallikreins may be decreased in conversion to active hormones by ACE inhibitors, thus reducing blood pressure

Contraindications Hypersensitivity to fosinopril or any component of the formulation; angioedema related to previous treatment with an ACE inhibitor; idiopathic or hereditary angioedema; bilateral renal artery stenosis; pregnancy (2nd and 3rd trimesters)

Warnings/Precautions Anaphylactic reactions can occur. Angioedema can occur at any time during treatment (especially following first dose). It may involve head and neck (potentially affecting the airway) or the intestine (presenting with abdominal pain). Prolonged monitoring may be required especially if tongue, glottis, or larynx are involved as they are associated with airway obstruction. Those with a history of airway surgery in this situation have a higher risk. Careful blood pressure monitoring (hypotension can occur especially in volume-depleted patients). Dosage adjustment needed in severe renal impairment (Cl_{cr} <10 mL/minute). Use with caution in hypovolemia; collagen vascular diseases; valvular stenosis (particularly aortic stenosis); hyperkalemia; or before, during, or immediately after anesthesia. Avoid rapid dosage escalation which may lead to renal insufficiency. Rare toxicities associated with ACE inhibitors include cholestatic jaundice (which may progress to hepatic necrosis) and neutropenia/agranulocytosis with myeloid hyperplasia. Hypersensitivity reactions may be seen during hemodialysis with high-flux dialysis membranes (eg, AN69). Hyperkalemia may rarely occur. If patient has renal impairment, then a baseline WBC with differential and serum creatinine should be evaluated and monitored closely during initial therapy. Use with caution in unilateral renal artery stenosis and pre-existing renal insufficiency.

Drug Interactions

Increased Effect/Toxicity: Potassium supplements, co-trimoxazole (high dose), angiotensin II receptor antagonists (eg, candesartan, losartan, irbesartan), or potassium-sparing diuretics (amiloride, spironolactone, triamterene) may result in elevated serum potassium levels when combined with fosinopril. ACE inhibitor effects may be increased by phenothiazines or probenecid (increases levels of captopril). ACE inhibitors may increase serum concentrations/effects of lithium.

Diuretics have additive hypotensive effects with ACE inhibitors, and hypovolemia increases the potential for adverse renal effects of ACE inhibitors. In patients with compromised renal function, coadministration with NSAIDs may result in further deterioration of renal function. Allopurinol and ACE inhibitors may cause a higher risk of hypersensitivity reaction when taken concurrently.

Decreased Effect: Aspirin (high dose) may reduce the therapeutic effects of ACE inhibitors; at low dosages this does not appear to be significant. Rifampin may decrease the effect of ACE inhibitors. Antacids may decrease the bioavailability of ACE inhibitors (may be more likely to occur with captopril); separate administration times by 1-2 hours. NSAIDs, specifically indomethacin, may reduce the hypotensive effects of ACE inhibitors. More likely to occur in low renin or volume dependent hypertensive patients.

Ethanol/Nutrition/Herb Interactions Herb/Nutraceutical: Avoid dong quai if using for hypertension (has estrogenic activity). Avoid ephedra, garlic, yohimbe, ginseng (may worsen hypertension).

Dietary Considerations Should not take a potassium salt supplement without the advice of healthcare provider.

Pharmacodynamics/Kinetics

Onset of action: 1 hour
Duration: 24 hours
Absorption: 36%
Protein binding: 95%
Metabolism: Prodrug, hydrolyzed to its active metabolite fosinoprilat by intestinal wall and hepatic esterases
Bioavailability: 36%
Half-life elimination, serum (fosinoprilat): 12 hours
Time to peak, serum: ~3 hours
Excretion: Urine and feces (as fosinoprilat and other metabolites in roughly equal proportions, 45% to 50%)

Pregnancy Risk Factor C (1st trimester)/D (2nd and 3rd trimesters)

Dosage Forms TAB: 10 mg, 20 mg, 40 mg

Fosinopril and Hydrochlorothiazide
(foe SIN oh pril & hye droe klor oh THYE a zide)

Related Information
Fosinopril *on page 707*
Hydrochlorothiazide *on page 776*

U.S. Brand Names Monopril-HCT®

Canadian Brand Names Monopril-HCT®

Generic Available Yes

Synonyms Hydrochlorothiazide and Fosinopril

Pharmacologic Category Antihypertensive Agent, Combination

Use Treatment of hypertension; not indicated for first-line treatment

Local Anesthetic/Vasoconstrictor Precautions No information available to require special precautions

Effects on Dental Treatment No significant effects or complications reported

Common Adverse Effects

2% to 10%:

Central nervous system: Headache (7%, less than placebo), fatigue (4%), dizziness (3%), orthostatic hypotension (2%)

Neuromuscular & skeletal: Musculoskeletal pain (2%)

Respiratory: Cough (6%), upper respiratory infection (2%, less than placebo)

<2%: Abdominal pain, angioedema, breast mass, BUN elevation (similar to placebo), chest pain, creatinine elevation (similar to placebo), depression, diarrhea, dyspepsia, dysuria, edema, eosinophilia, esophagitis, fever, flushing, gastritis, gout, heartburn, hepatic necrosis, leukopenia, libido change, liver function test elevations (transaminases, LDH, alkaline phosphatase, serum bilirubin), muscle cramps, myalgia, nausea, neutropenia, numbness, paresthesia, pharyngitis, pruritus, rash, rhinitis, sexual dysfunction, sinus congestion, somnolence, syncope, tinnitus, urinary frequency, urinary tract infection, viral infection, vomiting, weakness

Other adverse events reported with **ACE inhibitors:** Aplastic anemia, bullous pemphigus, cardiac arrest, cholestatic jaundice, exfoliative dermatitis, hemolytic anemia, hyperkalemia, pancreatitis, pancytopenia, photosensitivity; syndrome that may include one or more of arthralgia/arthritis, vasculitis, serositis, myalgia, fever, rash or other dermopathy, positive ANA titer, leukocytosis, eosinophilia, and elevated ESR; thrombocytopenia

Other adverse events reported with **hydrochlorothiazide:** Agranulocytosis, anaphylactic reactions, anorexia, blurred vision (transient), constipation, cramping, glucosuria, hemolytic anemia, hypercalcemia, hyperglycemia, hyperuricemia, hypokalemia, jaundice (intrahepatic cholestatic), lightheadedness, muscle spasm, necrotizing angiitis, pancreatitis, photosensitivity, pneumonitis, pulmonary edema, purpura, respiratory distress, restlessness, sialadenitis, SLE, Stevens-Johnson syndrome, urticaria, vertigo, xanthopsia

Mechanism of Action Fosinopril is a competitive inhibitor of angiotensin-converting enzyme (ACE); prevents conversion of angiotensin I to angiotensin II, a potent vasoconstrictor; results in lower levels of angiotensin II which causes an increase in plasma renin activity and a reduction in aldosterone secretion; a CNS mechanism may also be involved in hypotensive effect as angiotensin II increases adrenergic outflow from CNS; vasoactive kallikreins may be decreased in conversion to active hormones by ACE inhibitors, thus reducing blood pressure. Hydrochlorothiazide inhibits sodium reabsorption in the distal tubules causing increased excretion of sodium and water as well as potassium and hydrogen ions.

Drug Interactions

Increased Effect/Toxicity: Alpha$_1$ blockers, diuretics increase hypotension. Beta blockers may increase hyperglycemic effect. Cyclosporine may increase risk of gout or renal toxicity. Risk of lithium toxicity may be increased. Mercaptopurine may increase risk of neutropenia. Digoxin and neuromuscular-blocking agents: Effects may be increased with hypokalemia. Potassium-sparing diuretics, potassium supplements, trimethoprim may increase risk of hyperkalemia.

Decreased Effect: Aspirin, NSAIDs may decrease antihypertensive effect. Antacids, cholestyramine, colestipol may decrease absorption.

Pharmacodynamics/Kinetics See individual agents.

Pregnancy Risk Factor C (1st trimester); D (2nd and 3rd trimester)

Fosinopril Sodium *see* Fosinopril *on page 707*

Fosphenytoin (FOS fen i toyn)

Related Information
Phenytoin *on page 1228*
U.S. Brand Names Cerebyx®
Canadian Brand Names Cerebyx®
Generic Available No
Synonyms Fosphenytoin Sodium
Pharmacologic Category Anticonvulsant, Hydantoin
Use Used for the control of generalized convulsive status epilepticus and prevention and treatment of seizures occurring during neurosurgery; indicated for short-term parenteral administration when other means of phenytoin administration are unavailable, inappropriate or deemed less advantageous (the safety and effectiveness of fosphenytoin in this use has not been systematically evaluated for more than 5 days)

Local Anesthetic/Vasoconstrictor Precautions No information available to require special precautions

Effects on Dental Treatment No significant effects or complications reported

Common Adverse Effects The more important adverse clinical events caused by the I.V. use of fosphenytoin or phenytoin are cardiovascular collapse and/or central nervous system depression. Hypotension can occur when either drug is administered rapidly by the I.V. route. Do not exceed a rate of 150 mg phenytoin equivalent/minute when administering fosphenytoin.

The adverse clinical events most commonly observed with the use of fosphenytoin in clinical trials were nystagmus, dizziness, pruritus, paresthesia, headache, somnolence, and ataxia. Paresthesia and pruritus were seen more often following fosphenytoin (versus phenytoin) administration and occurred more often with I.V. fosphenytoin than with I.M. administration. These events were dose- and rate-related (doses ≥15 mg/kg at a rate of 150 mg/minute). These sensations, generally described as itching, burning, or tingling is usually not at the infusion site. The location of the discomfort varied with the groin mentioned most frequently. The paresthesia and pruritus were transient events that occurred within several minutes of the start of infusion and generally resolved within 10 minutes after completion of infusion.

Transient pruritus, tinnitus, nystagmus, somnolence, and ataxia occurred 2-3 times more often at doses ≥15 mg/kg and rates ≥150 mg/minute.

I.V. administration (maximum dose/rate):
>10%:
Central nervous system: Nystagmus, dizziness, somnolence, ataxia
Dermatologic: Pruritus
1% to 10%:
Cardiovascular: Hypotension, vasodilation, tachycardia
Central nervous system: Stupor, incoordination, paresthesia, extrapyramidal syndrome, tremor, agitation, hypoesthesia, dysarthria, vertigo, brain edema, headache
Gastrointestinal: Nausea, tongue disorder, dry mouth, vomiting
Neuromuscular & skeletal: Pelvic pain, muscle weakness, back pain
Ocular: Diplopia, amblyopia
Otic: Tinnitus, deafness
Miscellaneous: Taste perversion
I.M. administration (substitute for oral phenytoin):
1% to 10%:
Central nervous system: Nystagmus, tremor, ataxia, headache, incoordination, somnolence, dizziness, paresthesia, reflexes decreased
Dermatologic: Pruritus
Gastrointestinal: Nausea, vomiting
Hematologic/lymphatic: Ecchymosis
Neuromuscular & skeletal: Muscle weakness

Mechanism of Action Diphosphate ester salt of phenytoin which acts as a water soluble prodrug of phenytoin; after administration, plasma esterases convert fosphenytoin to phosphate, formaldehyde and phenytoin as the active moiety; phenytoin works by stabilizing neuronal membranes and decreasing seizure activity by increasing efflux or decreasing influx of sodium ions across cell membranes in the motor cortex during generation of nerve impulses

Drug Interactions
Cytochrome P450 Effect: As phenytoin: **Substrate** of CYP2C9 (major), 2C19 (major), 3A4 (minor); **Induces** CYP2B6 (strong), 2C8 (strong), 2C9 (strong), 2C19 (strong), 3A4 (strong)
Increased Effect/Toxicity: The sedative effects of phenytoin may be additive with other CNS depressants including ethanol, barbiturates, sedatives,

antidepressants, narcotic analgesics, and benzodiazepines. Selected anticonvulsants (felbamate, gabapentin, and topiramate) have been reported to increase phenytoin levels/effects. In addition, serum phenytoin concentrations may be increased by allopurinol, amiodarone, calcium channel blockers (including diltiazem and nifedipine), cimetidine, disulfiram, methylphenidate, metronidazole, omeprazole, selective serotonin reuptake inhibitors (SSRIs), ticlopidine, tricyclic antidepressants, trazodone, and trimethoprim. Case reports indicate ciprofloxacin may increase or decrease serum phenytoin concentrations.

The levels/effects of phenytoin may be increased by delavirdine, fluconazole, fluvoxamine, gemfibrozil, isoniazid, ketoconazole, nicardipine, NSAIDs, omeprazole, pioglitazone, sulfonamides, ticlopidine, and other CYP2C9 or 2C19 inhibitors.

Phenytoin enhances the conversion of primidone to phenobarbital resulting in elevated phenobarbital serum concentrations. Concurrent use of acetazolamide with phenytoin may result in an increased risk of osteomalacia. Concurrent use of phenytoin and lithium has resulted in lithium intoxication. Valproic acid (and sulfisoxazole) may displace phenytoin from binding sites; valproic acid may increase, decrease, or have no effect on phenytoin serum concentrations. Phenytoin transiently increased the response to warfarin initially; this is followed by an inhibition of the hypoprothrombinemic response. Phenytoin may enhance the hepatotoxic potential of acetaminophen overdoses. Concurrent use of dopamine and intravenous phenytoin may lead to an increased risk of hypotension.

Decreased Effect: Phenytoin may enhance the metabolism of estrogen and/or oral contraceptives, decreasing their clinical effect; an alternative method of contraception should be considered. Phenytoin may increase the metabolism of anticonvulsants including barbiturates, carbamazepine, ethosuximide, felbamate, lamotrigine, tiagabine, topiramate, and zonisamide. Valproic acid may increase, decrease, or have no effect on phenytoin serum concentrations. Phenytoin may also decrease the serum concentrations/effects of some antiarrhythmics (disopyramide, propafenone, quinidine, quetiapine) and tricyclic antidepressants may be reduced by phenytoin. Phenytoin may enhance the metabolism of doxycycline, decreasing its clinical effect; higher dosages may be required. Phenytoin may increase the metabolism of chloramphenicol or itraconazole.

Phenytoin may decrease the levels/effects of amiodarone, benzodiazepines, bupropion, calcium channel blockers, carbamazepine, citalopram, clarithromycin, cyclosporine, efavirenz, erythromycin, estrogens, fluoxetine, glimepiride, glipizide, losartan, methsuximide, mirtazapine, nateglinide, nefazodone, nevirapine, phenytoin, pioglitazone, promethazine, propranolol, protease inhibitors, proton pump inhibitors, rosiglitazone, selegiline, sertraline, sulfonamides, tacrolimus, venlafaxine. voriconazole, warfarin, zafirlukast, and other CYP2B6, 2C8, 2C9, 2C19, or 3A4 substrates.

The levels/effects of phenytoin may be decreased by aminoglutethimide, carbamazepine, phenobarbital, rifampin, rifapentine, secobarbital, and other CYP2C8/9 or 2C19 inducers. Clozapine and vigabatrin may reduce phenytoin serum concentrations. Case reports indicate ciprofloxacin may increase or decrease serum phenytoin concentrations. Dexamethasone may decrease serum phenytoin concentrations. Replacement of folic acid has been reported to increase the metabolism of phenytoin, decreasing its serum concentrations and/or increasing seizures.

Initially, phenytoin increases the response to warfarin; this is followed by a decrease in response to warfarin. Phenytoin may inhibit the anti-Parkinson effect of levodopa. The duration of neuromuscular blockade from neuromuscular-blocking agents may be decreased by phenytoin. Phenytoin may enhance the metabolism of methadone resulting in methadone withdrawal. Phenytoin may decrease serum levels/effects of digitalis glycosides, theophylline, and thyroid hormones.

Several chemotherapeutic agents have been associated with a decrease in serum phenytoin levels; includes cisplatin, bleomycin, carmustine, methotrexate, and vinblastine. Enzyme-inducing anticonvulsant therapy may reduce the effectiveness of some chemotherapy regimens (specifically in ALL). Teniposide and methotrexate may be cleared more rapidly in these patients.

Pharmacodynamics/Kinetics Also refer to Phenytoin monograph for additional information.

Protein binding: Fosphenytoin: 95% to 99% to albumin; can displace phenytoin and increase free fraction (up to 30% unbound) during the period required for conversion of fosphenytoin to phenytoin

(Continued)

Fosphenytoin *(Continued)*

Metabolism: Fosphenytoin is rapidly converted via hydrolysis to phenytoin; phenytoin is metabolized in the liver and forms metabolites

Bioavailability: I.M.: Fosphenytoin: 100%

Half-life elimination:

Fosphenytoin: 15 minutes

Phenytoin: Variable (mean: 12-29 hours); kinetics of phenytoin are saturable

Time to peak: Conversion to phenytoin: Following I.V. administration (maximum rate of administration): 15 minutes; following I.M. administration, peak phenytoin levels are reached in 3 hours

Excretion: Phenytoin: Urine (as inactive metabolites)

Pregnancy Risk Factor D

Fosphenytoin Sodium see Fosphenytoin on page 710

Fosrenol™ see Lanthanum on page 899

Fostex® 10% BPO [OTC] see Benzoyl Peroxide on page 194

Fototar® [OTC] see Coal Tar on page 383

Fragmin® see Dalteparin on page 418

Freezone® [OTC] see Salicylic Acid on page 1374

Frova® see Frovatriptan on page 712

Frovatriptan *(froe va TRIP tan)*

U.S. Brand Names Frova®

Generic Available No

Synonyms Frovatriptan Succinate

Pharmacologic Category Antimigraine Agent; Serotonin 5-HT$_{1B, 1D}$ Receptor Agonist

Use Acute treatment of migraine with or without aura in adults

Local Anesthetic/Vasoconstrictor Precautions No information available to require special precautions

Effects on Dental Treatment Key adverse event(s) related to dental treatment: Xerostomia (normal salivary flow resumes upon discontinuation).

Common Adverse Effects 1% to 10%:

Cardiovascular: Chest pain (2%), flushing (4%), palpitation (1%)

Central nervous system: Dizziness (8%), fatigue (5%), headache (4%), hot or cold sensation (3%), anxiety (1%), dysesthesia (1%), hypoesthesia (1%), insomnia (1%), pain (1%)

Gastrointestinal: Hyposalivation (3%), dyspepsia (2%), abdominal pain (1%), diarrhea (1%), vomiting (1%)

Neuromuscular & skeletal: Paresthesia (4%), skeletal pain (3%)

Ocular: Visual abnormalities (1%)

Otic: Tinnitus (1%)

Respiratory: Rhinitis (1%), sinusitis (1%)

Miscellaneous: Diaphoresis (1%)

Dosage Oral: Adults: Migraine: 2.5 mg; if headache recurs, a second dose may be given if first dose provided some relief and at least 2 hours have elapsed since the first dose (maximum daily dose: 7.5 mg)

Dosage adjustment in renal impairment: No adjustment necessary

Dosage adjustment in hepatic impairment: No adjustment necessary in mild to moderate hepatic impairment; use with caution in severe impairment

Mechanism of Action Selective agonist for serotonin (5-HT$_{1B}$ and 5-HT$_{1D}$ receptor) in cranial arteries to cause vasoconstriction and reduces sterile inflammation associated with antidromic neuronal transmission correlating with relief of migraine.

Contraindications Hypersensitivity to frovatriptan or any component of the formulation; patients with ischemic heart disease or signs or symptoms of ischemic heart disease (including Prinzmetal's angina, angina pectoris, myocardial infarction, silent myocardial ischemia); cerebrovascular syndromes (including strokes, transient ischemic attacks); peripheral vascular syndromes (including ischemic bowel disease); uncontrolled hypertension; use within 24 hours of ergotamine derivatives; use within 24 hours of another 5-HT$_1$ agonist; management of hemiplegic or basilar migraine; prophylactic treatment of migraine; severe hepatic impairment

Warnings/Precautions Not intended for migraine prophylaxis, or treatment of cluster headaches, hemiplegic or basilar migraines. Cardiac events, cerebral/subarachnoid hemorrhage, and stroke have been reported with 5-HT$_1$ agonist administration. May cause vasospastic reactions resulting in colonic, peripheral, or coronary ischemia. Do not give to patients with risk factors for CAD until a cardiovascular evaluation has been performed; if evaluation is satisfactory, the healthcare provider should administer the first dose and cardiovascular status should be periodically evaluated. Significant elevation in blood pressure, including hypertensive crisis, has also been reported on rare occasions in patients using other 5-HT$_{1D}$ agonists with and without a history of hypertension. Use with caution in patients with history of seizure disorder. Safety and efficacy in pediatric patients have not been established

Drug Interactions
  Cytochrome P450 Effect: **Substrate** of CYP1A2 (minor)
  Increased Effect/Toxicity: The effects of frovatriptan may be increased by estrogen derivatives and propranolol. Ergot derivatives may increase the effects of frovatriptan (do not use within 24 hours of each other). SSRIs may exhibit additive toxicity with frovatriptan or other serotonin agonists (eg, antidepressants, dextromethorphan, tramadol) leading to serotonin syndrome.
Ethanol/Nutrition/Herb Interactions Food: Food does not affect frovatriptan bioavailability.
Pharmacodynamics/Kinetics
  Distribution: Male: 4.2 L/kg; Female: 3.0 L/kg
  Protein binding: 15%
  Metabolism: Primarily hepatic via CYP1A2
  Bioavailability: 20% to 30%
  Half-life elimination: 26 hours
  Time to peak: 2-4 hours
  Excretion: Feces (62%); urine (32%)
Pregnancy Risk Factor C
Dosage Forms TAB: 2.5 mg

Frovatriptan Succinate *see* Frovatriptan *on page 712*

Fructose, Dextrose, and Phosphoric Acid
(FRUK tose, DEKS trose, & foss FOR ik AS id)

U.S. Brand Names Emetrol® [OTC]; Especol® [OTC]; Formula EM [OTC]; Kalmz [OTC]; Nausea Relief [OTC]; Nausetrol® [OTC]
Generic Available Yes
Synonyms Dextrose, Levulose and Phosphoric Acid; Levulose, Dextrose and Phosphoric Acid; Phosphorated Carbohydrate Solution; Phosphoric Acid, Levulose and Dextrose
Pharmacologic Category Antiemetic
Use Relief of nausea associated with upset stomach that occurs with intestinal flu, food indiscretions, and emotional upsets
Unlabeled/Investigational Use Relief of nausea associated with pregnancy
Local Anesthetic/Vasoconstrictor Precautions No information available to require special precautions
Effects on Dental Treatment No significant effects or complications reported
Common Adverse Effects 1% to 10%: Gastrointestinal: Abdominal pain, diarrhea

Frusemide *see* Furosemide *on page 715*
FS *see* Fibrin Sealant Kit *on page 653*
FTC *see* Emtricitabine *on page 536*
FU *see* Fluorouracil *on page 674*
5-FU *see* Fluorouracil *on page 674*
FUDR® *see* Floxuridine *on page 659*
5-FUDR *see* Floxuridine *on page 659*

Fulvestrant (fool VES trant)

U.S. Brand Names Faslodex®
Generic Available No
Synonyms ICI-182,780; Zeneca 182,780; ZM-182,780
Pharmacologic Category Antineoplastic Agent, Estrogen Receptor Antagonist
Use Treatment of hormone receptor positive metastatic breast cancer in postmenopausal women with disease progression following antiestrogen therapy.
Unlabeled/Investigational Use Endometriosis; uterine bleeding
Local Anesthetic/Vasoconstrictor Precautions No information available to require special precautions
Effects on Dental Treatment No significant effects or complications reported
Common Adverse Effects
  >10%:
    Cardiovascular: Vasodilation (18%)
    Central nervous system: Pain (19%), headache (15%)
  (Continued)

Fulvestrant *(Continued)*

Endocrine & metabolic: Hot flushes (19% to 24%)

Gastrointestinal: Nausea (26%), vomiting (13%), constipation (13%), diarrhea (12%), abdominal pain (12%)

Local: Injection site reaction (11%)

Neuromuscular & skeletal: Weakness (23%), bone pain (16%), back pain (14%)

Respiratory: Pharyngitis (16%), dyspnea (15%)

1% to 10%:

Cardiovascular: Edema (9%), chest pain (7%)

Central nervous system: Dizziness (7%), insomnia (7%), paresthesia (6%), fever (6%), depression (6%), anxiety (5%)

Dermatologic: Rash (7%)

Gastrointestinal: Anorexia (9%), weight gain (1% to 2%)

Genitourinary: Pelvic pain (10%), urinary tract infection (6%), vaginitis (2% to 3%)

Hematologic: Anemia (5%)

Neuromuscular and skeletal: Arthritis (3%)

Respiratory: Cough (10%)

Miscellaneous: Diaphoresis increased (5%)

Mechanism of Action Steroidal compound which competitively binds to estrogen receptors on tumors and other tissue targets, producing a nuclear complex that decreases DNA synthesis and inhibits estrogen effects. Fulvestrant has no estrogen-receptor agonist activity. Causes down-regulation of estrogen receptors and inhibits tumor growth.

Drug Interactions

Cytochrome P450 Effect: Substrate of CYP3A4 (minor)

Pharmacodynamics/Kinetics

Duration: I.M.: Plasma levels maintained for at least 1 month

Distribution: V_d: 3-5 L/kg

Protein binding: 99%

Metabolism: Hepatic via multiple pathways (CYP3A4 substrate, relative contribution to metabolism unknown)

Bioavailability: Oral: Poor

Half-life elimination: ~40 days

Time to peak, plasma: I.M.: 7-9 days

Excretion: Feces (>90%); urine (<1%)

Pregnancy Risk Factor D

Fungi-Guard [OTC] *see* Tolnaftate *on page 1506*

Fungi-Nail® [OTC] *see* Undecylenic Acid and Derivatives *on page 1550*

Fung-O® [OTC] *see* Salicylic Acid *on page 1374*

Fungoid® Tincture [OTC] *see* Miconazole *on page 1039*

Furadantin® *see* Nitrofurantoin *on page 1119*

Furazolidone *(fyoor a ZOE li done)*

Canadian Brand Names Furoxone®

Mexican Brand Names Furoxona®; Fuxol®; Salmocide®

Generic Available No

Synonyms Furoxone

Pharmacologic Category Antiprotozoal

Use Treatment of bacterial or protozoal diarrhea and enteritis caused by susceptible organisms *Giardia lamblia* and *Vibrio cholerae*

Local Anesthetic/Vasoconstrictor Precautions No information available to require special precautions

Effects on Dental Treatment No significant effects or complications reported

Common Adverse Effects

>10%: Genitourinary: Discoloration of urine (dark yellow to brown)

1% to 10%:

Central nervous system: Headache

Gastrointestinal: Abdominal pain, diarrhea, nausea, vomiting

Restrictions Not available in U.S.

Mechanism of Action Inhibits several vital enzymatic reactions causing antibacterial and antiprotozoal action

Drug Interactions

Increased Effect/Toxicity: Increased effect with sympathomimetic amines, tricyclic antidepressants, tyramine-containing foods, MAO inhibitors, meperidine, anorexiants, dextromethorphan, fluoxetine, paroxetine, sertraline, and trazodone. Increased effect/toxicity of levodopa. Disulfiram-like reaction with alcohol.

Pharmacodynamics/Kinetics
Absorption: Poor
Excretion: Urine (33% as active drug and metabolites)

Pregnancy Risk Factor C

Furazosin *see Prazosin on page 1267*

Furosemide (fyoor OH se mide)

Related Information
Cardiovascular Diseases *on page 1636*

U.S. Brand Names Lasix®

Canadian Brand Names Apo-Furosemide®; Lasix®; Lasix® Special; Novo-Semide

Mexican Brand Names Edenol®; Lasix®; Selectofur®[tabs]; Zafimida®

Generic Available Yes

Synonyms Frusemide

Pharmacologic Category Diuretic, Loop

Use Management of edema associated with congestive heart failure and hepatic or renal disease; alone or in combination with antihypertensives in treatment of hypertension

Local Anesthetic/Vasoconstrictor Precautions No information available to require special precautions

Effects on Dental Treatment No significant effects or complications reported

Common Adverse Effects Frequency not defined.

Cardiovascular: Orthostatic hypotension, necrotizing angiitis, thrombophlebitis, chronic aortitis, acute hypotension, sudden death from cardiac arrest (with I.V. or I.M. administration)

Central nervous system: Paresthesias, vertigo, dizziness, lightheadedness, headache, blurred vision, xanthopsia , fever, restlessness

Dermatologic: Exfoliative dermatitis, erythema multiforme, purpura, photosensitivity, urticaria, rash, pruritus, cutaneous vasculitis

Endocrine & metabolic: Hyperglycemia, hyperuricemia, hypokalemia, hypochloremia, metabolic alkalosis, hypocalcemia, hypomagnesemia, gout, hyponatremia

Gastrointestinal: Nausea, vomiting, anorexia, oral and gastric irritation, cramping, diarrhea, constipation, pancreatitis, intrahepatic cholestatic jaundice, ischemia hepatitis

Genitourinary: Urinary bladder spasm, urinary frequency

Hematological: Aplastic anemia (rare), thrombocytopenia, agranulocytosis (rare), hemolytic anemia, leukopenia, anemia, purpura

Neuromuscular & skeletal: Muscle spasm, weakness

Otic: Hearing impairment (reversible or permanent with rapid I.V. or I.M. administration), tinnitus, reversible deafness (with rapid I.V. or I.M. administration)

Renal: Vasculitis, allergic interstitial nephritis, glycosuria, fall in glomerular filtration rate and renal blood flow (due to overdiuresis), transient rise in BUN

Miscellaneous: Anaphylaxis (rare), exacerbate or activate systemic lupus erythematosus

Dosage
Infants and Children:
Oral: 1-2 mg/kg/dose increased in increments of 1 mg/kg/dose with each succeeding dose until a satisfactory effect is achieved to a maximum of 6 mg/kg/dose no more frequently than 6 hours.

I.M., I.V.: 1 mg/kg/dose, increasing by each succeeding dose at 1 mg/kg/dose at intervals of 6-12 hours until a satisfactory response up to 6 mg/kg/dose.

Adults:
Oral: 20-80 mg/dose initially increased in increments of 20-40 mg/dose at intervals of 6-8 hours; usual maintenance dose interval is twice daily or every day; may be titrated up to 600 mg/day with severe edematous states.

Hypertension (JNC 7): 20-80 mg/day in 2 divided doses

I.M., I.V.: 20-40 mg/dose, may be repeated in 1-2 hours as needed and increased by 20 mg/dose until the desired effect has been obtained. Usual dosing interval: 6-12 hours; for acute pulmonary edema, the usual dose is 40 mg I.V. over 1-2 minutes. If not adequate, may increase dose to 80 mg. **Note:** ACC/AHA 2005 guidelines for chronic congestive heart failure recommend a maximum single dose of 160-200 mg.

Continuous I.V. infusion: Initial I.V. bolus dose of 0.1 mg/kg followed by continuous I.V. infusion doses of 0.1 mg/kg/hour doubled every 2 hours to a maximum of 0.4 mg/kg/hour if urine output is <1 mL/kg/hour have been found to be effective and result in a lower daily requirement of furosemide than with intermittent dosing. Other studies have used a rate of ≤4 mg/minute as a continuous I.V. infusion. **Note:** ACC/AHA 2005 guidelines for

(Continued)

715

Furosemide *(Continued)*

chronic congestive heart failure recommend 40 mg I.V. load then 10-40 mg/hour infusion.

Refractory heart failure: Oral, I.V.: Doses up to 8 g/day have been used.

Elderly: Oral, I.M., I.V.: Initial: 20 mg/day; increase slowly to desired response.

Dosing adjustment/comments in renal impairment: Acute renal failure: High doses (up to 1-3 g/day - oral/I.V.) have been used to initiate desired response; avoid use in oliguric states.

Dialysis: Not removed by hemo- or peritoneal dialysis; supplemental dose is not necessary.

Dosing adjustment/comments in hepatic disease: Diminished natriuretic effect with increased sensitivity to hypokalemia and volume depletion in cirrhosis; monitor effects, particularly with high doses.

Mechanism of Action Inhibits reabsorption of sodium and chloride in the ascending loop of Henle and distal renal tubule, interfering with the chloride-binding cotransport system, thus causing increased excretion of water, sodium, chloride, magnesium, and calcium

Contraindications Hypersensitivity to furosemide, any component, or sulfonylureas; anuria; patients with hepatic coma or in states of severe electrolyte depletion until the condition improves or is corrected

Warnings/Precautions Loop diuretics are potent diuretics; close medical supervision and dose evaluation is required to prevent fluid and electrolyte imbalance; use caution with other nephrotoxic or ototoxic drugs; use caution in patients with known hypersensitivity to sulfonamides or thiazides (due to possible cross-sensitivity; avoid in history of severe reactions).

Chemical similarities are present among sulfonamides, sulfonylureas, carbonic anhydrase inhibitors, thiazides, and loop diuretics (except ethacrynic acid). Use in patients with sulfonylurea allergy is specifically contraindicated in product labeling, however, a risk of cross-reaction exists in patients with allergy to any of these compounds; avoid use when previous reaction has been severe.

Drug Interactions

Increased Effect/Toxicity: Furosemide-induced hypokalemia may predispose to digoxin toxicity and may increase the risk of arrhythmia with drugs which may prolong QT interval, including type Ia and type III antiarrhythmic agents, cisapride, and some quinolones (sparfloxacin, gatifloxacin, and moxifloxacin). The risk of toxicity from lithium and salicylates (high dose) may be increased by loop diuretics. Hypotensive effects and/or adverse renal effects of ACE inhibitors and NSAIDs are potentiated by furosemide-induced hypovolemia. The effects of peripheral adrenergic-blocking drugs or ganglionic blockers may be increased by furosemide.

Furosemide may increase the risk of ototoxicity with other ototoxic agents (aminoglycosides, cis-platinum), especially in patients with renal dysfunction. Synergistic diuretic effects occur with thiazide-type diuretics. Diuretics tend to be synergistic with other antihypertensive agents, and hypotension may occur.

Decreased Effect: Indomethacin, aspirin, phenobarbital, phenytoin, and NSAIDs may reduce natriuretic and hypotensive effects of furosemide. Colestipol, cholestyramine, and sucralfate may reduce the effect of furosemide; separate administration by 2 hours. Furosemide may antagonize the effect of skeletal muscle relaxants (tubocurarine). Glucose tolerance may be decreased by furosemide, requiring an adjustment in the dose of hypoglycemic agents. Metformin may decrease furosemide concentrations.

Ethanol/Nutrition/Herb Interactions

Food: Furosemide serum levels may be decreased if taken with food.

Herb/Nutraceutical: Avoid dong quai if using for hypertension (has estrogenic activity). Avoid ephedra, yohimbe, ginseng (may worsen hypertension). Limit intake of natural licorice. Avoid garlic (may have increased antihypertensive effect).

Dietary Considerations May cause a potassium loss; potassium supplement or dietary changes may be required. Administer on an empty stomach. May be administered with food or milk if GI distress occurs. Do not mix with acidic solutions.

Pharmacodynamics/Kinetics

Onset of action: Diuresis: Oral: 30-60 minutes; I.M.: 30 minutes; I.V.: ~5 minutes

Peak effect: Oral: 1-2 hours

Duration: Oral: 6-8 hours; I.V.: 2 hours

Absorption: Oral: 60% to 67%

Protein binding: >98%

Metabolism: Minimally hepatic

Half-life elimination: Normal renal function: 0.5-1.1 hours; End-stage renal disease: 9 hours

Excretion: Urine (Oral: 50%, I.V.: 80%) within 24 hours; feces (as unchanged drug); nonrenal clearance prolonged in renal impairment

Pregnancy Risk Factor C

Dosage Forms INJ, solution: 10 mg/mL (2 mL, 4 mL, 8 mL, 10 mL). **SOLN, oral:** 10 mg/mL (60 mL, 120 mL); 40 mg/5 mL (5 mL, 500 mL). **TAB** (Lasix®): 20 mg, 40 mg, 80 mg

Furoxone *see* Furazolidone *on page 714*

Fuzeon™ *see* Enfuvirtide *on page 541*

Gabapentin (GA ba pen tin)

U.S. Brand Names Neurontin®
Canadian Brand Names Apo-Gabapentin®; Gen-Gabapentin; Neurontin®; Novo-Gabapentin; Nu-Gabapentin; PMS-Gabapentin
Mexican Brand Names Neurontin®
Generic Available Yes: Capsule, tablet
Pharmacologic Category Anticonvulsant, Miscellaneous
Dental Use Neuropathic pain (consult with physician)
Use Adjunct for treatment of partial seizures with and without secondary generalized seizures in patients >12 years of age with epilepsy; adjunct for treatment of partial seizures in pediatric patients 3-12 years of age; management of postherpetic neuralgia (PHN) in adults
Unlabeled/Investigational Use Social phobia; chronic pain
Local Anesthetic/Vasoconstrictor Precautions No information available to require special precautions
Effects on Dental Treatment Key adverse event(s) related to dental treatment: Xerostomia (normal salivary flow resumes upon discontinuation), dry throat, and dental abnormalities.
Significant Adverse Effects As reported in patients >12 years of age, unless otherwise noted in children (3-12 years)

>10%:
Central nervous system: Somnolence (20%; children 8%), dizziness (17% to 28%; children 3%), ataxia (13%), fatigue (11%)
Miscellaneous: Viral infection (children 11%)

1% to 10%:
Cardiovascular: Peripheral edema (2% to 8%), vasodilatation (1%)
Central nervous system: Fever (children 10%), hostility (children 8%), emotional lability (children 4%), fatigue (children 3%), headache (3%), ataxia (3%), abnormal thinking (2% to 3%; children 2%), amnesia (2%), depression (2%), dysarthria (2%), nervousness (2%), abnormal coordination (1% to 2%), twitching (1%), hyperesthesia (1%)
Dermatologic: Pruritus (1%), rash (1%)
Endocrine & metabolic: Hyperglycemia (1%)
Gastrointestinal: Diarrhea (6%), nausea/vomiting (3% to 4%; children 8%), abdominal pain (3%), weight gain (adults and children 2% to 3%), dyspepsia (2%), flatulence (2%), dry throat (2%), xerostomia (2% to 5%), constipation (2% to 4%), dental abnormalities (2%), appetite stimulation (1%)
Genitourinary: Impotence (2%)
Hematologic: Leukopenia (1%), decreased WBC (1%)
Neuromuscular & skeletal: Tremor (7%), weakness (6%), hyperkinesia (children 3%), abnormal gait (2%), back pain (2%), myalgia (2%), fracture (1%)
Ocular: Nystagmus (8%), diplopia (1% to 6%), blurred vision (3% to 4%), conjunctivitis (1%)
Otic: Otitis media (1%)
Respiratory: Rhinitis (4%), bronchitis (children 3%), respiratory infection (children 3%), pharyngitis (1% to 3%), cough (2%)
Miscellaneous: Infection (5%)
Postmarketing and additional clinical reports (limited to important or life-threatening): Acute renal failure, anemia, angina, angioedema, aphasia, arrhythmias (various), aspiration pneumonia, blindness, bradycardia, bronchospasm, cerebrovascular accident, CNS tumors, coagulation defect, colitis, Cushingoid appearance, dyspnea, encephalopathy, facial paralysis, fecal incontinence, glaucoma, glycosuria, heart block, hearing loss, hematemesis, hematuria, hemiplegia, hemorrhage, hepatitis, hepatomegaly, hyper-/hypotension, hyperlipidemia, hyper-/hypothyroidism, hyper-/hypoventilation, gastroenteritis, heart failure, leukocytosis, liver function tests increased, local myoclonus, lymphadenopathy, lymphocytosis, meningismus, MI, migraine, nephrosis, nerve palsy, non-Hodgkin's lymphoma, ovarian failure, pulmonary
(Continued)

Gabapentin *(Continued)*

thrombosis, pericardial rub, pulmonary embolus, pericardial effusion, pericarditis, pancreatitis, peptic ulcer, purpura, paresthesia, palpitation, peripheral vascular disorder, pneumonia, psychosis, renal stone, retinopathy, skin necrosis, status epilepticus, subdural hematoma, syncope, tachycardia, thrombocytopenia, thrombophlebitis

Dental Usual Dosing

Pain (unlabeled use): Children >12 years and Adults: Oral: 300-1800 mg/day given in 3 divided doses has been the most common dosage range

Postherpetic neuralgia or neuropathic pain: Adults: Oral: Day 1: 300 mg, Day 2: 300 mg twice daily, Day 3: 300 mg 3 times/day; dose may be titrated as needed for pain relief (range: 1800-3600 mg/day, daily doses >1800 mg do not generally show greater benefit)

Dosage Oral:

Children: Anticonvulsant:

3-12 years: Initial: 10-15 mg/kg/day in 3 divided doses; titrate to effective dose over ~3 days; dosages of up to 50 mg/kg/day have been tolerated in clinical studies

3-4 years: Effective dose: 40 mg/kg/day in 3 divided doses

≥5-12 years: Effective dose: 25-35 mg/kg/day in 3 divided doses

See "Note" in Adults dosing.

Children >12 years and Adults:

Anticonvulsant: Initial: 300 mg 3 times/day; if necessary the dose may be increased up to 1800 mg/day. Doses of up to 2400 mg/day have been tolerated in long-term clinical studies; up to 3600 mg/day has been tolerated in short-term studies.

Note: If gabapentin is discontinued or if another anticonvulsant is added to therapy, it should be done slowly over a minimum of 1 week

Pain (unlabeled use): 300-1800 mg/day given in 3 divided doses has been the most common dosage range

Adults: Postherpetic neuralgia or neuropathic pain: Day 1: 300 mg, Day 2: 300 mg twice daily, Day 3: 300 mg 3 times/day; dose may be titrated as needed for pain relief (range: 1800-3600 mg/day, daily doses >1800 mg do not generally show greater benefit)

Elderly: Studies in elderly patients have shown a decrease in clearance as age increases. This is most likely due to age-related decreases in renal function; dose reductions may be needed.

Dosing adjustment in renal impairment: Children ≥12 years and Adults: See table.

Hemodialysis: Dialyzable

Gabapentin Dosing Adjustments in Renal Impairment

Creatinine Clearance (mL/min)	Daily Dose Range
≥60	300-1200 mg tid
>30-59	200-700 mg bid
>15-29	200-700 mg daily
15[1]	100-300 mg daily
Hemodialysis[2]	125-350 mg

[1]Cl$_{cr}$<15 mL/minute: Reduce daily dose in proportion to creatinine clearance.
[2]Single supplemental dose administered after each 4 hours of hemodialysis

Mechanism of Action Gabapentin is structurally related to GABA. However, it does not bind to GABA$_A$ or GABA$_B$ receptors, and it does not appear to influence synthesis or uptake of GABA. High affinity gabapentin binding sites have been located throughout the brain; these sites correspond to the presence of voltage-gated calcium channels specifically possessing the alpha-2-delta-1 subunit. This channel appears to be located presynaptically, and may modulate the release of excitatory neurotransmitters which participate in epileptogenesis and nociception.

Contraindications Hypersensitivity to gabapentin or any component of the formulation

Warnings/Precautions Avoid abrupt withdrawal, may precipitate seizures; use cautiously in patients with severe renal dysfunction; male rat studies demonstrated an association with pancreatic adenocarcinoma (clinical implication unknown). May cause CNS depression, which may impair physical or mental abilities. Patients must be cautioned about performing tasks which require mental alertness (eg, operating machinery or driving). Effects with other sedative drugs or ethanol may be potentiated. Pediatric patients (3-12 years of age) have shown increased incidence of CNS-related adverse effects, including emotional lability, hostility, thought disorder, and hyperkinesia. Safety and efficacy in children <3 years of age have not been established.

Drug Interactions CNS depressants: Sedative effects may be additive with CNS depressants; includes ethanol, barbiturates, narcotic analgesics, and other sedative agents. Monitor for increased effect.

Ethanol/Nutrition/Herb Interactions

Ethanol: Avoid ethanol (may increase CNS depression).

Food: Does not change rate or extent of absorption.

Herb/Nutraceutical: Avoid evening primrose (seizure threshold decreased). Avoid valerian, St John's wort, kava kava, gotu kola (may increase CNS depression).

Dietary Considerations May be taken without regard to meals.

Pharmacodynamics/Kinetics

Absorption: 50% to 60% from proximal small bowel by L-amino transport system

Distribution: V_d: 0.6-0.8 L/kg

Protein binding: <3%

Bioavailability: Inversely proportional to dose due to saturable absorption:

900 mg/day: 60%

1200 mg/day: 47%

2400 mg/day: 34%

3600 mg/day: 33%

4800 mg/day: 27%

Half-life elimination: 5-7 hours; anuria 132 hours; during dialysis 3.8 hours

Excretion: Proportional to renal function; urine (as unchanged drug)

Pregnancy Risk Factor C

Lactation Enters breast milk/use caution

Breast-Feeding Considerations Gabapentin is excreted in human breast milk. A nursed infant could be exposed to ~1 mg/kg/day of gabapentin; the effect on the child is not known. Use in breast-feeding women only if the benefits to the mother outweigh the potential risk to the infant.

Dosage Forms

Capsule (Neurontin®): 100 mg, 300 mg, 400 mg

Solution, oral (Neurontin®): 250 mg/5 mL (480 mL) [cool strawberry anise flavor]

Tablet: 100 mg, 300 mg, 400 mg

Neurontin®: 600 mg, 800 mg

Selected Readings

Laird MA and Gidal BE, "Use of Gabapentin in the Treatment of Neuropathic Pain," *Ann Pharmacother*, 2000, 34(6):802-7.

Rose MA and Kam PCA, "Gabapentin: Pharmacology and Its Use in Pain Management," *Anaesthesia*, 2002, 57:451-62.

Rosenberg JM, Harrell C, Ristic H, et al, "The Effect of Gabapentin on Neuropathic Pain," *Clin J Pain*, 1997, 13(3):251-5.

Rowbotham M, Harden N, Stacey B, et al, "Gabapentin for the Treatment of Postherpetic Neuralgia: A Randomized Controlled Trial," *JAMA*, 1998, 280(21):1837-42.

Gabitril® *see* Tiagabine *on page 1483*

Gadopentetate Dimeglumine
(gad oh PEN te tate dye MEG loo meen)

U.S. Brand Names Magnevist®

Generic Available No

Synonyms Gd-DTPA

Pharmacologic Category Radiological/Contrast Media, Paramagnetic Agent

Use Contrast medium for magnetic resonance imaging (MRI) to visualize lesions with abnormal vascularity in the brain, spine and associated tissues, head and neck, and body (excluding the heart)

Local Anesthetic/Vasoconstrictor Precautions No information available to require special precautions

Effects on Dental Treatment No significant effects or complications reported

Mechanism of Action Exposure to an external magnetic field induces a large local magnetic field in gadopentetate exposed tissues. This local magnetism disrupts water protons in the vicinity, resulting in a change in proton density and spin characteristics, which can be detected by the imaging device.

Pregnancy Risk Factor C

Gadoteridol (gad oh TER i dol)

U.S. Brand Names ProHance®

Generic Available No

(Continued)

Gadoteridol *(Continued)*

Synonyms Gd-HP-DO3A

Pharmacologic Category Radiological/Contrast Media, Nonionic

Use Contrast medium for magnetic resonance imaging (MRI)

Local Anesthetic/Vasoconstrictor Precautions No information available to require special precautions

Effects on Dental Treatment No significant effects or complications reported

Pregnancy Risk Factor C

Galantamine *(ga LAN ta meen)*

U.S. Brand Names Razadyne™; Razadyne™ ER; Reminyl® [DSC]

Canadian Brand Names Reminyl®

Generic Available No

Synonyms Galantamine Hydrobromide

Pharmacologic Category Acetylcholinesterase Inhibitor (Central)

Use Treatment of mild-to-moderate dementia of Alzheimer's disease

Local Anesthetic/Vasoconstrictor Precautions No information available to require special precautions

Effects on Dental Treatment No significant effects or complications reported

Common Adverse Effects

>10%: Gastrointestinal: Nausea (6% to 24%), vomiting (4% to 13%), diarrhea (6% to 12%)

1% to 10%:

Cardiovascular: Bradycardia (2% to 3%), syncope (0.4% to 2.2%: dose related), chest pain (≥1%)

Central nervous system: Dizziness (9%), headache (8%), depression (7%), fatigue (5%), insomnia (5%), somnolence (4%)

Gastrointestinal: Anorexia (7% to 9%), weight loss (5% to 7%), abdominal pain (5%), dyspepsia (5%), flatulence (≥1%)

Genitourinary: Urinary tract infection (8%), hematuria (<1% to 3%), incontinence (≥1%)

Hematologic: Anemia (3%)

Neuromuscular & skeletal: Tremor (3%)

Respiratory: Rhinitis (4%)

Mechanism of Action Centrally-acting cholinesterase inhibitor (competitive and reversible). It elevates acetylcholine in cerebral cortex by slowing the degradation of acetylcholine. Modulates nicotinic acetylcholine receptor to increase acetylcholine from surviving presynaptic nerve terminals. May increase glutamate and serotonin levels.

Drug Interactions

Cytochrome P450 Effect: Substrate (minor) of CYP2D6, 3A4

Increased Effect/Toxicity: Succinylcholine: increased neuromuscular blockade. Amiodarone, beta-blockers without ISA activity, diltiazem, verapamil may increase bradycardia. NSAIDs increase risk of peptic ulcer. Other CYP3A4 inhibitors and other CYP2D6 inhibitors increase levels of galantamine. Concurrent cholinergic agents may have synergistic effects. Digoxin may lead to AV block. Acetylcholinesterase inhibitors (central) may increase the risk of antipsychotic-related extrapyramidal symptoms.

Decreased Effect: Anticholinergic agents are antagonized by galantamine. CYP inducers may decrease galantamine levels.

Pharmacodynamics/Kinetics

Duration: 3 hours; maximum inhibition of erythrocyte acetylcholinesterase ~40% at 1 hour post 8 mg oral dose; levels return to baseline at 30 hours

Absorption: Rapid and complete

Distribution: 175 L; levels in the brain are 2-3 times higher than in plasma

Protein binding: 18%

Metabolism: Hepatic; linear, CYP2D6 and 3A4; metabolized to epigalanthaminone and galanthaminone both of which have acetylcholinesterase inhibitory activity 130 times less than galantamine

Bioavailability: ~90%

Half-life elimination: 7 hours

Time to peak: Immediate release: 1 hour (2.5 hours with food); extended release: 4.5-5 hours

Excretion: Urine (25%)

Pregnancy Risk Factor B

Galantamine Hydrobromide *see* Galantamine *on page 720*

Gallium Nitrate (GAL ee um NYE trate)

U.S. Brand Names Ganite™
Generic Available No
Synonyms NSC-15200
Pharmacologic Category Calcium-Lowering Agent
Use Treatment of hypercalcemia
Local Anesthetic/Vasoconstrictor Precautions No information available to require special precautions
Effects on Dental Treatment No significant effects or complications reported
Mechanism of Action Inhibits bone resorption by inhibiting osteoclast function
Pregnancy Risk Factor C

Galsulfase (gal SUL fase)

U.S. Brand Names Naglazyme™
Generic Available No
Synonyms Recombinant N-Acetylgalactosamine 4-Sulfatase; rhASB
Pharmacologic Category Enzyme
Use Replacement therapy in mucopolysaccharidosis VI (MPS VI; Maroteaux-Lamy Syndrome) for improvement of walking and stair-climbing capacity
Local Anesthetic/Vasoconstrictor Precautions No information available to require special precautions
Effects on Dental Treatment No significant effects or complications reported
Common Adverse Effects
Note: Percentages reported are from a placebo-controlled study (39 patients, 19 on galsulfase); also included are adverse effects noted during other clinical studies.
Cardiovascular: Chest pain (16%), facial edema (11%), hypertension (11%)
Central nervous system: Pain (26%), malaise (11%), fever, headache
Gastrointestinal: Abdominal pain (53%), gastroenteritis (11%), diarrhea, vomiting
Neuromuscular & skeletal: Rigors (21%), areflexia (11%), arthralgia
Ocular: Conjunctivitis (21%), corneal opacification increased (11%)
Otic: Ear pain (42%), otitis media
Respiratory: Dyspnea (21%), pharyngitis (16%), nasal congestion (11%), cough, upper respiratory tract infections
Miscellaneous: Antigalsulfase antibodies (98%), umbilical hernia (11%)
Infusion-related reactions: Angioedema, apnea, bronchospasm, chills, facial and neck urticaria, hypotension, rash, respiratory distress
Mechanism of Action Galsulfase is a recombinant form of N-acetylgalactosamine 4-sulfatase, produced in Chinese hamster cells. A deficiency of this enzyme leads to accumulation of the glycosaminoglycan dermatan sulfate in various tissues, causing progressive disease which includes decreased growth, skeletal deformities, upper airway obstruction, clouding of the cornea, heart disease, and coarse facial features. Replacement of this enzyme has been shown to improve mobility and physical function (measured by walking and stair-climbing).
Pharmacodynamics/Kinetics
Half-life elimination: Week 1: Median 9 hours (range: 6-21 hours); Week 24: Median 26 hours (range: 8-40 hours)
Pregnancy Risk Factor B

Gamma Benzene Hexachloride see Lindane on page 933
Gamma E-Gems® [OTC] see Vitamin E on page 1581
Gamma-E Plus [OTC] see Vitamin E on page 1581
Gammagard® Liquid see Immune Globulin (Intravenous) on page 824
Gammagard® S/D see Immune Globulin (Intravenous) on page 824
Gamma Globulin see Immune Globulin (Intramuscular) on page 823
Gamma Hydroxybutyric Acid see Sodium Oxybate on page 1402
Gammaphos see Amifostine on page 83
Gammar®-P I.V. see Immune Globulin (Intravenous) on page 824
Gamunex® see Immune Globulin (Intravenous) on page 824

Ganciclovir (gan SYE kloe veer)

Related Information
Systemic Viral Diseases *on page 1675*
Valganciclovir *on page 1555*

U.S. Brand Names Cytovene®; Vitrasert®
Canadian Brand Names Cytovene®; Vitrasert®
Mexican Brand Names Cymevene®
Generic Available Yes: Capsule
Synonyms DHPG Sodium; GCV Sodium; Nordeoxyguanosine
Pharmacologic Category Antiviral Agent

Use
Parenteral: Treatment of CMV retinitis in immunocompromised individuals, including patients with acquired immunodeficiency syndrome; prophylaxis of CMV infection in transplant patients

Oral: Alternative to the I.V. formulation for maintenance treatment of CMV retinitis in immunocompromised patients, including patients with AIDS, in whom retinitis is stable following appropriate induction therapy and for whom the risk of more rapid progression is balanced by the benefit associated with avoiding daily I.V. infusions.

Implant: Treatment of CMV retinitis

Unlabeled/Investigational Use May be given in combination with foscarnet in patients who relapse after monotherapy with either drug

Local Anesthetic/Vasoconstrictor Precautions No information available to require special precautions

Effects on Dental Treatment Key adverse event(s) related to dental treatment: Xerostomia (normal salivary flow resumes upon discontinuation).

Common Adverse Effects
>10%:
Central nervous system: Fever (38% to 48%)
Dermatologic: Rash (15% oral, 10% I.V.)
Gastrointestinal: Abdominal pain (17% to 19%), diarrhea (40%), nausea (25%), anorexia (15%), vomiting (13%)
Hematologic: Anemia (20% to 25%), leukopenia (30% to 40%)

1% to 10%:
Central nervous system: Confusion, neuropathy (8% to 9%), headache (4%)
Dermatologic: Pruritus (5%)
Hematologic: Thrombocytopenia (6%), neutropenia with ANC <500/mm³ (5% oral, 14% I.V.)
Neuromuscular & skeletal: Paresthesia (6% to 10%), weakness (6%)
Ocular: Retinal detachment (8% oral, 11% I.V.; relationship to ganciclovir not established)
Miscellaneous: Sepsis (4% oral, 15% I.V.)

Dosage
CMV retinitis: Slow I.V. infusion (dosing is based on total body weight):
Children >3 months and Adults:
Induction therapy: 5 mg/kg/dose every 12 hours for 14-21 days followed by maintenance therapy
Maintenance therapy: 5 mg/kg/day as a single daily dose for 7 days/week or 6 mg/kg/day for 5 days/week

CMV retinitis: Oral: 1000 mg 3 times/day with food **or** 500 mg 6 times/day with food

Prevention of CMV disease in patients with advanced HIV infection and normal renal function: Oral: 1000 mg 3 times/day with food

Prevention of CMV disease in transplant patients: Same initial and maintenance dose as CMV retinitis except duration of initial course is 7-14 days, duration of maintenance therapy is dependent on clinical condition and degree of immunosuppression

Intravitreal implant: One implant for 5- to 8-month period; following depletion of ganciclovir, as evidenced by progression of retinitis, implant may be removed and replaced

Elderly: Refer to adult dosing; in general, dose selection should be cautious, reflecting greater frequency of organ impairment

Dosing adjustment in renal impairment:
I.V. (Induction):
Cl_{cr} 50-69 mL/minute: Administer 2.5 mg/kg/dose every 12 hours
Cl_{cr} 25-49 mL/minute: Administer 2.5 mg/kg/dose every 24 hours
Cl_{cr} 10-24 mL/minute: Administer 1.25 mg/kg/dose every 24 hours
Cl_{cr} <10 mL/minute: Administer 1.25 mg/kg/dose 3 times/week following hemodialysis

I.V. (Maintenance):
Cl$_{cr}$ 50-69 mL/minute: Administer 2.5 mg/kg/dose every 24 hours
Cl$_{cr}$ 25-49 mL/minute: Administer 1.25 mg/kg/dose every 24 hours
Cl$_{cr}$ 10-24 mL/minute: Administer 0.625 mg/kg/dose every 24 hours
Cl$_{cr}$ <10 mL/minute: Administer 0.625 mg/kg/dose 3 times/week following hemodialysis

Oral:
Cl$_{cr}$ 50-69 mL/minute: Administer 1500 mg/day or 500 mg 3 times/day
Cl$_{cr}$ 25-49 mL/minute: Administer 1000 mg/day or 500 mg twice daily
Cl$_{cr}$ 10-24 mL/minute: Administer 500 mg/day
Cl$_{cr}$ <10 mL/minute: Administer 500 mg 3 times/week following hemodialysis

Hemodialysis effects: Dialyzable (50%) following hemodialysis; administer dose postdialysis. During peritoneal dialysis, dose as for Cl$_{cr}$ <10 mL/minute. During continuous arteriovenous or venovenous hemofiltration, administer 2.5 mg/kg/dose every 24 hours.

Mechanism of Action Ganciclovir is phosphorylated to a substrate which competitively inhibits the binding of deoxyguanosine triphosphate to DNA polymerase resulting in inhibition of viral DNA synthesis

Contraindications Hypersensitivity to ganciclovir, acyclovir, or any component of the formulation; absolute neutrophil count <500/mm^3; platelet count <25,000/mm^3

Warnings/Precautions Hazardous agent - use appropriate precautions for handling and disposal. Dosage adjustment or interruption of ganciclovir therapy may be necessary in patients with neutropenia and/or thrombocytopenia and patients with impaired renal function. Use with extreme caution in children since long-term safety has not been determined and due to ganciclovir's potential for long-term carcinogenic and adverse reproductive effects; ganciclovir may adversely affect spermatogenesis and fertility; due to its mutagenic potential, contraceptive precautions for female and male patients need to be followed during and for at least 90 days after therapy with the drug; take care to administer only into veins with good blood flow.

Drug Interactions
Increased Effect/Toxicity: Immunosuppressive agents may increase hematologic toxicity of ganciclovir. Imipenem/cilastatin may increase seizure potential. Oral ganciclovir increases blood levels of zidovudine, although zidovudine decreases steady-state levels of ganciclovir. Since both drugs have the potential to cause neutropenia and anemia, some patients may not tolerate concomitant therapy with these drugs at full dosage. Didanosine levels are increased with concurrent ganciclovir. Other nephrotoxic drugs (eg, amphotericin and cyclosporine) may have additive nephrotoxicity with ganciclovir.
Decreased Effect: A decrease in blood levels of ganciclovir AUC may occur when used with didanosine.

Dietary Considerations Sodium content of 500 mg vial: 46 mg

Pharmacodynamics/Kinetics
Distribution: V$_d$: 15.26 L/1.73 m^2; widely to all tissues including CSF and ocular tissue
Protein binding: 1% to 2%
Bioavailability: Oral: Fasting: 5%; Following food: 6% to 9%; Following fatty meal: 28% to 31%
Half-life elimination: 1.7-5.8 hours; prolonged with renal impairment; End-stage renal disease: 5-28 hours
Excretion: Urine (80% to 99% as unchanged drug)

Pregnancy Risk Factor C

Dosage Forms CAP: 250 mg, 500 mg. **IMPLANT, intravitreal** (Vitrasert®): 4.5 mg. **INJ, powder for reconstitution** (Cytovene®): 500 mg

Ganidin NR see Guaifenesin on page 752

Ganirelix (ga ni REL ix)

U.S. Brand Names Antagon®
Canadian Brand Names Antagon®; Orgalutran®
Generic Available No
Synonyms Ganirelix Acetate
Pharmacologic Category Gonadotropin Releasing Hormone Antagonist
Use Inhibits premature luteinizing hormone (LH) surges in women undergoing controlled ovarian hyperstimulation in fertility clinics.
Local Anesthetic/Vasoconstrictor Precautions No information available to require special precautions
Effects on Dental Treatment No significant effects or complications reported
Common Adverse Effects 1% to 10%:
Central nervous system: Headache (3%)
(Continued)

Ganirelix (Continued)

Endocrine & metabolic: Ovarian hyperstimulation syndrome (2%)
Gastrointestinal: Abdominal pain (5%), nausea (1%), and abdominal pain (1%)
Genitourinary: Vaginal bleeding (2%)
Local: Injection site reaction (1%)

Mechanism of Action Competitively blocks the gonadotropin-release hormone receptors on the pituitary gonadotroph and transduction pathway. This suppresses gonadotropin secretion and luteinizing hormone secretion preventing ovulation until the follicles are of adequate size.

Drug Interactions
Increased Effect/Toxicity: No formal studies have been performed.
Decreased Effect: No formal studies have been performed.

Pharmacodynamics/Kinetics
Absorption: SubQ: Rapid
Distribution: Mean V_d: 43.7 L
Protein binding: 81.9%
Metabolism: Hepatic to two primary metabolites (1-4 and 1-6 peptide)
Bioavailability: 91.1%
Half-life elimination: 16.2 hours
Time to peak: 1.1 hours
Excretion: Feces (75%) within 288 hours; urine (22%) within 24 hours

Pregnancy Risk Factor X

Ganirelix Acetate *see* Ganirelix *on page 723*

Ganite™ *see* Gallium Nitrate *on page 721*

Gani-Tuss DM NR *see* Guaifenesin and Dextromethorphan *on page 754*

Gani-Tuss® NR *see* Guaifenesin and Codeine *on page 753*

Gantrisin® *see* SulfiSOXAZOLE *on page 1429*

GAR-936 *see* Tigecycline *on page 1487*

Gas-X® [OTC] *see* Simethicone *on page 1394*

Gas-X® Extra Strength [OTC] *see* Simethicone *on page 1394*

Gas-X® Maximum Strength [OTC] *see* Simethicone *on page 1394*

GasAid [OTC] *see* Simethicone *on page 1394*

Gas Ban™ [OTC] *see* Calcium Carbonate and Simethicone *on page 249*

Gastrocrom® *see* Cromolyn *on page 397*

Gastrografin® *see* Diatrizoate Meglumine and Diatrizoate Sodium *on page 453*

Gatifloxacin (gat i FLOKS a sin)

Related Information
Bacterial Infections *on page 1697*
Respiratory Diseases *on page 1656*
Sexually-Transmitted Diseases *on page 1674*
U.S. Brand Names Tequin® [DSC]; Zymar™
Canadian Brand Names Tequin®; Zymar™
Generic Available No
Pharmacologic Category Antibiotic, Ophthalmic; Antibiotic, Quinolone
Use
Oral, I.V.: Treatment of the following infections when caused by susceptible bacteria: Acute bacterial exacerbation of chronic bronchitis; acute sinusitis; community-acquired pneumonia including pneumonia caused by multi-drug-resistant *S. pneumoniae* (MDRSP); uncomplicated skin and skin structure infection; uncomplicated urinary tract infections (cystitis); complicated urinary tract infections; pyelonephritis; uncomplicated urethral and cervical gonorrhea; acute, uncomplicated rectal infections in women
Ophthalmic: Bacterial conjunctivitis

Local Anesthetic/Vasoconstrictor Precautions No information available to require special precautions (see Dental Comment)
Effects on Dental Treatment Key adverse event(s) related to dental treatment: Taste disturbance.

Common Adverse Effects
Systemic therapy:
3% to 10%:
Central nervous system: Headache (3%), dizziness (3%)
Gastrointestinal: Nausea (8%), diarrhea (4%)
Genitourinary: Vaginitis (6%)
Local: Injection site reactions (5%)
0.1% to ≤3%: Abdominal pain, abnormal dreams, abnormal vision, agitation, alkaline phosphatase increased, allergic reaction, anorexia, anxiety, arthralgia, back pain, chest pain, chills, confusion, constipation, diaphoresis,

dry skin, dyspepsia, dyspnea, dysuria, electrolyte abnormalities, facial edema, fever, flatulence, gastritis, glossitis, hematuria, hyperglycemia, hypertension, insomnia, leg cramps, mouth ulceration, nervousness, neutropenia, oral candidiasis, palpitation, paresthesia, peripheral edema, pharyngitis, pruritus, rash, serum amylase increased, serum bilirubin increased, serum transaminases increased, somnolence, stomatitis, taste perversion, thirst, tinnitus, tremor, weakness, vasodilation, vertigo, vomiting

Ophthalmic therapy:
5% to 10%: Ocular: Conjunctival irritation, keratitis, lacrimation increased, papillary conjunctivitis

1% to 4%:
Central nervous system: Headache
Gastrointestinal: Taste disturbance
Ocular: Chemosis, conjunctival hemorrhage, discharge, dry eye, edema, irritation, pain, visual acuity decreased

Dosage
Usual dosage range:
Adults: Oral, I.V.: 400 mg once daily

Indication-specific dosing:
Children ≥1 year and Adults:
Bacterial conjunctivitis: Ophthalmic:
Days 1 and 2: Instill 1 drop into affected eye(s) every 2 hours while awake (maximum: 8 times/day)
Days 3-7: Instill 1 drop into affected eye(s) up to 4 times/day while awake
Adults: Oral, I.V.:
Acute bacterial exacerbation of chronic bronchitis: 400 mg every 24 hours for 5 days
Acute sinusitis: 400 mg every 24 hours for 10 days
Community-acquired pneumonia (including atypical organisms): 400 mg every 24 hours for 7-14 days
Pyelonephritis (acute): 400 mg every 24 hours for 7-10 days
Skin/skin structure infections (uncomplicated): 400 mg every 24 hours for 7-10 days
Traveler's diarrhea (unlabeled use): 400 mg once daily for 3 days
Urinary tract infections:
Complicated: 400 mg every 24 hours for 7-10 days
Uncomplicated, cystitis: 400 mg single dose or 200 mg every 24 hours for 3 days
Urethral gonorrhea in men (uncomplicated), cervical or rectal gonorrhea in women and pharyngitis (gonococcal): 400 mg single dose
Elderly: No dosage adjustment is required based on age, however, assessment of renal function is particularly important in this population.

Dosage adjustment in renal impairment: Creatinine clearance <40 mL/minute (or patients on hemodialysis/CAPD) should receive an initial dose of 400 mg, followed by a subsequent dose of 200 mg every 24 hours. Patients receiving single-dose or 3-day therapy for appropriate indications do not require dosage adjustment. Administer after hemodialysis.

Dosage adjustment in hepatic impairment: No dosage adjustment is required in mild-moderate hepatic disease. No data are available in severe hepatic impairment (Child-Pugh Class C).

Mechanism of Action Gatifloxacin is a DNA gyrase inhibitor, and also inhibits topoisomerase IV. DNA gyrase (topoisomerase II) is an essential bacterial enzyme that maintains the superhelical structure of DNA. DNA gyrase is required for DNA replication and transcription, DNA repair, recombination, and transposition; inhibition is bactericidal.

Contraindications Hypersensitivity to gatifloxacin, other quinolone antibiotics, or any component of the formulation; diabetes mellitus

Warnings/Precautions Use with caution in patients with significant bradycardia or acute myocardial ischemia. May prolong QT interval (concentration related). Use caution in patients with known prolongation of QT interval, uncorrected hypokalemia, or concurrent administration of other medications known to prolong the QT interval (including Class Ia and Class III antiarrhythmics, cisapride, erythromycin, antipsychotics, and tricyclic antidepressants). May cause increased CNS stimulation, increased intracranial pressure, convulsions, or psychosis. Use with caution in individuals at risk of seizures. Discontinue in patients who experience significant CNS adverse effects. Use caution in renal dysfunction (dosage adjustment required) and in severe hepatic insufficiency (no data available). Serious disruptions in glucose regulation (including hyperglycemia and severe hypoglycemia) may occur, usually (but not always) in patients with diabetes. Other risk factors for glucose dysregulation include advanced age, renal insufficiency, and use of concurrent medications which alter glucose utilization. Hypoglycemia may be more prevalent in the initial 3
(Continued)

Gatifloxacin *(Continued)*

days of therapy while a greater risk of hyperglycemia may be present after the initial 3 days (particularly days 4-10). Monitor closely and discontinue if hyper- or hypoglycemia occur. Tendon inflammation and/or rupture has been reported with this and other quinolone antibiotics. Discontinue at first signs or symptoms of tendon or pain. Quinolones may exacerbate myasthenia gravis. May cause peripheral neuropathy (rare); discontinue if symptoms of sensory or sensori-motor neuropathy occur.

Severe hypersensitivity reactions, including anaphylaxis, have occurred with quinolone therapy. Prolonged use may result in superinfection; pseudomembranous colitis may occur and should be considered in all patients who present with diarrhea. Do not inject ophthalmic solution subconjunctivally or introduce directly into the anterior chamber of the eye.

Safety and efficacy for ophthalmic use have not been established in children <1 year of age. Safety and efficacy for systemic use have not been established in patients <18 years of age.

Drug Interactions

Increased Effect/Toxicity: Gatifloxacin may increase the effects/toxicity of hypoglycemic agents and warfarin. Concomitant use with corticosteroids may increase the risk of tendon rupture. Concomitant use with other QT_c-prolonging agents (eg, Class Ia and Class III antiarrhythmics, erythromycin, cisapride, antipsychotics, and cyclic antidepressants) may result in arrhythmias, such as torsade de pointes. Probenecid may increase gatifloxacin levels. Atypical antipsychotics and protease inhibitors may cause hyperglycemia; use with caution and monitor.

Decreased Effect: Concurrent administration of metal cations, including most antacids (not calcium carbonate), oral electrolyte supplements, quinapril, sucralfate, some didanosine formulations (chewable/buffered tablets and pediatric powder for oral suspension), and other highly-buffered oral drugs, may decrease quinolone levels; separate doses.

Ethanol/Nutrition/Herb Interactions

Ethanol: Caution with ethanol (may cause hypoglycemia).

Herb/Nutraceutical: Avoid dong quai, St John's wort (may also cause photosensitization); caution with chromium, garlic, gymnema (may cause hypoglycemia).

Dietary Considerations May take tablets with or without food, milk, or calcium supplements. Gatifloxacin should be taken 4 hours before supplements (including multivitamins) containing iron, zinc, or magnesium.

Pharmacodynamics/Kinetics

Absorption: Oral: Well absorbed; Ophthalmic: Not measurable

Distribution: V_d: 1.5-2.0 L/kg; concentrates in alveolar macrophages and lung parenchyma

Protein binding: 20%

Metabolism: Only 1%; no interaction with CYP

Bioavailability: 96%

Half-life elimination: 7.1-13.9 hours; ESRD/CAPD: 30-40 hours

Time to peak: Oral: 1 hour

Excretion: Urine (70% as unchanged drug, <1% as metabolites); feces (5%)

Pregnancy Risk Factor C

Dosage Forms SOLN, ophthalmic (Zymar™): 0.3% (2.5 mL, 5 mL).

Dental Comment

This drug is known to prolong the QT interval. The QT interval is measured as the time and distance between the Q point of the QRS complex and the end of the T wave in the ECG tracing. After adjustment for heart rate, the QT interval is defined as prolonged if it is more than 450 msec in men and 460 msec in women. A long QT syndrome was first described in the 1950s and 60s as a congenital syndrome involving QT interval prolongation and syncope and sudden death. Some of the congenital long QT syndromes were characterized by a peculiar electrocardiographic appearance of the QRS complex involving a premature atria beat followed by a pause, then a subsequent sinus beat showing marked QT prolongation and deformity. This type of cardiac arrhythmia was originally termed "torsade de pointes" (translated from the French as "twisting of the points").

Prolongation of the QT interval is thought to result from delayed ventricular repolarization. The repolarization process within the myocardial cell is due to the efflux of intracellular potassium. The channels associated with this current can be blocked by many drugs and predisposes the electrical propagation cycle to torsade de pointes.

Gatifloxacin is one of the drugs confirmed to prolong the QT interval and is accepted as having a risk of causing torsade de pointes. The risk of drug-induced torsade de pointes is extremely low when a single QT interval prolonging drug is prescribed. In terms of epinephrine, it is not known what effect vasoconstrictors in the local anesthetic regimen will have in patients with a known history of congenital prolonged QT interval or in patients taking any medication that prolongs the QT interval. Until more information is obtained, it is suggested that the clinician consult with the physician prior to the use of a vasoconstrictor in suspected patients, and that the vasoconstrictor (epinephrine, levonordefrin [Neo-Cobefrin®]) be used with caution.

Gaviscon® Extra Strength [OTC] see Aluminum Hydroxide and Magnesium Carbonate on page 79

Gaviscon® Liquid [OTC] see Aluminum Hydroxide and Magnesium Carbonate on page 79

Gaviscon® Tablet [OTC] see Aluminum Hydroxide and Magnesium Trisilicate on page 80

G-CSF see Filgrastim on page 654

G-CSF (PEG Conjugate) see Pegfilgrastim on page 1195

GCV Sodium see Ganciclovir on page 722

Gd-DTPA see Gadopentetate Dimeglumine on page 719

Gd-HP-DO3A see Gadoteridol on page 719

Gebauer's Ethyl Chloride® see Ethyl Chloride on page 620

Gebauer's Instant Ice™ [OTC] see Pentafluoropropane and Tetrafluoroethane on page 1206

Gebauer's Pain Ease® see Pentafluoropropane and Tetrafluoroethane on page 1206

Gebauer's Spray and Stretch® see Pentafluoropropane and Tetrafluoroethane on page 1206

Gefitinib (ge FI tye nib)

U.S. Brand Names IRESSA®
Generic Available No
Synonyms NSC-715055; ZD1839
Pharmacologic Category Antineoplastic Agent, Tyrosine Kinase Inhibitor
Use

U.S. Labeling: Monotherapy for continued treatment of locally advanced or metastatic nonsmall cell lung cancer after failure of platinum-based and docetaxel therapies. Treatment is limited to patients who are benefiting or have benefited from treatment with gefitinib.

Note: Due to the lack of improved survival data from clinical trials of gefitinib, and in response to positive survival data with another EGFR inhibitor, physicians are advised to use other treatment options in advanced nonsmall cell lung cancer patients following one or two prior chemotherapy regimens when they are refractory/intolerant to their most recent regimen.

Canada labeling: Approved indication is limited to NSCLC patients with epidermal growth factor receptor (EGFR) expression status positive or unknown.

Local Anesthetic/Vasoconstrictor Precautions No information available to require special precautions

Effects on Dental Treatment Key adverse event(s) related to dental treatment: Mouth ulceration.

Common Adverse Effects
>10%:
Dermatologic: Rash (43% to 54%), acne (25% to 33%), dry skin (13% to 26%)
Gastrointestinal: Diarrhea (48% to 76%), nausea (13% to 18%), vomiting (9% to 12%)
1% to 10%:
Cardiovascular: Peripheral edema (2%)
Dermatologic: Pruritus (8% to 9%)
Gastrointestinal: Anorexia (7% to 10%), weight loss (3% to 5%), mouth ulceration (1%)
Neuromuscular & skeletal: Weakness (4% to 6%)
Ocular: Amblyopia (2%), conjunctivitis (1%)
Respiratory: Dyspnea (2%), interstitial lung disease (1% to 2%)

Restrictions As of September 15, 2005, distribution will be limited to patients enrolled in the Iressa Access Program. This has been developed as part of a risk-management plan by AstraZeneca and the FDA. Under this program, access to gefitinib will be limited to the following groups:
Patients who are currently receiving and benefitting from gefitinib (IRESSA®)
Patients who have previously received and benefited from gefitinib (IRESSA®)
(Continued)

Gefitinib *(Continued)*

Previously-enrolled patients or new patients in non-Investigational New Drug (IND) clinical trials involving gefitinib (IRESSA®) if these protocols were approved by an IRB prior to June 17, 2005

New patients may also receive Iressa if the manufacturer (AstraZeneca) decides to make it available under IND, and the patients meet the criteria for enrollment under the IND

Additional information on the IRESSA® Access Program, including enrollment forms, may be obtained by calling AstraZeneca at 1-800-601-8933 or via the web at www.Iressa-access.com

Mechanism of Action The mechanism of antineoplastic action is not fully understood. Gefitinib inhibits tyrosine kinases (TK) associated with transmembrane cell surface receptors found on both normal and cancer cells. One such receptor is epidermal growth factor receptor. TK activity appears to be vitally important to cell proliferation and survival.

Drug Interactions

Cytochrome P450 Effect: Substrate of CYP3A4 (major); **Inhibits** CYP2C19 (weak), 2D6 (weak)

Increased Effect/Toxicity: Gefitinib may increase the effects of warfarin. CYP3A4 inhibitors may increase the levels/effects of gefitinib; example inhibitors include azole antifungals, clarithromycin, diclofenac, doxycycline, erythromycin, imatinib, isoniazid, nefazodone, nicardipine, propofol, protease inhibitors, quinidine, telithromycin, and verapamil.

Decreased Effect: Gefitinib effects may be decreased by H_2-receptor blockers and sodium bicarbonate. CYP3A4 inducers may decrease the levels/effects of gefitinib; example inducers include aminoglutethimide, carbamazepine, nafcillin, nevirapine, phenobarbital, phenytoin, and rifamycins.

Pharmacodynamics/Kinetics

Absorption: Oral: slow

Distribution: I.V.: 1400 L

Protein binding: 90%, albumin and alpha$_1$-acid glycoprotein

Metabolism: Hepatic, primarily via CYP3A4; forms metabolites

Bioavailability: 60%

Half-life elimination: I.V.: 48 hours

Time to peak, plasma: Oral: 3-7 hours

Excretion: Feces (86%); urine (<4%)

Pregnancy Risk Factor D

Gelatin (Absorbable) *(JEL a tin, ab SORB a ble)*

U.S. Brand Names Gelfilm®; Gelfoam®

Generic Available No

Synonyms Absorbable Gelatin Sponge

Pharmacologic Category Hemostatic Agent

Dental Use Adjunct to provide hemostasis in oral and dental surgery

Use Adjunct to provide hemostasis in surgery; open prostatic surgery

Local Anesthetic/Vasoconstrictor Precautions No information available to require special precautions

Effects on Dental Treatment Key adverse event(s) related to dental treatment: Local infection and abscess formation.

Significant Adverse Effects 1% to 10%: Local: Infection and abscess formation

Dosage Hemostasis: Apply packs or sponges dry or saturated with sodium chloride. When applied dry, hold in place with moderate pressure. When applied wet, squeeze to remove air bubbles. The powder is applied as a paste prepared by adding approximately 4 mL of sterile saline solution to the powder.

Contraindications Should not be used in closure of skin incisions since they may interfere with the healing of skin edges

Warnings/Precautions Do not sterilize by heat; do not use in the presence of infection

Drug Interactions No data reported

Pregnancy Risk Factor No data reported

Dosage Forms

Film, ophthalmic (Gelfilm®): 25 mm x 50 mm (6s)

Film, topical (Gelfilm®): 100 mm x 125 mm (1s)

Powder, topical (Gelfoam®): 1 g

Sponge, dental (Gelfoam®): Size 4 (12s)

Sponge, topical (Gelfoam®):

Size 50 (4s)

Size 100 (6s)

Size 200 (6s)
Size 2 cm (1s)
Size 6 cm (6s)
Size 12-7 mm (12s)

Gelclair® *see* Maltodextrin *on page 963*

Gelfilm® *see* Gelatin (Absorbable) *on page 728*

Gelfoam® *see* Gelatin (Absorbable) *on page 728*

Gel-Kam® [OTC] *see* Fluoride *on page 671*

Gel-Kam® Rinse *see* Fluoride *on page 671*

Gelucast® *see* Zinc Gelatin *on page 1597*

Gelusil® [OTC] *see* Aluminum Hydroxide, Magnesium Hydroxide, and Simethicone *on page 81*

Gemcitabine (jem SITE a been)

U.S. Brand Names Gemzar®
Canadian Brand Names Gemzar®
Mexican Brand Names Gemzar®
Generic Available No
Synonyms Gemcitabine Hydrochloride
Pharmacologic Category Antineoplastic Agent, Antimetabolite (Pyrimidine Antagonist)
Use
Adenocarcinoma of the pancreas: First-line therapy in locally-advanced (nonresectable stage II or stage III) or metastatic (stage IV) adenocarcinoma of the pancreas

Breast cancer: First-line therapy in metastatic breast cancer

Nonsmall-cell lung cancer: First-line therapy in locally-advanced (stage IIIA or IIIB) or metastatic (stage IV) nonsmall-cell lung cancer
Unlabeled/Investigational Use Bladder cancer, ovarian cancer
Local Anesthetic/Vasoconstrictor Precautions No information available to require special precautions
Effects on Dental Treatment Key adverse event(s) related to dental treatment: Stomatitis.
Common Adverse Effects Percentages reported with single-agent therapy for pancreatic cancer and other malignancies.
>10%:
Central nervous system: Pain (42% to 48%; grades 3 and 4: <1% to 9%), fever (38% to 41%; grades 3 and 4: ≤2%), somnolence (11%; grades 3 and 4: <1%). Fever was reported to occur in the absence of infection in pancreatic cancer treatment.

Dermatologic: Rash (28% to 30%; grades 3 and 4: <1%), alopecia (15% to 16%; grades 3 and 4: <1%). Rash in pancreatic cancer treatment was typically a macular or finely-granular maculopapular pruritic eruption of mild-to-moderate severity involving the trunk and extremities.

Gastrointestinal: Nausea and vomiting (69% to 71%; grades 3 and 4: 1% to 13%), constipation (23% to 31%; grades 3 and 4: <1% to 3%), diarrhea (19% to 30%; grades 3 and 4: ≤3%), stomatitis (10% to 11%; grades 3 and 4: <1%)

Hematologic: Anemia (73% to 68%; grades 3 and 4: 1% to 8%), leukopenia (62% to 64%; grades 3 and 4: <1% to 9%), neutropenia (61% to 63%; grades 3 and 4: 6% to 19%), thrombocytopenia (24% to 36%; grades 3 and 4: <1% to 7%), hemorrhage (4% to 17%; grades 3 or 4: <1%). Myelosuppression may be the dose-limiting toxicity with pancreatic cancer

Hepatic: Transaminases increased (68% to 78%; grades 3 and 4: 1% to 12%), alkaline phosphatase increased (55% to 77%; grades 3 and 4: 2% to 16%), bilirubin increased (13% to 26%; grades 3 or 4: <1% to 6%). Serious hepatotoxicity was reported rarely in pancreatic cancer treatment.

Renal: Proteinuria (32% to 45%; grades 3 and 4: <1%), hematuria (23% to 35%; grades 3 and 4: <1%), BUN increased (15% to 16%; grades 3 and 4: 0%)

Respiratory: Dyspnea (10% to 23%; grades 3 and 4: <1% to 3%)

Miscellaneous: Infection (10% to 16%; grades 3 or 4: <1% to 2%)

1% to 10%:
Local: Injection site reactions (4%)
Neuromuscular & skeletal: Paresthesias (10%)
Renal: Creatinine increased (6% to 8%)
Respiratory: Bronchospasm (<2%)
(Continued)

Gemcitabine *(Continued)*

Mechanism of Action A pyrimidine antimetabolite that inhibits DNA synthesis by inhibition of DNA polymerase and ribonucleotide reductase, specific for the S-phase of the cycle.

Drug Interactions

Decreased Effect: No confirmed interactions have been reported. No specific drug interaction studies have been conducted.

Pharmacodynamics/Kinetics

Distribution: Infusions <70 minutes: 50 L/m²; Long infusion times: 370 L/m²

Protein binding: Low

Metabolism: Hepatic, metabolites: di- and triphosphates (active); uridine derivative (inactive)

Half-life elimination:

Gemcitabine: Infusion time ≤1 hour: 32-94 minutes; infusion time 3-4 hours: 4-10.5 hours

Metabolite (gemcitabine triphosphate), terminal phase: 1.7-19.4 hours

Time to peak, plasma: 30 minutes

Excretion: Urine (99%, 92% to 98% as intact drug or inactive uridine metabolite); feces (<1%)

Pregnancy Risk Factor D

Gemcitabine Hydrochloride *see* Gemcitabine *on page 729*

Gemfibrozil *(jem FI broe zil)*

Related Information

Cardiovascular Diseases *on page 1636*

U.S. Brand Names Lopid®

Canadian Brand Names Apo-Gemfibrozil®; Gen-Gemfibrozil; Lopid®; Novo-Gemfibrozil; Nu-Gemfibrozil; PMS-Gemfibrozil

Mexican Brand Names Lopid®

Generic Available Yes

Synonyms CI-719

Pharmacologic Category Antilipemic Agent, Fibric Acid

Use Treatment of hypertriglyceridemia in types IV and V hyperlipidemia for patients who are at greater risk for pancreatitis and who have not responded to dietary intervention

Local Anesthetic/Vasoconstrictor Precautions No information available to require special precautions

Effects on Dental Treatment No significant effects or complications reported

Common Adverse Effects

>10%: Gastrointestinal: Dyspepsia (20%)

1% to 10%:

Central nervous system: Fatigue (4%), vertigo (2%), headache (1%)

Dermatologic: Eczema (2%), rash (2%)

Gastrointestinal: Abdominal pain (10%), diarrhea (7%), nausea/vomiting (3%), constipation (1%)

Reports where causal relationship has not been established: Weight loss, extrasystoles, pancreatitis, hepatoma, colitis, confusion, seizure, syncope, retinal edema, decreased fertility (male), renal dysfunction, positive ANA, drug-induced lupus-like syndrome, thrombocytopenia, anaphylaxis, vasculitis, alopecia, photosensitivity

Dosage Adults: Oral: 1200 mg/day in 2 divided doses, 30 minutes before breakfast and dinner

Hemodialysis: Not removed by hemodialysis; supplemental dose is not necessary

Mechanism of Action The exact mechanism of action of gemfibrozil is unknown, however, several theories exist regarding the VLDL effect; it can inhibit lipolysis and decrease subsequent hepatic fatty acid uptake as well as inhibit hepatic secretion of VLDL; together these actions decrease serum VLDL levels; increases HDL-cholesterol; the mechanism behind HDL elevation is currently unknown

Contraindications Hypersensitivity to gemfibrozil or any component of the formulation; significant hepatic or renal dysfunction; primary biliary cirrhosis; pre-existing gallbladder disease

Warnings/Precautions Abnormal elevation of AST, ALT, LDH, bilirubin, and alkaline phosphatase has occurred; if no appreciable triglyceride or cholesterol lowering effect occurs after 3 months, the drug should be discontinued; not useful for type I hyperlipidemia; myositis may be more common in patients with poor renal function

Drug Interactions

Cytochrome P450 Effect: Substrate of CYP3A4 (minor); **Inhibits** CYP1A2 (moderate), 2C8 (strong), 2C9 (strong), 2C19 (strong)

Increased Effect/Toxicity: Gemfibrozil may potentiate the effects of bexarotene (avoid concurrent use), sulfonylureas (including glyburide, chlorpropamide), and warfarin. HMG-CoA reductase inhibitors (atorvastatin, fluvastatin, lovastatin, pravastatin, simvastatin) may increase the risk of myopathy and rhabdomyolysis. The manufacturer warns against the concurrent use of lovastatin (if unavoidable, limit lovastatin to <20 mg/day). Combination therapy with statins has been used in some patients with resistant hyperlipidemias (with great caution). Gemfibrozil may increase the serum concentration of repaglinide (resulting in severe, prolonged hypoglycemia); the addition of itraconazole may augment the effects of gemfibrozil on repaglinide (consider alternative therapy). Gemfibrozil may increase the levels/effects of aminophylline, amiodarone, bosentan, citalopram, dapsone, diazepam, fluoxetine, fluvoxamine, glimepiride, glipizide, losartan, methsuximide, mexiletine, mirtazapine, montelukast, nateglinide, paclitaxel, phenytoin, pioglitazone, propranolol, repaglinide, ropinirole, rosiglitazone, sertraline, theophylline, trifluoperazine, warfarin, zafirlukast, and other substrates of CYP1A2, 2C8, 2C9, or 2C19.

Decreased Effect: Cyclosporine's blood levels may be reduced during concurrent therapy. Rifampin may decrease gemfibrozil blood levels.

Ethanol/Nutrition/Herb Interactions Ethanol: Avoid ethanol to decrease triglycerides.

Dietary Considerations Before initiation of therapy, patients should be placed on a standard cholesterol-lowering diet for 3-6 months and the diet should be continued during drug therapy.

Pharmacodynamics/Kinetics

Onset of action: May require several days

Absorption: Well absorbed

Protein binding: 99%

Metabolism: Hepatic via oxidation to two inactive metabolites; undergoes enterohepatic recycling

Half-life elimination: 1.4 hours

Time to peak, serum: 1-2 hours

Excretion: Urine (70% primarily as conjugated drug); feces (6%)

Pregnancy Risk Factor C

Dosage Forms TAB, film coated: 600 mg

Gemifloxacin (je mi FLOKS a sin)

Related Information

Bacterial Infections *on page 1697*

U.S. Brand Names Factive®

Generic Available No

Synonyms DW286; Gemifloxacin Mesylate; LA 20304a; SB-265805

Pharmacologic Category Antibiotic, Quinolone

Use Treatment of acute exacerbation of chronic bronchitis; treatment of community-acquired pneumonia, including pneumonia caused by multidrug-resistant strains of *S. pneumoniae* (MDRSP)

Unlabeled/Investigational Use Acute sinusitis, uncomplicated urinary tract infection

Local Anesthetic/Vasoconstrictor Precautions No information available to require special precautions

Effects on Dental Treatment No significant effects or complications reported

Common Adverse Effects

1% to 10%:

Central nervous system: Headache (1%), dizziness (1%)

Dermatologic: Rash (3%)

Gastrointestinal: Diarrhea (4%), nausea (3%), abdominal pain (1%), vomiting (1%)

Hepatic: Transaminases increased (1% to 2%)

Important adverse effects reported with other agents in this drug class include (not reported for gemifloxacin): Allergic reactions, CNS stimulation, hepatitis, jaundice, peripheral neuropathy, pneumonitis (eosinophilic), seizure; sensorimotor-axonal neuropathy (paresthesia, hypoesthesias, dysesthesias, weakness); severe dermatologic reactions (toxic epidermal necrolysis, Stevens-Johnson syndrome); tendon rupture, torsade de pointes, vasculitis

Dosage

Usual dosage range:

Adults: Oral: 320 mg once daily

(Continued)

Gemifloxacin *(Continued)*

Indication-specific dosing:
Adults: Oral:

Acute exacerbations of chronic bronchitis: 320 mg once daily for 5 days
Community-acquired pneumonia (mild to moderate): 320 mg once daily for 7 days
Sinusitis (unlabeled use): 320 mg once daily for 10 days

Dosage adjustment in renal impairment: Cl_{cr} ≤40 mL/minute (or patients on hemodialysis/CAPD): 160 mg once daily (administer dose following hemodialysis)

Dosage adjustment in hepatic impairment: No adjustment required.

Mechanism of Action Gemifloxacin is a DNA gyrase inhibitor and also inhibits topoisomerase IV. DNA gyrase (topoisomerase IV) is an essential bacterial enzyme that maintains the superhelical structure of DNA. DNA gyrase is required for DNA replication and transcription, DNA repair, recombination, and transposition; bactericidal

Contraindications Hypersensitivity to gemifloxacin, other fluoroquinolones, or any component of the formulation

Warnings/Precautions Fluoroquinolones may prolong QT_c interval; avoid use of gemifloxacin in patients with uncorrected hypokalemia, hypomagnesemia, or concurrent administration of other medications known to prolong the QT interval (including class Ia and class III antiarrhythmics, cisapride, erythromycin, antipsychotics, and tricyclic antidepressants). Use with caution in patients with significant bradycardia or acute myocardial ischemia. Use with caution in individuals at risk of seizures; discontinue in patients who experience significant CNS adverse effects. Use caution in renal dysfunction (dosage adjustment required).

Severe hypersensitivity reactions, including anaphylaxis, have occurred with quinolone therapy. Tendon inflammation and/or rupture has been reported with other quinolone antibiotics; risk may increase with concurrent corticosteroids, particularly in the elderly. Discontinue at first sign of tendon inflammation or pain. Peripheral neuropathy has been linked to the use of quinolones; these cases were rare. Experience with quinolones in immature animals has resulted in permanent arthropathy. Safety and effectiveness in pediatric patients (<18 years of age) have not been established.

Drug Interactions

Increased Effect/Toxicity: Gemifloxacin may increase the effects/toxicity of glyburide and warfarin. Concomitant use with corticosteroids may increase the risk of tendon rupture. Concomitant use with other QT_c-prolonging agents (eg, Class Ia and Class III antiarrhythmics, erythromycin, cisapride, antipsychotics, and cyclic antidepressants) may result in arrhythmias, such as torsade de pointes. Probenecid may increase gemifloxacin levels.

Decreased Effect: Concurrent administration of metal cations, including most antacids, oral electrolyte supplements, quinapril, sucralfate, some didanosine formulations (chewable/buffered tablets and pediatric powder for oral suspension), and other highly-buffered oral drugs, may decrease quinolone levels; separate doses.

Ethanol/Nutrition/Herb Interactions Herb/Nutraceutical: Avoid dong quai, St John's wort (may also cause photosensitization).

Dietary Considerations May take tablets with or without food, milk, or calcium supplements. Gemifloxacin should be taken 3 hours before or 2 hours after supplements (including multivitamins) containing iron, zinc, or magnesium.

Pharmacodynamics/Kinetics
Absorption: Well absorbed from the GI tract
Bioavailability: 71%
Metabolism: Hepatic (minor); forms metabolites (CYP isoenzymes are not involved)
Time to peak, plasma: 1-2 hours
Protein binding: 60% to 70%
Half-life elimination: 7 hours (range 4-12 hours)
Excretion: Urine (30% to 40%); feces (60%)

Pregnancy Risk Factor C
Dosage Forms TAB, as mesylate: 320 mg

Gemifloxacin Mesylate *see* Gemifloxacin *on page 731*

Gemtuzumab Ozogamicin (gem TOO zoo mab oh zog a MY sin)

U.S. Brand Names Mylotarg®
Canadian Brand Names Mylotarg®
Generic Available No

Synonyms CMA-676; NSC-720568

Pharmacologic Category Antineoplastic Agent, Monoclonal Antibody

Use Treatment of relapsed CD33 positive acute myeloid leukemia (AML) in patients ≥60 years of age who are not candidates for cytotoxic chemotherapy

Unlabeled/Investigational Use Salvage therapy for acute promyelocytic leukemia (APL), relapsed/ refractory CD33 positive acute myeloid leukemia in children and adults <60 years

Local Anesthetic/Vasoconstrictor Precautions No information available to require special precautions

Effects on Dental Treatment Key adverse event(s) related to dental treatment: Stomatitis and mucositis.

Common Adverse Effects Percentages established in adults ≥60 years of age. **Note:** A postinfusion symptom complex (fever, chills, less commonly hypertension, and/or dyspnea) may occur within 24 hours of administration; the incidence of infusion-related events decreases with repeat administration.

>10%:
Cardiovascular: Peripheral edema (19%), hypotension (18%), hypertension (17%), tachycardia (11%)

Central nervous system: Fever (78%), chills (64%), headache (27%), pain (18%), insomnia (11%)

Dermatologic: Petechiae (19%), cutaneous herpes simplex (18%), rash (18%), bruising (11%)

Endocrine & metabolic: Hypokalemia (24%), hyperglycemia (11%)

Gastrointestinal: Nausea (63%), vomiting (53%), diarrhea (30%), anorexia (27%), abdominal pain (26%), constipation (23%), stomatitis/mucositis (22%)

Hematologic: Neutropenia (grades 3/4: 98%; median recovery 40.5 days), lymphopenia (grades 3/4: 93%), thrombocytopenia (49%; grades 3/4: 48%; median recovery 39 days), hemoglobin decreased (grades 3/4: 50%), leukopenia (grades 3/4: 43%), anemia (22%, grades 3/4: 12%)

Hepatic: Abnormal liver function tests (20%; grade 3/4: 7%), LDH increased (18%), hyperbilirubinemia (11%)

Local: Local reaction (17%)

Neuromuscular & skeletal: Weakness (36%), back pain (12%)

Respiratory: Dyspnea (26%), epistaxis (24%; grade 3/4: 3%), cough (18%), pneumonia (13%)

Miscellaneous: Sepsis (25%), neutropenic fever (19%)

1% to 10%:
Central nervous system: Anxiety (10%), depression (10%), dizziness (10%), cerebral hemorrhage (2%), intracranial hemorrhage (1%)

Dermatologic: Pruritus (4%)

Endocrine & metabolic: Hypocalcemia (10%), hypophosphatemia (6%) hypomagnesemia (3%)

Gastrointestinal: Dyspepsia (8%), gingival hemorrhage (5%)

Genitourinary: Vaginal hemorrhage (5%), vaginal bleeding 2%, hematuria (grade 3/4: 1%)

Hematologic: Hemorrhage (9%), disseminated intravascular coagulation (DIC) (1%)

Hepatic: Alkaline phosphatase increased (10%), PT/PTT increased, veno-occlusive disease (5% to 10%; up to 20% in relapsed patients; higher frequency in patients with prior history of subsequent hematopoietic stem cell transplant)

Neuromuscular & skeletal: Arthralgia (10%), myalgia (3%)

Respiratory: Pharyngitis (10%), rhinitis (7%), hypoxia (5%)

Miscellaneous: Infection (10%)

Mechanism of Action Antibody to CD33 antigen. Binding results in internalization of the antibody-antigen complex. Following internalization, the calicheamicin derivative is released inside the myeloid cell. The calicheamicin derivative binds to DNA resulting in double strand breaks and cell death. Pluripotent stem cells and nonhematopoietic cells are not affected.

Drug Interactions

Increased Effect/Toxicity: Monoclonal antibodies may increase the risk for allergic reactions to gemtuzumab due to the presence of HACA antibodies

Pharmacodynamics/Kinetics

Distribution: V_{ss}: Adults: Initial dose: 21 L; Repeat dose: 10 L

Half-life elimination: Total calicheamicin: Initial: 41-45 hours, Repeat dose: 60-64 hours; Unconjugated: 100-143 hours (no change noted in repeat dosing)

Time to peak, plasma: Immediate; higher concentrations observed after repeat dose

Pregnancy Risk Factor D

Gemzar® *see* Gemcitabine *on page 729*

Genac® [OTC] *see* Triprolidine and Pseudoephedrine *on page 1542*

Genaced™ [OTC] *see* Acetaminophen, Aspirin, and Caffeine *on page 41*

Genahist® [OTC] *see* DiphenhydrAMINE *on page 483*

Genapap™ [OTC] *see* Acetaminophen *on page 31*

Genapap™ Children [OTC] *see* Acetaminophen *on page 31*

Genapap™ Extra Strength [OTC] *see* Acetaminophen *on page 31*

Genapap™ Infant [OTC] *see* Acetaminophen *on page 31*

Genapap™ Sinus Maximum Strength [OTC] *see* Acetaminophen and Pseudoephedrine *on page 38*

Genaphed® [OTC] *see* Pseudoephedrine *on page 1309*

Genasal [OTC] *see* Oxymetazoline *on page 1172*

Genasoft® [OTC] *see* Docusate *on page 496*

Genasoft® Plus [DSC] [OTC] *see* Docusate and Casanthranol *on page 496*

Genasyme® [OTC] *see* Simethicone *on page 1394*

Genaton Tablet [OTC] *see* Aluminum Hydroxide and Magnesium Trisilicate *on page 80*

Genatuss DM® [OTC] *see* Guaifenesin and Dextromethorphan *on page 754*

Genebs [OTC] *see* Acetaminophen *on page 31*

Genebs Extra Strength [OTC] *see* Acetaminophen *on page 31*

Generlac *see* Lactulose *on page 893*

Genesec® [OTC] *see* Acetaminophen and Phenyltoloxamine *on page 38*

Geneye® [OTC] *see* Tetrahydrozoline *on page 1470*

Genfiber® [OTC] *see* Psyllium *on page 1313*

Gengraf® *see* CycloSPORINE *on page 406*

Genoptic® [DSC] *see* Gentamicin *on page 734*

Genotropin® *see* Somatropin *on page 1406*

Genotropin Miniquick® *see* Somatropin *on page 1406*

Genpril® [OTC] *see* Ibuprofen *on page 808*

Gentak® *see* Gentamicin *on page 734*

Gentamicin (jen ta MYE sin)

Related Information
Cardiovascular Diseases *on page 1636*
Treatment of Sexually-Transmitted Infections *on page 1674*

U.S. Brand Names Genoptic® [DSC]; Gentak®

Canadian Brand Names Alcomicin®; Diogent®; Garamycin®; SAB-Gentamicin

Mexican Brand Names Garamicina®; Genemicin®; Genkova®; Genrex®; Gentabac®; Gentacin®; Genta Grin®; Gentarim®; Gentazaf®; G.I.®; Ikatin®; Servigenta®; Tondex®; Yectamicina®

Generic Available Yes

Synonyms Gentamicin Sulfate

Pharmacologic Category Antibiotic, Aminoglycoside; Antibiotic, Ophthalmic; Antibiotic, Topical

Dental Use Prevention of bacterial endocarditis prior to dental or surgical procedures

Use Treatment of susceptible bacterial infections, normally gram-negative organisms including *Pseudomonas*, *Proteus*, *Serratia*, and gram-positive *Staphylococcus*; treatment of bone infections, respiratory tract infections, skin and soft tissue infections, as well as abdominal and urinary tract infections, endocarditis, and septicemia; used topically to treat superficial infections of the skin or ophthalmic infections caused by susceptible bacteria; prevention of bacterial endocarditis prior to dental or surgical procedures

Local Anesthetic/Vasoconstrictor Precautions No information available to require special precautions

Effects on Dental Treatment No significant effects or complications reported

Common Adverse Effects
>10%:
Central nervous system: Neurotoxicity (vertigo, ataxia)
Neuromuscular & skeletal: Gait instability
Otic: Ototoxicity (auditory), ototoxicity (vestibular)
Renal: Nephrotoxicity, decreased creatinine clearance
1% to 10%:
Cardiovascular: Edema
Dermatologic: Skin itching, reddening of skin, rash

Mechanism of Action Interferes with bacterial protein synthesis by binding to 30S and 50S ribosomal subunits resulting in a defective bacterial cell membrane

Drug Interactions

Increased Effect/Toxicity: Penicillins, cephalosporins, amphotericin B, loop diuretics may increase nephrotoxic potential. Aminoglycosides may potentiate the effects of neuromuscular blocking agents.

Pharmacodynamics/Kinetics

Absorption: Oral: None

Distribution: Crosses placenta

V_d: Increased by edema, ascites, fluid overload; decreased with dehydration

Neonates: 0.4-0.6 L/kg

Children: 0.3-0.35 L/kg

Adults: 0.2-0.3 L/kg

Relative diffusion from blood into CSF: Minimal even with inflammation

CSF:blood level ratio: Normal meninges: Nil; Inflamed meninges: 10% to 30%

Protein binding: <30%

Half-life elimination:

Infants: <1 week old: 3-11.5 hours; 1 week to 6 months old: 3-3.5 hours

Adults: 1.5-3 hours; End-stage renal disease: 36-70 hours

Time to peak, serum: I.M.: 30-90 minutes; I.V.: 30 minutes after 30-minute infusion

Excretion: Urine (as unchanged drug)

Clearance: Directly related to renal function

Pregnancy Risk Factor C

Gentamicin and Prednisolone *see* Prednisolone and Gentamicin *on page 1271*

Gentamicin Sulfate *see* Gentamicin *on page 734*

GenTeal® [OTC] *see* Hydroxypropyl Methylcellulose *on page 800*

GenTeal® Mild [OTC] *see* Hydroxypropyl Methylcellulose *on page 800*

Gentian Violet (JEN shun VYE oh let)

Generic Available Yes

Synonyms Crystal Violet; Methylrosaniline Chloride

Pharmacologic Category Antibiotic, Topical; Antifungal Agent, Topical

Use Treatment of cutaneous or mucocutaneous infections caused by *Candida albicans* and other superficial skin infections

Local Anesthetic/Vasoconstrictor Precautions No information available to require special precautions

Effects on Dental Treatment No significant effects or complications reported

Common Adverse Effects Frequency not defined.

Dermatologic: Vesicle formation

Gastrointestinal: Esophagitis, ulceration of mucous membranes

Local: Burning, irritation

Respiratory: Laryngitis, laryngeal obstruction, tracheitis

Miscellaneous: Sensitivity reactions

Mechanism of Action Topical antiseptic/germicide effective against some vegetative gram-positive bacteria, particularly *Staphylococcus* sp, and some yeast; it is much less effective against gram-negative bacteria and is ineffective against acid-fast bacteria

Pregnancy Risk Factor C

Gentlax® [OTC] [DSC] *see* Bisacodyl *on page 209*

Gentran® *see* Dextran *on page 447*

Geocillin® *see* Carbenicillin *on page 265*

Geodon® *see* Ziprasidone *on page 1598*

Geref® Diagnostic *see* Sermorelin Acetate *on page 1384*

Geriation [OTC] *see* Vitamins (Multiple/Oral) *on page 1582*

Geri-Hydrolac™ [OTC] *see* Lactic Acid and Ammonium Hydroxide *on page 893*

Geri-Hydrolac™-12 [OTC] *see* Lactic Acid and Ammonium Hydroxide *on page 893*

Geritol Complete® [OTC] *see* Vitamins (Multiple/Oral) *on page 1582*

Geritol Extend® [OTC] *see* Vitamins (Multiple/Oral) *on page 1582*

Geritol® Tonic [OTC] *see* Vitamins (Multiple/Oral) *on page 1582*

German Measles Vaccine *see* Rubella Virus Vaccine (Live) *on page 1372*

Gevrabon® [OTC] *see* Vitamin B Complex Combinations *on page 1581*

GF196960 *see* Tadalafil *on page 1441*

GG *see* Guaifenesin *on page 752*

GHB *see* Sodium Oxybate *on page 1402*

GI87084B *see* Remifentanil *on page 1338*

Giltuss® *see* Guaifenesin, Dextromethorphan, and Phenylephrine *on page 756*

Giltuss HC® *see* Hydrocodone, Phenylephrine, and Guaifenesin *on page 791*

Giltuss Pediatric® *see* Guaifenesin, Dextromethorphan, and Phenylephrine *on page 756*

Giltuss TR® *see* Guaifenesin, Dextromethorphan, and Phenylephrine *on page 756*

Gladase® *see* Papain and Urea *on page 1186*

Glargine Insulin *see* Insulin Glargine *on page 837*

Glatiramer Acetate (gla TIR a mer AS e tate)

U.S. Brand Names Copaxone®
Canadian Brand Names Copaxone®
Generic Available No
Synonyms Copolymer-1
Pharmacologic Category Biological, Miscellaneous
Use Treatment of relapsing-remitting type multiple sclerosis; studies indicate that it reduces the frequency of attacks and the severity of disability; appears to be most effective for patients with minimal disability

Local Anesthetic/Vasoconstrictor Precautions No information available to require special precautions

Effects on Dental Treatment Key adverse event(s) related to dental treatment: Ulcerative stomatitis and salivary gland enlargement.

Common Adverse Effects Reported in >2% of patients in placebo-controlled trials:

>10%:
Cardiovascular: Chest pain (21%), vasodilation (27%), palpitation (17%)
Central nervous system: Pain (28%), anxiety (23%)
Dermatologic: Pruritus (18%), rash (18%), diaphoresis (15%)
Gastrointestinal: Nausea (22%), diarrhea (12%)
Local: Injection site reactions: Pain (73%), erythema (66%), inflammation (49%), pruritus (40%), mass (27%), induration (13%), welt (11%)
Neuromuscular & skeletal: Weakness (41%), arthralgia (24%), hypertonia (22%), back pain (16%)
Respiratory: Dyspnea (19%), rhinitis (14%)
Miscellaneous: Infection (50%), flu-like syndrome (19%), lymphadenopathy (12%)

1% to 10%:
Cardiovascular: Peripheral edema (7%), facial edema (6%), edema (3%), tachycardia (5%)
Central nervous system: Fever (8%), vertigo (6%), migraine (5%), syncope (5%), agitation (4%), chills (4%), confusion (2%), nervousness (2%), speech disorder (2%)
Dermatologic: Bruising (8%), erythema (4%), urticaria (4%), skin nodule (2%)
Endocrine & metabolic: Dysmenorrhea (6%)
Gastrointestinal: Anorexia (8%), vomiting (6%), gastrointestinal disorder (5%), gastroenteritis (3%), weight gain (3%)
Genitourinary: Urinary urgency (10%), vaginal moniliasis (8%)
Local: Injection site reactions: Hemorrhage (5%), urticaria (5%)
Neuromuscular & skeletal: Tremor (7%), foot drop (3%)
Ocular: Eye disorder (4%), nystagmus (2%)
Otic: Ear pain (7%)
Respiratory: Bronchitis (9%), laryngismus (5%)
Miscellaneous: Neck pain (8%), bacterial infection (5%), herpes simplex (4%), cyst (2%)

Mechanism of Action Glatiramer is a mixture of random polymers of four amino acids; L-alanine, L-glutamic acid, L-lysine and L-tyrosine, the resulting mixture is antigenically similar to myelin basic protein, which is an important component of the myelin sheath of nerves; glatiramer is thought to suppress T-lymphocytes specific for a myelin antigen, it is also proposed that glatiramer interferes with the antigen-presenting function of certain immune cells opposing pathogenic T-cell function

Pharmacodynamics/Kinetics
Distribution: Small amounts of intact and partial hydrolyzed drug enter lymphatic circulation
Metabolism: SubQ: Large percentage hydrolyzed locally

Pregnancy Risk Factor B

Gleevec® *see* Imatinib *on page 817*

Gliadel® *see* Carmustine *on page 273*

Glibenclamide *see* GlyBURIDE *on page 744*

Gliclazide (GLYE kla zide)

Canadian Brand Names Apo-Gliclazide®; Diamicron®; Diamicron® MR; Novo-Gliclazide; Rhoxal-gliclazide; Sandoz-Gliclazide

Generic Available Yes: 80 mg tablet

Pharmacologic Category Antidiabetic Agent, Sulfonylurea

Use Management of type 2 diabetes mellitus (noninsulin dependent, NIDDM)

Local Anesthetic/Vasoconstrictor Precautions No information available to require special precautions

Effects on Dental Treatment Gliclazide-dependent diabetics (noninsulin dependent, type 2) should be appointed for dental treatment in morning in order to minimize chance of stress-induced hypoglycemia.

Common Adverse Effects Frequency not defined.

Central nervous system: Headache, nervousness, dizziness

Dermatologic: Rash, erythema, pruritus, urticaria. Sulfonylureas have also been associated with rare photosensitivity and porphyria cutanea tarda

Endocrine & metabolic: Hypoglycemia (dose dependent), hyponatremia (rare)

Gastrointestinal: Nausea, vomiting, diarrhea, epigastric fullness, gastritis

Hematologic: Agranulocytosis, leukopenia, thrombocytopenia, anemia

Hepatic: Jaundice, LDH increased, transaminases increased

Miscellaneous: Disulfiram reaction (very low potential)

Restrictions Not available in U.S.

Dosage Oral: Adults:

Immediate release tablet: Initial: 80-160 mg/day; typical dose range 80-320 mg/day; dosage of ≥160 mg should be divided into 2 equal parts for twice-daily administration; maximum dose: 320 mg/day; should be taken with meals

Sustained release tablet: 30-120 mg once daily

Note: There is no fixed dosage regimen for the management of diabetes mellitus with gliclazide or any other hypoglycemic agent. Dose must be individualized based on frequent determinations of blood glucose during dose titration and throughout maintenance.

Dosage adjustment in renal/hepatic impairment: Contraindicated in severe impairment

Mechanism of Action Stimulates insulin release from the pancreatic beta cells; reduces glucose output from the liver; lowers plasma glucose concentrations. Gliclazide has also been shown to decrease platelet aggregation at therapeutic doses.

Contraindications Hypersensitivity to gliclazide, sulfonylureas, or any component of the formulation; type 1 diabetes mellitus (insulin dependent, IDDM), diabetic ketoacidosis with or without coma; renal or hepatic impairment; pregnancy (per manufacturer); breast-feeding

Warnings/Precautions All sulfonylurea drugs are capable of producing severe hypoglycemia. Hypoglycemia is more likely to occur when caloric intake is deficient, after severe or prolonged exercise, when ethanol is ingested, or when more than one glucose-lowering drug is used. Hypoglycemia is also more likely in elderly patients, or in impaired renal or hepatic function.

Chemical similarities are present among sulfonamides, sulfonylureas, carbonic anhydrase inhibitors, thiazides, and loop diuretics (except ethacrynic acid). Use in patients with sulfonamide allergy is specifically contraindicated in product labeling, however, a risk of cross-reaction exists in patients with allergy to any of these compounds; avoid use when previous reaction has been severe. Safety and efficacy have not been established in pediatric patients.

Product labeling of sulfonylureas (in U.S.) states oral hypoglycemic drugs may be associated with an increased cardiovascular mortality as compared to treatment with diet alone or diet plus insulin. Data to support this association are limited, and several studies, including a large prospective trial (UKPDS), have not supported an association.

Drug Interactions

Increased Effect/Toxicity: Anabolic steroids, ACE inhibitors, H$_2$ antagonists, antacids, oral sodium bicarbonate, salicylates, and sulfonamides may increase the hypoglycemic effect of gliclazide. A possible interaction between sulfonylureas and fluoroquinolone antibiotics has been reported resulting in a potentiation of hypoglycemic action of sulfonylureas. Warfarin's anticoagulant effects may be increased by sulfonylureas. Rare disulfiram reactions may occur with ethanol. Gliclazide may increase serum concentrations of cyclosporine.

Decreased Effect: Beta-blockers may decrease gliclazide's hypoglycemic effect, mask most hypoglycemic symptoms, and decrease glycogenolysis; avoid use in patients with diabetes with frequent hypoglycemic episodes

(Continued)

Gliclazide *(Continued)*

(particularly nonselective beta-blockers). Corticosteroids and thiazide diuretics may cause hyperglycemia; adjustment of hypoglycemic agent may be necessary. Ethanol (large amounts) and/or rifampin may decrease gliclazide's hypoglycemic effect; avoid concurrent use.

Ethanol/Nutrition/Herb Interactions

Ethanol: Avoid ethanol (may cause hypoglycemia and/or rare disulfiram reactions).

Herb/Nutraceutical: Avoid chromium, garlic, gymnema (may cause hypoglycemia).

Dietary Considerations Should be taken with meals. Dietary modification based on ADA recommendations is a part of therapy. Decreases blood glucose concentration. Hypoglycemia may occur. Must be able to recognize symptoms of hypoglycemia (palpitations, sweaty palms, lightheadedness).

Pharmacodynamics/Kinetics

Absorption: Rapid

Protein binding: 94%

Metabolism: Hepatic, to inactive metabolites

Half-life elimination: 10 hours

Time to peak: 4-6 hours

Excretion: Urine (60% to 70%) and feces (10% to 20%) as metabolites

Pregnancy Risk Factor Not available (similar agents rated C); manufacturer contraindicates use

Dosage Forms TAB 80 mg. **TAB, sustained-release:** 30 mg

Glimepiride *(GLYE me pye ride)*

Related Information

Endocrine Disorders and Pregnancy *on page 1659*

U.S. Brand Names Amaryl®

Canadian Brand Names Amaryl®; ratio-Glimepiride; Sandoz-Glimepiride

Mexican Brand Names Amaryl®

Generic Available Yes

Pharmacologic Category Antidiabetic Agent, Sulfonylurea

Use Management of type 2 diabetes mellitus (noninsulin dependent, NIDDM) as an adjunct to diet and exercise to lower blood glucose; may be used in combination with metformin or insulin in patients whose hyperglycemia cannot be controlled by diet and exercise in conjunction with a single oral hypoglycemic agent

Local Anesthetic/Vasoconstrictor Precautions No information available to require special precautions

Effects on Dental Treatment Glimepiride-dependent diabetics (noninsulin dependent, type 2) should be appointed for dental treatment in morning in order to minimize chance of stress-induced hypoglycemia.

Common Adverse Effects

1% to 10%:

Central nervous system: Dizziness (2%), headache (2%)

Endocrine & metabolic: Hypoglycemia (1% to 2%)

Gastrointestinal: Nausea (1%)

Neuromuscular & skeletal: Weakness (2%)

Dosage Oral:

Children 10-18 years (unlabeled use): Initial: 1 mg once daily; maintenance: 1-4 mg once daily

Adults: Initial: 1-2 mg once daily, administered with breakfast or the first main meal; usual maintenance dose: 1-4 mg once daily; after a dose of 2 mg once daily, increase in increments of 2 mg at 1- to 2-week intervals based upon the patient's blood glucose response to a maximum of 8 mg once daily. If inadequate response to maximal dose, combination therapy with metformin may be considered.

Combination with insulin therapy (fasting glucose level for instituting combination therapy is in the range of >150 mg/dL in plasma or serum depending on the patient): initial recommended dose: 8 mg once daily with the first main meal

After starting with low-dose insulin, upward adjustments of insulin can be done approximately weekly as guided by frequent measurements of fasting blood glucose. Once stable, combination-therapy patients should monitor their capillary blood glucose on an ongoing basis, preferably daily.

Conversion from therapy with long half-life agents: Observe patient carefully for 1-2 weeks when converting from a longer half-life agent (eg, chlorpropamide) to glimepiride due to overlapping hypoglycemic effects.

Dosing adjustment/comments in renal impairment: Cl_{cr} <22 mL/minute: Initial starting dose should be 1 mg and dosage increments should be based on fasting blood glucose levels

Dosing adjustment in hepatic impairment: No data available

Elderly: Initial: 1 mg/day; dose titration and maintenance dosing should be conservative to avoid hypoglycemia

Mechanism of Action Stimulates insulin release from the pancreatic beta cells; reduces glucose output from the liver; insulin sensitivity is increased at peripheral target sites

Contraindications Hypersensitivity to glimepiride, any component of the formulation, or sulfonamides; diabetic ketoacidosis (with or without coma)

Warnings/Precautions All sulfonylurea drugs are capable of producing severe hypoglycemia. Hypoglycemia is more likely to occur when caloric intake is deficient, after severe or prolonged exercise, when ethanol is ingested, or when more than one glucose-lowering drug is used.

Chemical similarities are present among sulfonamides, sulfonylureas, carbonic anhydrase inhibitors, thiazides, and loop diuretics (except ethacrynic acid). Use in patients with sulfonamide allergy is specifically contraindicated in product labeling, however, a risk of cross-reaction exists in patients with allergy to any of these compounds; avoid use when previous reaction has been severe.

Product labeling states oral hypoglycemic drugs may be associated with an increased cardiovascular mortality as compared to treatment with diet alone or diet plus insulin. Data to support this association are limited, and several studies, including a large prospective trial (UKPDS) have not supported an association. Safety and efficacy in pediatric patients have not been established.

Drug Interactions

Cytochrome P450 Effect: Substrate of CYP2C9 (major)

Increased Effect/Toxicity: CYP2C9 inhibitors may increase the levels/effects of glimepiride; example inhibitors include delavirdine, ketoconazole, nicardipine, NSAIDs, sulfonamides, and tolbutamide. Beta-blockers, chloramphenicol, cimetidine, fibric acid derivatives, fluconazole, pegvisomant, salicylates, sulfonamides, and tricyclic antidepressants may increase the hypoglycemic effects of glimepiride. Glimepiride may increase effects of cyclosporine. Sulfonylureas may induce a disulfiram-like reaction with ethanol.

Decreased Effect: CYP2C9 inducers may decrease the levels/effects of glimepiride; example inducers include carbamazepine, phenobarbital, phenytoin, rifampin, rifapentine, and secobarbital. There may be a decreased effect of glimepiride with corticosteroids, estrogens, oral contraceptives, thiazide and other diuretics, phenothiazines, NSAIDs, thyroid products, nicotinic acid, isoniazid, sympathomimetics, urinary alkalinizers, and charcoal. **Note:** However, pooled data did **not** demonstrate drug interactions with calcium channel blockers, estrogens, NSAIDs, HMG-CoA reductase inhibitors, sulfonamides, or thyroid hormone.

Ethanol/Nutrition/Herb Interactions

Ethanol: Caution with ethanol (may cause hypoglycemia).

Herb/Nutraceutical: Caution with chromium, garlic, gymnema (may cause hypoglycemia).

Dietary Considerations Administer with breakfast or the first main meal of the day. Dietary modification based on ADA recommendations is a part of therapy. Decreases blood glucose concentration. Hypoglycemia may occur. Must be able to recognize symptoms of hypoglycemia (palpitations, sweaty palms, lightheadedness).

Pharmacodynamics/Kinetics

Onset of action: Peak effect: Blood glucose reductions: 2-3 hours

Duration: 24 hours

Absorption: 100%; delayed when given with food

Distribution: V_d: 8.8 L

Protein binding: >99.5%

Metabolism: Hepatic oxidation via CYP2C9 to M1 metabolite (~33% activity of parent compound); further oxidative metabolism to inactive M2 metabolite

Half-life elimination: 5-9 hours

Time to peak, plasma: 2-3 hours

Excretion: Urine (60%, 80% to 90% M1 and M2); feces (40%, 70% M1 and M2)

Pregnancy Risk Factor C

Dosage Forms TAB: 1 mg, 2 mg, 4 mg

Glimepiride and Rosiglitazone Maleate *see* Rosiglitazone and Glimepiride *on page 1369*

GlipiZIDE (GLIP i zide)

Related Information
  Endocrine Disorders and Pregnancy *on page 1659*
U.S. Brand Names Glucotrol®; Glucotrol® XL
Mexican Brand Names Glupitel®; Minodiab®
Generic Available Yes
Synonyms Glydiazinamide
Pharmacologic Category Antidiabetic Agent, Sulfonylurea
Use Management of type 2 diabetes mellitus (noninsulin dependent, NIDDM)
Local Anesthetic/Vasoconstrictor Precautions No information available to require special precautions
Effects on Dental Treatment Glipizide-dependent diabetics (noninsulin dependent, type 2) should be appointed for dental treatment in morning in order to minimize chance of stress-induced hypoglycemia.
Common Adverse Effects Frequency not defined.
  Cardiovascular: Edema, syncope
  Central nervous system: Anxiety, depression, dizziness, headache, insomnia, nervousness
  Dermatologic: Rash, urticaria, photosensitivity, pruritus
  Endocrine & metabolic: Hypoglycemia, hyponatremia, SIADH (rare)
  Gastrointestinal: Anorexia, nausea, vomiting, diarrhea, epigastric fullness, constipation, heartburn, flatulence
  Hematologic: Blood dyscrasias, aplastic anemia, hemolytic anemia, bone marrow suppression, thrombocytopenia, agranulocytosis
  Hepatic: Cholestatic jaundice, hepatic porphyria
  Neuromuscular & skeletal: Arthralgia, leg cramps, myalgia, tremor
  Ocular: Blurred vision
  Renal: Diuretic effect (minor)
  Miscellaneous: Diaphoresis, disulfiram-like reaction
Dosage Oral (allow several days between dose titrations): Adults: Initial: 5 mg/day; adjust dosage at 2.5-5 mg daily increments as determined by blood glucose response at intervals of several days.
  Immediate release tablet: Maximum recommended once-daily dose: 15 mg; maximum recommended total daily dose: 40 mg
  Extended release tablet (Glucotrol® XL): Maximum recommended dose: 20 mg
  When transferring from insulin to glipizide:
    Current insulin requirement ≤20 units: Discontinue insulin and initiate glipizide at usual dose
    Current insulin requirement >20 units: Decrease insulin by 50% and initiate glipizide at usual dose; gradually decrease insulin dose based on patient response. Several days should elapse between dosage changes.
  Elderly: Initial: 2.5 mg/day; increase by 2.5-5 mg/day at 1- to 2-week intervals
Dosing adjustment/comments in renal impairment: Cl_{cr} <10 mL/minute: Some investigators recommend not using
Dosing adjustment in hepatic impairment: Initial dosage should be 2.5 mg/day
Mechanism of Action Stimulates insulin release from the pancreatic beta cells; reduces glucose output from the liver; insulin sensitivity is increased at peripheral target sites
Contraindications Hypersensitivity to glipizide or any component of the formulation, other sulfonamides; type 1 diabetes mellitus (insulin dependent, IDDM)
Warnings/Precautions Use with caution in patients with severe hepatic disease.

Chemical similarities are present among sulfonamides, sulfonylureas, carbonic anhydrase inhibitors, thiazides, and loop diuretics (except ethacrynic acid). Use in patients with sulfonamide allergy is specifically contraindicated in product labeling, however, a risk of cross-reaction exists in patients with allergy to any of these compounds; avoid use when previous reaction has been severe.

Product labeling states oral hypoglycemic drugs may be associated with an increased cardiovascular mortality as compared to treatment with diet alone or diet plus insulin. Data to support this association are limited, and several studies, including a large prospective trial (UKPDS) have not supported an association.

At higher dosages, sulfonylureas may block the ATP-sensitive potassium channels, which have been suggested to increase the risk of cardiovascular events. In May, 2000, the National Diabetes Center (a patient advocacy group, not a government agency) issued a warning to avoid the use of sulfonylureas at higher dosages. The clinical data supporting an association is inconsistent, and there is no consensus within the medical community to support this assertion. Avoid use of extended release tablets (Glucotrol® XL) in patients with known stricture/narrowing of the GI tract.

Drug Interactions
Cytochrome P450 Effect: Substrate of 2C8/9 (major)
Increased Effect/Toxicity: CYP2C8/9 inhibitors may increase the levels/effects of glipizide; example inhibitors include delavirdine, fluconazole, gemfibrozil, ketoconazole, nicardipine, NSAIDs, pioglitazone, and sulfonamides. Increased effects/hypoglycemic effects of glipizide with H_2 antagonists, anticoagulants, androgens, cimetidine, salicylates, tricyclic antidepressants, probenecid, MAO inhibitors, methyldopa, digitalis glycosides, and urinary acidifiers.
Decreased Effect: CYP2C8/9 inducers may decrease the levels/effects of glipizide; example inducers include carbamazepine, phenobarbital, phenytoin, rifampin, rifapentine, and secobarbital. Decreased effect of glipizide with beta-blockers, cholestyramine, hydantoins, thiazide diuretics, urinary alkalinizers, and charcoal.

Ethanol/Nutrition/Herb Interactions
Ethanol: Caution with ethanol (may cause hypoglycemia or rare disulfiram reaction).
Food: A delayed release of insulin may occur if glipizide is taken with food. Immediate release tablets should be administered 30 minutes before meals to avoid erratic absorption.
Herb/Nutraceutical: Caution with chromium, garlic, gymnema (may cause hypoglycemia).

Dietary Considerations Take immediate release tablets 30 minutes before meals; extended release tablets should be taken with breakfast. Dietary modification based on ADA recommendations is a part of therapy. Decreases blood glucose concentration. Hypoglycemia may occur. Must be able to recognize symptoms of hypoglycemia (palpitations, sweaty palms, lightheadedness).

Pharmacodynamics/Kinetics
Onset of action: Peak effect: Blood glucose reductions: 1.5-2 hours
Duration: 12-24 hours
Absorption: Delayed with food
Protein binding: 92% to 99%
Metabolism: Hepatic with metabolites
Half-life elimination: 2-4 hours
Excretion: Urine (60% to 80%, 91% to 97% as metabolites); feces (11%)
Pregnancy Risk Factor C
Dosage Forms TAB (Glucotrol®): 5 mg, 10 mg. **TAB, extended release:** 5 mg, 10 mg; (Glucotrol® XL): 2.5 mg, 5 mg, 10 mg

---

Glipizide and Metformin (GLIP i zide & met FOR min)

Related Information
GlipiZIDE on page 740
Metformin on page 1001
U.S. Brand Names Metaglip™
Generic Available No
Synonyms Glipizide and Metformin Hydrochloride; Metformin and Glipizide
Pharmacologic Category Antidiabetic Agent, Biguanide; Antidiabetic Agent, Sulfonylurea
Use Initial therapy for management of type 2 diabetes mellitus (noninsulin dependent, NIDDM) when hyperglycemia cannot be managed with diet and exercise alone. Second-line therapy for management of type 2 diabetes (NIDDM) when hyperglycemia cannot be managed with a sulfonylurea or metformin along with diet and exercise.
Local Anesthetic/Vasoconstrictor Precautions No information available to require special precautions
Effects on Dental Treatment Key adverse event(s) related to dental treatment: Upper respiratory tract infection (8% to 10%). Dependent diabetics (noninsulin dependent, type 2) should be appointed for dental treatment in the morning in order to minimize chance of stress-induced hypoglycemia.
Common Adverse Effects Also see individual agents.
>10%:
Central nervous system: Headache (12%)
Endocrine & metabolic: Hypoglycemia (8% to 13%)
Gastrointestinal: Diarrhea (2% to 18%)
1% to 10%:
Cardiovascular: Hypertension (3%)
(Continued)

Glipizide and Metformin *(Continued)*

Central nervous system: Dizziness (2% to 5%)
Gastrointestinal: Nausea/vomiting (<1% to 8%), abdominal pain (6%)
Neuromuscular & skeletal: Musculoskeletal pain (8%)
Renal: Urinary tract infection (1%)
Respiratory: Upper respiratory tract infection (8% to 10%)

Mechanism of Action The combination of glipizide and metformin is used to improve glycemic control in patients with type 2 diabetes mellitus (noninsulin dependent, NIDDM) by using two different, but complementary, mechanisms of action:

Glipizide: Stimulates insulin release from the pancreatic beta cells; reduces glucose output from the liver; insulin sensitivity is increased at peripheral target sites

Metformin: Decreases hepatic glucose production, decreasing intestinal absorption of glucose and improves insulin sensitivity (increases peripheral glucose uptake and utilization)

Drug Interactions
Cytochrome P450 Effect: Glipizide: **Substrate** of 2C8/9 (major)
Increased Effect/Toxicity: See individual agents.
Decreased Effect: See individual agents.
Pharmacodynamics/Kinetics See individual agents.
Pregnancy Risk Factor C

Glipizide and Metformin Hydrochloride *see* Glipizide and Metformin *on page 741*

Glivec *see* Imatinib *on page 817*

Gln *see* Glutamine *on page 743*

GlucaGen® *see* Glucagon *on page 742*

GlucaGen® Diagnostic Kit *see* Glucagon *on page 742*

GlucaGen® HypoKit™ *see* Glucagon *on page 742*

Glucagon *(GLOO ka gon)*

U.S. Brand Names GlucaGen®; GlucaGen® Diagnostic Kit; GlucaGen® HypoKit™; Glucagon Diagnostic Kit [DSC]; Glucagon Emergency Kit
Generic Available No
Synonyms Glucagon Hydrochloride
Pharmacologic Category Antidote; Diagnostic Agent
Use Management of hypoglycemia; diagnostic aid in radiologic examinations to temporarily inhibit GI tract movement
Unlabeled/Investigational Use Used with some success as a cardiac stimulant in management of severe cases of beta-adrenergic blocking agent overdosage; treatment of myocardial depression due to calcium channel blocker overdose
Local Anesthetic/Vasoconstrictor Precautions No information available to require special precautions
Effects on Dental Treatment No significant effects or complications reported
Common Adverse Effects Frequency not defined.
Cardiovascular: Hypotension (up to 2 hours after GI procedures), hypertension, tachycardia
Gastrointestinal: Nausea, vomiting (high incidence with rapid administration of high doses)
Miscellaneous: Hypersensitivity reactions, anaphylaxis
Mechanism of Action Stimulates adenylate cyclase to produce increased cyclic AMP, which promotes hepatic glycogenolysis and gluconeogenesis, causing a raise in blood glucose levels
Drug Interactions
Increased Effect/Toxicity: Oral anticoagulant: Hypoprothrombinemic effects may be increased possibly with bleeding; effect seen with glucagon doses of 50 mg administered over 1-2 days
Pharmacodynamics/Kinetics
Onset of action: Peak effect: Blood glucose levels: Parenteral:
I.V.: 5-20 minutes
I.M.: 30 minutes
SubQ: 30-45 minutes
Duration: Hyperglycemia: 60-90 minutes
Metabolism: Primarily hepatic; some inactivation occurring renally and in plasma
Half-life elimination, plasma: 3-10 minutes
Pregnancy Risk Factor B

Glucagon Diagnostic Kit [DSC] *see* Glucagon *on page 742*
Glucagon Emergency Kit *see* Glucagon *on page 742*
Glucagon Hydrochloride *see* Glucagon *on page 742*
Glucocerebrosidase *see* Alglucerase *on page 68*
Glucophage® *see* Metformin *on page 1001*
Glucophage® XR *see* Metformin *on page 1001*
Glucose *see* Dextrose *on page 452*
Glucose Monohydrate *see* Dextrose *on page 452*

Glucose Polymers (GLOO kose POL i merz)

U.S. Brand Names Moducal® [OTC]; Polycose® [OTC]
Generic Available No
Pharmacologic Category Nutritional Supplement
Use Supplies calories for those persons not able to meet the caloric requirement with usual food intake
Local Anesthetic/Vasoconstrictor Precautions No information available to require special precautions
Effects on Dental Treatment No significant effects or complications reported

Glucotrol® *see* GlipiZIDE *on page 740*
Glucotrol® XL *see* GlipiZIDE *on page 740*
Glucovance® *see* Glyburide and Metformin *on page 745*
Glu-K® [OTC] *see* Potassium Gluconate *on page 1259*
Glulisine Insulin *see* Insulin Glulisine *on page 837*

Glutamic Acid (gloo TAM ik AS id)

Generic Available Yes
Synonyms Glutamic Acid Hydrochloride
Pharmacologic Category Gastrointestinal Agent, Miscellaneous
Use Treatment of hypochlorhydria and achlorhydria
Local Anesthetic/Vasoconstrictor Precautions No information available to require special precautions
Effects on Dental Treatment No significant effects or complications reported
Pregnancy Risk Factor C

Glutamic Acid Hydrochloride *see* Glutamic Acid *on page 743*

Glutamine (GLOO ta meen)

U.S. Brand Names Enterex® Glutapak-10® [OTC]; NutreStore™; Resource® GlutaSolve® [OTC]; Sympt-X [OTC]; Sympt-X G.I. [OTC]
Synonyms Gln; L-Glutamine
Pharmacologic Category Amino Acid
Use Treatment of short bowel syndrome when used in combination with nutritional support and growth hormone therapy; a medical food used to promote GI tract healing and nutritional supplementation with GI disorders, HIV/AIDS, cancer, and other critical illnesses
Local Anesthetic/Vasoconstrictor Precautions No information available to require special precautions
Effects on Dental Treatment No significant effects or complications reported
Common Adverse Effects Frequency not defined.
  Cardiovascular: Facial edema, peripheral edema
  Central nervous system: Dizziness, fever, headache, pain
  Dermatologic: Pruritus, rash
  Gastrointestinal: Abdominal pain, flatulence, nausea, pancreatitis, tenesmus, vomiting
  Neuromuscular & skeletal: Arthralgia, back pain, hypoesthesia
  Otic: Ear or hearing symptoms
  Respiratory: Rhinitis
  Miscellaneous: Flu-like syndrome, infection, sepsis
Mechanism of Action Glutamine regulates gastrointestinal cell growth, function, and regeneration. Considered a "conditionally essential" amino acid during metabolic stress and injury.
Pharmacodynamics/Kinetics As reported in healthy adults; parameters may vary following oral administration in patients with short bowel syndrome.
  Distribution: I.V.: V_d: 200 mL/kg
  Metabolism: Via splanchnic tissue, lymphocytes, kidney, and liver to glutamate and ammonia
  (Continued)

Glutamine (Continued)

Half-life elimination: I.V.: 1 hour
Pregnancy Risk Factor C

Glutofac®-MX *see* Vitamins (Multiple/Oral) *on page 1582*
Glutofac®-ZX *see* Vitamins (Multiple/Oral) *on page 1582*
Glutol™ [OTC] *see* Dextrose *on page 452*
Glutose™ [OTC] *see* Dextrose *on page 452*
Glybenclamide *see* GlyBURIDE *on page 744*
Glybenzcyclamide *see* GlyBURIDE *on page 744*

GlyBURIDE (GLYE byoor ide)

Related Information
Endocrine Disorders and Pregnancy *on page 1659*
U.S. Brand Names Diaβeta®; Glynase® PresTab®; Micronase®
Canadian Brand Names Albert® Glyburide; Apo-Glyburide®; Diaβeta®; Euglucon®; Gen-Glybe; Novo-Glyburide; Nu-Glyburide; PMS-Glyburide; ratio-Glyburide; Sandoz-Glyburide
Mexican Brand Names Daonil®; Euglucon®; Glibenil®; Glucal®; Glucoven®; Nadib®; Norboral®
Generic Available Yes
Synonyms Diabeta; Glibenclamide; Glybenclamide; Glybenzcyclamide
Pharmacologic Category Antidiabetic Agent, Sulfonylurea
Use Management of type 2 diabetes mellitus (noninsulin dependent, NIDDM)
Unlabeled/Investigational Use Alternative to insulin in women for the treatment of gestational diabetes (11-33 weeks gestation)
Local Anesthetic/Vasoconstrictor Precautions No information available to require special precautions
Effects on Dental Treatment Glyburide-dependent diabetics (noninsulin dependent, type 2) should be appointed for dental treatment in morning in order to minimize chance of stress-induced hypoglycemia.
Common Adverse Effects Frequency not defined.
Central nervous system: Headache, dizziness
Dermatologic: Pruritus, rash, urticaria, photosensitivity reaction
Endocrine & metabolic: Hypoglycemia, hyponatremia (SIADH reported with other sulfonylureas)
Gastrointestinal: Nausea, epigastric fullness, heartburn, constipation, diarrhea, anorexia
Genitourinary: Nocturia
Hematologic: Leukopenia, thrombocytopenia, hemolytic anemia, aplastic anemia, bone marrow suppression, agranulocytosis
Hepatic: Cholestatic jaundice, hepatitis
Neuromuscular & skeletal: Arthralgia, paresthesia
Ocular: Blurred vision
Renal: Diuretic effect (minor)
Mechanism of Action Stimulates insulin release from the pancreatic beta cells; reduces glucose output from the liver; insulin sensitivity is increased at peripheral target sites
Drug Interactions
Cytochrome P450 Effect: Inhibits CYP2C8 (weak), 3A4 (weak)
Increased Effect/Toxicity: Increased hypoglycemic effects of glyburide may occur with oral anticoagulants (warfarin), phenytoin, other hydantoins, salicylates, NSAIDs, sulfonamides, and beta-blockers. Ethanol ingestion may cause disulfiram reactions.
Decreased Effect: Thiazides and other diuretics, corticosteroids may decrease effectiveness of glyburide.
Pharmacodynamics/Kinetics
Onset of action: Serum insulin levels begin to increase 15-60 minutes after a single dose
Duration: ≤24 hours
Protein binding, plasma: >99%
Metabolism: To one moderately active and several inactive metabolites
Half-life elimination: 5-16 hours; may be prolonged with renal or hepatic impairment
Time to peak, serum: Adults: 2-4 hours
Excretion: Feces (50%) and urine (50%) as metabolites
Pregnancy Risk Factor C

Glyburide and Metformin (GLYE byoor ide & met FOR min)

Related Information

Endocrine Disorders and Pregnancy *on page 1659*
GlyBURIDE *on page 744*
Metformin *on page 1001*

U.S. Brand Names Glucovance®

Generic Available Yes

Synonyms Glyburide and Metformin Hydrochloride; Metformin and Glyburide

Pharmacologic Category Antidiabetic Agent, Biguanide; Antidiabetic Agent, Sulfonylurea

Use Initial therapy for management of type 2 diabetes mellitus (noninsulin dependent, NIDDM). Second-line therapy for management of type 2 diabetes (NIDDM) when hyperglycemia cannot be managed with a sulfonylurea or metformin; combination therapy with a thiazolidinedione may be required to achieve additional control.

Local Anesthetic/Vasoconstrictor Precautions No information available to require special precautions

Effects on Dental Treatment Glyburide-dependent diabetics (noninsulin dependent, type 2) should be appointed for dental treatment in morning in order to minimize chance of stress-induced hypoglycemia. Metformin-dependent diabetics (noninsulin dependent, type 2) should be appointed for dental treatment in morning in order to minimize chance of stress-induced hypoglycemia.

Common Adverse Effects (Also refer to individual agents)

>10%:

Endocrine & metabolic: Hypoglycemia (11% to 38%, effects higher when increased doses were used as initial therapy)

Gastrointestinal: Diarrhea (17%)

Respiratory: Upper respiratory infection (17%)

1% to 10%:

Central nervous system: Headache (9%), dizziness (6%)

Gastrointestinal: Nausea (8%), vomiting (8%), abdominal pain (7%) (combined GI effects increased to 38% in patients taking high doses as initial therapy)

Dosage Note: Dose must be individualized. Dosages expressed as glyburide/metformin components.

Adults: Oral:

Initial therapy (no prior treatment with sulfonylurea or metformin): 1.25 mg/250 mg once daily with a meal; patients with Hb A_{1c} >9% or fasting plasma glucose (FPG) >200 mg/dL may start with 1.25 mg/250 mg twice daily

Dosage may be increased in increments of 1.25 mg/250 mg, at intervals of not less than 2 weeks; maximum daily dose: 10 mg/2000 mg (limited experience with higher doses)

Previously treated with a sulfonylurea or metformin alone: Initial: 2.5 mg/500 mg or 5 mg/500 mg twice daily; increase in increments no greater than 5 mg/500 mg; maximum daily dose: 20 mg/2000 mg

When switching patients previously on a sulfonylurea and metformin together, do not exceed the daily dose of glyburide (or glyburide equivalent) or metformin.

Note: May combine with a thiazolidinedione in patients with an inadequate response to glyburide/metformin therapy (risk of hypoglycemia may be increased).

Elderly: Oral: Conservative doses are recommended in the elderly due to potentially decreased renal function; **do not titrate to maximum dose;** should not be used in patients ≥80 years of age unless renal function is verified as normal

Dosage adjustment in renal impairment: Risk of lactic acidosis increases with degree of renal impairment; contraindicated in renal disease or renal dysfunction (see Contraindications)

Dosage adjustment in hepatic impairment: Use conservative initial and maintenance doses and avoid use in severe hepatic disease

Mechanism of Action The combination of glyburide and metformin is used to improve glycemic control in patients with type 2 diabetes mellitus by using two different, but complementary, mechanisms of action:

Glyburide: Stimulates insulin release from the pancreatic beta cells; reduces glucose output from the liver; insulin sensitivity is increased at peripheral target sites

Metformin: Decreases hepatic glucose production, decreasing intestinal absorption of glucose and improves insulin sensitivity (increases peripheral glucose uptake and utilization)

(Continued)

Glyburide and Metformin *(Continued)*

Contraindications Hypersensitivity to glyburide or other sulfonamides, metformin, or any component of the formulation; renal disease or renal dysfunction (serum creatinine ≥1.5 mg/dL in males or ≥1.4 mg/dL in females, or abnormal creatinine clearance which may also result from conditions such as cardiovascular collapse, acute myocardial infarction, and septicemia); acute or chronic metabolic acidosis with or without coma (including diabetic ketoacidosis); congestive heart failure requiring pharmacologic treatment

Note: Temporarily discontinue in patients undergoing radiologic studies in which intravascular iodinated contrast materials are utilized.

Warnings/Precautions Age, hepatic and renal impairment are independent risk factors for hypoglycemia. Use with caution in patients with hepatic impairment, malnourished or debilitated conditions, or adrenal or pituitary insufficiency. Use caution in patients with renal impairment. Lactic acidosis is a rare, but potentially severe consequence of therapy with metformin. Withhold therapy in hypoxia, dehydration, or sepsis. The risk of lactic acidosis is increased in any patient with CHF requiring pharmacologic management. This risk is particularly high during acute or unstable CHF because of the risk of hypoperfusion and hypoxemia.

Metformin is substantially excreted by the kidney. The risk of accumulation and lactic acidosis increases with the degree of impairment of renal function. Patients with renal function below the limit of normal for their age should not receive metformin. In elderly patients, renal function should be monitored regularly; should not be used in any patient ≥80 years of age unless measurement of creatinine clearance verifies normal renal function. Use of concomitant medications that may affect renal function (ie, affect tubular secretion) may also affect metformin disposition. Metformin should be suspended in patients with dehydration and/or prerenal azotemia. Therapy should be suspended for any surgical procedures (resume only after normal intake resumed and normal renal function is verified).Intravascular iodinated contrast materials used for radiologic studies are associated with alteration of renal function and may increase risk of lactic acidosis. Discontinue Glucovance® at the time of or prior to the procedure and withhold for 48 hours subsequent to the procedure; reinstitute only after renal function has been re-evaluated and found to be normal.

Chemical similarities are present among sulfonamides, sulfonylureas, carbonic anhydrase inhibitors, thiazides, and loop diuretics (except ethacrynic acid). Use in patients with sulfonamide allergy is specifically contraindicated in product labeling, however a risk of cross-reaction exists in patients with allergy to any of these compounds; avoid use when previous reaction has been severe.

Product labeling states oral hypoglycemic drugs may be associated with an increased cardiovascular mortality as compared to treatment with diet alone or diet plus insulin. Data to support this association are limited, and several studies, including a large prospective trial (UKPDS), have not supported an association.

Drug Interactions
  Increased Effect/Toxicity: See individual agents.
  Decreased Effect: See individual agents.

Ethanol/Nutrition/Herb Interactions
  Ethanol: May cause hypoglycemia; incidence of lactic acidosis may be increased; a disulfiram-like reaction characterized by flushing, headache, nausea, vomiting, sweating, or tachycardia has been reported with sulfonylureas; avoid or limit use.
  Food: Metformin decreases absorption of vitamin B_{12}. Metformin decreases absorption of folic acid.

Dietary Considerations May cause GI upset; take with food to decrease GI upset. Dietary modification based on ADA recommendations is a part of therapy. Decreases blood glucose concentration. Hypoglycemia may occur. Must be able to recognize symptoms of hypoglycemia (palpitations, sweaty palms, lightheadedness). Monitor for signs and symptoms of vitamin B_{12} deficiency. Monitor for signs and symptoms of folic acid deficiency.

Pharmacodynamics/Kinetics
  Glucovance®:
    Bioavailability: 18% with 2.5 mg glyburide/500 mg metformin dose; 7% with 5 mg glyburide/500 mg metformin dose; bioavailability is greater than that of Micronase® brand of glyburide and therefore not bioequivalent
    Time to peak: 2.75 hours when taken with food
  Glyburide: See Glyburide monograph.
  Metformin: This component of Glucovance® is bioequivalent to metformin coadministration with glyburide.

Pregnancy Risk Factor B (manufacturer); C (expert analysis)

Dosage Forms TAB, film coated: 1.25 mg/250 mg: Glyburide 1.25 mg and metformin 250 mg; 2.5 mg/500 mg: Glyburide 2.5 mg and metformin 500 mg; 5 mg/500 mg: Glyburide 5 mg and metformin 500 mg

Glyburide and Metformin Hydrochloride see Glyburide and Metformin on page 745

Glycerin (GLIS er in)

U.S. Brand Names Bausch & Lomb® Computer Eye Drops [OTC]; Colace® Adult/Children Suppositories [OTC]; Colace® Infant/Children Suppositories [OTC]; Fleet® Babylax® [OTC]; Fleet® Glycerin Suppositories [OTC]; Fleet® Glycerin Suppositories Maximum Strength [OTC]; Fleet® Liquid Glycerin Suppositories [OTC]; Osmoglyn® [DSC]; Sani-Supp® [OTC]

Mexican Brand Names Supositorios Senosiain®

Generic Available Yes: Suppositories

Synonyms Glycerol

Pharmacologic Category Laxative, Osmotic; Ophthalmic Agent, Miscellaneous

Use Constipation; reduction of intraocular pressure; reduction of corneal edema; glycerin has been administered orally to reduce intracranial pressure

Local Anesthetic/Vasoconstrictor Precautions No information available to require special precautions

Effects on Dental Treatment No significant effects or complications reported

Common Adverse Effects Frequency not defined.

Cardiovascular: Arrhythmias

Central nervous system: Headache, confusion, dizziness, hyperosmolar nonketotic coma

Endocrine: Polydipsia, hyperglycemia, dehydration

Gastrointestinal: Nausea, vomiting, tenesmus, rectal irritation, cramping pain, diarrhea, dry mouth

Mechanism of Action Osmotic dehydrating agent which increases osmotic pressure; draws fluid into colon and thus stimulates evacuation

Pharmacodynamics/Kinetics

Onset of action:

Decrease in intraocular pressure: Oral: 10-30 minutes

Reduction of intracranial pressure: Oral: 10-60 minutes

Constipation: Suppository: 15-30 minutes

Peak effect:

Decrease in intraocular pressure: Oral: 60-90 minutes

Reduction of intracranial pressure: Oral: 60-90 minutes

Duration:

Decrease in intraocular pressure: Oral: 4-8 hours

Reduction of intracranial pressure: Oral: ~2-3 hours

Absorption: Oral: Well absorbed; Rectal: Poorly absorbed

Half-life elimination, serum: 30-45 minutes

Pregnancy Risk Factor C

Glycerol see Glycerin on page 747

Glycerol Guaiacolate see Guaifenesin on page 752

Glycerol Triacetate see Triacetin on page 1526

Glyceryl Trinitrate see Nitroglycerin on page 1120

GlycoLax™ see Polyethylene Glycol 3350 on page 1253

Glycopyrrolate (glye koe PYE roe late)

U.S. Brand Names Robinul®; Robinul® Forte

Generic Available Yes: Injection

Synonyms Glycopyrronium Bromide

Pharmacologic Category Anticholinergic Agent

Use Inhibit salivation and excessive secretions of the respiratory tract preoperatively; reversal of neuromuscular blockade; control of upper airway secretions; adjunct in treatment of peptic ulcer

Local Anesthetic/Vasoconstrictor Precautions No information available to require special precautions

Effects on Dental Treatment Key adverse event(s) related to dental treatment: Dysphagia, significant xerostomia (normal salivary flow resumes upon discontinuation), and dry throat.

Common Adverse Effects Frequency not defined. **Note:** Includes adverse effects which may occur as an extension of the pharmacologic action of (Continued)

Glycopyrrolate *(Continued)*

anticholinergics (including glycopyrrolate) and adverse effects reported postmarketing with glycopyrrolate.

Cardiovascular: Arrhythmias, cardiac arrest, heart block, hyper-/hypotension, malignant hyperthermia, palpitation, QT_c interval prolongation, tachycardia

Central nervous system: Confusion, dizziness, drowsiness, excitement, headache, insomnia, nervousness, seizures

Dermatologic: Dry skin, pruritus, sensitivity to light increased

Endocrine & metabolic: Lactation suppression

Gastrointestinal: Bloated feeling, constipation, loss of taste, nausea, vomiting, xerostomia

Genitourinary: Impotence, urinary hesitancy, urinary retention

Local: Irritation at injection site

Neuromuscular & skeletal: Weakness

Ocular: Blurred vision, cycloplegia, mydriasis, ocular tension increased, photophobia, sensitivity to light increased

Respiratory: Respiratory depression

Miscellaneous: Anaphylactoid reactions, diaphoresis decreased, hypersensitivity reactions

Mechanism of Action Blocks the action of acetylcholine at parasympathetic sites in smooth muscle, secretory glands, and the CNS

Drug Interactions

Increased Effect/Toxicity: Effects of other anticholinergic agents or medications with anticholinergic activity may be increased by glycopyrrolate. Severity of potassium chloride-induced gastrointestinal lesions (when potassium is given in a wax matrix formulation, eg, Klor-Con®) may be increased by glycopyrrolate. Pramlinitide may enhance the anticholinergic effects of anticholinergics (effects are specific to the GI tract).

Pharmacodynamics/Kinetics

Onset of action: Oral: 50 minutes; I.M.: 15-30 minutes; I.V.: ~1 minute
Peak effect: Oral: ~1 hour; I.M.: 30-45 minutes

Duration: Vagal effect: 2-3 hours; Inhibition of salivation: Up to 7 hours; Anticholinergic: Oral: 8-12 hours

Absorption: Oral: Poor and erratic

Distribution: V_d: 0.2-0.62 L/kg

Metabolism: Hepatic (minimal)

Bioavailability: ~10%

Half-life elimination: Infants: 22-130 minutes; Children 19-99 minutes; Adults: ~30-75 minutes

Excretion: Urine (as unchanged drug, I.M.: 80%, I.V.: 85%); bile (as unchanged drug)

Pregnancy Risk Factor B

Glycopyrronium Bromide *see* Glycopyrrolate *on page 747*

Glycosum *see* Dextrose *on page 452*

Glydiazinamide *see* GlipiZIDE *on page 740*

Glynase® PresTab® *see* GlyBURIDE *on page 744*

Gly-Oxide® [OTC] *see* Carbamide Peroxide *on page 264*

Glyquin® *see* Hydroquinone *on page 798*

Glyquin-XM™ *see* Hydroquinone *on page 798*

Glyset® *see* Miglitol *on page 1046*

GM-CSF *see* Sargramostim *on page 1378*

GnRH *see* Gonadorelin *on page 749*

GnRH Agonist *see* Histrelin *on page 772*

Gold Bond® Antifungal [OTC] *see* Tolnaftate *on page 1506*

Gold Sodium Thiomalate *(gold SOW dee um thye oh MAL ate)*

Related Information
Rheumatoid Arthritis, Osteoarthritis, and Osteoporosis *on page 1668*

U.S. Brand Names Aurolate®

Canadian Brand Names Myochrysine®

Generic Available No

Pharmacologic Category Gold Compound

Use Treatment of progressive rheumatoid arthritis

Local Anesthetic/Vasoconstrictor Precautions No information available to require special precautions

Effects on Dental Treatment Key adverse event(s) related to dental treatment: Stomatitis, gingivitis, and glossitis.

Common Adverse Effects
>10%:
Dermatologic: Itching, rash
Gastrointestinal: Stomatitis, gingivitis, glossitis
Ocular: Conjunctivitis
1% to 10%:
Dermatologic: Urticaria, alopecia
Hematologic: Eosinophilia, leukopenia, thrombocytopenia
Renal: Proteinuria, hematuria
Mechanism of Action Unknown, may decrease prostaglandin synthesis or may alter cellular mechanisms by inhibiting sulfhydryl systems
Drug Interactions
Decreased Effect: Penicillamine and acetylcysteine may decrease effect of gold sodium thiomalate.
Pharmacodynamics/Kinetics
Onset of action: Delayed; may require up to 3 months
Half-life elimination: 5 days; may be prolonged with multiple doses
Time to peak, serum: 4-6 hours
Excretion: Urine (60% to 90%); feces (10% to 40%)
Pregnancy Risk Factor C

GoLYTELY® *see* Polyethylene Glycol-Electrolyte Solution *on page 1253*

Gonadorelin (goe nad oh RELL in)

U.S. Brand Names Factrel®
Canadian Brand Names Lutrepulse™
Mexican Brand Names Relisorm L®
Generic Available No
Synonyms GnRH; Gonadorelin Acetate; Gonadorelin Hydrochloride; Gonadotropin Releasing Hormone; LHRH; LRH; Luteinizing Hormone Releasing Hormone
Pharmacologic Category Diagnostic Agent; Gonadotropin
Use Evaluation of functional capacity and response of gonadotrophic hormones; evaluate abnormal gonadotropin regulation as in precocious puberty and delayed puberty.
Orphan drug: Lutrepulse®: Induction of ovulation in females with hypothalamic amenorrhea
Local Anesthetic/Vasoconstrictor Precautions No information available to require special precautions
Effects on Dental Treatment No significant effects or complications reported
Common Adverse Effects 1% to 10%: Local: Pain at injection site
Mechanism of Action Stimulates the release of luteinizing hormone (LH) from the anterior pituitary gland
Drug Interactions
Increased Effect/Toxicity: Increased levels/effect with androgens, estrogens, progestins, glucocorticoids, spironolactone, and levodopa.
Decreased Effect: Decreased levels/effect with oral contraceptives, digoxin, phenothiazines, and dopamine antagonists.
Pharmacodynamics/Kinetics
Onset of action: Peak effect: Maximal LH release: ~20 minutes
Duration: 3-5 hours
Half-life elimination: 4 minutes
Pregnancy Risk Factor B

Gonadorelin Acetate *see* Gonadorelin *on page 749*
Gonadorelin Hydrochloride *see* Gonadorelin *on page 749*
Gonadotropin Releasing Hormone *see* Gonadorelin *on page 749*
Gonak™ [OTC] *see* Hydroxypropyl Methylcellulose *on page 800*
Gonal-f® *see* Follitropins *on page 698*
Gonal-f® RFF *see* Follitropins *on page 698*
Gonioscopic Ophthalmic Solution *see* Hydroxypropyl Methylcellulose *on page 800*
Goniosoft™ *see* Hydroxypropyl Methylcellulose *on page 800*
Goniosol® [OTC] [DSC] *see* Hydroxypropyl Methylcellulose *on page 800*
Good Sense Sleep Aid [OTC] *see* Doxylamine *on page 517*
Goody's® Extra Strength Headache Powder [OTC] *see* Acetaminophen, Aspirin, and Caffeine *on page 41*
Goody's® Extra Strength Pain Relief [OTC] *see* Acetaminophen, Aspirin, and Caffeine *on page 41*

Goody's PM® Powder [OTC] *see* Acetaminophen and Diphenhydramine *on page 38*

Gordofilm® [OTC] *see* Salicylic Acid *on page 1374*

Gordon Boro-Packs [OTC] *see* Aluminum Sulfate and Calcium Acetate *on page 81*

Gormel® [OTC] *see* Urea *on page 1551*

Goserelin (GOE se rel in)

U.S. Brand Names Zoladex®
Canadian Brand Names Zoladex®; Zoladex® LA
Mexican Brand Names Zoladex®
Generic Available No
Synonyms D-Ser(Bu^t)^6,Azgly^{10}-LHRH; Goserelin Acetate; ICI-118630; NSC-606864
Pharmacologic Category Gonadotropin Releasing Hormone Agonist
Use Palliative treatment of advanced breast cancer and carcinoma of the prostate; treatment of endometriosis, including pain relief and reduction of endometriotic lesions; endometrial thinning agent as part of treatment for dysfunctional uterine bleeding
Local Anesthetic/Vasoconstrictor Precautions No information available to require special precautions
Effects on Dental Treatment Key adverse event(s) related to dental treatment: Taste disturbances.
Common Adverse Effects Percentages reported in males with prostatic carcinoma and females with endometriosis using the 1-month implant:

>10%:

Central nervous system: Headache (female 75%, male 1% to 5%), emotional lability (female 60%), depression (female 54%, male 1% to 5%), pain (female 17%, male 8%), insomnia (female 11%, male 5%)

Endocrine & metabolic: Hot flashes (female 96%, male 62%), sexual dysfunction (21%), erections decreased (18%), libido decreased (female 61%), breast enlargement (male 18%)

Genitourinary: Lower urinary symptoms (male 13%), vaginitis (75%), dyspareunia (female 14%)

Miscellaneous: Diaphoresis (female 45%, male 6%); infection (female 13%)

1% to 10%:

Cardiovascular: CHF (male 5%), arrhythmia, cerebrovascular accident, hypertension, MI, peripheral vascular disorder, chest pain, palpitation, tachycardia, edema

Central nervous system: Lethargy (male 8%), dizziness (female 6%, male 5%), abnormal thinking, anxiety, chills, fever, malaise, migraine, somnolence

Dermatologic: Rash (female >1%, male 6%), alopecia, bruising, dry skin, skin discoloration

Endocrine & metabolic: Breast pain (female 7%), breast swelling/tenderness (male 1% to 5%), dysmenorrhea, gout, hyperglycemia

Gastrointestinal: Anorexia (female >1%, male 5%), nausea (male 5%), constipation, diarrhea, flatulence, dyspepsia, ulcer, vomiting, weight increased, xerostomia

Genitourinary: Renal insufficiency, urinary frequency, urinary obstruction, urinary tract infection, vaginal hemorrhage

Hematologic: Anemia, hemorrhage

Neuromuscular & skeletal: Arthralgia, bone mineral density decreased (female; ~4% decrease in 6 months), joint disorder, paresthesia

Ocular: Amblyopia, dry eyes

Respiratory: Upper respiratory tract infection (male 7%), COPD (male 5%), pharyngitis (female 5%), bronchitis, cough, epistaxis, rhinitis, sinusitis

Miscellaneous: Allergic reaction

Mechanism of Action Goserelin is a synthetic analog of luteinizing-hormone-releasing hormone (LHRH). Following an initial increase in luteinizing hormone (LH) and follicle stimulating hormone (FSH), chronic administration of goserelin results in a sustained suppression of pituitary gonadotropins. Serum testosterone falls to levels comparable to surgical castration. The exact mechanism of this effect is unknown, but may be related to changes in the control of LH or down-regulation of LH receptors.

Pharmacodynamics/Kinetics Note: Data reported using the 1-month implant.

Absorption: SubQ: Rapid and can be detected in serum in 10 minutes

Distribution: V$_d$: Male: 44.1 L; Female: 20.3 L

Time to peak, serum: SubQ: Male: 12-15 days, Female: 8-22 days

Half-life elimination: SubQ: Male: ~4 hours, Female: ~2 hours; Renal impairment: Male: 12 hours

Excretion: Urine (90%)

Pregnancy Risk Factor X (endometriosis, endometrial thinning); D (advanced breast cancer)

Goserelin Acetate *see* Goserelin *on page 750*

GP 47680 *see* Oxcarbazepine *on page 1159*

G-Phed *see* Guaifenesin and Pseudoephedrine *on page 755*

GR38032R *see* Ondansetron *on page 1147*

Gramicidin, Neomycin, and Polymyxin B *see* Neomycin, Polymyxin B, and Gramicidin *on page 1101*

Granisetron (gra NI se tron)

U.S. Brand Names Kytril®
Canadian Brand Names Kytril®
Mexican Brand Names Kytril®
Generic Available No
Synonyms BRL 43694
Pharmacologic Category Antiemetic; Selective 5-HT$_3$ Receptor Antagonist
Use Prophylaxis of nausea and vomiting associated with emetogenic chemotherapy and radiation therapy, (including total body irradiation and fractionated abdominal radiation); prophylaxis and treatment of postoperative nausea and vomiting (PONV)

Generally **not** recommended for treatment of existing chemotherapy-induced emesis (CIE) or for prophylaxis of nausea from agents with a low emetogenic potential.

Local Anesthetic/Vasoconstrictor Precautions No information available to require special precautions

Effects on Dental Treatment No significant effects or complications reported

Common Adverse Effects

>10%:

Central nervous system: Headache (9% to 21%)

Gastrointestinal: Constipation (3% to 18%)

Neuromuscular & skeletal: Weakness (5% to 18%)

1% to 10%:

Cardiovascular: Hypertension (1% to 2%)

Central nervous system: Pain (10%), fever (3% to 9%), dizziness (4% to 5%), insomnia (<2% to 5%), somnolence (1% to 4%), anxiety (2%), agitation (<2%), CNS stimulation (<2%)

Dermatologic: Rash (1%)

Gastrointestinal: Diarrhea (3% to 9%), abdominal pain (4% to 6%), dyspepsia (3% to 6%), taste perversion (2%)

Hepatic: Liver enzymes increased (5% to 6%)

Renal: Oliguria (2%)

Respiratory: Cough (2%)

Miscellaneous: Infection (3%)

Mechanism of Action Selective 5-HT$_3$-receptor antagonist, blocking serotonin, both peripherally on vagal nerve terminals and centrally in the chemoreceptor trigger zone

Drug Interactions

Cytochrome P450 Effect: Substrate of CYP3A4 (minor)

Increased Effect/Toxicity: Granisetron may enhance the hypotensive effect of apomorphine.

Pharmacodynamics/Kinetics

Duration: Generally up to 24 hours

Absorption: Tablets and oral solution are bioequivalent

Distribution: V$_d$: 2-4 L/kg; widely throughout body

Protein binding: 65%

Metabolism: Hepatic via N-demethylation, oxidation, and conjugation; some metabolites may have 5-HT$_3$ antagonist activity

Half-life elimination: Terminal: 5-9 hours

Excretion: Urine (12% as unchanged drug, 48% to 49% as metabolites); feces (34% to 38% as metabolites)

Pregnancy Risk Factor B

Granulex® *see* Trypsin, Balsam Peru, and Castor Oil *on page 1547*

Granulocyte Colony Stimulating Factor *see* Filgrastim *on page 654*

Granulocyte Colony Stimulating Factor (PEG Conjugate) *see* Pegfilgrastim *on page 1195*

Granulocyte-Macrophage Colony Stimulating Factor *see* Sargramostim *on page 1378*

Grifulvin® V *see* Griseofulvin *on page 752*

Griseofulvin (gri see oh FUL vin)

U.S. Brand Names Grifulvin® V; Gris-PEG®

Mexican Brand Names Grisovin®

Generic Available Yes: Suspension, ultramicrosized product

Synonyms Griseofulvin Microsize; Griseofulvin Ultramicrosize

Pharmacologic Category Antifungal Agent, Oral

Use Treatment of susceptible tinea infections of the skin, hair, and nails

Local Anesthetic/Vasoconstrictor Precautions No information available to require special precautions

Effects on Dental Treatment Key adverse event(s) related to dental treatment: May cause soreness or irritation of mouth or tongue.

Common Adverse Effects Frequency not defined.

Central nervous system: Headache, fatigue, dizziness, insomnia, mental confusion

Dermatologic: Rash (most common), urticaria (most common), photosensitivity, erythema multiforme, angioneurotic edema (rare)

Gastrointestinal: Nausea, vomiting, epigastric distress, diarrhea, GI bleeding

Genitourinary: Menstrual irregularities (rare)

Hematologic: Leukopenia, granulocytopenia

Neuromuscular & skeletal: Paresthesia (rare)

Renal: Hepatotoxicity, proteinuria, nephrosis

Miscellaneous: Oral thrush, drug-induced lupus-like syndrome (rare)

Mechanism of Action Inhibits fungal cell mitosis at metaphase; binds to human keratin making it resistant to fungal invasion

Drug Interactions

Cytochrome P450 Effect: Induces CYP1A2 (weak), 2C8 (weak), 2C9 (weak), 3A4 (weak)

Increased Effect/Toxicity: Increased toxicity with ethanol, may cause tachycardia and flushing.

Decreased Effect: Barbiturates may decrease levels. Decreased warfarin activity. Decreased oral contraceptive effectiveness.

Pharmacodynamics/Kinetics

Absorption: Ultramicrosize griseofulvin absorption is almost complete; absorption of microsize griseofulvin is variable (25% to 70% of an oral dose); enhanced by ingestion of a fatty meal (GI absorption of ultramicrosize is ~1.5 times that of microsize)

Distribution: Crosses placenta

Metabolism: Extensively hepatic

Half-life elimination: 9-22 hours

Excretion: Urine (<1% as unchanged drug); feces; perspiration

Pregnancy Risk Factor C

Griseofulvin Microsize *see* Griseofulvin *on page 752*

Griseofulvin Ultramicrosize *see* Griseofulvin *on page 752*

Gris-PEG® *see* Griseofulvin *on page 752*

Guaicon DM [OTC] *see* Guaifenesin and Dextromethorphan *on page 754*

Guaicon DMS [OTC] *see* Guaifenesin and Dextromethorphan *on page 754*

Guaifed® *see* Guaifenesin and Phenylephrine *on page 754*

Guaifed-PD® *see* Guaifenesin and Phenylephrine *on page 754*

Guaifen-C *see* Guaifenesin and Codeine *on page 753*

Guaifenesin (gwye FEN e sin)

U.S. Brand Names Allfen Jr; Diabetic Tussin® EX [OTC]; Ganidin NR; Guiatuss™ [OTC]; Humibid® e [OTC]; Iophen NR; Mucinex® [OTC]; Naldecon Senior EX® [OTC] [DSC]; Organ-1 NR; Organidin® NR; Phanasin® [OTC]; Phanasin® Diabetic Choice [OTC]; Q-Tussin [OTC]; Robitussin® [OTC]; Scot-Tussin® Expectorant [OTC]; Siltussin DAS [OTC]; Siltussin SA [OTC]; Tussin [OTC]; Vicks® Casero™ [OTC]

Canadian Brand Names Balminil Expectorant; Benylin® E Extra Strength; Koffex Expectorant; Robitussin®

Mexican Brand Names Tukol®

Generic Available Yes: Excludes extended release

Synonyms GG; Glycerol Guaiacolate

Pharmacologic Category Expectorant

Use Help loosen phlegm and thin bronchial secretions to make coughs more productive

Local Anesthetic/Vasoconstrictor Precautions No information available to require special precautions

Effects on Dental Treatment No significant effects or complications reported

Common Adverse Effects Frequency not defined.

Central nervous system: Dizziness, drowsiness, headache

Dermatologic: Rash

Endocrine & metabolic: Uric acid levels decreased

Gastrointestinal: Nausea, vomiting, stomach pain

Postmarketing and/or case reports: Kidney stone formation (with consumption of large quantities)

Mechanism of Action Thought to act as an expectorant by irritating the gastric mucosa and stimulating respiratory tract secretions, thereby increasing respiratory fluid volumes and decreasing mucus viscosity

Pharmacodynamics/Kinetics

Absorption: Well absorbed

Half-life elimination: ~1 hour

Excretion: Urine (as unchanged drug and metabolites)

Pregnancy Risk Factor C

Guaifenesin AC *see* Guaifenesin and Codeine *on page 753*

Guaifenesin and Codeine (gwye FEN e sin & KOE deen)

Related Information

Codeine *on page 385*

Guaifenesin *on page 752*

U.S. Brand Names Brontex®; Cheracol®; Cheratussin AC; Diabetic Tussin C®; Gani-Tuss® NR; Guaifen-C; Guaifenesin AC; Guaituss AC; Iophen-C NR; Kolephrin® #1; Mytussin® AC; Robafen® AC; Romilar® AC; Tussi-Organidin® NR; Tussi-Organidin® S-NR

Generic Available Yes

Synonyms Codeine and Guaifenesin

Pharmacologic Category Antitussive; Cough Preparation; Expectorant

Use Temporary control of cough due to minor throat and bronchial irritation

Local Anesthetic/Vasoconstrictor Precautions No information available to require special precautions

Effects on Dental Treatment Key adverse event(s) related to dental treatment: Xerostomia (normal salivary flow resumes upon discontinuation).

Common Adverse Effects

Based on **guaifenesin** component:

Central nervous system: Drowsiness, headache

Dermatologic: Rash

Gastrointestinal: Nausea, vomiting, stomach pain

Based on **codeine** component:

>10%:

Central nervous system: Drowsiness

Gastrointestinal: Constipation

1% to 10%:

Cardiovascular: Tachycardia or bradycardia, hypotension

Central nervous system: Dizziness, lightheadedness, false feeling of well being, malaise, headache, restlessness, paradoxical CNS stimulation, confusion

Dermatologic: Rash, urticaria

Gastrointestinal: Xerostomia, anorexia, nausea, vomiting,

Genitourinary: Decreased urination, ureteral spasm

Hepatic: Increased LFTs

Local: Burning at injection site

Neuromuscular & skeletal: Weakness

Ocular: Blurred vision

Respiratory: Dyspnea

Miscellaneous: Histamine release

Percentage unknown: Increased AST, ALT

Restrictions C-V

Mechanism of Action

Guaifenesin is thought to act as an expectorant by irritating the gastric mucosa and stimulating respiratory tract secretions, thereby increasing respiratory fluid volumes and decreasing phlegm viscosity

(Continued)

Guaifenesin and Codeine (Continued)

Codeine is an antitussive that controls cough by depressing the medullary cough center

Drug Interactions

Increased Effect/Toxicity: See individual agents.

Decreased Effect: See individual agents.

Pharmacodynamics/Kinetics See individual agents.

Pregnancy Risk Factor C

Guaifenesin and Dextromethorphan
(gwye FEN e sin & deks troe meth OR fan)

Related Information

Dextromethorphan on page 451

Guaifenesin on page 752

U.S. Brand Names Allfen-DM; Altarussin DM [OTC]; Amibid DM; Benylin® Expectorant [OTC] [DSC]; Cheracol® D [OTC]; Cheracol® Plus [OTC]; Coricidin HBP® Chest Congestion and Cough [OTC]; Diabetic Tussin® DM [OTC]; Diabetic Tussin® DM Maximum Strength [OTC]; Drituss DM; Duratuss® DM; Gani-Tuss DM NR; Genatuss DM® [OTC]; Guaicon DM [OTC]; Guaicon DMS [OTC]; Guaifenex® DM; Guia-D; Guiatuss-DM® [OTC]; Humibid® CS [OTC] [DSC]; Hydro-Tussin™ DM; Iophen DM NR; Kolephrin® GG/DM [OTC]; Mindal DM [DSC]; Mintab DM; Mucinex® DM [OTC]; Phanatuss® DM [OTC]; Q-Bid DM; Q-Tussin DM [OTC]; Respa-DM®; Robafen DM [OTC]; Robitussin® Cough and Congestion [OTC]; Robitussin® DM [OTC]; Robitussin® DM Infant [OTC]; Robitussin® Sugar Free Cough [OTC]; Safe Tussin® [OTC]; Scot-Tussin® Senior [OTC]; Silexin [OTC]; Siltussin DM [OTC]; Siltussin DM DAS [OTC]; Su-Tuss DM; Touro® DM; Vicks® 44E [OTC]; Vicks® Pediatric Formula 44E [OTC]; Z-Cof LA™

Canadian Brand Names Balminil DM E; Benylin® DM-E; Koffex DM-Expectorant; Robitussin® DM

Generic Available Yes

Synonyms Dextromethorphan and Guaifenesin

Pharmacologic Category Antitussive; Cough Preparation; Expectorant

Use Temporary control of cough due to minor throat and bronchial irritation

Local Anesthetic/Vasoconstrictor Precautions No information available to require special precautions

Effects on Dental Treatment No significant effects or complications reported

Common Adverse Effects See individual agents.

Mechanism of Action

Guaifenesin is thought to act as an expectorant by irritating the gastric mucosa and stimulating respiratory tract secretions, thereby increasing respiratory fluid volumes and decreasing phlegm viscosity

Dextromethorphan is a chemical relative of morphine lacking narcotic properties except in overdose; controls cough by depressing the medullary cough center

Drug Interactions

Cytochrome P450 Effect: Dextromethorphan: **Substrate** of CYP2B6 (minor), 2C9 (minor), 2C19 (minor), 2D6 (major), 2E1 (minor), 3A4 (minor); **Inhibits** CYP2D6 (weak)

Increased Effect/Toxicity: See individual agents.

Decreased Effect: See individual agents.

Pharmacodynamics/Kinetics See individual agents.

Pregnancy Risk Factor C

Guaifenesin and Hydrocodone see Hydrocodone and Guaifenesin on page 785

Guaifenesin and Phenylephrine (gwye FEN e sin & fen il EF rin)

Related Information

Guaifenesin on page 752

Phenylephrine on page 1226

U.S. Brand Names Aldex™; Amidal; Ami-Tex LA; Crantex ER; Crantex LA; Deconsal® II; Endal®; Entex®; Entex® ER; Entex® LA; Guaifed®; Guaifed-PD®; Liquibid-D; Liquibid-PD; PhenaVent™; PhenaVent™ D; PhenaVent™ Ped; Prolex™-D; Rescon GG; Sil-Tex; Sina-12X; SINUvent® PE

Generic Available Yes: Excludes suspension

Synonyms Guaifenesin and Phenylephrine Tannate; Phenylephrine Hydrochloride and Guaifenesin

Pharmacologic Category Decongestant; Expectorant

Use Temporary relief of nasal congestion, sinusitis, rhinitis and hay fever; temporary relief of cough associated with upper respiratory tract conditions, especially when associated with dry, nonproductive cough

Local Anesthetic/Vasoconstrictor Precautions Use with caution since phenylephrine is a sympathomimetic amine which could interact with epinephrine to cause a pressor response

Effects on Dental Treatment Key adverse event(s) related to dental treatment:

Guaifenesin: No significant effects or complications reported

Phenylephrine: Up to 10% of patients could experience tachycardia, palpitations, and xerostomia (normal salivary flow resumes upon discontinuation); use vasoconstrictor with caution

Common Adverse Effects See individual agents.

Mechanism of Action See individual agents.

Drug Interactions

Increased Effect/Toxicity: See individual agents.

Decreased Effect: See individual agents.

Pharmacodynamics/Kinetics See individual agents.

Pregnancy Risk Factor C

Guaifenesin and Phenylephrine Tannate *see* Guaifenesin and Phenylephrine *on page 754*

Guaifenesin and Potassium Guaiacolsulfonate
(gwye FEN e sin & poe TASS ee um gwye a kole SUL foe nate)

Related Information

Guaifenesin *on page 752*

U.S. Brand Names Allfen *(reformulation)*; Humibid® LA *(reformulation)*

Generic Available No

Synonyms Potassium Guaiacolsulfonate and Guaifenesin

Pharmacologic Category Expectorant

Use Temporary control of cough associated with respiratory tract infections and related conditions which are complicated by tenacious mucus and/or mucus plugs and congestion

Local Anesthetic/Vasoconstrictor Precautions No information available to require special precautions

Effects on Dental Treatment No significant effects or complications reported

Mechanism of Action Guaifenesin and potassium guaiacolsulfonate are both expectorants. Guaifenesin is thought to act as an expectorant by irritating the gastric mucosa and stimulating respiratory tract secretions, thereby increasing respiratory fluid volumes and decreasing mucus viscosity.

Pregnancy Risk Factor C

Guaifenesin and Pseudoephedrine
(gwye FEN e sin & soo doe e FED rin)

Related Information

Guaifenesin *on page 752*

Pseudoephedrine *on page 1309*

U.S. Brand Names Ambifed-G; Ami-Tex PSE; Congestac® [OTC]; Dynex; Entex® PSE; Eudal®-SR; G-Phed; Guaifenex® GP; Guaifenex® PSE; Guaimax-D®; Levall G; Maxifed®; Maxifed-G®; Miraphen PSE; Mucinex®-D [OTC]; Nasatab® LA; PanMist®-JR; PanMist®-LA; PanMist®-S; Profen Forte®; Profen II®; Pseudo GG TR; Pseudovent™; Pseudovent™ 400; Pseudovent™-Ped; Refenesen Plus [OTC]; Respaire®-60 SR; Respaire®-120 SR; Robitussin-PE® [OTC]; Robitussin® Severe Congestion [OTC]; Sudafed® Non-Drying Sinus [OTC]; Touro LA®; Zephrex®; Zephrex LA®

Canadian Brand Names Contac® Cold-Chest Congestion, Non Drowsy, Regular Strength; Entex® LA; Novahistex® Expectorant with Decongestant

Generic Available Yes

Synonyms Pseudoephedrine and Guaifenesin

Pharmacologic Category Alpha/Beta Agonist; Expectorant

Use Temporary relief of nasal congestion and to help loosen phlegm and thin bronchial secretions in the treatment of cough

Local Anesthetic/Vasoconstrictor Precautions Use with caution since pseudoephedrine is a sympathomimetic amine which could interact with epinephrine to cause a pressor response

(Continued)

Guaifenesin and Pseudoephedrine *(Continued)*

Effects on Dental Treatment Key adverse event(s) related to dental treatment:

Guaifenesin: No significant effects or complications reported

Pseudoephedrine: Xerostomia (normal salivary flow resumes upon discontinuation).

Common Adverse Effects See individual agents.

Drug Interactions

Increased Effect/Toxicity: See individual agents.

Decreased Effect: See individual agents.

Pharmacodynamics/Kinetics See individual agents.

Pregnancy Risk Factor C

Guaifenesin and Theophylline *see* Theophylline and Guaifenesin *on page 1475*

Guaifenesin, Dextromethorphan, and Phenylephrine
(gwye FEN e sin, deks troe meth OR fan, & fen il EF rin)

Related Information

Dextromethorphan *on page 451*

Guaifenesin *on page 752*

Phenylephrine *on page 1226*

U.S. Brand Names Anextuss; Certuss-D®; Dacex-DM; Dexcon-DM; Dexcon-PE; Duraphen™ DM; Duraphen™ Forte; Duraphen™ II DM; Giltuss®; Giltuss Pediatric®; Giltuss TR®; Maxiphen DM

Generic Available Yes

Synonyms Guaifenesin, Dextromethorphan Hydrobromide, and Phenylephrine Hydrochloride; Phenylephrine Hydrochloride, Guaifenesin, and Dextromethorphan Hydrobromide

Pharmacologic Category Antitussive; Decongestant

Use Symptomatic relief of dry nonproductive coughs and upper respiratory symptoms associated with hay fever, colds, or the flu

Local Anesthetic/Vasoconstrictor Precautions Use with caution since phenylephrine is a sympathomimetic amine which could interact with epinephrine to cause a pressor response

Effects on Dental Treatment Key adverse event(s) related to dental treatment:

Dextromethorphan: No significant effects or complications reported

Guaifenesin: No significant effects or complications reported

Phenylephrine: Up to 10% of patients could experience tachycardia, palpitations, and xerostomia (normal salivary flow resumes upon discontinuation); use vasoconstrictor with caution

Mechanism of Action See individual agents.

Drug Interactions

Cytochrome P450 Effect: Dextromethorphan: **Substrate** of CYP2B6 (minor), 2C9 (minor), 2C19 (minor), 2D6 (major), 2E1 (minor), 3A4 (minor); **Inhibits** CYP2D6 (weak)

Pharmacodynamics/Kinetics See individual agents.

Pregnancy Risk Factor C

Guaifenesin, Dextromethorphan Hydrobromide, and Phenylephrine Hydrochloride *see* Guaifenesin, Dextromethorphan, and Phenylephrine *on page 756*

Guaifenesin, Dihydrocodeine, and Pseudoephedrine *see* Dihydrocodeine, Pseudoephedrine, and Guaifenesin *on page 476*

Guaifenesin, Hydrocodone, and Pseudoephedrine *see* Hydrocodone, Pseudoephedrine, and Guaifenesin *on page 792*

Guaifenesin, Hydrocodone Bitartrate, and Phenylephrine Hydrochloride *see* Hydrocodone, Phenylephrine, and Guaifenesin *on page 791*

Guaifenesin, Pseudoephedrine, and Codeine
(gwye FEN e sin, soo doe e FED rin, & KOE deen)

Related Information

Codeine *on page 385*

Guaifenesin *on page 752*

Pseudoephedrine *on page 1309*

U.S. Brand Names Guiatuss™ DAC®; Mytussin® DAC; Nucofed® Expectorant; Nucofed® Pediatric Expectorant

Canadian Brand Names Benylin® 3.3 mg-D-E; Calmylin with Codeine

Generic Available Yes

Synonyms Codeine, Guaifenesin, and Pseudoephedrine; Pseudoephedrine, Guaifenesin, and Codeine

Pharmacologic Category Antitussive/Decongestant/Expectorant

Use Temporarily relieves nasal congestion and controls cough due to minor throat and bronchial irritation; helps loosen phlegm and thin bronchial secretions to make coughs more productive

Local Anesthetic/Vasoconstrictor Precautions Use with caution since pseudoephedrine is a sympathomimetic amine which could interact with epinephrine to cause a pressor response

Effects on Dental Treatment Key adverse event(s) related to dental treatment:

Codeine: Xerostomia (normal salivary flow resumes upon discontinuation).

Guaifenesin: No significant effects or complications reported

Pseudoephedrine: Xerostomia (normal salivary flow resumes upon discontinuation).

Common Adverse Effects See individual agents.

Restrictions C-III; C-V

Drug Interactions

Increased Effect/Toxicity: See individual agents.

Decreased Effect: See individual agents.

Pharmacodynamics/Kinetics See individual agents.

Pregnancy Risk Factor C

Guaifenesin, Pseudoephedrine, and Dextromethorphan

(gwye FEN e sin, soo doe e FED rin, & deks troe meth OR fan)

Related Information

Dextromethorphan *on page 451*

Guaifenesin *on page 752*

Pseudoephedrine *on page 1309*

U.S. Brand Names Ambifed-G DM; Dimetapp® Cold and Congestion [OTC]; Maxifed DM; PanMist®-DM [DSC]; Profen Forte™ DM; Profen II DM®; Pseudovent™ DM; Relacon-DM; Robitussin® CF [OTC]; Robitussin® Cold and Congestion [OTC]; Robitussin® Cough and Cold Infant [OTC]; Touro™ CC; Tri-Vent™ DM; Z-Cof DM

Canadian Brand Names Balminil DM + Decongestant + Expectorant; Benylin® DM-D-E; Koffex DM + Decongestant + Expectorant; Novahistex® DM Decongestant Expectorant; Novahistine® DM Decongestant Expectorant; Robitussin® Cough & Cold®

Generic Available Yes

Synonyms Dextromethorphan, Guaifenesin, and Pseudoephedrine; Pseudoephedrine, Dextromethorphan, and Guaifenesin

Pharmacologic Category Antitussive/Decongestant/Expectorant

Use Temporarily relieves nasal congestion and controls cough due to minor throat and bronchial irritation; helps loosen phlegm and thin bronchial secretions to make coughs more productive

Local Anesthetic/Vasoconstrictor Precautions Use with caution since pseudoephedrine is a sympathomimetic amine which could interact with epinephrine to cause a pressor response

Effects on Dental Treatment Key adverse event(s) related to dental treatment:

Dextromethorphan: No significant effects or complications reported

Guaifenesin: No significant effects or complications reported

Pseudoephedrine: Xerostomia (normal salivary flow resumes upon discontinuation).

Common Adverse Effects See individual agents.

Mechanism of Action See individual agents.

Drug Interactions

Cytochrome P450 Effect: Dextromethorphan: **Substrate** of CYP2B6 (minor), 2C9 (minor), 2C19 (minor), 2D6 (major), 2E1 (minor), 3A4 (minor); **Inhibits** CYP2D6 (weak)

Increased Effect/Toxicity: See individual agents.

Decreased Effect: See individual agents.

Pharmacodynamics/Kinetics See individual agents.

Pregnancy Risk Factor C

Guaifenex® DM *see* Guaifenesin and Dextromethorphan *on page 754*

Guaifenex® GP *see* Guaifenesin and Pseudoephedrine *on page 755*

Guaifenex® PSE *see* Guaifenesin and Pseudoephedrine *on page 755*

Guaimax-D® *see* Guaifenesin and Pseudoephedrine *on page 755*

Guaituss AC *see* Guaifenesin and Codeine *on page 753*

Guanabenz (GWAHN a benz)

Related Information
Cardiovascular Diseases *on page 1636*
Canadian Brand Names Wytensin®
Generic Available Yes
Synonyms Guanabenz Acetate
Pharmacologic Category Alpha₂-Adrenergic Agonist
Use Management of hypertension
Local Anesthetic/Vasoconstrictor Precautions No information available to require special precautions
Effects on Dental Treatment Key adverse event(s) related to dental treatment: Taste disorder, nasal congestion, dyspnea, significant xerostomia (normal salivary flow resumes upon discontinuation).
Common Adverse Effects Higher rates with larger doses
>5% (at doses of 16 mg/day):
  Cardiovascular: Orthostasis
  Central nervous system: Drowsiness or sedation (39%), dizziness (12% to 17%), headache (5%)
  Gastrointestinal: Xerostomia (28% to 38%)
  Neuromuscular & skeletal: Weakness (~10%)
≤3% (may be similar to placebo):
  Cardiovascular: Arrhythmias, palpitation, chest pain, edema
  Central nervous system: Anxiety, ataxia, depression, sleep disturbances
  Dermatologic: Rash, pruritus
  Endocrine & metabolic: Disturbances of sexual function, gynecomastia, decreased sexual function
  Gastrointestinal: Diarrhea, vomiting, constipation, nausea
  Genitourinary: Polyuria
  Neuromuscular & skeletal: Myalgia
  Ocular: Blurring of vision
  Respiratory: Nasal congestion, dyspnea
  Miscellaneous: Taste disorders
Mechanism of Action Stimulates alpha₂-adrenoreceptors in the brain stem, thus activating an inhibitory neuron, resulting in reduced sympathetic outflow, producing a decrease in vasomotor tone and heart rate
Drug Interactions
Cytochrome P450 Effect: Substrate of CYP1A2 (major)
Increased Effect/Toxicity: CYP1A2 inhibitors may increase the levels/effects of guanabenz; example inhibitors include amiodarone, ciprofloxacin, fluvoxamine, ketoconazole, norfloxacin, ofloxacin, and rofecoxib. Nitroprusside and guanabenz have additive hypotensive effects. Noncardioselective beta-blockers (nadolol, propranolol, timolol) may exacerbate rebound hypertension when guanabenz is withdrawn. The beta-blocker should be withdrawn first. The gradual withdrawal of guanabenz or a cardioselective beta-blocker could be substituted.

Hypoglycemic agents: Hypoglycemic symptoms may be reduced. Educate patient about decreased signs and symptoms of hypoglycemia or avoid use in patients with frequent episodes of hypoglycemia.
Decreased Effect: CYP1A2 inducers may decrease the levels/effects of guanabenz; example inducers include aminoglutethimide, carbamazepine, phenobarbital, and rifampin. TCAs decrease the hypotensive effect of guanabenz.
Pharmacodynamics/Kinetics
Onset of action: Antihypertensive: ~1 hour
Absorption: ~75%
Half-life elimination, serum: 7-10 hours
Pregnancy Risk Factor C

Guanabenz Acetate *see* Guanabenz *on page 758*

Guanfacine (GWAHN fa seen)

Related Information
Cardiovascular Diseases *on page 1636*
U.S. Brand Names Tenex®
Canadian Brand Names Tenex®
Generic Available Yes

Synonyms Guanfacine Hydrochloride

Pharmacologic Category Alpha$_2$-Adrenergic Agonist

Use Management of hypertension

Unlabeled/Investigational Use ADHD, tic disorder, aggression

Local Anesthetic/Vasoconstrictor Precautions No information available to require special precautions

Effects on Dental Treatment Key adverse event(s) related to dental treatment: Xerostomia and changes in salivation (normal salivary flow resumes upon discontinuation).

Common Adverse Effects

>10%:

Central nervous system: Somnolence (5% to 40%), headache (3% to 13%), dizziness (2% to 15%)

Gastrointestinal: Xerostomia (10% to 54%), constipation (2% to 15%)

1% to 10%:

Central nervous system: Fatigue (2% to 10%)

Endocrine & metabolic: Impotence (up to 7%)

Mechanism of Action Stimulates alpha$_2$-adrenoreceptors in the brain stem, thus activating an inhibitory neuron, resulting in reduced sympathetic outflow, producing a decrease in vasomotor tone and heart rate

Drug Interactions

Increased Effect/Toxicity: Nitroprusside and guanfacine have additive hypotensive effects. Noncardioselective beta-blockers (nadolol, propranolol, timolol) may exacerbate rebound hypertension when guanfacine is withdrawn. The beta-blocker should be withdrawn first. The gradual withdrawal of guanfacine or a cardioselective beta-blocker could be substituted.

Decreased Effect: TCAs decrease the hypotensive effect of guanfacine.

Pharmacodynamics/Kinetics

Onset of action: Peak effect: 8-11 hours

Duration: 24 hours following single dose

Half-life elimination, serum: 17 hours

Time to peak, serum: 1-4 hours

Pregnancy Risk Factor B

Guanfacine Hydrochloride *see* Guanfacine *on page 758*

Guanidine (GWAHN i deen)

Generic Available No

Synonyms Guanidine Hydrochloride

Pharmacologic Category Cholinergic Agonist

Use Reduction of the symptoms of muscle weakness associated with the myasthenic syndrome of Eaton-Lambert, not for myasthenia gravis

Local Anesthetic/Vasoconstrictor Precautions No information available to require special precautions

Effects on Dental Treatment No significant effects or complications reported

Guanidine Hydrochloride *see* Guanidine *on page 759*

Guia-D *see* Guaifenesin and Dextromethorphan *on page 754*

Guiatuss™ [OTC] *see* Guaifenesin *on page 752*

Guiatuss™ DAC® *see* Guaifenesin, Pseudoephedrine, and Codeine *on page 756*

Guiatuss-DM® [OTC] *see* Guaifenesin and Dextromethorphan *on page 754*

Gum Benjamin *see* Benzoin *on page 193*

GW506U78 *see* Nelarabine *on page 1097*

GW-1000-02 *see* Tetrahydrocannabinol and Cannabidiol *on page 1469*

GW433908G *see* Fosamprenavir *on page 702*

Gynazole-1® *see* Butoconazole *on page 242*

Gyne-Lotrimin® 3 [OTC] *see* Clotrimazole *on page 379*

Gynodiol® *see* Estradiol *on page 574*

Gynol II® [OTC] *see* Nonoxynol 9 *on page 1124*

Gynovite® Plus [OTC] *see* Vitamins (Multiple/Oral) *on page 1582*

Habitrol *see* Nicotine *on page 1109*

Haemophilus b Oligosaccharide Conjugate Vaccine *see* Haemophilus b Conjugate Vaccine *on page 534*

Haemophilus b Polysaccharide Vaccine *see* Haemophilus b Conjugate Vaccine *on page 534*

Halcinonide (hal SIN oh nide)

U.S. Brand Names Halog®
Canadian Brand Names Halog®
Mexican Brand Names Dermalog®
Generic Available No
Pharmacologic Category Corticosteroid, Topical
Use Inflammation of corticosteroid-responsive dermatoses [high potency topical corticosteroid]
Local Anesthetic/Vasoconstrictor Precautions No information available to require special precautions
Effects on Dental Treatment No significant effects or complications reported
Common Adverse Effects Frequency not defined: Itching; dry skin; folliculitis; hypertrichosis; acneiform eruptions; hypopigmentation; perioral dermatitis; allergic contact dermatitis; skin maceration; striae; local burning, irritation, miliaria; secondary infection
Mechanism of Action Decreases inflammation by suppression of migration of polymorphonuclear leukocytes and reversal of increased capillary permeability
Pharmacodynamics/Kinetics
  Absorption: Percutaneous absorption varies by location of topical application and use of occlusive dressings
  Metabolism: Primarily hepatic
  Excretion: Urine
Pregnancy Risk Factor C

Halcion® *see* Triazolam *on page 1531*
Haldol® *see* Haloperidol *on page 762*
Haldol® Decanoate *see* Haloperidol *on page 762*
Haley's M-O *see* Magnesium Hydroxide and Mineral Oil *on page 961*
Halfprin® [OTC] *see* Aspirin *on page 145*

Halobetasol (hal oh BAY ta sol)

U.S. Brand Names Ultravate®
Canadian Brand Names Ultravate®
Generic Available Yes
Synonyms Halobetasol Propionate
Pharmacologic Category Corticosteroid, Topical
Dental Use Relief of inflammatory and pruritic manifestations (super high potency topical corticosteroid)
Use Relief of inflammatory and pruritic manifestations of corticosteroid-response dermatoses [super high potency topical corticosteroid]
Local Anesthetic/Vasoconstrictor Precautions No information available to require special precautions
Effects on Dental Treatment No significant effects or complications reported
Significant Adverse Effects
  1% to 4%: Dermatologic: Burning, itching, stinging
  <1% (Limited to important or life-threatening): Acneiform eruptions, allergic contact dermatitis, dry skin, erythema, HPA axis suppression, hypopigmentation, leukoderma, miliaria, perioral dermatitis, pustulation, rash, secondary infection, skin atrophy, striae, vesicles
Dental Usual Dosing Inflammatory and pruritic manifestations: Children ≥12 years and Adults: Topical: Cream: Apply sparingly to lesion twice daily. Treatment should not exceed 2 consecutive weeks and total dosage should not exceed 50 g/week. Therapy should be discontinued when control is achieved; if no improvement is seen, reassessment of diagnosis may be necessary.
Dosage Children ≥12 years and Adults: Topical:
  Inflammatory and pruritic manifestations (dental use): Cream: Apply sparingly to lesion twice daily. Treatment should not exceed 2 consecutive weeks and total dosage should not exceed 50g/week. Therapy should be discontinued when control is achieved; if no improvement is seen, reassessment of diagnosis may be necessary.
  Steroid-responsive dermatoses: Apply sparingly to skin twice daily, rub in gently and completely; treatment should not exceed 2 consecutive weeks and total dosage should not exceed 50 g/week. Therapy should be discontinued when control is achieved; if no improvement is seen, reassessment of diagnosis may be necessary.
Mechanism of Action Corticosteroids inhibit the initial manifestations of the inflammatory process (ie, capillary dilation and edema, fibrin deposition, and migration and diapedesis of leukocytes into the inflamed site) as well as later sequelae (angiogenesis, fibroblast proliferation)

Contraindications Hypersensitivity to halobetasol or any component of the formulation; viral, fungal, or tubercular skin lesions

Warnings/Precautions Not for ophthalmic use. May cause suppression of hypothalamic-pituitary-adrenal (HPA) axis, particularly in younger children or in patients receiving high doses for prolonged periods; use should be limited to <50 g/week. Application to abraded or inflamed areas or too large of areas of the body may increase the risk of systemic absorption and the risk of adrenal suppression. Topical halobetasol should not be used for the treatment of rosacea or perioral dermatitis. Not recommended for application to the face, groin, or axillae. Safety and efficacy have not been established in pediatric patients; use in children <12 years of age is not recommended.

Drug Interactions No data reported

Pharmacodynamics/Kinetics

Absorption: Percutaneous absorption varies by location of topical application; ~6% of a topically applied dose of ointment enters circulation within 96 hours

Metabolism: Primarily hepatic

Excretion: Urine

Pregnancy Risk Factor C

Lactation Excretion in breast milk unknown/use caution

Breast-Feeding Considerations Systemically administered corticosteroids appear in human milk and may cause adverse effects in a nursing infant. It is not known if the systemic absorption of topical halobetasol results in detectable quantities in human milk.

Dosage Forms

Cream, as propionate: 0.05% (15 g, 50 g)

Ointment, as propionate: 0.05% (15 g, 50 g)

Halobetasol Propionate *see* Halobetasol *on page 760*

Halofantrine (ha loe FAN trin)

Generic Available No

Synonyms Halofantrine Hydrochloride

Pharmacologic Category Antimalarial Agent

Use Treatment of mild to moderate acute malaria caused by susceptible strains of *Plasmodium falciparum* and *Plasmodium vivax*

Local Anesthetic/Vasoconstrictor Precautions No information available to require special precautions (see Dental Comment)

Effects on Dental Treatment No significant effects or complications reported

Common Adverse Effects

1% to 10%:

Cardiovascular: Edema

Central nervous system: Malaise, headache (3%), dizziness (5%)

Dermatologic: Pruritus (3%)

Gastrointestinal: Nausea (3%), vomiting (4%), abdominal pain (9%), diarrhea (6%), anorexia (5%)

Hematologic: Leukocytosis

Hepatic: Elevated LFTs

Local: Tenderness

Neuromuscular & skeletal: Myalgia (1%), rigors (2%)

Respiratory: Cough

Miscellaneous: Lymphadenopathy

Restrictions Not available in U.S.

Mechanism of Action Exact mechanism unknown; destruction of asexual blood forms, possible inhibition of proton pump

Drug Interactions

Cytochrome P450 Effect: **Substrate** of CYP2C9 (minor), 2D6 (minor), 3A4 (major); **Inhibits** CYP2D6 (weak)

Increased Effect/Toxicity: CYP3A4 inhibitors may increase the levels/ effects of halofantrine; example inhibitors include azole antifungals, clarithromycin, diclofenac, doxycycline, erythromycin, imatinib, isoniazid, nefazodone, nicardipine, propofol, protease inhibitors, quinidine, telithromycin, and verapamil. Increased toxicity (QT_c interval prolongation) with other agents that cause QT_c interval prolongation, especially mefloquine.

Decreased Effect: CYP3A4 inducers may decrease the levels/effects of halofantrine; example inducers include aminoglutethimide, carbamazepine, nafcillin, nevirapine, phenobarbital, phenytoin, and rifamycins.

Pharmacodynamics/Kinetics

Absorption: Erratic and variable; serum levels are proportional to dose up to 1000 mg; smaller doses should be divided; may be increased 60% with high fat meals

Distribution: V_d: 570 L/kg; widely to most tissues

(Continued)

Halofantrine (Continued)

Metabolism: Hepatic to active metabolite

Half-life elimination: 6-10 days; Metabolite: 3-4 days; may be prolonged in active disease

Excretion: Primarily in feces (hepatobiliary)

Clearance: Parasite: Mean: 40-84 hours

Pregnancy Risk Factor C

Dental Comment

This drug is known to prolong the QT interval. The QT interval is measured as the time and distance between the Q point of the QRS complex and the end of the T wave in the ECG tracing. After adjustment for heart rate, the QT interval is defined as prolonged if it is more than 450 msec in men and 460 msec in women. A long QT syndrome was first described in the 1950s and 60s as a congenital syndrome involving QT interval prolongation and syncope and sudden death. Some of the congenital long QT syndromes were characterized by a peculiar electrocardiographic appearance of the QRS complex involving a premature atria beat followed by a pause, then a subsequent sinus beat showing marked QT prolongation and deformity. This type of cardiac arrhythmia was originally termed "torsade de pointes" (translated from the French as "twisting of the points").

Prolongation of the QT interval is thought to result from delayed ventricular repolarization. The repolarization process within the myocardial cell is due to the efflux of intracellular potassium. The channels associated with this current can be blocked by many drugs and predisposes the electrical propagation cycle to torsade de pointes.

Halofantrine is one of the drugs confirmed to prolong the QT interval and is accepted as having a risk of causing torsade de pointes. The risk of drug-induced torsade de pointes is extremely low when a single QT interval prolonging drug is prescribed. In terms of epinephrine, it is not known what effect vasoconstrictors in the local anesthetic regimen will have in patients with a known history of congenital prolonged QT interval or in patients taking any medication that prolongs the QT interval. Until more information is obtained, it is suggested that the clinician consult with the physician prior to the use of a vasoconstrictor in suspected patients, and that the vasoconstrictor (epinephrine, levonordefrin [Neo-Cobefrin®]) be used with caution.

Halofantrine Hydrochloride see Halofantrine on page 761

Halog® see Halcinonide on page 760

Haloperidol (ha loe PER i dole)

U.S. Brand Names Haldol®; Haldol® Decanoate

Canadian Brand Names Apo-Haloperidol®; Apo-Haloperidol LA®; Haloperidol-LA Omega; Haloperidol Long Acting; Novo-Peridol; Peridol; PMS-Haloperidol LA

Mexican Brand Names Haldol®; Haldol decanoas®; Haloperil®

Generic Available Yes

Synonyms Haloperidol Decanoate; Haloperidol Lactate

Pharmacologic Category Antipsychotic Agent, Typical

Use Management of schizophrenia; control of tics and vocal utterances of Tourette's disorder in children and adults; severe behavioral problems in children

Unlabeled/Investigational Use Treatment of psychosis; may be used for the emergency sedation of severely-agitated or delirious patients; adjunctive treatment of ethanol dependence; antiemetic

Local Anesthetic/Vasoconstrictor Precautions Manufacturer's information states that haloperidol may block vasopressor activity of epinephrine. This has not been observed during use of epinephrine as a vasoconstrictor in local anesthesia. See Dental Comment.

Effects on Dental Treatment Key adverse event(s) related to dental treatment: Orthostatic hypotension, and nasal congestion are possible; since the drug is a dopamine antagonist, extrapyramidal symptoms of the TMJ are a possibility.

Common Adverse Effects Frequency not defined.

Cardiovascular: Hyper-/hypotension, tachycardia, arrhythmia, abnormal T waves with prolonged ventricular repolarization, torsade de pointes (case-control study ~4%)

Central nervous system: Restlessness, anxiety, extrapyramidal symptoms, dystonic reactions, pseudoparkinsonian signs and symptoms, tardive dyskinesia, neuroleptic malignant syndrome (NMS), altered central temperature regulation, akathisia, tardive dystonia, insomnia, euphoria, agitation, drowsiness, depression, lethargy, headache, confusion, vertigo, seizure

Dermatologic: Hyperpigmentation, pruritus, rash, contact dermatitis, alopecia, photosensitivity (rare)

Endocrine & metabolic: Amenorrhea, galactorrhea, gynecomastia, sexual dysfunction, lactation, breast engorgement, mastalgia, menstrual irregularities, hyperglycemia, hypoglycemia, hyponatremia

Gastrointestinal: Nausea, vomiting, anorexia, constipation, diarrhea, hypersalivation, dyspepsia, xerostomia

Genitourinary: Urinary retention, priapism

Hematologic: Cholestatic jaundice, obstructive jaundice

Ocular: Blurred vision

Respiratory: Laryngospasm, bronchospasm

Miscellaneous: Heat stroke, diaphoresis

Mechanism of Action Haloperidol is a butyrophenone antipsychotic which blocks postsynaptic mesolimbic dopaminergic D_1 and D_2 receptors in the brain; depresses the release of hypothalamic and hypophyseal hormones; believed to depress the reticular activating system thus affecting basal metabolism, body temperature, wakefulness, vasomotor tone, and emesis

Drug Interactions

Cytochrome P450 Effect: Substrate of CYP1A2 (minor), 2D6 (major), 3A4 (major); **Inhibits** CYP2D6 (moderate), 3A4 (moderate)

Increased Effect/Toxicity: Haloperidol concentrations/effects may be increased by chloroquine, propranolol, and sulfadoxine-pyridoxine. The levels/effects of haloperidol may be increased by azole antifungals, chlorpromazine, clarithromycin, delavirdine, diclofenac, doxycycline, erythromycin, fluoxetine, imatinib, isoniazid, miconazole, nefazodone, nicardipine, paroxetine, pergolide, propofol, protease inhibitors, quinidine, quinine, ritonavir, ropinirole, telithromycin, verapamil, and other CYP2D6 or 3A4 inhibitors.

Haloperidol may increase the levels/effects of amphetamines, selected beta-blockers, selected benzodiazepines, calcium channel blockers, cisapride, cyclosporine, dextromethorphan, ergot alkaloids, fluoxetine, selected HMG-CoA reductase inhibitors, lidocaine, mesoridazine, mirtazapine, nateglinide, nefazodone, paroxetine, risperidone, ritonavir, sildenafil (and other PDE-5 inhibitors), tacrolimus, thioridazine, tricyclic antidepressants, venlafaxine, and other substrates of CYP2D6 or 3A4.

Haloperidol may increase the effects of antihypertensives, CNS depressants (ethanol, narcotics, sedative-hypnotics), lithium, trazodone, and TCAs. Haloperidol in combination with indomethacin may result in drowsiness, tiredness, and confusion. Metoclopramide may increase risk of extrapyramidal symptoms (EPS). Acetylcholinesterase inhibitors (central) may increase the risk of antipsychotic-related EPS.

Decreased Effect: Haloperidol may inhibit the ability of bromocriptine to lower serum prolactin concentrations. Benztropine (and other anticholinergics) may inhibit the therapeutic response to haloperidol and excess anticholinergic effects may occur. Barbiturates, carbamazepine, and cigarette smoking may enhance the hepatic metabolism of haloperidol. Haloperidol may inhibit the antiparkinsonian effect of levodopa; avoid this combination. The levels/effects of haloperidol may be decreased by aminoglutethimide, carbamazepine, nafcillin, nevirapine, phenobarbital, phenytoin, rifamycins, and other CYP3A4 inducers. Haloperidol may decrease the levels/effects of CYP2D6 prodrug substrates (eg, codeine, hydrocodone, oxycodone, tramadol).

Pharmacodynamics/Kinetics

Onset of action: Sedation: I.V.: ~1 hour

Duration: Decanoate: ~3 weeks

Distribution: Crosses placenta; enters breast milk

Protein binding: 90%

Metabolism: Hepatic to inactive compounds

Bioavailability: Oral: 60%

Half-life elimination: 20 hours

Time to peak, serum: 20 minutes

Excretion: Urine (33% to 40% as metabolites) within 5 days; feces (15%)

Pregnancy Risk Factor C

Dental Comment

This drug is known to prolong the QT interval. The QT interval is measured as the time and distance between the Q point of the QRS complex and the end of the T wave in the ECG tracing. After adjustment for heart rate, the QT interval is defined as prolonged if it is more than 450 msec in men and 460 msec in women. A long QT syndrome was first described in the 1950s and 60s as a congenital syndrome involving QT interval prolongation and syncope and sudden death. Some of the congenital long QT syndromes were characterized

(Continued)

Haloperidol *(Continued)*

by a peculiar electrocardiographic appearance of the QRS complex involving a premature atria beat followed by a pause, then a subsequent sinus beat showing marked QT prolongation and deformity. This type of cardiac arrhythmia was originally termed "torsade de pointes" (translated from the French as "twisting of the points").

Prolongation of the QT interval is thought to result from delayed ventricular repolarization. The repolarization process within the myocardial cell is due to the efflux of intracellular potassium. The channels associated with this current can be blocked by many drugs and predisposes the electrical propagation cycle to torsade de pointes.

Haloperidol is one of the drugs confirmed to prolong the QT interval and is accepted as having a risk of causing torsade de pointes. The risk of drug-induced torsade de pointes is extremely low when a single QT interval prolonging drug is prescribed. In terms of epinephrine, it is not known what effect vasoconstrictors in the local anesthetic regimen will have in patients with a known history of congenital prolonged QT interval or in patients taking any medication that prolongs the QT interval. Until more information is obtained, it is suggested that the clinician consult with the physician prior to the use of a vasoconstrictor in suspected patients, and that the vasoconstrictor (epinephrine, levonordefrin [Neo-Cobefrin®]) be used with caution.

Haloperidol Decanoate *see* Haloperidol *on page 762*

Haloperidol Lactate *see* Haloperidol *on page 762*

Halotestin® *see* Fluoxymesterone *on page 679*

HandClens® [OTC] *see* Benzalkonium Chloride *on page 188*

Havrix® *see* Hepatitis A Vaccine *on page 767*

Havrix® and Engerix-B® *see* Hepatitis A Inactivated and Hepatitis B (Recombinant) Vaccine *on page 766*

HbCV *see* Haemophilus b Conjugate Vaccine *on page 534*

HBIG *see* Hepatitis B Immune Globulin *on page 768*

hBNP *see* Nesiritide *on page 1103*

HbOC *see* Haemophilus b Conjugate Vaccine *on page 534*

hCG *see* Chorionic Gonadotropin (Human) *on page 336*

HCTZ (error-prone abbreviation) *see* Hydrochlorothiazide *on page 776*

HD 85® *see* Barium *on page 179*

HD 200® Plus *see* Barium *on page 179*

HDA® Toothache [OTC] *see* Benzocaine *on page 190*

HDCV *see* Rabies Virus Vaccine *on page 1329*

Head & Shoulders® Citrus Breeze [OTC] *see* Pyrithione Zinc *on page 1318*

Head & Shoulders® Classic Clean [OTC] *see* Pyrithione Zinc *on page 1318*

Head & Shoulders® Classic Clean 2-In-1 [OTC] *see* Pyrithione Zinc *on page 1318*

Head & Shoulders® Dry Scalp Care [OTC] *see* Pyrithione Zinc *on page 1318*

Head & Shoulders® Extra Volume [OTC] *see* Pyrithione Zinc *on page 1318*

Head & Shoulders® Leave-in Treatment [OTC] *see* Pyrithione Zinc *on page 1318*

Head & Shoulders® Refresh [OTC] *see* Pyrithione Zinc *on page 1318*

Head & Shoulders® Sensitive Care [OTC] *see* Pyrithione Zinc *on page 1318*

Head & Shoulders® Smooth & Silky 2-In-1 [OTC] *see* Pyrithione Zinc *on page 1318*

Healon® *see* Hyaluronate and Derivatives *on page 773*

Healon®5 *see* Hyaluronate and Derivatives *on page 773*

Healon GV® *see* Hyaluronate and Derivatives *on page 773*

Hectorol® *see* Doxercalciferol *on page 508*

Helidac® *see* Bismuth Subsalicylate, Metronidazole, and Tetracycline *on page 210*

Helistat® *see* Collagen Hemostat *on page 392*

Helitene® *see* Collagen Hemostat *on page 392*

Helixate® FS *see* Antihemophilic Factor (Recombinant) *on page 130*

Hemabate® *see* Carboprost Tromethamine *on page 270*

Hemiacidrin *see* Citric Acid, Magnesium Carbonate, and Glucono-Delta-Lactone *on page 353*

Hemin *(HEE min)*

U.S. Brand Names Panhematin®
Generic Available No

Pharmacologic Category Blood Modifiers
Use Orphan drug: Treatment of recurrent attacks of acute intermittent porphyria (AIP) only after an appropriate period of alternate therapy has been tried
Local Anesthetic/Vasoconstrictor Precautions No information available to require special precautions
Effects on Dental Treatment No significant effects or complications reported
Common Adverse Effects Frequency not defined.
  Central nervous system: Mild pyrexia
  Hematologic: Leukocytosis
  Local: Phlebitis
  Case report: Coagulopathy

Hemocyte® [OTC] see Ferrous Fumarate on page 650
Hemocyte Plus® see Vitamins (Multiple/Oral) on page 1582
Hemodent™ see Aluminum Chloride on page 78
Hemofil® M see Antihemophilic Factor (Human) on page 129
Hemorrhoidal HC see Hydrocortisone on page 793
Hemril®-30 see Hydrocortisone on page 793
HepaGam B™ see Hepatitis B Immune Globulin on page 768

Heparin (HEP a rin)

U.S. Brand Names HepFlush®-10; Hep-Lock®
Canadian Brand Names Hepalean®; Hepalean® Leo; Hepalean®-LOK
Generic Available Yes
Synonyms Heparin Calcium; Heparin Lock Flush; Heparin Sodium
Pharmacologic Category Anticoagulant
Use Prophylaxis and treatment of thromboembolic disorders
  Note: Heparin lock flush solution is intended only to maintain patency of I.V. devices and is **not** to be used for anticoagulant therapy.
Unlabeled/Investigational Use Acute MI — combination regimen of heparin (unlabeled dose), tenecteplase (half dose), and abciximab (full dose)
Local Anesthetic/Vasoconstrictor Precautions No information available to require special precautions
Effects on Dental Treatment Key adverse event(s) related to dental treatment: Bleeding from the gums.
Common Adverse Effects
  Cardiovascular: Chest pain, vasospasm (possibly related to thrombosis), hemorrhagic shock
  Central nervous system: Fever, headache, chills
  Dermatologic: Unexplained bruising, urticaria, alopecia, dysesthesia pedis, purpura, eczema, cutaneous necrosis (following deep SubQ injection), erythematous plaques (case reports)
  Endocrine & metabolic: Hyperkalemia (supression of aldosterone), rebound hyperlipidemia on discontinuation
  Gastrointestinal: Nausea, vomiting, constipation, hematemesis
  Genitourinary: Frequent or persistent erection
  Hematologic: Hemorrhage, blood in urine, bleeding from gums, epistaxis, adrenal hemorrhage, ovarian hemorrhage, retroperitoneal hemorrhage, thrombocytopenia (see note)
  Hepatic: Elevated liver enzymes (AST/ALT)
  Local: Irritation, ulceration, cutaneous necrosis have been rarely reported with deep SubQ injections, I.M. injection (not recommended) is associated with a high incidence of these effects
  Neuromuscular & skeletal: Peripheral neuropathy, osteoporosis (chronic therapy effect)
  Ocular: Conjunctivitis (allergic reaction)
  Respiratory: Hemoptysis, pulmonary hemorrhage, asthma, rhinitis, bronchospasm (case reports)
  Miscellaneous: Allergic reactions, anaphylactoid reactions

  Note: Thrombocytopenia has been reported to occur at an incidence between 0% and 30%. It is often of no clinical significance. However, immunologically mediated heparin-induced thrombocytopenia has been estimated to occur in 1% to 2% of patients, and is marked by a progressive fall in platelet counts and, in some cases, thromboembolic complications (skin necrosis, pulmonary embolism, gangrene of the extremities, stroke or MI). For recommendations regarding platelet monitoring during heparin therapy, consult "Seventh ACCP Consensus Conference on Antithrombotic and Thrombolytic Therapy."
Mechanism of Action Potentiates the action of antithrombin III and thereby inactivates thrombin (as well as activated coagulation factors IX, X, XI, XII, and
(Continued)

Heparin *(Continued)*

plasmin) and prevents the conversion of fibrinogen to fibrin; heparin also stimulates release of lipoprotein lipase (lipoprotein lipase hydrolyzes triglycerides to glycerol and free fatty acids)

Drug Interactions

Increased Effect/Toxicity: The risk of hemorrhage associated with heparin may be increased by oral anticoagulants (warfarin), thrombolytics, dextran, and drugs which affect platelet function (eg, aspirin, NSAIDs, dipyridamole, ticlopidine, clopidogrel, IIb/IIIa antagonists). However, heparin is often used in conjunction with thrombolytic therapy or during the initiation of warfarin therapy to assure anticoagulation and to protect against possible transient hypercoagulability. Cephalosporins which contain the MTT side chain and parenteral penicillins (may inhibit platelet aggregation) may increase the risk of hemorrhage. Other drugs reported to increase heparin's anticoagulant effect include antihistamines, tetracycline, quinine, nicotine, and cardiac glycosides (digoxin).

Decreased Effect: Nitroglycerin (I.V.) may decrease heparin's anticoagulant effect. This interaction has not been validated in some studies, and may only occur at high nitroglycerin dosages.

Pharmacodynamics/Kinetics

Onset of action: Anticoagulation: I.V.: Immediate; SubQ: ~20-30 minutes

Absorption: Oral, rectal, I.M.: Erratic at best from all these routes of administration; SubQ absorption is also erratic, but considered acceptable for prophylactic use

Distribution: Does not cross placenta; does not enter breast milk

Metabolism: Hepatic; may be partially metabolized in the reticuloendothelial system

Half-life elimination: Mean: 1.5 hours; Range: 1-2 hours; affected by obesity, renal function, hepatic function, malignancy, presence of pulmonary embolism, and infections

Excretion: Urine (small amounts as unchanged drug)

Pregnancy Risk Factor C

Heparin Calcium *see* Heparin *on page 765*

Heparin Cofactor I *see* Antithrombin III *on page 131*

Heparin Lock Flush *see* Heparin *on page 765*

Heparin Sodium *see* Heparin *on page 765*

Hepatitis A Inactivated and Hepatitis B (Recombinant) Vaccine

(hep a TYE tis aye in ak ti VAY ted & hep a TYE tis bee ree KOM be nant vak SEEN)

Related Information

Immunizations (Vaccines) *on page 1786*
Systemic Viral Diseases *on page 1675*

U.S. Brand Names Twinrix®

Canadian Brand Names Twinrix®

Generic Available No

Synonyms Engerix-B® and Havrix®; Havrix® and Engerix-B®; Hepatitis B (Recombinant) and Hepatitis A Inactivated Vaccine

Pharmacologic Category Vaccine

Use Active immunization against disease caused by hepatitis A virus and hepatitis B virus (all known subtypes) in populations desiring protection against or at high risk of exposure to these viruses.

Populations include travelers to areas of intermediate/high endemicity for **both** HAV and HBV; those at increased risk of HBV infection due to behavioral or occupational factors; patients with chronic liver disease; laboratory workers who handle live HAV and HBV; healthcare workers, police, and other personnel who render first-aid or medical assistance; workers who come in contact with sewage; employees of day care centers and correctional facilities; patients/staff of hemodialysis units; male homosexuals; patients frequently receiving blood products; military personnel; users of injectable illicit drugs; close household contacts of patients with hepatitis A and hepatitis B infection.

Local Anesthetic/Vasoconstrictor Precautions No information available to require special precautions

Effects on Dental Treatment Key adverse event(s) related to dental treatment: Flu-like syndrome and upper respiratory tract infection.

Common Adverse Effects All serious adverse reactions must be reported to the U.S. Department of Health and Human Services (DHHS) Vaccine Adverse Event Reporting System (VAERS) 1-800-822-7967.

Incidence of adverse effects of the combination product were similar to those occurring after administration of hepatitis A vaccine and hepatitis B vaccine alone. (Incidence reported is not versus placebo.)

>10%:
   Central nervous system: Headache (13% to 22%), fatigue (11% to 14%)
   Local: Injection site reaction: Soreness (37% to 41%), redness (9% to 11%)

1% to 10%:
   Central nervous system: Fever (2% to 3%)
   Gastrointestinal: Diarrhea (4% to 6%), nausea (2% to 4%), vomiting (≤1%)
   Local: Injection site reaction: Swelling (4% to 6%), induration
   Respiratory: Upper respiratory tract infection
   Miscellaneous: Flu-like syndrome

Mechanism of Action
   Hepatitis A vaccine (Havrix®), an inactivated virus vaccine, offers active immunization against hepatitis A virus infection at an effective immune response rate in up to 99% of subjects.
   Recombinant hepatitis B vaccine (Engerix-B®) is a noninfectious subunit viral vaccine. The vaccine is derived from hepatitis B surface antigen (HB$_s$Ag) produced through recombinant DNA techniques from yeast cells. The portion of the hepatitis B gene which codes for HB$_s$Ag is cloned into yeast which is then cultured to produce hepatitis B vaccine.

   In immunocompetent people, Twinrix® provides active immunization against hepatitis A virus infection (at an effective immune response rate >99% of subjects) and against hepatitis B virus infection (at an effective immune response rate of 93% to 97%) 30 days after completion of the 3-dose series. This is comparable to using hepatitis A vaccine (Havrix®) and hepatitis B vaccine (Engerix-B®) concomitantly.

Drug Interactions
   Decreased Effect: Immunosuppressant agents: May decrease immune response to vaccine

Pharmacodynamics/Kinetics
   Onset of action: Seroconversion for antibodies against HAV and HBV were detected 1 month after completion of the 3-dose series.
   Duration: Patients remained seropositive for at least 4 years during clinical studies.

Pregnancy Risk Factor C

Hepatitis A Vaccine (hep a TYE tis aye vak SEEN)

Related Information
   Immunizations (Vaccines) *on page 1786*
   Systemic Viral Diseases *on page 1675*

U.S. Brand Names Havrix®; VAQTA®
Canadian Brand Names Avaxim®; Avaxim®-Pediatric; Havrix®; VAQTA®
Generic Available No
Pharmacologic Category Vaccine
Use
   Active immunization against disease caused by hepatitis A virus in populations desiring protection against or at high risk of exposure
   Populations at high risk of exposure to hepatitis A virus may include children and adolescents in selected states and regions, travelers to developing countries, household and sexual contacts of persons infected with hepatitis A, child day care employees, patients with chronic liver disease, illicit drug users, male homosexuals, institutional workers (eg, institutions for the mentally and physically handicapped persons, prisons), and healthcare workers who may be exposed to hepatitis A virus (eg, laboratory employees)

Local Anesthetic/Vasoconstrictor Precautions No information available to require special precautions

Effects on Dental Treatment No significant effects or complications reported

Common Adverse Effects All serious adverse reactions must be reported to the U.S. Department of Health and Human Services (DHHS) Vaccine Adverse Event Reporting System (VAERS) 1-800-822-7967.

Frequency dependant upon age, product used, and concomitant vaccine administration. In general, injection site reactions were less common in younger children.

>10%:
   Central nervous system: Irritability (11% to 36%), drowsiness (15% to 17%), headache (2% to 16%), fever ≥100.4°F (9% to 11%)

(Continued)

Hepatitis A Vaccine *(Continued)*

Gastrointestinal: Anorexia (1% to 19%)

Local: Injection site: Pain, soreness, tenderness (3% to 56%), erythema (1% to 22%), warmth (<1% to 17%), swelling (1% to 14%)

1% to 10%:

Central nervous system: Fever ≥102°F (3% to 4%)

Dermatologic: Rash (≤1% to 5%)

Endocrine & metabolic: Menstrual disorder (1%)

Gastrointestinal: Diarrhea (<1% to 6%), vomiting (<1% to 4%), nausea (2%), abdominal pain (<1% to 2%), anorexia (1%)

Local: Injection site bruising (1% to 2%)

Neuromuscular & skeletal: Weakness/fatigue (4%), myalgia (<1% to 2%), arm pain (1%), back pain (1%), stiffness (1%)

Ocular: Conjunctivitis (1%)

Otic: Otitis media (8%), otitis (2%)

Respiratory: Upper respiratory tract infection (<1% to 10%), rhinorrhea (6%), cough (1% to 5%), pharnyngitis (<1% to 3%), respiratory congestion (2%), nasal congestion (1%), laryngotracheobronchitis (1%)

Miscellaneous: Crying (2%), viral exanthema (1%)

Mechanism of Action As an inactivated virus vaccine, hepatitis A vaccine offers active immunization against hepatitis A virus infection at an effective immune response rate in up to 99% of subjects

Pharmacodynamics/Kinetics

Onset of action (protection): 4 weeks after a single dose

Duration: Neutralizing antibodies have persisted for up to 8 years; based on kinetic models, antibodies may be present >20 years

Pregnancy Risk Factor C

Hepatitis B Immune Globulin

(hep a TYE tis bee i MYUN GLOB yoo lin)

Related Information

Immunizations (Vaccines) *on page 1786*

Occupational Exposure to Bloodborne Pathogens (Standard / Universal Precautions) *on page 1770*

Systemic Viral Diseases *on page 1675*

U.S. Brand Names BayHep B®; HepaGam B™; Nabi-HB®

Canadian Brand Names BayHep B®; HyperHep B®

Generic Available No

Synonyms HBIG

Pharmacologic Category Immune Globulin

Use Passive prophylactic immunity to hepatitis B following: Acute exposure to blood containing hepatitis B surface antigen (HBsAg); perinatal exposure of infants born to HBsAg-positive mothers; sexual exposure to HBsAg-positive persons; household exposure to persons with acute HBV infection

Note: Hepatitis B immune globulin is not indicated for treatment of active hepatitis B infection and is ineffective in the treatment of chronic active hepatitis B infection.

Unlabeled/Investigational Use

Prevention of hepatitis B virus recurrence after liver transplantation

Local Anesthetic/Vasoconstrictor Precautions No information available to require special precautions

Effects on Dental Treatment No significant effects or complications reported

Common Adverse Effects Frequency not defined.

Central nervous system: Chills, dizziness, fever, headache, lethargy, malaise

Dermatologic: Angioedema, erythema, rash, urticaria

Gastrointestinal: Nausea, vomiting

Genitourinary: Nephrotic syndrome

Local: Muscular stiffness, pain, and tenderness at injection site

Neuromuscular & skeletal: Arthralgia, back pain, myalgia

Miscellaneous: Anaphylaxis, flu-like syndrome

Mechanism of Action Hepatitis B immune globulin (HBIG) is a nonpyrogenic sterile solution containing immunoglobulin G (IgG) specific to hepatitis B surface antigen (HB$_s$Ag). HBIG differs from immune globulin in the amount of anti-HB$_s$. Immune globulin is prepared from plasma that is not preselected for anti-HB$_s$ content. HBIG is prepared from plasma preselected for high titer anti-HB$_s$. In the U.S., HBIG has an anti-HB$_s$ high titer >1:100,000 by IRA.

Drug Interactions

Decreased Effect:

Interferes with immune response of live virus vaccines; defer live virus vaccine for about 3 months after immune globulin

Note: HBIG may be administered at the same time (but at a different site) or up to 1 month preceding hepatitis B vaccination without impairing the active immune response

Pharmacodynamics/Kinetics
Absorption: Slow
Half-life: 17-25 days
Distribution: V_d: 7-15 L
Time to peak, serum: 2-10 days

Pregnancy Risk Factor C

Hepatitis B Inactivated Virus Vaccine (plasma derived) *see* Hepatitis B Vaccine *on page 769*

Hepatitis B Inactivated Virus Vaccine (recombinant DNA) *see* Hepatitis B Vaccine *on page 769*

Hepatitis B (Recombinant) and Hepatitis A Inactivated Vaccine *see* Hepatitis A Inactivated and Hepatitis B (Recombinant) Vaccine *on page 766*

Hepatitis B Vaccine (hep a TYE tis bee vak SEEN)

Related Information
Immunizations (Vaccines) *on page 1786*
Systemic Viral Diseases *on page 1675*
U.S. Brand Names Engerix-B®; Recombivax HB®
Canadian Brand Names Engerix-B®; Recombivax HB®
Generic Available No
Synonyms Hepatitis B Inactivated Virus Vaccine (plasma derived); Hepatitis B Inactivated Virus Vaccine (recombinant DNA)
Pharmacologic Category Vaccine
Dental Use Immunization is recommended for dentists, oral surgeons, dental hygienists, dental nurses, and dental students
Use Immunization against infection caused by all known subtypes of hepatitis B virus, in individuals considered at high risk of potential exposure to hepatitis B virus or HB_sAg-positive materials: See table.

Pre-exposure Prophylaxis for Hepatitis B

Healthcare workers[1]

Special patient groups (eg, adolescents, infants born to HB_sAg-positive mothers, children born after 11/21/91, military personnel, etc)

  Hemodialysis patients[2] (see dosing recommendations)

  Recipients of certain blood products[3]

Lifestyle factors

  Homosexual and bisexual men

  Intravenous drug abusers

  Heterosexually-active persons with multiple sexual partners or recently acquired sexually-transmitted diseases

Environmental factors

  Household and sexual contacts of HBV carriers

  Prison inmates

  Clients and staff of institutions for the mentally handicapped

  Residents, immigrants, and refugees from areas with endemic HBV infection

  International travelers at increased risk of acquiring HBV infection

---

[1]The risk of hepatitis B virus (HBV) infection for healthcare workers varies both between hospitals and within hospitals. Hepatitis B vaccination is recommended for all healthcare workers with blood exposure.

[2]Hemodialysis patients often respond poorly to hepatitis B vaccination; higher vaccine doses or increased number of doses are required. A special formulation of one vaccine is now available for such persons (Recombivax HB®, 40 mcg/mL). The anti-HB_s (antibody to hepatitis B surface antigen) response of such persons should be tested after they are vaccinated, and those who have not responded should be revaccinated with 1-3 additional doses.

Patients with chronic renal disease should be vaccinated as early as possible, ideally before they require hemodialysis. In addition, their anti-HB_s levels should be monitored at 6- to 12-month intervals to assess the need for revaccination.

[3]Patients with hemophilia should be immunized subcutaneously, not intramuscularly.

Local Anesthetic/Vasoconstrictor Precautions No information available to require special precautions
Effects on Dental Treatment No significant effects or complications reported
Common Adverse Effects All serious adverse reactions must be reported to the U.S. Department of Health and Human Services (DHHS) Vaccine Adverse Event Reporting System (VAERS) 1-800-822-7967.

(Continued)

Hepatitis B Vaccine *(Continued)*

Frequency not defined. The most common adverse effects reported with both products included injection site reactions (>10%).

Cardiovascular: Hypotension

Central nervous system: Agitation, chills, dizziness, fatigue, fever (≥37.5°C / 100°F), flushing, headache, insomnia, irritability, lightheadedness, malaise, vertigo

Dermatologic: Angioedema, petechiae, pruritus, rash, urticaria

Gastrointestinal: Abdominal pain, appetite decreased, cramps, diarrhea, dyspepsia, nausea, vomiting

Genitourinary: Dysuria

Local: Injection site reactions: Ecchymosis, erythema, induration, pain, nodule formation, soreness, swelling, tenderness, warmth

Neuromuscular & skeletal: Achiness, arthralgia, back pain, myalgia, neck pain, neck stiffness, paresthesia, shoulder pain, weakness

Otic: Earache

Respiratory: Cough, pharyngitis, rhinitis, upper respiratory tract infection

Miscellaneous: Lymphadenopathy, diaphoresis

Mechanism of Action Recombinant hepatitis B vaccine is a noninfectious subunit viral vaccine. The vaccine is derived from hepatitis B surface antigen (HB$_s$Ag) produced through recombinant DNA techniques from yeast cells. The portion of the hepatitis B gene which codes for HB$_s$Ag is cloned into yeast which is then cultured to produce hepatitis B vaccine.

Drug Interactions

Decreased Effect: Decreased effect: Immunosuppressive agents

Pharmacodynamics/Kinetics Duration of action: Following a 3-dose series, immunity lasts ~5-7 years

Pregnancy Risk Factor C

HepFlush®-10 *see* Heparin *on page 765*

Hep-Lock® *see* Heparin *on page 765*

Hepsera™ *see* Adefovir *on page 54*

Herceptin® *see* Trastuzumab *on page 1520*

HES *see* Hetastarch *on page 770*

Hespan® *see* Hetastarch *on page 770*

Hetastarch *(HET a starch)*

U.S. Brand Names Hespan®; Hextend®

Canadian Brand Names Hextend®; Voluven®

Mexican Brand Names HAES-steril®

Generic Available Yes: Sodium chloride infusion

Synonyms HES; Hydroxyethyl Starch

Pharmacologic Category Plasma Volume Expander, Colloid

Use Blood volume expander used in treatment of hypovolemia

Hespan®: Adjunct in leukapheresis to improve harvesting and increasing the yield of granulocytes by centrifugal means

Unlabeled/Investigational Use Hextend®: Priming fluid in pump oxygenators during cardiopulmonary bypass, and as a plasma volume expander during cardiopulmonary bypass

Local Anesthetic/Vasoconstrictor Precautions No information available to require special precautions

Effects on Dental Treatment No significant effects or complications reported

Common Adverse Effects Frequency not defined.

Cardiovascular: Circulatory overload, heart failure, peripheral edema

Central nervous system: Chills, fever, headache, intracranial bleeding

Dermatologic: Itching, pruritus, rash

Endocrine & metabolic: Amylase levels increased, parotid gland enlargement, indirect bilirubin increased, metabolic acidosis

Gastrointestinal: Vomiting

Hematologic: Bleeding, factor VIII:C plasma levels decreased, decreased plasma aggregation decreased, von Willebrand factor decreased, dilutional coagulopathy; prolongation of PT, PTT, clotting time, and bleeding time; thrombocytopenia, anemia, disseminated intravascular coagulopathy (rare), hemolysis (rare)

Neuromuscular & skeletal: Myalgia

Miscellaneous: Anaphylactoid reactions, hypersensitivity, flu-like symptoms (mild)

Mechanism of Action Produces plasma volume expansion by virtue of its highly colloidal starch structure, similar to albumin

Pharmacodynamics/Kinetics
Onset of action: Volume expansion: I.V.: ~30 minutes
Duration: 24-36 hours
Metabolism: Molecules >50,000 daltons require enzymatic degradation by the reticuloendothelial system or amylases in the blood
Excretion: Urine (~40%) within 24 hours; smaller molecular weight molecules readily excreted

Pregnancy Risk Factor C

Hexabrix™ *see* Ioxaglate Meglumine and Ioxaglate Sodium *on page 856*

Hexachlorocyclohexane *see* Lindane *on page 933*

Hexachlorophene (heks a KLOR oh feen)

U.S. Brand Names pHisoHex®
Canadian Brand Names pHisoHex®
Generic Available No
Pharmacologic Category Antibiotic, Topical
Use Surgical scrub and as a bacteriostatic skin cleanser; control an outbreak of gram-positive infection when other procedures have been unsuccessful
Local Anesthetic/Vasoconstrictor Precautions No information available to require special precautions
Effects on Dental Treatment No significant effects or complications reported
Mechanism of Action Bacteriostatic polychlorinated biphenyl which inhibits membrane-bound enzymes and disrupts the cell membrane
Pharmacodynamics/Kinetics
Absorption: Percutaneously through inflamed, excoriated, and intact skin
Distribution: Crosses placenta
Half-life elimination: Infants: 6.1-44.2 hours
Pregnancy Risk Factor C

Hexalen® *see* Altretamine *on page 78*

Hexamethylenetetramine *see* Methenamine *on page 1007*

Hexamethylmelamine *see* Altretamine *on page 78*

HEXM *see* Altretamine *on page 78*

Hextend® *see* Hetastarch *on page 770*

Hexylresorcinol (heks il re ZOR si nole)

U.S. Brand Names S.T. 37® [OTC]; Sucrets® Original [OTC]
Generic Available No
Pharmacologic Category Antiseptic, Topical; Local Anesthetic
Use Minor antiseptic and local anesthetic for sore throat; topical antiseptic for minor cuts or abrasions
Local Anesthetic/Vasoconstrictor Precautions No information available to require special precautions
Effects on Dental Treatment No significant effects or complications reported

Hibiclens® [OTC] *see* Chlorhexidine Gluconate *on page 316*

Hibistat® [OTC] *see* Chlorhexidine Gluconate *on page 316*

Hib Polysaccharide Conjugate *see* Haemophilus b Conjugate Vaccine *on page 534*

HibTITER® *see* Haemophilus b Conjugate Vaccine *on page 534*

High Gamma Vitamin E Complete™ [OTC] *see* Vitamin E *on page 1581*

Hi-Kovite [OTC *see* Vitamins (Multiple/Oral) *on page 1582*

Hiprex® *see* Methenamine *on page 1007*

Hirulog *see* Bivalirudin *on page 213*

Histade™ *see* Chlorpheniramine and Pseudoephedrine *on page 325*

Hista-Vent® DA *see* Chlorpheniramine, Phenylephrine, and Methscopolamine *on page 327*

Histex™ *see* Chlorpheniramine and Pseudoephedrine *on page 325*

Histex™ I/E *see* Carbinoxamine *on page 268*

Histex™ CT *see* Carbinoxamine *on page 268*

Histex™ HC *see* Hydrocodone, Carbinoxamine, and Pseudoephedrine *on page 789*

Histex™ PD *see* Carbinoxamine *on page 268*

Histex™ PD-12 *see* Carbinoxamine *on page 268*

Histex™ SR *see* Brompheniramine and Pseudoephedrine *on page 223*

Histrelin (his TREL in)

U.S. Brand Names Vantas™
Canadian Brand Names Vantas™
Generic Available No
Synonyms GnRH Agonist; Histrelin Acetate; LH-RH Agonist
Pharmacologic Category Gonadotropin Releasing Hormone Agonist
Use Palliative treatment of advanced prostate cancer
Local Anesthetic/Vasoconstrictor Precautions No information available to require special precautions
Effects on Dental Treatment No significant effects or complications reported
Common Adverse Effects
>10%: Endocrine & metabolic: Expected pharmacological consequence of testosterone suppression: Hot flashes (66%)
2% to 10%:
  Central nervous system: Fatigue (10%), headache (3%), insomnia (3%)
  Endocrine & metabolic: Expected pharmacological consequences of testosterone suppression: Gynecomastia (4%), sexual dysfunction (4%), libido decreased (2%)
  Gastrointestinal: Constipation (4%), weight gain (2%)
  Genitourinary: Expected pharmacological consequence of testosterone suppression: Testicular atrophy (5%)
  Local: Implant site reaction (6%)
  Renal: Renal impairment (5%)
Mechanism of Action Potent inhibitor of gonadotropin secretion; continuous administration results in, after an initiation phase, the suppression of luteinizing hormone (LH), follicle-stimulating hormone (FSH), and a subsequent decrease in testosterone.
Drug Interactions
  Increased Effect/Toxicity: Not studied
Pharmacodynamics/Kinetics
  Onset: Chemical castration: 14 days
  Duration: 1 year
  Distribution: V_d: ~58 L
  Protein binding: 70% ± 9%
  Metabolism: Hepatic via C-terminal dealkylation and hydrolysis
  Bioavailability: 92%
  Half-life elimination: Terminal: ~4 hours
  Time to peak, serum: 12 hours
Pregnancy Risk Factor X

Histrelin Acetate see Histrelin on page 772
Histussin D® see Hydrocodone and Pseudoephedrine on page 788
Hi-Vegi-Lip [OTC] see Pancreatin on page 1183
Hivid® see Zalcitabine on page 1590
HMM see Altretamine on page 78
HMR 3647 see Telithromycin on page 1448
HMS Liquifilm® [DSC] see Medrysone on page 973
Hold® DM [OTC] see Dextromethorphan on page 451

Homatropine (hoe MA troe peen)

U.S. Brand Names Isopto® Homatropine
Generic Available No
Synonyms Homatropine Hydrobromide
Pharmacologic Category Anticholinergic Agent, Ophthalmic; Ophthalmic Agent, Mydriatic
Use Producing cycloplegia and mydriasis for refraction; treatment of acute inflammatory conditions of the uveal tract
Local Anesthetic/Vasoconstrictor Precautions No information available to require special precautions
Effects on Dental Treatment Key adverse event(s) related to dental treatment: Nasal congestion.
Mechanism of Action Blocks response of iris sphincter muscle and the accommodative muscle of the ciliary body to cholinergic stimulation resulting in dilation and loss of accommodation
Pregnancy Risk Factor C

Homatropine and Hydrocodone see Hydrocodone and Homatropine on page 786

Homatropine Hydrobromide *see* Homatropine *on page 772*

Horse Antihuman Thymocyte Gamma Globulin *see* Antithymocyte Globulin (Equine) *on page 131*

H.P. Acthar® Gel *see* Corticotropin *on page 395*

HTF919 *see* Tegaserod *on page 1448*

hu1124 *see* Efalizumab *on page 529*

Humalog® *see* Insulin Lispro *on page 839*

Humalog® Mix 50/50™ *see* Insulin Lispro Protamine and Insulin Lispro *on page 839*

Humalog® Mix 75/25™ *see* Insulin Lispro Protamine and Insulin Lispro *on page 839*

Human Antitumor Necrosis Factor Alpha *see* Adalimumab *on page 52*

Human Diploid Cell Cultures Rabies Vaccine *see* Rabies Virus Vaccine *on page 1329*

Human Growth Hormone *see* Somatropin *on page 1406*

Humanized IgG1 Anti-CD52 Monoclonal Antibody *see* Alemtuzumab *on page 63*

Human LFA-3/IgG(1) Fusion Protein *see* Alefacept *on page 62*

Human Thyroid Stimulating Hormone *see* Thyrotropin Alpha *on page 1483*

Humate-P® *see* Antihemophilic Factor (Human) *on page 129*

Humatin® *see* Paromomycin *on page 1188*

Humatrope® *see* Somatropin *on page 1406*

Humibid® CS [OTC] [DSC] *see* Guaifenesin and Dextromethorphan *on page 754*

Humibid® e [OTC] *see* Guaifenesin *on page 752*

Humibid® LA *(reformulation)* *see* Guaifenesin and Potassium Guaiacolsulfonate *on page 755*

Humira® *see* Adalimumab *on page 52*

Humulin® 50/50 *see* Insulin NPH and Insulin Regular *on page 840*

Humulin® 70/30 *see* Insulin NPH and Insulin Regular *on page 840*

Humulin® N *see* Insulin NPH *on page 840*

Humulin® R *see* Insulin Regular *on page 841*

Humulin® R (Concentrated) U-500 *see* Insulin Regular *on page 841*

Hurricaine® [OTC] *see* Benzocaine *on page 190*

HXM *see* Altretamine *on page 78*

Hyalgan® *see* Hyaluronate and Derivatives *on page 773*

Hyaluronan *see* Hyaluronate and Derivatives *on page 773*

Hyaluronate and Derivatives
(hye al yoor ON ate & dah RIV ah tives)

U.S. Brand Names Biolon™; Euflexxa™; Healon®; Healon®5; Healon GV®; Hyalgan®; Hylaform®; Hylaform® Plus; IPM Wound Gel™ [OTC]; Orthovisc®; Provisc®; Restylane®; Supartz™; Synvisc®; Vitrax®

Canadian Brand Names Cystistat®; Durolane®; Eyestil; Healon®; Healon GV®; OrthoVisc®; Suplasyn®

Mexican Brand Names Biolon™; Healon®

Generic Available No

Synonyms Hyaluronan; Hyaluronic Acid; Hylan Polymers; Sodium Hyaluronate

Pharmacologic Category Antirheumatic Miscellaneous; Ophthalmic Agent, Viscoelastic; Skin and Mucous Membrane Agent, Miscellaneous

Use

Intra-articular injection: Treatment of pain in osteoarthritis in knee in patients who have failed nonpharmacologic treatment and simple analgesics

Intradermal: Correction of moderate-to-severe facial wrinkles or folds

Ophthalmic: Surgical aid in cataract extraction, intraocular implantation, corneal transplant, glaucoma filtration, and retinal attachment surgery

Topical: Management of skin ulcers and wounds

Local Anesthetic/Vasoconstrictor Precautions No information available to require special precautions

Effects on Dental Treatment No significant effects or complications reported

Common Adverse Effects Not all frequencies are defined. Frequencies and/or type of local reaction may vary by formulation and site of application/injection.

Cardiovascular: Blood pressure increased (2% to 4%), edema, flushing, hypotension, tachycardia

Central nervous system: Dizziness, fatigue (1%), headache

Dermatologic: Itching, rash

Gastrointestinal: Nausea (≤2%)

(Continued)

Hyaluronate and Derivatives *(Continued)*

Local: Injection site: Arthralgia, bruising, desquamation, erythema, pain, rash, swelling; nodule, pruritus, skin discoloration

Neuromuscular & skeletal: Back pain (<1% to 6%), tendonitis (2%), parasthesia (1%), hypokinesia (knee)

Ocular (with ophthalmic formulation): Postoperative inflammatory reactions (iritis, hypopyon), corneal edema, corneal decompensation, transient postoperative increase in IOP

Respiratory: Infection (12%), rhinitis (3%)

Miscellaneous: Abscess formation, allergic reactions, anaphylaxis, respiratory difficulties

Mechanism of Action Sodium hyaluronate is a polysaccharide which is distributed widely in the extracellular matrix of connective tissue in man (vitreous and aqueous humor of the eye, synovial fluid, skin, and umbilical cord). Sodium hyaluronate and its derivatives form a viscoelastic solution in water (at physiological pH and ionic strength) which makes it suitable for aqueous and vitreous humor in ophthalmic surgery, and functions as a tissue and/or joint lubricant which plays an important role in modulating the interactions between adjacent tissues. Intradermal injection may decrease the depth of facial wrinkles.

Drug Interactions

Increased Effect/Toxicity: Anticoagulants or antiplatelet agents may increase the risk of injection site bleeding or hematoma.

Pharmacodynamics/Kinetics

Distribution: Intravitreous injection: Diffusion occurs slowly

Excretion: Ophthalmic: Via Canal of Schlemm

Pregnancy Risk Factor C

Hyaluronic Acid *see* Hyaluronate and Derivatives *on page 773*

Hyaluronidase (hye al yoor ON i dase)

U.S. Brand Names Amphadase™; Hydase™; Hylenex™; Vitrase®

Generic Available No

Pharmacologic Category Enzyme

Use Increase the dispersion and absorption of other drugs; increase rate of absorption of parenteral fluids given by hypodermoclysis; adjunct in subcutaneous urography for improving resorption of radiopaque agents

Unlabeled/Investigational Use Management of drug extravasations

Local Anesthetic/Vasoconstrictor Precautions No information available to require special precautions

Effects on Dental Treatment No significant effects or complications reported

Common Adverse Effects

Frequency not defined:

Cardiovascular: Edema

Local: Injection site reactions

Mechanism of Action Modifies the permeability of connective tissue through hydrolysis of hyaluronic acid, one of the chief components of tissue cement which offers resistance to diffusion of liquids through tissues; hyaluronidase increases both the distribution and absorption of locally injected substances.

Drug Interactions

Increased Effect/Toxicity: Absorption and toxicity of local anesthetics may be increased.

Pharmacodynamics/Kinetics

Onset of action: SubQ: Immediate

Duration: 24-48 hours

Pregnancy Risk Factor C

Hycamtamine *see* Topotecan *on page 1511*

Hycamtin® *see* Topotecan *on page 1511*

hycet™ *see* Hydrocodone and Acetaminophen *on page 779*

Hycoclear Tuss *see* Hydrocodone and Guaifenesin *on page 785*

Hycodan® *see* Hydrocodone and Homatropine *on page 786*

Hycomine® Compound *see* Hydrocodone, Chlorpheniramine, Phenylephrine, Acetaminophen, and Caffeine *on page 790*

Hycotuss® *see* Hydrocodone and Guaifenesin *on page 785*

Hydase™ *see* Hyaluronidase *on page 774*

Hydergine [DSC] *see* Ergoloid Mesylates *on page 557*

HydrALAZINE (hye DRAL a zeen)

Related Information
Cardiovascular Diseases *on page 1636*
Canadian Brand Names Apo-Hydralazine®; Apresoline®; Novo-Hylazin; Nu-Hydral
Generic Available Yes
Synonyms Apresoline [DSC]; Hydralazine Hydrochloride
Pharmacologic Category Vasodilator
Use Management of moderate to severe hypertension, congestive heart failure, hypertension secondary to pre-eclampsia/eclampsia; treatment of primary pulmonary hypertension
Local Anesthetic/Vasoconstrictor Precautions No information available to require special precautions
Effects on Dental Treatment No significant effects or complications reported
Common Adverse Effects Frequency not defined.
Cardiovascular: Tachycardia, angina pectoris, orthostatic hypotension (rare), dizziness (rare), paradoxical hypertension, peripheral edema, vascular collapse (rare), flushing
Central nervous system: Increased intracranial pressure (I.V., in patient with pre-existing increased intracranial pressure), fever (rare), chills (rare), anxiety*, disorientation*, depression*, coma*
Dermatologic: Rash (rare), urticaria (rare), pruritus (rare)
Gastrointestinal: Anorexia, nausea, vomiting, diarrhea, constipation, adynamic ileus
Genitourinary: Difficulty in micturition, impotence
Hematologic: Hemolytic anemia (rare), eosinophilia (rare), decreased hemoglobin concentration (rare), reduced erythrocyte count (rare), leukopenia (rare), agranulocytosis (rare), thrombocytopenia (rare)
Neuromuscular & skeletal: Rheumatoid arthritis, muscle cramps, weakness, tremor, peripheral neuritis (rare)
Ocular: Lacrimation, conjunctivitis
Respiratory: Nasal congestion, dyspnea
Miscellaneous: Drug-induced lupus-like syndrome (dose related; fever, arthralgia, splenomegaly, lymphadenopathy, asthenia, myalgia, malaise, pleuritic chest pain, edema, positive ANA, positive LE cells, maculopapular facial rash, positive direct Coombs' test, pericarditis, pericardial tamponade), diaphoresis
*Seen in uremic patients and severe hypertension where rapidly escalating doses may have caused hypotension leading to these effects.
Mechanism of Action Direct vasodilation of arterioles (with little effect on veins) with decreased systemic resistance
Drug Interactions
Cytochrome P450 Effect: Inhibits CYP3A4 (weak)
Increased Effect/Toxicity: Hydralazine may increase levels of beta-blockers (metoprolol, propranolol). Some beta-blockers (acebutolol, atenolol, and nadolol) are unlikely to be affected due to limited hepatic metabolism. Concurrent use of hydralazine with MAO inhibitors may cause a significant decrease in blood pressure. Propranolol may increase hydralazine serum concentrations.
Decreased Effect: NSAIDs (eg, indomethacin) may decrease the hemodynamic effects of hydralazine.
Pharmacodynamics/Kinetics
Onset of action: Oral: 20-30 minutes; I.V.: 5-20 minutes
Duration: Oral: Up to 8 hours; I.V.: 1-4 hours; **Note:** May vary depending on acetylator status of patient
Distribution: Crosses placenta; enters breast milk
Protein binding: 85% to 90%
Metabolism: Hepatically acetylated; extensive first-pass effect (oral)
Bioavailability: 30% to 50%; increased with food
Half-life elimination: Normal renal function: 2-8 hours; End-stage renal disease: 7-16 hours
Excretion: Urine (14% as unchanged drug)
Pregnancy Risk Factor C

Hydralazine and Hydrochlorothiazide
(hye DRAL a zeen & hye droe klor oh THYE a zide)

Related Information
HydrALAZINE *on page 775*
(Continued)

Hydralazine and Hydrochlorothiazide *(Continued)*

Hydrochlorothiazide *on page 776*

Generic Available Yes

Synonyms Apresazide [DSC]; Hydrochlorothiazide and Hydralazine

Pharmacologic Category Antihypertensive Agent, Combination

Use Management of moderate to severe hypertension and treatment of congestive heart failure

Local Anesthetic/Vasoconstrictor Precautions No information available to require special precautions

Effects on Dental Treatment No significant effects or complications reported

Common Adverse Effects See individual agents.

Drug Interactions

Cytochrome P450 Effect: Hydralazine: **Inhibits** CYP3A4 (weak)

Increased Effect/Toxicity: See individual agents.

Pharmacodynamics/Kinetics See individual agents.

Pregnancy Risk Factor C

Hydralazine and Isosorbide Dinitrate *see* Isosorbide Dinitrate and Hydralazine *on page 867*

Hydralazine Hydrochloride *see* HydrALAZINE *on page 775*

Hydramine® [OTC] *see* DiphenhydrAMINE *on page 483*

Hydrated Chloral *see* Chloral Hydrate *on page 312*

Hydrea® *see* Hydroxyurea *on page 800*

Hydrisalic™ [OTC] *see* Salicylic Acid *on page 1374*

Hydrochlorothiazide *(hye droe klor oh THYE a zide)*

Related Information

Cardiovascular Diseases *on page 1636*

U.S. Brand Names Microzide™

Canadian Brand Names Apo-Hydro®; Novo-Hydrazide; PMS-Hydrochlorothiazide

Mexican Brand Names Diclotride®

Generic Available Yes

Synonyms HCTZ (error-prone abbreviation)

Pharmacologic Category Diuretic, Thiazide

Use Management of mild to moderate hypertension; treatment of edema in congestive heart failure and nephrotic syndrome

Unlabeled/Investigational Use Treatment of lithium-induced diabetes insipidus

Local Anesthetic/Vasoconstrictor Precautions No information available to require special precautions

Effects on Dental Treatment Key adverse event(s) related to dental treatment: Orthostatic hypotension and hypotension.

Common Adverse Effects

1% to 10%:

Cardiovascular: Orthostatic hypotension, hypotension

Dermatologic: Photosensitivity

Endocrine & metabolic: Hypokalemia

Gastrointestinal: Anorexia, epigastric distress

Dosage Oral (effect of drug may be decreased when used every day):

Children (in pediatric patients, chlorothiazide may be preferred over hydrochlorothiazide as there are more dosage formulations [eg, suspension] available):

<6 months: 2-3 mg/kg/day in 2 divided doses

>6 months: 2 mg/kg/day in 2 divided doses

Adults:

Edema: 25-100 mg/day in 1-2 doses; maximum: 200 mg/day

Hypertension: 12.5-50 mg/day; minimal increase in response and more electrolyte disturbances are seen with doses >50 mg/day

Elderly: 12.5-25 mg once daily

Dosing adjustment/comments in renal impairment: Cl_{cr} <10 mL/minute: Avoid use. Usually ineffective with GFR <30 mL/minute. Effective at lower GFR in combination with a loop diuretic.

Mechanism of Action Inhibits sodium reabsorption in the distal tubules causing increased excretion of sodium and water as well as potassium and hydrogen ions

Contraindications Hypersensitivity to hydrochlorothiazide or any component of the formulation, thiazides, or sulfonamide-derived drugs; anuria; renal decompensation; pregnancy

Warnings/Precautions Avoid in severe renal disease (ineffective). Electrolyte disturbances (hypokalemia, hypochloremic alkalosis, hyponatremia) can occur. Use with caution in severe hepatic dysfunction; hepatic encephalopathy can be caused by electrolyte disturbances. Gout can be precipitate in certain patients with a history of gout, a familial predisposition to gout, or chronic renal failure. Cautious use in diabetics; may see a change in glucose control. Hypersensitivity reactions can occur. Can cause SLE exacerbation or activation. Use with caution in patients with moderate or high cholesterol concentrations. Photosensitization may occur. Correct hypokalemia before initiating therapy.

Chemical similarities are present among sulfonamides, sulfonylureas, carbonic anhydrase inhibitors, thiazides, and loop diuretics (except ethacrynic acid). Use in patients with sulfonamide allergy is specifically contraindicated in product labeling, however, a risk of cross-reaction exists in patients with allergy to any of these compounds; avoid use when previous reaction has been severe.

Drug Interactions

Increased Effect/Toxicity: Increased effect of hydrochlorothiazide with furosemide and other loop diuretics. Increased hypotension and/or renal adverse effects of ACE inhibitors may result in aggressively diuresed patients. Beta-blockers increase hyperglycemic effects of thiazides in type 2 diabetes mellitus. Cyclosporine and thiazides can increase the risk of gout or renal toxicity. Digoxin toxicity can be exacerbated if a thiazide induces hypokalemia or hypomagnesemia. Lithium toxicity can occur with thiazides due to reduced renal excretion of lithium. Thiazides may prolong the duration of action with neuromuscular blocking agents.

Decreased Effect: Effects of oral hypoglycemics may be decreased. Decreased absorption of hydrochlorothiazide with cholestyramine and colestipol. NSAIDs can decrease the efficacy of thiazides, reducing the diuretic and antihypertensive effects.

Ethanol/Nutrition/Herb Interactions

Food: Hydrochlorothiazide peak serum levels may be decreased if taken with food. This product may deplete potassium, sodium, and magnesium.

Herb/Nutraceutical: Avoid dong quai if using for hypertension (has estrogenic activity). Dong quai may also cause photosensitization. Avoid ephedra, ginseng, yohimbe (may worsen hypertension). Avoid garlic (may have increased antihypertensive effect).

Pharmacodynamics/Kinetics

Onset of action: Diuresis: ~2 hours

Peak effect: 4-6 hours

Duration: 6-12 hours

Absorption: ~50% to 80%

Distribution: 3.6-7.8 L/kg

Protein binding: 68%

Metabolism: Not metabolized

Bioavailability: 50% to 80%

Half-life elimination: 5.6-14.8 hours

Time to peak: 1-2.5 hours

Excretion: Urine (as unchanged drug)

Pregnancy Risk Factor B (manufacturer); D (expert analysis)

Dosage Forms CAP (Microzide™): 12.5 mg. **TAB:** 25 mg, 50 mg

Hydrochlorothiazide and Amiloride *see* Amiloride and Hydrochlorothiazide *on page 85*

Hydrochlorothiazide and Benazepril *see* Benazepril and Hydrochlorothiazide *on page 187*

Hydrochlorothiazide and Bisoprolol *see* Bisoprolol and Hydrochlorothiazide *on page 212*

Hydrochlorothiazide and Captopril *see* Captopril and Hydrochlorothiazide *on page 259*

Hydrochlorothiazide and Enalapril *see* Enalapril and Hydrochlorothiazide *on page 541*

Hydrochlorothiazide and Eprosartan *see* Eprosartan and Hydrochlorothiazide *on page 555*

Hydrochlorothiazide and Fosinopril *see* Fosinopril and Hydrochlorothiazide *on page 709*

Hydrochlorothiazide and Hydralazine *see* Hydralazine and Hydrochlorothiazide *on page 775*

Hydrochlorothiazide and Irbesartan *see* Irbesartan and Hydrochlorothiazide *on page 860*

Hydrochlorothiazide and Lisinopril *see* Lisinopril and Hydrochlorothiazide *on page 938*

Hydrochlorothiazide and Losartan *see* Losartan and Hydrochlorothiazide *on page 952*

Hydrochlorothiazide and **Methyldopa** *see* Methyldopa and Hydrochlorothiazide *on page 1022*

Hydrochlorothiazide and **Metoprolol** *see* Metoprolol and Hydrochlorothiazide *on page 1032*

Hydrochlorothiazide and **Metoprolol Tartrate** *see* Metoprolol and Hydrochlorothiazide *on page 1032*

Hydrochlorothiazide and **Moexipril** *see* Moexipril and Hydrochlorothiazide *on page 1059*

Hydrochlorothiazide and **Olmesartan Medoxomil** *see* Olmesartan and Hydrochlorothiazide *on page 1143*

Hydrochlorothiazide and **Propranolol** *see* Propranolol and Hydrochlorothiazide *on page 1305*

Hydrochlorothiazide and **Quinapril** *see* Quinapril and Hydrochlorothiazide *on page 1323*

Hydrochlorothiazide and Spironolactone
(hye droe klor oh THYE a zide & speer on oh LAK tone)

Related Information
Cardiovascular Diseases *on page 1636*
Hydrochlorothiazide *on page 776*
Spironolactone *on page 1413*
U.S. Brand Names Aldactazide®
Canadian Brand Names Aldactazide 25®; Aldactazide 50®; Novo-Spirozine
Generic Available Yes
Synonyms Spironolactone and Hydrochlorothiazide
Pharmacologic Category Antihypertensive Agent, Combination
Use Management of mild to moderate hypertension; treatment of edema in congestive heart failure and nephrotic syndrome, and cirrhosis of the liver accompanied by edema and/or ascites
Local Anesthetic/Vasoconstrictor Precautions No information available to require special precautions
Effects on Dental Treatment No significant effects or complications reported
Common Adverse Effects See individual agents.
Drug Interactions
Increased Effect/Toxicity: See individual agents.
Pharmacodynamics/Kinetics See individual agents.
Pregnancy Risk Factor C

Hydrochlorothiazide and **Telmisartan** *see* Telmisartan and Hydrochlorothiazide *on page 1452*

Hydrochlorothiazide and Triamterene
(hye droe klor oh THYE a zide & trye AM ter een)

Related Information
Cardiovascular Diseases *on page 1636*
Hydrochlorothiazide *on page 776*
Triamterene *on page 1531*
U.S. Brand Names Dyazide®; Maxzide®; Maxzide®-25
Canadian Brand Names Apo-Triazide®; Novo-Triamzide; Nu-Triazide; Penta-Triamterene HCTZ; Riva-Zide
Generic Available Yes
Synonyms Triamterene and Hydrochlorothiazide
Pharmacologic Category Antihypertensive Agent, Combination; Diuretic, Potassium-Sparing; Diuretic, Thiazide
Use Management of mild to moderate hypertension; treatment of edema in congestive heart failure and nephrotic syndrome
Local Anesthetic/Vasoconstrictor Precautions No information available to require special precautions
Effects on Dental Treatment No significant effects or complications reported
Common Adverse Effects Also see individual agents. Frequency not defined.
Central nervous system: Dizziness, fatigue
Dermatologic: Purpura, cracked corners of mouth
Endocrine & metabolic: Electrolyte disturbances
Gastrointestinal: Bright orange tongue, burning of tongue, loss of appetite, nausea, vomiting, stomach cramps, diarrhea, upset stomach
Hematologic: Aplastic anemia, agranulocytosis, hemolytic anemia, leukopenia, thrombocytopenia, megaloblastic anemia
Neuromuscular & skeletal: Muscle cramps
Ocular: Xanthopsia, transient blurred vision

Respiratory: Allergic pneumonitis, pulmonary edema, respiratory distress

Dosage Adults: Oral:

Hydrochlorothiazide 25 mg and triamterene 37.5 mg: 1-2 tablets/capsules once daily

Hydrochlorothiazide 50 mg and triamterene 75 mg: $1/_2$-1 tablet daily

Mechanism of Action

Based on **triamterene** component: Competes with aldosterone for receptor sites in the distal renal tubules, increasing sodium, chloride, and water excretion while conserving potassium and hydrogen ions; may block the effect of aldosterone on arteriolar smooth muscle as well

Based on **hydrochlorothiazide** component: Inhibits sodium reabsorption in the distal tubules causing increased excretion of sodium and water as well as potassium and hydrogen ions

Contraindications

Based on **hydrochlorothiazide** component: Hypersensitivity to hydrochlorothiazide or any component of the formulation, thiazides, or sulfonamide-derived drugs; anuria; renal decompensation; pregnancy

Based on **triamterene** component: Hypersensitivity to triamterene or any component of the formulation; patients receiving other potassium-sparing diuretics; anuria; severe hepatic disease; hyperkalemia or history of hyperkalemia; severe or progressive renal disease

Drug Interactions

Increased Effect/Toxicity: See individual agents.

Ethanol/Nutrition/Herb Interactions Food: Avoid food with high potassium content and potassium-containing salt substitutes.

Dietary Considerations Should be taken after meals.

Pharmacodynamics/Kinetics See individual agents.

Pregnancy Risk Factor C (per manufacturer)

Dosage Forms CAP: (Dyazide®): Hydrochlorothiazide 25 mg and triamterene 37.5 mg. **TAB:** (Maxzide®): Hydrochlorothiazide 50 mg and triamterene 75 mg; (Maxzide®-25): Hydrochlorothiazide 25 mg and triamterene 37.5 mg

Hydrochlorothiazide and Valsartan see Valsartan and Hydrochlorothiazide on page 1562

Hydrocil® Instant [OTC] see Psyllium on page 1313

Hydrocodone and Acetaminophen

(hye droe KOE done & a seet a MIN oh fen)

Related Information

Acetaminophen on page 31

Oral Pain on page 1692

Related Sample Prescriptions

Moderate/Moderately Severe Oral Pain on page 1734

U.S. Brand Names Anexsia®; Bancap HC®; Ceta-Plus®; Co-Gesic®; hycet™; Lorcet® 10/650; Lorcet®-HD [DSC]; Lorcet® Plus; Lortab®; Margesic® H; Maxidone™; Norco®; Stagesic®; Vicodin®; Vicodin® ES; Vicodin® HP; Zydone®

Generic Available Yes

Synonyms Acetaminophen and Hydrocodone

Pharmacologic Category Analgesic Combination (Narcotic)

Dental Use Treatment of postoperative pain

Use Relief of moderate to severe pain

Local Anesthetic/Vasoconstrictor Precautions No information available to require special precautions

Effects on Dental Treatment Key adverse event(s) related to dental treatment: Xerostomia (normal salivary flow resumes upon discontinuation). See Dental Comment.

Significant Adverse Effects Frequency not defined.

Cardiovascular: Bradycardia, cardiac arrest, circulatory collapse, coma, hypotension

Central nervous system: Anxiety, dizziness, drowsiness, dysphoria, euphoria, fear, lethargy, lightheadedness, malaise, mental clouding, mental impairment, mood changes, physiological dependence, sedation, somnolence, stupor

Dermatologic: Pruritus, rash

Endocrine & metabolic: Hypoglycemic coma

Gastrointestinal: Abdominal pain, constipation, gastric distress, heartburn, nausea, peptic ulcer, vomiting

Genitourinary: Ureteral spasm, urinary retention, vesical sphincter spasm

Hematologic: Agranulocytosis, bleeding time prolonged, hemolytic anemia, iron deficiency anemia, occult blood loss, thrombocytopenia

Hepatic: Hepatic necrosis, hepatitis

Neuromuscular & skeletal: Skeletal muscle rigidity

(Continued)

Hydrocodone and Acetaminophen *(Continued)*

Otic: Hearing impairment or loss (chronic overdose)

Renal: Renal toxicity, renal tubular necrosis

Respiratory: Acute airway obstruction, apnea, dyspnea, respiratory depression (dose related)

Miscellaneous: Allergic reactions, clamminess, diaphoresis

Restrictions C-III

Dental Usual Dosing Postoperative pain: Oral:

Children and Adults ≥50 kg: Average starting dose in opioid naive patients: Hydrocodone 5-10 mg 4 times/day; the dosage of acetaminophen should be limited to ≤4 g/day (and possibly less in patients with hepatic impairment or ethanol use).

Dosage ranges (based on specific product labeling): Hydrocodone 2.5-10 mg every 4-6 hours; maximum: 60 mg hydrocodone/day (maximum dose of hydrocodone may be limited by the acetaminophen content of specific product)

Elderly: Doses should be titrated to appropriate analgesic effect; 2.5-5 mg of the hydrocodone component every 4-6 hours. Do not exceed 4 g/day of acetaminophen.

Dosage Oral (doses should be titrated to appropriate analgesic effect): Analgesic:

Children 2-13 years or <50 kg: Hydrocodone 0.135 mg/kg/dose every 4-6 hours; do not exceed 6 doses/day or the maximum recommended dose of acetaminophen

Children and Adults ≥50 kg: Average starting dose in opioid naive patients: Hydrocodone 5-10 mg 4 times/day; the dosage of acetaminophen should be limited to ≤4 g/day (and possibly less in patients with hepatic impairment or ethanol use).

Dosage ranges (based on specific product labeling): Hydrocodone 2.5-10 mg every 4-6 hours; maximum: 60 mg hydrocodone/day (maximum dose of hydrocodone may be limited by the acetaminophen content of specific product)

Elderly: Doses should be titrated to appropriate analgesic effect; 2.5-5 mg of the hydrocodone component every 4-6 hours. Do not exceed 4 g/day of acetaminophen.

Dosage adjustment in hepatic impairment: Use with caution. Limited, low-dose therapy usually well tolerated in hepatic disease/cirrhosis; however, cases of hepatotoxicity at daily acetaminophen dosages <4 g/day have been reported. Avoid chronic use in hepatic impairment.

Mechanism of Action Hydrocodone, as with other narcotic (opiate) analgesics, blocks pain perception in the cerebral cortex by binding to specific receptor molecules (opiate receptors) within the neuronal membranes of synapses. This binding results in a decreased synaptic chemical transmission throughout the CNS thus inhibiting the flow of pain sensations into the higher centers. Mu and kappa are the two subtypes of the opiate receptor which hydrocodone binds to cause analgesia.

Acetaminophen inhibits the synthesis of prostaglandins in the CNS and peripherally blocks pain impulse generation; produces antipyresis from inhibition of hypothalamic heat-regulating center.

Contraindications Hypersensitivity to hydrocodone, acetaminophen, or any component of the formulation; CNS depression; severe respiratory depression

Warnings/Precautions Use with caution in patients with hypersensitivity reactions to other phenanthrene derivative opioid agonists (morphine, hydromorphone, levorphanol, oxycodone, oxymorphone); tolerance or drug dependence may result from extended use.

Respiratory depressant effects may be increased with head injuries. Use caution with acute abdominal conditions; clinical course may be obscured. Use caution with thyroid dysfunction, prostatic hyperplasia, hepatic or renal disease, and in the elderly. Causes sedation; caution must be used in performing tasks which require alertness (eg, operating machinery or driving).

Limit acetaminophen to <4 g/day. May cause severe hepatic toxicity in acute overdose; in addition, chronic daily dosing in adults has resulted in liver damage in some patients. Use with caution in patients with alcoholic liver disease; consuming ≥3 alcoholic drinks/day may increase the risk of liver damage. Use caution in patients with known G6PD deficiency.

Drug Interactions

Hydrocodone: **Substrate** of CYP2D6 (major)

Acetaminophen: **Substrate** (minor) of CYP1A2, 2A6, 2C9, 2D6, 2E1, 3A4; **Inhibits** CYP3A4 (weak)

Acetaminophen component: Refer to Acetaminophen monograph.

Hydrocodone component:

CYP2D6 inhibitors may decrease the effects of hydrocodone. Example inhibitors include chlorpromazine, delavirdine, fluoxetine, miconazole, paroxetine, pergolide, quinidine, quinine, ritonavir, and ropinirole.

CNS depressants (including antianxiety agents, antihistamines, antipsychotics, narcotics): CNS depression is additive; dose adjustment may be needed

MAO inhibitors: May see increased effects of MAO inhibitor and hydrocodone.

Tricyclic antidepressants (TCAs): May see increased effects of TCA and hydrocodone.

Ethanol/Nutrition/Herb Interactions

Ethanol: Avoid ethanol (may increase CNS depression); consuming ≥3 alcoholic drinks/day may increase the risk of liver damage

Herb/Nutraceutical: Avoid valerian, St John's wort, SAMe, kava kava (may increase risk of excessive sedation).

Pharmacodynamics/Kinetics

Acetaminophen: See Acetaminophen monograph.

Hydrocodone:

Onset of action: Narcotic analgesic: 10-20 minutes

Duration: 4-8 hours

Distribution: Crosses placenta

Metabolism: Hepatic; O-demethylation; N-demethylation and 6-ketosteroid reduction

Half-life elimination: 3.3-4.4 hours

Excretion: Urine

Pregnancy Risk Factor C/D (prolonged use or high doses near term)

Lactation Excretion in breast milk unknown/contraindicated

Breast-Feeding Considerations Acetaminophen is excreted in breast milk. The AAP considers it to be "compatible" with breast-feeding. Information is not available for hydrocodone; codeine and other opioids are excreted in breast milk and the AAP considers codeine to be "compatible" with breast-feeding. The manufacturers recommend discontinuing the medication or to discontinue nursing during therapy.

Dosage Forms

Capsule (Bancap HC®, Ceta-Plus®, Margesic® H, Stagesic®): Hydrocodone bitartrate 5 mg and acetaminophen 500 mg

Elixir: Hydrocodone bitartrate 7.5 mg and acetaminophen 500 mg per 15 mL (480 mL)

Lortab®: Hydrocodone bitartrate 7.5 mg and acetaminophen 500 mg per 15 mL (480 mL) [contains alcohol 7%; tropical fruit punch flavor]

Solution, oral (hycet™): Hydrocodone bitartrate 7.5 mg and acetaminophen 325 mg per 15 mL (480 mL) [contains alcohol 7%; tropical fruit punch flavor]

Tablet:

Hydrocodone bitartrate 2.5 mg and acetaminophen 500 mg

Hydrocodone bitartrate 5 mg and acetaminophen 325 mg

Hydrocodone bitartrate 5 mg and acetaminophen 500 mg

Hydrocodone bitartrate 7.5 mg and acetaminophen 325 mg

Hydrocodone bitartrate 7.5 mg and acetaminophen 500 mg

Hydrocodone bitartrate 7.5 mg and acetaminophen 650 mg

Hydrocodone bitartrate 7.5 mg and acetaminophen 750 mg

Hydrocodone bitartrate 10 mg and acetaminophen 325 mg

Hydrocodone bitartrate 10 mg and acetaminophen 500 mg

Hydrocodone bitartrate 10 mg and acetaminophen 650 mg

Hydrocodone bitartrate 10 mg and acetaminophen 660 mg

Anexsia®:

5/500: Hydrocodone bitartrate 5 mg and acetaminophen 500 mg

7.5/650: Hydrocodone bitartrate 7.5 mg and acetaminophen 650 mg

Co-Gesic® 5/500: Hydrocodone bitartrate 5 mg and acetaminophen 500 mg

Lorcet® 10/650: Hydrocodone bitartrate 10 mg and acetaminophen 650 mg

Lorcet® Plus: Hydrocodone bitartrate 7.5 mg and acetaminophen 650 mg

Lortab®:

2.5/500: Hydrocodone bitartrate 2.5 mg and acetaminophen 500 mg

5/500: Hydrocodone bitartrate 5 mg and acetaminophen 500 mg

7.5/500: Hydrocodone bitartrate 7.5 mg and acetaminophen 500 mg

10/500: Hydrocodone bitartrate 10 mg and acetaminophen 500 mg

Maxidone™: Hydrocodone bitartrate 10 mg and acetaminophen 750 mg

Norco®:

Hydrocodone bitartrate 5 mg and acetaminophen 325 mg

Hydrocodone bitartrate 7.5 mg and acetaminophen 325 mg

Hydrocodone bitartrate 10 mg and acetaminophen 325 mg

Vicodin®: Hydrocodone bitartrate 5 mg and acetaminophen 500 mg

Vicodin® ES: Hydrocodone bitartrate 7.5 mg and acetaminophen 750 mg

(Continued)

Hydrocodone and Acetaminophen *(Continued)*

Vicodin® HP: Hydrocodone bitartrate 10 mg and acetaminophen 660 mg

Zydone®:

Hydrocodone bitartrate 5 mg and acetaminophen 400 mg

Hydrocodone bitartrate 7.5 mg and acetaminophen 400 mg

Hydrocodone bitartrate 10 mg and acetaminophen 400 mg

Dental Comment Neither hydrocodone nor acetaminophen elicit anti-inflammatory effects. Because of addiction liability of opiate analgesics, the use of hydrocodone should be limited to 2-3 days postoperatively for treatment of dental pain. Nausea is the most common adverse effect seen after use in dental patients; sedation and constipation are second. Nausea elicited by narcotic analgesics is centrally mediated and the presence or absence of food will not affect the degree nor incidence of nausea.

Acetaminophen:

A study by Hylek, et al, suggested that the combination of acetaminophen with warfarin (Coumadin®) may cause enhanced anticoagulation. The following recommendations have been made by Hylek, et al, and supported by an editorial in *JAMA* by Bell.

Dose and duration of acetaminophen should be as low as possible, individualized and monitored

The study by Hylek reported the following:

For patients who reported taking the equivalent of at least 4 regular strength (325 mg) tablets for longer than a week, the odds of having an INR >6.0 were increased 10-fold above those not taking acetaminophen. Risk decreased with lower intakes of acetaminophen reaching a background level of risk at a dose of 6 or fewer 325 mg tablets per week.

Selected Readings

Bell WR, "Acetaminophen and Warfarin: Undesirable Synergy," *JAMA*, 1998, 279(9):702-3.

Botting RM, "Mechanism of Action of Acetaminophen: Is There a Cyclooxygenase 3?" *Clin Infect Dis*, 2000, Suppl 5:S202-10.

Dart RC, Kuffner EK, and Rumack BH, "Treatment of Pain or Fever With Paracetamol (Acetaminophen) in the Alcoholic Patient: A Systematic Review," *Am J Ther*, 2000, 7(2):123-34.

Dionne RA, "New Approaches to Preventing and Treating Postoperative Pain," *J Am Dent Assoc*, 1992, 123(6):26-34.

Gobetti JP, "Controlling Dental Pain," *J Am Dent Assoc*, 1992, 123(6):47-52.

Grant JA and Weiler JM, "A Report of a Rare Immediate Reaction After Ingestion of Acetaminophen," *Ann Allergy Asthma Immunol*, 2001, 87(3):227-9.

Hylek EM, Heiman H, Skates SJ, et al, "Acetaminophen and Other Risk factors for excessive warfarin anticoagulation," *JAMA*, 1998, 279(9):657-62.

Kwan D, Bartle WR, and Walker SE, "The Effects of Acetaminophen on Pharmacokinetics and Pharmacodynamics of Warfarin," *J Clin Pharmacol*, 1999, 39(1):68-75.

McClain CJ, Price S, Barve S, et al, "Acetaminophen Hepatotoxicity: An Update," *Curr Gastroenterol Rep*, 1999, 1(1):42-9.

Shek KL, Chan LN, and Nutescu E, "Warfarin-Acetaminophen Drug Interaction Revisited," *Pharmacotherapy*, 1999, 19(10):1153-8.

Tanaka E, Yamazaki K, and Misawa S, "Update: The Clinical Importance of Acetaminophen Hepatotoxicity in Nonalcoholic and Alcoholic Subjects," *J Clin Pharm Ther*, 2000, 25(5):325-32.

Wynn RL, "Narcotic Analgesics for Dental Pain: Available Products, Strengths, and Formulations," *Gen Dent*, 2001, 49(2):126-8, 130, 132 passim.

Hydrocodone and Aspirin *(hye droe KOE done & AS pir in)*

Related Information

Aspirin *on page 145*

U.S. Brand Names Damason-P®

Generic Available No

Synonyms Aspirin and Hydrocodone

Pharmacologic Category Analgesic Combination (Narcotic)

Dental Use Treatment of postoperative pain

Use Relief of moderate to moderately severe pain

Local Anesthetic/Vasoconstrictor Precautions No information available to require special precautions

Effects on Dental Treatment Key adverse event(s) related to dental treatment: Nausea is the most common adverse effect seen after use in dental patients. Sedation and constipation are second. Aspirin component affects bleeding times and could influence wound-healing time. Elderly are a high-risk population for adverse effects from NSAIDs. As many as 60% of elderly patients with GI complications from NSAIDs can develop peptic ulceration and/or hemorrhage asymptomatically. Concomitant disease and drug use contribute to the risk of GI adverse effects. See Dental Comment.

Significant Adverse Effects

>10%:

Cardiovascular: Hypotension

Central nervous system: Lightheadedness, dizziness, sedation, drowsiness, fatigue

Gastrointestinal: Nausea, heartburn, stomach pain, heartburn, epigastric discomfort

Neuromuscular & skeletal: Weakness

1% to 10%:

Cardiovascular: Bradycardia

Central nervous system: Confusion

Dermatologic: Rash

Gastrointestinal: Vomiting, gastrointestinal ulceration

Genitourinary: Decreased urination

Hematologic: Hemolytic anemia

Respiratory: Dyspnea

Miscellaneous: Anaphylactic shock

<1% (Limited to important or life-threatening): Biliary tract spasm, broncho-spasm, hallucinations, hepatotoxicity, histamine release, leukopenia, occult bleeding, physical and psychological dependence with prolonged use, prolon-gated bleeding time, thrombocytopenia, urinary tract spasm

Restrictions C-III

Dental Usual Dosing Postoperative pain: Adults: Oral: 1-2 tablets every 4-6 hours as needed for pain

Dosage Adults: Oral: 1-2 tablets every 4-6 hours as needed for pain

Mechanism of Action

Based on **hydrocodone** component: Binds to opiate receptors in the CNS, altering the perception of and response to pain; suppresses cough in medul-lary center; produces generalized CNS depression

Based on **aspirin** component: Inhibits prostaglandin synthesis, acts on the hypothalamus heat-regulating center to reduce fever, blocks prostaglandin synthetase action which prevents formation of the platelet-aggregating substance thromboxane A_2

Contraindications

Based on **hydrocodone** component: Hypersensitivity to hydrocodone or any component of the formulation

Based on **aspirin** component: Hypersensitivity to salicylates, other NSAIDs, or any component of the formulation; asthma; rhinitis; nasal polyps; inherited or acquired bleeding disorders (including factor VII and factor IX deficiency); pregnancy (in 3rd trimester especially); do not use in children (<16 years) for viral infections (chickenpox or flu symptoms), with or without fever, due to a potential association with Reye's syndrome

Warnings/Precautions Use with caution in patients with impaired renal func-tion, erosive gastritis, or peptic ulcer disease; children and teenagers should not use for chickenpox or flu symptoms before a physician is consulted about Reye's syndrome; tolerance or drug dependence may result from extended use

Based on **hydrocodone** component: Use with caution in patients with hyper-sensitivity reactions to other phenanthrene-derivative opioid agonists (morphine, codeine, hydromorphone, levorphanol, oxycodone, oxymorphone); should be used with caution in elderly or debilitated patients, and those with severe impairment of hepatic or renal function, prostatic hyperplasia, or urethral stricture. Also use caution in patients with head injury, increased intracranial pressure, acute abdomen, or impaired thyroid function. Hydrocodone suppresses the cough reflex; caution should be exercised when this agent is used postoperatively and in patients with pulmonary diseases (including asthma, emphysema, COPD)

Based on **aspirin** component: Use with caution in patients with platelet and bleeding disorders, renal dysfunction, dehydration, erosive gastritis, or peptic ulcer disease. Heavy ethanol use (>3 drinks/day) can increase bleeding risks. Avoid use in severe renal failure or in severe hepatic failure. Discontinue use if tinnitus or impaired hearing occurs. Caution in mild-moderate renal failure (only at high dosages). Patients with sensitivity to tartrazine dyes, nasal polyps and asthma may have an increased risk of salicylate sensitivity. Surgical patients should avoid ASA if possible, for 1-2 weeks prior to surgery, to reduce the risk of excessive bleeding.

Drug Interactions

Based on **hydrocodone** component: **Substrate** of CYP2D6 (major)

CNS depressants, MAO inhibitors, general anesthetics, and tricyclic antide-pressants: May potentiate the effects of opiate agonists; dextroampheta-mine may enhance the analgesic effect of opiate agonists.

CYP2D6 inhibitors: May decrease the effects of hydrocodone. Example inhibi-tors include chlorpromazine, delavirdine, fluoxetine, miconazole, paroxetine, pergolide, quinidine, quinine, ritonavir, and ropinirole.

Based on **aspirin** component: **Substrate** of CYP2C9 (minor)

(Continued)

Hydrocodone and Aspirin *(Continued)*

ACE inhibitors: The effects of ACE inhibitors may be blunted by aspirin administration, particularly at higher dosages.

Buspirone increases aspirin's free % *in vitro*.

Carbonic anhydrase inhibitors and corticosteroids have been associated with alteration in salicylate serum concentrations.

Heparin and low molecular weight heparins: Concurrent use may increase the risk of bleeding

Methotrexate serum levels may be increased; consider discontinuing aspirin 2-3 days before high-dose methotrexate treatment or avoid concurrent use.

NSAIDs may increase the risk of gastrointestinal adverse effects and bleeding. Serum concentrations of some NSAIDs may be decreased by aspirin.

Platelet inhibitors (IIb/IIIa antagonists): Risk of bleeding may be increased.

Probenecid effects may be antagonized by aspirin.

Sulfonylureas: The effects of older sulfonylurea agents (tolazamide, tolbutamide) may be potentiated due to displacement from plasma proteins. This effect does not appear to be clinically significant for newer sulfonylurea agents (glyburide, glipizide, glimepiride).

Valproic acid may be displaced from its binding sites which can result in toxicity.

Verapamil may potentiate the prolongation of bleeding time associated with aspirin.

Warfarin and oral anticoagulants may increase the risk of bleeding.

Ethanol/Nutrition/Herb Interactions

Based on **hydrocodone** component: Ethanol: Avoid or limit ethanol (may increase CNS depression). Watch for sedation.

Based on **aspirin** component:

Ethanol: Avoid ethanol (may enhance gastric mucosal damage).

Food: Food may decrease the rate but not the extent of oral absorption. Take with food or large volume of water or milk to minimize GI upset.

Herb/Nutraceutical: Avoid cat's claw, dong quai, evening primrose, feverfew, garlic, ginger, ginkgo, red clover, horse chestnut, green tea, ginseng (all have additional antiplatelet activity).

Pharmacodynamics/Kinetics

Aspirin: See Aspirin monograph.

Hydrocodone:

Onset of action: Narcotic analgesic: 10-20 minutes

Duration: 4-8 hours

Distribution: Crosses placenta

Metabolism: Hepatic; O-demethylation; N-demethylation and 6-ketosteroid reduction

Half-life elimination: 3.3-4.4 hours

Excretion: Urine

Pregnancy Risk Factor D

Lactation Enters breast milk/contraindicated

Breast-Feeding Considerations

Hydrocodone: No data reported.

Aspirin: Cautious use due to potential adverse effects in nursing infants.

Dosage Forms Tablet: Hydrocodone bitartrate 5 mg and aspirin 500 mg

Dental Comment Because of addiction liability of opiate analgesics, the use of hydrocodone should be limited to 2-3 days postoperatively for treatment of dental pain; nausea is the most common adverse effect seen after use in dental patients; sedation and constipation are second; aspirin component affects bleeding times and could influence time of wound healing

Selected Readings

Dionne RA, "New Approaches to Preventing and Treating Postoperative Pain," *J Am Dent Assoc*, 1992, 123(6):26-34.

Gobetti JP, "Controlling Dental Pain," *J Am Dent Assoc*, 1992, 123(6):47-52.

Wynn RL, "Narcotic Analgesics for Dental Pain: Available Products, Strengths, and Formulations," *Gen Dent*, 2001, 49(2):126-8, 130, 132 passim.

Hydrocodone and Chlorpheniramine
(hye droe KOE done & klor fen IR a meen)

Related Information

Chlorpheniramine *on page 323*

U.S. Brand Names HyTan™; Tussionex®

Generic Available No

Synonyms Chlorpheniramine Maleate and Hydrocodone Bitartrate; Hydrocodone Tannate and Chlorpheniramine Tannate

Pharmacologic Category Antihistamine/Antitussive

Use Symptomatic relief of cough and upper respiratory symptoms associated with cold and allergy

Local Anesthetic/Vasoconstrictor Precautions No information available to require special precautions

Effects on Dental Treatment Key adverse event(s) related to dental treatment: Prolonged use will cause significant xerostomia (normal salivary flow resumes upon discontinuation).

Common Adverse Effects Frequency not defined.

Central nervous system: Anxiety, dizziness, drowsiness, dysphoria, euphoria, fear, lethargy, mental impairment, mood changes, sedation

Dermatologic: Pruritus, rash

Gastrointestinal: Constipation, nausea, vomiting

Genitourinary: Ureteral spasm, urinary retention, vesicle sphincter spasm

Respiratory: Dryness of pharynx, respiratory depression

Restrictions C-III

Mechanism of Action

Hydrocodone binds to opiate receptors in the CNS, altering the perception of and response to pain; suppresses cough in medullary center; produces generalized CNS depression

Chlorpheniramine competes with histamine for H_1-receptor sites on effector cells in the gastrointestinal tract, blood vessels, and respiratory tract

Drug Interactions

Cytochrome P450 Effect:

Hydrocodone: **Substrate** of CYP2D6 (major)

Chlorpheniramine: **Substrate** of CYP2D6 (minor), 3A4 (major); **Inhibits** CYP2D6 (weak)

Increased Effect/Toxicity: Anticholinergics may enhance the adverse/toxic effect of chlorpheniramine; CNS depressants may enhance the adverse/toxic effects of hydrocodone and chlorpheniramine

Pharmacodynamics/Kinetics

Chlorpheniramine: See Chlorpheniramine monograph.

Hydrocodone:

Onset of action: Narcotic analgesic: 10-20 minutes

Duration: 4-8 hours

Distribution: Crosses placenta

Metabolism: Hepatic; O-demethylation; N-demethylation and 6-ketosteroid reduction

Half-life elimination: 3.3-4.4 hours

Excretion: Urine

Pregnancy Risk Factor C

Hydrocodone and Guaifenesin
(hye droe KOE done & gwye FEN e sin)

Related Information

Guaifenesin on page 752

U.S. Brand Names Codiclear® DH; Hycotuss®; Kwelcof®; Maxi-Tuss HCG; Pneumotussin®; Vitussin

Generic Available Yes: Liquid

Synonyms Guaifenesin and Hydrocodone; Hycoclear Tuss

Pharmacologic Category Antitussive/Expectorant

Use Symptomatic relief of nonproductive coughs associated with upper and lower respiratory tract congestion

Local Anesthetic/Vasoconstrictor Precautions No information available to require special precautions

Effects on Dental Treatment Key adverse event(s) related to dental treatment: Xerostomia (normal salivary flow resumes upon discontinuation).

Common Adverse Effects Frequency not defined.

Cardiovascular: Hypertension, postural hypotension, palpitation

Central nervous system: Drowsiness, sedation, mental clouding, mental and physical impairment, anxiety, fear, dysphoria, dizziness, psychotic dependence, mood changes

Gastrointestinal: Nausea, vomiting, constipation with prolonged use

Genitourinary: Ureteral spasm, urinary retention

Ocular: Blurred vision

Respiratory: Respiratory depression (dose related)

Restrictions C-III

(Continued)

Hydrocodone and Guaifenesin *(Continued)*

Mechanism of Action

Hydrocodone binds to opiate receptors in the CNS, altering the perception of and response to pain; suppresses cough in medullary center; produces generalized CNS depression

Guaifenesin is thought to act as an expectorant by irritating the gastric mucosa and stimulating respiratory tract secretions, thereby increasing respiratory fluid volumes and decreasing phlegm viscosity

Drug Interactions

Cytochrome P450 Effect: Hydrocodone: **Substrate** of CYP2D6 (major)

Increased Effect/Toxicity:

Based on **hydrocodone** component: CNS depressants, MAO inhibitors, general anesthetics, and tricyclic antidepressants may potentiate the effects of opiate agonists; dextroamphetamine may enhance the analgesic effect of opiate agonists

Also refer to individual monograph for Guaifenesin.

Pharmacodynamics/Kinetics

Guaifenesin: See Guaifenesin monograph.

Hydrocodone:

Onset of action: Narcotic analgesic: 10-20 minutes

Duration: 4-8 hours

Distribution: Crosses placenta

Metabolism: Hepatic; O-demethylation; N-demethylation and 6-ketosteroid reduction

Half-life elimination: 3.3-4.4 hours

Excretion: Urine

Pregnancy Risk Factor C

Hydrocodone and Homatropine
(hye droe KOE done & hoe MA troe peen)

Related Information

Homatropine *on page 772*

U.S. Brand Names Hycodan®; Hydromet®; Hydropane®; Tussigon®

Generic Available Yes: Syrup

Synonyms Homatropine and Hydrocodone

Pharmacologic Category Antitussive

Use Symptomatic relief of cough

Local Anesthetic/Vasoconstrictor Precautions No information available to require special precautions

Effects on Dental Treatment Key adverse event(s) related to dental treatment: Xerostomia (normal salivary flow resumes upon discontinuation).

Common Adverse Effects Frequency not defined.

Cardiovascular: Bradycardia, tachycardia, hyper-/hypotension

Central nervous system: Lightheadedness, dizziness, sedation, drowsiness, fatigue, confusion, hallucinations

Gastrointestinal: Nausea, vomiting, xerostomia, anorexia, impaired GI motility

Genitourinary: Decreased urination, urinary tract spasm

Hepatic: Biliary tract spasm

Neuromuscular & skeletal: Weakness

Ocular: Diplopia, miosis, mydriasis, blurred vision

Respiratory: Dyspnea

Miscellaneous: Histamine release, physical and psychological dependence with prolonged use

Restrictions C-III

Mechanism of Action

Based on **hydrocodone** component: Binds to opiate receptors in the CNS, altering the perception of and response to pain; suppresses cough in medullary center; produces generalized CNS depression

Based on **homatropine** component: Blocks response of iris sphincter muscle and the accommodative muscle of the ciliary body to cholinergic stimulation resulting in dilation and loss of accommodation

Drug Interactions

Cytochrome P450 Effect: Hydrocodone: **Substrate** of CYP2D6 (major)

Increased Effect/Toxicity:

Based on **hydrocodone** component: Increased toxicity: CNS depressants, MAO inhibitors, general anesthetics, and tricyclic antidepressants may potentiate the effects of opiate agonists; dextroamphetamine may enhance the analgesic effect of opiate agonists

Based on **homatropine** component:

Phenothiazine and TCAs may increase anticholinergic effects when used concurrently.

Sympathomimetic amines may cause tachyarrhythmias; avoid concurrent use

Pharmacodynamics/Kinetics Duration: Hydrocodone: 4-6 hours

Pregnancy Risk Factor C

Hydrocodone and Ibuprofen
(hye droe KOE done & eye byoo PROE fen)

Related Information
Ibuprofen *on page 808*
Oral Pain *on page 1692*

Related Sample Prescriptions
Moderate/Moderately Severe Oral Pain *on page 1734*

U.S. Brand Names Reprexain™; Vicoprofen®

Canadian Brand Names Vicoprofen®

Generic Available Yes

Synonyms Ibuprofen and Hydrocodone

Pharmacologic Category Analgesic, Narcotic; Nonsteroidal Anti-inflammatory Drug (NSAID), Oral

Dental Use Short-term management (generally <10 days) of moderate-to-severe acute postoperative dental pain where an anti-inflammatory effect is desired

Use Short-term (generally <10 days) management of moderate to severe acute pain; is not indicated for treatment of such conditions as osteoarthritis or rheumatoid arthritis

Local Anesthetic/Vasoconstrictor Precautions No information available to require special precautions

Effects on Dental Treatment Key adverse event(s) related to dental treatment: Xerostomia (normal salivary flow resumes upon discontinuation).

Significant Adverse Effects
>10%:
Central nervous system: Headache (27%), dizziness (14%), sedation (22%)
Dermatologic: Rash, urticaria
Gastrointestinal: Constipation (22%), nausea (21%), dyspepsia (12%)
1% to 10%:
Cardiovascular: Bradycardia, palpitation (<3%), vasodilation (<3%), edema (3% to 9%)
Central nervous system: Nervousness, confusion, fever (<3%), pain (3% to 9%), anxiety (3% to 9%), thought abnormalities
Dermatologic: Itching (3% to 9%)
Endocrine & metabolic: Fluid retention
Gastrointestinal: Vomiting (3% to 9%), anorexia, diarrhea (3% to 9%), xerostomia (3% to 9%), flatulence (3% to 9%), gastritis (<3%), melena (<3%), mouth ulcers (<3%)
Genitourinary: Polyuria (<3%)
Neuromuscular & skeletal: Weakness (3% to 9%)
Otic: Tinnitus
Respiratory: Dyspnea, hiccups, pharyngitis, rhinitis
Miscellaneous: Flu syndrome (<3%), infection (3% to 9%)
<1% (Limited to important or life-threatening): Acute renal failure, agranulocytosis, anemia, arrhythmia, aseptic meningitis, biliary tract spasm, bone marrow suppression, CHF, depression, diplopia, erythema multiforme, hallucinations, hemolytic anemia, hepatitis, histamine release, inhibition of platelet aggregation, leukopenia, neutropenia, peripheral neuropathy, physical and psychological dependence with prolonged use, Stevens-Johnson syndrome, thrombocytopenia, toxic amblyopia, toxic epidermal necrolysis, urinary tract spasm, urticaria

Restrictions C-III

Dental Usual Dosing Moderate-to-severe acute postoperative dental pain: Adults: Oral: 1-2 tablets every 4-6 hours as needed for pain; maximum: 5 tablets/day

Dosage Adults: Oral: 1-2 tablets every 4-6 hours as needed for pain; maximum: 5 tablets/day

Mechanism of Action
Based on **hydrocodone** component: Binds to opiate receptors in the CNS, altering the perception of and response to pain; suppresses cough in medullary center; produces generalized CNS depression
(Continued)

Hydrocodone and Ibuprofen *(Continued)*

Based on **ibuprofen** component: Inhibits prostaglandin synthesis by decreasing the activity of the enzyme, cyclooxygenase, which results in decreased formation of prostaglandin precursors

Contraindications Hypersensitivity to hydrocodone, ibuprofen, aspirin, other NSAIDs, or any component of the formulation; pregnancy (3rd trimester)

Warnings/Precautions NSAIDs are associated with an increased risk of adverse cardiovascular events, including MI, stroke, and new onset or worsening of pre-existing hypertension. Risk may be increased with duration of use or pre-existing cardiovascular risk-factors or disease. Use caution with fluid retention, CHF, or hypertension. Use of NSAIDs can compromise existing renal function. Rehydrate patient before starting therapy. Monitor renal function closely. Ibuprofen is not recommended for patients with advanced renal disease. NSAIDs may increase risk of gastrointestinal irritation, ulceration, bleeding, and perforation. NSAIDs may cause serious skin adverse events. Anaphylactoid reactions may occur, even without prior exposure. Do not use in patients who experience bronchospasm, asthma, rhinitis, or urticaria with NSAID or aspirin therapy. The elderly are at increased risk for adverse effects (especially peptic ulceration, CNS effects, renal toxicity) from NSAIDs even at low doses.

Drug Interactions

Hydrocodone: **Substrate** of CYP2D6 (major)
Ibuprofen: **Substrate** (minor) of CYP2C8/9, 2C19; **Inhibits** CYP2C8/9 (strong)

Also see individual agents.

Ethanol/Nutrition/Herb Interactions

Based on **hydrocodone** component: Ethanol: Avoid or limit ethanol (may increase CNS depression). Watch for sedation.

Based on **ibuprofen** component:

Ethanol: Avoid ethanol (may enhance gastric mucosal irritation).

Food: Ibuprofen peak serum levels may be decreased if taken with food.

Herb/Nutraceutical: Avoid alfalfa, anise, bilberry, bladderwrack, bromelain, cat's claw, celery, coleus, cordyceps, dong quai, evening primrose, feverfew, fenugreek, garlic, ginger, ginkgo biloboa, red clover, horse chestnut, grapeseed, green tea, ginseng, guggul, horse chestnut seed, horseradish, licorice, prickly ash, red clover, reishi, SAMe, sweet clover, turmeric, white willow (all have additional antiplatelet activity).

Pharmacodynamics/Kinetics

Ibuprofen: See Ibuprofen monograph.

Hydrocodone:

Onset of action: Narcotic analgesic: 10-20 minutes

Duration: 4-8 hours

Distribution: Crosses placenta

Protein binding: 19% to 45%

Metabolism: Hepatic; O-demethylation; N-demethylation and 6-ketosteroid reduction

Half-life elimination: 3.3-4.4 hours

Time to peak: 1.7 hours

Excretion: Urine

Pregnancy Risk Factor C/D (3rd trimester)

Lactation Excretion in breast milk unknown/contraindicated

Dosage Forms

Tablet: Hydrocodone bitartrate 5 mg and ibuprofen 200 mg; hydrocodone bitartrate 7.5 mg and ibuprofen 200 mg

Reprexain™: Hydrocodone bitartrate 5 mg and ibuprofen 200 mg

Vicoprofen®: Hydrocodone bitartrate 7.5 mg and ibuprofen 200 mg

Selected Readings

Dionne R, "To Tame the Pain?" *Compend Contin Educ Dent*, 1998, 19(4):426-8, 430-1.

Hargreaves KM, "Management of Pain in Endodontic Patients," *Tex Dent J*, 1997, 114(10):27-31.

Sunshine A, Olson NZ, O'Neill E, et al, "Analgesic Efficacy of a Hydrocodone With Ibuprofen Combination Compared With Ibuprofen Alone for the Treatment of Acute Postoperative Pain," *J Clin Pharmacol*, 1997, 37(10):908-15.

Wynn RL, "Narcotic Analgesics for Dental Pain: Available Products, Strengths, and Formulations," *Gen Dent*, 2001, 49(2):126-8, 130, 132 passim.

Hydrocodone and Pseudoephedrine

(hye droe KOE done & soo doe e FED rin)

Related Information

Pseudoephedrine *on page 1309*

U.S. Brand Names Histussin D®; P-V Tussin Tablet

Generic Available Yes: Syrup

Synonyms Pseudoephedrine and Hydrocodone
Pharmacologic Category Antitussive/Decongestant
Use Symptomatic relief of cough due to colds, nasal congestion, and cough
Local Anesthetic/Vasoconstrictor Precautions Use with caution since
pseudoephedrine is a sympathomimetic amine which could interact with
epinephrine to cause a pressor response
Effects on Dental Treatment Key adverse event(s) related to dental treat-
ment: Pseudoephedrine: Xerostomia (normal salivary flow resumes upon
discontinuation).
Common Adverse Effects See individual agents.
Restrictions C-III
Mechanism of Action
Based on **hydrocodone** component: Binds to opiate receptors in the CNS,
altering the perception of and response to pain; suppresses cough in medul-
lary center; produces generalized CNS depression
Based on **pseudoephedrine** component: Directly stimulates alpha-adrenergic
receptors of respiratory mucosa causing vasoconstriction; directly stimulates
beta-adrenergic receptors causing bronchial relaxation, increased heart rate
and contractility
Drug Interactions
Cytochrome P450 Effect: Hydrocodone: **Substrate** of CYP2D6 (major)
Increased Effect/Toxicity:
Based on **hydrocodone** component: Increased toxicity: CNS depressants,
MAO inhibitors, general anesthetics, and tricyclic antidepressants may
potentiate the effects of opiate agonists; dextroamphetamine may enhance
the analgesic effect of opiate agonists
Based on **pseudoephedrine** component: Increased toxicity: MAO inhibitors
may increase blood pressure effects of pseudoephedrine; propranolol,
sympathomimetic agents may increase toxicity
Decreased Effect: Based on **pseudoephedrine** component: Decreased
effect of methyldopa, reserpine
Pharmacodynamics/Kinetics
Pseudoephedrine: See Pseudoephedrine monograph.
Hydrocodone:
Onset of action: Narcotic analgesic: 10-20 minutes
Duration: 4-8 hours
Distribution: Crosses placenta
Metabolism: Hepatic; O-demethylation; N-demethylation and 6-ketosteroid
reduction
Half-life elimination: 3.3-4.4 hours
Excretion: Urine

Hydrocodone Bitartrate, Carbinoxamine Maleate, and Pseudoephedrine
Hydrochloride see Hydrocodone, Carbinoxamine, and Pseudoephedrine on
page 789

Hydrocodone Bitartrate, Phenylephrine Hydrochloride, and Diphenhydramine Hydrochloride see Hydrocodone, Phenylephrine, and Diphenhydramine on
page 791

Hydrocodone, Carbinoxamine, and Pseudoephedrine
(hye droe KOE done, kar bi NOKS a meen, & soo doe e FED rin)

Related Information
Carbinoxamine on page 268
Pseudoephedrine on page 1309
U.S. Brand Names Histex™ HC; Tri-Vent™ HC
Generic Available Yes
Synonyms Carbinoxamine, Pseudoephedrine, and Hydrocodone; Hydrocodone
Bitartrate, Carbinoxamine Maleate, and Pseudoephedrine Hydrochloride; Pseu-
doephedrine, Hydrocodone, and Carbinoxamine
Pharmacologic Category Antihistamine/Decongestant/Antitussive
Use Symptomatic relief of cough, congestion, and rhinorrhea associated with the
common cold, influenza, bronchitis, or sinusitis
Local Anesthetic/Vasoconstrictor Precautions Use with caution since
pseudoephedrine is a sympathomimetic amine which could interact with
epinephrine to cause a pressor response
Effects on Dental Treatment Key adverse event(s) related to dental treat-
ment: Pseudoephedrine: Xerostomia (normal salivary flow resumes upon
discontinuation).
Common Adverse Effects See individual agents.
Restrictions C-III
(Continued)

Hydrocodone, Carbinoxamine, and Pseudoephedrine
(Continued)

Mechanism of Action
Hydrocodone binds to opiate receptors in the CNS, altering the perception of and response to pain; suppresses cough in medullary center; produces generalized CNS depression.

Carbinoxamine competes with histamine for H₁-receptor sites on effector cells in the gastrointestinal tract, blood vessels, and respiratory tract.

Pseudoephedrine is a sympathomimetic amine and isomer of ephedrine; acts as a decongestant in respiratory tract mucous membranes with less vasoconstrictor action than ephedrine in normotensive individuals.

Pharmacodynamics/Kinetics See individual agents.

Pregnancy Risk Factor C

Hydrocodone, Chlorpheniramine, Phenylephrine, Acetaminophen, and Caffeine

(hye droe KOE done, klor fen IR a meen, fen il EF rin, a seet a MIN oh fen, & KAF een)

Related Information
Acetaminophen *on page 31*
Caffeine *on page 245*
Chlorpheniramine *on page 323*
Phenylephrine *on page 1226*

U.S. Brand Names Hycomine® Compound

Generic Available No

Synonyms Acetaminophen, Caffeine, Hydrocodone, Chlorpheniramine, and Phenylephrine; Caffeine, Hydrocodone, Chlorpheniramine, Phenylephrine, and Acetaminophen; Chlorpheniramine, Hydrocodone, Phenylephrine, Acetaminophen, and Caffeine; Phenylephrine, Hydrocodone, Chlorpheniramine, Acetaminophen, and Caffeine

Pharmacologic Category Antitussive/Decongestant

Use Symptomatic relief of cough and symptoms of upper respiratory infection

Local Anesthetic/Vasoconstrictor Precautions Use with caution since phenylephrine is a sympathomimetic amine which could interact with epinephrine to cause a pressor response

Effects on Dental Treatment Key adverse event(s) related to dental treatment:
Acetaminophen: No significant effects or complications reported.
Chlorpheniramine: Prolonged use will cause significant xerostomia (normal salivary flow resumes upon discontinuation).
Phenylephrine: Up to 10% of patients could experience tachycardia, palpitations, and xerostomia; use vasoconstrictor with caution.

Common Adverse Effects Frequency not defined.
Cardiovascular: Hypertension, postural hypotension, tachycardia, palpitation
Central nervous system: Sedation, drowsiness, mental clouding, lethargy, impairment of mental and physical performance, anxiety, fear, dysphoria, dizziness, psychic dependence, mood changes
Dermatologic: Rash, pruritus
Gastrointestinal: Nausea, vomiting, constipation with prolonged use
Genitourinary: Ureteral spasms, spasm of vesical sphincters and urinary retention
Ocular: Blurred vision
Respiratory: Respiratory depression

Restrictions C-III

Drug Interactions
Cytochrome P450 Effect:
Hydrocodone: **Substrate** of CYP2D6 (major)
Chlorpheniramine: **Substrate** of CYP2D6 (minor), 3A4 (major); **Inhibits** CYP2D6 (weak)
Acetaminophen: **Substrate** (minor) of CYP1A2, 2A6, 2C9, 2D6, 2E1, 3A4;
Caffeine: **Substrate** of CYP1A2 (major), 2C9 (minor), 2D6 (minor), 2E1 (minor), 3A4 (minor); **Inhibits** CYP1A2 (weak), 3A4 (moderate)
Increased Effect/Toxicity: See individual agents.

Pharmacodynamics/Kinetics
See Chlorpheniramine, Phenylephrine, and Acetaminophen monographs.
Hydrocodone:
Onset of action: Narcotic analgesic: 10-20 minutes
Duration: 4-8 hours

Distribution: Crosses placenta
Metabolism: Hepatic; O-demethylation; N-demethylation and 6-ketosteroid reduction
Half-life elimination: 3.3-4.4 hours
Excretion: Urine
Pregnancy Risk Factor C

Hydrocodone, Phenylephrine, and Diphenhydramine
(hye droe KOE done, fen il EF rin, & dye fen HYE dra meen)

Related Information
DiphenhydrAMINE *on page 483*
Phenylephrine *on page 1226*
U.S. Brand Names Endal® HD; Hydro DP; TussiNate™
Generic Available Yes
Synonyms Diphenhydramine, Hydrocodone, and Phenylephrine; Hydrocodone Bitartrate, Phenylephrine Hydrochloride, and Diphenhydramine Hydrochloride; Phenylephrine, Diphenhydramine, and Hydrocodone
Pharmacologic Category Antihistamine/Decongestant/Antitussive; Antitussive; Decongestant; Histamine H_1 Antagonist
Use Symptomatic relief of cough and congestion associated with the common cold, sinusitis, or acute upper respiratory tract infections
Local Anesthetic/Vasoconstrictor Precautions Use with caution since phenylephrine is a sympathomimetic amine which could interact with epinephrine to cause a pressor response
Effects on Dental Treatment Key adverse event(s) related to dental treatment: Xerostomia (normal salivary flow resumes upon discontinuation).
Common Adverse Effects See individual agents.
Restrictions C-III
Mechanism of Action
Hydrocodone binds to opiate receptors in the CNS; suppresses cough in medullary center.
Phenylephrine is a potent, direct-acting alpha-adrenergic stimulator.
Diphenhydramine is an H_1-receptor antagonist.
Pharmacodynamics/Kinetics See individual agents.
Pregnancy Risk Factor C

Hydrocodone, Phenylephrine, and Guaifenesin
(hye droe KOE done, fen il EF rin, & gwye FEN e sin)

Related Information
Guaifenesin *on page 752*
Phenylephrine *on page 1226*
U.S. Brand Names Crantex HC; De-Chlor G; Giltuss HC®; Hydro-GP; Levall 5.0; Quintex HC; Tussafed® HC
Generic Available Yes
Synonyms Guaifenesin, Hydrocodone Bitartrate, and Phenylephrine Hydrochloride; Phenylephrine, Guaifenesin, and Hydrocodone
Pharmacologic Category Antitussive/Decongestant/Expectorant
Use Temporary relief of cough, congestion, and other symptoms associated with colds or allergies
Local Anesthetic/Vasoconstrictor Precautions Use with caution since pseudoephedrine is a sympathomimetic amine which could interact with epinephrine to cause a pressor response
Effects on Dental Treatment Key adverse event(s) related to dental treatment: Tachycardia, palpitations, and xerostomia (normal salivary flow resumes upon discontinuation).
Common Adverse Effects Frequency not defined.
Central nervous system: Drowsiness, giddiness, lassitude
Gastrointestinal: Constipation, GI upset, nausea
Restrictions C-III
Mechanism of Action
Hydrocodone binds to opiate receptors in the CNS, altering the perception of and response to pain; suppresses cough in medullary center; produces generalized CNS depression.
Phenylephrine is a direct-acting alpha-adrenergic stimulator with weak beta-adrenergic activity; causes vasoconstriction of the arterioles of the nasal mucosa and conjunctiva; activates the dilator muscle of the pupil to cause contraction; produces vasoconstriction of arterioles in the body; produces systemic arterial vasoconstriction.
(Continued)

Hydrocodone, Phenylephrine, and Guaifenesin
(Continued)

Guaifenesin is thought to act as an expectorant by irritating the gastric mucosa and stimulating respiratory tract secretions, thereby increasing respiratory fluid volumes and decreasing phlegm viscosity.

Drug Interactions

Cytochrome P450 Effect: Hydrocodone: **Substrate** of CYP2D6 (major)

Increased Effect/Toxicity: CNS depressants, MAO inhibitors, general anesthetics, and tricyclic antidepressants may potentiate the effects of opiate agonists. Dextroamphetamine may enhance the analgesic effect of opiate agonists.

Also refer to individual monographs for Phenylephrine and Guaifenesin.

Decreased Effect: CYP2D6 inhibitors may decrease the effects of hydrocodone (example inhibitors include chlorpromazine, delavirdine, fluoxetine, miconazole, paroxetine, pergolide, quinidine, quinine, ritonavir, and ropinirole).

Also refer to individual monographs for Phenylephrine and Guaifenesin.

Pregnancy Risk Factor C

Hydrocodone, Pseudoephedrine, and Guaifenesin
(hye droe KOE done, soo doe e FED rin & gwye FEN e sin)

Related Information
Guaifenesin *on page 752*
Pseudoephedrine *on page 1309*

U.S. Brand Names Hydro-Tussin™ HD; Hydro-Tussin™ XP; Su-Tuss®-HD; Tussend® Expectorant; Ztuss™ Tablet

Generic Available Yes: Excludes tablet

Synonyms Guaifenesin, Hydrocodone, and Pseudoephedrine; Pseudoephedrine, Hydrocodone, and Guaifenesin

Pharmacologic Category Antitussive/Decongestant/Expectorant

Use Symptomatic relief of irritating, nonproductive cough associated with upper respiratory conditions and allergies

Local Anesthetic/Vasoconstrictor Precautions Use with caution since pseudoephedrine is a sympathomimetic amine which could interact with epinephrine to cause a pressor response

Effects on Dental Treatment Key adverse event(s) related to dental treatment:

Guaifenesin: No significant effects or complications reported

Pseudoephedrine: Xerostomia (normal salivary flow resumes upon discontinuation).

Common Adverse Effects Frequency not defined.

Cardiovascular: Arrhythmias, tachycardia, hypertension

Central nervous system: Drowsiness, fear, anxiety, tenseness, restlessness, pallor, insomnia, hallucinations, CNS depression

Gastrointestinal: GI upset, nausea, constipation with prolonged use

Genitourinary: Dysuria

Hepatic: Transaminases increased (slight)

Neuromuscular & skeletal: Weakness, tremor

Respiratory: Respiratory difficulty

Patients hyper-reactive to pseudoephedrine may display ephedrine-like reactions such as tachycardia, palpitation, headache, dizziness, or nausea; patient idiosyncrasy to adrenergic agents may be manifested by insomnia, dizziness, weakness, tremor, or arrhythmia.

Restrictions C-III

Mechanism of Action

Hydrocodone binds to opiate receptors in the CNS, altering the perception of and response to pain; suppresses cough in medullary center; produces generalized CNS depression.

Pseudoephedrine directly stimulates alpha-adrenergic receptors of respiratory mucosa causing vasoconstriction; directly stimulates beta-adrenergic receptors causing bronchial relaxation, increased heart rate and contractility.

Guaifenesin is thought to act as an expectorant by irritating the gastric mucosa and stimulating respiratory tract secretions, thereby increasing respiratory fluid volumes and decreasing phlegm viscosity.

Drug Interactions

Cytochrome P450 Effect: Hydrocodone: **Substrate** of CYP2D6 (major)

Increased Effect/Toxicity: CNS depressants, MAO inhibitors, general anesthetics, and tricyclic antidepressants may potentiate the effects of opiate agonists. Dextroamphetamine may enhance the analgesic effect of opiate agonists.

Also refer to individual monographs for Pseudoephedrine and Guaifenesin.

Decreased Effect: CYP2D6 inhibitors may decrease the effects of hydrocodone (example inhibitors include chlorpromazine, delavirdine, fluoxetine, miconazole, paroxetine, pergolide, quinidine, quinine, ritonavir, and ropinirole).

Also refer to individual monographs for Pseudoephedrine and Guaifenesin.

Pharmacodynamics/Kinetics

See Guaifenesin and Pseudoephedrine monographs.

Hydrocodone:

Onset of action: Narcotic analgesic: 10-20 minutes

Duration: 4-8 hours

Distribution: Crosses placenta

Metabolism: Hepatic; O-demethylation; N-demethylation and 6-ketosteroid reduction

Half-life elimination: 3.3-4.4 hours

Excretion: Urine

Pregnancy Risk Factor C

Hydrocodone Tannate and Chlorpheniramine Tannate *see* Hydrocodone and Chlorpheniramine *on page 784*

Hydrocortisone (hye droe KOR ti sone)

U.S. Brand Names Anucort-HC®; Anusol-HC®; Anusol® HC-1 [OTC]; Aquanil™ HC [OTC]; Beta-HC®; Caldecort® [OTC]; Cetacort®; Colocort®; Cortaid® Intensive Therapy [OTC]; Cortaid® Maximum Strength [OTC]; Cortaid® Sensitive Skin [OTC]; Cortef®; Corticool® [OTC]; Cortifoam®; Cortizone®-10 Maximum Strength [OTC]; Cortizone®-10 Plus Maximum Strength [OTC]; Cortizone®-10 Quick Shot [OTC]; Dermarest Dricort® [OTC]; Dermtex® HC [OTC]; EarSol® HC; Encort™; Hemril®-30; HydroZone Plus [OTC]; Hytone®; IvySoothe® [OTC]; Locoid®; Locoid Lipocream®; Nupercainal® Hydrocortisone Cream [OTC]; Nutracort®; Pandel®; Post Peel Healing Balm [OTC]; Preparation H® Hydrocortisone [OTC]; Proctocort®; ProctoCream® HC; Procto-Kit™; Procto-Pak™; Proctosert; Proctosol-HC®; Proctozone-HC™; Sarnol®-HC [OTC]; Solu-Cortef®; Summer's Eve® SpecialCare™ Medicated Anti-Itch Cream [OTC]; Texacort®; Tucks® Anti-Itch [OTC]; Westcort®

Canadian Brand Names Aquacort®; Cortamed®; Cortef®; Cortenema®; Cortifoam™; Emo-Cort®; Hycort™; Hyderm; HydroVal®; Locoid®; Prevex® HC; Sarna® HC; Solu-Cortef®; Westcort®

Mexican Brand Names Aquanil™ HC; LactiCare-HC®; Nutracort®

Generic Available Yes: Excludes acetate foam, butyrate cream and ointment, gel as base, otic drops as base, probutate cream, sodium succinate injection

Synonyms A-hydroCort; Compound F; Cortisol; Hemorrhoidal HC; Hydrocortisone Acetate; Hydrocortisone Butyrate; Hydrocortisone Probutate; Hydrocortisone Sodium Succinate; Hydrocortisone Valerate

Pharmacologic Category Corticosteroid, Rectal; Corticosteroid, Systemic; Corticosteroid, Topical

Dental Use Treatment of a variety of oral diseases of allergic, inflammatory, or autoimmune origin

Use Management of adrenocortical insufficiency; relief of inflammation of corticosteroid-responsive dermatoses (low and medium potency topical corticosteroid); adjunctive treatment of ulcerative colitis

Local Anesthetic/Vasoconstrictor Precautions No information available to require special precautions

Effects on Dental Treatment No significant effects or complications reported

Significant Adverse Effects

Systemic:

>10%:

Central nervous system: Insomnia, nervousness

Gastrointestinal: Increased appetite, indigestion

1% to 10%:

Dermatologic: Hirsutism

Endocrine & metabolic: Diabetes mellitus

Neuromuscular & skeletal: Arthralgia

Ocular: Cataracts

Respiratory: Epistaxis

<1% (Limited to important or life-threatening): Hypertension, edema, euphoria, headache, delirium, hallucinations, seizure, mood swings, acne, dermatitis, skin atrophy, bruising, hyperpigmentation, hypokalemia, hyperglycemia, Cushing's syndrome, sodium and water retention, bone growth suppression, (Continued)

Hydrocortisone *(Continued)*

amenorrhea, peptic ulcer, abdominal distention, ulcerative esophagitis, pancreatitis, muscle wasting, hypersensitivity reactions, immunosuppression

Topical:

>10%: Dermatologic: Eczema (12.5%)

1% to 10%: Dermatologic: Pruritus (6%), stinging (2%), dry skin (2%)

<1% (Limited to important or life-threatening): Allergic contact dermatitis, burning, dermal atrophy, folliculitis, HPA axis suppression, hypopigmentation; metabolic effects (hyperglycemia, hypokalemia); striae

Dental Usual Dosing Treatment of a variety of oral diseases of allergic, inflammatory, or autoimmune origin: Children >2 years and Adults: Topical: Apply to affected area 2-4 times/day (Buteprate: Apply once or twice daily). Therapy should be discontinued when control is achieved; if no improvement is seen, reassessment of diagnosis may be necessary.

Dosage Dose should be based on severity of disease and patient response

Acute adrenal insufficiency: I.M., I.V.:

Infants and young Children: Succinate: 1-2 mg/kg/dose bolus, then 25-150 mg/day in divided doses every 6-8 hours

Older Children: Succinate: 1-2 mg/kg bolus then 150-250 mg/day in divided doses every 6-8 hours

Adults: Succinate: 100 mg I.V. bolus, then 300 mg/day in divided doses every 8 hours or as a continuous infusion for 48 hours; once patient is stable change to oral, 50 mg every 8 hours for 6 doses, then taper to 30-50 mg/day in divided doses

Chronic adrenal corticoid insufficiency: Adults: Oral: 20-30 mg/day

Anti-inflammatory or immunosuppressive:

Infants and Children:

Oral: 2.5-10 mg/kg/day **or** 75-300 mg/m^2/day every 6-8 hours

I.M., I.V.: Succinate: 1-5 mg/kg/day **or** 30-150 mg/m^2/day divided every 12-24 hours

Adolescents and Adults: Oral, I.M., I.V.: Succinate: 15-240 mg every 12 hours

Congenital adrenal hyperplasia: Oral: Initial: 10-20 mg/m^2/day in 3 divided doses; a variety of dosing schedules have been used. **Note:** Inconsistencies have occurred with liquid formulations; tablets may provide more reliable levels. Doses must be individualized by monitoring growth, bone age, and hormonal levels. Mineralocorticoid and sodium supplementation may be required based upon electrolyte regulation and plasma renin activity.

Physiologic replacement: Children:

Oral: 0.5-0.75 mg/kg/day **or** 20-25 mg/m^2/day every 8 hours

I.M.: Succinate: 0.25-0.35 mg/kg/day **or** 12-15 mg/m^2/day once daily

Shock: I.M., I.V.: Succinate:

Children: Initial: 50 mg/kg, then repeated in 4 hours and/or every 24 hours as needed

Adolescents and Adults: 500 mg to 2 g every 2-6 hours

Status asthmaticus: Children and Adults: I.V.: Succinate: 1-2 mg/kg/dose every 6 hours for 24 hours, then maintenance of 0.5-1 mg/kg every 6 hours

Adults:

Rheumatic diseases:

Intralesional, intra-articular, soft tissue injection: Acetate:

Large joints: 25 mg (up to 37.5 mg)

Small joints: 10-25 mg

Tendon sheaths: 5-12.5 mg

Soft tissue infiltration: 25-50 mg (up to 75 mg)

Bursae: 25-37.5 mg

Ganglia: 12.5-25 mg

Stress dosing (surgery) in patients known to be adrenally-suppressed or on chronic systemic steroids: I.V.:

Minor stress (ie, inguinal herniorrhaphy): 25 mg/day for 1 day

Moderate stress (ie, joint replacement, cholecystectomy): 50-75 mg/day (25 mg every 8-12 hours) for 1-2 days

Major stress (pancreatoduodenectomy, esophagogastrectomy, cardiac surgery): 100-150 mg/day (50 mg every 8-12 hours) for 2-3 days

Dermatosis: Children >2 years and Adults: Topical: Apply to affected area 2-4 times/day (Buteprate: Apply once or twice daily). Therapy should be discontinued when control is achieved; if no improvement is seen, reassessment of diagnosis may be necessary.

Ulcerative colitis: Adults: Rectal: 10-100 mg 1-2 times/day for 2-3 weeks

Mechanism of Action Decreases inflammation by suppression of migration of polymorphonuclear leukocytes and reversal of increased capillary permeability

Contraindications Hypersensitivity to hydrocortisone or any component of the formulation; serious infections, except septic shock or tuberculous meningitis; viral, fungal, or tubercular skin lesions

Warnings/Precautions

Use with caution in patients with hyperthyroidism, cirrhosis, nonspecific ulcerative colitis, hypertension, osteoporosis, thromboembolic tendencies, CHF, convulsive disorders, myasthenia gravis, thrombophlebitis, peptic ulcer, diabetes, glaucoma, cataracts, or tuberculosis. Use caution in hepatic impairment.

May cause HPA axis suppression. Acute adrenal insufficiency may occur with abrupt withdrawal after long-term therapy or with stress; young pediatric patients may be more susceptible to adrenal axis suppression from topical therapy. Avoid use of topical preparations with occlusive dressings or on weeping or exudative lesions.

Because of the risk of adverse effects, systemic corticosteroids should be used cautiously in the elderly, in the smallest possible dose, and for the shortest possible time

Drug Interactions Substrate of CYP3A4 (minor); **Induces** CYP3A4 (weak)

Decreased effect:

Insulin decreases hypoglycemic effect

Phenytoin, phenobarbital, ephedrine, and rifampin increase metabolism of hydrocortisone and decrease steroid blood level

Increased toxicity:

Oral anticoagulants change prothrombin time

Potassium-depleting diuretics increase risk of hypokalemia

Cardiac glucosides increase risk of arrhythmias or digitalis toxicity secondary to hypokalemia

Ethanol/Nutrition/Herb Interactions

Ethanol: Avoid ethanol (may enhance gastric mucosal irritation).

Food: Hydrocortisone interferes with calcium absorption.

Herb/Nutraceutical: St John's wort may decrease hydrocortisone levels. Avoid cat's claw, echinacea (have immunostimulant properties).

Dietary Considerations Systemic use of corticosteroids may require a diet with increased potassium, vitamins A, B_6, C, D, folate, calcium, zinc, phosphorus, and decreased sodium. Sodium content of 1 g (sodium succinate injection): 47.5 mg (2.07 mEq)

Pharmacodynamics/Kinetics

Onset of action:

Hydrocortisone acetate: Slow

Hydrocortisone sodium succinate (water soluble): Rapid

Duration: Hydrocortisone acetate: Long

Absorption: Rapid by all routes, except rectally

Metabolism: Hepatic

Half-life elimination: Biologic: 8-12 hours

Excretion: Urine (primarily as 17-hydroxysteroids and 17-ketosteroids)

Pregnancy Risk Factor C

Lactation Excretion in breast milk unknown/use caution

Breast-Feeding Considerations It is not known if hydrocortisone is excreted in breast milk, however, other corticosteroids are excreted. Prednisone and prednisolone are excreted in breast milk; the AAP considers them to be "usually compatible" with breast-feeding. Hypertension was reported in a nursing infant when a topical corticosteroid was applied to the nipples of the mother.

Dosage Forms [DSC] = Discontinued product

Aerosol, rectal, as acetate (Cortifoam®): 10% (15 g) [90 mg/applicator]

Cream, rectal, as acetate (Nupercainal® Hydrocortisone Cream): 1% (30 g) [strength expressed as base]

Cream, rectal, as base:

Cortizone®-10: 1% (30 g) [contains aloe]

Preparation H® Hydrocortisone: 1% (27 g)

Cream, topical, as acetate: 0.5% (9 g, 30 g, 60 g) [available with aloe]; 1% (30 g, 454 g) [available with aloe]

Cream, topical, as base: 0.5% (30 g); 1% (1.5 g, 30 g, 114 g, 454 g); 2.5% (20 g, 30 g, 454 g)

Anusol-HC®: 2.5% (30 g) [contains benzyl alcohol]

Caldecort®: 1% (30 g) [contains aloe vera gel]

Cortaid® Intensive Therapy: 1% (60 g)

Cortaid® Maximum Strength: 1% (15 g, 30 g, 40 g, 60 g) [contains aloe vera gel and benzyl alcohol]

Cortaid® Sensitive Skin: 0.5% (15 g) [contains aloe vera gel]

Cortizone®-10 Maximum Strength: 1% (15 g, 30 g, 60 g) [contains aloe]

Cortizone®-10 Plus Maximum Strength: 1% (30 g, 60 g) [contains vitamins A, D, E and aloe]

(Continued)

Hydrocortisone *(Continued)*

Dermarest® Dricort®: 1% (15 g, 30 g)
HydroZone Plus, Proctocort®, Procto-Pak™: 1% (30 g)
Hytone®: 2.5% (30 g, 60 g)
IvySoothe®: 1% (30 g) [contains aloe]
Post Peel Healing Balm: 1% (23 g)
ProctoCream® HC: 2.5% (30 g) [contains benzyl alcohol]
Procto-Kit™: 1% (30 g) [packaged with applicator tips and finger cots]; 2.5% (30 g) [packaged with applicator tips and finger cots]
Proctosol-HC®, Proctozone-HC™: 2.5% (30 g)
Summer's Eve® SpecialCare™ Medicated Anti-Itch Cream: 1% (30 g)
Cream, topical, as butyrate (Locoid®, Locoid Lipocream®): 0.1% (15 g, 45 g)
Cream, topical, as probutate (Pandel®): 0.1% (15 g, 45 g, 80 g)
Cream, topical, as valerate (Westcort®): 0.2% (15 g, 45 g, 60 g)
Gel, topical, as base (Corticool®): 1% (45 g)
Injection, powder for reconstitution, as sodium succinate (Solu-Cortef®): 100 mg, 250 mg, 500 mg, 1 g [diluent contains benzyl alcohol; strength expressed as base]
Lotion, topical, as base: 1% (120 mL); 2.5% (60 mL)
Aquanil™ HC: 1% (120 mL)
Beta-HC®, Cetacort®, Sarnol®-HC: 1% (60 mL)
HydroZone Plus: 1% (120 mL)
Hytone®: 2.5% (60 mL)
Nutracort®: 1% (60 mL, 120 mL); 2.5% (60 mL, 120 mL)
Ointment, topical, as acetate: 1% (30 g) [strength expressed as base; available with aloe]
Anusol® HC-1: 1% (21 g) [strength expressed as base]
Cortaid® Maximum Strength: 1% (15 g, 30 g) [strength expressed as base]
Ointment, topical, as base: 0.5% (30 g); 1% (30 g, 454 g); 2.5% (20 g, 30 g, 454 g)
Cortizone®-10 Maximum Strength: 1% (30 g, 60 g)
Hytone®: 2.5% (30 g) [DSC]
Ointment, topical, as butyrate (Locoid®): 0.1% (15 g, 45 g)
Ointment, topical, as valerate (Westcort®): 0.2% (15 g, 45 g, 60 g)
Solution, otic, as base (EarSol® HC): 1% (30 mL) [contains alcohol 44%, benzyl benzoate, yerba santa]
Solution, topical, as base (Texacort®): 2.5% (30 mL) [contains alcohol]
Solution, topical, as butyrate (Locoid®): 0.1% (20 mL, 60 mL) [contains alcohol 50%]
Solution, topical spray, as base:
Cortaid® Intensive Therapy: 1% (60 mL) [contains alcohol]
Cortizone®-10 Quick Shot: 1% (44 mL) [contains benzyl alcohol]
Dermtex® HC: 1% (52 mL) [contains menthol 1%]
Suppository, rectal, as acetate: 25 mg (12s, 24s, 100s)
Anucort-HC®, Tucks® Anti-Itch: 25 mg (12s, 24s, 100s) [strength expressed as base; Anucort-HC® renamed Tucks® Anti-Itch]
Anusol-HC®, Proctosol-HC®: 25 mg (12s, 24s)
Encort™: 30 mg (12s)
Hemril®-30, Proctocort®, Proctosert: 30 mg (12s, 24s)
Suspension, rectal, as base: 100 mg/60 mL (7s)
Colocort®: 100 mg/60 mL (1s, 7s)
Tablet, as base: 20 mg
Cortef®: 5 mg, 10 mg, 20 mg

Hydrocortisone Acetate see Hydrocortisone on page 793

Hydrocortisone, Acetic Acid, and Propylene Glycol Diacetate see Acetic Acid, Propylene Glycol Diacetate, and Hydrocortisone on page 45

Hydrocortisone and Benzoyl Peroxide see Benzoyl Peroxide and Hydrocortisone on page 195

Hydrocortisone and Ciprofloxacin see Ciprofloxacin and Hydrocortisone on page 348

Hydrocortisone and Iodoquinol see Iodoquinol and Hydrocortisone on page 853

Hydrocortisone and Lidocaine see Lidocaine and Hydrocortisone on page 928

Hydrocortisone and Pramoxine see Pramoxine and Hydrocortisone on page 1264

Hydrocortisone and Urea see Urea and Hydrocortisone on page 1551

Hydrocortisone, Bacitracin, Neomycin, and Polymyxin B see Bacitracin, Neomycin, Polymyxin B, and Hydrocortisone on page 177

Hydrocortisone Butyrate see Hydrocortisone on page 793

Hydrocortisone, Neomycin, and Polymyxin B see Neomycin, Polymyxin B, and Hydrocortisone on page 1101

Hydrocortisone Probutate *see* Hydrocortisone *on page 793*
Hydrocortisone Sodium Succinate *see* Hydrocortisone *on page 793*
Hydrocortisone Valerate *see* Hydrocortisone *on page 793*
Hydro DP *see* Hydrocodone, Phenylephrine, and Diphenhydramine *on page 791*
Hydro-GP *see* Hydrocodone, Phenylephrine, and Guaifenesin *on page 791*
Hydromet® *see* Hydrocodone and Homatropine *on page 786*

Hydromorphone (hye droe MOR fone)

Related Information
Oxymorphone *on page 1174*

U.S. Brand Names Dilaudid®; Dilaudid-HP®; Palladone™ *[Withdrawn]*

Canadian Brand Names Dilaudid®; Dilaudid-HP®; Dilaudid-HP-Plus®; Dilaudid® Sterile Powder; Dilaudid-XP®; Hydromorph Contin®; Hydromorph-IR®; Hydromorphone HP; PMS-Hydromorphone

Generic Available Yes: Excludes capsule, liquid, powder for injection

Synonyms Dihydromorphinone; Hydromorphone Hydrochloride

Pharmacologic Category Analgesic, Narcotic

Use Management of moderate-to-severe pain

Unlabeled/Investigational Use Antitussive

Local Anesthetic/Vasoconstrictor Precautions No information available to require special precautions

Effects on Dental Treatment Key adverse event(s) related to dental treatment: Xerostomia (normal salivary flow resumes upon discontinuation).

Common Adverse Effects Frequency not defined.
Cardiovascular: Palpitations, hypotension, peripheral vasodilation, tachycardia, bradycardia, flushing of face
Central nervous system: CNS depression, increased intracranial pressure, fatigue, headache, nervousness, restlessness, dizziness, lightheadedness, drowsiness, hallucinations, mental depression, seizure
Dermatologic: Pruritus, rash, urticaria
Endocrine & metabolic: Antidiuretic hormone release
Gastrointestinal: Nausea, vomiting, constipation, stomach cramps, xerostomia, anorexia, biliary tract spasm, paralytic ileus
Genitourinary: Decreased urination, ureteral spasm, urinary tract spasm
Hepatic: LFTs increased, AST increased, ALT increased
Local: Pain at injection site (I.M.)
Neuromuscular & skeletal: Trembling, weakness, myoclonus
Ocular: Miosis
Respiratory: Respiratory depression, dyspnea
Miscellaneous: Histamine release, physical and psychological dependence

Restrictions C-II

Mechanism of Action Binds to opiate receptors in the CNS, causing inhibition of ascending pain pathways, altering the perception of and response to pain; causes cough supression by direct central action in the medulla; produces generalized CNS depression

Drug Interactions
Increased Effect/Toxicity: Effects may be additive with CNS depressants; hypotensive effects may be increased with phenothiazines; serotonergic effects may be additive with SSRIs

Decreased Effect: Hydromorphone may diminish the effects of pegvisomant.

Pharmacodynamics/Kinetics
Onset of action: Analgesic: Immediate release formulations:
Oral: 15-30 minutes
Peak effect: Oral: 30-60 minutes
Duration: Immediate release formulations: 4-5 hours
Absorption: I.M.: Variable and delayed; Palladone™: Biphasic
Distribution: V_d: 4 L/kg
Protein binding: ~20%
Metabolism: Hepatic; to inactive metabolites
Bioavailability: 62%
Half-life elimination:
Immediate release formulations: 1-3 hours
Palladone™: 18.6 hours
Excretion: Urine (primarily as glucuronide conjugates)

Pregnancy Risk Factor C/D (prolonged use or high doses at term)

Hydromorphone Hydrochloride *see* Hydromorphone *on page 797*
Hydropane® *see* Hydrocodone and Homatropine *on page 786*
Hydroquinol *see* Hydroquinone *on page 798*

Hydroquinone (HYE droe kwin one)

U.S. Brand Names Alphaquin HP®; Claripel™; Dermarest® Skin Correction Cream Plus [OTC]; Eldopaque® [OTC]; Eldopaque Forte®; Eldoquin® [OTC]; Eldoquin Forte®; EpiQuin™ Micro; Esoterica® Regular [OTC]; Glyquin®; Glyquin-XM™; Lustra®; Lustra-AF™; Melanex®; Melpaque HP®; Melquin-3®; Melquin HP®; NeoStrata® AHA [OTC]; Nuquin HP®; Palmer's® Skin Success Eventone® Fade Cream [OTC]; Solaquin® [OTC]; Solaquin Forte®

Canadian Brand Names Eldopaque®; Eldoquin®; Glyquin® XM; Lustra®; NeoStrata® HQ; Solaquin®; Solaquin Forte®; Ultraquin™

Mexican Brand Names Crema Blanca®; Eldopaque®; Eldoquin®; Hidroquin®

Generic Available Yes

Synonyms Hydroquinol; Quinol

Pharmacologic Category Depigmenting Agent

Use Gradual bleaching of hyperpigmented skin conditions

Local Anesthetic/Vasoconstrictor Precautions No information available to require special precautions

Effects on Dental Treatment No significant effects or complications reported

Common Adverse Effects Frequency not defined.

Dermatologic: Dermatitis, dryness, erythema, stinging, inflammatory reaction, sensitization

Local: Irritation

Mechanism of Action Produces reversible depigmentation of the skin by suppression of melanocyte metabolic processes, in particular the inhibition of the enzymatic oxidation of tyrosine to DOPA (3,4-dihydroxyphenylalanine); sun exposure reverses this effect and will cause repigmentation.

Pharmacodynamics/Kinetics Onset and duration of depigmentation produced by hydroquinone varies among individuals

Pregnancy Risk Factor C

Hydroquinone, Fluocinolone Acetonide, and Tretinoin see Fluocinolone, Hydroquinone, and Tretinoin on page 669

Hydro-Tussin™-CBX see Carbinoxamine and Pseudoephedrine on page 268

Hydro-Tussin™ DHC see Pseudoephedrine, Dihydrocodeine, and Chlorpheniramine on page 1312

Hydro-Tussin™ DM see Guaifenesin and Dextromethorphan on page 754

Hydro-Tussin™ EXP see Dihydrocodeine, Pseudoephedrine, and Guaifenesin on page 476

Hydro-Tussin™ HD see Hydrocodone, Pseudoephedrine, and Guaifenesin on page 792

Hydro-Tussin™ XP see Hydrocodone, Pseudoephedrine, and Guaifenesin on page 792

Hydroxocobalamin (hye droks oh koe BAL a min)

Mexican Brand Names Axofor®; Duradoce®

Generic Available Yes

Synonyms Vitamin B_{12}

Pharmacologic Category Vitamin, Water Soluble

Use Treatment of pernicious anemia, vitamin B_{12} deficiency, increased B_{12} requirements due to pregnancy, thyrotoxicosis, hemorrhage, malignancy, liver or kidney disease

Unlabeled/Investigational Use Neuropathies, multiple sclerosis

Local Anesthetic/Vasoconstrictor Precautions No information available to require special precautions

Effects on Dental Treatment No significant effects or complications reported

Common Adverse Effects Frequency not defined.

Cardiovascular: Peripheral vascular thrombosis

Dermatologic: Itching, urticaria

Gastrointestinal: Diarrhea

Miscellaneous: Hypersensitivity reactions

Mechanism of Action Coenzyme for various metabolic functions, including fat and carbohydrate metabolism and protein synthesis, used in cell replication and hematopoiesis

Pregnancy Risk Factor A/C (dose exceeding RDA recommendation)

Hydroxyamphetamine and Tropicamide
(hye droks ee am FET a meen & troe PIK a mide)

Related Information
Tropicamide *on page 1545*
U.S. Brand Names Paremyd®
Generic Available No
Synonyms Hydroxyamphetamine Hydrobromide and Tropicamide; Tropicamide and Hydroxyamphetamine
Pharmacologic Category Adrenergic Agonist Agent, Ophthalmic
Use Short-term pupil dilation for diagnostic procedures and exams
Local Anesthetic/Vasoconstrictor Precautions No information available to require special precautions
Effects on Dental Treatment No significant effects or complications reported
Mechanism of Action Hydroxyamphetamine hydrobromide is an indirect acting sympathomimetic agent which causes the release of norepinephrine from adrenergic nerve terminals, resulting in mydriasis. Tropicamide is a parasympatholytic agent which produces mydriasis and paralysis by blocking the sphincter muscle in the iris and the ciliary muscle.
Pregnancy Risk Factor C

Hydroxyamphetamine Hydrobromide and Tropicamide *see* Hydroxyamphetamine and Tropicamide *on page 799*

4-Hydroxybutyrate *see* Sodium Oxybate *on page 1402*

Hydroxycarbamide *see* Hydroxyurea *on page 800*

Hydroxychloroquine (hye droks ee KLOR oh kwin)

Related Information
Rheumatoid Arthritis, Osteoarthritis, and Osteoporosis *on page 1668*
U.S. Brand Names Plaquenil®
Canadian Brand Names Apo-Hydroxyquine®; Gen-Hydroxychloroquine; Plaquenil®
Generic Available Yes
Synonyms Hydroxychloroquine Sulfate
Pharmacologic Category Aminoquinoline (Antimalarial)
Use Suppression and treatment of acute attacks of malaria; treatment of systemic lupus erythematosus and rheumatoid arthritis
Unlabeled/Investigational Use Porphyria cutanea tarda, polymorphous light eruptions
Local Anesthetic/Vasoconstrictor Precautions No information available to require special precautions
Effects on Dental Treatment No significant effects or complications reported
Common Adverse Effects Frequency not defined.
Cardiovascular: Cardiomyopathy (rare, relationship to hydroxychloroquine unclear)
Central nervous system: Irritability, nervousness, emotional changes, nightmares, psychosis, headache, dizziness, vertigo, seizure, ataxia, lassitude
Dermatologic: Bleaching of hair, alopecia, pigmentation changes (skin and mucosal; black-blue color), rash (urticarial, morbilliform, lichenoid, maculopapular, purpuric, erythema annulare centrifugum, Stevens-Johnson syndrome, acute generalized exanthematous pustulosis, and exfoliative dermatitis)
Endocrine & metabolic: Weight loss
Gastrointestinal: Anorexia, nausea, vomiting, diarrhea, abdominal cramping
Hematologic: Aplastic anemia, agranulocytosis, leukopenia, thrombocytopenia, hemolysis (in patients with glucose-6-phosphate deficiency)
Hepatic: Abnormal liver function/hepatic failure (isolated cases)
Neuromuscular & skeletal: Myopathy, palsy, or neuromyopathy leading to progressive weakness and atrophy of proximal muscle groups (may be associated with mild sensory changes, loss of deep tendon reflexes, and abnormal nerve conduction)
Ocular: Disturbance in accommodation, keratopathy, corneal changes/deposits (visual disturbances, blurred vision, photophobia - reversible on discontinuation), macular edema, atrophy, abnormal pigmentation, retinopathy (early changes reversible - may progress despite discontinuation if advanced), optic disc pallor/atrophy, attenuation of retinal arterioles, pigmentary retinopathy, scotoma, decreased visual acuity, nystagmus
Otic: Tinnitus, deafness
Miscellaneous: Exacerbation of porphyria and nonlight sensitive psoriasis
(Continued)

Hydroxychloroquine *(Continued)*

Mechanism of Action Interferes with digestive vacuole function within sensitive malarial parasites by increasing the pH and interfering with lysosomal degradation of hemoglobin; inhibits locomotion of neutrophils and chemotaxis of eosinophils; impairs complement-dependent antigen-antibody reactions

Drug Interactions

Increased Effect/Toxicity: Cimetidine increases levels of chloroquine and probably other 4-aminoquinolones.

Decreased Effect: Chloroquine and other 4-aminoquinolones absorption may be decreased due to GI binding with kaolin or magnesium trisilicate.

Pharmacodynamics/Kinetics

Onset of action: Rheumatic disease: May require 4-6 weeks to respond

Absorption: Complete

Protein binding: 55%

Metabolism: Hepatic

Half-life elimination: 32-50 days

Time to peak: Rheumatic disease: Several months

Excretion: Urine (as metabolites and unchanged drug); may be enhanced by urinary acidification

Pregnancy Risk Factor C

Hydroxychloroquine Sulfate *see Hydroxychloroquine on page 799*

Hydroxydaunomycin Hydrochloride *see DOXOrubicin on page 509*

1α-Hydroxyergocalciferol *see Doxercalciferol on page 508*

Hydroxyethylcellulose *see Artificial Tears on page 143*

Hydroxyethyl Starch *see Hetastarch on page 770*

Hydroxyldaunorubicin Hydrochloride *see DOXOrubicin on page 509*

Hydroxypropyl Cellulose *(hye droks ee PROE pil SEL yoo lose)*

Related Information

Hydroxypropyl Methylcellulose *on page 800*

U.S. Brand Names Lacrisert®

Canadian Brand Names Lacrisert®

Generic Available No

Pharmacologic Category Ophthalmic Agent, Miscellaneous

Use Dry eyes (moderate to severe)

Local Anesthetic/Vasoconstrictor Precautions No information available to require special precautions

Effects on Dental Treatment No significant effects or complications reported

---

Hydroxypropyl Methylcellulose

(hye droks ee PROE pil meth il SEL yoo lose)

Related Information

Hydroxypropyl Cellulose *on page 800*

U.S. Brand Names Cellugel®; GenTeal® [OTC]; GenTeal® Mild [OTC]; Gonak™ [OTC]; Goniosoft™; Goniosol® [OTC] [DSC]; Isopto® Tears [OTC]; Tearisol® [OTC]; Tears Again® MC [OTC]

Canadian Brand Names Genteal®; Isopto® Tears

Mexican Brand Names Celuvisc Grin®; Meticel Ofteno®

Generic Available Yes: Solution

Synonyms Gonioscopic Ophthalmic Solution; Hypromellose

Pharmacologic Category Diagnostic Agent, Ophthalmic; Lubricant, Ocular

Use Relief of burning and minor irritation due to dry eyes; diagnostic agent in gonioscopic examination

Local Anesthetic/Vasoconstrictor Precautions No information available to require special precautions

Effects on Dental Treatment No significant effects or complications reported

Pregnancy Risk Factor C

Hydroxyurea *(hye droks ee yoor EE a)*

U.S. Brand Names Droxia®; Hydrea®; Mylocel™

Canadian Brand Names Apo-Hydroxyurea®; Gen-Hydroxyurea; Hydrea®

Mexican Brand Names Hydrea®

Generic Available Yes: Capsule

Synonyms Hydroxycarbamide

Pharmacologic Category Antineoplastic Agent, Antimetabolite

Use Treatment of melanoma, refractory chronic myelocytic leukemia (CML), relapsed and refractory metastatic ovarian cancer; radiosensitizing agent in the treatment of squamous cell head and neck cancer (excluding lip cancer); adjunct in the management of sickle cell patients who have had at least three painful crises in the previous 12 months (to reduce frequency of these crises and the need for blood transfusions)

Unlabeled/Investigational Use Treatment of HIV; treatment of psoriasis, treatment of hematologic conditions such as essential thrombocythemia, polycythemia vera, hypereosinophilia, and hyperleukocytosis due to acute leukemia; treatment of uterine, cervix and nonsmall cell lung cancers; radiosensitizing agent in the treatment of primary brain tumors; has shown activity against renal cell cancer and prostate cancer

Local Anesthetic/Vasoconstrictor Precautions No information available to require special precautions

Effects on Dental Treatment No significant effects or complications reported

Common Adverse Effects Frequency not defined.

Cardiovascular: Edema

Central nervous system: Chills, disorientation, dizziness, drowsiness (dose-related), fever, hallucinations, headache, malaise, seizure

Dermatologic: Alopecia (rare), cutaneous vasculitic toxicities, dermatomyositis-like skin changes, dry skin, facial erythema, gangrene, hyperpigmentation, maculopapular rash, nail atrophy, nail pigmentation, peripheral erythema, scaling, skin atrophy, skin cancer, vasculitis ulcerations, violet papules

Endocrine & metabolic: Hyperuricemia

Gastrointestinal: Anorexia, constipation, diarrhea, gastrointestinal irritation and mucositis, (potentiated with radiation therapy), nausea, pancreatitis, stomatitis, vomiting

Genitourinary: Dysuria (rare)

Hematologic: Myelosuppression (primarily leukopenia; onset: 24-48 hours; nadir: 10 days; recovery: 7 days after stopping drug; reversal of WBC count occurs rapidly but the platelet count may take 7-10 days to recover); thrombocytopenia and anemia, megaloblastic erythropoiesis, macrocytosis, hemolysis, serum iron decreased, persistent cytopenias, secondary leukemias (long-term use)

Hepatic: Hepatic enzymes increased, hepatotoxicity

Neuromuscular & skeletal: Weakness, peripheral neuropathy

Renal: BUN increased, creatinine increased

Respiratory: Acute diffuse pulmonary infiltrates (rare), dyspnea, pulmonary fibrosis (rare)

Mechanism of Action Thought to interfere (unsubstantiated hypothesis) with synthesis of DNA, during the S phase of cell division, without interfering with RNA synthesis; inhibits ribonucleoside diphosphate reductase, preventing conversion of ribonucleotides to deoxyribonucleotides; cell-cycle specific for the S phase and may hold other cells in the G_1 phase of the cell cycle.

Drug Interactions

Increased Effect/Toxicity: Hydroxyurea may increase the toxicity of didanosine.

Pharmacodynamics/Kinetics

Absorption: Readily ($\geq 80\%$)

Distribution: Readily crosses blood-brain barrier; distributes into intestine, brain, lung, kidney tissues, effusions and ascites

Metabolism: 60% via hepatic and GI tract

Half-life elimination: 3-4 hours

Time to peak: 1-4 hours

Excretion: Urine (80%, 50% as unchanged drug, 30% as urea); exhaled gases (as CO_2)

Pregnancy Risk Factor D

HydrOXYzine (hye DROKS i zeen)

Related Information

Sedation *on page 1727*

Related Sample Prescriptions

Sedation (Prior to Dental Treatment) *on page 1746*

U.S. Brand Names Vistaril®

Canadian Brand Names Apo-Hydroxyzine®; Atarax®; Atarax® IM; Atarax® Syrup; Novo-Hydroxyzin; PMS-Hydroxyzine; Vistaril®

Generic Available Yes

(Continued)

HydrOXYzine *(Continued)*

Synonyms Hydroxyzine Hydrochloride; Hydroxyzine Pamoate

Pharmacologic Category Antiemetic; Antihistamine

Dental Use Treatment of anxiety, as a preoperative sedative in pediatric dentistry

Use Treatment of anxiety; preoperative sedative; antipruritic

Unlabeled/Investigational Use Antiemetic; ethanol withdrawal symptoms

Local Anesthetic/Vasoconstrictor Precautions No information available to require special precautions

Effects on Dental Treatment Key adverse event(s) related to dental treatment: Xerostomia (normal salivary flow resumes upon discontinuation).

Significant Adverse Effects Frequency not defined.

Central nervous system: Drowsiness, headache, fatigue, nervousness, dizziness, hallucination

Dermatologic: Pruritus, rash, urticaria

Gastrointestinal: Xerostomia

Neuromuscular & skeletal: Tremor, paresthesia, seizure, involuntary movements

Ocular: Blurred vision

Respiratory: Thickening of bronchial secretions

Miscellaneous: Allergic reaction

Dental Usual Dosing

Anxiety: Adults: Oral: 25-100 mg 4 times/day; maximum dose: 600 mg/day

Preoperative sedation:

Children:

Oral: 0.6 mg/kg/dose every 6 hours

I.M.: 0.5-1.1 mg/kg/dose every 4-6 hours as needed

Adults:

Oral: 50-100 mg

I.M.: 25-100 mg

Dosage

Children:

Preoperative sedation:

Oral: 0.6 mg/kg/dose every 6 hours

I.M.: 0.5-1.1 mg/kg/dose every 4-6 hours as needed

Manufacturer labeling: Pruritus, anxiety:

<6 years: 50 mg daily in divided doses

≥6 years: 50-100 mg daily in divided doses

Adults:

Antiemetic: I.M.: 25-100 mg/dose every 4-6 hours as needed

Anxiety: Oral: 25-100 mg 4 times/day; maximum dose: 600 mg/day

Preoperative sedation:

Oral: 50-100 mg

I.M.: 25-100 mg

Management of pruritus: Oral: 25 mg 3-4 times/day

Dosing interval in hepatic impairment: Change dosing interval to every 24 hours in patients with primary biliary cirrhosis

Mechanism of Action Competes with histamine for H_1-receptor sites on effector cells in the gastrointestinal tract, blood vessels, and respiratory tract. Possesses skeletal muscle relaxing, bronchodilator, antihistamine, antiemetic, and analgesic properties.

Contraindications Hypersensitivity to hydroxyzine or any component of the formulation; early pregnancy

Warnings/Precautions Causes sedation, caution must be used in performing tasks which require alertness (eg, operating machinery or driving). Sedative effects of CNS depressants or ethanol are potentiated. SubQ and intra-arterial administration are not recommended since thrombosis and digital gangrene can occur; should be used with caution in patients with narrow-angle glaucoma, prostatic hyperplasia, and bladder neck obstruction; should also be used with caution in patients with asthma or COPD.

Anticholinergic effects are not well tolerated in the elderly. Hydroxyzine may be useful as a short-term antipruritic, but it is not recommended for use as a sedative or anxiolytic in the elderly.

Drug Interactions Inhibits CYP2D6 (weak)

Amantadine, rimantadine: Central and/or peripheral anticholinergic syndrome can occur when administered with amantadine or rimantadine

Anticholinergic agents: Central and/or peripheral anticholinergic syndrome can occur when administered with narcotic analgesics, phenothiazines and other antipsychotics (especially with high anticholinergic activity), tricyclic antidepressants, quinidine and some other antiarrhythmics, and antihistamines

Antipsychotics: Hydroxyzine may antagonize the therapeutic effects of antipsychotics

CNS depressants: Sedative effects of hydroxyzine may be additive with CNS depressants; includes ethanol, benzodiazepines, barbiturates, narcotic analgesics, and other sedative agents; monitor for increased effect

Ethanol/Nutrition/Herb Interactions

Ethanol: Avoid ethanol (may increase CNS depression).

Herb/Nutraceutical: Avoid valerian, St John's wort, kava kava, gotu kola (may increase CNS depression).

Pharmacodynamics/Kinetics

Onset of action: 15-30 minutes

Duration: 4-6 hours

Absorption: Oral: Rapid

Metabolism: Exact fate unknown

Half-life elimination: 3-7 hours

Time to peak: ~2 hours

Pregnancy Risk Factor C

Lactation Enters breast milk/contraindicated

Dosage Forms

Capsule, as pamoate: 25 mg, 50 mg, 100 mg

Vistaril®: 25 mg, 50 mg

Injection, solution, as hydrochloride: 25 mg/mL (1 mL); 50 mg/mL (1 mL, 2 mL, 10 mL)

Suspension, oral, as pamoate:

Vistaril®: 25 mg/5 mL (120 mL, 480 mL) [lemon flavor]

Syrup, as hydrochloride: 10 mg/5 mL (120 mL, 480 mL)

Tablet, as hydrochloride: 10 mg, 25 mg, 50 mg

Hydroxyzine Hydrochloride *see* HydrOXYzine *on page 801*

Hydroxyzine Pamoate *see* HydrOXYzine *on page 801*

HydroZone Plus [OTC] *see* Hydrocortisone *on page 793*

Hygroton *see* Chlorthalidone *on page 332*

Hylaform® *see* Hyaluronate and Derivatives *on page 773*

Hylaform® Plus *see* Hyaluronate and Derivatives *on page 773*

Hylan Polymers *see* Hyaluronate and Derivatives *on page 773*

Hylenex™ *see* Hyaluronidase *on page 774*

Hyoscine Butylbromide *see* Scopolamine *on page 1380*

Hyoscine Hydrobromide *see* Scopolamine *on page 1380*

Hyoscyamine (hye oh SYE a meen)

U.S. Brand Names Anaspaz®; Cystospaz®; Cystospaz-M® [DSC]; Hyosine; Levbid®; Levsin®; Levsinex®; Levsin/SL®; NuLev™; Spacol [DSC]; Spacol T/S [DSC]; Symax SL; Symax SR

Canadian Brand Names Cystospaz®; Levsin®

Generic Available Yes

Synonyms Hyoscyamine Sulfate; *l*-Hyoscyamine Sulfate

Pharmacologic Category Anticholinergic Agent

Use

Oral: Adjunctive therapy for peptic ulcers, irritable bowel, neurogenic bladder/bowel; treatment of infant colic, GI tract disorders caused by spasm; to reduce rigidity, tremors, sialorrhea, and hyperhidrosis associated with parkinsonism; as a drying agent in acute rhinitis

Injection: Preoperative antimuscarinic to reduce secretions and block cardiac vagal inhibitory reflexes; to improve radiologic visibility of the kidneys; symptomatic relief of biliary and renal colic; reduce GI motility to facilitate diagnostic procedures (ie, endoscopy, hypotonic duodenography); reduce pain and hypersecretion in pancreatitis, certain cases of partial heart block associated with vagal activity; reversal of neuromuscular blockade

Local Anesthetic/Vasoconstrictor Precautions No information available to require special precautions

Effects on Dental Treatment Key adverse event(s) related to dental treatment: Xerostomia (normal salivary flow resumes upon discontinuation).

Mechanism of Action Blocks the action of acetylcholine at parasympathetic sites in smooth muscle, secretory glands and the CNS; increases cardiac output, dries secretions, antagonizes histamine and serotonin

Pregnancy Risk Factor C

Hyoscyamine, Atropine, Scopolamine, and Phenobarbital

(hye oh SYE a meen, A troe peen, skoe POL a meen, & fee noe BAR bi tal)

Related Information

Atropine *on page 161*
Hyoscyamine *on page 803*
Phenobarbital *on page 1221*
Scopolamine *on page 1380*

U.S. Brand Names Donnatal®; Donnatal Extentabs®

Generic Available Yes: Elixir, tablet

Synonyms Atropine, Hyoscyamine, Scopolamine, and Phenobarbital; Belladonna Alkaloids With Phenobarbital; Phenobarbital, Hyoscyamine, Atropine, and Scopolamine; Scopolamine, Hyoscyamine, Atropine, and Phenobarbital

Pharmacologic Category Anticholinergic Agent; Antispasmodic Agent, Gastrointestinal

Use Adjunct in treatment of irritable bowel syndrome, acute enterocolitis, duodenal ulcer

Local Anesthetic/Vasoconstrictor Precautions No information available to require special precautions

Effects on Dental Treatment Key adverse event(s) related to dental treatment: Xerostomia, dry throat (normal salivary flow resumes upon discontinuation).

Common Adverse Effects Frequency not defined.

Cardiovascular: Palpitation, tachycardia

Central nervous system: Dizziness, drowsiness, headache, insomnia, nervousness

Dermatologic: Urticaria

Gastrointestinal: Bloating, constipation, nausea, taste loss, vomiting, xerostomia

Genitourinary: Impotence, urinary hesitancy, urinary retention

Neuromuscular & skeletal: Musculoskeletal pain, weakness

Ocular: Blurred vision, cycloplegia, mydriasis, ocular tension increased

Miscellaneous: Allergic reaction (may be severe), anaphylaxis, lactation suppressed, diaphoresis decreased

Mechanism of Action A fixed combination of belladonna alkaloids and phenobarbital which provides anticholinergic/antispasmodic action and mild sedation.

Drug Interactions

Cytochrome P450 Effect: Phenobarbital: **Substrate** (minor) of CYP2C8/9, 2C19, 2E1; **Induces** CYP1A2 (strong), 2A6 (strong), 2B6 (strong), 2C8/9 (strong), 3A4 (strong)

Increased Effect/Toxicity: Anticholinergic effects may be additive with other anticholinergic agents, or drugs with significant anticholinergic activity (antihistamine, tricyclic antidepressants, phenothiazines). When combined with other CNS depressants, ethanol, narcotic analgesics, antidepressants, or benzodiazepines, additive respiratory and CNS depression may occur. Barbiturates may enhance the hepatotoxic potential of acetaminophen overdoses. Chloramphenicol, MAO inhibitors, valproic acid, and felbamate may inhibit barbiturate metabolism. Barbiturates may impair the absorption of griseofulvin, and may enhance the nephrotoxic effects of methoxyflurane. Concurrent use of phenobarbital with meperidine may result in increased CNS depression. Concurrent use of phenobarbital with primidone may result in elevated phenobarbital serum concentrations. The levels/effects of phenobarbital may be increased by delavirdine, fluconazole, fluvoxamine, gemfibrozil, isoniazid, omeprazole, ticlopidine, and other CYP2C19 inhibitors.

Decreased Effect: Barbiturates may increase the metabolism of estrogens and reduce the efficacy of oral contraceptives; an alternative method of contraception should be considered. Barbiturates inhibit the hypoprothrombinemic effects of oral anticoagulants via increased metabolism. Barbiturates may enhance the metabolism of methadone resulting in methadone withdrawal. The levels/effects of phenobarbital may be decreased by aminoglutethimide, carbamazepine, phenytoin, rifampin, and other CYP2C19 inducers.

Phenobarbital may decrease the levels/effects of aminophylline, amiodarone, benzodiazepines, bupropion, calcium channel blockers, carbamazepine, citalopram, clarithromycin, cyclosporine diazepam, efavirenz, erythromycin, estrogens, fluoxetine, fluvoxamine, glimepiride, glipizide, ifosfamide, losartan, methsuximide, mirtazapine, nateglinide, nefazodone, nevirapine, phenytoin, pioglitazone, promethazine, propranolol, protease inhibitors, proton pump inhibitors, rifampin, ropinirole, rosiglitazone, selegiline, sertraline, sulfonamides, tacrolimus, theophylline, venlafaxine. voriconazole warfarin, zafirlukast, and other CYP1A2, 2A6, 2B6, 2C8/9, or 3A4 substrates.

Pregnancy Risk Factor C

Hyoscyamine, Methenamine, Sodium Biphosphate, Phenyl Salicylate, and Methylene Blue *see* Methenamine, Sodium Biphosphate, Phenyl Salicylate, Methylene Blue, and Hyoscyamine *on page 1008*

Hyoscyamine Sulfate *see* Hyoscyamine *on page 803*

Hyosine *see* Hyoscyamine *on page 803*

Hypaque™-76 *see* Diatrizoate Meglumine and Diatrizoate Sodium *on page 453*

Hypaque-Cysto™ *see* Diatrizoate Meglumine *on page 453*

Hypaque™ Meglumine *see* Diatrizoate Meglumine *on page 453*

Hypaque™ Sodium *see* Diatrizoate Sodium *on page 454*

Hyperstat® *see* Diazoxide *on page 457*

HypoTears [OTC] *see* Artificial Tears *on page 143*

HypoTears PF [OTC] *see* Artificial Tears *on page 143*

Hypromellose *see* Hydroxypropyl Methylcellulose *on page 800*

Hytakerol® [DSC] *see* Dihydrotachysterol *on page 478*

HyTan™ *see* Hydrocodone and Chlorpheniramine *on page 784*

Hytinic® [OTC] *see* Polysaccharide-Iron Complex *on page 1254*

Hytone® *see* Hydrocortisone *on page 793*

Hytrin® *see* Terazosin *on page 1458*

Hyzaar® *see* Losartan and Hydrochlorothiazide *on page 952*

Ibandronate (eye BAN droh nate)

U.S. Brand Names Boniva®
Canadian Brand Names Bondronat®
Generic Available No
Synonyms Ibandronate Sodium
Pharmacologic Category Bisphosphonate Derivative
Use Treatment and prevention of osteoporosis in postmenopausal females
Unlabeled/Investigational Use Hypercalcemia of malignancy; corticosteroid-induced osteoporosis; Paget's disease; reduce bone pain and skeletal complications from metastatic bone disease
Local Anesthetic/Vasoconstrictor Precautions No information available to require special precautions
Effects on Dental Treatment Osteonecrosis of the jaw (ONJ), generally associated with local infection and/or tooth extraction and often with delayed healing, has been reported in patients taking bisphosphonates. Most reported cases of bisphosphonate-associated osteonecrosis have been in cancer patients treated with intravenous bisphosphonates. However, some have occurred in patients with postmenopausal osteoporosis taking oral bisphosphonates. Dental surgery may exacerbate ONJ. For patients requiring dental procedures, there are no data available to suggest whether discontinuation of bisphosphonate treatment reduces the risk of ONJ. See Dental Comment.
Common Adverse Effects Percentages vary based on frequency of administration (daily vs monthly). Unless specified, percentages are reported with oral use.
>10%:
  Gastrointestinal: Dyspepsia (6% to 12%)
  Neuromuscular & skeletal: Back pain (4% to 14%)
1% to 10%:
  Central nervous system: Headache (3% to 7%), dizziness (1% to 4%), insomnia (1% to 2%)
  Dermatologic: Rash (1% to 2%)
  Endocrine & metabolic: Hypercholesterolemia (5%)
  Gastrointestinal: Abdominal pain (5% to 8%), diarrhea (4% to 7%), nausea (5%), tooth disorder (4%), vomiting (3%), constipation (3% to 4%)
  Genitourinary: Urinary tract infection (2% to 6%)
  Hepatic: Alkaline phosphatase decreased (frequency not defined)
  Local: Injection-site reaction (<2%)
  Neuromuscular & skeletal: Pain in extremity (8%), myalgia (1% to 6%), joint disorder (4%), weakness (4%), muscle cramp (2%)
  Respiratory: Bronchitis (3% to 10%), pneumonia (6%), pharyngitis/nasopharyngitis (3% to 4%), upper respiratory infection (2%)
  Miscellaneous: Acute phase reaction (I.V. 10%; oral 4%), allergic reaction (3%), flu-like syndrome (1% to 3%)
(Continued)

Ibandronate *(Continued)*

Dosage

Oral:

Treatment of postmenopausal osteoporosis: 2.5 mg/day or 150 mg once a month

Prevention of postmenopausal osteoporosis: 2.5 mg/day; 150 mg once a month may be considered

I.V.: Treatment of postmenopausal osteoporosis: 3 mg every 3 months

Dosage adjustment in renal impairment:

Mild or moderate impairment: Dosing adjustment not needed

Severe impairment (Cl_{cr} <30 mL/minute): Use not recommended

Dosage adjustment in hepatic impairment: Dosing adjustment not needed

Mechanism of Action
A bisphosphonate which inhibits bone resorption via actions on osteoclasts or on osteoclast precursors; decreases the rate of bone resorption, leading to an indirect increase in bone mineral density.

Contraindications
Hypersensitivity to ibandronate, other bisphosphonates, or any component of the formulation; hypocalcemia; oral tablets are also contraindicated in patients unable to stand or sit upright for at least 60 minutes

Warnings/Precautions
Hypocalcemia must be corrected before therapy initiation. Ensure adequate calcium and vitamin D intake. Bisphosphonate therapy has been associated with osteonecrosis, primarily of the jaw; this has been observed mostly in cancer patients, but also in patients with postmenopausal osteoporosis and other diagnoses. Dental exams and preventative dentistry should be performed prior to placing patients with risk factors on chronic bisphosphonate therapy. Invasive dental procedures should be avoided during treatment.

Oral bisphosphonates may cause dysphagia, esophagitis, esophageal or gastric ulcer; risk may increase in patients unable to comply with dosing instructions. Intravenous bisphosphonates may cause transient decreases in serum calcium and have also been associated with renal toxicity.

Use not recommended with severe renal impairment (Cl_{cr} <30 mL/minute or serum creatinine >2.3 mg/dL). Safety and efficacy have not been established in patients <18 years of age.

Drug Interactions

Increased Effect/Toxicity: Aminoglycosides may lower serum calcium levels with prolonged administration; concomitant use may have an additive hypocalcemic effect. Nonsteroidal anti-inflammatory drugs may enhance the gastrointestinal adverse/toxic effects (increased incidence of GI ulcers) of bisphosphonate derivatives. Bisphosphonate derivatives may enhance the hypocalcemic effect of phosphate supplements.

Decreased Effect: The following agents may decrease the absorption of oral bisphosphonate derivatives: Antacids (aluminum, calcium, magnesium), oral calcium salts, oral iron salts, and oral magnesium salts

Ethanol/Nutrition/Herb Interactions

Ethanol: Avoid ethanol (may increase risk of osteoporosis).

Food: May reduce absorption; mean oral bioavailability is decreased up to 90% when given with food.

Dietary Considerations
Supplemental calcium or vitamin D may be required if dietary intake is not adequate. Tablet should be taken with a full glass (6-8 oz) of plain water, at least 60 minutes prior to any food, beverages, or medications. Mineral water with a high calcium content should be avoided.

Pharmacodynamics/Kinetics

Distribution: Terminal V_d: 90 L; 40% to 50% of circulating ibandronate binds to bone

Protein binding: 85% to 99%

Bioavailability: Oral: Reduced by 90% following standard breakfast

Half-life elimination:

Oral: 150 mg dose: Terminal: 37-157 hours

I.V.: Terminal: ~5-25 hours

Time to peak, plasma: Oral: 0.5-2 hours

Excretion: Urine (50% to 60% of absorbed dose, excreted as unchanged drug); feces (unabsorbed drug)

Pregnancy Risk Factor C

Dosage Forms
INJ, solution: 1 mg/mL (3 mL) [prefilled syringe].**TAB:** 2.5 mg, 150 mg

Dental Comment Novartis Pharmaceuticals Corporation has notified dental health professionals of the risk of osteonecrosis of the jaw (ONJ) and the use of the bisphosphonates, pamidronate, and zoledronic acid. This warning has not be issued for ibandronate.

Previously, Novartis and the Food and Drug Administration (FDA) had notified healthcare providers of a serious adverse event related to the use of bisphosphonates. Osteonecrosis of the jaw has been reported in patients with cancer who were receiving chemotherapy, corticosteroids, and chronic bisphosphonate therapy. The bisphosphonates involved were pamidronate and zoledronic acid. To date, there are no reported associations between iban-dronate and osteonecrosis of the jaw. Dental exams and preventative dentistry should be performed prior to placing patients with risk factors (chemotherapy, corticosteroids, poor oral hygiene) on chronic bisphosphonate therapy. Invasive dental procedures should be avoided during treatment. Product labelings for pamidronate (Aredia®) and zoledronic acid (Zometa®) have been updated. Recently, 63 cases of osteonecrosis associated with the use of bisphosphonates were published (Ruggiero, 2004). In a retrospective review, 56 of the patients received intravenous bisphosphonates for at least one year and 7 patients were on chronic oral therapy. The presenting symptom was a nonhealing extraction socket or an exposed jawbone. These lesions did not show evidence of metastatic disease and required removal of involved bone in most cases.

Bisphosphonates are widely used in the management of metastatic bone disease to treat hypercalcemia associated with malignancies and to treat osteo-porosis. In the report by Ruggiero et al, the cluster of patients observed to have necrotic lesions in the jaw shared only one common clinical feature, all received chronic bisphosphonate therapy. The necrosis detected was typical of osteora-dionecrosis. It was suggested that because of the trend in the use of chronic bisphosphonate therapy, the observation of an associated risk of osteonecrosis of the jaw should alert practitioners to monitor for this previously unrecognized potential complication.

Selected Readings

Barrett J, Worth E, Bauss F, et al, "Ibandronate: A Clinical Pharmacological and Pharmacokinetic Update," *J Clin Pharmacol*, 2004, 44(9):951-65.

French AE, Kaplan N, Lishner M, et al, "Taking Bisphosphonates During Pregnancy," *Can Fam Physician*, 2003, 49:1281-2.

Ruggiero SL, Mehrotra B, Rosenberg TJ, et al, "Osteonecrosis of the Jaws Associated With the Use of Bisphosphonates: A Review of 63 Cases," *J Oral Maxillofac Surg*, 2004, 62(5):527-34.

Ibandronate Sodium *see* Ibandronate *on page 805*

Iberet® [OTC] *see* Vitamins (Multiple/Oral) *on page 1582*

Iberet®-500 [OTC] *see* Vitamins (Multiple/Oral) *on page 1582*

Ibidomide Hydrochloride *see* Labetalol *on page 891*

Ibritumomab (ib ri TYOO mo mab)

U.S. Brand Names Zevalin®

Generic Available No

Synonyms Ibritumomab Tiuxetan; In-111 Zevalin; Y-90 Zevalin

Pharmacologic Category Antineoplastic Agent, Monoclonal Antibody; Radio-pharmaceutical

Use Treatment of relapsed or refractory low-grade, follicular, or transformed B-cell non-Hodgkin's lymphoma

Local Anesthetic/Vasoconstrictor Precautions No information available to require special precautions

Effects on Dental Treatment Key adverse event(s) related to dental treatment: Hypotension, cough, throat irritation, rhinitis.

Common Adverse Effects Severe, potentially life-threatening allergic reactions have occurred in association with infusions. Also refer to Rituximab monograph.

>10%:

Central nervous system: Chills (24%), fever (17%), pain (13%), headache (12%)

Gastrointestinal: Nausea (31%), abdominal pain (16%), vomiting (12%)

Hematologic: Thrombocytopenia (95%), neutropenia (77%), anemia (61%)

Myelosuppressive:

WBC: Severe

Platelets: Severe

Nadir: 7-9 weeks

Recovery: 22-35 days

Neuromuscular & skeletal: Weakness (43%)

Respiratory: Dyspnea (14%)

Miscellaneous: Infection (29%)

1% to 10%:

Cardiovascular: Peripheral edema (8%), hypotension (6%), flushing (6%), angioedema (5%)

Central nervous system: Dizziness (10%), insomnia (5%), anxiety (4%)

(Continued)

Ibritumomab *(Continued)*

Dermatologic: Pruritus (9%), rash (8%), urticaria (4%), petechia (3%)

Gastrointestinal: Diarrhea (9%), anorexia (8%), abdominal distension (5%), constipation (5%), dyspepsia (4%), melena (2%; life threatening in 1%), gastrointestinal hemorrhage (1%)

Hematologic: Bruising (7%), pancytopenia (2%), secondary malignancies (2%)

Neuromuscular & skeletal: Back pain (8%), arthralgia (7%), myalgia (7%)

Respiratory: Cough (10%), throat irritation (10%), rhinitis (6%), bronchospasm (5%), epistaxis (3%), apnea (1%)

Miscellaneous: Diaphoresis (4%), allergic reaction (2%; life-threatening in 1%)

Mechanism of Action Ibritumomab is a monoclonal antibody directed against the CD20 antigen found on B lymphocytes (normal and malignant). Ibritumomab binding induces apoptosis in B lymphocytes *in vitro*. It is combined with the chelator tiuxetan, which acts as a specific chelation site for either Indium-111 (In-111) or Yttrium-90 (Y-90). The monoclonal antibody acts as a delivery system to direct the radioactive isotope to the targeted cells, however, binding has been observed in lymphoid cells throughout the body and in lymphoid nodules in organs such as the large and small intestines. Indium-111 is a gamma-emitter used to assess biodistribution of ibritumomab, while Y-90 emits beta particles. Beta-emission induces cellular damage through the formation of free radicals (in both target cells and surrounding cells).

Drug Interactions

Increased Effect/Toxicity: Due to the high incidence of thrombocytopenia associated with ibritumomab, the use of agents which decrease platelet function may be associated with a higher risk of bleeding (includes aspirin, NSAIDs, glycoprotein IIb/IIIa antagonists, clopidogrel and ticlopidine). In addition, the risk of bleeding may be increased with anticoagulant agents, including heparin, low molecular weight heparins, thrombolytics, and warfarin. The safety of live viral vaccines has not been established.

Decreased Effect: Response to vaccination may be impaired.

Pharmacodynamics/Kinetics

Duration: Beta cell recovery begins in ~12 weeks; generally in normal range within 9 months

Distribution: To lymphoid cells throughout the body and in lymphoid nodules in organs such as the large and small intestines, spleen, testes, and liver

Metabolism: Has not been characterized; the product of yttrium-90 radioactive decay is zirconium-90 (nonradioactive); Indium-111 decays to cadmium-111 (nonradioactive)

Half-life elimination: Y-90 ibritumomab: 30 hours; Indium-111 decays with a physical half-life of 67 hours; Yttrium-90 decays with a physical half-life of 64 hours

Excretion: A median of 7.2% of the radiolabeled activity was excreted in urine over 7 days

Pregnancy Risk Factor D

Ibritumomab Tiuxetan *see* Ibritumomab *on page 807*

Ibu-200 [OTC] *see* Ibuprofen *on page 808*

Ibuprofen *(eye byoo PROE fen)*

Related Information

Oral Pain *on page 1692*

Rheumatoid Arthritis, Osteoarthritis, and Osteoporosis *on page 1668*

Temporomandibular Dysfunction (TMD) *on page 1724*

Related Sample Prescriptions

Mild/Moderate Oral Pain *on page 1734*

Moderate/Moderately Severe Oral Pain *on page 1734*

U.S. Brand Names Advil® [OTC]; Advil® Children's [OTC]; Advil® Infants' [OTC]; Advil® Junior [OTC]; Advil® Migraine [OTC]; ElixSure™ IB [OTC]; Genpril® [OTC]; Ibu-200 [OTC]; I-Prin [OTC]; Midol® Cramp and Body Aches [OTC]; Motrin®; Motrin® Children's [OTC]; Motrin® IB [OTC]; Motrin® Infants' [OTC]; Motrin® Junior Strength [OTC]; Proprinal [OTC]; Ultraprin [OTC]

Canadian Brand Names Advil®; Apo-Ibuprofen®; Motrin® (Children's); Motrin® IB; Novo-Profen; Nu-Ibuprofen

Generic Available Yes: Caplet, suspension, tablet

Synonyms *p*-Isobutylhydratropic Acid

Pharmacologic Category Nonsteroidal Anti-inflammatory Drug (NSAID), Oral

Dental Use Management of pain and swelling

Use Inflammatory diseases and rheumatoid disorders including juvenile rheumatoid arthritis, mild to moderate pain, fever, dysmenorrhea

Unlabeled/Investigational Use Cystic fibrosis, gout, ankylosing spondylitis, acute migraine headache

Local Anesthetic/Vasoconstrictor Precautions No information available to require special precautions

Effects on Dental Treatment NSAID formulations are known to reversibly decrease platelet aggregation via mechanisms different than observed with aspirin. The dentist should be aware of the potential of abnormal coagulation. Caution should also be exercised in the use of NSAIDs in patients already on anticoagulant therapy with drugs such as warfarin (Coumadin®). See Dental Comment.

Significant Adverse Effects

1% to 10%:

Cardiovascular: Edema (1% to 3%)

Central nervous system: Dizziness (3% to 9%), headache (1% to 3%), nervousness (1% to 3%)

Dermatologic: Itching (1% to 3%), rash (3% to 9%)

Endocrine & metabolic: Fluid retention (1% to 3%)

Gastrointestinal: Dyspepsia (1% to 3%), vomiting (1% to 3%), abdominal pain/cramps/distress (1% to 3%), heartburn (3% to 9%), nausea (3% to 9%), diarrhea (1% to 3%), constipation (1% to 3%), flatulence (1% to 3%), epigastric pain (3% to 9%), appetite decreased (1% to 3%)

Otic: Tinnitus (3% to 9%)

<1% (Limited to important or life-threatening): Acute renal failure, agranulocytosis, anaphylaxis, aplastic anemia, azotemia, blurred vision, bone marrow suppression, confusion, creatinine clearance decreased, duodenal ulcer, edema, eosinophilia, epistaxis, erythema multiforme, gastric ulcer, GI bleed, GI hemorrhage, GI ulceration, hallucinations, hearing decreased, hematuria, hematocrit decreased, hemoglobin decreased, hemolytic anemia, hepatitis, hypertension, inhibition of platelet aggregation, jaundice, liver function tests abnormal, leukopenia, melena, neutropenia, pancreatitis, photosensitivity, Stevens-Johnson syndrome, thrombocytopenia, toxic amblyopia, toxic epidermal necrolysis, urticaria, vesiculobullous eruptions, vision changes

Restrictions A medication guide should be dispensed with each prescription. A template for the required MedGuide can be found on the FDA website at: http://www.fda.gov/medwatch/SAFETY/2005/safety05.htm#NSAID

Dental Usual Dosing

Analgesic/pain/fever: Oral:

Children: 4-10 mg/kg/dose every 6-8 hours

Adults: 200-400 mg/dose every 4-6 hours (maximum daily dose: 1.2 g, unless directed by physician)

OTC labeling (analgesic, antipyretic): Oral:

Children 6 months to 11 years: See table; use of weight to select dose is preferred; doses may be repeated every 6-8 hours (maximum: 4 doses/day)

Children ≥12 years and Adults: 200 mg every 4-6 hours as needed (maximum: 1200 mg/24 hours)

Ibuprofen Dosing

Weight (lb)	Age	Dosage (mg)
12-17	6-11 mo	50
18-23	12-23 mo	75
24-35	2-3 y	100
35-47	4-5 y	150
48-59	6-8 y	200
60-71	9-10 y	250
72-95	11 y	300

Dosage Oral:

Children:

Antipyretic: 6 months to 12 years: Temperature <102.5°F (39°C): 5 mg/kg/dose; temperature >102.5°F: 10 mg/kg/dose given every 6-8 hours (maximum daily dose: 40 mg/kg/day)

Juvenile rheumatoid arthritis: 30-50 mg/kg/24 hours divided every 8 hours; start at lower end of dosing range and titrate upward (maximum: 2.4 g/day)

Analgesic: 4-10 mg/kg/dose every 6-8 hours

Cystic fibrosis (unlabeled use): Chronic (>4 years) twice daily dosing adjusted to maintain serum levels of 50-100 mcg/mL has been associated with slowing of disease progression in younger patients with mild lung disease

(Continued)

Ibuprofen *(Continued)*

OTC labeling (analgesic, antipyretic):

Children 6 months to 11 years: See table on previous page. Use of weight to select dose is preferred; doses may be repeated every 6-8 hours (maximum: 4 doses/day)

Children ≥12 years: 200 mg every 4-6 hours as needed (maximum: 1200 mg/24 hours)

Adults:

Inflammatory disease: 400-800 mg/dose 3-4 times/day (maximum dose: 3.2 g/day)

Analgesia/pain/fever/dysmenorrhea: 200-400 mg/dose every 4-6 hours (maximum daily dose: 1.2 g, unless directed by physician)

OTC labeling (analgesic, antipyretic): 200 mg every 4-6 hours as needed (maximum: 1200 mg/24 hours)

Dosing adjustment/comments in severe hepatic impairment: Avoid use

Mechanism of Action Inhibits prostaglandin synthesis by decreasing the activity of the enzyme, cyclooxygenase, which results in decreased formation of prostaglandin precursors

Contraindications Hypersensitivity to ibuprofen, aspirin, other NSAIDs, or any component of the formulation; perioperative pain in the setting of coronary artery bypass surgery (CABG); pregnancy (3rd trimester)

Warnings/Precautions NSAIDs are associated with an increased risk of adverse cardiovascular events, including MI, stroke, and new onset or worsening of pre-existing hypertension. Risk may be increased with duration of use or pre-existing cardiovascular risk-factors or disease. Carefully evaluate individual cardiovascular risk profiles prior to prescribing. Use caution with fluid retention, CHF or hypertension.

Use of NSAIDs can compromise existing renal function. Renal toxicity can occur in patient with impaired renal function, dehydration, heart failure, liver dysfunction, those taking diuretics and ACEI and the elderly. Rehydrate patient before starting therapy. Monitor renal function closely. Ibuprofen is not recommended for patients with advanced renal disease.

NSAIDs may increase risk of gastrointestinal irritation, ulceration, bleeding, and perforation. These events may occur at any time during therapy and without warning. Use caution with a history of GI disease (bleeding or ulcers), concurrent therapy with aspirin, anticoagulants and/or corticosteroids, smoking, use of alcohol, the elderly or debilitated patients.

Use the lowest effective dose for the shortest duration of time, consistent with individual patient goals, to reduce risk of cardiovascular or GI adverse events. Alternate therapies should be considered for patients at high risk.

NSAIDs may cause serious skin adverse events including exfoliative dermatitis, Stevens-Johnson syndrome (SJS) and toxic epidermal necrolysis (TEN). Anaphylactoid reactions may occur, even without prior exposure; patients with "aspirin triad" (bronchial asthma, aspirin intolerance, rhinitis) may be at increased risk. Do not use in patients who experience bronchospasm, asthma, rhinitis, or urticaria with NSAID or aspirin therapy.

Use with caution in patients with decreased hepatic function. Closely monitor patients with any abnormal LFT. Severe hepatic reactions (eg, fulminant hepatitis, liver failure) have occurred with NSAID use, rarely; discontinue if signs or symptoms of liver disease develop, or if systemic manifestations occur.

The elderly are at increased risk for adverse effects (especially peptic ulceration, CNS effects, renal toxicity) from NSAIDs even at low doses.

Withhold for at least 4-6 half-lives prior to surgical or dental procedures.

OTC labeling: Prior to self-medication, patients should contact health care provider if they have had recurring stomach pain or upset, ulcers, bleeding problems, high blood pressure, heart or kidney disease, other serious medical problems, are currently taking a diuretic, or are ≥60 years of age. Recommended dosages should not be exceeded, due to an increased risk of GI bleeding. Consuming ≥3 alcoholic beverages/day or taking longer than recommended may increase the risk of GI bleeding. When used for self-medication, patients should contact healthcare provider if used for fever lasting >3 days or for pain lasting >10 days in adults or >3 days in children. In children with a sore throat, do not use for >2 days or administer to children <3 years of age unless instructed by healthcare provider. Consult healthcare provider when sore throat pain is severe, persistent, or accompanied by fever, headache, nausea, and/or vomiting.

Drug Interactions Substrate (minor) of CYP2C8/9, 2C19; **Inhibits** CYP2C8/9 (strong)

ACE inhibitors: Antihypertensive effects may be decreased by concurrent therapy with NSAIDs; monitor blood pressure.

Angiotensin II antagonists: Antihypertensive effects may be decreased by concurrent therapy with NSAIDs; monitor blood pressure.

Anticoagulants (warfarin, heparin, LMWHs) in combination with NSAIDs can cause increased risk of bleeding.

Antiplatelet drugs (ticlopidine, clopidogrel, aspirin, abciximab, dipyridamole, eptifibatide, tirofiban) can cause an increased risk of bleeding.

Aspirin: Ibuprofen and other COX-1 inhibitors may reduce the cardioprotective effects of aspirin. Avoid giving prior to aspirin therapy or on a regular basis in patients with CAD.

Beta-blockers: NSAIDs may decrease the antihypertensive effect of beta-blockers. Monitor.

Cholestyramine (and other bile acid sequestrants): May decrease the absorption of NSAIDs. Separate by at least 2 hours.

Corticosteroids: May increase the risk of GI ulceration; avoid concurrent use

Cyclosporine: NSAIDs may increase serum creatinine, potassium, blood pressure, and cyclosporine levels; monitor cyclosporine levels and renal function carefully.

CYP2C8/9 substrates: Ibuprofen may increase the levels/effects of CYP2C8/9 substrates. Example substrates include amiodarone, fluoxetine, glimepiride, glipizide, nateglinide, phenytoin, pioglitazone, rosiglitazone, sertraline, and warfarin.

Hydralazine's antihypertensive effect is decreased; avoid concurrent use

Lithium levels can be increased; avoid concurrent use if possible or monitor lithium levels and adjust dose. Sulindac may have the least effect. When NSAID is stopped, lithium will need adjustment again.

Loop diuretics efficacy (diuretic and antihypertensive effect) is reduced. Indomethacin reduces this efficacy, however, it may be anticipated with any NSAID.

Methotrexate: Severe bone marrow suppression, aplastic anemia, and GI toxicity have been reported with concomitant NSAID therapy. Avoid use during moderate or high-dose methotrexate (increased and prolonged methotrexate levels). NSAID use during low-dose treatment of rheumatoid arthritis has not been fully evaluated; extreme caution is warranted.

Warfarin's INRs may be increased by piroxicam. Other NSAIDs may have the same effect depending on dose and duration. Monitor INR closely. Use the lowest dose of NSAIDs possible and for the briefest duration. May alter the anticoagulant effects of warfarin; concurrent use with other antiplatelet agents or anticoagulants may increase risk of bleeding.

Ethanol/Nutrition/Herb Interactions

Ethanol: Avoid ethanol (may enhance gastric mucosal irritation).

Food: Ibuprofen peak serum levels may be decreased if taken with food.

Herb/Nutraceutical: Avoid alfalfa, anise, bilberry, bladderwrack, bromelain, cat's claw, celery, coleus, cordyceps, dong quai, evening primrose, feverfew, fenugreek, garlic, ginger, ginkgo biloba, red clover, horse chestnut, grapeseed, green tea, ginseng, guggul, horse chestnut seed, horseradish, licorice, prickly ash, red clover, reishi, SAMe, sweet clover, turmeric, white willow (all have additional antiplatelet activity).

Dietary Considerations Should be taken with food. Chewable tablets may contain phenylalanine; amount varies by product, consult manufacturers labeling.

Pharmacodynamics/Kinetics

Onset of action: Analgesic: 30-60 minutes; Anti-inflammatory: ≤7 days
  Peak effect: 1-2 weeks
Duration: 4-6 hours
Absorption: Oral: Rapid (85%)
Protein binding: 90% to 99%
Metabolism: Hepatic via oxidation
(Continued)

Ibuprofen *(Continued)*

Half-life elimination: 2-4 hours; End-stage renal disease: Unchanged
Time to peak: ~1-2 hours
Excretion: Urine (1% as free drug); some feces

Pregnancy Risk Factor C/D (3rd trimester)

Lactation Enters breast milk/use caution (AAP rates "compatible")

Breast-Feeding Considerations Limited data suggests minimal excretion in breast milk.

Dosage Forms [DSC] = Discontinued product

Caplet: 200 mg [OTC]
    Advil®: 200 mg [contains sodium benzoate]
    Ibu-200, Motrin® IB: 200 mg
    Motrin® Junior Strength: 100 mg

Capsule, liqui-gel:
    Advil®: 200 mg
    Advil® Migraine: 200 mg [solubilized ibuprofen; contains potassium 20 mg]

Gelcap:
    Advil®: 200 mg [contains coconut oil]
    Motrin® IB: 200 mg [contains benzyl alcohol] [DSC]

Suspension, oral: 100 mg/5 mL (5 mL, 120 mL, 480 mL)
    Advil® Children's: 100 mg/5 mL (60 mL, 120 mL) [contains sodium benzoate; blue raspberry, fruit, and grape flavors]
    ElixSure™ IB: 100 mg/5 mL (120 mL) [berry flavor]
    Motrin® Children's: 100 mg/5 mL (60 mL, 120 mL) [contains sodium benzoate; berry, dye free berry, bubble gum, and grape flavors]

Suspension, oral drops: 40 mg/mL (15 mL)
    Advil® Infants': 40 mg/mL (15 mL) [contains sodium benzoate; fruit and grape flavors]
    Motrin® Infants': 40 mg/mL (15 mL, 30 mL) [contains sodium benzoate; berry and dye-free berry flavors]

Tablet: 200 mg [OTC], 400 mg, 600 mg, 800 mg
    Advil®: 200 mg [contains sodium benzoate]
    Advil® Junior: 100 mg [contains sodium benzoate; coated tablets]
    Genpril®, I-Prin, Midol® Cramp and Body Aches, Motrin® IB, Proprinal, Ultraprin: 200 mg
    Motrin®: 400 mg, 600 mg, 800 mg

Tablet, chewable:
    Advil® Children's: 50 mg [contains phenylalanine 2.1 mg; grape flavors]
    Advil® Junior: 100 mg [contains phenylalanine 4.2 mg; grape flavors]
    Motrin® Children's: 50 mg [contains phenylalanine 1.4 mg; grape and orange flavor]
    Motrin® Junior Strength: 100 mg [contains phenylalanine 2.1 mg; grape and orange flavors]

Dental Comment Preoperative use of ibuprofen at a dose of 400-600 mg every 6 hours 24 hours before the appointment decreases postoperative edema and hastens healing time.

Selected Readings

Ahmad N, Grad HA, Haas DA, et al, "The Efficacy of Nonopioid Analgesics for Postoperative Dental Pain: A Meta-Analysis," *Anesth Prog,* 1997, 44(4):119-26.

Beaver WT, "Review of the Analgesic Efficacy of Ibuprofen," *Int J Clin Pract,* 2003, (Suppl 135):13-7.

Dionne R, "Additive Analgesia Without Opioid Side Effects," *Compend Contin Educ Dent,* 2000, 21(7):572-4, 576-7.

Dionne R, "Relative Efficacy of Selective COX-2 Inhibitors Compared With Over-The-Counter Ibuprofen," *Int J Clin Pract Suppl,* 2003, (135):18-22.

Dionne RA and Berthold CW, "Therapeutic Uses of Nonsteroidal Anti-inflammatory Drugs in Dentistry," *Crit Rev Oral Biol Med,* 2001, 12(4):315-30.

Doyle G, Jayawardena S, Ashraf E, et al, "Efficacy and Tolerability of Nonprescription Ibuprofen Versus Celecoxib for Dental Pain," *J Clin Pharmacol,* 2002, 42(8):912-9.

Gobetti JP, "Controlling Dental Pain," *J Am Dent Assoc,* 1992, 123(6):47-52.

Hersh EV, Levin LM, Cooper SA, et al, "Ibuprofen Liquigel for Oral Surgery Pain," *Clin Ther,* 2000, 22(11):1306-18.

Nguyen AM, Graham DY, Gage T, et al, "Nonsteroidal Anti-inflammatory Drug Use in Dentistry: Gastrointestinal Implications," *Gen Dent,* 1999, 47(6):590-6.

Olson NZ, Otero AM, Marrero I, et al, "Onset of Analgesia for Liquigel Ibuprofen 400 mg, Acetaminophen 1000 mg, Ketoprofen 25 mg, and Placebo in the Treatment of Postoperative Dental Pain," *J Clin Pharmacol,* 2001, 41(11):1238-47.

Pearlman B, Boyatzis S, Daly C, et al, "The Analgesic Efficacy of Ibuprofen in Periodontal Surgery: A Multicentre Study," *Aust Dent J,* 1997, 42(5):328-34.

Wynn RL, "Update on Nonprescription Pain Relievers for Dental Pain," *Gen Dent,* 2004, 52(2):94-8.

Ibuprofen and Hydrocodone see Hydrocodone and Ibuprofen *on page 787*

Ibuprofen and Oxycodone see Oxycodone and Ibuprofen *on page 1170*

Ibuprofen and Pseudoephedrine see Pseudoephedrine and Ibuprofen *on page 1311*

Ibutilide (i BYOO ti lide)

Related Information
Cardiovascular Diseases *on page 1636*
U.S. Brand Names Corvert®
Generic Available No
Synonyms Ibutilide Fumarate
Pharmacologic Category Antiarrhythmic Agent, Class III
Use Acute termination of atrial fibrillation or flutter of recent onset; the effectiveness of ibutilide has not been determined in patients with arrhythmias >90 days in duration
Local Anesthetic/Vasoconstrictor Precautions No information available to require special precautions (see Dental Comment)
Effects on Dental Treatment No significant effects or complications reported
Common Adverse Effects 1% to 10%:

Cardiovascular: Sustained polymorphic ventricular tachycardia (ie, torsade de pointes) (1.7%, often requiring cardioversion), nonsustained polymorphic ventricular tachycardia (2.7%), nonsustained monomorphic ventricular tachycardia (4.9%), ventricular extrasystoles (5.1%), nonsustained monomorphic VT (4.9%), tachycardia/supraventricular tachycardia (2.7%), hypotension (2%), bundle branch block (1.9%), AV block (1.5%), bradycardia (1.2%), QT segment prolongation, hypertension (1.2%), palpitation (1%)

Central nervous system: Headache (3.6%)

Gastrointestinal: Nausea (>1%)

Mechanism of Action Exact mechanism of action is unknown; prolongs the action potential in cardiac tissue

Drug Interactions

Increased Effect/Toxicity: Class Ia antiarrhythmic drugs (disopyramide, quinidine, and procainamide) and other class III drugs such as amiodarone and sotalol should not be given concomitantly with ibutilide due to their potential to prolong refractoriness. Signs of digoxin toxicity may be masked when coadministered with ibutilide. Toxicity of ibutilide is potentiated by concurrent administration of other drugs which may prolong QT interval: phenothiazines, tricyclic and tetracyclic antidepressants, cisapride, sparfloxacin, gatifloxacin, moxifloxacin, and erythromycin.

Pharmacodynamics/Kinetics

Onset of action: ~90 minutes after start of infusion ($\frac{1}{2}$ of conversions to sinus rhythm occur during infusion)

Distribution: V_d: 11 L/kg

Protein binding: 40%

Metabolism: Extensively hepatic; oxidation

Half-life elimination: 2-12 hours (average: 6 hours)

Excretion: Urine (82%, 7% as unchanged drug and metabolites); feces (19%)

Pregnancy Risk Factor C

Dental Comment

This drug is known to prolong the QT interval. The QT interval is measured as the time and distance between the Q point of the QRS complex and the end of the T wave in the ECG tracing. After adjustment for heart rate, the QT interval is defined as prolonged if it is more than 450 msec in men and 460 msec in women. A long QT syndrome was first described in the 1950s and 60s as a congenital syndrome involving QT interval prolongation and syncope and sudden death. Some of the congenital long QT syndromes were characterized by a peculiar electrocardiographic appearance of the QRS complex involving a premature atria beat followed by a pause, then a subsequent sinus beat showing marked QT prolongation and deformity. This type of cardiac arrhythmia was originally termed "torsade de pointes" (translated from the French as "twisting of the points").

Prolongation of the QT interval is thought to result from delayed ventricular repolarization. The repolarization process within the myocardial cell is due to the efflux of intracellular potassium. The channels associated with this current can be blocked by many drugs and predisposes the electrical propagation cycle to torsade de pointes.

Ibutilide is one of the drugs confirmed to prolong the QT interval and is accepted as having a risk of causing torsade de pointes. The risk of drug-induced torsade de pointes is extremely low when a single QT interval prolonging drug is prescribed. In terms of epinephrine, it is not known what effect vasoconstrictors in the local anesthetic regimen will have in patients with a known history of congenital prolonged QT interval or in patients taking any medication that prolongs the QT interval. Until more information is obtained, it is suggested that the clinician consult with the physician prior to the use of a vasoconstrictor in (Continued)

Ibutilide *(Continued)*

suspected patients, and that the vasoconstrictor (epinephrine, levonordefrin [Neo-Cobefrin®]) be used with caution.

Ibutilide Fumarate *see* Ibutilide *on page 813*

IC-Green® *see* Indocyanine Green *on page 830*

ICI-182,780 *see* Fulvestrant *on page 713*

ICI-204,219 *see* Zafirlukast *on page 1590*

ICI-46474 *see* Tamoxifen *on page 1443*

ICI-118630 *see* Goserelin *on page 750*

ICI-176334 *see* Bicalutamide *on page 207*

ICI-D1033 *see* Anastrozole *on page 126*

ICL670 *see* Deferasirox *on page 427*

Icodextrin *(eye KOE dex trin)*

U.S. Brand Names Extraneal®
Generic Available No
Pharmacologic Category Peritoneal Dialysate, Osmotic
Use Daily exchange for the long dwell (8- to 16-hour) during continuous ambulatory peritoneal dialysis (CAPD) or automated peritoneal dialysis (APD) for the management of end-stage renal disease (ESRD); improvement of long-dwell ultrafiltration and clearance of creatinine and urea nitrogen (compared to 4.25% dextrose) in patients with high/average or greater transport characteristics as measured by peritoneal equilibration test (PET)
Local Anesthetic/Vasoconstrictor Precautions No information available to require special precautions
Effects on Dental Treatment No significant effects or complications reported
Mechanism of Action Exerts osmotic pressure across small intercellular pores resulting in transcapillary ultrafiltration throughout the dwell while providing electrolytes and lactate for the maintenance of both the electrolyte and acid-base balance.
Pregnancy Risk Factor C

ICRF-187 *see* Dexrazoxane *on page 446*

Idamycin PFS® *see* Idarubicin *on page 814*

Idarubicin *(eye da ROO bi sin)*

U.S. Brand Names Idamycin PFS®
Canadian Brand Names Idamycin®
Mexican Brand Names Idamycin®
Generic Available Yes
Synonyms 4-Demethoxydaunorubicin; 4-DMDR; Idarubicin Hydrochloride; IDR; IMI 30; NSC-256439; SC 33428
Pharmacologic Category Antineoplastic Agent, Anthracycline; Antineoplastic Agent, Antibiotic
Use Treatment of acute leukemias (AML, ANLL, ALL), accelerated phase or blast crisis of chronic myelogenous leukemia (CML), breast cancer
Unlabeled/Investigational Use Autologous hematopoietic stem cell transplantation
Local Anesthetic/Vasoconstrictor Precautions No information available to require special precautions
Effects on Dental Treatment Key adverse event(s) related to dental treatment: Stomatitis.
Common Adverse Effects
>10%:
  Cardiovascular: Transient ECG abnormalities (supraventricular tachycardia, S-T wave changes, atrial or ventricular extrasystoles); generally asymptomatic and self-limiting. CHF, dose related. The relative cardiotoxicity of idarubicin compared to doxorubicin is unclear. Some investigators report no increase in cardiac toxicity at cumulative oral idarubicin doses up to 540 mg/m^2; other reports suggest a maximum cumulative intravenous dose of 150 mg/m^2.
  Central nervous system: Headache
  Dermatologic: Alopecia (25% to 30%), radiation recall, skin rash (11%), urticaria
  Gastrointestinal: Nausea, vomiting (30% to 60%); diarrhea (9% to 22%); stomatitis (11%); GI hemorrhage (30%)
  Genitourinary: Discoloration of urine (darker yellow)

Hematologic: Myelosuppression, primarily leukopenia; thrombocytopenia and anemia. Effects are generally less severe with oral dosing.
Nadir: 10-15 days
Recovery: 21-28 days
Hepatic: Bilirubin and transaminases increased (44%)
1% to 10%:
Central nervous system: Seizures
Neuromuscular & skeletal: Peripheral neuropathy

Mechanism of Action Similar to doxorubicin and daunorubicin; inhibition of DNA and RNA synthesis by intercalation between DNA base pairs

Drug Interactions
Decreased Effect: Patients may experience impaired immune response to vaccines; possible infection after administration of live vaccines in patients receiving immunosuppressants.

Pharmacodynamics/Kinetics
Absorption: Oral: Variable (4% to 77%; mean: ~30%)
Distribution: V_d: 64 L/kg (some reports indicate 2250 L); extensive tissue binding; CSF
Protein binding: 94% to 97%
Metabolism: Hepatic to idarubicinol (pharmacologically active)
Half-life elimination: Oral: 14-35 hours; I.V.: 12-27 hours
Time to peak, serum: 1-5 hours
Excretion:
Oral: Urine (~5% of dose; 0.5% to 0.7% as unchanged drug, 4% as idarubicinol); hepatic (8%)
I.V.: Urine (13% as idarubicinol, 3% as unchanged drug); hepatic (17%)

Pregnancy Risk Factor D

Idarubicin Hydrochloride see Idarubicin on page 814

IDEC-C2B8 see Rituximab on page 1360

IDR see Idarubicin on page 814

Ifex® see Ifosfamide on page 815

IFLrA see Interferon Alfa-2a on page 842

Ifosfamide (eye FOSS fa mide)

U.S. Brand Names Ifex®
Canadian Brand Names Ifex®
Mexican Brand Names Alquimid®; Ifolem®; Ifoxan®
Generic Available Yes
Synonyms Isophosphamide; NSC-109724; Z4942
Pharmacologic Category Antineoplastic Agent, Alkylating Agent; Antineoplastic Agent, Alkylating Agent (Nitrogen Mustard)
Use Treatment of lung cancer, Hodgkin's and non-Hodgkin's lymphoma, breast cancer, acute and chronic lymphocytic leukemias, ovarian cancer, sarcomas, pancreatic and gastric carcinomas
Orphan drug: Treatment of testicular cancer
Local Anesthetic/Vasoconstrictor Precautions No information available to require special precautions
Effects on Dental Treatment No significant effects or complications reported
Common Adverse Effects
>10%:
Central nervous system: Somnolence, confusion, hallucinations (12%)
Dermatologic: Alopecia (75% to 100%)
Endocrine & metabolic: Metabolic acidosis (31%)
Gastrointestinal: Nausea and vomiting (58%), may be more common with higher doses or bolus infusions; constipation
Genitourinary: Hemorrhagic cystitis (40% to 50%), patients should be vigorously hydrated (at least 2 L/day) and receive mesna
Hematologic: Myelosuppression, leukopenia (65% to 100%), thrombocytopenia (10%) - dose related
Onset: 7-14 days
Nadir: 21-28 days
Recovery: 21-28 days
Renal: Hematuria (6% to 92%)
1% to 10%:
Central nervous system: Hallucinations, depressive psychoses, polyneuropathy
Dermatologic: Dermatitis, nail banding/ridging, hyperpigmentation
Endocrine & metabolic: SIADH, sterility
Hematologic: Anemia
(Continued)

Ifosfamide (Continued)

> Hepatic: Transaminases increased (3%)
> Local: Phlebitis
> Renal: BUN/creatinine increased (6%)
> Respiratory: Nasal stuffiness

Mechanism of Action Causes cross-linking of strands of DNA by binding with nucleic acids and other intracellular structures; inhibits protein synthesis and DNA synthesis

Drug Interactions

Cytochrome P450 Effect: Substrate of CYP2A6 (minor), 2B6 (minor), 2C8/9 (minor), 2C19 (minor), 3A4 (major); **Inhibits** CYP3A4 (weak); **Induces** CYP2C8/9 (weak)

Increased Effect/Toxicity: CYP3A4 inducers may increase the levels/effects of acrolein (the active metabolite of ifosfamide); example inducers include aminoglutethimide, carbamazepine, nafcillin, nevirapine, phenobarbital, phenytoin, and rifamycins.

Decreased Effect: CYP3A4 inhibitors may decrease the levels/effects of acrolein (the active metabolite of ifosfamide); example inhibitors include azole antifungals, clarithromycin, diclofenac, doxycycline, erythromycin, imatinib, isoniazid, nefazodone, nicardipine, propofol, protease inhibitors, quinidine, telithromycin, and verapamil.

Pharmacodynamics/Kinetics Pharmacokinetics are dose dependent

Distribution: V_d: 5.7-49 L; does penetrate CNS, but not in therapeutic levels

Protein binding: Negligible

Metabolism: Hepatic to active metabolites phosphoramide mustard, acrolein, and inactive dichloroethylated and carboxy metabolites; acrolein is the agent implicated in development of hemorrhagic cystitis

Bioavailability: Estimated at 100%

Half-life elimination: Beta: High dose: 11-15 hours (3800-5000 mg/m^2); Lower dose: 4-7 hours (1800 mg/m^2)

Time to peak, plasma: Oral: Within 1 hour

Excretion: Urine (15% to 50% as unchanged drug, 41% as metabolites)

Pregnancy Risk Factor D

IG *see* Immune Globulin (Intramuscular) *on page 823*

IgG4-Kappa Monoclonal Antibody *see* Natalizumab *on page 1093*

IGIM *see* Immune Globulin (Intramuscular) *on page 823*

IL-1Ra *see* Anakinra *on page 125*

IL-2 *see* Aldesleukin *on page 61*

IL-11 *see* Oprelvekin *on page 1149*

Iloprost (EYE loe prost)

U.S. Brand Names Ventavis™

Generic Available No

Synonyms Iloprost Tromethamine; Prostacyclin PGI$_2$

Pharmacologic Category Prostaglandin

Use Treatment of idiopathic pulmonary arterial hypertension in patients with NYHA Class III or IV symptoms

Local Anesthetic/Vasoconstrictor Precautions No information available to require special precautions

Effects on Dental Treatment Key adverse event(s) related to dental treatment: Jaw pain (reported in >10% of patients).

Common Adverse Effects

>10%:
> Cardiovascular: Flushing (27%), hypotension (11%)
> Central nervous system: Headache (30%)
> Gastrointestinal: Nausea (13%)
> Neuromuscular & skeletal: Trismus (12%)
> Respiratory: Cough increased (39%)
> Miscellaneous: Flu-like syndrome (14%), jaw pain (12%)

1% to 10%:
> Cardiovascular: Syncope (8%), palpitation (7%)
> Central nervous system: Insomnia (8%)
> Gastrointestinal: Vomiting (7%)
> Hepatic: Alkaline phosphatase increased (6%), GGT increased (6%)
> Neuromuscular & skeletal: Back pain (7%), muscle cramps (6%)
> Respiratory: Hemoptysis (5%), pneumonia (4%)

Mechanism of Action Acutely, iloprost dilates systemic and pulmonary arterial vascular beds. In longer-term use, alters pulmonary vascular resistance and suppresses vascular smooth muscle proliferation. In addition, it is a potent endogenous inhibitor of platelet aggregation.

Drug Interactions

Increased Effect/Toxicity: Vasodilators and antihypertensives may increase the hypotensive effects; anticoagulants and antiplatelet medications may increase the risk of bleeding.

Pharmacodynamics/Kinetics

Duration: 30-90 minutes

Protein binding: ~60%, primarily to albumin

Metabolism: Hepatic via beta oxidation of the carboxyl side chain; main metabolite, tetranor-iloprost (inactive in animal studies)

Half-life elimination: 20-30 minutes

Pregnancy Risk Factor C

Iloprost Tromethamine *see* Iloprost *on page 816*

Imatinib (eye MAT eh nib)

U.S. Brand Names Gleevec®
Canadian Brand Names Gleevec®
Mexican Brand Names Gleevec®
Generic Available No
Synonyms CGP-57148B; Glivec; Imatinib Mesylate; STI571
Pharmacologic Category Antineoplastic Agent, Tyrosine Kinase Inhibitor
Use Treatment of adult patients with Philadelphia chromosome-positive (Ph+) chronic myeloid leukemia (CML) in chronic phase; treatment of patients with Ph+ CML in blast crisis, accelerated phase or chronic phase after failure of interferon therapy; treatment of pediatric patients with Ph+ CML (chronic phase) recurring following stem cell transplant or who are resistant to interferon-alpha therapy; treatment of Kit-positive (CD117) unresectable and/or (metastatic) malignant gastrointestinal stromal tumors (GIST)

Local Anesthetic/Vasoconstrictor Precautions No information available to require special precautions

Effects on Dental Treatment Key adverse event(s) related to dental treatment: Taste disturbance.

Common Adverse Effects Adverse reactions listed were established in patients with a wide variation in level of illness or specific diagnosis. In many cases, other medications were used concurrently (relationship to imatinib not specific). Effects reported in children were similar to adults, except that musculoskeletal pain was less frequent (21%) and peripheral edema was not reported in children.

>10%:

Cardiovascular: Chest pain (7% to 11%)

Central nervous system: Fatigue (30% to 53%), pyrexia (15% to 41%), headache (27% to 39%), insomnia (10% to 19%), dizziness (11% to 16%), depression (13%), anxiety (7% to 12%)

Dermatologic: Rash (36% to 53%), pruritus (8% to 14%)

Endocrine & metabolic: Fluid retention (7% to 81% includes aggravated edema, anasarca, ascites, pericardial effusion, pleural effusion, pulmonary edema); hypokalemia (6% to 13%)

Gastrointestinal: Nausea (47% to 74%), diarrhea (39% to 70%), vomiting (21% to 58%), abdominal pain (30% to 40%), flatulence (30% to 34%), weight gain (5% to 32%), dyspepsia (12% to 27%), anorexia (7% to 17%), constipation (9% to 16%), sore throat (10% to 15%), loose stools (10% to 12%)

Hematologic: Hemorrhage (24% to 53%; grade 3 or 4: 11% to 19%), neutropenia (grade 3 or 4: 3% to 48%), anemia (grade 3 or 4: <1% to 42%), thrombocytopenia (grade 3 or 4: <1% to 33%)

Hepatic: Hepatotoxicity (6% to 12%)

Neuromuscular & skeletal: Muscle cramps (28% to 62%), musculoskeletal pain (30% to 49%), arthralgia (25% to 40%), joint pain (11 to 30%), myalgia (9% to 27%), back pain (23% to 26%), weakness (15% to 21%), rigors (10% to 12%)

Ocular: Lacrimation increased (16% to 18%)

Respiratory: Cough (14% to 27%), nasopharyngitis (10% to 27%), dyspnea (12% to 21%), upper respiratory tract infection (3% to 19%), pharyngolaryngeal pain (7% to 17%), pneumonia (4% to 13%)

Miscellaneous: Superficial edema (58% to 81%), night sweats (13% to 17%), influenza (1% to 11%)

1% to 10%:

Central nervous system: CNS hemorrhage (1% to 9%), paresthesia

Dermatologic: Alopecia, dry skin

(Continued)

Imatinib *(Continued)*

Gastrointestinal: Gastrointestinal hemorrhage (1% to 8%), abdominal distension, gastroesophageal reflux, mouth ulceration

Hepatic: Ascites or pleural effusion (GIST: 4% to 6%), alkaline phosphatase increased (grade 3 or 4: <1% to 6%), ALT increased (grade 3 or 4: <1% to 7%), bilirubin increased (grade 3 or 4: <1% to 3%), AST increased (grade 3 or 4: <1% to 5%)

Neuromuscular & skeletal: Joint swelling

Ocular: Blurred vision, conjunctivitis

Renal: Albumin decreased (grade 3 or 4: 3% to 4%), creatine increased (grade 3 or 4: <1% to 2%)

Miscellaneous: Flu-like syndrome (<1% to 10%)

Mechanism of Action Inhibits Bcr-Abl tyrosine kinase, the constitutive abnormal gene product of the Philadelphia chromosome in chronic myeloid leukemia (CML). Inhibition of this enzyme blocks proliferation and induces apoptosis in Bcr-Abl positive cell lines as well as in fresh leukemic cells in Philadelphia chromosome positive CML. Also inhibits tyrosine kinase for platelet-derived growth factor (PDGF), stem cell factor (SCF), c-kit, and events mediated by PDGF and SCF.

Drug Interactions

Cytochrome P450 Effect: Substrate of CYP1A2 (minor), 2D6 (minor), 2C8/9 (minor), 2C19 (minor), 3A4 (major), **Inhibits** CYP2C8/9 (weak), 2D6 (weak), 3A4 (strong)

Increased Effect/Toxicity: Note: Drug interaction data are limited. Few clinical studies have been conducted. Many interactions listed here are derived by extrapolation from *in vitro* inhibition of cytochrome P450 isoenzymes. Chronic use of acetaminophen may increase potential for hepatotoxic reaction with imatinib (case report of hepatic failure with concurrent therapy).

Imatinib may increase the levels/effects of amiodarone, selected benzodiazepines, calcium channel blockers, cisapride, cyclosporine, ergot derivatives, fluoxetine, glimepiride, glipizide, HMG-CoA reductase inhibitors, nateglinide, phenytoin, phenytoin, propranolol, sertraline, mirtazapine, nateglinide, nefazodone, pioglitazone, rosiglitazone, sertraline, sildenafil (and other PDE-5 inhibitors), tacrolimus, telithromycin, venlafaxine, warfarin, and other substrates of CYP2C8/9 or 3A4. Selected benzodiazepines (midazolam and triazolam), cisapride, ergot alkaloids, selected HMG-CoA reductase inhibitors (lovastatin and simvastatin), mesoridazine, pimozide, and thioridazine are generally contraindicated with strong CYP3A4 inhibitors. When used with strong CYP3A4 inhibitors, dosage adjustment/limits are recommended for sildenafil and other PDE-5 inhibitors; consult individual monographs.

The levels/effects of imatinib may be increased by azole antifungals, clarithromycin, diclofenac, doxycycline, erythromycin, isoniazid, nefazodone, nicardipine, propofol, protease inhibitors, quinidine, telithromycin, verapamil, and other CYP3A4 inhibitors. Lansoprazole may enhance the dermatologic adverse effects of Imatinib.

Decreased Effect: The levels/effects of imatinib may be decreased by aminoglutethimide, carbamazepine, nafcillin, nevirapine, phenobarbital, phenytoin, rifamycins, and other CYP3A4 inducers. Dosage of imatinib should be increased by at least 50% (with careful monitoring) when used concurrently with a strong inducer. Imatinib may decrease the absorption of digoxin (tablet formulation). Imatinib may decrease the effects of levothyroxine replacement therapy.

Pharmacodynamics/Kinetics

Protein binding: 95% to albumin and alpha$_1$-acid glycoprotein

Metabolism: Hepatic via CYP3A4 (minor metabolism via CYP1A2, CYP2D6, CYP2C9, CYP2C19); primary metabolite (active): N-demethylated piperazine derivative; severe hepatic impairment (bilirubin >3-10 times ULN) increases AUC by 45% to 55% for imatinib and its active metabolite, respectively

Bioavailability: 98%

Half-life elimination: Parent drug: 18 hours; N-demethyl metabolite: 40 hours

Time to peak: 2-4 hours

Excretion: Feces (68% primarily as metabolites, 20% as unchanged drug); urine (13% primarily as metabolites, 5% as unchanged drug)

Clearance: Highly variable; Mean: 8-14 L/hour (for 50 kg and 100 kg male, respectively)

Pregnancy Risk Factor D

Imatinib Mesylate *see* Imatinib *on page 817*

IMC-C225 *see* Cetuximab *on page 308*

Imdur® *see* Isosorbide Mononitrate *on page 868*

IMI 30 *see* Idarubicin *on page 814*

IMid-3 *see* Lenalidomide *on page 903*
Imidazole Carboxamide *see* Dacarbazine *on page 415*
Imidazole Carboxamide Dimethyltriazene *see* Dacarbazine *on page 415*

Imiglucerase (i mi GLOO ser ace)

U.S. Brand Names Cerezyme®
Canadian Brand Names Cerezyme®
Generic Available No
Pharmacologic Category Enzyme
Use Long-term enzyme replacement therapy for patients with Type 1 Gaucher's disease
Local Anesthetic/Vasoconstrictor Precautions No information available to require special precautions
Effects on Dental Treatment No significant effects or complications reported
Common Adverse Effects
1% to 10%: Miscellaneous: Hypersensitivity reaction (7%; symptoms may include pruritus, flushing, urticaria, angioedema, bronchospasm)
Individual frequency not defined, but <1.5%:
  Cardiovascular: Tachycardia
  Central nervous system: Headache, dizziness, fatigue, fever
  Dermatologic: Rash, pruritus
  Gastrointestinal: Nausea, abdominal discomfort, vomiting, diarrhea
Local: Injection site burning, swelling, or sterile abscess (<1%)
  Neuromuscular & skeletal: Backache
  Miscellaneous: Anaphylactoid reactions (<1%)
Mechanism of Action Imiglucerase is an analogue of glucocerebrosidase; it is produced by recombinant DNA technology using mammalian cell culture. Glucocerebrosidase is an enzyme deficient in Gaucher's disease. It is needed to catalyze the hydrolysis of glucocerebroside to glucose and ceramide.
Pharmacodynamics/Kinetics
Distribution: V_d: 0.09-0.15 L/kg
Half-life elimination: 3.6-10.4 minutes
Pregnancy Risk Factor C

Imipemide *see* Imipenem and Cilastatin *on page 819*

Imipenem and Cilastatin (i mi PEN em & sye la STAT in)

U.S. Brand Names Primaxin®
Canadian Brand Names Primaxin®
Generic Available No
Synonyms Imipemide
Pharmacologic Category Antibiotic, Carbapenem
Use Treatment of respiratory tract, urinary tract, intra-abdominal, gynecologic, bone and joint, skin structure, and polymicrobic infections as well as bacterial septicemia and endocarditis. Antibacterial activity includes resistant gram-negative bacilli (*Pseudomonas aeruginosa* and *Enterobacter* sp), gram-positive bacteria (methicillin-sensitive *Staphylococcus aureus* and *Streptococcus* sp) and anaerobes.
Local Anesthetic/Vasoconstrictor Precautions No information available to require special precautions
Effects on Dental Treatment No significant effects or complications reported
Common Adverse Effects 1% to 10%:
Gastrointestinal: Nausea/diarrhea/vomiting (1% to 2%)
Local: Phlebitis (3%), pain at I.M. injection site (1.2%)
Mechanism of Action Inhibits bacterial cell wall synthesis by binding to one or more of the penicillin binding proteins (PBPs); which in turn inhibits the final transpeptidation step of peptidoglycan synthesis in bacterial cell walls, thus inhibiting cell wall biosynthesis. Bacteria eventually lyse due to ongoing activity of cell wall autolytic enzymes (autolysins and murein hydrolases) while cell wall assembly is arrested. Cilastatin prevents renal metabolism of imipenem by competitive inhibition of dehydropeptidase along the brush border of the renal tubules.
Drug Interactions
Decreased Effect: Imipenem may decrease valproic acid concentrations to subtherapeutic levels; monitor.
Pharmacodynamics/Kinetics
Absorption: I.M.: Imipenem: 60% to 75%; cilastatin: 95% to 100%
(Continued)

Imipenem and Cilastatin *(Continued)*

Distribution: Rapidly and widely to most tissues and fluids including sputum, pleural fluid, peritoneal fluid, interstitial fluid, bile, aqueous humor, reproductive organs, and bone; highest concentrations in pleural fluid, interstitial fluid, peritoneal fluid, and reproductive organs; low concentrations in CSF; crosses placenta; enters breast milk

Metabolism: Renally by dehydropeptidase; activity is blocked by cilastatin; cilastatin is partially metabolized renally

Half-life elimination: Both drugs: 60 minutes; prolonged with renal impairment

Excretion: Both drugs: Urine (~70% as unchanged drug)

Pregnancy Risk Factor C

Imipramine *(im IP ra meen)*

U.S. Brand Names Tofranil®; Tofranil-PM®

Canadian Brand Names Apo-Imipramine®; Novo-Pramine; Tofranil®

Mexican Brand Names Talpramin®; Tofranil®; Tofranil-PM®

Generic Available Yes: Tablet

Synonyms Imipramine Hydrochloride; Imipramine Pamoate

Pharmacologic Category Antidepressant, Tricyclic (Tertiary Amine)

Use Treatment of depression; treatment of nocturnal enuresis in children

Unlabeled/Investigational Use Analgesic for certain chronic and neuropathic pain; panic disorder; attention-deficit/hyperactivity disorder (ADHD)

Local Anesthetic/Vasoconstrictor Precautions Use with caution; epinephrine and levonordefrin have been shown to have an increased pressor response in combination with TCAs (see Dental Comment)

Effects on Dental Treatment Key adverse event(s) related to dental treatment: Xerostomia and changes in salivation (normal salivary flow resumes upon discontinuation). Long-term treatment with TCAs, such as imipramine, increases the risk of caries by reducing salivation and salivary buffer capacity. In a study by Rundergren, et al, pathological alterations were observed in the oral mucosa of 72% of 58 patients; 55% had new carious lesions after taking TCAs for a median of $5\frac{1}{2}$ years. Current research is investigating the use of the salivary stimulant pilocarpine to overcome the xerostomia from imipramine.

Common Adverse Effects Frequency not defined.

Cardiovascular: Orthostatic hypotension, arrhythmia, tachycardia, hypertension, palpitation, MI, heart block, ECG changes, CHF, stroke

Central nervous system: Dizziness, drowsiness, headache, agitation, insomnia, nightmares, hypomania, psychosis, fatigue, confusion, hallucinations, disorientation, delusions, anxiety, restlessness, seizure

Endocrine & metabolic: Gynecomastia, breast enlargement, galactorrhea, increase or decrease in libido, increase or decrease in blood sugar, SIADH

Gastrointestinal: Nausea, unpleasant taste, weight gain, xerostomia, constipation, ileus, stomatitis, abdominal cramps, vomiting, anorexia, epigastric disorders, diarrhea, black tongue, weight loss

Genitourinary: Urinary retention, impotence

Neuromuscular & skeletal: Weakness, numbness, tingling, paresthesia, incoordination, ataxia, tremor, peripheral neuropathy, extrapyramidal symptoms

Ocular: Blurred vision, disturbances of accommodation, mydriasis

Otic: Tinnitus

Miscellaneous: Diaphoresis

Restrictions A medication guide concerning the use of antidepressants in children and teenagers can be found on the FDA website at http://www.fda.gov/cder/Offices/ODS/labeling.htm. It should be dispensed to parents or guardians of children and teenagers receiving this medication.

Mechanism of Action Traditionally believed to increase the synaptic concentration of serotonin and/or norepinephrine in the central nervous system by inhibition of their reuptake by the presynaptic neuronal membrane. However, additional receptor effects have been found including desensitization of adenyl cyclase, down regulation of beta-adrenergic receptors, and down regulation of serotonin receptors.

Drug Interactions

Cytochrome P450 Effect: Substrate of CYP1A2 (minor), 2B6 (minor), 2C19 (major), 2D6 (major), 3A4 (minor); Inhibits CYP1A2 (weak), 2C19 (weak), 2D6 (moderate), 2E1 (weak)

Increased Effect/Toxicity: When used with MAO inhibitors, hyperpyrexia, hypertension, tachycardia, confusion, seizures, and **deaths have been reported** (serotonin syndrome). Serotonin syndrome has also been reported with ritonavir (rare). Use of lithium with a TCA may increase the risk for neurotoxicity.

CYP2C19 inhibitors may increase the levels/effects of imipramine; example inhibitors include delavirdine, fluconazole, fluvoxamine, gemfibrozil, isoniazid, omeprazole, and ticlopidine. Imipramine increases the effects of amphetamines, anticholinergics, other CNS depressants (sedatives, hypnotics, or ethanol), chlorpropamide, tolazamide, and warfarin. CYP2D6 inhibitors may increase the levels/effects of imipramine; example inhibitors include chlorpromazine, delavirdine, fluoxetine, miconazole, paroxetine, pergolide, quinidine, quinine, ritonavir, and ropinirole.

Phenothiazines may increase concentration of some TCAs and TCAs may increase concentration of phenothiazines. Pressor response to I.V. epinephrine, norepinephrine, and phenylephrine may be enhanced in patients receiving TCAs (**Note:** Effect is unlikely with epinephrine or levonordefrin dosages typically administered as infiltration in combination with local anesthetics).

Combined use of beta-agonists or drugs which prolong QT_c (including quinidine, procainamide, disopyramide, cisapride, sparfloxacin, gatifloxacin, moxifloxacin) with TCAs may predispose patients to cardiac arrhythmias.

Decreased Effect: CYP2C19 inducers may decrease the levels/effects of imipramine; example inducers include aminoglutethimide, carbamazepine, phenytoin, and rifampin. Imipramine inhibits the antihypertensive response to bethanidine, clonidine, debrisoquin, guanadrel, guanethidine, guanabenz, and guanfacine. Cholestyramine and colestipol may bind TCAs and reduce their absorption; monitor for altered response.

Pharmacodynamics/Kinetics
Onset of action: Peak antidepressant effect: Usually after ≥2 weeks
Absorption: Well absorbed
Distribution: Crosses placenta
Metabolism: Hepatic via CYP to desipramine (active) and other metabolites; significant first-pass effect
Half-life elimination: 6-18 hours
Excretion: Urine (as metabolites)

Pregnancy Risk Factor D

Dental Comment
This drug is known to prolong the QT interval. The QT interval is measured as the time and distance between the Q point of the QRS complex and the end of the T wave in the ECG tracing. After adjustment for heart rate, the QT interval is defined as prolonged if it is more than 450 msec in men and 460 msec in women. A long QT syndrome was first described in the 1950s and 60s as a congenital syndrome involving QT interval prolongation and syncope and sudden death. Some of the congenital long QT syndromes were characterized by a peculiar electrocardiographic appearance of the QRS complex involving a premature atria beat followed by a pause, then a subsequent sinus beat showing marked QT prolongation and deformity. This type of cardiac arrhythmia was originally termed "torsade de pointes" (translated from the French as "twisting of the points").

Prolongation of the QT interval is thought to result from delayed ventricular repolarization. The repolarization process within the myocardial cell is due to the efflux of intracellular potassium. The channels associated with this current can be blocked by many drugs and predisposes the electrical propagation cycle to torsade de pointes.

Imipramine is one of the drugs confirmed to prolong the QT interval and is accepted as having a risk of causing torsade de pointes. The risk of drug-induced torsade de pointes is extremely low when a single QT interval prolonging drug is prescribed. In terms of epinephrine, it is not known what effect vasoconstrictors in the local anesthetic regimen will have in patients with a known history of congenital prolonged QT interval or in patients taking any medication that prolongs the QT interval. Until more information is obtained, it is suggested that the clinician consult with the physician prior to the use of a vasoconstrictor in suspected patients, and that the vasoconstrictor (epinephrine, levonordefrin [Neo-Cobefrin®]) be used with caution.

Imipramine Hydrochloride see Imipramine on page 820
Imipramine Pamoate see Imipramine on page 820

Imiquimod (i mi KWI mod)

Related Information
Systemic Viral Diseases on page 1675
Viral Infections on page 1709
(Continued)

Imiquimod *(Continued)*

U.S. Brand Names Aldara™

Canadian Brand Names Aldara™

Mexican Brand Names Aldara®

Generic Available No

Pharmacologic Category Skin and Mucous Membrane Agent; Topical Skin Product

Dental Use Treatment of oral worts

Use Treatment of external genital and perianal warts/condyloma acuminata; nonhyperkeratotic, nonhypertrophic actinic keratosis on face or scalp; superficial basal cell carcinoma (sBCC) with a maximum tumor diameter of 2 cm located on the trunk, neck, or extremities (excluding hands or feet)

Unlabeled/Investigational Use Treatment of common warts

Local Anesthetic/Vasoconstrictor Precautions No information available to require special precautions

Effects on Dental Treatment No significant effects or complications reported

Significant Adverse Effects

>10%:

Local: Application site reactions are common. Frequency of reactions vary, and are related to the degree of inflammation associated with the treated disease, number of weekly applications, and individual sensitivity. Symptoms of local reaction include burning, edema, erosion, erythema, excoriation/flaking, pain, pruritus, vesicles, and scabbing. In some cases, systemic symptoms (fever, malaise, myalgia, flu-like symptoms) occur, which should prompt consideration of an interruption of therapy.

Respiratory: Upper respiratory infection (15%)

1% to 10%:

Cardiovascular: Hypertension (1% to 3%), atrial fibrillation (1%)

Central nervous system: Pain (2% to 8%), headache (4% to 8%), fatigue (1% to 2%), fever (1% to 2%), dizziness (1%)

Dermatologic: Hyperkeratosis (2% to 9%), eczema (2%), alopecia (1%), hypopigmentation (1%), rash (<1% to 2%)

Endocrine & metabolic: Hypercholesterolemia (2%), gout (1%)

Gastrointestinal: Diarrhea (3%), dyspepsia (2% to 3%), nausea (1%)

Neuromuscular & skeletal: Myalgia (1%), back pain (<1% to 4%)

Respiratory: Sinusitis (7%), rhinitis (3%), pharyngitis (2%), coughing (2%)

Miscellaneous: Influenza-like symptoms (also see Local reactions; 1% to 3%), squamous cell carcinoma (4%)

Postmarketing and/or case reports (limited to important and/or life-threatening): Agitation, angioedema, arrhythmias, capillary leak syndrome, cardiac failure, cardiomyopathy, depression, dyspnea, exfoliative dermatitis, insomnia, ischemia, liver function abnormal, MI, multiple sclerosis aggravated, paresis, proteinuria, pulmonary edema, seizure, stroke, syncope, thyroiditis

Dental Usual Dosing Common oral warts: Adults: Topical: Apply once daily prior to bedtime

Dosage Topical:

Children ≥12 years and Adults: Perianal warts/condyloma acuminata: Apply a thin layer 3 times/week prior to bedtime and leave on skin for 6-10 hours. Remove with mild soap and water. Examples of 3 times/week application schedules are: Monday, Wednesday, Friday; or Tuesday, Thursday, Saturday. Continue imiquimod treatment until there is total clearance of the genital/perianal warts for ≤16 weeks. A rest period of several days may be taken if required by the patient's discomfort or severity of the local skin reaction. Treatment may resume once the reaction subsides.

Adults:

Actinic keratosis: Apply twice weekly for 16 weeks to a treatment area on face or scalp; apply prior to bedtime and leave on skin for 8 hours. Remove with mild soap and water.

Common oral warts (dental use): Apply once daily prior to bedtime

Common warts (unlabeled use): Apply once daily prior to bedtime

Superficial basal cell carcinoma: Apply once daily prior to bedtime, 5 days/week for 6 weeks. Treatment area should include a 1 cm margin of skin around the tumor. Leave on skin for 8 hours. Remove with mild soap and water.

Mechanism of Action Mechanism of action is unknown; however, induces cytokines, including interferon-alpha and others

Contraindications Hypersensitivity to imiquimod or any component of the formulation

Warnings/Precautions Imiquimod has not been evaluated for the treatment of urethral, intravaginal, cervical, rectal, or intra-anal human papilloma viral disease and is not recommended for these conditions. Topical imiquimod is not intended for ophthalmic use. Topical imiquimod administration is not recommended until genital/perianal tissue is healed from any previous drug or surgical treatment. Imiquimod has the potential to exacerbate inflammatory conditions of the skin. Intense inflammatory reactions may occur, and may be accompanied by systemic symptoms (fever, malaise, myalgia); interruption of therapy should be considered. May increase sunburn susceptibility; patients should protect themselves from the sun. Use in basal cell carcinoma should be limited to superficial carcinomas with a maximum diameter of 2 cm. Efficacy in treatment of SBCC lesions of the face, head, and anogenital area, or other subtypes of basal cell carcinoma, have not been established. Safety and efficacy in immunosuppressed patients have not been established. Treatment of actinic keratosis should be limited to areas ≤5 cm^2. Safety and efficacy of repeated use in the same 25 cm^2 area has not been established. Safety and efficacy in patients <12 years of age have not been established.

Drug Interactions Substrate (minor) of CYP1A2, 3A4

Pharmacodynamics/Kinetics

Absorption: Minimal

Excretion: Urine and feces (<0.9%)

Pregnancy Risk Factor C

Lactation Excretion in breast milk unknown/consult prescriber

Dosage Forms Cream: 5% (12s) [contains benzyl alcohol; single-dose packets]

Imitrex® see Sumatriptan on page 1432

Immune Globulin (Intramuscular)
(i MYUN GLOB yoo lin, IN tra MUS kyoo ler)

Related Information

Immunizations (Vaccines) on page 1786
Systemic Viral Diseases on page 1675

U.S. Brand Names BayGam®

Canadian Brand Names BayGam®

Generic Available No

Synonyms Gamma Globulin; IG; IGIM; Immune Serum Globulin; ISG

Pharmacologic Category Immune Globulin

Use Household and sexual contacts of persons with hepatitis A, measles, varicella, and possibly rubella; travelers to high-risk areas outside tourist routes; staff, attendees, and parents of diapered attendees in day-care center outbreaks

For travelers, IG is not an alternative to careful selection of foods and water; immune globulin can interfere with the antibody response to parenterally administered live virus vaccines. Frequent travelers should be tested for hepatitis A antibody, immune hemolytic anemia, and neutropenia (with ITP, I.V. route is usually used).

Local Anesthetic/Vasoconstrictor Precautions No information available to require special precautions

Effects on Dental Treatment No significant effects or complications reported

Common Adverse Effects Frequency not defined.

Cardiovascular: Flushing, angioedema
Central nervous system: Chills, lethargy, fever
Dermatologic: Urticaria, erythema
Gastrointestinal: Nausea, vomiting
Local: Pain, tenderness, muscle stiffness at I.M. site
Neuromuscular & skeletal: Myalgia
Miscellaneous: Hypersensitivity reactions

Dosage I.M.:

Hepatitis A:

Pre-exposure prophylaxis upon travel into endemic areas (hepatitis A vaccine preferred):

0.02 mL/kg for anticipated risk 1-3 months

0.06 mL/kg for anticipated risk >3 months

Repeat approximate dose every 4-6 months if exposure continues

Postexposure prophylaxis: 0.02 mL/kg given within 7 days of exposure

Measles:

Prophylaxis: 0.25 mL/kg/dose (maximum dose: 15 mL) given within 6 days of exposure followed by live attenuated measles vaccine in 3 months or at 15 months of age (whichever is later)

For patients with leukemia, lymphoma, immunodeficiency disorders, generalized malignancy, or receiving immunosuppressive therapy: 0.5 mL/kg (maximum dose: 15 mL)

Poliomyelitis: Prophylaxis: 0.3 mL/kg/dose as a single dose

Rubella: Prophylaxis: 0.55 mL/kg/dose within 72 hours of exposure

(Continued)

Immune Globulin (Intramuscular) *(Continued)*

Varicella: Prophylaxis: 0.6-1.2 mL/kg (varicella zoster immune globulin preferred) within 72 hours of exposure

IgG deficiency: 1.3 mL/kg, then 0.66 mL/kg in 3-4 weeks

Hepatitis B: Prophylaxis: 0.06 mL/kg/dose (HBIG preferred)

Mechanism of Action Provides passive immunity by increasing the antibody titer and antigen-antibody reaction potential

Contraindications Hypersensitivity to immune globulin, thimerosal, or any component of the formulation; IgA deficiency; I.M. injections in patients with thrombocytopenia or coagulation disorders

Warnings/Precautions Skin testing should not be performed as local irritation can occur and be misinterpreted as a positive reaction; IG should **not** be used to control outbreaks of measles. As a product of human plasma, this product may potentially transmit disease; screening of donors, as well as testing and/or inactivation of certain viruses reduces this risk. Epidemiologic and laboratory data indicate current IMIG products do not have a discernible risk of transmitting HIV. Use caution in patients with thrombocytopenia or coagulation disorders (I.M. injections may be contraindicated). Not for I.V. administration.

Drug Interactions

Increased Effect/Toxicity: Increased toxicity: Live virus, vaccines (measles, mumps, rubella); do not administer within 3 months after administration of these vaccines.

Pharmacodynamics/Kinetics

Duration: Immune effect: Usually 3-4 weeks

Half-life elimination: 23 days

Time to peak, serum: I.M.: ~24-48 hours

Pregnancy Risk Factor C

Dosage Forms INJ, solution [preservative free]: 15% to 18% (2 mL, 10 mL)

Selected Readings

ASHP Commission on Therapeutics, "ASHP Therapeutic Guidelines for Intravenous Immune Globulin," *Clin Pharm*, 1992, 11(2):117-36.

Berkman SA, Lee ML, and Gale RP, "Clinical Uses of Intravenous Immunoglobulins," *Ann Intern Med*, 1990, 112(4):278-92.

Immune Globulin (Intravenous)

(i MYUN GLOB yoo lin, IN tra VEE nus)

Related Information

Systemic Viral Diseases *on page 1675*

U.S. Brand Names Carimune™ NF; Gammagard® Liquid; Gammagard® S/D; Gammar®-P I.V.; Gamunex®; Iveegam EN; Octagam®; Panglobulin® NF; Polygam® S/D

Canadian Brand Names Gamimune® N; Gammagard® Liquid; Gammagard® S/D; Gamunex®; Iveegam Immuno®

Generic Available No

Synonyms IVIG

Pharmacologic Category Immune Globulin

Use

Treatment of primary immunodeficiency syndromes (congenital agammaglobulinemia, severe combined immunodeficiency syndromes [SCIDS], common variable immunodeficiency, X-linked immunodeficiency, Wiskott-Aldrich syndrome); idiopathic thrombocytopenic purpura (ITP); Kawasaki disease (in combination with aspirin)

Prevention of bacterial infection in B-cell chronic lymphocytic leukemia (CLL); pediatric HIV infection; bone marrow transplant (BMT)

Unlabeled/Investigational Use Autoimmune diseases (myasthenia gravis, SLE, bullous pemphigoid, severe rheumatoid arthritis), Guillain-Barré syndrome; used in conjunction with appropriate anti-infective therapy to prevent or modify acute bacterial or viral infections in patients with iatrogenically-induced or disease-associated immunodepression; autoimmune hemolytic anemia or neutropenia, refractory dermatomyositis/polymyositis

Local Anesthetic/Vasoconstrictor Precautions No information available to require special precautions

Effects on Dental Treatment No significant effects or complications reported

Common Adverse Effects Frequency not defined.

Cardiovascular: Flushing of the face, tachycardia, hyper-/hypotension, chest tightness, angioedema, lightheadedness, chest pain, MI, CHF, pulmonary embolism

Central nervous system: Anxiety, chills, dizziness, drowsiness, fatigue, fever, headache, irritability, lethargy, malaise, aseptic meningitis syndrome

Dermatologic: Pruritus, rash, urticaria

Gastrointestinal: Abdominal cramps, diarrhea, nausea, sore throat, vomiting

Hematologic: Autoimmune hemolytic anemia, hematocrit decreased, leukopenia, mild hemolysis

Hepatic: Liver function test increased

Local: Pain or irritation at the infusion site

Neuromuscular & skeletal: Arthralgia, back or hip pain, myalgia, nuchal rigidity

Ocular: Photophobia, painful eye movements

Renal: Acute renal failure, acute tubular necrosis, anuria, BUN increased, creatinine increased, nephrotic syndrome, oliguria, proximal tubular nephropathy, osmotic nephrosis

Respiratory: Cough, dyspnea, wheezing, nasal congestion, pharyngeal pain, rhinorrhea, sinusitis

Miscellaneous: Diaphoresis, hypersensitivity reactions, anaphylaxis

Dosage Approved doses and regimens may vary between brands; check manufacturer guidelines. **Note:** Some clinicians dose IVIG on ideal body weight or an adjusted ideal body weight in morbidly obese patients.

Infants and Children: Prevention of gastroenteritis (unlabeled use): Oral: 50 mg/kg/day divided every 6 hours

Children: I.V.:

Pediatric HIV: 400 mg/kg every 28 days

Severe systemic viral and bacterial infections (unlabeled use): 500-1000 mg/kg/week

Children and Adults: I.V.:

Primary immunodeficiency disorders: 200-400 mg/kg every 4 weeks or as per monitored serum IgG concentrations

Gammagard® Liquid, Gamunex®, Octagam®: 300-600 mg/kg every 3-4 weeks; adjusted based on dosage and interval in conjunction with monitored serum IgG concentrations.

B-cell chronic lymphocytic leukemia (CLL): 400 mg/kg/dose every 3 weeks

Idiopathic thrombocytopenic purpura (ITP):

Acute: 400 mg/kg/day for 5 days or 1000 mg/kg/day for 1-2 days

Chronic: 400 mg/kg as needed to maintain platelet count >30,000/mm³; may increase dose to 800 mg/kg (1000 mg/kg if needed)

Kawasaki disease: Initiate therapy within 10 days of disease onset: 2 g/kg as a single dose administered over 10 hours, or 400 mg/kg/day for 4 days. **Note:** Must be used in combination with aspirin: 80-100 mg/kg/day in 4 divided doses for 14 days; when fever subsides, dose aspirin at 3-5 mg/kg once daily for ≥6-8 weeks

Acquired immunodeficiency syndrome (patients must be symptomatic) (unlabeled use): Various regimens have been used, including:

200-250 mg/kg/dose every 2 weeks

or

400-500 mg/kg/dose every month or every 4 weeks

Autoimmune hemolytic anemia and neutropenia (unlabeled use): 1000 mg/kg/dose for 2-3 days

Autoimmune diseases (unlabeled use): 400 mg/kg/day for 4 days

Bone marrow transplant: 500 mg/kg beginning on days 7 and 2 pretransplant, then 500 mg/kg/week for 90 days post-transplant

Adjuvant to severe cytomegalovirus infections (unlabeled use): 500 mg/kg/dose every other day for 7 doses

Guillain-Barré syndrome (unlabeled use): Various regimens have been used, including:

400 mg/kg/day for 4 days

or

1000 mg/kg/day for 2 days

or

2000 mg/kg/day for one day

Refractory dermatomyositis (unlabeled use): 2 g/kg/dose every month x 3-4 doses

Refractory polymyositis (unlabeled use): 1 g/kg/day x 2 days every month x 4 doses

Chronic inflammatory demyelinating polyneuropathy (unlabeled use): Various regimens have been used, including:

400 mg/kg/day for 5 doses once each month

or

800 mg/kg/day for 3 doses once each month

or

1000 mg/kg/day for 2 days once each month

Dosing adjustment/comments in renal impairment: Cl_{cr} <10 mL/minute: Avoid use; in patients at risk of renal dysfunction, consider infusion at a rate less than maximum.

(Continued)

Immune Globulin (Intravenous) *(Continued)*

Mechanism of Action Replacement therapy for primary and secondary immunodeficiencies; interference with F_c receptors on the cells of the reticuloendothelial system for autoimmune cytopenias and ITP; possible role of contained antiviral-type antibodies

Contraindications Hypersensitivity to immune globulin or any component of the formulation; selective IgA deficiency

Warnings/Precautions Anaphylactic hypersensitivity reactions can occur, especially in IgA-deficient patients; studies indicate that the currently available products have no discernible risk of transmitting HIV or hepatitis B; aseptic meningitis may occur with high doses (≥2 g/kg). Use with caution in the elderly, patients with renal disease, diabetes mellitus, volume depletion, sepsis, paraproteinemia, and nephrotoxic medications due to risk of renal dysfunction. Patients should be adequately hydrated prior to therapy. Acute renal dysfunction (increased serum creatinine, oliguria, acute renal failure) can rarely occur; usually within 7 days of use (more likely with products stabilized with sucrose). Use caution in patients with a history of thrombotic events or cardiovascular disease; there is clinical evidence of a possible association between thrombotic events and administration of intravenous immune globulin. For intravenous administration only.

Drug Interactions

Decreased Effect: Decreased effect of live virus vaccines (eg, measles, mumps, rubella); separate administration by at least 3 months

Dietary Considerations Octagam® contains sodium 30 mmol/L

Pharmacodynamics/Kinetics

Onset of action: I.V.: Provides immediate antibody levels

Duration: Immune effect: 3-4 weeks (variable)

Distribution: V_d: 0.09-0.13 L/kg

Intravascular portion (primarily): Healthy subjects: 41% to 57%; Patients with congenital humoral immunodeficiencies: ~70%

Half-life elimination: IgG (variable among patients): Healthy subjects: 14-24 days; Patients with congenital humoral immunodeficiencies: 26-40 days; hypermetabolism associated with fever and infection have coincided with a shortened half-life

Pregnancy Risk Factor C

Dosage Forms INJ, powder for reconstitution [preservative free] (Gammar®-P I.V.): 5 g, 10 g; (Iveegam EN): 5 g; (Panglobulin®): 6 g, 12 g. **INJ, powder for reconstitution** [preservative free, nanofiltered] (Panglobulin® NF): 6 g, 12 g. **INJ, powder for reconstitution** [preservative free, solvent detergent treated] (Gammagard® S/D): 2.5 g, 5 g, 10 g; (Polygam® S/D): 5 g, 10 g. **SOLN, injection** [preservative free, solvent detergent-treated] (Gammagard® Liquid): 10% [100 mg/mL] (10 mL, 25 mL, 50 mL, 100 mL, 200 mL); (Octagam®): 5% [50 mg/mL] (20 mL, 50 mL, 100 mL, 200 mL). **SOLN, injection** [preservative free]: (Gamunex®): 10% (10 mL, 25 mL, 50 mL, 100 mL, 200 mL) [caprylate/chromatography purified]

Selected Readings

ASHP Commission on Therapeutics, "ASHP Therapeutic Guidelines for Intravenous Immune Globulin," *Am J Hosp Pharm*, 1992, 49(3):652-4.

Blanchette VS, Luke B, Andrew M, et al, "A Prospective Randomized Trial of High-Dose Intravenous Immune Globulin G Therapy, Oral Prednisone Therapy, and No Therapy in Childhood Acute Immune Thrombocytopenic Purpura," *J Pediatr*, 1993, 123(6):989-95.

Grillo JA, Gorson, KC, Ropper AH, et al, "Rapid Infusion of Intravenous Immune Globulin in Patients With Neuromuscular Disorders," *Neurology*, 2001; 57:1699-1701.

Morrell A, "Pharmacokinetics of Intravenous Immunoglobulin Preparations," *Intravenous Immunoglobulins in Clinical Practice*, Lee ML and Strand V eds, New York, NY: Marcel Dekker, Inc, 1997, 1-18.

NIH Consensus Conference, "Intravenous Immunoglobulin, Prevention and Treatment of Disease," *JAMA*, 1990, 264(24):3189-93.

Skvaril F and Gardi A, "Differences Among Available Immunoglobulin Preparations for Intravenous Use," *Pediatr Infect Dis J*, 1988, 7:543-48.

"University Hospital Consortium Expert Panel for Off-Label Use of Polyvalent Intravenously Administered Immunoglobulin Preparations Consensus Statement," *JAMA*, 1995, 273(23):1865-70.

Immune Globulin (Subcutaneous)
(i MYUN GLOB yoo lin sub kyoo TAY nee us)

U.S. Brand Names Vivaglobin®

Generic Available No

Synonyms Immune Globulin Subcutaneous (Human); SCIG

Pharmacologic Category Immune Globulin

Use Treatment of primary immune deficiency (PID)

Local Anesthetic/Vasoconstrictor Precautions No information available to require special precautions

Effects on Dental Treatment No significant effects or complications reported

Common Adverse Effects Adverse reactions can be expected to be similar to those experienced with other immune globulin products; percentages are reported as adverse events per patient; injection-site reactions decreased with subsequent infusions

>10%:

Central nervous system: Headache (32% to 48%), fever (3% to 25%)

Dermatologic: Rash (6% to 17%)

Gastrointestinal: Gastrointestinal disorder (5% to 37%), nausea (11% to 18%), sore throat (17%)

Local: Injection-site reactions (swelling, redness, itching; 92%)

Miscellaneous: Allergic reaction (11%)

1% to 10%:

Cardiovascular: Tachycardia (3%)

Central nervous system: Pain (10%)

Dermatologic: Skin disorder (3%)

Gastrointestinal: Diarrhea (10%)

Genitourinary: Urine abnormality (3%)

Neuromuscular & skeletal: Weakness (5%)

Respiratory: Cough (10%)

Mechanism of Action Immune globulin replacement therapy of IgG antibodies against bacteria and viral agents.

Drug Interactions

Decreased Effect: Immune globulin may decrease the efficacy of immune response to live vaccines.

Pharmacodynamics/Kinetics

Bioavailability: 73% (compared to I.V.)

Time to peak, plasma: 2.5 days

Pregnancy Risk Factor C

Immune Globulin Subcutaneous (Human) *see* Immune Globulin (Subcutaneous) *on page 826*

Immune Serum Globulin *see* Immune Globulin (Intramuscular) *on page 823*

Imodium® A-D [OTC] *see* Loperamide *on page 942*

Imodium® Advanced *see* Loperamide and Simethicone *on page 943*

Imogam® Rabies-HT *see* Rabies Immune Globulin (Human) *on page 1328*

Imovax® Rabies *see* Rabies Virus Vaccine *on page 1329*

Imuran® *see* Azathioprine *on page 168*

In-111 Zevalin *see* Ibritumomab *on page 807*

Inamrinone (eye NAM ri none)

Related Information

Cardiovascular Diseases *on page 1636*

Generic Available Yes

Synonyms Amrinone Lactate

Pharmacologic Category Phosphodiesterase Enzyme Inhibitor

Use Infrequently used as a last resort, short-term therapy in patients with intractable heart failure

Local Anesthetic/Vasoconstrictor Precautions No information available to require special precautions

Effects on Dental Treatment No significant effects or complications reported

Common Adverse Effects

1% to 10%:

Cardiovascular: Arrhythmias (3%, especially in high-risk patients), hypotension (1% to 2%), (may be infusion rate-related)

Gastrointestinal: Nausea (1% to 2%)

Hematologic: Thrombocytopenia (may be dose related)

Mechanism of Action Inhibits myocardial cyclic adenosine monophosphate (cAMP) phosphodiesterase activity and increases cellular levels of cAMP resulting in a positive inotropic effect and increased cardiac output; also possesses systemic and pulmonary vasodilator effects resulting in pre- and afterload reduction; slightly increases atrioventricular conduction

Drug Interactions

Increased Effect/Toxicity: Diuretics may cause significant hypovolemia and decrease filling pressure. Inotropic effects with digitalis are additive.

Pharmacodynamics/Kinetics

Onset of action: I.V.: 2-5 minutes

Peak effect: ~10 minutes

Duration (dose dependent): Low dose: ~30 minutes; Higher doses: ~2 hours

(Continued)

Inamrinone *(Continued)*

Half-life elimination, serum: Adults: Healthy volunteers: 3.6 hours, Congestive heart failure: 5.8 hours

Pregnancy Risk Factor C

Inapsine® *see* Droperidol *on page 519*

Increlex™ *see* Mecasermin *on page 968*

Indapamide *(in DAP a mide)*

Related Information
Cardiovascular Diseases *on page 1636*

U.S. Brand Names Lozol®

Canadian Brand Names Apo-Indapamide®; Gen-Indapamide; Lozide®; Lozol®; Novo-Indapamide; Nu-Indapamide; PMS-Indapamide

Generic Available Yes

Pharmacologic Category Diuretic, Thiazide-Related

Use Management of mild to moderate hypertension; treatment of edema in congestive heart failure and nephrotic syndrome

Local Anesthetic/Vasoconstrictor Precautions No information available to require special precautions (see Dental Comment)

Effects on Dental Treatment Key adverse event(s) related to dental treatment: Orthostatic hypotension, palpitations, flushing, xerostomia (normal salivary flow resumes upon discontinuation), and rhinorrhea.

Common Adverse Effects 1% to 10%:

Cardiovascular: Orthostatic hypotension, palpitation (<5%), flushing

Central nervous system: Dizziness (<5%), lightheadedness (<5%), vertigo (<5%), headache (≥5%), restlessness (<5%), drowsiness (<5%), fatigue, lethargy, malaise, lassitude, anxiety, agitation, depression, nervousness (≥5%)

Dermatologic: Rash (<5%), pruritus (<5%), hives (<5%)

Endocrine & metabolic: Hyperglycemia (<5%), hyperuricemia (<5%)

Gastrointestinal: Anorexia, gastric irritation, nausea, vomiting, abdominal pain, cramping, bloating, diarrhea, constipation, dry mouth, weight loss

Genitourinary: Nocturia, frequent urination, polyuria, impotence (<5%), reduced libido (<5%), glycosuria (<5%)

Neuromuscular & skeletal: Muscle cramps, spasm, weakness (≥5%)

Ocular: Blurred vision (<5%)

Renal: Necrotizing angiitis, vasculitis, cutaneous vasculitis (<5%)

Respiratory: Rhinorrhea (<5%)

Mechanism of Action Diuretic effect is localized at the proximal segment of the distal tubule of the nephron; it does not appear to have significant effect on glomerular filtration rate nor renal blood flow; like other diuretics, it enhances sodium, chloride, and water excretion by interfering with the transport of sodium ions across the renal tubular epithelium

Drug Interactions

Increased Effect/Toxicity: The diuretic effect of indapamide is synergistic with furosemide and other loop diuretics. Increased hypotension and/or renal adverse effects of ACE inhibitors may result in aggressively diuresed patients. Cyclosporine and thiazide-type diuretics can increase the risk of gout or renal toxicity. Digoxin toxicity can be exacerbated if a diuretic induces hypokalemia or hypomagnesemia. Lithium toxicity can occur with thiazide-type diuretics due to reduced renal excretion of lithium. Thiazide-type diuretics may prolong the duration of action of neuromuscular blocking agents.

Decreased Effect: Effects of oral hypoglycemics may be decreased. Decreased absorption of indapamide with cholestyramine and colestipol. NSAIDs can decrease the efficacy of thiazide-type diuretics, reducing the diuretic and antihypertensive effects.

Pharmacodynamics/Kinetics

Onset of action: 1-2 hours

Duration: ≤36 hours

Absorption: Complete

Protein binding, plasma: 71% to 79%

Metabolism: Extensively hepatic

Half-life elimination: 14-18 hours

Time to peak: 2-2.5 hours

Excretion: Urine (~60%) within 48 hours; feces (~16% to 23%)

Pregnancy Risk Factor B (manufacturer); D (expert analysis)

Dental Comment

This drug is known to prolong the QT interval. The QT interval is measured as the time and distance between the Q point of the QRS complex and the end of the T wave in the ECG tracing. After adjustment for heart rate, the QT interval is defined as prolonged if it is more than 450 msec in men and 460 msec in women. A long QT syndrome was first described in the 1950s and 60s as a congenital syndrome involving QT interval prolongation and syncope and sudden death. Some of the congenital long QT syndromes were characterized by a peculiar electrocardiographic appearance of the QRS complex involving a premature atria beat followed by a pause, then a subsequent sinus beat showing marked QT prolongation and deformity. This type of cardiac arrhythmia was originally termed "torsade de pointes" (translated from the French as "twisting of the points").

Prolongation of the QT interval is thought to result from delayed ventricular repolarization. The repolarization process within the myocardial cell is due to the efflux of intracellular potassium. The channels associated with this current can be blocked by many drugs and predisposes the electrical propagation cycle to torsade de pointes.

Indapamide is one of the drugs confirmed to prolong the QT interval and is accepted as having a risk of causing torsade de pointes. The risk of drug-induced torsade de pointes is extremely low when a single QT interval prolonging drug is prescribed. In terms of epinephrine, it is not known what effect vasoconstrictors in the local anesthetic regimen will have in patients with a known history of congenital prolonged QT interval or in patients taking any medication that prolongs the QT interval. Until more information is obtained, it is suggested that the clinician consult with the physician prior to the use of a vasoconstrictor in suspected patients, and that the vasoconstrictor (epinephrine, levonordefrin [Neo-Cobefrin®]) be used with caution.

Inderal® *see* Propranolol *on page 1301*

Inderal® LA *see* Propranolol *on page 1301*

Inderide® *see* Propranolol and Hydrochlorothiazide *on page 1305*

Indinavir (in DIN a veer)

Related Information
HIV Infection and AIDS *on page 1662*
Tuberculosis *on page 1673*
U.S. Brand Names Crixivan®
Canadian Brand Names Crixivan®
Mexican Brand Names Crixivan®
Generic Available No
Synonyms Indinavir Sulfate
Pharmacologic Category Antiretroviral Agent, Protease Inhibitor
Use Treatment of HIV infection; should always be used as part of a multidrug regimen (at least three antiretroviral agents)
Local Anesthetic/Vasoconstrictor Precautions No information available to require special precautions
Effects on Dental Treatment Key adverse event(s) related to dental treatment: Abnormal taste.
Common Adverse Effects Protease inhibitors cause dyslipidemia which includes elevated cholesterol and triglycerides and a redistribution of body fat centrally to cause increased abdominal girth, buffalo hump, facial atrophy, and breast enlargement. These agents also cause hyperglycemia (exacerbation or new-onset diabetes).

>10%:
    Gastrointestinal: Nausea (12%)
    Hepatic: Hyperbilirubinemia (14%)
    Renal: Nephrolithiasis/urolithiasis (29%, pediatric patients; 12% adult patients)
1% to 10%:
    Central nervous system: Headache (6%), insomnia (3%)
    Gastrointestinal: Abdominal pain (9%), diarrhea/vomiting (4% to 5%), taste perversion (3%)
    Neuromuscular & skeletal: Weakness (4%), flank pain (3%)
    Renal: Hematuria

Mechanism of Action Indinavir is a human immunodeficiency virus protease inhibitor, binding to the protease activity site and inhibiting the activity of this enzyme. HIV protease is an enzyme required for the cleavage of viral polyprotein precursors into individual functional proteins found in infectious HIV. Inhibition prevents cleavage of these polyproteins resulting in the formation of immature noninfectious viral particles.

Drug Interactions
Cytochrome P450 Effect: Substrate of CYP2D6 (minor), 3A4 (major); **Inhibits** CYP2C8/9 (weak), 2C19 (weak), 2D6 (weak), 3A4 (strong)
(Continued)

Indinavir *(Continued)*

Increased Effect/Toxicity: Indinavir may increase the levels/effects of selected benzodiazepines, calcium channel blockers, cyclosporine, mirtazapine, nateglinide, nefazodone, quinidine, sildenafil (and other PDE-5 inhibitors), tacrolimus, venlafaxine, and other CYP3A4 substrates. Selected benzodiazepines (midazolam, triazolam), cisapride, ergot alkaloids, selected HMG-CoA reductase inhibitors (lovastatin and simvastatin), mesoridazine, pimozide, and thioridazine are generally contraindicated with strong CYP3A4 inhibitors. When used with strong CYP3A4 inhibitors, dosage adjustment/limits are recommended for sildenafil and other PDE-5 inhibitors; refer to individual monographs.

Itraconazole or ketoconazole may increase the serum concentrations of indinavir; dosage adjustment is recommended. The levels/effects of indinavir may be increased by azole antifungals, clarithromycin, diclofenac, doxycycline, erythromycin, imatinib, isoniazid, nefazodone, nicardipine, propofol, protease inhibitors, quinidine, telithromycin, verapamil, and other CYP3A4 inhibitors.

When used with delavirdine, serum levels of indinavir are increased; dosage adjustment of indinavir may be required for this combination. Serum levels of both nelfinavir and indinavir are increased with concurrent use. Serum concentrations of indinavir may be increased by ritonavir; serum levels of ritonavir and saquinavir may be increased; dosage adjustments of indinavir are required during concurrent therapy. Rifabutin serum concentrations has been increased when coadministered with indinavir; dosage adjustments of both agents required. Concurrent use or atazanavir with indinavir may increase the risk of hyperbilirubinemia.

Decreased Effect: The levels/effects of indinavir may be decreased by aminoglutethimide, carbamazepine, nafcillin, nevirapine, phenobarbital, phenytoin, rifamycins, and other CYP3A4 inducers; dosage adjustment may be recommended (see individual agents). Rifampin and/or St John's wort (*Hypericum perforatum*); should not be used with indinavir.

Pharmacodynamics/Kinetics

Absorption: Administration with a high fat, high calorie diet resulted in a reduction in AUC and in maximum serum concentration (77% and 84% respectively); lighter meal resulted in little or no change in these parameters.

Protein binding, plasma: 60%

Metabolism: Hepatic via CYP3A4; seven metabolites of indinavir identified

Bioavailability: Good

Half-life elimination: 1.8 ± 0.4 hour

Time to peak: 0.8 ± 0.3 hour

Excretion: Urine and feces

Pregnancy Risk Factor C

Indinavir Sulfate *see* Indinavir *on page 829*

Indocin® *see* Indomethacin *on page 830*

Indocin® I.V. *see* Indomethacin *on page 830*

Indocin® SR *see* Indomethacin *on page 830*

Indocyanine Green *(in doe SYE a neen green)*

U.S. Brand Names IC-Green®

Generic Available No

Pharmacologic Category Diagnostic Agent

Use Determining hepatic function, cardiac output and liver blood flow and for ophthalmic angiography

Local Anesthetic/Vasoconstrictor Precautions No information available to require special precautions

Effects on Dental Treatment No significant effects or complications reported

Common Adverse Effects 1% to 10%:

Central nervous system: Headache

Dermatologic: Pruritus, skin discoloration

Miscellaneous: Diaphoresis, anaphylactoid reactions

Pregnancy Risk Factor C

Indometacin *see* Indomethacin *on page 830*

Indomethacin *(in doe METH a sin)*

Related Information

Rheumatoid Arthritis, Osteoarthritis, and Osteoporosis *on page 1668*

Temporomandibular Dysfunction (TMD) *on page 1724*

U.S. Brand Names Indocin®; Indocin® I.V.; Indocin® SR

Canadian Brand Names Apo-Indomethacin®; Indocid® P.D.A.; Indocin®; Indo-Lemmon; Indotec; Novo-Methacin; Nu-Indo; Rhodacine®

Generic Available Yes: Capsule, suspension

Synonyms Indometacin; Indomethacin Sodium Trihydrate

Pharmacologic Category Nonsteroidal Anti-inflammatory Drug (NSAID), Oral; Nonsteroidal Anti-inflammatory Drug (NSAID), Parenteral

Use Acute gouty arthritis, acute bursitis/tendonitis, moderate to severe osteoarthritis, rheumatoid arthritis, ankylosing spondylitis; I.V. form used as alternative to surgery for closure of patent ductus arteriosus in neonates

Local Anesthetic/Vasoconstrictor Precautions No information available to require special precautions

Effects on Dental Treatment NSAID formulations are known to reversibly decrease platelet aggregation via mechanisms different than observed with aspirin. The dentist should be aware of the potential of abnormal coagulation. Caution should also be exercised in the use of NSAIDs in patients already on anticoagulant therapy with drugs such as warfarin (Coumadin®).

Common Adverse Effects

>10%: Central nervous system: Headache (12%)

1% to 10%:

Central nervous system: Dizziness (3% to 9%), drowsiness (<1%), fatigue (<3%), vertigo (<3%), depression (<3%), malaise (<3%), somnolence (<3%)

Gastrointestinal: Nausea (3% to 9%), epigastric pain (3% to 9%), abdominal pain/cramps/distress (<3%), heartburn (3% to 9%), indigestion (3% to 9%), constipation (<3%), diarrhea (<3%), dyspepsia (3% to 9%), vomiting

Otic: Tinnitus (<3%)

Restrictions A medication guide should be dispensed with each prescription. A template for the required MedGuide can be found on the FDA website at: http://www.fda.gov/medwatch/SAFETY/2005/safety05.htm#NSAID

Dosage

Patent ductus arteriosus:

Neonates: I.V.: Initial: 0.2 mg/kg, followed by 2 doses depending on postnatal age (PNA):

PNA at time of first dose <48 hours: 0.1 mg/kg at 12- to 24-hour intervals

PNA at time of first dose 2-7 days: 0.2 mg/kg at 12- to 24-hour intervals

PNA at time of first dose >7 days: 0.25 mg/kg at 12- to 24-hour intervals

In general, may use 12-hour dosing interval if urine output >1 mL/kg/hour after prior dose; use 24-hour dosing interval if urine output is <1 mL/kg/hour but >0.6 mL/kg/hour; doses should be withheld if patient has oliguria (urine output <0.6 mL/kg/hour) or anuria

Inflammatory/rheumatoid disorders: Oral: Use lowest effective dose.

Children >2 years: 1-2 mg/kg/day in 2-4 divided doses; maximum dose: 4 mg/kg/day; not to exceed 150-200 mg/day

Adults: 25-50 mg/dose 2-3 times/day; maximum dose: 200 mg/day; extended release capsule should be given on a 1-2 times/day schedule; maximum dose for sustained release is 150 mg/day. In patients with arthritis and persistent night pain and/or morning stiffness may give the larger portion (up to 100 mg) of the total daily dose at bedtime.

Bursitis/tendonitis: Oral: Adults: Initial dose: 75-150 mg/day in 3-4 divided doses; usual treatment is 7-14 days

Acute gouty arthritis: Oral: Adults: 50 mg 3 times daily until pain is tolerable then reduce dose; usual treatment <3-5 days

Elderly: Refer to Adults dosing; best to start older adults on 25 mg dose given 2-3 times/day

Dosage adjustment in renal impairment: Not recommended in patients with advanced renal disease

Mechanism of Action Inhibits prostaglandin synthesis by decreasing the activity of the enzyme, cyclooxygenase, which results in decreased formation of prostaglandin precursors

Contraindications Hypersensitivity to indomethacin, aspirin, other NSAIDs, or any component of the formulation; perioperative pain in the setting of coronary artery bypass surgery (CABG); pregnancy (3rd trimester)

Neonates: Necrotizing enterocolitis, impaired renal function, active bleeding, thrombocytopenia, coagulation defects, untreated infection

Warnings/Precautions NSAIDs are associated with an increased risk of adverse cardiovascular events, including MI, stroke, and new onset or worsening of pre-existing hypertension. Risk may be increased with duration of use or pre-existing cardiovascular risk-factors or disease. Use caution with fluid retention, CHF or hypertension.

Use of NSAIDs can compromise existing renal function. Indomethacin is not recommended for patients with advanced renal disease. Use with caution in patients with decreased hepatic function.

(Continued)

Indomethacin *(Continued)*

NSAIDs may increase risk of gastrointestinal irritation, ulceration, bleeding, and perforation. Use caution with a history of GI disease (bleeding or ulcers), concurrent therapy with aspirin, anticoagulants and/or corticosteroids, smoking, use of alcohol, the elderly or debilitated patients.

Use the lowest effective dose for the shortest duration of time, consistent with individual patient goals, to reduce risk of cardiovascular or GI adverse events.

NSAIDs may cause serious skin adverse events including exfoliative dermatitis, Stevens-Johnson syndrome (SJS) and toxic epidermal necrolysis (TEN). Do not use in patients who experience bronchospasm, asthma, rhinitis, or urticaria with NSAID or aspirin therapy.

Withhold for at least 4-6 half-lives prior to surgical or dental procedures.

Drug Interactions
Cytochrome P450 Effect: Substrate (minor) of CYP2C8/9, 2C19; **Inhibits** CYP2C8/9 (strong), 2C19 (weak)

Increased Effect/Toxicity: Indomethacin may increase effect/toxicity of anti-coagulants (bleeding), antiplatelet agents (bleeding), aminoglycosides, biphosphonates (GI irritation), corticosteroids (GI irritation), cyclosporine (nephrotoxicity), lithium, methotrexate, pemetrexed, treprostinil (bleeding), vancomycin. Tilundronate serum concentrations may be increased. CYP2C8/9 substrates (eg, amiodarone, fluoxetine, glimepiride, glipizide, nateglinide, phenytoin, pioglitazone, rosiglitazone, sertraline, and warfarin) serum concentrations may be increased with concurrent use.

Decreased Effect: May reduce effect of some diuretics and antihypertensive effect of beta-blockers, ACE inhibitors, angiotensin II inhibitors, hydralazine Cholestyramine and colestipol may reduce absorption of indomethacin.

Ethanol/Nutrition/Herb Interactions
Ethanol: Avoid ethanol (may enhance gastric mucosal irritation).

Food: Food may decrease the rate but not the extent of absorption. Indomethacin peak serum levels may be delayed if taken with food.

Herb/Nutraceutical: Avoid alfalfa, anise, bilberry, bladderwrack, bromelain, cat's claw, celery, coleus, cordyceps, dong quai, evening primrose, feverfew, fenugreek, garlic, ginger, ginkgo biloba, red clover, horse chestnut, grapeseed, green tea, ginseng, guggul, horse chestnut seed, horseradish, licorice, prickly ash, red clover, reishi, SAMe, sweet clover, turmeric, white willow (all have additional antiplatelet activity).

Dietary Considerations
May cause GI upset; take with food or milk to minimize

Pharmacodynamics/Kinetics
Onset of action: ~30 minutes

Duration: 4-6 hours

Absorption: Prompt and extensive

Distribution: V_d: 0.34-1.57 L/kg; crosses blood brain barrier and placenta; enters breast milk

Protein binding: 99%

Metabolism: Hepatic; significant enterohepatic recirculation

Bioavailability: 100%

Half-life elimination: 4.5 hours; prolonged in neonates

Time to peak: Oral: 2 hours

Excretion: Urine (60%, primarily as glucuronide conjugates); feces (33%, primarily as metabolites)

Pregnancy Risk Factor
C/D (3rd trimester)

Dosage Forms
CAP (Indocin®): 25 mg, 50 mg. **CAP, sustained release** (Indocin® SR): 75 mg. **INJ, powder for reconstitution** (Indocin® I.V.): 1 mg. **SUSP, oral** (Indocin®): 25 mg/5 mL (237 mL)

Indomethacin Sodium Trihydrate see Indomethacin on page 830

INF-alpha 2 see Interferon Alfa-2b on page 844

Infantaire [OTC] see Acetaminophen on page 31

Infantaire Gas Drops [OTC] see Simethicone on page 1394

Infants' Tylenol® Cold Plus Cough Concentrated Drops [OTC] see Acetaminophen, Dextromethorphan, and Pseudoephedrine on page 44

Infasurf® see Calfactant on page 251

INFeD® see Iron Dextran Complex on page 862

Infliximab *(in FLIKS e mab)*

U.S. Brand Names Remicade®
Canadian Brand Names Remicade®
Generic Available No

Synonyms Infliximab, Recombinant

Pharmacologic Category Antirheumatic, Disease Modifying; Gastrointestinal Agent, Miscellaneous; Monoclonal Antibody; Tumor Necrosis Factor (TNF) Blocking Agent

Use

Ankylosing spondylitis: Improving signs and symptoms of disease

Crohn's disease: Induction and maintenance of remission in patients with moderate to severe disease who have an inadequate response to conventional therapy; to reduce the number of draining enterocutaneous and rectovaginal fistulas and to maintain fistula closure

Psoriatic arthritis: Improving signs and symptoms of active arthritis in patients with psoriatic arthritis

Rheumatoid arthritis: Inhibits the progression of structural damage and improves physical function in patients with moderate to severe disease; used with methotrexate

Ulcerative colitis (UC): To reduce signs and symptoms, achieve clinical remission and mucosal healing and eliminate corticosteroid use in moderately to severely active UC inadequately responsive to conventional therapy

Local Anesthetic/Vasoconstrictor Precautions No information available to require special precautions

Effects on Dental Treatment No significant effects or complications reported

Common Adverse Effects Note: Although profile is similar, frequency of adverse effects may vary with disease state. Except where noted, percentages reported with rheumatoid arthritis:

>10%:

Central nervous system: Headache (18%)

Dermatologic: Rash (10%)

Gastrointestinal: Nausea (21%), diarrhea (12%), abdominal pain (12%, Crohn's 26%)

Genitourinary: Urinary tract infection (8%)

Hepatic: ALT increased (risk increased with concomitant methotrexate)

Local: Infusion reactions (20%)

Neuromuscular & skeletal: Arthralgia (8%), back pain (8%)

Respiratory: Upper respiratory tract infection (32%), cough (12%), sinusitis (14%), pharyngitis (12%)

Miscellaneous: Development of antinuclear antibodies (~50%), infection (36%), development of antibodies to double-stranded DNA (17%); Crohn's patients with fistulizing disease: Development of new abscess (15%)

5% to 10%:

Cardiovascular: Hypertension (7%)

Central nervous system: Pain (8%), fatigue (9%), fever (7%)

Dermatologic: Pruritus (7%)

Gastrointestinal: Dyspepsia (10%)

Respiratory: Bronchitis (10%), dyspnea (6%), rhinitis (8%)

Miscellaneous: Moniliasis (5%)

Mechanism of Action Infliximab is a chimeric monoclonal antibody that binds to human tumor necrosis factor alpha (TNFα), thereby interfering with endogenous TNFα activity. Biological activities of TNFα include the induction of proinflammatory cytokines (interleukins), enhancement of leukocyte migration, activation of neutrophils and eosinophils, and the induction of acute phase reactants and tissue degrading enzymes. Animal models have shown TNFα expression causes polyarthritis, and infliximab can prevent disease as well as allow diseased joints to heal.

Drug Interactions

Increased Effect/Toxicity: Specific drug interaction studies have not been conducted. Anti-TNF agents may be associated with increased risk of serious infection when used in combination with anakinra. Abciximab may increase potential for hypersensitivity reaction to infliximab, and may increase risk of thrombocytopenia and/or reduced therapeutic efficacy of infliximab.

Decreased Effect: Specific drug interaction studies have not been conducted.

Pharmacodynamics/Kinetics

Onset of action: Crohn's disease: ~2 weeks

Half-life elimination: 8-9.5 days

Pregnancy Risk Factor B (manufacturer)

Infliximab, Recombinant *see* Infliximab *on page 832*

Influenza Virus Vaccine (in floo EN za VYE rus vak SEEN)

Related Information

Immunizations (Vaccines) *on page 1786*

(Continued)

Influenza Virus Vaccine *(Continued)*

U.S. Brand Names Fluarix™; fluMist®; Fluvirin®; Fluzone®

Canadian Brand Names Fluviral S/F®; Vaxigrip®

Generic Available No

Synonyms Influenza Virus Vaccine (Purified Surface Antigen); Influenza Virus Vaccine (Split-Virus); Influenza Virus Vaccine (Trivalent, Live); Live Attenuated Influenza Vaccine (LAIV); Trivalent Inactivated Influenza Vaccine (TIV)

Pharmacologic Category Vaccine

Use Provide active immunity to influenza virus strains contained in the vaccine

Groups at Increased Risk for Influenza-Related Complications: Recommendations for vaccination:

- Persons ≥65 years of age
- Residents of nursing homes and other chronic-care facilities that house persons of any age with chronic medical conditions
- Adults and children with chronic disorders of the pulmonary or cardiovascular systems, including children with asthma
- Adults and children who have required regular medical follow-up or hospitalization during the preceding year because of chronic metabolic diseases (including diabetes mellitus), renal dysfunction, hemoglobinopathies, or immunosuppression (including immunosuppression caused by medications or HIV)
- Adults and children with conditions which may compromise respiratory function, the handling of respiratory secretions, or that can increase the risk of aspiration (eg, cognitive dysfunction, spinal; cord injuries, seizure disorders, other neuromuscular disorders)
- Children and adolescents (6 months to 18 years of age) who are receiving long-term aspirin therapy and therefore, may be at risk for developing Reye's syndrome after influenza
- Women who will be pregnant during the influenza season
- Children 6-23 months of age

Vaccination is also recommended for persons 50-64 years of age, close contacts of children 0-23 months of age, healthy persons who may transmit influenza to those at risk, all healthcare workers, and persons who smoke.

Local Anesthetic/Vasoconstrictor Precautions No information available to require special precautions

Effects on Dental Treatment No significant effects or complications reported

Common Adverse Effects All serious adverse reactions must be reported to the U.S. Department of Health and Human Services (DHHS) Vaccine Adverse Event Reporting System (VAERS) 1-800-822-7967.

Injection: Frequency not defined:

Central nervous system: Fever and malaise (may start within 6-12 hours and last 1-2 days; incidence equal to placebo in adults; occurs more frequently than placebo in children); GBS (previously reported with older vaccine formulations; relationship to current formulations not known, however, patients with history of GBS have a greater likelihood of developing GBS than those without)

Dermatologic: Angioedema, urticaria

Local: Tenderness, redness, or induration at the site of injection (10% to 64%; may last up to 2 days); injection site pain

Neuromuscular & skeletal: Myalgia (may start within 6-12 hours and last 1-2 days; incidence equal to placebo in adults; occurs more frequently than placebo in children)

Miscellaneous: Allergic or anaphylactoid reactions (most likely to residual egg protein; includes allergic asthma, angioedema, hives, systemic anaphylaxis)

Nasal spray: **Note:** Frequency of events reported within 10 days

>10%:

Central nervous system: Headache (children 18% after first dose, < placebo after second dose; adults 40%) irritability (children 10% to 19%)

Neuromuscular & skeletal: Tiredness/weakness (adults 26%), muscle aches (children 5% to 6%; adults 17%)

Respiratory: Cough, nasal congestion/ runny nose (children 46% to 48%; adults 9% to 45%), sore throat (children < placebo; adults 28%)

Miscellaneous: Activity decreased (children 14% after first dose, < placebo after second dose)

1% to 10%:

Central nervous system: Chills

Gastrointestinal: Abdominal pain, diarrhea, vomiting

Otic: Otitis media

Mechanism of Action Promotes immunity to influenza virus by inducing specific antibody production. Each year the formulation is standardized according to the U.S. Public Health Service. Preparations from previous seasons must not be used.

Drug Interactions
  Increased Effect/Toxicity: Concomitant use of aspirin and the nasal spray formulation may increase the risk of Reye syndrome in patients 5-17 years; concomitant use in this age group is contraindicated.
  Decreased Effect: Decreased effect with immunosuppressive agents; some manufacturers and clinicians recommend that the flu vaccine not be administered concomitantly with DTP due to the potential for increased febrile reactions (specifically whole-cell pertussis) and that one should wait at least 3 days. However, ACIP recommends that children at high risk for influenza may get the vaccine concomitantly with DTP. Safety and efficacy of nasal spray with other vaccines have not been established; do not give within 1 month of other live virus vaccines or within 2 weeks of inactivated or subunit vaccines.

Pharmacodynamics/Kinetics
  Onset: Protective antibody levels achieved ~2 weeks after vaccination
  Duration: Protective antibody levels persist approximately ≥6 months

Pregnancy Risk Factor C

Influenza Virus Vaccine (Purified Surface Antigen) *see* Influenza Virus Vaccine *on page 833*

Influenza Virus Vaccine (Split-Virus) *see* Influenza Virus Vaccine *on page 833*

Influenza Virus Vaccine (Trivalent, Live) *see* Influenza Virus Vaccine *on page 833*

Infumorph® *see* Morphine Sulfate *on page 1065*

INH *see* Isoniazid *on page 864*

Inhaled Insulin *see* Insulin Inhalation *on page 837*

Innohep® *see* Tinzaparin *on page 1492*

InnoPran XL™ *see* Propranolol *on page 1301*

INOmax® *see* Nitric Oxide *on page 1118*

Insect Sting Kit *see* Epinephrine and Chlorpheniramine *on page 549*

Insoluble Prussian Blue *see* Ferric Hexacyanoferrate *on page 650*

Inspra™ *see* Eplerenone *on page 551*

Insta-Glucose® [OTC] *see* Dextrose *on page 452*

Instat™ *see* Collagen Hemostat *on page 392*

Instat™ MCH *see* Collagen Hemostat *on page 392*

Insulin Aspart (IN soo lin AS part)

Related Information
  Insulin Regular *on page 841*
U.S. Brand Names NovoLog®
Canadian Brand Names NovoRapid®
Generic Available No
Synonyms Aspart Insulin
Pharmacologic Category Antidiabetic Agent, Insulin
Use Treatment of type 1 diabetes mellitus (insulin dependent, IDDM); type 2 diabetes mellitus (noninsulin dependent, NIDDM) to control hyperglycemia
  Local Anesthetic/Vasoconstrictor Precautions No information available to require special precautions
  Effects on Dental Treatment Type 1 diabetics (insulin dependent) should be appointed for dental treatment in the morning in order to minimize chance of stress-induced hypoglycemia.
Mechanism of Action Refer to Insulin Regular *on page 841*. Insulin aspart is a rapid-acting insulin analog.
Drug Interactions
  Increased Effect/Toxicity: Refer to Insulin Regular *on page 841*.
Pharmacodynamics/Kinetics
  Onset of action: 0.2-0.5 hours
  Duration: 3-5 hours
  Time to peak: 1-3 hours
  Excretion: Urine
Pregnancy Risk Factor C

Insulin Aspart and Insulin Aspart Protamine *see* Insulin Aspart Protamine and Insulin Aspart *on page 836*

Insulin Aspart Protamine and Insulin Aspart
(IN soo lin AS part PROE ta meen & IN soo lin AS part)

Related Information
Insulin Regular *on page 841*

U.S. Brand Names NovoLog® Mix 70/30

Generic Available No

Synonyms Insulin Aspart and Insulin Aspart Protamine

Pharmacologic Category Antidiabetic Agent, Insulin

Use Treatment of type 1 diabetes mellitus (insulin dependent, IDDM); type 2 diabetes mellitus (noninsulin dependent, NIDDM) to control hyperglycemia

Local Anesthetic/Vasoconstrictor Precautions No information available to require special precautions

Effects on Dental Treatment Type 1 diabetics (insulin dependent) should be appointed for dental treatment in the morning in order to minimize chance of stress-induced hypoglycemia.

Common Adverse Effects Refer to Insulin Regular *on page 841*.

Mechanism of Action Refer to Insulin Regular *on page 841*. Insulin aspart protamine and insulin aspart is a combination insulin product with intermediate-acting characteristics. Normally administered twice daily.

Pharmacodynamics/Kinetics
Onset of action: 0.2 hours

Duration: 18-24 hours

Half-life: 8-9 hours

Time to peak: 1-4 hours

Excretion: Urine

Pregnancy Risk Factor C

Insulin Detemir (IN soo lin DE te mir)

Related Information
Insulin Regular *on page 841*

U.S. Brand Names Levemir®

Canadian Brand Names Levemir®

Generic Available No

Synonyms Detemir Insulin

Pharmacologic Category Antidiabetic Agent, Insulin

Use Treatment of type 1 diabetes mellitus (insulin dependent, IDDM); type 2 diabetes mellitus (noninsulin dependent, NIDDM) to control hyperglycemia

Local Anesthetic/Vasoconstrictor Precautions No information available to require special precautions

Effects on Dental Treatment Type 1 diabetics (insulin dependent) should be appointed for dental treatment in the morning in order to minimize chance of stress-induced hypoglycemia.

Common Adverse Effects Refer to Insulin Regular *on page 841*.

Mechanism of Action Refer to Insulin Regular *on page 841*. The product labeling identifies this product as a long-acting insulin analog; however, at lower dosages (<0.6 units/kg) its pharmacodynamic characteristics and dosing are consistent with intermediate insulin forms. In some patients, or at higher dosages, it may have a duration of action approaching 24 hours, which is consistent with a long-acting insulin.

Drug Interactions
Cytochrome P450 Effect: Refer to Insulin Regular *on page 841*.

Increased Effect/Toxicity: Refer to Insulin Regular *on page 841*.

Pharmacodynamics/Kinetics
Onset of action: 3-4 hours

Duration: Dose dependent: 6-23 hours

Note: Duration is dose-dependent. At lower dosages (0.1-0.2 units/kg), mean duration is variable (5.7-12.1 hours). At 0.6 units/kg, the mean duration was 19.9 hours. At high dosages (>0.6 units/kg) the duration is longer and less variable (mean of 22-23 hours).

Bioavailability: 60%

Half-life: 5-7 hours (dose dependent)

Protein binding: >98% (albumin)

Distribution: V_d: 0.1 L/kg

Time to peak: 6-8 hours

Excretion: Urine

Pregnancy Risk Factor C

Insulin Glargine (IN soo lin GLAR jeen)

Related Information
Insulin Regular *on page 841*
U.S. Brand Names Lantus®
Canadian Brand Names Lantus®; Lantus® OptiSet®
Generic Available No
Synonyms Glargine Insulin
Pharmacologic Category Antidiabetic Agent, Insulin
Use Treatment of type 1 diabetes mellitus (insulin dependent, IDDM); type 2 diabetes mellitus (noninsulin dependent, NIDDM) requiring basal (long-acting) insulin to control hyperglycemia
Local Anesthetic/Vasoconstrictor Precautions No information available to require special precautions
Effects on Dental Treatment Type 1 diabetics (insulin dependent) should be appointed for dental treatment in the morning in order to minimize chance of stress-induced hypoglycemia.
Common Adverse Effects Refer to Insulin Regular *on page 841*.
Mechanism of Action Refer to Insulin Regular *on page 841*. Insulin glargine is a long-acting insulin analog.
Drug Interactions
Cytochrome P450 Effect: Refer to Insulin Regular *on page 841*.
Increased Effect/Toxicity: Refer to Insulin Regular *on page 841*.
Pharmacodynamics/Kinetics
Onset of action: 3-4 hours
Duration: 24 hours
Absorption: Slow; forms microprecipitates which allow small amounts to release over time
Metabolism: Partially metabolized in the skin to form teo active metabolites
Time to peak: No pronounced peak
Excretion: Urine
Pregnancy Risk Factor C

Insulin Glulisine (IN soo lin gloo LIS een)

Related Information
Insulin Regular *on page 841*
U.S. Brand Names Apidra®
Canadian Brand Names Apidra®
Generic Available No
Synonyms Glulisine Insulin
Pharmacologic Category Antidiabetic Agent, Insulin
Use Treatment of type 1 diabetes mellitus (insulin dependent, IDDM); type 2 diabetes mellitus (noninsulin dependent, NIDDM) to control hyperglycemia
Local Anesthetic/Vasoconstrictor Precautions No information available to require special precautions
Effects on Dental Treatment Type 1 diabetics (insulin dependent) should be appointed for dental treatment in the morning in order to minimize chance of stress-induced hypoglycemia.
Common Adverse Effects Refer to Insulin Regular *on page 841*.
Mechanism of Action Refer to Insulin Regular *on page 841*. Insulin glulisine is a rapid-acting insulin analog.
Drug Interactions
Increased Effect/Toxicity: Refer to Insulin Regular *on page 841*.
Pharmacodynamics/Kinetics
Onset of action: 0.2-0.5 hours
Duration: 3-4 hours
Time to Peak: 30-90 minutes
Excretion: Urine
Pregnancy Risk Factor C

Insulin Inhalation (IN soo lin in ha LAY shun)

Related Information
Insulin Regular *on page 841*
(Continued)

Insulin Inhalation *(Continued)*

U.S. Brand Names Exubera®

Synonyms Inhaled Insulin

Pharmacologic Category Antidiabetic Agent, Insulin

Use Treatment of type 1 diabetes mellitus (insulin dependent, IDDM); type 2 diabetes mellitus (noninsulin dependent, NIDDM)

Local Anesthetic/Vasoconstrictor Precautions No information available to require special precautions

Effects on Dental Treatment Key adverse event(s) related to dental treatment: Xerostomia and changes in salivation (normal salivary flow resumes upon discontinuation). Type 1 diabetics (insulin dependent) should be appointed for dental treatment in the morning in order to minimize chance of stress-induced hypoglycemia.

Common Adverse Effects Also refer to Insulin Regular *on page 841*.

Cardiovascular: Chest pain (5%; usually mild to moderate)

Dermatologic: Rash (rare)

Endocrine & metabolic: Hypoglycemia

Gastrointestinal: Xerostomia (2%)

Otic: Otitis media (pediatric patients 7%), ear pain (4%), ear disorder (1%)

Respiratory: Respiratory infection (30% to 43%), cough increased (22% to 30%), pharyngitis (10% to 18%), rhinitis (9% to 15%), sinusitis (5% to 10%), dyspnea (4%), sputum increased (3% to 4%), bronchitis (3% to 5%), epistaxis (1%), laryngitis (1%), voice alteration (1%), bronchospasm (rare)

> Note: Decreases in pulmonary function (reduced FEV1, DLco) have been associated with use, usually noted in the initial weeks of therapy; declines from baseline of 20% in, respectively, FEV1 and DLco, were reported in 5.1% and 1.5% of patients as compared to 3.6% and 1.3% in comparator-treated patients.

Miscellaneous: Allergic reactions, anaphylaxis (including tachycardia and hypotension), diaphoresis increased

Restrictions A medication guide must be distributed to each patient to whom this medication is dispensed.

Dosage Inhalation: Children ≥6 years and Adults:

Initial: 0.05 mg/kg (rounded down to nearest whole milligram) 3 times/daily administered within 10 minutes of a meal

Adjustment: Dosage may be increased or decreased based on serum glucose monitoring, meal size, nutrient composition, time of day, and exercise patterns.

> Note: A 1 mg blister is approximately equivalent to 3 units of regular insulin, while a 3 mg blister is approximately equivalent to 8 units of regular insulin administered subcutaneously. Patients should combine 1 mg and 3 mg blisters so that the fewest blisters are required to achieve the prescribed dose. Consecutive inhalation of three 1 mg blisters results in significantly higher insulin levels as compared to inhalation of a single 3 mg blister (do not substitute). In a patient stabilized on a dosage which uses 3 mg blisters, if 3 mg blister is temporarily unavailable, inhalation of two 1 mg blisters may be substituted.

Dosing adjustment in renal impairment: Insulin requirements are reduced due to changes in insulin clearance or metabolism.

Mechanism of Action Refer to Insulin Regular *on page 841*. Insulin inhalation is a rapid-acting form of human insulin.

Contraindications Hypersensitivity to any component of the formulation; smokers or patients who have discontinued smoking for <6 months; poorly-controlled or unstable lung disease

Warnings/Precautions Also refer to Insulin Regular *on page 841*.

Due to increased systemic absorption, the risk of hypoglycemia is greatly increased in patients who smoke or who have stopped smoking for less than 6 months. The effect of passive exposure to smoke has not been fully evaluated but may result in alteration in absorption and/or hypoglycemia. Insulin inhalation should be immediately discontinued in any patient who resumes smoking.

Decreases in pulmonary function have been associated with use. Due the potential impact on pulmonary function, testing should be performed prior to the initiation of inhaled insulin therapy. Not recommended for use in patients with lung disease (asthma, COPD). Monitor closely during periods of intercurrent respiratory illness.

In type 1 diabetes mellitus (insulin dependent, IDDM), rapid-acting insulins including insulin inhalation should be used in combination with a long-acting insulin. However, in type 2 diabetes mellitus (noninsulin dependent, NIDDM), rapid-acting agents may be used without a long-acting insulin when used as monotherapy or combined with an oral antidiabetic agent.

Use caution in renal and/or hepatic impairment.

Drug Interactions
  Cytochrome P450 Effect: Refer to Insulin Regular *on page 841*.
  Increased Effect/Toxicity: Refer to Insulin Regular *on page 841*.
  Decreased Effect: Refer to Insulin Regular *on page 841*.

Ethanol/Nutrition/Herb Interactions Refer to Insulin Regular *on page 841*.

Dietary Considerations Dietary modification based on ADA recommendations is a key component of therapy.

Pharmacodynamics/Kinetics
  Onset of action: 0.2-0.4 hours
  Duration: 6-8 hours
  Absorption: Rapid
  Bioavailability: Absolute bioavailability not defined (depends on inspiratory flow characteristics); systemic exposure may be up to 2-5 times higher in smokers
  Time to peak, plasma: 30-90 minutes
  Excretion: Urine

Pregnancy Risk Factor C

Dosage Forms
  POWDER for oral inhalation [prefilled blister pack]: 1 mg (90s), 3 mg (90s).
  COMB PACK [prefilled blister pack]: Powder for inhalation: 1 mg (90s); powder for inhalation: 3 mg (90s)

Selected Readings
  Skyler JS, Weinstock RS, and Raskin P, "Use of Inhaled Insulin in a Basal/Bolus Insulin Regimen in Type 1 Diabetic Subjects: A 6-Month, Randomized, Comparative Trial," *Diabetes Care*, 2005, 28(7):1630-5.

Insulin Lispro (IN soo lin LYE sproe)

Related Information
  Insulin Regular *on page 841*

U.S. Brand Names Humalog®

Canadian Brand Names Humalog®

Generic Available No

Synonyms Lispro Insulin

Pharmacologic Category Antidiabetic Agent, Insulin

Use Treatment of type 1 diabetes mellitus (insulin dependent, IDDM); type 2 diabetes mellitus (noninsulin dependent, NIDDM) to control hyperglycemia
  Note: In type 1 diabetes mellitus (insulin dependent, IDDM), insulin lispro (Humalog®) should be used in combination with a long-acting insulin. However, in type 2 diabetes mellitus (noninsulin dependent, NIDDM), insulin lispro (Humalog®) may be used without a long-acting insulin when used in combination with a sulfonylurea.

Local Anesthetic/Vasoconstrictor Precautions No information available to require special precautions

Effects on Dental Treatment Type 1 diabetics (insulin dependent) should be appointed for dental treatment in the morning in order to minimize chance of stress-induced hypoglycemia.

Common Adverse Effects Refer to Insulin Regular *on page 841*.

Mechanism of Action Refer to Insulin Regular *on page 841*. Insulin lispro is a rapid-acting form of insulin.

Drug Interactions
  Cytochrome P450 Effect: Refer to Insulin Regular *on page 841*.
  Increased Effect/Toxicity: Refer to Insulin Regular *on page 841*.

Pharmacodynamics/Kinetics
  Onset of action: 0.2-0.5 hours
  Duration: 3-4 hours
  Distribution: 0.26-0.36 L/kg
  Bioavailability: 55% to 77%
  Time to peak: 30-90 minutes
  Excretion: Urine

Pregnancy Risk Factor B

Insulin Lispro and Insulin Lispro Protamine *see* Insulin Lispro Protamine and Insulin Lispro *on page 839*

Insulin Lispro Protamine and Insulin Lispro
  (IN soo lin LYE sproe PROE ta meen & IN soo lin LYE sproe)

Related Information
  Insulin Regular *on page 841*
  (Continued)

Insulin Lispro Protamine and Insulin Lispro
(Continued)

U.S. Brand Names Humalog® Mix 50/50™; Humalog® Mix 75/25™
Canadian Brand Names Humalog® Mix 25
Generic Available No
Synonyms Insulin Lispro and Insulin Lispro Protamine
Pharmacologic Category Antidiabetic Agent, Insulin
Use Treatment of type 1 diabetes mellitus (insulin dependent, IDDM); type 2 diabetes mellitus (noninsulin dependent, NIDDM) to control hyperglycemia
Local Anesthetic/Vasoconstrictor Precautions No information available to require special precautions
Effects on Dental Treatment Type 1 diabetics (insulin-dependent) should be appointed for dental treatment in the morning in order to minimize chance of stress-induced hypoglycemia.
Common Adverse Effects Refer to Insulin Regular *on page 841.*
Mechanism of Action Refer to Insulin Regular *on page 841.* Insulin lispro protamine and insulin lispro is a combination product with a rapid onset, and a duration of action which is similar to intermediate-acting insulin products.
Drug Interactions
  Increased Effect/Toxicity: Refer to Insulin Regular *on page 841.*
Pharmacodynamics/Kinetics
  Onset of action: 0.2-0.5 hours
  Duration: 18-24 hours
  Time to peak: 2-12 hours
  Excretion: Urine
Pregnancy Risk Factor B

Insulin NPH (IN soo lin N P H)

Related Information
  Insulin Regular *on page 841*
U.S. Brand Names Humulin® N; Novolin® N
Canadian Brand Names Humulin® N; Novolin® ge NPH
Generic Available No
Synonyms Isophane Insulin; NPH Insulin
Pharmacologic Category Antidiabetic Agent, Insulin
Use Treatment of type 1 diabetes mellitus (insulin dependent, IDDM); type 2 diabetes mellitus (noninsulin dependent, NIDDM) to control hyperglycemia
Local Anesthetic/Vasoconstrictor Precautions No information available to require special precautions
Effects on Dental Treatment Type 1 diabetics (insulin dependent) should be appointed for dental treatment in the morning in order to minimize chance of stress-induced hypoglycemia.
Common Adverse Effects Refer to Insulin Regular *on page 841.*
Mechanism of Action Refer to Insulin Regular *on page 841.* Insulin NPH is an intermediate-acting form of insulin.
Drug Interactions
  Cytochrome P450 Effect: Refer to Insulin Regular *on page 841.*
  Increased Effect/Toxicity: Refer to Insulin Regular *on page 841.*
Pharmacodynamics/Kinetics
  Onset of action: 1-2 hours
  Duration: 18-24 hours
  Time to peak: 6-12 hours
  Excretion: Urine
Pregnancy Risk Factor B

Insulin NPH and Insulin Regular
(IN soo lin N P H & IN soo lin REG yoo ler)

Related Information
  Insulin Regular *on page 841*
U.S. Brand Names Humulin® 50/50; Humulin® 70/30; Novolin® 70/30
Canadian Brand Names Humulin® 20/80; Humulin® 70/30; Novolin® ge 10/90; Novolin® ge 20/80; Novolin® ge 30/70; Novolin® ge 40/60; Novolin® ge 50/50
Generic Available No
Synonyms Insulin Regular and Insulin NPH; Isophane Insulin and Regular Insulin; NPH Insulin and Regular Insulin

Pharmacologic Category Antidiabetic Agent, Insulin

Use Treatment of type 1 diabetes mellitus (insulin dependent, IDDM); type 2 diabetes mellitus (noninsulin dependent, NIDDM) to control hyperglycemia

Local Anesthetic/Vasoconstrictor Precautions No information available to require special precautions

Effects on Dental Treatment Type 1 diabetics (insulin dependent) should be appointed for dental treatment in the morning in order to minimize chance of stress-induced hypoglycemia.

Mechanism of Action Refer to Insulin Regular *on page 841*. Insulin NPH and insulin regular is a combination insulin product with intermediate-acting characteristics. It may be administered once or twice daily.

Pharmacodynamics/Kinetics
Onset of action: 0.5 hours
Duration: 18-24 hours
Time to peak: 2-12 hours
Excretion: Urine

Pregnancy Risk Factor C

Insulin Regular (IN soo lin REG yoo ler)

Related Information
Insulin Aspart *on page 835*
Insulin Aspart Protamine and Insulin Aspart *on page 836*
Insulin Detemir *on page 836*
Insulin Glargine *on page 837*
Insulin Glulisine *on page 837*
Insulin Lispro *on page 839*
Insulin Lispro Protamine and Insulin Lispro *on page 839*
Insulin NPH *on page 840*
Insulin NPH and Insulin Regular *on page 840*

U.S. Brand Names Humulin® R; Humulin® R (Concentrated) U-500; Novolin® R

Canadian Brand Names Humulin® R; Novolin® ge Toronto

Generic Available No

Synonyms Regular Insulin

Pharmacologic Category Antidiabetic Agent, Insulin; Antidote

Use Treatment of type 1 diabetes mellitus (insulin dependent, IDDM); type 2 diabetes mellitus (noninsulin dependent, NIDDM) unresponsive to treatment with diet and/or oral hypoglycemics, to control hyperglycemia; adjunct to parenteral nutrition; diabetic ketoacidosis (DKA)

Unlabeled/Investigational Use Hyperkalemia (regular insulin only; use with glucose to shift potassium into cells to lower serum potassium levels)

Local Anesthetic/Vasoconstrictor Precautions No information available to require special precautions

Effects on Dental Treatment Type 1 diabetics (insulin dependent) should be appointed for dental treatment in the morning in order to minimize chance of stress-induced hypoglycemia.

Common Adverse Effects Frequency not defined.
Cardiovascular: Palpitation, pallor, tachycardia
Central nervous system: Fatigue, headache, hypothermia, loss of consciousness, mental confusion
Dermatologic: Urticaria, redness
Endocrine & metabolic: Hypoglycemia
Gastrointestinal: Hunger, nausea, numbness of mouth
Local: Atrophy or hypertrophy of SubQ fat tissue; edema, itching, pain or warmth at injection site; stinging
Neuromuscular & skeletal: Muscle weakness, paresthesia, tremor
Ocular: Transient presbyopia or blurred vision
Miscellaneous: Anaphylaxis, diaphoresis, local allergy, systemic allergic symptoms

Mechanism of Action Insulin acts via specific membrane-bound receptors on target tissues to regulate metabolism of carbohydrate, protein, and fats. Insulin facilitates entry of glucose into muscle, adipose, and other tissues via hexose transporters, including GLUT4. Insulin stimulates the cellular uptake of amino acids and increases cellular permeability to several ions, including potassium, magnesium, and phosphate. By activating sodium-potassium ATPases, insulin promotes the intracellular movement of potassium.

Target organs for insulin include the liver, skeletal muscle, and adipose tissue. Within the liver, insulin stimulates hepatic glycogen synthesis through the activation of the enzymes hexokinase, phosphofructokinase, and glycogen synthase as well as the inhibition of glucose-6 phosphatase. Insulin promotes hepatic synthesis of fatty acids, which are released into the circulation as
(Continued)

Insulin Regular *(Continued)*

lipoproteins. Skeletal muscle effects of insulin include increased protein synthesis and increased glycogen synthesis. Within adipose tissue, insulin stimulates the processing of circulating lipoproteins to provide free fatty acids, facilitating triglyceride synthesis and storage by adipocytes. Insulin also directly inhibits the hydrolysis of triglycerides.

Normally secreted by the pancreas, insulin products are manufactured for pharmacologic use through recombinant DNA technology using either *E. coli* or *Saccharomyces cerevisiae*. Insulins are categorized based on promptness and duration of effect, including rapid-, short-, intermediate-, and long-acting insulins.

Drug Interactions

Cytochrome P450 Effect: Induces CYP1A2 (weak)

Increased Effect/Toxicity: Increased hypoglycemic effect of insulin with alcohol, alpha-blockers, anabolic steroids, beta-blockers (nonselective beta-blockers may delay recovery from hypoglycemic episodes and mask signs/symptoms of hypoglycemia; cardioselective beta-blocker agents may be alternatives), clofibrate, guanethidine, MAO inhibitors, pentamidine, phenylbutazone, salicylates, sulfinpyrazone, and tetracyclines.

Insulin increases the risk of hypoglycemia associated with oral hypoglycemic agents (including sulfonylureas, metformin, pioglitazone, rosiglitazone, and troglitazone).

Decreased Effect: Decreased hypoglycemic effect of insulin with corticosteroids, dextrothyroxine, diltiazem, dobutamine, epinephrine, niacin, oral contraceptives, thiazide diuretics, thyroid hormone, and smoking.

Pharmacodynamics/Kinetics

Onset of action: 0.5 hours

Duration: 6-8 hours (may increase with dose)

Time to peak: 2-4 hours

Excretion: Urine

Pregnancy Risk Factor B

Insulin Regular and Insulin NPH *see* Insulin NPH and Insulin Regular *on page 840*

Intal® *see* Cromolyn *on page 397*

Integrilin® *see* Eptifibatide *on page 556*

α-2-interferon *see* Interferon Alfa-2b *on page 844*

Interferon Alfa-2a *(in ter FEER on AL fa too aye)*

Related Information

Systemic Viral Diseases *on page 1675*

U.S. Brand Names Roferon-A®

Canadian Brand Names Roferon-A®

Generic Available No

Synonyms IFLrA; rIFN-A

Pharmacologic Category Interferon

Use

Patients >18 years of age: Hairy cell leukemia, AIDS-related Kaposi's sarcoma, chronic hepatitis C

Children and Adults: Chronic myelogenous leukemia (CML), Philadelphia chromosome positive, within 1 year of diagnosis (limited experience in children)

Unlabeled/Investigational Use Adjuvant therapy for malignant melanoma, AIDS-related thrombocytopenia, cutaneous ulcerations of Behçet's disease, brain tumors, metastatic ileal carcinoid tumors, cervical and colorectal cancers, genital warts, idiopathic mixed cryoglobulinemia, hemangioma, hepatitis D, hepatocellular carcinoma, idiopathic hypereosinophilic syndrome, mycosis fungoides, Sézary syndrome, low-grade non-Hodgkin's lymphoma, macular degeneration, multiple myeloma, renal cell carcinoma, basal and squamous cell skin cancer, essential thrombocythemia, cutaneous T-cell lymphoma

Local Anesthetic/Vasoconstrictor Precautions No information available to require special precautions

Effects on Dental Treatment Key adverse event(s) related to dental treatment: Significant xerostomia (normal salivary flow resumes upon discontinuation), metallic taste, taste change, loss of taste, cough, irritation of oropharynx.

Common Adverse Effects Note: A flu-like syndrome (fever, chills, tachycardia, malaise, myalgia, arthralgia, headache) occurs within 1-2 hours of administration; may last up to 24 hours and may be dose-limiting (symptoms in up to 92% of patients). For the listing below, the percentage of incidence noted generally corresponds to highest reported ranges. Incidence depends upon dosage and indication.

>10%:
Cardiovascular: Chest pain (4% to 11%), edema (11%), hypertension (11%)
Central nervous system: Psychiatric disturbances (including depression and suicidal behavior/ideation; reported incidence highly variable, generally >15%), fatigue (90%), headache (52%), dizziness (21%), irritability (15%), insomnia (14%), somnolence, lethargy, confusion, mental impairment, and motor weakness (most frequently seen at high doses [>100 million units], usually reverses within a few days); vertigo (19%); mental status changes (12%)
Dermatologic: Rash (usually maculopapular) on the trunk and extremities (7% to 18%), alopecia (19% to 22%), pruritus (13%), dry skin
Endocrine & metabolic: Hypocalcemia (10% to 51%), hyperglycemia (33% to 39%), transaminases increased (25% to 30%), alkaline phosphatase increased (48%)
Gastrointestinal: Loss of taste, anorexia (30% to 70%), nausea (28% to 53%), vomiting (10% to 30%, usually mild), diarrhea (22% to 34%, may be severe), taste change (13%), dry throat, xerostomia, abdominal cramps, abdominal pain
Hematologic (often due to underlying disease): Myelosuppression; neutropenia (32% to 70%); thrombocytopenia (22% to 70%); anemia (24% to 65%, may be dose-limiting, usually seen only during the first 6 months of therapy)
  Onset: 7-10 days
  Nadir: 14 days, may be delayed 20-40 days in hairy cell leukemia
  Recovery: 21 days
Hepatic: Elevation of AST (SGOT) (77% to 80%), LDH (47%), bilirubin (31%)
Local: Injection site reaction (29%)
Neuromuscular & skeletal: Weakness (may be severe at doses >20,000,000 units/day); arthralgia and myalgia (5% to 73%, usually during the first 72 hours of treatment); rigors
Renal: Proteinuria (15% to 25%)
Respiratory: Cough (27%), irritation of oropharynx (14%)
Miscellaneous: Flu-like syndrome (up to 92% of patients), diaphoresis (15%)

1% to 10%:
Cardiovascular: Hypotension (6%), supraventricular tachyarrhythmia, palpitation (<3%), acute MI (<1% to 1%)
Central nervous system: Confusion (10%), delirium
Dermatologic: Erythema (diffuse), urticaria
Endocrine & metabolic: Hyperphosphatemia (2%)
Gastrointestinal: Stomatitis, pancreatitis (<5%), flatulence, liver pain
Genitourinary: Impotence (6%), menstrual irregularities
Neuromuscular & skeletal: Leg cramps; peripheral neuropathy, paresthesia (7%), and numbness (4%) are more common in patients previously treated with vinca alkaloids or receiving concurrent vinblastine
Ocular: Conjunctivitis (4%)
Respiratory: Dyspnea (7.5%), epistaxis (4%), rhinitis (3%)
Miscellaneous: Antibody production to interferon (10%)

Restrictions An FDA-approved medication guide is available at http://www.fda.gov/cder/Offices/ODS/labeling.htm; distribute to each patient to whom this medication is dispensed.

Mechanism of Action Following activation, multiple effects can be detected including induction of gene transcription. Inhibits cellular growth, alters the state of cellular differentiation, interferes with oncogene expression, alters cell surface antigen expression, increases phagocytic activity of macrophages, and augments cytotoxicity of lymphocytes for target cells

Drug Interactions
Cytochrome P450 Effect: Inhibits CYP1A2 (weak)
Increased Effect/Toxicity: Note: May exacerbate the toxicity of other agents with respect to CNS, myelotoxicity, or cardiotoxicity. Theophylline clearance has been reported to be decreased in hepatitis patients receiving interferon. Interferons may increase the adverse/toxic effects of ACE inhibitors, specifically the development of granulocytopenia. Agranulocytosis has been reported with concurrent use of clozapine (case report). Interferons may increase the anticoagulant effects of warfarin, and interferons may increase serum levels of zidovudine. Concurrent therapy with ribavirin may increase the risk of hemolytic anemia.
Decreased Effect: Prednisone may decrease the therapeutic effects of interferon alpha. A decreased response to erythropoietin has been reported (case reports) in patients receiving interferons. Interferon alpha may decrease the serum concentrations of melphalan (may or may not decrease toxicity of melphalan).
(Continued)

Interferon Alfa-2a (Continued)

Pharmacodynamics/Kinetics

Absorption: Filtered and absorbed at the renal tubule

Distribution: V_d: 0.223-0.748 L/kg

Metabolism: Primarily renal; filtered through glomeruli and undergoes rapid proteolytic degradation during tubular reabsorption

Bioavailability: I.M.: 83%; SubQ: 90%

Half-life elimination: I.V.: 3.7-8.5 hours (mean ~5 hours)

Time to peak, serum: I.M., SubQ: ~6-8 hours

Pregnancy Risk Factor C

Interferon Alfa-2a (PEG Conjugate) see Peginterferon Alfa-2a on page 1195

Interferon Alfa-2b (in ter FEER on AL fa too bee)

Related Information

Systemic Viral Diseases on page 1675

U.S. Brand Names Intron® A

Canadian Brand Names Intron® A

Generic Available No

Synonyms α-2-interferon; INF-alpha 2; rLFN-α2

Pharmacologic Category Interferon

Dental Use

Patients ≥1 year of age: Chronic hepatitis B

Patients ≥18 years of age: Condyloma acuminata, chronic hepatitis C, hairy cell leukemia, malignant melanoma, AIDS-related Kaposi's sarcoma, follicular non-Hodgkin's lymphoma

Use

Patients ≥1 year of age: Chronic hepatitis B

Patients ≥18 years of age: Condyloma acuminata, chronic hepatitis C, hairy cell leukemia, malignant melanoma, AIDS-related Kaposi's sarcoma, follicular non-Hodgkin's lymphoma

Unlabeled/Investigational Use AIDS-related thrombocytopenia, cutaneous ulcerations of Behçet's disease, carcinoid syndrome, cervical cancer, lymphomatoid granulomatosis, genital herpes, hepatitis D, chronic myelogenous leukemia (CML), non-Hodgkin's lymphomas (other than follicular lymphoma, see approved use), polycythemia vera, medullary thyroid carcinoma, multiple myeloma, renal cell carcinoma, basal and squamous cell skin cancers, essential thrombocytopenia, thrombocytopenic purpura

Investigational: West Nile virus

Local Anesthetic/Vasoconstrictor Precautions No information available to require special precautions

Effects on Dental Treatment Key adverse event(s) related to dental treatment: Xerostomia (normal salivary flow resumes upon discontinuation) and metallic taste.

Significant Adverse Effects Flu-like symptoms are common (up to 79%)

>10%:

Cardiovascular: Chest pain (2% to 28%)

Central nervous system: Fatigue (8% to 96%), headache (21% to 62%), fever (34% to 94%), depression (4% to 40%), somnolence (1% to 33%), irritability (1% to 22%), paresthesia (1% to 21%, more common in patients previously treated with vinca alkaloids or receiving concurrent vinblastine), dizziness (7% to 23%), confusion (1% to 12%), malaise (3% to 14%), pain (3% to 15%), insomnia (1% to 12%), impaired concentration (1% to 14%, usually reverses within a few days), amnesia (1% to 14%), chills (45% to 54%)

Dermatologic: Alopecia (8% to 38%), rash (usually maculopapular) on the trunk and extremities (1% to 25%), pruritus (3% to 11%), dry skin (1% to 10%)

Endocrine & metabolic: Hypocalcemia (10% to 51%), hyperglycemia (33% to 39%), amenorrhea (up to 12% in lymphoma), alkaline phosphatase increased (48%)

Gastrointestinal: Anorexia (1% to 69%), nausea (19% to 66%), vomiting (2% to 32%, usually mild), diarrhea (2% to 45%, may be severe), taste change (2% to 24%), xerostomia (1% to 28%), abdominal pain (2% to 23%), gingivitis (2% to 14%), constipation (1% to 14%)

Hematologic: Myelosuppression; neutropenia (30% to 66%); thrombocytopenia (5% to 15%); anemia (15% to 32%, may be dose-limiting, usually seen only during the first 6 months of therapy)

Onset: 7-10 days

Nadir: 14 days, may be delayed 20-40 days in hairy cell leukemia

Recovery: 21 days

Hepatic: Right upper quadrant pain (15% in hepatitis C), transaminases increased (increased SGOT in up to 63%)

Local: Injection site reaction (1% to 20%)

Neuromuscular & skeletal: Weakness (5% to 63%) may be severe at doses >20,000,000 units/day; mild arthralgia and myalgia (5% to 75% - usually during the first 72 hours of treatment), rigors (2% to 42%), back pain (1% to 19%), musculoskeletal pain (1% to 21%), paresthesia (1% to 21%)

Renal: Urinary tract infection (up to 5% in hepatitis C)

Respiratory: Dyspnea (1% to 34%), cough (1% to 31%), pharyngitis (1% to 31%),

Miscellaneous: Loss of smell, flu-like symptoms (5% to 79%), diaphoresis (2% to 21%)

5% to 10%:
Cardiovascular: Hypertension (9% in hepatitis C)

Central nervous system: Anxiety (1% to 9%), nervousness (1% to 3%), vertigo (up to 8% in lymphoma)

Dermatologic: Dermatitis (1% to 8%)

Endocrine & metabolic: Decreased libido (1% to 5%)

Gastrointestinal: Loose stools (1% to 21%), dyspepsia (2% to 8%)

Neuromuscular & skeletal: Hypoesthesia (1% to 10%)

Respiratory: Nasal congestion (1% to 10%)

<5% (Limited to important or life-threatening): Acute hypersensitivity reactions, allergic reactions, angina, aphasia, arrhythmia, ataxia, atrial fibrillation, Bell's palsy, bronchospasm, cardiomyopathy, CHF, coma, depression, epidermal necrolysis, extrapyramidal disorder, gastrointestinal hemorrhage, gingival hyperplasia, granulocytopenia, hallucinations, hemolytic anemia, hemoptysis, hepatic encephalopathy (rare), hepatic failure (rare), hepatotoxic reaction, hypoventilation, jaundice, lupus erythematosus, mania, MI, nephrotic syndrome, pancreatitis, polyarteritis nodosa, psychosis, pulmonary embolism, pulmonary fibrosis, Raynaud's phenomenon, renal failure, seizure, stroke, suicidal ideation, suicide attempt, syncope, tendonitis, thrombocytopenic purpura, thrombosis, vasculitis

Dental Usual Dosing

Chronic hepatitis B:
Children 1-17 years: SubQ: 3 million units/m^2 3 times/week for 1 week; then 6 million units/m^2 3 times/week; maximum: 10 million units 3 times/week; total duration of therapy 16-24 weeks

Adults: I.M., SubQ: 5 million units/day or 10 million units 3 times/week for 16 weeks

Chronic hepatitis C: Adults: I.M., SubQ: 3 million units 3 times/week for 16 weeks. In patients with normalization of ALT at 16 weeks, continue treatment for 18-24 months; consider discontinuation if normalization does not occur at 16 weeks. Note: May be used in combination therapy with ribavirin in previously untreated patients or in patients who relapse following alpha interferon therapy; refer to Interferon Alfa-2b and Ribavirin Combination Pack monograph.

Dosage Refer to individual protocols

Children 1-17 years: Chronic hepatitis B: SubQ: 3 million units/m^2 3 times/week for 1 week; then 6 million units/m^2 3 times/week; maximum: 10 million units 3 times/week; total duration of therapy 16-24 weeks

Adults:
Hairy cell leukemia: I.M., SubQ: 2 million units/m^2 3 times/week for 2-6 months

Lymphoma (follicular): SubQ: 5 million units 3 times/week for up to 18 months

Malignant melanoma: 20 million units/m^2 I.V. for 5 consecutive days per week for 4 weeks, then 10 million units/m^2 SubQ 3 times/week for 48 weeks

AIDS-related Kaposi's sarcoma: I.M., SubQ: 30 million units/m^2 3 times/week

Chronic hepatitis B: I.M., SubQ: 5 million units/day or 10 million units 3 times/week for 16 weeks

Chronic hepatitis C: I.M., SubQ: 3 million units 3 times/week for 16 weeks. In patients with normalization of ALT at 16 weeks, continue treatment for 18-24 months; consider discontinuation if normalization does not occur at 16 weeks. Note: May be used in combination therapy with ribavirin in previously untreated patients or in patients who relapse following alpha interferon therapy; refer to Interferon Alfa-2b and Ribavirin Combination Pack monograph.

Condyloma acuminata: Intralesionally: 1 million units/lesion (maximum: 5 lesions/treatment) 3 times/week (on alternate days) for 3 weeks; may administer a second course at 12-16 weeks

Dosage adjustment in renal impairment: Combination therapy with ribavirin (hepatitis C) should not be used in patients with reduced renal function (Cl$_{cr}$ <50 mL/minute).

Not removed by peritoneal or hemodialysis

(Continued)

Interferon Alfa-2b *(Continued)*

Dosage adjustment for toxicity: Manufacturer-recommended adjustments, listed according to indication:

Lymphoma (follicular):
Severe toxicity (neutrophils <1000 cells/mm^3 or platelets <50,000 cells/mm^3): Reduce dose by 50% or temporarily discontinue
AST/ALT >5 times ULN: Permanently discontinue

Hairy cell leukemia:
Severe toxicity: Reduce dose by 50% or temporarily discontinue; permanently discontinue if persistent or recurrent severe toxicity is noted

Hepatitis B or C:
WBC <1500 cells/mm^3, granulocytes <750 cells/mm^3, or platelet count <50,000 cells/mm^3: Reduce dose by 50%
WBC <1000 cells/mm^3, granulocytes <500 cells/mm^3, or platelet count <25,000 cells/mm^3: Permanently discontinue

Kaposi sarcoma: Severe toxicity: Reduce dose by 50% or temporarily discontinue

Malignant melanoma:
Severe toxicity (neutrophils <500 cells/mm^3 or AST/ALT >5 times ULN): Reduce dose by 50% or temporarily discontinue
Neutrophils <250 cells/mm^3 or AST/ALT >10 times ULN: Permanently discontinue

Mechanism of Action Following activation, multiple effects can be detected including induction of gene transcription. Inhibits cellular growth, alters the state of cellular differentiation, interferes with oncogene expression, alters cell surface antigen expression, increases phagocytic activity of macrophages, and augments cytotoxicity of lymphocytes for target cells

Contraindications Hypersensitivity to interferon alfa or any component of the formulation; decompensated liver disease; autoimmune hepatitis; history of autoimmune disease; immunosuppressed transplant patients

Warnings/Precautions Suicidal ideation or attempts may occur more frequently in pediatric patients when compared to adults. May cause severe psychiatric adverse events (psychosis, mania, depression, suicidal behavior/ideation) in patients with and without previous psychiatric symptoms, avoid use in severe psychiatric disorders or in patients with a history of depression; careful neuropsychiatric monitoring is required during therapy. Use with caution in patients with a history of seizures, brain metastases, multiple sclerosis, cardiac disease (ischemic or thromboembolic), arrhythmias, myelosuppression, hepatic impairment, or renal dysfunction (use is not recommended if Cl$_{cr}$<50 mL/minute). Use caution in patients with a history of pulmonary disease, coagulopathy, thyroid disease (monitor thyroid function), hypertension, or diabetes mellitus (particularly if prone to DKA). Caution in patients receiving drugs that may cause lactic acidosis (eg, nucleoside analogues).

Avoid use in patients with autoimmune disorders; worsening of psoriasis and/or development of autoimmune disorders has been associated with alpha interferons. Higher doses in elderly patients, or diseases other than hairy cell leukemia, may result in increased CNS toxicity. Treatment should be discontinued in patients who develop severe pulmonary symptoms with chest x-ray changes, autoimmune disorders, worsening of hepatic function, psychiatric symptoms (including depression and/or suicidal thoughts/behaviors), ischemic and/or infectious disorders. Ophthalmologic disorders (including retinal hemorrhages, cotton wool spots and retinal artery or vein obstruction) have occurred in patients receiving alpha interferons. Hypertriglyceridemia has been reported (discontinue if severe).

Safety and efficacy in children <1 year of age have not been established. Do not treat patients with visceral AIDS-related Kaposi's sarcoma associated with rapidly-progressing or life-threatening disease. A transient increase in SGOT (>2x baseline) is common in patients treated with interferon alfa-2b for chronic hepatitis. Therapy generally may continue, however, functional indicators (albumin, prothrombin time, bilirubin) should be monitored at 2-week intervals. **Due to differences in dosage, patients should not change brands of interferons without the prescribers knowledge.**

Intron® A may cause bone marrow suppression, including very rarely, aplastic anemia. Hemolytic anemia (hemoglobin <10 g/dL) was observed in up to 10% of treated patients in clinical trials when combined with ribavirin; anemia occurred within 1-2 weeks of initiation of therapy.

Drug Interactions Inhibits CYP1A2 (weak)
ACE inhibitors: Interferons may increase the adverse/toxic effects of ACE inhibitors, specifically the development of granulocytopenia; monitor.
Clozapine: A case report of agranulocytosis with concurrent use.
Erythropoietin: Case reports of decreased hematopoietic effect.

Melphalan: Interferon alfa may decrease the serum concentrations of melphalan; this may or may not decrease the potential toxicity of melphalan; monitor.

Prednisone: Prednisone may decrease the therapeutic effects of interferon alfa. Risk: Moderate

Ribavirin: Concurrent therapy may increase the risk of hemolytic anemia.

Theophylline: Interferon alfa may decrease the P450 isoenzyme metabolism of theophylline. Risk: Moderate

Warfarin: Interferons may increase the anticoagulant effects of warfarin; monitor.

Zidovudine: Interferons may decrease the metabolism of zidovudine; monitor.

Pharmacodynamics/Kinetics

Distribution: V_d: 31 L; but has been noted to be much greater (370-720 L) in leukemia patients receiving continuous infusion IFN; IFN does not penetrate the CSF

Metabolism: Primarily renal

Bioavailability: I.M.: 83%; SubQ: 90%

Half-life elimination: I.M., I.V.: 2 hours; SubQ: 3 hours

Time to peak, serum: I.M., SubQ: ~3-12 hours

Pregnancy Risk Factor C

Lactation Enters breast milk/not recommended (AAP rates "compatible")

Breast-Feeding Considerations Women with hepatitis C should be instructed that there is a theoretical risk the virus may be transmitted in breast milk. HIV-infected mothers are discouraged from breast-feeding to decrease potential transmission of HIV.

Dosage Forms

Injection, powder for reconstitution: 10 million units; 18 million units; 50 million units [contains human albumin]

Injection, solution [multidose prefilled pen]:
Delivers 3 million units/0.2 mL (1.5 mL) [delivers 6 doses; 18 million units]
Delivers 5 million units/0.2 mL (1.5 mL) [delivers 6 doses; 30 million units]
Delivers 10 million units/0.2 mL (1.5 mL) [delivers 6 doses; 60 million units]

Injection, solution [multidose vial]: 6 million units/mL (3 mL); 10 million units/mL (2.5 mL)

Injection, solution [single-dose vial]: 10 million units/ mL (1 mL)

Interferon Alfa-2b and Ribavirin
(in ter FEER on AL fa too bee & rye ba VYE rin)

Related Information

Interferon Alfa-2b *on page 844*

Ribavirin *on page 1343*

U.S. Brand Names Rebetron®

Generic Available No

Synonyms Interferon Alfa-2b and Ribavirin Combination Pack; Ribavirin and Interferon Alfa-2b Combination Pack

Pharmacologic Category Antiviral Agent; Interferon

Use Combination therapy for the treatment of chronic hepatitis C in patients with compensated liver disease previously untreated with alpha interferon or who have relapsed after alpha interferon therapy

Local Anesthetic/Vasoconstrictor Precautions No information available to require special precautions

Effects on Dental Treatment Key adverse event(s) related to dental treatment: Xerostomia (normal salivary flow resumes upon discontinuation), metallic taste, and taste perversion.

Common Adverse Effects Note: Adverse reactions listed are specific to combination regimen in previously untreated hepatitis patients. See individual agents for additional adverse reactions reported with each agent during therapy for other diseases.

>10%:

Central nervous system: Fatigue (children 61%; adults 68%), headache (63%), insomnia (children 14%; adults 39%), fever (children 61%; adults 37%), depression (children 13%; adults 32% to 36%), irritability (children 10%; adults 23% to 32%), dizziness (17% to 23%), emotional lability (children 16%; adults 7% to 11%), impaired concentration (5% to 14%)

Dermatologic: Alopecia (23% to 32%), pruritus (children 12%; adults 19% to 21%), rash (17% to 28%)

Gastrointestinal: Nausea (33% to 46%), anorexia (children 51%; adults 25% to 27%), dyspepsia (children <1%; adults 14% to 16%), vomiting (children 42%; adults 9% to 11%)

Hematologic: Leukopenia, neutropenia (usually recovers within 4 weeks of treatment discontinuation), anemia

Hepatic: Hyperbilirubinemia (27%; only 0.9% to 2% >3.0-6 mg/dL)

Local: Injection site inflammation (13%)

(Continued)

Interferon Alfa-2b and Ribavirin *(Continued)*

Neuromuscular & skeletal: Myalgia (children 32%; adults 61% to 64%), rigors (40%), arthralgia (children 15%; adults 30% to 33%), musculoskeletal pain (20% to 28%)

Respiratory: Dyspnea (children 5%; adults 18% to 19%)

Miscellaneous: Flu-like syndrome (children 31%; adults 14% to 18%)

1% to 10%:

Cardiovascular: Chest pain (5% to 9%)

Central nervous system: Nervousness (3% to 4%)

Endocrine & metabolic: Thyroid abnormalities (hyper- or hypothyroidism), serum uric acid increased, hyperglycemia

Gastrointestinal: Taste perversion (children <1%; adults 7% to 8%)

Hematologic: Hemolytic anemia (10%), thrombocytopenia, anemia

Local: Injection site reaction (7%)

Neuromuscular & skeletal: Weakness (5% to 9%)

Respiratory: Sinusitis (children <1%; adults 9% to 10%)

Restrictions An FDA-approved medication guide is available at http://www.fda.gov/cder/Offices/ODS/labeling.htm; distribute to each patient to whom this medication is dispensed.

Mechanism of Action

Interferon Alfa-2b: Alpha interferons are a family of proteins, produced by nucleated cells, that have antiviral, antiproliferative, and immune-regulating activity. There are 16 known subtypes of alpha interferons. Interferons interact with cells through high affinity cell surface receptors. Following activation, multiple effects can be detected including induction of gene transcription. Inhibits cellular growth, alters the state of cellular differentiation, interferes with oncogene expression, alters cell surface antigen expression, increases phagocytic activity of macrophages, and augments cytotoxicity of lymphocytes for target cells

Ribavirin: Inhibits replication of RNA and DNA viruses; inhibits influenza virus RNA polymerase activity and inhibits the initiation and elongation of RNA fragments resulting in inhibition of viral protein synthesis

Drug Interactions

Cytochrome P450 Effect: Interferon Alfa-2b: **Inhibits** CYP1A2 (weak)

Increased Effect/Toxicity: Interferon alpha: Cimetidine may augment the antitumor effects of interferon in melanoma. Theophylline clearance has been reported to be decreased in hepatitis patients receiving interferon. Vinblastine enhances interferon toxicity in several patients; increased incidence of paresthesia has also been noted. Interferons may increase the adverse/toxic effects of ACE inhibitors, specifically the development of granulocytopenia. Agranulocytosis has been reported with concurrent use of clozapine (case report). Interferons may increase the anticoagulant effects of warfarin, and interferons may increase serum levels of zidovudine. Concurrent therapy with ribavirin may increase the risk of hemolytic anemia. Concomitant use of ribavirin and nucleoside analogues may increase the risk of developing lactic acidosis. Concomitant therapy of interferon (alfa) and ribavirin may increase the risk of hemolytic anemia.

Decreased Effect:

Interferon alpha: Prednisone may decrease the therapeutic effects of interferon alpha. A decreased response to erythropoietin has been reported (case reports) in patients receiving interferons. Interferon alpha may decrease the serum concentrations of melphalan (may or may not decrease toxicity of melphalan). Thyroid dysfunction has been reported during treatment; monitor response to thyroid hormones.

Ribavirin: Decreased effect of stavudine and zidovudine.

Pharmacodynamics/Kinetics See individual agents.

Pregnancy Risk Factor X

Interferon Alfa-2b and Ribavirin Combination Pack *see* Interferon Alfa-2b and Ribavirin *on page 847*

Interferon Alfa-2b (PEG Conjugate) *see* Peginterferon Alfa-2b *on page 1197*

Interferon Alfa-n3 *(in ter FEER on AL fa en three)*

Related Information

Systemic Viral Diseases *on page 1675*

U.S. Brand Names Alferon® N

Canadian Brand Names Alferon® N

Generic Available No

Pharmacologic Category Interferon

Use Patients ≥18 years of age: Intralesional treatment of refractory or recurring genital or venereal warts (condylomata acuminata)

Local Anesthetic/Vasoconstrictor Precautions No information available to require special precautions

Effects on Dental Treatment Key adverse event(s) related to dental treatment: Xerostomia (normal salivary flow resumes upon discontinuation), metallic taste, tongue hyperesthesia, abnormal taste, thirst, rhinitis, pharyngitis, nosebleed, and increased diaphoresis.

Common Adverse Effects Note: Adverse reaction incidence noted below is specific to intralesional administration in patients with condylomata acuminata. Flu-like reactions, consisting of headache, fever, and/or myalgia, was reported in 30% of patients, and abated with repeated dosing.

>10%:
Central nervous system: Fever (40%), headache (31%), chills (14%), fatigue (14%)
Hematologic: Decreased WBC (11%)
Neuromuscular & skeletal: Myalgia (45%)
Miscellaneous: Flu-like syndrome (30%)

1% to 10%:
Central nervous system: Malaise (9%), dizziness (9%), depression (2%), insomnia (2%), thirst (1%)
Dermatologic: Pruritus (2%)
Gastrointestinal: Nausea (45), vomiting (3%), dyspepsia (3%), diarrhea (2%), tongue hyperesthesia (1%), taste disturbance (1%)
Genitourinary: Groin lymph node swelling (1%)
Neuromuscular & skeletal: Arthralgia (5%), back pain (4%), cramps (1%), paresthesia (1%)
Ocular: Visual disturbance (1%)
Respiratory: Rhinitis (2%), pharyngitis (1%), nosebleed (1%)
Miscellaneous: Diaphoresis increased (2%), vasovagal reaction (2%)

Mechanism of Action Interferons interact with cells through high affinity cell surface receptors. Following activation, multiple effects can be detected including induction of gene transcription. Inhibits cellular growth, alters the state of cellular differentiation, interferes with oncogene expression, alters cell surface antigen expression, increases phagocytic activity of macrophages, and augments cytotoxicity of lymphocytes for target cells

Drug Interactions

Increased Effect/Toxicity: Interferons may increase the adverse/toxic effects of ACE inhibitors, specifically the development of granulocytopenia. Risk: Monitor A case report of agranulocytosis has been reported with concurrent use of clozapine. Case reports of decreased hematopoietic effect with erythropoietin. Interferon alpha may decrease the P450 isoenzyme metabolism of theophylline. Interferons may increase the anticoagulant effects of warfarin. Interferons may decrease the metabolism of zidovudine.

Decreased Effect: Interferon alpha may decrease the serum concentrations of melphalan; this may or may not decrease the potential toxicity of melphalan. Prednisone may decrease the therapeutic effects of Interferon alpha.

Pregnancy Risk Factor C

Interferon Beta-1a (in ter FEER on BAY ta won aye)

U.S. Brand Names Avonex®; Rebif®
Canadian Brand Names Avonex®; Rebif®
Generic Available No
Synonyms rIFN beta-1a
Pharmacologic Category Interferon
Use Treatment of relapsing forms of multiple sclerosis (MS)

Local Anesthetic/Vasoconstrictor Precautions No information available to require special precautions

Effects on Dental Treatment No significant effects or complications reported

Common Adverse Effects
>10%:
Central nervous system: Headache (Avonex® 58%; Rebif® 65% to 70%), fatigue (Rebif® 33% to 41%), fever (Avonex® 20%; Rebif® 25% to 28%), pain (Avonex® 23%), chills (Avonex® 19%), depression (Avonex® 18%), dizziness (Avonex® 14%)
Gastrointestinal: Nausea (Avonex® 23%), abdominal pain (Avonex® 8%; Rebif® 20% to 22%)
Genitourinary: Urinary tract infection (Avonex® 17%)

(Continued)

Interferon Beta-1a *(Continued)*

Hematologic: Leukopenia (Rebif® 28% to 36%)

Hepatic: ALT increased (Rebif® 20% to 27%), AST increased (Rebif® 10% to 17%)

Local: Injection site reaction (Avonex® 3%; Rebif® 89% to 92%)

Neuromuscular & skeletal: Myalgia (Avonex® 29%; Rebif® 25%), back pain (Rebif® 23% to 25%), weakness (Avonex® 24%), skeletal pain (Rebif® 10% to 15%), rigors (Rebif® 6% to 13%)

Ocular: Vision abnormal (Rebif® 7% to 13%)

Respiratory: Sinusitis (Avonex® 14%), upper respiratory tract infection (Avonex® 14%)

Miscellaneous: Flu-like symptoms (Avonex® 49%; Rebif® 56% to 59%), neutralizing antibodies (significance not known; Avonex® 5%; Rebif® 24%), lymphadenopathy (Rebif® 11% to 12%)

1% to 10% (reported with one or both products):

Cardiovascular: Chest pain, vasodilation

Central nervous system: Convulsions, malaise, migraine, somnolence

Dermatologic: Alopecia, erythematous rash, maculopapular rash, urticaria

Endocrine & metabolic: Thyroid disorder

Gastrointestinal: Toothache, xerostomia

Genitourinary: Micturition frequency, urinary incontinence

Hematologic: Anemia, thrombocytopenia

Hepatic: Bilirubinemia, hepatic function abnormal

Local: Injection site bruising, injection site inflammation, injection site necrosis, injection site pain

Neuromuscular & skeletal: Arthralgia, coordination abnormal, hypertonia

Ocular: Eye disorder, xerophthalmia

Respiratory: Bronchitis

Miscellaneous: Infection

Restrictions An FDA-approved medication guide is available at http://www.fda.gov/cder/Offices/ODS/labeling.htm; distribute to each patient to whom this medication is dispensed.

Mechanism of Action Interferon beta differs from naturally occurring human protein by a single amino acid substitution and the lack of carbohydrate side chains; alters the expression and response to surface antigens and can enhance immune cell activities. Properties of interferon beta that modify biologic responses are mediated by cell surface receptor interactions; mechanism in the treatment of MS is unknown.

Drug Interactions

Increased Effect/Toxicity: Interferons may increase the adverse/toxic effects of ACE inhibitors, specifically the development of granulocytopenia. Agranulocytosis has been reported with concurrent use of clozapine (case report). Interferons may increase the anticoagulant effects of warfarin, and interferons may increase serum levels of zidovudine. Concurrent use of hepatotoxic drugs may increase the risk of hepatic injury in patients receiving interferon beta-1a.

Pharmacodynamics/Kinetics Limited data due to small doses used

Half-life elimination: Avonex®: 10 hours; Rebif®: 69 hours

Time to peak, serum: Avonex® (I.M.): 3-15 hours; Rebif® (SubQ): 16 hours

Pregnancy Risk Factor C

Interferon Beta-1b *(in ter FEER on BAY ta won bee)*

U.S. Brand Names Betaseron®

Canadian Brand Names Betaseron®

Generic Available No

Synonyms rIFN beta-1b

Pharmacologic Category Interferon

Use Treatment of relapsing forms of multiple sclerosis (MS)

Local Anesthetic/Vasoconstrictor Precautions No information available to require special precautions

Effects on Dental Treatment No significant effects or complications reported

Common Adverse Effects Note: Flu-like symptoms (including at least two of the following - headache, fever, chills, malaise, diaphoresis, and myalgia) are reported in the majority of patients (60%) and decrease over time (average duration ~1 week).

>10%:

Cardiovascular: Peripheral edema (15%), chest pain (11%)

Central nervous system: Headache (57%), fever (36%), pain (51%), chills (25%), dizziness (24%), insomnia (24%)

Dermatologic: Rash (24%), skin disorder (12%)

Endocrine & metabolic: Metrorrhagia (11%)

Gastrointestinal: Nausea (27%), diarrhea (19%), abdominal pain (19%), constipation (20%), dyspepsia (14%)

Genitourinary: Urinary urgency (13%)

Hematologic: Lymphopenia (88%), neutropenia (14%), leukopenia (14%)

Local: Injection site reaction (85%), inflammation (53%), pain (18%)

Neuromuscular & skeletal: Weakness (61%), myalgia (27%), hypertonia (50%), myasthenia (46%), arthralgia (31%), incoordination (21%)

Miscellaneous: Flu-like symptoms (60%)

1% to 10%:

Cardiovascular: Palpitation (4%), vasodilation (8%), hypertension (7%), tachycardia (4%), peripheral vascular disorder (6%)

Central nervous system: Anxiety (10%), malaise (8%), nervousness (7%)

Dermatologic: Alopecia (4%)

Endocrine & metabolic: Menorrhagia (8%), dysmenorrhea (7%)

Gastrointestinal: Weight gain (7%)

Genitourinary: Impotence (9%), pelvic pain (6%), cystitis (8%), urinary frequency (7%), prostatic disorder (3%)

Hematologic: Lymphadenopathy (8%)

Hepatic: SGPT increased >5x baseline (10%), SGOT increased >5x baseline (3%)

Local: Injection site necrosis (5%), edema (3%), mass (2%)

Neuromuscular & skeletal: Leg cramps (4%)

Respiratory: Dyspnea (7%)

Miscellaneous: Diaphoresis (8%), hypersensitivity (3%)

Mechanism of Action Interferon beta-1b differs from naturally occurring human protein by a single amino acid substitution and the lack of carbohydrate side chains; mechanism in the treatment of MS is unknown; however, immunomodulatory effects attributed to interferon beta-1b include enhancement of suppressor T cell activity, reduction of proinflammatory cytokines, down-regulation of antigen presentation, and reduced trafficking of lymphocytes into the central nervous system.

Drug Interactions

Increased Effect/Toxicity: Interferons may increase the adverse/toxic effects of ACE inhibitors, specifically the development of granulocytopenia. Risk: Monitor A case report of agranulocytosis has been reported with concurrent use of clozapine. Case reports of decreased hematopoietic effect with erythropoietin. Interferon alpha may decrease the P450 isoenzyme metabolism of theophylline. Interferons may increase the anticoagulant effects of warfarin. Interferons may decrease the metabolism of zidovudine.

Pharmacodynamics/Kinetics Limited data due to small doses used

Half-life elimination: 8 minutes to 4.3 hours

Time to peak, serum: 1-8 hours

Pregnancy Risk Factor C

Interferon Gamma-1b (in ter FEER on GAM ah won bee)

U.S. Brand Names Actimmune®

Canadian Brand Names Actimmune®

Generic Available No

Pharmacologic Category Interferon

Use Reduce frequency and severity of serious infections associated with chronic granulomatous disease; delay time to disease progression in patients with severe, malignant osteopetrosis

Local Anesthetic/Vasoconstrictor Precautions No information available to require special precautions

Effects on Dental Treatment No significant effects or complications reported

Common Adverse Effects Based on 50 mcg/m² dose administered 3 times weekly for chronic granulomatous disease

>10%:

Central nervous system: Fever (52%), headache (33%), chills (14%), fatigue (14%)

Dermatologic: Rash (17%)

Gastrointestinal: Diarrhea (14%), vomiting (13%)

Local: Injection site erythema or tenderness (14%)

1% to 10%:

Central nervous system: Depression (3%)

Gastrointestinal: Nausea (10%), abdominal pain (8%)

Neuromuscular & skeletal: Myalgia (6%), arthralgia (2%), back pain (2%)

(Continued)

Interferon Gamma-1b *(Continued)*

Drug Interactions
Cytochrome P450 Effect: Inhibits CYP1A2 (weak), 2E1 (weak)

Increased Effect/Toxicity: Interferon gamma-1b may increase hepatic enzymes or enhance myelosuppression when taken with other myelosuppressive agents. May decrease cytochrome P450 concentrations leading to increased serum concentrations of drugs metabolized by this pathway.

Pharmacodynamics/Kinetics
Absorption: I.M., SubQ: Slowly

Half-life elimination: I.V.: 38 minutes; I.M., SubQ: 3-6 hours

Time to peak, plasma: I.M.: 4 hours (1.5 ng/mL); SubQ: 7 hours (0.6 ng/mL)

Pregnancy Risk Factor C

Interleukin-1 Receptor Antagonist *see* Anakinra *on page 125*

Interleukin-2 *see* Aldesleukin *on page 61*

Interleukin-11 *see* Oprelvekin *on page 1149*

Intralipid® *see* Fat Emulsion *on page 637*

Intravenous Fat Emulsion *see* Fat Emulsion *on page 637*

Intrifiban *see* Eptifibatide *on page 556*

Intron® A *see* Interferon Alfa-2b *on page 844*

Intropaste *see* Barium *on page 179*

Invanz® *see* Ertapenem *on page 561*

Inversine® *see* Mecamylamine *on page 968*

Invirase® *see* Saquinavir *on page 1377*

Iodex [OTC] *see* Iodine *on page 852*

Iodine *(EYE oh dyne)*

Related Information
Trace Metals *on page 1513*

U.S. Brand Names Iodex [OTC]; Iodoflex™; Iodosorb®

Generic Available Yes: Tincture

Pharmacologic Category Antiseptic, Topical

Use Used topically as an antiseptic in the management of minor, superficial skin wounds and has been used to disinfect the skin preoperatively

Local Anesthetic/Vasoconstrictor Precautions No information available to require special precautions

Effects on Dental Treatment No significant effects or complications reported

Common Adverse Effects Reactions reported following topical application: Frequency not defined:

Endocrine & metabolic: TSH increased

Local: Eczema, edema, irritation, pain, redness

Miscellaneous: Allergic reaction

Reactions reported more likely observed following large doses or chronic iodine intoxication; Frequency not defined:

Central nervous system: Fever, headache

Dermatologic: Skin rash, angioedema, urticaria, acne

Endocrine & metabolic: Hypothyroidism

Gastrointestinal: Metallic taste, diarrhea

Hematologic: Eosinophilia, hemorrhage (mucosal)

Neuromuscular & skeletal: Arthralgia

Ocular: Swelling of eyelids

Respiratory: Pulmonary edema

Miscellaneous: Ioderma, lymph node enlargement

Mechanism of Action Iodine is required for thyroid hormone synthesis. Iodine is also known to be a powerful broad spectrum germicidal agent effective against a wide range of bacteria, viruses, fungi, protozoa, and spores. Iodosorb® and Iodoflex™ contain iodine in hydrophilic beads of cadexomer which allows a slow release of iodine into the wound and absorption of fluid, bacteria, and other substances from the wound

Pharmacodynamics/Kinetics
Absorption: Topical: Amount absorbed systemically depends upon concentration and characteristics of skin

Distribution: Primarily trapped by the thyroid

Bioavailability: Oral: >90%

Excretion: Urine (>90%)

Iodipamide Meglumine (eye oh DI pa mide MEG loo meen)

U.S. Brand Names Cholografin® Meglumine
Generic Available No
Pharmacologic Category Iodinated Contrast Media; Radiological/Contrast Media, Ionic
Use Contrast medium for intravenous cholangiography and cholecystography
Local Anesthetic/Vasoconstrictor Precautions No information available to require special precautions
Effects on Dental Treatment No significant effects or complications reported

Iodipamide Meglumine and Diatrizoate Meglumine *see* Diatrizoate Meglumine and Iodipamide Meglumine *on page 453*

Iodixanol (EYE oh dix an ole)

U.S. Brand Names Visipaque™
Generic Available No
Pharmacologic Category Iodinated Contrast Media; Radiological/Contrast Media, Nonionic
Use
Intra-arterial: Digital subtraction angiography, angiocardiography, peripheral arteriography, visceral arteriography, cerebral arteriography
Intravenous: Contrast enhanced computed tomography imaging, excretory urography, and peripheral venography
Local Anesthetic/Vasoconstrictor Precautions No information available to require special precautions
Effects on Dental Treatment No significant effects or complications reported
Mechanism of Action Opacifies vessels in the path of flow permitting radiographic imaging of internal structures.
Pregnancy Risk Factor B

Iodoflex™ *see* Iodine *on page 852*
Iodopen® *see* Trace Metals *on page 1513*

Iodoquinol (eye oh doe KWIN ole)

U.S. Brand Names Yodoxin®
Canadian Brand Names Diodoquin®
Generic Available No
Synonyms Diiodohydroxyquin
Pharmacologic Category Amebicide
Use Treatment of acute and chronic intestinal amebiasis; asymptomatic cyst passers; *Blastocystis hominis* infections; ineffective for amebic hepatitis or hepatic abscess
Local Anesthetic/Vasoconstrictor Precautions No information available to require special precautions
Effects on Dental Treatment No significant effects or complications reported
Common Adverse Effects Frequency not defined.
Central nervous system: Fever, chills, agitation, retrograde amnesia, headache
Dermatologic: Rash, urticaria, pruritus
Endocrine & metabolic: Thyroid gland enlargement
Gastrointestinal: Diarrhea, nausea, vomiting, stomach pain, abdominal cramps
Neuromuscular & skeletal: Peripheral neuropathy, weakness
Ocular: Optic neuritis, optic atrophy, visual impairment
Miscellaneous: Itching of rectal area
Mechanism of Action Contact amebicide that works in the lumen of the intestine by an unknown mechanism
Pharmacodynamics/Kinetics
Absorption: Poor and erratic
Metabolism: Hepatic
Excretion: Feces (high percentage)
Pregnancy Risk Factor C

Iodoquinol and Hydrocortisone
(eye oh doe KWIN ole & hye droe KOR ti sone)

Related Information
Hydrocortisone *on page 793*
Iodoquinol *on page 853*
(Continued)

Iodoquinol and Hydrocortisone *(Continued)*

Related Sample Prescriptions

Angular Cheilitis *on page 1741*

U.S. Brand Names Dermazene®; Vytone®

Generic Available Yes

Synonyms Hydrocortisone and Iodoquinol

Pharmacologic Category Antifungal Agent, Topical; Corticosteroid, Topical

Dental Use Reported to be useful in the treatment of angular cheilitis

Use Treatment of eczema; infectious dermatitis; chronic eczematoid otitis externa; mycotic dermatoses

Local Anesthetic/Vasoconstrictor Precautions No information available to require special precautions

Effects on Dental Treatment No significant effects or complications reported

Significant Adverse Effects See individual agents.

Dental Usual Dosing Angular cheilitis: Adults: Topical: Apply 3-4 times/day

Dosage Apply 3-4 times/day

Contraindications

Based on **iodoquinol** component: Hypersensitivity to iodine or iodoquinol or any component of the formulation; hepatic damage; pre-existing optic neuropathy

Based on **hydrocortisone** component: Hypersensitivity to hydrocortisone or any component of the formulation; serious infections, except septic shock or tuberculous meningitis; viral, fungal, or tubercular skin lesions

Warnings/Precautions

Based on **iodoquinol** component: Optic neuritis, optic atrophy, and peripheral neuropathy have occurred following prolonged use; avoid long-term therapy

Based on **hydrocortisone** component:

Use with caution in patients with hyperthyroidism, cirrhosis, nonspecific ulcerative colitis, hypertension, osteoporosis, thromboembolic tendencies, CHF, convulsive disorders, myasthenia gravis, thrombophlebitis, peptic ulcer, diabetes

Acute adrenal insufficiency may occur with abrupt withdrawal (depending on degree of systemic absorption) after long-term therapy or with stress; young pediatric patients may be more susceptible to adrenal axis suppression from topical therapy

Drug Interactions Hydrocortisone: **Substrate** of CYP3A4 (minor); **Induces** CYP3A4 (weak)

Also see individual agents.

Pharmacodynamics/Kinetics See individual agents.

Pregnancy Risk Factor C

Lactation Excretion in breast milk unknown

Dosage Forms

Cream: Iodoquinol 1% and hydrocortisone acetate 1% (30 g)

Dermazene®: Iodoquinol 1% and hydrocortisone acetate 1% (30 g, 45 g)

Vytone®: Iodoquinol 1% and hydrocortisone acetate 1% (30 g)

Iodosorb® *see* Iodine *on page 852*

Iohexol *(eye oh HEX ole)*

U.S. Brand Names Omnipaque™

Generic Available No

Pharmacologic Category Polypeptide Hormone; Radiological/Contrast Media, Nonionic

Use

Intrathecal: Myelography; contrast enhancement for computerized tomography

Intravascular: Angiocardiography, aortography, digital subtraction angiography, peripheral arteriography, excretory urography; contrast enhancement for computed tomographic imaging

Oral/body cavity: Arthrography, GI tract examination, hysterosalpingography, pancreatography, cholangiopancreatography, herniography, cystourethrography; enhanced computed tomography of the abdomen

Local Anesthetic/Vasoconstrictor Precautions No information available to require special precautions

Effects on Dental Treatment No significant effects or complications reported

Pregnancy Risk Factor B

Ionamin® *see* Phentermine *on page 1224*

Ionil® [OTC] *see* Salicylic Acid *on page 1374*

Ionil® Plus [OTC] *see* Salicylic Acid *on page 1374*

Ionil T® [OTC] *see* Coal Tar *on page 383*

Ionil T® Plus [OTC] see Coal Tar on page 383

Iopamidol (eye oh PA mi dole)

U.S. Brand Names Isovue®; Isovue-M®; Isovue Multipack®
Generic Available No
Pharmacologic Category Iodinated Contrast Media; Radiological/Contrast Media, Nonionic
Use
    Intrathecal (Isovue-M®): Neuroradiology; contrast enhancement of computed tomographic cisternography and ventriculography; thoraco-lumbar myelography
    Intravascular (Isovue®, Isovue Multipack®): Angiography, excretory urography; contrast enhancement of computed tomographic imaging; evaluation of certain malignancies; image enhancement of non-neoplastic lesions
Local Anesthetic/Vasoconstrictor Precautions No information available to require special precautions
Effects on Dental Treatment No significant effects or complications reported
Pregnancy Risk Factor B

Iophen-C NR see Guaifenesin and Codeine on page 753
Iophen DM NR see Guaifenesin and Dextromethorphan on page 754
Iophen NR see Guaifenesin on page 752
Iopidine® see Apraclonidine on page 133

Iopromide (eye oh PROE mide)

U.S. Brand Names Ultravist®
Generic Available No
Pharmacologic Category Radiological/Contrast Media, Nonionic
Use Enhance imaging in cerebral arteriography and peripheral arteriography; coronary arteriography and left ventriculography, visceral angiography and aortography; contrast-enhanced computed tomographic imaging of the head and body, excretory urography, intra-arterial digital subtraction angiography, peripheral venography
Local Anesthetic/Vasoconstrictor Precautions No information available to require special precautions
Effects on Dental Treatment No significant effects or complications reported
Mechanism of Action Iopromide opacifies vessels in its path of flow, permitting radiographic visualization of internal structures.
Pregnancy Risk Factor B

Iosat™ [OTC] see Potassium Iodide on page 1260

Iothalamate Meglumine (eye oh thal A mate MEG loo meen)

U.S. Brand Names Conray®; Conray® 30; Conray® 43; Cysto-Conray® II
Generic Available No
Pharmacologic Category Iodinated Contrast Media; Radiological/Contrast Media, Ionic
Use
    Solution for injection: Arthrography, cerebral angiography, cranial computerized angiotomography, digital subtraction angiography, direct cholangiography, endoscopic retrograde cholangiopancreatography, excretory urography, peripheral arteriography, urography, venography; contrast enhancement of computed tomographic images
    Solution for instillation: Retrograde cystography and cystourethrography
Local Anesthetic/Vasoconstrictor Precautions No information available to require special precautions
Effects on Dental Treatment No significant effects or complications reported
Pregnancy Risk Factor B/C (product dependent)

Iothalamate Sodium (eye oh thal A mate SOW dee um)

U.S. Brand Names Conray® 400
Generic Available No
Pharmacologic Category Iodinated Contrast Media; Radiological/Contrast Media, Ionic
Use Excretory urography, angiocardiography, aortography; contrast enhancement of computed tomographic brain images
(Continued)

Iothalamate Sodium *(Continued)*

Local Anesthetic/Vasoconstrictor Precautions No information available to require special precautions

Effects on Dental Treatment No significant effects or complications reported

Pregnancy Risk Factor B

Ioversol *(EYE oh ver sole)*

U.S. Brand Names Optiray®

Generic Available No

Pharmacologic Category Iodinated Contrast Media; Radiological/Contrast Media, Nonionic

Use Arteriography, angiography, angiocardiography, ventriculography, excretory urography, and venography procedures; contrast enhanced tomographic imaging

Pregnancy Risk Factor B

Ioxaglate Meglumine and Ioxaglate Sodium
(eye ox AG late MEG loo meen & eye ox AG late SOW dee um)

U.S. Brand Names Hexabrix™

Generic Available No

Synonyms Ioxaglate Sodium and Ioxaglate Meglumine

Pharmacologic Category Iodinated Contrast Media; Radiological/Contrast Media, Ionic

Use Angiocardiography, arteriography, aortography, arthrography, angiography, hysterosalpingography, venography, and urography procedures; contrast enhancement of computed tomographic imaging

Local Anesthetic/Vasoconstrictor Precautions No information available to require special precautions

Effects on Dental Treatment No significant effects or complications reported

Pregnancy Risk Factor B

Ioxaglate Sodium and Ioxaglate Meglumine *see* Ioxaglate Meglumine and Ioxaglate Sodium *on page 856*

Ipecac Syrup *(IP e kak SIR up)*

Generic Available Yes

Synonyms Syrup of Ipecac

Pharmacologic Category Antidote

Use Treatment of acute oral drug overdosage and in certain poisonings

Local Anesthetic/Vasoconstrictor Precautions No information available to require special precautions

Effects on Dental Treatment No significant effects or complications reported

Common Adverse Effects Frequency not defined.

Cardiovascular: Cardiotoxicity

Central nervous system: Lethargy

Gastrointestinal: Protracted vomiting, diarrhea

Neuromuscular & skeletal: Myopathy

Mechanism of Action Irritates the gastric mucosa and stimulates the medullary chemoreceptor trigger zone to induce vomiting

Drug Interactions

Increased Effect/Toxicity: Phenothiazines (chlorpromazine has been associated with serious dystonic reactions).

Decreased Effect: Activated charcoal, milk, carbonated beverages decrease the effect of ipecac syrup.

Pharmacodynamics/Kinetics

Onset of action: 15-30 minutes

Duration: 20-25 minutes; 60 minutes in some cases

Absorption: Significant amounts, mainly when it does not produce emesis

Excretion: Urine; emetine (alkaloid component) may be detected in urine 60 days after excess dose or chronic use

Pregnancy Risk Factor C

Iplex™ *see* Mecasermin *on page 968*
IPM Wound Gel™ [OTC] *see* Hyaluronate and Derivatives *on page 773*
IPOL® *see* Poliovirus Vaccine (Inactivated) *on page 1252*

Ipratropium (i pra TROE pee um)

Related Information
Respiratory Diseases *on page 1656*
U.S. Brand Names Atrovent®; Atrovent® HFA
Canadian Brand Names Alti-Ipratropium; Apo-Ipravent®; Atrovent®; Atrovent®
HFA; Gen-Ipratropium; Novo-Ipramide; Nu-Ipratropium; PMS-Ipratropium
Mexican Brand Names Atrovent®
Generic Available Yes: Excludes solution for oral inhalation
Synonyms Ipratropium Bromide
Pharmacologic Category Anticholinergic Agent
Use Anticholinergic bronchodilator used in bronchospasm associated with
COPD, bronchitis, and emphysema; symptomatic relief of rhinorrhea associated
with the common cold and allergic and nonallergic rhinitis
Local Anesthetic/Vasoconstrictor Precautions No information available to
require special precautions
Effects on Dental Treatment Key adverse event(s) related to dental treat-
ment: Xerostomia and changes in salivation (normal salivary flow resumes upon
discontinuation), and dry mucous membranes.
Common Adverse Effects
Inhalation aerosol and inhalation solution:
>10%: Bronchitis (10% to 23%), upper respiratory tract infection (13%)
1% to 10%:
Cardiovascular: Palpitation
Central nervous system: Dizziness (2% to 3%)
Dermatologic: Rash (1%)
Gastrointestinal: Nausea, xerostomia, stomach upset, dry mucous
membranes
Renal: Urinary tract infection
Respiratory: Nasal congestion, dyspnea (10%), sputum increased (1%), bron-
chospasm (2%), pharyngitis (3%), rhinitis (2%), sinusitis (5%)
Miscellaneous: Flu-like syndrome

Nasal spray: Respiratory: Epistaxis (8%), nasal dryness (5%), nausea (2%)
Mechanism of Action Blocks the action of acetylcholine at parasympathetic
sites in bronchial smooth muscle causing bronchodilation
Drug Interactions
Increased Effect/Toxicity: Increased toxicity with anticholinergics or drugs
with anticholinergic properties.
Pharmacodynamics/Kinetics
Onset of action: Bronchodilation: 1-3 minutes
Peak effect: 1.5-2 hours
Duration: ≤4 hours
Absorption: Negligible
Distribution: Inhalation: 15% of dose reaches lower airways
Pregnancy Risk Factor B

Ipratropium and Albuterol (i pra TROE pee um & al BYOO ter ole)

Related Information
Albuterol *on page 58*
Ipratropium *on page 857*
U.S. Brand Names Combivent®; DuoNeb™
Canadian Brand Names Apo-Salvent®; CO Ipra-Sal; Combivent®; Gen-Combo
Sterinebs
Generic Available No
Synonyms Albuterol and Ipratropium; Salbutamol and Ipratropium
Pharmacologic Category Bronchodilator
Use Treatment of COPD in those patients that are currently on a regular broncho-
dilator who continue to have bronchospasms and require a second bronchodi-
lator
Local Anesthetic/Vasoconstrictor Precautions No information available to
require special precautions
Effects on Dental Treatment Key adverse event(s) related to dental treat-
ment: Xerostomia (normal salivary flow resumes upon discontinuation) and dry
mucous membrane.
Common Adverse Effects
Based on **ipratropium** component: **Note:** Ipratropium is poorly absorbed from
the lung, so systemic effects are rare.
(Continued)

Ipratropium and Albuterol *(Continued)*

Inhalation aerosol and inhalation solution:
<10%: Respiratory: Upper respiratory infection (13%), bronchitis (15%)
1% to 10%:
 Cardiovascular: Palpitations (2%)
 Central nervous system: Nervousness (3%), dizziness (2%), fatigue, headache (6%), pain (4%)
 Dermatologic: Rash (1%)
 Gastrointestinal: Nausea, xerostomia, stomach upset, dry mucous membranes
 Respiratory: Nasal congestion, dyspnea (10%), increased sputum (1%), bronchospasm (2%), pharyngitis (3%), rhinitis (2%), sinusitis (5%)
 Miscellaneous: Influenza-like symptoms

Based on **albuterol** component:
>10%:
 Cardiovascular: Tachycardia, palpitation, pounding heartbeat
 Gastrointestinal: GI upset, nausea
1% to 10%:
 Cardiovascular: Flushing of face, hypertension or hypotension
 Central nervous system: Nervousness, CNS stimulation, hyperactivity, insomnia, dizziness, lightheadedness, drowsiness, headache
 Gastrointestinal: Xerostomia, heartburn, vomiting, unusual taste
 Genitourinary: Dysuria
 Neuromuscular & skeletal: Muscle cramping, tremor, weakness
 Respiratory: Coughing
 Miscellaneous: Diaphoresis (increased)

Dosage Adults:
 Inhalation: 2 inhalations 4 times/day (maximum: 12 inhalations/24 hours)
 Inhalation via nebulization: Initial: 3 mL every 6 hours (maximum: 3 mL every 4 hours)
Mechanism of Action See individual agents.
Contraindications
 Based on **ipratropium** component: Hypersensitivity to atropine, its derivatives, or any component of the formulation
  In addition, Combivent® inhalation aerosol is contraindicated in patients with hypersensitivity to soya lecithin or related food products (eg, soybean and peanut). **Note:** Other formulations may include these components; refer to product-specific labeling.
 Based on **albuterol** component: Hypersensitivity to albuterol, adrenergic amines, or any component of the formulation
Drug Interactions
 Cytochrome P450 Effect: Albuterol: **Substrate** of CYP3A4 (major)
 Increased Effect/Toxicity: See individual agents.
 Decreased Effect: See individual agents.
Dietary Considerations Some dosage forms may contain soya lecithin. Do not use in patients allergic to soya lecithin or related food products such as soybean and peanut.
Pharmacodynamics/Kinetics See individual agents.
Pregnancy Risk Factor C
Dosage Forms AERO, oral inhalation (Combivent®): Ipratropium 18 mcg and albuterol 103 mcg per actuation (14.7 g). **SOLN, nebulization** (DuoNeb™): Ipratropium 0.5 mg [0.017%] and albuterol base 2.5 mg [0.083%] per 3 mL vial (30s, 60s)

Ipratropium Bromide *see Ipratropium on page 857*

I-Prin [OTC] *see Ibuprofen on page 808*

Iproveratril Hydrochloride *see Verapamil on page 1571*

IPV *see Poliovirus Vaccine (Inactivated) on page 1252*

Iquix® *see Levofloxacin on page 913*

Irbesartan *(ir be SAR tan)*

Related Information
 Cardiovascular Diseases *on page 1636*
U.S. Brand Names Avapro®
Canadian Brand Names Avapro®
Mexican Brand Names Aprovel®; Avapro®
Generic Available No

Pharmacologic Category Angiotensin II Receptor Blocker

Use Treatment of hypertension alone or in combination with other antihypertensives; treatment of diabetic nephropathy in patients with type 2 diabetes mellitus (noninsulin dependent, NIDDM) and hypertension

Local Anesthetic/Vasoconstrictor Precautions No information available to require special precautions

Effects on Dental Treatment Key adverse event(s) related to dental treatment: Orthostatic hypotension.

Common Adverse Effects Unless otherwise indicated, percentage of incidence is reported for patients with hypertension.

>10%: Endocrine & metabolic: Hyperkalemia (19%, diabetic nephropathy; rarely seen in HTN)

1% to 10%:

Cardiovascular: Orthostatic hypotension (5%, diabetic nephropathy)

Central nervous system: Fatigue (4%), dizziness (10%, diabetic nephropathy)

Gastrointestinal: Diarrhea (3%), dyspepsia (2%)

Respiratory: Upper respiratory infection (9%), cough (2.8% versus 2.7% in placebo)

>1% but frequency ≤ placebo: Abdominal pain, anxiety, chest pain, edema, headache, influenza, musculoskeletal pain, nausea, nervousness, pharyngitis, rash, rhinitis, sinus abnormality, syncope, tachycardia, urinary tract infection, vertigo, vomiting

Dosage Oral:

Hypertension:

Children:

<6 years: Safety and efficacy have not been established.

≥6-12 years: Initial: 75 mg once daily; may be titrated to a maximum of 150 mg once daily

Children ≥13 years and Adults: 150 mg once daily; patients may be titrated to 300 mg once daily

Note: Starting dose in volume-depleted patients should be 75 mg

Nephropathy in patients with type 2 diabetes and hypertension: Adults: Target dose: 300 mg once daily

Dosage adjustment in renal impairment: No dosage adjustment necessary with mild to severe impairment unless the patient is also volume depleted.

Mechanism of Action Irbesartan is an angiotensin receptor antagonist. Angiotensin II acts as a vasoconstrictor. In addition to causing direct vasoconstriction, angiotensin II also stimulates the release of aldosterone. Once aldosterone is released, sodium as well as water are reabsorbed. The end result is an elevation in blood pressure. Irbesartan binds to the AT1 angiotensin II receptor. This binding prevents angiotensin II from binding to the receptor thereby blocking the vasoconstriction and the aldosterone secreting effects of angiotensin II.

Contraindications Hypersensitivity to irbesartan or any component of the formulation; hypersensitivity to other A-II receptor antagonists; bilateral renal artery stenosis; pregnancy (2nd and 3rd trimesters)

Warnings/Precautions Safety and efficacy have not been established in pediatric patients <6 years of age. Avoid use or use a much smaller dose in patients who are intravascularly volume-depleted; use caution in patients with unilateral or bilateral renal artery stenosis to avoid a decrease in renal function; AUCs of irbesartan (not the active metabolite) are about 50% greater in patients with Cl_{cr} <30 mL/minute and are doubled in hemodialysis patients

Drug Interactions

Cytochrome P450 Effect: Substrate of CYP2C8/9 (minor); **Inhibits** CYP2C8/9 (moderate), 2D6 (weak), 3A4 (weak)

Increased Effect/Toxicity: Potassium salts/supplements, co-trimoxazole (high dose), ACE inhibitors, and potassium-sparing diuretics (amiloride, spironolactone, triamterene) may increase the risk of hyperkalemia. Irbesartan may increase the levels/effects of amiodarone, fluoxetine, glimepiride, glipizide, nateglinide, phenytoin, pioglitazone, rosiglitazone, sertraline, warfarin, and other CYP2C8/9 substrates.

Ethanol/Nutrition/Herb Interactions Herb/Nutraceutical: Avoid dong quai if using for hypertension (has estrogenic activity). Avoid ephedra, yohimbe, ginseng (may worsen hypertension). Avoid garlic (may have increased antihypertensive effect).

Dietary Considerations May be taken with or without food.

Pharmacodynamics/Kinetics

Onset of action: Peak effect: 1-2 hours

Duration: >24 hours

Distribution: V_d: 53-93 L

Protein binding, plasma: 90%

Metabolism: Hepatic, primarily CYP2C9

Bioavailability: 60% to 80%

(Continued)

Irbesartan *(Continued)*

Half-life elimination: Terminal: 11-15 hours
Time to peak, serum: 1.5-2 hours
Excretion: Feces (80%); urine (20%)
Pregnancy Risk Factor C/D (2nd and 3rd trimesters)
Dosage Forms TAB: 75 mg, 150 mg, 300 mg

Irbesartan and Hydrochlorothiazide

(ir be SAR tan & hye droe klor oh THYE a zide)

Related Information
Cardiovascular Diseases *on page 1636*
Hydrochlorothiazide *on page 776*
Irbesartan *on page 858*
U.S. Brand Names Avalide®
Canadian Brand Names Avalide®
Generic Available No
Synonyms Avapro® HCT; Hydrochlorothiazide and Irbesartan
Pharmacologic Category Angiotensin II Receptor Blocker Combination; Anti-hypertensive Agent, Combination; Diuretic, Thiazide
Use Combination therapy for the management of hypertension
Local Anesthetic/Vasoconstrictor Precautions No information available to require special precautions
Effects on Dental Treatment No significant effects or complications reported
Common Adverse Effects See individual agents.
Mechanism of Action
Irbesartan: Irbesartan is an angiotensin receptor antagonist. Angiotensin II acts as a vasoconstrictor. In addition to causing direct vasoconstriction, angiotensin II also stimulates the release of aldosterone. Once aldosterone is released, sodium as well as water are reabsorbed. The end result is an elevation in blood pressure. Irbesartan binds to the AT1 angiotensin II receptor. This binding prevents angiotensin II from binding to the receptor thereby blocking the vasoconstriction and the aldosterone secreting effects of angiotensin II.
Hydrochlorothiazide: Inhibits sodium reabsorption in the distal tubules causing increased excretion of sodium and water as well as potassium and hydrogen ions
Drug Interactions
Cytochrome P450 Effect: Irbesartan: **Substrate** of CYP2C8/9 (minor); **Inhibits** CYP2C8/9 (moderate), 2D6 (weak), 3A4 (weak)
Increased Effect/Toxicity: See individual agents.
Decreased Effect: See individual agents.
Pregnancy Risk Factor C/D (2nd and 3rd trimesters)

Ircon® [OTC] *see* Ferrous Fumarate *on page 650*
IRESSA® *see* Gefitinib *on page 727*

Irinotecan (eye rye no TEE kan)

U.S. Brand Names Camptosar®
Canadian Brand Names Camptosar®
Mexican Brand Names Camptosar®
Generic Available No
Synonyms Camptothecin-11; CPT-11; NSC-616348
Pharmacologic Category Antineoplastic Agent, Natural Source (Plant) Derivative
Use Treatment of metastatic carcinoma of the colon or rectum
Unlabeled/Investigational Use Lung cancer (small cell and nonsmall cell), cervical cancer, gastric cancer, pancreatic cancer, leukemia, lymphoma, breast cancer
Local Anesthetic/Vasoconstrictor Precautions No information available to require special precautions
Effects on Dental Treatment No significant effects or complications reported
Common Adverse Effects Frequency of adverse reactions reported for single-agent use of irinotecan only. Frequencies vary with alternative dosage regimens or combination therapy.
>10%:
Cardiovascular: Vasodilatation (9% to 11%)

Central nervous system: Pain (23% to 62%), fever (26% to 45%; neutropenic grade 3/4: <1% to 6%), dizziness (15% to 21%), headache (17%), chills (14%), insomnia (19%)

Dermatologic: Rash (13% to 14%), alopecia (17% to 60%, grade 2), hand/foot syndrome (13%), cutaneous reactions (20%)

Gastrointestinal: Gastrointestinal: Diarrhea, early (43% to 51%; grade 3/4: 7% to 22%), diarrhea, late (45% to 88%; grade 3/4: 6% to 31%), nausea (55% to 86%), abdominal pain (17% to 68%), vomiting (32% to 67%), anorexia (19% to 55%), constipation (25% to 32%), mucositis (29% to 30%), flatulence (12%), stomatitis (12%), dyspepsia (10%), abdominal cramping (57%), weight loss (30%), dehydration (15%)

Hepatic: Bilirubin increased (36% to 84%), alkaline phosphatase increased (13%)

Neuromuscular & skeletal: Weakness (48% to 76%), back pain (14%)

Respiratory: Dyspnea (5% to 22%), cough (17% to 20%), rhinitis (16%)

Miscellaneous: Infection (14% to 34%), diaphoresis (16%)

1% to 10%:

Cardiovascular: Hypotension (<1% to 6%), thromboembolic events (5% to 6%), edema (10%)

Central nervous system: Somnolence (9%), confusion (3%)

Gastrointestinal: Abdominal enlargement (10%)

Hepatic: SGOT increased (10%), ascites and/or jaundice (9%)

Respiratory: Pneumonia (4%)

Note: In limited pediatric experience, dehydration (often associated with severe hypokalemia and hyponatremia) was among the most significant grade 3/4 adverse events, with a frequency up to 29%. In addition, grade 3/4 infection was reported in 24%.

Mechanism of Action Irinotecan and its active metabolite (SN-38) bind reversibly to topoisomerase I and stabilize the cleavable complex so that religation of the cleaved DNA strand cannot occur. This results in the accumulation of cleavable complexes and single-strand DNA breaks. This interaction results in single-stranded DNA breaks and cell death consistent with S-phase cell cycle specificity.

Drug Interactions

Cytochrome P450 Effect: Substrate (major) of CYP2B6, 3A4

Increased Effect/Toxicity: CYP2B6 inhibitors may increase the levels/ effects of irinotecan; example inhibitors include desipramine, paroxetine, and sertraline. CYP3A4 inhibitors may increase the levels/effects of irinotecan; example inhibitors include azole antifungals, clarithromycin, diclofenac, doxycycline, erythromycin, imatinib, isoniazid, nefazodone, nicardipine, propofol, protease inhibitors, quinidine, telithromycin, and verapamil. Bevacizumab may increase the adverse effects of irinotecan (eg, diarrhea, neutropenia). Ketoconazole increases the levels/effects of irinotecan and active metabolite; discontinue ketoconazole 1 week prior to irinotecan therapy; **concurrent use is contraindicated.**

Decreased Effect: CYP2B6 inducers may decrease the levels/effects of irinotecan; example inducers include carbamazepine, nevirapine, phenobarbital, phenytoin, and rifampin. CYP3A4 inducers may decrease the levels/ effects of irinotecan; example inducers include aminoglutethimide, carbamazepine, nafcillin, nevirapine, phenobarbital, phenytoin, and rifamycins. St John's wort decreases therapeutic effect of irinotecan; discontinue ≥2 weeks prior to irinotecan therapy; **concurrent use is contraindicated.**

Pharmacodynamics/Kinetics

Distribution: V_d: 33-150 L/m^2

Protein binding, plasma: Predominantly albumin; Parent drug: 30% to 68%, SN-38 (active drug): ~95%

Metabolism: Primarily hepatic to SN-38 (active metabolite) by carboxylesterase enzymes; SN-38 undergoes conjugation by UDP- glucuronosyl transferase 1A1 (UGT1A1) to form a glucuronide metabolite. SN-38 is increased by UGT1A1*28 polymorphism (10% of North Americans are homozygous for UGT1A1*28 allele). The lactones of both irinotecan and SN-38 undergo hydrolysis to inactive hydroxy acid forms.

Half-life elimination: SN-38: Mean terminal: 10-20 hours

Time to peak: SN-38: Following 90-minute infusion: ~1 hour

Excretion: Within 24 hours: Urine: Irinotecan (11% to 20%), metabolites (SN-38 <1%, SN-38 glucuronide, 3%)

Pregnancy Risk Factor D

Iron Dextran Complex (EYE ern DEKS tran KOM pleks)

U.S. Brand Names Dexferrum®; INFeD®
Canadian Brand Names Dexiron™; Infufer®
Generic Available No
Pharmacologic Category Iron Salt
Use Treatment of microcytic hypochromic anemia resulting from iron deficiency in patients in whom oral administration is infeasible or ineffective
Local Anesthetic/Vasoconstrictor Precautions No information available to require special precautions
Effects on Dental Treatment Key adverse event(s) related to dental treatment: Metallic taste.
Common Adverse Effects
>10%:
Cardiovascular: Flushing
Central nervous system: Dizziness, fever, headache, pain
Gastrointestinal: Nausea, vomiting, metallic taste
Local: Staining of skin at the site of I.M. injection
Miscellaneous: Diaphoresis
1% to 10%:
Cardiovascular: Hypotension (1% to 2%)
Dermatologic: Urticaria (1% to 2%), phlebitis (1% to 2%)
Gastrointestinal: Diarrhea
Genitourinary: Discoloration of urine
Note: Diaphoresis, urticaria, arthralgia, fever, chills, dizziness, headache, and nausea may be delayed 24-48 hours after I.V. administration or 3-4 days after I.M. administration.
Anaphylactoid reactions: Respiratory difficulties and cardiovascular collapse have been reported and occur most frequently within the first several minutes of administration.
Mechanism of Action The released iron, from the plasma, eventually replenishes the depleted iron stores in the bone marrow where it is incorporated into hemoglobin
Drug Interactions
Decreased Effect: Decreased effect with chloramphenicol.
Pharmacodynamics/Kinetics
Absorption:
I.M.: 50% to 90% is promptly absorbed, balance is slowly absorbed over month
I.V.: Uptake of iron by the reticuloendothelial system appears to be constant at about 10-20 mg/hour
Excretion: Urine and feces via reticuloendothelial system
Pregnancy Risk Factor C

Iron Fumarate see Ferrous Fumarate on page 650
Iron Gluconate see Ferrous Gluconate on page 651
Iron-Polysaccharide Complex see Polysaccharide-Iron Complex on page 1254

Iron Sucrose (EYE ern SOO krose)

U.S. Brand Names Venofer®
Canadian Brand Names Venofer®
Generic Available No
Pharmacologic Category Iron Salt
Use Treatment of iron-deficiency anemia in chronic renal failure, including nondialysis-dependent patients (with or without erythropoietin therapy) and dialysis-dependent patients receiving erythropoietin therapy
Local Anesthetic/Vasoconstrictor Precautions No information available to require special precautions
Effects on Dental Treatment No significant effects or complications reported
Common Adverse Effects
>10%:
Cardiovascular: Hypotension (1% to 7%; 39% in hemodialysis patients; may be related to total dose or rate of administration), peripheral edema (2% to 13%)
Central nervous system: Headache (3% to 13%)
Gastrointestinal: Nausea (1% to 15%)
Neuromuscular & skeletal: Muscle cramps (1% to 3%; 29% in hemodialysis patients)

1% to 10%:
  Cardiovascular: Hypertension (6% to 8%), edema (1% to 7%), chest pain (1% to 6%), murmur (<1% to 3%), CHF
  Central nervous system: Dizziness (1% to 10%), fatigue (2% to 5%), fever (1% to 3%), anxiety
  Dermatologic: Pruritus (1% to 7%), rash (<1% to 2%)
  Endocrine & metabolic: Gout (2% to 7%), hypoglycemia (<1% to 4%), hyperglycemia (3% to 4%), fluid overload (1% to 3%)
  Gastrointestinal: Diarrhea (1% to 10%), vomiting (5% to 9%), taste perversion (1% to 9%), peritoneal infection (8%), constipation (1% to 7%), abdominal pain (1% to 4%), positive fecal occult blood (1% to 3%)
  Genitourinary: Urinary tract infection (≤1%)
  Local: Injection site reaction (2% to 4%), catheter site infection (4%)
  Neuromuscular & skeletal: Muscle pain (1% to 7%), extremity pain (3% to 6%), arthralgia (1% to 4%), weakness (1% to 3%), back pain (1% to 3%)
  Ocular: Conjunctivitis (<1% to 3%)
  Otic: Ear pain (1% to 7%)
  Respiratory: Dyspnea (1% to 10%), pharyngitis (<1% to 7%), cough (1% to 7%), sinusitis (1% to 4%), rhinitis (1% to 3%), upper respiratory infection (1% to 3%), nasal congestion (1%)
  Miscellaneous: Graft complication (1% to 10%), hypersensitivity, sepsis
Mechanism of Action Iron sucrose is dissociated by the reticuloendothelial system into iron and sucrose. The released iron increases serum iron concentrations and is incorporated into hemoglobin.
Drug Interactions
  Increased Effect/Toxicity: Iron sucrose injection may reduce the absorption of oral iron preparations.
  Decreased Effect: Ace inhibitors may enhance the adverse/toxic effects (erythema, abdominal cramps, nausea, vomiting, hypotension) of iron sucrose.
Pharmacodynamics/Kinetics
  Distribution: V_{dss}: Healthy adults: 7.9 L
  Metabolism: Dissociated into iron and sucrose by the reticuloendothelial system
  Half-life elimination: Healthy adults: 6 hours
  Excretion: Healthy adults: Urine (5%) within 24 hours
Pregnancy Risk Factor B

Iron Sulfate see Ferrous Sulfate on page 651
Iron Sulfate and Vitamin C see Ferrous Sulfate and Ascorbic Acid on page 651
ISD see Isosorbide Dinitrate on page 866
ISDN see Isosorbide Dinitrate on page 866
ISG see Immune Globulin (Intramuscular) on page 823
ISMN see Isosorbide Mononitrate on page 868
Ismo® see Isosorbide Mononitrate on page 868
Isoamyl Nitrite see Amyl Nitrite on page 124
Isobamate see Carisoprodol on page 271

Isocarboxazid (eye soe kar BOKS a zid)

U.S. Brand Names Marplan®
Generic Available No
Pharmacologic Category Antidepressant, Monoamine Oxidase Inhibitor
Use Treatment of depression
Local Anesthetic/Vasoconstrictor Precautions Attempts should be made to avoid use of vasoconstrictor due to possibility of hypertensive episodes with monoamine oxidase inhibitors
Effects on Dental Treatment Key adverse event(s) related to dental treatment: Orthostatic hypotension, xerostomia (normal salivary flow resumes upon discontinuation).
Common Adverse Effects
  >10%:
    Cardiovascular: Orthostatic hypotension
    Central nervous system: Drowsiness
    Endocrine & metabolic: Decreased sexual ability
    Neuromuscular & skeletal: Weakness, trembling
    Ocular: Blurred vision
  1% to 10%:
    Cardiovascular: Tachycardia, peripheral edema
    Central nervous system: Nervousness, chills
    Dermatologic: Xerostomia
    Gastrointestinal: Diarrhea, anorexia, constipation, xerostomia
  (Continued)

Isocarboxazid (Continued)

Restrictions A medication guide concerning the use of antidepressants in children and teenagers can be found on the FDA website at http://www.fda.gov/cder/Offices/ODS/labeling.htm. It should be dispensed to parents or guardians of children and teenagers receiving this medication.

Mechanism of Action Thought to act by increasing endogenous concentrations of epinephrine, norepinephrine, dopamine, and serotonin through inhibition of the enzyme (monoamine oxidase) responsible for the breakdown of these neurotransmitters

Drug Interactions

Increased Effect/Toxicity: In general, the combined use with TCAs, venlafaxine, trazodone, dexfenfluramine, sibutramine, lithium, meperidine, fenfluramine, dextromethorphan, and SSRIs should be avoided due to the potential for severe adverse reactions (serotonin syndrome, death). MAO inhibitors (including isocarboxazid) may inhibit the metabolism of barbiturates and prolong their effect. Isocarboxazid in combination with amphetamines, other stimulants (methylphenidate), levodopa, metaraminol, reserpine, and decongestants (pseudoephedrine) may result in severe hypertensive reactions. Foods (eg, cheese) and beverages (eg, ethanol) containing tyramine should be avoided; hypertensive crisis may result. Isocarboxazid may increase the pressor response of norepinephrine and may prolong neuromuscular blockade produced by succinylcholine. Tramadol may increase the risk of seizures and serotonin syndrome in patients receiving an MAO inhibitor. Isocarboxazid may produce additive hypoglycemic effect in patients receiving hypoglycemic agents and may produce delirium in patients receiving disulfiram.

Decreased Effect: MAO inhibitors may inhibit the antihypertensive response to guanadrel or guanethidine.

Pregnancy Risk Factor C

Isochron™ *see* Isosorbide Dinitrate *on page 866*

Isometheptene, Acetaminophen, and Dichloralphenazone *see* Acetaminophen, Isometheptene, and Dichloralphenazone *on page 44*

Isometheptene, Dichloralphenazone, and Acetaminophen *see* Acetaminophen, Isometheptene, and Dichloralphenazone *on page 44*

Isoniazid (eye soe NYE a zid)

Related Information
Tuberculosis *on page 1673*

U.S. Brand Names Nydrazid® [DSC]

Canadian Brand Names Isotamine®; PMS-Isoniazid

Generic Available Yes

Synonyms INH; Isonicotinic Acid Hydrazide

Pharmacologic Category Antitubercular Agent

Use Treatment of susceptible tuberculosis infections; treatment of latent tuberculosis infection (LTBI)

Local Anesthetic/Vasoconstrictor Precautions No information available to require special precautions

Effects on Dental Treatment Key adverse event(s) related to dental treatment: Xerostomia (normal salivary flow resumes upon discontinuation).

Common Adverse Effects Frequency not defined.

Cardiovascular: Hypertension, palpitation, tachycardia, vasculitis

Central nervous system: Dizziness, encephalopathy, memory impairment, slurred speech, lethargy, fever, depression, psychosis, seizure

Dermatologic: Rash (morbilliform, maculopapular, pruritic, or exfoliative), flushing

Endocrine & metabolic: Hyperglycemia, metabolic acidosis, gynecomastia, pellagra, pyridoxine deficiency

Gastrointestinal: Anorexia, nausea, vomiting, stomach pain

Hematologic: Agranulocytosis, anemia (sideroblastic, hemolytic, or aplastic), thrombocytopenia, eosinophilia, lymphadenopathy

Hepatic: LFTs mildly increased (10% to 20%); hyperbilirubinemia, jaundice, hepatitis (may involve progressive liver damage; risk increases with age; 2.3% in patients >50 years)

Neuromuscular & skeletal: Weakness, peripheral neuropathy (dose-related incidence, 10% to 20% incidence with 10 mg/kg/day), hyper-reflexia, arthralgia, lupus-like syndrome

Ocular: Blurred vision, loss of vision, optic neuritis and atrophy

Mechanism of Action Unknown, but may include the inhibition of myocolic acid synthesis resulting in disruption of the bacterial cell wall

Drug Interactions

Cytochrome P450 Effect: Substrate of CYP2E1 (major); **Inhibits** CYP1A2 (weak), 2A6 (moderate), 2C9 (weak), 2C19 (strong), 2D6 (moderate), 2E1 (moderate), 3A4 (strong); **Induces** CYP2E1 (after discontinuation) (weak)

Increased Effect/Toxicity: Concurrent use of disulfiram may result in acute intolerance reactions. Isoniazid may increase the levels/effects of amphetamines, benzodiazepines, beta-blockers, calcium channel blockers, citalopram, dexmedetomidine, dextromethorphan, diazepam, fluoxetine, ifosfamide, inhalational anesthetics, lidocaine, methsuximide, mirtazapine, nateglinide, nefazodone, phenytoin, propranolol, risperidone, ritonavir, sertraline, tacrolimus, theophylline, thioridazine, tricyclic antidepressants, trimethadione, venlafaxine, and other substrates of CYP2A6, 2C19, 2D6, 2E1, or 3A4. Selected benzodiazepines (midazolam and triazolam), cisapride, ergot alkaloids, selected HMG-CoA reductase inhibitors (lovastatin and simvastatin), and pimozide are generally contraindicated with strong CYP3A4 inhibitors. Mesoridazine and thioridazine are generally contraindicated with strong CYP2D6 inhibitors. When used with strong CYP3A4 inhibitors, dosage adjustment/limits are recommended for sildenafil and other PDE-5 inhibitors; consult individual monographs.

Decreased Effect: Decreased effect/levels of isoniazid with aluminum salts or antacids. Isoniazid may decrease the levels/effects of CYP2D6 prodrug substrates (eg, codeine, hydrocodone, oxycodone, tramadol).

Pharmacodynamics/Kinetics

Absorption: Rapid and complete; rate can be slowed with food

Distribution: All body tissues and fluids including CSF; crosses placenta; enters breast milk

Protein binding: 10% to 15%

Metabolism: Hepatic with decay rate determined genetically by acetylation phenotype

Half-life elimination: Fast acetylators: 30-100 minutes; Slow acetylators: 2-5 hours; may be prolonged with hepatic or severe renal impairment

Time to peak, serum: 1-2 hours

Excretion: Urine (75% to 95%); feces; saliva

Pregnancy Risk Factor C

Isoniazid and Rifampin *see* Rifampin and Isoniazid *on page 1348*

Isoniazid, Rifampin, and Pyrazinamide *see* Rifampin, Isoniazid, and Pyrazinamide *on page 1348*

Isonicotinic Acid Hydrazide *see* Isoniazid *on page 864*

Isonipecaine Hydrochloride *see* Meperidine *on page 983*

Isophane Insulin *see* Insulin NPH *on page 840*

Isophane Insulin and Regular Insulin *see* Insulin NPH and Insulin Regular *on page 840*

Isophosphamide *see* Ifosfamide *on page 815*

Isopropyl Alcohol Tincture of Benzylkonium Chloride *see* Benzalkonium Chloride and Isopropyl Alcohol *on page 189*

Isoproterenol (eye soe proe TER e nole)

Related Information

Cardiovascular Diseases *on page 1636*

U.S. Brand Names Isuprel®

Generic Available Yes

Synonyms Isoproterenol Hydrochloride

Pharmacologic Category Beta$_1$- & Beta$_2$-Adrenergic Agonist Agent

Use Ventricular arrhythmias due to AV nodal block; hemodynamically compromised bradyarrhythmias or atropine- and dopamine-resistant bradyarrhythmias (when transcutaneous/venous pacing is not available); temporary use in third-degree AV block until pacemaker insertion

Unlabeled/Investigational Use Pharmacologic overdrive pacing for torsade de pointes; diagnostic aid (vasovagal syncope)

Local Anesthetic/Vasoconstrictor Precautions Isoproterenol is selective for beta-adrenergic receptors and not alpha receptors; therefore, there is no precaution in the use of vasoconstrictor such as epinephrine

Effects on Dental Treatment Key adverse event(s) related to dental treatment: Xerostomia and changes in salivation (normal salivary flow resumes upon discontinuation).

Common Adverse Effects Frequency not defined.

Cardiovascular: Premature ventricular beats, bradycardia, hyper-/hypotension, chest pain, palpitation, tachycardia, ventricular arrhythmia, MI size increased

Central nervous system: Headache, nervousness or restlessness

(Continued)

Isoproterenol *(Continued)*

Endocrine & metabolic: Serum glucose increased, serum potassium decreased, hypokalemia

Gastrointestinal: Nausea, vomiting

Respiratory: Dyspnea

Mechanism of Action Stimulates beta$_1$- and beta$_2$-receptors resulting in relaxation of bronchial, GI, and uterine smooth muscle, increased heart rate and contractility, vasodilation of peripheral vasculature

Drug Interactions

Increased Effect/Toxicity: Sympathomimetic agents may cause headaches and elevate blood pressure. General anesthetics may cause arrhythmias.

Pharmacodynamics/Kinetics

Onset of action: Bronchodilation: I.V.: Immediate

Duration: I.V.: 10-15 minutes

Metabolism: Via conjugation in many tissues including hepatic and pulmonary

Half-life elimination: 2.5-5 minutes

Excretion: Urine (primarily as sulfate conjugates)

Pregnancy Risk Factor C

Isoproterenol Hydrochloride *see* Isoproterenol *on page 865*

Isoptin® SR *see* Verapamil *on page 1571*

Isopto® Atropine *see* Atropine *on page 161*

Isopto® Carbachol *see* Carbachol *on page 260*

Isopto® Carpine *see* Pilocarpine (Ophthalmic) *on page 1234*

Isopto® Homatropine *see* Homatropine *on page 772*

Isopto® Hyoscine *see* Scopolamine *on page 1380*

Isopto® Tears [OTC] *see* Artificial Tears *on page 143*

Isordil® *see* Isosorbide Dinitrate *on page 866*

Isosorbide Dinitrate *(eye soe SOR bide dye NYE trate)*

Related Information

Cardiovascular Diseases *on page 1636*

Isosorbide Mononitrate *on page 868*

U.S. Brand Names Dilatrate®-SR; Isochron™; Isordil®

Canadian Brand Names Apo-ISDN®; Cedocard®-SR; Coronex®; Novo-Sorbide; PMS-Isosorbide

Mexican Brand Names Isoket®; Isorbid®

Generic Available Yes: Tablet, sublingual tablet

Synonyms ISD; ISDN

Pharmacologic Category Vasodilator

Use Prevention and treatment of angina pectoris; for congestive heart failure; to relieve pain, dysphagia, and spasm in esophageal spasm with GE reflux

Unlabeled/Investigational Use Esophageal spastic disorders

Local Anesthetic/Vasoconstrictor Precautions No information available to require special precautions

Effects on Dental Treatment No significant effects or complications reported

Common Adverse Effects Frequency not defined.

Cardiovascular: Hypotension (infrequent), postural hypotension, crescendo angina (uncommon), rebound hypertension (uncommon), pallor, cardiovascular collapse, tachycardia, shock, flushing, peripheral edema

Central nervous system: Headache (most common), lightheadedness (related to blood pressure changes), syncope (uncommon), dizziness, restlessness

Gastrointestinal: Nausea, vomiting, bowel incontinence, xerostomia

Genitourinary: Urinary incontinence

Hematologic: Methemoglobinemia (rare, overdose)

Neuromuscular & skeletal: Weakness

Ocular: Blurred vision

Miscellaneous: Cold sweat

The incidence of hypotension and adverse cardiovascular events may be increased when used in combination with sildenafil (Viagra®).

Mechanism of Action Stimulation of intracellular cyclic-GMP results in vascular smooth muscle relaxation of both arterial and venous vasculature. Increased venous pooling decreases left ventricular pressure (preload) and arterial dilatation decreases arterial resistance (afterload). Therefore, this reduces cardiac oxygen demand by decreasing left ventricular pressure and systemic vascular resistance by dilating arteries. Additionally, coronary artery dilation improves collateral flow to ischemic regions; esophageal smooth muscle is relaxed via the same mechanism.

Drug Interactions

Cytochrome P450 Effect: Substrate of CYP3A4 (major)

Increased Effect/Toxicity: CYP3A4 inhibitors may increase the levels/ effects of isosorbide dinitrate; example inhibitors include azole antifungals, clarithromycin, diclofenac, doxycycline, erythromycin, imatinib, isoniazid, nefazodone, nicardipine, propofol, protease inhibitors, quinidine, telithro-mycin, and verapamil. Significant reduction of systolic and diastolic blood pressure with concurrent use of sildenafil, tadalafil, or vardenafil (contraindi-cated). Do not administer sildenafil, tadalafil, or vardenafil within 24 hours of a nitrate preparation.

Decreased Effect: CYP3A4 inducers may decrease the levels/effects of isosorbide dinitrate; example inducers include aminoglutethimide, carbamaz-epine, nafcillin, nevirapine, phenobarbital, phenytoin, and rifamycins.

Pharmacodynamics/Kinetics

Onset of action: Sublingual tablet: 2-10 minutes; Chewable tablet: 3 minutes; Oral tablet: 45-60 minutes

Duration: Sublingual tablet: 1-2 hours; Chewable tablet: 0.5-2 hours; Oral tablet: 4-6 hours

Metabolism: Extensively hepatic to conjugated metabolites, including isosorbide 5-mononitrate (active) and 2-mononitrate (active)

Half-life elimination: Parent drug: 1-4 hours; Metabolite (5-mononitrate): 4 hours

Excretion: Urine and feces

Pregnancy Risk Factor C

Isosorbide Dinitrate and Hydralazine
(eye soe SOR bide dye NYE trate & hye DRAL a zeen)

U.S. Brand Names BiDil®

Generic Available No

Synonyms Hydralazine and Isosorbide Dinitrate

Pharmacologic Category Vasodilator

Use Treatment of heart failure, adjunct to standard therapy, in self-identified African-Americans

Local Anesthetic/Vasoconstrictor Precautions No information available to require special precautions

Effects on Dental Treatment No significant effects or complications reported

Common Adverse Effects The following events were reported in the A-HeFT Study using the combination isosorbide dinitrate/hydralazine product. See indi-vidual drug monographs for additional information.

>10%:

Cardiovascular: Chest pain (16%)

Central nervous system: Headache (50%), dizziness (32%)

Neuromuscular & skeletal: Weakness (14%)

1% to 10%:

Cardiovascular: Hypotension (8%), ventricular tachycardia (4%), palpitations (4%), tachycardia (2%)

Dermatologic: Alopecia (1%), angioedema (1%)

Endocrine & metabolic: Hyperglycemia (4%), hyperlipidemia (3%), hypercho-lesterolemia (1%)

Gastrointestinal: Nausea (10%), vomiting (4%)

Hepatic: Cholecystitis (1%)

Neuromuscular & skeletal: Paresthesia (4%), arthralgia (1%), myalgia (1%), tendon disorder (1%)

Respiratory: Bronchitis (8%), sinusitis (4%), rhinitis (4%)

Miscellaneous: Allergic reaction (1%), diaphoresis (1%)

Dosage Oral: Adults: Initial: 1 tablet 3 times/day; titrate to a maximum dose of 2 tablets 3 times/day

Dosage adjustment for toxicity: If patient experiences persistent headache, adjust dosing to twice daily.

Mechanism of Action

Hydralazine: Direct vasodilation of arterioles (with little effect on veins) resulting in decreased systemic resistance

Isosorbide Dinitrate: Nitric oxide release causes stimulation of intracellular guanylyl cyclase leading to increased cyclic GMP. This results in vascular smooth muscle relaxation of both arterial and venous vasculature. Increased venous pooling decreases left ventricular pressure (preload) and arterial dila-tation decreases arterial resistance (afterload). Therefore, this reduces cardiac oxygen demand by decreasing left ventricular pressure and systemic vascular resistance by dilating arteries. Additionally, coronary artery dilation improves collateral flow to ischemic regions.

(Continued)

Isosorbide Dinitrate and Hydralazine *(Continued)*

Contraindications Hypersensitivity to isosorbide dinitrate, hydralazine, or any component of the formulation; hypersensitivity to organic nitrates; concurrent use with phosphodiesterase-5 inhibitors (sildenafil, tadalafil, or vardenafil); angle-closure glaucoma (intraocular pressure may be increased); head trauma or cerebral hemorrhage (increase intracranial pressure); severe anemia; mitral valve rheumatic heart disease

Warnings/Precautions May cause a drug-induced lupus-like syndrome (more likely on larger doses, longer duration). Adjust dose in severe renal dysfunction. Use with caution in CAD (increase in tachycardia may increase myocardial oxygen demand). Use with caution in pulmonary hypertension; severe hypotension can occur. Use with caution in volume depletion, hypotension, and right ventricular infarctions. Paradoxical bradycardia and increased angina pectoris can accompany hypotension. Postural hypotension can also occur. Nitrates may aggravate angina caused by hypertrophic cardiomyopathy. Tolerance may develop to nitrates and appropriate dosing is needed to minimize this. Safety and efficacy have not been established in pediatric patients.

Drug Interactions
    Cytochrome P450 Effect: Hydralazine: **Inhibits** CYP3A4 (weak); Isosorbide dinitrate: **Substrate** of CYP3A4 (major)
    Increased Effect/Toxicity: See individual agents.

Pharmacodynamics/Kinetics The following values are from administration of isosorbide dinitrate 40 mg and hydralazine 75 mg in healthy adults. Also see individual drug monographs.

    Half-life elimination: Hydralazine: 4 hours; Isosorbide dinitrate: 2 hours
    Time to peak, plasma: 1 hour (both agents)

Pregnancy Risk Factor C

Dosage Forms TAB: Isosorbide dinitrate 20 mg and hydralazine 37.5 mg

Selected Readings

Cohn JN, Archibald DG, Francis GS, et al, "Effect of Vasodilator Therapy on Mortality in Chronic Congestive Heart Failure: Results of a Veterans Administration Cooperative Study," *N Engl J Med*, 1986, 314 (24):1547-52.

Cohn JN, Johnson G, Ziesche S, et al, "A Comparison of Enalapril With Hydralazine " Isosorbide Dinitrate in the Treatment of Chronic Congestive Heart Failure," *N Engl J Med*, 1991, 325(5):303-10.

Hunt SA, Abraham WT, Chin MH, et al, "ACC/AHA 2005 Guideline Update for the Diagnosis and Management of Chronic Heart Failure in the Adult-Summary Article A Report of the American College of Cardiology/American Heart Association Task Force on Practice Guidelines (Writing Committee to Update the 2001 Guidelines for the Evaluation and Management of Heart Failure)," *J Am Coll Cardiol*, 2005, 46(6):1116-43.

Taylor AL, Ziesche S, Yancy C, et al, "Combination of Isosorbide Dinitrate and Hydralazine in Blacks With Heart Failure," *N Engl J Med*, 2004, 351(20):2049-57.

Isosorbide Mononitrate *(eye soe SOR bide mon oh NYE trate)*

Related Information
    Cardiovascular Diseases *on page 1636*
    Isosorbide Dinitrate *on page 866*

U.S. Brand Names Imdur®; Ismo®; Monoket®

Canadian Brand Names Imdur®

Mexican Brand Names Elantan®; Imdur®; Mono Mack®

Generic Available Yes

Synonyms ISMN

Pharmacologic Category Vasodilator

Use Long-acting metabolite of the vasodilator isosorbide dinitrate used for the prophylactic treatment of angina pectoris

Local Anesthetic/Vasoconstrictor Precautions No information available to require special precautions

Effects on Dental Treatment No significant effects or complications reported

Common Adverse Effects
    >10%: Central nervous system: Headache (19% to 38%)
    1% to 10%:
        Central nervous system: Dizziness (3% to 5%)
        Gastrointestinal: Nausea/vomiting (2% to 4%)

The incidence of hypotension and adverse cardiovascular events may be increased when used in combination with sildenafil (Viagra®).

Dosage Adults and Geriatrics (start with lowest recommended dose): Oral:
    Regular tablet: 5-10 mg twice daily with the two doses given 7 hours apart (eg, 8 AM and 3 PM) to decrease tolerance development; then titrate to 10 mg twice daily in first 2-3 days.

Extended release tablet: Initial: 30-60 mg given in morning as a single dose; titrate upward as needed, giving at least 3 days between increases; maximum daily single dose: 240 mg

Dosing adjustment in renal impairment: Not necessary for elderly or patients with altered renal or hepatic function.

Tolerance to nitrate effects develops with chronic exposure. Dose escalation does not overcome this effect. Tolerance can only be overcome by short periods of nitrate absence from the body. Short periods (10-12 hours) of nitrate withdrawal help minimize tolerance. Recommended dosage regimens incorporate this interval. General recommendations are to take the last dose of short-acting agents no later than 7 PM; administer 2 times/day rather than 4 times/day. Administer sustained release tablet once daily in the morning.

Mechanism of Action Prevailing mechanism of action for nitroglycerin (and other nitrates) is systemic venodilation, decreasing preload as measured by pulmonary capillary wedge pressure and left ventricular end diastolic volume and pressure; the average reduction in left ventricular end diastolic volume is 25% at rest, with a corresponding increase in ejection fractions of 50% to 60%. This effect improves congestive symptoms in heart failure and improves the myocardial perfusion gradient in patients with coronary artery disease.

Contraindications Hypersensitivity to isosorbide or any component of the formulation; hypersensitivity to organic nitrates; concurrent use with phosphodiesterase-5 (PDE-5) inhibitors (sildenafil, tadalafil, or vardenafil); angle-closure glaucoma (intraocular pressure may be increased); head trauma or cerebral hemorrhage (increase intracranial pressure); severe anemia

Warnings/Precautions Postural hypotension, transient episodes of weakness, dizziness, or syncope may occur even with small doses; ethanol accentuates these effects; tolerance and cross-tolerance to nitrate antianginal and hemodynamic effects may occur during prolonged isosorbide mononitrate therapy; (minimized by using the smallest effective dose, by alternating coronary vasodilators or offering drug-free intervals of as little as 12 hours). Excessive doses may result in severe headache, blurred vision, or xerostomia; increased anginal symptoms may be a result of dosage increases. Avoid use with sildenafil.

Drug Interactions

Cytochrome P450 Effect: Substrate of CYP3A4 (major)

Increased Effect/Toxicity: CYP3A4 inhibitors may increase the levels/effects of isosorbide dinitrate; example inhibitors include azole antifungals, clarithromycin, diclofenac, doxycycline, erythromycin, imatinib, isoniazid, nefazodone, nicardipine, propofol, protease inhibitors, quinidine, telithromycin, and verapamil. Significant reduction of systolic and diastolic blood pressure with concurrent use of sildenafil, tadalafil, or vardenafil (contraindicated). Do not administer sildenafil, tadalafil, or vardenafil within 24 hours of a nitrate preparation.

Ethanol/Nutrition/Herb Interactions Ethanol: Caution with ethanol (may increase risk of hypotension).

Pharmacodynamics/Kinetics

Onset of action: 30-60 minutes

Absorption: Nearly complete and low intersubject variability in its pharmacokinetic parameters and plasma concentrations

Metabolism: Hepatic

Half-life elimination: Mononitrate: ~4 hours

Excretion: Urine and feces

Pregnancy Risk Factor C

Dosage Forms TAB: 10 mg, 20 mg; (Ismo®): 20 mg; (Monoket®): 10 mg, 20 mg.
TAB, extended release (Imdur®): 30 mg, 60 mg, 120 mg

Isotretinoin (eye soe TRET i noyn)

U.S. Brand Names Accutane®; Amnesteem™; Claravis™; Sotret®

Canadian Brand Names Accutane®; Isotrex®

Mexican Brand Names Isotrex®; Roaccutan®

Generic Available Yes

Synonyms 13-*cis*-Retinoic Acid

Pharmacologic Category Acne Products; Retinoic Acid Derivative

Use Treatment of severe recalcitrant nodular acne unresponsive to conventional therapy

Unlabeled/Investigational Use Investigational: Treatment of children with metastatic neuroblastoma or leukemia that does not respond to conventional therapy

Local Anesthetic/Vasoconstrictor Precautions No information available to require special precautions
(Continued)

Isotretinoin *(Continued)*

Effects on Dental Treatment Key adverse event(s) related to dental treatment: Xerostomia and changes in salivation (normal salivary flow resumes upon discontinuation).

Common Adverse Effects Frequency not defined.

Cardiovascular: Palpitation, tachycardia, vascular thrombotic disease, stroke, chest pain, syncope, flushing

Central nervous system: Edema, fatigue, pseudotumor cerebri, dizziness, drowsiness, headache, insomnia, lethargy, malaise, nervousness, paresthesia, seizure, stroke, suicidal ideation, suicide attempts, suicide, depression, psychosis, aggressive or violent behavior, emotional instability

Dermatologic: Cutaneous allergic reactions, purpura, acne fulminans, alopecia, bruising, cheilitis, dry mouth, dry nose, dry skin, epistaxis, eruptive xanthomas, fragility of skin, hair abnormalities, hirsutism, hyperpigmentation, hypopigmentation, peeling of palms, peeling of soles, photoallergic reactions, photosensitizing reactions, pruritus, rash, dystrophy, paronychia, facial erythema, seborrhea, eczema, increased sunburn susceptibility, diaphoresis, urticaria, abnormal wound healing

Endocrine & metabolic: Triglycerides increased (25%), abnormal menses, blood glucose increased, cholesterol increased, HDL decreased

Gastrointestinal: Weight loss, inflammatory bowel disease, regional ileitis, pancreatitis, bleeding and inflammation of the gums, colitis, nausea, nonspecific gastrointestinal symptoms

Genitourinary: Nonspecific urogenital findings

Hematologic: Anemia, thrombocytopenia, neutropenia, agranulocytosis, pyogenic granuloma

Hepatic: Hepatitis

Neuromuscular & skeletal: Skeletal hyperostosis, calcification of tendons and ligaments, premature epiphyseal closure, arthralgia, CPK elevations, arthritis, tendonitis, bone abnormalities, weakness, back pain (29% in pediatric patients), rhabdomyolysis (rare), bone mineral density decreased

Ocular: Corneal opacities, decreased night vision, cataracts, color vision disorder, conjunctivitis, dry eyes, eyelid inflammation, keratitis, optic neuritis, photophobia, visual disturbances

Otic: Hearing impairment, tinnitus

Renal: Vasculitis, glomerulonephritis,

Respiratory: Bronchospasms, respiratory infection, voice alteration, Wegener's granulomatosis

Miscellaneous: Allergic reactions, anaphylactic reactions, lymphadenopathy, infection, disseminated herpes simplex, diaphoresis

Restrictions A new program for risk minimization (iPLEDGE) is being designed by the FDA and the manufacturers of isotretinoin. The program will be implemented December 31, 2005. Details may be found on the FDA website at Additional details may be found on the FDA website at http://www.fda.gov/cder/drug/infopage/accutane/default.htm, last accessed August 12, 2005. When implemented, iPLEDGE will strengthen the current prescribing and dispensing requirements. All patients, prescribers, wholesalers and dispensing pharmacists must be registered. Registration will be possible via internet at www.ipledgeprogram.com or by calling 866-495-0654.

Under the current guidelines, prescriptions for isotretinoin may not be dispensed unless they are affixed with a yellow, self-adhesive, qualification sticker filled out by the prescriber. Telephone, fax, or computer-generated prescriptions are no longer valid. Prescriptions may not be written for more than a 1-month supply and must be dispensed with a patient education guide every month. In addition, prescriptions for females must be filled within 7 days of the qualification date noted on the yellow sticker; prescriptions filled after 7 days of the noted date are considered to be expired and cannot be honored. Pharmacists may call the manufacturer to confirm the prescriber's authority to write for this medication; however, this is not mandatory.

Prescribers will be provided with qualification stickers after they have read the details of the program and have signed (and mailed to the manufacturer) their agreement to participate. Audits of pharmacies will be conducted to monitor program compliance.

An FDA-approved medication guide is available at http://www.fda.gov/cder/Offices/ODS/labeling.htm; distribute to each patient to whom this medication is dispensed.

Mechanism of Action Reduces sebaceous gland size and reduces sebum production; regulates cell proliferation and differentiation

Drug Interactions

Increased Effect/Toxicity: Increased toxicity: Corticosteroids may cause osteoporosis; interactive effect with isotretinoin unknown; use with caution.

Phenytoin may cause osteomalacia; interactive effect with isotretinoin unknown; use with caution. Cases of pseudotumor cerebri have been reported in concurrent use with tetracycline; avoid combination.

Decreased Effect: Isotretinoin may increase clearance of carbamazepine resulting in reduced carbamazepine levels. Retinoic acid derivatives may diminish the therapeutic effect of oral contraceptives (two forms of contraception are recommended in females of childbearing potential during retinoic acid therapy).

Pharmacodynamics/Kinetics
Distribution: Crosses placenta
Protein binding: 99% to 100%; primarily albumin
Metabolism: Hepatic via CYP2B6, 2C8, 2C9, 2D6, 3A4; forms metabolites; major metabolite: 4-oxo-isotretinoin (active)
Half-life elimination: Terminal: Parent drug: 21 hours; Metabolite: 21-24 hours
Time to peak, serum: 3-5 hours
Excretion: Urine and feces (equal amounts)

Pregnancy Risk Factor X

Isovue® *see* Iopamidol *on page 855*
Isovue-M® *see* Iopamidol *on page 855*
Isovue Multipack® *see* Iopamidol *on page 855*

Isoxsuprine (eye SOKS syoo preen)

U.S. Brand Names Vasodilan® [DSC]
Generic Available Yes
Synonyms Isoxsuprine Hydrochloride
Pharmacologic Category Vasodilator
Use Treatment of peripheral vascular diseases, such as arteriosclerosis obliterans and Raynaud's disease
Local Anesthetic/Vasoconstrictor Precautions No information available to require special precautions
Effects on Dental Treatment May enhance effects of other vasodilators.
Common Adverse Effects Frequency not defined.
Cardiovascular: Hypotension, tachycardia, chest pain
Central nervous system: Dizziness
Dermatologic: Rash
Gastrointestinal: Nausea, vomiting
Neuromuscular & skeletal: Weakness
Mechanism of Action In studies on normal human subjects, isoxsuprine increases muscle blood flow, but skin blood flow is usually unaffected. Rather than increasing muscle blood flow by beta-receptor stimulation, isoxsuprine probably has a direct action on vascular smooth muscle. The generally accepted mechanism of action of isoxsuprine on the uterus is beta-adrenergic stimulation. Isoxsuprine was shown to inhibit prostaglandin synthetase at high serum concentrations, with low concentrations there was an increase in the P-G synthesis.
Drug Interactions
Increased Effect/Toxicity: May enhance effects of other vasodilators/hypotensive agents.
Pharmacodynamics/Kinetics
Absorption: Nearly complete
Half-life elimination, serum: Mean: 1.25 hours
Time to peak, serum: ~1 hour
Pregnancy Risk Factor C

Isoxsuprine Hydrochloride *see* Isoxsuprine *on page 871*

Isradipine (iz RA di peen)

Related Information
Cardiovascular Diseases *on page 1636*
U.S. Brand Names DynaCirc® [DSC]; DynaCirc® CR
Canadian Brand Names DynaCirc®
Mexican Brand Names DynaCirc®
Generic Available No
Pharmacologic Category Calcium Channel Blocker
Use Treatment of hypertension
Local Anesthetic/Vasoconstrictor Precautions No information available to require special precautions (see Dental Comment)
Effects on Dental Treatment No significant effects or complications reported
(Continued)

Isradipine (Continued)

Common Adverse Effects

>10%: Central nervous system: Headache (dose related 2% to 22%)

1% to 10%:

Cardiovascular: Edema (dose related 1% to 9%), palpitation (dose related 1% to 5%), flushing (dose related 1% to 5%), tachycardia (1% to 3%), chest pain (2% to 3%)

Central nervous system: Dizziness (2% to 8%), fatigue (dose related 1% to 9%), flushing (9%)

Dermatologic: Rash (1.5% to 2%)

Gastrointestinal: Nausea (1% to 5%), abdominal discomfort (≤3%), vomiting (≤1%), diarrhea (≤3%)

Renal: Urinary frequency (1% to 3%)

Respiratory: Dyspnea (1% to 3%)

Mechanism of Action

Inhibits calcium ion from entering the "slow channels" or select voltage-sensitive areas of vascular smooth muscle and myocardium during depolarization, producing a relaxation of coronary vascular smooth muscle and coronary vasodilation; increases myocardial oxygen delivery in patients with vasospastic angina

Drug Interactions

Cytochrome P450 Effect: Substrate of CYP3A4 (major); Inhibits CYP3A4 (weak)

Increased Effect/Toxicity: Isradipine may increase cardiovascular adverse effects of beta-blockers. Isradipine may minimally increase cyclosporine levels. CYP3A4 inhibitors may increase the levels/effects of isradipine; example inhibitors include azole antifungals, clarithromycin, diclofenac, doxycycline, erythromycin, imatinib, isoniazid, nefazodone, nicardipine, propofol, protease inhibitors, quinidine, telithromycin, and verapamil. Blood pressure-lowering effects may be additive with sildenafil, tadalafil, and vardenafil (use caution).

Decreased Effect: NSAIDs (diclofenac) may decrease the antihypertensive response of isradipine. Isradipine may cause a decrease in lovastatin effect. CYP3A4 inducers may decrease the levels/effects of isradipine; example inducers include aminoglutethimide, carbamazepine, nafcillin, nevirapine, phenobarbital, phenytoin, and rifamycins.

Pharmacodynamics/Kinetics

Onset of action: Immediate release: 20 minutes

Duration: Immediate release: >12 hours

Absorption: 90% to 95%

Distribution: V_d: 3 L/kg

Protein binding: 95%

Metabolism: Hepatic; CYP3A4 substrate (major); extensive first-pass effect

Bioavailability: 15% to 24%

Half-life elimination: 8 hours

Time to peak, serum: 1-1.5 hours

Excretion: Urine (as metabolites)

Pregnancy Risk Factor C

Dental Comment

This drug is known to prolong the QT interval. The QT interval is measured as the time and distance between the Q point of the QRS complex and the end of the T wave in the ECG tracing. After adjustment for heart rate, the QT interval is defined as prolonged if it is more than 450 msec in men and 460 msec in women. A long QT syndrome was first described in the 1950s and 60s as a congenital syndrome involving QT interval prolongation and syncope and sudden death. Some of the congenital long QT syndromes were characterized by a peculiar electrocardiographic appearance of the QRS complex involving a premature atria beat followed by a pause, then a subsequent sinus beat showing marked QT prolongation and deformity. This type of cardiac arrhythmia was originally termed "torsade de pointes" (translated from the French as "twisting of the points").

Prolongation of the QT interval is thought to result from delayed ventricular repolarization. The repolarization process within the myocardial cell is due to the efflux of intracellular potassium. The channels associated with this current can be blocked by many drugs and predisposes the electrical propagation cycle to torsade de pointes.

Isradipine is one of the drugs confirmed to prolong the QT interval and is accepted as having a risk of causing torsade de pointes. The risk of drug-induced torsade de pointes is extremely low when a single QT interval prolonging drug is prescribed. In terms of epinephrine, it is not known what effect vasoconstrictors in the local anesthetic regimen will have in patients with a known history of congenital prolonged QT interval or in patients taking any medication that prolongs the QT interval. Until more information is obtained, it is suggested that the clinician consult with the physician prior to the use of a vasoconstrictor in suspected patients, and that the vasoconstrictor (epinephrine, levonordefrin [Neo-Cobefrin®]) be used with caution.

Istalol™ see Timolol on page 1489
Isuprel® see Isoproterenol on page 865
Itch-X® [OTC] see Pramoxine on page 1264

Itraconazole (i tra KOE na zole)

Related Information
Fungal Infections on page 1707
U.S. Brand Names Sporanox®
Canadian Brand Names Sporanox®
Mexican Brand Names Carexan®; Isox®; Itranax®; Sporanox®
Generic Available No
Pharmacologic Category Antifungal Agent, Oral
Dental Use Treatment of susceptible fungal infections in immunocompromised and immunocompetent patients including blastomycosis and histoplasmosis; has activity against *Aspergillus, Candida, Coccidioides, Cryptococcus, Sporothrix*, and chromomycosis. Useful in superficial mycoses including dermatophytoses (eg, tinea capitis), pityriasis versicolor, sebopsoriasis, vaginal and chronic mucocutaneous candidiases; systemic mycoses including candidiasis, meningeal and disseminated cryptococcal infections, paracoccidioidomycosis, coccidioidomycoses; miscellaneous mycoses such as sporotrichosis, chromomycosis, leishmaniasis, fungal keratitis, alternariosis, zygomycosis.
Use Treatment of susceptible fungal infections in immunocompromised and immunocompetent patients including blastomycosis and histoplasmosis; indicated for aspergillosis, and onychomycosis of the toenail; treatment of onychomycosis of the fingernail without concomitant toenail infection via a pulse-type dosing regimen; has activity against *Aspergillus, Candida, Coccidioides, Cryptococcus, Sporothrix*, tinea unguium

Oral: Useful in superficial mycoses including dermatophytoses (eg, tinea capitis), pityriasis versicolor, sebopsoriasis, vaginal and chronic mucocutaneous candidiases; systemic mycoses including candidiasis, meningeal and disseminated cryptococcal infections, paracoccidioidomycosis, coccidioidomycoses; miscellaneous mycoses such as sporotrichosis, chromomycosis, leishmaniasis, fungal keratitis, alternariosis, zygomycosis
Oral solution: Treatment of oral and esophageal candidiasis
Intravenous solution: Indicated in the treatment of blastomycosis, histoplasmosis (nonmeningeal), and aspergillosis (in patients intolerant or refractory to amphotericin B therapy); empiric therapy of febrile neutropenic fever

Local Anesthetic/Vasoconstrictor Precautions No information available to require special precautions
Effects on Dental Treatment No significant effects or complications reported
Significant Adverse Effects Listed incidences are for higher doses appropriate for systemic fungal infection.

>10%: Gastrointestinal: Nausea (11%)
1% to 10%:
Cardiovascular: Edema (4%), hypertension (3%)
Central nervous system: Headache (4%), fatigue (2% to 3%), malaise (1%), fever (3%), dizziness (2%)
Dermatologic: Rash (9%), pruritus (3%)
Endocrine & metabolic: Decreased libido (1%), hypertriglyceridemia, hypokalemia (2%)
Gastrointestinal: Abdominal pain (2%), anorexia (1%), vomiting (5%), diarrhea (3%)
Hepatic: Abnormal LFTs (3%), hepatitis
Renal: Albuminuria (1%)
<1% (Limited to important or life-threatening): Adrenal suppression; allergic reactions (urticaria, angioedema); alopecia, anaphylactoid reactions, anaphylaxis, arrhythmia, CHF, constipation, gastritis, gynecomastia, hepatic failure, impotence, neutropenia, peripheral neuropathy, photosensitivity, pulmonary edema, somnolence, Stevens-Johnson syndrome, tinnitus

Dental Usual Dosing Oropharyngeal candidiasis: Adults: Oral solution: 200 mg once daily for 1-2 weeks; in patients unresponsive or refractory to fluconazole: 100 mg twice daily (clinical response expected in 1-2 weeks)
(Continued)

Itraconazole *(Continued)*

Dosage

Usual dosage ranges:

Children: Efficacy and safety have not been established; a small number of patients 3-16 years of age have been treated with 100 mg/day for systemic fungal infections with no serious adverse effects reported. A dose of 5 mg/kg once daily was used in a pharmacokinetic study using the oral solution in patients 6 months to 12 years; duration of study was 2 weeks.

Adults: Oral, I.V.: 100-400 mg/day; doses >200 mg/day are given in 2 divided doses; length of therapy varies from 1 day to >6 months depending on the condition and mycological response

Indication-specific dosing:

Adults:

Aspergillosis:

Oral: 200-400 mg/day

I.V.: 200 mg twice daily for 4 doses, followed by 200 mg daily

Blastomycosis/histoplasmosis:

Oral: 200 mg once daily, if no obvious improvement or there is evidence of progressive fungal disease, increase the dose in 100 mg increments to a maximum of 400 mg/day; doses >200 mg/day are given in 2 divided doses; length of therapy varies from 1 day to >6 months depending on the condition and mycological response

I.V.: 200 mg twice daily for 4 doses, followed by 200 mg/day

Brain abscess: Cerebral phaeohyphomycosis (dematiaceous): Oral: 200 mg twice daily for at least 6 months with amphotericin

Candidiasis:

Oropharyngeal: Oral solution: 200 mg once daily for 1-2 weeks; in patients unresponsive or refractory to fluconazole: 100 mg twice daily (clinical response expected in 1-2 weeks)

Esophageal: Oral solution: 100-200 mg once daily for a minimum of 3 weeks; continue dosing for 2 weeks after resolution of symptoms

Coccidioides: Oral: 200 mg twice daily

Infections, life-threatening:

Oral: 200 mg 3 times/day (600 mg/day) should be given for the first 3 days of therapy

I.V.: 200 mg twice daily for 4 doses, followed by 200 mg/day

Meningitis:

Coccidioides: Oral: 400-800 mg/day

Cryptococcal: HIV positive (unlabeled use): Induction: Oral: 400 mg/day for 10-12 weeks; maintenance: 200 mg twice daily lifelong

Onychomycosis: Oral: 200 mg once daily for 12 consecutive weeks

Pneumonia:

Coccidioides: Mild to moderate: Oral, I.V.: 200 mg twice daily

Cryptococcal: Mild to moderate (unlabeled use): 200-400 mg/day for 6-12 months (lifelong for HIV positive)

Protothecal infection: 200 mg once daily for 2 months

Sporotrichosis: Oral:

Lymphocutaneous: 100-200 mg/day for 3-6 months

Osteoarticular and pulmonary: 200 mg twice daily for 1-2 years (may use amphotericin B initially for stabilization)

Dosing adjustment in renal impairment: Not necessary; itraconazole injection is not recommended in patients with Cl_{cr} <30 mL/minute; hydroxypropyl-β-cyclodextrin (the excipient) is eliminated primarily by the kidneys. Hemodialysis: Not dialyzable

Dosing adjustment in hepatic impairment: May be necessary, but specific guidelines are not available. Risk-to-benefit evaluation should be undertaken in patients who develop liver function abnormalities during treatment.

Mechanism of Action Interferes with cytochrome P450 activity, decreasing ergosterol synthesis (principal sterol in fungal cell membrane) and inhibiting cell membrane formation

Contraindications Hypersensitivity to itraconazole, any component of the formulation, or to other azoles; concurrent administration with cisapride, dofetilide, ergot derivatives, levomethadyl, lovastatin, midazolam, pimozide, quinidine, simvastatin, or triazolam; treatment of onychomycosis in patients with evidence of left ventricular dysfunction, CHF, or a history of CHF

Warnings/Precautions Discontinue if signs or symptoms of CHF or neuropathy occur during treatment. Rare cases of serious cardiovascular adverse events (including death), ventricular tachycardia, and torsade de pointes have been observed due to increased cisapride concentrations induced by itraconazole. Use with caution in patients with left ventricular dysfunction or a history of CHF. Not recommended for use in patients with active liver disease, elevated liver enzymes, or prior hepatotoxic reactions to other drugs. Itraconazole has been associated with rare cases of serious hepatotoxicity (including fatal cases and cases within the first week of treatment); treatment should be discontinued in patients who develop clinical symptoms of liver dysfunction or abnormal liver function tests during itraconazole therapy except in cases where expected benefit exceeds risk. Large differences in itraconazole pharmacokinetic parameters have been observed in cystic fibrosis patients receiving the solution; if a patient with cystic fibrosis does not respond to therapy, alternate therapies should be considered. **Due to differences in bioavailability, oral capsules and oral solution cannot be used interchangeably.** Intravenous formulation should be used with caution in renal impairment; consider conversion to oral therapy if renal dysfunction/toxicity is noted. Initiation of treatment with oral solution is not recommended in patients at immediate risk for systemic candidiasis (eg, patients with severe neutropenia).

Drug Interactions Substrate of CYP3A4 (major); **Inhibits** CYP3A4 (strong)

Antacids: May decrease serum concentration of itraconazole. Administer antacids 1 hour before or 2 hours after itraconazole capsules.

Alfentanil: Serum concentrations may be increased; monitor.

Anticonvulsants: Itraconazole may increase the serum concentration of carbamazepine; carbamazepine, phenobarbital, and phenytoin may decrease the serum concentration of itraconazole.

Benzodiazepines: Alprazolam, diazepam, temazepam, triazolam, and midazolam serum concentrations may be increased; consider a benzodiazepine not metabolized by CYP3A4 (such as lorazepam) or another antifungal that is metabolized by CYP3A4

Buspirone: Serum concentrations may be increased; monitor for sedation

Busulfan: Serum concentrations may be increased; avoid concurrent use

Calcium channel blockers: Serum concentrations may be increased (applies to those agents metabolized by CYP3A4, including felodipine, nifedipine, and verapamil); consider another agent instead of a calcium channel blocker, another antifungal, or reduce the dose of the calcium channel blocker; monitor blood pressure

Cisapride; Serum concentration is increased which may lead to malignant arrhythmias; concurrent use is contraindicated

Corticosteroids: Serum levels/effects of the corticosteroid may be increased; use caution.

CYP3A4 inducers: CYP3A4 inducers may decrease the levels/effects of itraconazole. Example inducers include aminoglutethimide, carbamazepine, nafcillin, nevirapine, phenobarbital, phenytoin, and rifamycins.

CYP3A4 substrates: Itraconazole may increase the levels/effects of CYP3A4 substrates. Example substrates include benzodiazepines, calcium channel blockers, mirtazapine, nateglinide, nefazodone, tacrolimus, and venlafaxine. Selected benzodiazepines (midazolam and triazolam), cisapride, ergot alkaloids, selected HMG-CoA reductase inhibitors (lovastatin and simvastatin), and pimozide are generally contraindicated with strong CYP3A4 inhibitors.

Didanosine: May decrease absorption of itraconazole (due to buffering capacity of oral solution); applies only to oral solution formulation of didanosine

Digoxin: Serum concentrations may be increased; monitor.

Disopyramide: Serum levels/effects (including QT_c prolongation) may be increased; use caution.

Docetaxel: Serum concentrations may be increased; avoid concurrent use

Dofetilide: Serum levels/toxicity may be increased; concurrent use is contraindicated.

Eletriptan: Serum level/toxicity of eletriptan may be increased; use caution.

Ergot alkaloids: Toxicity (vasospasm, ischemia) may be significantly increased by itraconazole; concurrent use is contraindicated.

Erythromycin (and clarithromycin): May increase serum concentrations of itraconazole.

H_2 blockers: May decrease itraconazole absorption. Itraconazole depends on gastric acidity for absorption. Avoid concurrent use.

Halofantrine: Serum levels/effects (including QT_c prolongation) may be increased; use caution.

HMG-CoA reductase inhibitors (except pravastatin and fluvastatin): Serum concentrations may be increased. The risk of myopathy/rhabdomyolysis may be increased. Switch to pravastatin/fluvastatin or suspend treatment during course of itraconazole therapy.

Hypoglycemic agents, oral: Serum concentrations may be increased; monitor.

Immunosuppressants: Cyclosporine, sirolimus, and tacrolimus: Serum concentrations may be increased; monitor serum concentrations and renal function.

Levomethadyl: Serum levels/effects may be increased by itraconazole, potentially resulting in malignant arrhythmia; concurrent use is contraindicated.

Nevirapine: May decrease serum concentrations of itraconazole; monitor

(Continued)

Itraconazole *(Continued)*

Oral contraceptives: Efficacy may be reduced by itraconazole (limited data); use barrier birth control method during concurrent use

Pimozide: Serum levels/toxicity may be increased; concurrent use is contraindicated.

Protease inhibitors: May increase serum concentrations of itraconazole. Includes amprenavir, indinavir, nelfinavir, ritonavir, and saquinavir; monitor. Serum concentrations of indinavir, ritonavir, or saquinavir may be increased by itraconazole.

Proton pump inhibitors: May decrease itraconazole absorption. Itraconazole depends on gastric acidity for absorption. Avoid concurrent use (includes omeprazole, lansoprazole).

Quinidine: Serum levels may be increased. Concurrent use is contraindicated.

Rifabutin: Serum concentrations may be increased; monitor.

Sildenafil: Serum concentrations may be increased by itraconazole; consider dosage reduction. A maximum sildenafil dose of 25 mg in 48 hours is recommended with other strong CYP3A4 inhibitors.

Tadalafil: Serum concentrations may be increased by itraconazole. A maximum tadalafil dose of 10 mg in 72 hours is recommended with strong CYP3A4 inhibitors.

Trimetrexate: Serum concentrations may be increased; monitor

Vardenafil: Serum concentrations may be increased by itraconazole. If itraconazole dose is 200 mg/day, limit vardenafil dose to a maximum of 5 mg/24 hours. If itraconazole dose is 400 mg/day, limit vardenafil dose to a maximum of 2.5 mg/24 hours.

Warfarin: Anticoagulant effects may be increased; monitor INR and adjust warfarin's dose as needed

Vinca alkaloids: Serum concentrations may be increased; avoid concurrent use

Zolpidem: Serum levels may be increased; monitor

Ethanol/Nutrition/Herb Interactions

Food:

Capsules: Enhanced by food and possibly by gastric acidity. cola drinks have been shown to increase the absorption of the capsules in patients with achlorhydria or those taking H_2-receptor antagonists or other gastric acid suppressors. Avoid grapefruit juice.

Solution: Decreased by food, time to peak concentration prolonged by food.

Herb/Nutraceutical: St John's wort may decrease itraconazole levels.

Dietary Considerations

Capsule: Administer with food.

Solution: Take without food, if possible.

Pharmacodynamics/Kinetics

Absorption: Requires gastric acidity; capsule better absorbed with food, solution better absorbed on empty stomach

Distribution: V_d (average): 796 ± 185 L or 10 L/kg; highly lipophilic and tissue concentrations are higher than plasma concentrations. The highest concentrations: adipose, omentum, endometrium, cervical and vaginal mucus, and skin/nails. Aqueous fluids (eg, CSF and urine) contain negligible amounts.

Protein binding, plasma: 99.9%; metabolite hydroxy-itraconazole: 99.5%

Metabolism: Extensively hepatic via CYP3A4 into >30 metabolites including hydroxy-itraconazole (major metabolite); appears to have *in vitro* antifungal activity. Main metabolic pathway is oxidation; may undergo saturation metabolism with multiple dosing.

Bioavailability: Variable, ~55% (oral solution) in 1 small study; **Note:** Oral solution has a higher degree of bioavailability (149% ± 68%) relative to oral capsules; should not be interchanged

Half-life elimination: Oral: After single 200 mg dose: 21 ± 5 hours; 64 hours at steady-state; I.V.: steady-state: 35 hours; steady-state concentrations are achieved in 13 days with multiple administration of itraconazole 100-400 mg/day.

Excretion: Feces (~3% to 18%); urine (~0.03% as parent drug, 40% as metabolites)

Pregnancy Risk Factor C

Lactation Enters breast milk/not recommended

Dosage Forms

Capsule: 100 mg

Injection, solution: 10 mg/mL (25 mL) [packaged in a kit containing sodium chloride 0.9% (50 mL); filtered infusion set (1)]

Solution, oral: 100 mg/10 mL (150 mL) [cherry flavor]

Iveegam EN *see* Immune Globulin (Intravenous) *on page 824*

Ivermectin (eye ver MEK tin)

U.S. Brand Names Stromectol®
Generic Available No
Pharmacologic Category Anthelmintic
Use Treatment of the following infections: Strongyloidiasis of the intestinal tract due to the nematode parasite *Strongyloides stercoralis*. Onchocerciasis due to the nematode parasite *Onchocerca volvulus*. Ivermectin is only active against the immature form of *Onchocerca volvulus*, and the intestinal forms of *Strongyloides stercoralis*.
Unlabeled/Investigational Use Has been used for other parasitic infections including *Ascaris lumbricoides*, Bancroftian filariasis, *Brugia malayi*, scabies, *Enterobius vermicularis*, *Mansonella ozzardi*, *Trichuris trichiura*.
Local Anesthetic/Vasoconstrictor Precautions No information available to require special precautions
Effects on Dental Treatment No significant effects or complications reported
Common Adverse Effects Frequency not defined.
  Cardiovascular: Hypotension, mild ECG changes, orthostasis, peripheral and facial edema, transient tachycardia
  Central nervous system: Dizziness, encephalopathy (rare; associated with loiasis), headache, hyperthermia, insomnia, seizure, somnolence, vertigo
  Dermatologic: Pruritus, rash, Stevens-Johnson syndrome, toxic epidermal necrolysis, urticaria
  Gastrointestinal: Abdominal pain, anorexia, constipation, diarrhea, nausea, vomiting
  Hematologic: Anemia, eosinophilia, leukopenia
  Hepatic: ALT/AST increased, bilirubin increased
  Neuromuscular & skeletal: Limbitis, myalgia, tremor, weakness
  Ocular: Blurred vision, mild conjunctivitis, punctate opacity
  Respiratory: Asthma exacerbation
  Miscellaneous: Mazzotti reaction (with onchocerciasis): Arthralgia, edema, fever, lymphadenopathy, ocular damage, pruritus, rash, synovitis
Mechanism of Action Ivermectin is a semisynthetic antihelminthic agent; it binds selectively and with strong affinity to glutamate-gated chloride ion channels which occur in invertebrate nerve and muscle cells. This leads to increased permeability of cell membranes to chloride ions then hyperpolarization of the nerve or muscle cell, and death of the parasite.
Drug Interactions
  Cytochrome P450 Effect: Substrate of CYP3A4 (minor)
Pharmacodynamics/Kinetics
  Onset of action: Peak effect: 3-6 months
  Absorption: Well absorbed
  Distribution: Does not cross blood-brain barrier
  Half-life elimination: 16-35 hours
  Metabolism: Hepatic (>97%)
  Excretion: Urine (<1%); feces
Pregnancy Risk Factor C

IVIG see Immune Globulin (Intravenous) *on page 824*
IvyBlock® [OTC] *see* Bentoquatam *on page 188*
Ivy-Rid® [OTC] *see* Benzocaine *on page 190*
IvySoothe® [OTC] *see* Hydrocortisone *on page 793*
Jantoven™ *see* Warfarin *on page 1585*

Japanese Encephalitis Virus Vaccine (Inactivated)
(jap a NEESE en sef a LYE tis VYE rus vak SEEN, in ak ti VAY ted)

Related Information
  Immunizations (Vaccines) *on page 1786*
U.S. Brand Names JE-VAX®
Canadian Brand Names JE-VAX®
Generic Available No
Pharmacologic Category Vaccine
Use Active immunization against Japanese encephalitis for persons 1 year of age and older who plan to spend 1 month or more in endemic areas in Asia, especially persons traveling during the transmission season or visiting rural areas; consider vaccination for shorter trips to epidemic areas or extensive outdoor activities in rural endemic areas; elderly (>55 years of age) individuals should be considered for vaccination, since they have increased risk of developing symptomatic illness after infection; those planning travel to or residence in
(Continued)

Japanese Encephalitis Virus Vaccine (Inactivated)
(Continued)

endemic areas should consult the Travel Advisory Service (Central Campus) for specific advice

Local Anesthetic/Vasoconstrictor Precautions No information available to require special precautions

Effects on Dental Treatment No significant effects or complications reported

Common Adverse Effects Report allergic or unusual adverse reactions to the Vaccine Adverse Event Reporting System (VAERS) 1-800-822-7967.

Frequency not defined, common:
Cardiovascular: Hypotension
Central nervous system: Fever, headache, malaise, chills, dizziness
Dermatologic: Rash, urticaria, itching with or without accompanying rash
Gastrointestinal: Nausea, vomiting, abdominal pain
Local: Tenderness, redness, and swelling at injection site
Neuromuscular & skeletal: Myalgia
Frequency not defined, rare:
Cardiovascular: Angioedema
Central nervous system: Seizure, encephalitis, encephalopathy
Dermatologic: Erythema multiforme, erythema nodosum
Neuromuscular & skeletal: Peripheral neuropathy, joint swelling
Respiratory: Dyspnea
Miscellaneous: Anaphylactic reaction

Pregnancy Risk Factor C

JE-VAX® *see* Japanese Encephalitis Virus Vaccine (Inactivated) *on page 877*

Jolivette™ *see* Norethindrone *on page 1125*

Junel™ *see* Ethinyl Estradiol and Norethindrone *on page 608*

Junel™ Fe *see* Ethinyl Estradiol and Norethindrone *on page 608*

Just for Kids™ [OTC] *see* Fluoride *on page 671*

Kadian® *see* Morphine Sulfate *on page 1065*

Kala® [OTC] *see* Lactobacillus *on page 535*

Kaletra® *see* Lopinavir and Ritonavir *on page 943*

Kalmz [OTC] *see* Fructose, Dextrose, and Phosphoric Acid *on page 713*

Kanamycin (kan a MYE sin)

Related Information
Tuberculosis *on page 1673*
U.S. Brand Names Kantrex®
Canadian Brand Names Kantrex®
Mexican Brand Names Koptin®
Generic Available No
Synonyms Kanamycin Sulfate
Pharmacologic Category Antibiotic, Aminoglycoside
Use Treatment of serious infections caused by susceptible strains of *E. coli*, *Proteus* species, *Enterobacter aerogenes*, *Klebsiella pneumoniae*, *Serratia marcescens*, and *Acinetobacter* species; second-line treatment of *Mycobacterium tuberculosis*

Local Anesthetic/Vasoconstrictor Precautions No information available to require special precautions

Effects on Dental Treatment No significant effects or complications reported

Common Adverse Effects Frequency not defined.
Cardiovascular: Edema
Central nervous system: Neurotoxicity, drowsiness, headache, pseudomotor cerebri
Dermatologic: Skin itching, redness, rash, photosensitivity, erythema
Gastrointestinal: Nausea, vomiting, diarrhea, malabsorption syndrome (with prolonged and high-dose therapy of hepatic coma), anorexia, weight loss, salivation increased, enterocolitis
Hematologic: Granulocytopenia, agranulocytosis, thrombocytopenia
Local: Burning, stinging
Neuromuscular & skeletal: Weakness, tremor, muscle cramps
Otic: Ototoxicity (auditory), ototoxicity (vestibular)
Renal: Nephrotoxicity
Respiratory: Dyspnea

Mechanism of Action Interferes with protein synthesis in bacterial cell by binding to ribosomal subunit

Drug Interactions
Increased Effect/Toxicity: Increased toxicity may occur with amphotericin B, cisplatin, loop diuretics, neuromuscular-blocking agents. Use with bisphosphonate derivatives may lead to hypocalcemia.

Pharmacodynamics/Kinetics
Distribution:
Relative diffusion from blood into CSF: Good only with inflammation (exceeds usual MICs)
CSF:blood level ratio: Normal meninges: Nil; Inflamed meninges: 43%
Half-life elimination: 2-4 hours; Anuria: 80 hours; End-stage renal disease: 40-96 hours
Time to peak, serum: I.M.: 1-2 hours (decreased in burn patients)
Excretion: Urine (entire amount)

Pregnancy Risk Factor D

Kanamycin Sulfate *see* Kanamycin *on page 878*
Kanka® Soft Brush™ [OTC] *see* Benzocaine *on page 190*
Kantrex® *see* Kanamycin *on page 878*
Kaodene® NN [OTC] [DSC] *see* Kaolin and Pectin *on page 879*

Kaolin and Pectin (KAY oh lin & PEK tin)

U.S. Brand Names Kaodene® NN [OTC] [DSC]; Kao-Spen® [OTC] [DSC]; Kapectolin® [OTC] [DSC]
Generic Available Yes
Synonyms Pectin and Kaolin
Pharmacologic Category Antidiarrheal
Use Treatment of uncomplicated diarrhea
Local Anesthetic/Vasoconstrictor Precautions No information available to require special precautions
Effects on Dental Treatment No significant effects or complications reported
Common Adverse Effects Gastrointestinal: Constipation, fecal impaction
Drug Interactions
Decreased Effect: May decrease absorption of many drugs, including chloroquine, atenolol, metoprolol, propranolol, diflunisal, isoniazid, penicillamine, clindamycin, digoxin (give kaolin/pectin 2 hours before or 4 hours after medication).

Pregnancy Risk Factor C

Kaon-Cl-10® *see* Potassium Chloride *on page 1258*
Kaon-Cl® 20 *see* Potassium Chloride *on page 1258*
Kao-Paverin® [OTC] *see* Loperamide *on page 942*
Kaopectate® [OTC] *see* Bismuth *on page 210*
Kaopectate® Advanced Formula [OTC] [DSC] *see* Attapulgite *on page 165*
Kaopectate® Extra Strength [OTC] *see* Bismuth *on page 210*
Kaopectate® Maximum Strength Caplets [OTC] [DSC] *see* Attapulgite *on page 165*
Kaopectolin *(new formulation)* [OTC] *see* Bismuth *on page 210*
Kao-Spen® [OTC] [DSC] *see* Kaolin and Pectin *on page 879*
Kapectolin® [OTC] [DSC] *see* Kaolin and Pectin *on page 879*
Kariva™ *see* Ethinyl Estradiol and Desogestrel *on page 592*
Kay Ciel® *see* Potassium Chloride *on page 1258*
KCl *see* Potassium Chloride *on page 1258*
K-Dur® 10 *see* Potassium Chloride *on page 1258*
K-Dur® 20 *see* Potassium Chloride *on page 1258*
Keflex® *see* Cephalexin *on page 301*
Kelnor™ *see* Ethinyl Estradiol and Ethynodiol Diacetate *on page 597*
Kemadrin® *see* Procyclidine *on page 1288*
Kenalog® *see* Triamcinolone *on page 1526*
Kenalog-10® *see* Triamcinolone *on page 1526*
Kenalog-40® *see* Triamcinolone *on page 1526*
Keoxifene Hydrochloride *see* Raloxifene *on page 1329*
Kepivance™ *see* Palifermin *on page 1178*
Keppra® *see* Levetiracetam *on page 908*
Keralac™ *see* Urea *on page 1551*
Keralac™ Nailstik *see* Urea *on page 1551*
Keralyt® [OTC] *see* Salicylic Acid *on page 1374*
Kerlone® *see* Betaxolol *on page 203*
Kerr Insta-Char® [OTC] *see* Charcoal *on page 311*

Ketalar® *see* Ketamine *on page 880*

Ketamine (KEET a meen)

U.S. Brand Names Ketalar®
Canadian Brand Names Ketalar®
Mexican Brand Names Ketalin®
Generic Available Yes
Synonyms Ketamine Hydrochloride
Pharmacologic Category General Anesthetic
Use Induction and maintenance of general anesthesia, especially when cardiovascular depression must be avoided (ie, hypotension, hypovolemia, cardiomyopathy, constrictive pericarditis); sedation; analgesia
Local Anesthetic/Vasoconstrictor Precautions No information available to require special precautions
Effects on Dental Treatment Key adverse event(s) related to dental treatment: Increased salivation.
Common Adverse Effects
>10%:
Cardiovascular: Hypertension, increased cardiac output, paradoxical direct myocardial depression, tachycardia
Central nervous system: Increased intracranial pressure, visual hallucinations, vivid dreams
Neuromuscular & skeletal: Tonic-clonic movements, tremor
Miscellaneous: Emergence reactions, vocalization
1% to 10%:
Cardiovascular: Bradycardia, hypotension
Dermatologic: Pain at injection site, skin rash
Gastrointestinal: Anorexia, nausea, vomiting
Ocular: Diplopia, nystagmus
Respiratory: Respiratory depression
Restrictions C-III
Mechanism of Action Produces a cataleptic-like state in which the patient is dissociated from the surrounding environment by direct action on the cortex and limbic system. Releases endogenous catecholamines (epinephrine, norepinephrine) which maintain blood pressure and heart rate. Reduces polysynaptic spinal reflexes.
Drug Interactions
Cytochrome P450 Effect: Substrate (major) of CYP2B6, 2C8/9, 3A4
Increased Effect/Toxicity: CYP2B6 inhibitors may increase the levels/effects of ketamine; example inhibitors include desipramine, paroxetine, and sertraline. CYP2C8/9 inhibitors may increase the levels/effects of ketamine; example inhibitors include delavirdine, fluconazole, gemfibrozil, ketoconazole, nicardipine, NSAIDs, pioglitazone, and sulfonamides. CYP3A4 inhibitors may increase the levels/effects of ketamine; example inhibitors include azole antifungals, clarithromycin, diclofenac, doxycycline, erythromycin, imatinib, isoniazid, nefazodone, nicardipine, propofol, protease inhibitors, quinidine, telithromycin, and verapamil. Barbiturates, narcotics, hydroxyzine increase prolonged recovery; nondepolarizing neuromuscular blockers may increase effects. Muscle relaxants, thyroid hormones may increase blood pressure and heart rate. Halothane may decrease BP.
Pharmacodynamics/Kinetics
Onset of action:
I.V.: General anesthesia: 1-2 minutes; Sedation: 1-2 minutes
I.M.: General anesthesia: 3-8 minutes
Duration: I.V.: 5-15 minutes; I.M.: 12-25 minutes
Metabolism: Hepatic via hydroxylation and N-demethylation; the metabolite norketamine is 25% as potent as parent compound
Half-life elimination: 11-17 minutes; Elimination: 2.5-3.1 hours
Excretion: Clearance: 18 mL/kg/minute
Pregnancy Risk Factor D

Ketamine Hydrochloride *see* Ketamine *on page 880*
Ketek® *see* Telithromycin *on page 1448*

Ketoconazole (kee toe KOE na zole)

Related Information
Fungal Infections *on page 1707*
Respiratory Diseases *on page 1656*

Related Sample Prescriptions
Systemic Fungal Infections *on page 1740*
Topical Fungal Infections *on page 1740*

U.S. Brand Names Nizoral®; Nizoral® A-D [OTC]

Canadian Brand Names Apo-Ketoconazole®; Ketoderm®; Novo-Ketoconazole

Mexican Brand Names Akorazol®; Conazol®; Cremosan®; Fungoral®; Konaderm®; Mi-Ke-Son's®; Mycodib®; Nizoral®; Onofin-K®; Termizol®; Tiniazol®

Generic Available Yes

Pharmacologic Category Antifungal Agent, Oral; Antifungal Agent, Topical

Dental Use Treatment of susceptible fungal infections in the oral cavity including candidiasis, oral thrush, and chronic mucocutaneous candidiasis

Use Treatment of susceptible fungal infections, including candidiasis, oral thrush, blastomycosis, histoplasmosis, paracoccidioidomycosis, coccidioidomycosis, chromomycosis, candiduria, chronic mucocutaneous candidiasis, as well as certain recalcitrant cutaneous dermatophytoses; used topically for treatment of tinea corporis, tinea cruris, tinea versicolor, and cutaneous candidiasis, seborrheic dermatitis

Unlabeled/Investigational Use Treatment of prostate cancer (androgen synthesis inhibitor)

Local Anesthetic/Vasoconstrictor Precautions No information available to require special precautions

Effects on Dental Treatment No significant effects or complications reported

Significant Adverse Effects
Oral:
1% to 10%:
Dermatologic: Pruritus (2%)
Gastrointestinal: Nausea/vomiting (3% to 10%), abdominal pain (1%)
<1% (Limited to important or life-threatening): Bulging fontanelles, chills, depression, diarrhea, dizziness, fever, gynecomastia, headache, hemolytic anemia, hepatotoxicity, impotence, leukopenia, photophobia, somnolence, thrombocytopenia
Cream: Severe irritation, pruritus, stinging (~5%)
Shampoo: Increases in normal hair loss, irritation (<1%), abnormal hair texture, scalp pustules, mild dryness of skin, itching, oiliness/dryness of hair

Dental Usual Dosing Oral fungal infections: Oral:
Children ≥2 years: 3.3-6.6 mg/kg/day as a single dose for 1-2 weeks for candidiasis, for at least 4 weeks in recalcitrant dermatophyte infections, and for up to 6 months for other systemic mycoses
Adults: 200-400 mg/day as a single daily dose for durations as stated above

Dosage
Fungal infections:
Oral:
Children ≥2 years: 3.3-6.6 mg/kg/day as a single dose for 1-2 weeks for candidiasis, for at least 4 weeks in recalcitrant dermatophyte infections, and for up to 6 months for other systemic mycoses
Adults: 200-400 mg/day as a single daily dose for durations as stated above
Shampoo: Apply twice weekly for 4 weeks with at least 3 days between each shampoo
Topical: Rub gently into the affected area once daily to twice daily
Prostate cancer (unlabeled use): Oral: Adults: 400 mg 3 times/day
Dosing adjustment in hepatic impairment: Dose reductions should be considered in patients with severe liver disease
Hemodialysis: Not dialyzable (0% to 5%)

Mechanism of Action Alters the permeability of the cell wall by blocking fungal cytochrome P450; inhibits biosynthesis of triglycerides and phospholipids by fungi; inhibits several fungal enzymes that results in a build-up of toxic concentrations of hydrogen peroxide; also inhibits androgen synthesis

Contraindications Hypersensitivity to ketoconazole or any component of the formulation; CNS fungal infections (due to poor CNS penetration); coadministration with ergot derivatives or cisapride is contraindicated due to risk of potentially fatal cardiac arrhythmias

Warnings/Precautions Use with caution in patients with impaired hepatic function; has been associated with hepatotoxicity, including some fatalities; perform periodic liver function tests; high doses of ketoconazole may depress adrenocortical function.

Drug Interactions Substrate of CYP3A4 (major); **Inhibits** CYP1A2 (strong), 2A6 (moderate), 2B6 (weak), 2C8 (weak), 2C9 (strong), 2C19 (moderate), 2D6 (moderate), 3A4 (strong)
Benzodiazepines: Alprazolam, diazepam, temazepam, triazolam, and midazolam serum concentrations may be increased; consider a benzodiazepine not metabolized by CYP3A4 (such as lorazepam) or another antifungal that is metabolized by CYP3A4. Concurrent use is contraindicated.
(Continued)

Ketoconazole *(Continued)*

Buspirone: Serum concentrations may be increased; monitor for sedation

Busulfan: Serum concentrations may be increased; avoid concurrent use

Calcium channel blockers: Serum concentrations may be increased (applies to those agents metabolized by CYP3A4, including felodipine, nifedipine, and verapamil); consider another agent instead of a calcium channel blocker, another antifungal, or reduce the dose of the calcium channel blocker; monitor blood pressure

Cisapride: Serum concentration is increased which may lead to malignant arrhythmias; concurrent use is contraindicated

CYP1A2 substrates: Ketoconazole may increase the levels/effects of CYP1A2 substrates. Example substrates include aminophylline, fluvoxamine, mexiletine, mirtazapine, ropinirole, theophylline, and trifluoperazine.

CYP2A6 substrates: Ketoconazole may increase the levels/effects of CYP2A6 substrates. Example substrates include dexmedetomidine and ifosfamide.

CYP2C9 substrates: Ketoconazole may increase the levels/effects of CYP2C9 substrates. Example substrates include bosentan, dapsone, fluoxetine, glimepiride, glipizide, losartan, montelukast, nateglinide, paclitaxel, phenytoin, warfarin, and zafirlukast.

CYP2C19 substrates: Ketoconazole may increase the levels/effects of CYP2C19 substrates. Example substrates include citalopram, diazepam, methsuximide, phenytoin, propranolol, and sertraline.

CYP2D6 substrates: Ketoconazole may increase the levels/effects of CYP2D6 substrates. Example substrates include amphetamines, selected beta-blockers, dextromethorphan, fluoxetine, lidocaine, mirtazapine, nefazodone, paroxetine, risperidone, ritonavir, thioridazine, tricyclic antidepressants, and venlafaxine.

CYP2D6 prodrug substrates: Ketoconazole may decrease the levels/effects of CYP2D6 prodrug substrates. Example prodrug substrates include codeine, hydrocodone, oxycodone, and tramadol.

CYP3A4 inducers: CYP3A4 inducers may decrease the levels/effects of ketoconazole. Example inducers include aminoglutethimide, carbamazepine, nafcillin, nevirapine, phenobarbital, phenytoin, and rifamycins.

CYP3A4 substrates: Ketoconazole may increase the levels/effects of CYP3A4 substrates. Example substrates include benzodiazepines, calcium channel blockers, mirtazapine, nateglinide, nefazodone, tacrolimus, and venlafaxine. Selected benzodiazepines (midazolam and triazolam), cisapride, ergot alkaloids, selected HMG-CoA reductase inhibitors (lovastatin and simvastatin), and pimozide are generally contraindicated with strong CYP3A4 inhibitors.

Didanosine: May decrease absorption of ketoconazole (due to buffering capacity of oral solution); applies only to oral solution formulation of didanosine

Docetaxel: Serum concentrations may be increased; avoid concurrent use

Erythromycin (and clarithromycin): May increase serum concentrations of ketoconazole.

H_2 blockers: May decrease ketoconazole absorption. Ketoconazole depends on gastric acidity for absorption. Avoid concurrent use.

HMG-CoA reductase inhibitors (except pravastatin and fluvastatin): Serum concentrations may be increased. The risk of myopathy/rhabdomyolysis may be increased. Switch to pravastatin/fluvastatin or suspend treatment during course of ketoconazole therapy.

Immunosuppressants: Cyclosporine, sirolimus, and tacrolimus: Serum concentrations may be increased; monitor serum concentrations and renal function

Methylprednisolone: Serum concentrations may be increased; monitor

Nevirapine: May decrease serum concentrations of ketoconazole; monitor

Oral contraceptives: Efficacy may be reduced by ketoconazole (limited data); use barrier birth control method during concurrent use

Phenytoin: Serum concentrations may be increased; monitor phenytoin levels and adjust dose as needed

Protease inhibitors: May increase serum concentrations of ketoconazole. Includes amprenavir, indinavir, nelfinavir, ritonavir, and saquinavir; monitor

Proton pump inhibitors: May decrease ketoconazole absorption. Ketoconazole depends on gastric acidity for absorption. Avoid concurrent use (includes omeprazole, lansoprazole).

Quinidine: Serum levels may be increased; monitor

Rifampin: Rifampin decreases ketoconazole's serum concentration to levels which are no longer effective; avoid concurrent use.

Sildenafil: Serum concentrations may be increased by ketoconazole; consider dosage reduction. A maximum sildenafil dose of 25 mg in 48 hours is recommended with other strong CYP3A4 inhibitors.

Tadalafil: Serum concentrations may be increased by ketoconazole. A maximum tadalafil dose of 10 mg in 72 hours is recommended with strong CYP3A4 inhibitors.

Trimetrexate: Serum concentrations may be increased; monitor

Vardenafil: Serum concentrations may be increased by ketoconazole. If ketoconazole dose is 200 mg/day, limit vardenafil to a maximum of 5 mg/24 hours. If ketoconazole dose is 400 mg/day, limit vardenafil dose to a maximum of 2.5 mg/24 hours.

Warfarin: Anticoagulant effects may be increased; monitor INR and adjust warfarin's dose as needed

Vinca alkaloids: Serum concentrations may be increased; avoid concurrent use

Zolpidem: Serum levels may be increased; monitor

Ethanol/Nutrition/Herb Interactions

Food: Ketoconazole peak serum levels may be prolonged if taken with food.

Herb/Nutraceutical: St John's wort may decrease ketoconazole levels.

Dietary Considerations May be taken with food or milk to decrease GI adverse effects.

Pharmacodynamics/Kinetics

Absorption: Oral: Rapid (~75%); Shampoo: None

Distribution: Well into inflamed joint fluid, saliva, bile, urine, breast milk, sebum, cerumen, feces, tendons, skin and soft tissues, and testes; crosses blood-brain barrier poorly; only negligible amounts reach CSF

Protein binding: 93% to 96%

Metabolism: Partially hepatic via CYP3A4 to inactive compounds

Bioavailability: Decreases as gastric pH increases

Half-life elimination: Biphasic: Initial: 2 hours; Terminal: 8 hours

Time to peak, serum: 1-2 hours

Excretion: Feces (57%); urine (13%)

Pregnancy Risk Factor C

Lactation Enters breast milk/not recommended

Dosage Forms

Cream, topical: 2% (15 g, 30 g, 60 g)

Shampoo, topical (Nizoral® A-D): 1% (6 mL, 120 mL, 210 mL)

Tablet (Nizoral®): 200 mg

Ketoprofen (kee toe PROE fen)

Related Information

Oral Pain *on page 1692*

Rheumatoid Arthritis, Osteoarthritis, and Osteoporosis *on page 1668*

Temporomandibular Dysfunction (TMD) *on page 1724*

U.S. Brand Names Orudis® KT [OTC] [DSC]

Canadian Brand Names Apo-Keto®; Apo-Keto-E®; Apo-Keto SR®; Novo-Keto; Novo-Keto-EC; Nu-Ketoprofen; Nu-Ketoprofen-E; Oruvail®; Rhodis™; Rhodis-EC™; Rhodis SR™

Generic Available Yes: Capsule

Pharmacologic Category Nonsteroidal Anti-inflammatory Drug (NSAID), Oral

Dental Use Management of pain and swelling

Use Acute and long-term treatment of rheumatoid arthritis and osteoarthritis; primary dysmenorrhea; mild to moderate pain

Local Anesthetic/Vasoconstrictor Precautions No information available to require special precautions

Effects on Dental Treatment Key adverse event(s) related to dental treatment: Stomatitis.

NSAID formulations are known to reversibly decrease platelet aggregation via mechanisms different than observed with aspirin. The dentist should be aware of the potential of abnormal coagulation. Caution should also be exercised in the use of NSAIDs in patients already on anticoagulant therapy with drugs such as warfarin (Coumadin®).

Significant Adverse Effects

>10%: Gastrointestinal: Dyspepsia (11%)

1% to 10%:

Central nervous system: Headache (3% to 9%), depression, dizziness (>1%), dreams, insomnia, malaise, nervousness, somnolence

Dermatologic: Rash

Gastrointestinal: Abdominal pain (3% to 9%), constipation (3% to 9%), diarrhea (3% to 9%), flatulence (3% to 9%), nausea (3% to 9%), anorexia (>1%), stomatitis (>1%), vomiting (>1%)

Genitourinary: Urinary tract infection (>1%)

Ocular: Visual disturbances

Otic: Tinnitus

(Continued)

Ketoprofen *(Continued)*

Renal: Renal dysfunction (3% to 9%)

<1% (Limited to important or life-threatening): Agranulocytosis, allergic reaction, allergic rhinitis, alopecia, anaphylaxis, anemia, angioedema, arrhythmia, aseptic meningitis, blurred vision, bone marrow suppression, buccal necrosis, bullous rash, cholestatic hepatitis, confusion, CHF, conjunctivitis, cystitis, diabetes mellitus (aggravated), drowsiness, dry eyes, dysphoria, dyspnea, eczema, epistaxis, erythema multiforme, exfoliative dermatitis, gastritis, gastrointestinal perforation, GI ulceration, gynecomastia, hallucinations, hearing decreased, hemolytic anemia, hepatic dysfunction, hepatitis, hot flashes, hypertension, hyponatremia, impotence, interstitial nephritis, intestinal ulceration, jaundice, leukopenia, microvesicular steatosis, migraine, myocardial infarction, nephrotic syndrome, nightmares, onycholysis, pancreatitis, peptic ulcer, peripheral neuropathy, peripheral vascular disease, photosensitivity, polydipsia, polyuria, purpura, renal failure, retinal hemorrhage, Stevens-Johnson syndrome, tachycardia, taste perversion, thrombocytopenia, toxic amblyopia, toxic epidermal necrolysis, tubulopathy, ulcerative colitis, urticaria

Restrictions A medication guide should be dispensed with each prescription. A template for the required MedGuide can be found on the FDA website at: http://www.fda.gov/medwatch/SAFETY/2005/safety05.htm#NSAID

Dental Usual Dosing Mild-to-moderate pain: Children ≥16 years and Adults:
Oral: Capsule: 25-50 mg every 6-8 hours up to a maximum of 300 mg/day
OTC labeling: 12.5 mg every 4-6 hours, up to a maximum of 6 tablets/24 hours

Dosage Oral:

Children ≥16 years and Adults:

Rheumatoid arthritis or osteoarthritis (lower doses may be used in small patients or in the elderly, or debilitated):
Capsule: 50-75 mg 3-4 times/day up to a maximum of 300 mg/day
Capsule, extended release: 200 mg once daily

Mild-to-moderate pain: Capsule: 25-50 mg every 6-8 hours up to a maximum of 300 mg/day

OTC labeling: 12.5 mg every 4-6 hours, up to a maximum of 6 tablets/24 hours

Elderly: Initial dose should be decreased in patients >75 years; use caution when dosage changes are made

Dosage adjustment in renal impairment: In general, NSAIDs are not recommended for use in patients with advanced renal disease, but the manufacturer of ketoprofen does provide some guidelines for adjustment in renal dysfunction:

Mild impairment: Maximum dose: 150 mg/day
Severe impairment: Cl_{cr}<25 mL/minute: Maximum dose: 100 mg/day

Dosage adjustment in hepatic impairment and serum albumin <3.5 g/dL: Maximum dose: 100 mg/day

Mechanism of Action Inhibits prostaglandin synthesis by decreasing the activity of the enzyme, cyclooxygenase, which results in decreased formation of prostaglandin precursors

Contraindications Hypersensitivity to ketoprofen, aspirin, other NSAIDs, or any component of the formulation; perioperative pain in the setting of coronary artery bypass surgery (CABG); pregnancy (3rd trimester)

Warnings/Precautions NSAIDs are associated with an increased risk of adverse cardiovascular events, including MI, stroke, and new onset or worsening of pre-existing hypertension. Risk may be increased with duration of use or pre-existing cardiovascular risk-factors or disease. Carefully evaluate individual cardiovascular risk profiles prior to prescribing. Use caution with fluid retention, CHF or hypertension.

Use of NSAIDs can compromise existing renal function. Renal toxicity can occur in patient with impaired renal function, dehydration, heart failure, liver dysfunction, those taking diuretics and ACEI and the elderly. Rehydrate patient before starting therapy. Monitor renal function closely. Ketoprofen is not recommended for patients with advanced renal disease.

NSAIDs may increase risk of gastrointestinal irritation, ulceration, bleeding, and perforation. These events may occur at any time during therapy and without warning. Use caution with a history of GI disease (bleeding or ulcers), concurrent therapy with aspirin, anticoagulants and/or corticosteroids, smoking, use of alcohol, the elderly or debilitated patients.

Use the lowest effective dose for the shortest duration of time, consistent with individual patient goals, to reduce risk of cardiovascular or GI adverse events. Alternate therapies should be considered for patients at high risk.

NSAIDs may cause serious skin adverse events including exfoliative dermatitis, Stevens-Johnson syndrome (SJS) and toxic epidermal necrolysis (TEN). Anaphylactoid reactions may occur, even without prior exposure; patients with "aspirin triad" (bronchial asthma, aspirin intolerance, rhinitis) may be at increased risk. Do not use in patients who experience bronchospasm, asthma, rhinitis, or urticaria with NSAID or aspirin therapy.

Use with caution in patients with decreased hepatic function. Closely monitor patients with any abnormal LFT. Severe hepatic reactions (eg, fulminant hepatitis, liver failure) have occurred with NSAID use, rarely; discontinue if signs or symptoms of liver disease develop, or if systemic manifestations occur.

Withhold for at least 4-6 half-lives prior to surgical or dental procedures. Safety and efficacy have not been established in pediatric patients.

Drug Interactions Inhibits CYP2C8/9 (weak)

ACE inhibitors: Antihypertensive effects may be decreased by concurrent therapy with NSAIDs; monitor blood pressure

Aminoglycosides: NSAIDs may decrease the excretion of aminoglycosides.

Angiotensin II antagonists: Antihypertensive effects may be decreased by concurrent therapy with NSAIDs; monitor blood pressure

Anticoagulants (warfarin, heparin, LMWHs): In combination with NSAIDs can cause increased risk of bleeding.

Antiplatelet agents (ticlopidine, clopidogrel, aspirin, abciximab, dipyridamole, eptifibatide, tirofiban): In combination with NSAIDs can cause an increased risk of bleeding.

Beta-blockers: NSAIDs may decrease the antihypertensive effect of beta-blockers. Monitor.

Bisphosphonates: NSAIDs may increase the risk of gastrointestinal ulceration.

Cholestyramine (and other bile acid sequestrants): May decrease the absorption of NSAIDs. Separate by at least 2 hours.

Corticosteroids: May increase the risk of GI ulceration; avoid concurrent use.

Cyclosporine: NSAIDs may increase serum creatinine, potassium, blood pressure, and cyclosporine levels; monitor cyclosporine levels and renal function carefully.

Hydralazine: Antihypertensive effect is decreased; avoid concurrent use.

Lithium: Lithium levels can be increased; avoid concurrent use if possible or monitor lithium levels and adjust dose. Sulindac may have the least effect. When NSAID is stopped, lithium will need adjustment again.

Loop diuretics: Antihypertensive and diuretic effects may be diminished. Indomethacin reduces this efficacy, however, it may be anticipated with any NSAID.

Methotrexate: Severe bone marrow suppression, aplastic anemia, and GI toxicity have been reported with concomitant NSAID therapy. Avoid use during moderate or high-dose methotrexate (increased and prolonged methotrexate levels). NSAID use during low-dose treatment of rheumatoid arthritis has not been fully evaluated; extreme caution is warranted.

Pemetrexed: NSAIDs may decrease the excretion of pemetrexed. Patients with Cl_{cr} 45-79 mL/minute should avoid long acting NSAIDs for 5 days before and 2 days after pemetrexed treatment.

Probenecid: May increase the serum concentration of ketoprofen.

Thiazides: Antihypertensive effects may be decreased; avoid concurrent use.

Treprostinil: May enhance the risk of bleeding with concurrent use.

Vancomycin: NSAIDs may decrease the excretion of vancomycin.

Ethanol/Nutrition/Herb Interactions

Ethanol: Avoid ethanol (due to GI irritation).

Food: Food slows rate of absorption resulting in delayed and reduced peak serum concentrations.

Herb/Nutraceutical: Avoid alfalfa, anise, bilberry, bladderwrack, bromelain, cat's claw, celery, coleus, cordyceps, dong quai, evening primrose, feverfew, fenugreek, garlic, ginger, ginkgo biloba, red clover, horse chestnut, grapeseed, green tea, ginseng, guggul, horse chestnut seed, horseradish, licorice, prickly ash, red clover, reishi, SAMe, sweet clover, turmeric, white willow (all have additional antiplatelet activity).

Dietary Considerations In order to minimize gastrointestinal effects, ketoprofen can be prescribed to be taken with food or milk.

Pharmacodynamics/Kinetics

Absorption: Almost complete

Protein binding: >99%, primarily albumin

Metabolism: Hepatic via glucuronidation; metabolite can be converted back to parent compound; may have enterohepatic recirculation

Half-life elimination:

Capsule: 2-4 hours; moderate-severe renal impairment: 5-9 hours

Capsule, extended release: ~3-7.5 hours

(Continued)

Ketoprofen (Continued)

Time to peak, serum:
  Capsule: 0.5-2 hours
  Capsule, extended release: 6-7 hours
Excretion: Urine (~80%, primarily as glucuronide conjugates)

Pregnancy Risk Factor C/D (3rd trimester)

Lactation Excretion in breast milk unknown/not recommended

Dosage Forms [DSC] = Discontinued product
  Capsule: 50 mg, 75 mg
  Capsule, extended release: 200 mg
  Tablet (Orudis® KT): 12.5 mg [contains tartrazine and sodium benzoate] [DSC]

Selected Readings
Brooks PM and Day RO, "Nonsteroidal Anti-inflammatory Drugs - Differences and Similarities," *N Engl J Med*, 1991, 324(24):1716-25.
Cooper SA, "Ketoprofen in Oral Surgery Pain: A Review," *J Clin Pharmacol*, 1988, 28(12 Suppl):S40-6.
Hersh EV, "The Efficacy and Safety of Ketoprofen in Postsurgical Dental Pain," *Compendium*, 1991, 12(4):234.

Ketorolac (KEE toe role ak)

Related Information
Rheumatoid Arthritis, Osteoarthritis, and Osteoporosis *on page 1668*
Temporomandibular Dysfunction (TMD) *on page 1724*

U.S. Brand Names Acular®; Acular LS™; Acular® PF; Toradol®

Canadian Brand Names Acular®; Acular LS™; Apo-Ketorolac®; Apo-Ketorolac Injectable®; Novo-Ketorolac; ratio-Ketorolac; Toradol®; Toradol® IM

Generic Available Yes: Injection, tablet

Synonyms Ketorolac Tromethamine

Pharmacologic Category Nonsteroidal Anti-inflammatory Drug (NSAID), Ophthalmic; Nonsteroidal Anti-inflammatory Drug (NSAID), Oral; Nonsteroidal Anti-inflammatory Drug (NSAID), Parenteral

Dental Use Oral, injection: Short-term (≤5 days) management of moderately-severe acute pain requiring analgesia at the opioid level

Use
Oral, injection: Short-term (≤5 days) management of moderately-severe acute pain requiring analgesia at the opioid level
Ophthalmic: Temporary relief of ocular itching due to seasonal allergic conjunctivitis; postoperative inflammation following cataract extraction; reduction of ocular pain and photophobia following incisional refractive surgery, reduction of ocular pain, burning and stinging following corneal refractive surgery

Local Anesthetic/Vasoconstrictor Precautions No information available to require special precautions

Effects on Dental Treatment Key adverse event(s) related to dental treatment: Xerostomia (normal salivary flow resumes upon discontinuation).
NSAID formulations are known to reversibly decrease platelet aggregation via mechanisms different than observed with aspirin. The dentist should be aware of the potential of abnormal coagulation. Caution should also be exercised in the use of NSAIDs in patients already on anticoagulant therapy with drugs such as warfarin (Coumadin®). See Dental Comment.

Significant Adverse Effects
Systemic:
>10%:
  Central nervous system: Headache (17%)
  Gastrointestinal: Gastrointestinal pain (13%), dyspepsia (12%), nausea (12%)
>1% to 10%:
  Cardiovascular: Edema (4%), hypertension
  Central nervous system: Dizziness (7%), drowsiness (6%)
  Dermatologic: Pruritus, purpura, rash
  Gastrointestinal: Diarrhea (7%), constipation, flatulence, gastrointestinal fullness, vomiting, stomatitis
  Local: Injection site pain (2%)
  Miscellaneous: Diaphoresis
≤1% (Limited to important or life-threatening): Abnormal vision, acute renal failure, anaphylactoid reaction, anaphylaxis, asthma, azotemia, bronchospasm, cholestatic jaundice, convulsions, eosinophilia, epistaxis, esophagitis, extrapyramidal symptoms, GI hemorrhage, GI perforation, hallucinations, hearing loss, hematemesis, hematuria, hepatitis, hypersensitivity reactions, liver failure, Lyell's syndrome, maculopapular rash, nephritis, peptic ulceration, Stevens-Johnson syndrome, tinnitus, toxic epidermal necrolysis, urticaria, vertigo, wound hemorrhage (postoperative)

Ophthalmic solution:
>10%: Ocular: Transient burning/stinging (Acular®: 40%; Acular® PF: 20%)
>1% to 10%:
Central nervous system: Headache
Ocular: Conjunctival hyperemia, corneal infiltrates, iritis, ocular edema, ocular inflammation, ocular irritation, ocular pain, superficial keratitis, superficial ocular infection
Miscellaneous: Allergic reactions
≤1% (Limited to important or life-threatening): Blurred vision corneal ulcer, corneal erosion, corneal perforation, corneal thinning, dry eyes, epithelial breakdown

Restrictions A medication guide should be dispensed with each prescription. A template for the required MedGuide can be found on the FDA website at: http://www.fda.gov/medwatch/SAFETY/2005/safety05.htm#NSAID

Dental Usual Dosing Short-term (≤5 days) management of moderately-severe acute pain requiring analgesia at the opioid level (**Note:** The maximum combined duration of treatment (for parenteral and oral) is 5 days; do not increase dose or frequency; supplement with low-dose opioids if needed for breakthrough pain). For patients <50 kg and/or ≥65 years, see Elderly dosing.
Adults:
  I.M.: 60 mg as a single dose or 30 mg every 6 hours (maximum daily dose: 120 mg)
  I.V.: 30 mg as a single dose or 30 mg every 6 hours (maximum daily dose: 120 mg)
  Oral: 20 mg, followed by 10 mg every 4-6 hours; do not exceed 40 mg/day; oral dosing is intended to be a continuation of I.M. or I.V. therapy only
Elderly >65 years: Renal insufficiency or weight <50 kg: **Note:** Ketorolac has decreased clearance and increased half-life in the elderly. In addition, the elderly have reported increased incidence of GI bleeding, ulceration, and perforation. The maximum combined duration of treatment (for parenteral and oral) is 5 days.
  I.M.: 30 mg as a single dose or 15 mg every 6 hours (maximum daily dose: 60 mg)
  I.V.: 15 mg as a single dose or 15 mg every 6 hours (maximum daily dose: 60 mg)
  Oral: 10 mg every 4-6 hours; do not exceed 40 mg/day; oral dosing is intended to be a continuation of I.M. or I.V. therapy only

Dosage
Children 2-16 years: **Do not exceed adult doses**
Single-dose treatment:
  I.M.: 1 mg/kg (maximum: 30 mg)
  I.V.: 0.5 mg/kg (maximum: 15 mg)
  Oral (unlabeled): 1 mg/kg as a single dose reported in one study
Multiple-dose treatment (unlabeled): Limited pediatric studies. The maximum combined duration of treatment (for parenteral and oral) is 5 days.
  I.V.: Initial dose: 0.5 mg/kg, followed by 0.25-1 mg/kg every 6 hours for up to 48 hours (maximum daily dose: 90 mg)
  Oral: 0.25 mg/kg every 6 hours
Adults (pain relief usually begins within 10 minutes with parenteral forms): **Note:** The maximum combined duration of treatment (for parenteral and oral) is 5 days; do not increase dose or frequency; supplement with low-dose opioids if needed for breakthrough pain. For patients <50 kg and/or ≥65 years, see Elderly dosing.
  I.M.: 60 mg as a single dose or 30 mg every 6 hours (maximum daily dose: 120 mg)
  I.V.: 30 mg as a single dose or 30 mg every 6 hours (maximum daily dose: 120 mg)
  Oral: 20 mg, followed by 10 mg every 4-6 hours; do not exceed 40 mg/day; oral dosing is intended to be a continuation of I.M. or I.V. therapy only
Ophthalmic: Children ≥3 years and Adults:
  Allergic conjunctivitis (relief of ocular itching) (Acular®): Instill 1 drop (0.25 mg) 4 times/day for seasonal allergic conjunctivitis
  Inflammation following cataract extraction (Acular®): Instill 1 drop (0.25 mg) to affected eye(s) 4 times/day beginning 24 hours after surgery; continue for 2 weeks
  Pain and photophobia following incisional refractive surgery (Acular® PF): Instill 1 drop (0.25 mg) 4 times/day to affected eye for up to 3 days
  Pain following corneal refractive surgery (Acular LS™): Instill 1 drop 4 times/day as needed to affected eye for up to 4 days
Elderly >65 years: Renal insufficiency or weight <50 kg: **Note:** Ketorolac has decreased clearance and increased half-life in the elderly. In addition, the elderly have reported increased incidence of GI bleeding, ulceration, and
(Continued)

Ketorolac *(Continued)*

perforation. The maximum combined duration of treatment (for parenteral and oral) is 5 days.

I.M.: 30 mg as a single dose or 15 mg every 6 hours (maximum daily dose: 60 mg)

I.V.: 15 mg as a single dose or 15 mg every 6 hours (maximum daily dose: 60 mg)

Oral: 10 mg every 4-6 hours; do not exceed 40 mg/day; oral dosing is intended to be a continuation of I.M. or I.V. therapy only

Dosage adjustment in renal impairment: Do not use in patients with advanced renal impairment. Patients with moderately-elevated serum creatinine should use half the recommended dose, not to exceed 60 mg/day I.M./I.V.

Dosage adjustment in hepatic impairment: Use with caution, may cause elevation of liver enzymes

Mechanism of Action Inhibits prostaglandin synthesis by decreasing the activity of the enzyme, cyclooxygenase, which results in decreased formation of prostaglandin precursors

Contraindications Hypersensitivity to ketorolac, aspirin, other NSAIDs, or any component of the formulation; active or history of peptic ulcer disease; recent or history of GI bleeding or perforation; patients with advanced renal disease or risk of renal failure; labor and delivery; nursing mothers; prophylaxis before major surgery; suspected or confirmed cerebrovascular bleeding; hemorrhagic diathesis; concurrent ASA or other NSAIDs; epidural or intrathecal administration; concomitant probenecid; perioperative pain in the setting of coronary artery bypass surgery (CABG); pregnancy (3rd trimester)

Warnings/Precautions

Systemic: Treatment should be started with I.V./I.M. administration then changed to oral only as a continuation of treatment. Total therapy is not to exceed 5 days. Should not be used for minor or chronic pain.

May prolong bleeding time; do not use when hemostasis is critical. Patients should be euvolemic prior to treatment. Low doses of narcotics may be needed for breakthrough pain.

NSAIDs are associated with an increased risk of adverse cardiovascular events, including MI, stroke, and new onset or worsening of pre-existing hypertension. Risk may be increased with duration of use or pre-existing cardiovascular risk-factors or disease. Carefully evaluate individual cardiovascular risk profiles prior to prescribing. Use caution with fluid retention, CHF or hypertension.

Use of NSAIDs can compromise existing renal function. Renal toxicity can occur in patient with impaired renal function, dehydration, heart failure, liver dysfunction, those taking diuretics and ACEI and the elderly. Rehydrate patient before starting therapy. Monitor renal function closely. Ketorolac is not recommended for patients with advanced renal disease.

NSAIDs may increase risk of gastrointestinal irritation, ulceration, bleeding, and perforation. These events may occur at any time during therapy and without warning. Use caution with a history of GI disease (bleeding or ulcers), concurrent therapy with aspirin, anticoagulants and/or corticosteroids, smoking, use of alcohol, the elderly or debilitated patients.

Use the lowest effective dose for the shortest duration of time, consistent with individual patient goals, to reduce risk of cardiovascular or GI adverse events. Alternate therapies should be considered for patients at high risk.

NSAIDs may cause serious skin adverse events including exfoliative dermatitis, Stevens-Johnson syndrome (SJS) and toxic epidermal necrolysis (TEN). Anaphylactoid reactions may occur, even without prior exposure; patients with "aspirin triad" (bronchial asthma, aspirin intolerance, rhinitis) may be at increased risk. Do not use in patients who experience bronchospasm, asthma, rhinitis, or urticaria with NSAID or aspirin therapy.

Use with caution in patients with decreased hepatic function. Closely monitor patients with any abnormal LFT. Severe hepatic reactions (eg, fulminant hepatitis, liver failure) have occurred with NSAID use, rarely; discontinue if signs or symptoms of liver disease develop, or if systemic manifestations occur.

The elderly are at increased risk for adverse effects (especially peptic ulceration, CNS effects, renal toxicity) from NSAIDs even at low doses.

Withhold for at least 4-6 half-lives prior to surgical or dental procedures.

Ophthalmic: May increase bleeding time associated with ocular surgery. Use with caution in patients with known bleeding tendencies or those receiving anticoagulants. Healing time may be slowed or delayed. Corneal thinning, erosion, or ulceration have been reported with topical NSAIDs; discontinue if corneal epithelial breakdown occurs. Use caution with complicated ocular surgery, corneal denervation, corneal epithelial defects, diabetes, rheumatoid arthritis, ocular surface disease, or ocular surgeries repeated within short periods of time; risk of corneal epithelial breakdown may be increased. Use for >24 hours prior to or for >14 days following surgery also increases risk of corneal adverse effects. Do not administer while wearing soft contact lenses. Safety and efficacy in pediatric patients <3 years of age have not been established.

Drug Interactions

ACE inhibitors: Antihypertensive effects may be decreased by concurrent therapy with NSAIDs; monitor blood pressure.

Angiotensin II antagonists: Antihypertensive effects may be decreased by concurrent therapy with NSAIDs; monitor blood pressure.

Anticoagulants: Increased risk of bleeding complications with concomitant use; monitor closely.

Antiepileptic drugs (carbamazepine, phenytoin): Sporadic cases of seizures have been reported with concomitant use.

Beta-blockers: NSAIDs may decrease the antihypertensive effect of beta-blockers. Monitor.

Cholestyramine (and other bile acid sequestrants): May decrease the absorption of NSAIDs. Separate by at least 2 hours.

Diuretics: May see decreased effect of diuretics.

Hydralazine's antihypertensive effect may be reduced; monitor.

Lithium: May increase lithium levels; monitor.

Methotrexate: Severe bone marrow suppression, aplastic anemia, and GI toxicity have been reported with concomitant NSAID therapy. Avoid use during moderate or high-dose methotrexate (increased and prolonged methotrexate levels). NSAID use during low-dose treatment of rheumatoid arthritis has not been fully evaluated; extreme caution is warranted.

Nondepolarizing muscle relaxants: Concomitant use has resulted in apnea.

NSAIDs, salicylates: Concomitant use increases NSAID-induced adverse effects; contraindicated.

Probenecid: Probenecid significantly decreases ketorolac clearance, increases ketorolac plasma levels, and doubles the half-life of ketorolac; concomitant use is contraindicated.

Psychoactive drugs (alprazolam, fluoxetine, thiothixene): Hallucinations have been reported with concomitant use.

Ethanol/Nutrition/Herb Interactions

Ethanol: Avoid ethanol (may enhance gastric mucosal irritation).

Food: Oral: High-fat meals may delay time to peak (by ~1 hour) and decrease peak concentrations.

Herb/Neutraceuticals: Avoid alfalfa, anise, bilberry, bladderwrack, bromelain, cat's claw, celery, coleus, cordyceps, dong quai, evening primrose, feverfew, fenugreek, garlic, ginger, ginkgo biloboa, red clover, horse chestnut, grapeseed, green tea, ginseng, guggul, horse chestnut seed, horseradish, licorice, prickly ash, red clover, reishi, SAMe, sweet clover, turmeric, white willow (all have additional antiplatelet activity).

Dietary Considerations Administer tablet with food or milk to decrease gastrointestinal distress.

Pharmacodynamics/Kinetics

Onset of action: Analgesic: I.M.: ~10 minutes

Peak effect: Analgesic: 2-3 hours

Duration: Analgesic: 6-8 hours

Absorption: Oral: Well absorbed

Distribution: Poor penetration into CSF; crosses placenta; enters breast milk

Protein binding: 99%

Metabolism: Hepatic

Half-life elimination: 2-8 hours; prolonged 30% to 50% in elderly

Time to peak, serum: I.M.: 30-60 minutes

Excretion: Urine (61% as unchanged drug)

Pregnancy Risk Factor C/D (3rd trimester)

Lactation Enters breast milk/contraindicated (AAP rates "compatible")

Dosage Forms [DSC] = Discontinued product

Injection, solution, as tromethamine: 15 mg/mL (1 mL); 30 mg/mL (1 mL, 2 mL, 10 mL) [contains alcohol]

Solution, ophthalmic, as tromethamine:

Acular®: 0.5% (3 mL, 5 mL, 10 mL) [contains benzalkonium chloride]

Acular LS™: 0.4% (5 mL) [contains benzalkonium chloride]

Acular® P.F. [preservative free]: 0.5% (0.4 mL)

Tablet, as tromethamine: 10 mg

Toradol®: 10 mg [DSC]

(Continued)

Ketorolac *(Continued)*

Dental Comment According to the manufacturer, ketorolac has been used inappropriately by physicians in the past. The drug had been prescribed to NSAID-sensitive patients, patients with GI bleeding, and for long-term use; a warning has been issued regarding increased incidence and severity of GI complications with increasing doses and duration of use. Labeling now includes the statement that ketorolac inhibits platelet function and is indicated for up to 5 days use only.

Selected Readings
Ahmad N, Grad HA, Haas DA, et al, "The Efficacy of Nonopioid Analgesics for Postoperative Dental Pain: A Meta-Analysis," *Anesth Prog*, 1997, 44(4):119-26.

Balevi B, "Ketorolac Versus Ibuprofen: A Simple Cost-Efficacy Comparison for Dental Use," *J Can Dent Assoc*, 1994, 60(1):31-2.

Forbes JA, Butterworth GA, Burchfield WH, et al, "Evaluation of Ketorolac, Aspirin, and an Aceta-minophen-Codeine Combination in Postoperative Oral Surgery Pain," *Pharmacotherapy*, 1990, 10(6 Pt 2): 77S-93S.

Forbes JA, Kehm CJ, Grodin CD, et al, "Evaluation of Ketorolac, Ibuprofen, Acetaminophen, and an Acetaminophen-Codeine Combination in Postoperative Oral Surgery Pain," *Pharmacotherapy*, 1990, 10(6 Pt 2):94S-105S.

Fricke JR Jr, Angelocci D, Fox K, et al, "Comparison of the Efficacy and Safety of Ketorolac and Meperidine in the Relief of Dental Pain," *J Clin Pharmacol*, 1992, 32(4):376-84.

Fricke J, Halladay SC, Bynum L, et al, "Pain Relief After Dental Impaction Surgery Using Ketorolac, Hydrocodone Plus Acetaminophen, or Placebo," *Clin Ther*, 1993, 15(3):500-9.

Pendeville PE, Van Boven MJ, Contreras V, et al, "Ketorolac Tromethamine for Postoperative Analgesia in Oral Surgery," *Acta Anaesthesiol Belg*, 1995, 46(1):25-30.

Swift JQ, Roszkowski MT, Alton T, "Effect of Intra-articular Versus Systemic Anti-inflammatory Drugs in a Rabbit Model of Temporomandibular Joint Inflammation," *J Oral Maxillofac Surg*, 1998, 56(11):1288-95; discussion 1295-6.

Walton GM, Rood JP, Snowdon AT, et al, "Ketorolac and Diclofenac for Postoperative Pain Relief Following Oral Surgery," *Br J Oral Maxillofac Surg*, 1993, 31(3):158-60.

Wynn RL, "Ketorolac (Toradol®) for Dental Pain," *Gen Dent*, 1992, 40(6):476-9.

Ketorolac Tromethamine *see* Ketorolac *on page 886*

Ketotifen *(kee toe TYE fen)*

U.S. Brand Names Zaditor™
Canadian Brand Names Apo-Ketotifen®; Novo-Ketotifen; Zaditen®; Zaditor™
Mexican Brand Names Kasmal®; Ventisol®; Zaditen®
Generic Available No
Synonyms Ketotifen Fumarate
Pharmacologic Category Antihistamine, H₁ Blocker, Ophthalmic
Use Temporary prevention of eye itching due to allergic conjunctivitis
Local Anesthetic/Vasoconstrictor Precautions No information available to require special precautions
Effects on Dental Treatment Key adverse event(s) related to dental treatment: Pharyngitis.
Mechanism of Action Relatively selective, noncompetitive H_1-receptor antagonist and mast cell stabilizer, inhibiting the release of mediators from cells involved in hypersensitivity reactions
Pregnancy Risk Factor C

Ketotifen Fumarate *see* Ketotifen *on page 890*

Key-E® [OTC] *see* Vitamin E *on page 1581*

Key-E® Kaps [OTC] *see* Vitamin E *on page 1581*

Keygesic [OTC] *see* Magnesium Salicylate *on page 962*

KI *see* Potassium Iodide *on page 1260*

Kidkare Decongestant [OTC] *see* Pseudoephedrine *on page 1309*

Kineret® *see* Anakinra *on page 125*

Kinevac® *see* Sincalide *on page 1396*

Klaron® *see* Sulfacetamide *on page 1423*

Klonopin® *see* Clonazepam *on page 371*

K-Lor® *see* Potassium Chloride *on page 1258*

Klor-Con® *see* Potassium Chloride *on page 1258*

Klor-Con® 8 *see* Potassium Chloride *on page 1258*

Klor-Con® 10 *see* Potassium Chloride *on page 1258*

Klor-Con®/25 *see* Potassium Chloride *on page 1258*

Klor-Con® M *see* Potassium Chloride *on page 1258*

Klor-Con®/EF *see* Potassium Bicarbonate and Potassium Citrate *on page 1258*

K-Lyte® *see* Potassium Bicarbonate and Potassium Citrate *on page 1258*

K-Lyte/Cl® *see* Potassium Bicarbonate and Potassium Chloride *on page 1258*

K-Lyte/Cl® 50 [DSC] *see* Potassium Bicarbonate and Potassium Chloride *on page 1258*

K-Lyte® DS *see* Potassium Bicarbonate and Potassium Citrate *on page 1258*

Kodet SE [OTC] *see* Pseudoephedrine *on page 1309*

Kogenate® FS *see* Antihemophilic Factor (Recombinant) *on page 130*

Kolephrin® [OTC] *see* Acetaminophen, Chlorpheniramine, and Pseudoephedrine *on page 43*

Kolephrin® #1 *see* Guaifenesin and Codeine *on page 753*

Kolephrin® GG/DM [OTC] *see* Guaifenesin and Dextromethorphan *on page 754*

Konsyl® [OTC] *see* Psyllium *on page 1313*

Konsyl-D® [OTC] *see* Psyllium *on page 1313*

Konsyl® Easy Mix [OTC] *see* Psyllium *on page 1313*

Konsyl® Fiber Tablets [OTC] *see* Polycarbophil *on page 1252*

Konsyl® Orange [OTC] *see* Psyllium *on page 1313*

Kovia® *see* Papain and Urea *on page 1186*

Koāte®-DVI *see* Antihemophilic Factor (Human) *on page 129*

K-Pek II [OTC] *see* Loperamide *on page 942*

K-Phos® MF *see* Potassium Phosphate and Sodium Phosphate *on page 1261*

K-Phos® Neutral *see* Potassium Phosphate and Sodium Phosphate *on page 1261*

K-Phos® No. 2 *see* Potassium Phosphate and Sodium Phosphate *on page 1261*

K-Phos® Original *see* Potassium Acid Phosphate *on page 1257*

K+ Potassium *see* Potassium Chloride *on page 1258*

Kristalose™ *see* Lactulose *on page 893*

Kronofed-A® *see* Chlorpheniramine and Pseudoephedrine *on page 325*

Kronofed-A®-Jr *see* Chlorpheniramine and Pseudoephedrine *on page 325*

K-Tab® *see* Potassium Chloride *on page 1258*

kutrase® *see* Pancreatin *on page 1183*

ku-zyme® *see* Pancreatin *on page 1183*

ku-zyme® HP *see* Pancrelipase *on page 1183*

Kwelcof® *see* Hydrocodone and Guaifenesin *on page 785*

Kytril® *see* Granisetron *on page 751*

L-749,345 *see* Ertapenem *on page 561*

L-M-X™ 4 [OTC] *see* Lidocaine *on page 920*

L-M-X™ 5 [OTC] *see* Lidocaine *on page 920*

L 754030 *see* Aprepitant *on page 134*

LA 20304a *see* Gemifloxacin *on page 731*

Labetalol (la BET a lole)

Related Information
Cardiovascular Diseases *on page 1636*

U.S. Brand Names Trandate®

Canadian Brand Names Apo-Labetalol®; Normodyne®; Trandate®

Generic Available Yes

Synonyms Ibidomide Hydrochloride; Labetalol Hydrochloride

Pharmacologic Category Beta Blocker With Alpha-Blocking Activity

Use Treatment of mild to severe hypertension; I.V. for hypertensive emergencies

Local Anesthetic/Vasoconstrictor Precautions Use with caution; epinephrine has interacted with nonselective beta-blockers to result in initial hypertensive episode followed by bradycardia

Effects on Dental Treatment Key adverse event(s) related to dental treatment: Taste disorder.

Noncardioselective beta-blockers enhance the pressor response to epinephrine, resulting in hypertension and bradycardia. Many nonsteroidal anti-inflammatory drugs, such as ibuprofen and indomethacin, can reduce the hypotensive effect of beta-blockers after 3 or more weeks of therapy with the NSAID. Short-term NSAID use (ie, 3 days) requires no special precautions in patients taking beta-blockers.

Common Adverse Effects
>10%:
  Central nervous system: Dizziness (1% to 16%)
  Gastrointestinal: Nausea (0% to 19%)

1% to 10%:
  Cardiovascular: Edema (0% to 2%), hypotension (1% to 5%); with IV use, hypotension may occur in up to 58%
  Central nervous system: Fatigue (1% to 10%), paresthesia (1% to 5%), headache (2%), vertigo (2%)
  Dermatologic: Rash (1%), scalp tingling (1% to 5%)
  Gastrointestinal: Vomiting (<1% to 3%), dyspepsia (1% to 4%)
  Genitourinary: Ejaculatory failure (0% to 5%), impotence (1% to 4%)
  Hepatic: Transaminases increased (4%)

(Continued)

Labetalol *(Continued)*

Neuromuscular & skeletal: Weakness (1%)
Respiratory: Nasal congestion (1% to 6%), dyspnea (2%)
Miscellaneous: Taste disorder (1%), abnormal vision (1%)

Other adverse reactions noted with beta-adrenergic blocking agents include mental depression, catatonia, disorientation, short-term memory loss, emotional lability, clouded sensorium, intensification of pre-existing AV block, laryngospasm, respiratory distress, agranulocytosis, thrombocytopenic purpura, nonthrombocytopenic purpura, mesenteric artery thrombosis, and ischemic colitis.

Mechanism of Action Blocks alpha-, beta$_1$-, and beta$_2$-adrenergic receptor sites; elevated renins are reduced

Drug Interactions

Cytochrome P450 Effect: Substrate of CYP2D6 (major); **Inhibits** CYP2D6 (weak)

Increased Effect/Toxicity: CYP2D6 inhibitors may increase the levels/effects of labetalol; example inhibitors include chlorpromazine, delavirdine, fluoxetine, miconazole, paroxetine, pergolide, quinidine, quinine, ritonavir, and ropinirole. Cimetidine increases the bioavailability of labetalol. Labetalol has additive hypotensive effects with other antihypertensive agents. Concurrent use with alpha-blockers (prazosin, terazosin) and beta-blockers increases the risk of orthostasis. Concurrent use with diltiazem, verapamil, or digoxin may increase the risk of bradycardia with beta-blocking agents. Halothane, enflurane, isoflurane, and potentially other inhalation anesthetics may cause synergistic hypotension. Beta-blockers may affect the action or levels of ethanol, disopyramide, nondepolarizing muscle relaxants, and theophylline although the effects are difficult to predict.

Decreased Effect: Decreased effect of beta-blockers with aluminum salts, barbiturates, calcium salts, cholestyramine, colestipol, NSAIDs, penicillins (ampicillin), rifampin, salicylates, and sulfinpyrazone due to decreased bioavailability and plasma levels. Beta-blockers may decrease the effect of sulfonylureas.

Pharmacodynamics/Kinetics

Onset of action: Oral: 20 minutes to 2 hours; I.V.: 2-5 minutes
Peak effect: Oral: 1-4 hours; I.V.: 5-15 minutes
Duration: Oral: 8-24 hours (dose dependent); I.V.: 2-4 hours
Distribution: V$_d$: Adults: 3-16 L/kg; mean: <9.4 L/kg; moderately lipid soluble, therefore, can enter CNS; crosses placenta; small amounts enter breast milk
Protein binding: 50%
Metabolism: Hepatic, primarily via glucuronide conjugation; extensive first-pass effect
Bioavailability: Oral: 25%; increased with liver disease, elderly, and concurrent cimetidine
Half-life elimination: Normal renal function: 2.5-8 hours
Excretion: Urine (<5% as unchanged drug)
Clearance: Possibly decreased in neonates/infants

Pregnancy Risk Factor C (manufacturer); D (2nd and 3rd trimesters - expert analysis)

Labetalol Hydrochloride *see* Labetalol *on page 891*

Lac-Hydrin® *see* Lactic Acid and Ammonium Hydroxide *on page 893*

Lac-Hydrin® Five [OTC] *see* Lactic Acid and Ammonium Hydroxide *on page 893*

LAClotion™ *see* Lactic Acid and Ammonium Hydroxide *on page 893*

Lacrisert® *see* Hydroxypropyl Cellulose *on page 800*

Lactaid® Extra Strength [OTC] [DSC] *see* Lactase *on page 892*

Lactaid® Fast Act [OTC] *see* Lactase *on page 892*

Lactaid® Original [OTC] *see* Lactase *on page 892*

Lactaid® Ultra [OTC] [DSC] *see* Lactase *on page 892*

Lactase *(LAK tase)*

U.S. Brand Names Lactaid® Extra Strength [OTC] [DSC]; Lactaid® Fast Act [OTC]; Lactaid® Original [OTC]; Lactaid® Ultra [OTC] [DSC]; Lactrase® [OTC]
Canadian Brand Names Dairyaid®
Generic Available No
Pharmacologic Category Enzyme
Use Help digest lactose in milk for patients with lactose intolerance
Local Anesthetic/Vasoconstrictor Precautions No information available to require special precautions
Effects on Dental Treatment No significant effects or complications reported

Lactic Acid (LAK tik AS id)

U.S. Brand Names LactiCare® [OTC]; Lactinol®; Lactinol-E®
Generic Available Yes
Synonyms Sodium-PCA and Lactic Acid
Pharmacologic Category Topical Skin Product
Use Lubricate and moisturize the skin counteracting dryness and itching
Local Anesthetic/Vasoconstrictor Precautions No information available to require special precautions
Effects on Dental Treatment No significant effects or complications reported
Common Adverse Effects Frequency not defined.
  Dermatologic: Burning, mild stinging, peeling

Lactic Acid and Ammonium Hydroxide
(LAK tik AS id with a MOE nee um hye DROKS ide)

U.S. Brand Names AmLactin® [OTC]; Geri-Hydrolac™ [OTC]; Geri-Hydrolac™-12 [OTC]; Lac-Hydrin®; Lac-Hydrin® Five [OTC]; LAClotion™
Generic Available Yes
Synonyms Ammonium Lactate
Pharmacologic Category Topical Skin Product
Use Treatment of moderate to severe xerosis and ichthyosis vulgaris
Local Anesthetic/Vasoconstrictor Precautions No information available to require special precautions
Effects on Dental Treatment No significant effects or complications reported
Common Adverse Effects
  >10%: Dermatologic: Rash, including erythema and irritation (2% to 15%); burning/stinging (2% to 15%)
  1% to 10%: Dermatologic: Itching (5%), dry skin (2%)
Mechanism of Action Exact mechanism of action unknown; lactic acid is a normal component in blood and tissues. When applied topically to the skin, acts as a humectant.
Pharmacodynamics/Kinetics Absorption: 6%
Pregnancy Risk Factor B

LactiCare® [OTC] see Lactic Acid on page 893
Lactinex™ [OTC] see Lactobacillus on page 535
Lactinol® see Lactic Acid on page 893
Lactinol-E® see Lactic Acid on page 893
Lactobacillus acidophilus see Lactobacillus on page 535
Lactobacillus bifidus see Lactobacillus on page 535
Lactobacillus bulgaricus see Lactobacillus on page 535
Lactobacillus casei see Lactobacillus on page 535
Lactobacillus paracasei see Lactobacillus on page 535
Lactobacillus reuteri see Lactobacillus on page 535
Lactobacillus rhamnosus GG see Lactobacillus on page 535
Lacto-Bifidus [OTC] see Lactobacillus on page 535
Lactoflavin see Riboflavin on page 1345
Lacto-Key [OTC] see Lactobacillus on page 535
Lacto-Pectin [OTC] see Lactobacillus on page 535
Lacto-TriBlend [OTC] see Lactobacillus on page 535
Lactrase® [OTC] see Lactase on page 892

Lactulose (LAK tyoo lose)

U.S. Brand Names Constulose®; Enulose®; Generlac; Kristalose™
Canadian Brand Names Acilac; Apo-Lactulose®; Laxilose; PMS-Lactulose
Mexican Brand Names Lactulax®; Regulact®
Generic Available Yes
Pharmacologic Category Ammonium Detoxicant; Laxative, Osmotic
Use Adjunct in the prevention and treatment of portal-systemic encephalopathy; treatment of chronic constipation
Local Anesthetic/Vasoconstrictor Precautions No information available to require special precautions
Effects on Dental Treatment No significant effects or complications reported
  (Continued)

Lactulose (Continued)

Common Adverse Effects Frequency not defined: Gastrointestinal: Flatulence, diarrhea (excessive dose), abdominal discomfort, nausea, vomiting, cramping

Mechanism of Action The bacterial degradation of lactulose resulting in an acidic pH inhibits the diffusion of NH_3 into the blood by causing the conversion of NH_3 to NH_4+; also enhances the diffusion of NH_3 from the blood into the gut where conversion to NH_4+ occurs; produces an osmotic effect in the colon with resultant distention promoting peristalsis

Drug Interactions
Decreased Effect: Oral neomycin, laxatives, antacids

Pharmacodynamics/Kinetics
Absorption: Not appreciable
Metabolism: Via colonic flora to lactic acid and acetic acid; requires colonic flora for drug activation
Excretion: Primarily feces and urine (~3%)

Pregnancy Risk Factor B

Ladakamycin *see* Azacitidine *on page 167*
L-AmB *see* Amphotericin B (Liposomal) *on page 116*
Lamictal® *see* Lamotrigine *on page 895*
Lamisil® *see* Terbinafine *on page 1459*
Lamisil® AT™ [OTC] *see* Terbinafine *on page 1459*

Lamivudine (la MI vyoo deen)

Related Information
HIV Infection and AIDS *on page 1662*
U.S. Brand Names Epivir®; Epivir-HBV®
Canadian Brand Names Heptovir®; 3TC®
Mexican Brand Names 3TC®
Generic Available No
Synonyms 3TC
Pharmacologic Category Antiretroviral Agent, Reverse Transcriptase Inhibitor (Nucleoside)

Use
Epivir®: Treatment of HIV infection when antiretroviral therapy is warranted; should always be used as part of a multidrug regimen (at least three antiretroviral agents)
Epivir-HBV®: Treatment of chronic hepatitis B associated with evidence of hepatitis B viral replication and active liver inflammation

Unlabeled/Investigational Use Prevention of HIV following needlesticks (with or without protease inhibitor)

Local Anesthetic/Vasoconstrictor Precautions No information available to require special precautions

Effects on Dental Treatment No significant effects or complications reported

Common Adverse Effects (As reported in adults treated for HIV infection)
>10%:
Central nervous system: Headache, fatigue
Gastrointestinal: Nausea, diarrhea, vomiting, pancreatitis (range: 0.5% to 18%; higher percentage in pediatric patients)
Neuromuscular & skeletal: Peripheral neuropathy, paresthesia, musculoskeletal pain
1% to 10%:
Central nervous system: Dizziness, depression, fever, chills, insomnia
Dermatologic: Rash
Gastrointestinal: Anorexia, abdominal pain, heartburn, elevated amylase
Hematologic: Neutropenia
Hepatic: Elevated AST, ALT
Neuromuscular & skeletal: Myalgia, arthralgia
Respiratory: Nasal signs and symptoms, cough

Mechanism of Action Lamivudine is a cytosine analog. After lamivudine is triphosphorylated, the principle mode of action is inhibition of HIV reverse transcription via viral DNA chain termination; inhibits RNA- and DNA-dependent DNA polymerase activities of reverse transcriptase. The monophosphate form of lamivudine is incorporated into the viral DNA by hepatitis B virus polymerase, resulting in DNA chain termination.

Drug Interactions
Increased Effect/Toxicity: Zidovudine concentrations increase significantly (~39%) with lamivudine coadministration. sulfamethoxazole/trimethoprim

increases lamivudine's blood levels. Concomitant use of ribavirin and nucleoside analogues may increase the risk of developing lactic acidosis (includes adefovir, didanosine, lamivudine, stavudine, zalcitabine, zidovudine). Trimethoprim (and other drugs excreted by organic cation transport) may increase serum levels/effects of lamivudine.

Decreased Effect: Zalcitabine and lamivudine may inhibit the intracellular phosphorylation of each other; concomitant use should be avoided.

Pharmacodynamics/Kinetics
Absorption: Rapid
Distribution: V_d: 1.3 L/kg
Protein binding, plasma: <36%
Metabolism: 5.6% to trans-sulfoxide metabolite
Bioavailability: Absolute; Cp_{max} decreased with food although AUC not significantly affected
  Children: 66%
  Adults: 87%
Half-life elimination: Children: 2 hours; Adults: 5-7 hours
Excretion: Primarily urine (as unchanged drug)

Pregnancy Risk Factor C

Lamivudine, Abacavir, and Zidovudine *see* Abacavir, Lamivudine, and Zidovudine *on page 23*

Lamivudine and Abacavir *see* Abacavir and Lamivudine *on page 23*

Lamivudine and Zidovudine *see* Zidovudine and Lamivudine *on page 1596*

Lamotrigine (la MOE tri jeen)

U.S. Brand Names Lamictal®
Canadian Brand Names Apo-Lamotrigine®; Lamictal®; Novo-Lamotrigine; PMS-Lamotrigine; ratio-Lamotrigine
Mexican Brand Names Lamictal®
Generic Available No
Synonyms BW-430C; LTG
Pharmacologic Category Anticonvulsant, Miscellaneous
Use Adjunctive therapy in the treatment of generalized seizures of Lennox-Gastaut syndrome and partial seizures in adults and children ≥2 years of age; conversion to monotherapy in adults with partial seizures who are receiving treatment with valproate or a single enzyme-inducing antiepileptic drug; maintenance treatment of bipolar disorder

Local Anesthetic/Vasoconstrictor Precautions No information available to require special precautions

Effects on Dental Treatment No significant effects or complications reported

Common Adverse Effects Percentages reported in adults receiving adjunctive therapy:
>10%:
  Central nervous system: Headache (29%), dizziness (38%), ataxia (22%), somnolence (14%)
  Gastrointestinal: Nausea (19%)
  Ocular: Diplopia (28%), blurred vision (16%)
  Respiratory: Rhinitis (14%)
1% to 10%:
  Cardiovascular: Peripheral edema
  Central nervous system: Depression (4%), anxiety (4%), irritability (3%), confusion, speech disorder (3%), difficulty concentrating (2%), malaise, seizure (includes exacerbations) (2% to 3%), incoordination (6%), insomnia (6%), pain, amnesia, hostility, memory decreased, nervousness, vertigo
  Dermatologic: Hypersensitivity rash (10%; serious rash requiring hospitalization - adults 0.3%, children 0.8%), pruritus (3%)
  Gastrointestinal: Abdominal pain (5%), vomiting (9%), diarrhea (6%), dyspepsia (5%), xerostomia, constipation (4%), anorexia (2%), tooth disorder (3%)
  Genitourinary: Vaginitis (4%), dysmenorrhea (7%), amenorrhea (2%)
  Neuromuscular & skeletal: Tremor (4%), arthralgia (2%), neck pain (2%)
  Ocular: Nystagmus (2%), visual abnormality
  Respiratory: Epistaxis, bronchitis, dyspnea
  Miscellaneous: Flu syndrome (7%), fever (6%)

Mechanism of Action A triazine derivative which inhibits release of glutamate (an excitatory amino acid) and inhibits voltage-sensitive sodium channels, which stabilizes neuronal membranes. Lamotrigine has weak inhibitory effect on the 5-HT$_3$ receptor; *in vitro* inhibits dihydrofolate reductase.
(Continued)

Lamotrigine *(Continued)*

Drug Interactions

Increased Effect/Toxicity: Lamotrigine may increase the epoxide metabolite of carbamazepine resulting in toxicity. Valproic acid increases blood levels of lamotrigine. Valproic acid inhibits the clearance of lamotrigine, dosage adjustment required when adding or withdrawing valproic acid; inhibition appears maximal at valproic acid 250-500 mg/day; the incidence of serious rash may be increased by valproic acid. Toxicity has been reported following addition of sertraline (limited documentation).

Decreased Effect: Acetaminophen (chronic administration), carbamazepine, oral contraceptives (estrogens), phenytoin, phenobarbital may decrease concentrations of lamotrigine; dosage adjustments may be needed when adding or withdrawing agent; monitor

Pharmacodynamics/Kinetics

Distribution: V_d: 1.1 L/kg

Protein binding: 55%

Metabolism: Hepatic and renal; metabolized by glucuronic acid conjugation to inactive metabolites

Bioavailability: 98%

Half-life elimination: Adults: 25-33 hours; Concomitant valproic acid therapy: 59-70 hours; Concomitant phenytoin or carbamazepine therapy: 13-14 hours

Time to peak, plasma: 1-4 hours

Excretion: Urine (94%, ~90% as glucuronide conjugates and ~10% unchanged); feces (2%)

Pregnancy Risk Factor C

Lamprene® [DSC] *see* Clofazimine *on page 369*

Lanacane® [OTC] *see* Benzocaine *on page 190*

Lanacane® Maximum Strength [OTC] *see* Benzocaine *on page 190*

Lanaphilic® [OTC] *see* Urea *on page 1551*

Lanolin, Cetyl Alcohol, Glycerin, Petrolatum, and Mineral Oil

(LAN oh lin, SEE til AL koe hol, GLIS er in, pe troe LAY tum, & MIN er al oyl)

Related Information

Glycerin *on page 747*

U.S. Brand Names Lubriderm® [OTC]; Lubriderm® Fragrance Free [OTC]

Generic Available Yes

Synonyms Mineral Oil, Petrolatum, Lanolin, Cetyl Alcohol, and Glycerin

Pharmacologic Category Topical Skin Product

Use Treatment of dry skin

Local Anesthetic/Vasoconstrictor Precautions No information available to require special precautions

Effects on Dental Treatment No significant effects or complications reported

Common Adverse Effects 1% to 10%: Local irritation

Pregnancy Risk Factor C

Lanoxicaps® *see* Digoxin *on page 471*

Lanoxin® *see* Digoxin *on page 471*

Lansoprazole *(lan SOE pra zole)*

Related Information

Gastrointestinal Disorders *on page 1654*

U.S. Brand Names Prevacid®; Prevacid® SoluTab™

Canadian Brand Names Prevacid®

Mexican Brand Names Ilsatec®; Ogastro®; Ulpax®

Generic Available No

Pharmacologic Category Proton Pump Inhibitor; Substituted Benzimidazole

Use

Oral: Short-term treatment of active duodenal ulcers; maintenance treatment of healed duodenal ulcers; as part of a multidrug regimen for *H. pylori* eradication to reduce the risk of duodenal ulcer recurrence; short-term treatment of active benign gastric ulcer; treatment of NSAID-associated gastric ulcer; to reduce the risk of NSAID-associated gastric ulcer in patients with a history of gastric ulcer who require an NSAID; short-term treatment of symptomatic GERD; short-term treatment for all grades of erosive esophagitis; to maintain

healing of erosive esophagitis; long-term treatment of pathological hypersecretory conditions, including Zollinger-Ellison syndrome
I.V.: Short-term treatment (≤7 days) of erosive esophagitis in adults unable to
take oral medications

Unlabeled/Investigational Use Active ulcer bleeding (parenteral formulation)

Local Anesthetic/Vasoconstrictor Precautions No information available to
require special precautions

Effects on Dental Treatment No significant effects or complications reported

Common Adverse Effects 1% to 10%:
Central nervous system: Headache (children 1-11 years 3%, 12-17 years 7%)
Gastrointestinal: Abdominal pain (children 12-17 years 5%; adults 2%), constipation (children 1-11 years 5%; adults 1%), diarrhea (4%; 4% to 7% at doses
of 30-60 mg/day), nausea (children 12-17 years 3%; adults 1%)

Dosage
Children 1-11 years: GERD, erosive esophagitis: Oral:
≤30 kg: 15 mg once daily
>30 kg: 30 mg once daily
Note: Doses were increased in some pediatric patients if still symptomatic
after 2 or more weeks of treatment (maximum dose: 30 mg twice daily)
Children 12-17 years: Oral:
Nonerosive GERD: 15 mg once daily for up to 8 weeks
Erosive esophagitis: 30 mg once daily for up to 8 weeks
Adults:
Duodenal ulcer: Oral: Short-term treatment: 15 mg once daily for 4 weeks;
maintenance therapy: 15 mg once daily
Gastric ulcer: Oral: Short-term treatment: 30 mg once daily for up to 8 weeks
NSAID-associated gastric ulcer (healing): Oral: 30 mg once daily for 8 weeks;
controlled studies did not extend past 8 weeks of therapy
NSAID-associated gastric ulcer (to reduce risk): Oral: 15 mg once daily for up
to 12 weeks; controlled studies did not extend past 12 weeks of therapy
Symptomatic GERD: Oral: Short-term treatment: 15 mg once daily for up to 8
weeks
Erosive esophagitis:
Oral: Short-term treatment: 30 mg once daily for up to 8 weeks; continued
treatment for an additional 8 weeks may be considered for recurrence or
for patients that do not heal after the first 8 weeks of therapy; maintenance
therapy: 15 mg once daily
I.V.: 30 mg once daily for up to 7 days; patients should be switched to an
oral formulation as soon as they can take oral medications
Hypersecretory conditions: Oral: Initial: 60 mg once daily; adjust dose based
upon patient response and to reduce acid secretion to <10 mEq/hour (5
mEq/hour in patients with prior gastric surgery); doses of 90 mg twice daily
have been used; administer doses >120 mg/day in divided doses
Helicobacter pylori eradication: Oral: Currently accepted recommendations
(may differ from product labeling): Dose varies with regimen: 30 mg once
daily or 60 mg/day in 2 divided doses; requires combination therapy with
antibiotics
Prevention of rebleeding in peptic ulcer bleed (unlabeled use): I.V.: 60 mg,
followed by 6 mg/hour infusion for 72 hours
Elderly: No dosage adjustment is needed in elderly patients with normal hepatic
function

Dosage adjustment in renal impairment: No dosage adjustment is needed
Dosing adjustment in hepatic impairment: Dose reduction is necessary for
severe hepatic impairment

Mechanism of Action A proton pump inhibitor which decreases acid secretion
in gastric parietal cells

Contraindications Hypersensitivity to lansoprazole, substituted
benzimidazoles (ie, esomeprazole, omeprazole, pantoprazole, rabeprazole), or
any component of the formulation

Warnings/Precautions Severe liver dysfunction may require dosage reductions. Symptomatic response does not exclude malignancy. Safety and efficacy
have not been established in children <1 year of age.

Drug Interactions
Cytochrome P450 Effect: Substrate of CYP2C8/9 (minor), 2C19 (major),
3A4 (major); Inhibits CYP2C8/9 (weak), 2C19 (moderate), 2D6 (weak), 3A4
(weak); Induces CYP1A2 (weak)
Increased Effect/Toxicity: Lansoprazole may increase the levels/effects of
citalopram, diazepam, methsuximide, phenytoin, propranolol, sertraline, and
other CYP2C19 substrates.
Decreased Effect: Proton pump inhibitors may decrease the absorption of
atazanavir, indinavir, itraconazole, and ketoconazole. The levels/effects of
lansoprazole may be decreased by aminoglutethimide, carbamazepine,
(Continued)

Lansoprazole *(Continued)*

nafcillin, nevirapine, phenobarbital, phenytoin, rifamycins, and other CYP2C19 or 3A4 inducers.

Ethanol/Nutrition/Herb Interactions
Ethanol: Avoid ethanol (may cause gastric mucosal irritation).
Food: Lansoprazole serum concentrations may be decreased if taken with food.

Dietary Considerations Should be taken before eating; best if taken before breakfast. Prevacid® SoluTab™ contains phenylalanine 2.5 mg per 15 mg tablet; phenylalanine 5.1 mg per 30 mg tablet.

Pharmacodynamics/Kinetics
Duration: >1 day
Absorption: Rapid
Protein binding: 97%
Metabolism: Hepatic via CYP2C19 and 3A4, and in parietal cells to two inactive metabolites
Bioavailability: 80%; decreased 50% to 70% if given 30 minutes after food
Half-life elimination: 2 hours; Elderly: 2-3 hours; Hepatic impairment: ≤7 hours
Time to peak, plasma: 1.7 hours
Excretion: Feces (67%); urine (33%)

Pregnancy Risk Factor B

Dosage Forms CAP, delayed release (Prevacid®): 15 mg, 30 mg. **GRAN, for oral suspension, delayed release** (Prevacid®): 15 mg/packet (30s), 30 mg/packet (30s). **INJ, powder for reconstitution** (Prevacid®): 30 mg. **TAB, orally-disintegrating** (Prevacid® SoluTab™): 15 mg, 30 mg

Lansoprazole, Amoxicillin, and Clarithromycin

(lan SOE pra zole, a moks i SIL in, & kla RITH roe mye sin)

Related Information
Amoxicillin *on page 106*
Clarithromycin *on page 355*
Gastrointestinal Disorders *on page 1654*
Lansoprazole *on page 896*

U.S. Brand Names Prevpac®

Canadian Brand Names Hp-PAC®; Prevpac®

Generic Available No

Synonyms Amoxicillin, Lansoprazole, and Clarithromycin; Clarithromycin, Lansoprazole, and Amoxicillin

Pharmacologic Category Antibiotic, Macrolide Combination; Antibiotic, Penicillin; Gastrointestinal Agent, Miscellaneous

Use Eradication of *H. pylori* to reduce the risk of recurrent duodenal ulcer

Local Anesthetic/Vasoconstrictor Precautions No information available to require special precautions

Effects on Dental Treatment No significant effects or complications reported

Common Adverse Effects Note: Frequencies noted refer to experience with combination therapy for 14 days with all components. Refer to individual monographs for more extensive information on adverse reactions reported with each component.
3% to 10%:
Central nervous system: Headache (6%)
Gastrointestinal: Diarrhea (7%), taste perversion (5%)

Drug Interactions
Cytochrome P450 Effect:
Lansoprazole: **Substrate** of CYP2C8/9 (minor), 2C19 (major), 3A4 (major); **Inhibits** CYP2C8/9 (weak), 2C19 (moderate), 2D6 (weak), 3A4 (weak); **Induces** CYP1A2 (weak)
Clarithromycin: **Substrate** of CYP3A4 (major); **Inhibits** CYP1A2 (weak), 3A4 (strong)
Increased Effect/Toxicity: See individual agents.
Decreased Effect: See individual agents.

Pharmacodynamics/Kinetics See individual agents.

Pregnancy Risk Factor C (clarithromycin)

Lansoprazole and Naproxen (lan SOE pra zole & na PROKS en)

Related Information
Gastrointestinal Disorders *on page 1654*
Lansoprazole *on page 896*
Naproxen *on page 1089*
Oral Pain *on page 1692*

U.S. Brand Names Prevacid® NapraPAC™

Generic Available No

Synonyms NapraPAC™; Naproxen and Lansoprazole

Pharmacologic Category Nonsteroidal Anti-inflammatory Drug (NSAID), Oral; Proton Pump Inhibitor

Use Reduction of the risk of NSAID-associated gastric ulcers in patients with history of gastric ulcer who require an NSAID for the treatment of rheumatoid arthritis, osteoarthritis, and ankylosing spondylitis

Local Anesthetic/Vasoconstrictor Precautions No information available to require special precautions

Effects on Dental Treatment No significant effects or complications reported

Common Adverse Effects See individual agents.

Mechanism of Action Lansoprazole is a proton pump inhibitor which decreases acid secretion in gastric parietal cells; naproxen inhibits prostaglandin synthesis by decreasing the activity of the enzyme (cyclooxygenase) which results in decreased formation of prostaglandin precursors.

Drug Interactions

Cytochrome P450 Effect:

Lansoprazole: **Substrate** of CYP2C8/9 (minor), 2C19 (major), 3A4 (major); **Inhibits** CYP2C8/9 (weak), 2C19 (moderate), 2D6 (weak), 3A4 (weak); **Induces** CYP1A2 (weak)

Naproxen: **Substrate** (minor) of CYP1A2, 2C8/9

Increased Effect/Toxicity: See individual agents.

Decreased Effect: See individual agents.

Pharmacodynamics/Kinetics See individual agents.

Pregnancy Risk Factor B (naproxen: D/third trimester)

Lanthanum (LAN tha num)

U.S. Brand Names Fosrenol™

Generic Available No

Synonyms Lanthanum Carbonate

Pharmacologic Category Phosphate Binder

Use Reduction of serum phosphate in patients with stage 5 chronic kidney disease (kidney failure: GFR <15 mL/minute/1.73 m^2 or dialysis)

Local Anesthetic/Vasoconstrictor Precautions No information available to require special precautions

Effects on Dental Treatment No significant effects or complications reported

Common Adverse Effects

>10%:

Cardiovascular: Hypotension (8% to 16%)

Central nervous system: Headache (5% to 21%)

Gastrointestinal: Nausea (11% to 36%), vomiting (9% to 26%), diarrhea (13% to 23%), abdominal pain (5% to 17%), constipation (6% to 14%)

Miscellaneous: Dialysis graft occlusion (8% to 21%), dialysis graft complication (3% to 26%)

1% to 10%: Endocrine & metabolic: Hypercalcemia (≤4%)

Mechanism of Action Disassociates in the upper gastrointestinal tract to lanthanum ions (La^{3+}) which bind to dietary phosphate resulting in insoluble lanthanum phosphate complexes and a net decrease in serum phosphate and calcium levels.

Drug Interactions

Decreased Effect: Lanthanum may bind to some drugs in the gastrointestinal tract and decrease their absorption. It is recommended that compounds known to interact with antacids, especially those with significant clinical consequences (eg, antiarrhythmic and antiseizure medications), not be administered within 2 hours of the administration of lanthanum.

Pharmacodynamics/Kinetics

Absorption: <0.002%

Protein binding: 99%

Metabolism: Not metabolized

Half-life elimination: Plasma: 53 hours; Bone: 2-3.6 years

Excretion: Feces primarily; urine <2%

Pregnancy Risk Factor C

Lanthanum Carbonate *see* Lanthanum *on page 899*

Lantus® *see* Insulin Glargine *on page 837*

Lapase *see* Pancrelipase *on page 1183*

Lariam® *see* Mefloquine *on page 975*

Laronidase (lair OH ni days)

U.S. Brand Names Aldurazyme®
Canadian Brand Names Aldurazyme®
Generic Available No
Synonyms Recombinant α-L-Iduronidase (Glycosaminoglycan α-L-Idurono-hydrolase)
Pharmacologic Category Enzyme
Use Treatment of Hurler and Hurler-Scheie forms of mucopolysaccharidosis I (MPS I); treatment of Scheie form of MPS I in patients with moderate to severe symptoms
Local Anesthetic/Vasoconstrictor Precautions No information available to require special precautions
Effects on Dental Treatment No significant effects or complications reported
Common Adverse Effects
>10%:
  Cardiovascular: Vein disorder (14%)
  Dermatologic: Rash (36%)
  Local: Infusion reactions [31%; may be severe; includes flushing (23%), fever, and headache; frequency decreased over time during open-label extension period], injection site reaction (18%)
  Neuromuscular & skeletal: Hyper-reflexia (14%), paresthesia (14%)
  Respiratory: Upper respiratory tract infection (32%)
  Miscellaneous: Antibody development to laronidase (91%; significance unknown)
1% to 10%:
  Cardiovascular: Chest pain (9%), edema (9%), facial edema (9%), hypotension (9%)
  Hematologic: Thrombocytopenia (9%)
  Hepatic: Bilirubinemia
  Local: Abscess (9%), injection site pain (9%)
  Ocular: Corneal opacity (9%)
Mechanism of Action Laronidase is a recombinant (replacement) form of α-L-iduronidase derived from Chinese hamster cells. α-L-iduronidase is an enzyme needed to break down endogenous glycosaminoglycans (GAGs) within lysosomes. A deficiency of α-L-iduronidase leads to an accumulation of GAGs, causing cellular, tissue, and organ dysfunction as seen in MPS I. Improved pulmonary function and walking capacity have been demonstrated with the administration of laronidase to patients with Hurler, Hurler-Scheie, or Scheie (with moderate to severe symptoms) forms of MPS.
Pharmacodynamics/Kinetics
Distribution: V_d: 0.24-0.6 L/kg
Half-life elimination: 1.5-3.6 hours
Excretion: Clearance: 1.7 to 2.7 mL/minute/kg; during the first 12 weeks of therapy the clearance of laronidase increases proportionally to the amount of antibodies a given patient develops against the enzyme. However, with long-term use (≥26 weeks) antibody titers have no effect on laronidase clearance.
Pregnancy Risk Factor B

Lasix® see Furosemide on page 715
L-asparaginase see Asparaginase on page 144
Lassar's Zinc Paste see Zinc Oxide on page 1597

Latanoprost (la TA noe prost)

U.S. Brand Names Xalatan®
Canadian Brand Names Xalatan®
Mexican Brand Names Xalatan®
Generic Available No
Pharmacologic Category Ophthalmic Agent, Antiglaucoma; Prostaglandin, Ophthalmic
Use Reduction of elevated intraocular pressure in patients with open-angle glaucoma or ocular hypertension
Local Anesthetic/Vasoconstrictor Precautions No information available to require special precautions
Effects on Dental Treatment No significant effects or complications reported

Common Adverse Effects

>10%: Ocular: Blurred vision, burning and stinging, conjunctival hyperemia, foreign body sensation, itching, increased pigmentation of the iris, and punctate epithelial keratopathy

1% to 10%:

Cardiovascular: Chest pain, angina pectoris

Dermatologic: Rash, allergic skin reaction

Neuromuscular & skeletal: Myalgia, arthralgia, back pain

Ocular: Dry eye, excessive tearing, eye pain, lid crusting, lid edema, lid erythema, lid discomfort/pain, photophobia

Respiratory: Upper respiratory tract infection, cold, flu

Dosage Adults: Ophthalmic: 1 drop (1.5 mcg) in the affected eye(s) once daily in the evening; do not exceed the once daily dosage because it has been shown that more frequent administration may decrease the IOP lowering effect

Note: A medication delivery device (Xal-Ease™) is available for use with Xalatan®.

Mechanism of Action Latanoprost is a prostaglandin F_2-alpha analog believed to reduce intraocular pressure by increasing the outflow of the aqueous humor

Contraindications Hypersensitivity to latanoprost or any component of the formulation

Warnings/Precautions Latanoprost may gradually change eye color, increasing the amount of brown pigment in the iris by increasing the number of melanosome in melanocytes. The long-term effects on the melanocytes and the consequences of potential injury to the melanocytes or deposition of pigment granules to other areas of the eye is currently unknown. Patients should be examined regularly, and depending on the clinical situation, treatment may be stopped if increased pigmentation ensues.

There have been reports of bacterial keratitis associated with the use of multiple-dose containers of topical ophthalmic products. Do not administer while wearing contact lenses.

Drug Interactions

Increased Effect/Toxicity:

Combination therapy with bimatoprost may result in higher IOP than either agent alone.

Decreased Effect: Precipitation occurs when eye drops containing thimerosal are mixed with latanoprost. If such drugs are used, administer with an interval of at least 5 minutes between applications. May be used concomitantly with other topical ophthalmic drugs if administration is separated by at least 5 minutes.

Pharmacodynamics/Kinetics

Onset of action: 3-4 hours

Peak effect: Maximum: 8-12 hours

Absorption: Through the cornea where the isopropyl ester prodrug is hydrolyzed by esterases to the biologically active acid. Peak concentration is reached in 2 hours after topical administration in the aqueous humor.

Distribution: V_d: 0.16 L/kg

Metabolism: Primarily hepatic via fatty acid beta-oxidation

Half-life elimination: 17 minutes

Excretion: Urine (as metabolites)

Pregnancy Risk Factor C

Dosage Forms SOLN, ophthalmic: 0.005% (2.5 mL)

l-Bunolol Hydrochloride see Levobunolol on page 909

L-Carnitine see Levocarnitine on page 910

LCD see Coal Tar on page 383

LCR see VinCRIStine on page 1576

L-Deprenyl see Selegiline on page 1382

LDP-341 see Bortezomib on page 215

Leena™ see Ethinyl Estradiol and Norethindrone on page 608

Leflunomide (le FLOO noh mide)

Related Information

Rheumatoid Arthritis, Osteoarthritis, and Osteoporosis on page 1668

U.S. Brand Names Arava®

Canadian Brand Names Apo-Leflunomide®; Arava®; Novo-Leflunomide

Generic Available Yes

Pharmacologic Category Antirheumatic, Disease Modifying

Use Treatment of active rheumatoid arthritis; indicated to reduce signs and symptoms, and to retard structural damage and improve physical function

(Continued)

Leflunomide *(Continued)*

Orphan drug: Prevention of acute and chronic rejection in recipients of solid organ transplants

Unlabeled/Investigational Use

Treatment of cytomegalovirus (CMV) disease

Local Anesthetic/Vasoconstrictor Precautions No information available to require special precautions

Effects on Dental Treatment Key adverse event(s) related to dental treatment: Stomatitis, oral candidiasis, and abnormal taste.

Common Adverse Effects

>10%:

Gastrointestinal: Diarrhea (17%)

Respiratory: Respiratory tract infection (15%)

1% to 10%:

Cardiovascular: Hypertension (10%), chest pain (2%), palpitation, tachycardia, vasculitis, vasodilation, varicose vein, edema (peripheral)

Central nervous system: Headache (7%), dizziness (4%), pain (2%), fever, malaise, migraine, anxiety, depression, insomnia, sleep disorder

Dermatologic: Alopecia (10%), rash (10%), pruritus (4%), dry skin (2%), eczema (2%), acne, dermatitis, hair discoloration, hematoma, herpes infection, nail disorder, subcutaneous nodule, skin disorder/discoloration, skin ulcer, bruising

Endocrine & metabolic: Hypokalemia (1%), diabetes mellitus, hyperglycemia, hyperlipidemia, hyperthyroidism, menstrual disorder

Gastrointestinal: Nausea (9%), abdominal pain (5%), dyspepsia (5%), weight loss (4%), anorexia (3%), gastroenteritis (3%), stomatitis (3%), vomiting (3%), cholelithiasis, colitis, constipation, esophagitis, flatulence, gastritis, gingivitis, melena, candidiasis (oral), enlarged salivary gland, tooth disorder, xerostomia, taste disturbance

Genitourinary: Urinary tract infection (5%), albuminuria, cystitis, dysuria, hematuria, vaginal candidiasis, prostate disorder, urinary frequency

Hematologic: Anemia

Hepatic: Abnormal LFTs (5%)

Neuromuscular & skeletal: Back pain (5%), joint disorder (4%), weakness (3%), tenosynovitis (3%), synovitis (2%), arthralgia (1%), paresthesia (2%), muscle cramps (1%), neck pain, pelvic pain, increased CPK, arthrosis, bursitis, myalgia, bone necrosis, bone pain, tendon rupture, neuralgia, neuritis

Ocular: Blurred vision, cataract, conjunctivitis, eye disorder

Respiratory: Bronchitis (7%), cough (3%), pharyngitis (3%), pneumonia (2%), rhinitis (2%), sinusitis (2%), asthma, dyspnea, epistaxis

Miscellaneous: Infection (4%), accidental injury (5%), allergic reactions (2%), diaphoresis

Mechanism of Action Inhibits pyrimidine synthesis, resulting in antiproliferative and anti-inflammatory effects. For CMV, may interfere with virion assembly.

Drug Interactions

Cytochrome P450 Effect: Inhibits CYP2C8/9 (weak)

Increased Effect/Toxicity: Leflunomide may increase the risk of hepatotoxicity when combined with drugs which may cause hepatic injury. Concomitant treatment of methotrexate with leflunomide may increase the risk of hepatotoxicity or hematologic toxicity. Rifampin may increase the serum concentration of leflunomide's active metabolite. Leflunomide may increase the effects of warfarin.

Decreased Effect: Bile acid sequestrants (cholestyramine) may interfere with enterohepatic recycling of leflunomide; this is used emergently to remove drug from the circulation, but may decrease levels inadvertently if used concomitantly.

Pharmacodynamics/Kinetics

Distribution: V_d: 0.13 L/kg

Metabolism: Hepatic to A77 1726 (MI) which accounts for nearly all pharmacologic activity; further metabolism to multiple inactive metabolites; undergoes enterohepatic recirculation

Bioavailability: 80%

Half-life elimination: Mean: 14-15 days; enterohepatic recycling appears to contribute to the long half-life of this agent, since activated charcoal and cholestyramine substantially reduce plasma half-life

Time to peak: 6-12 hours

Excretion: Feces (48%); urine (43%)

Pregnancy Risk Factor X

Legatrin PM® [OTC] see Acetaminophen and Diphenhydramine *on page 38*

Lenalidomide (le na LID oh mide)

U.S. Brand Names Revlimid®
Generic Available No
Synonyms CC-5013; IMid-3
Pharmacologic Category Angiogenesis Inhibitor; Immunosuppressant Agent; Tumor Necrosis Factor (TNF) Blocking Agent
Use Treatment of transfusion-dependent anemia in myelodysplastic syndrome (MDS) patients with deletion 5q (del 5q) cytogenetic abnormality with or without additional cytogenetic abnormalities
Unlabeled/Investigational Use Treatment of multiple myeloma
Local Anesthetic/Vasoconstrictor Precautions No information available to require special precautions
Effects on Dental Treatment Key adverse event(s) related to dental treatment: Xerostomia (normal salivary flow resumes upon discontinuation), taste perversion.
Common Adverse Effects Note: Myelosuppression is dose-dependent and reversible with treatment interruption or dose reduction.
>10%:
  Cardiovascular: Edema (peripheral 8% to 20%)
  Central nervous system: Fatigue (31%), pyrexia (21%), dizziness (20%), headache (20%)
  Dermatologic: Pruritus (42%), rash (36%), dry skin (14%)
  Endocrine & metabolic: Hypokalemia (11%)
  Gastrointestinal: Diarrhea (49%), constipation (24%), nausea (24%), abdominal pain (8% to 12%)
  Genitourinary: Urinary tract infection (11%)
  Hematologic: Thrombocytopenia (62%; grades 3/4: 50%), neutropenia (59%; grades 3/4: 53%), anemia (12%)
  Neuromuscular & skeletal: Arthralgia (22%), back pain (21%), muscle cramp (18%), weakness (15%), limb pain (11%)
  Respiratory: Nasopharyngitis (23%), cough (20%), dyspnea (17%), pharyngitis (16%), epistaxis (15%), upper respiratory infection (15%), pneumonia (12%)
1% to 10%:
  Cardiovascular: Hypertension (6%), chest pain (5%), palpitations (5%)
  Central nervous system: Insomnia (10%), hypoesthesia (7%), pain (7%), depression (5%)
  Dermatologic: Bruising (5% to 8%), cellulitis (5%), erythema (5%)
  Endocrine & metabolic: Hypothyroidism (7%), hypomagnesemia (6%)
  Gastrointestinal: Anorexia (10%), vomiting (10%), xerostomia (7%), loose stools (6%), taste perversion (6%)
  Genitourinary: Dysuria (7%)
  Hematologic: Leukopenia (8%), febrile neutropenia (5%)
  Hepatic: ALT increased (8%)
  Neuromuscular & skeletal: Myalgia (9%), rigors (6%), neuropathy (peripheral 5%)
  Respiratory: Sinusitis (8%), dyspnea (on exertion 7%), rhinitis (7%), bronchitis (6%)
  Miscellaneous: Night sweats (8%), diaphoresis increased (7%)
Restrictions Lenalidomide is approved for marketing only under a Food and Drug Administration (FDA) approved, restricted distribution program called RevAssist℠ (www.REVLIMID.com or 1-888-423-5436). Physicians, pharmacies, and patients must be registered; a maximum 28-day supply may be dispensed; a new prescription is required each time it is filled; pregnancy testing is required for females of childbearing potential.
Mechanism of Action Not fully characterized; immunomodulatory and antiangiogenic characteristics via multiple mechanisms. Selectively inhibits secretion of proinflammatory cytokines (potent inhibitor of tumor necrosis factor-alpha secretion); enhances cell-mediated immunity by stimulating proliferation of anti-CD3 stimulated T cells (resulting in increased IL-2 and interferon gamma secretion); inhibits trophic signals to angiogenic factors in cells.
Drug Interactions
  Increased Effect/Toxicity: Abatacept and anakinra may increase the risk of serious infection when used in combination with lenalidomide. Lenalidomide may increase the risk of infections associated with vaccines (live organism).
Pharmacodynamics/Kinetics
  Absorption: Rapid
  Protein binding: ~30%
  Half-life elimination: ~3 hours
  Excretion: Urine (~67% as unchanged drug)
Pregnancy Risk Factor X

Lepirudin (leh puh ROO din)

Related Information
Cardiovascular Diseases *on page 1636*
U.S. Brand Names Refludan®
Canadian Brand Names Refludan®
Generic Available No
Synonyms Lepirudin (rDNA); Recombinant Hirudin
Pharmacologic Category Anticoagulant, Thrombin Inhibitor
Use Indicated for anticoagulation in patients with heparin-induced thrombocytopenia (HIT) and associated thromboembolic disease in order to prevent further thromboembolic complications
Unlabeled/Investigational Use Investigational: Prevention or reduction of ischemic complications associated with unstable angina
Local Anesthetic/Vasoconstrictor Precautions No information available to require special precautions
Effects on Dental Treatment No significant effects or complications reported
Common Adverse Effects As with all anticoagulants, bleeding is the most common adverse event associated with lepirudin. Hemorrhage may occur at virtually any site. Risk is dependent on multiple variables.
HIT patients:
>10%: Hematologic: Anemia (12%), bleeding from puncture sites (11%), hematoma (11%)
1% to 10%:
Cardiovascular: Heart failure (3%), pericardial effusion (1%), ventricular fibrillation (1%)
Central nervous system: Fever (7%)
Dermatologic: Eczema (3%), maculopapular rash (4%)
Gastrointestinal: GI bleeding/rectal bleeding (5%)
Genitourinary: Vaginal bleeding (2%)
Hepatic: Transaminases increased (6%)
Renal: Hematuria (4%)
Respiratory: Epistaxis (4%)
Non-HIT populations (including those receiving thrombolytics and/or contrast media):
1% to 10%: Respiratory: Bronchospasm/stridor/dyspnea/cough
Mechanism of Action Lepirudin is a highly specific direct inhibitor of thrombin; lepirudin is a recombinant hirudin derived from yeast cells
Drug Interactions
Increased Effect/Toxicity: Thrombolytics may enhance anticoagulant properties of lepirudin on aPTT and can increase the risk of bleeding complications. Bleeding risk may also be increased by oral anticoagulants (warfarin) and platelet function inhibitors (NSAIDs, dipyridamole, ticlopidine, clopidogrel, IIb/IIIa antagonists, and aspirin).
Pharmacodynamics/Kinetics
Distribution: Two-compartment model; confined to extracellular fluids.
Metabolism: Via release of amino acids via catabolic hydrolysis of parent drug
Half-life elimination: Initial: ~10 minutes: Terminal: Healthy volunteers: 1.3 hours; Marked renal impairment (Cl_{cr} <15 mL/minute and on hemodialysis): ≤2 days
Excretion: Urine (~48%, 35% as unchanged drug and unchanged drug fragments of parent drug); systemic clearance is proportional to glomerular filtration rate or creatinine clearance
Pregnancy Risk Factor B

Lepirudin (rDNA) *see Lepirudin on page 904*

Lescol® *see Fluvastatin on page 693*

Lescol® XL *see Fluvastatin on page 693*

Lessina™ *see Ethinyl Estradiol and Levonorgestrel on page 602*

Letrozole (LET roe zole)

U.S. Brand Names Femara®
Canadian Brand Names Femara®
Generic Available No

Synonyms CGS-20267; NSC-719345

Pharmacologic Category Antineoplastic Agent, Aromatase Inhibitor

Use First-line treatment of hormone receptor positive or hormone receptor unknown, locally advanced, or metastatic breast cancer in postmenopausal women; treatment of advanced breast cancer in postmenopausal women with disease progression following antiestrogen therapy; adjuvant treatment of post-menopausal hormone receptor positive early breast cancer; extended adjuvant treatment of early breast cancer in postmenopausal women who have received 5 years of adjuvant tamoxifen therapy

Local Anesthetic/Vasoconstrictor Precautions No information available to require special precautions

Effects on Dental Treatment No significant effects or complications reported

Common Adverse Effects

>10%:
  Central nervous system: Headache (8% to 12%), fatigue (6% to 13%)
  Endocrine & metabolic: Hot flashes (5% to 19%)
  Gastrointestinal: Nausea (13% to 17%)
  Neuromuscular & skeletal: Musculoskeletal pain, bone pain (22%), back pain (18%), arthralgia (8% to 16%)
  Respiratory: Dyspnea (7% to 18%), cough (5% to 13%)

2% to 10%:
  Cardiovascular: Chest pain (3% to 8%), peripheral edema (5%), hypertension (5% to 8%)
  Central nervous system: Pain (5%), insomnia (7%), dizziness (3% to 5%), somnolence (2% to 3%), depression (<5%), anxiety (<5%), vertigo (<5%)
  Dermatologic: Rash (4% to 5%), alopecia (<5%), pruritus (1% to 2%)
  Endocrine & metabolic: Breast pain (7%), hypercholesterolemia (3%), hyper-calcemia (<5%)
  Gastrointestinal: Vomiting (7%), constipation (6% to 10%), diarrhea (5% to 8%), abdominal pain (5% to 6%), anorexia (3% to 5%), dyspepsia (3% to 4%), weight loss (7%), weight gain (2%)
  Neuromuscular & skeletal: Limb pain (10%), arthritis (7%), myalgia (6% to 7%), bone fractures (6%), bone mineral density decreased (3% to 5%), osteoporosis (2%)
  Miscellaneous: Flu (6%)

Mechanism of Action Competitive inhibitor of the aromatase enzyme system which binds to the heme group of aromatase, a cytochrome P450 enzyme which catalyzes conversion of androgens to estrogens (specifically, androstene-dione to estrone and testosterone to estradiol). This leads to inhibition of the enzyme and a significant reduction in plasma estrogen levels. Does not affect synthesis of adrenal or thyroid hormones, aldosterone, or androgens.

Drug Interactions

Cytochrome P450 Effect: Substrate (minor) of CYP2A6, 3A4; **Inhibits** CYP2A6 (strong), 2C19 (weak)

Increased Effect/Toxicity: Letrozole may increase the levels/effects of CYP2A6 substrates; example substrates include dexmedetomidine and ifos-famide.

Pharmacodynamics/Kinetics

Absorption: Rapid and well absorbed; not affected by food

Distribution: V_d: ~1.9 L/kg

Protein binding, plasma: Weak

Metabolism: Hepatic via CYP3A4 and 2A6 to an inactive carbinol metabolite

Half-life elimination: Terminal: ~2 days

Time to steady state, plasma: 2-6 weeks

Excretion: Urine (90%; 6% as unchanged drug, 75% as glucuronide carbinol metabolite, 9% as unidentified metabolites)

Pregnancy Risk Factor D

Leucovorin (loo koe VOR in)

Mexican Brand Names Dalisol®; Flynoken®

Generic Available Yes

Synonyms Calcium Leucovorin; Citrovorum Factor; Folinic Acid; 5-Formyl Tetrahydrofolate; Leucovorin Calcium

Pharmacologic Category Antidote; Vitamin, Water Soluble

Use Antidote for folic acid antagonists (methotrexate, trimethoprim, pyrimetha-mine); treatment of megaloblastic anemias when folate is deficient as in infancy, sprue, pregnancy, and nutritional deficiency when oral folate therapy is not possible; in combination with fluorouracil in the treatment of colon cancer

Local Anesthetic/Vasoconstrictor Precautions No information available to require special precautions

(Continued)

Leucovorin (Continued)

Effects on Dental Treatment No significant effects or complications reported

Common Adverse Effects Frequency not defined.

Dermatologic: Rash, pruritus, erythema, urticaria

Hematologic: Thrombocytosis

Respiratory: Wheezing

Miscellaneous: Anaphylactoid reactions

Mechanism of Action A reduced form of folic acid, leucovorin supplies the necessary cofactor blocked by methotrexate, enters the cells via the same active transport system as methotrexate. Stabilizes the binding of 5-dUMP and thymidylate synthetase, enhancing the activity of fluorouracil.

Drug Interactions

Decreased Effect: May decrease efficacy of co-trimoxazole against *Pneumocystis carinii* pneumonitis

Pharmacodynamics/Kinetics

Onset of action: Oral: ~30 minutes; I.V.: ~5 minutes

Absorption: Oral, I.M.: Rapid and well absorbed

Metabolism: Intestinal mucosa and hepatically to 5-methyl-tetrahydrofolate (5MTHF; active)

Bioavailability: 31% following 200 mg dose; 98% following doses ≤25 mg

Half-life elimination: Leucovorin: 15 minutes; 5MTHF: 33-35 minutes

Excretion: Urine (80% to 90%); feces (5% to 8%)

Pregnancy Risk Factor C

Leucovorin Calcium *see* Leucovorin *on page 905*

Leukeran® *see* Chlorambucil *on page 313*

Leukine® *see* Sargramostim *on page 1378*

Leuprolide (loo PROE lide)

U.S. Brand Names Eligard®; Lupron®; Lupron Depot®; Lupron Depot-Ped®; Viadur®

Canadian Brand Names Eligard®; Lupron®; Lupron® Depot®; Viadur®

Generic Available Yes: Injection (solution)

Synonyms Abbott-43818; Leuprolide Acetate; Leuprorelin Acetate; NSC-377526; TAP-144

Pharmacologic Category Gonadotropin Releasing Hormone Agonist

Use Palliative treatment of advanced prostate carcinoma; management of endometriosis; treatment of anemia caused by uterine leiomyomata (fibroids); central precocious puberty

Unlabeled/Investigational Use Treatment of breast, ovarian, and endometrial cancer; infertility; prostatic hyperplasia

Local Anesthetic/Vasoconstrictor Precautions No information available to require special precautions

Effects on Dental Treatment No significant effects or complications reported

Common Adverse Effects

Children: 2% to 10%:

Central nervous system: Pain (2%)

Dermatologic: Acne (2%), rash (2% including erythema multiforme), seborrhea (2%)

Genitourinary: Vaginitis (2%), vaginal bleeding (2%), vaginal discharge (2%)

Local: Injection site reaction (5%)

Adults (frequency dependent upon formulation and indication):

Cardiovascular: Angina, atrial fibrillation, CHF, deep vein thrombosis, edema, hot flashes, hypertension, MI, peripheral edema, syncope, tachycardia

Central nervous system: Abnormal thinking, agitation, amnesia, anxiety, chills, confusion, convulsion, dementia, depression, dizziness, fatigue, fever, headache, insomnia, malaise, pain, vertigo

Dermatologic: Alopecia, bruising, burning, cellulitis, pruritus

Endocrine & metabolic: Bone density decreased, breast enlargement, breast tenderness, dehydration, hirsutism, hyperglycemia, hyperlipidemia, hyperphosphatemia, libido decreased, menstrual disorders, potassium decreased

Gastrointestinal: Anorexia, appetite increased, constipation, diarrhea, dry mucous membranes, dysphagia, eructation, GI hemorrhage, gingivitis, gum hemorrhage, intestinal obstruction, nausea, peptic ulcer, vomiting, weight gain/loss

Genitourinary: Balanitis, impotence, nocturia, penile shrinkage, testicular atrophy; urinary disorder (eg, urgency, incontinence, retention); UTI, vaginitis

Hematologic: Anemia, platelets decreased, PT prolonged, WBC increased

Hepatic: Hepatomegaly, liver function tests abnormal

Local: Abscess, injection site reaction

Neuromuscular & skeletal: Arthritis, bone pain, leg cramps, myalgia, paresthesia, tremor, weakness

Renal: BUN increased

Respiratory: Allergic reaction, dyspnea, emphysema, hemoptysis, hypoxia, lung edema, pulmonary embolism

Miscellaneous: Body odor, diaphoresis, flu-like syndrome, neoplasm, night sweats, voice alteration

Mechanism of Action Potent inhibitor of gonadotropin secretion; continuous daily administration results in suppression of ovarian and testicular steroidogenesis due to decreased levels of LH and FSH with subsequent decrease in testosterone (male) and estrogen (female) levels. Leuprolide may also have a direct inhibitory effect on the testes, and act by a different mechanism not directly related to reduction in serum testosterone.

Pharmacodynamics/Kinetics

Onset of action: Following transient increase, testosterone suppression occurs in ~2-4 weeks of continued therapy

Distribution: Males: V_d: 27 L

Protein binding: 43% to 49%

Metabolism: Major metabolite, pentapeptide (M-1)

Bioavailability: Oral: None; SubQ: 94%

Half-life elimination: I.V.: 3 hours

Excretion: Urine (<5% as parent and major metabolite)

Pregnancy Risk Factor X

Leuprolide Acetate *see* Leuprolide *on page 906*

Leuprorelin Acetate *see* Leuprolide *on page 906*

Leurocristine Sulfate *see* VinCRIStine *on page 1576*

Leustatin® *see* Cladribine *on page 354*

Levalbuterol (leve al BYOO ter ole)

U.S. Brand Names Xopenex®; Xopenex HFA™

Canadian Brand Names Xopenex®

Generic Available No

Synonyms Levalbuterol Hydrochloride; Levalbuterol Tartrate; R-albuterol

Pharmacologic Category Beta₂-Adrenergic Agonist

Use Treatment or prevention of bronchospasm in children and adults with reversible obstructive airway disease

Local Anesthetic/Vasoconstrictor Precautions No information available to require special precautions

Effects on Dental Treatment No significant effects or complications reported

Common Adverse Effects

>10%:

Endocrine & metabolic: Serum glucose increased, serum potassium decreased

Respiratory: Viral infection (7% to 12%), rhinitis (3% to 11%)

>2% to 10%:

Central nervous system: Nervousness (3% to 10%), tremor (≤7%), anxiety (≤3%), dizziness (1% to 3%), migraine (≤3%), pain (1% to 3%)

Cardiovascular: Tachycardia (~3%)

Gastrointestinal: Dyspepsia (1% to 3%)

Neuromuscular & skeletal: Leg cramps (≤3%)

Respiratory: Asthma (9%), pharyngitis (8%), cough (1% to 4%), nasal edema (1% to 3%), sinusitis (1% to 3%)

Miscellaneous: Flu-like syndrome (1% to 4%), accidental injury (≤3%)

Mechanism of Action Relaxes bronchial smooth muscle by action on beta-2 receptors with little effect on heart rate

Drug Interactions

Increased Effect/Toxicity: May add to effects of medications which deplete potassium (eg, loop or thiazide diuretics). Cardiac effects of levalbuterol may be potentiated in patients receiving MAO inhibitors, tricyclic antidepressants, sympathomimetics (eg, amphetamine, dobutamine), or inhaled anesthetics (eg, enflurane).

Decreased Effect: Beta-blockers (particularly nonselective agents) block the effect of levalbuterol. Digoxin levels may be decreased.

Pharmacodynamics/Kinetics

Onset of action:

Aerosol: 5.5-10.2 minutes

Peak effect: ~77 minutes

Nebulization: 10-17 minutes (measured as a 15% increase in FEV_1)

(Continued)

Levalbuterol (Continued)

Peak effect: 1.5 hours
Duration:
Aerosol: 3-4 hours (up to 6 hours in some patients)
Nebulization: 5-6 hours (up to 8 hours in some patients)
Absorption: A portion of inhaled dose is absorbed to systemic circulation
Half-life elimination: 3.3-4 hours
Time to peak, serum:
Aerosol: 0.5 hours
Nebulization: 0.2 hours

Pregnancy Risk Factor C

Levalbuterol Hydrochloride see Levalbuterol on page 907
Levalbuterol Tartrate see Levalbuterol on page 907
Levall 5.0 see Hydrocodone, Phenylephrine, and Guaifenesin on page 791
Levall G see Guaifenesin and Pseudoephedrine on page 755
Levaquin® see Levofloxacin on page 913
Levarterenol Bitartrate see Norepinephrine on page 1125
Levatol® see Penbutolol on page 1199
Levbid® see Hyoscyamine on page 803
Levemir® see Insulin Detemir on page 836

Levetiracetam (lee va tye RA se tam)

U.S. Brand Names Keppra®
Canadian Brand Names Keppra®
Generic Available No
Pharmacologic Category Anticonvulsant, Miscellaneous
Use Adjunctive therapy in the treatment of partial onset seizures
Unlabeled/Investigational Use Bipolar disorder
Local Anesthetic/Vasoconstrictor Precautions No information available to require special precautions
Effects on Dental Treatment No significant effects or complications reported
Common Adverse Effects
>10%:
Central nervous system: Behavioral symptoms (agitation, aggression, anger, anxiety, apathy, depersonalization, depression, emotional lability, hostility, hyperkinesias, irritability, nervousness, neurosis and personality disorder: adults 13%; children 38%), somnolence (15% to 23%), headache (14%), hostility (2% to 12%)
Gastrointestinal: Vomiting (15%), anorexia (13%)
Neuromuscular & skeletal: Weakness (9% to 15%)
Respiratory: Rhinitis (4% to 13%), cough (2% to 11%)
Miscellaneous: Accidental injury (17%), infection (2% to 13%)
1% to 10%:
Cardiovascular: Facial edema (2%)
Central nervous system: Nervousness (4% to 10%), dizziness (7% to 9%), personality disorder (8%), pain (6% to 7%), agitation (6%), emotional lability (2% to 6%), depression (3% to 4%), ataxia (3%), vertigo (3%), amnesia (2%), anxiety (2%), confusion (2%)
Dermatologic: Bruising (4%), pruritus (2%), rash (2%), skin discoloration (2%)
Gastrointestinal: Diarrhea (8%), gastroenteritis (4%), anorexia (3%), constipation (3%), dehydration (2%)
Hematologic: Decreased leukocytes (2% to 3%)
Neuromuscular & skeletal: Neck pain (2%), paresthesia (2%), reflexes increased (2%)
Ocular: Conjunctivitis (3%), diplopia (2%), amblyopia (2%)
Otic: Ear pain (2%)
Renal: Albuminuria (4%), urine abnormality (2%)
Respiratory: Pharyngitis (6% to 10%), asthma (2%), sinusitis (2%)
Miscellaneous: Flu-like symptoms (3%), viral infection (2%)
Mechanism of Action The precise mechanism by which levetiracetam exerts its antiepileptic effect is unknown. However, several studies have suggested the mechanism may involve one or more of the following central pharmacologic effects: inhibition of voltage-dependent N-type calcium channels; blockade of GABA-ergic inhibitory transmission through displacement of negative modulators; reduction of delayed rectifier potassium current; and/or binding to synaptic proteins which modulate neurotransmitter release.

Drug Interactions
  Increased Effect/Toxicity: CNS depressants may enhance the adverse/toxic effect of levetiracetam.
Pharmacodynamics/Kinetics
  Onset of action: Peak effect: 1 hour
  Absorption: Rapid and complete
  Distribution: V_d: Similar to total body water
  Protein binding: <10%
  Metabolism: Not extensive; primarily by enzymatic hydrolysis; forms metabolites (inactive)
  Bioavailability: 100%
  Half-life elimination: 6-8 hours
  Excretion: Urine (66% as unchanged drug)
Pregnancy Risk Factor C

Levitra® see Vardenafil on page 1565

Levlen® see Ethinyl Estradiol and Levonorgestrel on page 602

Levlite™ see Ethinyl Estradiol and Levonorgestrel on page 602

Levobunolol (lee voe BYOO noe lole)

U.S. Brand Names Betagan®
Canadian Brand Names Apo-Levobunolol®; Betagan®; Novo-Levobunolol; Optho-Bunolol®; PMS-Levobunolol
Mexican Brand Names Betagan®
Generic Available Yes
Synonyms l-Bunolol Hydrochloride; Levobunolol Hydrochloride
Pharmacologic Category Beta-Adrenergic Blocker, Nonselective; Ophthalmic Agent, Antiglaucoma
Use To lower intraocular pressure in chronic open-angle glaucoma or ocular hypertension
Local Anesthetic/Vasoconstrictor Precautions No information available to require special precautions
Effects on Dental Treatment Key adverse event(s) related to dental treatment: Levobunolol is a nonselective beta-blocker and may enhance the pressor response to epinephrine, resulting in hypertension and bradycardia. Many nonsteroidal anti-inflammatory drugs, such as ibuprofen and indomethacin, can reduce the hypotensive effect of beta-blockers after 3 or more weeks of therapy with the NSAID. Short-term NSAID use (ie, 3 days) requires no special precautions in patients taking beta-blockers.
Mechanism of Action A nonselective beta-adrenergic blocking agent that lowers intraocular pressure by reducing aqueous humor production and possibly increases the outflow of aqueous humor
Pregnancy Risk Factor C

Levobunolol Hydrochloride see Levobunolol on page 909

Levobupivacaine (LEE voe byoo PIV a kane)

Related Information
  Oral Pain on page 1692
U.S. Brand Names Chirocaine® [DSC]
Canadian Brand Names Chirocaine®
Generic Available No
Pharmacologic Category Local Anesthetic
Use Production of local or regional anesthesia for surgery and obstetrics, and for postoperative pain management
Local Anesthetic/Vasoconstrictor Precautions No information available to require special precautions
Effects on Dental Treatment No significant effects or complications reported
Common Adverse Effects
  >10%:
    Cardiovascular: Hypotension (20% to 31%)
    Central nervous system: Pain (postoperative) (7% to 18%), fever (7% to 17%)
    Gastrointestinal: Nausea (12% to 21%), vomiting (8% to 14%)
    Hematologic: Anemia (10% to 12%)
  1% to 10%:
    Cardiovascular: Abnormal ECG (3%), bradycardia (2%), tachycardia (2%), hypertension (1%)
(Continued)

Levobupivacaine *(Continued)*

Central nervous system: Pain (4% to 8%), headache (5% to 7%), dizziness (5% to 6%), hypoesthesia (3%), somnolence (1%), anxiety (1%), hypothermia (2%)

Dermatologic: Pruritus (4% to 9%), purpura (1%)

Endocrine & metabolic: Breast pain - female (1%)

Gastrointestinal: Constipation (3% to 7%), enlarged abdomen (3%), flatulence (2%), abdominal pain (2%), dyspepsia (2%), diarrhea (1%)

Genitourinary: Urinary incontinence (1%), urine flow decreased (1%), urinary tract infection (1%)

Hematologic: Leukocytosis (1%)

Local: Anesthesia (1%)

Neuromuscular & skeletal: Back pain (6%), rigors (3%), paresthesia (2%)

Ocular: Diplopia (3%)

Renal: Albuminuria (3%), hematuria (2%)

Respiratory: Cough (1%)

Miscellaneous: Fetal distress (5% to 10%), delayed delivery (6%), hemorrhage in pregnancy (2%), uterine abnormality (2%), increased wound drainage (1%)

Mechanism of Action Levobupivacaine is the S-enantiomer of bupivacaine. It blocks both the initiation and transmission of nerve impulses by decreasing the neuronal membrane's permeability to sodium ions, which results in inhibition of depolarization with resultant blockade of conduction. Local anesthetics reversibly prevent generation and conduction of electrical impulses in neurons by decreasing the transient increase in permeability to sodium. The differential sensitivity generally depends on the size of the fiber; small fibers are more sensitive than larger fibers and require a longer period for recovery. Sensory pain fibers are usually blocked first, followed by fibers that transmit sensations of temperature, touch, and deep pressure. High concentrations block sympathetic somatic sensory and somatic motor fibers. The spread of anesthesia depends upon the distribution of the solution. This is primarily dependent on the site of administration and volume of drug injected.

Drug Interactions

Cytochrome P450 Effect: Substrate (minor) of CYP1A2, 3A4

Pharmacodynamics/Kinetics

Onset of action: Epidural: 10-14 minutes

Duration (dose dependent): 1-8 hours

Absorption: Dependent on route of administration and dose

Distribution: 67 L

Protein binding, plasma: >97%

Metabolism: Extensively hepatic via CYP3A4 and CYP1A2

Half-life elimination: 1.3 hours

Time to peak: Epidural: 30 minutes

Excretion: Urine (71%) and feces (24%) as metabolites

Pregnancy Risk Factor B

Levocabastine *(LEE voe kab as teen)*

U.S. Brand Names Livostin® [DSC]

Canadian Brand Names Livostin®

Mexican Brand Names Livostin®

Generic Available No

Synonyms Levocabastine Hydrochloride

Pharmacologic Category Antihistamine, H₁ Blocker, Ophthalmic

Use Treatment of allergic conjunctivitis

Local Anesthetic/Vasoconstrictor Precautions No information available to require special precautions

Effects on Dental Treatment Key adverse event(s) related to dental treatment: Xerostomia (normal salivary flow resumes upon discontinuation).

Mechanism of Action Potent, selective histamine H₁-receptor antagonist for topical ophthalmic use

Pregnancy Risk Factor C

Levocabastine Hydrochloride *see* Levocabastine *on page 910*

Levocarnitine *(lee voe KAR ni teen)*

U.S. Brand Names Carnitor®

Canadian Brand Names Carnitor®

Mexican Brand Names Cardispan®

Generic Available Yes

Synonyms L-Carnitine

Pharmacologic Category Dietary Supplement

Use Orphan drug:

Oral: Primary systemic carnitine deficiency; acute and chronic treatment of patients with an inborn error of metabolism which results in secondary carnitine deficiency

I.V.: Acute and chronic treatment of patients with an inborn error of metabolism which results in secondary carnitine deficiency; prevention and treatment of carnitine deficiency in patients with end-stage renal disease (ESRD) who are undergoing hemodialysis.

Local Anesthetic/Vasoconstrictor Precautions No information available to require special precautions

Effects on Dental Treatment No significant effects or complications reported

Common Adverse Effects Frequencies noted with I.V. therapy (hemodialysis patients):

Cardiovascular: Hypertension (18% to 21%), peripheral edema (3% to 6%)

Central nervous system: Dizziness (10% to 18%), fever (5% to 12%), paresthesia (3% to 12%), depression (5% to 6%)

Endocrine & metabolic: Hypercalcemia (6% to 15%)

Gastrointestinal: Diarrhea (9% to 35%), abdominal pain (5% to 21%), vomiting (9% to 21%), nausea (5% to 12%)

Neuromuscular & skeletal: Weakness (9% to 12%)

Miscellaneous: Allergic reaction (2% to 6%)

Mechanism of Action Carnitine is a naturally occurring metabolic compound which functions as a carrier molecule for long-chain fatty acids within the mitochondria, facilitating energy production. Carnitine deficiency is associated with accumulation of excess acyl CoA esters and disruption of intermediary metabolism. Carnitine supplementation increases carnitine plasma concentrations. The effects on specific metabolic alterations have not been evaluated. ESRD patients on maintenance HD may have low plasma carnitine levels because of reduced intake of meat and dairy products, reduced renal synthesis, and dialytic losses. Certain clinical conditions (malaise, muscle weakness, cardiomyopathy and arrhythmias) in HD patients may be related to carnitine deficiency.

Pharmacodynamics/Kinetics

Metabolism: Hepatic (limited with moderate renal impairment), to trimethylamine (TMA) and trimethylamine N-oxide (TMAO)

Bioavailability: Tablet/solution: 15% to 16%

Half-life elimination: 17.4 hours

Time to peak: Tablet/solution: 3.3 hours

Excretion: Urine (4% to 9% as unchanged drug); metabolites also eliminated in urine

Pregnancy Risk Factor B

Levodopa and Carbidopa (lee voe DOE pa & kar bi DOE pa)

Related Information

Carbidopa *on page 267*

U.S. Brand Names Parcopa™; Sinemet®; Sinemet® CR

Canadian Brand Names Apo-Levocarb®; Apo-Levocarb® CR; Endo®-Levodopa/Carbidopa; Novo-Levocarbidopa; Nu-Levocarb; Sinemet®; Sinemet® CR

Generic Available Yes: Excludes orally-disintegrating tablet

Synonyms Carbidopa and Levodopa

Pharmacologic Category Anti-Parkinson's Agent, Dopamine Agonist

Use Idiopathic Parkinson's disease; postencephalitic parkinsonism; symptomatic parkinsonism

Unlabeled/Investigational Use Restless leg syndrome

Local Anesthetic/Vasoconstrictor Precautions No information available to require special precautions

Effects on Dental Treatment Key adverse event(s) related to dental treatment: Xerostomia (normal salivary flow resumes upon discontinuation). Dopaminergic therapy in Parkinson's disease (ie, treatment with levodopa and carbidopa combination) is associated with orthostatic hypotension. Patients medicated with this drug combination should be carefully assisted from the chair and observed for signs of orthostatic hypotension.

Common Adverse Effects Frequency not defined.

Cardiovascular: Orthostatic hypotension, arrhythmia, chest pain, hypertension, syncope, palpitation, phlebitis

Central nervous system: Dizziness, anxiety, confusion, nightmares, headache, hallucinations, on-off phenomenon, decreased mental acuity, memory impairment, disorientation, delusions, euphoria, agitation, somnolence, insomnia, (Continued)

Levodopa and Carbidopa (Continued)

gait abnormalities, nervousness, ataxia, EPS, falling, psychosis, peripheral neuropathy, seizure (causal relationship not established)

Dermatologic: Rash, alopecia, malignant melanoma, hypersensitivity (angioedema, urticaria, pruritus, bullous lesions, Henoch-Schönlein purpura)

Endocrine & metabolic: Increased libido

Gastrointestinal: Anorexia, nausea, vomiting, constipation, GI bleeding, duodenal ulcer, diarrhea, dyspepsia, taste alterations, sialorrhea, heartburn

Genitourinary: Discoloration of urine, urinary frequency

Hematologic: Hemolytic anemia, agranulocytosis, thrombocytopenia, leukopenia; decreased hemoglobin and hematocrit; abnormalities in AST and ALT, LDH, bilirubin, BUN, Coombs' test

Neuromuscular & skeletal: Choreiform and involuntary movements, paresthesia, bone pain, shoulder pain, muscle cramps, weakness

Ocular: Blepharospasm, oculogyric crises (may be associated with acute dystonic reactions)

Renal: Difficult urination

Respiratory: Dyspnea, cough

Miscellaneous: Hiccups, discoloration of sweat, diaphoresis (increased)

Mechanism of Action Parkinson's symptoms are due to a lack of striatal dopamine; levodopa circulates in the plasma to the blood-brain-barrier (BBB), where it crosses, to be converted by striatal enzymes to dopamine; carbidopa inhibits the peripheral plasma breakdown of levodopa by inhibiting its decarboxylation, and thereby increases available levodopa at the BBB

Drug Interactions

Increased Effect/Toxicity: Concurrent use of levodopa with nonselective MAO inhibitors may result in hypertensive reactions via an increased storage and release of dopamine, norepinephrine, or both. Use with carbidopa to minimize reactions if combination is necessary; otherwise avoid combination.

Decreased Effect: Antipsychotics, benzodiazepines, L-methionine, phenytoin, pyridoxine, spiramycin, and tacrine may inhibit the antiparkinsonian effects of levodopa; monitor for reduced effect. Antipsychotics may inhibit the antiparkinsonian effects of levodopa via dopamine receptor blockade. Use antipsychotics with low dopamine blockade (clozapine, olanzapine, quetiapine). High-protein diets may inhibit levodopa's efficacy; avoid high protein foods. Iron binds levodopa and reduces its bioavailability; separate doses of iron and levodopa.

Pharmacodynamics/Kinetics

Duration: Variable, 6-12 hours; longer with sustained release forms

See individual agents.

Pregnancy Risk Factor C

Levodopa, Carbidopa, and Entacapone
(lee voe DOE pa, kar bi DOE pa, & en TA ka pone)

Related Information

Carbidopa *on page 267*

Entacapone *on page 543*

U.S. Brand Names Stalevo™

Generic Available No

Synonyms Carbidopa, Levodopa, and Entacapone; Entacapone, Carbidopa, and Levodopa

Pharmacologic Category Anti-Parkinson's Agent, COMT Inhibitor; Anti-Parkinson's Agent, Dopamine Agonist

Use Treatment of idiopathic Parkinson's disease

Local Anesthetic/Vasoconstrictor Precautions No information available to require special precautions

Effects on Dental Treatment No significant effects or complications reported

Common Adverse Effects See individual agents.

Mechanism of Action

Levodopa: The metabolic precursor of dopamine, a chemical depleted in Parkinson's disease. Levodopa is able to circulate in the plasma and cross the blood-brain-barrier (BBB), where it is converted by striatal enzymes to dopamine.

Carbidopa: Inhibits the peripheral plasma breakdown of levodopa by inhibiting its decarboxylation; increases available levodopa at the BBB

Entacapone: A reversible and selective inhibitor of catechol-O-methyltransferase (COMT). Alters the pharmacokinetics of levodopa, resulting in more sustained levodopa serum levels and increased concentrations available for absorption across the BBB.

Pharmacodynamics/Kinetics See individual agents.

Pregnancy Risk Factor C

Levo-Dromoran® *see* Levorphanol *on page 916*

Levofloxacin (lee voe FLOKS a sin)

Related Information
Sexually-Transmitted Diseases *on page 1674*
Tuberculosis *on page 1673*
Related Sample Prescriptions
Bacterial Infections and Periodontal Diseases *on page 1736*
U.S. Brand Names Iquix®; Levaquin®; Quixin™
Canadian Brand Names Levaquin®; Novo-Levofloxacin
Generic Available No
Pharmacologic Category Antibiotic, Quinolone
Use
> Systemic: Treatment of mild, moderate, or severe infections caused by susceptible organisms. Includes the treatment of community-acquired pneumonia, including multidrug resistant strains of *S. pneumoniae* (MDRSP); nosocomial pneumonia; chronic bronchitis (acute bacterial exacerbation); acute bacterial sinusitis; urinary tract infection (uncomplicated or complicated), including acute pyelonephritis caused by *E. coli*; prostatitis (chronic bacterial); skin or skin structure infections (uncomplicated or complicated); prevention of inhalational anthrax (postexposure)
>
> Ophthalmic: Treatment of bacterial conjunctivitis caused by susceptible organisms (Quixin™ 0.5% ophthalmic solution); treatment of corneal ulcer caused by susceptible organisms (Iquix® 1.5% ophthalmic solution)

Unlabeled/Investigational Use Diverticulitis, enterocolitis, (*Shigella* sp), gonococcal infections, Legionnaires' disease, peritonitis, PID
Local Anesthetic/Vasoconstrictor Precautions No information available to require special precautions (see Dental Comment)
Effects on Dental Treatment No significant effects or complications reported
Common Adverse Effects 1% to 10%:
> Cardiovascular: Chest pain (1%)
> Central nervous system: Headache (6%), insomnia (5%), dizziness (2%), fatigue (1%), pain (1%), fever
> Dermatologic: Pruritus (1%), rash (1%)
> Gastrointestinal: Nausea (7%), diarrhea (5%), abdominal pain (3%), constipation (3%), dyspepsia (2%), vomiting (2%), flatulence (1%)
> Genitourinary: Vaginitis (1%)
> Hematologic: Lymphopenia (2%)
> Ocular (with ophthalmic solution use): Decreased vision (transient), foreign body sensation, transient ocular burning, ocular pain or discomfort, photophobia
> Respiratory: Pharyngitis (4%), dyspnea (1%), rhinitis (1%), sinusitis (1%)

Dosage Note: Sequential therapy (intravenous to oral) may be instituted based on prescriber's discretion.
Usual dosage range:
> Children ≥1 year: Ophthalmic: 1-2 drops every 2-6 hours
> Adults:
>> Ophthalmic: 1-2 drops every 2-6 hours
>> Oral, I.V.: 500 mg every 24 hours; severe or complicated infections: 750 mg every 24 hours

Indication-specific dosing:
> Children ≥1 year and Adults: Ophthalmic:
>> **Conjunctivitis** (0.5% ophthalmic solution):
>>> Treatment day 1 and day 2: Instill 1-2 drops into affected eye(s) every 2 hours while awake, up to 8 times/day
>>> Treatment day 3 through day 7: Instill 1-2 drops into affected eye(s) every 4 hours while awake, up to 4 times/day
> Children ≥6 years and Adults: Ophthalmic:
>> **Corneal ulceration** (1.5% ophthalmic solution): Treatment day 1 through day 3: Instill 1-2 drops into affected eye(s) every 30 minutes to 2 hours while awake and 4-6 hours after retiring.
> Adults: Oral, I.V.:
>> **Anthrax (inhalational):** 500 mg every 24 hours for 60 days, beginning as soon as possible after exposure
>> **Chronic bronchitis (acute bacterial exacerbation):** 500 mg every 24 hours for at least 7 days
>> **Diverticulitis, peritonitis (unlabeled use):** 750 mg every 24 hours for 7-10 days; use adjunctive metronidazole therapy

(Continued)

Levofloxacin *(Continued)*

Dysenteric enterocolitis, *Shigella spp.* **(unlabeled use):** 500 mg every 24 hours for 3-5 days

Gonococcal infection (unlabeled use):

Cervicitis, urethritis: 250 mg for one dose with azithromycin or doxycycline

Disseminated infection: 250 mg I.V. once daily; 24 hours after symptoms improve may change to 500 mg orally every 24 hours to complete total therapy of 7 days

Epididymo-orchitis: 750 mg once daily for 10-14 days

***Legionella* (unlabeled use):** 500 mg every 24 hours for 10-21 days or 750 mg every 24 hours for 5 days

Pelvic inflammatory disease (unlabeled use): 500 mg every 24 hours for 14 days with adjunctive metronidazole

Pneumonia:

Community-acquired: 500 mg every 24 hours for 7-14 days or 750 mg every 24 hours for 5 days (efficacy of 5-day regimen for MDRSP not established)

Nosocomial: 750 mg every 24 hours for 7-14 days

Prostatitis (chronic bacterial): 500 mg every 24 hours for 28 days

Sinusitis (bacterial, acute): 500 mg every 24 hours for 10-14 days or 750 mg every 24 hours for 5 days

Skin and skin structure infections:

Uncomplicated: 500 mg every 24 hours for 7-10 days

Complicated: 750 mg every 24 hours for 7-14 days

Traveler's diarrhea (unlabeled use): 500 mg for one dose

Urinary tract infections:

Uncomplicated: 250 mg once daily for 3 days

Complicated, including pyelonephritis: 250 mg once daily for 10 days

Dosing adjustment in renal impairment:

Chronic bronchitis, acute bacterial sinusitis, uncomplicated skin infection, community-acquired pneumonia, chronic bacterial prostatitis, or inhalational anthrax: Initial: 500 mg, then as follows:

Cl_{cr} 20-49 mL/minute: 250 mg every 24 hours

Cl_{cr} 10-19 mL/minute: 250 mg every 48 hours

Hemodialysis/CAPD: 250 mg every 48 hours

Uncomplicated UTI: No dosage adjustment required

Complicated UTI, acute pyelonephritis: Cl_{cr} 10-19 mL/minute: 250 mg every 48 hours

Complicated skin infection, acute bacterial sinusitis, community-acquired pneumonia, or nosocomial pneumonia: Initial: 750 mg, then as follows:

Cl_{cr} 20-49 mL/minute: 750 mg every 48 hours

Cl_{cr} 10-19 mL/minute: 500 mg every 48 hours

Hemodialysis/CAPD: 500 mg every 48 hours

Mechanism of Action As the S (-) enantiomer of the fluoroquinolone, ofloxacin, levofloxacin, inhibits DNA-gyrase in susceptible organisms thereby inhibits relaxation of supercoiled DNA and promotes breakage of DNA strands. DNA gyrase (topoisomerase II), is an essential bacterial enzyme that maintains the superhelical structure of DNA and is required for DNA replication and transcription, DNA repair, recombination, and transposition.

Contraindications Hypersensitivity to levofloxacin, any component of the formulation, or other quinolones

Warnings/Precautions

Systemic: Not recommended in children <18 years of age; CNS stimulation may occur (tremor, restlessness, confusion, and very rarely hallucinations or seizures); use with caution in patients with known or suspected CNS disorders or renal dysfunction; use caution to avoid possible photosensitivity reactions during and for several days following fluoroquinolone therapy

Rare cases of torsade de pointes have been reported in patients receiving levofloxacin. Use caution in patients with known prolongation of QT interval, bradycardia, hypokalemia, hypomagnesemia, or in those receiving concurrent therapy with Class Ia or Class III antiarrhythmics.

Severe hypersensitivity reactions, including anaphylaxis, have occurred with quinolone therapy. If an allergic reaction occurs (itching, urticaria, dyspnea or facial edema, loss of consciousness, tingling, cardiovascular collapse), discontinue drug immediately. Prolonged use may result in superinfection; pseudomembranous colitis may occur and should be considered in all patients who present with diarrhea. Tendon inflammation and/or rupture has been reported; risk may be increased with concurrent corticosteroids, particularly in the elderly. Discontinue at first sign of tendon inflammation or pain. Peripheral neuropathies have been linked to levofloxacin use; discontinue if numbness, tingling, or weakness develops. Quinolones may exacerbate myasthenia gravis.

Ophthalmic solution: For topical use only. Do not inject subconjunctivally or introduce into anterior chamber of the eye. Contact lenses should not be worn during treatment for bacterial conjunctivitis. Safety and efficacy in children <1 year of age (Quixin™) or <6 years of age (Iquix®) have not been established. **Note:** Indications for ophthalmic solutions are product concentration-specific and should not be used interchangeably.

Drug Interactions

Increased Effect/Toxicity: Levofloxacin may increase the effects/toxicity of glyburide and warfarin. Concomitant use with corticosteroids may increase the risk of tendon rupture. Concomitant use with other QT_c-prolonging agents (eg, Class Ia and Class III antiarrhythmics, erythromycin, cisapride, antipsychotics, and cyclic antidepressants) may result in arrhythmias, such as torsade de pointes. Probenecid may increase levofloxacin levels.

Decreased Effect: Concurrent administration of metal cations, including most antacids, oral electrolyte supplements, quinapril, sucralfate, some didanosine formulations (chewable/buffered tablets and pediatric powder for oral suspension), and other highly-buffered oral drugs, may decrease quinolone levels; separate doses.

Dietary Considerations Tablets may be taken without regard to meals. Oral solution should be administered on an empty stomach (1 hour before or 2 hours after a meal).

Pharmacodynamics/Kinetics

Absorption: Rapid and complete

Distribution: V_d: 1.25 L/kg; CSF concentrations ~15% of serum levels; high concentrations are achieved in prostate, lung, and gynecological tissues, sinus, saliva

Protein binding: 50%

Metabolism: Minimally hepatic

Bioavailability: 99%

Half-life elimination: 6-8 hours

Time to peak, serum: 1-2 hours

Excretion: Primarily urine (as unchanged drug)

Pregnancy Risk Factor C

Dosage Forms INF [premixed in D₅W] (Levaquin®): 250 mg (50 mL); 500 mg (100 mL); 750 mg (150 mL). **INJ, solution** [preservative free] (Levaquin®): 25 mg/mL (20 mL, 30 mL). **SOLN, ophthalmic:** (Iquix®): 1.5% (5 mL); (Quixin™): 0.5% (5 mL). **SOLN, oral** (Levaquin®): 25 mg/mL (480 mL). **TAB** (Levaquin®): 250 mg, 500 mg, 750 mg; (Levaquin® Leva-Pak): 750 mg (5s)

Dental Comment

This drug is known to prolong the QT interval. The QT interval is measured as the time and distance between the Q point of the QRS complex and the end of the T wave in the ECG tracing. After adjustment for heart rate, the QT interval is defined as prolonged if it is more than 450 msec in men and 460 msec in women. A long QT syndrome was first described in the 1950s and 60s as a congenital syndrome involving QT interval prolongation and syncope and sudden death. Some of the congenital long QT syndromes were characterized by a peculiar electrocardiographic appearance of the QRS complex involving a premature atria beat followed by a pause, then a subsequent sinus beat showing marked QT prolongation and deformity. This type of cardiac arrhythmia was originally termed "torsade de pointes" (translated from the French as "twisting of the points").

Prolongation of the QT interval is thought to result from delayed ventricular repolarization. The repolarization process within the myocardial cell is due to the efflux of intracellular potassium. The channels associated with this current can be blocked by many drugs and predisposes the electrical propagation cycle to torsade de pointes.

Levofloxacin is one of the drugs confirmed to prolong the QT interval and is accepted as having a risk of causing torsade de pointes. The risk of drug-induced torsade de pointes is extremely low when a single QT interval prolonging drug is prescribed. In terms of epinephrine, it is not known what effect vasoconstrictors in the local anesthetic regimen will have in patients with a known history of congenital prolonged QT interval or in patients taking any medication that prolongs the QT interval. Until more information is obtained, it is suggested that the clinician consult with the physician prior to the use of a vasoconstrictor in suspected patients, and that the vasoconstrictor (epinephrine, levonordefrin [Neo-Cobefrin®]) be used with caution.

Levomepromazine *see* Methotrimeprazine *on page 1016*

Levonordefrin and Mepivacaine Hydrochloride *see* Mepivacaine and Levonordefrin *on page 991*

Levonorgestrel (LEE voe nor jes trel)

Related Information
Endocrine Disorders and Pregnancy *on page 1659*
U.S. Brand Names Mirena®; Plan B®
Canadian Brand Names Mirena®; Norplant® Implant; Plan B™
Mexican Brand Names Microlut®
Generic Available No
Synonyms LNg 20
Pharmacologic Category Contraceptive; Progestin
Use Prevention of pregnancy
Local Anesthetic/Vasoconstrictor Precautions No information available to require special precautions
Effects on Dental Treatment No significant effects or complications reported
Common Adverse Effects
Intrauterine system:
>5%:
Cardiovascular: Hypertension
Central nervous system: Headache, depression, nervousness
Dermatologic: Acne
Endocrine & metabolic: Breast pain, dysmenorrhea, decreased libido, abnormal Pap smear, amenorrhea (20% at 1 year), enlarged follicles (12%)
Gastrointestinal: Abdominal pain, nausea, weight gain
Genitourinary: Leukorrhea, vaginitis
Neuromuscular & skeletal: Back pain
Respiratory: Upper respiratory tract infection, sinusitis
<3% and postmarketing reports: Alopecia, anemia, cervicitis, dyspareunia, eczema, failed insertion, migraine, sepsis, vomiting
Oral tablets:
>10%:
Central nervous system: Fatigue (17%), headache (17%), dizziness (11%)
Endocrine & metabolic: Heavier menstrual bleeding (14%), lighter menstrual bleeding (12%), breast tenderness (11%)
Gastrointestinal: Nausea (23%), abdominal pain (18%)
1% to 10%: Gastrointestinal: Vomiting (6%), diarrhea (5%)
Mechanism of Action Pregnancy may be prevented through several mechanisms: Thickening of cervical mucus, which inhibits sperm passage through the uterus and sperm survival; inhibition of ovulation, from a negative feedback mechanism on the hypothalamus, leading to reduced secretion of follicle stimulating hormone (FSH) and luteinizing hormone (LH); inhibition of implantation. Levonorgestrel is not effective once the implantation process has begun.
Drug Interactions
Cytochrome P450 Effect: Substrate of CYP3A4 (major)
Decreased Effect: CYP3A4 inducers may decrease the levels/effects of levonorgestrel; example inducers include aminoglutethimide, carbamazepine, nafcillin, nevirapine, phenobarbital, phenytoin, and rifamycins.
Pharmacodynamics/Kinetics
Duration: Intrauterine system: Up to 5 years
Absorption: Rapid and complete
Protein binding: Highly bound to albumin and sex hormone-binding globulin
Metabolism: To inactive metabolites
Bioavailability: 100%
Half-life elimination: Oral tablet: ~24 hours
Excretion: Primarily urine
Pregnancy Risk Factor X

Levonorgestrel and Ethinyl Estradiol *see* Ethinyl Estradiol and Levonorgestrel *on page 602*

Levophed® *see* Norepinephrine *on page 1125*

Levora® *see* Ethinyl Estradiol and Levonorgestrel *on page 602*

Levorphanol (lee VOR fa nole)

U.S. Brand Names Levo-Dromoran®
Generic Available Yes: Tablet
Synonyms Levorphanol Tartrate; Levorphan Tartrate
Pharmacologic Category Analgesic, Narcotic
Use Relief of moderate to severe pain; also used parenterally for preoperative sedation and an adjunct to nitrous oxide/oxygen anesthesia

No information available to require special precautions

Effects on Dental Treatment Key adverse event(s) related to dental treatment: Xerostomia (normal salivary flow resumes upon discontinuation).

Common Adverse Effects Frequency not defined.

Cardiovascular: Palpitations, hypotension, bradycardia, peripheral vasodilation, cardiac arrest, shock, tachycardia

Central nervous system: CNS depression, fatigue, drowsiness, dizziness, nervousness, headache, restlessness, anorexia, malaise, confusion, coma, convulsion, insomnia, amnesia, mental depression, hallucinations, paradoxical CNS stimulation, intracranial pressure (increased)

Dermatologic: Pruritus, urticaria, rash

Endocrine & metabolic: Antidiuretic hormone release

Gastrointestinal: Nausea, vomiting, dyspepsia, stomach cramps, xerostomia, constipation, abdominal pain, dry mouth, biliary tract spasm, paralytic ileus

Genitourinary: Decreased urination, urinary tract spasm, urinary retention

Local: Pain at injection site

Neuromuscular & skeletal: Weakness

Ocular: Miosis, diplopia

Respiratory: Respiratory depression, apnea, hypoventilation, cyanosis

Miscellaneous: Histamine release, physical and psychological dependence

Restrictions C-II

Mechanism of Action Levorphanol tartrate is a synthetic opioid agonist that is classified as a morphinan derivative. Opioids interact with stereospecific opioid receptors in various parts of the central nervous system and other tissues. Analgesic potency parallels the affinity for these binding sites. These drugs do not alter the threshold or responsiveness to pain, but the perception of pain.

Drug Interactions

Increased Effect/Toxicity: CNS depression is enhanced with coadministration of other CNS depressants.

Pharmacodynamics/Kinetics

Onset of action: Oral: 10-60 minutes

Duration: 4-8 hours

Metabolism: Hepatic

Half-life elimination: 11-16 hours

Excretion: Urine (as inactive metabolite)

Pregnancy Risk Factor B/D (prolonged use or high doses at term)

Levorphanol Tartrate *see* Levorphanol *on page 916*

Levorphan Tartrate *see* Levorphanol *on page 916*

Levothroid® *see* Levothyroxine *on page 917*

Levothyroxine (lee voe thye ROKS een)

Related Information

Endocrine Disorders and Pregnancy *on page 1659*

U.S. Brand Names Levothroid®; Levoxyl®; Synthroid®; Unithroid®

Canadian Brand Names Eltroxin®; Synthroid®

Mexican Brand Names Eutirox®; Tiroidine®

Generic Available Yes

Synonyms Levothyroxine Sodium; *L*-Thyroxine Sodium; T_4

Pharmacologic Category Thyroid Product

Use Replacement or supplemental therapy in hypothyroidism; pituitary TSH suppression

Local Anesthetic/Vasoconstrictor Precautions No precautions with vasoconstrictor are necessary if patient is well controlled with levothyroxine

Effects on Dental Treatment No significant effects or complications reported

Common Adverse Effects Frequency not defined.

Cardiovascular: Angina, arrhythmia, blood pressure increased, cardiac arrest, flushing, heart failure, MI, palpitation, pulse increased, tachycardia

Central nervous system: Anxiety, emotional lability, fatigue, fever, headache, hyperactivity, insomnia, irritability, nervousness, pseudotumor cerebri (children), seizure (rare)

Dermatologic: Alopecia

Endocrine & metabolic: Fertility impaired, menstrual irregularities

Gastrointestinal: Abdominal cramps, appetite increased, diarrhea, vomiting, weight loss

Hepatic: Liver function tests increased

Neuromuscular & skeletal: Bone mineral density decreased, muscle weakness, tremor, slipped capital femoral epiphysis (children)

Respiratory: Dyspnea

(Continued)

Levothyroxine *(Continued)*

Miscellaneous: Diaphoresis, heat intolerance, hypersensitivity (to inactive ingredients, symptoms include urticaria, pruritus, rash, flushing, angioedema, GI symptoms, fever, arthralgia, serum sickness, wheezing)

Levoxyl®: Choking, dysphagia, gagging

Dosage Doses should be adjusted based on clinical response and laboratory parameters.

Oral:

Children: Hypothyroidism:

Newborns: Initial: 10-15 mcg/kg/day. Lower doses of 25 mcg/day should be considered in newborns at risk for cardiac failure. Newborns with T$_4$ levels <5 mcg/dL should be started at 50 mcg/day. Adjust dose at 4- to 6-week intervals.

Infants and Children: Dose based on body weight and age as listed below. Children with severe or chronic hypothyroidism should be started at 25 mcg/day; adjust dose by 25 mcg every 2-4 weeks. In older children, hyperactivity may be decreased by starting with ¼ of the recommended dose and increasing by ¼ dose each week until the full replacement dose is reached. Refer to adult dosing once growth and puberty are complete.

0-3 months: 10-15 mcg/kg/day

3-6 months: 8-10 mcg/kg/day

6-12 months: 6-8 mcg/kg/day

1-5 years: 5-6 mcg/kg/day

6-12 years: 4-5 mcg/kg/day

>12 years: 2-3 mcg/kg/day

Adults:

Hypothyroidism: 1.7 mcg/kg/day in otherwise healthy adults <50 years old, children in whom growth and puberty are complete, and older adults who have been recently treated for hyperthyroidism or who have been hypothyroid for only a few months. Titrate dose every 6 weeks. Average starting dose ~100 mcg; usual doses are ≤200 mcg/day; doses ≥300 mcg/day are rare (consider poor compliance, malabsorption, and/or drug interactions). **Note:** For patients >50 years or patients with cardiac disease, refer to Elderly dosing.

Severe hypothyroidism: Initial: 12.5-25 mcg/day; adjust dose by 25 mcg/day every 2-4 weeks as appropriate; **Note:** Oral agents are not recommended for myxedema (see I.V. dosing).

Subclinical hypothyroidism (if treated): 1 mcg/kg/day

TSH suppression:

Well-differentiated thyroid cancer: Highly individualized; Doses >2 mcg/kg/day may be needed to suppress TSH to <0.1 mU/L.

Benign nodules and nontoxic multinodular goiter: Goal TSH suppression: 0.1-0.3 mU/L

Elderly: Hypothyroidism:

>50 years without cardiac disease **or** <50 years with cardiac disease: Initial: 25-50 mcg/day; adjust dose at 6- to 8-week intervals as needed

>50 years with cardiac disease: Initial: 12.5-25 mcg/day; adjust dose by 12.5-25 mcg increments at 4- to 6-week intervals. (**Note:** Many clinicians prefer to adjust at 6- to 8-week intervals.)

Note: Elderly patients may require <1 mcg/kg/day

I.M., I.V.: Children, Adults, Elderly: Hypothyroidism: 50% of the oral dose

I.V.:

Adults: Myxedema coma or stupor: 200-500 mcg, then 100-300 mcg the next day if necessary; smaller doses should be considered in patients with cardiovascular disease

Elderly: Myxedema coma: Refer to Adults dosing; lower doses may be needed

Mechanism of Action Exact mechanism of action is unknown; however, it is believed the thyroid hormone exerts its many metabolic effects through control of DNA transcription and protein synthesis; involved in normal metabolism, growth, and development; promotes gluconeogenesis, increases utilization and mobilization of glycogen stores, and stimulates protein synthesis, increases basal metabolic rate

Contraindications Hypersensitivity to levothyroxine sodium or any component of the formulation; recent MI or thyrotoxicosis; uncorrected adrenal insufficiency

Warnings/Precautions Ineffective and potentially toxic for weight reduction; high doses may produce serious or even life-threatening toxic effects particularly when used with some anorectic drugs. Use with caution and reduce dosage in patients with angina pectoris or other cardiovascular disease; use cautiously in elderly since they may be more likely to have compromised cardiovascular functions. Patients with adrenal insufficiency, myxedema, diabetes mellitus and insipidus may have symptoms exaggerated or aggravated; thyroid replacement requires periodic assessment of thyroid status. Chronic hypothyroidism predisposes patients to coronary artery disease. Levoxyl® may rapidly swell and disintegrate causing choking or gagging (should be administered with a full glass of water); use caution in patients with dysphagia or other swallowing disorders.

Drug Interactions

Increased Effect/Toxicity: Levothyroxine may potentiate the hypoprothrombinemic effect of warfarin (and other oral anticoagulants). Tricyclic antidepressants (TCAs) coadministered with levothyroxine may increase potential for toxicity of both drugs. Coadministration with ketamine may lead to hypertension and tachycardia.

Decreased Effect: Some medications may decrease absorption of levothyroxine: Cholestyramine, colestipol (separate administration by at least 2 hours); aluminum- and magnesium-containing antacids, iron preparations, sucralfate, Kayexalate® (separate administration by at least 4 hours). Enzyme inducers (phenytoin, phenobarbital, carbamazepine, and rifampin/rifabutin) may decrease levothyroxine levels. Levothyroxine may decrease effect of oral sulfonylureas. Serum levels of digoxin and theophylline may be altered by thyroid function. Estrogens may decrease serum free-thyroxine concentrations. Imatinib may decrease the effects of thyroid replacement therapy.

Ethanol/Nutrition/Herb Interactions Food: Taking levothyroxine with enteral nutrition may cause reduced bioavailability and may lower serum thyroxine levels leading to signs or symptoms of hypothyroidism. Limit intake of goitrogenic foods (eg, asparagus, cabbage, peas, turnip greens, broccoli, spinach, Brussels sprouts, lettuce, soybeans). Soybean flour (infant formula), cottonseed meal, walnuts, and dietary fiber may decrease absorption of levothyroxine from the GI tract.

Dietary Considerations Should be taken on an empty stomach, at least 30 minutes before food.

Pharmacodynamics/Kinetics

Onset of action: Therapeutic: Oral: 3-5 days; I.V. 6-8 hours
Peak effect: I.V.: ~24 hours
Absorption: Oral: Erratic (40% to 80%); decreases with age
Protein binding: >99%
Metabolism: Hepatic to triiodothyronine (active)
Time to peak, serum: 2-4 hours
Half-life elimination: Euthyroid: 6-7 days; Hypothyroid: 9-10 days; Hyperthyroid: 3-4 days
Excretion: Urine and feces; decreases with age

Pregnancy Risk Factor A

Dosage Forms INJ, powder for reconstitution: 0.2 mg, 0.5 mg. **TAB**: 25 mcg, 50 mcg, 75 mcg, 88 mcg, 100 mcg, 112 mcg, 125 mcg, 150 mcg, 175 mcg, 200 mcg, 300 mcg; (Levothroid®): 25 mcg, 50 mcg, 75 mcg, 88 mcg, 100 mcg, 112 mcg, 125 mcg, 150 mcg, 175 mcg, 200 mcg, 300 mcg; (Levoxyl®, Synthroid®): 25 mcg, 50 mcg, 75 mcg, 88 mcg, 100 mcg, 112 mcg, 125 mcg, 137 mcg, 150 mcg, 175 mcg, 200 mcg, 300 mcg; (Unithroid®): 25 mcg, 50 mcg, 75 mcg, 88 mcg, 100 mcg, 112 mcg, 125 mcg, 150 mcg, 175 mcg, 200 mcg, 300 mcg

Levothyroxine Sodium see Levothyroxine on page 917

Levoxyl® see Levothyroxine on page 917

Levsin® see Hyoscyamine on page 803

Levsinex® see Hyoscyamine on page 803

Levsin/SL® see Hyoscyamine on page 803

Levulan® Kerastick® see Aminolevulinic Acid on page 88

Levulose, Dextrose and Phosphoric Acid see Fructose, Dextrose, and Phosphoric Acid on page 713

Lexapro® see Escitalopram on page 568

Lexiva™ see Fosamprenavir on page 702

Lexxel® see Enalapril and Felodipine on page 540

LFA-3/IgG(1) Fusion Protein, Human see Alefacept on page 62

L-Glutamine see Glutamine on page 743

LHRH see Gonadorelin on page 749

LH-RH Agonist see Histrelin on page 772

l-Hyoscyamine Sulfate see Hyoscyamine on page 803

Librax® [original formulation] see Clidinium and Chlordiazepoxide on page 360

Librium® see Chlordiazepoxide on page 315

Lice-Aid [OTC] see Pyrethrins and Piperonyl Butoxide on page 1315

Licide® [OTC] see Pyrethrins and Piperonyl Butoxide on page 1315

LidaMantle® see Lidocaine on page 920

Lida-Mantle® HC *see* Lidocaine and Hydrocortisone *on page 928*

Lidex® *see* Fluocinonide *on page 670*

Lidex-E® *see* Fluocinonide *on page 670*

Lidocaine (LYE doe kane)

Related Information
Cardiovascular Diseases *on page 1636*
Management of Patients Undergoing Cancer Therapy *on page 1728*
Oral Pain *on page 1692*
Viral Infections *on page 1709*
U.S. Brand Names Anestacon®; Band-Aid® Hurt-Free™ Antiseptic Wash [OTC]; Burnamycin [OTC]; Burn Jel [OTC]; Burn-O-Jel [OTC]; LidaMantle®; Lidoderm®; L-M-X™ 4 [OTC]; L-M-X™ 5 [OTC]; LTA® 360; Premjact® [OTC]; Solarcaine® Aloe Extra Burn Relief [OTC]; Topicaine® [OTC]; Xylocaine®; Xylocaine® MPF; Xylocaine® Viscous; Zilactin-L® [OTC]

Canadian Brand Names Betacaine®; Lidodan™; Lidoderm®; Xylocaine®; Xylocard®; Zilactin®

Mexican Brand Names Xylocaina®

Generic Available Yes: Cream, infusion, injection, jelly, lotion, ointment, solution

Synonyms Lidocaine Hydrochloride; Lignocaine Hydrochloride

Pharmacologic Category Analgesic, Topical; Antiarrhythmic Agent, Class Ib; Local Anesthetic

Dental Use Amide-type injectable local anesthetic and topical local anesthetic; Patch: Production of mild topical anesthesia of accessible mucous membranes of the mouth prior to superficial dental procedures

Use Local anesthetic and acute treatment of ventricular arrhythmias from myocardial infarction, or cardiac manipulation
Rectal: Temporary relief of pain and itching due to anorectal disorders
Topical: Local anesthetic for use in laser, cosmetic, and outpatient surgeries; minor burns, cuts, and abrasions of the skin
Lidoderm® Patch: Relief of allodynia (painful hypersensitivity) and chronic pain in postherpetic neuralgia

Unlabeled/Investigational Use ACLS guidelines (not considered drug of choice): Stable monomorphic VT (preserved ventricular function), polymorphic VT (preserved ventricular function), drug-induced monomorphic VT

Local Anesthetic/Vasoconstrictor Precautions No information available to require special precautions

Effects on Dental Treatment No significant effects or complications reported

Significant Adverse Effects Effects vary with route of administration. Many effects are dose related.
Frequency not defined.
Cardiovascular: Arrhythmia, bradycardia, arterial spasms, cardiovascular collapse, defibrillator threshold increased, edema, flushing, heart block, hypotension, sinus node supression, vascular insufficiency (periarticular injections)
Central nervous system: Agitation, anxiety, apprehension, coma, confusion, disorientation, dizziness, drowsiness, euphoria, hallucinations, headache, hyperesthesia, hypoesthesia, lethargy, lightheadedness, nervousness, psychosis, seizure, slurred speech, somnolence, unconsciousness
Dermatologic: Angioedema, bruising (transdermal system), contact dermatitis, depigmentation (transdermal system), edema of the skin, itching, petechia (transdermal system), pruritus, rash, urticaria
Gastrointestinal: Metallic taste, nausea, vomiting
Local: Irritation (transdermal system), thrombophlebitis
Neuromuscular & skeletal: Pain exacerbation (transdermal system), paresthesia, transient radicular pain (subarachnoid administration; up to 1.9%), tremor, twitching, weakness
Ocular: Diplopia, visual changes
Otic: Tinnitus
Respiratory: Bronchospasm, dyspnea, respiratory depression or arrest
Miscellaneous: Allergic reactions, anaphylactoid reaction, sensitivity to temperature extremes

Following spinal anesthesia positional headache (3%), shivering (2%) nausea, peripheral nerve symptoms, respiratory inadequacy and double vision (<1%), hypotension, cauda equina syndrome
Postmarketing and/or case reports: ARDS (inhalation), asystole, disorientation, methemoglobinemia, skin reaction

Dental Usual Dosing Anesthesia, topical:

Cold sores and fever blisters: Children ≥5 years and Adults: Liquid: Apply to affected area every 6 hours as needed

Postherpetic neuralgia: Adults: Patch: Apply patch to most painful area. Up to 3 patches may be applied in a single application. Patch may remain in place for up to 12 hours in any 24-hour period.

Dosage

Antiarrhythmic:

Children:

I.V., I.O.: **Note:** For use in pulseless VT or VF, give after defibrillation, CPR, and epinephrine:

Loading dose: 1 mg/kg (maximum 100 mg); follow with continuous infusion; may administer second bolus of 0.5-1 mg/kg if delay between bolus and start of infusion is >15 minutes

Continuous infusion: 20-50 mcg/kg/minute. Use 20 mcg/kg/minute in patients with shock, hepatic disease, cardiac arrest, mild CHF; moderate-to-severe CHF may require ½ loading dose and lower infusion rates to avoid toxicity.

E.T. (loading dose only): 2-10 times the I.V. bolus dose; dilute with NS to a volume of 3-5 mL and follow with several positive-pressure ventilations

Adults:

Ventricular fibrillation or pulseless ventricular tachycardia (after defibrillation, CPR, and vasopressor administration): I.V.: Initial: 1-1.5 mg/kg. Refractory ventricular tachycardia or ventricular fibrillation, a repeat 0.5-0.75 mg/kg bolus may be given every 5-10 minutes after initial dose for a maximum of 3 doses. Total dose should not exceed 3 mg/kg. Follow with continuous infusion (1-4 mg/minute) after return of perfusion. Reappearance of arrhythmia during constant infusion: 0.5 mg/kg bolus and reassessment of infusion.

E.T. (loading dose only): 2-2.5 times the recommended I.V. dose; dilute in 10 mL NS or distilled water. **Note:** Absorption is greater with distilled water, but causes more adverse effects on PaO$_2$.

Hemodynamically stable VT: 0.5-0.75 mg/kg followed by synchronized cardioversion

Note: Decrease dose in patients with CHF, shock, or hepatic disease.

Anesthesia, topical:

Cream:

LidaMantle®: Skin irritation: Children and Adults: Apply to affected area 2-3 times/day as needed

L-M-X™ 4: Children ≥2 years and Adults: Apply ¼ inch thick layer to intact skin. Leave on until adequate anesthetic effect is obtained. Remove cream and cleanse area before beginning procedure.

L-M-X™ 5: Relief of anorectal pain and itching: Children ≥12 years and Adults: Rectal: Apply topically to clean, dry area or using applicator, insert rectally, up to 6 times/day

Gel, ointment, solution: Adults: Apply to affected area ≤3 times/day as needed (maximum dose: 4.5 mg/kg, not to exceed 300 mg)

Jelly:

Children ≥10 years: Dose varies with age and weight (maximum dose: 4.5 mg/kg)

Adults (maximum dose: 30 mL [600 mg] in any 12-hour period):

Anesthesia of male urethra: 5-30 mL

Anesthesia of female urethra: 3-5 mL

Lubrication of endotracheal tube: Apply a moderate amount to external surface only

Liquid: Cold sores and fever blisters: Children ≥5 years and Adults: Apply to affected area every 6 hours as needed

Patch: Postherpetic neuralgia: Adults: Apply patch to most painful area. Up to 3 patches may be applied in a single application. Patch may remain in place for up to 12 hours in any 24-hour period.

Anesthetic, local injectable: Children and Adults: Varies with procedure, degree of anesthesia needed, vascularity of tissue, duration of anesthesia required, and physical condition of patient; maximum: 4.5 mg/kg/dose; do not repeat within 2 hours.

Dosage adjustment in renal impairment: Not dialyzable (0% to 5%) by hemo- or peritoneal dialysis; supplemental dose is not necessary.

Dosage adjustment in hepatic impairment: Reduce dose in acute hepatitis and decompensated cirrhosis by 50%.

Mechanism of Action Class Ib antiarrhythmic; suppresses automaticity of conduction tissue, by increasing electrical stimulation threshold of ventricle, His-Purkinje system, and spontaneous depolarization of the ventricles during (Continued)

Lidocaine *(Continued)*

diastole by a direct action on the tissues; blocks both the initiation and conduction of nerve impulses by decreasing the neuronal membrane's permeability to sodium ions, which results in inhibition of depolarization with resultant blockade of conduction

Contraindications Hypersensitivity to lidocaine or any component of the formulation; hypersensitivity to another local anesthetic of the amide type; Adam-Stokes syndrome; severe degrees of SA, AV, or intraventricular heart block (except in patients with a functioning artificial pacemaker); premixed injection may contain corn-derived dextrose and its use is contraindicated in patients with allergy to corn-related products

Warnings/Precautions

Intravenous: Constant ECG monitoring is necessary during I.V. administration. Use cautiously in hepatic impairment, any degree of heart block, Wolff-Parkinson-White syndrome, CHF, marked hypoxia, severe respiratory depression, hypovolemia, history of malignant hyperthermia, or shock. Increased ventricular rate may be seen when administered to a patient with atrial fibrillation. Correct any underlying causes of ventricular arrhythmias. Monitor closely for signs and symptoms of CNS toxicity. The elderly may be prone to increased CNS and cardiovascular side effects. Reduce dose in hepatic dysfunction and CHF.

Injectable anesthetic: Follow appropriate administration techniques so as not to administer any intravascularly. Solutions containing antimicrobial preservatives should not be used for epidural or spinal anesthesia. Some solutions contain a bisulfite; avoid in patients who are allergic to bisulfite. Resuscitative equipment, medicine and oxygen should be available in case of emergency. Use products containing epinephrine cautiously in patients with significant vascular disease, compromised blood flow, or during or following general anesthesia (increased risk of arrhythmias). Adjust the dose for the elderly, pediatric, acutely ill, and debilitated patients.

Topical: L-M-X™ 4 cream: Do not leave on large body areas for >2 hours. Observe young children closely to prevent accidental ingestion. Not for use ophthalmic use or for use on mucous membranes.

Transdermal patch: May contain conducting metal (eg, aluminum); remove patch prior to MRI.

Drug Interactions Substrate of CYP1A2 (minor), 2A6 (minor), 2B6 (minor), 2C8/9 (minor), 2D6 (major), 3A4 (major); **Inhibits** CYP1A2 (strong), 2D6 (moderate), 3A4 (moderate)

Cimetidine increases lidocaine blood levels; monitor levels or use an alternative H_2 antagonist.

CYP1A2 substrates: Lidocaine may increase the levels/effects of CYP1A2 substrates. Example substrates include aminophylline, fluvoxamine, mexiletine, mirtazapine, ropinirole, theophylline, and trifluoperazine.

CYP2D6 inhibitors: May increase the levels/effects of lidocaine. Example inhibitors include chlorpromazine, delavirdine, fluoxetine, miconazole, paroxetine, pergolide, quinidine, quinine, ritonavir, and ropinirole.

CYP2D6 substrates: Lidocaine may increase the levels/effects of CYP2D6 substrates. Example substrates include amphetamines, selected beta-blockers, dextromethorphan, fluoxetine, mirtazapine, nefazodone, paroxetine, risperidone, ritonavir, thioridazine, tricyclic antidepressants, and venlafaxine.

CYP2D6 prodrug substrates: Lidocaine may decrease the levels/effects of CYP2D6 prodrug substrates. Example prodrug substrates include codeine, hydrocodone, oxycodone, and tramadol.

CYP3A4 inducers: CYP3A4 inducers may decrease the levels/effects of lidocaine. Example inducers include aminoglutethimide, carbamazepine, nafcillin, nevirapine, phenobarbital, phenytoin, and rifamycins.

CYP3A4 inhibitors: May increase the levels/effects of lidocaine. Example inhibitors include amiodarone (doses >400 mg/day), azole antifungals, clarithromycin, diclofenac, doxycycline, erythromycin, imatinib, isoniazid, nefazodone, nicardipine, propofol, protease inhibitors, quinidine, telithromycin, and verapamil.

CYP3A4 substrates: Lidocaine may increase the levels/effects of CYP3A4 substrates. Example substrates include benzodiazepines, calcium channel blockers, cyclosporine, mirtazapine, nateglinide, nefazodone, sildenafil (and other PDE-5 inhibitors), tacrolimus, and venlafaxine. Selected benzodiazepines (midazolam and triazolam), cisapride, ergot alkaloids, selected HMG-CoA reductase inhibitors (lovastatin and simvastatin), and pimozide are generally contraindicated with strong CYP3A4 inhibitors.

Propranolol: Increases lidocaine blood levels.

Protease inhibitors (eg, amprenavir, ritonavir): May increase lidocaine blood levels.

Ethanol/Nutrition/Herb Interactions Herb/Nutraceutical: St John's wort may decrease lidocaine levels; avoid concurrent use.

Dietary Considerations Premixed injection may contain corn-derived dextrose and its use is contraindicated in patients with allergy to corn-related products.

Pharmacodynamics/Kinetics

Onset of action: Single bolus dose: 45-90 seconds

Duration: 10-20 minutes

Distribution: V_d: 1.1-2.1 L/kg; alterable by many patient factors; decreased in CHF and liver disease; crosses blood-brain barrier

Protein binding: 60% to 80% to alpha$_1$ acid glycoprotein

Metabolism: 90% hepatic; active metabolites monoethylglycinexylidide (MEGX) and glycinexylidide (GX) can accumulate and may cause CNS toxicity

Half-life elimination: Biphasic: Prolonged with congestive heart failure, liver disease, shock, severe renal disease; Initial: 7-30 minutes; Terminal: Infants, premature: 3.2 hours, Adults: 1.5-2 hours

Pregnancy Risk Factor B

Lactation Enters breast milk (small amounts)/use caution (AAP rates "compatible")

Dosage Forms [DSC] = Discontinued product

Cream, rectal (L-M-X™ 5): 5% (15 g) [contains benzyl alcohol; packaged with applicator]; (30 g) [contains benzyl alcohol]

Cream, topical (L-M-X™ 4): 4% (5 g) [contains benzyl alcohol; packaged with Tegaderm™ dressing]; (15 g, 30 g) [contains benzyl alcohol]

Cream, topical, as hydrochloride: 3% (30 g)

LidaMantle®: 3% (30 g, 85 g)

Gel, topical:

Burn-O-Jel: 0.5% (90 g)

Topicaine: 4% (10 g, 30 g, 113 g) [contains alcohol 35%, benzyl alcohol, aloe vera, and jojoba]

Gel, topical, as hydrochloride:

Burn Jel: 2% (3.5 g, 120 g)

Solarcaine® Aloe Extra Burn Relief: 0.5% (113 g, 226 g) [contains aloe vera gel and tartrazine]

Infusion, as hydrochloride [premixed in D$_5$W]: 0.4% [4 mg/mL] (250 mL, 500 mL); 0.8% [8 mg/mL] (250 mL, 500 mL)

Injection, solution, as hydrochloride: 0.5% [5 mg/mL] (50 mL); 1% [10 mg/mL] (2 mL, 10 mL, 20 mL, 30 mL, 50 mL); 2% [20 mg/mL] (2 mL, 5 mL, 20 mL, 50 mL)

Xylocaine®: 0.5% [5 mg/mL] (50 mL); 1% [10 mg/mL] (10 mL, 20 mL, 50 mL); 2% [20 mg/mL] (1.8 mL, 10 mL, 20 mL, 50 mL)

Injection, solution, as hydrochloride [preservative free]: 0.5% [5 mg/mL] (50 mL); 1% [10 mg/mL] (2 mL, 5 mL, 30 mL); 1.5% [15 mg/mL] (20 mL); 2% [20 mg/mL] (2 mL, 5 mL, 10 mL); 4% [40 mg/mL] (5 mL)

Xylocaine®: 10% [100 mg/mL] (5 mL) [for ventricular arrhythmias]

Xylocaine® MPF: 0.5% [5 mg/mL] (50 mL); 1% [10 mg/mL] (2 mL, 5 mL, 10 mL, 30 mL); 1.5% [15 mg/mL] (10 mL, 20 mL); 2% [20 mg/mL] (2 mL, 5 mL, 10 mL); 4% [40 mg/mL] (5 mL)

Injection, solution, as hydrochloride [premixed in D$_{7.5}$W, preservative free]: 5% (2 mL)

Xylocaine® MPF: 1.5% (2 mL) [DSC]

Jelly, topical, as hydrochloride: 2% (5 mL, 30 mL)

Anestacon®: 2% (15 mL) [contains benzalkonium chloride]

Xylocaine®: 2% (5 mL, 30 mL)

Liquid, topical (Zilactin®-L): 2.5% (7.5 mL)

Lotion, topical, as hydrochloride (LidaMantle®): 3% (177 mL)

Ointment, topical: 5% (37 g, 50 g)

Solution, topical, as hydrochloride: 4% [40 mg/mL] (50 mL)

Band-Aid® Hurt-Free™ Antiseptic Wash: 2% (180 mL)

LTA® 360: 4% [40 mg/mL] (4 mL) [packaged with cannula for laryngotracheal administration]

Xylocaine®: 4% [40 mg/mL] (50 mL)

Solution, viscous, as hydrochloride: 2% [20 mg/mL] (20 mL, 100 mL)

Xylocaine® Viscous: 2% [20 mg/mL] (100 mL, 450 mL)

Spray, topical:

Burnamycin: 0.5% (60 mL) [contains aloe vera gel and menthol]

Premjact®: 9.6% (13 mL)

Solarcaine® Aloe Extra Burn Relief: 0.5% (127 g) [contains aloe vera]

Transdermal system, topical (Lidoderm®): 5% (30s)

Lidocaine and Bupivacaine (LYE doe kane & byoo PIV a kane)

Related Information
Bupivacaine *on page 228*
Lidocaine *on page 920*
U.S. Brand Names Duocaine™
Generic Available No
Synonyms Bupivacaine and Lidocaine; Lidocaine Hydrochloride and Bupivacaine Hydrochloride
Pharmacologic Category Local Anesthetic
Use Local or regional anesthesia in ophthalmologic surgery by peripheral nerve block techniques such as peribulbar, retrobulbar, and facial blocks; may be used with or without epinephrine
Local Anesthetic/Vasoconstrictor Precautions No information available to require special precautions
Effects on Dental Treatment No significant effects or complications reported
Common Adverse Effects Frequency not defined; reactions may be dose related or due to unintentional intravascular injection.
Cardiovascular: Bradycardia, cardiac arrest, cardiac output decreased, heart block, hypotension, myocardium depression, ventricular arrhythmia
Central nervous system: Anxiety, chills, convulsions, depression, dizziness, drowsiness, excitation, restlessness
Gastrointestinal: Nausea, vomiting
Neuromuscular & skeletal: Tremors
Ocular: Blurred vision, pupil constriction, permanent injury to extraocular muscle
Otic: Tinnitus
Respiratory: Respiratory arrest
Miscellaneous: Allergic reaction

Following unintentional subarachnoid injection: Backache, cranial nerve palsies, headache, incontinence (fecal or urinary), meningismus, paralysis, paresthesia, perineal sensation loss, persistent anesthesia, septic meningitis, sexual function loss, spinal block, urinary retention, weakness
Mechanism of Action Blocks both the initiation and conduction of nerve impulses by decreasing the neuronal membrane's permeability to sodium ions, which results in inhibition of depolarization with resultant blockade of conduction.
Drug Interactions
Cytochrome P450 Effect: Lidocaine: **Substrate** of CYP1A2 (minor), 2A6 (minor), 2B6 (minor), 2C8/9 (minor), 2D6 (major), 3A4 (major); **Inhibits** CYP1A2 (strong), 2D6 (moderate), 3A4 (moderate)
Decreased Effect: Epinephrine may be used to decrease systemic absorption of lidocaine/bupivacaine; if used, see Epinephrine monograph for Drug Interactions.
Pharmacodynamics/Kinetics Also see individual agents.
Protein binding: Lidocaine: Fraction bound decreases with increased concentration; also dependent upon plasma concentration of alpha$_1$-acid glycoprotein
Metabolism: Lidocaine: Hepatic, forms metabolites; Bupivacaine: hepatic, forms metabolites
Half-life elimination: Lidocaine: I.V.: 1.5-2 hours; Bupivacaine: I.V.: 2.7 hours
Time to peak, plasma: Following peribulbar block: Lidocaine: 20 minutes; Bupivacaine: 21 minutes
Excretion: Urine
Pregnancy Risk Factor C

Lidocaine and Epinephrine (LYE doe kane & ep i NEF rin)

Related Information
Epinephrine *on page 546*
Lidocaine *on page 920*
Oral Pain *on page 1692*
U.S. Brand Names LidoSite™; Xylocaine® MPF With Epinephrine; Xylocaine® With Epinephrine
Canadian Brand Names Xylocaine® With Epinephrine
Generic Available Yes: Excludes transdermal system
Synonyms Epinephrine and Lidocaine
Pharmacologic Category Local Anesthetic
Dental Use Amide-type anesthetic used for local infiltration anesthesia injection near nerve trunks to produce nerve block
Use Local infiltration anesthesia; AVS for nerve block; topical local analgesia for superficial dermatologic procedures

Local Anesthetic/Vasoconstrictor Precautions No information available to require special precautions

Effects on Dental Treatment It is common to misinterpret psychogenic responses to local anesthetic injection as an allergic reaction. Intraoral injections are perceived by many patients as a stressful procedure in dentistry. Common symptoms to this stress are diaphoresis, palpitations, hyperventilation. Patients may exhibit hypersensitivity to bisulfites contained in local anesthetic solution to prevent oxidation of epinephrine. In general, patients reacting to bisulfites have a history of asthma and their airways are hyper-reactive to asthmatic syndrome.

Degree of adverse effects in the CNS and cardiovascular system is directly related to the blood levels of lidocaine: Bradycardia, hypersensitivity reactions (rare; may be manifest as dermatologic reactions and edema at injection site), asthmatic syndromes

High blood levels: Anxiety, restlessness, disorientation, confusion, dizziness, tremors, seizures, CNS depression (resulting in somnolence, unconsciousness and possible respiratory arrest), nausea, and vomiting.

Significant Adverse Effects Degree of adverse effects in the central nervous system and cardiovascular system are directly related to the blood levels of lidocaine. The effects below are more likely to occur after systemic administration rather than infiltration.

Cardiovascular: Myocardial effects include a decrease in contraction force as well as a decrease in electrical excitability and myocardial conduction rate resulting in bradycardia and reduction in cardiac output.

Central nervous system: High blood levels result in anxiety, restlessness, disorientation, confusion, dizziness, tremor, and seizure. This is followed by depression of CNS resulting in somnolence, unconsciousness and possible respiratory arrest. In some cases, symptoms of CNS stimulation may be absent and the primary CNS effects are somnolence and unconsciousness.

Gastrointestinal: Nausea and vomiting may occur

Hypersensitivity reactions: Extremely rare, but may be manifest as dermatologic reactions and edema at injection site. Asthmatic syndromes have occurred. Patients may exhibit hypersensitivity to bisulfites contained in local anesthetic solution to prevent oxidation of epinephrine. In general, patients reacting to bisulfites have a history of asthma and their airways are hyper-reactive to asthmatic syndrome.

Psychogenic reactions: It is common to misinterpret psychogenic responses to local anesthetic injection as an allergic reaction. Intraoral injections are perceived by many patients as a stressful procedure in dentistry. Common symptoms to this stress are diaphoresis, palpitation, hyperventilation, generalized pallor and a fainting feeling

Topical formulation:
>10%: Dermatologic: Papules (up to 12%)
1% to 10%: Dermatologic: Burns (up to 8%), rash (5%), skin irritation, burning sensation, blanching
<1% (Limited to important or life-threatening): Erythema, hematoma, urticaria

Dental Usual Dosing Dosage varies with the anesthetic procedure, degree of anesthesia needed, vascularity of tissue, duration of anesthesia required, and physical condition of patient.

Dental anesthesia, infiltration, or conduction block:
Children <10 years: 20-30 mg (1-1.5 mL) of lidocaine hydrochloride as a 2% solution with epinephrine 1:100,000; maximum: 4-5 mg of lidocaine hydrochloride/kg of body weight or 100-150 mg as a single dose

# of Cartridges (1.8 mL)	Lidocaine HCl (2%) (mg)	Epinephrine 1:100,000 (mg)
1	36	0.018
2	72	0.036
3	108	0.054
4	144	0.072
5	180	0.090
6	216	0.108
7	252	0.126
8	288	0.144
9	324	0.162
10	360	0.180

(Continued)

Lidocaine and Epinephrine *(Continued)*

Children >10 years and Adults: Do not exceed 6.6 mg/kg body weight or 300 mg of lidocaine hydrochloride and 3 mcg (0.003 mg) of epinephrine/kg of body weight or 0.2 mg epinephrine per dental appointment. The effective anesthetic dose varies with procedure, intensity of anesthesia needed, duration of anesthesia required, and physical condition of the patient. Always use the lowest effective dose along with careful aspiration.

The following numbers of dental carpules (1.8 mL) provide the indicated amounts of lidocaine hydrochloride 2% and epinephrine 1:100,000 (see table on previous page)

For most routine dental procedures, lidocaine hydrochloride 2% with epinephrine 1:100,000 is preferred. When a more pronounced hemostasis is required, a 1:50,000 epinephrine concentration should be used. The following numbers of dental carpules (1.8 mL) provide the indicated amounts of lidocaine hydrochloride 2% and epinephrine 1:50,000 (see table):

# of Cartridges (1.8 mL)	Lidocaine HCl (2%) (mg)	Epinephrine 1:50,000 (mg)
1	36	0.036
2	72	0.072
3	108	0.108
4	144	0.144
5	180	0.180
6	216	0.216

Dermatologic procedure: Children ≥5 and Adults: Topical: Place 1 transdermal patch over area requiring analgesia; attach patch to iontophoretic controller and leave on for 10 minutes. Remove patch and perform procedure within 10-20 minutes of patch removal. Do not use another patch for 30 minutes.

Dosage Dosage varies with the anesthetic procedure, degree of anesthesia needed, vascularity of tissue, duration of anesthesia required, and physical condition of patient.

Dental anesthesia, infiltration, or conduction block:

Children <10 years: 20-30 mg (1-1.5 mL) of lidocaine hydrochloride as a 2% solution with epinephrine 1:100,000; maximum: 4-5 mg of lidocaine hydrochloride/kg of body weight or 100-150 mg as a single dose

Children >10 years and Adults: Do not exceed 6.6 mg/kg body weight or 300 mg of lidocaine hydrochloride and 3 mcg (0.003 mg) of epinephrine/kg of body weight or 0.2 mg epinephrine per dental appointment. The effective anesthetic dose varies with procedure, intensity of anesthesia needed, duration of anesthesia required, and physical condition of the patient. Always use the lowest effective dose along with careful aspiration.

For most routine dental procedures, lidocaine hydrochloride 2% with epinephrine 1:100,000 is preferred. When a more pronounced hemostasis is required, a 1:50,000 epinephrine concentration should be used.

Dermatologic procedure: Children ≥5 and Adults: Topical: Place 1 transdermal patch over area requiring analgesia; attach patch to iontophoretic controller and leave on for 10 minutes. Remove patch and perform procedure within 10-20 minutes of patch removal. Do not use another patch for 30 minutes.

Mechanism of Action Lidocaine blocks both the initiation and conduction of nerve impulses via decreased permeability of sodium ions; epinephrine increases the duration of action of lidocaine by causing vasoconstriction (via alpha effects) which slows the vascular absorption of lidocaine

Contraindications Hypersensitivity to lidocaine, epinephrine, or any component of the formulation; hypersensitivity to other local anesthetics of the amide type; myasthenia gravis; shock; cardiac conduction disease; angle-closure glaucoma

LidoSite™: Hypersensitivity to lidocaine, epinephrine, other local anesthetics of the amide type, or any component of the formulation; patients with electrically-sensitive devices (eg, pacemakers, implantable defibrillators)

Warnings/Precautions Aspirate the syringe (injection solution for infiltration formulation) after tissue penetration and before injection to minimize chance of direct vascular injection. Use caution in endocrine, hepatic, or thyroid disease. Avoid use in presence of flammable anesthetics. Avoid in patients with uncontrolled hyperthyroidism. Use minimal amounts in patients with significant cardiovascular problems (because of epinephrine component). May contain sodium metabisulfite; use caution in patients with a sulfite allergy. Avoid application of topical formulation to distal portions of body (eg, digits, nose, ears, penis).

Transdermal patch may contain conducting metal (eg, aluminum); remove patch prior to MRI.

LidoSite™: Do not use near flammable anesthetics. Use with caution in patients with peripheral vascular disease; may have exaggerated vasoconstriction. Use with caution in patients with severe coronary artery disease, hypertension, cardiac dysrhythmias, or patients taking MAO inhibitors or tricyclic antidepressants. Use caution in patients with skin susceptible to injury.

Drug Interactions Lidocaine: **Substrate** of CYP1A2 (minor), 2A6 (minor), 2B6 (minor), 2C8/9 (minor), 2D6 (major), 3A4 (major); **Inhibits** CYP1A2 (strong), 2D6 (strong), 3A4 (moderate)

Also see individual agents. **Note:** Significance of interaction may depend on route of drug delivery and systemic exposure.

Beta-blockers, nonselective: Combination treatment may increase blood pressure.

Epinephrine (and other direct alpha-agonists): Pressor response to I.V. epinephrine, norepinephrine, and phenylephrine may be enhanced in patients receiving TCAs (**Note:** Effect is unlikely with epinephrine or levonordefrin dosages typically administered as infiltration in combination with local anesthetics)

General Anesthetics: May increase sensitivity of myocardium to dysrhythmic effects of epinephrine.

Tricyclic Antidepressants: Combination treatment may increase blood pressure.

Pharmacodynamics/Kinetics

Onset of action: Peak effect: ~5 minutes

Duration: ~2 hours; dose and anesthetic procedure dependent

Absorption: Topical: Lidocaine: Minimal; Epinephrine: Minimal

See individual agents.

Pregnancy Risk Factor B

Lactation Enters breast milk/compatible

Breast-Feeding Considerations Usual infiltration doses of lidocaine with epinephrine given to nursing mothers has not been shown to affect the health of the nursing infant.

Dosage Forms

Injection, solution:

0.5% / 1:200,000: Lidocaine hydrochloride 0.5% and epinephrine 1:200,000 (50 mL)

1% / 1:100,000: Lidocaine hydrochloride 1% and epinephrine 1:100,000 (20 mL, 30 mL, 50 mL)

1% / 1:200,000: Lidocaine hydrochloride 1% and epinephrine 1:200,000 (30 mL)

1.5% / 1:200,000: Lidocaine hydrochloride 1.5% and epinephrine 1:200,000 (30 mL)

2% / 1:50,000: Lidocaine hydrochloride 2% and epinephrine 1:50,000 (1.8 mL)

2% / 1:100,000: Lidocaine hydrochloride 2% and epinephrine 1:100,000 (1.8 mL, 30 mL, 50 mL)

2% / 1:200,000: Lidocaine hydrochloride 2% and epinephrine 1:200,000 (20 mL)

Xylocaine® with Epinephrine:

0.5% / 1:200,000: Lidocaine hydrochloride 0.5% and epinephrine 1:200,000 (50 mL) [contains methylparaben]

1% / 1:100,000: Lidocaine hydrochloride 1% and epinephrine 1:100,000 (10 mL, 20 mL, 50 mL) [contains methylparaben]

2% / 1:50,000: Lidocaine hydrochloride 2% and epinephrine 1:50,000 (1.8 mL) [contains sodium metabisulfite]

2% / 1:100,000: Lidocaine hydrochloride 2% and epinephrine 1:100,000 (1.8 mL) [contains sodium metabisulfite]; (10 mL, 20 mL, 50 mL) [contains methylparaben]

Xylocaine®-MPF with Epinephrine:

1% / 1:200,000: Lidocaine hydrochloride 1% and epinephrine 1:200,000 (5 mL, 10 mL, 30 mL) [contains sodium metabisulfite]

1.5% / 1:200,000: Lidocaine hydrochloride 1.5% and epinephrine 1:200,000 (5 mL, 10 mL, 30 mL) [contains sodium metabisulfite]

2% / 1:200,000: Lidocaine hydrochloride 2% and epinephrine 1:200,000 (5 mL, 10 mL, 20 mL) [contains sodium metabisulfite]

Transdermal system (LidoSite™): Lidocaine hydrochloride 10% and epinephrine 0.1% (25s) [contains sodium metabisulfite; for use only with LidoSite™ controller]

Selected Readings

Ayoub ST and Coleman AE, "A Review of Local Anesthetics," *Gen Dent*, 1992, 40(4):285-7, 289-90.

Budenz AW, "Local Anesthetics in Dentistry: Then and Now," *J Calif Dent Assoc*, 2003, 31(5):388-96.

(Continued)

Lidocaine and Epinephrine *(Continued)*

Dower JS Jr, "A Review of Paresthesia in Association With Administration of Local Anesthesia," *Dent Today*, 2003, 22(2):64-9.

Finder RL and Moore PA, "Adverse Drug Reactions to Local Anesthesia," *Dent Clin North Am*, 2002, 46(4):747-57, x.

Haas DA, "An Update on Local Anesthetics in Dentistry," *J Can Dent Assoc*, 2002, 68(9):546-51.

Hawkins JM and Moore PA, "Local Anesthesia: Advances in Agents and Techniques," *Dent Clin North Am*, 2002, 46(4):719-32, ix.

"Injectable Local Anesthetics," *J Am Dent Assoc*, 2003, 134(5):628-9.

Jastak JT and Yagiela JA, "Vasoconstrictors and Local Anesthesia: A Review and Rationale for Use," *J Am Dent Assoc*, 1983, 107(4):623-30.

MacKenzie TA and Young ER, "Local Anesthetic Update," *Anesth Prog*, 1993, 40(2):29-34.

Malamed SF, "Allergy and Toxic Reactions to Local Anesthetics," *Dent Today*, 2003, 22(4):114-6, 118-21.

Nusstein J, Reader A, and Beck FM, "Anesthetic Efficacy of Different Volumes of Lidocaine With Epinephrine for Inferior Alveolar Nerve Blocks," *Gen Dent*, 2002, 50(4):372-5.

Wynn RL, "Epinephrine Interactions With Beta-Blockers," *Gen Dent*, 1994, 42(1):16, 18.

Wynn RL, "Recent Research on Mechanisms of Local Anesthetics," *Gen Dent*, 1995, 43(4):316-8.

Yagiela JA, "Local Anesthetics," *Anesth Prog*, 1991, 38(4-5):128-41.

Lidocaine and Hydrocortisone
(LYE doe kane & hye droe KOR ti sone)

Related Information
Hydrocortisone *on page 793*
Lidocaine *on page 920*

U.S. Brand Names AnaMantle® HC; Lida-Mantle® HC

Generic Available Yes: Topical cream

Synonyms Hydrocortisone and Lidocaine

Pharmacologic Category Anesthetic/Corticosteroid

Use Topical anti-inflammatory and anesthetic for skin disorders; rectal for the treatment of hemorrhoids, anal fissures, pruritus ani, or similar conditions

Local Anesthetic/Vasoconstrictor Precautions No information available to require special precautions

Effects on Dental Treatment No significant effects or complications reported

Drug Interactions

Cytochrome P450 Effect:
Lidocaine: **Substrate** of CYP1A2 (minor), 2A6 (minor), 2B6 (minor), 2C8/9 (minor), 2D6 (major), 3A4 (major); **Inhibits** CYP1A2 (strong), 2D6 (strong), 3A4 (moderate)
Hydrocortisone: **Substrate** of CYP3A4 (minor); **Induces** CYP3A4 (weak)

Increased Effect/Toxicity: See individual agents.

Decreased Effect: See individual agents.

Pharmacodynamics/Kinetics See individual agents.

Pregnancy Risk Factor B

Lidocaine and Prilocaine (LYE doe kane & PRIL oh kane)

Related Information
Lidocaine *on page 920*
Prilocaine *on page 1277*

U.S. Brand Names EMLA®; Oraquix®

Canadian Brand Names EMLA®

Generic Available Yes: Cream

Synonyms Prilocaine and Lidocaine

Pharmacologic Category Local Anesthetic

Dental Use
Periodontal gel (Oraqix®): Use in adults who require localized anesthesia in periodontal pockets during scaling and/or root planning.
Topical: Amide-type topical anesthetic for use on normal intact skin to provide local analgesia for minor procedures such as I.V. cannulation or venipuncture

Use Topical anesthetic for use on normal intact skin to provide local analgesia for minor procedures such as I.V. cannulation or venipuncture; has also been used for painful procedures such as lumbar puncture and skin graft harvesting; for superficial minor surgery of genital mucous membranes and as an adjunct for local infiltration anesthesia in genital mucous membranes.

Local Anesthetic/Vasoconstrictor Precautions No information available to require special precautions

Effects on Dental Treatment Key adverse event(s) related to dental treatment: Application site reactions in the oral cavity in 52/391 patients (13%) included pain, soreness, irritation, numbness, ulcerations, vesicles, edema, abscess and/or redness in the treated area. The 13% represented adverse effects occurring in more than one patient. Each patient was counted only once per adverse event. Taste perversion also reported (2%) including complaints of bad or bitter taste for up to 4 hours after administration.

Significant Adverse Effects Frequency not defined.

Cardiovascular: Hypotension, angioedema

Central nervous system: Shock

Dermatologic: Hyperpigmentation, erythema, itching, rash, burning, urticaria

Genitourinary: Blistering of foreskin (rare)

Local: Burning, stinging, edema

Respiratory: Bronchospasm

Miscellaneous: Alteration in temperature sensation, hypersensitivity reactions

Dental Usual Dosing Oraqix®: Gel: Apply on gingival margin around selected teeth using the blunt-tipped applicator included in package. Wait 30 seconds, then fill the periodontal pockets using the blunt-tipped applicator until gel becomes visible at the gingival margin. Wait another 30 seconds before starting treatment. Maximum recommended dose: One treatment session: 5 cartridges (8.5 g)

Dosage Although the incidence of systemic adverse effects with EMLA® is very low, caution should be exercised, particularly when applying over large areas and leaving on for >2 hours

Children (intact skin): EMLA® should **not** be used in neonates with a gestation age <37 weeks nor in infants <12 months of age who are receiving treatment with methemoglobin-inducing agents

Dosing is based on child's age and weight:

Age 0-3 months or <5 kg: Apply a maximum of 1 g over no more than 10 cm^2 of skin; leave on for no longer than 1 hour

Age 3 months to 12 months and >5 kg: Apply no more than a maximum 2 g total over no more than 20 cm^2 of skin; leave on for no longer than 4 hours

Age 1-6 years and >10 kg: Apply no more than a maximum of 10 g total over no more than 100 cm^2 of skin; leave on for no longer than 4 hours.

Age 7-12 years and >20 kg: Apply no more than a maximum 20 g total over no more than 200 cm^2 of skin; leave on for no longer than 4 hours.

Note: If a patient greater than 3 months old does not meet the minimum weight requirement, the maximum total dose should be restricted to the corresponding maximum based on patient weight.

Adults (intact skin):

EMLA® cream and EMLA® anesthetic disc: A thick layer of EMLA® cream is applied to intact skin and covered with an occlusive dressing, or alternatively, an EMLA® anesthetic disc is applied to intact skin

Minor dermal procedures (eg, I.V. cannulation or venipuncture): Apply 2.5 g of cream (1/2 of the 5 g tube) over 20-25 cm of skin surface area, or 1 anesthetic disc (1 g over 10 cm^2) for at least 1 hour. **Note:** In clinical trials, 2 sites were usually prepared in case there was a technical problem with cannulation or venipuncture at the first site.

Major dermal procedures (eg, more painful dermatological procedures involving a larger skin area such as split thickness skin graft harvesting): Apply 2 g of cream per 10 cm^2 of skin and allow to remain in contact with the skin for at least 2 hours.

Adult male genital skin (eg, pretreatment prior to local anesthetic infiltration): Apply a thick layer of cream (1 g/10 cm^2) to the skin surface for 15 minutes. Local anesthetic infiltration should be performed immediately after removal of EMLA® cream.

Note: Dermal analgesia can be expected to increase for up to 3 hours under occlusive dressing and persist for 1-2 hours after removal of the cream

Adult females: Genital mucous membranes: Minor procedures (eg, removal of condylomata acuminata, pretreatment for local anesthetic infiltration): Apply 5-10 g (thick layer) of cream for 5-10 minutes

Periodontal gel (Oraqix®): Adults: Apply on gingival margin around selected teeth using the blunt-tipped applicator included in package. Wait 30 seconds, then fill the periodontal pockets using the blunt-tipped applicator until gel becomes visible at the gingival margin. Wait another 30 seconds before starting treatment. Maximum recommended dose: One treatment session: 5 cartridges (8.5 g)

Mechanism of Action Local anesthetic action occurs by stabilization of neuronal membranes and inhibiting the ionic fluxes required for the initiation and conduction of impulses

Contraindications Hypersensitivity to amide-type anesthetic agents (eg, lidocaine, prilocaine, dibucaine, mepivacaine, bupivacaine, etidocaine); hypersensitivity to any component of the formulation selected; application on mucous membranes or broken or inflamed skin; infants <1 month of age if gestational age is <37 weeks; infants <12 months of age receiving therapy with methemoglobin-inducing agents; children with congenital or idiopathic methemoglobinemia, or in children who are receiving medications associated with (Continued)

Lidocaine and Prilocaine *(Continued)*

drug-induced methemoglobinemia (eg, acetaminophen [overdosage], benzocaine, chloroquine, dapsone, nitrofurantoin, nitroglycerin, nitroprusside, phenazopyridine, phenelzine, phenobarbital, phenytoin, quinine, sulfonamides)

Warnings/Precautions Use with caution in patients receiving class I and III antiarrhythmic drugs, since systemic absorption occurs and synergistic toxicity is possible. Although the incidence of systemic adverse reactions with EMLA® is very low, caution should be exercised, particularly when applying over large areas and leaving on for longer than 2 hours. Avoid use on open wounds or near the eyes.

Drug Interactions Lidocaine: **Substrate** of CYP1A2 (minor), 2A6 (minor), 2B6 (minor), 2C8/9 (minor), 2D6 (major), 3A4 (major); **Inhibits** CYP1A2 (strong), 2D6 (strong), 3A4 (moderate)

Also see individual agents.

Increased toxicity:

Class I antiarrhythmic drugs (eg, mexiletine): Effects are additive and potentially synergistic

Class III antiarrhythmic drugs (eg, amiodarone, sotalol, dofetilide): Cardiac ffects may be additive. Consider ECG monitoring.

Drugs known to induce methemoglobinemia

Pharmacodynamics/Kinetics

EMLA®:

Onset of action: 1 hour

Peak effect: 2-3 hours

Duration: 1-2 hours after removal

Absorption: Related to duration of application and area where applied

3-hour application: 3.6% lidocaine and 6.1% prilocaine

24-hour application: 16.2% lidocaine and 33.5% prilocaine

See individual agents.

Pregnancy Risk Factor B

Lactation Enters breast milk/compatible

Breast-Feeding Considerations Usual infiltration doses of lidocaine and prilocaine given to nursing mothers has not been shown to affect the health of the nursing infant.

Dosage Forms

Cream, topical: Lidocaine 2.5% and prilocaine 2.5% (5 g, 30 g)

EMLA®: Lidocaine 2.5% and prilocaine 2.5% (5 g, 30 g) [each packaged with Tegaderm® dressings]

Disc, topical: Lidocaine 2.5% and prilocaine 2.5% per disc (2s, 10s) [each 1 g disc is 10 cm^2]

Gel, periodontal: Lidocaine 2.5% and prilocaine 2.5% (1.7 g) [cartridge]

Selected Readings

Broadman LM, Soliman IE, Hannallah RS, et al, "Analgesic Efficacy of Eutectic Mixture of Local Anesthetics (EMLA®) vs Intradermal Infiltration Prior to Venous Cannulation in Children," *Am J Anaesth*, 1987, 34:S56.

Friskopp J and Huledal G, "Plasma Levels of Lidocaine and Prilocaine After Application of Oraqix, a New Intrapocket Anesthetic, in Patients With Advanced Periodontitis," *J Clin Periodontol*, 2001, 28(5):425-9.

Friskopp J, Nilsson M, and Isacsson G, "The Anesthetic Onset and Duration of a New Lidocaine/Prilocaine Gel Intra-Pocket Anesthetic (Oraqix) for Periodontal Scaling/Root Planing," *J Clin Periodontol*, 2001, 28(5):453-8.

Halperin DL, Koren G, Attias D, et al, "Topical Skin Anesthesia for Venous Subcutaneous Drug Reservoir and Lumbar Puncture in Children," *Pediatrics*, 1989, 84(2):281-4.

Robieux I, Kumar R, Radhakrishnan S, et al, "Assessing Pain and Analgesia With a Lidocaine-Prilocaine Emulsion in Infants and Toddlers During Venipuncture," *J Pediatr*, 1991, 118(6):971-3.

Taddio A, Shennan AT, Stevens B, et al, "Safety of Lidocaine-Prilocaine Cream in the Treatment of Preterm Neonates," *J Pediatr*, 1995, 127(6):1002-5.

Vickers ER, Mazbani N, Gerzina TM, et al, "Pharmacokinetics of EMLA Cream 5% Application to Oral Mucosa," *Anesth Prog*, 1997, 44:32-7.

Lidocaine and Tetracaine *(LYE doe kane & TET ra kane)*

U.S. Brand Names Synera™

Synonyms Tetracaine and Lidocaine

Pharmacologic Category Analgesic, Topical; Local Anesthetic

Use Topical anesthetic for use on normal intact skin for minor procedures (eg, I.V. cannulation or venipuncture) and superficial dermatologic procedures

Local Anesthetic/Vasoconstrictor Precautions No information available to require special precautions

Effects on Dental Treatment No significant effects or complications reported

Common Adverse Effects

>10%: Dermatologic: Erythema (71%), blanching (12%), edema (12%)

1% to 10%: Dermatologic: Application site reactions (contact dermatitis, rash, skin discoloration 4%)

Dosage Transdermal patch: Children ≥3 years and Adults:

Venipuncture or intravenous cannulation: Prior to procedure, apply to intact skin for 20-30 minutes

Superficial dermatological procedures: Prior to procedure, apply to intact skin for 30 minutes

Note: Adults can use another patch at a new location to facilitate venous access after a failed attempt; remove previous patch.

Dosage adjustment in hepatic impairment: Use caution in patients with severe hepatic dysfunction.

Mechanism of Action

Local anesthetic action occurs by stabilization of neuronal membranes and inhibiting the ionic fluxes required for the initiation and conduction of impulses. A heating mechanism within the patch enhances drug delivery.

Contraindications Hypersensitivity to amide or ester type anesthetic agents, para-aminobenzoid acid (PABA), or any other component of the formulation

Warnings/Precautions Use with caution in patients receiving class I antiarrhythmic drugs, since systemic absorption occurs and synergistic toxicity is possible. Although the incidence of systemic adverse reactions is very low, caution should be exercised when applying simultaneous or sequential application of multiple patches to adults; this practice is not recommended with children. Use with caution in patients who may be sensitive to systemic effects (eg, acutely ill, debilitated). If being used with other products containing local anesthetic, consider potential for additive effects. Avoid contact with eye; loss of protective reflexes may predispose to corneal irritation and/or abrasion. Application to broken or inflamed skin or mucous membranes may lead to increased systemic absorption. Use caution in patients with severe hepatic disease or pseudocholinesterase deficiency. Remove patch prior to MRI. Not for use at home.

Drug Interactions

Cytochrome P450 Effect: Lidocaine: **Substrate** of CYP1A2 (minor), 2A6 (minor), 2B6 (minor), 2C8/9 (minor), 2D6 (major), 3A4 (major); **Inhibits** CYP1A2 (strong), 2D6 (strong), 3A4 (moderate)

Increased Effect/Toxicity: See individual agents. With administration with class I antiarrhythmic agents (eg, mexiletine), effects are additive and potentially synergistic.

Pharmacodynamics/Kinetics

Also see individual agents.

Absorption: Related to duration of application and area where applied.

Pregnancy Risk Factor B

Dosage Forms PATCH, transdermal system: Lidocaine 70 mg and tetracaine 70 mg (2s, 10s)

Lidocaine Hydrochloride see Lidocaine on page 920

Lidocaine Hydrochloride and Bupivacaine Hydrochloride see Lidocaine and Bupivacaine on page 924

Lidocaine (Transoral) (LYE doe kane trans OR al)

Related Information

Lidocaine on page 920
Oral Pain on page 1692

U.S. Brand Names DentiPatch®

Generic Available No

Pharmacologic Category Local Anesthetic, Transoral

Dental Use

Local anesthesia of the oral mucosa prior to oral injections and soft-tissue dental procedures

Use Local anesthesia of the oral mucosa prior to oral injections and soft-tissue dental procedures

Local Anesthetic/Vasoconstrictor Precautions No information available to require special precautions

Effects on Dental Treatment No significant effects or complications reported (see Dental Comment)

Significant Adverse Effects No data reported

Dental Usual Dosing Local anesthesia of the oral mucosa (prior to oral injections): Adults: Topical: One patch on selected area of oral mucosa

Dosage One patch on selected area of oral mucosa

(Continued)

Lidocaine (Transoral) (Continued)

Mechanism of Action Blocks both the initiation and conduction of nerve impulses by decreasing the neuronal membrane's permeability to sodium ions, which results in inhibition of depolarization with resultant blockade of conduction

Contraindications Hypersensitivity to lidocaine or any of component of the formulation

Dietary Considerations Oral patch with lidocaine 46.1 mg/2 cm^2 contains phenylalanine 0.62 mg.

Pharmacodynamics/Kinetics

Onset of action: 2 minutes

Duration: Anesthesia: 40 minutes after 15-minute wear period

Dosage Forms Patch, oral: 46.1 mg/2 cm^2 (50s, 100s) [contains phenylalanine 0.62 mg/patch; spearmint flavor]

Dental Comment Peak plasma levels were 10% of those seen following local infiltration anesthesia with 1.8 mL lidocaine and 1:100,000 epinephrine.

The manufacturer claims DentiPatch® is safe, with "negligible systemic absorption" of lidocaine. The agent is "clinically proven to prevent injection pain from 25-gauge needles that are inserted to the level of the bone." Data from controlled studies (235 patients) have shown no serious adverse effects with the application of lidocaine patch to the oral mucosa for 15 minutes.

Selected Readings

Hersh EV, Houpt MI, Cooper SA, et al, "Analgesic Efficacy and Safety of an Intraoral Lidocaine Patch," *J Am Dent Assoc*, 1996, 127(11):1626-34.

Houpt MI, Heins P, Lamster I, et al, "An Evaluation of Intraoral Lidocaine Patches in Reducing Needle-Insertion Pain," *Compend Contin Educ Dent*, 1997, 18(4):309-10, 312-4, 316.

"The Lidocaine Patch: A New Delivery System," *Biolog Ther Dent*, 1997, 13:17-22.

Lidoderm® *see* Lidocaine *on page 920*

LidoSite™ *see* Lidocaine and Epinephrine *on page 924*

Lignocaine Hydrochloride *see* Lidocaine *on page 920*

Lilly CT-3231 *see* Vindesine *on page 1577*

Limbitrol® *see* Amitriptyline and Chlordiazepoxide *on page 97*

Limbitrol® DS *see* Amitriptyline and Chlordiazepoxide *on page 97*

Limbrel™ *see* Flavocoxid *on page 656*

Lincocin® *see* Lincomycin *on page 932*

Lincomycin (lin koe MYE sin)

U.S. Brand Names Lincocin®

Canadian Brand Names Lincocin®

Mexican Brand Names Lincocin®; Princol®; Rimsalin®

Generic Available No

Synonyms Lincomycin Hydrochloride

Pharmacologic Category Antibiotic, Lincosamide

Use Treatment of serious susceptible bacterial infections, mainly those caused by streptococci and staphylococci resistant to other agents

Local Anesthetic/Vasoconstrictor Precautions No information available to require special precautions

Effects on Dental Treatment No significant effects or complications reported

Common Adverse Effects Frequency not defined.

Cardiovascular: Cardiopulmonary arrest and hypotension (I.V. infusion, rate related)

Central nervous system: Vertigo

Dermatologic: Dermatitis (exfoliative, vesiculobullous); erythema multiforme, rash, urticaria

Gastrointestinal: Colitis, diarrhea, glossitis, nausea, pruritus ani, stomatitis, vomiting

Genitourinary: Vaginitis

Hematologic: Agranulocytosis, aplastic anemia, leukopenia, neutropenia, pancytopenia, thrombocytopenic purpura

Hepatic: Jaundice, liver function test abnormalities

Otic: Tinnitus

Renal: Azotemia, proteinuria, oliguria

Miscellaneous: Hypersensitivity reactions (anaphylaxis, angioneurotic edema, serum sickness)

Mechanism of Action Lincosamide antibiotic which was isolated from a strain of *Streptomyces lincolnensis*; lincomycin, like clindamycin, inhibits bacterial protein synthesis by specifically binding on the 50S subunit and affecting the process of peptide chain initiation. Other macrolide antibiotics (erythromycin) also bind to the 50S subunit. Since only one molecule of antibiotic can bind to a single ribosome, the concomitant use of erythromycin and lincomycin is not recommended.

Drug Interactions
  Increased Effect/Toxicity: Lincomycin may enhance the neuromuscular-blocking effect; use with caution.
  Decreased Effect: Lincomycin may diminish the therapeutic effect of erythromycin; concomitant use is not recommended.

Pharmacodynamics/Kinetics
  Metabolism: Hepatic
  Half-life elimination, serum: ~5 hours; prolonged with renal or hepatic impairment
  Time to peak, serum: I.M.: 1 hour
  Excretion: Urine (2% to 30%); bile

Pregnancy Risk Factor C

Lincomycin Hydrochloride *see* Lincomycin *on page 932*

Lindane (LIN dane)

Canadian Brand Names Hexit™; PMS-Lindane
Mexican Brand Names Herklin Shampoo®; Scabisan®
Generic Available Yes
Synonyms Benzene Hexachloride; Gamma Benzene Hexachloride; Hexachlorocyclohexane
Pharmacologic Category Antiparasitic Agent, Topical; Pediculocide; Scabicidal Agent
Use Treatment of *Sarcoptes scabiei* (scabies), *Pediculus capitis* (head lice), and *Phthirus pubis* (crab lice); FDA recommends reserving lindane as a second-line agent or with inadequate response to other therapies
Local Anesthetic/Vasoconstrictor Precautions No information available to require special precautions
Effects on Dental Treatment No significant effects or complications reported
Common Adverse Effects Frequency not defined (includes postmarketing and/or case reports).
  Cardiovascular: Cardiac arrhythmia
  Central nervous system: Ataxia, dizziness, headache, restlessness, seizure, pain
  Dermatologic: Alopecia, contact dermatitis, skin and adipose tissue may act as repositories, eczematous eruptions, pruritus, urticaria
  Gastrointestinal: Nausea, vomiting
  Hematologic: Aplastic anemia
  Hepatic: Hepatitis
  Local: Burning and stinging
  Neuromuscular & skeletal: Paresthesias
  Renal: Hematuria
  Respiratory: Pulmonary edema
Restrictions An FDA-approved medication guide is available at http://www.fda.gov/cder/Offices/ODS/labeling.htm; distribute to each patient to whom this medication is dispensed.
Mechanism of Action Directly absorbed by parasites and ova through the exoskeleton; stimulates the nervous system resulting in seizures and death of parasitic arthropods
Drug Interactions
  Increased Effect/Toxicity: Increased toxicity: Drugs which lower seizure threshold
Pharmacodynamics/Kinetics
  Absorption: ≤13% systemically
  Distribution: Stored in body fat; accumulates in brain; skin and adipose tissue may act as repositories
  Metabolism: Hepatic
  Half-life elimination: Children: 17-22 hours
  Time to peak, serum: Children: 6 hours
  Excretion: Urine and feces
Pregnancy Risk Factor C

Linezolid (li NE zoh lid)

U.S. Brand Names Zyvox™
Canadian Brand Names Zyvoxam®
Generic Available No
(Continued)

Linezolid *(Continued)*

Pharmacologic Category Antibiotic, Oxazolidinone

Use Treatment of vancomycin-resistant *Enterococcus faecium* (VRE) infections, nosocomial pneumonia caused by *Staphylococcus aureus* including MRSA or *Streptococcus pneumoniae* (including multidrug-resistant strains [MDRSP]), complicated and uncomplicated skin and skin structure infections (including diabetic foot infections without concomitant osteomyelitis), and community-acquired pneumonia caused by susceptible gram-positive organisms

Local Anesthetic/Vasoconstrictor Precautions Linezolid has mild monoamine oxidase inhibitor properties. The clinician is reminded that vasoconstrictors have the potential to interact with MAOIs to result in elevation of blood pressure. Caution is suggested.

Effects on Dental Treatment Key adverse event(s) related to dental treatment: Oral moniliasis, taste alteration, and tongue discoloration.

Common Adverse Effects Percentages as reported in adults; frequency similar in pediatric patients

>10%:
Central nervous system: Headache (<1% to 11%)
Gastrointestinal: Diarrhea (3% to 11%)

1% to 10%:
Central nervous system: Insomnia (3%), dizziness (0.4% to 2%), fever (2%)
Dermatologic: Rash (2%)
Gastrointestinal: Nausea (3% to 10%), vomiting (1% to 4%), pancreatic enzymes increased (<1% to 4%), constipation (2%), taste alteration (1% to 2%), tongue discoloration (0.2% to 1%), oral moniliasis (0.4% to 1%), pancreatitis
Genitourinary: Vaginal moniliasis (1% to 2%)
Hematologic: Thrombocytopenia (0.3% to 10%), hemoglobin decreased (0.9% to 7%), anemia, leukopenia, neutropenia; **Note:** Myelosuppression (including anemia, leukopenia, pancytopenia, and thrombocytopenia; may be more common in patients receiving linezolid for >2 weeks)
Hepatic: Abnormal LFTs (0.4% to 1%)
Renal: BUN increased (<1% to 2%)
Miscellaneous: Fungal infection (0.1% to 2%), lactate dehydrogenase increased (<1% to 2%)

Mechanism of Action Inhibits bacterial protein synthesis by binding to bacterial 23S ribosomal RNA of the 50S subunit. This prevents the formation of a functional 70S initiation complex that is essential for the bacterial translation process. Linezolid is bacteriostatic against enterococci and staphylococci and bactericidal against most strains of streptococci.

Drug Interactions

Increased Effect/Toxicity: Linezolid is a reversible, nonselective inhibitor of MAO. Serotonergic agents (eg, TCAs, venlafaxine, trazodone, sibutramine, meperidine, dextromethorphan, and SSRIs) may cause a serotonin syndrome (eg, hyperpyrexia, cognitive dysfunction) when used concomitantly. Adrenergic agents (eg, phenylpropanolamine, pseudoephedrine, sympathomimetic agents, vasopressor or dopaminergic agents) may cause hypertension. Tramadol may increase the risk of seizures when used concurrently with linezolid. Myelosuppressive medications may increase risk of myelosuppression when used concurrently with linezolid.

Pharmacodynamics/Kinetics

Absorption: Rapid and extensive
Distribution: V_{dss}: Adults: 40-50 L
Protein binding: Adults: 31%
Metabolism: Hepatic via oxidation of the morpholine ring, resulting in two inactive metabolites (aminoethoxyacetic acid, hydroxyethyl glycine); does not involve CYP
Bioavailability: 100%
Half-life elimination: Children ≥1 week (full-term) to 11 years: 1.5-3 hours; Adults: 4-5 hours
Time to peak: Adults: Oral: 1-2 hours
Excretion: Urine (30% as parent drug, 50% as metabolites); feces (9% as metabolites)
Nonrenal clearance: 65%; increased in children ≥1 week to 11 years

Pregnancy Risk Factor C

Lioresal® *see Baclofen on page 178*

Liothyronine *(lye oh THYE roe neen)*

Related Information
Endocrine Disorders and Pregnancy *on page 1659*

U.S. Brand Names Cytomel®; Triostat®
Canadian Brand Names Cytomel®
Mexican Brand Names Triyotex®
Generic Available No
Synonyms Liothyronine Sodium; Sodium *L*-Triiodothyronine; T_3 Sodium (error-prone abbreviation)
Pharmacologic Category Thyroid Product
Use
 Oral: Replacement or supplemental therapy in hypothyroidism; management of nontoxic goiter; a diagnostic aid
 I.V.: Treatment of myxedema coma/precoma
Local Anesthetic/Vasoconstrictor Precautions No precautions with vaso-constrictor are necessary if patient is well controlled with liothyronine
Effects on Dental Treatment No significant effects or complications reported
Common Adverse Effects 1% to 10%: Cardiovascular: Arrhythmia (6%), tach-ycardia (3%), cardiopulmonary arrest (2%), hypotension (2%), MI (2%)
Mechanism of Action Exact mechanism of action is unknown; however, it is believed the thyroid hormone exerts its many metabolic effects through control of DNA transcription and protein synthesis; involved in normal metabolism, growth, and development; promotes gluconeogenesis, increases utilization and mobilization of glycogen stores, and stimulates protein synthesis, increases basal metabolic rate
Drug Interactions
 Increased Effect/Toxicity: Thyroid products may potentiate the hypopro-thrombinemic effect of warfarin (and other oral anticoagulants). Tricyclic anti-depressants (TCAs) may increase potential for toxicity of both drugs. Coadministration with ketamine may lead to hypertension and tachycardia.
 Decreased Effect: Some medications may decrease absorption of liothyro-nine: Cholestyramine, colestipol (separate administration by at least 2 hours); aluminum- and magnesium-containing antacids, iron preparations, sucralfate, Kayexalate® (separate administration by at least 4 hours). Enzyme inducers (phenytoin, phenobarbital, carbamazepine, and rifampin/rifabutin) may decrease thyroid hormone levels. Thyroid hormone may decrease effect of oral sulfonylureas. Serum levels of digoxin and theophylline may be altered by thyroid function. Estrogens may decrease serum free-thyroxine concentra-tions.
Pharmacodynamics/Kinetics
 Onset of action: 2-4 hours
 Peak response: 2-3 days
 Absorption: Oral: Well absorbed (95% in 4 hours)
 Half-life elimination: 2.5 days
 Excretion: Urine
Pregnancy Risk Factor A

Liothyronine Sodium see Liothyronine on page 934

Liotrix (LYE oh triks)

Related Information
 Endocrine Disorders and Pregnancy on page 1659
U.S. Brand Names Thyrolar®
Canadian Brand Names Thyrolar®
Generic Available No
Synonyms T_3/T_4 Liotrix
Pharmacologic Category Thyroid Product
Use Replacement or supplemental therapy in hypothyroidism (uniform mixture of T_4:T_3 in 4:1 ratio by weight); little advantage to this product exists and cost is not justified
Local Anesthetic/Vasoconstrictor Precautions No precautions with vaso-constrictor are necessary if patient is well controlled with liotrix
Effects on Dental Treatment No significant effects or complications reported
Common Adverse Effects Frequency not defined.
 Cardiovascular: Palpitations, cardiac arrhythmia, tachycardia, chest pain
 Central nervous system: Nervousness, headache, insomnia, fever, ataxia
 Dermatologic: Alopecia
 Endocrine & metabolic: Changes in menstrual cycle, weight loss, increased appetite
 Gastrointestinal: Diarrhea, abdominal cramps, constipation, vomiting
 Neuromuscular & skeletal: Myalgia, hand tremor, tremor
 Respiratory: Dyspnea
 Miscellaneous: Diaphoresis, allergic skin reactions (rare)
 (Continued)

Liotrix *(Continued)*

Mechanism of Action The primary active compound is T_3 (triiodothyronine), which may be converted from T_4 (thyroxine) and then circulates throughout the body to influence growth and maturation of various tissues. Liotrix is uniform mixture of synthetic T_4 and T_3 in 4:1 ratio; exact mechanism of action is unknown; however, it is believed the thyroid hormone exerts its many metabolic effects through control of DNA transcription and protein synthesis; involved in normal metabolism, growth, and development; promotes gluconeogenesis, increases utilization and mobilization of glycogen stores and stimulates protein synthesis, increases basal metabolic rate

Drug Interactions

Increased Effect/Toxicity: Thyroid products may potentiate the hypoprothrombinemic effect of warfarin (and other oral anticoagulants). Effect of warfarin may be dramatically increased when thyroid is added. However, the addition of warfarin in a patient previously receiving a stable dose of thyroid hormone does not require a significantly different dosing strategy. Tricyclic antidepressants (TCAs) may increase potential for toxicity of both drugs. Excessive thyroid replacement in patients receiving growth hormone may lead to accelerated epiphyseal closure; inadequate replacement interferes with growth response. Coadministration with ketamine may lead to hypertension and tachycardia.

Decreased Effect: Aluminum- and magnesium-containing antacids, iron preparations, sucralfate, cholestyramine, colestipol, and Kayexalate® may decrease absorption (separate administration by 8 hours). Thyroid hormone may decrease effect of oral sulfonylureas. Dosage of thyroid hormone may need to be increased when SSRIs are added. Serum levels of digoxin and theophylline may be altered by thyroid function.

Pharmacodynamics/Kinetics
Absorption: 50% to 95%
Metabolism: Partially hepatic, renal, and in intestines
Half-life elimination: 6-7 days
Time to peak, serum: 12-48 hours
Excretion: Partially feces (as conjugated metabolites)

Pregnancy Risk Factor A

Lipancreatin *see* Pancrelipase *on page 1183*

Lipitor® *see* Atorvastatin *on page 158*

Lipofen™ *see* Fenofibrate *on page 639*

Liposyn® III *see* Fat Emulsion *on page 637*

Lipram 4500 *see* Pancrelipase *on page 1183*

Lipram-CR *see* Pancrelipase *on page 1183*

Lipram-PN *see* Pancrelipase *on page 1183*

Lipram-UL *see* Pancrelipase *on page 1183*

Liquibid-D *see* Guaifenesin and Phenylephrine *on page 754*

Liquibid-PD *see* Guaifenesin and Phenylephrine *on page 754*

Liqui-Coat HD® *see* Barium *on page 179*

Liquid Antidote *see* Charcoal *on page 311*

Liquid Barosperse® *see* Barium *on page 179*

Liquifilm® Tears [OTC] *see* Artificial Tears *on page 143*

Lisinopril *(lyse IN oh pril)*

Related Information
Cardiovascular Diseases *on page 1636*
U.S. Brand Names Prinivil®; Zestril®
Canadian Brand Names Apo-Lisinopril®; Prinivil®; Zestril®
Mexican Brand Names Alfaken®; Prinivil®; Zestril®
Generic Available Yes
Pharmacologic Category Angiotensin-Converting Enzyme (ACE) Inhibitor
Use Treatment of hypertension, either alone or in combination with other antihypertensive agents; adjunctive therapy in treatment of CHF (afterload reduction); treatment of acute myocardial infarction within 24 hours in hemodynamically-stable patients to improve survival; treatment of left ventricular dysfunction after myocardial infarction
Local Anesthetic/Vasoconstrictor Precautions No information available to require special precautions
Effects on Dental Treatment Key adverse event(s) related to dental treatment: Orthostatic effects.
Common Adverse Effects Note: Frequency ranges include data from hypertension and heart failure trials. Higher rates of adverse reactions have generally

been noted in patients with CHF. However, the frequency of adverse effects associated with placebo is also increased in this population.

1% to 10%:
  Cardiovascular: Orthostatic effects (1%), hypotension (1% to 4%)
  Central nervous system: Headache (4% to 6%), dizziness (5% to 12%), fatigue (3%)
  Dermatologic: Rash (1% to 2%)
  Endocrine & metabolic: Hyperkalemia (2% to 5%)
  Gastrointestinal: Diarrhea (3% to 4%), nausea (2%), vomiting (1%), abdominal pain (2%)
  Genitourinary: Impotence (1%)
  Hematologic: Decreased hemoglobin (small)
  Neuromuscular & skeletal: Chest pain (3%), weakness (1%)
  Renal: BUN increased (2%); deterioration in renal function (in patients with bilateral renal artery stenosis or hypovolemia); serum creatinine increased (often transient)
  Respiratory: Cough (4% to 9%), upper respiratory infection (2% to 2%)

Dosage Oral:
  Hypertension:
    Children ≥6 years: Initial: 0.07 mg/kg once daily (up to 5 mg); increase dose at 1- to 2-week intervals; doses >0.61 mg/kg or >40 mg have not been evaluated.
    Adults: Usual dosage range (JNC 7): 10-40 mg/day
    Not maintained on diuretic: Initial: 10 mg/day
    Maintained on diuretic: Initial: 5 mg/day
    Note: Antihypertensive effect may diminish toward the end of the dosing interval especially with doses of 10 mg/day. An increased dose may aid in extending the duration of antihypertensive effect. Doses up to 80 mg/day have been used, but do not appear to give greater effect (Zestoril® Product Information, 12/04).
    Elderly: Initial: 2.5-5 mg/day; increase doses 2.5-5 mg/day at 1- to 2-week intervals; maximum daily dose: 40 mg
    Patients taking diuretics should have them discontinued 2-3 days prior to initiating lisinopril if possible. Restart diuretic after blood pressure is stable if needed. If diuretic cannot be discontinued prior to therapy, begin with 5 mg with close supervision until stable blood pressure. In patients with hyponatremia (<130 mEq/L), start dose at 2.5 mg/day
  Congestive heart failure: Adults: Initial: 2.5-5 mg once daily; then increase by no more than 10 mg increments at intervals no less than 2 weeks to a maximum daily dose of 40 mg. Usual maintenance: 5-40 mg/day as a single dose. Target dose: 20-40 mg once daily (ACC/AHA 2005 Heart Failure Guidelines)
    Note: If patient has hyponatremia (serum sodium <130 meq/L) or renal impairment (Cl$_{cr}$ <30 mL/minute or creatinine >3 mg/dL), then initial dose should be 2.5 mg/day
  Acute myocardial infarction (within 24 hours in hemodynamically stable patients): Oral: 5 mg immediately, then 5 mg at 24 hours, 10 mg at 48 hours, and 10 mg every day thereafter for 6 weeks. Patients should continue to receive standard treatments such as thrombolytics, aspirin, and beta-blockers.

  Dosing adjustment in renal impairment:
    Hypertension:
      Adults: Initial doses should be modified and upward titration should be cautious, based on response (maximum: 40 mg/day)
        Cl$_{cr}$ >30 mL/minute: Initial: 10 mg/day
        Cl$_{cr}$ 10-30 mL/minute: Initial: 5 mg/day
      Hemodialysis: Initial: 2.5 mg/day; dialyzable (50%)
      Children: Use in not recommended in pediatric patients with GFR <30 mL/minute/1.73 m^2
    Congestive heart failure: Adults: Cl$_{cr}$ <30 mL/minute or creatinine >3 mg/dL): Initial: 2.5 mg/day

Mechanism of Action Competitive inhibitor of angiotensin-converting enzyme (ACE); prevents conversion of angiotensin I to angiotensin II, a potent vasoconstrictor; results in lower levels of angiotensin II which causes an increase in plasma renin activity and a reduction in aldosterone secretion; a CNS mechanism may also be involved in hypotensive effect as angiotensin II increases adrenergic outflow from CNS; vasoactive kallikreins may be decreased in conversion to active hormones by ACE inhibitors, thus reducing blood pressure

Contraindications Hypersensitivity to lisinopril or any component of the formulation; angioedema related to previous treatment with an ACE inhibitor; bilateral renal artery stenosis; pregnancy (2nd and 3rd trimesters)

Warnings/Precautions Anaphylactic reactions can occur. Angioedema can occur at any time during treatment (especially following first dose). It may (Continued)

Lisinopril *(Continued)*

involve head and neck (potentially affecting the airway) or the intestine (presenting with abdominal pain). Prolonged monitoring may be required especially if tongue, glottis, or larynx are involved as they are associated with airway obstruction. Those with a history of airway surgery in this situation have a higher risk. Careful blood pressure monitoring with first dose (hypotension can occur especially in volume depleted patients). Dosage adjustment needed in renal impairment. Use with caution in hypovolemia; collagen vascular diseases; valvular stenosis (particularly aortic stenosis); hyperkalemia; or before, during, or immediately after anesthesia. Avoid rapid dosage escalation, which may lead to renal insufficiency. Rare toxicities associated with ACE inhibitors include cholestatic jaundice (which may progress to hepatic necrosis) and neutropenia/ agranulocytosis with myeloid hyperplasia. If patient has renal impairment then a baseline WBC with differential and serum creatinine should be evaluated and monitored closely during the first 3 months of therapy. Hypersensitivity reactions may be seen during hemodialysis with high-flux dialysis membranes (eg, AN69). Deterioration in renal function can occur with initiation. Use with caution in unilateral renal artery stenosis and pre-existing renal insufficiency. Safety and efficacy have not been established in children <6 years of age.

Drug Interactions

Increased Effect/Toxicity: Potassium supplements, co-trimoxazole (high dose), angiotensin II receptor antagonists (eg, candesartan, losartan, irbesartan), or potassium-sparing diuretics (amiloride, spironolactone, triamterene) may result in elevated serum potassium levels when combined with lisinopril. ACE inhibitor effects may be increased by phenothiazines or probenecid (increases levels of captopril). ACE inhibitors may increase serum concentrations/effects of lithium.

Diuretics have additive hypotensive effects with ACE inhibitors, and hypovolemia increases the potential for adverse renal effects of ACE inhibitors. In patients with compromised renal function, coadministration with NSAIDs may result in further deterioration of renal function. Allopurinol and ACE inhibitors may cause a higher risk of hypersensitivity reaction when taken concurrently.

Decreased Effect: Aspirin (high dose) may reduce the therapeutic effects of ACE inhibitors; at low dosages this does not appear to be significant. Rifampin may decrease the effect of ACE inhibitors. Antacids may decrease the bioavailability of ACE inhibitors (may be more likely to occur with captopril); separate administration times by 1-2 hours. NSAIDs, specifically indomethacin, may reduce the hypotensive effects of ACE inhibitors. More likely to occur in low renin or volume dependent hypertensive patients.

Ethanol/Nutrition/Herb Interactions Herb/Nutraceutical: Avoid dong quai if using for hypertension (has estrogenic activity). Avoid ephedra, yohimbe, ginseng (may worsen hypertension). Avoid garlic (may have increased antihypertensive effect).

Pharmacodynamics/Kinetics

Onset of action: 1 hour

Peak effect: Hypotensive: Oral: ~6 hours

Duration: 24 hours

Absorption: Well absorbed; unaffected by food

Protein binding: 25%

Half-life elimination: 11-12 hours

Excretion: Primarily urine (as unchanged drug)

Pregnancy Risk Factor C (1st trimester)/D (2nd and 3rd trimesters)

Dosage Forms TAB: 2.5 mg, 5 mg, 10 mg, 20 mg, 30 mg, 40 mg; (Prinivil®): 5 mg, 10 mg, 20 mg, 30 mg; (Zestril®): 2.5 mg, 5 mg, 10 mg, 20 mg, 30 mg, 40 mg

---

Lisinopril and Hydrochlorothiazide

(lyse IN oh pril & hye droe klor oh THYE a zide)

Related Information

Cardiovascular Diseases *on page 1636*
Hydrochlorothiazide *on page 776*
Lisinopril *on page 936*

U.S. Brand Names Prinzide®; Zestoretic®

Canadian Brand Names Prinzide®; Zestoretic®

Generic Available Yes

Synonyms Hydrochlorothiazide and Lisinopril

Pharmacologic Category Antihypertensive Agent, Combination

Use Treatment of hypertension

Local Anesthetic/Vasoconstrictor Precautions No information available to require special precautions

Effects on Dental Treatment No significant effects or complications reported

Common Adverse Effects See individual agents.

Drug Interactions
Increased Effect/Toxicity: See individual agents.
Decreased Effect: See individual agents.

Pharmacodynamics/Kinetics See individual agents.

Pregnancy Risk Factor C/D (2nd and 3rd trimesters)

Lispro Insulin *see* Insulin Lispro *on page 839*

Lithium (LITH ee um)

U.S. Brand Names Eskalith® [DSC]; Eskalith CR®; Lithobid®
Canadian Brand Names Apo-Lithium®; Apo-Lithium® Carbonate SR; Carbo-lith™; Duralith®; Lithane™; PMS-Lithium Carbonate; PMS-Lithium Citrate
Mexican Brand Names Carbolit®; Litheum®
Generic Available Yes
Synonyms Lithium Carbonate; Lithium Citrate
Pharmacologic Category Lithium
Use Management of bipolar disorders; treatment of mania in individuals with bipolar disorder (maintenance treatment prevents or diminishes intensity of subsequent episodes)
Unlabeled/Investigational Use Potential augmenting agent for antidepressants; aggression, post-traumatic stress disorder, conduct disorder in children
Local Anesthetic/Vasoconstrictor Precautions No information available to require special precautions
Effects on Dental Treatment Avoid NSAIDs if analgesics are required since lithium toxicity has been reported with concomitant administration; acetaminophen products (ie, singly or with narcotics) are recommended.
Common Adverse Effects Frequency not defined.
Cardiovascular: Cardiac arrhythmia, hypotension, sinus node dysfunction, flattened or inverted T waves (reversible), edema, bradycardia, syncope
Central nervous system: Dizziness, vertigo, slurred speech, blackout spells, seizure, sedation, restlessness, confusion, psychomotor retardation, stupor, coma, dystonia, fatigue, lethargy, headache, pseudotumor cerebri, slowed intellectual functioning, tics
Dermatologic: Dry or thinning of hair, folliculitis, alopecia, exacerbation of psoriasis, rash
Endocrine & metabolic: Euthyroid goiter and/or hypothyroidism, hyperthyroidism, hyperglycemia, diabetes insipidus
Gastrointestinal: Polydipsia, anorexia, nausea, vomiting, diarrhea, xerostomia, metallic taste, weight gain, salivary gland swelling, excessive salivation
Genitourinary: Incontinence, polyuria, glycosuria, oliguria, albuminuria
Hematologic: Leukocytosis
Neuromuscular & skeletal: Tremor, muscle hyperirritability, ataxia, choreoathetoid movements, hyperactive deep tendon reflexes, myasthenia gravis (rare)
Ocular: Nystagmus, blurred vision, transient scotoma
Miscellaneous: Coldness and painful discoloration of fingers and toes
Mechanism of Action Alters cation transport across cell membrane in nerve and muscle cells and influences reuptake of serotonin and/or norepinephrine; second messenger systems involving the phosphatidylinositol cycle are inhibited; postsynaptic D2 receptor supersensitivity is inhibited
Drug Interactions
Increased Effect/Toxicity: Concurrent use of lithium with carbamazepine, diltiazem, SSRIs (fluoxetine, fluvoxamine), haloperidol, methyldopa, metronidazole (rare), phenothiazines, phenytoin, TCAs, and verapamil may increase the risk for neurotoxicity. A rare encephalopathic syndrome has been reported in association with haloperidol (causal relationship not established). Lithium concentrations/toxicity may be increased by diuretics, NSAIDs (sulindac and aspirin may be exceptions), ACE inhibitors, angiotensin receptor antagonists (losartan), tetracyclines, or COX-2 inhibitors (celecoxib).

Lithium and MAO inhibitors should generally be avoided due to use reports of fatal malignant hyperpyrexia; risk with selective MAO type B inhibitors (selegiline) appears to be lower. Potassium iodide may enhance the hypothyroid effects of lithium. Combined use of lithium with tricyclic antidepressants or sibutramine may increase the risk of serotonin syndrome; this combination is best avoided. Lithium may potentiate effect of neuromuscular blockers.
Decreased Effect: Combined use of lithium and chlorpromazine may lower serum concentrations of both drugs. Lithium may blunt the pressor response

(Continued)

Lithium *(Continued)*

to sympathomimetics (epinephrine, norepinephrine). Caffeine (xanthine derivatives) may lower lithium serum concentrations by increasing urinary lithium excretion (monitor).

Pharmacodynamics/Kinetics

Absorption: Rapid and complete

Distribution: V_d: Initial: 0.3-0.4 L/kg; V_{dss}: 0.7-1 L/kg; crosses placenta; enters breast milk at 35% to 50% the concentrations in serum; distribution is complete in 6-10 hours

CSF, liver concentrations: $1/3$ to $1/2$ of serum concentration

Erythrocyte concentration: ~$1/2$ of serum concentration

Heart, lung, kidney, muscle concentrations: Equivalent to serum concentration

Saliva concentration: 2-3 times serum concentration

Thyroid, bone, brain tissue concentrations: Increase 50% over serum concentrations

Protein binding: Not protein bound

Metabolism: Not metabolized

Bioavailability: Not affected by food; Capsule, immediate release tablet: 95% to 100%; Extended release tablet: 60% to 90%; Syrup: 100%

Half-life elimination: 18-24 hours; can increase to more than 36 hours in elderly or with renal impairment

Time to peak, serum: Nonsustained release: ~0.5-2 hours; slow release: 4-12 hours; syrup: 15-60 minutes

Excretion: Urine (90% to 98% as unchanged drug); sweat (4% to 5%); feces (1%)

Clearance: 80% of filtered lithium is reabsorbed in the proximal convoluted tubules; therefore, clearance approximates 20% of GFR or 20-40 mL/minute

Pregnancy Risk Factor D

Lithium Carbonate *see* Lithium *on page 939*

Lithium Citrate *see* Lithium *on page 939*

Lithobid® *see* Lithium *on page 939*

Lithostat® *see* Acetohydroxamic Acid *on page 46*

Live Attenuated Influenza Vaccine (LAIV) *see* Influenza Virus Vaccine *on page 833*

Livostin® [DSC] *see* Levocabastine *on page 910*

L-Lysine Hydrochloride *see* L-Lysine *on page 959*

LMD® *see* Dextran *on page 447*

LNg 20 *see* Levonorgestrel *on page 916*

Locoid® *see* Hydrocortisone *on page 793*

Locoid Lipocream® *see* Hydrocortisone *on page 793*

Lodine® [DSC] *see* Etodolac *on page 623*

Lodine® XL [DSC] *see* Etodolac *on page 623*

Lodosyn® *see* Carbidopa *on page 267*

Lodoxamide *(loe DOKS a mide)*

U.S. Brand Names Alomide®

Canadian Brand Names Alomide®

Generic Available No

Synonyms Lodoxamide Tromethamine

Pharmacologic Category Mast Cell Stabilizer

Use Treatment of vernal keratoconjunctivitis, vernal conjunctivitis, and vernal keratitis

Local Anesthetic/Vasoconstrictor Precautions No information available to require special precautions

Effects on Dental Treatment No significant effects or complications reported

Common Adverse Effects

>10%: Local: Transient burning, stinging, discomfort

1% to 10%:

Central nervous system: Headache

Ocular: Blurred vision, corneal erosion/ulcer, eye pain, corneal abrasion, blepharitis

Mechanism of Action Mast cell stabilizer that inhibits the *in vivo* type I immediate hypersensitivity reaction to increase cutaneous vascular permeability associated with IgE and antigen-mediated reactions

Pharmacodynamics/Kinetics Absorption: Topical: Negligible

Pregnancy Risk Factor B

Lodoxamide Tromethamine *see* Lodoxamide *on page 940*

Lodrane® *see* Brompheniramine and Pseudoephedrine *on page 223*

Lodrane® 12D *see* Brompheniramine and Pseudoephedrine *on page 223*

Lodrane® LD *see* Brompheniramine and Pseudoephedrine *on page 223*

Loestrin® *see* Ethinyl Estradiol and Norethindrone *on page 608*

Loestrin® 24 Fe *see* Ethinyl Estradiol and Norethindrone *on page 608*

Loestrin® Fe *see* Ethinyl Estradiol and Norethindrone *on page 608*

Lofibra™ *see* Fenofibrate *on page 639*

LoHist-D *see* Chlorpheniramine and Pseudoephedrine *on page 325*

L-OHP *see* Oxaliplatin *on page 1154*

LoKara™ *see* Desonide *on page 437*

Lomefloxacin (loe me FLOKS a sin)

Related Information
Sexually-Transmitted Diseases *on page 1674*
U.S. Brand Names Maxaquin® [DSC]
Mexican Brand Names Lomacin®; Maxaquin®
Generic Available No
Synonyms Lomefloxacin Hydrochloride
Pharmacologic Category Antibiotic, Quinolone
Use Acute bacterial exacerbation of chronic bronchitis caused by susceptible gram-negative organisms; urinary tract infections (uncomplicated and complicated) caused by susceptible organisms; surgical prophylaxis (transrectal prostate biopsy or transurethral procedures)
Local Anesthetic/Vasoconstrictor Precautions No information available to require special precautions
Effects on Dental Treatment No significant effects or complications reported
Common Adverse Effects 1% to 10%:
Central nervous system: Headache (4%), dizziness (2%)
Dermatologic: Photosensitivity (2%)
Gastrointestinal: Nausea (4%), abdominal pain (1%), diarrhea (1%)
Mechanism of Action Inhibits DNA-gyrase in susceptible organisms thereby inhibits relaxation of supercoiled DNA and promotes breakage of DNA strands. DNA gyrase (topoisomerase II), is an essential bacterial enzyme that maintains the superhelical structure of DNA and is required for DNA replication and transcription, DNA repair, recombination, and transposition.
Drug Interactions
Cytochrome P450 Effect: Inhibits CYP1A2 (weak)
Increased Effect/Toxicity: Concomitant use with corticosteroids may increase the risk of tendon rupture. Probenecid may increase lomefloxacin levels.
Decreased Effect: Concurrent administration of metal cations, including most antacids, oral electrolyte supplements, quinapril, sucralfate, some didanosine formulations (chewable/buffered tablets and pediatric powder for oral suspension), and other highly-buffered oral drugs, may decrease quinolone level; separate doses.
Pharmacodynamics/Kinetics
Absorption: Well absorbed (95% to 98%)
Distribution: V_d: 2.4-3.5 L/kg; into bronchus, prostatic tissue, and urine
Protein binding: 10%
Half-life elimination: 7.8 hours
Time to peak, plasma: 1.5 hours
Excretion: Urine (65% as unchanged drug, 9% as metabolite); feces (10% as unchanged drug)
Pregnancy Risk Factor C

Lomefloxacin Hydrochloride *see* Lomefloxacin *on page 941*

Lomotil® *see* Diphenoxylate and Atropine *on page 487*

Lomustine (loe MUS teen)

U.S. Brand Names CeeNU®
Canadian Brand Names CeeNU®
Mexican Brand Names CeeNU®
Generic Available No
Synonyms CCNU
Pharmacologic Category Antineoplastic Agent, Alkylating Agent
Use Treatment of brain tumors and Hodgkin's disease, non-Hodgkin's lymphoma, melanoma, renal carcinoma, lung cancer, colon cancer
(Continued)

Lomustine (Continued)

Local Anesthetic/Vasoconstrictor Precautions No information available to require special precautions

Effects on Dental Treatment No significant effects or complications reported

Common Adverse Effects

>10%:

Gastrointestinal: Nausea and vomiting, usually within 3-6 hours after oral administration. Administration of the dose at bedtime, with an antiemetic, significantly reduces both the incidence and severity of nausea.

Hematologic: Myelosuppression, common, dose-limiting, may be cumulative and irreversible

Onset: 10-14 days

Nadir: Leukopenia: 6 weeks

Thrombocytopenia: 4 weeks

Recovery: 6-8 weeks

1% to 10%:

Dermatologic: Rash

Gastrointestinal: Anorexia, stomatitis, diarrhea

Genitourinary: Progressive azotemia, renal failure, decrease in kidney size

Hematologic: Anemia

Hepatic: Elevated liver enzymes, transient, reversible

Mechanism of Action Inhibits DNA and RNA synthesis via carbamylation of DNA polymerase, alkylation of DNA, and alteration of RNA, proteins, and enzymes

Drug Interactions

Cytochrome P450 Effect: Substrate of CYP2D6 (major); **Inhibits** CYP2D6 (weak), 3A4 (weak)

Increased Effect/Toxicity: CYP2D6 inhibitors may increase the levels/effects of lomustine; example inhibitors include chlorpromazine, delavirdine, fluoxetine, miconazole, paroxetine, pergolide, quinidine, quinine, ritonavir, and ropinirole. Increased toxicity with cimetidine, reported to cause bone marrow depression or to potentiate the myelosuppressive effects of lomustine.

Decreased Effect: Decreased effect with phenobarbital, resulting in reduced efficacy of both drugs.

Pharmacodynamics/Kinetics

Duration: Marrow recovery: ≤6 weeks

Absorption: Complete; appears in plasma within 3 minutes after administration

Distribution: Crosses blood-brain barrier to a greater degree than BCNU; CNS concentrations are equal to that of plasma

Protein binding: 50%

Metabolism: Rapidly hepatic via hydroxylation producing at least two active metabolites; enterohepatically recycled

Half-life elimination: Parent drug: 16-72 hours; Active metabolite: Terminal: 1.3-2 days

Time to peak, serum: Active metabolite: ~3 hours

Excretion: Urine; feces (<5%); expired air (<10%)

Pregnancy Risk Factor D

Loniten® see Minoxidil on page 1051

Lonox® see Diphenoxylate and Atropine on page 487

Lo/Ovral® see Ethinyl Estradiol and Norgestrel on page 616

Loperamide (loe PER a mide)

U.S. Brand Names Diamode [OTC]; Imodium® A-D [OTC]; Kao-Paverin® [OTC]; K-Pek II [OTC]

Canadian Brand Names Apo-Loperamide®; Diarr-Eze; Imodium®; Loperacap; Novo-Loperamide; PMS-Loperamine; Rho®-Loperamine; Riva-Loperamine

Mexican Brand Names Acanol®; Cryoperacid®; Pramidal®; Top-Dal®[tabs]

Generic Available Yes

Synonyms Loperamide Hydrochloride

Pharmacologic Category Antidiarrheal

Use Treatment of chronic diarrhea associated with inflammatory bowel disease; acute nonspecific diarrhea; increased volume of ileostomy discharge

OTC labeling: Control of symptoms of diarrhea, including Traveler's diarrhea

Unlabeled/Investigational Use Cancer treatment-induced diarrhea (eg, irinotecan induced); chronic diarrhea caused by bowel resection

Local Anesthetic/Vasoconstrictor Precautions No information available to require special precautions

Effects on Dental Treatment No significant effects or complications reported

Common Adverse Effects 1% to 10%:
Central nervous system: Dizziness (1%)
Gastrointestinal: Constipation (2% to 5%), abdominal cramping (<1% to 3%), nausea (<1% to 3%)
Postmarketing and/or case reports: Abdominal distention, abdominal pain, allergic reactions, anaphylactic shock, anaphylactoid reactions, angioedema, bullous eruption (rare), drowsiness, dry mouth, dyspepsia, erythema multiforme (rare), fatigue, flatulence, paralytic ileus, megacolon, pruritus, rash, Stevens-Johnson syndrome, toxic epidermal necrolysis, toxic megacolon, urinary retention, urticaria, vomiting

Mechanism of Action Acts directly on circular and longitudinal intestinal muscles, through the opioid receptor, to inhibit peristalsis and prolong transit time; reduces fecal volume, increases viscosity, and diminishes fluid and electrolyte loss; demonstrates antisecretory activity. Loperamide increases tone on the anal sphincter

Drug Interactions
Cytochrome P450 Effect: Substrate (minor) of CYP2B6
Increased Effect/Toxicity: P-glycoprotein Inhibitors may increase CNS depressant effects.
Decreased Effect: Loperamide may decrease levels/effects of saquinavir.

Pharmacodynamics/Kinetics
Absorption: Poor
Distribution: Poor penetration into brain; low amounts enter breast milk
Metabolism: Hepatic via oxidative N-demethylation
Half-life elimination: 7-14 hours
Time to peak, plasma: Liquid: 2.5 hours; Capsule: 5 hours
Excretion: Urine and feces (1% as metabolites, 30% to 40% as unchanged drug)

Pregnancy Risk Factor C

Loperamide and Simethicone
(loe PER a mide & sye METH i kone)

U.S. Brand Names Imodium® Advanced
Generic Available No
Synonyms Simethicone and Loperamide Hydrochloride
Pharmacologic Category Antidiarrheal; Antiflatulent
Use Control of symptoms of diarrhea and gas (bloating, pressure, and cramps)
Local Anesthetic/Vasoconstrictor Precautions No information available to require special precautions
Effects on Dental Treatment No significant effects or complications reported
Common Adverse Effects See individual agents.
Mechanism of Action
Loperamide acts by slowing intestinal motility and by affecting water and electrolyte movement through the bowel.
Simethicone acts in the stomach and intestines by altering the surface tension of gas bubbles enabling them to coalesce thereby freeing and eliminating the gas more easily by belching or passing flatus.
Drug Interactions
Increased Effect/Toxicity: CNS depressants, phenothiazines, tricyclic antidepressants may potentiate adverse effects. Also see individual agents.
Pharmacodynamics/Kinetics See individual agents.

Loperamide Hydrochloride *see* Loperamide *on page 942*
Lopid® *see* Gemfibrozil *on page 730*

Lopinavir and Ritonavir (loe PIN a veer & rit ON uh veer)

Related Information
HIV Infection and AIDS *on page 1662*
Ritonavir *on page 1359*
U.S. Brand Names Kaletra®
Canadian Brand Names Kaletra®
Generic Available No
Synonyms Ritonavir and Lopinavir
Pharmacologic Category Antiretroviral Agent, Protease Inhibitor
Use Treatment of HIV infection in combination with other antiretroviral agents
Local Anesthetic/Vasoconstrictor Precautions No information available to require special precautions
Effects on Dental Treatment No significant effects or complications reported
(Continued)

Lopinavir and Ritonavir *(Continued)*

Common Adverse Effects Protease inhibitors cause dyslipidemia which includes elevated cholesterol and triglycerides and a redistribution of body fat centrally to cause increased abdominal girth, buffalo hump, facial atrophy, and breast enlargement. These agents also cause hyperglycemia.

>10%:

Endocrine & metabolic: Hypercholesterolemia (3% to 39%), triglycerides increased (4% to 36%)

Gastrointestinal: Diarrhea (5% to 27%), nausea (5% to 16%)

Hepatic: GGT increased (6% to 29%)

2% to 10%:

Cardiovascular: Hypertension (up to 2%), vein distension (up to 2%)

Central nervous system: Headache (2% to 7%), chills (up to 2%), depression (up to 2%), fever (2%), insomnia (up to 2%)

Dermatologic: Rash (up to 4%)

Endocrine & metabolic: Amylase increased (3% to 8%), amenorrhea (up to 5%), hyperglycemia (1% to 5%), hyperuricemia (up to 3%), sodium decreased or increased (3% children), hypogonadism (up to 2%), inorganic phosphorus decreased (up to 2%), libido decreased (up to 2%)

Gastrointestinal: Abdominal pain (2% to 10%), abnormal stools (up to 6%), vomiting (2% to 6%), dyspepsia (up to 5%), flatulence (1% to 4%), weight loss (up to 3%), dysphagia (up to 2%), anorexia (1% to 2%)

Hematologic: Platelets decreased (4% children), neutrophils decreased (1% to 5%)

Hepatic: ALT increased (3% to 10%), AST increased (2% to 9%), bilirubin increased (children 3%)

Neuromuscular & skeletal: Weakness (up to 9%), myalgia (up to 2%), paresthesia (up to 2%)

Respiratory: Bronchitis (up to 2%)

Mechanism of Action A coformulation of lopinavir and ritonavir. The lopinavir component is the active inhibitor of HIV protease. Lopinavir inhibits HIV protease and renders the enzyme incapable of processing polyprotein precursor which leads to production of noninfectious immature HIV particles. The ritonavir component inhibits the CYP3A metabolism of lopinavir, allowing increased plasma levels of lopinavir.

Drug Interactions

Cytochrome P450 Effect:

Lopinavir: **Substrate** of 3A4 (minor)

Ritonavir: **Substrate** of CYP1A2 (minor), 2B6 (minor), 2D6 (major), 3A4 (major); **Inhibits** CYP2C8 (strong), 2C9 (weak), 2C19 (weak), 2D6 (strong), 2E1 (weak), 3A4 (strong); **Induces** CYP1A2 (weak), 2C8 (weak), 2C9 (weak), 3A4 (weak)

Increased Effect/Toxicity: Concurrent use of cisapride, ergot alkaloids, (dihydroergotamine, ergonovine, methylergonovine), lovastatin, midazolam, pimozide, simvastatin, and triazolam is contraindicated. Alfuzosin serum level may be increased by ritonavir; concurrent use is contraindicated (by the manufacturer of ritonavir). Antiarrhythmic agents (including amiodarone, bepridil, flecainide, propafenone, lidocaine (systemic), and quinidine) should be used with caution; life-threatening arrhythmias may result from concurrent use.

Ritonavir may increase the levels/effects of amiodarone, amphetamines, selected beta-blockers, selected benzodiazepines (midazolam and triazolam contraindicated), calcium channel blockers, dextromethorphan, fluoxetine, lidocaine, HMG-CoA reductase inhibitors (lovastatin and simvastatin are not recommended), mesoridazine, mirtazapine, nateglinide, nefazodone, paclitaxel, paroxetine, pioglitazone, repaglinide, risperidone, rosiglitazone, sildenafil (and other PDE-5 inhibitors), thioridazine, tricyclic antidepressants, venlafaxine, and other substrates of CYP2D6 or 3A4. Mesoridazine and thioridazine are generally contraindicated with strong CYP2D6 inhibitors. When used with strong CYP3A4 inhibitors, dosage adjustment/limits are recommended for sildenafil and other PDE-5 inhibitors; refer to individual monographs. Warfarin levels/effects may also be increased. High dosages of itraconazole or ketoconazole (>200 mg/day) are not recommended.

Serum levels of protease inhibitors may be altered during concurrent therapy. Ritonavir may increase serum concentrations of amprenavir, indinavir, or saquinavir. Delavirdine increases levels of lopinavir; dosing recommendations are not yet established. Serum concentrations of corticosteroids (eg, budesonide, dexamethasone, fluticasone, prednisone) may be increased by lopinavir/ritonavir, resulting in decreased serum cortisol, HPA axis suppression; concurrent use is not recommended.

Lopinavir/ritonavir solution contains alcohol, concurrent use with disulfiram or metronidazole should be avoided. May cause disulfiram-like reaction. Serum concentrations of meperidine's neuroexcitatory metabolite (normeperidine) are increased by ritonavir, which may increase the risk of CNS toxicity/seizures. Rifabutin and rifabutin metabolite serum concentrations may be increased by ritonavir; reduce rifabutin dose to 150 mg every other day. Tenofovir serum concentration/effects may be increased by lopinavir/ritonavir. Trazodone serum concentration/effects may be increased by lopinavir/ritonavir; use caution and reduce trazodone dose.

Decreased Effect: The levels/effects of ritonavir may be decreased by aminoglutethimide, carbamazepine, nafcillin, nevirapine, phenobarbital, phenytoin, rifamycins, and other CYP3A4 inducers. Concurrent use of rifampin is not recommended. Ritonavir may decrease the levels/effects of CYP2D6 prodrug substrates (eg, codeine, hydrocodone, oxycodone, tramadol). Non-nucleoside reverse transcriptase inhibitors (efavirenz, nevirapine) may decrease levels of lopinavir. To avoid incompatibility with didanosine, administer didanosine 1 hour before or 2 hours after lopinavir/ritonavir. Decreased levels of ethinyl estradiol may result from concurrent use (alternative contraception is recommended). Lopinavir/ritonavir may decrease levels of abacavir, atovaquone, or zidovudine. Voriconazole serum levels are reduced by ritonavir. Lopinavir/ritonavir may decrease the concentration and effect of amprenavir when administered as fosamprenavir.

Pharmacodynamics/Kinetics
Ritonavir: See Ritonavir monograph.
Lopinavir:
Protein binding: 98% to 99%; decreased with mild-to-moderate hepatic dysfunction
Metabolism: Hepatic via CYP3A; 13 metabolites identified
Half-life elimination: 5-6 hours
Time to peak, plasma: ~4 hours
Excretion: Feces (83%, 20% as unchanged drug); urine (2%)

Pregnancy Risk Factor C

Lopremone see Protirelin on page 1307
Lopressor® see Metoprolol on page 1030
Lopressor HCT® see Metoprolol and Hydrochlorothiazide on page 1032
Loprox® see Ciclopirox on page 338
Lorabid® see Loracarbef on page 945

Loracarbef (lor a KAR bef)

U.S. Brand Names Lorabid®
Canadian Brand Names Lorabid®
Mexican Brand Names Carbac®; Lorabid®
Generic Available No
Pharmacologic Category Antibiotic, Carbacephem
Use Treatment of infections caused by susceptible organisms involving the upper and lower respiratory tract, uncomplicated skin and skin structure, and urinary tract (including uncomplicated pyelonephritis)
Local Anesthetic/Vasoconstrictor Precautions No information available to require special precautions
Effects on Dental Treatment No significant effects or complications reported
Common Adverse Effects
1% to 10%:
Central nervous system: Headache (1% to 3%), somnolence (<1% to 2%)
Dermatologic: Rash (1% to 3%)
Gastrointestinal: Diarrhea (4% to 6%), nausea (2% to 3%), vomiting (1% to 3%), anorexia (<1% to 2%), abdominal pain (1%)
Genitourinary: Vaginitis (1%), vaginal moniliasis (1%)
Respiratory: Rhinitis (2% to 6%)
Miscellaneous: Hypersensitivity reactions (1%; eg, urticaria, pruritus, erythema multiforme)
Other adverse reactions observed with beta-lactam antibiotics: Agranulocytosis, allergic reactions, aplastic anemia, hemolytic anemia, hemorrhage, interstitial nephritis, LDH increased, neutropenia, pancytopenia, positive direct Coombs' test, pseudomembranous colitis, seizure (with high doses and renal dysfunction), toxic epidermal necrolysis
Mechanism of Action Inhibits bacterial cell wall synthesis by binding to one or more of the penicillin binding proteins (PBPs); inhibits the final transpeptidation step of peptidoglycan synthesis in bacterial cell walls, thus inhibiting cell wall biosynthesis. It is thought that beta-lactam antibiotics inactivate transpeptidase via acylation of the enzyme with cleavage of the CO-N bond of the beta-lactam
(Continued)

Loracarbef *(Continued)*

ring. Upon exposure to beta-lactam antibiotics, bacteria eventually lyse due to ongoing activity of cell wall autolytic enzymes (autolysins and murein hydrolases) while cell wall assembly is arrested.

Drug Interactions

Increased Effect/Toxicity: Loracarbef serum levels are increased with coadministered probenecid.

Pharmacodynamics/Kinetics

Absorption: Rapid

Protein binding: ~25%

Bioavailability: ~90%; decreased by food

Half-life elimination: ~1 hour

Time to peak, serum: ~1 hour

Excretion: Clearance: Plasma: ~200-300 mL/minute

Pregnancy Risk Factor B

Loratadine *(lor AT a deen)*

U.S. Brand Names Alavert® [OTC]; Claritin® 24 Hour Allergy [OTC]; Claritin® Hives Relief [OTC]; Tavist® ND [OTC]; Triaminic® Allerchews™ [OTC]

Canadian Brand Names Apo-Loratadine®; Claritin®; Claritin® Kids

Mexican Brand Names Clarityne®; Lertamine®; Sensibit®

Generic Available Yes

Pharmacologic Category Antihistamine, Nonsedating

Use Relief of nasal and non-nasal symptoms of seasonal allergic rhinitis; treatment of chronic idiopathic urticaria

Local Anesthetic/Vasoconstrictor Precautions No information available to require special precautions

Effects on Dental Treatment Key adverse event(s) related to dental treatment: Xerostomia (normal salivary flow resumes upon discontinuation).

Common Adverse Effects

Adults:

Central nervous system: Headache (12%), somnolence (8%), fatigue (4%)

Gastrointestinal: Xerostomia (3%)

Children:

Central nervous system: Nervousness (4% ages 6-12 years), fatigue (3% ages 6-12 years, 2% to 3% ages 2-5 years), malaise (2% ages 6-12 years)

Dermatologic: Rash (2% to 3% ages 2-5 years)

Gastrointestinal: Abdominal pain (2% ages 6-12 years), stomatitis (2% to 3% ages 2-5 years)

Neuromuscular & skeletal: Hyperkinesia (3% ages 6-12 years)

Ocular: Conjunctivitis (2% ages 6-12 years)

Respiratory: Wheezing (4% ages 6-12 years), dysphonia (2% ages 6-12 years), upper respiratory infection (2% ages 6-12 years), epistaxis (2% to 3% ages 2-5 years), pharyngitis (2% to 3% ages 2-5 years), flu-like symptoms (2% to 3% ages 2-5 years)

Miscellaneous: Viral infection (2% to 3% ages 2-5 years)

Mechanism of Action Long-acting tricyclic antihistamine with selective peripheral histamine H_1-receptor antagonist properties

Drug Interactions

Cytochrome P450 Effect: Substrate (minor) of CYP2D6, 3A4; **Inhibits** CYP2C19 (moderate), 2D6 (weak)

Increased Effect/Toxicity: Increased toxicity with procarbazine, other antihistamines. Protease inhibitors (amprenavir, ritonavir, nelfinavir) may increase the serum levels of loratadine. Loratadine may increase the levels/effects of citalopram, diazepam, methsuximide, phenytoin, propranolol, sertraline, and other CYP2C19 substrates.

Pharmacodynamics/Kinetics

Onset of action: 1-3 hours

Peak effect: 8-12 hours

Duration: >24 hours

Absorption: Rapid

Distribution: Significant amounts enter breast milk

Metabolism: Extensively hepatic via CYP2D6 and 3A4 to active metabolite

Half-life elimination: 12-15 hours

Excretion: Urine (40%) and feces (40%) as metabolites

Pregnancy Risk Factor B

Loratadine and Pseudoephedrine
(lor AT a deen & soo doe e FED rin)

Related Information
Bacterial Infections *on page 1697*
Loratadine *on page 946*
Pseudoephedrine *on page 1309*

U.S. Brand Names Alavert™ Allergy and Sinus [OTC]; Claritin-D® 12-Hour [OTC]; Claritin-D® 24-Hour [OTC]

Canadian Brand Names Chlor-Tripolon ND®; Claritin® Extra; Claritin® Liberator

Generic Available Yes

Synonyms Pseudoephedrine and Loratadine

Pharmacologic Category Antihistamine/Decongestant Combination

Use Temporary relief of symptoms of seasonal allergic rhinitis, other upper respiratory allergies, or the common cold

Local Anesthetic/Vasoconstrictor Precautions Use with caution since pseudoephedrine is a sympathomimetic amine which could interact with epinephrine to cause a pressor response

Effects on Dental Treatment Key adverse event(s) related to dental treatment: Pseudoephedrine: Xerostomia (normal salivary flow resumes upon discontinuation).

Common Adverse Effects See individual agents.

Dosage Children ≥12 years and Adults: Oral:
Claritin-D® 12-Hour: 1 tablet every 12 hours
Alavert™ Allergy and Sinus, Claritin-D® 24-Hour: 1 tablet daily

Dosage adjustment in renal impairment: Cl_{cr} ≤30 mL/minute:
Claritin-D® 12-Hour: 1 tablet daily
Claritin-D® 24-Hour: 1 tablet every other day

Dosage adjustment in hepatic impairment: Should be avoided

Contraindications Hypersensitivity to loratadine, pseudoephedrine, or any component of the formulation; use with or within 14 days of MAO inhibitors

Warnings/Precautions Patients with renal impairment (Cl_{cr} <30 mL/minute) should start with a lower dose since their ability to clear the drug will be reduced. Avoid use in hepatic dysfunction. Use with caution in lactation. Safety and efficacy in children <12 years of age have not been established. Use with caution in hypertension, diabetes mellitus, ischemic heart disease, increased intraocular pressure, hyperthyroidism, and prostatic hyperplasia. Do not take with MAO inhibitors and for 2 weeks after stopping MAO inhibitors. Patients with swallowing difficulties (eg, upper GI narrowing or abnormal esophageal peristalsis) should not use Claritin-D® 24-Hour.

Drug Interactions
Cytochrome P450 Effect: Loratadine: **Substrate** (minor) of CYP2D6, 3A4; **Inhibits** CYP2C19, 2D6

Increased Effect/Toxicity: See individual agents.

Pharmacodynamics/Kinetics See individual agents.

Pregnancy Risk Factor B

Dosage Forms TAB, extended release: Loratadine 10 mg and pseudoephedrine 240 mg; (Alavert™ Allergy and Sinus, Claritin-D® 12-hour): Loratadine 5 mg and pseudoephedrine 120 mg; Claritin-D® 24-hour: Loratadine 10 mg and pseudoephedrine 240 mg

---

Lorazepam (lor A ze pam)

Related Information
Sedation *on page 1727*
Temporomandibular Dysfunction (TMD) *on page 1724*

Related Sample Prescriptions
Sedation (Prior to Dental Treatment) *on page 1746*

U.S. Brand Names Ativan®; Lorazepam Intensol®

Canadian Brand Names Apo-Lorazepam®; Ativan®; Novo-Lorazepam; Nu-Loraz; PMS-Lorazepam; Riva-Lorazepam

Mexican Brand Names Ativan®; Sinestron®

Generic Available Yes

Pharmacologic Category Benzodiazepine

Dental Use Short-term relief of anxiety prior to dental appointment

Use
Oral: Management of anxiety disorders or short-term relief of the symptoms of anxiety or anxiety associated with depressive symptoms
(Continued)

Lorazepam *(Continued)*

I.V.: Status epilepticus, preanesthesia for desired amnesia, antiemetic adjunct

Unlabeled/Investigational Use Ethanol detoxification; insomnia; psychogenic catatonia; partial complex seizures; agitation (I.V.)

Local Anesthetic/Vasoconstrictor Precautions No information available to require special precautions

Effects on Dental Treatment Key adverse event(s) related to dental treatment: Xerostomia (normal salivary flow resumes upon discontinuation).

Significant Adverse Effects

>10%:

Central nervous system: Sedation

Respiratory: Respiratory depression

1% to 10%:

Cardiovascular: Hypotension

Central nervous system: Confusion, dizziness, akathisia, unsteadiness, headache, depression, disorientation, amnesia

Dermatologic: Dermatitis, rash

Gastrointestinal: Weight gain/loss, nausea, changes in appetite

Neuromuscular & skeletal: Weakness

Respiratory: Nasal congestion, hyperventilation, apnea

<1% (Limited to important or life-threatening): Menstrual irregularities, increased salivation, blood dyscrasias, reflex slowing, physical and psychological dependence with prolonged use, polyethylene glycol or propylene glycol poisoning (prolonged I.V. infusion)

Restrictions C-IV

Dental Usual Dosing

Anxiety and sedation: Adults: Oral: 1-10 mg/day in 2-3 divided doses; usual dose: 2-6 mg/day in divided doses

Preoperative: Adults:

I.M.: 0.05 mg/kg administered 2 hours before surgery (maximum: 4 mg/dose)

I.V.: 0.044 mg/kg 15-20 minutes before surgery (usual maximum: 2 mg/dose)

Preprocedural anxiety: Adults: Oral: 1-2 mg 1 hour before procedure

Dosage

Antiemetic:

Children 2-15 years: I.V.: 0.05 mg/kg (up to 2 mg/dose) prior to chemotherapy

Adults: Oral, I.V. **(Note:** May be administered sublingually; not a labeled route): 0.5-2 mg every 4-6 hours as needed

Anxiety and sedation:

Infants and Children: Oral, I.M., I.V.: Usual: 0.05 mg/kg/dose (range: 0.02-0.09 mg/kg) every 4-8 hours

I.V.: May use smaller doses (eg, 0.01-0.03 mg/kg) and repeat every 20 minutes, as needed to titrate to effect

Adults: Oral: 1-10 mg/day in 2-3 divided doses; usual dose: 2-6 mg/day in divided doses

Elderly: 0.5-4 mg/day; initial dose not to exceed 2 mg

Insomnia: Adults: Oral: 2-4 mg at bedtime

Preoperative: Adults:

I.M.: 0.05 mg/kg administered 2 hours before surgery (maximum: 4 mg/dose)

I.V.: 0.044 mg/kg 15-20 minutes before surgery (usual maximum: 2 mg/dose)

Preprocedural anxiety (dental use): Adults: Oral: 1-2 mg 1 hour before procedure

Operative amnesia: Adults: I.V.: Up to 0.05 mg/kg (maximum: 4 mg/dose)

Sedation (preprocedure): Infants and Children:

Oral, I.M., I.V.: Usual: 0.05 mg/kg (range: 0.02-0.09 mg/kg);

I.V.: May use smaller doses (eg, 0.01-0.03 mg/kg) and repeat every 20 minutes, as needed to titrate to effect

Status epilepticus: I.V.:

Infants and Children: 0.1 mg/kg slow I.V. over 2-5 minutes; do not exceed 4 mg/single dose; may repeat second dose of 0.05 mg/kg slow I.V. in 10-15 minutes if needed

Adolescents: 0.07 mg/kg slow I.V. over 2-5 minutes; maximum: 4 mg/dose; may repeat in 10-15 minutes

Adults: 4 mg/dose slow I.V. over 2-5 minutes; may repeat in 10-15 minutes; usual maximum dose: 8 mg

Rapid tranquilization of agitated patient (administer every 30-60 minutes):

Oral: 1-2 mg

I.M.: 0.5-1 mg

Average total dose for tranquilization: Oral, I.M.: 4-8 mg

Agitation in the ICU patient (unlabeled):

I.V.: 0.02-0.06 mg/kg every 2-6 hours

I.V. infusion: 0.01-0.1 mg/kg/hour

Mechanism of Action Binds to stereospecific benzodiazepine receptors on the postsynaptic GABA neuron at several sites within the central nervous system, including the limbic system, reticular formation. Enhancement of the inhibitory effect of GABA on neuronal excitability results by increased neuronal membrane permeability to chloride ions. This shift in chloride ions results in hyperpolarization (a less excitable state) and stabilization.

Contraindications Hypersensitivity to lorazepam or any component of the formulation (cross-sensitivity with other benzodiazepines may exist); acute narrow-angle glaucoma; sleep apnea (parenteral); intra-arterial injection of parenteral formulation; severe respiratory insufficiency (except during mechanical ventilation); pregnancy

Warnings/Precautions Use with caution in elderly or debilitated patients, patients with hepatic disease (including alcoholics) or renal impairment. Use with caution in patients with respiratory disease or impaired gag reflex. Initial doses in elderly or debilitated patients should not exceed 2 mg. Prolonged lorazepam use may have a possible relationship to GI disease, including esophageal dilation.

The parenteral formulation of lorazepam contains polyethylene glycol and propylene glycol. Also contains benzyl alcohol - avoid in neonates. Concurrent administration with scopolamine results in an increased risk of hallucinations, sedation, and irrational behavior.

Causes CNS depression (dose-related) resulting in sedation, dizziness, confusion, or ataxia which may impair physical and mental capabilities. Patients must be cautioned about performing tasks which require mental alertness (eg, operating machinery or driving). Use with caution in patients receiving other CNS depressants or psychoactive agents. Effects with other sedative drugs or ethanol may be potentiated. Benzodiazepines have been associated with falls and traumatic injury and should be used with extreme caution in patients who are at risk of these events (especially the elderly).

Lorazepam may cause anterograde amnesia. Paradoxical reactions, including hyperactive or aggressive behavior have been reported with benzodiazepines, particularly in adolescent/pediatric or psychiatric patients. Does not have analgesic, antidepressant, or antipsychotic properties.

Use caution in patients with depression, particularly if suicidal risk may be present. Use with caution in patients with a history of drug dependence. Benzodiazepines have been associated with dependence and acute withdrawal symptoms on discontinuation or reduction in dose. Acute withdrawal, including seizures, may be precipitated after administration of flumazenil to patients receiving long-term benzodiazepine therapy.

As a hypnotic agent, should be used only after evaluation of potential causes of sleep disturbance. Failure of sleep disturbance to resolve after 7-10 days may indicate psychiatric or medical illness. A worsening of insomnia or the emergence of new abnormalities of thought or behavior may represent unrecognized psychiatric or medical illness and requires immediate and careful evaluation.

Drug Interactions

CNS depressants: Sedative effects and/or respiratory depression may be additive with CNS depressants; includes ethanol, barbiturates, narcotic analgesics, and other sedative agents; monitor for increased effect

Levodopa: Lorazepam may decrease the antiparkinsonian efficacy of levodopa (limited documentation); monitor

Loxapine: There are rare reports of significant respiratory depression, stupor, and/or hypotension with concomitant use of loxapine and lorazepam; use caution if concomitant administration of loxapine and CNS drugs is required

Scopolamine: May increase the incidence of sedation, hallucinations, and irrational behavior; reported only with parenteral lorazepam

Theophylline: May partially antagonize some of the effects of benzodiazepines; monitor for decreased response; may require higher doses for sedation

Ethanol/Nutrition/Herb Interactions

Ethanol: Avoid or limit ethanol (may increase CNS depression).

Herb/Nutraceutical: Avoid valerian, St John's wort, kava kava, gotu kola (may increase CNS depression).

Pharmacodynamics/Kinetics

Onset of action:

Hypnosis: I.M.: 20-30 minutes

Sedation: I.V.: 5-20 minutes

Anticonvulsant: I.V.: 5 minutes, oral: 30-60 minutes

Duration: 6-8 hours

Absorption: Oral, I.M.: Prompt

Distribution:

V_d: Neonates: 0.76 L/kg, Adults: 1.3 L/kg; crosses placenta; enters breast milk

Protein binding: 85%; free fraction may be significantly higher in elderly

Metabolism: Hepatic to inactive compounds

(Continued)

Lorazepam *(Continued)*

Half-life elimination: Neonates: 40.2 hours; Older children: 10.5 hours; Adults: 12.9 hours; Elderly: 15.9 hours; End-stage renal disease: 32-70 hours

Excretion: Urine; feces (minimal)

Pregnancy Risk Factor D

Lactation Enters breast milk/contraindicated (AAP rates "of concern")

Breast-Feeding Considerations Crosses into breast milk and no data on clinical effects on the infant. AAP states MAY BE OF CONCERN.

Dosage Forms

Injection, solution (Ativan®): 2 mg/mL (1 mL, 10 mL); 4 mg/mL (1 mL, 10 mL) [contains benzyl alcohol]

Solution, oral concentrate (Lorazepam Intensol®): 2 mg/mL (30 mL) [alcohol free, dye free]

Tablet (Ativan®): 0.5 mg, 1 mg, 2 mg

Lorazepam Intensol® *see* Lorazepam *on page 947*

Lorcet® 10/650 *see* Hydrocodone and Acetaminophen *on page 779*

Lorcet®-HD [DSC] *see* Hydrocodone and Acetaminophen *on page 779*

Lorcet® Plus *see* Hydrocodone and Acetaminophen *on page 779*

Loroxide® [OTC] *see* Benzoyl Peroxide *on page 194*

Lortab® *see* Hydrocodone and Acetaminophen *on page 779*

Losartan *(loe SAR tan)*

Related Information

Cardiovascular Diseases *on page 1636*

U.S. Brand Names Cozaar®

Canadian Brand Names Cozaar®

Mexican Brand Names Cozaar®

Generic Available No

Synonyms DuP 753; Losartan Potassium; MK594

Pharmacologic Category Angiotensin II Receptor Blocker

Use Treatment of hypertension (HTN); treatment of diabetic nephropathy in patients with type 2 diabetes mellitus (noninsulin dependent, NIDDM) and a history of hypertension; stroke risk reduction in patients with HTN and left ventricular hypertrophy (LVH)

Local Anesthetic/Vasoconstrictor Precautions No information available to require special precautions

Effects on Dental Treatment No significant effects or complications reported

Common Adverse Effects

>10%:

Cardiovascular: Chest pain (12% diabetic nephropathy)

Central nervous system: Fatigue (14% diabetic nephropathy)

Endocrine: Hypoglycemia (14% diabetic nephropathy)

Gastrointestinal: Diarrhea (2% hypertension to 15% diabetic nephropathy)

Genitourinary: Urinary tract infection (13% diabetic nephropathy)

Hematologic: Anemia (14% diabetic nephropathy)

Neuromuscular & skeletal: Weakness (14% diabetic nephropathy), back pain (2% hypertension to 12% diabetic nephropathy)

Respiratory: Cough (≤3% to 11%; similar to placebo; incidence higher in patients with previous cough related to ACE inhibitor therapy)

1% to 10%:

Cardiovascular: Hypotension (7% diabetic nephropathy), orthostatic hypotension (4% hypertension to 4% diabetic nephropathy), first-dose hypotension (dose related: <1% with 50 mg, 2% with 100 mg)

Central nervous system: Dizziness (4%), hypoesthesia (5% diabetic nephropathy), fever (4% diabetic nephropathy), insomnia (1%)

Dermatology: Cellulitis (7% diabetic nephropathy)

Endocrine: Hyperkalemia (<1% hypertension to 7% diabetic nephropathy)

Gastrointestinal: Gastritis (5% diabetic nephropathy), weight gain (4% diabetic nephropathy), dyspepsia (1% to 4%), abdominal pain (2%), nausea (2%)

Neuromuscular & skeletal: Muscular weakness (7% diabetic nephropathy), knee pain (5% diabetic nephropathy), leg pain (1% to 5%), muscle cramps (1%), myalgia (1%)

Respiratory: Bronchitis (10% diabetic nephropathy), upper respiratory infection (8%), nasal congestion (2%), sinusitis (1% hypertension to 6% diabetic nephropathy)

Miscellaneous: Infection (5% diabetic nephropathy), flu-like syndrome (10% diabetic nephropathy)

Dosage Oral:

Hypertension:

Children 6-16 years: 0.7 mg/kg once daily (maximum: 50 mg/day); adjust dose based on response; doses >1.4 mg/kg (maximum: 100 mg) have not been studied

Adults: Usual starting dose: 50 mg once daily; can be administered once or twice daily with total daily doses ranging from 25-100 mg

Patients receiving diuretics or with intravascular volume depletion: Usual initial dose: 25 mg

Nephropathy in patients with type 2 diabetes and hypertension: Adults: Initial: 50 mg once daily; can be increased to 100 mg once daily based on blood pressure response

Stroke reduction (HTN with LVH): Adults: 50 mg once daily (maximum daily dose: 100 mg); may be used in combination with a thiazide diuretic

Dosing adjustment in renal impairment:

Children: Use is not recommended if Cl_{cr} <30 mL/minute.

Adults: No adjustment necessary.

Dosing adjustment in hepatic impairment: Reduce the initial dose to 25 mg/day; divide dosage intervals into two.

Mechanism of Action As a selective and competitive, nonpeptide angiotensin II receptor antagonist, losartan blocks the vasoconstrictor and aldosterone-secreting effects of angiotensin II; losartan interacts reversibly at the AT1 and AT2 receptors of many tissues and has slow dissociation kinetics; its affinity for the AT1 receptor is 1000 times greater than the AT2 receptor. Angiotensin II receptor antagonists may induce a more complete inhibition of the renin-angiotensin system than ACE inhibitors, they do not affect the response to bradykinin, and are less likely to be associated with nonrenin-angiotensin effects (eg, cough and angioedema). Losartan increases urinary flow rate and in addition to being natriuretic and kaliuretic, increases excretion of chloride, magnesium, uric acid, calcium, and phosphate.

Contraindications Hypersensitivity to losartan or any component of the formulation; hypersensitivity to other A-II receptor antagonists; bilateral renal artery stenosis; pregnancy (2nd and 3rd trimesters)

Warnings/Precautions Avoid use or use a much smaller dose in patients who are volume-depleted; correct depletion first. Use with caution in patients with pre-existing renal insufficiency or significant aortic/mitral stenosis. May cause hyperkalemia; avoid potassium supplementation unless specifically required by healthcare provider. Use caution in patients with unilateral or bilateral renal artery stenosis to avoid a decrease in renal function. AUCs of losartan (not the active metabolite) are about 50% greater in patients with Cl_{cr} <30 mL/minute and are doubled in hemodialysis patients. When used to reduce the risk of stroke in patients with HTN and LVH, may not be effective in African-American population. Use caution with hepatic dysfunction, dose adjustment may be needed. Safety and efficacy in children <6 years of age have not been established.

Drug Interactions

Cytochrome P450 Effect: Substrate (major) of CYP2C8/9, 3A4; **Inhibits** CYP1A2 (weak), 2C8/9 (moderate), 2C19 (weak), 3A4 (weak)

Increased Effect/Toxicity: Cimetidine may increase the absorption of losartan by 18% (clinical effect is unknown). Potassium salts/supplements, co-trimoxazole (high dose), ACE inhibitors, and potassium-sparing diuretics (amiloride, spironolactone, triamterene) may increase the risk of hyperkalemia. Risk of lithium toxicity may be increased by losartan. Losartan may increase the levels/effects of amiodarone, fluoxetine, glimepiride, glipizide, nateglinide, phenytoin, pioglitazone, rosiglitazone, sertraline, warfarin, and other CYP2C8/9 substrates. Fluconazole may increase the levels/effects of losartan.

Decreased Effect: The levels/effects of losartan may be decreased by aminoglutethimide, carbamazepine, nafcillin, nevirapine, phenobarbital, phenytoin, rifampin, rifapentine, secobarbital, and other CYP2C8/9 or 3A4 inducers. NSAIDs may decrease the efficacy of losartan.

Ethanol/Nutrition/Herb Interactions Herb/Nutraceutical: St John's wort may decrease levels. Avoid dong quai if using for hypertension (has estrogenic activity). Avoid ephedra, yohimbe, ginseng (may worsen hypertension). Avoid garlic (may have increased antihypertensive effect).

Dietary Considerations May be taken with or without food.

Pharmacodynamics/Kinetics

Onset of action: 6 hours

Distribution: V_d: Losartan: 34 L; E-3174: 12 L; does not cross blood brain barrier

Protein binding, plasma: High

Metabolism: Hepatic (14%) via CYP2C9 and 3A4 to active metabolite, E-3174 (40 times more potent than losartan); extensive first-pass effect

(Continued)

Losartan *(Continued)*

Bioavailability: 25% to 33%; AUC of E-3174 is four times greater than that of losartan

Half-life elimination: Losartan: 1.5-2 hours; E-3174: 6-9 hours

Time to peak, serum: Losartan: 1 hour; E-3174: 3-4 hours

Excretion: Urine (4% as unchanged drug, 6% as active metabolite)

Clearance: Plasma: Losartan: 600 mL/minute; Active metabolite: 50 mL/minute

Pregnancy Risk Factor C/D (2nd and 3rd trimesters)

Dosage Forms TAB, film coated: 25 mg, 50 mg, 100 mg

Losartan and Hydrochlorothiazide
(loe SAR tan & hye droe klor oh THYE a zide)

Related Information

Hydrochlorothiazide *on page 776*

Losartan *on page 950*

U.S. Brand Names Hyzaar®

Canadian Brand Names Hyzaar®; Hyzaar® DS

Generic Available No

Synonyms Hydrochlorothiazide and Losartan

Pharmacologic Category Angiotensin II Receptor Blocker Combination; Antihypertensive Agent, Combination; Diuretic, Thiazide

Use Treatment of hypertension; stroke risk reduction in patients with HTN and left ventricular hypertrophy (LVH)

Local Anesthetic/Vasoconstrictor Precautions No information available to require special precautions

Effects on Dental Treatment No significant effects or complications reported

Common Adverse Effects Based on clinical trials of the combination product in patients with essential hypertension. Also see individual agents.

1% to 10%:

Cardiovascular: Edema (1%), palpitation (1%)

Central nervous system: Dizziness (6%)

Dermatologic: Skin rash (1%)

Gastrointestinal: Abdominal pain (1%)

Neuromuscular & skeletal: Back pain (2%)

Respiratory: Upper respiratory infection (6%), cough (3%), sinusitis (1%)

Dosage

Oral: Adults: Dose is individualized (combination substituted for individual components); dose may be titrated after 2-4 weeks of therapy

Hypertension/stroke reduction in hypertension (with LVH): Usual recommended starting dose of losartan: 50 mg once daily when used as monotherapy in patients who are not volume depleted

Dosage adjustment in renal impairment: Cl_{cr} ≤30 mL/minute: Use of combination formulation not recommended

Dosage adjustment in hepatic impairment: Use is not recommended

Contraindications

Hypersensitivity to hydrochlorothiazide, thiazides, sulfonamide-derived drugs, losartan,or any component of the formulation; hypersensitivity to other A-II receptor antagonists; bilateral renal artery stenosis, anuria, renal decompensation; pregnancy (2nd and 3rd trimesters)

Warnings/Precautions See individual agents.

Drug Interactions

Cytochrome P450 Effect: Losartan: **Substrate** (major) of CYP2C8/9, 3A4; **Inhibits** CYP1A2 (weak), 2C8/9 (moderate), 2C19 (weak), 3A4 (weak)

Increased Effect/Toxicity: See individual agents.

Pharmacodynamics/Kinetics See individual agents.

Pregnancy Risk Factor C/D (2nd and 3rd trimesters)

Dosage Forms TAB, film coated: 50-12.5: Losartan potassium 50 mg and hydrochlorothiazide 12.5 mg; 100-12.5: Losartan potassium 100 mg and hydrochlorothiazide 12.5 mg; 100-25: Losartan potassium 100 mg and hydrochlorothiazide 25 mg

Losartan Potassium see Losartan *on page 950*

Lotemax® see Loteprednol *on page 953*

Lotensin® see Benazepril *on page 185*

Lotensin® HCT see Benazepril and Hydrochlorothiazide *on page 187*

Loteprednol (loe te PRED nol)

U.S. Brand Names Alrex®; Lotemax®
Canadian Brand Names Alrex®; Lotemax®
Generic Available No
Synonyms Loteprednol Etabonate
Pharmacologic Category Corticosteroid, Ophthalmic
Use

Suspension, 0.2% (Alrex®): Temporary relief of signs and symptoms of seasonal allergic conjunctivitis

Suspension, 0.5% (Lotemax®): Inflammatory conditions (treatment of steroid-responsive inflammatory conditions of the palpebral and bulbar conjunctiva, cornea, and anterior segment of the globe such as allergic conjunctivitis, acne rosacea, superficial punctate keratitis, herpes zoster keratitis, iritis, cyclitis, selected infective conjunctivitis, when the inherent hazard of steroid use is accepted to obtain an advisable diminution in edema and inflammation) and treatment of postoperative inflammation following ocular surgery

Local Anesthetic/Vasoconstrictor Precautions No information available to require special precautions

Effects on Dental Treatment No significant effects or complications reported

Mechanism of Action Corticosteroids inhibit the inflammatory response including edema, capillary dilation, leukocyte migration, and scar formation. Loteprednol is highly lipid soluble and penetrates cells readily to induce the production of lipocortins. These proteins modulate the activity of prostaglandins and leukotrienes.

Pregnancy Risk Factor C

Loteprednol and Tobramycin (loe te PRED nol & toe bra MYE sin)

U.S. Brand Names Zylet™
Generic Available No
Synonyms Loteprednol Etabonate and Tobramycin; Tobramycin and Loteprednol Etabonate
Pharmacologic Category Antibiotic/Corticosteroid, Ophthalmic
Use Treatment of steroid-responsive ocular inflammatory conditions where either a superficial bacterial ocular infection or the risk of a superficial bacterial ocular infection exists

Local Anesthetic/Vasoconstrictor Precautions No information available to require special precautions

Effects on Dental Treatment No significant effects or complications reported

Mechanism of Action See individual agents.

Pregnancy Risk Factor C

Loteprednol Etabonate *see* Loteprednol *on page 953*

Loteprednol Etabonate and Tobramycin *see* Loteprednol and Tobramycin *on page 953*

Lotrel® *see* Amlodipine and Benazepril *on page 102*

Lotrimin® AF Athlete's Foot Cream [OTC] *see* Clotrimazole *on page 379*

Lotrimin® AF Athlete's Foot Solution [OTC] *see* Clotrimazole *on page 379*

Lotrimin® AF Jock Itch Cream [OTC] *see* Clotrimazole *on page 379*

Lotrimin® AF Jock Itch Powder Spray [OTC] *see* Miconazole *on page 1039*

Lotrimin® AF Powder/Spray [OTC] *see* Miconazole *on page 1039*

Lotrimin® Ultra™ [OTC] *see* Butenafine *on page 242*

Lotrisone® *see* Betamethasone and Clotrimazole *on page 202*

Lotronex® *see* Alosetron *on page 72*

Lovastatin (LOE va sta tin)

Related Information
Cardiovascular Diseases *on page 1636*
U.S. Brand Names Altoprev™; Mevacor®
Canadian Brand Names Apo-Lovastatin®; CO Lovastatin; Gen-Lovastatin; Mevacor®; Novo-Lovastatin; Nu-Lovastatin; PMS-Lovastatin; ratio-Lovastatin; Sandoz-Lovastatin
Generic Available Yes: Immediate release tablet
(Continued)

Lovastatin *(Continued)*

Synonyms Mevinolin; Monacolin K

Pharmacologic Category Antilipemic Agent, HMG-CoA Reductase Inhibitor

Use

Adjunct to dietary therapy to decrease elevated serum total and LDL-cholesterol concentrations in primary hypercholesterolemia

Primary prevention of coronary artery disease (patients without symptomatic disease with average to moderately elevated total and LDL-cholesterol and below average HDL-cholesterol); slow progression of coronary atherosclerosis in patients with coronary heart disease

Adjunct to dietary therapy in adolescent patients (10-17 years of age, females >1 year postmenarche) with heterozygous familial hypercholesterolemia having LDL >189 mg/dL, **or** LDL >160 mg/dL with positive family history of premature cardiovascular disease (CVD), **or** LDL >160 mg/dL with the presence of at least two other CVD risk factors

Local Anesthetic/Vasoconstrictor Precautions No information available to require special precautions

Effects on Dental Treatment No significant effects or complications reported

Common Adverse Effects Percentages as reported with immediate release tablets; similar adverse reactions seen with extended release tablets.

>10%: Neuromuscular & skeletal: Increased CPK (>2x normal) (11%)

1% to 10%:

Central nervous system: Headache (2% to 3%), dizziness (0.5% to 1%)

Dermatologic: Rash (0.8% to 1%)

Gastrointestinal: Abdominal pain (2% to 3%), constipation (2% to 4%), diarrhea (2% to 3%), dyspepsia (1% to 2%), flatulence (4% to 5%), nausea (2% to 3%)

Neuromuscular & skeletal: Myalgia (2% to 3%), weakness (1% to 2%), muscle cramps (0.6% to 1%)

Ocular: Blurred vision (0.8% to 1%)

Dosage Oral:

Adolescents 10-17 years: Immediate release tablet:

LDL reduction <20%: Initial: 10 mg/day with evening meal

LDL reduction ≥20%: Initial: 20 mg/day with evening meal

Usual range: 10-40 mg with evening meal, then adjust dose at 4-week intervals

Adults: Initial: 20 mg with evening meal, then adjust at 4-week intervals; maximum dose: 80 mg/day immediate release tablet **or** 60 mg/day extended release tablet

Dosage modification/limits based on concurrent therapy:

Cyclosporine and other immunosuppressant drugs: Initial dose: 10 mg/day with a maximum recommended dose of 20 mg/day

Concurrent therapy with fibrates, danazol, and/or lipid-lowering doses of niacin (>1 g/day): Maximum recommended dose: 20 mg/day. Concurrent use with fibrates should be avoided unless risk to benefit favors use.

Concurrent therapy with amiodarone or verapamil: Maximum recommended dose: 40 mg/day of regular release or 20 mg/day with extended release.

Dosage adjustment in renal impairment: Cl_{cr} <30 mL/minute: Use doses >20 mg/day with caution.

Mechanism of Action Lovastatin acts by competitively inhibiting 3-hydroxy-3-methylglutaryl-coenzyme A (HMG-CoA) reductase, the enzyme that catalyzes the rate-limiting step in cholesterol biosynthesis

Contraindications Hypersensitivity to lovastatin or any component of the formulation; active liver disease; unexplained persistent elevations of serum transaminases; pregnancy; breast-feeding

Warnings/Precautions Liver function tests should be assessed before initiation of therapy in patients with a history of liver disease, prior to upwards dosage adjustment to ≥40 mg daily or when otherwise indicated; enzyme levels should be followed periodically thereafter as clinically warranted. Rhabdomyolysis with or without acute renal failure has occurred. Risk is dose-related and is increased with concurrent use of lipid-lowering agents which may cause rhabdomyolysis (gemfibrozil, fibric acid derivatives, or niacin at doses ≥1 g/day) or during concurrent use with potent CYP3A4 inhibitors. Avoid concurrent use of azole antifungals, macrolide antibiotics, and protease inhibitors. Use caution/limit dose with amiodarone, cyclosporine, danazol, gemfibrozil (or other fibrates), lipid-lowering doses of niacin, or verapamil. Patients should be instructed to report unexplained muscle pain or weakness; lovastatin should be discontinued if myopathy is suspected/confirmed. Temporarily discontinue in any patient experiencing an acute or serious condition predisposing to renal failure secondary to rhabdomyolysis. Use with caution in patients who consume large amounts of ethanol or have a history of liver disease. Safety and efficacy of the immediate release tablet have not been evaluated in prepubertal patients, patients <10 years of age, or doses >40 mg/day in appropriately-selected adolescents; extended release tablets have not been studied in patients <20 years of age.

Drug Interactions

Cytochrome P450 Effect: Substrate of CYP3A4 (major); **Inhibits** CYP2C8/ 9 (weak), 2D6 (weak), 3A4 (weak)

Increased Effect/Toxicity: CYP3A4 inhibitors may increase the levels/ effects of lovastatin; example inhibitors include azole antifungals, clarithromycin, diclofenac, doxycycline, erythromycin, imatinib, isoniazid, nefazodone, nicardipine, propofol, protease inhibitors, quinidine, telithromycin, and verapamil. Suspend lovastatin therapy during concurrent clarithromycin, erythromycin, itraconazole, or ketoconazole therapy. Concurrent use of danazol may increase risk of myopathy (limit dose of lovastatin). Cyclosporine, clofibrate, fenofibrate, gemfibrozil, and niacin also may increase the risk of myopathy and rhabdomyolysis. The effect/toxicity of warfarin (elevated PT) and levothyroxine may be increased by lovastatin. Digoxin, norethindrone, and ethinyl estradiol levels may be increased. Effects are additive with other lipid-lowering therapies.

Decreased Effect: Cholestyramine taken with lovastatin reduces lovastatin absorption and effect.

Ethanol/Nutrition/Herb Interactions

Ethanol: Avoid excessive ethanol consumption (due to potential hepatic effects).

Food: Food **decreases** the bioavailability of lovastatin extended release tablets and **increases** the bioavailability of lovastatin immediate release tablets. Lovastatin serum concentrations may be increased if taken with grapefruit juice; avoid concurrent intake of large quantities (>1 quart/day). Red yeast rice contains an estimated 2.4 mg lovastatin per 600 mg rice.

Herb/Nutraceutical: St John's wort may decrease lovastatin levels.

Dietary Considerations Before initiation of therapy, patients should be placed on a standard cholesterol-lowering diet for 6 weeks and the diet should be continued during drug therapy. Avoid intake of large quantities of grapefruit juice (≥1 quart/day); may increase toxicity. Red yeast rice contains an estimated 2.4 mg lovastatin per 600 mg rice.

Pharmacodynamics/Kinetics

Onset of action: LDL-cholesterol reductions: 3 days

Absorption: 30%; increased with extended release tablets when taken in the fasting state

Protein binding: 95%

Metabolism: Hepatic; extensive first-pass effect; hydrolyzed to B-hydroxy acid (active)

Bioavailability: Increased with extended release tablets

Half-life elimination: 1.1-1.7 hours

Time to peak, serum: 2-4 hours

Excretion: Feces (~80% to 85%); urine (10%)

Pregnancy Risk Factor X

Dosage Forms TAB: 10 mg, 20 mg, 40 mg; (Mevacor®): 20 mg, 40 mg. **TAB, extended release:** (Altoprev™) 10 mg, 20 mg, 40 mg, 60 mg

Lovastatin and Niacin see Niacin and Lovastatin on page 1107

Lovenox® see Enoxaparin on page 542

Low-Ogestrel® see Ethinyl Estradiol and Norgestrel on page 616

Loxapine (LOKS a peen)

U.S. Brand Names Loxitane®

Canadian Brand Names Apo-Loxapine®; Nu-Loxapine; PMS-Loxapine

Generic Available Yes

Synonyms Loxapine Succinate; Oxilapine Succinate

Pharmacologic Category Antipsychotic Agent, Typical

Use Management of psychotic disorders

Local Anesthetic/Vasoconstrictor Precautions Most pharmacology textbooks state that in presence of phenothiazines, systemic doses of epinephrine paradoxically decrease the blood pressure. This is the so called "epinephrine reversal" phenomenon. This has never been observed when epinephrine is given by infiltration as part of the anesthesia procedure. See Dental Comment.

Effects on Dental Treatment Key adverse event(s) related to dental treatment:

Xerostomia and changes in salivation (normal salivary flow resumes upon discontinuation).

(Continued)

Loxapine *(Continued)*

Significant hypotension may occur, especially when the drug is administered parenterally; orthostatic hypotension is due to alpha-receptor blockade, the elderly are at greater risk for orthostatic hypotension.

Tardive dyskinesia: Prevalence rate may be 40% in elderly; development of the syndrome and the irreversible nature are proportional to duration and total cumulative dose over time. Extrapyramidal reactions are more common in elderly with up to 50% developing these reactions after 60 years of age. Drug-induced Parkinson's syndrome occurs often; akathisia is the most common extrapyramidal reaction in elderly.

Increased confusion, memory loss, psychotic behavior, and agitation frequently occur as a consequence of anticholinergic effects. Antipsychotic associated sedation in nonpsychotic patients is extremely unpleasant due to feelings of depersonalization, derealization, and dysphoria.

Common Adverse Effects Frequency not defined.

Cardiovascular: Orthostatic hypotension, tachycardia, arrhythmia, abnormal T-waves with prolonged ventricular repolarization, hyper-/hypotension, light-headedness, syncope

Central nervous system: Drowsiness, extrapyramidal symptoms (dystonia, akathisia, pseudoparkinsonism, tardive dyskinesia, akinesia), dizziness, faintness, ataxia, insomnia, agitation, tension, seizure, slurred speech, confusion, headache, neuroleptic malignant syndrome (NMS), altered central temperature regulation

Dermatologic: Rash, pruritus, photosensitivity, dermatitis, alopecia, seborrhea

Endocrine & metabolic: Enlargement of breasts, galactorrhea, amenorrhea, gynecomastia, menstrual irregularity

Gastrointestinal: Xerostomia, constipation, nausea, vomiting, weight gain/loss, adynamic ileus, polydipsia

Genitourinary: Urinary retention, sexual dysfunction

Hematologic: Agranulocytosis, leukopenia, thrombocytopenia

Neuromuscular & skeletal: Weakness

Ocular: Blurred vision

Respiratory: Nasal congestion

Mechanism of Action Loxapine is a dibenzoxazepine antipsychotic which blocks postsynaptic mesolimbic D_1 and D_2 receptors in the brain, and also possesses serotonin 5-HT$_2$ blocking activity

Drug Interactions

Increased Effect/Toxicity: Loxapine concentrations may be increased by chloroquine, propranolol, sulfadoxine-pyrimethamine. Loxapine may increased the effect and/or toxicity of antihypertensives, lithium, TCAs, CNS depressants (ethanol, narcotics), and trazodone. There are rare reports of significant respiratory depression, stupor, and/or hypotension with the concomitant use of loxapine and lorazepam. Use caution if the concomitant administration of loxapine and CNS drugs is required. Metoclopramide may increase risk of extrapyramidal symptoms (EPS). Acetylcholinesterase inhibitors (central) may increase the risk of antipsychotic-related EPS. Effects on QT$_c$ interval may be additive with antipsychotics, increasing the risk of malignant arrhythmias; other QT$_c$-prolonging agents include type Ia antiarrhythmics, TCAs, and some quinolone antibiotics (sparfloxacin, moxifloxacin and gatifloxacin). Concomitant use with thioridazine is contraindicated.

Decreased Effect: Antipsychotics inhibit the activity of bromocriptine and levodopa. Benztropine (and other anticholinergics) may inhibit the therapeutic response to loxapine and excess anticholinergic effects may occur. Loxapine and possibly other low potency antipsychotic may reverse the pressor effects of epinephrine.

Pharmacodynamics/Kinetics

Onset of action: Neuroleptic: Oral: 20-30 minutes

Peak effect: 1.5-3 hours

Duration: ~12 hours

Metabolism: Hepatic to glucuronide conjugates

Half-life elimination: Biphasic: Initial: 5 hours; Terminal: 12-19 hours

Excretion: Urine; feces (small amounts)

Pregnancy Risk Factor C

Dental Comment

This drug is known to prolong the QT interval. The QT interval is measured as the time and distance between the Q point of the QRS complex and the end of the T wave in the ECG tracing. After adjustment for heart rate, the QT interval is defined as prolonged if it is more than 450 msec in men and 460 msec in women. A long QT syndrome was first described in the 1950s and 60s as a congenital syndrome involving QT interval prolongation and syncope and sudden death. Some of the congenital long QT syndromes were characterized by a peculiar electrocardiographic appearance of the QRS complex involving a premature atria beat followed by a pause, then a subsequent sinus beat showing marked QT prolongation and deformity. This type of cardiac arrhythmia was originally termed "torsade de pointes" (translated from the French as "twisting of the points").

Prolongation of the QT interval is thought to result from delayed ventricular repolarization. The repolarization process within the myocardial cell is due to the efflux of intracellular potassium. The channels associated with this current can be blocked by many drugs and predisposes the electrical propagation cycle to torsade de pointes.

Loxapine is one of the drugs confirmed to prolong the QT interval and is accepted as having a risk of causing torsade de pointes. The risk of drug-induced torsade de pointes is extremely low when a single QT interval prolonging drug is prescribed. In terms of epinephrine, it is not known what effect vasoconstrictors in the local anesthetic regimen will have in patients with a known history of congenital prolonged QT interval or in patients taking any medication that prolongs the QT interval. Until more information is obtained, it is suggested that the clinician consult with the physician prior to the use of a vasoconstrictor in suspected patients, and that the vasoconstrictor (epinephrine, levonordefrin [Neo-Cobefrin®]) be used with caution.

Loxapine Succinate see Loxapine on page 955

Loxitane® see Loxapine on page 955

Lozi-Flur™ see Fluoride on page 671

Lozol® see Indapamide on page 828

L-PAM see Melphalan on page 979

LRH see Gonadorelin on page 749

L-Sarcolysin see Melphalan on page 979

LTA® 360 see Lidocaine on page 920

LTG see Lamotrigine on page 895

Lu-26-054 see Escitalopram on page 568

Lubiprostone (loo bi PROS tone)

U.S. Brand Names Amitiza™
Generic Available No
Synonyms RU 0211; SPI 0211
Pharmacologic Category Gastrointestinal Agent, Miscellaneous
Use Treatment of chronic idiopathic constipation
Local Anesthetic/Vasoconstrictor Precautions No information available to require special precautions
Effects on Dental Treatment Key adverse event(s) related to dental treatment: Xerostomia (normal salivary flow resumes upon discontinuation).
Common Adverse Effects
>10%:
  Central nervous system: Headache (13%)
  Gastrointestinal: Nausea (31%; dose related), diarrhea (13%; severe 3%)
1% to 10%:
  Cardiovascular: Peripheral edema (4%), chest discomfort (2%), chest pain (1%), hypertension (1%)
  Central nervous system: Dizziness (4%), fatigue (2%), fever (1%), depression (1%), anxiety (1%), insomnia (1%)
  Gastrointestinal: Abdominal distention (7%), abdominal pain (7%), flatulence (6%), vomiting (5%), loose stools (3%), dyspepsia (3%), gastroesophageal reflux disease (2%), xerostomia (2%), weight gain (1%)
  Neuromuscular & skeletal: Arthralgia (3%), back pain (2%), muscle cramp (1%)
  Renal: Urinary tract infection (4%)
  Respiratory: Sinusitis (5%), upper respiratory tract infection (4%), nasopharyngitis (3%), bronchitis (2%), dyspnea (2%), cough (2%)
  Miscellaneous: Influenza (2%)
Mechanism of Action Bicyclic fatty acid that acts locally at the apical portion of the intestine as a chloride channel activator, increasing intestinal water secretion.
Pharmacodynamics/Kinetics
  Absorption: Systemic: Parent drug: Poor (below levels of detection); Active metabolite (M3): Low
  Distribution: Gastrointestinal tissue
  Metabolism: Within stomach and jejunum by carbonyl reductase to M3 (active metabolite) and others
  Bioavailability: Minimal
  (Continued)

Lubiprostone (Continued)

Half-life elimination: M3: 0.9-1.4 hours
Excretion: M3: Feces (trace amounts)

Pregnancy Risk Factor C

Lubriderm® [OTC] *see* Lanolin, Cetyl Alcohol, Glycerin, Petrolatum, and Mineral Oil *on page 896*

Lubriderm® Fragrance Free [OTC] *see* Lanolin, Cetyl Alcohol, Glycerin, Petrolatum, and Mineral Oil *on page 896*

Lucidex [OTC] *see* Caffeine *on page 245*

Ludiomil *see* Maprotiline *on page 964*

Lufyllin® *see* Dyphylline *on page 526*

Lugol's Solution *see* Potassium Iodide and Iodine *on page 1260*

Lumigan® *see* Bimatoprost *on page 208*

Luminal® Sodium *see* Phenobarbital *on page 1221*

Lumitene™ *see* Beta-Carotene *on page 198*

Lunesta™ *see* Eszopiclone *on page 587*

LupiCare™ II Psoriasis [OTC] *see* Salicylic Acid *on page 1374*

LupiCare™ Dandruff [OTC] *see* Salicylic Acid *on page 1374*

LupiCare™ Psoriasis [OTC] *see* Salicylic Acid *on page 1374*

Lupron® *see* Leuprolide *on page 906*

Lupron Depot® *see* Leuprolide *on page 906*

Lupron Depot-Ped® *see* Leuprolide *on page 906*

Luride® *see* Fluoride *on page 671*

Luride® Lozi-Tab® *see* Fluoride *on page 671*

Lustra® *see* Hydroquinone *on page 798*

Lustra-AF™ *see* Hydroquinone *on page 798*

Luteinizing Hormone Releasing Hormone *see* Gonadorelin *on page 749*

Lutera™ *see* Ethinyl Estradiol and Levonorgestrel *on page 602*

Lutropin Alfa (LOO troe pin AL fa)

U.S. Brand Names Luveris®
Generic Available No
Synonyms Recombinant Human Luteinizing Hormone; r-hLH
Pharmacologic Category Gonadotropin; Ovulation Stimulator
Use Stimulation of follicular development in infertile hypogonadotropic hypogonadal (HH) women with profound luteinizing hormone (LH) deficiency; to be used in combination with follitropin alfa
Local Anesthetic/Vasoconstrictor Precautions No information available to require special precautions
Effects on Dental Treatment No significant effects or complications reported
Common Adverse Effects
1% to 10%:
Central nervous system: Headache (10%), fatigue (2% to 3%)
Endocrine & metabolic: Ovarian hyperstimulation (6%)
Gastrointestinal: Nausea (7%), constipation (2% to 3%), diarrhea (2% to 3%)
Adverse events reported with gonadotropin or menotropin therapy: Adnexal torsion, arterial thromboembolism, congenital abnormalities, ectopic pregnancy, hemoperitoneum, ovarian enlargement (mild-to-moderate), ovarian neoplasms (infrequent), postpartum fever, premature labor, pulmonary complications, spontaneous abortion, vascular complications
Mechanism of Action Lutropin alfa is a recombinant luteinizing hormone prepared using Chinese hamster cell ovaries. Administration leads to increased follicular estradiol secretion needed for follicle stimulating hormone induced follicular development.
Pharmacodynamics/Kinetics
Distribution: V_d: 10
Bioavailability: 56% ± 23%
Half-life elimination: Terminal: ~18 hours
Time to peak, serum: 4-16 hours
Excretion: Urine (<5% unchanged)
Pregnancy Risk Factor X

Luveris® *see* Lutropin Alfa *on page 958*

Luvox *see* Fluvoxamine *on page 694*

Luxiq® *see* Betamethasone *on page 199*

LY139603 *see* Atomoxetine *on page 156*

LY146032 *see* Daptomycin *on page 423*

LY170053 *see* Olanzapine *on page 1139*

LY231514 *see* Pemetrexed *on page 1198*

LY248686 *see* Duloxetine *on page 523*

LY303366 *see* Anidulafungin *on page 128*

LY2148568 *see* Exenatide *on page 629*

Lymphocyte Immune Globulin *see* Antithymocyte Globulin (Equine) *on page 131*

Lymphocyte Mitogenic Factor *see* Aldesleukin *on page 61*

Lyrica® *see* Pregabalin *on page 1274*

L-Lysine (el LYE seen)

U.S. Brand Names Lysinyl [OTC]
Generic Available Yes
Synonyms L-Lysine Hydrochloride
Pharmacologic Category Nutritional Supplement
Dental Use Prevention of recurrent herpes simplex infection
Use Improves utilization of vegetable proteins
Local Anesthetic/Vasoconstrictor Precautions No information available to require special precautions
Effects on Dental Treatment No significant effects or complications reported
Dental Usual Dosing Recurrent herpes simplex infection: Adults: Oral: 2000 mg every 4 hours until symptoms subside. Begin treatment during early stage of recurrence.
Dosage Oral: Adults: 334-1500 mg/day
Recurrent herpes simplex infection (dental use): 2000 mg every 4 hours until symptoms subside. Begin treatment during early stage of recurrence.
Pregnancy Risk Factor C
Dosage Forms
Capsule (Lysinyl): 500 mg
Tablet: 500 mg, 1000 mg

Lysinyl [OTC] *see* L-Lysine *on page 959*

Lysodren® *see* Mitotane *on page 1055*

M-M-R® II *see* Measles, Mumps, and Rubella Vaccines (Combined) *on page 966*

Maalox® [OTC] *see* Aluminum Hydroxide, Magnesium Hydroxide, and Simethicone *on page 81*

Maalox® Max [OTC] *see* Aluminum Hydroxide, Magnesium Hydroxide, and Simethicone *on page 81*

Maalox® Quick Dissolve [OTC] *see* Calcium Carbonate *on page 248*

Maalox® Total Stomach Relief® [OTC] *see* Bismuth *on page 210*

Macrobid® *see* Nitrofurantoin *on page 1119*

Macrodantin® *see* Nitrofurantoin *on page 1119*

Macugen® *see* Pegaptanib *on page 1193*

Mafenide (MA fe nide)

U.S. Brand Names Sulfamylon®
Generic Available No
Synonyms Mafenide Acetate
Pharmacologic Category Antibiotic, Topical
Use Adjunct in the treatment of second- and third-degree burns to prevent septicemia caused by susceptible organisms such as *Pseudomonas aeruginosa*
Orphan drug: Prevention of graft loss of meshed autografts on excised burn wounds
Local Anesthetic/Vasoconstrictor Precautions No information available to require special precautions
Effects on Dental Treatment No significant effects or complications reported
Mechanism of Action Interferes with bacterial folic acid synthesis through competitive inhibition of para-aminobenzoic acid
Pregnancy Risk Factor C

Mafenide Acetate *see* Mafenide *on page 959*

Magaldrate and Simethicone (MAG al drate & sye METH i kone)

Related Information
Simethicone *on page 1394*
U.S. Brand Names Riopan Plus® [OTC] [DSC]; Riopan Plus® Double Strength [OTC] [DSC]
Generic Available Yes
Synonyms Simethicone and Magaldrate
Pharmacologic Category Antacid; Antiflatulent
Use Relief of hyperacidity associated with peptic ulcer, gastritis, peptic esophagitis and hiatal hernia which are accompanied by symptoms of gas
Local Anesthetic/Vasoconstrictor Precautions No information available to require special precautions
Effects on Dental Treatment No significant effects or complications reported
Common Adverse Effects Frequency not defined.
Based on **magaldrate** component:
Central nervous system: Encephalopathy
Gastrointestinal: Constipation, chalky taste, stomach cramps, fecal impaction, diarrhea, nausea, vomiting, discoloration of feces (white speckles), rebound hyperacidity
Endocrine & metabolic: Hypophosphatemia, hypermagnesemia, milk-alkali syndrome
Neuromuscular & metabolic: Osteomalacia
Miscellaneous: Aluminum intoxication
Based on **simethicone** component: No data reported
Drug Interactions
Increased Effect/Toxicity: See individual agents.
Pregnancy Risk Factor C

Mag Delay® [OTC] *see* Magnesium Chloride *on page 960*
Mag G® [OTC] *see* Magnesium Gluconate *on page 961*
Maginex™ [OTC] *see* Magnesium L-aspartate Hydrochloride *on page 962*
Maginex™ DS [OTC] *see* Magnesium L-aspartate Hydrochloride *on page 962*
Magnesia Magma *see* Magnesium Hydroxide *on page 961*
Magnesium Carbonate and Aluminum Hydroxide *see* Aluminum Hydroxide and Magnesium Carbonate *on page 79*

Magnesium Chloride (mag NEE zhum KLOR ide)

U.S. Brand Names Chloromag®; Mag Delay® [OTC]; Mag-SR® [OTC]; Slow-Mag® [OTC]
Generic Available Yes: Injection
Pharmacologic Category Magnesium Salt
Use Correction or prevention of hypomagnesemia
Local Anesthetic/Vasoconstrictor Precautions No information available to require special precautions
Effects on Dental Treatment Key adverse event(s) related to dental treatment: Magnesium products may prevent GI absorption of tetracyclines by forming a large ionized chelated molecule with the tetracyclines in the stomach. Tetracyclines should be given at least 1 hour before magnesium.
Pregnancy Risk Factor D

Magnesium Citrate (mag NEE zhum SIT rate)

Canadian Brand Names Citro-Mag®
Generic Available Yes
Synonyms Citrate of Magnesia
Pharmacologic Category Laxative, Saline; Magnesium Salt
Use Evacuation of bowel prior to certain surgical and diagnostic procedures or overdose situations
Local Anesthetic/Vasoconstrictor Precautions No information available to require special precautions
Effects on Dental Treatment Key adverse event(s) related to dental treatment: Magnesium products may prevent GI absorption of tetracyclines by forming a large ionized chelated molecule with the tetracyclines in the stomach. Tetracyclines should be given at least 1 hour before magnesium.
Mechanism of Action Promotes bowel evacuation by causing osmotic retention of fluid which distends the colon with increased peristaltic activity
Pregnancy Risk Factor B

Magnesium Gluconate (mag NEE zhum GLOO koe nate)

U.S. Brand Names Almora® [OTC]; Mag G® [OTC]; Magonate® [OTC]; Magonate® Sport [OTC] [DSC]; Magtrate® [OTC]

Generic Available Yes: Tablet

Pharmacologic Category Magnesium Salt

Use Dietary supplement for treatment of magnesium deficiencies

Local Anesthetic/Vasoconstrictor Precautions No information available to require special precautions

Effects on Dental Treatment Key adverse event(s) related to dental treatment: Magnesium products may prevent GI absorption of tetracyclines by forming a large ionized chelated molecule with the tetracyclines in the stomach. Tetracyclines should be given at least 1 hour before magnesium.

Mechanism of Action Magnesium is important as a cofactor in many enzymatic reactions in the body involving protein synthesis and carbohydrate metabolism (at least 300 enzymatic reactions require magnesium). Actions on lipoprotein lipase have been found to be important in reducing serum cholesterol and on sodium/potassium ATPase in promoting polarization (ie, neuromuscular functioning).

Magnesium Hydroxide (mag NEE zhum hye DROKS ide)

U.S. Brand Names Dulcolax® Milk of Magnesia [OTC]; Phillips'® Milk of Magnesia [OTC]

Generic Available Yes: Liquid

Synonyms Magnesia Magma; Milk of Magnesia; MOM

Pharmacologic Category Antacid; Magnesium Salt

Use Short-term treatment of occasional constipation and symptoms of hyperacidity, magnesium replacement therapy

Local Anesthetic/Vasoconstrictor Precautions No information available to require special precautions

Effects on Dental Treatment Key adverse event(s) related to dental treatment: Magnesium products may prevent GI absorption of tetracyclines by forming a large ionized chelated molecule with the tetracyclines in the stomach. Tetracyclines should be given at least 1 hour before magnesium.

Mechanism of Action Promotes bowel evacuation by causing osmotic retention of fluid which distends the colon with increased peristaltic activity; reacts with hydrochloric acid in stomach to form magnesium chloride

Pregnancy Risk Factor B

Magnesium Hydroxide, Aluminum Hydroxide, and Simethicone *see* Aluminum Hydroxide, Magnesium Hydroxide, and Simethicone *on page 81*

Magnesium Hydroxide and Aluminum Hydroxide *see* Aluminum Hydroxide and Magnesium Hydroxide *on page 80*

Magnesium Hydroxide and Calcium Carbonate *see* Calcium Carbonate and Magnesium Hydroxide *on page 249*

Magnesium Hydroxide and Mineral Oil
(mag NEE zhum hye DROKS ide & MIN er al oyl)

Related Information
Magnesium Hydroxide *on page 961*

U.S. Brand Names Phillips'® M-O [OTC]

Generic Available No

Synonyms Haley's M-O; MOM/Mineral Oil Emulsion

Pharmacologic Category Laxative

Use Short-term treatment of occasional constipation

Local Anesthetic/Vasoconstrictor Precautions No information available to require special precautions

Effects on Dental Treatment Key adverse event(s) related to dental treatment: Magnesium products may prevent GI absorption of tetracyclines by forming a large ionized chelated molecule with the tetracyclines in the stomach. Tetracyclines should be given at least 1 hour before magnesium.

Pregnancy Risk Factor B

Magnesium Hydroxide, Famotidine, and Calcium Carbonate *see* Famotidine, Calcium Carbonate, and Magnesium Hydroxide *on page 636*

Magnesium L-aspartate Hydrochloride
(mag NEE zhum el as PAR tate hye droe KLOR ide)

U.S. Brand Names Maginex™ [OTC]; Maginex™ DS [OTC]
Synonyms MAH
Pharmacologic Category Electrolyte Supplement, Oral
Use Dietary supplement
Local Anesthetic/Vasoconstrictor Precautions No information available to require special precautions
Effects on Dental Treatment Key adverse event(s) related to dental treatment: Magnesium ions prevent GI absorption of tetracycline by forming a large, ionized, chelated molecule with the magnesium ion and tetracyclines in the stomach. Magnesium supplement should not be taken within 2-4 hours of oral tetracycline or other members of the tetracycline family.
Common Adverse Effects Frequency not defined: Gastrointestinal: Diarrhea, loose stools

Magnesium Oxide (mag NEE zhum OKS ide)

U.S. Brand Names Mag-Ox® 400 [OTC]; Uro-Mag® [OTC]
Generic Available Yes: Tablet
Pharmacologic Category Electrolyte Supplement, Oral
Use Electrolyte replacement
Local Anesthetic/Vasoconstrictor Precautions No information available to require special precautions
Effects on Dental Treatment Key adverse event(s) related to dental treatment: Magnesium products may prevent GI absorption of tetracycline by forming a large ionized chelated molecule with the tetracyclines in the stomach. Tetracyclines should be given at least 1 hour before magnesium.
Pregnancy Risk Factor B

Magnesium Salicylate (mag NEE zhum sa LIS i late)

Related Information
Rheumatoid Arthritis, Osteoarthritis, and Osteoporosis *on page 1668*
Temporomandibular Dysfunction (TMD) *on page 1724*
U.S. Brand Names Doan's® [OTC]; Doan's® Extra Strength [OTC]; Keygesic [OTC]; Momentum® [OTC]
Mexican Brand Names Myoflex®
Generic Available Yes
Pharmacologic Category Salicylate
Use Mild to moderate pain, fever, various inflammatory conditions
Local Anesthetic/Vasoconstrictor Precautions No information available to require special precautions
Effects on Dental Treatment NSAID formulations are known to reversibly decrease platelet aggregation via mechanisms different than observed with aspirin. The dentist should be aware of the potential of abnormal coagulation. Caution should also be exercised in the use of NSAIDs in patients already on anticoagulant therapy with drugs such as warfarin (Coumadin®).
Dosage Oral: Children ≥12 years and Adults:
Doan's®: Two caplets every 4 hours as needed (maximum: 12 caplets/24 hours)
Doan's® Extra Strength, Momentum®: Two caplets every 6 hours (maximum: 8 caplets/24 hours)
Keygesic: One caplet every 4 hours as needed (maximum 4 caplets/24 hours)
Warnings/Precautions Use with caution with bleeding disorders, renal dysfunction, dehydration, gastritis, or peptic ulcer disease. Heavy ethanol use (>3 drinks/day) can increase bleeding risks. Avoid use in renal or hepatic failure. Discontinue use if tinnitus or impaired hearing occurs. Patients with sensitivity to tartrazine dyes, nasal polyps, and asthma may have an increased risk of salicylate sensitivity. Surgical patients should avoid ASA if possible, for 1-2 weeks prior to surgery, to reduce the risk of excessive bleeding. Children and teenagers who have or are recovering from chickenpox or flu-like symptoms should not use this product. Changes in behavior (along with nausea and vomiting) may be an early sign of Reye's syndrome; patients should be instructed to contact their healthcare provider if these occur.
Drug Interactions
Decreased Effect: Decreased absorption of aminoquinolones, digoxin, nitrofurantoin, penicillamine, and tetracyclines may occur with magnesium salts.

Dosage Forms CAPLET, as anhydrous magnesium salicylate: 467 mg; (Doan's®): 304 mg; (Doan's® Extra Strength, Momentum®): 467 mg; (Keygesic): 650 mg

Magnesium Sulfate (mag NEE zhum SUL fate)

Generic Available Yes

Synonyms Epsom Salts; $MgSO_4$ (error-prone abbreviation)

Pharmacologic Category Antacid; Anticonvulsant, Miscellaneous; Electrolyte Supplement, Parenteral; Laxative, Saline; Magnesium Salt

Use Treatment and prevention of hypomagnesemia; seizure prevention in severe pre-eclampsia or eclampsia, pediatric acute nephritis; short-term treatment torsade de pointes; treatment of cardiac arrhythmias (VT/VF) caused by hypomagnesemia; short-term treatment of constipation or soaking aid

Local Anesthetic/Vasoconstrictor Precautions No information available to require special precautions

Effects on Dental Treatment Key adverse event(s) related to dental treatment: Magnesium products may prevent GI absorption of tetracyclines by forming a large ionized chelated molecule with the tetracyclines in the stomach. Tetracyclines should be given at least 1 hour before magnesium.

Mechanism of Action When taken orally, magnesium promotes bowel evacuation by causing osmotic retention of fluid which distends the colon with increased peristaltic activity; parenterally, magnesium decreases acetylcholine in motor nerve terminals and acts on myocardium by slowing rate of S-A node impulse formation and prolonging conduction time

Pregnancy Risk Factor B

Magnesium Trisilicate and Aluminum Hydroxide *see* Aluminum Hydroxide and Magnesium Trisilicate *on page 80*

Magnevist® *see* Gadopentetate Dimeglumine *on page 719*

Magonate® [OTC] *see* Magnesium Gluconate *on page 961*

Magonate® Sport [OTC] [DSC] *see* Magnesium Gluconate *on page 961*

Mag-Ox® 400 [OTC] *see* Magnesium Oxide *on page 962*

Mag-SR® [OTC] *see* Magnesium Chloride *on page 960*

Magtrate® [OTC] *see* Magnesium Gluconate *on page 961*

MAH *see* Magnesium L-aspartate Hydrochloride *on page 962*

Malarone® *see* Atovaquone and Proguanil *on page 160*

Maltodextrin (mal toe DEK strin)

U.S. Brand Names Gelclair®; Multidex® [OTC]; OraRinse™ [OTC]

Generic Available No

Pharmacologic Category Anti-inflammatory, Locally Applied

Dental Use Oral: Management and relief of pain due to oral lesions (including mucositis/stomatitis), oral ulcers, or irritation; treatment of aphthous ulcers

Use Topical: Treatment of infected or noninfected wounds

Local Anesthetic/Vasoconstrictor Precautions No information available to require special precautions

Effects on Dental Treatment No significant effects or complications reported (see Dental Comment)

Dental Usual Dosing Management of pain due to oral lesions: Adults: Oral:
   Gelclair®: Using contents of 1 reconstituted packet, rinse around mouth for ~1 minute, 3 times/day or more if needed; gargle and expectorate. May be used undiluted or with less dilution if adequate pain relief is not achieved.
   OraRinse™: 1 tablespoonful, swish or gargle for ~1 minute, 4 times/day or more if needed

Dosage Adults:
   Oral: Management of pain due to oral lesions:
      Gelclair®: Using contents of 1 reconstituted packet, rinse around mouth for ~1 minute, 3 times/day or more if needed; gargle and expectorate. May be used undiluted or with less dilution if adequate pain relief is not achieved.
      OraRinse™: 1 tablespoonful, swish or gargle for ~1 minute, 4 times/day or more if needed
   Topical: Wound dressing: Multidex®: After debridement and irrigation of wound, apply and cover with a nonadherent, nonocclusive dressing. May be applied to moist or dry, infected or noninfected wounds.

Mechanism of Action Forms a protective barrier over wound providing an environment which promotes tissue growth.

Contraindications Hypersensitivity to maltodextrin or any component of the formulation
(Continued)

Maltodextrin *(Continued)*

Warnings/Precautions Oral: Avoid eating or drinking for 1 hour; products are not harmful if accidentally swallowed; notify healthcare provider if improvement is not seen within 7 days

Dosage Forms

Gel, oral [concentrate] (Gelclair®): 15 mL/packet (21s) [contains benzalkonium chloride and sodium benzoate]

Gel, topical dressing (Multidex®): (4 mL, 7 mL, 14 mL, 85 mL)

Powder, for oral suspension (OraRinse™): (19 g) [contains phenylalanine; also contains aloe vera, fructose, and sodium benzoate; vanilla flavor]

Powder, topical dressing (Multidex®): (6 g, 12 g, 25 g, 45 g)

Dental Comment

Gelclair®: Store at room temperature away from direct sunlight. Do not refrigerate. Gel may become darker or thicker over time; efficacy and safety are not affected if used prior to labeled expiration date. Mix contents of one packet with 40 mL of water. Stir and use at once. Product may be used undiluted if water is unavailable.

OraRinse™: Fill bottle with water to first arrow; shake vigorously until suspended; continue to fill to second arrow; shake well

m-AMSA *see Amsacrine on page 123*

Mandelamine® *see Methenamine on page 1007*

Mandrake *see Podophyllum Resin on page 1251*

Manganese *see Trace Metals on page 1513*

Mantoux *see Tuberculin Tests on page 1548*

Mapap [OTC] *see Acetaminophen on page 31*

Mapap Children's [OTC] *see Acetaminophen on page 31*

Mapap Extra Strength [OTC] *see Acetaminophen on page 31*

Mapap Infants [OTC] *see Acetaminophen on page 31*

Mapap Sinus Maximum Strength [OTC] *see Acetaminophen and Pseudoephedrine on page 38*

Maprotiline *(ma PROE ti leen)*

Canadian Brand Names Novo-Maprotiline

Mexican Brand Names Ludiomil®

Generic Available Yes

Synonyms Ludiomil; Maprotiline Hydrochloride

Pharmacologic Category Antidepressant, Tetracyclic

Use Treatment of depression and anxiety associated with depression

Unlabeled/Investigational Use Bulimia; duodenal ulcers; enuresis; urinary symptoms of multiple sclerosis; pain; panic attacks; tension headache; cocaine withdrawal

Local Anesthetic/Vasoconstrictor Precautions Although maprotiline is not a tricyclic antidepressant, it does block norepinephrine reuptake within CNS synapses as part of its mechanisms. It has been suggested that vasoconstrictor be administered with caution and to monitor vital signs in dental patients taking antidepressants that affect norepinephrine in this way, including maprotiline. Epinephrine and levonordefrin have been shown to have an increased pressor response in combination with TCAs.

Effects on Dental Treatment Key adverse event(s) related to dental treatment: Xerostomia and changes in salivation (normal salivary flow resumes upon discontinuation).

Common Adverse Effects

>10%:

Central nervous system: Drowsiness

Gastrointestinal: Xerostomia

1% to 10%:

Central nervous system: Insomnia, nervousness, anxiety, agitation, dizziness, fatigue, headache

Gastrointestinal: Constipation, nausea

Neuromuscular & skeletal: Tremor, weakness

Ocular: Blurred vision

Restrictions A medication guide concerning the use of antidepressants in children and teenagers can be found on the FDA website at http://www.fda.gov/cder/Offices/ODS/labeling.htm. It should be dispensed to parents or guardians of children and teenagers receiving this medication.

Mechanism of Action Traditionally believed to increase the synaptic concentration of norepinephrine in the central nervous system by inhibition of their reuptake by the presynaptic neuronal membrane. However, additional receptor effects have been found including desensitization of adenyl cyclase, down regulation of beta-adrenergic receptors, and down regulation of serotonin receptors.

Drug Interactions

Cytochrome P450 Effect: Substrate of CYP2D6 (major)

Increased Effect/Toxicity: Maprotiline may increase the effects of amphetamines, anticholinergics, other CNS depressants (sedatives, hypnotics, or ethanol), carbamazepine, tolazamide, chlorpropamide, and warfarin. When used with MAO inhibitors, hyperpyrexia, hypertension, tachycardia, confusion, seizures, and **deaths have been reported** (serotonin syndrome). CYP2D6 inhibitors may increase the levels/effects of maprotiline; example inhibitors include chlorpromazine, delavirdine, fluoxetine, miconazole, paroxetine, pergolide, quinidine, quinine, ritonavir, and ropinirole. Cimetidine, fenfluramine, grapefruit juice, indinavir, methylphenidate, diltiazem, valproate, and verapamil may increase the serum concentrations of cyclic antidepressants. Use of lithium with a cyclic antidepressant may increase the risk for neurotoxicity. Phenothiazines may increase concentration of some cyclic antidepressants and cyclic antidepressants may increase the concentration of phenothiazines. Pressor response to I.V. epinephrine, norepinephrine, and phenylephrine may be enhanced in patients receiving cyclic antidepressants (**Note:** Effect is unlikely with epinephrine or levonordefrin dosages typically administered as infiltration in combination with local anesthetics). Combined use of beta-agonists or drugs which prolong QT_c (including quinidine, procainamide, disopyramide, cisapride, sparfloxacin, gatifloxacin, moxifloxacin) with cyclic antidepressants may predispose patients to cardiac arrhythmias.

Decreased Effect: Maprotiline inhibits the antihypertensive response to bethanidine, clonidine, debrisoquin, guanadrel, guanethidine, guanabenz, or guanfacine. Cholestyramine and colestipol may bind cyclic antidepressants and reduce their absorption.

Pharmacodynamics/Kinetics

Absorption: Slow
Protein binding: 88%
Metabolism: Hepatic to active and inactive compounds
Half-life elimination, serum: 27-58 hours (mean: 43 hours)
Time to peak, serum: Within 12 hours
Excretion: Urine (70%); feces (30%)

Pregnancy Risk Factor B

Maprotiline Hydrochloride see Maprotiline on page 964

Marcaine® see Bupivacaine on page 228

Marcaine® Spinal see Bupivacaine on page 228

Marcaine® with Epinephrine see Bupivacaine and Epinephrine on page 228

Marezine® [OTC] see Cyclizine on page 400

Margesic® H see Hydrocodone and Acetaminophen on page 779

Marinol® see Dronabinol on page 518

Marplan® see Isocarboxazid on page 863

Matulane® see Procarbazine on page 1284

3M™ Avagard™ [OTC] see Chlorhexidine Gluconate on page 316

Mavik® see Trandolapril on page 1517

Maxair™ Autohaler™ see Pirbuterol on page 1248

Maxalt® see Rizatriptan on page 1363

Maxalt-MLT® see Rizatriptan on page 1363

Maxaquin® [DSC] see Lomefloxacin on page 941

Maxidex® see Dexamethasone on page 439

Maxidone™ see Hydrocodone and Acetaminophen on page 779

Maxifed® see Guaifenesin and Pseudoephedrine on page 755

Maxifed DM see Guaifenesin, Pseudoephedrine, and Dextromethorphan on page 757

Maxifed-G® see Guaifenesin and Pseudoephedrine on page 755

Maxiphen DM see Guaifenesin, Dextromethorphan, and Phenylephrine on page 756

Maxipime® see Cefepime on page 287

Maxitrol® see Neomycin, Polymyxin B, and Dexamethasone on page 1101

Maxi-Tuss HCG see Hydrocodone and Guaifenesin on page 785

Maxivate® see Betamethasone on page 199

Maxzide® see Hydrochlorothiazide and Triamterene on page 778

Maxzide®-25 see Hydrochlorothiazide and Triamterene on page 778

May Apple see Podophyllum Resin on page 1251

3M™ Cavilon™ Skin Cleanser [OTC] see Benzalkonium Chloride on page 188

MCH see Collagen Hemostat on page 392

m-Cresyl Acetate (em-KREE sil AS e tate)

U.S. Brand Names Cresylate®
Generic Available No
Pharmacologic Category Otic Agent, Anti-infective
Use Provides an acid medium; for external otitis infections caused by susceptible bacteria or fungus
Local Anesthetic/Vasoconstrictor Precautions No information available to require special precautions
Effects on Dental Treatment No significant effects or complications reported

MCT *see* Medium Chain Triglycerides *on page 972*

MCT Oil® [OTC] *see* Medium Chain Triglycerides *on page 972*

MCV4 *see* Meningococcal Polysaccharide (Groups A / C / Y and W-135) Diphtheria Toxoid Conjugate Vaccine *on page 980*

MD-76®R *see* Diatrizoate Meglumine and Diatrizoate Sodium *on page 453*

MD-Gastroview® *see* Diatrizoate Meglumine and Diatrizoate Sodium *on page 453*

MDL 73,147EF *see* Dolasetron *on page 498*

Measles, Mumps, and Rubella Vaccines (Combined)
(MEE zels, mumpz & roo BEL a vak SEENS, kom BINED)

Related Information
Immunizations (Vaccines) *on page 1786*
U.S. Brand Names M-M-R® II
Canadian Brand Names M-M-R® II; Priorix™
Generic Available No
Synonyms MMR; Mumps, Measles and Rubella Vaccines, Combined; Rubella, Measles and Mumps Vaccines, Combined
Pharmacologic Category Vaccine, Live Virus
Use Measles, mumps, and rubella prophylaxis
Local Anesthetic/Vasoconstrictor Precautions No information available to require special precautions
Effects on Dental Treatment No significant effects or complications reported
Common Adverse Effects All serious adverse reactions must be reported to the U.S. Department of Health and Human Services (DHHS) Vaccine Adverse Event Reporting System (VAERS) 1-800-822-7967.
Frequency not defined:
Cardiovascular: Syncope, vasculitis
Central nervous system: Ataxia, dizziness, febrile convulsions, fever, encephalitis, encephalopathy, Guillain-Barré syndrome, headache, irritability, malaise, measles inclusion body encephalitis, polyneuritis, polyneuropathy, seizure, subacute sclerosing panencephalitis,
Dermatologic: Angioneurotic edema, erythema multiforme, purpura, rash, Stevens-Johnson syndrome, urticaria
Endocrine & metabolic: Diabetes mellitus, parotitis
Gastrointestinal: Diarrhea, nausea, pancreatitis, sore throat, vomiting
Genitourinary: Orchitis
Hematologic: Leukocytosis, thrombocytopenia
Local: Injection site reactions which include burning, induration, redness, stinging, swelling, tenderness, wheal and flare, vesiculation
Neuromuscular & skeletal: Arthralgia/arthritis (variable; highest rates in women, 12% to 26% versus children, up to 3%), myalgia, paresthesia
Ocular: Ocular palsies
Otic: Otitis media
Renal: Conjunctivitis, retinitis, optic neuritis, papillitis, retrobulbar neuritis
Respiratory: Bronchospasm, cough, pneumonitis, rhinitis
Miscellaneous: Anaphylactoid reactions, anaphylaxis, atypical measles, panniculitis, regional lymphadenopathy
Mechanism of Action As a live, attenuated vaccine, MMR vaccine offers active immunity to disease caused by the measles, mumps, and rubella viruses.
Drug Interactions
Decreased Effect: The effect of the vaccine may be decreased in individuals who are receiving immunosuppressant drugs (including high dose systemic corticosteroids). Effect of vaccine may be decreased when given with immune globulin; do not administer with vaccine. Effectiveness of MMR may be decreased if given within 30 days of varicella vaccine (effectiveness not decreased when administered simultaneously).
Pregnancy Risk Factor C

Measles, Mumps, Rubella, and Varicella Virus Vaccine
(MEE zels, mumpz, roo BEL a, & var i SEL a VYE rus vak SEEN)

U.S. Brand Names ProQuad®

Generic Available No

Synonyms Mumps, Rubella, Varicella, and Measles Vaccine; Rubella, Varicella, Measles, and Mumps Vaccine; Varicella, Measles, Mumps, and Rubella Vaccine

Pharmacologic Category Vaccine, Live Virus

Use To provide simultaneous active immunization against measles, mumps, rubella, and varicella

Local Anesthetic/Vasoconstrictor Precautions No information available to require special precautions

Effects on Dental Treatment No significant effects or complications reported

Common Adverse Effects All serious adverse reactions must be reported to the U.S. Department of Health and Human Services (DHHS) Vaccine Adverse Event Reporting System (VAERS) 1-800-822-7967.

With the exception of fever and measles-like rash, incidence of adverse events was generally lower in patients receiving ProQuad® compared to those receiving M-M-R® II and Varivax®. Also refer to M-M-R® II and Varivax® monographs for additional adverse reactions reported with those agents.

>10%:
Central nervous system: Fever ≥38.9°C (≥102°F) (22%)
Local: Injection site reaction including pain, tenderness, soreness (22%); erythema (14%)

1% to 10%:
Central nervous system: Irritability (7%)
Dermatologic: Measles-like rash (3%), varicella-like rash (2%), rash (2%), viral exanthema (1%)
Gastrointestinal: Diarrhea (1%)
Local: Injection site reaction: Swelling (8%), bruising (2%)
Respiratory: Upper respiratory tract infection (1%)

Mechanism of Action A live, attenuated virus; offers active immunity to disease caused by the measles, mumps, rubella, and varicella-zoster virus.

Drug Interactions
Increased Effect/Toxicity: Salicylates may increase the risk of Reye's syndrome following varicella vaccination; avoid use of salicylates for 6 weeks following vaccination.

Decreased Effect:
In patients receiving high doses of systemic corticosteroids for ≥14 days, wait at least 1 month between discontinuing steroid therapy and administering vaccine. Do not administer with immune globulin (including varicella zoster immune globulin); vaccination should be deferred for at least 5 months following immune globulin administration; immune globulins should not be given for at least 2 months following vaccination (unless benefits of use outweigh benefits of vaccination). The effect of the vaccine may be decreased and the risk of varicella disease in individuals who are receiving immunosuppressant drugs may be increased.

Pregnancy Risk Factor C

Measles Virus Vaccine (Live) (MEE zels VYE rus vak SEEN, live)

Related Information
Immunizations (Vaccines) *on page 1786*

U.S. Brand Names Attenuvax®

Generic Available No

Synonyms More Attenuated Enders Strain; Rubeola Vaccine

Pharmacologic Category Vaccine, Live Virus

Use Adults born before 1957 are generally considered to be immune. All those born in or after 1957 without documentation of live vaccine on or after first birthday, physician-diagnosed measles, or laboratory evidence of immunity should be vaccinated, ideally with two doses of vaccine separated by no less than 1 month. For those previously vaccinated with one dose of measles vaccine, revaccination is recommended for students entering colleges and other institutions of higher education, for healthcare workers at the time of employment, and for international travelers who visit endemic areas.

MMR is the vaccine of choice if recipients are likely to be susceptible to rubella and/or mumps as well as to measles. Persons vaccinated between 1963 and 1967 with a killed measles vaccine, followed by live vaccine
(Continued)

Measles Virus Vaccine (Live) *(Continued)*

within 3 months, or with a vaccine of unknown type should be revaccinated with live measles virus vaccine.

Local Anesthetic/Vasoconstrictor Precautions No information available to require special precautions

Effects on Dental Treatment No significant effects or complications reported

Common Adverse Effects All serious adverse reactions must be reported to the U.S. Department of Health and Human Services (DHHS) Vaccine Adverse Event Reporting System (VAERS) 1-800-822-7967.

>10%:

Cardiovascular: Edema

Central nervous system: Fever (<100°F)

Local: Burning or stinging, induration

1% to 10%:

Central nervous system: Fever between 100°F and 103°F usually between 5th and 12th days postvaccination

Dermatologic: Rash (rarely generalized)

Mechanism of Action Promotes active immunity to measles virus by inducing specific measles IgG and IgM antibodies.

Pregnancy Risk Factor X

Mebaral® *see* Mephobarbital *on page 986*

Mebendazole *(me BEN da zole)*

U.S. Brand Names Vermox® [DSC]

Canadian Brand Names Vermox®

Mexican Brand Names Revapol®; Vermicol®; Vermidil®; Vermin®

Generic Available Yes

Pharmacologic Category Anthelmintic

Use Treatment of pinworms (*Enterobius vermicularis*), whipworms (*Trichuris trichiura*), roundworms (*Ascaris lumbricoides*), and hookworms (*Ancylostoma duodenale*)

Local Anesthetic/Vasoconstrictor Precautions No information available to require special precautions

Effects on Dental Treatment No significant effects or complications reported

Mechanism of Action Selectively and irreversibly blocks glucose uptake and other nutrients in susceptible adult intestine-dwelling helminths

Pregnancy Risk Factor C

Mecamylamine *(mek a MIL a meen)*

U.S. Brand Names Inversine®

Canadian Brand Names Inversine®

Generic Available No

Synonyms Mecamylamine Hydrochloride

Pharmacologic Category Ganglionic Blocking Agent

Use Treatment of moderately severe to severe hypertension and in uncomplicated malignant hypertension

Unlabeled/Investigational Use Tourette's syndrome

Local Anesthetic/Vasoconstrictor Precautions No information available to require special precautions

Effects on Dental Treatment Key adverse event(s) related to dental treatment: Xerostomia (normal salivary flow resumes upon discontinuation).

Mechanism of Action Mecamylamine is a ganglionic blocker. This agent inhibits acetylcholine at the autonomic ganglia, causing a decrease in blood pressure. Mecamylamine also blocks central nicotinic cholinergic receptors, which inhibits the effects of nicotine and may suppress the desire to smoke.

Pregnancy Risk Factor C

Mecamylamine Hydrochloride *see* Mecamylamine *on page 968*

Mecasermin *(mek a SER min)*

U.S. Brand Names Increlex™; Iplex™

Generic Available No

Synonyms Mecasermin (rDNA Origin); Mecasermin Rinfabate; Recombinant Human Insulin-Like Growth Factor-1; rhIGF-1; rhIGF-1/rhIGFBP-3

Pharmacologic Category Growth Hormone

Use Treatment of growth failure in children with severe primary insulin-like growth factor-1 deficiency (IGF-1 deficiency; primary IGFD), or with growth hormone (GH) gene deletions who have developed neutralizing antibodies to GH

Local Anesthetic/Vasoconstrictor Precautions No information available to require special precautions

Effects on Dental Treatment No significant effects or complications reported

Common Adverse Effects

≥5%:

Cardiovascular: Cardiac murmur

Central nervous system: Convulsion, dizziness, headache (Iplex™: 22%)

Endocrine & metabolic: Hyper-/hypoglycemia (Increlex™: 42%; Iplex™ 31%), iron-deficiency anemia, ovarian cysts, thymus hypertrophy, thyromegaly

Gastrointestinal: Vomiting

Hepatic: Liver enzymes increased

Local: Injection site reactions: Erythema, bruising, hair growth, lipohypertrophy

Neuromuscular & skeletal: Arthralgia, bone pain, extremity pain, muscular atrophy

Ocular: Papilledema

Otic: Ear pain, hypoacusis, middle ear fluid, otitis media, serous otitis media, tympanometry abnormal

Renal: Hematuria

Respiratory: Snoring, tonsillar hypertrophy (Increlex™: 15%; Iplex™ 19%)

Miscellanous: Lymphadenopathy

<5% or frequency not defined: Hypoglycemic seizure, intracranial hypertension, loss of consciousness secondary to hypoglycemia, thickening of soft facial tissue

Mechanism of Action Mecasermin is an insulin-like growth factor (IGF-1) produced using recombinant DNA technology to replace endogenous IGF-1. Endogenous IGF-1 circulates predominately bound to insulin-like growth factor-binding protein-3 (IGFBP-3) and a growth hormone-dependent acid-labile subunit (ALS). Acting at receptors in the liver and other tissues, endogenous growth hormone (GH) stimulates the synthesis and secretion of IGF-1. In patients with primary severe IGF-1 deficiency, growth hormone receptors in the liver are unresponsive to GH, leading to reduced endogenous IGF-I concentrations and decreased growth (skeletal, cell, and organ). Endogenous IGF-1 also suppresses liver glucose production, stimulates peripheral glucose utilization and has an inhibitory effect on insulin secretion.

Mecasermin rinfabate is a complex of IGF-1 and IGFBP-3, both produced by recombinant DNA technology.

Pharmacodynamics/Kinetics

Distribution: V_d: Severe primary IGFD: 0.184-0.33 L/kg

Protein binding: >80% bound to IGFBP-3 and an acid-labile subunit (IGFBP-3 reduced with severe primary IGFD)

Metabolism: Hepatic and renal

Half-life elimination: Severe primary IGFD: Mecasermin: 5.8 hours; Mecasermin rinfabate: >12 hours

Pregnancy Risk Factor C

Mecasermin (rDNA Origin) *see* Mecasermin *on page 968*

Mecasermin Rinfabate *see* Mecasermin *on page 968*

Meclizine (MEK li zeen)

U.S. Brand Names Antivert®; Bonine® [OTC]; Dramamine® Less Drowsy Formula [OTC]

Canadian Brand Names Bonamine™; Bonine®

Generic Available Yes

Synonyms Meclizine Hydrochloride; Meclozine Hydrochloride

Pharmacologic Category Antiemetic; Antihistamine

Use Prevention and treatment of symptoms of motion sickness; management of vertigo with diseases affecting the vestibular system

Local Anesthetic/Vasoconstrictor Precautions No information available to require special precautions

Effects on Dental Treatment Key adverse event(s) related to dental treatment: Slight to moderate drowsiness, thickening of bronchial secretions, significant xerostomia (normal salivary flow resumes upon discontinuation).

Common Adverse Effects

>10%:

Central nervous system: Slight to moderate drowsiness

Respiratory: Thickening of bronchial secretions

(Continued)

Meclizine (Continued)

1% to 10%:

Central nervous system: Headache, fatigue, nervousness, dizziness

Gastrointestinal: Appetite increase, weight gain, nausea, diarrhea, abdominal pain, xerostomia

Neuromuscular & skeletal: Arthralgia

Respiratory: Pharyngitis

Mechanism of Action Has central anticholinergic action by blocking chemoreceptor trigger zone; decreases excitability of the middle ear labyrinth and blocks conduction in the middle ear vestibular-cerebellar pathways

Drug Interactions

Increased Effect/Toxicity: Increased toxicity with CNS depressants, neuroleptics, and anticholinergics.

Pharmacodynamics/Kinetics

Onset of action: ~1 hour

Duration: 8-24 hours

Metabolism: Hepatic

Half-life elimination: 6 hours

Excretion: Urine (as metabolites); feces (as unchanged drug)

Pregnancy Risk Factor B

Meclizine Hydrochloride see Meclizine on page 969

Meclofenamate (me kloe fen AM ate)

Related Information

Rheumatoid Arthritis, Osteoarthritis, and Osteoporosis on page 1668

Temporomandibular Dysfunction (TMD) on page 1724

Canadian Brand Names Meclomen®

Generic Available Yes

Synonyms Meclofenamate Sodium

Pharmacologic Category Nonsteroidal Anti-inflammatory Drug (NSAID), Oral

Use Treatment of inflammatory disorders, arthritis, mild to moderate pain, dysmenorrhea

Local Anesthetic/Vasoconstrictor Precautions No information available to require special precautions

Effects on Dental Treatment NSAID formulations are known to reversibly decrease platelet aggregation via mechanisms different than observed with aspirin. The dentist should be aware of the potential of abnormal coagulation. Caution should also be exercised in the use of NSAIDs in patients already on anticoagulant therapy with drugs such as warfarin (Coumadin®). Recovery of platelet function usually occurs 1-2 days after discontinuation of NSAIDs.

Common Adverse Effects

>10%:

Central nervous system: Dizziness

Dermatologic: Rash

Gastrointestinal: Abdominal cramps, heartburn, indigestion, nausea

1% to 10%:

Central nervous system: Headache, nervousness

Dermatologic: Itching

Endocrine & metabolic: Fluid retention

Gastrointestinal: Vomiting

Otic: Tinnitus

Restrictions A medication guide should be dispensed with each prescription. A template for the required MedGuide can be found on the FDA website at: http://www.fda.gov/medwatch/SAFETY/2005/safety05.htm#NSAID

Dosage Children >14 years and Adults: Oral:

Mild to moderate pain: 50 mg every 4-6 hours; increases to 100 mg may be required; maximum dose: 400 mg

Rheumatoid arthritis and osteoarthritis: 50 mg every 4-6 hours; increase, over weeks, to 200-400 mg/day in 3-4 divided doses; do not exceed 400 mg/day; maximal benefit for any dose may not be seen for 2-3 weeks

Mechanism of Action Inhibits prostaglandin synthesis by decreasing the activity of the enzyme, cyclooxygenase, which results in decreased formation of prostaglandin precursors

Contraindications Hypersensitivity to meclofenamate, aspirin, other NSAIDs, or any component of the formulation; perioperative pain in the setting of coronary artery bypass surgery (CABG); active GI bleeding, ulcer disease; pregnancy (3rd trimester)

Warnings/Precautions NSAIDs are associated with an increased risk of adverse cardiovascular events, including MI, stroke, and new onset or worsening of pre-existing hypertension. Risk may be increased with duration of use or pre-existing cardiovascular risk-factors or disease. Carefully evaluate individual cardiovascular risk profiles prior to prescribing. Use caution with fluid retention, CHF or hypertension.

Use of NSAIDs can compromise existing renal function. Renal toxicity can occur in patient with impaired renal function, dehydration, heart failure, liver dysfunction, those taking diuretics and ACEI and the elderly. Rehydrate patient before starting therapy. Monitor renal function closely. Use caution in patients with advanced renal disease.

NSAIDs may increase risk of gastrointestinal irritation, ulceration, bleeding, and perforation. These events may occur at any time during therapy and without warning. Use caution with a history of GI disease (bleeding or ulcers), concurrent therapy with aspirin, anticoagulants and/or corticosteroids, smoking, use of alcohol, the elderly or debilitated patients.

Use the lowest effective dose for the shortest duration of time, consistent with individual patient goals, to reduce risk of cardiovascular or GI adverse events. Alternate therapies should be considered for patients at high risk.

NSAIDs may cause serious skin adverse events including exfoliative dermatitis, Stevens-Johnson syndrome (SJS) and toxic epidermal necrolysis (TEN). Anaphylactoid reactions may occur, even without prior exposure; patients with "aspirin triad" (bronchial asthma, aspirin intolerance, rhinitis) may be at increased risk. Do not use in patients who experience bronchospasm, asthma, rhinitis, or urticaria with NSAID or aspirin therapy.

Use with caution in patients with decreased hepatic function. Closely monitor patients with any abnormal LFT. Severe hepatic reactions (eg, fulminant hepatitis, liver failure) have occurred with NSAID use, rarely; discontinue if signs or symptoms of liver disease develop, or if systemic manifestations occur.

The elderly are at increased risk for adverse effects (especially peptic ulceration, CNS effects, renal toxicity) from NSAIDs even at low doses

Withhold for at least 4-6 half-lives prior to surgical or dental procedures. Safety and efficacy have not been established in children <14 years of age.

Drug Interactions
Increased Effect/Toxicity: Anticoagulants (warfarin, heparin, LMWHs) in combination with NSAIDs can cause increased risk of bleeding. Other antiplatelet drugs (ticlopidine, clopidogrel, aspirin, abciximab, dipyridamole, eptifibatide, tirofiban) can cause an increased risk of bleeding. NSAIDs may increase serum creatinine, potassium, blood pressure, and cyclosporine levels during concurrent therapy; monitor cyclosporine levels and renal function carefully. Lithium levels can be increased; avoid concurrent use if possible or monitor lithium levels and adjust dose. Sulindac may have the least effect. When NSAID is stopped, lithium will need adjustment again. Corticosteroids may increase the risk of GI ulceration; avoid concurrent use. Serum concentration/toxicity of methotrexate may be increased.
Decreased Effect: Antihypertensive effects of ACE inhibitors, angiotensin antagonists, beta-blockers, diuretics, and hydralazine may be decreased by concurrent therapy with NSAIDs; monitor blood pressure. Cholestyramine (and other bile acid sequestrants) may decrease the absorption of NSAIDs; separate by at least 2 hours.

Ethanol/Nutrition/Herb Interactions
Ethanol: Avoid ethanol (may enhance gastric mucosal irritation).
Herb/Nutraceutical: Avoid alfalfa, anise, bilberry, bladderwrack, bromelain, cat's claw, celery, coleus, cordyceps, dong quai, evening primrose, feverfew, fenugreek, garlic, ginger, ginkgo biloboa, red clover, horse chestnut, grapeseed, green tea, ginseng, guggul, horse chestnut seed, horseradish, licorice, prickly ash, red clover, reishi, SAMe, sweet clover, turmeric, white willow (all have additional antiplatelet activity).

Dietary Considerations May be taken with food, milk, or antacids.

Pharmacodynamics/Kinetics
Duration: 2-4 hours
Distribution: Crosses placenta
Protein binding: 99%
Half-life elimination: 2-3.3 hours
Time to peak, serum: 0.5-1.5 hours
Excretion: Primarily urine and feces (as metabolites)

Pregnancy Risk Factor C/D (3rd trimester)

Dosage Forms CAP: 50 mg, 100 mg

Meclofenamate Sodium *see* Meclofenamate *on page 970*

Meclozine Hydrochloride *see* Meclizine *on page 969*

Medebar® Plus *see* Barium *on page 179*

Medescan *see* Barium *on page 179*

Medicinal Carbon *see* Charcoal *on page 311*

Medicinal Charcoal *see* Charcoal *on page 311*

Medicone® [OTC] *see* Phenylephrine *on page 1226*

Medigesic® *see* Butalbital, Acetaminophen, and Caffeine *on page 239*

Mediplast® [OTC] *see* Salicylic Acid *on page 1374*

Medi-Synal [OTC] *see* Acetaminophen and Pseudoephedrine *on page 38*

Medium Chain Triglycerides
(mee DEE um chane trye GLIS er ides)

U.S. Brand Names MCT Oil® [OTC]
Canadian Brand Names MCT Oil®
Generic Available No
Synonyms MCT; Triglycerides, Medium Chain
Pharmacologic Category Nutritional Supplement
Use Dietary supplement for those who cannot digest long chain fats; malabsorption associated with disorders such as pancreatic insufficiency, bile salt deficiency, short bowel syndrome, and bacterial overgrowth of the small bowel; induce ketosis as a prevention for seizures
Local Anesthetic/Vasoconstrictor Precautions No information available to require special precautions
Effects on Dental Treatment No significant effects or complications reported
Common Adverse Effects Frequency not defined.
  Endocrine & metabolic: HDL serum levels decreased and triglycerides serum levels increased (>6 months daily use)
  Gastrointestinal: Abdominal pain, bloating, cramping, diarrhea, nausea
Mechanism of Action MCTs are saturated fatty acids in chains of 6-12 carbon atoms. They are water soluble and can pass directly through intestinal cell membranes and blood stream. Once taken up by the liver, they are used for metabolic energy before being stored.

Medrol® *see* MethylPREDNISolone *on page 1025*

MedroxyPROGESTERone (me DROKS ee proe JES te rone)

Related Information
  Endocrine Disorders and Pregnancy *on page 1659*
U.S. Brand Names Depo-Provera®; Depo-Provera® Contraceptive; depo-subQ provera 104™; Provera®
Canadian Brand Names Alti-MPA; Apo-Medroxy®; Depo-Prevera®; Depo-Provera®; Gen-Medroxy; Novo-Medrone; Provera®
Generic Available Yes
Synonyms Acetoxymethylprogesterone; Medroxyprogesterone Acetate; Methylacetoxyprogesterone; MPA
Pharmacologic Category Contraceptive; Progestin
Use Endometrial carcinoma or renal carcinoma; secondary amenorrhea or abnormal uterine bleeding due to hormonal imbalance; reduction of endometrial hyperplasia in nonhysterectomized postmenopausal women receiving conjugated estrogens; prevention of pregnancy; management of endometriosis-associated pain
Local Anesthetic/Vasoconstrictor Precautions No information available to require special precautions
Effects on Dental Treatment Progestins may predispose the patient to gingival bleeding.
Common Adverse Effects Adverse effects as reported with any dosage form; percent ranges presented are noted with the MPA contraceptive injection:
  >5%:
    Central nervous system: Dizziness, headache, nervousness
    Endocrine & metabolic: Libido decreased, menstrual irregularities (includes bleeding, amenorrhea, or both)
    Gastrointestinal: Abdominal pain/discomfort, weight changes (average 3-5 pounds after 1 year, 8 pounds after 2 years)
    Neuromuscular & skeletal: Weakness
  1% to 5%:
    Cardiovascular: Edema
    Central nervous system: Depression, fatigue, insomnia, irritability, pain
    Dermatologic: Acne, alopecia, rash

Endocrine & metabolic: Anorgasmia, breast pain, hot flashes

Gastrointestinal: Bloating, nausea

Genitourinary: Cervical smear abnormal, leukorrhea, menometrorrhagia, menorrhagia, pelvic pain, urinary tract infection, vaginitis, vaginal infection, vaginal hemorrhage

Local: Injection site atrophy, injection site reaction, injection site pain

Neuromuscular & skeletal: Arthralgia, backache, leg cramp

Respiratory: Respiratory tract infections

Mechanism of Action Inhibits secretion of pituitary gonadotropins, which prevents follicular maturation and ovulation; causes endometrial thinning

Drug Interactions

Cytochrome P450 Effect: Substrate of CYP3A4 (major); **Induces** CYP3A4 (weak)

Decreased Effect: Acitretin, and griseofulvin may diminish the therapeutic effect of progestin contraceptives (contraceptive failure is possible). CYP3A4 inducers may decrease the levels/effects of medroxyprogesterone; example inducers include aminoglutethimide, carbamazepine, nafcillin, nevirapine, phenobarbital, phenytoin, and rifamycins. Progestins may diminish the anticoagulant effect of coumarin derivatives; and in contrast, enhanced anticoagulant effects have also been noted with some products.

Pharmacodynamics/Kinetics

Absorption: Oral: Well absorbed; I.M.: Slow

Protein binding: 86% to 90% primarily to albumin; does not bind to sex hormone-binding globulin

Metabolism: Extensively hepatic via hydroxylation and conjugation; forms metabolites

Time to peak: Oral: 2-4 hours

Half-life elimination: Oral: 12-17 hours; I.M. (Depo-Provera® Contraceptive): 50 days; SubQ: ~40 days

Excretion: Urine

Pregnancy Risk Factor X

Medroxyprogesterone Acetate *see* MedroxyPROGESTERone *on page 972*

Medroxyprogesterone and Estrogens (Conjugated) *see* Estrogens (Conjugated/Equine) and Medroxyprogesterone *on page 583*

Medrysone (ME dri sone)

U.S. Brand Names HMS Liquifilm® [DSC]

Generic Available No

Pharmacologic Category Corticosteroid, Ophthalmic

Use Treatment of allergic conjunctivitis, vernal conjunctivitis, episcleritis, ophthalmic epinephrine sensitivity reaction

Local Anesthetic/Vasoconstrictor Precautions No information available to require special precautions

Effects on Dental Treatment No significant effects or complications reported

Mechanism of Action Decreases inflammation by suppression of migration of polymorphonuclear leukocytes and reversal of increased capillary permeability

Pregnancy Risk Factor C

Mefenamic Acid (me fe NAM ik AS id)

Related Information

Rheumatoid Arthritis, Osteoarthritis, and Osteoporosis *on page 1668*

Temporomandibular Dysfunction (TMD) *on page 1724*

U.S. Brand Names Ponstel®

Canadian Brand Names Apo-Mefenamic®; Dom-Mefenamic Acid; Mefenamic-250; Nu-Mefenamic; PMS-Mefenamic Acid

Generic Available No

Pharmacologic Category Nonsteroidal Anti-inflammatory Drug (NSAID), Oral

Use Short-term relief of mild to moderate pain including primary dysmenorrhea

Local Anesthetic/Vasoconstrictor Precautions No information available to require special precautions

Effects on Dental Treatment NSAID formulations are known to reversibly decrease platelet aggregation via mechanisms different than observed with aspirin. The dentist should be aware of the potential of abnormal coagulation. Caution should also be exercised in the use of NSAIDs in patients already on anticoagulant therapy with drugs such as warfarin (Coumadin®). Recovery of platelet function usually occurs 1-2 days after discontinuation of NSAIDs.

Common Adverse Effects 1% to 10%:

Central nervous system: Headache, nervousness, dizziness (3% to 9%)

(Continued)

Mefenamic Acid *(Continued)*

Dermatologic: Itching, rash

Endocrine & metabolic: Fluid retention

Gastrointestinal: Abdominal cramps, heartburn, indigestion, nausea (1% to 10%), vomiting (1% to 10%), diarrhea (1% to 10%), constipation (1% to 10%), abdominal distress/cramping/pain (1% to 10%), dyspepsia (1% to 10%), flatulence (1% to 10%), gastric or duodenal ulcer with bleeding or perforation (1% to 10%), gastritis (1% to 10%)

Hematologic: Bleeding (1% to 10%)

Hepatic: Elevated LFTs (1% to 10%)

Otic: Tinnitus (1% to 10%)

Restrictions A medication guide should be dispensed with each prescription. A template for the required MedGuide can be found on the FDA website at: http://www.fda.gov/medwatch/SAFETY/2005/safety05.htm#NSAID

Dosage Children >14 years and Adults: Oral: 500 mg to start then 250 mg every 4 hours as needed; maximum therapy: 1 week

Dosing adjustment/comments in renal impairment: Not recommended for use

Mechanism of Action Inhibits prostaglandin synthesis by decreasing the activity of the enzyme, cyclooxygenase, which results in decreased formation of prostaglandin precursors

Contraindications Hypersensitivity to mefenamic acid, aspirin, other NSAIDs, or any component of the formulation; perioperative pain in the setting of coronary artery bypass surgery (CABG); active ulceration or chronic inflammation of the GI tract; renal disease; pregnancy (3rd trimester)

Warnings/Precautions NSAIDs are associated with an increased risk of adverse cardiovascular events, including MI, stroke, and new onset or worsening of pre-existing hypertension. Risk may be increased with duration of use or pre-existing cardiovascular risk-factors or disease. Carefully evaluate individual cardiovascular risk profiles prior to prescribing. Use caution with fluid retention, CHF or hypertension.

Use of NSAIDs can compromise existing renal function. Renal toxicity can occur in patient with impaired renal function, dehydration, heart failure, liver dysfunction, those taking diuretics and ACEI and the elderly. Rehydrate patient before starting therapy. Monitor renal function closely. Mefenamic acid is not recommended for patients with advanced renal disease.

NSAIDs may increase risk of gastrointestinal irritation, ulceration, bleeding, and perforation. These events may occur at any time during therapy and without warning. Use caution with a history of GI disease (bleeding or ulcers), concurrent therapy with aspirin, anticoagulants and/or corticosteroids, smoking, use of alcohol, the elderly or debilitated patients.

Use the lowest effective dose for the shortest duration of time, consistent with individual patient goals, to reduce risk of cardiovascular or GI adverse events. Alternate therapies should be considered for patients at high risk.

NSAIDs may cause serious skin adverse events including exfoliative dermatitis, Stevens-Johnson syndrome (SJS) and toxic epidermal necrolysis (TEN). Anaphylactoid reactions may occur, even without prior exposure; patients with "aspirin triad" (bronchial asthma, aspirin intolerance, rhinitis) may be at increased risk. Do not use in patients who experience bronchospasm, asthma, rhinitis, or urticaria with NSAID or aspirin therapy.

Use with caution in patients with decreased hepatic function. Closely monitor patients with any abnormal LFT. Severe hepatic reactions (eg, fulminant hepatitis, liver failure) have occurred with NSAID use, rarely; discontinue if signs or symptoms of liver disease develop, or if systemic manifestations occur.

The elderly are at increased risk for adverse effects (especially peptic ulceration, CNS effects, renal toxicity) from NSAIDs even at low doses.

Withhold for at least 4-6 half-lives prior to surgical or dental procedures. Safety and efficacy have not been established in children <14 years of age.

Drug Interactions

Cytochrome P450 Effect: Substrate of CYP2C8/9 (minor); **Inhibits** CYP2C8/9 (strong)

Increased Effect/Toxicity: Anticoagulants (warfarin, heparin, LMWHs) in combination with NSAIDs can cause increased risk of bleeding. Other antiplatelet drugs (ticlopidine, clopidogrel, aspirin, abciximab, dipyridamole, eptifibatide, tirofiban) can cause an increased risk of bleeding. Mefenamic acid may increase the levels/effects of CYP2C8/9 substrates (eg, amiodarone, fluoxetine, glimepiride, glipizide, nateglinide, phenytoin, pioglitazone, rosiglitazone, sertraline, warfarin). NSAIDs may increase serum creatinine, potassium, blood pressure, and cyclosporine levels during concurrent therapy; monitor cyclosporine levels and renal function carefully. Lithium levels can be increased; avoid concurrent use if possible or monitor lithium levels and adjust dose. Sulindac may have the least effect. When NSAID is stopped, lithium will need adjustment again. Corticosteroids may increase the risk of GI ulceration; avoid concurrent use. Serum concentration/toxicity of methotrexate may be increased.

Decreased Effect: Antihypertensive effects of ACE inhibitors, angiotensin antagonists, beta-blockers, diuretics, and hydralazine may be decreased by concurrent therapy with NSAIDs; monitor blood pressure. Cholestyramine (and other bile acid sequestrants) may decrease the absorption of NSAIDs; separate by at least 2 hours.

Ethanol/Nutrition/Herb Interactions

Ethanol: Avoid ethanol (may enhance gastric mucosal irritation).

Herb/Nutraceutical: Avoid alfalfa, anise, bilberry, bladderwrack, bromelain, cat's claw, celery, coleus, cordyceps, dong quai, evening primrose, feverfew, fenugreek, garlic, ginger, ginkgo biloboa, red clover, horse chestnut, grapeseed, green tea, ginseng, guggul, horse chestnut seed, horseradish, licorice, prickly ash, red clover, reishi, SAMe, sweet clover, turmeric, white willow (all have additional antiplatelet activity).

Pharmacodynamics/Kinetics

Onset of action: Peak effect: 2-4 hours

Duration: ≤6 hours

Protein binding: High

Metabolism: Conjugated hepatically

Half-life elimination: 3.5 hours

Excretion: Urine (50%) and feces as unchanged drug and metabolites

Pregnancy Risk Factor C/D (3rd trimester)

Dosage Forms CAP: 250 mg

Mefloquine (ME floe kwin)

U.S. Brand Names Lariam®

Canadian Brand Names Apo-Mefloquine®; Lariam®

Generic Available Yes

Synonyms Mefloquine Hydrochloride

Pharmacologic Category Antimalarial Agent

Use Treatment of acute malarial infections and prevention of malaria

Local Anesthetic/Vasoconstrictor Precautions No information available to require special precautions

Effects on Dental Treatment No significant effects or complications reported

Common Adverse Effects

Frequency not defined: Neuropsychiatric events

1% to 10%:

Central nervous system: Headache, fever, chills, fatigue

Dermatologic: Rash

Gastrointestinal: Vomiting (3%), diarrhea, stomach pain, nausea, appetite decreased

Neuromuscular & skeletal: Myalgia

Otic: Tinnitus

Restrictions A medication guide and wallet card must be provided to patients when mefloquine is dispensed for malaria. An FDA-approved medication guide is available at http://www.fda.gov/cder/Offices/ODS/labeling.htm.

Mechanism of Action Mefloquine is a quinoline-methanol compound structurally similar to quinine; mefloquine's effectiveness in the treatment and prophylaxis of malaria is due to the destruction of the asexual blood forms of the malarial pathogens that affect humans, *Plasmodium falciparum*, *P. vivax*, *P. malariae*, *P. ovale*

Drug Interactions

Cytochrome P450 Effect: Substrate of CYP3A4 (major); **Inhibits** CYP2D6 (weak), 3A4 (weak)

Increased Effect/Toxicity: Use caution with drugs that alter cardiac conduction; increased toxicity with chloroquine, quinine, and quinidine (hold treatment until at least 12 hours after these later drugs); increased toxicity with halofantrine (concurrent use is contraindicated). CYP3A4 inhibitors may increase the levels/effects of mefloquine; example inhibitors include azole antifungals, clarithromycin, diclofenac, doxycycline, erythromycin, imatinib, isoniazid, nefazodone, nicardipine, propofol, protease inhibitors, quinidine, telithromycin, and verapamil.

Decreased Effect: Mefloquine may decrease the effect of valproic acid, carbamazepine, phenobarbital, and phenytoin. CYP3A4 inducers may

(Continued)

Mefloquine (Continued)

decrease the levels/effects of mefloquine; example inducers include amino-glutethimide, carbamazepine, nafcillin, nevirapine, phenobarbital, phenytoin, and rifamycins. Vaccination with oral live attenuated Ty21a vaccine should be delayed for at least 24 hours after the administration of mefloquine.

Pharmacodynamics/Kinetics

Absorption: Well absorbed

Distribution: V_d: 19 L/kg; blood, urine, CSF, tissues; enters breast milk

Protein binding: 98%

Metabolism: Extensively hepatic; main metabolite is inactive

Bioavailability: Increased by food

Half-life elimination: 21-22 days

Time to peak, plasma: 6-24 hours (median: ~17 hours)

Excretion: Primarily bile and feces; urine (9% as unchanged drug, 4% as primary metabolite)

Pregnancy Risk Factor C

Mefloquine Hydrochloride see Mefloquine on page 975

Mefoxin® see Cefoxitin on page 290

Megace® see Megestrol on page 976

Megace® ES see Megestrol on page 976

Megadophilus® [OTC] see Lactobacillus on page 535

Megestrol (me JES trole)

U.S. Brand Names Megace®; Megace® ES

Canadian Brand Names Apo-Megestrol®; Megace®; Megace® OS; Nu-Megestrol

Generic Available Yes

Synonyms 5071-1DL(6); Megestrol Acetate; NSC-10363

Pharmacologic Category Antineoplastic Agent, Hormone; Appetite Stimulant; Progestin

Use Palliative treatment of breast and endometrial carcinoma; treatment of anorexia, cachexia, or unexplained significant weight loss in patients with AIDS

Local Anesthetic/Vasoconstrictor Precautions No information available to require special precautions

Effects on Dental Treatment No significant effects or complications reported

Common Adverse Effects

Cardiovascular: Edema, hypertension (≤8%), cardiomyopathy, palpitation

Central nervous system: Insomnia, fever (2% to 6%), headache (≤10%), pain (≤6%, similar to placebo), confusion (1% to 3%), convulsions (1% to 3%), depression (1% to 3%)

Dermatologic: Allergic rash (2% to 12%) with or without pruritus, alopecia

Endocrine & metabolic: Breakthrough bleeding and amenorrhea, spotting, changes in menstrual flow, changes in cervical erosion and secretions, increased breast tenderness, changes in vaginal bleeding pattern, edema, fluid retention, hyperglycemia (≤6%), diabetes, HPA axis suppression, adrenal insufficiency, Cushing's syndrome

Gastrointestinal: Weight gain (not attributed to edema or fluid retention), nausea, vomiting (7%), diarrhea (8% to 15%, similar to placebo), flatulence (≤10%), constipation (1% to 3%)

Genitourinary: Impotence (4% to 14%), decreased libido (≤5%)

Hepatic: Cholestatic jaundice, hepatotoxicity, hepatomegaly (1% to 3%)

Local: Thrombophlebitis

Neuromuscular & skeletal: Carpal tunnel syndrome, weakness, paresthesia (1% to 3%)

Respiratory: Hyperpnea, dyspnea (1% to 3%), cough (1% to 3%)

Miscellaneous: Diaphoresis

Mechanism of Action A synthetic progestin with antiestrogenic properties which disrupt the estrogen receptor cycle. Megestrol interferes with the normal estrogen cycle and results in a lower LH titer. May also have a direct effect on the endometrium. Megestrol is an antineoplastic progestin thought to act through an antileutenizing effect mediated via the pituitary. May stimulate appetite by antagonizing the metabolic effects of catabolic cytokines.

Pharmacodynamics/Kinetics

Absorption: Well absorbed orally

Metabolism: Completely hepatic to free steroids and glucuronide conjugates

Time to peak, serum: 1-3 hours

Half-life elimination: 15-100 hours

Excretion: Urine (57% to 78% as steroid metabolites and inactive compound); feces (8% to 30%)

Pregnancy Risk Factor X

Megestrol Acetate *see* Megestrol *on page 976*

Melanex® *see* Hydroquinone *on page 798*

Melfiat® *see* Phendimetrazine *on page 1220*

Meloxicam (mel OKS i kam)

U.S. Brand Names Mobic®

Canadian Brand Names Apo-Meloxicam®; CO Meloxicam; Gen-Meloxicam; Mobic®; Mobicox®; Novo-Meloxicam; PMS-Meloxicam

Generic Available No

Pharmacologic Category Nonsteroidal Anti-inflammatory Drug (NSAID), Oral

Use Relief of signs and symptoms of osteoarthritis, rheumatoid arthritis, and juvenile rheumatoid arthritis (JRA)

Local Anesthetic/Vasoconstrictor Precautions No information available to require special precautions

Effects on Dental Treatment Key adverse event(s) related to dental treatment: Taste perversion, ulcerative stomatitis, and xerostomia (normal salivary flow resumes upon discontinuation).

Common Adverse Effects Percentages reported in adult patients; abdominal pain, diarrhea, headache, pyrexia, and vomiting were reported more commonly in pediatric patients

2% to 10%:

Cardiovascular: Edema (<1% to 4%)

Central nervous system: Headache (2% to 8%), dizziness (<1% to 4%), insomnia (<1% to 4%)

Dermatologic: Pruritus (<1% to 2%), rash (<1% to 3%)

Gastrointestinal: Diarrhea (3% to 8%), dyspepsia (4% to 9%), abdominal pain (2% to 5%), nausea (2% to 7%), constipation (<1% to 3%), flatulence (<1% to 3%), vomiting (<1% to 3%)

Hematologic: Anemia (<1% to 4%)

Neuromuscular & skeletal: Arthralgia (<1% to 5%), back pain (<1% to 3%)

Respiratory: Cough (<1% to 2%), pharyngitis (<1% to 3%), upper respiratory infection (2% to 8%)

Miscellaneous: Flu-like symptoms (2% to 6%), falls (3%)

Restrictions A medication guide should be dispensed with each prescription. A template for the required MedGuide can be found on the FDA website at: http://www.fda.gov/medwatch/SAFETY/2005/safety05.htm#NSAID

Dosage Oral:

Children ≥2 years: JRA: 0.125 mg/kg/day; maximum dose: 7.5 mg/day

Adults: Osteoarthritis, rheumatoid arthritis: Initial: 7.5 mg once daily; some patients may receive additional benefit from an increased dose of 15 mg once daily; maximum dose: 15 mg/day

Elderly: Increased concentrations may occur in elderly patients (particularly in females); however, no specific dosage adjustment is recommended

Dosage adjustment in renal impairment:

Mild-to-moderate impairment: No specific dosage recommendations

Significant impairment (Cl_{cr} ≤15 mL/minute): Avoid use

Hemodialysis: Supplemental dose after dialysis not necessary

Dosage adjustment in hepatic impairment:

Mild (Child-Pugh class A) to moderate (Child-Pugh class B) hepatic dysfunction: No dosage adjustment is necessary

Severe hepatic impairment: Patients with severe hepatic impairment have not been adequately studied

Mechanism of Action Inhibits prostaglandin synthesis by decreasing the activity of the enzyme, cyclooxygenase, which results in decreased formation of prostaglandin precursors

Contraindications Hypersensitivity to meloxicam, aspirin, other NSAIDs, or any component of the formulation; perioperative pain in the setting of coronary artery bypass surgery (CABG); pregnancy (3rd trimester)

Warnings/Precautions NSAIDs are associated with an increased risk of adverse cardiovascular events, including MI, stroke, and new onset or worsening of pre-existing hypertension. Risk may be increased with duration of use or pre-existing cardiovascular risk-factors or disease. Carefully evaluate individual cardiovascular risk profiles prior to prescribing. Use caution with fluid retention, CHF or hypertension.

Use of NSAIDs can compromise existing renal function. Renal toxicity can occur in patient with impaired renal function, dehydration, heart failure, liver dysfunction, those taking diuretics and ACEI and the elderly. Rehydrate patient before (Continued)

Meloxicam *(Continued)*

starting therapy. Monitor renal function closely. Meloxicam is not recommended for patients with advanced renal disease

NSAIDs may increase risk of gastrointestinal irritation, ulceration, bleeding, and perforation. These events may occur at any time during therapy and without warning. Use caution with a history of GI disease (bleeding or ulcers), concurrent therapy with aspirin, anticoagulants and/or corticosteroids, smoking, use of alcohol, the elderly or debilitated patients.

Use the lowest effective dose for the shortest duration of time, consistent with individual patient goals, to reduce risk of cardiovascular or GI adverse events. Alternate therapies should be considered for patients at high risk.

NSAIDs may cause serious skin adverse events including exfoliative dermatitis, Stevens-Johnson syndrome (SJS) and toxic epidermal necrolysis (TEN). Anaphylactoid reactions may occur, even without prior exposure; patients with "aspirin triad" (bronchial asthma, aspirin intolerance, rhinitis) may· be at increased risk. Do not use in patients who experience bronchospasm, asthma, rhinitis, or urticaria with NSAID or aspirin therapy.

Use with caution in patients with decreased hepatic function. Closely monitor patients with any abnormal LFT. Severe hepatic reactions (eg, fulminant hepatitis, liver failure) have occurred with NSAID use, rarely; discontinue if signs or symptoms of liver disease develop, or if systemic manifestations occur.

The elderly are at increased risk for adverse effects (especially peptic ulceration, CNS effects, renal toxicity) from NSAIDs even at low doses.

Withhold for at least 4-6 half-lives prior to surgical or dental procedures. Safety and efficacy have not been established in pediatric patients <2 years of age.

Drug Interactions

Cytochrome P450 Effect: Substrate (minor) of CYP2C8/9, 3A4; **Inhibits** CYP2C8/9 (weak)

Increased Effect/Toxicity: Anticoagulants (warfarin, heparin, LMWHs) in combination with NSAIDs can cause increased risk of bleeding. Antiplatelet drugs (ticlopidine, clopidogrel, aspirin, abciximab, dipyridamole, eptifibatide, tirofiban) can cause an increased risk of bleeding. Aspirin increases serum concentrations (AUC) of meloxicam (in addition to potential for additive adverse effects); concurrent use is not recommended. Corticosteroids may increase the risk of GI ulceration; avoid concurrent use. NSAIDs may increase serum creatinine, potassium, blood pressure, and cyclosporine levels; monitor cyclosporine levels and renal function carefully. Lithium levels can be increased; avoid concurrent use if possible or monitor lithium levels and adjust dose. When NSAID is stopped, lithium will need adjustment again. Serum concentration/toxicity of methotrexate may be increased. Warfarin INRs may be increased by meloxicam. Monitor INR closely, particularly during initiation or change in dose. May increase risk of bleeding. Use lowest possible dose for shortest duration possible.

Decreased Effect: Cholestyramine (and possibly colestipol) increases the clearance of meloxicam. Hydralazine's antihypertensive effect is decreased; avoid concurrent use. Loop diuretic efficacy (diuretic and antihypertensive effect) may be reduced by NSAIDs. Antihypertensive effects of thiazide diuretics are decreased; avoid concurrent use. NSAIDs may decrease the antihypertensive effect of beta-blockers, ACE inhibitors, and angiotensin antagonists. Cholestyramine (and other bile acid sequestrants) may decrease the absorption of NSAIDs; separate by at least 2 hours.

Ethanol/Nutrition/Herb Interactions

Ethanol: Avoid ethanol (may enhance gastric mucosal irritation).

Herb/Nutraceutical: Avoid alfalfa, anise, bilberry, bladderwrack, bromelain, cat's claw, celery, coleus, cordyceps, dong quai, evening primrose, feverfew, fenugreek, garlic, ginger, ginkgo biloboa, red clover, horse chestnut, grapeseed, green tea, ginseng, guggul, horse chestnut seed, horseradish, licorice, prickly ash, red clover, reishi, SAMe, sweet clover, turmeric, white willow (all have additional antiplatelet activity).

Dietary Considerations Should be taken with food or milk to minimize gastrointestinal irritation.

Pharmacodynamics/Kinetics

Distribution: 10 L

Protein binding: 99.4%

Metabolism: Hepatic via CYP2C9 and CYP3A4 (minor); forms 4 metabolites (inactive)

Bioavailability: 89%

Half-life elimination: Adults: 15-20 hours

Time to peak: Initial: 5-10 hours; Secondary: 12-14 hours

Excretion: Urine and feces (as inactive metabolites)
Pregnancy Risk Factor C/D (3rd trimester)
Dosage Forms SUSP: 7.5 mg/5 mL (100 mL). **TAB:** 7.5 mg, 15 mg

Melpaque HP® *see Hydroquinone on page 798*

Melphalan (MEL fa lan)

U.S. Brand Names Alkeran®
Canadian Brand Names Alkeran®
Mexican Brand Names Alkeran®
Generic Available No
Synonyms L-PAM; L-Sarcolysin; Phenylalanine Mustard
Pharmacologic Category Antineoplastic Agent, Alkylating Agent
Use Palliative treatment of multiple myeloma and nonresectable epithelial ovarian carcinoma; neuroblastoma, rhabdomyosarcoma, breast cancer
Local Anesthetic/Vasoconstrictor Precautions No information available to require special precautions
Effects on Dental Treatment Key adverse event(s) related to dental treatment: Stomatitis.
Common Adverse Effects
>10%: Hematologic: Myelosuppressive: Leukopenia and thrombocytopenia are the most common effects of melphalan; irreversible bone marrow failure has been reported
WBC: Moderate
Platelets: Moderate
Onset: 7 days
Nadir: 8-10 days and 27-32 days
Recovery: 42-50 days
1% to 10%:
Cardiovascular: Vasculitis
Dermatologic: Vesiculation of skin, alopecia, pruritus, rash
Endocrine & metabolic: SIADH, sterility, amenorrhea
Gastrointestinal: Nausea and vomiting are mild; stomatitis and diarrhea are infrequent
Genitourinary: Hemorrhagic cystitis, bladder irritation
Hematologic: Anemia, agranulocytosis, hemolytic anemia
Hepatic: Transaminases increased (hepatitis, jaundice have been reported)
Respiratory: Pulmonary fibrosis, interstitial pneumonitis
Miscellaneous: Hypersensitivity, secondary malignancy
Mechanism of Action Alkylating agent which is a derivative of mechlorethamine that inhibits DNA and RNA synthesis via formation of carbonium ions; cross-links strands of DNA
Drug Interactions
Increased Effect/Toxicity: Risk of nephrotoxicity of cyclosporine is increased by melphalan. Concomitant use of I.V. melphalan may cause serious GI toxicity.
Decreased Effect: Cimetidine and other H_2 antagonists: The reduction in gastric pH has been reported to decrease bioavailability of melphalan by 30%.
Pharmacodynamics/Kinetics
Absorption: Oral: Variable and incomplete
Distribution: V_d: 0.5-0.6 L/kg throughout total body water
Bioavailability: Unpredictable, decreasing from 85% to 58% with repeated doses
Half-life elimination: Terminal: 1.5 hours
Time to peak, serum: ~2 hours
Excretion: Oral: Feces (20% to 50%); urine (10% to 30% as unchanged drug)
Pregnancy Risk Factor D

Melquin-3® *see Hydroquinone on page 798*
Melquin HP® *see Hydroquinone on page 798*

Memantine (me MAN teen)

U.S. Brand Names Namenda™
Canadian Brand Names Ebixa®
Generic Available No
Synonyms Memantine Hydrochloride
Pharmacologic Category N-Methyl-D-Aspartate Receptor Antagonist
Use Treatment of moderate-to-severe dementia of the Alzheimer's type
(Continued)

Memantine *(Continued)*

Unlabeled/Investigational Use Treatment of mild-to-moderate vascular dementia

Local Anesthetic/Vasoconstrictor Precautions No information available to require special precautions

Effects on Dental Treatment No significant effects or complications reported

Common Adverse Effects

1% to 10%:

Cardiovascular: Hypertension (4%), cardiac failure, syncope, cerebrovascular accident, transient ischemic attack

Central nervous system: Dizziness (7%), confusion (6%), headache (6%), hallucinations (3%), pain (3%), somnolence (3%), fatigue (2%), aggressive reaction, ataxia, vertigo

Dermatologic: Rash

Gastrointestinal: Constipation (5%), vomiting (3%), weight loss

Genitourinary: Micturition

Hematologic: Anemia

Hepatic: Alkaline phosphatase increased

Neuromuscular & skeletal: Back pain (3%), hypokinesia

Ocular: Cataract, conjunctivitis

Respiratory: Cough (4%), dyspnea (2%), pneumonia

Mechanism of Action Glutamate, the primary excitatory amino acid in the CNS, may contribute to the pathogenesis of Alzheimer's disease (AD) by over-stimulating various glutamate receptors leading to excitotoxicity and neuronal cell death. Memantine is an uncompetitive antagonist of the N-methyl-D-aspartate (NMDA) type of glutamate receptors, located ubiquitously throughout the brain. Under normal physiologic conditions, the (unstimulated) NMDA receptor ion channel is blocked by magnesium ions, which are displaced after agonist-induced depolarization. Pathologic or excessive receptor activation, as postulated to occur during AD, prevents magnesium from reentering and blocking the channel pore resulting in a chronically open state and excessive calcium influx. Memantine binds to the intra-pore magnesium site, but with longer dwell time, and thus functions as an effective receptor blocker only under conditions of excessive stimulation; memantine does not affect normal neurotransmission.

Drug Interactions

Increased Effect/Toxicity: Clearance of memantine is decreased 80% at urinary pH 8; use caution with medications (carbonic anhydrase inhibitors, sodium bicarbonate) which may increase urinary pH.

Pharmacodynamics/Kinetics

Distribution: 9-11 L/kg

Protein binding: 45%

Metabolism: Forms 3 metabolites (minimal activity)

Half-life elimination: Terminal: 60-80 hours; severe renal impairment (Cl_{cr} 5-29 mL/minute): 117-156 hours

Time to peak, serum: 3-7 hours

Excretion: Urine (57% to 82% unchanged); excretion reduced by alkaline urine pH

Pregnancy Risk Factor B

Memantine Hydrochloride *see* Memantine *on page 979*

Menactra® *see* Meningococcal Polysaccharide (Groups A / C / Y and W-135) Diphtheria Toxoid Conjugate Vaccine *on page 980*

Menest® *see* Estrogens (Esterified) *on page 584*

Meningococcal Polysaccharide (Groups A / C / Y and W-135) Diphtheria Toxoid Conjugate Vaccine

(me NIN joe kok al pol i SAK a ride groops aye, see, why & dubl yoo won thur tee fyve dif THEER ee a TOKS oyds KON joo gate vak SEEN)

Related Information

Immunizations (Vaccines) *on page 1786*

U.S. Brand Names Menactra®

Canadian Brand Names Meningitec®

Generic Available No

Synonyms MCV4

Pharmacologic Category Vaccine

Use Provide active immunization of adolescents and adults (11-55 years of age) against invasive meningococcal disease caused by *N. meningitidis* serogroups A, C, Y and W-135

The ACIP recommends routine vaccination of all adolescents at age 11-12 years. For adolescents not previously vaccinated, vaccine should be administered prior to high school entry (~15 years of age).

The ACIP also recommends routine vaccination for persons at increased risk for meningococcal disease. (MCV4 is preferred for persons aged 11-55 years; MPSV4 may be used if MCV4 is not available). Persons at increased risk include:

College freshmen living in dormitories

Microbiologists routinely exposed to isolates of *N. meningitides*

Military recruits

Persons traveling to or who reside in countries where *N. meningitides* is hyperendemic or epidemic, particularly if contact with local population will be prolonged

Persons with terminal complement component deficiencies

Persons with anatomic or functional asplenia

Use is also recommended during meningococcal outbreaks caused by vaccine preventable serogroups.

Local Anesthetic/Vasoconstrictor Precautions No information available to require special precautions

Effects on Dental Treatment No significant effects or complications reported

Common Adverse Effects All serious adverse reactions must be reported to the U.S. Department of Health and Human Services Vaccine Adverse Event Reporting System (VAERS) 1-800-822-7967 or www.vaers.org.

>10%:

Central nervous system: Pain (54% to 59%), headache (36% to 41%), fatigue (30% to 35%), malaise (22% to 24%)

Gastrointestinal: Diarrhea (12% to 16%), anorexia (11% to 12%)

Local: Redness (11% to 14%), swelling (11% to 13%), induration (16% to 17%)

Neuromuscular & skeletal: Arthralgia (17% to 20%)

1% to 10%:

Central nervous system: Chills (7% to 10%), fever (2% to 5%)

Gastrointestinal: Vomiting (2%)

Local: Rash (1% to 2%)

Postmarketing and/or case reports: Guillain-Barré syndrome, transverse myelitis

Mechanism of Action Induces immunity against meningococcal disease via the formation of bactericidal antibodies directed toward the polysaccharide capsular components of *Neisseria meningitidis* serogroups A, C, Y and W-135.

Pharmacodynamics/Kinetics

Onset: Protective antibody levels achieved within 7-10 days of vaccination.

Pregnancy Risk Factor C

Meningococcal Polysaccharide Vaccine (Groups A, C, Y, and W-135)

(me NIN joe kok al pol i SAK a ride vak SEEN groops aye, see, why & dubl yoo won thur tee fyve)

U.S. Brand Names Menomune®-A/C/Y/W-135

Generic Available No

Synonyms MPSV4

Pharmacologic Category Vaccine

Use Provide active immunity to meningococcal serogroups contained in the vaccine

The ACIP recommends routine vaccination for persons at increased risk for meningococcal disease. (Use of MPSV4 is recommended in children 2-10 years and adults >55 years. MCV4 is preferred for persons aged 11-55 years; MPSV4 may be used if MCV4 is not available). Persons at increased risk include:

College freshmen living in dormitories

Microbiologists routinely exposed to isolates of *N. meningitides*

Military recruits

Persons traveling to or who reside in countries where *N. meningitides* is hyperendemic or epidemic, particularly if contact with local population will be prolonged

Persons with terminal complement component deficiencies

Persons with anatomic or functional asplenia

Use is also recommended during meningococcal outbreaks caused by vaccine preventable serogroups.

(Continued)

Meningococcal Polysaccharide Vaccine (Groups A, C, Y, and W-135) *(Continued)*

Local Anesthetic/Vasoconstrictor Precautions No information available to require special precautions

Effects on Dental Treatment No significant effects or complications reported

Common Adverse Effects All serious adverse reactions must be reported to the U.S. Department of Health and Human Services (DHHS) Vaccine Adverse Event Reporting System (VAERS) 1-800-822-7967. Percentages reported in adults; incidence of erythema, swelling, or tenderness may be higher in children

>10%: Local: Tenderness (9% to 36%)

1% to 10%:
  Central nervous system: Headache (2% to 5%), malaise (2%), fever (100°F to 106°F: 3%), chills (2%)
  Local: Pain at injection site (2% to 3%), erythema (1% to 4%), induration (1% to 4%)

Mechanism of Action Induces the formation of bactericidal antibodies to meningococcal antigens; the presence of these antibodies is strongly correlated with immunity to meningococcal disease caused by *Neisseria meningitidis* groups A, C, Y and W-135.

Drug Interactions
  Increased Effect/Toxicity: Should not be administered with whole-cell pertussis or whole-cell typhoid vaccines due to combined endotoxin content.
  Decreased Effect: Decreased effect with administration of immunoglobulin within 1 month.

Pharmacodynamics/Kinetics
  Onset of action: Antibody levels: 7-10 days
  Duration: Antibodies against group A and C polysaccharides decline markedly (to prevaccination levels) over the first 3 years following a single dose of vaccine, especially in children <4 years of age

Pregnancy Risk Factor C

Menomune®-A/C/Y/W-135 *see* Meningococcal Polysaccharide Vaccine (Groups A, C, Y, and W-135) *on page 981*

Menopur® *see* Menotropins *on page 982*

Menostar™ *see* Estradiol *on page 574*

Menotropins (men oh TROE pins)

U.S. Brand Names Menopur®; Pergonal® [DSC]; Repronex®
Canadian Brand Names Repronex®
Mexican Brand Names HMG Massone®; Humegon®
Generic Available No
Pharmacologic Category Gonadotropin; Ovulation Stimulator
Use
  Female:
    In conjunction with hCG to induce ovulation and pregnancy in infertile females experiencing oligoanovulation or anovulation when the cause of anovulation is functional and not caused by primary ovarian failure (Pergonal®, Repronex®)
    Stimulation of multiple follicle development in ovulatory patients as part of an assisted reproductive technology (ART) (Menopur®, Pergonal®, Repronex®)
  Male: Stimulation of spermatogenesis in primary or secondary hypogonadotropic hypogonadism (Pergonal®)

Local Anesthetic/Vasoconstrictor Precautions No information available to require special precautions

Effects on Dental Treatment No significant effects or complications reported

Common Adverse Effects Adverse effects may vary according to specific product, route, and/or dosage.

Male:
  >10%: Endocrine & metabolic: Gynecomastia
  1% to 10%: Erythrocytosis (dyspnea, dizziness, anorexia, syncope, epistaxis)
Female:
  >10%:
    Central nervous system: Headache (up to 34%)
    Gastrointestinal: Abdominal pain (up to 18%), nausea (up to 12%)
    Genitourinary: OHSS (up to 13%, dose related)
    Local: Injection site reaction (4% to 12%)
  1% to 10%:
    Cardiovascular: Flushing

Central nervous system: Dizziness, malaise, migraine

Endocrine & metabolic: Breast tenderness, hot flashes, menstrual irregularities

Gastrointestinal: Abdominal cramping, abdominal fullness, constipation, diarrhea, enlarged abdomen, vomiting

Genitourinary: Ectopic pregnancy, ovarian disease, vaginal hemorrhage

Local: Injection site edema/pain

Neuromuscular & skeletal: Back pain

Respiratory: Cough increased, respiratory disorder

Miscellaneous: Infection, flu-like syndrome

Frequency not defined:

Cardiovascular: Stroke, tachycardia, thrombosis (venous or arterial)

Central nervous system: Dizziness

Dermatologic: Angioedema, urticaria

Genitourinary: Adnexal torsion, hemoperitoneum, ovarian enlargement

Neuromuscular & skeletal: Limb necrosis

Respiratory: Acute respiratory distress syndrome, atelectasis, dyspnea, embolism, laryngeal edema pulmonary infarction tachypnea

Miscellaneous: Allergic reaction, anaphylaxis, rash

Mechanism of Action Actions occur as a result of both follicle stimulating hormone (FSH) effects and luteinizing hormone (LH) effects; menotropins stimulate the development and maturation of the ovarian follicle (FSH), cause ovulation (LH), and stimulate the development of the corpus luteum (LH); in males it stimulates spermatogenesis (LH)

Pharmacodynamics/Kinetics Excretion: Urine (~10% as unchanged drug)

Pregnancy Risk Factor X

Mentax® *see* Butenafine *on page 242*

Mepenzolate (me PEN zoe late)

U.S. Brand Names Cantil® [DSC]

Canadian Brand Names Cantil®

Generic Available No

Synonyms Mepenzolate Bromide

Pharmacologic Category Anticholinergic Agent; Antispasmodic Agent, Gastrointestinal

Use Adjunctive treatment of peptic ulcer disease

Local Anesthetic/Vasoconstrictor Precautions No information available to require special precautions

Effects on Dental Treatment Key adverse event(s) related to dental treatment: Xerostomia (normal salivary flow resumes upon discontinuation) and dry throat.

Common Adverse Effects Frequency not defined.

Cardiovascular: Palpitations, tachycardia

Central nervous system: Headache, nervousness, drowsiness, dizziness, CNS stimulation may be produced with large doses, confusion, insomnia

Dermatologic: Dry skin, urticaria

Gastrointestinal: Constipation, xerostomia, dysphagia, nausea, vomiting, delayed gastric emptying, loss of taste

Genitourinary: Impotence, urinary hesitation, urinary retention

Neuromuscular & skeletal: Weakness

Ophthalmic: Cycloplegia, blurred vision, ocular tension increased, pupil dilation

Miscellaneous: Diaphoresis decreased, hypersensitivity reactions, anaphylaxis, lactation suppressed

Mechanism of Action Mepenzolate is a postganglionic parasympathetic inhibitor. It decreases gastric acid and pepsin secretion and suppresses spontaneous contractions of the colon.

Pharmacodynamics/Kinetics

Absorption: Oral: Low

Excretion: Urine (3% to 33%); feces

Pregnancy Risk Factor B

Mepenzolate Bromide *see* Mepenzolate *on page 983*

Mepergan *see* Meperidine and Promethazine *on page 986*

Meperidine (me PER i deen)

Related Information

Oral Pain *on page 1692*

(Continued)

Meperidine *(Continued)*

Related Sample Prescriptions
Severe Oral Pain *on page 1735*

U.S. Brand Names Demerol®; Meperitab®

Canadian Brand Names Demerol®

Generic Available Yes

Synonyms Isonipecaine Hydrochloride; Meperidine Hydrochloride; Pethidine Hydrochloride

Pharmacologic Category Analgesic, Narcotic

Dental Use Adjunct in preoperative intravenous conscious sedation in patients undergoing dental surgery; alternate oral narcotic in patients allergic to codeine to treat moderate to moderate-severe pain

Use Management of moderate to severe pain; adjunct to anesthesia and preoperative sedation

Unlabeled/Investigational Use
Reduce postoperative shivering; reduce rigors from amphotericin

Local Anesthetic/Vasoconstrictor Precautions No information available to require special precautions

Effects on Dental Treatment Key adverse event(s) related to dental treatment: Xerostomia (normal salivary flow resumes upon discontinuation). See Dental Comment.

Significant Adverse Effects Frequency not defined.

Cardiovascular: Hypotension

Central nervous system: Fatigue, drowsiness, dizziness, nervousness, headache, restlessness, malaise, confusion, mental depression, hallucinations, paradoxical CNS stimulation, increased intracranial pressure, seizure (associated with metabolite accumulation), serotonin syndrome

Dermatologic: Rash, urticaria

Gastrointestinal: Nausea, vomiting, constipation, anorexia, stomach cramps, xerostomia, biliary spasm, paralytic ileus, sphincter of Oddi spasm

Genitourinary: Ureteral spasms, decreased urination

Local: Pain at injection site

Neuromuscular & skeletal: Weakness

Respiratory: Dyspnea

Miscellaneous: Histamine release, physical and psychological dependence

Restrictions C-II

Dental Usual Dosing Pain (analgesic): Adults: Oral: Initial: Opiate-naive: 50 mg every 3-4 hours as needed; usual dosage range: 50-150 mg every 2-4 hours as needed (manufacturers recommendation; oral route is not recommended for acute pain)

Dosage Note: Doses should be titrated to necessary analgesic effect. When changing route of administration, note that oral doses are about half as effective as parenteral dose. Not recommended for chronic pain. These are guidelines and do not represent the maximum doses that may be required in all patients. In patients with normal renal function, doses of ≤600 mg/24 hours and use for ≤48 hours are recommended (American Pain Society, 1999).

Children: Pain: Oral, I.M., I.V., SubQ: 1-1.5 mg/kg/dose every 3-4 hours as needed; 1-2 mg/kg as a single dose preoperative medication may be used; maximum 100 mg/dose (Note: Oral route is not recommended for acute pain.)

Adults: Pain:

Oral: Initial: Opiate-naive: 50 mg every 3-4 hours as needed; usual dosage range: 50-150 mg every 2-4 hours as needed (manufacturers recommendation; oral route is not recommended for acute pain)

I.M., SubQ: Initial: Opiate-naive: 50-75 mg every 3-4 hours as needed; patients with prior opiate exposure may require higher initial doses

Preoperatively: 50-100 mg given 30-90 minutes before the beginning of anesthesia

Slow I.V.: Initial: 5-10 mg every 5 minutes as needed

Patient-controlled analgesia (PCA): Usual concentration: 10 mg/mL

Initial dose: 10 mg

Demand dose: 1-5 mg (manufacturer recommendations); range 5-25 mg (American Pain Society, 1999).

Lockout interval: 5-10 minutes

Elderly:

Oral: 50 mg every 4 hours

I.M.: 25 mg every 4 hours

Dosing adjustment in renal impairment: Avoid repeated administration of meperidine in renal dysfunction:

Cl_{cr} 10-50 mL/minute: Administer at 75% of normal dose

Cl_{cr} <10 mL/minute: Administer at 50% of normal dose

Dosing adjustment/comments in hepatic disease: Increased narcotic effect in cirrhosis; reduction in dose more important for oral than I.V. route

Mechanism of Action Binds to opiate receptors in the CNS, causing inhibition of ascending pain pathways, altering the perception of and response to pain; produces generalized CNS depression

Contraindications Hypersensitivity to meperidine or any component of the formulation; use with or within 14 days of MAO inhibitors; pregnancy (prolonged use or high doses near term)

Warnings/Precautions Meperidine is not recommended for the management of chronic pain. When used for acute pain (in patients without renal or CNS disease), treatment should be limited to 48 hours and doses should not exceed 600 mg/24 hours. Oral meperidine is not recommended for acute pain management. Normeperidine (an active metabolite and CNS stimulant) may accumulate and precipitate anxiety, tremors, or seizures; risk increases with renal dysfunction and cumulative dose.

Use only with extreme caution (if at all) in patients with head injury or increased intracranial pressure (ICP); potential to elevate ICP may be greatly exaggerated in these patients. Use caution with pulmonary, hepatic, or renal disorders, supraventricular tachycardias, acute abdominal conditions, hypothyroidism, Addison's disease, BPH, or urethral stricture.

An opioid-containing analgesic regimen should be tailored to each patient's needs and based upon the type of pain being treated (acute versus chronic), the route of administration, degree of tolerance for opioids (naive versus chronic user), age, weight, and medical condition. The optimal analgesic dose varies widely among patients. Doses should be titrated to pain relief/prevention.

Some preparations contain sulfites which may cause allergic reaction. Tolerance or drug dependence may result from extended use.

Drug Interactions

Substrate (minor) of CYP2B6, 2C19, 3A4

Acyclovir: May increase meperidine metabolite concentrations. Use caution.

Barbiturates: May decrease analgesic efficacy and increase sedative and/or respiratory depressive effects of meperidine.

Cimetidine: May increase meperidine metabolite concentrations; use caution.

CNS depressants (including benzodiazepines): May potentiate the sedative and/or respiratory depressive effects of meperidine.

MAO inhibitors: May enhance the serotonergic effect of meperidine, which may cause serotonin syndrome. Concurrent use with or within 14 days of an MAO inhibitor is contraindicated.

Phenothiazines: May potentiate the sedative and/or respiratory depressive effects of meperidine; may increase the incidence of hypotension.

Phenytoin: May decrease the analgesic effects of meperidine

Ritonavir: May increase meperidine metabolite concentrations; use caution.

Serotonin agonists: Serotonin agonists and meperidine may enhance serotonin levels in the brain. Serotonin syndrome may occur.

Serotonin reuptake inhibitors: May potentiate the effects of meperidine, increasing serotonin levels in the brain. Serotonin syndrome may occur.

Sibutramine: May enhance the serotonergic effect of meperidine. Serotonin syndrome may occur.

Tricyclic antidepressants: May potentiate the sedative and/or respiratory depressive effects of meperidine. In addition, potentially may increase the risk of serotonin syndrome.

Ethanol/Nutrition/Herb Interactions

Ethanol: Avoid or limit ethanol (may increase CNS depression). Watch for sedation.

Herb/Nutraceutical: Avoid valerian, St John's wort, kava kava, gotu kola (may increase CNS depression).

Pharmacodynamics/Kinetics

Onset of action: Analgesic: Oral, SubQ: 10-15 minutes; I.V.: ~5 minutes

Peak effect: SubQ.: ~1 hour; Oral: 2 hours

Duration: Oral, SubQ.: 2-4 hours

Absorption: I.M.: Erratic and highly variable

Distribution: Crosses placenta; enters breast milk

Protein binding: 65% to 75%

Metabolism: Hepatic; hydrolyzed to meperidinic acid (inactive) or undergoes N-demethylation to normeperidine (active; has 1/2 the analgesic effect and 2-3 times the CNS effects of meperidine)

Bioavailability: ~50% to 60%; increased with liver disease

Half-life elimination:

Parent drug: Terminal phase: Adults: 2.5-4 hours, Liver disease: 7-11 hours

Normeperidine (active metabolite): 15-30 hours; can accumulate with high doses or with decreased renal function

(Continued)

Meperidine *(Continued)*

Excretion: Urine (as metabolites)

Pregnancy Risk Factor C/D (prolonged use or high doses at term)

Lactation Enters breast milk/contraindicated (AAP rates "compatible")

Breast-Feeding Considerations Meperidine is excreted in breast milk and may cause CNS and/or respiratory depression in the nursing infant.

Dosage Forms

Injection, solution, as hydrochloride [ampul]: 25 mg/0.5 mL (0.5 mL); 25 mg/mL (1 mL); 50 mg/mL (1 mL, 1.5 mL, 2 mL); 75 mg/mL (1 mL); 100 mg/mL (1 mL)

Injection, solution, as hydrochloride [prefilled syringe]: 25 mg/mL (1 mL); 50 mg/mL (1 mL); 75 mg/mL (1 mL); 100 mg/mL (1 mL)

Injection, solution, as hydrochloride [for PCA pump]: 10 mg/mL (30 mL, 50 mL, 60 mL)

Injection, solution, as hydrochloride [vial]: 25 mg/mL (1 mL); 50 mg/mL (1 mL, 30 mL); 75 mg/mL (1 mL); 100 mg/mL (1 mL, 20 mL) [may contain sodium metabisulfite]

Syrup, as hydrochloride: 50 mg/5 mL (500 mL) [contains sodium benzoate]

Demerol®: 50 mg/5 mL (480 mL) [contains benzoic acid; banana flavor]

Tablet, as hydrochloride (Demerol®, Meperitab®): 50 mg, 100 mg

Dental Comment Meperidine is not to be used as the narcotic drug of first choice. It is recommended only to be used in codeine-allergic patients when a narcotic analgesic is indicated. Meperidine is not an anti-inflammatory agent. Meperidine, as with other narcotic analgesics, is recommended only for limited acute dosing (ie, 3 days or less); common adverse effects in the dental patient are nausea, sedation, and constipation. Meperidine has a significant addiction liability, especially when given long-term.

Meperidine and Promethazine

(me PER i deen & proe METH a zeen)

Related Information

Meperidine *on page 983*

Promethazine *on page 1290*

Generic Available Yes

Synonyms Mepergan; Promethazine and Meperidine

Pharmacologic Category Analgesic Combination (Narcotic)

Use Management of moderate pain

Local Anesthetic/Vasoconstrictor Precautions No information available to require special precautions

Effects on Dental Treatment Key adverse event(s) related to dental treatment: Xerostomia (normal salivary flow resumes upon discontinuation).

Common Adverse Effects See individual agents.

Restrictions C-II

Drug Interactions

Cytochrome P450 Effect: Promethazine: **Substrate** (major) of CYP2B6, 2D6; **Inhibits** CYP2D6 (weak)

Pharmacodynamics/Kinetics See individual agents.

Meperidine Hydrochloride *see* Meperidine *on page 983*

Meperitab® *see* Meperidine *on page 983*

Mephobarbital (me foe BAR bi tal)

U.S. Brand Names Mebaral®

Canadian Brand Names Mebaral®

Generic Available No

Synonyms Methylphenobarbital

Pharmacologic Category Barbiturate

Use Sedative; treatment of grand mal and petit mal epilepsy

Local Anesthetic/Vasoconstrictor Precautions No information available to require special precautions

Effects on Dental Treatment No significant effects or complications reported

Common Adverse Effects

>10%: Central nervous system: Dizziness, lightheadedness, drowsiness, "hangover" effect

1% to 10%:

Central nervous system: Confusion, mental depression, unusual excitement, nervousness, faint feeling, headache, insomnia, nightmares

Gastrointestinal: Constipation, nausea, vomiting

Restrictions C-IV

Mechanism of Action Increases seizure threshold in the motor cortex; depresses monosynaptic and polysynaptic transmission in the CNS

Drug Interactions

Cytochrome P450 Effect: Substrate of CYP2B6 (minor), 2C8/9 (minor), 2C19 (major); **Inhibits** CYP2C19 (weak); **Induces** CYP2A6 (weak)

Increased Effect/Toxicity: When combined with other CNS depressants, ethanol, narcotic analgesics, antidepressants, or benzodiazepines, additive respiratory and CNS depression may occur. Barbiturates may enhance the hepatotoxic potential of acetaminophen overdoses. Chloramphenicol, MAO inhibitors, valproic acid, and felbamate may inhibit barbiturate metabolism. Barbiturates may impair the absorption of griseofulvin, and may enhance the nephrotoxic effects of methoxyflurane. Concurrent use of phenobarbital with meperidine may result in increased CNS depression. CYP2C19 inhibitors may increase the levels/effects of mephobarbital; example inhibitors include delavirdine, fluconazole, fluvoxamine, gemfibrozil, isoniazid, omeprazole, and ticlopidine.

Decreased Effect: Barbiturates are hepatic enzyme inducers, and may increase the metabolism of antipsychotics, some beta-blockers (unlikely with atenolol and nadolol), calcium channel blockers, chloramphenicol, cimetidine, corticosteroids, cyclosporine, disopyramide, doxycycline, ethosuximide, felbamate, furosemide, griseofulvin, lamotrigine, phenytoin, propafenone, quinidine, tacrolimus, TCAs, and theophylline. Barbiturates may increase the metabolism of estrogens and reduce the efficacy of oral contraceptives; an alternative method of contraception should be considered. Barbiturates inhibit the hypoprothrombinemic effects of oral anticoagulants via increased metabolism. Barbiturates may enhance the metabolism of methadone resulting in methadone withdrawal. CYP2C19 inducers may decrease the levels/effects of mephobarbital; example inducers include aminoglutethimide, carbamazepine, phenytoin, and rifampin.

Pharmacodynamics/Kinetics

Onset of action: 20-60 minutes

Duration: 6-8 hours

Absorption: ~50%

Half-life elimination, serum: 34 hours

Pregnancy Risk Factor D

Mephyton® *see* Phytonadione *on page 1233*

Mepivacaine (me PIV a kane)

U.S. Brand Names Carbocaine®; Polocaine®; Polocaine® Dental; Polocaine® MPF

Canadian Brand Names Carbocaine®; Polocaine®

Generic Available No

Synonyms Mepivacaine Hydrochloride

Pharmacologic Category Local Anesthetic

Dental Use Local anesthesia by nerve block, infiltration in dental procedures

Use Local or regional analgesia; anesthesia by local infiltration, peripheral and central neural techniques including epidural and caudal blocks; **not** for use in spinal anesthesia

Local Anesthetic/Vasoconstrictor Precautions No information available to require special precautions

Effects on Dental Treatment Key adverse event(s) related to dental treatment: Degree of adverse effects in the CNS and cardiovascular system is directly related to blood levels of mepivacaine (frequency not defined; more likely to occur after systemic administration rather than infiltration): Bradycardia, cardiovascular collapse, hypotension, myocardial depression, ventricular arrhythmias, nausea, vomiting, respiratory arrest, anaphylactoid reactions, blurred vision, heart block, transient stinging or burning at injection site

High blood levels: Anxiety, restlessness, disorientation, confusion, dizziness, and seizures, followed by CNS depression resulting in somnolence, unconsciousness, and possible respiratory arrest.

In some cases, symptoms of CNS stimulation may be absent and the primary CNS effects are somnolence and unconsciousness.

Significant Adverse Effects Degree of adverse effects in the CNS and cardiovascular system is directly related to the blood levels of mepivacaine, route of administration, and physical status of the patient. The effects below are more likely to occur after systemic administration rather than infiltration.

Cardiovascular: Bradycardia, cardiac arrest, cardiac output decreased, heart block, hyper-/hypotension, myocardial depression, syncope, tachycardia, ventricular arrhythmias

(Continued)

Mepivacaine *(Continued)*

Central nervous system: Anxiety, chills, convulsions, depression, dizziness, excitation, restlessness, tremors

Dermatologic: Angioneurotic edema, diaphoresis, erythema, pruritus, urticaria

Gastrointestinal: Fecal incontinence, nausea, vomiting

Genitourinary: Incontinence, urinary retention

Neuromuscular & skeletal: Paralysis

Ocular: Blurred vision, pupil constriction

Otic: Tinnitus

Respiratory: Apnea, hypoventilation, sneezing

Miscellaneous: Allergic reaction, anaphylactoid reaction

Dental Usual Dosing Injectable local anesthetic: Children and Adults: Dose varies with procedure, degree of anesthesia needed, vascularity of tissue, duration of anesthesia required, and physical condition of patient. The smallest dose and concentration required to produce the desired effect should be used.

Children: Maximum dose: 5-6 mg/kg; only concentrations <2% should be used in children <3 years or <14 kg (30 lbs)

Adults: Dental anesthesia:

Single site in upper or lower jaw: 54 mg (1.8 mL) as a 3% solution

Infiltration and nerve block of entire oral cavity: 270 mg (9 mL) as a 3% solution. Manufacturer's maximum recommended dose is not more than 400 mg to normal healthy adults.

Dosage

Injectable local anesthetic: Dose varies with procedure, degree of anesthesia needed, vascularity of tissue, duration of anesthesia required, and physical condition of patient. The smallest dose and concentration required to produce the desired effect should be used.

Children: Maximum dose: 5-6 mg/kg; only concentrations <2% should be used in children <3 years or <14 kg (30 lbs)

Adults: Maximum dose: 400 mg; do not exceed 1000 mg/24 hours

Cervical, brachial, intercostal, pudenal nerve block: 5-40 mL of a 1% solution (maximum: 400 mg) **or** 5-20 mL of a 2% solution (maximum: 400 mg). For pudenal block, inject ¹/₂ the total dose each side.

Transvaginal block (paracervical plus pudenal): Up to 30 mL (both sides) of a 1% solution (maximum: 300 mg). Inject ¹/₂ the total dose each side.

Paracervical block: Up to 20 mL (both sides) of a 1% solution (maximum: 200 mg). Inject ¹/₂ the total dose to each side. This is the maximum recommended dose per 90-minute procedure; inject slowly with 5 minutes between sides.

Caudal and epidural block (preservative free solutions only): 15-30 mL of a 1% solution (maximum: 300 mg) **or** 10-25 mL of a 1.5% solution (maximum: 375 mg) **or** 10-20 mL of a 2% solution (maximum: 400 mg)

Infiltration: Up to 40 mL of a 1% solution (maximum: 400 mg)

Therapeutic block (pain management): 1-5 mL of a 1% solution (maximum: 50 mg) **or** 1-5 mL of a 2% solution (maximum: 100 mg)

Dental anesthesia: Adults:

Single site in upper or lower jaw: 54 mg (1.8 mL) as a 3% solution

Infiltration and nerve block of entire oral cavity: 270 mg (9 mL) as a 3% solution. Manufacturer's maximum recommended dose is not more than 400 mg to normal healthy adults.

Mechanism of Action Mepivacaine is an amide local anesthetic similar to lidocaine; like all local anesthetics, mepivacaine acts by preventing the generation and conduction of nerve impulses

Contraindications Hypersensitivity to mepivacaine, other amide-type local anesthetics, or any component of the formulation

Warnings/Precautions Use with caution in patients with cardiac disease, hepatic or renal disease, or hyperthyroidism. Local anesthetics have been associated with rare occurrences of sudden respiratory arrest; convulsions due to systemic toxicity leading to cardiac arrest have been reported presumably due to intravascular injection. A test dose is recommended prior to epidural administration and all reinforcing doses with continuous catheter technique. Do not use solutions containing preservatives for caudal or epidural block. Use caution in debilitated, elderly, or acutely-ill patients; dose reduction may be required.

Pharmacodynamics/Kinetics

Onset of action (route and dose dependent): Range: 3-20 minutes

Duration (route and dose dependent): 2-2.5 hours

Protein binding: ~75%

Metabolism: Primarily hepatic via N-demethylation, hydroxylation, and glucuronidation

Half-life elimination: Neonates: 8.7-9 hours; Adults: 1.9-3 hours

Excretion: Urine (95% as metabolites)

Pregnancy Risk Factor C

Lactation Excretion in breast milk unknown/use caution

Dosage Forms

Injection, solution, as hydrochloride [contains methylparabens]:

Carbocaine®: 1% (50 mL); 2% (50 mL)

Polocaine®: 1% (50 mL); 2% (50 mL)

Injection, solution, as hydrochloride [preservative free]:

Carbocaine®: 1% (30 mL); 1.5% (30 mL); 2% (20 mL); 3% (1.8 mL) [dental cartridge]

Polocaine® Dental: 3% (1.8 mL) [dental cartridge]

Polocaine® MPF: 1% (30 mL); 1.5% (30 mL); 2% (20 mL)

Mepivacaine (Dental Anesthetic) (me PIV a kane)

Related Information

Mepivacaine *on page 987*

Oral Pain *on page 1692*

U.S. Brand Names Carbocaine®; Polocaine®

Canadian Brand Names Polocaine®

Generic Available No

Pharmacologic Category Local Anesthetic

Dental Use Amide-type anesthetic used for local infiltration anesthesia; injection near nerve trunks to produce nerve block

Local Anesthetic/Vasoconstrictor Precautions No information available to require special precautions

Effects on Dental Treatment It is common to misinterpret psychogenic responses to local anesthetic injection as an allergic reaction. Intraoral injections are perceived by many patients as a stressful procedure in dentistry. Common symptoms to this stress are diaphoresis, palpitations, hyperventilation, generalized pallor, and a fainting feeling.

Degree of adverse effects in the CNS and cardiovascular system is directly related to the blood levels of mepivacaine.

Frequency not defined: Bradycardia and reduction in cardiac output, nausea, vomiting, tremors, asthmatic syndromes, hypersensitivity reactions (may manifest as dermatologic reactions and edema at injection site)

High blood levels: Anxiety, restlessness, disorientation, confusion, dizziness, tremors and seizures, followed by CNS depression resulting in somnolence, unconsciousness and possible respiratory arrest. In some cases, symptoms of CNS stimulation may be absent and the primary CNS effects are somnolence and unconsciousness.

Significant Adverse Effects Degree of adverse effects in the CNS and cardiovascular system is directly related to the blood levels of local anesthetic.

Cardiovascular: Myocardial effects include a decrease in contraction force as well as a decrease in electrical excitability and myocardial conduction rate resulting in bradycardia and reduction in cardiac output

Central nervous system: High blood levels result in anxiety, restlessness, disorientation, confusion, dizziness, and seizure. This is followed by depression of CNS resulting in somnolence, unconsciousness and possible respiratory arrest. In some cases, symptoms of CNS stimulation may be absent and the primary CNS effects are somnolence and unconsciousness.

Gastrointestinal: Nausea and vomiting may occur

Hypersensitivity reactions: May manifest as dermatologic reactions and edema at injection site. Asthmatic syndromes have occurred.

Neuromuscular & skeletal: Tremors

Psychogenic reactions: It is common to misinterpret psychogenic responses to local anesthetic injection as an allergic reaction. Intraoral injection is perceived by many patients as a stressful procedure in dentistry. Common symptoms to this stress are diaphoresis, palpitation, hyperventilation, generalized pallor and a fainting feeling.

Dental Usual Dosing

Children <10 years: Up to 5-6 mg/kg of body weight; maximum pediatric dosage must be carefully calculated on the basis of patient's weight but must not exceed 270 mg (9 mL) of the 3% solution

Children >10 years and Adults:

Dental anesthesia, single site in upper or lower jaw: 54 mg (1.8 mL) as a 3% solution

Infiltration and nerve block of entire oral cavity: 270 mg (9 mL) as a 3% solution; up to a maximum of 6.6 mg/kg of body weight but not to exceed 300 mg per appointment. Manufacturer's maximum recommended dose is not more than 400 mg to normal healthy adults. The effective anesthetic dose varies with procedure, intensity of anesthesia needed, duration of anesthesia required, and physical condition of the patient. Always use the lowest effective dose along with careful aspiration.

(Continued)

Mepivacaine (Dental Anesthetic) *(Continued)*

The following number of dental carpules (1.8 mL) provide the indicated amounts of mepivacaine dental anesthetic 3%. See table.

# of Cartridges (1.8 mL)	mg Mepivacaine (3%)
1	54
2	108
3	162
4	216
5	270
6	324
7	378
8	432

Note: Adult and children doses of mepivacaine dental anesthetic cited from USP Dispensing Information (USP DI), 17th ed, The United States Pharmacopeial Convention, Inc, Rockville, MD, 1997, 138-9.

Dosage

Children <10 years: Up to 5-6 mg/kg of body weight; maximum pediatric dosage must be carefully calculated on the basis of patient's weight but must not exceed 270 mg (9 mL) of the 3% solution

Children >10 years and Adults:

Dental anesthesia, single site in upper or lower jaw: 54 mg (1.8 mL) as a 3% solution

Infiltration and nerve block of entire oral cavity: 270 mg (9 mL) as a 3% solution; up to a maximum of 6.6 mg/kg of body weight but not to exceed 300 mg per appointment. Manufacturer's maximum recommended dose is not more than 400 mg to normal healthy adults. The effective anesthetic dose varies with procedure, intensity of anesthesia needed, duration of anesthesia required, and physical condition of the patient. Always use the lowest effective dose along with careful aspiration.

Note: Adult and children doses of mepivacaine dental anesthetic cited from USP Dispensing Information (USP DI), 17th ed, The United States Pharmacopeial Convention, Inc, Rockville, MD, 1997, 138-9.

Mechanism of Action Local anesthetics bind selectively to the intracellular surface of sodium channels to block influx of sodium into the axon. As a result, depolarization necessary for action potential propagation and subsequent nerve function is prevented. The block at the sodium channel is reversible. When drug diffuses away from the axon, sodium channel function is restored and nerve propagation returns.

Contraindications Hypersensitivity to local anesthetics of the amide type or any component of the formulation

Warnings/Precautions Aspirate the syringe after tissue penetration and before injection to minimize chance of direct vascular injection

Drug Interactions No data reported

Pharmacodynamics/Kinetics

Onset of action: Upper jaw: 30-120 seconds; Lower jaw: 1-4 minutes

Duration: Upper jaw: 20 minutes; Lower jaw: 40 minutes

Half-life elimination, serum: 1.9 hours

Pregnancy Risk Factor C

Breast-Feeding Considerations Usual infiltration doses of mepivacaine dental anesthetic given to nursing mothers has not been shown to affect the health of the nursing infant.

Dosage Forms Injection, solution, as hydrochloride: 3% (1.8 mL) [dental cartridges]

Selected Readings

Ayoub ST and Coleman AE, "A Review of Local Anesthetics," *Gen Dent*, 1992, 40(4):285-7, 289-90.

Budenz AW, "Local Anesthetics in Dentistry: Then and Now," *J Calif Dent Assoc*, 2003, 31(5):388-96.

Dower JS Jr, "A Review of Paresthesia in Association With Administration of Local Anesthesia," *Dent Today*, 2003, 22(2):64-9.

Finder RL and Moore PA, "Adverse Drug Reactions to Local Anesthesia," *Dent Clin North Am*, 2002, 46(4):747-57, x.

Haas DA, "An Update on Local Anesthetics in Dentistry," *J Can Dent Assoc*, 2002, 68(9):546-51.

Hawkins JM and Moore PA, "Local Anesthesia: Advances in Agents and Techniques," *Dent Clin North Am*, 2002, 46(4):719-32, ix.

"Injectable Local Anesthetics," *J Am Dent Assoc*, 2003, 134(5):628-9.

Malamed SF, "Allergy and Toxic Reactions to Local Anesthetics," *Dent Today*, 2003, 22(4):114-6, 118-21.

Wynn RL, "Recent Research on Mechanisms of Local Anesthetics," *Gen Dent*, 1995, 43(4):316-8.

Mepivacaine and Levonordefrin
(me PIV a kane & lee voe nor DEF rin)

Related Information
Mepivacaine *on page 987*
Oral Pain *on page 1692*

U.S. Brand Names Carbocaine® 2% with Neo-Cobefrin®

Canadian Brand Names Polocaine® 2% and Levonordefrin 1:20,000

Generic Available No

Synonyms Levonordefrin and Mepivacaine Hydrochloride

Pharmacologic Category Local Anesthetic

Dental Use Amide-type anesthetic used for local infiltration anesthesia; injection near nerve trunks to produce nerve block

Local Anesthetic/Vasoconstrictor Precautions No information available to require special precautions

Effects on Dental Treatment It is common to misinterpret psychogenic responses to local anesthetic injection as an allergic reaction. Intraoral injections are perceived by many patients as a stressful procedure in dentistry. Common symptoms to this stress are diaphoresis, palpitations, hyperventilation, generalized pallor and a fainting feeling. Patients may exhibit hypersensitivity to bisulfites contained in local anesthetic solution to prevent oxidation of levonordefrin. In general, patients reacting to bisulfites have a history of asthma and their airways are hyper-reactive to asthmatic syndrome.

Degree of adverse effects in the CNS and cardiovascular system is directly related to the blood levels of mepivacaine (frequency not defined; more likely to occur after systemic administration rather than infiltration): Bradycardia and reduction in cardiac output, nausea, vomiting, tremors, hypersensitivity reactions (extremely rare; may be manifest as dermatologic reactions and edema at injection site), asthmatic syndromes

High blood levels: Anxiety, restlessness, disorientation, confusion, dizziness, and seizures, followed by CNS depression resulting in somnolence, unconsciousness and possible respiratory arrest.

In some cases, symptoms of CNS stimulation may be absent and the primary CNS effects are somnolence and unconsciousness.

Significant Adverse Effects Degree of adverse effects in the CNS and cardiovascular system is directly related to the blood levels of mepivacaine. The effects below are more likely to occur after systemic administration rather than infiltration.

Cardiovascular: Myocardial effects include a decrease in contraction force as well as a decrease in electrical excitability and myocardial conduction rate resulting in bradycardia and reduction in cardiac output.

Central nervous system: High blood levels result in anxiety, restlessness, disorientation, confusion, dizziness, and seizure. This is followed by depression of CNS resulting in somnolence, unconsciousness and possible respiratory arrest. In some cases, symptoms of CNS stimulation may be absent and the primary CNS effects are somnolence and unconsciousness.

Gastrointestinal: Nausea and vomiting may occur

Hypersensitivity reactions: Extremely rare, but may be manifest as dermatologic reactions and edema at injection site. Asthmatic syndromes have occurred. Patients may exhibit hypersensitivity to bisulfites contained in local anesthetic solution to prevent oxidation of levonordefrin. In general, patients reacting to bisulfites have a history of asthma and their airways are hyper-reactive to asthmatic syndrome.

Neuromuscular & skeletal: Tremors

Psychogenic reactions: It is common to misinterpret psychogenic responses to local anesthetic injection as an allergic reaction. Intraoral injections are perceived by many patients as a stressful procedure in dentistry. Common symptoms to this stress are diaphoresis, palpitation, hyperventilation, generalized pallor and a fainting feeling.

Dental Usual Dosing

Children <10 years: Maximum pediatric dosage must be carefully calculated on the basis of patient's weight but should not exceed 6.6 mg/kg of body weight or 180 mg of mepivacaine hydrochloride as a 2% solution with levonordefrin 1:20,000

Children >10 years and Adults:
Dental infiltration and nerve block, single site: 36 mg (1.8 mL) of mepivacaine hydrochloride as a 2% solution with levonordefrin 1:20,000

Entire oral cavity: 180 mg (9 mL) of mepivacaine hydrochloride as a 2% solution with levonordefrin 1:20,000; up to a maximum of 6.6 mg/kg of body

(Continued)

Mepivacaine and Levonordefrin *(Continued)*

weight but not to exceed 400 mg of mepivacaine hydrochloride per appointment. The effective anesthetic dose varies with procedure, intensity of anesthesia needed, duration of anesthesia required, and physical condition of the patient. Always use the lowest effective dose along with careful aspiration.

The following numbers of dental carpules (1.8 mL) provide the indicated amounts of mepivacaine hydrochloride 2% and levonordefrin 1:20,000. See table.

# of Cartridges (1.8 mL)	mg Mepivacaine (2%)	mg Vasoconstrictor (Levonordefrin 1:20,000)
1	36	0.090
2	72	0.180
3	108	0.270
4	144	0.360
5	180	0.450
6	216	0.540
7	252	0.630
8	288	0.720
9	324	0.810
10	360	0.900

Note: Adult and children doses of mepivacaine hydrochloride with levonordefrin cited from USP Dispensing Information (USP DI), 17th ed, The United States Pharmacopeial Convention, Inc, Rockville, MD, 1997, 139.

Dosage

Children <10 years: Maximum pediatric dosage must be carefully calculated on the basis of patient's weight but should not exceed 6.6 mg/kg of body weight or 180 mg of mepivacaine hydrochloride as a 2% solution with levonordefrin 1:20,000

Children >10 years and Adults:

Dental infiltration and nerve block, single site: 36 mg (1.8 mL) of mepivacaine hydrochloride as a 2% solution with levonordefrin 1:20,000

Entire oral cavity: 180 mg (9 mL) of mepivacaine hydrochloride as a 2% solution with levonordefrin 1:20,000; up to a maximum of 6.6 mg/kg of body weight but not to exceed 400 mg of mepivacaine hydrochloride per appointment. The effective anesthetic dose varies with procedure, intensity of anesthesia needed, duration of anesthesia required, and physical condition of the patient. Always use the lowest effective dose along with careful aspiration.

Note: Adult and children doses of mepivacaine hydrochloride with levonordefrin cited from USP Dispensing Information (USP DI), 17th ed, The United States Pharmacopeial Convention, Inc, Rockville, MD, 1997, 139.

Mechanism of Action Local anesthetics bind selectively to the intracellular surface of sodium channels to block influx of sodium into the axon. As a result, depolarization necessary for action potential propagation and subsequent nerve function is prevented. The block at the sodium channel is reversible. When drug diffuses away from the axon, sodium channel function is restored and nerve propagation returns.

Levonordefrin prolongs the duration of the anesthetic actions of mepivacaine by causing vasoconstriction (alpha adrenergic receptor agonist) of the vasculature surrounding the nerve axons. This prevents the diffusion of mepivacaine away from the nerves resulting in a longer retention in the axon.

Contraindications Hypersensitivity to local anesthetics of the amide-type or any component of the formulation

Warnings/Precautions Should be avoided in patients with uncontrolled hyperthyroidism. Should be used in minimal amounts in patients with significant cardiovascular problems (because of levonordefrin component). Aspirate the syringe after tissue penetration and before injection to minimize chance of direct vascular injection. Contains sodium bisulfite which may cause allergic reactions in some individuals.

Drug Interactions Due to levonordefrin component, use with tricyclic antidepressants or MAO inhibitors could result in increased pressor response; use with nonselective beta-blockers (ie, propranolol) could result in serious hypertension and reflex bradycardia

Pharmacodynamics/Kinetics
Duration: Upper jaw: 1-2.5 hours; Lower jaw: 2.5-5.5 hours
Infiltration: 50 minutes
Inferior alveolar block: 60-75 minutes

Pregnancy Risk Factor C

Breast-Feeding Considerations Usual infiltration doses of mepivacaine with levonordefrin given to nursing mothers has not been shown to affect the health of the nursing infant.

Dosage Forms Injection, solution: Mepivacaine hydrochloride 2% and levonordefrin 1:20,000 (1.8 mL) [dental cartridges; contains sodium bisulfite]

Selected Readings
Ayoub ST and Coleman AE, "A Review of Local Anesthetics," *Gen Dent*, 1992, 40(4):285-7, 289-90.
Jastak JT and Yagiela JA, "Vasoconstrictors and Local Anesthesia: A Review and Rationale for Use," *J Am Dent Assoc*, 1983, 107(4):623-30.
MacKenzie TA and Young ER, "Local Anesthetic Update," *Anesth Prog*, 1993, 40(2):29-34.
Wynn RL, "Epinephrine Interactions With Beta-Blockers," *Gen Dent*, 1994, 42(1):16, 18.
Wynn RL, "Recent Research on Mechanisms of Local Anesthetics," *Gen Dent*, 1995, 43(4):316-8.
Yagiela JA, "Local Anesthetics," *Anesth Prog*, 1991, 38(4-5):128-41.

Mepivacaine Hydrochloride *see* Mepivacaine *on page 987*

Meprobamate (me proe BA mate)

U.S. Brand Names Miltown® [DSC]
Canadian Brand Names Novo-Mepro
Generic Available Yes
Synonyms Equanil
Pharmacologic Category Antianxiety Agent, Miscellaneous
Dental Use Treatment of muscle spasm associated with acute temporomandibular joint (TMJ) pain; management of dental anxiety disorders
Use Management of anxiety disorders
Unlabeled/Investigational Use Demonstrated value for muscle contraction, headache, premenstrual tension, external sphincter spasticity, muscle rigidity, opisthotonos-associated with tetanus
Local Anesthetic/Vasoconstrictor Precautions No information available to require special precautions
Effects on Dental Treatment No significant effects or complications reported
Significant Adverse Effects Frequency not defined.
Cardiovascular: Syncope, peripheral edema, palpitation, tachycardia, arrhythmia
Central nervous system: Drowsiness, ataxia, dizziness, paradoxical excitement, confusion, slurred speech, headache, euphoria, chills, vertigo, paresthesia, overstimulation
Dermatologic: Rashes, purpura, dermatitis, Stevens-Johnson syndrome, petechiae, ecchymosis
Gastrointestinal: Diarrhea, vomiting, nausea
Hematologic: Leukopenia, eosinophilia, agranulocytosis, aplastic anemia
Neuromuscular & skeletal: Weakness
Ocular: Blurred vision, impairment of accommodation
Renal: Renal failure
Respiratory: Wheezing, dyspnea, bronchospasm, angioneurotic edema
Restrictions C-IV
Dental Usual Dosing Muscle spasm (TMJ) pain or anxiety: Adults: Oral: 400 mg 3-4 times/day, up to 2400 mg/day
Dosage Oral:
Children 6-12 years: Anxiety: 100-200 mg 2-3 times/day
Adults: Anxiety: 400 mg 3-4 times/day, up to 2400 mg/day
Dosing interval in renal impairment:
Cl_{cr} 10-50 mL/minute: Administer every 9-12 hours
Cl_{cr} <10 mL/minute: Administer every 12-18 hours
Hemodialysis: Moderately dialyzable (20% to 50%)
Dosing adjustment in hepatic impairment: Probably necessary in patients with liver disease
Mechanism of Action Affects the thalamus and limbic system; also appears to inhibit multineuronal spinal reflexes
Contraindications Hypersensitivity to meprobamate, related compounds (including carisoprodol), or any component of the formulation; acute intermittent porphyria; pre-existing CNS depression; narrow-angle glaucoma; severe uncontrolled pain; pregnancy
Warnings/Precautions Physical and psychological dependence and abuse may occur; abrupt cessation may precipitate withdrawal. Use with caution in patients with depression or suicidal tendencies, or in patients with a history of drug abuse. May cause CNS depression, which may impair physical or mental
(Continued)

Meprobamate (Continued)

abilities. Patients must be cautioned about performing tasks which require mental alertness (eg, operating machinery or driving). Effects with other sedative drugs or ethanol may be potentiated. Not recommended in children <6 years of age; allergic reaction may occur in patients with history of dermatological condition (usually by fourth dose). Use with caution in patients with renal or hepatic impairment, or with a history of seizures. Use caution in the elderly as it may cause confusion, cognitive impairment, or excessive sedation.

Drug Interactions CNS depressants: Sedative effects may be additive with other CNS depressants; monitor for increased effect; includes barbiturates, benzodiazepines, narcotic analgesics, ethanol, and other sedative agents

Ethanol/Nutrition/Herb Interactions

Ethanol: Avoid ethanol (may increase CNS depression).

Herb/Nutraceutical: Avoid valerian, St John's wort, kava kava, gotu kola (may increase CNS depression).

Pharmacodynamics/Kinetics

Onset of action: Sedation: ~1 hour

Distribution: Crosses placenta; enters breast milk

Metabolism: Hepatic

Half-life elimination: 10 hours

Excretion: Urine (8% to 20% as unchanged drug); feces (10% as metabolites)

Pregnancy Risk Factor D

Lactation Enters breast milk/not recommended

Breast-Feeding Considerations Breast milk concentrations are higher than plasma; effects are unknown.

Dosage Forms

[DSC] = Discontinued product

Tablet: 200 mg, 400 mg

Miltown®: 200 mg, 400 mg [DSC]

Meprobamate and Aspirin see Aspirin and Meprobamate on page 151

Mepron® see Atovaquone on page 160

Mequinol and Tretinoin (ME kwi nole & TRET i noyn)

U.S. Brand Names Solagé™

Canadian Brand Names Solagé™

Generic Available No

Synonyms Tretinoin and Mequinol

Pharmacologic Category Retinoic Acid Derivative; Vitamin A Derivative; Vitamin, Topical

Use Treatment of solar lentigines; the efficacy of using Solagé™ daily for >24 weeks has not been established. The local cutaneous safety of Solagé™ in non-Caucasians has not been adequately established.

Local Anesthetic/Vasoconstrictor Precautions No information available to require special precautions

Effects on Dental Treatment No significant effects or complications reported

Common Adverse Effects

>10%: Dermatologic: Erythema (49%), burning, stinging or tingling (26%), desquamation (14%), pruritus (12%)

1% to 10%: Dermatologic: Skin irritation (5%), hypopigmentation (5%), halo hypopigmentation (7%), rash (3%), dry skin (3%), crusting (3%), vesicular bullae rash (2%), contact allergic reaction (1%)

Mechanism of Action Solar lentigines are localized, pigmented, macular lesions of the skin on areas of the body chronically exposed to the sun. Mequinol is a substrate for the enzyme tyrosinase and acts as a competitive inhibitor of the formation of melanin precursors. The mechanisms of depigmentation for both drugs is unknown.

Drug Interactions

Cytochrome P450 Effect: Tretinoin: **Substrate** (minor) of CYP2A6, 2B6, 2C8/9; **Inhibits** CYP2C8/9 (weak); **Induces** CYP2E1 (weak)

Increased Effect/Toxicity:

Topical products with skin drying effects (eg, those containing alcohol, astringents, spices, or lime; medicated soaps or shampoos; permanent wave solutions; hair depilatories or waxes; and others) may increase skin irritation. Avoid concurrent use.

Photosensitizing drugs (eg, thiazides, tetracyclines, fluoroquinolones, phenothiazines, sulfonamides) can further increase sun sensitivity. Avoid concurrent use.

Pharmacodynamics/Kinetics

Absorption: Percutaneous absorption was 4.4% of tretinoin when applied as 0.8 mL of Solagé™ to a 400 cm² area of the back

Time to peak: Mequinol: 2 hours

Pregnancy Risk Factor X

Mercaptopurine (mer kap toe PYOOR een)

U.S. Brand Names Purinethol®
Canadian Brand Names Purinethol®
Mexican Brand Names Purinethol®
Generic Available Yes
Synonyms 6-Mercaptopurine; 6-MP; NSC-755
Pharmacologic Category Antineoplastic Agent, Antimetabolite
Use Treatment (maintenance and induction) of acute lymphoblastic leukemia (ALL)
Local Anesthetic/Vasoconstrictor Precautions No information available to require special precautions
Effects on Dental Treatment Key adverse event(s) related to dental treatment: Stomatitis and mucositis.
Common Adverse Effects

>10%:

Hematologic: Myelosuppression; leukopenia, thrombocytopenia, anemia
Onset: 7-10 days
Nadir: 14-16 days
Recovery: 21-28 days

Hepatic: Intrahepatic cholestasis and focal centralobular necrosis (40%), characterized by hyperbilirubinemia, increased alkaline phosphatase and AST, jaundice, ascites, encephalopathy; more common at doses >2.5 mg/kg/day. Usually occurs within 2 months of therapy but may occur within 1 week, or be delayed up to 8 years.

1% to 10%:

Central nervous system: Drug fever
Dermatologic: Hyperpigmentation, rash
Endocrine & metabolic: Hyperuricemia
Gastrointestinal: Nausea, vomiting, diarrhea, stomatitis, anorexia, stomach pain, mucositis
Renal: Renal toxicity

Restrictions Note: I.V. formulation is not commercially available in the U.S.
Mechanism of Action Purine antagonist which inhibits DNA and RNA synthesis; acts as false metabolite and is incorporated into DNA and RNA, eventually inhibiting their synthesis; specific for the S phase of the cell cycle
Drug Interactions

Increased Effect/Toxicity: Allopurinol can cause increased levels of mercaptopurine by inhibition of xanthine oxidase. Decrease dose of mercaptopurine by 75% when both drugs are used concomitantly. Seen only with oral mercaptopurine usage, not with I.V. May potentiate effect of bone marrow suppression (reduce mercaptopurine to 25% of dose). Synergistic liver toxicity between doxorubicin and mercaptopurine has been reported. Any agent which could potentially alter the metabolic function of the liver could produce higher drug levels and greater toxicities from either mercaptopurine or thioguanine (6-TG). Aminosalicylates (eg, olsalazine, mesalamine, sulfasalazine) may inhibit TPMT, increasing toxicity/myelosuppression of mercaptopurine.

Decreased Effect: Mercaptopurine inhibits the anticoagulation effect of warfarin by an unknown mechanism.

Pharmacodynamics/Kinetics

Absorption: Variable and incomplete (16% to 50%)
Distribution: V_d = total body water; CNS penetration is poor
Protein binding: 19%
Metabolism: Hepatic and in GI mucosa; hepatically via xanthine oxidase and methylation via TPMT to sulfate conjugates, 6-thiouric acid, and other inactive compounds; first-pass effect
Half-life elimination (age dependent): Children: 21 minutes; Adults: 47 minutes
Time to peak, serum: ~2 hours
Excretion: Urine; following high (1 g/m²) I.V. doses, 20% to 40% excreted unchanged; at lower doses renal elimination minor

Pregnancy Risk Factor D

6-Mercaptopurine see Mercaptopurine on page 995
Mercapturic Acid see Acetylcysteine on page 46
Meridia® see Sibutramine on page 1389

Meropenem (mer oh PEN em)

U.S. Brand Names Merrem® I.V.
Canadian Brand Names Merrem®
Mexican Brand Names Merrem®
Generic Available No
Pharmacologic Category Antibiotic, Carbapenem
Use Treatment of intra-abdominal infections (complicated appendicitis and perito-nitis); treatment of bacterial meningitis in pediatric patients ≥3 months of age caused by *S. pneumoniae*, *H. influenzae*, and *N. meningitidis*; treatment of complicated skin and skin structure infections caused by susceptible organisms
Unlabeled/Investigational Use
Febrile neutropenia, urinary tract infections
Local Anesthetic/Vasoconstrictor Precautions No information available to require special precautions
Effects on Dental Treatment Key adverse event(s) related to dental treat-ment: Oral moniliasis (pediatric patients) and glossitis.
Common Adverse Effects
1% to 10%:
Cardiovascular: Peripheral vascular disorder (<1%)
Central nervous system: Headache (2% to 8%), pain (5%)
Dermatologic: Rash (2% to 3%, includes diaper-area moniliasis in pediatrics), pruritus (1%)
Gastrointestinal: Diarrhea (4% to 5%), nausea/vomiting (1% to 8%), constipa-tion (1% to 7%), oral moniliasis (up to 2% in pediatric patients), glossitis
Hematologic: Anemia (up to 6%)
Local: Inflammation at the injection site (2%), phlebitis/thrombophlebitis (1%), injection site reaction (1%)
Respiratory: Apnea (1%)
Miscellaneous: Sepsis (2%), septic shock (1%)
Mechanism of Action Inhibits bacterial cell wall synthesis by binding to several of the penicillin-binding proteins, which in turn inhibit the final transpeptidation step of peptidoglycan synthesis in bacterial cell walls, thus inhibiting cell wall biosynthesis; bacteria eventually lyse due to ongoing activity of cell wall auto-lytic enzymes (autolysins and murein hydrolases) while cell wall assembly is arrested
Drug Interactions
Increased Effect/Toxicity: Probenecid may increase meropenem serum concentrations.
Decreased Effect: Meropenem may decrease valproic acid serum concentra-tions to subtherapeutic levels.
Pharmacodynamics/Kinetics
Distribution: V_d: Adults: ~0.3 L/kg, Children: 0.4-0.5 L/kg; penetrates well into most body fluids and tissues; CSF concentrations approximate those of the plasma
Protein binding: 2%
Metabolism: Hepatic; metabolized to open beta-lactam form (inactive)
Half-life elimination:
Normal renal function: 1-1.5 hours
Cl_{cr} 30-80 mL/minute: 1.9-3.3 hours
Cl_{cr} 2-30 mL/minute: 3.82-5.7 hours
Time to peak, tissue: 1 hour following infusion
Excretion: Urine (~25% as inactive metabolites)
Pregnancy Risk Factor B

Merrem® I.V. *see* Meropenem *on page 996*
Meruvax® II *see* Rubella Virus Vaccine (Live) *on page 1372*

Mesalamine (me SAL a meen)

U.S. Brand Names Asacol®; Canasa™; Pentasa®; Rowasa®
Canadian Brand Names Asacol®; Mesasal®; Novo-5 ASA; Pentasa®; Quintasa®; Rowasa®; Salofalk®
Mexican Brand Names Salofalk®
Generic Available Yes: Rectal suspension
Synonyms 5-Aminosalicylic Acid; 5-ASA; Fisalamine; Mesalazine
Pharmacologic Category 5-Aminosalicylic Acid Derivative
Use
Oral: Treatment and maintenance of remission of mildly to moderately active ulcerative colitis

Rectal: Treatment of active mild to moderate distal ulcerative colitis, proctosigmoiditis, or proctitis

Local Anesthetic/Vasoconstrictor Precautions No information available to require special precautions

Effects on Dental Treatment Key adverse event(s) related to dental treatment: Pharyngitis.

Common Adverse Effects Adverse effects vary depending upon dosage form. Effects as reported with tablets, unless otherwise noted:

>10%:
  Central nervous system: Headache (suppository 14%), pain (14%)
  Gastrointestinal: Abdominal pain (18%; enema 8%)
  Genitourinary: Eructation (16%)
  Respiratory: Pharyngitis (11%)

1% to 10%:
  Cardiovascular: Chest pain (3%), peripheral edema (3%)
  Central nervous system: Chills (3%), dizziness (suppository 3%), fever (enema 3%; suppository 1%), insomnia (2%), malaise (2%)
  Dermatologic: Rash (6%; suppository 1%), pruritus (3%; enema 1%), acne (2%; suppository 1%)
  Gastrointestinal: Abdominal pain (enema 8%; suppository 5%), colitis exacerbation (3%; suppository 1%), constipation (5%), diarrhea (suppository 3%), dyspepsia (6%), flatulence (enema 6%; suppository 5%), hemorrhoids (enema 1%), nausea (capsule/suppository 3%), nausea and vomiting (capsule 1%), rectal pain (enema 1%; suppository 2%), vomiting (5%)
  Local: Pain on insertion of enema tip (enema 1%)
  Neuromuscular & skeletal: Back pain (7%; enema 1%), arthralgia (5%), hypertonia (5%), myalgia (3%), arthritis (2%), leg/joint pain (enema 2%)
  Ocular: Conjunctivitis (2%)
  Respiratory: Flu-like syndrome (3%; enema 5%), cough increased (2%)
  Miscellaneous: Diaphoresis (3%)

Mechanism of Action Mesalamine (5-aminosalicylic acid) is the active component of sulfasalazine; the specific mechanism of action of mesalamine is unknown; however, it is thought that it modulates local chemical mediators of the inflammatory response, especially leukotrienes, and is also postulated to be a free radical scavenger or an inhibitor of tumor necrosis factor (TNF); action appears topical rather than systemic

Drug Interactions
  Increased Effect/Toxicity: Mesalamine may increase the risk of myelosuppression from azathioprine, mercaptopurine, and thioguanine.
  Decreased Effect: Decreased digoxin bioavailability.

Pharmacodynamics/Kinetics
  Absorption: Rectal: Variable and dependent upon retention time, underlying GI disease, and colonic pH; Oral: Tablet: ~28%, Capsule: ~20% to 30%
  Metabolism: Hepatic and via GI tract to acetyl-5-aminosalicylic acid
  Half-life elimination: 5-ASA: 0.5-1.5 hours; acetyl-5-ASA: 5-10 hours
  Time to peak, serum: 4-7 hours
  Excretion: Urine (as metabolites); feces (<2%)

Pregnancy Risk Factor B

Mesalazine see Mesalamine on page 996

Mesoridazine (mez oh RID a zeen)

U.S. Brand Names Serentil® [DSC]
Canadian Brand Names Serentil®
Generic Available No
Synonyms Mesoridazine Besylate
Pharmacologic Category Antipsychotic Agent, Typical, Phenothiazine
Use Management of schizophrenic patients who fail to respond adequately to treatment with other antipsychotic drugs, either because of insufficient effectiveness or the inability to achieve an effective dose due to intolerable adverse effects from these drugs

Unlabeled/Investigational Use Psychosis

Local Anesthetic/Vasoconstrictor Precautions No information available to require special precautions (see Dental Comment)

Effects on Dental Treatment Key adverse event(s) related to dental treatment: Orthostatic hypotension.

Common Adverse Effects Frequency not defined.
  Cardiovascular: Hypotension, orthostatic hypotension, tachycardia, QT prolongation (dose dependent, up to 100% of patients at higher dosages), syncope, edema

(Continued)

Mesoridazine *(Continued)*

Central nervous system: Pseudoparkinsonism, akathisia, dystonias, tardive dyskinesia, dizziness, drowsiness, restlessness, ataxia, slurred speech, neuroleptic malignant syndrome (NMS), impairment of temperature regulation, lowering of seizure threshold

Dermatologic: Increased sensitivity to sun, rash, itching, angioneurotic edema, dermatitis, discoloration of skin (blue-gray)

Endocrine & metabolic: Changes in menstrual cycle, libido (changes in), gynecomastia, lactation, galactorrhea

Gastrointestinal: Constipation, xerostomia, weight gain, nausea, vomiting, stomach pain

Genitourinary: Difficulty in urination, ejaculatory disturbances, impotence, enuresis, incontinence, priapism, urinary retention

Hematologic: Agranulocytosis, leukopenia, eosinophilia, thrombocytopenia, anemia, aplastic anemia

Hepatic: Cholestatic jaundice, hepatotoxicity

Neuromuscular & skeletal: Weakness, tremor, rigidity

Ocular: Pigmentary retinopathy, photophobia, blurred vision, cornea and lens changes

Respiratory: Nasal congestion

Miscellaneous: Diaphoresis (decreased), lupus-like syndrome

Mechanism of Action Mesoridazine is a piperidine phenothiazine antipsychotic which blocks postsynaptic CNS dopamine$_2$ receptors in the mesolimbic and mesocortical areas

Drug Interactions

Increased Effect/Toxicity: Use of mesoridazine with other agents known to prolong QT$_c$ may increase the risk of malignant arrhythmias; concurrent use is contraindicated - includes type I and type III antiarrhythmics, TCAs, and some quinolone antibiotics (sparfloxacin, moxifloxacin, gatifloxacin). Mesoridazine may increase the effect and/or toxicity of antihypertensives, anticholinergics, lithium, CNS depressants (ethanol, narcotics), and trazodone. Metoclopramide may increase risk of extrapyramidal symptoms (EPS). Acetylcholinesterase inhibitors (central) may increase the risk of antipsychotic-related EPS.

Decreased Effect: Mesoridazine may inhibit the activity of bromocriptine and levodopa. Benztropine (and other anticholinergics) may inhibit the therapeutic response to mesoridazine and excess anticholinergic effects may occur. Mesoridazine and possibly other low potency antipsychotic may reverse the pressor effects of epinephrine.

Pharmacodynamics/Kinetics

Duration: 4-6 hours

Absorption: Tablet: Erratic; Liquid: More dependable

Protein binding: 91% to 99%

Half-life elimination: 24-48 hours

Time to peak, serum: 2-4 hours; Steady-state serum: 4-7 days

Excretion: Urine

Pregnancy Risk Factor C

Dental Comment

This drug is known to prolong the QT interval. The QT interval is measured as the time and distance between the Q point of the QRS complex and the end of the T wave in the ECG tracing. After adjustment for heart rate, the QT interval is defined as prolonged if it is more than 450 msec in men and 460 msec in women. A long QT syndrome was first described in the 1950s and 60s as a congenital syndrome involving QT interval prolongation and syncope and sudden death. Some of the congenital long QT syndromes were characterized by a peculiar electrocardiographic appearance of the QRS complex involving a premature atria beat followed by a pause, then a subsequent sinus beat showing marked QT prolongation and deformity. This type of cardiac arrhythmia was originally termed "torsade de pointes" (translated from the French as "twisting of the points").

Prolongation of the QT interval is thought to result from delayed ventricular repolarization. The repolarization process within the myocardial cell is due to the efflux of intracellular potassium. The channels associated with this current can be blocked by many drugs and predisposes the electrical propagation cycle to torsade de pointes.

Mesoridazine is one of the drugs confirmed to prolong the QT interval and is accepted as having a risk of causing torsade de pointes. The risk of drug-induced torsade de pointes is extremely low when a single QT interval prolonging drug is prescribed. In terms of epinephrine, it is not known what effect vasoconstrictors in the local anesthetic regimen will have in patients with a known history of congenital prolonged QT interval or in patients taking any medication that prolongs the QT interval. Until more information is obtained, it is suggested that the clinician consult with the physician prior to the use of a vasoconstrictor in suspected patients, and that the vasoconstrictor (epinephrine, levonordefrin [Neo-Cobefrin®]) be used with caution.

Mesoridazine Besylate *see* Mesoridazine *on page 997*

Mestinon® *see* Pyridostigmine *on page 1315*

Mestinon® Timespan® *see* Pyridostigmine *on page 1315*

Mestranol and Norethindrone (MES tra nole & nor eth IN drone)

Related Information
Endocrine Disorders and Pregnancy *on page 1659*
Norethindrone *on page 1125*
U.S. Brand Names Necon® 1/50; Norinyl® 1+50; Ortho-Novum® 1/50
Canadian Brand Names Ortho-Novum® 1/50
Generic Available Yes
Synonyms Norethindrone and Mestranol; Ortho Novum 1/50
Pharmacologic Category Contraceptive; Estrogen and Progestin Combination

Use Prevention of pregnancy
Unlabeled/Investigational Use Treatment of hypermenorrhea (menorrhagia); pain associated with endometriosis; dysmenorrhea; dysfunctional uterine bleeding
Local Anesthetic/Vasoconstrictor Precautions No information available to require special precautions
Effects on Dental Treatment When prescribing antibiotics, patient must be advised to use additional methods of birth control if on hormonal contraceptives.
Common Adverse Effects Frequency not defined.
Cardiovascular: Arterial thromboembolism, cerebral hemorrhage, cerebral thrombosis, edema, hypertension, mesenteric thrombosis, MI
Central nervous system: Depression, dizziness, headache, migraine, nervousness, premenstrual syndrome, stroke
Dermatologic: Acne, erythema multiforme, erythema nodosum, hirsutism, loss of scalp hair, melasma (may persist), rash (allergic)
Endocrine & metabolic: Amenorrhea, breakthrough bleeding, breast enlargement, breast secretion, breast tenderness, carbohydrate intolerance, lactation decreased (postpartum), glucose tolerance decreased, libido changes, menstrual flow changes, sex hormone-binding globulins (SHBG) increased, spotting, temporary infertility (following discontinuation), thyroid-binding globulin increased, triglycerides increased
Gastrointestinal: Abdominal cramps, appetite changes, bloating, cholestasis, colitis, gallbladder disease, jaundice, nausea, vomiting, weight gain/loss
Genitourinary: Cervical erosion changes, cervical secretion changes, cystitis-like syndrome, vaginal candidiasis, vaginitis
Hematologic: Antithrombin III decreased, folate levels decreased, hemolytic uremic syndrome, norepinephrine induced platelet aggregability increased, porphyria, prothrombin increased; factors VII, VIII, IX, and X increased
Hepatic: Benign liver tumors, Budd-Chiari syndrome, cholestatic jaundice, hepatic adenomas
Local: Thrombophlebitis
Ocular: Cataracts, change in corneal curvature (steepening), contact lens intolerance, optic neuritis, retinal thrombosis
Renal: Impaired renal function
Respiratory: Pulmonary thromboembolism
Miscellaneous: Hemorrhagic eruption
Mechanism of Action Combination oral contraceptives inhibit ovulation via a negative feedback mechanism on the hypothalamus, which alters the normal pattern of gonadotropin secretion of a follicle-stimulating hormone (FSH) and luteinizing hormone by the anterior pituitary. The follicular phase FSH and midcycle surge of gonadotropins are inhibited. In addition, combination hormonal contraceptives produce alterations in the genital tract, including changes in the cervical mucus, rendering it unfavorable for sperm penetration even if ovulation occurs. Changes in the endometrium may also occur, producing an unfavorable environment for nidation. Combination hormonal contraceptive drugs may alter the tubal transport of the ova through the fallopian tubes. Progestational agents may also alter sperm fertility.
Drug Interactions
Cytochrome P450 Effect:
Mestranol: **Substrate** of CYP2C19 (major); Based on active metabolite ethinyl estradiol: **Substrate** of CYP3A4 (major), 3A5-7 (minor); **Inhibits** CYP1A2 (weak), 2B6 (weak), 2C19 (weak), 3A4 (weak)
Norethindrone: **Substrate** of CYP3A4 (major); **Induces** CYP2C19 (weak)
(Continued)

Mestranol and Norethindrone *(Continued)*

Increased Effect/Toxicity: Acetaminophen and ascorbic acid may increase plasma levels of estrogen component. Atorvastatin and indinavir increase plasma levels of combination hormonal contraceptives. Combination hormonal contraceptives increase the plasma levels of alprazolam, chlordiazepoxide, cyclosporine, diazepam, prednisolone, selegiline, theophylline, tricyclic antidepressants. Combination hormonal contraceptives may increase (or decrease) the effects of coumarin derivatives.

Decreased Effect: CYP2C8/9 inhibitors may decrease the levels of ethinyl estradiol (active metabolite of mestranol); example inhibitors include delavirdine, fluconazole, gemfibrozil, ketoconazole, nicardipine, NSAIDs, pioglitazone, and sulfonamides. CYP3A4 inducers may decrease the levels of ethinyl estradiol (active metabolite of mestranol); example inducers include aminoglutethimide, carbamazepine, nafcillin, nevirapine, phenobarbital, phenytoin, and rifamycins. Combination hormonal contraceptives may decrease plasma levels of acetaminophen, clofibric acid, lorazepam, morphine, oxazepam, salicylic acid, temazepam. Contraceptive effect decreased by acitretin, aminoglutethimide, amprenavir, griseofulvin, lopinavir, nelfinavir, nevirapine, penicillins (effect not consistent), ritonavir, tetracyclines (effect not consistent) troglitazone. Combination hormonal contraceptives may decrease (or increase) the effects of coumarin derivatives.

Pharmacodynamics/Kinetics
Mestranol: Metabolism: Hepatic via demethylation to ethinyl estradiol
Norethindrone: See Norethindrone monograph for additional information.

Pregnancy Risk Factor X

Metacortandralone *see* PrednisoLONE *on page 1268*
Metadate® CD *see* Methylphenidate *on page 1023*
Metadate® ER *see* Methylphenidate *on page 1023*
Metaglip™ *see* Glipizide and Metformin *on page 741*
Metamucil® [OTC] *see* Psyllium *on page 1313*
Metamucil® Plus Calcium [OTC] *see* Psyllium *on page 1313*
Metamucil® Smooth Texture [OTC] *see* Psyllium *on page 1313*

Metaproterenol (met a proe TER e nol)

Related Information
Respiratory Diseases *on page 1656*
U.S. Brand Names Alupent®
Generic Available Yes: Excludes inhaler
Synonyms Metaproterenol Sulfate; Orciprenaline Sulfate
Pharmacologic Category Beta$_2$-Adrenergic Agonist
Use Bronchodilator in reversible airway obstruction due to asthma or COPD; because of its delayed onset of action (1 hour) and prolonged effect (4 or more hours), this may not be the drug of choice for assessing response to a bronchodilator

Local Anesthetic/Vasoconstrictor Precautions No information available to require special precautions

Effects on Dental Treatment Key adverse event(s) related to dental treatment: Bad taste and xerostomia (normal salivary flow resumes upon discontinuation).

Common Adverse Effects
>10%:
Cardiovascular: Tachycardia (<17%)
Central nervous system: Nervousness (3% to 14%)
Endocrine & metabolic: Serum glucose increased, serum potassium decreased
Neuromuscular & skeletal: Tremor (1% to 33%)
1% to 10%:
Cardiovascular: Palpitations (<4%)
Central nervous system: Headache (<4%), dizziness (1% to 4%), insomnia (2%)
Gastrointestinal: Nausea, vomiting, bad taste, heartburn (≥4%), xerostomia
Neuromuscular & skeletal: Trembling, muscle cramps, weakness (1%)
Respiratory: Coughing, pharyngitis (≤4%)
Miscellaneous: Diaphoresis (increased) (≤4%)

Mechanism of Action Relaxes bronchial smooth muscle by action on beta$_2$-receptors with very little effect on heart rate

Drug Interactions
Increased Effect/Toxicity: Sympathomimetics, TCAs, MAO inhibitors taken with metaproterenol may result in toxicity. Inhaled ipratropium may increase

duration of bronchodilation. Halothane may increase risk of malignant arrhythmias; avoid concurrent use.

Decreased Effect: Decreased effect of beta-blockers.

Pharmacodynamics/Kinetics
Onset of action: Bronchodilation: Oral: ~15 minutes; Inhalation: ~60 seconds
Peak effect: Oral: ~1 hour
Duration: ~1-5 hours

Pregnancy Risk Factor C

Metaproterenol Sulfate *see* Metaproterenol *on page 1000*

Metaxalone (me TAKS a lone)

U.S. Brand Names Skelaxin®
Canadian Brand Names Skelaxin®
Generic Available No
Pharmacologic Category Skeletal Muscle Relaxant
Use Relief of discomfort associated with acute, painful musculoskeletal conditions
Local Anesthetic/Vasoconstrictor Precautions No information available to require special precautions
Effects on Dental Treatment No significant effects or complications reported
Common Adverse Effects Frequency not defined.
Central nervous system: Paradoxical stimulation, headache, drowsiness, dizziness, irritability
Dermatologic: Allergic dermatitis
Gastrointestinal: Nausea, vomiting, stomach cramps
Hematologic: Leukopenia, hemolytic anemia
Hepatic: Hepatotoxicity
Miscellaneous: Anaphylaxis
Dosage Children >12 years and Adults: Oral: 800 mg 3-4 times/day
Mechanism of Action Does not have a direct effect on skeletal muscle; most of its therapeutic effect comes from actions on the central nervous system
Contraindications Hypersensitivity to metaxalone or any component of the formulation; impaired hepatic or renal function, history of drug-induced hemolytic anemias or other anemias
Warnings/Precautions Use with caution in patients with impaired hepatic function
Drug Interactions
Increased Effect/Toxicity: Additive effects with ethanol or CNS depressants
Ethanol/Nutrition/Herb Interactions Ethanol: Avoid ethanol (may increase CNS depression).
Dietary Considerations Administration with food may increase serum concentrations.
Pharmacodynamics/Kinetics
Onset of action: ~1 hour
Duration: ~4-6 hours
Metabolism: Hepatic
Bioavailability: Not established; food may increase
Half-life elimination: 9 hours
Time to peak: T_{max}: 3 hours
Excretion: Urine (as metabolites)
Pregnancy Risk Factor C
Dosage Forms TAB: 800 mg

Metformin (met FOR min)

Related Information
Endocrine Disorders and Pregnancy *on page 1659*
U.S. Brand Names Fortamet™; Glucophage®; Glucophage® XR; Riomet™
Canadian Brand Names Alti-Metformin; Apo-Metformin®; Gen-Metformin; Glucophage®; Glumetza®; Glycon; Novo-Metformin; Nu-Metformin; PMS-Metformin; Rho®-Metformin; Sandoz-Metformin FC
Mexican Brand Names Dabex®; Dimefor®; Glucophage®
Generic Available Yes: Excludes solution
Synonyms Metformin Hydrochloride
Pharmacologic Category Antidiabetic Agent, Biguanide
Use Management of type 2 diabetes mellitus (noninsulin dependent, NIDDM) as monotherapy when hyperglycemia cannot be managed on diet alone. May be used concomitantly with a sulfonylurea or insulin to improve glycemic control.
(Continued)

Metformin *(Continued)*

Unlabeled/Investigational Use Treatment of HIV lipodystrophy syndrome

Local Anesthetic/Vasoconstrictor Precautions No information available to require special precautions

Effects on Dental Treatment No significant effects or complications reported

Common Adverse Effects

>10%:

Gastrointestinal: Nausea/vomiting (6% to 25%), diarrhea (10% to 53%), flatulence (12%)

Neuromuscular & skeletal: Weakness (9%)

1% to 10%:

Cardiovascular: Chest discomfort, flushing, palpitation

Central nervous system: Headache (6%), chills, dizziness, lightheadedness

Dermatologic: Rash

Endocrine & metabolic: Hypoglycemia

Gastrointestinal: Indigestion (7%), abdominal discomfort (6%), abdominal distention, abnormal stools, constipation, dyspepsia/ heartburn, taste disorder

Neuromuscular & skeletal: Myalgia

Respiratory: Dyspnea, upper respiratory tract infection

Miscellaneous: Decreased vitamin B_{12} levels (7%), increased diaphoresis, flu-like syndrome, nail disorder

Dosage Note: Allow 1-2 weeks between dose titrations: Generally, clinically significant responses are not seen at doses <1500 mg daily; however, a lower recommended starting dose and gradual increased dosage is recommended to minimize gastrointestinal symptoms

Children 10-16 years: Management of type 2 diabetes mellitus: Oral (500 mg tablet or oral solution): Initial: 500 mg twice daily (given with the morning and evening meals); increases in daily dosage should be made in increments of 500 mg at weekly intervals, given in divided doses, up to a maximum of 2000 mg/day

Adults ≥17 years: Management of type 2 diabetes mellitus: Oral:

Immediate release tablet or oral solution: Initial: 500 mg twice daily (give with the morning and evening meals) **or** 850 mg once daily; increase dosage incrementally.

Incremental dosing recommendations based on dosage form:

500 mg tablet: One tablet/day at weekly intervals

850 mg tablet: One tablet/day every other week

Oral solution: 500 mg twice daily every other week

Doses of up to 2000 mg/day may be given twice daily. If a dose >2000 mg/day is required, it may be better tolerated in three divided doses. Maximum recommended dose 2550 mg/day.

Extended release tablet: Initial: 500 mg once daily (with the evening meal); dosage may be increased by 500 mg weekly; maximum dose: 2000 mg once daily. If glycemic control is not achieved at maximum dose, may divide dose to 1000 mg twice daily. If doses >2000 mg/day are needed, switch to regular release tablets and titrate to maximum dose of 2550 mg/day.

Elderly: The initial and maintenance dosing should be conservative, due to the potential for decreased renal function. Generally, elderly patients should not be titrated to the maximum dose of metformin. Do not use in patients ≥80 years of age unless normal renal function has been established.

Transfer from other antidiabetic agents: No transition period is generally necessary except when transferring from chlorpropamide. When transferring from chlorpropamide, care should be exercised during the first 2 weeks because of the prolonged retention of chlorpropamide in the body, leading to overlapping drug effects and possible hypoglycemia.

Concomitant metformin and oral sulfonylurea therapy: If patients have not responded to 4 weeks of the maximum dose of metformin monotherapy, consider a gradual addition of an oral sulfonylurea, even if prior primary or secondary failure to a sulfonylurea has occurred. Continue metformin at the maximum dose.

Failed sulfonylurea therapy: Patients with prior failure on glyburide may be treated by gradual addition of metformin. Initiate with glyburide 20 mg and metformin 500 mg daily. Metformin dosage may be increased by 500 mg/day at weekly intervals, up to a maximum of 2500 mg/day (dosage of glyburide maintained at 20 mg/day).

Concomitant metformin and insulin therapy: Initial: 500 mg metformin once daily, continue current insulin dose; increase by 500 mg metformin weekly until adequate glycemic control is achieved

Maximum dose: 2500 mg metformin; 2000 mg metformin extended release

Decrease insulin dose 10% to 25% when FPG <120 mg/dL; monitor and make further adjustments as needed

Dosing adjustment/comments in renal impairment: The plasma and blood half-life of metformin is prolonged and the renal clearance is decreased in proportion to the decrease in creatinine clearance. Per the manufacturer, metformin is contraindicated in the presence of renal dysfunction defined as a serum creatinine >1.5 mg/dL in males, or >1.4 mg/dL in females and in patients with abnormal clearance. Clinically, it has been recommended that metformin be avoided in patients with Cl_{cr} <60-70 mL/minute (DeFronzo, 1999).

Dosing adjustment in hepatic impairment: Avoid metformin; liver disease is a risk factor for the development of lactic acidosis during metformin therapy.

Mechanism of Action Decreases hepatic glucose production, decreasing intestinal absorption of glucose and improves insulin sensitivity (increases peripheral glucose uptake and utilization)

Contraindications Hypersensitivity to metformin or any component of the formulation; renal disease or renal dysfunction (serum creatinine ≥1.5 mg/dL in males or ≥1.4 mg/dL in females or abnormal creatinine clearance from any cause, including shock, acute myocardial infarction, or septicemia); congestive heart failure requiring pharmacological management; acute or chronic metabolic acidosis with or without coma (including diabetic ketoacidosis)

Note: Temporarily discontinue in patients undergoing radiologic studies in which intravascular iodinated contrast materials are utilized.

Warnings/Precautions Lactic acidosis is a rare, but potentially severe consequence of therapy with metformin. Lactic acidosis should be suspected in any diabetic patient receiving metformin who has evidence of acidosis when evidence of ketoacidosis is lacking. Discontinue metformin in clinical situations predisposing to hypoxemia, including conditions such as cardiovascular collapse, respiratory failure, acute myocardial infarction, acute congestive heart failure, and septicemia.

Metformin is substantially excreted by the kidney. The risk of accumulation and lactic acidosis increases with the degree of impairment of renal function. Patients with renal function below the limit of normal for their age should not receive metformin. In elderly patients, renal function should be monitored regularly; should not be used in any patient ≥80 years of age unless measurement of creatinine clearance verifies normal renal function. Use of concomitant medications that may affect renal function (ie, affect tubular secretion) may also affect metformin disposition. Metformin should be suspended in patients with dehydration and/or prerenal azotemia. Therapy should be suspended for any surgical procedures (resume only after normal intake resumed and normal renal function is verified). Metformin should also be temporarily discontinued for 48 hours in patients undergoing radiologic studies involving the intravascular administration of iodinated contrast materials (potential for acute alteration in renal function).

Avoid use in patients with impaired liver function. Patient must be instructed to avoid excessive acute or chronic ethanol use. Administration of oral antidiabetic drugs has been reported to be associated with increased cardiovascular mortality; metformin does not appear to share this risk. Safety and efficacy of metformin have been established for use in children ≥10 years of age; the extended release preparation is for use in patients ≥17 years of age.

Drug Interactions

Increased Effect/Toxicity: Furosemide and cimetidine may increase metformin blood levels. Cationic drugs (eg, amiloride, digoxin, morphine, procainamide, quinidine, quinine, ranitidine, triamterene, trimethoprim, and vancomycin) which are eliminated by renal tubular secretion have the potential to increase metformin levels by competing for common renal tubular transport systems. Contrast agents may increase the risk of metformin-induced lactic acidosis; discontinue metformin prior to exposure and withhold for 48 hours.

Decreased Effect: Drugs which tend to produce hyperglycemia (eg, diuretics, corticosteroids, phenothiazines, thyroid products, estrogens, oral contraceptives, phenytoin, nicotinic acid, sympathomimetics, calcium channel blocking drugs, isoniazid) may lead to a loss of glucose control.

Ethanol/Nutrition/Herb Interactions

Ethanol: Avoid or limit ethanol (incidence of lactic acidosis may be increased; may cause hypoglycemia).

Food: Food decreases the extent and slightly delays the absorption. May decrease absorption of vitamin B_{12} and/or folic acid.

Herb/Nutraceutical: Caution with chromium, garlic, gymnema (may cause hypoglycemia).

Dietary Considerations Drug may cause GI upset; take with food (to decrease GI upset). Take at the same time each day. Dietary modification based on ADA (Continued)

Metformin *(Continued)*

recommendations is a part of therapy. Monitor for signs and symptoms of vitamin B_{12} and/or folic acid deficiency; supplementation may be required.

Pharmacodynamics/Kinetics

Onset of action: Within days; maximum effects up to 2 weeks

Distribution: V_d: 654 ± 358 L

Protein binding: Negligible

Bioavailability: Absolute: Fasting: 50% to 60%

Half-life elimination, plasma: 6.2 hours

Excretion: Urine (90% as unchanged drug)

Pregnancy Risk Factor B

Dosage Forms SOLN, oral (Riomet™): 100 mg/mL (118 mL, 473 mL). **TAB** (Glucophage®): 500 mg, 850 mg, 1000 mg. **TAB, extended release:** 500 mg; (Fortamet™): 500 mg, 1000 mg; (Glucophage® XR): 500 mg, 750 mg

Metformin and Glipizide *see* Glipizide and Metformin *on page 741*

Metformin and Glyburide *see* Glyburide and Metformin *on page 745*

Metformin and Rosiglitazone *see* Rosiglitazone and Metformin *on page 1369*

Metformin Hydrochloride *see* Metformin *on page 1001*

Metformin Hydrochloride and Pioglitazone Hydrochloride *see* Pioglitazone and Metformin *on page 1242*

Metformin Hydrochloride and Rosiglitazone Maleate *see* Rosiglitazone and Metformin *on page 1369*

Methadone *(METH a done)*

U.S. Brand Names Dolophine®; Methadone Diskets®; Methadone Intensol™; Methadose®

Canadian Brand Names Dolophine®; Metadol™; Methadose®

Generic Available Yes

Synonyms Methadone Hydrochloride

Pharmacologic Category Analgesic, Narcotic

Use Management of severe pain; detoxification and maintenance treatment of narcotic addiction (if used for detoxification and maintenance treatment of narcotic addiction, it must be part of an FDA-approved program)

Local Anesthetic/Vasoconstrictor Precautions No information available to require special precautions

Effects on Dental Treatment Key adverse event(s) related to dental treatment: Significant xerostomia (normal salivary flow resumes upon discontinuation).

Common Adverse Effects Frequency not defined. During prolonged administration, adverse effects may decrease over several weeks; however, constipation and sweating may persist.

Cardiovascular: Bradycardia, peripheral vasodilation, cardiac arrest, syncope, faintness, shock, hypotension, edema, arrhythmia, bigeminal rhythms, extrasystoles, tachycardia, torsade de pointes, ventricular fibrillation, ventricular tachycardia, ECG changes, QT interval prolonged, T-wave inversion, cardiomyopathy, flushing, heart failure, palpitation, phlebitis, orthostatic hypotension

Central nervous system: Euphoria, dysphoria, headache, insomnia, agitation, disorientation, drowsiness, dizziness, lightheadedness, sedation, confusion, seizure

Dermatologic: Pruritus, urticaria, rash, hemorrhagic urticaria

Endocrine & metabolic: Libido decreased, hypokalemia, hypomagnesemia, antidiuretic effect, amenorrhea

Gastrointestinal: Nausea, vomiting, constipation, anorexia, stomach cramps, xerostomia, biliary tract spasm, abdominal pain, glossitis, weight gain

Genitourinary: Urinary retention or hesitancy, impotence

Hematologic: Thrombocytopenia (reversible, reported in patients with chronic hepatitis)

Neuromuscular & skeletal: Weakness

Local: I.M./SubQ injection: Pain, erythema, swelling; I.V. injection: pruritus, urticaria, rash, hemorrhagic urticaria (rare)

Ocular: Miosis, visual disturbances

Respiratory: Respiratory depression, respiratory arrest, pulmonary edema

Miscellaneous: Physical and psychological dependence, death, diaphoresis

Restrictions C-II

When used for treatment of narcotic addiction: May only be dispensed in accordance to guidelines established by the Substance Abuse and Mental Health Services Administration's (SAMHSA) Center for Substance Abuse Treatment (CSAT).

Mechanism of Action Binds to opiate receptors in the CNS, causing inhibition of ascending pain pathways, altering the perception of and response to pain; produces generalized CNS depression

Drug Interactions

Cytochrome P450 Effect: Substrate of CYP2C8/9 (minor), 2C19 (minor), 2D6 (minor), 3A4 (major); **Inhibits** CYP2D6 (moderate), 3A4 (weak)

Increased Effect/Toxicity: CYP3A4 inhibitors may increase the levels/effects of methadone (eg, azole antifungals, clarithromycin, diclofenac, doxycycline, erythromycin, imatinib, isoniazid, nefazodone, nicardipine, propofol, protease inhibitors, quinidine, telithromycin, verapamil). Methadone may increase the levels/effects of CYP2D6 substrates (eg, amphetamines, selected beta-blockers, dextromethorphan, fluoxetine, lidocaine, mirtazapine, nefazodone, paroxetine, risperidone, ritonavir, thioridazine, tricyclic antidepressants, venlafaxine). Methadone may increase bioavailability and toxic effects of zidovudine. CNS depressants (including but not limited to opioid analgesics, general anesthetics, sedatives, hypnotics, ethanol) may cause respiratory depression, hypotension, profound sedation, or coma. Levels of desipramine may be increased by methadone. Effects/toxicity of QT_c interval-prolonging agents may be increased; use with caution (including but may not be limited to amitriptyline, astemizole, bepridil, disopyramide, erythromycin, haloperidol, imipramine, quinidine, pimozide, procainamide, sotalol, thioridazine). Ritonavir may increase levels/effects of methadone shortly after initiation.

Decreased Effect: Agonist/antagonist analgesics (buprenorphine, butorphanol, nalbuphine, pentazocine) may decrease analgesic effect of methadone and precipitate withdrawal symptoms; use is not recommended. Efavirenz and nevirapine may decrease levels of methadone (opioid withdrawal syndrome has been reported). Methadone may decrease bioavailability of didanosine and stavudine. Ritonavir (and combinations) may decrease levels of methadone; withdrawal symptoms have inconsistently been observed, monitor. CYP3A4 inducers may decrease the levels/effects of methadone (eg, aminoglutethimide, carbamazepine, nafcillin, nevirapine, phenobarbital, phenytoin, rifamycins). Monitor for methadone withdrawal. Larger doses of methadone may be required. Methadone may decrease the levels/effects of CYP2D6 prodrug substrates (eg, codeine, hydrocodone, oxycodone, tramadol). Ritonavir may decrease levels/effects of methadone with continued dosing.

Pharmacodynamics/Kinetics

Onset of action: Oral: Analgesic: 0.5-1 hour; Parenteral: 10-20 minutes
Peak effect: Parenteral: 1-2 hours

Duration: Oral: 4-8 hours, increases to 22-48 hours with repeated doses

Distribution: V_{dss}: 1-8 L/kg

Protein binding: 85% to 90%

Metabolism: Hepatic; N-demethylation primarily via CYP3A4, CYP2B6, and CYP2C19 to inactive metabolites

Bioavailability: Oral: 36% to 100%

Half-life elimination: 7-59 hours; may be prolonged with alkaline pH, decreased during pregnancy

Excretion: Urine (<10% as unchanged drug); increased with urine pH <6

Pregnancy Risk Factor C/D (prolonged use or high doses at term)

Methadone Diskets® *see Methadone on page 1004*

Methadone Hydrochloride *see Methadone on page 1004*

Methadone Intensol™ *see Methadone on page 1004*

Methadose® *see Methadone on page 1004*

Methaminodiazepoxide Hydrochloride *see Chlordiazepoxide on page 315*

Methamphetamine (meth am FET a meen)

U.S. Brand Names Desoxyn®

Canadian Brand Names Desoxyn®

Generic Available Yes

Synonyms Desoxyephedrine Hydrochloride; Methamphetamine Hydrochloride

Pharmacologic Category Stimulant

Use Treatment of attention-deficit/hyperactivity disorder (ADHD); exogenous obesity (short-term adjunct)

Unlabeled/Investigational Use Narcolepsy

Local Anesthetic/Vasoconstrictor Precautions Use vasoconstrictor with caution in patients taking methamphetamine. Amphetamines enhance the sympathomimetic response of epinephrine and norepinephrine leading to potential hypertension and cardiotoxicity.

(Continued)

Methamphetamine *(Continued)*

Effects on Dental Treatment Key adverse event(s) related to dental treatment: Xerostomia (normal salivary flow resumes upon discontinuation). Up to 10% of patients taking methamphetamine may present with hypertension. Monitor blood pressure prior to using local anesthetic with vasoconstrictors.

Common Adverse Effects Frequency not defined.

Cardiovascular: Hypertension, tachycardia, palpitation

Central nervous system: Restlessness, headache, exacerbation of motor and phonic tics and Tourette's syndrome, dizziness, psychosis, dysphoria, overstimulation, euphoria, insomnia

Dermatologic: Rash, urticaria

Endocrine & metabolic: Change in libido

Gastrointestinal: Diarrhea, nausea, vomiting, stomach cramps, constipation, anorexia, weight loss, xerostomia, unpleasant taste

Genitourinary: Impotence

Neuromuscular & skeletal: Tremor

Miscellaneous: Suppression of growth in children, tolerance and withdrawal with prolonged use

Restrictions C-II

Mechanism of Action A sympathomimetic amine related to ephedrine and amphetamine with CNS stimulant activity; peripheral actions include elevation of systolic and diastolic blood pressure and weak bronchodilator and respiratory stimulant action

Drug Interactions

Cytochrome P450 Effect: **Substrate** of CYP2D6 (major)

Increased Effect/Toxicity: Amphetamines may precipitate hypertensive crisis or serotonin syndrome in patients receiving MAO inhibitors (selegiline >10 mg/day, isocarboxazid, phenelzine, tranylcypromine, furazolidone). Serotonin syndrome has also been associated with combinations of amphetamines and SSRIs; these combinations should be avoided. TCAs may enhance the effects of amphetamines, potentially leading to hypertensive crisis. CYP2D6 inhibitors may increase the levels/effects of methamphetamine; example inhibitors include chlorpromazine, delavirdine, fluoxetine, miconazole, paroxetine, pergolide, quinidine, quinine, ritonavir, and ropinirole. Large doses of antacids or urinary alkalinizers increase the half-life and duration of action of amphetamines. May precipitate arrhythmias in patients receiving general anesthetics. Inhibitors of CYP2D6 may increase the effects of amphetamines (includes amiodarone, cimetidine, delavirdine, fluoxetine, paroxetine, propafenone, quinidine, and ritonavir).

Decreased Effect: Amphetamines inhibit the antihypertensive response to guanethidine, methyldopa, and guanadrel. Enzyme inducers (barbiturates, carbamazepine, phenytoin, and rifampin) may decrease serum concentrations of amphetamines.

Pharmacodynamics/Kinetics

Absorption: Rapid from GI tract

Metabolism: Hepatic; forms metabolite

Half-life elimination: 4-5 hours

Excretion: Urine primarily (dependent on urine pH)

Pregnancy Risk Factor C

Methamphetamine Hydrochloride *see* Methamphetamine *on page 1005*

Methazolamide *(meth a ZOE la mide)*

Canadian Brand Names Apo-Methazolamide®

Generic Available Yes

Pharmacologic Category Carbonic Anhydrase Inhibitor; Diuretic, Carbonic Anhydrase Inhibitor; Ophthalmic Agent, Antiglaucoma

Use Adjunctive treatment of open-angle or secondary glaucoma; short-term therapy of narrow-angle glaucoma when delay of surgery is desired

Local Anesthetic/Vasoconstrictor Precautions No information available to require special precautions

Effects on Dental Treatment No significant effects or complications reported

Common Adverse Effects Frequency not defined.

Central nervous system: Malaise, fever, mental depression, drowsiness, dizziness, nervousness, headache, confusion, seizure, fatigue, trembling, unsteadiness

Dermatologic: Urticaria, pruritus, photosensitivity, rash, Stevens-Johnson syndrome

Endocrine & metabolic: Hyperchloremic metabolic acidosis, hypokalemia, hyperglycemia

Gastrointestinal: Metallic taste, anorexia, nausea, vomiting, diarrhea, constipation, weight loss, GI irritation, xerostomia, black tarry stools

Genitourinary: Polyuria, crystalluria, hematuria, polyuria, renal calculi, impotence

Hematologic: Bone marrow depression, thrombocytopenia, thrombocytopenic purpura, hemolytic anemia, leukopenia, pancytopenia, agranulocytosis

Hepatic: Hepatic insufficiency

Neuromuscular & skeletal: Weakness, ataxia, paresthesia

Miscellaneous: Hypersensitivity

Mechanism of Action Noncompetitive inhibition of the enzyme carbonic anhydrase; thought that carbonic anhydrase is located at the luminal border of cells of the proximal tubule. When the enzyme is inhibited, there is an increase in urine volume and a change to an alkaline pH with a subsequent decrease in the excretion of titratable acid and ammonia.

Drug Interactions

Increased Effect/Toxicity: Methazolamide may induce hypokalemia which would sensitize a patient to digitalis toxicity. Hypokalemia may be compounded with concurrent diuretic use or steroids. Methazolamide may increase the potential for salicylate toxicity. Primidone absorption may be delayed.

Decreased Effect: Increased lithium excretion and altered excretion of other drugs by alkalinization of the urine, such as amphetamines, quinidine, procainamide, methenamine, phenobarbital, and salicylates.

Pharmacodynamics/Kinetics

Onset of action: Slow in comparison with acetazolamide (2-4 hours)

Peak effect: 6-8 hours

Duration: 10-18 hours

Absorption: Slow

Distribution: Well into tissue

Protein binding: ~55%

Metabolism: Slowly from GI tract

Half-life elimination: ~14 hours

Excretion: Urine (~25% as unchanged drug)

Pregnancy Risk Factor C

Methenamine (meth EN a meen)

U.S. Brand Names Hiprex®; Mandelamine®; Urex®

Canadian Brand Names Dehydral®; Hiprex®; Mandelamine®; Urasal®; Urex®

Generic Available Yes

Synonyms Hexamethylenetetramine; Methenamine Hippurate; Methenamine Mandelate

Pharmacologic Category Antibiotic, Miscellaneous

Use Prophylaxis or suppression of recurrent urinary tract infections; urinary tract discomfort secondary to hypermotility

Local Anesthetic/Vasoconstrictor Precautions No information available to require special precautions

Effects on Dental Treatment No significant effects or complications reported

Common Adverse Effects 1% to 10%:

Dermatologic: Rash (<4%)

Gastrointestinal: Nausea, dyspepsia (<4%)

Genitourinary: Dysuria (<4%)

Mechanism of Action Methenamine is hydrolyzed to formaldehyde and ammonia in acidic urine; formaldehyde has nonspecific bactericidal action

Drug Interactions

Increased Effect/Toxicity: Sulfonamides may precipitate in the urine; concurrent use is contraindicated.

Decreased Effect: Sodium bicarbonate and acetazolamide will decrease effect secondary to alkalinization of urine.

Pharmacodynamics/Kinetics

Absorption: Readily

Metabolism: Gastric juices: Hydrolyze 10% to 30% unless protected via enteric coating; Hepatic: ~10% to 25%

Half-life elimination: 3-6 hours

Excretion: Urine (~70% to 90% as unchanged drug) within 24 hours

Pregnancy Risk Factor C

Methenamine Hippurate see Methenamine on page 1007

Methenamine Mandelate see Methenamine on page 1007

Methenamine, Sodium Biphosphate, Phenyl Salicylate, Methylene Blue, and Hyoscyamine

(meth EN a meen, SOW dee um bye FOS fate, fen nil sa LIS i late, METH i leen bloo, & hye oh SYE a meen)

Related Information
Hyoscyamine *on page 803*
Methenamine *on page 1007*

U.S. Brand Names Urimar-T; Urimax® [DSC]

Generic Available No

Synonyms Hyoscyamine, Methenamine, Sodium Biphosphate, Phenyl Salicylate, and Methylene Blue; Methylene Blue, Methenamine, Sodium Biphosphate, Phenyl Salicylate, and Hyoscyamine; Phenyl Salicylate, Methenamine, Methylene Blue, Sodium Biphosphate, and Hyoscyamine; Sodium Biphosphate, Methenamine, Methylene Blue, Phenyl Salicylate, and Hyoscyamine

Pharmacologic Category Antibiotic, Miscellaneous

Use Treatment of symptoms of irritative voiding; relief of local symptoms associated with urinary tract infections; relief of urinary tract symptoms caused by diagnostic procedures

Local Anesthetic/Vasoconstrictor Precautions No information available to require special precautions

Effects on Dental Treatment No significant effects or complications reported

Common Adverse Effects Frequency not defined.

Cardiovascular: Tachycardia, flushing

Central nervous system: Dizziness

Gastrointestinal: Xerostomia, nausea, vomiting

Genitourinary: Urinary retention (acute), micturition difficulty, discoloration of urine (blue)

Ocular: Blurred vision

Respiratory: Dyspnea, shortness of breath

Drug Interactions

Increased Effect/Toxicity: Refer to individual monographs for Hyoscyamine and Methenamine.

Decreased Effect: Refer to individual monographs for Hyoscyamine and Methenamine.

Pregnancy Risk Factor C

Methergine® *see Methylergonovine on page 1022*

Methimazole (meth IM a zole)

Related Information
Endocrine Disorders and Pregnancy *on page 1659*

U.S. Brand Names Tapazole®

Canadian Brand Names Dom-Methimazole; Tapazole®

Generic Available Yes

Synonyms Thiamazole

Pharmacologic Category Antithyroid Agent

Use Palliative treatment of hyperthyroidism, return the hyperthyroid patient to a normal metabolic state prior to thyroidectomy, and to control thyrotoxic crisis that may accompany thyroidectomy. The use of antithyroid thioamides is as effective in elderly as they are in younger adults; however, the expense, potential adverse effects, and inconvenience (compliance, monitoring) make them undesirable. The use of radioiodine due to ease of administration and less concern for long-term side effects and reproduction problems (some older males) makes it a more appropriate therapy.

Local Anesthetic/Vasoconstrictor Precautions No information available to require special precautions

Effects on Dental Treatment No significant effects or complications reported

Common Adverse Effects Frequency not defined.

Cardiovascular: Edema

Central nervous system: Headache, vertigo, drowsiness, CNS stimulation, depression

Dermatologic: Skin rash, urticaria, pruritus, erythema nodosum, skin pigmentation, exfoliative dermatitis, alopecia

Endocrine & metabolic: Goiter

Gastrointestinal: Nausea, vomiting, stomach pain, abnormal taste, constipation, weight gain, salivary gland swelling

Hematologic: Leukopenia, agranulocytosis, granulocytopenia, thrombocytopenia, aplastic anemia, hypoprothrombinemia

Hepatic: Cholestatic jaundice, jaundice, hepatitis

Neuromuscular & skeletal: Arthralgia, paresthesia

Renal: Nephrotic syndrome

Miscellaneous: SLE-like syndrome

Mechanism of Action Inhibits the synthesis of thyroid hormones by blocking the oxidation of iodine in the thyroid gland, blocking iodine's ability to combine with tyrosine to form thyroxine and triiodothyronine (T_3), does not inactivate circulating T_4 and T_3

Drug Interactions

Cytochrome P450 Effect: Inhibits CYP1A2 (weak), 2A6 (weak), 2B6 (weak), 2C8/9 (weak), 2C19 (weak), 2D6 (moderate), 2E1 (weak), 3A4 (weak)

Increased Effect/Toxicity: Dosage of some drugs (including beta-blockers, digoxin, and theophylline) require adjustment during treatment of hyperthyroidism. Methimazole may increase the levels/effects of CYP2D6 substrates (eg, amphetamines, selected beta-blockers, dextromethorphan, fluoxetine, lidocaine, mirtazapine, nefazodone, paroxetine, risperidone, ritonavir, thioridazine, tricyclic antidepressants, venlafaxine).

Decreased Effect: Anticoagulant effect of warfarin may be decreased. Methimazole may decrease the levels/effects of CYP2D6 prodrug substrates (eg, codeine, hydrocodone, oxycodone, tramadol).

Pharmacodynamics/Kinetics

Onset of action: Antithyroid: Oral: 12-18 hours

Duration: 36-72 hours

Distribution: Concentrated in thyroid gland; crosses placenta; enters breast milk (1:1)

Protein binding, plasma: None

Metabolism: Hepatic

Bioavailability: 80% to 95%

Half-life elimination: 4-13 hours

Excretion: Urine (80%)

Pregnancy Risk Factor D

Methitest™ *see* MethylTESTOSTERone *on page 1028*

Methocarbamol (meth oh KAR ba mole)

Related Information

Temporomandibular Dysfunction (TMD) *on page 1724*

U.S. Brand Names Robaxin®

Canadian Brand Names Robaxin®

Generic Available Yes: Tablet

Pharmacologic Category Skeletal Muscle Relaxant

Dental Use Treatment of muscle spasm associated with acute temporomandibular joint pain (TMJ)

Use Treatment of muscle spasm associated with acute painful musculoskeletal conditions; supportive therapy in tetanus

Local Anesthetic/Vasoconstrictor Precautions No information available to require special precautions

Effects on Dental Treatment Key adverse event(s) related to dental treatment: Metallic taste.

Significant Adverse Effects Frequency not defined.

Cardiovascular: Flushing of face, bradycardia, hypotension, syncope

Central nervous system: Drowsiness, dizziness, lightheadedness, convulsion, vertigo, headache, fever, amnesia, confusion, insomnia, sedation, coordination impaired (mild)

Dermatologic: Allergic dermatitis, urticaria, pruritus, rash, angioneurotic edema

Gastrointestinal: Nausea, vomiting, metallic taste, dyspepsia

Hematologic: Leukopenia

Hepatic: Jaundice

Local: Pain at injection site, thrombophlebitis

Ocular: Nystagmus, blurred vision, diplopia, conjunctivitis

Renal: Renal impairment

Respiratory: Nasal congestion

Miscellaneous: Allergic manifestations, anaphylactic reaction

Dental Usual Dosing Muscle spasm associated with acute TMJ pain: Children ≥16 years and Adults: Oral: 1.5 g 4 times/day for 2-3 days (up to 8 g/day may be given in severe conditions), then decrease to 4-4.5 g/day in 3-6 divided doses (Continued)

Methocarbamol *(Continued)*

Dosage

Tetanus: I.V.:

Children: Recommended **only** for use in tetanus: 15 mg/kg/dose or 500 mg/m²/dose, may repeat every 6 hours if needed; maximum dose: 1.8 g/m²/day for 3 days only

Adults: Initial dose: 1-3 g; may repeat dose every 6 hours until oral dosing is possible; injection should not be used for more than 3 consecutive days

Muscle spasm: Children ≥16 years and Adults:

Oral: 1.5 g 4 times/day for 2-3 days (up to 8 g/day may be given in severe conditions), then decrease to 4-4.5 g/day in 3-6 divided doses

I.M., I.V.: 1 g every 8 hours if oral not possible; injection should not be used for more than 3 consecutive days. If condition persists, may repeat course of therapy after a drug-free interval of 48 hours.

Elderly: Muscle spasm: Oral: Initial: 500 mg 4 times/day; titrate to response

Dosing adjustment/comments in renal impairment: Do not administer parenteral formulation to patients with renal dysfunction.

Dosing adjustment in hepatic impairment: Specific dosing guidelines are not available; plasma protein binding and clearance are decreased; half-life is increased

Mechanism of Action Causes skeletal muscle relaxation by general CNS depression

Contraindications Hypersensitivity to methocarbamol or any component of the formulation; renal impairment (injection formulation)

Warnings/Precautions

Oral: Use caution with renal or hepatic impairment.

Injection: Rate of injection should not exceed 3 mL/minute; solution is hypertonic; avoid extravasation. Use with caution in patients with a history of seizures. Use caution with hepatic impairment.

Drug Interactions Increased effect/toxicity with CNS depressants; pyridostigmine (a single case of worsening myasthenia has been reported following methocarbamol administration)

Ethanol/Nutrition/Herb Interactions

Ethanol: Avoid ethanol (may increase CNS depression).

Herb/Nutraceutical: Avoid valerian, St John's wort, kava kava, gotu kola (may increase CNS depression).

Pharmacodynamics/Kinetics

Onset of action: Muscle relaxation: Oral: ~30 minutes

Protein binding: 46% to 50%

Metabolism: Hepatic via dealkylation and hydroxylation

Half-life elimination: 1-2 hours

Time to peak, serum: ~2 hours

Excretion: Urine (as metabolites)

Pregnancy Risk Factor C

Lactation Excretion in breast milk unknown/use caution

Dosage Forms

Injection, solution: 100 mg/mL (10 mL) [in polyethylene glycol; vial stopper contains latex]

Tablet: 500 mg, 750 mg

Methohexital *(meth oh HEKS i tal)*

U.S. Brand Names Brevital® Sodium

Canadian Brand Names Brevital®

Generic Available No

Synonyms Methohexital Sodium

Pharmacologic Category Barbiturate

Dental Use Induction and maintenance of general anesthesia for short procedures

Use Induction and maintenance of general anesthesia for short procedures

Can be used in pediatric patients ≥1 month of age as follows: For rectal or intramuscular induction of anesthesia prior to the use of other general anesthetic agents, as an adjunct to subpotent inhalational anesthetic agents for short surgical procedures, or for short surgical, diagnostic, or therapeutic procedures associated with minimal painful stimuli

Unlabeled/Investigational Use Wada test

Local Anesthetic/Vasoconstrictor Precautions No information available to require special precautions

Effects on Dental Treatment No significant effects or complications reported

Significant Adverse Effects Frequency not defined.

Cardiovascular: Hypotension, peripheral vascular collapse

Central nervous system: Seizures, headache

Gastrointestinal: Cramping, diarrhea, rectal bleeding, nausea, vomiting, abdominal pain

Hematologic: Hemolytic anemia, thrombophlebitis

Hepatic: Transaminases increased

Local: Pain on I.M. injection

Neuromuscular & skeletal: Tremor, twitching, rigidity, involuntary muscle movement, radial nerve palsy

Respiratory: Apnea, respiratory depression, laryngospasm, cough, hiccups

Restrictions C-IV

Dental Usual Dosing Induction and maintenance of general anesthesia for short procedures: Doses must be titrated to effect: Adults: I.V.: Induction: 50-120 mg to start; 20-40 mg every 4-7 minutes

Dosage Doses must be titrated to effect

Manufacturer's recommendations:

Infants <1 month: Safety and efficacy not established

Infants ≥1 month and Children:

I.M.: Induction: 6.6-10 mg/kg of a 5% solution

Rectal: Induction: Usual: 25 mg/kg of a 1% solution

Alternative pediatric dosing:

Children 3-12 years:

I.M.: Preoperative: 5-10 mg/kg/dose

I.V.: Induction: 1-2 mg/kg/dose

Rectal: Preoperative/induction: 20-35 mg/kg/dose; usual: 25 mg/kg/dose; maximum dose: 500 mg/dose; give as 10% aqueous solution

Adults: I.V.:

Induction: 50-120 mg to start; 20-40 mg every 4-7 minutes

Wada test (unlabeled): 3-4 mg over 3 second; following signs of recovery, administer a second dose of 2 mg over 2 seconds

Dosing adjustment/comments in hepatic impairment: Lower dosage and monitor closely

Mechanism of Action Ultra short-acting I.V. barbiturate anesthetic

Contraindications Hypersensitivity to methohexital or any component of the formulation; porphyria

Warnings/Precautions Use with extreme caution in patients with liver impairment, asthma, cardiovascular instability

Drug Interactions

Acetaminophen: Barbiturates may enhance the hepatotoxic potential of acetaminophen overdoses

Antiarrhythmics: Barbiturates may increase the metabolism of antiarrhythmics, decreasing their clinical effect; includes disopyramide, propafenone, and quinidine

Anticonvulsants: Barbiturates may increase the metabolism of anticonvulsants; includes ethosuximide, felbamate (possibly), lamotrigine, phenytoin, tiagabine, topiramate, and zonisamide; does not appear to affect gabapentin or levetiracetam

Antineoplastics: Limited evidence suggests that enzyme-inducing anticonvulsant therapy may reduce the effectiveness of some chemotherapy regimens (specifically in ALL); teniposide and methotrexate may be cleared more rapidly in these patients

Antipsychotics: Barbiturates may enhance the metabolism (decrease the efficacy) of antipsychotics; monitor for altered response; dose adjustment may be needed

Beta-blockers: Metabolism of beta-blockers may be increased and clinical effect decreased; atenolol and nadolol are unlikely to interact given their renal elimination

Calcium channel blockers: Barbiturates may enhance the metabolism of calcium channel blockers, decreasing their clinical effect

Chloramphenicol: Barbiturates may increase the metabolism of chloramphenicol and chloramphenicol may inhibit barbiturate metabolism; monitor for altered response

Cimetidine: Barbiturates may enhance the metabolism of cimetidine, decreasing its clinical effect

CNS depressants: Sedative effects and/or respiratory depression with barbiturates may be additive with other CNS depressants; monitor for increased effect; includes ethanol, sedatives, antidepressants, narcotic analgesics, and benzodiazepines

Corticosteroids: Barbiturates may enhance the metabolism of corticosteroids, decreasing their clinical effect

Cyclosporine: Levels may be decreased by barbiturates; monitor

(Continued)

Methohexital *(Continued)*

Doxycycline: Barbiturates may enhance the metabolism of doxycycline, decreasing its clinical effect; higher dosages may be required

Estrogens: Barbiturates may increase the metabolism of estrogens and reduce their efficacy

Felbamate may inhibit the metabolism of barbiturates and barbiturates may increase the metabolism of felbamate

Griseofulvin: Barbiturates may impair the absorption of griseofulvin, and griseofulvin metabolism may be increased by barbiturates, decreasing clinical effect

Guanfacine: Effect may be decreased by barbiturates

Immunosuppressants: Barbiturates may enhance the metabolism of immunosuppressants, decreasing its clinical effect; includes both cyclosporine and tacrolimus

Loop diuretics: Metabolism may be increased and clinical effects decreased; established for furosemide, effect with other loop diuretics not established

MAO inhibitors: Metabolism of barbiturates may be inhibited, increasing clinical effect or toxicity of the barbiturates

Methadone: Barbiturates may enhance the metabolism of methadone resulting in methadone withdrawal

Methoxyflurane: Barbiturates may enhance the nephrotoxic effects of methoxyflurane

Oral contraceptives: Barbiturates may enhance the metabolism of oral contraceptives, decreasing their clinical effect; an alternative method of contraception should be considered

Theophylline: Barbiturates may increase metabolism of theophylline derivatives and decrease their clinical effect

Tricyclic antidepressants: Barbiturates may increase metabolism of tricyclic antidepressants and decrease their clinical effect; sedative effects may be additive

Valproic acid: Metabolism of barbiturates may be inhibited by valproic acid; monitor for excessive sedation; a dose reduction may be needed

Warfarin: Barbiturates inhibit the hypoprothrombinemic effects of oral anticoagulants via increased metabolism; this combination should generally be avoided

Dietary Considerations Should not be given to patients with food in stomach because of danger of vomiting during anesthesia.

Pharmacodynamics/Kinetics

Onset of action: I.V.: Immediately

Duration: Single dose: 10-20 minutes

Pregnancy Risk Factor C

Dosage Forms Injection, powder for reconstitution, as sodium: 500 mg, 2.5 g, 5 g

Selected Readings

Buchtel HA, Passaro EA, Selwa LM, et al, "Sodium Methohexital (Brevital) as an Anesthetic in the Wada Test," *Epilepsia*, 2002, 43(9):1056-61.

Cote' CJ, "Sedation for the Pediatric Patient," *Pediatr Clin North Am*, 1994, 41(1):31-58.

Dionne RA, Yagiela JA, Moore PA, et al, "Comparing Efficacy and Safety of Four Intravenous Sedation Regimens in Dental Outpatients," *Am Dent Assoc*, 2001, 132(6):740-51.

Methohexital Sodium *see* Methohexital *on page 1010*

Methotrexate *(meth oh TREKS ate)*

Related Information

Rheumatoid Arthritis, Osteoarthritis, and Osteoporosis *on page 1668*

U.S. Brand Names Rheumatrex®; Trexall™

Canadian Brand Names Apo-Methotrexate®; ratio-Methotrexate

Mexican Brand Names Ledertrexate®; Texate®; Trixilem®

Generic Available Yes

Synonyms Amethopterin; Methotrexate Sodium; MTX (error-prone abbreviation); NSC-740

Pharmacologic Category Antineoplastic Agent, Antimetabolite (Antifolate)

Use Treatment of trophoblastic neoplasms; leukemias; psoriasis; rheumatoid arthritis (RA), including polyarticular-course juvenile rheumatoid arthritis (JRA); breast, head and neck, and lung carcinomas; osteosarcoma; soft-tissue sarcomas; carcinoma of gastrointestinal tract, esophagus, testes; lymphomas

Unlabeled/Investigational Use

Treatment and maintenance of remission in Crohn's disease

Local Anesthetic/Vasoconstrictor Precautions No information available to require special precautions

Effects on Dental Treatment Key adverse event(s) related to dental treatment: Ulcerative stomatitis, gingivitis, glossitis, and mucositis (dose dependent; appears 3-7 days post-therapy and resolves within 2 weeks).

Common Adverse Effects Note: Adverse reactions vary by route and dosage. Hematologic and/or gastrointestinal toxicities may be common at dosages used in chemotherapy; these reactions are much less frequent when used at typical dosages for rheumatic diseases.

>10%:

Central nervous system (with I.T. administration or very high-dose therapy):

Arachnoiditis: Acute reaction manifested as severe headache, nuchal rigidity, vomiting, and fever; may be alleviated by reducing the dose

Subacute toxicity: 10% of patients treated with 12-15 mg/m^2 of I.T. methotrexate may develop this in the second or third week of therapy; consists of motor paralysis of extremities, cranial nerve palsy, seizure, or coma. This has also been seen in pediatric cases receiving very high-dose I.V. methotrexate.

Demyelinating encephalopathy: Seen months or years after receiving methotrexate; usually in association with cranial irradiation or other systemic chemotherapy

Dermatologic: Reddening of skin

Endocrine & metabolic: Hyperuricemia, defective oogenesis or spermatogenesis

Gastrointestinal: Ulcerative stomatitis, glossitis, gingivitis, nausea, vomiting, diarrhea, anorexia, intestinal perforation, mucositis (dose dependent; appears in 3-7 days after therapy, resolving within 2 weeks)

Hematologic: Leukopenia, thrombocytopenia

Renal: Renal failure, azotemia, nephropathy

Respiratory: Pharyngitis

1% to 10%:

Cardiovascular: Vasculitis

Central nervous system: Dizziness, malaise, encephalopathy, seizure, fever, chills

Dermatologic: Alopecia, rash, photosensitivity, depigmentation or hyperpigmentation of skin

Endocrine & metabolic: Diabetes

Genitourinary: Cystitis

Hematologic: Hemorrhage

Myelosuppressive: This is the primary dose-limiting factor (along with mucositis) of methotrexate; occurs about 5-7 days after methotrexate therapy, and should resolve within 2 weeks

WBC: Mild

Platelets: Moderate

Onset: 7 days

Nadir: 10 days

Recovery: 21 days

Hepatic: Cirrhosis and portal fibrosis have been associated with chronic methotrexate therapy; acute elevation of liver enzymes are common after high-dose methotrexate, and usually resolve within 10 days.

Neuromuscular & skeletal: Arthralgia

Ocular: Blurred vision

Renal: Renal dysfunction: Manifested by an abrupt rise in serum creatinine and BUN and a fall in urine output; more common with high-dose methotrexate, and may be due to precipitation of the drug.

Respiratory: Pneumonitis: Associated with fever, cough, and interstitial pulmonary infiltrates; treatment is to withhold methotrexate during the acute reaction; interstitial pneumonitis has been reported to occur with an incidence of 1% in patients with RA (dose 7.5-15 mg/week)

Dosage Refer to individual protocols.

Note: Doses between 100-500 mg/m^2 **may require** leucovorin rescue. Doses >500 mg/m^2 **require** leucovorin rescue: Oral, I.M., I.V.: Leucovorin 10-15 mg/m^2 every 6 hours for 8 or 10 doses, starting 24 hours after the start of methotrexate infusion. Continue until the methotrexate level is ≤0.1 micromolar (10^{-7}M). Some clinicians continue leucovorin until the methotrexate level is <0.05 micromolar (5 x 10^{-8}M) or 0.01 micromolar (10^{-8}M).

If the 48-hour methotrexate level is >1 micromolar (10^{-7}M) or the 72-hour methotrexate level is >0.2 micromolar (2 x 10^{-7}M): I.V., I.M, Oral: Leucovorin 100 mg/m^2 every 6 hours until the methotrexate level is ≤0.1 micromolar (10^{-7}M). Some clinicians continue leucovorin until the methotrexate level is <0.05 micromolar (5 x 10^{-8}M) or 0.01 micromolar (10^{-8}M).

(Continued)

Methotrexate *(Continued)*

Children:

Dermatomyositis: Oral: 15-20 mg/m^2/week as a single dose once weekly **or** 0.3-1 mg/kg/dose once weekly

Juvenile rheumatoid arthritis: Oral, I.M.: 10 mg/m^2 once weekly, then 5-15 mg/m^2/week as a single dose **or** as 3 divided doses given 12 hours apart

Antineoplastic dosage range:

Oral, I.M.: 7.5-30 mg/m^2/week **or** every 2 weeks

I.V.: 10-18,000 mg/m^2 bolus dosing **or** continuous infusion over 6-42 hours For dosing schedules, see table.

Methotrexate Dosing Schedules

Dose	Route	Frequency
Conventional		
15-20 mg/m^2	P.O.	Twice weekly
30-50 mg/m^2	P.O., I.V.	Weekly
15 mg/day for 5 days	P.O., I.M.	Every 2-3 weeks
Intermediate		
50-150 mg/m^2*	I.V. push	Every 2-3 weeks
240 mg/m^2*	I.V. infusion	Every 4-7 days
0.5-1 g/m^2**	I.V. infusion	Every 2-3 weeks
High		
1-25 g/m^2*	I.V. infusion	Every 1-3 weeks

*Doses between 100-500 mg/m^2 may require leucovorin rescue in some patients.

**Followed with leucovorin rescue - refer to Leucovorin monograph for details.

Pediatric solid tumors (high-dose): I.V.:

<12 years: 12-25 g/m^2

≥12 years: 8 g/m^2

Acute lymphocytic leukemia (intermediate-dose): I.V.: Loading: 100 mg/m^2 bolus dose, followed by 900 mg/m^2/day infusion over 23-41 hours.

Meningeal leukemia: I.T.: 10-15 mg/m^2 (maximum dose: 15 mg) **or** an age-based dosing regimen; one possible system is:

≤3 months: 3 mg/dose

4-11 months: 6 mg/dose

1 year: 8 mg/dose

2 years: 10 mg/dose

≥3 years: 12 mg/dose

Adults: I.V.: Range is wide from 30-40 mg/m^2/week to 100-12,000 mg/m^2 with leucovorin rescue

Trophoblastic neoplasms:

Oral, I.M.: 15-30 mg/day for 5 days; repeat in 7 days for 3-5 courses

I.V.: 11 mg/m^2 days 1 through 5 every 3 weeks

Head and neck cancer: Oral, I.M., I.V.: 25-50 mg/m^2 once weekly

Mycosis fungoides (cutaneous T-cell lymphoma): Oral, I.M.: Initial (early stages):

5-50 mg once weekly **or**

15-37.5 mg twice weekly

Bladder cancer: I.V.:

30 mg/m^2 day 1 and 8 every 3 weeks **or**

30 mg/m^2 day 1, 15, and 22 every 4 weeks

Breast cancer: I.V.: 30-60 mg/m^2 days 1 and 8 every 3-4 weeks

Gastric cancer: I.V.:1500 mg/m^2 every 4 weeks

Lymphoma, non-Hodgkin's: I.V.:

30 mg/m^2 days 3 and 10 every 3 weeks **or**

120 mg/m^2 day 8 and 15 every 3-4 weeks **or**

200 mg/m^2 day 8 and 15 every 3-4 weeks **or**

400 mg/m^2 every 4 weeks for 3 cycles **or**

1 g/m^2 every 3 weeks **or**

1.5 g/m^2 every 4 weeks

Sarcoma: I.V.: 8-12 g/m^2 weekly for 2-4 weeks

Rheumatoid arthritis: Oral: 7.5 mg once weekly **or** 2.5 mg every 12 hours for 3 doses/week, not to exceed 20 mg/week

Psoriasis:

Oral: 2.5-5 mg/dose every 12 hours for 3 doses given weekly **or**

Oral, I.M.: 10-25 mg/dose given once weekly

Ectopic pregnancy: I.M., I.V.: 50 mg/m^2 as a single dose

Active Crohn's disease (unlabeled use): Induction of remission: I.M., SubQ: 15-25 mg once weekly; remission maintenance: 15 mg once weekly

Note: Oral dosing has been reported as effective but oral absorption is highly variable. If patient relapses after a switch to oral, may consider returning to injectable.

Elderly: Rheumatoid arthritis/psoriasis: Oral: Initial: 5-7.5 mg/week, not to exceed 20 mg/week

Dosing adjustment in renal impairment:

Cl$_{cr}$ 61-80 mL/minute: Reduce dose to 75% of usual dose

Cl$_{cr}$ 51-60 mL/minute: Reduce dose to 70% of usual dose

Cl$_{cr}$ 10-50 mL/minute: Reduce dose to 30% to 50% of usual dose

Cl$_{cr}$ <10 mL/minute: Avoid use

Hemodialysis: Not dialyzable (0% to 5%); supplemental dose is not necessary

Peritoneal dialysis: Supplemental dose is not necessary

Dosage adjustment in hepatic impairment:

Bilirubin 3.1-5 mg/dL **or** AST >180 units: Administer 75% of usual dose

Bilirubin >5 mg/dL: Do not use

Mechanism of Action Methotrexate is a folate antimetabolite that inhibits DNA synthesis. Methotrexate irreversibly binds to dihydrofolate reductase, inhibiting the formation of reduced folates, and thymidylate synthetase, resulting in inhibition of purine and thymidylic acid synthesis. Methotrexate is cell cycle specific for the S phase of the cycle.

The MOA in the treatment of rheumatoid arthritis is unknown, but may affect immune function. In psoriasis, methotrexate is thought to target rapidly proliferating epithelial cells in the skin.

In Crohn's disease, it may have immune modulator and anti-inflammatory activity

Contraindications Hypersensitivity to methotrexate or any component of the formulation; severe renal or hepatic impairment; pre-existing profound bone marrow suppression in patients with psoriasis or rheumatoid arthritis, alcoholic liver disease, AIDS, pre-existing blood dyscrasias; pregnancy (in patients with psoriasis or rheumatoid arthritis); breast-feeding

Warnings/Precautions Hazardous agent - use appropriate precautions for handling and disposal. May cause potentially life-threatening pneumonitis (may occur at any time during therapy and at any dosage); monitor closely for pulmonary symptoms, particularly dry, nonproductive cough. Methotrexate may cause photosensitivity and/or severe dermatologic reactions which are not dose-related. Methotrexate has been associated with acute and chronic hepatotoxicity, fibrosis, and cirrhosis. Risk is related to cumulative dose and prolonged exposure. Ethanol abuse, obesity, advanced age, and diabetes may increase the risk of hepatotoxic reactions.

Methotrexate may cause renal failure, gastrointestinal toxicity, or bone marrow depression. Use with caution in patients with renal impairment, peptic ulcer disease, ulcerative colitis, or pre-existing bone marrow suppression. Diarrhea and ulcerative stomatitis may require interruption of therapy; death from hemorrhagic enteritis or intestinal perforation has been reported. Methotrexate penetrates slowly into 3rd space fluids, such as pleural effusions or ascites, and exits slowly from these compartments (slower than from plasma). Dosage reduction may be necessary in patients with renal or hepatic impairment, ascites, and pleural effusion. Toxicity from methotrexate or any immunosuppressive is increased in the elderly.

Severe bone marrow suppression, aplastic anemia, and GI toxicity have occurred during concomitant administration with NSAIDs. Use caution when used with other hepatotoxic agents (azathioprine, retinoids, sulfasalazine). Methotrexate given concomitantly with radiotherapy may increase the risk of soft tissue necrosis and osteonecrosis. Immune suppression may lead to opportunistic infections.

For rheumatoid arthritis and psoriasis, immunosuppressive therapy should only be used when disease is active and less toxic; traditional therapy is ineffective. Discontinue therapy in RA or psoriasis if a significant decrease in hematologic components is noted. Methotrexate formulations and/or diluents containing preservatives should not be used for intrathecal or high-dose therapy. Methotrexate injection may contain benzyl alcohol and should not be used in neonates.

Drug Interactions

Increased Effect/Toxicity: Concurrent therapy with NSAIDs has resulted in severe bone marrow suppression, aplastic anemia, and GI toxicity. NSAIDs should not be used during moderate or high-dose methotrexate due to increased and prolonged methotrexate levels (may increase toxicity); NSAID use during treatment of rheumatoid arthritis has not been fully explored, but (Continued)

Methotrexate *(Continued)*

continuation of prior regimen has been allowed in some circumstances, with cautious monitoring. Salicylates may increase methotrexate levels, however salicylate doses used for prophylaxis of cardiovascular events are not likely to be of concern.

Penicillins, probenecid, sulfonamides, tetracyclines may increase methotrexate concentrations due to a reduction in renal tubular secretion; primarily a concern with high doses of methotrexate. Hepatotoxic agents (acitretin, azathioprine, retinoids, sulfasalazine) may increase the risk of hepatotoxic reactions with methotrexate.

Concomitant administration of cyclosporine with methotrexate may increase levels and toxicity of each. Methotrexate may increase mercaptopurine or theophylline levels. Methotrexate, when administered prior to cytarabine, may enhance the efficacy and toxicity of cytarabine; some combination treatment regimens (eg, hyper-CVAD) have been designed to take advantage of this interaction.

Concurrent use of live virus vaccines may result in infections.

Decreased Effect: Cholestyramine may decrease levels of methotrexate. Corticosteroids may decrease uptake of methotrexate into leukemia cells. Administration of these drugs should be separated by 12 hours. Dexamethasone has been reported to not affect methotrexate influx into cells.

Ethanol/Nutrition/Herb Interactions
Ethanol: Avoid ethanol (may be associated with increased liver injury).
Food: Methotrexate peak serum levels may be decreased if taken with food. Milk-rich foods may decrease methotrexate absorption. Folate may decrease drug response.
Herb/Nutraceutical: Avoid echinacea (has immunostimulant properties).

Dietary Considerations
Sodium content of 100 mg injection: 20 mg (0.86 mEq)
Sodium content of 100 mg (low sodium) injection: 15 mg (0.65 mEq)

Pharmacodynamics/Kinetics
Onset of action: Antirheumatic: 3-6 weeks; additional improvement may continue longer than 12 weeks
Absorption: Oral: Rapid; well absorbed at low doses (<30 mg/m^2), incomplete after large doses; I.M.: Complete
Distribution: Penetrates slowly into 3rd space fluids (eg, pleural effusions, ascites), exits slowly from these compartments (slower than from plasma); crosses placenta; small amounts enter breast milk; sustained concentrations retained in kidney and liver
Protein binding: 50%
Metabolism: <10%; degraded by intestinal flora to DAMPA by carboxypeptidase; hepatic aldehyde oxidase converts methotrexate to 7-OH methotrexate; polyglutamates are produced intracellularly and are just as potent as methotrexate; their production is dose- and duration-dependent and they are slowly eliminated by the cell once formed
Half-life elimination: Low dose: 3-10 hours; High dose: 8-12 hours
Time to peak, serum: Oral: 1-2 hours; I.M.: 30-60 minutes
Excretion: Urine (44% to 100%); feces (small amounts)

Pregnancy Risk Factor X (psoriasis, rheumatoid arthritis)
Dosage Forms INJ, powder for reconstitution [preservative free]: 20 mg, 1 g. **INJ, solution:** 25 mg/mL (2 mL, 10 mL). **INJ, solution** [preservative free]: 25 mg/mL (2 mL, 4 mL, 8 mL, 10 mL). **TAB:** 2.5 mg; (Trexall™): 5 mg, 7.5 mg, 10 mg, 15 mg. **TAB** [dose pack] (Rheumatrex® Dose Pack): 2.5 mg (4 cards with 2, 3, 4, 5, or 6 tablets each)

Methotrexate Sodium *see* Methotrexate *on page 1012*

Methotrimeprazine *(meth oh trye MEP ra zeen)*

Canadian Brand Names Apo-Methopradine®; Nozinan®
Mexican Brand Names Levocina®; Sinogan®
Generic Available No
Synonyms Levomepromazine; Methotrimeprazine Hydrochloride
Pharmacologic Category Analgesic, Non-narcotic
Use Treatment of schizophrenia or psychosis; management of pain, including pain caused by neuralgia or cancer; adjunct to general anesthesia; management of nausea and vomiting; sedation
Unlabeled/Investigational Use Bipolar disorder, agitation
Local Anesthetic/Vasoconstrictor Precautions No information available to require special precautions (see Dental Comment)

Effects on Dental Treatment Key adverse event(s) related to dental treatment: Anticholinergic side effects can cause a reduction of saliva production or secretion, contributing to discomfort and dental disease (ie, caries, oral candidiasis, and periodontal disease). Phenothiazines can cause extrapyramidal reactions which may appear as muscle twitching or increased motor activity of the face, neck, or head.

Common Adverse Effects Note: Frequencies not defined; some reactions listed are based on reports for other agents in this same pharmacologic class, and may not be specifically reported for methotrimeprazine.

Cardiovascular: Hypotension, orthostatic hypotension, tachycardia, QT_c prolongation (rare)

Central nervous system: Extrapyramidal symptoms (pseudoparkinsonism, akathisia, dystonias, tardive dyskinesia), dizziness, seizure, headache, drowsiness, neuroleptic malignant syndrome (NMS), impairment of temperature regulation

Dermatologic: Photosensitivity (rare), rash

Endocrine & metabolic: Gynecomastia, weight gain, menstrual irregularity, libido (changes in)

Gastrointestinal: Constipation, vomiting, nausea, xerostomia, ileus

Genitourinary: Difficulty in urination, ejaculatory disturbances, incontinence, polyuria, ejaculating dysfunction, priapism

Hematologic: Agranulocytosis (rare), leukopenia, eosinophilia, hemolytic anemia, thrombocytopenic purpura, pancytopenia

Hepatic: Cholestatic jaundice, hepatotoxicity

Miscellaneous: Diaphoresis

Restrictions Not available in U.S.

Mechanism of Action Dopamine antagonist; also binds alpha-1, alpha-2, and serotonin receptors

Drug Interactions

Cytochrome P450 Effect: **Inhibits CYP2D6**

Increased Effect/Toxicity: Concurrent use of MAO inhibitors may result in toxicity; these combinations are best avoided. Methotrimeprazine may produce additive CNS depressant effects with CNS depressants (ethanol, narcotics). If a patient is receiving methotrimeprazine, the dose of a barbiturate or narcotic should be reduced by 50%. Chloroquine, propranolol, and sulfadoxine-pyrimethamine may increase methotrimeprazine concentrations. Concurrent use with TCA may produce increased toxicity or altered therapeutic response. A phenothiazine plus lithium may rarely produce neurotoxicity. Metoclopramide may increase risk of extrapyramidal symptoms (EPS). Acetylcholinesterase inhibitors (central) may increase the risk of antipsychotic-related EPS.

Methotrimeprazine may increase the levels/effects of amphetamines, selected beta blockers, dextromethorphan, fluoxetine, lidocaine, mesoridazine, mirtazapine, nefazodone, paroxetine, risperidone, ritonavir, thioridazine, tricyclic antidepressants, venlafaxine, and other CYP2D6 substrates.

Decreased Effect: Benztropine (and other anticholinergics) may inhibit the therapeutic response to phenothiazines. Antipsychotics such as methotrimeprazine inhibit the ability of bromocriptine to lower serum prolactin concentrations. The antihypertensive effects of guanethidine and guanadrel may be inhibited by phenothiazines. Methotrimeprazine may inhibit the antiparkinsonian effect of levodopa. Low potency antipsychotics may reverse the pressor effects of epinephrine. Methotrimeprazine may decrease the levels/effects of CYP2D6 prodrug substrates (eg, codeine, hydrocodone, oxycodone, tramadol).

Pharmacodynamics/Kinetics

Onset of action: Injection: 1 hour

Duration of action: 2-4 hours

Bioavailability: 50%

Time to peak, serum: I.M.: 0.5-1.5 hours; Oral: 1-3 hours

Half-life elimination: 30 hours

Pregnancy Risk Factor C

Dental Comment

This drug is known to prolong the QT interval. The QT interval is measured as the time and distance between the Q point of the QRS complex and the end of the T wave in the ECG tracing. After adjustment for heart rate, the QT interval is defined as prolonged if it is more than 450 msec in men and 460 msec in women. A long QT syndrome was first described in the 1950s and 60s as a congenital syndrome involving QT interval prolongation and syncope and sudden death. Some of the congenital long QT syndromes were characterized by a peculiar electrocardiographic appearance of the QRS complex involving a premature atria beat followed by a pause, then a subsequent sinus beat showing marked QT prolongation and deformity. This type of cardiac
(Continued)

Methotrimeprazine *(Continued)*

arrhythmia was originally termed "torsade de pointes" (translated from the French as "twisting of the points").

Prolongation of the QT interval is thought to result from delayed ventricular repolarization. The repolarization process within the myocardial cell is due to the efflux of intracellular potassium. The channels associated with this current can be blocked by many drugs and predisposes the electrical propagation cycle to torsade de pointes.

Methotrimeprazine is one of the drugs confirmed to prolong the QT interval and is accepted as having a risk of causing torsade de pointes. The risk of drug-induced torsade de pointes is extremely low when a single QT interval prolonging drug is prescribed. In terms of epinephrine, it is not known what effect vasoconstrictors in the local anesthetic regimen will have in patients with a known history of congenital prolonged QT interval or in patients taking any medication that prolongs the QT interval. Until more information is obtained, it is suggested that the clinician consult with the physician prior to the use of a vasoconstrictor in suspected patients, and that the vasoconstrictor (epinephrine, levonordefrin [Neo-Cobefrin®]) be used with caution.

Methotrimeprazine Hydrochloride *see* Methotrimeprazine *on page 1016*

Methoxsalen *(meth OKS a len)*

U.S. Brand Names 8-MOP®; Oxsoralen®; Oxsoralen-Ultra®; Uvadex®
Canadian Brand Names 8-MOP®; Oxsoralen®; Oxsoralen-Ultra®; Ultramop™; Uvadex®
Mexican Brand Names Dermox®; Meladinina®; Oxsoralen®
Generic Available No
Synonyms Methoxypsoralen; 8-Methoxypsoralen; 8-MOP
Pharmacologic Category Psoralen
Use
Oral: Symptomatic control of severe, recalcitrant disabling psoriasis; repigmentation of idiopathic vitiligo; palliative treatment of skin manifestations of cutaneous T-cell lymphoma (CTCL)
Topical: Repigmentation of idiopathic vitiligo
Extracorporeal: Palliative treatment of skin manifestations of CTCL

Local Anesthetic/Vasoconstrictor Precautions No information available to require special precautions

Effects on Dental Treatment No significant effects or complications reported
Common Adverse Effects Frequency not always defined.
Cardiovascular: Severe edema, hypotension
Central nervous system: Nervousness, vertigo, depression, dizziness, headache, malaise
Dermatologic: Painful blistering, burning, and peeling of skin; pruritus (10%), freckling, hypopigmentation, rash, cheilitis, erythema, itching, urticaria
Gastrointestinal: Nausea (10%)
Neuromuscular & skeletal: Loss of muscle coordination, leg cramps
Miscellaneous: Miliaria
Mechanism of Action Bonds covalently to pyrimidine bases in DNA, inhibits the synthesis of DNA, and suppresses cell division. The augmented sunburn reaction involves excitation of the methoxsalen molecule by radiation in the long-wave ultraviolet light (UVA), resulting in transference of energy to the methoxsalen molecule producing an excited state ("triplet electronic state"). The molecule, in this "triplet state", then reacts with cutaneous DNA.

Drug Interactions
Cytochrome P450 Effect: Substrate of CYP2A6 (minor); **Inhibits** CYP1A2 (strong), 2A6 (strong), 2C8/9 (weak), 2C19 (weak), 2D6 (weak), 2E1 (weak), 3A4 (weak)

Increased Effect/Toxicity: Methoxsalen may increase the levels/effects of CYP1A2 substrates (eg, aminophylline, fluvoxamine, mexiletine, mirtazapine, ropinirole, theophylline, trifluoperazine) and CYP2A6 substrates (eg, dexmedetomidine, ifosfamide).

Pharmacodynamics/Kinetics
Protein binding: Reversibly bound to albumin
Metabolism: Hepatic; forms metabolites
Bioavailability: Bioavailability increased with soft-gelatin capsules compared to hard-gelatin capsules; exposure using UVAR® system is ~200 times less than with oral administration
Time to peak, serum:
Hard-gelatin capsules: 1.5-6 hours (peak photosensitivity: ~4 hours)
Soft-gelatin capsules: 0.5-4 hours (peak photosensitivity: 1.5-2 hours)

Half-life elimination: ~2 hours
Excretion: Urine (~95% as metabolites)
Pregnancy Risk Factor C/D (Uvadex®)

Methoxypsoralen *see* Methoxsalen *on page 1018*
8-Methoxypsoralen *see* Methoxsalen *on page 1018*

Methscopolamine (meth skoe POL a meen)

U.S. Brand Names Pamine®; Pamine® Forte
Canadian Brand Names Pamine®
Generic Available No
Synonyms Methscopolamine Bromide
Pharmacologic Category Anticholinergic Agent
Use Adjunctive therapy in the treatment of peptic ulcer
Local Anesthetic/Vasoconstrictor Precautions No information available to require special precautions
Effects on Dental Treatment Key adverse event(s) related to dental treatment: Xerostomia and changes in salivation (normal salivary flow resumes upon discontinuation), and dry throat and nose. Anticholinergic side effects can cause a reduction of saliva production or secretion, contributing to discomfort and dental disease (ie, caries, oral candidiasis and periodontal disease).
Common Adverse Effects Frequency not defined.
Cardiovascular: Palpitations, tachycardia
Central nervous system: Headache, insomnia, flushing, nervousness, drowsiness, dizziness, confusion, fever, CNS stimulation may be produced with large doses
Dermatologic: Dry skin, urticaria
Endocrine & metabolic: Lactation suppressed
Gastrointestinal: Constipation, xerostomia, dry throat, dysphagia, nausea, vomiting, loss of taste
Genitourinary: Impotence, urinary hesitancy, urinary retention
Neuromuscular & skeletal: Weakness
Ocular: Blurred vision, cycloplegia, ocular tension increased, pupil dilation
Respiratory: Dry nose
Miscellaneous: Allergic reaction, diaphoresis decreased, hypersensitivity reactions, anaphylaxis
Mechanism of Action Methscopolamine is a peripheral anticholinergic agent with limited ability to cross the blood-brain barrier and provides a peripheral blockade of muscarinic receptors. This agent reduces the volume and the total acid content of gastric secretions, inhibits salivation, and reduces gastrointestinal motility.
Drug Interactions
Increased Effect/Toxicity: Antipsychotic agents and TCAs may produce additive anticholinergic effects.
Decreased Effect: Antacids may decrease the absorption of methscopolamine.
Pharmacodynamics/Kinetics
Onset: 1 hour
Duration: 4-6 hours
Excretion: Bile, urine
Pregnancy Risk Factor C

Methscopolamine Bromide *see* Methscopolamine *on page 1019*
Methscopolamine, Chlorpheniramine, and Phenylephrine *see* Chlorpheniramine, Phenylephrine, and Methscopolamine *on page 327*
Methscopolamine Nitrate and Chlordiazepoxide Hydrochloride *see* Chlordiazepoxide and Methscopolamine *on page 316*

Methsuximide (meth SUKS i mide)

U.S. Brand Names Celontin®
Canadian Brand Names Celontin®
Generic Available No
Pharmacologic Category Anticonvulsant, Succinimide
Use Control of absence (petit mal) seizures that are refractory to other drugs
Unlabeled/Investigational Use Partial complex (psychomotor) seizures
Local Anesthetic/Vasoconstrictor Precautions No information available to require special precautions
Effects on Dental Treatment No significant effects or complications reported
Common Adverse Effects Frequency not defined.
(Continued)

Methsuximide (Continued)

Cardiovascular: Hyperemia

Central nervous system: Ataxia, dizziness, drowsiness, headache, aggressiveness, mental depression, irritability, nervousness, insomnia, confusion, psychosis, suicidal behavior, auditory hallucinations

Dermatologic: Stevens-Johnson syndrome, rash, urticaria, pruritus

Gastrointestinal: Anorexia, nausea, vomiting, weight loss, diarrhea, epigastric and abdominal pain, constipation

Genitourinary: Proteinuria, hematuria (microscopic); cases of blood dyscrasias have been reported with succinimides

Hematologic: Leukopenia, pancytopenia, eosinophilia, monocytosis

Neuromuscular & skeletal: Cases of systemic lupus erythematosus have been reported

Ocular: Blurred vision, photophobia, peripheral edema

Mechanism of Action Increases the seizure threshold and suppresses paroxysmal spike-and-wave pattern in absence seizures; depresses nerve transmission in the motor cortex

Drug Interactions

Cytochrome P450 Effect: Substrate of CYP2C19 (major); **Inhibits** CYP2C19 (weak)

Increased Effect/Toxicity: CYP2C19 inhibitors may increase the levels/effects of methsuximide; example inhibitors include delavirdine, fluconazole, fluvoxamine, gemfibrozil, isoniazid, omeprazole, and ticlopidine. Sedative effects and/or respiratory depression may be additive with CNS depressants; includes ethanol, benzodiazepines, barbiturates, narcotic analgesics, and other sedative agents. Methsuximide may increase phenobarbital and/or phenytoin concentration.

Decreased Effect: CYP2C19 inducers may decrease the levels/effects of methsuximide; example inducers include aminoglutethimide, carbamazepine, phenytoin, and rifampin.

Pharmacodynamics/Kinetics

Metabolism: Hepatic; rapidly demethylated to N-desmethylmethsuximide (active metabolite)

Half-life elimination: 2-4 hours

Time to peak, serum: Within 1-3 hours

Excretion: Urine (<1% as unchanged drug)

Pregnancy Risk Factor C

Methyclothiazide (meth i kloe THYE a zide)

Related Information

Cardiovascular Diseases on page 1636

U.S. Brand Names Enduron® [DSC]

Canadian Brand Names Aquatensen®; Enduron®

Generic Available Yes

Pharmacologic Category Diuretic, Thiazide

Use Management of mild to moderate hypertension; treatment of edema in congestive heart failure and nephrotic syndrome

Local Anesthetic/Vasoconstrictor Precautions No information available to require special precautions

Effects on Dental Treatment No significant effects or complications reported

Common Adverse Effects 1% to 10%:

Cardiovascular: Orthostatic hypotension

Dermatologic: Photosensitivity

Endocrine & metabolic: Hypokalemia

Gastrointestinal: Anorexia, epigastric distress

Mechanism of Action Inhibits sodium reabsorption in the distal tubules causing increased excretion of sodium and water, as well as, potassium and hydrogen ions

Drug Interactions

Increased Effect/Toxicity: Increased effect of methyclothiazide with furosemide and other loop diuretics. Increased hypotension and/or renal adverse effects of ACE inhibitors may result in aggressively diuresed patients. Beta-blockers increase hyperglycemic effects of thiazides in Type 2 diabetes mellitus. Cyclosporine and thiazides can increase the risk of gout or renal toxicity. Digoxin toxicity can be exacerbated if a thiazide induces hypokalemia or hypomagnesemia. Lithium toxicity can occur with thiazides due to reduced renal excretion of lithium. Thiazides may prolong the duration of action with neuromuscular blocking agents.

Decreased Effect: Effects of oral hypoglycemics may be decreased. Decreased absorption of thiazides with cholestyramine and colestipol. NSAIDs can decrease the efficacy of thiazides, reducing the diuretic and antihypertensive effects.

Pharmacodynamics/Kinetics
Onset of action: Diuresis: 2 hours
  Peak effect: 6 hours
Duration: ~1 day
Distribution: Crosses placenta; enters breast milk
Excretion: Urine (as unchanged drug)

Pregnancy Risk Factor B

Methylacetoxyprogesterone see MedroxyPROGESTERone on page 972

Methylcellulose (meth il SEL yoo lose)

U.S. Brand Names Citrucel® [OTC]; FiberEase™ [OTC]
Generic Available No
Pharmacologic Category Laxative
Use Adjunct in treatment of constipation
Local Anesthetic/Vasoconstrictor Precautions No information available to require special precautions
Effects on Dental Treatment No significant effects or complications reported
Pregnancy Risk Factor C

Methyldopa (meth il DOE pa)

Related Information
Cardiovascular Diseases on page 1636
Canadian Brand Names Apo-Methyldopa®; Nu-Medopa
Mexican Brand Names Aldomet®
Generic Available Yes
Synonyms Aldomet; Methyldopate Hydrochloride
Pharmacologic Category Alpha-Adrenergic Inhibitor
Use Management of moderate to severe hypertension
Local Anesthetic/Vasoconstrictor Precautions No information available to require special precautions
Effects on Dental Treatment Key adverse event(s) related to dental treatment: Xerostomia (normal salivary flow resumes upon discontinuation). Anticholinergic side effects can cause a reduction of saliva production or secretion, contributing to discomfort and dental disease (ie, caries, oral candidiasis, and periodontal disease).

Common Adverse Effects
>10%: Cardiovascular: Peripheral edema
1% to 10%:
  Central nervous system: Drug fever, mental depression, anxiety, nightmares, drowsiness, headache
  Gastrointestinal: Dry mouth

Mechanism of Action Stimulation of central alpha-adrenergic receptors by a false transmitter that results in a decreased sympathetic outflow to the heart, kidneys, and peripheral vasculature

Drug Interactions
  Increased Effect/Toxicity: Beta-blockers, MAO inhibitors, phenothiazines, and sympathomimetics (including epinephrine) may result in hypertension (sometimes severe) when combined with methyldopa. Methyldopa may increase lithium serum levels resulting in lithium toxicity. Levodopa may cause enhanced blood pressure lowering; methyldopa may also potentiate the effect of levodopa. Tolbutamide, haloperidol, and anesthetics effects/toxicity are increased with methyldopa.
  Decreased Effect: Iron supplements can interact and cause a significant increase in blood pressure. Ferrous sulfate and ferrous gluconate decrease bioavailability. Barbiturates and TCAs may reduce response to methyldopa.

Pharmacodynamics/Kinetics
Onset of action: Peak effect: Hypotensive: Oral/parenteral: 3-6 hours
Duration: 12-24 hours
Distribution: Crosses placenta; enters breast milk
Protein binding: <15%
Metabolism: Intestinal and hepatic
Half-life elimination: 75-80 minutes; End-stage renal disease: 6-16 hours
Excretion: Urine (85% as metabolites) within 24 hours

Pregnancy Risk Factor B

Methyldopa and Hydrochlorothiazide
(meth il DOE pa & hye droe klor oh THYE a zide)

Related Information
Hydrochlorothiazide *on page 776*
Methyldopa *on page 1021*
U.S. Brand Names Aldoril®
Canadian Brand Names Apo-Methazide®
Generic Available Yes
Synonyms Hydrochlorothiazide and Methyldopa
Pharmacologic Category Antihypertensive Agent, Combination
Use Management of moderate to severe hypertension
Local Anesthetic/Vasoconstrictor Precautions No information available to require special precautions
Effects on Dental Treatment Key adverse event(s) related to dental treatment: Anticholinergic side effects can cause a reduction of saliva production or secretion, contributing to discomfort and dental disease (ie, caries, oral candidiasis, and periodontal disease).
Common Adverse Effects See individual agents.
Drug Interactions
Increased Effect/Toxicity: See individual agents.
Decreased Effect: See individual agents.
Pharmacodynamics/Kinetics See individual agents.
Pregnancy Risk Factor C

Methyldopate Hydrochloride *see Methyldopa on page 1021*

Methylene Blue, Methenamine, Sodium Biphosphate, Phenyl Salicylate, and Hyoscyamine *see Methenamine, Sodium Biphosphate, Phenyl Salicylate, Methylene Blue, and Hyoscyamine on page 1008*

Methylergometrine Maleate *see Methylergonovine on page 1022*

Methylergonovine (meth il er goe NOE veen)

U.S. Brand Names Methergine®
Canadian Brand Names Methergine®
Generic Available No
Synonyms Methylergometrine Maleate; Methylergonovine Maleate
Pharmacologic Category Ergot Derivative
Use Prevention and treatment of postpartum and postabortion hemorrhage caused by uterine atony or subinvolution
Local Anesthetic/Vasoconstrictor Precautions No information available to require special precautions
Effects on Dental Treatment No significant effects or complications reported
Common Adverse Effects Frequency not defined.
Cardiovascular: Acute MI, hypertension, temporary chest pain, palpitation
Central nervous system: Hallucinations, dizziness, seizure, headache
Endocrine & metabolic: Water intoxication
Gastrointestinal: Nausea, vomiting, diarrhea, foul taste
Local: Thrombophlebitis
Neuromuscular & skeletal: Leg cramps
Otic: Tinnitus
Renal: Hematuria
Respiratory: Dyspnea, nasal congestion
Miscellaneous: Diaphoresis
Mechanism of Action Similar smooth muscle actions as seen with ergotamine; however, it affects primarily uterine smooth muscles producing sustained contractions and thereby shortens the third stage of labor
Drug Interactions
Cytochrome P450 Effect: Substrate of CYP3A4 (major)
Increased Effect/Toxicity: CYP3A4 inhibitors may increase the levels/effects of methylergonovine; example inhibitors include azole antifungals, clarithromycin, diclofenac, doxycycline, erythromycin, imatinib, isoniazid, nefazodone, nicardipine, nicardipine, propofol, protease inhibitors, quinidine, telithromycin, and verapamil. Ergot alkaloids are contraindicated with potent CYP3A4 inhibitors. Methylergonovine may increase the effects of 5-HT₁ agonists (eg, sumatriptan), MAO inhibitors, sibutramine, and other serotonin agonists (serotonin syndrome). Severe vasoconstriction may occur when peripheral vasoconstrictors or beta-blockers are used in patients receiving ergot alkaloids; concurrent use is contraindicated.

Decreased Effect: Effects of methylergonovine may be diminished by anti-psychotics, metoclopramide/

Pharmacodynamics/Kinetics

Onset of action: Oxytocic: Oral: 5-10 minutes; I.M.: 2-5 minutes; I.V.: Immediately

Duration: Oral: ~3 hours; I.M.: ~3 hours; I.V.: 45 minutes

Absorption: Rapid

Distribution: V_d: 39-73 L

Rapid; primarily to plasma and extracellular fluid following I.V. administration; tissues

Metabolism: Hepatic

Bioavailability: Oral: 60%; I.M.: 78%

Half-life elimination: Biphasic: Initial: 1-5 minutes; Terminal: 0.5-2 hours

Time to peak, serum: Oral: 0.3-2 hours; I.M.: 0.2-0.6 hours

Excretion: Urine and feces

Pregnancy Risk Factor C

Methylergonovine Maleate *see* Methylergonovine *on page 1022*

Methylin® *see* Methylphenidate *on page 1023*

Methylin® ER *see* Methylphenidate *on page 1023*

Methylmorphine *see* Codeine *on page 385*

Methylphenidate (meth il FEN i date)

U.S. Brand Names Concerta®; Daytrana™; Metadate® CD; Metadate® ER; Methylin®; Methylin® ER; Ritalin®; Ritalin® LA; Ritalin-SR®

Canadian Brand Names Apo-Methylphenidate® SR; Concerta®; PMS-Methylphenidate; Riphenidate; Ritalin®; Ritalin® SR

Mexican Brand Names Ritalin®

Generic Available Yes: Tablet

Synonyms Methylphenidate Hydrochloride

Pharmacologic Category Central Nervous System Stimulant

Use Treatment of attention-deficit/hyperactivity disorder (ADHD); symptomatic management of narcolepsy

Unlabeled/Investigational Use Depression (especially elderly or medically ill)

Local Anesthetic/Vasoconstrictor Precautions No information available to require special precautions

Effects on Dental Treatment Key adverse event(s) related to dental treatment: Up to 10% of patients taking amphetamine-like drugs may present with hypertension. Monitor blood pressure prior to using local anesthetic with vasoconstrictors.

Common Adverse Effects

Transdermal system: Frequency of adverse events as reported in trials of 7-week duration. Incidence of some events reportedly higher with extended use.

>10%:

Central nervous system: Insomnia (13%)

Endocrine and metabolic: Appetite decreased (26%)

Gastrointestinal: Nausea (12%)

1% to 10%:

Central nervous system: Tic (7%), emotional instability (6%)

Gastrointestinal: Vomiting (10%), anorexia (5%)

Respiratory: Nasal congestion (6%), nasopharyngitis (5%)

Endocrine and metabolic: Weight loss (9%)

All dosage forms: Frequency not defined:

Cardiovascular: Angina, cardiac arrhythmia, cerebral arteritis, cerebral occlusion, hyper-/hypotension, MI, necrotizing vasculitis, palpitation, pulse increase/decrease, tachycardia

Central nervous system: Depression, dizziness, drowsiness, fever, headache, insomnia, nervousness, neuroleptic malignant syndrome (NMS), Tourette's syndrome, toxic psychosis

Dermatologic: Erythema multiforme, exfoliative dermatitis, hair loss, rash, urticaria

Endocrine & metabolic: Growth retardation

Gastrointestinal: Abdominal pain, anorexia, diarrhea, nausea, vomiting, weight loss

Hematologic: Anemia, leukopenia, thrombocytopenic purpura

Hepatic: Liver function tests abnormal, hepatic coma, transaminases increased

Neuromuscular & skeletal: Arthralgia, dyskinesia

Ocular: Blurred vision

Renal: Necrotizing vasculitis

(Continued)

Methylphenidate *(Continued)*

Respiratory: Cough increased, pharyngitis, sinusitis, upper respiratory tract infection

Miscellaneous: Accidental injury, hypersensitivity reactions

Restrictions C-II

Dosage ADHD:

Oral (discontinue periodically to re-evaluate or if no improvement occurs within 1 month): Children ≥6 years and Adults: Initial: 0.3 mg/kg/dose or 2.5-5 mg/dose given before breakfast and lunch; increase by 0.1 mg/kg/dose or by 5-10 mg/day at weekly intervals; usual dose: 0.5-1 mg/kg/day; maximum dose: 2 mg/kg/day or 90 mg/day

Extended release products:

Metadate® ER, Methylin® ER, Ritalin® SR: Duration of action is 8 hours. May be given in place of regular tablets, once the daily dose is titrated using the regular tablets and the titrated 8-hour dosage corresponds to sustained release tablet size.

Metadate® CD, Ritalin® LA: Initial: 20 mg once daily; may be adjusted in 10-20 mg increments at weekly intervals; maximum: 60 mg/day

Concerta®: Duration of action is 12 hours:

Initial dose:

Children not currently taking methylphenidate: 18 mg once daily in the morning

Children currently taking methylphenidate: **Note:** Dosing based on current regimen and clinical judgment; suggested dosing listed below:

Patients taking methylphenidate 5 mg 2-3 times/day or 20 mg/day sustained release formulation: 18 mg once every morning

Patients taking methylphenidate 10 mg 2-3 times/day or 40 mg/day sustained release formulation: 36 mg once every morning

Patients taking methylphenidate 15 mg 2-3 times/day or 60 mg/day sustained release formulation: 54 mg once every morning

Dose adjustment: May increase dose in increments of 18 mg; dose may be adjusted at weekly intervals. A dosage strength of 27 mg is available for situations in which a dosage between 18-36 mg is desired. Maximum dose should not exceed 2 mg/kg/day **or** 54 mg/day in children 6-12 years or 72 mg/day in children 13-17 years.

Transdermal (Daytrana™): Children 6-12 years: Initial: 10 mg patch once daily; remove up to 9 hours after application. Titrate based on response and tolerability; may increase to next transdermal dose no more frequently than every week. **Note:** Application should occur 2 hours prior to desired effect. Drug absorption may continue for a period of time after patch removal.

Adults:

Narcolepsy: 10 mg 2-3 times/day, up to 60 mg/day

Depression (unlabeled use): Initial: 2.5 mg every morning before 9 AM; dosage may be increased by 2.5-5 mg every 2-3 days as tolerated to a maximum of 20 mg/day; may be divided (ie, 7 AM and 12 noon), but should not be given after noon; do not use sustained release product

Mechanism of Action Mild CNS stimulant; blocks the reuptake of norepinephrine and dopamine into presynaptic neurons; appears to stimulate the cerebral cortex and subcortical structures similar to amphetamines

Contraindications Hypersensitivity to methylphenidate, any component of the formulation, or idiosyncratic reactions to sympathomimetic amines; marked anxiety, tension, and agitation; glaucoma; use during or within 14 days following MAO inhibitor therapy; Tourette's syndrome or tics

Warnings/Precautions Methylphenidate has a high potential for abuse; avoid abrupt discontinuation in patients who have received for prolonged periods. Has demonstrated value as part of a comprehensive treatment program for ADHD. May have value in selected patients as an antidepressant.

Safety and efficacy in children <6 years of age not established. Use with caution in patients with bipolar disorder, diabetes mellitus, cardiovascular disease, seizure disorders, insomnia, porphyria, or mild hypertension (stage I). Do not use in patients with known structural cardiac abnormalities; sudden death associated with CNS stimulant use has been reported in these patients. May exacerbate symptoms of behavior and thought disorder in psychotic patients. Do not use to treat severe depression or fatigue states. Stimulant use has been associated with growth suppression; growth should be monitored during treatment. Concerta® should not be used in patients with pre-existing severe gastrointestinal narrowing (small bowel disease, short gut syndrome, history of peritonitis, cystic fibrosis, chronic intestinal pseudo-obstruction, Meckel's diverticulum). Transdermal system may cause allergic contact sensitization, characterized by intense local reactions (edema, papules); sensitization may subsequently manifest systemically with other routes of methylphenidate administration; monitor closely. Efficacy of transdermal methylphenidate therapy for >7 weeks has not been established.

Drug Interactions
  Cytochrome P450 Effect: Substrate of CYP2D6 (major); **Inhibits** CYP2D6 (weak)
  Increased Effect/Toxicity: Methylphenidate may cause hypertensive effects when used in combination with MAO inhibitors or drugs with MAO-inhibiting activity (linezolid). Risk may be less with selegiline (MAO type B selective at low doses); it is best to avoid this combination. CYP2D6 inhibitors may increase the levels/effects of methylphenidate; example inhibitors include chlorpromazine, delavirdine, fluoxetine, miconazole, paroxetine, pergolide, quinidine, quinine, ritonavir, and ropinirole. Methylphenidate may increase levels of phenytoin, phenobarbital, and TCAs. Increased toxicity with clonidine and sibutramine.
  Decreased Effect: Effectiveness of antihypertensive agents may be decreased. Carbamazepine may decrease the effect of methylphenidate.

Ethanol/Nutrition/Herb Interactions
  Ethanol: Avoid ethanol (may cause CNS depression).
  Food: Food may increase oral absorption; Concerta® formulation is not affected. Food delays early peak and high-fat meals increase C_{max} and AUC of Metadate® CD formulation.
  Herb/Nutraceutical: Avoid ephedra (may cause hypertension or arrhythmias) and yohimbe (also has CNS stimulatory activity).

Dietary Considerations Should be taken 30-45 minutes before meals. Concerta® is not affected by food and should be taken with water, milk, or juice. Metadate® CD should be taken before breakfast. Metadate™ ER should be taken before breakfast and lunch.

Pharmacodynamics/Kinetics
  Onset of action: Peak effect:
    Immediate release tablet: Cerebral stimulation: ~2 hours
    Extended release capsule (Metadate® CD): Biphasic; initial peak similar to immediate release product, followed by second rising portion (corresponding to extended release portion)
    Sustained release tablet: 4-7 hours
    Osmotic release tablet (Concerta®): Initial: 1-2 hours
    Transdermal: ~2 hours
  Duration: Immediate release tablet: 3-6 hours; Sustained release tablet: 8 hours
  Absorption:
    Oral: Readily absorbed
    Transdermal: Absorption increased when applied to inflamed skin or exposed to heat.
  Metabolism: Hepatic via de-esterification to minimally active metabolite
  Half-life elimination: *d*-methylphenidate: 3-4 hours; *l*-methylphenidate: 1-3 hours
  Time to peak (Concerta®): C_{max}: 6-8 hours
  Excretion: Urine (90% as metabolites and unchanged drug)

Pregnancy Risk Factor C

Dosage Forms CAP, extended release (Metadate® CD): 10 mg, 20 mg, 30 mg, 40 mg, 50 mg, 60 mg; (Ritalin® LA): 10 mg, 20 mg, 30 mg, 40 mg. **PATCH, transdermal system** [once-daily]: (Daytrana™): 10 mg/9 hours (10s, 30s); 15 mg/9 hours (10s, 30s); 20 mg/9 hours (10s, 30s); 30 mg/9 hours (10s, 30s). **SOLN, oral** Methylin®: 5 mg/5 mL (500 mL).**TAB, chewable** (Methylin®): 2.5 mg, 5 mg,10 mg. **TAB** (Methylin®, Ritalin®): 5 mg, 10 mg, 20 mg. **TAB, extended release:** 20 mg; (Concerta®): 18 mg, 27 mg, 36 mg, 54 mg; (Metadate® ER, Methylin® ER): 10 mg, 20 mg. **TAB, sustained release** (Ritalin-SR®): 20 mg.

Methylphenidate Hydrochloride *see* Methylphenidate *on page 1023*
Methylphenobarbital *see* Mephobarbital *on page 986*
Methylphenoxy-Benzene Propanamine *see* Atomoxetine *on page 156*
Methylphenyl Isoxazolyl Penicillin *see* Oxacillin *on page 1153*
Methylphytyl Napthoquinone *see* Phytonadione *on page 1233*

MethylPREDNISolone (meth il pred NIS oh lone)

Related Information
  Respiratory Diseases *on page 1656*
Related Sample Prescriptions
  Erosive Lichen Planus and Major Aphthae *on page 1745*
U.S. Brand Names Depo-Medrol®; Medrol®; Solu-Medrol®
Canadian Brand Names Depo-Medrol®; Medrol®; Solu-Medrol®
Generic Available Yes: Sodium succinate injection, tablet
  (Continued)

MethylPREDNISolone (Continued)

Synonyms 6-α-Methylprednisolone; A-Methapred; Methylprednisolone Acetate; Methylprednisolone Sodium Succinate

Pharmacologic Category Corticosteroid, Systemic

Dental Use Treatment of a variety of oral diseases of allergic, inflammatory, or autoimmune origin

Use Primarily as an anti-inflammatory or immunosuppressant agent in the treatment of a variety of diseases including those of hematologic, allergic, inflammatory, neoplastic, and autoimmune origin. Prevention and treatment of graft-versus-host disease following allogeneic bone marrow transplantation.

Unlabeled/Investigational Use Treatment of fibrosing-alveolitis phase of adult respiratory distress syndrome (ARDS)

Local Anesthetic/Vasoconstrictor Precautions No information available to require special precautions

Effects on Dental Treatment No significant effects or complications reported

Significant Adverse Effects Frequency not defined.

Cardiovascular: Edema, hypertension, arrhythmia

Central nervous system: Insomnia, nervousness, vertigo, seizure, psychoses, pseudotumor cerebri, headache, mood swings, delirium, hallucinations, euphoria

Dermatologic: Hirsutism, acne, skin atrophy, bruising, hyperpigmentation

Endocrine & metabolic: Diabetes mellitus, adrenal suppression, hyperlipidemia, Cushing's syndrome, pituitary-adrenal axis suppression, growth suppression, glucose intolerance, hypokalemia, alkalosis, amenorrhea, sodium and water retention, hyperglycemia

Gastrointestinal: Increased appetite, indigestion, peptic ulcer, nausea, vomiting, abdominal distention, ulcerative esophagitis, pancreatitis

Hematologic: Transient leukocytosis

Neuromuscular & skeletal: Arthralgia, muscle weakness, osteoporosis, fractures

Ocular: Cataracts, glaucoma

Miscellaneous: Infections, hypersensitivity reactions, avascular necrosis, secondary malignancy, intractable hiccups

Dental Usual Dosing Anti-inflammatory or immunosuppressive: Adults: Oral: 2-60 mg/day in 1-4 divided doses to start, followed by gradual reduction in dosage to the lowest possible level consistent with maintaining an adequate clinical response.

Dosage Dosing should be based on the lesser of ideal body weight or actual body weight

Only sodium succinate may be given I.V.; methylprednisolone sodium succinate is highly soluble and has a rapid effect by I.M. and I.V. routes. Methylprednisolone acetate has a low solubility and has a sustained I.M. effect.

Children:

Anti-inflammatory or immunosuppressive: Oral, I.M., I.V. (sodium succinate): 0.5-1.7 mg/kg/day **or** 5-25 mg/m²/day in divided doses every 6-12 hours; "Pulse" therapy: 15-30 mg/kg/dose over ≥30 minutes given once daily for 3 days

Status asthmaticus: I.V. (sodium succinate): Loading dose: 2 mg/kg/dose, then 0.5-1 mg/kg/dose every 6 hours for up to 5 days

Acute spinal cord injury: I.V. (sodium succinate): 30 mg/kg over 15 minutes, followed in 45 minutes by a continuous infusion of 5.4 mg/kg/hour for 23 hours

Lupus nephritis: I.V. (sodium succinate): 30 mg/kg over ≥30 minutes every other day for 6 doses

Adults: **Only sodium succinate may be given I.V.**; methylprednisolone sodium succinate is highly soluble and has a rapid effect by I.M. and I.V. routes. Methylprednisolone acetate has a low solubility and has a sustained I.M. effect.

Acute spinal cord injury: I.V. (sodium succinate): 30 mg/kg over 15 minutes, followed in 45 minutes by a continuous infusion of 5.4 mg/kg/hour for 23 hours

Anti-inflammatory or immunosuppressive:

Oral: 2-60 mg/day in 1-4 divided doses to start, followed by gradual reduction in dosage to the lowest possible level consistent with maintaining an adequate clinical response.

I.M. (sodium succinate): 10-80 mg/day once daily

I.M. (acetate): 10-80 mg every 1-2 weeks

I.V. (sodium succinate): 10-40 mg over a period of several minutes and repeated I.V. or I.M. at intervals depending on clinical response; when high dosages are needed, give 30 mg/kg over a period ≥30 minutes and may be repeated every 4-6 hours for 48 hours.

Status asthmaticus: I.V. (sodium succinate): Loading dose: 2 mg/kg/dose, then 0.5-1 mg/kg/dose every 6 hours for up to 5 days

Lupus nephritis: High-dose "pulse" therapy: I.V. (sodium succinate): 1 g/day for 3 days

Aplastic anemia: I.V. (sodium succinate): 1 mg/kg/day or 40 mg/day (whichever dose is higher), for 4 days. After 4 days, change to oral and continue until day 10 or until symptoms of serum sickness resolve, then rapidly reduce over approximately 2 weeks.

Pneumocystis pneumonia in AIDs patients: I.V.: 40-60 mg every 6 hours for 7-10 days

Intra-articular (acetate): Administer every 1-5 weeks.

Large joints: 20-80 mg

Small joints: 4-10 mg

Intralesional (acetate): 20-60 mg every 1-5 weeks

Mechanism of Action In a tissue-specific manner, corticosteroids regulate gene expression subsequent to binding specific intracellular receptors and translocation into the nucleus. Corticosteroids exert a wide array of physiologic effects including modulation of carbohydrate, protein, and lipid metabolism and maintenance of fluid and electrolyte homeostasis. Moreover cardiovascular, immunologic, musculoskeletal, endocrine, and neurologic physiology are influenced by corticosteroids. Decreases inflammation by suppression of migration of polymorphonuclear leukocytes and reversal of increased capillary permeability.

Contraindications Hypersensitivity to methylprednisolone or any component of the formulation; viral, fungal, or tubercular skin lesions; administration of live virus vaccines; serious infections, except septic shock or tuberculous meningitis. Methylprednisolone formulations containing benzyl alcohol preservative are contraindicated in infants.

Warnings/Precautions Use with caution in patients with hyperthyroidism, cirrhosis, nonspecific ulcerative colitis, hypertension, osteoporosis, thromboembolic tendencies, CHF, convulsive disorders, myasthenia gravis, thrombophlebitis, peptic ulcer, diabetes, glaucoma, cataracts, or tuberculosis. Use caution in hepatic impairment. Because of the risk of adverse effects, systemic corticosteroids should be used cautiously in the elderly, in the smallest possible dose, and for the shortest possible time

Acute adrenal insufficiency may occur with abrupt withdrawal after long-term therapy or with stress; young pediatric patients may be more susceptible to adrenal axis suppression from topical therapy

Drug Interactions Substrate of CYP3A4 (minor); **Inhibits** CYP3A4 (weak)

Decreased effect:

Phenytoin, phenobarbital, rifampin increase clearance of methylprednisolone

Potassium depleting diuretics enhance potassium depletion

Increased toxicity:

Skin test antigens, immunizations decrease response and increase potential infections

Methylprednisolone may increase circulating glucose levels and may need adjustments of insulin or oral hypoglycemics

Ethanol/Nutrition/Herb Interactions

Ethanol: Avoid ethanol (may increase gastric mucosal irritation).

Food: Methylprednisolone interferes with calcium absorption. Limit caffeine.

Herb/Nutraceutical: St John's wort may decrease methylprednisolone levels. Avoid cat's claw, echinacea (have immunostimulant properties).

Dietary Considerations Should be taken after meals or with food or milk; need diet rich in pyridoxine, vitamin C, vitamin D, folate, calcium, phosphorus, and protein.

Sodium content of 1 g sodium succinate injection: 2.01 mEq; 53 mg of sodium succinate salt is equivalent to 40 mg of methylprednisolone base

Methylprednisolone acetate: Depo-Medrol®

Methylprednisolone sodium succinate: Solu-Medrol®

Pharmacodynamics/Kinetics

Onset of action: Peak effect (route dependent): Oral: 1-2 hours; I.M.: 4-8 days; Intra-articular: 1 week; methylprednisolone sodium succinate is highly soluble and has a rapid effect by I.M. and I.V. routes

Duration (route dependent): Oral: 30-36 hours; I.M.: 1-4 weeks; Intra-articular: 1-5 weeks; methylprednisolone acetate has a low solubility and has a sustained I.M. effect

Distribution: V_d: 0.7-1.5 L/kg

Half-life elimination: 3-3.5 hours; reduced in obese

Excretion: Clearance: Reduced in obese

Pregnancy Risk Factor C

Lactation Excretion in breast milk unknown

(Continued)

MethylPREDNISolone *(Continued)*

Dosage Forms

Injection, powder for reconstitution, as sodium succinate: 125 mg [strength expressed as base]

Solu-Medrol®: 40 mg, 125 mg, 500 mg, 1 g, 2 g [packaged with diluent; diluent contains benzyl alcohol; strength expressed as base]

Solu-Medrol®: 500 mg, 1 g

Injection, suspension, as acetate (Depo-Medrol®): 20 mg/mL (5 mL); 40 mg/mL (5 mL); 80 mg/mL (5 mL) [contains benzyl alcohol; strength expressed as base]

Injection, suspension, as acetate [single-dose vial] (Depo-Medrol®): 40 mg/mL (1 mL, 10 mL); 80 mg/mL (1 mL)

Tablet: 4 mg

Medrol®: 2 mg, 4 mg, 8 mg, 16 mg, 32 mg

Tablet, dose-pack: 4 mg (21s)

Medrol® Dosepack™: 4 mg (21s)

6-α-Methylprednisolone *see* MethylPREDNISolone *on page 1025*

Methylprednisolone Acetate *see* MethylPREDNISolone *on page 1025*

Methylprednisolone Sodium Succinate *see* MethylPREDNISolone *on page 1025*

4-Methylpyrazole *see* Fomepizole *on page 699*

Methylrosaniline Chloride *see* Gentian Violet *on page 735*

MethylTESTOSTERone *(meth il tes TOS te rone)*

U.S. Brand Names Android®; Methitest™; Testred®; Virilon®

Generic Available No

Pharmacologic Category Androgen

Use

Male: Hypogonadism; delayed puberty; impotence and climacteric symptoms

Female: Palliative treatment of metastatic breast cancer

Local Anesthetic/Vasoconstrictor Precautions No information available to require special precautions

Effects on Dental Treatment No significant effects or complications reported

Common Adverse Effects Frequency not defined.

Male: Virilism, priapism, prostatic hyperplasia, prostatic carcinoma, impotence, testicular atrophy, gynecomastia

Female: Virilism, menstrual problems (amenorrhea), breast soreness, hirsutism (increase in pubic hair growth) atrophy

Cardiovascular: Edema

Central nervous system: Headache, anxiety, depression

Dermatologic: Acne, "male pattern" baldness, seborrhea

Endocrine & metabolic: Hypercalcemia, hypercholesterolemia

Gastrointestinal: GI irritation, nausea, vomiting

Hematologic: Leukopenia, polycythemia

Hepatic: Hepatic dysfunction, hepatic necrosis, cholestatic hepatitis

Miscellaneous: Hypersensitivity reactions

Restrictions C-III

Mechanism of Action Stimulates receptors in organs and tissues to promote growth and development of male sex organs and maintains secondary sex characteristics in androgen-deficient males

Drug Interactions

Increased Effect/Toxicity: Effects of oral anticoagulants and hypoglycemic agents may be increased. Toxicity may occur with cyclosporine; avoid concurrent use.

Decreased Effect: Decreased oral anticoagulant effect

Pharmacodynamics/Kinetics

Metabolism: Hepatic

Excretion: Urine

Pregnancy Risk Factor X

Metipranolol *(met i PRAN oh lol)*

U.S. Brand Names OptiPranolol®

Canadian Brand Names OptiPranolol®

Generic Available Yes

Synonyms Metipranolol Hydrochloride

Pharmacologic Category Beta-Adrenergic Blocker, Nonselective; Ophthalmic Agent, Antiglaucoma

Use Agent for lowering intraocular pressure in patients with chronic open-angle glaucoma

Local Anesthetic/Vasoconstrictor Precautions No information available to require special precautions

Effects on Dental Treatment Metipranolol is a nonselective beta-blocker and may enhance the pressor response to epinephrine, resulting in hypertension and bradycardia. Many nonsteroidal anti-inflammatory drugs, such as ibuprofen and indomethacin, can reduce the hypotensive effect of beta-blockers after 3 or more weeks of therapy with the NSAID. Short-term NSAID use (ie, 3 days) requires no special precautions in patients taking beta-blockers.

Mechanism of Action Beta-adrenoceptor-blocking agent; lacks intrinsic sympathomimetic activity and membrane-stabilizing effects and possesses only slight local anesthetic activity; mechanism of action of metipranolol in reducing intraocular pressure appears to be via reduced production of aqueous humor. This effect may be related to a reduction in blood flow to the iris root-ciliary body. It remains unclear if the reduction in intraocular pressure observed with beta-blockers is actually secondary to beta-adrenoceptor blockade.

Pregnancy Risk Factor C

Metipranolol Hydrochloride see Metipranolol on page 1028

Metoclopramide (met oh kloe PRA mide)

Related Information
Endocrine Disorders and Pregnancy *on page 1659*
U.S. Brand Names Reglan®
Canadian Brand Names Apo-Metoclop®; Nu-Metoclopramide
Mexican Brand Names Carnotprim®; Clorimet®; Meclomid®; Plasil®
Generic Available Yes
Pharmacologic Category Antiemetic; Gastrointestinal Agent, Prokinetic
Use

Oral: Symptomatic treatment of diabetic gastric stasis; gastroesophageal reflux

I.V., I.M.: Symptomatic treatment of diabetic gastric stasis; postpyloric placement of enteral feeding tubes; prevention and/or treatment of nausea and vomiting associated with chemotherapy, or postsurgery; to stimulate gastric emptying and intestinal transit of barium during radiological examination

Local Anesthetic/Vasoconstrictor Precautions No information available to require special precautions

Effects on Dental Treatment Key adverse event(s) related to dental treatment: Xerostomia (normal salivary flow resumes upon discontinuation).

Common Adverse Effects Frequency not always defined.

Cardiovascular: AV block, bradycardia, CHF, fluid retention, flushing (following high I.V. doses), hyper-/hypotension, supraventricular tachycardia

Central nervous system: Drowsiness (~10% to 70%; dose related), fatigue (~10%), restlessness (~10%), acute dystonic reactions (<1% to 25%; dose and age related), akathisia, confusion, depression, dizziness, hallucinations (rare), headache, insomnia, neuroleptic malignant syndrome (rare), Parkinsonian-like symptoms, suicidal ideation, seizures, tardive dyskinesia

Dermatologic: Angioneurotic edema (rare), rash, urticaria

Endocrine & metabolic: Amenorrhea, galactorrhea, gynecomastia, impotence

Gastrointestinal: Diarrhea, nausea

Genitourinary: Incontinence, urinary frequency

Hematologic: Agranulocytosis, leukopenia, neutropenia, porphyria

Hepatic: Hepatotoxicity (rare)

Ocular: Visual disturbance

Respiratory: Bronchospasm, laryngeal edema (rare)

Miscellaneous: Allergic reactions, methemoglobinemia, sulfhemoglobinemia

Mechanism of Action Blocks dopamine receptors and (when given in higher doses) also blocks serotonin receptors in chemoreceptor trigger zone of the CNS; enhances the response to acetylcholine of tissue in upper GI tract causing enhanced motility and accelerated gastric emptying without stimulating gastric, biliary, or pancreatic secretions; increases lower esophageal sphincter tone

Drug Interactions

Cytochrome P450 Effect: Substrate (minor) of CYP1A2, 2D6; **Inhibits** CYP2D6 (weak)

Increased Effect/Toxicity: Opiate analgesics may increase CNS depression. Metoclopramide may increase extrapyramidal symptoms (EPS) or risk when used concurrently with antipsychotic agents. Metoclopramide may increase cyclosporine levels.

Decreased Effect: Anticholinergic agents antagonize metoclopramide's actions.

(Continued)

Metoclopramide *(Continued)*

Pharmacodynamics/Kinetics

Onset of action: Oral: 0.5-1 hour; I.V.: 1-3 minutes; I.M.: 10-15 minutes

Duration: Therapeutic: 1-2 hours, regardless of route

Distribution: V_d: 2-4 L/kg

Protein binding: 30%

Bioavailability: Oral: 65% to 95%

Half-life elimination: Normal renal function: 4-6 hours (may be dose dependent)

Time to peak, serum: Oral: 1-2 hours

Excretion: Urine (~85%)

Pregnancy Risk Factor B

Metolazone *(me TOLE a zone)*

Related Information

Cardiovascular Diseases *on page 1636*

U.S. Brand Names Zaroxolyn®

Canadian Brand Names Mykrox®; Zaroxolyn®

Generic Available Yes

Pharmacologic Category Diuretic, Thiazide-Related

Use Management of mild to moderate hypertension; treatment of edema in congestive heart failure and nephrotic syndrome, impaired renal function

Local Anesthetic/Vasoconstrictor Precautions No information available to require special precautions

Effects on Dental Treatment No significant effects or complications reported

Mechanism of Action Inhibits sodium reabsorption in the distal tubules causing increased excretion of sodium and water, as well as, potassium and hydrogen ions

Pregnancy Risk Factor B (manufacturer); D (expert analysis)

Metoprolol *(me toe PROE lole)*

Related Information

Cardiovascular Diseases *on page 1636*

U.S. Brand Names Lopressor®; Toprol-XL®

Canadian Brand Names Apo-Metoprolol®; Betaloc®; Betaloc® Durules®; Lopressor®; Novo-Metoprolol; Nu-Metop; PMS-Metoprolol; Sandoz-Metoprolol; Toprol-XL®

Mexican Brand Names Lopresor®; Proken M®; Prolaken®; Ritmolol®; Selectadril®; Seloken®

Generic Available Yes: Injection, tablet (nonextended release)

Synonyms Metoprolol Succinate; Metoprolol Tartrate

Pharmacologic Category Beta Blocker, Beta₁ Selective

Use Treatment of hypertension and angina pectoris; prevention of myocardial infarction, atrial fibrillation, flutter, symptomatic treatment of hypertrophic subaortic stenosis; to reduce mortality/hospitalization in patients with congestive heart failure (stable NYHA Class II or III) in patients already receiving ACE inhibitors, diuretics, and/or digoxin (sustained-release only)

Unlabeled/Investigational Use Treatment of ventricular arrhythmias, atrial ectopy, migraine prophylaxis, essential tremor, aggressive behavior

Local Anesthetic/Vasoconstrictor Precautions No information available to require special precautions

Effects on Dental Treatment Metoprolol is a cardioselective beta-blocker. Local anesthetic with vasoconstrictor can be safely used in patients medicated with metoprolol. Nonselective beta-blockers (ie, propranolol, nadolol) enhance the pressor response to epinephrine, resulting in hypertension and bradycardia; this has not been reported for metoprolol. Many nonsteroidal anti-inflammatory drugs, such as ibuprofen and indomethacin, can reduce the hypotensive effect of beta-blockers after 3 or more weeks of therapy with the NSAID. Short-term NSAID use (ie, 3 days) requires no special precautions in patients taking beta-blockers.

Common Adverse Effects

>10%:

Central nervous system: Drowsiness, insomnia

Endocrine & metabolic: Decreased sexual ability

1% to 10%:

Cardiovascular: Bradycardia, palpitation, edema, CHF, reduced peripheral circulation

Central nervous system: Mental depression

Gastrointestinal: Diarrhea or constipation, nausea, stomach discomfort

Respiratory: Bronchospasm
Miscellaneous: Cold extremities

Dosage

Children: Oral: 1-5 mg/kg/24 hours divided twice daily; allow 3 days between dose adjustments

Adults:

Hypertension: Oral: 100-450 mg/day in 2-3 divided doses, begin with 50 mg twice daily and increase doses at weekly intervals to desired effect; usual dosage range (JNC 7): 50-100 mg/day

Extended release: Initial: 25-100 mg/day (maximum: 400 mg/day)

Angina, SVT, MI prophylaxis: Oral: 100-450 mg/day in 2-3 divided doses, begin with 50 mg twice daily and increase doses at weekly intervals to desired effect

Extended release: Initial: 100 mg/day (maximum: 400 mg/day)

Hypertension/ventricular rate control: I.V. (in patients having nonfunctioning GI tract): Initial: 1.25-5 mg every 6-12 hours; titrate initial dose to response. Initially, low doses may be appropriate to establish response; however, up to 15 mg every 3-6 hours has been employed.

Congestive heart failure: Oral (extended release): Initial: 25 mg once daily (reduce to 12.5 mg once daily in NYHA class higher than class II); may double dosage every 2 weeks as tolerated, up to 200 mg/day

Myocardial infarction (acute): I.V.: 5 mg every 2 minutes for 3 doses in early treatment of myocardial infarction; thereafter give 50 mg orally every 6 hours 15 minutes after last I.V. dose and continue for 48 hours; then administer a maintenance dose of 100 mg twice daily.

Elderly: Oral: Initial: 25 mg/day; usual range: 25-300 mg/day

Extended release: 25-50 mg/day initially as a single dose; increase at 1- to 2-week intervals.

Hemodialysis: Administer dose posthemodialysis or administer 50 mg supplemental dose; supplemental dose is not necessary following peritoneal dialysis

Dosing adjustment/comments in hepatic disease: Reduced dose probably necessary

Mechanism of Action
Selective inhibitor of beta$_1$-adrenergic receptors; competitively blocks beta$_1$-receptors, with little or no effect on beta$_2$-receptors at doses <100 mg; does not exhibit any membrane stabilizing or intrinsic sympathomimetic activity

Contraindications
Hypersensitivity to metoprolol or any component of the formulation; sinus bradycardia; heart block greater than first degree (except in patients with a functioning artificial pacemaker); cardiogenic shock; uncompensated cardiac failure; pregnancy (2nd and 3rd trimesters)

Warnings/Precautions
Abrupt withdrawal of the drug should be avoided (may result in an exaggerated cardiac beta-adrenergic response, tachycardia, hypertension, ischemia, angina, myocardial infarction, and sudden death), drug should be discontinued over 1-2 weeks. Must use care in compensated heart failure and monitor closely for a worsening of the condition (efficacy has not been established for metoprolol). Avoid abrupt discontinuation in patients with a history of CAD; slowly wean while monitoring for signs and symptoms of ischemia. Use caution in patients with PVD (can aggravate arterial insufficiency). Use caution with concurrent use of beta-blockers and either verapamil or diltiazem; bradycardia or heart block can occur. Avoid concurrent I.V. use of both agents. In general, beta-blockers should be avoided in patients with bronchospastic disease. Metoprolol, with B1 selectivity, should be used cautiously in bronchospastic disease with close monitoring, since selectivity can be lost with higher doses. Beta-blockers may increase the risk of anaphylaxis (in predisposed patients) and blunt response to epinephrine. Use cautiously in diabetics because it can mask prominent hypoglycemic symptoms. Can mask signs of thyrotoxicosis. Can cause fetal harm when administered in pregnancy. Use cautiously in the hepatically impaired. Use care with anesthetic agents which decrease myocardial function. Avoid use of extended release tablets (Toprol-XL®) in patients with known stricture/narrowing of the GI tract.

Drug Interactions

Cytochrome P450 Effect: Substrate of CYP2C19 (minor), 2D6 (major); Inhibits CYP2D6 (weak)

Increased Effect/Toxicity: CYP2D6 inhibitors may increase the levels/effects of metoprolol; example inhibitors include chlorpromazine, delavirdine, fluoxetine, miconazole, paroxetine, pergolide, quinidine, quinine, ritonavir, and ropinirole. Metoprolol may increase the effects of other drugs which slow AV conduction (digoxin, verapamil, diltiazem), alpha-blockers (prazosin, terazosin), and alpha-adrenergic stimulants (epinephrine, phenylephrine). Metoprolol may mask the tachycardia from hypoglycemia caused by insulin and oral hypoglycemics. In patients receiving concurrent therapy, the risk of hypertensive crisis is increased when either clonidine or the beta-blocker is

(Continued)

Metoprolol *(Continued)*

withdrawn. Reserpine has been shown to enhance the effect of beta-blockers. Beta-blockers may increase the action or levels of ethanol, disopyramide, nondepolarizing muscle relaxants, and theophylline although the effects are difficult to predict.

Decreased Effect: Decreased effect of beta-blockers with aluminum salts, barbiturates, calcium salts, cholestyramine, colestipol, NSAIDs, penicillins (ampicillin), rifampin, salicylates, and sulfinpyrazone due to decreased bioavailability and plasma levels. Beta-blockers may decrease the effect of sulfonylureas.

Ethanol/Nutrition/Herb Interactions

Food: Food increases absorption. Metoprolol serum levels may be increased if taken with food.

Herb/Nutraceutical: Avoid dong quai if using for hypertension (has estrogenic activity). Avoid ephedra, yohimbe, ginseng (may worsen hypertension). Avoid garlic (may have increased antihypertensive effect).

Dietary Considerations Regular tablets should be taken with food. Extended release tablets may be taken without regard to meals.

Pharmacodynamics/Kinetics

Onset of action: Peak effect: Antihypertensive: Oral: 1.5-4 hours

Duration: 10-20 hours

Absorption: 95%

Protein binding: 8%

Metabolism: Extensively hepatic; significant first-pass effect

Bioavailability: Oral: 40% to 50%

Half-life elimination: 3-4 hours; End-stage renal disease: 2.5-4.5 hours

Excretion: Urine (3% to 10% as unchanged drug)

Pregnancy Risk Factor C (manufacturer); D (2nd and 3rd trimesters - expert analysis)

Dosage Forms INJ, solution, as tartrate (Lopressor®): 1 mg/mL (5 mL). **TAB, as tartrate:** 25 mg, 50 mg, 100 mg; (Lopressor®): 50 mg, 100 mg. **TAB, extended release, as succinate** (Toprol-XL®): 25 mg, 50 mg, 100 mg, 200 mg

Selected Readings

Foster CA and Aston SJ, "Propranolol-Epinephrine Interaction: A Potential Disaster," *Plast Reconstr Surg*, 1983, 72(1):74-8.

Wong DG, Spence JD, Lamki L, et al, "Effect of Nonsteroidal Anti-inflammatory Drugs on Control of Hypertension of Beta-Blockers and Diuretics," *Lancet*, 1986, 1(8488):997-1001.

Wynn RL, "Dental Nonsteroidal Anti-inflammatory Drugs and Prostaglandin-Based Drug Interactions, Part Two," *Gen Dent*, 1992, 40(2):104, 106, 108.

Wynn RL, "Epinephrine Interactions With Beta-Blockers," *Gen Dent*, 1994, 42(1):16, 18.

Metoprolol and Hydrochlorothiazide
(me toe PROE lole & hye droe klor oh THYE a zide)

U.S. Brand Names Lopressor HCT®

Generic Available Yes

Synonyms Hydrochlorothiazide and Metoprolol; Hydrochlorothiazide and Metoprolol Tartrate; Metoprolol Tartrate and Hydrochlorothiazide

Pharmacologic Category Beta Blocker, Beta$_1$ Selective; Diuretic, Thiazide

Use Treatment of hypertension

Local Anesthetic/Vasoconstrictor Precautions No information available to require special precautions

Effects on Dental Treatment

Metoprolol: Treatment of oral soft tissue infections due to anaerobic bacteria including all anaerobic cocci, anaerobic gram-negative bacilli (*Bacteroides*), and gram-positive spore-forming bacilli (*Clostridium*). Useful as single agent or in combination with amoxicillin, Augmentin®, or ciprofloxacin in the treatment of periodontitis associated with the presence of *Actinobacillus actinomycetemcomitans* (AA).

Hydrochlorothiazide: Key adverse event(s) related to dental treatment: Orthostatic hypotension and hypotension.

Common Adverse Effects Reactions noted here have been reported with the combination product; see individual drug monographs for additional adverse reactions that may be expected from each agent.

1% to 10%:

Cardiovascular: Bradycardia (6%), edema (1%)

Central nervous system: Fatigue (10%), dizziness (10%), drowsiness (10%), headache (10%), vertigo (10%), abnormal dreams (1%)

Dermatologic: Purpura (1%)

Endocrine & metabolic: Hypokalemia, gout (1%)

Gastrointestinal: Anorexia (1%), constipation (1%), diarrhea (1%), nausea (1%), vomiting (1%), xerostomia (1%)

Genitourinary: Impotence (1%)
Neuromuscular & skeletal: Myalgia
Ocular: Blurred vision (1%)
Otic: Earache (1%), tinnitus (1%)
Respiratory: Dyspnea (1%)
Miscellaneous: Flu-like syndrome (10%), diaphoresis (1%), exercise tolerance decreased (1%)

Mechanism of Action See individual agents.

Drug Interactions
Cytochrome P450 Effect: Metoprolol: **Substrate** of CYP2C19 (minor), 2D6 (major); Inhibits CYP2D6 (weak)

Pharmacodynamics/Kinetics See individual agents.

Pregnancy Risk Factor C/D (expert analysis)

Metoprolol Succinate *see* Metoprolol *on page 1030*
Metoprolol Tartrate *see* Metoprolol *on page 1030*
Metoprolol Tartrate and Hydrochlorothiazide *see* Metoprolol and Hydrochlorothiazide *on page 1032*
MetroCream® *see* Metronidazole *on page 1033*
MetroGel® *see* Metronidazole *on page 1033*
MetroGel-Vaginal® *see* Metronidazole *on page 1033*
MetroLotion® *see* Metronidazole *on page 1033*

Metronidazole (me troe NI da zole)

Related Information
Bacterial Infections *on page 1697*
Gastrointestinal Disorders *on page 1654*
Periodontal Diseases *on page 1705*
Sexually-Transmitted Diseases *on page 1674*
Ulcerative and Erosive Disorders *on page 1712*

Related Sample Prescriptions
Bacterial Infections and Periodontal Diseases *on page 1736*

U.S. Brand Names Flagyl®; Flagyl ER®; Flagyl® I.V. RTU™; MetroCream®; MetroGel®; MetroGel-Vaginal®; MetroLotion®; Noritate®; Vandazole™

Canadian Brand Names Apo-Metronidazole®; Flagyl®; Florazole® ER; MetroCream®; Metrogel®; Nidagel™; Noritate®; Trikacide

Mexican Brand Names Ameblin®; Flagenase®; Flagyl®; Fresenizol®; MetroGel®; Nidrozol®; Selegil®; Servizol®; Vertisal®

Generic Available Yes: Cream, gel, infusion, tablet

Synonyms Metronidazole Hydrochloride

Pharmacologic Category Amebicide; Antibiotic, Miscellaneous; Antibiotic, Topical; Antiprotozoal, Nitroimidazole

Dental Use Treatment of oral soft tissue infections due to anaerobic bacteria including all anaerobic cocci, anaerobic gram-negative bacilli (*Bacteroides*), and gram-positive spore-forming bacilli (*Clostridium*). Useful as single agent or in combination with amoxicillin, Augmentin®, or ciprofloxacin in the treatment of periodontitis associated with the presence of *Actinobacillus actinomycetemcomitans* (AA).

Use Treatment of susceptible anaerobic bacterial and protozoal infections in the following conditions: Amebiasis, symptomatic and asymptomatic trichomoniasis; skin and skin structure infections; CNS infections; intra-abdominal infections (as part of combination regimen); systemic anaerobic infections; treatment of antibiotic-associated pseudomembranous colitis (AAPC), bacterial vaginosis; as part of a multidrug regimen for *H. pylori* eradication to reduce the risk of duodenal ulcer recurrence
Topical: Treatment of inflammatory lesions and erythema of rosacea

Unlabeled/Investigational Use Crohn's disease

Local Anesthetic/Vasoconstrictor Precautions No information available to require special precautions

Effects on Dental Treatment Key adverse event(s) related to dental treatment: Unusual/metallic taste, glossitis, stomatitis, and xerostomia (normal salivary flow resumes upon discontinuation).

Significant Adverse Effects
Systemic: Frequency not defined:
Cardiovascular: Flattening of the T-wave, flushing
Central nervous system: Ataxia, confusion, coordination impaired, dizziness, fever, headache, insomnia, irritability, seizure, vertigo
Dermatologic: Erythematous rash, urticaria
Endocrine & metabolic: Disulfiram-like reaction, dysmenorrhea, libido decreased
(Continued)

Metronidazole *(Continued)*

Gastrointestinal: Nausea (~12%), anorexia, abdominal cramping, constipation, diarrhea, furry tongue, glossitis, proctitis, stomatitis, unusual/metallic taste, vomiting, xerostomia

Genitourinary: Cystitis, darkened urine (rare), dysuria, incontinence, polyuria, vaginitis

Hematologic: Neutropenia (reversible), thrombocytopenia (reversible, rare)

Neuromuscular & skeletal: Peripheral neuropathy, weakness

Respiratory: Nasal congestion, rhinitis, sinusitis, pharyngitis

Miscellaneous: Flu-like syndrome, moniliasis

Topical: Frequency not defined:

Central nervous system: Headache

Dermatologic: Burning, contact dermatitis, dryness, erythema, irritation, pruritus, rash

Gastrointestinal: Unusual/metallic taste, nausea, constipation

Local: Local allergic reaction

Neuromuscular & skeletal: Tingling/numbness of extremities

Ocular: Eye irritation

Vaginal:

>10%: Genitourinary: Vaginal discharge (12%)

1% to 10%:

Central nervous system: Headache (5%), dizziness (2%)

Gastrointestinal: Gastrointestinal discomfort (7%), nausea and/or vomiting (4%), unusual/metallic taste (2%), diarrhea (1%)

Genitourinary: Vaginitis (10%), vulva/vaginal irritation (9%), pelvic discomfort (3%)

Hematologic: WBC increased (2%)

<1%: Abdominal bloating, abdominal gas, darkened urine, depression, fatigue, itching, rash, thirst, xerostomia

Dental Usual Dosing Anaerobic infections/abscess: Adults: Oral, I.V.: 500 mg every 6-8 hours, not to exceed 4 g/day

Dosage

Infants and Children:

Amebiasis: Oral: 35-50 mg/kg/day in divided doses every 8 hours for 10 days

Trichomoniasis: Oral: 15-30 mg/kg/day in divided doses every 8 hours for 7 days

Anaerobic infections:

Oral: 15-35 mg/kg/day in divided doses every 8 hours

I.V.: 30 mg/kg/day in divided doses every 6 hours

Clostridium difficile (antibiotic-associated colitis): Oral: 20 mg/kg/day divided every 6 hours

Maximum dose: 2 g/day

Adults:

Anaerobic infections (diverticulitis, intra-abdominal, peritonitis, cholangitis, or abscess): Oral, I.V.: 500 mg every 6-8 hours, not to exceed 4 g/day

Acne rosacea: Topical:

0.75%: Apply and rub a thin film twice daily, morning and evening, to entire affected areas after washing. Significant therapeutic results should be noticed within 3 weeks. Clinical studies have demonstrated continuing improvement through 9 weeks of therapy.

1%: Apply thin film to affected area once daily

Amebiasis: Oral: 500-750 mg every 8 hours for 5-10 days

Antibiotic-associated pseudomembranous colitis: Oral: 250-500 mg 3-4 times/day for 10-14 days

Giardiasis: 500 mg twice daily for 5-7 days

Helicobacter pylori eradication: Oral: 250-500 mg with meals and at bedtime for 14 days; requires combination therapy with at least one other antibiotic and an acid-suppressing agent (proton pump inhibitor or H$_2$ blocker)

Bacterial vaginosis or vaginitis due to *Gardnerella, Mobiluncus*:

Oral: 500 mg twice daily (regular release) or 750 mg once daily (extended release tablet) for 7 days

Vaginal: 1 applicatorful (~37.5 mg metronidazole) intravaginally once or twice daily for 5 days; apply once in morning and evening if using twice daily, if daily, use at bedtime

Trichomoniasis: Oral: 250 mg every 8 hours for 7 days **or** 375 mg twice daily for 7 days **or** 2 g as a single dose

Elderly: Use lower end of dosing recommendations for adults, do not administer as a single dose

Dosing adjustment in renal impairment: Cl$_{cr}$ <10 mL/minute: Administer 50% of dose or every 12 hours

Hemodialysis: Extensively removed by hemodialysis and peritoneal dialysis (50% to 100%); administer dose posthemodialysis

Peritoneal dialysis: Dose as for Cl_{cr} <10 mL/minute

Continuous arteriovenous or venovenous hemofiltration: Administer usual dose

Dosing adjustment/comments in hepatic disease: Unchanged in mild liver disease; reduce dosage in severe liver disease

Mechanism of Action After diffusing into the organism, interacts with DNA to cause a loss of helical DNA structure and strand breakage resulting in inhibition of protein synthesis and cell death in susceptible organisms

Contraindications Hypersensitivity to metronidazole, nitroimidazole derivatives, or any component of the formulation; pregnancy (1st trimester - found to be carcinogenic in rats)

Warnings/Precautions Use with caution in patients with liver impairment due to potential accumulation, blood dyscrasias; history of seizures, CHF, or other sodium retaining states; reduce dosage in patients with severe liver impairment, CNS disease, and severe renal failure (Cl_{cr} <10 mL/minute); if *H. pylori* is not eradicated in patients being treated with metronidazole in a regimen, it should be assumed that metronidazole-resistance has occurred and it should not again be used; seizures and neuropathies have been reported especially with increased doses and chronic treatment; if this occurs, discontinue therapy

Drug Interactions Inhibits CYP2C8/9 (weak), 3A4 (moderate)

Cimetidine may increase metronidazole levels.

Cisapride: May inhibit metabolism of cisapride, causing potential arrhythmias; avoid concurrent use

CYP3A4 substrates: Metronidazole may increase the levels/effects of CYP3A4 substrates. Example substrates include benzodiazepines, calcium channel blockers, cyclosporine, mirtazapine, nateglinide, nefazodone, sildenafil (and other PDE-5 inhibitors), tacrolimus, and venlafaxine. Selected benzodiazepines (midazolam and triazolam), cisapride, ergot alkaloids, selected HMG-CoA reductase inhibitors (lovastatin and simvastatin), and pimozide are generally contraindicated with strong CYP3A4 inhibitors.

Ethanol: Ethanol results in disulfiram-like reactions.

Lithium: Metronidazole may increase lithium levels/toxicity; monitor lithium levels.

Phenytoin, phenobarbital may increase metabolism of metronidazole, potentially decreasing its effect.

Warfarin: Metronidazole increases P-T prolongation with warfarin.

Ethanol/Nutrition/Herb Interactions

Ethanol: The manufacturer recommends to avoid all ethanol or any ethanol-containing drugs (may cause disulfiram-like reaction characterized by flushing, headache, nausea, vomiting, sweating or tachycardia).

Food: Peak antibiotic serum concentration lowered and delayed, but total drug absorbed not affected.

Dietary Considerations Take on an empty stomach. Drug may cause GI upset; if GI upset occurs, take with food. Extended release tablets should be taken on an empty stomach (1 hour before or 2 hours after meals). Sodium content of 500 mg (I.V.): 322 mg (14 mEq). The manufacturer recommends that ethanol be avoided during treatment and for 3 days after therapy is complete.

Pharmacodynamics/Kinetics

Absorption: Oral: Well absorbed; Topical: Concentrations achieved systemically after application of 1 g topically are 10 times less than those obtained after a 250 mg oral dose

Distribution: To saliva, bile, seminal fluid, breast milk, bone, liver, and liver abscesses, lung and vaginal secretions; crosses placenta and blood-brain barrier

CSF:blood level ratio: Normal meninges: 16% to 43%; Inflamed meninges: 100%

Protein binding: <20%

Metabolism: Hepatic (30% to 60%)

Half-life elimination: Neonates: 25-75 hours; Others: 6-8 hours; prolonged with hepatic impairment; End-stage renal disease: 21 hours

Time to peak, serum: Oral: Immediate release: 1-2 hours

Excretion: Urine (20% to 40% as unchanged drug); feces (6% to 15%)

Pregnancy Risk Factor B (may be contraindicated in 1st trimester)

Lactation Enters breast milk/not recommended (AAP rates "of concern")

Breast-Feeding Considerations It is suggested to stop breast-feeding for 12-24 hours following single dose therapy to allow excretion of dose.

Dosage Forms [DSC] = Discontinued product

Capsule (Flagyl®): 375 mg

Cream, topical: 0.75% (45 g)

MetroCream®: 0.75% (45 g) [contains benzyl alcohol]

Noritate®: 1% (60 g)

(Continued)

Metronidazole *(Continued)*

Gel, topical (MetroGel®): 0.75% (45 g) [DSC], 1% (45 g)

Gel, vaginal (MetroGel-Vaginal®, Vandazole™): 0.75% (70 g)

Infusion (Flagyl® I.V. RTU™) [premixed iso-osmotic sodium chloride solution]: 500 mg (100 mL) [contains sodium 14 mEq]

Lotion, topical (MetroLotion®): 0.75% (60 mL) [contains benzyl alcohol]

Tablet (Flagyl®): 250 mg, 500 mg

Tablet, extended release (Flagyl® ER): 750 mg

Selected Readings

Eisenberg L, Suchow R, Coles RS, et al, "The Effects of Metronidazole Administration on Clinical and Microbiologic Parameters of Periodontal Disease," *Clin Prev Dent*, 1991, 13(1):28-34.

Herrera D, Sanz M, Jepsen S, et al, "A Systematic Review on the Effect of Systemic Antimicrobials as an Adjunct to Scaling and Root Planing in Periodontitis Patients," *J Clin Periodontol*, 2002, 29(Suppl 3):136-59, discussion 160-2.

Jansson H, Bratthall G, and Soderholm G, "Clinical Outcome Observed in Subjects With Recurrent Periodontal Disease Following Local Treatment With 25% Metronidazole Gel," *J Periodontol*, 2003, 74(3):372-7.

Jenkins WM, MacFarlane TW, Gilmour WH, et al, "Systemic Metronidazole in the Treatment of Periodontitis," *J Clin Periodontol*, 1989, 16(7):433-50.

Loesche WJ, Giordano JR, Hujoel P, et al, "Metronidazole in Periodontitis: Reduced Need for Surgery," *J Clin Periodontol*, 1992, 19(2):103-12.

Loesche WJ, Schmidt E, Smith BA, et al, "Effects of Metronidazole on Periodontal Treatment Needs," *J Periodontol*, 1991, 62(4):247-57.

Noiri Y, Okami Y, Narimatsu M, et al, "Effects of Chlorhexidine, Minocycline, and Metronidazole on Porphyromonas Gingivalis Strain 381 in Biofilms," *J Periodontol*, 2003, 74(11):1647-51.

Soder PO, Frithiof L, Wikner S, et al, "The Effect of Systemic Metronidazole After Nonsurgical Treatment in Moderate and Advanced Periodontitis in Young Adults," *J Periodontol*, 1990, 61(5):281-8.

Wynn RL, Bergman SA, Meiller TF, et al, "Antibiotics in Treating Oral-Facial Infections of Odontogenic Origin: An Update," *Gen Dent*, 2001, 49(3):238-40, 242, 244 passim.

Metronidazole and Nystatin (me troe NI da zole & nye STAT in)

Related Information

Metronidazole *on page 1033*

Nystatin *on page 1133*

Canadian Brand Names Flagystatin®

Pharmacologic Category Antifungal Agent, Vaginal; Antiprotozoal, Nitroimidazole

Use Treatment of mixed vaginal infection due to *T. vaginalis* and *C. albicans*

Local Anesthetic/Vasoconstrictor Precautions No information available to require special precautions

Effects on Dental Treatment Key adverse event(s) related to dental treatment: Taste disturbances (bitter).

Common Adverse Effects Note: Adverse effects are infrequent and generally minor.

Central nervous system: Headache

Dermatologic: Pruritus, spots on skin (around knees), welts on body

Gastrointestinal: Coated tongue, nausea, taste disturbance (bitter), vomiting

Genitourinary: Vaginal: Burning, granular sensation

Neuromuscular & skeletal: Fatigue, swelling/aching or wrists

Restrictions Not available in U.S.

Mechanism of Action See individual agents.

Drug Interactions

Increased Effect/Toxicity: See individual agents. Due to low systemic absorption, the risk for interaction with other drugs is considered very low.

Metronidazole, Bismuth Subsalicylate, and Tetracycline *see* Bismuth Subsalicylate, Metronidazole, and Tetracycline *on page 210*

Metronidazole Hydrochloride *see* Metronidazole *on page 1033*

Metyrosine (me TYE roe seen)

U.S. Brand Names Demser®

Canadian Brand Names Demser®

Generic Available No

Synonyms AMPT; OGMT

Pharmacologic Category Tyrosine Hydroxylase Inhibitor

Use Short-term management of pheochromocytoma before surgery, long-term management when surgery is contraindicated or when chronic malignant pheochromocytoma exists

Local Anesthetic/Vasoconstrictor Precautions No information available to require special precautions

Effects on Dental Treatment Key adverse event(s) related to dental treatment: Xerostomia (normal salivary flow resumes upon discontinuation).

Common Adverse Effects

>10%:

Central nervous system: Drowsiness, extrapyramidal symptoms

Gastrointestinal: Diarrhea

1% to 10%:

Endocrine & metabolic: Galactorrhea, edema of the breasts

Gastrointestinal: Nausea, vomiting, xerostomia

Genitourinary: Impotence

Respiratory: Nasal congestion

Mechanism of Action Blocks the rate-limiting step in the biosynthetic pathway of catecholamines. It is a tyrosine hydroxylase inhibitor, blocking the conversion of tyrosine to dihydroxyphenylalanine. This inhibition results in decreased levels of endogenous catecholamines. Catecholamine biosynthesis is reduced by 35% to 80% in patients treated with metyrosine 1-4 g/day.

Drug Interactions

Increased Effect/Toxicity: Phenothiazines, haloperidol may potentiate EPS

Pharmacodynamics/Kinetics

Half-life elimination: 7.2 hours

Excretion: Primarily urine (as unchanged drug)

Pregnancy Risk Factor C

Mevacor® see Lovastatin on page 953

Mevinolin see Lovastatin on page 953

Mexiletine (MEKS i le teen)

Related Information

Cardiovascular Diseases on page 1636

U.S. Brand Names Mexitil® [DSC]

Canadian Brand Names Novo-Mexiletine

Generic Available Yes

Pharmacologic Category Antiarrhythmic Agent, Class Ib

Use Management of serious ventricular arrhythmias; suppression of PVCs

Unlabeled/Investigational Use Diabetic neuropathy

Local Anesthetic/Vasoconstrictor Precautions No information available to require special precautions

Effects on Dental Treatment Key adverse event(s) related to dental treatment: Xerostomia (normal salivary flow resumes upon discontinuation).

Common Adverse Effects

>10%:

Central nervous system: Lightheadedness (11% to 25%), dizziness (20% to 25%), nervousness (5% to 10%), incoordination (10%)

Gastrointestinal: GI distress (41%), nausea/vomiting (40%)

Neuromuscular & skeletal: Trembling, unsteady gait, tremor (13%), ataxia (10% to 20%)

1% to 10%:

Cardiovascular: Chest pain (3% to 8%), premature ventricular contractions (1% to 2%), palpitation (4% to 8%), angina (2%), proarrhythmic (10% to 15% in patients with malignant arrhythmia)

Central nervous system: Confusion, headache, insomnia (5% to 7%), depression (2%)

Dermatologic: Rash (4%)

Gastrointestinal: Constipation or diarrhea (4% to 5%), xerostomia (3%), abdominal pain (1%)

Neuromuscular & skeletal: Weakness (5%), numbness of fingers or toes (2% to 4%), paresthesia (2%), arthralgia (1%)

Ocular: Blurred vision (5% to 7%), nystagmus (6%)

Otic: Tinnitus (2% to 3%)

Respiratory: Dyspnea (3%)

Mechanism of Action Class IB antiarrhythmic, structurally related to lidocaine, which inhibits inward sodium current, decreases rate of rise of phase 0, increases effective refractory period/action potential duration ratio

Drug Interactions

Cytochrome P450 Effect: Substrate (major) of CYP1A2, 2D6; **Inhibits** CYP1A2 (strong)

Increased Effect/Toxicity: Mexiletine may increase the levels/effects of aminophylline, fluvoxamine, mirtazapine, ropinirole, trifluoperazine, or other CYP1A2 substrates. The levels/effects of mexiletine may be increased by inhibitors of CYP1A2 or 2D6; example inhibitors include amiodarone, chlorpromazine, ciprofloxacin, delavirdine, fluoxetine, fluvoxamine, ketoconazole, (Continued)

Mexiletine *(Continued)*

miconazole, norfloxacin, ofloxacin, paroxetine, pergolide, quinidine, quinine, ritonavir, rofecoxib, ropinirole, and other CYP1A2 or 2D6 inhibitors. Mexiletine may increase levels of theophylline and caffeine. Quinidine and urinary alkalinizers (antacids, sodium bicarbonate, acetazolamide) may increase mexiletine blood levels.

Decreased Effect: The levels/effects of mexiletine may be decreased by aminoglutethimide, carbamazepine, phenobarbital, rifampin, and other CYP1A2 inducers. Urinary acidifying agents may decrease mexiletine levels.

Pharmacodynamics/Kinetics
Absorption: Elderly have a slightly slower rate, but extent of absorption is the same as young adults
Distribution: V_d: 5-7 L/kg
Protein binding: 50% to 70%
Metabolism: Hepatic; low first-pass effect
Half-life elimination: Adults: 10-14 hours (average: elderly: 14.4 hours, younger adults: 12 hours); prolonged with hepatic impairment or heart failure
Time to peak: 2-3 hours
Excretion: Urine (10% to 15% as unchanged drug); urinary acidification increases excretion, alkalinization decreases excretion

Pregnancy Risk Factor C

Mexitil® [DSC] *see* Mexiletine *on page 1037*

M-FA-142 *see* Amonafide *on page 104*

MG 217® [OTC] *see* Coal Tar *on page 383*

MG 217® Medicated Tar [OTC] *see* Coal Tar *on page 383*

MG217 Sal-Acid® [OTC] *see* Salicylic Acid *on page 1374*

MgSO₄ (error-prone abbreviation) *see* Magnesium Sulfate *on page 963*

Miacalcin® *see* Calcitonin *on page 246*

Mi-Acid [OTC] *see* Aluminum Hydroxide, Magnesium Hydroxide, and Simethicone *on page 81*

Mi-Acid™ Double Strength [OTC] *see* Calcium Carbonate and Magnesium Hydroxide *on page 249*

Mi-Acid Maximum Strength [OTC] *see* Aluminum Hydroxide, Magnesium Hydroxide, and Simethicone *on page 81*

Micaderm® [OTC] *see* Miconazole *on page 1039*

Micafungin *(mi ka FUN gin)*

U.S. Brand Names Mycamine™
Synonyms Micafungin Sodium
Pharmacologic Category Antifungal Agent, Parenteral; Echinocandin
Use Esophageal candidiasis; *Candida* prophylaxis in patients undergoing hematopoietic stem cell transplant
Unlabeled/Investigational Use Treatment of infections due to *Aspergillus* spp; prophylaxis of HIV-related esophageal candidiasis
Local Anesthetic/Vasoconstrictor Precautions No information available to require special precautions
Effects on Dental Treatment No significant effects or complications reported
Common Adverse Effects 1% to 10%:
Cardiovascular: Phlebitis (2%), hypertension (1%), flushing (1%)
Central nervous system: Headache (2%), pyrexia (2%), delirium (1%), dizziness (1%), somnolence (1%)
Dermatologic: Rash (2%), pruritus (1%), febrile neutropenia (1%)
Endocrine & metabolic: Hypokalemia (1%), hypocalcemia (1%), hypomagnesemia (1%), hypophosphatemia (1%)
Gastrointestinal: Nausea (3%), diarrhea (2%), vomiting (2%), abdominal pain (1%), appetite decreased (1%), dysgeusia (1%), dyspepsia (1%)
Hematologic: Leukopenia (2%), neutropenia (1%), thrombocytopenia (1%), anemia (1%), lymphopenia (1%), eosinophilia (1%)
Hepatic: Transaminase increased (2% to 3%), serum alkaline phosphatase increased (2%), hyperbilirubinemia (1%)
Local: Infusion site inflammation (1%)
Neuromuscular & skeletal: Rigors (1%), lactate dehydrogenase increased (1%)
Renal: Serum creatinine increased (1%), serum urea increased (1%)
Mechanism of Action Concentration-dependent inhibition of 1,3-beta-D-glucan synthase resulting in reduced formation of 1,3-beta-D-glucan, an essential polysaccharide comprising 30% to 60% of *Candida* cell walls (absent in mammalian cells); decreased glucan content leads to osmotic instability and cellular lysis

Drug Interactions
Cytochrome P450 Effect:
Substrate of CYP3A4 (minor); **Inhibits** CYP3A4 (weak)
Increased Effect/Toxicity:
No clinically-significant interactions have been identified.
Decreased Effect:
No clinically-signficant interactions have been identified.
Pharmacodynamics/Kinetics
Distribution: 0.28-0.5 L/kg
Protein binding: >99%
Metabolism: Hepatic; forms M-1 (catechol) and M-2 (methoxy) metabolites (activity unknown)
Half-life elimination: 11-21 hours
Excretion: Primarily feces (71%), urine (<15%, unchanged drug)
Pregnancy Risk Factor C

Micafungin Sodium *see* Micafungin *on page 1038*
Micardis® *see* Telmisartan *on page 1451*
Micardis® HCT *see* Telmisartan and Hydrochlorothiazide *on page 1452*
Micatin® Athlete's Foot [OTC] *see* Miconazole *on page 1039*
Micatin® Jock Itch [OTC] *see* Miconazole *on page 1039*

Miconazole (mi KON a zole)

Related Information
Sexually-Transmitted Diseases *on page 1674*
U.S. Brand Names Aloe Vesta® 2-n-1 Antifungal [OTC]; Baza® Antifungal [OTC]; Carrington Antifungal [OTC]; DermaFungal [OTC]; Dermagran® AF [OTC]; DiabetAid™ Antifungal Foot Bath [OTC]; Fungoid® Tincture [OTC]; Lotrimin® AF Jock Itch Powder Spray [OTC]; Lotrimin® AF Powder/Spray [OTC]; Micaderm® [OTC]; Micatin® Athlete's Foot [OTC]; Micatin® Jock Itch [OTC]; Micro-Guard® [OTC]; Mitrazol™ [OTC]; Monistat® 1 Combination Pack [OTC]; Monistat® 3 [OTC]; Monistat® 7 [OTC]; Monistat-Derm®; Neosporin® AF [OTC]; Podactin Cream [OTC]; Secura® Antifungal [OTC]; Zeasorb®-AF [OTC]
Canadian Brand Names Dermazole; Micatin®; Micozole; Monistat®; Monistat® 3
Mexican Brand Names Aloid®; Daktarin®; Dermifun®; Lotrimin AF®; Neomicol®
Generic Available Yes
Synonyms Miconazole Nitrate
Pharmacologic Category Antifungal Agent, Topical; Antifungal Agent, Vaginal
Use Treatment of vulvovaginal candidiasis and a variety of skin and mucous membrane fungal infections
Local Anesthetic/Vasoconstrictor Precautions No information available to require special precautions
Effects on Dental Treatment No significant effects or complications reported
Common Adverse Effects Frequency not defined.
Topical: Allergic contact dermatitis, burning, maceration
Vaginal: Abdominal cramps, burning, irritation, itching
Mechanism of Action Inhibits biosynthesis of ergosterol, damaging the fungal cell wall membrane, which increases permeability causing leaking of nutrients
Drug Interactions
Cytochrome P450 Effect: Substrate of CYP3A4 (major); **Inhibits** CYP1A2 (moderate), 2A6 (strong), 2B6 (weak), 2C8/9 (strong), 2C19 (strong), 2D6 (strong), 2E1 (moderate), 3A4 (strong)
Increased Effect/Toxicity: Note: The majority of reported drug interactions were observed following intravenous miconazole administration. Although systemic absorption following topical and/or vaginal administration is low, potential interactions due to CYP isoenzyme inhibition may occur (rarely). This may be particularly true in situations where topical absorption may be increased (ie, inflamed tissue).

Miconazole coadministered with warfarin has increased the anticoagulant effect of warfarin (including reports associated with vaginal miconazole therapy of as little as 3 days). Concurrent administration of cisapride is contra-indicated due to an increased risk of cardiotoxicity. Miconazole may increase the serum levels/effects of amiodarone, amphetamines, benzodiazepines, beta-blockers, buspirone, busulfan, calcium channel blockers, citalopram, dexmedetomidine, dextromethorphan, diazepam, digoxin, docetaxel, fluoxetine, fluvoxamine, glimepiride, glipizide, ifosfamide, inhalational anesthetics, lidocaine, mesoridazine, methsuximide, mexiletine, mirtazapine, nateglinide, nefazodone, paroxetine, phenytoin, pioglitazone, propranolol, risperidone,
(Continued)

Miconazole *(Continued)*

ritonavir, ropinirole, rosiglitazone, sertraline, sirolimus, tacrolimus, theophylline, thioridazine, tricyclic antidepressants, trifluoperazine, trimetrexate, venlafaxine, vincristine, vinblastine, warfarin, zolpidem, and other substrates of CYP1A2, 2A6, 2C8/9, 2C19, 2D6, or 3A4. Selected benzodiazepines (midazolam and triazolam), cisapride, ergot alkaloids, selected HMG-CoA reductase inhibitors (lovastatin and simvastatin), and pimozide are generally contraindicated with strong CYP3A4 inhibitors. Mesoridazine and thioridazine are generally contraindicated with strong CYP2D6 inhibitors. When used with strong CYP3A4 inhibitors, dosage adjustment/limits are recommended for sildenafil and other PDE-5 inhibitors; consult individual monographs.

Decreased Effect: Amphotericin B may decrease antifungal effect of both agents. The levels/effects of miconazole may be decreased by aminoglutethimide, carbamazepine, nafcillin, nevirapine, phenobarbital, phenytoin, rifamycins or other CYP3A4 inducers. Miconazole may decrease the levels/effects of CYP2D6 prodrug substrates (eg, codeine, hydrocodone, oxycodone, tramadol).

Pharmacodynamics/Kinetics

Absorption: Topical: Negligible

Distribution: Widely to body tissues; penetrates well into inflamed joints, vitreous humor of eye, and peritoneal cavity, but poorly into saliva and sputum; crosses blood-brain barrier but only to a small extent

Protein binding: 91% to 93%

Metabolism: Hepatic

Half-life elimination: Multiphasic: Initial: 40 minutes; Secondary: 126 minutes; Terminal: 24 hours

Excretion: Feces (~50%); urine (<1% as unchanged drug)

Pregnancy Risk Factor C

Miconazole and Zinc Oxide *(mi KON a zole & zink OKS ide)*

U.S. Brand Names Vusion™

Generic Available No

Synonyms Zinc Oxide and Miconazole Nitrate

Pharmacologic Category Antifungal Agent, Topical

Use Adjunctive treatment of diaper dermatitis complicated by *Candida albicans* infection

Local Anesthetic/Vasoconstrictor Precautions No information available to require special precautions

Effects on Dental Treatment No significant effects or complications reported

Mechanism of Action

Miconazole inhibits the biosynthesis of ergosterol, damaging the fungal cell wall membrane.

Zinc oxide is a mild astringent with weak antiseptic properties.

Pharmacodynamics/Kinetics Absorption: Topical: Miconazole: Undetectable to 3.8 ng/mL in infants with dermatitis

Pregnancy Risk Factor C

Miconazole Nitrate *see* Miconazole *on page 1039*

MICRhoGAM® *see* Rh$_o$(D) Immune Globulin *on page 1342*

Microfibrillar Collagen Hemostat *see* Collagen Hemostat *on page 392*

Microgestin™ *see* Ethinyl Estradiol and Norethindrone *on page 608*

Microgestin™ Fe *see* Ethinyl Estradiol and Norethindrone *on page 608*

Micro-Guard® [OTC] *see* Miconazole *on page 1039*

microK® *see* Potassium Chloride *on page 1258*

microK® 10 *see* Potassium Chloride *on page 1258*

Micronase® *see* GlyBURIDE *on page 744*

microNefrin® *see* Epinephrine (Racemic) *on page 549*

Micronor® *see* Norethindrone *on page 1125*

Microzide™ *see* Hydrochlorothiazide *on page 776*

Midamor® [DSC] *see* Amiloride *on page 85*

Midazolam *(MID aye zoe lam)*

Canadian Brand Names Apo-Midazolam®

Mexican Brand Names Dormicum®

Generic Available Yes

Synonyms Midazolam Hydrochloride; Versed

Pharmacologic Category Benzodiazepine

Dental Use Sedation component in I.V. conscious sedation in oral surgery patients; syrup formulation is used for children to help alleviate anxiety before a dental procedure

Use Preoperative sedation and provides conscious sedation prior to diagnostic or radiographic procedures; ICU sedation (continuous infusion); intravenous anesthesia (induction); intravenous anesthesia (maintenance)

Unlabeled/Investigational Use Anxiety, status epilepticus

Local Anesthetic/Vasoconstrictor Precautions No information available to require special precautions

Effects on Dental Treatment No significant effects or complications reported

Significant Adverse Effects As reported in adults unless otherwise noted:

>10%: Respiratory: Decreased tidal volume and/or respiratory rate decrease, apnea (3% children)

1% to 10%:

Cardiovascular: Hypotension (3% children)

Central nervous system: Drowsiness (1%), oversedation, headache (1%), seizure-like activity (1% children)

Gastrointestinal: Nausea (3%), vomiting (3%)

Local: Pain and local reactions at injection site (4% I.M., 5% I.V.; severity less than diazepam)

Ocular: Nystagmus (1% children)

Respiratory: Cough (1%)

Miscellaneous: Physical and psychological dependence with prolonged use, hiccups (4%, 1% children), paradoxical reaction (2% children)

<1% (Limited to important or life-threatening): Agitation, amnesia, bigeminy, bronchospasm, emergence delirium, euphoria, hallucinations, laryngospasm, rash

Restrictions C-IV

Dental Usual Dosing Adults:

Preoperative sedation:

I.M.: 0.07-0.08 mg/kg 30-60 minutes prior to surgery/procedure; usual dose: 5 mg; **Note:** Reduce dose in patients with COPD, high-risk patients, patients ≥60 years of age, and patients receiving other narcotics or CNS depressants

I.V.: 0.02-0.04 mg/kg; repeat every 5 minutes as needed to desired effect or up to 0.1-0.2 mg/kg

Intranasal (not an approved route): 0.2 mg/kg (up to 0.4 mg/kg in some studies); administer 30-45 minutes prior to surgery/procedure

Conscious sedation: I.V.: Initial: 0.5-2 mg slow I.V. over at least 2 minutes; slowly titrate to effect by repeating doses every 2-3 minutes if needed; usual total dose: 2.5-5 mg; use decreased doses in elderly.

Healthy Adults <60 years: Initial: Some patients respond to doses as low as 1 mg; no more than 2.5 mg should be administered over a period of 2 minutes. Additional doses of midazolam may be administered after a 2-minute waiting period and evaluation of sedation after each dose increment. A total dose >5 mg is generally not needed. If narcotics or other CNS depressants are administered concomitantly, the midazolam dose should be reduced by 30%.

Dosage The dose of midazolam needs to be individualized based on the patient's age, underlying diseases, and concurrent medications. Decrease dose (by ~30%) if narcotics or other CNS depressants are administered concomitantly. **Personnel and equipment needed for standard respiratory resuscitation should be immediately available during midazolam administration.**

Children <6 years may require higher doses and closer monitoring than older children; calculate dose on ideal body weight

Conscious sedation for procedures or preoperative sedation:

Oral: 0.25-0.5 mg/kg as a single dose preprocedure, up to a maximum of 20 mg; administer 30-45 minutes prior to procedure. Children <6 years or less cooperative patients may require as much as 1 mg/kg as a single dose; 0.25 mg/kg may suffice for children 6-16 years of age.

Intranasal (not an approved route): 0.2 mg/kg (up to 0.4 mg/kg in some studies), to a maximum of 15 mg; may be administered 30-45 minutes prior to procedure

I.M.: 0.1-0.15 mg/kg 30-60 minutes before surgery or procedure; range 0.05-0.15 mg/kg; doses up to 0.5 mg/kg have been used in more anxious patients; maximum total dose: 10 mg

I.V.:

Infants <6 months: Limited information is available in nonintubated infants; dosing recommendations not clear; infants <6 months are at higher risk

(Continued)

Midazolam *(Continued)*

for airway obstruction and hypoventilation; titrate dose in small increments to desired effect; monitor carefully

Infants 6 months to Children 5 years: Initial: 0.05-0.1 mg/kg; titrate dose carefully; total dose of 0.6 mg/kg may be required; usual maximum total dose: 6 mg

Children 6-12 years: Initial: 0.025-0.05 mg/kg; titrate dose carefully; total doses of 0.4 mg/kg may be required; usual maximum total dose: 10 mg

Children 12-16 years: Dose as adults; usual maximum total dose: 10 mg

Conscious sedation during mechanical ventilation: Children: Loading dose: 0.05-0.2 mg/kg, followed by initial continuous infusion: 0.06-0.12 mg/kg/ hour (1-2 mcg/kg/minute); titrate to the desired effect; usual range: 0.4-6 mcg/kg/minute

Status epilepticus refractory to standard therapy (unlabeled use): Infants >2 months and Children: Loading dose: 0.15 mg/kg followed by a continuous infusion of 1 mcg/kg/minute; titrate dose upward every 5 minutes until clinical seizure activity is controlled; mean infusion rate required in 24 children was 2.3 mcg/kg/minute with a range of 1-18 mcg/kg/minute

Adults:

Preoperative sedation:

I.M.: 0.07-0.08 mg/kg 30-60 minutes prior to surgery/procedure; usual dose: 5 mg; **Note:** Reduce dose in patients with COPD, high-risk patients, patients ≥60 years of age, and patients receiving other narcotics or CNS depressants

I.V.: 0.02-0.04 mg/kg; repeat every 5 minutes as needed to desired effect or up to 0.1-0.2 mg/kg

Intranasal (not an approved route): 0.2 mg/kg (up to 0.4 mg/kg in some studies); administer 30-45 minutes prior to surgery/procedure

Conscious sedation: I.V.: Initial: 0.5-2 mg slow I.V. over at least 2 minutes; slowly titrate to effect by repeating doses every 2-3 minutes if needed; usual total dose: 2.5-5 mg; use decreased doses in elderly

Healthy Adults <60 years: Some patients respond to doses as low as 1 mg; no more than 2.5 mg should be administered over a period of 2 minutes. Additional doses of midazolam may be administered after a 2-minute waiting period and evaluation of sedation after each dose increment. A total dose >5 mg is generally not needed. If narcotics or other CNS depressants are administered concomitantly, the midazolam dose should be reduced by 30%.

Anesthesia: I.V.:

Induction:

Unpremedicated patients: 0.3-0.35 mg/kg (up to 0.6 mg/kg in resistant cases)

Premedicated patients: 0.15-0.35 mg/kg

Maintenance: 0.05-0.3 mg/kg as needed, or continuous infusion 0.25-1.5 mcg/kg/minute

Sedation in mechanically-ventilated patients: I.V. continuous infusion: 100 mg in 250 mL D_5W or NS (if patient is fluid-restricted, may concentrate up to a maximum of 0.5 mg/mL); initial dose: 0.02-0.08 mg/kg (~1 mg to 5 mg in 70 kg adult) initially and either repeated at 5-15 minute intervals until adequate sedation is achieved or continuous infusion rates of 0.04-0.2 mg/kg/hour and titrate to reach desired level of sedation

Elderly: I.V.: Conscious sedation: Initial: 0.5 mg slow I.V.; give no more than 1.5 mg in a 2-minute period; if additional titration is needed, give no more than 1 mg over 2 minutes, waiting another 2 or more minutes to evaluate sedative effect; a total dose of >3.5 mg is rarely necessary

Dosage adjustment in renal impairment:

Hemodialysis: Supplemental dose is not necessary

Peritoneal dialysis: Significant drug removal is unlikely based on physiochemical characteristics

Mechanism of Action Binds to stereospecific benzodiazepine receptors on the postsynaptic GABA neuron at several sites within the central nervous system, including the limbic system, reticular formation. Enhancement of the inhibitory effect of GABA on neuronal excitability results by increased neuronal membrane permeability to chloride ions. This shift in chloride ions results in hyperpolarization (a less excitable state) and stabilization.

Contraindications Hypersensitivity to midazolam or any component of the formulation, including benzyl alcohol (cross-sensitivity with other benzodiazepines may exist); parenteral form is not for intrathecal or epidural injection; narrow-angle glaucoma; concurrent use of potent inhibitors of CYP3A4 (amprenavir, atazanavir, or ritonavir); pregnancy

Warnings/Precautions May cause severe respiratory depression, respiratory arrest, or apnea. Use with extreme caution, particularly in noncritical care settings. Appropriate resuscitative equipment and qualified personnel must be available for administration and monitoring. Initial dosing must be cautiously titrated and individualized, particularly in elderly or debilitated patients, patients with hepatic impairment (including alcoholics), or in renal impairment, particularly if other CNS depressants (including opiates) are used concurrently. Initial doses in elderly or debilitated patients should not exceed 2.5 mg. Use with caution in patients with respiratory disease or impaired gag reflex. Use during upper airway procedures may increase risk of hypoventilation. Prolonged responses have been noted following extended administration by continuous infusion (possibly due to metabolite accumulation) or in the presence of drugs which inhibit midazolam metabolism.

May cause hypotension - hemodynamic events are more common in pediatric patients or patients with hemodynamic instability. Hypotension and/or respiratory depression may occur more frequently in patients who have received narcotic analgesics. Use with caution in obese patients, chronic renal failure, and CHF. Parenteral form contains benzyl alcohol - avoid rapid injection in neonates or prolonged infusions. Does not protect against increases in heart rate or blood pressure during intubation. Should not be used in shock, coma, or acute alcohol intoxication. Avoid intra-arterial administration or extravasation of parenteral formulation.

Causes CNS depression (dose-related) resulting in sedation, dizziness, confusion, or ataxia which may impair physical and mental capabilities. Patients must be cautioned about performing tasks which require mental alertness (eg, operating machinery or driving). A minimum of 1 day should elapse after midazolam administration before attempting these tasks. Use with caution in patients receiving other CNS depressants or psychoactive agents. Effects with other sedative drugs or ethanol may be potentiated. Benzodiazepines have been associated with falls and traumatic injury and should be used with extreme caution in patients who are at risk of these events (especially the elderly).

Midazolam causes anterograde amnesia. Paradoxical reactions, including hyperactive or aggressive behavior have been reported with benzodiazepines, particularly in adolescent/pediatric or psychiatric patients. Does not have analgesic, antidepressant, or antipsychotic properties.

Benzodiazepines have been associated with dependence and acute withdrawal symptoms on discontinuation or reduction in dose. Acute withdrawal, including seizures, may be precipitated after administration of flumazenil to patients receiving long-term benzodiazepine therapy.

Drug Interactions Substrate of CYP2B6 (minor), 3A4 (major); **Inhibits** CYP2C8/9 (weak), 3A4 (weak)

CNS depressants: Sedative effects and/or respiratory depression may be additive with CNS depressants; includes ethanol, barbiturates, narcotic analgesics, and other sedative agents; monitor for increased effect. **If narcotics or other CNS depressants are administered concomitantly, the midazolam dose should be reduced by 30% if <65 years of age, or by at least 50% if >65 years of age.**

CYP3A4 inducers: CYP3A4 inducers may decrease the levels/effects of midazolam. Example inducers include aminoglutethimide, carbamazepine, nafcillin, nevirapine, phenobarbital, phenytoin, and rifamycins.

CYP3A4 inhibitors: May increase the levels/effects of midazolam. Example inhibitors include azole antifungals, clarithromycin, diclofenac, doxycycline, erythromycin, imatinib, isoniazid, nefazodone, nicardipine, propofol, protease inhibitors, quinidine, telithromycin, and verapamil.

Levodopa: Therapeutic effects may be diminished in some patients following the addition of a benzodiazepine; limited/inconsistent data

Oral contraceptives: May decrease the clearance of some benzodiazepines (those which undergo oxidative metabolism); monitor for increased benzodiazepine effect

Saquinavir: A 56% reduction in clearance and a doubling of midazolam's half-life were seen with concurrent administration with saquinavir.

Theophylline: May partially antagonize some of the effects of benzodiazepines; monitor for decreased response; may require higher doses for sedation

Ethanol/Nutrition/Herb Interactions

Ethanol: Avoid ethanol (may increase CNS depression).

Food: Grapefruit juice may increase serum concentrations of midazolam; avoid concurrent use with oral form.

Herb/Nutraceutical: Avoid concurrent use with St John's wort (may decrease midazolam levels, may increase CNS depression). Avoid concurrent use with valerian, kava kava, gotu kola (may increase CNS depression).

Dietary Considerations Injection: Sodium content of 1 mL: 0.14 mEq

(Continued)

Midazolam *(Continued)*

Pharmacodynamics/Kinetics

Onset of action: I.M.: Sedation: ~15 minutes; I.V.: 1-5 minutes
 Peak effect: I.M.: 0.5-1 hour

Duration: I.M.: Up to 6 hours; Mean: 2 hours

Absorption: Oral: Rapid

Distribution: V_d: 0.8-2.5 L/kg; increased with congestive heart failure (CHF) and chronic renal failure

Protein binding: 95%

Metabolism: Extensively hepatic via CYP3A4

Bioavailability: Mean: 45%

Half-life elimination: 1-4 hours; prolonged with cirrhosis, congestive heart failure, obesity, and elderly

Excretion: Urine (as glucuronide conjugated metabolites); feces (~2% to 10%)

Pregnancy Risk Factor D

Lactation Enters breast milk/not recommended (AAP rates "of concern")

Dosage Forms

Injection, solution: 1 mg/mL (2 mL, 5 mL, 10 mL); 5 mg/mL (1 mL, 2 mL, 5 mL, 10 mL) [contains benzyl alcohol 1%]

Injection, solution [preservative free]: 1 mg/mL (2 mL, 5 mL); 5 mg/mL (1 mL, 2 mL)

Syrup: 2 mg/mL (118 mL) [contains sodium benzoate; cherry flavor]

Selected Readings

Dionne RA, Yagiela JA, Moore PA, et al, "Comparing Efficacy and Safety of Four Intravenous Sedation Regimens in Dental Outpatients," *Am Dent Assoc*, 2001, 132(6):740-51.

Midazolam Hydrochloride *see* Midazolam *on page 1040*

Midodrine *(MI doe dreen)*

U.S. Brand Names Orvaten™; ProAmatine®

Canadian Brand Names Amatine®

Generic Available Yes

Synonyms Midodrine Hydrochloride

Pharmacologic Category Alpha$_1$ Agonist

Use Orphan drug: Treatment of symptomatic orthostatic hypotension

Unlabeled/Investigational Use Investigational: Management of urinary incontinence

Local Anesthetic/Vasoconstrictor Precautions No information available to require special precautions

Effects on Dental Treatment Key adverse event(s) related to dental treatment: Xerostomia (normal salivary flow resumes upon discontinuation).

Causes of Orthostatic Hypotension

Primary Autonomic Causes
Pure autonomic failure (Bradbury-Eggleston syndrome, idiopathic orthostatic hypotension)
Autonomic failure with multiple system atrophy (Shy-Drager syndrome)
Familial dysautonomia (Riley-Day syndrome)
Dopamine beta-hydroxylase deficiency
Secondary Autonomic Causes
Chronic alcoholism
Parkinson's disease
Diabetes mellitus
Porphyria
Amyloidosis
Various carcinomas
Vitamin B_1 or B_{12} deficiency
Nonautonomic Causes
Hypovolemia (such as associated with hemorrhage, burns, or hemodialysis) and dehydration
Diminished homeostatic regulation (such as associated with aging, pregnancy, fever, or prolonged bedrest)
Medications (eg, antihypertensives, insulin, tricyclic antidepressants)

Common Adverse Effects

>10%:
 Cardiovascular: Supine hypertension (7% to 13%)

Dermatologic: Piloerection (13%), pruritus (12%)
Genitourinary: Urinary urgency, retention, or polyuria, dysuria (up to 13%)
Neuromuscular & skeletal: Paresthesia (18%)
1% to 10%:
Central nervous system: Chills (5%), pain (5%)
Dermatologic: Rash (2%)
Gastrointestinal: Abdominal pain

Mechanism of Action Midodrine forms an active metabolite, desglymidodrine, that is an alpha$_1$-agonist. This agent increases arteriolar and venous tone resulting in a rise in standing, sitting, and supine systolic and diastolic blood pressure in patients with orthostatic hypotension. See table on previous page.

Drug Interactions
Increased Effect/Toxicity: Concomitant fludrocortisone results in hypernatremia or an increase in intraocular pressure and glaucoma. Bradycardia may be accentuated with concomitant administration of cardiac glycosides, psychotherapeutics, and beta-blockers. Alpha agonists may increase the pressure effects and alpha antagonists may negate the effects of midodrine.

Pharmacodynamics/Kinetics
Onset of action: ~1 hour
Duration: 2-3 hours
Absorption: Rapid
Distribution: V$_d$ (desglymidodrine): <1.6 L/kg; poorly across membrane (eg, blood brain barrier)
Protein binding: Minimal
Metabolism: Hepatic; midodrine is a prodrug which undergoes rapid deglycination to desglymidodrine (active metabolite); metabolism occurs in many tissues and plasma
Bioavailability: Desglymidodrine: 93%
Half-life elimination: Desglymidodrine: ~3-4 hours; Midodrine: 25 minutes
Time to peak, serum: Desglymidodrine: 1-2 hours; Midodrine: 30 minutes
Excretion: Urine (2% to 4%)
Clearance: Desglymidodrine: 385 mL/minute (predominantly by renal secretion)

Pregnancy Risk Factor C

Midodrine Hydrochloride *see* Midodrine *on page 1044*
Midol® Cramp and Body Aches [OTC] *see* Ibuprofen *on page 808*
Midol® Extended Relief *see* Naproxen *on page 1089*
Midrin® *see* Acetaminophen, Isometheptene, and Dichloralphenazone *on page 44*
Mifeprex® *see* Mifepristone *on page 1045*

Mifepristone (mi FE pris tone)

Related Information
Endocrine Disorders and Pregnancy *on page 1659*
U.S. Brand Names Mifeprex®
Generic Available No
Synonyms RU-486; RU-38486
Pharmacologic Category Abortifacient; Antineoplastic Agent, Hormone Antagonist; Antiprogestin
Use Medical termination of intrauterine pregnancy, through day 49 of pregnancy. Patients may need treatment with misoprostol and possibly surgery to complete therapy
Unlabeled/Investigational Use Treatment of unresectable meningioma; has been studied in the treatment of breast cancer, ovarian cancer, and adrenal cortical carcinoma
Local Anesthetic/Vasoconstrictor Precautions No information available to require special precautions
Effects on Dental Treatment No significant effects or complications reported
Common Adverse Effects Vaginal bleeding and uterine cramping are expected to occur when this medication is used to terminate a pregnancy; 90% of women using this medication for this purpose also report adverse reactions. Bleeding or spotting occurs in most women for a period of 9-16 days. Up to 8% of women will experience some degree of bleeding or spotting for 30 days or more. In some cases, bleeding may be prolonged and heavy, potentially leading to hypovolemic shock.

>10%:
Central nervous system: Headache (2% to 31%), dizziness (1% to 12%)
Gastrointestinal: Abdominal pain (cramping) (96%), nausea (43% to 61%), vomiting (18% to 26%), diarrhea (12% to 20%)
(Continued)

Mifepristone *(Continued)*

Genitourinary: Uterine cramping (83%)

1% to 10%:

Cardiovascular: Syncope (1%)

Central nervous system: Fatigue (10%), fever (4%), insomnia (3%), anxiety (2%), fainting (2%)

Gastrointestinal: Dyspepsia (3%)

Genitourinary: Uterine hemorrhage (5%), vaginitis (3%), pelvic pain (2%), endometriosis/salpingitis/pelvic inflammatory disease (1%)

Hematologic: Decreased hemoglobin >2 g/dL (6%), anemia (2%), leukorrhea (2%)

Neuromuscular & skeletal: Back pain (9%), rigors (3%), leg pain (2%), weakness (2%)

Respiratory: Sinusitis (2%)

Miscellaneous: Viral infection (4%)

Restrictions Investigators wishing to obtain the agent for use in oncology patients must apply for a patient-specific IND from the FDA. Mifepristone will be supplied only to licensed physicians who sign and return a "Prescriber's Agreement." Distribution of mifepristone will be subject to specific requirements imposed by the distributor. Mifepristone will **not** be available to the public through licensed pharmacies. A patient medication guide is available and must be dispensed with the medication; the FDA-approved medication guide is available at http://www.fda.gov/cder/Offices/ODS/labeling.htm.

Not available in Canada

Mechanism of Action Mifepristone, a synthetic steroid, competitively binds to the intracellular progesterone receptor, blocking the effects of progesterone. When used for the termination of pregnancy, this leads to contraction-inducing activity in the myometrium. In the absence of progesterone, mifepristone acts as a partial progesterone agonist. Mifepristone also has weak antiglucocorticoid and antiandrogenic properties; it blocks the feedback effect of cortisol on corticotropin secretion.

Drug Interactions

Cytochrome P450 Effect: Substrate of CYP3A4 (minor); **Inhibits** CYP2D6 (weak), 3A4 (weak)

Increased Effect/Toxicity: There are no reported interactions. It might be anticipated that the concurrent administration of mifepristone and a progestin would result in an attenuation of the effects of one or both agents.

Pharmacodynamics/Kinetics

Absorption: Oral: rapid

Protein binding: 98% to albumin and α_1-acid glycoprotein

Metabolism: Hepatic via CYP3A4 to three metabolites (may possess some antiprogestin and antiglucocorticoid activity)

Bioavailability: Oral: 69%

Half-life elimination: Terminal: 18 hours following a slower phase where 50% eliminated between 12-72 hours

Time to peak: Oral: 90 minutes

Excretion: Feces (83%); urine (9%)

Pregnancy Risk Factor X

Miglitol *(MIG li tol)*

Related Information

Endocrine Disorders and Pregnancy *on page 1659*

U.S. Brand Names Glyset®

Canadian Brand Names Glyset®

Generic Available No

Pharmacologic Category Antidiabetic Agent, Alpha-Glucosidase Inhibitor

Use Type 2 diabetes mellitus (noninsulin-dependent, NIDDM):

Monotherapy adjunct to diet to improve glycemic control in patients with type 2 diabetes mellitus (noninsulin-dependent, NIDDM) whose hyperglycemia cannot be managed with diet alone

Combination therapy with a sulfonylurea when diet plus either miglitol or a sulfonylurea alone do not result in adequate glycemic control. The effect of miglitol to enhance glycemic control is additive to that of sulfonylureas when used in combination.

Local Anesthetic/Vasoconstrictor Precautions No information available to require special precautions

Effects on Dental Treatment No significant effects or complications reported

Common Adverse Effects
>10%: Gastrointestinal: Flatulence (42%), diarrhea (29%), abdominal pain (12%)

1% to 10%: Dermatologic: Rash

Mechanism of Action In contrast to sulfonylureas, miglitol does not enhance insulin secretion; the antihyperglycemic action of miglitol results from a reversible inhibition of membrane-bound intestinal alpha-glucosidases which hydrolyze oligosaccharides and disaccharides to glucose and other monosaccharides in the brush border of the small intestine; in diabetic patients, this enzyme inhibition results in delayed glucose absorption and lowering of postprandial hyperglycemia

Drug Interactions
Decreased Effect: Miglitol may decrease the absorption and bioavailability of digoxin, propranolol, and ranitidine. Digestive enzymes (amylase, pancreatin, charcoal) may reduce the effect of miglitol and should **not** be taken concomitantly.

Pharmacodynamics/Kinetics
Absorption: Saturable at high doses: 25 mg dose: Completely absorbed; 100 mg dose: 50% to 70% absorbed

Distribution: V_d: 0.18 L/kg

Protein binding: <4%

Metabolism: None

Half-life elimination: ~2 hours

Time to peak: 2-3 hours

Excretion: Urine (as unchanged drug)

Pregnancy Risk Factor B

Miglustat (MIG loo stat)

U.S. Brand Names Zavesca®

Canadian Brand Names Zavesca®

Generic Available No

Synonyms OGT-918

Pharmacologic Category Enzyme Inhibitor

Use Treatment of mild-to-moderate type 1 Gaucher disease when enzyme replacement therapy is not a therapeutic option

Local Anesthetic/Vasoconstrictor Precautions No information available to require special precautions

Effects on Dental Treatment No significant effects or complications reported

Common Adverse Effects Percentages reported from open-label, uncontrolled monotherapy trials.

>10%:
Central nervous system: Headache (21% to 22%), dizziness (up to 11%)

Gastrointestinal: Diarrhea (89%; up to 100% in other studies), weight loss (39% to 67%), abdominal pain (18% to 50%), flatulence (29% to 44%), nausea (14% to 22%), vomiting (4% to 11%), cramps (up to 11%)

Neuromuscular & skeletal: Tremor (11%; up to 30% in other studies), leg cramps (4% to 11%),

Ocular: visual disturbances (up to 17%)

1% to 10%:
Central nervous system: headache (up to 6%)

Endocrine & metabolic: Menstrual disorder (up to 6%)

Gastrointestinal: Anorexia (up to 7%), dyspepsia (up to 7%), epigastric pain (up to 6%)

Hematologic: Thrombocytopenia (6% to 7%)

Neuromuscular & skeletal: Paresthesia (up to 7%)

Mechanism of Action Miglustat inhibits the enzyme needed to produce glycosphingolipids and decreases the rate of glycosphingolipid glucosylceramide formation. Glucosylceramide accumulates in type 1 Gaucher disease, causing complications specific to this disease.

Drug Interactions
Decreased Effect: Miglustat increases the clearance of imiglucerase; combination therapy is not indicated.

Pharmacodynamics/Kinetics
Distribution: V_d: 83-105 L

Protein binding: No binding to plasma proteins

Bioavailability: 97%

Half-life elimination: 6-7 hours

Time to peak, plasma: 2-2.5 hours

Excretion: Urine (as unchanged drug)

Pregnancy Risk Factor X

Migquin *see* Acetaminophen, Isometheptene, and Dichloralphenazone *on page 44*

Migranal® *see* Dihydroergotamine *on page 477*

Migratine *see* Acetaminophen, Isometheptene, and Dichloralphenazone *on page 44*

Migrazone® *see* Acetaminophen, Isometheptene, and Dichloralphenazone *on page 44*

Migrin-A *see* Acetaminophen, Isometheptene, and Dichloralphenazone *on page 44*

Milk of Magnesia *see* Magnesium Hydroxide *on page 961*

Milrinone (MIL ri none)

Related Information
Cardiovascular Diseases *on page 1636*
U.S. Brand Names Primacor®
Canadian Brand Names Primacor®
Generic Available Yes
Synonyms Milrinone Lactate
Pharmacologic Category Phosphodiesterase Enzyme Inhibitor
Use Short-term I.V. therapy of congestive heart failure; calcium antagonist intoxication
Local Anesthetic/Vasoconstrictor Precautions No information available to require special precautions
Effects on Dental Treatment No significant effects or complications reported
Common Adverse Effects
>10%: Cardiovascular: Ventricular arrhythmia (ectopy 9%, NSVT 3%, sustained ventricular tachycardia 1%, ventricular fibrillation <1%); life-threatening arrhythmia are infrequent, often associated with underlying factors (eg, pre-existing arrhythmia, electrolyte disturbances, catheter insertion)
1% to 10%:
Cardiovascular: Supraventricular arrhythmia (4%), hypotension
Central nervous system: Headache
Mechanism of Action Phosphodiesterase inhibitor resulting in vasodilation
Pharmacodynamics/Kinetics
Onset of action: I.V.: 5-15 minutes
Serum level: I.V.: Following a 125 mcg/kg dose, peak plasma concentrations ~1000 ng/mL were observed at 2 minutes postinjection, decreasing to <100 ng/mL in 2 hours
Drug concentration levels:
Therapeutic:
Serum levels of 166 ng/mL, achieved during I.V. infusions of 0.25-1 mcg/kg/minute, were associated with sustained hemodynamic benefit in severe congestive heart failure patients over a 24-hour period
Maximum beneficial effects on cardiac output and pulmonary capillary wedge pressure following I.V. infusion have been associated with plasma milrinone concentrations of 150-250 ng/mL
Toxic: Serum concentrations >250-300 ng/mL have been associated with marked reductions in mean arterial pressure and tachycardia; however, more studies are required to determine the toxic serum levels for milrinone
Distribution: V_{dss}: 0.32 L/kg; Severe congestive heart failure (CHF): V_d: 0.33-0.47 L/kg; not significantly bound to tissues; excretion in breast milk unknown
Protein binding, plasma: ~70%
Metabolism: Hepatic (12%)
Half-life elimination: I.V.: 136 minutes in patients with CHF; patients with severe CHF have a more prolonged half-life, with values ranging from 1.7-2.7 hours. Patients with CHF have a reduction in the systemic clearance of milrinone, resulting in a prolonged elimination half-life. Alternatively, one study reported that 1 month of therapy with milrinone did not change the pharmacokinetic parameters for patients with CHF despite improvement in cardiac function.
Excretion: I.V.: Urine (85% as unchanged drug) within 24 hours; active tubular secretion is a major elimination pathway for milrinone
Clearance: I.V. bolus: 25.9 ± 5.7 L/hour (0.37 L/hour/kg); Severe congestive heart failure: 0.11-0.13 L/hour/kg. The reduction in clearance may be a result of reduced renal function. Creatinine clearance values were $\frac{1}{2}$ those reported for healthy adults in patients with severe congestive heart failure (52 vs 119 mL/minute).
Pregnancy Risk Factor C

Milrinone Lactate *see* Milrinone *on page 1048*
Miltown® [DSC] *see* Meprobamate *on page 993*

Mindal DM [DSC] *see* Guaifenesin and Dextromethorphan *on page 754*

Mineral Oil, Petrolatum, Lanolin, Cetyl Alcohol, and Glycerin *see* Lanolin, Cetyl Alcohol, Glycerin, Petrolatum, and Mineral Oil *on page 896*

Minidyne® [OTC] *see* Povidone-Iodine *on page 1262*

Minipress® *see* Prazosin *on page 1267*

Minitran™ *see* Nitroglycerin *on page 1120*

Minizide® *see* Prazosin and Polythiazide *on page 1268*

Minocin® *see* Minocycline *on page 1049*

Minocycline (mi noe SYE kleen)

Related Information
Sexually-Transmitted Diseases *on page 1674*

U.S. Brand Names Dynacin®; Minocin®; myrac™; Solodyn™

Canadian Brand Names Alti-Minocycline; Apo-Minocycline®; Gen-Minocycline; Minocin®; Novo-Minocycline; PMS-Minocycline; Rhoxal-minocycline

Mexican Brand Names Minocin®

Generic Available Yes: Excludes extended release tablet

Synonyms Minocycline Hydrochloride

Pharmacologic Category Antibiotic, Tetracycline Derivative

Use Treatment of susceptible bacterial infections of both gram-negative and gram-positive organisms; treatment of anthrax (inhalational, cutaneous, and gastrointestinal); acne; meningococcal (asymptomatic) carrier state; Rickettsial diseases (including Rocky Mountain spotted fever, Q fever); nongonococcal urethritis, gonorrhea; acute intestinal amebiasis

Local Anesthetic/Vasoconstrictor Precautions No information available to require special precautions

Effects on Dental Treatment Key adverse event(s) related to dental treatment: Discoloration of teeth (children). Opportunistic "superinfection" with *Candida albicans*; tetracyclines are not recommended for use during pregnancy or in children ≤8 years of age since they have been reported to cause enamel hypoplasia and permanent teeth discoloration. The use of tetracycline's should only be used in these patients if other agents are contraindicated or alternative antimicrobials will not eradicate the organism. Long-term use associated with oral candidiasis.

Common Adverse Effects Frequency not defined.

Cardiovascular: Myocarditis, pericarditis, vasculitis

Central nervous system: Bulging fontanels, dizziness, fatigue, fever, headache, hypoesthesia, malaise, mood changes, paresthesia, pseudotumor cerebri, sedation, seizure, somnolence, vertigo

Dermatologic: Alopecia, angioedema, erythema multiforme, erythema nodosum, erythematous rash, exfoliative dermatitis, hyperpigmentation of nails, maculopapular rash, photosensitivity, pigmentation of the skin and mucous membranes, pruritus, Stevens-Johnson syndrome, toxic epidermal necrolysis, urticaria

Endocrine & metabolic: Thyroid discoloration, thyroid dysfunction

Gastrointestinal: Anorexia, diarrhea, dyspepsia, dysphagia, enamel hypoplasia, enterocolitis, esophageal ulcerations, esophagitis, glossitis, inflammatory lesions (oral/anogenital), moniliasis, nausea, oral cavity discoloration, pancreatitis, pseudomembranous colitis, stomatitis, tooth discoloration, vomiting, xerostomia

Genitourinary: Balanitis, vulvovaginitis

Hematologic: Agranulocytosis, eosinophilia, hemolytic anemia, leukopenia, neutropenia, pancytopenia, thrombocytopenia

Hepatic: Hepatic cholestasis, hepatic failure, hepatitis, hyperbilirubinemia, jaundice, liver enzyme increases

Neuromuscular & skeletal: Arthralgia, arthritis, bone discoloration, joint stiffness, joint swelling, myalgia

Otic: Hearing loss, tinnitus

Renal: Acute renal failure, BUN increased, interstitial nephritis

Respiratory: Asthma, bronchospasm, cough, dyspnea, pneumonitis, pulmonary infiltrate (with eosinophilia)

Miscellaneous: Anaphylaxis, hypersensitivity, lupus erythematosus, lupus-like syndrome, serum sickness

Mechanism of Action Inhibits bacterial protein synthesis by binding with the 30S and possibly the 50S ribosomal subunit(s) of susceptible bacteria; cell wall synthesis is not affected

Drug Interactions
Increased Effect/Toxicity: Minocycline may increase the effect of warfarin. Retinoic acid derivatives may increase risk of pseudotumor cerebri.
(Continued)

Minocycline *(Continued)*

Decreased Effect: Calcium-, magnesium-, or aluminum-containing antacids, bile acid sequestrants, bismuth, oral contraceptives, iron, zinc, sodium bicarbonate, penicillins, cimetidine, quinapril may decrease absorption of tetracyclines. Methoxyflurane anesthesia (when concurrent with tetracyclines) may cause fatal nephrotoxicity. Tetracyclines may reduce bactericidal efficacy of penicillins and cephalosporins. Tetracycline may reduce the efficacy of the live, attenuated typhoid vaccine (Ty21a).

Pharmacodynamics/Kinetics

Absorption: Well absorbed

Distribution: Majority deposits for extended periods in fat; crosses placenta; enters breast milk

Protein binding: 70% to 75%

Half-life elimination: 16 hours (range: 11-23 hours)

Time to peak: Capsule, pellet filled: 1-4 hours; Extended release tablet: 3.5-4 hours

Excretion: Urine

Pregnancy Risk Factor D

Minocycline Hydrochloride *see* Minocycline *on page 1049*

Minocycline Hydrochloride (Periodontal)

(mi noe SYE kleen hye droe KLOR ide pair ee oh DON tol)

Related Information

Minocycline *on page 1049*

U.S. Brand Names Arestin™

Generic Available No

Pharmacologic Category Antibiotic, Tetracycline Derivative

Dental Use Adjunct to scaling and root planing procedures for reduction of pocket depth in patients with adult periodontitis. May be used as part of a periodontal maintenance program which includes good oral hygiene, scaling, and root planing.

Local Anesthetic/Vasoconstrictor Precautions No information available to require special precautions

Effects on Dental Treatment Key adverse event(s) related to dental treatment: Patients should avoid the following postadministration: Eating hard, crunchy, or sticky foods for 1 week; brushing for a 12-hour period; touching treated areas; use of interproximal cleaning devices for 10 days.

Significant Adverse Effects Frequency not defined.

Central nervous system: Headache, pain

Gastrointestinal: Periodontitis, tooth disorder, dental caries, dental pain, gingivitis, stomatitis, mouth ulceration, dyspepsia, dental infection, mucous membrane disorder

Respiratory: Pharyngitis

Miscellaneous: Infection, flu syndrome

Dental Usual Dosing Arestin™ is a variable-dose product; dependent upon the size, shape, and number of pockets being treated.

Administration of Arestin™ does not require local anesthesia. Professional subgingival administration is accomplished by inserting the unit-dose cartridge to the base of the periodontal pocket and then pressing the thumb ring in the handle mechanism to expel the powder while gradually withdrawing the tip from the base of the pocket. The handle mechanism should be sterilized between patients. Arestin™ does not have to be removed (it is bioresorbable) nor is an adhesive dressing required.

Mechanism of Action Minocycline, a member of the tetracycline class of antibiotics, has a broad spectrum of activity. It is bacteriostatic and exerts its antimicrobial activity by inhibiting protein synthesis.

Contraindications Known hypersensitivity to minocycline, tetracyclines, or any component of the formulation; pregnancy

Warnings/Precautions The use of the tetracycline class during tooth development (last half of pregnancy, infancy, and childhood to 8 years of age) may cause permanent discoloration of the teeth (yellow-gray brown). This adverse reaction is more common during long-term use of the drugs, but has been observed following repeated short-term courses. Enamel hypoplasia has also been reported. Tetracycline drugs, therefore, should not be used in this age group, or in pregnant or nursing women, unless the potential benefits are considered to outweigh the potential risks. Results of animal studies indicate that tetracyclines cross the placenta, are found in fetal tissues, and can have toxic effects on the developing fetus (often related to retardation of skeletal development). Evidence of embryotoxicity has also been noted in animals treated early in pregnancy. If any tetracyclines are used during pregnancy, or if the patient becomes pregnant while taking this drug, the patient should be apprised of the potential hazard to the fetus. Photosensitivity manifested by an exaggerated sunburn reaction has been observed in some individuals taking tetracyclines. Patients apt to be exposed to direct sunlight or ultraviolet light should be advised that this reaction can occur with tetracycline drugs, and treatment should be discontinued at the first evidence of skin erythema.

The use of Arestin™ in an acutely abscessed periodontal pocket has not been studied and is not recommended. While no overgrowth by opportunistic microorganisms, such as yeast, were noted during clinical studies, as with other antimicrobials, the use of Arestin™ may result in overgrowth of nonsusceptible microorganisms including fungi. The effects of treatment for >6 months have not been studied. Arestin™ should be used with caution in patients having a history of predisposition to oral candidiasis. The safety and effectiveness of Arestin™ have not been established for the treatment of periodontitis in patients with coexistent oral candidiasis. Arestin™ has not been clinically tested in immunocompromised patients (such as those immunocompromised by diabetes, chemotherapy, radiation therapy, or infection with HIV). If superinfection is suspected, appropriate measures should be taken. Arestin™ has not been clinically tested for use in the regeneration of alveolar bone, either in preparation for or in conjunction with the placement of endosseous (dental) implants or in the treatment of failing implants.

Pregnancy Risk Factor D

Dosage Forms Injection, powder, sustained release [microspheres for subgingival application]: 1 mg (12s) [each unit-dose cartridge delivers minocycline hydrochloride equivalent to minocycline free base 1 mg]

Minoxidil (mi NOKS i dil)

Related Information
Cardiovascular Diseases *on page 1636*

U.S. Brand Names Loniten®; Rogaine® Extra Strength for Men [OTC]; Rogaine® for Men [OTC]; Rogaine® for Women [OTC]

Canadian Brand Names Apo-Gain®; Minox; Rogaine®

Mexican Brand Names Regaine®

Generic Available Yes

Pharmacologic Category Topical Skin Product; Vasodilator

Use Management of severe hypertension (usually in combination with a diuretic and beta-blocker); treatment (topical formulation) of alopecia androgenetica in males and females

Local Anesthetic/Vasoconstrictor Precautions No information available to require special precautions

Effects on Dental Treatment No significant effects or complications reported

Common Adverse Effects

Oral: Incidence of reactions not always reported.
Cardiovascular: Peripheral edema (7%), sodium and water retention, CHF, tachycardia, angina pectoris, pericardial effusion with or without tamponade, pericarditis, ECG changes (T-wave changes, 60%), rebound hypertension (in children after a gradual withdrawal)
Central nervous system: Headache (rare), fatigue
Dermatologic: Hypertrichosis (common, 80%), transient pruritus, changes in pigmentation (rare), serosanguineous bullae (rare), rash (rare), Stevens-Johnson syndrome
Hepatic: Increased alkaline phosphatase
Renal: Transient increase in serum BUN and creatinine
Respiratory: Pulmonary edema

Topical: Incidence of adverse events is not always reported.
Cardiovascular: Increased left ventricular end-diastolic volume, increased cardiac output, increased left ventricular mass, dizziness, tachycardia, edema, transient chest pain, palpitation, increase or decrease in blood pressure, increase or decrease in pulse rate (1.5%, placebo 1.6%)
Central nervous system: Headache, dizziness, taste alterations, faintness, lightheadedness (3.4%, placebo 3.5%), vertigo (1.2%, placebo 1.2%), anxiety (rare), mental depression (rare), fatigue (rare 0.4%, placebo 1%)
Dermatologic: Local irritation, dryness, erythema, allergic contact dermatitis (7.4%, placebo 5.4%), pruritus, scaling/flaking, eczema, seborrhea, papular rash, folliculitis, local erythema, flushing, exacerbation of hair loss, alopecia, hypertrichosis, increased hair growth outside the area of application (face, beard, eyebrows, ear, arm)
Gastrointestinal: Diarrhea, nausea, vomiting (4.3%, placebo 6.6%), weight gain (1.2%, placebo 1.3%)

(Continued)

Minoxidil *(Continued)*

Neuromuscular & skeletal: Fractures, back pain, retrosternal chest pain of muscular origin, tendonitis (2.6%, placebo 2.2%), weakness

Ocular: Conjunctivitis, visual disturbances, decreased visual acuity

Respiratory: Bronchitis, upper respiratory infection, sinusitis (7.2%, placebo 8.6%)

Mechanism of Action Produces vasodilation by directly relaxing arteriolar smooth muscle, with little effect on veins; effects may be mediated by cyclic AMP; stimulation of hair growth is secondary to vasodilation, increased cutaneous blood flow and stimulation of resting hair follicles

Drug Interactions

Increased Effect/Toxicity: Concurrent use of guanethidine can cause severe orthostasis; avoid concurrent use - discontinue 1-3 weeks prior to initiating minoxidil. Effects of other antihypertensives may be additive with minoxidil.

Pharmacodynamics/Kinetics

Onset of action: Hypotensive: Oral: ~30 minutes

Peak effect: 2-8 hours

Duration: 2-5 days

Protein binding: None

Metabolism: 88%, primarily via glucuronidation

Bioavailability: Oral: 90%

Half-life elimination: Adults: 3.5-4.2 hours

Excretion: Urine (12% as unchanged drug)

Pregnancy Risk Factor C

Mintab DM *see* Guaifenesin and Dextromethorphan *on page 754*

Mintezol® *see* Thiabendazole *on page 1475*

Mintox Extra Strength [OTC] *see* Aluminum Hydroxide, Magnesium Hydroxide, and Simethicone *on page 81*

Mintox Plus [OTC] *see* Aluminum Hydroxide, Magnesium Hydroxide, and Simethicone *on page 81*

Miochol-E® *see* Acetylcholine *on page 46*

Miostat® *see* Carbachol *on page 260*

MiraLax™ *see* Polyethylene Glycol 3350 *on page 1253*

Mirapex® *see* Pramipexole *on page 1262*

Miraphen PSE *see* Guaifenesin and Pseudoephedrine *on page 755*

Mircette® *see* Ethinyl Estradiol and Desogestrel *on page 592*

Mirena® *see* Levonorgestrel *on page 916*

Mirtazapine *(mir TAZ a peen)*

U.S. Brand Names Remeron®; Remeron SolTab®

Canadian Brand Names CO Mirtazapine; Gen-Mirtazapine; Novo-Mirtazapine; PMS-Mirtazapine; Remeron®; Remeron® RD; Rhoxal-mirtazapine; Sandoz-Mirtazapine; Sandoz-Mirtazapine FC

Mexican Brand Names Remeron®

Generic Available Yes

Pharmacologic Category Antidepressant, Alpha-2 Antagonist

Use Treatment of depression

Local Anesthetic/Vasoconstrictor Precautions Although mirtazapine is not a tricyclic antidepressant, it does block norepinephrine reuptake within CNS synapses as part of its mechanisms. It has been suggested that vasoconstrictor be administered with caution and to monitor vital signs in dental patients taking antidepressants that affect norepinephrine in this way, including mirtazapine.

Effects on Dental Treatment Key adverse event(s) related to dental treatment: Significant xerostomia (normal salivary flow resumes upon discontinuation).

Common Adverse Effects

>10%:

Central nervous system: Somnolence (54%)

Endocrine & metabolic: Increased cholesterol

Gastrointestinal: Constipation (13%), xerostomia (25%), increased appetite (17%), weight gain (12%; weight gain of >7% reported in 8% of adults, ≤49% of pediatric patients)

1% to 10%:

Cardiovascular: Hypertension, vasodilatation, peripheral edema (2%), edema (1%)

Central nervous system: Dizziness (7%), abnormal dreams (4%), abnormal thoughts (3%), confusion (2%), malaise

Endocrine & metabolic: Increased triglycerides
Gastrointestinal: Vomiting, anorexia, abdominal pain
Genitourinary: Urinary frequency (2%)
Neuromuscular & skeletal: Myalgia (2%), back pain (2%), arthralgia, tremor (2%), weakness (8%)
Respiratory: Dyspnea (1%)
Miscellaneous: Flu-like symptoms (5%), thirst

Restrictions A medication guide concerning the use of antidepressants in children and teenagers can be found on the FDA website at http://www.fda.gov/cder/Offices/ODS/labeling.htm. It should be dispensed to parents or guardians of children and teenagers receiving this medication.

Mechanism of Action Mirtazapine is a tetracyclic antidepressant that works by its central presynaptic alpha$_2$-adrenergic antagonist effects, which results in increased release of norepinephrine and serotonin. It is also a potent antagonist of 5-HT$_2$ and 5-HT$_3$ serotonin receptors and H1 histamine receptors and a moderate peripheral alpha$_1$-adrenergic and muscarinic antagonist; it does not inhibit the reuptake of norepinephrine or serotonin.

Drug Interactions
 Cytochrome P450 Effect: Substrate of CYP1A2 (major), 2C8/9 (minor), 2D6 (major), 3A4 (major); Inhibits CYP1A2 (weak), 3A4 (weak)
 Increased Effect/Toxicity: Contraindicated with drugs which inhibit MAO (including linezolid, selegiline, sibutramine, and MAOIs); severe/fatal reactions may occur. CYP1A2 inhibitors may increase the levels/effects of mirtazapine; example inhibitors include amiodarone, ciprofloxacin, fluvoxamine, ketoconazole, norfloxacin, ofloxacin, and rofecoxib. CYP2D6 inhibitors may increase the levels/effects of mirtazapine; example inhibitors include chlorpromazine, delavirdine, fluoxetine, miconazole, paroxetine, pergolide, quinidine, quinine, ritonavir, and ropinirole. CYP3A4 inhibitors may increase the levels/effects of mirtazapine; example inhibitors include azole antifungals, clarithromycin, diclofenac, doxycycline, erythromycin, imatinib, isoniazid, nefazodone, nicardipine, propofol, protease inhibitors, quinidine, telithromycin, and verapamil. Increased sedative effect seen with CNS depressants.
 Decreased Effect: CYP1A2 inducers may decrease the levels/effects of mirtazapine; example inducers include aminoglutethimide, carbamazepine, phenobarbital, and rifampin. Decreased effect seen with clonidine. CYP3A4 inducers may decrease the levels/effects of mirtazapine; example inducers include aminoglutethimide, carbamazepine, nafcillin, nevirapine, phenobarbital, phenytoin, and rifamycins.

Pharmacodynamics/Kinetics
 Protein binding: 85%
 Metabolism: Extensively hepatic via CYP1A2, 2C9, 2D6, 3A4 and via demethylation and hydroxylation
 Bioavailability: 50%
 Half-life elimination: 20-40 hours; hampered with renal or hepatic impairment
 Time to peak, serum: 2 hours
 Excretion: Urine (75%) and feces (15%) as metabolites
Pregnancy Risk Factor C

Misoprostol (mye soe PROST ole)

U.S. Brand Names Cytotec®
Canadian Brand Names Apo-Misoprostol®; Novo-Misoprostol
Mexican Brand Names Cytotec®
Generic Available Yes
Pharmacologic Category Prostaglandin
Use Prevention of NSAID-induced gastric ulcers; medical termination of pregnancy of ≤49 days (in conjunction with mifepristone)
Unlabeled/Investigational Use Cervical ripening and labor induction; NSAID-induced nephropathy; fat malabsorption in cystic fibrosis
Local Anesthetic/Vasoconstrictor Precautions No information available to require special precautions
Effects on Dental Treatment No significant effects or complications reported
Common Adverse Effects
 >10%: Gastrointestinal: Diarrhea, abdominal pain
 1% to 10%:
  Central nervous system: Headache
  Gastrointestinal: Constipation, flatulence, nausea, dyspepsia, vomiting
Mechanism of Action Misoprostol is a synthetic prostaglandin E$_1$ analog that replaces the protective prostaglandins consumed with prostaglandin-inhibiting therapies (eg, NSAIDs); has been shown to induce uterine contractions
(Continued)

Misoprostol (Continued)

Drug Interactions
Increased Effect/Toxicity: Misoprostol may increase the effect of oxytocin; wait 6-12 hours after misoprostol administration before initiating oxytocin.

Pharmacodynamics/Kinetics
Absorption: Rapid

Metabolism: Hepatic; rapidly de-esterified to misoprostol acid (active)

Half-life elimination: Metabolite: 20-40 minutes

Time to peak, serum: Active metabolite: Fasting: 15-30 minutes

Excretion: Urine (64% to 73%) and feces (15%) within 24 hours

Pregnancy Risk Factor X

Misoprostol and Diclofenac *see* Diclofenac and Misoprostol *on page 462*

Mitomycin (mye toe MYE sin)

U.S. Brand Names Mutamycin®

Canadian Brand Names Mutamycin®

Mexican Brand Names Mitocin®

Generic Available Yes

Synonyms Mitomycin-C; Mitomycin-X; MTC; NSC-26980

Pharmacologic Category Antineoplastic Agent, Antibiotic

Use Treatment of adenocarcinoma of stomach or pancreas, bladder cancer, breast cancer, or colorectal cancer

Unlabeled/Investigational Use Prevention of excess scarring in glaucoma filtration procedures in patients at high risk of bleb failure

Local Anesthetic/Vasoconstrictor Precautions No information available to require special precautions

Effects on Dental Treatment Key adverse event(s) related to dental treatment: Stomatitis.

Common Adverse Effects
>10%:

Cardiovascular: CHF (3% to 15%) (doses >30 mg/m^2)

Central nervous system: Fever (14%)

Dermatologic: Alopecia, nail banding/discoloration

Gastrointestinal: Nausea, vomiting and anorexia (14%)

Hematologic: Anemia (19% to 24%); myelosuppression, common, dose-limiting, delayed

Onset: 3 weeks

Nadir: 4-6 weeks

Recovery: 6-8 weeks

1% to 10%:

Dermatologic: Rash

Gastrointestinal: Stomatitis

Neuromuscular: Paresthesias

Renal: Creatinine increase (2%)

Respiratory: Interstitial pneumonitis, infiltrates, dyspnea, cough (7%)

Mechanism of Action Acts like an alkylating agent and produces DNA cross-linking (primarily with guanine and cytosine pairs); cell-cycle nonspecific; inhibits DNA and RNA synthesis; degrades preformed DNA, causes nuclear lysis and formation of giant cells. While not phase-specific *per se*, mitomycin has its maximum effect against cells in late G and early S phases.

Drug Interactions
Increased Effect/Toxicity: *Vinca* alkaloids or doxorubicin may enhance cardiac toxicity when coadministered with mitomycin.

Pharmacodynamics/Kinetics
Distribution: V_d: 22 L/m^2; high drug concentrations found in kidney, tongue, muscle, heart, and lung tissue; probably not distributed into the CNS

Metabolism: Hepatic

Half-life elimination: 23-78 minutes; Terminal: 50 minutes

Excretion: Urine (<10% as unchanged drug), with elevated serum concentrations

Pregnancy Risk Factor D

Mitomycin-X *see* Mitomycin *on page 1054*

Mitomycin-C *see* Mitomycin *on page 1054*

Mitotane (MYE toe tane)

U.S. Brand Names Lysodren®
Canadian Brand Names Lysodren®
Generic Available No
Synonyms NSC-38721; o,p'-DDD
Pharmacologic Category Antineoplastic Agent, Miscellaneous
Use Treatment of adrenocortical carcinoma
Unlabeled/Investigational Use Treatment of Cushing's syndrome
Local Anesthetic/Vasoconstrictor Precautions No information available to require special precautions
Effects on Dental Treatment No significant effects or complications reported
Common Adverse Effects
>10%:
  Central nervous system: CNS depression (32%), dizziness (15%)
  Dermatologic: Skin rash (12%)
  Gastrointestinal: Anorexia (24%), nausea (39%), vomiting (37%), diarrhea (13%)
  Neuromuscular & skeletal: Weakness (12%)
1% to 10%:
  Central nervous system: Headache (5%), confusion (3%)
  Neuromuscular & skeletal: Muscle tremor (3%)
Mechanism of Action Causes adrenal cortical atrophy; drug affects mitochondria in adrenal cortical cells and decreases production of cortisol; also alters the peripheral metabolism of steroids
Drug Interactions
  Increased Effect/Toxicity: CNS depressants taken with mitotane may enhance CNS depression.
  Decreased Effect: Mitotane may enhance the clearance of barbiturates and warfarin by induction of the hepatic microsomal enzyme system resulting in a decreased effect. Coadministration of spironolactone has resulted in negation of mitotane's effect. Mitotane may increase clearance of phenytoin by microsomal enzyme stimulation.
Pharmacodynamics/Kinetics
  Absorption: Oral: ~35% to 40%
  Distribution: Stored mainly in fat tissue but is found in all body tissues
  Metabolism: Hepatic and other tissues
  Half-life elimination: 18-159 days
  Time to peak, serum: 3-5 hours
  Excretion: Urine and feces (as metabolites)
Pregnancy Risk Factor C

Mitoxantrone (mye toe ZAN trone)

U.S. Brand Names Novantrone®
Canadian Brand Names Novantrone®
Mexican Brand Names Mitroxone®; Novantrone®
Generic Available Yes
Synonyms DAD; DHAD; DHAQ; Dihydroxyanthracenedione Dihydrochloride; Mitoxantrone Hydrochloride CL-232315; Mitozantrone; NSC-301739
Pharmacologic Category Antineoplastic Agent, Anthracenedione
Use Treatment of acute leukemias, lymphoma, breast cancer, pediatric sarcoma, progressive or relapsing-remitting multiple sclerosis, prostate cancer
Local Anesthetic/Vasoconstrictor Precautions No information available to require special precautions
Effects on Dental Treatment Key adverse event(s) related to dental treatment: Mucositis and stomatitis.
Common Adverse Effects Reported with any indication; incidence varies based on treatment/dose
>10%:
  Cardiovascular: Arrhythmia (3% to 18%), edema (10% to 31%), nail bed changes (11%)
  Central nervous system: Fatigue (up to 39%), fever (7% to 78%), headache (6% to 13%)
  Dermatologic: Alopecia (22% to 61%)
  Endocrine & metabolic: Amenorrhea (28% to 53%), menstrual disorder (26% to 61%)
  Gastrointestinal: Abdominal pain (9% to 15%), anorexia (24% to 25%), nausea (29% to 76%), constipation (10% to 16%), diarrhea (16% to 47%),
(Continued)

Mitoxantrone *(Continued)*

GI bleeding (2% to 16%), mucositis (10% to 29%), stomatitis (8% to 29%), vomiting (6% to 12%), weight gain/loss (13% to 18%)

Genitourinary: Abnormal urine (6% to 11%), urinary tract infection (7% to 32%)

Hematologic: Hemoglobin decreased, leukopenia, lymphopenia, petechiae/bruising; myelosuppressive effects of chemotherapy:

WBC: Mild

Platelets: Mild

Onset: 7-10 days

Nadir: 14 days

Recovery: 21 days

Hepatic: GGT increased (3% to 15%)

Neuromuscular & skeletal: Weakness (24%)

Respiratory: Cough (5% to 13%), dyspnea (6% to 18%), upper respiratory tract infection (7% to 53%)

Miscellaneous: Fungal infection (9% to 15%), infection (4% to 18%), sepsis (ANLL 31% to 34%)

1% to 10%:

Cardiovascular: CHF (2% to 3%; risk is much lower with anthracyclines, some reports suggest cumulative doses >160 mg/mL cause CHF in ~10% of patients), ECG changes, hypertension, ischemia, LVEF decreased (≤5%)

Central nervous system: Chills, anxiety, depression, seizure

Dermatologic: Skin infection

Endocrine & metabolic: Hypocalcemia, hypokalemia, hyponatremia, hyperglycemia

Gastrointestinal: Dyspepsia, aphthosis

Genitourinary: Impotence, proteinuria, renal failure, sterility

Hematologic: Anemia, granulocytopenia, hemorrhage

Hepatic: Jaundice, increased SGOT, increased SGPT

Neuromuscular & skeletal: Back pain, myalgia, arthralgia

Ocular: Blurred vision, conjunctivitis

Renal: Hematuria

Respiratory: Pneumonia, rhinitis, sinusitis

Miscellaneous: Systemic infection, sweats, development of secondary leukemia

Mechanism of Action Analogue of the anthracyclines, mitoxantrone intercalates DNA; binds to nucleic acids and inhibits DNA and RNA synthesis by template disordering and steric obstruction; replication is decreased by binding to DNA topoisomerase II and seems to inhibit the incorporation of uridine into RNA and thymidine into DNA; active throughout entire cell cycle

Drug Interactions

Cytochrome P450 Effect: Inhibits CYP3A4 (weak)

Decreased Effect: Patients may experience impaired immune response to vaccines; possible infection after administration of live vaccines in patients receiving immunosuppressants.

Pharmacodynamics/Kinetics

Absorption: Oral: Poor

Distribution: V_d: 14 L/kg; distributes into pleural fluid, kidney, thyroid, liver, heart, and red blood cells

Protein binding: >95%, 76% to albumin

Metabolism: Hepatic; pathway not determined

Half-life elimination: Terminal: 23-215 hours; may be prolonged with hepatic impairment

Excretion: Urine (6% to 11%) and feces as unchanged drug and metabolites

Pregnancy Risk Factor D

Mitoxantrone Hydrochloride CL-232315 *see* Mitoxantrone *on page 1055*

Mitozantrone *see* Mitoxantrone *on page 1055*

Mitrazol™ [OTC] *see* Miconazole *on page 1039*

MK383 *see* Tirofiban *on page 1496*

MK462 *see* Rizatriptan *on page 1363*

MK594 *see* Losartan *on page 950*

MK0826 *see* Ertapenem *on page 561*

MK 869 *see* Aprepitant *on page 134*

MLN341 *see* Bortezomib *on page 215*

MMF *see* Mycophenolate *on page 1075*

MMR *see* Measles, Mumps, and Rubella Vaccines (Combined) *on page 966*

Moban® *see* Molindone *on page 1059*

Mobic® *see* Meloxicam *on page 977*

Mobisyl® [OTC] *see* Triethanolamine Salicylate *on page 1535*

Modafinil (moe DAF i nil)

U.S. Brand Names Provigil®
Canadian Brand Names Alertec®; Provigil®
Generic Available No
Pharmacologic Category Stimulant
Use Improve wakefulness in patients with excessive daytime sleepiness associated with narcolepsy and shift work sleep disorder (SWSD); adjunctive therapy for obstructive sleep apnea/hypopnea syndrome (OSAHS)
Unlabeled/Investigational Use Attention-deficit/hyperactivity disorder (ADHD); treatment of fatigue in MS and other disorders
Local Anesthetic/Vasoconstrictor Precautions No information available to require special precautions
Effects on Dental Treatment Key adverse event(s) related to dental treatment: Xerostomia (normal salivary flow resumes upon discontinuation), oral ulceration, and gingivitis.
Common Adverse Effects
>10%:
    Central nervous system: Headache (34%, dose related)
    Gastrointestinal: Nausea (11%)
1% to 10%:
    Cardiovascular: Chest pain (3%), hypertension (3%), palpitation (2%), tachycardia (2%), vasodilation (2%), edema (1%)
    Central nervous system: Nervousness (7%), dizziness (5%), depression (2%), anxiety (5%, dose related), insomnia (5%), somnolence (2%), chills (1%), agitation (1%), confusion (1%), emotional lability (1%), vertigo (1%)
    Gastrointestinal: Diarrhea (6%), dyspepsia (5%), xerostomia (4%), anorexia (4%), constipation (2%), flatulence (1%), mouth ulceration (1%), taste perversion (1%)
    Genitourinary: Abnormal urine (1%), hematuria (1%), pyuria (1%)
    Hematologic: Eosinophilia (1%)
    Hepatic: Abnormal LFTs (2%)
    Neuromuscular & skeletal: Back pain (6%), paresthesia (2%), dyskinesia (1%), hyperkinesia (1%), hypertonia (1%), neck rigidity (1%), tremor (1%)
    Ocular: Amblyopia (1%), abnormal vision (1%), eye pain (1%)
    Respiratory: Pharyngitis (4%), rhinitis (7%), lung disorder (2%), asthma (1%), epistaxis (1%)
    Miscellaneous: Diaphoresis
    Postmarketing and/or case reports: Agranulocytosis, mania, psychosis
Restrictions C-IV
Mechanism of Action The exact mechanism of action is unclear, it does not appear to alter the release of dopamine or norepinephrine, it may exert its stimulant effects by decreasing GABA-mediated neurotransmission, although this theory has not yet been fully evaluated; several studies also suggest that an intact central alpha-adrenergic system is required for modafinil's activity; the drug increases high-frequency alpha waves while decreasing both delta and theta wave activity, and these effects are consistent with generalized increases in mental alertness
Drug Interactions
    Cytochrome P450 Effect: Substrate of CYP3A4 (major); **Inhibits** CYP1A2 (weak), 2A6 (weak), 2C8/9 (weak), 2C19 (strong), 2E1 (weak), 3A4 (weak); **Induces** CYP1A2 (weak), 2B6 (weak), 3A4 (weak)
    Increased Effect/Toxicity: Modafinil may increase the levels/effects of citalopram, diazepam, methsuximide, phenytoin, propranolol, sertraline, or other CYP2C19 substrates. Modafinil may increase levels of warfarin. In populations deficient in the CYP2D6 isoenzyme, where CYP2C19 acts as a secondary metabolic pathway, concentrations of tricyclic antidepressants and selective serotonin reuptake inhibitors may be increased during coadministration. The levels/effects of modafinil may be increased by azole antifungals, clarithromycin, diclofenac, doxycycline, erythromycin, imatinib, isoniazid, nefazodone, nicardipine, propofol, protease inhibitors, quinidine, telithromycin, verapamil, or other CYP3A4 inhibitors.
    Decreased Effect: Modafinil may decrease serum concentrations of oral contraceptives, cyclosporine, and to a lesser degree, theophylline. The levels/effects of modafinil may be decreased by aminoglutethimide, carbamazepine, nafcillin, nevirapine, phenobarbital, phenytoin, rifamycins, and other CYP3A4 inducers. There is also evidence to suggest that modafinil may induce its own metabolism.
Pharmacodynamics/Kinetics Modafinil is a racemic compound (10% d-isomer and 90% l-isomer at steady state) whose enantiomers have different pharmacokinetics
(Continued)

Modafinil (Continued)

Distribution: V_d: 0.9 L/kg
Protein binding: 60%, primarily to albumin
Metabolism: Hepatic; multiple pathways including CYP3A4
Half-life elimination: Effective half-life: 15 hours; Steady-state: 2-4 days
Time to peak, serum: 2-4 hours
Excretion: Urine (as metabolites, <10% as unchanged drug)

Pregnancy Risk Factor C

Modane® Bulk [OTC] *see* Psyllium *on page 1313*

Modane Tablets® [OTC] *see* Bisacodyl *on page 209*

Modicon® *see* Ethinyl Estradiol and Norethindrone *on page 608*

Modified Dakin's Solution *see* Sodium Hypochlorite Solution *on page 1402*

Modified Shohl's Solution *see* Sodium Citrate and Citric Acid *on page 1401*

Moducal® [OTC] *see* Glucose Polymers *on page 743*

Moexipril (mo EKS i pril)

Related Information
Cardiovascular Diseases *on page 1636*

U.S. Brand Names Univasc®

Generic Available No

Synonyms Moexipril Hydrochloride

Pharmacologic Category Angiotensin-Converting Enzyme (ACE) Inhibitor

Use Treatment of hypertension, alone or in combination with thiazide diuretics; treatment of left ventricular dysfunction after myocardial infarction

Local Anesthetic/Vasoconstrictor Precautions No information available to require special precautions

Effects on Dental Treatment No significant effects or complications reported

Common Adverse Effects 1% to 10%:
Cardiovascular: Hypotension, peripheral edema
Central nervous system: Headache, dizziness, fatigue
Dermatologic: Rash, alopecia, flushing, rash
Endocrine & metabolic: Hyperkalemia, hyponatremia
Gastrointestinal: Diarrhea, nausea, heartburn
Genitourinary: Polyuria
Neuromuscular & skeletal: Myalgia
Renal: Reversible increases in creatinine or BUN
Respiratory: Cough, pharyngitis, upper respiratory infection, sinusitis

Mechanism of Action Competitive inhibitor of angiotensin-converting enzyme (ACE); prevents conversion of angiotensin I to angiotensin II, a potent vasoconstrictor; results in lower levels of angiotensin II which causes an increase in plasma renin activity and a reduction in aldosterone secretion

Drug Interactions
Increased Effect/Toxicity: Potassium supplements, co-trimoxazole (high dose), angiotensin II receptor antagonists (eg, candesartan, losartan, irbesartan), or potassium-sparing diuretics (amiloride, spironolactone, triamterene) may result in elevated serum potassium levels when combined with moexipril. ACE inhibitor effects may be increased by probenecid (increases levels of captopril). ACE inhibitors may increase serum concentrations/effects of lithium.

Diuretics have additive hypotensive effects with ACE inhibitors, and hypovolemia increases the potential for adverse renal effects of ACE inhibitors. In patients with compromised renal function, coadministration with NSAIDs may result in further deterioration of renal function. Allopurinol and ACE inhibitors may cause a higher risk of hypersensitivity reaction when taken concurrently.

Decreased Effect: Aspirin (high dose) may reduce the therapeutic effects of ACE inhibitors; at low dosages this does not appear to be significant. Rifampin may decrease the effect of ACE inhibitors. Antacids may decrease the bioavailability of ACE inhibitors (may be more likely to occur with captopril); separate administration times by 1-2 hours. NSAIDs, specifically indomethacin, may reduce the hypotensive effects of ACE inhibitors. More likely to occur in low renin or volume dependent hypertensive patients.

Pharmacodynamics/Kinetics
Onset of action: Peak effect: 1-2 hours
Duration: >24 hours
Distribution: V_d (moexiprilat): 180 L
Protein binding, plasma: Moexipril: 90%; Moexiprilat: 50% to 70%
Metabolism: Parent drug: Hepatic and via GI tract to moexiprilat, 1000 times more potent than parent

Bioavailability: Moexiprilat: 13%; reduced with food (AUC decreased by ~40%)
Half-life elimination: Moexipril: 1 hour; Moexiprilat: 2-9 hours
Time to peak: 1.5 hours
Excretion: Feces (50%)
Pregnancy Risk Factor C (1st trimester)/D (2nd and 3rd trimesters)

Moexipril and Hydrochlorothiazide
(mo EKS i pril & hye droe klor oh THYE a zide)

Related Information
Hydrochlorothiazide on page 776
Moexipril on page 1058
U.S. Brand Names Uniretic®
Canadian Brand Names Uniretic®
Generic Available No
Synonyms Hydrochlorothiazide and Moexipril
Pharmacologic Category Antihypertensive Agent, Combination
Use Combination therapy for hypertension, however, not indicated for initial treatment of hypertension; replacement therapy in patients receiving separate dosage forms (for patient convenience); when monotherapy with one component fails to achieve desired antihypertensive effect, or when dose-limiting adverse effects limit upward titration of monotherapy
Local Anesthetic/Vasoconstrictor Precautions No information available to require special precautions
Effects on Dental Treatment No significant effects or complications reported
Common Adverse Effects See individual agents.
Mechanism of Action See individual agents.
Drug Interactions
Increased Effect/Toxicity: See individual agents.
Decreased Effect: See individual agents.
Pharmacodynamics/Kinetics See individual agents.
Pregnancy Risk Factor C/D (2nd and 3rd trimesters)

Moexipril Hydrochloride see Moexipril on page 1058
Moi-Stir® [OTC] see Saliva Substitute on page 1374
Moisture® Eyes [OTC] see Artificial Tears on page 143
Moisture® Eyes PM [OTC] see Artificial Tears on page 143

Molindone (moe LIN done)

U.S. Brand Names Moban®
Canadian Brand Names Moban®
Generic Available No
Synonyms Molindone Hydrochloride
Pharmacologic Category Antipsychotic Agent, Typical
Use Management of schizophrenia
Unlabeled/Investigational Use Management of psychotic disorders
Local Anesthetic/Vasoconstrictor Precautions No information available to require special precautions
Effects on Dental Treatment Key adverse event(s) related to dental treatment: Xerostomia and changes in salivation (normal salivary flow resumes upon discontinuation). Anticholinergic side effects can cause a reduction of saliva production or secretion, contributing to discomfort and dental disease (ie, caries, oral candidiasis, and periodontal disease). Molindone can cause extrapyramidal reactions which may appear as muscle twitching or increased motor activity of the face, neck, or head.
Common Adverse Effects Frequency not defined.
Cardiovascular: Orthostatic hypotension, tachycardia, arrhythmia
Central nervous system: Extrapyramidal reactions (akathisia, pseudoparkinsonism, dystonia, tardive dyskinesia), mental depression, altered central temperature regulation, sedation, drowsiness, restlessness, anxiety, hyperactivity, euphoria, seizure, neuroleptic malignant syndrome (NMS)
Dermatologic: Pruritus, rash, photosensitivity
Endocrine & metabolic: Change in menstrual periods, edema of breasts, amenorrhea, galactorrhea, gynecomastia
Gastrointestinal: Constipation, xerostomia, nausea, salivation, weight gain (minimal compared to other antipsychotics), weight loss
Genitourinary: Urinary retention, priapism
Hematologic: Leukopenia, leukocytosis
Ocular: Blurred vision, retinal pigmentation
(Continued)

Molindone *(Continued)*

Miscellaneous: Diaphoresis (decreased)

Mechanism of Action Molindone is a dihydroindoline antipsychotic whose mechanism of action mimics that of chlorpromazine; however, it produces more extrapyramidal symptoms and less sedation than chlorpromazine

Drug Interactions

Increased Effect/Toxicity: Molindone concentrations may be increased by chloroquine, propranolol, sulfadoxine-pyrimethamine. Molindone may increase the effect and/or toxicity of antihypertensives, lithium, TCAs, CNS depressants (ethanol, narcotics), and trazodone. Metoclopramide may increase risk of extrapyramidal symptoms (EPS). Acetylcholinesterase inhibitors (central) may increase the risk of antipsychotic-related EPS.

Decreased Effect: Antipsychotics inhibit the activity of bromocriptine and levodopa. Benztropine (and other anticholinergics) may inhibit the therapeutic response to molindone and excess anticholinergic effects may occur. Barbiturates and cigarette smoking may enhance the hepatic metabolism of molindone. Molindone and possibly other low potency antipsychotic may reverse the pressor effects of epinephrine.

Pharmacodynamics/Kinetics

Metabolism: Hepatic

Half-life elimination: 1.5 hours

Time to peak, serum: ~1.5 hours

Excretion: Urine and feces (90%) within 24 hours

Pregnancy Risk Factor C

Molindone Hydrochloride *see Molindone on page 1059*

Molybdenum *see Trace Metals on page 1513*

Molypen® *see Trace Metals on page 1513*

MOM *see Magnesium Hydroxide on page 961*

Momentum® [OTC] *see Magnesium Salicylate on page 962*

Mometasone Furoate *(moe MET a sone FYOOR oh ate)*

Related Information

Respiratory Diseases on page 1656

U.S. Brand Names Asmanex® Twisthaler®; Elocon®; Nasonex®

Canadian Brand Names Elocom®; Nasonex®; ratio-Mometasone

Generic Available Yes: Ointment

Pharmacologic Category Corticosteroid, Inhalant (Oral); Corticosteroid, Nasal; Corticosteroid, Topical

Use Relief of the inflammatory and pruritic manifestations of corticosteroid-responsive dermatoses (medium potency topical corticosteroid); treatment of nasal symptoms of seasonal and perennial allergic rhinitis; prevention of nasal symptoms associated with seasonal allergic rhinitis; treatment of nasal polyps in adults; maintenance treatment of asthma as prophylactic therapy or as a supplement in asthma patients requiring oral corticosteroids for the purpose of decreasing or eliminating the oral corticosteroid requirement

Local Anesthetic/Vasoconstrictor Precautions No information available to require special precautions

Effects on Dental Treatment No significant effects or complications reported

Common Adverse Effects

Nasal/oral inhalation:

>10%:

Central nervous system: Headache (17% to 22%), fatigue (oral inhalation 1% to 13%), depression (oral inhalation 11%)

Neuromuscular & skeletal: Musculoskeletal pain (1% to 22%), arthralgia (oral inhalation 13%)

Respiratory: Sinusitis (oral inhalation 22%), rhinitis (2% to 20%), upper respiratory infection (8% to 15%), pharyngitis (8% to 13%), cough (nasal inhalation 7% to 13%), epistaxis (1% to 11%)

Miscellaneous: Viral infection (nasal inhalation 8% to 14%), oral candidiasis (oral inhalation 4% to 22%)

1% to 10%:

Cardiovascular: Chest pain

Gastrointestinal: Abdominal pain, dry throat (oral inhalation), vomiting (1% to 5%), diarrhea, dyspepsia, flatulence, gastroenteritis, nausea, vomiting

Genitourinary: Dysmenorrhea

Neuromuscular & skeletal: Back pain, myalgia

Ocular: Conjunctivitis

Otic: Earache, otitis media

Respiratory: Asthma, bronchitis, dysphonia, epistaxis, nasal irritation, rhinitis, wheezing

Miscellaneous: Accidental injury, flu-like symptoms

Topical:

1% to 10%: Dermatologic: Bacterial skin infection, burning, furunculosis, pruritus, skin atrophy, tingling/stinging

Cataract formation, reduction in growth velocity, and HPA axis suppression have been reported with other corticosteroids

Dosage

Oral inhalation: Children ≥12 years and Adults: Previous therapy:

Bronchodilators or inhaled corticosteroids: Initial: 1 inhalation (220 mcg) daily (maximum 2 inhalations or 440 mcg/day); may be given in the evening or in divided doses twice daily

Oral corticosteroids: Initial: 440 mcg twice daily (maximum 880 mcg/day); prednisone should be reduced no faster than 2.5 mg/day on a weekly basis, beginning after at least 1 week of mometasone furoate use

Note: Maximum effects may not be evident for 1-2 weeks or longer; dose should be titrated to effect, using the lowest possible dose

Nasal spray:

Allergic rhinitis:

Children 2-11 years: 1 spray (50 mcg) in each nostril daily

Children ≥12 years and Adults: 2 sprays (100 mcg) in each nostril daily; when used for the prevention of allergic rhinitis, treatment should begin 2-4 weeks prior to pollen season

Nasal polyps: Adults: 2 sprays (100 mcg) in each nostril twice daily; 2 sprays (100 mcg) once daily may be effective in some patients

Topical: Apply sparingly, do not use occlusive dressings. Therapy should be discontinued when control is achieved; if no improvement is seen in 2 weeks, reassessment of diagnosis may be necessary.

Cream, ointment: Children ≥2 years and Adults: Apply a thin film to affected area once daily; do not use in pediatric patients for longer than 3 weeks

Lotion: Children ≥12 years and Adults: Apply a few drops to affected area once daily

Mechanism of Action May depress the formation, release, and activity of endogenous chemical mediators of inflammation (kinins, histamine, liposomal enzymes, prostaglandins). Leukocytes and macrophages may have to be present for the initiation of responses mediated by the above substances. Inhibits the margination and subsequent cell migration to the area of injury, and also reverses the dilatation and increased vessel permeability in the area resulting in decreased access of cells to the sites of injury.

Contraindications Hypersensitivity to mometasone or any component of the formulation; treatment of acute bronchospasm (oral inhaler)

Warnings/Precautions

May cause suppression of hypothalamic-pituitary-adrenal (HPA) axis, particularly in younger children, or in patients receiving high doses for prolonged periods, or when used topically on large areas of the body, denuded areas, or with an occlusive dressing. Use caution if replacing systemic corticosteroid with nasal or oral inhaler; may cause symptoms of withdrawal or acute adrenal insufficiency. Transfer to oral inhaler may unmask previously-suppressed allergic conditions (rhinitis, conjunctivitis, eczema).

Controlled clinical studies have shown that corticosteroids may cause a reduction in growth velocity in pediatric patients; titrate to the lowest effective dose. Decreases in bone mineral density have been observed. May suppress the immune system, patients may be more susceptible to infection; monitor for signs of oropharyngeal candidiasis. Use with caution, if at all, in patients with systemic infections, active or quiescent tuberculosis infection, or ocular herpes simplex. Avoid exposure to chickenpox and measles. Rare instances of glaucoma have been reported with inhaled steroids.

Drug Interactions

Cytochrome P450 Effect: Substrate of CYP3A4 (minor)

Increased Effect/Toxicity:

Concomitant use with ketoconazole may result in increased mometasone furoate plasma levels.

Dietary Considerations

Asmanex® Twisthaler® contains lactose.

Pharmacodynamics/Kinetics

Absorption:

Nasal inhalation: Mometasone furoate monohydrate: Undetectable in plasma

Ointment: 0.7%; increased by occlusive dressings

Oral inhalation: <1%

Protein binding: Mometasone furoate: 98% to 99%

(Continued)

Mometasone Furoate *(Continued)*

Metabolism: Mometasone furoate: Hepatic via CYP3A4; forms metabolite
Half-life elimination: Oral inhalation: 5 hours
Excretion: Feces, bile, urine
Pregnancy Risk Factor C
Dosage Forms CRM, topical (Elocon®): 0.1% (15 g, 45 g). **LOTION, topical**
(Elocon®): 0.1% (30 mL, 60 mL). **OINT, topical:** 0.1% (15 g, 45 g); (Elocon®):
0.1% (15 g, 45 g). **POWDER for oral inhalation** (Asmanex® Twisthaler®): 220
mcg (14 units, 30 units, 60 units, 120 units). **SUSP, intranasal [spray]**
(Nasonex®): 50 mcg/spray (17 g)

MOM/Mineral Oil Emulsion *see* Magnesium Hydroxide and Mineral Oil *on page 961*

Monacolin K *see* Lovastatin *on page 953*

Monarc® M *see* Antihemophilic Factor (Human) *on page 129*

Monistat® 1 Combination Pack [OTC] *see* Miconazole *on page 1039*

Monistat® 3 [OTC] *see* Miconazole *on page 1039*

Monistat® 7 [OTC] *see* Miconazole *on page 1039*

Monistat-Derm® *see* Miconazole *on page 1039*

Monobenzone *(mon oh BEN zone)*

U.S. Brand Names Benoquin®
Generic Available No
Pharmacologic Category Topical Skin Product
Use Final depigmentation in extensive vitiligo
Local Anesthetic/Vasoconstrictor Precautions No information available to require special precautions
Effects on Dental Treatment No significant effects or complications reported
Common Adverse Effects Frequency not defined.
   Local: Burning sensation, depigmentation of skin distant to application site, dermatitis, irritation
Mechanism of Action Increases excretion of melanin from melanocytes; causes melanocyte destruction and permanent depigmentation
Pharmacodynamics/Kinetics Onset of action: 1-4 months
Pregnancy Risk Factor C

Monocaps [OTC] *see* Vitamins (Multiple/Oral) *on page 1582*

Monoclate-P® *see* Antihemophilic Factor (Human) *on page 129*

Monoclonal Antibody *see* Muromonab-CD3 *on page 1074*

Monodox® *see* Doxycycline (Systemic) *on page 514*

Monoethanolamine *see* Ethanolamine Oleate *on page 591*

Monoket® *see* Isosorbide Mononitrate *on page 868*

MonoNessa™ *see* Ethinyl Estradiol and Norgestimate *on page 613*

Mononine® *see* Factor IX *on page 632*

Monopril® *see* Fosinopril *on page 707*

Monopril-HCT® *see* Fosinopril and Hydrochlorothiazide *on page 709*

Montelukast *(mon te LOO kast)*

Related Information
   Respiratory Diseases *on page 1656*
U.S. Brand Names Singulair®
Canadian Brand Names Singulair®
Mexican Brand Names Singulair®
Generic Available No
Synonyms Montelukast Sodium
Pharmacologic Category Leukotriene-Receptor Antagonist
Use Prophylaxis and chronic treatment of asthma; relief of symptoms of seasonal allergic rhinitis and perennial allergic rhinitis
Unlabeled/Investigational Use Acute asthma
Local Anesthetic/Vasoconstrictor Precautions No information available to require special precautions
Effects on Dental Treatment No significant effects or complications reported
Common Adverse Effects (As reported in adults)
   1% to 10%:
      Central nervous system: Dizziness (2%), fatigue (2%), fever (2%)
      Dermatologic: Rash (2%)

Gastrointestinal: Abdominal pain (3%), dyspepsia (2%), dental pain (2%), gastroenteritis (2%)

Neuromuscular & skeletal: Weakness (2%)

Respiratory: Cough (3%), nasal congestion (2%), upper respiratory infection (2%)

Miscellaneous: Flu-like symptoms (4%), trauma (1%)

Dosage Oral:

Children:

6-11 months: Asthma (unlabeled use): 4 mg (oral granules) once daily, taken in the evening

6-23 months: Perennial allergic rhinitis: 4 mg (oral granules) once daily

12-23 months: Asthma: 4 mg (oral granules) once daily, taken in the evening

2-5 years: Asthma, seasonal or perennial allergic rhinitis: 4 mg (chewable tablet or oral granules) once daily, taken in the evening

6-14 years: Asthma, seasonal or perennial allergic rhinitis: Chew one 5 mg chewable tablet/day, taken in the evening

Children ≥15 years and Adults:

Asthma, seasonal or perennial allergic rhinitis: 10 mg/day, taken in the evening

Asthma, acute (unlabeled use): 10 mg as a single dose administered with first-line therapy

Dosing adjustment in renal impairment: No adjustment necessary

Dosing adjustment in hepatic impairment: Mild-to-moderate: No adjustment necessary. Patients with severe hepatic disease were **not** studied.

Mechanism of Action Selective leukotriene receptor antagonist that inhibits the cysteinyl leukotriene receptor. Cysteinyl leukotrienes and leukotriene receptor occupation have been correlated with the pathophysiology of asthma, including airway edema, smooth muscle contraction, and altered cellular activity associated with the inflammatory process, which contribute to the signs and symptoms of asthma.

Contraindications Hypersensitivity to montelukast or any component of the formulation

Warnings/Precautions Montelukast is not FDA approved for use in the reversal of bronchospasm in acute asthma attacks; some clinicians, however, support its use (Cylly, 2003; Camargo, 2003; Ferreira, 2001). Should not be used as monotherapy for the treatment and management of exercise-induced bronchospasm. Advise patients to have appropriate rescue medication available. Appropriate clinical monitoring and caution are recommended when systemic corticosteroid reduction is considered in patients receiving montelukast. Inform phenylketonuric patients that the chewable tablet contains phenylalanine. Safety and efficacy in children <6 months of age have not been established.

In rare cases, patients on therapy with montelukast may present with systemic eosinophilia, sometimes presenting with clinical features of vasculitis consistent with Churg-Strauss syndrome, a condition which is often treated with systemic corticosteroid therapy. Healthcare providers should be alert to eosinophilia, vasculitic rash, worsening pulmonary symptoms, cardiac complications, and/or neuropathy presenting in their patients. A causal association between montelukast and these underlying conditions has not been established.

Drug Interactions

Cytochrome P450 Effect: Substrate (major) of CYP2C9, 3A4; **Inhibits** CYP2C8 (weak), 2C9 (weak)

Decreased Effect: CYP2C9 inducers may decrease the levels/effects of montelukast; example inducers include carbamazepine, phenobarbital, phenytoin, rifampin, rifapentine, and secobarbital. CYP3A4 inducers may decrease the levels/effects of montelukast; example inducers include aminoglutethimide, carbamazepine, nafcillin, nevirapine, phenobarbital, phenytoin, and rifamycins.

Ethanol/Nutrition/Herb Interactions Herb/Nutraceutical: St John's wort may decrease montelukast levels.

Dietary Considerations Tablet, chewable: 4 mg strength contains phenylalanine 0.674 mg; 5 mg strength contains phenylalanine 0.842 mg

Pharmacodynamics/Kinetics

Duration: >24 hours

Absorption: Rapid

Distribution: V_d: 8-11 L

Protein binding, plasma: >99%

Metabolism: Extensively hepatic via CYP3A4 and 2C8/9

Bioavailability: Tablet: 10 mg: Mean: 64%; 5 mg: 63% to 73%

Half-life elimination, plasma: Mean: 2.7-5.5 hours

Time to peak, serum: Tablet: 10 mg: 3-4 hours; 5 mg: 2-2.5 hours; 4 mg: 2 hours

(Continued)

Montelukast (Continued)

Excretion: Feces (86%); urine (<0.2%)
Pregnancy Risk Factor B
Dosage Forms GRAN: 4 mg/packet. **TAB:** 10 mg. **TAB, chewable:** 4 mg, 5 mg

Montelukast Sodium *see* Montelukast *on page 1062*

Monurol™ *see* Fosfomycin *on page 706*

8-MOP® *see* Methoxsalen *on page 1018*

More Attenuated Enders Strain *see* Measles Virus Vaccine (Live) *on page 967*

MoreDophilus® [OTC] *see* Lactobacillus *on page 535*

Moricizine (mor I siz een)

Related Information
Cardiovascular Diseases *on page 1636*
U.S. Brand Names Ethmozine®
Canadian Brand Names Ethmozine®
Generic Available No
Synonyms Moricizine Hydrochloride
Pharmacologic Category Antiarrhythmic Agent, Class I
Use Treatment of ventricular tachycardia and life-threatening ventricular arrhythmias
Unlabeled/Investigational Use PVCs, complete and nonsustained ventricular tachycardia, atrial arrhythmias
Local Anesthetic/Vasoconstrictor Precautions No information available to require special precautions
Effects on Dental Treatment No significant effects or complications reported
Common Adverse Effects
>10%: Central nervous system: Dizziness
1% to 10%:
Cardiovascular: Proarrhythmia, palpitation, cardiac death, ECG abnormalities, CHF
Central nervous system: Headache, fatigue, insomnia
Endocrine & metabolic: Decreased libido
Gastrointestinal: Nausea, diarrhea, ileus
Ocular: Blurred vision, periorbital edema
Respiratory: Dyspnea
Mechanism of Action Class I antiarrhythmic agent; reduces the fast inward current carried by sodium ions, shortens Phase I and Phase II repolarization, resulting in decreased action potential duration and effective refractory period
Drug Interactions
Cytochrome P450 Effect: Substrate of CYP3A4 (major); **Induces** CYP1A2 (weak), 3A4 (weak)
Increased Effect/Toxicity: CYP3A4 inhibitors may increase the levels/effects of moricizine; example inhibitors include azole antifungals, clarithromycin, diclofenac, doxycycline, erythromycin, imatinib, isoniazid, nefazodone, nicardipine, propofol, protease inhibitors, quinidine, telithromycin, and verapamil. Moricizine levels may be increased by cimetidine and diltiazem. Digoxin may result in additive prolongation of the PR interval when combined with moricizine (but not rate of second- and third-degree AV block). Drugs which may prolong QT interval (including cisapride, erythromycin, phenothiazines, cyclic antidepressants, and some quinolones) are contraindicated with type Ia antiarrhythmics. Moricizine has some type Ia activity, and caution should be used.
Decreased Effect: Moricizine may decrease levels of theophylline (50%) and diltiazem. CYP3A4 inducers may decrease the levels/effects of moricizine; example inducers include aminoglutethimide, carbamazepine, nafcillin, nevirapine, phenobarbital, phenytoin, and rifamycins.
Pharmacodynamics/Kinetics
Protein binding, plasma: 95%
Metabolism: Significant first-pass effect; some enterohepatic recycling
Bioavailability: 38%
Half-life elimination: Healthy volunteers: 3-4 hours; Cardiac disease: 6-13 hours
Excretion: Feces (56%); urine (39%)
Pregnancy Risk Factor B

Moricizine Hydrochloride *see* Moricizine *on page 1064*

Morning After Pill *see* Ethinyl Estradiol and Norgestrel *on page 616*

Morphine Sulfate (MOR feen SUL fate)

Related Information
Oxymorphone *on page 1174*

U.S. Brand Names Astramorph/PF™; Avinza®; DepoDur™; Duramorph®; Infumorph®; Kadian®; MS Contin®; Oramorph SR®; RMS®; Roxanol™; Roxanol 100™; Roxanol™-T [DSC]

Canadian Brand Names Kadian®; M-Eslon®; Morphine HP®; Morphine LP® Epidural; M.O.S.-Sulfate®; MS Contin®; MS-IR®; PMS-Morphine Sulfate SR; ratio-Morphine SR; Statex®

Generic Available Yes: Excludes capsule, controlled release tablet, sustained release tablet, extended release liposomal suspension for injection

Synonyms MSO₄ (error-prone abbreviation and should not be used)

Pharmacologic Category Analgesic, Narcotic

Use Relief of moderate to severe acute and chronic pain; relief of pain of myocardial infarction; relief of dyspnea of acute left ventricular failure and pulmonary edema; preanesthetic medication

DepoDur™: Epidural (lumbar) single-dose management of surgical pain

Infumorph®: Used in microinfusion devices for intraspinal administration in treatment of intractable chronic pain

Local Anesthetic/Vasoconstrictor Precautions No information available to require special precautions

Effects on Dental Treatment Key adverse event(s) related to dental treatment: Xerostomia (normal salivary flow resumes upon discontinuation). Anticholinergic side effects can cause a reduction of saliva production or secretion, contributing to discomfort and dental disease (ie, caries, oral candidiasis, and periodontal disease).

Common Adverse Effects Note: Individual patient differences are unpredictable, and percentage may differ in acute pain (surgical) treatment.

Frequency not defined: Flushing, CNS depression, sedation, antidiuretic hormone release, physical and psychological dependence, diaphoresis

>10%:
Cardiovascular: Palpitations, hypotension, bradycardia
Central nervous system: Drowsiness (48%, tolerance usually develops to drowsiness with regular dosing for 1-2 weeks); dizziness (20%), confusion, headache (following epidural or intrathecal use)
Dermatologic: Pruritus (may be secondary to histamine release)
Note: Pruritus may be dose-related, but not confined to the site of administration.
Gastrointestinal: Nausea (28%, tolerance usually develops to nausea and vomiting with chronic use); constipation (40%, tolerance develops very slowly if at all); xerostomia (78%)
Genitourinary: Urinary retention (16%; may be prolonged, up to 20 hours, following epidural or intrathecal use)
Local: Pain at injection site
Neuromuscular & skeletal: Weakness
Miscellaneous: Histamine release

1% to 10%:
Cardiovascular: Atrial fibrillation (<3%), chest pain (<3%), edema (<3%), syncope (<3%), tachycardia (<3%)
Central nervous system: Amnesia, anxiety, apathy, ataxia, chills, depression, euphoria, false feeling of well being, fever, headache, hypoesthesia, insomnia, lethargy, malaise, restlessness, seizure, vertigo
Endocrine & metabolic: Gynecomastia (<3%), hyponatremia (<3%)
Gastrointestinal: Anorexia, biliary colic, dyspepsia, dysphagia, GERD, GI irritation, paralytic ileus, vomiting (9%)
Genitourinary: Decreased urination
Hematologic: Anemia (<3%), leukopenia (<3%), thrombocytopenia (<3%)
Neuromuscular & skeletal: Arthralgia, back pain, bone pain, paresthesia, trembling
Ocular: Vision problems
Respiratory: Asthma, atelectasis, dyspnea, hiccups, hypoxia, noncardiogenic pulmonary edema, respiratory depression, rhinitis
Miscellaneous: Diaphoresis, flu-like syndrome, withdrawal syndrome

Restrictions C-II

Dosage Note: These are guidelines and do not represent the doses that may be required in all patients. Doses should be titrated to pain relief/prevention.
Children >6 months and <50 kg: Acute pain (moderate-to-severe):
Oral (prompt release): 0.15-0.3 mg/kg every 3-4 hours as needed
I.M.: 0.1 mg/kg every 3-4 hours as needed
I.V.: 0.05-0.1 mg/kg every 3-4 hours as needed
(Continued)

Morphine Sulfate *(Continued)*

I.V. infusion: Range: 10-30 mcg/kg/hour

Adolescents >12 years: Sedation/analgesia for procedures: I.V.: 3-4 mg and repeat in 5 minutes if necessary

Adults:

Acute pain (moderate-to-severe):

Oral: Prompt release formulations: Opiate-naive: Initial: 10 mg every 3-4 hours as needed; patients with prior opiate exposure may require higher initial doses: usual dosage range: 10-30 mg every 3-4 hours as needed

I.M., SubQ: **Note:** Repeated SubQ administration causes local tissue irritation, pain, and induration.

Initial: Opiate-naive: 5-10 mg every 3-4 hours as needed; patients with prior opiate exposure may require higher initial doses; usual dosage range: 5-20 mg every 3-4 hours as needed

Rectal: 10-20 mg every 3-4 hours

I.V.: Initial: Opiate-naive: 2.5-5 mg every 3-4 hours; patients with prior opiate exposure may require higher initial doses. **Note:** Repeated doses (up to every 5 minutes if needed) in small increments (eg, 1-4 mg) may be preferred to larger and less frequent doses.

I.V., SubQ continuous infusion: 0.8-10 mg/hour; usual range: Up to 80 mg/hour

Mechanically-ventilated patients (based on 70 kg patient): 0.7-10 mg every 1-2 hours as needed; infusion: 5-35 mg/hour

Patient-controlled analgesia (PCA): (Opiate-naive: Consider lower end of dosing range):

Usual concentration: 1 mg/mL

Demand dose: Usual: 1 mg; range: 0.5-2.5 mg

Lockout interval: 5-10 minutes

Intrathecal (I.T.): **Note:** Administer with extreme caution and in reduced dosage to geriatric or debilitated patients.

Opioid-naive: 0.2-0.25 mg/dose (may provide adequate relief for 24 hours); repeat doses are **not** recommended.

Epidural: **Note:** Administer with extreme caution and in reduced dosage to geriatric or debilitated patients. Vigilant monitoring is particularly important in these patients.

Pain management:

Single-dose (Duramorph®): Initial: 3-5 mg

Infusion:

Bolus dose: 1-6 mg

Infusion rate: 0.1-0.2 mg/hour

Maximum dose: 10 mg/24 hours

Surgical anesthesia: Epidural: Single-dose (extended release, Depo-Dur™): Lumbar epidural only; not recommended in patients <18 years of age:

Cesarean section: 10 mg

Lower abdominal/pelvic surgery: 10-15 mg

Major orthopedic surgery of lower extremity: 15 mg

For Depo-Dur™: To minimize the pharmacokinetic interaction resulting in higher peak serum concentrations of morphine, administer the test dose of the local anesthetic at least 15 minutes prior to Depo-Dur™ administration. Use of Depo-Dur™ with epidural local anesthetics has not been studied.

Note: Some patients may benefit from a 20 mg dose, however, the incidence of adverse effects may be increased.

Chronic pain: Note: Patients taking opioids chronically may become tolerant and require doses higher than the usual dosage range to maintain the desired effect. Tolerance can be managed by appropriate dose titration. There is no optimal or maximal dose for morphine in chronic pain. The appropriate dose is one that relieves pain throughout its dosing interval without causing unmanageable side effects.

Oral: Controlled-, extended-, or sustained-release formulations: A patient's morphine requirement should be established using prompt-release formulations. Conversion to long-acting products may be considered when chronic, continuous treatment is required. Higher dosages should be reserved for use only in opioid-tolerant patients.

Capsules, extended release (Avinza™): Daily dose administered once daily (for best results, administer at same time each day)

Capsules, sustained release (Kadian®): Daily dose administered once daily or in 2 divided doses daily (every 12 hours)

Tablets, controlled release (MS Contin®), sustained release (Oramorph SR®), or extended release: Daily dose divided and administered every 8 or every 12 hours

Elderly or debilitated patients: Use with caution; may require dose reduction

Dosing adjustment in renal impairment:
Cl$_{cr}$ 10-50 mL/minute: Administer at 75% of normal dose
Cl$_{cr}$ <10 mL/minute: Administer at 50% of normal dose

Dosing adjustment/comments in hepatic disease: Unchanged in mild liver disease; substantial extrahepatic metabolism may occur; excessive sedation may occur in cirrhosis

Mechanism of Action Binds to opiate receptors in the CNS, causing inhibition of ascending pain pathways, altering the perception of and response to pain; produces generalized CNS depression

Contraindications Hypersensitivity to morphine sulfate or any component of the formulation; increased intracranial pressure; severe respiratory depression; acute or severe asthma; known or suspected paralytic ileus; sustained release products are not recommended with gastrointestinal obstruction or in acute/postoperative pain; pregnancy (prolonged use or high doses at term)

Warnings/Precautions An opioid-containing analgesic regimen should be tailored to each patient's needs and based upon the type of pain being treated (acute versus chronic), the route of administration, degree of tolerance for opioids (naive versus chronic user), age, weight, and medical condition. The optimal analgesic dose varies widely among patients. Doses should be titrated to pain relief/prevention. When used as an epidural injection, monitor for delayed sedation.

May cause respiratory depression; use with caution in patients (particularly elderly or debilitated) with impaired respiratory function or severe hepatic dysfunction and in patients with hypersensitivity reactions to other phenanthrene derivative opioid agonists (codeine, hydrocodone, hydromorphone, levorphanol, oxycodone, oxymorphone). Some preparations contain sulfites which may cause allergic reactions; infants <3 months of age are more susceptible to respiratory depression, use with caution and generally in reduced doses in this age group. Extended or sustained release dosage forms should not be crushed or chewed. Do not administer Avinza® with alcoholic beverages or ethanol-containing products, which may disrupt extended-release characteristic of product. Morphine shares the toxic potential of opiate agonists and usual precautions of opiate agonist therapy should be observed; may cause hypotension in patients with acute myocardial infarction, volume depletion, or concurrent drug therapy which may exaggerate vasodilation. Tolerance or drug dependence may result from extended use. MS Contin® 200 mg tablets are for use only in opioid-tolerant patients requiring >400 mg/day. Infumorph® solutions **are for use in microinfusion devices only**; not for I.V., I.M., or SubQ administration.

Elderly may be particularly susceptible to the CNS depressant and constipating effects of narcotics.

Drug Interactions

Cytochrome P450 Effect: Substrate of CYP2D6 (minor)

Increased Effect/Toxicity: Antipsychotic agents may increase the hypotensive effects of morphine. Use of selective serotonin reuptake inhibitors (SSRIs) or meperidine may lead to additive serotonergic effects with concomitant morphine, possibly precipitating serotonin syndrome. CNS depressants and tricyclic antidepressants may potentiate the effects of morphine. Concurrent use of MAO inhibitors and meperidine has been associated with significant adverse effects; use caution with morphine. Some manufacturers recommend avoiding use within 14 days of MAO inhibitors.

Decreased Effect: The therapeutic efficacy of pegvisomant may be decreased by concomitant opiates, possibly requiring dosage adjustment of pegvisomant. Rifamycin derivatives may decrease levels or effects of morphine.

Ethanol/Nutrition/Herb Interactions

Ethanol: Avoid ethanol (may increase CNS depression).

Avinza®: Alcoholic beverages or ethanol-containing products may disrupt extended-release formulation resulting in rapid release of entire morphine dose.

Food: Administration of oral morphine solution with food may increase bioavailability (ie, a report of 34% increase in morphine AUC when morphine oral solution followed a high-fat meal). The bioavailability of Oramorph SR® or Kadian® does not appear to be affected by food.

Herb/Nutraceutical: Avoid valerian, St John's wort, kava kava, gotu kola (may increase CNS depression).

Dietary Considerations Morphine may cause GI upset; take with food if GI upset occurs. Be consistent when taking morphine with or without meals.

Pharmacodynamics/Kinetics

Onset of action: Oral (immediate release): ~30 minutes; I.V.: 5-10 minutes
(Continued)

Morphine Sulfate *(Continued)*

Duration: Pain relief:
Immediate release formulations: 4 hours
Extended release epidural injection (DepoDur™): >48 hours
Absorption: Variable
Distribution: V_d: 3-4 L/kg; binds to opioid receptors in the CNS and periphery (eg, GI tract)
Protein binding: 30% to 35%
Metabolism: Hepatic via conjugation with glucuronic acid to morphine-3-glucuronide (inactive), morphine-6-glucuronide (active), and in lesser amounts, morphine-3,6-diglucuronide; other minor metabolites include normorphine (active) and the 3-ethereal sulfate
Bioavailability: Oral: 17% to 33% (first-pass effect limits oral bioavailability; oral:parenteral effectiveness reportedly varies from 1:6 in opioid naive patients to 1:3 with chronic use)
Half-life elimination: Adults: 2-4 hours (immediate release forms)
Time to peak, plasma: Kadian®: ~10 hours
Excretion: Urine (primarily as morphine-3-glucuronide, ~2% to 12% excreted unchanged); feces (~7% to 10%). It has been suggested that accumulation of morphine-6-glucuronide might cause toxicity with renal insufficiency. All of the metabolites (ie, morphine-3-glucuronide, morphine-6-glucuronide, and normorphine) have been suggested as possible causes of neurotoxicity (eg, myoclonus).
Pregnancy Risk Factor C/D (prolonged use or high doses at term)
Dosage Forms CAP, extended release (Avinza®): 30 mg, 60 mg, 90 mg, 120 mg. **CAP, sustained release** (Kadian®): 20 mg, 30 mg, 50 mg, 60 mg, 100 mg. **INF** [premixed in D_5W]: 1 mg/mL (100 mL, 250 mL, 500 mL). **INJ, solution:** 2 mg/mL (1 mL); 4 mg/mL (1 mL); 5 mg/mL (1 mL); 8 mg/mL (1 mL); 10 mg/mL (1 mL, 10 mL); 15 mg/mL (1 mL, 20 mL); 25 mg/mL (4 mL, 10 mL, 20 mL, 40 mL,50 mL, 100 mL, 250 mL); 50 mg/mL (20 mL, 40 mL). **INJ, solution** [epidural, intrathecal, or I.V. infusion; preservative free] (Astramorph/PF™): 0.5 mg/mL (2 mL, 10 mL); 1 mg/mL (2 mL, 10 mL); (Duramorph®): 0.5 mg/mL (10 mL); 1 mg/mL (10 mL). **INJ, solution** [epidural or intrathecal infusion via microinfusion device; preservative free] (Infumorph®): 10 mg/mL (20 mL); 25 mg/mL (20 mL). **INJ, extended release liposomal suspension** [lumbar epidural injection, preservative free] (DepoDur™): 10 mg/mL (1 mL, 1.5 mL, 2 mL). **INJ, solution** [I.V. infusion via PCA pump]: 1 mg/mL (50 mL); 5 mg/mL (50 mL). **INJ, solution** [preservative free]: 0.5 mg/mL (30 mL); 1 mg/mL (30 mL, 50 mL); 2 mg/mL (30 mL); 5 mg/mL (30 mL, 50 mL). **SOLN, oral:** 10 mg/5 mL (5 mL, 10 mL, 100 mL, 500 mL); 20 mg/mL (30 mL, 120 mL, 240 mL); 20 mg/5 mL (100 mL, 500 mL); (Roxanol™): 20 mg/mL (30 mL, 120 mL); (Roxanol 100™): 100 mg/5 mL (240 mL). **SUPP, rectal** (RMS®): 5 mg (12s), 10 mg (12s), 20 mg (12s), 30 mg (12s). **TAB, controlled release** (MS Contin®): 15 mg, 30 mg, 60 mg, 100 mg, 200 mg. **TAB, extended release:** 15 mg, 30 mg, 60 mg, 100 mg, 200 mg. **TAB, sustained release** (Oramorph SR®): 15 mg, 30 mg, 60 mg, 100 mg

---

Morrhuate Sodium *(MOR yoo ate SOW dee um)*

U.S. Brand Names Scleromate®
Generic Available Yes
Pharmacologic Category Sclerosing Agent
Use Treatment of small, uncomplicated varicose veins of the lower extremities
Local Anesthetic/Vasoconstrictor Precautions No information available to require special precautions
Effects on Dental Treatment No significant effects or complications reported
Mechanism of Action Both varicose veins and esophageal varices are treated by the thrombotic action of morrhuate sodium. By causing inflammation of the vein's intima, a thrombus is formed. Occlusion secondary to the fibrous tissue and the thrombus results in the obliteration of the vein.
Pregnancy Risk Factor C

Mosco® Corn and Callus Remover [OTC] *see* Salicylic Acid *on page 1374*

Motofen® *see* Difenoxin and Atropine *on page 467*

Motrin® *see* Ibuprofen *on page 808*

Motrin® Children's [OTC] *see* Ibuprofen *on page 808*

Motrin® Cold and Sinus [OTC] *see* Pseudoephedrine and Ibuprofen *on page 1311*

Motrin® Cold, Children's [OTC] *see* Pseudoephedrine and Ibuprofen *on page 1311*

Motrin® IB [OTC] *see* Ibuprofen *on page 808*

Motrin® Infants' [OTC] *see* Ibuprofen *on page 808*
Motrin® Junior Strength [OTC] *see* Ibuprofen *on page 808*
Mouthkote® [OTC] *see* Saliva Substitute *on page 1374*

Mouthwash (Antiseptic) (MOUTH wosh)

Related Information
Bacterial Infections *on page 1697*
Dentin Hypersensitivity, High Caries Index, and Xerostomia *on page 1714*
Oral Rinse Products *on page 1831*
Periodontal Diseases *on page 1705*
Ulcerative and Erosive Disorders *on page 1712*
Related Sample Prescriptions
Antimicrobial Oral Rinse *on page 1739*
Synonyms Antiseptic Mouthwash
Pharmacologic Category Antimicrobial Mouth Rinse; Antiplaque Agent; Mouthwash
Dental Use Aid in prevention and reduction of plaque and gingivitis; halitosis
Local Anesthetic/Vasoconstrictor Precautions No information available to require special precautions
Effects on Dental Treatment No significant effects or complications reported (see Dental Comment)
Significant Adverse Effects No data reported
Dental Usual Dosing Plaque/gingivitis prevention: Adults: Oral: Rinse full strength for 30 seconds with 20 mL (²/₃ fluid ounce or 4 teaspoonfuls) morning and night
Dosage Rinse full strength for 30 seconds with 20 mL (²/₃ fluid ounce or 4 teaspoonfuls) morning and night
Contraindications Hypersensitivity to any component of the formulation
Dosage Forms Rinse: 250 mL, 500 mL, 1000 mL
Dental Comment Active ingredients:
Listerine® Antiseptic: Thymol 0.064%, eucalyptus 0.092%, methyl salicylate 0.060%, menthol 0.042%, alcohol 26.9%, water, benzoic acid, poloxamer 407, sodium benzoate, caramel
Fresh Burst Listerine® Antiseptic: Thymol 0.064%, eucalyptus 0.092%, methyl salicylate 0.060%, menthol 0.042%, alcohol 26.9%, water, benzoic acid, poloxamer 407, sodium benzoate, flavoring, sodium, saccharin, sodium citrate, citric acid, D&C yellow #10, FD&C green #3
Cool Mint Listerine® Antiseptic: Thymol 0.064%, eucalyptus 0.092%, methyl salicylate 0.060%, menthol 0.042%, alcohol 26.9%, water, benzoic acid, poloxamer 407, sodium benzoate, flavoring, sodium, saccharin, sodium citrate, citric acid, FD&C green #3
The following information is endorsed on the label of the Listerine® products by the Council on Scientific Affairs, American Dental Association: "Listerine® Antiseptic has been shown to help prevent and reduce supragingival plaque accumulation and gingivitis when used in a conscientiously applied program of oral hygiene and regular professional care. Its effect on periodontitis has not been determined."

Moxifloxacin (moxs i FLOKS a sin)

Related Information
Bacterial Infections *on page 1697*
Respiratory Diseases *on page 1656*
U.S. Brand Names Avelox®; Avelox® I.V.; Vigamox™
Canadian Brand Names Avelox®; Avelox® I.V.; Vigamox™
Generic Available No
Synonyms Moxifloxacin Hydrochloride
Pharmacologic Category Antibiotic, Ophthalmic; Antibiotic, Quinolone
Use Treatment of mild-to-moderate community-acquired pneumonia, including multidrug-resistant *Streptococcus pneumoniae* (MDRSP); acute bacterial exacerbation of chronic bronchitis; acute bacterial sinusitis; complicated and uncomplicated skin and skin structure infections; complicated intra-abdominal infections; bacterial conjunctivitis (ophthalmic formulation)
Unlabeled/Investigational Use Legionella
Local Anesthetic/Vasoconstrictor Precautions No information available to require special precautions (see Dental Comment)
Effects on Dental Treatment No significant effects or complications reported
(Continued)

Moxifloxacin *(Continued)*

Common Adverse Effects

Systemic:

3% to 10%: Gastrointestinal: Nausea (6%), diarrhea (5%)

0.1% to 3%:

Cardiovascular: Hypertension, palpitation, QT_c prolongation, tachycardia, vasodilation

Central nervous system: Anxiety, chills, dizziness, headache, insomnia, nervousness, pain, somnolence, tremor, vertigo

Dermatologic: Dry skin, pruritus, rash (maculopapular, purpuric, pustular)

Endocrine & metabolic: Serum chloride increased (≥2%), serum ionized calcium increased (≥2%), serum glucose decreased (≥2%)

Gastrointestinal: Abdominal pain, amylase increased, amylase decreased (≥2%), anorexia, constipation, dry mouth, dyspepsia, flatulence, glossitis, lactic dehydrogenase increased, stomatitis, taste perversion, vomiting

Genitourinary: Vaginal moniliasis, vaginitis

Hematologic: Eosinophilia, leukopenia, prothrombin time prolonged, increased INR, thrombocythemia

Increased serum levels of the following (≥2%): MCH, neutrophils, WBC

Decreased serum levels of the following (≥2%): Basophils, eosinophils, hemoglobin, RBC, neutrophils

Hepatic: Bilirubin decreased or increased (≥2%), GGTP increased, liver function test abnormal

Local: Injection site reaction

Neuromuscular & skeletal: Arthralgia, myalgia, weakness

Renal: Kidney function abnormal, serum albumin increased (≥2%)

Respiratory: Pharyngitis, pneumonia, rhinitis, sinusitis, pO_2 increased (≥2%)

Additional reactions with **ophthalmic** preparation: 1% to 6%: Conjunctivitis, dry eye, ocular discomfort, ocular hyperemia, ocular pain, ocular pruritus, subconjunctival hemorrhage, tearing, visual acuity decreased

Dosage

Usual dosage range:

Children ≥1 year and Adults: Ophthalmic: Instill 1 drop into affected eye(s) 3 times/day for 7 days

Adults: Oral, I.V.: 400 mg every 24 hours

Indication-specific dosing:

Children ≥1 year and Adults: Ophthalmic:

Bacterial conjunctivitis: Instill 1 drop into affected eye(s) 3 times/day for 7 days

Adults: Oral, I.V.:

Acute bacterial sinusitis: 400 mg every 24 hours for 10 days

Chronic bronchitis, acute bacterial exacerbation: 400 mg every 24 hours for 5 days

Intra-abdominal infections (complicated): 400 mg every 24 hours for 5-14 days (initiate with I.V.)

***Legionella* (unlabeled use):** 400 mg every 24 hours for 10-21 days

Pneumonia, community-acquired (including MDRSP): 400 mg every 24 hours for 7-14 days

Skin and skin structure infections:

Complicated: 400 mg every 24 hours for 7-21 days

Uncomplicated: 400 mg every 24 hours for 7 days

Elderly: No dosage adjustments are required based on age

Dosage adjustment in renal impairment: No dosage adjustment is required, including patients on hemodialysis or CAPD

Dosage adjustment in hepatic impairment: No dosage adjustment is required in mild to moderate hepatic insufficiency (Child-Pugh Class A and B). Not recommended in patients with severe hepatic insufficiency.

Mechanism of Action Moxifloxacin is a DNA gyrase inhibitor, and also inhibits topoisomerase IV. DNA gyrase (topoisomerase II) is an essential bacterial enzyme that maintains the superhelical structure of DNA. DNA gyrase is required for DNA replication and transcription, DNA repair, recombination, and transposition; inhibition is bactericidal.

Contraindications Hypersensitivity to moxifloxacin, other quinolone antibiotics, or any component of the formulation

Warnings/Precautions Use with caution in patients with significant bradycardia or acute myocardial ischemia. Moxifloxacin causes a concentration-dependent QT prolongation. Do not exceed recommended dose or infusion rate. Avoid use with uncorrected hypokalemia, with other drugs that prolong the QT interval or induce bradycardia, or with class IA or III antiarrhythmic agents. Use with caution in individuals at risk of seizures (CNS disorders or concurrent therapy with medications which may lower seizure threshold). Discontinue in patients who experience significant CNS adverse effects (dizziness, hallucinations, suicidal ideation or actions). Not recommended in patients with moderate to severe hepatic insufficiency. Use with caution in diabetes; glucose regulation may be altered. Tendon inflammation and/or rupture have been reported with quinolone antibiotics. Risk may be increased with concurrent corticosteroids, particularly in the elderly. Discontinue at first signs or symptoms of tendon pain.

Severe hypersensitivity reactions, including anaphylaxis, have occurred with quinolone therapy. If an allergic reaction occurs (itching, urticaria, dyspnea or facial edema, loss of consciousness, tingling, cardiovascular collapse) discontinue drug immediately. May cause photosensitivity. Prolonged use may result in superinfection; pseudomembranous colitis may occur and should be considered in all patients who present with diarrhea. Quinolones may exacerbate myasthenia gravis. Peripheral neuropathy may rarely occur. Safety and efficacy of systemically administered moxifloxacin (oral, intravenous) in patients <18 years of age have not been established.

Ophthalmic: Eye drops should not be injected subconjunctivally or introduced directly into the anterior chamber of the eye. Contact lenses should not be worn during therapy.

Drug Interactions

Increased Effect/Toxicity: Moxifloxacin may increase the effects/toxicity of glyburide and warfarin. Concomitant use with corticosteroids may increase the risk of tendon rupture. Concomitant use with other QT_c-prolonging agents (eg, Class Ia and Class III antiarrhythmics, erythromycin, cisapride, antipsychotics, and cyclic antidepressants) may result in arrhythmias, such as torsade de pointes.

Decreased Effect: Concurrent administration of metal cations, including most antacids, oral electrolyte supplements, quinapril, sucralfate, some didanosine formulations (chewable/buffered tablets and pediatric powder for oral suspension), and other higly-buffered oral drugs, may decrease quinolone levels; separate doses.

Ethanol/Nutrition/Herb Interactions Food: Absorption is not affected by administration with a high-fat meal or yogurt.

Dietary Considerations May be taken with or without food. Take 4 hours before or 8 hours after multiple vitamins, antacids, or other products containing magnesium, aluminum, iron, or zinc.

Pharmacodynamics/Kinetics

Absorption: Well absorbed; not affected by high fat meal or yogurt

Distribution: V_d: 1.7 to 2.7 L/kg; tissue concentrations often exceed plasma concentrations in respiratory tissues, alveolar macrophages, abdominal tissues/fluids, and sinus tissues

Protein binding: 30% to 50%

Metabolism: Hepatic (52% of dose) via glucuronide (14%) and sulfate (38%) conjugation

Bioavailability: 90%

Half-life elimination: Oral: 12 hours; I.V.: 15 hours

Excretion: Approximately 45% of a dose is excreted in feces (25%) and urine (20%) as unchanged drug

Metabolites: Sulfate conjugates in feces, glucuronide conjugates in urine

Pregnancy Risk Factor C

Dosage Forms INF [premixed in sodium chloride 0.8%] (Avelox® I.V.): 400 mg (250 mL). **SOLN, ophthalmic** (Vigamox™): 0.5% (3 mL). **TAB, film coated** (Avelox®): 400 mg. **TAB, film coated, unit-dose pack** (Avelox® ABC Pack): 400 mg (5s)

Dental Comment

This drug is known to prolong the QT interval. The QT interval is measured as the time and distance between the Q point of the QRS complex and the end of the T wave in the ECG tracing. After adjustment for heart rate, the QT interval is defined as prolonged if it is more than 450 msec in men and 460 msec in women. A long QT syndrome was first described in the 1950s and 60s as a congenital syndrome involving QT interval prolongation and syncope and sudden death. Some of the congenital long QT syndromes were characterized by a peculiar electrocardiographic appearance of the QRS complex involving a premature atria beat followed by a pause, then a subsequent sinus beat showing marked QT prolongation and deformity. This type of cardiac arrhythmia was originally termed "torsade de pointes" (translated from the French as "twisting of the points").

Prolongation of the QT interval is thought to result from delayed ventricular repolarization. The repolarization process within the myocardial cell is due to the efflux of intracellular potassium. The channels associated with this current can be blocked by many drugs and predisposes the electrical propagation cycle to torsade de pointes.

(Continued)

Moxifloxacin *(Continued)*

Moxifloxacin is one of the drugs confirmed to prolong the QT interval and is accepted as having a risk of causing torsade de pointes. The risk of drug-induced torsade de pointes is extremely low when a single QT interval prolonging drug is prescribed. In terms of epinephrine, it is not known what effect vasoconstrictors in the local anesthetic regimen will have in patients with a known history of congenital prolonged QT interval or in patients taking any medication that prolongs the QT interval. Until more information is obtained, it is suggested that the clinician consult with the physician prior to the use of a vasoconstrictor in suspected patients, and that the vasoconstrictor (epinephrine, levonordefrin [Neo-Cobefrin®]) be used with caution.

Moxifloxacin Hydrochloride *see* Moxifloxacin *on page 1069*

Moxilin® *see* Amoxicillin *on page 106*

4-MP *see* Fomepizole *on page 699*

6-MP *see* Mercaptopurine *on page 995*

MPA *see* MedroxyPROGESTERone *on page 972*

MPA and Estrogens (Conjugated) *see* Estrogens (Conjugated/Equine) and Medroxyprogesterone *on page 583*

MPSV4 *see* Meningococcal Polysaccharide Vaccine (Groups A, C, Y, and W-135) *on page 981*

MS Contin® *see* Morphine Sulfate *on page 1065*

MSO₄ (error-prone abbreviation and should not be used) *see* Morphine Sulfate *on page 1065*

MTA *see* Pemetrexed *on page 1198*

MTC *see* Mitomycin *on page 1054*

M.T.E.-4® *see* Trace Metals *on page 1513*

M.T.E.-5® *see* Trace Metals *on page 1513*

M.T.E.-6® *see* Trace Metals *on page 1513*

M.T.E.-7® *see* Trace Metals *on page 1513*

MTX (error-prone abbreviation) *see* Methotrexate *on page 1012*

Mucinex® [OTC] *see* Guaifenesin *on page 752*

Mucinex®-D [OTC] *see* Guaifenesin and Pseudoephedrine *on page 755*

Mucinex® DM [OTC] *see* Guaifenesin and Dextromethorphan *on page 754*

Mucomyst *see* Acetylcysteine *on page 46*

Multidex® [OTC] *see* Maltodextrin *on page 963*

Multiple Vitamins *see* Vitamins (Multiple/Oral) *on page 1582*

Multiret Folic 500 *see* Vitamins (Multiple/Oral) *on page 1582*

Multitargeted Antifolate *see* Pemetrexed *on page 1198*

Multitrace™-4 *see* Trace Metals *on page 1513*

Multitrace™-4 Neonatal *see* Trace Metals *on page 1513*

Multitrace™-4 Pediatric *see* Trace Metals *on page 1513*

Multitrace™-5 *see* Trace Metals *on page 1513*

Mumps, Measles and Rubella Vaccines, Combined *see* Measles, Mumps, and Rubella Vaccines (Combined) *on page 966*

Mumps, Rubella, Varicella, and Measles Vaccine *see* Measles, Mumps, Rubella, and Varicella Virus Vaccine *on page 967*

Mumpsvax® *see* Mumps Virus Vaccine (Live/Attenuated) *on page 1072*

Mumps Virus Vaccine (Live/Attenuated)
(mumpz VYE rus vak SEEN, live, a ten YOO ate ed)

Related Information
Immunizations (Vaccines) *on page 1786*

U.S. Brand Names Mumpsvax®

Generic Available No

Pharmacologic Category Vaccine

Use Mumps prophylaxis by promoting active immunity

Note: Trivalent measles-mumps-rubella (MMR) vaccine is the preferred agent for most children and many adults; persons born prior to 1957 are generally considered immune and need not be vaccinated

Local Anesthetic/Vasoconstrictor Precautions No information available to require special precautions

Effects on Dental Treatment No significant effects or complications reported

Common Adverse Effects All serious adverse reactions must be reported to the U.S. Department of Health and Human Services (DHHS) Vaccine Adverse Event Reporting System (VAERS) 1-800-822-7967.

Frequency not defined.

Cardiovascular: Syncope, vasculitis

Central nervous system: Encephalitis, febrile seizures, fever, Guillain-Barré syndrome, irritability

Dermatologic: Angioneurotic edema, erythema multiforme, purpura, Stevens-Johnson syndrome, urticaria

Endocrine & metabolic: Diabetes mellitus, parotitis

Gastrointestinal: Diarrhea, pancreatitis

Genitourinary: Orchitis

Hematologic: Leukocytosis, thrombocytopenia

Local: Burning/stinging at injection site, wheal and flare at injection site

Ocular: Conjunctivitis, ocular palsies, optic neuritis, papillitis, retrobulbar neuritis

Otic: Nerve deafness, otitis media

Respiratory: Bronchial spasm, cough, rhinitis

Miscellaneous: Anaphylaxis, anaphylactoid reactions, lymphadenopathy

Mechanism of Action Promotes active immunity to mumps virus by inducing specific antibodies.

Drug Interactions

Decreased Effect:

In patients receiving high doses of systemic corticosteroids for ≥14 days, wait at least 1 month between discontinuing steroid therapy and administering vaccine. Do not administer this vaccine with Immune globulin, whole blood, plasma; immune response may be compromised (defer vaccine administration for ≥3 months). The effect of the vaccine may be decreased with Immunosuppressant medications. Do not give within 1 month of other live virus vaccine.

Pregnancy Risk Factor C

Mupirocin (myoo PEER oh sin)

U.S. Brand Names Bactroban®; Bactroban® Nasal; Centany™

Canadian Brand Names Bactroban®

Mexican Brand Names Bactroban®

Generic Available Yes: Topical ointment

Synonyms Mupirocin Calcium; Pseudomonic Acid A

Pharmacologic Category Antibiotic, Topical

Use

Intranasal: Eradication of nasal colonization with MRSA in adult patients and healthcare workers

Topical treatment of impetigo due to *Staphylococcus aureus*, beta-hemolytic *Streptococcus*, and *S. pyogenes*

Unlabeled/Investigational Use Intranasal: Surgical prophylaxis to prevent wound infections

Local Anesthetic/Vasoconstrictor Precautions No information available to require special precautions

Effects on Dental Treatment No significant effects or complications reported

Common Adverse Effects Frequency not defined.

Central nervous system: Dizziness, headache

Dermatologic: Pruritus, rash, erythema, dry skin, cellulitis, dermatitis

Gastrointestinal: Nausea, taste perversion

Local: Burning, stinging, tenderness, edema, pain

Respiratory: Rhinitis, upper respiratory tract infection, pharyngitis, cough

Mechanism of Action Binds to bacterial isoleucyl transfer-RNA synthetase resulting in the inhibition of protein and RNA synthesis

Pharmacodynamics/Kinetics

Absorption: Topical: Penetrates outer layers of skin; systemic absorption minimal through intact skin

Protein binding: 95%

Metabolism: Skin: 3% to monic acid

Half-life elimination: 17-36 minutes

Excretion: Urine

Pregnancy Risk Factor B

Mupirocin Calcium *see* Mupirocin *on page 1073*

Murine® Ear Wax Removal System [OTC] *see* Carbamide Peroxide *on page 264*

Murine® Tears [OTC] *see* Artificial Tears *on page 143*

Murine® Tears Plus [OTC] *see* Tetrahydrozoline *on page 1470*

Muro 128® [OTC] *see* Sodium Chloride *on page 1400*

Murocel® [OTC] *see* Artificial Tears *on page 143*

Murocoll-2® *see* Phenylephrine and Scopolamine *on page 1227*

Muromonab-CD3 (myoo roe MOE nab see dee three)

U.S. Brand Names Orthoclone OKT® 3
Canadian Brand Names Orthoclone OKT® 3
Mexican Brand Names Orthoclone®
Generic Available No
Synonyms Monoclonal Antibody; OKT3
Pharmacologic Category Immunosuppressant Agent
Use Treatment of acute allograft rejection in renal transplant patients; treatment of acute hepatic, kidney, and pancreas rejection episodes resistant to conventional treatment. Acute graft-versus-host disease following bone marrow transplantation resistant to conventional treatment.
Local Anesthetic/Vasoconstrictor Precautions No information available to require special precautions
Effects on Dental Treatment No significant effects or complications reported
Common Adverse Effects Note: Signs and symptoms of Cytokine Release Syndrome (characterized by pyrexia, chills, dyspnea, nausea, vomiting, chest pain, diarrhea, tremor, wheezing, headache, tachycardia, rigor, hypertension, pulmonary edema and/or other cardiorespiratory manifestations) occurs in a significant proportion of patients following the first couple of doses of muromonab-CD3. Additionally, some patients have experienced immediate hypersensitivity reactions to muromonab-CD3 (characterized by cardiovascular collapse, cardiorespiratory arrest, loss of consciousness, hypotension/shock, tachycardia, tingling, angioedema (including laryngeal, pharyngeal, or facial edema), airway obstruction, bronchospasm, dyspnea, urticaria, and/or pruritus) upon initial exposure and re-exposure.

>10%:
   Cardiovascular: Tachycardia (26%), hypotension (25%), hypertension (19%), edema (12%)
   Central nervous system: Pyrexia (77%), chills (43%), headache (28%)
   Dermatologic: Rash (14%; erythematous 2%)
   Gastrointestinal: Diarrhea (37%), nausea (32%), vomiting (25%)
   Respiratory: Dyspnea (16%)

1% to 10%:
   Cardiovascular: Chest pain (9%), vasodilation (7%), arrhythmia (4%), bradycardia (4%), vascular occlusion (2%)
   Central nervous system: Fatigue (9%), confusion (6%), dizziness (6%), lethargy (6%), pain trunk (6%), malaise (5%), nervousness (5%), depression (3%), somnolence (2%), meningitis (1%), seizures (1%)
   Dermatologic: Pruritus (7%)
   Gastrointestinal: Gastrointestinal pain (7%), abdominal pain (6%), anorexia (4%)
   Hematologic: Leukopenia (7%), anemia (2%), thrombocytopenia (2%), leukocytosis (1%)
   Neuromuscular & skeletal: Weakness (10%), arthralgia (7%), myalgia (1%), tremor (14%)
   Ocular: Photophobia (1%)
   Otic: Tinnitus (1%)
   Renal: Renal dysfunction (3%)
   Respiratory: Abnormal chest sound (10%), hyperventilation (7%), wheezing (6%), respiratory congestion (4%), pulmonary edema (2%), hypoxia (1%), pneumonia (1%)
   Miscellaneous: Diaphoresis (7%), infections (various)

Mechanism of Action Reverses graft rejection by binding to T cells and interfering with their function by binding T-cell receptor-associated CD3 glycoprotein
Drug Interactions
   Increased Effect/Toxicity: Recommend decreasing dose of prednisone to 0.5 mg/kg, azathioprine to 0.5 mg/kg (approximate 50% decrease in dose), and discontinuing cyclosporine while patient is receiving OKT3.
   Decreased Effect: Decreased effect with immunosuppressive drugs.
Pharmacodynamics/Kinetics
   Duration: 7 days after discontinuation
   Time to peak: Steady-state: Trough: 3-14 days
Pregnancy Risk Factor C

Muse® see Alprostadil on page 76
Mutamycin® see Mitomycin on page 1054
Myambutol® see Ethambutol on page 591
Mycamine™ see Micafungin on page 1038
Mycelex® see Clotrimazole on page 379

Mycelex®-3 [OTC] see Butoconazole on page 242
Mycelex®-7 [OTC] see Clotrimazole on page 379
Mycelex® Twin Pack [OTC] see Clotrimazole on page 379
Mycinaire™ [OTC] see Sodium Chloride on page 1400
Mycinettes® [OTC] see Benzocaine on page 190
Mycobutin® see Rifabutin on page 1345
Mycolog®-II [DSC] see Nystatin and Triamcinolone on page 1134
Myco-Nail [OTC] see Triacetin on page 1526

Mycophenolate (mye koe FEN oh late)

U.S. Brand Names CellCept®; Myfortic®
Canadian Brand Names CellCept®; Myfortic®
Generic Available No
Synonyms MMF; MPA; Mycophenolate Mofetil; Mycophenolate Sodium; Mycophenolic Acid
Pharmacologic Category Immunosuppressant Agent
Use Prophylaxis of organ rejection concomitantly with cyclosporine and corticosteroids in patients receiving allogenic renal (CellCept®, Myfortic®), cardiac (CellCept®), or hepatic (CellCept®) transplants
Unlabeled/Investigational Use Treatment of rejection in liver transplant patients unable to tolerate tacrolimus or cyclosporine due to neurotoxicity; mild rejection in heart transplant patients; treatment of moderate-severe psoriasis; treatment of proliferative lupus nephritis; treatment of myasthenia gravis
Local Anesthetic/Vasoconstrictor Precautions No information available to require special precautions
Effects on Dental Treatment No significant effects or complications reported
Common Adverse Effects As reported in adults following oral dosing of CellCept® alone in renal, cardiac, and hepatic allograft rejection studies. In general, lower doses used in renal rejection patients had less adverse effects than higher doses. Rates of adverse effects were similar for each indication, except for those unique to the specific organ involved. The type of adverse effects observed in pediatric patients was similar to those seen in adults; abdominal pain, anemia, diarrhea, fever, hypertension, infection, pharyngitis, respiratory tract infection, sepsis, and vomiting were seen in higher proportion; lymphoproliferative disorder was the only type of malignancy observed. Percentages of adverse reactions were similar in studies comparing CellCept® to Myfortic® in patients following renal transplant.

>20%:
  Cardiovascular: Hypertension (28% to 77%), hypotension (up to 33%), peripheral edema (27% to 64%), edema (27% to 28%), tachycardia (20% to 22%)
  Central nervous system: Pain (31% to 76%), headache (16% to 54%), insomnia (41% to 52%), fever (21% to 52%), dizziness (up to 29%), anxiety (28%)
  Dermatologic: Rash (up to 22%)
  Endocrine & metabolic: Hyperglycemia (44% to 47%), hypercholesterolemia (41%), hypokalemia (32% to 37%), hypocalcemia (up to 30%), hypomagnesemia (up to 39%), hyperkalemia (up to 22%)
  Gastrointestinal: Abdominal pain (25% to 62%), nausea (20% to 54%), diarrhea (31% to 52%), constipation (18% to 41%), vomiting (33% to 34%), anorexia (up to 25%), dyspepsia (22%)
  Genitourinary: Urinary tract infection (37%)
  Hematologic: Leukopenia (23% to 46%), leukocytosis (22% to 40%), hypochromic anemia (26% to 43%), thrombocytopenia (24% to 36%)
  Hepatic: Liver function tests abnormal (up to 25%), ascites (24%)
  Neuromuscular & skeletal: Back pain (35% to 47%), weakness (35% to 43%), tremor (24% to 34%), paresthesia (21%)
  Renal: BUN increased (up to 35%), creatinine increased (up to 39%)
  Respiratory: Dyspnea (31% to 37%), respiratory tract infection (22% to 37%), cough (31%), lung disorder (22% to 30%)
  Miscellaneous: Infection (18% to 27%), Candida (11% to 22%), herpes simplex (10% to 21%)
3% to <20%:
  Cardiovascular: Angina, arrhythmia, arterial thrombosis, atrial fibrillation, atrial flutter, bradycardia, cardiac arrest, cardiac failure, CHF, extrasystole, facial edema, hypervolemia, pallor, palpitation, pericardial effusion, peripheral vascular disorder, postural hypotension, supraventricular extrasystoles, supraventricular tachycardia, syncope, thrombosis, vasodilation, vasospasm, venous pressure increased, ventricular extrasystole, ventricular tachycardia

(Continued)

Mycophenolate *(Continued)*

Central nervous system: Agitation, chills with fever, confusion, convulsion, delirium, depression, emotional lability, hallucinations, hypoesthesia, malaise, nervousness, psychosis, somnolence, thinking abnormal, vertigo

Dermatologic: Acne, alopecia, bruising, cellulitis, hirsutism, petechia, pruritus, skin carcinoma, skin hypertrophy, skin ulcer, vesiculobullous rash

Endocrine & metabolic: Acidosis, Cushing's syndrome, dehydration, diabetes mellitus, gout, hypercalcemia, hyperlipemia, hyperphosphatemia, hyperuricemia, hypochloremia, hypoglycemia, hyponatremia, hypoproteinemia, hypothyroidism, parathyroid disorder, weight gain/loss

Gastrointestinal: Abdomen enlarged, dry mouth, dysphagia, esophagitis, flatulence, gastritis, gastroenteritis, gastrointestinal hemorrhage, gastrointestinal moniliasis, gingivitis, gum hyperplasia, ileus, melena, mouth ulceration, oral moniliasis, stomach disorder, stomatitis

Genitourinary: Impotence, nocturia, pelvic pain, prostatic disorder, scrotal edema, urinary frequency, urinary incontinence, urinary retention, urinary tract disorder

Hematologic: Coagulation disorder, hemorrhage, neutropenia, pancytopenia, polycythemia, prothrombin time increased, thromboplastin increased

Hepatic: Alkaline phosphatase increased, alkalosis, bilirubinemia, cholangitis, cholestatic jaundice, GGT increased, hepatitis, jaundice, liver damage, transaminases increased

Local: Abscess

Neuromuscular & skeletal: Arthralgia, hypertonia, joint disorder, leg cramps, myalgia, myasthenia, neck pain, neuropathy, osteoporosis

Ocular: Amblyopia, cataract, conjunctivitis, eye hemorrhage, lacrimation disorder, vision abnormal

Otic: Deafness, ear disorder, ear pain, tinnitus

Renal: Albuminuria, creatinine increased, dysuria, hematuria, hydronephrosis, kidney failure, kidney tubular necrosis, oliguria

Respiratory: Apnea, asthma, atelectasis, bronchitis, epistaxis, hemoptysis, hiccup, hyperventilation, hypoxia, respiratory acidosis, lung edema, pharyngitis, pleural effusion, pneumonia, pneumothorax, pulmonary hypertension, respiratory moniliasis, rhinitis, sinusitis, sputum increased, voice alteration

Miscellaneous: *Candida* (mucocutaneous 15% to 18%), CMV viremia/syndrome (12% to 14%), CMV tissue invasive disease (6% to 11%), herpes zoster cutaneous disease (4% to 10%), cyst, diaphoresis, flu-like syndrome, fungal dermatitis, healing abnormal, hernia, ileus infection, lactic dehydrogenase increased, peritonitis, pyelonephritis, thirst

Mechanism of Action MPA exhibits a cytostatic effect on T and B lymphocytes. It is an inhibitor of inosine monophosphate dehydrogenase (IMPDH) which inhibits *de novo* guanosine nucleotide synthesis. T and B lymphocytes are dependent on this pathway for proliferation.

Drug Interactions

Increased Effect/Toxicity: Acyclovir, valacyclovir, ganciclovir, and valganciclovir levels may increase due to competition for tubular secretion of these drugs. Probenecid may increase mycophenolate levels due to inhibition of tubular secretion. High doses of salicylates may increase free fraction of mycophenolic acid. Azathioprine's bone marrow suppression may be potentiated; do not administer together.

Decreased Effect: Antacids decrease serum levels (C_{max} and AUC); **do not administer together**. Cholestyramine resin decreases serum levels; **do not administer together**. Avoid use of live vaccines; vaccinations may be less effective. Influenza vaccine may be of value. During concurrent use of oral contraceptives, progesterone levels are not significantly affected, however, effect on estrogen component varies; an additional form of contraception should be used.

Pharmacodynamics/Kinetics

Onset of action: Peak effect: Correlation of toxicity or efficacy is still being developed, however, one study indicated that 12-hour AUCs >40 mcg/mL/hour were correlated with efficacy and decreased episodes of rejection

T_{max}: Oral: MPA:

CellCept®: 1-1.5 hours

Myfortic®: 1.5-2.5 hours

Absorption: AUC values for MPA are lower in the early post-transplant period versus later (>3 months) post-transplant period. The extent of absorption in pediatrics is similar to that seen in adults, although there was wide variability reported.

Oral: Myfortic®: 93%

Distribution:

CellCept®: MPA: Oral: 4 L/kg; I.V.: 3.6 L/kg

Myfortic®: MPA: Oral: 54 L (at steady state); 112 L (elimination phase)

Protein binding: MPA: 97%, MPAG 82%

Metabolism: Hepatic and via GI tract; CellCept® is completely hydrolyzed in the liver to mycophenolic acid (MPA; active metabolite); enterohepatic recirculation of MPA may occur; MPA is glucuronidated to MPAG (inactive metabolite)

Bioavailability: Oral: CellCept®: 94%; Myfortic®: 72%

Half-life elimination:

CellCept®: MPA: Oral: 18 hours; I.V.: 17 hours

Myfortic®: MPA: Oral: 8-16 hours; MPAG: 13-17 hours

Excretion:

CellCept®: MPA: Urine (<1%), feces (6%); MPAG: Urine (87%)

Myfortic®: MPA: Urine (3%), feces; MPAG: Urine (>60%)

Pregnancy Risk Factor C (manufacturer)

Mycophenolate Mofetil *see* Mycophenolate *on page 1075*

Mycophenolate Sodium *see* Mycophenolate *on page 1075*

Mycophenolic Acid *see* Mycophenolate *on page 1075*

Mycostatin® *see* Nystatin *on page 1133*

Mydfrin® *see* Phenylephrine *on page 1226*

Mydral™ *see* Tropicamide *on page 1545*

Mydriacyl® *see* Tropicamide *on page 1545*

Myfortic® *see* Mycophenolate *on page 1075*

Mylanta® Children's [OTC] *see* Calcium Carbonate *on page 248*

Mylanta® Gas [OTC] *see* Simethicone *on page 1394*

Mylanta® Gas Maximum Strength [OTC] *see* Simethicone *on page 1394*

Mylanta® Gelcaps® [OTC] *see* Calcium Carbonate and Magnesium Hydroxide *on page 249*

Mylanta® Liquid [OTC] *see* Aluminum Hydroxide, Magnesium Hydroxide, and Simethicone *on page 81*

Mylanta® Maximum Strength Liquid [OTC] *see* Aluminum Hydroxide, Magnesium Hydroxide, and Simethicone *on page 81*

Mylanta® Supreme [OTC] *see* Calcium Carbonate and Magnesium Hydroxide *on page 249*

Mylanta® Ultra [OTC] *see* Calcium Carbonate and Magnesium Hydroxide *on page 249*

Myleran® *see* Busulfan *on page 237*

Mylicon® Infants [OTC] *see* Simethicone *on page 1394*

Mylocel™ *see* Hydroxyurea *on page 800*

Mylotarg® *see* Gemtuzumab Ozogamicin *on page 732*

Myobloc® *see* Botulinum Toxin Type B *on page 218*

Myoflex® [OTC] *see* Triethanolamine Salicylate *on page 1535*

myrac™ *see* Minocycline *on page 1049*

Mysoline® *see* Primidone *on page 1281*

Mytelase® *see* Ambenonium *on page 82*

Mytussin® AC *see* Guaifenesin and Codeine *on page 753*

Mytussin® DAC *see* Guaifenesin, Pseudoephedrine, and Codeine *on page 756*

N-9 *see* Nonoxynol 9 *on page 1124*

Na2EDTA *see* Edetate Disodium *on page 527*

Nabi-HB® *see* Hepatitis B Immune Globulin *on page 768*

NAB-Paclitaxel *see* Paclitaxel (Protein Bound) *on page 1177*

Nabumetone (na BYOO me tone)

Related Information

Rheumatoid Arthritis, Osteoarthritis, and Osteoporosis *on page 1668*

Temporomandibular Dysfunction (TMD) *on page 1724*

U.S. Brand Names Relafen®

Canadian Brand Names Apo-Nabumetone®; Gen-Nabumetone; Novo-Nabumetone; Relafen™; Rhoxal-nabumetone; Sandoz-Nabumetone

Generic Available Yes

Pharmacologic Category Nonsteroidal Anti-inflammatory Drug (NSAID), Oral

Use Management of osteoarthritis and rheumatoid arthritis

Unlabeled/Investigational Use Moderate pain

Local Anesthetic/Vasoconstrictor Precautions No information available to require special precautions

Effects on Dental Treatment Key adverse event(s) related to dental treatment: Xerostomia (normal salivary flow resumes upon discontinuation). NSAID formulations are known to reversibly decrease platelet aggregation via mechanisms different than observed with aspirin. The dentist should be aware of the potential of abnormal coagulation. Caution should also be exercised in the use (Continued)

Nabumetone *(Continued)*

of NSAIDs in patients already on anticoagulant therapy with drugs such as warfarin (Coumadin®).

Common Adverse Effects

>10%: Gastrointestinal: Abdominal pain (12%), diarrhea (14%), dyspepsia (13%)

1% to 10%:

Cardiovascular: Edema (3% to 9%)

Central nervous system: Dizziness (3% to 9%), headache (3% to 9%), fatigue (1% to 3%), insomnia (1% to 3%), nervousness (1% to 3%), somnolence (1% to 3%)

Dermatologic: Pruritus (3% to 9%), rash (3% to 9%)

Gastrointestinal: Constipation (3% to 9%), flatulence (3% to 9%), guaic positive (3% to 9%), nausea (3% to 9%), gastritis (1% to 3%), stomatitis (1% to 3%), vomiting (1% to 3%), xerostomia (1% to 3%)

Otic: Tinnitus

Miscellaneous: Diaphoresis (1% to 3%)

Restrictions A medication guide should be dispensed with each prescription. A template for the required MedGuide can be found on the FDA website at: http://www.fda.gov/medwatch/SAFETY/2005/safety05.htm#NSAID

Dosage Adults: Oral: 1000 mg/day; an additional 500-1000 mg may be needed in some patients to obtain more symptomatic relief; may be administered once or twice daily (maximum dose: 2000 mg/day)

Note: Patients <50 kg are less likely to require doses >1000 mg/day.

Dosage adjustment in renal impairment: In general, NSAIDs are not recommended for use in patients with advanced renal disease, but the manufacturer of nabumetone does provide some guidelines for adjustment in renal dysfunction:

Moderate impairment (Cl_{cr} 30-49 mL/minute): Initial dose: 750 mg/day; maximum dose: 1500 mg/day

Severe impairment (Cl_{cr} <30 mL/minute): Initial dose: 500 mg/day; maximum dose: 1000 mg/day

Mechanism of Action Nabumetone is a nonacidic NSAID that is rapidly metabolized after absorption to a major active metabolite, 6-methoxy-2-naphthylacetic acid. As found with previous NSAIDs, nabumetone's active metabolite inhibits the cyclooxygenase enzyme which is indirectly responsible for the production of inflammation and pain during arthritis by way of enhancing the production of endoperoxides and prostaglandins E_2 and I_2 (prostacyclin). The active metabolite of nabumetone is felt to be the compound primarily responsible for therapeutic effect. Comparatively, the parent drug is a poor inhibitor of prostaglandin synthesis.

Contraindications Hypersensitivity to nabumetone, aspirin, other NSAIDs, or any component of the formulation; perioperative pain in the setting of coronary artery bypass surgery (CABG); pregnancy (3rd trimester)

Warnings/Precautions NSAIDs are associated with an increased risk of adverse cardiovascular events, including MI, stroke, and new onset or worsening of pre-existing hypertension. Risk may be increased with duration of use or pre-existing cardiovascular risk-factors or disease. Carefully evaluate individual cardiovascular risk profiles prior to prescribing. Use caution with fluid retention, CHF or hypertension.

Use of NSAIDs can compromise existing renal function. Renal toxicity can occur in patient with impaired renal function, dehydration, heart failure, liver dysfunction, those taking diuretics and ACEI and the elderly. Rehydrate patient before starting therapy. Monitor renal function closely. Not recommended for use in patients with advanced renal disease.

NSAIDs may increase risk of gastrointestinal irritation, ulceration, bleeding, and perforation. These events may occur at any time during therapy and without warning. Use caution with a history of GI disease (bleeding or ulcers), concurrent therapy with aspirin, anticoagulants and/or corticosteroids, smoking, use of alcohol, the elderly or debilitated patients.

Use the lowest effective dose for the shortest duration of time, consistent with individual patient goals, to reduce risk of cardiovascular or GI adverse events. Alternate therapies should be considered for patients at high risk.

NSAIDs may cause serious skin adverse events including exfoliative dermatitis, Stevens-Johnson syndrome (SJS) and toxic epidermal necrolysis (TEN). Anaphylactoid reactions may occur, even without prior exposure; patients with "aspirin triad" (bronchial asthma, aspirin intolerance, rhinitis) may be at increased risk. Do not use in patients who experience bronchospasm, asthma, rhinitis, or urticaria with NSAID or aspirin therapy.

Use with caution in patients with decreased hepatic function. Closely monitor patients with any abnormal LFT. Severe hepatic reactions (eg, fulminant hepatitis, liver failure) have occurred with NSAID use, rarely; discontinue if signs or symptoms of liver disease develop, or if systemic manifestations occur.

The elderly are at increased risk for adverse effects (especially peptic ulceration, CNS effects, renal toxicity) from NSAIDs even at low doses

Withhold for at least 4-6 half-lives prior to surgical or dental procedures. May cause photosensitivity reactions. Safety and efficacy have not been established in pediatric patients.

Drug Interactions

Increased Effect/Toxicity: NSAIDs may increase digoxin, methotrexate, and lithium serum concentrations. The renal adverse effects of ACE inhibitors may be potentiated by NSAIDs. Potential for bleeding may be increased with anticoagulants or antiplatelet agents. Concurrent use of corticosteroids may increase the risk of GI ulceration.

Decreased Effect: NSAIDs may decrease the effect of some antihypertensive agents, including ACE inhibitors, angiotensin receptor antagonists, beta-blockers, and hydralazine. The efficacy of diuretics (loop and/or thiazide) may be decreased. Cholestyramine (and other bile acid sequestrants) may decrease the absorption of NSAIDs; separate by at least 2 hours.

Ethanol/Nutrition/Herb Interactions

Ethanol: Avoid ethanol (may enhance gastric mucosal irritation).

Food: Nabumetone peak serum concentrations may be increased if taken with food or dairy products.

Herb/Nutraceutical: Avoid alfalfa, anise, bilberry, bladderwrack, bromelain, cat's claw, celery, coleus, cordyceps, dong quai, evening primrose, feverfew, fenugreek, garlic, ginger, ginkgo biloboa, red clover, horse chestnut, grapeseed, green tea, ginseng, guggul, horse chestnut seed, horseradish, licorice, prickly ash, red clover, reishi, SAMe, sweet clover, turmeric, white willow (all have additional antiplatelet activity).

Pharmacodynamics/Kinetics

Onset of action: Several days

Distribution: Diffusion occurs readily into synovial fluid

V_d: 6MNA: 29-82 L

Protein binding: 6MNA: >99%

Metabolism: Prodrug, rapidly metabolized in the liver to an active metabolite [6-methoxy-2-naphthylacetic acid (6MNA)] and inactive metabolites; extensive first-pass effect

Half-life elimination: 6MNA: ~24 hours

Time to peak, serum: 6MNA: Oral: 2.5-4 hours; Synovial fluid: 4-12 hours

Excretion: 6MNA: Urine (80%) and feces (9%)

Pregnancy Risk Factor C/D (3rd trimester)

Dosage Forms TAB: 500 mg, 750 mg

NAC *see* Acetylcysteine *on page 46*

N-Acetyl-L-cysteine *see* Acetylcysteine *on page 46*

N-Acetylcysteine *see* Acetylcysteine *on page 46*

N-Acetyl-P-Aminophenol *see* Acetaminophen *on page 31*

NaCl *see* Sodium Chloride *on page 1400*

Nadolol (nay DOE lole)

Related Information

Cardiovascular Diseases *on page 1636*

U.S. Brand Names Corgard®

Canadian Brand Names Alti-Nadolol; Apo-Nadol®; Corgard®; Novo-Nadolol

Generic Available Yes

Pharmacologic Category Beta-Adrenergic Blocker, Nonselective

Use Treatment of hypertension and angina pectoris; prophylaxis of migraine headaches

Local Anesthetic/Vasoconstrictor Precautions Use with caution; epinephrine has interacted with nonselective beta-blockers to result in initial hypertensive episode followed by bradycardia

Effects on Dental Treatment Nadolol is a nonselective beta-blocker and may enhance the pressor response to epinephrine, resulting in hypertension and bradycardia. Many nonsteroidal anti-inflammatory drugs, such as ibuprofen and indomethacin, can reduce the hypotensive effect of beta-blockers after 3 or more weeks of therapy with the NSAID. Short-term NSAID use (ie, 3 days) requires no special precautions in patients taking beta-blockers.

(Continued)

Nadolol *(Continued)*

Common Adverse Effects

>10%:

Central nervous system: Drowsiness, insomnia

Endocrine & metabolic: Decreased sexual ability

1% to 10%:

Cardiovascular: Bradycardia, palpitation, edema, CHF, reduced peripheral circulation

Central nervous system: Mental depression

Gastrointestinal: Diarrhea or constipation, nausea, vomiting, stomach discomfort

Respiratory: Bronchospasm

Miscellaneous: Cold extremities

Mechanism of Action Competitively blocks response to beta$_1$- and beta$_2$-adrenergic stimulation; does not exhibit any membrane stabilizing or intrinsic sympathomimetic activity

Drug Interactions

Increased Effect/Toxicity: The heart rate lowering effects of nadolol are additive with other drugs which slow AV conduction (digoxin, verapamil, diltiazem). Concurrent use of alpha-blockers (prazosin, terazosin) with beta-blockers may increase risk of orthostasis. Nadolol may mask the tachycardia from hypoglycemia caused by insulin and oral hypoglycemics. In patients receiving concurrent therapy, the risk of hypertensive crisis is increased when either clonidine or the beta-blocker is withdrawn. Reserpine has been shown to enhance the effect of beta-blockers. Avoid using with alpha-adrenergic stimulants (phenylephrine, epinephrine, etc) which may have exaggerated hypertensive responses. Beta-blockers may affect the action or levels of ethanol, disopyramide, nondepolarizing muscle relaxants, and theophylline although the effects are difficult to predict. The vasoconstrictive effects of ergot alkaloids may be enhanced.

Decreased Effect: Decreased effect of beta-blockers with aluminum salts, barbiturates, calcium salts, cholestyramine, colestipol, NSAIDs, penicillins (ampicillin), rifampin, salicylates, and sulfinpyrazone due to decreased bioavailability and plasma levels. Beta-blockers may decrease the effect of sulfonylureas (possibly hyperglycemia). Nonselective beta-blockers blunt the effect of beta-2 adrenergic agonists (albuterol).

Pharmacodynamics/Kinetics

Duration: 17-24 hours

Absorption: 30% to 40%

Distribution: Concentration in human breast milk is 4.6 times higher than serum

Protein binding: 28%

Half-life elimination: Adults: 10-24 hours; prolonged with renal impairment; End-stage renal disease: 45 hours

Time to peak, serum: 2-4 hours

Excretion: Urine (as unchanged drug)

Pregnancy Risk Factor C

Nadolol and Bendroflumethiazide

(nay DOE lole & ben droe floo meth EYE a zide)

U.S. Brand Names Corzide®

Generic Available No

Synonyms Bendroflumethiazide and Nadolol

Pharmacologic Category Antihypertensive Agent, Combination; Beta-Adrenergic Blocker, Nonselective; Diuretic, Thiazide

Use Treatment of hypertension; combination product should not be used for initial therapy

Local Anesthetic/Vasoconstrictor Precautions Use with caution; epinephrine has interacted with nonselective beta-blockers to result in initial hypertensive episode followed by bradycardia

Effects on Dental Treatment Nadolol is a nonselective beta-blocker and may enhance the pressor response to epinephrine, resulting in hypertension and bradycardia. Many nonsteroidal anti-inflammatory drugs, such as ibuprofen and indomethacin, can reduce the hypotensive effect of beta-blockers after 3 or more weeks of therapy with the NSAID. Short-term NSAID use (ie, 3 days) requires no special precautions in patients taking beta-blockers.

Common Adverse Effects See individual agents.

Mechanism of Action See individual agents.

Drug Interactions
  Increased Effect/Toxicity: See individual agents.
  Decreased Effect: See individual agents.
Pharmacodynamics/Kinetics Also see individual agents.
  Bioavailability: Bendroflumethiazide: When used in this combination, bioavailability is increased 30% compared to single agent administration.
Pregnancy Risk Factor C

Nafarelin (NAF a re lin)

U.S. Brand Names Synarel®
Canadian Brand Names Synarel®
Mexican Brand Names Synarel®
Generic Available No
Synonyms Nafarelin Acetate
Pharmacologic Category Gonadotropin Releasing Hormone Agonist
Use Treatment of endometriosis, including pain and reduction of lesions; treatment of central precocious puberty (CPP; gonadotropin-dependent precocious puberty) in children of both sexes
Local Anesthetic/Vasoconstrictor Precautions No information available to require special precautions
Effects on Dental Treatment No significant effects or complications reported
Common Adverse Effects Note: Adverse events may be more frequent in the first 6 weeks of treatment due to stimulation of the pituitary-gonadal axis. Sensitivity reactions included chest pain, pruritus, shortness of breath, rash.
  CPP: 1% to 10%:
    Central nervous system: Emotional lability (6%)
    Dermatologic: Acne (10%), seborrhea (3%)
    Endocrine & metabolic: Breast enlargement (8%; transient), vaginal bleeding (8%), hot flashes (3%; transient), vaginal discharge (3%)
    Respiratory: Rhinitis (5%)
    Miscellaneous: Pubic hair increased (5%; transient), body odor (4%), sensitivity reactions (3%)
  Endometriosis:
    >10%:
      Central nervous system: Headache, emotional lability
      Dermatologic: Acne
      Endocrine & metabolic: Hot flashes (90%), hyperphosphatemia, hypertriglyceridemia, hypocalcemia, libido decreased
      Genitourinary: Vaginal dryness
      Hematologic: Leukopenia
    1% to 10%:
      Cardiovascular: Edema
      Central nervous system: Depression, insomnia
      Dermatologic: Hirsutism, seborrhea
      Endocrine & metabolic: Breast size reduced, cholesterol increased, hyperlipidemia, libido increased
      Gastrointestinal: Weight gain/loss
      Neuromuscular & skeletal: Bone mineral density decreased, myalgia
      Respiratory: Nasal irritation
Mechanism of Action Potent synthetic decapeptide analogue of gonadotropin-releasing hormone (GnRH; LHRH) which is approximately 200 times more potent than GnRH in terms of pituitary release of luteinizing hormone (LH) and follicle-stimulating hormone (FSH). Effects on the pituitary gland and sex hormones are dependent upon its length of administration. After acute administration, an initial stimulation of the release of LH and FSH from the pituitary is observed; an increase in androgens and estrogens subsequently follows. Continued administration of nafarelin, however, suppresses gonadotrope responsiveness to endogenous GnRH resulting in reduced secretion of LH and FSH and, secondarily, decreased ovarian and testicular steroid production.
Pharmacodynamics/Kinetics
  Protein binding, plasma: 80%
  Metabolism: Degraded by peptidase; forms metabolites
  Bioavailability: ~1% to 6%
  Half-life elimination: ~3 hours; Metabolites: ~86 hours
  Time to peak, serum: 10-45 minutes
  Excretion: Urine (44% to 55%, ~3% as unchanged drug); feces (19% to 44%)
Pregnancy Risk Factor X

Nafarelin Acetate see Nafarelin on page 1081

Nafcillin (naf SIL in)

Canadian Brand Names Nallpen®; Unipen®

Generic Available Yes

Synonyms Ethoxynaphthamido Penicillin Sodium; Nafcillin Sodium; Nallpen; Sodium Nafcillin

Pharmacologic Category Antibiotic, Penicillin

Use Treatment of infections such as osteomyelitis, septicemia, endocarditis, and CNS infections caused by susceptible strains of staphylococci species

Local Anesthetic/Vasoconstrictor Precautions No information available to require special precautions

Effects on Dental Treatment Key adverse event(s) related to dental treatment: Prolonged use of penicillins may lead to the development of oral candidiasis.

Common Adverse Effects Frequency not defined.

Central nervous system: Pain, fever

Dermatologic: Rash

Gastrointestinal: Nausea, diarrhea

Hematologic: Agranulocytosis, bone marrow depression, neutropenia

Local: Pain, swelling, inflammation, phlebitis, skin sloughing, and thrombophlebitis at the injection site; oxacillin (less likely to cause phlebitis) is often preferred in pediatric patients

Renal: Interstitial nephritis (acute)

Miscellaneous: Hypersensitivity reactions

Mechanism of Action Interferes with bacterial cell wall synthesis during active multiplication, causing cell wall death and resultant bactericidal activity against susceptible bacteria

Drug Interactions

Cytochrome P450 Effect: Induces CYP3A4 (strong)

Increased Effect/Toxicity: Probenecid may cause an increase in nafcillin levels. Penicillins may increase the exposure to methotrexate during concurrent therapy; monitor.

Decreased Effect: Chloramphenicol may decrease nafcillin efficacy. If taken concomitantly with warfarin, nafcillin may inhibit the anticoagulant response to warfarin. This effect may persist for up to 30 days after nafcillin has been discontinued. Subtherapeutic cyclosporine levels may result when taken concomitantly with nafcillin. Although anecdotal reports suggest oral contraceptive efficacy could be reduced by penicillins, this has been refuted by more rigorous scientific and clinical data. Nafcillin may decrease the levels/effects of benzodiazepines, calcium channel blockers, clarithromycin, cyclosporine, erythromycin, estrogens, mirtazapine, nateglinide, nefazodone, nevirapine, protease inhibitors, tacrolimus, venlafaxine, and other CYP3A4 substrates.

Pharmacodynamics/Kinetics

Distribution: Widely distributed; CSF penetration is poor but enhanced by meningeal inflammation; crosses placenta

Protein binding: 70% to 90%

Metabolism: Primarily hepatic; undergoes enterohepatic recirculation

Half-life elimination:

Neonates: <3 weeks: 2.2-5.5 hours; 4-9 weeks: 1.2-2.3 hours

Children 3 months to 14 years: 0.75-1.9 hours

Adults: 30 minutes to 1.5 hours with normal renal and hepatic function

Time to peak, serum: I.M.: 30-60 minutes

Excretion: Primarily feces; urine (10% to 30% as unchanged drug)

Pregnancy Risk Factor B

Nafcillin Sodium *see* Nafcillin *on page 1082*

Nafidimide *see* Amonafide *on page 104*

Naftifine (NAF ti feen)

Related Information

Fungal Infections *on page 1707*

U.S. Brand Names Naftin®

Generic Available No

Synonyms Naftifine Hydrochloride

Pharmacologic Category Antifungal Agent, Topical

Use Topical treatment of tinea cruris (jock itch), tinea corporis (ringworm), and tinea pedis (athlete's foot)

Local Anesthetic/Vasoconstrictor Precautions No information available to require special precautions

Effects on Dental Treatment No significant effects or complications reported

Common Adverse Effects

>10%: Local: Burning, stinging

1% to 10%:
Dermatologic: Erythema, itching
Local: Dryness, irritation

Mechanism of Action Synthetic, broad-spectrum antifungal agent in the allyla-mine class; appears to have both fungistatic and fungicidal activity. Exhibits antifungal activity by selectively inhibiting the enzyme squalene epoxidase in a dose-dependent manner which results in the primary sterol, ergosterol, within the fungal membrane not being synthesized.

Pharmacodynamics/Kinetics

Absorption: Systemic: Cream: 6%; Gel: ≤4%
Half-life elimination: 2-3 days
Excretion: Urine and feces (as metabolites)

Pregnancy Risk Factor B

Naftifine Hydrochloride *see* Naftifine *on page 1082*

Naftin® *see* Naftifine *on page 1082*

Naglazyme™ *see* Galsulfase *on page 721*

NaHCO₃ *see* Sodium Bicarbonate *on page 1400*

Nalbuphine (NAL byoo feen)

U.S. Brand Names Nubain®
Mexican Brand Names Bufigen®; Nalcryn®; Nubain®
Generic Available Yes
Synonyms Nalbuphine Hydrochloride
Pharmacologic Category Analgesic, Narcotic
Use Relief of moderate to severe pain; preoperative analgesia, postoperative and surgical anesthesia, and obstetrical analgesia during labor and delivery

Local Anesthetic/Vasoconstrictor Precautions No information available to require special precautions

Effects on Dental Treatment Key adverse event(s) related to dental treatment: Anticholinergic side effects can cause a reduction of saliva production or secretion, contributing to discomfort and dental disease (ie, caries, oral candidiasis, and periodontal disease).

Common Adverse Effects

>10%: Central nervous system: Sedation (36%)

1% to 10%:
Central nervous system: Dizziness (5%), headache (3%)
Gastrointestinal: Nausea/vomiting (6%), xerostomia (4%)
Miscellaneous: Clamminess (9%)

Mechanism of Action Agonist of kappa opiate receptors and partial antagonist of mu opiate receptors in the CNS, causing inhibition of ascending pain pathways, altering the perception of and response to pain; produces generalized CNS depression

Drug Interactions

Increased Effect/Toxicity: Barbiturate anesthetics may increase CNS depression.

Pharmacodynamics/Kinetics

Onset of action: Peak effect: SubQ, I.M.: <15 minutes; I.V.: 2-3 minutes
Metabolism: Hepatic
Half-life elimination: 5 hours
Excretion: Feces; urine (~7% as metabolites)

Pregnancy Risk Factor B/D (prolonged use or high doses at term)

Nalbuphine Hydrochloride *see* Nalbuphine *on page 1083*

Naldecon Senior EX® [OTC] [DSC] *see* Guaifenesin *on page 752*

Nalex®-A *see* Chlorpheniramine, Phenylephrine, and Phenyltoloxamine *on page 328*

Nalfon® *see* Fenoprofen *on page 642*

Nalidixic Acid (nal i DIKS ik AS id)

U.S. Brand Names NegGram® [DSC]
Canadian Brand Names NegGram®
Generic Available No
Synonyms Nalidixinic Acid
Pharmacologic Category Antibiotic, Quinolone
Use Treatment of urinary tract infections
(Continued)

Nalidixic Acid *(Continued)*

Local Anesthetic/Vasoconstrictor Precautions No information available to require special precautions

Effects on Dental Treatment No significant effects or complications reported

Mechanism of Action Inhibits DNA polymerization in late stages of chromosomal replication

Pregnancy Risk Factor C

Nalidixinic Acid *see Nalidixic Acid on page 1083*

Nallpen *see Nafcillin on page 1082*

N-allylnoroxymorphine Hydrochloride *see Naloxone on page 1084*

Nalmefene *(NAL me feen)*

U.S. Brand Names Revex®
Generic Available No
Synonyms Nalmefene Hydrochloride
Pharmacologic Category Antidote
Use Complete or partial reversal of opioid drug effects, including respiratory depression induced by natural or synthetic opioids; reversal of postoperative opioid depression; management of known or suspected opioid overdose

Local Anesthetic/Vasoconstrictor Precautions No information available to require special precautions

Effects on Dental Treatment No significant effects or complications reported

Common Adverse Effects
>10%: Gastrointestinal: Nausea (18%)
1% to 10%:
Cardiovascular: Tachycardia (5%), hypertension (5%), hypotension (1%), vasodilation (1%)
Central nervous system: Fever (3%), dizziness (3%), headache (1%), chills (1%)
Gastrointestinal: Vomiting (9%)
Miscellaneous: Postoperative pain (4%)

Mechanism of Action As a 6-methylene analog of naltrexone, nalmefene acts as a competitive antagonist at opioid receptor sites, preventing or reversing the respiratory depression, sedation, and hypotension induced by opiates; no pharmacologic activity of its own (eg, opioid agonist activity) has been demonstrated

Drug Interactions
Increased Effect/Toxicity: Potential increased risk of seizures may exist with use of flumazenil and nalmefene coadministration.

Pharmacodynamics/Kinetics
Onset of action: I.M., SubQ: 5-15 minutes
Distribution: V_d: 8.6 L/kg; rapid
Protein binding: 45%
Metabolism: Hepatic via glucuronide conjugation to metabolites with little or no activity
Bioavailability: I.M., SubQ: 100%
Half-life elimination: 10.8 hours
Time to peak, serum: Serum: I.M.: 2.3 hours; I.V.: <2 minutes; SubQ: 1.5 hours
Excretion: Feces (17%); urine (<5% as unchanged drug)
Clearance: 0.8 L/hour/kg

Pregnancy Risk Factor B

Nalmefene Hydrochloride *see Nalmefene on page 1084*

Naloxone *(nal OKS one)*

U.S. Brand Names Narcan® [DSC]
Mexican Brand Names Narcanti®
Generic Available Yes
Synonyms *N*-allylnoroxymorphine Hydrochloride; Naloxone Hydrochloride
Pharmacologic Category Antidote
Dental Use Reverse overdose effects of the two narcotic agents, fentanyl and meperidine, used in the technique of I.V. conscious sedation
Use
Complete or partial reversal of opioid depression, including respiratory depression, induced by natural and synthetic opioids, including propoxyphene, methadone, and certain mixed agonist-antagonist analgesics: nalbuphine, pentazocine, and butorphanol
Diagnosis of suspected opioid tolerance or acute opioid overdose
Adjunctive agent to increase blood pressure in the management of septic shock

Unlabeled/Investigational Use PCP and ethanol ingestion

Local Anesthetic/Vasoconstrictor Precautions No information available to require special precautions

Effects on Dental Treatment No significant effects or complications reported

Significant Adverse Effects Frequency not defined.

Cardiovascular: Hyper-/hypotension, tachycardia, ventricular arrhythmia, cardiac arrest

Central nervous system: Irritability, anxiety, narcotic withdrawal, restlessness, seizure

Gastrointestinal: Nausea, vomiting, diarrhea

Neuromuscular & skeletal: Tremulousness

Respiratory: Dyspnea, pulmonary edema, runny nose, sneezing

Miscellaneous: Diaphoresis

Dental Usual Dosing Narcotic overdose: Adults: I.V.: 0.4-2 mg every 2-3 minutes as needed; may need to repeat doses every 20-60 minutes, if no response is observed after 10 mg, question the diagnosis. **Note:** Use 0.1-0.2 mg increments in patients who are opioid dependent and in postoperative patients to avoid large cardiovascular changes.

Dosage I.M., I.V. (preferred), intratracheal, SubQ:

Postanesthesia narcotic reversal: Infants and Children: 0.01 mg/kg; may repeat every 2-3 minutes, as needed based on response

Opiate intoxication:

Children:

Birth (including premature infants) to 5 years or <20 kg: 0.1 mg/kg; repeat every 2-3 minutes if needed; may need to repeat doses every 20-60 minutes

>5 years or ≥20 kg: 2 mg/dose; if no response, repeat every 2-3 minutes; may need to repeat doses every 20-60 minutes

Children and Adults: Continuous infusion: I.V.: If continuous infusion is required, calculate dosage/hour based on effective intermittent dose used and duration of adequate response seen, titrate dose 0.04-0.16 mg/kg/hour for 2-5 days in children, adult dose typically 0.25-6.25 mg/hour (short-term infusions as high as 2.4 mg/kg/hour have been tolerated in adults during treatment for septic shock); alternatively, continuous infusion utilizes $^2/_3$ of the initial naloxone bolus on an hourly basis; add 10 times this dose to each liter of D_5W and infuse at a rate of 100 mL/hour; $^1/_2$ of the initial bolus dose should be readministered 15 minutes after initiation of the continuous infusion to prevent a drop in naloxone levels; increase infusion rate as needed to assure adequate ventilation

Narcotic overdose: Adults: I.V.: 0.4-2 mg every 2-3 minutes as needed; may need to repeat doses every 20-60 minutes, if no response is observed after 10 mg, question the diagnosis. **Note:** Use 0.1-0.2 mg increments in patients who are opioid dependent and in postoperative patients to avoid large cardiovascular changes.

Mechanism of Action Pure opioid antagonist that competes and displaces narcotics at opioid receptor sites

Contraindications Hypersensitivity to naloxone or any component of the formulation

Warnings/Precautions Due to an association between naloxone and acute pulmonary edema, use with caution in patients with cardiovascular disease or in patients receiving medications with potential adverse cardiovascular effects (eg, hypotension, pulmonary edema or arrhythmias). Excessive dosages should be avoided after use of opiates in surgery. Abrupt postoperative reversal may result in nausea, vomiting, sweating, tachycardia, hypertension, seizures, and other cardiovascular events (including pulmonary edema and arrhythmias). May precipitate withdrawal symptoms in patients addicted to opiates, including pain, hypertension, sweating, agitation, irritability; in neonates: shrill cry, failure to feed. Recurrence of respiratory depression is possible if the opioid involved is long-acting; observe patients until there is no reasonable risk of recurrent respiratory depression.

Drug Interactions Narcotic analgesics: Decreased effect of narcotic analgesics; may precipitate acute withdrawal reaction in physically dependent patients

Pharmacodynamics/Kinetics

Onset of action: Endotracheal, I.M., SubQ: 2-5 minutes; I.V.: ~2 minutes

Duration: 20-60 minutes; since shorter than that of most opioids, repeated doses are usually needed

Distribution: Crosses placenta

Metabolism: Primarily hepatic via glucuronidation

Half-life elimination: Neonates: 1.2-3 hours; Adults: 1-1.5 hours

Excretion: Urine (as metabolites)

Pregnancy Risk Factor C

Lactation Excretion in breast milk unknown/not recommended

(Continued)

Naloxone *(Continued)*

Breast-Feeding Considerations No data reported. Since naloxone is used for opiate reversal the concern should be on opiate drug levels in a breast-feeding mother and transfer to the infant rather than naloxone exposure. The safest approach would be **not** to breast-feed.

Dosage Forms

Injection, solution, as hydrochloride: 0.4 mg/mL (1 mL, 10 mL)
  Narcan®: 0.4 mg/mL (1 mL) [DSC]

Naloxone and Buprenorphine see Buprenorphine and Naloxone on page 232

Naloxone Hydrochloride see Naloxone on page 1084

Naloxone Hydrochloride and Pentazocine Hydrochloride see Pentazocine on page 1208

Naloxone Hydrochloride Dihydrate and Buprenorphine Hydrochloride see Buprenorphine and Naloxone on page 232

Naltrexone *(nal TREKS one)*

U.S. Brand Names Depade®; ReVia®; Vivitrol™
Canadian Brand Names ReVia®
Generic Available Yes: Tablet
Synonyms Naltrexone Hydrochloride
Pharmacologic Category Antidote
Use Treatment of ethanol dependence; blockade of the effects of exogenously administered opioids
Local Anesthetic/Vasoconstrictor Precautions No information available to require special precautions
Effects on Dental Treatment No significant effects or complications reported
Common Adverse Effects Combined reporting of adverse events from oral and injectable formulations:

>10%:

Cardiovascular: Syncope (13%)

Central nervous system: Headache (25%), insomnia (14%), dizziness (13%), anxiety (12%), somnolence (4%), nervousness, fatigue

Gastrointestinal: Nausea (33%), vomiting (14%), appetite decreased (14%), diarrhea (13%), abdominal pain (11%), abdominal cramping

Local: Injection-site reaction (69%)

Neuromuscular & skeletal: Arthralgia (12%), CPK increased (11%)

Respiratory: Upper respiratory tract infection (13%), pharyngitis (11%)

1% to 10%:

Central nervous system: Depression (8%), suicidal thoughts (1%), energy increased, feeling down

Dermatologic: Rash (6%)

Endocrine & metabolic: Polydipsia

Gastrointestinal: Dry mouth (5%)

Genitourinary: Delayed ejaculation, impotency

Hepatic: AST increased (2%)

Neuromuscular & skeletal: Muscle cramps (8%), back pain (6%)

Mechanism of Action Naltrexone (a pure opioid antagonist) is a cyclopropyl derivative of oxymorphone similar in structure to naloxone and nalorphine (a morphine derivative); it acts as a competitive antagonist at opioid receptor sites, showing the highest affinity for mu receptors.

Drug Interactions

Increased Effect/Toxicity: Lethargy and somnolence have been reported with the combination of naltrexone and thioridazine.

Decreased Effect: Naltrexone decreases effects of opioid-containing products.

Pharmacodynamics/Kinetics

Duration: Oral: 50 mg: 24 hours; 100 mg: 48 hours; 150 mg: 72 hours; I.M.: 4 weeks

Absorption: Oral: Almost complete

Distribution: V_d: 19 L/kg; widely throughout the body but considerable inter-individual variation exists

Protein binding: 21%

Metabolism: Noncytochrome-mediated dehydrogenase conversion to 6-β-naltrexol and related minor metabolites; Oral: Extensive first-pass effect

Half-life elimination: Oral: 4 hours; 6-β-naltrexol: 13 hours; I.M.: naltrexone and 6-β-naltrexol: 5-10 days

Time to peak, serum: Oral: ~60 minutes; I.M.: Biphasic: 2 hours (first peak), 2-3 days (second peak)

Excretion: Primarily urine (as metabolites and unchanged drug)

Pregnancy Risk Factor C

Naltrexone Hydrochloride *see* Naltrexone *on page 1086*

Namenda™ *see* Memantine *on page 979*

Nandrolone (NAN droe lone)

Canadian Brand Names Deca-Durabolin®; Durabolin®
Mexican Brand Names Deca-Durabolin®
Generic Available Yes
Synonyms Nandrolone Decanoate; Nandrolone Phenpropionate
Pharmacologic Category Androgen
Use Control of metastatic breast cancer; management of anemia of renal insufficiency
Local Anesthetic/Vasoconstrictor Precautions No information available to require special precautions
Effects on Dental Treatment No significant effects or complications reported
Common Adverse Effects
Male:
Postpubertal:
>10%:
Dermatologic: Acne
Endocrine & metabolic: Gynecomastia
Genitourinary: Bladder irritability, priapism
1% to 10%:
Central nervous system: Insomnia, chills
Endocrine & metabolic: Decreased libido, hepatic dysfunction
Gastrointestinal: Nausea, diarrhea
Genitourinary: Prostatic hyperplasia (elderly)
Hematologic: Iron deficiency anemia, suppression of clotting factors
Prepubertal:
>10%:
Dermatologic: Acne
Endocrine & metabolic: Virilism
1% to 10%:
Central nervous system: Chills, insomnia
Dermatologic: Hyperpigmentation
Gastrointestinal: Diarrhea, nausea
Hematologic: Iron deficiency anemia, suppression of clotting
Female:
>10%: Endocrine & metabolic: Virilism
1% to 10%:
Central nervous system: Chills, insomnia
Endocrine & metabolic: Hypercalcemia
Gastrointestinal: Nausea, diarrhea
Hematologic: Iron deficiency anemia, suppression of clotting factors
Hepatic: Hepatic dysfunction
Restrictions C-III
Mechanism of Action Promotes tissue-building processes, increases production of erythropoietin, causes protein anabolism; increases hemoglobin and red blood cell volume
Drug Interactions
Increased Effect/Toxicity: Nandrolone may increase the effect of oral anticoagulants, insulin, oral hypoglycemic agents, adrenal steroids, or ACTH when taken together.
Pharmacodynamics/Kinetics
Onset of action: 3-6 months
Duration: Up to 30 days
Absorption: I.M.: 77%
Metabolism: Hepatic
Excretion: Urine
Pregnancy Risk Factor X

Nandrolone Decanoate *see* Nandrolone *on page 1087*

Nandrolone Phenpropionate *see* Nandrolone *on page 1087*

Naphazoline (naf AZ oh leen)

U.S. Brand Names AK-Con™; Albalon®; Allersol®; Clear Eyes® ACR [OTC]; Clear Eyes® Extra Relief [OTC]; Naphcon® [OTC]; Privine® [OTC]
(Continued)

Naphazoline *(Continued)*

Canadian Brand Names Naphcon Forte®; Vasocon®
Mexican Brand Names Afazol Grin®; Alphadinal®
Generic Available Yes: Ophthalmic solution
Synonyms Naphazoline Hydrochloride
Pharmacologic Category Alpha₁ Agonist; Ophthalmic Agent, Vasoconstrictor
Use Topical ocular vasoconstrictor; will temporarily relieve congestion, itching, and minor irritation, and to control hyperemia in patients with superficial corneal vascularity; treatment of nasal congestion; adjunct for sinusitis
Local Anesthetic/Vasoconstrictor Precautions No information available to require special precautions
Effects on Dental Treatment No significant effects or complications reported
Common Adverse Effects Frequency not defined.
  Cardiovascular: Systemic cardiovascular stimulation
  Central nervous system: Dizziness, headache, nervousness
  Gastrointestinal: Nausea
  Local: Transient stinging, nasal mucosa irritation, dryness, rebound congestion
  Ocular: Mydriasis, increased intraocular pressure, blurred vision
  Respiratory: Sneezing
Mechanism of Action Stimulates alpha-adrenergic receptors in the arterioles of the conjunctiva and the nasal mucosa to produce vasoconstriction
Drug Interactions
  Increased Effect/Toxicity: Anesthetics (discontinue mydriatic prior to use of anesthetics that sensitize the myocardium to sympathomimetics, ie, cyclopropane, halothane), MAO inhibitors, tricyclic antidepressants may cause hypertensive reactions.
Pharmacodynamics/Kinetics
  Onset of action: Decongestant: Topical: ~10 minutes
  Duration: 2-6 hours
Pregnancy Risk Factor C

Naphazoline and Antazoline (naf AZ oh leen & an TAZ oh leen)

Related Information
  Naphazoline *on page 1087*
U.S. Brand Names Vasocon®-A [OTC] [DSC]
Canadian Brand Names Albalon®-A Liquifilm; Vasocon®-A
Generic Available No
Synonyms Antazoline and Naphazoline
Pharmacologic Category Ophthalmic Agent, Vasoconstrictor
Use Topical ocular congestion, irritation and itching
Local Anesthetic/Vasoconstrictor Precautions No information available to require special precautions
Effects on Dental Treatment No significant effects or complications reported
Pregnancy Risk Factor C

Naphazoline and Pheniramine (naf AZ oh leen & fen NIR a meen)

Related Information
  Naphazoline *on page 1087*
U.S. Brand Names Naphcon-A® [OTC]; Opcon-A® [OTC]; Visine-A™ [OTC]
Canadian Brand Names Naphcon-A®; Visine® Advanced Allergy
Generic Available Yes
Synonyms Pheniramine and Naphazoline
Pharmacologic Category Ophthalmic Agent, Vasoconstrictor
Use Treatment of ocular congestion, irritation, and itching
Local Anesthetic/Vasoconstrictor Precautions No information available to require special precautions
Effects on Dental Treatment No significant effects or complications reported
Pregnancy Risk Factor C

Naphazoline Hydrochloride *see* Naphazoline *on page 1087*
Naphcon® [OTC] *see* Naphazoline *on page 1087*
Naphcon-A® [OTC] *see* Naphazoline and Pheniramine *on page 1088*
NapraPAC™ *see* Lansoprazole and Naproxen *on page 898*
Naprelan® *see* Naproxen *on page 1089*
Naprosyn® *see* Naproxen *on page 1089*

Naproxen (na PROKS en)

Related Information
Oral Pain *on page 1692*
Rheumatoid Arthritis, Osteoarthritis, and Osteoporosis *on page 1668*
Temporomandibular Dysfunction (TMD) *on page 1724*

Related Sample Prescriptions
Mild/Moderate Oral Pain *on page 1734*

U.S. Brand Names Aleve® [OTC]; Anaprox®; Anaprox® DS; EC-Naprosyn®; Midol® Extended Relief; Naprelan®; Naprosyn®; Pamprin® Maximum Strength All Day Relief [OTC]

Canadian Brand Names Anaprox®; Anaprox® DS; Apo-Napro-Na®; Apo-Napro-Na DS®; Apo-Naproxen®; Apo-Naproxen SR®; Gen-Naproxen EC; Naprosyn®; Naxen®; Novo-Naproc EC; Novo-Naprox; Novo-Naprox Sodium; Novo-Naprox Sodium DS; Novo-Naprox SR; Nu-Naprox; Riva-Naproxen

Generic Available Yes

Synonyms Naproxen Sodium

Pharmacologic Category Nonsteroidal Anti-inflammatory Drug (NSAID), Oral

Dental Use Management of pain and swelling

Use Management of ankylosing spondylitis, osteoarthritis, and rheumatoid disorders (including juvenile rheumatoid arthritis); acute gout; mild-to-moderate pain; tendonitis, bursitis; dysmenorrhea; fever

Local Anesthetic/Vasoconstrictor Precautions No information available to require special precautions

Effects on Dental Treatment Key adverse event(s) related to dental treatment: Stomatitis. NSAID formulations are known to reversibly decrease platelet aggregation via mechanisms different than observed with aspirin. The dentist should be aware of the potential of abnormal coagulation. Caution should also be exercised in the use of NSAIDs in patients already on anticoagulant therapy with drugs such as warfarin (Coumadin®).

Significant Adverse Effects
1% to 10%:
  Cardiovascular: Edema (3% to 9%), palpitations (<3%)
  Central nervous system: Dizziness (3% to 9%), drowsiness (3% to 9%), headache (3% to 9%), lightheadedness (<3%), vertigo (<3%)
  Dermatologic: Pruritus (3% to 9%), skin eruption (3% to 9%), ecchymosis (3% to 9%), purpura (<3%), rash
  Endocrine & metabolic: Fluid retention (3% to 9%)
  Gastrointestinal: Abdominal pain (3% to 9%), constipation (3% to 9%), nausea (3% to 9%), heartburn (3% to 9%), diarrhea (<3%), dyspepsia (<3%), stomatitis (<3%), heartburn (<3%), flatulence, gross bleeding/perforation, indigestion, ulcers, vomiting
  Genitourinary: Abnormal renal function
  Hematologic: Hemolysis (3% to 9%), ecchymosis (3% to 9%), anemia, bleeding time increased
  Hepatic: LFTs increased
  Ocular: Visual disturbances (<3%)
  Otic: Tinnitus (3% to 9%), hearing disturbances (<3%)
  Respiratory: Dyspnea (3% to 9%)
  Miscellaneous: Diaphoresis (<3%), thirst (<3%)
<1% (Limited to important or life-threatening): Agranulocytosis, alopecia, anaphylactic/anaphylactoid reaction, angioneurotic edema, arrhythmia, aseptic meningitis, asthma, blurred vision, cognitive dysfunction, colitis, coma, confusion, CHF, conjunctivitis, cystitis, depression, dream abnormalities, dysuria, eosinophilia, eosinophilic pneumonitis, erythema multiforme, exfoliative dermatitis, glossitis, granulocytopenia, hallucinations, hematemesis, hepatitis, hyper-/hypoglycemia, hyper-/hypotension, infection, interstitial nephritis, melena, jaundice, leukopenia, liver failure, lymphadenopathy, menstrual disorders, malaise, MI, muscle weakness, myalgia, oliguria, pancreatitis, pancytopenia, paresthesia, photosensitivity, pneumonia, polyuria, proteinuria, pyrexia, rectal bleeding, renal failure, renal papillary necrosis, respiratory depression, sepsis, Stevens-Johnson syndrome, tachycardia, seizure, syncope, thrombocytopenia, toxic epidermal necrolysis ulcerative stomatitis, vasculitis

Restrictions A medication guide should be dispensed with each prescription. A template for the required MedGuide can be found on the FDA website at: http://www.fda.gov/medwatch/SAFETY/2005/safety05.htm#NSAID

Dental Usual Dosing Mild-to-moderate pain: Adults: Initial: 500 mg, then 250 mg every 6-8 hours; maximum: 1250 mg/day naproxen base
(Continued)

Naproxen *(Continued)*

Pain/fever (OTC labeling):

Children ≥12 years and Adults ≤65 years: 200 mg naproxen base every 8-12 hours; if needed, may take 400 mg naproxen base for the initial dose; maximum: 600 mg naproxen base/24 hours

Adults >65 years: 200 mg naproxen base every 12 hours

Dosage Note: Dosage expressed as naproxen base; 200 mg naproxen base is equivalent to 220 mg naproxen sodium.

Oral:

Children >2 years: Juvenile arthritis: 10 mg/kg/day in 2 divided doses

Adults:

Gout, acute: Initial: 750 mg, followed by 250 mg every 8 hours until attack subsides. **Note:** EC-Naprosyn® is not recommended.

Migraine, acute (unlabeled use): Initial: 500-750 mg.; an additional 250-500 mg may be given if needed (maximum: 1250 mg in 24 hours). **Note:** EC-Naprosyn® is not recommended.

Pain (mild-to-moderate), dysmenorrhea, acute tendonitis, bursitis: Initial: 500 mg, then 250 mg every 6-8 hours; maximum: 1250 mg/day naproxen base

Rheumatoid arthritis, osteoarthritis, and ankylosing spondylitis: 500-1000 mg/day in 2 divided doses; may increase to 1.5 g/day of naproxen base for limited time period

OTC labeling: Pain/fever:

Children ≥12 years and Adults ≤65 years: 200 mg naproxen base every 8-12 hours; if needed, may take 400 mg naproxen base for the initial dose; maximum: 600 mg naproxen base/24 hours

Adults >65 years: 200 mg naproxen base every 12 hours

Dosing adjustment in renal impairment: Cl_{cr} <30 mL/minute: use is not recommended

Mechanism of Action Inhibits prostaglandin synthesis by decreasing the activity of the enzyme, cyclooxygenase, which results in decreased formation of prostaglandin precursors

Contraindications Hypersensitivity to naproxen, aspirin, other NSAIDs, or any component of the formulation; perioperative pain in the setting of coronary artery bypass surgery (CABG); pregnancy (3rd trimester)

Warnings/Precautions

NSAIDs are associated with an increased risk of adverse cardiovascular events, including MI, stroke, and new onset or worsening of pre-existing hypertension. Risk may be increased with duration of use or pre-existing cardiovascular risk-factors or disease. Carefully evaluate individual cardiovascular risk profiles prior to prescribing. Use caution with fluid retention, CHF, or hypertension. Use the lowest effective dose for the shortest duration of time, consistent with individual patient goals, to reduce risk of cardiovascular or GI adverse events. Alternate therapies should be considered for patients at high risk.

Use of NSAIDs can compromise existing renal function. Renal toxicity can occur in patient with impaired renal function, dehydration, heart failure, liver dysfunction, those taking diuretics and ACEI and the elderly. Rehydrate patient before starting therapy. Monitor renal function closely. Naproxen is not recommended for patients with advanced renal disease.

NSAIDs may increase risk of gastrointestinal irritation, ulceration, bleeding, and perforation. These events may occur at any time during therapy and without warning. Use caution with a history of GI disease (bleeding or ulcers), concurrent therapy with aspirin, anticoagulants and/or corticosteroids, smoking, use of alcohol, the elderly or debilitated patients.

NSAIDs may cause serious skin adverse events including exfoliative dermatitis, Stevens-Johnson Syndrome (SJS) and toxic epidermal necrolysis (TEN). Anaphylactoid reactions may occur, even without prior exposure; patients with "aspirin triad" (bronchial asthma, aspirin intolerance, rhinitis) may be at increased risk. Do not use in patients who experience bronchospasm, asthma, rhinitis, or urticaria with NSAID or aspirin therapy.

Use with caution in patients with decreased hepatic function. Closely monitor patients with any abnormal LFT. Severe hepatic reactions (eg, fulminant hepatitis, liver failure) have occurred with NSAID use, rarely; discontinue if signs or symptoms of liver disease develop, or if systemic manifestations occur.

The elderly are at increased risk for adverse effects (especially peptic ulceration, CNS effects, renal toxicity) from NSAIDs even at low doses.

Withhold for at least 4-6 half-lives prior to surgical or dental procedures. Safety and efficacy have not been established in children <2 years of age.

OTC labeling: Prior to self-medication, patients should contact health care provider if they have had recurring stomach pain or upset, ulcers, bleeding problems, high blood pressure, heart or kidney disease, other serious medical problems, are currently taking a diuretic, or are ≥60 years of age. Recommended dosages should not be exceeded, due to an increased risk of GI bleeding. Consuming ≥3 alcoholic beverages/day or taking longer than recommended may increase the risk of GI bleeding. When used for self-medication, patients should be instructed to contact healthcare provider if used for fever lasting >3 days or for pain lasting >10 days in adults or >3 days in children. Not for self-medication (OTC use) in children <12 years of age.

Drug Interactions Substrate (minor) of CYP1A2, 2C8/9

ACE inhibitors: Antihypertensive effects may be decreased by concurrent therapy with NSAIDs; monitor blood pressure.

Angiotensin II antagonists: Antihypertensive effects may be decreased by concurrent therapy with NSAIDs; monitor blood pressure.

Anticoagulants (warfarin, heparin, LMWHs) in combination with NSAIDs can cause increased risk of bleeding.

Antiplatelet drugs (ticlopidine, clopidogrel, aspirin, abciximab, dipyridamole, eptifibatide, tirofiban) can cause an increased risk of bleeding.

Beta-blockers: NSAIDs may decrease the antihypertensive effect of beta-blockers. Monitor.

Cholestyramine (and other bile acid sequestrants): May decrease the absorption of NSAIDs. Separate by at least 2 hours.

Corticosteroids may increase the risk of GI ulceration; avoid concurrent use.

Cyclosporine: NSAIDs may increase serum creatinine, potassium, blood pressure, and cyclosporine levels; monitor cyclosporine levels and renal function carefully.

Hydralazine's antihypertensive effect is decreased; avoid concurrent use.

Lithium levels can be increased; avoid concurrent use if possible or monitor lithium levels and adjust dose. Sulindac may have the least effect. When NSAID is stopped, lithium will need adjustment again.

Loop diuretics efficacy (diuretic and antihypertensive effect) is reduced. Indomethacin reduces this efficacy, however, it may be anticipated with any NSAID.

Methotrexate: Severe bone marrow suppression, aplastic anemia, and GI toxicity have been reported with concomitant NSAID therapy. Avoid use during moderate or high-dose methotrexate (increased and prolonged methotrexate levels). NSAID use during low-dose treatment of rheumatoid arthritis has not been fully evaluated; extreme caution is warranted.

Thiazides antihypertensive effects are decreased; avoid concurrent use.

Warfarin's INRs may be increased by naproxen. Other NSAIDs may have the same effect depending on dose and duration. Monitor INR closely. Use the lowest dose of NSAIDs possible and for the briefest duration.

Ethanol/Nutrition/Herb Interactions

Ethanol: Avoid ethanol (may enhance gastric mucosal irritation).

Food: Naproxen absorption ratelevels may be decreased if taken with food.

Herb/Nutraceutical: Avoid alfalfa, anise, bilberry, bladderwrack, bromelain, cat's claw, celery, coleus, cordyceps, dong quai, evening primrose, feverfew, fenugreek, garlic, ginger, ginkgo biloboa, red clover, horse chestnut, grapeseed, green tea, ginseng, guggul, horse chestnut seed, horseradish, licorice, prickly ash, red clover, reishi, SAMe, sweet clover, turmeric, white willow (all have additional antiplatelet activity).

Dietary Considerations Drug may cause GI upset, bleeding, ulceration, perforation; take with food or milk to minimize GI upset.

Pharmacodynamics/Kinetics

Onset of action: Analgesic: 1 hour; Anti-inflammatory: ~2 weeks

Peak effect: Anti-inflammatory: 2-4 weeks

Duration: Analgesic: ≤7 hours; Anti-inflammatory: ≤12 hours

Absorption: Almost 100%

Protein binding: >99%; increased free fraction in elderly

Half-life elimination: Normal renal function: 12-17 hours; End-stage renal disease: No change

Time to peak, serum: 1-4 hours

Excretion: Urine (95%)

Pregnancy Risk Factor C/D (3rd trimester)

Lactation Enters breast milk/not recommended (AAP rates "compatible")

Dosage Forms

Caplet, as sodium (Aleve®, Midol® Extended Relief, Pamprin® Maximum Strength All Day Relief): 220 mg [equivalent to naproxen 200 mg and sodium 20 mg]

Gelcap, as sodium (Aleve®): 220 mg [equivalent to naproxen 200 mg and sodium 20 mg]

Suspension, oral (Naprosyn®): 125 mg/5 mL (480 mL) [contains sodium 0.3 mEq/mL; orange-pineapple flavor]

(Continued)

Naproxen *(Continued)*

Tablet (Naprosyn®): 250 mg, 375 mg, 500 mg

Tablet, as sodium: 220 mg [equivalent to naproxen 200 mg and sodium 20 mg]; 275 mg [equivalent to naproxen 250 mg and sodium 25 mg]; 550 mg [equivalent to naproxen 500 mg and sodium 50 mg]

Aleve®: 220 mg [equivalent to naproxen 200 mg and sodium 20 mg]

Anaprox®: 275 mg [equivalent to naproxen 250 mg and sodium 25 mg]

Anaprox® DS: 550 mg [equivalent to naproxen 500 mg and sodium 50 mg]

Tablet, controlled release, as sodium: 550 mg [equivalent to naproxen 500 mg and sodium 50 mg]

Naprelan®: 421.5 mg [equivalent to naproxen 375 mg and sodium 37.5 mg]; 550 mg [equivalent to naproxen 500 mg and sodium 50 mg]

Tablet, delayed release (EC-Naprosyn®): 375 mg, 500 mg

Selected Readings

Ahmad N, Grad HA, Haas DA, et al, "The Efficacy of Nonopioid Analgesics for Postoperative Dental Pain: A Meta-Analysis," *Anesth Prog*, 1997, 44(4):119-26.

Brooks PM and Day RO, "Nonsteroidal Anti-inflammatory Drugs - Differences and Similarities," *N Engl J Med*, 1991, 324(24):1716-25.

Dionne R, "Additive Analgesia Without Opioid Side Effects," *Compend Contin Educ Dent*, 2000, 21(7):572-4, 576-7.

Dionne RA and Berthold CW, "Therapeutic Uses of Nonsteroidal Anti-inflammatory Drugs in Dentistry," *Crit Rev Oral Biol Med*, 2001, 12(4):315-30.

Forbes JA, Keller CK, Smith JW, et al, "Analgesic Effect of Naproxen Sodium, Codeine, a Naproxen-Codeine Combination and Aspirin on the Postoperative Pain of Oral Surgery," *Pharmacotherapy*, 1986, 6(5):211-8.

Nguyen AM, Graham DY, Gage T, et al, "Nonsteroidal Anti-inflammatory Drug Use in Dentistry: Gastrointestinal Implications," *Gen Dent*, 1999, 47(6):590-6.

Naproxen and Lansoprazole *see* Lansoprazole and Naproxen *on page 898*

Naproxen Sodium *see* Naproxen *on page 1089*

Naratriptan *(NAR a trip tan)*

U.S. Brand Names Amerge®

Canadian Brand Names Amerge®

Mexican Brand Names Naramig®

Generic Available No

Synonyms Naratriptan Hydrochloride

Pharmacologic Category Serotonin 5-HT$_{1D}$ Receptor Agonist

Use Treatment of acute migraine headache with or without aura

Local Anesthetic/Vasoconstrictor Precautions No information available to require special precautions

Effects on Dental Treatment No significant effects or complications reported

Common Adverse Effects 1% to 10%:

Central nervous system: Dizziness, drowsiness, malaise/fatigue

Gastrointestinal: Nausea, vomiting

Neuromuscular & skeletal: Paresthesias

Miscellaneous: Pain or pressure in throat or neck

Mechanism of Action The therapeutic effect for migraine is due to serotonin agonist activity

Drug Interactions

Increased Effect/Toxicity: Ergot-containing drugs (dihydroergotamine or methysergide) may cause vasospastic reactions when taken with naratriptan. Avoid concomitant use with ergots; separate dose of naratriptan and ergots by at least 24 hours. Oral contraceptives taken with naratriptan reduced the clearance of naratriptan ~30% which may contribute to adverse effects. Selective serotonin reuptake inhibitors (SSRIs) (eg, fluoxetine, fluvoxamine, paroxetine, sertraline) may cause lack of coordination, hyper-reflexia, or weakness and should be avoided when taking naratriptan.

Decreased Effect: Smoking increases the clearance of naratriptan.

Pharmacodynamics/Kinetics

Onset of action: 30 minutes

Absorption: Well absorbed

Protein binding, plasma: 28% to 31%

Metabolism: Hepatic via CYP

Bioavailability: 70%

Time to peak: 2-3 hours

Excretion: Urine

Pregnancy Risk Factor C

Naratriptan Hydrochloride *see* Naratriptan *on page 1092*

Narcan® [DSC] *see* Naloxone *on page 1084*

Nardil® *see* Phenelzine *on page 1221*

Naropin® *see* Ropivacaine *on page 1366*

Nasacort® AQ *see* Triamcinolone *on page 1526*
NaSal™ [OTC] *see* Sodium Chloride *on page 1400*
NasalCrom® [OTC] *see* Cromolyn *on page 397*
Nasal Moist® [OTC] *see* Sodium Chloride *on page 1400*
Nasarel® *see* Flunisolide *on page 667*
Nasatab® LA *see* Guaifenesin and Pseudoephedrine *on page 755*
Nascobal® *see* Cyanocobalamin *on page 399*
Nasonex® *see* Mometasone Furoate *on page 1060*
Natacyn® *see* Natamycin *on page 1093*

Natalizumab (na ta LIZ u mab)

U.S. Brand Names Tysabri®
Generic Available No
Synonyms AN100226; Anti-4 Alpha Integrin; IgG4-Kappa Monoclonal Antibody
Pharmacologic Category Monoclonal Antibody, Selective Adhesion-Molecule Inhibitor
Use Treatment of relapsing forms of multiple sclerosis
Unlabeled/Investigational Use Crohn's disease
Local Anesthetic/Vasoconstrictor Precautions No information available to require special precautions
Effects on Dental Treatment No significant effects or complications reported
Common Adverse Effects
>10%:
Central nervous system: Headache (35%), fatigue (24%), depression (17%)
Genitourinary: Urinary tract infection (18%)
Neuromuscular & skeletal: Arthralgia (15%)
Respiratory: Lower respiratory infection (15%)
Miscellaneous: Infusion-related reaction (22%)
1% to 10%:
Cardiovascular: Chest discomfort (4%)
Central nervous system: Syncope (2%), suicidal ideation (1%)
Dermatologic: Rash (9%), dermatitis (5%), pruritus (4%), urticaria (2%)
Endocrine & metabolic: Menstrual irregularities (7%), amenorrhea (2%)
Gastrointestinal: Abdominal discomfort (10%), gastroenteritis (9%), cholelithiasis (1%)
Genitourinary: Urinary frequency (7%), vaginitis (8%)
Hepatic: Transaminase abnormal (5%)
Local: Bleeding at injection site (3%)
Neuromuscular & skeletal: Rigors (3%), tremor (3%)
Respiratory: Tonsillitis (5%), pneumonia (1%)
Miscellaneous: Allergic reaction (7%), infection (2%), anaphylaxis (1%)
Mechanism of Action Natalizumab is a monoclonal antibody to the alpha-4 subunit of integrin molecules. These molecules are important to adhesion and migration of cells from the vasculature into inflamed tissue. Natalizumab blocks integrin association with vascular receptors, limiting adhesion and transmigration of leukocytes. Efficacy in specific disorders may be related to reduction in specific inflammatory cell populations in target tissues. In multiple sclerosis, efficacy may be related to blockade of T-lymphocyte migration into the central nervous system; treatment results in a decreased frequency of relapse.
Drug Interactions
Increased Effect/Toxicity: Concomitant immunosuppressant therapy may increase the risk of infection. Interferon beta-1a may increase the levels of natalizumab (no dosage adjustment necessary).
Pharmacodynamics/Kinetics
Distribution: 3.8-7.6 L
Half-life elimination: 7-15 days
Excretion: Clearance: 11-21 mL/hour
Pregnancy Risk Factor C

Natamycin (na ta MYE sin)

U.S. Brand Names Natacyn®
Canadian Brand Names Natacyn®
Generic Available No
Synonyms Pimaricin
Pharmacologic Category Antifungal Agent, Ophthalmic
Use Treatment of blepharitis, conjunctivitis, and keratitis caused by susceptible fungi (*Aspergillus, Candida*), *Cephalosporium, Curvularia, Fusarium, Penicillium, Microsporum, Epidermophyton, Blastomyces dermatitidis, Coccidioides*
(Continued)

Natamycin *(Continued)*

immitis, *Cryptococcus neoformans*, *Histoplasma capsulatum*, *Sporothrix schenckii*, and *Trichomonas vaginalis*

Local Anesthetic/Vasoconstrictor Precautions No information available to require special precautions

Effects on Dental Treatment No significant effects or complications reported

Mechanism of Action Increases cell membrane permeability in susceptible fungi

Pregnancy Risk Factor C

Nateglinide *(na te GLYE nide)*

Related Information

Endocrine Disorders and Pregnancy *on page 1659*

U.S. Brand Names Starlix®

Canadian Brand Names Starlix®

Generic Available No

Pharmacologic Category Antidiabetic Agent, Meglitinide Derivative

Use Management of type 2 diabetes mellitus (noninsulin dependent, NIDDM) as monotherapy when hyperglycemia cannot be managed by diet and exercise alone; in combination with metformin or a thiazolidinedione to lower blood glucose in patients whose hyperglycemia cannot be controlled by exercise, diet, or a single agent alone

Local Anesthetic/Vasoconstrictor Precautions No information available to require special precautions

Effects on Dental Treatment No significant effects or complications reported

Common Adverse Effects As reported with nateglinide monotherapy:

1% to 10%:
Central nervous system: Dizziness (4%)
Endocrine & metabolic: Hypoglycemia (2%), increased uric acid
Gastrointestinal: Weight gain
Neuromuscular & skeletal: Arthropathy (3%)
Respiratory: Upper respiratory infection (10%)
Miscellaneous: Flu-like symptoms (4%)

Mechanism of Action A phenylalanine derivative, nonsulfonylurea hypoglycemic agent used in the management of type 2 diabetes mellitus (noninsulin dependent, NIDDM); stimulates insulin release from the pancreatic beta cells to reduce postprandial hyperglycemia; amount of insulin release is dependent upon existing glucose levels

Drug Interactions

Cytochrome P450 Effect: Substrate (major) of CYP2C8/9, 3A4; **Inhibits** CYP2C8/9 (weak)

Increased Effect/Toxicity: CYP2C8/9 inhibitors may increase the levels/effects of nateglinide; example inhibitors include delavirdine, fluconazole, gemfibrozil, ketoconazole, nicardipine, NSAIDs, pioglitazone, and sulfonamides. CYP3A4 inhibitors may increase the levels/effects of nateglinide; example inhibitors include azole antifungals, clarithromycin, diclofenac, doxycycline, erythromycin, imatinib, isoniazid, nefazodone, nicardipine, propofol, protease inhibitors, quinidine, telithromycin, and verapamil. Possible increased hypoglycemic effect may be seen with salicylates, MAO inhibitors, and nonselective beta-adrenergic blocking agents; monitor glucose closely when agents are initiated, modified, or discontinued.

Decreased Effect: CYP2C8/9 inducers may decrease the levels/effects of nateglinide; example inducers include carbamazepine, phenobarbital, phenytoin, rifampin, rifapentine, and secobarbital. CYP3A4 inducers may decrease the levels/effects of nateglinide; example inducers include aminoglutethimide, carbamazepine, nafcillin, nevirapine, phenobarbital, phenytoin, and rifamycins. Possible decreased hypoglycemic effect may be seen with thiazides, corticosteroids, thyroid products, and sympathomimetic drugs; monitor glucose closely when agents are initiated, modified, or discontinued.

Pharmacodynamics/Kinetics

Onset of action: Insulin secretion: ~20 minutes
Peak effect: 1 hour
Duration: 4 hours
Absorption: Rapid
Distribution: 10 L
Protein binding: 98%, primarily to albumin
Metabolism: Hepatic via hydroxylation followed by glucuronide conjugation via CYP2C9 (70%) and CYP3A4 (30%) to metabolites
Bioavailability: 73%

Half-life elimination: 1.5 hours
Time to peak: ≤1 hour
Excretion: Urine (83%, 16% as unchanged drug); feces (10%)
Pregnancy Risk Factor C

Natrecor® *see* Nesiritide *on page 1103*
Natriuretic Peptide *see* Nesiritide *on page 1103*
Natural Fiber Therapy [OTC] *see* Psyllium *on page 1313*
Natural Lung Surfactant *see* Beractant *on page 198*
Nature's Tears® [OTC] *see* Artificial Tears *on page 143*
Nature-Throid® NT *see* Thyroid *on page 1482*
Nausea Relief [OTC] *see* Fructose, Dextrose, and Phosphoric Acid *on page 713*
Nausetrol® [OTC] *see* Fructose, Dextrose, and Phosphoric Acid *on page 713*
Navane® *see* Thiothixene *on page 1480*
Navelbine® *see* Vinorelbine *on page 1578*
Na-Zone® [OTC] *see* Sodium Chloride *on page 1400*
NC-722665 *see* Bicalutamide *on page 207*
n-Docosanol *see* Docosanol *on page 495*
NebuPent® *see* Pentamidine *on page 1207*
Necon® 0.5/35 *see* Ethinyl Estradiol and Norethindrone *on page 608*
Necon® 1/35 *see* Ethinyl Estradiol and Norethindrone *on page 608*
Necon® 1/50 *see* Mestranol and Norethindrone *on page 999*
Necon® 7/7/7 *see* Ethinyl Estradiol and Norethindrone *on page 608*
Necon® 10/11 *see* Ethinyl Estradiol and Norethindrone *on page 608*

Nedocromil (ne doe KROE mil)

Related Information
  Respiratory Diseases *on page 1656*
U.S. Brand Names Alocril®; Tilade®
Canadian Brand Names Alocril®; Tilade®
Mexican Brand Names Irtan®; Tilaire®
Generic Available No
Synonyms Nedocromil Sodium
Pharmacologic Category Mast Cell Stabilizer
Use
  Aerosol: Maintenance therapy in patients with mild to moderate bronchial asthma
  Ophthalmic: Treatment of itching associated with allergic conjunctivitis
Local Anesthetic/Vasoconstrictor Precautions No information available to require special precautions
Effects on Dental Treatment No significant effects or complications reported
Common Adverse Effects
  Inhalation aerosol:
  >10%: Gastrointestinal: Unpleasant taste
  1% to 10%:
    Cardiovascular: Chest pain
    Central nervous system: Dizziness, dysphonia, headache, fatigue
    Dermatologic: Rash
    Gastrointestinal: Nausea, vomiting, dyspepsia, diarrhea, abdominal pain, xerostomia, unpleasant taste
    Hepatic: Increased ALT
    Neuromuscular & skeletal: Arthritis, tremor
    Respiratory: Cough, pharyngitis, rhinitis, bronchitis, upper respiratory infection, bronchospasm, increased sputum production
  Ophthalmic solution:
  >10%:
    Central nervous system: Headache (40%)
    Gastrointestinal: Unpleasant taste
    Ocular: Burning, irritation, stinging
    Respiratory: Nasal congestion
  1% to 10%:
    Ocular: Conjunctivitis, eye redness, photophobia
    Respiratory: Asthma, rhinitis
Mechanism of Action Inhibits the activation of and mediator release from a variety of inflammatory cell types associated with asthma including eosinophils, neutrophils, macrophages, mast cells, monocytes, and platelets; it inhibits the release of histamine, leukotrienes, and slow-reacting substance of anaphylaxis; it inhibits the development of early and late bronchoconstriction responses to inhaled antigen
(Continued)

Nedocromil (Continued)

Pharmacodynamics/Kinetics

Duration: Therapeutic effect: 2 hours
Protein binding, plasma: 89%
Bioavailability: 7% to 9%
Half-life elimination: 1.5-2 hours
Excretion: Urine (as unchanged drug)

Pregnancy Risk Factor B

Nedocromil Sodium see Nedocromil on page 1095

Nefazodone (nef AY zoe done)

Generic Available Yes

Synonyms Nefazodone Hydrochloride; Serzone

Pharmacologic Category Antidepressant, Serotonin Reuptake Inhibitor/ Antagonist

Use Treatment of depression

Unlabeled/Investigational Use Post-traumatic stress disorder

Local Anesthetic/Vasoconstrictor Precautions Nefazodone inhibits reuptake of both serotonin and norepinephrine and also blocks some serotonin receptors. No precautions with vasoconstrictors appear to be necessary.

Effects on Dental Treatment Key adverse event(s) related to dental treatment: Significant xerostomia (normal salivary flow resumes upon discontinuation).

Common Adverse Effects

>10%:

Central nervous system: Headache, drowsiness, insomnia, agitation, dizziness

Gastrointestinal: Xerostomia, nausea, constipation

Neuromuscular & skeletal: Weakness

1% to 10%:

Cardiovascular: Bradycardia, hypotension, peripheral edema, postural hypotension, vasodilation

Central nervous system: Chills, fever, incoordination, lightheadedness, confusion, memory impairment, abnormal dreams, decreased concentration, ataxia, psychomotor retardation, tremor

Dermatologic: Pruritus, rash

Endocrine & metabolic: Breast pain, impotence, libido decreased

Gastrointestinal: Gastroenteritis, vomiting, dyspepsia, diarrhea, increased appetite, thirst, taste perversion

Genitourinary: Urinary frequency, urinary retention

Hematologic: Hematocrit decreased

Neuromuscular & skeletal: Arthralgia, hypertonia, paresthesia, neck rigidity, tremor

Ocular: Blurred vision (9%), abnormal vision (7%), eye pain, visual field defect

Otic: Tinnitus

Respiratory: Bronchitis, cough, dyspnea, pharyngitis

Miscellaneous: Flu syndrome, infection

Restrictions A medication guide concerning the use of antidepressants in children and teenagers can be found on the FDA website at http://www.fda.gov/ cder/Offices/ODS/labeling.htm. It should be dispensed to parents or guardians of children and teenagers receiving this medication.

Mechanism of Action Inhibits neuronal reuptake of serotonin and norepinephrine; also blocks 5-HT$_2$ and alpha$_1$ receptors; has no significant affinity for alpha$_2$, beta-adrenergic, 5-HT$_{1A}$, cholinergic, dopaminergic, or benzodiazepine receptors

Drug Interactions

Cytochrome P450 Effect: Substrate (major) of CYP2D6, 3A4; **Inhibits** CYP1A2 (weak), 2B6 (weak), 2D6 (weak), 3A4 (strong)

Increased Effect/Toxicity: Concurrent use of carbamazepine, cisapride, or pimozide is contraindicated. Concurrent therapy with triazolam or alprazolam is generally contraindicated (dosage must be reduced by 75% for triazolam and 50% for alprazolam; such reductions may not be possible with available dosage forms). Concurrent use of ergot alkaloids and/or selected HMG-CoA reductase inhibitors (lovastatin and simvastatin) is generally contraindicated with strong CYP3A4 inhibitors.

Concurrent use of MAO inhibitors may lead to serotonin syndrome; avoid concurrent use or use within 14 days (includes phenelzine, isocarboxazid, and linezolid). Selegiline may increase the risk of serotonin syndrome, particularly at higher doses (>10 mg/day, where selectivity for MAO type B is decreased). Theoretically, concurrent use of buspirone, meperidine, serotonin agonists (sumatriptan and rizatriptan), SSRIs, and venlafaxine may result in serotonin syndrome.

Nefazodone may increase the serum levels/effects of antiarrhythmics (amiodarone, lidocaine, propafenone, quinidine), some antipsychotics (clozapine, haloperidol, mesoridazine, quetiapine, and risperidone), some benzodiazepines (triazolam is contraindicated; decrease alprazolam dose by 50%), buspirone (limit buspirone dose to <2.5 mg/day), Nefazodone may increase the levels/effects of calcium channel blockers, cyclosporine, mirtazapine, nateglinide, nefazodone, quinidine, sildenafil (and other PDE-5 inhibitors), tacrolimus, venlafaxine, and other CYP3A4 substrates. When used with strong CYP3A4 inhibitors, dosage adjustment/limits are recommended for sildenafil and other PDE-5 inhibitors; refer to individual monographs.

The levels/effects of nefazodone may be increased by azole antifungals, chlorpromazine, clarithromycin, delavirdine, diclofenac, doxycycline, erythromycin, fluoxetine, imatinib, isoniazid, miconazole, nicardipine, paroxetine, pergolide, propofol, protease inhibitors, quinidine, quinine, ritonavir, ropinirole, telithromycin, verapamil, and other CYP2D6 or 3A4 inhibitors.

Decreased Effect: Carbamazepine may reduce serum concentrations of nefazodone; concurrent administration should be avoided. The levels/effects of nefazodone may be decreased by aminoglutethimide, nafcillin, nevirapine, phenobarbital, phenytoin, and rifamycins and other CYP3A4 inducers.

Pharmacodynamics/Kinetics

Onset of action: Therapeutic: Up to 6 weeks

Metabolism: Hepatic to three active metabolites: Triazoledione, hydroxynefazodone, and m-chlorophenylpiperazine (mCPP)

Bioavailability: 20% (variable)

Half-life elimination: Parent drug: 2-4 hours; active metabolites persist longer

Time to peak, serum: 1 hour, prolonged in presence of food

Excretion: Primarily urine (as metabolites); feces

Pregnancy Risk Factor C

Nefazodone Hydrochloride see Nefazodone on page 1096

NegGram® [DSC] see Nalidixic Acid on page 1083

Nelarabine (nel AY re been)

U.S. Brand Names Arranon®

Generic Available No

Synonyms 2-Amino-6-Methoxypurine Arabinoside; GW506U78; 506U78

Pharmacologic Category Antineoplastic Agent, Antimetabolite

Use Treatment of relapsed or refractory T-cell acute lymphoblastic leukemia (ALL) and T-cell lymphoblastic lymphoma

Unlabeled/Investigational Use CML (Philadelphia chromosome positive) T-Cell blast phase

Local Anesthetic/Vasoconstrictor Precautions No information available to require special precautions

Effects on Dental Treatment Key adverse event(s) related to dental treatment: Taste perversion and stomatitis.

Common Adverse Effects Note: Adverse drug reactions listed regardless of grade. Grade 4 toxicities (grade 2 or higher for neurotoxicity) noted when applicable. Pediatric adverse reactions fell within a range similar to adults except where noted.

>10%:

Cardiovascular: Peripheral edema (15%), edema (11%)

Central nervous system: Fatigue (50%), fever (23%), somnolence (7% to 22%; grades 2-4: 3% to 6%), dizziness (21%; grade 2: 8% adults), headache (15% to 17%; grades 2-4: 4% to 8%), hypoesthesia (6% to 17%; grades 2-4: children 5%, adults 12%), pain (11%)

Dermatologic: Petechiae (12%)

Endocrine & metabolic: Hypokalemia (12%)

Gastrointestinal: Nausea (41%), diarrhea (22%), vomiting (10% to 22%), constipation (21%)

Hematologic: Anemia (95% to 99%; grade 4: 10% to 14%; grade 4: children 62%, adults 49%), neutropenia (81% to 94%; grade 4: children 62%, adults 49%), thrombocytopenia (86% to 88%; grade 4: 22% to 32%), leukopenia (38%; grade 4: 7%), febrile neutropenia (12%; grade 4: 1%)

Hepatic: Transaminases increased (12%)

Neuromuscular & skeletal: Peripheral neuropathy (12% to 21%; grades 2-4: 11% to 14%; grade 4: 1%), weakness (6% to 17%; grade 4: 1%), paresthesia (4% to 15%; grades 2-4: 3% to 4%), myalgia (13%)

(Continued)

Nelarabine *(Continued)*

Respiratory: Cough (25%), dyspnea (7% to 20%)

1% to 10%:

Cardiovascular: Hypotension (8%), tachycardia (8%), chest pain (5%)

Central nervous system: Ataxia (2% to 9%; grades 2-4: children 1%, adults 8%), confusion (8%), insomnia (7%), depressed level of consciousness (6%; grades 2-4: 2%), depression (6%), seizure (grade 4: 6% children), motor dysfunction (4%; grades 2-4: 2%), amnesia (3%; grades 2-4: 1%), balance disorder (2%; grades 2-4: 1%), nerve paralysis (2%), sensory loss (1% to 2%), aphasia (1%), cerebral hemorrhage (1%), coma (1%), encephalopathy (1%), hemiparesis (1%), hydrocephalus (1%), lethargy (1%), leukoencephalopathy (1%), loss of consciousness (1%), mental impairment (1%), neuropathic pain (1%), nerve palsy (1%), nystagmus (1%), paralysis (1%), sciatica (1%), sensory disturbance (1%), speech disorder (1%), demyelination, ascending peripheral neuropathy

Endocrine & Metabolic: Hypocalcemia (8%), dehydration (7%), hyper-/hypoglycemia (6%), hypomagnesemia (6%)

Gastrointestinal: Abdominal pain (9%), anorexia (9%), stomatitis (8%), abdominal distension (6%), taste perversion (3%)

Hepatic: Albumin decreased (10%), bilirubin increased (10%), AST increased (6%)

Neuromuscular & skeletal: Arthralgia (9%), back pain (8%), muscle weakness (8%), rigors (8%), limb pain (7%), abnormal gait (6%), noncardiac chest pain (5%), tremor (4% to 5%; grades 2-4: 2% to 3%), dysarthria (1%), hyporeflexia (1%), hypertonia (1%), incoordination (1%)

Ocular: Blurred vision (4%)

Renal: Creatinine increased (6%)

Respiratory: Pleural effusion (10%), epistaxis (8%), pneumonia (8%), sinusitis (7%), wheezing (5%), sinus headache (1%)

Miscellaneous: Infection (5% to 9%)

Mechanism of Action Nelarabine is a prodrug of ara-G. It is demethylated by adenosine deaminase to ara-G and then converted to ara-GTP. Ara-GTP is incorporated into the DNA of the leukemic blasts, leading to inhibition of DNA synthesis and inducing apoptosis. Ara-GTP appears to accumulate at higher levels in T-cells, which correlates to clinical response.

Drug Interactions

Increased Effect/Toxicity: Vaccines: Avoid administration of live vaccines in immunosuppressive therapy.

Pharmacodynamics/Kinetics

Distribution: Nelarabine: 197-213 L/m^2; ara-G: 33-50 L/m^2

Protein binding: Nelarabine and ara-G: <25%

Metabolism: Hepatic; demethylated by adenosine deaminase to form ara-G (active); also hydrolyzed to form methylguanine. Both ara-G and methylguanine metabolized to guanine. Guanine is deaminated into xanthine, which is further oxidized to form uric acid, which is then oxidized to form allantoin.

Half-life elimination: Nelarabine: 30 minutes; ara-G: 3 hours

Excretion: Urine (nelarabine 7%, ara-G 27%) within 24 hours of infusion on day 1

Pregnancy Risk Factor D

Nelfinavir *(nel FIN a veer)*

Related Information

HIV Infection and AIDS *on page 1662*

Tuberculosis *on page 1673*

Viral Infections *on page 1709*

U.S. Brand Names Viracept®

Canadian Brand Names Viracept®

Generic Available No

Synonyms NFV

Pharmacologic Category Antiretroviral Agent, Protease Inhibitor

Use In combination with other antiretroviral therapy in the treatment of HIV infection

Local Anesthetic/Vasoconstrictor Precautions No information available to require special precautions

Effects on Dental Treatment Key adverse event(s) related to dental treatment: Mouth ulcers.

Common Adverse Effects

>10%: Gastrointestinal: Diarrhea

2% to 10%:
Dermatologic: Rash
Gastrointestinal: Nausea, flatulence
Hematologic: Abnormal creatine kinase, hemoglobin, lymphocytes, neutrophils
Hepatic: Abnormal ALT, AST

Dosage Oral:
Children 2-13 years: 45-55 mg/kg twice daily **or** 25-35 mg/kg 3 times/day (maximum: 2500 mg/day); all doses should be taken with a meal. If tablets are unable to be taken, use oral powder in small amount of water, milk, formula, or dietary supplements; do not use acidic food/juice or store for >6 hours.
Adults: 750 mg 3 times/day with meals or 1250 mg twice daily with meals in combination with other antiretroviral therapies
Dosing adjustment in renal impairment: No adjustment needed
Dosing adjustment in hepatic impairment: Use caution

Mechanism of Action Inhibits the HIV-1 protease; inhibition of the viral protease prevents cleavage of the gag-pol polyprotein resulting in the production of immature, noninfectious virus

Contraindications Hypersensitivity to nelfinavir or any component of the formulation; concurrent therapy with amiodarone, ergot derivatives, midazolam, pimozide, quinidine, triazolam; additional medications which should not be coadministered (per manufacturer) include lovastatin and simvastatin

Warnings/Precautions Nelfinavir is hepatically metabolized and has multiple drug interactions. A listing of medications that should not be used is available with each bottle and patients should be provided with this information. Use caution with hepatic impairment. Warn patients that redistribution of body fat can occur. New onset diabetes mellitus, exacerbation of diabetes, and hyperglycemia have been reported in HIV-infected patients receiving protease inhibitors. Immune reconstitution syndrome has been reported; may require additional evaluation and treatment. The oral powder contains phenylalanine; use caution in patients with phenylketonuria.

Drug Interactions
Cytochrome P450 Effect: Substrate of CYP2C8/9 (minor), 2C19 (major), 2D6 (minor), 3A4 (major); **Inhibits** CYP1A2 (weak), 2B6 (weak), 2C8/9 (weak), 2C19 (weak), 2D6 (weak), 3A4 (strong)
Increased Effect/Toxicity: Nelfinavir effects may be increased by azithromycin, delavirdine, and protease inhibitors. Nelfinavir may increase the levels/effects of selected benzodiazepines, calcium channel blockers, corticosteroids (eg, fluticasone), cyclosporine, mirtazapine, nateglinide, nefazodone, quinidine, sildenafil (and other PDE-5 inhibitors), tacrolimus, venlafaxine, and other CYP3A4 substrates. Selected benzodiazepines (midazolam, triazolam), cisapride, ergot alkaloids, selected HMG-CoA reductase inhibitors (lovastatin and simvastatin), and pimozide are generally contraindicated with strong CYP3A4 inhibitors. When used with strong CYP3A4 inhibitors, dosage adjustment/limits are recommended for sildenafil and other PDE-5 inhibitors; refer to individual monographs.
Decreased Effect: The levels/effects of nelfinavir may be decreased by aminoglutethimide, carbamazepine, nafcillin, nevirapine, phenobarbital, phenytoin, rifamycins, or other inducers of CYP2C19 or 3A4. Nelfinavir effects may be decreased by St John's wort. Nelfinavir may decrease the effects of delavirdine, methadone, and oral contraceptives

Ethanol/Nutrition/Herb Interactions
Food: Nelfinavir taken with food increases plasma concentration time curve (AUC) by two- to threefold. Do not administer with acidic food or juice (orange juice, apple juice, or applesauce) since the combination may have a bitter taste.
Herb/Nutraceutical: St John's wort may decrease nelfinavir serum concentrations; avoid concurrent use.

Dietary Considerations Should be taken as scheduled with food. Oral powder contains phenylalanine 11.2 mg/g.

Pharmacodynamics/Kinetics
Absorption: Food increases plasma concentration-time curve (AUC) by two- to threefold
Distribution: V_d: 2-7 L/kg
Protein binding: 98%
Metabolism: Hepatic via CYP2C19 and 3A4; major metabolite has activity comparable to parent drug
Half-life elimination: 3.5-5 hours
Time to peak, serum: 2-4 hours
Excretion: Feces (98% to 99%, 78% as metabolites, 22% as unchanged drug); urine (1% to 2%)

Pregnancy Risk Factor B
(Continued)

Nelfinavir (Continued)

Dosage Forms POWDER, oral: 50 mg/g (144 g). **TAB, film coated:** 250 mg, 625 mg

Nembutal® see Pentobarbital on page 1210

NeoCeuticals™ Acne Spot Treatment [OTC] see Salicylic Acid on page 1374

Neo-Fradin™ see Neomycin on page 1100

Neomycin (nee oh MYE sin)

U.S. Brand Names Neo-Fradin™; Neo-Rx

Generic Available Yes

Synonyms Neomycin Sulfate

Pharmacologic Category Ammonium Detoxicant; Antibiotic, Aminoglycoside; Antibiotic, Topical

Use Orally to prepare GI tract for surgery; topically to treat minor skin infections; treatment of diarrhea caused by *E. coli*; adjunct in the treatment of hepatic encephalopathy; bladder irrigation; ocular infections

Local Anesthetic/Vasoconstrictor Precautions No information available to require special precautions

Effects on Dental Treatment No significant effects or complications reported

Common Adverse Effects

Oral: >10%: Gastrointestinal: Nausea, diarrhea, vomiting, irritation or soreness of the mouth or rectal area

Topical: >10%: Dermatologic: Contact dermatitis

Mechanism of Action Interferes with bacterial protein synthesis by binding to 30S ribosomal subunits

Drug Interactions

Increased Effect/Toxicity: Oral neomycin may potentiate the effects of oral anticoagulants. Neomycin may increase the adverse effects with other neurotoxic, ototoxic, or nephrotoxic drugs.

Decreased Effect: May decrease GI absorption of digoxin and methotrexate.

Pharmacodynamics/Kinetics

Absorption: Oral, percutaneous: Poor (3%)

Distribution: V_d: 0.36 L/kg

Metabolism: Slightly hepatic

Half-life elimination (age and renal function dependent): 3 hours

Time to peak, serum: Oral: 1-4 hours

Excretion: Feces (97% of oral dose as unchanged drug); urine (30% to 50% of absorbed drug as unchanged drug)

Pregnancy Risk Factor D

Neomycin and Polymyxin B (nee oh MYE sin & pol i MIKS in bee)

Related Information

Neomycin on page 1100

Polymyxin B on page 1253

U.S. Brand Names Neosporin® G.U. Irrigant

Canadian Brand Names Neosporin® Irrigating Solution

Generic Available No

Synonyms Polymyxin B and Neomycin

Pharmacologic Category Antibiotic, Topical

Use Short-term as a continuous irrigant or rinse in the urinary bladder to prevent bacteriuria and gram-negative rod septicemia associated with the use of indwelling catheters; to help prevent infection in minor cuts, scrapes, and burns

Local Anesthetic/Vasoconstrictor Precautions No information available to require special precautions

Effects on Dental Treatment No significant effects or complications reported

Common Adverse Effects Frequency not defined.

Dermatologic: Contact dermatitis, erythema, rash, urticaria

Genitourinary: Bladder irritation

Local: Burning

Neuromuscular & skeletal: Neuromuscular blockade

Otic: Ototoxicity

Renal: Nephrotoxicity

Mechanism of Action See individual agents.

Pharmacodynamics/Kinetics

Absorption: Topical: Not absorbed following application to intact skin; absorbed through denuded or abraded skin, peritoneum, wounds, or ulcers

See individual agents.

Pregnancy Risk Factor C/D (for G.U. irrigant)

Neomycin, Bacitracin, and Polymyxin B *see* Bacitracin, Neomycin, and Polymyxin B *on page 176*

Neomycin, Bacitracin, Polymyxin B, and Hydrocortisone *see* Bacitracin, Neomycin, Polymyxin B, and Hydrocortisone *on page 177*

Neomycin, Bacitracin, Polymyxin B, and Pramoxine *see* Bacitracin, Neomycin, Polymyxin B, and Pramoxine *on page 177*

Neomycin, Polymyxin B, and Dexamethasone
(nee oh MYE sin, pol i MIKS in bee, & deks a METH a sone)

Related Information
Dexamethasone *on page 439*
Neomycin *on page 1100*
Polymyxin B *on page 1253*

U.S. Brand Names AK-Trol® [DSC]; Maxitrol®; Poly-Dex™

Canadian Brand Names Dioptrol®; Maxitrol®

Generic Available Yes

Synonyms Dexamethasone, Neomycin, and Polymyxin B; Polymyxin B, Neomycin, and Dexamethasone

Pharmacologic Category Antibiotic/Corticosteroid, Ophthalmic

Use Steroid-responsive inflammatory ocular conditions in which a corticosteroid is indicated and where bacterial infection or a risk of bacterial infection exists

Local Anesthetic/Vasoconstrictor Precautions No information available to require special precautions

Effects on Dental Treatment No significant effects or complications reported

Mechanism of Action See individual agents.

Pregnancy Risk Factor C

Neomycin, Polymyxin B, and Gramicidin
(nee oh MYE sin, pol i MIKS in bee, & gram i SYE din)

Related Information
Neomycin *on page 1100*
Polymyxin B *on page 1253*

U.S. Brand Names Neosporin® Ophthalmic Solution

Canadian Brand Names Neosporin®; Optimyxin Plus®

Generic Available Yes

Synonyms Gramicidin, Neomycin, and Polymyxin B; Polymyxin B, Neomycin, and Gramicidin

Pharmacologic Category Antibiotic, Ophthalmic

Use Treatment of superficial ocular infection

Local Anesthetic/Vasoconstrictor Precautions No information available to require special precautions

Effects on Dental Treatment No significant effects or complications reported

Mechanism of Action Interferes with bacterial protein synthesis by binding to 30S ribosomal subunits; binds to phospholipids, alters permeability, and damages the bacterial cytoplasmic membrane permitting leakage of intracellular constituents

Pregnancy Risk Factor C

Neomycin, Polymyxin B, and Hydrocortisone
(nee oh MYE sin, pol i MIKS in bee, & hye droe KOR ti sone)

Related Information
Hydrocortisone *on page 793*
Neomycin *on page 1100*
Polymyxin B *on page 1253*

U.S. Brand Names Cortisporin® Cream; Cortisporin® Ophthalmic; Cortisporin® Otic; PediOtic®

Canadian Brand Names Cortimyxin®; Cortisporin® Otic

Generic Available Yes

Synonyms Hydrocortisone, Neomycin, and Polymyxin B; Polymyxin B, Neomycin, and Hydrocortisone

Pharmacologic Category Antibiotic/Corticosteroid, Ophthalmic; Antibiotic/Corticosteroid, Otic; Topical Skin Product

Use Steroid-responsive inflammatory condition for which a corticosteroid is indicated and where bacterial infection or a risk of bacterial infection exists
(Continued)

Neomycin, Polymyxin B, and Hydrocortisone
(Continued)

Local Anesthetic/Vasoconstrictor Precautions No information available to require special precautions

Effects on Dental Treatment No significant effects or complications reported

Common Adverse Effects Frequency not defined.

Dermatologic: Contact dermatitis, erythema, rash, urticaria

Local: Burning, itching, swelling, pain, stinging

Ocular: Intraocular pressure increased, glaucoma, cataracts, conjunctival erythema, transient irritation, burning, stinging, itching, inflammation, angioneurotic edema, urticaria, vesicular and maculopapular dermatitis

Otic: Ototoxicity

Miscellaneous: Hypersensitivity, sensitization to neomycin, secondary infection

Mechanism of Action See individual agents.

Drug Interactions

Cytochrome P450 Effect: Hydrocortisone: **Substrate** of CYP3A4 (minor); **Induces** CYP3A4 (weak)

Pharmacodynamics/Kinetics See individual agents.

Pregnancy Risk Factor C

Neomycin, Polymyxin B, and Prednisolone
(nee oh MYE sin, pol i MIKS in bee, & pred NIS oh lone)

Related Information
Neomycin on page 1100
Polymyxin B on page 1253
PrednisoLONE on page 1268

U.S. Brand Names Poly-Pred®

Generic Available No

Synonyms Polymyxin B, Neomycin, and Prednisolone; Prednisolone, Neomycin, and Polymyxin B

Pharmacologic Category Antibiotic/Corticosteroid, Ophthalmic

Use Steroid-responsive inflammatory ocular condition in which bacterial infection or a risk of bacterial ocular infection exists

Local Anesthetic/Vasoconstrictor Precautions No information available to require special precautions

Effects on Dental Treatment No significant effects or complications reported

Mechanism of Action See individual agents.

Pregnancy Risk Factor C

Neomycin Sulfate see Neomycin on page 1100

Neonatal Trace Metals see Trace Metals on page 1513

Neoral® see CycloSPORINE on page 406

Neo-Rx see Neomycin on page 1100

Neosporin® AF [OTC] see Miconazole on page 1039

Neosporin® G.U. Irrigant see Neomycin and Polymyxin B on page 1100

Neosporin® Neo To Go® [OTC] see Bacitracin, Neomycin, and Polymyxin B on page 176

Neosporin® Ophthalmic Ointment [DSC] see Bacitracin, Neomycin, and Polymyxin B on page 176

Neosporin® Ophthalmic Solution see Neomycin, Polymyxin B, and Gramicidin on page 1101

Neosporin® + Pain Ointment [OTC] see Bacitracin, Neomycin, Polymyxin B, and Pramoxine on page 177

Neosporin® Topical [OTC] see Bacitracin, Neomycin, and Polymyxin B on page 176

NeoStrata® AHA [OTC] see Hydroquinone on page 798

Neo-Synephrine® 12 Hour [OTC] see Oxymetazoline on page 1172

Neo-Synephrine® 12 Hour Extra Moisturizing [OTC] see Oxymetazoline on page 1172

Neo-Synephrine® Extra Strength [OTC] see Phenylephrine on page 1226

Neo-Synephrine® Mild [OTC] see Phenylephrine on page 1226

Neo-Synephrine® Ophthalmic [DSC] see Phenylephrine on page 1226

Neo-Synephrine® Regular Strength [OTC] see Phenylephrine on page 1226

Neotrace-4® see Trace Metals on page 1513

Nepafenac (ne pa FEN ak)

U.S. Brand Names Nevanac™
Generic Available No
Pharmacologic Category Nonsteroidal Anti-inflammatory Drug (NSAID), Ophthalmic
Use Treatment of pain and inflammation associated with cataract surgery
Local Anesthetic/Vasoconstrictor Precautions No information available to require special precautions
Effects on Dental Treatment No significant effects or complications reported
Mechanism of Action Nepafenac is a prodrug which once converted to amfenac inhibits prostaglandin synthesis by decreasing the activity of the enzyme, cyclooxygenase, which results in decreased formation of prostaglandin precursors.
Pregnancy Risk Factor C/D (3rd trimester)

NephPlex® Rx *see* Vitamin B Complex Combinations *on page 1581*
Nephro-Calci® [OTC] *see* Calcium Carbonate *on page 248*
Nephrocaps® *see* Vitamin B Complex Combinations *on page 1581*
Nephro-Fer® [OTC] *see* Ferrous Fumarate *on page 650*
Nephron FA® *see* Vitamin B Complex Combinations *on page 1581*
Nephro-Vite® *see* Vitamin B Complex Combinations *on page 1581*
Nephro-Vite® Rx *see* Vitamin B Complex Combinations *on page 1581*
Nesacaine® *see* Chloroprocaine *on page 320*
Nesacaine®-MPF *see* Chloroprocaine *on page 320*

Nesiritide (ni SIR i tide)

U.S. Brand Names Natrecor®
Generic Available No
Synonyms B-type Natriuretic Peptide (Human); hBNP; Natriuretic Peptide
Pharmacologic Category Natriuretic Peptide, B-Type, Human; Vasodilator
Use Treatment of acutely decompensated congestive heart failure (CHF) in patients with dyspnea at rest or with minimal activity
Local Anesthetic/Vasoconstrictor Precautions No information available to require special precautions
Effects on Dental Treatment No significant effects or complications reported
Common Adverse Effects Note: Frequencies cited below were recorded in VMAC trial at dosages similar to approved labeling. Higher frequencies have been observed in trials using higher dosages of nesiritide.
>10%:
  Cardiovascular: Hypotension (total: 11%; symptomatic: 4% at recommended dose, up to 17% at higher doses)
  Renal: Increased serum creatinine (28% with >0.5 mg/dL increase over baseline)
1% to 10%:
  Cardiovascular: Ventricular tachycardia (3%)*, ventricular extrasystoles (3%)*, angina (2%)*, bradycardia (1%), tachycardia, atrial fibrillation, AV node conduction abnormalities
  Central nervous system: Headache (8%)*, dizziness (3%)*, insomnia (2%), anxiety (3%), fever, confusion, paresthesia, somnolence, tremor
  Dermatologic: Pruritus, rash
  Gastrointestinal: Nausea (4%)*, abdominal pain (1%)*, vomiting (1%)*
  Hematologic: Anemia
  Local: Injection site reaction
  Neuromuscular & skeletal: Back pain (4%), leg cramps
  Ocular: Amblyopia
  Respiratory: Cough (increased), hemoptysis, apnea
  Miscellaneous: Increased diaphoresis
  *Frequency less than or equal to placebo or other standard therapy
Mechanism of Action Binds to guanylate cyclase receptor on vascular smooth muscle and endothelial cells, increasing intracellular cyclic GMP, resulting in smooth muscle cell relaxation. Has been shown to produce dose-dependent reductions in pulmonary capillary wedge pressure (PCWP) and systemic arterial pressure.
Drug Interactions
  Increased Effect/Toxicity: An increased frequency of symptomatic hypotension was observed with concurrent administration of ACE inhibitors. Other hypotensive agents are likely to have additive effects on hypotension. In patients receiving diuretic therapy leading to depletion of intravascular (Continued)

Nesiritide *(Continued)*

volume, the risk of hypotension and/or renal impairment may be increased. Nesiritide should be avoided in patients with low filling pressures.

Pharmacodynamics/Kinetics

Onset of action: 15 minutes (60% of 3-hour effect achieved)

Duration: >60 minutes (up to several hours) for systolic blood pressure; hemodynamic effects persist longer than serum half-life would predict

Distribution: V_{ss}: 0.19 L/kg

Metabolism: Proteolytic cleavage by vascular endopeptidases and proteolysis following receptor binding and cellular internalization

Half-life elimination: Initial (distribution) 2 minutes; Terminal: 18 minutes

Time to peak: 1 hour

Excretion: Urine

Pregnancy Risk Factor C

Neulasta® *see* Pegfilgrastim *on page 1195*

Neumega® *see* Oprelvekin *on page 1149*

Neupogen® *see* Filgrastim *on page 654*

Neurontin® *see* Gabapentin *on page 717*

Neut® *see* Sodium Bicarbonate *on page 1400*

NeutraCare® *see* Fluoride *on page 671*

NeutraGard® [OTC] *see* Fluoride *on page 671*

NeutraGard® Advanced *see* Fluoride *on page 671*

NeutraGard® Plus *see* Fluoride *on page 671*

Neutra-Phos® [OTC] *see* Potassium Phosphate and Sodium Phosphate *on page 1261*

Neutra-Phos®-K [OTC] *see* Potassium Phosphate *on page 1261*

NeuTrexin® *see* Trimetrexate *on page 1539*

Neutrogena® Acne Mask [OTC] *see* Benzoyl Peroxide *on page 194*

Neutrogena® Acne Wash [OTC] *see* Salicylic Acid *on page 1374*

Neutrogena® Body Clear™ [OTC] *see* Salicylic Acid *on page 1374*

Neutrogena® Clear Pore [OTC] *see* Salicylic Acid *on page 1374*

Neutrogena® Clear Pore Shine Control [OTC] *see* Salicylic Acid *on page 1374*

Neutrogena® Healthy Scalp [OTC] *see* Salicylic Acid *on page 1374*

Neutrogena® Maximum Strength T/Sal® [OTC] *see* Salicylic Acid *on page 1374*

Neutrogena® On The Spot® Acne Patch [OTC] *see* Salicylic Acid *on page 1374*

Neutrogena® On The Spot® Acne Treatment [OTC] *see* Benzoyl Peroxide *on page 194*

Neutrogena® T/Gel [OTC] *see* Coal Tar *on page 383*

Neutrogena® T/Gel Extra Strength [OTC] *see* Coal Tar *on page 383*

Neutrogena® T/Gel Stubborn Itch Control [OTC] *see* Coal Tar *on page 383*

Nevanac™ *see* Nepafenac *on page 1103*

Nevirapine *(ne VYE ra peen)*

Related Information

HIV Infection and AIDS *on page 1662*

Tuberculosis *on page 1673*

U.S. Brand Names Viramune®

Canadian Brand Names Viramune®

Mexican Brand Names Viramune®

Generic Available No

Synonyms NVP

Pharmacologic Category Antiretroviral Agent, Reverse Transcriptase Inhibitor (Non-nucleoside)

Use In combination therapy with other antiretroviral agents for the treatment of HIV-1

Local Anesthetic/Vasoconstrictor Precautions No information available to require special precautions

Effects on Dental Treatment Key adverse event(s) related to dental treatment: Ulcerative stomatitis and oral lesions.

Common Adverse Effects Note: Potentially life-threatening nevirapine-associated adverse effects may present with the following symptoms: Abrupt onset of flu-like symptoms, abdominal pain, jaundice, or fever with or without rash; may progress to hepatic failure with encephalopathy. Skin rash is present in ~50% of cases.

Percentages of adverse effects vary by clinical trial:

>10%:

Dermatologic: Rash (grade 1/2: 13%; grade 3/4: 1.5%) is the most common toxicity; occurs most frequently within the first 6 weeks of therapy; women may be at higher risk than men

Hepatic: ALT >250 units/L (5% to 14%); symptomatic hepatic events (4%, range: up to 11%) are more common in women, women with CD4+ cell counts >250 cells/mm^3, and men with CD4+ cell counts >400 cells/mm^3

1% to 10%:

Central nervous system: Headache (1% to 4%), fatigue (up to 5%)

Gastrointestinal: Nausea (<1% to 9%), abdominal pain (<1% to 2%), diarrhea (up to 2%)

Hepatic: AST >250 units/L (4% to 8%); coinfection with hepatitis B or C and/or increased liver function tests at the beginning of therapy are associated with a greater risk of asymptomatic transaminase elevations (ALT or AST >5 times ULN: 6%, range: up to 9%) or symptomatic events occurring ≥6 weeks after beginning treatment

Restrictions An FDA-approved medication guide is available at http://www.fda.gov/cder/Offices/ODS/labeling.htm

Mechanism of Action As a non-nucleoside reverse transcriptase inhibitor, nevirapine has activity against HIV-1 by binding to reverse transcriptase. It consequently blocks the RNA-dependent and DNA-dependent DNA polymerase activities including HIV-1 replication. It does not require intracellular phosphorylation for antiviral activity.

Drug Interactions

Cytochrome P450 Effect: Substrate of CYP2B6 (minor), 2D6 (minor), 3A4 (major); **Inhibits** CYP1A2 (weak), 2D6 (weak), 3A4 (weak); **Induces** CYP2B6 (strong), 3A4 (strong)

Increased Effect/Toxicity: Cimetidine, itraconazole, ketoconazole, and some macrolide antibiotics may increase nevirapine plasma concentrations. Concurrent administration of prednisone for the initial 14 days of nevirapine therapy was associated with an increased incidence and severity of rash. Rifabutin concentrations are increased by nevirapine.

Decreased Effect: The levels/effects of nevirapine may be decreased by aminoglutethimide, carbamazepine, nafcillin, nevirapine, phenobarbital, phenytoin, and rifamycins, and other CYP3A4 inducers; avoid concurrent use. Nevirapine may decrease the levels/effects of benzodiazepines, bupropion, calcium channel blockers, clarithromycin, cyclosporine, efavirenz, erythromycin, estrogens, mirtazapine, nateglinide, nefazodone, promethazine, selegiline, sertraline, tacrolimus, venlafaxine, and other CYP2B6 or 3A4 substrates. Nevirapine may decrease serum concentrations of some protease inhibitors (AUC of indinavir, lopinavir, nelfinavir, and saquinavir may be decreased, however, no effect noted with ritonavir); specific dosage adjustments have not been recommended; no adjustment recommended for ritonavir, unless combined with lopinavir (Kaletra™). Nevirapine may decrease the effectiveness of oral contraceptives; suggest alternate method or additional form of birth control. Nevirapine also decreases the effect of ketoconazole and methadone.

Pharmacodynamics/Kinetics

Absorption: >90%

Distribution: Widely; V_d: 1.2-1.4 L/kg; CSF penetration approximates 40% to 50% of plasma

Protein binding, plasma: 60%

Metabolism: Extensively hepatic via CYP3A4 (hydroxylation to inactive compounds); may undergo enterohepatic recycling

Half-life elimination: Decreases over 2- to 4-week time with chronic dosing due to autoinduction (ie, half-life = 45 hours initially and decreases to 25-30 hours)

Time to peak, serum: 2-4 hours

Excretion: Urine (~81%, primarily as metabolites, <3% as unchanged drug); feces (~10%)

Pregnancy Risk Factor C

New-Fill® see Poly-L-Lactic Acid on page 1253

Nexavar® see Sorafenib on page 1407

Nexium® see Esomeprazole on page 572

NFV see Nelfinavir on page 1098

Niacin (NYE a sin)

Related Information

Cardiovascular Diseases on page 1636
(Continued)

Niacin *(Continued)*

U.S. Brand Names Niacor®; Niaspan®; Slo-Niacin® [OTC]

Canadian Brand Names Niaspan®

Mexican Brand Names Hipocol®; Pepevit®

Generic Available Yes

Synonyms Nicotinic Acid; Vitamin B_3

Pharmacologic Category Antilipemic Agent, Miscellaneous; Vitamin, Water Soluble

Use Adjunctive treatment of dyslipidemias (types IIa and IIb or primary hypercholesterolemia) to lower the risk of recurrent MI and/or slow progression of coronary artery disease, including combination therapy with other antidyslipidemic agents when additional triglyceride-lowering or HDL-increasing effects are desired; treatment of hypertriglyceridemia in patients at risk of pancreatitis; treatment of peripheral vascular disease and circulatory disorders; treatment of pellagra; dietary supplement

Local Anesthetic/Vasoconstrictor Precautions No information available to require special precautions

Effects on Dental Treatment No significant effects or complications reported

Common Adverse Effects Frequency not defined.

Cardiovascular: Arrhythmias, atrial fibrillation, edema, flushing, hypotension, orthostasis, palpitation, syncope (rare), tachycardia

Central nervous system: Chills, dizziness, headache, insomnia, migraine

Dermatologic: Acanthosis nigricans, dry skin, hyperpigmentation, maculopapular rash, pruritus, rash, urticaria

Endocrine & metabolic: Glucose tolerance decreased, gout, phosphorous levels decreased, uric acid level increased

Gastrointestinal: Abdominal pain, dyspepsia, eructation, flatulence, nausea, peptic ulcers, vomiting

Hematologic: Platelet counts decreased, prothrombin time increased

Hepatic: Hepatic necrosis (rare), jaundice, liver enzymes increased

Neuromuscular & skeletal: Leg cramps, myalgia, myasthenia, myopathy (with concurrent HMG-CoA reductase inhibitor), pain, rhabdomyolysis (with concurrent HMG-CoA reductase inhibitor; rare), weakness

Ocular: Cystoid macular edema, toxic amblyopia

Respiratory: Dyspnea

Miscellaneous: Diaphoresis, hypersensitivity reactions (rare)

Mechanism of Action Component of two coenzymes which is necessary for tissue respiration, lipid metabolism, and glycogenolysis; inhibits the synthesis of very low density lipoproteins

Drug Interactions

Decreased Effect: Bile acid sequestrants may decrease the absorption of niacin; separate administration by 4-6 hours.

Pharmacodynamics/Kinetics

Absorption: Rapid and extensive (60% to 76%)

Distribution: Mainly to hepatic, renal, and adipose tissue

Metabolism: Extensive first-pass effects; converted to nicotinamide adenine dinucleotide, nicotinuric acid, and other metabolites

Half-life elimination: 45 minutes

Time to peak, serum: Immediate release formulation: ~45 minutes; extended release formulation: 4-5 hours

Excretion: Urine 60% to 88% (unchanged drug and metabolites)

Pregnancy Risk Factor A/C (dose exceeding RDA recommendation)

Niacinamide *(nye a SIN a mide)*

U.S. Brand Names Nicomide-T™

Generic Available Yes: Tablet

Synonyms Nicotinamide; Nicotinic Acid Amide; Vitamin B_3

Pharmacologic Category Vitamin, Water Soluble

Use

Oral: Prophylaxis and treatment of pellagra

Topical: Improve the appearance of acne and decrease visible inflammation and irritation caused by acne medications

Local Anesthetic/Vasoconstrictor Precautions No information available to require special precautions

Effects on Dental Treatment No significant effects or complications reported

Common Adverse Effects Frequency not defined.

Cardiovascular: Tachycardia

Dermatologic: Increased sebaceous gland activity, rash

Endocrine & metabolic: Hyperglycemia, hyperuricemia

Gastrointestinal: Bloating, flatulence, nausea
Neuromuscular & skeletal: Paresthesia in extremities
Ocular: Blurred vision
Respiratory: Wheezing

Mechanism of Action Used by the body as a source of niacin; is a component of two coenzymes which is necessary for tissue respiration, lipid metabolism, and glycogenolysis; does not have hypolipidemia or vasodilating effects. Niacinamide has anti-inflammatory properties which are believed to help decrease inflammatory acne lesions.

Pharmacodynamics/Kinetics
Absorption: Oral: Rapid; Topical: Absorbed systemically
Metabolism: Hepatic
Half-life elimination: 45 minutes
Time to peak, serum: 20-70 minutes
Excretion: Urine (as metabolites)

Pregnancy Risk Factor A/C (dose exceeding RDA recommendation)

Niacin and Lovastatin (NYE a sin & LOE va sta tin)

Related Information
Lovastatin *on page 953*
Niacin *on page 1105*

U.S. Brand Names Advicor®

Canadian Brand Names Advicor®

Generic Available No

Synonyms Lovastatin and Niacin

Pharmacologic Category Antilipemic Agent, HMG-CoA Reductase Inhibitor; Antilipemic Agent, Miscellaneous

Use Treatment of primary hypercholesterolemia (heterozygous familial and nonfamilial) and mixed dyslipidemia (Fredrickson types IIa and IIb) in patients previously treated with either agent alone (patients who require further lowering of triglycerides (TG) or increase in HDL-cholesterol (HDL-C) from addition of niacin or further lowering of LDL-cholesterol (LDL-C) from addition of lovastatin). Combination product; not intended for initial treatment.

Local Anesthetic/Vasoconstrictor Precautions No information available to require special precautions

Effects on Dental Treatment No significant effects or complications reported

Common Adverse Effects
>10%: Cardiovascular: Flushing (71%)
1% to 10%:
Central nervous system: Headache (9%), pain (8%)
Dermatologic: Pruritus (7%), rash (5%)
Endocrine & metabolic: Hyperglycemia (4%)
Gastrointestinal: Nausea (7%), diarrhea (6%), abdominal pain (4%), dyspepsia (3%), vomiting (3%)
Neuromuscular & skeletal: Back pain (5%), weakness (5%), myalgia (3%)
Miscellaneous: Flu-like syndrome (6%)

Mechanism of Action Lovastatin acts by competitively inhibiting 3-hydroxyl-3-methylglutaryl-coenzyme A (HMG-CoA) reductase, the enzyme that catalyzes the rate-limiting step in cholesterol biosynthesis. Niacin is a component of two coenzymes which is necessary for tissue respiration, lipid metabolism, and glycogenolysis; inhibits the synthesis of very low density lipoproteins.

Drug Interactions
Cytochrome P450 Effect: Lovastatin: **Substrate** of CYP3A4 (major); **Inhibits** CYP2C8/9 (weak), 2D6 (weak), 3A4 (weak)
Increased Effect/Toxicity: See individual agents.
Decreased Effect: See individual agents.

Pharmacodynamics/Kinetics See individual agents.
Bioavailability: Tablet strengths (eg, two tablets of 500 mg/20 mg and one tablet of 1000 mg/40 mg) are not interchangeable; bioavailability varies.

Pregnancy Risk Factor X

Niacor® *see* Niacin *on page 1105*
Niaspan® *see* Niacin *on page 1105*

NiCARdipine (nye KAR de peen)

Related Information
Cardiovascular Diseases *on page 1636*
(Continued)

NiCARdipine *(Continued)*

U.S. Brand Names Cardene®; Cardene® I.V.; Cardene® SR
Mexican Brand Names Ridene®
Generic Available Yes: Capsule
Synonyms Nicardipine Hydrochloride
Pharmacologic Category Calcium Channel Blocker
Use Chronic stable angina (immediate-release product only); management of essential hypertension (immediate and sustained release; parenteral only for short time that oral treatment is not feasible)
Unlabeled/Investigational Use Congestive heart failure
Local Anesthetic/Vasoconstrictor Precautions No information available to require special precautions
Effects on Dental Treatment Key adverse event(s) related to dental treatment: Xerostomia (normal salivary flow resumes upon discontinuation). Other drugs of this class can cause gingival hyperplasia (ie, nifedipine). The first case of nicardipine-induced gingival hyperplasia has been reported in a child taking 40-50 mg daily for 20 months.
Common Adverse Effects
1% to 10%:
  Cardiovascular: Flushing (6% to 10%), palpitation (3% to 4%), tachycardia (1% to 4%), peripheral edema (dose related 7% to 8%), increased angina (dose related 6%), hypotension (I.V. 6%), orthostasis (I.V. 1%)
  Central nervous system: Headache (6% to 15%), dizziness (4% to 7%), somnolence (4% to 6%), paresthesia (1%)
  Dermatologic: Rash (1%)
  Gastrointestinal: Nausea (2% to 5%), dry mouth (1%)
  Genitourinary: Polyuria (1%)
  Local: Injection site reaction (I.V. 1%)
  Neuromuscular & skeletal: Weakness (4% to 6%), myalgia (1%)
  Miscellaneous: Diaphoresis
Mechanism of Action Inhibits calcium ion from entering the "slow channels" or select voltage-sensitive areas of vascular smooth muscle and myocardium during depolarization, producing a relaxation of coronary vascular smooth muscle and coronary vasodilation; increases myocardial oxygen delivery in patients with vasospastic angina
Drug Interactions
  Cytochrome P450 Effect: Substrate of CYP1A2 (minor), 2C8/9 (minor), 2D6 (minor), 2E1 (minor), 3A4 (major); **Inhibits** CYP2C8/9 (strong), 2C19 (moderate), 2D6 (moderate), 3A4 (strong)
  Increased Effect/Toxicity: H_2 blockers (cimetidine) may increase the bioavailability of nicardipine. The levels/effects of nicardipine may be increased by azole antifungals, clarithromycin, diclofenac, doxycycline, erythromycin, imatinib, isoniazid, nefazodone, propofol, protease inhibitors, quinidine, telithromycin, verapamil and other CYP3A4 inhibitors.

  Nicardipine may increase the effect of vecuronium (reduce dose 25%). Nicardipine increase the levels/effects of amiodarone, amphetamines, selected benzodiazepines, selected beta-blockers, calcium channel blockers, cisapride, citalopram, cyclosporine, dextromethorphan, diazepam, ergot derivatives, fluoxetine, glimepiride, glipizide, HMG-CoA reductase inhibitors, lidocaine, methsuximide, mirtazapine, nateglinide, nefazodone, paroxetine, phenytoin, pioglitazone, propranolol, risperidone, ritonavir, rosiglitazone, sertraline, sildenafil (and other PDE-5 inhibitors), tacrolimus, thioridazine, tricyclic antidepressants, venlafaxine, warfarin, and other substrates of CYP2C8/9, 2C19, 2D6, or 3A4.
  Decreased Effect: The levels/effects of nicardipine may be decreased by aminoglutethimide, carbamazepine, nafcillin, nevirapine, phenobarbital, phenytoin, rifamycins, and other CYP3A4 inducers. Nicardipine may decrease the levels/effects of CYP2D6 prodrug substrates (eg, codeine, hydrocodone, oxycodone, tramadol). Calcium may reduce the calcium channel blocker's effects, particularly hypotension.
Pharmacodynamics/Kinetics
  Onset of action: Oral: 0.5-2 hours; I.V.: 10 minutes; Hypotension: ~20 minutes
  Duration: ≤8 hours
  Absorption: Oral: ~100%
  Protein binding: >95%
  Metabolism: Hepatic; CYP3A4 substrate (major); extensive first-pass effect (saturable)
  Bioavailability: 35%
  Half-life elimination: 2-4 hours
  Time to peak, serum: 30-120 minutes
  Excretion: Urine (60% as metabolites); feces (35%)
Pregnancy Risk Factor C

Nicardipine Hydrochloride *see* NiCARdipine *on page 1107*

NicoDerm® CQ® [OTC] *see* Nicotine *on page 1109*

Nicomide-T™ *see* Niacinamide *on page 1106*

Nicorette® [OTC] *see* Nicotine *on page 1109*

Nicotinamide *see* Niacinamide *on page 1106*

Nicotine (nik oh TEEN)

U.S. Brand Names Commit™ [OTC]; NicoDerm® CQ® [OTC]; Nicorette® [OTC]; Nicotrol® Inhaler; Nicotrol® NS; Nicotrol® Patch [OTC]

Canadian Brand Names Habitrol®; Nicoderm®; Nicorette®; Nicorette® Plus; Nicotrol®

Mexican Brand Names Nicotinell TTS®

Generic Available Yes: Transdermal patch and gum

Synonyms Habitrol

Pharmacologic Category Smoking Cessation Aid

Dental Use Treatment to aid smoking cessation for the relief of nicotine withdrawal symptoms (including nicotine craving)

Use Treatment to aid smoking cessation for the relief of nicotine withdrawal symptoms (including nicotine craving)

Unlabeled/Investigational Use Management of ulcerative colitis (transdermal)

Local Anesthetic/Vasoconstrictor Precautions No information available to require special precautions

Effects on Dental Treatment Key adverse event(s) related to dental treatment: Chewing gum: Excessive salivation, mouth/throat soreness, jaw muscle ache, hiccups, tachycardia, headache (mild), vomiting, belching, nausea, xerostomia (normal salivary flow resumes upon discontinuation), dizziness, nervousness, GI distress, hoarseness, hiccups, and muscle pain.

Significant Adverse Effects

Nasal spray/inhaler:

>10%:

Central nervous system: Headache (18% to 26%)

Gastrointestinal: Inhaler: Mouth/throat irritation (66%), dyspepsia (18%)

Respiratory: Inhaler: Cough (32%), rhinitis (23%)

1% to 10%:

Dermatologic: Acne (3%)

Endocrine & metabolic: Dysmenorrhea (3%)

Gastrointestinal: Flatulence (4%), gum problems (4%), diarrhea, hiccup, nausea, taste disturbance, tooth disorder

Neuromuscular & skeletal: Back pain (6%), arthralgia (5%), jaw/neck pain

Respiratory: Sinusitis

Miscellaneous: Withdrawal symptoms

<1% (Limited to important or life-threatening): Allergy, amnesia, aphasia, bronchitis, bronchospasm, edema, migraine, numbness, pain, purpura, rash, sputum increased, vision abnormalities, xerostomia

Adverse events previously reported in prescription labeling for chewing gum, lozenge and/or transdermal systems. Frequency not defined; may be product or dose specific:

Central nervous system: Concentration impaired, depression, dizziness, headache, insomnia, nervousness, pain

Gastrointestinal: Aphthous stomatitis, constipation, cough, diarrhea, dyspepsia, flatulence, gingival bleeding, glossitis, hiccups, jaw pain, nausea, salivation increased, stomatitis, taste perversion, tooth disorder, ulcerative stomatitis, xerostomia

Dermatologic: Rash

Local: Application site reaction, local edema, local erythema

Neuromuscular & skeletal: Arthralgia, myalgia, paresthesia

Respiratory: Cough, sinusitis

Miscellaneous: Allergic reaction, diaphoresis

Dental Usual Dosing Tobacco cessation (patients should be advised to completely stop smoking upon initiation of therapy): Adults:

Gum: Oral: Chew 1 piece of gum when urge to smoke, up to 30 pieces/day; most patients require 10-12 pieces of gum/day

Inhaler: Oral: Usually 6 to 16 cartridges per day; best effect was achieved by frequent continuous puffing (20 minutes); recommended duration of treatment is 3 months, after which patients may be weaned from the inhaler by gradual reduction of the daily dose over 6-12 weeks

(Continued)

Nicotine *(Continued)*

Lozenge: Oral: Patients who smoke their first cigarette within 30 minutes of waking should use the 4 mg strength; otherwise the 2 mg strength is recommended.

Weeks 1-6: One lozenge every 1-2 hours

Weeks 7-9: One lozenge every 2-4 hours

Weeks 10-12: One lozenge every 4-8 hours

Note: Use at least 9 lozenges/day during first 6 weeks to improve chances of quitting; do not use more than one lozenge at a time (maximum: 5 lozenges every 6 hours, 20 lozenges/day)

Spray: Nasal: 1-2 sprays/hour; do not exceed more than 5 doses (10 sprays) per hour [maximum: 40 doses/day (80 sprays); each dose (2 sprays) contains 1 mg of nicotine

Transdermal patch: Topical: Apply new patch every 24 hours to nonhairy, clean, dry skin on the upper body or upper outer arm; each patch should be applied to a different site. **Note:** Adjustment may be required during initial treatment (move to higher dose if experiencing withdrawal symptoms; lower dose if side effects are experienced).

NicoDerm CQ®:

Patients smoking ≥10 cigarettes/day: Begin with step 1 (21 mg/day) for 4-6 weeks, **followed by** step 2 (14 mg/day) for 2 weeks; **finish with** step 3 (7 mg/day) for 2 weeks

Patients smoking <10 cigarettes/day: Begin with step 2 (14 mg/day) for 6 weeks, **followed by** step 3 (7 mg/day) for 2 weeks

Note: Initial starting dose for patients <100 pounds, history of cardiovascular disease: 14 mg/day for 4-6 weeks, **followed by** 7 mg/day for 2-4 weeks

Note: Patients who are receiving >600 mg/day of cimetidine: Decrease to the next lower patch size

Nicotrol®: One patch daily for 6 weeks

Benefits of use of nicotine transdermal patches beyond 3 months have not been demonstrated

Dosage

Smoking deterrent: Patients should be advised to completely stop smoking upon initiation of therapy.

Oral:

Gum: Chew 1 piece of gum when urge to smoke, up to 30 pieces/day; most patients require 10-12 pieces of gum/day

Inhaler: Usually 6 to 16 cartridges per day; best effect was achieved by frequent continuous puffing (20 minutes); recommended duration of treatment is 3 months, after which patients may be weaned from the inhaler by gradual reduction of the daily dose over 6-12 weeks

Lozenge: Patients who smoke their first cigarette within 30 minutes of waking should use the 4 mg strength; otherwise the 2 mg strength is recommended.

Weeks 1-6: One lozenge every 1-2 hours

Weeks 7-9: One lozenge every 2-4 hours

Weeks 10-12: One lozenge every 4-8 hours

Note: Use at least 9 lozenges/day during first 6 weeks to improve chances of quitting; do not use more than one lozenge at a time (maximum: 5 lozenges every 6 hours, 20 lozenges/day)

Topical:

Transdermal patch: Apply new patch every 24 hours to nonhairy, clean, dry skin on the upper body or upper outer arm; each patch should be applied to a different site. **Note:** Adjustment may be required during initial treatment (move to higher dose if experiencing withdrawal symptoms; lower dose if side effects are experienced).

NicoDerm CQ®:

Patients smoking ≥10 cigarettes/day: Begin with **step 1** (21 mg/day) for 4-6 weeks, followed by **step 2** (14 mg/day) for 2 weeks; finish with **step 3** (7 mg/day) for 2 weeks

Patients smoking <10 cigarettes/day: Begin with **step 2** (14 mg/day) for 6 weeks, followed by **step 3** (7 mg/day) for 2 weeks

Note: Initial starting dose for patients <100 pounds, history of cardiovascular disease: 14 mg/day for 4-6 weeks, followed by 7 mg/day for 2-4 weeks

Note: Patients receiving >600 mg/day of cimetidine: Decrease to the next lower patch size

Nicotrol®: One patch daily for 6 weeks

Note: Benefits of use of nicotine transdermal patches beyond 3 months have not been demonstrated.

Ulcerative colitis (unlabeled use): Transdermal: Titrated to 22-25 mg/day

Nasal: Spray: 1-2 sprays/hour; do not exceed more than 5 doses (10 sprays) per hour [maximum: 40 doses/day (80 sprays); each dose (2 sprays) contains 1 mg of nicotine

Mechanism of Action Nicotine is one of two naturally-occurring alkaloids which exhibit their primary effects via autonomic ganglia stimulation. The other alkaloid is lobeline which has many actions similar to those of nicotine but is less potent. Nicotine is a potent ganglionic and central nervous system stimulant, the actions of which are mediated via nicotine-specific receptors. Biphasic actions are observed depending upon the dose administered. The main effect of nicotine in small doses is stimulation of all autonomic ganglia; with larger doses, initial stimulation is followed by blockade of transmission. Biphasic effects are also evident in the adrenal medulla; discharge of catecholamines occurs with small doses, whereas prevention of catecholamines release is seen with higher doses as a response to splanchnic nerve stimulation. Stimulation of the central nervous system (CNS) is characterized by tremors and respiratory excitation. However, convulsions may occur with higher doses, along with respiratory failure secondary to both central paralysis and peripheral blockade to respiratory muscles.

Contraindications Hypersensitivity to nicotine or any component of the formulation; patients who are smoking during the postmyocardial infarction period; patients with life-threatening arrhythmias, or severe or worsening angina pectoris; active temporomandibular joint disease (gum); pregnancy; not for use in nonsmokers

Warnings/Precautions The risk versus the benefits must be weighed for each of these groups: patients with CAD, serious cardiac arrhythmias, vasospastic disease. Use caution in patients with hyperthyroidism, pheochromocytoma, or insulin-dependent diabetes. Use with caution in oropharyngeal inflammation and in patients with history of esophagitis, peptic ulcer, coronary artery disease, vasospastic disease, angina, hypertension, pheochromocytoma, severe renal dysfunction, and hepatic dysfunction. The inhaler should be used with caution in patients with bronchospastic disease (other forms of nicotine replacement may be preferred). Use of nasal product is not recommended with chronic nasal disorders (eg, allergy, rhinitis, nasal polyps, and sinusitis). Transdermal patch may contain conducting metal (eg, aluminum); remove patch prior to MRI. Cautious use of topical nicotine in patients with certain skin diseases. Hypersensitivity to the topical products can occur. Dental problems may be worsened by chewing the gum. Urge patients to stop smoking completely when initiating therapy. Safety and efficacy have not been established in pediatric patients.

Drug Interactions Substrate (minor) of CYP1A2, 2A6, 2B6, 2C8/9, 2C19, 2D6, 2E1, 3A4; **Inhibits** CYP2A6 (weak), 2E1 (weak)

Adenosine: Nicotine increases the hemodynamic and AV blocking effects of adenosine; monitor

Bupropion: Monitor for treatment-emergent hypertension in patients treated with the combination of nicotine patch and bupropion

Cimetidine: May increases nicotine concentrations; therefore, may decrease amount of gum or patches needed

Ethanol/Nutrition/Herb Interactions Food: Lozenge: Acidic foods/beverages decrease absorption of nicotine.

Dietary Considerations Commit™: Each lozenge contains phenylalanine 3.4 mg.

Pharmacodynamics/Kinetics

Onset of action: Intranasal: More closely approximate the time course of plasma nicotine levels observed after cigarette smoking than other dosage forms

Duration: Transdermal: 24 hours

Absorption: Transdermal: Slow

Metabolism: Hepatic, primarily to cotinine ($\frac{1}{5}$ as active)

Half-life elimination: 4 hours

Time to peak, serum: Transdermal: 8-9 hours

Excretion: Urine

Clearance: Renal: pH dependent

Pregnancy Risk Factor D (nasal)

Lactation Excretion in breast milk unknown/use caution

Breast-Feeding Considerations Nicotine from cigarette smoke is found in breast milk at 1.5-3 times the maternal plasma concentrations. The amount from nicotine replacement products is not known. Women who are breast-feeding are encouraged not to smoke.

Dosage Forms

Gum, chewing, as polacrilex: 2 mg (48s, 108s); 4 mg (48s, 108s)

Nicorette®: 2 mg (48s, 50s, 110s, 168s, 170s, 192s, 200s, 216s); 4 mg (48s, 108s, 168s) [mint, fresh mint, orange, and original flavors]

(Continued)

Nicotine *(Continued)*

Lozenge, as polacrilex (Commit™): 2 mg (48s, 72s) [contains phenylalanine 3.4 mg/lozenge; mint flavor]; 4 mg (48s, 72s) [contains phenylalanine 3.4 mg/lozenge; mint flavor]

Oral inhalation system (Nicotrol® Inhaler): 10 mg cartridge [delivering 4 mg nicotine] (168s) [each unit consists of 5 mouthpieces, 28 storage trays each containing 6 cartridges, and 1 storage case]

Patch, transdermal: 7 mg/24 (30s); 14 mg/24 hours (30s); 21 mg/24 hours (30s)

NicoDerm® CQ®: 7 mg/24 hours (14s); 14 mg/24 hours (14s); 21 mg/24 hours (14s) [available in tan or clear patch]

Nicotrol®: 15 mg/16 hours (7s, 14s) [step 1]; 10 mg/16 hours (14s) [step 2]; 5 mg/16 hours (14s) [step 3]

Solution, intranasal spray (Nicotrol® NS): 10 mg/mL (10 mL) [delivers 0.5 mg/spray; 200 sprays]

Selected Readings

Christen AG and Christen JA, "The Prescription of Transdermal Nicotine Patches for Tobacco-Using Dental Patients: Current Status in Indiana," *J Indiana Dent Assoc*, 1992, 71(6):12-8.

Davies GM, Willner P, James DL, et al, "Influence of Nicotine Gum on Acute Cravings for Cigarettes," *J Psychopharmacol*, 2004, 18(1):83-7.

Li Wan Po A, "Transdermal Nicotine in Smoking Cessation. A Meta-Analysis," *Eur J Clin Pharmacol*, 1993, 45(6):519-28.

Stafne EE, "The Nicotine Transdermal Patch: Use in the Dental Office Tobacco Cessation Program," *Northwest Dent*, 1994, 73(3):19-22.

Tonstad S and Johnston JA, "Does Bupropion Have Advantages Over Other Medical Therapies in the Cessation of Smoking?" *Expert Opin Pharmacother*, 2004, 5(4):727-34.

Transdermal Nicotine Study Group, "Transdermal Nicotine for Smoking Cessation. Six-Month Results From Two Multicenter Controlled Clinical Trials," *JAMA*, 1991, 266(22):3133-8.

Westman EC, Levin ED, and Rose JE, "The Nicotine Patch in Smoking Cessation," *Arch Intern Med*, 1993, 153(16):1917-23.

Wynn RL, "Nicotine Patches in Smoking Cessation," *AGD Impact*, 1994, 22:14.

Nicotinic Acid *see Niacin on page 1105*

Nicotinic Acid Amide *see Niacinamide on page 1106*

Nicotrol® Inhaler *see Nicotine on page 1109*

Nicotrol® NS *see Nicotine on page 1109*

Nicotrol® Patch [OTC] *see Nicotine on page 1109*

Nicoumalone *see Acenocoumarol on page 30*

Nifediac™ CC *see NIFEdipine on page 1112*

Nifedical™ XL *see NIFEdipine on page 1112*

NIFEdipine *(nye FED i peen)*

Related Information

Cardiovascular Diseases *on page 1636*

U.S. Brand Names Adalat® CC; Afeditab™ CR; Nifediac™ CC; Nifedical™ XL; Procardia®; Procardia XL®

Canadian Brand Names Adalat® XL®; Apo-Nifed®; Apo-Nifed PA®; Novo-Nifedin; Nu-Nifed; Procardia®

Mexican Brand Names Adalat®; Adalat CC®; Adalat Oros®; Adalat Retard®; Corotrend®; Nifedipres®

Generic Available Yes

Pharmacologic Category Calcium Channel Blocker

Use Angina and hypertension (sustained release only), pulmonary hypertension

Local Anesthetic/Vasoconstrictor Precautions No information available to require special precautions

Effects on Dental Treatment Nifedipine has been reported to cause 10% incidence of gingival hyperplasia; effects from 30-100 mg/day have appeared after 1-9 months. Discontinuance results in complete disappearance or marked regression of symptoms; symptoms will reappear upon remedication. Marked regression occurs after 1 week and complete disappearance of symptoms has occurred within 15 days. If a gingivectomy is performed and use of the drug is continued or resumed, hyperplasia usually will recur. The success of the gingivectomy usually requires that the medication be discontinued or that a switch to a noncalcium channel blocker be made. If for some reason nifedipine cannot be discontinued, hyperplasia has not recurred after gingivectomy when extensive plaque control was performed. If nifedipine is changed to another class of cardiovascular agent, the gingival hyperplasia will probably regress and resolve. Switching to another calcium channel blocker may result in continued hyperplasia.

Common Adverse Effects

>10%:

Cardiovascular: Flushing (10% to 25%), peripheral edema (dose related 7% to 10%; up to 50%)

Central nervous system: Dizziness/lightheadedness/giddiness (10% to 27%), headache (10% to 23%)

Gastrointestinal: Nausea/heartburn (10% to 11%)

Neuromuscular & skeletal: Weakness (10% to 12%)

≥1% to 10%:

Cardiovascular: Palpitations (≤2% to 7%), transient hypotension (dose related 5%), CHF (2%)

Central nervous system: Nervousness/mood changes (≤2% to 7%), shakiness (≤2%), jitteriness (≤2%), sleep disturbances (≤2%), difficulties in balance (≤2%), fever (≤2%), chills (≤2%)

Dermatologic: Dermatitis (≤2%), pruritus (≤2%), urticaria (≤2%)

Endocrine & metabolic: Sexual difficulties (≤2%)

Gastrointestinal: Diarrhea (≤2%), constipation (≤2%), cramps (≤2%), flatulence (≤2%), gingival hyperplasia (≤10%)

Neuromuscular & skeletal: Muscle cramps/tremor (≤2% to 8%), weakness (10%), inflammation (≤2%), joint stiffness (≤2%)

Ocular: Blurred vision (≤2%)

Respiratory: Dyspnea/cough/wheezing (6%), nasal congestion/sore throat (≤2% to 6%), chest congestion (≤2%), dyspnea (≤2%)

Miscellaneous: Diaphoresis (≤2%)

Dosage Oral:

Children: Hypertrophic cardiomyopathy: 0.6-0.9 mg/kg/24 hours in 3-4 divided doses

Adolescents and Adults: (**Note:** When switching from immediate release to sustained release formulations, total daily dose will start the same)

Initial: 30 mg once daily as sustained release formulation, or if indicated, 10 mg 3 times/day as capsules

Usual dose: 10-30 mg 3 times/day as capsules or 30-60 mg once daily as sustained release

Maximum dose: 120-180 mg/day

Increase sustained release at 7- to 14-day intervals

Hemodialysis: Supplemental dose is not necessary.

Peritoneal dialysis effects: Supplemental dose is not necessary.

Dosing adjustment in hepatic impairment: Reduce oral dose by 50% to 60% in patients with cirrhosis.

Mechanism of Action Inhibits calcium ion from entering the "slow channels" or select voltage-sensitive areas of vascular smooth muscle and myocardium during depolarization, producing a relaxation of coronary vascular smooth muscle and coronary vasodilation; increases myocardial oxygen delivery in patients with vasospastic angina

Contraindications Hypersensitivity to nifedipine or any component of the formulation; immediate release preparation for treatment of urgent or emergent hypertension; acute MI

Warnings/Precautions The routine use of short-acting nifedipine capsules in hypertensive emergencies and pseudoemergencies is not recommended. **The use of sublingual short-acting nifedipine in hypertensive emergencies is neither safe or effective and SHOULD BE ABANDONED!** Serious adverse events (cerebrovascular ischemia, syncope, heart block, stroke, sinus arrest, severe hypotension, acute myocardial infarction, ECG changes, and fetal distress) have been reported in relation to the administration of short-acting nifedipine in hypertensive emergencies.

Severe hypotension may occur in patients taking immediate release nifepine concurrently with beta blockers when undergoing CABG with high dose fentanyl anesthesia. When considering surgery with high dose fentanyl, may consider withdrawing nifedipine (>36 hours) before surgery if possible.

Increased angina may be seen upon starting or increasing doses; may increase frequency, duration, and severity of angina during initiation of therapy; use with caution in patients with CHF or aortic stenosis (especially with concomitant beta-adrenergic blocker); severe left ventricular dysfunction, hepatic or renal impairment, hypertrophic cardiomyopathy (especially obstructive), concomitant therapy with beta-blockers or digoxin, edema

Mild and transient elevations in liver function enzymes may be apparent within 8 weeks of therapy initiation.

Avoid use of extended release tablets (Procardia XL®) in patients with known stricture/narrowing of the GI tract. Therapeutic potential of sustained-release formulation (elementary osmotic pump, gastrointestinal therapeutic system [GITS]) may be decreased in patients with certain GI disorders that accelerate intestinal transit time (eg, short bowel syndrome, inflammatory bowel disease, severe diarrhea).

Note: Elderly patients may experience a greater hypotensive response and the use of the immediate release formulation in patients >71 years of age has been (Continued)

NIFEdipine *(Continued)*

associated with a nearly fourfold increased risk for all-cause mortality when compared to beta-blockers, ACE inhibitors, or other classes of calcium channel blockers

Drug Interactions

Cytochrome P450 Effect: Substrate of CYP2D6 (minor), 3A4 (major); Inhibits CYP1A2 (moderate), 2C8/9 (weak), 2D6 (weak), 3A4 (weak)

Increased Effect/Toxicity: The levels/effects of nifedipine may be increased by alpha-1 blockers, azole antifungals, cisapride, clarithromycin, cyclosporine, diclofenac, doxycycline, erythromycin, grapefruit juice, imatinib, isoniazid, nefazodone, nicardipine, propofol, protease inhibitors, quinidine, quinupristin/dalfopristin, telithromycin, verapamil, and other CYP3A4 inhibitors. Cimetidine may also increase nifedipine levels. Nifedipine may increase the levels/effects of aminophylline, digoxin, fluvoxamine, mexiletine, mirtazapine, ropinirole, trifluoperazine, vincristine, and other CYP1A2 substrates. Digoxin, phenytoin, and vincristine levels may also be increased by nifedipine.

Blood pressure-lowering effects may be additive with sildenafil, tadalafil, and vardenafil (use caution). Concurrent use with magnesium salts may enhance the adverse/toxic effects of magnesium and enhance the hypotensive effects of the calcium channel blocker. Calcium channel blockers may enhance the neuromuscular blocking effect from nondepolarizing neuromuscular blockers. Calcium channel blocker (nondihydropyridine) may enhance the hypotensive effects of calcium channel blocker (dihydropyridine).

Decreased Effect: Nifedipine may decrease quinidine serum levels. Calcium may reduce the hypotension from of calcium channel blockers. The levels/effects of nifedipine may be decreased by aminoglutethimide, barbiturates, carbamazepine, nafcillin, nevirapine, phenobarbital, phenytoin, rifamycins, and other CYP3A4 inducers.

Ethanol/Nutrition/Herb Interactions

Ethanol: Avoid ethanol (may increase CNS depression and may increase the effects of nifedipine). Monitor.

Food: Nifedipine serum levels may be decreased if taken with food. Food may decrease the rate but not the extent of absorption of Procardia XL®. Increased therapeutic and vasodilator side effects, including severe hypotension and myocardial ischemia, may occur if nifedipine is taken by patients ingesting grapefruit.

Herb/Nutraceutical: St John's wort may decrease nifedipine levels. Avoid dong quai if using for hypertension (has estrogenic activity). Avoid ephedra, yohimbe, ginseng (may worsen hypertension). Avoid garlic (may have increased antihypertensive effect).

Dietary Considerations Capsule is rapidly absorbed orally if it is administered without food, but may result in vasodilator side effects; administration with low-fat meals may decrease flushing. Avoid grapefruit juice.

Pharmacodynamics/Kinetics

Onset of action: Immediate release: ~20 minutes

Protein binding (concentration dependent): 92% to 98%

Metabolism: Hepatic to inactive metabolites

Bioavailability: Capsule: 40% to 77%; Sustained release: 65% to 89% relative to immediate release capsules

Half-life elimination: Adults: Healthy: 2-5 hours, Cirrhosis: 7 hours; Elderly: 6.7 hours

Excretion: Urine (as metabolites)

Pregnancy Risk Factor C

Dosage Forms CAP, liquid-filled: 10 mg, 20 mg; {Procardia®): 10 mg. **TAB, extended release:** 30 mg, 60 mg, 90 mg; (Adalat® CC, Nifediac™ CC, Procardia XL®): 30 mg, 60 mg, 90 mg; (Afeditab™ CR, Nifedical™ XL): 30 mg, 60 mg

Selected Readings

Deen-Duggins L, Fry HR, Clay JR, et al, "Nifedipine-Associated Gingival Overgrowth: A Survey of the Literature and Report of Four Cases," *Quintessence Int*, 1996, 27(3):163-70.

Desai P and Silver JG, "Drug-Induced Gingival Enlargements," *J Can Dent Assoc*, 1998, 64(4):263-8.

Harel-Raviv M, Eckler M, Lalani K, et al, "Nifedipine-Induced Gingival Hyperplasia. A Comprehensive Review and Analysis," *Oral Surg Oral Med Oral Pathol Oral Radiol Endod*, 1995, 79(6):715-22.

Lederman D, Lumerman H, Reuben S, et al, "Gingival Hyperplasia Associated With Nifedipine Therapy," *Oral Surg Oral Med Oral Pathol*, 1984, 57(6):620-2.

Lucas RM, Howell LP, and Wall BA, "Nifedipine-Induced Gingival Hyperplasia: A Histochemical and Ultrastructural Study," *J Periodontol*, 1985, 56(4):211-5.

Nery EB, Edson RG, Lee KK, et al, "Prevalence of Nifedipine-Induced Gingival Hyperplasia," *J Periodontol*, 1995, 66(7):572-8.

Nishikawa SJ, Tada H, Hamasaki A, et al, "Nifedipine-Induced Gingival Hyperplasia: A Clinical and In Vitro Study," *J Periodontol*, 1991, 62(1):30-5.

Pilloni A, Camargo PM, Carere M, et al, "Surgical Treatment of Cyclosporine A- and Nifedipine-Induced Gingival Enlargement: Gingivectomy Versus Periodontal Flap," *J Periodontol*, 1998, 69(7):791-7.

Saito K, Mori S, Iwakura M, et al, "Immunohistochemical Localization of Transforming Growth Factor Beta, Basic Fibroblast Growth Factor and Heparin Sulphate Glycosaminoglycan in Gingival Hyperplasia Induced by Nifedipine and Phenytoin," *J Periodontal Res*, 1996, 31(8):545-5.

Silverstein LH, Koch JP, Lefkove MD, et al, "Nifedipine-Induced Gingival Enlargement Around Dental Implants: A Clinical Report," *J Oral Implantol*, 1995, 21(2):116-20.

Westbrook P, Bednarczyk EM, Carlson M, et al, "Regression of Nifedipine-Induced Gingival Hyperplasia Following Switch to a Same Class Calcium Channel Blocker, Isradipine," *J Periodontol*, 1997, 68(7):645-50.

Wynn RL, "Calcium Channel Blockers and Gingival Hyperplasia," *Gen Dent*, 1991, 39(4):240-3.

Wynn RL, "Update on Calcium Channel Blocker-Induced Gingival Hyperplasia," *Gen Dent*, 1995, 43(3):218-22.

Niferex® [OTC] *see* Polysaccharide-Iron Complex *on page 1254*

Niferex® 150 [OTC] *see* Polysaccharide-Iron Complex *on page 1254*

Niftolid *see* Flutamide *on page 686*

Nilandron® *see* Nilutamide *on page 1115*

Nilutamide (ni LOO ta mide)

U.S. Brand Names Nilandron®
Canadian Brand Names Anandron®
Generic Available No
Synonyms RU-23908
Pharmacologic Category Antiandrogen; Antineoplastic Agent, Antiandrogen
Use Treatment of metastatic prostate cancer
Local Anesthetic/Vasoconstrictor Precautions No information available to require special precautions
Effects on Dental Treatment Key adverse event(s) related to dental treatment: Xerostomia (normal salivary flow resumes upon discontinuation).
Common Adverse Effects
>10%:
    Central nervous system: Headache, insomnia
    Endocrine & metabolic: Hot flashes (30% to 67%), gynecomastia (10%)
    Gastrointestinal: Nausea (mild - 10% to 32%), abdominal pain (10%), constipation, anorexia
    Genitourinary: Testicular atrophy (16%), libido decreased
    Hepatic: Transaminases increased (8% to 13%; transient)
    Ocular: Impaired dark adaptation (13% to 57%), usually reversible with dose reduction, may require discontinuation of the drug in 1% to 2% of patients
    Respiratory: Dyspnea (11%)
1% to 10%:
    Cardiovascular: Chest pain, edema, heart failure, hypertension, syncope
    Central nervous system: Dizziness, drowsiness, malaise, hypoesthesia, depression
    Dermatologic: Pruritus, alopecia, dry skin, rash
    Endocrine & metabolic: Disulfiram-like reaction (hot flashes, rash) (5%); Flu-like syndrome, fever
    Gastrointestinal: Vomiting, diarrhea, dyspepsia, GI hemorrhage, melena, weight loss, xerostomia
    Genitourinary: Hematuria, nocturia
    Hematologic: Anemia
    Hepatic: Hepatitis (1%)
    Neuromuscular & skeletal: Arthritis, paresthesia
    Ocular: Chromatopsia (9%), abnormal vision (6% to 7%), cataracts, photophobia
    Respiratory: Interstitial pneumonitis (2% - typically exertional dyspnea, cough, chest pain, and fever; most often occurring within the first 3 months of treatment); rhinitis
    Miscellaneous: Diaphoresis
Mechanism of Action Nonsteroidal antiandrogen that inhibits androgen uptake or inhibits binding of androgen in target tissues. It specifically blocks the action of androgens by interacting with cytosolic androgen receptor F sites in target tissue
Drug Interactions
    Cytochrome P450 Effect: Substrate of CYP2C19 (major); **Inhibits** CYP2C19 (weak)
    Increased Effect/Toxicity: CYP2C19 inhibitors may increase the levels/effects of nilutamide; example inhibitors include delavirdine, fluconazole, fluvoxamine, gemfibrozil, isoniazid, omeprazole, and ticlopidine.
    (Continued)

Nilutamide *(Continued)*

Decreased Effect: CYP2C19 inducers may decrease the levels/effects of nilutamide; example inducers include aminoglutethimide, carbamazepine, phenytoin, and rifampin.

Pharmacodynamics/Kinetics

Absorption: Rapid and complete

Protein binding: 72% to 85%

Metabolism: Hepatic, forms active metabolites

Half-life elimination: Terminal: 23-87 hours; Metabolites: 35-137 hours

Excretion: Urine (up to 78% at 120 hours; <1% as unchanged drug); feces (1% to 7%)

Pregnancy Risk Factor C

Nimodipine *(nye MOE di peen)*

Related Information

Cardiovascular Diseases *on page 1636*

U.S. Brand Names Nimotop®

Canadian Brand Names Nimotop®

Mexican Brand Names Nimotop®

Generic Available No

Pharmacologic Category Calcium Channel Blocker

Use Spasm following subarachnoid hemorrhage from ruptured intracranial aneurysms regardless of the patients neurological condition postictus (Hunt and Hess grades I-V)

Local Anesthetic/Vasoconstrictor Precautions No information available to require special precautions

Effects on Dental Treatment Other drugs of this class can cause gingival hyperplasia (ie, nifedipine) but there have been no reports for nimodipine.

Common Adverse Effects 1% to 10%:

Cardiovascular: Reductions in systemic blood pressure (1% to 8%)

Central nervous system: Headache (1% to 4%)

Dermatologic: Rash (1% to 2%)

Gastrointestinal: Diarrhea (2% to 4%), abdominal discomfort (2%)

Mechanism of Action Nimodipine shares the pharmacology of other calcium channel blockers; animal studies indicate that nimodipine has a greater effect on cerebral arterials than other arterials; this increased specificity may be due to the drug's increased lipophilicity and cerebral distribution as compared to nifedipine; inhibits calcium ion from entering the "slow channels" or select voltage sensitive areas of vascular smooth muscle and myocardium during depolarization

Drug Interactions

Cytochrome P450 Effect: Substrate of CYP3A4 (major)

Increased Effect/Toxicity: Calcium channel blockers and nimodipine may result in enhanced cardiovascular effects of other calcium channel blockers. Cimetidine, omeprazole, and valproic acid may increase serum nimodipine levels. The effects of antihypertensive agents may be increased by nimodipine. Blood pressure-lowering effects may be additive with sildenafil, tadalafil, and vardenafil (use caution). CYP3A4 inhibitors may increase the levels/effects of nimodipine; example inhibitors include azole antifungals, clarithromycin, diclofenac, doxycycline, erythromycin, imatinib, isoniazid, nefazodone, nicardipine, propofol, protease inhibitors, quinidine, telithromycin, and verapamil.

Decreased Effect: CYP3A4 inducers may decrease the levels/effects of nimodipine; example inducers include aminoglutethimide, carbamazepine, nafcillin, nevirapine, phenobarbital, phenytoin, and rifamycins.

Pharmacodynamics/Kinetics

Protein binding: >95%

Metabolism: Extensively hepatic

Bioavailability: 13%

Half-life elimination: 1-2 hours; prolonged with renal impairment

Time to peak, serum: ~1 hour

Excretion: Urine (50%) and feces (32%) within 4 days

Pregnancy Risk Factor C

Nimotop® *see* Nimodipine *on page 1116*

Nipent® *see* Pentostatin *on page 1211*

Niravam™ *see* Alprazolam *on page 73*

Nisoldipine (NYE sole di peen)

Related Information
Cardiovascular Diseases on page 1636
U.S. Brand Names Sular®
Mexican Brand Names Sular®; Syscor®
Generic Available No
Pharmacologic Category Calcium Channel Blocker
Use Management of hypertension, alone or in combination with other antihypertensive agents
Local Anesthetic/Vasoconstrictor Precautions No information available to require special precautions
Effects on Dental Treatment Key adverse event(s) related to dental treatment: Xerostomia (normal salivary flow resumes upon discontinuation).
Common Adverse Effects
>10%:
 Cardiovascular: Peripheral edema (dose related 7% to 29%)
 Central nervous system: Headache (22%)
1% to 10%:
 Cardiovascular: Chest pain (2%), palpitation (3%), vasodilation (4%)
 Central nervous system: Dizziness (3% to 10%)
 Dermatologic: Rash (2%)
 Gastrointestinal: Nausea (2%)
 Respiratory: Pharyngitis (5%), sinusitis (3%), dyspnea (3%), cough (5%)
Mechanism of Action As a dihydropyridine calcium channel blocker, structurally similar to nifedipine, nisoldipine impedes the movement of calcium ions into vascular smooth muscle and cardiac muscle. Dihydropyridines are potent vasodilators and are not as likely to suppress cardiac contractility and slow cardiac conduction as other calcium antagonists such as verapamil and diltiazem; nisoldipine is 5-10 times as potent a vasodilator as nifedipine.
Drug Interactions
 Cytochrome P450 Effect: Substrate of CYP3A4 (major); **Inhibits** CYP1A2 (weak), 3A4 (weak)
 Increased Effect/Toxicity: CYP3A4 inhibitors may increase the levels/effects of nisoldipine; example inhibitors include azole antifungals, clarithromycin, diclofenac, doxycycline, erythromycin, imatinib, isoniazid, nefazodone, nicardipine, propofol, protease inhibitors, quinidine, telithromycin, and verapamil. Calcium may reduce the calcium channel blocker's effects, particularly hypotension. Blood pressure-lowering effects may be additive with sildenafil, tadalafil, and vardenafil (use caution). Digoxin and nisoldipine may increase digoxin effect.
 Decreased Effect: CYP3A4 inducers may decrease the levels/effects of nisoldipine; example inducers include aminoglutethimide, carbamazepine, nafcillin, nevirapine, phenobarbital, phenytoin, and rifamycins. Calcium may decrease the hypotension from calcium channel blockers.
Pharmacodynamics/Kinetics
Duration: >24 hours
Absorption: Well absorbed
Protein binding: >99%
Metabolism: Extensively hepatic; 1 active metabolite (10% of parent); first-pass effect
Bioavailability: 5%
Half-life elimination: 7-12 hours
Time to peak: 6-12 hours
Excretion: Urine (as metabolites)
Pregnancy Risk Factor C

Nitalapram see Citalopram on page 351

Nitazoxanide (nye ta ZOX a nide)

U.S. Brand Names Alinia®
Mexican Brand Names Colufase®; NTZ®
Generic Available No
Synonyms NTZ
Pharmacologic Category Antiprotozoal
Use Treatment of diarrhea caused by Cryptosporidium parvum or Giardia lamblia
Local Anesthetic/Vasoconstrictor Precautions No information available to require special precautions
Effects on Dental Treatment No significant effects or complications reported
(Continued)

Nitazoxanide (Continued)

Common Adverse Effects Rates of adverse effects were similar to those reported with placebo.

1% to 10%:

Central nervous system: Headache (1% to 3%)

Gastrointestinal: Abdominal pain (7% to 8%), diarrhea (2% to 4%), nausea (3%), vomiting (1%)

Mechanism of Action Nitazoxanide is rapidly metabolized to the active metabolite tizoxanide *in vivo*. Activity may be due to interference with the pyruvate:ferredoxin oxidoreductase (PFOR) enzyme-dependent electron transfer reaction which is essential to anaerobic metabolism. *In vitro*, nitazoxanide and tizoxanide inhibit the growth of sporozoites and oocysts of *Cryptosporidium parvum* and trophozoites of *Giardia lamblia*.

Pharmacodynamics/Kinetics

Protein binding: Tizoxanide: >99%

Bioavailability: Relative bioavailability of suspension compared to tablet: 70%

Metabolism: Hepatic, to an active metabolite, tizoxanide. Tizoxanide undergoes conjugation to form tizoxanide glucuronide. Nitazoxanide is not detectable in the serum following oral administration.

Time to peak, plasma: Tizoxanide and tizoxanide glucuronide: 1-4 hours

Excretion: Tizoxanide: Urine, bile, and feces; Tizoxanide glucuronide: Urine and bile

Pregnancy Risk Factor B

Nitisinone (ni TIS i known)

U.S. Brand Names Orfadin®

Generic Available No

Pharmacologic Category 4-Hydroxyphenylpyruvate Dioxygenase Inhibitor

Use Treatment of hereditary tyrosinemia type 1 (HT-1); to be used with dietary restriction of tyrosine and phenylalanine

Local Anesthetic/Vasoconstrictor Precautions No information available to require special precautions

Effects on Dental Treatment No significant effects or complications reported

Mechanism of Action In patients with HT-1, tyrosine metabolism is interrupted due to a lack of the enzyme (fumarylacetoacetate hydrolase) needed in the last step of tyrosine degradation. Toxic metabolites of tyrosine accumulate and cause liver and kidney toxicity. Nitisinone competitively inhibits 4-hydroxyphenyl-pyruvate dioxygenase, an enzyme needed earlier in the tyrosine degradation pathway, and therefore prevents the build-up of the damaging metabolites.

Pregnancy Risk Factor C

Nitrek® see Nitroglycerin on page 1120

Nitric Oxide (NYE trik OKS ide)

U.S. Brand Names INOmax®

Canadian Brand Names INOmax®

Generic Available No

Pharmacologic Category Vasodilator, Pulmonary

Use Treatment of term and near-term (>34 weeks) neonates with hypoxic respiratory failure associated with pulmonary hypertension; used concurrently with ventilatory support and other agents

Unlabeled/Investigational Use Treatment of adult respiratory distress syndrome (ARDS)

Local Anesthetic/Vasoconstrictor Precautions No information available to require special precautions

Effects on Dental Treatment No significant effects or complications reported

Common Adverse Effects

>10%:

Cardiovascular: Hypotension (13%)

Miscellaneous: Withdrawal syndrome (12%)

1% to 10%:

Dermatologic: Cellulitis (5%)

Endocrine & metabolic: Hyperglycemia (8%)

Genitourinary: Hematuria (8%)

Respiratory: Atelectasis (9% - same as placebo), stridor (5%)

Miscellaneous: Sepsis (7%), infection (6%)

Mechanism of Action In neonates with persistent pulmonary hypertension, nitric oxide improves oxygenation. Nitric oxide relaxes vascular smooth muscle by binding to the heme moiety of cytosolic guanylate cyclase, activating guanylate cyclase and increasing intracellular levels of cyclic guanosine 3',5'-monophosphate, which leads to vasodilation. When inhaled, pulmonary vasodilation occurs and an increase in the partial pressure of arterial oxygen results. Dilation of pulmonary vessels in well ventilated lung areas redistributes blood flow away from lung areas where ventilation/perfusion ratios are poor.

Drug Interactions
  Increased Effect/Toxicity: Concurrent use of sodium nitroprusside, nitroglycerin, or prilocaine may result in an increased risk of developing methemoglobinemia.

Pharmacodynamics/Kinetics
  Absorption: Systemic after inhalation
  Metabolism: Nitric oxide combines with hemoglobin that is 60% to 100% oxygenated. Nitric oxide combines with oxyhemoglobin to produce methemoglobin and nitrate. Within the pulmonary system, nitric oxide can combine with oxygen and water to produce nitrogen dioxide and nitrite respectively, which interact with oxyhemoglobin to then produce methemoglobin and nitrate. At 80 ppm the methemoglobin percent is ~5% after 8 hours of administration. Methemoglobin levels >7% were attained only in patients receiving 80 ppm.
  Excretion: Urine (as nitrate)
    Clearance: Nitrate: At a rate approaching the glomerular filtration rate
Pregnancy Risk Factor C

4'-Nitro-3'-Trifluoromethylisobutyrantide *see* Flutamide *on page 686*
Nitro-Bid® *see* Nitroglycerin *on page 1120*
Nitro-Dur® *see* Nitroglycerin *on page 1120*

Nitrofurantoin (nye troe fyoor AN toyn)

U.S. Brand Names Furadantin®; Macrobid®; Macrodantin®
Canadian Brand Names Apo-Nitrofurantoin®; Macrobid®; Macrodantin®; Novo-Furantoin
Mexican Brand Names Macrodantina®
Generic Available Yes: Excludes suspension
Pharmacologic Category Antibiotic, Miscellaneous
Use Prevention and treatment of urinary tract infections caused by susceptible gram-negative and some gram-positive organisms; *Pseudomonas*, *Serratia*, and most species of *Proteus* are generally resistant to nitrofurantoin
Local Anesthetic/Vasoconstrictor Precautions No information available to require special precautions
Effects on Dental Treatment No significant effects or complications reported
Common Adverse Effects Frequency not defined.
  Cardiovascular: Chest pain, cyanosis, ECG changes (associated with pulmonary toxicity)
  Central nervous system: Chills, depression, dizziness, drowsiness, fatigue, fever, headache, pseudotumor cerebri, psychotic reaction
  Dermatologic: Alopecia, erythema multiforme, exfoliative dermatitis, pruritus, rash, Stevens-Johnson syndrome
  Gastrointestinal: Abdominal pain, *C. difficile*-colitis, constipation, diarrhea, dyspepsia, loss of appetite, nausea (most common), pancreatitis, sore throat, vomiting
  Hematologic: Agranulocytosis, aplastic anemia, eosinophilia, hemolytic anemia, methemoglobinemia, thrombocytopenia
  Hepatic: Cholestasis, hepatitis, hepatic necrosis, transaminases increased, jaundice (cholestatic)
  Neuromuscular & skeletal: Arthralgia, numbness, paresthesia, peripheral neuropathy, weakness
  Ocular: Amblyopia, nystagmus, optic neuritis (rare)
  Respiratory: Cough, dyspnea, pneumonitis, pulmonary fibrosis
  Miscellaneous: Hypersensitivity (including acute pulmonary hypersensitivity), lupus-like syndrome
Mechanism of Action Inhibits several bacterial enzyme systems including acetyl coenzyme A interfering with metabolism and possibly cell wall synthesis
Drug Interactions
  Increased Effect/Toxicity: Probenecid decreases renal excretion of nitrofurantoin.
  Decreased Effect: Antacids decrease absorption of nitrofurantoin.
Pharmacodynamics/Kinetics
  Absorption: Well absorbed; macrocrystalline form absorbed more slowly due to slower dissolution (causes less GI distress)
  (Continued)

Nitrofurantoin *(Continued)*

Distribution: V_d: 0.8 L/kg; crosses placenta; enters breast milk

Protein binding: 60% to 90%

Metabolism: Body tissues (except plasma) metabolize 60% of drug to inactive metabolites

Bioavailability: Increased with food

Half-life elimination: 20-60 minutes; prolonged with renal impairment

Excretion:

Suspension: Urine (40%) and feces (small amounts) as metabolites and unchanged drug

Macrocrystals: Urine (20% to 25% as unchanged drug)

Pregnancy Risk Factor B (contraindicated at term)

Nitroglycerin *(nye troe GLI ser in)*

Related Information

Cardiovascular Diseases *on page 1636*

U.S. Brand Names Minitran™; Nitrek®; Nitro-Bid®; Nitro-Dur®; Nitrolingual®; NitroQuick®; Nitrostat®; Nitro-Tab®; NitroTime®

Canadian Brand Names Gen-Nitro; Minitran™; Nitro-Dur®; Nitrol®; Nitrostat™; Rho®-Nitro; Transderm-Nitro®; Trinipatch® 0.2; Trinipatch® 0.4; Trinipatch® 0.6

Mexican Brand Names Anglix®; Cardinit®; Minitran®; Nitradisc®; Nitroderm TTS®; Nitro-Dur®

Generic Available Yes: Capsule, injection, patch, tablet

Synonyms Glyceryl Trinitrate; Nitroglycerol; NTG

Pharmacologic Category Vasodilator

Use Treatment of angina pectoris; I.V. for congestive heart failure (especially when associated with acute myocardial infarction); pulmonary hypertension; hypertensive emergencies occurring perioperatively (especially during cardiovascular surgery)

Unlabeled/Investigational Use Esophageal spastic disorders (sublingual)

Local Anesthetic/Vasoconstrictor Precautions No information available to require special precautions

Effects on Dental Treatment No significant effects or complications reported

Common Adverse Effects

Spray or patch:

>10%: Central nervous system: Headache (patch 63%, spray 50%)

1% to 10%:

Cardiovascular: Hypotension (patch 4%), increased angina (patch 2%)

Central nervous system: Lightheadedness (patch 6%), syncope (patch 4%)

Topical, sublingual, intravenous: Frequency not defined:

Cardiovascular: Hypotension (infrequent), postural hypotension, crescendo angina (uncommon), rebound hypertension (uncommon), pallor, cardiovascular collapse, tachycardia, shock, flushing, peripheral edema

Central nervous system: Headache (most common), lightheadedness (related to blood pressure changes), syncope (uncommon), dizziness, restlessness

Gastrointestinal: Nausea, vomiting, bowel incontinence, xerostomia

Genitourinary: Urinary incontinence

Hematologic: Methemoglobinemia (rare, overdose)

Neuromuscular & skeletal: Weakness

Ocular: Blurred vision

Miscellaneous: Cold sweat

The incidence of hypotension and adverse cardiovascular events may be increased when used in combination with sildenafil (Viagra®).

Dosage Note: Hemodynamic and antianginal tolerance often develop within 24-48 hours of continuous nitrate administration. Nitrate-free interval (10-12 hours/day) is recommended to avoid tolerance development; gradually decrease dose in patients receiving NTG for prolonged period to avoid withdrawal reaction.

Children: Pulmonary hypertension: Continuous infusion: Start 0.25-0.5 mcg/kg/minute and titrate by 1 mcg/kg/minute at 20- to 60-minute intervals to desired effect; usual dose: 1-3 mcg/kg/minute; maximum: 5 mcg/kg/minute

Adults:

Oral: 2.5-9 mg 2-4 times/day (up to 26 mg 4 times/day)

I.V.: 5 mcg/minute, increase by 5 mcg/minute every 3-5 minutes to 20 mcg/minute; if no response at 20 mcg/minute increase by 10 mcg/minute every 3-5 minutes, up to 200 mcg/minute

Ointment: 1/2" upon rising and 1/2" 6 hours later; the dose may be doubled and even doubled again as needed

Patch, transdermal: Initial: 0.2-0.4 mg/hour, titrate to doses of 0.4-0.8 mg/hour; tolerance is minimized by using a patch-on period of 12-14 hours and patch-off period of 10-12 hours

Sublingual: 0.2-0.6 mg every 5 minutes for maximum of 3 doses in 15 minutes; may also use prophylactically 5-10 minutes prior to activities which may provoke an attack

Esophageal spastic disorders (unlabeled use): 0.3-0.4 mg 5 minutes before meals

Translingual: 1-2 sprays into mouth under tongue every 3-5 minutes for maximum of 3 doses in 15 minutes, may also be used 5-10 minutes prior to activities which may provoke an attack prophylactically

Hemodialysis: Supplemental dose is not necessary

Peritoneal dialysis: Supplemental dose is not necessary

Elderly: In general, dose selection should be cautious, usually starting at the low end of the dosing range

Mechanism of Action Works by relaxation of smooth muscle, producing a vasodilator effect on the peripheral veins and arteries with more prominent effects on the veins. Primarily reduces cardiac oxygen demand by decreasing preload (left ventricular end-diastolic pressure); may modestly reduce afterload; dilates coronary arteries and improves collateral flow to ischemic regions

Contraindications Hypersensitivity to organic nitrates; hypersensitivity to isosorbide, nitroglycerin, or any component of the formulation; concurrent use with phosphodiesterase-5 (PDE-5) inhibitors (sildenafil, tadalafil, or vardenafil); angle-closure glaucoma (intraocular pressure may be increased); head trauma or cerebral hemorrhage (increase intracranial pressure); severe anemia; allergy to adhesive (transdermal product)

Additional contraindications for I.V. product: Hypotension; uncorrected hypovolemia; inadequate cerebral circulation; constrictive pericarditis; pericardial tamponade

Warnings/Precautions Do not use extended release preparations in patients with GI hypermotility or malabsorptive syndrome; use with caution in patients with hepatic impairment, CHF, or acute myocardial infarction; available preparations of I.V. nitroglycerin differ in concentration or volume; pay attention to dilution and dosage; I.V. preparations contain alcohol and/or propylene glycol; avoid loss of nitroglycerin in standard PVC tubing; dosing instructions must be followed with care when the appropriate infusion sets are used

Hypotension may occur, use with caution in patients who are volume-depleted, are hypotensive, have inadequate circulation; nitrate therapy may aggravate angina caused by hypertrophic cardiomyopathy. Nitroglycerin transdermal patches should be removed prior to defibrillation or MRI study.

Drug Interactions

Increased Effect/Toxicity: Significant reduction of systolic and diastolic blood pressure with concurrent use of sildenafil, tadalafil, or vardenafil (contraindicated); do not administer sildenafil, tadalafil, or vardenafil within 24 hours of a nitrate preparation. Ethanol can cause hypotension when nitrates are taken 1 hour or more after ethanol ingestion.

Decreased Effect: I.V. nitroglycerin may antagonize the anticoagulant effect of heparin (possibly only at high nitroglycerin dosages); monitor closely. May need to decrease heparin dosage when nitroglycerin is discontinued. Alteplase (tissue plasminogen activator) has a lesser effect when used with I.V. nitroglycerin; avoid concurrent use. Ergot alkaloids may cause an increase in blood pressure and decrease in antianginal effects; avoid concurrent use.

Pharmacodynamics/Kinetics

Onset of action: Sublingual tablet: 1-3 minutes; Translingual spray: 2 minutes; Sustained release: 20-45 minutes; Topical: 15-60 minutes; Transdermal: 40-60 minutes; I.V. drip: Immediate

Peak effect: Sublingual tablet: 4-8 minutes; Translingual spray: 4-10 minutes; Sustained release: 45-120 minutes; Topical: 30-120 minutes; Transdermal: 60-180 minutes; I.V. drip: Immediate

Duration: Sublingual tablet: 30-60 minutes; Translingual spray: 30-60 minutes; Sustained release: 4-8 hours; Topical: 2-12 hours; Transdermal: 18-24 hours; I.V. drip: 3-5 minutes

Protein binding: 60%

Metabolism: Extensive first-pass effect

Half-life elimination: 1-4 minutes

Excretion: Urine (as inactive metabolites)

Pregnancy Risk Factor C

Dosage Forms **CAP,** extended release (Nitro-Time®): 2.5 mg, 6.5 mg, 9 mg. **INF** [premixed in D_5W]: 0.1 mg/mL (250 mL, 500 mL); 0.2 mg/mL (250 mL); 0.4 mg/mL (250 mL, 500 mL). **INJ, solution:** 5 mg/mL (5 mL, 10 mL). **OINT, topical** (Continued)

Nitroglycerin *(Continued)*

(Nitro-Bid®): 2% [20 mg/g] (1 g, 30 g, 60 g). **PATCH, transdermal:** Systems deliver 0.1 mg/hour (30s), 0.2 mg/hour (30s), 0.4 mg/hour (30s), 0.6 mg/hour (30s); (Minitran™): 0.1 mg/hour (30s), 0.2 mg/hour (30s), 0.4 mg/hour (30s), 0.6 mg/hour (30s); (Nitrek®): 0.2 mg/hour (30s), 0.4 mg/hour (30s), 0.6 mg/hour (30s); (Nitro-Dur®): 0.1 mg/hour (30s), 0.2 mg/hour (30s), 0.3 mg/hour (30s), 0.4 mg/hour (30s), 0.6 mg/hour (30s), 0.8 mg/hour (30s). **SOLN, translingual spray** (Nitrolingual®): 0.4 mg/metered spray (4.9 g, 12 g). **TAB, sublingual** (NitroQuick®, Nitrostat®, NitroTab®): 0.3 mg, 0.4 mg, 0.6 mg.

Nitroglycerol *see* Nitroglycerin *on page 1120*

Nitrolingual® *see* Nitroglycerin *on page 1120*

Nitropress® *see* Nitroprusside *on page 1122*

Nitroprusside *(nye troe PRUS ide)*

Related Information
Cardiovascular Diseases *on page 1636*
U.S. Brand Names Nitropress®
Generic Available Yes
Synonyms Nitroprusside Sodium; Sodium Nitroferricyanide; Sodium Nitroprusside
Pharmacologic Category Vasodilator
Use Management of hypertensive crises; congestive heart failure; used for controlled hypotension to reduce bleeding during surgery
Local Anesthetic/Vasoconstrictor Precautions No information available to require special precautions
Effects on Dental Treatment No significant effects or complications reported
Common Adverse Effects 1% to 10%:
Cardiovascular: Excessive hypotensive response, palpitation, substernal distress
Central nervous system: Disorientation, psychosis, headache, restlessness
Endocrine & metabolic: Thyroid suppression
Gastrointestinal: Nausea, vomiting
Neuromuscular & skeletal: Weakness, muscle spasm
Otic: Tinnitus
Respiratory: Hypoxia
Miscellaneous: Diaphoresis, thiocyanate toxicity
Mechanism of Action Causes peripheral vasodilation by direct action on venous and arteriolar smooth muscle, thus reducing peripheral resistance; will increase cardiac output by decreasing afterload; reduces aortal and left ventricular impedance
Pharmacodynamics/Kinetics
Onset of action: BP reduction <2 minutes
Duration: 1-10 minutes
Metabolism: Nitroprusside is converted to cyanide ions in the bloodstream; decomposes to prussic acid which in the presence of sulfur donor is converted to thiocyanate (hepatic and renal rhodanase systems)
Half-life elimination: Parent drug: <10 minutes; Thiocyanate: 2.7-7 days
Excretion: Urine (as thiocyanate)
Pregnancy Risk Factor C

Nitroprusside Sodium *see* Nitroprusside *on page 1122*

NitroQuick® *see* Nitroglycerin *on page 1120*

Nitrostat® *see* Nitroglycerin *on page 1120*

Nitro-Tab® *see* Nitroglycerin *on page 1120*

NitroTime® *see* Nitroglycerin *on page 1120*

Nitrous Oxide *(NYE trus OKS ide)*

Related Information
Sedation *on page 1727*
Generic Available Yes
Pharmacologic Category Dental Gases; General Anesthetic
Dental Use Induction of sedation and analgesia in anxious dental patients
Use Produces sedation and analgesia; principal adjunct to inhalation and intravenous general anesthesia

Local Anesthetic/Vasoconstrictor Precautions No information available to require special precautions

Effects on Dental Treatment No significant effects or complications reported

Significant Adverse Effects Frequency not defined.

Cardiovascular: Hypotension

Central nervous system: Headache, dizziness, confusion, CNS excitation

Gastrointestinal: Possibly nausea and vomiting

Respiratory: Apnea

Miscellaneous: Personnel exposed to unscavenged nitrous oxide have an increased risk of renal and hepatic diseases and peripheral neuropathy similar to that of vitamin B_{12} deficiency. Female dental personnel who were exposed to unscavenged nitrous oxide for more than 5 hours/week were significantly less fertile than women who were not exposed, or who were exposed to lower levels of scavenged or unscavenged nitrous oxide.

Dental Usual Dosing Sedation and analgesia: Children and Adults: Concentrations of 25% to 50% nitrous oxide with oxygen

Dosage Children and Adults:

Surgical: For sedation and analgesia: Concentrations of 25% to 50% nitrous oxide with oxygen. For general anesthesia, concentrations of 40% to 70% via mask or endotracheal tube. Minimal alveolar concentration (MAC), which can be considered the ED_{50} of inhalational anesthetics, is 105%; therefore delivery in a hyperbaric chamber is necessary to use as a complete anesthetic. When administered at 70%, reduces the MAC of other anesthetics by half.

Dental: For sedation and analgesia: Concentrations of 25% to 50% nitrous oxide with oxygen

Mechanism of Action General CNS depressant action; may act similarly as inhalant general anesthetics by stabilizing axonal membranes to partially inhibit action potentials leading to sedation; may partially act on opiate receptor systems to cause mild analgesia; central sympathetic stimulating action supports blood pressure, systemic vascular resistance, and cardiac output; it does not depress carbon dioxide drive to breath. Nitrous oxide increases cerebral blood flow and intracranial pressure while decreasing hepatic and renal blood flow; has analgesic action similar to morphine.

Contraindications Hypersensitivity to nitrous oxide or any component of the formulation; nitrous oxide should not be administered without oxygen; should not be given to patients after a full meal

Warnings/Precautions Nausea and vomiting occurs postoperatively in ~15% of patients. Prolonged use may produce bone marrow suppression and/or neurologic dysfunction. Oxygen should be briefly administered during emergence from prolonged anesthesia with nitrous oxide to prevent diffusion hypoxia. Patients with vitamin B_{12} deficiency (pernicious anemia) and those with other nutritional deficiencies (alcoholics) are at increased risk of developing neurologic disease and bone marrow suppression with exposure to nitrous oxide. May be addictive.

Drug Interactions No data reported

Pharmacodynamics/Kinetics

Onset of action: Inhalation: 2-5 minutes

Absorption: Rapid via lungs; blood/gas partition coefficient is 0.47

Metabolism: Body: <0.004%

Excretion: Primarily exhaled gases; skin (minimal amounts)

Pregnancy Risk Factor No data reported

Dosage Forms Supplied in blue cylinders

Nix® [OTC] see Permethrin on page 1218

Nizatidine (ni ZA ti deen)

Related Information

Gastrointestinal Disorders on page 1654

U.S. Brand Names Axid®; Axid® AR [OTC]

Canadian Brand Names Apo-Nizatidine®; Axid®; Gen-Nizatidine; Novo-Nizatidine; Nu-Nizatidine; PMS-Nizatidine

Mexican Brand Names Axid®

Generic Available Yes: Capsule

Pharmacologic Category Histamine H_2 Antagonist

Use Treatment and maintenance of duodenal ulcer; treatment of benign gastric ulcer; treatment of gastroesophageal reflux disease (GERD); OTC tablet used for the prevention of meal-induced heartburn, acid indigestion, and sour stomach

Unlabeled/Investigational Use Part of a multidrug regimen for *H. pylori* eradication to reduce the risk of duodenal ulcer recurrence

(Continued)

Nizatidine (Continued)

Local Anesthetic/Vasoconstrictor Precautions No information available to require special precautions

Effects on Dental Treatment Key adverse event(s) related to dental treatment: Xerostomia (normal salivary flow resumes upon discontinuation).

Common Adverse Effects

>10%: Central nervous system: Headache (16%)

1% to 10%:

Central nervous system: Anxiety, dizziness, fever (reported in children), insomnia, irritability (reported in children), somnolence, nervousness

Dermatologic: Pruritus, rash

Gastrointestinal: Abdominal pain, anorexia, constipation, diarrhea, dry mouth, flatulence, heartburn, nausea, vomiting

Respiratory: Reported in children: Cough, nasal congestion, nasopharyngitis

Mechanism of Action Competitive inhibition of histamine at H_2-receptors of the gastric parietal cells resulting in reduced gastric acid secretion, gastric volume and hydrogen ion concentration reduced. In healthy volunteers, nizatidine suppresses gastric acid secretion induced by pentagastrin infusion or food.

Drug Interactions

Cytochrome P450 Effect: Inhibits 3A4 (weak)

Decreased Effect: May decrease the absorption of itraconazole or ketoconazole.

Pharmacodynamics/Kinetics

Distribution: V_d: 0.8-1.5 L/kg

Protein binding: 35% to α_1-acid glycoprotein

Metabolism: Partially hepatic; forms metabolites

Bioavailability: >70%

Half-life elimination: 1-2 hours; prolonged with renal impairment

Time to peak, plasma: 0.5-3.0 hours

Excretion: Urine (90%; ~60% as unchanged drug); feces (<6%)

Pregnancy Risk Factor B

Nizoral® see Ketoconazole on page 880

Nizoral® A-D [OTC] see Ketoconazole on page 880

N-Methylhydrazine see Procarbazine on page 1284

No Doz® Maximum Strength [OTC] see Caffeine on page 245

Nolahist® [OTC] [DSC] see Phenindamine on page 1221

Nolvadex® [DSC] see Tamoxifen on page 1443

Nonoxynol 9 (non OKS i nole nine)

U.S. Brand Names Advantage-S™ [OTC]; Conceptrol® [OTC]; Delfen® [OTC]; Emko® [OTC] [DSC]; Encare® [OTC]; Gynol II® [OTC]; Shur-Seal® [OTC] [DSC]; Today® Sponge [OTC]; VCF™ [OTC]

Generic Available No

Synonyms N-9

Pharmacologic Category Contraceptive; Spermicide

Use Prevention of pregnancy

Local Anesthetic/Vasoconstrictor Precautions No information available to require special precautions

Effects on Dental Treatment No significant effects or complications reported

Common Adverse Effects Frequency not defined: Genitourinary: Irritation, burning, or itching of mucous membranes (including vaginal/urethral)

Mechanism of Action

Nonoxynol 9 is a surfactant which prevents pregnancy by damaging the cell membrane of sperm; some product formulations may also provide a physical barrier

Nora-BE™ see Norethindrone on page 1125

Noradrenaline see Norepinephrine on page 1125

Noradrenaline Acid Tartrate see Norepinephrine on page 1125

Norco® see Hydrocodone and Acetaminophen on page 779

Nordeoxyguanosine see Ganciclovir on page 722

Nordette® see Ethinyl Estradiol and Levonorgestrel on page 602

Norditropin® see Somatropin on page 1406

Norditropin® NordiFlex® see Somatropin on page 1406

Norelgestromin and Ethinyl Estradiol see Ethinyl Estradiol and Norelgestromin on page 605

Norepinephrine (nor ep i NEF rin)

U.S. Brand Names Levophed®
Canadian Brand Names Levophed®
Generic Available Yes
Synonyms Levarterenol Bitartrate; Noradrenaline; Noradrenaline Acid Tartrate; Norepinephrine Bitartrate
Pharmacologic Category Alpha/Beta Agonist
Use Treatment of shock which persists after adequate fluid volume replacement
Local Anesthetic/Vasoconstrictor Precautions No information available to require special precautions
Effects on Dental Treatment No significant effects or complications reported
Mechanism of Action Stimulates beta₁-adrenergic receptors and alpha-adrenergic receptors causing increased contractility and heart rate as well as vasoconstriction, thereby increasing systemic blood pressure and coronary blood flow; clinically alpha effects (vasoconstriction) are greater than beta effects (inotropic and chronotropic effects)
Pregnancy Risk Factor C

Norepinephrine Bitartrate see Norepinephrine on page 1125

Norethindrone (nor eth IN drone)

Related Information
Endocrine Disorders and Pregnancy *on page 1659*
U.S. Brand Names Aygestin®; Camila™; Errin™; Jolivette™; Micronor®; Nora-BE™; Nor-QD®
Canadian Brand Names Micronor®
Generic Available Yes
Synonyms Norethindrone Acetate; Norethisterone
Pharmacologic Category Contraceptive; Progestin
Use Treatment of amenorrhea; abnormal uterine bleeding; endometriosis, oral contraceptive; **higher rate of failure with progestin only contraceptives**
Local Anesthetic/Vasoconstrictor Precautions No information available to require special precautions
Effects on Dental Treatment Until we know more about the mechanism of interaction, caution is required in prescribing antibiotics to female dental patients taking progestin-only hormonal contraceptives.
Common Adverse Effects
>10%:
Cardiovascular: Edema
Endocrine & metabolic: Breakthrough bleeding, spotting, changes in menstrual flow, amenorrhea
Gastrointestinal: Anorexia
Local: Pain at injection site
Neuromuscular & skeletal: Weakness
1% to 10%:
Cardiovascular: Edema
Central nervous system: Mental depression, fever, insomnia
Dermatologic: Melasma or chloasma, allergic rash with or without pruritus
Endocrine & metabolic: Increased breast tenderness
Gastrointestinal: Weight gain/loss
Genitourinary: Changes in cervical erosion and secretions
Hepatic: Cholestatic jaundice
Mechanism of Action Inhibits secretion of pituitary gonadotropin (LH) which prevents follicular maturation and ovulation
Drug Interactions
Cytochrome P450 Effect: Substrate of CYP3A4 (major); **Induces** CYP2C19 (weak)
Decreased Effect: Nelfinavir decreases the pharmacologic effect of norethindrone. CYP3A4 inducers may decrease the levels/effects of norethindrone; example inducers include aminoglutethimide, carbamazepine, nafcillin, nevirapine, phenobarbital, phenytoin, and rifamycins.
Pharmacodynamics/Kinetics
Absorption: Oral, transdermal: Rapidly absorbed
Distribution: V_d: 2-4 L/kg
Protein binding: 61% to albumin; 36% to sex hormone-binding globulin (SHBG); SHBG capacity affected by plasma ethinyl estradiol levels
Metabolism: Oral: Hepatic via reduction and conjugation; first-pass effect
Bioavailability: 64%
(Continued)

Norethindrone *(Continued)*

Half-life elimination: 5-14 hours
Time to peak: 1-2 hours
Excretion: Primarily urine (as metabolites)
Pregnancy Risk Factor X

Norethindrone Acetate *see* Norethindrone *on page 1125*

Norethindrone Acetate and Ethinyl Estradiol *see* Ethinyl Estradiol and Norethindrone *on page 608*

Norethindrone and Estradiol *see* Estradiol and Norethindrone *on page 575*

Norethindrone and Mestranol *see* Mestranol and Norethindrone *on page 999*

Norethisterone *see* Norethindrone *on page 1125*

Norflex™ *see* Orphenadrine *on page 1151*

Norfloxacin *(nor FLOKS a sin)*

Related Information
Sexually-Transmitted Diseases *on page 1674*

U.S. Brand Names Noroxin®

Canadian Brand Names Apo-Norflox®; Norfloxacine®; Novo-Norfloxacin; PMS-Norfloxacin; Riva-Norfloxacin

Mexican Brand Names Difoxacil®; Floxacin®; Noroxin®; Oranor®

Generic Available No

Pharmacologic Category Antibiotic, Quinolone

Use Uncomplicated urinary tract infections and cystitis caused by susceptible gram-negative and gram-positive bacteria; sexually-transmitted disease (eg, uncomplicated urethral and cervical gonorrhea) caused by *N. gonorrhoeae*; prostatitis due to *E. coli*

Local Anesthetic/Vasoconstrictor Precautions No information available to require special precautions (see Dental Comment)

Effects on Dental Treatment No significant effects or complications reported

Common Adverse Effects 1% to 10%:
Central nervous system: Headache (3%), dizziness (3%)
Gastrointestinal: Nausea (4%)
Neuromuscular & skeletal: Weakness (1%)

Mechanism of Action Norfloxacin is a DNA gyrase inhibitor. DNA gyrase is an essential bacterial enzyme that maintains the superhelical structure of DNA. DNA gyrase is required for DNA replication and transcription, DNA repair, recombination, and transposition; bactericidal

Drug Interactions
Cytochrome P450 Effect: Inhibits CYP1A2 (strong), 3A4 (moderate)

Increased Effect/Toxicity: Norfloxacin may increase the effects/toxicity of cyclosporine, CYP1A2 substrates (eg, aminophylline, fluvoxamine, mexiletine, mirtazapine, ropinirole, and trifluoperazine), CYP3A4 substrates (such as benzodiazepines, calcium channel blockers, cisapride, ergot alkaloids, selected HMG-CoA reductase inhibitors, mirtazapine, nateglinide, nefazodone, pimozide, sildenafil (and other PDE-5 inhibitors), tacrolimus, and venlafaxine), glyburide, theophylline, and warfarin. Concomitant use with corticosteroids may increase the risk of tendon rupture. Concomitant use with other QT$_c$-prolonging agents (eg, Class Ia and Class III antiarrhythmics, erythromycin, cisapride, antipsychotics, and cyclic antidepressants) may result in arrhythmias such as torsade de pointes. Probenecid may increase norfloxacin levels.

Decreased Effect: Concurrent administration of metal cations, including most antacids, oral electrolyte supplements, quinapril, sucralfate, some didanosine formulations (chewable/buffered tablets and pediatric powder for oral suspension), and other highly-buffered oral drugs, may decrease quinolone levels; separate doses.

Pharmacodynamics/Kinetics
Absorption: Oral: Rapid, up to 40%
Distribution: Crosses placenta; small amounts enter breast milk
Protein binding: 15%
Metabolism: Hepatic
Half-life elimination: 3-4 hours; Renal impairment (Cl$_{cr}$ ≤30 mL/minute): 6.5 hours; Elderly: 4 hours
Time to peak, serum: 1-2 hours
Excretion: Urine (26% to 36%); feces (30%)
Pregnancy Risk Factor C

Dental Comment

This drug is known to prolong the QT interval. The QT interval is measured as the time and distance between the Q point of the QRS complex and the end of the T wave in the ECG tracing. After adjustment for heart rate, the QT interval is defined as prolonged if it is more than 450 msec in men and 460 msec in women. A long QT syndrome was first described in the 1950s and 60s as a congenital syndrome involving QT interval prolongation and syncope and sudden death. Some of the congenital long QT syndromes were characterized by a peculiar electrocardiographic appearance of the QRS complex involving a premature atria beat followed by a pause, then a subsequent sinus beat showing marked QT prolongation and deformity. This type of cardiac arrhythmia was originally termed "torsade de pointes" (translated from the French as "twisting of the points").

Prolongation of the QT interval is thought to result from delayed ventricular repolarization. The repolarization process within the myocardial cell is due to the efflux of intracellular potassium. The channels associated with this current can be blocked by many drugs and predisposes the electrical propagation cycle to torsade de pointes.

Norfloxacin is one of the drugs confirmed to prolong the QT interval and is accepted as having a risk of causing torsade de pointes. The risk of drug-induced torsade de pointes is extremely low when a single QT interval prolonging drug is prescribed. In terms of epinephrine, it is not known what effect vasoconstrictors in the local anesthetic regimen will have in patients with a known history of congenital prolonged QT interval or in patients taking any medication that prolongs the QT interval. Until more information is obtained, it is suggested that the clinician consult with the physician prior to the use of a vasoconstrictor in suspected patients, and that the vasoconstrictor (epinephrine, levonordefrin [Neo-Cobefrin®]) be used with caution.

Norgesic™ [DSC] *see* Orphenadrine, Aspirin, and Caffeine *on page 1152*

Norgesic™ Forte [DSC] *see* Orphenadrine, Aspirin, and Caffeine *on page 1152*

Norgestimate and Estradiol *see* Estradiol and Norgestimate *on page 576*

Norgestimate and Ethinyl Estradiol *see* Ethinyl Estradiol and Norgestimate *on page 613*

Norgestrel (nor JES trel)

Related Information
Endocrine Disorders and Pregnancy *on page 1659*

U.S. Brand Names Ovrette® [DSC]

Canadian Brand Names Ovrette®

Generic Available No

Pharmacologic Category Contraceptive; Progestin

Use Prevention of pregnancy; **progestin only products have higher risk of failure in contraceptive use**

Local Anesthetic/Vasoconstrictor Precautions No information available to require special precautions

Effects on Dental Treatment Until we know more about the mechanism of interaction, caution is required in prescribing antibiotics to female dental patients taking progestin-only hormonal contraceptives.

Common Adverse Effects Frequency not defined.
Cardiovascular: Embolism, cerebral thrombosis, edema
Central nervous system: Mental depression, fever, insomnia
Dermatologic: Melasma or chloasma, allergic rash with or without pruritus
Endocrine & metabolic: Breakthrough bleeding, spotting, changes in menstrual flow, amenorrhea, changes in cervical erosion and secretions, increased breast tenderness
Gastrointestinal: Weight gain/loss, anorexia
Hepatic: Cholestatic jaundice
Local: Thrombophlebitis
Neuromuscular & skeletal: Weakness

Mechanism of Action Inhibits secretion of pituitary gonadotropin (LH) which prevents follicular maturation and ovulation

Drug Interactions
Cytochrome P450 Effect: Substrate of CYP3A4 (major)

Increased Effect/Toxicity: Oral contraceptives may increase toxicity of acetaminophen, anticoagulants, benzodiazepines, caffeine, corticosteroids, metoprolol, theophylline, and tricyclic antidepressants.

Decreased Effect: CYP3A4 inducers may decrease the levels/effects of norgestrel; example inducers include aminoglutethimide, carbamazepine, nafcillin, nevirapine, phenobarbital, phenytoin, and rifamycins. Antibiotics *(Continued)*

Norgestrel (Continued)

(penicillins, tetracyclines, griseofulvin) were reported to decrease efficacy of oral contraceptives, but this has not been validated in more rigorous investigations.

Pharmacodynamics/Kinetics

Absorption: Oral: Well absorbed

Protein binding: >97% to sex hormone-binding globulin

Metabolism: Primarily hepatic via reduction and conjugation

Half-life elimination: ~20 hours

Excretion: Urine (as metabolites)

Pregnancy Risk Factor X

Norgestrel and Ethinyl Estradiol see Ethinyl Estradiol and Norgestrel on page 616

Norinyl® 1+35 see Ethinyl Estradiol and Norethindrone on page 608

Norinyl® 1+50 see Mestranol and Norethindrone on page 999

Noritate® see Metronidazole on page 1033

Normal Saline see Sodium Chloride on page 1400

Noroxin® see Norfloxacin on page 1126

Norpace® see Disopyramide on page 491

Norpace® CR see Disopyramide on page 491

Norpramin® see Desipramine on page 434

Nor-QD® see Norethindrone on page 1125

Nortemp Children's [OTC] see Acetaminophen on page 31

Nortrel™ see Ethinyl Estradiol and Norethindrone on page 608

Nortrel™ 7/7/7 see Ethinyl Estradiol and Norethindrone on page 608

Nortriptyline (nor TRIP ti leen)

U.S. Brand Names Pamelor®

Canadian Brand Names Alti-Nortriptyline; Apo-Nortriptyline®; Aventyl®; Gen-Nortriptyline; Norventyl; Novo-Nortriptyline; Nu-Nortriptyline; PMS-Nortriptyline

Generic Available Yes: Excludes solution

Synonyms Nortriptyline Hydrochloride

Pharmacologic Category Antidepressant, Tricyclic (Secondary Amine)

Dental Use Treatment of myofascial pain, neuralgia, burning mouth syndrome

Use Treatment of symptoms of depression

Unlabeled/Investigational Use Chronic pain, anxiety disorders, enuresis, attention-deficit/hyperactivity disorder (ADHD); adjunctive therapy for smoking cessation

Local Anesthetic/Vasoconstrictor Precautions Use with caution; epinephrine and levonordefrin have been shown to have an increased pressor response in combination with TCAs

Effects on Dental Treatment Key adverse event(s) related to dental treatment: Xerostomia (normal salivary flow resumes upon discontinuation). Long-term treatment with TCAs, such as nortriptyline, increases the risk of caries by reducing salivation and salivary buffer capacity.

Significant Adverse Effects Frequency not defined.

Cardiovascular: Postural hypotension, arrhythmia, hypertension, heart block, tachycardia, palpitation, MI

Central nervous system: Confusion, delirium, hallucinations, restlessness, insomnia, disorientation, delusions, anxiety, agitation, panic, nightmares, hypomania, exacerbation of psychosis, incoordination, ataxia, extrapyramidal symptoms, seizure

Dermatologic: Alopecia, photosensitivity, rash, petechiae, urticaria, itching

Endocrine & metabolic: Sexual dysfunction, gynecomastia, breast enlargement, galactorrhea, increase or decrease in libido, increase in blood sugar, SIADH

Gastrointestinal: Xerostomia, constipation, vomiting, anorexia, diarrhea, abdominal cramps, black tongue, nausea, unpleasant taste, weight gain/loss

Genitourinary: Urinary retention, delayed micturition, impotence, testicular edema

Hematologic: Rarely agranulocytosis, eosinophilia, purpura, thrombocytopenia

Hepatic: Increased liver enzymes, cholestatic jaundice

Neuromuscular & skeletal: Tremor, numbness, tingling, paresthesia, peripheral neuropathy

Ocular: Blurred vision, eye pain, disturbances in accommodation, mydriasis

Otic: Tinnitus

Miscellaneous: Diaphoresis (excessive), allergic reactions

Restrictions A medication guide concerning the use of antidepressants in children and teenagers can be found on the FDA website at http://www.fda.gov/cder/Offices/ODS/labeling.htm. It should be dispensed to parents or guardians of children and teenagers receiving this medication.

Dental Usual Dosing Myofascial pain, neuralgia, burning mouth syndrome: Adults: Initial: 10-25 mg at bedtime; dosage may be increased by 25 mg/day weekly, if tolerated; usual maintenance dose: 75 mg as a single bedtime dose or 2 divided doses

Dosage Oral:

Nocturnal enuresis: Children (unlabeled use): 10-20 mg/day; titrate to a maximum of 40 mg/day

Depression (unlabeled use): Children: 1-3 mg/kg/day

Depression:

Adults: 25 mg 3-4 times/day up to 150 mg/day

Elderly (**Note:** Nortriptyline is one of the best tolerated TCAs in the elderly)

Initial: 10-25 mg at bedtime

Dosage can be increased by 25 mg every 3 days for inpatients and weekly for outpatients if tolerated

Usual maintenance dose: 75 mg as a single bedtime dose or 2 divided doses; however, lower or higher doses may be required to stay within the therapeutic window

Myofascial pain, neuralgia, burning mouth syndrome (dental use): Initial: 10-25 mg at bedtime; dosage may be increased by 25 mg/day weekly, if tolerated; usual maintenance dose: 75 mg as a single bedtime dose or 2 divided doses

Chronic urticaria, angioedema, nocturnal pruritus (unlabeled use): Adults: Oral: 75 mg/day

Smoking cessation (unlabeled use): Adults: 25-75 mg/day beginning 10-14 days before "quit" day; continue therapy for ≥12 weeks after "quit" day

Dosing adjustment in hepatic impairment: Lower doses and slower titration dependent on individualization of dosage is recommended

Mechanism of Action Traditionally believed to increase the synaptic concentration of serotonin and/or norepinephrine in the central nervous system by inhibition of their reuptake by the presynaptic neuronal membrane. However, additional receptor effects have been found including desensitization of adenyl cyclase, down regulation of beta-adrenergic receptors, and down regulation of serotonin receptors.

Contraindications Hypersensitivity to nortriptyline and similar chemical class, or any component of the formulation; use of MAO inhibitors within 14 days; use in a patient during the acute recovery phase of MI; pregnancy

Warnings/Precautions Antidepressants increase the risk of suicidal thinking and behavior in children and adolescents with major depressive disorder (MDD) and other depressive disorders; consider risk prior to prescribing. Closely monitor for clinical worsening, suicidality, or unusual changes in behavior; the child's family or caregiver should be instructed to closely observe the patient and communicate condition with healthcare provider. Such observation would generally include at least weekly face-to-face contact with patients or their family members or caregivers during the first 4 weeks of treatment, then every other week visits for the next 4 weeks, then at 12 weeks, and as clinically indicated beyond 12 weeks. Additional contact by telephone may be appropriate between face-to-face visits. Adults treated with antidepressants should be observed similarly for clinical worsening and suicidality, especially during the initial few months of a course of drug therapy, or at times of dose changes, either increases or decreases. A medication guide should be dispensed with each prescription. **Nortriptyline is not FDA approved for use in children.**

The possibility of a suicide attempt is inherent in major depression and may persist until remission occurs. Monitor for worsening of depression or suicidality, especially during initiation of therapy or with dose increases or decreases. Worsening depression and severe abrupt suicidality that are not part of the presenting symptoms may require discontinuation or modification of drug therapy. Use caution in high-risk patients during initiation of therapy. Prescriptions should be written for the smallest quantity consistent with good patient care. The patient's family or caregiver should be alerted to monitor patients for the emergence of suicidality and associated behaviors such as anxiety, agitation, panic attacks, insomnia, irritability, hostility, impulsivity, akathisia, hypomania, and mania; patients should be instructed to notify their healthcare provider if any of these symptoms or worsening depression occur.

May worsen psychosis in some patients or precipitate a shift to mania or hypomania in patients with bipolar disorder. Monotherapy in patients with bipolar disorder should be avoided. Patients presenting with depressive symptoms should be screened for bipolar disorder. **Nortriptyline is not FDA approved for the treatment of bipolar depression.**
(Continued)

Nortriptyline *(Continued)*

May cause sedation, resulting in impaired performance of tasks requiring alertness (eg, operating machinery or driving). Sedative effects may be additive with other CNS depressants and/or ethanol. The degree of sedation is low-moderate relative to other antidepressants. May increase the risks associated with electroconvulsive therapy. Consider discontinuing, when possible, prior to elective surgery. Therapy should not be abruptly discontinued in patients receiving high doses for prolonged periods. May alter glucose regulation - use caution in patients with diabetes.

May cause orthostatic hypotension (risk is low relative to other antidepressants) - use with caution in patients at risk of hypotension or in patients where transient hypotensive episodes would be poorly tolerated (cardiovascular disease or cerebrovascular disease). The degree of anticholinergic blockade produced by this agent is moderate relative to other cyclic antidepressants, however, caution should still be used in patients with urinary retention, benign prostatic hyperplasia, narrow-angle glaucoma, xerostomia, visual problems, constipation, or history of bowel obstruction.

Use with caution in patients with a history of cardiovascular disease (including previous MI, stroke, tachycardia, or conduction abnormalities). The risk conduction abnormalities with this agent is moderate relative to other antidepressants. Use caution in patients with a previous seizure disorder or condition predisposing to seizures such as brain damage, alcoholism, or concurrent therapy with other drugs which lower the seizure threshold. Use with caution in hyperthyroid patients or those receiving thyroid supplementation. Use with caution in patients with hepatic or renal dysfunction and in elderly patients.

Drug Interactions Substrate of CYP1A2 (minor), 2C19 (minor), 2D6 (major), 3A4 (minor); **Inhibits** CYP2D6 (weak), 2E1 (weak)

Altretamine: Concurrent use may cause orthostatic hypertension

Amphetamines: TCAs may enhance the effect of amphetamines; monitor for adverse CV effects

Anticholinergics: Combined use with TCAs may produce additive anticholinergic effects

Antihypertensives: TCAs may inhibit the antihypertensive response to bethanidine, clonidine, debrisoquin, guanadrel, guanethidine, guanabenz, guanfacine; monitor BP; consider alternate antihypertensive agent

Beta-agonists: When combined with TCAs may predispose patients to cardiac arrhythmias

Bupropion: May increase the levels of tricyclic antidepressants; based on limited information; monitor response

Carbamazepine: Tricyclic antidepressants may increase carbamazepine levels; monitor

Cholestyramine and colestipol: May bind TCAs and reduce their absorption; monitor for altered response

Clonidine: Abrupt discontinuation of clonidine may cause hypertensive crisis, amitriptyline may enhance the response

CNS depressants: Sedative effects may be additive with TCAs; monitor for increased effect; includes benzodiazepines, barbiturates, antipsychotics, ethanol and other sedative medications

CYP2D6 inhibitors: May increase the levels/effects of nortriptyline. Example inhibitors include chlorpromazine, delavirdine, fluoxetine, miconazole, paroxetine, pergolide, quinidine, quinine, ritonavir, and ropinirole.

Epinephrine (and other direct alpha-agonists): Pressor response to I.V. epinephrine, norepinephrine, and phenylephrine may be enhanced in patients receiving TCAs (**Note:** Effect is unlikely with epinephrine or levonordefrin dosages typically administered as infiltration in combination with local anesthetics)

Fenfluramine: May increase tricyclic antidepressant levels/effects

Hypoglycemic agents (including insulin): TCAs may enhance the hypoglycemic effects of tolazamide, chlorpropamide, or insulin; monitor for changes in blood glucose levels; reported with chlorpropamide, tolazamide, and insulin

Levodopa: Tricyclic antidepressants may decrease the absorption (bioavailability) of levodopa; rare hypertensive episodes have also been attributed to this combination

Linezolid: Hyperpyrexia, hypertension, tachycardia, confusion, seizures, and **deaths have been reported** with agents which inhibit MAO (serotonin syndrome); this combination should be avoided

Lithium: Concurrent use with a TCA may increase the risk for neurotoxicity

MAO inhibitors: Hyperpyrexia, hypertension, tachycardia, confusion, seizures, and **deaths have been reported** (serotonin syndrome); this combination should be avoided

Methylphenidate: Metabolism of TCAs may be decreased

Phenothiazines: Serum concentrations of some TCAs may be increased; in addition, TCAs may increase concentration of phenothiazines; monitor for altered clinical response

QT_c-prolonging agents: Concurrent use of tricyclic agents with other drugs which may prolong QT_c interval may increase the risk of potentially fatal arrhythmias; includes type Ia and type III antiarrhythmics agents, selected quinolones (sparfloxacin, gatifloxacin, moxifloxacin, grepafloxacin), cisapride, and other agents

Ritonavir: Combined use of high-dose tricyclic antidepressants with ritonavir may cause serotonin syndrome in HIV-positive patients; monitor

Sucralfate: Absorption of tricyclic antidepressants may be reduced with coadministration

Sympathomimetics, indirect-acting: Tricyclic antidepressants may result in a decreased sensitivity to indirect-acting sympathomimetics; includes dopamine and ephedrine; also see interaction with epinephrine (and direct-acting sympathomimetics)

Tramadol: Tramadol's risk of seizures may be increased with TCAs

Valproic acid: May increase serum concentrations/adverse effects of some tricyclic antidepressants

Warfarin (and other oral anticoagulants): TCAs may increase the anticoagulant effect in patients stabilized on warfarin; monitor INR

Ethanol/Nutrition/Herb Interactions

Ethanol: Avoid ethanol (may increase CNS depression).

Food: Grapefruit juice may inhibit the metabolism of some TCAs and clinical toxicity may result.

Herb/Nutraceutical: Avoid valerian, St John's wort, SAMe, kava kava (may increase risk of serotonin syndrome and/or excessive sedation).

Pharmacodynamics/Kinetics

Onset of action: Therapeutic: 1-3 weeks

Distribution: V_d: 21 L/kg

Protein binding: 93% to 95%

Metabolism: Primarily hepatic; extensive first-pass effect

Half-life elimination: 28-31 hours

Time to peak, serum: 7-8.5 hours

Excretion: Urine (as metabolites and small amounts of unchanged drug); feces (small amounts)

Pregnancy Risk Factor D

Lactation Enters breast milk/contraindicated (AAP rates "of concern")

Dosage Forms

Capsule, as hydrochloride: 10 mg, 25 mg, 50 mg, 75 mg

Pamelor®: 10 mg, 25 mg, 50 mg, 75 mg [may contain benzyl alcohol; 50 mg may also contain sodium bisulfite]

Solution, as hydrochloride (Pamelor®): 10 mg/5 mL (473 mL) [contains alcohol 4% and benzoic acid]

Selected Readings

Friedlander AH and Mahler ME, "Major Depressive Disorder. Psychopathology, Medical Management, and Dental Implications," *J Am Dent Assoc*, 2001, 132(5):629-38.

Ganzberg S, "Psychoactive Drugs," *ADA Guide to Dental Therapeutics*, 2nd ed, Chicago, IL: ADA Publishing, a Division of ADA Business Enterprises, Inc, 2000, 376-405.

Jastak JT and Yagiela JA, "Vasoconstrictors and Local Anesthesia: A Review and Rationale for Use," *J Am Dent Assoc*, 1983, 107(4):623-30.

Rundegren J, van Dijken J, Mörnstad H, et al, "Oral Conditions in Patients Receiving Long-Term Treatment With Cyclic Antidepressant Drugs," *Swed Dent J*, 1985, 9(2):55-64.

Yagiela JA, "Adverse Drug Interactions in Dental Practice: Interactions Associated With Vasoconstrictors. Part V of a Series," *J Am Dent Assoc*, 1999, 130(5):701-9.

Nortriptyline Hydrochloride *see* Nortriptyline *on page 1128*

Norvasc® *see* Amlodipine *on page 100*

Norvir® *see* Ritonavir *on page 1359*

Novantrone® *see* Mitoxantrone *on page 1055*

Novarel™ *see* Chorionic Gonadotropin (Human) *on page 336*

Novocain® *see* Procaine *on page 1284*

Novolin® 70/30 *see* Insulin NPH and Insulin Regular *on page 840*

Novolin® N *see* Insulin NPH *on page 840*

Novolin® R *see* Insulin Regular *on page 841*

NovoLog® *see* Insulin Aspart *on page 835*

NovoLog® Mix 70/30 *see* Insulin Aspart Protamine and Insulin Aspart *on page 836*

NovoSeven® *see* Factor VIIa (Recombinant) *on page 632*

NPH Insulin *see* Insulin NPH *on page 840*

NPH Insulin and Regular Insulin *see* Insulin NPH and Insulin Regular *on page 840*

NRS® [OTC] *see* Oxymetazoline *on page 1172*

NSC-740 *see* Methotrexate *on page 1012*
NSC-752 *see* Thioguanine *on page 1476*
NSC-755 *see* Mercaptopurine *on page 995*
NSC-3053 *see* Dactinomycin *on page 417*
NSC-3088 *see* Chlorambucil *on page 313*
NSC-10363 *see* Megestrol *on page 976*
NSC-13875 *see* Altretamine *on page 78*
NSC-15200 *see* Gallium Nitrate *on page 721*
NSC-26271 *see* Cyclophosphamide *on page 403*
NSC-26980 *see* Mitomycin *on page 1054*
NSC-27640 *see* Floxuridine *on page 659*
NSC-38721 *see* Mitotane *on page 1055*
NSC-49842 *see* VinBLAStine *on page 1575*
NSC-63878 *see* Cytarabine *on page 413*
NSC-66847 *see* Thalidomide *on page 1471*
NSC-67574 *see* VinCRIStine *on page 1576*
NSC-77213 *see* Procarbazine *on page 1284*
NSC-82151 *see* DAUNOrubicin Hydrochloride *on page 426*
NSC-85998 *see* Streptozocin *on page 1418*
NSC-89199 *see* Estramustine *on page 578*
NSC-102816 *see* Azacitidine *on page 167*
NSC-106977 *(Erwinia) see* Asparaginase *on page 144*
NSC-109229 *(E. coli) see* Asparaginase *on page 144*
NSC-109724 *see* Ifosfamide *on page 815*
NSC-122758 *see* Tretinoin (Oral) *on page 1524*
NSC-123127 *see* DOXOrubicin *on page 509*
NSC-125066 *see* Bleomycin *on page 214*
NSC-125973 *see* Paclitaxel *on page 1176*
NSC-147834 *see* Flutamide *on page 686*
NSC-180973 *see* Tamoxifen *on page 1443*
NSC-218321 *see* Pentostatin *on page 1211*
NSC-245467 *see* Vindesine *on page 1577*
NSC-249992 *see* Amsacrine *on page 123*
NSC-256439 *see* Idarubicin *on page 814*
NSC-266046 *see* Oxaliplatin *on page 1154*
NSC-301739 *see* Mitoxantrone *on page 1055*
NSC-308847 *see* Amonafide *on page 104*
NSC-352122 *see* Trimetrexate *on page 1539*
NSC-362856 *see* Temozolomide *on page 1454*
NSC-373364 *see* Aldesleukin *on page 61*
NSC-377526 *see* Leuprolide *on page 906*
NSC-409962 *see* Carmustine *on page 273*
NSC-603071 *see* Aminocamptothecin *on page 86*
NSC-606864 *see* Goserelin *on page 750*
NSC606869 *see* Clofarabine *on page 367*
NSC-609699 *see* Topotecan *on page 1511*
NSC-616348 *see* Irinotecan *on page 860*
NSC-628503 *see* Docetaxel *on page 494*
NSC-644954 *see* Pegaspargase *on page 1194*
NSC-673089 *see* Paclitaxel *on page 1176*
NSC-687451 *see* Rituximab *on page 1360*
NSC-698037 *see* Pemetrexed *on page 1198*
NSC-704865 *see* Bevacizumab *on page 204*
NSC-706725 *see* Raloxifene *on page 1329*
NSC-712807 *see* Capecitabine *on page 255*
NSC-714692 *see* Cetuximab *on page 308*
NSC-714744 *see* Denileukin Diftitox *on page 432*
NSC-715055 *see* Gefitinib *on page 727*
NSC-718781 *see* Erlotinib *on page 560*
NSC-719345 *see* Letrozole *on page 904*
NSC-720568 *see* Gemtuzumab Ozogamicin *on page 732*
NSC736511 *see* Sunitinib *on page 1434*
NTG *see* Nitroglycerin *on page 1120*
N-trifluoroacetyladriamycin-14-valerate *see* Valrubicin *on page 1560*
NTZ *see* Nitazoxanide *on page 1117*

Nubain® see Nalbuphine on page 1083

Nucofed® Expectorant see Guaifenesin, Pseudoephedrine, and Codeine on page 756

Nucofed® Pediatric Expectorant see Guaifenesin, Pseudoephedrine, and Codeine on page 756

Nu-Iron® 150 [OTC] see Polysaccharide-Iron Complex on page 1254

NuLev™ see Hyoscyamine on page 803

Nullo® [OTC] see Chlorophyll on page 319

NuLYTELY® see Polyethylene Glycol-Electrolyte Solution on page 1253

Numorphan® see Oxymorphone on page 1174

Nupercainal® [OTC] see Dibucaine on page 458

Nupercainal® Hydrocortisone Cream [OTC] see Hydrocortisone on page 793

Nuquin HP® see Hydroquinone on page 798

Nu-Tears® [OTC] see Artificial Tears on page 143

Nu-Tears® II [OTC] see Artificial Tears on page 143

Nutracort® see Hydrocortisone on page 793

Nutralox® [OTC] see Calcium Carbonate on page 248

Nutraplus® [OTC] see Urea on page 1551

NutreStore™ see Glutamine on page 743

Nutropin® see Somatropin on page 1406

Nutropin AQ® see Somatropin on page 1406

NuvaRing® see Ethinyl Estradiol and Etonogestrel on page 600

NVB see Vinorelbine on page 1578

NVP see Nevirapine on page 1104

Nyamyc™ see Nystatin on page 1133

Nydrazid® [DSC] see Isoniazid on page 864

Nylidrin (NYE li drin)

Canadian Brand Names Arlidin®

Pharmacologic Category Vasodilator, Peripheral

Use Considered "possibly effective" for increasing blood supply to treat peripheral disease (arteriosclerosis obliterans, diabetic vascular disease, nocturnal leg cramps, Raynaud's disease, frost bite, ischemic ulcer, thrombophlebitis) and circulatory disturbances of the inner ear (cochlear ischemia, macular or ampullar ischemia, etc)

Local Anesthetic/Vasoconstrictor Precautions No information available to require special precautions

Effects on Dental Treatment No significant effects or complications reported

Common Adverse Effects

1% to 10%:
Central nervous system: Nervousness
Neuromuscular & skeletal: Trembling

Mechanism of Action Nylidrin is a peripheral vasodilator; this results from direct relaxation of vascular smooth muscle and beta agonist action. Nylidrin does not appear to affect cutaneous blood flow; it reportedly increases heart rate and cardiac output; cutaneous blood flow is not enhanced to any appreciable extent.

Pregnancy Risk Factor C

Nystatin (nye STAT in)

Related Information
Fungal Infections on page 1707
Management of Patients Undergoing Cancer Therapy on page 1728
Sexually-Transmitted Diseases on page 1674

Related Sample Prescriptions
Topical Fungal Infections on page 1740

U.S. Brand Names Bio-Statin®; Mycostatin®; Nyamyc™; Nystat-Rx®; Nystop®; Pedi-Dri®

Canadian Brand Names Candistatin®; Nilstat; Nyaderm; PMS-Nystatin

Mexican Brand Names Micostatin®

Generic Available Yes: Cream, ointment, powder, suspension, tablet

Pharmacologic Category Antifungal Agent, Oral Nonabsorbed; Antifungal Agent, Topical; Antifungal Agent, Vaginal

Dental Use Treatment of susceptible cutaneous, mucocutaneous, and oral cavity fungal infections normally caused by the *Candida* species

(Continued)

Nystatin *(Continued)*

Use Treatment of susceptible cutaneous, mucocutaneous, and oral cavity fungal infections normally caused by the *Candida* species

Local Anesthetic/Vasoconstrictor Precautions No information available to require special precautions

Effects on Dental Treatment No significant effects or complications reported

Significant Adverse Effects

Frequency not defined: Dermatologic: Contact dermatitis, Stevens-Johnson syndrome

1% to 10%: Gastrointestinal: Nausea, vomiting, diarrhea, stomach pain

<1% (Limited to important or life-threatening): Hypersensitivity reactions

Dental Usual Dosing

Oral candidiasis:

Suspension (swish and swallow orally):

Premature infants: 100,000 units 4 times/day

Infants: 200,000 units 4 times/day or 100,000 units to each side of mouth 4 times/day

Children and Adults: 400,000-600,000 units 4 times/day

Mucocutaneous infections: Children and Adults: Topical: Apply 2-3 times/day to affected areas; very moist topical lesions are treated best with powder

Dosage

Oral candidiasis:

Suspension (swish and swallow orally):

Premature infants: 100,000 units 4 times/day

Infants: 200,000 units 4 times/day or 100,000 units to each side of mouth 4 times/day

Children and Adults: 400,000-600,000 units 4 times/day

Powder for compounding: Children and Adults: 1/8 teaspoon (500,000 units) to equal approximately 1/2 cup of water; give 4 times/day

Mucocutaneous infections: Children and Adults: Topical: Apply 2-3 times/day to affected areas; very moist topical lesions are treated best with powder

Intestinal infections: Adults: Oral: 500,000-1,000,000 units every 8 hours

Vaginal infections: Adults: Vaginal tablets: Insert 1 tablet/day at bedtime for 2 weeks

Mechanism of Action Binds to sterols in fungal cell membrane, changing the cell wall permeability allowing for leakage of cellular contents

Contraindications Hypersensitivity to nystatin or any component of the formulation

Drug Interactions No data reported

Pharmacodynamics/Kinetics

Onset of action: Symptomatic relief from candidiasis: 24-72 hours

Absorption: Topical: None through mucous membranes or intact skin; Oral: Poorly absorbed

Excretion: Feces (as unchanged drug)

Pregnancy Risk Factor B/C (oral)

Lactation Does not enter breast milk/compatible (not absorbed orally)

Dosage Forms

Capsule (Bio-Statin®): 500,000 units, 1 million units

Cream: 100,000 units/g (15 g, 30 g)

Mycostatin®: 100,000 units/g (30 g)

Ointment, topical: 100,000 units/g (15 g, 30 g)

Powder, for prescription compounding: 50 million units (10 g); 150 million units (30 g); 500 million units (100 g); 2 billion units (400 g)

Nystat-Rx®: 50 million units (10 g); 150 million units (30 g); 500 million units (100 g); 1 billion units (190 g); 2 billion units (350 g)

Powder, topical:

Mycostatin®: 100,000 units/g (15 g)

Nyamyc™: 100,000 units/g (15 g, 30 g)

Nystop®: 100,000 units/g (15 g, 30 g, 60 g)

Pedi-Dri®: 100,000 units/g (56.7 g)

Suspension, oral: 100,000 units/mL (5 mL, 60 mL, 480 mL)

Tablet: 500,000 units

Tablet, vaginal: 100,000 units (15s) [packaged with applicator]

Nystatin and Triamcinolone *(nye STAT in & trye am SIN oh lone)*

Related Information

Fungal Infections *on page 1707*
Nystatin *on page 1133*
Triamcinolone *on page 1526*

Related Sample Prescriptions

Angular Cheilitis *on page 1741*

U.S. Brand Names Mycolog®-II [DSC]

Generic Available Yes

Synonyms Triamcinolone and Nystatin

Pharmacologic Category Antifungal Agent, Topical; Corticosteroid, Topical

Dental Use Treatment of angular cheilitis and cutaneous candidiasis

Use Treatment of cutaneous candidiasis

Local Anesthetic/Vasoconstrictor Precautions No information available to require special precautions

Effects on Dental Treatment No significant effects or complications reported

Significant Adverse Effects 1% to 10%:

Dermatologic: Dryness, folliculitis, hypertrichosis, acne, hypopigmentation, allergic dermatitis, maceration of the skin, skin atrophy

Local: Burning, itching, irritation

Miscellaneous: Increased incidence of secondary infection

Dental Usual Dosing Angular cheilitis and cutaneous candidiasis: Children and Adults: Topical: Apply sparingly 2-4 times/day. Therapy should be discontinued when control is achieved; if no improvement is seen, reassessment of diagnosis may be necessary.

Dosage Children and Adults: Topical: Apply sparingly 2-4 times/day. Therapy should be discontinued when control is achieved; if no improvement is seen, reassessment of diagnosis may be necessary.

Mechanism of Action Nystatin is an antifungal agent that binds to sterols in fungal cell membrane, changing the cell wall permeability allowing for leakage of cellular contents. Triamcinolone is a synthetic corticosteroid; it decreases inflammation by suppression of migration of polymorphonuclear leukocytes and reversal of increased capillary permeability. It suppresses the immune system reducing activity and volume of the lymphatic system. It suppresses adrenal function at high doses.

Contraindications Hypersensitivity to nystatin, triamcinolone, or any component of the formulation

Warnings/Precautions Avoid use of occlusive dressings; limit therapy to least amount necessary for effective therapy, pediatric patients may be more susceptible to HPA axis suppression due to larger BSA to weight ratio

Drug Interactions No data reported

Pharmacodynamics/Kinetics See individual agents.

Pregnancy Risk Factor C

Lactation Excretion in breast milk unknown

Breast-Feeding Considerations

Nystatin: Compatible

Triamcinolone: No data reported

Dosage Forms [DSC] = Discontinued product

Cream (Mycolog®-II [DSC]): Nystatin 100,000 units and triamcinolone acetonide 0.1% (15 g, 30 g, 60 g)

Ointment: Nystatin 100,000 units and triamcinolone acetonide 0.1% (15 g, 30 g, 60 g)

Mycolog®-II: Nystatin 100,000 units and triamcinolone acetonide 0.1% (15 g, 30 g, 60 g) [DSC]

Nystat-Rx® *see* Nystatin *on page 1133*

Nystop® *see* Nystatin *on page 1133*

Nytol® Quick Caps [OTC] *see* DiphenhydrAMINE *on page 483*

Nytol® Quick Gels [OTC] *see* DiphenhydrAMINE *on page 483*

NaSop™ *see* Phenylephrine *on page 1226*

Nostrilla® [OTC] *see* Oxymetazoline *on page 1172*

Obezine® [DSC] *see* Phendimetrazine *on page 1220*

OCBZ *see* Oxcarbazepine *on page 1159*

Occlusal®-HP [OTC] *see* Salicylic Acid *on page 1374*

Ocean® [OTC] *see* Sodium Chloride *on page 1400*

Oceant® for Kids [OTC] *see* Sodium Chloride *on page 1400*

Octagam® *see* Immune Globulin (Intravenous) *on page 824*

Octreotide (ok TREE oh tide)

U.S. Brand Names Sandostatin®; Sandostatin LAR®

Canadian Brand Names Octreotide Acetate Omega; Sandostatin®; Sandostatin LAR®

Generic Available Yes: Solution

(Continued)

Octreotide *(Continued)*

Synonyms Octreotide Acetate

Pharmacologic Category Antidiarrheal; Somatostatin Analog

Use Control of symptoms in patients with metastatic carcinoid and vasoactive intestinal peptide-secreting tumors (VIPomas); acromegaly

Unlabeled/Investigational Use AIDS-associated secretory diarrhea (including *Cryptosporidiosis*), control of bleeding of esophageal varices, breast cancer, cryptosporidiosis, Cushing's syndrome (ectopic), insulinomas, small bowel fistulas, pancreatic tumors, gastrinoma, postgastrectomy dumping syndrome, chemotherapy-induced diarrhea, graft-versus-host disease (GVHD) induced diarrhea, Zollinger-Ellison syndrome, congenital hyperinsulinism

Local Anesthetic/Vasoconstrictor Precautions No information available to require special precautions (see Dental Comment)

Effects on Dental Treatment No significant effects or complications reported

Common Adverse Effects Adverse reactions vary by route of administration. Frequency of cardiac, endocrine, and gastrointestinal adverse reactions were generally higher in acromegalics.

>16%:
　Cardiovascular: Sinus bradycardia (19% to 25%), chest pain (16% to 20%)
　Central nervous system: Fatigue (1% to 20%), malaise (16% to 20%), dizziness (5% to 20%), headache (6% to 20%), fever (16% to 20%)
　Endocrine & metabolic: Hyperglycemia (2% to 27%)
　Gastrointestinal: Diarrhea (5% to 61%), abdominal discomfort (5% to 61%), flatulence (<10% to 38%), constipation (9% to 21%), nausea (5% to 61%), cholelithiasis (27%; length of therapy dependent), biliary duct dilatation (12%), biliary sludge (24%; length of therapy dependent), loose stools (5% to 61%), vomiting (4% to 21%)
　Hematologic: Antibodies to octreotide (up to 25%; no efficacy change)
　Local: Injection pain (2% to 50%; dose- and formulation-related)
　Neuromuscular & skeletal: Backache (1% to 20%), arthropathy (16% to 20%)
　Respiratory: Dyspnea (16% to 20%), upper respiratory infection (16% to 20%)
　Miscellaneous: Flu symptoms (1% to 20%)

5% to 15%:
　Cardiovascular: Conduction abnormalities (9% to 10%), arrhythmia (3% to 9%), hypertension, palpitations, peripheral edema
　Central nervous system: Anxiety, confusion, depression, hypoesthesia, insomnia, vertigo
　Dermatologic: Pruritus, rash
　Endocrine & metabolic: Hypothyroidism (2% to 12%), goiter (2% to 8%)
　Gastrointestinal: Abdominal pain, anorexia, cramping, dehydration, discomfort, hemorrhoids, tenesmus (4% to 6%), dyspepsia (4% to 6%), steatorrhea (4% to 6%), feces discoloration (4% to 6%), weight loss
　Genitourinary: UTI
　Hematologic: Anemia
　Hepatic: Hepatitis
　Neuromuscular & skeletal: Arthralgia, leg cramps, myalgia, paresthesia, rigors, weakness
　Otic: Ear ache, otitis media
　Renal: Renal calculus
　Respiratory: coughing, pharyngitis, sinusitis, rhinitis
　Miscellaneous: Allergy, diaphoresis

1% to 4%:
　Cardiovascular: Angina, cardiac failure, cerebral vascular disorder, edema, flushing, hematoma, phlebitis, tachycardia
　Central nervous system: Abnormal gait, amnesia, dysphonia, hallucinations, nervousness, neuralgia, neuropathy, somnolence, tremor, vertigo
　Dermatologic: Acne, alopecia, bruising, cellulitis, urticaria
　Endocrine & metabolic: Hypoglycemia (2% to 4%), hypokalemia, hypoproteinemia, gout, cachexia, menstrual irregularities, breast pain, impotence
　Gastrointestinal: Colitis, diverticulitis, dysphagia, fat malabsorption, gastritis, gastroenteritis, gingivitis, glossitis, melena, rectal bleeding, stomatitis, taste perversion, xerostomia
　Genitourinary: Incontinence
　Hematologic: Epistaxis
　Hepatic: Ascites, jaundice
　Local: Injection hematoma
　Neuromuscular & skeletal: Hyperkinesia, hypertonia, joint pain
　Ocular: Blurred vision, visual disturbance
　Otic: Tinnitus
　Renal: Albuminuria, renal abscess
　Respiratory: Bronchitis, pleural effusion, pneumonia, pulmonary embolism
　Miscellaneous: Bacterial infection, cold symptoms, moniliasis

Mechanism of Action Mimics natural somatostatin by inhibiting serotonin release, and the secretion of gastrin, VIP, insulin, glucagon, secretin, motilin, and pancreatic polypeptide. Decreases growth hormone and IGF-1 in acromegaly.

Drug Interactions

Decreased Effect: Octreotide may lower cyclosporine serum levels (case reports of transplant rejection due to reduction of serum cyclosporine levels when cyclosporine was given orally in conjunction with a somatostatin analogue).

Pharmacodynamics/Kinetics

Duration: SubQ: 6-12 hours

Absorption: SubQ: Rapid

Distribution: V_d: 14 L (13-30 L in acromegaly)

Protein binding: 65%

Metabolism: Extensively hepatic

Bioavailability: SubQ: 100%

Half-life elimination: 1.7-1.9 hours; up to 3.7 hours with cirrhosis

Time to peak, plasma: SubQ: 0.4 hours (0.7 hours acromegaly)

Excretion: Urine (32%)

Pregnancy Risk Factor B

Dental Comment

This drug is known to prolong the QT interval. The QT interval is measured as the time and distance between the Q point of the QRS complex and the end of the T wave in the ECG tracing. After adjustment for heart rate, the QT interval is defined as prolonged if it is more than 450 msec in men and 460 msec in women. A long QT syndrome was first described in the 1950s and 60s as a congenital syndrome involving QT interval prolongation and syncope and sudden death. Some of the congenital long QT syndromes were characterized by a peculiar electrocardiographic appearance of the QRS complex involving a premature atria beat followed by a pause, then a subsequent sinus beat showing marked QT prolongation and deformity. This type of cardiac arrhythmia was originally termed "torsade de pointes" (translated from the French as "twisting of the points").

Prolongation of the QT interval is thought to result from delayed ventricular repolarization. The repolarization process within the myocardial cell is due to the efflux of intracellular potassium. The channels associated with this current can be blocked by many drugs and predisposes the electrical propagation cycle to torsade de pointes.

Octreotide is one of the drugs confirmed to prolong the QT interval and is accepted as having a risk of causing torsade de pointes. The risk of drug-induced torsade de pointes is extremely low when a single QT interval prolonging drug is prescribed. In terms of epinephrine, it is not known what effect vasoconstrictors in the local anesthetic regimen will have in patients with a known history of congenital prolonged QT interval or in patients taking any medication that prolongs the QT interval. Until more information is obtained, it is suggested that the clinician consult with the physician prior to the use of a vasoconstrictor in suspected patients, and that the vasoconstrictor (epinephrine, levonordefrin [Neo-Cobefrin®]) be used with caution.

Octreotide Acetate *see* Octreotide *on page 1135*

OcuCoat® [OTC] *see* Artificial Tears *on page 143*

OcuCoat® PF [OTC] *see* Artificial Tears *on page 143*

Ocufen® *see* Flurbiprofen *on page 683*

Ocuflox® *see* Ofloxacin *on page 1137*

Ocupress® [DSC] *see* Carteolol *on page 274*

Ocuvite® [OTC] *see* Vitamins (Multiple/Oral) *on page 1582*

Ocuvite® Extra® [OTC] *see* Vitamins (Multiple/Oral) *on page 1582*

Ocuvite® Lutein [OTC] *see* Vitamins (Multiple/Oral) *on page 1582*

Ofloxacin (oh FLOKS a sin)

Related Information

Sexually-Transmitted Diseases *on page 1674*

Tuberculosis *on page 1673*

U.S. Brand Names Floxin®; Ocuflox®

Canadian Brand Names Apo-Oflox®; Apo-Ofloxacin®; Floxin®; Novo-Ofloxacin; Ocuflox®; PMS-Ofloxacin

Generic Available Yes: Tablet, ophthalmic solution

(Continued)

Ofloxacin *(Continued)*

Synonyms Floxin Otic Singles

Pharmacologic Category Antibiotic, Quinolone

Use Quinolone antibiotic for the treatment of acute exacerbations of chronic bronchitis, community-acquired pneumonia, skin and skin structure infections (uncomplicated), urethral and cervical gonorrhea (acute, uncomplicated), urethritis and cervicitis (nongonococcal), mixed infections of the urethra and cervix, pelvic inflammatory disease (acute), cystitis (uncomplicated), urinary tract infections (complicated), prostatitis

Ophthalmic: Treatment of superficial ocular infections involving the conjunctiva or cornea due to strains of susceptible organisms

Otic: Otitis externa, chronic suppurative otitis media, acute otitis media

Unlabeled/Investigational Use Epididymitis (gonorrhea), leprosy, Traveler's diarrhea

Local Anesthetic/Vasoconstrictor Precautions No information available to require special precautions

Effects on Dental Treatment No significant effects or complications reported

Common Adverse Effects

Systemic:

1% to 10%:

Cardiovascular: Chest pain (1% to 3%)

Central nervous system: Headache (1% to 9%), insomnia (3% to 7%), dizziness (1% to 5%), fatigue (1% to 3%), somnolence (1% to 3%), sleep disorders (1% to 3%), nervousness (1% to 3%), pyrexia (1% to 3%)

Dermatologic: Rash/pruritus (1% to 3%)

Gastrointestinal: Diarrhea (1% to 4%), vomiting (1% to 4%), GI distress (1% to 3%), abdominal cramps (1% to 3%), flatulence (1% to 3%), abnormal taste (1% to 3%), xerostomia (1% to 3%), decreased appetite (1% to 3%), nausea (3% to 10%), constipation (1% to 3%)

Genitourinary: Vaginitis (1% to 5%), external genital pruritus in women (1% to 3%)

Ocular: Visual disturbances (1% to 3%)

Respiratory: Pharyngitis (1% to 3%)

Miscellaneous: Trunk pain

Ophthalmic: Frequency not defined:

Central nervous system: Dizziness

Gastrointestinal: Nausea

Ocular: Blurred vision, burning, chemical conjunctivitis/keratitis, discomfort, dryness, edema, eye pain, foreign body sensation, itching, photophobia, redness, stinging, tearing

Otic:

>10%: Local: Application site reaction (<1% to 17%)

1% to 10%:

Central nervous system: Dizziness (≤1%), vertigo (≤1%)

Dermatologic: Pruritus (1% to 4%), rash (1%)

Gastrointestinal: Taste perversion (7%)

Neuromuscular & skeletal: Paresthesia (1%)

Mechanism of Action Ofloxacin is a DNA gyrase inhibitor. DNA gyrase is an essential bacterial enzyme that maintains the superhelical structure of DNA. DNA gyrase is required for DNA replication and transcription, DNA repair, recombination, and transposition; bactericidal

Drug Interactions

Cytochrome P450 Effect: Inhibits CYP1A2 (strong)

Increased Effect/Toxicity: Ofloxacin may increase the effects/toxicity of CYP1A2 substrates (eg, aminophylline, fluvoxamine, mexiletine, mirtazapine, ropinirole, and trifluoperazine), glyburide, theophylline and warfarin. Concomitant use with corticosteroids may increase the risk of tendon rupture. Concomitant use with other QT_c-prolonging agents (eg, Class Ia and Class III antiarrhythmics, erythromycin, cisapride, antipsychotics, and cyclic antidepressants) may result in arrhythmias such as torsade de pointes. Probenecid may increase ofloxacin levels.

Decreased Effect: Concurrent administration of metal cations, including most antacids, oral electrolyte supplements, quinapril, sucralfate, some didanosine formulations (chewable/buffered tablets and pediatric powder for oral suspension), and other highly-buffered oral drugs, may decrease quinolone levels; separate doses.

Pharmacodynamics/Kinetics

Absorption: Well absorbed; food causes only minor alterations

Distribution: V_d: 2.4-3.5 L/kg

Protein binding: 20%

Bioavailability: Oral: 98%

Half-life elimination: Biphasic: 5-7.5 hours and 20-25 hours (accounts for <5%); prolonged with renal impairment

Excretion: Primarily urine (as unchanged drug)

Pregnancy Risk Factor C

Ogen® see Estropipate on page 586

Ogestrel® see Ethinyl Estradiol and Norgestrel on page 616

OGMT see Metyrosine on page 1036

OGT-918 see Miglustat on page 1047

OKT3 see Muromonab-CD3 on page 1074

Olanzapine (oh LAN za peen)

U.S. Brand Names Zyprexa®; Zyprexa® Zydis®

Canadian Brand Names Zyprexa®; Zyprexa® Zydis®

Generic Available No

Synonyms LY170053; Zyprexa Zydis

Pharmacologic Category Antipsychotic Agent, Atypical

Use Treatment of the manifestations of schizophrenia; treatment of acute or mixed mania episodes associated with Bipolar I Disorder (as monotherapy or in combination with lithium or valproate); maintenance treatment of bipolar disorder; acute agitation (patients with schizophrenia or bipolar mania)

Unlabeled/Investigational Use Treatment of psychotic symptoms; chronic pain

Local Anesthetic/Vasoconstrictor Precautions No information available to require special precautions

Effects on Dental Treatment No significant effects or complications reported

Common Adverse Effects

>10%:

Central nervous system: Somnolence (6% to 39% dose-dependent), extrapyramidal symptoms (15% to 32% dose-dependent), insomnia (up to 12%), dizziness (4% to 18%)

Gastrointestinal: Dyspepsia (7% to 11%), constipation (9% to 11%), weight gain (5% to 6%, has been reported as high as 40%), xerostomia (9% to 22% dose-dependent)

Neuromuscular & skeletal: Weakness (2% to 20% dose-dependent)

Miscellaneous: Accidental injury (12%)

1% to 10%:

Cardiovascular: Postural hypotension (1% to 5%), tachycardia (up to 3%), peripheral edema (up to 3%), chest pain (up to 3%), hyper-/hypotension (up to 2%)

Central nervous system: Personality changes (8%), speech disorder (7%), fever (up to 6%), abnormal dreams, euphoria, amnesia, delusions, emotional lability, mania, schizophrenia

Dermatologic: Bruising (up to 5%)

Endocrine & metabolic: Cholesterol increased, prolactin increased

Gastrointestinal: Nausea (up to 9% dose-dependent), appetite increased (3% to 6%), vomiting (up to 4%), flatulence, salivation increased, thirst

Genitourinary: Incontinence (up to 2%), UTI (up to 2%), vaginitis

Local: Injection site pain (I.M. administration)

Neuromuscular & skeletal: Twitching, hypertonia (up to 3%), tremor (up to 7% dose-dependent), back pain (up to 5%), abnormal gait (6%), joint/extremity pain (up to 5%) akathisia (3% to 5%), articulation impairment (up to 2%), falling (particularly in older patients), joint stiffness

Ocular: Amblyopia (up to 3%), conjunctivitis

Respiratory: Rhinitis (up to 7%), cough (up to 6%), pharyngitis (up to 4%), dyspnea

Miscellaneous: Dental pain, diaphoresis, flu-like symptoms

Dosage

Children: Schizophrenia/bipolar disorder: Oral: Initial: 2.5 mg/day; titrate as necessary to 20 mg/day (0.12-0.29 mg/kg/day)

Adults:

Schizophrenia: Oral:

Initial: 5-10 mg once daily (increase to 10 mg once daily within 5-7 days); thereafter, adjust by 5 mg/day at 1-week intervals, up to a recommended maximum of 20 mg/day. Maintenance: 10-20 mg once daily. **Note:** Doses of 30-50 mg/day have been used; however, doses >10 mg/day have not demonstrated better efficacy, and safety and efficacy of doses >20 mg/day have not been evaluated.

(Continued)

Olanzapine *(Continued)*

Bipolar I acute mixed or manic episodes: Oral:

Monotherapy: Initial: 10-15 mg once daily; increase by 5 mg/day at intervals of not less than 24 hours. Maintenance: 5-20 mg/day; recommended maximum dose: 20 mg/day

Combination therapy (with lithium or valproate): Initial: 10 mg once daily; dosing range: 5-20 mg/day

Agitation (acute, associated with bipolar I mania or schizophrenia): I.M.: Initial dose: 5-10 mg (a lower dose of 2.5 mg may be considered when clinical factors warrant); additional doses (2.5-10 mg) may be considered; however, 2-4 hours should be allowed between doses to evaluate response (maximum total daily dose: 30 mg, per manufacturer's recommendation)

Elderly: Oral, I.M.: Consider lower starting dose of 2.5-5 mg/day for elderly or debilitated patients; may increase as clinically indicated and tolerated with close monitoring of orthostatic blood pressure

Dosage adjustment in renal impairment: No adjustment required. Not removed by dialysis

Mechanism of Action Olanzapine is a thienobenzodiazepine antipsychotic which is a potent selective antagonist of serotonin 5-HT$_{2A}$ and 5-HT$_{2C}$, dopamine D$_{1-4}$, muscarinic M$_{1-5}$, histamine H$_1$- and alpha$_1$-adrenergic receptors. Olanzapine shows moderate antagonism of 5-HT$_3$ and muscarinic M$_{1-5}$ receptors, and weak binding to GABA-A, BZD, and beta-adrenergic receptors. Although the precise mechanism of action in schizophrenia and bipolar disorder is not known, the efficacy of olanzapine is thought to be mediated through combined antagonism of dopamine and serotonin type 2 receptor sites.

Contraindications Hypersensitivity to olanzapine or any component of the formulation

Warnings/Precautions Patients with dementia-related behavioral disorders treated with atypical antipsychotics are at an increased risk of cerebrovascular adverse events and death compared to placebo. Olanzapine is not approved for this indication.

Moderate to highly sedating, use with caution in disorders where CNS depression is a feature; patients must be cautioned about performing tasks which require mental alertness (eg, operating machinery or driving). Use with caution in Parkinson's disease; in patients with bone marrow suppression; predisposition to seizures; subcortical brain damage; severe hepatic, renal, or respiratory disease. Life-threatening arrhythmias have occurred some neuroleptics. May induce orthostatic hypotension; use caution with history of cardiovascular disease. Esophageal dysmotility and aspiration have been associated with antipsychotic use; use with caution in patients at risk of aspiration pneumonia. Caution in breast cancer or other prolactin-dependent tumors. Significant weight gain may occur. Impaired core body temperature regulation may occur; caution with strenuous exercise, heat exposure, dehydration, and concomitant medication possessing anticholinergic effects.

May cause anticholinergic effects; use with caution in patients with decreased gastrointestinal motility, urinary retention, BPH, xerostomia, glaucoma, or myasthenia gravis. Relative to other neuroleptics, olanzapine has a moderate potency of cholinergic blockade. May cause extrapyramidal symptoms, although risk of these reactions is lower relative to other neuroleptics). May be associated with neuroleptic malignant syndrome (NMS). May cause extreme and life-threatening hyperglycemia; use with caution in patients with diabetes or other disorders of glucose regulation; monitor. Olanzapine levels may be lower in patients who smoke, requiring dosage adjustment.

The possibility of a suicide attempt is inherent in psychotic illness or bipolar disorder; use caution in high-risk patients during initiation of therapy. Prescriptions should be written for the smallest quantity consistent with good patient care. Safety and efficacy in pediatric patients have not been established.

Drug Interactions

Cytochrome P450 Effect: Substrate of CYP1A2 (major), 2D6 (minor); Inhibits CYP1A2 (weak), 2C8/9 (weak), 2C19 (weak), 2D6 (weak), 3A4 (weak)

Increased Effect/Toxicity: Olanzapine levels may be increased by CYP1A2 inhibitors such as cimetidine and fluvoxamine. Sedation from olanzapine is increased with ethanol or other CNS depressants. Concomitant use with pramlintide and other anticholinergic agents may result in increased anticholinergic adverse effects. Concomitant use with ciprofloxacin may increase the levels/effects of olanzapine. Use of acetylcholinesterase inhibitors (central) or lithium may increase the risk of antipsychotic-related EPS.

Decreased Effect: Olanzapine levels may be decreased by CYP1A2 inducers such as rifampin, omeprazole, and carbamazepine (also cigarette smoking).

Ethanol/Nutrition/Herb Interactions

Ethanol: Avoid ethanol (may increase CNS depression).

Herb/Nutraceutical: Avoid dong quai, St John's wort (may also cause photosensitization). Avoid kava kava, gotu kola, valerian, St John's wort (may increase CNS depression).

Dietary Considerations Tablets may be taken with or without food/meals. Zyprexa® Zydis®: 5 mg tablet contains phenylalanine 0.34 mg; 10 mg tablet contains phenylalanine 0.45 mg; 15 mg tablet contains phenylalanine 0.67 mg; 20 mg tablet contains phenylalanine 0.9 mg

Pharmacodynamics/Kinetics

Absorption:

I.M.: Rapidly absorbed

Oral: Well absorbed; not affected by food; tablets and orally-disintegrating tablets are bioequivalent

Distribution: V_d: Extensive, 1000 L

Protein binding, plasma: 93% bound to albumin and alpha$_1$-glycoprotein

Metabolism: Highly metabolized via direct glucuronidation and cytochrome P450 mediated oxidation (CYP1A2, CYP2D6); 40% removed via first pass metabolism

Bioavailability: >57%

Half-life elimination: 21-54 hours; ~1.5 times greater in elderly

Time to peak, plasma: Maximum plasma concentrations after I.M. administration are 5 times higher than maximum plasma concentrations produced by an oral dose.

I.M.: 15-45 minutes

Oral: ~6 hours

Excretion: Urine (57%, 7% as unchanged drug); feces (30%); feces (30%)

Clearance: 40% increase in olanzapine clearance in smokers; 30% decrease in females

Pregnancy Risk Factor C

Dosage Forms INJ, powder for reconstitution (Zyprexa® IntraMuscular): 10 mg. **TAB** (Zyprexa®): 2.5 mg, 5 mg, 7.5 mg, 10 mg, 15 mg, 20 mg. **TAB, orally-disintegrating** (Zyprexa® Zydis®): 5 mg, 10 mg, 15 mg, 20 mg

---

Olanzapine and Fluoxetine (oh LAN za peen & floo OKS e teen)

Related Information

Fluoxetine *on page 675*

Olanzapine *on page 1139*

U.S. Brand Names Symbyax™

Generic Available No

Synonyms Fluoxetine and Olanzapine; Olanzapine and Fluoxetine Hydrochloride

Pharmacologic Category Antidepressant, Selective Serotonin Reuptake Inhibitor; Antipsychotic Agent, Atypical

Use Treatment of depressive episodes associated with bipolar disorder

Local Anesthetic/Vasoconstrictor Precautions No information available to require special precautions

Effects on Dental Treatment Key adverse event(s) related to dental treatment: Xerostomia or salivation increased (normal salivary flow resumes upon discontinuation), tooth disorder, and taste perversion.

Common Adverse Effects As reported with combination product (also see individual agents):

>10%:

Central nervous system: Somnolence (21% to 22%)

Gastrointestinal: Weight gain (17% to 21%), diarrhea (8% to 19%), appetite increased (13% to 16%), xerostomia (11% to 16%)

Neuromuscular & skeletal: Weakness (13% to 15%)

1% to 10%:

Cardiovascular: Peripheral edema (4% to 8%), edema (up to 5%), hypertension (2%), tachycardia (2%), vasodilation

Central nervous system: Thinking abnormal (6%), fever (3% to 4%), amnesia (1% to 3%), personality disorder (1% to 2%), sleep disorder (1% to 2%), speech disorder (up to 2%), chills, migraine

Dermatologic: Photosensitivity

Endocrine & metabolic: Ejaculation abnormal (2% to 7%), impotence (2% to 4%), libido decreased (2% to 4%), anorgasmia (1% to 3%), breast pain, menorrhagia

Gastrointestinal: Tooth disorder (1% to 2%), salivation increased, taste perversion, thirst, weight loss

Genitourinary: Urinary frequency, urinary incontinence, urinary tract infection

(Continued)

Olanzapine and Fluoxetine *(Continued)*

Neuromuscular & skeletal: Tremor (8% to 9%), twitching (2% to 6%), arthralgia (3% to 5%), hyperkinesias (1% to 2%), joint disorder (1% to 2%), bruising, neck pain/rigidity

Ocular: Amblyopia (4% to 5%), vision abnormal

Otic: Ear pain (1% to 2%), otitis media (up to 2%), tinnitus

Respiratory: Pharyngitis (4% to 6%), dyspnea (1% to 2%), bronchitis, lung disorder

Frequency not defined: Alkaline phosphate increased, cholesterol increased, GGT increased, hemoglobin decreased, prolactin increased, uric acid increased

Restrictions A medication guide concerning the use of antidepressants in children and teenagers can be found on the FDA website at http://www.fda.gov/cder/Offices/ODS/labeling.htm. It should be dispensed to parents or guardians of children and teenagers receiving this medication.

Mechanism of Action Olanzapine is a thienobenzodiazepine antipsychotic (neuroleptic) which is thought to work by antagonizing dopamine and serotonin activities. It is a selective monoaminergic antagonist with high affinity binding to serotonin 5-HT$_{2A}$ and 5-HT$_{2C}$, dopamine D$_{1-4}$, muscarinic M$_{1-5}$, histamine H$_1$- and alpha$_1$-adrenergic receptor sites. Olanzapine binds weakly to GABA-A, BZD, and beta-adrenergic receptors. Fluoxetine inhibits CNS neuron serotonin reuptake; minimal or no effect on reuptake of norepinephrine or dopamine; does not significantly bind to alpha-adrenergic, histamine, or cholinergic receptors. The enhanced antidepressant effect of the combination may be due to synergistic increases in serotonin, norepinephrine and dopamine.

Pharmacodynamics/Kinetics See individual agents.

Pregnancy Risk Factor C

Olanzapine and Fluoxetine Hydrochloride *see* Olanzapine and Fluoxetine *on page 1141*

Olay® Vitamins Complete Women's [OTC] *see* Vitamins (Multiple/Oral) *on page 1582*

Olay® Vitamins Complete Women's 50+[OTC] *see* Vitamins (Multiple/Oral) *on page 1582*

Olay® Vitamins Even Complexion [OTC] *see* Vitamins (Multiple/Oral) *on page 1582*

Oleovitamin A *see* Vitamin A *on page 1580*

Oleum Ricini *see* Castor Oil *on page 279*

Olmesartan *(ole me SAR tan)*

U.S. Brand Names Benicar®

Generic Available No

Synonyms Olmesartan Medoxomil

Pharmacologic Category Angiotensin II Receptor Blocker

Use Treatment of hypertension with or without concurrent use of other antihypertensive agents

Local Anesthetic/Vasoconstrictor Precautions No information available to require special precautions

Effects on Dental Treatment No significant effects or complications reported

Common Adverse Effects 1% to 10%:

Central nervous system: Dizziness (3%), headache

Endocrine & metabolic: Hyperglycemia, hypertriglyceridemia

Gastrointestinal: Diarrhea

Neuromuscular & skeletal: Back pain, CPK increased

Renal: Hematuria

Respiratory: Bronchitis, pharyngitis, rhinitis, sinusitis

Miscellaneous: Flu-like syndrome

Mechanism of Action As a selective and competitive, nonpeptide angiotensin II receptor antagonist, olmesartan blocks the vasoconstrictor and aldosterone-secreting effects of angiotensin II; olmesartan interacts reversibly at the AT1 and AT2 receptors of many tissues and has slow dissociation kinetics; its affinity for the AT1 receptor is 12,500 times greater than the AT2 receptor. Angiotensin II receptor antagonists may induce a more complete inhibition of the renin-angiotensin system than ACE inhibitors, they do not affect the response to bradykinin, and are less likely to be associated with nonrenin-angiotensin effects (eg, cough and angioedema). Olmesartan increases urinary flow rate and, in addition to being natriuretic and kaliuretic, increases excretion of chloride, magnesium, uric acid, calcium, and phosphate.

Drug Interactions
Increased Effect/Toxicity: The risk of hyperkalemia may be increased during concomitant use with potassium-sparing diuretics, potassium supplements, and trimethoprim; may increase risk of lithium toxicity.
Decreased Effect: NSAIDs may decrease the efficacy of olmesartan.
Pharmacodynamics/Kinetics
Distribution: 17 L; does not cross the blood-brain barrier (animal studies)
Protein binding: 99%
Metabolism: Olmesartan medoxomil is hydrolyzed in the GI tract to active olmesartan. No further metabolism occurs.
Bioavailability: 26%
Half-life elimination: Terminal: 13 hours
Time to peak: 1-2 hours
Excretion: All as unchanged drug: Feces (50% to 65%); urine (35% to 50%)
Pregnancy Risk Factor C/D (2nd and 3rd trimesters)

Olmesartan and Hydrochlorothiazide
(ole me SAR tan & hye droe klor oh THYE a zide)

Related Information
Hydrochlorothiazide *on page 776*
Olmesartan *on page 1142*
U.S. Brand Names Benicar HCT®
Generic Available No
Synonyms Hydrochlorothiazide and Olmesartan Medoxomil; Olmesartan Medoxomil and Hydrochlorothiazide
Pharmacologic Category Angiotensin II Receptor Blocker Combination; Antihypertensive Agent, Combination; Diuretic, Thiazide
Use Treatment of hypertension (not recommended for initial treatment)
Local Anesthetic/Vasoconstrictor Precautions No information available to require special precautions
Effects on Dental Treatment No significant effects or complications reported
Common Adverse Effects Frequencies reported with combination product. See individual monographs for additional adverse effects reported with each agent.
Cardiovascular: Chest pain, peripheral edema
Central nervous system: Dizziness (9%), vertigo
Dermatologic: Rash
Endocrine & metabolic: Hyperuricemia (4%), hyperglycemia
Gastrointestinal: Nausea (3%), abdominal pain, dyspepsia, gastroenteritis, diarrhea
Genitourinary: Hematuria
Hepatic: Transaminases increased
Neuromuscular & skeletal: Back pain, arthritis, arthralgia, myalgia
Respiratory: Upper respiratory infection (7%), cough
Miscellaneous: CPK increased

Angioedema and rhabdomyolysis have been reported with angiotensin-receptor blockers. Severe dermatologic reactions, hypokalemia, and pancreatitis have been reported with hydrochlorothiazide.
Mechanism of Action Olmesartan blocks the vasoconstrictor and aldosterone-secreting effects of angiotensin II. Hydrochlorothiazide inhibits sodium reabsorption in the distal tubules causing increased excretion of sodium and water as well as potassium and hydrogen ions.
Pharmacodynamics/Kinetics See individual agents.
Pregnancy Risk Factor C/D (2nd and 3rd trimesters)

Olmesartan Medoxomil *see Olmesartan on page 1142*

Olmesartan Medoxomil and Hydrochlorothiazide *see Olmesartan and Hydrochlorothiazide on page 1143*

Olopatadine (oh loe pa TA deen)

U.S. Brand Names Patanol®
Canadian Brand Names Patanol®
Generic Available No
Pharmacologic Category Antihistamine; Ophthalmic Agent, Miscellaneous
Use Treatment of the signs and symptoms of allergic conjunctivitis
Local Anesthetic/Vasoconstrictor Precautions No information available to require special precautions
Effects on Dental Treatment No significant effects or complications reported
Pregnancy Risk Factor C

Olsalazine (ole SAL a zeen)

U.S. Brand Names Dipentum®
Canadian Brand Names Dipentum®
Generic Available No
Synonyms Olsalazine Sodium
Pharmacologic Category 5-Aminosalicylic Acid Derivative
Use Maintenance of remission of ulcerative colitis in patients intolerant to sulfasalazine
Local Anesthetic/Vasoconstrictor Precautions No information available to require special precautions
Effects on Dental Treatment No significant effects or complications reported
Common Adverse Effects
>10%: Gastrointestinal: Diarrhea, cramps, abdominal pain
1% to 10%:
Central nervous system: Headache, fatigue, depression
Dermatologic: Rash, itching
Gastrointestinal: Nausea, heartburn, bloating, anorexia
Neuromuscular & skeletal: Arthralgia
Mechanism of Action The mechanism of action appears to be topical rather than systemic
Drug Interactions
Increased Effect/Toxicity: Olsalazine has been reported to increase the prothrombin time in patients taking warfarin. Olsalazine may increase the risk of myelosuppression with azathioprine, mesalamine, or sulfasalazine.
Pharmacodynamics/Kinetics
Absorption: <3%; very little intact olsalazine is systemically absorbed
Protein binding, plasma: >99%
Metabolism: Primarily via colonic bacteria to active drug, 5-aminosalicylic acid
Half-life elimination: 56 minutes
Time to peak: ~1 hour
Excretion: Primarily feces
Pregnancy Risk Factor C

Olsalazine Sodium *see* Olsalazine *on page 1144*
Olux® *see* Clobetasol *on page 365*

Omalizumab (oh mah lye ZOO mab)

U.S. Brand Names Xolair®
Canadian Brand Names Xolair®
Generic Available No
Synonyms rhuMAb-E25
Pharmacologic Category Monoclonal Antibody, Anti-Asthmatic
Use Treatment of moderate-to-severe, persistent allergic asthma not adequately controlled with inhaled corticosteroids
Local Anesthetic/Vasoconstrictor Precautions No information available to require special precautions
Effects on Dental Treatment No significant effects or complications reported
Common Adverse Effects
>10%:
Central nervous system: Headache (15%)
Local: Injection site reaction (45%; placebo 43%), severe injection site reactions (12%; placebo 9%). Most reactions occurred within 1 hour, lasted <8 days, and decreased in frequency with additional dosing.
Respiratory: Upper respiratory tract infection (23%), sinusitis (16%), pharyngitis (11%)
Miscellaneous: Viral infection (23%)
1% to 10%:
Central nervous system: Pain (7%), fatigue (3%), dizziness (3%)
Dermatologic: Dermatitis (2%), pruritus (2%)
Neuromuscular & skeletal: Arthralgia (8%), leg pain (4%), arm pain (2%), fracture (2%)
Otic: Earache (2%)
Mechanism of Action Omalizumab is an IgG monoclonal antibody (recombinant DNA-derived) which inhibits IgE binding to the high-affinity IgE receptor on mast cells and basophils. By decreasing bound IgE, the activation and release of mediators in the allergic response (early and late phase) is limited. Serum free IgE levels and the number of high-affinity IgE receptors are decreased.

Long-term treatment in patients with allergic asthma showed a decrease in asthma exacerbations and corticosteroid usage.

Pharmacodynamics/Kinetics
Absorption: Slow following SubQ injection
Distribution: V_d: 78 ± 32 mL/kg
Metabolism: Hepatic; IgG degradation by reticuloendothelial system and endothelial cells
Bioavailability: 62%
Half-life elimination: 26 days
Time to peak: 7-8 days
Excretion: Primarily via hepatic degradation; intact IgG may be secreted in bile

Pregnancy Risk Factor B

Omeprazole (oh ME pray zol)

Related Information
Esomeprazole *on page 572*
Gastrointestinal Disorders *on page 1654*

U.S. Brand Names Prilosec®; Prilosec OTC™ [OTC]

Canadian Brand Names Apo-Omeprazole®; Losec®; Losec MUPS®

Mexican Brand Names Alboz®; Aleprozil®; Inhibitron®; Losec®; Olexin®; Osiren®; Prazidec®; Prazolit®; Ulsen®

Generic Available Yes: Delayed release capsule

Pharmacologic Category Proton Pump Inhibitor; Substituted Benzimidazole

Use Short-term (4-8 weeks) treatment of active duodenal ulcer disease or active benign gastric ulcer; treatment of heartburn and other symptoms associated with gastroesophageal reflux disease (GERD); short-term (4-8 weeks) treatment of endoscopically-diagnosed erosive esophagitis; maintenance healing of erosive esophagitis; long-term treatment of pathological hypersecretory conditions; as part of a multidrug regimen for *H. pylori* eradication to reduce the risk of duodenal ulcer recurrence

OTC labeling: Short-term treatment of frequent, uncomplicated heartburn occurring ≥2 days/week

Unlabeled/Investigational Use Healing NSAID-induced ulcers; prevention of NSAID-induced ulcers

Local Anesthetic/Vasoconstrictor Precautions No information available to require special precautions

Effects on Dental Treatment Key adverse event(s) related to dental treatment: Taste perversion, dry mouth, esophageal candidiasis, and mucosal atrophy (tongue).

Common Adverse Effects 1% to 10%:
Central nervous system: Headache (3% to 7%), dizziness (2%)
Dermatologic: Rash (2%)
Gastrointestinal: Diarrhea (3% to 4%), abdominal pain (2% to 5%), nausea (2% to 4%), vomiting (2% to 3%), flatulence (3%), acid regurgitation (2%), constipation (1% to 2%), taste perversion
Neuromuscular & skeletal: Weakness (1%), back pain (1%)
Respiratory: Upper respiratory infection (2%), cough (1%)

Dosage Oral:
Children ≥2 years: GERD or other acid-related disorders:
<20 kg: 10 mg once daily
≥20 kg: 20 mg once daily
Adults:
Active duodenal ulcer: 20 mg/day for 4-8 weeks
Gastric ulcers: 40 mg/day for 4-8 weeks
Symptomatic GERD: 20 mg/day for up to 4 weeks
Erosive esophagitis: 20 mg/day for 4-8 weeks; maintenance of healing: 20 mg/day for up to 12 months total therapy (including treatment period of 4-8 weeks)
Helicobacter pylori eradication: Dose varies with regimen: 20 mg once daily **or** 40 mg/day as single dose or in 2 divided doses; requires combination therapy with antibiotics
Pathological hypersecretory conditions: Initial: 60 mg once daily; doses up to 120 mg 3 times/day have been administered; administer daily doses >80 mg in divided doses
Frequent heartburn (OTC labeling): 20 mg/day for 14 days; treatment may be repeated after 4 months if needed
Dosage adjustment in hepatic impairment: Specific guidelines are not available; bioavailability is increased with chronic liver disease

Mechanism of Action Suppresses gastric basal and stimulated acid secretion by inhibiting the parietal cell H+/K+ ATP pump
(Continued)

Omeprazole *(Continued)*

Contraindications Hypersensitivity to omeprazole, substituted benzimidazoles (ie, esomeprazole, lansoprazole, pantoprazole, rabeprazole), or any component of the formulation

Warnings/Precautions In long-term (2-year) studies in rats, omeprazole produced a dose-related increase in gastric carcinoid tumors. While available endoscopic evaluations and histologic examinations of biopsy specimens from human stomachs have not detected a risk from short-term exposure to omeprazole, further human data on the effect of sustained hypochlorhydria and hypergastrinemia are needed to rule out the possibility of an increased risk for the development of tumors in humans receiving long-term therapy. Bioavailability may be increased in the elderly, Asian population, and with hepatic dysfunction. Safety and efficacy have not been established in children <2 years of age. When used for self-medication (OTC), do not use for >14 days; treatment should not be repeated more often than every 4 months; OTC and oral suspension are not approved for use in children <18 years of age.

Drug Interactions

Cytochrome P450 Effect: Substrate of CYP2A6 (minor), 2C9 (minor), 2C19 (major), 2D6 (minor), 3A4 (minor); **Inhibits** CYP1A2 (weak), 2C9 (moderate), 2C19 (strong), 2D6 (weak), 3A4 (weak); **Induces** CYP1A2 (weak)

Increased Effect/Toxicity: Esomeprazole and omeprazole may increase the levels of benzodiazepines metabolized by oxidation (eg, diazepam, midazolam, triazolam), methotrexate, and carbamazepine. Elimination of phenytoin or warfarin may be prolonged when used concomitantly with omeprazole. Omeprazole may increase the levels/effects of amiodarone, citalopram, diazepam, fluoxetine, glimepiride, glipizide, methsuximide, nateglinide, phenytoin, pioglitazone, propranolol, rosiglitazone, sertraline, warfarin, and other CYP2C9 or 2C19 substrates. Omeprazole may alter the concentrations/effects of clozapine.

Decreased Effect: Proton pump inhibitors may decrease the absorption of atazanavir, indinavir, itraconazole, and ketoconazole; avoid concurrent use. The levels/effects of omeprazole may be decreased by aminoglutethimide, carbamazepine, phenytoin, rifampin, and other CYP2C19 inducers. Omeprazole may alter the concentrations/effects of clozapine.

Ethanol/Nutrition/Herb Interactions

Ethanol: Avoid ethanol (may cause gastric mucosal irritation).

Food: Food delays absorption.

Herb/Nutraceutical: St John's wort may decrease omeprazole levels.

Dietary Considerations Should be taken on an empty stomach; best if taken before breakfast.

Pharmacodynamics/Kinetics

Onset of action: Antisecretory: ~1 hour

Peak effect: 2 hours

Duration: 72 hours

Protein binding: 95%

Metabolism: Extensively hepatic to inactive metabolites

Bioavailability: Oral: 30% to 40%; increased in Asian patients and patients with hepatic dysfunction

Half-life elimination: Delayed release capsule: 0.5-1 hour

Excretion: Urine (77% as metabolites, very small amount as unchanged drug); feces

Pregnancy Risk Factor C

Dosage Forms CAP, delayed release: 10 mg, 20 mg; (Prilosec®): 10 mg, 20 mg, 40 mg. **TAB, delayed release** (Prilosec OTC™): 20 mg

Omeprazole and Sodium Bicarbonate

(oh ME pray zol & SOW dee um bye KAR bun ate)

U.S. Brand Names Zegerid®

Generic Available No

Pharmacologic Category Proton Pump Inhibitor; Substituted Benzimidazole

Use Short-term (4-8 weeks) treatment of active duodenal ulcer disease or active benign gastric ulcer; treatment of heartburn and other symptoms associated with gastroesophageal reflux disease (GERD); short-term (4-8 weeks) treatment of endoscopically-diagnosed erosive esophagitis; maintenance healing of erosive esophagitis; reduction of risk of upper gastrointestinal bleeding in critically-ill patients

Local Anesthetic/Vasoconstrictor Precautions No information available to require special precautions

Effects on Dental Treatment Key adverse event(s) related to dental treatment: Oral candidiasis.

Common Adverse Effects

Frequency of adverse events reported for 40 mg dose of oral powder for suspension.

>10%:

Central nervous system: Pyrexia (20%)

Endocrine & metabolic: Hypokalemia (12%), hyperglycemia (11%)

Respiratory: Nosocomial pneumonia (11%)

1% to 10%:

Cardiovascular: Hypotension (10%), hypertension (8%), atrial fibrillation (6%), ventricular tachycardia (5%), bradycardia (4%), tachycardia (3%), supraventricular tachycardia (3%), edema (3%)

Central nervous system: Hyperpyrexia (5%), agitation (3%)

Dermatological: Rash (6%), decubitus ulcer (3%)

Endocrine & metabolic: Hypomagnesemia (10%), hypocalcemia (6%), hypophosphatemia (6%), fluid overload (5%), hypoglycemia (3%), hyponatremia (4%), hypernatremia (2%), hyperkalemia (2%)

Gastrointestinal: Constipation (5%), diarrhea (4%), hypomotility (2%)

Genitourinary: Urinary tract infection (2%)

Hematological: Thrombocytopenia (10%), anemia (8%), anemia increased (2%)

Hepatic: LFTs increased (2%)

Respiratory: ARDS (3%), respiratory failure (2%)

Miscellaneous: Sepsis (5%), oral candidiasis (4%), candidal infection (2%)

Mechanism of Action Suppresses gastric basal and stimulated acid secretion by inhibiting the parietal cell H+/K+ ATP pump

Drug Interactions

Cytochrome P450 Effect: Substrate of CYP2A6 (minor), 2C9 (minor), 2C19 (major), 2D6 (minor), 3A4 (minor); **Inhibits** CYP1A2 (weak), 2C9 (moderate), 2C19 (strong), 2D6 (weak), 3A4 (weak); **Induces** CYP1A2 (weak)

Increased Effect/Toxicity: Esomeprazole and omeprazole may increase the levels of benzodiazepines metabolized by oxidation (eg, diazepam, midazolam, triazolam), methotrexate, and carbamazepine. Elimination of phenytoin or warfarin may be prolonged when used concomitantly with omeprazole. Omeprazole may increase the levels/effects of amiodarone, citalopram, diazepam, fluoxetine, glimepiride, glipizide, methsuximide, nateglinide, phenytoin, pioglitazone, propranolol, rosiglitazone, sertraline, warfarin, and other CYP2C9 or 2C19 substrates. Omeprazole may alter the concentrations/effects of clozapine.

Decreased Effect: Proton pump inhibitors may decrease the absorption of atazanavir, indinavir, itraconazole, and ketoconazole. The levels/effects of omeprazole may be decreased by aminoglutethimide, carbamazepine, phenytoin, rifampin, and other CYP2C19 inducers. Omeprazole may alter the concentrations/effects of clozapine.

Pharmacodynamics/Kinetics

Onset of action: Antisecretory: ~1 hour

Peak effect: 2 hours

Duration: 72 hours

Protein binding: 95%

Metabolism: Extensively hepatic to inactive metabolites

Bioavailability: Oral: 30% to 40%; increased in Asian patients and patients with hepatic dysfunction

Half-life elimination: 0.4-3.2 hours

Excretion: Urine (77% as metabolites, very small amount as unchanged drug); feces

Pregnancy Risk Factor C

Omnicef® see Cefdinir on page 284

Omnii Gel™ [OTC] see Fluoride on page 671

Omnipaque™ see Iohexol on page 854

Oncaspar® see Pegaspargase on page 1194

Ondansetron (on DAN se tron)

U.S. Brand Names Zofran®; Zofran® ODT

Canadian Brand Names Zofran®; Zofran® ODT

Mexican Brand Names Zofran®

Generic Available No

Synonyms GR38032R; Ondansetron Hydrochloride

Pharmacologic Category Antiemetic; Selective 5-HT₃ Receptor Antagonist

Use Prevention of nausea and vomiting associated with moderately- to highly-emetogenic cancer chemotherapy [not recommended for treatment of **existing** chemotherapy-induced emesis (CIE)]; radiotherapy in patients

(Continued)

Ondansetron *(Continued)*

receiving total body irradiation or fractions to the abdomen; prevention of post-operative nausea and vomiting (PONV); treatment of PONV if no prophylactic dose received

Unlabeled/Investigational Use Treatment of early-onset alcoholism; hyperemesis gravidarum

Local Anesthetic/Vasoconstrictor Precautions No information available to require special precautions

Effects on Dental Treatment Key adverse event(s) related to dental treatment: Xerostomia (normal salivary flow resumes upon discontinuation).

Common Adverse Effects

Note: Percentages reported in adult patients.

>10%:

Central nervous system: Headache (9% to 27%), malaise/fatigue (9% to 13%)

Gastrointestinal: Constipation (6% to 11%)

1% to 10%:

Central nervous system: Drowsiness (8%), fever (2% to 8%), dizziness (4% to 7%), anxiety (6%), cold sensation (2%)

Dermatologic: Pruritus (2% to 5%), rash (1%)

Gastrointestinal: Diarrhea (2% to 7%)

Genitourinary: Gynecological disorder (7%), urinary retention (5%)

Hepatic: ALT/AST increased (1% to 5%)

Local: Injection site reaction (4%; pain, redness, burning)

Neuromuscular & skeletal: Paresthesia (2%)

Respiratory: Hypoxia (9%)

Mechanism of Action Selective 5-HT$_3$-receptor antagonist, blocking serotonin, both peripherally on vagal nerve terminals and centrally in the chemoreceptor trigger zone

Drug Interactions

Cytochrome P450 Effect: Substrate of CYP1A2 (minor), 2C8/9 (minor), 2D6 (minor), 2E1 (minor), 3A4 (major); **Inhibits** CYP1A2 (weak), 2C8/9 (weak), 2D6 (weak)

Increased Effect/Toxicity: Ondansetron may enhance the hypotensive effect of apomorphine; concurrent use is contraindicated.

Decreased Effect: CYP3A4 inducers may decrease the levels/effects of ondansetron; example inducers include aminoglutethimide, carbamazepine, nafcillin, nevirapine, phenobarbital, phenytoin, and rifamycins. The manufacturer does not recommend dosage adjustment in patients receiving CYP3A4 inducers.

Pharmacodynamics/Kinetics

Onset of action: ~30 minutes

Distribution: V$_d$: Children: 1.7-3.7 L/kg; Adults: 2.2-2.5 L/kg

Protein binding, plasma: 70% to 76%

Metabolism: Extensively hepatic via hydroxylation, followed by glucuronide or sulfate conjugation; CYP1A2, CYP2D6, and CYP3A4 substrate; some demethylation occurs

Bioavailability: Oral: 56% to 71%; Rectal: 58% to 74%

Half-life elimination: Children <15 years: 2-7 hours; Adults: 3-6 hours

Mild-to-moderate hepatic impairment: Adults: 12 hours

Severe hepatic impairment (Child-Pugh C): Adults: 20 hours

Time to peak: Oral: ~2 hours

Excretion: Urine (44% to 60% as metabolites, 5% to 10% as unchanged drug); feces (~25%)

Pregnancy Risk Factor B

Ondansetron Hydrochloride *see* Ondansetron *on page 1147*

One-A-Day® 50 Plus Formula [OTC] *see* Vitamins (Multiple/Oral) *on page 1582*

One-A-Day® Active Formula [OTC] *see* Vitamins (Multiple/Oral) *on page 1582*

One-A-Day® Carb Smart [OTC] *see* Vitamins (Multiple/Oral) *on page 1582*

One-A-Day® Cholesterol Plus™ [OTC] *see* Vitamins (Multiple/Oral) *on page 1582*

One-A-Day® Essential Formula [OTC] *see* Vitamins (Multiple/Oral) *on page 1582*

One-A-Day® Maximum Formula [OTC] *see* Vitamins (Multiple/Oral) *on page 1582*

One-A-Day® Men's Formula [OTC] *see* Vitamins (Multiple/Oral) *on page 1582*

One-A-Day® Today [OTC] *see* Vitamins (Multiple/Oral) *on page 1582*

One-A-Day® Weight Smart [OTC *see* Vitamins (Multiple/Oral) *on page 1582*

One-A-Day® Women's Formula [OTC] *see* Vitamins (Multiple/Oral) *on page 1582*

ONTAK® *see* Denileukin Diftitox *on page 432*

Onxol™ see Paclitaxel on page 1176

Ony-Clear [OTC] [DSC] see Benzalkonium Chloride on page 188

OPC-13013 see Cilostazol on page 340

OPC-14597 see Aripiprazole on page 138

OP-CCK see Sincalide on page 1396

Opcon-A® [OTC] see Naphazoline and Pheniramine on page 1088

Operand® [OTC] see Povidone-Iodine on page 1262

Operand® Chlorhexidine Gluconate [OTC] see Chlorhexidine Gluconate on page 316

Ophthetic® see Proparacaine on page 1296

Opium and Belladonna see Belladonna and Opium on page 184

Opium Tincture (OH pee um TING chur)

Generic Available Yes

Synonyms DTO (error-prone abbreviation); Opium Tincture, Deodorized

Pharmacologic Category Analgesic, Narcotic; Antidiarrheal

Use Treatment of diarrhea or relief of pain

Local Anesthetic/Vasoconstrictor Precautions No information available to require special precautions

Effects on Dental Treatment No significant effects or complications reported

Mechanism of Action Contains many narcotic alkaloids including morphine; its mechanism for gastric motility inhibition is primarily due to this morphine content; it results in a decrease in digestive secretions, an increase in GI muscle tone, and therefore a reduction in GI propulsion

Pregnancy Risk Factor B/D (prolonged use or high doses at term)

Opium Tincture, Deodorized see Opium Tincture on page 1149

Oprelvekin (oh PREL ve kin)

U.S. Brand Names Neumega®

Generic Available No

Synonyms IL-11; Interleukin-11; Recombinant Human Interleukin-11; Recombinant Interleukin-11; rhIL-11; rIL-11

Pharmacologic Category Biological Response Modulator; Human Growth Factor

Use Prevention of severe thrombocytopenia and the reduction of the need for platelet transfusions following myelosuppressive chemotherapy

Local Anesthetic/Vasoconstrictor Precautions No information available to require special precautions

Effects on Dental Treatment No significant effects or complications reported

Common Adverse Effects

>10%:

Cardiovascular: Tachycardia (19% to 30%), palpitation (14% to 24%), atrial arrhythmia (12%), peripheral edema (60% to 75%), syncope (6% to 13%)

Central nervous system: Headache (41%), dizziness (38%), insomnia (33%), fatigue (30%), fever (36%)

Dermatologic: Rash (25%)

Endocrine & metabolic: Fluid retention

Gastrointestinal: Nausea (50% to 77%), vomiting, anorexia

Hematologic: Anemia (100%), probably a dilutional phenomena; appears within 3 days of initiation of therapy, resolves in about 1 week after cessation of oprelvekin

Neuromuscular & skeletal: Arthralgia, myalgia

Ocular: Papilledema (children 16%, adults 1%)

Respiratory: Dyspnea (48%), pleural effusion (10%)

1% to 10%: Gastrointestinal: Weight gain (5%)

Mechanism of Action Oprelvekin stimulates multiple stages of megakaryocytopoiesis and thrombopoiesis, resulting in proliferation of megakaryocyte progenitors and megakaryocyte maturation

Drug Interactions

Increased Effect/Toxicity: Oprelvekin may increase the risk of hypokalemia in patients receiving chronic diuretic therapy.

Pharmacodynamics/Kinetics

Metabolism: Uncertain

Half-life elimination: Terminal: 5-8 hours

Time to peak, serum: 1-6 hours

Excretion: Urine (primarily as metabolites)

Pregnancy Risk Factor C

Opticrom® *see* Cromolyn *on page 397*

Optigene® 3 [OTC] *see* Tetrahydrozoline *on page 1470*

OptiPranolol® *see* Metipranolol *on page 1028*

Optiray® *see* Ioversol *on page 856*

Optivar® *see* Azelastine *on page 170*

Optivite® P.M.T. [OTC] *see* Vitamins (Multiple/Oral) *on page 1582*

o,p'-DDD *see* Mitotane *on page 1055*

Orabase® with Benzocaine [OTC] *see* Benzocaine *on page 190*

Oracit® *see* Sodium Citrate and Citric Acid *on page 1401*

Orajel® Baby Daytime and Nighttime [OTC] *see* Benzocaine *on page 190*

Orajel® Baby Teething [OTC] *see* Benzocaine *on page 190*

Orajel® Baby Teething Nighttime [OTC] *see* Benzocaine *on page 190*

Orajel® Denture Plus [OTC] *see* Benzocaine *on page 190*

Orajel® Maximum Strength [OTC] *see* Benzocaine *on page 190*

Orajel® Medicated Toothache [OTC] *see* Benzocaine *on page 190*

Orajel® Mouth Sore [OTC] *see* Benzocaine *on page 190*

Orajel® Multi-Action Cold Sore [OTC] *see* Benzocaine *on page 190*

Orajel® Perioseptic® Spot Treatment [OTC] *see* Carbamide Peroxide *on page 264*

Orajel PM® [OTC] *see* Benzocaine *on page 190*

Orajel® Ultra Mouth Sore [OTC] *see* Benzocaine *on page 190*

Oramorph SR® *see* Morphine Sulfate *on page 1065*

Oranyl [OTC] *see* Pseudoephedrine *on page 1309*

Orap® *see* Pimozide *on page 1238*

Orapred® *see* PrednisoLONE *on page 1268*

Oraquix® *see* Lidocaine and Prilocaine *on page 928*

OraRinse™ [OTC] *see* Maltodextrin *on page 963*

Orazinc® [OTC] *see* Zinc Sulfate *on page 1598*

Orciprenaline Sulfate *see* Metaproterenol *on page 1000*

Orencia® *see* Abatacept *on page 25*

Orfadin® *see* Nitisinone *on page 1118*

Organ-1 NR *see* Guaifenesin *on page 752*

Organidin® NR *see* Guaifenesin *on page 752*

Orlistat (OR li stat)

U.S. Brand Names Xenical®
Canadian Brand Names Xenical®
Mexican Brand Names Xenical®
Generic Available No
Pharmacologic Category Lipase Inhibitor
Use Management of obesity, including weight loss and weight management when used in conjunction with a reduced-calorie diet; reduce the risk of weight regain after prior weight loss; indicated for obese patients with an initial body mass index (BMI) ≥ 30 kg/m^2 or ≥ 27 kg/m^2 in the presence of other risk factors

Local Anesthetic/Vasoconstrictor Precautions No information available to require special precautions

Effects on Dental Treatment No significant effects or complications reported

Common Adverse Effects
>10%:
  Central nervous system: Headache (31%)
  Gastrointestinal: Oily spotting (27%), abdominal pain/discomfort (26%), flatus with discharge (24%), fatty/oily stool (20%), fecal urgency (22%), oily evacuation (12%), increased defecation (11%)
  Neuromuscular & skeletal: Back pain (14%)
  Respiratory: Upper respiratory infection (38%)
1% to 10%:
  Central nervous system: Fatigue (7%), anxiety (5%), sleep disorder (4%)
  Dermatologic: Dry skin (2%)
  Endocrine & metabolic: Menstrual irregularities (10%)
  Gastrointestinal: Fecal incontinence (8%), nausea (8%), infectious diarrhea (5%), rectal pain/discomfort (5%), vomiting (4%)
  Neuromuscular & skeletal: Arthritis (5%), myalgia (4%)
  Otic: Otitis (4%)
Mechanism of Action A reversible inhibitor of gastric and pancreatic lipases thus inhibiting absorption of dietary fats by 30% (at doses of 120 mg 3 times/day).

Drug Interactions

Decreased Effect: Orlistat may decrease amiodarone absorption (monitor). Coadministration with cyclosporine may decrease plasma levels of cyclosporine (administer cyclosporine 2 hours before or after orlistat and monitor). Orlistat does not alter the pharmacokinetics of warfarin, however, vitamin K absorption may be decreased during orlistat therapy (patients stabilized on warfarin should be monitored for changes in warfarin effects).

Pharmacodynamics/Kinetics

Absorption: Minimal

Metabolism: Metabolized within the gastrointestinal wall; forms inactive metabolites

Excretion: Feces (83% as unchanged drug)

Pregnancy Risk Factor B

Ornex® [OTC] *see* Acetaminophen and Pseudoephedrine *on page 38*

Ornex® Maximum Strength [OTC] *see* Acetaminophen and Pseudoephedrine *on page 38*

Orphenadrine (or FEN a dreen)

Related Information

Temporomandibular Dysfunction (TMD) *on page 1724*

U.S. Brand Names Norflex™

Canadian Brand Names Norflex™; Orphenace®; Rhoxal-orphenadrine

Generic Available Yes

Synonyms Orphenadrine Citrate

Pharmacologic Category Anti-Parkinson's Agent, Anticholinergic; Skeletal Muscle Relaxant

Use Treatment of muscle spasm associated with acute painful musculoskeletal conditions; supportive therapy in tetanus

Local Anesthetic/Vasoconstrictor Precautions No information available to require special precautions

Effects on Dental Treatment The peripheral anticholinergic effects of orphenadrine may decrease or inhibit salivary flow; normal salivation will return with cessation of drug therapy.

Common Adverse Effects

>10%:

Central nervous system: Drowsiness, dizziness

Ocular: Blurred vision

1% to 10%:

Cardiovascular: Flushing of face, tachycardia, syncope

Dermatologic: Rash

Gastrointestinal: Nausea, vomiting, constipation

Genitourinary: Decreased urination

Neuromuscular & skeletal: Weakness

Ocular: Nystagmus, increased intraocular pressure

Respiratory: Nasal congestion

Dosage Adults:

Oral: 100 mg twice daily

I.M., I.V.: 60 mg every 12 hours

Mechanism of Action Indirect skeletal muscle relaxant thought to work by central atropine-like effects; has some euphorigenic and analgesic properties

Contraindications Hypersensitivity to orphenadrine or any component of the formulation; glaucoma; GI obstruction; cardiospasm; myasthenia gravis

Warnings/Precautions Use with caution in patients with CHF or cardiac arrhythmias; some products contain sulfites

Drug Interactions

Cytochrome P450 Effect: Substrate (minor) of CYP1A2, 2B6, 2D6, 3A4; Inhibits CYP1A2 (weak), 2A6 (weak), 2B6 (weak), 2C9 (weak), 2C19 (weak), 2D6 (weak), 2E1 (weak), 3A4 (weak)

Increased Effect/Toxicity: Orphenadrine may increase potential for anticholinergic adverse effects of anticholinergic agents; includes drugs with high anticholinergic activity (diphenhydramine, TCAs, phenothiazines). Sedative effects of may be additive in concurrent use of orphenadrine and CNS depressants (monitor). Effects of levodopa may be decreased by orphenadrine. Monitor.

Ethanol/Nutrition/Herb Interactions

Ethanol: Avoid ethanol (may increase CNS depression).

Herb/Nutraceutical: St John's wort may decrease orphenadrine levels. Avoid valerian, St John's wort, kava kava, gotu kola (may increase CNS depression).

(Continued)

Orphenadrine (Continued)

Pharmacodynamics/Kinetics
Onset of effect: Peak effect: Oral: 2-4 hours
Duration: 4-6 hours
Protein binding: 20%
Metabolism: Extensively hepatic
Half-life elimination: 14-16 hours
Excretion: Primarily urine (8% as unchanged drug)

Pregnancy Risk Factor C

Dosage Forms INJ, solution: 30 mg/mL (2 mL). **TAB, extended release:** 100 mg

Orphenadrine, Aspirin, and Caffeine
(or FEN a dreen, AS pir in, & KAF een)

Related Information
Aspirin *on page 145*
Caffeine *on page 245*
Orphenadrine *on page 1151*

U.S. Brand Names Norgesic™ [DSC]; Norgesic™ Forte [DSC]; Orphengesic [DSC]; Orphengesic Forte [DSC]

Canadian Brand Names Norgesic™; Norgesic™ Forte

Generic Available Yes

Synonyms Aspirin, Orphenadrine, and Caffeine; Caffeine, Orphenadrine, and Aspirin

Pharmacologic Category Skeletal Muscle Relaxant

Use Relief of discomfort associated with skeletal muscular conditions

Local Anesthetic/Vasoconstrictor Precautions No information available to require special precautions

Effects on Dental Treatment The peripheral anticholinergic effects of orphenadrine may decrease or inhibit salivary flow; normal salivation will return with cessation of drug therapy.

Drug Interactions
Cytochrome P450 Effect:
Orphenadrine: **Substrate** (minor) of CYP1A2, 2B6, 2D6, 3A4; **Inhibits** CYP1A2 (weak), 2A6 (weak), 2B6 (weak), 2C9 (weak), 2C19 (weak), 2D6 (weak), 2E1 (weak), 3A4 (weak)
Aspirin: **Substrate** of CYP2C9 (minor)
Caffeine: **Substrate** of CYP1A2 (major), 2C9 (minor), 2D6 (minor), 2E1 (minor), 3A4 (minor); **Inhibits** CYP1A2 (weak), 3A4 (moderate)

Pharmacodynamics/Kinetics See individual agents.

Pregnancy Risk Factor D

Orphenadrine Citrate *see* Orphenadrine *on page 1151*
Orphengesic [DSC] *see* Orphenadrine, Aspirin, and Caffeine *on page 1152*
Orphengesic Forte [DSC] *see* Orphenadrine, Aspirin, and Caffeine *on page 1152*
Ortho-Cept® *see* Ethinyl Estradiol and Desogestrel *on page 592*
Orthoclone OKT® 3 *see* Muromonab-CD3 *on page 1074*
Ortho-Cyclen® *see* Ethinyl Estradiol and Norgestimate *on page 613*
Ortho-Est® *see* Estropipate *on page 586*
Ortho Evra® *see* Ethinyl Estradiol and Norelgestromin *on page 605*
Ortho-Novum® *see* Ethinyl Estradiol and Norethindrone *on page 608*
Ortho-Novum® 1/50 *see* Mestranol and Norethindrone *on page 999*
Ortho Prefest *see* Estradiol and Norgestimate *on page 576*
Ortho Tri-Cyclen® *see* Ethinyl Estradiol and Norgestimate *on page 613*
Ortho Tri-Cyclen® Lo *see* Ethinyl Estradiol and Norgestimate *on page 613*
Orthovisc® *see* Hyaluronate and Derivatives *on page 773*
Orudis® KT [OTC] [DSC] *see* Ketoprofen *on page 883*
Orvaten™ *see* Midodrine *on page 1044*
Os-Cal® 500 [OTC] *see* Calcium Carbonate *on page 248*

Oseltamivir (oh sel TAM i vir)

Related Information
Systemic Viral Diseases *on page 1675*

U.S. Brand Names Tamiflu®

Canadian Brand Names Tamiflu®

Generic Available No

Pharmacologic Category Antiviral Agent; Neuraminidase Inhibitor

Use Treatment of uncomplicated acute illness due to influenza (A or B) infection in children ≥1 year of age and adults who have been symptomatic for no more than 2 days; prophylaxis against influenza (A or B) infection in children ≥1 year of age and adults

Local Anesthetic/Vasoconstrictor Precautions No information available to require special precautions

Effects on Dental Treatment No significant effects or complications reported

Common Adverse Effects

>10%: Gastrointestinal: Vomiting (2% to 15%)

1% to 10%: Gastrointestinal: Nausea (3% to 10%), abdominal pain (2% to 5%)

Mechanism of Action Oseltamivir, a prodrug, is hydrolyzed to the active form, oseltamivir carboxylate. It is thought to inhibit influenza virus neuraminidase, with the possibility of alteration of virus particle aggregation and release.

Drug Interactions

Decreased Effect: Influenza virus vaccine nasal spray (fluMist™): Safety and efficacy for use with influenza virus vaccine nasal spray have not been established. Do not administer nasal spray until 48 hours after stopping antiviral; do not administer antiviral for 2 weeks after receiving influenza virus vaccine nasal spray.

Pharmacodynamics/Kinetics

Absorption: Well absorbed

Distribution: V_d: 23-26 L (oseltamivir carboxylate)

Protein binding, plasma: Oseltamivir carboxylate: 3%; Oseltamivir: 42%

Metabolism: Hepatic (90%) to oseltamivir carboxylate; neither the parent drug nor active metabolite has any effect on CYP

Bioavailability: 75% as oseltamivir carboxylate

Half-life elimination: Oseltamivir: 1-3 hours; Oseltamivir carboxylate: 6-10 hours

Excretion: Urine (>90% as oseltamivir carboxylate); feces

Pregnancy Risk Factor C

OSI-774 *see* Erlotinib *on page 560*

Osmoglyn® [DSC] *see* Glycerin *on page 747*

OsmoPrep™ *see* Sodium Phosphates *on page 1403*

Oticaine *see* Benzocaine *on page 190*

Otocaine™ *see* Benzocaine *on page 190*

Otrivin® [OTC] [DSC] *see* Xylometazoline *on page 1588*

Otrivin® Pediatric [OTC] [DSC] *see* Xylometazoline *on page 1588*

Outgro® [OTC] *see* Benzocaine *on page 190*

Ovace™ *see* Sulfacetamide *on page 1423*

Ovcon® *see* Ethinyl Estradiol and Norethindrone *on page 608*

Ovidrel® *see* Chorionic Gonadotropin (Recombinant) *on page 337*

Ovrette® [DSC] *see* Norgestrel *on page 1127*

Oxacillin (oks a SIL in)

Generic Available Yes

Synonyms Methylphenyl Isoxazolyl Penicillin; Oxacillin Sodium

Pharmacologic Category Antibiotic, Penicillin

Use Treatment of infections such as osteomyelitis, septicemia, endocarditis, and CNS infections caused by susceptible strains of *Staphylococcus*

Local Anesthetic/Vasoconstrictor Precautions No information available to require special precautions

Effects on Dental Treatment Key adverse event(s) related to dental treatment: Prolonged use of penicillins may lead to development of oral candidiasis.

Common Adverse Effects Frequency not defined.

Central nervous system: Fever

Dermatologic: Rash

Gastrointestinal: Nausea, diarrhea, vomiting

Hematologic: Eosinophilia, leukopenia, neutropenia, thrombocytopenia, agranulocytosis

Hepatic: Hepatotoxicity, AST increased

Renal: Acute interstitial nephritis, hematuria

Miscellaneous: Serum sickness-like reactions

Mechanism of Action Inhibits bacterial cell wall synthesis by binding to one or more of the penicillin binding proteins (PBPs); which in turn inhibits the final transpeptidation step of peptidoglycan synthesis in bacterial cell walls, thus inhibiting cell wall biosynthesis. Bacteria eventually lyse due to ongoing activity of cell wall autolytic enzymes (autolysins and murein hydrolases) while cell wall assembly is arrested.

(Continued)

Oxacillin *(Continued)*

Drug Interactions

Increased Effect/Toxicity: Probenecid increases penicillin levels. Penicillins and anticoagulants may increase the effect of anticoagulants. Penicillins may increase the exposure to methotrexate during concurrent therapy; monitor.

Decreased Effect: Although anecdotal reports suggest oral contraceptive efficacy could be reduced by penicillins, this has been refuted by more rigorous scientific and clinical data.

Pharmacodynamics/Kinetics

Distribution: Into bile, synovial and pleural fluids, bronchial secretions, peritoneal, and pericardial fluids; crosses placenta; enters breast milk; penetrates the blood-brain barrier only when meninges are inflamed

Protein binding: ~94%

Metabolism: Hepatic to active metabolites

Half-life elimination: Children 1 week to 2 years: 0.9-1.8 hours; Adults: 23-60 minutes; prolonged in neonates and with renal impairment

Time to peak, serum: I.M.: 30-60 minutes

Excretion: Urine and feces (small amounts as unchanged drug and metabolites)

Pregnancy Risk Factor B

Oxacillin Sodium *see* Oxacillin *on page 1153*

Oxaliplatin *(ox AL i pla tin)*

U.S. Brand Names Eloxatin™

Generic Available No

Synonyms Diaminocyclohexane Oxalatoplatinum; L-OHP; NSC-266046

Pharmacologic Category Antineoplastic Agent, Alkylating Agent

Use Treatment of advanced colon cancer and advanced rectal carcinoma

Unlabeled/Investigational Use Head and neck cancer, nonsmall cell lung cancer, non-Hodgkin's lymphoma, ovarian cancer

Local Anesthetic/Vasoconstrictor Precautions No information available to require special precautions

Effects on Dental Treatment No significant effects or complications reported

Common Adverse Effects Based on clinical trial data using oxaliplatin alone. Some adverse effects (eg, thrombocytopenia, hemorrhagic events, neutropenia) may be increased when therapy is combined with fluorouracil/leucovorin.

>10%:

Central nervous system: Fatigue (61%), fever (25%), pain (14%), headache (13%), insomnia (11%)

Gastrointestinal: Nausea (64%), diarrhea (46%), vomiting (37%), abdominal pain (31%), constipation (31%), anorexia (20%), stomatitis (14%)

Hematologic: Anemia (64%), thrombocytopenia (30%), leukopenia (13%)

Hepatic: SGOT increased (54%), SGPT increased (36%); total bilirubin increased (13%)

Neuromuscular & skeletal: Neuropathy (may be dose-limiting), peripheral (acute 56%, persistent 48%), back pain (11%)

Respiratory: Dyspnea (13%), cough (11%)

1% to 10%:

Cardiovascular: Edema (10%), chest pain (5%), flushing (3%), thrombosis (2% to 6%), thromboembolism (6% to 9%)

Central nervous system: Rigors (9%), dizziness (7%), hand-foot syndrome (1%)

Dermatologic: Rash (5%), alopecia (3%)

Endocrine & metabolic: Dehydration (5%), hypokalemia (3%)

Gastrointestinal: Dyspepsia (7%), taste perversion (5%), flatulence (3%), mucositis (2%), gastroesophageal reflux (1%), dysphagia (acute 1% to 2%)

Genitourinary: Dysuria (1%)

Hematologic: Neutropenia (7%)

Local: Injection site reaction (9%)

Neuromuscular & skeletal: Arthralgia (7%)

Ocular: Abnormal lacrimation (1%)

Renal: Serum creatinine increased (10%)

Respiratory: URI (7%), rhinitis (6%), epistaxis (2%), pharyngitis (2%), pharyngolaryngeal dysesthesia (1% to 2%)

Miscellaneous: Allergic reactions (3%), hiccup (2%)

Mechanism of Action Oxaliplatin is an alkylating agent. Following intracellular hydrolysis, the platinum compound binds to DNA, RNA, or proteins. Cytotoxicity is cell-cycle nonspecific.

Drug Interactions

Increased Effect/Toxicity: Taxane derivatives may increase oxaliplatin toxicity if administered before the platin as a sequential infusion. Nephrotoxic agents may increase oxaliplatin toxicity. Prolonged prothrombin time and increased INR associated with hemorrhage have been reported in patients receiving oxaliplatin/fluorouracil/leucovorin concomitantly with oral anticoagulants.

Pharmacodynamics/Kinetics

Distribution: V_d: 440 L

Protein binding: >90% primarily albumin and gamma globulin (irreversible binding to platinum)

Metabolism: Nonenzymatic (rapid and extensive), forms active and inactive derivatives

Half-life elimination: 391 hours; Distribution: Alpha phase: 0.4 hours, Beta phase: 16.8 hours

Excretion: Primarily urine

Pregnancy Risk Factor D

Oxandrin® *see* Oxandrolone *on page 1155*

Oxandrolone (oks AN droe lone)

U.S. Brand Names Oxandrin®

Generic Available No

Pharmacologic Category Androgen

Use Adjunctive therapy to promote weight gain after weight loss following extensive surgery, chronic infections, or severe trauma, and in some patients who, without definite pathophysiologic reasons, fail to gain or to maintain normal weight; to offset protein catabolism with prolonged corticosteroid administration; relief of bone pain associated with osteoporosis

Local Anesthetic/Vasoconstrictor Precautions No information available to require special precautions

Effects on Dental Treatment No significant effects or complications reported

Common Adverse Effects Frequency not defined.

Cardiovascular: Edema

Central nervous system: Depression, excitation, insomnia

Dermatologic: Acne (females and prepubertal males)

Also reported in females: Hirsutism, male-pattern baldness

Endocrine & metabolic: Electrolyte imbalances, glucose intolerance, gonadotropin secretion inhibited, gynecomastia, HDL decreased, LDL increased

Also reported in females: Clitoral enlargement, menstrual irregularities

Genitourinary:

Prepubertal males: Increased or persistent erections, penile enlargement

Postpubertal males: Bladder irritation, epididymitis, impotence, oligospermia, priapism (chronic), testicular atrophy, testicular function

Hepatic: Alkaline phosphatase increased, ALT/AST increased, bilirubin increased, cholestatic jaundice, hepatic necrosis (rare), hepatocellular neoplasms, peliosis hepatitis (with long-term therapy)

Neuromuscular & skeletal: CPK increased, premature closure of epiphyses (in children)

Renal: Creatinine excretion increased

Miscellaneous: Bromsulfophthalein retention, habituation, voice alteration (deepening, in females)

Restrictions C-III

Mechanism of Action Synthetic testosterone derivative with similar androgenic and anabolic actions

Drug Interactions

Increased Effect/Toxicity: ACTH, adrenal steroids may increase risk of edema and acne. Oxandrolone enhances the hypoprothrombinemic effects of oral anticoagulants, and enhances the hypoglycemic effects of insulin and sulfonylureas (oral hypoglycemics).

Pharmacodynamics/Kinetics Half-life elimination: 10-13 hours

Pregnancy Risk Factor X

Oxaprozin (oks a PROE zin)

Related Information

Rheumatoid Arthritis, Osteoarthritis, and Osteoporosis *on page 1668*

Temporomandibular Dysfunction (TMD) *on page 1724*

(Continued)

Oxaprozin *(Continued)*

U.S. Brand Names Daypro®

Canadian Brand Names Apo-Oxaprozin®; Daypro®

Generic Available Yes

Pharmacologic Category Nonsteroidal Anti-inflammatory Drug (NSAID), Oral

Use Acute and long-term use in the management of signs and symptoms of osteoarthritis and rheumatoid arthritis; juvenile rheumatoid arthritis

Local Anesthetic/Vasoconstrictor Precautions No information available to require special precautions

Effects on Dental Treatment NSAID formulations are known to reversibly decrease platelet aggregation via mechanisms different than observed with aspirin. The dentist should be aware of the potential of abnormal coagulation. Caution should also be exercised in the use of NSAIDs in patients already on anticoagulant therapy with drugs such as warfarin (Coumadin®).

Common Adverse Effects

1% to 10%:

Cardiovascular: Edema

Central nervous system: Confusion, depression, dizziness, headache, sedation, sleep disturbance, somnolence

Dermatologic: Pruritus, rash

Gastrointestinal: Abdominal distress, abdominal pain, anorexia, constipation, diarrhea, flatulence, gastrointestinal ulcer, gross bleeding with perforation, heartburn, nausea, vomiting

Hematologic: Anemia, bleeding time increased

Hepatic: Liver enzyme elevation

Otic: Tinnitus

Renal: Dysuria, renal function abnormal, urinary frequency

Restrictions A medication guide should be dispensed with each prescription. A template for the required MedGuide can be found on the FDA website at: http://www.fda.gov/medwatch/SAFETY/2005/safety05.htm#NSAID

Dosage Oral (individualize dosage to lowest effective dose to minimize adverse effects):

Children 6-16 years: Juvenile rheumatoid arthritis:

22-31 kg: 600 mg once daily

32-54 kg: 900 mg once daily

≥55 kg: 1200 mg once daily

Adults:

Osteoarthritis: 600-1200 mg once daily; patients should be titrated to lowest dose possible; patients with low body weight should start with 600 mg daily

Rheumatoid arthritis: 1200 mg once daily; a one-time loading dose of up to 1800 mg/day or 26 mg/kg (whichever is lower) may be given

Maximum doses:

Patient <50 kg: Maximum: 1200 mg/day

Patient >50 kg with normal renal/hepatic function and low risk of peptic ulcer: Maximum: 1800 mg or 26 mg/kg (whichever is lower) in divided doses

Dosing adjustment in renal impairment: In general NSAIDs are not recommended for use in patients with advanced renal disease but the manufacturer of oxaprozin does provide some guidelines for adjustment in renal dysfunction.

Severe renal impairment or on dialysis: 600 mg once daily, may increase cautiously to 1200 mg/day with close monitoring

Dosing adjustment in hepatic impairment: Use caution in patients with severe dysfunction

Mechanism of Action Inhibits prostaglandin synthesis by decreasing the activity of the enzyme, cyclooxygenase, which results in decreased formation of prostaglandin precursors

Contraindications Hypersensitivity to oxaprozin, aspirin, other NSAIDs, or any component of the formulation; perioperative pain in the setting of coronary artery bypass surgery (CABG); pregnancy (3rd trimester)

Warnings/Precautions NSAIDs are associated with an increased risk of adverse cardiovascular events, including MI, stroke, and new onset or worsening of pre-existing hypertension. Risk may be increased with duration of use or pre-existing cardiovascular risk-factors or disease. Carefully evaluate individual cardiovascular risk profiles prior to prescribing. Use caution with fluid retention, CHF or hypertension.

Use of NSAIDs can compromise existing renal function. Renal toxicity can occur in patient with impaired renal function, dehydration, heart failure, liver dysfunction, those taking diuretics and ACEI and the elderly. Rehydrate patient before starting therapy. Monitor renal function closely. Oxaprozin is not recommended for patients with advanced renal disease.

NSAIDs may increase risk of gastrointestinal irritation, ulceration, bleeding, and perforation. These events may occur at any time during therapy and without warning. Use caution with a history of GI disease (bleeding or ulcers), concurrent therapy with aspirin, anticoagulants and/or corticosteroids, smoking, use of alcohol, the elderly or debilitated patients.

Use the lowest effective dose for the shortest duration of time, consistent with individual patient goals, to reduce risk of cardiovascular or GI adverse events. Alternate therapies should be considered for patients at high risk.

NSAIDs may cause serious skin adverse events including exfoliative dermatitis, Stevens-Johnson syndrome (SJS) and toxic epidermal necrolysis (TEN). Anaphylactoid reactions may occur, even without prior exposure; patients with "aspirin triad" (bronchial asthma, aspirin intolerance, rhinitis) may be at increased risk. Do not use in patients who experience bronchospasm, asthma, rhinitis, or urticaria with NSAID or aspirin therapy.

Use with caution in patients with decreased hepatic function. Closely monitor patients with any abnormal LFT. Severe hepatic reactions (eg, fulminant hepatitis, liver failure) have occurred with NSAID use, rarely; discontinue if signs or symptoms of liver disease develop, or if systemic manifestations occur.

The elderly are at increased risk for adverse effects (especially peptic ulceration, CNS effects, renal toxicity) from NSAIDs even at low doses.

Withhold for at least 4-6 half-lives prior to surgical or dental procedures. May cause mild photosensitivity reactions. Safety and efficacy have not been established in children <6 years of age.

Drug Interactions
Increased Effect/Toxicity: Oxaprozin may increase cyclosporine, digoxin, lithium, and methotrexate serum concentrations. The renal adverse effects of ACE inhibitors may be potentiated by NSAIDs. Corticosteroids may increase the risk of GI ulceration. The risk of bleeding with anticoagulants (warfarin, antiplatelet agents, low molecular weight heparins) may be increased.

Decreased Effect: Oxaprozin may decrease the effect of some antihypertensive agents (including ACE inhibitors, beta-blockers, hydralazine, and angiotensin antagonists) and diuretics. Cholestyramine (and other bile acid sequestrants) may decrease the absorption of NSAIDs; separate by at least 2 hours.

Ethanol/Nutrition/Herb Interactions
Ethanol: Avoid ethanol (may enhance gastric mucosal irritation).
Herb/Nutraceutical: Avoid alfalfa, anise, bilberry, bladderwrack, bromelain, cat's claw, celery, coleus, cordyceps, dong quai, evening primrose, feverfew, fenugreek, garlic, ginger, ginkgo biloboa, red clover, horse chestnut, grapeseed, green tea, ginseng, guggul, horse chestnut seed, horseradish, licorice, prickly ash, red clover, reishi, SAMe, sweet clover, turmeric, white willow (all have additional antiplatelet activity).

Pharmacodynamics/Kinetics
Absorption: Almost complete
Protein binding: >99%
Metabolism: Hepatic via oxidation and glucuronidation; no active metabolites
Half-life elimination: 40-50 hours
Time to peak: 2-4 hours
Excretion: Urine (5% unchanged, 65% as metabolites); feces (35% as metabolites)

Pregnancy Risk Factor C/D (3rd trimester)
Dosage Forms TAB: 600 mg

Oxazepam (oks A ze pam)

Related Information
Sedation on page 1727
Related Sample Prescriptions
Sedation (Prior to Dental Treatment) on page 1746
U.S. Brand Names Serax®
Canadian Brand Names Apo-Oxazepam®; Novoxapram®; Oxpram®; PMS-Oxazepam; Riva-Oxazepam
Generic Available Yes: Capsule
Pharmacologic Category Benzodiazepine
Use Treatment of anxiety; management of ethanol withdrawal
Unlabeled/Investigational Use Anticonvulsant in management of simple partial seizures; hypnotic
Local Anesthetic/Vasoconstrictor Precautions No information available to require special precautions
(Continued)

Oxazepam *(Continued)*

Effects on Dental Treatment Key adverse event(s) related to dental treatment: Xerostomia (normal salivary flow resumes upon discontinuation).

Common Adverse Effects Frequency not defined.

Cardiovascular: Syncope (rare), edema

Central nervous system: Drowsiness, ataxia, dizziness, vertigo, memory impairment, headache, paradoxical reactions (excitement, stimulation of effect), lethargy, amnesia, euphoria

Dermatologic: Rash

Endocrine & metabolic: Decreased libido, menstrual irregularities

Genitourinary: Incontinence

Hematologic: Leukopenia, blood dyscrasias

Hepatic: Jaundice

Neuromuscular & skeletal: Dysarthria, tremor, reflex slowing

Ocular: Blurred vision, diplopia

Miscellaneous: Drug dependence

Restrictions C-IV

Dosage Oral:

Children: Anxiety: 1 mg/kg/day has been administered

Adults:

Anxiety: 10-30 mg 3-4 times/day

Ethanol withdrawal: 15-30 mg 3-4 times/day

Hypnotic: 15-30 mg

Elderly: Oral: Anxiety: 10 mg 2-3 times/day; increase gradually as needed to a total of 30-45 mg/day. Dose titration should be slow to evaluate sensitivity.

Hemodialysis: Not dialyzable (0% to 5%)

Mechanism of Action Binds to stereospecific benzodiazepine receptors on the postsynaptic GABA neuron at several sites within the central nervous system, including the limbic system, reticular formation. Enhancement of the inhibitory effect of GABA on neuronal excitability results by increased neuronal membrane permeability to chloride ions. This shift in chloride ions results in hyperpolarization (a less excitable state) and stabilization.

Contraindications Hypersensitivity to oxazepam or any component of the formulation (cross-sensitivity with other benzodiazepines may exist); narrow-angle glaucoma (not in product labeling, however, benzodiazepines are contraindicated); not indicated for use in the treatment of psychosis; pregnancy

Warnings/Precautions May cause hypotension (rare) - use with caution in patients with cardiovascular or cerebrovascular disease, or in patients who would not tolerate transient decreases in blood pressure. Serax® 15 contains tartrazine; use is not recommended in pediatric patients <6 years of age; dose has not been established between 6-12 years of age.

Use with caution in elderly or debilitated patients, patients with hepatic disease (including alcoholics), or renal impairment. Use with caution in patients with respiratory disease or impaired gag reflex. Avoid use in patients with sleep apnea.

Causes CNS depression (dose-related) resulting in sedation, dizziness, confusion, or ataxia which may impair physical and mental capabilities. Patients must be cautioned about performing tasks which require mental alertness (eg, operating machinery or driving). Use with caution in patients receiving other CNS depressants or psychoactive agents. Effects with other sedative drugs or ethanol may be potentiated. Benzodiazepines have been associated with falls and traumatic injury and should be used with extreme caution in patients who are at risk of these events (especially the elderly).

Use caution in patients with suicidal risk. Use with caution in patients with a history of drug dependence. Benzodiazepines have been associated with dependence and acute withdrawal symptoms on discontinuation or reduction in dose. Acute withdrawal, including seizures, may be precipitated after administration of flumazenil to patients receiving long-term benzodiazepine therapy.

Benzodiazepines have been associated with anterograde amnesia. Paradoxical reactions, including hyperactive or aggressive behavior have been reported with benzodiazepines, particularly in adolescent/pediatric or psychiatric patients. Does not have analgesic, antidepressant, or antipsychotic properties.

Drug Interactions

Increased Effect/Toxicity: Ethanol and other CNS depressants may increase the CNS effects of oxazepam. Oxazepam may decrease the antiparkinsonian efficacy of levodopa. Flumazenil may cause seizures if administered following long-term benzodiazepine treatment.

Decreased Effect: Oral contraceptives may increase the clearance of oxazepam. Theophylline and other CNS stimulants may antagonize the sedative effects of oxazepam. Phenytoin may increase the clearance of oxazepam.

Ethanol/Nutrition/Herb Interactions
Ethanol: Avoid ethanol (may increase CNS depression).
Herb/Nutraceutical: Avoid valerian, St John's wort, kava kava, gotu kola (may increase CNS depression).

Pharmacodynamics/Kinetics
Absorption: Almost complete
Protein binding: 86% to 99%
Metabolism: Hepatic to inactive compounds (primarily as glucuronides)
Half-life elimination: 2.8-5.7 hours
Time to peak, serum: 2-4 hours
Excretion: Urine (as unchanged drug (50%) and metabolites)

Pregnancy Risk Factor D

Dosage Forms CAP: 10 mg, 15 mg, 30 mg. TAB: 15 mg

Oxcarbazepine (ox car BAZ e peen)

U.S. Brand Names Trileptal®
Canadian Brand Names Trileptal®
Generic Available No
Synonyms GP 47680; OCBZ
Pharmacologic Category Anticonvulsant, Miscellaneous
Use Monotherapy or adjunctive therapy in the treatment of partial seizures in adults and children ≥4 years of age with epilepsy; adjunctive therapy in the treatment of partial seizures in children ≥2 years of age with epilepsy.
Unlabeled/Investigational Use Bipolar disorder; treatment of neuropathic pain
Local Anesthetic/Vasoconstrictor Precautions No information available to require special precautions
Effects on Dental Treatment No significant effects or complications reported
Common Adverse Effects As reported in adults with doses of up to 2400 mg/day (includes patients on monotherapy, adjunctive therapy, and those not previously on AEDs); incidence in children was similar.

>10%:
Central nervous system: Dizziness (22% to 49%), somnolence (20% to 36%), headache (13% to 32%, placebo 23%), ataxia (5% to 31%), fatigue (12% to 15%), vertigo (6% to 15%)
Gastrointestinal: Vomiting (7% to 36%), nausea (15% to 29%), abdominal pain (10% to 13%)
Neuromuscular & skeletal: Abnormal gait (5% to 17%), tremor (3% to 16%)
Ocular: Diplopia (14% to 40%), nystagmus (7% to 26%), abnormal vision (4% to 14%)

1% to 10%:
Cardiovascular: Hypotension (1% to 2%), leg edema (1% to 2%, placebo 1%)
Central nervous system: Nervousness (2% to 5%, placebo 1% to 2%), amnesia (4%), abnormal thinking (2% to 4%), insomnia (2% to 4%), speech disorder (1% to 3%), EEG abnormalities (2%), abnormal feelings (1% to 2%), agitation (1% to 2%, placebo 1%), confusion (1% to 2%, placebo 1%)
Dermatologic: Rash (4%), acne (1% to 2%)
Endocrine & metabolic: Hyponatremia (1% to 3%, placebo 1%)
Gastrointestinal: Diarrhea (5% to 7%), dyspepsia (5% to 6%), constipation (2% to 6%, placebo 0% to 4%), gastritis (1% to 2%, placebo 1%), weight gain (1% to 2%, placebo 1%)
Neuromuscular & skeletal: Weakness (3% to 6%, placebo 5%), back pain (4%), falling down (4%), abnormal coordination (1% to 4%, placebo 1% to 2%), dysmetria (1% to 3%), sprains/strains (2%), muscle weakness (1% to 2%)
Ocular: Abnormal accommodation (2%)
Respiratory: Upper respiratory tract infection (7%), rhinitis (2% to 5%, placebo 4%), chest infection (4%), epistaxis (4%), sinusitis (4%)

Mechanism of Action Pharmacological activity results from both oxcarbazepine and its monohydroxy metabolite (MHD). Precise mechanism of anticonvulsant effect has not been defined. Oxcarbazepine and MHD block voltage sensitive sodium channels, stabilizing hyperexcited neuronal membranes, inhibiting repetitive firing, and decreasing the propagation of synaptic impulses. These actions are believed to prevent the spread of seizures. Oxcarbazepine and MHD also increase potassium conductance and modulate the activity of high-voltage activated calcium channels.

Drug Interactions
Cytochrome P450 Effect: Inhibits CYP2C19 (weak); Induces CYP3A4 (strong)
(Continued)

Oxcarbazepine (Continued)

Increased Effect/Toxicity: Serum concentrations of phenytoin and phenobarbital are increased by oxcarbazepine.

Decreased Effect: Oxcarbazepine serum concentrations may be reduced by carbamazepine, phenytoin, phenobarbital, valproic acid and verapamil (decreases levels of active oxcarbazepine metabolite). Oxcarbazepine reduces the serum concentrations of hormonal contraceptives; use alternative contraceptive measures. Oxcarbazepine may decrease the levels/effects of benzodiazepines, calcium channel blockers, clarithromycin, cyclosporine, erythromycin, estrogens, mirtazapine, nateglinide, nefazodone, nevirapine, protease inhibitors, tacrolimus, venlafaxine, and other CYP3A4 substrates.

Pharmacodynamics/Kinetics

Absorption: Complete; food has no affect on rate or extent

Distribution: MHD: V_d: 49 L

Protein binding, serum: MHD: 40%

Metabolism: Hepatic to 10-monohydroxy metabolite (MHD; active); MHD is further conjugated to DHD (inactive)

Bioavailability: Decreased in children <8 years; increased in elderly >60 years

Half-life elimination: Parent drug: 2 hours; MHD: 9 hours; renal impairment (Cl_{cr} 30 mL/minute): MHD: 19 hours

Clearance of MHD is increased in younger children (~80% in children 2-4 years of age) and approaches that of adults by ~13 years of age

Time to peak, serum: 4.5 hours (3-13 hours)

Excretion: Urine (95%, <1% as unchanged oxcarbazepine, 27% as unchanged MHD, 49% as MHD glucuronides); feces (<4%)

Pregnancy Risk Factor C

Oxiconazole (oks i KON a zole)

Related Information
Fungal Infections on page 1707

U.S. Brand Names Oxistat®

Canadian Brand Names Oxistat®

Mexican Brand Names Gyno-Myfungar®; Myfungar®; Oxistat®

Generic Available No

Synonyms Oxiconazole Nitrate

Pharmacologic Category Antifungal Agent, Topical

Use Treatment of tinea pedis (athlete's foot), tinea cruris (jock itch), and tinea corporis (ringworm)

Local Anesthetic/Vasoconstrictor Precautions No information available to require special precautions

Effects on Dental Treatment No significant effects or complications reported

Common Adverse Effects 1% to 10%:

Dermatologic: Itching, erythema

Local: Transient burning, local irritation, stinging, dryness

Mechanism of Action The cytoplasmic membrane integrity of fungi is destroyed by oxiconazole which exerts a fungicidal activity through inhibition of ergosterol synthesis. Effective for treatment of tinea pedis, tinea cruris, tinea corporis, and tinea versicolor. Active against *Trichophyton rubrum, Trichophyton mentagrophytes, Trichophyton violaceum, Microsporum canis, Microsporum audouinii, Microsporum gypseum, Epidermophyton floccosum, Candida albicans,* and *Malassezia furfur.*

Pharmacodynamics/Kinetics

Absorption: In each layer of the dermis; very little systemically after one topical dose

Distribution: To each layer of the dermis; enters breast milk

Excretion: Urine (<0.3%)

Pregnancy Risk Factor B

Oxiconazole Nitrate see Oxiconazole on page 1160

Oxidized Regenerated Cellulose see Cellulose (Oxidized/Regenerated) on page 300

Oxilapine Succinate see Loxapine on page 955

Oxipor® VHC [OTC] see Coal Tar on page 383

Oxistat® see Oxiconazole on page 1160

Oxpentifylline see Pentoxifylline on page 1212

Oxprenolol (ox PREN oh lole)

Canadian Brand Names Slow-Trasicor®; Trasicor®

Generic Available No

Synonyms Oxprenolol Hydrochloride

Pharmacologic Category Antihypertensive; Beta-Adrenergic Blocker, Noncardioselective

Use Treatment of mild or moderate hypertension

Unlabeled/Investigational Use Treatment of nonsevere hypertension in pregnancy (second-line agent)

Local Anesthetic/Vasoconstrictor Precautions No information available to require special precautions

Effects on Dental Treatment Nonselective beta-blockers may enhance the pressor response to epinephrine, resulting in hypertension and bradycardia. Many nonsteroidal anti-inflammatory drugs, such as ibuprofen and indomethacin, can reduce the hypotensive effect of beta-blockers after 3 or more weeks of therapy with the NSAID. Short-term NSAID use (ie, 3 days) requires no special precautions in patients taking beta-blockers.

Common Adverse Effects Frequency not defined.

Cardiovascular: CHF, pulmonary edema, cardiac enlargement, postural hypotension, severe bradycardia, lengthening of PR interval, second- and third-degree AV block, sinus arrest, palpitation, chest pain; peripheral vascular disorders, Raynaud's phenomenon, claudication, hot flashes, syncope

Central nervous system: Vertigo, lightheadedness, headache, dizziness, anxiety, mental depression, nervousness, irritability, hallucinations, sleep disturbances, nightmares, insomnia, weakness, sedation, vivid dreams, slurred speech

Dermatological: Dry skin, rash, pruritus

Endocrine & metabolic: Libido decreased, impotence, weight gain, hypoglycemia

Gastrointestinal: Diarrhea, constipation, flatulence, heartburn, anorexia, nausea, vomiting, abdominal pain, dry mouth

Hematological: Thrombocytopenia, leukopenia

Hepatic: Alkaline phosphatase increased, bilirubin increased, transaminases increased

Neuromuscular & skeletal: Paresthesia

Ocular: Keratoconjunctivitis, dry eyes, itching eyes, blurred vision

Otic: Tinnitus

Renal: BUN increased

Respiratory: Dyspnea, wheezing, bronchospasm, nasal congestion, status asthmaticus

Miscellaneous: Diaphoresis, exertional tiredness

Restrictions Not available in U.S.

Mechanism of Action Oxprenolol has a competitive ability to antagonize catecholamine-induced tachycardia at the beta-receptor sites in the heart, thus decreasing cardiac output, inhibits of renin release by the kidneys, and inhibits the vasomotor centers.

Drug Interactions

Cytochrome P450 Effect: Inhibits CYP2D6 (weak)

Increased Effect/Toxicity: Antiarrhythmic agents (eg, quinidine, amiodarone) may potentiate the negative inotropic and dromotropic effect of antiarrhythmic agents (quinidine, amiodarone) may be potentiated by oxprenolol. Concomitant use of I.V. calcium channel blockers with AV-blocking potential (eg, diltiazem and verapamil) may lead to severe hypotension, cardiac arrhythmias and cardiac arrest may occur. Catecholamine-depleting drugs (reserpine, guanethidine) may produce any excessive reduction of sympathetic activity, leading to severe bradycardia and hypotension.

Ergot alkaloids may cause deterioration in peripheral blood flow, leading to peripheral ischemia. Inhalational anesthetics may cause cardiodepressant effects in patients receiving oxprenolol. Oxprenolol may potentiate hypoglycemic effects of insulin and hypoglycemic agents. Concomitant use of MAO inhibitors may produce any excessive reduction of sympathetic activity. CNS depressants (opiate analgesics, antihistamines, ethanol, and psycho-active drugs) may potentiate CNS depressant effects of oxprenolol.

Decreased Effect: Concomitant use of NSAIDs (indomethacin) may decrease antihypertensive effect of oxprenolol. Concomitant use of sympathomimetic agents (eg, epinephrine) may cause hypertensive reactions.

(Continued)

Oxprenolol (Continued)

Pharmacodynamics/Kinetics

Duration of beta-blocking effects: Immediate-release tablet: 8-12 hours; Slow-release tablet: Up to 24 hours

Absorption: 20% to 70%

Distribution: 1.3 L/kg

Protein binding: 80%

Metabolism: Hepatic first-pass effect

Half-life elimination: 1.3-1.5 hours

Time to peak, serum: Immediate-release tablet: 0.5-1.5 hours; Slow-release tablet: 2-4 hours

Excretion: Urine (as inactive metabolites, <5% as unchanged drug); major metabolite is glucuronide

Pregnancy Risk Factor Not assigned (similar agents rated C/D)

Oxprenolol Hydrochloride see Oxprenolol on page 1161

Oxsoralen® see Methoxsalen on page 1018

Oxsoralen-Ultra® see Methoxsalen on page 1018

Oxy 10® Balanced Medicated Face Wash [OTC] see Benzoyl Peroxide on page 194

Oxy 10® Balance Spot Treatment [OTC] see Benzoyl Peroxide on page 194

Oxy Balance® [OTC] see Salicylic Acid on page 1374

Oxy Balance® Deep Pore [OTC] see Salicylic Acid on page 1374

Oxybutynin (oks i BYOO ti nin)

U.S. Brand Names Ditropan®; Ditropan® XL; Oxytrol®

Canadian Brand Names Ditropan®; Ditropan® XL; Gen-Oxybutynin; Novo-Oxybutynin; Nu-Oxybutyn; Oxytrol®; PMS-Oxybutynin

Mexican Brand Names Tavor®

Generic Available Yes: Excludes extended release formulation and transdermal patch

Synonyms Oxybutynin Chloride

Pharmacologic Category Antispasmodic Agent, Urinary

Use Antispasmodic for neurogenic bladder (urgency, frequency, urge incontinence) and uninhibited bladder

Local Anesthetic/Vasoconstrictor Precautions No information available to require special precautions

Effects on Dental Treatment Key adverse event(s) related to dental treatment: Xerostomia and changes in salivation (normal salivary flow resumes upon discontinuation), and taste perversion.

Common Adverse Effects

Oral:

>10%:

Central nervous system: Dizziness (6% to 16%), somnolence (12% to 13%)

Gastrointestinal: Xerostomia (61% to 71%), constipation (13%)

Genitourinary: Urination impaired (11%)

1% to 10%:

Cardiovascular: Palpitation (2% to <5%), peripheral edema (2% to <5%), hypertension (2% to <5%), vasodilation (2% to <5%)

Central nervous system: Headache (6% to 10%), pain (7%), confusion (2% to <5%), insomnia (2% to <5%), nervousness (2% to <5%)

Dermatologic: Dry skin (2% to <5%), skin rash (2% to <5%)

Gastrointestinal: Nausea (9% to 10%), dyspepsia (7%), abdominal pain (2% to 6%), diarrhea (5% to 9%), flatulence (2% to <5%), gastrointestinal reflux (2% to <5%), taste perversion (2% to <5%)

Genitourinary: Postvoid residuals increased (2% to 9%), urinary tract infection (5%)

Neuromuscular & skeletal: Weakness (2% to 7%)

Ocular: Blurred vision (8% to 9%), dry eyes (2% to 6%)

Respiratory: Rhinitis (6%), dry nasal and sinus membranes (2% to <5%)

Transdermal:

>10%: Local: Application site reaction (17%), pruritus (14%)

1% to 10%:

Gastrointestinal: Xerostomia (4% to 10%), diarrhea (3%), constipation (3%)

Genitourinary: Dysuria (2%)

Local: Erythema (6% to 8%), vesicles (3%), rash (3%)

Ocular: Vision changes (3%)

Mechanism of Action Direct antispasmodic effect on smooth muscle, also inhibits the action of acetylcholine on smooth muscle (exhibits $\frac{1}{5}$ the anticholinergic activity of atropine, but is 4-10 times the antispasmodic activity); does not block effects at skeletal muscle or at autonomic ganglia; increases bladder capacity, decreases uninhibited contractions, and delays desire to void; therefore, decreases urgency and frequency

Drug Interactions

Cytochrome P450 Effect: Substrate of CYP3A4 (minor); **Inhibits** CYP2D6 (weak), 3A4 (weak)

Increased Effect/Toxicity: Additive sedation with CNS depressants and ethanol. Additive anticholinergic effects with antihistamines and anticholinergic agents.

Pharmacodynamics/Kinetics

Onset of action: Oral: 30-60 minutes

Peak effect: 3-6 hours

Duration: 6-10 hours (up to 24 hours for extended release oral formulation)

Absorption: Oral: Rapid and well absorbed; Transdermal: High

Distribution: V_d: 193 L

Metabolism: Hepatic via CYP3A4; Oral: High first-pass metabolism; I.V.: Forms active and inactive metabolites

Half-life elimination: I.V.: ~2 hours (parent drug), 7-8 hours (metabolites)

Time to peak, serum: Oral: ~60 minutes; Transdermal: 24-48 hours

Excretion: Urine (<0.1%)

Pregnancy Risk Factor B

Oxybutynin Chloride *see* Oxybutynin *on page 1162*

Oxychlorosene (oks i KLOR oh seen)

U.S. Brand Names Clorpactin® WCS-90 [OTC]

Generic Available No

Synonyms Oxychlorosene Sodium

Pharmacologic Category Antibiotic, Topical

Use Treatment of localized infections

Local Anesthetic/Vasoconstrictor Precautions No information available to require special precautions

Effects on Dental Treatment No significant effects or complications reported

Oxychlorosene Sodium *see* Oxychlorosene *on page 1163*

Oxycodone (oks i KOE done)

Related Information

Oral Pain *on page 1692*

U.S. Brand Names OxyContin®; Oxydose™; OxyFast®; OxyIR®; Roxicodone™; Roxicodone™ Intensol™

Canadian Brand Names OxyContin®; Oxy.IR®; Supeudol®

Mexican Brand Names Oxycontin®

Generic Available Yes

Synonyms Dihydrohydroxycodeinone; Oxycodone Hydrochloride

Pharmacologic Category Analgesic, Narcotic

Dental Use Treatment of postoperative pain

Use Management of moderate to severe pain, normally used in combination with non-narcotic analgesics

OxyContin® is indicated for around-the-clock management of moderate to severe pain when an analgesic is needed for an extended period of time. **Note:** OxyContin® is not intended for use as an "as needed" analgesic or for immediately-postoperative pain management (should be used postoperatively only if the patient has received it prior to surgery or if severe, persistent pain is anticipated).

Local Anesthetic/Vasoconstrictor Precautions No information available to require special precautions

Effects on Dental Treatment Key adverse event(s) related to dental treatment: Xerostomia (normal salivary flow resumes upon discontinuation).

Significant Adverse Effects

>10%:

Central nervous system: Fatigue, drowsiness, dizziness, somnolence

Dermatologic: Pruritus

Gastrointestinal: Nausea, vomiting, constipation

Neuromuscular & skeletal: Weakness

1% to 10%:

Cardiovascular: Postural hypotension

Central nervous system: Nervousness, headache, restlessness, malaise, confusion, anxiety, abnormal dreams, euphoria, thought abnormalities

(Continued)

Oxycodone *(Continued)*

Dermatologic: Rash

Gastrointestinal: Anorexia, stomach cramps, xerostomia, biliary spasm, abdominal pain, dyspepsia, gastritis

Genitourinary: Ureteral spasms, decreased urination

Local: Pain at injection site

Respiratory: Dyspnea, hiccups

Miscellaneous: Diaphoresis

<1% (Limited to important or life-threatening): Anaphylaxis, anaphylactoid reaction, dysphagia, exfoliative dermatitis, hallucinations, histamine release, hyponatremia, ileus, intracranial pressure increased, mental depression, paradoxical CNS stimulation, paralytic ileus, physical and psychological dependence, SIADH, syncope, urinary retention, urticaria, vasodilation, withdrawal syndrome (may include seizure)

Note: Deaths due to overdose have been reported due to misuse/abuse after crushing the sustained release tablets.

Restrictions C-II

Dental Usual Dosing Postoperative pain: Adults: Oral: 5 mg every 6 hours as needed

Dosage Oral:

Immediate release:

Children:

6-12 years: 1.25 mg every 6 hours as needed

>12 years: 2.5 mg every 6 hours as needed

Adults: 5 mg every 6 hours as needed

Controlled release: Adults:

Opioid naive (not currently on opioid): 10 mg every 12 hours

Currently on opioid/ASA or acetaminophen or NSAID combination:

1-5 tablets: 10-20 mg every 12 hours

6-9 tablets: 20-30 mg every 12 hours

10-12 tablets: 30-40 mg every 12 hours

May continue the nonopioid as a separate drug.

Currently on opioids: Use standard conversion chart to convert daily dose to oxycodone equivalent. Divide daily dose in 2 (for every 12-hour dosing) and round down to nearest dosage form.

Note: 80 mg or 160 mg tablets are for use **only** in opioid-tolerant patients. Special safety considerations must be addressed when converting to OxyContin® doses ≥160 mg every 12 hours. Dietary caution must be taken when patients are initially titrated to 160 mg tablets.

Dosing adjustment in hepatic impairment: Reduce dosage in patients with severe liver disease

Mechanism of Action Binds to opiate receptors in the CNS, causing inhibition of ascending pain pathways, altering the perception of and response to pain; produces generalized CNS depression

Contraindications Hypersensitivity to oxycodone or any component of the formulation; significant respiratory depression; hypercarbia; acute or severe bronchial asthma; OxyContin® is also contraindicated in paralytic ileus (known or suspected); pregnancy (prolonged use or high doses at term)

Warnings/Precautions Use with caution in patients with hypersensitivity reactions to other phenanthrene derivative opioid agonists (morphine, hydrocodone, hydromorphone, levorphanol, oxycodone, oxymorphone), respiratory diseases including asthma, emphysema, or COPD. Use with caution in pancreatitis or biliary tract disease, acute alcoholism (including delirium tremens), adrenocortical insufficiency, CNS depression/coma, kyphoscoliosis (or other skeletal disorder which may alter respiratory function), hypothyroidism (including myxedema), prostatic hyperplasia, urethral stricture, and toxic psychosis.

Use with caution in the elderly, debilitated, severe hepatic or renal function. Hemodynamic effects (hypotension, orthostasis) may be exaggerated in patients with hypovolemia, concurrent vasodilating drugs, or in patients with head injury. Respiratory depressant effects and capacity to elevate CSF pressure may be exaggerated in presence of head injury, other intracranial lesion, or pre-existing intracranial pressure. Tolerance or drug dependence may result from extended use. Healthcare provider should be alert to problems of abuse, misuse, and diversion. Do **not** crush controlled-release tablets. Some preparations contain sulfites which may cause allergic reactions. OxyContin® 80 mg and 160 mg strengths are for use only in opioid-tolerant patients requiring high daily dosages >160 mg (80 mg formulation) or >320 mg (160 mg formulation).

Drug Interactions Substrate of CYP2D6 (major)

CNS depressants, MAO inhibitors, general anesthetics, and tricyclic antidepressants: May potentiate the effects of opiate agonists; dextroamphetamine may enhance the analgesic effect of opiate agonists

CYP2D6 inhibitors: May decrease the effects of oxycodone. Example inhibitors include chlorpromazine, delavirdine, fluoxetine, miconazole, paroxetine, pergolide, quinidine, quinine, ritonavir, and ropinirole.

Ethanol/Nutrition/Herb Interactions

Ethanol: Avoid ethanol (may increase CNS depression).

Food: When taken with a high-fat meal, peak concentration is 25% greater following a single OxyContin® 160 mg tablet as compared to two 80 mg tablets.

Herb/Nutraceutical: Avoid valerian, St John's wort, kava kava, gotu kola (may increase CNS depression).

Dietary Considerations Instruct patient to avoid high-fat meals when taking OxyContin® 160 mg tablets.

Pharmacodynamics/Kinetics

Onset of action: Pain relief: 10-15 minutes

Peak effect: 0.5-1 hour

Duration: 3-6 hours; Controlled release: ≤12 hours

Metabolism: Hepatic

Half-life elimination: 2-3 hours

Excretion: Urine

Pregnancy Risk Factor B/D (prolonged use or high doses at term)

Lactation Enters breast milk/use caution

Dosage Forms

Capsule, immediate release, as hydrochloride (OxyIR®): 5 mg

Solution, oral, as hydrochloride: 5 mg/5 mL (500 mL)

Roxicodone™: 5 mg/5 mL (5 mL, 500 mL) [contains alcohol]

Solution, oral concentrate, as hydrochloride: 20 mg/mL (30 mL)

Oxydose™: 20 mg/mL (30 mL) [contains sodium benzoate; berry flavor]

OxyFast®, Roxicodone™ Intensol™: 20 mg/mL (30 mL) [contains sodium benzoate]

Tablet, as hydrochloride: 5 mg, 15 mg, 30 mg

Roxicodone™: 5 mg, 15 mg, 30 mg

Tablet, controlled release, as hydrochloride (OxyContin®): 10 mg, 20 mg, 40 mg, 80 mg, 160 mg

Tablet, extended release, as hydrochloride: 10 mg, 20 mg, 40 mg, 80 mg

Selected Readings

Wynn RL, "Narcotic Analgesics for Dental Pain: Available Products, Strengths, and Formulations," *Gen Dent*, 2001, 49(2)126-36.

Oxycodone and Acetaminophen

(oks i KOE done & a seet a MIN oh fen)

Related Information

Acetaminophen *on page 31*

Oral Pain *on page 1692*

Oxycodone *on page 1163*

Related Sample Prescriptions

Severe Oral Pain *on page 1735*

U.S. Brand Names Endocet®; Percocet®; Roxicet™; Roxicet™ 5/500; Tylox®

Canadian Brand Names Endocet®; Oxycocet®; Percocet®; Percocet®-Demi; PMS-Oxycodone-Acetaminophen

Generic Available Yes: Excludes caplet and solution

Synonyms Acetaminophen and Oxycodone

Pharmacologic Category Analgesic, Narcotic

Dental Use Treatment of postoperative pain

Use Management of moderate to severe pain

Local Anesthetic/Vasoconstrictor Precautions No information available to require special precautions

Effects on Dental Treatment Key adverse event(s) related to dental treatment: Nausea, sedation, constipation, and xerostomia (normal salivary flow resumes upon discontinuation). See Dental Comment.

Significant Adverse Effects Frequency not defined (also see individual agents): Allergic reaction, constipation, dizziness, dysphoria, euphoria, lightheadedness, nausea, pruritus, respiratory depression, sedation, skin rash, vomiting

Restrictions C-II

Dental Usual Dosing Note: Initial dose is based on the **oxycodone** content; however, the maximum daily dose is based on the **acetaminophen** content.

Management of pain: Doses should be given every 4-6 hours as needed and titrated to appropriate analgesic effects.

Mild to moderate pain:

Children: Initial dose, **based on oxycodone content:** 0.05-0.1 mg/kg/dose

(Continued)

Oxycodone and Acetaminophen *(Continued)*

Maximum acetaminophen dose: Children <45 kg: 90 mg/kg/day; children >45 kg: 4 g/day

Adults: Initial dose, **based on oxycodone content:** 5 mg

Severe pain:

Children: Initial dose, **based on oxycodone content:** 0.3 mg/kg/dose

Adults: Initial dose, **based on oxycodone content:** 15-30 mg. Do not exceed acetaminophen 4 g/day.

Elderly: Doses should be titrated to appropriate analgesic effects: Initial dose, **based on oxycodone content:** 2.5-5 mg every 6 hours. Do not exceed acetaminophen 4 g/day.

Dosage adjustment in hepatic impairment: Dose should be reduced in patients with severe liver disease.

Dosage Oral: Doses should be given every 4-6 hours as needed and titrated to appropriate analgesic effects. **Note:** Initial dose is based on the **oxycodone** content; however, the maximum daily dose is based on the **acetaminophen** content.

Children: Maximum acetaminophen dose: Children <45 kg: 90 mg/kg/day; children >45 kg: 4 g/day

Mild to moderate pain: Initial dose, **based on oxycodone content:** 0.05-0.1 mg/kg/dose

Severe pain: Initial dose, **based on oxycodone content:** 0.3 mg/kg/dose

Adults:

Mild to moderate pain: Initial dose, **based on oxycodone content:** 5 mg

Severe pain: Initial dose, **based on oxycodone content:** 15-30 mg. Do not exceed acetaminophen 4 g/day.

Elderly: Doses should be titrated to appropriate analgesic effects: Initial dose, **based on oxycodone content:** 2.5-5 mg every 6 hours. Do not exceed acetaminophen 4 g/day.

Dosage adjustment in hepatic impairment: Dose should be reduced in patients with severe liver disease.

Mechanism of Action

Oxycodone, as with other narcotic (opiate) analgesics, blocks pain perception in the cerebral cortex by binding to specific receptor molecules (opiate receptors) within the neuronal membranes of synapses. This binding results in a decreased synaptic chemical transmission throughout the CNS thus inhibiting the flow of pain sensations into the higher centers. Mu and kappa are the two subtypes of the opiate receptor to which oxycodone binds to cause analgesia.

Acetaminophen inhibits the synthesis of prostaglandins in the CNS and peripherally blocks pain impulse generation; produces antipyresis from inhibition of hypothalamic heat-regulating center

Contraindications Hypersensitivity to oxycodone, acetaminophen, or any component of the formulation; severe respiratory depression (in absence of resuscitative equipment or ventilatory support); pregnancy (prolonged periods or high doses at term)

Warnings/Precautions Use with caution in patients with hypersensitivity reactions to other phenanthrene-derivative opioid agonists (morphine, codeine, hydrocodone, hydromorphone, levorphanol, oxymorphone); respiratory diseases including asthma, emphysema, COPD, or severe liver or renal insufficiency, hypothyroidism, Addison's disease, prostatic hypertrophy, or urethral stricture; some preparations contain sulfites which may cause allergic reactions; may be habit-forming

Use with caution in patients with head injury and increased intracranial pressure (respiratory depressant effects increased and may also elevate CSF pressure). May mask diagnosis or clinical course in patients with acute abdominal conditions.

Enhanced analgesia has been seen in elderly patients on therapeutic doses of narcotics; duration of action may be increased in the elderly; the elderly may be particularly susceptible to the CNS depressant and constipating effects of narcotics

Drug Interactions Also see individual agents.

Oxycodone: **Substrate** of CYP2D6 (major)

Acetaminophen: **Substrate** (minor) of CYP1A2, 2A6, 2C9, 2D6, 2E1, 3A4

Anesthetics, general: May have additive CNS depression; consider lowering dose of one or both agents

Anticholinergics: Concomitant use may lead to paralytic ileus

CNS depressants: May have additive CNS depression; consider lowering dose of one or both agents

CYP2D6 inhibitors: May decrease the effects of oxycodone. Example inhibitors include chlorpromazine, delavirdine, fluoxetine, miconazole, paroxetine, pergolide, quinidine, quinine, ritonavir, and ropinirole.

Phenothiazines: May have additive CNS depression with phenothiazine and other tranquilizers; consider lowering dose of one or both agents

Sedative hypnotics: May have additive CNS depression; consider lowering dose of one or both agents

Ethanol/Nutrition/Herb Interactions Ethanol: May have additive CNS depression. In addition, excessive intake of ethanol may increase the risk of acetaminophen-induced hepatotoxicity. Avoid ethanol or limit to <3 drinks/day.

Pharmacodynamics/Kinetics See individual agents.

Pregnancy Risk Factor C/D (prolonged periods or high doses at term)

Lactation Enters breast milk/use caution

Breast-Feeding Considerations

Oxycodone: Excreted in breast milk. If occasional doses are used during breast-feeding, monitor infant for sedation, GI effects and changes in feeding pattern.

Acetaminophen: May be taken while breast-feeding

Dosage Forms

Caplet:

Roxicet™ 5/500: Oxycodone hydrochloride 5 mg and acetaminophen 500 mg

Capsule: 5/500: Oxycodone hydrochloride 5 mg and acetaminophen 500 mg

Tylox®: 5/500: Oxycodone hydrochloride 5 mg and acetaminophen 500 mg [contains sodium benzoate and sodium metabisulfite]

Solution, oral:

Roxicet™: Oxycodone hydrochloride 5 mg and acetaminophen 325 mg per 5 mL (5 mL, 500 mL) [contains alcohol <0.5%]

Tablet: 5/325: Oxycodone hydrochloride 5 mg and acetaminophen 325 mg; 7.5/325: Oxycodone hydrochloride 7.5 mg and acetaminophen 325 mg; 7.5/500: Oxycodone hydrochloride 7.5 mg and acetaminophen 500 mg; 10/325: Oxycodone hydrochloride 10 mg and acetaminophen 325 mg; 10/650: Oxycodone hydrochloride 10 mg and acetaminophen 650 mg

Endocet® 5/325 [scored]: Oxycodone hydrochloride 5 mg and acetaminophen 325 mg

Endocet® 7.5/325: Oxycodone hydrochloride 7.5 mg and acetaminophen 325 mg

Endocet® 7.5/500: Oxycodone hydrochloride 7.5 mg and acetaminophen 500 mg

Endocet® 10/325: Oxycodone hydrochloride 10 mg and acetaminophen 325 mg

Endocet® 10/650: Oxycodone hydrochloride 10 mg and acetaminophen 650 mg

Percocet® 2.5/325: Oxycodone hydrochloride 2.5 mg and acetaminophen 325 mg

Percocet® 5/325 [scored]: Oxycodone hydrochloride 5 mg and acetaminophen 325 mg

Percocet® 7.5/325: Oxycodone hydrochloride 7.5 mg and acetaminophen 325 mg

Percocet® 7.5/500: Oxycodone hydrochloride 7.5 mg and acetaminophen 500 mg

Percocet® 10/325: Oxycodone hydrochloride 10 mg and acetaminophen 325 mg

Percocet® 10/650: Oxycodone hydrochloride 10 mg and acetaminophen 650 mg

Roxicet™ [scored]: Oxycodone hydrochloride 5 mg and acetaminophen 325 mg

Dental Comment Oxycodone, as with other narcotic analgesics, is recommended only for limited acute dosing (ie, 3 days or less). Oxycodone has an addictive liability, especially when given long-term. The acetaminophen component requires use with caution in patients with alcoholic liver disease.

Acetaminophen: A study by Hylek, et al, suggested that the combination of acetaminophen with warfarin (Coumadin®) may cause enhanced anticoagulation. The following recommendations have been made by Hylek, et al, and supported by an editorial in *JAMA* by Bell.

Dose and duration of acetaminophen should be as low as possible, individualized and monitored

For patients who reported taking the equivalent of at least 4 regular strength (325 mg) tablets for longer than a week, the odds of having an INR >6.0 were increased 10-fold above those not taking acetaminophen. Risk decreased with lower intakes of acetaminophen reaching a background level of risk at a dose of 6 or fewer 325 mg tablets per week.

(Continued)

Oxycodone and Acetaminophen (Continued)

Selected Readings

Bell WR, "Acetaminophen and Warfarin: Undesirable Synergy," *JAMA*, 1998, 279(9):702-3.

Botting RM, "Mechanism of Action of Acetaminophen: Is There a Cyclooxygenase 3?" *Clin Infect Dis*, 2000, Suppl 5:S202-10.

Cooper SA, Precheur H, Rauch D, et al, "Evaluation of Oxycodone and Acetaminophen in Treatment of Postoperative Pain," *Oral Surg Oral Med Oral Pathol*, 1980, 50(6):496-501.

Dart RC, Kuffner EK, and Rumack BH, "Treatment of Pain or Fever With Paracetamol (Acetaminophen) in the Alcoholic Patient: A Systematic Review," *Am J Ther*, 2000, 7(2):123-34.

Dionne RA, "New Approaches to Preventing and Treating Postoperative Pain," *J Am Dent Assoc*, 1992, 123(6):26-34.

Gobetti JP, "Controlling Dental Pain," *J Am Dent Assoc*, 1992, 123(6):47-52.

Grant JA and Weiler JM, "A Report of a Rare Immediate Reaction After Ingestion of Acetaminophen," *Ann Allergy Asthma Immunol*, 2001, 87(3):227-9.

Hylek EM, Heiman H, Skates SJ, et al, "Acetaminophen and Other Risk Factors for Excessive Warfarin Anticoagulation 1998," *JAMA*, 1998, 279(9):702-3.

Kwan D, Bartle WR, and Walker SE, "The Effects of Acetaminophen on Pharmacokinetics and Pharmacodynamics of Warfarin," *J Clin Pharmacol*, 1999, 39(1):68-75.

McClain CJ, Price S, Barve S, et al, "Acetaminophen Hepatotoxicity: An Update," *Curr Gastroenterol Rep*, 1999, 1(1):42-9.

Shek KL, Chan LN, and Nutescu E, "Warfarin-Acetaminophen Drug Interaction Revisited," *Pharmacotherapy*, 1999, 19(10):1153-8.

Tanaka E, Yamazaki K, and Misawa S, "Update: The Clinical Importance of Acetaminophen Hepatotoxicity in Nonalcoholic and Alcoholic Subjects," *J Clin Pharm Ther*, 2000, 25(5):325-32.

Wynn RL, "Narcotic Analgesics for Dental Pain: Available Products, Strengths, and Formulations," *Gen Dent*, 2001, 49(2):126-8, 130, 132 passim.

Oxycodone and Aspirin (oks i KOE done & AS pir in)

Related Information

Aspirin *on page 145*
Oral Pain *on page 1692*
Oxycodone *on page 1163*

U.S. Brand Names Endodan® [DSC]; Percodan®

Canadian Brand Names Endodan®; Oxycodan®; Percodan®

Generic Available Yes

Synonyms Aspirin and Oxycodone

Pharmacologic Category Analgesic, Narcotic

Dental Use Treatment of postoperative pain

Use Management of moderate to severe pain

Local Anesthetic/Vasoconstrictor Precautions No information available to require special precautions

Effects on Dental Treatment Key adverse event(s) related to dental treatment: Nausea, sedation, constipation, and xerostomia (normal salivary flow resumes upon discontinuation). May have anticoagulant effects which may affect bleeding time. The elderly are a high-risk population for adverse effects from NSAIDs. As many as 60% of elderly patients with GI complications from NSAIDs can develop peptic ulceration and/or hemorrhage asymptomatically. Concomitant disease and drug use contribute to the risk of GI adverse effects. Enhanced analgesia has been seen with therapeutic doses of narcotics; duration of action may be increased. Elderly may also be particularly susceptible to the CNS depressant effects of narcotics. See Dental Comment.

Significant Adverse Effects Note: Also refer to individual agents

Common (frequency not defined):

Central nervous system: Dizziness, drowsiness, lightheadedness, sedation

Dermatologic: Pruritus

Gastrointestinal: Nausea, vomiting, constipation

<1%, postmarketing, and/or case reports (limited to important or life-threatening): Allergic reaction, anaphylaxis, anaphylactoid reaction, angioedema, apnea, asthma, bradycardia, bronchospasm, circulatory depression, confusion, duodenal ulcer, dysphoria, dyspnea, ecchymosis, euphoria, gastric ulcer, gastrointestinal bleeding, hallucination, hemorrhage, hepatitis, hepatotoxicity, hypotension, hypoglycemia, hyperglycemia, ileus, interstitial nephritis, intestinal obstruction, laryngeal edema, metabolic acidosis, pancreatitis, papillary necrosis, paresthesia, purpura, pulmonary edema, proteinuria, rash, renal failure, respiratory alkalosis, respiratory depression, Reye syndrome, rhabdomyolysis, seizure, shock, thrombocytopenia, tinnitus

Restrictions C-II

Dental Usual Dosing Analgesic: Oral (based on oxycodone combined salts):

Children: Maximum oxycodone: 5 mg/dose; maximum aspirin dose should not exceed 4 g/day. Doses should be given every 6 hours as needed.

Mild-to-moderate pain: Initial dose, **based on oxycodone content:** 0.05-0.1 mg/kg/dose

Severe pain: Initial dose, **based on oxycodone content:** 0.3 mg/kg/dose

Adults: Percodan®: 1 tablet every 6 hours as needed for pain; maximum aspirin dose should not exceed 4 g/day.

Dosage Oral (based on oxycodone combined salts):

Children: Maximum oxycodone: 5 mg/dose; maximum aspirin dose should not exceed 4 g/day. Doses should be given every 6 hours as needed.

Mild-to-moderate pain: Initial dose, **based on oxycodone content:** 0.05-0.1 mg/kg/dose

Severe pain: Initial dose, **based on oxycodone content:** 0.3 mg/kg/dose

Adults: Percodan®: 1 tablet every 6 hours as needed for pain; maximum aspirin dose should not exceed 4 g/day.

Dosing adjustment in hepatic impairment: Dose should be reduced in patients with severe liver disease.

Mechanism of Action

Oxycodone, as with other narcotic (opiate) analgesics, blocks pain perception in the cerebral cortex by binding to specific receptor molecules (opiate receptors) within the neuronal membranes of synapses. This binding results in a decreased synaptic chemical transmission throughout the CNS thus inhibiting the flow of pain sensations into the higher centers. Mu and kappa are the two subtypes of the opiate receptor to which oxycodone binds to cause analgesia.

Aspirin inhibits prostaglandin synthesis by decreasing the activity of the enzyme, cyclooxygenase, which results in decreased formation of prostaglandin precursors, acts on the hypothalamic heat-regulating center to reduce fever, blocks thromboxane synthetase action which prevents formation of the platelet-aggregating substance thromboxane A_2

Contraindications Hypersensitivity to oxycodone, salicylates, other NSAIDs, or any component of the formulation; patients with the syndrome of asthma, rhinitis, and nasal polyps; inherited or acquired bleeding disorders (including factor VII and factor IX deficiency); do not use in children (<16 years of age) in the presence of viral infections (chickenpox or flu symptoms), with or without fever, due to a potential association with Reye's syndrome; significant respiratory depression; hypercarbia; known or suspected paralytic ileus; acute or severe bronchial asthma; pregnancy (3rd trimester)

Warnings/Precautions Use with caution in patients with hypersensitivity reactions to other phenanthrene derivative opioid agonists (morphine, hydrocodone, hydromorphone, levorphanol, oxycodone, oxymorphone), respiratory diseases including asthma, emphysema, or COPD. Use with caution in pancreatitis or biliary tract disease, acute alcoholism (including delirium tremens), adrenocortical insufficiency, CNS depression/coma, kyphoscoliosis (or other skeletal disorder which may alter respiratory function), hypothyroidism (including myxedema), prostatic hyperplasia, urethral stricture, and toxic psychosis.

Use with caution in the elderly, debilitated, severe hepatic or renal dysfunction. Hemodynamic effects (hypotension, orthostasis) may be exaggerated in patients with dehydration, hypovolemia, concurrent vasodilating drugs, or in patients with head injury. Respiratory depressant effects and capacity to elevate CSF pressure may be exaggerated in presence of head injury, other intracranial lesion, or pre-existing elevation of intracranial pressure. Tolerance or drug dependence may result from extended use. Healthcare provider should be alert to problems of abuse, misuse, and diversion. Taper dose gradually to avoid withdrawal symptoms in physically dependent patients.

Use with caution in patients with platelet and bleeding disorders, erosive gastritis, or peptic ulcer disease. Heavy ethanol use (>3 drinks/day) can increase bleeding risks. Discontinue use if tinnitus or impaired hearing occurs. Patients with sensitivity to tartrazine dyes, nasal polyps and asthma may have an increased risk of salicylate sensitivity. Surgical patients should avoid ASA if possible, for 1-2 weeks prior to surgery, to reduce the risk of excessive bleeding.

Drug Interactions

Oxycodone: **Substrate** of CYP2D6 (major)

Aspirin: **Substrate** of CYP2C9 (minor)

Also see individual agents.

CYP2D6 inhibitors: May decrease the effects of oxycodone. Example inhibitors include chlorpromazine, delavirdine, fluoxetine, miconazole, paroxetine, pergolide, quinidine, quinine, ritonavir, and ropinirole.

Increased effect/toxicity with CNS depressants, TCAs, dextroamphetamine

Dietary Considerations May be taken with food or water.

Pharmacodynamics/Kinetics See individual agents.

Pregnancy Risk Factor D

Lactation Enters breast milk/use caution

Breast-Feeding Considerations

Aspirin: Caution is suggested due to potential adverse effects in nursing infants.

Oxycodone: No data reported.

(Continued)

Oxycodone and Aspirin *(Continued)*

Dosage Forms [DSC] = Discontinued product

Tablet: Oxycodone hydrochloride 4.5 mg, oxycodone terephthalate 0.38 mg, and aspirin 325 mg

Endodan® [DSC], Percodan®: Oxycodone hydrochloride 4.5 mg, oxycodone terephthalate 0.38 mg, and aspirin 325 mg

Dental Comment Oxycodone, as with other narcotic analgesics, is recommended only for limited acute dosing (ie, 3 days or less). Oxycodone has an addictive liability, especially when given long-term. The oxycodone with aspirin could have anticoagulant effects and could possibly affect bleeding times.

Selected Readings

Dionne RA, "New Approaches to Preventing and Treating Postoperative Pain," *J Am Dent Assoc*, 1992, 123(6):26-34.

Gobetti JP, "Controlling Dental Pain," *J Am Dent Assoc*, 1992, 123(6):47-52.

Wynn RL, "Narcotic Analgesics for Dental Pain: Available Products, Strengths, and Formulations," *Gen Dent*, 2001, 49(2):126-8, 130, 132 passim.

Oxycodone and Ibuprofen (oks i KOE done & eye byoo PROE fen)

Related Sample Prescriptions

Severe Oral Pain *on page 1735*

U.S. Brand Names Combunox™

Generic Available No

Synonyms Ibuprofen and Oxycodone

Pharmacologic Category Analgesic, Narcotic; Nonsteroidal Anti-inflammatory Drug (NSAID), Oral

Dental Use Short-term (≤3-5 days) management of acute, moderate-to-severe pain

Use Short-term (≤7 days) management of acute, moderate-to-severe pain

Local Anesthetic/Vasoconstrictor Precautions No information available to require special precautions

Effects on Dental Treatment Key adverse event(s) related to dental treatment: Nausea, sedation, dizziness. See Dental Comment.

Significant Adverse Effects

>10%:

Central nervous system: Dizziness (5% to 19%), somnolence (7% to 17%)

Gastrointestinal: Nausea (9% to 25%)

2% to 10%:

Cardiovascular: Vasodilation (<1% to 3%)

Central nervous system: Headache (10%), fever (3%)

Gastrointestinal: Constipation (<1% to 5%), vomiting (5%), diarrhea (2%), dyspepsia (<1% to 2%), flatulence (1%)

Neuromuscular & skeletal: Weakness (3%)

Miscellaneous: Diaphoresis (2%)

<2% (Limited to important or life-threatening): Abdominal enlargement/pain, anemia, amblyopia, anxiety, arthritis, back pain, chest pain, chills, edema, euphoria, hyperkinesias, hypertonia, hypokalemia, hypotension, hypoxia, ileus, infection, LFTs increased, lung disorder, pharyngitis, syncope, rash, tachycardia, taste perversion, thrombophlebitis, urinary retention

Restrictions C-II

Dental Usual Dosing Pain: Adults: Oral: Take 1 tablet every 6 hours as needed (maximum: 4 tablets/24 hours); do not take for longer than 7 days

Dosage Oral: Adults: Pain: Take 1 tablet every 6 hours as needed (maximum: 4 tablets/24 hours); do not take for longer than 7 days

Mechanism of Action

Based on **oxycodone** component: Binds to opiate receptors in the CNS, altering the perception of and response to pain; suppresses cough in medullary center; produces generalized CNS depression

Based on **ibuprofen** component: Inhibits prostaglandin synthesis by decreasing the activity of the enzyme, cyclooxygenase, which results in decreased formation of prostaglandin precursors

Contraindications Hypersensitivity to oxycodone, other opioids, ibuprofen, aspirin, other NSAIDs, or any component of the formulation; patients with suspected paralytic ileus; pregnancy (3rd trimester)

Warnings/Precautions Use with caution in elderly or debilitated patients, and those with severe hepatic or renal dysfunction, hypothyroidism, Addison's disease, prostatic hyperplasia, or urethral stricture. Respiratory depression is possible; use with caution in patients with underlying respiratory depression, acute or severe asthma, or hypercarbia. Oxycodone suppresses the cough reflex; use caution postoperatively and in patients with pulmonary disease.

Patients with head injury, increased intracranial pressure, acute abdominal condition, or impaired thyroid function should use this agent cautiously. Tolerance or drug dependence may result from extended use.

NSAIDs are associated with an increased risk of adverse cardiovascular events, including MI, stroke, and new onset or worsening of pre-existing hypertension. Risk may be increased with duration of use or pre-existing cardiovascular risk-factors or disease. Use caution with fluid retention, CHF, or hypertension. Use of NSAIDs can compromise existing renal function. Rehydrate patient before starting therapy. Monitor renal function closely. Ibuprofen is not recommended for patients with advanced renal disease.NSAIDs may increase risk of gastrointestinal irritation, ulceration, bleeding, and perforation. Use caution with a history of GI disease (bleeding or ulcers), concurrent therapy with aspirin, anticoagulants and/or corticosteroids, smoking, use of alcohol, the elderly or debilitated patients. NSAIDs may cause serious skin adverse events. Anaphylactoid reactions may occur, even without prior exposure. Do not use in patients who experience bronchospasm, asthma, rhinitis, or urticaria with NSAID or aspirin therapy. The elderly are at increased risk for adverse effects (especially peptic ulceration, CNS effects, renal toxicity) from NSAIDs even at low doses.

Safety and efficacy in pediatric patients have not been established.

Drug Interactions
Oxycodone: **Substrate** of CYP2D6
Ibuprofen: **Substrate** (minor) of CYP2C8/9, 2C19; **Inhibits** CYP2C8/9 (strong)

See individual agents.

Ethanol/Nutrition/Herb Interactions
Based on **oxycodone** component:
Ethanol: Avoid or limit ethanol (may increase CNS depression). Watch for sedation.
Based on **ibuprofen** component:
Ethanol: Avoid ethanol (may enhance gastric mucosal irritation).
Food: Food or milk are recommended to decrease gastric irritation.
Herb/Nutraceutical: Avoid alfalfa, anise, bilberry, bladderwrack, bromelain, cat's claw, celery, coleus, cordyceps, dong quai, evening primrose, feverfew, fenugreek, garlic, ginger, ginkgo biloboa, red clover, horse chestnut, grapeseed, green tea, ginseng, guggul, horse chestnut seed, horseradish, licorice, prickly ash, red clover, reishi, SAMe, sweet clover, turmeric, white willow (all have additional antiplatelet activity).

Dietary Considerations Take with or without food.

Pharmacodynamics/Kinetics Also see individual agents.
Absorption: Ibuprofen, oxycodone: rapidly absorbed
Protein binding: Ibuprofen: 99%; Oxycodone: 45%
Metabolism: Oxycodone: Hepatic to metabolites, noroxycodone (major), and oxymorphone (minor)
Bioavailability: Oxycodone: increased with food (25%)
Half-life elimination: Ibuprofen: 1.8-2.6 hours; Oxycodone: 3.1-3.7 hours
Time to peak, serum: Ibuprofen: 1.6-3.1 hours; Oxycodone 1.3-2.1 hours
Excretion: Ibuprofen: Urine (<0.2% unchanged); Oxycodone: Urine (~4 % unchanged)

Pregnancy Risk Factor C/D (3rd trimester)

Lactation Enters breast milk/contraindicated

Breast-Feeding Considerations Ibuprofen is not transferred to milk in significant quantities and is considered compatible with breast-feeding by AAP Oxycodone, however, is excreted in breast milk and withdrawal may occur in breast-fed infants when maternal opioid administration is discontinued. Discontinuation of either the opioid-containing medication (Combunox™) or breast-feeding is recommended.

Dosage Forms
Tablet:
Combunox™: 5/400: Oxycodone 5 mg and ibuprofen 400 mg

Dental Comment The combination of oxycodone and ibuprofen in this dose form is appropriate for the management of moderate-to-severe pain when the concomitant anti-inflammatory action of ibuprofen is desired. Oxycodone is recommended only for limited acute dosing (ie, ≤3 days). Oxycodone has an addictive liability, especially when given long term.

Oxycodone Hydrochloride *see* Oxycodone *on page 1163*

OxyContin® *see* Oxycodone *on page 1163*

Oxydose™ *see* Oxycodone *on page 1163*

OxyFast® *see* Oxycodone *on page 1163*

Oxygen (OKS i jen)

Generic Available Yes

Pharmacologic Category Dental Gases

Dental Use Administered as a supplement with nitrous oxide to ensure adequate ventilation during sedation; a resuscitative agent for medical emergencies in dental office

Use Treatment of various clinical disorders, both respiratory and nonrespiratory; relief of arterial hypoxia and secondary complications; treatment of pulmonary hypertension, polycythemia secondary to hypoxemia, chronic disease states complicated by anemia, cancer, migraine headaches, coronary artery disease, seizure disorders, sickle-cell crisis, and sleep apnea

Local Anesthetic/Vasoconstrictor Precautions No information available to require special precautions

Effects on Dental Treatment No significant effects or complications reported

Significant Adverse Effects No data reported

Dental Usual Dosing Administered as a supplement with nitrous oxide to ensure adequate ventilation during sedation: Children and Adults: Average rate of 2 L/minute

Dosage Children and Adults: Average rate of 2 L/minute

Mechanism of Action Increased oxygen in tidal volume and oxygenation of tissues at molecular level

Contraindications No data reported

Warnings/Precautions Oxygen-induced hypoventilation is the greatest potential hazard of oxygen therapy. In patients with severe COPD, the respiratory drive results from hypoxic stimulation of the carotid chemoreceptors. If this hypoxic drive is diminished by excessive oxygen therapy, hypoventilation may occur and further carbon dioxide retention with possible cessation of ventilation.

Drug Interactions No data reported

Pregnancy Risk Factor No data reported

Dosage Forms Liquid system with large reservoir holding 75-100 lb of liquid oxygen; compressed gas system consisting of high-pressure tank; tank sizes are "H" (6900 L of oxygen), "E" (622 L of oxygen) and "D" (356 L of oxygen)

OxyIR® see Oxycodone on page 1163

Oxymetazoline (oks i met AZ oh leen)

Related Information
Bacterial Infections on page 1697

Related Sample Prescriptions
Sinus Infection Treatment on page 1738

U.S. Brand Names Afrin® Extra Moisturizing [OTC]; Afrin® Original [OTC]; Afrin® Severe Congestion [OTC]; Afrin® Sinus [OTC]; Duramist® Plus [OTC]; Duration® [OTC]; Genasal [OTC]; Neo-Synephrine® 12 Hour [OTC]; Neo-Synephrine® 12 Hour Extra Moisturizing [OTC]; Nöstrilla® [OTC]; NRS® [OTC]; Vicks Sinex® 12 Hour [OTC]; Vicks Sinex® 12 Hour Ultrafine Mist [OTC]; Visine® L.R. [OTC]; 4-Way® 12 Hour [OTC]

Canadian Brand Names Claritin® Allergic Decongestant; Dristan® Long Lasting Nasal; Drixoral® Nasal

Mexican Brand Names Afrin®; Iliadin®; Ocuclear®; Oxylin®; Visine A.D.®

Generic Available Yes: Nasal spray

Synonyms Oxymetazoline Hydrochloride

Pharmacologic Category Adrenergic Agonist Agent; Vasoconstrictor

Dental Use Symptomatic relief of nasal mucosal congestion

Use Adjunctive therapy of middle ear infections, associated with acute or chronic rhinitis, the common cold, sinusitis, hay fever, or other allergies
Ophthalmic: Relief of redness of eye due to minor eye irritations

Local Anesthetic/Vasoconstrictor Precautions No information available to require special precautions

Effects on Dental Treatment No significant effects or complications reported

Significant Adverse Effects Frequency not defined.
Cardiovascular: Hypertension, palpitation
Local: Transient burning, stinging
Respiratory: Dryness of the nasal mucosa, rebound congestion with prolonged use, sneezing

Dental Usual Dosing Symptomatic relief of nasal mucosal congestion: Children ≥6 years and Adults: Intranasal (therapy should not exceed 3 days): 0.05% solution: Instill 2-3 sprays into each nostril twice daily

Dosage

Intranasal (therapy should not exceed 3 days): Children ≥6 years and Adults: 0.05% solution: Instill 2-3 sprays into each nostril twice daily

Ophthalmic: Children ≥6 years and Adults: 0.025% solution: Instill 1-2 drops in affected eye(s) every 6 hours as needed or as directed by healthcare provider

Mechanism of Action Stimulates alpha-adrenergic receptors in the arterioles of the nasal mucosa to produce vasoconstriction

Contraindications Hypersensitivity to oxymetazoline or any component of the formulation

Warnings/Precautions

Nasal: Rebound congestion may occur with extended use (>3 days). Prior to self-medication (OTC use), contact healthcare provider in the presence of hypertension, diabetes, hyperthyroidism, heart disease, coronary artery disease, cerebral arteriosclerosis, or long-standing bronchial asthma.

Ophthalmic: Prior to OTC use, contact healthcare provider in the presence of glaucoma or if needed for >72 hours.

Drug Interactions Increased toxicity with MAO inhibitors

Pharmacodynamics/Kinetics

Onset of action: Intranasal: 5-10 minutes

Duration: 5-6 hours

Dosage Forms

Solution, intranasal, as hydrochloride [spray]: 0.05% (15 mL, 30 mL)

Afrin® Extra Moisturizing: 0.05% (15 mL) [contains benzyl alcohol and glycerin; regular or no drip formula]

Afrin® Original: 0.05% (15 mL, 30 mL) [contains benzalkonium chloride]

Afrin® Original: 0.05% (15 mL) [contains benzyl alcohol and benzalkonium chloride; no drip formula]

Afrin® Severe Congestion: 0.05% (15 mL) [contains benzyl alcohol and menthol; regular or no drip formula]

Afrin® Sinus: 0.05% (15 mL) [contains benzyl alcohol, benzalkonium chloride, camphor, phenol; regular or no drip formula]

Duramist® Plus, Neo-Synephrine® 12 Hour, Nōstrilla®, Vicks Sinex® 12 Hour Ultrafine Mist, Vicks Sinex® 12 Hour, 4-Way® 12 Hour: 0.05% (15 mL) [contains benzalkonium chloride]

Duration®: 0.05% (30 mL) [contains benzalkonium chloride]

Genasal, NRS®: 0.05% (15 mL, 30 mL) [contains benzalkonium chloride]

Neo-Synephrine® 12 Hour Extra Moisturizing: 0.05% (15 mL) [contains glycerin]

Solution, ophthalmic, as hydrochloride (Visine® L.R.): 0.025% (15 mL, 30 mL) [contains benzalkonium chloride]

Oxymetazoline Hydrochloride *see* Oxymetazoline *on page 1172*

Oxymetholone (oks i METH oh lone)

U.S. Brand Names Anadrol®

Generic Available No

Pharmacologic Category Anabolic Steroid

Use Treatment of anemias caused by deficient red cell production

Local Anesthetic/Vasoconstrictor Precautions No information available to require special precautions

Effects on Dental Treatment No significant effects or complications reported

Common Adverse Effects Frequency not defined.

Cardiovascular: Coronary artery disease, peripheral edema

Central nervous system: Excitation, insomnia

Dermatologic: Acne (prepubertal males, women); hirsutism (women), hypercalcemia, hyperchloremia, hyperkalemia, hyperphosphatemia, hyperpigmentation; male-pattern baldness (postpubertal males, women)

Endocrine & metabolic: Amenorrhea, cholesterol increased, clitoromegaly, creatinine phosphokinase increased, glucose tolerance decreased, gynecomastia, HDL-cholesterol decreased, hoarseness (women), hypernatremia, impotence (postpubertal males), LDL-cholesterol decreased, libido increased/decreased, menstrual irregularities, oligospermia, phallic enlargement (prepubertal males), priapism (postpubertal males), testicular atrophy (postpubertal males), testicular dysfunction (postpubertal males); virilism (women, high dose); voice deepening (women)

Gastrointestinal: Diarrhea, nausea, vomiting

Genitourinary: Bladder irritability (postpubertal males), epididymitis (postpubertal males), prostatic hyperplasia (elderly males), seminal volume decreased (postpubertal males)

Hematologic: Iron-deficiency anemia, polycythemia, suppression of clotting factors

(Continued)

Oxymetholone *(Continued)*

Hepatic: Cholestatic hepatitis, hepatic necrosis, hepatocellular carcinoma jaundice, liver cell tumors, peliosis hepatic, transaminases increased

Neuromuscular & skeletal: Premature closure of epiphysis (children)

Restrictions C-III

Mechanism of Action Enhances the production and urinary excretion of erythropoietin in patients with anemias due to bone marrow failure; stimulates erythropoiesis in anemias due to deficient red cell production.

Drug Interactions

Increased Effect/Toxicity: Androgens may enhance the hepatotoxic effect of cyclosporine; may enhance the anticoagulant effect of warfarin

Pregnancy Risk Factor X

Oxymorphone *(oks i MOR fone)*

U.S. Brand Names Numorphan®

Generic Available No

Synonyms Oxymorphone Hydrochloride

Pharmacologic Category Analgesic, Narcotic

Use Management of moderate to severe pain and preoperatively as a sedative and a supplement to anesthesia

Local Anesthetic/Vasoconstrictor Precautions No information available to require special precautions

Effects on Dental Treatment Key adverse event(s) related to dental treatment: Anticholinergic side effects can cause a reduction of saliva production or secretion, contributing to discomfort and dental disease (ie, caries, oral candidiasis, and periodontal disease).

Common Adverse Effects

>10%:

Cardiovascular: Hypotension

Central nervous system: Fatigue, drowsiness, dizziness

Gastrointestinal: Nausea, vomiting, constipation

Neuromuscular & skeletal: Weakness

Miscellaneous: Histamine release

1% to 10%:

Central nervous system: Nervousness, headache, restlessness, malaise, confusion

Gastrointestinal: Anorexia, stomach cramps, xerostomia, biliary spasm

Genitourinary: Decreased urination, ureteral spasms

Local: Pain at injection site

Respiratory: Dyspnea

Restrictions C-II

Mechanism of Action Oxymorphone hydrochloride (Numorphan®) is a potent narcotic analgesic with uses similar to those of morphine. The drug is a semisynthetic derivative of morphine (phenanthrene derivative) and is closely related to hydromorphone chemically (Dilaudid®).

Drug Interactions

Increased Effect/Toxicity: Increased effect/toxicity with CNS depressants (phenothiazines, tranquilizers, anxiolytics, sedatives, hypnotics, alcohol), tricyclic antidepressants, and dextroamphetamine.

Decreased Effect: Decreased effect with phenothiazines.

Pharmacodynamics/Kinetics

Onset of action: Analgesic: I.V., I.M., SubQ: 5-10 minutes; Rectal: 15-30 minutes

Duration: Analgesic: Parenteral, rectal: 3-4 hours

Metabolism: Hepatic via glucuronidation

Excretion: Urine

Pregnancy Risk Factor B/D (prolonged use or high doses at term)

Oxymorphone Hydrochloride *see* Oxymorphone *on page 1174*

Oxytetracycline *(oks i tet ra SYE kleen)*

U.S. Brand Names Terramycin® I.M. [DSC]

Canadian Brand Names Terramycin®

Mexican Brand Names Oxitraklin®; Terramicina®

Generic Available No

Synonyms Oxytetracycline Hydrochloride

Pharmacologic Category Antibiotic, Tetracycline Derivative

Use Treatment of susceptible bacterial infections; both gram-positive and gram-negative, as well as, *Rickettsia* and *Mycoplasma* organisms

Local Anesthetic/Vasoconstrictor Precautions No information available to require special precautions

Effects on Dental Treatment Tetracyclines are not recommended for use during pregnancy or in children ≤8 years of age since they have been reported to cause enamel hypoplasia and permanent teeth discoloration. Tetracyclines should only be used in these patients if other agents are contraindicated or alternative antimicrobials will not eradicate the organism. Long-term use associated with oral candidiasis.

Common Adverse Effects Frequency not defined; also refer to Tetracycline monograph

Cardiovascular: Pericarditis

Central nervous system: Bulging fontanels (infants), intracranial hypertension (adults)

Dermatologic: Angioneurotic edema, erythematous rash, exfoliative dermatitis (uncommon), maculopapular rash, photosensitivity, urticaria

Gastrointestinal: Anogenital inflammatory lesions, diarrhea, dysphagia, enamel hypoplasia, enterocolitis, glossitis, nausea, tooth discoloration, vomiting

Hematologic: Anemia, eosinophilia, neutropenia, thrombocytopenia

Local: Irritation

Renal: BUN increased

Miscellaneous: Anaphylactoid purpura, anaphylaxis, hypersensitivity reaction, SLE exacerbation

Mechanism of Action Inhibits bacterial protein synthesis by binding with the 30S and possibly the 50S ribosomal subunit(s) of susceptible bacteria, cell wall synthesis is not affected

Drug Interactions

Increased Effect/Toxicity: Oral anticoagulant (warfarin) effects may be increased.

Decreased Effect: Barbiturates, phenytoin, and carbamazepine decrease serum levels of tetracyclines. Although anecdotal reports suggest oral contraceptive efficacy could be reduced by tetracyclines, this has been refuted by more rigorous scientific and clinical data.

Pharmacodynamics/Kinetics

Absorption: Poor

Distribution: Crosses placenta

Metabolism: Hepatic (small amounts)

Half-life elimination: 8.5-9.6 hours; prolonged with renal impairment

Excretion: Urine; feces

Pregnancy Risk Factor D

Oxytetracycline Hydrochloride *see* Oxytetracycline *on page 1174*

Oxytocin (oks i TOE sin)

U.S. Brand Names Pitocin®

Canadian Brand Names Pitocin®; Syntocinon®

Mexican Brand Names Syntocinon®; Xitocin®

Generic Available Yes

Synonyms Pit

Pharmacologic Category Oxytocic Agent

Use Induction of labor at term; control of postpartum bleeding; adjunctive therapy in management of abortion

Local Anesthetic/Vasoconstrictor Precautions No information available to require special precautions

Effects on Dental Treatment No significant effects or complications reported

Common Adverse Effects Frequency not defined.

Fetus or neonate:

Cardiovascular: Arrhythmias (including premature ventricular contractions), bradycardia

Central nervous system: Brain or CNS damage (permanent), neonatal seizure

Hepatic: Neonatal jaundice

Ocular: Neonatal retinal hemorrhage

Miscellaneous: Fetal death, low Apgar score (5 minute)

Mother:

Cardiovascular: Arrhythmias, hypertensive episodes, premature ventricular contractions

Gastrointestinal: Nausea, vomiting

(Continued)

Oxytocin *(Continued)*

Genitourinary: Pelvic hematoma, postpartum hemorrhage, uterine hypertonicity, tetanic contraction of the uterus, uterine rupture, uterine spasm

Hematologic: Afibrinogenemia (fatal)

Miscellaneous: Anaphylactic reaction, subarachnoid hemorrhage

Mechanism of Action Produces the rhythmic uterine contractions characteristic to delivery

Drug Interactions

Increased Effect/Toxicity: Dinoprostone and misoprostol may increase the effect of oxytocin; wait 6-12 hours after dinoprostone or misoprostol administration before initiating oxytocin.

Pharmacodynamics/Kinetics

Onset of action: Uterine contractions: I.M.: 3-5 minutes; I.V.: ~1 minute

Duration: I.M.: 2-3 hour; I.V.: 1 hour

Metabolism: Rapidly hepatic and via plasma (by oxytocinase) and to a smaller degree the mammary gland

Half-life elimination: 1-5 minutes

Excretion: Urine

Pregnancy Risk Factor X

Oxytrol® *see* Oxybutynin *on page 1162*

Oysco 500 [OTC] *see* Calcium Carbonate *on page 248*

Oyst-Cal 500 [OTC] *see* Calcium Carbonate *on page 248*

P-V Tussin Tablet *see* Hydrocodone and Pseudoephedrine *on page 788*

P-071 *see* Cetirizine *on page 306*

Pacerone® *see* Amiodarone *on page 90*

Paclitaxel *(PAK li taks el)*

U.S. Brand Names Onxol™; Taxol®

Canadian Brand Names Taxol®

Generic Available Yes

Synonyms NSC-125973; NSC-673089

Pharmacologic Category Antineoplastic Agent, Antimicrotubular; Antineoplastic Agent, Natural Source (Plant) Derivative

Use Treatment of breast, lung (small cell and nonsmall cell), and ovarian cancers; treatment of AIDS-related Kaposi's sarcoma (KS)

Unlabeled/Investigational Use Treatment of bladder, cervical, prostate, and head and neck cancers

Local Anesthetic/Vasoconstrictor Precautions No information available to require special precautions

Effects on Dental Treatment Key adverse event(s) related to dental treatment: Severe, potentially dose-limiting mucositis and stomatitis.

Common Adverse Effects Percentages reported with single-agent therapy, first- or second-line treatment. **Note:** Myelosuppression is dose related, schedule related, and infusion-rate dependent (increased incidences with higher doses, more frequent doses, and longer infusion times) and, in general, rapidly reversible upon discontinuation.

>10%:

Cardiovascular: Flushing (28%), ECG abnormal (14% to 23%), edema (21%), hypotension (4% to 12%),

Dermatologic: Alopecia (87%), rash (12%)

Gastrointestinal: Nausea/vomiting (52%), diarrhea (38%), mucositis (17% to 35%; grades 3/4: up to 3%), stomatitis (15%; most common at doses >390 mg/m^2), abdominal pain (with intraperitoneal paclitaxel)

Hematologic: Neutropenia (78% to 98%; grade 4: 14% to 75%; onset 8-10 days, median nadir 11 days, recovery 15-21 days), leukopenia (90%; grade 4: 17%), anemia (47% to 90%; grades 3/4: 2% to 16%), thrombocytopenia (4% to 20%; grades 3/4: 1% to 7%), bleeding (14%)

Hepatic: Alkaline Phosphatase increased (22%), AST increased (19%)

Local: Injection site reaction (erythema, tenderness, skin discoloration, swelling: 13%)

Neuromuscular & skeletal: Peripheral neuropathy (42% to 70%; grades 3/4: up to 7%), arthralgia/myalgia (60%), weakness (17%)

Renal: Creatinine increased (observed in KS patients only: 18% to 34%; severe: 5% to 7%)

Miscellaneous: Hypersensitivity reaction (31% to 45%; grades 3/4: up to 2%), infection (15% to 30%)

1% to 10%:

Cardiovascular: Bradycardia (3%), tachycardia (2%), hypertension (1%), rhythm abnormalities (1%), syncope (1%), venous thrombosis (1%)

Dermatologic: Nail changes (2%)
Hematologic: Febrile neutropenia (2%)
Hepatic: Bilirubin increased (7%)
Respiratory: Dyspnea (2%)

Mechanism of Action Paclitaxel promotes microtubule assembly by enhancing the action of tubulin dimers, stabilizing existing microtubules, and inhibiting their disassembly, interfering with the late G_2 mitotic phase, and inhibiting cell replication. In addition, the drug can distort mitotic spindles, resulting in the breakage of chromosomes. Paclitaxel may also suppress cell proliferation and modulate immune response.

Drug Interactions

Cytochrome P450 Effect: Substrate (major) of CYP2C8/9, 3A4; **Induces** CYP3A4 (weak)

Increased Effect/Toxicity: CYP2C8/9 inhibitors may increase the levels/ effects of paclitaxel; example inhibitors include delavirdine, fluconazole, gemfibrozil, ketoconazole, nicardipine, NSAIDs, pioglitazone, and sulfonamides. CYP3A4 inhibitors may increase the levels/effects of paclitaxel; example inhibitors include azole antifungals, clarithromycin, diclofenac, doxycycline, erythromycin, imatinib, isoniazid, nefazodone, nicardipine, propofol, protease inhibitors, quinidine, telithromycin, and verapamil. In Phase I trials, myelosuppression was more profound when given after cisplatin than with alternative sequence. administered as sequential infusions, studies indicate a potential for increased toxicity when platinum derivatives (carboplatin, cisplatin) are administered before taxane derivatives (docetaxel, paclitaxel). Paclitaxel may increase doxorubicin levels/toxicity.

Decreased Effect: CYP2C8/9 inducers may decrease the levels/effects of paclitaxel; example inducers include carbamazepine, phenobarbital, phenytoin, rifampin, rifapentine, and secobarbital. CYP3A4 inducers may decrease the levels/effects of paclitaxel; example inducers include aminoglutethimide, carbamazepine, nafcillin, nevirapine, phenobarbital, phenytoin, and rifamycins.

Pharmacodynamics/Kinetics

Distribution:

V_d: Widely distributed into body fluids and tissues; affected by dose and duration of infusion

V_{dss}:
1- to 6-hour infusion: 67.1 L/m^2
24-hour infusion: 227-688 L/m^2

Protein binding: 89% to 98%

Metabolism: Hepatic via CYP2C8 and 3A4; forms metabolites (primarily 6α-hydroxypaclitaxel)

Half-life elimination:
1- to 6-hour infusion: Mean (beta): 6.4 hours
3-hour infusion: Mean (terminal): 13.1-20.2 hours
24-hour infusion: Mean (terminal): 15.7-52.7 hours

Excretion: Feces (~70%, 5% as unchanged drug); urine (14%)

Clearance: Mean: Total body: After 1- and 6-hour infusions: 5.8-16.3 L/hour/ m^2; After 24-hour infusions: 14.2-17.2 L/hour/m^2

Pregnancy Risk Factor D

Paclitaxel (Protein Bound) (PAK li taks el PROE teen bownd)

U.S. Brand Names Abraxane™

Generic Available No

Synonyms BI-007; NAB-Paclitaxel; Protein-Bound Paclitaxel

Pharmacologic Category Antineoplastic Agent, Antimicrotubular; Antineoplastic Agent, Natural Source (Plant) Derivative

Use Treatment of breast cancer (second-line)

Local Anesthetic/Vasoconstrictor Precautions No information available to require special precautions

Effects on Dental Treatment Key adverse event(s) related to dental treatment: Mucositis.

Common Adverse Effects

>10%:
Cardiovascular: EKG abnormal (60%)
Dermatologic: Alopecia (90%)
Gastrointestinal: Nausea (30%; severe 3%), diarrhea (26%; severe <1%), vomiting (18%; severe 4%)
Hematologic: Neutropenia (80%; grade 4 - 9%), anemia (33%; severe 1%)
Hepatic: AST increased (39%), alkaline phosphatase increased (36%)

(Continued)

Paclitaxel (Protein Bound) *(Continued)*

Neuromuscular & skeletal: Sensory neuropathy (71%; severe 10%), asthenia (47%; severe 8%), myalgia/arthralgia (44%; severe 8%)

Ocular: Vision disturbance (13%; severe 1%)

Respiratory: Dyspnea (12%)

Miscellaneous: Infections (24%; primarily included oral candidiasis, respiratory tract infections, and pneumonia)

1% to 10%:

Cardiovascular: Edema (10%; severe 0%), hypotension (5%), cardiovascular events (grade 3 - 3%; included chest pain, cardiac arrest, supraventricular tachycardia, edema, thrombosis, pulmonary thromboembolism, pulmonary emboli, and hypertension)

Central nervous system: Febrile neutropenia (2%)

Gastrointestinal: Mucositis (7%; severe <1%)

Hematologic: Thrombocytopenia (2%), bleeding (2%)

Hepatic: Bilirubin increased (7%)

Local: Injection site reaction (1%)

Renal: Creatinine increased (11%; severe 1%)

Respiratory: Cough (6%)

Miscellaneous: Hypersensitivity reaction (4%)

Mechanism of Action Paclitaxel promotes microtubule assembly by enhancing the action of tubulin dimers, stabilizing existing microtubules, and inhibiting their disassembly, interfering with the late G_2 mitotic phase, and inhibiting cell replication. In addition, the drug can distort mitotic spindles, resulting in the breakage of chromosomes. Paclitaxel may also suppress cell proliferation and modulate immune response.

Drug Interactions

Cytochrome P450 Effect: Substrate (major) of CYP2C8/9, 3A4; Induces CYP3A4 (weak)

Increased Effect/Toxicity: CYP2C8/9 inhibitors may increase the levels/effects of paclitaxel; example inhibitors include delavirdine, fluconazole, gemfibrozil, ketoconazole, nicardipine, NSAIDs, pioglitazone, and sulfonamides. CYP3A4 inhibitors may increase the levels/effects of paclitaxel; example inhibitors include azole antifungals, clarithromycin, diclofenac, doxycycline, erythromycin, imatinib, isoniazid, nefazodone, nicardipine, propofol, protease inhibitors, quinidine, telithromycin, and verapamil. In Phase I trials, myelosuppression was more profound when given after cisplatin than with alternative sequence. administered as sequential infusions, studies indicate a potential for increased toxicity when platinum derivatives (carboplatin, cisplatin) are administered before taxane derivatives (docetaxel, paclitaxel). Paclitaxel may increase doxorubicin levels/toxicity.

Decreased Effect: CYP2C8/9 inducers may decrease the levels/effects of paclitaxel; example inducers include carbamazepine, phenobarbital, phenytoin, rifampin, rifapentine, and secobarbital. CYP3A4 inducers may decrease the levels/effects of paclitaxel; example inducers include aminoglutethimide, carbamazepine, nafcillin, nevirapine, phenobarbital, phenytoin, and rifamycins.

Pharmacodynamics/Kinetics

Distribution: V_d: 632 L/m^2

Protein binding: 89% to 98%

Metabolism: Hepatic via CYP3A4 and 2C8

Half-life elimination: Terminal: 27 hours

Excretion: Urine (4% as unchanged drug, 1% as metabolites); feces (20%)

Clearance 15 L/hour/m^2

Pregnancy Risk Factor D

Pain-A-Lay® [OTC] *see* Phenol *on page 1223*

Pain Eze [OTC] *see* Acetaminophen *on page 31*

Pain-Off [OTC] *see* Acetaminophen, Aspirin, and Caffeine *on page 41*

Palgic *see* Carbinoxamine *on page 268*

Palgic®-D *see* Carbinoxamine and Pseudoephedrine *on page 268*

Palgic®-DS *see* Carbinoxamine and Pseudoephedrine *on page 268*

Palifermin *(pal ee FER min)*

U.S. Brand Names Kepivance™

Generic Available No

Synonyms AMJ 9701; rHu-KGF

Pharmacologic Category Keratinocyte Growth Factor

Dental Use Decrease the incidence and severity of severe oral mucositis associated with hematologic malignancies in patients receiving myelotoxic therapy requiring hematopoietic stem cell support

Use Decrease the incidence and severity of severe oral mucositis associated with hematologic malignancies in patients receiving myelotoxic therapy requiring hematopoietic stem cell support

Local Anesthetic/Vasoconstrictor Precautions No information available to require special precautions

Effects on Dental Treatment Key adverse event(s) related to dental treatment: Taste alteration, mouth/tongue discoloration or thickness. See Dental Comment.

Significant Adverse Effects

>10%:

Cardiovascular: Edema (28%), hypertension (7% to 14%)

Central nervous system: Fever (39%), pain (16%), dysesthesia (12%)

Dermatologic: Rash (62%), pruritus (35%), erythema (32%)

Gastrointestinal: Mouth/tongue discoloration or thickness (17%), taste alteration (16%)

Miscellaneous: Serum amylase increased (grade 3/4, 38%); serum lipase increased (grade 3/4, 11%)

1% to 10%: Neuromuscular & skeletal: Arthralgia (10%)

Dental Usual Dosing Oral mucositis: Adults: I.V.: 60 mcg/kg/day for 3 consecutive days before and after myelotoxic therapy; total of 6 doses

Dosage I.V.: Adults: 60 mcg/kg/day for 3 consecutive days before and after myelotoxic therapy; total of 6 doses. **Note:** Administer first 3 doses prior to myelotoxic therapy, with the 3rd dose given 24-48 hours before therapy begins. The last 3 doses should be administered after myelotoxic therapy, with the first of these doses after but on the same day of hematopoietic stem cell infusion and at least 4 days after the most recent dose of palifermin.

Mechanism of Action Palifermin is a recombinant keratinocyte growth factor (KGF) produced in *E. coli*. Endogenous KGF is produced by mesenchymal cells in response to epithelial tissue injury. KGF binds to the KGF receptor resulting in proliferation, differentiation and migration of epithelial cells in multiple tissues, including (but not limited to) the tongue, buccal mucosa, esophagus, and salivary gland.

Contraindications Hypersensitivity to palifermin, *E. coli*-derived proteins, or any component of the formulation

Warnings/Precautions Safety and efficacy have not been established with nonhematologic malignancies; effect on the growth of nonhematopoietic human tumors is not known. Palifermin should be administered prior to and following, but not with, chemotherapy. If administered within 24 hours of chemotherapy, palifermin may increase the severity and duration of mucositis due to the increased sensitivity of rapidly-dividing epithelial cells. Safety and efficacy have not been established in children.

Drug Interactions Drug interaction studies have not been conducted.

Pharmacodynamics/Kinetics Half-life elimination: 4.5 hours (range: 3.3-5.7 hours)

Pregnancy Risk Factor C

Lactation Excretion in breast milk unknown/use caution

Dosage Forms Injection, powder for reconstitution [preservative free]: 6.25 mg [contains mannitol 50 mg, sucrose 25 mg]

Dental Comment Palifermin works at the cellular level by protecting the epithelial cells lining the mouth and throat from damage caused by chemotherapy and radiation and by stimulating the growth and development of new epithelial cells to build up the mucosal barrier.

Palivizumab (pah li VIZ u mab)

U.S. Brand Names Synagis®

Canadian Brand Names Synagis®

Generic Available No

Pharmacologic Category Monoclonal Antibody

Use Prevention of serious lower respiratory tract disease caused by respiratory syncytial virus (RSV) in infants and children <2 years of age at high risk of RSV disease

Local Anesthetic/Vasoconstrictor Precautions No information available to require special precautions

Effects on Dental Treatment No significant effects or complications reported

(Continued)

Palivizumab (Continued)

Common Adverse Effects The incidence of adverse events was similar between the palivizumab and placebo groups.

>1%:

Central nervous system: Nervousness, fever

Dermatologic: Fungal dermatitis, eczema, seborrhea, rash

Gastrointestinal: Diarrhea, vomiting, gastroenteritis

Hematologic: Anemia

Hepatic: ALT increase, abnormal LFTs

Local: Injection site reaction, erythema, induration

Ocular: Conjunctivitis

Otic: Otitis media

Respiratory: Cough, wheezing, bronchiolitis, pneumonia, bronchitis, asthma, croup, dyspnea, sinusitis, apnea, upper respiratory infection, rhinitis

Miscellaneous: Oral moniliasis, failure to thrive, viral infection, flu syndrome

Postmarketing and/or case reports: Hypersensitivity reactions, anaphylaxis (very rare)

Mechanism of Action Exhibits neutralizing and fusion-inhibitory activity against RSV; these activities inhibit RSV replication in laboratory and clinical studies

Pharmacodynamics/Kinetics

Half-life elimination: Children <24 months: 20 days; Adults: 18 days

Time to peak, serum: 48 hours

Pregnancy Risk Factor C

Palladone™ *[Withdrawn]* see Hydromorphone on page 797

Palmer's® Skin Success Acne [OTC] *see* Benzoyl Peroxide on page 194

Palmer's® Skin Success Acne Cleanser [OTC] *see* Salicylic Acid on page 1374

Palmer's® Skin Success Eventone® Fade Cream [OTC] *see* Hydroquinone on page 798

Palmitate-A® [OTC] *see* Vitamin A on page 1580

Palonosetron (pal oh NOE se tron)

U.S. Brand Names Aloxi®

Generic Available No

Synonyms Palonosetron Hydrochloride; RS-25259; RS-25259-197

Pharmacologic Category Antiemetic; Selective 5-HT$_3$ Receptor Antagonist

Use Prevention of acute (within 24 hours) and delayed (2-5 days) chemotherapy-induced nausea and vomiting

Note: Not recommended for treatment of existing chemotherapy-induced emesis (CIE)

Unlabeled/Investigational Use Prevention of postoperative vomiting

Local Anesthetic/Vasoconstrictor Precautions No information available to require special precautions

Effects on Dental Treatment No significant effects or complications reported

Common Adverse Effects

>10%: Dermatologic: Pruritus (8% to 22%)

1% to 10%:

Cardiovascular: Bradycardia (1%), hypotension (1%), tachycardia (nonsustained) (1%)

Central nervous system: Headache (6% to 9%), anxiety (1% to 5%), dizziness (1%)

Endocrine & metabolic: Hyperkalemia (1%)

Gastrointestinal: Constipation (5% to 10%), diarrhea (1%)

Neuromuscular & skeletal: Weakness (1%)

Mechanism of Action Selective 5-HT$_3$ receptor antagonist, blocking serotonin, both peripherally on vagal nerve terminals and centrally in the chemoreceptor trigger zone

Drug Interactions

Cytochrome P450 Effect: Substrate (minor) of CYP1A2, 2D6, 3A4

Increased Effect/Toxicity: Palonosetron may enhance the hypotensive effect of apomorphine; concurrent use is contraindicated.

Pharmacodynamics/Kinetics

Distribution: V$_d$: 8.3 ± 2.5 L/kg

Protein binding: 62%

Metabolism: ~50% metabolized via CYP enzymes (and likely other pathways) to relatively inactive metabolites (N-oxide-palonosetron and 6-S-hydroxy-palonosetron); CYP1A2, 2D6, and 3A4 contribute to its metabolism

Half-life elimination: Terminal: 40 hours
Excretion: Urine (80%, 40% as unchanged drug)
Pregnancy Risk Factor B

Palonosetron Hydrochloride *see* Palonosetron *on page 1180*

Pamelor® *see* Nortriptyline *on page 1128*

Pamidronate (pa mi DROE nate)

U.S. Brand Names Aredia®
Canadian Brand Names Aredia®; Pamidronate Disodium®
Generic Available Yes
Synonyms Pamidronate Disodium
Pharmacologic Category Antidote; Bisphosphonate Derivative
Use Treatment of hypercalcemia associated with malignancy; treatment of osteo-lytic bone lesions associated with multiple myeloma or metastatic breast cancer; moderate to severe Paget's disease of bone
Unlabeled/Investigational Use Treatment of pediatric osteoporosis, treatment of osteogenesis imperfecta
Local Anesthetic/Vasoconstrictor Precautions No information available to require special precautions
Effects on Dental Treatment Osteonecrosis of the jaw (ONJ), generally asso-ciated with local infection and/or tooth extraction and often with delayed healing, has been reported in patients taking bisphosphonates. Most reported cases of bisphosphonate-associated osteonecrosis have been in cancer patients treated with intravenous bisphosphonates. However, some have occurred in patients with postmenopausal osteoporosis taking oral bisphosphonates. Dental surgery may exacerbate ONJ. For patients requiring dental procedures, there are no data available to suggest whether discontinuation of bisphosphonate treatment reduces the risk of ONJ. See Dental Comment.
Common Adverse Effects Percentage of adverse effect varies upon dose and duration of infusion.
>10%:
  Central nervous system: Fatigue (12% to 40%), fever (18% to 39%), head-ache (24% to 27%), anxiety (8% to 18%), insomnia (1% to 25%), pain (13% to 15%)
  Endocrine & metabolic: Hypophosphatemia (9% to 18%), hypokalemia (4% to 18%), hypomagnesemia (4% to 12%), hypocalcemia (1% to 12%)
  Gastrointestinal: Nausea (4% to 64%), vomiting (4% to 46%), anorexia (1% to 31%), abdominal pain (1% to 24%), dyspepsia (4% to 23%)
  Genitourinary: Urinary tract infection (15% to 20%)
  Hematologic: Anemia (6% to 48%), leukopenia (4% to 21%)
  Local: Infusion site reaction (4% to 18%)
  Neuromuscular & skeletal: Weakness (16% to 26%), myalgia (1% to 26%), arthralgia (11% to 15%)
  Renal: Serum creatinine increased (19%)
  Respiratory: Dyspnea (22% to 35%), cough (25% to 26%), upper respiratory tract infection (3% to 20%), sinusitis (15% to 16%), pleural effusion (3% to 15%)
1% to 10%:
  Cardiovascular: Atrial fibrillation (6%), hypertension (6%), syncope (6%), tach-ycardia (6%), atrial flutter (1%), cardiac failure (1%), edema (1%)
  Central nervous system: Somnolence (1% to 6%), psychosis (4%)
  Endocrine & metabolic: Hypothyroidism (6%)
  Gastrointestinal: Constipation (4% to 6%), gastrointestinal hemorrhage (6%), diarrhea (1%), stomatitis (1%)
  Hematologic: Neutropenia (1%), thrombocytopenia (1%)
  Neuromuscular & skeletal: Back pain (5%), bone pain (5%)
  Renal: Uremia (4%)
  Respiratory: Rales (6%), rhinitis (6%)
  Miscellaneous: Moniliasis (6%)
Mechanism of Action A bisphosphonate which inhibits bone resorption via actions on osteoclasts or on osteoclast precursors. Does not appear to produce any significant effects on renal tubular calcium handling and is poorly absorbed following oral administration (high oral doses have been reported effective); therefore, I.V. therapy is preferred.

Drug Interactions
  Increased Effect/Toxicity: Aminoglycosides may lower serum calcium levels with prolonged administration; concomitant use may have an additive hypocalcemic effect. NSAIDs may enhance the gastrointestinal adverse/toxic effects (increased incidence of GI ulcers) of bisphosphonate derivatives. (Continued)

Pamidronate *(Continued)*

Bisphosphonate derivatives may enhance the hypocalcemic effect of phosphate supplements.

Decreased Effect: The following agents may decrease the absorption of oral bisphosphonate derivatives: Antacids (aluminum, calcium, magnesium), oral calcium salts, oral iron salts, and oral magnesium salts.

Pharmacodynamics/Kinetics

Onset of action: 24-48 hours

Peak effect: Maximum: 5-7 days

Absorption: Poor; pharmacokinetic studies lacking

Metabolism: Not metabolized

Half-life elimination: 21-35 hours

Excretion: Biphasic; urine (~50% as unchanged drug) within 120 hours

Pregnancy Risk Factor D

Dental Comment

"Dear Dental Health Professional" Letter Issued for Intravenous Bisphosphonates, Pamidronate and Zoledronic Acid, Regarding the Risk of Osteonecrosis of the Jaw (ONJ) in Cancer Patients - May 2005

Novartis Pharmaceuticals Corporation has notified dental health professionals of the risk of **osteonecrosis of the jaw (ONJ)** and the use of the bisphosphonates, pamidronate, and zoledronic acid. Often observed in patients receiving chemotherapy and corticosteroids, reports of ONJ (the majority being associated with dental procedures) have been documented in cancer patients. Consequently, the manufacturer recommends that a dental examination precede therapy in cancer patients beginning I.V. bisphosphonate therapy. Additionally, invasive dental procedures should be avoided during therapy; patients developing ONJ while on bisphosphonate therapy should not have invasive dental procedures because the condition may be exacerbated. It has not been determined whether the discontinuation of bisphosphonate therapy in patients requiring dental surgery decreases the risk of ONJ. The treating healthcare professional is encouraged to assess the benefits and risks.

Additional information is available at: http://www.fda.gov/medwatch/SAFETY/ 2005/safety05.htm#zometa2, or by contacting Novartis Oncology Medical Services at 1-888-669-6682.

Previously, Novartis and the Food and Drug Administration (FDA) had notified healthcare providers of a serious adverse event related to the use of bisphosphonates. Osteonecrosis of the jaw has been reported in patients with cancer who were receiving chemotherapy, corticosteroids, and chronic bisphosphonate therapy. Dental exams and preventative dentistry should be performed prior to placing patients with risk factors (chemotherapy, corticosteroids, poor oral hygiene) on chronic bisphosphonate therapy. Invasive dental procedures should be avoided during treatment. Product labeling for pamidronate (Aredia®) and zoledronic acid (Zometa®) have been updated. Recently, 63 cases of osteonecrosis associated with the use of bisphosphonates were published (Ruggiero, 2004). In a retrospective review, 56 of the patients received intravenous bisphosphonates for at least 1 year and 7 patients were on chronic oral therapy. The presenting symptom was a nonhealing extraction socket or an exposed jawbone. These lesions did not show evidence of metastatic disease and required removal of involved bone in most cases.

Bisphosphonates are widely used in the management of metastatic bone disease to treat hypercalcemia associated with malignancies and to treat osteoporosis. In the report by Ruggiero et al, the cluster of patients observed to have necrotic lesions in the jaw shared only one common clinical feature, all received chronic bisphosphonate therapy. The necrosis detected was typical of osteoradionecrosis. It was suggested that because of the trend in the use of chronic bisphosphonate therapy, the observation of an associated risk of osteonecrosis of the jaw should alert practitioners to monitor for this previously unrecognized potential complication.

Selected Readings

Ruggiero SL, Mehrotra B, Rosenberg TJ, et al, "Osteonecrosis of the Jaws Associated With the Use of Bisphosphonates: A Review of 63 Cases," *J Oral Maxillofac Surg*, 2004, 62(5):527-34.

Pamidronate Disodium *see* Pamidronate *on page 1181*

Pamine® *see* Methscopolamine *on page 1019*

Pamine® Forte *see* Methscopolamine *on page 1019*

p-Aminoclonidine *see* Apraclonidine *on page 133*

Pamix™ [OTC] *see* Pyrantel Pamoate *on page 1314*

Pamprin® Maximum Strength All Day Relief [OTC] *see* Naproxen *on page 1089*

Pan-2400™ [OTC] *see* Pancreatin *on page 1183*

Panafil® *see* Chlorophyllin, Papain, and Urea *on page 319*

Pan-B Antibody *see* Rituximab *on page 1360*

Pancof® *see* Pseudoephedrine, Dihydrocodeine, and Chlorpheniramine *on page 1312*

Pancof®-EXP *see* Dihydrocodeine, Pseudoephedrine, and Guaifenesin *on page 476*

Pancof®-PD *see* Dihydrocodeine, Chlorpheniramine, and Phenylephrine *on page 476*

Pancrease® [DSC] *see* Pancrelipase *on page 1183*

Pancrease® MT *see* Pancrelipase *on page 1183*

Pancreatin (PAN kree a tin)

U.S. Brand Names Hi-Vegi-Lip [OTC]; kutrase®; ku-zyme®; Pan-2400™ [OTC]; Pancreatin 4X [OTC]; Pancreatin 8X [OTC]; Veg-Pancreatin 4X [OTC]

Mexican Brand Names Creon®; Optifree®; Pancrease®; Selecto®

Generic Available Yes

Pharmacologic Category Enzyme

Use Relief of functional indigestion due to enzyme deficiency or imbalance

Local Anesthetic/Vasoconstrictor Precautions No information available to require special precautions

Effects on Dental Treatment No significant effects or complications reported

Common Adverse Effects Frequency not defined.

Gastrointestinal: Loose stools (decrease dose)

Respiratory: Mucous membrane irritation or precipitation of asthma attack (due to inhalation of airborne powder)

Mechanism of Action An enzyme supplement, not a replacement, which contains a combination of lipase, amylase and protease. Enhances the digestion of proteins, starch and fat in the stomach and intestines.

Pregnancy Risk Factor C

Pancreatin 4X [OTC] *see* Pancreatin *on page 1183*

Pancreatin 8X [OTC] *see* Pancreatin *on page 1183*

Pancrecarb MS® *see* Pancrelipase *on page 1183*

Pancrelipase (pan kre LI pase)

U.S. Brand Names Creon®; Dygase; ku-zyme® HP; Lapase; Lipram 4500; Lipram-CR; Lipram-PN; Lipram-UL; Pancrease® [DSC]; Pancrease® MT; Pancrecarb MS®; Pangestyme™ CN; Pangestyme™ EC; Pangestyme™ MT; Pangestyme™ UL; Panokase®; Panokase® 16; Plaretase® 8000; Ultrase®; Ultrase® MT; Viokase®

Canadian Brand Names Cotazym®; Creon® 5; Creon® 10; Creon® 20; Creon® 25; Pancrease®; Pancrease® MT; Ultrase®; Ultrase® MT; Viokase®

Generic Available Yes

Synonyms Lipancreatin

Pharmacologic Category Enzyme

Use Replacement therapy in symptomatic treatment of malabsorption syndrome caused by pancreatic insufficiency

Unlabeled/Investigational Use Treatment of occluded feeding tubes

Local Anesthetic/Vasoconstrictor Precautions No information available to require special precautions

Effects on Dental Treatment No significant effects or complications reported

Common Adverse Effects Frequency not defined; occurrence of events may be dose related.

Central nervous system: Pain

Dermatologic: Rash

Endocrine & metabolic: Hyperuricemia

Gastrointestinal: Nausea, cramps, constipation, diarrhea, perianal irritation/inflammation (large doses), irritation of the mouth, abdominal pain, intestinal obstruction, vomiting, flatulence, melena, weight loss, fibrotic strictures, greasy stools

Ocular: Lacrimation

Renal: Hyperuricosuria

Respiratory: Sneezing, dyspnea, bronchospasm

Miscellaneous: Allergic reactions

Mechanism of Action Pancrelipase is a natural product harvested from the hog pancreas. It contains a combination of lipase, amylase, and protease. Products are formulated to dissolve in the more basic pH of the duodenum so that they may act locally to break down fats, protein, and starch.

Pharmacodynamics/Kinetics

Absorption: None; acts locally in GI tract

Excretion: Feces

Pregnancy Risk Factor B/C (product specific)

Pandel® *see* Hydrocortisone *on page 793*

Pangestyme™ CN *see* Pancrelipase *on page 1183*

Pangestyme™ EC *see* Pancrelipase *on page 1183*

Pangestyme™ MT *see* Pancrelipase *on page 1183*

Pangestyme™ UL *see* Pancrelipase *on page 1183*

Panglobulin® NF *see* Immune Globulin (Intravenous) *on page 824*

Panhematin® *see* Hemin *on page 764*

Panixine DisperDose™ [DSC] *see* Cephalexin *on page 301*

Panlor® DC *see* Acetaminophen, Caffeine, and Dihydrocodeine *on page 42*

Panlor® SS *see* Acetaminophen, Caffeine, and Dihydrocodeine *on page 42*

PanMist®-DM [DSC] *see* Guaifenesin, Pseudoephedrine, and Dextromethorphan *on page 757*

PanMist®-JR *see* Guaifenesin and Pseudoephedrine *on page 755*

PanMist®-LA *see* Guaifenesin and Pseudoephedrine *on page 755*

PanMist®-S *see* Guaifenesin and Pseudoephedrine *on page 755*

Panokase® *see* Pancrelipase *on page 1183*

Panokase® 16 *see* Pancrelipase *on page 1183*

PanOxyl® *see* Benzoyl Peroxide *on page 194*

PanOxyl®-AQ *see* Benzoyl Peroxide *on page 194*

PanOxyl® Aqua Gel *see* Benzoyl Peroxide *on page 194*

PanOxyl® Bar [OTC] *see* Benzoyl Peroxide *on page 194*

Panretin® *see* Alitretinoin *on page 69*

Panthoderm® [OTC] *see* Dexpanthenol *on page 446*

Pantoprazole (pan TOE pra zole)

Related Information
  Gastrointestinal Disorders *on page 1654*
U.S. Brand Names Protonix®
Canadian Brand Names Panto™ IV; Pantoloc™; Protonix®
Mexican Brand Names Pantozol®; Zurcal®
Generic Available No
Pharmacologic Category Proton Pump Inhibitor; Substituted Benzimidazole
Use
  Oral: Treatment and maintenance of healing of erosive esophagitis associated with GERD; reduction in relapse rates of daytime and nighttime heartburn symptoms in GERD; hypersecretory disorders associated with Zollinger-Ellison syndrome or other neoplastic disorders
  I.V.: Short-term treatment (7-10 days) of patients with gastroesophageal reflux disease (GERD) and a history of erosive esophagitis; hypersecretory disorders associated with Zollinger-Ellison syndrome or other neoplastic disorders
Unlabeled/Investigational Use Peptic ulcer disease, active ulcer bleeding (parenteral formulation); adjunct treatment with antibiotics for *Helicobacter pylori* eradication
Local Anesthetic/Vasoconstrictor Precautions No information available to require special precautions
Effects on Dental Treatment No significant effects or complications reported
Common Adverse Effects
  ≥1%:
    Cardiovascular: Chest pain
    Central nervous system: Headache (5% to 9%), insomnia (<1% to 1%), dizziness, migraine, anxiety
    Dermatologic: Rash (<1% to 2%)
    Endocrine and metabolic: Hyperglycemia (<1% to 1%), hyperlipidemia
    Gastrointestinal: Diarrhea (4% to 6%), flatulence (2% to 4%), abdominal pain (1% to 4%), nausea (≤2%), vomiting (≤2%), eructation (≤1%), constipation, dyspepsia, gastroenteritis, rectal disorder
    Genitourinary: Urinary frequency, UTI
    Hepatic: Liver function abnormal (up to 2%)
    Local: Injection site reaction (includes thrombophlebitis and abscess)
    Neuromuscular & skeletal: Arthralgia, back pain, hypertonia, neck pain, weakness
    Respiratory: Bronchitis, cough, dyspnea, pharyngitis, rhinitis, sinusitis, upper respiratory tract infection
    Miscellaneous: Flu syndrome, infection, pain

Dosage Adults:

Oral:

Erosive esophagitis associated with GERD:

Treatment: 40 mg once daily for up to 8 weeks; an additional 8 weeks may be used in patients who have not healed after an 8-week course

Maintenance of healing: 40 mg once daily

Note: Lower doses (20 mg once daily) have been used successfully in mild GERD treatment and maintenance of healing

Hypersecretory disorders (including Zollinger-Ellison): Initial: 40 mg twice daily; adjust dose based on patient needs; doses up to 240 mg/day have been administered

Helicobacter pylori eradication (unlabeled use): Doses up to 40 mg twice daily have been used as part of combination therapy

I.V.:

Erosive esophagitis associated with GERD: 40 mg once daily for 7-10 days

Hypersecretory disorders: 80 mg twice daily; adjust dose based on acid output measurements; 160-240 mg/day in divided doses has been used for a limited period (up to 7 days)

Prevention of rebleeding in peptic ulcer bleed (unlabeled use): 80 mg, followed by 8 mg/hour infusion for 72 hours. **Note:** A daily infusion of 40 mg does not raise gastric pH sufficiently to enhance coagulation in active GI bleeds.

Elderly: Dosage adjustment not required

Dosage adjustment in renal impairment: Not required; pantoprazole is not removed by hemodialysis

Dosage adjustment in hepatic impairment: Not required

Mechanism of Action Suppresses gastric acid secretin by inhibiting the parietal cell H^+/K^+ ATP pump

Contraindications Hypersensitivity to pantoprazole, substituted benzamidazoles (ie, esomeprazole, lansoprazole, omeprazole, rabeprazole), or any component of the formulation

Warnings/Precautions Symptomatic response does not preclude gastric malignancy. Not indicated for maintenance therapy; safety and efficacy for use beyond 16 weeks have not been established. Prolonged treatment (typically >3 years) may lead to vitamin B_{12} malabsorption. Intravenous preparation contains edetate sodium (EDTA); use caution in patients who are risk for zinc deficiency if other EDTA-containing solutions are coadministered. Safety and efficacy in pediatric patients have not been established.

Drug Interactions

Cytochrome P450 Effect: Substrate of CYP2C19 (major), 3A4 (minor); **Inhibits** 2C8/9 (moderate); **Induces** CYP1A2 (weak), 3A4 (weak)

Increased Effect/Toxicity: Pantoprazole may increase the levels/effects of amiodarone, fluoxetine, glimepiride, glipizide, nateglinide, phenytoin, pioglitazone, rosiglitazone, sertraline, warfarin, and other CYP2C8/9 substrates.

Decreased Effect: Proton pump inhibitors may decrease the absorption of atazanavir, indinavir, iron salts, itraconazole, and ketoconazole. The levels/effects of pantoprazole may be decreased by aminoglutethimide, carbamazepine, phenytoin, rifampin, and other CYP2C19 inducers.

Ethanol/Nutrition/Herb Interactions

Ethanol: Avoid ethanol (may cause gastric mucosal irritation).

Herb/Nutraceutical: Prolonged treatment (typically >3 years) may lead to vitamin B_{12} malabsorption.

Dietary Considerations

Oral: May be taken with or without food; best if taken before breakfast.

I.V.: Due to EDTA in preparation, zinc supplementation may be needed in patients prone to zinc deficiency.

Pharmacodynamics/Kinetics

Absorption: Well absorbed

Distribution: V_d: 11-24 L

Protein binding: 98%, primarily to albumin

Metabolism: Extensively hepatic; CYP2C19 (demethylation), CYP3A4; no evidence that metabolites have pharmacologic activity

Bioavailability: 77%

Half-life elimination: 1 hour; increased to 3.5-10 hours with CYP2C19 deficiency

Time to peak: Oral: 2.5 hours

Excretion: Urine (71%); feces (18%)

Pregnancy Risk Factor B

Dosage Forms Strength expressed as base: **INJ, powder for reconstitution:** 40 mg. **TAB, delayed release:** 20 mg, 40 mg

Pantothenic Acid (pan toe THEN ik AS id)

Generic Available Yes
Synonyms Calcium Pantothenate; Vitamin B$_5$
Pharmacologic Category Vitamin, Water Soluble
Use Pantothenic acid deficiency
Local Anesthetic/Vasoconstrictor Precautions No information available to require special precautions
Effects on Dental Treatment No significant effects or complications reported
Pregnancy Risk Factor A/C (dose exceeding RDA recommendation)

Pantothenyl Alcohol *see* Dexpanthenol *on page 446*

Papain and Urea (pa PAY in & yoor EE a)

U.S. Brand Names Accuzyme®; Ethezyme™; Ethezyme™ 830; Gladase®; Kovia®
Generic Available Yes: Ointment
Pharmacologic Category Enzyme, Topical Debridement
Use Debridement of necrotic tissue and liquefaction of slough in acute and chronic lesions such as pressure ulcers, varicose and diabetic ulcers, burns, postoperative wounds, pilonidal cyst wounds, carbuncles, and miscellaneous traumatic or infected wounds
Local Anesthetic/Vasoconstrictor Precautions No information available to require special precautions
Effects on Dental Treatment No significant effects or complications reported
Common Adverse Effects Frequency not defined: Local: Burning sensation, skin irritation
Mechanism of Action
Papain: Potent digestant of nonviable protein matter; harmless to viable tissue. Requires activation to exert its function.
Urea: Exposes papain activators (sulfhydryl groups) and denatures nonviable protein matter making it more susceptible to enzymatic digestion.
Drug Interactions
Decreased Effect: Heavy metals, hydrogen peroxide

Papain, Urea, and Chlorophyllin *see* Chlorophyllin, Papain, and Urea *on page 319*

Papaverine (pa PAV er een)

U.S. Brand Names Para-Time SR®
Generic Available Yes
Synonyms Papaverine Hydrochloride; Pavabid [DSC]
Pharmacologic Category Vasodilator
Use Oral: Relief of peripheral and cerebral ischemia associated with arterial spasm and myocardial ischemia complicated by arrhythmias
Unlabeled/Investigational Use Investigational: Parenteral: Various vascular spasms associated with muscle spasms as in myocardial infarction, angina, peripheral and pulmonary embolism, peripheral vascular disease, angiospastic states, and visceral spasm (ureteral, biliary, and GI colic); testing for impotence
Local Anesthetic/Vasoconstrictor Precautions No information available to require special precautions
Effects on Dental Treatment No significant effects or complications reported
Common Adverse Effects Frequency not defined.
Cardiovascular: Arrhythmias (with rapid I.V. use), flushing of the face, mild hypertension, tachycardia
Central nervous system: Drowsiness, headache, lethargy, sedation, vertigo
Gastrointestinal: Abdominal distress, anorexia, constipation, diarrhea, nausea
Hepatic: Chronic hepatitis, hepatic hypersensitivity
Respiratory: Apnea (with rapid I.V. use)
Mechanism of Action Smooth muscle spasmolytic producing a generalized smooth muscle relaxation including: vasodilatation, gastrointestinal sphincter relaxation, bronchiolar muscle relaxation, and potentially a depressed myocardium (with large doses); muscle relaxation may occur due to inhibition or cyclic nucleotide phosphodiesterase, increasing cyclic AMP; muscle relaxation is unrelated to nerve innervation; papaverine increases cerebral blood flow in normal subjects; oxygen uptake is unaltered

Drug Interactions
Decreased Effect: Papaverine decreases the effects of levodopa.
Pharmacodynamics/Kinetics
Onset of action: Oral: Rapid
Protein binding: 90%
Metabolism: Rapidly hepatic
Half-life elimination: 0.5-1.5 hours
Excretion: Primarily urine (as metabolites)
Pregnancy Risk Factor C

Papaverine Hydrochloride *see* Papaverine *on page 1186*
Para-Aminosalicylate Sodium *see* Aminosalicylic Acid *on page 89*
Paracetamol *see* Acetaminophen *on page 31*
Parafon Forte® DSC *see* Chlorzoxazone *on page 333*
Paraplatin® *see* Carboplatin *on page 270*
Parathyroid Hormone (1-34) *see* Teriparatide *on page 1461*
Para-Time SR® *see* Papaverine *on page 1186*
Parcopa™ *see* Levodopa and Carbidopa *on page 911*

Paregoric (par e GOR ik)

Generic Available Yes
Synonyms Camphorated Tincture of Opium (error-prone synonym)
Pharmacologic Category Analgesic, Narcotic
Use Treatment of diarrhea or relief of pain; neonatal opiate withdrawal
Local Anesthetic/Vasoconstrictor Precautions No information available to require special precautions
Effects on Dental Treatment No significant effects or complications reported
Mechanism of Action Increases smooth muscle tone in GI tract, decreases motility and peristalsis, diminishes digestive secretions
Pregnancy Risk Factor B/D (prolonged use or high doses)

Paremyd® *see* Hydroxyamphetamine and Tropicamide *on page 799*

Paricalcitol (pah ri KAL si tole)

U.S. Brand Names Zemplar®
Canadian Brand Names Zemplar®
Generic Available No
Pharmacologic Category Vitamin D Analog
Use
I.V.: Prevention and treatment of secondary hyperparathyroidism associated with stage 5 chronic kidney disease (CKD)
Oral: Prevention and treatment of secondary hyperparathyroidism associated with stage 3 and 4 CKD
Local Anesthetic/Vasoconstrictor Precautions No information available to require special precautions
Effects on Dental Treatment No significant effects or complications reported
Common Adverse Effects
>10%: Gastrointestinal: Nausea (6% to 13%)
1% to 10%:
Cardiovascular: Edema (7%), hypertension (7%), hypotension (5%), palpitation (3%), chest pain (3%), syncope (3%), cardiomyopathy (2%), MI (2%), postural hypotension (2%)
Central nervous system: Pain (8%), chills (5%), dizziness (5%), headache (5%), lightheadedness (5%), vertigo (5%), fever (3% to 5%), depression (3%), insomnia (2%)
Dermatologic: Rash (2% to 6%), skin ulcer (3%), pruritus (3%), skin hypertrophy (2%)
Endocrine & metabolic: Dehydration (3%), acidosis (2%), hypokalemia (2%)
Gastrointestinal: Vomiting (6% to 8%), diarrhea (7%), GI bleeding (5%), abdominal pain (4%), xerostomia (3%), constipation (4%), gastroenteritis (3%), dyspepsia (2%), gastritis (2%), rectal disorder (2%)
Genitourinary: Urinary tract infection (3%), kidney function abnormal (2%)
Neuromuscular & skeletal: Arthritis (5%), back pain (4%), leg cramps (3%), weakness (3%), neuropathy (2%)
Ocular: Amblyopia (2%), retinal disorder (2%)
Respiratory: Pneumonia (2% to 5%), rhinitis (5%), sinusitis (3%), bronchitis (3%), cough (3%), epistaxis (2%)
Miscellaneous: Infection (bacterial, fungal, viral: 2% to 8%); allergic reaction (6%), flu-like syndrome (2% to 5%), sepsis (5%), cyst (2%)
(Continued)

Paricalcitol (Continued)

Mechanism of Action Decreased renal conversion of vitamin D to its primary active metabolite (1,25-hydroxyvitamin D) in chronic renal failure leads to reduced activation of vitamin D receptor (VDR), which subsequently removes inhibitory suppression of parathyroid hormone (PTH) release; increased serum PTH (secondary hyperparathyroidism) reduces calcium excretion and enhances bone resorption. Paricalcitol is a synthetic vitamin D analog which binds to and activates the VDR in kidney, parathyroid gland, intestine and bone, thus reducing PTH levels and improving calcium and phosphate homeostasis.

Drug Interactions

Cytochrome P450 Effect:
Substrate of CYP3A4 (major)

Increased Effect/Toxicity:
CYP3A4 inhibitors (strong) may increase the levels/effects of paricalcitol; example CYP3A4 inhibitors include azole antifungals, ciprofloxacin, clarithromycin, diclofenac, doxycycline, erythromycin, imatinib, isoniazid, nefazodone, nicardipine, propofol, protease inhibitors, quinidine, and verapamil. Ketoconazole may increase paricalcitol levels/effects.

Pharmacodynamics/Kinetics

Distribution: V_d:
Healthy subjects: Oral: 34 L; I.V.: 24 L
Stage 3 and 4 CKD: Oral: 44-46 L;
Stage 5 CKD: I.V.: 31-35 L

Protein binding: >99%

Metabolism: Hydroxylation and glucuronidation via hepatic and nonhepatic enzymes, including CYP24, CYP3A4, UGT1A4; forms metabolites (at least one active)

Bioavailability: Oral: ~72% in healthy subjects

Half-life elimination:
Healthy subjects: Oral: 4-6 hours
Stage 3 and 4 CKD: Oral: 17-20 hours
Stage 5 CKD: I.V.: 14-15 hours

Excretion: Healthy subjects: Feces (oral: 70% to 74%; I.V.: 63%); urine (oral: 16% to 18%, I.V.: 19%); 51% to 59% as metabolites

Pregnancy Risk Factor C

Pariprazole see Rabeprazole on page 1327

Parlodel® see Bromocriptine on page 222

Parnate® see Tranylcypromine on page 1519

Paromomycin (par oh moe MYE sin)

U.S. Brand Names Humatin®
Canadian Brand Names Humatin®
Generic Available Yes
Synonyms Paromomycin Sulfate
Pharmacologic Category Amebicide
Use Treatment of acute and chronic intestinal amebiasis; hepatic coma
Unlabeled/Investigational Use Treatment of cryptosporidiosis
Local Anesthetic/Vasoconstrictor Precautions No information available to require special precautions
Effects on Dental Treatment No significant effects or complications reported
Common Adverse Effects
1% to 10%: Gastrointestinal: Diarrhea, abdominal cramps, nausea, vomiting, heartburn

Mechanism of Action Acts directly on ameba; has antibacterial activity against normal and pathogenic organisms in the GI tract; interferes with bacterial protein synthesis by binding to 30S ribosomal subunits

Pharmacodynamics/Kinetics
Absorption: None
Excretion: Feces (100% as unchanged drug)

Pregnancy Risk Factor C

Paromomycin Sulfate see Paromomycin on page 1188

Paroxetine (pa ROKS e teen)

U.S. Brand Names Paxil®; Paxil CR®; Pexeva®
Canadian Brand Names Apo-Paroxetine®; CO Paroxetine; Gen-Paroxetine; Novo-Paroxetine; Paxil®; Paxil CR®; PMS-Paroxetine; ratio-Paroxetine; Rhoxal-paroxetine; Sandoz-Paroxetine

Mexican Brand Names Aropax®; Paxil®

Generic Available Yes: Tablet, as hydrochloride

Synonyms Paroxetine Hydrochloride; Paroxetine Mesylate

Pharmacologic Category Antidepressant, Selective Serotonin Reuptake Inhibitor

Use Treatment of depression in adults; treatment of panic disorder with or without agoraphobia; obsessive-compulsive disorder (OCD) in adults; social anxiety disorder (social phobia); generalized anxiety disorder (GAD); post-traumatic stress disorder (PTSD)

Paxil CR®: Treatment of depression; panic disorder; premenstrual dysphoric disorder (PMDD); social anxiety disorder (social phobia)

Unlabeled/Investigational Use May be useful in eating disorders, impulse control disorders, self-injurious behavior; premenstrual disorders, vasomotor symptoms of menopause; treatment of depression and obsessive-compulsive disorder (OCD) in children

Local Anesthetic/Vasoconstrictor Precautions Although caution should be used in patients taking tricyclic antidepressants, no interactions have been reported with vasoconstrictor and paroxetine, a nontricyclic antidepressant which acts to increase serotonin; no precautions appear to be needed

Effects on Dental Treatment Key adverse event(s) related to dental treatment: Xerostomia and changes in salivation (normal salivary flow resumes upon discontinuation), postural hypotension, and abnormal taste. Problems with SSRI-induced bruxism have been reported and may preclude their use; clinicians attempting to evaluate any patient with bruxism or involuntary muscle movement, who is simultaneously being treated with an SSRI drug, should be aware of the potential association. Prolonged use may decrease or inhibit salivary flow; normal salivation resumes upon discontinuation.

Common Adverse Effects Frequency varies by dose and indication. Adverse reactions reported as a composite of all indications.

>10%:
Central nervous system: Somnolence (15% to 24%), insomnia (11% to 24%), headache (17% to 18%), dizziness (6% to 14%)
Endocrine & metabolic: Libido decreased (6% to 15%)
Gastrointestinal: Nausea (19% to 26%), xerostomia (9% to 18%), constipation (5% to 16%), diarrhea (9% to 12%)
Genitourinary: Ejaculatory disturbances (10% to 28%)
Neuromuscular & skeletal: Weakness (12% to 22%), tremor (4% to 11%)
Miscellaneous: Diaphoresis (5% to 14%)

1% to 10%:
Cardiovascular: Vasodilation (2% to 4%), chest pain (3%), palpitations (2% to 3%), hypertension (≥1%), tachycardia (≥1%)
Central nervous system: Nervousness (4% to 9%), anxiety (5%), agitation (3% to 5%), abnormal dreams (3% to 4%), concentration impaired (3% to 4%), yawning (2% to 4%), depersonalization (up to 3%), amnesia (2%), emotional lability (≥1%), vertigo (≥1%), confusion (1%), chills (2%)
Dermatologic: Rash (2% to 3%), pruritus (≥1%)
Endocrine & metabolic: Orgasmic disturbance (2% to 9%), dysmenorrhea (5%)
Gastrointestinal: Anorexia, appetite decreased (5% to 9%), dyspepsia (2% to 5%), flatulence (4%), abdominal pain (4%), appetite increased (2% to 4%), vomiting (2% to 3%), taste perversion (2%), weight gain (≥1%)
Genitourinary: Impotence (2% to 9%), genital disorder (female 2% to 9%), urinary frequency (2% to 3%), urinary tract infection (2%)
Neuromuscular & skeletal: Paresthesia (4%), myalgia (2% to 4%), back pain (3%), myoclonus (2% to 3%), myopathy (2%), myasthenia (1%), arthralgia (≥1%)
Ocular: Blurred vision (4%), abnormal vision (2% to 3%)
Otic: Tinnitus (≥1%)
Respiratory: Respiratory disorder (up to 7%), pharyngitis (4%), sinusitis (up to 4%), rhinitis (3%)
Miscellaneous: Infection (5% to 6%)

Restrictions A medication guide concerning the use of antidepressants in children and teenagers can be found on the FDA website at http://www.fda.gov/cder/Offices/ODS/labeling.htm. It should be dispensed to parents or guardians of children and teenagers receiving this medication.

Dosage Oral:
Children:
Depression (unlabeled use; not recommended by FDA): Initial: 10 mg/day and adjusted upward on an individual basis to 20 mg/day
OCD (unlabeled use): Initial: 10 mg/day and titrate up as necessary to 60 mg/day
Self-injurious behavior (unlabeled use): 20 mg/day
(Continued)

Paroxetine *(Continued)*

Social phobia (unlabeled use): 2.5-15 mg/day

Adults:

Depression:

Paxil®, Pexeva®: Initial: 20 mg once daily, preferably in the morning; increase if needed by 10 mg/day increments at intervals of at least 1 week; maximum dose: 50 mg/day

Paxil CR®: Initial: 25 mg once daily; increase if needed by 12.5 mg/day increments at intervals of at least 1 week; maximum dose: 62.5 mg/day

GAD (Paxil®): Initial: 20 mg once daily, preferably in the morning; doses of 20-50 mg/day were used in clinical trials, however, no greater benefit was seen with doses >20 mg. If dose is increased, adjust in increments of 10 mg/day at 1-week intervals.

OCD (Paxil®, Pexeva™): Initial: 20 mg once daily, preferably in the morning; increase if needed by 10 mg/day increments at intervals of at least 1 week; recommended dose: 40 mg/day; range: 20-60 mg/day; maximum dose: 60 mg/day

Panic disorder:

Paxil®, Pexeva®: Initial: 10 mg once daily, preferably in the morning; increase if needed by 10 mg/day increments at intervals of at least 1 week; recommended dose: 40 mg/day; range: 10-60 mg/day; maximum dose: 60 mg/day

Paxil CR®: Initial: 12.5 mg once daily; increase if needed by 12.5 mg/day at intervals of at least 1 week; maximum dose: 75 mg/day

PMDD (Paxil CR®): Initial: 12.5 mg once daily in the morning; may be increased to 25 mg/day; dosing changes should occur at intervals of at least 1 week. May be given daily throughout the menstrual cycle or limited to the luteal phase.

PTSD (Paxil®): Initial: 20 mg once daily, preferably in the morning; increase if needed by 10 mg/day increments at intervals of at least 1 week; range: 20-50 mg. Limited data suggest doses of 40 mg/day were not more efficacious than 20 mg/day.

Social anxiety disorder:

Paxil®: Initial: 20 mg once daily, preferably in the morning; recommended dose: 20 mg/day; range: 20-60 mg/day; doses >20 mg may not have additional benefit

Paxil CR®: Initial: 12.5 mg once daily, preferably in the morning; may be increased by 12.5 mg/day at intervals of at least 1 week; maximum dose: 37.5 mg/day

Vasomotor symptoms of menopause (unlabeled use, Paxil CR®): 12.5-25 mg/day

Elderly:

Paxil®, Pexeva®: Initial: 10 mg/day; increase if needed by 10 mg/day increments at intervals of at least 1 week; maximum dose: 40 mg/day

Paxil CR®; Initial: 12.5 mg/day; increase if needed by 12.5 mg/day increments at intervals of at least 1 week; maximum dose: 50 mg/day

Note: Upon discontinuation of paroxetine therapy, gradually taper dose:

Paxil®: 10 mg/day at weekly intervals; when 20 mg/day dose is reached, continue for 1 week before treatment is discontinued. Some patients may need to be titrated to 10 mg/day for 1 week before discontinuation.

Paxil CR®: Patients receiving 37.5 mg/day in clinical trials had their dose decreased by 12.5 mg/day to a dose of 25 mg/day and remained at a dose of 25 mg/day for 1 week before treatment was discontinued.

Dosage adjustment in severe renal/hepatic impairment: Adults:

Cl_{cr} <30 mL/minute: Mean plasma concentration is ~4 times that seen in normal function.

Cl_{cr} 30-60 mL/minute and hepatic dysfunction: Plasma concentration is 2 times that seen in normal function.

Paxil®, Pexeva®: Initial: 10 mg/day; increase if needed by 10 mg/day increments at intervals of at least 1 week; maximum dose: 40 mg/day

Paxil CR®: Initial: 12.5 mg/day; increase if needed by 12.5 mg/day increments at intervals of at least 1 week; maximum dose: 50 mg/day

Mechanism of Action Paroxetine is a selective serotonin reuptake inhibitor, chemically unrelated to tricyclic, tetracyclic, or other antidepressants; presumably, the inhibition of serotonin reuptake from brain synapse stimulated serotonin activity in the brain

Contraindications Hypersensitivity to paroxetine or any component of the formulation; use of MAO inhibitors or within 14 days; concurrent use with thioridazine or pimozide

Warnings/Precautions Antidepressants increase the risk of suicidal thinking and behavior in children and adolescents with major depressive disorder (MDD)

and other depressive disorders; consider risk prior to prescribing. All patients must be closely monitored for clinical worsening, suicidality, or unusual changes in behavior, especially during the initiation of therapy or following an increase or decrease in dosage. When used in children, the child's family or caregiver should be instructed to closely observe the patient and communicate condition with healthcare provider. A medication guide should be dispensed with each prescription. **Paroxetine is not FDA approved for use in children.**

The possibility of a suicide attempt is inherent in major depression and may persist until remission occurs. Use caution in high-risk patients. Worsening depression and severe abrupt suicidality that are not part of the presenting symptoms may require discontinuation or modification of drug therapy. The patient's family or caregiver should be alerted to monitor patients for the emergence of suicidality and associated behaviors (such as agitation, irritability, hostility, impulsivity, and hypomania) and call healthcare provider.

May worsen psychosis in some patients or precipitate a shift to mania or hypomania in patients with bipolar disorder. Patients presenting with depressive symptoms should be screened for bipolar disorder. Monotherapy in patients with bipolar disorder should be avoided. **Paroxetine is not FDA approved for the treatment of bipolar depression.**

Potential for severe reaction when used with MAO inhibitors - serotonin syndrome (hyperthermia, muscular rigidity, mental status changes/agitation, autonomic instability) may occur; concurrent use contraindicated. May increase the risks associated with electroconvulsive therapy. Has a low potential to impair cognitive or motor performance - caution operating hazardous machinery or driving. Symptoms of agitation and/or restlessness may occur during initial few weeks of therapy. Low potential for sedation or anticholinergic effects relative to cyclic antidepressants.

Use caution in patients with a previous seizure disorder or condition predisposing to seizures such as brain damage, alcoholism, or concurrent therapy with other drugs which lower the seizure threshold. Use with caution in patients with hepatic dysfunction and in elderly patients. May cause hyponatremia/SIADH. Use with caution in patients at risk of bleeding or receiving anticoagulant therapy - may cause impairment in platelet aggregation. Use with caution in patients with renal insufficiency or other concurrent illness (due to limited experience); dose reduction recommended with severe renal impairment. May cause or exacerbate sexual dysfunction. Use caution in patients with narrow-angle glaucoma. Avoid use in the first trimester of pregnancy.

Upon discontinuation of paroxetine therapy, gradually taper dose and monitor for discontinuation symptoms (eg, dizziness, dysphoric mood, irritability, agitation, confusion, paresthesias). If intolerable symptoms occur following a decrease in dosage or upon discontinuation of therapy, then resuming the previous dose with a more gradual taper should be considered.

Drug Interactions

Cytochrome P450 Effect: Substrate of CYP2D6 (major); **Inhibits** CYP1A2 (weak), 2B6 (moderate), 2C8/9 (weak), 2C19 (weak), 2D6 (strong), 3A4 (weak)

Increased Effect/Toxicity: Paroxetine should not be used with nonselective MAO inhibitors (phenelzine, isocarboxazid) or other drugs with MAO inhibition (linezolid); fatal reactions have been reported. Wait 5 weeks after stopping fluoxetine before starting a nonselective MAO inhibitor and 2 weeks after stopping an MAO inhibitor before starting paroxetine. Concurrent selegiline has been associated with mania, hypertension, or serotonin syndrome (risk may be reduced relative to nonselective MAO inhibitors). Serum levels of atomoxetine, carbamazepine, and galantamine may be increased by paroxetine.

Paroxetine may inhibit the metabolism of thioridazine or mesoridazine, resulting in increased plasma levels and increasing the risk of QT_c interval prolongation. This may lead to serious ventricular arrhythmias, such as torsade de pointes-type arrhythmias and sudden death. Do not use together. Wait at least 5 weeks after discontinuing paroxetine prior to starting thioridazine.

The levels/effects of paroxetine may be increased by chlorpromazine, delavirdine, fluoxetine, miconazole, pergolide, quinidine, quinine, ritonavir, ropinirole, and other CYP2D6 inhibitors. Paroxetine may increase the levels/effects of amphetamines, selected beta-blockers, bupropion, dextromethorphan, fluoxetine, lidocaine, mirtazapine, nefazodone, promethazine, propofol, risperidone, ritonavir, sertraline, tricyclic antidepressants, venlafaxine, and other CYP2B6 or 2D6 substrates.

(Continued)

Paroxetine *(Continued)*

Concomitant use of paroxetine and NSAIDs, aspirin, or other drugs affecting coagulation has been associated with an increased risk of bleeding. Paroxetine may increase the hypoprothrombinemic response to warfarin. Paroxetine increases levels of procyclidine; this may result in increased anticholinergic effects; procyclidine dose reduction may be necessary.

Combined use of SSRIs and amphetamines, buspirone, meperidine, nefazodone, serotonin agonists (such as sumatriptan), sibutramine, other SSRIs, sympathomimetics, ritonavir, tramadol, and venlafaxine may increase the risk of serotonin syndrome. Combined use of sumatriptan (and other serotonin agonists) may result in toxicity; weakness, hyper-reflexia, and incoordination have been observed with sumatriptan and SSRIs. In addition, concurrent use may theoretically increase the risk of serotonin syndrome; includes sumatriptan, naratriptan, rizatriptan, and zolmitriptan. Concurrent lithium may increase risk of nephrotoxicity. Risk of hyponatremia may increase with concurrent use of loop diuretics (bumetanide, furosemide, torsemide).

Decreased Effect: Cyproheptadine, a serotonin antagonist, may inhibit the effects of serotonin reuptake inhibitors (paroxetine). Paroxetine may decrease the levels/effects of CYP2D6 prodrug substrates (eg, codeine, hydrocodone, oxycodone, tramadol).

Ethanol/Nutrition/Herb Interactions

Ethanol: Avoid ethanol.

Food: Peak concentration is increased, but bioavailability is not significantly altered by food.

Herb/Nutraceutical: Avoid valerian, St John's wort, SAMe, kava kava.

Dietary Considerations May be taken with or without food.

Pharmacodynamics/Kinetics

Absorption: Completely absorbed following oral administration

Distribution: V_d: 8.7 L/kg (3-28 L/kg)

Protein binding: 93% to 95%

Metabolism: Extensively hepatic via CYP enzymes via oxidation and methylation; nonlinear pharmacokinetics may be seen with higher doses and longer duration of therapy. Saturation of CYP2D6 appears to account for the nonlinearity. C_{min} concentrations 70% to 80% greater in the elderly compared to nonelderly patients; clearance is also decreased.

Half-life elimination: 21 hours (3-65 hours)

Time to peak, serum: Immediate release: 5.2 hours; controlled release: 6-10 hours

Excretion: Urine (64%, 2% as unchanged drug); feces (36% primarily via bile)

Pregnancy Risk Factor D

Dosage Forms SUSP, oral, as hydrochloride (Paxil®): 10 mg/5 mL (250 mL). **TAB, as hydrochloride** (Paxil®): 10 mg, 20 mg, 30 mg, 40 mg. **TAB, as mesylate** (Pexeva®): 10 mg, 20 mg, 30 mg, 40 mg. **TAB, controlled release, as hydrochloride** (Paxil CR®): 12.5 mg, 25 mg, 37.5 mg

Paroxetine Hydrochloride *see* Paroxetine *on page 1188*

Paroxetine Mesylate *see* Paroxetine *on page 1188*

PAS *see* Aminosalicylic Acid *on page 89*

Paser® *see* Aminosalicylic Acid *on page 89*

Patanol® *see* Olopatadine *on page 1143*

Pavabid [DSC] *see* Papaverine *on page 1186*

Paxil® *see* Paroxetine *on page 1188*

Paxil CR® *see* Paroxetine *on page 1188*

PBZ® *see* Tripelennamine *on page 1541*

PBZ-SR® *see* Tripelennamine *on page 1541*

PCA (error-prone abbreviation) *see* Procainamide *on page 1283*

PCE® *see* Erythromycin *on page 562*

PCEC *see* Rabies Virus Vaccine *on page 1329*

PCM *see* Chlorpheniramine, Phenylephrine, and Methscopolamine *on page 327*

PCM Allergy *see* Chlorpheniramine, Phenylephrine, and Methscopolamine *on page 327*

PCV7 *see* Pneumococcal Conjugate Vaccine (7-Valent) *on page 1250*

Pectin and Kaolin *see* Kaolin and Pectin *on page 879*

PediaCare® Children's Long Acting Cough Plus Cold [OTC] *see* Pseudoephedrine and Dextromethorphan *on page 1311*

PediaCare® Children's Medicated Freezer Pops Long Acting Cough [OTC] *see* Dextromethorphan *on page 451*

PediaCare® Cold and Allergy [OTC] *see* Chlorpheniramine and Pseudoephedrine *on page 325*

PediaCare® Decongestant Infants [OTC] see Pseudoephedrine on page 1309

PediaCare® Infants' Decongestant & Cough [OTC] see Pseudoephedrine and Dextromethorphan on page 1311

PediaCare® Infants' Long-Acting Cough [OTC] see Dextromethorphan on page 451

Pediacof [DSC] see Chlorpheniramine, Phenylephrine, Codeine, and Potassium Iodide on page 328

Pediaflor® [DSC] see Fluoride on page 671

Pediapred® see PrednisoLONE on page 1268

Pedia Relief Cough and Cold [OTC] see Pseudoephedrine and Dextromethorphan on page 1311

Pedia Relief Infants [OTC] see Pseudoephedrine and Dextromethorphan on page 1311

Pediarix™ see Diphtheria, Tetanus Toxoids, Acellular Pertussis, Hepatitis B (Recombinant), and Poliovirus (Inactivated) Vaccine on page 488

Pediatex™ see Carbinoxamine on page 268

Pediatex™ 12 see Carbinoxamine on page 268

Pediatex™-D see Carbinoxamine and Pseudoephedrine on page 268

Pediatex™ DM [DSC] see Carbinoxamine, Pseudoephedrine, and Dextromethorphan on page 269

Pediazole® see Erythromycin and Sulfisoxazole on page 568

Pedi-Boro® [OTC] see Aluminum Sulfate and Calcium Acetate on page 81

Pedi-Dri® see Nystatin on page 1133

PediOtic® see Neomycin, Polymyxin B, and Hydrocortisone on page 1101

Pedisilk® [OTC] see Salicylic Acid on page 1374

Pedtrace-4® see Trace Metals on page 1513

PedvaxHIB® see Haemophilus b Conjugate Vaccine on page 534

PEG see Polyethylene Glycol 3350 on page 1253

PEG-L-asparaginase see Pegaspargase on page 1194

Pegademase Bovine (peg A de mase BOE vine)

U.S. Brand Names Adagen®
Canadian Brand Names Adagen®
Generic Available No
Pharmacologic Category Enzyme
Use Orphan drug: Enzyme replacement therapy for adenosine deaminase (ADA) deficiency in patients with severe combined immunodeficiency disease (SCID) who can not benefit from bone marrow transplant; not a cure for SCID, unlike bone marrow transplants, injections must be used the rest of the child's life, therefore is not really an alternative
Local Anesthetic/Vasoconstrictor Precautions No information available to require special precautions
Effects on Dental Treatment No significant effects or complications reported
Mechanism of Action Adenosine deaminase is an enzyme that catalyzes the deamination of both adenosine and deoxyadenosine. Hereditary lack of adenosine deaminase activity results in severe combined immunodeficiency disease, a fatal disorder of infancy characterized by profound defects of both cellular and humoral immunity. It is estimated that 25% of patients with the autosomal recessive form of severe combined immunodeficiency lack adenosine deaminase.
Pharmacodynamics/Kinetics
Absorption: Rapid
Half-life elimination: 48-72 hours
Time to peak: Plasma adenosine deaminase activity: 2-3 weeks
Pregnancy Risk Factor C

Peganone® see Ethotoin on page 619

Pegaptanib (peg AP ta nib)

U.S. Brand Names Macugen®
Generic Available No
Synonyms EYE001; Pegaptanib Sodium
Pharmacologic Category Ophthalmic Agent; Vascular Endothelial Growth Factor (VEGF) Inhibitor
Use Treatment of neovascular (wet) age-related macular degeneration (AMD)
Local Anesthetic/Vasoconstrictor Precautions No information available to require special precautions
(Continued)

Pegaptanib *(Continued)*

Effects on Dental Treatment No significant effects or complications reported

Common Adverse Effects

10% to 40%:

Cardiovascular: Hypertension

Ocular: Anterior chamber inflammation, blurred vision, cataract, conjunctival hemorrhage, corneal edema, eye discharge, eye irritation, eye pain, intraocular pressure increased, ocular discomfort, punctate keratitis, visual acuity decreased, visual disturbance, vitreous floaters, vitreous opacities

1% to 10%:

Cardiovascular: Carotid artery occlusion (1% to 5%), cerebrovascular accident (1% to 5%), chest pain (1% to 5%), transient ischemic attack (1% to 5%)

Central nervous system: Dizziness (6% to 10%), headache (6% to 10%), vertigo (1% to 5%)

Dermatologic: Contact dermatitis (1% to 5%)

Endocrine & metabolic: Diabetes mellitus (1% to 5%)

Gastrointestinal: Diarrhea (6% to 10%), nausea (6% to 10%), dyspepsia (1% to 5%), vomiting (1% to 5%)

Genitourinary: Urinary retention (1% to 5%)

Neuromuscular & skeletal: Arthritis (1% to 5%), bone spur (1% to 5%)

Ocular: Blepharitis (6% to 10%), conjunctivitis (6% to 10%), photopsia (6% to 10%), vitreous disorder (6% to 10%), allergic conjunctivitis (1% to 5%), conjunctival edema (1% to 5%), corneal abrasion (1% to 5%), corneal deposits (1% to 5%), corneal epithelium disorder (1% to 5%), endophthalmitis (1% to 5%), eye inflammation (1% to 5%), eye swelling (1% to 5%), eyelid irritation (1% to 5%), meibomianitis (1% to 5%), mydriasis (1% to 5%), periorbital hematoma (1% to 5%), retinal edema (1% to 5%), vitreous hemorrhage (1% to 5%)

Otic: Hearing loss (1% to 5%)

Renal: Urinary tract infection (6% to 10%)

Respiratory: Bronchitis (6% to 10%), pleural effusion (1% to 5%)

Miscellaneous: Contusion (1% to 5%)

Mechanism of Action Pegaptanib is an apatamer, an oligonucleotide covalently bound to polyethylene glycol, which can adopt a three-dimensional shape and bind to vascular endothelial growth factor (VEGF). Pegaptanib binds to extracellular VEGF, inhibiting VEGF from binding to its receptors and thereby suppressing neovascularization and slowing vision loss.

Pharmacodynamics/Kinetics

Absorption: Slow systemic absorption following intravitreous injection

Metabolism: Metabolized by endo- and exonucleases

Half-life elimination: Plasma: 6-14 days

Pregnancy Risk Factor B

Pegaptanib Sodium *see* Pegaptanib *on page 1193*

Pegaspargase *(peg AS par jase)*

Related Information

Asparaginase *on page 144*

U.S. Brand Names Oncaspar®

Generic Available No

Synonyms NSC-644954; PEG-L-asparaginase

Pharmacologic Category Antineoplastic Agent, Miscellaneous

Use Treatment of acute lymphocytic leukemia when L-asparaginase is required in treatment regimen but previous hypersensitivity to native L-asparaginase exists

Local Anesthetic/Vasoconstrictor Precautions No information available to require special precautions

Effects on Dental Treatment No significant effects or complications reported

Common Adverse Effects In general, pegaspargase toxicities tend to be less frequent and appear somewhat later than comparable toxicities of asparaginase. Intramuscular rather than intravenous injection may decrease the incidence of coagulopathy; GI, hepatic, and renal toxicity. Except for hypersensitivity reactions, adults tend to have a higher incidence than children.

>10%:

Cardiovascular: Edema

Central nervous system: Fever, malaise

Gastrointestinal: Nausea, vomiting (50% to 60%), generally mild to moderate, but may be severe and protracted in some patients; anorexia (33%); abdominal pain (38%); diarrhea (28%); increased serum lipase and amylase

Hematologic: Hypofibrinogenemia and depression of clotting factors V and VII, variable decreases in factors VII and IX, severe protein C deficiency and decrease in antithrombin III - overt bleeding is uncommon, but may be dose-limiting, or fatal in some patients

Hypersensitivity: Acute allergic reactions, including fever, rash, urticaria, arthralgia, hypotension, angioedema, bronchospasm, anaphylaxis (10% to 30%) - dose-limiting in some patients

Neuromuscular & skeletal: Weakness (33%)

1% to 10%:

Cardiovascular: Hypotension, tachycardia, thrombosis

Dermatologic: Urticaria, erythema, lip edema

Endocrine & metabolic: Hyperglycemia (3%)

Gastrointestinal: Acute pancreatitis (1%)

Mechanism of Action Pegaspargase is a modified version of asparaginase. Leukemic cells, especially lymphoblasts, require exogenous asparagine; normal cells can synthesize asparagine. Asparaginase contains L-asparaginase amidohydrolase type EC-2 which inhibits protein synthesis by deaminating asparagine to aspartic acid and ammonia in the plasma and extracellular fluid and therefore deprives tumor cells of the amino acid for protein synthesis. Asparaginase is cycle-specific for the G_1 phase of the cell cycle.

Pharmacodynamics/Kinetics

Duration: Asparaginase was measurable for at least 15 days following initial treatment with pegaspargase

Distribution: V_d: 4-5 L/kg; 70% to 80% of plasma volume; does not penetrate the CSF

Metabolism: Systemically degraded

Half-life elimination: 5.7 days; unaffected by age, renal or hepatic function; half life decreased to 3.2 days in patients with previous hypersensitivity to native L-asparaginase

Excretion: Urine (trace amounts)

Pregnancy Risk Factor C

Pegasys® see Peginterferon Alfa-2a on page 1195

Pegfilgrastim (peg fil GRA stim)

U.S. Brand Names Neulasta®

Canadian Brand Names Neulasta®

Generic Available No

Synonyms G-CSF (PEG Conjugate); Granulocyte Colony Stimulating Factor (PEG Conjugate)

Pharmacologic Category Colony Stimulating Factor

Use Decrease the incidence of infection, by stimulation of granulocyte production, in patients with nonmyeloid malignancies receiving myelosuppressive therapy associated with a significant risk of febrile neutropenia

Local Anesthetic/Vasoconstrictor Precautions No information available to require special precautions

Effects on Dental Treatment No significant effects or complications reported

Common Adverse Effects >10%:

Cardiovascular: Peripheral edema (12%)

Central nervous system: Headache (16%)

Gastrointestinal: Vomiting (13%), constipation (12%)

Neuromuscular & skeletal: Bone pain (31% to 57%), myalgia (21%), arthralgia (16%), weakness (13%)

Mechanism of Action Stimulates the production, maturation, and activation of neutrophils, pegfilgrastim activates neutrophils to increase both their migration and cytotoxicity. Pegfilgrastim has a prolonged duration of effect relative to filgrastim and a reduced renal clearance.

Drug Interactions

Increased Effect/Toxicity: No formal drug interactions studies have been conducted. Lithium may potentiate release of neutrophils.

Pharmacodynamics/Kinetics Half-life elimination: SubQ: 15-80 hours

Pregnancy Risk Factor C

Peginterferon Alfa-2a (peg in ter FEER on AL fa too aye)

U.S. Brand Names Pegasys®

Canadian Brand Names Pegasys®

Generic Available No

(Continued)

Peginterferon Alfa-2a *(Continued)*

Synonyms Interferon Alfa-2a (PEG Conjugate); Pegylated Interferon Alfa-2a

Pharmacologic Category Interferon

Use Treatment of chronic hepatitis C (CHC), alone or in combination with ribavirin, in patients with compensated liver disease and histological evidence of cirrhosis (Child-Pugh class A) and patients with clinically-stable HIV disease; treatment of patients with HBeAg positive and HBeAg negative chronic hepatitis B with compensated liver disease and evidence of viral replication and liver inflammation

Local Anesthetic/Vasoconstrictor Precautions No information available to require special precautions

Effects on Dental Treatment No significant effects or complications reported

Common Adverse Effects Note: Percentages are reported for peginterferon alfa-2a in chronic hepatitis C (CHC) patients. Other percentages indicated as "with ribavirin" or "in HIV/CHC" are those which significantly exceed incidence reported for peginterferon monotherapy in CHC patients.

>10%:

Central nervous system: Headache (54%), fatigue (50%), pyrexia (37%; 41% with ribavirin; 54% in hepatitis B), insomnia (19%; 30% with ribavirin), depression (18%), dizziness (16%), irritability/anxiety/nervousness (19%; 33% with ribavirin), pain (11%)

Dermatologic: Alopecia (23%; 28% with ribavirin), pruritus (12%; 19% with ribavirin), dermatitis (16% with ribavirin)

Gastrointestinal: Nausea/vomiting (24%), anorexia (17%; 24% with ribavirin), diarrhea (16%), weight loss (16% in HIV/CHC), abdominal pain (15%)

Hematologic: Neutropenia (21%; 27% with ribavirin; 40% in HIV/CHC), lymphopenia (14% with ribavirin), anemia (11% with ribavirin; 14% in HIV/CHC)

Hepatic: ALT increases 5-10 x ULN during treatment (25% to 27% in hepatitis B); ALT increases >10 x ULN during treatment (12% to 18% in hepatitis B); ALT increases 5-10 x ULN after treatment (13% to 16% in hepatitis B); ALT increases >10 x ULN after treatment (7% to 12% in hepatitis B)

Local: Injection site reaction (22%)

Neuromuscular & skeletal: Weakness (56%; 65% with ribavirin), myalgia (37%), rigors (32%; 25% to 27% in hepatitis B), arthralgia (28%)

Respiratory: Dyspnea (13% with ribavirin)

1% to 10%:

Central nervous system: Concentration impaired (8%), memory impaired (5%), mood alteration (3%; 9% in HIV/CHC)

Dermatologic: Dermatitis (8%), rash (5%), dry skin (4%; 10% with ribavirin), eczema (5% with ribavirin)

Endocrine & metabolic: Hypothyroidism (4%), hyperthyroidism (1%)

Gastrointestinal: Xerostomia (6%), dyspepsia (6% with ribavirin), weight loss (4%; 10% with ribavirin)

Hematologic: Thrombocytopenia (5%), platelets decreased <50,000/mm³ (5%), lymphopenia (3%), anemia (2%)

Hepatic: Hepatic decompensation (2% CHC/HIV patients)

Neuromuscular & skeletal: Back pain (9%)

Ocular: Blurred vision (4%)

Respiratory: Cough (4%; 10% with ribavirin), dyspnea (4%), exertional dyspnea (4% with ribavirin)

Miscellaneous: Diaphoresis (6%), bacterial infection (3%; 5% in HIV/CHC)

Restrictions An FDA-approved medication guide is available at http://www.fda.gov/cder/Offices/ODS/labeling.htm; distribute to each patient to whom this medication is dispensed.

Mechanism of Action Alpha interferons are a family of proteins, produced by nucleated cells, that have antiviral, antiproliferative, and immune-regulating activity. There are 16 known subtypes of alpha interferons. Interferons interact with cells through high affinity cell surface receptors. Following activation, multiple effects can be detected including induction of gene transcription. Inhibits cellular growth, alters the state of cellular differentiation, interferes with oncogene expression, alters cell surface antigen expression, increases phagocytic activity of macrophages, and augments cytotoxicity of lymphocytes for target cells.

Drug Interactions

Cytochrome P450 Effect: Inhibits CYP1A2 (weak)

Increased Effect/Toxicity: Interferons may increase the risk of neutropenia when used with ACE inhibitors; fluorouracil concentrations doubled with interferon alfa-2b; interferon alfa may decrease the metabolism of theophylline and zidovudine; interferons may increase the anticoagulant effects of warfarin. Concurrent therapy with ribavirin may increase the risk of hemolytic anemia.

Decreased Effect: Prednisone may decrease the therapeutic effects of interferon alfa; interferon alfa may decrease the serum concentrations of melphalan

Pharmacodynamics/Kinetics
Half-life elimination: Terminal: 50-140 hours; increased with renal dysfunction
Time to peak, serum: 72-96 hours

Pregnancy Risk Factor C; X when used with ribavirin

Peginterferon Alfa-2b (peg in ter FEER on AL fa too bee)

Related Information
Systemic Viral Diseases *on page 1675*

U.S. Brand Names PEG-Intron®

Canadian Brand Names PEG-Intron®

Generic Available No

Synonyms Interferon Alfa-2b (PEG Conjugate); Pegylated Interferon Alfa-2b

Pharmacologic Category Interferon

Use Treatment of chronic hepatitis C (as monotherapy or in combination with ribavirin) in adult patients who have never received interferon alpha and have compensated liver disease

Local Anesthetic/Vasoconstrictor Precautions No information available to require special precautions

Effects on Dental Treatment No significant effects or complications reported

Common Adverse Effects
>10%:
Central nervous system: Headache (56%), fatigue (52%), depression (16% to 29%), anxiety/emotional liability/irritability (28%), insomnia (23%), fever (22%), dizziness (12%), impaired concentration (5% to 12%), pain (12%)
Dermatologic: Alopecia (22%), pruritus (11%), dry skin (11%)
Gastrointestinal: Nausea (26%), anorexia (20%), diarrhea (18%), abdominal pain (15%), weight loss (11%)
Local: Injection site inflammation/reaction (47%),
Neuromuscular & skeletal: Musculoskeletal pain (56%), myalgia (38% to 42%), rigors (23% to 45%)
Respiratory: Epistaxis (14%), nasopharyngitis (11%)
Miscellaneous: Flu-like syndrome (46%), viral infection (11%)
>1% to 10%:
Cardiovascular: Flushing (6%)
Central nervous system: Malaise (8%)
Dermatologic: Rash (6%), dermatitis (7%)
Endocrine & metabolic: Hypothyroidism (5%)
Gastrointestinal: Vomiting (7%), dyspepsia (6%), taste perversion
Hematologic: Neutropenia, thrombocytopenia
Hepatic: Hepatomegaly (6%), transaminases increased (10%; transient)
Local: Injection site pain (2%)
Neuromuscular & skeletal: Hypertonia (5%)
Respiratory: Pharyngitis (10%), sinusitis (7%), cough (6%)
Miscellaneous: Diaphoresis (6%)

Restrictions An FDA-approved medication guide is available at http://www.fda.gov/cder/Offices/ODS/labeling.htm; distribute to each patient to whom this medication is dispensed.

Mechanism of Action Alpha interferons are a family of proteins, produced by nucleated cells, that have antiviral, antiproliferative, and immune-regulating activity. There are 16 known subtypes of alpha interferons. Interferons interact with cells through high affinity cell surface receptors. Following activation, multiple effects can be detected including induction of gene transcription. Inhibits cellular growth, alters the state of cellular differentiation, interferes with oncogene expression, alters cell surface antigen expression, increases phagocytic activity of macrophages, and augments cytotoxicity of lymphocytes for target cells.

Drug Interactions
Cytochrome P450 Effect: Inhibits CYP1A2 (weak)
Increased Effect/Toxicity: ACE inhibitors, clozapine, erythropoietin may increase risk of bone marrow suppression. Fluorouracil, theophylline, zidovudine concentrations may increase. Warfarin's anticoagulant effect may increase. Concurrent therapy with ribavirin may increase the risk of hemolytic anemia.
Decreased Effect: Melphalan concentrations may decrease. Prednisone may decrease effects of interferon alfa.
(Continued)

Peginterferon Alfa-2b *(Continued)*

Pharmacodynamics/Kinetics
Bioavailability: Increases with chronic dosing
Half-life elimination: 40 hours
Time to peak: 15-44 hours
Excretion: Urine (30%)

Pregnancy Risk Factor C (manufacturer) as monotherapy; X in combination with ribavirin

PEG-Intron® see Peginterferon Alfa-2b on page 1197

Pegylated Interferon Alfa-2a see Peginterferon Alfa-2a on page 1195

Pegylated Interferon Alfa-2b see Peginterferon Alfa-2b on page 1197

PemADD® [DSC] see Pemoline on page 1199

PemADD® CT [DSC] see Pemoline on page 1199

Pemetrexed (pem e TREKS ed)

U.S. Brand Names Alimta®

Canadian Brand Names Alimta®

Synonyms LY231514; MTA; Multitargeted Antifolate; NSC-698037; Pemetrexed Disodium

Pharmacologic Category Antineoplastic Agent, Antimetabolite; Antineoplastic Agent, Antimetabolite (Antifolate)

Use Treatment of malignant pleural mesothelioma in combination with cisplatin; treatment of nonsmall cell lung cancer

Unlabeled/Investigational Use Bladder, breast, cervical, colorectal, esophageal, gastric, head and neck, ovarian, pancreatic, and renal cell cancers

Local Anesthetic/Vasoconstrictor Precautions No information available to require special precautions

Effects on Dental Treatment No significant effects or complications reported

Common Adverse Effects Note: Reported frequencies of adverse effects vary by indication/population and concurrent therapy.

>10%:
Cardiovascular: Chest pain (38% to 40%), edema (19%)
Central nervous system: Fatigue (80% to 87%), fever (17% to 26%), depression (11% to 14%)
Dermatologic: Rash (17% to 22%), alopecia (11%)
Gastrointestinal: Nausea (39% to 84%; grade 3/4 in 12%), vomiting (25% to 58%; grade 3/4 in 11%), constipation (30% to 44%), anorexia (35% to 62%), stomatitis/pharyngitis (20% to 28%), diarrhea (21% to 26%)
Hematologic: Neutropenia (11% to 58%), leukopenia (13% to 55%), anemia (33%), thrombocytopenia (9% to 27%)
Nadir: 8-10 days
Recovery: 12-17 days
Neuromuscular & skeletal: Neuropathy (17% to 29%), myalgia (13%)
Renal: Creatinine increased (3% to 16%)
Respiratory: Dyspnea (66%)
Miscellaneous: Infection (17% to 23%)

1% to 10%:
Cardiovascular: Thrombosis/embolism (4% to 7%), cardiac ischemia (3%)
Endocrine & metabolic: Dehydration (3% to 7%)
Gastrointestinal: Dysphagia/esophagitis/odynophagia (5% to 6%)
Renal: Renal failure (<1% to 2%)
Miscellaneous: Allergic reaction (2% to 8%)
Neuromuscular & skeletal: Arthralgia (8%)

Mechanism of Action Inhibits thymidylate synthase (TS), dihydrofolate reductase (DHFR), glycinamide ribonucleotide formyltransferase (GARFT), and aminoimidazole carboxamide ribonucleotide formyltransferase (AICARFT), the enzymes involved in folate metabolism and DNA synthesis, resulting in inhibition of purine and thymidine nucleotide and protein synthesis.

Drug Interactions
Increased Effect/Toxicity: NSAIDs may increase the toxicity of pemetrexed.

Pharmacodynamics/Kinetics
Duration: V_{dss}: 16.1 L
Protein binding: ~81%
Metabolism: Minimal
Half-life elimination: Normal renal function: 3.5 hours
Excretion: Urine (70% to 90% as unchanged drug)

Pregnancy Risk Factor D

Pemetrexed Disodium see Pemetrexed on page 1198

Pemirolast (pe MIR oh last)

U.S. Brand Names Alamast®
Canadian Brand Names Alamast®
Generic Available No
Pharmacologic Category Mast Cell Stabilizer; Ophthalmic Agent, Miscellaneous
Use Prevention of itching of the eye due to allergic conjunctivitis
Local Anesthetic/Vasoconstrictor Precautions No information available to require special precautions
Effects on Dental Treatment No significant effects or complications reported
Mechanism of Action Mast cell stabilizer that inhibits the *in vivo* type I immediate hypersensitivity reaction; in addition, inhibits chemotaxis of eosinophils into the ocular tissue and blocks their release of mediators; also reported to prevent calcium influx into mast cells following antigen stimulation
Pregnancy Risk Factor C

Pemoline (PEM oh leen)

U.S. Brand Names Cylert® [DSC]; PemADD® [DSC]; PemADD® CT [DSC]
Generic Available Yes
Synonyms Phenylisohydantoin; PIO
Pharmacologic Category Stimulant
Use Treatment of attention-deficit/hyperactivity disorder (ADHD) (not first-line)
Unlabeled/Investigational Use Narcolepsy
Local Anesthetic/Vasoconstrictor Precautions Pemoline has minimal sympathomimetic effects; there are no precautions in using vasoconstrictors
Effects on Dental Treatment No significant effects or complications reported
Common Adverse Effects Frequency not defined.
  Central nervous system: Insomnia, dizziness, drowsiness, mental depression, increased irritability, seizure, precipitation of Tourette's syndrome, hallucinations, headache, movement disorders
  Dermatologic: Rash
  Endocrine & metabolic: Suppression of growth in children
  Gastrointestinal: Anorexia, weight loss, stomach pain, nausea
  Hematologic: Aplastic anemia
  Hepatic: Increased liver enzyme (usually reversible upon discontinuation), hepatitis, jaundice, hepatic failure
Restrictions C-IV
Mechanism of Action Blocks the reuptake mechanism of dopaminergic neurons, appears to act at the cerebral cortex and subcortical structures; CNS and respiratory stimulant with weak sympathomimetic effects; actions may be mediated via increase in CNS dopamine
Drug Interactions
  Increased Effect/Toxicity: Use caution when pemoline is used with other CNS-acting medications.
  Decreased Effect: Pemoline in combination with antiepileptic medications may decrease seizure threshold.
Pharmacodynamics/Kinetics
  Onset of action: Peak effect: 4 hours
  Duration: 8 hours
  Protein binding: 50%
  Metabolism: Partially hepatic
  Half-life elimination: Children: 7-8.6 hours; Adults: 12 hours
  Time to peak, serum: 2-4 hours
  Excretion: Urine; feces (negligible amounts)
Pregnancy Risk Factor B

Penbutolol (pen BYOO toe lole)

Related Information
  Cardiovascular Diseases *on page 1636*
U.S. Brand Names Levatol®
Canadian Brand Names Levatol®
Generic Available No
Synonyms Penbutolol Sulfate
Pharmacologic Category Beta Blocker With Intrinsic Sympathomimetic Activity
Use Treatment of mild to moderate arterial hypertension
  (Continued)

Penbutolol *(Continued)*

Local Anesthetic/Vasoconstrictor Precautions No information available to require special precautions

Effects on Dental Treatment Key adverse event(s) related to dental treatment: Xerostomia (normal salivary flow resumes upon discontinuation). Penbutolol is a nonselective beta-blocker and may enhance the pressor response to epinephrine, resulting in hypertension and bradycardia. Many nonsteroidal anti-inflammatory drugs, such as ibuprofen and indomethacin, can reduce the hypotensive effect of beta-blockers after 3 or more weeks of therapy with the NSAID. Short-term NSAID use (ie, 3 days) requires no special precautions in patients taking beta-blockers.

Common Adverse Effects 1% to 10%:

Cardiovascular: CHF, arrhythmia

Central nervous system: Mental depression, headache, dizziness, fatigue

Gastrointestinal: Nausea, diarrhea, dyspepsia

Neuromuscular & skeletal: Arthralgia

Mechanism of Action Blocks both beta$_1$- and beta$_2$-receptors and has mild intrinsic sympathomimetic activity; has negative inotropic and chronotropic effects and can significantly slow AV nodal conduction

Drug Interactions

Increased Effect/Toxicity: The heart rate lowering effects of propranolol are beta-blockers are additive with other drugs which slow AV conduction (digoxin, verapamil, diltiazem). Concurrent use of beta-blockers may increase the effects of alpha-blockers (prazosin, terazosin), alpha-adrenergic stimulants (epinephrine, phenylephrine), and the vasoconstrictive effects of ergot alkaloids. Beta-blockers may mask the tachycardia from hypoglycemia caused by insulin and oral hypoglycemics. In patients receiving concurrent therapy, the risk of hypertensive crisis is increased when either clonidine or the beta-blocker is withdrawn. Beta-blockers may increase the action or levels of ethanol, disopyramide, nondepolarizing muscle relaxants, and theophylline although the effects are difficult to predict.

Beta-blocker effects may be enhanced by oral contraceptives, flecainide, haloperidol (hypotensive effects), H$_2$-antagonists (cimetidine, possibly ranitidine), hydralazine, loop diuretics, possibly MAO inhibitors, phenothiazines, propafenone, quinidine (in extensive metabolizers), ciprofloxacin, thyroid hormones (when hypothyroid patient is converted to euthyroid state). Beta-blockers may increase the effect/toxicity of flecainide, haloperidol (hypotensive effects), hydralazine, phenothiazines, acetaminophen, anticoagulants (warfarin), and benzodiazepines.

Decreased Effect: Aluminum salts, barbiturates, calcium salts, cholestyramine, colestipol, NSAIDs, penicillins (ampicillin), rifampin, salicylates, and sulfinpyrazone decrease effect of beta-blockers due to decreased bioavailability and plasma levels. Beta-blockers may decrease the effect of sulfonylureas. Nonselective beta-blockers blunt the response to beta-2 adrenergic agonists (albuterol).

Pharmacodynamics/Kinetics

Absorption: ~100%

Protein binding: 80% to 98%

Metabolism: Extensively hepatic (oxidation and conjugation)

Bioavailability: ~100%

Half-life elimination: 5 hours

Excretion: Urine

Pregnancy Risk Factor C (manufacturer); D (2nd and 3rd trimester - expert analysis)

Penbutolol Sulfate *see* Penbutolol *on page 1199*

Penciclovir *(pen SYE kloe veer)*

Related Information

Systemic Viral Diseases *on page 1675*

Viral Infections *on page 1709*

Related Sample Prescriptions

Herpes Simplex (Recurrent) *on page 1742*

U.S. Brand Names Denavir®

Generic Available No

Pharmacologic Category Antiviral Agent

Dental Use Topical treatment of herpes simplex labialis (cold sores)

Use Topical treatment of herpes simplex labialis (cold sores)

Local Anesthetic/Vasoconstrictor Precautions No information available to require special precautions

Effects on Dental Treatment No significant effects or complications reported

Significant Adverse Effects

>10%: Dermatologic: Mild erythema (50%)

1% to 10%: Central nervous system: Headache (5.3%)

<1%: Local anesthesia (0.9%)

Postmarketing and/or case reports: Application site reaction, local edema, urticaria, pain, pruritus, paresthesia, skin discoloration, erythematous rash, oropharyngeal edema, parosmia

Dental Usual Dosing Treatment of herpes simplex labialis (cold sores): Children ≥12 years and Adults: Topical: Apply cream at the first sign or symptom of cold sore (eg, tingling, swelling); apply every 2 hours during waking hours for 4 days

Dosage Children ≥12 years and Adults: Topical: Apply cream at the first sign or symptom of cold sore (eg, tingling, swelling); apply every 2 hours during waking hours for 4 days

Mechanism of Action In cells infected with HSV-1 or HSV-2, viral thymidine kinase phosphorylates penciclovir to a monophosphate form which, in turn, is converted to penciclovir triphosphate by cellular kinases. Penciclovir triphosphate inhibits HSV polymerase competitively with deoxyguanosine triphosphate. Consequently, herpes viral DNA synthesis and, therefore, replication are selectively inhibited

Contraindications Hypersensitivity to the penciclovir or any component of the formulation; previous and significant adverse reactions to famciclovir

Warnings/Precautions Penciclovir should only be used on herpes labialis on the lips and face; because no data are available, application to mucous membranes is not recommended. Avoid application in or near eyes since it may cause irritation. The effect of penciclovir has not been established in immunocompromised patients.

Drug Interactions No data reported

Pharmacodynamics/Kinetics Absorption: Topical: None

Pregnancy Risk Factor B

Lactation Excretion in breast milk unknown

Dosage Forms Cream: 1% (1.5 g)

Penicillamine (pen i SIL a meen)

U.S. Brand Names Cuprimine®; Depen®

Canadian Brand Names Cuprimine®; Depen®

Mexican Brand Names Adalken®; Sufortan®; Sufortanon®

Generic Available No

Synonyms β,β-Dimethylcysteine; D-3-Mercaptovaline; D-Penicillamine

Pharmacologic Category Chelating Agent

Use Treatment of Wilson's disease, cystinuria; adjunctive treatment of rheumatoid arthritis

Unlabeled/Investigational Use Lead, mercury, copper, arsenic, and possibly gold poisoning (Note: Oral succimer [DMSA] is preferable for lead or mercury poisoning)

Local Anesthetic/Vasoconstrictor Precautions No information available to require special precautions

Effects on Dental Treatment No significant effects or complications reported

Common Adverse Effects Frequency not defined, may vary by indication. Adverse effects requiring discontinuation of treatment have been reported in 20% to 30% of patients with Wilson's disease.

Cardiovascular: Vasculitis

Central nervous system: Anxiety, agitation, fever, hyperpyrexia, psychiatric disturbances; worsening neurologic symptoms (10% to 50% patients with Wilson's disease)

Dermatologic: Alopecia, cheilosis, dermatomyositis, exfoliative dermatitis, lichen planus, rash (early and late 5%), pemphigus, pruritus, skin friability increased, toxic epidermal necrolysis, urticaria, wrinkling (excessive), yellow nail syndrome

Endocrine & metabolic: Hypoglycemia, thyroiditis

Gastrointestinal: Anorexia, diarrhea (17%), epigastric pain, gingivostomatitis, glossitis, nausea, oral ulcerations, pancreatitis, peptic ulcer reactivation, taste alteration (12%), vomiting

Hematologic: Eosinophilia, hemolytic anemia, leukocytosis, leukopenia (2% to 5%), monocytosis, red cell aplasia, thrombocytopenia (4% to 5%), thrombotic thrombocytopenia purpura, thrombocytosis

Hepatic: Alkaline phosphatase increased, hepatic failure, intrahepatic cholestasis, toxic hepatitis

Local: Thrombophlebitis, white papules at venipuncture and surgical sites

(Continued)

Penicillamine *(Continued)*

Neuromuscular & skeletal: Arthralgia, dystonia, myasthenia gravis, muscle weakness, neuropathies, polyarthralgia (migratory, often with objective synovitis), polymyositis

Ocular: Diplopia, extraocular muscle weakness, optic neuritis, ptosis, visual disturbances

Otic: Tinnitus

Renal: Goodpasture's syndrome, hematuria, nephrotic syndrome, proteinuria (6%), renal failure, renal vasculitis

Respiratory: Asthma, interstitial pneumonitis, pulmonary fibrosis, obliterative bronchiolitis

Miscellaneous: Allergic alveolitis, anetoderma, elastosis perforans serpiginosa, lupus-like syndrome, lactic dehydrogenase increased, lymphadenopathy, mammary hyperplasia, positive ANA test

Mechanism of Action Chelates with lead, copper, mercury and other heavy metals to form stable, soluble complexes that are excreted in urine; depresses circulating IgM rheumatoid factor, depresses T-cell but not B-cell activity; combines with cystine to form a compound which is more soluble, thus cystine calculi are prevented

Drug Interactions

Decreased Effect: Antacids, iron salts may decrease the effects of penicillamine. Penicillamine may decrease the levels of digoxin.

Pharmacodynamics/Kinetics

Onset of action: Rheumatoid arthritis: 2-3 months; Wilson's disease: 1-3 months

Absorption: 40% to 70%

Protein binding: 80% to albumin

Metabolism: Hepatic (small amounts)

Half-life elimination: 1.7-3.2 hours

Time to peak, serum: ~2 hours

Excretion: Urine (30% to 60% as unchanged drug)

Pregnancy Risk Factor D

Penicillin G Benzathine (pen i SIL in jee BENZ a theen)

Related Information

Sexually-Transmitted Diseases *on page 1674*

U.S. Brand Names Bicillin® L-A

Mexican Brand Names Bencelin®; Benzanil®; Benzetacil®

Generic Available No

Synonyms Benzathine Benzylpenicillin; Benzathine Penicillin G; Benzylpenicillin Benzathine

Pharmacologic Category Antibiotic, Penicillin

Use Active against some gram-positive organisms, few gram-negative organisms such as *Neisseria gonorrhoeae*, and some anaerobes and spirochetes; used in the treatment of syphilis; used only for the treatment of mild to moderately severe infections caused by organisms susceptible to low concentrations of penicillin G or for prophylaxis of infections caused by these organisms

Local Anesthetic/Vasoconstrictor Precautions No information available to require special precautions

Effects on Dental Treatment No significant effects or complications reported

Common Adverse Effects Frequency not defined.

Central nervous system: Convulsions, confusion, drowsiness, myoclonus, fever

Dermatologic: Rash

Endocrine & metabolic: Electrolyte imbalance

Hematologic: Positive Coombs' reaction, hemolytic anemia

Local: Pain, thrombophlebitis

Renal: Acute interstitial nephritis

Miscellaneous: Anaphylaxis, hypersensitivity reactions, Jarisch-Herxheimer reaction

Mechanism of Action Interferes with bacterial cell wall synthesis during active multiplication, causing cell wall death and resultant bactericidal activity against susceptible bacteria

Drug Interactions

Increased Effect/Toxicity: Probenecid increases penicillin levels. Aminoglycosides may lead to synergistic efficacy. Penicillins may increase the exposure to methotrexate during concurrent therapy; monitor.

Decreased Effect: Tetracyclines may decrease penicillin effectiveness. Although anecdotal reports suggest oral contraceptive efficacy could be reduced by penicillins, this has been refuted by more rigorous scientific and clinical data.

Pharmacodynamics/Kinetics

Duration: 1-4 weeks (dose dependent); larger doses result in more sustained levels

Absorption: I.M.: Slow

Time to peak, serum: 12-24 hours

Pregnancy Risk Factor B

Penicillin G Benzathine and Penicillin G Procaine

(pen i SIL in jee BENZ a theen & pen i SIL in jee PROE kane)

Related Information

Penicillin G Benzathine *on page 1202*

Penicillin G Procaine *on page 1204*

U.S. Brand Names Bicillin® C-R; Bicillin® C-R 900/300

Generic Available No

Synonyms Penicillin G Procaine and Benzathine Combined

Pharmacologic Category Antibiotic, Penicillin

Use May be used in specific situations in the treatment of streptococcal infections

Local Anesthetic/Vasoconstrictor Precautions No information available to require special precautions

Effects on Dental Treatment No significant effects or complications reported

Common Adverse Effects Frequency not defined.

Central nervous system: CNS toxicity (convulsions, confusion, drowsiness, myoclonus)

Hematologic: Positive Coombs' reaction, hemolytic anemia

Renal: Interstitial nephritis

Miscellaneous: Hypersensitivity reactions, Jarisch-Herxheimer reaction

Mechanism of Action Inhibits bacterial cell wall synthesis by binding to one or more of the penicillin binding proteins (PBPs); which in turn inhibits the final transpeptidation step of peptidoglycan synthesis in bacterial cell walls, thus inhibiting cell wall biosynthesis. Bacteria eventually lyse due to ongoing activity of cell wall autolytic enzymes (autolysins and murein hydrolases) while cell wall assembly is arrested.

Drug Interactions

Increased Effect/Toxicity: Probenecid increases penicillin levels. Aminoglycosides may lead to synergistic efficacy. Warfarin effects may be increased. Penicillins may increase the exposure to methotrexate during concurrent therapy; monitor.

Decreased Effect: Tetracyclines may decrease penicillin effectiveness. Although anecdotal reports suggest oral contraceptive efficacy could be reduced by penicillins, this has been refuted by more rigorous scientific and clinical data.

Pregnancy Risk Factor B

Penicillin G (Parenteral/Aqueous)

(pen i SIL in jee, pa REN ter al, AYE kwee us)

Related Information

Sexually-Transmitted Diseases *on page 1674*

U.S. Brand Names Pfizerpen®

Canadian Brand Names Pfizerpen®

Generic Available Yes

Synonyms Benzylpenicillin Potassium; Benzylpenicillin Sodium; Crystalline Penicillin; Penicillin G Potassium; Penicillin G Sodium

Pharmacologic Category Antibiotic, Penicillin

Use Active against some gram-positive organisms, generally not *Staphylococcus aureus*; some gram-negative organisms such as *Neisseria gonorrhoeae*, and some anaerobes and spirochetes

Local Anesthetic/Vasoconstrictor Precautions No information available to require special precautions

Effects on Dental Treatment No significant effects or complications reported

Common Adverse Effects Frequency not defined.

Central nervous system: Convulsions, confusion, drowsiness, myoclonus, fever

Dermatologic: Rash

Endocrine & metabolic: Electrolyte imbalance

Hematologic: Positive Coombs' reaction, hemolytic anemia

Local: Injection site reaction, thrombophlebitis

Renal: Acute interstitial nephritis

Miscellaneous: Anaphylaxis, hypersensitivity reactions, Jarisch-Herxheimer reaction

(Continued)

Penicillin G (Parenteral/Aqueous) *(Continued)*

Mechanism of Action Interferes with bacterial cell wall synthesis during active multiplication, causing cell wall death and resultant bactericidal activity against susceptible bacteria

Drug Interactions

Increased Effect/Toxicity: Probenecid increases penicillin levels. Aminoglycosides may lead to synergistic efficacy. Penicillins may increase the exposure to methotrexate during concurrent therapy; monitor.

Decreased Effect: Tetracyclines may decrease penicillin effectiveness. Although anecdotal reports suggest oral contraceptive efficacy could be reduced by penicillins, this has been refuted by more rigorous scientific and clinical data.

Pharmacodynamics/Kinetics

Distribution: Poor penetration across blood-brain barrier, despite inflamed meninges; crosses placenta; enters breast milk

Relative diffusion from blood into CSF: Good only with inflammation (exceeds usual MICs)

CSF:blood level ratio: Normal meninges: <1%; Inflamed meninges: 3% to 5%

Protein binding: 65%

Metabolism: Hepatic (30%) to penicilloic acid

Half-life elimination:

Neonates: <6 days old: 3.2-3.4 hours; 7-13 days old: 1.2-2.2 hours; >14 days old: 0.9-1.9 hours

Children and Adults: Normal renal function: 20-50 minutes

End-stage renal disease: 3.3-5.1 hours

Time to peak, serum: I.M.: ~30 minutes; I.V. ~1 hour

Excretion: Urine

Pregnancy Risk Factor B

Penicillin G Potassium *see* Penicillin G (Parenteral/Aqueous) *on page 1203*

Penicillin G Procaine *(pen i SIL in jee PROE kane)*

Related Information

Sexually-Transmitted Diseases *on page 1674*

Canadian Brand Names Pfizerpen-AS®; Wycillin®

Generic Available Yes

Synonyms APPG; Aqueous Procaine Penicillin G; Procaine Benzylpenicillin; Procaine Penicillin G; Wycillin [DSC]

Pharmacologic Category Antibiotic, Penicillin

Use Moderately severe infections due to *Treponema pallidum* and other penicillin G-sensitive microorganisms that are susceptible to low, but prolonged serum penicillin concentrations; anthrax due to *Bacillus anthracis* (postexposure) to reduce the incidence or progression of disease following exposure to aerolized *Bacillus anthracis*

Local Anesthetic/Vasoconstrictor Precautions No information available to require special precautions

Effects on Dental Treatment No significant effects or complications reported

Common Adverse Effects Frequency not defined.

Cardiovascular: Myocardial depression, vasodilation, conduction disturbances

Central nervous system: Confusion, drowsiness, myoclonus, CNS stimulation, seizure

Hematologic: Positive Coombs' reaction, hemolytic anemia, neutropenia

Local: Pain at injection site, thrombophlebitis, sterile abscess at injection site

Renal: Interstitial nephritis

Miscellaneous: Pseudoanaphylactic reactions, hypersensitivity reactions, Jarisch-Herxheimer reaction, serum sickness

Mechanism of Action Inhibits bacterial cell wall synthesis by binding to one or more of the penicillin binding proteins (PBPs); which in turn inhibits the final transpeptidation step of peptidoglycan synthesis in bacterial cell walls, thus inhibiting cell wall biosynthesis. Bacteria eventually lyse due to ongoing activity of cell wall autolytic enzymes (autolysins and murein hydrolases) while cell wall assembly is arrested.

Drug Interactions

Increased Effect/Toxicity: Probenecid increases penicillin levels. Aminoglycosides may lead to synergistic efficacy. Penicillins may increase the exposure to methotrexate during concurrent therapy; monitor.

Decreased Effect: Tetracyclines may decrease penicillin effectiveness. Although anecdotal reports suggest oral contraceptive efficacy could be reduced by penicillins, this has been refuted by more rigorous scientific and clinical data.

Pharmacodynamics/Kinetics
Duration: Therapeutic: 15-24 hours
Absorption: I.M.: Slow
Distribution: Penetration across the blood-brain barrier is poor, despite inflamed meninges; enters breast milk
Protein binding: 65%
Metabolism: ~30% hepatically inactivated
Time to peak, serum: 1-4 hours
Excretion: Urine (60% to 90% as unchanged drug)
  Clearance: Renal: Delayed in neonates, young infants, and with impaired renal function

Pregnancy Risk Factor B

Penicillin G Procaine and Benzathine Combined see Penicillin G Benzathine and Penicillin G Procaine on page 1203

Penicillin G Sodium see Penicillin G (Parenteral/Aqueous) on page 1203

Penicillin V Potassium (pen i SIL in vee poe TASS ee um)

Related Information
Antibiotic Prophylaxis on page 1680
Bacterial Infections on page 1697
Viral Infections on page 1709
Related Sample Prescriptions
Bacterial Infections and Periodontal Diseases on page 1736
U.S. Brand Names Veetids®
Canadian Brand Names Apo-Pen VK®; Novo-Pen-VK; Nu-Pen-VK
Generic Available Yes
Synonyms Pen VK; Phenoxymethyl Penicillin
Pharmacologic Category Antibiotic, Penicillin
Dental Use Antibiotic of first choice in treatment of common orofacial infections caused by aerobic gram-positive cocci and anaerobes. These orofacial infections include cellulitis, periapical abscess, periodontal abscess, acute suppurative pulpitis, oronasal fistula, pericoronitis, osteitis, osteomyelitis, postsurgical and post-traumatic infection. **Note: This agent is no longer recommended for dental procedure prophylaxis.**
Use Treatment of infections caused by susceptible organisms involving the respiratory tract, otitis media, sinusitis, skin, and urinary tract; prophylaxis in rheumatic fever
Local Anesthetic/Vasoconstrictor Precautions No information available to require special precautions
Effects on Dental Treatment Key adverse event(s) related to dental treatment: Oral candidiasis (prolonged use).
Significant Adverse Effects
>10%: Gastrointestinal: Mild diarrhea, vomiting, nausea, oral candidiasis
<1% (Limited to important or life-threatening): Acute interstitial nephritis, convulsions, hemolytic anemia, positive Coombs' reaction
Dental Usual Dosing Note: No longer recommended for dental procedure prophylaxis
Orofacial infections: Oral:
  Children <12 years: 25-50 mg/kg/day in divided doses every 6-8 hours (maximum dose: 3 g/day)
  Children ≥12 years and Adults: 125-500 mg every 6-8 hours

Dosage
Usual dosage range:
  Children <12 years: Oral: 25-50 mg/kg/day in divided doses every 6-8 hours (maximum dose: 3 g/day)
  Children ≥12 years and Adults: Oral: 125-500 mg every 6-8 hours
Indication-specific dosing:
  Children: Oral:
    Pharyngitis (streptococcal): 250 mg 2-3 times/day for 10 days
    Prophylaxis of pneumococcal infections:
      Children <5 years: 125 mg twice daily
      Children ≥5 years: 250 mg twice daily
    Prophylaxis of recurrent rheumatic fever:
      Children <5 years: 125 mg twice daily
      Children ≥5 years: 250 mg twice daily
  Adults: Oral:
    Acintomycosis:
      Mild: 2-4 g/day in 4 divided doses for 8 weeks
      Surgical: 2-4 g/day in 4 divided doses for 6-12 months (after I.V. penicillin G therapy of 4-6 weeks)

(Continued)

Penicillin V Potassium *(Continued)*

Erysipelas: 500 mg 4 times/day

Pharyngitis (streptococcal): 500 mg 3-4 times/day for 10 days

Prophylaxis of pneumococcal or recurrent rheumatic fever infections: 250 mg twice daily

Dosing interval in renal impairment: Cl_{cr} <10 mL/minute: Administer 250 mg every 6 hours

Mechanism of Action Inhibits bacterial cell wall synthesis by binding to one or more of the penicillin binding proteins (PBPs); which in turn inhibits the final transpeptidation step of peptidoglycan synthesis in bacterial cell walls, thus inhibiting cell wall biosynthesis. Bacteria eventually lyse due to ongoing activity of cell wall autolytic enzymes (autolysins and murein hydrolases) while cell wall assembly is arrested.

Contraindications Hypersensitivity to penicillin or any component of the formulation

Warnings/Precautions Use with caution in patients with severe renal impairment (modify dosage), history of seizures, or hypersensitivity to cephalosporins

Drug Interactions

Aminoglycosides: May be synergistic against selected organisms

Methotrexate: Penicillins may increase the exposure to methotrexate during concurrent therapy; monitor.

Oral contraceptives: Anecdotal reports suggesting decreased contraceptive efficacy with penicillins have been refuted by more rigorous scientific and clinical data.

Probenecid, disulfiram: May increase penicillin levels

Tetracyclines: May decrease penicillin effectiveness

Warfarin: Effects of warfarin may be increased

Ethanol/Nutrition/Herb Interactions Food: Decreases drug absorption rate; decreases drug serum concentration.

Dietary Considerations Take on an empty stomach 1 hour before or 2 hours after meals.

Pharmacodynamics/Kinetics

Absorption: 60% to 73%

Distribution: Enters breast milk

Protein binding, plasma: 80%

Half-life elimination: 30 minutes; prolonged with renal impairment

Time to peak, serum: 0.5-1 hour

Excretion: Urine (as unchanged drug and metabolites)

Pregnancy Risk Factor B

Lactation Enters breast milk (other penicillins are compatible with breast-feeding)

Breast-Feeding Considerations No data reported; however, other penicillins may be taken while breast-feeding.

Dosage Forms Note: 250 mg = 400,000 units

Powder for oral solution: 125 mg/5 mL (100 mL, 200 mL); 250 mg/5 mL (100 mL, 200 mL)

Tablet: 250 mg, 500 mg

Selected Readings

Wynn RL and Bergman SA, "Antibiotics and Their Use in the Treatment of Orofacial Infections, Part I," *Gen Dent*, 1994, 42(5):398, 400, 402.

Wynn RL and Bergman SA, "Antibiotics and Their Use in the Treatment of Orofacial Infections, Part II," *Gen Dent*, 1994, 42(6):498-502.

Wynn RL, Bergman SA, Meiller TF, et al, "Antibiotics in Treating Oral-Facial Infections of Odontogenic Origin: An Update," *Gen Dent*, 2001, 49(3):238-40, 242, 244 passim.

Penicilloyl-polylysine *see* Benzylpenicilloyl-polylysine *on page 198*

Penlac® *see* Ciclopirox *on page 338*

Pentafluoropropane and Tetrafluoroethane

(pen ta flure oh PRO pane & tet ra flure oh ETH ane)

U.S. Brand Names Gebauer's Instant Ice™ [OTC]; Gebauer's Pain Ease®; Gebauer's Spray and Stretch®

Generic Available No

Synonyms Tetrafluoroethane and Pentafluoropropane

Pharmacologic Category Anesthetic, Topical

Use

Treatment of myofascial pain, restricted motion due to muscle tension, muscle spasm and minor sports injuries (eg, bruises, contusions, swelling, minor sprains); pain associated with injections or minor surgical procedures

Local Anesthetic/Vasoconstrictor Precautions No information available to require special precautions

Effects on Dental Treatment No significant effects or complications reported
Common Adverse Effects
Frequency not defined.
Dermatologic: Skin irritation, skin pigmentation change, frostbite
Mechanism of Action
Vapocoolant and counterirritant

Pentahydrate *see* Sodium Thiosulfate *on page 1404*
Pentam-300® *see* Pentamidine *on page 1207*

Pentamidine (pen TAM i deen)

U.S. Brand Names NebuPent®; Pentam-300®
Generic Available No
Synonyms Pentamidine Isethionate
Pharmacologic Category Antibiotic, Miscellaneous
Use Treatment and prevention of pneumonia caused by *Pneumocystis carinii* (PCP)
Unlabeled/Investigational Use Treatment of trypanosomiasis and visceral leishmaniasis
Local Anesthetic/Vasoconstrictor Precautions No information available to require special precautions (see Dental Comment)
Effects on Dental Treatment No significant effects or complications reported
Common Adverse Effects Injection (I); Aerosol (A)
>10%:
Cardiovascular: Chest pain (A - 10% to 23%)
Central nervous system: Fatigue (A - 50% to 70%); dizziness (A - 31% to 47%)
Dermatologic: Rash (31% to 47%)
Endocrine & metabolic: Hyperkalemia
Gastrointestinal: Anorexia (A - 50% to 70%), nausea (A - 10% to 23%)
Local: Local reactions at injection site
Renal: Increased creatinine (I - 23%)
Respiratory: Wheezing (A - 10% to 23%), dyspnea (A - 50% to 70%), cough (A - 31% to 47%), pharyngitis (10% to 23%)
1% to 10%:
Cardiovascular: Hypotension (I - 4%)
Central nervous system: Confusion/hallucinations (1% to 2%), headache (A - 1% to 5%)
Dermatologic: Rash (I - 3.3%)
Endocrine & metabolic: Hypoglycemia <25 mg/dL (I - 2.4%)
Gastrointestinal: Nausea/anorexia (I - 6%), diarrhea (A - 1% to 5%), vomiting
Hematologic: Severe leukopenia (I - 2.8%), thrombocytopenia <20,000/mm^3 (I - 1.7%), anemia (A - 1% to 5%)
Hepatic: Increased LFTs (I - 8.7%)
Mechanism of Action Interferes with RNA/DNA, phospholipids and protein synthesis, through inhibition of oxidative phosphorylation and/or interference with incorporation of nucleotides and nucleic acids into RNA and DNA, in protozoa
Drug Interactions
Cytochrome P450 Effect: **Substrate** of CYP2C19 (major); **Inhibits** CYP2C8/9 (weak), 2C19 (weak), 2D6 (weak), 3A4 (weak)
Increased Effect/Toxicity: CYP2C19 inhibitors may increase the levels/effects of pentamidine; example inhibitors include delavirdine, fluconazole, fluvoxamine, gemfibrozil, isoniazid, omeprazole, and ticlopidine. Pentamidine may potentiate the effect of other drugs which prolong QT interval (cisapride, sparfloxacin, gatifloxacin, moxifloxacin, pimozide, and type Ia and type III antiarrhythmics).
Decreased Effect: CYP2C19 inducers may decrease the levels/effects of pentamidine; example inducers include aminoglutethimide, carbamazepine, phenytoin, and rifampin.
Pharmacodynamics/Kinetics
Absorption: I.M.: Well absorbed; Inhalation: Limited systemic absorption
Half-life elimination: Terminal: 6.4-9.4 hours; may be prolonged with severe renal impairment
Excretion: Urine (33% to 66% as unchanged drug)
Pregnancy Risk Factor C
Dental Comment
This drug is known to prolong the QT interval. The QT interval is measured as the time and distance between the Q point of the QRS complex and the end of the T wave in the ECG tracing. After adjustment for heart rate, the QT interval is defined as prolonged if it is more than 450 msec in men and 460 msec in
(Continued)

Pentamidine *(Continued)*

women. A long QT syndrome was first described in the 1950s and 60s as a congenital syndrome involving QT interval prolongation and syncope and sudden death. Some of the congenital long QT syndromes were characterized by a peculiar electrocardiographic appearance of the QRS complex involving a premature atria beat followed by a pause, then a subsequent sinus beat showing marked QT prolongation and deformity. This type of cardiac arrhythmia was originally termed "torsade de pointes" (translated from the French as "twisting of the points").

Prolongation of the QT interval is thought to result from delayed ventricular repolarization. The repolarization process within the myocardial cell is due to the efflux of intracellular potassium. The channels associated with this current can be blocked by many drugs and predisposes the electrical propagation cycle to torsade de pointes.

Pentamidine is one of the drugs confirmed to prolong the QT interval and is accepted as having a risk of causing torsade de pointes. The risk of drug-induced torsade de pointes is extremely low when a single QT interval prolonging drug is prescribed. In terms of epinephrine, it is not known what effect vasoconstrictors in the local anesthetic regimen will have in patients with a known history of congenital prolonged QT interval or in patients taking any medication that prolongs the QT interval. Until more information is obtained, it is suggested that the clinician consult with the physician prior to the use of a vasoconstrictor in suspected patients, and that the vasoconstrictor (epinephrine, levonordefrin [Neo-Cobefrin®]) be used with caution.

Pentamidine Isethionate *see* Pentamidine *on page 1207*
Pentasa® *see* Mesalamine *on page 996*
Pentaspan® *see* Pentastarch *on page 1208*

Pentastarch *(PEN ta starch)*

U.S. Brand Names Pentaspan®
Canadian Brand Names Pentaspan®
Mexican Brand Names Pentaspan®
Generic Available No
Pharmacologic Category Blood Modifiers
Use Orphan drug: Adjunct in leukapheresis to improve harvesting and increase yield of leukocytes by centrifugal means
Local Anesthetic/Vasoconstrictor Precautions No information available to require special precautions
Effects on Dental Treatment No significant effects or complications reported

Pentavalent Human-Bovine Reassortant Rotavirus Vaccine *see* Rotavirus Vaccine *on page 1371*

Pentazocine *(pen TAZ oh seen)*

U.S. Brand Names Talwin®; Talwin® NX
Canadian Brand Names Talwin®
Generic Available Yes: Tablet
Synonyms Naloxone Hydrochloride and Pentazocine Hydrochloride; Pentazocine Hydrochloride; Pentazocine Hydrochloride and Naloxone Hydrochloride; Pentazocine Lactate
Pharmacologic Category Analgesic, Narcotic
Use Relief of moderate to severe pain; has also been used as a sedative prior to surgery and as a supplement to surgical anesthesia
Local Anesthetic/Vasoconstrictor Precautions No information available to require special precautions
Effects on Dental Treatment No significant effects or complications reported
Common Adverse Effects Frequency not defined.
Cardiovascular: Circulatory depression, facial edema, flushing, hypotension, shock, syncope, tachycardia
Central nervous system: Chills, CNS depression, confusion, disorientation, dizziness, drowsiness, euphoria, excitement, hallucinations, headache, insomnia, irritability, lightheadedness, malaise, nightmares, sedation
Dermatologic: dermatitis, erythema multiforme, pruritus, rash, Stevens-Johnson syndrome, toxic epidermal necrolysis, urticaria
Gastrointestinal: Abdominal distress, anorexia, constipation, diarrhea, nausea, vomiting, xerostomia
Genitourinary: Urinary retention

Hematologic: Decreased WBCs, eosinophilia

Local: Tissue damage and irritation with I.M./SubQ use

Neuromuscular & skeletal: Paresthesia, tremor, weakness

Ocular: Blurred vision, miosis

Otic: Tinnitus

Respiratory: Dyspnea, respiratory depression (rare)

Miscellaneous: Anaphylaxis, diaphoresis, physical and psychological dependence

Restrictions C-IV

Mechanism of Action Binds to opiate receptors in the CNS, causing inhibition of ascending pain pathways, altering the perception of and response to pain; produces generalized CNS depression; partial agonist-antagonist

Drug Interactions

Increased Effect/Toxicity: Increased effect/toxicity with tripelennamine (can be lethal), CNS depressants (eg, phenothiazines, tranquilizers, anxiolytics, sedatives, hypnotics, alcohol).

Decreased Effect: May potentiate or reduce analgesic effect of opiate agonist (eg, morphine) depending on patients tolerance to opiates; can precipitate withdrawal in narcotic addicts.

Pharmacodynamics/Kinetics

Onset of action: Oral, I.M., SubQ: 15-30 minutes; I.V.: 2-3 minutes

Duration: Oral: 4-5 hours; Parenteral: 2-3 hours

Protein binding: 60%

Metabolism: Hepatic via oxidative and glucuronide conjugation pathways; extensive first-pass effect

Bioavailability: Oral: ~20%; increased to 60% to 70% with cirrhosis

Half-life elimination: 2-3 hours; prolonged with hepatic impairment

Excretion: Urine (small amounts as unchanged drug)

Pregnancy Risk Factor C/D (prolonged use or high doses at term)

Pentazocine and Acetaminophen

(pen TAZ oh seen & a seet a MIN oh fen)

Related Information

Acetaminophen *on page 31*

Pentazocine *on page 1208*

U.S. Brand Names Talacen®

Generic Available Yes

Synonyms Acetaminophen and Pentazocine; Pentazocine Hydrochloride and Acetaminophen

Pharmacologic Category Analgesic Combination (Narcotic)

Dental Use Relief of mild to moderate pain

Use Relief of mild to moderate pain

Local Anesthetic/Vasoconstrictor Precautions No information available to require special precautions

Effects on Dental Treatment No significant effects or complications reported

Significant Adverse Effects Frequency not defined.

Cardiovascular: Tachycardia, hypotension, syncope, flushing

Central nervous system: Headache, dizziness, drowsiness, lightheadedness, sedation, insomnia, hallucinations, euphoria, depression, confusion, disorientation, chills, irritability, excitement

Dermatologic: Rash, urticaria, erythema multiforme, Stevens-Johnson syndrome, toxic epidermal necrolysis

Gastrointestinal: Nausea, vomiting, biliary spasm, constipation, anorexia, diarrhea, abdominal distress

Genitourinary: Urinary retention

Hematologic: WBCs decreased, eosinophilia, thrombocytopenic purpura, hemolytic anemia, agranulocytosis

Neuromuscular & skeletal: Weakness, tremor, paresthesia

Ocular: Blurred vision

Otic: Tinnitus

Respiratory: Respiratory depression

Miscellaneous: Diaphoresis, facial edema, anaphylaxis

Restrictions C-IV

Dental Usual Dosing Analgesic: Adults: Oral: 1 caplet every 4 hours, up to maximum of 6 caplets

Dosage Oral: Adults: Analgesic: 1 caplet every 4 hours, up to a maximum of 6 caplets

(Continued)

Pentazocine and Acetaminophen *(Continued)*

Mechanism of Action

Pentazocine: Binds to opiate receptors in the CNS, causing inhibition of ascending pain pathways, altering the perception of and response to pain; produces generalized CNS depression; partial agonist-antagonist

Acetaminophen: Inhibits the synthesis of prostaglandins in the central nervous system and peripherally blocks pain impulse generation

Contraindications Hypersensitivity to pentazocine, acetaminophen, or any component of the formulation; pregnancy (prolonged use or high doses at term)

Warnings/Precautions Contains sodium metasulfite; may cause allergic-type reactions; potential for elevating CSF pressure due to respiratory effects which may be exaggerated in presence of head injury, intracranial lesions, or pre-existing increase in intracranial lesions. May experience hallucinations, disorientation, and confusion. May cause psychological and physical dependence. Use with caution in patients with myocardial infarction who have nausea or vomiting, patients with respiratory depression, severely limited respiratory reserve, severe bronchial asthma, other obstructive respiratory conditions or cyanosis, impaired renal or hepatic function, patients prone to seizures. Abrupt discontinuation may result in withdrawal symptoms. Pentazocine may precipitate opiate withdrawal symptoms in patients who have been receiving opiates regularly.

Ethanol/Nutrition/Herb Interactions

Ethanol: Avoid ethanol (may increase CNS depression).

Herb/Nutraceutical: Avoid valerian, St John's wort, kava kava, gotu kola (may increase CNS depression).

Pharmacodynamics/Kinetics See individual agents.

Pregnancy Risk Factor C/D (prolonged use or high doses at term)

Lactation Excretion in breast milk unknown/use caution

Breast-Feeding Considerations Excretion of pentazocine in breast milk is unknown; acetaminophen is excreted in breast milk

Dosage Forms Caplet: Pentazocine 25 mg and acetaminophen 650 mg [contains sodium metabisulfite]

Pentazocine Hydrochloride *see* Pentazocine *on page 1208*

Pentazocine Hydrochloride and Acetaminophen *see* Pentazocine and Acetaminophen *on page 1209*

Pentazocine Hydrochloride and Naloxone Hydrochloride *see* Pentazocine *on page 1208*

Pentazocine Lactate *see* Pentazocine *on page 1208*

Pentetate Calcium Trisodium *see* Diethylene Triamine Penta-Acetic Acid *on page 466*

Pentetate Zinc Trisodium *see* Diethylene Triamine Penta-Acetic Acid *on page 466*

Pentobarbital *(pen toe BAR bi tal)*

U.S. Brand Names Nembutal®

Canadian Brand Names Nembutal® Sodium

Generic Available No

Synonyms Pentobarbital Sodium

Pharmacologic Category Anticonvulsant, Barbiturate; Barbiturate

Use Sedative/hypnotic; preanesthetic; high-dose barbiturate coma for treatment of increased intracranial pressure or status epilepticus unresponsive to other therapy

Local Anesthetic/Vasoconstrictor Precautions No information available to require special precautions

Effects on Dental Treatment No significant effects or complications reported

Mechanism of Action Short-acting barbiturate with sedative, hypnotic, and anticonvulsant properties. Barbiturates depress the sensory cortex, decrease motor activity, alter cerebellar function, and produce drowsiness, sedation, and hypnosis. In high doses, barbiturates exhibit anticonvulsant activity; barbiturates produce dose-dependent respiratory depression.

Pregnancy Risk Factor D

Pentobarbital Sodium *see* Pentobarbital *on page 1210*

Pentosan Polysulfate Sodium
(PEN toe san pol i SUL fate SOW dee um)

U.S. Brand Names Elmiron®
Canadian Brand Names Elmiron®
Generic Available No
Synonyms PPS
Pharmacologic Category Analgesic, Urinary
Use Orphan drug: Relief of bladder pain or discomfort due to interstitial cystitis
Local Anesthetic/Vasoconstrictor Precautions No information available to require special precautions
Effects on Dental Treatment No significant effects or complications reported
Common Adverse Effects 1% to 10%:
  Central nervous system: Headache (3%), dizziness (1%)
  Dermatologic: Alopecia (4%), rash (3%)
  Gastrointestinal: Rectal hemorrhage (6%), diarrhea (4%), nausea (4%), dyspepsia (2%), abdominal pain (2%)
  Hepatic: Liver function test abnormalities (1%)
Mechanism of Action Although pentosan polysulfate sodium is a low-molecular weight heparinoid, it is not known whether these properties play a role in its mechanism of action in treating interstitial cystitis; the drug appears to adhere to the bladder wall mucosa where it may act as a buffer to protect the tissues from irritating substances in the urine.
Drug Interactions
  Increased Effect/Toxicity: Concomitant therapy with anticoagulants, antiplatelet agents, or salicylates may increase the risk of bleeding.
Pharmacodynamics/Kinetics
  Absorption: ~3%
  Metabolism: Hepatic and via spleen; some metabolism occurs in renal parenchyma
  Half-life elimination: 4.8 hours
  Excretion: Urine (3% as unchanged drug)
Pregnancy Risk Factor B

Pentostatin (PEN toe stat in)

U.S. Brand Names Nipent®
Canadian Brand Names Nipent®
Generic Available No
Synonyms CL-825; Co-Vidarabine; dCF; Deoxycoformycin; NSC-218321; 2'-Deoxycoformycin
Pharmacologic Category Antineoplastic Agent, Antibiotic; Antineoplastic Agent, Antimetabolite (Purine Antagonist)
Use Treatment of hairy cell leukemia; non-Hodgkin's lymphoma, cutaneous T-cell lymphoma
Local Anesthetic/Vasoconstrictor Precautions No information available to require special precautions
Effects on Dental Treatment Key adverse event(s) related to dental treatment: Stomatitis.
Common Adverse Effects
  >10%:
    Central nervous system: Fever, chills, headache
    Dermatologic: Skin rash (25% to 30%), alopecia (10%)
    Gastrointestinal: Mild to moderate nausea, vomiting (60%), stomatitis, diarrhea (13%), anorexia
    Genitourinary: Acute renal failure (35%)
    Hematologic: Thrombocytopenia (50%), dose-limiting in 25% of patients; anemia (40% to 45%), neutropenia, mild to moderate, not dose-limiting (11%)
      Nadir: 7 days
      Recovery: 10-14 days
    Hepatic: Transaminases increased, mild-moderate, usually transient (30%); hepatitis (19%), usually reversible
    Respiratory: Pulmonary edema (15%), may be exacerbated by fludarabine
    Miscellaneous: Infection (57%; 35% severe, life-threatening)
  1% to 10%:
    Cardiovascular: Chest pain, arrhythmia, peripheral edema
    Central nervous system: Opportunistic infection (8%); anxiety, confusion, depression, dizziness, insomnia, nervousness, somnolence, myalgia, malaise
(Continued)

Pentostatin *(Continued)*

Dermatologic: Dry skin, eczema, pruritus
Gastrointestinal: Constipation, flatulence, weight loss
Neuromuscular & skeletal: Paresthesia, weakness
Ocular: Moderate to severe keratoconjunctivitis, abnormal vision, eye pain
Otic: Ear pain
Respiratory: Dyspnea, pneumonia, bronchitis, pharyngitis, rhinitis, epistaxis, sinusitis (3% to 7%)

Mechanism of Action Pentostatin is a purine antimetabolite that inhibits adenosine deaminase, preventing the deamination of adenosine to inosine. Accumulation of deoxyadenosine (dAdo) and deoxyadenosine 5'-triphosphate (dATP) results in a reduction of purine metabolism and DNA synthesis and cell death.

Drug Interactions

Increased Effect/Toxicity: Increased toxicity with vidarabine and allopurinol; combined use with fludarabine may lead to severe, even fatal, pulmonary toxicity

Pharmacodynamics/Kinetics

Distribution: I.V.: V_d: 36.1 L (20.1 L/m²); rapidly to body tissues
Half-life elimination: Distribution half-life: 30-85 minutes; Terminal: 5-15 hours
Excretion: Urine (~50% to 96%) within 24 hours (30% to 90% as unchanged drug)

Pregnancy Risk Factor D

Pentothal® *see* Thiopental *on page 1477*

Pentoxifylline *(pen toks I fi leen)*

U.S. Brand Names Pentoxil®; Trental®
Canadian Brand Names Albert® Pentoxifylline; Apo-Pentoxifylline SR®; Nu-Pentoxifylline SR; ratio-Pentoxifylline; Trental®
Mexican Brand Names Fixoten®; Kentadin®; Peridane®; Sufisal®; Trental®; Vasofyl®
Generic Available Yes
Synonyms Oxpentifylline
Pharmacologic Category Blood Viscosity Reducer Agent
Use Treatment of intermittent claudication on the basis of chronic occlusive arterial disease of the limbs; may improve function and symptoms, but not intended to replace more definitive therapy
Unlabeled/Investigational Use AIDS patients with increased TNF, CVA, cerebrovascular diseases, diabetic atherosclerosis, diabetic neuropathy, gangrene, hemodialysis shunt thrombosis, vascular impotence, cerebral malaria, septic shock, sickle cell syndromes, and vasculitis
Local Anesthetic/Vasoconstrictor Precautions No information available to require special precautions
Effects on Dental Treatment No significant effects or complications reported
Common Adverse Effects
1% to 10%: Gastrointestinal: Nausea (2%), vomiting (1%)
Mechanism of Action Reduces blood viscosity via increased leukocyte and erythrocyte deformability and decreased neutrophil adhesion/activation; improves peripheral tissue oxygenation presumably through enhanced blood flow.
Drug Interactions
Cytochrome P450 Effect: Inhibits CYP1A2 (weak)
Increased Effect/Toxicity:
Pentoxifylline may increase the serum levels of theophylline.
Pharmacodynamics/Kinetics
Absorption: Well absorbed
Metabolism: Hepatic and via erythrocytes; extensive first-pass effect
Half-life elimination: Parent drug: 24-48 minutes; Metabolites: 60-96 minutes
Time to peak, serum: 2-4 hours
Excretion: Primarily urine (active metabolites); feces (4%)
Pregnancy Risk Factor C

Pentoxil® *see* Pentoxifylline *on page 1212*
Pen VK *see* Penicillin V Potassium *on page 1205*
Pepcid® *see* Famotidine *on page 635*
Pepcid® AC [OTC] *see* Famotidine *on page 635*
Pepcid® Complete [OTC] *see* Famotidine, Calcium Carbonate, and Magnesium Hydroxide *on page 636*
Pepto-Bismol® [OTC] *see* Bismuth *on page 210*
Pepto-Bismol® Maximum Strength [OTC] *see* Bismuth *on page 210*

Perchloracap® [DSC] *see* Potassium Perchlorate *on page 1261*

Percocet® *see* Oxycodone and Acetaminophen *on page 1165*

Percodan® *see* Oxycodone and Aspirin *on page 1168*

Percogesic® [OTC] *see* Acetaminophen and Phenyltoloxamine *on page 38*

Percogesic® Extra Strength [OTC] *see* Acetaminophen and Diphenhydramine *on page 38*

Perdiem® Overnight Relief [OTC] *see* Senna *on page 1384*

Pergolide (PER go lide)

U.S. Brand Names Permax®
Canadian Brand Names Permax®
Mexican Brand Names Permax®
Generic Available Yes
Synonyms Pergolide Mesylate
Pharmacologic Category Anti-Parkinson's Agent, Dopamine Agonist; Ergot Derivative
Use Adjunctive treatment to levodopa/carbidopa in the management of Parkinson's disease
Unlabeled/Investigational Use Tourette's disorder, chronic motor or vocal tic disorder
Local Anesthetic/Vasoconstrictor Precautions No information available to require special precautions
Effects on Dental Treatment Key adverse event(s) related to dental treatment: Xerostomia (normal salivary flow resumes upon discontinuation). Prolonged use may decrease or inhibit salivary flow, contributing to discomfort and dental disease (ie, oral candidiasis and periodontal disease).
Common Adverse Effects
>10%:
Central nervous system: Dizziness (19%), hallucinations (14%), dystonia (12%), somnolence (10%), confusion (10%)
Gastrointestinal: Nausea (24%), constipation (11%)
Neuromuscular & skeletal: Dyskinesia (62%)
Respiratory: Rhinitis (12%)
1% to 10%:
Cardiovascular: Hypotension or postural hypotension (10%), peripheral edema (7%), chest pain (4%), vasodilation (3%), palpitation (2%), syncope (2%), arrhythmia (1%), hypertension (2%), MI (1%)
Central nervous system: Insomnia (8%), pain (7%), anxiety (6%), psychosis (2%), EPS (2%), incoordination (2%), chills (1%)
Dermatologic: Rash (3%)
Gastrointestinal: Diarrhea (6%), dyspepsia (6%), abdominal pain (6%), anorexia (5%), xerostomia (4%), vomiting (3%), dysphagia (1%), nausea (1%)
Hematologic: Anemia (1%)
Neuromuscular & skeletal: Myalgia (1%), neuralgia (1%)
Ocular: Abnormal vision (6%), diplopia (2%)
Respiratory: Dyspnea (5%), epistaxis (2%)
Miscellaneous: Flu syndrome (3%), hiccups (1%)
Mechanism of Action Pergolide is a semisynthetic ergot alkaloid similar to bromocriptine but stated to be more potent (10-1000 times) and longer-acting; it is a centrally-active dopamine agonist stimulating both D_1 and D_2 receptors. Pergolide is believed to exert its therapeutic effect by directly stimulating postsynaptic dopamine receptors in the nigrostriatal system.
Drug Interactions
Cytochrome P450 Effect: Substrate of CYP3A4 (major); **Inhibits** CYP2D6 (strong), 3A4 (weak)
Increased Effect/Toxicity: Effects of pergolide may be increased by levodopa (hallucinations) and MAO inhibitors. Pergolide may increase the levels/effects of amphetamines, selected beta-blockers, dextromethorphan, fluoxetine, lidocaine, mirtazapine, nefazodone, paroxetine, risperidone, ritonavir, thioridazine, tricyclic antidepressants, venlafaxine, and other CYP2D6 substrates. Pergolide may increase the levels/effects of sibutramine and other serotonin agonists (serotonin syndrome). Macrolide antibiotics may increase the effects of pergolide. The levels/effects of pergolide may be increased by azole antifungals, clarithromycin, diclofenac, doxycycline, erythromycin, imatinib, isoniazid, nefazodone, nicardipine, propofol, protease inhibitors, quinidine, telithromycin, verapamil, and other CYP3A4 inhibitors.
Decreased Effect: Effects of pergolide may be diminished by antipsychotics, metoclopramide. Pergolide may decrease the levels/effects of CYP2D6 prodrug substrates (eg, codeine, hydrocodone, oxycodone, tramadol).
(Continued)

Pergolide *(Continued)*

Pharmacodynamics/Kinetics
Absorption: Well absorbed
Protein binding, plasma: 90%
Metabolism: Extensively hepatic
Half-life elimination: 27 hours
Excretion: Urine (~50%); feces (50%)

Pregnancy Risk Factor B

Pergolide Mesylate *see* Pergolide *on page 1213*

Pergonal® [DSC] *see* Menotropins *on page 982*

Periactin *see* Cyproheptadine *on page 412*

Peri-Colace® [DSC] [OTC] *see* Docusate and Casanthranol *on page 496*

Pericyazine *(per ee CYE ah zeen)*

Canadian Brand Names Neuleptil®

Pharmacologic Category Antipsychotic Agent, Typical, Phenothiazine, Piperidine

Use Adjunctive therapy in selected psychotic patients to control prevailing hostility, impulsivity, or aggression

Local Anesthetic/Vasoconstrictor Precautions Most pharmacology textbooks state that in presence of phenothiazines, systemic doses of epinephrine paradoxically decrease the blood pressure. This is the so called "epinephrine reversal" phenomenon. This has never been observed when epinephrine is given by infiltration as part of the anesthesia procedure. See Dental Comment.

Effects on Dental Treatment Key adverse event(s) related to dental treatment:

Significant hypotension may occur, especially when the drug is administered parenterally. Orthostatic hypotension is due to alpha-receptor blockade; elderly are at greater risk.

Tardive dyskinesia: Prevalence rate may be 40% in elderly; development of the syndrome and the irreversible nature are proportional to duration and total cumulative dose over time. Extrapyramidal reactions are more common in elderly with up to 50% developing these reactions after 60 years of age. Drug-induced Parkinson's syndrome occurs often; akathisia is the most common extrapyramidal reaction in elderly.

Increased confusion, memory loss, psychotic behavior, and agitation frequently occur as a consequence of anticholinergic effects. Antipsychotic-associated sedation in nonpsychotic patients is extremely unpleasant due to feelings of depersonalization, derealization, and dysphoria.

Common Adverse Effects Frequency not defined; listing includes adverse reactions reported with other agents from the phenothiazine class.

Cardiovascular: AV block, cardiac arrest, ECG changes, edema, hypotension, paroxysmal atrial tachycardia, QT_c prolongation, syncope, tachycardia

Central nervous system; Aggressive behavior, agitation, anxiety, bizarre dreams, cerebral edema, depression, dizziness, drowsiness, EEG changes, excitement; extrapyramidal symptoms (tremor, akathisia, dystonia, dyskinesia, oculogyric, opisthotonos, hyper-reflexia, pseudo-Parkinsonism, rigidity, sialorrhea); fatigue, fever, headache, insomnia, paradoxical psychosis, restlessness, seizures, sleep disturbance, tardive dyskinesia

Dermatologic: Angioedema, dermatitis, eczema, epithelial keratopathy, erythema, exfoliative dermatitis, photosensitivity, pruritus, rash, seborrhea, skin pigmentation (prolonged therapy), urticaria

Endocrine & metabolic: Anorexia, appetite increased, delayed ovulation, galactorrhea, gynecomastia, libido changes, menstrual irregularities, thirst, weight changes

Gastrointestinal: Adynamic ileus, constipation, fecal impaction, nausea, salivation, vomiting, xerostomia

Genitourinary: Bladder paralysis, impotence, incontinence, polyuria, urinary retention

Hematologic: Agranulocytosis, anemia, eosinophilia, leukopenia, pancytopenia, thrombocytopenia

Hepatic: Cholestasis, cholestatic jaundice, jaundice

Ocular: Blurred vision, corneal deposits (prolonged therapy), glaucoma, lenticular deposits, pigmentary retinopathy (prolonged therapy)

Respiratory: Nasal congestion, pneumonia, pneumonitis

Miscellaneous: Diaphoresis increased, Lupus-like syndrome

Restrictions Not available in U.S.

Dosage Oral:

Children >5 years: 2.5-10 mg in the morning, followed by 5-30 mg in the evening. In general, lower dosage should be used on initiation and gradually increased based on effect and tolerance.

Adults: 5-20 mg in the morning, followed by 10-40 mg in the evening. In dividing doses, it is suggested that the larger dose should be administered in the evening. In general, lower dosage should be used on initiation and gradually increased based on effect and tolerance.

Elderly: Initial daily dose should be ~5 mg/day. May be increased gradually based on effect and tolerance. Also see adult dosing.

Dosage adjustment in renal impairment: No dosage adjustment required.

Mechanism of Action Blocks postsynaptic mesolimbic dopaminergic receptors in the brain; depresses the release of hypothalamic and hypophyseal hormones.

Contraindications Hypersensitivity to pericyazine, phenothiazine derivatives, or any component of the formulation; severe CNS depression including acute intoxication with CNS depressant medications; subcortical brain damage; hepatic dysfunction; circulatory collapse; severely-depressed patients; bone marrow suppression; blood dyscrasias; coma; patients receiving spinal or regional anesthesia

Warnings/Precautions Cross-reactivity with other phenothiazine derivatives may occur. May be sedating; use with caution in disorders where CNS depression is a feature (risk may be lower than with other phenothiazines). Use with caution in Parkinson's disease, hemodynamic instability, predisposition to seizures, and severe disease. Esophageal dysmotility and aspiration have been associated with antipsychotic use; use with caution in patients at risk of pneumonia (eg, Alzheimer's disease). Caution in breast cancer or other prolactin-dependent tumors (may elevate prolactin levels). May alter temperature regulation or mask toxicity of other drugs due to antiemetic effects.

Use caution in cardiovascular disease (other piperidine phenothiazines have been associated with QT_c prolongation; relative risk with pericyazine has not been established, although rare cases of QT_c prolongation have been reported). May cause orthostatic hypotension; use with caution in patients at risk of this effect or those who would not tolerate transient hypotensive episodes (cerebrovascular disease, cardiovascular disease, or other medications which may predispose). Phenothiazines have been associated with worsening of pheochromocytoma and mitral valve prolapse; use caution.

Phenothiazines may cause anticholinergic effects (confusion, agitation, constipation, xerostomia, blurred vision, urinary retention); therefore, use with caution in patients with decreased gastrointestinal motility, urinary retention, BPH, xerostomia, or visual problems. Conditions which also may be exacerbated by cholinergic blockade include narrow-angle glaucoma (screening is recommended) and worsening of myasthenia gravis.

May cause extrapyramidal symptoms, including pseudoparkinsonism, acute dystonic reactions, akathisia, and tardive dyskinesia. May be associated with neuroleptic malignant syndrome (NMS). Prolonged therapy may cause pigmentary retinopathy, corneal deposits, and/or changes in skin pigmentation.

Drug Interactions

Cytochrome P450 Effect: No published data on CYP metabolism. Based on structural analysis, may be a substrate of CYP2D6 and 3A4.

Increased Effect/Toxicity: The levels/effects of pericyazine may be increased by azole antifungals, chlorpromazine, ciprofloxacin, clarithromycin, delavirdine, diclofenac, doxycycline, erythromycin, fluoxetine, imatinib, isoniazid, miconazole, nefazodone, nicardipine, paroxetine, pergolide, propofol, protease inhibitors, quinidine, quinine, ritonavir, ropinirole, verapamil and other CYP2D6 or 3A4 inhibitors.

Drugs which alter the QT_c interval may be additive with pericyazine, increasing the risk of malignant arrhythmias; includes type Ia antiarrhythmics, TCAs, and some quinolone antibiotics (sparfloxacin, moxifloxacin, and gatifloxacin). **These agents are contraindicated with other piperidine phenothiazines (thioridazine).** Potassium-depleting agents may increase the risk of serious arrhythmias with pericyazine (includes many diuretics, aminoglycosides, and amphotericin).

Phenothiazines inhibit the ability of bromocriptine to lower serum prolactin concentrations. The sedative effects of CNS depressants or ethanol may be additive with phenothiazines. Phenothiazines and trazodone may produce additive hypotensive effects. Metoclopramide may increase risk of extrapyramidal symptoms (EPS). Concurrent use of antihypertensives may result in additive hypotensive effects (particularly orthostasis).

Phenothiazines may produce neurotoxicity with lithium; this is a rare effect. Rare cases of respiratory paralysis have been reported with concurrent use

(Continued)

Pericyazine *(Continued)*

of phenothiazines and polypeptide antibiotics (eg, bacitracin). Naltrexone in combination with some phenothiazines has been reported to cause lethargy and somnolence.

Decreased Effect:
Aluminum salts may decrease the absorption of phenothiazines. The efficacy of amphetamines may be diminished by antipsychotics; in addition, amphetamines may increase psychotic symptoms; avoid concurrent use. Anticholinergics may inhibit the therapeutic response to phenothiazines and excess anticholinergic effects may occur (includes benztropine, trihyxyphenidyl, biperiden, and drugs with significant anticholinergic activity). Low potency antipsychotics (such as pericyazine) may diminish the pressor effects of epinephrine. The antihypertensive effects of guanethidine or guanadrel may be inhibited by phenothiazines. Phenothiazines may inhibit the antiparkinsonian effect of levodopa. Enzyme inducers may enhance the hepatic metabolism of phenothiazines; larger doses may be required; includes rifampin, rifabutin, barbiturates, and phenytoin.

Ethanol/Nutrition/Herb Interactions
Ethanol: Avoid ethanol (may increase CNS depression).
Herb/Nutraceutical: Avoid kava kava, valerian, St John's wort, gotu kola (may increase CNS depression). Avoid dong quai, St John's wort (may also cause photosensitization). Cigarette smoking may decrease the serum concentrations of pericyazine.

Dental Comment
This drug is known to prolong the QT interval. The QT interval is measured as the time and distance between the Q point of the QRS complex and the end of the T wave in the ECG tracing. After adjustment for heart rate, the QT interval is defined as prolonged if it is more than 450 msec in men and 460 msec in women. A long QT syndrome was first described in the 1950s and 60s as a congenital syndrome involving QT interval prolongation and syncope and sudden death. Some of the congenital long QT syndromes were characterized by a peculiar electrocardiographic appearance of the QRS complex involving a premature atria beat followed by a pause, then a subsequent sinus beat showing marked QT prolongation and deformity. This type of cardiac arrhythmia was originally termed "torsade de pointes" (translated from the French as "twisting of the points").

Prolongation of the QT interval is thought to result from delayed ventricular repolarization. The repolarization process within the myocardial cell is due to the efflux of intracellular potassium. The channels associated with this current can be blocked by many drugs and predisposes the electrical propagation cycle to torsade de pointes.

Periyazine is one of the drugs confirmed to prolong the QT interval and is accepted as having a risk of causing torsade de pointes. The risk of drug-induced torsade de pointes is extremely low when a single QT interval prolonging drug is prescribed. In terms of epinephrine, it is not known what effect vasoconstrictors in the local anesthetic regimen will have in patients with a known history of congenital prolonged QT interval or in patients taking any medication that prolongs the QT interval. Until more information is obtained, it is suggested that the clinician consult with the physician prior to the use of a vasoconstrictor in suspected patients, and that the vasoconstrictor (epinephrine, levonordefrin [Neo-Cobefrin®]) be used with caution.

Selected Readings

Buckley NA, Whyte IM, and Dawson AH, "Cardiotoxicity More Common in Thioridazine Overdose Than With Other Neuroleptics," *J Toxicol Clin Toxicol*, 1995, 33(3):199-204.

Jaworowsky S and Zamir S, "Cardiac Arrhythmia in a Child Receiving Pericyazine," *Isr J Psychiatry Relat Sci*, 1995, 32(4):299-300.

Johnson A, Giuffre RM, and O'Malley K, "ECG Changes in Pediatric Patients on Tricyclic Antidepressants, Desipramine, and Imipramine," *Can J Psychiatry*, 1996, 41(2):102-6.

Peridex® *see Chlorhexidine Gluconate on page 316*

Perindopril Erbumine *(per IN doe pril er BYOO meen)*

Related Information
Cardiovascular Diseases *on page 1636*
U.S. Brand Names Aceon®
Canadian Brand Names Coversyl®
Mexican Brand Names Coversyl®
Generic Available No
Pharmacologic Category Angiotensin-Converting Enzyme (ACE) Inhibitor
Use Treatment of essential hypertension; reduction of cardiovascular mortality or nonfatal myocardial infarction in patients with stable coronary artery disease

Unlabeled/Investigational Use As a class, ACE inhibitors are recommended in the treatment of congestive heart failure with left ventricular dysfunction.

Local Anesthetic/Vasoconstrictor Precautions No information available to require special precautions

Effects on Dental Treatment No significant effects or complications reported

Common Adverse Effects

>10%:
Central nervous system: Headache (24%)
Respiratory: Cough (incidence is higher in women, 3:1) (12%)

1% to 10%:
Cardiovascular: Edema (4%), chest pain (2%)), ECG abnormal (2%), palpitation (1%)
Central nervous system: Dizziness (8%, less than placebo), sleep disorders (3%), depression (2%), fever (2%), nervousness (1%), somnolence (1%)
Dermatologic: Rash (2%)
Endocrine & metabolic: Hyperkalemia (1%, less than placebo), triglycerides increased (1%), menstrual disorder (1%)
Gastrointestinal: Nausea (2%), diarrhea (4%), vomiting (2%), dyspepsia (2%), abdominal pain (3%), flatulence (1%)
Genitourinary: Urinary tract infection (3%), sexual dysfunction (male 1%)
Hepatic: Increased ALT (2%)
Neuromuscular & skeletal: Weakness (8%), back pain (6%), lower extremity pain (5%), upper extremity pain (3%), hypertonia (3%), paresthesia (2%), joint pain (1%), myalgia (1%), arthritis (1%), neck pain (1%)
Renal: Proteinuria (2%)
Respiratory: Upper respiratory tract infection (9%), sinusitis (5%), rhinitis (5%), pharyngitis (3%)
Otic: Tinnitus (2%), ear infection (1%)
Miscellaneous: Viral infection (3%%), allergy (2%)
Note: Some reactions occurred at an incidence >1% but ≤ placebo.

Additional adverse effects that have been reported with **ACE inhibitors** include agranulocytosis (especially in patients with renal impairment or collagen vascular disease), neutropenia, anemia, bullous pemphigus, cardiac arrest, eosinophilic pneumonitis, exfoliative dermatitis, hepatic failure, hyponatremia, jaundice, pancreatitis (acute), pancytopenia, thrombocytopenia; decreases in creatinine clearance in some elderly hypertensive patients or those with chronic renal failure, and worsening of renal function in patients with bilateral renal artery stenosis or hypovolemic patients (diuretic therapy). In addition, a syndrome which may include fever, myalgia, arthralgia, interstitial nephritis, vasculitis, rash, eosinophilia and positive ANA, and elevated ESR has been reported with ACE inhibitors.

Mechanism of Action Perindopril is a prodrug for perindoprilat, which acts as a competitive inhibitor of angiotensin-converting enzyme (ACE); prevents conversion of angiotensin I to angiotensin II, a potent vasoconstrictor; results in lower levels of angiotensin II which, in turn, causes an increase in plasma renin activity and a reduction in aldosterone secretion

Drug Interactions

Increased Effect/Toxicity: Potassium supplements, co-trimoxazole (high dose), angiotensin II receptor antagonists (eg, candesartan, losartan, irbesartan), or potassium-sparing diuretics (amiloride, eplerenone, spironolactone, triamterene) may result in elevated serum potassium levels when combined with perindopril. ACE inhibitor effects may be increased by phenothiazines or probenecid (increases levels of captopril). ACE inhibitors may increase serum concentrations/effects of lithium.

Diuretics have additive hypotensive effects with ACE inhibitors, and hypovolemia increases the potential for adverse renal effects of ACE inhibitors. ACE inhibitors may increase nephrotoxicity of cyclosporine. In patients with compromised renal function, coadministration with NSAIDs may result in further deterioration of renal function. Allopurinol and ACE inhibitors may cause a higher risk of hypersensitivity reaction when taken concurrently.

Decreased Effect: Aspirin (high dose) may reduce the therapeutic effects of ACE inhibitors; at low dosages this does not appear to be significant. Rifampin may decrease the effect of ACE inhibitors. Antacids may decrease the bioavailability of ACE inhibitors (may be more likely to occur with captopril); separate administration times by 1-2 hours. NSAIDs, specifically indomethacin, may reduce the hypotensive effects of ACE inhibitors. More likely to occur in low renin or volume dependent hypertensive patients.

Pharmacodynamics/Kinetics

Onset of action: Peak effect: 1-2 hours
Distribution: Small amounts enter breast milk
Protein binding: Perindopril: 60%; Perindoprilat: 10% to 20%
(Continued)

Perindopril Erbumine *(Continued)*

Metabolism: Hepatically hydrolyzed to active metabolite, perindoprilat (~17% to 20% of a dose) and other inactive metabolites

Bioavailability: Perindopril: 75%; Perindoprilat ~25% (~16% with food)

Half-life elimination: Parent drug: 1.5-3 hours; Metabolite: Effective: 3-10 hours, Terminal: 30-120 hours

Time to peak: Chronic therapy: Perindopril: 1 hour; Perindoprilat: 3-7 hours (maximum perindoprilat serum levels are 2-3 times higher and T_{max} is shorter following chronic therapy); CHF: Perindoprilat: 6 hours

Excretion: Urine (75%, 4% to 12% as unchanged drug)

Pregnancy Risk Factor C (1st trimester) / D (2nd and 3rd trimesters)

PerioChip® *see* Chlorhexidine Gluconate *on page 316*

PerioGard® *see* Chlorhexidine Gluconate *on page 316*

PerioMed™ *see* Fluoride *on page 671*

Periostat® *see* Doxycycline (Subantimicrobial) *on page 514*

Permax® *see* Pergolide *on page 1213*

Permethrin *(per METH rin)*

U.S. Brand Names A200® Lice [OTC]; Acticin®; Elimite®; Nix® [OTC]; Rid® Spray [OTC]

Canadian Brand Names Kwellada-P™; Nix®

Mexican Brand Names Novo-Herklin 2000®

Generic Available Yes: Excludes spray

Pharmacologic Category Antiparasitic Agent, Topical; Scabicidal Agent

Use Single-application treatment of infestation with *Pediculus humanus capitis* (head louse) and its nits or *Sarcoptes scabiei* (scabies); indicated for prophylactic use during epidemics of lice

Local Anesthetic/Vasoconstrictor Precautions No information available to require special precautions

Effects on Dental Treatment No significant effects or complications reported

Common Adverse Effects 1% to 10%:

Dermatologic: Pruritus, erythema, rash of the scalp

Local: Burning, stinging, tingling, numbness or scalp discomfort, edema

Mechanism of Action Inhibits sodium ion influx through nerve cell membrane channels in parasites resulting in delayed repolarization and thus paralysis and death of the pest

Pharmacodynamics/Kinetics

Absorption: <2%

Metabolism: Hepatic via ester hydrolysis to inactive metabolites

Excretion: Urine

Pregnancy Risk Factor B

Perphenazine *(per FEN a zeen)*

Canadian Brand Names Apo-Perphenazine®

Mexican Brand Names Leptopsique®

Generic Available Yes

Pharmacologic Category Antipsychotic Agent, Typical, Phenothiazine

Use Treatment of schizophrenia; nausea and vomiting

Unlabeled/Investigational Use Ethanol withdrawal; dementia in elderly; Tourette's syndrome; Huntington's chorea; spasmodic torticollis; Reye's syndrome; psychosis

Local Anesthetic/Vasoconstrictor Precautions Most pharmacology textbooks state that in presence of phenothiazines, systemic doses of epinephrine paradoxically decrease the blood pressure. This is the so called "epinephrine reversal" phenomenon. This has never been observed when epinephrine is given by infiltration as part of the anesthesia procedure.

Effects on Dental Treatment Key adverse event(s) related to dental treatment:

Significant hypotension may occur, especially when the drug is administered parenterally; orthostatic hypotension is due to alpha-receptor blockade, the elderly are at greater risk for orthostatic hypotension.

Tardive dyskinesia: Prevalence rate may be 40% in elderly; development of the syndrome and the irreversible nature are proportional to duration and total cumulative dose over time. Extrapyramidal reactions are more common in elderly with up to 50% developing these reactions after 60 years of age. Drug-induced Parkinson's syndrome occurs often; akathisia is the most common extrapyramidal reaction in elderly.

Common Adverse Effects Frequency not defined.

Cardiovascular: Hyper-/hypotension, orthostatic hypotension, tachycardia, bradycardia, dizziness, cardiac arrest

Central nervous system: Extrapyramidal symptoms (pseudoparkinsonism, akathisia, dystonias, tardive dyskinesia), dizziness, cerebral edema, seizure, headache, drowsiness, paradoxical excitement, restlessness, hyperactivity, insomnia, neuroleptic malignant syndrome (NMS), impairment of temperature regulation

Dermatologic: Rash, discoloration of skin (blue-gray), photosensitivity

Endocrine & metabolic: Hypoglycemia, hyperglycemia, galactorrhea, lactation, breast enlargement, gynecomastia, menstrual irregularity, amenorrhea, SIADH, libido (changes in)

Gastrointestinal: Constipation, weight gain, vomiting, stomach pain, nausea, xerostomia, salivation, diarrhea, anorexia, ileus

Genitourinary: Difficulty in urination, ejaculatory disturbances, incontinence, polyuria, ejaculating dysfunction, priapism

Hematologic: Agranulocytosis, leukopenia, eosinophilia, hemolytic anemia, thrombocytopenic purpura, pancytopenia

Hepatic: Cholestatic jaundice, hepatotoxicity

Neuromuscular & skeletal: Tremor

Ocular: Pigmentary retinopathy, blurred vision, cornea and lens changes

Respiratory: Nasal congestion

Miscellaneous: Diaphoresis

Mechanism of Action Perphenazine is a piperazine phenothiazine antipsychotic which blocks postsynaptic mesolimbic dopaminergic receptors in the brain; exhibits alpha-adrenergic blocking effect and depresses the release of hypothalamic and hypophyseal hormones

Drug Interactions

Cytochrome P450 Effect: Substrate of CYP1A2 (minor), 2C9 (minor), 2C19 (minor), 2D6 (major), 3A4 (minor); **Inhibits** CYP1A2 (weak), 2D6 (weak)

Increased Effect/Toxicity: CYP2D6 inhibitors may increase the levels/effects of perphenazine; example inhibitors include chlorpromazine, delavirdine, fluoxetine, miconazole, paroxetine, pergolide, quinidine, quinine, ritonavir, and ropinirole. Effects on CNS depression may be additive when perphenazine is combined with CNS depressants (narcotic analgesics, ethanol, barbiturates, cyclic antidepressants, antihistamines, or sedative-hypnotics). Perphenazine may increase the effects/toxicity of anticholinergics, antihypertensives, lithium (rare neurotoxicity), trazodone, or valproic acid. Concurrent use with TCA may produce increased toxicity or altered therapeutic response. Chloroquine and propranolol may increase perphenazine concentrations. Hypotension may occur when perphenazine is combined with epinephrine. May increase the risk of arrhythmia when combined with antiarrhythmics, cisapride, pimozide, sparfloxacin, or other drugs which prolong QT interval. Metoclopramide may increase risk of extrapyramidal symptoms (EPS). Acetylcholinesterase inhibitors (central) may increase the risk of antipsychotic-related EPS.

Decreased Effect: Phenothiazines inhibit the ability of bromocriptine to lower serum prolactin concentrations. Benztropine (and other anticholinergics) may inhibit the therapeutic response to perphenazine and excess anticholinergic effects may occur. Cigarette smoking and barbiturates may enhance the hepatic metabolism of chlorpromazine. Antihypertensive effects of guanethidine and guanadrel may be inhibited by perphenazine. Perphenazine may inhibit the antiparkinsonian effect of levodopa. Perphenazine and possibly other low potency antipsychotics may reverse the pressor effects of epinephrine.

Pharmacodynamics/Kinetics

Absorption: Oral: Well absorbed

Distribution: Crosses placenta

Metabolism: Extensively hepatic to metabolites via sulfoxidation, hydroxylation, dealkylation, and glucuronidation

Half-life elimination: Perphenazine: 9-12 hours; 7-hydroxyperphenazine: 11.3 hours

Time to peak, serum: Perphenazine: 1-3 hours; 7-hydroxyperphenazine: 2-4 hours

Excretion: Urine and feces

Pregnancy Risk Factor C

Perphenazine and Amitriptyline Hydrochloride *see* Amitriptyline and Perphenazine *on page 97*

Persantine® *see* Dipyridamole *on page 489*

Pethidine Hydrochloride *see* Meperidine *on page 983*

Pexeva® *see* Paroxetine *on page 1188*

PFA see Foscarnet on page 703

Pfizerpen® see Penicillin G (Parenteral/Aqueous) on page 1203

PGE₁ see Alprostadil on page 76

PGE₂ see Dinoprostone on page 482

PGI₂ see Epoprostenol on page 553

PGX see Epoprostenol on page 553

Phanasin® [OTC] see Guaifenesin on page 752

Phanasin® Diabetic Choice [OTC] see Guaifenesin on page 752

Phanatuss® DM [OTC] see Guaifenesin and Dextromethorphan on page 754

Pharmaflur® see Fluoride on page 671

Pharmaflur® 1.1 see Fluoride on page 671

Phazyme® Quick Dissolve [OTC] see Simethicone on page 1394

Phazyme® Ultra Strength [OTC] see Simethicone on page 1394

Phenabid DM® see Chlorpheniramine, Phenylephrine, and Dextromethorphan on page 326

Phenadoz™ see Promethazine on page 1290

Phenaseptic [OTC] see Phenol on page 1223

PhenaVent™ see Guaifenesin and Phenylephrine on page 754

PhenaVent™ D see Guaifenesin and Phenylephrine on page 754

PhenaVent™ Ped see Guaifenesin and Phenylephrine on page 754

Phenazopyridine (fen az oh PEER i deen)

U.S. Brand Names AZO-Gesic® [OTC]; AZO-Standard® [OTC]; Baridium® [OTC]; Pyridium®; ReAzo [OTC]; Uristat® [OTC]; UTI Relief® [OTC]

Canadian Brand Names Phenazo™

Generic Available Yes

Synonyms Phenazopyridine Hydrochloride; Phenylazo Diamino Pyridine Hydrochloride

Pharmacologic Category Analgesic, Urinary

Use Symptomatic relief of urinary burning, itching, frequency and urgency in association with urinary tract infection or following urologic procedures

Local Anesthetic/Vasoconstrictor Precautions No information available to require special precautions

Effects on Dental Treatment No significant effects or complications reported

Common Adverse Effects 1% to 10%:
Central nervous system: Headache, dizziness
Gastrointestinal: Stomach cramps

Mechanism of Action An azo dye which exerts local anesthetic or analgesic action on urinary tract mucosa through an unknown mechanism

Pharmacodynamics/Kinetics
Metabolism: Hepatic and via other tissues
Excretion: Urine (65% as unchanged drug)

Pregnancy Risk Factor B

Phenazopyridine Hydrochloride see Phenazopyridine on page 1220

Phendimetrazine (fen dye ME tra zeen)

U.S. Brand Names Bontril PDM®; Bontril® Slow-Release; Melfiat®; Obezine® [DSC]; Prelu-2® [DSC]

Canadian Brand Names Bontril®; Plegine®; Statobex®

Generic Available Yes

Synonyms Phendimetrazine Tartrate

Pharmacologic Category Anorexiant

Use Appetite suppressant during the first few weeks of dieting to help establish new eating habits; its effectiveness lasts only for short periods (3-12 weeks)

Local Anesthetic/Vasoconstrictor Precautions Use vasoconstrictor with caution in patients taking phendimetrazine. Phendimetrazine can enhance the sympathomimetic response to epinephrine leading to potential hypertension and cardiotoxicity.

Effects on Dental Treatment No significant effects or complications reported

Common Adverse Effects Frequency not defined.
Cardiovascular: Hypertension, tachycardia, arrhythmia
Central nervous system: Euphoria, nervousness, insomnia, confusion, mental depression, restlessness, headache
Dermatologic: Alopecia
Endocrine & metabolic: Changes in libido
Gastrointestinal: Nausea, vomiting, constipation, diarrhea, abdominal cramps

Genitourinary: Dysuria
Hematologic: Blood dyscrasias
Neuromuscular & skeletal: Tremor, myalgia
Ocular: Blurred vision
Renal: Polyuria
Respiratory: Dyspnea
Miscellaneous: Diaphoresis (increased)
Restrictions C-III
Pregnancy Risk Factor C

Phendimetrazine Tartrate *see* Phendimetrazine *on page 1220*

Phenelzine (FEN el zeen)

U.S. Brand Names Nardil®
Canadian Brand Names Nardil®
Generic Available No
Synonyms Phenelzine Sulfate
Pharmacologic Category Antidepressant, Monoamine Oxidase Inhibitor
Use Symptomatic treatment of atypical, nonendogenous, or neurotic depression
Unlabeled/Investigational Use Selective mutism
Local Anesthetic/Vasoconstrictor Precautions Attempts should be made to avoid use of vasoconstrictor due to possibility of hypertensive episodes with monoamine oxidase inhibitors
Effects on Dental Treatment Key adverse event(s) related to dental treatment: Orthostatic hypotension, xerostomia and changes in salivation (normal salivary flow resumes upon discontinuation). Avoid use as an analgesic due to toxic reactions with MAO inhibitors.
Mechanism of Action Thought to act by increasing endogenous concentrations of norepinephrine, dopamine, and serotonin through inhibition of the enzyme (monoamine oxidase) responsible for the breakdown of these neurotransmitters
Pregnancy Risk Factor C

Phenelzine Sulfate *see* Phenelzine *on page 1221*
Phenergan® *see* Promethazine *on page 1290*

Phenindamine (fen IN dah meen)

U.S. Brand Names Nolahist® [OTC] [DSC]
Canadian Brand Names Nolahist®
Generic Available No
Synonyms Phenindamine Tartrate
Pharmacologic Category Antihistamine
Use Treatment of perennial and seasonal allergic rhinitis and chronic urticaria
Local Anesthetic/Vasoconstrictor Precautions No information available to require special precautions
Effects on Dental Treatment No significant effects or complications reported

Phenindamine Tartrate *see* Phenindamine *on page 1221*
Pheniramine and Naphazoline *see* Naphazoline and Pheniramine *on page 1088*

Phenobarbital (fee noe BAR bi tal)

U.S. Brand Names Luminal® Sodium
Canadian Brand Names PMS-Phenobarbital
Mexican Brand Names Alepsal®
Generic Available Yes
Synonyms Phenobarbital Sodium; Phenobarbitone; Phenylethylmalonylurea
Pharmacologic Category Anticonvulsant, Barbiturate; Barbiturate
Use Management of generalized tonic-clonic (grand mal) and partial seizures; sedative
Unlabeled/Investigational Use Febrile seizures in children; may also be used for prevention and treatment of neonatal hyperbilirubinemia and lowering of bilirubin in chronic cholestasis; neonatal seizures; management of sedative/hypnotic withdrawal
Local Anesthetic/Vasoconstrictor Precautions No information available to require special precautions
Effects on Dental Treatment No significant effects or complications reported
Common Adverse Effects Frequency not defined.
Cardiovascular: Bradycardia, hypotension, syncope
(Continued)

Phenobarbital *(Continued)*

Central nervous system: Drowsiness, lethargy, CNS excitation or depression, impaired judgment, "hangover" effect, confusion, somnolence, agitation, hyperkinesia, ataxia, nervousness, headache, insomnia, nightmares, hallucinations, anxiety, dizziness

Dermatologic: Rash, exfoliative dermatitis, Stevens-Johnson syndrome

Gastrointestinal: Nausea, vomiting, constipation

Hematologic: Agranulocytosis, thrombocytopenia, megaloblastic anemia

Local: Pain at injection site, thrombophlebitis with I.V. use

Renal: Oliguria

Respiratory: Laryngospasm, respiratory depression, apnea (especially with rapid I.V. use), hypoventilation

Miscellaneous: Gangrene with inadvertent intra-arterial injection

Restrictions C-IV

Dosage

Children:

Sedation: Oral: 2 mg/kg 3 times/day

Hypnotic: I.M., I.V., SubQ: 3-5 mg/kg at bedtime

Preoperative sedation: Oral, I.M., I.V.: 1-3 mg/kg 1-1.5 hours before procedure

Adults:

Sedation: Oral, I.M., I.V.: 30-120 mg/day in 2-3 divided doses

Hypnotic: Oral, I.M., I.V., SubQ: 100-320 mg at bedtime

Preoperative sedation: I.M.: 100-200 mg 1-1.5 hours before procedure

Anticonvulsant: Status epilepticus: Loading dose: I.V.:

Infants and Children: 10-20 mg/kg in a single or divided dose; in select patients may administer additional 5 mg/kg/dose every 15-30 minutes until seizure is controlled or a total dose of 40 mg/kg is reached

Adults: 300-800 mg initially followed by 120-240 mg/dose at 20-minute intervals until seizures are controlled or a total dose of 1-2 g

Anticonvulsant maintenance dose: Oral, I.V.:

Infants: 5-8 mg/kg/day in 1-2 divided doses

Children:

1-5 years: 6-8 mg/kg/day in 1-2 divided doses

5-12 years: 4-6 mg/kg/day in 1-2 divided doses

Children >12 years and Adults: 1-3 mg/kg/day in divided doses or 50-100 mg 2-3 times/day

Sedative/hypnotic withdrawal (unlabeled use): Initial daily requirement is determined by substituting phenobarbital 30 mg for every 100 mg pentobarbital used during tolerance testing; then daily requirement is decreased by 10% of initial dose

Dosing interval in renal impairment: Cl_{cr} <10 mL/minute: Administer every 12-16 hours

Hemodialysis: Moderately dialyzable (20% to 50%)

Dosing adjustment/comments in hepatic disease: Increased side effects may occur in severe liver disease; monitor plasma levels and adjust dose accordingly

Mechanism of Action Short-acting barbiturate with sedative, hypnotic, and anticonvulsant properties. Barbiturates depress the sensory cortex, decrease motor activity, alter cerebellar function, and produce drowsiness, sedation, and hypnosis. In high doses, barbiturates exhibit anticonvulsant activity; barbiturates produce dose-dependent respiratory depression.

Contraindications Hypersensitivity to barbiturates or any component of the formulation; marked hepatic impairment; dyspnea or airway obstruction; porphyria; pregnancy

Warnings/Precautions Use with caution in patients with hypovolemic shock, CHF, hepatic impairment, respiratory dysfunction or depression, previous addiction to the sedative/hypnotic group, chronic or acute pain, renal dysfunction, and the elderly, due to its long half-life and risk of dependence, phenobarbital is not recommended as a sedative in the elderly; tolerance or psychological and physical dependence may occur with prolonged use. Use with caution in patients with depression or suicidal tendencies, or in patients with a history of drug abuse. **Abrupt withdrawal in patients with epilepsy may precipitate status epilepticus.**

Drug Interactions

Cytochrome P450 Effect: Substrate of CYP2C8/9 (minor), 2C19 (major), 2E1 (minor); **Induces** CYP1A2 (strong), 2A6 (strong), 2B6 (strong), 2C8/9 (strong), 3A4 (strong)

Increased Effect/Toxicity: When combined with other CNS depressants, ethanol, narcotic analgesics, antidepressants, or benzodiazepines, additive respiratory and CNS depression may occur. Barbiturates may enhance the hepatotoxic potential of acetaminophen overdoses. Chloramphenicol, MAO inhibitors, valproic acid, and felbamate may inhibit barbiturate metabolism. Barbiturates may impair the absorption of griseofulvin, and may enhance the nephrotoxic effects of methoxyflurane. Concurrent use of phenobarbital with meperidine may result in increased CNS depression. Concurrent use of phenobarbital with primidone may result in elevated phenobarbital serum concentrations. The levels/effects of phenobarbital may be increased by delavirdine, fluconazole, fluvoxamine, gemfibrozil, isoniazid, omeprazole, ticlopidine, and other CYP2C19 inhibitors.

Decreased Effect: Barbiturates may increase the metabolism of estrogens and reduce the efficacy of oral contraceptives; an alternative method of contraception should be considered. Barbiturates inhibit the hypoprothrom-binemic effects of oral anticoagulants via increased metabolism. Barbiturates may enhance the metabolism of methadone resulting in methadone with-drawal. The levels/effects of phenobarbital may be decreased by aminoglu-tethimide, carbamazepine, phenytoin, rifampin, and other CYP2C19 inducers.

Phenobarbital may decrease the levels/effects of aminophylline, amiodarone, benzodiazepines, bupropion, calcium channel blockers, carbamazepine, citalopram, clarithromycin, cyclosporine, diazepam, efavirenz, erythromycin, estrogens, fluoxetine, fluvoxamine, glimepiride, glipizide, ifosfamide, losartan, methsuximide, mirtazapine, nateglinide, nefazodone, nevirapine, phenytoin, pioglitazone, promethazine, propranolol, protease inhibitors, proton pump inhibitors, rifampin, ropinirole, rosiglitazone, selegiline, sertraline, sulfona-mides, tacrolimus, theophylline, venlafaxine, voriconazole, warfarin, zafirlukast, and other CYP1A2, 2A6, 2B6, 2C8/9, or 3A4 substrates.

Ethanol/Nutrition/Herb Interactions
Ethanol: Avoid ethanol (may increase CNS depression).
Food: May cause decrease in vitamin D and calcium.
Herb/Nutraceutical: Avoid evening primrose (seizure threshold decreased). Avoid valerian, St John's wort, kava kava, gotu kola (may increase CNS depression).

Dietary Considerations Vitamin D: Loss in vitamin D due to malabsorption; increase intake of foods rich in vitamin D. Supplementation of vitamin D and/or calcium may be necessary. Sodium content of injection (65 mg, 1 mL): 6 mg (0.3 mEq).

Pharmacodynamics/Kinetics
Onset of action: Oral: Hypnosis: 20-60 minutes; I.V.: ~5 minutes
Peak effect: I.V.: ~30 minutes
Duration: Oral: 6-10 hours; I.V.: 4-10 hours
Absorption: Oral: 70% to 90%
Protein binding: 20% to 45%; decreased in neonates
Metabolism: Hepatic via hydroxylation and glucuronide conjugation
Half-life elimination: Neonates: 45-500 hours; Infants: 20-133 hours; Children: 37-73 hours; Adults: 53-140 hours
Time to peak, serum: Oral: 1-6 hours
Excretion: Urine (20% to 50% as unchanged drug)

Pregnancy Risk Factor D

Dosage Forms ELIX: 20 mg/5 mL (473 mL). **INJ, solution, as sodium:** 65 mg/mL (1 mL); 130 mg/mL (1 mL); (Luminal® Sodium): 60 mg/mL (1 mL); 130 mg/mL (1 mL). **TAB:** 15 mg, 30 mg, 32 mg, 60 mg, 65 mg, 100 mg

Phenobarbital, Belladonna, and Ergotamine Tartrate see Belladonna, Phenobar-bital, and Ergotamine on page 185

Phenobarbital, Hyoscyamine, Atropine, and Scopolamine see Hyoscyamine, Atropine, Scopolamine, and Phenobarbital on page 804

Phenobarbital Sodium see Phenobarbital on page 1221

Phenobarbitone see Phenobarbital on page 1221

Phenol (FEE nol)

Related Information
Mouth Pain, Cold Sore, and Canker Sore Products on page 1828
U.S. Brand Names Castellani Paint Modified [OTC]; Cepastat® [OTC]; Cepastat® Extra Strength [OTC]; Cheracol® [OTC]; Chloraseptic® Gargle [OTC]; Chloraseptic® Mouth Pain [OTC]; Chloraseptic® Rinse [OTC]; Chloraseptic® Spray [OTC]; Chloraseptic® Spray for Kids [OTC]; Pain-A-Lay® [OTC]; Phenaseptic [OTC]; Phenol EZ® [OTC]; Ulcerease® [OTC]
Canadian Brand Names P & S™ Liquid Phenol
Generic Available Yes: Oral spray
(Continued)

Phenol *(Continued)*

Synonyms Carbolic Acid

Pharmacologic Category Anesthetic, Topical

Use Relief of sore throat pain, mouth, gum, and throat irritations; antiseptic; topical anesthetic

Local Anesthetic/Vasoconstrictor Precautions No information available to require special precautions

Effects on Dental Treatment No significant effects or complications reported

Phenol and Camphor *see* Camphor and Phenol *on page 252*

Phenol EZ® [OTC] *see* Phenol *on page 1223*

Phenoxybenzamine (fen oks ee BEN za meen)

U.S. Brand Names Dibenzyline®

Canadian Brand Names Dibenzyline®

Generic Available No

Synonyms Phenoxybenzamine Hydrochloride

Pharmacologic Category Alpha$_1$ Blocker

Use Symptomatic management of pheochromocytoma; treatment of hypertensive crisis caused by sympathomimetic amines

Unlabeled/Investigational Use Micturition problems associated with neurogenic bladder, functional outlet obstruction, and partial prostate obstruction

Local Anesthetic/Vasoconstrictor Precautions No information available to require special precautions

Effects on Dental Treatment No significant effects or complications reported

Common Adverse Effects Frequency not defined.

Cardiovascular: Postural hypotension, tachycardia, syncope, shock

Central nervous system: Lethargy, headache, confusion, fatigue

Gastrointestinal: Vomiting, nausea, diarrhea, xerostomia

Genitourinary: Inhibition of ejaculation

Neuromuscular & skeletal: Weakness

Ocular: Miosis

Respiratory: Nasal congestion

Mechanism of Action Produces long-lasting noncompetitive alpha-adrenergic blockade of postganglionic synapses in exocrine glands and smooth muscle; relaxes urethra and increases opening of the bladder

Drug Interactions

Increased Effect/Toxicity: Beta-blockers may result in increased toxicity (hypotension, tachycardia). Blood pressure-lowering effects are additive with sildenafil (use with extreme caution at a dose ≤25 mg), tadalafil (use is contraindicated by the manufacturer), and vardenafil (use is contraindicated by the manufacturer).

Decreased Effect: Alpha adrenergic agonists decrease the effect of phenoxybenzamine.

Pharmacodynamics/Kinetics

Onset of action: ~2 hours

Peak effect: 4-6 hours

Duration: ≥4 days

Half-life elimination: 24 hours

Excretion: Primarily urine and feces

Pregnancy Risk Factor C

Phenoxybenzamine Hydrochloride *see* Phenoxybenzamine *on page 1224*

Phenoxymethyl Penicillin *see* Penicillin V Potassium *on page 1205*

Phentermine (FEN ter meen)

U.S. Brand Names Adipex-P®; Ionamin®

Canadian Brand Names Ionamin®

Mexican Brand Names Ifa Reduccing "S"®

Generic Available Yes: Capsule (excludes resin complex capsule), tablet

Synonyms Phentermine Hydrochloride

Pharmacologic Category Anorexiant

Use Short-term adjunct in a regimen of weight reduction based on exercise, behavioral modification, and caloric reduction in the management of exogenous obesity for patients with an initial body mass index ≥30 kg/m^2 or ≥27 kg/m^2 in the presence of other risk factors (diabetes, hypertension)

Local Anesthetic/Vasoconstrictor Precautions Use vasoconstrictor with caution in patients taking phentermine. Amphetamines enhance the sympathomimetic response of epinephrine and norepinephrine leading to potential hypertension and cardiotoxicity.

Effects on Dental Treatment Key adverse event(s) related to dental treatment: Up to 10% of patients may present with hypertension. The use of local anesthetic without vasoconstrictor is recommended in these patients. See Dental Comment.

Common Adverse Effects Frequency not defined.

Cardiovascular: Hypertension, palpitation, tachycardia, primary pulmonary hypertension and/or regurgitant cardiac valvular disease

Central nervous system: Euphoria, insomnia, overstimulation, dizziness, dysphoria, headache, restlessness, psychosis

Dermatologic: Urticaria

Endocrine & metabolic: Changes in libido, impotence

Gastrointestinal: Nausea, constipation, xerostomia, unpleasant taste, diarrhea

Hematologic: Blood dyscrasias

Neuromuscular & skeletal: Tremor

Ocular: Blurred vision

Restrictions C-IV

Mechanism of Action Phentermine is structurally similar to dextroamphetamine and is comparable to dextroamphetamine as an appetite suppressant, but is generally associated with a lower incidence and severity of CNS side effects. Phentermine, like other anorexiants, stimulates the hypothalamus to result in decreased appetite; anorexiant effects are most likely mediated via norepinephrine and dopamine metabolism. However, other CNS effects or metabolic effects may be involved.

Drug Interactions

Increased Effect/Toxicity: Dosage of hypoglycemic agents may need to be adjusted when phentermine is used in a diabetic receiving a special diet. Concurrent use of MAO inhibitors and drugs with MAO activity (furazolidone, linezolid) may be associated with hypertensive episodes. Concurrent use of SSRIs may be associated with a risk of serotonin syndrome.

Decreased Effect: Phentermine may decrease the effect of antihypertensive medications The efficacy of anorexiants may be decreased by antipsychotics; in addition, amphetamines or related compounds may induce an increase in psychotic symptoms in some patients. Amphetamines (and related compounds) inhibit the antihypertensive response to guanethidine; probably also may occur with guanadrel.

Pharmacodynamics/Kinetics

Duration: Resin produces more prolonged clinical effects

Absorption: Well absorbed; resin absorbed slower

Half-life elimination: 20 hours

Excretion: Primarily urine (as unchanged drug)

Pregnancy Risk Factor C

Dental Comment Many diet physicians have prescribed fenfluramine ("fen") and phentermine ("phen"). When taken together the combination is known as "fen-phen". The diet drug dexfenfluramine (Redux®) is chemically similar to fenfluramine (Pondimin®) and was also used in combination with phentermine called "Redux-phen". While each of the three drugs alone had approval from the FDA for sale in the treatment of obesity, neither combination had an official approval. The use of the combinations in the treatment of obesity was considered an "off-label" use. Reports in medical literature have been accumulating for some years about significant side effects associated with fenfluramine and dexfenfluramine. In 1997, the manufacturers, at the urging of the FDA, agreed to voluntarily withdraw the drugs from the market. The action was based on findings from physicians who evaluated patients taking fenfluramine and dexfenfluramine with echocardiograms. The findings indicated that approximately 30% of patients had abnormal echocardiograms, even though they had no symptoms. This was a much higher than expected percentage of abnormal test results. This conclusion was based on a sample of 291 patients examined by five different physicians. Under normal conditions, fewer than 1% of patients would be expected to show signs of heart valve disease. The findings suggested that fenfluramine and dexfenfluramine were the likely cause of heart valve problems of the type that promoted FDA's earlier warnings concerning "fen-phen". The earlier warning included the following: The mitral valve and other valves in the heart are damaged by a strange white coating and allow blood to flow back, causing heart muscle damage. In several cases, valve replacement surgery has been done. As a rule, the person must, thereafter for life, be on a blood thinner to prevent clots from the mechanical valve. This type of valve damage had only been seen before in persons who were exposed to (Continued)

Phentermine *(Continued)*

large amounts of serotonin. The fenfluramine increases the availability of sero-tonin.

Phentermine Hydrochloride *see* Phentermine *on page 1224*

Phentolamine *(fen TOLE a meen)*

Canadian Brand Names Regitine®; Rogitine®
Mexican Brand Names Z-Max®
Generic Available Yes
Synonyms Phentolamine Mesylate; Regitine [DSC]
Pharmacologic Category Alpha₁ Blocker

Use Diagnosis of pheochromocytoma and treatment of hypertension associated with pheochromocytoma or other forms of hypertension caused by excess sympathomimetic amines; as treatment of dermal necrosis after extravasation of drugs with alpha-adrenergic effects (norepinephrine, dopamine, epinephrine)

Unlabeled/Investigational Use Treatment of pralidoxime-induced hypertension

Local Anesthetic/Vasoconstrictor Precautions Although the alpha-adrenergic blocking effects could antagonize epinephrine, there is no information available to require special precautions

Effects on Dental Treatment No significant effects or complications reported

Common Adverse Effects Frequency not defined.
Cardiovascular: Hypotension, tachycardia, arrhythmia, flushing, orthostatic hypotension
Central nervous system: Dizziness
Gastrointestinal: Nausea, vomiting, diarrhea
Neuromuscular & skeletal: Weakness
Respiratory: Nasal congestion
Case report: Pulmonary hypertension

Mechanism of Action Competitively blocks alpha-adrenergic receptors to produce brief antagonism of circulating epinephrine and norepinephrine to reduce hypertension caused by alpha effects of these catecholamines; also has a positive inotropic and chronotropic effect on the heart

Drug Interactions
Increased Effect/Toxicity: Phentolamine's toxicity is increased with ethanol (disulfiram reaction). Blood pressure-lowering effects are additive with sildenafil (use with extreme caution at a dose ≤25 mg), tadalafil (use is contraindicated by the manufacturer), and vardenafil (use is contraindicated by the manufacturer).
Decreased Effect: Decreased effect of phentolamine with epinephrine and ephedrine.

Pharmacodynamics/Kinetics
Onset of action: I.M.: 15-20 minutes; I.V.: Immediate
Duration: I.M.: 30-45 minutes; I.V.: 15-30 minutes
Metabolism: Hepatic
Half-life elimination: 19 minutes
Excretion: Urine (10% as unchanged drug)
Pregnancy Risk Factor C

Phentolamine Mesylate *see* Phentolamine *on page 1226*

Phenylalanine Mustard *see* Melphalan *on page 979*

Phenylazo Diamino Pyridine Hydrochloride *see* Phenazopyridine *on page 1220*

Phenylephrine *(fen il EF rin)*

U.S. Brand Names AH-chew® D [OTC] [DSC]; AK-Dilate®; Altafrin; Anu-Med [OTC]; Formulation R™ [OTC]; Medicone® [OTC]; Mydfrin®; NāSop™; Neo-Synephrine® Extra Strength [OTC]; Neo-Synephrine® Mild [OTC]; Neo-Synephrine® Ophthalmic [DSC]; Neo-Synephrine® Regular Strength [OTC]; Rectacaine [OTC]; Relief® [OTC]; Rhinall [OTC]; Sudafed PE™ [OTC]; Tronolane® Suppository [OTC]; Vicks® Sinex® Nasal Spray [OTC]; Vicks® Sinex® UltraFine Mist [OTC]

Canadian Brand Names Dionephrine®; Mydfrin®; Neo-Synephrine®
Generic Available Yes: Excludes cream, suspension, tablet
Synonyms Phenylephrine Hydrochloride; Phenylephrine Tannate
Pharmacologic Category Alpha/Beta Agonist; Ophthalmic Agent, Antiglaucoma; Ophthalmic Agent, Mydriatic

Use Treatment of hypotension, vascular failure in shock; as a vasoconstrictor in regional analgesia; as a mydriatic in ophthalmic procedures and treatment of wide-angle glaucoma; supraventricular tachycardia

For OTC use as symptomatic relief of nasal and nasopharyngeal mucosal congestion, treatment of hemorrhoids, relief of redness of the eye due to irritation

Local Anesthetic/Vasoconstrictor Precautions Use with caution since phenylephrine is a sympathomimetic amine which could interact with epinephrine to cause a pressor response

Effects on Dental Treatment Key adverse event(s) related to dental treatment: Tachycardia, palpitations (use vasoconstrictor with caution), and xerostomia (normal salivary flow resumes upon discontinuation).

Common Adverse Effects Frequency not defined.

Cardiovascular: Reflex bradycardia, excitability, restlessness, arrhythmia (rare), precordial pain or discomfort, pallor, hypertension, severe peripheral and visceral vasoconstriction, decreased cardiac output

Central nervous system: Headache, anxiety, dizziness, tremor, paresthesia, restlessness

Endocrine & metabolic: Metabolic acidosis

Local: I.V.: Extravasation which may lead to necrosis and sloughing of surrounding tissue, blanching of skin

Neuromuscular & skeletal: Pilomotor response, weakness

Renal: Decreased renal perfusion, reduced urine output, reduced urine output

Respiratory: Respiratory distress

Mechanism of Action Potent, direct-acting alpha-adrenergic stimulator with weak beta-adrenergic activity; causes vasoconstriction of the arterioles of the nasal mucosa and conjunctiva; activates the dilator muscle of the pupil to cause contraction; produces vasoconstriction of arterioles in the body; produces systemic arterial vasoconstriction

Drug Interactions

Increased Effect/Toxicity: Phenylephrine, taken with sympathomimetics, may induce tachycardia or arrhythmias. If taken with MAO inhibitors or oxytocic agents, actions may be potentiated. Nonselective beta-blockers may increase hypertensive effects; MAO inhibitors may potentiate hypertension and hypertensive crisis; TCAs may enhance vasopressor effect; avoid concurrent use with these agents. Methyldopa may increase pressor response.

Pharmacodynamics/Kinetics

Onset of action: I.M., SubQ: 10-15 minutes; I.V.: Immediate; Ophthalmic: 10-15 minutes

Duration: I.M.: 0.5-2 hours; I.V.: 15-30 minutes; SubQ: 1 hour; Ophthalmic: Maximal mydriasis: 1 hour, recover time: 3-6 hours

Metabolism: Hepatic, via intestinal monoamine oxidase to phenolic conjugates

Excretion: Urine (90%)

Pregnancy Risk Factor C

Phenylephrine and Chlorpheniramine *see* Chlorpheniramine and Phenylephrine *on page 324*

Phenylephrine and Cyclopentolate *see* Cyclopentolate and Phenylephrine *on page 403*

Phenylephrine and Promethazine *see* Promethazine and Phenylephrine *on page 1292*

Phenylephrine and Scopolamine
(fen il EF rin & skoe POL a meen)

Related Information
Phenylephrine *on page 1226*
Scopolamine *on page 1380*

U.S. Brand Names Murocoll-2®

Generic Available No

Synonyms Scopolamine and Phenylephrine

Pharmacologic Category Anticholinergic/Adrenergic Agonist

Use Mydriasis, cycloplegia, and to break posterior synechiae in iritis

Local Anesthetic/Vasoconstrictor Precautions Use with caution since phenylephrine is a sympathomimetic amine which could interact with epinephrine to cause a pressor response

Effects on Dental Treatment This form of phenylephrine will have no effect on dental treatment when given as eye drops.

Pharmacodynamics/Kinetics See individual agents.

Pregnancy Risk Factor C

Phenylephrine and Zinc Sulfate (fen il EF rin & zingk SUL fate)

Related Information
 Phenylephrine *on page 1226*
 Zinc Sulfate *on page 1598*
U.S. Brand Names Zincfrin® [OTC]
Canadian Brand Names Zincfrin®
Generic Available No
Synonyms Zinc Sulfate and Phenylephrine
Pharmacologic Category Adrenergic Agonist Agent
Use Soothe, moisturize, and remove redness due to minor eye irritation
Local Anesthetic/Vasoconstrictor Precautions No information available to require special precautions
Effects on Dental Treatment No significant effects or complications reported
Pharmacodynamics/Kinetics See individual agents.

Phenylephrine, Chlorpheniramine, and Dextromethorphan *see* Chlorpheniramine, Phenylephrine, and Dextromethorphan *on page 326*

Phenylephrine, Chlorpheniramine, and Dihydrocodeine *see* Dihydrocodeine, Chlorpheniramine, and Phenylephrine *on page 476*

Phenylephrine, Chlorpheniramine, and Methscopolamine *see* Chlorpheniramine, Phenylephrine, and Methscopolamine *on page 327*

Phenylephrine, Chlorpheniramine, and Phenyltoloxamine *see* Chlorpheniramine, Phenylephrine, and Phenyltoloxamine *on page 328*

Phenylephrine, Chlorpheniramine, Codeine, and Potassium Iodide *see* Chlorpheniramine, Phenylephrine, Codeine, and Potassium Iodide *on page 328*

Phenylephrine, Diphenhydramine, and Hydrocodone *see* Hydrocodone, Phenylephrine, and Diphenhydramine *on page 791*

Phenylephrine, Ephedrine, Chlorpheniramine, and Carbetapentane *see* Chlorpheniramine, Ephedrine, Phenylephrine, and Carbetapentane *on page 325*

Phenylephrine, Guaifenesin, and Hydrocodone *see* Hydrocodone, Phenylephrine, and Guaifenesin *on page 791*

Phenylephrine Hydrochloride *see* Phenylephrine *on page 1226*

Phenylephrine Hydrochloride and Guaifenesin *see* Guaifenesin and Phenylephrine *on page 754*

Phenylephrine Hydrochloride, Guaifenesin, and Dextromethorphan Hydrobromide *see* Guaifenesin, Dextromethorphan, and Phenylephrine *on page 756*

Phenylephrine, Hydrocodone, Chlorpheniramine, Acetaminophen, and Caffeine *see* Hydrocodone, Chlorpheniramine, Phenylephrine, Acetaminophen, and Caffeine *on page 790*

Phenylephrine, Promethazine, and Codeine *see* Promethazine, Phenylephrine, and Codeine *on page 1293*

Phenylephrine Tannate *see* Phenylephrine *on page 1226*

Phenylephrine Tannate, Carbetapentane Tannate, and Pyrilamine Tannate *see* Carbetapentane, Phenylephrine, and Pyrilamine *on page 267*

Phenylethylmalonylurea *see* Phenobarbital *on page 1221*

Phenylgesic® [OTC] *see* Acetaminophen and Phenyltoloxamine *on page 38*

Phenylisohydantoin *see* Pemoline *on page 1199*

Phenyl Salicylate, Methenamine, Methylene Blue, Sodium Biphosphate, and Hyoscyamine *see* Methenamine, Sodium Biphosphate, Phenyl Salicylate, Methylene Blue, and Hyoscyamine *on page 1008*

Phenyltoloxamine and Acetaminophen *see* Acetaminophen and Phenyltoloxamine *on page 38*

Phenyltoloxamine, Chlorpheniramine, and Phenylephrine *see* Chlorpheniramine, Phenylephrine, and Phenyltoloxamine *on page 328*

Phenytek™ *see* Phenytoin *on page 1228*

Phenytoin (FEN i toyn)

Related Information
 Cardiovascular Diseases *on page 1636*
 Fosphenytoin *on page 710*
U.S. Brand Names Dilantin®; Phenytek™
Canadian Brand Names Dilantin®
Mexican Brand Names Epamin®; Fenidantoin®; Fenitron® Hidantoina®
Generic Available Yes: Excludes chewable tablet
Synonyms Diphenylhydantoin; DPH; Phenytoin Sodium; Phenytoin Sodium, Extended; Phenytoin Sodium, Prompt

Pharmacologic Category Antiarrhythmic Agent, Class Ib; Anticonvulsant, Hydantoin

Use Management of generalized tonic-clonic (grand mal), complex partial seizures; prevention of seizures following head trauma/neurosurgery

Unlabeled/Investigational Use Ventricular arrhythmias, including those associated with digitalis intoxication, prolonged QT interval and surgical repair of congenital heart diseases in children; epidermolysis bullosa

Local Anesthetic/Vasoconstrictor Precautions No information available to require special precautions

Effects on Dental Treatment Gingival hyperplasia is a common problem observed during the first 6 months of phenytoin therapy appearing as gingivitis or gum inflammation. To minimize severity and growth rate of gingival tissue begin a program of professional cleaning and patient plaque control within 10 days of starting anticonvulsant therapy.

Common Adverse Effects I.V. effects: Hypotension, bradycardia, cardiac arrhythmia, cardiovascular collapse (especially with rapid I.V. use), venous irritation and pain, thrombophlebitis

Effects not related to plasma phenytoin concentrations: Hypertrichosis, gingival hypertrophy, thickening of facial features, carbohydrate intolerance, folic acid deficiency, peripheral neuropathy, vitamin D deficiency, osteomalacia, systemic lupus erythematosus

Concentration-related effects: Nystagmus, blurred vision, diplopia, ataxia, slurred speech, dizziness, drowsiness, lethargy, coma, rash, fever, nausea, vomiting, gum tenderness, confusion, mood changes, folic acid depletion, osteomalacia, hyperglycemia

Related to elevated concentrations:

>20 mcg/mL: Far lateral nystagmus

>30 mcg/mL: 45° lateral gaze nystagmus and ataxia

>40 mcg/mL: Decreased mentation

>100 mcg/mL: Death

Cardiovascular: Hypotension, bradycardia, cardiac arrhythmia, cardiovascular collapse

Central nervous system: Psychiatric changes, slurred speech, dizziness, drowsiness, headache, insomnia

Dermatologic: Rash

Gastrointestinal: Constipation, nausea, vomiting, gingival hyperplasia, enlargement of lips

Hematologic: Leukopenia, thrombocytopenia, agranulocytosis

Hepatic: Hepatitis

Local: Thrombophlebitis

Neuromuscular & skeletal: Tremor, peripheral neuropathy, paresthesia

Ocular: Diplopia, nystagmus, blurred vision

Rarely seen effects: SLE-like syndrome, lymphadenopathy, hepatitis, Stevens-Johnson syndrome, blood dyscrasias, dyskinesias, pseudolymphoma, lymphoma, venous irritation and pain, coarsening of the facial features, hypertrichosis

Dosage

Status epilepticus: I.V.:

Infants and Children: Loading dose: 15-20 mg/kg in a single or divided dose; maintenance dose: Initial: 5 mg/kg/day in 2 divided doses; usual doses:

6 months to 3 years: 8-10 mg/kg/day

4-6 years: 7.5-9 mg/kg/day

7-9 years: 7-8 mg/kg/day

10-16 years: 6-7 mg/kg/day, some patients may require every 8 hours dosing

Adults: Loading dose: Manufacturer recommends 10-15 mg/kg, however, 15-25 mg/kg has been used clinically; maintenance dose: 300 mg/day or 5-6 mg/kg/day in 3 divided doses or 1-2 divided doses using extended release

Anticonvulsant: Children and Adults: Oral:

Loading dose: 15-20 mg/kg; based on phenytoin serum concentrations and recent dosing history; administer oral loading dose in 3 divided doses given every 2-4 hours to decrease GI adverse effects and to ensure complete oral absorption; maintenance dose: same as I.V.

Neurosurgery (prophylactic): 100-200 mg at approximately 4-hour intervals during surgery and during the immediate postoperative period

Dosing adjustment/comments in renal impairment or hepatic disease: Safe in usual doses in mild liver disease; clearance may be substantially reduced in cirrhosis and plasma level monitoring with dose adjustment advisable. Free phenytoin levels should be monitored closely.

Mechanism of Action Stabilizes neuronal membranes and decreases seizure activity by increasing efflux or decreasing influx of sodium ions across cell

(Continued)

Phenytoin (Continued)

membranes in the motor cortex during generation of nerve impulses; prolongs effective refractory period and suppresses ventricular pacemaker automaticity, shortens action potential in the heart

Contraindications Hypersensitivity to phenytoin, other hydantoins, or any component of the formulation; pregnancy

Warnings/Precautions May increase frequency of petit mal seizures; I.V. form may cause hypotension, skin necrosis at I.V. site; avoid I.V. administration in small veins; use with caution in patients with porphyria; discontinue if rash or lymphadenopathy occurs; use with caution in patients with hepatic dysfunction, sinus bradycardia, S-A block, or AV block; use with caution in elderly or debilitated patients, or in any condition associated with low serum albumin levels, which will increase the free fraction of phenytoin in the serum and, therefore, the pharmacologic response. Sedation, confusional states, or cerebellar dysfunction (loss of motor coordination) may occur at higher total serum concentrations, or at lower total serum concentrations when the free fraction of phenytoin is increased. Abrupt withdrawal may precipitate status epilepticus.

Drug Interactions

Cytochrome P450 Effect: Substrate of CYP2C8/9 (major), 2C19 (major), 3A4 (minor); Induces CYP2B6 (strong), 2C8/9 (strong), 2C19 (strong), 3A4 (strong)

Increased Effect/Toxicity: The sedative effects of phenytoin may be additive with other CNS depressants including ethanol, barbiturates, sedatives, antidepressants, narcotic analgesics, and benzodiazepines. Selected anticonvulsants (felbamate, gabapentin, and topiramate) have been reported to increase phenytoin levels/effects. In addition, serum phenytoin concentrations may be increased by allopurinol, amiodarone, calcium channel blockers (including diltiazem and nifedipine), cimetidine, disulfiram, methylphenidate, metronidazole, omeprazole, selective serotonin reuptake inhibitors (SSRIs), ticlopidine, tricyclic antidepressants, trazodone, and trimethoprim.

The levels/effects of phenytoin may be increased by delavirdine, fluconazole, fluvoxamine, gemfibrozil, isoniazid, ketoconazole, nicardipine, NSAIDs, omeprazole, pioglitazone, sulfonamides, ticlopidine, and other CYP2C8/9 or 2C19 inhibitors.

Phenytoin enhances the conversion of primidone to phenobarbital resulting in elevated phenobarbital serum concentrations. Concurrent use of acetazolamide with phenytoin may result in an increased risk of osteomalacia. Concurrent use of phenytoin and lithium has resulted in lithium intoxication. Valproic acid (and sulfisoxazole) may displace phenytoin from binding sites; valproic acid may increase, decrease, or have no effect on phenytoin serum concentrations. Phenytoin transiently increased the response to warfarin initially; this is followed by an inhibition of the hypoprothrombinemic response. Phenytoin may enhance the hepatotoxic potential of acetaminophen overdoses. Concurrent use of dopamine and intravenous phenytoin may lead to an increased risk of hypotension.

Decreased Effect: Phenytoin may enhance the metabolism of estrogen and/or oral contraceptives, decreasing their clinical effect; an alternative method of contraception should be considered. Phenytoin may increase the metabolism of anticonvulsants including barbiturates, carbamazepine, ethosuximide, felbamate, lamotrigine, tiagabine, topiramate, and zonisamide. Valproic acid may increase, decrease, or have no effect on phenytoin serum concentrations. Phenytoin may also decrease the serum concentrations/effects of some antiarrhythmics (disopyramide, propafenone, quinidine, quetiapine) and tricyclic antidepressants may be reduced by phenytoin. Phenytoin may enhance the metabolism of doxycycline, decreasing its clinical effect; higher dosages may be required. Phenytoin may increase the metabolism of chloramphenicol or itraconazole.

Phenytoin may decrease the levels/effects of amiodarone, benzodiazepines, bupropion, calcium channel blockers, carbamazepine, citalopram, clarithromycin, clozapine, cyclosporine, efavirenz, erythromycin, estrogens, fluoxetine, glimepiride, glipizide, losartan, methsuximide, mirtazapine, nateglinide, nefazodone, nevirapine, phenytoin, pioglitazone, promethazine, propranolol, protease inhibitors, proton pump inhibitors, rosiglitazone, selegiline, sertraline, sulfonamides, tacrolimus, venlafaxine. voriconazole, warfarin, zafirlukast, and other CYP2B6, 2C8/9, 2C19, or 3A4 substrates.

The levels/effects of phenytoin may be decreased by aminoglutethimide, carbamazepine, phenobarbital, rifampin, rifapentine, secobarbital, and other CYP2C8/9 or 2C19 inducers. Clozapine and vigabatrin may reduce phenytoin serum concentrations. Ciprofloxacin may decrease serum phenytoin concentrations. Dexamethasone may decrease serum phenytoin concentrations.

Replacement of folic acid has been reported to increase the metabolism of phenytoin, decreasing its serum concentrations and/or increasing seizures.

Initially, phenytoin increases the response to warfarin; this is followed by a decrease in response to warfarin. Phenytoin may inhibit the anti-Parkinson effect of levodopa. The duration of neuromuscular blockade from neuromuscular-blocking agents may be decreased by phenytoin. Phenytoin may enhance the metabolism of methadone resulting in methadone withdrawal. Phenytoin may decrease serum levels/effects of digitalis glycosides, theophylline, and thyroid hormones.

Several chemotherapeutic agents have been associated with a decrease in serum phenytoin levels; includes cisplatin, bleomycin, carmustine, methotrexate, and vinblastine. Enzyme-inducing anticonvulsant therapy may reduce the effectiveness of some chemotherapy regimens (specifically in ALL). Teniposide and methotrexate may be cleared more rapidly in these patients.

Ethanol/Nutrition/Herb Interactions

Ethanol:

Acute use: Avoid or limit ethanol (inhibits metabolism of phenytoin). Watch for sedation.

Chronic use: Avoid or limit ethanol (stimulates metabolism of phenytoin).

Food: Phenytoin serum concentrations may be altered if taken with food. If taken with enteral nutrition, phenytoin serum concentrations may be decreased. Tube feedings decrease bioavailability; hold tube feedings 2 hours before and 2 hours after phenytoin administration. May decrease calcium, folic acid, and vitamin D levels.

Herb/Nutraceutical: Avoid evening primrose (seizure threshold decreased). Avoid valerian, St John's wort, kava kava, gotu kola (may increase CNS depression).

Dietary Considerations

Folic acid: Phenytoin may decrease mucosal uptake of folic acid; to avoid folic acid deficiency and megaloblastic anemia, some clinicians recommend giving patients on anticonvulsants prophylactic doses of folic acid and cyanocobalamin. However, folate supplementation may increase seizures in some patients (dose dependent). Discuss with healthcare provider prior to using any supplements.

Calcium: Hypocalcemia has been reported in patients taking prolonged high-dose therapy with an anticonvulsant. Some clinicians have given an additional 4000 units/week of vitamin D (especially in those receiving poor nutrition and getting no sun exposure) to prevent hypocalcemia.

Vitamin D: Phenytoin interferes with vitamin D metabolism and osteomalacia may result; may need to supplement with vitamin D

Tube feedings: Tube feedings decrease phenytoin absorption. To avoid decreased serum levels with continuous NG feeds, hold feedings for 2 hours prior to and 2 hours after phenytoin administration, if possible. There is a variety of opinions on how to administer phenytoin with enteral feedings. Be **consistent** throughout therapy.

Sodium content of 1 g injection: 88 mg (3.8 mEq)

Pharmacodynamics/Kinetics

Onset of action: I.V.: ~0.5-1 hour

Absorption: Oral: Slow

Distribution: V_d:

Neonates: Premature: 1-1.2 L/kg; Full-term: 0.8-0.9 L/kg

Infants: 0.7-0.8 L/kg

Children: 0.7 L/kg

Adults: 0.6-0.7 L/kg

Protein binding:

Neonates: ≥80% (≤20% free)

Infants: ≥85% (≤15% free)

Adults: 90% to 95%

Others: Decreased protein binding

Disease states resulting in a decrease in serum albumin concentration: Burns, hepatic cirrhosis, nephrotic syndrome, pregnancy, cystic fibrosis

Disease states resulting in an apparent decrease in affinity of phenytoin for serum albumin: Renal failure, jaundice (severe), other drugs (displacers), hyperbilirubinemia (total bilirubin >15 mg/dL), Cl_{cr} <25 mL/minute (unbound fraction is increased two- to threefold in uremia)

Metabolism: Follows dose-dependent capacity-limited (Michaelis-Menten) pharmacokinetics with increased V_{max} in infants >6 months of age and children versus adults; major metabolite (via oxidation), HPPA, undergoes enterohepatic recirculation

Bioavailability: Form dependent

Half-life elimination: Oral: 22 hours (range: 7-42 hours)

(Continued)

Phenytoin (Continued)

Time to peak, serum (form dependent): Oral: Extended-release capsule: 4-12 hours; Immediate release preparation: 2-3 hours

Excretion: Urine (<5% as unchanged drug); as glucuronides

Clearance: Highly variable, dependent upon intrinsic hepatic function and dose administered; increased clearance and decreased serum concentrations with febrile illness

Pregnancy Risk Factor D

Dosage Forms CAP, extended release: 100 mg; (Dilantin®): 30 mg, 100 mg; (Phenytek™): 200 mg, 300 mg. **CAP, prompt release:** 100 mg. **INJ, solution:** 50 mg/mL (2 mL, 5 mL). **SUSP, oral** (Dilantin®): 125 mg/5 mL (240 mL). **TAB, chewable** (Dilantin®): 50 mg

Selected Readings

Dooley G and Vasan N, "Dilantin® Hyperplasia: A Review of the Literature," *J N Z Soc Periodontol*, 1989, 68:19-22.

Iacopino AM, Doxey D, Cutler CW, et al, "Phenytoin and Cyclosporine A Specifically Regulate Macrophage Phenotype and Expression of Platelet-Derived Growth Factor and Interleukin-1 *In Vitro* and *In Vivo*: Possible Molecular Mechanism of Drug-Induced Gingival Hyperplasia," *J Periodontol*, 1997, 68(1):73-83.

Pihlstrom BL, "Prevention and Treatment of Dilantin®-Associated Gingival Enlargement," *Compendium*, 1990, 14:S506-10.

Saito K, Mori S, Iwakura M, et al, "Immunohistochemical Localization of Transforming Growth Factor Beta, Basic Fibroblast Growth Factor and Heparin Sulphate Glycosaminoglycan in Gingival Hyperplasia Induced by Nifedipine and Phenytoin," *J Periodontal Res*, 1996, 31(8):545-5.

Zhou LX, Pihlstrom B, Hardwick JP, et al, "Metabolism of Phenytoin by the Gingiva of Normal Humans: The Possible Role of Reactive Metabolites of Phenytoin in the Initiation of Gingival Hyperplasia," *Clin Pharmacol Ther*, 1996, 60(2):191-8.

Phenytoin Sodium *see* Phenytoin *on page 1228*

Phenytoin Sodium, Extended *see* Phenytoin *on page 1228*

Phenytoin Sodium, Prompt *see* Phenytoin *on page 1228*

Phillips'® Fibercaps [OTC] *see* Polycarbophil *on page 1252*

Phillips'® Milk of Magnesia [OTC] *see* Magnesium Hydroxide *on page 961*

Phillips'® M-O [OTC] *see* Magnesium Hydroxide and Mineral Oil *on page 961*

Phillips'® Stool Softener Laxative [OTC] *see* Docusate *on page 496*

pHisoHex® *see* Hexachlorophene *on page 771*

Phos-Flur® *see* Fluoride *on page 671*

Phos-Flur® Rinse [OTC] *see* Fluoride *on page 671*

PhosLo® *see* Calcium Acetate *on page 248*

Phos-NaK *see* Potassium Phosphate and Sodium Phosphate *on page 1261*

Phospha 250™ Neutral *see* Potassium Phosphate and Sodium Phosphate *on page 1261*

Phosphate, Potassium *see* Potassium Phosphate *on page 1261*

Phospholine Iodide® *see* Echothiophate Iodide *on page 526*

Phosphonoformate *see* Foscarnet *on page 703*

Phosphonoformic Acid *see* Foscarnet *on page 703*

Phosphorated Carbohydrate Solution *see* Fructose, Dextrose, and Phosphoric Acid *on page 713*

Phosphoric Acid, Levulose and Dextrose *see* Fructose, Dextrose, and Phosphoric Acid *on page 713*

Photofrin® *see* Porfimer *on page 1256*

Phrenilin® With Caffeine and Codeine *see* Butalbital, Aspirin, Caffeine, and Codeine *on page 241*

p-Hydroxyampicillin *see* Amoxicillin *on page 106*

Phylloquinone *see* Phytonadione *on page 1233*

Physostigmine (fye zoe STIG meen)

Canadian Brand Names Eserine®; Isopto® Eserine

Generic Available Yes

Synonyms Eserine Salicylate; Physostigmine Salicylate; Physostigmine Sulfate

Pharmacologic Category Acetylcholinesterase Inhibitor

Use Reverse toxic CNS effects caused by anticholinergic drugs

Local Anesthetic/Vasoconstrictor Precautions No information available to require special precautions

Effects on Dental Treatment Key adverse event(s) related to dental treatment: Salivation.

Common Adverse Effects Frequency not defined.

Cardiovascular: Palpitations, bradycardia

Central nervous system: Restlessness, nervousness, hallucinations, seizure

Gastrointestinal: Nausea, salivation, diarrhea, stomach pain

Genitourinary: Frequent urge to urinate

Neuromuscular & skeletal: Muscle twitching

Ocular: Lacrimation, miosis

Respiratory: Dyspnea, bronchospasm, respiratory paralysis, pulmonary edema

Miscellaneous: Diaphoresis

Mechanism of Action Inhibits destruction of acetylcholine by acetylcholines-terase which facilitates transmission of impulses across myoneural junction and prolongs the central and peripheral effects of acetylcholine

Drug Interactions

Increased Effect/Toxicity: Increased toxicity with bethanechol, methacho-line. Succinylcholine may increase neuromuscular blockade with systemic administration.

Pharmacodynamics/Kinetics

Onset of action: ~5 minutes

Duration: 0.5-5 hours

Absorption: I.M., SubQ: Readily absorbed

Distribution: Crosses blood-brain barrier readily and reverses both central and peripheral anticholinergic effects

Metabolism: Hepatic and via hydrolysis by cholinesterases

Half-life elimination: 15-40 minutes

Pregnancy Risk Factor C

Physostigmine Salicylate *see* Physostigmine *on page 1232*

Physostigmine Sulfate *see* Physostigmine *on page 1232*

Phytomenadione *see* Phytonadione *on page 1233*

Phytonadione (fye toe na DYE one)

U.S. Brand Names Mephyton®

Canadian Brand Names AquaMEPHYTON®; Konakion; Mephyton®

Mexican Brand Names Konakion®

Generic Available Yes: Injection

Synonyms Methylphytyl Napthoquinone; Phylloquinone; Phytomenadione; Vitamin K_1

Pharmacologic Category Vitamin, Fat Soluble

Use Prevention and treatment of hypoprothrombinemia caused by coumarin derivative-induced or other drug-induced vitamin K deficiency, hypoprothrom-binemia caused by malabsorption or inability to synthesize vitamin K; hemor-rhagic disease of the newborn

Local Anesthetic/Vasoconstrictor Precautions No information available to require special precautions

Effects on Dental Treatment No significant effects or complications reported

Common Adverse Effects Parenteral administration: Frequency not defined.

Cardiovascular: Cyanosis, flushing, hypotension

Central nervous system: Dizziness

Dermatologic: Scleroderma-like lesions

Endocrine & metabolic: Hyperbilirubinemia (newborn; greater than recom-mended doses)

Gastrointestinal: Abnormal taste

Local: Injection site reactions

Respiratory: Dyspnea

Miscellaneous: Anaphylactoid reactions, diaphoresis, hypersensitivity reactions

Mechanism of Action Promotes liver synthesis of clotting factors (II, VII, IX, X); however, the exact mechanism as to this stimulation is unknown. Menadiol is a water soluble form of vitamin K; phytonadione has a more rapid and prolonged effect than menadione; menadiol sodium diphosphate (K_4) is half as potent as menadione (K_3).

Drug Interactions

Decreased Effect:

Phytonadione may diminish the anticoagulant effect of coumarin derivatives (monitor INR). Phytonadione (oral) may not be properly absorbed when administered concurrently with orlistat (separate doses by at least 2 hours).

Pharmacodynamics/Kinetics

Onset of action: Increased coagulation factors: Oral: 6-10 hours; I.V.: 1-2 hours

Peak effect: INR values return to normal: Oral: 24-48 hours; I.V.: 12-14 hours

Absorption: Oral: From intestines in presence of bile; SubQ: Variable

Metabolism: Rapidly hepatic

Excretion: Urine and feces

Pregnancy Risk Factor C

α_1-PI *see* Alpha$_1$-Proteinase Inhibitor *on page 73*

Pidorubicin *see* Epirubicin *on page 550*

Pidorubicin Hydrochloride *see* Epirubicin *on page 550*

Pilocar® *see* Pilocarpine (Ophthalmic) *on page 1234*

Pilocarpine Hydrochloride *see* Pilocarpine (Ophthalmic) *on page 1234*

Pilocarpine Nitrate *see* Pilocarpine (Ophthalmic) *on page 1234*

Pilocarpine (Ophthalmic) (pye loe KAR peen)

U.S. Brand Names Isopto® Carpine; Pilocar®; Pilopine HS®; Piloptic®

Canadian Brand Names Diocarpine; Isopto® Carpine; Pilopine HS®

Generic Available Yes: Hydrochloride solution

Synonyms Pilocarpine Hydrochloride; Pilocarpine Nitrate

Pharmacologic Category Cholinergic Agonist; Ophthalmic Agent, Antiglaucoma; Ophthalmic Agent, Miotic

Use Ophthalmic: Management of chronic simple glaucoma, chronic and acute angle-closure glaucoma

Unlabeled/Investigational Use Counter effects of cycloplegics

Local Anesthetic/Vasoconstrictor Precautions No information available to require special precautions

Effects on Dental Treatment No significant effects or complications reported

Significant Adverse Effects Ophthalmic (frequency not defined):
Gastrointestinal: Diarrhea
Ocular: Burning, ciliary spasm, conjunctival vascular congestion, corneal granularity (gel 10%), lacrimation, lens opacity, myopia, retinal detachment,
Respiratory: Pulmonary edema

Dosage Adults:
Ophthalmic:
Glaucoma:
Solution: Instill 1-2 drops up to 6 times/day; adjust the concentration and frequency as required to control elevated intraocular pressure
Gel: Instill 0.5" ribbon into lower conjunctival sac once daily at bedtime.
Ocular systems: Systems are labeled in terms of mean rate of release of pilocarpine over 7 days; begin with 20 mcg/hour at night and adjust based on response.
To counteract the mydriatic effects of sympathomimetic agents (unlabeled use): Solution: Instill 1 drop of a 1% solution into the affected eye(s).

Mechanism of Action Directly stimulates cholinergic receptors in the eye causing miosis (by contraction of the iris sphincter), loss of accommodation (by constriction of ciliary muscle), and lowering of intraocular pressure (with decreased resistance to aqueous humor outflow)

Contraindications Hypersensitivity to pilocarpine or any component of the formulation; acute inflammatory disease of the anterior chamber of the eye

Warnings/Precautions Ophthalmic products may cause decreased visual acuity, especially at night or with reduced lighting. Use caution with cardiovascular disease; patients may have difficulty compensating for transient changes in hemodynamics or rhythm induced by pilocarpine.

Drug Interactions Inhibits CYP2A6 (weak), 2E1 (weak), 3A4 (weak)
Concurrent use with beta-blockers may cause conduction disturbances. Pilocarpine may antagonize the effects of anticholinergic drugs.

Pharmacodynamics/Kinetics Ophthalmic:
Onset of action:
Miosis: 10-30 minutes
Intraocular pressure reduction: 1 hour
Duration:
Miosis: 4-8 hours
Intraocular pressure reduction: 4-12 hours

Pregnancy Risk Factor C

Lactation Excretion in breast milk unknown/not recommended

Breast-Feeding Considerations The excretion in breast milk is unknown; however, breast-feeding in women receiving this medication is not recommended.

Dosage Forms

Gel, ophthalmic, as hydrochloride (Pilopine HS®): 4% (3.5 g) [contains benzalkonium chloride]

Solution, ophthalmic, as hydrochloride: 1% (15 mL); 2% (15 mL); 4% (15 mL); 6% (15 mL) [may contain benzalkonium chloride]

Isopto® Carpine: 1% (15 mL); 2% (15 mL, 30 mL); 4% (15 mL, 30 mL); 6% (15 mL); 8% (15 mL) [contains benzalkonium chloride]

Pilocar®: 0.5% (15 mL); 1% (1 mL, 15 mL); 2% (1 mL, 15 mL); 3% (15 mL); 4% (1 mL, 15 mL); 6% (15 mL) [contains benzalkonium chloride]

Piloptic®: 0.5% (15 mL); 1% (15 mL); 2% (15 mL); 3% (15 mL); 4% (15 mL); 6% (15 mL) [contains benzalkonium chloride]

Pilocarpine (Oral) (pye loe KAR peen)

Related Information

Dentin Hypersensitivity, High Caries Index, and Xerostomia *on page 1714*

Pilocarpine (Ophthalmic) *on page 1234*

U.S. Brand Names Salagen®

Canadian Brand Names Salagen®

Generic Available No

Pharmacologic Category Cholinergic Agonist

Dental Use Treatment of xerostomia caused by radiation therapy in patients with head and neck cancer and from Sjögren's syndrome

Use Treatment of xerostomia caused by radiation therapy in patients with head and neck cancer and from Sjögren's syndrome

Local Anesthetic/Vasoconstrictor Precautions No information available to require special precautions

Effects on Dental Treatment Key adverse event(s) related to dental treatment: Increased salivation (therapeutic effect). See Dental Comment.

Significant Adverse Effects Oral (frequency varies by indication and dose):

>10%: Genitourinary: Urinary frequency (9% to 12%)

1% to 10%:

Cardiovascular: Edema (<1% to 5%)

Dermatologic: Pruritus, rash

Gastrointestinal: Diarrhea (4% to 7%), constipation, flatulence

Genitourinary: Vaginitis, urinary incontinence

Neuromuscular & skeletal: Myalgias

Ocular: Lacrimation (6%), amblyopia (4%), conjunctivitis

Otic: Tinnitus

Miscellaneous: Allergic reaction, voice alteration

<1%: Abnormal dreams, abnormal thinking, alopecia, angina pectoris, anorexia, anxiety, aphasia, appetite increased, arrhythmia, arthralgia, arthritis, bilirubinemia, body odor, bone disorder, bradycardia, breast pain, bronchitis, cataract, cholelithiasis, colitis, confusion, contact dermatitis, cyst, deafness, depression, dry eyes, dry mouth, dry skin, dyspnea, dysuria, ear pain, ECG abnormality, eczema, emotional lability, eructation, erythema nodosum, esophagitis, exfoliative dermatitis, eye hemorrhage, eye pain, gastritis, gastroenteritis, gastrointestinal disorder, gingivitis, glaucoma, hematuria, hepatitis, herpes simplex, hiccup, hyperkinesias, hypesthesia, hypoglycemia, hypotension, hypothermia, insomnia, intracranial hemorrhage, laryngismus, laryngitis, leg cramps, leukopenia, liver function test abnormal, lymphadenopathy, mastitis, melena, menorrhagia, metrorrhagia, migraine, moniliasis, myasthenia, MI, neck pain, photosensitivity reaction, nervousness, ovarian disorder, pancreatitis, paresthesias, parotid gland enlargement, peripheral edema, platelet abnormality, pneumonia, pyuria, salivary gland enlargement, salpingitis, seborrhea, skin ulcer, speech disorder, sputum increased, stridor, syncope, taste loss, tendon disorder, tenosynovitis, thrombocythemia, thrombocytopenia, thrombosis, tongue disorder, twitching, urethral pain, urinary impairment, urinary urgency, vaginal hemorrhage, vaginal moniliasis, vesiculobullous rash, WBC abnormality, yawning

(Continued)

Pilocarpine (Oral) *(Continued)*

Dental Usual Dosing Treatment of xerostomia: Adults: Oral: 1-2 tablets 3-4 times/day not to exceed 30 mg/day (minimum 90-day therapy required for optimum effects)

Dosage Oral: Adults: 1-2 tablets 3-4 times/day not to exceed 30 mg/day (minimum 90-day therapy required for optimum effects)

Mechanism of Action Stimulates the muscarinic-type acetylcholine receptors in the salivary glands within the parasympathetic division of the autonomic nervous system to cause an increase in serous-type saliva

Contraindications Hypersensitivity to pilocarpine or any component of the formulation; uncontrolled asthma, angle-closure glaucoma, severe hepatic impairment

Warnings/Precautions Use caution with cardiovascular disease (patients may have difficulty compensating for transient changes in hemodynamics or rhythm induced by pilocarpine); controlled asthma, chronic bronchitis, or COPD (may increase airway resistance, bronchial smooth muscle tone, bronchial secretions); cholelithiasis, biliary tract disease, and nephrolithiasis. Adjust dose with moderate hepatic impairment.

Drug Interactions Increased Effect/Toxicity: Concurrent use with anticholinergics may cause antagonism of pilocarpine's cholinergic effect; medications with cholinergic actions may result in additive cholinergic effects. Beta-adrenergic receptor blocking drugs when used with pilocarpine may increase the possibility of myocardial conduction disturbances.

Pharmacodynamics/Kinetics

Onset of action: 20 minutes after single dose

Duration: 3-5 hours

Half-life, elimination: 0.76 hours

Time to peak: 1.25 hours

Pregnancy Risk Factor C

Breast-Feeding Considerations The excretion in breast milk is unknown; however, breast-feeding in women receiving this medication is not recommended.

Dosage Forms Tablet, as hydrochloride (Salagen®): 5 mg, 7.5 mg

Dental Comment Pilocarpine may have potential as a salivary stimulant in individuals suffering from xerostomia induced by antidepressants and other medications. At the present time however, the FDA has not approved pilocarpine for use in drug-induced xerostomia (clinical studies required). In an attempt to discern the efficacy of pilocarpine as a salivary stimulant in patients suffering from Sjögren's syndrome (SS), Rhodus and Schuh studied 9 patients with SS given daily doses of pilocarpine over a 6-week period. A dose of 5 mg daily produced a significant overall increase in both whole unstimulated salivary flow and parotid stimulated salivary flow. These results support the use of pilocarpine to increase salivary flow in patients with SS.

Selected Readings

Davies AN and Singer I, "A Comparison of Artificial Saliva and Pilocarpine in Radiation-Induced Xerostomia," *J Laryngol Otol*, 1994, 108(8):663-5.

Fox PC, "Management of Dry Mouth," *Dent Clin North Am*, 1997, 41(4):863-75.

Fox PC, Atkinson JC, Macynski AA, et al, "Pilocarpine Treatment of Salivary Gland Hypofunction and Dry Mouth (Xerostomia)," *Arch Intern Med*, 1991, 151(6):1149-52.

Fox PC, "Salivary Enhancement Therapies," *Caries Res*, 2004, 38(3):241-6.

Garg AK and Malo M, "Manifestations and Treatment of Xerostomia and Associated Oral Effects Secondary to Head and Neck Radiation Therapy," *J Am Dent Assoc*, 1997, 128(8):1128-33.

Gotrick B, Akerman S, Ericson D, et al, "Oral Pilocarpine for Treatment of Opioid-Induced Oral Dryness in Healthy Adults," *J Dent Res*, 2004, 83(5):393-7.

Hendrickson RG, Morocco AP, and Greenberg MI, "Pilocarpine Toxicity and the Treatment of Xerostomia," *J Emerg Med*, 2004, 26(4):429-32.

Johnson JT, Ferretti GA, Nethery WJ, et al, "Oral Pilocarpine for Postirradiation Xerostomia in Patients With Head and Neck Cancer," *N Engl J Med*, 1993, 329(6):390-5.

Mosqueda-Taylor A, Luna-Ortiz K, Irigoyen-Camacho ME, et al, "Effect of Pilocarpine Hydrochloride on Salivary Production in Previously Irradiated Head and Neck Cancer Patients," *Med Oral*, 2004, 9(3):204-11.

Nagler RM and Laufer D, "Protection Against Irradiation-Induced Damage to Salivary Glands by Adrenergic Agonist Administration," *Int J Radiat Oncol Biol Phys*, 1998, 40(2):477-81.

Nelson JD, Friedlaender M, Yeatts RP, et al, "Oral Pilocarpine for Symptomatic Relief of Keratoconjunctivitis Sicca in Patients With Sjögren's Syndrome. The MGI PHARMA Sjögren's Syndrome Study Group," *Adv Exp Med Biol*, 1998, 438:979-83.

Rhodus NL and Schuh MJ, "Effects of Pilocarpine on Salivary Flow in Patients With Sjögren's Syndrome," *Oral Surg Oral Med Oral Pathol*, 1991, 72(5):545-9.

Rieke JW, Hafermann MD, Johnson JT, et al, "Oral Pilocarpine for Radiation-Induced Xerostomia: Integrated Efficacy and Safety Results From Two Prospective Randomized Clinical Trials," *Int J Radiat Oncol Biol Phys*, 1995, 31(3):661-9.

Rousseau P, "Pilocarpine in Radiation-Induced Xerostomia," *Am J Hosp Palliat Care*, 1995, 12(2):38-9.

Schuller DE, Stevens P, Clausen KP, et al, "Treatment of Radiation Side Effects With Pilocarpine," *J Surg Oncol*, 1989, 42(4):272-6.

Singhal S, Mehta J, Rattenbury H, et al, "Oral Pilocarpine Hydrochloride for the Treatment of Refractory Xerostomia Associated With Chronic Graft-Versus-Host Disease," *Blood*, 1995, 85(4):1147-8.

Valdez IH, Wolff A, Atkinson JC, et al, "Use of Pilocarpine During Head and Neck Radiation Therapy to Reduce Xerostomia Salivary Dysfunction," *Cancer*, 1993, 71(5):1848-51.

Wiseman LR and Faulds D, "Oral Pilocarpine: A Review of Its Pharmacological Properties and Clinical Potential in Xerostomia," *Drugs*, 1995, 49(1):143-55.

Wynn RL, "Oral Pilocarpine (Salagen®) - A Recently Approved Salivary Stimulant," *Gen Dent*, 1996, 44(1):26,29-30.

Zimmerman RP, Mark RJ, Tran LM, et al, "Concomitant Pilocarpine During Head and Neck Irradiation Is Associated With Decreased Post-Treatment Xerostomia," *Int J Radiat Oncol Biol Phys*, 1997, 37(3):571-5.

Pilopine HS® *see* Pilocarpine (Ophthalmic) *on page 1234*

Piloptic® *see* Pilocarpine (Ophthalmic) *on page 1234*

Pima® *see* Potassium Iodide *on page 1260*

Pimaricin *see* Natamycin *on page 1093*

Pimecrolimus (pim e KROE li mus)

U.S. Brand Names Elidel®

Canadian Brand Names Elidel®

Generic Available No

Pharmacologic Category Immunosuppressant Agent; Topical Skin Product

Use Short-term and intermittent long-term treatment of mild to moderate atopic dermatitis in patients not responsive to conventional therapy or when conventional therapy is not appropriate

Local Anesthetic/Vasoconstrictor Precautions No information available to require special precautions

Effects on Dental Treatment No significant effects or complications reported

Common Adverse Effects

>10%:

Central nervous system: Headache (7% to 25%), pyrexia (1% to 13%)

Local: Burning at application site (2% to 26%; tends to resolve/improve as lesions resolve)

Respiratory: Nasopharyngitis (8% to 27%), cough (2% to 16%), upper respiratory tract infection (4% to 19%), bronchitis (0.4% to 11%)

Miscellaneous: Influenza (3% to 13%)

1% to 10%:

Dermatologic: Skin papilloma (warts) (up to 3%), molluscum contagiosum (0.7% to 2%), herpes simplex dermatitis (up to 2%)

Gastrointestinal: Diarrhea (0.6% to 8%), constipation (up to 4%)

Local: Irritation at application site (0.4% to 6%), erythema at application site (0.4% to 2%), pruritus at application site (0.6% to 6%)

Ocular: Eye infection (up to 1%)

Otic: Ear infection (0.6% to 6%)

Respiratory: Pharyngitis (0.7% to 8%), sinusitis (0.6% to 3%), nasal congestion (0.6% to 3%)

Miscellaneous: Viral infection (up to 7%), herpes simplex infection (0.4% to 4%), tonsillitis (0.4% to 6%)

Restrictions An FDA-approved medication guide is available at http://www.fda.gov/cder/Offices/ODS/labeling.htm; distribute to each patient to whom this medication is dispensed.

Dosage Children ≥2 years and Adults: Topical: Apply thin layer to affected area twice daily; rub in gently and completely. **Note:** Limit application to involved areas. Continue as long as signs and symptoms persist; discontinue if resolution occurs; re-evaluate if symptoms persist >6 weeks.

Mechanism of Action Penetrates inflamed epidermis to inhibit T cell activation by blocking transcription of proinflammatory cytokine genes such as interleukin-2, interferon gamma (Th1-type), interleukin-4, and interleukin-10 (Th2-type). Blocks catalytic function of calcineurin. Prevents release of inflammatory cytokines and mediators from mast cells *in vitro* after stimulation by antigen/IgE.

Contraindications Hypersensitivity to pimecrolimus or any component of the formulation; Netherton's syndrome

Warnings/Precautions Topical calcineurin inhibitors have been associated with rare cases of malignancy. Avoid use on malignant or premalignant skin conditions (eg, cutaneous T-cell lymphoma). Topical calcineurin agents are considered second-line therapies in the treatment of atopic dermatitis/eczema, and should be limited to use in patients who have failed treatment with other therapies. They should be used for short-term and intermittent treatment using the minimum amount necessary for the control of symptoms should be used. Application should be limited to involved areas. Safety of intermittent use for >1 year has not been established.

(Continued)

Pimecrolimus *(Continued)*

Should not be used in immunocompromised patients. Do not apply to areas of active viral infection; infections at the treatment site should be cleared prior to therapy. Patients with atopic dermatitis are predisposed to skin infections, and tacrolimus therapy has been associated with risk of developing eczema herpeticum, varicella zoster, and herpes simplex. May be associated with development of lymphadenopathy; possible infectious causes should be investigated. Discontinue use in patients with unknown cause of lymphadenopathy or acute infectious mononucleosis. Not recommended for use in patients with skin disease which may increase systemic absorption (eg, Netherton's syndrome). Avoid artificial or natural sunlight exposure, even when Elidel® is not on the skin. Safety not established in patients with generalized erythroderma. The use of Elidel® in children <2 years of age is not recommended, particularly since the effect on immune system development is unknown.

Drug Interactions
Cytochrome P450 Effect: Substrate of CYP3A4 (minor)
Increased Effect/Toxicity: CYP3A inhibitors may increase pimecrolimus levels in patients where increased absorption expected.
Pharmacodynamics/Kinetics Absorption: Poor when applied to 13% to 62% body surface area for up to a year
Pregnancy Risk Factor C
Dosage Forms CRM, topical: 1% (30 g, 60 g, 100 g)

Pimozide *(PI moe zide)*

U.S. Brand Names Orap®
Canadian Brand Names Apo-Pimozide®; Orap®
Generic Available No
Pharmacologic Category Antipsychotic Agent, Typical
Use Suppression of severe motor and phonic tics in patients with Tourette's disorder who have failed to respond satisfactorily to standard treatment
Unlabeled/Investigational Use Psychosis; reported use in individuals with delusions focused on physical symptoms (ie, preoccupation with parasitic infestation); Huntington's chorea
Local Anesthetic/Vasoconstrictor Precautions No information available to require special precautions (see Dental Comment)
Effects on Dental Treatment Key adverse event(s) related to dental treatment: Tourette's disorder: Xerostomia and increased salivation (normal salivary flow resumes upon discontinuation), and taste disturbance.
Common Adverse Effects
Frequencies >1% reported in adults (limited data) and/or children with Tourette's disorder:
Cardiovascular: Abnormal ECG (3%)
Central nervous system: Somnolence (up to 28% in children), sedation (14%), akathisia (8%), drowsiness (7%), hyperkinesias (6%), insomnia (2%), depression (2%), headache (1%), nervousness (1% to 8%)
Dermatologic: Rash (8%)
Gastrointestinal: Xerostomia (25%), constipation (20%), increased salivation (14%), diarrhea (5%), thirst (5%), appetite increased (5%), taste disturbance (5%), dysphagia (3%)
Genitourinary: Impotence (15%)
Neuromuscular & skeletal: Weakness (22%), muscle tightness (15%), rigidity (10%), myalgia (3%), torticollis (3%), tremor (3%)
Ocular: Visual disturbance (6% to 20%), accommodation decreased (20%)
Miscellaneous: Speech disorder (10%)
Frequency not established (reported in disorders other than Tourette's disorder): Blood dyscrasias, breast edema, chest pain, dizziness, extrapyramidal symptoms (akathisia, akinesia, dystonia, pseudoparkinsonism, tardive dyskinesia); facial edema, gingival hyperplasia (case report), hyper-/hypotension, hyponatremia, jaundice, libido decreased, neuroleptic malignant syndrome, orthostatic hypotension, palpitation, periorbital edema, postural hypotension, QT_c prolongation, seizure, tachycardia, ventricular arrhythmia, vomiting, weight gain/loss
Mechanism of Action Pimozide, a diphenylbutylperidine antipsychotic, is a potent centrally-acting dopamine-receptor antagonist resulting in its characteristic neuroleptic effects
Drug Interactions
Cytochrome P450 Effect: Substrate (major) of CYP1A2, 3A4; **Inhibits** CYP2C19 (weak), 2D6 (weak), 2E1 (weak), 3A4 (weak)

Increased Effect/Toxicity: Concurrent use with QT$_c$-prolonging agents is contraindicated including Class Ia and Class III antiarrhythmics, arsenic trioxide, chlorpromazine, dolasetron, droperidol, halofantrine, levomethadyl, mefloquine, pentamidine, probucol, tacrolimus, ziprasidone, mesoridazine, thioridazine, tricyclic antidepressants, and some quinolone antibiotics (sparfloxacin, moxifloxacin, and gatifloxacin).

CYP1A2 inhibitors may increase the levels/effects of pimozide; example inhibitors include amiodarone, ciprofloxacin, fluvoxamine, ketoconazole, norfloxacin, ofloxacin, and rofecoxib. Chloroquine, propranolol, and sulfadoxine-pyrimethamine also may increase pimozide concentrations. Concurrent use with TCA may produce increased toxicity or altered therapeutic response. Pimozide plus lithium may (rarely) produce neurotoxicity. Pimozide and CNS depressants (ethanol, narcotics) may produce additive CNS depressant effects. Pimozide with fluoxetine has been associated with the development of bradycardia (case report). Metoclopramide may increase risk of extrapyramidal symptoms (EPS). Acetylcholinesterase inhibitors (central) may increase the risk of antipsychotic-related EPS. Macrolide antibiotics may increase the effects of pimozide.

CYP3A4 inhibitors may increase the levels/effects of pimozide; example inhibitors include azole antifungals, clarithromycin, diclofenac, doxycycline, erythromycin, imatinib, isoniazid, nefazodone, nicardipine, propofol, protease inhibitors, quinidine, telithromycin, and verapamil. Concurrent use of strong CYP3A4 inhibitors with pimozide is contraindicated.

Decreased Effect: CYP1A2 inducers may decrease the levels/effects of pimozide; example inducers include aminoglutethimide, carbamazepine, phenobarbital, and rifampin. CYP3A4 inducers may decrease the levels/effects of pimozide; example inducers include aminoglutethimide, carbamazepine, nafcillin, nevirapine, phenobarbital, phenytoin, and rifamycins. Benztropine (and other anticholinergics) may inhibit the therapeutic response to pimozide. Antipsychotics such as pimozide inhibit the ability of bromocriptine to lower serum prolactin concentrations. The antihypertensive effects of guanethidine and guanadrel may be inhibited by pimozide. Pimozide may inhibit the antiparkinsonian effect of levodopa. Pimozide (and possibly other low potency antipsychotics) may reverse the pressor effects of epinephrine.

Pharmacodynamics/Kinetics

Absorption: 50%
Protein binding: 99%
Metabolism: Hepatic; significant first-pass effect
Half-life elimination: 50 hours
Time to peak, serum: 6-8 hours
Excretion: Urine

Pregnancy Risk Factor C

Dental Comment

This drug is known to prolong the QT interval. The QT interval is measured as the time and distance between the Q point of the QRS complex and the end of the T wave in the ECG tracing. After adjustment for heart rate, the QT interval is defined as prolonged if it is more than 450 msec in men and 460 msec in women. A long QT syndrome was first described in the 1950s and 60s as a congenital syndrome involving QT interval prolongation and syncope and sudden death. Some of the congenital long QT syndromes were characterized by a peculiar electrocardiographic appearance of the QRS complex involving a premature atria beat followed by a pause, then a subsequent sinus beat showing marked QT prolongation and deformity. This type of cardiac arrhythmia was originally termed "torsade de pointes" (translated from the French as "twisting of the points")

Prolongation of the QT interval is thought to result from delayed ventricular repolarization. The repolarization process within the myocardial cell is due to the efflux of intracellular potassium. The channels associated with this current can be blocked by many drugs and predisposes the electrical propagation cycle to torsade de pointes.

Pimozide is one of the drugs confirmed to prolong the QT interval and is accepted as having a risk of causing torsade de pointes. The risk of drug-induced torsade de pointes is extremely low when a single QT interval prolonging drug is prescribed. In terms of epinephrine, it is not known what effect vasoconstrictors in the local anesthetic regimen will have in patients with a known history of congenital prolonged QT interval or in patients taking any medication that prolongs the QT interval. Until more information is obtained, it is suggested that the clinician consult with the physician prior to the use of a vasoconstrictor in suspected patients, and that the vasoconstrictor (epinephrine, levonordefrin [Neo-Cobefrin®]) be used with caution.

Pin-X® [OTC] see Pyrantel Pamoate on page 1314

Pindolol (PIN doe lole)

Related Information
Cardiovascular Diseases *on page 1636*
Canadian Brand Names Apo-Pindol®; Gen-Pindolol; Novo-Pindol; Nu-Pindol;
PMS-Pindolol; Visken®
Generic Available Yes
Pharmacologic Category Beta Blocker With Intrinsic Sympathomimetic
Activity
Use Management of hypertension
Unlabeled/Investigational Use Potential augmenting agent for antidepressants; ventricular arrhythmias/tachycardia, antipsychotic-induced akathisia, situational anxiety; aggressive behavior associated with dementia
Local Anesthetic/Vasoconstrictor Precautions Use with caution; epinephrine has interacted with nonselective beta-blockers to result in initial hypertensive episode followed by bradycardia
Effects on Dental Treatment Pindolol is a nonselective beta-blocker and may enhance the pressor response to epinephrine, resulting in hypertension and bradycardia. Many nonsteroidal anti-inflammatory drugs, such as ibuprofen and indomethacin, can reduce the hypotensive effect of beta-blockers after 3 or more weeks of therapy with the NSAID. Short-term NSAID use (ie, 3 days) requires no special precautions in patients taking beta-blockers.
Common Adverse Effects 1% to 10%:
Cardiovascular: Chest pain (3%), edema (6%)
Central nervous system: Nightmares/vivid dreams (5%), dizziness (9%), insomnia (10%), fatigue (8%), nervousness (7%), anxiety (<2%)
Dermatologic: Rash, itching (4%)
Gastrointestinal: Nausea (5%), abdominal discomfort (4%)
Neuromuscular & skeletal: Weakness (4%), paresthesia (3%), arthralgia (7%), muscle pain (10%)
Respiratory: Dyspnea (5%)
Mechanism of Action Blocks both beta$_1$- and beta$_2$-receptors and has mild intrinsic sympathomimetic activity; pindolol has negative inotropic and chronotropic effects and can significantly slow AV nodal conduction. Augmentive action of antidepressants thought to be mediated via a serotonin 1A autoreceptor antagonism.
Drug Interactions
Cytochrome P450 Effect: Substrate of CYP2D6 (major); **Inhibits** CYP2D6 (weak)
Increased Effect/Toxicity: CYP2D6 inhibitors may increase the levels/ effects of pindolol; example inhibitors include chlorpromazine, delavirdine, fluoxetine, miconazole, paroxetine, pergolide, quinidine, quinine, ritonavir, and ropinirole. Pindolol may increase the effects of other drugs which slow AV conduction (digoxin, verapamil, diltiazem), alpha-blockers (prazosin, terazosin), and alpha-adrenergic stimulants (epinephrine, phenylephrine). Pindolol may mask the tachycardia from hypoglycemia caused by insulin and oral hypoglycemics. In patients receiving concurrent therapy, the risk of hypertensive crisis is increased when either clonidine or the beta-blocker is withdrawn. Reserpine has been shown to enhance the effect of beta-blockers. Beta-blockers may increase the action or levels of ethanol, disopyramide, nondepolarizing muscle relaxants, and theophylline although the effects are difficult to predict.
Decreased Effect: Decreased levels/effect of pindolol with aluminum salts, barbiturates, calcium salts, cholestyramine, colestipol, NSAIDs, penicillins (ampicillin), rifampin, salicylates, and sulfinpyrazone due to decreased bioavailability and plasma levels. Beta-blockers may decrease the effect of sulfonylureas (possibly hyperglycemia). Nonselective beta-blockers blunt the effect of beta-2 adrenergic agonists (albuterol).
Pharmacodynamics/Kinetics
Absorption: Rapid, 50% to 95%
Protein binding: 50%
Metabolism: Hepatic (60% to 65%) to conjugates
Half-life elimination: 2.5-4 hours; prolonged with renal impairment, age, and cirrhosis
Time to peak, serum: 1-2 hours
Excretion: Urine (35% to 50% as unchanged drug)
Pregnancy Risk Factor B

Pink Bismuth *see* Bismuth *on page 210*
PIO *see* Pemoline *on page 1199*

Pioglitazone (pye oh GLI ta zone)

U.S. Brand Names Actos®
Canadian Brand Names Actos®
Generic Available No
Pharmacologic Category Antidiabetic Agent, Thiazolidinedione
Use

Type 2 diabetes mellitus (noninsulin dependent, NIDDM), monotherapy: Adjunct to diet and exercise, to improve glycemic control

Type 2 diabetes mellitus (noninsulin dependent, NIDDM), combination therapy with sulfonylurea, metformin, or insulin: When diet, exercise, and a single agent alone does not result in adequate glycemic control

Local Anesthetic/Vasoconstrictor Precautions No information available to require special precautions

Effects on Dental Treatment Pioglitazone-dependent diabetics should be appointed for dental treatment in morning in order to minimize chance of stress-induced hypoglycemia.

Common Adverse Effects

>10%:

Endocrine & metabolic: Serum triglycerides decreased, HDL-cholesterol increased

Gastrointestinal: Weight gain

Respiratory: Upper respiratory tract infection (13%)

1% to 10%:

Cardiovascular: Edema (5%) (in combination trials with sulfonylureas or insulin, the incidence of edema was as high as 15%)

Central nervous system: Headache (9%), fatigue (4%)

Endocrine & metabolic: Aggravation of diabetes mellitus (5%), hypoglycemia (range 2% to 15% when used in combination with sulfonylureas or insulin)

Hematologic: Anemia (1%)

Neuromuscular & skeletal: Myalgia (5%)

Respiratory: Sinusitis (6%), pharyngitis (5%)

Dosage Oral:

Adults:

Monotherapy: Initial: 15-30 mg once daily; if response is inadequate, the dosage may be increased in increments up to 45 mg once daily; maximum recommended dose: 45 mg once daily

Combination therapy: Maximum recommended dose: 45 mg/day

With sulfonylureas: Initial: 15-30 mg once daily; dose of sulfonylurea should be reduced if the patient reports hypoglycemia

With metformin: Initial: 15-30 mg once daily; it is unlikely that the dose of metformin will need to be reduced due to hypoglycemia

With insulin: Initial: 15-30 mg once daily; dose of insulin should be reduced by 10% to 25% if the patient reports hypoglycemia or if the plasma glucose falls to <100 mg/dL.

Dosage adjustment in patients with CHF (NYHA Class II) in mono- or combination therapy: Initial: 15 mg once daily; may be increased after several months of treatment, with close attention to heart failure symptoms

Elderly: No dosage adjustment is recommended in elderly patients.

Dosage adjustment in renal impairment: No dosage adjustment is required.

Dosage adjustment in hepatic impairment: Clearance is significantly lower in hepatic impairment. Therapy should not be initiated if the patient exhibits active liver disease or increased transaminases (>2.5 times the upper limit of normal) at baseline.

Mechanism of Action Thiazolidinedione antidiabetic agent that lowers blood glucose by improving target cell response to insulin, without increasing pancreatic insulin secretion. It has a mechanism of action that is dependent on the presence of insulin for activity. Pioglitazone is a potent and selective agonist for peroxisome proliferator-activated receptor-gamma (PPARgamma). Activation of nuclear PPARgamma receptors influences the production of a number of gene products involved in glucose and lipid metabolism.

Contraindications Hypersensitivity to pioglitazone or any component of the formulation; active liver disease (transaminases >2.5 times the upper limit of normal at baseline); patients who have experienced jaundice during troglitazone therapy

Warnings/Precautions Should not be used in diabetic ketoacidosis. Mechanism requires the presence of insulin, therefore use in type 1 diabetes is not recommended. May potentiate hypoglycemia when used in combination with sulfonylureas or insulin. Use with caution in premenopausal, anovulatory women - may result in a resumption of ovulation, increasing the risk of pregnancy. Use with caution in patients with anemia (may reduce hemoglobin and (Continued)

Pioglitazone (Continued)

hematocrit). Use with caution in patients with edema; may increase plasma volume and/or increase cardiac hypertrophy. Monitor closely for signs and symptoms of heart failure (including weight gain, edema, or dyspnea). Not recommended for use in patients with NYHA Class III or IV heart failure, unless serum glucose control outweighs the risk of excessive fluid retention. Discontinue if heart failure develops. Use with caution in patients with minor elevations in transaminases (AST or ALT). Idiosyncratic hepatotoxicity has been reported with another thiazolidinedione agent (troglitazone) and postmarketing case reports of hepatitis (with rare hepatic failure) have been received for pioglitazone. Monitoring should include periodic determinations of liver function. Not for use in children <18 years of age.

Drug Interactions

Cytochrome P450 Effect: Substrate of CYP2C8 (major), 3A4 (minor); **Inhibits** CYP2C8 (moderate), 2C9 (weak), 2C19 (weak), 2D6 (moderate); **Induces** CYP3A4 (weak)

Increased Effect/Toxicity: Concomitant use with thioridazine is contraindicated, due to a risk of arrhythmias. The levels/effects of pioglitazone may be increased by atazanavir, gemfibrozil, ritonavir, and other CYP2C8 inhibitors.

Pioglitazone may increase the levels/effects of amiodarone, amphetamines, selected beta-blockers, dextromethorphan, fluoxetine, lidocaine, mirtazapine, nefazodone, paclitaxel, paroxetine, risperidone, repaglinide, ritonavir, rosiglitazone, thioridazine, and other CYP2D6 or 2C8 substrates.

Decreased Effect: The levels/effects of pioglitazone may be decreased by carbamazepine, phenobarbital, phenytoin, rifampin, rifapentine, secobarbital, and other CYP2C8 inducers. Pioglitazone may decrease the levels/effects of CYP2D6 prodrug substrates (eg, codeine, hydrocodone, oxycodone, tramadol). Effects of oral contraceptives (hormonal) may be decreased, based on data from a related compound. This has not been specifically evaluated for pioglitazone. Bile acid sequestrants may decrease pioglitazone levels.

Ethanol/Nutrition/Herb Interactions

Ethanol: Caution with ethanol (may cause hypoglycemia).

Food: Peak concentrations are delayed when administered with food, but the extent of absorption is not affected. Pioglitazone may be taken without regard to meals.

Herb/Nutraceutical: St John's wort may decrease levels. Caution with chromium, garlic, gymnema (may cause hypoglycemia).

Dietary Considerations Management of type 2 diabetes mellitus (noninsulin dependent, NIDDM) should include diet control. May be taken without regard to meals.

Pharmacodynamics/Kinetics

Onset of action: Delayed

Peak effect: Glucose control: Several weeks

Distribution: V_{ss} (apparent): 0.63 L/kg

Protein binding: 99.8%

Metabolism: Hepatic (99%) via CYP2C8/9 and 3A4 to both active and inactive metabolites

Half-life elimination: Parent drug: 3-7 hours; Total: 16-24 hours

Time to peak: ~2 hours

Excretion: Urine (15% to 30%) and feces as metabolites

Pregnancy Risk Factor C

Dosage Forms TAB: 15 mg, 30 mg, 45 mg

Pioglitazone and Metformin (pye oh GLI ta zone & met FOR min)

U.S. Brand Names Actoplus Met™

Generic Available No

Synonyms Metformin Hydrochloride and Pioglitazone Hydrochloride

Pharmacologic Category Antidiabetic Agent, Biguanide; Antidiabetic Agent, Thiazolidinedione

Use Management of type 2 diabetes mellitus (noninsulin dependent, NIDDM)

Local Anesthetic/Vasoconstrictor Precautions Patients with pioglitazone-dependent diabetes (noninsulin dependent, type 2) or metformin-dependent diabetes (noninsulin dependent, type 2) should be appointed for dental treatment in morning in order to minimize chance of stress-induced hypoglycemia.

Effects on Dental Treatment No significant effects or complications reported

Common Adverse Effects Also see individual agents. Percentages of adverse effects as reported with the combination product.

>10%:
Cardiovascular: Edema (lower limb, 3% to 11%)
Respiratory: Upper respiratory infection (12% to 14%)
1% to 10%:
Central nervous system: Headache (5%), dizziness (4% to 5%)
Endocrine & metabolic: Weight gain (3% to 7%)
Gastrointestinal: Diarrhea (5% to 6%), nausea (4% to 6%)
Genitourinary: Urinary tract infection (5% to 6%)
Respiratory: Sinusitis (4% to 5%)

Dosage Oral: Type 2 diabetes mellitus:
Adults: Initial dose should be based on current dose of pioglitazone and/or metformin; daily dose should be divided and given with meals
Patients inadequately controlled on **metformin alone:** Initial dose: Pioglitazone 15-30 mg/day plus current dose of metformin
Patients inadequately controlled on **pioglitazone alone:** Initial dose: Metformin 1000-1700 mg/day plus current dose of pioglitazone
Note: When switching from combination pioglitazone and metformin as separate tablets: Use current dose.
Dosing adjustment: Doses may be increased as increments of pioglitazone 15 mg and/or metformin 500-850 mg, up to the maximum dose; doses should be titrated gradually. Guidelines for frequency of adjustment (adapted from rosiglitazone/metformin combination labeling):
After a change in the **metformin** dosage, titration can be done after 1-2 weeks
After a change in the **pioglitazone** dosage, titration can be done after 8-12 weeks
Maximum dose: Pioglitazone 45 mg/metformin 2550 mg daily
Elderly: The initial and maintenance dosing should be conservative, due to the potential for decreased renal function (monitor). Generally, elderly patients should not be titrated to the maximum; do not use in patients ≥80 years of age unless normal renal function has been established.

Dosage adjustment in renal impairment: Do not use with renal disease or renal dysfunction (serum creatinine ≥1.5 mg/dL in males or ≥1.4 mg/dL in females or abnormal clearance).
Dosage adjustment in hepatic impairment: Do not use with active liver disease or ALT >2.5 times the upper limit of normal.

Mechanism of Action Pioglitazone is a thiazolidinedione antidiabetic agent that lowers blood glucose by improving target cell response to insulin, without increasing pancreatic insulin secretion. It has a mechanism of action that is dependent on the presence of insulin for activity. Metformin decreases hepatic glucose production, decreasing intestinal absorption of glucose, and improves insulin sensitivity (increases peripheral glucose uptake and utilization).

Contraindications Hypersensitivity to pioglitazone, metformin, or any component of the formulation; renal disease or renal dysfunction (serum creatinine ≥1.5 mg/dL in males or ≥1.4 mg/dL in females, or abnormal creatinine clearance which may also result from conditions such as cardiovascular collapse, acute myocardial infarction, and septicemia); acute or chronic metabolic acidosis with or without coma (including diabetic ketoacidosis). Metformin is also contraindicated in CHF requiring pharmacologic management (not included in labeling of the combination product).
Note: Temporarily discontinue in patients undergoing radiologic studies in which intravascular iodinated contrast materials are used.

Warnings/Precautions Lactic acidosis is a rare, but potentially severe consequence of therapy with metformin. Lactic acidosis should be suspected in any diabetic patient receiving metformin who has evidence of acidosis when evidence of ketoacidosis is lacking. Discontinue metformin in clinical situations predisposing to hypoxemia, including conditions such as cardiovascular collapse, respiratory failure, acute myocardial infarction, acute congestive heart failure, and septicemia.

Metformin is substantially excreted by the kidney. The risk of accumulation and lactic acidosis increases with the degree of impairment of renal function. Patients with renal function below the limit of normal for their age should not receive metformin. In elderly patients, renal function should be monitored regularly; should not be used in any patient ≥80 years of age unless measurement of creatinine clearance verifies normal renal function. Use of concomitant medications that may affect renal function (ie, affect tubular secretion) may also affect metformin disposition. Metformin should be suspended in patients with dehydration and/or prerenal azotemia. Therapy should be suspended for any surgical procedures (resume only after normal intake resumed and normal renal function is verified). Metformin should also be temporarily discontinued for 48 hours in patients undergoing radiologic studies involving the intravascular administration of iodinated contrast materials (potential for acute alteration in renal function). (Continued)

Pioglitazone and Metformin *(Continued)*

Avoid use in patients with impaired liver function. Pioglitazone must be used with caution in patients with elevated transaminases (AST or ALT); avoid use in patients where hepatic dysfunction presents a risk of lactic acidosis. Idiosyncratic hepatotoxicity has been reported with another thiazolidinedione agent (troglitazone) and (rarely) with pioglitazone; discontinue if jaundice occurs. Monitoring should include periodic determinations of liver function. Patient must be instructed to avoid excessive acute or chronic ethanol use.

Pioglitazone may cause fluid retention which could exacerbate or lead to heart failure; monitor closely for signs and symptoms of heart failure; not recommended for use in patients with NYHA Class III or IV heart failure. May increase plasma volume and/or increase cardiac hypertrophy. Discontinue if heart failure develops. Use caution in patients with edema. Pioglitazone requires the presence of endogenous insulin to be active; therefore, use in type 1 diabetes (insulin dependent, IDDM) is not recommended. Use pioglitazone with caution in patients with anemia or depressed leukocyte counts (may reduce hemoglobin, hematocrit, and/or WBC). Use pioglitazone with caution in premenopausal, anovulatory women; may result in resumption of ovulation, increasing the risk of pregnancy. May result in hormonal imbalance; development of menstrual irregularities should prompt reconsideration of therapy. Safety and efficacy of this combination have not been established in pediatric patients.

Drug Interactions

Cytochrome P450 Effect: Pioglitazone: **Substrate** of CYP2C8 (major), 3A4 (minor); **Inhibits** CYP2C8 (moderate), 2C9 (weak), 2C19 (weak), 2D6 (moderate); **Induces** CYP3A4 (weak)

Increased Effect/Toxicity: See individual agents.

Ethanol/Nutrition/Herb Interactions

Ethanol: Avoid or limit ethanol (incidence of lactic acidosis may be increased; may cause hypoglycemia).

Food: Food decreases the extent and slightly delays the absorption. May decrease absorption of vitamin B_{12} and/or folic acid.

Herb/Nutraceutical: Caution with chromium, garlic, gymnema (may cause hypoglycemia).

Dietary Considerations Should be taken with meals. Avoid ethanol. Dietary modification based on ADA recommendations is a part of therapy. Monitor for signs and symptoms of vitamin B_{12} and/or folic acid deficiency; supplementation may be required.

Pharmacodynamics/Kinetics See individual agents.

Pregnancy Risk Factor C

Dosage Forms TAB: (15/500): Pioglitazone 15 mg and metformin hydrochloride 500 mg; (15/850): Pioglitazone 15 mg and metformin hydrochloride 850 mg

---

Piperacillin *(pi PER a sil in)*

Generic Available Yes

Synonyms Piperacillin Sodium

Pharmacologic Category Antibiotic, Penicillin

Use Treatment of susceptible infections such as septicemia, acute and chronic respiratory tract infections, skin and soft tissue infections, and urinary tract infections due to susceptible strains of *Pseudomonas*, *Proteus*, and *Escherichia coli* and *Enterobacter*; active against some streptococci and some anaerobic bacteria; febrile neutropenia (as part of combination regimen)

Local Anesthetic/Vasoconstrictor Precautions No information available to require special precautions

Effects on Dental Treatment Key adverse event(s) related to dental treatment: Prolonged use of penicillins may lead to development of oral candidiasis.

Common Adverse Effects Frequency not defined.

Central nervous system: Confusion, convulsions, drowsiness, fever, Jarisch-Herxheimer reaction

Dermatologic: Rash, toxic epidermal necrolysis, urticaria

Endocrine & metabolic: Electrolyte imbalance, hypokalemia

Hematologic: Abnormal platelet aggregation and prolonged PT (high doses), agranulocytosis, Coombs' reaction (positive), hemolytic anemia, pancytopenia

Local: Thrombophlebitis

Neuromuscular & skeletal: Myoclonus

Renal: Acute interstitial nephritis, acute renal failure

Miscellaneous: Anaphylaxis, hypersensitivity reactions

Mechanism of Action Inhibits bacterial cell wall synthesis by binding to one or more of the penicillin binding proteins (PBPs); which in turn inhibits the final transpeptidation step of peptidoglycan synthesis in bacterial cell walls, thus inhibiting cell wall biosynthesis. Bacteria eventually lyse due to ongoing activity of cell wall autolytic enzymes (autolysins and murein hydrolases) while cell wall assembly is arrested.

Drug Interactions

Increased Effect/Toxicity: Probenecid may increase penicillin levels. Neuromuscular blockers may increase duration of blockade. Penicillins may increase the exposure to methotrexate during concurrent therapy; monitor.

Decreased Effect: Tetracyclines may decrease penicillin effectiveness. High concentrations of piperacillin may cause physical inactivation of aminoglycosides and lead to potential toxicity in patients with mild-moderate renal dysfunction. Although anecdotal reports suggest oral contraceptive efficacy could be reduced by penicillins, this has been refuted by more rigorous scientific and clinical data.

Pharmacodynamics/Kinetics

Absorption: I.M.: 70% to 80%

Distribution: Crosses placenta; low concentrations enter breast milk

Protein binding: 22%

Half-life elimination (dose dependent; prolonged with moderately severe renal or hepatic impairment):

Neonates: 1-5 days old: 3.6 hours; >6 days old: 2.1-2.7 hours

Children: 1-6 months: 0.79 hour; 6 months to 12 years: 0.39-0.5 hour

Adults: 36-80 minutes

Time to peak, serum: I.M.: 30-50 minutes

Excretion: Primarily urine; partially feces

Pregnancy Risk Factor B

Piperacillin and Tazobactam Sodium
(pi PER a sil in & ta zoe BAK tam SOW dee um)

Related Information

Piperacillin *on page 1244*

U.S. Brand Names Zosyn®

Canadian Brand Names Tazocin®

Generic Available No

Synonyms Piperacillin Sodium and Tazobactam Sodium

Pharmacologic Category Antibiotic, Penicillin

Use Treatment of moderate-to-severe infections caused by susceptible organisms, including infections of the lower respiratory tract (community-acquired pneumonia, nosocomial pneumonia); urinary tract; uncomplicated and complicated skin and skin structures; gynecologic (endometritis, pelvic inflammatory disease); bone and joint infections; intra-abdominal infections (appendicitis with rupture/abscess, peritonitis); and septicemia. Tazobactam expands activity of piperacillin to include beta-lactamase producing strains of *S. aureus*, *H. influenzae*, *Bacteroides*, and other gram-negative bacteria.

Local Anesthetic/Vasoconstrictor Precautions No information available to require special precautions

Effects on Dental Treatment Key adverse event(s) related to dental treatment: Prolonged use of penicillins may lead to development of oral candidiasis.

Common Adverse Effects

>10%: Gastrointestinal: Diarrhea (11%)

>1% to 10%:

Cardiovascular: Hypertension (2%), chest pain, edema

Central nervous system: Insomnia (7%), headache (7% to 8%), agitation (2%), fever (2%), pain (2%), anxiety, dizziness

Dermatologic: Rash (4%), pruritus (3%)

Gastrointestinal: Constipation (7% to 8%), nausea (7%), vomiting (3%), dyspepsia (3%), stool changes (2%), abdominal pain

Hepatic: Transaminases increased

Respiratory: Dyspnea, rhinitis

Miscellaneous: Moniliasis (2%)

Mechanism of Action Inhibits bacterial cell wall synthesis by binding to one or more of the penicillin binding proteins (PBPs); which in turn inhibits the final transpeptidation step of peptidoglycan synthesis in bacterial cell walls, thus inhibiting cell wall biosynthesis. Bacteria eventually lyse due to ongoing activity of cell wall autolytic enzymes (autolysins and murein hydrolases) while cell wall assembly is arrested. Tazobactam inhibits many beta-lactamases, including staphylococcal penicillinase and Richmond and Sykes types II, III, IV, and V, including extended spectrum enzymes; it has only limited activity against class I beta-lactamases other than class Ic types.

(Continued)

Piperacillin and Tazobactam Sodium *(Continued)*

Drug Interactions

Increased Effect/Toxicity: Probenecid may increase penicillin levels. Neuro-muscular blockers may increase duration of blockade. Penicillins may increase methotrexate exposure; clinical significance has not been established.

Decreased Effect: Tetracyclines may decrease penicillin effectiveness. Aminoglycosides may cause physical inactivation of aminoglycosides in the presence of high concentrations of piperacillin and potential toxicity in patients with mild-moderate renal dysfunction. Although anecdotal reports suggest oral contraceptive efficacy could be reduced by penicillins, this has been refuted by more rigorous scientific and clinical data.

Pharmacodynamics/Kinetics Both AUC and peak concentrations are dose proportional; hepatic impairment does not affect kinetics

Distribution: Well into lungs, intestinal mucosa, skin, muscle, uterus, ovary, prostate, gallbladder, and bile; penetration into CSF is low in subject with noninflamed meninges

Protein binding: Piperacillin and tazobactam: ~30%

Metabolism:

Piperacillin: 6% to 9% to desethyl metabolite (weak activity)

Tazobactam: ~26% to inactive metabolite

Half-life elimination: Piperacillin and tazobactam: 0.7-1.2 hours

Time to peak, plasma: Immediately following infusion of 30 minutes

Excretion: Clearance of both piperacillin and tazobactam are directly proportional to renal function

Piperacillin: Urine (68% as unchanged drug); feces (10% to 20%)

Tazobactam: Urine (80% as inactive metabolite)

Pregnancy Risk Factor B

Piperacillin Sodium *see* Piperacillin *on page 1244*

Piperacillin Sodium and Tazobactam Sodium *see* Piperacillin and Tazobactam Sodium *on page 1245*

Piperazine *(PI per a zeen)*

Canadian Brand Names Entacyl®

Mexican Brand Names Desparasil®

Generic Available Yes

Synonyms Piperazine Citrate

Pharmacologic Category Anthelmintic

Use Treatment of pinworm and roundworm infections (used as an alternative to first-line agents, mebendazole, or pyrantel pamoate)

Local Anesthetic/Vasoconstrictor Precautions No information available to require special precautions

Effects on Dental Treatment No significant effects or complications reported

Mechanism of Action Causes muscle paralysis of the roundworm by blocking the effects of acetylcholine at the neuromuscular junction

Drug Interactions

Decreased Effect: Pyrantel pamoate (antagonistic mode of action).

Pharmacodynamics/Kinetics

Absorption: Well absorbed

Time to peak, serum: 1 hour

Excretion: Urine (as unchanged drug and metabolites)

Pregnancy Risk Factor B

Piperazine Citrate *see* Piperazine *on page 1246*

Piperazine Estrone Sulfate *see* Estropipate *on page 586*

Piperonyl Butoxide and Pyrethrins *see* Pyrethrins and Piperonyl Butoxide *on page 1315*

Pipotiazine *(pip oh TYE a zeen)*

Canadian Brand Names Piportil® L₄

Mexican Brand Names Piportil L4®

Generic Available No

Synonyms Pipotiazine Palmitate

Pharmacologic Category Antipsychotic Agent, Typical, Phenothiazine, Piperidine

Use Management of schizophrenia

Local Anesthetic/Vasoconstrictor Precautions No information available to require special precautions

Effects on Dental Treatment No significant effects or complications reported

Common Adverse Effects Frequency not defined.

Cardiovascular: Tachycardia, hypotension, syncope, edema, ECG changes, QT_c prolongation, cardiac arrest

Central nervous system; Extrapyramidal symptoms (tremor, akathisia, dystonia, dyskinesia, oculogyric crisis, opisthotonos, hyper-reflexia, pseudo-Parkinsonism, rigidity, sialorrhea); tardive dyskinesia, sleep disturbance, dizziness, drowsiness, fatigue, insomnia, depression, agitation, anxiety, restlessness, excitement, bizarre dreams, fever, headache, cerebral edema, EEG changes, seizure, paradoxical psychosis

Dermatologic: Pruritus, dermatitis, rash, erythema, urticaria, seborrhea, eczema, exfoliative dermatitis, photosensitivity, skin pigmentation (prolonged therapy), epithelial keratopathy

Endocrine & metabolic: Anorexia, menstrual irregularities, thirst, weight changes, appetite increased, galactorrhea, gynecomastia, libido (changes in)

Gastrointestinal: Nausea, constipation, xerostomia, vomiting, salivation, adynamic ileus, fecal impaction, cholestasis, jaundice

Genitourinary: Urinary retention, bladder paralysis, incontinence, polyuria, impotence

Hematologic: Agranulocytosis, anemia, eosinophilia, leukopenia, pancytopenia, thrombocytopenia

Ocular: Blurred vision, glaucoma, corneal deposits (prolonged therapy), lenticular deposits, pigmentary retinopathy (prolonged therapy)

Respiratory: Nasal congestion, pneumonia, pneumonitis

Miscellaneous: Angioedema, diaphoresis increased, Lupus-like syndrome

Restrictions Not available in U.S.

Mechanism of Action Blocks postsynaptic mesolimbic dopaminergic receptors in the brain; depresses the release of hypothalamic and hypophyseal hormones. Relative to other piperidine phenothiazines, pipotiazine appears to be less sedating, with less potential to potentiate other CNS depressants, and may possess a lower propensity to cause hypotension. However, it has a relatively high propensity for cause extrapyramidal reactions.

Drug Interactions

Cytochrome P450 Effect: No published data on CYP metabolism. Based on structural analysis, pipotiazine may be a substrate of CYP2D6 and 3A4.

Increased Effect/Toxicity: The levels/effects of pipotiazine may be increased by azole antifungals, chlorpromazine, clarithromycin, delavirdine, diclofenac, doxycycline, erythromycin, fluoxetine, imatinib, isoniazid, miconazole, nefazodone, nicardipine, paroxetine, pergolide, propofol, protease inhibitors, quinidine, quinine, ritonavir, ropinirole, telithromycin, verapamil and other CYP2D6 or 3A4 inhibitors.

Drugs which alter the QT_c interval may be additive with pipotiazine, increasing the risk of malignant arrhythmias; includes type Ia antiarrhythmics, TCAs, and some quinolone antibiotics (sparfloxacin, moxifloxacin and gatifloxacin). **These agents are contraindicated with other piperadine phenothiazines (thioridazine)** Potassium depleting agents may increase the risk of serious arrhythmias with pipotiazine (includes many diuretics, aminoglycosides, and amphotericin).

Phenothiazines inhibit the ability of bromocriptine to lower serum prolactin concentrations. The sedative effects of CNS depressants or ethanol may be additive with phenothiazines. Phenothiazines and trazodone may produce additive hypotensive effects. Metoclopramide may increase risk of extrapyramidal symptoms (EPS). Concurrent use of antihypertensives may result in additive hypotensive effects (particularly orthostasis).

Phenothiazines may produce neurotoxicity with lithium; this is a rare effect. Rare cases of respiratory paralysis have been reported with concurrent use of phenothiazines and polypeptide antibiotics. Naltrexone in combination with pipotiazine has been reported to cause lethargy and somnolence. Phenylpropanolamine has been reported to result in cardiac arrhythmias when combined with some phenothiazines.

Decreased Effect: Aluminum salts may decrease the absorption of phenothiazines. The efficacy of amphetamines may be diminished by antipsychotics; in addition, amphetamines may increase psychotic symptoms; avoid concurrent use. Anticholinergics may inhibit the therapeutic response to phenothiazines and excess anticholinergic effects may occur (includes benztropine, trihexyphenidyl, biperiden, and drugs with significant anticholinergic activity). Low potency antipsychotics (such as pipotiazine) may diminish the pressor effects of epinephrine. The antihypertensive effects of guanethidine or guanadrel may be inhibited by phenothiazines. Phenothiazines may inhibit the

(Continued)

Pipotiazine *(Continued)*

antiparkinsonian effect of levodopa. Enzyme inducers may enhance the hepatic metabolism of phenothiazines; larger doses may be required; includes rifampin, rifabutin, barbiturates, phenytoin, and cigarette smoking.

Pharmacodynamics/Kinetics
Onset: I.M.: 2-3 days
Duration: 3-6 weeks

Pipotiazine Palmitate *see* Pipotiazine *on page 1246*

Pirbuterol *(peer BYOO ter ole)*

Related Information
Respiratory Diseases *on page 1656*
U.S. Brand Names Maxair™ Autohaler™
Generic Available No
Synonyms Pirbuterol Acetate
Pharmacologic Category Beta$_2$-Adrenergic Agonist
Use Prevention and treatment of reversible bronchospasm including asthma
Local Anesthetic/Vasoconstrictor Precautions No information available to require special precautions
Effects on Dental Treatment Key adverse event(s) related to dental treatment: Xerostomia (normal salivary flow resumes upon discontinuation).

Common Adverse Effects
>10%:
Central nervous system: Nervousness (7%)
Endocrine & metabolic: Serum glucose increased, serum potassium decreased
Neuromuscular & skeletal: Trembling (6%)
1% to 10%:
Cardiovascular: Palpitations (2%), tachycardia (1%)
Central nervous system: Headache (2%), dizziness (1%)
Gastrointestinal: Nausea (2%)
Respiratory: Cough (1%)

Mechanism of Action Pirbuterol is a beta$_2$-adrenergic agonist with a similar structure to albuterol, specifically a pyridine ring has been substituted for the benzene ring in albuterol. The increased beta$_2$ selectivity of pirbuterol results from the substitution of a tertiary butyl group on the nitrogen of the side chain, which additionally imparts resistance of pirbuterol to degradation by monoamine oxidase and provides a lengthened duration of action in comparison to the less selective previous beta-agonist agents.

Drug Interactions
Increased Effect/Toxicity: Increased toxicity with other beta agonists, MAO inhibitors, tricyclic antidepressants.
Decreased Effect: Decreased effect with beta-blockers.

Pharmacodynamics/Kinetics
Onset of action: Peak effect: Therapeutic: Oral: 2-3 hours with peak serum concentration of 6.2-9.8 mcg/L; Inhalation: 0.5-1 hour
Half-life elimination: 2-3 hours
Metabolism: Hepatic
Excretion: Urine (10% as unchanged drug)

Pregnancy Risk Factor C

Pirbuterol Acetate *see* Pirbuterol *on page 1248*

Piroxicam *(peer OKS i kam)*

Related Information
Rheumatoid Arthritis, Osteoarthritis, and Osteoporosis *on page 1668*
Temporomandibular Dysfunction (TMD) *on page 1724*
U.S. Brand Names Feldene®
Canadian Brand Names Apo-Piroxicam®; Gen-Piroxicam; Novo-Pirocam; Nu-Pirox; Pexicam®
Generic Available Yes
Pharmacologic Category Nonsteroidal Anti-inflammatory Drug (NSAID), Oral
Use Symptomatic treatment of acute and chronic rheumatoid arthritis and osteoarthritis
Unlabeled/Investigational Use Ankylosing spondylitis
Local Anesthetic/Vasoconstrictor Precautions No information available to require special precautions

Effects on Dental Treatment NSAID formulations are known to reversibly decrease platelet aggregation via mechanisms different than observed with aspirin. The dentist should be aware of the potential of abnormal coagulation. Caution should also be exercised in the use of NSAIDs in patients already on anticoagulant therapy with drugs such as warfarin (Coumadin®).

Common Adverse Effects

>10%:

Central nervous system: Dizziness

Dermatologic: Rash

Gastrointestinal: Abdominal cramps, heartburn, indigestion, nausea

1% to 10%:

Central nervous system: Headache, nervousness

Dermatologic: Itching

Endocrine & metabolic: Fluid retention

Gastrointestinal: Vomiting

Otic: Tinnitus

Restrictions A medication guide should be dispensed with each prescription. A template for the required MedGuide can be found on the FDA website at: http://www.fda.gov/medwatch/SAFETY/2005/safety05.htm#NSAID

Dosage Oral:

Children (unlabeled use): 0.2-0.3 mg/kg/day once daily; maximum dose: 15 mg/day

Adults: 10-20 mg/day once daily; although associated with increase in GI adverse effects, doses >20 mg/day have been used (ie, 30-40 mg/day)

Dosing adjustment in renal impairment: Not recommended in patients with advanced renal disease

Dosing adjustment in hepatic impairment: Reduction of dosage is necessary

Mechanism of Action Inhibits prostaglandin synthesis, acts on the hypothalamus heat-regulating center to reduce fever, blocks prostaglandin synthetase action which prevents formation of the platelet-aggregating substance thromboxane A_2; decreases pain receptor sensitivity. Other proposed mechanisms of action for salicylate anti-inflammatory action are lysosomal stabilization, kinin and leukotriene production, alteration of chemotactic factors, and inhibition of neutrophil activation. This latter mechanism may be the most significant pharmacologic action to reduce inflammation.

Contraindications Hypersensitivity to piroxicam, aspirin, other NSAIDs or any component of the formulation; perioperative pain in the setting of coronary artery bypass surgery (CABG); pregnancy (3rd trimester or near term)

Warnings/Precautions NSAIDs are associated with an increased risk of adverse cardiovascular events, including MI, stroke, and new onset or worsening of pre-existing hypertension. Risk may be increased with duration of use or pre-existing cardiovascular risk-factors or disease. Carefully evaluate individual cardiovascular risk profiles prior to prescribing. Use caution with fluid retention, CHF or hypertension.

Use of NSAIDs can compromise existing renal function. Renal toxicity can occur in patient with impaired renal function, dehydration, heart failure, liver dysfunction, those taking diuretics and ACEI and the elderly. Rehydrate patient before starting therapy. Monitor renal function closely. Not recommended for use in patients with advanced renal disease.

NSAIDs may increase risk of gastrointestinal irritation, ulceration, bleeding, and perforation. These events may occur at any time during therapy and without warning. Use caution with a history of GI disease (bleeding or ulcers), concurrent therapy with aspirin, anticoagulants and/or corticosteroids, smoking, use of alcohol, the elderly or debilitated patients.

Use the lowest effective dose for the shortest duration of time, consistent with individual patient goals, to reduce risk of cardiovascular or GI adverse events. Alternate therapies should be considered for patients at high risk.

NSAIDs may cause serious skin adverse events including exfoliative dermatitis, Stevens-Johnson syndrome (SJS) and toxic epidermal necrolysis (TEN). Anaphylactoid reactions may occur, even without prior exposure; patients with "aspirin triad" (bronchial asthma, aspirin intolerance, rhinitis) may be at increased risk. Do not use in patients who experience bronchospasm, asthma, rhinitis, or urticaria with NSAID or aspirin therapy. A serum sickness-like reaction can rarely occur; watch for arthralgias, pruritus, fever, fatigue, and rash.

Use with caution in patients with decreased hepatic function. Closely monitor patients with any abnormal LFT. Severe hepatic reactions (eg, fulminant hepatitis, liver failure) have occurred with NSAID use, rarely; discontinue if signs or symptoms of liver disease develop, or if systemic manifestations occur.

The elderly are at increased risk for adverse effects (especially peptic ulceration, CNS effects, renal toxicity) from NSAIDs even at low doses
(Continued)

Piroxicam *(Continued)*

Withhold for at least 4-6 half-lives prior to surgical or dental procedures.

Drug Interactions

Cytochrome P450 Effect: Substrate of CYP2C8/9 (minor); **Inhibits** CYP2C8/9 (strong)

Increased Effect/Toxicity: Increased effect/toxicity of lithium and methotrexate (controversial). Piroxicam may increase the levels/effects of amiodarone, fluoxetine, glimepiride, glipizide, nateglinide, pioglitazone, rosiglitazone, sertraline, warfarin, and other CYP2C8/9 substrates.

Decreased Effect: Decreased effect of diuretics, ACE inhibitors, angiotensin antagonists, beta-blockers, and hydralazine. Decreased effect with aspirin, antacids. Cholestyramine (and other bile acid sequestrants) may decrease the absorption of NSAIDs; separate by at least 2 hours.

Ethanol/Nutrition/Herb Interactions

Ethanol: Avoid ethanol (may enhance gastric mucosal irritation).

Food: Onset of effect may be delayed if piroxicam is taken with food.

Herb/Nutraceutical: Avoid alfalfa, anise, bilberry, bladderwrack, bromelain, cat's claw, celery, coleus, cordyceps, dong quai, evening primrose, feverfew, fenugreek, garlic, ginger, ginkgo biloboa, red clover, horse chestnut, grapeseed, green tea, ginseng, guggul, horse chestnut seed, horseradish, licorice, prickly ash, red clover, reishi, SAMe, sweet clover, turmeric, white willow (all have additional antiplatelet activity).

Dietary Considerations May be taken with food to decrease GI adverse effect.

Pharmacodynamics/Kinetics

Onset of action: Analgesic: ~1 hour

Peak effect: 3-5 hours

Protein binding: 99%

Metabolism: Hepatic

Half-life elimination: 45-50 hours

Excretion: Primarily urine and feces (small amounts) as unchanged drug (5%) and metabolites

Pregnancy Risk Factor C/D (3rd trimester)

Dosage Forms CAP: 10 mg, 20 mg

p-Isobutylhydratropic Acid *see* Ibuprofen *on page 808*

Pit *see* Oxytocin *on page 1175*

Pitocin® *see* Oxytocin *on page 1175*

Pitressin® *see* Vasopressin *on page 1567*

Pix Carbonis *see* Coal Tar *on page 383*

PLA *see* Poly-L-Lactic Acid *on page 1253*

Plan B® *see* Levonorgestrel *on page 916*

Plantago Seed *see* Psyllium *on page 1313*

Plantain Seed *see* Psyllium *on page 1313*

Plaquenil® *see* Hydroxychloroquine *on page 799*

Plaretase® 8000 *see* Pancrelipase *on page 1183*

Platinol®-AQ [DSC] *see* Cisplatin *on page 350*

Plavix® *see* Clopidogrel *on page 376*

Plenaxis™ [DSC] *see* Abarelix *on page 24*

Plendil® *see* Felodipine *on page 638*

Pletal® *see* Cilostazol *on page 340*

PMPA *see* Tenofovir *on page 1457*

Pneumococcal 7-Valent Conjugate Vaccine *see* Pneumococcal Conjugate Vaccine (7-Valent) *on page 1250*

Pneumococcal Conjugate Vaccine (7-Valent)
(noo moe KOK al KON ju gate vak SEEN, seven vay lent)

Related Information

Immunizations (Vaccines) *on page 1786*

U.S. Brand Names Prevnar®

Canadian Brand Names Prevnar®

Generic Available No

Synonyms Diphtheria CRM$_{197}$ Protein; PCV7; Pneumococcal 7-Valent Conjugate Vaccine

Pharmacologic Category Vaccine

Use Immunization of infants and toddlers against *Streptococcus pneumoniae* infection caused by serotypes included in the vaccine

Advisory Committee on Immunization Practices (ACIP) guidelines also recommend PCV7 for use in:

All children 2-23 months

Children ≥2-59 months with cochlear implants

Children ages 24-59 months with: Sickle cell disease (including other sickle cell hemoglobinopathies, asplenia, splenic dysfunction), HIV infection, immunocompromising conditions (congenital immunodeficiencies, renal failure, nephrotic syndrome, diseases associated with immunosuppressive or radiation therapy, solid organ transplant), chronic illnesses (cardiac disease, cerebrospinal fluid leaks, diabetes mellitus, pulmonary disease excluding asthma unless on high dose corticosteroids)

Consider use in all children 24-59 months with priority given to:

Children 24-35 months

Children 24-59 months who are of Alaska native, American Indian, or African-American descent

Children 24-59 months who attend group day care centers

Local Anesthetic/Vasoconstrictor Precautions No information available to require special precautions

Effects on Dental Treatment No significant effects or complications reported

Common Adverse Effects All serious adverse reactions must be reported to the U.S. Department of Health and Human Services (DHHS) Vaccine Adverse Event Reporting System (VAERS) 1-800-822-7967.

>10%:

Central nervous system: Fever, irritability, drowsiness, restlessness

Dermatologic: Erythema

Gastrointestinal: Decreased appetite, vomiting, diarrhea

Local: Induration, tenderness, nodule

1% to 10%: Dermatologic: Rash

Mechanism of Action Promotes active immunization against invasive disease caused by *S. pneumoniae* capsular serotypes 4, 6B, 9V, 18C, 19F, and 23F, all which are individually conjugated to CRM197 protein

Drug Interactions

Decreased Effect: Immunosuppressants may decrease response to active immunizations.

Pregnancy Risk Factor C

Pneumotussin® *see* Hydrocodone and Guaifenesin *on page 785*

PNU-140690E *see* Tipranavir *on page 1495*

Podactin Cream [OTC] *see* Miconazole *on page 1039*

Podactin Powder [OTC] *see* Tolnaftate *on page 1506*

Podocon-25® *see* Podophyllum Resin *on page 1251*

Podofilox (po do FIL oks)

U.S. Brand Names Condylox®

Canadian Brand Names Condyline™; Wartec®

Generic Available Yes: Topical solution

Pharmacologic Category Keratolytic Agent; Topical Skin Product

Use Treatment of external genital warts

Local Anesthetic/Vasoconstrictor Precautions No information available to require special precautions

Effects on Dental Treatment No significant effects or complications reported

Pregnancy Risk Factor C

Podophyllin *see* Podophyllum Resin *on page 1251*

Podophyllum Resin (po DOF il um REZ in)

U.S. Brand Names Podocon-25®

Canadian Brand Names Podofilm®

Generic Available No

Synonyms Mandrake; May Apple; Podophyllin

Pharmacologic Category Keratolytic Agent

Use Topical treatment of benign growths including external genital and perianal warts, papillomas, fibroids; compound benzoin tincture generally is used as the medium for topical application

Local Anesthetic/Vasoconstrictor Precautions No information available to require special precautions

Effects on Dental Treatment No significant effects or complications reported

Common Adverse Effects 1% to 10%:

Dermatologic: Pruritus

(Continued)

Podophyllum Resin *(Continued)*

Gastrointestinal: Nausea, vomiting, abdominal pain, diarrhea

Mechanism of Action Directly affects epithelial cell metabolism by arresting mitosis through binding to a protein subunit of spindle microtubules (tubulin)

Pregnancy Risk Factor X

Poliovirus Vaccine (Inactivated)
(POE lee oh VYE rus vak SEEN, in ak ti VAY ted)

Related Information

Immunizations (Vaccines) *on page 1786*

U.S. Brand Names IPOL®

Canadian Brand Names IPOL®

Generic Available No

Synonyms Enhanced-potency Inactivated Poliovirus Vaccine; IPV; Salk Vaccine

Pharmacologic Category Vaccine

Use

As the global eradication of poliomyelitis continues, the risk for importation of wild-type poliovirus into the United States decreases dramatically. To eliminate the risk for vaccine-associated paralytic poliomyelitis (VAPP), an all-IPV schedule is recommended for routine childhood vaccination in the United States. All children should receive four doses of IPV (at age 2 months, age 4 months, between ages 6-18 months, and between ages 4-6 years). Oral poliovirus vaccine (OPV), if available, may be used only for the following special circumstances:

Mass vaccination campaigns to control outbreaks of paralytic polio

Unvaccinated children who will be traveling within 4 weeks to areas where polio is endemic or epidemic

Children of parents who do not accept the recommended number of vaccine injections; these children may receive OPV only for the third or fourth dose or both. In this situation, healthcare providers should administer OPV only after discussing the risk for VAPP with parents or caregivers.

OPV supplies are expected to be very limited in the United States after inventories are depleted. ACIP reaffirms its support for the global eradication initiative and use of OPV as the vaccine of choice to eradicate polio where it is endemic.

Local Anesthetic/Vasoconstrictor Precautions No information available to require special precautions

Effects on Dental Treatment No significant effects or complications reported

Common Adverse Effects All serious adverse reactions must be reported to the U.S. Department of Health and Human Services (DHHS) Vaccine Adverse Event Reporting System (VAERS) 1-800-822-7967.

1% to 10%:

Central nervous system: Fever (>101.3°F)

Dermatologic: Rash

Local: Tenderness or pain at injection site

Pregnancy Risk Factor C

Polocaine® *see* Mepivacaine *on page 987*

Polocaine® Dental *see* Mepivacaine *on page 987*

Polocaine® MPF *see* Mepivacaine *on page 987*

Polycarbophil *(pol i KAR boe fil)*

U.S. Brand Names Equalactin® [OTC]; FiberCon® [OTC]; Fiber-Lax® [OTC]; Konsyl® Fiber Tablets [OTC]; Phillips'® Fibercaps [OTC]

Mexican Brand Names Fibercon®

Generic Available Yes: Tablet

Pharmacologic Category Antidiarrheal; Laxative, Bulk-Producing

Use Treatment of constipation or diarrhea

Local Anesthetic/Vasoconstrictor Precautions No information available to require special precautions

Effects on Dental Treatment Oral medication should be given at least 1 hour prior to taking the bulk-producing laxative in order to prevent decreased absorption of medication.

Mechanism of Action Restoring a more normal moisture level and providing bulk in the patient's intestinal tract

Pregnancy Risk Factor C

Polycitra® *see* Citric Acid, Sodium Citrate, and Potassium Citrate *on page 354*

Polycitra®-K *see* Potassium Citrate and Citric Acid *on page 1259*

Polycitra®-LC see Citric Acid, Sodium Citrate, and Potassium Citrate on page 354

Polycose® [OTC] see Glucose Polymers on page 743

Poly-Dex™ see Neomycin, Polymyxin B, and Dexamethasone on page 1101

Polyethylene Glycol 3350 (pol i ETH i leen GLY kol 3350)

U.S. Brand Names GlycoLax™; MiraLax™
Generic Available Yes
Synonyms PEG
Pharmacologic Category Laxative, Osmotic
Use Treatment of occasional constipation in adults
Unlabeled/Investigational Use Treatment of constipation in children
Local Anesthetic/Vasoconstrictor Precautions No information available to require special precautions
Effects on Dental Treatment No significant effects or complications reported
Common Adverse Effects Frequency not defined.
Dermatologic: Urticaria
Gastrointestinal: Abdominal bloating, cramping, diarrhea, flatulence, nausea
Mechanism of Action An osmotic agent, polyethylene glycol 3350 causes water retention in the stool; increases stool frequency and consistency
Pharmacodynamics/Kinetics Onset of action: Oral: 48-96 hours
Pregnancy Risk Factor C

Polyethylene Glycol-Electrolyte Solution
(pol i ETH i leen GLY kol ee LEK troe lite soe LOO shun)

U.S. Brand Names Colyte®; GoLYTELY®; NuLYTELY®; TriLyte™
Canadian Brand Names Colyte™; Klean-Prep®; Peglyte™
Generic Available Yes
Synonyms Electrolyte Lavage Solution
Pharmacologic Category Laxative, Osmotic
Use Bowel cleansing prior to GI examination or following toxic ingestion
Local Anesthetic/Vasoconstrictor Precautions No information available to require special precautions
Effects on Dental Treatment No significant effects or complications reported
Common Adverse Effects Frequency not defined.
Dermatologic: Dermatitis, rash, urticaria
Gastrointestinal: Nausea, abdominal fullness, bloating, abdominal cramps, vomiting, anal irritation, diarrhea, flatulence
Mechanism of Action Induces catharsis by strong electrolyte and osmotic effects
Drug Interactions
Decreased Effect: Oral medications should not be administered within 1 hour of start of therapy.
Pharmacodynamics/Kinetics Onset of effect: Oral: ~1-2 hours
Pregnancy Risk Factor C

Polygam® S/D see Immune Globulin (Intravenous) on page 824

Poly-L-Lactic Acid (POL i el LAK tik AS id)

U.S. Brand Names Sculptra™
Generic Available No
Synonyms New-Fill®; PLA
Pharmacologic Category Cosmetic Agent, Implant
Use Restoration and/or correction of facial lipoatrophy in patients with HIV
Local Anesthetic/Vasoconstrictor Precautions No information available to require special precautions
Effects on Dental Treatment No significant effects or complications reported
Mechanism of Action Poly-L-lactic acid is an immunologically inert synthetic polymer. It increases dermal thickness by causing a local reaction leading to an increase in collagen deposits. It is eventually degraded and undergoes resorption.

Polymyxin B (pol i MIKS in bee)

U.S. Brand Names Poly-Rx
Generic Available Yes
(Continued)

Polymyxin B *(Continued)*

Synonyms Polymyxin B Sulfate

Pharmacologic Category Antibiotic, Irrigation; Antibiotic, Miscellaneous

Use Treatment of acute infections caused by susceptible strains of *Pseudomonas aeruginosa*; used occasionally for gut decontamination; parenteral use of polymyxin B has mainly been replaced by less toxic antibiotics, reserved for life-threatening infections caused by organisms resistant to the preferred drugs (eg, pseudomonal meningitis - intrathecal administration)

Local Anesthetic/Vasoconstrictor Precautions No information available to require special precautions

Effects on Dental Treatment No significant effects or complications reported

Common Adverse Effects Frequency not defined.

Cardiovascular: Facial flushing

Central nervous system: Neurotoxicity (irritability, drowsiness, ataxia, perioral paresthesia, numbness of the extremities, and blurred vision); dizziness, drug fever, meningeal irritation with intrathecal administration

Dermatologic: Urticarial rash

Endocrine & metabolic: Hypocalcemia, hyponatremia, hypokalemia, hypochloremia

Local: Pain at injection site

Neuromuscular & skeletal: Neuromuscular blockade, weakness

Renal: Nephrotoxicity

Respiratory: Respiratory arrest

Miscellaneous: Anaphylactoid reaction

Mechanism of Action Binds to phospholipids, alters permeability, and damages the bacterial cytoplasmic membrane permitting leakage of intracellular constituents

Drug Interactions

Increased Effect/Toxicity: Increased/prolonged effect of neuromuscular blocking agents.

Pharmacodynamics/Kinetics

Absorption: Well absorbed from peritoneum; minimal from GI tract (except in neonates) from mucous membranes or intact skin

Distribution: Minimal into CSF; does not cross placenta

Half-life elimination: 4.5-6 hours; prolonged with renal impairment

Time to peak, serum: I.M.: ~2 hours

Excretion: Urine (>60% primarily as unchanged drug)

Pregnancy Risk Factor B (per expert opinion)

Polymyxin B and Bacitracin *see* Bacitracin and Polymyxin B *on page 176*

Polymyxin B and Neomycin *see* Neomycin and Polymyxin B *on page 1100*

Polymyxin B and Trimethoprim *see* Trimethoprim and Polymyxin B *on page 1539*

Polymyxin B, Bacitracin, and Neomycin *see* Bacitracin, Neomycin, and Polymyxin B *on page 176*

Polymyxin B, Bacitracin, Neomycin, and Hydrocortisone *see* Bacitracin, Neomycin, Polymyxin B, and Hydrocortisone *on page 177*

Polymyxin B, Neomycin, and Dexamethasone *see* Neomycin, Polymyxin B, and Dexamethasone *on page 1101*

Polymyxin B, Neomycin, and Gramicidin *see* Neomycin, Polymyxin B, and Gramicidin *on page 1101*

Polymyxin B, Neomycin, and Hydrocortisone *see* Neomycin, Polymyxin B, and Hydrocortisone *on page 1101*

Polymyxin B, Neomycin, and Prednisolone *see* Neomycin, Polymyxin B, and Prednisolone *on page 1102*

Polymyxin B, Neomycin, Bacitracin, and Pramoxine *see* Bacitracin, Neomycin, Polymyxin B, and Pramoxine *on page 177*

Polymyxin B Sulfate *see* Polymyxin B *on page 1253*

Poly-Pred® *see* Neomycin, Polymyxin B, and Prednisolone *on page 1102*

Poly-Rx *see* Polymyxin B *on page 1253*

Polysaccharide-Iron Complex
(pol i SAK a ride-EYE ern KOM pleks)

U.S. Brand Names Ferrex 150 [OTC]; Fe-Tinic™ 150 [OTC] [DSC]; Hytinic® [OTC]; Niferex® [OTC]; Niferex® 150 [OTC]; Nu-Iron® 150 [OTC]

Generic Available Yes: Capsule

Synonyms Iron-Polysaccharide Complex

Pharmacologic Category Iron Salt

Use Prevention and treatment of iron-deficiency anemias

Local Anesthetic/Vasoconstrictor Precautions No information available to require special precautions
Effects on Dental Treatment No significant effects or complications reported

Common Adverse Effects

>10%: Gastrointestinal: Stomach cramping, constipation, nausea, vomiting, dark stools, GI irritation, epigastric pain, nausea

1% to 10%:

Gastrointestinal: Heartburn, diarrhea

Genitourinary: Discolored urine

Miscellaneous: Staining of teeth

Pregnancy Risk Factor A

Polysporin® Ophthalmic see Bacitracin and Polymyxin B on page 176

Polysporin® Topical [OTC] see Bacitracin and Polymyxin B on page 176

Polytar® [OTC] see Coal Tar on page 383

Polythiazide (pol i THYE a zide)

Related Information

Cardiovascular Diseases on page 1636

U.S. Brand Names Renese®

Generic Available No

Pharmacologic Category Diuretic, Thiazide

Use Adjunctive therapy in treatment of edema and hypertension

Local Anesthetic/Vasoconstrictor Precautions No information available to require special precautions

Effects on Dental Treatment No significant effects or complications reported

Mechanism of Action The diuretic mechanism of action of the thiazides is primarily inhibition of sodium, chloride, and water reabsorption in the renal distal tubules, thereby producing diuresis with a resultant reduction in plasma volume. The antihypertensive mechanism of action of the thiazides is unknown. It is known that doses of thiazides produce greater reductions in blood pressure than equivalent diuretic doses of loop diuretics (eg, furosemide). There has been speculation that the thiazides may have some influence on vascular tone mediated through sodium depletion, but this remains to be proven.

Pregnancy Risk Factor D

Polythiazide and Prazosin see Prazosin and Polythiazide on page 1268

Polytrim® see Trimethoprim and Polymyxin B on page 1539

Polyvinyl Alcohol see Artificial Tears on page 143

Polyvinylpyrrolidone with Iodine see Povidone-Iodine on page 1262

Ponstel® see Mefenamic Acid on page 973

Pontocaine® see Tetracaine on page 1466

Pontocaine® Niphanoid® see Tetracaine on page 1466

Pontocaine® With Dextrose see Tetracaine and Dextrose on page 1467

Poractant Alfa (por AKT ant AL fa)

U.S. Brand Names Curosurf®

Canadian Brand Names Curosurf®

Generic Available No

Pharmacologic Category Lung Surfactant

Use Orphan drug: Treatment and prevention of respiratory distress syndrome (RDS) in premature infants

Local Anesthetic/Vasoconstrictor Precautions No information available to require special precautions

Effects on Dental Treatment No significant effects or complications reported

Common Adverse Effects Frequency not defined.

Cardiovascular: Bradycardia, hypotension

Gastrointestinal: Endotracheal tube blockage

Respiratory: Oxygen desaturation

Mechanism of Action Endogenous pulmonary surfactant reduces surface tension at the air-liquid interface of the alveoli during ventilation and stabilizes the alveoli against collapse at resting transpulmonary pressures. A deficiency of pulmonary surfactant in preterm infants results in respiratory distress syndrome characterized by poor lung expansion, inadequate gas exchange, and atelectasis. Poractant alpha compensates for the surfactant deficiency and restores surface activity to the infant's lungs. It reduces mortality and pneumothoraces associated with RDS.

Pharmacodynamics/Kinetics Information limited to animal models. No human information about pharmacokinetics exists.

Porfimer (POR fi mer)

U.S. Brand Names Photofrin®
Canadian Brand Names Photofrin®
Generic Available No
Synonyms CL-184116; Dihematoporphyrin Ether; Porfimer Sodium
Pharmacologic Category Antineoplastic Agent, Miscellaneous
Use Adjunct to laser light therapy for obstructing esophageal cancer, obstructing endobronchial nonsmall cell lung cancer (NSCLC), ablation of high-grade dysplasia in Barrett's esophagus
Unlabeled/Investigational Use Transitional cell carcinoma *in situ* of the urinary bladder; gastric and rectal cancers
Local Anesthetic/Vasoconstrictor Precautions No information available to require special precautions
Effects on Dental Treatment No significant effects or complications reported
Common Adverse Effects
>10%:
  Cardiovascular: Atrial fibrillation (10%), chest pain (5% to 22%)
  Central nervous system: Insomnia (14%), hyperthermia (31%)
  Dermatologic: Photosensitivity reaction (10% to 80%, minor reactions may occur in up to 100%)
  Gastrointestinal: Abdominal pain (20%), constipation (23%), dysphagia, nausea (24%), vomiting (17%)
  Genitourinary: Urinary tract irritation including frequency, urgency, nocturia, painful urination, or bladder spasm (~100% of bladder cancer patients)
  Hematologic: Anemia (26% of esophageal cancer patients)
  Neuromuscular & skeletal: Back pain
  Respiratory: Dyspnea (20%), pharyngitis (11%), pleural effusion (32% of esophageal cancer patients), pneumonia (18%), respiratory insufficiency
  Miscellaneous: Mild-moderate allergic-type reactions (34% of lung cancer patients)
1% to 10%:
  Cardiovascular: Hyper-/hypotension (6% to 7%), edema, cardiac failure (6% to 7%), tachycardia (6%), chest pain (substernal)
  Central nervous system: Anxiety (7%), confusion (8%)
  Dermatologic: Increased hair growth, skin discoloration, skin wrinkles, skin nodules, increased skin fragility
  Endocrine & metabolic: Dehydration
  Gastrointestinal: Diarrhea (5%), dyspepsia (6%), eructation (5%), esophageal edema (8%), esophageal tumor bleeding, esophageal stricture, esophagitis, hematemesis, melena, weight loss, anorexia
  Genitourinary: Urinary tract infection
  Neuromuscular & skeletal: Weakness
  Respiratory: Coughing, tracheoesophageal fistula
  Miscellaneous: Moniliasis, surgical complication
Mechanism of Action Porfimer's cytotoxic activity is dependent on light and oxygen. Following administration, the drug is selectively retained in neoplastic tissues. Exposure of the drug to laser light at wavelengths >630 nm results in the production of oxygen free-radicals. Release of thromboxane A$_2$, leading to vascular occlusion and ischemic necrosis, may also occur.
Drug Interactions
  Increased Effect/Toxicity: Concomitant administration of other photosensitizing agents (eg, tetracyclines, sulfonamides, phenothiazines, sulfonylureas, thiazide diuretics, griseofulvin) could increase the photosensitivity reaction.
  Decreased Effect: Compounds that quench active oxygen species or scavenge radicals (eg, dimethyl sulfoxide, beta-carotene, ethanol, mannitol) would be expected to decrease photodynamic therapy (PDT) activity. Allopurinol, calcium channel blockers, and some prostaglandin synthesis inhibitors could interfere with porfimer. Drugs that decrease clotting, vasoconstriction, or platelet aggregation could decrease the efficacy of PDT. Glucocorticoid hormones may decrease the efficacy of the treatment.
Pharmacodynamics/Kinetics
  Distribution: V$_{dss}$: 0.49 L/kg
  Protein binding, plasma: 90%
  Half-life elimination: Mean: 21.5 days (range: 11-28 days)
  Time to peak, serum: ~2 hours
  Excretion: Feces; Clearance: Plasma: Total: 0.051 mL/minute/kg
Pregnancy Risk Factor C

Porfimer Sodium *see* Porfimer *on page 1256*
Portia™ *see* Ethinyl Estradiol and Levonorgestrel *on page 602*

Post Peel Healing Balm [OTC] *see* Hydrocortisone *on page 793*
Posture® [OTC] *see* Calcium Phosphate (Tribasic) *on page 251*
Potaba® *see* Potassium P-Aminobenzoate *on page 1261*

Potassium Acetate (poe TASS ee um AS e tate)

Generic Available Yes
Pharmacologic Category Electrolyte Supplement, Parenteral
Use Potassium deficiency; to avoid chloride when high concentration of potassium is needed, source of bicarbonate
Local Anesthetic/Vasoconstrictor Precautions No information available to require special precautions
Effects on Dental Treatment No significant effects or complications reported
Mechanism of Action Potassium is the major cation of intracellular fluid and is essential for the conduction of nerve impulses in heart, brain, and skeletal muscle; contraction of cardiac, skeletal and smooth muscles; maintenance of normal renal function, acid-base balance, carbohydrate metabolism, and gastric secretion
Pregnancy Risk Factor C

Potassium Acetate, Potassium Bicarbonate, and Potassium Citrate
(poe TASS ee um AS e tate, poe TASS ee um bye KAR bun ate, & poe TASS ee um SIT rate)

Related Information
Potassium Acetate *on page 1257*
Potassium Bicarbonate *on page 1257*
Potassium Citrate *on page 1259*
U.S. Brand Names Tri-K®
Generic Available No
Synonyms Potassium Acetate, Potassium Citrate, and Potassium Bicarbonate; Potassium Bicarbonate, Potassium Acetate, and Potassium Citrate; Potassium Bicarbonate, Potassium Citrate, and Potassium Acetate; Potassium Citrate, Potassium Acetate, and Potassium Bicarbonate; Potassium Citrate, Potassium Bicarbonate, and Potassium Acetate
Pharmacologic Category Electrolyte Supplement, Oral
Use Treatment or prevention of hypokalemia
Local Anesthetic/Vasoconstrictor Precautions No information available to require special precautions
Effects on Dental Treatment No significant effects or complications reported
Pregnancy Risk Factor C

Potassium Acetate, Potassium Citrate, and Potassium Bicarbonate *see* Potassium Acetate, Potassium Bicarbonate, and Potassium Citrate *on page 1257*

Potassium Acid Phosphate (poe TASS ee um AS id FOS fate)

U.S. Brand Names K-Phos® Original
Generic Available No
Pharmacologic Category Urinary Acidifying Agent
Use Acidifies urine and lowers urinary calcium concentration; reduces odor and rash caused by ammoniacal urine; increases the antibacterial activity of methenamine
Local Anesthetic/Vasoconstrictor Precautions No information available to require special precautions
Effects on Dental Treatment No significant effects or complications reported
Mechanism of Action The principal intracellular cation; involved in transmission of nerve impulses, muscle contractions, enzyme activity, and glucose utilization
Pregnancy Risk Factor C

Potassium Bicarbonate (poe TASS ee um bye KAR bun ate)

Mexican Brand Names Kaliolite®; K-Dur®
Generic Available Yes
Pharmacologic Category Electrolyte Supplement, Oral
Use Potassium deficiency, hypokalemia
(Continued)

Potassium Bicarbonate *(Continued)*

Local Anesthetic/Vasoconstrictor Precautions No information available to require special precautions

Effects on Dental Treatment No significant effects or complications reported

Pregnancy Risk Factor C

Potassium Bicarbonate and Potassium Chloride

(poe TASS ee um bye KAR bun ate & poe TASS ee um KLOR ide)

Related Information
Potassium Bicarbonate *on page 1257*
Potassium Chloride *on page 1258*

U.S. Brand Names K-Lyte/Cl®; K-Lyte/Cl® 50 [DSC]

Generic Available No

Synonyms Potassium Bicarbonate and Potassium Chloride (Effervescent)

Pharmacologic Category Electrolyte Supplement, Oral

Use Treatment or prevention of hypokalemia

Local Anesthetic/Vasoconstrictor Precautions No information available to require special precautions

Effects on Dental Treatment No significant effects or complications reported

Pregnancy Risk Factor C

Potassium Bicarbonate and Potassium Chloride (Effervescent) *see* Potassium Bicarbonate and Potassium Chloride *on page 1258*

Potassium Bicarbonate and Potassium Citrate

(poe TASS ee um bye KAR bun ate & poe TASS ee um SIT rate)

Related Information
Potassium Bicarbonate *on page 1257*
Potassium Citrate *on page 1259*

U.S. Brand Names Effer-K™; Klor-Con®/EF; K-Lyte®; K-Lyte® DS

Generic Available Yes

Synonyms Potassium Bicarbonate and Potassium Citrate (Effervescent)

Pharmacologic Category Electrolyte Supplement, Oral

Use Treatment or prevention of hypokalemia

Local Anesthetic/Vasoconstrictor Precautions No information available to require special precautions

Effects on Dental Treatment No significant effects or complications reported

Mechanism of Action Needed for the conduction of nerve impulses in heart, brain, and skeletal muscle; contraction of cardiac, skeletal and smooth muscles; maintenance of normal renal function

Pregnancy Risk Factor C

Potassium Bicarbonate and Potassium Citrate (Effervescent) *see* Potassium Bicarbonate and Potassium Citrate *on page 1258*

Potassium Bicarbonate, Potassium Acetate, and Potassium Citrate *see* Potassium Acetate, Potassium Bicarbonate, and Potassium Citrate *on page 1257*

Potassium Bicarbonate, Potassium Citrate, and Potassium Acetate *see* Potassium Acetate, Potassium Bicarbonate, and Potassium Citrate *on page 1257*

Potassium Chloride (poe TASS ee um KLOR ide)

U.S. Brand Names Kaon-Cl-10®; Kaon-Cl® 20; Kay Ciel®; K-Dur® 10; K-Dur® 20; K-Lor®; Klor-Con®; Klor-Con® 8; Klor-Con® 10; Klor-Con®/25; Klor-Con® M; K+ Potassium; K-Tab®; microK®; microK® 10; Rum-K®

Canadian Brand Names Apo-K®; K-10®; K-Dur®; K-Lor®; K-Lyte®/Cl; Micro-K Extencaps®; Roychlor®; Slow-K®

Generic Available Yes

Synonyms KCl

Pharmacologic Category Electrolyte Supplement, Oral; Electrolyte Supplement, Parenteral

Use Treatment or prevention of hypokalemia

Local Anesthetic/Vasoconstrictor Precautions No information available to require special precautions

Effects on Dental Treatment No significant effects or complications reported

Mechanism of Action Potassium is the major cation of intracellular fluid and is essential for the conduction of nerve impulses in heart, brain, and skeletal muscle; contraction of cardiac, skeletal and smooth muscles; maintenance of normal renal function, acid-base balance, carbohydrate metabolism, and gastric secretion

Pregnancy Risk Factor A

Potassium Citrate (poe TASS ee um SIT rate)

U.S. Brand Names Urocit®-K

Canadian Brand Names K-Citra®; K-Lyte®; Polycitra®-K

Generic Available No

Pharmacologic Category Alkalinizing Agent, Oral

Use Prevention of uric acid nephrolithiasis; prevention of calcium renal stones in patients with hypocitraturia; urinary alkalinizer when sodium citrate is contraindicated

Local Anesthetic/Vasoconstrictor Precautions No information available to require special precautions

Effects on Dental Treatment No significant effects or complications reported

Pregnancy Risk Factor Not available

Potassium Citrate and Citric Acid
(poe TASS ee um SIT rate & SI trik AS id)

Related Information
Potassium Citrate on page 1259

U.S. Brand Names Cytra-K; Polycitra®-K

Generic Available Yes

Synonyms Citric Acid and Potassium Citrate

Pharmacologic Category Alkalinizing Agent, Oral

Use Treatment of metabolic acidosis; alkalinizing agent in conditions where long-term maintenance of an alkaline urine is desirable

Local Anesthetic/Vasoconstrictor Precautions No information available to require special precautions

Effects on Dental Treatment No significant effects or complications reported

Drug Interactions
Increased Effect/Toxicity: Concurrent administration with potassium-containing medications, potassium-sparing diuretics, ACE inhibitors, or cardiac glycosides could lead to toxicity.

Pharmacodynamics/Kinetics
Metabolism: To potassium bicarbonate; citric acid is metabolized to CO_2 and H_2O
Excretion: Urine

Pregnancy Risk Factor A

Potassium Citrate, Citric Acid, and Sodium Citrate see Citric Acid, Sodium Citrate, and Potassium Citrate on page 354

Potassium Citrate, Potassium Acetate, and Potassium Bicarbonate see Potassium Acetate, Potassium Bicarbonate, and Potassium Citrate on page 1257

Potassium Citrate, Potassium Bicarbonate, and Potassium Acetate see Potassium Acetate, Potassium Bicarbonate, and Potassium Citrate on page 1257

Potassium Gluconate (poe TASS ee um GLOO coe nate)

U.S. Brand Names Glu-K® [OTC]

Generic Available Yes

Pharmacologic Category Electrolyte Supplement, Oral

Use Treatment or prevention of hypokalemia

Local Anesthetic/Vasoconstrictor Precautions No information available to require special precautions

Effects on Dental Treatment No significant effects or complications reported

Mechanism of Action Potassium is the major cation of intracellular fluid and is essential for the conduction of nerve impulses in heart, brain, and skeletal muscle; contraction of cardiac, skeletal and smooth muscles; maintenance of normal renal function, acid-base balance, carbohydrate metabolism, and gastric secretion

Pregnancy Risk Factor A

Potassium Guaiacolsulfonate and Guaifenesin see Guaifenesin and Potassium Guaiacolsulfonate on page 755

Potassium Iodide (poe TASS ee um EYE oh dide)

Related Information
Endocrine Disorders and Pregnancy *on page 1659*

U.S. Brand Names Iosat™ [OTC]; Pima®; SSKI®; ThyroSafe™ [OTC]; ThyroShield™ [OTC]

Synonyms KI

Pharmacologic Category Antithyroid Agent; Expectorant

Use Expectorant for the symptomatic treatment of chronic pulmonary diseases complicated by mucous; reduce thyroid vascularity prior to thyroidectomy and management of thyrotoxic crisis; block thyroidal uptake of radioactive isotopes of iodine in a radiation emergency or other exposure to radioactive iodine

Unlabeled/Investigational Use Lymphocutaneous and cutaneous sporotrichosis

Local Anesthetic/Vasoconstrictor Precautions No information available to require special precautions

Effects on Dental Treatment No significant effects or complications reported

Common Adverse Effects Frequency not defined.

Cardiovascular: Irregular heart beat

Central nervous system: Confusion, tiredness, fever

Dermatologic: Skin rash

Endocrine & metabolic: Goiter, salivary gland swelling/tenderness, thyroid adenoma, swelling of neck/throat, myxedema, lymph node swelling, hyper-/hypothyroidism

Gastrointestinal: Diarrhea, gastrointestinal bleeding, metallic taste, nausea, stomach pain, stomach upset, vomiting

Neuromuscular & skeletal: Numbness, tingling, weakness, joint pain

Miscellaneous: Chronic iodine poisoning (with prolonged treatment/high doses); iodism, hypersensitivity reactions (angioedema, cutaneous and mucosal hemorrhage, serum sickness-like symptoms)

Mechanism of Action Reduces viscosity of mucus by increasing respiratory tract secretions; inhibits secretion of thyroid hormone, fosters colloid accumulation in thyroid follicles. Following radioactive iodine exposure, potassium iodide blocks uptake of radioiodine by the thyroid, reducing the risk of thyroid cancer.

Drug Interactions

Increased Effect/Toxicity: Lithium may cause additive hypothyroid effects; ACE inhibitors, potassium-sparing diuretics, and potassium/potassium-containing products may lead to hyperkalemia, cardiac arrhythmias, or cardiac arrest

Pharmacodynamics/Kinetics

Onset of action: Hyperthyroidism: 24-48 hours

Peak effect: 10-15 days after continuous therapy

Duration: Radioactive iodine exposure: ~ 24 hours

Pregnancy Risk Factor D

Potassium Iodide and Iodine
(poe TASS ee um EYE oh dide & EYE oh dine)

Generic Available Yes

Synonyms Lugol's Solution; Strong Iodine Solution

Pharmacologic Category Antithyroid Agent

Use Reduce thyroid vascularity prior to thyroidectomy and management of thyrotoxic crisis; block thyroidal uptake of radioactive isotopes of iodine in a radiation emergency or other exposure to radioactive iodine

Local Anesthetic/Vasoconstrictor Precautions No information available to require special precautions

Effects on Dental Treatment No significant effects or complications reported

Common Adverse Effects Frequency not defined.

Cardiovascular: Irregular heart beat

Central nervous system: Confusion, tiredness, fever

Dermatologic: Skin rash

Endocrine & metabolic: Goiter, salivary gland swelling/tenderness, thyroid adenoma, swelling of neck/throat, myxedema, lymph node swelling, hyper-/hypothyroidism

Gastrointestinal: Diarrhea, gastrointestinal bleeding, metallic taste, nausea, stomach pain, stomach upset, vomiting

Neuromuscular & skeletal: Numbness, tingling, weakness, joint pain

Miscellaneous: Chronic iodine poisoning (with prolonged treatment/high doses); iodism, hypersensitivity reactions (angioedema, cutaneous and mucosal hemorrhage, serum sickness-like symptoms)

Mechanism of Action Inhibits secretion of thyroid hormone, fosters colloid accumulation in thyroid follicles. Following radioactive iodine exposure, potassium iodide blocks uptake of radioiodine by the thyroid, reducing the risk of thyroid cancer.

Drug Interactions

Increased Effect/Toxicity: Concurrent use of ACE inhibitors, potassium-sparing diuretics, or potassium (and potassium-containing products) may lead to hyperkalemia, cardiac arrhythmias or cardiac arrest. Lithium may cause additive hypothyroid effects.

Pharmacodynamics/Kinetics

Onset of action: Hyperthyroidism: 24-48 hours

Peak effect: 10-15 days after continuous therapy

Pregnancy Risk Factor D (potassium iodide)

Potassium Iodide, Chlorpheniramine, Phenylephrine, and Codeine *see* Chlorpheniramine, Phenylephrine, Codeine, and Potassium Iodide *on page 328*

Potassium P-Aminobenzoate (poe TASS ee um pe a mee noe BEN zoe ate)

U.S. Brand Names Potaba®

Generic Available Yes

Pharmacologic Category Vitamin, Water Soluble

Use Presently, all indications are classified by the FDA as "possibly effective." Treatment of scleroderma, dermatomyositis, morphea, linear scleroderma, pemphigus, Peyronie's disease

Local Anesthetic/Vasoconstrictor Precautions No information available to require special precautions

Effects on Dental Treatment No significant effects or complications reported

Mechanism of Action P-aminobenzoate is a member of the vitamin B complex family. It may have an antifibrotic effect due to increased oxygen uptake at the tissue level.

Potassium Perchlorate (poe TASS ee um per KLOR ate)

U.S. Brand Names Perchloracap® [DSC]

Generic Available No

Pharmacologic Category Diagnostic Agent

Use Minimizes accumulation of pertechnetate Tc 99m in imaging studies

Local Anesthetic/Vasoconstrictor Precautions No information available to require special precautions

Effects on Dental Treatment No significant effects or complications reported

Pregnancy Risk Factor C

Potassium Phosphate (poe TASS ee um FOS fate)

U.S. Brand Names Neutra-Phos®-K [OTC]

Generic Available Yes: Injection

Synonyms Phosphate, Potassium

Pharmacologic Category Electrolyte Supplement, Oral; Electrolyte Supplement, Parenteral

Use Treatment and prevention of hypophosphatemia or hypokalemia

Local Anesthetic/Vasoconstrictor Precautions No information available to require special precautions

Effects on Dental Treatment No significant effects or complications reported

Pregnancy Risk Factor C

Potassium Phosphate and Sodium Phosphate (poe TASS ee um FOS fate & SOW dee um FOS fate)

Related Information

Potassium Phosphate *on page 1261*

Sodium Phosphates *on page 1403*

U.S. Brand Names K-Phos® MF; K-Phos® Neutral; K-Phos® No. 2; Neutra-Phos® [OTC]; Phos-NaK; Phospha 250™ Neutral; Uro-KP-Neutral®

Generic Available Yes

Synonyms Sodium Phosphate and Potassium Phosphate

Pharmacologic Category Electrolyte Supplement, Oral

Use Treatment of conditions associated with excessive renal phosphate loss or inadequate GI absorption of phosphate; to acidify the urine to lower calcium

(Continued)

Potassium Phosphate and Sodium Phosphate
(Continued)

concentrations; to increase the antibacterial activity of methenamine; reduce odor and rash caused by ammonia in urine

Local Anesthetic/Vasoconstrictor Precautions No information available to require special precautions

Effects on Dental Treatment No significant effects or complications reported

Pregnancy Risk Factor C

Povidine™ [OTC] see Povidone-Iodine on page 1262

Povidone-Iodine (POE vi done EYE oh dyne)

Related Information
Management of Patients Undergoing Cancer Therapy on page 1728

U.S. Brand Names Betadine® [OTC]; Betadine® Ophthalmic; Minidyne® [OTC]; Operand® [OTC]; Povidine™ [OTC]; Summer's Eve® Medicated Douche [OTC]; Vagi-Gard® [OTC]

Canadian Brand Names Betadine®; Proviodine

Mexican Brand Names Isodine®; Yodine®

Generic Available Yes

Synonyms Polyvinylpyrrolidone with Iodine; PVP-I

Pharmacologic Category Antiseptic, Ophthalmic; Antiseptic, Topical; Antiseptic, Vaginal; Topical Skin Product

Use External antiseptic with broad microbicidal spectrum for the prevention or treatment of topical infections associated with surgery, burns, minor cuts/scrapes; relief of minor vaginal irritation

Local Anesthetic/Vasoconstrictor Precautions No information available to require special precautions

Effects on Dental Treatment No significant effects or complications reported

Common Adverse Effects Frequency not defined. Also refer to Iodine on page 852.
Local: Edema, irritation, pruritus, rash

Mechanism of Action Povidone-iodine is known to be a powerful broad spectrum germicidal agent effective against a wide range of bacteria, viruses, fungi, protozoa, and spores.

Pharmacodynamics/Kinetics Absorption: Topical: Absorbed systemically as iodine; amount depends upon concentration, route of administration, characteristics of skin

Pregnancy Risk Factor C (ophthalmic)

PPD see Tuberculin Tests on page 1548
PPI-149 see Abarelix on page 24
PPL see Benzylpenicilloyl-polylysine on page 198
PPS see Pentosan Polysulfate Sodium on page 1211

Pramipexole (pra mi PEKS ole)

U.S. Brand Names Mirapex®

Canadian Brand Names Mirapex®

Generic Available No

Pharmacologic Category Anti-Parkinson's Agent, Dopamine Agonist

Use Treatment of the signs and symptoms of idiopathic Parkinson's disease

Unlabeled/Investigational Use Treatment of depression

Local Anesthetic/Vasoconstrictor Precautions No information available to require special precautions

Effects on Dental Treatment No significant effects or complications reported

Common Adverse Effects
>10%:
Cardiovascular: Postural hypotension
Central nervous system: Asthenia, dizziness, somnolence, insomnia, hallucinations, abnormal dreams
Gastrointestinal: Nausea, constipation
Neuromuscular & skeletal: Weakness, dyskinesia, EPS
1% to 10%:
Cardiovascular: Edema, syncope, tachycardia, chest pain
Central nervous system: Malaise, confusion, amnesia, dystonias, akathisia, thinking abnormalities, myoclonus, hyperesthesia, paranoia, fever
Endocrine & metabolic: Decreased libido
Gastrointestinal: Anorexia, weight loss, xerostomia, dysphagia

Genitourinary: Urinary frequency, impotence, urinary incontinence

Neuromuscular & skeletal: Muscle twitching, leg cramps, arthritis, bursitis, myasthenia, gait abnormalities, hypertonia

Ocular: Vision abnormalities

Respiratory: Dyspnea, rhinitis

Mechanism of Action Pramipexole is a nonergot dopamine agonist with specificity for the D_2 subfamily dopamine receptor, and has also been shown to bind to D_3 and D_4 receptors. By binding to these receptors, it is thought that pramipexole can stimulate dopamine activity on the nerves of the striatum and substantia nigra.

Drug Interactions

Increased Effect/Toxicity: Cimetidine in combination with pramipexole produced a 50% increase in AUC and a 40% increase in half-life. Drugs secreted by the cationic transport system (diltiazem, triamterene, verapamil, quinidine, quinine, ranitidine) decrease the clearance of pramipexole by ~20%.

Decreased Effect: Dopamine antagonists (antipsychotics, metoclopramide) may decrease the efficiency of pramipexole.

Pharmacodynamics/Kinetics

Protein binding: 15%

Bioavailability: 90%

Half-life elimination: ~8 hours; Elderly: 12-14 hours

Time to peak, serum: ~2 hours

Excretion: Urine (90% as unchanged drug)

Pregnancy Risk Factor C

Pramlintide (PRAM lin tide)

U.S. Brand Names Symlin®

Generic Available No

Synonyms Pramlintide Acetate

Pharmacologic Category Amylinomimetic; Antidiabetic Agent

Use

Adjunctive treatment with mealtime insulin in type 1 diabetes mellitus (insulin dependent, IDDM) patients who have failed to achieve desired glucose control despite optimal insulin therapy

Adjunctive treatment with mealtime insulin in type 2 diabetes mellitus (noninsulin dependent, NIDDM) patients who have failed to achieve desired glucose control despite optimal insulin therapy, with or without concurrent sulfonylurea and/or metformin

Local Anesthetic/Vasoconstrictor Precautions No information available to require special precautions

Effects on Dental Treatment No significant effects or complications reported

Common Adverse Effects

>10%:

Central nervous system: Headache (5% to 13%)

Gastrointestinal: Nausea (28% to 48%), vomiting (7% to 11%), anorexia (<1% to 17%)

Endocrine & metabolic: Severe hypoglycemia (type 1 diabetes: <1% to 17%)

Miscellaneous: Inflicted injury (8% to 14%)

1% to 10%:

Central nervous system: Fatigue (3% to 7%), dizziness (2% to 6%)

Endocrine & metabolic: Severe hypoglycemia (type 2 diabetes: <1% to 8%)

Gastrointestinal: Abdominal pain (2% to 8%)

Respiratory: Pharyngitis (3% to 5%), cough (2% to 6%)

Neuromuscular & skeletal: Arthralgia (2% to 7%)

Miscellaneous: Allergic reaction (<1% to 6%)

Restrictions An FDA-approved medication guide is available at http://www.fda.gov/cder/Offices/ODS/labeling.htm; distribute to each patient to whom this medication is dispensed.

Mechanism of Action Synthetic analog of human amylin cosecreted with insulin by pancreatic beta cells; reduces postprandial glucose increases via the following mechanisms: 1) prolongation of gastric emptying time, 2) reduction of postprandial glucagon secretion, and 3) reduction of caloric intake through centrally-mediated appetite suppression

Drug Interactions

Increased Effect/Toxicity: Medications which may induce or exacerbate hypoglycemia include ACE inhibitors, alcohol, alpha-blockers, anabolic steroids, beta-blockers, clofibrate, clonidine, disopyramide, fenfluramine, fibrates, fluoxetine, guanethidine, MAO inhibitors, pentamidine, pentoxifylline, (Continued)

Pramlintide (Continued)

phenylbutazone, propoxyphene, reserpine, salicylates, sulfinpyrazone, sulfon-amides, and tetracyclines. Nonselective beta-blockers may delay recovery from hypoglycemic episodes and mask signs/symptoms of hypoglycemia. Anticholinergic agents may cause synergistic impairment of gastric motility.

Decreased Effect: Pramlintide may delay absorption of concomitantly admin-istered medication due to increased gastric emptying time; coadministration with agents in which a rapid onset of action is desired (eg, analgesics) may delay drug response.

Pharmacodynamics/Kinetics
Duration: 3 hours
Protein binding: 60%
Metabolism: Primarily renal to des-lys[1] pramlintide (active metabolite)
Bioavailability: 30% to 40%
Half-life elimination: 48 minutes
Time to peak, plasma: 20 minutes
Excretion: Primarily urine

Pregnancy Risk Factor C

Pramlintide Acetate *see* Pramlintide *on page 1263*

Pramosone® *see* Pramoxine and Hydrocortisone *on page 1264*

Pramoxine (pra MOKS een)

U.S. Brand Names Anusol® Ointment [OTC]; Caladryl® Clear [OTC]; CalaMycin® Cool and Clear [OTC]; Callergy Clear [OTC]; Curasore® [OTC]; Itch-X® [OTC]; Prax® [OTC]; ProctoFoam® NS [OTC]; Sarna® Sensitive; Trono-lane® Cream [OTC]; Tucks® Hemorrhoidal [OTC]

Generic Available Yes: Lotion

Synonyms Pramoxine Hydrochloride

Pharmacologic Category Local Anesthetic

Use Temporary relief of pain and itching associated with anogenital pruritus or irritation; dermatosis, minor burns, or hemorrhoids

Local Anesthetic/Vasoconstrictor Precautions No information available to require special precautions

Effects on Dental Treatment No significant effects or complications reported

Common Adverse Effects 1% to 10%:
Dermatologic: Angioedema
Local: Contact dermatitis, burning, stinging

Mechanism of Action Pramoxine, like other anesthetics, decreases the neuronal membrane's permeability to sodium ions; both initiation and conduc-tion of nerve impulses are blocked, thus depolarization of the neuron is inhibited

Pharmacodynamics/Kinetics
Onset of action: Therapeutic: 2-5 minutes
Peak effect: 3-5 minutes
Duration: Several days

Pregnancy Risk Factor C

Pramoxine and Hydrocortisone
(pra MOKS een & hye droe KOR ti sone)

Related Information
Hydrocortisone *on page 793*
Pramoxine *on page 1264*

U.S. Brand Names Analpram-HC®; Enzone®; Epifoam®; Pramosone®; ProctoFoam®-HC; Zone-A®; Zone-A Forte®

Canadian Brand Names Pramox® HC; Proctofoam™-HC

Generic Available No

Synonyms Hydrocortisone and Pramoxine

Pharmacologic Category Anesthetic/Corticosteroid

Use Relief of inflammatory and pruritic manifestations of corticoste-roid-responsive dermatoses

Local Anesthetic/Vasoconstrictor Precautions No information available to require special precautions

Effects on Dental Treatment No significant effects or complications reported

Common Adverse Effects See individual agents.

Drug Interactions
Cytochrome P450 Effect: Hydrocortisone: **Substrate** of CYP3A4 (minor); **Induces** CYP3A4 (weak)

Increased Effect/Toxicity: See individual agents.
Decreased Effect: See individual agents.
Pharmacodynamics/Kinetics See individual agents.
Pregnancy Risk Factor C

Pramoxine Hydrochloride *see* Pramoxine *on page 1264*

Pramoxine, Neomycin, Bacitracin, and Polymyxin B *see* Bacitracin, Neomycin, Polymyxin B, and Pramoxine *on page 177*

Prandin® *see* Repaglinide *on page 1339*

Pravachol® *see* Pravastatin *on page 1265*

Pravastatin (PRA va stat in)

Related Information
Cardiovascular Diseases *on page 1636*
U.S. Brand Names Pravachol®
Canadian Brand Names Apo-Pravastatin®; CO Pravastatin; Novo-Pravastatin; PMS-Pravastatin; Pravachol®; ratio-Pravastatin; Sandoz-Pravastatin
Mexican Brand Names Pravacol®
Generic Available No
Synonyms Pravastatin Sodium
Pharmacologic Category Antilipemic Agent, HMG-CoA Reductase Inhibitor
Use Use with dietary therapy for the following:

Primary prevention of coronary events: In hypercholesterolemic patients without established coronary heart disease to reduce cardiovascular morbidity (myocardial infarction, coronary revascularization procedures) and mortality.

Secondary prevention of cardiovascular events in patients with established coronary heart disease: To slow the progression of coronary atherosclerosis; to reduce cardiovascular morbidity (myocardial infarction, coronary vascular procedures) and to reduce mortality; to reduce the risk of stroke and transient ischemic attacks

Hyperlipidemias: Reduce elevations in total cholesterol, LDL-C, apolipoprotein B, and triglycerides (elevations of 1 or more components are present in Fredrickson type IIa, IIb, III, and IV hyperlipidemias)

Heterozygous familial hypercholesterolemia (HeFH): In pediatric patients, 8-18 years of age, with HeFH having LDL-C ≥190 mg/dL **or** LDL ≥160 mg/dL with positive family history of premature cardiovascular disease (CVD) or 2 or more CVD risk factors in the pediatric patient

Local Anesthetic/Vasoconstrictor Precautions No information available to require special precautions

Effects on Dental Treatment No significant effects or complications reported

Common Adverse Effects As reported in short-term trials; safety and tolerability with long-term use were similar to placebo
1% to 10%:

Cardiovascular: Chest pain (4%)

Central nervous system: Headache (2% to 6%), fatigue (4%), dizziness (1% to 3%)

Dermatologic: Rash (4%)

Gastrointestinal: Nausea/vomiting (7%), diarrhea (6%), heartburn (3%)

Hepatic: Transaminases increased (>3x normal on two occasions - 1%)

Neuromuscular & skeletal: Myalgia (2%)

Respiratory: Cough (3%)

Miscellaneous: Influenza (2%)

Additional class-related events or case reports (not necessarily reported with pravastatin therapy): Angioedema, cataracts, depression, dyspnea, eosinophilia, erectile dysfunction, facial paresis, hypersensitivity reaction, impaired extraocular muscle movement, impotence, leukopenia, malaise, memory loss, ophthalmoplegia, paresthesia, peripheral neuropathy, photosensitivity, psychic disturbance, skin discoloration, thrombocytopenia, thyroid dysfunction, toxic epidermal necrolysis, transaminases increased, vomiting

Dosage Oral: **Note:** Doses should be individualized according to the baseline LDL-cholesterol levels, the recommended goal of therapy, and patient response; adjustments should be made at intervals of 4 weeks or more; doses may need adjusted based on concomitant medications
Children: HeFH:

8-13 years: 20 mg/day

14-18 years: 40 mg/day

Dosage adjustment for pravastatin based on concomitant immunosuppressants (ie, cyclosporine): Refer to Adults dosing section

Adults: Hyperlipidemias, primary prevention of coronary events, secondary prevention of cardiovascular events: Initial: 40 mg once daily; titrate dosage to response; usual range: 10-80 mg; (maximum dose: 80 mg once daily)
(Continued)

Pravastatin *(Continued)*

Dosage adjustment for pravastatin based on concomitant immunosuppressants (ie, cyclosporine): Initial: 10 mg/day, titrate with caution (maximum dose: 20 mg/day)

Elderly: No specific dosage recommendations. Clearance is reduced in the elderly, resulting in an increase in AUC between 25% to 50%. However, substantial accumulation is not expected.

Dosing adjustment in renal impairment: Initial: 10 mg/day

Dosing adjustment in hepatic impairment: Initial: 10 mg/day

Mechanism of Action Pravastatin is a competitive inhibitor of 3-hydroxy-3-methylglutaryl coenzyme A (HMG-CoA) reductase, which is the rate-limiting enzyme involved in *de novo* cholesterol synthesis.

Contraindications Hypersensitivity to pravastatin or any component of the formulation; active liver disease; unexplained persistent elevations of serum transaminases; pregnancy; breast-feeding

Warnings/Precautions Secondary causes of hyperlipidemia should be ruled out prior to therapy. Liver function must be monitored by periodic laboratory assessment. Rhabdomyolysis with acute renal failure has occurred. Risk may be increased with concurrent use of other drugs which may cause rhabdomyolysis (including gemfibrozil, fibric acid derivatives, or niacin at doses ≥1 g/day). Temporarily discontinue in any patient experiencing an acute or serious condition predisposing to renal failure secondary to rhabdomyolysis. Use caution in patients with previous liver disease or heavy ethanol use. Treatment in patients <8 years of age is not recommended.

Drug Interactions

Cytochrome P450 Effect: Substrate of CYP3A4 (minor); **Inhibits** CYP2C9 (weak), 2D6 (weak), 3A4 (weak)

Increased Effect/Toxicity: Clofibrate, cyclosporine, fenofibrate, gemfibrozil, and niacin may increase the risk of myopathy and rhabdomyolysis. Imidazole antifungals (itraconazole, ketoconazole), P-glycoprotein inhibitors may increase pravastatin concentrations.

Decreased Effect: Concurrent administration of cholestyramine or colestipol can decrease pravastatin absorption.

Ethanol/Nutrition/Herb Interactions

Ethanol: Consumption of large amounts of ethanol may increase the risk of liver damage with HMG-CoA reductase inhibitors.

Food: Red yeast rice contains an estimated 2.4 mg lovastatin per 600 mg rice.

Herb/Nutraceutical: St John's wort may decrease pravastatin levels.

Dietary Considerations May be taken without regard to meals. Before initiation of therapy, patients should be placed on a standard cholesterol-lowering diet for 6 weeks and the diet should be continued during drug therapy. Red yeast rice contains an estimated 2.4 mg lovastatin per 600 mg rice.

Pharmacodynamics/Kinetics

Onset of action: Several days

Peak effect: 4 weeks

Absorption: Rapidly absorbed; average absorption 34%

Protein binding: 50%

Metabolism: Hepatic to at least two metabolites

Bioavailability: 17%

Half-life elimination: ~2-3 hours

Time to peak, serum: 1-1.5 hours

Excretion: Feces (70%); urine (≤20%, 8% as unchanged drug)

Pregnancy Risk Factor X

Dosage Forms TAB: 10 mg, 20 mg, 40 mg, 80 mg

Pravastatin and Aspirin *see* Aspirin and Pravastatin *on page 151*

Pravastatin Sodium *see* Pravastatin *on page 1265*

Pravigard™ PAC [DSC] *see* Aspirin and Pravastatin *on page 151*

Prax® [OTC] *see* Pramoxine *on page 1264*

Praziquantel *(pray zi KWON tel)*

U.S. Brand Names Biltricide®

Canadian Brand Names Biltricide®

Mexican Brand Names Cesol®; Cisticid®

Generic Available No

Pharmacologic Category Anthelmintic

Use All stages of schistosomiasis caused by all *Schistosoma* species pathogenic to humans; clonorchiasis and opisthorchiasis

Unlabeled/Investigational Use Cysticercosis and many intestinal tapeworms

Local Anesthetic/Vasoconstrictor Precautions No information available to require special precautions

Effects on Dental Treatment No significant effects or complications reported

Common Adverse Effects 1% to 10%:

Central nervous system: Dizziness, drowsiness, headache, malaise, CSF reaction syndrome in patients being treated for neurocysticercosis

Gastrointestinal: Abdominal pain, loss of appetite, nausea, vomiting

Miscellaneous: Diaphoresis

Mechanism of Action Increases the cell permeability to calcium in schistosomes, causing strong contractions and paralysis of worm musculature leading to detachment of suckers from the blood vessel walls and to dislodgment

Drug Interactions

Cytochrome P450 Effect: Inhibits CYP2D6 (weak)

Pharmacodynamics/Kinetics

Absorption: Oral: ~80%

Distribution: CSF concentration is 14% to 20% of plasma concentration; enters breast milk

Protein binding: ~80%

Metabolism: Extensive first-pass effect

Half-life elimination: Parent drug: 0.8-1.5 hours; Metabolites: 4.5 hours

Time to peak, serum: 1-3 hours

Excretion: Urine (99% as metabolites)

Pregnancy Risk Factor B

Prazosin (PRA zoe sin)

Related Information

Cardiovascular Diseases *on page 1636*

U.S. Brand Names Minipress®

Canadian Brand Names Apo-Prazo®; Minipress™; Novo-Prazin; Nu-Prazo

Mexican Brand Names Minipres®; Sinozzard®

Generic Available Yes

Synonyms Furazosin; Prazosin Hydrochloride

Pharmacologic Category Alpha₁ Blocker

Use Treatment of hypertension

Unlabeled/Investigational Use Benign prostatic hyperplasia; Raynaud's syndrome

Local Anesthetic/Vasoconstrictor Precautions No information available to require special precautions

Effects on Dental Treatment Key adverse event(s) related to dental treatment: Significant xerostomia (normal salivary flow resumes upon discontinuation). Significant orthostatic hypotension is a possibility; monitor patient when getting out of dental chair.

Common Adverse Effects

>10%: Central nervous system: Dizziness (10%)

1% to 10%:

Cardiovascular: Palpitations (5%), edema, orthostatic hypotension, syncope (1%)

Central nervous system: Headache (8%), drowsiness (8%), weakness (7%), vertigo, depression, nervousness

Dermatologic: Rash (1% to 4%)

Endocrine & metabolic: Decreased energy (7%)

Gastrointestinal: Nausea (5%), vomiting, diarrhea, constipation

Genitourinary: Urinary frequency (1% to 5%)

Ocular: Blurred vision, reddened sclera, xerostomia

Respiratory: Dyspnea, epistaxis, nasal congestion

Mechanism of Action Competitively inhibits postsynaptic alpha-adrenergic receptors which results in vasodilation of veins and arterioles and a decrease in total peripheral resistance and blood pressure

Drug Interactions

Increased Effect/Toxicity: Prazosin's hypotensive effect may be increased with beta-blockers, diuretics, ACE inhibitors, calcium channel blockers, other antihypertensive medications, sildenafil (use with extreme caution at a dose ≤25 mg), tadalafil (use is contraindicated by the manufacturer), and vardenafil (use is contraindicated by the manufacturer). Concurrent use with tricyclic antidepressants (TCAs) and low-potency antipsychotics may increase risk of orthostasis.

Decreased Effect: Decreased antihypertensive effect if taken with NSAIDs.

Pharmacodynamics/Kinetics

Onset of action: BP reduction: ~2 hours

Maximum decrease: 2-4 hours

(Continued)

Prazosin *(Continued)*

Duration: 10-24 hours
Distribution: Hypertensive adults: V_d: 0.5 L/kg
Protein binding: 92% to 97%
Metabolism: Extensively hepatic
Bioavailability: 43% to 82%
Half-life elimination: 2-4 hours; prolonged with congestive heart failure
Excretion: Urine (6% to 10% as unchanged drug)
Pregnancy Risk Factor C

Prazosin and Polythiazide *(PRA zoe sin & pol i THYE a zide)*

Related Information
Polythiazide on page 1255
Prazosin on page 1267
U.S. Brand Names Minizide®
Generic Available No
Synonyms Polythiazide and Prazosin
Pharmacologic Category Antihypertensive Agent, Combination
Use Management of mild to moderate hypertension
Local Anesthetic/Vasoconstrictor Precautions No information available to require special precautions
Effects on Dental Treatment Key adverse event(s) related to dental treatment: Significant xerostomia (normal salivary flow resumes upon discontinuation). Significant orthostatic hypotension is a possibility; monitor patient when getting out of dental chair.
Common Adverse Effects See individual agents.
Pharmacodynamics/Kinetics See individual agents.
Pregnancy Risk Factor C

Prazosin Hydrochloride see Prazosin on page 1267
Precedex™ see Dexmedetomidine on page 444
Precose® see Acarbose on page 28
Pred Forte® see PrednisoLONE on page 1268
Pred-G® see Prednisolone and Gentamicin on page 1271
Pred Mild® see PrednisoLONE on page 1268

Prednicarbate *(PRED ni kar bate)*

U.S. Brand Names Dermatop®
Canadian Brand Names Dermatop®
Generic Available No
Pharmacologic Category Corticosteroid, Topical
Use Relief of the inflammatory and pruritic manifestations of corticosteroid-responsive dermatoses (medium potency topical corticosteroid)
Local Anesthetic/Vasoconstrictor Precautions No information available to require special precautions
Effects on Dental Treatment No significant effects or complications reported
Mechanism of Action Topical corticosteroids have anti-inflammatory, antipruritic, vasoconstrictive, and antiproliferative actions
Pregnancy Risk Factor C

PrednisoLONE *(pred NISS oh lone)*

Related Information
PredniSONE on page 1271
Respiratory Diseases on page 1656
U.S. Brand Names AK-Pred®; Bubbli-Pred™ [DSC]; Econopred® Plus; Orapred®; Pediapred®; Pred Forte®; Pred Mild®; Prelone®
Canadian Brand Names Diopred®; Hydeltra T.B.A.®; Inflamase® Mild; Novo-Prednisolone; Ophtho-Tate®; Pediapred®; Pred Forte®; Pred Mild®; Sab-Prenase
Generic Available Yes
Synonyms Deltahydrocortisone; Metacortandralone; Prednisolone Acetate; Prednisolone Acetate, Ophthalmic; Prednisolone Sodium Phosphate; Prednisolone Sodium Phosphate, Ophthalmic
Pharmacologic Category Corticosteroid, Ophthalmic; Corticosteroid, Systemic

Dental Use Treatment of a variety of oral diseases of allergic, inflammatory, or autoimmune origin

Use Treatment of palpebral and bulbar conjunctivitis; corneal injury from chemical, radiation, thermal burns, or foreign body penetration; endocrine disorders, rheumatic disorders, collagen diseases, dermatologic diseases, allergic states, ophthalmic diseases, respiratory diseases, hematologic disorders, neoplastic diseases, edematous states, and gastrointestinal diseases; resolution of acute exacerbations of multiple sclerosis

Local Anesthetic/Vasoconstrictor Precautions No information available to require special precautions

Effects on Dental Treatment No significant effects or complications reported

Significant Adverse Effects Frequency not defined.

Ophthalmic formulation:

Endocrine & metabolic: Hypercorticoidism (rare)

Ocular: Conjunctival hyperemia, conjunctivitis, corneal ulcers, delayed wound healing, glaucoma, intraocular pressure increased, keratitis, loss of accommodation, optic nerve damage, mydriasis, posterior subcapsular cataract formation, ptosis, secondary ocular infection

Oral formulation:

Cardiovascular: CHF, edema, hypertension

Central nervous system: Convulsions, headache, insomnia, malaise, nervousness, psychic disorders, vertigo

Dermatologic: Bruising, diaphoresis increased, facial erythema, hirsutism, petechiae, skin test reaction suppression, thin fragile skin, urticaria

Endocrine & metabolic: Carbohydrate tolerance decreased, Cushing's syndrome, diabetes mellitus, growth suppression, hyperglycemia, hypokalemic alkalosis, menstrual irregularities, negative nitrogen balance, pituitary adrenal axis suppression, potassium loss

Gastrointestinal: Abdominal distention, increased appetite, indigestion, nausea, peptic ulcer, ulcerative esophagitis, weight gain

Hepatic: LFTs increased (usually reversible)

Neuromuscular & skeletal: Arthralgia, fractures, intracranial pressure with papilledema (usually after discontinuation), muscle mass decreased, muscle weakness, osteoporosis, steroid myopathy, tendon rupture, weakness

Ocular: Cataracts, exophthalmus, glaucoma, intraocular pressure increased

Respiratory: Epistaxis

Miscellaneous: Impaired wound healing

Dental Usual Dosing Anti-inflammatory or immunosuppressive dose: Oral:

Children: 0.1-2 mg/kg/day in divided doses 1-4 times/day

Adults: Usual range: 5-60 mg/day

Dosage Dose depends upon condition being treated and response of patient; dosage for infants and children should be based on severity of the disease and response of the patient rather than on strict adherence to dosage indicated by age, weight, or body surface area. Consider alternate day therapy for long-term therapy. Discontinuation of long-term therapy requires gradual withdrawal by tapering the dose. Patients undergoing unusual stress while receiving corticosteroids, should receive increased doses prior to, during, and after the stressful situation.

Children: Oral:

Acute asthma: 1-2 mg/kg/day in divided doses 1-2 times/day for 3-5 days

Anti-inflammatory or immunosuppressive dose: 0.1-2 mg/kg/day in divided doses 1-4 times/day

Nephrotic syndrome:

Initial (first 3 episodes): 2 mg/kg/day **or** 60 mg/m^2/day (maximum: 80 mg/day) in divided doses 3-4 times/day until urine is protein free for 3 consecutive days (maximum: 28 days); followed by 1-1.5 mg/kg/dose **or** 40 mg/m^2/dose given every other day for 4 weeks

Maintenance (long-term maintenance dose for frequent relapses): 0.5-1 mg/kg/dose given every other day for 3-6 months

Adults: Oral:

Usual range: 5-60 mg/day

Multiple sclerosis: 200 mg/day for 1 week followed by 80 mg every other day for 1 month

Rheumatoid arthritis: Initial: 5-7.5 mg/day; adjust dose as necessary

Ophthalmic suspension/solution: Conjunctivitis, corneal injury: Children and Adults: Instill 1-2 drops into conjunctival sac every hour during day, every 2 hours at night until favorable response is obtained, then use 1 drop every 4 hours.

Elderly: Use lowest effective dose

Dosing adjustment in hyperthyroidism: Prednisolone dose may need to be increased to achieve adequate therapeutic effects

(Continued)

PrednisoLONE *(Continued)*

Hemodialysis: Slightly dialyzable (5% to 20%); administer dose posthemodialysis

Peritoneal dialysis: Supplemental dose is not necessary

Mechanism of Action Decreases inflammation by suppression of migration of polymorphonuclear leukocytes and reversal of increased capillary permeability; suppresses the immune system by reducing activity and volume of the lymphatic system

Contraindications Hypersensitivity to prednisolone or any component of the formulation; acute superficial herpes simplex keratitis; live or attenuated virus vaccines; systemic fungal infections; varicella

Warnings/Precautions Use with caution in patients with hyperthyroidism, cirrhosis, nonspecific ulcerative colitis, hypertension, osteoporosis, thromboembolic tendencies, CHF, convulsive disorders, myasthenia gravis, thrombophlebitis, peptic ulcer, diabetes, or tuberculosis; acute adrenal insufficiency may occur with abrupt withdrawal after long-term therapy or with stress; young pediatric patients may be more susceptible to adrenal axis suppression from topical therapy.

Prolonged use of corticosteroids may result in glaucoma; damage to the optic nerve (not indicated for treatment of optic neuritis), defects in visual acuity and fields of vision, and posterior subcapsular cataract formation may occur. Prolonged use of corticosteroids may also increase the incidence of secondary infection, mask acute infection (including fungal infections) or prolong or exacerbate viral infections. Exposure to chickenpox should be avoided; corticosteroids should not be used to treat ocular herpes simplex. Use following cataract surgery may delay healing or increase the incidence of bleb formation.

Corticosteroids should not be used for cerebral malaria. Because of the risk of adverse effects, systemic corticosteroids should be used cautiously in the elderly, in the smallest possible dose, and for the shortest possible time.

Drug Interactions Substrate of CYP3A4 (minor); **Inhibits** CYP3A4 (weak)

Aminoglutethimide: May reduce the serum levels/effects of prednisolone; likely via induction of microsomal isoenzymes.

Antacids: May increase the absorption of corticosteroids; separate administration by ≥2 hours.

Anticholinesterases: Concurrent use may lead to severe weakness in patients with myasthenia gravis.

Azole antifungals: May increase the serum levels of corticosteroids; monitor.

Barbiturates: May decrease prednisolone levels; monitor.

Calcium channel blockers (nondihydropyridine): May increase the serum levels of corticosteroids; monitor.

CYP3A4 inducers: May decrease the levels/effects of prednisolone. Example inducers include aminoglutethimide, carbamazepine, nafcillin, nevirapine, phenobarbital, and phenytoin.

Cyclosporine: Corticosteroids may increase the serum levels of cyclosporine. In addition, cyclosporine may increase levels of corticosteroids; monitor.

Estrogens: May increase the serum levels of corticosteroids; monitor.

Fluoroquinolones: Concurrent use may increase the risk of tendon rupture, particularly in elderly patients (overall incidence rare).

Isoniazid: Serum concentrations may be decreased by corticosteroids.

Ketoconazole: May decrease metabolism of certain corticosteroids leading to increased levels (up to 60%) and increased risk of adverse effects; monitor.

Neuromuscular-blocking agents: Concurrent use with corticosteroids may increase the risk of myopathy.

Nonsteroidal anti-inflammatory drugs (NSAIDs), aspirin: Concurrent use with corticosteroids may lead to an increased incidence of gastrointestinal adverse effects; use caution.

Phenytoin: May decrease serum levels/effects of prednisolone; monitor

Potassium depleting agents (eg, diuretics, amphotericin B): Concurrent use increases risk of hypokalemia (especially if digitalized); monitor.

Rifampin: May decrease serum levels/effects of prednisolone; monitor.

Salicylates: Salicylates may increase the gastrointestinal adverse effects of corticosteroids.

Skin tests: Corticosteroids may suppress reactions to skin tests.

Vaccines, toxoids: Corticosteroids may suppress the response to vaccinations. The use of live vaccines is contraindicated in immunosuppressed patients. In patients receiving high doses of systemic corticosteroids for ≥14 days, wait at least 1 month between discontinuing steroid therapy and administering immunization.

Warfarin: Corticosteroids may lead to a reduction in warfarin effect; monitor.

Ethanol/Nutrition/Herb Interactions

Ethanol: Avoid ethanol (may increase gastric mucosal irritation).

Food: Prednisolone interferes with calcium absorption. Limit caffeine.

Herb/Nutraceutical: St John's wort may decrease prednisolone levels. Avoid cat's claw, echinacea (have immunostimulant properties).

Dietary Considerations Should be taken after meals or with food or milk to decrease GI effects; increase dietary intake of pyridoxine, vitamin C, vitamin D, folate, calcium, and phosphorus.

Pharmacodynamics/Kinetics

Duration: 18-36 hours

Protein binding (concentration dependent): 65% to 91%; decreased in elderly

Metabolism: Primarily hepatic, but also metabolized in most tissues, to inactive compounds

Half-life elimination: 3.6 hours; End-stage renal disease: 3-5 hours

Excretion: Primarily urine (as glucuronides, sulfates, and unconjugated metabolites)

Pregnancy Risk Factor C

Lactation Enters breast milk/use caution (AAP rates "compatible")

Dosage Forms [DSC] = Discontinued product

Solution, ophthalmic, as sodium phosphate: 1% (5 mL, 10 mL, 15 mL) [contains benzalkonium chloride]

AK-Pred®: 1% (5 mL, 15 mL) [contains benzalkonium chloride]

Solution, oral, as sodium phosphate: Prednisolone base 5 mg/5 mL (120 mL)

Bubbli-Pred™: Prednisolone base 5 mg/5 mL (120 mL) [bubble gum flavor] [DSC]

Orapred®: 20 mg/5 mL (240 mL) [equivalent to prednisolone base 15 mg/5 mL; dye free; contains alcohol 2%, sodium benzoate; grape flavor]

Pediapred®: 6.7 mg/5 mL (120 mL) [equivalent to prednisolone base 5 mg/5 mL; dye free; raspberry flavor]

Suspension, ophthalmic, as acetate: 1% (5 mL, 10 mL, 15 mL) [contains benzalkonium chloride]

Econopred® Plus: 1% (5 mL, 10 mL) [contains benzalkonium chloride]

Pred Forte®: 1% (1 mL, 5 mL, 10 mL, 15 mL) [contains benzalkonium chloride and sodium bisulfite]

Pred Mild®: 0.12% (5 mL, 10 mL) [contains benzalkonium chloride and sodium bisulfite]

Syrup, as base: 5 mg/5 mL (120 mL); 15 mg/5 mL (240 mL, 480 mL)

Prelone®: 15 mg/5 mL (240 mL, 480 mL) [contains alcohol 5%, benzoic acid; cherry flavor]

Tablet, as base: 5 mg

Prednisolone Acetate see PrednisoLONE on page 1268

Prednisolone Acetate, Ophthalmic see PrednisoLONE on page 1268

Prednisolone and Gentamicin
(pred NIS oh lone & jen ta MYE sin)

Related Information

Gentamicin on page 734
PrednisoLONE on page 1268

U.S. Brand Names Pred-G®

Generic Available No

Synonyms Gentamicin and Prednisolone

Pharmacologic Category Antibiotic/Corticosteroid, Ophthalmic

Use Treatment of steroid responsive inflammatory conditions and superficial ocular infections due to microorganisms susceptible to gentamicin

Local Anesthetic/Vasoconstrictor Precautions No information available to require special precautions

Effects on Dental Treatment No significant effects or complications reported

Pregnancy Risk Factor C

Prednisolone and Sulfacetamide see Sulfacetamide and Prednisolone on page 1424

Prednisolone, Neomycin, and Polymyxin B see Neomycin, Polymyxin B, and Prednisolone on page 1102

Prednisolone Sodium Phosphate see PrednisoLONE on page 1268

Prednisolone Sodium Phosphate, Ophthalmic see PrednisoLONE on page 1268

PredniSONE (PRED ni sone)

Related Information

PrednisoLONE on page 1268
Respiratory Diseases on page 1656
(Continued)

PredniSONE *(Continued)*

Rheumatoid Arthritis, Osteoarthritis, and Osteoporosis *on page 1668*
Ulcerative and Erosive Disorders *on page 1712*

Related Sample Prescriptions

Erosive Lichen Planus and Major Aphthae *on page 1745*

U.S. Brand Names Prednisone Intensol™; Sterapred®; Sterapred® DS

Canadian Brand Names Apo-Prednisone®; Novo-Prednisone; Winpred™

Mexican Brand Names Meticorten®; Prednidib®

Generic Available Yes

Synonyms Deltacortisone; Deltadehydrocortisone

Pharmacologic Category Corticosteroid, Systemic

Dental Use Treatment of a variety of oral diseases of allergic, inflammatory, or autoimmune origin

Use Treatment of a variety of diseases including adrenocortical insufficiency, hypercalcemia, rheumatic, and collagen disorders; dermatologic, ocular, respiratory, gastrointestinal, and neoplastic diseases; organ transplantation and a variety of diseases including those of hematologic, allergic, inflammatory, and autoimmune in origin; not available in injectable form, prednisolone must be used

Unlabeled/Investigational Use Investigational: Prevention of postherpetic neuralgia and relief of acute pain in the early stages

Local Anesthetic/Vasoconstrictor Precautions No information available to require special precautions

Effects on Dental Treatment No significant effects or complications reported

Significant Adverse Effects

>10%:

Central nervous system: Insomnia, nervousness

Gastrointestinal: Increased appetite, indigestion

1% to 10%:

Central nervous system: Dizziness or lightheadedness, headache

Dermatologic: Hirsutism, hypopigmentation

Endocrine & metabolic: Diabetes mellitus, glucose intolerance, hyperglycemia

Neuromuscular & skeletal: Arthralgia

Ocular: Cataracts, glaucoma

Respiratory: Epistaxis

Miscellaneous: Diaphoresis

<1% (Limited to important or life-threatening): Cushing's syndrome, edema, fractures, hallucinations, hypertension, muscle-wasting, osteoporosis, pancreatitis, pituitary-adrenal axis suppression, seizure

Dental Usual Dosing

Anti-inflammatory or immunosuppressive dose: Children: Oral: 0.05-2 mg/kg/day divided 1-4 times/day

Immunosuppression/chemotherapy adjunct: Adults: Oral: Range: 5-60 mg/day in divided doses 1-4 times/day

Dosage Oral: Dose depends upon condition being treated and response of patient; dosage for infants and children should be based on severity of the disease and response of the patient rather than on strict adherence to dosage indicated by age, weight, or body surface area. Consider alternate day therapy for long-term therapy. Discontinuation of long-term therapy requires gradual withdrawal by tapering the dose.

Children:

Anti-inflammatory or immunosuppressive dose: 0.05-2 mg/kg/day divided 1-4 times/day

Acute asthma: 1-2 mg/kg/day in divided doses 1-2 times/day for 3-5 days

Alternatively (for 3- to 5-day "burst"):

<1 year: 10 mg every 12 hours

1-4 years: 20 mg every 12 hours

5-13 years: 30 mg every 12 hours

>13 years: 40 mg every 12 hours

Asthma long-term therapy (alternative dosing by age):

<1 year: 10 mg every other day

1-4 years: 20 mg every other day

5-13 years: 30 mg every other day

>13 years: 40 mg every other day

Nephrotic syndrome:

Initial (first 3 episodes): 2 mg/kg/day **or** 60 mg/m^2/day (maximum: 80 mg/day) in divided doses 3-4 times/day until urine is protein free for 3 consecutive days (maximum: 28 days); followed by 1-1.5 mg/kg/dose **or** 40 mg/m^2/dose given every other day for 4 weeks

Maintenance dose (long-term maintenance dose for frequent relapses): 0.5-1 mg/kg/dose given every other day for 3-6 months

Children and Adults: Physiologic replacement: 4-5 mg/m^2/day

Children ≥5 years and Adults: Asthma:

    Moderate persistent: Inhaled corticosteroid (medium dose) or inhaled corticosteroid (low-medium dose) with a long-acting bronchodilator

    Severe persistent: Inhaled corticosteroid (high dose) and corticosteroid tablets or syrup long term: 2 mg/kg/day, generally not to exceed 60 mg/day

Adults:

    Immunosuppression/chemotherapy adjunct: Range: 5-60 mg/day in divided doses 1-4 times/day

    Allergic reaction (contact dermatitis):

        Day 1: 30 mg divided as 10 mg before breakfast, 5 mg at lunch, 5 mg at dinner, 10 mg at bedtime

        Day 2: 5 mg at breakfast, 5 mg at lunch, 5 mg at dinner, 10 mg at bedtime

        Day 3: 5 mg 4 times/day (with meals and at bedtime)

        Day 4: 5 mg 3 times/day (breakfast, lunch, bedtime)

        Day 5: 5 mg 2 times/day (breakfast, bedtime)

        Day 6: 5 mg before breakfast

    Pneumocystis carinii pneumonia (PCP):

        40 mg twice daily for 5 days **followed by**

        40 mg once daily for 5 days **followed by**

        20 mg once daily for 11 days or until antimicrobial regimen is completed

    Thyrotoxicosis: Oral: 60 mg/day

    Chemotherapy (refer to individual protocols): Oral: Range: 20 mg/day to 100 mg/m^2/day

    Rheumatoid arthritis: Oral: Use lowest possible daily dose (often ≤7.5 mg/day)

    Idiopathic thrombocytopenia purpura (ITP): Oral: 60 mg daily for 4-6 weeks, gradually tapered over several weeks

    Systemic lupus erythematosus (SLE): Oral:

        Acute: 1-2 mg/kg/day in 2-3 divided doses

        Maintenance: Reduce to lowest possible dose, usually <1 mg/kg/day as single dose (morning)

Elderly: Use the lowest effective dose

Dosing adjustment in hepatic impairment: Prednisone is inactive and must be metabolized by the liver to prednisolone. This conversion may be impaired in patients with liver disease, however, prednisolone levels are observed to be higher in patients with severe liver failure than in normal patients. Therefore, compensation for the inadequate conversion of prednisone to prednisolone occurs.

Dosing adjustment in hyperthyroidism: Prednisone dose may need to be increased to achieve adequate therapeutic effects

Hemodialysis: Supplemental dose is not necessary

Peritoneal dialysis: Supplemental dose is not necessary

Mechanism of Action Decreases inflammation by suppression of migration of polymorphonuclear leukocytes and reversal of increased capillary permeability; suppresses the immune system by reducing activity and volume of the lymphatic system; suppresses adrenal function at high doses. Antitumor effects may be related to inhibition of glucose transport, phosphorylation, or induction of cell death in immature lymphocytes. Antiemetic effects are thought to occur due to blockade of cerebral innervation of the emetic center via inhibition of prostaglandin synthesis.

Contraindications Hypersensitivity to prednisone or any component of the formulation; serious infections, except tuberculous meningitis; systemic fungal infections; varicella

Warnings/Precautions Withdraw therapy with gradual tapering of dose, may retard bone growth. Use with caution in patients with hypothyroidism, cirrhosis, CHF, ulcerative colitis, thromboembolic disorders, and patients at increased risk for peptic ulcer disease. Corticosteroids should be used with caution in patients with diabetes, hypertension, osteoporosis, glaucoma, cataracts, or tuberculosis. Use caution in hepatic impairment. Because of the risk of adverse effects, systemic corticosteroids should be used cautiously in the elderly, in the smallest possible dose, and for the shortest possible time.

Drug Interactions Substrate of CYP3A4 (minor); **Induces** CYP2C19 (weak), 3A4 (weak)

Decreased effect:

    Barbiturates, phenytoin, rifampin decrease corticosteroid effectiveness

    Decreases salicylates

    Decreases vaccines

    Decreases toxoids effectiveness

Increased effect/toxicity: NSAIDs: Concurrent use of prednisone may increase the risk of GI ulceration

Ethanol/Nutrition/Herb Interactions

Ethanol: Avoid ethanol (may increase gastric mucosal irritation)

Food: Prednisone interferes with calcium absorption, Limit caffeine.

(Continued)

PredniSONE *(Continued)*

Herb/Nutraceutical: St John's wort may decrease prednisone levels. Avoid cat's claw, echinacea (have immunostimulant properties).

Dietary Considerations Should be taken after meals or with food or milk; increase dietary intake of pyridoxine, vitamin C, vitamin D, folate, calcium, and phosphorus.

Pharmacodynamics/Kinetics

Protein binding (concentration dependent): 65% to 91%

Metabolism: Hepatically converted from prednisone (inactive) to prednisolone (active); may be impaired with hepatic dysfunction

Half-life elimination: Normal renal function: 2.5-3.5 hours

See Prednisolone monograph for complete information.

Pregnancy Risk Factor B

Lactation Enters breast milk/compatible

Breast-Feeding Considerations Crosses into breast milk. No data on clinical effects on the infant. AAP considers **compatible** with breast-feeding.

Dosage Forms

Solution, oral: 1 mg/mL (5 mL, 120 mL, 500 mL) [contains alcohol 5%, sodium benzoate; vanilla flavor]

Solution, oral concentrate (Prednisone Intensol™): 5 mg/mL (30 mL) [contains alcohol 30%]

Tablet: 1 mg, 2.5 mg, 5 mg, 10 mg, 20 mg, 50 mg

Sterapred®: 5 mg [supplied as 21 tablet 6-day unit-dose package or 48 tablet 12-day unit-dose package]

Sterapred® DS: 10 mg [supplied as 21 tablet 6-day unit-dose package or 48 tablet 12-day unit-dose package]

Prednisone Intensol™ see PredniSONE on page 1271

Prefest™ see Estradiol and Norgestimate on page 576

Pregabalin *(pre GAB a lin)*

U.S. Brand Names Lyrica®

Canadian Brand Names Lyrica®

Generic Available No

Synonyms CI-1008; S-(+)-3-isobutylgaba

Pharmacologic Category Analgesic, Miscellaneous; Anticonvulsant, Miscellaneous

Use Management of pain associated with diabetic peripheral neuropathy; management of postherpetic neuralgia; adjunctive therapy for partial-onset seizure disorder in adults

Local Anesthetic/Vasoconstrictor Precautions No information available to require special precautions

Effects on Dental Treatment Key adverse event(s) related to dental treatment: Xerostomia and changes in salivation (normal salivary flow resumes upon discontinuation).

Common Adverse Effects Note: Frequency of adverse effects may be influenced by dose or concurrent therapy. In add-on trials in epilepsy, frequency of CNS and visual adverse effects were higher than those reported in pain management trials. Range noted below is inclusive of all trials.

>10%:

Cardiovascular: Peripheral edema (up to 16%)

Central nervous system: Dizziness (8% to 38%), somnolence (4% to 28%), ataxia (1% to 20%)

Gastrointestinal: Weight gain (up to 16%), xerostomia (1% to 15%)

Neuromuscular & skeletal: Tremor (1% to 11%)

Ocular: Blurred vision (1% to 12%), diplopia (up to 12%)

Miscellaneous: Infection (up to 14%), accidental injury (2% to 11%)

1% to 10%:

Cardiovascular: Chest pain (up to 4%), edema (up to 6%)

Central nervous system: Neuropathy (up to 9%), headache (up to 9%), thinking abnormal (up to 9%), confusion (up to 7%), speech disorder (up to 7%), incoordination (up to 6%), amnesia (up to 6%), pain (up to 5%), vertigo (up to 4%), nervousness (>2%), euphoria (up to 3%), fever (≥1%), anxiety (≥1%), depersonalization (≥1%), hypertonia (≥1%), hypoesthesia (≥1%), stupor (≥1%)

Dermatologic: Facial edema (up to 3%), ecchymosis (≥1%), pruritus (≥1%)

Endocrine & metabolic: Appetite increased (up to 6%), hypoglycemia (up to 3%), libido decreased (≥1%)

Gastrointestinal: Constipation (up to 7%), flatulence (up to 3%), vomiting (up to 3%), abdominal pain (≥1%), gastroenteritis (≥1%)

Genitourinary: Anorgasmia (≥1%), impotence (≥1%), urinary frequency (≥1%), incontinence (≥1%)

Neuromuscular & skeletal: Abnormal gait (up to 8%), weakness (up to 7%), twitching (up to 5%), myoclonus (up to 4%), back pain (up to 2%), paresthesia (>2%), CPK increased (2%), arthralgia (≥1%), leg cramps (≥1%), myalgia (≥1%), myasthenia (≥1%)

Ocular: Visual abnormalities (up to 5%), visual field defect (≥2%), eye disorder (up to 2%), nystagmus (>2%), conjunctivitis (≥1%)

Otic: Otitis media (≥1%), tinnitus (≥1%)

Respiratory: Dyspnea (up to 3%), bronchitis (up to 3%)

Miscellaneous: Flu-like syndrome (up to 2%), allergic reaction (≥1%)

Restrictions C-V

Dosage Oral: Adults:

Neuropathic pain (diabetes-associated): Initial: 150 mg/day in divided doses (50 mg 3 times/day); may be increased within 1 week based on tolerability and effect; maximum dose: 300 mg/day (dosages up to 600 mg/day were evaluated with no significant additional benefit and an increase in adverse effects)

Postherpetic neuralgia: Initial: 150 mg/day in divided doses (75 mg 2 times/day or 50 mg 3 times/day); may be increased to 300 mg/day within 1 week based on tolerability and effect; further titration (to 600 mg/day) after 2-4 weeks may be considered in patients who do not experience sufficient relief of pain provided they are able to tolerate pregabalin. Maximum dose: 600 mg/day

Partial-onset seizures (adjunctive therapy): Initial: 150 mg per day in divided doses (75 mg 2 times/day or 50 mg 3 times/day); may be increased based on tolerability and effect (optimal titration schedule has not been defined). Maximum dose: 600 mg/day

Discontinuing therapy: Pregabalin should not be abruptly discontinued; taper dosage over at least 1 week

Dosage adjustment in renal impairment: Cl_{cr} ≥60 mL/minute: No dosage adjustment required. In renally-impaired patients, dosage adjustment depends on renal function and daily dosage:

Cl_{cr} 30-60 mL/minute: Total daily dose:
  75 mg in 2-3 divided doses **or**
  150 mg in 2-3 divided doses **or**
  300 mg in 2-3 divided doses

Cl_{cr} 15-30 mL/minute: Total daily dose:
  25-50 mg in once daily or in 2 divided doses **or**
  75 mg once daily or in 2 divided doses **or**
  150 mg once daily or in 2 divided doses

Cl_{cr} <15 mL/minute: Total daily dose:
  25 mg once daily **or**
  25-50 mg once daily **or**
  75 mg once daily

Hemodialysis: Total daily dose:
  25 mg: Single supplementary dose of 25 mg **or** 50 mg
  25-50 mg: Single supplementary dose of 50 mg **or** 75 mg
  75 mg: Single supplementary dose of 100 mg **or** 150 mg

Mechanism of Action Binds to alpha$_2$-delta subunit of voltage-gated calcium channels within the CNS, inhibiting excitatory neurotransmitter release. Although structurally related to GABA, it does not bind to GABA or benzodiazepine receptors. Exerts antinociceptive and anticonvulsant activity. Decreases symptoms of painful peripheral neuropathies and, as adjunctive therapy in partial seizures, decreases the frequency of seizures.

Contraindications Hypersensitivity to pregabalin or any component of the formulation

Warnings/Precautions May cause CNS depression and/or dizziness, which may impair physical or mental abilities. Patients must be cautioned about performing tasks which require mental alertness (eg, operating machinery or driving). Effects with other sedative drugs or ethanol may be potentiated. Visual disturbances (blurred vision, decreased acuity and visual field changes) have been associated with pregabalin therapy; patients should be instructed to notify their physician if these effects are noted.

Pregabalin has been associated with increases in CPK and rare cases of rhabdomyolysis. Patients should be instructed to notify their prescriber if unexplained muscle pain, tenderness, or weakness, particularly if fever and/or malaise are associated with these symptoms. Use may be associated with weight gain and peripheral edema; use caution in patients with congestive heart failure, hypertension, or diabetes. Effect on weight gain/edema may be additive to thiazolidinedione antidiabetic agent; particularly in patients with prior cardiovascular disease. May decrease platelet count or prolong PR interval.
(Continued)

Pregabalin *(Continued)*

Has been noted to be tumorigenic (increased incidence of hemangiosarcoma) in animal studies; significance of these findings in humans is unknown. Pregabalin has been associated with discontinuation symptoms following abrupt cessation, and increases in seizure frequency (when used as an antiepileptic) may occur. Should not be discontinued abruptly; dosage tapering over at least 1 week is recommended. Use caution in renal impairment; dosage adjustment required. Safety and efficacy have not been established in pediatric patients.

Drug Interactions

Increased Effect/Toxicity:

Sedative effects may be additive with CNS depressants (includes ethanol, barbiturates, narcotic analgesics, and other sedative agents). Pregabalin's effect on weight gain/edema may be additive with thiazolidinedione antidiabetic agents (includes pioglitazone, rosiglitazone).

Ethanol/Nutrition/Herb Interactions

Ethanol: Avoid ethanol (may increase CNS depression).

Herb/Nutraceutical: Avoid valerian, St John's wort, kava kava, gotu kola (may increase CNS depression).

Dietary Considerations May be taken with or without food.

Pharmacodynamics/Kinetics

Onset: Pain management: Effects may be noted as early as the first week of therapy.

Distribution: V_d: 0.5 L/kg

Protein binding: 0%

Metabolism: Negligible

Bioavailability: >90%

Half-life elimination: 6.3 hours

Time to peak, plasma: 1.5 hours (3 hours with food)

Excretion: Urine (90% as unchanged drug; minor metabolites)

Pregnancy Risk Factor C

Dosage Forms CAP: 25 mg, 50 mg, 75 mg, 100 mg, 150 mg, 200 mg, 225 mg, 300 mg

Selected Readings

Hill CM, Balkenohl M, Thomas DW, et al, "Pregabalin in Patients With Postoperative Dental Pain," *Eur J Pain*, 2001, 5(2):119-24.

Pregnenedione *see* Progesterone *on page 1289*

Pregnyl® *see* Chorionic Gonadotropin (Human) *on page 336*

Prelone® *see* PrednisoLONE *on page 1268*

Prelu-2® [DSC] *see* Phendimetrazine *on page 1220*

Premarin® *see* Estrogens (Conjugated/Equine) *on page 580*

Premjact® [OTC] *see* Lidocaine *on page 920*

Premphase® *see* Estrogens (Conjugated/Equine) and Medroxyprogesterone *on page 583*

Prempro™ *see* Estrogens (Conjugated/Equine) and Medroxyprogesterone *on page 583*

Preparation H® Hydrocortisone [OTC] *see* Hydrocortisone *on page 793*

Prepcat *see* Barium *on page 179*

Pre-Pen® [DSC] *see* Benzylpenicilloyl-polylysine *on page 198*

Prepidil® *see* Dinoprostone *on page 482*

PreserVision® AREDS [OTC] *see* Vitamins (Multiple/Oral) *on page 1582*

PreserVision® Lutein [OTC] *see* Vitamins (Multiple/Oral) *on page 1582*

Pretz® [OTC] *see* Sodium Chloride *on page 1400*

Pretz-D® [OTC] *see* Ephedrine *on page 545*

Prevacid® *see* Lansoprazole *on page 896*

Prevacid® NapraPAC™ *see* Lansoprazole and Naproxen *on page 898*

Prevacid® SoluTab™ *see* Lansoprazole *on page 896*

Prevalite® *see* Cholestyramine Resin *on page 334*

PREVEN® *see* Ethinyl Estradiol and Levonorgestrel *on page 602*

PreviDent® *see* Fluoride *on page 671*

PreviDent® 5000 Plus™ *see* Fluoride *on page 671*

Previfem™ *see* Ethinyl Estradiol and Norgestimate *on page 613*

Prevnar® *see* Pneumococcal Conjugate Vaccine (7-Valent) *on page 1250*

Prevpac® *see* Lansoprazole, Amoxicillin, and Clarithromycin *on page 898*

Prialt® *see* Ziconotide *on page 1594*

Priftin® *see* Rifapentine *on page 1349*

Prilocaine (PRIL oh kane)

Related Information
Oral Pain *on page 1692*

U.S. Brand Names Citanest® Plain

Canadian Brand Names Citanest® Plain

Generic Available No

Pharmacologic Category Local Anesthetic

Dental Use Amide-type anesthetic used for local infiltration anesthesia; injection near nerve trunks to produce nerve block

Local Anesthetic/Vasoconstrictor Precautions No information available to require special precautions

Effects on Dental Treatment It is common to misinterpret psychogenic responses to local anesthetic injection as an allergic reaction. Intraoral injections are perceived by many patients as a stressful procedure in dentistry. Common symptoms to this stress are diaphoresis, palpitations, hyperventilation, generalized pallor and a fainting feeling.

Degree of adverse effects in the CNS and cardiovascular system is directly related to blood levels of prilocaine (frequency not defined; more likely to occur after systemic administration rather than infiltration): Bradycardia and reduction in cardiac output, hypersensitivity reactions (may be manifest as dermatologic reactions and edema at injection site), asthmatic syndromes

High blood levels: Anxiety, restlessness, disorientation, confusion, dizziness, tremors, and seizures, followed by CNS depression, resulting in somnolence, unconsciousness and possible respiratory arrest; nausea and vomiting

In some cases, symptoms of CNS stimulation may be absent and the primary CNS effects are somnolence and unconsciousness.

Significant Adverse Effects

1% to 10%: Cardiovascular: Hypotension

<1% (Limited to important or life-threatening): Anaphylactoid reaction, aseptic meningitis resulting in paralysis, chills, CNS stimulation followed by CNS depression, miosis, nausea, skin discoloration, tinnitus, vomiting

Dental Usual Dosing

Children <10 years: Doses >40 mg (1 mL) as a 4% solution per procedure rarely needed

Children >10 years and Adults: Dental anesthesia, infiltration, or conduction block: Initial: 40-80 mg (1-2 mL) as a 4% solution; up to a maximum of 400 mg (10 mL) as a 4% solution within a 2-hour period. Manufacturer's maximum recommended dose is not more than 600 mg to normal healthy adults. The effective anesthetic dose varies with procedure, intensity of anesthesia needed, duration of anesthesia required and physical condition of the patient. Always use the lowest effective dose along with careful aspiration.

The following numbers of dental carpules (1.8 mL) provide the indicated amounts of prilocaine hydrochloride 4%. See table.

Prilocaine

# of Cartridges (1.8 mL)	mg Prilocaine (4%)
1	72
2	144
3	216
4	288
5	360
6	432
7	504
8	576

Note: Adult and children doses of prilocaine hydrochloride cited from USP Dispensing Information (USP DI), 17th ed, The United States Pharmacopeial Convention, Inc, Rockville, MD, 1997, 139.

Dosage

Children <10 years: Doses >40 mg (1 mL) as a 4% solution per procedure rarely needed

Children >10 years and Adults: Dental anesthesia, infiltration, or conduction block: Initial: 40-80 mg (1-2 mL) as a 4% solution; up to a maximum of 400 mg (10 mL) as a 4% solution within a 2-hour period. Manufacturer's maximum recommended dose is not more than 600 mg to normal healthy adults. The effective anesthetic dose varies with procedure, intensity of anesthesia
(Continued)

Prilocaine *(Continued)*

needed, duration of anesthesia required and physical condition of the patient. Always use the lowest effective dose along with careful aspiration.

Note: Adult and children doses of prilocaine hydrochloride cited from USP Dispensing Information (USP DI), 17th ed, The United States Pharmacopeial Convention, Inc, Rockville, MD, 1997, 139.

Mechanism of Action Local anesthetics bind selectively to the intracellular surface of sodium channels to block influx of sodium into the axon. As a result, depolarization necessary for action potential propagation and subsequent nerve function is prevented. The block at the sodium channel is reversible. When drug diffuses away from the axon, sodium channel function is restored and nerve propagation returns.

Contraindications Hypersensitivity to local anesthetics of the amide type or any component of the formulation

Warnings/Precautions Aspirate the syringe after tissue penetration and before injection to minimize chance of direct vascular injection

Drug Interactions No data reported

Pharmacodynamics/Kinetics

Onset of action: Infiltration: ~2 minutes; Inferior alveolar nerve block: ~3 minutes

Duration: Infiltration: Complete anesthesia for procedures lasting 20 minutes; Inferior alveolar nerve block: ~2.5 hours

Distribution: V_d: 0.7-4.4 L/kg; crosses blood-brain barrier

Protein binding: 55%

Metabolism: Hepatic and renal

Half-life elimination: 10-150 minutes; prolonged with hepatic or renal impairment

Pregnancy Risk Factor B

Breast-Feeding Considerations Usual infiltration doses of prilocaine given to nursing mothers has not been shown to affect the health of the nursing infant.

Dosage Forms Injection, solution: Prilocaine hydrochloride 4% (1.8 mL) [prefilled cartridge]

Selected Readings

Budenz AW, "Local Anesthetics in Dentistry: Then and Now," *J Calif Dent Assoc*, 2003, 31(5):388-96.

Dower JS Jr, "A Review of Paresthesia in Association With Administration of Local Anesthesia," *Dent Today*, 2003, 22(2):64-9.

Finder RL and Moore PA, "Adverse Drug Reactions to Local Anesthesia," *Dent Clin North Am*, 2002, 46(4):747-57, x.

Haas DA, "An Update on Local Anesthetics in Dentistry," *J Can Dent Assoc*, 2002, 68(9):546-51.

Hawkins JM and Moore PA, "Local Anesthesia: Advances in Agents and Techniques," *Dent Clin North Am*, 2002, 46(4):719-32, ix.

"Injectable Local Anesthetics," *J Am Dent Assoc*, 2003, 134(5):628-9.

Jastak JT and Yagiela JA, "Vasoconstrictors and Local Anesthesia: A Review and Rationale for Use," *J Am Dent Assoc*, 1983, 107(4):623-30.

MacKenzie TA and Young ER, "Local Anesthetic Update," *Anesth Prog*, 1993, 40(2):29-34.

Malamed SF, "Allergy and Toxic Reactions to Local Anesthetics," *Dent Today*, 2003, 22(4):114-6, 118-21.

Wahl MJ, Schmitt MM, Overton DA, et al, "Injection Pain of Bupivacaine With Epinephrine vs. Prilocaine Plain," *J Am Dent Assoc*, 2002, 133(12):1652-6.

Wynn RL, "Epinephrine Interactions With Beta-Blockers," *Gen Dent*, 1994, 42(1):16, 18.

Yagiela JA, "Local Anesthetics," *Anesth Prog*, 1991, 38(4-5):128-41.

Prilocaine and Epinephrine *(PRIL oh kane with ep i NEF rin)*

Related Information

Epinephrine *on page 546*
Oral Pain *on page 1692*
Prilocaine *on page 1277*

U.S. Brand Names Citanest® Forte Dental

Canadian Brand Names Citanest® Forte

Generic Available No

Synonyms Epinephrine and Prilocaine (Dental)

Pharmacologic Category Local Anesthetic

Dental Use Amide-type anesthetic used for local infiltration anesthesia; injection near nerve trunks to produce nerve block

Local Anesthetic/Vasoconstrictor Precautions No information available to require special precautions

Effects on Dental Treatment It is common to misinterpret psychogenic responses to local anesthetic injection as an allergic reaction. Intraoral injections are perceived by many patients as a stressful procedure in dentistry. Common symptoms to this stress are diaphoresis, palpitations, hyperventilation, generalized pallor and a fainting feeling. Patients may exhibit hypersensitivity to bisulfites contained in local anesthetic solution to prevent oxidation of epineph-rine. In general, patients reacting to bisulfites have a history of asthma and their airways are hyper-reactive to asthmatic syndrome.

Degree of adverse effects in the CNS and cardiovascular system is directly related to blood levels of prilocaine (frequency not defined; more likely to occur after systemic administration rather than infiltration): Bradycardia and reduction in cardiac output, hypersensitivity reactions (extremely rare; may be manifest as dermatologic reactions and edema at injection site), asthmatic syndromes

High blood levels: Anxiety, restlessness, disorientation, confusion, dizziness, tremors, and seizures, followed by CNS depression, resulting in somnolence, unconsciousness and possible respiratory arrest; nausea and vomiting

In some cases, symptoms of CNS stimulation may be absent and the primary CNS effects are somnolence and unconsciousness.

Significant Adverse Effects Degree of adverse effects in the CNS and cardio-vascular system are directly related to the blood levels of prilocaine. The effects below are more likely to occur after systemic administration rather than infiltra-tion.

Cardiovascular: Myocardial effects include a decrease in contraction force as well as a decrease in electrical excitability and myocardial conduction rate resulting in bradycardia and reduction in cardiac output.

Central nervous system: High blood levels result in anxiety, restlessness, disori-entation, confusion, dizziness, tremor and seizure. This is followed by depres-sion of CNS resulting in somnolence, unconsciousness and possible respiratory arrest. Nausea and vomiting may also occur. In some cases, symptoms of CNS stimulation may be absent and the primary CNS effects are somnolence and unconsciousness.

Hypersensitivity reactions: Extremely rare, but may be manifest as dermatologic reactions and edema at injection site. Asthmatic syndromes have occurred. Patients may exhibit hypersensitivity to bisulfites contained in local anesthetic solution to prevent oxidation of epinephrine. In general, patients reacting to bisulfites have a history of asthma and their airways are hyper-reactive to asthmatic syndrome.

Psychogenic reactions: It is common to misinterpret psychogenic responses to local anesthetic injection as an allergic reaction. Intraoral injections are perceived by many patients as a stressful procedure in dentistry. Common symptoms to this stress are diaphoresis, palpitation, hyperventilation, general-ized pallor, and a fainting feeling.

Dental Usual Dosing

Children <10 years: Doses >40 mg (1 mL) of prilocaine hydrochloride as a 4% solution with epinephrine 1:200,000 are rarely needed

Children >10 years and Adults: Dental anesthesia, infiltration, or conduction block: Initial: 40-80 mg (1-2 mL) of prilocaine hydrochloride as a 4% solution with epinephrine 1:200,000; up to a maximum of 400 mg (10 mL) of prilocaine hydrochloride within a 2-hour period. The effective anesthetic dose varies with procedure, intensity of anesthesia needed, duration of anesthesia required, and physical condition of the patient. Always use the lowest effective dose along with careful aspiration.

The following numbers of dental carpules (1.8 mL) provide the indicated amounts of prilocaine hydrochloride 4% and epinephrine 1:200,000. See table.

Prilocaine With Epinephrine

# of Cartridges (1.8 mL)	mg Prilocaine (4%)	mg Vasoconstrictor (Epinephrine 1:200,000)
1	72	0.009
2	144	0.018
3	216	0.027
4	288	0.036
5	360	0.045
6	432	0.054
7	504	0.063
8	576	0.072

Note: Adult and pediatric doses of prilocaine hydrochloride with epinephrine cited from USP Dispensing Information (USP DI), 17th ed, The United States Pharmacopeial Convention, Inc, Rockville, MD, 1997, 140.

Dosage

Children <10 years: Doses >40 mg (1 mL) of prilocaine hydrochloride as a 4% solution with epinephrine 1:200,000 are rarely needed

(Continued)

Prilocaine and Epinephrine *(Continued)*

Children >10 years and Adults: Dental anesthesia, infiltration, or conduction block: Initial: 40-80 mg (1-2 mL) of prilocaine hydrochloride as a 4% solution with epinephrine 1:200,000; up to a maximum of 400 mg (10 mL) of prilocaine hydrochloride within a 2-hour period. The effective anesthetic dose varies with procedure, intensity of anesthesia needed, duration of anesthesia required, and physical condition of the patient. Always use the lowest effective dose along with careful aspiration.

Note: Adult and pediatric doses of prilocaine hydrochloride with epinephrine cited from USP Dispensing Information (USP DI), 17th ed, The United States Pharmacopeial Convention, Inc, Rockville, MD, 1997, 140.

Mechanism of Action Local anesthetics bind selectively to the intracellular surface of sodium channels to block influx of sodium into the axon. As a result, depolarization necessary for action potential propagation and subsequent nerve function is prevented. The block at the sodium channel is reversible. When drug diffuses away from the axon, sodium channel function is restored and nerve propagation returns.

Epinephrine prolongs the duration of the anesthetic actions of prilocaine by causing vasoconstriction (alpha adrenergic receptor agonist) of the vasculature surrounding the nerve axons. This prevents the diffusion of prilocaine away from the nerves resulting in a longer retention in the axon.

Contraindications Hypersensitivity to local anesthetics of the amide-type or any component of the formulation

Warnings/Precautions Should be avoided in patients with uncontrolled hyperthyroidism. Should be used in minimal amounts in patients with significant cardiovascular problems (because of epinephrine component). Aspirate the syringe after tissue penetration and before injection to minimize chance of direct vascular injection

Drug Interactions

Beta-blockers, nonselective (ie, propranolol): Concurrent use could result in serious hypertension and reflex bradycardia

MAO inhibitors: Administration of local anesthetic solutions containing epinephrine may produce severe, prolonged hypertension

Tricyclic antidepressants: Pressor response to I.V. epinephrine, norepinephrine, and phenylephrine may be enhanced in patients receiving TCAs **(Note:** Effect is unlikely with epinephrine or levonordefrin dosages typically administered as infiltration in combination with local anesthetics)

Pharmacodynamics/Kinetics

Onset of action: Infiltration: <2 minutes; Inferior alveolar nerve block: <3 minutes

Duration: Infiltration: 2.25 hours; Inferior alveolar nerve block: 3 hours

Pregnancy Risk Factor C

Breast-Feeding Considerations Usual infiltration doses of prilocaine with epinephrine given to nursing mothers has not been shown to affect the health of the nursing infant.

Dosage Forms Injection, solution: Prilocaine hydrochloride 4% and epinephrine bitartrate 1:200,000 (1.8 mL)

Selected Readings

Ayoub ST and Coleman AE, "A Review of Local Anesthetics," *Gen Dent*, 1992, 40(4):285-7, 289-90.

Blanton PL and Roda RS, "The Anatomy of Local Anesthesia," *J Calif Dent Assoc*, 1995, 23(4):55-65.

Budenz AW, "Local Anesthetics in Dentistry: Then and Now," *J Calif Dent Assoc*, 2003, 31(5):388-96.

Dower JS Jr, "A Review of Paresthesia in Association With Administration of Local Anesthesia," *Dent Today*, 2003, 22(2):64-9.

Finder RL and Moore PA, "Adverse Drug Reactions to Local Anesthesia," *Dent Clin North Am*, 2002, 46(4):747-57, x.

Haas DA, "An Update on Local Anesthetics in Dentistry," *J Can Dent Assoc*, 2002, 68(9):546-51.

Hawkins JM and Moore PA, "Local Anesthesia: Advances in Agents and Techniques," *Dent Clin North Am*, 2002, 46(4):719-32, ix.

"Injectable Local Anesthetics," *J Am Dent Assoc*, 2003, 134(5):628-9.

Jastak JT and Yagiela JA, "Vasoconstrictors and Local Anesthesia: A Review and Rationale for Use," *J Am Dent Assoc*, 1983, 107(4):623-30.

MacKenzie TA and Young ER, "Local Anesthetic Update," *Anesth Prog*, 1993, 40(2):29-34.

Malamed SF, "Allergy and Toxic Reactions to Local Anesthetics," *Dent Today*, 2003, 22(4):114-6, 118-21.

Wynn RL, "Epinephrine Interactions With Beta-Blockers," *Gen Dent*, 1994, 42(1):16, 18.

Yagiela JA, "Local Anesthetics," *Anesth Prog*, 1991, 38(4-5):128-41.

Yagiela JA, "Vasoconstrictor Agents for Local Anesthesia," *Anesth Prog*, 1995, 42(3-4):116-20.

Prilocaine and Lidocaine *see* Lidocaine and Prilocaine *on page 928*

Prilosec® *see* Omeprazole *on page 1145*

Prilosec OTC™ [OTC] *see* Omeprazole *on page 1145*

Primaclone *see* Primidone *on page 1281*

Primacor® *see* Milrinone *on page 1048*

Primaquine (PRIM a kween)

Generic Available Yes
Synonyms Primaquine Phosphate; Prymaccone
Pharmacologic Category Aminoquinoline (Antimalarial)
Use Treatment of malaria
Unlabeled/Investigational Use Prevention of malaria; treatment *Pneumocystis carinii* pneumonia
Local Anesthetic/Vasoconstrictor Precautions No information available to require special precautions
Effects on Dental Treatment No significant effects or complications reported
Common Adverse Effects Frequency not defined.
  Cardiovascular: Arrhythmias
  Central nervous system: Headache
  Dermatologic: Pruritus
  Gastrointestinal: Abdominal pain, nausea, vomiting
  Hematologic: Agranulocytosis, hemolytic anemia in G6PD deficiency, leukopenia, leukocytosis, methemoglobinemia in NADH-methemoglobin reductase-deficient individuals
  Ocular: Interference with visual accommodation
Mechanism of Action Eliminates the primary tissue exoerythrocytic forms of *P. falciparum*; disrupts mitochondria and binds to DNA
Drug Interactions
  Cytochrome P450 Effect: Substrate of CYP3A4 (major); **Inhibits** CYP1A2 (strong), 2D6 (weak), 3A4 (weak); **Induces** CYP1A2 (weak)
  Increased Effect/Toxicity: Increased toxicity/levels with quinacrine. Primaquine may increase the levels/effects of aminophylline, fluvoxamine, mexiletine, mirtazapine, ropinirole, theophylline, trifluoperazine, and other CYP1A2 substrates.
  Decreased Effect: The levels/effects of primaquine may be decreased by aminoglutethimide, carbamazepine, nafcillin, nevirapine, phenobarbital, phenytoin, rifamycins, and other CYP3A4 inducers.
Pharmacodynamics/Kinetics
  Absorption: Well absorbed
  Metabolism: Hepatic to carboxyprimaquine (active)
  Half-life elimination: 3.7-9.6 hours
  Time to peak, serum: 1-2 hours
  Excretion: Urine (small amounts as unchanged drug)
Pregnancy Risk Factor C

Primaquine Phosphate see Primaquine on page 1281
Primatene® Mist [OTC] see Epinephrine on page 546
Primaxin® see Imipenem and Cilastatin on page 819

Primidone (PRI mi done)

U.S. Brand Names Mysoline®
Canadian Brand Names Apo-Primidone®
Mexican Brand Names Mysoline®
Generic Available Yes
Synonyms Desoxyphenobarbital; Primaclone
Pharmacologic Category Anticonvulsant, Miscellaneous; Barbiturate
Use Management of grand mal, psychomotor, and focal seizures
Unlabeled/Investigational Use Benign familial tremor (essential tremor)
Local Anesthetic/Vasoconstrictor Precautions No information available to require special precautions
Effects on Dental Treatment No significant effects or complications reported
Common Adverse Effects Frequency not defined.
  Central nervous system: Drowsiness, vertigo, ataxia, lethargy, behavior change, fatigue, hyperirritability
  Dermatologic: Rash
  Gastrointestinal: Nausea, vomiting, anorexia
  Genitourinary: Impotence
  Hematologic: Agranulocytopenia, agranulocytosis, anemia
  Ocular: Diplopia, nystagmus
Mechanism of Action Decreases neuron excitability, raises seizure threshold similar to phenobarbital; primidone has two active metabolites, phenobarbital and phenylethylmalonamide (PEMA); PEMA may enhance the activity of phenobarbital
(Continued)

Primidone (Continued)

Drug Interactions

Cytochrome P450 Effect: Metabolized to phenobarbital; **Induces** CYP1A2 (strong), 2B6 (strong), 2C8/9 (strong), 3A4 (strong)

Increased Effect/Toxicity: When combined with other CNS depressants, ethanol, narcotic analgesics, antidepressants, or benzodiazepines, additive respiratory and CNS depression may occur. Barbiturates may enhance the hepatotoxic potential of acetaminophen overdoses. Chloramphenicol, MAO inhibitors, valproic acid, and felbamate may inhibit barbiturate metabolism. Barbiturates may impair the absorption of griseofulvin, and may enhance the nephrotoxic effects of methoxyflurane. Concurrent use of phenobarbital with meperidine may result in increased CNS depression. Concurrent use of phenobarbital with primidone may result in elevated phenobarbital serum concentrations. CYP2C19 inhibitors may increase the levels/effects of primidone; example inhibitors include delavirdine, fluconazole, fluvoxamine, gemfibrozil, isoniazid, omeprazole, and ticlopidine.

Decreased Effect: Barbiturates may increase the metabolism of estrogens and reduce the efficacy of oral contraceptives; an alternative method of contraception should be considered. Barbiturates inhibit the hypoprothrombinemic effects of oral anticoagulants via increased metabolism. Barbiturates may enhance the metabolism of methadone resulting in methadone withdrawal. The levels/effects of primidone may be decreased by aminoglutethimide, carbamazepine, phenytoin, rifampin, and other CYP2C19 inducers.

Primidone may decrease the levels/effects of aminophylline, amiodarone, benzodiazepines, bupropion, calcium channel blockers, carbamazepine, citalopram, clarithromycin, cyclosporine, diazepam, efavirenz, erythromycin, estrogens, fluoxetine, fluvoxamine, glimepiride, glipizide, ifosfamide, losartan, methsuximide, mirtazapine, nateglinide, nefazodone, nevirapine, phenytoin, pioglitazone, promethazine, propranolol, protease inhibitors, proton pump inhibitors, rifampin, ropinirole, rosiglitazone, selegiline, sertraline, sulfonamides, tacrolimus, theophylline, venlafaxine. voriconazole, warfarin, zafirlukast, and other CYP1A2, 2A6, 2B6, 2C8/9, or 3A4 substrates.

Pharmacodynamics/Kinetics

Distribution: Adults: V_d: 2-3 L/kg

Protein binding: 99%

Metabolism: Hepatic to phenobarbital (active) and phenylethylmalonamide (PEMA)

Bioavailability: 60% to 80%

Half-life elimination (age dependent): Primidone: 10-12 hours; PEMA: 16 hours; Phenobarbital: 52-118 hours

Time to peak, serum: ~4 hours

Excretion: Urine (15% to 25% as unchanged drug and active metabolites)

Pregnancy Risk Factor D

Primsol® *see* Trimethoprim *on page 1538*
Principen® *see* Ampicillin *on page 117*
Prinivil® *see* Lisinopril *on page 936*
Prinzide® *see* Lisinopril and Hydrochlorothiazide *on page 938*
Priscoline® [DSC] *see* Tolazoline *on page 1501*
Pristinamycin *see* Quinupristin and Dalfopristin *on page 1326*
Privine® [OTC] *see* Naphazoline *on page 1087*
ProAmatine® *see* Midodrine *on page 1044*

Probenecid (proe BEN e sid)

Related Information

Sexually-Transmitted Diseases *on page 1674*

Canadian Brand Names Benuryl™

Mexican Brand Names Benecid®

Generic Available Yes

Synonyms Benemid [DSC]

Pharmacologic Category Uricosuric Agent

Use Prevention of gouty arthritis; hyperuricemia; prolongation of beta-lactam effect (ie, serum levels)

Local Anesthetic/Vasoconstrictor Precautions No information available to require special precautions

Effects on Dental Treatment No significant effects or complications reported

Common Adverse Effects Frequency not defined.

Cardiovascular: Flushing of face

Central nervous system: Headache, dizziness

Dermatologic: Rash, itching
Gastrointestinal: Anorexia, nausea, vomiting, sore gums
Genitourinary: Painful urination
Hematologic: Aplastic anemia, hemolytic anemia, leukopenia
Hepatic: Hepatic necrosis
Neuromuscular & skeletal: Gouty arthritis (acute)
Renal: Renal calculi, nephrotic syndrome, urate nephropathy
Miscellaneous: Anaphylaxis

Mechanism of Action Competitively inhibits the reabsorption of uric acid at the proximal convoluted tubule, thereby promoting its excretion and reducing serum uric acid levels; increases plasma levels of weak organic acids (penicillins, cephalosporins, or other beta-lactam antibiotics) by competitively inhibiting their renal tubular secretion

Drug Interactions

Cytochrome P450 Effect: Inhibits CYP2C19 (weak)

Increased Effect/Toxicity: Increases methotrexate toxic potential. Probenecid increases the serum concentrations of quinolones and beta-lactams such as penicillins and cephalosporins. Also increases levels/toxicity of acyclovir, diflunisal, ketorolac, thiopental, benzodiazepines, dapsone, fluoroquinolones, methotrexate, NSAIDs, sulfonylureas, zidovudine.

Decreased Effect: Salicylates (high-dose) may decrease uricosuria. Decreased urinary levels of nitrofurantoin may decrease efficacy.

Pharmacodynamics/Kinetics
Onset of action: Effect on penicillin levels: 2 hours
Absorption: Rapid and complete
Metabolism: Hepatic
Half-life elimination (dose dependent): Normal renal function: 6-12 hours
Time to peak, serum: 2-4 hours
Excretion: Urine

Pregnancy Risk Factor B

Probenecid and Colchicine see Colchicine and Probenecid on page 388

Procainamide (proe kane A mide)

Related Information
Cardiovascular Diseases on page 1636

U.S. Brand Names Procanbid®

Canadian Brand Names Apo-Procainamide®; Procan® SR; Pronestyl®-SR

Generic Available Yes

Synonyms PCA (error-prone abbreviation); Procainamide Hydrochloride; Procaine Amide Hydrochloride

Pharmacologic Category Antiarrhythmic Agent, Class Ia

Use Treatment of ventricular tachycardia (VT), premature ventricular contractions, paroxysmal atrial tachycardia (PSVT), and atrial fibrillation (AF); prevent recurrence of ventricular tachycardia, paroxysmal supraventricular tachycardia, atrial fibrillation or flutter

Unlabeled/Investigational Use ACLS guidelines:
Stable monomorphic VT (EF >40%, no CHF)
Stable wide complex tachycardia, likely VT (EF >40%, no CHF, patient stable)
Atrial fibrillation or flutter, including pre-excitation syndrome (EF >40%, no CHF)
AV reentrant, narrow complex tachycardia (eg, reentrant SVT) [preserved ventricular function]
PALS guidelines: Tachycardia with pulses and poor perfusion (possible VT)

Local Anesthetic/Vasoconstrictor Precautions No information available to require special precautions (see Dental Comment)

Effects on Dental Treatment No significant effects or complications reported

Mechanism of Action Decreases myocardial excitability and conduction velocity and may depress myocardial contractility, by increasing the electrical stimulation threshold of ventricle, His-Purkinje system and through direct cardiac effects

Pregnancy Risk Factor C

Dental Comment
This drug is known to prolong the QT interval. The QT interval is measured as the time and distance between the Q point of the QRS complex and the end of the T wave in the ECG tracing. After adjustment for heart rate, the QT interval is defined as prolonged if it is more than 450 msec in men and 460 msec in women. A long QT syndrome was first described in the 1950s and 60s as a congenital syndrome involving QT interval prolongation and syncope and sudden death. Some of the congenital long QT syndromes were characterized by a peculiar electrocardiographic appearance of the QRS complex involving a
(Continued)

Procainamide *(Continued)*

premature atria beat followed by a pause, then a subsequent sinus beat showing marked QT prolongation and deformity. This type of cardiac arrhythmia was originally termed "torsade de pointes" (translated from the French as "twisting of the points").

Prolongation of the QT interval is thought to result from delayed ventricular repolarization. The repolarization process within the myocardial cell is due to the efflux of intracellular potassium. The channels associated with this current can be blocked by many drugs and predisposes the electrical propagation cycle to torsade de pointes.

Procainamide is one of the drugs confirmed to prolong the QT interval and is accepted as having a risk of causing torsade de pointes. The risk of drug-induced torsade de pointes is extremely low when a single QT interval prolonging drug is prescribed. In terms of epinephrine, it is not known what effect vasoconstrictors in the local anesthetic regimen will have in patients with a known history of congenital prolonged QT interval or in patients taking any medication that prolongs the QT interval. Until more information is obtained, it is suggested that the clinician consult with the physician prior to the use of a vasoconstrictor in suspected patients, and that the vasoconstrictor (epinephrine, levonordefrin [Neo-Cobefrin®]) be used with caution.

Procainamide Hydrochloride *see* Procainamide *on page 1283*

Procaine (PROE kane)

U.S. Brand Names Novocain®
Generic Available No
Synonyms Procaine Hydrochloride
Pharmacologic Category Local Anesthetic
Use Produces spinal anesthesia and epidural and peripheral nerve block by injection and infiltration methods
Local Anesthetic/Vasoconstrictor Precautions No information available to require special precautions
Effects on Dental Treatment This is no longer a useful anesthetic in dentistry due to high incidence of allergic reactions.
Mechanism of Action Blocks both the initiation and conduction of nerve impulses by decreasing the neuronal membrane's permeability to sodium ions, which results in inhibition of depolarization with resultant blockade of conduction
Pregnancy Risk Factor C

Procaine Amide Hydrochloride *see* Procainamide *on page 1283*
Procaine Benzylpenicillin *see* Penicillin G Procaine *on page 1204*
Procaine Hydrochloride *see* Procaine *on page 1284*
Procaine Penicillin G *see* Penicillin G Procaine *on page 1204*
Procanbid® *see* Procainamide *on page 1283*

Procarbazine (proe KAR ba zeen)

U.S. Brand Names Matulane®
Canadian Brand Names Matulane®; Natulan®
Mexican Brand Names Natulan®
Generic Available No
Synonyms Benzmethyzin; N-Methylhydrazine; NSC-77213; Procarbazine Hydrochloride
Pharmacologic Category Antineoplastic Agent, Alkylating Agent
Use Treatment of Hodgkin's disease
Unlabeled/Investigational Use Treatment of non-Hodgkin's lymphoma, brain tumors, melanoma, lung cancer, multiple myeloma
Local Anesthetic/Vasoconstrictor Precautions No information available to require special precautions
Effects on Dental Treatment No significant effects or complications reported
Common Adverse Effects Frequency not defined.
Central nervous system: Reports of neurotoxicity with procarbazine generally originate from early usage with single agent oral (continuous) or I.V. dosing; CNS depression is commonly reported to be additive with other CNS depressants
Hematologic: Myelosuppression, hemolysis in patients with G6PD deficiency
Gastrointestinal: Nausea and vomiting (60% to 90%); increasing the dose in a stepwise fashion over several days may minimize this

Genitourinary: Reproductive dysfunction >10% (in animals, hormone treatment has prevented azoospermia)

Respiratory: Pulmonary toxicity (<1%); the most commonly reported pulmonary toxicity is a hypersensitivity pneumonitis which responds to steroids and discontinuation of the drug. At least one report of persistent pulmonary fibrosis has been reported, however, a higher incidence (18%) of pulmonary toxicity (fibrosis) was reported when procarbazine was given prior to BCNU (BCNU alone does cause pulmonary fibrosis).

Miscellaneous: Second malignancies (cumulative incidence 2% to 15% reported with MOPP combination therapy)

Mechanism of Action Mechanism of action is not clear, methylating of nucleic acids; inhibits DNA, RNA, and protein synthesis; may damage DNA directly and suppresses mitosis; metabolic activation required by host

Drug Interactions

Increased Effect/Toxicity: Procarbazine exhibits weak MAO inhibitor activity. Foods containing high amounts of tyramine should, therefore, be avoided. When an MAO inhibitor is given with food high in tyramine, hypertensive crisis, intracranial bleeding, and headache have been reported.

Sympathomimetic amines (epinephrine and amphetamines) and antidepressants (tricyclics) should be used cautiously with procarbazine. Barbiturates, narcotics, phenothiazines, and other CNS depressants can cause somnolence, ataxia, and other symptoms of CNS depression. Ethanol has caused a disulfiram-like reaction with procarbazine. May result in headache, respiratory difficulties, nausea, vomiting, sweating, thirst, hypotension, and flushing.

Pharmacodynamics/Kinetics
Absorption: Rapid and complete
Distribution: Crosses blood-brain barrier; distributes into CSF
Metabolism: Hepatic and renal
Half-life elimination: 1 hour
Excretion: Urine and respiratory tract (<5% as unchanged drug, 70% as metabolites)

Pregnancy Risk Factor D

Procarbazine Hydrochloride see Procarbazine on page 1284

Procardia® see NIFEdipine on page 1112

Procardia XL® see NIFEdipine on page 1112

Procetofene see Fenofibrate on page 639

Prochieve™ see Progesterone on page 1289

Prochlorperazine (proe klor PER a zeen)

U.S. Brand Names Compro™

Canadian Brand Names Apo-Prochlorperazine®; Compazine®; Nu-Prochlor; Stemetil®

Generic Available Yes: Injection, tablet, suppository

Synonyms Chlormeprazine; Compazine; Prochlorperazine Edisylate; Prochlorperazine Maleate

Pharmacologic Category Antiemetic; Antipsychotic Agent, Typical, Phenothiazine

Use Management of nausea and vomiting; psychotic disorders including schizophrenia; anxiety

Unlabeled/Investigational Use Behavioral syndromes in dementia

Local Anesthetic/Vasoconstrictor Precautions Most pharmacology textbooks state that in presence of phenothiazines, systemic doses of epinephrine paradoxically decrease the blood pressure. This is the so called "epinephrine reversal" phenomenon. This has never been observed when epinephrine is given by infiltration as part of the anesthesia procedure.

Effects on Dental Treatment Key adverse event(s) related to dental treatment: Xerostomia and changes in salivation (normal salivary flow resumes upon discontinuation). Significant hypotension may occur, especially when the drug is administered parenterally; orthostatic hypotension is due to alpha-receptor blockade, the elderly are at greater risk for orthostatic hypotension.

Tardive dyskinesia: Prevalence rate may be 40% in elderly; development of the syndrome and the irreversible nature are proportional to duration and total cumulative dose over time. Extrapyramidal reactions are more common in elderly with up to 50% developing these reactions after 60 years of age. Drug-induced Parkinson's syndrome occurs often; akathisia is the most common extrapyramidal reaction in elderly.

Common Adverse Effects Reported with prochlorperazine or other phenothiazines. Frequency not defined
(Continued)

Prochlorperazine *(Continued)*

Cardiovascular: Cardiac arrest, hypotension, peripheral edema, Q-wave distortions, T-wave distortions

Central nervous system: Agitation, catatonia, cerebral edema, cough reflex suppressed, dizziness, drowsiness, fever (mild-I.M.), headache, hyperactivity, hyperpyrexia, impairment of temperature regulation. insomnia, neuroleptic malignant syndrome (NMS), paradoxical excitement, restlessness, seizure

Dermatologic: Angioedema, contact dermatitis, discoloration of skin (blue-gray), epithelial keratopathy, erythema, eczema, exfoliative dermatitis (injectable), itching, photosensitivity, rash, skin pigmentation, urticaria

Endocrine & metabolic: Amenorrhea, breast enlargement, galactorrhea, gynecomastia, glucosuria, hyperglycemia, hypoglycemia, lactation, libido (changes in), menstrual irregularity, SIADH

Gastrointestinal: Appetite increased, atonic colon, constipation, ileus, nausea, weight gain, xerostomia

Genitourinary: Ejaculating dysfunction, ejaculatory disturbances, impotence, incontinence, polyuria, priapism, urinary retention, urination difficulty

Hematologic: Agranulocytosis, aplastic anemia, eosinophilia, hemolytic anemia, leukopenia, pancytopenia, thrombocytopenic purpura

Hepatic: Biliary stasis, cholestatic jaundice, hepatotoxicity

Neuromuscular & skeletal: Dystonias (torticollis, opisthotonos, carpopedal spasm, trismus, oculogyric crisis, protusion of tongue); extrapyramidal symptoms (pseudoparkinsonism, akathisia, dystonias, tardive dyskinesia); SLE-like syndrome, tremor

Ocular: blurred vision, cornea and lens changes, lenticular/corneal deposits, miosis, mydriasis, pigmentary retinopathy

Respiratory: Asthma, laryngeal edema, nasal congestion

Miscellaneous: Allergic reactions, diaphoresis

Dosage

Antiemetic: Children (therapy >1 day usually not required): Note: Not recommended for use in children <9 kg or <2 years:

Oral, rectal: >9 kg: 0.4 mg/kg/24 hours in 3-4 divided doses; or
9-13 kg: 2.5 mg every 12-24 hours as needed; maximum: 7.5 mg/day
13.1-17 kg: 2.5 mg every 8-12 hours as needed; maximum: 10 mg/day
17.1-37 kg: 2.5 mg every 8 hours or 5 mg every 12 hours as needed; maximum: 15 mg/day

I.M.: 0.13 mg/kg/dose; change to oral as soon as possible

Antiemetic: Adults:

Oral (tablet): 5-10 mg 3-4 times/day; usual maximum: 40 mg/day; larger doses may rarely be required

I.M. (deep): 5-10 mg every 3-4 hours; usual maximum: 40 mg/day

I.V.: 2.5-10 mg; maximum 10 mg/dose or 40 mg/day; may repeat dose every 3-4 hours as needed

Rectal: 25 mg twice daily

Surgical nausea/vomiting: Adults: Note: Should not exceed 40 mg/day

I.M.: 5-10 mg 1-2 hours before induction or to control symptoms during or after surgery; may repeat once if necessary

I.V. (administer slow IVP <5 mg/minute): 5-10 mg 15-30 minutes before induction or to control symptoms during or after surgery; may repeat once if necessary

Rectal (unlabeled use): 25 mg

Antipsychotic:

Children 2-12 years (not recommended in children <9 kg or <2 years):

Oral, rectal: 2.5 mg 2-3 times/day; do not give more than 10 mg the first day; increase dosage as needed to maximum daily dose of 20 mg for 2-5 years and 25 mg for 6-12 years

I.M.: 0.13 mg/kg/dose; change to oral as soon as possible

Adults:

Oral: 5-10 mg 3-4 times/day; titrate dose slowly every 2-3 days; doses up to 150 mg/day may be required in some patients for treatment of severe disturbances

I.M.: Initial: 10-20 mg; if necessary repeat initial dose every 1-4 hours to gain control; more than 3-4 doses are rarely needed. If parenteral administration is still required; give 10-20 mg every 4-6 hours; change to oral as soon as possible.

Nonpsychotic anxiety: Oral (tablet): Adults: Usual dose: 15-20 mg/day in divided doses; do not give doses >20 mg/day or for longer than 12 weeks

Elderly: Behavioral symptoms associated with dementia (unlabeled use): Initial: 2.5-5 mg 1-2 times/day; increase dose at 4- to 7-day intervals by 2.5-5 mg/day; increase dosing intervals (twice daily, 3 times/day, etc) as necessary to control response or side effects; maximum daily dose should probably not exceed 75 mg in elderly; gradual increases (titration) may prevent some side effects or decrease their severity

Mechanism of Action Prochlorperazine is a piperazine phenothiazine antipsychotic which blocks postsynaptic mesolimbic dopaminergic D_1 and D_2 receptors in the brain, including the chemoreceptor trigger zone; exhibits a strong alpha-adrenergic and anticholinergic blocking effect and depresses the release of hypothalamic and hypophyseal hormones; believed to depress the reticular activating system, thus affecting basal metabolism, body temperature, wakefulness, vasomotor tone and emesis

Contraindications Hypersensitivity to prochlorperazine or any component of the formulation (cross-reactivity between phenothiazines may occur); severe CNS depression; coma; pediatric surgery; Reye's syndrome; should not be used in children <2 years of age or <9 kg

Warnings/Precautions May be sedating; use with caution in disorders where CNS depression is a feature. May obscure intestinal obstruction or brain tumor. May impair physical or mental abilities. Effects with other sedative drugs or ethanol may be potentiated. Use with caution in Parkinson's disease; hemodynamic instability; bone marrow suppression; predisposition to seizures; subcortical brain damage; and in severe cardiac, hepatic, renal or respiratory disease. Caution in breast cancer or other prolactin-dependent tumors. May alter temperature regulation or mask toxicity of other drugs. Use caution with exposure to heat. May alter cardiac conduction. May cause orthostatic hypotension. Hypotension may occur following administration, particularly when parenteral form is used or in high dosages.

Phenothiazines may cause anticholinergic effects; therefore, they should be used with caution in patients with decreased gastrointestinal motility, urinary retention, BPH, xerostomia, or visual problems. Conditions which also may be exacerbated by cholinergic blockade include narrow-angle glaucoma (screening is recommended) and worsening of myasthenia gravis. May cause extrapyramidal symptoms. Use caution in the the elderly. Children with acute illness or dehydration are more susceptible to neuromuscular reactions; use cautiously. May be associated with neuroleptic malignant syndrome (NMS).

Drug Interactions

Increased Effect/Toxicity: Prochlorperazine plus lithium may rarely produce neurotoxicity. Prochlorperazing may produce additive CNS depressant effects with other CNS depressants. Acetylcholinesterase inhibitors may increase the risk of EPS. Alpha-/beta-agonists, antihistamines, QT_c-prolonging agents may enhance the arrhythmogenic effects of phenothiazines. Concurrent use may enhance the hypotensive effects of narcotics and beta blockers. SSRIs may increase risk of hypotension. Antimalarials and beta blockers may increase serum levels of prochlorperazine. Pramlintide may increase anticholinergic effects of prochlorperazine.

Decreased Effect: The antihypertensive effects of methyldopa and guanadrel may be inhibited by prochlorperazine. Prochlorperazine may inhibit the antiparkinsonian effect of levodopa. Prochlorperazine may reverse the pressor effects of epinephrine. Antacids and attapulgite may decreased absorption of phenothiazines. Anticholinertics may decrease the therapeutic response to phenothiazines.

Ethanol/Nutrition/Herb Interactions

Ethanol: Avoid ethanol (may increase CNS depression).

Food: Limit caffeine.

Herb/Nutraceutical: Avoid dong quai, St John's wort (may also cause photosensitization). Avoid kava kava, gotu kola, valerian, St John's wort (may increase CNS depression).

Dietary Considerations Increase dietary intake of riboflavin; should be administered with food or water. Rectal suppositories may contain coconut and palm oil.

Pharmacodynamics/Kinetics

Onset of action: Oral: 30-40 minutes; I.M.: 10-20 minutes; Rectal: ~60 minutes Peak antiemetic effect: I.V.: 30-60 minutes

Duration: Rectal: 12 hours; Oral: 3-4 hours; I.M., I.V.: Adults: 4-6 hours; I.M.: Children: 12 hours

Distribution: V_d: 1400-1548 L; crosses placenta; enters breast milk

Metabolism: Primarily hepatic; N-desmethyl prochlorperazine (major active metabolite)

Bioavailability: Oral: 12.5%

Half-life elimination: Oral: 3-5 hours; I.V.: ~7 hours

Dosage Forms INJ, solution, as edisylate: 5 mg/mL (2 mL). **SUPP,** rectal: 2.5 mg (12s), 5 mg (12s), 25 mg (12s); (Compro™): 25 mg (12s). **TAB, as maleate:** 5 mg, 10 mg

Prochlorperazine Edisylate *see* Prochlorperazine *on page 1285*

Prochlorperazine Maleate *see* Prochlorperazine *on page 1285*

Procrit® *see* Epoetin Alfa *on page 552*

Proctocort® *see* Hydrocortisone *on page 793*

ProctoCream® HC *see* Hydrocortisone *on page 793*

Proctofene *see* Fenofibrate *on page 639*

ProctoFoam®-HC *see* Pramoxine and Hydrocortisone *on page 1264*

ProctoFoam® NS [OTC] *see* Pramoxine *on page 1264*

Procto-Kit™ *see* Hydrocortisone *on page 793*

Procto-Pak™ *see* Hydrocortisone *on page 793*

Proctosert *see* Hydrocortisone *on page 793*

Proctosol-HC® *see* Hydrocortisone *on page 793*

Proctozone-HC™ *see* Hydrocortisone *on page 793*

Procyclidine (proe SYE kli deen)

U.S. Brand Names Kemadrin®

Canadian Brand Names PMS-Procyclidine

Generic Available No

Synonyms Procyclidine Hydrochloride

Pharmacologic Category Anti-Parkinson's Agent, Anticholinergic; Anticholinergic Agent

Use Relieves symptoms of parkinsonian syndrome and drug-induced extrapyramidal symptoms

Local Anesthetic/Vasoconstrictor Precautions No information available to require special precautions

Effects on Dental Treatment Key adverse event(s) related to dental treatment: Xerostomia (normal salivary flow resumes upon discontinuation) and dry throat and nose. Prolonged use of antidyskinetics may decrease or inhibit salivary flow, contributing to discomfort and dental disease (ie, caries, oral candidiasis, and periodontal disease).

Common Adverse Effects Frequency not defined.

Cardiovascular: Tachycardia, palpitation

Central nervous system: Confusion, drowsiness, headache, loss of memory, fatigue, ataxia, giddiness, lightheadedness

Dermatologic: Dry skin, increased sensitivity to light, rash

Gastrointestinal: Constipation, xerostomia, dry throat, nausea, vomiting, epigastric distress

Genitourinary: Difficult urination

Neuromuscular & skeletal: Weakness

Ocular: Increased intraocular pain, blurred vision, mydriasis

Respiratory: Dry nose

Miscellaneous: Diaphoresis (decreased)

Mechanism of Action Thought to act by blocking excess acetylcholine at cerebral synapses; many of its effects are due to its pharmacologic similarities with atropine; it exerts an antispasmodic effect on smooth muscle, is a potent mydriatic; inhibits salivation

Drug Interactions

Increased Effect/Toxicity: Central and/or peripheral anticholinergic syndrome can occur when administered with amantadine, rimantadine, narcotic analgesics, phenothiazines and other antipsychotics (especially with high anticholinergic activity), tricyclic antidepressants, quinidine and some other antiarrhythmics, and antihistamines.

Decreased Effect: May increase gastric degradation of levodopa and decrease the amount of levodopa absorbed by delaying gastric emptying; the opposite may be true for digoxin. Therapeutic effects of cholinergic agents (tacrine, donepezil) and neuroleptics may be antagonized.

Pharmacodynamics/Kinetics

Onset of action: 30-40 minutes

Duration: 4-6 hours

Pregnancy Risk Factor C

Procyclidine Hydrochloride *see* Procyclidine *on page 1288*

Profen II® *see* Guaifenesin and Pseudoephedrine *on page 755*

Profen II DM® *see* Guaifenesin, Pseudoephedrine, and Dextromethorphan *on page 757*

Profen Forte® *see* Guaifenesin and Pseudoephedrine *on page 755*

Profen Forte™ DM *see* Guaifenesin, Pseudoephedrine, and Dextromethorphan *on page 757*

Profilnine® SD *see* Factor IX Complex (Human) *on page 633*

Progesterone (proe JES ter one)

U.S. Brand Names Crinone®; Prochieve™; Prometrium®
Canadian Brand Names Crinone®; Prometrium®
Mexican Brand Names Crinone®
Generic Available Yes: Injection
Synonyms Pregnenedione; Progestin
Pharmacologic Category Progestin
Use

Oral: Prevention of endometrial hyperplasia in nonhysterectomized, postmeno-pausal women who are receiving conjugated estrogen tablets; secondary amenorrhea

I.M.: Amenorrhea; abnormal uterine bleeding due to hormonal imbalance

Intravaginal gel: Part of assisted reproductive technology (ART) for infertile women with progesterone deficiency; secondary amenorrhea

Local Anesthetic/Vasoconstrictor Precautions No information available to require special precautions

Effects on Dental Treatment Key adverse event(s) related to dental treatment: Progestins may predispose the patient to gingival bleeding.

Common Adverse Effects

Injection (I.M.):

Cardiovascular: Edema

Central nervous system: Depression, fever, insomnia, somnolence

Dermatologic: Acne, allergic rash (rare), alopecia, hirsutism, pruritus, rash, urticaria

Endocrine & metabolic: Amenorrhea, breakthrough bleeding, breast tender-ness, galactorrhea, menstrual flow changes, spotting

Gastrointestinal: Nausea, weight gain, weight loss

Genitourinary: Cervical erosion changes, cervical secretion changes

Hepatic: Cholestatic jaundice

Local: Pain at the injection site

Miscellaneous: Anaphylactoid reactions

Oral capsule (percentages reported when used in combination with or cycled with conjugated estrogens):

>10%:

Central nervous system: Headache (10% to 31%), dizziness (15% to 24%), depression (19%)

Endocrine & metabolic: Breast tenderness (27%), breast pain (6% to 16%)

Gastrointestinal: Abdominal pain (6% to 12%), abdominal bloating (10% to 20%)

Genitourinary: Urinary problems (11%)

Neuromuscular & skeletal: Joint pain (20%), musculoskeletal pain (6% to 12%)

Miscellaneous: Viral infection (7% to 12%)

5% to 10%:

Cardiovascular: Chest pain (7%)

Central nervous system: Fatigue (8% to 9%), emotional lability (6%), irritability (5% to 8%), worry (8%)

Gastrointestinal: Nausea/vomiting (8%), diarrhea (8%)

Respiratory: Upper respiratory tract infection (5%), cough (8%)

Miscellaneous: Night sweats (7%)

Vaginal gel (percentages reported with ART); also refer to oral capsule reac-tions listing for additional effects noted with progesterone:

>10%:

Central nervous system: Somnolence (27%), headache (13% to 17%), nervousness (16%), depression (11%)

Endocrine & metabolic: Breast enlargement (40%), breast pain (13%), libido decreased (11%)

Gastrointestinal: Constipation (27%), nausea (7% to 22%), cramps (15%), abdominal pain (12%)

Genitourinary: Perineal pain (17%), nocturia (13%)

5% to 10%:

Central nervous system: Pain (8%), dizziness (5%)

Gastrointestinal: Diarrhea (8%), bloating (7%), vomiting (5%)

Genitourinary: Vaginal discharge (7%), dyspareunia (6%), genital moniliasis (5%), genital pruritus (5%)

Neuromuscular & skeletal: Arthralgia (8%)

Mechanism of Action Natural steroid hormone that induces secretory changes in the endometrium, promotes mammary gland development, relaxes uterine
(Continued)

Progesterone (Continued)

smooth muscle, blocks follicular maturation and ovulation, and maintains pregnancy

Drug Interactions

Cytochrome P450 Effect: Substrate of CYP1A2 (minor), 2A6 (minor), 2C8/9 (minor), 2C19 (major), 2D6 (minor), 3A4 (major); **Inhibits** CYP2C8/9 (weak), 2C19 (weak), 3A4 (weak)

Increased Effect/Toxicity: Ketoconazole may increase the bioavailability of progesterone. Progesterone may increase concentrations of estrogenic compounds during concurrent therapy with conjugated estrogens.

Decreased Effect: CYP2C19 inducers may decrease the levels/effects of progesterone; example inducers include aminoglutethimide, carbamazepine, phenytoin, and rifampin. CYP3A4 inducers may decrease the levels/effects of progesterone; example inducers include aminoglutethimide, carbamazepine, nafcillin, nevirapine, phenobarbital, phenytoin, and rifamycins.

Pharmacodynamics/Kinetics

Absorption: Vaginal gel: Prolonged

Absorption half-life: 25-50 hours

Protein binding: 96% to 99%

Metabolism: Hepatic to metabolites

Half-life elimination: Vaginal gel: 5-20 minutes

Time to peak: Oral: Within 3 hours

Excretion: Urine, bile, feces

Pregnancy Risk Factor B (Prometrium®, per manufacturer); none established for vaginal gel or injection (contraindicated)

Progestin see Progesterone on page 1289

Proglycem® see Diazoxide on page 457

Prograf® see Tacrolimus on page 1437

Proguanil and Atovaquone see Atovaquone and Proguanil on page 160

ProHance® see Gadoteridol on page 719

Prolastin® see Alpha₁-Proteinase Inhibitor on page 73

Proleukin® see Aldesleukin on page 61

Prolex™-D see Guaifenesin and Phenylephrine on page 754

Prolixin® [DSC] see Fluphenazine on page 680

Prolixin Decanoate® see Fluphenazine on page 680

Proloprim® see Trimethoprim on page 1538

Promethazine (proe METH a zeen)

U.S. Brand Names Phenadoz™; Phenergan®; Promethegan™

Canadian Brand Names Phenergan®

Generic Available Yes

Synonyms Promethazine Hydrochloride

Pharmacologic Category Antiemetic; Antihistamine; Phenothiazine Derivative; Sedative

Use Symptomatic treatment of various allergic conditions; antiemetic; motion sickness; sedative; postoperative pain (adjunctive therapy); anesthetic (adjunctive therapy); anaphylactic reactions (adjunctive therapy)

Local Anesthetic/Vasoconstrictor Precautions Most pharmacology textbooks state that in presence of phenothiazines, systemic doses of epinephrine paradoxically decrease the blood pressure. This is the so called "epinephrine reversal" phenomenon. This has never been observed when epinephrine is given by infiltration as part of the anesthesia procedure.

Effects on Dental Treatment Key adverse event(s) related to dental treatment: Xerostomia (normal salivary flow resumes upon discontinuation). Significant hypotension may occur, especially when the drug is administered parenterally; orthostatic hypotension is due to alpha-receptor blockade, the elderly are at greater risk for orthostatic hypotension.

Tardive dyskinesia: Prevalence rate may be 40% in elderly; development of the syndrome and the irreversible nature are proportional to duration and total cumulative dose over time. Extrapyramidal reactions are more common in elderly with up to 50% developing these reactions after 60 years of age. Drug-induced Parkinson's syndrome occurs often; akathisia is the most common extrapyramidal reaction in elderly.

Increased confusion, memory loss, psychotic behavior, and agitation frequently occur as a consequence of anticholinergic effects. Antipsychotic associated sedation in nonpsychotic patients is extremely unpleasant due to feelings of depersonalization, derealization, and dysphoria.

Common Adverse Effects

Cardiovascular: Bradycardia, hypertension, nonspecific QT changes, postural hypotension, tachycardia

Central nervous system: Akathisia, catatonic states, confusion, delirium, disorientation, dizziness, drowsiness, dystonias, euphoria, excitation, extrapyramidal symptoms, fatigue, hallucinations, hysteria, insomnia, lassitude, nervousness, neuroleptic malignant syndrome, nightmares, pseudoparkinsonism, sedation, seizure, somnolence, tardive dyskinesia

Dermatologic: Angioneurotic edema, dermatitis, photosensitivity, skin pigmentation (slate gray), urticaria

Endocrine & metabolic: Amenorrhea, breast engorgement, gynecomastia, hyper-/hypoglycemia, lactation

Gastrointestinal: Constipation, nausea, vomiting, xerostomia

Genitourinary: Ejaculatory disorder, impotence, urinary retention

Hematologic: Agranulocytosis, aplastic anemia, eosinophilia, hemolytic anemia, leukopenia, thrombocytopenia, thrombocytopenic purpura

Hepatic: Jaundice

Neuromuscular & skeletal: Incoordination, tremor

Ocular: Blurred vision, corneal and lenticular changes, diplopia, epithelial keratopathy, pigmentary retinopathy

Otic: Tinnitus

Respiratory: Apnea, asthma, nasal congestion, respiratory depression

Mechanism of Action Blocks postsynaptic mesolimbic dopaminergic receptors in the brain; exhibits a strong alpha-adrenergic blocking effect and depresses the release of hypothalamic and hypophyseal hormones; competes with histamine for the H_1-receptor; reduces stimuli to the brainstem reticular system

Drug Interactions

Cytochrome P450 Effect: Substrate (major) of CYP2B6, 2D6; **Inhibits** CYP2D6 (weak)

Increased Effect/Toxicity: CYP2B6 inhibitors may increase the levels/effects of promethazine; example inhibitors include desipramine, paroxetine, and sertraline. CYP2D6 inhibitors may increase the levels/effects of promethazine; example inhibitors include chlorpromazine, delavirdine, fluoxetine, miconazole, paroxetine, pergolide, quinidine, quinine, ritonavir, and ropinirole. Chloroquine, propranolol, and sulfadoxine-pyrimethamine also may increase promethazine concentrations. Concurrent use with TCA may produce increased toxicity or altered therapeutic response. Promethazine plus lithium may rarely produce neurotoxicity. Concurrent use of promethazine and CNS depressants (ethanol, narcotics) may produce additive depressant effects.

Decreased Effect: CYP2B6 inducers may decrease the levels/effects of promethazine; example inducers include carbamazepine, nevirapine, phenobarbital, phenytoin, and rifampin. Benztropine (and other anticholinergics) may inhibit the therapeutic response to promethazine. Promethazine may inhibit the ability of bromocriptine to lower serum prolactin concentrations. The antihypertensive effects of guanethidine and guanadrel may be inhibited by promethazine. Promethazine may inhibit the antiparkinsonian effect of levodopa. Promethazine (and possibly other low potency antipsychotics) may reverse the pressor effects of epinephrine.

Pharmacodynamics/Kinetics

Onset of action: I.M.: ~20 minutes; I.V.: 3-5 minutes

Peak effect: C_{max}: 9.04 ng/mL (suppository); 19.3 ng/mL (syrup)

Duration: 2-6 hours

Absorption:

I.M.: Bioavailability may be greater than with oral or rectal administration

Oral: Rapid and complete; large first pass effect limits systemic bioavailability

Distribution: V_d: 171 L

Protein binding: 93%

Metabolism: Hepatic; primarily oxidation; forms metabolites

Half-life elimination: 9-16 hours

Time to maximum serum concentration: 4.4 hours (syrup); 6.7-8.6 hours (suppositories)

Excretion: Primarily urine and feces (as inactive metabolites)

Pregnancy Risk Factor C

Promethazine and Codeine (proe METH a zeen & KOE deen)

Related Information

Codeine on page 385

Promethazine on page 1290

Generic Available Yes

(Continued)

Promethazine and Codeine *(Continued)*

Synonyms Codeine and Promethazine

Pharmacologic Category Antihistamine/Antitussive

Use Temporary relief of coughs and upper respiratory symptoms associated with allergy or the common cold

Local Anesthetic/Vasoconstrictor Precautions No information available to require special precautions

Effects on Dental Treatment Although promethazine is a phenothiazine derivative, extrapyramidal reactions or tardive dyskinesias are not seen with the use of this drug.

Restrictions C-V

Drug Interactions

Cytochrome P450 Effect: Promethazine: **Substrate** (major) of CYP2B6, 2D6; **Inhibits** CYP2D6 (weak)

Pharmacodynamics/Kinetics See individual agents.

Pregnancy Risk Factor C

Promethazine and Dextromethorphan

(proe METH a zeen & deks troe meth OR fan)

Related Information

Dextromethorphan *on page 451*

Promethazine *on page 1290*

Generic Available Yes

Synonyms Dextromethorphan and Promethazine

Pharmacologic Category Antihistamine/Antitussive

Use Temporary relief of coughs and upper respiratory symptoms associated with allergy or the common cold

Local Anesthetic/Vasoconstrictor Precautions No information available to require special precautions

Effects on Dental Treatment Although promethazine is a phenothiazine derivative, extrapyramidal reactions or tardive dyskinesias are not seen with the use of this drug.

Drug Interactions

Cytochrome P450 Effect:

Promethazine: **Substrate** (major) of CYP2B6, 2D6; **Inhibits** CYP2D6 (weak)

Dextromethorphan: **Substrate** of CYP2B6 (minor), 2C9 (minor), 2C19 (minor), 2D6 (major), 2E1 (minor), 3A4 (minor); **Inhibits** CYP2D6 (weak)

Pharmacodynamics/Kinetics See individual agents.

Pregnancy Risk Factor C

Promethazine and Meperidine *see* Meperidine and Promethazine *on page 986*

Promethazine and Phenylephrine

(proe METH a zeen & fen il EF rin)

Related Information

Phenylephrine *on page 1226*

Promethazine *on page 1290*

Generic Available Yes

Synonyms Phenylephrine and Promethazine

Pharmacologic Category Antihistamine/Decongestant Combination

Use Temporary relief of upper respiratory symptoms associated with allergy or the common cold

Local Anesthetic/Vasoconstrictor Precautions

Phenylephrine: Use with caution since phenylephrine is a sympathomimetic amine which could interact with epinephrine to cause a pressor response

Promethazine: No information available to require special precautions

Effects on Dental Treatment Key adverse event(s) related to dental treatment: Phenylephrine: Tachycardia, palpitations, xerostomia (normal salivary flow resumes upon discontinuation); use vasoconstrictor with caution. Although promethazine is a phenothiazine derivative, extrapyramidal reactions or tardive dyskinesias are not seen with the use of this drug.

Drug Interactions

Cytochrome P450 Effect: Promethazine: **Substrate** (major) of CYP2B6, 2D6; **Inhibits** CYP2D6 (weak)

Pharmacodynamics/Kinetics See individual agents.

Pregnancy Risk Factor C

Promethazine Hydrochloride *see* Promethazine *on page 1290*

Promethazine, Phenylephrine, and Codeine
(proe METH a zeen, fen il EF rin, & KOE deen)

Related Information
Codeine *on page 385*
Phenylephrine *on page 1226*
Promethazine *on page 1582*

Generic Available Yes

Synonyms Codeine, Promethazine, and Phenylephrine; Phenylephrine, Promethazine, and Codeine

Pharmacologic Category Antihistamine/Decongestant/Antitussive

Use Temporary relief of coughs and upper respiratory symptoms including nasal congestion associated with allergy or the common cold

Local Anesthetic/Vasoconstrictor Precautions
Phenylephrine: Use with caution since phenylephrine is a sympathomimetic amine which could interact with epinephrine to cause a pressor response
Promethazine: No information available to require special precautions

Effects on Dental Treatment Key adverse event(s) related to dental treatment: Phenylephrine: Tachycardia, palpitations, xerostomia (normal salivary flow resumes upon discontinuation); use vasoconstrictor with caution. Although promethazine is a phenothiazine derivative, extrapyramidal reactions or tardive dyskinesias are not seen with the use of this drug.

Restrictions C-V

Drug Interactions
Cytochrome P450 Effect:
Promethazine: **Substrate** (major) of CYP2B6, 2D6; **Inhibits** CYP2D6 (weak)
Codeine: **Substrate** of CYP2D6 (major), 3A4 (minor); **Inhibits** CYP2D6 (weak)

Pharmacodynamics/Kinetics See individual agents.

Pregnancy Risk Factor C

Promethegan™ *see Promethazine on page 1290*

Prometrium® *see Progesterone on page 1289*

Promit® *see Dextran 1 on page 447*

Pronap-100® *see Propoxyphene and Acetaminophen on page 1298*

Pronto® Complete Lice Killing Kit [OTC] *see Pyrethrins and Piperonyl Butoxide on page 1315*

Pronto® Plus Hair and Scalp Masque [OTC] *see Pyrethrins and Piperonyl Butoxide on page 1315*

Pronto® Plus Mousse [OTC] *see Pyrethrins and Piperonyl Butoxide on page 1315*

Pronto® Plus Warm Oil Treatment and Conditioner [OTC] *see Pyrethrins and Piperonyl Butoxide on page 1315*

Pronto® Plus with Natural Extracts and Oils [OTC] *see Pyrethrins and Piperonyl Butoxide on page 1315*

Propafenone (proe pa FEEN one)

Related Information
Cardiovascular Diseases *on page 1636*

U.S. Brand Names Rythmol®; Rythmol® SR

Canadian Brand Names Apo-Propafenone®; Rythmol® Gen-Propafenone

Mexican Brand Names Nistaken®; Norfenon®

Generic Available Yes: Tablet

Synonyms Propafenone Hydrochloride

Pharmacologic Category Antiarrhythmic Agent, Class Ic

Use Treatment of life-threatening ventricular arrhythmias
Rythmol® SR: Maintenance of normal sinus rhythm in patients with symptomatic atrial fibrillation

Unlabeled/Investigational Use Supraventricular tachycardias, including those patients with Wolff-Parkinson-White syndrome

Local Anesthetic/Vasoconstrictor Precautions In some patients, propafenone has been reported to induce new or worsened arrhythmias (proarrhythmic effect). It is suggested that vasoconstrictors be used with caution since epinephrine has the potential to stimulate the heart rate when given in the anesthetic regimen. See Dental Comment.

Effects on Dental Treatment Key adverse event(s) related to dental treatment: Unusual taste and significant xerostomia (normal salivary flow resumes upon discontinuation).
(Continued)

Propafenone *(Continued)*

Common Adverse Effects 1% to 10%:

Cardiovascular: New or worsened arrhythmia (proarrhythmic effect) (2% to 10%), angina (2% to 5%), CHF (1% to 4%), ventricular tachycardia (1% to 3%), palpitation (1% to 3%), AV block (first-degree) (1% to 3%), syncope (1% to 2%), increased QRS interval (1% to 2%), chest pain (1% to 2%), PVCs (1% to 2%), bradycardia (1% to 2%), edema (0% to 1%), bundle branch block (0% to 1%), atrial fibrillation (1%), hypotension (0% to 1%), intraventricular conduction delay (0% to 1%)

Central nervous system: Dizziness (4% to 15%), fatigue (2% to 6%), headache (2% to 5%), ataxia (0% to 2%), insomnia (0% to 2%), anxiety (1% to 2%), drowsiness (1%)

Dermatologic: Rash (1% to 3%)

Gastrointestinal: Nausea/vomiting (2% to 11%), unusual taste (3% to 23%), constipation (2% to 7%), dyspepsia (1% to 3%), diarrhea (1% to 3%), xerostomia (1% to 2%), anorexia (1% to 2%), abdominal pain (1% to 2%), flatulence (0% to 1%)

Neuromuscular & skeletal: Tremor (0% to 1%), arthralgia (0% to 1%), weakness (1% to 2%)

Ocular: Blurred vision (1% to 6%)

Respiratory: Dyspnea (2% to 5%)

Miscellaneous: Diaphoresis (1%)

Mechanism of Action
Propafenone is a class 1c antiarrhythmic agent which possesses local anesthetic properties, blocks the fast inward sodium current, and slows the rate of increase of the action potential. Prolongs conduction and refractoriness in all areas of the myocardium, with a slightly more pronounced effect on intraventricular conduction; it prolongs effective refractory period, reduces spontaneous automaticity and exhibits some beta-blockade activity.

Drug Interactions

Cytochrome P450 Effect: Substrate of CYP1A2 (minor), 2D6 (major), 3A4 (minor); Inhibits CYP1A2 (weak), 2C8/9 (weak), 2D6 (weak)

Increased Effect/Toxicity: Cimetidine and quinidine may increase propafenone levels. Ritonavir may increase propafenone levels; concurrent use is contraindicated. CYP2D6 inhibitors may increase the levels/effects of propafenone; example inhibitors include chlorpromazine, delavirdine, fluoxetine, miconazole, paroxetine, pergolide, quinine, and ropinirole. Digoxin (reduce dose by 25%), metoprolol, propranolol, theophylline, and warfarin blood levels are increased by propafenone. Use caution with Class Ia and Class III antiarrhythmics, erythromycin, cisapride, antipsychotics, and cyclic antidepressants; QT_c-prolonging effects may be additive with propafenone.

Decreased Effect: Enzyme inducers (phenobarbital, phenytoin, rifabutin, rifampin) may decrease propafenone blood levels.

Pharmacodynamics/Kinetics

Absorption: Well absorbed

Metabolism: Hepatic; two genetically determined metabolism groups exist: fast or slow metabolizers; 10% of Caucasians are slow metabolizers; exhibits nonlinear pharmacokinetics; when dose is increased from 300-900 mg/day, serum concentrations increase tenfold; this nonlinearity is thought to be due to saturable first-pass effect

Bioavailability: 150 mg: 3.4%; 300 mg: 10.6%

Half-life elimination: Single dose (100-300 mg): 2-8 hours; Chronic dosing: 10-32 hours

Time to peak: 150 mg dose: 2 hours, 300 mg dose: 3 hours

Pregnancy Risk Factor C

Dental Comment

This drug is known to prolong the QT interval. The QT interval is measured as the time and distance between the Q point of the QRS complex and the end of the T wave in the ECG tracing. After adjustment for heart rate, the QT interval is defined as prolonged if it is more than 450 msec in men and 460 msec in women. A long QT syndrome was first described in the 1950s and 60s as a congenital syndrome involving QT interval prolongation and syncope and sudden death. Some of the congenital long QT syndromes were characterized by a peculiar electrocardiographic appearance of the QRS complex involving a premature atria beat followed by a pause, then a subsequent sinus beat showing marked QT prolongation and deformity. This type of cardiac arrhythmia was originally termed "torsade de pointes" (translated from the French as "twisting of the points").

Prolongation of the QT interval is thought to result from delayed ventricular repolarization. The repolarization process within the myocardial cell is due to the efflux of intracellular potassium. The channels associated with this current can be blocked by many drugs and predisposes the electrical propagation cycle to torsade de pointes.

Propafenone is one of the drugs confirmed to prolong the QT interval and is accepted as having a risk of causing torsade de pointes. The risk of drug-induced torsade de pointes is extremely low when a single QT interval prolonging drug is prescribed. In terms of epinephrine, it is not known what effect vasoconstrictors in the local anesthetic regimen will have in patients with a known history of congenital prolonged QT interval or in patients taking any medication that prolongs the QT interval. Until more information is obtained, it is suggested that the clinician consult with the physician prior to the use of a vasoconstrictor in suspected patients, and that the vasoconstrictor (epinephrine, levonordefrin [Neo-Cobefrin®]) be used with caution.

Propafenone Hydrochloride *see* Propafenone *on page 1293*

Propantheline (proe PAN the leen)

Generic Available Yes

Synonyms Propantheline Bromide

Pharmacologic Category Anticholinergic Agent

Dental Use Induce dry field (xerostomia) in oral cavity

Use Adjunctive treatment of peptic ulcer, irritable bowel syndrome, pancreatitis, ureteral and urinary bladder spasm; reduce duodenal motility during diagnostic radiologic procedures

Local Anesthetic/Vasoconstrictor Precautions No information available to require special precautions

Effects on Dental Treatment Key adverse event(s) related to dental treatment: Significant xerostomia (therapeutic effect; normal salivary flow resumes upon discontinuation), dry throat, nasal dryness, and dysphagia.

Significant Adverse Effects Frequency not defined.
Dermatologic: Dry skin
Gastrointestinal: Constipation, dry mouth and throat, dysphagia
Respiratory: Dry nose
Miscellaneous: Diaphoresis (decreased)

Dental Usual Dosing Antisecretory: Oral:
Children: 1-2 mg/kg/day in 3-4 divided doses
Adults: 15 mg 3 times/day before meals or food and 30 mg at bedtime
Elderly: 7.5 mg 3 times/day before meals and at bedtime

Dosage Oral:
Antisecretory:
Children: 1-2 mg/kg/day in 3-4 divided doses
Adults: 15 mg 3 times/day before meals or food and 30 mg at bedtime
Elderly: 7.5 mg 3 times/day before meals and at bedtime
Antispasmodic:
Children: 2-3 mg/kg/day in divided doses every 4-6 hours and at bedtime
Adults: 15 mg 3 times/day before meals or food and 30 mg at bedtime

Mechanism of Action Competitively blocks the action of acetylcholine at post-ganglionic parasympathetic receptor sites

Contraindications Hypersensitivity to propantheline or any component of the formulation; ulcerative colitis, toxic megacolon, obstructive disease of the GI or urinary tract; narrow-angle glaucoma; myasthenia gravis

Warnings/Precautions Use with caution in patients with hyperthyroidism, hepatic, cardiac, or renal disease, hypertension, GI infections, or other endocrine diseases.

Drug Interactions
Decreased effect with antacids (decreased absorption); decreased effect of sustained release dosage forms (decreased absorption)
Increased effect/toxicity with anticholinergics, disopyramide, narcotic analgesics, bretylium, type I antiarrhythmics, antihistamines, phenothiazines, TCAs, corticosteroids (increased IOP), CNS depressants (sedation), adenosine, amiodarone, beta-blockers, amoxapine

Dietary Considerations Should be taken 30 minutes before meals so that the drug's peak effect occurs at the proper time. The tablet (15 mg) contains lactose 23.2 mg.

Pharmacodynamics/Kinetics
Onset of action: 30-45 minutes
Duration: 4-6 hours
Half-life elimination, serum: Average: 1.6 hours

Pregnancy Risk Factor C

Lactation Excretion in breast milk unknown
(Continued)

Propantheline *(Continued)*

Breast-Feeding Considerations No data reported; however, atropine may be taken while breast-feeding.

Dosage Forms Tablet, as bromide: 15 mg [contains lactose 23.2 mg]

Propantheline Bromide *see* Propantheline *on page 1295*
Propa pH [OTC] *see* Salicylic Acid *on page 1374*

Proparacaine *(proe PAR a kane)*

U.S. Brand Names Alcaine®; Ophthetic®
Canadian Brand Names Alcaine®; Diocaine®
Generic Available Yes
Synonyms Proparacaine Hydrochloride; Proxymetacaine
Pharmacologic Category Local Anesthetic, Ophthalmic
Use Anesthesia for tonometry, gonioscopy; suture removal from cornea; removal of corneal foreign body; cataract extraction, glaucoma surgery; short operative procedure involving the cornea and conjunctiva
Local Anesthetic/Vasoconstrictor Precautions No information available to require special precautions
Effects on Dental Treatment No significant effects or complications reported
Mechanism of Action Prevents initiation and transmission of impulse at the nerve cell membrane by decreasing ion permeability through stabilizing
Pregnancy Risk Factor C

Proparacaine and Fluorescein
(proe PAR a kane & FLURE e seen)

Related Information
Proparacaine *on page 1296*
U.S. Brand Names Flucaine®; Fluoracaine®
Generic Available Yes
Synonyms Fluorescein and Proparacaine
Pharmacologic Category Diagnostic Agent; Local Anesthetic
Use Anesthesia for tonometry, gonioscopy; suture removal from cornea; removal of corneal foreign body; cataract extraction, glaucoma surgery
Local Anesthetic/Vasoconstrictor Precautions No information available to require special precautions
Effects on Dental Treatment No significant effects or complications reported
Common Adverse Effects 1% to 10%: Local: Burning, stinging of eye
Mechanism of Action Prevents initiation and transmission of impulse at the nerve cell membrane by decreasing ion permeability through stabilizing
Pharmacodynamics/Kinetics
Onset of action: ~20 seconds
Duration: 15-20 minutes
Pregnancy Risk Factor C

Proparacaine Hydrochloride *see* Proparacaine *on page 1296*
Propecia® *see* Finasteride *on page 655*
Propine® *see* Dipivefrin *on page 489*
Proplex® T *see* Factor IX Complex (Human) *on page 633*

Propofol *(PROE po fole)*

U.S. Brand Names Diprivan®
Canadian Brand Names Diprivan®
Mexican Brand Names Diprivan®; Fresofol®; Recofol®
Generic Available Yes
Pharmacologic Category General Anesthetic
Use Induction of anesthesia for inpatient or outpatient surgery in patients ≥3 years of age; maintenance of anesthesia for inpatient or outpatient surgery in patients >2 months of age; in adults, for the induction and maintenance of monitored anesthesia care sedation during diagnostic procedures; treatment of agitation in intubated, mechanically-ventilated ICU patients
Unlabeled/Investigational Use Postoperative antiemetic; refractory delirium tremens (case reports); conscious sedation
Local Anesthetic/Vasoconstrictor Precautions No information available to require special precautions
Effects on Dental Treatment No significant effects or complications reported

Common Adverse Effects

>10%:

Cardiovascular: Hypotension (children 17%, adults 3% to 26%)

Central nervous system: Dystonic or choreiform movement (children 17%)

Local: Injection site burning, stinging, or pain (children 10%, adults 18%)

Respiratory: Apnea lasting 30-60 seconds (children 10%, adults 24%); apnea lasting >60 seconds (children 5%, adults 12%)

1% to 10%:

Cardiovascular: Hypertension (children 8%), arrhythmia, bradycardia, cardiac output decreased, tachycardia

Central nervous system: Movement (adults)

Dermatologic: Pruritus (children 2%), rash (children 5%)

Endocrine & metabolic: Hyperlipidemia, hypertriglyceridemia

Respiratory: Respiratory acidosis during weaning

Mechanism of Action Propofol is a hindered phenolic compound with intravenous general anesthetic properties. The drug is unrelated to any of the currently used barbiturate, opioid, benzodiazepine, arylcyclohexylamine, or imidazole intravenous anesthetic agents.

Drug Interactions

Cytochrome P450 Effect: Substrate of CYP1A2 (minor), 2A6 (minor), 2B6 (major), 2C8/9 (major), 2C19 (minor), 2D6 (minor), 2E1 (minor), 3A4 (minor); **Inhibits** CYP1A2 (moderate), 2C8/9 (weak), 2C19 (moderate), 2D6 (weak), 2E1 (weak), 3A4 (strong)

Increased Effect/Toxicity: Additive CNS depression and respiratory depression may necessitate dosage reduction when used with anesthetics, benzodiazepines, opiates, ethanol, narcotics, phenothiazines. The levels/effects of propofol may be increased by delavirdine, desipramine, fluconazole, gemfibrozil, ketoconazole, nicardipine, NSAIDs, paroxetine, sertraline, sulfonamides, and other inhibitors of CYP2B6 or 2C8/9.

Propofol may potentiate the neuromuscular blockade of vecuronium (and possibly other neuromuscular-blocking agents). Propofol may increase the levels/effects of aminophylline, benzodiazepines, calcium channel blockers, cyclosporine, fluvoxamine, selected HMG-CoA reductase inhibitors, mexiletine, mirtazapine, nateglinide, nefazodone, ropinirole, sildenafil (and other PDE-5 inhibitors) tacrolimus, theophylline, trifluoperazine, venlafaxine, and other CYP1A2 or 3A4 substrates. Selected benzodiazepines (midazolam and triazolam), cisapride, ergot alkaloids, selected HMG-CoA reductase inhibitors (lovastatin and simvastatin), and pimozide are generally contraindicated with strong CYP3A4 inhibitors.

Pharmacodynamics/Kinetics

Onset of action: Anesthetic: Bolus infusion (dose dependent): 9-51 seconds (average 30 seconds)

Duration (dose and rate dependent): 3-10 minutes

Distribution: V_d: 2-10 L/kg; highly lipophilic

Protein binding: 97% to 99%

Metabolism: Hepatic to water-soluble sulfate and glucuronide conjugates

Half-life elimination: Biphasic: Initial: 40 minutes; Terminal: 4-7 hours (up to 1-3 days)

Excretion: Urine (~88% as metabolites, 40% as glucuronide metabolite); feces (<2%)

Clearance: 20-30 mL/kg/minute; total body clearance exceeds liver blood flow

Pregnancy Risk Factor B

Propoxyphene (proe POKS i feen)

U.S. Brand Names Darvon®; Darvon-N®

Canadian Brand Names Darvon-N®; 642® Tablet

Generic Available Yes: Capsule

Synonyms Dextropropoxyphene; Propoxyphene Hydrochloride; Propoxyphene Napsylate

Pharmacologic Category Analgesic, Narcotic

Use Management of mild to moderate pain

Local Anesthetic/Vasoconstrictor Precautions No information available to require special precautions

Effects on Dental Treatment Key adverse event(s) related to dental treatment: Xerostomia (normal salivary flow resumes upon discontinuation).

Common Adverse Effects Frequency not defined.

Cardiovascular: Hypotension, bundle branch block

(Continued)

Propoxyphene *(Continued)*

Central nervous system: Dizziness, lightheadedness, sedation, paradoxical excitement and insomnia, fatigue, drowsiness, mental depression, hallucinations, paradoxical CNS stimulation, increased intracranial pressure, nervousness, headache, restlessness, malaise, confusion, dysphoria, vertigo

Dermatologic: Rash, urticaria

Endocrine & metabolic: Hypoglycemia, urinary 17-OHCS decreased

Gastrointestinal: Anorexia, stomach cramps, xerostomia, biliary spasm, nausea, vomiting, constipation, paralytic ileus, abdominal pain

Genitourinary: Urination decreased, ureteral spasms

Hepatic: LFTs increased, jaundice

Neuromuscular & skeletal: Weakness

Ocular: Visual disturbances

Respiratory: Dyspnea

Miscellaneous: Psychologic and physical dependence with prolonged use, histamine release, hypersensitivity reaction

Restrictions C-IV

Mechanism of Action Propoxyphene is a weak narcotic analgesic which acts through binding to opiate receptors to inhibit ascending pain pathways. Propoxyphene, as with other narcotic (opiate) analgesics, blocks pain perception in the cerebral cortex by binding to specific receptor molecules (opiate receptors) within the neuronal membranes of synapses. This binding results in a decreased synaptic chemical transmission throughout the CNS thus inhibiting the flow of pain sensations into the higher centers. Mu and kappa are the two subtypes of the opiate receptor which propoxyphene binds to cause analgesia.

Drug Interactions

Cytochrome P450 Effect: Inhibits CYP2C9 (weak), 2D6 (weak), 3A4 (weak)

Increased Effect/Toxicity: CNS depressants (phenothiazines, tranquilizers, anxiolytics, sedatives, hypnotics, or alcohol) may potentiate pharmacologic effects. Propoxyphene may inhibit the metabolism and increase the serum concentrations of carbamazepine, phenobarbital, MAO inhibitors, tricyclic antidepressants, and warfarin.

Decreased Effect: Decreased effect with cigarette smoking.

Pharmacodynamics/Kinetics

Onset of action: 0.5-1 hour

Duration: 4-6 hours

Metabolism: Hepatic to active metabolite (norpropoxyphene) and inactive metabolites; first-pass effect

Half-life elimination: Adults: Parent drug: 6-12 hours; Norpropoxyphene: 30-36 hours

Excretion: Urine (primarily as metabolites)

Pregnancy Risk Factor C/D (prolonged use)

Propoxyphene and Acetaminophen

(proe POKS i feen & a seet a MIN oh fen)

Related Information

Acetaminophen *on page 31*

Propoxyphene *on page 1297*

Related Sample Prescriptions

Moderate/Moderately Severe Oral Pain *on page 1734*

U.S. Brand Names Balacet 325™; Darvocet A500™; Darvocet-N® 50; Darvocet-N® 100; Pronap-100®

Canadian Brand Names Darvocet-N® 50; Darvocet-N® 100

Generic Available Yes

Synonyms Acetaminophen and Propoxyphene; Propoxyphene Hydrochloride and Acetaminophen; Propoxyphene Napsylate and Acetaminophen

Pharmacologic Category Analgesic Combination (Narcotic)

Dental Use Management of postoperative pain

Use Management of mild to moderate pain

Local Anesthetic/Vasoconstrictor Precautions No information available to require special precautions

Effects on Dental Treatment Key adverse event(s) related to dental treatment: Xerostomia (normal salivary flow resumes upon discontinuation). See Dental Comment.

Significant Adverse Effects See individual agents.

Restrictions C-IV

Dental Usual Dosing Postoperative pain: Adults: Oral:

Darvocet A500™, Darvocet-N® 100: 1 tablet every 4 hours as needed; maximum: 600 mg propoxyphene napsylate/day

Darvocet-N® 50: 1-2 tablets every 4 hours as needed; maximum: 600 mg propoxyphene napsylate/day

Note: Dosage of acetaminophen should not exceed 4 g/day (6 tablets of Darvocet-N® 100); possibly less in patients with ethanol

Dosage Oral: Adults:

Darvocet A500™, Darvocet-N® 100: 1 tablet every 4 hours as needed; maximum: 600 mg propoxyphene napsylate/day

Darvocet-N® 50: 1-2 tablets every 4 hours as needed; maximum: 600 mg propoxyphene napsylate/day

Note: Dosage of acetaminophen should not exceed 4 g/day (6 tablets of Darvocet-N® 100); possibly less in patients with ethanol

Elderly: Refer to Adults dosing

Dosing adjustment in renal/hepatic impairment: Serum concentrations of propoxyphene may be increased or elimination may be delayed; specific dosing recommendations not available.

Mechanism of Action

Propoxyphene is a weak narcotic analgesic which acts through binding to opiate receptors to inhibit ascending pain pathways

Propoxyphene, as with other narcotic (opiate) analgesics, blocks pain perception in the cerebral cortex by binding to specific receptor molecules (opiate receptors) within the neuronal membranes of synapses. This binding results in a decreased synaptic chemical transmission throughout the CNS thus inhibiting the flow of pain sensations into the higher centers. Mu and kappa are the two subtypes of the opiate receptor to which propoxyphene binds to cause analgesia.

Acetaminophen inhibits the synthesis of prostaglandins in the CNS and peripherally blocks pain impulse generation; produces antipyresis from inhibition of hypothalamic heat-regulating center

Contraindications Hypersensitivity to propoxyphene, acetaminophen, or any component of the formulation

Warnings/Precautions When given in excessive doses, either alone or in combination with other CNS depressants, propoxyphene is a major cause of drug-related deaths; do not exceed recommended dosage; give with caution in patients dependent on opiates, substitution may result in acute opiate withdrawal symptoms. Avoid use in severely-depressed or suicidal patients. Tolerance or drug dependence may result from extended use.

Propoxyphene should be used with caution in patients with renal or hepatic dysfunction or in the elderly; consider dosing adjustment. Acetaminophen should be used with caution in patients with liver disease; consuming ≥3 alcoholic drinks/day may increase risk of liver damage. Use caution in patients with known G6PD deficiency. Safety and efficacy of this combination have not been established in pediatric patients.

Drug Interactions

Propoxyphene: **Inhibits** CYP2C9 (weak), 2D6 (weak), 3A4 (weak)

Acetaminophen: **Substrate** (minor) of CYP1A2, 2A6, 2C9, 2D6, 2E1, 3A4; **Inhibits** CYP3A4 (weak)

Also see individual agents.

Ethanol/Nutrition/Herb Interactions

Based on **propoxyphene** component:

Ethanol: Avoid or limit ethanol (may increase CNS depression). Watch for sedation.

Food: May decrease rate of absorption, but may slightly increase bioavailability.

Based on **acetaminophen** component:

Ethanol: Excessive intake of ethanol may increase the risk of acetaminophen-induced hepatotoxicity. Avoid ethanol or limit to <3 drinks/day.

Food: Rate of absorption may be decreased when given with food.

Herb/Nutraceutical: St John's wort may decrease acetaminophen levels.

Dietary Considerations May be taken with food if gastrointestinal distress occurs.

Pharmacodynamics/Kinetics See individual agents.

Pregnancy Risk Factor C

Lactation Enters breast milk/compatible

Breast-Feeding Considerations Propoxyphene, norpropoxyphene and acetaminophen are excreted in breast milk. The AAP considers propoxyphene and acetaminophen to be "compatible" with breast-feeding.

Dosage Forms

Tablet: Propoxyphene hydrochloride 65 mg and acetaminophen 650 mg, propoxyphene napsylate 100 mg, and acetaminophen 650 mg

(Continued)

Propoxyphene and Acetaminophen (Continued)

Balacet 325™: Propoxyphene napsylate 100 mg and acetaminophen 325 mg

Darvocet A500™: Propoxyphene napsylate 100 mg and acetaminophen 500 mg [contains lactose]

Darvocet-N® 50: Propoxyphene napsylate 50 mg and acetaminophen 325 mg

Darvocet-N® 100, Pronap-100®: Propoxyphene napsylate 100 mg and acetaminophen 650 mg

Dental Comment Propoxyphene is a narcotic analgesic and shares many properties including addiction liability. The acetaminophen component requires use with caution in patients with alcoholic liver disease.

Selected Readings

Botting RM, "Mechanism of Action of Acetaminophen: Is There a Cyclooxygenase 3?" *Clin Infect Dis*, 2000, Suppl 5:S202-10.

Dart RC, Kuffner EK, and Rumack BH, "Treatment of Pain or Fever with Paracetamol (Acetaminophen) in the Alcoholic Patient: A Systematic Review," *Am J Ther*, 2000, 7(2):123-34.

Grant JA and Weiler JM, "A Report of a Rare Immediate Reaction After Ingestion of Acetaminophen," *Ann Allergy Asthma Immunol*, 2001, 87(3):227-9.

Kwan D, Bartle WR, and Walker SE, "The Effects of Acetaminophen on Pharmacokinetics and Pharmacodynamics of Warfarin," *J Clin Pharmacol*, 1999, 39(1):68-75.

McClain CJ, Price S, Barve S, et al, "Acetaminophen Hepatotoxicity: An Update," *Curr Gastroenterol Rep*, 1999, 1(1):42-9.

Shek KL, Chan LN, and Nutescu E, "Warfarin-Acetaminophen Drug Interaction Revisited," *Pharmacotherapy*, 1999, 19(10):1153-8.

Tanaka E, Yamazaki K, and Misawa S, "Update: The Clinical Importance of Acetaminophen Hepatotoxicity in Nonalcoholic and Alcoholic Subjects," *J Clin Pharm Ther*, 2000, 25(5):325-32.

Propoxyphene, Aspirin, and Caffeine

(proe POKS i feen, AS pir in, & KAF een)

Related Information

Aspirin *on page 145*
Caffeine *on page 245*
Propoxyphene *on page 1297*

U.S. Brand Names Darvon® Compound [DSC]

Generic Available No

Synonyms Aspirin, Caffeine, and Propoxyphene; Caffeine, Propoxyphene, and Aspirin; Propoxyphene Hydrochloride, Aspirin, and Caffeine

Pharmacologic Category Analgesic Combination (Narcotic)

Dental Use Treatment of mild-to-moderate pain

Use Treatment of mild-to-moderate pain

Local Anesthetic/Vasoconstrictor Precautions No information available to require special precautions

Effects on Dental Treatment Key adverse event(s) related to dental treatment: As with all drugs which may affect hemostasis, bleeding is associated with aspirin. Hemorrhage may occur at virtually any site; risk is dependent on multiple variables including dosage, concurrent use of multiple agents which alter hemostasis, and patient susceptibility. Many adverse effects of aspirin are dose-related, and are rare at low dosages. Other serious reactions are idiosyncratic, related to allergy or individual sensitivity. See Dental Comment.

Elderly are a high-risk population for adverse effects from nonsteroidal anti-inflammatory agents. As many as 60% of elderly patients with GI complications from NSAIDs can develop peptic ulceration and/or hemorrhage asymptomatically. Concomitant disease and drug use contribute to the risk of GI adverse effects. Use lowest effective dose for shortest period possible. Consider renal function decline with age.

Significant Adverse Effects See individual agents.

Restrictions C-IV

Dental Usual Dosing Pain: Adults: Oral: One capsule (providing propoxyphene 65 mg) every 4 hours as needed; maximum propoxyphene 390 mg/day. This will also provide aspirin 389 mg and caffeine 32.4 mg per capsule.

Dosage Oral: Adults: Pain: One capsule (providing propoxyphene 65 mg) every 4 hours as needed; maximum propoxyphene 390 mg/day. This will also provide aspirin 389 mg and caffeine 32.4 mg per capsule.

Elderly: Refer to Adults dosing; consider increasing dosing interval

Dosage adjustment in renal impairment: Serum concentrations of propoxyphene may be increased or elimination may be delayed; specific dosing recommendations not available. Avoid use with Cl_{cr} <10 mL/minute.

Dosage adjustment in hepatic impairment: Serum concentrations or propoxyphene may be increased or elimination may be delayed; specific dosing recommendations not available.

Mechanism of Action Propoxyphene is a weak narcotic analgesic which acts through binding to opiate receptors to inhibit ascending pain pathways. Propoxyphene, as with other narcotic (opiate) analgesics, blocks pain perception in the cerebral cortex by binding to specific receptor molecules (opiate receptors) within the neuronal membranes of synapses. This binding results in a decreased synaptic chemical transmission throughout the CNS thus inhibiting the flow of pain sensations into the higher centers. Mu and kappa are the two subtypes of the opiate receptor to which propoxyphene binds to cause analgesia.

Aspirin inhibits prostaglandin synthesis, acts on the hypothalamus heat-regulating center to reduce fever, blocks prostaglandin synthetase action which prevents formation of the platelet-aggregating substance thromboxane A_2.

Caffeine is a CNS stimulant; use with propoxyphene and aspirin increases the level of analgesia provided by each agent.

Contraindications Hypersensitivity to propoxyphene, aspirin, caffeine, or any component of the formulation

Warnings/Precautions When given in excessive doses, either alone or in combination with other CNS depressants, propoxyphene is a major cause of drug-related deaths; do not exceed recommended dosage; give with caution in patients dependent on opiates, substitution may result in acute opiate withdrawal symptoms. Avoid use in severely-depressed or suicidal patients. Tolerance or drug dependence may result from extended use. Propoxyphene should be used with caution in patients with renal or hepatic dysfunction or in the elderly; consider dosing adjustment

Aspirin should be used with caution in patients with ulcers or coagulation abnormalities. Patients with sensitivity to tartrazine dyes, nasal polyps and asthma may have an increased risk of salicylate sensitivity. Surgical patients should avoid ASA if possible, for 1-2 weeks prior to surgery, to reduce the risk of excessive bleeding. Heavy ethanol use (≥3 drinks/day) can increase bleeding risks. Aspirin should be avoided in children (<16 years of age) with viral infections (chickenpox or flu symptoms), with or without fever, due to a potential association with Reye's syndrome. Safety and efficacy of this combination product in children have not been established.

Drug Interactions See individual agents for Propoxyphene and Aspirin.

Ethanol/Nutrition/Herb Interactions Based on **propoxyphene** component:
Ethanol: Avoid or limit ethanol (may increase CNS depression). Watch for sedation.
Food: May decrease rate of absorption, but may slightly increase bioavailability.

Pharmacodynamics/Kinetics See individual agents.

Pregnancy Risk Factor C

Lactation Enters breast milk/use caution

Breast-Feeding Considerations Propoxyphene, norpropoxyphene, aspirin, and caffeine are excreted in breast milk. The AAP recommends that aspirin be used "with caution" during breast-feeding; propoxyphene and caffeine (moderate intake) are considered "compatible."

Dosage Forms [DSC] = Discontinued product
Capsule (Darvon® Compound 65): Propoxyphene hydrochloride 65 mg, aspirin 389 mg, and caffeine 32.4 mg [DSC]

Dental Comment Propoxyphene is a narcotic analgesic and shares many properties including addiction liability. The aspirin component could have anticoagulant effects and could possibly affect bleeding times.

Propoxyphene Hydrochloride see Propoxyphene on page 1297

Propoxyphene Hydrochloride and Acetaminophen see Propoxyphene and Acetaminophen on page 1298

Propoxyphene Hydrochloride, Aspirin, and Caffeine see Propoxyphene, Aspirin, and Caffeine on page 1300

Propoxyphene Napsylate see Propoxyphene on page 1297

Propoxyphene Napsylate and Acetaminophen see Propoxyphene and Acetaminophen on page 1298

Propranolol (proe PRAN oh lole)

Related Information
Cardiovascular Diseases on page 1636
Endocrine Disorders and Pregnancy on page 1659

U.S. Brand Names Inderal®; Inderal® LA; InnoPran XL™

Canadian Brand Names Apo-Propranolol®; Inderal®; Inderal®-LA; Novo-Pranol; Nu-Propranolol

Generic Available Yes: Excludes capsule

(Continued)

Propranolol *(Continued)*

Synonyms Propranolol Hydrochloride

Pharmacologic Category Antiarrhythmic Agent, Class II; Beta-Adrenergic Blocker, Nonselective

Use Management of hypertension; angina pectoris; pheochromocytoma; essential tremor; tetralogy of Fallot cyanotic spells; arrhythmias (such as atrial fibrillation and flutter, AV nodal re-entrant tachycardias, and catecholamine-induced arrhythmias); prevention of myocardial infarction; migraine headache; symptomatic treatment of hypertrophic subaortic stenosis

Unlabeled/Investigational Use Tremor due to Parkinson's disease; ethanol withdrawal; aggressive behavior; antipsychotic-induced akathisia; prevention of bleeding esophageal varices; anxiety; schizophrenia; acute panic; gastric bleeding in portal hypertension; thyrotoxicosis

Local Anesthetic/Vasoconstrictor Precautions Use with caution; epinephrine has interacted with nonselective beta-blockers to result in initial hypertensive episode followed by bradycardia

Effects on Dental Treatment Propranolol is a nonselective beta-blocker and may enhance the pressor response to epinephrine, resulting in hypertension and bradycardia. Many nonsteroidal anti-inflammatory drugs, such as ibuprofen and indomethacin, can reduce the hypotensive effect of beta-blockers after 3 or more weeks of therapy with the NSAID. Short-term NSAID use (ie, 3 days) requires no special precautions in patients taking beta-blockers.

Common Adverse Effects Frequency not defined.

Cardiovascular: Bradycardia, CHF, reduced peripheral circulation, chest pain, hypotension, impaired myocardial contractility, worsening of AV conduction disturbance, cardiogenic shock, Raynaud's syndrome, mesenteric thrombosis (rare)

Central nervous system: Mental depression, lightheadedness, amnesia, emotional lability, confusion, hallucinations, dizziness, insomnia, fatigue, vivid dreams, lethargy, cold extremities, vertigo, syncope, cognitive dysfunction, psychosis, hypersomnolence

Dermatologic: Alopecia, contact dermatitis, eczematous eruptions, erythema multiforme, exfoliative dermatitis, hyperkeratosis, nail changes, pruritus, psoriasiform eruptions, rash, ulcerative lichenoid, urticaria, Stevens-Johnson syndrome, toxic epidermal necrolysis

Endocrine & metabolic: Hypoglycemia, hyperglycemia, hyperlipidemia, hyperkalemia

Gastrointestinal: Diarrhea, nausea, vomiting, stomach discomfort, constipation, anorexia

Genitourinary: Impotence, proteinuria (rare), oliguria (rare), interstitial nephritis (rare), Peyronie's disease

Hematologic: Agranulocytosis, thrombocytopenia, thrombocytopenic purpura

Neuromuscular & skeletal: Weakness, carpal tunnel syndrome (rare), paresthesia, myotonus, polyarthritis, arthropathy

Ocular: Hyperemia of the conjunctiva, decreased tear production, decreased visual acuity, mydriasis

Respiratory: Wheezing, pharyngitis, bronchospasm, pulmonary edema, respiratory distress, laryngospasm

Miscellaneous: Lupus-like syndrome (rare), anaphylactic/anaphylactoid allergic reaction

Dosage

Akathisia: Oral: Adults: 30-120 mg/day in 2-3 divided doses

Angina: Oral: Adults: 80-320 mg/day in doses divided 2-4 times/day

Long-acting formulation: Initial: 80 mg once daily; maximum dose: 320 mg once daily

Essential tremor: Oral: Adults: 20-40 mg twice daily initially; maintenance doses: usually 120-320 mg/day

Hypertension:

Oral:

Children: Initial: 0.5-1 mg/kg/day in divided doses every 6-12 hours; increase gradually every 5-7 days; maximum: 16 mg/kg/24 hours

Adults: Initial: 40 mg twice daily; increase dosage every 3-7 days; usual dose: ≤320 mg divided in 2-3 doses/day; maximum daily dose: 640 mg; usual dosage range (JNC 7): 40-160 mg/day in 2 divided doses

Long-acting formulation: Initial: 80 mg once daily; usual maintenance: 120-160 mg once daily; maximum daily dose: 640 mg; usual dosage range (JNC 7): 60-180 mg/day once daily

I.V.: Children: 0.01-0.05 mg/kg over 1 hour; maximum dose: 10 mg

Hypertrophic subaortic stenosis: Oral: Adults: 20-40 mg 3-4 times/day

Long-acting formulation: 80-160 mg once daily

Migraine headache prophylaxis: Oral:

Children: Initial: 2-4 mg/kg/day **or**

≤35 kg: 10-20 mg 3 times/day
>35 kg: 20-40 mg 3 times/day

Adults: Initial: 80 mg/day divided every 6-8 hours; increase by 20-40 mg/dose every 3-4 weeks to a maximum of 160-240 mg/day given in divided doses every 6-8 hours; if satisfactory response not achieved within 6 weeks of starting therapy, drug should be withdrawn gradually over several weeks
Long-acting formulation: Initial: 80 mg once daily; effective dose range: 160-240 mg once daily

Myocardial infarction prophylaxis: Oral: Adults: 180-240 mg/day in 3-4 divided doses

Pheochromocytoma: Oral: Adults: 30-60 mg/day in divided doses

Tachyarrhythmias:
Oral:
Children: Initial: 0.5-1 mg/kg/day in divided doses every 6-8 hours; titrate dosage upward every 3-7 days; usual dose: 2-6 mg/kg/day; higher doses may be needed; do not exceed 16 mg/kg/day or 60 mg/day
Adults: 10-30 mg/dose every 6-8 hours
Elderly: Initial: 10 mg twice daily; increase dosage every 3-7 days; usual dosage range: 10-320 mg given in 2 divided doses
I.V.:
Children: 0.01-0.1 mg/kg/dose slow IVP over 10 minutes; maximum dose: 1 mg for infants; 3 mg for children
Adults (in patients having nonfunctional GI tract): 1 mg/dose slow IVP; repeat every 5 minutes up to a total of 5 mg; titrate initial dose to desired response

Tetralogy spells: Children:
Oral: Palliation: Initial: 1 mg/kg/day every 6 hours; if ineffective, may increase dose after 1 week by 1 mg/kg/day to a maximum of 5 mg/kg/day; if patient becomes refractory, may increase slowly to a maximum of 10-15 mg/kg/day. Allow 24 hours between dosing changes.
I.V.: 0.01-0.2 mg/kg/dose infused over 10 minutes; maximum initial dose: 1 mg

Thyrotoxicosis:
Oral:
Children: 2 mg/kg/day, divided every 6-8 hours, titrate to effective dose
Adolescents and Adults: Oral: 10-40 mg/dose every 6 hours
I.V.: Adults: 1-3 mg/dose slow IVP as a single dose

Dosing adjustment/comments in renal impairment:
Not dialyzable (0% to 5%); supplemental dose is not necessary.
Peritoneal dialysis effects: Supplemental dose is not necessary.

Dosing adjustment/comments in hepatic disease: Marked slowing of heart rate may occur in cirrhosis with conventional doses; low initial dose and regular heart rate monitoring

Mechanism of Action Nonselective beta-adrenergic blocker (class II antiarrhythmic); competitively blocks response to beta$_1$- and beta$_2$-adrenergic stimulation which results in decreases in heart rate, myocardial contractility, blood pressure, and myocardial oxygen demand

Contraindications Hypersensitivity to propranolol, beta-blockers, or any component of the formulation; uncompensated congestive heart failure (unless the failure is due to tachyarrhythmias being treated with propranolol); cardiogenic shock, bradycardia or heart block (2nd or 3rd degree), pulmonary edema, severe hyperactive airway disease (asthma or COPD), Raynaud's disease; pregnancy (2nd and 3rd trimesters)

Warnings/Precautions Administer cautiously in compensated heart failure and monitor for a worsening of the condition (efficacy of propranolol in CHF has not been demonstrated). Beta-blocker therapy should not be withdrawn abruptly (particularly in patients with CAD), but gradually tapered (over 2 weeks) to avoid acute tachycardia, hypertension, and/or ischemia. Use caution in patient with PVD. Use caution with concurrent use of beta-blockers and either verapamil or diltiazem; bradycardia or heart block can occur. Avoid concurrent I.V. use of both agents. Use cautiously in diabetics because it can mask prominent hypoglycemic symptoms. Can mask signs of thyrotoxicosis. Can cause fetal harm when administered in pregnancy. Use cautiously in hepatic dysfunction (dosage adjustment required). Use care with anesthetic agents which decrease myocardial function. Not indicated for hypertensive emergencies.

Drug Interactions
Cytochrome P450 Effect: Substrate of CYP1A2 (major), 2C19 (minor), 2D6 (major), 3A4 (minor); **Inhibits** CYP1A2 (weak), 2D6 (weak)
Increased Effect/Toxicity: CYP1A2 inhibitors may increase the levels/effects of propranolol; example inhibitors include amiodarone, ciprofloxacin, fluvoxamine, ketoconazole, norfloxacin, ofloxacin, and rofecoxib. CYP2D6 inhibitors may increase the levels/effects of propranolol; example inhibitors
(Continued)

Propranolol *(Continued)*

include chlorpromazine, delavirdine, fluoxetine, miconazole, paroxetine, pergolide, quinidine, quinine, ritonavir, and ropinirole. The heart rate-lowering effects of propranolol are additive with other drugs which slow AV conduction (digoxin, verapamil, diltiazem). Reserpine increases the effects of propranolol. Concurrent use of propranolol may increase the effects of alpha-blockers (prazosin, terazosin), alpha-adrenergic stimulants (epinephrine, phenylephrine), and the vasoconstrictive effects of ergot alkaloids. Propranolol may mask the tachycardia from hypoglycemia caused by insulin and oral hypoglycemics. In patients receiving concurrent therapy, the risk of hypertensive crisis is increased when either clonidine or the beta-blocker is withdrawn. Beta-blockers may increase the action or levels of ethanol, disopyramide, nondepolarizing muscle relaxants, and theophylline although the effects are difficult to predict. Propranolol may increase the bioavailability of serotonin 5-HT$_{1D}$ receptor agonists. Propranolol may decrease the metabolism of lidocaine.

Beta-blocker effects may be enhanced by oral contraceptives, flecainide, haloperidol (hypotensive effects), cimetidine, hydralazine, phenothiazines, propafenone, thyroid hormones (when hypothyroid patient is converted to euthyroid state). Beta-blockers may increase the effect/toxicity of flecainide, haloperidol (hypotensive effects), hydralazine, phenothiazines, acetaminophen, anticoagulants (warfarin), and benzodiazepines.

Decreased Effect: CYP1A2 inducers may decrease the levels/effects of propranolol; example inducers include aminoglutethimide, carbamazepine, phenobarbital, and rifampin. Aluminum salts, calcium salts, cholestyramine, colestipol, NSAIDs, penicillins (ampicillin), salicylates, and sulfinpyrazone decrease effect of beta-blockers due to decreased bioavailability and plasma levels. Beta-blockers may decrease the effect of sulfonylureas. Ascorbic acid decreases propranolol Cp_{max} and AUC and increases the T_{max} significantly resulting in a greater decrease in the reduction of heart rate, possibly due to decreased absorption and first pass metabolism (n=5). Nefazodone decreased peak plasma levels and AUC of propranolol and increases time to reach steady-state; monitoring of clinical response is recommended. Nonselective beta-blockers blunt the response to beta-2 adrenergic agonists (albuterol).

Ethanol/Nutrition/Herb Interactions

Ethanol: Ethanol may decrease plasma levels of propranolol by increasing metabolism.

Food: Propranolol serum levels may be increased if taken with food. Protein-rich foods may increase bioavailability; a change in diet from high carbohydrate/low protein to low carbohydrate/high protein may result in increased oral clearance.

Cigarette: Smoking may decrease plasma levels of propranolol by increasing metabolism.

Herb/Nutraceutical: Avoid dong quai if using for hypertension (has estrogenic activity). Avoid ephedra, yohimbe, ginseng (may worsen hypertension or arrhythmia). Avoid natural licorice (causes sodium and water retention and increases potassium loss). Avoid garlic (may have increased antihypertensive effect).

Dietary Considerations Tablets should be taken on an empty stomach; capsules may be taken with or without food, but should always be taken consistently (with food or on an empty stomach)

Pharmacodynamics/Kinetics

Onset of action: Beta-blockade: Oral: 1-2 hours

Duration: ~6 hours

Distribution: V_d: 3.9 L/kg in adults; crosses placenta; small amounts enter breast milk

Protein binding: Newborns: 68%; Adults: 93%

Metabolism: Hepatic to active and inactive compounds; extensive first-pass effect

Bioavailability: 30% to 40%; may be increased in Down syndrome

Half-life elimination: Neonates and Infants: Possible increased half-life; Children: 3.9-6.4 hours; Adults: 4-6 hours

Excretion: Urine (96% to 99%)

Pregnancy Risk Factor C (manufacturer); D (2nd and 3rd trimesters - expert analysis)

Dosage Forms CAP, extended release (InnPran™): 80 mg, 120 mg. **CAP, sustained release** (Inderal® LA): 60 mg, 80 mg, 120 mg, 160 mg. **INJ, solution** (Inderal®): 1 mg/mL (1 mL). **SOLN, oral:** 4 mg/mL (5 mL, 500 mL); 8 mg/mL (500 mL). **TAB** (Inderal®): 10 mg, 20 mg, 40 mg, 60 mg, 80 mg

Selected Readings

Foster CA and Aston SJ, "Propranolol-Epinephrine Interaction: A Potential Disaster," *Plast Reconstr Surg*, 1983, 72(1):74-8.

Wong DG, Spence JD, Lamki L, et al, "Effect of Nonsteroidal Anti-Inflammatory Drugs on Control of Hypertension of Beta-Blockers and Diuretics," *Lancet*, 1986, 1(8488):997-1001.

Wynn RL, "Dental Nonsteroidal Anti-Inflammatory Drugs and Prostaglandin-Based Drug Interactions, Part Two," *Gen Dent*, 1992, 40(2):104, 106, 108.

Wynn RL, "Epinephrine Interactions With Beta-Blockers," *Gen Dent*, 1994, 42(1):16, 18.

Propranolol and Hydrochlorothiazide
(proe PRAN oh lole & hye droe klor oh THYE a zide)

Related Information
Hydrochlorothiazide *on page 776*
Propranolol *on page 1301*

U.S. Brand Names Inderide®

Generic Available Yes

Synonyms Hydrochlorothiazide and Propranolol

Pharmacologic Category Antihypertensive Agent, Combination

Use Management of hypertension

Local Anesthetic/Vasoconstrictor Precautions Use with caution; epinephrine has interacted with nonselective beta-blockers to result in initial hypertensive episode followed by bradycardia

Effects on Dental Treatment Noncardioselective beta-blockers (ie, propranolol, nadolol) enhance the pressor response to epinephrine, resulting in hypertension and bradycardia. Many nonsteroidal anti-inflammatory drugs, such as ibuprofen and indomethacin, can reduce the hypotensive effect of beta-blockers after 3 or more weeks of therapy with the NSAID. Short-term NSAID use (ie, 3 days) requires no special precautions in patients taking beta-blockers.

Common Adverse Effects See individual agents.

Drug Interactions
Cytochrome P450 Effect: Propranolol: **Substrate** of CYP1A2 (major), 2C19 (major), 2D6 (major), 3A4 (minor); **Inhibits** CYP1A2 (weak), 2D6 (weak)

Pharmacodynamics/Kinetics See individual agents.

Pregnancy Risk Factor C

Propranolol Hydrochloride *see Propranolol on page 1301*

Proprinal [OTC] *see Ibuprofen on page 808*

Proprinal® Cold and Sinus [OTC] *see Pseudoephedrine and Ibuprofen on page 1311*

Propulsid® *see Cisapride on page 348*

Propylene Glycol Diacetate, Acetic Acid, and Hydrocortisone *see Acetic Acid, Propylene Glycol Diacetate, and Hydrocortisone on page 45*

Propylhexedrine (proe pil HEKS e dreen)

U.S. Brand Names Benzedrex® [OTC]

Generic Available No

Pharmacologic Category Adrenergic Agonist Agent

Use Topical nasal decongestant

Local Anesthetic/Vasoconstrictor Precautions No information available to require special precautions

Effects on Dental Treatment No significant effects or complications reported

2-Propylpentanoic Acid *see Valproic Acid and Derivatives on page 1556*

Propylthiouracil (proe pil thye oh YOOR a sil)

Related Information
Endocrine Disorders and Pregnancy *on page 1659*

Canadian Brand Names Propyl-Thyracil®

Generic Available Yes

Synonyms PTU (error-prone abbreviation)

Pharmacologic Category Antithyroid Agent

Use Palliative treatment of hyperthyroidism as an adjunct to ameliorate hyperthyroidism in preparation for surgical treatment or radioactive iodine therapy; management of thyrotoxic crisis

Local Anesthetic/Vasoconstrictor Precautions No information available to require special precautions

Effects on Dental Treatment No significant effects or complications reported

Common Adverse Effects Frequency not defined.

(Continued)

Propylthiouracil (Continued)

Cardiovascular: Edema, cutaneous vasculitis, leukocytoclastic vasculitis, ANCA-positive vasculitis

Central nervous system: Fever, drowsiness, vertigo, headache, drug fever, dizziness, neuritis

Dermatologic: Skin rash, urticaria, pruritus, exfoliative dermatitis, alopecia, erythema nodosum

Endocrine & metabolic: Goiter, weight gain, swollen salivary glands

Gastrointestinal: Nausea, vomiting, loss of taste perception, stomach pain, constipation

Hematologic: Leukopenia, agranulocytosis, thrombocytopenia, bleeding, aplastic anemia

Hepatic: Cholestatic jaundice, hepatitis

Neuromuscular & skeletal: Arthralgia, paresthesia

Renal: Nephritis, glomerulonephritis, acute renal failure

Respiratory: Interstitial pneumonitis, alveolar hemorrhage

Miscellaneous: SLE-like syndrome

Mechanism of Action Inhibits the synthesis of thyroid hormones by blocking the oxidation of iodine in the thyroid gland; blocks synthesis of thyroxine and triiodothyronine

Drug Interactions

Increased Effect/Toxicity: Propylthiouracil may increase the anticoagulant activity of warfarin.

Decreased Effect: Oral anticoagulant activity is increased only until metabolic effect stabilizes. Anticoagulants may be potentiated by antivitamin K effect of propylthiouracil. Correction of hyperthyroidism may alter disposition of beta-blockers, digoxin, and theophylline, necessitating a dose reduction of these agents.

Pharmacodynamics/Kinetics

Onset of action: Therapeutic: 24-36 hours

Peak effect: Remission: 4 months of continued therapy

Duration: 2-3 hours

Distribution: Concentrated in the thyroid gland

Protein binding: 75% to 80%

Metabolism: Hepatic

Bioavailability: 80% to 95%

Half-life elimination: 1.5-5 hours; End-stage renal disease: 8.5 hours

Time to peak, serum: ~1 hour

Excretion: Urine (35%)

Pregnancy Risk Factor D

2-Propylvaleric Acid see Valproic Acid and Derivatives on page 1556

ProQuad® see Measles, Mumps, Rubella, and Varicella Virus Vaccine on page 967

Proquin® XR see Ciprofloxacin on page 343

Proscar® see Finasteride on page 655

ProSom® see Estazolam on page 573

Prostacyclin see Epoprostenol on page 553

Prostacyclin PGI₂ see Iloprost on page 816

Prostaglandin E₁ see Alprostadil on page 76

Prostaglandin E₂ see Dinoprostone on page 482

Prostin E₂® see Dinoprostone on page 482

Prostin VR Pediatric® see Alprostadil on page 76

Protamine Sulfate (PROE ta meen SUL fate)

Generic Available Yes

Pharmacologic Category Antidote

Use Treatment of heparin overdosage; neutralize heparin during surgery or dialysis procedures

Unlabeled/Investigational Use Treatment of low molecular weight heparin (LMWH) overdose

Local Anesthetic/Vasoconstrictor Precautions No information available to require special precautions

Effects on Dental Treatment No significant effects or complications reported

Common Adverse Effects Frequency not defined.

Cardiovascular: Sudden fall in blood pressure, bradycardia, flushing, hypotension

Central nervous system: Lassitude

Gastrointestinal: Nausea, vomiting

Hematologic: Hemorrhage
Respiratory: Dyspnea, pulmonary hypertension
Miscellaneous: Hypersensitivity reactions

Mechanism of Action Combines with strongly acidic heparin to form a stable complex (salt) neutralizing the anticoagulant activity of both drugs

Pharmacodynamics/Kinetics Onset of action: I.V.: Heparin neutralization: ~5 minutes

Pregnancy Risk Factor C

Protein C (Activated), Human, Recombinant see Drotrecogin Alfa on page 522

Protein-Bound Paclitaxel see Paclitaxel (Protein Bound) on page 1177

Prothrombin Complex Concentrate see Factor IX Complex (Human) on page 633

Protirelin (proe TYE re lin)

U.S. Brand Names Thyrel® TRH [DSC]
Canadian Brand Names Relefact® TRH
Generic Available No
Synonyms Lopremone; Thyrotropin Releasing Hormone; TRH
Pharmacologic Category Diagnostic Agent
Use Adjunct in the diagnostic assessment of thyroid function, and an adjunct to other diagnostic procedures in patients with pituitary or hypothalamic dysfunction; also causes release of prolactin from the pituitary and is used to detect defective control of prolactin secretion

Local Anesthetic/Vasoconstrictor Precautions No information available to require special precautions

Effects on Dental Treatment Key adverse event(s) related to dental treatment: Xerostomia (normal salivary flow resumes upon discontinuation).

Common Adverse Effects
>10%:
  Central nervous system: Headache, lightheadedness
  Dermatologic: Flushing of face
  Gastrointestinal: Nausea, xerostomia
  Genitourinary: Urge to urinate
1% to 10%:
  Central nervous system: Anxiety
  Endocrine & metabolic: Breast enlargement and leaking in lactating women
  Gastrointestinal: Bad taste in mouth, abdominal discomfort
  Neuromuscular & skeletal: Tingling
  Miscellaneous: Diaphoresis

Mechanism of Action Increase release of thyroid stimulating hormone from the anterior pituitary

Drug Interactions
  Decreased Effect: Aspirin, levodopa, thyroid hormones, adrenocorticoid drugs

Pharmacodynamics/Kinetics
  Onset of action: Peak effect: TSH: 20-30 minutes
  Duration: TSH returns to baseline after ~3 hours
  Half-life elimination, serum: Mean plasma: 5 minutes

Pregnancy Risk Factor C

Protonix® see Pantoprazole on page 1184
Protopic® see Tacrolimus on page 1437

Protriptyline (proe TRIP ti leen)

U.S. Brand Names Vivactil®
Generic Available No
Synonyms Protriptyline Hydrochloride
Pharmacologic Category Antidepressant, Tricyclic (Secondary Amine)
Use Treatment of depression

Local Anesthetic/Vasoconstrictor Precautions Use with caution; epinephrine and levonordefrin have been shown to have an increased pressor response in combination with TCAs

Effects on Dental Treatment Key adverse event(s) related to dental treatment: Xerostomia and changes in salivation (normal salivary flow resumes upon discontinuation). Long-term treatment with TCAs, such as protriptyline, increases the risk of caries by reducing salivation and salivary buffer capacity.

Common Adverse Effects Frequency not defined.

(Continued)

Protriptyline *(Continued)*

Cardiovascular: Arrhythmias, hyper-/hypotension, MI, stroke, heart block, tachycardia, palpitation

Central nervous system: Dizziness, drowsiness, headache, confusion, delirium, hallucinations, restlessness, insomnia, nightmares, fatigue, delusions, anxiety, agitation, hypomania, exacerbation of psychosis, panic, seizure, incoordination, ataxia, EPS

Dermatologic: Alopecia, photosensitivity, rash, petechiae, urticaria, itching

Endocrine & metabolic: Breast enlargement, galactorrhea, SIADH, gynecomastia, increased or decreased libido

Gastrointestinal: Xerostomia, constipation, unpleasant taste, weight gain/loss, increased appetite, nausea, diarrhea, heartburn, vomiting, anorexia, trouble with gums, decreased lower esophageal sphincter tone may cause GE reflux

Genitourinary: Difficult urination, impotence, testicular edema

Hematologic: Agranulocytosis, leukopenia, eosinophilia, thrombocytopenia, purpura

Hepatic: Cholestatic jaundice, increased liver enzymes

Neuromuscular & skeletal: Fine muscle tremor, weakness, tremor, numbness, tingling

Ocular: Blurred vision, eye pain, increased intraocular pressure

Otic: Tinnitus

Miscellaneous: Diaphoresis (excessive), allergic reactions

Restrictions A medication guide concerning the use of antidepressants in children and teenagers can be found on the FDA website at http://www.fda.gov/cder/Offices/ODS/labeling.htm. It should be dispensed to parents or guardians of children and teenagers receiving this medication.

Mechanism of Action Increases the synaptic concentration of serotonin and/or norepinephrine in the central nervous system by inhibition of their reuptake by the presynaptic neuronal membrane

Drug Interactions

Cytochrome P450 Effect: Substrate of CYP2D6 (major)

Increased Effect/Toxicity: Protriptyline increases the effects of amphetamines, anticholinergics, other CNS depressants (sedatives, hypnotics, or ethanol), chlorpropamide, tolazamide, and warfarin. When used with MAO inhibitors, hyperpyrexia, hypertension, tachycardia, confusion, seizures, and **deaths have been reported** (serotonin syndrome). The SSRIs (to varying degrees), cimetidine, grapefruit juice, indinavir, methylphenidate, ritonavir, quinidine, diltiazem, and verapamil inhibit the metabolism of TCAs. Levels/effects of protriptyline may be increased by chlorpromazine, delavirdine, fluoxetine, miconazole, paroxetine, pergolide, quinidine, quinine, ritonavir, ropinirole, and other CYP2D6 inhibitors. Use of lithium with a TCA may increase the risk for neurotoxicity. Phenothiazines may increase concentration of some TCAs and TCAs may increase concentration of phenothiazines. Pressor response to I.V. epinephrine, norepinephrine, and phenylephrine may be enhanced in patients receiving TCAs (**Note:** Effect is unlikely with epinephrine or levonordefrin dosages typically administered as infiltration in combination with local anesthetics). Combined use of beta-agonists or drugs which prolong QT$_c$ (including quinidine, procainamide, disopyramide, cisapride, sparfloxacin, gatifloxacin, moxifloxacin) with TCAs may predispose patients to cardiac arrhythmias.

Decreased Effect: Carbamazepine, phenobarbital, and rifampin may increase the metabolism of protriptyline, decreasing its effects. Protriptyline inhibits the antihypertensive response to bethanidine, clonidine, debrisoquin, guanadrel, guanethidine, guanabenz, guanfacine. Cimetidine and methylphenidate may decrease the metabolism of protriptyline. Cholestyramine and colestipol may bind TCAs and reduce their absorption.

Pharmacodynamics/Kinetics

Distribution: Crosses placenta

Protein binding: 92%

Metabolism: Extensively hepatic via N-oxidation, hydroxylation, and glucuronidation; first-pass effect (10% to 25%)

Half-life elimination: 54-92 hours (average: 74 hours)

Time to peak, serum: 24-30 hours

Excretion: Urine

Pregnancy Risk Factor C

Protriptyline Hydrochloride *see* Protriptyline *on page 1307*

Proventil® *see* Albuterol *on page 58*

Proventil® HFA *see* Albuterol *on page 58*

Provera® *see* MedroxyPROGESTERone *on page 972*

Provigil® *see* Modafinil *on page 1057*

Provisc® *see* Hyaluronate and Derivatives *on page 773*

Proxymetacaine *see* Proparacaine *on page 1296*

Prozac® *see* Fluoxetine *on page 675*

Prozac® Weekly™ *see* Fluoxetine *on page 675*

PRP-OMP *see Haemophilus* b Conjugate Vaccine *on page 534*

PRP-T *see Haemophilus* b Conjugate Vaccine *on page 534*

Prudoxin™ *see* Doxepin *on page 505*

Prussian Blue *see* Ferric Hexacyanoferrate *on page 650*

Prymaccone *see* Primaquine *on page 1281*

PS-341 *see* Bortezomib *on page 215*

Pseudoephedrine (soo doe e FED rin)

Related Information
Bacterial Infections *on page 1697*

U.S. Brand Names Biofed [OTC]; Contact® Cold [OTC]; Dimetapp® 12-Hour Non-Drowsy Extentabs® [OTC]; Dimetapp® Decongestant Infant [OTC]; Elix-Sure™ Congestion [OTC]; Genaphed® [OTC]; Kidkare Decongestant [OTC]; Kodet SE [OTC]; Oranyl [OTC]; PediaCare® Decongestant Infants [OTC]; Silfedrine Children's [OTC]; Simply Stuffy™ [OTC]; Sudafed® [OTC]; Sudafed® 12 Hour [OTC]; Sudafed® 24 Hour [OTC]; Sudafed® Children's [OTC]; Sudodrin [OTC]; SudoGest [OTC]; Sudo-Tab® [OTC]

Canadian Brand Names Balminil Decongestant; Benylin® D for Infants; Contac® Cold 12 Hour Relief Non Drowsy; Drixoral® ND; Eltor®; PMS-Pseudoephedrine; Pseudofrin; Robidrine®; Sudafed® Decongestant

Mexican Brand Names Lertamine-D®; Sudafed®

Generic Available Yes: Liquid, syrup, tablet

Synonyms *d*-Isoephedrine Hydrochloride; Pseudoephedrine Hydrochloride; Pseudoephedrine Sulfate

Pharmacologic Category Alpha/Beta Agonist

Dental Use Temporary symptomatic relief of nasal congestion due to common cold, upper respiratory allergies, and sinusitis; also promotes nasal or sinus drainage

Use Temporary symptomatic relief of nasal congestion due to common cold, upper respiratory allergies, and sinusitis; also promotes nasal or sinus drainage

Local Anesthetic/Vasoconstrictor Precautions Use with caution since pseudoephedrine is a sympathomimetic amine which could interact with epinephrine to cause a pressor response

Effects on Dental Treatment Key adverse event(s) related to dental treatment: Xerostomia (normal salivary flow resumes upon discontinuation).

Significant Adverse Effects Frequency not defined.
Cardiovascular: Tachycardia, palpitation, arrhythmia
Central nervous system: Nervousness, transient stimulation, insomnia, excitability, dizziness, drowsiness, convulsions, hallucinations, headache
Gastrointestinal: Nausea, vomiting
Genitourinary: Dysuria
Neuromuscular & skeletal: Weakness, tremor
Respiratory: Dyspnea
Miscellaneous: Diaphoresis

Dosage Oral: General dosing guidelines:
Children:
    <2 years: 4 mg/kg/day in divided doses every 6 hours
    2-5 years: 15 mg every 4-6 hours; maximum: 60 mg/24 hours
    6-12 years: 30 mg every 4-6 hours; maximum: 120 mg/24 hours
Adults: 30-60 mg every 4-6 hours, sustained release: 120 mg every 12 hours; maximum: 240 mg/24 hours
Dosing adjustment in renal impairment: Reduce dose

Mechanism of Action Directly stimulates alpha-adrenergic receptors of respiratory mucosa causing vasoconstriction; directly stimulates beta-adrenergic receptors causing bronchial relaxation, increased heart rate and contractility

Contraindications Hypersensitivity to pseudoephedrine or any component of the formulation; with or within 14 days of MAO inhibitor therapy

Warnings/Precautions Use with caution in patients >60 years of age; administer with caution to patients with hypertension, hyperthyroidism, diabetes mellitus, cardiovascular disease, ischemic heart disease, increased intraocular pressure, or prostatic hyperplasia. Elderly patients are more likely to experience adverse reactions to sympathomimetics. Overdosage may cause hallucinations, seizures, CNS depression, and death. When used for self-medication (OTC), notify healthcare provider if symptoms do not improve within 7 days or are accompanied by fever.
(Continued)

Pseudoephedrine *(Continued)*

Drug Interactions

Decreased effect of methyldopa, reserpine

Increased toxicity: MAO inhibitors may increase blood pressure effects of pseudoephedrine; propranolol, sympathomimetic agents may increase toxicity

Ethanol/Nutrition/Herb Interactions

Food: Onset of effect may be delayed if pseudoephedrine is taken with food.

Herb/Nutraceutical: Avoid ephedra, yohimbe (may cause hypertension).

Dietary Considerations Should be taken with water or milk to decrease GI distress.

Pharmacodynamics/Kinetics

Onset of action: Decongestant: Oral: 15-30 minutes

Duration: Immediate release tablet: 4-6 hours; Extended release: ≤12 hours

Absorption: Rapid

Metabolism: Partially hepatic

Half-life elimination: 9-16 hours

Excretion: Urine (70% to 90% as unchanged drug, 1% to 6% as active norpseudoephedrine); dependent on urine pH and flow rate; alkaline urine decreases renal elimination of pseudoephedrine

Pregnancy Risk Factor C

Lactation Enters breast milk/use caution (AAP rates "compatible")

Dosage Forms

Caplet, extended release, as hydrochloride (Contact® Cold, Sudafed® 12 Hour): 120 mg

Liquid, as hydrochloride: 30 mg/5 mL (120 mL, 480 mL)

Silfedrine Children's: 15 mg/5 mL (120 mL, 480 mL) [alcohol and sugar free; grape flavor]

Simply Stuffy™: 15 mg/5 mL (120 mL) [alcohol free; contains sodium benzoate; cherry berry flavor]

Sudafed® Children's: 15 mg/5 mL (120 mL) [alcohol and sugar free; contains sodium benzoate; grape flavor]

Liquid, oral drops, as hydrochloride:

Dimetapp® Decongestant Infant Drops: 7.5 mg/0.8 mL (15 mL) [alcohol free; contains sodium benzoate; grape flavor]

Kidkare Decongestant: 7.5 mg/0.8 mL (30 mL) [alcohol free; contains benzoic acid and sodium benzoate; cherry flavor]

PediaCare® Decongestant: 7.5 mg/0.8 mL (15 mL) [alcohol free, dye free; contains benzoic acid, sodium benzoate; fruit flavor]

Syrup, as hydrochloride:

Biofed: 30 mg/5 mL (120 mL, 240 mL, 480 mL, 3840 mL) [alcohol free; contains sodium benzoate]

ElixSure™ Congestion: 15 mg/5 mL (120 mL) [grape bubble gum flavor]

Tablet, as hydrochloride: 30 mg, 60 mg

Genaphed®, Kodet SE, Oranyl, Sudafed®, Sudodrin, Sudo-Tab®: 30 mg

SudoGest: 30 mg, 60 mg

Tablet, chewable, as hydrochloride (Sudafed® Children's): 15 mg [sugar free; contains phenylalanine 0.78 mg/tablet; orange flavor]

Tablet, extended release, as hydrochloride:

Dimetapp® 12-Hour Non-Drowsy Extentabs®: 120 mg

Sudafed® 24 Hour: 240 mg

Pseudoephedrine, Acetaminophen, and Chlorpheniramine *see* Acetaminophen, Chlorpheniramine, and Pseudoephedrine *on page 43*

Pseudoephedrine, Acetaminophen, and Dextromethorphan *see* Acetaminophen, Dextromethorphan, and Pseudoephedrine *on page 44*

Pseudoephedrine and Acetaminophen *see* Acetaminophen and Pseudoephedrine *on page 38*

Pseudoephedrine and Brompheniramine *see* Brompheniramine and Pseudoephedrine *on page 223*

Pseudoephedrine and Carbinoxamine *see* Carbinoxamine and Pseudoephedrine *on page 268*

Pseudoephedrine and Chlorpheniramine *see* Chlorpheniramine and Pseudoephedrine *on page 325*

Pseudoephedrine and Desloratadine *see* Desloratadine and Pseudoephedrine *on page 436*

Pseudoephedrine and Dexbrompheniramine *see* Dexbrompheniramine and Pseudoephedrine *on page 442*

Pseudoephedrine and Dextromethorphan
(soo doe e FED rin & deks troe meth OR fan)

Related Information
Dextromethorphan *on page 451*
Pseudoephedrine *on page 1309*

U.S. Brand Names Dimetapp® Infant Decongestant Plus Cough [OTC]; Pedia-Care® Children's Long Acting Cough Plus Cold [OTC]; PediaCare® Infants' Decongestant & Cough [OTC]; Pedia Relief Cough and Cold [OTC]; Pedia Relief Infants [OTC]; Robitussin® Maximum Strength Cough & Cold [OTC]; Robitussin® Pediatric Cough & Cold [OTC]; Sudafed® Children's Cold & Cough [OTC]; SudoGest Children's [OTC]; Triaminic® Cough [OTC]; Triaminic® Cough & Nasal Congestion [OTC]; Vicks® 44D Cough & Head Congestion [OTC]

Canadian Brand Names Balminil DM D; Benylin® DM-D; Koffex DM-D; Novahistex® DM Decongestant; Novahistine® DM Decongestant; Robitussin® Childrens Cough & Cold

Generic Available Yes: Excludes chewable tablet

Synonyms Dextromethorphan and Pseudoephedrine

Pharmacologic Category Antitussive/Decongestant

Use Temporary symptomatic relief of nasal congestion and cough due to common cold, hay fever, upper respiratory allergies

Local Anesthetic/Vasoconstrictor Precautions Use with caution since pseudoephedrine is a sympathomimetic amine which could interact with epinephrine to cause a pressor response

Effects on Dental Treatment Key adverse event(s) related to dental treatment: Pseudoephedrine: Xerostomia (normal salivary flow resumes upon discontinuation).

Common Adverse Effects See individual agents.

Drug Interactions
Cytochrome P450 Effect: Dextromethorphan: **Substrate** of CYP2B6 (minor), 2C9 (minor), 2C19 (minor), 2D6 (major), 2E1 (minor), 3A4 (minor); **Inhibits** CYP2D6 (weak)

Increased Effect/Toxicity: Based on **pseudoephedrine** component: MAO inhibitors may increase blood pressure effects of pseudoephedrine. Sympathomimetic agents may increase toxicity.

Decreased Effect: Based on **pseudoephedrine** component: Decreased effect of methyldopa, reserpine.

Pharmacodynamics/Kinetics See individual agents.

Pseudoephedrine and Diphenhydramine *see* Diphenhydramine and Pseudoephedrine *on page 487*

Pseudoephedrine and Fexofenadine *see* Fexofenadine and Pseudoephedrine *on page 653*

Pseudoephedrine and Guaifenesin *see* Guaifenesin and Pseudoephedrine *on page 755*

Pseudoephedrine and Hydrocodone *see* Hydrocodone and Pseudoephedrine *on page 788*

Pseudoephedrine and Ibuprofen
(soo doe e FED rin & eye byoo PROE fen)

Related Information
Ibuprofen *on page 808*
Pseudoephedrine *on page 1309*

U.S. Brand Names Advil® Cold & Sinus [OTC]; Advil® Cold, Children's [OTC]; Dristan® Sinus [OTC]; Motrin® Cold and Sinus [OTC]; Motrin® Cold, Children's [OTC]; Proprinal® Cold and Sinus [OTC]

Canadian Brand Names Advil® Cold & Sinus; Children's Advil® Cold; Sudafed® Sinus Advance

Generic Available Yes: Caplet

Synonyms Ibuprofen and Pseudoephedrine

Pharmacologic Category Decongestant/Analgesic

Use For temporary relief of cold, sinus and flu symptoms (including nasal congestion, headache, sore throat, minor body aches and pains, and fever)

Local Anesthetic/Vasoconstrictor Precautions Use with caution since pseudoephedrine is a sympathomimetic amine which could interact with epinephrine to cause a pressor response

Effects on Dental Treatment Key adverse event(s) related to dental treatment: Pseudoephedrine: Xerostomia (normal salivary flow resumes upon discontinuation).
(Continued)

Pseudoephedrine and Ibuprofen *(Continued)*

Common Adverse Effects See individual agents.

Drug Interactions

Cytochrome P450 Effect: Ibuprofen: **Substrate** (minor) of CYP2C8/9, 2C19; **Inhibits** CYP2C8/9 (strong)

Increased Effect/Toxicity: See individual agents.

Decreased Effect: See individual agents.

Pharmacodynamics/Kinetics See individual agents.

Pregnancy Risk Factor Ibuprofen: B/D (3rd trimester)

Pseudoephedrine and Loratadine *see* Loratadine and Pseudoephedrine *on page 947*

Pseudoephedrine and Triprolidine *see* Triprolidine and Pseudoephedrine *on page 1542*

Pseudoephedrine, Carbinoxamine, and Dextromethorphan *see* Carbinoxamine, Pseudoephedrine, and Dextromethorphan *on page 269*

Pseudoephedrine, Chlorpheniramine, and Acetaminophen *see* Acetaminophen, Chlorpheniramine, and Pseudoephedrine *on page 43*

Pseudoephedrine, Chlorpheniramine, and Codeine *see* Chlorpheniramine, Pseudoephedrine, and Codeine *on page 329*

Pseudoephedrine, Chlorpheniramine, and Dihydrocodeine *see* Pseudoephedrine, Dihydrocodeine, and Chlorpheniramine *on page 1312*

Pseudoephedrine, Codeine, and Triprolidine *see* Triprolidine, Pseudoephedrine, and Codeine *on page 1543*

Pseudoephedrine, Dextromethorphan, and Acetaminophen *see* Acetaminophen, Dextromethorphan, and Pseudoephedrine *on page 44*

Pseudoephedrine, Dextromethorphan, and Carbinoxamine *see* Carbinoxamine, Pseudoephedrine, and Dextromethorphan *on page 269*

Pseudoephedrine, Dextromethorphan, and Guaifenesin *see* Guaifenesin, Pseudoephedrine, and Dextromethorphan *on page 757*

Pseudoephedrine, Dihydrocodeine, and Chlorpheniramine

(soo doe e FED rin, dye hye droe KOE, & klor fen IR a meen)

Related Information

Chlorpheniramine *on page 323*

Pseudoephedrine *on page 1309*

U.S. Brand Names DiHydro-CP; Hydro-Tussin™ DHC; Pancof®; Uni-Cof

Generic Available Yes

Synonyms Chlorpheniramine, Pseudoephedrine, and Dihydrocodeine; Dihydrocodeine Bitartrate, Pseudoephedrine Hydrochloride, and Chlorpheniramine Maleate; Pseudoephedrine, Chlorpheniramine, and Dihydrocodeine

Pharmacologic Category Antihistamine/Decongestant/Antitussive

Use Temporary relief of cough, congestion, and sneezing due to colds, respiratory infections, or hay fever

Local Anesthetic/Vasoconstrictor Precautions Use with caution since pseudoephedrine is a sympathomimetic amine which could interact with epinephrine to cause a pressor response

Effects on Dental Treatment Key adverse event(s) related to dental treatment:

Chlorpheniramine: Prolonged use will cause significant xerostomia (normal salivary flow resumes upon discontinuation).

Pseudoephedrine: Xerostomia (prolonged use worsens; normal salivary flow resumes upon discontinuation).

Common Adverse Effects See individual agents.

Restrictions C-III

Mechanism of Action

Pseudoephedrine: Directly stimulates alpha-adrenergic receptors of respiratory mucosa causing vasoconstriction; directly stimulates beta-adrenergic receptors causing bronchial relaxation

Dihydrocodeine: Binds to opiate receptors in the CNS; suppresses cough in medullary center

Chlorpheniramine: Competes with histamine for H_1-receptor sites on effector cells in the gastrointestinal tract, blood vessels, and respiratory tract

Drug Interactions

Cytochrome P450 Effect:

Dihydrocodeine: **Substrate** of CYP2D6 (major)

Chlorpheniramine: **Substrate** of CYP2D6 (minor), 3A4 (major); **Inhibits** CYP2D6 (weak).

Increased Effect/Toxicity: Also see individual agents. CYP3A4 inhibitors may increase the levels/effects of chlorpheniramine (example inhibitors include azole antifungals, clarithromycin, diclofenac, doxycycline, erythromycin, imatinib, isoniazid, nefazodone, nicardipine, propofol, protease inhibitors, quinidine, telithromycin, and verapamil).

Decreased Effect: Also see individual agents. CYP2D6 inhibitors may decrease the effects of dihydrocodeine (example inhibitors include chlorpromazine, delavirdine, fluoxetine, miconazole, paroxetine, pergolide, quinidine, quinine, ritonavir, and ropinirole).

Pharmacodynamics/Kinetics See individual agents.

Pregnancy Risk Factor C

Pseudoephedrine, Guaifenesin, and Codeine *see* Guaifenesin, Pseudoephedrine, and Codeine *on page 756*

Pseudoephedrine Hydrochloride *see* Pseudoephedrine *on page 1309*

Pseudoephedrine Hydrochloride and Acrivastine *see* Acrivastine and Pseudoephedrine *on page 47*

Pseudoephedrine Hydrochloride and Cetirizine Hydrochloride *see* Cetirizine and Pseudoephedrine *on page 307*

Pseudoephedrine Hydrochloride, Guaifenesin, and Dihydrocodeine Bitartrate *see* Dihydrocodeine, Pseudoephedrine, and Guaifenesin *on page 476*

Pseudoephedrine, Hydrocodone, and Carbinoxamine *see* Hydrocodone, Carbinoxamine, and Pseudoephedrine *on page 789*

Pseudoephedrine, Hydrocodone, and Guaifenesin *see* Hydrocodone, Pseudoephedrine, and Guaifenesin *on page 792*

Pseudoephedrine Sulfate *see* Pseudoephedrine *on page 1309*

Pseudoephedrine Tannate and Dexchlorpheniramine Tannate *see* Dexchlorpheniramine and Pseudoephedrine *on page 443*

Pseudoephedrine, Triprolidine, and Codeine *see* Triprolidine, Pseudoephedrine, and Codeine *on page 1543*

Pseudo GG TR *see* Guaifenesin and Pseudoephedrine *on page 755*

Pseudomonic Acid A *see* Mupirocin *on page 1073*

Pseudovent™ *see* Guaifenesin and Pseudoephedrine *on page 755*

Pseudovent™ 400 *see* Guaifenesin and Pseudoephedrine *on page 755*

Pseudovent™ DM *see* Guaifenesin, Pseudoephedrine, and Dextromethorphan *on page 757*

Pseudovent™-Ped *see* Guaifenesin and Pseudoephedrine *on page 755*

Psorcon® e™ *see* Diflorasone *on page 468*

Psoriatec™ *see* Anthralin *on page 128*

PsoriGel® [OTC] [DSC] *see* Coal Tar *on page 383*

Psyllium (SIL i yum)

U.S. Brand Names Fiberall®; Fibro-Lax [OTC]; Fibro-XL [OTC]; Genfiber® [OTC]; Hydrocil® Instant [OTC]; Konsyl® [OTC]; Konsyl-D® [OTC]; Konsyl® Easy Mix [OTC]; Konsyl® Orange [OTC]; Metamucil® [OTC]; Metamucil® Plus Calcium [OTC]; Metamucil® Smooth Texture [OTC]; Modane® Bulk [OTC]; Natural Fiber Therapy [OTC]; Reguloid® [OTC]; Serutan® [OTC]

Canadian Brand Names Metamucil®

Generic Available Yes: Capsule, powder

Synonyms Plantago Seed; Plantain Seed; Psyllium Hydrophilic Mucilloid

Pharmacologic Category Antidiarrheal; Laxative, Bulk-Producing

Use Treatment of chronic atonic or spastic constipation and in constipation associated with rectal disorders; management of irritable bowel syndrome; labeled for OTC use as fiber supplement, treatment of constipation

Local Anesthetic/Vasoconstrictor Precautions No information available to require special precautions

Effects on Dental Treatment No significant effects or complications reported

Common Adverse Effects Frequency not defined.

Gastrointestinal: Esophageal or bowel obstruction, diarrhea, constipation, abdominal cramps

Respiratory: Bronchospasm

Miscellaneous: Anaphylaxis upon inhalation in susceptible individuals, rhinoconjunctivitis

Mechanism of Action Adsorbs water in the intestine to form a viscous liquid which promotes peristalsis and reduces transit time

Drug Interactions

Decreased Effect: Decreased effect of warfarin, digitalis, potassium-sparing diuretics, salicylates, tetracyclines, nitrofurantoin when taken together. Separate administration times to reduce potential for drug-drug interaction.

(Continued)

Psyllium *(Continued)*

Pharmacodynamics/Kinetics
Onset of action: 12-24 hours
Peak effect: 2-3 days
Absorption: None; small amounts of grain extracts present in the preparation have been reportedly absorbed following colonic hydrolysis

Pregnancy Risk Factor B

Psyllium Hydrophilic Mucilloid *see* Psyllium *on page 1313*

P.T.E.-4® *see* Trace Metals *on page 1513*

P.T.E.-5® *see* Trace Metals *on page 1513*

Pteroylglutamic Acid *see* Folic Acid *on page 697*

PTU (error-prone abbreviation) *see* Propylthiouracil *on page 1305*

Pulmicort Respules® *see* Budesonide *on page 224*

Pulmicort Turbuhaler® *see* Budesonide *on page 224*

Pulmozyme® *see* Dornase Alfa *on page 501*

Puralube® Tears [OTC] *see* Artificial Tears *on page 143*

Purge® [OTC] *see* Castor Oil *on page 279*

Purified Chick Embryo Cell *see* Rabies Virus Vaccine *on page 1329*

Purinethol® *see* Mercaptopurine *on page 995*

PVP-I *see* Povidone-Iodine *on page 1262*

Pyrantel Pamoate *(pi RAN tel PAM oh ate)*

U.S. Brand Names Pamix™ [OTC]; Pin-X® [OTC]; Reese's® Pinworm Medicine [OTC]

Canadian Brand Names Combantrin™

Mexican Brand Names Combantrin®

Generic Available No

Pharmacologic Category Anthelmintic

Use Treatment of pinworms (*Enterobius vermicularis*) and roundworms (*Ascaris lumbricoides*)

Unlabeled/Investigational Use Treatment of whipworms (*Trichuris trichiura*) and hookworms (*Ancylostoma duodenale*)

Local Anesthetic/Vasoconstrictor Precautions No information available to require special precautions

Effects on Dental Treatment No significant effects or complications reported

Common Adverse Effects Frequency not defined.
Central nervous system: Dizziness, drowsiness, insomnia, headache
Dermatologic: Rash
Gastrointestinal: Anorexia, nausea, vomiting, abdominal cramps, diarrhea, tenesmus
Hepatic: Elevated liver enzymes
Neuromuscular & skeletal: Weakness

Mechanism of Action Causes the release of acetylcholine and inhibits cholinesterase; acts as a depolarizing neuromuscular blocker, paralyzing the helminths

Drug Interactions
Decreased Effect: Decreased effect with piperazine

Pharmacodynamics/Kinetics
Absorption: Oral: Poor
Metabolism: Partially hepatic
Time to peak, serum: 1-3 hours
Excretion: Feces (50% as unchanged drug); urine (7% as unchanged drug)

Pregnancy Risk Factor C

Pyrazinamide *(peer a ZIN a mide)*

Related Information
Tuberculosis *on page 1673*

Canadian Brand Names Tebrazid™

Generic Available Yes

Synonyms Pyrazinoic Acid Amide

Pharmacologic Category Antitubercular Agent

Use Adjunctive treatment of tuberculosis in combination with other antituberculosis agents

Local Anesthetic/Vasoconstrictor Precautions No information available to require special precautions

Effects on Dental Treatment No significant effects or complications reported

Common Adverse Effects 1% to 10%:
Central nervous system: Malaise
Gastrointestinal: Nausea, vomiting, anorexia
Neuromuscular & skeletal: Arthralgia, myalgia

Mechanism of Action Converted to pyrazinoic acid in susceptible strains of *Mycobacterium* which lowers the pH of the environment; exact mechanism of action has not been elucidated

Drug Interactions
Increased Effect/Toxicity: Combination therapy with rifampin and pyrazinamide has been associated with severe and fatal hepatotoxic reactions.

Pharmacodynamics/Kinetics Bacteriostatic or bactericidal depending on drug's concentration at infection site

Absorption: Well absorbed
Distribution: Widely into body tissues and fluids including liver, lung, and CSF
Relative diffusion from blood into CSF: Adequate with or without inflammation (exceeds usual MICs)
CSF:blood level ratio: Inflamed meninges: 100%
Protein binding: 50%
Metabolism: Hepatic
Half-life elimination: 9-10 hours
Time to peak, serum: Within 2 hours
Excretion: Urine (4% as unchanged drug)

Pregnancy Risk Factor C

Pyrazinamide, Rifampin, and Isoniazid see Rifampin, Isoniazid, and Pyrazinamide on page 1348

Pyrazinoic Acid Amide see Pyrazinamide on page 1314

Pyrethrins and Piperonyl Butoxide
(pye RE thrins & pi PER oh nil byo TOKS ide)

U.S. Brand Names A-200® Maximum Strength [OTC]; Lice-Aid [OTC]; Licide® [OTC]; Pronto® Complete Lice Killing Kit [OTC]; Pronto® Plus Hair and Scalp Masque [OTC]; Pronto® Plus Mousse [OTC]; Pronto® Plus Warm Oil Treatment and Conditioner [OTC]; Pronto® Plus with Natural Extracts and Oils [OTC]; Pyrinyl Plus® [OTC]; RID® Maximum Strength [OTC]; Tisit® [OTC]; Tisit® Blue Gel [OTC]

Canadian Brand Names Pronto® Lice Control; R & C™ II; R & C™ Shampoo/Conditioner; RID® Mousse

Generic Available Yes: Shampoo

Synonyms Piperonyl Butoxide and Pyrethrins

Pharmacologic Category Antiparasitic Agent, Topical; Pediculocide; Shampoo, Pediculocide

Use Treatment of *Pediculus humanus* infestations (head lice, body lice, pubic lice and their eggs)

Local Anesthetic/Vasoconstrictor Precautions No information available to require special precautions

Effects on Dental Treatment No significant effects or complications reported

Common Adverse Effects Frequency not defined.
Dermatologic: Pruritus
Local: Burning, stinging, irritation with repeat use

Mechanism of Action Pyrethrins are derived from flowers that belong to the chrysanthemum family. The mechanism of action on the neuronal membranes of lice is similar to that of DDT. Piperonyl butoxide is usually added to pyrethrin to enhance the product's activity by decreasing the metabolism of pyrethrins in arthropods.

Pharmacodynamics/Kinetics
Onset of action: ~30 minutes
Absorption: Minimal
Metabolism: Via ester hydrolysis and hydroxylation

Pregnancy Risk Factor C

Pyridium® see Phenazopyridine on page 1220

Pyridostigmine (peer id oh STIG meen)

U.S. Brand Names Mestinon®; Mestinon® Timespan®; Regonol®
Canadian Brand Names Mestinon®; Mestinon®-SR
Generic Available Yes: Tablet
(Continued)

Pyridostigmine *(Continued)*

Synonyms Pyridostigmine Bromide

Pharmacologic Category Acetylcholinesterase Inhibitor

Use Symptomatic treatment of myasthenia gravis; antidote for nondepolarizing neuromuscular blockers

Military use: Pretreatment for Soman nerve gas exposure

Local Anesthetic/Vasoconstrictor Precautions No information available to require special precautions

Effects on Dental Treatment No significant effects or complications reported

Common Adverse Effects Frequency not defined.

Cardiovascular: Arrhythmias (especially bradycardia), hypotension, decreased carbon monoxide, tachycardia, AV block, nodal rhythm, nonspecific ECG changes, cardiac arrest, syncope, flushing

Central nervous system: Convulsions, dysarthria, dysphonia, dizziness, loss of consciousness, drowsiness, headache

Dermatologic: Skin rash, thrombophlebitis (I.V.), urticaria

Gastrointestinal: Hyperperistalsis, nausea, vomiting, salivation, diarrhea, stomach cramps, dysphagia, flatulence, abdominal pain

Genitourinary: Urinary urgency

Neuromuscular & skeletal: Weakness, fasciculations, muscle cramps, spasms, arthralgia, myalgia

Ocular: Small pupils, lacrimation, amblyopia

Respiratory: Increased bronchial secretions, laryngospasm, bronchiolar constriction, respiratory muscle paralysis, dyspnea, respiratory depression, respiratory arrest, bronchospasm

Miscellaneous: Diaphoresis (increased), anaphylaxis, allergic reactions

Mechanism of Action Inhibits destruction of acetylcholine by acetylcholinesterase which facilitates transmission of impulses across myoneural junction

Drug Interactions

Increased Effect/Toxicity: Increased effect of depolarizing neuromuscular blockers (succinylcholine). Increased toxicity with edrophonium. Increased bradycardia/hypotension with beta-blockers.

Decreased Effect: Neuromuscular blockade reversal effect of pyridostigmine may be decreased by aminoglycosides, quinolones, tetracyclines, bacitracin, colistin, polymyxin B, sodium colistimethate, quinidine, elevated serum magnesium concentrations.

Pharmacodynamics/Kinetics

Onset of action: Oral, I.M.: 15-30 minutes; I.V. injection: 2-5 minutes

Duration: Oral: Up to 6-8 hours (due to slow absorption); I.V.: 2-3 hours

Absorption: Oral: Very poor

Distribution: 19 ± 12 L

Metabolism: Hepatic

Bioavailability: 10% to 20%

Half-life elimination: 1-2 hours; Renal failure: ≤ 6 hours

Excretion: Urine (80% to 90% as unchanged drug)

Pregnancy Risk Factor B

Pyridostigmine Bromide *see* Pyridostigmine *on page 1315*

Pyridoxine *(peer i DOKS een)*

U.S. Brand Names Aminoxin® [OTC]

Generic Available Yes

Synonyms Pyridoxine Hydrochloride; Vitamin B_6

Pharmacologic Category Vitamin, Water Soluble

Use Prevention and treatment of vitamin B_6 deficiency, pyridoxine-dependent seizures in infants; adjunct to treatment of acute toxicity from isoniazid, cycloserine, or hydrazine overdose

Local Anesthetic/Vasoconstrictor Precautions No information available to require special precautions

Effects on Dental Treatment No significant effects or complications reported

Common Adverse Effects Frequency not defined.

Central nervous system: Headache, seizure (following very large I.V. doses), sensory neuropathy

Endocrine & metabolic: Decreased serum folic acid secretions

Gastrointestinal: Nausea

Hepatic: Increased AST

Neuromuscular & skeletal: Paresthesia

Miscellaneous: Allergic reactions

Mechanism of Action Precursor to pyridoxal, which functions in the metabolism of proteins, carbohydrates, and fats; pyridoxal also aids in the release of liver and muscle-stored glycogen and in the synthesis of GABA (within the central nervous system) and heme

Drug Interactions

Decreased Effect: Pyridoxine may decrease serum levels of levodopa, phenobarbital, and phenytoin (patients taking levodopa without carbidopa should avoid supplemental vitamin B$_6$ >5 mg per day, which includes multivitamin preparations).

Pharmacodynamics/Kinetics

Absorption: Enteral, parenteral: Well absorbed

Metabolism: Via 4-pyridoxic acid (active form) and other metabolites

Half-life elimination: 15-20 days

Excretion: Urine

Pregnancy Risk Factor A/C (dose exceeding RDA recommendation)

Pyridoxine, Folic Acid, and Cyanocobalamin *see* Folic Acid, Cyanocobalamin, and Pyridoxine *on page 697*

Pyridoxine Hydrochloride *see* Pyridoxine *on page 1316*

Pyrilamine, Phenylephrine, and Carbetapentane *see* Carbetapentane, Phenylephrine, and Pyrilamine *on page 267*

Pyrimethamine (peer i METH a meen)

U.S. Brand Names Daraprim®

Canadian Brand Names Daraprim®

Mexican Brand Names Daraprim®

Generic Available No

Pharmacologic Category Antimalarial Agent

Use Prophylaxis of malaria due to susceptible strains of plasmodia; used in conjunction with quinine and sulfadiazine for the treatment of uncomplicated attacks of chloroquine-resistant *P. falciparum* malaria; used in conjunction with fast-acting schizonticide to initiate transmission control and suppression cure; synergistic combination with sulfonamide in treatment of toxoplasmosis

Local Anesthetic/Vasoconstrictor Precautions No information available to require special precautions

Effects on Dental Treatment Key adverse event(s) related to dental treatment: Atrophic glossitis has been reported.

Common Adverse Effects Frequency not defined.

Cardiovascular: Arrhythmias (large doses)

Central nervous system: Depression, fever, insomnia, lightheadedness, malaise, seizure

Dermatologic: Abnormal skin pigmentation, dermatitis, erythema multiforme, rash, Stevens-Johnson syndrome, toxic epidermal necrolysis

Gastrointestinal: Anorexia, abdominal cramps, vomiting, diarrhea, xerostomia, atrophic glossitis

Genitourinary: Hematuria

Hematologic: Megaloblastic anemia, leukopenia, pancytopenia, thrombocytopenia, pulmonary eosinophilia

Miscellaneous: Anaphylaxis

Mechanism of Action Inhibits parasitic dihydrofolate reductase, resulting in inhibition of vital tetrahydrofolic acid synthesis

Drug Interactions

Cytochrome P450 Effect: Inhibits CYP2C8/9 (moderate), 2D6 (moderate)

Increased Effect/Toxicity: Serum levels of antipsychotic agents may be increased by pyrimethamine. Sulfonamides (synergy), methotrexate, TMP/SMZ, and zidovudine may increase the risk of bone marrow suppression. Pyrimethamine may increase the levels/effects of amiodarone, amphetamines, selected beta-blockers, dextromethorphan, fluoxetine, glimepiride, glipizide, lidocaine, mirtazapine, nateglinide, nefazodone, paroxetine, phenytoin, pioglitazone, risperidone, ritonavir, rosiglitazone, sertraline, thioridazine, tricyclic antidepressants, venlafaxine, warfarin, and other CYP2C8/9 or 2D6 substrates.

Decreased Effect: Pyrimethamine may decrease the levels/effects of CYP2D6 prodrug substrates (eg, codeine, hydrocodone, oxycodone, tramadol).

Pharmacodynamics/Kinetics

Onset of action: ~1 hour

Absorption: Well absorbed

Distribution: Widely, mainly in blood cells, kidneys, lungs, liver, and spleen; crosses into CSF; crosses placenta; enters breast milk

Protein binding: 80% to 87%

Metabolism: Hepatic

Half-life elimination: 80-95 hours

(Continued)

Pyrimethamine *(Continued)*

Time to peak, serum: 1.5-8 hours
Excretion: Urine (20% to 30% as unchanged drug)

Pregnancy Risk Factor C

Pyrimethamine and Sulfadoxine *see* Sulfadoxine and Pyrimethamine *on page 1424*

Pyrinyl Plus® [OTC] *see* Pyrethrins and Piperonyl Butoxide *on page 1315*

Pyrithione Zinc *(peer i THYE one zingk)*

U.S. Brand Names BetaMed [OTC]; DermaZinc™ [OTC]; DHS™ Zinc [OTC]; Head & Shoulders® Citrus Breeze [OTC]; Head & Shoulders® Classic Clean [OTC]; Head & Shoulders® Classic Clean 2-In-1 [OTC]; Head & Shoulders® Dry Scalp Care [OTC]; Head & Shoulders® Extra Volume [OTC]; Head & Shoulders® Leave-in Treatment [OTC]; Head & Shoulders® Refresh [OTC]; Head & Shoulders® Sensitive Care [OTC]; Head & Shoulders® Smooth & Silky 2-In-1 [OTC]; Skin Care™ [OTC]; Zincon® [OTC]; ZNP® Bar [OTC]

Mexican Brand Names ZNP®

Generic Available No

Pharmacologic Category Topical Skin Product

Use Relieves the itching, irritation and scalp flaking associated with dandruff and/or seborrheal dermatitis

Local Anesthetic/Vasoconstrictor Precautions No information available to require special precautions

Effects on Dental Treatment No significant effects or complications reported

Q-Bid DM *see* Guaifenesin and Dextromethorphan *on page 754*

Q-Dryl [OTC] *see* DiphenhydrAMINE *on page 483*

Q-Naftate [OTC] *see* Tolnaftate *on page 1506*

Q-Tussin [OTC] *see* Guaifenesin *on page 752*

Q-Tussin DM [OTC] *see* Guaifenesin and Dextromethorphan *on page 754*

Quaternium-18 Bentonite *see* Bentoquatam *on page 188*

Quazepam *(KWAY ze pam)*

U.S. Brand Names Doral®

Canadian Brand Names Doral®

Generic Available No

Pharmacologic Category Benzodiazepine

Use Treatment of insomnia

Local Anesthetic/Vasoconstrictor Precautions No information available to require special precautions

Effects on Dental Treatment Key adverse event(s) related to dental treatment: Xerostomia (normal salivary flow resumes upon discontinuation).

Common Adverse Effects Frequency not defined.

Cardiovascular: Palpitations

Central nervous system: Drowsiness, fatigue, ataxia, memory impairment, anxiety, depression, headache, confusion, nervousness, dizziness, incoordination, hypo- and hyperkinesia, agitation, euphoria, paranoid reaction, nightmares, abnormal thinking

Dermatologic: Dermatitis, pruritus, rash

Endocrine & metabolic: Decreased libido, menstrual irregularities

Gastrointestinal: Xerostomia, constipation, diarrhea, dyspepsia, anorexia, abnormal taste perception, nausea, vomiting, increased or decreased appetite, abdominal pain

Genitourinary: Impotence, incontinence

Hematologic: Blood dyscrasias

Neuromuscular & skeletal: Dysarthria, rigidity, tremor, muscle cramps, reflex slowing

Ocular: Blurred vision

Miscellaneous: Drug dependence

Restrictions C-IV

Mechanism of Action Binds to stereospecific benzodiazepine receptors on the postsynaptic GABA neuron at several sites within the central nervous system, including the limbic system, reticular formation. Enhancement of the inhibitory effect of GABA on neuronal excitability results by increased neuronal membrane permeability to chloride ions. This shift in chloride ions results in hyperpolarization (a less excitable state) and stabilization.

Drug Interactions
Cytochrome P450 Effect: Substrate of CYP3A4 (minor)
Increased Effect/Toxicity: Serum levels and/or toxicity of quazepam may be increased by cimetidine, ciprofloxacin, clarithromycin, clozapine, CNS depressants, diltiazem, disulfiram, digoxin, erythromycin, ethanol, fluconazole, fluoxetine, fluvoxamine, grapefruit juice, isoniazid, itraconazole, ketoconazole, labetalol, levodopa, loxapine, metoprolol, metronidazole, miconazole, nefazodone, omeprazole, phenytoin, rifabutin, rifampin, troleandomycin, valproic acid, and verapamil.

Pharmacodynamics/Kinetics
Absorption: Rapid
Protein binding: 95%
Half-life elimination, serum: Parent drug: 25-41 hours; Active metabolite: 40-114 hours

Pregnancy Risk Factor X

Quelicin® *see* Succinylcholine *on page 1419*

Quenalin [OTC] *see* DiphenhydrAMINE *on page 483*

Questran® *see* Cholestyramine Resin *on page 334*

Questran® Light *see* Cholestyramine Resin *on page 334*

Quetiapine (kwe TYE a peen)

U.S. Brand Names Seroquel®
Canadian Brand Names Seroquel®
Generic Available No
Synonyms Quetiapine Fumarate
Pharmacologic Category Antipsychotic Agent, Atypical
Use Treatment of schizophrenia; treatment of acute manic episodes associated with bipolar disorder (as monotherapy or in combination with lithium or valproate)
Unlabeled/Investigational Use Autism, psychosis (children)
Local Anesthetic/Vasoconstrictor Precautions No information available to require special precautions (see Dental Comment)
Effects on Dental Treatment No significant effects or complications reported
Common Adverse Effects
>10%:
  Central nervous system: Agitation, dizziness, headache, somnolence
  Endocrine & metabolic: Cholesterol increased (11%), triglycerides increased (17%)
  Gastrointestinal: Weight gain (≥7% body weight, dose related), xerostomia
1% to 10%:
  Cardiovascular: Postural hypotension, tachycardia, palpitation, peripheral edema
  Central nervous system: Anxiety, fever, pain
  Dermatologic: Rash
  Gastrointestinal: Abdominal pain (dose related), constipation, dyspepsia (dose related), anorexia, vomiting, gastroenteritis
  Hematologic: Leukopenia
  Hepatic: AST increased, ALT increased, GGT increased
  Neuromuscular & skeletal: Dysarthria, back pain, weakness, tremor, hypertonia, dysarthria
  Ocular: Amblyopia
  Respiratory: Rhinitis, pharyngitis, cough, dyspnea
  Miscellaneous: Diaphoresis, flu-like syndrome
Dosage Oral:
  Children and Adolescents:
    Autism (unlabeled use): 100-350 mg/day (1.6-5.2 mg/kg/day)
    Psychosis and mania (unlabeled use): Initial: 25 mg twice daily; titrate as necessary to 450 mg/day
  Adults:
    Schizophrenia/psychoses: Initial: 25 mg twice daily; increase in increments of 25-50 mg 2-3 times/day on the second and third day, if tolerated, to a target dose of 300-400 mg in 2-3 divided doses by day 4. Make further adjustments as needed at intervals of at least 2 days in adjustments of 25-50 mg twice daily. Usual maintenance range: 300-800 mg/day
    Mania: Initial: 50 mg twice daily on day 1, increase dose in increments of 100 mg/day to 200 mg twice daily on day 4; may increase to a target dose of 800 mg/day by day 6 at increments of ≤200 mg/day. Usual dosage range: 400-800 mg/day
  Note: Dose reductions should be attempted periodically to establish lowest effective dose in patients with psychosis or to establish need to continue
(Continued)

Quetiapine *(Continued)*

treating agitated symptoms in demented older adults. Patients being restarted after 1 week of no drug need to be titrated as above.

Elderly: 40% lower mean oral clearance of quetiapine in adults >65 years of age; higher plasma levels expected and, therefore, dosage adjustment may be needed; elderly patients usually require 50-200 mg/day. See "Note" in Adults dosing.

Dosing comments in renal insufficiency: 25% lower mean oral clearance of quetiapine than normal subjects; however, plasma concentrations similar to normal subjects receiving the same dose; no dosage adjustment required

Dosing comments in hepatic insufficiency: 30% lower mean oral clearance of quetiapine than normal subjects; higher plasma levels expected in hepatically impaired subjects; dosage adjustment may be needed

Initial: 25 mg/day, increase dose by 25-50 mg/day to effective dose, based on clinical response and tolerability to patient

Mechanism of Action Mechanism of action of quetiapine (dibenzothiazepine antipsychotic), as with other antipsychotic drugs, is unknown. However, it has been proposed that this drug's antipsychotic activity is mediated through a combination of dopamine type 2 (D_2) and serotonin type 2 (5-HT_2) antagonism. It is an antagonist at multiple neurotransmitter receptors in the brain: serotonin 5-HT_{1A} and 5-HT_2, dopamine D_1 and D_2, histamine H_1, and adrenergic alpha$_1$- and alpha$_2$- receptors; but appears to have no appreciable affinity at cholinergic muscarinic and benzodiazepine receptors.

Antagonism at receptors other than dopamine and 5-HT_2 with similar receptor affinities may explain some of the other effects of quetiapine. The drug's antagonism of histamine H_1-receptors may explain the somnolence observed with it. The drug's antagonism of adrenergic alpha$_1$-receptors may explain the orthostatic hypotension observed with it.

Contraindications Hypersensitivity to quetiapine or any component of the formulation; severe CNS depression; bone marrow suppression; blood dyscrasias; severe hepatic disease, coma

Warnings/Precautions Patients with dementia-related behavioral disorders treated with atypical antipsychotics are at an increased risk of death compared to placebo. Quetiapine is not approved for this indication.

May induce orthostatic hypotension associated with dizziness, tachycardia, and, in some cases, syncope, especially during the initial dose titration period. Should be used with particular caution in patients with known cardiovascular disease (history of MI or ischemic heart disease, heart failure, or conduction abnormalities), cerebrovascular disease, or conditions that predispose to hypotension. Development of cataracts has been observed in animal studies, therefore, lens examinations should be made upon initiation of therapy and every 6 months thereafter.

Neuroleptic malignant syndrome (NMS) is a potentially fatal symptom complex that has been reported in association with administration of antipsychotic drugs. Clinical manifestations of NMS are hyperpyrexia, muscle rigidity, altered mental status, and evidence of autonomic instability (irregular pulse or blood pressure, tachycardia, diaphoresis, and cardiac dysrhythmia). Management of NMS should include immediate discontinuation of antipsychotic drugs and other drugs not essential to concurrent therapy, intensive symptomatic treatment and medication monitoring, and treatment of any concomitant medical problems for which specific treatment are available.

Tardive dyskinesia; caution in patients with a history of seizures, decreases in total free thyroxine, pre-existing hyperprolactinemia, elevations of liver enzymes, cholesterol levels and/or triglyceride increases.

May cause hyperglycemia; in some cases may be extreme and associated with ketoacidosis, hyperosmolar coma, or death. Use with caution in patients with diabetes or other disorders of glucose regulation; monitor for worsening of glucose control.

The possibility of a suicide attempt is inherent in psychotic illness or bipolar disorder; use caution in high-risk patients during initiation of therapy. Prescriptions should be written for the smallest quantity consistent with good patient care.

Drug Interactions

Cytochrome P450 Effect: Substrate of CYP2D6 (minor), 3A4 (major)

Increased Effect/Toxicity: Quetiapine increases levels of lorazepam. The effects of other centrally-acting drugs, sedatives, or ethanol may be potentiated by quetiapine. Quetiapine may enhance the effects of antihypertensive agents. CYP3A4 inhibitors may increase the levels/effects of quetiapine;

example inhibitors include azole antifungals, clarithromycin, diclofenac, doxy-cycline, erythromycin, imatinib, isoniazid, nefazodone, nicardipine, propofol, protease inhibitors, quinidine, telithromycin, and verapamil; ketoconazole increased serum concentrations of quetiapine by 335%. Concomitant use of quetiapine and divalproex increased the mean maximum plasma concentration of quetiapine by 17% at steady state (the mean oral clearance of valproic acid was increased by 11%). Cimetidine increases blood levels of quetiapine (quetiapine's clearance is reduced by by 20%). Metoclopramide may increase risk of extrapyramidal symptoms (EPS). Acetylcholinesterase inhibitors (central) may increase the risk of antipsychotic-related EPS.

Decreased Effect: Thioridazine increases quetiapine's clearance (by 65%), decreasing serum levels. CYP3A4 inducers may decrease the levels/effects of quetiapine. Example inducers include aminoglutethimide, carbamazepine, nafcillin, nevirapine, phenobarbital, phenytoin, and rifamycins.

Ethanol/Nutrition/Herb Interactions

Ethanol: Avoid ethanol (may cause excessive impairment in cognition/motor function).

Food: In healthy volunteers, administration of quetiapine with food resulted in an increase in the peak serum concentration and AUC (each by ~15%) compared to the fasting state.

Herb/Nutraceutical: St John's wort may decrease quetiapine levels. Avoid valerian, St John's wort, kava kava, gotu kola (may increase CNS depression).

Dietary Considerations May be taken with or without food.

Pharmacodynamics/Kinetics

Absorption: Rapidly absorbed following oral administration

Distribution: V_d: 10 ± 4 L/kg; V_{dss}: ~2 days

Protein binding, plasma: 83%

Metabolism: Primarily hepatic; via CYP3A4; forms two inactive metabolites

Bioavailability: 9% ± 4%; tablet is 100% bioavailable relative to solution

Half-life elimination: Mean: Terminal: ~6 hours

Time to peak, plasma: 1.5 hours

Excretion: Urine (73% as metabolites, <1% as unchanged drug); feces (20%)

Pregnancy Risk Factor C

Dosage Forms TAB: (Seroquel®): 25 mg, 50 mg, 100 mg, 200 mg, 300 mg, 400 mg

Dental Comment

This drug is known to prolong the QT interval. The QT interval is measured as the time and distance between the Q point of the QRS complex and the end of the T wave in the ECG tracing. After adjustment for heart rate, the QT interval is defined as prolonged if it is more than 450 msec in men and 460 msec in women. A long QT syndrome was first described in the 1950s and 60s as a congenital syndrome involving QT interval prolongation and syncope and sudden death. Some of the congenital long QT syndromes were characterized by a peculiar electrocardiographic appearance of the QRS complex involving a premature atria beat followed by a pause, then a subsequent sinus beat showing marked QT prolongation and deformity. This type of cardiac arrhythmia was originally termed "torsade de pointes" (translated from the French as "twisting of the points").

Prolongation of the QT interval is thought to result from delayed ventricular repolarization. The repolarization process within the myocardial cell is due to the efflux of intracellular potassium. The channels associated with this current can be blocked by many drugs and predisposes the electrical propagation cycle to torsade de pointes.

Quetiapine is one of the drugs confirmed to prolong the QT interval and is accepted as having a risk of causing torsade de pointes. The risk of drug-induced torsade de pointes is extremely low when a single QT interval prolonging drug is prescribed. In terms of epinephrine, it is not known what effect vasoconstrictors in the local anesthetic regimen will have in patients with a known history of congenital prolonged QT interval or in patients taking any medication that prolongs the QT interval. Until more information is obtained, it is suggested that the clinician consult with the physician prior to the use of a vasoconstrictor in suspected patients, and that the vasoconstrictor (epinephrine, levonordefrin [Neo-Cobefrin®]) be used with caution.

Quetiapine Fumarate see Quetiapine on page 1319

Quibron® see Theophylline and Guaifenesin on page 1475

Quibron®-T see Theophylline on page 1473

Quibron®-T/SR see Theophylline on page 1473

Quinalbarbitone Sodium see Secobarbital on page 1381

Quinapril (KWIN a pril)

Related Information
Cardiovascular Diseases *on page 1636*

U.S. Brand Names Accupril®

Canadian Brand Names Accupril®

Mexican Brand Names Acupril®

Generic Available Yes

Synonyms Quinapril Hydrochloride

Pharmacologic Category Angiotensin-Converting Enzyme (ACE) Inhibitor

Use Management of hypertension; treatment of congestive heart failure

Unlabeled/Investigational Use Treatment of left ventricular dysfunction after myocardial infarction

Local Anesthetic/Vasoconstrictor Precautions No information available to require special precautions

Effects on Dental Treatment No significant effects or complications reported

Common Adverse Effects Note: Frequency ranges include data from hypertension and heart failure trials. Higher rates of adverse reactions have generally been noted in patients with CHF. However, the frequency of adverse effects associated with placebo is also increased in this population.

1% to 10%:

Cardiovascular: Hypotension (3%), chest pain (2%), first-dose hypotension (up to 3%)

Central nervous system: Dizziness (4% to 8%), headache (2% to 6%), fatigue (3%)

Dermatologic: Rash (1%)

Endocrine & metabolic: Hyperkalemia (2%)

Gastrointestinal: Vomiting/nausea (1% to 2%), diarrhea (2%)

Neuromuscular & skeletal: Myalgias (2% to 5%), back pain (1%)

Renal: Increased BUN/serum creatinine (2%, transient elevations may occur with a higher frequency), worsening of renal function (in patients with bilateral renal artery stenosis or hypovolemia)

Respiratory: Upper respiratory symptoms, cough (2% to 4%; up to 13% in some studies), dyspnea (2%)

Dosage

Adults: Oral:

Hypertension: Initial: 10-20 mg once daily, adjust according to blood pressure response at peak and trough blood levels; initial dose may be reduced to 5 mg in patients receiving diuretic therapy if the diuretic is continued; usual dose range (JNC 7): 10-40 mg once daily

Congestive heart failure or post-MI: Initial: 5 mg once or twice daily, titrated at weekly intervals to 20-40 mg daily in 2 divided doses; target dose (heart failure): 20 mg twice daily (ACC/AHA 2005 Heart Failure Guidelines)

Elderly: Initial: 2.5-5 mg/day; increase dosage at increments of 2.5-5 mg at 1- to 2-week intervals.

Dosing adjustment in renal impairment: Lower initial doses should be used; after initial dose (if tolerated), administer initial dose twice daily; may be increased at weekly intervals to optimal response:

Hypertension: Initial:

Cl_{cr} >60 mL/minute: Administer 10 mg/day

Cl_{cr} 30-60 mL/minute: Administer 5 mg/day

Cl_{cr} 10-30 mL/minute: Administer 2.5 mg/day

Congestive heart failure: Initial:

Cl_{cr} >30 mL/minute: Administer 5 mg/day

Cl_{cr} 10-30 mL/minute: Administer 2.5 mg/day

Dosing comments in hepatic impairment: In patients with alcoholic cirrhosis, hydrolysis of quinapril to quinaprilat is impaired; however, the subsequent elimination of quinaprilat is unaltered.

Mechanism of Action Competitive inhibitor of angiotensin-converting enzyme (ACE); prevents conversion of angiotensin I to angiotensin II, a potent vasoconstrictor; results in lower levels of angiotensin II which causes an increase in plasma renin activity and a reduction in aldosterone secretion; a CNS mechanism may also be involved in hypotensive effect as angiotensin II increases adrenergic outflow from CNS; vasoactive kallikreins may be decreased in conversion to active hormones by ACE inhibitors, thus reducing blood pressure

Contraindications Hypersensitivity to quinapril or any component of the formulation; angioedema related to previous treatment with an ACE inhibitor; bilateral renal artery stenosis; patients with idiopathic or hereditary angioedema; pregnancy (2nd and 3rd trimesters)

Warnings/Precautions Use with caution in patients with renal insufficiency, autoimmune disease, renal artery stenosis; excessive hypotension may be more likely in volume-depleted patients, the elderly, and following the first dose (first dose phenomenon); quinapril should be discontinued if laryngeal stridor or angioedema is observed. Angioedema can occur at any time during treatment (especially following first dose). It may involve head and neck (potentially affecting the airway) or the intestine (presenting with abdominal pain). Prolonged monitoring may be required especially if tongue, glottis, or larynx are involved as they are associated with airway obstruction. Those with a history of airway surgery in this situation have a higher risk. Rare toxicities associated with ACE inhibitors include cholestatic jaundice (which may progress to hepatic necrosis) and neutropenia/agranulocytosis with myeloid hyperplasia.

Drug Interactions

Increased Effect/Toxicity: Potassium supplements, co-trimoxazole (high dose), angiotensin II receptor antagonists (eg, candesartan, losartan, irbesartan), or potassium-sparing diuretics (amiloride, spironolactone, triamterene) may result in elevated serum potassium levels when combined with quinapril. ACE inhibitor effects may be increased by phenothiazines or probenecid (increases levels of captopril). ACE inhibitors may increase serum concentrations/effects of lithium.

Diuretics have additive hypotensive effects with ACE inhibitors, and hypovolemia increases the potential for adverse renal effects of ACE inhibitors. In patients with compromised renal function, coadministration with NSAIDs may result in further deterioration of renal function. Allopurinol and ACE inhibitors may cause a higher risk of hypersensitivity reaction when taken concurrently.

Decreased Effect: Quinapril may reduce the absorption of quinolones and tetracycline antibiotics. Aspirin (high dose) may reduce the therapeutic effects of ACE inhibitors; at low dosages this does not appear to be significant. Rifampin may decrease the effect of ACE inhibitors. Antacids may decrease the bioavailability of ACE inhibitors (may be more likely to occur with captopril); separate administration times by 1-2 hours. NSAIDs, specifically indomethacin, may reduce the hypotensive effects of ACE inhibitors.

Ethanol/Nutrition/Herb Interactions Herb/Nutraceutical: Avoid dong quai if using for hypertension (has estrogenic activity). Avoid ephedra, yohimbe, ginseng (may worsen hypertension). Avoid garlic (may have increased antihypertensive effect).

Pharmacodynamics/Kinetics
Onset of action: 1 hour
Duration: 24 hours
Absorption: Quinapril: ≥60%
Protein binding: Quinapril: 97%; Quinaprilat: 97%
Metabolism: Rapidly hydrolyzed to quinaprilat, the active metabolite
Half-life elimination: Quinapril: 0.8 hours; Quinaprilat: 3 hours; increases as Cl_{cr} decreases
Time to peak, serum: Quinapril: 1 hour; Quinaprilat: ~2 hours
Excretion: Urine (50% to 60% primarily as quinaprilat)
Pregnancy Risk Factor C (1st trimester)/D (2nd and 3rd trimesters)
Dosage Forms TAB: 5 mg, 10 mg, 20 mg, 40 mg

Quinapril and Hydrochlorothiazide
(KWIN a pril & hye droe klor oh THYE a zide)

Related Information
Hydrochlorothiazide *on page 776*
Quinapril *on page 1322*
U.S. Brand Names Accuretic®; Quinaretic
Canadian Brand Names Accuretic®
Generic Available Yes
Synonyms Hydrochlorothiazide and Quinapril
Pharmacologic Category Angiotensin-Converting Enzyme (ACE) Inhibitor; Antihypertensive; Diuretic, Thiazide
Use Treatment of hypertension (not for initial therapy)
Local Anesthetic/Vasoconstrictor Precautions No information available to require special precautions
Effects on Dental Treatment No significant effects or complications reported
Common Adverse Effects
1% to 10%:
Central nervous system: Dizziness (5%), somnolence (1%)
Neuromuscular & skeletal: Weakness (1%)
Renal: Serum creatinine increase (3%), blood urea nitrogen increase (4%)
Respiratory: Cough (3%), bronchitis (1%)
(Continued)

Quinapril and Hydrochlorothiazide *(Continued)*

Drug Interactions
Increased Effect/Toxicity: See individual agents.
Decreased Effect: See individual agents.
Pharmacodynamics/Kinetics See individual agents.
Pregnancy Risk Factor C (1st trimester); D (2nd and 3rd trimesters)

Quinapril Hydrochloride *see* Quinapril *on page 1322*

Quinaretic *see* Quinapril and Hydrochlorothiazide *on page 1323*

Quinidine *(KWIN i deen)*

Related Information
Cardiovascular Diseases *on page 1636*

Canadian Brand Names Apo-Quin-G®; Apo-Quinidine®; BioQuin® Durules™; Novo-Quinidin; Quinate®

Generic Available Yes

Synonyms Quinidine Gluconate; Quinidine Polygalacturonate; Quinidine Sulfate

Pharmacologic Category Antiarrhythmic Agent, Class Ia

Use Prophylaxis after cardioversion of atrial fibrillation and/or flutter to maintain normal sinus rhythm; prevent recurrence of paroxysmal supraventricular tachycardia, paroxysmal AV junctional rhythm, paroxysmal ventricular tachycardia, paroxysmal atrial fibrillation, and atrial or ventricular premature contractions; has activity against *Plasmodium falciparum* malaria

Local Anesthetic/Vasoconstrictor Precautions No information available to require special precautions (see Dental Comment)

Effects on Dental Treatment When taken over a long period of time, the anticholinergic side effects from quinidine can cause a reduction of saliva production or secretion contributing to discomfort and dental disease (ie, caries, oral candidiasis and periodontal disease).

Common Adverse Effects
Frequency not defined: Hypotension, syncope
>10%:
Cardiovascular: QT_c prolongation (modest prolongation is common, however, excessive prolongation is rare and indicates toxicity)
Central nervous system: Lightheadedness (15%)
Gastrointestinal: Diarrhea (35%), upper GI distress, bitter taste, diarrhea, anorexia, nausea, vomiting, stomach cramping (22%)
1% to 10%:
Cardiovascular: Angina (6%), palpitation (7%), new or worsened arrhythmia (proarrhythmic effect)
Central nervous system: Syncope (1% to 8%), headache (7%), fatigue (7%), sleep disturbance (3%), tremor (2%), nervousness (2%), incoordination (1%)
Dermatologic: Rash (5%)
Neuromuscular & skeletal: Weakness (5%)
Ocular: Blurred vision
Otic: Tinnitus
Respiratory: Wheezing

Note: Cinchonism, a syndrome which may include tinnitus, high-frequency hearing loss, deafness, vertigo, blurred vision, diplopia, photophobia, headache, confusion, and delirium has been associated with quinidine use. Usually associated with chronic toxicity, this syndrome has also been described after brief exposure to a moderate dose in sensitive patients. Vomiting and diarrhea may also occur as isolated reactions to therapeutic quinidine levels.

Mechanism of Action Class 1a antiarrhythmic agent; depresses phase O of the action potential; decreases myocardial excitability and conduction velocity, and myocardial contractility by decreasing sodium influx during depolarization and potassium efflux in repolarization; also reduces calcium transport across cell membrane

Drug Interactions
Cytochrome P450 Effect: Substrate of CYP2C8/9 (minor), 2E1 (minor), 3A4 (major); **Inhibits** CYP2C8/9 (weak), 2D6 (strong), 3A4 (strong)
Increased Effect/Toxicity: Effects may be additive with drugs which prolong the QT interval, including amiodarone, amitriptyline, bepridil, cisapride (use is contraindicated), disopyramide, erythromycin, haloperidol, imipramine, pimozide, procainamide, sotalol, thioridazine, and some quinolones (sparfloxacin, gatifloxacin, moxifloxacin - concurrent use is contraindicated). Concurrent use of amprenavir, or ritonavir is contraindicated. Quinidine increases digoxin serum concentrations; digoxin dosage may need to be reduced (by 50%)

when quinidine is initiated; new steady-state digoxin plasma concentrations occur in 5-7 days.

Quinidine may increase the levels/effects of amphetamines, selected beta-blockers, selected benzodiazepines, calcium channel blockers, cisapride, cyclosporine, dextromethorphan, ergot alkaloids, fluoxetine, selected HMG-CoA reductase inhibitors, lidocaine, mesoridazine, mirtazapine, nateglinide, nefazodone, paroxetine, risperidone, ritonavir, sildenafil (and other PDE-5 inhibitors), tacrolimus, thioridazine, tricyclic antidepressants, venlafaxine, and other substrates of CYP2D6 or 3A4. Selected benzodiazepines (midazolam and triazolam), cisapride, ergot alkaloids, selected HMG-CoA reductase inhibitors (lovastatin and simvastatin), mesoridazine, pimozide, and thioridazine are generally contraindicated with strong CYP3A4 inhibitors. When used with strong CYP3A4 inhibitors, dosage adjustment/limits are recommended for sildenafil and other PDE-5 inhibitors; refer to individual monographs.

The levels/effects of quinidine may be increased by azole antifungals, clarithromycin, diclofenac, doxycycline, erythromycin, imatinib, isoniazid, nefazodone, nicardipine, propofol, protease inhibitors (amprenavir and ritonavir are contraindicated), telithromycin, verapamil, and other CYP3A4 inhibitors. Quinidine potentiates nondepolarizing and depolarizing muscle relaxants. When combined with quinidine, amiloride may cause prolonged ventricular conduction leading to arrhythmias. Urinary alkalinizers (antacids, sodium bicarbonate, acetazolamide) increase quinidine blood levels. Warfarin effects may be increased by quinidine.

Decreased Effect: The levels/effects of quinidine may be decreased by aminoglutethimide, carbamazepine, nafcillin, nevirapine, phenobarbital, phenytoin, rifamycins, and other CYP3A4 inducers. Quinidine may decrease the levels/effects of CYP2D6 prodrug substrates (eg, codeine, hydrocodone, oxycodone, tramadol).

Pharmacodynamics/Kinetics

Distribution: V_d: Adults: 2-3.5 L/kg, decreased with congestive heart failure, malaria; increased with cirrhosis; crosses placenta; enters breast milk

Protein binding:
  Newborns: 60% to 70%; decreased protein binding with cyanotic congenital heart disease, cirrhosis, or acute myocardial infarction
  Adults: 80% to 90%

Metabolism: Extensively hepatic (50% to 90%) to inactive compounds

Bioavailability: Sulfate: 80%; Gluconate: 70%

Half-life elimination, plasma: Children: 2.5-6.7 hours; Adults: 6-8 hours; prolonged with elderly, cirrhosis, and congestive heart failure

Excretion: Urine (15% to 25% as unchanged drug)

Pregnancy Risk Factor C

Dental Comment

This drug is known to prolong the QT interval. The QT interval is measured as the time and distance between the Q point of the QRS complex and the end of the T wave in the ECG tracing. After adjustment for heart rate, the QT interval is defined as prolonged if it is more than 450 msec in men and 460 msec in women. A long QT syndrome was first described in the 1950s and 60s as a congenital syndrome involving QT interval prolongation and syncope and sudden death. Some of the congenital long QT syndromes were characterized by a peculiar electrocardiographic appearance of the QRS complex involving a premature atria beat followed by a pause, then a subsequent sinus beat showing marked QT prolongation and deformity. This type of cardiac arrhythmia was originally termed "torsade de pointes" (translated from the French as "twisting of the points").

Prolongation of the QT interval is thought to result from delayed ventricular repolarization. The repolarization process within the myocardial cell is due to the efflux of intracellular potassium. The channels associated with this current can be blocked by many drugs and predisposes the electrical propagation cycle to torsade de pointes.

Quinidine is one of the drugs confirmed to prolong the QT interval and is accepted as having a risk of causing torsade de pointes. The risk of drug-induced torsade de pointes is extremely low when a single QT interval prolonging drug is prescribed. In terms of epinephrine, it is not known what effect vasoconstrictors in the local anesthetic regimen will have in patients with a known history of congenital prolonged QT interval or in patients taking any medication that prolongs the QT interval. Until more information is obtained, it is suggested that the clinician consult with the physician prior to the use of a vasoconstrictor in suspected patients, and that the vasoconstrictor (epinephrine, levonordefrin [Neo-Cobefrin®]) be used with caution.

Quinidine Gluconate *see* Quinidine *on page 1324*

Quinidine Polygalacturonate *see* Quinidine *on page 1324*

Quinidine Sulfate *see* Quinidine *on page 1324*

Quinine (KWYE nine)

Canadian Brand Names Apo-Quinine®; Novo-Quinine; Quinine-Odan™

Generic Available Yes

Synonyms Quinine Sulfate

Pharmacologic Category Antimalarial Agent

Use In conjunction with other antimalarial agents, suppression or treatment of chloroquine-resistant *P. falciparum* malaria; treatment of *Babesia microti* infection in conjunction with clindamycin

Unlabeled/Investigational Use Prevention and treatment of nocturnal recumbency leg muscle cramps

Local Anesthetic/Vasoconstrictor Precautions No information available to require special precautions

Effects on Dental Treatment No significant effects or complications reported

Common Adverse Effects Frequency not defined.

Central nervous system: Severe headache

Gastrointestinal: Nausea, vomiting, diarrhea

Ocular: Blurred vision

Otic: Tinnitus

Miscellaneous: Cinchonism (risk of cinchonism is directly related to dose and duration of therapy)

Mechanism of Action Depresses oxygen uptake and carbohydrate metabolism; intercalates into DNA, disrupting the parasite's replication and transcription; affects calcium distribution within muscle fibers and decreases the excitability of the motor end-plate region; cardiovascular effects similar to quinidine

Drug Interactions

Cytochrome P450 Effect: Substrate (minor) of CYP1A2, 2C19, 3A4; **Inhibits** CYP2C8/9 (moderate); 2D6 (strong); 3A4 (weak)

Increased Effect/Toxicity: Quinine may increase the levels/effects of CYP2D6 substrates (eg, amphetamines, selected beta-blockers, dextromethorphan, fluoxetine, lidocaine, mirtazapine, nefazodone, paroxetine, risperidone, ritonavir, thioridazine, tricyclic antidepressants, venlafaxine). Beta-blockers with quinine may increase bradycardia. Quinine may enhance warfarin anticoagulant effect. Quinine potentiates nondepolarizing and depolarizing muscle relaxants. Quinine may increase plasma concentration of digoxin. Closely monitor digoxin concentrations. Digoxin dosage may need to be reduced (by one-half) when quinine is initiated. New steady-state digoxin plasma concentrations occur in 5-7 days. Verapamil, amiodarone, alkalinizing agents, and cimetidine may increase quinine serum concentrations.

Decreased Effect: Phenobarbital, phenytoin, and rifampin may decrease quinine serum concentrations. Quinine may decrease the levels/effects of CYP2D6 prodrug substrates (eg, codeine, hydrocodone, oxycodone, tramadol).

Pharmacodynamics/Kinetics

Absorption: Readily, mainly from upper small intestine

Protein binding: 70% to 95%

Metabolism: Primarily hepatic

Half-life elimination: Children: 6-12 hours; Adults: 8-14 hours

Time to peak, serum: 1-3 hours

Excretion: Feces and saliva; urine (<5% as unchanged drug)

Pregnancy Risk Factor X

Quinine Sulfate *see* Quinine *on page 1326*

Quinol *see* Hydroquinone *on page 798*

Quintabs [OTC] *see* Vitamins (Multiple/Oral) *on page 1582*

Quintabs-M [OTC] *see* Vitamins (Multiple/Oral) *on page 1582*

Quintex HC *see* Hydrocodone, Phenylephrine, and Guaifenesin *on page 791*

Quinupristin and Dalfopristin
(kwi NYOO pris tin & dal FOE pris tin)

U.S. Brand Names Synercid®

Canadian Brand Names Synercid®

Generic Available No

Synonyms Pristinamycin; RP-59500
Pharmacologic Category Antibiotic, Streptogramin
Use Treatment of serious or life-threatening infections associated with vanco-mycin-resistant *Enterococcus faecium* bacteremia; treatment of complicated skin and skin structure infections caused by methicillin-susceptible *Staphylococcus aureus* or *Streptococcus pyogenes*

Has been studied in the treatment of a variety of infections caused by *Enterococcus faecium* (not *E. fecalis*) including vancomycin-resistant strains. May also be effective in the treatment of serious infections caused by *Staphylococcus* species including those resistant to methicillin.

Local Anesthetic/Vasoconstrictor Precautions No information available to require special precautions
Effects on Dental Treatment No significant effects or complications reported
Common Adverse Effects
>10%:
  Hepatic: Hyperbilirubinemia (3% to 35%)
  Local: Inflammation at infusion site (38% to 42%), local pain (40% to 44%), local edema (17% to 18%), infusion site reaction (12% to 13%)
  Neuromuscular & skeletal: Arthralgia (up to 47%), myalgia (up to 47%)
1% to 10%:
  Central nervous system: Pain (2% to 3%), headache (2%)
  Dermatologic: Pruritus (2%), rash (3%)
  Endocrine & metabolic: Hyperglycemia (1%)
  Gastrointestinal: Nausea (3% to 5%), diarrhea (3%), vomiting (3% to 4%)
  Hematologic: Anemia (3%)
  Hepatic: GGT increased (2%), LDH increased (3%)
  Local: Thrombophlebitis (2%)
  Neuromuscular & skeletal: CPK increased (2%)
Mechanism of Action Quinupristin/dalfopristin inhibits bacterial protein synthesis by binding to different sites on the 50S bacterial ribosomal subunit thereby inhibiting protein synthesis
Drug Interactions
  Cytochrome P450 Effect: Quinupristin: **Inhibits** CYP3A4 (weak)
  Increased Effect/Toxicity: The manufacturer states that quinupristin/dalfopristin may increase cisapride concentrations and cause QT_c prolongation, and recommends to avoid concurrent use with cisapride. Quinupristin/dalfopristin may increase cyclosporine concentrations; monitor.
Pharmacodynamics/Kinetics
  Distribution: Quinupristin: 0.45 L/kg; Dalfopristin: 0.24 L/kg
  Protein binding: Moderate
  Metabolism: To active metabolites via nonenzymatic reactions
  Half-life elimination: Quinupristin: 0.85 hour; Dalfopristin: 0.7 hour (mean elimination half-lives, including metabolites: 3 and 1 hours, respectively)
  Excretion: Feces (75% to 77% as unchanged drug and metabolites); urine (15% to 19%)
Pregnancy Risk Factor B

Quixin™ *see* Levofloxacin *on page 913*
QVAR® *see* Beclomethasone *on page 183*
R 14-15 *see* Erlotinib *on page 560*
R-3827 *see* Abarelix *on page 24*
RabAvert® *see* Rabies Virus Vaccine *on page 1329*

Rabeprazole (ra BE pray zole)

U.S. Brand Names AcipHex®
Canadian Brand Names AcipHex®; Pariet®
Mexican Brand Names Pariet®
Generic Available No
Synonyms Pariprazole
Pharmacologic Category Proton Pump Inhibitor; Substituted Benzimidazole
Use Short-term (4-8 weeks) treatment and maintenance of erosive or ulcerative gastroesophageal reflux disease (GERD); symptomatic GERD; short-term (up to 4 weeks) treatment of duodenal ulcers; long-term treatment of pathological hypersecretory conditions, including Zollinger-Ellison syndrome; *H. pylori* eradication (in combination with amoxicillin and clarithromycin)
Unlabeled/Investigational Use Maintenance of duodenal ulcer
Local Anesthetic/Vasoconstrictor Precautions No information available to require special precautions
Effects on Dental Treatment No significant effects or complications reported
Common Adverse Effects 1% to 10%: Central nervous system: Headache
(Continued)

Rabeprazole (Continued)

Dosage Oral: Adults >18 years and Elderly:

GERD: 20 mg once daily for 4-8 weeks; maintenance: 20 mg once daily

Duodenal ulcer: 20 mg/day before breakfast for 4 weeks

H. pylori eradication: 20 mg twice daily for 7 days; to be administered with amoxicillin 1000 mg and clarithromycin 500 mg, also given twice daily for 7 days.

Hypersecretory conditions: 60 mg once daily; dose may need to be adjusted as necessary. Doses as high as 100 mg once daily and 60 mg twice daily have been used.

Dosage adjustment in renal impairment: No dosage adjustment required

Dosage adjustment in hepatic impairment:

Mild to moderate: Elimination decreased; no dosage adjustment required

Severe: Use caution

Mechanism of Action Potent proton pump inhibitor; suppresses gastric acid secretion by inhibiting the parietal cell H+/K+ ATP pump

Contraindications Hypersensitivity to rabeprazole, substituted benzimidazoles (ie, esomeprazole, lansoprazole, omeprazole, pantoprazole), or any component of the formulation

Warnings/Precautions Use caution in severe hepatic impairment; relief of symptoms with rabeprazole does not preclude the presence of a gastric malignancy

Drug Interactions

Cytochrome P450 Effect: Substrate (major) of CYP2C19, 3A4; **Inhibits** CYP2C19 (moderate), 2DC (weak), 3A4 (weak)

Increased Effect/Toxicity: Rabeprazole may increase the levels/effects of citalopram, diazepam, methsuximide, phenytoin, propranolol, sertraline, or other CYP2C19 substrates.

Decreased Effect: Proton pump inhibitors may decrease the absorption of atazanavir, indinavir, itraconazole, and ketoconazole. The levels/effects of rabeprazole may be decreased by aminoglutethimide, carbamazepine, nafcillin, nevirapine, phenobarbital, phenytoin, rifampin, and other CYP2C19 or 3A4 inducers.

Ethanol/Nutrition/Herb Interactions

Ethanol: Avoid ethanol (may cause gastric mucosal irritation).

Food: High-fat meals may delay absorption, but C_{max} and AUC are not altered.

Dietary Considerations May be taken with or without food; best if taken before breakfast.

Pharmacodynamics/Kinetics

Onset of action: 1 hour

Duration: 24 hours

Absorption: Oral: Well absorbed within 1 hour

Distribution: 96.3%

Protein binding, serum: 94.8% to 97.5%

Metabolism: Hepatic via CYP3A and 2C19 to inactive metabolites

Bioavailability: Oral: 52%

Half-life elimination (dose dependent): 0.85-2 hours

Time to peak, plasma: 2-5 hours

Excretion: Urine (90% primarily as thioether carboxylic acid); remainder in feces

Pregnancy Risk Factor B

Dosage Forms TAB, delayed release, enteric coated: 20 mg

Rabies Immune Globulin (Human)

(RAY beez i MYUN GLOB yoo lin, HYU man)

Related Information

Immunizations (Vaccines) *on page 1786*

U.S. Brand Names BayRab®; Imogam® Rabies-HT

Canadian Brand Names BayRab™; Imogam® Rabies Pasteurized

Generic Available No

Synonyms RIG

Pharmacologic Category Immune Globulin

Use Part of postexposure prophylaxis of persons with rabies exposure who lack a history of pre-exposure or postexposure prophylaxis with rabies vaccine or a recently documented neutralizing antibody response to previous rabies vaccination; although it is preferable to administer RIG with the first dose of vaccine, it can be given up to 8 days after vaccination

Local Anesthetic/Vasoconstrictor Precautions No information available to require special precautions

Effects on Dental Treatment No significant effects or complications reported

Common Adverse Effects 1% to 10%:
Central nervous system: Fever (mild)
Local: Soreness at injection site
Mechanism of Action Rabies immune globulin is a solution of globulins dried from the plasma or serum of selected adult human donors who have been immunized with rabies vaccine and have developed high titers of rabies antibody. It generally contains 10% to 18% of protein of which not less than 80% is monomeric immunoglobulin G.
Pregnancy Risk Factor C

Rabies Virus Vaccine (RAY beez VYE rus vak SEEN)

Related Information
Immunizations (Vaccines) *on page 1786*
U.S. Brand Names Imovax® Rabies; RabAvert®
Canadian Brand Names Imovax® Rabies; RabAvert®
Generic Available No
Synonyms HDCV; Human Diploid Cell Cultures Rabies Vaccine; PCEC; Purified Chick Embryo Cell
Pharmacologic Category Vaccine
Use Pre-exposure immunization: Vaccinate persons with greater than usual risk due to occupation or avocation including veterinarians, rangers, animal handlers, certain laboratory workers, and persons living in or visiting countries for longer than 1 month where rabies is a constant threat.

Postexposure prophylaxis: If a bite from a carrier animal is unprovoked, if it is not captured and rabies is present in that species and area, administer rabies immune globulin (RIG) and the vaccine as indicated
Local Anesthetic/Vasoconstrictor Precautions No information available to require special precautions
Effects on Dental Treatment No significant effects or complications reported
Common Adverse Effects All serious adverse reactions must be reported to the U.S. Department of Health and Human Services (DHHS) Vaccine Adverse Event Reporting System (VAERS) 1-800-822-7967.
Frequency not defined.
Cardiovascular: Edema
Central nervous system: Dizziness, malaise, encephalomyelitis, transverse myelitis, fever, pain, headache, neuroparalytic reactions
Gastrointestinal: Nausea, abdominal pain
Local: Local discomfort, pain at injection site, itching, erythema, swelling or pain
Neuromuscular & skeletal: Myalgia
Mechanism of Action Rabies vaccine is an inactivated virus vaccine which promotes immunity by inducing an active immune response. The production of specific antibodies requires about 7-10 days to develop. Rabies immune globulin or antirabies serum, equine (ARS) is given in conjunction with rabies vaccine to provide immune protection until an antibody response can occur.
Pharmacodynamics/Kinetics
Onset of action: I.M.: Rabies antibody: ~7-10 days
Peak effect: ~30-60 days
Duration: ≥1 year
Pregnancy Risk Factor C

Racepinephrine *see* Epinephrine *on page 546*
Radiogardase™ *see* Ferric Hexacyanoferrate *on page 650*
rAHF *see* Antihemophilic Factor (Recombinant) *on page 130*
R-albuterol *see* Levalbuterol *on page 907*

Raloxifene (ral OKS i feen)

Related Information
Endocrine Disorders and Pregnancy *on page 1659*
Rheumatoid Arthritis, Osteoarthritis, and Osteoporosis *on page 1668*
U.S. Brand Names Evista®
Canadian Brand Names Evista®
Mexican Brand Names Evista®
Generic Available No
Synonyms Keoxifene Hydrochloride; NSC-706725; Raloxifene Hydrochloride
Pharmacologic Category Selective Estrogen Receptor Modulator (SERM)
Use Prevention and treatment of osteoporosis in postmenopausal women
Unlabeled/Investigational Use Risk reduction for invasive breast cancer in postmenopausal women at increased risk for breast cancer
(Continued)

Raloxifene *(Continued)*

Local Anesthetic/Vasoconstrictor Precautions No information available to require special precautions

Effects on Dental Treatment No significant effects or complications reported

Common Adverse Effects Note: Raloxifene has been associated with increased risk of thromboembolism (DVT, PE) and superficial thrombophlebitis; risk is similar to reported risk of HRT

>10%:

Endocrine & metabolic: Hot flashes (10% to 29%)

Neuromuscular & skeletal: Arthralgia (11% to 16%)

Miscellaneous: Flu syndrome (14% to 15%), infection (11% to 15%)

1% to 10%:

Cardiovascular: Peripheral edema (3% to 5%), chest pain (3% to 4%), syncope (2%), varicose vein (2%)

Central nervous system: Headache (9%), depression (6%), insomnia (6%), vertigo (4%), fever (3% to 4%), migraine (3%)

Dermatologic: Rash (6%)

Endocrine & metabolic: Breast pain (4%)

Gastrointestinal: Nausea (8% to 9%), weight gain (9%), abdominal pain (7%), diarrhea (7%), dyspepsia (6%), vomiting (3% to 5%), flatulence (2% to 3%), gastroenteritis (≤3%)

Genitourinary: Vaginal bleeding (6%), cystitis (3% to 5%), urinary tract infection (4%), vaginitis (4%), leukorrhea (3%), urinary tract disorder (3%), uterine disorder (3%), vaginal hemorrhage (3%), endometrial disorder (≤3%)

Neuromuscular & skeletal: Myalgia (7%), leg cramps (6% to 7%), arthritis (4%), tendon disorder (4%), hypoesthesia (≤2%), neuralgia (≤2%)

Ocular: Conjunctivitis (2%)

Respiratory: Bronchitis (10%), rhinitis (10%), sinusitis (8% to 10%), cough (6% to 9%), pharyngitis (5% to 8%), pneumonia (3%), laryngitis (≤2%)

Miscellaneous: Diaphoresis (3%)

Dosage Adults: Female: Oral:

Osteoporosis: 60 mg/day

Invasive breast cancer risk reduction (investigational use): 60 mg/day for 5 years

Dosage adjustment in hepatic impairment: Child-Pugh class A: Plasma concentrations were higher and correlated with total bilirubin. Safety and efficacy in hepatic insufficiency have not been established.

Mechanism of Action A selective estrogen receptor modulator, meaning that it affects some of the same receptors that estrogen does, but not all, and in some instances, it antagonizes or blocks estrogen; it acts like estrogen to prevent bone loss and improve lipid profiles (decreases total and LDL-cholesterol but does not raise triglycerides), but it has the potential to block some estrogen effects such as those that lead to breast cancer and uterine cancer

Contraindications Hypersensitivity to raloxifene or any component of the formulation; active or history of venous thromboembolic events; pregnancy; breast-feeding

Warnings/Precautions Use caution in patients at high risk for venous thromboembolism (deep vein thrombosis, pulmonary embolism); patients with cardiovascular disease; history of cervical/uterine carcinoma; renal/hepatic insufficiency (however, pharmacokinetic data are lacking); concurrent use of estrogens; women with a history of elevated triglycerides in response to treatment with oral estrogens (or estrogen/progestin). Safety and efficacy in premenopausal women or men have not been established.

Drug Interactions

Decreased Effect: Cholestyramine decreases raloxifene absorption; raloxifene decreases levothyroxine absorption

Ethanol/Nutrition/Herb Interactions Ethanol: Avoid ethanol (may increase risk of osteoporosis).

Dietary Considerations Supplemental calcium or vitamin D may be required if dietary intake is not adequate.

Pharmacodynamics/Kinetics

Onset of action: 8 weeks

Absorption: ~60%

Distribution: 2348 L/kg

Protein binding: >95% to albumin and α-glycoprotein

Metabolism: Hepatic, extensive first-pass effect; metabolized to glucuronide conjugates

Bioavailability: ~2%

Half-life elimination: 27.7-32.5 hours

Excretion: Primarily feces; urine (0.2%)

Pregnancy Risk Factor X
Dosage Forms TAB: 60 mg

Raloxifene Hydrochloride *see* Raloxifene *on page 1329*

Ramelteon (ra MEL tee on)

U.S. Brand Names Rozerem™
Generic Available No
Synonyms TAK-375
Pharmacologic Category Hypnotic, Nonbenzodiazepine
Use Treatment of insomnia characterized by difficulty with sleep onset
Local Anesthetic/Vasoconstrictor Precautions No information available to require special precautions
Effects on Dental Treatment Key adverse event(s) related to dental treatment: Taste perversion.
Common Adverse Effects 1% to 10%:
Central nervous system: Headache (7%, same as placebo), somnolence (5%), dizziness (5%), fatigue (4%), insomnia worsened (3%), depression (2%)
Endocrine & metabolic: Serum cortisol decreased (1%)
Gastrointestinal: Nausea (3%), diarrhea (2%, same as placebo), taste perversion (2%)
Neuromuscular & skeletal: Myalgia (2%), arthralgia (2%)
Respiratory: Upper respiratory infection (3%; 2 % with placebo)
Miscellaneous: Influenza (1%)

Dosage
Oral: Adults: One 8 mg tablet within 30 minutes of bedtime
Dosage adjustment in renal impairment: No dosage adjustment required
Dosage adjustment in hepatic impairment: No adjustment required for mild-to-moderate impairment. Avoid use with severe impairment.

Mechanism of Action Potent, selective agonist of melatonin receptors MT_1 and MT_2 (with little affinity for MT_3) within the suprachiasmic nucleus of the hypothalamus, an area responsible for determination of circadian rhythms and synchronization of the sleep-wake cycle. Agonism of MT_1 is thought to preferentially induce sleepiness, while MT_2 receptor activation preferentially influences regulation of circadian rhythms. Ramelteon is eightfold more selective for MT_1 than MT_2 and exhibits nearly sixfold higher affinity for MT_1 than melatonin, presumably allowing for enhanced effects on sleep induction.

Contraindications Hypersensitivity to ramelteon or any component of the formulation; severe hepatic impairment; concurrent use with fluvoxamine

Warnings/Precautions
Use caution with pre-existing depression or other psychiatric conditions. Caution when using with other CNS depressants; avoid engaging in hazardous activities or activities requiring mental alertness. Not recommended for use in patients with severe sleep apnea or COPD. Use caution with moderate hepatic impairment. Do not take with a high-fat meal. May cause disturbances of hormonal regulation. Use caution when administered concomitantly with strong CYP1A2 inhibitors. Safety and efficacy in pediatric patients have not been established.

Drug Interactions
Cytochrome P450 Effect: Substrate of CYP1A2 (major), CYP3A4 (minor), CYP2C family (minor)
Increased Effect/Toxicity: The following agents may increase the levels/effects of ramelteon: CNS depressants, CYP1A2 inhibitors (example inhibitors include amiodarone, ciprofloxacin, fluvoxamine (concomitant use not recommended), ketoconazole, norfloxacin, ofloxacin, and rofecoxib), fluvoxamine, fluconazole, and ketoconazole.
Decreased Effect: Rifampin may decrease the levels/effects of ramelteon.

Ethanol/Nutrition/Herb Interactions
Ethanol: Avoid ethanol (may increase CNS depression).

Dietary Considerations Taking with high-fat meal delays T_{max} and increases AUC (~31%); do not take with high-fat meal.

Pharmacodynamics/Kinetics
Onset of action: 30 minutes
Absorption: Rapid
Distribution: 74 L
Protein binding: 82%
Metabolism: Extensive first-pass effect; oxidative metabolism primarily through CYP1A2 and to a lesser extent through CYP2C and CYP3A4; forms active metabolite (M-II)
Bioavailability: Absolute: 1.8%
Half-life elimination: Ramelteon: 1-2.6 hours; M-II: 2-5 hours
(Continued)

Ramelteon *(Continued)*

Time to peak, plasma: Median: 0.5-1.5 hours

Excretion: Primarily as metabolites: Urine (84%); feces (4%)

Pregnancy Risk Factor C

Dosage Forms TAB: 8 mg

Selected Readings

Kato K, Hirai K, Nishiyama K, et al, "Neurochemical Properties of Ramelteon (TAK-375), A Selective MT1/MT2 Receptor Agonist," *Neuropharmacology.* 2005, 48(2):301-10.

Nguyen NN, Uy SS, and Song JC, "Ramelteon: A Novel Melatonin Receptor Agonist for the Treatment of Insomnia," *Formulary*, 2005, 40:146-55.

Ramipril *(ra MI pril)*

Related Information

Cardiovascular Diseases *on page 1636*

U.S. Brand Names Altace®

Canadian Brand Names Altace®

Mexican Brand Names Ramace®; Tritace®

Generic Available No

Pharmacologic Category Angiotensin-Converting Enzyme (ACE) Inhibitor

Use Treatment of hypertension, alone or in combination with thiazide diuretics; treatment of left ventricular dysfunction after myocardial infarction; to reduce risk of heart attack, stroke, and death in patients at increased risk for these problems

Unlabeled/Investigational Use Treatment of heart failure

Local Anesthetic/Vasoconstrictor Precautions No information available to require special precautions

Effects on Dental Treatment No significant effects or complications reported

Common Adverse Effects Note: Frequency ranges include data from hypertension and heart failure trials. Higher rates of adverse reactions have generally been noted in patients with CHF. However, the frequency of adverse effects associated with placebo is also increased in this population.

>10%: Respiratory: Cough (increased) (7% to 12%)

1% to 10%:

Cardiovascular: Hypotension (11%), angina (3%), postural hypotension (2%), syncope (2%)

Central nervous system: Headache (1% to 5%), dizziness (2% to 4%), fatigue (2%), vertigo (2%)

Endocrine & metabolic: Hyperkalemia (1% to 10%)

Gastrointestinal: Nausea/vomiting (1% to 2%)

Neuromuscular & skeletal: Chest pain (noncardiac) (1%)

Renal: Renal dysfunction (1%), elevation in serum creatinine (1% to 2%), increased BUN (<1% to 3%); transient elevations of creatinine and/or BUN may occur more frequently

Respiratory: Cough (estimated 1% to 10%)

Worsening of renal function may occur in patients with bilateral renal artery stenosis or in hypovolemia. In addition, a syndrome which may include fever, myalgia, arthralgia, interstitial nephritis, vasculitis, rash, eosinophilia and positive ANA, and elevated ESR has been reported with ACE inhibitors. Risk of pancreatitis and agranulocytosis may be increased in patients with collagen vascular disease or renal impairment.

Dosage Adults: Oral:

Hypertension: 2.5-5 mg once daily, maximum: 20 mg/day

Reduction in risk of MI, stroke, and death from cardiovascular causes: Initial: 2.5 mg once daily for 1 week, then 5 mg once daily for the next 3 weeks, then increase as tolerated to 10 mg once daily (may be given as divided dose)

Heart failure postmyocardial infarction: Initial: 2.5 mg twice daily titrated upward, if possible, to 5 mg twice daily.

Heart failure (unlabeled use): Initial: 1.25-2.5 mg once daily; target dose: 10 mg once daily (ACC/AHA 2005 Heart Failure Guidelines)

Note: The dose of any concomitant diuretic should be reduced. If the diuretic cannot be discontinued, initiate therapy with 1.25 mg. After the initial dose, the patient should be monitored carefully until blood pressure has stabilized.

Dosing adjustment in renal impairment:

Cl_{cr} <40 mL/minute: Administer 25% of normal dose.

Renal failure and hypertension: Administer 1.25 mg once daily, titrated upward as possible.

Renal failure and heart failure: Administer 1.25 mg once daily, increasing to 1.25 mg twice daily up to 2.5 mg twice daily as tolerated.

Mechanism of Action Ramipril is an ACE inhibitor which prevents the formation of angiotensin II from angiotensin I and exhibits pharmacologic effects that are similar to captopril. Ramipril must undergo enzymatic saponification by esterases in the liver to its biologically active metabolite, ramiprilat. The pharmacodynamic effects of ramipril result from the high-affinity, competitive, reversible binding of ramiprilat to angiotensin-converting enzyme thus preventing the formation of the potent vasoconstrictor angiotensin II. This isomerized enzyme-inhibitor complex has a slow rate of dissociation, which results in high potency and a long duration of action; a CNS mechanism may also be involved in the hypotensive effect as angiotensin II increases adrenergic outflow from CNS; vasoactive kallikreins may be decreased in conversion to active hormones by ACE inhibitors, thus reducing blood pressure

Contraindications Hypersensitivity to ramipril or any component of the formulation; prior hypersensitivity (including angioedema) to ACE inhibitors; bilateral renal artery stenosis; pregnancy (2nd and 3rd trimesters)

Warnings/Precautions Anaphylactic or anaphylactoid reactions can occur. Use with caution and modify dosage in patients with renal impairment (especially renal artery stenosis), severe CHF. Severe hypotension may occur in the elderly and patients who are sodium and/or volume depleted, initiate lower doses and monitor closely when starting therapy in these patients. Angioedema can occur at any time during treatment (especially following first dose). It may involve head and neck (potentially affecting the airway) or the intestine (presenting with abdominal pain). Prolonged monitoring may be required especially if tongue, glottis, or larynx are involved as they are associated with airway obstruction. Those with a history of airway surgery in this situation have a higher risk. Careful blood pressure monitoring with first dose (hypotension can occur especially in volume-depleted patients). Use with caution in hypovolemia; collagen vascular diseases; valvular stenosis (particularly aortic stenosis); hyperkalemia; or before, during, or immediately after anesthesia. Avoid rapid dosage escalation, which may lead to renal insufficiency. Rare toxicities associated with ACE inhibitors include cholestatic jaundice (which may progress to hepatic necrosis) and neutropenia/agranulocytosis with myeloid hyperplasia. If patient has renal impairment then a baseline WBC with differential and serum creatinine should be evaluated and monitored closely during the first 3 months of therapy. Hypersensitivity reactions may be seen during hemodialysis with high-flux dialysis membranes (eg, AN69).

Drug Interactions

Increased Effect/Toxicity: Potassium supplements, co-trimoxazole (high dose), angiotensin II receptor antagonists (eg, candesartan, losartan, irbesartan), or potassium-sparing diuretics (amiloride, spironolactone, triamterene) may result in elevated serum potassium levels when combined with ramipril. ACE inhibitor effects may be increased by phenothiazines or probenecid (increases levels of captopril). ACE inhibitors may increase serum concentrations/effects of lithium.

Diuretics have additive hypotensive effects with ACE inhibitors, and hypovolemia increases the potential for adverse renal effects of ACE inhibitors. In patients with compromised renal function, coadministration with NSAIDs may result in further deterioration of renal function. Allopurinol and ACE inhibitors may cause a higher risk of hypersensitivity reaction when taken concurrently.

Decreased Effect: Aspirin (high dose) may reduce the therapeutic effects of ACE inhibitors; at low dosages this does not appear to be significant. Rifampin may decrease the effect of ACE inhibitors. Antacids may decrease the bioavailability of ACE inhibitors (may be more likely to occur with captopril); separate administration times by 1-2 hours. NSAIDs, specifically indomethacin, may reduce the hypotensive effects of ACE inhibitors. More likely to occur in low renin or volume dependent hypertensive patients.

Ethanol/Nutrition/Herb Interactions Herb/Nutraceutical: Avoid dong quai if using for hypertension (has estrogenic activity). Avoid ephedra, yohimbe, ginseng (may worsen hypertension). Avoid garlic (may have increased antihypertensive effect).

Pharmacodynamics/Kinetics

Onset of action: 1-2 hours

Duration: 24 hours

Absorption: Well absorbed (50% to 60%)

Distribution: Plasma levels decline in a triphasic fashion; rapid decline is a distribution phase to peripheral compartment, plasma protein and tissue ACE (half-life 2-4 hours); 2nd phase is an apparent elimination phase representing the clearance of free ramiprilat (half-life: 9-18 hours); and final phase is the terminal elimination phase representing the equilibrium phase between tissue binding and dissociation

Metabolism: Hepatic to the active form, ramiprilat

Half-life elimination: Ramiprilat: Effective: 13-17 hours; Terminal: >50 hours

Time to peak, serum: ~1 hour

Excretion: Urine (60%) and feces (40%) as parent drug and metabolites

(Continued)

Ramipril (Continued)

Pregnancy Risk Factor C (1st trimester)/D (2nd and 3rd trimesters)
Dosage Forms CAP: 1.25 mg, 2.5 mg, 5 mg, 10 mg

Ranexa™ see Ranolazine on page 1336
Raniclor™ see Cefaclor on page 279

Ranitidine (ra NI ti deen)

Related Information
Gastrointestinal Disorders on page 1654
U.S. Brand Names Zantac®; Zantac 75® [OTC]; Zantac 150™ [OTC]; Zantac® EFFERdose®

Canadian Brand Names Alti-Ranitidine; Apo-Ranitidine®; CO Ranitidine; Gen-Ranidine; Novo-Ranidine; Nu-Ranit; PMS-Ranitidine; Rhoxal-ranitidine; Zantac®; Zantac 75®

Mexican Brand Names Acloral®; Alter-H!2®; Alvidina®; Anistal®; Azanplus®; Azantac®; Credaxol®; Galidrin®; Neugal®; Ranifur®; Ranifur®; Ranisen®; Raudil®; Serviradine®; Ulcedin®; Ulsaven®; Ultran®

Generic Available Yes: Excludes effervescent tablet

Synonyms Ranitidine Hydrochloride

Pharmacologic Category Histamine H_2 Antagonist

Use
Zantac®: Short-term and maintenance therapy of duodenal ulcer, gastric ulcer, gastroesophageal reflux, active benign ulcer, erosive esophagitis, and pathological hypersecretory conditions; as part of a multidrug regimen for *H. pylori* eradication to reduce the risk of duodenal ulcer recurrence
Zantac® 75 [OTC]: Relief of heartburn, acid indigestion, and sour stomach

Unlabeled/Investigational Use Recurrent postoperative ulcer, upper GI bleeding, prevention of acid-aspiration pneumonitis during surgery, and prevention of stress-induced ulcers

Local Anesthetic/Vasoconstrictor Precautions No information available to require special precautions

Effects on Dental Treatment No significant effects or complications reported

Common Adverse Effects Frequency not defined.
Cardiovascular: Atrioventricular block, bradycardia, premature ventricular beats, tachycardia, vasculitis
Central nervous system: Agitation, dizziness, depression, hallucinations, headache, insomnia, malaise, mental confusion, somnolence, vertigo
Dermatologic: Alopecia, erythema multiforme, rash
Endocrine & metabolic: Gynecomastia, impotence, increased prolactin levels, loss of libido
Gastrointestinal: Abdominal discomfort/pain, constipation, diarrhea, nausea, pancreatitis, vomiting
Hematologic: Acquired hemolytic anemia, agranulocytosis, aplastic anemia, granulocytopenia, leukopenia, pancytopenia, thrombocytopenia
Hepatic: Hepatic failure, hepatitis
Local: Transient pain, burning or itching at the injection site
Neuromuscular & skeletal: Arthralgia, involuntary motor disturbance, myalgia
Ocular: Blurred vision
Renal: Increased serum creatinine
Miscellaneous: Anaphylaxis, angioneurotic edema, hypersensitivity reactions

Dosage
Children 1 month to 16 years:
Duodenal and gastric ulcer:
Oral:
Treatment: 2-4 mg/kg/day divided twice daily; maximum treatment dose: 300 mg/day
Maintenance: 2-4 mg/kg once daily; maximum maintenance dose: 150 mg/day
I.V.: 2-4 mg/kg/day divided every 6-8 hours; maximum: 150 mg/day
GERD and erosive esophagitis:
Oral: 5-10 mg/kg/day divided twice daily; maximum: GERD 300 mg/day, erosive esophagitis: 600 mg/day
I.V.: 2-4 mg/kg/day divided every 6-8 hours; maximum: 150 mg/day **or as an alternative**
Continuous infusion: Initial: 1 mg/kg/dose for one dose followed by infusion of 0.08-0.17 mg/kg/hour or 2-4 mg/kg/day
Children ≥12 years: Prevention of heartburn: Oral: Zantac® 75 [OTC]: 75 mg 30-60 minutes before eating food or drinking beverages which cause heartburn; maximum: 150 mg/24 hours; do not use for more than 14 days

Adults:

Duodenal ulcer: Oral: Treatment: 150 mg twice daily, or 300 mg once daily after the evening meal or at bedtime; maintenance: 150 mg once daily at bedtime

Helicobacter pylori eradication: 150 mg twice daily; requires combination therapy

Pathological hypersecretory conditions:

Oral: 150 mg twice daily; adjust dose or frequency as clinically indicated; doses of up to 6 g/day have been used

I.V.: Continuous infusion for Zollinger-Ellison: 1 mg/kg/hour; measure gastric acid output at 4 hours, if >10 mEq or if patient is symptomatic, increase dose in increments of 0.5 mg/kg/hour; doses of up to 2.5 mg/kg/hour have been used

Gastric ulcer, benign: Oral: 150 mg twice daily; maintenance: 150 mg once daily at bedtime

Erosive esophagitis: Oral: Treatment: 150 mg 4 times/day; maintenance: 150 mg twice daily

Prevention of heartburn: Oral: Zantac® 75 [OTC]: 75 mg 30-60 minutes before eating food or drinking beverages which cause heartburn; maximum: 150 mg in 24 hours; do not use for more than 14 days

Patients not able to take oral medication:

I.M.: 50 mg every 6-8 hours

I.V.: Intermittent bolus or infusion: 50 mg every 6-8 hours

Continuous I.V. infusion: 6.25 mg/hour

Elderly: Ulcer healing rates and incidence of adverse effects are similar in the elderly, when compared to younger patients; dosing adjustments not necessary based on age alone

Dosing adjustment in renal impairment: Adults: Cl_{cr} <50 mL/minute:

Oral: 150 mg every 24 hours; adjust dose cautiously if needed

I.V.: 50 mg every 18-24 hours; adjust dose cautiously if needed

Hemodialysis: Adjust dosing schedule so that dose coincides with the end of hemodialysis

Dosing adjustment/comments in hepatic disease: Patients with hepatic impairment may have minor changes in ranitidine half-life, distribution, clearance, and bioavailability; dosing adjustments not necessary, monitor

Mechanism of Action Competitive inhibition of histamine at H_2-receptors of the gastric parietal cells, which inhibits gastric acid secretion, gastric volume, and hydrogen ion concentration are reduced. Does not affect pepsin secretion, pentagastrin-stimulated intrinsic factor secretion, or serum gastrin.

Contraindications Hypersensitivity to ranitidine or any component of the formulation

Warnings/Precautions Use with caution in patients with hepatic impairment; use with caution in renal impairment, dosage modification required; avoid use in patients with history of acute porphyria (may precipitate attacks); long-term therapy may be associated with vitamin B_{12} deficiency; EFFERdose® formulations contain phenylalanine; safety and efficacy have not been established for pediatric patients <1 month of age

Drug Interactions

Cytochrome P450 Effect: Substrate (minor) of CYP1A2, 2C19, 2D6; **Inhibits** CYP1A2 (weak), 2D6 (weak)

Increased Effect/Toxicity: Increased the effect/toxicity of cyclosporine (increased serum creatinine), gentamicin (neuromuscular blockade), glipizide, glyburide, midazolam (increased concentrations), metoprolol, pentoxifylline, phenytoin, quinidine, and triazolam.

Decreased Effect:

Decreased effect: Variable effects on warfarin; antacids may decrease absorption of ranitidine; ketoconazole and itraconazole absorptions are decreased; may produce altered serum levels of procainamide and ferrous sulfate; decreased effect of nondepolarizing muscle relaxants, cefpodoxime, cyanocobalamin (decreased absorption), diazepam, oxaprozin

Decreased toxicity of atropine

Ethanol/Nutrition/Herb Interactions

Ethanol: Avoid ethanol (may cause gastric mucosal irritation).

Food: Does not interfere with absorption of ranitidine.

Dietary Considerations Oral dosage forms may be taken with or without food.

Zantac® EFFERdose®:

Effervescent tablet 25 mg contains sodium 1.33 mEq/tablet and phenylalanine 2.81 mg/tablet

Effervescent tablet 150 mg contains sodium 7.96 mEq/tablet and phenylalanine 16.84 mg/tablet

(Continued)

Ranitidine *(Continued)*

Pharmacodynamics/Kinetics

Absorption: Oral: 50%

Distribution: Normal renal function: V_d: 1.7 L/kg; Cl_{cr} 25-35 mL/minute: 1.76 L/kg minimally penetrates the blood-brain barrier; enters breast milk

Protein binding: 15%

Metabolism: Hepatic to N-oxide, S-oxide, and N-desmethyl metabolites

Bioavailability: Oral: 48%

Half-life elimination:

Oral: Normal renal function: 2.5-3 hours; Cl_{cr} 25-35 mL/minute: 4.8 hours

I.V.: Normal renal function: 2-2.5 hours

Time to peak, serum: Oral: 2-3 hours; I.M.: ≤15 minutes

Excretion: Urine: Oral: 30%, I.V.: 70% (as unchanged drug); feces (as metabolites)

Pregnancy Risk Factor B

Dosage Forms CAP: 150 mg, 300 mg. INF [premixed in NaCl 0.45%; preservative free] (Zantac®): 50 mg (50 mL). INJ, solution: 25 mg/mL (2 mL, 6 mL); (Zantac®): 25 mg/mL (2 mL, 6 mL, 40 mL). SYR: 15 mg/mL (10 mL); (Zantac®): 15 mg/mL (473 mL). TAB: 75 mg [OTC], 150 mg, 300 mg; (Zantac®): 150 mg, 300 mg; (Zantac® 75): 75 mg; (Zantac 150™): 150 mg. TAB, effervescent (Zantac® EFFERdose®): 25 mg, 150 mg

Ranitidine Hydrochloride *see* Ranitidine *on page 1334*

Ranolazine *(ra NOE la zeen)*

U.S. Brand Names Ranexa™

Generic Available No

Pharmacologic Category Cardiovascular Agent, Miscellaneous

Use Treatment of chronic angina in combination with amlodipine, beta-blockers, or nitrates

Local Anesthetic/Vasoconstrictor Precautions Ranolazine is known to prolong QT interval. It is not known what effect vasoconstrictors in the local anesthetic regimen will have in patients taking medications that prolong QT interval. Until more information is obtained, it is suggested that the clinician consult with the physician prior to the use of vasoconstrictor and that the vasoconstrictor be used with caution. See Dental Comment.

Effects on Dental Treatment Key adverse event(s) related to dental treatment: Xerostomia (normal salivary flow resumes upon discontinuation).

Common Adverse Effects

>10%: Gastrointestinal: Constipation (5% to 8%; 19% in the elderly)

>0.5% to 10%:

Cardiovascular: Syncope (0.7%), palpitations, peripheral edema

Central nervous system: Dizziness (5% to 6%), headache (3% to 6%), vertigo

Gastrointestinal: Nausea (4% to 6%), abdominal pain, vomiting, xerostomia

Hematologic: Hematocrit decreased

Neuromuscular & skeletal: Weakness

Respiratory: Dyspnea

Mechanism of Action A proposed mechanism suggests ranolazine is a partial fatty acid oxidation inhibitor; may change myocardial energy metabolism from fatty acids to glucose, increasing the efficiency of ATP production under hypoxic conditions. Exerts antianginal and anti-ischemic effects without changing hemodynamic parameters. In addition, it is a late sodium channel inhibitor.

Drug Interactions

Cytochrome P450 Effect: Substrate of CYP3A4 (major), 2D6 (minor); Inhibits CYP3A4 (weak), 2D6 (weak)

Increased Effect/Toxicity: CYP3A4 inhibitors (eg, diltiazem, ketoconazole, verapamil) may increase the effects of ranolazine. Ranolazine may increase the effects of simvastatin and digoxin. Concurrent use of QT_c-prolonging agents may further increase QT interval.

Decreased Effect: CYP3A4 inducers may decrease the effect of ranolazine.

Pharmacodynamics/Kinetics

Absorption: Highly variable; ranolazine is a substrate of P-glycoprotein; concurrent use of P-glycoprotein inhibitors may increase absorption

Protein binding: 62%

Metabolism: Hepatic via CYP3A (major) and 2D6 (minor)

Half-life elimination: Terminal: 7 hours

Time to peak, plasma: 2-5 hours

Excretion: Primarily urine (75% mostly as metabolites, <5% to 7% excreted unchanged); feces (25% mostly as metabolites)

Dental Comment

This drug is known to prolong the QT interval. The QT interval is measured as the time and distance between the Q point of the QRS complex and the end of the T wave in the ECG tracing. After adjustment for heart rate, the QT interval is defined as prolonged if it is more than 450 msec in men and 460 msec in women. A long QT syndrome was first described in the 1950s and 60s as a congenital syndrome involving QT interval prolongation and syncope and sudden death. Some of the congenital long QT syndromes were characterized by a peculiar electrocardiographic appearance of the QRS complex involving a premature atria beat followed by a pause, then a subsequent sinus beat showing marked QT prolongation and deformity. This type of cardiac arrhythmia was originally termed "torsade de pointes" (translated from the French as "twisting of the points").

Prolongation of the QT interval is thought to result from delayed ventricular repolarization. The repolarization process within the myocardial cell is due to the efflux of intracellular potassium. The channels associated with this current can be blocked by many drugs and predisposes the electrical propagation cycle to torsade de pointes.

Ranolazine is one of the drugs confirmed to prolong the QT interval and is accepted as having a risk of causing torsade de pointes. The risk of drug-induced torsade de pointes is extremely low when a single QT interval prolonging drug is prescribed. In terms of epinephrine, it is not known what effect vasoconstrictors in the local anesthetic regimen will have in patients with a known history of congenital prolonged QT interval or in patients taking any medication that prolongs the QT interval. Until more information is obtained, it is suggested that the clinician consult with the physician prior to the use of a vasoconstrictor in suspected patients, and that the vasoconstrictor (epinephrine, levonordefrin [Neo-Cobefrin®]) be used with caution.

Rapamune® *see* Sirolimus *on page 1397*

Raphon [OTC] *see* Epinephrine *on page 546*

Raptiva® *see* Efalizumab *on page 529*

Rasburicase (ras BYOOR i kayse)

U.S. Brand Names Elitek™
Canadian Brand Names Fasturtec®
Generic Available No
Pharmacologic Category Enzyme; Enzyme, Urate-Oxidase (Recombinant)
Use Initial management of uric acid levels in pediatric patients with leukemia, lymphoma, and solid tumor malignancies receiving anticancer therapy expected to result in tumor lysis and elevation of plasma uric acid
Local Anesthetic/Vasoconstrictor Precautions No information available to require special precautions
Effects on Dental Treatment No significant effects or complications reported
Common Adverse Effects As reported in patients receiving rasburicase with antitumor therapy versus active-control:

>10%:
    Central nervous system: Fever (5% to 46%), headache (26%)
    Dermatologic: Rash (13%)
    Gastrointestinal: Vomiting (50%), nausea (27%), abdominal pain (20%), constipation (20%), mucositis (2% to 15%), diarrhea (≤1% to 20%)

1% to 10%:
    Hematologic: Neutropenia with fever (4%), neutropenia (2%)
    Respiratory: Respiratory distress (3%)
    Miscellaneous: Sepsis (3%)

Mechanism of Action Rasburicase is a recombinant urate-oxidase enzyme, which converts uric acid to allantoin (an inactive and soluble metabolite of uric acid); it does not inhibit the formation of uric acid.

Pharmacodynamics/Kinetics
Distribution: Pediatric patients: 110-127 mL/kg
Half-life elimination: Pediatric patients: 18 hours

Pregnancy Risk Factor C

Razadyne™ *see* Galantamine *on page 720*

Razadyne™ ER *see* Galantamine *on page 720*

Rea-Lo® [OTC] *see* Urea *on page 1551*

ReAzo [OTC] *see* Phenazopyridine *on page 1220*

Rebetol® *see* Ribavirin *on page 1343*

Rebetron® *see* Interferon Alfa-2b and Ribavirin *on page 847*

Rebif® *see* Interferon Beta-1a *on page 849*

Reclipsen™ *see* Ethinyl Estradiol and Desogestrel *on page 592*

Recombinant α-L-Iduronidase (Glycosaminoglycan α-L-Iduronohydrolase) *see* Laronidase *on page 900*

Recombinant Hirudin *see* Lepirudin *on page 904*

Recombinant Human Deoxyribonuclease *see* Dornase Alfa *on page 501*

Recombinant Human Follicle Stimulating Hormone *see* Follitropins *on page 698*

Recombinant Human Insulin-Like Growth Factor-1 *see* Mecasermin *on page 968*

Recombinant Human Interleukin-11 *see* Oprelvekin *on page 1149*

Recombinant Human Luteinizing Hormone *see* Lutropin Alfa *on page 958*

Recombinant Human Parathyroid Hormone (1-34) *see* Teriparatide *on page 1461*

Recombinant Human Platelet-Derived Growth Factor B *see* Becaplermin *on page 182*

Recombinant Interleukin-11 *see* Oprelvekin *on page 1149*

Recombinant N-Acetylgalactosamine 4-Sulfatase *see* Galsulfase *on page 721*

Recombinant Plasminogen Activator *see* Reteplase *on page 1341*

Recombinate™ *see* Antihemophilic Factor (Recombinant) *on page 130*

Recombivax HB® *see* Hepatitis B Vaccine *on page 769*

Rectacaine [OTC] *see* Phenylephrine *on page 1226*

Red Cross™ Canker Sore [OTC] *see* Benzocaine *on page 190*

Reese's® Pinworm Medicine [OTC] *see* Pyrantel Pamoate *on page 1314*

ReFacto® *see* Antihemophilic Factor (Recombinant) *on page 130*

Refenesen Plus [OTC] *see* Guaifenesin and Pseudoephedrine *on page 755*

Refludan® *see* Lepirudin *on page 904*

Refresh® [OTC] *see* Artificial Tears *on page 143*

Refresh Liquigel™ [OTC] *see* Carboxymethylcellulose *on page 271*

Refresh Plus® [OTC] *see* Artificial Tears *on page 143*

Refresh Tears® [OTC] *see* Artificial Tears *on page 143*

Regitine [DSC] *see* Phentolamine *on page 1226*

Reglan® *see* Metoclopramide *on page 1029*

Regonol® *see* Pyridostigmine *on page 1315*

Regranex® *see* Becaplermin *on page 182*

Regular Insulin *see* Insulin Regular *on page 841*

Reguloid® [OTC] *see* Psyllium *on page 1313*

Relacon-DM *see* Guaifenesin, Pseudoephedrine, and Dextromethorphan *on page 757*

Relafen® *see* Nabumetone *on page 1077*

Relenza® *see* Zanamivir *on page 1592*

Relief® [OTC] *see* Phenylephrine *on page 1226*

Relpax® *see* Eletriptan *on page 533*

Remeron® *see* Mirtazapine *on page 1052*

Remeron SolTab® *see* Mirtazapine *on page 1052*

Reme-T™ [OTC] *see* Coal Tar *on page 383*

Remicade® *see* Infliximab *on page 832*

Remifentanil (rem i FEN ta nil)

U.S. Brand Names Ultiva®
Canadian Brand Names Ultiva®
Mexican Brand Names Ultiva®
Generic Available No
Synonyms GI87084B
Pharmacologic Category Analgesic, Narcotic
Use Analgesic for use during the induction and maintenance of general anesthesia; for continued analgesia into the immediate postoperative period; analgesic component of monitored anesthesia
Unlabeled/Investigational Use Management of pain in mechanically-ventilated patients
Local Anesthetic/Vasoconstrictor Precautions No information available to require special precautions
Effects on Dental Treatment No significant effects or complications reported
Common Adverse Effects
>10%: Gastrointestinal: Nausea, vomiting

1% to 10%:

Cardiovascular: Hypotension (dose dependent), bradycardia (dose dependent), tachycardia, hypertension

Central nervous system: Dizziness, headache, agitation, fever

Dermatologic: Pruritus

Neuromuscular & skeletal: Muscle rigidity (dose dependent)

Ocular: Visual disturbances

Respiratory: Respiratory depression, apnea, hypoxia

Miscellaneous: Shivering, postoperative pain

Restrictions C-II

Mechanism of Action Binds with stereospecific mu-opioid receptors at many sites within the CNS, increases pain threshold, alters pain reception, inhibits ascending pain pathways

Drug Interactions

Increased Effect/Toxicity: Additive effects with other CNS depressants. Synergistic with other anesthetics, may need to decrease thiopental, propofol, isoflurane, and midazolam by up to 75%.

Pharmacodynamics/Kinetics

Onset of action: I.V.: 1-3 minutes

Distribution: V_d: 100 mL/kg; increased in children

Protein binding: ~70% (primarily alpha$_1$ acid glycoprotein)

Metabolism: Rapid via blood and tissue esterases

Half-life elimination (dose dependent): Terminal: 10-20 minutes; effective: 3-10 minutes

Excretion: Urine

Pregnancy Risk Factor C

Reminyl® [DSC] *see* Galantamine *on page 720*

Remodulin® *see* Treprostinil *on page 1523*

Renacidin® *see* Citric Acid, Magnesium Carbonate, and Glucono-Delta-Lactone *on page 353*

Renagel® *see* Sevelamer *on page 1388*

Renese® *see* Polythiazide *on page 1255*

Reno-30® *see* Diatrizoate Meglumine *on page 453*

Reno-60® *see* Diatrizoate Meglumine *on page 453*

RenoCal-76® *see* Diatrizoate Meglumine and Diatrizoate Sodium *on page 453*

Reno-Dip® *see* Diatrizoate Meglumine *on page 453*

Renografin®-60 *see* Diatrizoate Meglumine and Diatrizoate Sodium *on page 453*

Renova® *see* Tretinoin (Topical) *on page 1525*

ReoPro® *see* Abciximab *on page 26*

Repaglinide (re pa GLI nide)

Related Information

Endocrine Disorders and Pregnancy *on page 1659*

U.S. Brand Names Prandin®

Canadian Brand Names GlucoNorm®; Prandin®

Generic Available No

Pharmacologic Category Antidiabetic Agent, Meglitinide Derivative

Use Management of type 2 diabetes mellitus (noninsulin dependent, NIDDM); may be used in combination with metformin or thiazolidinediones

Local Anesthetic/Vasoconstrictor Precautions No information available to require special precautions

Effects on Dental Treatment No significant effects or complications reported

Common Adverse Effects

>10%:

Central nervous system: Headache (9% to 11%)

Endocrine & metabolic: Hypoglycemia (16% to 31%)

Respiratory: Upper respiratory tract infection (10% to 16%)

1% to 10%:

Cardiovascular: Chest pain (2% to 3%), ischemia (4%)

Gastrointestinal: Nausea (3% to 5%), heartburn (2% to 4%), vomiting (2% to 3%) constipation (2% to 3%), diarrhea (4% to 5%), tooth disorder (<1% to 2%)

Genitourinary: Urinary tract infection (2% to 3%)

Neuromuscular & skeletal: Arthralgia (3% to 6%), back pain (5% to 6%), paresthesia (2% to 3%)

Respiratory: Sinusitis (3% to 6%), rhinitis (3% to 7%), bronchitis (2% to 6%)

Miscellaneous: Allergy (1% to 2%)

(Continued)

Repaglinide *(Continued)*

Mechanism of Action Nonsulfonylurea hypoglycemic agent of the meglitinide class (the nonsulfonylurea moiety of glyburide) used in the management of type 2 diabetes mellitus; stimulates insulin release from the pancreatic beta cells

Drug Interactions

Cytochrome P450 Effect: Substrate of CYP2C8/9 (major), 3A4 (major)

Increased Effect/Toxicity: Concurrent use of other hypoglycemic agents may increase risk of hypoglycemia. Gemfibrozil may increase the serum concentration of repaglinide (resulting in severe, prolonged hypoglycemia), and the addition of itraconazole may augment the effects of gemfibrozil on repaglinide. Macrolide antibiotics may increase the effects of repaglinide. CYP2C8/9 inhibitors may increase the levels/effects of repaglinide; example inhibitors include delavirdine, fluconazole, gemfibrozil, ketoconazole, nicardipine, NSAIDs, pioglitazone, and sulfonamides. CYP3A4 inhibitors may increase the levels/effects of repaglinide; example inhibitors include azole antifungals, clarithromycin, diclofenac, doxycycline, erythromycin, imatinib, isoniazid, nefazodone, nicardipine, propofol, protease inhibitors, quinidine, telithromycin, and verapamil.

Decreased Effect: CYP2C8/9 inducers may decrease the levels/effects of repaglinide; example inducers include carbamazepine, phenobarbital, phenytoin, rifampin, rifapentine, and secobarbital. CYP3A4 inducers may decrease the levels/effects of repaglinide; example inducers include aminoglutethimide, carbamazepine, nafcillin, nevirapine, phenobarbital, phenytoin, and rifamycins.

Pharmacodynamics/Kinetics

Onset of action: Single dose: Increased insulin levels: ~15-60 minutes

Duration: 4-6 hours

Absorption: Rapid and complete

Distribution: V_d: 31 L

Protein binding, plasma: >98%

Metabolism: Hepatic via CYP3A4 isoenzyme and glucuronidation to inactive metabolites

Bioavailability: Mean absolute: ~56%

Half-life elimination: 1 hour

Time to peak, plasma: ~1 hour

Excretion: Within 96 hours: Feces (~90%, <2% as parent drug); Urine (~8%)

Pregnancy Risk Factor C

Repan® *see* Butalbital, Acetaminophen, and Caffeine *on page 239*

Replace [OTC] *see* Vitamins (Multiple/Oral) *on page 1582*

Replace with Iron [OTC] *see* Vitamins (Multiple/Oral) *on page 1582*

Repliva 21/7™ *see* Vitamins (Multiple/Oral) *on page 1582*

Reprexain™ *see* Hydrocodone and Ibuprofen *on page 787*

Repronex® *see* Menotropins *on page 982*

Requip® *see* Ropinirole *on page 1365*

Rescon GG *see* Guaifenesin and Phenylephrine *on page 754*

Rescon-Jr *see* Chlorpheniramine and Phenylephrine *on page 324*

Rescriptor® *see* Delavirdine *on page 429*

Reserpine *(re SER peen)*

Related Information

Cardiovascular Diseases *on page 1636*

Generic Available Yes

Pharmacologic Category Central Monoamine-Depleting Agent; Rauwolfia Alkaloid

Use Management of mild-to-moderate hypertension; treatment of agitated psychotic states (schizophrenia)

Unlabeled/Investigational Use Management of tardive dyskinesia

Local Anesthetic/Vasoconstrictor Precautions No information available to require special precautions

Effects on Dental Treatment Key adverse event(s) related to dental treatment: Xerostomia and changes in salivation (normal salivary flow resumes upon discontinuation).

Mechanism of Action Reduces blood pressure via depletion of sympathetic biogenic amines (norepinephrine and dopamine); this also commonly results in sedative effects

Pregnancy Risk Factor C

Resource® GlutaSolve® [OTC] *see* Glutamine *on page 743*

Respa-DM® *see* Guaifenesin and Dextromethorphan *on page 754*

Respaire®-60 SR *see* Guaifenesin and Pseudoephedrine *on page 755*

Respaire®-120 SR *see* Guaifenesin and Pseudoephedrine *on page 755*

Restasis® *see* CycloSPORINE *on page 406*

Restoril® *see* Temazepam *on page 1453*

Restylane® *see* Hyaluronate and Derivatives *on page 773*

Retavase® *see* Reteplase *on page 1341*

Reteplase (RE ta plase)

Related Information
Cardiovascular Diseases *on page 1636*

U.S. Brand Names Retavase®

Canadian Brand Names Retavase®

Generic Available No

Synonyms Recombinant Plasminogen Activator; r-PA

Pharmacologic Category Thrombolytic Agent

Use Management of acute myocardial infarction (AMI); improvement of ventricular function; reduction of the incidence of CHF and the reduction of mortality following AMI

Local Anesthetic/Vasoconstrictor Precautions No information available to require special precautions

Effects on Dental Treatment No significant effects or complications reported

Common Adverse Effects Bleeding is the most frequent adverse effect associated with reteplase. Heparin and aspirin have been administered concurrently with reteplase in clinical trials. The incidence of adverse events is a reflection of these combined therapies, and are comparable with comparison thrombolytics.

>10%: Local: Injection site bleeding (4.6% to 48.6%)

1% to 10%:
Gastrointestinal: Bleeding (1.8% to 9.0%)
Genitourinary: Bleeding (0.9% to 9.5%)
Hematologic: Anemia (0.9% to 2.6%)

Other adverse effects noted are frequently associated with MI (and therefore may or may not be attributable to Retavase®) and include arrhythmia, hypotension, cardiogenic shock, pulmonary edema, cardiac arrest, reinfarction, pericarditis, tamponade, thrombosis, and embolism.

Mechanism of Action Reteplase is a nonglycosylated form of tPA produced by recombinant DNA technology using *E. coli*; it initiates local fibrinolysis by binding to fibrin in a thrombus (clot) and converts entrapped plasminogen to plasmin

Drug Interactions
Increased Effect/Toxicity: The risk of bleeding associated with reteplase may be increased by oral anticoagulants (warfarin), heparin, low molecular weight heparins, and drugs which affect platelet function (eg, NSAIDs, dipyridamole, ticlopidine, clopidogrel, IIb/IIIa antagonists). Concurrent use with aspirin and heparin may increase the risk of bleeding; however, aspirin and heparin were used concomitantly with reteplase in the majority of patients in clinical studies.

Decreased Effect: Aminocaproic acid (antifibrinolytic agent) may decrease effectiveness of thrombolytic agents.

Pharmacodynamics/Kinetics
Onset of action: Thrombolysis: 30-90 minutes
Half-life elimination: 13-16 minutes
Excretion: Feces and urine
Clearance: Plasma: 250-450 mL/minute

Pregnancy Risk Factor C

Retin-A® *see* Tretinoin (Topical) *on page 1525*

Retin-A® Micro *see* Tretinoin (Topical) *on page 1525*

Retinoic Acid *see* Tretinoin (Topical) *on page 1525*

Retisert™ *see* Fluocinolone *on page 667*

Retrovir® *see* Zidovudine *on page 1594*

Revatio™ *see* Sildenafil *on page 1390*

Reversol® *see* Edrophonium *on page 528*

Revex® *see* Nalmefene *on page 1084*

ReVia® *see* Naltrexone *on page 1086*

Revlimid® *see* Lenalidomide *on page 903*

Reyataz® *see* Atazanavir *on page 152*

rFSH-alpha *see* Follitropins *on page 698*

rFSH-beta *see* Follitropins *on page 698*

rFVIIa *see* Factor VIIa (Recombinant) *on page 632*

R-Gene® *see* Arginine *on page 137*

rGM-CSF *see* Sargramostim *on page 1378*

rhASB *see* Galsulfase *on page 721*

r-hCG *see* Chorionic Gonadotropin (Recombinant) *on page 337*

Rheumatrex® *see* Methotrexate *on page 1012*

rhFSH-alpha *see* Follitropins *on page 698*

rhFSH-beta *see* Follitropins *on page 698*

r-h α-GAL *see* Agalsidase Beta *on page 55*

RhIG *see* Rh_o(D) Immune Globulin *on page 1342*

rhIGF-1 *see* Mecasermin *on page 968*

rhIGF-1/rhIGFBP-3 *see* Mecasermin *on page 968*

rhIL-11 *see* Oprelvekin *on page 1149*

Rhinall [OTC] *see* Phenylephrine *on page 1226*

Rhinocort® Aqua® *see* Budesonide *on page 224*

r-hLH *see* Lutropin Alfa *on page 958*

Rho(D) Immune Globulin (Human) *see* Rh_o(D) Immune Globulin *on page 1342*

RhoGAM® *see* Rh_o(D) Immune Globulin *on page 1342*

RholGIV *see* Rh_o(D) Immune Globulin *on page 1342*

RholVIM *see* Rh_o(D) Immune Globulin *on page 1342*

Rhophylac® *see* Rh_o(D) Immune Globulin *on page 1342*

rhPTH(1-34) *see* Teriparatide *on page 1461*

Rh_o(D) Immune Globulin (ar aych oh (dee) i MYUN GLOB yoo lin)

Related Information

Immunizations (Vaccines) *on page 1786*

U.S. Brand Names BayRho-D® Full-Dose; BayRho-D® Mini-Dose; MICRhoGAM®; RhoGAM®; Rhophylac®; WinRho® SDF

Canadian Brand Names BayRho-D® Full-Dose

Generic Available No

Synonyms RhIG; Rho(D) Immune Globulin (Human); RholGIV; RholVIM

Pharmacologic Category Immune Globulin

Use

Suppression of Rh isoimmunization: Use in the following situations when an Rh_o(D)-negative individual is exposed to Rh_o(D)-positive blood: During delivery of an Rh_o(D)-positive infant; abortion; amniocentesis; chorionic villus sampling; ruptured tubal pregnancy; abdominal trauma; transplacental hemorrhage. Used when the mother is Rh_o(D) negative, the father of the child is either Rh_o(D) positive or Rh_o(D) unknown, the baby is either Rh_o(D) positive or Rh_o(D) unknown.

Transfusion: Suppression of Rh isoimmunization in Rh_o(D)-negative female children and female adults in their childbearing years transfused with Rh_o(D) antigen-positive RBCs or blood components containing Rh_o(D) antigen-positive RBCs

Treatment of idiopathic thrombocytopenic purpura (ITP): Used in the following nonsplenectomized Rh_o(D) positive individuals: Children with acute or chronic ITP, adults with chronic ITP, children and adults with ITP secondary to HIV infection

Local Anesthetic/Vasoconstrictor Precautions No information available to require special precautions

Effects on Dental Treatment No significant effects or complications reported

Common Adverse Effects Frequency not defined.

Cardiovascular: Hyper-/hypotension, pallor, tachycardia, vasodilation

Central nervous system: Chills, dizziness, fever, headache, malaise, somnolence

Dermatologic: Pruritus, rash

Gastrointestinal: Abdominal pain, diarrhea, nausea, vomiting

Hematologic: Hemoglobin decreased (patients with ITP), intravascular hemolysis (patients with ITP)

Hepatic: LDH increased

Local: Injection site reaction: Discomfort, induration, mild pain, redness, swelling

Neuromuscular & skeletal: Arthralgia, back pain, hyperkinesia, myalgia, weakness

Renal: Acute renal insufficiency

Miscellaneous: Anaphylaxis, diaphoresis, infusion-related reactions

Mechanism of Action

Rh suppression: Prevents isoimmunization by suppressing the immune response and antibody formation by $Rh_o(D)$ negative individuals to $Rh_o(D)$ positive red blood cells.

ITP: Not completely characterized; $Rh_o(D)$ immune globulin is thought to form anti-D-coated red blood cell complexes which bind to macrophage Fc receptors within the spleen; blocking or saturating the spleens ability to clear antibody-coated cells, including platelets. In this manner, platelets are spared from destruction.

Drug Interactions

Decreased Effect: $Rh_o(D)$ immune globulin may interfere with the response of live vaccines; vaccines should not be administered within 3 months after $Rh_o(D)$

Pharmacodynamics/Kinetics

Onset of platelet increase: ITP: Platelets should rise within 1-2 days

Peak effect: In 7-14 days

Duration: Suppression of Rh isoimmunization: ~12 weeks; Treatment of ITP: 30 days (variable)

Distribution: V_d: I.M.: 8.59 L

Half-life elimination: 21-30 days

Time to peak, plasma: I.M.: 5-10 days; I.V. (WinRho® SDF): ≤2 hours

Pregnancy Risk Factor C

rHuEPO-α *see* Epoetin Alfa *on page 552*

rHu-KGF *see* Palifermin *on page 1178*

rhuMAb-E25 *see* Omalizumab *on page 1144*

rhuMAb-VEGF *see* Bevacizumab *on page 204*

Ribasphere™ *see* Ribavirin *on page 1343*

Ribavirin (rye ba VYE rin)

Related Information

Systemic Viral Diseases *on page 1675*

U.S. Brand Names Copegus®; Rebetol®; Ribasphere™; Virazole®

Canadian Brand Names Virazole®

Generic Available Yes: Capsule, tablet

Synonyms RTCA; Tribavirin

Pharmacologic Category Antiviral Agent

Use

Inhalation: Treatment of patients with respiratory syncytial virus (RSV) infections; specially indicated for treatment of severe lower respiratory tract RSV infections in patients with an underlying compromising condition (prematurity, bronchopulmonary dysplasia and other chronic lung conditions, congenital heart disease, immunodeficiency, immunosuppression), and recent transplant recipients

Oral capsule:

In combination with interferon alfa-2b (Intron® A) injection for the treatment of chronic hepatitis C in patients with compensated liver disease who have relapsed after alpha interferon therapy or were previously untreated with alpha interferons

In combination with peginterferon alfa-2b (PEG-Intron®) injection for the treatment of chronic hepatitis C in patients with compensated liver disease who were previously untreated with alpha interferons

Oral solution: In combination with interferon alfa 2b (Intron® A) injection for the treatment of chronic hepatitis C in patients ≥3 years of age with compensated liver disease who were previously untreated with alpha interferons or patients ≥18 years of age who have relapsed after alpha interferon therapy

Oral tablet: In combination with peginterferon alfa-2a (Pegasys®) injection for the treatment of chronic hepatitis C in patients with compensated liver disease who were previously untreated with alpha interferons (includes patients with histological evidence of cirrhosis [Child-Pugh class A] and patients with clinically-stable HIV disease)

Unlabeled/Investigational Use Used in other viral infections including influenza A and B and adenovirus

Local Anesthetic/Vasoconstrictor Precautions No information available to require special precautions

Effects on Dental Treatment No significant effects or complications reported

Common Adverse Effects

Inhalation:

1% to 10%:

Central nervous system: Fatigue, headache, insomnia

(Continued)

Ribavirin *(Continued)*

Gastrointestinal: Nausea, anorexia

Hematologic: Anemia

Note: Incidence of adverse effects (approximate) in healthcare workers: Headache (51%); conjunctivitis (32%); rhinitis, nausea, rash, dizziness, pharyngitis, and lacrimation (10% to 20%)

Oral (all adverse reactions are documented while receiving combination therapy with interferon alpha-2b or interferon alpha-2a; percentages as reported in adults):

>10%:

Central nervous system: Fatigue (60% to 70%)*, headache (43% to 66%)*, fever (32% to 46%)*, insomnia (26% to 41%), depression (20% to 36%)*, irritability (23% to 32%), dizziness (14% to 26%), impaired concentration (10% to 14%)*, emotional lability (7% to 12%)*

Dermatologic: Alopecia (27% to 36%), pruritus (13% to 29%), dry skin (13% to 24%), rash (5% to 28%), dermatitis (up to 16%)

Gastrointestinal: Nausea (33% to 47%), anorexia (21% to 32%), weight decrease (10% to 29%), diarrhea (10% to 22%), dyspepsia (8% to 16%), vomiting (9% to 14%)*, abdominal pain (8% to 13%), xerostomia (up to 12%), RUQ pain (up to 12%)

Hematologic: Neutropenia (8% to 27%; 40% with HIV coinfection), hemoglobin decreased (25% to 36%), hyperbilirubinemia (24% to 34%), anemia (11% to 17%), lymphopenia (12% to 14%), absolute neutrophil count <0.5 x 10^9/L (5% to 11%), thrombocytopenia (<1% to 14%), hemolytic anemia (10% to 13%), WBC decreased

Neuromuscular & skeletal: Myalgia (40% to 64%)*, rigors (40% to 48%), arthralgia (22% to 34%)*, musculoskeletal pain (19% to 28%)

Respiratory: Dyspnea (13% to 26%), cough (7% to 23%), pharyngitis (up to 13%), sinusitis (up to 12%)*, nasal congestion

Miscellaneous: Flu-like syndrome (13% to 18%)*, viral infection (up to 12%), diaphoresis increased (up to 11%)

*Similar to interferon alone

1% to 10%:

Cardiovascular: Chest pain (5% to 9%)*, flushing (up to 4%)

Central nervous system: Mood alteration (up to 6%; 9% with HIV coinfection), memory impairment (up to 6%), malaise (up to 6%), nervousness (~5%)*

Dermatologic: Eczema (4% to 5%)

Endocrine & metabolic: Hypothyroidism (up to 5%)

Gastrointestinal: Taste perversion (4% to 9%), constipation (up to 5%)

Genitourinary: Menstrual disorder (up to 7%)

Hepatic: Hepatomegaly (up to 4%)

Neuromuscular & skeletal: Weakness (9% to 10%), back pain (5%)

Ocular: Conjunctivitis (up to 6%), blurred vision (up to 5%)

Respiratory: Rhinitis (up to 8%), exertional dyspnea (up to 7%)

Miscellaneous: Fungal infection (up to 6%)

*Similar to interferon alone

Note: Incidence of anorexia, headache, fever, suicidal ideation, and vomiting are higher in children.

Restrictions An FDA-approved medication guide is available at http://www.fda.gov/cder/Offices/ODS/labeling.htm; distribute to each patient to whom this medication is dispensed for the treatment of hepatitis C.

Mechanism of Action Inhibits replication of RNA and DNA viruses; inhibits influenza virus RNA polymerase activity and inhibits the initiation and elongation of RNA fragments resulting in inhibition of viral protein synthesis

Drug Interactions

Increased Effect/Toxicity: Concomitant use of ribavirin and nucleoside analogues may increase the risk of developing lactic acidosis (includes adefovir, didanosine, lamivudine, stavudine, zalcitabine, zidovudine). Concurrent therapy of zidovudine with ribavirin/interferon alfa-2a may cause increased risk of severe anemia and/or severe neutropenia. Concurrent use with didanosine has been noted to increase the risk of pancreatitis and/or peripheral neuropathy in addition to lactic acidosis. Suspend therapy if signs/symptoms of toxicity are present. Concurrent therapy with Interferons (alfa) may increase the risk of hemolytic anemia.

Decreased Effect: Decreased effect of lamivudine, stavudine, and zidovudine (*in vitro*).

Pharmacodynamics/Kinetics

Absorption: Inhalation: Systemic; dependent upon respiratory factors and method of drug delivery; maximal absorption occurs with the use of aerosol generator via endotracheal tube; highest concentrations in respiratory tract and erythrocytes

Distribution: Oral capsule: Single dose: V_d 2825 L; distribution significantly prolonged in the erythrocyte (16-40 days), which can be used as a marker for intracellular metabolism

Protein binding: Oral: None

Metabolism: Hepatically and intracellularly (forms active metabolites); may be necessary for drug action

Bioavailability: Oral: 64%

Half-life elimination, plasma:

Children: Inhalation: 6.5-11 hours

Adults: Oral:

Capsule, single dose (Rebetol®, Ribasphere™): 24 hours in healthy adults, 44 hours with chronic hepatitis C infection (increases to ~298 hours at steady state)

Tablet, single dose (Copegus®): 120-170 hours

Time to peak, serum: Inhalation: At end of inhalation period; Oral capsule: Multiple doses: 3 hours; Tablet: 2 hours

Excretion: Inhalation: Urine (40% as unchanged drug and metabolites); Oral capsule: Urine (61%), feces (12%)

Pregnancy Risk Factor X

Ribavirin and Interferon Alfa-2b Combination Pack *see* Interferon Alfa-2b and Ribavirin *on page 847*

Ribo-100 *see* Riboflavin *on page 1345*

Riboflavin (RYE boe flay vin)

U.S. Brand Names Ribo-100

Generic Available Yes

Synonyms Lactoflavin; Vitamin B_2; Vitamin G

Pharmacologic Category Vitamin, Water Soluble

Use Prevention of riboflavin deficiency and treatment of ariboflavinosis

Local Anesthetic/Vasoconstrictor Precautions No information available to require special precautions

Effects on Dental Treatment No significant effects or complications reported

Significant Adverse Effects Frequency not defined: Genitourinary: Discoloration of urine (yellow-orange)

Dosage Oral:

Riboflavin deficiency:

Children: 2.5-10 mg/day in divided doses

Adults: 5-30 mg/day in divided doses

Recommended daily allowance:

Children: 0.4-1.8 mg

Adults: 1.2-1.7 mg

Mechanism of Action Component of flavoprotein enzymes that work together, which are necessary for normal tissue respiration; also needed for activation of pyridoxine and conversion of tryptophan to niacin

Warnings/Precautions Riboflavin deficiency often occurs in the presence of other B vitamin deficiencies

Drug Interactions Decreased absorption with probenecid

Pharmacodynamics/Kinetics

Absorption: Readily via GI tract, however, food increases extent; decreased with hepatitis, cirrhosis, or biliary obstruction

Metabolism: None

Half-life elimination: Biologic: 66-84 minutes

Excretion: Urine (9%) as unchanged drug

Pregnancy Risk Factor A/C (dose exceeding RDA recommendation)

Lactation Enters breast milk/compatible

Dosage Forms

Tablet: 25 mg, 50 mg, 100 mg

Ribo-100: 100 mg

Rid-A-Pain Dental Drops [OTC] *see* Benzocaine *on page 190*

Ridaura® *see* Auranofin *on page 166*

RID® Maximum Strength [OTC] *see* Pyrethrins and Piperonyl Butoxide *on page 1315*

Rid® Spray [OTC] *see* Permethrin *on page 1218*

Rifabutin (rif a BYOO tin)

Related Information

Systemic Viral Diseases *on page 1675*

Tuberculosis *on page 1673*

(Continued)

Rifabutin *(Continued)*

U.S. Brand Names Mycobutin®

Canadian Brand Names Mycobutin®

Generic Available No

Synonyms Ansamycin

Pharmacologic Category Antibiotic, Miscellaneous; Antitubercular Agent

Use Prevention of disseminated *Mycobacterium avium* complex (MAC) in patients with advanced HIV infection

Unlabeled/Investigational Use Utilized in multidrug regimens for treatment of MAC

Local Anesthetic/Vasoconstrictor Precautions No information available to require special precautions

Effects on Dental Treatment No significant effects or complications reported

Common Adverse Effects

>10%:

Dermatologic: Rash (11%)

Genitourinary: Discoloration of urine (30%)

Hematologic: Neutropenia (25%), leukopenia (17%)

1% to 10%:

Central nervous system: Headache (3%)

Gastrointestinal: Vomiting/nausea (3%), abdominal pain (4%), diarrhea (3%), anorexia (2%), flatulence (2%), eructation (3%)

Hematologic: Anemia, thrombocytopenia (5%)

Hepatic: Increased AST/ALT (7% to 9%)

Neuromuscular & skeletal: Myalgia

Mechanism of Action Inhibits DNA-dependent RNA polymerase at the beta subunit which prevents chain initiation

Drug Interactions

Cytochrome P450 Effect: Substrate of CYP3A4 (major); Induces CYP3A4 (strong)

Increased Effect/Toxicity: Rifabutin may increase the therapeutic effect of clopidogrel; concurrent use with isoniazid may increase risk of hepatotoxicity; the levels/toxicity of rifabutin may be increased by imidazole antifungals, macrolide antibiotics, and protease inhibitors.

Decreased Effect: Rifabutin may decrease the levels/effects of alfentanil, amiodarone, angiotensin II receptor blockers (irbesartan, losartan), CYP3A4 substrates (eg, clarithromycin, erythromycin, mirtazapine, nefazodone, venlafaxine), 5-HT$_3$ antagonists, imidazole antifungals, aprepitant, barbiturates, benzodiazepines (metabolized by oxidation), beta blockers, buspirone, calcium channel blockers, chloramphenicol, corticosteroids, cyclosporine, dapsone, disopyramide, estrogen and progestin contraceptives, fluconazole, gefitinib, HMG-CoA reductase inhibitors, methadone, morphine, phenytoin, propafenone, protease inhibitors, quinidine, repaglinide, reverse transcriptase inhibitors (non-nucleoside), tacrolimus, tamoxifen, terbinafine, tocainide, tricyclic antidepressants, warfarin, zaleplon, zolpidem. The effects of rifabutin may be decreased by CYP3A4 inducers (eg, aminoglutethimide, carbamazepine, nafcillin, nevirapine, phenobarbital, phenytoin).

Pharmacodynamics/Kinetics

Absorption: Readily, 53%

Distribution: V$_d$: 9.32 L/kg; distributes to body tissues including the lungs, liver, spleen, eyes, and kidneys

Protein binding: 85%

Metabolism: To active and inactive metabolites

Bioavailability: Absolute: HIV: 20%

Half-life elimination: Terminal: 45 hours (range: 16-69 hours)

Time to peak, serum: 2-4 hours

Excretion: Urine (10% as unchanged drug, 53% as metabolites); feces (10% as unchanged drug, 30% as metabolites)

Pregnancy Risk Factor B

Rifadin® *see* Rifampin *on page 1346*

Rifamate® *see* Rifampin and Isoniazid *on page 1348*

Rifampicin *see* Rifampin *on page 1346*

Rifampin *(RIF am pin)*

Related Information

Rifapentine *on page 1349*

Tuberculosis *on page 1673*

U.S. Brand Names Rifadin®
Canadian Brand Names Rifadin®; Rofact™
Mexican Brand Names Pestarin®; Rifadin®; Rimactan®
Generic Available Yes
Synonyms Rifampicin
Pharmacologic Category Antibiotic, Miscellaneous; Antitubercular Agent
Use Management of active tuberculosis in combination with other agents; elimination of meningococci from the nasopharynx in asymptomatic carriers
Unlabeled/Investigational Use Prophylaxis of *Haemophilus influenzae* type b infection; *Legionella* pneumonia; used in combination with other anti-infectives in the treatment of staphylococcal infections; treatment of *M. leprae* infections
Local Anesthetic/Vasoconstrictor Precautions No information available to require special precautions
Effects on Dental Treatment No significant effects or complications reported
Common Adverse Effects
Frequency not defined:
  Cardiovascular: Edema, flushing
  Central nervous system: Ataxia, behavioral changes, concentration impaired, confusion, dizziness, drowsiness, fatigue, fever, headache, numbness, psychosis
  Dermatologic: Pemphigoid reaction, pruritus, urticaria
  Endocrine & metabolic: Adrenal insufficiency, menstrual disorders
  Hematologic: Agranulocytosis (rare), DIC, eosinophilia, hemoglobin decreased, hemolysis, hemolytic anemia, leukopenia, thrombocytopenia (especially with high-dose therapy)
  Hepatic: Hepatitis (rare), jaundice
  Neuromuscular & skeletal: Myalgia, osteomalacia, weakness
  Ocular: Exudative conjunctivitis, visual changes
  Renal: Acute renal failure, BUN increased, hemoglobinuria, hematuria, interstitial nephritis, uric acid increased
  Miscellaneous: Flu-like syndrome
1% to 10%:
  Dermatologic: Rash (1% to 5%)
  Gastrointestinal (1% to 2%): Anorexia, cramps, diarrhea, epigastric distress, flatulence, heartburn, nausea, pseudomembranous colitis, pancreatitis vomiting
  Hepatic: LFTs increased (up to 14%)
Mechanism of Action Inhibits bacterial RNA synthesis by binding to the beta subunit of DNA-dependent RNA polymerase, blocking RNA transcription
Drug Interactions
  Cytochrome P450 Effect: Induces CYP1A2 (strong), 2A6 (strong), 2B6 (strong), 2C8 (strong), 2C9 (strong), 2C19 (strong), 3A4 (strong)
  Increased Effect/Toxicity: Rifampin may increase the therapeutic effect of clopidogrel; concurrent use with isoniazid, pyrazinamide, or protease inhibitors (amprenavir, saquinavir/ritonavir) may increase risk of hepatotoxicity; macrolide antibiotics may increase levels/toxicity of rifampin
  Decreased Effect: Rifampin may decrease the levels/effects of the following drugs: Acetaminophen, alfentanil, amiodarone, angiotensin II receptor blockers (irbesartan and losartan), 5-HT$_3$ antagonists, imidazole antifungals, aprepitant, barbiturates, benzodiazepines (metabolized by oxidation), beta blockers, buspirone, calcium channel blockers, chloramphenicol, corticosteroids, cyclosporine; CYP1A2, 2A6, 2B6, 2C8, 2C9, 2C19, and 3A4 substrates (eg, aminophylline, amiodarone, bupropion, fluoxetine, fluvoxamine, ifosfamide, methsuximide, mirtazapine, nateglinide, pioglitazone, promethazine, proton pump inhibitors, ropinirole, rosiglitazone, selegiline, sertraline, theophylline, venlafaxine, and zafirlukast); dapsone, disopyramide, estrogen and progestin contraceptives, fexofenadine, fluconazole, fusidic acid, gefitinib, HMG-CoA reductase inhibitors, methadone, morphine, phenytoin, propafenone, protease inhibitors, quinidine, repaglinide, reverse transcriptase inhibitors (non-nucleoside), sulfonylureas, tacrolimus, tamoxifen, terbinafine, tocainide, tricyclic antidepressants, warfarin, zaleplon, zidovudine, zolpidem.
Pharmacodynamics/Kinetics
  Duration: ≤24 hours
  Absorption: Oral: Well absorbed; food may delay or slightly reduce peak
  Distribution: Highly lipophilic; crosses blood-brain barrier well
    Relative diffusion from blood into CSF: Adequate with or without inflammation (exceeds usual MICs)
    CSF:blood level ratio: Inflamed meninges: 25%
  Protein binding: 80%
  Metabolism: Hepatic; undergoes enterohepatic recirculation
  Half-life elimination: 3-4 hours; prolonged with hepatic impairment; End-stage renal disease: 1.8-11 hours
  (Continued)

Rifampin *(Continued)*

Time to peak, serum: Oral: 2-4 hours

Excretion: Feces (60% to 65%) and urine (~30%) as unchanged drug

Pregnancy Risk Factor C

Rifampin and Isoniazid (RIF am pin & eye soe NYE a zid)

Related Information
Isoniazid *on page 864*
Rifampin *on page 1346*

U.S. Brand Names Rifamate®

Canadian Brand Names Rifamate®

Generic Available No

Synonyms Isoniazid and Rifampin

Pharmacologic Category Antibiotic, Miscellaneous

Use Management of active tuberculosis; see individual agents for additional information

Local Anesthetic/Vasoconstrictor Precautions No information available to require special precautions

Effects on Dental Treatment No significant effects or complications reported

Drug Interactions

Cytochrome P450 Effect:
Rifampin: **Induces** CYP1A2 (strong), 2A6 (strong), 2B6 (strong), 2C8 (strong), 2C9 (strong), 2C19 (strong), 3A4 (strong)

Isoniazid: **Substrate** of CYP2E1 (major); **Inhibits** CYP1A2 (weak), 2A6 (moderate), 2C9 (weak), 2C19 (strong), 2D6 (moderate), 2E1 (moderate), 3A4 (strong); **Induces** CYP2E1 (after discontinuation) (weak)

Pharmacodynamics/Kinetics See individual agents.

Pregnancy Risk Factor C

Rifampin, Isoniazid, and Pyrazinamide
(RIF am pin, eye soe NYE a zid, & peer a ZIN a mide)

Related Information
Isoniazid *on page 864*
Pyrazinamide *on page 1314*
Rifampin *on page 1346*

U.S. Brand Names Rifater®

Canadian Brand Names Rifater®

Generic Available No

Synonyms Isoniazid, Rifampin, and Pyrazinamide; Pyrazinamide, Rifampin, and Isoniazid

Pharmacologic Category Antibiotic, Miscellaneous

Use Initial phase, short-course treatment of pulmonary tuberculosis; see individual agents for additional information

Local Anesthetic/Vasoconstrictor Precautions No information available to require special precautions

Effects on Dental Treatment No significant effects or complications reported

Common Adverse Effects Note: During clinical trial evaluation, the frequency of cardiorespiratory events (eg, chest pain, hemoptysis, palpitation, chest tightness, and pneumothorax) was higher with the combination product (7%) that that reported with individual agents (2%). Also see individual agents.

Drug Interactions

Cytochrome P450 Effect:
Rifampin: **Induces** CYP1A2 (strong), 2A6 (strong), 2B6 (strong), 2C8 (strong), 2C9 (strong), 2C19 (strong), 3A4 (strong)

Isoniazid: **Substrate** of CYP2E1 (major); **Inhibits** CYP1A2 (weak), 2A6 (moderate), 2C9 (weak), 2C19 (strong), 2D6 (moderate), 2E1 (moderate), 3A4 (strong); CYP2E1 (after discontinuation) (weak)

Increased Effect/Toxicity: Increased effect/toxicity: Combination therapy with rifampin and pyrazinamide has been associated with severe and fatal hepatotoxic reactions.

Based on **rifampin** component: Rifampin levels may be increased when given with co-trimoxazole, probenecid, or ritonavir. Rifampin given with halothane or isoniazid increases the potential for hepatotoxicity.

Pharmacodynamics/Kinetics See individual agents.

Pregnancy Risk Factor C

Rifapentine (RIF a pen teen)

Related Information
Rifampin *on page 1346*
U.S. Brand Names Priftin®
Canadian Brand Names Priftin®
Generic Available No
Pharmacologic Category Antitubercular Agent
Use Treatment of pulmonary tuberculosis; rifapentine must always be used in conjunction with at least one other antituberculosis drug to which the isolate is susceptible; it may also be necessary to add a third agent (either streptomycin or ethambutol) until susceptibility is known.

Local Anesthetic/Vasoconstrictor Precautions No information available to require special precautions

Effects on Dental Treatment No significant effects or complications reported

Common Adverse Effects
>10%: Endocrine & metabolic: Hyperuricemia (most likely due to pyrazinamide from initiation phase combination therapy)

1% to 10%:
Cardiovascular: Hypertension
Central nervous system: Headache, dizziness
Dermatologic: Rash, pruritus, acne
Gastrointestinal: Anorexia, nausea, vomiting, dyspepsia, diarrhea
Hematologic: Neutropenia, lymphopenia, anemia, leukopenia, thrombocytosis
Hepatic: Increased ALT/AST
Neuromuscular & skeletal: Arthralgia, pain
Renal: Pyuria, proteinuria, hematuria, urinary casts
Respiratory: Hemoptysis

Mechanism of Action Inhibits DNA-dependent RNA polymerase in susceptible strains of *Mycobacterium tuberculosis* (but not in mammalian cells). Rifapentine is bactericidal against both intracellular and extracellular MTB organisms. MTB resistant to other rifamycins including rifampin are likely to be resistant to rifapentine. Cross-resistance does not appear between rifapentine and other nonrifamycin antimycobacterial agents.

Drug Interactions
Cytochrome P450 Effect: Induces CYP2C8/9 (strong), 3A4 (strong)
Increased Effect/Toxicity: Rifapentine may increase the therapeutic effect of clopidogrel; concurrent use with isoniazid may increase risk of hepatotoxicity

Decreased Effect: Rifapentine may decrease the levels/effects of the following drugs: alfentanil, amiodarone, angiotensin II receptor blockers (irbesartan, losartan), 5-HT$_3$ antagonists, imidazole antifungals, aprepitant, barbiturates, benzodiazepines (metabolized by oxidation), beta blockers, buspirone, calcium channel blockers, corticosteroids, cyclosporine; CYP2C8/9 and 3A4 substrates (eg, amiodarone, clarithromycin, erythromycin, fluoxetine, mirtazapine, nateglinide, nefazodone, nevirapine, pioglitazone, rosiglitazone, sertraline, venlafaxine, and zafirlukast); dapsone, disopyramide, estrogen and progestin contraceptives, fluconazole, gefitinib, HMG-CoA reductase inhibitors, methadone, morphine, phenytoin, propafenone, protease inhibitors, quinidine, repaglinide, reverse transcriptase inhibitors (non-nucleoside), tacrolimus, tamoxifen, terbinafine, tocainide, tricyclic antidepressants, warfarin, zaleplon, zidovudine, and zolpidem.

Pharmacodynamics/Kinetics
Absorption: Food increases AUC and C$_{max}$ by 43% and 44% respectively.
Distribution: V$_d$: ~70.2 L; rifapentine and metabolite accumulate in human monocyte-derived macrophages with intracellular/extracellular ratios of 24:1 and 7:1 respectively
Protein binding: Rifapentine and 25-desacetyl metabolite: 97.7% and 93.2%, primarily to albumin
Metabolism: Hepatic; hydrolyzed by an esterase and esterase enzyme to form the active metabolite 25-desacetyl rifapentine
Bioavailability: ~70%
Half-life elimination: Rifapentine: 14-17 hours; 25-desacetyl rifapentine: 13 hours
Time to peak, serum: 5-6 hours
Excretion: Urine (17% primarily as metabolites)

Pregnancy Risk Factor C

Rifater® *see* Rifampin, Isoniazid, and Pyrazinamide *on page 1348*

Rifaximin (rif AX i min)

U.S. Brand Names Xifaxan™
Mexican Brand Names Redactiv®
Generic Available No
Pharmacologic Category Antibiotic, Miscellaneous
Use Treatment of travelers' diarrhea caused by noninvasive strains of *E. coli*
Local Anesthetic/Vasoconstrictor Precautions No information available to require special precautions
Effects on Dental Treatment No significant effects or complications reported
Common Adverse Effects Incidence of adverse effects reported as ≥2% occurred more in the placebo group than the rifaximin group except for headache.
   2% to 10%: Central nervous system: Headache (10%; placebo 9%)
Mechanism of Action Rifaximin inhibits bacterial RNA synthesis by binding to bacterial DNA-dependent RNA polymerase.
Drug Interactions
   Cytochrome P450 Effect: Induces CYP3A4 (minor)
Pharmacodynamics/Kinetics
   Absorption: Oral: <0.4%
   Distribution: 80% to 90% in the gut
   Half-life elimination: ~6 hours
   Excretion: Feces (~97% as unchanged drug); urine (<1%)
Pregnancy Risk Factor C

rIFN-A *see* Interferon Alfa-2a *on page 842*
rIFN beta-1a *see* Interferon Beta-1a *on page 849*
rIFN beta-1b *see* Interferon Beta-1b *on page 850*
RIG *see* Rabies Immune Globulin (Human) *on page 1328*
rIL-11 *see* Oprelvekin *on page 1149*
Rilutek® *see* Riluzole *on page 1350*

Riluzole (RIL yoo zole)

U.S. Brand Names Rilutek®
Canadian Brand Names Rilutek®
Mexican Brand Names Rilutek®
Generic Available No
Synonyms 2-Amino-6-Trifluoromethoxy-benzothiazole; RP-54274
Pharmacologic Category Glutamate Inhibitor
Use Treatment of amyotrophic lateral sclerosis (ALS); riluzole can extend survival or time to tracheostomy
Local Anesthetic/Vasoconstrictor Precautions No information available to require special precautions
Effects on Dental Treatment No significant effects or complications reported
Common Adverse Effects
   >10%:
      Gastrointestinal: Nausea (12% to 21%)
      Neuromuscular & skeletal: Weakness (15% to 20%)
      Respiratory: Lung function decreased (10% to 16%)
   1% to 10%:
      Cardiovascular: Edema, hypertension, tachycardia
      Central nervous system: Agitation, circumoral paresthesia, depression, dizziness, headache, insomnia, malaise, somnolence, tremor, vertigo
      Dermatologic: Alopecia, eczema, pruritus
      Gastrointestinal: Abdominal pain, anorexia, diarrhea, dyspepsia, flatulence, oral moniliasis, stomatitis, vomiting
      Hepatic: Liver function tests increased
      Neuromuscular & skeletal: Arthralgia, back pain
      Respiratory: Cough increased, rhinitis, sinusitis
      Miscellaneous: Aggravation reaction
Mechanism of Action Mechanism of action is not known. Pharmacologic properties include inhibitory effect on glutamate release, inactivation of voltage-dependent sodium channels; and ability to interfere with intracellular events that follow transmitter binding at excitatory amino acid receptors
Drug Interactions
   Cytochrome P450 Effect: Substrate of CYP1A2 (major)
   Increased Effect/Toxicity: CYP1A2 inhibitors may increase the levels/effects of riluzole; example inhibitors include amiodarone, ciprofloxacin, fluvoxamine, ketoconazole, norfloxacin, ofloxacin, and rofecoxib.

Decreased Effect: CYP1A2 inducers may decrease the levels/effects of riluzole; example inducers include aminoglutethimide, carbamazepine, phenobarbital, and rifampin.

Pharmacodynamics/Kinetics

Absorption: 90%; high-fat meal decreases AUC by 20% and peak blood levels by 45%

Protein binding, plasma: 96%, primarily to albumin and lipoproteins

Metabolism: Extensively hepatic to six major and a number of minor metabolites via CYP1A2 dependent hydroxylation and glucuronidation

Bioavailability: Oral: Absolute: 60%

Half-life elimination: 12 hours

Excretion: Urine (90%; 85% as metabolites, 2% as unchanged drug) and feces (5%) within 7 days

Pregnancy Risk Factor C

Rimantadine (ri MAN ta deen)

Related Information

Systemic Viral Diseases on page 1675

U.S. Brand Names Flumadine®

Canadian Brand Names Flumadine®

Generic Available Yes: Tablet

Synonyms Rimantadine Hydrochloride

Pharmacologic Category Antiviral Agent, Adamantane

Use Prophylaxis (adults and children >1 year of age) and treatment (adults) of influenza A viral infection

Unlabeled/Investigational Use Treatment of influenza A viral infection in children ≥13 years of age

Local Anesthetic/Vasoconstrictor Precautions No information available to require special precautions

Effects on Dental Treatment Key adverse event(s) related to dental treatment: Xerostomia (normal salivary flow resumes upon discontinuation).

Common Adverse Effects 1% to 10%:

Central nervous system: Dizziness (2%), insomnia (2%), anxiety (1%), fatigue (1%), headache (1%), nervousness (1%)

Gastrointestinal: Nausea (3%), anorexia (2%), vomiting (2%), xerostomia (2%), abdominal pain (1%)

Neuromuscular and skeletal: Weakness (1%)

Mechanism of Action Exerts its inhibitory effect on three antigenic subtypes of influenza A virus (H1N1, H2N2, H3N2) early in the viral replicative cycle, possibly inhibiting the uncoating process; it has no activity against influenza B virus and is two- to eightfold more active than amantadine

Drug Interactions

Increased Effect/Toxicity: Cimetidine increases blood levels/toxicity of rimantadine.

Decreased Effect: Acetaminophen may cause a small reduction in AUC and peak concentration of rimantadine. Peak plasma and AUC concentrations of rimantadine are slightly reduced by aspirin.

Pharmacodynamics/Kinetics

Onset of action: Antiviral activity: No data exist establishing a correlation between plasma concentration and antiviral effect

Absorption: Tablet and syrup formulations are equally absorbed

Metabolism: Extensively hepatic

Half-life elimination: 25.4 hours; prolonged in elderly

Time to peak: 6 hours

Excretion: Urine (<25% as unchanged drug)

Clearance: Hemodialysis does not contribute to clearance

Pregnancy Risk Factor C

Rimantadine Hydrochloride see Rimantadine on page 1351

Rimexolone (ri MEKS oh lone)

U.S. Brand Names Vexol®

Canadian Brand Names Vexol®

Generic Available No

Pharmacologic Category Corticosteroid, Ophthalmic

Use Treatment of inflammation after ocular surgery and the treatment of anterior uveitis

Local Anesthetic/Vasoconstrictor Precautions No information available to require special precautions

(Continued)

Rimexolone *(Continued)*

Effects on Dental Treatment No significant effects or complications reported

Mechanism of Action Decreases inflammation by suppression of migration of polymorphonuclear leukocytes and reversal of increased capillary permeability

Pregnancy Risk Factor C

Riomet™ *see* Metformin *on page 1001*

Riopan Plus® [OTC] [DSC] *see* Magaldrate and Simethicone *on page 960*

Riopan Plus® Double Strength [OTC] [DSC] *see* Magaldrate and Simethicone *on page 960*

Risedronate *(ris ED roe nate)*

Related Information
Rheumatoid Arthritis, Osteoarthritis, and Osteoporosis *on page 1668*

U.S. Brand Names Actonel®

Canadian Brand Names Actonel®

Mexican Brand Names Actonel®

Generic Available No

Synonyms Risedronate Sodium

Pharmacologic Category Bisphosphonate Derivative

Use Paget's disease of the bone; treatment and prevention of glucocorticoid-induced osteoporosis; treatment and prevention of osteoporosis in postmenopausal women

Local Anesthetic/Vasoconstrictor Precautions No information available to require special precautions

Effects on Dental Treatment Osteonecrosis of the jaw (ONJ), generally associated with local infection and/or tooth extraction and often with delayed healing, has been reported in patients taking bisphosphonates. Most reported cases of bisphosphonate-associated osteonecrosis have been in cancer patients treated with intravenous bisphosphonates. However, some have occurred in patients with postmenopausal osteoporosis taking oral bisphosphonates. Dental surgery may exacerbate ONJ. For patients requiring dental procedures, there are no data available to suggest whether discontinuation of bisphosphonate treatment reduces the risk of ONJ. See Dental Comment.

Common Adverse Effects Frequency may vary with dose and indication.

>10%:
Central nervous system: Headache (18%), pain (14%)
Dermatologic: Rash (8% to 12%)
Gastrointestinal: Diarrhea (11% to 20%), abdominal pain (12%), nausea (10% to 12%)
Genitourinary: Urinary tract infection (11%)
Neuromuscular & skeletal: Arthralgia (24% to 33%), back pain (26%)

1% to 10%:
Cardiovascular: Hypertension (10%), peripheral edema (8%), chest pain (5% to 7%), cardiovascular disorder (3%), angina (3%)
Central nervous system: Depression (7%), dizziness (6% to 7%), insomnia (5%), anxiety (4%), vertigo (3%)
Dermatologic: Bruising (4%), pruritus (3%), skin carcinoma (2%)
Gastrointestinal: Constipation (7%), flatulence (5%), belching (3%), colitis (3%), gastritis (3%), gastrointestinal disorder (2%), rectal disorder (2%), tooth disorder (2%)
Genitourinary: Cystitis (4%)
Hematologic: Anemia (2%)
Neuromuscular & skeletal: Joint disorder (7%), myalgia (7%), neck pain (5%), asthenia (5%), bone pain (5%), weakness (5%), bone disorder (4%), neuralgia (4%), leg cramps (4%), bursitis (3%), myasthenia (3%), tendon disorder (3%), hypertonia (2%), paresthesia (2%)
Ocular: Cataract (6%), conjunctivitis (3%), amblyopia (3%), dry eyes (3%)
Otic: Otitis media (3%), tinnitus (3%)
Respiratory: Pharyngitis (6%), rhinitis (6%), sinusitis (5%), dyspnea (4%), bronchitis (3%), pneumonia (3%)
Miscellaneous: Flu symptoms (10%), neoplasm (3%), hernia (3%)

Dosage Oral: Adults:
Paget's disease of bone: 30 mg once daily for 2 months
Retreatment may be considered (following post-treatment observation of at least 2 months) if relapse occurs, or if treatment fails to normalize serum alkaline phosphatase. For retreatment, the dose and duration of therapy are the same as for initial treatment. No data are available on more than one course of retreatment.

Osteoporosis (postmenopausal) prevention and treatment: 5 mg once daily or 35 mg once weekly

Osteoporosis (glucocorticoid-induced) prevention and treatment: 5 mg once daily

Dosage adjustment in renal impairment: Cl_{cr} <30 mL/minute: Not recommended for use

Mechanism of Action A bisphosphonate which inhibits bone resorption via actions on osteoclasts or on osteoclast precursors; decreases the rate of bone resorption, leading to an indirect increase in bone mineral density. In Paget's disease, characterized by disordered resorption and formation of bone, inhibition of resorption leads to an indirect decrease in bone formation; but the newly-formed bone has a more normal architecture.

Contraindications Hypersensitivity to risedronate, bisphosphonates, or any component of the formulation; hypocalcemia; abnormalities of the esophagus which delay esophageal emptying such as stricture or achalasia; inability to stand or sit upright for at least 30 minutes; severe renal impairment (Cl_{cr} <30 mL/minute)

Warnings/Precautions Bisphosphonates may cause upper gastrointestinal disorders such as dysphagia, esophageal ulcer, and gastric ulcer. Use caution in patients with renal impairment. Hypocalcemia must be corrected before therapy initiation with risedronate. Ensure adequate calcium and vitamin D intake, especially for patients with Paget's disease in whom the pretreatment rate of bone turnover may be greatly elevated.

Bisphosphonate therapy has been associated with osteonecrosis, primarily of the jaw; this has been observed mostly in cancer patients, but also in patients with postmenopausal osteoporosis and other diagnoses. There are no data addressing whether discontinuation of therapy reduces the risk of developing osteonecrosis. However, as a precautionary measure, dental exams and preventative dentistry should be performed prior to placing patients with risk factors (eg, chemotherapy, corticosteroids, poor oral hygiene) on chronic bisphosphonate therapy. Invasive dental procedures should be avoided during treatment.

Severe and potentially incapacitating musculoskeletal pain has been observed, with onset ranging from one day to several months after beginning therapy. Symptoms usually abate upon discontinuation, but may recur upon reinitiation of bisphosphonate treatment.

Safety and efficacy in pediatric patients have not been established.

Drug Interactions

Increased Effect/Toxicity:

Aminoglycosides may lower serum calcium levels with prolonged administration; concomitant use may have an additive hypocalcemic effect. NSAIDs may enhance the gastrointestinal adverse/toxic effects (increased incidence of GI ulcers) of bisphosphonate derivatives. Bisphosphonate derivatives may enhance the hypocalcemic effect of phosphate supplements.

Decreased Effect: The following agents may decrease the absorption of oral bisphosphonate derivatives: Antacids (aluminum, calcium, magnesium), oral calcium salts, oral iron salts, and oral magnesium salts

Ethanol/Nutrition/Herb Interactions

Ethanol: Avoid ethanol (may increase risk of osteoporosis).

Food: Food may reduce absorption (similar to other bisphosphonates); mean oral bioavailability is decreased when given with food.

Dietary Considerations Take ≥30 minutes before the first food or drink of the day other than water. Supplemental calcium or vitamin D may be required if dietary intake is not adequate.

Pharmacodynamics/Kinetics

Onset of action: May require weeks

Absorption: Rapid

Distribution: V_d: 6.3 L/kg

Protein binding: ~24%

Metabolism: None

Bioavailability: Poor, ~0.54% to 0.75%

Half-life elimination: Initial: 1.5 hours; Terminal: 480 hours

Excretion: Urine (up to 85%); feces (as unabsorbed drug)

Pregnancy Risk Factor C

Dosage Forms TAB: 5 mg, 30 mg, 35 mg

Dental Comment

Novartis Pharmaceuticals Corporation has notified dental health professionals of the risk of osteonecrosis of the jaw (ONJ) and the use of the bisphosphonates, pamidronate, and zoledronic acid. This warning has not be issued for risedronate.

(Continued)

Risedronate *(Continued)*

Previously, Novartis and the Food and Drug Administration (FDA) had notified healthcare providers of a serious adverse event related to the use of bisphosphonates. Osteonecrosis of the jaw has been reported in patients with cancer who were receiving chemotherapy, corticosteroids, and chronic bisphosphonate therapy. The bisphosphonates involved were pamidronate and zoledronic acid. To date, there are no reported associations between risedronate and osteonecrosis of the jaw. Dental exams and preventative dentistry should be performed prior to placing patients with risk factors (chemotherapy, corticosteroids, poor oral hygiene) on chronic bisphosphonate therapy. Invasive dental procedures should be avoided during treatment. Product labelings for pamidronate (Aredia®) and zoledronic acid (Zometa®) have been updated. Recently, 63 cases of osteonecrosis associated with the use of bisphosphonates were published (Ruggiero, 2004). In a retrospective review, 56 of the patients received intravenous bisphosphonates for at least one year and 7 patients were on chronic oral therapy. The presenting symptom was a nonhealing extraction socket or an exposed jawbone. These lesions did not show evidence of metastatic disease and required removal of involved bone in most cases.

Bisphosphonates are widely used in the management of metastatic bone disease to treat hypercalcemia associated with malignancies and to treat osteoporosis. In the report by Ruggiero et al, the cluster of patients observed to have necrotic lesions in the jaw shared only one common clinical feature, all received chronic bisphosphonate therapy. The necrosis detected was typical of osteoradionecrosis. It was suggested that because of the trend in the use of chronic bisphosphonate therapy, the observation of an associated risk of osteonecrosis of the jaw should alert practitioners to monitor for this previously unrecognized potential complication.

Selected Readings

Ruggiero SL, Mehrotra B, Rosenberg TJ, et al, "Osteonecrosis of the Jaws Associated With the Use of Bisphosphonates: A Review of 63 Cases," *J Oral Maxillofac Surg*, 2004, 62(5):527-34.

Risedronate and Calcium *(ris ED roe nate & KAL see um)*

U.S. Brand Names Actonel® and Calcium

Generic Available No

Synonyms Calcium and Risedronate; Risedronate Sodium and Calcium Carbonate

Pharmacologic Category Bisphosphonate Derivative; Calcium Salt

Use Treatment and prevention of osteoporosis in postmenopausal women

Local Anesthetic/Vasoconstrictor Precautions No information available to require special precautions

Effects on Dental Treatment No significant effects or complications reported (see Dental Comment)

Common Adverse Effects See individual agents.

Dosage

Oral: Adults: Osteoporosis in postmenopausal females:

Risedronate: 35 mg once weekly on day 1 of 7-day treatment cycle

Calcium carbonate: 1250 mg (elemental calcium 500 mg) once daily on days 2 through 7 of 7-day treatment cycle

Dosage adjustment in renal impairment: Cl_{cr} <30 mL/minute: Not recommended for use

Mechanism of Action

Risedronate inhibits bone resorption via actions on osteoclasts or on osteoclast precursors; decreases the rate of bone resorption, leading to an indirect increase in bone mineral density.

Calcium helps to prevent or decrease the rate of bone loss.

Contraindications Hypersensitivity to risedronate, bisphosphonates, or any component of the formulation; hypocalcemia, hypercalcemia; abnormalities of the esophagus which delay esophageal emptying (eg, stricture or achalasia); inability to stand or sit upright for at least 30 minutes; severe renal impairment (Cl_{cr} <30 mL/minute)

Warnings/Precautions Bisphosphonates may cause upper gastrointestinal disorders such as dysphagia, esophageal ulcer, and gastric ulcer. Use caution in patients with renal impairment. Hypocalcemia must be corrected before therapy initiation. Ensure adequate vitamin D intake. Severe bone pain has been reported (rare) with the use of bisphosphonates; onset varied from 1 day to several months following the onset of therapy.

Bisphosphonate therapy has been associated with osteonecrosis, primarily of the jaw; this has been observed mostly in cancer patients, but also in patients with postmenopausal osteoporosis and other diagnoses. Dental exams and preventative dentistry should be performed prior to placing patients with risk factors on chronic bisphosphonate therapy. Invasive dental procedures should be avoided during treatment.

Calcium carbonate absorption is impaired in achlorhydria. Calcium should be used with caution in patients with a history of kidney stones or hypercalciuria.

Safety and efficacy using the combination as packaged have not been established in pediatric patients or for the treatment of primary osteoporosis in men.

Drug Interactions
  Increased Effect/Toxicity: See individual agents.

Ethanol/Nutrition/Herb Interactions
  Ethanol: Avoid ethanol (may increase risk of osteoporosis).
  Food:
    Risedronate: Food may reduce absorption (similar to other bisphosphonates); mean oral bioavailability is decreased when given with food.
    Calcium: Food increases absorption. Calcium may decrease iron absorption. Bran, foods high in oxalates, or whole grain cereals may decrease calcium absorption

Dietary Considerations Take risedronate ≥30 minutes before the first food or drink of the day other than water. Calcium should be taken with food. Vitamin D supplementation may be needed.

Pharmacodynamics/Kinetics See individual agents.

Pregnancy Risk Factor C

Dosage Forms Combination package: (Actonel®): Risedronate 35 mg (4s) and calcium carbonate 1250 mg (24s)

Dental Comment Risedronate:

Novartis Pharmaceuticals Corporation has notified dental health professionals of the risk of osteonecrosis of the jaw (ONJ) and the use of the bisphosphonates, pamidronate, and zoledronic acid. This warning has not be issued for risedronate.

Previously, Novartis and the Food and Drug Administration (FDA) had notified healthcare providers of a serious adverse event related to the use of bisphosphonates. Osteonecrosis of the jaw has been reported in patients with cancer who were receiving chemotherapy, corticosteroids, and chronic bisphosphonate therapy. The bisphosphonates involved were pamidronate and zoledronic acid. To date, there are no reported associations between risedronate and osteonecrosis of the jaw. Dental exams and preventative dentistry should be performed prior to placing patients with risk factors (chemotherapy, corticosteroids, poor oral hygiene) on chronic bisphosphonate therapy. Invasive dental procedures should be avoided during treatment. Product labelings for pamidronate (Aredia®) and zoledronic acid (Zometa®) have been updated. Recently, 63 cases of osteonecrosis associated with the use of bisphosphonates were published (Ruggiero, 2004). In a retrospective review, 56 of the patients received intravenous bisphosphonates for at least one year and 7 patients were on chronic oral therapy. The presenting symptom was a nonhealing extraction socket or an exposed jawbone. These lesions did not show evidence of metastatic disease and required removal of involved bone in most cases.

Bisphosphonates are widely used in the management of metastatic bone disease to treat hypercalcemia associated with malignancies and to treat osteoporosis. In the report by Ruggiero et al, the cluster of patients observed to have necrotic lesions in the jaw shared only one common clinical feature, all received chronic bisphosphonate therapy. The necrosis detected was typical of osteoradionecrosis. It was suggested that because of the trend in the use of chronic bisphosphonate therapy, the observation of an associated risk of osteonecrosis of the jaw should alert practitioners to monitor for this previously unrecognized potential complication.

Selected Readings
Ruggiero SL, Mehrotra B, Rosenberg TJ, et al, "Osteonecrosis of the Jaws Associated With the Use of Bisphosphonates: A Review of 63 Cases," *J Oral Maxillofac Surg*, 2004, 62(5):527-34.

Risedronate Sodium *see* Risedronate *on page 1352*

Risedronate Sodium and Calcium Carbonate *see* Risedronate and Calcium *on page 1354*

Risperdal® *see* Risperidone *on page 1356*

Risperdal® M-Tab® *see* Risperidone *on page 1356*

Risperdal® Consta™ *see* Risperidone *on page 1356*

Risperidone (ris PER i done)

U.S. Brand Names Risperdal®; Risperdal® Consta™; Risperdal® M-Tab®

Canadian Brand Names Risperdal®; Risperdal® Consta™; Risperdal® M-Tab®

Generic Available No

Synonyms Risperdal M-Tab®

Pharmacologic Category Antipsychotic Agent, Atypical

Use Treatment of schizophrenia; treatment of acute mania or mixed episodes associated with bipolar I disorder (as monotherapy or in combination with lithium or valproate)

Unlabeled/Investigational Use Behavioral symptoms associated with dementia in elderly; treatment of Tourette's disorder; treatment of pervasive developmental disorder and autism in children and adolescents

Local Anesthetic/Vasoconstrictor Precautions No information available to require special precautions

Effects on Dental Treatment Key adverse event(s) related to dental treatment: Significant xerostomia (normal salivary flow resumes upon discontinuation).

Common Adverse Effects

Unless otherwise noted, frequency of adverse effects is reported for the oral formulation.

>10%:

Central nervous system: Extrapyramidal symptoms (17% to 34%; dose dependent), somnolence (3% to 28%), insomnia (13% to 26%), agitation (8% to 26%), anxiety (4% to 20%), headache (12% to 14%), dizziness (4% to 11%)

Gastrointestinal: Weight gain (>5% to 18%), constipation (7% to 13%), dyspepsia (5% to 11%), nausea (4% to 11%)

1% to 10%:

Cardiovascular: Tachycardia (3% to 5%), hypertension (3%), chest pain (2% to 3%), hypotension (2% — especially orthostatic)

Central nervous system: Mania (8%), pseudoparkinsonism (6%), dreaming increased (≥5%), sleep prolonged (≥5%) fatigue (4%), fever (2% to 3%), aggressiveness (1% to 3%), hypoesthesia (2%), tardive dyskinesia, neuroleptic malignant syndrome, altered central temperature regulation, nervousness, hallucination, restlessness

Dermatologic: Rash (2% to 5%), dry skin (2% to 4%), acne (2%), pruritus (2%), seborrhea (up to 1%)

Endocrine & metabolic: Sexual dysfunction (≥5%), menorrhagia (≥5%), galactorrhea, gynecomastia

Gastrointestinal: Xerostomia (≥5%), vomiting (5% to 7%), diarrhea (≥5%), salivation increased (2% to 5%), abdominal pain (1% to 4%), toothache (up to 2%), GI upset, anorexia

Genitourinary: Micturition disturbances (≥5%)

Hematologic: Anemia (≥1% I.M. injection)

Hepatic: Transaminases increased (≥1% I.M. injection)

Neuromuscular & skeletal: Myalgia (5%), arthralgia (2% to 3%), skeletal pain (2%), back pain (up to 2%)

Ocular: Abnormal vision (1% to 6%), accommodation disturbances (≥5%)

Respiratory: Rhinitis (3% to 10%), sinusitis (1% to 4%), upper respiratory infection (3%), cough (2% to 3%), pharyngitis (2% to 3%), dyspnea (up to 1%)

Miscellaneous: Injury (up to 2%)

Dosage

Oral:

Children and Adolescents:

Pervasive developmental disorder (unlabeled use): Initial: 0.25 mg twice daily; titrate up 0.25 mg/day every 5-7 days; optimal dose range: 0.75-3 mg/day

Autism (unlabeled use): Initial: 0.25 mg at bedtime; titrate to 1 mg/day (0.1 mg/kg/day)

Schizophrenia (unlabeled use): Initial: 0.5 mg once or twice daily; titrate as necessary up to 2-6 mg/day

Bipolar disorder (unlabeled use): Initial: 0.5 mg; titrate to 0.5-3 mg/day

Tourette's disorder (unlabeled use): Initial: 0.5 mg; titrate to 2-4 mg/day

Adults:

Schizophrenia:

Initial: 1 mg twice daily; may be increased by 2 mg/day to a target dose of 6 mg/day; usual range: 4-8 mg/day; may be given as a single daily dose once maintenance dose is achieved; daily dosages >6 mg do not appear to confer any additional benefit, and the incidence of extrapyramidal symptoms is higher than with lower doses. Further dose adjustments should be made in increments/decrements of 1-2 mg/day on a weekly basis. Dose range studied in clinical trials: 4-16 mg/day.

Maintenance: Target dose: 4 mg once daily (range 2-8 mg/day)

Bipolar mania:

Initial: 2-3 mg once daily; if needed, adjust dose by 1 mg/day in intervals ≥24 hours; dosing range: 1-6 mg/day

Maintenance: No dosing recommendation available for treatment >3 weeks duration.

Elderly: A starting dose of 0.5 mg twice daily, and titration should progress slowly in increments of no more than 0.5 mg twice daily; increases to dosages >1.5 mg twice daily should occur at intervals of ≥1 week.

Additional monitoring of renal function and orthostatic blood pressure may be warranted. If once-a-day dosing in the elderly or debilitated patient is considered, a twice daily regimen should be used to titrate to the target dose, and this dose should be maintained for 2-3 days prior to attempts to switch to a once-daily regimen.

I.M.: Adults: Schizophrenia (Risperdal® Consta™): 25 mg every 2 weeks; some patients may benefit from larger doses; maximum dose not to exceed 50 mg every 2 weeks. Dosage adjustments should not be made more frequently than every 4 weeks.

Note: Oral risperidone (or other antipsychotic) should be administered with the initial injection of Risperdal® Consta™ and continued for 3 weeks (then discontinued) to maintain adequate therapeutic plasma concentrations prior to main release phase of risperidone from injection site. When switching from depot administration to a short-acting formulation, administer short-acting agent in place of the next regularly-scheduled depot injection.

Dosing adjustment in renal impairment: Oral: Starting dose of 0.5 mg twice daily; clearance of the active moiety is decreased by 60% in patients with moderate to severe renal disease compared to healthy subjects.

Dosing adjustment in hepatic impairment: Oral: Starting dose of 0.5 mg twice daily; the mean free fraction of risperidone in plasma was increased by 35% compared to healthy subjects.

Mechanism of Action Risperidone is a benzisoxazole atypical antipsychotic with mixed serotonin-dopamine antagonist activity that binds to 5-HT$_2$-receptors in the CNS and in the periphery with a very high affinity; binds to dopamine-D$_2$ receptors with less affinity. The binding affinity to the dopamine-D$_2$ receptor is 20 times lower than the 5-HT$_2$ affinity. The addition of serotonin antagonism to dopamine antagonism (classic neuroleptic mechanism) is thought to improve negative symptoms of psychoses and reduce the incidence of extrapyramidal side effects. Alpha$_1$, alpha$_2$ adrenergic, and histaminergic receptors are also antagonized with high affinity. Risperidone has low to moderate affinity for 5-HT$_{1C}$, 5-HT$_{1D}$, and 5-HT$_{1A}$ receptors, weak affinity for D$_1$ and no affinity for muscarinics or beta$_1$ and beta$_2$ receptors

Contraindications Hypersensitivity to risperidone or any component of the formulation

Warnings/Precautions Elderly patients with dementia-related behavioral disorders treated with atypical antipsychotics are at an increased risk of cerebrovascular adverse events and death compared to placebo; risk may be increased with dehydration (increased risk of death observed with concurrent furosemide). Risperidone is not approved for the treatment of dementia-related psychosis.

Low to moderately sedating, use with caution in disorders where CNS depression is a feature. Use with caution in Parkinson's disease. Caution in patients with hemodynamic instability; bone marrow suppression; predisposition to seizures; subcortical brain damage; severe cardiac, hepatic, or respiratory disease. Use with caution in renal or hepatic dysfunction; dose reduction recommended. Esophageal dysmotility and aspiration have been associated with antipsychotic use; use with caution in patients at risk of aspiration pneumonia (ie, Alzheimer's disease). Caution in breast cancer or other prolactin-dependent tumors (elevates prolactin levels). May alter temperature regulation or mask toxicity of other drugs due to antiemetic effects.

May cause orthostasis. Use with caution in patients with cardiovascular diseases (eg, heart failure, history of myocardial infarction or ischemia, cerebrovascular disease, conduction abnormalities). Use caution in patients receiving medications for hypertension (orthostatic effects may be exacerbated) or in patients with hypovolemia or dehydration. May alter cardiac conduction (low risk relative to other neuroleptics); life-threatening arrhythmias have occurred with therapeutic doses of neuroleptics.

May cause anticholinergic effects (confusion, agitation, constipation, xerostomia, blurred vision, urinary retention); therefore, they should be used with (Continued)

Risperidone *(Continued)*

caution in patients with decreased gastrointestinal motility, urinary retention, BPH, xerostomia, or visual problems. Conditions which also may be exacerbated by cholinergic blockade include narrow-angle glaucoma (screening is recommended) and worsening of myasthenia gravis. Relative to other neuroleptics, risperidone has a low potency of cholinergic blockade.

May cause extrapyramidal symptoms, including pseudoparkinsonism, acute dystonic reactions, akathisia, and tardive dyskinesia (risk of these reactions is low relative to other neuroleptics, and is dose dependent). Risk of neuroleptic malignant syndrome (NMS) may be increased in patients with Parkinson's disease or Lewy Body Dementia; monitor for symptoms of confusion, obtundation, postural instability and extrapyramidal symptoms. May cause hyperglycemia; in some cases may be extreme and associated with ketoacidosis, hyperosmolar coma, or death. Use with caution in patients with diabetes or other disorders of glucose regulation; monitor for worsening of glucose control.

The possibility of a suicide attempt is inherent in psychotic illness or bipolar disorder; use caution in high-risk patients during initiation of therapy. Prescriptions should be written for the smallest quantity consistent with good patient care. Safety and efficacy in children have not been established.

Drug Interactions
Cytochrome P450 Effect: Substrate of CYP2D6 (major), 3A4 (minor); **Inhibits** CYP2D6 (weak), 3A4 (weak)

Increased Effect/Toxicity: CNS depressants may increase adverse effects/ toxicity of risperidone. CYP2D6 inhibitors may increase the levels/effects of risperidone; example inhibitors include chlorpromazine, delavirdine, fluoxetine, miconazole, paroxetine, pergolide, quinidine, quinine, ritonavir, and ropinirole. Clozapine decreases clearance of risperidone. Acetylcholinesterase inhibitors (central) may increase the risk of antipsychotic-related EPS. Pramlintide may increase anticholinergic effects of risperidone on the GI tract. Verapamil, SSRIs, and lithium may increase the levels and effects of risperidone.

Decreased Effect: Carbamazepine decreases risperidone serum concentrations.

Ethanol/Nutrition/Herb Interactions
Ethanol: Avoid ethanol (may increase CNS depression).
Herb/Nutraceutical: Avoid kava kava, gotu kola, valerian, St John's wort (may increase CNS depression).

Dietary Considerations
May be taken with or without food. Risperdal® M-Tabs™ contain phenylalanine.

Pharmacodynamics/Kinetics
Absorption:
Oral: Rapid and well absorbed; food does not affect rate or extent
Injection: <1% absorbed initially; main release occurs at ~3 weeks and is maintained from 4-6 weeks
Distribution: V_d: 1-2 L/kg
Protein binding, plasma: Risperidone 90%; 9-hydroxyrisperidone: 77%
Metabolism: Extensively hepatic via CYP2D6 to 9-hydroxyrisperidone (similar pharmacological activity as risperidone); *N*-dealkylation is a second minor pathway
Bioavailability: Solution: 70%; Tablet: 66%; orally-disintegrating tablets and oral solution are bioequivalent to tablets
Half-life elimination: Active moiety (risperidone and its active metabolite 9-hydroxyrisperidone)
Oral: 20 hours (mean)
Extensive metabolizers: Risperidone: 3 hours; 9-hydroxyrisperidone: 21 hours
Poor metabolizers: Risperidone: 20 hours; 9-hydroxyrisperidone: 30 hours
Injection: 3-6 days; related to microsphere erosion and subsequent absorption of risperidone
Time to peak, plasma: Oral: Risperidone: Within 1 hour; 9-hydroxyrisperidone: Extensive metabolizers: 3 hours; Poor metabolizers: 17 hours
Excretion: Urine (70%); feces (15%)

Pregnancy Risk Factor C

Dosage Forms
INJ, microspheres for reconstitution, extended release (Risperdal® Consta™): 25 mg, 37.5 mg, 50 mg. **SOLN, oral:** 1 mg/mL (30 mL). **TAB:** 0.25 mg, 0.5 mg, 1 mg, 2 mg, 3 mg, 4 mg. **TAB, orally disintegrating** (Risperdal® M-Tab™): 0.5 mg, 1 mg, 2 mg

Ritalin® *see* Methylphenidate *on page 1023*
Ritalin® LA *see* Methylphenidate *on page 1023*
Ritalin-SR® *see* Methylphenidate *on page 1023*

Ritonavir (ri TOE na veer)

Related Information
HIV Infection and AIDS *on page 1662*
Tuberculosis *on page 1673*

U.S. Brand Names Norvir®

Canadian Brand Names Norvir®; Norvir® SEC

Mexican Brand Names Norvir®

Generic Available No

Pharmacologic Category Antiretroviral Agent, Protease Inhibitor

Use Treatment of HIV infection; should always be used as part of a multidrug regimen (at least three antiretroviral agents); may be used as a pharmacokinetic "booster" for other protease inhibitors

Local Anesthetic/Vasoconstrictor Precautions No information available to require special precautions

Effects on Dental Treatment Key adverse event(s) related to dental treatment: Xerostomia (normal salivary flow resumes upon discontinuation).

Common Adverse Effects Protease inhibitors cause dyslipidemia which includes elevated cholesterol and triglycerides and a redistribution of body fat centrally to cause increased abdominal girth, buffalo hump, facial atrophy, and breast enlargement. These agents also cause hyperglycemia. Percentages as reported in adults:

>10%:
   Endocrine & metabolic: Hypercholesterolemia (>240 mg/dL: 37% to 45%), triglycerides increased (>800 mg/dL: 17% to 34%; >1500 mg/dL: 1% to 13%)
   Gastrointestinal: Nausea (26% to 30%), diarrhea (15% to 23%), vomiting (14% to 17%), taste perversion (7% to 11%)
   Hematologic: WBCs decreased
   Hepatic: GGT increased (5% to 20%)
   Neuromuscular & skeletal: Weakness (10% to 15%), creatine phosphokinase increased (9% to 12%)

2% to 10%:
   Cardiovascular: Syncope (<1% to 2%), vasodilation (2%)
   Central nervous system: Fever (4% to 5%), dizziness (3% to 4%), insomnia (2% to 3%), somnolence (2% to 3%), anxiety (2%),
   Dermatologic: Rash
   Endocrine & metabolic: Uric acid increased (up to 4%)
   Gastrointestinal: Abdominal pain (6% to 8%), anorexia (2% to 8%), dyspepsia (up to 6%), local throat irritation (2% to 3%)
   Hematologic: Eosinophilia, neutropenia, neutrophilia
   Hepatic: LFTs increased (6% to 10%)
   Neuromuscular & skeletal: Paresthesia (3% to 7%), arthralgia (up to 2%), myalgia (2%)
   Respiratory: Pharyngitis
   Miscellaneous: Circumoral paresthesia, diaphoresis (2% to 3%)

Mechanism of Action Ritonavir inhibits HIV protease and renders the enzyme incapable of processing of polyprotein precursor which leads to production of noninfectious immature HIV particles

Drug Interactions
Cytochrome P450 Effect: Substrate of CYP1A2 (minor), 2B6 (minor), 2D6 (major), 3A4 (major); **Inhibits** CYP2C8 (strong), 2C9 (weak), 2C19 (weak), 2D6 (strong), 2E1 (weak), 3A4 (strong); **Induces** CYP1A2 (weak), 2C8 (weak), 2C9 (weak), 3A4 (weak)

Increased Effect/Toxicity: Concurrent use of alfuzosin, amiodarone, cisapride, ergot alkaloids (including dihydroergotamine, ergonovine, methylergonovine), flecainide, midazolam, pimozide, propafenone, quinidine, and triazolam is contraindicated.

Saquinavir's serum concentrations are increased by ritonavir; the dosage of both agents should be reduced to 400 mg twice daily. Concurrent therapy with amprenavir may result in increased serum concentrations: dosage adjustment is recommended. Metronidazole or disulfiram may cause disulfiram reaction (oral solution contains 43% ethanol). Serum levels/effects of corticosteroids (eg, budesonide, fluticasone) and immunosuppressants (cyclosporine, sirolimus, tacrolimus; monitor) may be increased by ritonavir. Serum concentrations of the parent drug and/or metabolite(s) of several analgesics (eg, tramadol, meperidine, propoxyphene) may be increased by ritonavir; increased levels of normeperidine may increase the risk of CNS toxicity/seizures. Rifabutin and rifabutin metabolite serum concentrations may be increased by ritonavir; reduce rifabutin dose to 150 mg every other day.
(Continued)

Ritonavir *(Continued)*

Ritonavir may increase the levels/effects of amiodarone, amphetamines, selected beta-blockers, selected benzodiazepines (midazolam and triazolam contraindicated), calcium channel blockers, bupropion, carbamazepine, cisapride (contraindicated), delavirdine, dextromethorphan, digoxin, eplerenone, ergot alkaloids (contraindicated), ethosuximide, fentanyl, fluoxetine, lidocaine, HMG-CoA reductase inhibitors, mirtazapine, nateglinide, nefazodone, paclitaxel, paroxetine, perphenazine, pimozide (contraindicated), propafenone (contraindicated), repaglinide, risperidone, rosiglitazone, sildenafil (and other PDE-5 inhibitors), thioridazine, trazodone, tricyclic antidepressants, venlafaxine, zolpidem, and other substrates of CYP2D6 or 3A4. Thioridazine is generally contraindicated with strong CYP2D6 inhibitors. When used with strong CYP3A4 inhibitors, dosage adjustment/limits are recommended for sildenafil and other PDE-5 inhibitors; refer to individual monographs.

Decreased Effect: The administration of didanosine (buffered formulation) should be separated from ritonavir by 2.5 hours to limit interaction with ritonavir. Concurrent use of rifampin, rifabutin, dexamethasone, and many anticonvulsants may lower serum concentration of ritonavir. Ritonavir may reduce the concentration of ethinyl estradiol which may result in loss of contraception (including combination products). Theophylline concentrations may be reduced in concurrent therapy. Levels of didanosine and zidovudine may be decreased by ritonavir, however, no dosage adjustment is necessary. Voriconazole serum levels are reduced by ritonavir. In addition, ritonavir may decrease the serum concentrations of the following drugs: Atovaquone, divalproex, lamotrigine, methadone, phenytoin. The levels/effects of ritonavir may be decreased by aminoglutethimide, carbamazepine, nafcillin, nevirapine, phenobarbital, phenytoin, rifamycins, and other CYP3A4 inducers. Ritonavir may decrease the levels/effects of CYP2D6 prodrug substrates (eg, codeine, hydrocodone, oxycodone, tramadol).

Pharmacodynamics/Kinetics

Absorption: Variable; increased with food

Distribution: High concentrations in serum and lymph nodes

Protein binding: 98% to 99%

Metabolism: Hepatic via CYP3A4 and 2D6; five metabolites, low concentration of an active metabolite achieved in plasma (oxidative)

Half-life elimination: 3-5 hours

Time to peak, plasma: 2 hours (fasted); 4 hours (nonfasted)

Excretion: Urine (~11%); feces (~86%)

Pregnancy Risk Factor B

Ritonavir and Lopinavir see Lopinavir and Ritonavir on page 943
Rituxan® see Rituximab on page 1360

Rituximab *(ri TUK si mab)*

U.S. Brand Names Rituxan®

Canadian Brand Names Rituxan®

Mexican Brand Names Mabthera®

Generic Available No

Synonyms Anti-CD20 Monoclonal Antibody; C2B8; C2B8 Monoclonal Antibody; IDEC-C2B8; NSC-687451; Pan-B Antibody

Pharmacologic Category Antineoplastic Agent, Monoclonal Antibody; Monoclonal Antibody

Use Treatment of relapsed or refractory low-grade or follicular CD20-positive, B-cell non-Hodgkin's lymphoma (NHL); treatment of diffuse large B-cell CD20-positive NHL in combination with chemotherapy; treatment of rheumatoid arthritis (RA) in combination with methotrexate

Unlabeled/Investigational Use Treatment of autoimmune hemolytic anemia (AIHA) in children; chronic immune thrombocytopenic purpura (ITP); chronic lymphocytic leukemia (CLL) (in combination with chemotherapy); Waldenström's macroglobulinemia (WM)

Investigational: Treatment of systemic autoimmune diseases (in addition to rheumatoid arthritis)

Local Anesthetic/Vasoconstrictor Precautions No information available to require special precautions

Effects on Dental Treatment No significant effects or complications reported

Common Adverse Effects Note: Abdominal pain, anemia, dyspnea, hypotension, and neutropenia are more common in patients with bulky disease; percentages reported as monotherapy in NHL patients.

>10%:

    Central nervous system: Fever (53%), chills (33%), headache (19%), pain (12%)

    Dermatologic: Rash (15%), pruritus (14%), angioedema (11%)

    Gastrointestinal: Nausea (23%), abdominal pain (14%)

    Hematologic: Lymphopenia (48%; grade 3/4: 40%; median duration 14 days), leukopenia (14%; grade 3/4: 4%), neutropenia (14%; grade 3/4: 6%; median duration 13 days), thrombocytopenia (12%; grade 3/4: 2%)

    Neuromuscular & skeletal: Weakness (26%)

    Respiratory: Cough (13%), rhinitis (12%)

    Miscellaneous: Infection (31%; grade 3/4: 2%), night sweats (15%)

        Mild-to-moderate infusion-related reactions: Chills, fever, rigors, dizziness, hypertension, myalgia, nausea, pruritus, rash, and vomiting (lymphoma: first dose 77%; fourth dose 30%; eighth dose 14%); infusion-related reactions reported are lower in RA

1% to 10%:

    Cardiovascular: Hypotension (10%), peripheral edema (8%), hypertension (6%), flushing (5%), edema (<5%)

    Central nervous system: Dizziness (10%), anxiety (5%), agitation (<5%), depression (<5%), hypoesthesia (<5%), insomnia (<5%), malaise (<5%), nervousness (<5%), neuritis (<5%), somnolence (<5%), vertigo (<5%)

    Dermatologic: Urticaria (8%)

    Endocrine & metabolic: Hyperglycemia (9%), hypoglycemia (<5%)

    Gastrointestinal: Diarrhea (10%), vomiting (10%), anorexia (<5%), dyspepsia (<5%), weight loss (<5%)

    Hematologic: Anemia (8%; grade 3/4: 3%)

    Local: Pain at the injection site (<5%)

    Neuromuscular & skeletal: Arthralgia (10%), back pain (10%), myalgia (10%), arthritis (<5%), hyperkinesia (<5%), hypertonia (<5%), neuropathy (<5%), paresthesia (<5%)

    Ocular: Conjunctivitis (<5%), lacrimation disorder (<5%)

    Respiratory: Throat irritation (9%), bronchospasm (8%), dyspnea (7%), sinusitis (6%)

    Miscellaneous: LDH increased (7%)

Mechanism of Action Rituximab is a monoclonal antibody directed against the CD20 antigen on B-lymphocytes. CD20 regulates cell cycle initiation; and, possibly, functions as a calcium channel. Rituximab binds to the antigen on the cell surface, activating complement-dependent cytotoxicity; and to human Fc receptors, mediating cell killing through an antibody-dependent cellular toxicity. B-cells are believed to play a role in the development and progression of rheumatoid arthritis. Signs and symptoms of RA are reduced by targeting B-cells.

Drug Interactions

    Increased Effect/Toxicity: Monoclonal antibodies may increase the risk for allergic reactions to rituximab due to the presence of HACA antibody.

    Decreased Effect: Currently recommended not to administer live vaccines during rituximab treatment.

Pharmacodynamics/Kinetics

    Duration: Detectable in serum 3-6 months after completion of treatment; B-cell recovery begins ~6 months following completion of treatment; median B-cell levels return to normal by 12 months following completion of treatment

    Absorption: I.V.: Immediate and results in a rapid and sustained depletion of circulating and tissue-based B cells

    Distribution: 4.3 L (following two 1000 mg doses for rheumatoid arthritis)

    Half-life elimination:

        Cancer: Proportional to dose; wide ranges reflect variable tumor burden and changes in CD20 positive B-cell populations with repeated doses:

            >100 mg/m^2: 4.4 days (range 1.6-10.5 days)

            375 mg/m^2:

                Following first dose: Mean half-life: 3.2 days (range 1.3-6.4 days)

                Following fourth dose: Mean half-life: 8.6 days (range 3.5-17 days)

        RA: Mean terminal half-life: 19 days

    Excretion: Uncertain; may undergo phagocytosis and catabolism in the reticuloendothelial system (RES)

Pregnancy Risk Factor C

Rivastigmine (ri va STIG meen)

U.S. Brand Names Exelon®
Canadian Brand Names Exelon®
Mexican Brand Names Exelon®
Generic Available No
(Continued)

Rivastigmine *(Continued)*

Synonyms ENA 713; Rivastigmine Tartrate; SDZ ENA 713

Pharmacologic Category Acetylcholinesterase Inhibitor (Central)

Use Mild to moderate dementia from Alzheimer's disease

Local Anesthetic/Vasoconstrictor Precautions No information available to require special precautions

Effects on Dental Treatment No significant effects or complications reported

Common Adverse Effects

>10%:

Central nervous system: Dizziness (21%), headache (17%)

Gastrointestinal: Nausea (47%), vomiting (31%), diarrhea (19%), anorexia (17%), abdominal pain (13%)

2% to 10%:

Cardiovascular: Syncope (3%), hypertension (3%)

Central nervous system: Fatigue (9%), insomnia (9%), confusion (8%), depression (6%), anxiety (5%), malaise (5%), somnolence (5%), hallucinations (4%), aggressiveness (3%)

Gastrointestinal: Dyspepsia (9%), constipation (5%), flatulence (4%), weight loss (3%), eructation (2%)

Genitourinary: Urinary tract infection (7%)

Neuromuscular & skeletal: Weakness (6%), tremor (4%)

Respiratory: Rhinitis (4%)

Miscellaneous: Increased diaphoresis (4%), flu-like syndrome (3%)

>2% (but frequency equal to placebo): Chest pain, peripheral edema, vertigo, back pain, arthralgia, pain, bone fracture, agitation, nervousness, delusion, paranoid reaction, upper respiratory tract infection, infection, cough, pharyngitis, bronchitis, rash, urinary incontinence.

<2% (Limited to important or life-threatening symptoms; reactions may be at a similar frequency to placebo): Fever, edema, allergy, periorbital or facial edema, hypothermia, hypotension, postural hypotension, cardiac failure, ataxia, convulsions, apraxia, aphasia, dysphonia, hyperkinesia, hypertonia, hypokinesia, migraine, neuralgia, peripheral neuropathy, hypothyroidism, peptic ulcer, gastroesophageal reflux, GI hemorrhage, intestinal obstruction, pancreatitis, colitis, atrial fibrillation, bradycardia, AV block, bundle branch block, sick sinus syndrome, cardiac arrest, supraventricular tachycardia, tachycardia, abnormal hepatic function, cholecystitis, dehydration, arthritis, angina pectoris, MI, epistaxis, hematoma, thrombocytopenia, purpura, delirium, emotional lability, psychosis, anemia, bronchospasm, apnea, rash (maculopapular, eczema, bullous, exfoliative, psoriaform, erythematous), urticaria, acute renal failure, peripheral ischemia, pulmonary embolism, thrombosis, thrombophlebitis, intracranial hemorrhage, conjunctival hemorrhage, diplopia, glaucoma, lymphadenopathy, leukocytosis.

Mechanism of Action A deficiency of cortical acetylcholine is thought to account for some of the symptoms of Alzheimer's disease; rivastigmine increases acetylcholine in the central nervous system through reversible inhibition of its hydrolysis by cholinesterase

Drug Interactions

Increased Effect/Toxicity:

Acetylcholinesterase inhibitors (central) may increase the risk of antipsychotic-related extrapyramidal symptoms. Beta-blockers without ISA activity may increase risk of bradycardia. Calcium channel blockers (diltiazem or verapamil) may increase risk of bradycardia. Cholinergic agonists effects may be increased with rivastigmine. Cigarette use increases the clearance of rivastigmine by 23%. Depolarizing neuromuscular blocking agents effects may be increased with rivastigmine. Digoxin may increase risk of bradycardia.

Decreased Effect: Anticholinergic agents effects may be reduced with rivastigmine.

Pharmacodynamics/Kinetics

Absorption: Fasting: Rapid and complete within 1 hour

Distribution: V_d: 1.8-2.7 L/kg

Protein binding: 40%

Metabolism: Extensively via cholinesterase-mediated hydrolysis in the brain; metabolite undergoes N-demethylation and/or sulfate conjugation hepatically; CYP minimally involved; linear kinetics at 3 mg twice daily, but nonlinear at higher doses

Bioavailability: 40%

Half-life elimination: 1.5 hours

Time to peak: 1 hour

Excretion: Urine (97% as metabolites); feces (0.4%)

Pregnancy Risk Factor B

Rivastigmine Tartrate *see* Rivastigmine *on page 1361*

Rizatriptan (rye za TRIP tan)

U.S. Brand Names Maxalt®; Maxalt-MLT®
Canadian Brand Names Maxalt™; Maxalt RPD™
Mexican Brand Names Maxalt®
Generic Available No
Synonyms MK462
Pharmacologic Category Serotonin 5-HT$_{1D}$ Receptor Agonist
Use Acute treatment of migraine with or without aura
Local Anesthetic/Vasoconstrictor Precautions No information available to require special precautions
Effects on Dental Treatment Key adverse event(s) related to dental treatment: Xerostomia (normal salivary flow resumes upon discontinuation).
Common Adverse Effects 1% to 10%:
Cardiovascular: Systolic/diastolic blood pressure increases (5-10 mm Hg), chest pain (5%), palpitation
Central nervous system: Dizziness, drowsiness, fatigue (13% to 30%, dose related)
Dermatologic: Skin flushing
Endocrine & metabolic: Mild increase in growth hormone, hot flashes
Gastrointestinal: Nausea, abdominal pain, dry mouth (<5%)
Respiratory: Dyspnea
Dosage Note: In patients with risk factors for coronary artery disease, following adequate evaluation to establish the absence of coronary artery disease, the initial dose should be administered in a setting where response may be evaluated (physician's office or similarly staffed setting). ECG monitoring may be considered.
Oral: 5-10 mg, repeat after 2 hours if significant relief is not attained; maximum: 30 mg in a 24-hour period (use 5 mg dose in patients receiving propranolol with a maximum of 15 mg in 24 hours)
Note: For orally-disintegrating tablets (Maxalt-MLT®): Patient should be instructed to place tablet on tongue and allow to dissolve. Dissolved tablet will be swallowed with saliva.
Mechanism of Action Selective agonist for serotonin (5-HT$_{1D}$ receptor) in cranial arteries to cause vasoconstriction and reduce sterile inflammation associated with antidromic neuronal transmission correlating with relief of migraine
Contraindications Hypersensitivity to rizatriptan or any component of the formulation; documented ischemic heart disease or Prinzmetal's angina; uncontrolled hypertension; basilar or hemiplegic migraine; during or within 2 weeks of MAO inhibitors; during or within 24 hours of treatment with another 5-HT$_1$ agonist, or an ergot-containing or ergot-type medication (eg, methysergide, dihydroergotamine)
Warnings/Precautions Use only in patients with a clear diagnosis of migraine. May cause vasospastic reactions resulting in colonic, peripheral, or coronary ischemia. Use with caution in elderly or patients with hepatic or renal impairment (including dialysis patients), history of hypersensitivity to sumatriptan or adverse effects from sumatriptan, and in patients at risk of coronary artery disease (as predicted by presence of risk factors) unless cardiovascular evaluation provides evidence that the patient is free of cardiovascular disease. In patients with risk factors for coronary artery disease, following adequate evaluation to establish the absence of coronary artery disease, the initial dose should be administered in a setting where response may be evaluated (physician's office or similarly staffed setting). ECG monitoring may be considered. Do not use with ergotamines. May increase blood pressure transiently; may cause coronary vasospasm (less than sumatriptan); avoid in patients with signs/symptoms suggestive of reduced arterial flow (ischemic bowel, Raynaud's) which could be exacerbated by vasospasm.

Patients who experience sensations of chest pain/pressure/tightness or symptoms suggestive of angina following dosing should be evaluated for coronary artery disease or Prinzmetal's angina before receiving additional doses.

Reconsider diagnosis of migraine if no response to initial dose. Long-term effects on vision have not been evaluated.
Drug Interactions
Increased Effect/Toxicity: Use within 24 hours of another selective 5-HT$_1$ antagonist or ergot-containing drug should be avoided due to possible additive vasoconstriction. Use with propranolol increased plasma concentration of rizatriptan by 70%. Rarely, concurrent use with SSRIs results in weakness and incoordination; monitor closely. MAO inhibitors and nonselective MAO inhibitors increase concentration of rizatriptan.
(Continued)

Rizatriptan *(Continued)*

Ethanol/Nutrition/Herb Interactions Food: Food delays absorption.

Dietary Considerations Orally-disintegrating tablet contains phenylalanine (1.05 mg per 5 mg tablet, 2.10 mg per 10 mg tablet).

Pharmacodynamics/Kinetics

Onset of action: ~30 minutes

Duration: 14-16 hours

Protein binding: 14%

Metabolism: Via monoamine oxidase-A; first-pass effect

Bioavailability: 40% to 50%

Half-life elimination: 2-3 hours

Time to peak: 1-1.5 hours

Excretion: Urine (82%, 8% to 16% as unchanged drug); feces (12%)

Pregnancy Risk Factor C

Dosage Forms TAB (Maxalt®): 5 mg, 10 mg. TAB, orally-disintegrating (Maxalt-MLT®): 5 mg, 10 mg

rLFN-α2 *see* Interferon Alfa-2b *on page 844*

RMS® *see* Morphine Sulfate *on page 1065*

Ro 5488 *see* Tretinoin (Oral) *on page 1524*

Robafen® AC *see* Guaifenesin and Codeine *on page 753*

Robafen DM [OTC] *see* Guaifenesin and Dextromethorphan *on page 754*

Robaxin® *see* Methocarbamol *on page 1009*

Robinul® *see* Glycopyrrolate *on page 747*

Robinul® Forte *see* Glycopyrrolate *on page 747*

Robitussin® [OTC] *see* Guaifenesin *on page 752*

Robitussin® CF [OTC] *see* Guaifenesin, Pseudoephedrine, and Dextromethorphan *on page 757*

Robitussin® Cold and Congestion [OTC] *see* Guaifenesin, Pseudoephedrine, and Dextromethorphan *on page 757*

Robitussin® Cough and Cold Infant [OTC] *see* Guaifenesin, Pseudoephedrine, and Dextromethorphan *on page 757*

Robitussin® Cough and Congestion [OTC] *see* Guaifenesin and Dextromethorphan *on page 754*

Robitussin® CoughGels™ [OTC] *see* Dextromethorphan *on page 451*

Robitussin® DM [OTC] *see* Guaifenesin and Dextromethorphan *on page 754*

Robitussin® DM Infant [OTC] *see* Guaifenesin and Dextromethorphan *on page 754*

Robitussin® Honey Cough [OTC] *see* Dextromethorphan *on page 451*

Robitussin® Maximum Strength Cough [OTC] *see* Dextromethorphan *on page 451*

Robitussin® Maximum Strength Cough & Cold [OTC] *see* Pseudoephedrine and Dextromethorphan *on page 1311*

Robitussin-PE® [OTC] *see* Guaifenesin and Pseudoephedrine *on page 755*

Robitussin® Pediatric Cough [OTC] *see* Dextromethorphan *on page 451*

Robitussin® Pediatric Cough & Cold [OTC] *see* Pseudoephedrine and Dextromethorphan *on page 1311*

Robitussin® Severe Congestion [OTC] *see* Guaifenesin and Pseudoephedrine *on page 755*

Robitussin® Sugar Free Cough [OTC] *see* Guaifenesin and Dextromethorphan *on page 754*

Rocaltrol® *see* Calcitriol *on page 247*

Rocephin® *see* Ceftriaxone *on page 294*

Roferon-A® *see* Interferon Alfa-2a *on page 842*

Rogaine® Extra Strength for Men [OTC] *see* Minoxidil *on page 1051*

Rogaine® for Men [OTC] *see* Minoxidil *on page 1051*

Rogaine® for Women [OTC] *see* Minoxidil *on page 1051*

Rolaids® [OTC] *see* Calcium Carbonate and Magnesium Hydroxide *on page 249*

Rolaids® Extra Strength [OTC] *see* Calcium Carbonate and Magnesium Hydroxide *on page 249*

Rolaids® Softchews [OTC] *see* Calcium Carbonate *on page 248*

Romazicon® *see* Flumazenil *on page 665*

Romilar® AC *see* Guaifenesin and Codeine *on page 753*

Romycin® *see* Erythromycin *on page 562*

Rondec® *[reformulation] see* Chlorpheniramine and Phenylephrine *on page 324*

Rondec®-DM *[reformulation] see* Chlorpheniramine, Phenylephrine, and Dextromethorphan *on page 326*

Rondec®-DM Drops [DSC] *see* Carbinoxamine, Pseudoephedrine, and Dextromethorphan *on page 269*

Rondec® Drops [DSC] *see* Carbinoxamine and Pseudoephedrine *on page 268*
Rondec® Syrup [DSC] *see* Brompheniramine and Pseudoephedrine *on page 223*
Rondec® Tablets *see* Carbinoxamine and Pseudoephedrine *on page 268*
Rondec-TR® *see* Carbinoxamine and Pseudoephedrine *on page 268*

Ropinirole (roe PIN i role)

U.S. Brand Names Requip®
Canadian Brand Names Requip®
Generic Available No
Synonyms Ropinirole Hydrochloride
Pharmacologic Category Anti-Parkinson's Agent, Dopamine Agonist
Use Treatment of idiopathic Parkinson's disease; in patients with early Parkinson's disease who were not receiving concomitant levodopa therapy as well as in patients with advanced disease on concomitant levodopa; treatment of moderate-to-severe primary Restless Legs Syndrome (RLS)
Local Anesthetic/Vasoconstrictor Precautions No information available to require special precautions
Effects on Dental Treatment Key adverse event(s) related to dental treatment: Xerostomia and increased salivation (normal salivary flow resumes upon discontinuation).
Common Adverse Effects
Data inclusive of trials in early Parkinson's disease (without levodopa) and Restless Legs Syndrome:
>10%:
Cardiovascular: Syncope (1% to 12%)
Central nervous system: Somnolence (12% to 40%), dizziness (11% to 40%), fatigue (8% to 11%)
Gastrointestinal: Nausea (40% to 60%), vomiting (12%)
Miscellaneous: Viral infection (11%)
1% to 10%:
Cardiovascular: Dependent/leg edema (2% to 7%), orthostasis (1% to 6%), hypertension (5%), chest pain (4%), flushing (3%), palpitation (3%), peripheral ischemia (3%), hypotension (2%), tachycardia (2%)
Central nervous system: Pain (3% to 8%), confusion (5%), hallucinations (up to 5%, dose related), hypoesthesia (4%), amnesia (3%), malaise (3%), paresthesia (3%), vertigo (2%), yawning (3%)
Gastrointestinal: Constipation (>5%), dyspepsia (4% to 10%), abdominal pain (3% to 6%), xerostomia (3% to 5%), diarrhea (5%), anorexia (4%), flatulence (3%)
Genitourinary: Urinary tract infection (5%), impotence (3%)
Hepatic: Alkaline phosphatase increased (3%)
Neuromuscular & skeletal: Weakness (6%), arthralgia (4%), muscle cramps (3%)
Ocular: Abnormal vision (6%), xerophthalmia (2%)
Respiratory: Pharyngitis (6% to 9%), rhinitis (4%), sinusitis (4%), dyspnea (3%), influenza (3%), cough (3%), nasal congestion (2%)
Miscellaneous: Diaphoresis increased (3% to 6%)

Advanced Parkinson's disease (with levodopa):
>10%:
Central nervous system: Dizziness (26%), somnolence (20%), headache (17%)
Gastrointestinal: Nausea (30%)
Neuromuscular & skeletal: Dyskinesias (34%)
1% to 10%:
Cardiovascular: Syncope (3%), hypotension (2%)
Central nervous system: Hallucinations (10%, dose related), aggravated parkinsonism, confusion (9%), pain (5%), paresis (3%), amnesia (5%), anxiety (6%), abnormal dreaming (3%), insomnia
Gastrointestinal: Abdominal pain (9%), vomiting (7%), constipation (6%), diarrhea (5%), dysphagia (2%), flatulence (2%), increased salivation (2%), xerostomia, weight loss (2%)
Genitourinary: Urinary tract infection
Hematologic: Anemia (2%)
Neuromuscular & skeletal: Falls (10%), arthralgia (7%), tremor (6%), hypokinesia (5%), paresthesia (5%), arthritis (3%)
Respiratory: Upper respiratory tract infection (9%), dyspnea (3%)
Miscellaneous: Injury, diaphoresis increased (7%), viral infection, increased drug level (7%)
(Continued)

Ropinirole *(Continued)*

Other adverse effects (all phase 2/3 trials):
1% to 10%:
Central nervous system: Neuralgia (>1%)
Renal: BUN increased (>1%)

Mechanism of Action Ropinirole has a high relative *in vitro* specificity and full intrinsic activity at the D_2 and D_3 dopamine receptor subtypes, binding with higher affinity to D_3 than to D_2 or D_4 receptor subtypes; relevance of D_3 receptor binding in Parkinson's disease is unknown. Ropinirole has moderate *in vitro* affinity for opioid receptors. Ropinirole and its metabolites have negligible *in vitro* affinity for dopamine D_1, 5-HT$_1$, 5-HT$_2$, benzodiazepine, GABA, muscarinic, alpha$_1$-, alpha$_2$-, and beta-adrenoreceptors. Although precise mechanism of action of ropinirole is unknown, it is believed to be due to stimulation of postsynaptic dopamine D_2-type receptors within the caudate putamen in the brain. Ropinirole caused decreases in systolic and diastolic blood pressure at doses >0.25 mg. The mechanism of ropinirole-induced postural hypotension is believed to be due to D_2-mediated blunting of the noradrenergic response to standing and subsequent decrease in peripheral vascular resistance.

Drug Interactions
Cytochrome P450 Effect: Substrate of CYP1A2 (major), 3A4 (minor); **Inhibits** CYP1A2 (weak), 2D6 (strong)
Increased Effect/Toxicity: The levels/effects of ropinirole may be increased by amiodarone, ciprofloxacin, fluvoxamine, ketoconazole, norfloxacin, ofloxacin, rofecoxib, and other CYP1A2 inhibitors. Estrogens may also reduce the metabolism of ropinirole; dosage adjustments may be needed. Ropinirole may increase the levels/effects of amphetamines, selected beta-blockers, dextromethorphan, fluoxetine, lidocaine, mirtazapine, nefazodone, paroxetine, risperidone, ritonavir, thioridazine, tricyclic antidepressants, venlafaxine, and other CYP2D6 substrates.
Decreased Effect: The levels/effects of ropinirole may be decreased by aminoglutethimide, carbamazepine, phenobarbital, rifampin, and other CYP1A2 inducers. Antipsychotics, cigarette smoking, and metoclopramide may reduce the effect or serum concentrations of ropinirole. Ropinirole may decrease the levels/effects of CYP2D6 prodrug substrates (eg, codeine, hydrocodone, oxycodone, tramadol).

Pharmacodynamics/Kinetics
Absorption: Not affected by food
Distribution: V_d: 525 L
Metabolism: Extensively hepatic via CYP1A2 to inactive metabolites; first-pass effect
Bioavailability: Absolute: 55%
Half-life elimination: ~6 hours
Time to peak: ~1-2 hours; T_{max} increased by 2.5 hours when drug taken with food
Excretion: Clearance: Reduced by 30% in patients >65 years of age
Pregnancy Risk Factor C

Ropinirole Hydrochloride *see* Ropinirole *on page 1365*

Ropivacaine *(roe PIV a kane)*

Related Information
Oral Pain *on page 1692*
U.S. Brand Names Naropin®
Canadian Brand Names Naropin®
Mexican Brand Names Naropin®
Generic Available No
Synonyms Ropivacaine Hydrochloride
Pharmacologic Category Local Anesthetic
Use Local anesthetic for use in surgery, postoperative pain management, and obstetrical procedures when local or regional anesthesia is needed
Local Anesthetic/Vasoconstrictor Precautions No information available to require special precautions (see Dental Comment)
Effects on Dental Treatment No significant effects or complications reported
Common Adverse Effects
>5% (dose and route related):
Cardiovascular: Hypotension, bradycardia
Central nervous system: Headache
Dermatologic: Pruritus
Gastrointestinal: Nausea, vomiting
Hematologic: Anemia

Neuromuscular & skeletal: Back pain, paresthesia
1% to 5% (dose related):
Cardiovascular: Hypertension, tachycardia
Central nervous system: Dizziness, anxiety, lightheadedness
Endocrine & metabolic: Hypokalemia
Genitourinary: Urinary retention
Neuromuscular & skeletal: Hypoesthesia, rigors, circumoral paresthesia
Otic: Tinnitus
Renal: Oliguria
Respiratory: Dyspnea
Miscellaneous: Shivering

Mechanism of Action Blocks both the initiation and conduction of nerve impulses by decreasing the neuronal membrane's permeability to sodium ions, which results in inhibition of depolarization with resultant blockade of conduction

Drug Interactions

Cytochrome P450 Effect: Substrate of CYP1A2 (major), 2B6 (minor), 2D6 (minor), 3A4 (minor); may be major in cases of 1A2 inhibition/deficiency

Increased Effect/Toxicity: Cardiac effects may be additive with amiodarone and other class III antiarrhythmics. Amiodarone, ciprofloxacin, and fluvoxamine may increase ropivacaine levels/effects (monitor). Other CYP1A2 inhibitors may increase the levels/effects of ropivacaine; example inhibitors include ketoconazole, norfloxacin, ofloxacin, and rofecoxib.

Pharmacodynamics/Kinetics
Onset of action: Anesthesia (route dependent): 3-15 minutes
Duration (dose and route dependent): 3-15 hours
Metabolism: Hepatic
Half-life elimination: Epidural: 5-7 hours; I.V.: 2.4 hours
Excretion: Urine (86% as metabolites)

Pregnancy Risk Factor B
Dental Comment Not available with vasoconstrictor (epinephrine) and not available in dental (1.8 mL) carpules

Ropivacaine Hydrochloride see Ropivacaine on page 1366

Rosiglitazone (roh si GLI ta zone)

U.S. Brand Names Avandia®
Canadian Brand Names Avandia®
Generic Available No
Pharmacologic Category Antidiabetic Agent, Thiazolidinedione
Use Type 2 diabetes mellitus (noninsulin dependent, NIDDM):
Monotherapy: Improve glycemic control as an adjunct to diet and exercise
Combination therapy: In combination with a sulfonylurea, metformin, or insulin, or sulfonylurea plus metformin when diet, exercise, and a single agent do not result in adequate glycemic control

Local Anesthetic/Vasoconstrictor Precautions No information available to require special precautions

Effects on Dental Treatment Rosiglitazone-dependent diabetics should be appointed for dental treatment in morning in order to minimize chance of stress-induced hypoglycemia.

Common Adverse Effects Rare cases of hepatocellular injury have been reported in men in their 60s within 2-3 weeks after initiation of rosiglitazone therapy. LFTs in these patients revealed severe hepatocellular injury which responded with rapid improvement of liver function and resolution of symptoms upon discontinuation of rosiglitazone. Patients were also receiving other potentially hepatotoxic medications (Ann Intern Med, 2000, 132:121-4; 132:164-6). The rate of certain adverse reactions (eg, anemia, edema, hypoglycemia) may be higher with some combination therapies. Patients with Class I or II heart failure (EF ≤45%) have a higher frequency of cardiovascular adverse events (edema, dyspnea in ≥25%).

>10%: Endocrine & metabolic: Weight gain, increase in total cholesterol, increased LDL-cholesterol, increased HDL-cholesterol
1% to 10%:
Cardiovascular: Edema (5%)
Central nervous system: Headache (6%), fatigue (4%)
Endocrine & metabolic: Hyperglycemia (4%), hypoglycemia (1%; increased with insulin to 12% to 14%)
Gastrointestinal: Diarrhea (2%)
Hematologic: Anemia (2%)
Neuromuscular & skeletal: Back pain (4%)
Respiratory: Upper respiratory tract infection (10%), sinusitis (3%)
Miscellaneous: Injury (8%)
(Continued)

Rosiglitazone *(Continued)*

Dosage Oral:

Adults: **Note:** All patients should be initiated at the lowest recommended dose.

Monotherapy: Initial: 4 mg daily as a single daily dose or in divided doses twice daily. If response is inadequate after 8-12 weeks of treatment, the dosage may be increased to 8 mg daily as a single daily dose or in divided doses twice daily. In clinical trials, the 4 mg twice-daily regimen resulted in the greatest reduction in fasting plasma glucose and Hb A_{1c}.

Combination therapy: When adding rosiglitazone to existing therapy, continue current dose(s) of previous agents:

With sulfonylureas or metformin (or sulfonylurea plus metformin): Initial: 4 mg daily as a single daily dose or in divided doses twice daily. If response is inadequate after 8-12 weeks of treatment, the dosage may be increased to 8 mg daily as a single daily dose or in divided doses twice daily. Reduce dose of sulfonylurea if hypoglycemia occurs. It is unlikely that the dose of metformin will need to be reduced to hypoglycemia.

With insulin: Initial: 4 mg daily as a single daily dose or in divided doses twice daily. Dose of insulin should be reduced by 10% to 25% if the patient reports hypoglycemia or if the plasma glucose falls to <100 mg/dL. Doses of rosiglitazone >4 mg/day are not indicated in combination with insulin.

Elderly: No dosage adjustment is recommended

Dosage adjustment in renal impairment: No dosage adjustment is required

Dosage comment in hepatic impairment: Clearance is significantly lower in hepatic impairment. Therapy should not be initiated if the patient exhibits active liver disease of increased transaminases (>2.5 times the upper limit of normal) at baseline.

Mechanism of Action Thiazolidinedione antidiabetic agent that lowers blood glucose by improving target cell response to insulin, without increasing pancreatic insulin secretion. It has a mechanism of action that is dependent on the presence of insulin for activity.

Contraindications Hypersensitivity to rosiglitazone or any component of the formulation; active liver disease (transaminases >2.5 times the upper limit of normal at baseline); contraindicated in patients who previously experienced jaundice during troglitazone therapy

Warnings/Precautions Should not be used in diabetic ketoacidosis. Mechanism requires the presence of insulin, therefore use in type 1 diabetes (insulin dependent, IDDM) is not recommended.

May increase plasma volume and/or increase cardiac hypertrophy. Use with caution in patients with edema. Assess for fluid accumulation in patients with unusually rapid weight gain. Monitor closely for signs and symptoms of heart failure. Drug discontinuation is recommended if cardiovascular status worsens. A higher frequency of cardiovascular events has been noted in patients with NYHA Class I or II heart failure; up to 33% require adjustment of medications. Not recommended for use in patients with NYHA Class III or IV heart failure, unless serum glucose control outweighs the risk of excessive fluid retention. Use with caution in patients with anemia or depressed leukocyte counts (may reduce hemoglobin, hematocrit, and/or WBC).

Use with caution in patients with elevated transaminases (AST or ALT). Idiosyncratic hepatotoxicity has been reported with another thiazolidinedione agent (troglitazone) and (rarely) with rosiglitazone; discontinue if jaundice occurs. Monitoring should include periodic determinations of liver function. Rosiglitazone has been associated with new onset and/or worsening of macular edema in diabetic patients. Rosiglitazone should be used with caution in patients with a pre-existing macular edema or diabetic retinopathy. Discontinuation of rosiglitazone should be considered in any patient who reports visual deterioration. In addition, ophthalmological consultation should be initiated in these patients. May result in hormonal imbalance; development of menstrual irregularities should prompt reconsideration of therapy. Use with caution in premenopausal, anovulatory women; may result in resumption of ovulation, increasing the risk of pregnancy. Safety and efficacy in pediatric patients have not been established.

Drug Interactions

Cytochrome P450 Effect: **Substrate** of CYP2C8 (major), 2C9 (minor); **Inhibits** CYP2C8 (moderate), 2C9 (weak), 2C19 (weak), 2D6 (weak)

Increased Effect/Toxicity: The levels/effects of rosiglitazone may be increased by atazanavir, ritonavir, and other CYP2C8 inhibitors. Gemfibrozil may increase rosiglitazone levels; severe hypoglycemic episodes have been reported. Rosiglitazone may increase the levels/effects of amiodarone, paclitaxel, pioglitazone, repaglinide, rosiglitazone, and other CYP2C8 substrates.

Decreased Effect: The levels/effects of rosiglitazone may be decreased by carbamazepine, phenobarbital, phenytoin, rifampin, rifapentine, and secobarbital, and other CYP2C8 inducers. Bile acid sequestrants may decrease rosiglitazone levels.

Ethanol/Nutrition/Herb Interactions

Ethanol: Avoid ethanol (may cause hypoglycemia).

Food: Peak concentrations are lower by 28% and delayed when administered with food, but these effects are not believed to be clinically significant.

Herb/Nutraceutical: Avoid garlic, gymnema (may cause hypoglycemia).

Dietary Considerations Management of type 2 diabetes mellitus (noninsulin dependent, NIDDM) should include diet control. May be taken without regard to meals.

Pharmacodynamics/Kinetics

Onset of action: Delayed; Maximum effect: Up to 12 weeks

Distribution: V_{dss} (apparent): 17.6 L

Protein binding: 99.8%

Metabolism: Hepatic (99%) via CYP2C8; minor metabolism via CYP2C9

Bioavailability: 99%

Half-life elimination: 3-4 hours

Time to peak, plasma: 1 hour; delayed with food

Excretion: Urine (64%) and feces (23%) as metabolites

Pregnancy Risk Factor C

Dosage Forms TAB: 2 mg, 4 mg, 8 mg

Rosiglitazone and Glimepiride
(roh si GLI ta zone & GLYE me pye ride)

Related Information

Glimepiride on page 738

Rosiglitazone on page 1367

U.S. Brand Names Avandaryl™

Generic Available No

Synonyms Glimepiride and Rosiglitazone Maleate

Pharmacologic Category Antidiabetic Agent, Sulfonylurea; Antidiabetic Agent, Thiazolidinedione

Use Management of type 2 diabetes mellitus (noninsulin dependent, NIDDM) in patients who are already treated with the combination of rosiglitazone and a sulfonylurea, or who are not adequately controlled on a sulfonylurea alone, or who initially responded to rosiglitazone alone and require additional glycemic control; used as an adjunct to diet and exercise to lower the blood glucose when hyperglycemia cannot be controlled satisfactorily by diet and exercise alone

Local Anesthetic/Vasoconstrictor Precautions No information available to require special precautions

Effects on Dental Treatment Dependent diabetics (noninsulin dependent, type 2) should be appointed for dental treatment in the morning in order to minimize chance of stress-induced hypoglycemia.

Common Adverse Effects See individual agents.

Mechanism of Action

Rosiglitazone is a thiazolidinedione antidiabetic agent that lowers blood glucose by improving target cell response to insulin, without increasing pancreatic insulin secretion. It has a mechanism of action that is dependent on the presence of insulin for activity.

Glimepiride stimulates insulin release from the pancreatic beta cells; reduces glucose output from the liver; insulin sensitivity is increased at peripheral target sites.

Drug Interactions

Cytochrome P450 Effect:

Rosiglitazone: **Substrate** of CYP2C8 (major), 2C9 (minor); **Inhibits** CYP2C8 (moderate), 2C9 (weak), 2C19 (weak), 2D6 (weak)

Glimepiride: **Substrate** of CYP2C9 (major)

Increased Effect/Toxicity: See individual agents.

Decreased Effect: See individual agents.

Pharmacodynamics/Kinetics See individual agents.

Pregnancy Risk Factor C

Rosiglitazone and Metformin (roh si GLI ta zone & met FOR min)

Related Information

Metformin on page 1001

Rosiglitazone on page 1367

(Continued)

Rosiglitazone and Metformin *(Continued)*

U.S. Brand Names Avandamet™

Canadian Brand Names Avandamet™

Generic Available No

Synonyms Metformin and Rosiglitazone; Metformin Hydrochloride and Rosiglitazone Maleate; Rosiglitazone Maleate and Metformin Hydrochloride

Pharmacologic Category Antidiabetic Agent, Biguanide; Antidiabetic Agent, Thiazolidinedione

Use Management of type 2 diabetes mellitus (noninsulin dependent, NIDDM) in patients who are already treated with the combination of rosiglitazone and metformin, or who are not adequately controlled on metformin alone. Used as an adjunct to diet and exercise to lower the blood glucose when hyperglycemia cannot be controlled satisfactorily by diet and exercise alone

Local Anesthetic/Vasoconstrictor Precautions No information available to require special precautions

Effects on Dental Treatment Dependent diabetics (noninsulin dependent, type 2) should be appointed for dental treatment in the morning in order to minimize chance of stress-induced hypoglycemia.

Common Adverse Effects Also see individual agents. Percentages of adverse effects as reported with the combination product.

>10%:
  Gastrointestinal: Diarrhea (13%)
  Respiratory: Upper respiratory tract infection (16%)

1% to 10%:
  Cardiovascular: Edema (4%)
  Central nervous system: Headache (7%), fatigue (6%)
  Endocrine & metabolic: Hypoglycemia (3%), hyperglycemia (2%)
  Hematologic: Anemia (7%)
  Neuromuscular & skeletal: Arthralgia (5%), back pain (5%)
  Respiratory: Sinusitis (6%)
  Miscellaneous: Viral infection (5%)

Mechanism of Action Rosiglitazone is a thiazolidinedione antidiabetic agent that lowers blood glucose by improving target cell response to insulin, without increasing pancreatic insulin secretion. It has a mechanism of action that is dependent on the presence of insulin for activity. Metformin decreases hepatic glucose production, decreasing intestinal absorption of glucose, and improves insulin sensitivity (increases peripheral glucose uptake and utilization).

Drug Interactions

Cytochrome P450 Effect: Rosiglitazone: **Substrate** of CYP2C8 (major), 2C9 (minor); **Inhibits** CYP2C8 (moderate), 2C9 (weak), 2C19 (weak), 2D6 (weak)

Increased Effect/Toxicity: See individual agents.

Decreased Effect: See individual agents.

Pharmacodynamics/Kinetics See individual agents.

Pregnancy Risk Factor C

Rosiglitazone Maleate and Metformin Hydrochloride *see* Rosiglitazone and Metformin *on page 1369*

Rosuvastatin *(roe SOO va sta tin)*

U.S. Brand Names Crestor®

Canadian Brand Names Crestor®

Generic Available No

Synonyms Rosuvastatin Calcium

Pharmacologic Category Antilipemic Agent, HMG-CoA Reductase Inhibitor

Use Used with dietary therapy for hyperlipidemias to reduce elevations in total cholesterol (TC), LDL-C, apolipoprotein B, and triglycerides (TG) in patients with primary hypercholesterolemia (elevations of 1 or more components are present in Fredrickson type IIa, IIb, and IV hyperlipidemias); treatment of homozygous familial hypercholesterolemia (FH)

Local Anesthetic/Vasoconstrictor Precautions No information available to require special precautions

Effects on Dental Treatment No significant effects or complications reported

Common Adverse Effects

1% to 10%:
  Cardiovascular: Chest pain, hypertension, peripheral edema, palpitation
  Central nervous system: Headache (6%), depression, dizziness, insomnia, pain, anxiety, neuralgia, vertigo
  Dermatologic: Rash

Gastrointestinal: Pharyngitis (9%), diarrhea, dyspepsia, nausea, abdominal pain, constipation, gastroenteritis, vomiting

Hematologic: Anemia, bruising

Neuromuscular & skeletal: Myalgia (3%), weakness, back pain, arthritis, arthralgia, hypertonia, paresthesia

Respiratory: Bronchitis, rhinitis, sinusitis, cough

Miscellaneous: Flu-like syndrome

Adverse reactions reported with other HMG-CoA reductase inhibitors include a hypersensitivity syndrome (symptoms may include anaphylaxis, angioedema, arthralgia, erythema multiforme, eosinophilia, hemolytic anemia, lupus syndrome, photosensitivity, polymyalgia rheumatica, positive ANA, purpura, Stevens-Johnson syndrome, toxic epidermal necrolysis, urticaria, vasculitis)

Mechanism of Action Inhibitor of 3-hydroxy-3-methylglutaryl coenzyme A (HMG-CoA) reductase, the rate-limiting enzyme in cholesterol synthesis (reduces the production of mevalonic acid from HMG-CoA); this then results in a compensatory increase in the expression of LDL receptors on hepatocyte membranes and a stimulation of LDL catabolism

Drug Interactions

Cytochrome P450 Effect: Substrate (minor) of CYP2C9, 3A4

Increased Effect/Toxicity: Cyclosporine may increase serum concentrations of rosuvastatin (up to 10-fold); limit dose to 5 mg/day. Serum concentrations of rosuvastatin may be increased (doubled) during concurrent administration of gemfibrozil; combination should be avoided; limit dose to 10 mg/day. Clofibrate, fenofibrate, or niacin may increase the risk of myopathy and rhabdomyolysis with HMG-CoA reductase inhibitors; the effects on lipids may be additive. The anticoagulant effects of warfarin may be increased by rosuvastatin (monitor). Rosuvastatin increases serum concentrations of hormonal contraceptives (ethinyl estradiol and norgestrel).

Decreased Effect: Plasma concentrations of rosuvastatin may be decreased when given with magnesium/aluminum hydroxide-containing antacids; antacids should be administered at least 2 hours after rosuvastatin. Cholestyramine and colestipol (bile acid sequestrants) may reduce absorption of several HMG-CoA reductase inhibitors; separate administration times by at least 4 hours; cholesterol-lowering effects are additive.

Pharmacodynamics/Kinetics

Onset: Within 1 week; maximal at 4 weeks

Distribution: V_d: 134 L

Protein binding: 90%

Metabolism: Hepatic (10%), via CYP2C9 (1 active metabolite identified)

Bioavailability: 20% (high first-pass extraction by liver)

Asian patients have been noted to have increased bioavailability.

Half-life elimination: 19 hours

Time to peak, plasma: 3-5 hours

Excretion: Feces (90%), primarily as unchanged drug

Pregnancy Risk Factor X

Rosuvastatin Calcium *see* Rosuvastatin *on page 1370*

RotaTeq® *see* Rotavirus Vaccine *on page 1371*

Rotavirus Vaccine (ROE ta vye us vak SEEN)

U.S. Brand Names RotaTeq®

Generic Available No

Synonyms Pentavalent Human-Bovine Reassortant Rotavirus Vaccine; Rotavirus Vaccine, Pentavalent

Pharmacologic Category Vaccine

Use Prevention of rotavirus gastroenteritis in infants and children

Local Anesthetic/Vasoconstrictor Precautions No information available to require special precautions

Effects on Dental Treatment No significant effects or complications reported

Common Adverse Effects All serious adverse reactions must be reported to the U.S. Department of Health and Human Services (DHHS) Vaccine Adverse Event Reporting System (VAERS) 1-800-822-7967.

Note: An increased risk of intussusception was not noted in clinical trials

>10%:

Central nervous system: Fever (43%, equal to placebo)

Gastrointestinal: Diarrhea (4% to 24%), vomiting (3% to 15%)

Otic: Otitis media (14%)

1% to 10%:

Central nervous system: Irritability (3% to 8%)

Respiratory: Nasopharyngitis (7%), bronchospasm (1%)

(Continued)

Rotavirus Vaccine *(Continued)*

Mechanism of Action A live vaccine obtained from human and bovine sources; replicates in the small intestine and promotes active immunity to rotavirus gastroenteritis caused by serotypes G1, G2, G3, and G4.

Drug Interactions

Increased Effect/Toxicity: In clinical trials, rotavirus vaccine was administered with DTaP, IPV, HiB, hepatitis B vaccine, and pneumococcal conjugate vaccine. Antibody response was not decreased, with the exception of pertussis (insufficient data). Infants needing oral polio vaccine were excluded from clinical studies.

Decreased Effect: In clinical trials, rotavirus vaccine was administered with DTaP, IPV, HiB, hepatitis B vaccine and pneumococcal conjugate vaccine. Antibody response was not decreased, with the exception of pertussis (insufficient data). Infants needing oral polio vaccine were excluded from clinical studies. When used concurrently with immunosuppressant medications, the effect of the vaccine may be decreased.

Pharmacodynamics/Kinetics

Onset of action: A threefold increase in antirotavirus IgA was noted following completion of the 3-dose regimen in 93% to 100% of infants.

Duration: At least 2 years

Rotavirus Vaccine, Pentavalent *see* Rotavirus Vaccine *on page 1371*

Rowasa® *see* Mesalamine *on page 996*

Roxanol™ *see* Morphine Sulfate *on page 1065*

Roxanol 100™ *see* Morphine Sulfate *on page 1065*

Roxanol™-T [DSC] *see* Morphine Sulfate *on page 1065*

Roxicet™ *see* Oxycodone and Acetaminophen *on page 1165*

Roxicet™ 5/500 *see* Oxycodone and Acetaminophen *on page 1165*

Roxicodone™ *see* Oxycodone *on page 1163*

Roxicodone™ Intensol™ *see* Oxycodone *on page 1163*

Rozerem™ *see* Ramelteon *on page 1331*

RP-6976 *see* Docetaxel *on page 494*

RP-54274 *see* Riluzole *on page 1350*

RP-59500 *see* Quinupristin and Dalfopristin *on page 1326*

r-PA *see* Reteplase *on page 1341*

rPDGF-BB *see* Becaplermin *on page 182*

RS-25259 *see* Palonosetron *on page 1180*

RS-25259-197 *see* Palonosetron *on page 1180*

R-Tanna *see* Chlorpheniramine and Phenylephrine *on page 324*

RTCA *see* Ribavirin *on page 1343*

RU 0211 *see* Lubiprostone *on page 957*

RU-486 *see* Mifepristone *on page 1045*

RU-23908 *see* Nilutamide *on page 1115*

RU-38486 *see* Mifepristone *on page 1045*

Rubella, Measles and Mumps Vaccines, Combined *see* Measles, Mumps, and Rubella Vaccines (Combined) *on page 966*

Rubella, Varicella, Measles, and Mumps Vaccine *see* Measles, Mumps, Rubella, and Varicella Virus Vaccine *on page 967*

Rubella Virus Vaccine (Live) (rue BEL a VYE rus vak SEEN, live)

Related Information

Immunizations (Vaccines) *on page 1786*

U.S. Brand Names Meruvax® II

Generic Available No

Synonyms German Measles Vaccine

Pharmacologic Category Vaccine

Use Selective active immunization against rubella; vaccination is routinely recommended for persons from 12 months of age to puberty. All adults, both male and female, lacking documentation of live vaccine on or after first birthday, or laboratory evidence of immunity (particularly women of childbearing age and young adults who work in or congregate in hospitals, colleges, and on military bases) should be vaccinated. Susceptible travelers should be vaccinated.

Note: Trivalent measles - mumps - rubella (MMR) vaccine is the preferred immunizing agent for most children and many adults.

Local Anesthetic/Vasoconstrictor Precautions No information available to require special precautions

Effects on Dental Treatment No significant effects or complications reported

Common Adverse Effects All serious adverse reactions must be reported to the U.S. Department of Health and Human Services (DHHS) Vaccine Adverse Event Reporting System (VAERS) 1-800-822-7967.

Frequency not defined.

Cardiovascular: Syncope, vasculitis

Central nervous system: Dizziness, encephalitis, fever, Guillain-Barré syndrome, headache, irritability, malaise, polyneuritis, polyneuropathy

Dermatologic: Angioneurotic edema, erythema multiforme, purpura, rash, Stevens-Johnson syndrome, urticaria

Gastrointestinal: Diarrhea, nausea, sore throat, vomiting

Hematologic: Leukocytosis, thrombocytopenia

Local: Injection site reactions which include burning, induration, pain, redness, stinging, wheal and flare

Neuromuscular & skeletal: Arthralgia/arthritis (variable; highest rates in women, 12% to 26% versus children, up to 3%), myalgia, paresthesia

Ocular: Conjunctivitis, optic neuritis, papillitis, retrobulbar neuritis

Otic: Nerve deafness, otitis media

Respiratory: Bronchial spasm, cough, rhinitis

Miscellaneous: Anaphylactoid reactions, anaphylaxis, regional lymphadenopathy

Mechanism of Action Rubella vaccine is a live attenuated vaccine that contains the Wistar Institute RA 27/3 strain, which is adapted to and propagated in human diploid cell culture. Promotes active immunity by inducing rubella hemagglutination-inhibiting antibodies.

Drug Interactions

Decreased Effect: The effect of the vaccine may be decreased in individuals who are receiving immunosuppressant drugs (including high-dose systemic corticosteroids). Effect of vaccine may be decreased in given with immune globulin, whole blood or plasma; do not administer with vaccine. Effectiveness may be decreased if given within 30 days of varicella vaccine (effectiveness not decreased when administered simultaneously).

Pharmacodynamics/Kinetics Onset of action: Antibodies to vaccine: 2-4 weeks

Pregnancy Risk Factor C

Rubeola Vaccine *see* Measles Virus Vaccine (Live) *on page 967*

Rubex® *see* DOXOrubicin *on page 509*

Rubidomycin Hydrochloride *see* DAUNOrubicin Hydrochloride *on page 426*

Rulox [OTC] *see* Aluminum Hydroxide and Magnesium Hydroxide *on page 80*

Rulox No. 1 [DSC] *see* Aluminum Hydroxide and Magnesium Hydroxide *on page 80*

Rum-K® *see* Potassium Chloride *on page 1258*

Rynatan® *see* Chlorpheniramine and Phenylephrine *on page 324*

Rynatan® Pediatric Suspension *see* Chlorpheniramine and Phenylephrine *on page 324*

Rynatuss® *see* Chlorpheniramine, Ephedrine, Phenylephrine, and Carbetapentane *on page 325*

Rynatuss® Pediatric [DSC] *see* Chlorpheniramine, Ephedrine, Phenylephrine, and Carbetapentane *on page 325*

Rythmol® *see* Propafenone *on page 1293*

Rythmol® SR *see* Propafenone *on page 1293*

Rēv-Eyes™ *see* Dapiprazole *on page 421*

S-2® *see* Epinephrine (Racemic) *on page 549*

S-(+)-3-isobutylgaba *see* Pregabalin *on page 1274*

Sacrosidase (sak ROE si dase)

U.S. Brand Names Sucraid®

Canadian Brand Names Sucraid®

Generic Available No

Pharmacologic Category Enzyme, Gastrointestinal

Use Orphan drug: Oral replacement therapy in sucrase deficiency, as seen in congenital sucrase-isomaltase deficiency (CSID)

Local Anesthetic/Vasoconstrictor Precautions No information available to require special precautions

Effects on Dental Treatment No significant effects or complications reported

Common Adverse Effects 1% to 10%: Gastrointestinal: Abdominal pain, vomiting, nausea, diarrhea, constipation

Mechanism of Action Sacrosidase is a naturally-occurring gastrointestinal enzyme which breaks down the disaccharide sucrose to its monosaccharide components. Hydrolysis is necessary to allow absorption of these nutrients.

(Continued)

Sacrosidase *(Continued)*

Drug Interactions
Increased Effect/Toxicity: Drug-drug interactions have not been evaluated.
Pharmacodynamics/Kinetics
Absorption: Amino acids
Metabolism: GI tract to individual amino acids
Pregnancy Risk Factor C

Safe Tussin® [OTC] *see* Guaifenesin and Dextromethorphan *on page 754*

Saizen® *see* Somatropin *on page 1406*

SalAc® [OTC] *see* Salicylic Acid *on page 1374*

Sal-Acid® [OTC] *see* Salicylic Acid *on page 1374*

Salactic® [OTC] *see* Salicylic Acid *on page 1374*

Salagen® *see* Pilocarpine (Oral) *on page 1235*

Salbutamol *see* Albuterol *on page 58*

Salbutamol and Ipratropium *see* Ipratropium and Albuterol *on page 857*

Salicylazosulfapyridine *see* Sulfasalazine *on page 1428*

Salicylic Acid (sal i SIL ik AS id)

U.S. Brand Names Compound W® [OTC]; Compound W® One Step Wart Remover [OTC]; DHS™ Sal [OTC]; Dr. Scholl's® Callus Remover [OTC]; Dr. Scholl's® Clear Away [OTC]; DuoFilm® [OTC]; DuoPlant® [DSC] [OTC]; Freezone® [OTC]; Fung-O® [OTC]; Gordofilm® [OTC]; Hydrisalic™ [OTC]; Ionil® [OTC]; Ionil® Plus [OTC]; Keralyt® [OTC]; LupiCare™ Dandruff [OTC]; Lupi-Care™ II Psoriasis [OTC]; LupiCare™ Psoriasis [OTC]; Mediplast® [OTC]; MG217 Sal-Acid® [OTC]; Mosco® Corn and Callus Remover [OTC]; NeoCeuti-cals® Acne Spot Treatment [OTC]; Neutrogena® Acne Wash [OTC]; Neutrogena® Body Clear™ [OTC]; Neutrogena® Clear Pore [OTC]; Neutrogena® Clear Pore Shine Control [OTC]; Neutrogena® Healthy Scalp [OTC]; Neutrogena® Maximum Strength T/Sal® [OTC]; Neutrogena® On The Spot® Acne Patch [OTC]; Occlusal®-HP [OTC]; Oxy Balance® [OTC]; Oxy Balance® Deep Pore [OTC]; Palmer's® Skin Success Acne Cleanser [OTC]; Pedisilk® [OTC]; Propa pH [OTC]; SalAc® [OTC]; Sal-Acid® [OTC]; Salactic® [OTC]; Sal-Plant® [OTC]; Stri-dex® [OTC]; Stri-dex® Body Focus [OTC]; Stri-dex® Facewipes To Go™ [OTC]; Stri-dex® Maximum Strength [OTC]; Tinamed® [OTC]; Tiseb® [OTC]; Trans-Ver-Sal® [OTC]; Wart-Off® Maximum Strength [OTC]; Zapzyt® Acne Wash [OTC]; Zapzyt® Pore Treatment [OTC]
Canadian Brand Names Duofilm®; Duoforte® 27; Occlusal™-HP; Sebcur®; Soluver®; Soluver® Plus; Trans-Plantar®; Trans-Ver-Sal®
Mexican Brand Names DuoPlant®; Ionil; Ionil Plus®; Trans-Ver-Sal®
Generic Available Yes: Gel, soap
Pharmacologic Category Keratolytic Agent
Use Topically for its keratolytic effect in controlling seborrheic dermatitis or psori-asis of body and scalp, dandruff, and other scaling dermatoses; also used to remove warts, corns, and calluses; acne
Local Anesthetic/Vasoconstrictor Precautions No information available to require special precautions
Effects on Dental Treatment No significant effects or complications reported
Mechanism of Action Produces desquamation of hyperkeratotic epithelium via dissolution of the intercellular cement which causes the cornified tissue to swell, soften, macerate, and desquamate. Salicylic acid is keratolytic at concentra-tions of 3% to 6%; it becomes destructive to tissue at concentrations >6%. Concentrations of 6% to 60% are used to remove corns and warts and in the treatment of psoriasis and other hyperkeratotic disorders.
Pregnancy Risk Factor C

Salicylic Acid and Coal Tar *see* Coal Tar and Salicylic Acid *on page 383*

Salicylsalicylic Acid *see* Salsalate *on page 1376*

SalineX® [OTC] *see* Sodium Chloride *on page 1400*

Salivart® [OTC] *see* Saliva Substitute *on page 1374*

Saliva Substitute (sa LYE va SUB stee tute)

Related Information
Management of Patients Undergoing Cancer Therapy *on page 1728*
U.S. Brand Names Entertainer's Secret® [OTC]; Moi-Stir® [OTC]; Mouthkote® [OTC]; Salivart® [OTC]; Saliva Substitute™ [OTC]; Salix® [OTC]
Generic Available No

Pharmacologic Category Gastrointestinal Agent, Miscellaneous
Dental Use Relief of dry mouth and throat in xerostomia
Use Relief of dry mouth and throat in xerostomia
Local Anesthetic/Vasoconstrictor Precautions No information available to require special precautions
Effects on Dental Treatment No significant effects or complications reported
Dosage Use as needed
Dosage Forms
Lozenge (Salix®): Sorbitol, malic acid, sodium citrate, citric acid, dibasic calcium phosphate, sodium carboxymethylcellulose, propylene glycol, hydrogenated cottonseed oil, silicon dioxide, magnesium stearate [fruit flavor]
Solution, oral:
Entertainer's Secret®: Sodium carboxymethylcellulose, aloe vera gel, glycerin (60 mL) [honey-apple flavor]
Saliva Substitute®: Sorbitol, sodium carboxymethylcellulose, methylparaben (5 mL, 120 mL)
Spray, oral:
Moi-Stir®: Water, sorbitol, sodium carboxymethylcellulose, methylparaben, propylparaben, potassium chloride, dibasic sodium phosphate, calcium chloride, magnesium chloride, sodium chloride (120 mL)
Mouthkote®: Water, xylitol, sorbitol, yerba santa, citric acid, ascorbic acid, sodium saccharin, sodium benzoate (60 mL, 240 mL) [lemon-lime flavor]
Salivart®: Water, sodium carboxymethylcellulose, sorbitol, sodium chloride, potassium chloride, calcium chloride, magnesium chloride, potassium phosphate (70 mL)
Swabsticks, oral (Moi-Stir®): Water, sorbitol, sodium carboxymethylcellulose, methylparaben, propylparaben, potassium chloride, dibasic sodium phosphate, calcium chloride, magnesium chloride, sodium chloride (300s)

Salix® [OTC] *see* Saliva Substitute *on page 1374*
Salk Vaccine *see* Poliovirus Vaccine (Inactivated) *on page 1252*

Salmeterol (sal ME te role)

Related Information
Respiratory Diseases *on page 1656*
U.S. Brand Names Serevent® Diskus®
Canadian Brand Names Serevent®
Mexican Brand Names Serevent®
Generic Available No
Synonyms Salmeterol Xinafoate
Pharmacologic Category Beta$_2$-Adrenergic Agonist
Use Maintenance treatment of asthma and in prevention of bronchospasm with reversible obstructive airway disease, including patients with symptoms of nocturnal asthma; prevention of exercise-induced bronchospasm; maintenance treatment of bronchospasm associated with COPD
Local Anesthetic/Vasoconstrictor Precautions No information available to require special precautions
Effects on Dental Treatment No significant effects or complications reported
Common Adverse Effects
>10%:
Central nervous system: Headache (13% to 17%)
Neuromuscular & skeletal: Pain (1% to 12%)
1% to 10%:
Cardiovascular: Hypertension (4%), edema (1% to <3%)
Central nervous system: Dizziness (4%), sleep disturbance (1% to 3%), fever (1% to 3%), anxiety (1% to <3%), migraine (1% to <3%)
Dermatologic: Rash (1% to 4%), contact dermatitis (1% to 3%), eczema (1% to 3%), urticaria (3%), photodermatitis (1% to 2%)
Endocrine & metabolic: Hyperglycemia (1% to <3%)
Gastrointestinal: Nausea (1% to 3%), dyspepsia (1% to <3%), dental pain (1% to <3%), infections (1% to <3%), oropharyngeal candidiasis (1% to <3%), xerostomia (1% to <3%)
Neuromuscular & skeletal: Muscular cramps/spasm (3%), paresthesia (1% to 3%), arthralgia (1% to <3%), muscular stiffness, rigidity (1% to <3%)
Ocular: Keratitis/conjunctivitis (1% to <3%)
Respiratory: Tracheitis/bronchitis (7%), pharyngitis (up to 6%), cough (5%), influenza (5%), infection (5%), sinusitis (4% to 5%), rhinitis (4% to 5%), nasal congestion (4%), asthma (3% to 4%)
Restrictions An FDA-approved medication guide is available at http://www.fda.gov/cder/Offices/ODS/labeling.htm; distribute to each patient to whom this medication is dispensed.
(Continued)

Salmeterol *(Continued)*

Mechanism of Action Relaxes bronchial smooth muscle by selective action on $beta_2$-receptors with little effect on heart rate; because salmeterol acts locally in the lung, therapeutic effect is not predicted by plasma levels

Drug Interactions

Cytochrome P450 Effect: Substrate of CYP3A4 (major)

Increased Effect/Toxicity: CYP3A4 inhibitors may increase the levels/effects of fluticasone and salmeterol; example inhibitors include amprenavir, atazanavir, clarithromycin, delavirdine, diclofenac, fosamprenavir, imatinib, indinavir, isoniazid, itraconazole, ketoconazole, miconazole, nefazodone, nelfinavir, nicardipine, propofol, quinidine, ritonavir, and telithromycin. Atomoxetine may enhance the tachycardia effect of $beta_2$-agonists. Sympathomimetics may enhance the adverse/toxic effect of salmeterol.

Decreased Effect: Beta$_2$-agonists may diminish the bradycardia effect of beta-blockers (beta$_1$ selective). Beta-blockers (nonselective) may diminish the bronchodilator effect of beta$_2$-agonists.

Pharmacodynamics/Kinetics

Onset of action: Asthma: 30-48 minutes, COPD: 2 hours

Peak effect: 2-4 hours, COPD: 3.27-4.75 hours

Duration: 12 hours

Protein binding: 96%

Metabolism: Hepatically hydroxylated

Half-life elimination: 5.5 hours

Excretion: Feces (60%), urine (25%)

Pregnancy Risk Factor C

Salmeterol and Fluticasone *see* Fluticasone and Salmeterol *on page 690*

Salmeterol Xinafoate *see* Salmeterol *on page 1375*

Sal-Plant® [OTC] *see* Salicylic Acid *on page 1374*

Salsalate *(SAL sa late)*

Related Information

Rheumatoid Arthritis, Osteoarthritis, and Osteoporosis *on page 1668*

Temporomandibular Dysfunction (TMD) *on page 1724*

U.S. Brand Names Amigesic®

Canadian Brand Names Amigesic®; Salflex®

Generic Available Yes

Synonyms Disalicylic Acid; Salicylsalicylic Acid

Pharmacologic Category Salicylate

Use Treatment of minor pain or fever; arthritis

Local Anesthetic/Vasoconstrictor Precautions No information available to require special precautions

Effects on Dental Treatment NSAID formulations are known to reversibly decrease platelet aggregation via mechanisms different than observed with aspirin. The dentist should be aware of the potential of abnormal coagulation. Caution should also be exercised in the use of NSAIDs in patients already on anticoagulant therapy with drugs such as warfarin (Coumadin®).

Common Adverse Effects

>10%: Gastrointestinal: Nausea, heartburn, stomach pain, dyspepsia

1% to 10%:

Central nervous system: Fatigue

Dermatologic: Rash

Gastrointestinal: Gastrointestinal ulceration

Hematologic: Hemolytic anemia

Neuromuscular & skeletal: Weakness

Respiratory: Dyspnea

Miscellaneous: Anaphylactic shock

Dosage Adults: Oral: 3 g/day in 2-3 divided doses

Dosing comments in renal impairment: In patients with end-stage renal disease undergoing hemodialysis: 750 mg twice daily with an additional 500 mg after dialysis

Mechanism of Action Inhibits prostaglandin synthesis, acts on the hypothalamus heat-regulating center to reduce fever, blocks prostaglandin synthetase action which prevents formation of the platelet-aggregating substance thromboxane A$_2$

Contraindications Hypersensitivity to salsalate or any component of the formulation; GI ulcer or bleeding; pregnancy (3rd trimester)

Warnings/Precautions Use with caution in patients with platelet and bleeding disorders, dehydration, renal dysfunction, erosive gastritis, or peptic ulcer disease, previous nonreaction does not guarantee future safe taking of medication; do not use aspirin in children <16 years of age for chickenpox or flu symptoms due to the association with Reye's syndrome

Drug Interactions
Increased Effect/Toxicity: Increased effect/toxicity of oral anticoagulants, hypoglycemics, and methotrexate.
Decreased Effect: Decreased effect with urinary alkalinizers, antacids, and corticosteroids. Decreased effect of uricosurics and spironolactone.

Ethanol/Nutrition/Herb Interactions
Ethanol: Avoid ethanol (may enhance gastric mucosal irritation).
Food: Salsalate peak serum levels may be delayed if taken with food.
Herb/Nutraceutical: Avoid cat's claw, dong quai, evening primrose, feverfew, garlic, ginger, ginkgo, red clover, horse chestnut, green tea, ginseng (all have additional antiplatelet activity).

Dietary Considerations May be taken with food to decrease GI distress.

Pharmacodynamics/Kinetics
Onset of action: Therapeutic: 3-4 days of continuous dosing
Absorption: Complete from small intestine
Metabolism: Hepatically hydrolyzed to two moles of salicylic acid (active)
Half-life elimination: 7-8 hours
Excretion: Primarily urine

Pregnancy Risk Factor C/D (3rd trimester)

Dosage Forms TAB: 500 mg, 750 mg; (Amigesic®): 500 mg, 750 mg

Salt *see* Sodium Chloride *on page 1400*
Sal-Tropine™ *see* Atropine *on page 161*
Sanctura™ *see* Trospium *on page 1546*
Sandimmune® *see* CycloSPORINE *on page 406*
Sandostatin® *see* Octreotide *on page 1135*
Sandostatin LAR® *see* Octreotide *on page 1135*
Sani-Supp® [OTC] *see* Glycerin *on page 747*
Santyl® *see* Collagenase *on page 391*

Saquinavir (sa KWIN a veer)

Related Information
HIV Infection and AIDS *on page 1662*
Tuberculosis *on page 1673*

U.S. Brand Names Fortovase® [DSC]; Invirase®
Canadian Brand Names Fortovase®; Invirase®
Mexican Brand Names Invirase®
Generic Available No
Synonyms Saquinavir Mesylate
Pharmacologic Category Antiretroviral Agent, Protease Inhibitor
Use Treatment of HIV infection; used in combination with at least two other antiretroviral agents
Local Anesthetic/Vasoconstrictor Precautions No information available to require special precautions
Effects on Dental Treatment No significant effects or complications reported
Common Adverse Effects Protease inhibitors cause dyslipidemia which includes elevated cholesterol and triglycerides and a redistribution of body fat centrally to cause increased abdominal girth, buffalo hump, facial atrophy, and breast enlargement. These agents also cause hyperglycemia.

10%: Gastrointestinal: Diarrhea, nausea
1% to 10%:
Cardiovascular: Chest pain
Central nervous system: Anxiety, depression, fatigue, headache, insomnia, pain
Dermatologic: Rash, verruca
Endocrine & metabolic: Hyperglycemia, hypoglycemia, hyperkalemia, libido disorder, serum amylase increased
Gastrointestinal: Abdominal discomfort, abdominal pain, appetite decreased, buccal mucosa ulceration, constipation, dyspepsia, flatulence, taste alteration, vomiting
Hepatic: AST increased, ALT increased, bilirubin increased
Neuromuscular & skeletal: Paresthesia, weakness, CPK increased
Renal: Creatinine kinase increased

Mechanism of Action As an inhibitor of HIV protease, saquinavir prevents the cleavage of viral polyprotein precursors which are needed to generate functional proteins in and maturation of HIV-infected cells
(Continued)

Saquinavir *(Continued)*

Drug Interactions

Cytochrome P450 Effect: Substrate of CYP2D6 (minor), 3A4 (major); Inhibits CYP2C8/9 (weak), 2C19 (weak), 2D6 (weak), 3A4 (moderate)

Increased Effect/Toxicity: Concurrent use of amiodarone, bepridil, cisapride, flecainide, midazolam, pimozide, propafenone, quinidine, rifampin, triazolam, or ergot derivatives is contraindicated.

Saquinavir may increase the levels/effects of selected benzodiazepines, calcium channel blockers, cisapride, cyclosporine, ergot alkaloids, selected HMG-CoA reductase inhibitors, mirtazapine, nateglinide, nefazodone, pimozide, quinidine, sildenafil (and other PDE-5 inhibitors), tacrolimus, venlafaxine, and other CYP3A4 substrates. The effects of warfarin may also be increased.

Serum concentrations of saquinavir may be increased by azole antifungals (itraconazole, ketoconazole); dose adjustment was not needed at the study dose when used for a limited time (ketoconazole 400 mg once daily and Fortovase® 1200 mg 3 times/day). Saquinavir serum concentrations may be increased by delavirdine. Atazanavir, indinavir, and ritonavir may increase serum levels of saquinavir. Serum levels of saquinavir and nelfinavir may be increased with concurrent use. Lopinavir/ritonavir (combination product) may increase serum levels of saquinavir. Refer to Dosage (dosage adjustment recommendations with atazanavir have not been established).

Serum concentrations of saquinavir and clarithromycin may both be increased. Dose adjustment not was not needed at the study dose when used for 7 days (clarithromycin 500 mg twice daily and Fortovase® 1200 mg 3 times/day); dosage adjustment of clarithromycin is recommended in patients with renal impairment.

Serum concentrations of saquinavir are decreased and levels of rifabutin are increased when used together. Saquinavir should not be used as the sole protease inhibitor when given with rifabutin.

Decreased Effect: The levels/effects of saquinavir may be reduced by aminoglutethimide, carbamazepine, nafcillin, nevirapine, phenobarbital, phenytoin, rifamycins, and other CYP3A4 inducers. Loss of efficacy and potential resistance may occur. Concurrent use with rifampin is contraindicated.

Serum concentrations of methadone may be decreased; an increased dose may be needed when administered with saquinavir. Serum levels of the hormones in oral contraceptives may decrease significantly with administration of saquinavir. Patients should use alternative methods of contraceptives during saquinavir therapy.

Serum levels of saquinavir and efavirenz may be decreased with concurrent use; saquinavir should not be used as the sole protease inhibitor with efavirenz or nevirapine.

Dexamethasone may decrease serum concentrations of saquinavir; use with caution. Serum concentrations of saquinavir are decreased and levels of rifabutin are increased when used together. Saquinavir should not be used as the sole protease inhibitor when given with rifabutin.

Pharmacodynamics/Kinetics

Absorption: Poor; increased with high fat meal; Fortovase® has improved absorption over Invirase®

Distribution: V_d: 700 L; does not distribute into CSF

Protein binding, plasma: ~98%

Metabolism: Extensively hepatic via CYP3A4; extensive first-pass effect

Bioavailability: Invirase®: ~4%; Fortovase®: 12% to 15%

Excretion: Feces (81% to 88%), urine (1% to 3%) within 5 days

Pregnancy Risk Factor B

Saquinavir Mesylate *see* Saquinavir *on page 1377*

Sarafem® *see* Fluoxetine *on page 675*

Sargramostim *(sar GRAM oh stim)*

U.S. Brand Names Leukine®

Canadian Brand Names Leukine®

Generic Available No

Synonyms GM-CSF; Granulocyte-Macrophage Colony Stimulating Factor; rGM-CSF

Pharmacologic Category Colony Stimulating Factor

Use

Myeloid reconstitution after autologous bone marrow transplantation: Non-Hodgkin's lymphoma (NHL), acute lymphoblastic leukemia (ALL), Hodgkin's lymphoma, metastatic breast cancer

Myeloid reconstitution after allogeneic bone marrow transplantation

Peripheral stem cell transplantation: Metastatic breast cancer, non-Hodgkin's lymphoma, Hodgkin's lymphoma, multiple myeloma

Orphan drug:

Acute myelogenous leukemia (AML) following induction chemotherapy in older adults to shorten time to neutrophil recovery and to reduce the incidence of severe and life-threatening infections and infections resulting in death

Bone marrow transplant (allogeneic or autologous) failure or engraftment delay

Safety and efficacy of GM-CSF given simultaneously with cytotoxic chemotherapy have not been established. Concurrent treatment may increase myelosuppression.

Local Anesthetic/Vasoconstrictor Precautions No information available to require special precautions

Effects on Dental Treatment No significant effects or complications reported

Common Adverse Effects

>10%:

Cardiovascular: Hypotension, tachycardia, flushing, and syncope may occur with the first dose of a cycle ("first-dose effect"); peripheral edema (11%)

Central nervous system: Headache (26%)

Dermatologic: Rash, alopecia

Endocrine & metabolic: Polydypsia

Gastrointestinal: Diarrhea (52% to 89%), stomatitis, mucositis

Local: Local reactions at the injection site (~50%)

Neuromuscular & skeletal: Myalgia (18%), arthralgia (21%), bone pain

Renal: Increased serum creatinine (14%)

Respiratory: Dyspnea (28%)

1% to 10%:

Cardiovascular: Transient supraventricular arrhythmia; chest pain; capillary leak syndrome; pericardial effusion (4%)

Central nervous system: Headache

Gastrointestinal: Nausea, vomiting

Hematologic: Leukocytosis, thrombocytopenia

Neuromuscular & skeletal: Weakness

Respiratory: Cough; pleural effusion (1%)

Mechanism of Action Stimulates proliferation, differentiation and functional activity of neutrophils, eosinophils, monocytes, and macrophages, as indicated: See table.

Comparative Effects — G-CSF vs GM-CSF

Proliferation/Differentiation	G-CSF (Filgrastim)	GM-CSF (Sargramostim)
Neutrophils	Yes	Yes
Eosinophils	No	Yes
Macrophages	No	Yes
Neutrophil migration	Enhanced	Inhibited

Drug Interactions

Increased Effect/Toxicity: Lithium, corticosteroids may potentiate myeloproliferative effects.

Pharmacodynamics/Kinetics

Onset of action: Increase in WBC: 7-14 days

Duration: WBCs return to baseline within 1 week of discontinuing drug

Half-life elimination: 2 hours

Time to peak, serum: SubQ: 1-2 hours

Pregnancy Risk Factor C

Sarna® Sensitive see Pramoxine on page 1264

Sarnol®-HC [OTC] see Hydrocortisone on page 793

SB-265805 see Gemifloxacin on page 731

SC 33428 see Idarubicin on page 814

SCH 13521 see Flutamide on page 686

SCIG see Immune Globulin (Subcutaneous) on page 826

S-Citalopram see Escitalopram on page 568

Scleromate® see Morrhuate Sodium on page 1068

Scopace™ *see* Scopolamine *on page 1380*

Scopolamine (skoe POL a meen)

U.S. Brand Names Isopto® Hyoscine; Scopace™; Transderm Scōp®
Canadian Brand Names Buscopan®; Transderm-V®
Mexican Brand Names Buscapina®; Espacil®; Selpiran-S®
Generic Available Yes: Injection
Synonyms Hyoscine Butylbromide; Hyoscine Hydrobromide; Scopolamine Butylbromide; Scopolamine Hydrobromide
Pharmacologic Category Anticholinergic Agent
Use

Scopolamine hydrobromide:

Injection: Preoperative medication to produce amnesia, sedation, and decrease salivary and respiratory secretions

Ophthalmic: Produce cycloplegia and mydriasis; treatment of iridocyclitis

Oral: Symptomatic treatment of postencephalitic parkinsonism and paralysis agitans; inhibits excessive motility and hypertonus of the genitourinary or gastrointestinal tract in such conditions as the irritable colon syndrome, mild dysentery, diverticulitis, pylorospasm, and cardiospasm

Transdermal: Prevention of nausea/vomiting associated with anesthesia or opiate analgesia; prevention of motion sickness

Scopolamine butylbromide:

Oral/injection: Treatment of smooth muscle spasm of the genitourinary or gastrointestinal tract; injection may also be used to prior to radiological/diagnostic procedures to prevent spasm

Local Anesthetic/Vasoconstrictor Precautions No information available to require special precautions

Effects on Dental Treatment Key adverse event(s) related to dental treatment: Significant xerostomia (normal salivary flow resumes upon discontinuation) and dry throat (transdermal).

Common Adverse Effects Frequency not defined.

Ophthalmic: Note: Systemic adverse effects have been reported following ophthalmic administration.

Cardiovascular: Vascular congestion, edema

Central nervous system: Drowsiness

Dermatologic: Eczematoid dermatitis

Ocular: Blurred vision, photophobia, local irritation, increased intraocular pressure, follicular conjunctivitis, exudate

Respiratory: Congestion

Systemic:

Cardiovascular: Orthostatic hypotension, ventricular fibrillation, tachycardia, palpitation

Central nervous system: Confusion, drowsiness, headache, loss of memory, ataxia, fatigue

Dermatologic: Dry skin, increased sensitivity to light, rash

Endocrine & metabolic: Decreased flow of breast milk

Gastrointestinal: Constipation, xerostomia, dry throat, dysphagia, bloated feeling, nausea, vomiting

Genitourinary: Dysuria

Local: Irritation at injection site

Neuromuscular & skeletal: Weakness

Ocular: Increased intraocular pain, blurred vision

Respiratory: Dry nose

Miscellaneous: Diaphoresis (decreased)

Mechanism of Action Blocks the action of acetylcholine at parasympathetic sites in smooth muscle, secretory glands and the CNS; increases cardiac output, dries secretions, antagonizes histamine and serotonin

Drug Interactions

Increased Effect/Toxicity: Adverse anticholinergic effects may be additive with other anticholinergic agents (includes tricyclic antidepressants, antihistamines, and phenothiazines). Sedative effects of other CNS depressants may be additive with scopolamine.

Decreased Effect: Decreased effect of acetaminophen, levodopa, ketoconazole, digoxin, riboflavin, and potassium chloride in wax matrix preparations.

Pharmacodynamics/Kinetics

Onset of action: Oral, I.M.: 0.5-1 hour; I.V.: 10 minutes

Peak effect: 20-60 minutes; may take 3-7 days for full recovery; transdermal: 24 hours

Duration: Oral, I.M.: 4-6 hours; I.V.: 2 hours

Absorption: Tertiary salts (hydrobromide) are well absorbed; quaternary salts (butylbromide) are poorly absorbed (local concentrations in the GI tract following oral dosing may be high)

Metabolism: Hepatic

Half-life elimination: 4.8 hours

Excretion: Urine (as metabolites)

Pregnancy Risk Factor C

Scopolamine and Phenylephrine *see* Phenylephrine and Scopolamine *on page 1227*

Scopolamine Butylbromide *see* Scopolamine *on page 1380*

Scopolamine Hydrobromide *see* Scopolamine *on page 1380*

Scopolamine, Hyoscyamine, Atropine, and Phenobarbital *see* Hyoscyamine, Atropine, Scopolamine, and Phenobarbital *on page 804*

Scot-Tussin DM® Cough Chasers [OTC] *see* Dextromethorphan *on page 451*

Scot-Tussin® Expectorant [OTC] *see* Guaifenesin *on page 752*

Scot-Tussin® Senior [OTC] *see* Guaifenesin and Dextromethorphan *on page 754*

Sculptra™ *see* Poly-L-Lactic Acid *on page 1253*

SDZ ENA 713 *see* Rivastigmine *on page 1361*

Seasonale® *see* Ethinyl Estradiol and Levonorgestrel *on page 602*

Seba-Gel™ *see* Benzoyl Peroxide *on page 194*

Secobarbital (see koe BAR bi tal)

U.S. Brand Names Seconal®

Generic Available No

Synonyms Quinalbarbitone Sodium; Secobarbital Sodium

Pharmacologic Category Barbiturate

Use Preanesthetic agent; short-term treatment of insomnia

Local Anesthetic/Vasoconstrictor Precautions No information available to require special precautions

Effects on Dental Treatment No significant effects or complications reported

Mechanism of Action Depresses CNS activity by binding to barbiturate site at GABA-receptor complex enhancing GABA activity, depressing reticular activity system; higher doses may be gabamimetic

Pregnancy Risk Factor D

Secobarbital and Amobarbital *see* Amobarbital and Secobarbital *on page 104*

Secobarbital Sodium *see* Secobarbital *on page 1381*

Seconal® *see* Secobarbital *on page 1381*

SecreFlo™ *see* Secretin *on page 1381*

Secretin (SEE kre tin)

U.S. Brand Names SecreFlo™

Generic Available No

Synonyms Secretin, Human; Secretin, Porcine

Pharmacologic Category Diagnostic Agent

Use Secretin-stimulation testing to aid in diagnosis of pancreatic exocrine dysfunction; diagnosis of gastrinoma (Zollinger-Ellison syndrome); facilitation of ERCP visualization

Local Anesthetic/Vasoconstrictor Precautions No information available to require special precautions

Effects on Dental Treatment No significant effects or complications reported

Common Adverse Effects 1% to 10%:

Cardiovascular: Flushing (1%)

Gastrointestinal: Abdominal discomfort (1%), nausea (1%)

Miscellaneous: Bleeding (sphincterectomy, 1%)

Mechanism of Action Human and porcine secretin are both synthetically derived products and are equally potent on an osmolar basis. Secretin is a hormone which is normally secreted by duodenal mucosa and upper jejunal mucosa. It increases the volume and bicarbonate content of pancreatic juice; stimulates the flow of hepatic bile with a high bicarbonate concentration; stimulates gastrin release in patients with Zollinger-Ellison syndrome.

Drug Interactions

Decreased Effect: The response to secretin stimulation may be blunted by drugs with high anticholinergic activity such as tricyclic antidepressants, phenothiazines, and antihistamines as well as anticholinergic agents (ie, atropine, benztropine, biperiden).

(Continued)

Secretin (Continued)

Pharmacodynamics/Kinetics

Peak output of pancreatic secretions: ~30 minutes

Duration: At least 2 hours

Distribution: V_d: Human: 2.7 L; Porcine: 2 L

Half-life elimination: Human: 45 minutes; Porcine: 27 minutes

Pregnancy Risk Factor C

Secretin, Human see Secretin on page 1381

Secretin, Porcine see Secretin on page 1381

Sectral® see Acebutolol on page 28

Secura® Antifungal [OTC] see Miconazole on page 1039

Selegiline (se LE ji leen)

U.S. Brand Names Eldepryl®; Emsam®

Canadian Brand Names Apo-Selegiline®; Gen-Selegiline; Novo-Selegiline; Nu-Selegiline

Mexican Brand Names Niar®

Generic Available Yes: Excludes transdermal system

Synonyms Deprenyl; L-Deprenyl; Selegiline Hydrochloride

Pharmacologic Category Anti-Parkinson's Agent, MAO Type B Inhibitor; Antidepressant, Monoamine Oxidase Inhibitor

Use Adjunct in the management of parkinsonian patients in which levodopa/carbidopa therapy is deteriorating; treatment of major depressive disorder

Unlabeled/Investigational Use Early Parkinson's disease; attention-deficit/hyperactivity disorder (ADHD); negative symptoms of schizophrenia; extrapyramidal symptoms; Alzheimer's disease (studies have shown some improvement in behavioral and cognitive performance)

Local Anesthetic/Vasoconstrictor Precautions Selegiline in doses of 10 mg a day or less does not inhibit type-A MAO. Therefore, there are no precautions with the use of vasoconstrictors.

Effects on Dental Treatment Key adverse event(s) related to dental treatment: Xerostomia and changes in salivation (normal salivary flow resumes upon discontinuation). Anticholinergic side effects can cause a reduction of saliva production or secretion, contributing to discomfort and dental disease (ie, caries, oral candidiasis, and periodontal disease).

Common Adverse Effects Unless otherwise noted, the percentage of adverse events is reported for the transdermal patch:

> 10%:

Central nervous system: Headache (18%), insomnia (12%)

Local: Application site reaction (24%)

1% to 10%:

Cardiovascular: Hypotension (including postural 3% to 10%), chest pain (≥1%), hypertension (≥1%), peripheral edema (≥1%)

Central nervous system: Dizziness (7% oral), hallucinations (3% oral), confusion (3% oral), headache (2%) oral, agitation (≥1%), amnesia (≥1%), thinking abnormal (≥1%)

Dermatologic: Rash (4%), bruising (≥1%), pruritus (≥1%), acne (≥1%)

Endocrine and metabolic: Sexual side effects (≤1%), weight loss (5%)

Gastrointestinal: Nausea (10% oral), diarrhea (9%), xerostomia (8%), abdominal pain (4% oral), dyspepsia (4%), constipation (≥1%), flatulence (≥1%), anorexia (≥1%), gastroenteritis (≥1%), taste perversion (≥1%), vomiting (≥1%)

Genitourinary: Dysmenorrhea (≥1%), metrorrhagia (≥1%), UTI (≥1%), urinary frequency (≥1%)

Neuromuscular & skeletal: Myalgia (≥1%), neck pain (≥1%), paresthesia (≥1%)

Otic: Tinnitus (≥1%)

Respiratory: Pharyngitis (3%), sinusitis (3%), cough (≥1%), bronchitis (≥1%)

Miscellaneous: Diaphoresis (≥1%)

Mechanism of Action Potent, irreversible inhibitor of monoamine oxidase (MAO). When administered orally, the lower plasma concentrations achieved (due to an extensive first-pass effect) confer selective inhibition of MAO type B, which plays a major role in the metabolism of dopamine; selegiline may also increase dopaminergic activity by interfering with dopamine reuptake at the synapse. When administered transdermally, selegiline achieves higher blood levels and effectively inhibits both MAO-A and MAO-B, which blocks catabolism of other centrally-active biogenic amine neurotransmitters.

Drug Interactions
Cytochrome P450 Effect: Substrate of CYP1A2 (minor), 2A6 (minor), 2B6 (major), 2C9 (major), 2D6 (minor), 3A4 (minor); Inhibits CYP1A2 (weak), 2A6 (weak), 2C9 (weak), 2C19 (weak), 2D6 (weak), 2E1 (weak), 3A4 (weak)

Increased Effect/Toxicity: CYP2B6 inhibitors may increase the levels/ effects of selegiline; example inhibitors include desipramine, paroxetine, and sertraline. CYP2C9 inhibitors may increase the levels/effects of selegiline; example inhibitors include delavirdine, fluconazole, gemfibrozil, ketoconazole, nicardipine, NSAIDs, and sulfonamides. Concurrent use of oral selegiline (high dose) in combination with amphetamines, methylphenidate, dextremeth-orphan, fenfluramine, meperidine, nefazodone, sibutramine, tramadol, trazo-done, tricyclic antidepressants, and venlafaxine may result in serotonin syndrome; these combinations are best avoided. Concurrent use of selegiline with an SSRI or SNRI may result in mania or hypertension; it is generally best to avoid these combinations. Transdermal selegiline is contraindicated with amphetamines, sympathomimetics or other CNS stimulants, dextromethor-phan, meperidine, methadone, mirtazapine, propoxyphene, SSRIs/SNRIs, tramadol, tricyclic antidepressants. Oral selegiline (>10 mg/day) or trans-dermal doses ≥9 mg/24 hours in combination with tyramine (cheese, ethanol) may increase the pressor response; avoid high tyramine-containing foods in patients receiving >10 mg/day of oral selegiline or transdermal doses >6 mg/ 24 hours. The toxicity of levodopa (hypertension), lithium (hyperpyrexia), and reserpine may be increased by MAO inhibitors.

Decreased Effect: CYP2B6 inducers may decrease the levels/effects of selegiline; example inducers include carbamazepine, nevirapine, phenobar-bital, phenytoin, and rifampin. CYP2C9 inducers may decrease the levels/ effects of selegiline; example inducers include carbamazepine, phenobarbital, phenytoin, rifampin, rifapentine, and secobarbital.

Pharmacodynamics/Kinetics
Onset of action: Therapeutic: Oral: Within 1 hour

Duration: Oral: 24-72 hours

Absorption: Transdermal: 25% to 30% (of total selegiline content) over 24 hours

Half-life elimination: 18-25 hours

Protein binding: ~90%

Metabolism: Hepatic via CYP2D6, 2C9, and 3A4/5 to N-desmethylselegiline, methamphetamine and amphetamine

Excretion: Urine; feces

Pregnancy Risk Factor C

Selegiline Hydrochloride *see* Selegiline *on page 1382*

Selenicaps [OTC] *see* Selenium *on page 1383*

Selenimin [OTC] *see* Selenium *on page 1383*

Selenium (se LEE nee um)

Related Information
Trace Metals *on page 1513*

U.S. Brand Names Selenicaps [OTC]; Selenimin [OTC]; Selepen®

Generic Available Yes

Pharmacologic Category Trace Element, Parenteral

Use Trace metal supplement

Local Anesthetic/Vasoconstrictor Precautions No information available to require special precautions

Effects on Dental Treatment No significant effects or complications reported

Common Adverse Effects Frequency not defined.
Central nervous system: Lethargy
Dermatologic: Alopecia or hair discoloration
Gastrointestinal: Vomiting following long-term use on damaged skin; abdominal pain, garlic breath
Local: Irritation
Neuromuscular & skeletal: Tremor
Miscellaneous: Diaphoresis

Mechanism of Action Part of glutathione peroxidase which protects cell components from oxidative damage due to peroxidases produced in cellular metabolism

Pharmacodynamics/Kinetics Excretion: Urine, feces, lungs, skin

Pregnancy Risk Factor C

Selepen® *see* Selenium *on page 1383*

Semprex®-D *see* Acrivastine and Pseudoephedrine *on page 47*

Senexon [OTC] *see* Senna *on page 1384*

Senna (SEN na)

U.S. Brand Names Black Draught Tablets [OTC]; Evac-U-Gen [OTC]; ex-lax® [OTC]; ex-lax® Maximum Strength [OTC]; Fletcher's® Castoria® [OTC]; Perdiem® Overnight Relief [OTC]; Senexon [OTC]; Senna-Gen® [OTC]; Sennatural™ [OTC]; Senokot® [OTC]; Uni-Senna [OTC]; X-Prep® [OTC] [DSC]

Generic Available Yes

Pharmacologic Category Laxative, Stimulant

Use Short-term treatment of constipation; evacuate the colon for bowel or rectal examinations

Local Anesthetic/Vasoconstrictor Precautions No information available to require special precautions

Effects on Dental Treatment No significant effects or complications reported

Common Adverse Effects Frequency not defined: Gastrointestinal: Nausea, vomiting, diarrhea, abdominal cramps

Senna-Gen® [OTC] *see* Senna *on page 1384*

Sennatural™ [OTC] *see* Senna *on page 1384*

Senokot® [OTC] *see* Senna *on page 1384*

Sensipar™ *see* Cinacalcet *on page 342*

Sensorcaine® *see* Bupivacaine *on page 228*

Sensorcaine®-MPF *see* Bupivacaine *on page 228*

Sensorcaine®-MPF with Epinephrine *see* Bupivacaine and Epinephrine *on page 228*

Sensorcaine® with Epinephrine *see* Bupivacaine and Epinephrine *on page 228*

Septocaine™ *see* Articaine and Epinephrine *on page 139*

Septra® *see* Sulfamethoxazole and Trimethoprim *on page 1425*

Septra® DS *see* Sulfamethoxazole and Trimethoprim *on page 1425*

Serax® *see* Oxazepam *on page 1157*

Serentil® [DSC] *see* Mesoridazine *on page 997*

Serevent® Diskus® *see* Salmeterol *on page 1375*

Sermorelin Acetate (ser moe REL in AS e tate)

U.S. Brand Names Geref® Diagnostic

Mexican Brand Names Geref®

Generic Available No

Pharmacologic Category Diagnostic Agent; Growth Hormone

Use

Geref® Diagnostic: For evaluation of the ability of the pituitary gland to secrete growth hormone (GH)

Local Anesthetic/Vasoconstrictor Precautions No information available to require special precautions

Effects on Dental Treatment No significant effects or complications reported

Common Adverse Effects Frequency not defined.

Cardiovascular: Tightness in the chest

Central nervous system: Headache, dizziness, hyperactivity, somnolence

Dermatologic: Transient flushing of the face, urticaria

Gastrointestinal: Dysphagia, nausea, vomiting

Local: Pain, redness, and/or swelling at the injection site

Drug Interactions

Decreased Effect: The test should not be conducted in the presence of drugs that directly affect the pituitary secretion of somatotropin. These include preparations that contain or release somatostatin, insulin, glucocorticoids, or cyclooxygenase inhibitors such as ASA or indomethacin. Somatotropin levels may be transiently elevated by clonidine, levodopa, and insulin-induced hypoglycemia. Response to sermorelin may be blunted in patients who are receiving muscarinic antagonists (atropine) or who are hypothyroid or being treated with antithyroid medications such as propylthiouracil. Obesity, hyperglycemia, and elevated plasma fatty acids generally are associated with subnormal GH responses to sermorelin. Exogenous growth hormone therapy should be discontinued at least 1 week before administering the test.

Pharmacodynamics/Kinetics Onset of action: Peak response: Diagnostic: Children 30 ± 27 minutes; Adults: 35 ± 29 minutes

Pregnancy Risk Factor C

Seromycin® *see* CycloSERINE *on page 405*

Serophene® *see* ClomiPHENE *on page 369*

Seroquel® *see* Quetiapine *on page 1319*

Serostim® *see* Somatropin *on page 1406*

Sertaconazole (ser ta KOE na zole)

U.S. Brand Names Ertaczo™
Generic Available No
Synonyms Sertaconazole Nitrate
Pharmacologic Category Antifungal Agent, Topical
Use Topical treatment of tinea pedis (athlete's foot)
Local Anesthetic/Vasoconstrictor Precautions No information available to require special precautions
Effects on Dental Treatment No significant effects or complications reported
Common Adverse Effects 1% to 10%: Dermatologic: Burning, contact dermatitis, dry skin, tenderness
Mechanism of Action Alters fungal cell wall membrane permeability; inhibits the CYP450-dependent synthesis of ergosterol
Pharmacodynamics/Kinetics
Absorption: Topical: Minimal
Pregnancy Risk Factor C

Sertaconazole Nitrate *see* Sertaconazole *on page 1385*

Sertraline (SER tra leen)

U.S. Brand Names Zoloft®
Canadian Brand Names Apo-Sertraline®; Gen-Sertraline; GMD-Sertraline; Novo-Sertraline; Nu-Sertraline; PMS-Sertraline; ratio-Sertraline; Rhoxal-sertraline; Zoloft®
Generic Available No
Synonyms Sertraline Hydrochloride
Pharmacologic Category Antidepressant, Selective Serotonin Reuptake Inhibitor
Use Treatment of major depression; obsessive-compulsive disorder (OCD); panic disorder; post-traumatic stress disorder (PTSD); premenstrual dysphoric disorder (PMDD); social anxiety disorder
Unlabeled/Investigational Use Eating disorders; generalized anxiety disorder (GAD); impulse control disorders
Local Anesthetic/Vasoconstrictor Precautions Although caution should be used in patients taking tricyclic antidepressants, no interactions have been reported with vasoconstrictor and sertraline, a nontricyclic antidepressant which acts to increase serotonin; no precautions appear to be needed
Effects on Dental Treatment No significant effects or complications reported (see Dental Comment)
Common Adverse Effects
>10%:
Central nervous system: Insomnia, somnolence, dizziness, headache, fatigue
Gastrointestinal: Xerostomia, diarrhea, nausea
Genitourinary: Ejaculatory disturbances
1% to 10%:
Cardiovascular: Palpitations
Central nervous system: Agitation, anxiety, nervousness
Dermatologic: Rash
Endocrine & metabolic: Decreased libido
Gastrointestinal: Constipation, anorexia, dyspepsia, flatulence, vomiting, weight gain
Genitourinary: Micturition disorders
Neuromuscular & skeletal: Tremors, paresthesia
Ocular: Visual difficulty, abnormal vision
Otic: Tinnitus
Miscellaneous: Diaphoresis (increased)

Additional adverse reactions reported in pediatric patients (frequency >2%): Aggressiveness, epistaxis, hyperkinesia, purpura, sinusitis, urinary incontinence
Restrictions A medication guide concerning the use of antidepressants in children and teenagers can be found on the FDA website at http://www.fda.gov/cder/Offices/ODS/labeling.htm. It should be dispensed to parents or guardians of children and teenagers receiving this medication.
Dosage Oral:
Children and Adolescents: OCD:
6-12 years: Initial: 25 mg once daily
13-17 years: Initial: 50 mg once daily
(Continued)

Sertraline (Continued)

Note: May increase daily dose, at intervals of not less than 1 week, to a maximum of 200 mg/day. If somnolence is noted, give at bedtime.

Adults:

Depression/OCD: Oral: Initial: 50 mg/day (see "Note" above)

Panic disorder, PTSD, social anxiety disorder: Initial: 25 mg once daily; increase to 50 mg once daily after 1 week (see "Note" above)

PMDD: 50 mg/day either daily throughout menstrual cycle **or** limited to the luteal phase of menstrual cycle, depending on physician assessment. Patients not responding to 50 mg/day may benefit from dose increases (50 mg increments per menstrual cycle) up to 150 mg/day when dosing throughout menstrual cycle **or** up to 100 mg day when dosing during luteal phase only. If a 100 mg/day dose has been established with luteal phase dosing, a 50 mg/day titration step for 3 days should be utilized at the beginning of each luteal phase dosing period.

Elderly: Depression/OCD: Start treatment with 25 mg/day in the morning and increase by 25 mg/day increments every 2-3 days if tolerated to 50-100 mg/day; additional increases may be necessary; maximum dose: 200 mg/day

Dosage adjustment/comment in renal impairment: Multiple-dose pharmacokinetics are unaffected by renal impairment.

Hemodialysis: Not removed by hemodialysis

Dosage adjustment/comment in hepatic impairment: Sertraline is extensively metabolized by the liver; caution should be used in patients with hepatic impairment; a lower dose or less frequent dosing should be used.

Mechanism of Action Antidepressant with selective inhibitory effects on presynaptic serotonin (5-HT) reuptake and only very weak effects on norepinephrine and dopamine neuronal uptake. *In vitro* studies demonstrate no significant affinity for adrenergic, cholinergic, GABA, dopaminergic, histaminergic, serotonergic, or benzodiazepine receptors.

Contraindications Hypersensitivity to sertraline or any component of the formulation; use of MAO inhibitors within 14 days; concurrent use of pimozide; concurrent use of sertraline oral concentrate with disulfiram

Warnings/Precautions Antidepressants increase the risk of suicidal thinking and behavior in children and adolescents with major depressive disorder (MDD) and other depressive disorders; consider risk prior to prescribing. All patients must be closely monitored for clinical worsening, suicidality, or unusual changes in behavior, especially during the initiation of therapy or following an increase or decrease in dosage. When used in children, the child's family or caregiver should be instructed to closely observe the patient and communicate condition with healthcare provider. A medication guide should be dispensed with each prescription. **Sertraline is not FDA approved for use in children with major depressive disorder (MDD). However, it is approved for the treatment of obsessive-compulsive disorder (OCD) in children ≥6 years of age.**

The possibility of a suicide attempt is inherent in major depression and may persist until remission occurs. Use caution in high-risk patients. Worsening depression and severe abrupt suicidality that are not part of the presenting symptoms may require discontinuation or modification of drug therapy. The patient's family or caregiver should be alerted to monitor patients for the emergence of suicidality and associated behaviors (such as agitation, irritability, hostility, impulsivity, and hypomania) and call healthcare provider.

May worsen psychosis in some patients or precipitate a shift to mania or hypomania in patients with bipolar disorder. Patients presenting with depressive symptoms should be screened for bipolar disorder. Monotherapy in patients with bipolar disorder should be avoided. **Sertraline is not FDA approved for the treatment of bipolar depression.**

The potential for severe reaction exists when used with MAO inhibitors - serotonin syndrome (hyperthermia, muscular rigidity, mental status changes/agitation, autonomic instability) may occur. Has a very low potential to impair cognitive or motor performance. However, caution patients regarding activities requiring alertness until response to sertraline is known. Does not appear to potentiate the effects of alcohol, however, ethanol use is not advised.

Use caution in patients with a previous seizure disorder or condition predisposing to seizures such as brain damage, alcoholism, or concurrent therapy with other drugs which lower the seizure threshold. May increase the risks associated with electroconvulsive therapy. Use with caution in patients with hepatic or renal dysfunction and in elderly patients. May cause hyponatremia/SIADH. Use with caution in patients with renal insufficiency or other concurrent illness (due to limited experience). Sertraline acts as a mild uricosuric; use with caution in patients at risk of uric acid nephropathy. Use with caution in patients at risk of bleeding or receiving anticoagulant therapy; may cause impairment in platelet aggregation. Use with caution in patients where weight loss is undesirable. May cause or exacerbate sexual dysfunction.

Use oral concentrate formulation with caution in patients with latex sensitivity; dropper dispenser contains dry natural rubber. Monitor growth in pediatric patients. Discontinuation symptoms (eg, dysphoric mood, irritability, agitation, confusion, anxiety, insomnia, hypomania) may occur upon abrupt discontinuation. Taper dose when discontinuing therapy.

Drug Interactions

Cytochrome P450 Effect: Substrate of CYP2B6 (minor), 2C8/9 (minor), 2C19 (major), 2D6 (major), 3A4 (minor); **Inhibits** CYP1A2 (weak), 2B6 (moderate), 2C8/9 (weak), 2C19 (moderate), 2D6 (moderate), 3A4 (moderate)

Increased Effect/Toxicity: Sertraline should not be used with nonselective MAO inhibitors (phenelzine, isocarboxazid) or other drugs with MAO inhibition (linezolid); fatal reactions have been reported. Wait 5 weeks after stopping sertraline before starting a nonselective MAO inhibitor and 2 weeks after stopping an MAO inhibitor before starting sertraline. Concurrent selegiline has been associated with mania, hypertension, or serotonin syndrome (risk may be reduced relative to nonselective MAO inhibitors). Sertraline may increase serum concentrations of pimozide; concurrent use is contraindicated. Avoid use of oral concentrate with disulfiram.

Sertraline may inhibit the metabolism of thioridazine or mesoridazine, resulting in increased plasma levels and increasing the risk of QT_c interval prolongation. This may lead to serious ventricular arrhythmias, such as torsade de pointes-type arrhythmias and sudden death. Do not use together. Wait at least 5 weeks after discontinuing sertraline prior to starting thioridazine.

Sertraline may increase the levels/effects of levels/effects of amphetamines, selected beta-blockers, bupropion, selected benzodiazepines, calcium channel blockers, cisapride, cyclosporine, dextromethorphan, ergot alkaloids, fluoxetine, selected HMG-CoA reductase inhibitors, lidocaine, mesoridazine, mirtazapine, nateglinide, nefazodone, paroxetine, promethazine, propofol, risperidone, ritonavir, selegiline, sildenafil (and other PDE-5 inhibitors), tacrolimus, thioridazine, tricyclic antidepressants, venlafaxine, and other substrates of CYP2B6, 2D6 or 3A4. Sertraline may increase the hypoprothrombinemic response to warfarin.

The levels/effects of sertraline may be increased by chlorpromazine, delavirdine, fluconazole, fluoxetine, fluvoxamine, gemfibrozil, isoniazid, miconazole, omeprazole, paroxetine, pergolide, quinidine, quinine, ritonavir, ropinirole, ticlopidine, and other CYP2C19 or 2D6 inhibitors.

Combined use of SSRIs and amphetamines, buspirone, meperidine, nefazodone, serotonin agonists (such as sumatriptan), sibutramine, other SSRIs, sympathomimetics, ritonavir, tramadol, and venlafaxine may increase the risk of serotonin syndrome. Combined use of sumatriptan (and other serotonin agonists) may result in toxicity; weakness, hyper-reflexia, and incoordination have been observed with sumatriptan and SSRIs. In addition, concurrent use may theoretically increase the risk of serotonin syndrome; includes sumatriptan, naratriptan, rizatriptan, and zolmitriptan.

Concurrent lithium may increase risk of nephrotoxicity. Risk of hyponatremia may increase with concurrent use of loop diuretics (bumetanide, furosemide, torsemide). Concomitant use of sertraline and NSAIDs, aspirin, or other drugs affecting coagulation has been associated with an increased risk of bleeding; monitor.

Decreased Effect: The levels/effects of sertraline may be decreased by aminoglutethimide, carbamazepine, phenytoin, rifampin, and other CYP2C19 inducers. Sertraline may decrease the metabolism of tolbutamide; monitor for changes in glucose control. Sertraline may decrease the levels/effects of CYP2D6 prodrug substrates (eg, codeine, hydrocodone, oxycodone, tramadol).

Ethanol/Nutrition/Herb Interactions

Ethanol: Avoid ethanol (may increase CNS depression).

Food: Sertraline average peak serum levels may be increased if taken with food.

Herb/Nutraceutical: Avoid valerian, St John's wort, kava kava, gotu kola (may increase CNS depression).

Pharmacodynamics/Kinetics

Absorption: Slow

Protein binding: 98%

Metabolism: Hepatic; extensive first-pass metabolism

Bioavailability: 88%

(Continued)

Sertraline (Continued)

Half-life elimination: Parent drug: 26 hours; Metabolite N-desmethylsertraline: 66 hours (range: 62-104 hours)

Time to peak, plasma: 4.5-8.4 hours

Excretion: Urine and feces

Pregnancy Risk Factor C

Dosage Forms Note: Available as sertraline hydrochloride; mg strength refers to sertraline. **SOLN, oral concentrate:** 20 mg/mL (60 mL). **TAB:** 25 mg, 50 mg, 100 mg

Dental Comment Problems with SSRI-induced bruxism have been reported and may preclude their use; clinicians attempting to evaluate any patient with bruxism or involuntary muscle movement, who is simultaneously being treated with an SSRI drug, should be aware of the potential association.

Selected Readings

Gerber PE and Lynd LD, "Selective Serotonin Reuptake Inhibitor-Induced Movement Disorders," *Ann Pharmacother*, 1998, 32(6):692-8.

Sertraline Hydrochloride *see* Sertraline *on page 1385*

Serutan® [OTC] *see* Psyllium *on page 1313*

Serzone *see* Nefazodone *on page 1096*

Sevelamer (se VEL a mer)

U.S. Brand Names Renagel®

Canadian Brand Names Renagel®

Generic Available No

Synonyms Sevelamer Hydrochloride

Pharmacologic Category Phosphate Binder

Use Reduction of serum phosphorous in patients with chronic kidney disease on hemodialysis

Local Anesthetic/Vasoconstrictor Precautions No information available to require special precautions

Effects on Dental Treatment No significant effects or complications reported

Common Adverse Effects

>10%:

Dermatologic: Rash (13%)

Gastrointestinal: Vomiting (22%), nausea (7% to 20%), diarrhea (4% to 19%), dyspepsia (5% to 16%)

Neuromuscular & skeletal: Limb pain (13%), arthralgia (12%)

Respiratory: Nasopharyngitis (14%), bronchitis (11%)

1% to 10%:

Cardiovascular: Hypertension (10%)

Central nervous system: Headache (9%), pyrexia (5%)

Gastrointestinal: Constipation (2% to 8%), flatulence (4%)

Neuromuscular & skeletal: Back pain (4%)

Respiratory: Dyspnea (10%), cough (7%), upper respiratory tract infection (5%)

Postmarketing and/or case reports: Abdominal pain

Mechanism of Action Sevelamer (a polymeric compound) binds phosphate within the intestinal lumen, limiting absorption and decreasing serum phosphate concentrations without altering calcium, aluminum, or bicarbonate concentrations

Drug Interactions

Decreased Effect: Sevelamer may bind to some drugs in the gastrointestinal tract and decrease their absorption. When changes in absorption of oral medications may have significant clinical consequences (such as antiarrhythmic and antiseizure medications), these medications should be taken at least 1 hour before or 3 hours after a dose of sevelamer. Sevelamer may decrease the bioavailability of ciprofloxacin by 50%.

Pharmacodynamics/Kinetics

Absorption: None

Excretion: Feces

Pregnancy Risk Factor C

Sevelamer Hydrochloride *see* Sevelamer *on page 1388*

Shur-Seal® [OTC] [DSC] *see* Nonoxynol 9 *on page 1124*

Sibutramine (si BYOO tra meen)

U.S. Brand Names Meridia®
Canadian Brand Names Meridia®
Mexican Brand Names Raductil®; Reductil®
Generic Available No
Synonyms Sibutramine Hydrochloride Monohydrate
Pharmacologic Category Anorexiant
Use Management of obesity, including weight loss and maintenance of weight loss; should be used in conjunction with a reduced-calorie diet
Local Anesthetic/Vasoconstrictor Precautions No information available to require special precautions
Effects on Dental Treatment No significant effects or complications reported (see Dental Comment)

Common Adverse Effects

>10%:
  Central nervous system: Headache (30%), insomnia (11%)
  Gastrointestinal: Xerostomia (17%), anorexia (13%), constipation (12%)

1% to 10%:
  Cardiovascular: Tachycardia (3%), vasodilation (2%), hypertension (2%), palpitation (2%), chest pain (2%), edema (1%)
  Central nervous system: Dizziness (7%), nervousness (5%), anxiety (5%), depression (4%), migraine (2%), somnolence (2%), CNS stimulation (2%), emotional lability (1%)
  Dermatologic: Rash (4%), acne (1%), herpes simplex (1%)
  Endocrine & metabolic: Dysmenorrhea (4%), metrorrhagia (1%)
  Gastrointestinal: Appetite increased (9%), nausea (6%), abdominal pain (5%), dyspepsia (5%), gastritis (2%), vomiting (2%), taste perversion (2%), rectal disorder (1%)
  Genitourinary: Urinary tract infection (2%), vaginal Monilia (1%)
  Hepatic: Abnormal LFTs (2%)
  Neuromuscular & skeletal: Back pain (8%), weakness (6%), arthralgia (6%), neck pain (2%), myalgia (2%), paresthesia (2%), tenosynovitis (1%), joint disorder (1%)
  Otic: Ear disorder (2%), ear pain (1%)
  Respiratory: Pharyngitis (10%), rhinitis (10%), sinusitis (5%), cough (4%), laryngitis (1%)
  Miscellaneous: Flu-like syndrome (8%), diaphoresis (3%), allergic reactions (2), thirst (2%)

Frequency not defined:
  Cardiovascular: Peripheral edema
  Central nervous system: Thinking abnormal, agitation, fever
  Dermatologic: Pruritus
  Endocrine & metabolic: Menstrual disorders/irregularities
  Gastrointestinal: Diarrhea, flatulence, gastroenteritis, tooth disorder
  Neuromuscular & skeletal: Arthritis, hypertonia, leg cramps
  Ocular: Amblyopia
  Respiratory: Bronchitis, dyspnea

Restrictions C-IV; recommended only for obese patients with a body mass index ≥30 kg/m^2 or ≥27 kg/m^2 in the presence of other risk factors such as hypertension, diabetes, and/or dyslipidemia; rule out obesity due to untreated hypothyroidism

Mechanism of Action Sibutramine and its two primary metabolites block the neuronal uptake of norepinephrine, serotonin, and (to a lesser extent) dopamine. There is no monoamine-releasing (or depleting) activity.

Drug Interactions
  Cytochrome P450 Effect: Substrate of CYP3A4 (major)
  Increased Effect/Toxicity: Serotonergic agents such as buspirone, selective serotonin reuptake inhibitors (eg, citalopram, fluoxetine, fluvoxamine, paroxetine, sertraline), sumatriptan (and similar serotonin agonists), dihydroergotamine, lithium, tryptophan, some opioid/analgesics (eg, meperidine, tramadol), and venlafaxine, when combined with sibutramine may result in serotonin syndrome. Dextromethorphan, MAO inhibitors and other drugs that can raise the blood pressure (eg decongestants, centrally-acting weight loss products, amphetamines, and amphetamine-like compounds) can increase the possibility of sibutramine-associated cardiovascular complications. Sibutramine may increase serum levels of tricyclic antidepressants. CYP3A4 inhibitors may increase the levels/effects of sibutramine; example inhibitors
(Continued)

Sibutramine *(Continued)*

include azole antifungals, clarithromycin, diclofenac, doxycycline, erythromycin, imatinib, isoniazid, nefazodone, nicardipine, propofol, protease inhibitors, quinidine, telithromycin, and verapamil.

Decreased Effect: Inducers of CYP3A4 (including phenytoin, phenobarbital, carbamazepine, and rifampin) theoretically may reduce sibutramine serum concentrations.

Pharmacodynamics/Kinetics

Absorption: 77%; rapid

Protein binding, plasma: Parent drug and metabolites: >94%

Metabolism: Hepatic; undergoes first-pass metabolism via CYP3A4; forms two primary metabolites (active)

Half-life elimination: Sibutramine: 1 hour; Metabolites: M_1: 14 hours; M_2: 16 hours

Time to peak: Sibutramine: 1.2 hours; Metabolites (M_1 and M_2): 3-4 hours

Excretion: Primarily urine (77%); feces

Pregnancy Risk Factor C

Dental Comment The mechanism of action is thought to be different from the "fen" drugs. Sibutramine works to suppress the appetite by inhibiting the reuptake of norepinephrine and serotonin. Unlike dexfenfluramine and fenfluramine, it is not a serotonin releaser. Sibutramine is closer chemically to the widely used antidepressants such as fluoxetine (Prozac®). The FDA approved sibutramine over the objections of its own advisory panel, who called the drug too risky. FDA reported that the drug causes blood pressure to increase, generally by a small amount, though in some patients the increases were higher. It is now recommended that patients taking sibutramine have their blood pressure evaluated regularly.

Sibutramine Hydrochloride Monohydrate *see* Sibutramine *on page 1389*

Silace [OTC] *see* Docusate *on page 496*

Siladryl® Allergy [OTC] *see* DiphenhydrAMINE *on page 483*

Siladryl® DAS [OTC] *see* DiphenhydrAMINE *on page 483*

Silafed® [OTC] *see* Triprolidine and Pseudoephedrine *on page 1542*

Silapap® Children's [OTC] *see* Acetaminophen *on page 31*

Silapap® Infants [OTC] *see* Acetaminophen *on page 31*

Sildec *see* Carbinoxamine and Pseudoephedrine *on page 268*

Sildec-DM *see* Carbinoxamine, Pseudoephedrine, and Dextromethorphan *on page 269*

Sildenafil (sil DEN a fil)

U.S. Brand Names Revatio™; Viagra®

Canadian Brand Names Viagra®

Mexican Brand Names Viagra®

Generic Available No

Synonyms UK92480

Pharmacologic Category Phosphodiesterase-5 Enzyme Inhibitor

Use Treatment of erectile dysfunction; treatment of pulmonary arterial hypertension

Unlabeled/Investigational Use Psychotropic-induced sexual dysfunction; pulmonary arterial hypertension in children

Local Anesthetic/Vasoconstrictor Precautions No information available to require special precautions

Effects on Dental Treatment No significant effects or complications reported

Common Adverse Effects Based upon normal doses. (Adverse effects such as flushing, diarrhea, myalgia, and visual disturbances may be increased with doses >100 mg/24 hours.)

>10%:

Central nervous system: Headache (16% to 46%)

Gastrointestinal: Dyspepsia (7% to 17%)

1% to 10%:

Cardiovascular: Flushing (10%)

Central nervous system: Dizziness, insomnia, pyrexia

Dermatologic: Erythema, rash

Gastrointestinal: Diarrhea (3% to 9%), gastritis

Genitourinary: Urinary tract infection

Hematologic: Anemia, leukopenia

Hepatic: LFTs increased

Neuromuscular & skeletal: Myalgia, paresthesia

Ocular: Abnormal vision (color changes, blurred or increased sensitivity to light 3%; up to 11% with doses >100 mg)

Respiratory: Dyspnea exacerbated, epistaxis, nasal congestion, rhinitis, sinusitis

Dosage Adults: Oral:

Erectile dysfunction (Viagra®): For most patients, the recommended dose is 50 mg taken as needed, approximately 1 hour before sexual activity. However, sildenafil may be taken anywhere from 30 minutes to 4 hours before sexual activity. Based on effectiveness and tolerance, the dose may be increased to a maximum recommended dose of 100 mg or decreased to 25 mg. The maximum recommended dosing frequency is once daily.

Pulmonary arterial hypertension (Revatio™): 20 mg 3 times/day, taken 4-6 hours apart

Dosage adjustment for patients >65 years of age: Hepatic impairment (cirrhosis), severe renal impairment (creatinine clearance <30 mL/ minute): Higher plasma levels have been associated which may result in increase in efficacy and adverse effects; Viagra®: Starting dose of 25 mg should be considered

Dosage considerations for patients taking alpha blockers: Viagra®: Doses of 50 or 100 mg, should not be taken within 4 hours of an alpha blocker; doses of 25 mg may be given at any time

Dosage adjustment for concomitant use of potent CYP34A inhibitors:
Revatio™:

Erythromycin, saquinavir: No dosage adjustment

Itraconazole, ketoconazole, ritonavir: Not recommended

Viagra®:

Erythromycin, itraconazole, ketoconazole, saquinavir: Starting dose of 25 mg should be considered

Ritonavir: Maximum: 25 mg every 48 hours

Mechanism of Action

Erectile dysfunction: Does not directly cause penile erections, but affects the response to sexual stimulation. The physiologic mechanism of erection of the penis involves release of nitric oxide (NO) in the corpus cavernosum during sexual stimulation. NO then activates the enzyme guanylate cyclase, which results in increased levels of cyclic guanosine monophosphate (cGMP), producing smooth muscle relaxation and inflow of blood to the corpus cavernosum. Sildenafil enhances the effect of NO by inhibiting phosphodiesterase type 5 (PDE-5), which is responsible for degradation of cGMP in the corpus cavernosum; when sexual stimulation causes local release of NO, inhibition of PDE-5 by sildenafil causes increased levels of cGMP in the corpus cavernosum, resulting in smooth muscle relaxation and inflow of blood to the corpus cavernosum; at recommended doses, it has no effect in the absence of sexual stimulation.

Pulmonary arterial hypertension (PAH): Inhibits phosphodiesterase type 5 (PDE-5) in smooth muscle of pulmonary vasculature where PDE-5 is responsible for the degradation of cyclic guanosine monophosphate (cGMP). Increased cGMP concentration results in pulmonary vasculature relaxation; vasodilation in the pulmonary bed and the systemic circulation (to a lesser degree) may occur.

Contraindications Hypersensitivity to sildenafil or any component of the formulation; concurrent use of organic nitrates (nitroglycerin) in any form (potentiates the hypotensive effects)

Warnings/Precautions Decreases in blood pressure may occur due to vasodilator effects; use caution in patients with resting hypotension (BP <90/50), hypertension (BP >170/110), fluid depletion, severe left ventricular outflow obstruction, autonomic dysfunction, or taking alpha-blockers. Not recommended for use with pulmonary veno-occlusive disease.

Use caution in patients with cardiovascular disease, including cardiac failure, unstable angina, or a recent history (within the last 6 months) of myocardial infarction, stroke, or life-threatening arrhythmia. Use caution in patients receiving concurrent bosentan.

There is a degree of cardiac risk associated with sexual activity; therefore, physicians may wish to consider the cardiovascular status of their patients prior to initiating any treatment for erectile dysfunction. Sildenafil should be used with caution in patients with anatomical deformation of the penis (angulation, cavernosal fibrosis, or Peyronie's disease), or in patients who have conditions which may predispose them to priapism (sickle cell anemia, multiple myeloma, leukemia).

Rare cases of nonarteritic ischemic optic neuropathy (NAION) have been reported; risk may be increased with history of vision loss. Other risk factors for (Continued)

Sildenafil (Continued)

NAION include low cup-to-disc ratio ('crowded disc'), coronary artery disease, diabetes, hypertension, hyperlipidemia, smoking, and age >50 years.

The safety and efficacy of sildenafil with other treatments for erectile dysfunction have not been established; use is not recommended. May cause dose-related impairment of color discrimination. Use caution in patients with retinitis pigmentosa; a minority have generic disorders of retinal phosphodiesterases (no safety information available). Safety and efficacy in pediatric patients have not been established.

Drug Interactions

Cytochrome P450 Effect: Substrate of CYP2C8/9 (minor), 3A4 (major); Inhibits CYP1A2 (weak), 2C8/9 (weak), 2C19 (weak), 2D6 (weak), 2E1 (weak), 3A4 (weak)

Increased Effect/Toxicity: Sildenafil potentiates the hypotensive effects of nitrates (amyl nitrate, isosorbide dinitrate, isosorbide mononitrate, nitroglycerin); severe reactions have occurred and concurrent use is contraindicated. Concomitant use of alpha-blockers (doxazosin) may lead to symptomatic hypotension in some patients (sildenafil in doses >25 mg should not be given within 4 hours of administering an alpha-blocker). Macrolide antibiotics may increase the effects of sildenafil.

CYP3A4 inhibitors may increase the levels/effects of sildenafil; example inhibitors include azole antifungals, clarithromycin, diclofenac, doxycycline, erythromycin, imatinib, isoniazid, nefazodone, nicardipine, propofol, protease inhibitors, quinidine, telithromycin, and verapamil. Sildenafil may potentiate the effect of other antihypertensives. Sildenafil may potentiate bleeding in patients receiving heparin. Reduce sildenafil dose to 25 mg/24 hours in patients receiving azole antifungals or protease inhibitors (use of Revatio™ with concurrent protease inhibitors is not recommended).

Decreased Effect: Enzyme inducers (including phenytoin, carbamazepine, phenobarbital, rifampin) may decrease the serum concentration and efficacy of sildenafil. Bosentan may decrease serum concentration and effect of sildenafil.

Ethanol/Nutrition/Herb Interactions

Food: Amount and rate of absorption of sildenafil is reduced when taken with a high-fat meal. Serum concentrations/toxicity may be increased with grapefruit juice; avoid concurrent use.

Herb/Nutraceutical: St John's wort may decrease sildenafil levels.

Pharmacodynamics/Kinetics

Onset of action: ~60 minutes

Duration: 2-4 hours

Absorption: Rapid; slower with a high-fat meal

Distribution: V_{dss}: 105 L

Protein binding, plasma: ~96%

Metabolism: Hepatic via CYP3A4 (major) and CYP2C9 (minor route)

Bioavailability: 40%

Half-life elimination: 4 hours

Time to peak: 30-120 minutes; delayed by 60 minutes with a high-fat meal

Excretion: Feces (80%); urine (13%)

Pregnancy Risk Factor B

Dosage Forms TAB: (Revatio™): 20 mg; (Viagra®): 25 mg, 50 mg, 100 mg

Silexin [OTC] *see* Guaifenesin and Dextromethorphan *on page 754*

Silfedrine Children's [OTC] *see* Pseudoephedrine *on page 1309*

Silphen® [OTC] *see* DiphenhydrAMINE *on page 483*

Silphen DM® [OTC] *see* Dextromethorphan *on page 451*

Sil-Tex *see* Guaifenesin and Phenylephrine *on page 754*

Siltussin DAS [OTC] *see* Guaifenesin *on page 752*

Siltussin DM [OTC] *see* Guaifenesin and Dextromethorphan *on page 754*

Siltussin DM DAS [OTC] *see* Guaifenesin and Dextromethorphan *on page 754*

Siltussin SA [OTC] *see* Guaifenesin *on page 752*

Silvadene® *see* Silver Sulfadiazine *on page 1393*

Silver Nitrate (SIL ver NYE trate)

Generic Available Yes

Synonyms AgNO₃

Pharmacologic Category Antibiotic, Topical; Cauterizing Agent, Topical; Topical Skin Product, Antibacterial

Use Cauterization of wounds and sluggish ulcers, removal of granulation tissue and warts; aseptic prophylaxis of burns

Local Anesthetic/Vasoconstrictor Precautions No information available to require special precautions

Effects on Dental Treatment No significant effects or complications reported

Common Adverse Effects Frequency not defined.
Dermatologic: Burning and skin irritation, staining of the skin
Endocrine & metabolic: Hyponatremia
Hematologic: Methemoglobinemia

Dosage Children and Adults:
Sticks: Apply to mucous membranes and other moist skin surfaces only on area to be treated 2-3 times/week for 2-3 weeks
Topical solution: Apply a cotton applicator dipped in solution on the affected area 2-3 times/week for 2-3 weeks

Mechanism of Action Free silver ions precipitate bacterial proteins by combining with chloride in tissue forming silver chloride; coagulates cellular protein to form an eschar; silver ions or salts or colloidal silver preparations can inhibit the growth of both gram-positive and gram-negative bacteria. This germicidal action is attributed to the precipitation of bacterial proteins by liberated silver ions. Silver nitrate coagulates cellular protein to form an eschar, and this mode of action is the postulated mechanism for control of benign hematuria, rhinitis, and recurrent pneumothorax.

Contraindications Hypersensitivity to silver nitrate or any component of the formulation; not for use on broken skin, cuts, or wounds

Warnings/Precautions Do not use applicator sticks on the eyes. Prolonged use may result in skin discoloration.

Pharmacodynamics/Kinetics
Absorption: Because silver ions readily combine with protein, there is minimal GI and cutaneous absorption of the 0.5% and 1% preparations
Excretion: Highest amounts of silver noted on autopsy have been in kidneys, excretion in urine is minimal

Pregnancy Risk Factor C

Dosage Forms APPLICATOR STICKS, topical: Silver nitrate 75% and potassium nitrate 25% (6", 12", 18"). SOLN, topical: 10% (30 mL); 25% (30 mL); 50% (30 mL)

Selected Readings
Cushing AH and Smith S, "Methemoglobinemia With Silver Nitrate Therapy of a Burn: Report of a Case," *J Pediatr*, 1969, 74(4):613-5.
Hammerschlag MR, Cummings C, Roblin PM, et al, "Efficacy of Neonatal Ocular Prophylaxis for the Prevention of Chlamydial and Gonococcal Conjunctivitis," *N Engl J Med*, 1989, 320(12):769-72.
U.S. Department of Health and Human Services, "1993 Sexually Transmitted Diseases Treatment Guidelines," *MMWR Recomm Rep*, 1993, 42(RR-14).

Silver Sulfadiazine (SIL ver sul fa DYE a zeen)

U.S. Brand Names Silvadene®; SSD®; SSD® AF; Thermazene®
Canadian Brand Names Flamazine®
Generic Available Yes
Pharmacologic Category Antibiotic, Topical
Use Prevention and treatment of infection in second and third degree burns

Local Anesthetic/Vasoconstrictor Precautions No information available to require special precautions

Effects on Dental Treatment No significant effects or complications reported

Common Adverse Effects Frequency not defined.
Dermatologic: Itching, rash, erythema multiforme, discoloration of skin, photosensitivity
Hematologic: Hemolytic anemia, leukopenia, agranulocytosis, aplastic anemia
Hepatic: Hepatitis
Renal: Interstitial nephritis
Miscellaneous: Allergic reactions may be related to sulfa component

Mechanism of Action Acts upon the bacterial cell wall and cell membrane. Bactericidal for many gram-negative and gram-positive bacteria and is effective against yeast. Active against *Pseudomonas aeruginosa*, *Pseudomonas maltophilia*, *Enterobacter* species, *Klebsiella* species, *Serratia* species, *Escherichia coli*, *Proteus mirabilis*, *Morganella morganii*, *Providencia rettgeri*, *Proteus vulgaris*, *Providencia* species, *Citrobacter* species, *Acinetobacter calcoaceticus*, *Staphylococcus aureus*, *Staphylococcus epidermidis*, *Enterococcus* species, *Candida albicans*, *Corynebacterium diphtheriae*, and *Clostridium perfringens*

Drug Interactions
Decreased Effect: Topical proteolytic enzymes are inactivated by silver sulfadiazine.

Pharmacodynamics/Kinetics
Absorption: Significant percutaneous absorption of silver sulfadiazine can occur especially when applied to extensive burns
(Continued)

Silver Sulfadiazine (Continued)

Half-life elimination: 10 hours; prolonged with renal impairment
Time to peak, serum: 3-11 days of continuous therapy
Excretion: Urine (~50% as unchanged drug)
Pregnancy Risk Factor B

Simethicone (sye METH i kone)

U.S. Brand Names Equalizer Gas Relief [OTC]; GasAid [OTC]; Gas-X® [OTC]; Gas-X® Extra Strength [OTC]; Gas-X® Maximum Strength [OTC]; Genasyme® [OTC]; Infantaire Gas Drops [OTC]; Mylanta® Gas [OTC]; Mylanta® Gas Maximum Strength [OTC]; Mylicon® Infants [OTC]; Phazyme® Quick Dissolve [OTC]; Phazyme® Ultra Strength [OTC]

Canadian Brand Names Ovol®; Phazyme™
Generic Available Yes
Synonyms Activated Dimethicone; Activated Methylpolysiloxane
Pharmacologic Category Antiflatulent
Use Relieves flatulence and functional gastric bloating, and postoperative gas pains
Local Anesthetic/Vasoconstrictor Precautions No information available to require special precautions
Effects on Dental Treatment No significant effects or complications reported
Common Adverse Effects No data reported
Mechanism of Action Decreases the surface tension of gas bubbles thereby disperses and prevents gas pockets in the GI system
Pregnancy Risk Factor C

Simethicone, Aluminum Hydroxide, and Magnesium Hydroxide *see* Aluminum Hydroxide, Magnesium Hydroxide, and Simethicone *on page 81*

Simethicone and Calcium Carbonate *see* Calcium Carbonate and Simethicone *on page 249*

Simethicone and Loperamide Hydrochloride *see* Loperamide and Simethicone *on page 943*

Simethicone and Magaldrate *see* Magaldrate and Simethicone *on page 960*

Similac® Glucose *see* Dextrose *on page 452*

Simply Cough® [OTC] *see* Dextromethorphan *on page 451*

Simply Saline® [OTC] *see* Sodium Chloride *on page 1400*

Simply Saline® Baby [OTC] *see* Sodium Chloride *on page 1400*

Simply Saline® Nasal Moist® [OTC] *see* Sodium Chloride *on page 1400*

Simply Sleep® [OTC] *see* DiphenhydrAMINE *on page 483*

Simply Stuffy™ [OTC] *see* Pseudoephedrine *on page 1309*

Simulect® *see* Basiliximab *on page 180*

Simvastatin (SIM va stat in)

Related Information
Cardiovascular Diseases *on page 1636*
U.S. Brand Names Zocor®
Canadian Brand Names Apo-Simvastatin®; CO Simvastatin; Gen-Simvastatin; Novo-Simvastatin; PMS-Simvastatin; ratio-Simvastatin; Riva-Simvastatin; Sandoz-Simvastatin; Zocor®
Mexican Brand Names Zocor®
Generic Available No
Pharmacologic Category Antilipemic Agent, HMG-CoA Reductase Inhibitor
Use Used with dietary therapy for the following:

Secondary prevention of cardiovascular events in hypercholesterolemic patients with established coronary heart disease (CHD) or at high risk for CHD: To reduce cardiovascular morbidity (myocardial infarction, coronary revascularization procedures) and mortality; to reduce the risk of stroke and transient ischemic attacks

Hyperlipidemias: To reduce elevations in total cholesterol, LDL-C, apolipoprotein B, and triglycerides in patients with primary hypercholesterolemia (elevations of 1 or more components are present in Fredrickson type IIa, IIb, III, and IV hyperlipidemias); treatment of homozygous familial hypercholesterolemia
Heterozygous familial hypercholesterolemia (HeFH): In adolescent patients (10-17 years of age, females >1 year postmenarche) with HeFH having LDL-C ≥190 mg/dL **or** LDL ≥160 mg/dL with positive family history of premature cardiovascular disease (CVD), or 2 or more CVD risk factors in the adolescent patient

Local Anesthetic/Vasoconstrictor Precautions No information available to require special precautions

Effects on Dental Treatment No significant effects or complications reported

Common Adverse Effects 1% to 10%:

Gastrointestinal: Constipation (2%), dyspepsia (1%), flatulence (2%)

Neuromuscular & skeletal: CPK elevation (>3x normal on one or more occasions - 5%)

Respiratory: Upper respiratory infection (2%)

Additional class-related events or case reports (not necessarily reported with simvastatin therapy): Alopecia, alteration in taste, anaphylaxis, angioedema, anorexia, anxiety, arthritis, cataracts, chills, cholestatic jaundice, cirrhosis, decreased libido, depression, dermatomyositis, dryness of skin/mucous membranes, dyspnea, elevated transaminases, eosinophilia, erectile dysfunction/impotence, erythema multiforme, facial paresis, fatty liver, fever, flushing, fulminant hepatic necrosis, gynecomastia, hemolytic anemia, hepatitis, hepatoma, hyperbilirubinemia, hypersensitivity reaction, impaired extraocular muscle movement, increased alkaline phosphatase, increased CPK (>10x normal), increased ESR, increased GGT, leukopenia, malaise, memory loss, myopathy, nail changes, nodules, ophthalmoplegia, pancreatitis, paresthesia, peripheral nerve palsy, peripheral neuropathy, photosensitivity, polymyalgia rheumatica, positive ANA, pruritus, psychic disturbance, purpura, rash, renal failure (secondary to rhabdomyolysis), rhabdomyolysis, skin discoloration, Stevens-Johnson syndrome, systemic lupus erythematosus-like syndrome, thrombocytopenia, thyroid dysfunction, toxic epidermal necrolysis, tremor, urticaria, vasculitis, vertigo, vomiting

Dosage Oral: **Note:** Doses should be individualized according to the baseline LDL-cholesterol levels, the recommended goal of therapy, and the patient's response; adjustments should be made at intervals of 4 weeks or more; doses may need adjusted based on concomitant medications

Children 10-17 years (females >1 year postmenarche): HeFH: 10 mg once daily in the evening; range: 10-40 mg/day (maximum: 40 mg/day)

Dosage adjustment for simvastatin with concomitant cyclosporine, danazol, fibrates, niacin, amiodarone, or verapamil: Refer to drug-specific dosing in Adults dosing section

Adults:

Homozygous familial hypercholesterolemia: 40 mg once daily in the evening **or** 80 mg/day (given as 20 mg, 20 mg, and 40 mg evening dose)

Prevention of cardiovascular events, hyperlipidemias: 20-40 mg once daily in the evening; range: 5-80 mg/day

Patients requiring only moderate reduction of LDL-cholesterol may be started at 10 mg once daily

Patients requiring reduction of >45% in low-density lipoprotein (LDL) cholesterol may be started at 40 mg once daily in the evening

Patients with CHD or at high risk for CHD: Dosing should be started at 40 mg once daily in the evening; simvastatin may be started simultaneously with diet

Dosage adjustment with concomitant medications:

Cyclosporine or danazol (patient must first demonstrate tolerance to simvastatin ≥5 mg once daily): Initial: 5 mg simvastatin, should **not** exceed 10 mg/day

Fibrates or niacin: Simvastatin dose should **not** exceed 10 mg/day

Amiodarone or verapamil: Simvastatin dose should **not** exceed 20 mg/day

Dosing adjustment/comments in renal impairment: Because simvastatin does not undergo significant renal excretion, modification of dose should not be necessary in patients with mild to moderate renal insufficiency.

Severe renal impairment: Cl_{cr} <10 mL/minute: Initial: 5 mg/day with close monitoring.

Mechanism of Action Simvastatin is a methylated derivative of lovastatin that acts by competitively inhibiting 3-hydroxy-3-methylglutaryl-coenzyme A (HMG-CoA) reductase, the enzyme that catalyzes the rate-limiting step in cholesterol biosynthesis

Contraindications Hypersensitivity to simvastatin or any component of the formulation; acute liver disease; unexplained persistent elevations of serum transaminases; pregnancy; breast-feeding

Warnings/Precautions Secondary causes of hyperlipidemia should be ruled out prior to therapy. Liver function must be monitored by laboratory assessment. Rhabdomyolysis with acute renal failure has occurred. Risk is dose-related and is increased with concurrent use of lipid-lowering agents which may cause rhabdomyolysis (gemfibrozil, fibric acid derivatives, or niacin at doses ≥1 g/day), during concurrent use with danazol or strong CYP3A4 inhibitors (including amiodarone, clarithromycin, cyclosporine, erythromycin, telithromycin, itraconazole, ketoconazole, nefazodone, grapefruit juice in large quantities, (Continued)

Simvastatin *(Continued)*

verapamil, or protease inhibitors such as indinavir, nelfinavir, or ritonavir). Weigh the risk versus benefit when combining any of these drugs with simvastatin. Do not initiate simvastatin-containing treatment in a patient with pre-existing therapy of cyclosporine or danazol, unless the patient has previously demonstrated tolerance to ≥5 mg/day simvastatin. Temporarily discontinue in any patient experiencing an acute or serious major medical or surgical condition which may increase the risk of rhabdomyolysis. Discontinue temporarily for elective surgical procedures. Use caution in patients with renal insufficiency. Use with caution in patients who consume large amounts of ethanol or have a history of liver disease. Safety and efficacy have not been established in patients <10 years or in premenarcheal girls.

Drug Interactions

Cytochrome P450 Effect: Substrate of CYP3A4 (major); **Inhibits** CYP2C8/9 (weak), 2D6 (weak)

Increased Effect/Toxicity: Risk of myopathy/rhabdomyolysis may be increased by concurrent use of lipid-lowering agents which may cause rhabdomyolysis (gemfibrozil, fibric acid derivatives, or niacin at doses ≥1 g/day), or during concurrent use of strong CYP3A4 inhibitors.

CYP3A4 inhibitors may increase the levels/effects of simvastatin; example inhibitors include azole antifungals, clarithromycin, diclofenac, doxycycline, erythromycin, imatinib, isoniazid, nefazodone, nicardipine, propofol, protease inhibitors, quinidine, telithromycin, and verapamil. In large quantities (ie, >1 quart/day), grapefruit juice may also increase simvastatin serum concentrations, increasing the risk of rhabdomyolysis. In general, concurrent use with CYP3A4 inhibitors is not recommended; manufacturer recommends limiting simvastatin dose to 20 mg/day when used with amiodarone or verapamil, and 10 mg/day when used with cyclosporine, gemfibrozil, or fibric acid derivatives.

The anticoagulant effect of warfarin may be increased by simvastatin. Cholesterol-lowering effects are additive with bile-acid sequestrants (colestipol and cholestyramine).

Decreased Effect: When taken within 1 before or up to 2 hours after cholestyramine, a decrease in absorption of simvastatin can occur.

Ethanol/Nutrition/Herb Interactions

Ethanol: Avoid excessive ethanol consumption (due to potential hepatic effects).

Food: Simvastatin serum concentration may be increased when taken with grapefruit juice; avoid concurrent intake of large quantities (>1 quart/day). Red yeast rice contains an estimated 2.4 mg lovastatin per 600 mg rice.

Herb/Nutraceutical: St John's wort may decrease simvastatin levels.

Dietary Considerations Red yeast rice contains an estimated 2.4 mg lovastatin per 600 mg rice.

Pharmacodynamics/Kinetics

Onset of action: >3 days

Peak effect: 2 weeks

Absorption: 85%

Protein binding: ~95%

Metabolism: Hepatic via CYP3A4; extensive first-pass effect

Bioavailability: <5%

Half-life elimination: Unknown

Time to peak: 1.3-2.4 hours

Excretion: Feces (60%); urine (13%)

Pregnancy Risk Factor X

Dosage Forms TAB: 5 mg, 10 mg, 20 mg, 40 mg, 80 mg

Sina-12X *see* Guaifenesin and Phenylephrine *on page 754*

Sincalide *(SIN ka lide)*

U.S. Brand Names Kinevac®

Generic Available No

Synonyms C8-CCK; OP-CCK

Pharmacologic Category Diagnostic Agent

Use Postevacuation cholecystography; gallbladder bile sampling; stimulate pancreatic secretion for analysis; accelerate the transit of barium through the small bowel

Local Anesthetic/Vasoconstrictor Precautions No information available to require special precautions

Effects on Dental Treatment No significant effects or complications reported

Mechanism of Action Stimulates contraction of the gallbladder; inhibits gastric emptying by causing pyloric contraction, and increases intestinal motility; stimulates pancreatic secretion; causes smooth muscle contraction

Pregnancy Risk Factor B

Sinemet® *see* Levodopa and Carbidopa *on page 911*

Sinemet® CR *see* Levodopa and Carbidopa *on page 911*

Sinequan® [DSC] *see* Doxepin *on page 505*

Singulair® *see* Montelukast *on page 1062*

Sinografin® *see* Diatrizoate Meglumine and Iodipamide Meglumine *on page 453*

Sinus-Relief [OTC] *see* Acetaminophen and Pseudoephedrine *on page 38*

Sinutab® Sinus [OTC] *see* Acetaminophen and Pseudoephedrine *on page 38*

Sinutab® Sinus Allergy Maximum Strength [OTC] *see* Acetaminophen, Chlorpheniramine, and Pseudoephedrine *on page 43*

SINUvent® PE *see* Guaifenesin and Phenylephrine *on page 754*

Sirdalud® *see* Tizanidine *on page 1497*

Sirolimus (sir OH li mus)

U.S. Brand Names Rapamune®
Canadian Brand Names Rapamune®
Generic Available No
Pharmacologic Category Immunosuppressant Agent
Use Prophylaxis of organ rejection in patients receiving renal transplants, in combination with corticosteroids and cyclosporine (cyclosporine may be withdrawn in low-to-moderate immunological risk patients after 2-4 months, in conjunction with an increase in sirolimus dosage)
Unlabeled/Investigational Use Investigational: Immunosuppression in other forms of solid organ transplantation and peripheral stem cell/bone marrow transplantation
Local Anesthetic/Vasoconstrictor Precautions No information available to require special precautions
Effects on Dental Treatment No significant effects or complications reported
Common Adverse Effects Incidence of many adverse effects is dose related
>20%:
 Cardiovascular: Hypertension (39% to 49%), peripheral edema (54% to 64%), edema (16% to 24%), chest pain (16% to 24%)
 Central nervous system: Fever (23% to 34%), headache (23% to 34%), pain (24% to 33%), insomnia (13% to 22%)
 Dermatologic: Acne (20% to 31%)
 Endocrine & metabolic: Hypercholesterolemia (38% to 46%), hypophosphatemia (15% to 23%), hyperlipidemia (38% to 57%), hypokalemia (11% to 21%)
 Gastrointestinal: Abdominal pain (28% to 36%), nausea (25% to 36%), vomiting (19% to 25%), diarrhea (25% to 42%), constipation (28% to 38%), dyspepsia (17% to 25%), weight gain (8% to 21%)
 Genitourinary: Urinary tract infection (20% to 33%)
 Hematologic: Anemia (23% to 37%), thrombocytopenia (13% to 40%)
 Neuromuscular & skeletal: Arthralgia (25% to 31%), weakness (22% to 40%), back pain (16% to 26%), tremor (21% to 31%)
 Renal: Increased serum creatinine (35% to 40%)
 Respiratory: Dyspnea (22% to 30%), upper respiratory infection (20% to 26%), pharyngitis (16% to 21%)
3% to 20%:
 Cardiovascular: Atrial fibrillation, CHF, hypervolemia, hypotension, palpitation, peripheral vascular disorder, postural hypotension, syncope, tachycardia, thrombosis, vasodilation, venous thromboembolism
 Central nervous system: Chills, malaise, anxiety, confusion, depression, dizziness, emotional lability, hypoesthesia, hypotonia, insomnia, neuropathy, somnolence
 Dermatologic: Dermatitis (fungal), hirsutism, pruritus, skin hypertrophy, dermal ulcer, ecchymosis, cellulitis, rash (10% to 20%)
 Endocrine & metabolic: Cushing's syndrome, diabetes mellitus, glycosuria, acidosis, dehydration, hypercalcemia, hyperglycemia, hyperphosphatemia, hypocalcemia, hypoglycemia, hypomagnesemia, hyponatremia, hyperkalemia (12% to 17%)
 Gastrointestinal: Enlarged abdomen, anorexia, dysphagia, eructation, esophagitis, flatulence, gastritis, gastroenteritis, gingivitis, gingival hyperplasia, ileus, mouth ulceration, oral moniliasis, stomatitis, weight loss
 Genitourinary: Pelvic pain, scrotal edema, testis disorder, impotence
(Continued)

Sirolimus *(Continued)*

Hematologic: Leukocytosis, polycythemia, TTP, hemolytic-uremic syndrome, hemorrhage, leukopenia (9% to 15%)

Hepatic: Abnormal liver function tests, alkaline phosphatase increased, ascites, LDH increased, transaminases increased

Local: Thrombophlebitis

Neuromuscular & skeletal: Increased CPK, arthrosis, bone necrosis, leg cramps, myalgia, osteoporosis, tetany, hypertonia, paresthesia

Ocular: Abnormal vision, cataract, conjunctivitis

Otic: Ear pain, deafness, otitis media, tinnitus

Renal: Increased BUN, albuminuria, bladder pain, dysuria, hematuria, hydronephrosis, kidney pain, tubular necrosis, nocturia, oliguria, pyuria, nephropathy (toxic), urinary frequency, urinary incontinence, urinary retention

Respiratory: Asthma, atelectasis, bronchitis, cough, epistaxis, hypoxia, lung edema, pleural effusion, pneumonia, rhinitis, sinusitis

Miscellaneous: Abscess, diaphoresis, facial edema, flu-like syndrome, hernia, infection, lymphadenopathy, lymphocele, peritonitis, sepsis

Dosage

Oral:

Combination therapy with cyclosporine: For *de novo* transplant recipients, a loading dose of 3 times the daily maintenance dose should be administered on day 1 of dosing. Doses should be taken 4 hours after cyclosporine, and should be taken consistently either with or without food.

Children ≥13 years and Adults: Dosing by body weight:

<40 kg: Loading dose: Loading dose: 3 mg/m^2 on day 1, followed by a maintenance dosing of 1 mg/m^2/day

≥40 kg: Loading dose: 6 mg on day 1; maintenance: 2 mg/day

Maintenance therapy after withdrawal of cyclosporine:

Following 2-4 months of combined therapy, withdrawal of cyclosporine may be considered in low-to-moderate risk patients. Cyclosporine withdrawal in not recommended in high immunological risk patients. Cyclosporine should be discontinued over 4-8 weeks, and a necessary increase in the dosage of sirolimus (up to fourfold) should be anticipated due to removal of metabolic inhibition by cyclosporine and to maintain adequate immunosuppressive effects.

Sirolimus dosages should be adjusted to maintain trough concentrations of 12-24 ng/mL. Dosage should be adjusted at intervals of 7-14 days to account for the long half-life of sirolimus. Considerable increases in dosage may require an additional loading dose, calculated as the difference between the target concentration and the current concentration, multiplied by a factor of 3. Loading doses >40 mg may be administered over two days. Serum concentrations should not be used as the sole basis for dosage adjustment (monitor clinical signs/symptoms, tissue biopsy, and laboratory parameters).

Dosage adjustment in renal impairment: No dosage adjustment is necessary in renal impairment

Dosage adjustment in hepatic impairment: Reduce maintenance dose by approximately 33% in hepatic impairment. Loading dose is unchanged.

Mechanism of Action Sirolimus inhibits T-lymphocyte activation and proliferation in response to antigenic and cytokine stimulation. Its mechanism differs from other immunosuppressants. It inhibits acute rejection of allografts and prolongs graft survival.

Contraindications Hypersensitivity to sirolimus or any component of the formulation

Warnings/Precautions Immunosuppressive agents, including sirolimus, increase the risk of infection and may be associated with the development of lymphoma. May increase serum lipids (cholesterol and triglycerides). Use with caution in patients with hyperlipidemia. May increase serum creatinine and decrease GFR. Use caution in patients with renal impairment, or when used concurrently with medications which may alter renal function. Monitor renal function closely when combined with cyclosporine; consider dosage adjustment or discontinue in patients with increasing serum creatinine. Has been associated with an increased risk of lymphocele. Cases of interstitial lung disease (eg, pneumonitis, bronchiolitis obliterans organizing pneumonia, pulmonary fibrosis) have been observed; risk may be increased with higher trough levels. Avoid concurrent use of strong CYP3A4 inhibitors or strong inducers of either CYP3A4 or P-glycoprotein. Concurrent use with a calcineurin inhibitor (cyclosporine, tacrolimus) may increase the risk of calcineurin inhibitor-induced hemolytic uremic syndrome/thrombotic thrombocytopenic purpura/thrombotic microangiopathy (HUS/TTP/TMA). Anaphylactic reactions, angioedema and hypersensitivity vasculitis have been reported. May increase sensitivity to UV light; use appropriate sun protection.

Sirolimus is not recommended for use in liver transplant patients; studies indicate an association with an increase risk of hepatic artery thrombosis and graft failure in these patients. Cases of bronchial anastomotic dehiscence have been reported in lung transplant patients when sirolimus was used as part of an immunosuppressive regimen; most of these reactions were fatal. Use in patients with lung transplants is not recommended. Safety and efficacy of cyclosporine withdrawal in high-risk patients is not currently recommended. Safety and efficacy in children <13 years of age, or in adolescent patients <18 years of age considered at high immunological risk, have not been established.

Drug Interactions

Cytochrome P450 Effect: Substrate of CYP3A4 (major); Inhibits CYP3A4 (weak)

Increased Effect/Toxicity: Cyclosporine increases sirolimus concentrations during concurrent therapy, and cyclosporine levels may be increased; sirolimus should be taken 4 hours after cyclosporine oral solution (modified) and/or cyclosporine capsules (modified). CYP3A4 inhibitors may increase the levels/effects of sirolimus; example inhibitors include azole antifungals, clarithromycin, diclofenac, diltiazem, doxycycline, erythromycin, imatinib, isoniazid, nefazodone, nicardipine, propofol, protease inhibitors, quinidine, telithromycin, and verapamil; avoid concurrent use. Vaccination may be less effective and use of live vaccines should be avoided during sirolimus therapy. Concurrent therapy with calcineurin inhibitors (cyclosporine, tacrolimus) may increase the risk of HUS/TTP/TMA.

Decreased Effect: CYP3A4 inducers may decrease the levels/effects of sirolimus; example inducers include aminoglutethimide, carbamazepine, nafcillin, nevirapine, phenobarbital, phenytoin, and rifamycins.

Ethanol/Nutrition/Herb Interactions

Food: Do not administer with grapefruit juice; may decrease clearance of sirolimus. Ingestion with high-fat meals decreases peak concentrations but increases AUC by 35%. Sirolimus should be taken consistently either with or without food to minimize variability.

Herb/Nutraceutical: St John's wort may decrease sirolimus levels; avoid concurrent use. Avoid cat's claw, echinacea (have immunostimulant properties; consider therapy modifications).

Dietary Considerations Take consistently, with or without food, to minimize variability of absorption.

Pharmacodynamics/Kinetics

Absorption: Rapid

Distribution: 12 L/kg (range: 4-20 L/kg)

Protein binding: 92%, primarily to albumin

Metabolism: Extensively hepatic via CYP3A4; P-glycoprotein-mediated efflux into gut lumen

Bioavailability: Oral solution: 14%; Oral tablet: 18%

Half-life elimination: Mean: 62 hours

Time to peak: 1-2hours

Excretion: Feces (91%); urine (2%)

Pregnancy Risk Factor C

Dosage Forms SOLN, oral [bottle]: 1 mg/mL (60 mL). **TAB:** 1 mg, 2 mg

SK see Streptokinase on page 1417

SK and F 104864 see Topotecan on page 1511

Skeeter Stik [OTC] see Benzocaine on page 190

Skelaxin® see Metaxalone on page 1001

Skelid® see Tiludronate on page 1488

SKF 104864 see Topotecan on page 1511

SKF 104864-A see Topotecan on page 1511

Skin Care™ [OTC] see Pyrithione Zinc on page 1318

Sleep-ettes D [OTC] see DiphenhydrAMINE on page 483

Sleepinal® [OTC] see DiphenhydrAMINE on page 483

Slo-Niacin® [OTC] see Niacin on page 1105

Slow FE® [OTC] see Ferrous Sulfate on page 651

Slow-Mag® [OTC] see Magnesium Chloride on page 960

Smelling Salts see Ammonia Spirit (Aromatic) on page 103

SMZ-TMP see Sulfamethoxazole and Trimethoprim on page 1425

(+)-(S)-N-Methyl-γ-(1-naphthyloxy)-2-thiophenepropylamine Hydrochloride see Duloxetine on page 523

Sodium 4-Hydroxybutyrate see Sodium Oxybate on page 1402

Sodium L-Triiodothyronine see Liothyronine on page 934

Sodium Acid Carbonate see Sodium Bicarbonate on page 1400
Sodium Benzoate and Caffeine see Caffeine on page 245

Sodium Bicarbonate (SOW dee um bye KAR bun ate)

U.S. Brand Names Brioschi® [OTC]; Neut®
Generic Available Yes
Synonyms Baking Soda; NaHCO₃; Sodium Acid Carbonate; Sodium Hydrogen Carbonate
Pharmacologic Category Alkalinizing Agent; Antacid; Electrolyte Supplement, Oral; Electrolyte Supplement, Parenteral
Use Management of metabolic acidosis; gastric hyperacidity; as an alkalinization agent for the urine; treatment of hyperkalemia; management of overdose of certain drugs, including tricyclic antidepressants and aspirin
Local Anesthetic/Vasoconstrictor Precautions No information available to require special precautions
Effects on Dental Treatment No significant effects or complications reported
Common Adverse Effects Frequency not defined.
Cardiovascular: Cerebral hemorrhage, CHF (aggravated), edema
Central nervous system: Tetany
Gastrointestinal: Belching, flatulence (with oral), gastric distension
Endocrine & metabolic: Hypernatremia, hyperosmolality, hypocalcemia, hypokalemia, increased affinity of hemoglobin for oxygen-reduced pH in myocardial tissue necrosis when extravasated, intracranial acidosis, metabolic alkalosis, milk-alkali syndrome (especially with renal dysfunction)
Respiratory: Pulmonary edema
Mechanism of Action Dissociates to provide bicarbonate ion which neutralizes hydrogen ion concentration and raises blood and urinary pH
Drug Interactions
Increased Effect/Toxicity: Increased toxicity/levels of amphetamines, ephedrine, pseudoephedrine, flecainide, quinidine, and quinine due to urinary alkalinization.
Decreased Effect: Decreased effect/levels of lithium, chlorpropamide, and salicylates due to urinary alkalinization.
Pharmacodynamics/Kinetics
Onset of action: Oral: Rapid; I.V.: 15 minutes
Duration: Oral: 8-10 minutes; I.V.: 1-2 hours
Absorption: Oral: Well absorbed
Excretion: Urine (<1%)
Pregnancy Risk Factor C

Sodium Biphosphate, Methenamine, Methylene Blue, Phenyl Salicylate, and Hyoscyamine see Methenamine, Sodium Biphosphate, Phenyl Salicylate, Methylene Blue, and Hyoscyamine on page 1008
Sodium Cellulose Phosphate see Cellulose Sodium Phosphate on page 301

Sodium Chloride (SOW dee um KLOR ide)

U.S. Brand Names Altachlore [OTC]; Altamist [OTC]; Ayr® Baby Saline [OTC]; Ayr® Saline [OTC]; Ayr® Saline No-Drip [OTC]; Breathe Right® Saline [OTC]; Broncho Saline® [OTC]; Deep Sea [OTC]; Entsol® [OTC]; Muro 128® [OTC]; Mycinaire™ [OTC]; NaSal™ [OTC]; Nasal Moist® [OTC]; Na-Zone® [OTC]; Ocean® [OTC]; Oceant® for Kids [OTC]; Pretz® [OTC]; SalineX® [OTC]; Simply Saline® [OTC]; Simply Saline™ Baby [OTC]; Simply Saline® Nasal Moist® [OTC]; Syrex; 4-Way® Saline Moisturizing Mist [OTC]; Wound Saline™ [OTC]
Generic Available Yes
Synonyms NaCl; Normal Saline; Salt
Pharmacologic Category Electrolyte Supplement, Parenteral; Lubricant, Ocular; Sodium Salt
Use
Parenteral: Restores sodium ion in patients with restricted oral intake (especially hyponatremia states or low salt syndrome). In general, parenteral saline uses:
Bacteriostatic sodium chloride: Dilution or dissolving drugs for I.M., I.V., or SubQ injections
Concentrated sodium chloride: Additive for parenteral fluid therapy
Hypertonic sodium chloride: For severe hyponatremia and hypochloremia
Hypotonic sodium chloride: Hydrating solution
Normal saline: Restores water/sodium losses
Pharmaceutical aid/diluent for infusion of compatible drug additives
Ophthalmic: Reduces corneal edema

Inhalation: Restores moisture to pulmonary system; loosens and thins congestion caused by colds or allergies; diluent for bronchodilator solutions that require dilution before inhalation

Intranasal: Restores moisture to nasal membranes

Irrigation: Wound cleansing, irrigation, and flushing

Unlabeled/Investigational Use Traumatic brain injury (hypertonic sodium chloride)

Local Anesthetic/Vasoconstrictor Precautions No information available to require special precautions

Effects on Dental Treatment No significant effects or complications reported

Common Adverse Effects Frequency not defined.

Cardiovascular: Congestive conditions

Endocrine & metabolic: Extravasation, hypervolemia, hypernatremia, dilution of serum electrolytes, overhydration, hypokalemia

Local: Thrombosis, phlebitis, extravasation

Respiratory: Pulmonary edema

Mechanism of Action Principal extracellular cation; functions in fluid and electrolyte balance, osmotic pressure control, and water distribution

Drug Interactions

Decreased Effect: Lithium serum concentrations may be decreased.

Pharmacodynamics/Kinetics

Absorption: Oral, I.V.: Rapid

Distribution: Widely distributed

Excretion: Primarily urine; also sweat, tears, saliva

Pregnancy Risk Factor C

Sodium Citrate and Citric Acid
(SOW dee um SIT rate & SI trik AS id)

U.S. Brand Names Bicitra®; Cytra-2; Oracit®

Canadian Brand Names PMS-Dicitrate

Generic Available Yes

Synonyms Modified Shohl's Solution

Pharmacologic Category Alkalinizing Agent, Oral

Use Treatment of metabolic acidosis; alkalinizing agent in conditions where long-term maintenance of an alkaline urine is desirable

Local Anesthetic/Vasoconstrictor Precautions No information available to require special precautions

Effects on Dental Treatment No significant effects or complications reported

Common Adverse Effects Frequency not defined. Generally well tolerated with normal renal function.

Central nervous system: Tetany

Endocrine & metabolic: Metabolic alkalosis, hyperkalemia

Gastrointestinal: Diarrhea, nausea, vomiting

Drug Interactions

Increased Effect/Toxicity: Increased toxicity/levels of amphetamines, ephedrine, pseudoephedrine, flecainide, quinidine, and quinine due to urinary alkalinization.

Decreased Effect: Decreased effect/levels of lithium, chlorpropamide, and salicylates due to urinary alkalinization.

Pharmacodynamics/Kinetics

Metabolism: Oxidized to sodium bicarbonate

Excretion: Urine (<5% as sodium citrate)

Pregnancy Risk Factor Not established

Sodium Citrate, Citric Acid, and Potassium Citrate *see* Citric Acid, Sodium Citrate, and Potassium Citrate *on page 354*

Sodium Edetate *see* Edetate Disodium *on page 527*

Sodium Etidronate *see* Etidronate Disodium *on page 621*

Sodium Ferric Gluconate *see* Ferric Gluconate *on page 649*

Sodium Fluoride *see* Fluoride *on page 671*

Sodium Hyaluronate *see* Hyaluronate and Derivatives *on page 773*

Sodium Hyaluronate and Chondroitin Sulfate *see* Chondroitin Sulfate and Sodium Hyaluronate *on page 336*

Sodium Hydrogen Carbonate *see* Sodium Bicarbonate *on page 1400*

Sodium Hypochlorite Solution
(SOW dee um hye poe KLOR ite soe LOO shun)

U.S. Brand Names Dakin's Solution; Di-Dak-Sol
Generic Available No
Synonyms Modified Dakin's Solution
Pharmacologic Category Disinfectant, Antibacterial (Topical)
Use Treatment of athlete's foot (0.5%); wound irrigation (0.5%); disinfection of utensils and equipment (5%)
Local Anesthetic/Vasoconstrictor Precautions No information available to require special precautions
Effects on Dental Treatment No significant effects or complications reported
Common Adverse Effects Frequency not defined.
  Dermatologic: Irritating to skin
  Hematologic: Dissolves blood clots, delays clotting
Pregnancy Risk Factor C

Sodium Hyposulfate *see* Sodium Thiosulfate *on page 1404*
Sodium Nafcillin *see* Nafcillin *on page 1082*
Sodium Nitroferricyanide *see* Nitroprusside *on page 1122*
Sodium Nitroprusside *see* Nitroprusside *on page 1122*

Sodium Oxybate (SOW dee um ox i BATE)

U.S. Brand Names Xyrem®
Generic Available No
Synonyms Gamma Hydroxybutyric Acid; GHB; 4-Hydroxybutyrate; Sodium 4-Hydroxybutyrate
Pharmacologic Category Central Nervous System Depressant
Use Treatment of cataplexy and daytime sleepiness in patients with narcolepsy
Local Anesthetic/Vasoconstrictor Precautions No information available to require special precautions
Effects on Dental Treatment No significant effects or complications reported (see Dental Comment)
Common Adverse Effects
>10%:
  Central nervous system: Dizziness (8% to 37%), headache (9% to 37%), pain (9% to 20%), somnolence (1% to 14%), confusion (3% to 17%), sleep disorder (6% to 14%)
  Gastrointestinal: Nausea (8% to 40%), vomiting (2% to 23%), abdominal pain (3% to 11%)
  Genitourinary: Urinary incontinence (<1% to 14%, usually nocturnal), enuresis (3% to 17%), cystitis, metrorrhagia, urinary frequency
  Miscellaneous: Diaphoresis (3% to 11%)
1% to 10%:
  Cardiovascular: Hypertension (6%), chest pain, edema
  Central nervous system: Disorientation (up to 9%), inebriation (up to 9%), concentration decreased (3% to 9%), dream abnormality (3% to 9%), sleep-walking (4% to 7%), depression (3% to 6%), amnesia (3% to 6%), anxiety (3% to 6%), thinking abnormality (3% to 6%), lethargy (up to 6%), insomnia (5%), agitation, ataxia, chills, fatigue, malaise, memory impairment, nervousness, pyrexia, seizure, stupor, tremor, vertigo
  Dermatologic: Hyperhidrosis (3% to 6%), pruritus, rash
  Endocrine & metabolic: Dysmenorrhea (3% to 6%)
  Gastrointestinal: Dyspepsia (6% to 9%), diarrhea (6% to 8%), abdominal pain (6%), nausea and vomiting (6%), anorexia, constipation, tooth ache, weight gain
  Hepatic: Alkaline phosphatase increased, hypercholesteremia, hypocalcemia
  Neuromuscular & skeletal: Hypoesthesia (6%), weakness (6% to 8%), myasthenia (3% to 6%), pain (3% to 6%), arthritis, leg cramps, myalgia
  Ocular: Amblyopia (6%), blurred vision (6%)
  Otic: Tinnitus (6%), ear pain
  Renal: Albuminuria, hematuria
  Respiratory: Pharyngitis (6% to 8%), rhinitis (8%), nasopharyngitis (3% to 8%), infection (3% to 6%), bronchitis, cough, dyspnea
  Miscellaneous: Infection (3% to 6%), viral infection (3% to 9%), allergic reaction, flu-like syndrome
Restrictions C-I (illicit use); C-III (medical use)

Sodium oxybate oral solution will be available only to prescribers enrolled in the Xyrem® Patient Success Program® and dispensed to the patient through the designated centralized pharmacy (1-866-997-3688). Prior to dispensing the first prescription, prescribers will be sent educational materials to be reviewed with the patient and enrollment forms for the postmarketing surveillance program. Patients must be seen at least every 3 months; prescriptions can be written for a maximum of 3 months (the first prescription may only be written for a 1-month supply).

An FDA-approved medication guide is available at http://www.fda.gov/cder/Offices/ODS/labeling.htm; distribute to each patient to whom this medication is dispensed.

Mechanism of Action Sodium oxybate is derived from gamma aminobutyric acid (GABA) and acts as an inhibitory chemical transmitter in the brain. May function through specific receptors for gamma hydroxybutyrate (GHB) and GABA (B).

Drug Interactions
Increased Effect/Toxicity: CNS depressants: CNS depressant effects are potentiated; concomitant use with sodium oxybate is contraindicated.

Pharmacodynamics/Kinetics
Absorption: Rapid
Distribution: 190-384 mL/kg
Protein binding: <1%
Metabolism: Primarily via the Krebs cycle to form water and carbon dioxide; secondarily via beta oxidation; significant first-pass effect; no active metabolites; metabolic pathways are saturable
Bioavailability: 25%
Half-life elimination: 30-60 minutes
Time to peak: 30-75 minutes
Excretion: Primarily pulmonary (as carbon dioxide); urine (<5% unchanged drug)

Pregnancy Risk Factor B

Dental Comment Sodium oxybate is a known substance of abuse. When used illegally, it has been referred to as a "date-rape drug". The dentist should be aware of patients showing signs of CNS depression, as with all other drugs in this class.

Sodium PAS see Aminosalicylic Acid on page 89
Sodium-PCA and Lactic Acid see Lactic Acid on page 893

Sodium Phenylbutyrate (SOW dee um fen il BYOO ti rate)

U.S. Brand Names Buphenyl®
Generic Available No
Synonyms Ammonapse
Pharmacologic Category Urea Cycle Disorder (UCD) Treatment Agent
Use Orphan drug: Adjunctive therapy in the chronic management of patients with urea cycle disorder involving deficiencies of carbamoylphosphate synthetase, ornithine transcarbamylase, or argininosuccinic acid synthetase
Local Anesthetic/Vasoconstrictor Precautions No information available to require special precautions
Effects on Dental Treatment No significant effects or complications reported
Common Adverse Effects
>10%: Endocrine & metabolic: Amenorrhea, menstrual dysfunction
1% to 10%:
Gastrointestinal: Anorexia, abnormal taste
Miscellaneous: Offensive body odor
Mechanism of Action Sodium phenylbutyrate is a prodrug that, when given orally, is rapidly converted to phenylacetate, which is in turn conjugated with glutamine to form the active compound phenylacetylglutamine; phenylacetylglutamine serves as a substitute for urea and is excreted in the urine whereby it carries with it 2 moles of nitrogen per mole of phenylacetylglutamine and can thereby assist in the clearance of nitrogenous waste in patients with urea cycle disorders

Pregnancy Risk Factor C

Sodium Phosphate and Potassium Phosphate see Potassium Phosphate and Sodium Phosphate on page 1261

Sodium Phosphates (SOW dee um FOS fates)

U.S. Brand Names Fleet® Accu-Prep [OTC]; Fleet® Enema [OTC]; Fleet® Phospho-Soda® [OTC]; OsmoPrep™; Visicol®
(Continued)

Sodium Phosphates *(Continued)*

Canadian Brand Names Fleet Enema®; Fleet® Phospho-Soda® Oral Laxative

Generic Available Yes: Enema, injection

Pharmacologic Category Cathartic; Electrolyte Supplement, Oral; Electrolyte Supplement, Parenteral; Laxative, Bowel Evacuant

Use

Oral, rectal: Short-term treatment of constipation and to evacuate the colon for rectal and bowel exams

I.V.: Source of phosphate in large volume I.V. fluids and parenteral nutrition; treatment and prevention of hypophosphatemia

Local Anesthetic/Vasoconstrictor Precautions No information available to require special precautions

Effects on Dental Treatment No significant effects or complications reported

Mechanism of Action As a laxative, exerts osmotic effect in the small intestine by drawing water into the lumen of the gut, producing distention and promoting peristalsis and evacuation of the bowel; phosphorous participates in bone deposition, calcium metabolism, utilization of B complex vitamins, and as a buffer in acid-base equilibrium

Pregnancy Risk Factor C

Sodium Sulfacetamide *see* Sulfacetamide *on page 1423*

Sodium Tetradecyl *(SOW dee um tetra DEK il)*

U.S. Brand Names Sotradecol®

Canadian Brand Names Trombovar®

Generic Available No

Synonyms Sodium Tetradecyl Sulfate

Pharmacologic Category Sclerosing Agent

Use Treatment of small, uncomplicated varicose veins of the lower extremities

Local Anesthetic/Vasoconstrictor Precautions No information available to require special precautions

Effects on Dental Treatment No significant effects or complications reported

Common Adverse Effects Frequency not defined.

Central nervous system: Headache

Dermatologic: Discoloration at site of injection, sloughing and tissue necrosis following extravasation

Gastrointestinal: Nausea, vomiting

Local: Pain, itching, or ulceration at injection site

Miscellaneous: Allergic reaction (including hives, asthma, hay fever); anaphylactic shock

Mechanism of Action Acts by irritation of the vein intimal endothelium and causes thrombosis formation leading to occlusion of the injected vein

Pregnancy Risk Factor C

Sodium Tetradecyl Sulfate *see* Sodium Tetradecyl *on page 1404*

Sodium Thiosulfate *(SOW dee um thye oh SUL fate)*

U.S. Brand Names Versiclear™

Generic Available Yes: Injection

Synonyms Disodium Thiosulfate Pentahydrate; Pentahydrate; Sodium Hyposulfate; Sodium Thiosulphate; Thiosulfuric Acid Disodium Salt

Pharmacologic Category Antidote

Use

Parenteral: Used alone or with sodium nitrite or amyl nitrite in cyanide poisoning; reduce the risk of nephrotoxicity associated with cisplatin therapy

Topical: Treatment of tinea versicolor

Unlabeled/Investigational Use Management of I.V. extravasation

Local Anesthetic/Vasoconstrictor Precautions No information available to require special precautions

Effects on Dental Treatment No significant effects or complications reported

Common Adverse Effects 1% to 10%:

Cardiovascular: Hypotension

Central nervous system: Coma, CNS depression secondary to thiocyanate intoxication, psychosis, confusion

Dermatologic: Contact dermatitis, local irritation

Neuromuscular & skeletal: Weakness

Otic: Tinnitus

Mechanism of Action
Cyanide toxicity: Increases the rate of detoxification of cyanide by the enzyme rhodanese by providing an extra sulfur

Cisplatin toxicity: Complexes with cisplatin to form a compound that is nontoxic to either normal or cancerous cells

Pharmacodynamics/Kinetics
Absorption: Oral: Poor

Distribution: Extracellular fluid

Half-life elimination: 0.65 hour

Excretion: Urine (28.5% as unchanged drug)

Pregnancy Risk Factor C

Sodium Thiosulphate *see* Sodium Thiosulfate *on page 1404*

Solagé™ *see* Mequinol and Tretinoin *on page 994*

Solaquin® [OTC] *see* Hydroquinone *on page 798*

Solaquin Forte® *see* Hydroquinone *on page 798*

Solaraze® *see* Diclofenac *on page 459*

Solarcaine® Aloe Extra Burn Relief [OTC] *see* Lidocaine *on page 920*

Solia™ *see* Ethinyl Estradiol and Desogestrel *on page 592*

Solifenacin (sol i FEN a sin)

U.S. Brand Names VESIcare®

Generic Available No

Synonyms Solifenacin Succinate

Pharmacologic Category Anticholinergic Agent

Use Treatment of overactive bladder with symptoms of urinary frequency, urgency, or urge incontinence

Local Anesthetic/Vasoconstrictor Precautions No information available to require special precautions

Effects on Dental Treatment Key adverse event(s) related to dental treatment: Xerostomia (normal salivary flow resumes upon discontinuation). Prolonged xerostomia may contribute to discomfort and dental disease (eg, caries, periodontal disease, and oral candidiasis).

Common Adverse Effects Adverse reactions are dose related.

>10%: Gastrointestinal: Xerostomia (11% to 28%), constipation (5% to 13%)

1% to 10%:
 Cardiovascular: Edema (up to 1%), hypertension (up to 1%)
 Central nervous system: Dizziness (2%), fatigue (1% to 2%), depression (up to 1%)
 Gastrointestinal: Nausea (2% to 3%), dyspepsia (1% to 4%), upper abdominal pain (1% to 2%), vomiting (up to 1%)
 Genitourinary: Urinary tract infection (3% to 5%), urinary retention (up to 1%)
 Ocular: Blurred vision (4% to 5%), dry eyes (up to 2%)
 Respiratory: Cough (up to 1%), pharyngitis (up to 1%)
 Miscellaneous: Influenza (1% to 2%)

Mechanism of Action Inhibits muscarinic receptors resulting in decreased urinary bladder contraction, increased residual urine volume, and decreased detrusor muscle pressure.

Drug Interactions
Cytochrome P450 Effect: Substrate of CYP3A4 (major)

Increased Effect/Toxicity: CYP3A4 inhibitors may increase the levels/effects of solifenacin; example inhibitors include azole antifungals, clarithromycin, diclofenac, doxycycline, erythromycin, ketoconazole, imatinib, isoniazid, nefazodone, nicardipine, propofol, protease inhibitors, quinidine, telithromycin, and verapamil; solifenacin dose should not exceed 5 mg/day.

Decreased Effect: CYP3A4 inducers may decrease the levels/effects of solifenacin; example inducers include aminoglutethimide, carbamazepine, nafcillin, nevirapine, phenobarbital, and phenytoin.

Pharmacodynamics/Kinetics
Distribution: V_d: 600 L

Protein binding: 98% bound to alpha$_1$-acid glycoprotein

Metabolism: Extensively hepatic; via N-oxidation and 4 R-hydroxylation, forms one active and three inactive metabolites; primary pathway for elimination is via CYP3A4 route

Bioavailability: 90%

Half-life elimination: 45-68 hours following chronic dosing

Time to peak, plasma: 3-8 hours

Excretion: Urine 69% (<15% as unchanged drug); feces 23%

Pregnancy Risk Factor C

Solifenacin Succinate *see* Solifenacin *on page 1405*

Solodyn™ see Minocycline on page 1049

Soltamox™ see Tamoxifen on page 1443

Solu-Cortef® see Hydrocortisone on page 793

Solu-Medrol® see MethylPREDNISolone on page 1025

Soma® see Carisoprodol on page 271

Soma® Compound see Carisoprodol and Aspirin on page 272

Soma® Compound w/Codeine see Carisoprodol, Aspirin, and Codeine on page 273

Somatrem see Somatropin on page 1406

Somatropin (soe ma TROE pin)

U.S. Brand Names Genotropin®; Genotropin Miniquick®; Humatrope®; Norditropin®; Norditropin® NordiFlex®; Nutropin®; Nutropin AQ®; Saizen®; Serostim®; Tev-Tropin™; Zorbtive™

Canadian Brand Names Humatrope®; Nutropin® AQ; Nutropine®; Saizen®; Serostim®

Generic Available No

Synonyms Human Growth Hormone; Somatrem

Pharmacologic Category Growth Hormone

Use

Children:

Long-term treatment of growth failure due to inadequate endogenous growth hormone secretion (Genotropin®, Humatrope®, Norditropin®, Nutropin®, Nutropin AQ®, Saizen®, Tev-Tropin™)

Long-term treatment of short stature associated with Turner syndrome (Genotropin®, Humatrope®, Nutropin®, Nutropin AQ®)

Treatment of Prader-Willi syndrome (Genotropin®)

Treatment of growth failure associated with chronic renal insufficiency (CRI) up until the time of renal transplantation (Nutropin®, Nutropin AQ®)

Long-term treatment of growth failure in children born small for gestational age who fail to manifest catch-up growth by 2 years of age (Genotropin®)

Long-term treatment of idiopathic short stature (nongrowth hormone-deficient short stature) defined by height standard deviation score (SDS) less than or equal to -2.25 and growth rate not likely to attain normal adult height (Humatrope®, Nutropin®, Nutropin AQ®)

Adults:

AIDS-wasting or cachexia with concomitant antiviral therapy (Serostim®)

Replacement of endogenous growth hormone in patients with adult growth hormone deficiency who meet both of the following criteria (Genotropin®, Humatrope®, Norditropin®, Nutropin®, Nutropin AQ®, Saizen®):

Biochemical diagnosis of adult growth hormone deficiency by means of a subnormal response to a standard growth hormone stimulation test (peak growth hormone ≤5 mcg/L)

and

Adult-onset: Patients who have adult growth hormone deficiency whether alone or with multiple hormone deficiencies (hypopituitarism) as a result of pituitary disease, hypothalamic disease, surgery, radiation therapy, or trauma

or

Childhood-onset: Patients who were growth hormone deficient during childhood, confirmed as an adult before replacement therapy is initiated

Treatment of short-bowel syndrome (Zorbtive™)

Unlabeled/Investigational Use Investigational: Congestive heart failure; AIDS-wasting/cachexia in children (Serostim®)

Local Anesthetic/Vasoconstrictor Precautions No information available to require special precautions

Effects on Dental Treatment No significant effects or complications reported

Common Adverse Effects

Growth hormone deficiency: Antigrowth hormone antibodies, carpal tunnel syndrome (rare), fluid balance disturbances, glucosuria, gynecomastia (rare), headache, hematuria, hyperglycemia (mild), hypoglycemia, hypothyroidism, leukemia, lipoatrophy, muscle pain, increased growth of pre-existing nevi (rare), pain/ local reactions at the injection site, pancreatitis (rare), peripheral edema, exacerbation of psoriasis, rash, seizure, weakness

Idiopathic short stature: (From ISS NCGS Cohort; all frequencies <1%): Arthralgia, avascular necrosis, bone growth (abnormal), carpal tunnel syndrome, diabetes mellitus, edema, fracture, gynecomastia, injection site reaction, intracranial hypertension, neoplasm (new onset or recurring), scoliosis (new onset or progression), slipped capital femoral epiphysis, tumor (new onset or recurring). Additional adverse effects noted in product literature

(Humatrope®; frequency not established in large cohort): Hip pain, hyperlipidemia, hypertension, hypothyroidism, mylagia, otitis media.

Prader-Willi syndrome: Genotropin®: Aggressiveness, arthralgia, edema, hair loss, headache, benign intracranial hypertension, myalgia; fatalities associated with use in this population have been reported

Turner syndrome: Ear disorders, hypothyroidism, increased nevi, joint pain, otitis media, peripheral edema, surgical procedures

Adult growth hormone replacement: Increased ALT, increased AST, arthralgia, back pain, carpal tunnel syndrome, diabetes mellitus, fatigue, flu-like syndrome, gastritis, gastroenteritis, generalized edema, glucose intolerance, gynecomastia (rare), headache, hypertension, hypoesthesia, hypothyroidism, infection (nonviral), insomnia, joint disorder, laryngitis, myalgia, nausea, increased growth of pre-existing nevi, pain, pancreatitis (rare), paresthesia, peripheral edema, pharyngitis, rhinitis, stiffness in extremities, weakness

AIDS wasting or cachexia (limited): Serostim®: Musculoskeletal discomfort (54%), increased tissue turgor (27%), diarrhea (26%), neuropathy (26%), nausea (26%), fatigue (17%), albuminuria (15%), increased diaphoresis (14%), anorexia (12%), anemia (12%), increased AST (12%), insomnia (11%), tachycardia (11%), hyperglycemia (10%), increased ALT (10%)

Short-bowel syndrome: Zorbtive™: Peripheral edema (69% to 81%), edema (facial: 44% to 50%; peripheral 13%), arthralgia (13% to 44%), injection site reaction (19% to 31%), flatulence (25%), abdominal pain (20% to 25%), vomiting (19%), malaise (13%), nausea (13%), diaphoresis increased (13%), rhinitis (7%), dizziness (6%)

Small for gestational age: Genotropin®: Mild, transient hyperglycemia; benign intracranial hypertension (rare); central precocious puberty; jaw prominence (rare); aggravation of pre-existing scoliosis (rare); injection site reactions; progression of pigmented nevi

Mechanism of Action Somatropin is a purified polypeptide hormones of recombinant DNA origin; somatropin contains the identical sequence of amino acids found in human growth hormone; human growth hormone stimulates growth of linear bone, skeletal muscle, and organs; stimulates erythropoietin which increases red blood cell mass; exerts both insulin-like and diabetogenic effects; enhances the transmucosal transport of water, electrolytes, and nutrients across the gut

Drug Interactions
Decreased Effect: Glucocorticoid therapy may inhibit growth-promoting effects. Growth hormone may induce insulin resistance in patients with diabetes mellitus; monitor glucose and adjust insulin dose as necessary.

Pharmacodynamics/Kinetics
Duration: Maintains supraphysiologic levels for 18-20 hours
Absorption: I.M., SubQ: Well absorbed
Metabolism: Hepatic and renal (~90%)
Half-life elimination: Preparation and route of administration dependent
Excretion: Urine

Pregnancy Risk Factor B/C (depending upon manufacturer)

Sominex® [OTC] *see* DiphenhydrAMINE *on page 483*
Sominex® Maximum Strength [OTC] *see* DiphenhydrAMINE *on page 483*
Somnote™ *see* Chloral Hydrate *on page 312*
Sonata® *see* Zaleplon *on page 1591*

Sorafenib (sor AF e nib)

U.S. Brand Names Nexavar®
Generic Available No
Synonyms BAY 43-9006; Sorafenib Tosylate
Pharmacologic Category Antineoplastic Agent, Tyrosine Kinase Inhibitor; Vascular Endothelial Growth Factor (VEGF) Inhibitor
Use Treatment of advanced renal cell cancer
Unlabeled/Investigational Use Treatment of hepatocellular, breast, colon, colorectal, nonsmall cell lung, ovarian, pancreatic and thyroid cancers; melanoma, sarcoma
Local Anesthetic/Vasoconstrictor Precautions Sorafenib may cause hypertension; monitor blood pressure prior to vasoconstrictor use
Effects on Dental Treatment Key adverse event(s) related to dental treatment: Mouth pain, mucositis, stomatitis, and xerostomia (normal salivary flow resumes upon discontinuation)
Common Adverse Effects Note: Dose-limiting toxicities (diarrhea, fatigue, and hand-foot syndrome) were reversible upon discontinuation; rash and hand-foot syndrome are dose related; percentages not always reported.
(Continued)

Sorafenib (Continued)

>10%:
Cardiovascular: Hypertension (17%)
Central nervous system: Fatigue (32% to 33%; grade 3/4: 5% to <6%), sensory neuropathy (13%)
Dermatologic: Rash (38% to 40%), hand-foot syndrome (30% to 35%; grade 3/4: 6%), alopecia (27%), pruritus (19%), dry skin (11%), erythema
Endocrine & metabolic: Hypophosphatemia (45%; grade 3: 13%)
Gastrointestinal: Diarrhea (37% to 43%; grade 3/4: 2%), lipase increased (41%), amylase increased (30%), nausea (23%), anorexia (16%), vomiting (16%), constipation (15%), abdominal pain (11%), mouth pain
Hematologic: Lymphopenia (23%), neutropenia (<10% to 18%), hemorrhage (15%), thrombocytopenia (<10% to 12%), leukopenia
Neuromuscular & skeletal: Bone pain, muscle pain, weakness
Respiratory: Dyspnea (14%), cough (13%)

1% to 10%:
Cardiovascular: Flushing
Central nervous system: Headache (10%), depression, fever
Dermatologic: Acne, exfoliative dermatitis
Gastrointestinal: Weight loss (10%), appetite decreased, dyspepsia, dysphagia, glossodynia, mucositis, stomatitis, xerostomia
Genitourinary: Erectile dysfunction
Hematologic: Anemia
Hepatic: Transaminases increased
Neuromuscular & skeletal: Joint pain (10%), arthralgia, myalgia
Respiratory: Hoarseness
Miscellaneous: Influenza-like symptoms

Mechanism of Action Multikinase inhibitor; inhibits tumor growth and angiogenesis by inhibiting intracellular Raf kinases (CRAF, BRAF, and mutant BRAF), and cell surface kinase receptors (VEGFR-2, VEGFR-3, PDGFR-β, cKIT, and FLT-3)

Drug Interactions
Cytochrome P450 Effect: Substrate of CYP3A4 (minor); **Inhibits** CYP2B6 (weak) and 2C8/9 (weak)
Increased Effect/Toxicity: Sorafenib may increase the levels/effects of doxorubicin.

Pharmacodynamics/Kinetics
Absorption: Bioavailability decreased 29% with a high-fat meal (bioavailability similar to fasting state when administered with a moderate-fat meal).
Protein binding: 99.5%
Metabolism: Hepatic, via CYP3A4 (primarily oxidated to the pyridine N-oxide; active, minor) and UGT1A9 (glucuronidation)
Bioavailability: 38% to 49%
Half-life elimination: 25-48 hours
Time to peak, plasma: 3 hours
Excretion: Feces (77%, 51% as unchanged drug); urine (19%, as metabolites)
Pregnancy Risk Factor D

Sorafenib Tosylate see Sorafenib on page 1407

Sorbitol (SOR bi tole)

Generic Available Yes
Pharmacologic Category Genitourinary Irrigant; Laxative, Osmotic
Use Genitourinary irrigant in transurethral prostatic resection or other transurethral resection or other transurethral surgical procedures; diuretic; humectant; sweetening agent; hyperosmotic laxative; facilitate the passage of sodium polystyrene sulfonate through the intestinal tract
Local Anesthetic/Vasoconstrictor Precautions No information available to require special precautions
Effects on Dental Treatment No significant effects or complications reported
Common Adverse Effects Frequency not defined.
Cardiovascular: Edema
Endocrine & metabolic: Fluid and electrolyte losses, hyperglycemia, lactic acidosis
Gastrointestinal: Diarrhea, nausea, vomiting, abdominal discomfort, xerostomia
Mechanism of Action A polyalcoholic sugar with osmotic cathartic actions
Pharmacodynamics/Kinetics
Onset of action: 0.25-1 hour
Absorption: Oral, rectal: Poor
Metabolism: Primarily hepatic to fructose
Pregnancy Risk Factor C

Sorine® see Sotalol on page 1409

Sotalol (SOE ta lole)

Related Information
Cardiovascular Diseases on page 1636

U.S. Brand Names Betapace®; Betapace AF®; Sorine®

Canadian Brand Names Alti-Sotalol; Apo-Sotalol®; Betapace AF™; Gen-Sotalol; Lin-Sotalol; Novo-Sotalol; Nu-Sotalol; PMS-Sotalol; Rho®-Sotalol; Sotacor®

Generic Available Yes

Synonyms Sotalol Hydrochloride

Pharmacologic Category Antiarrhythmic Agent, Class II; Antiarrhythmic Agent, Class III; Beta-Adrenergic Blocker, Nonselective

Use Treatment of documented ventricular arrhythmias (ie, sustained ventricular tachycardia), that in the judgment of the physician are life-threatening; maintenance of normal sinus rhythm in patients with symptomatic atrial fibrillation and atrial flutter who are currently in sinus rhythm. Manufacturer states substitutions should not be made for Betapace AF® since Betapace AF® is distributed with a patient package insert specific for atrial fibrillation/flutter.

Local Anesthetic/Vasoconstrictor Precautions Use with caution; epinephrine has interacted with nonselective beta-blockers to result in initial hypertensive episode followed by bradycardia (see Dental Comment)

Effects on Dental Treatment Sotalol is a nonselective beta-blocker and may enhance the pressor response to epinephrine, resulting in hypertension and bradycardia. Many nonsteroidal anti-inflammatory drugs, such as ibuprofen and indomethacin, can reduce the hypotensive effect of beta-blockers after 3 or more weeks of therapy with the NSAID. Short-term NSAID use (ie, 3 days) requires no special precautions in patients taking beta-blockers.

Common Adverse Effects
>10%:
  Cardiovascular: Bradycardia (16%), chest pain (16%), palpitation (14%)
  Central nervous system: Fatigue (20%), dizziness (20%), lightheadedness (12%)
  Neuromuscular & skeletal: Weakness (13%)
  Respiratory: Dyspnea (21%)

1% to 10%:
  Cardiovascular: CHF (5%), peripheral vascular disorders (3%), edema (8%), abnormal ECG (7%), hypotension (6%), proarrhythmia (5%), syncope (5%)
  Central nervous system: Mental confusion (6%), anxiety (4%), headache (8%), sleep problems (8%), depression (4%)
  Dermatologic: Itching/rash (5%)
  Endocrine & metabolic: Sexual ability decreased (3%)
  Gastrointestinal: Diarrhea (7%), nausea/vomiting (10%), stomach discomfort (3% to 6%), flatulence (2%)
  Genitourinary: Impotence (2%)
  Hematologic: Bleeding (2%)
  Neuromuscular & skeletal: Paresthesia (4%), extremity pain (7%), back pain (3%)
  Ocular: Visual problems (5%)
  Respiratory: Upper respiratory problems (5% to 8%), asthma (2%)

Mechanism of Action
Beta-blocker which contains both beta-adrenoreceptor-blocking (Vaughan Williams Class II) and cardiac action potential duration prolongation (Vaughan Williams Class III) properties

Class II effects: Increased sinus cycle length, slowed heart rate, decreased AV nodal conduction, and increased AV nodal refractoriness

Class III effects: Prolongation of the atrial and ventricular monophasic action potentials, and effective refractory prolongation of atrial muscle, ventricular muscle, and atrioventricular accessory pathways in both the antegrade and retrograde directions

Sotalol is a racemic mixture of d- and l-sotalol; both isomers have similar Class III antiarrhythmic effects while the l-isomer is responsible for virtually all of the beta-blocking activity

Sotalol has both beta$_1$- and beta$_2$-receptor blocking activity

The beta-blocking effect of sotalol is a noncardioselective [half maximal at about 80 mg/day and maximal at doses of 320-640 mg/day]. Significant beta-blockade occurs at oral doses as low as 25 mg/day.

The Class III effects are seen only at oral doses ≥160 mg/day

(Continued)

Sotalol (Continued)

Drug Interactions

Increased Effect/Toxicity: Increased effect/toxicity of beta-blockers with calcium blockers since there may be additive effects on AV conduction or ventricular function. Other agents which prolong QT interval, including Class I antiarrhythmic agents, bepridil, cisapride, erythromycin, haloperidol, pimozide, phenothiazines, tricyclic antidepressants, and specific quinolones (including sparfloxacin, gatifloxacin, moxifloxacin) may increase the effect of sotalol on the prolongation of QT interval. Amiodarone may cause additive effects on QT_c prolongation as well as decreased heart rate, and has been associated with cardiac arrest in patients receiving some beta-blockers. When used concurrently with clonidine, sotalol may increase the risk of rebound hypertension after or during withdrawal of either agent. Beta-blocker and catecholamine depleting agents (reserpine or guanethidine) may result in additive hypotension or bradycardia. Beta-blockers may increase the action or levels of ethanol, nondepolarizing muscle relaxants, and theophylline although the effects are difficult to predict.

Decreased Effect: Decreased effect of sotalol may occur with aluminum-magnesium antacids (if taken within 2 hours), aluminum salts, barbiturates, calcium salts, cholestyramine, colestipol, NSAIDs, penicillins (ampicillin), rifampin, salicylates, and sulfinpyrazone due to decreased bioavailability and plasma levels. Beta-blockers may decrease the effect of sulfonylureas. Beta-agonists such as albuterol, terbutaline may have less of a therapeutic effect when administered concomitantly.

Pharmacodynamics/Kinetics

Onset of action: Rapid, 1-2 hours

Peak effect: 2.5-4 hours

Duration: 8-16 hours

Absorption: Decreased 20% to 30% by meals compared to fasting

Distribution: Low lipid solubility; enters milk of laboratory animals and is reported to be present in human milk

Protein binding: None

Metabolism: None

Bioavailability: 90% to 100%

Half-life elimination: 12 hours; Children: 9.5 hours; terminal half-life decreases with age <2 years (may by ≥1 week in neonates)

Excretion: Urine (as unchanged drug)

Pregnancy Risk Factor B

Dental Comment

This drug is known to prolong the QT interval. The QT interval is measured as the time and distance between the Q point of the QRS complex and the end of the T wave in the ECG tracing. After adjustment for heart rate, the QT interval is defined as prolonged if it is more than 450 msec in men and 460 msec in women. A long QT syndrome was first described in the 1950s and 60s as a congenital syndrome involving QT interval prolongation and syncope and sudden death. Some of the congenital long QT syndromes were characterized by a peculiar electrocardiographic appearance of the QRS complex involving a premature atria beat followed by a pause, then a subsequent sinus beat showing marked QT prolongation and deformity. This type of cardiac arrhythmia was originally termed "torsade de pointes" (translated from the French as "twisting of the points")

Prolongation of the QT interval is thought to result from delayed ventricular repolarization. The repolarization process within the myocardial cell is due to the efflux of intracellular potassium. The channels associated with this current can be blocked by many drugs and predisposes the electrical propagation cycle to torsade de pointes.

Sotalol is one of the drugs confirmed to prolong the QT interval and is accepted as having a risk of causing torsade de pointes. The risk of drug-induced torsade de pointes is extremely low when a single QT interval prolonging drug is prescribed. In terms of epinephrine, it is not known what effect vasoconstrictors in the local anesthetic regimen will have in patients with a known history of congenital prolonged QT interval or in patients taking any medication that prolongs the QT interval. Until more information is obtained, it is suggested that the clinician consult with the physician prior to the use of a vasoconstrictor in suspected patients, and that the vasoconstrictor (epinephrine, levonordefrin [Neo-Cobefrin®]) be used with caution.

Sotalol Hydrochloride see Sotalol on page 1409

Sotradecol® see Sodium Tetradecyl on page 1404

Sotret® see Isotretinoin on page 869

Spacol [DSC] see Hyoscyamine on page 803

Spacol T/S [DSC] *see* Hyoscyamine *on page 803*

Sparfloxacin (spar FLOKS a sin)

U.S. Brand Names Zagam® [DSC]
Generic Available No
Pharmacologic Category Antibiotic, Quinolone
Use Treatment of adults with community-acquired pneumonia caused by *C. pneumoniae*, *H. influenzae*, *H. parainfluenzae*, *M. catarrhalis*, *M. pneumoniae* or *S. pneumoniae*; treatment of acute bacterial exacerbations of chronic bronchitis caused by *C. pneumoniae*, *E. cloacae*, *H. influenzae*, *H. parainfluenzae*, *K. pneumoniae*, *M. catarrhalis*, *S. aureus* or *S. pneumoniae*
Local Anesthetic/Vasoconstrictor Precautions No information available to require special precautions (see Dental Comment)
Effects on Dental Treatment Key adverse event(s) related to dental treatment: Taste perversion.
Common Adverse Effects 1% to 10%:
  Cardiovascular: QT_c interval prolongation (1%), vasodilation (1%)
  Central nervous system: Insomnia (2%), dizziness (2%), headache (4%)
  Dermatologic: Photosensitivity reaction (8%; severe <1%), pruritus (2%)
  Gastrointestinal: Diarrhea (5%), dyspepsia (2%), nausea (4%), abdominal pain (2%), vomiting (1%), flatulence (1%), taste perversion (2%)
  Hepatic: Increased LFTs
Mechanism of Action Inhibits DNA-gyrase in susceptible organisms; inhibits relaxation of supercoiled DNA and promotes breakage of double-stranded DNA
Drug Interactions
  Increased Effect/Toxicity: Sparfloxacin may increase the effects/toxicity of glyburide and warfarin. Concomitant use with corticosteroids may increase the risk of tendon rupture. Concomitant use with other QT_c-prolonging agents (eg, Class Ia and Class III antiarrhythmics, erythromycin, cisapride, antipsychotics, and cyclic antidepressants) may result in arrhythmias such as torsade de pointes. Probenecid may increase sparfloxacin levels.
  Decreased Effect: Concurrent administration of metal cations, including most antacids, oral electrolyte supplements, quinapril, sucralfate, some didanosine formulations (chewable/buffered tablets and pediatric powder for oral suspension), and other highly-buffered oral drugs, may decrease quinolone levels; separate doses.
Pharmacodynamics/Kinetics
  Absorption: Unaffected by food or milk; reduced ~50% by concurrent administration of aluminum- and magnesium-containing antacids
  Distribution: Widely throughout the body; V_d: 3.9 L/kg
  Protein binding: 45%
  Metabolism: Hepatic, primarily by phase II glucuronidation
  Half-life elimination: Mean terminal: 20 hours (range: 16-30 hours)
  Time to peak, serum: 3-5 hours
  Excretion: Urine (50%; ~10% as unchanged drug); feces (50%)
Pregnancy Risk Factor C
Dental Comment
  This drug is known to prolong the QT interval. The QT interval is measured as the time and distance between the Q point of the QRS complex and the end of the T wave in the ECG tracing. After adjustment for heart rate, the QT interval is defined as prolonged if it is more than 450 msec in men and 460 msec in women. A long QT syndrome was first described in the 1950s and 60s as a congenital syndrome involving QT interval prolongation and syncope and sudden death. Some of the congenital long QT syndromes were characterized by a peculiar electrocardiographic appearance of the QRS complex involving a premature atria beat followed by a pause, then a subsequent sinus beat showing marked QT prolongation and deformity. This type of cardiac arrhythmia was originally termed "torsade de pointes" (translated from the French as "twisting of the points").

  Prolongation of the QT interval is thought to result from delayed ventricular repolarization. The repolarization process within the myocardial cell is due to the efflux of intracellular potassium. The channels associated with this current can be blocked by many drugs and predisposes the electrical propagation cycle to torsade de pointes.

  Sparfloxacin is one of the drugs confirmed to prolong the QT interval and is accepted as having a risk of causing torsade de pointes. The risk of drug-induced torsade de pointes is extremely low when a single QT interval prolonging drug is prescribed. In terms of epinephrine, it is not known what effect vasoconstrictors in the local anesthetic regimen will have in patients with a known history of congenital prolonged QT interval or in patients taking any
  (Continued)

Sparfloxacin *(Continued)*

medication that prolongs the QT interval. Until more information is obtained, it is suggested that the clinician consult with the physician prior to the use of a vasoconstrictor in suspected patients, and that the vasoconstrictor (epinephrine, levonordefrin [Neo-Cobefrin®]) be used with caution.

SPD417 *see* Carbamazepine *on page 260*
Spectazole® *see* Econazole *on page 526*

Spectinomycin *(spek ti noe MYE sin)*

Related Information
Sexually-Transmitted Diseases *on page 1674*
U.S. Brand Names Trobicin® [DSC]
Mexican Brand Names Trobicin®
Generic Available No
Synonyms Spectinomycin Hydrochloride
Pharmacologic Category Antibiotic, Miscellaneous
Use Treatment of uncomplicated gonorrhea
Local Anesthetic/Vasoconstrictor Precautions No information available to require special precautions
Effects on Dental Treatment No significant effects or complications reported
Mechanism of Action A bacteriostatic antibiotic that selectively binds to the 30s subunits of ribosomes, and thereby inhibiting bacterial protein synthesis
Pharmacodynamics/Kinetics
Duration: Up to 8 hours
Absorption: I.M.: Rapid and almost complete
Distribution: Concentrates in urine; does not distribute well into the saliva
Half-life elimination: 1.7 hours
Time to peak: ~1 hour
Excretion: Urine (70% to 100% as unchanged drug)
Pregnancy Risk Factor B

Spectinomycin Hydrochloride *see* Spectinomycin *on page 1412*
Spectracef™ *see* Cefditoren *on page 285*
Spectrocin Plus™ [OTC] *see* Bacitracin, Neomycin, Polymyxin B, and Pramoxine *on page 177*
SPI 0211 *see* Lubiprostone *on page 957*

Spiramycin *(speer a MYE sin)*

Generic Available No
Pharmacologic Category Antibiotic, Macrolide
Use Treatment of infections of the respiratory tract, buccal cavity, skin and soft tissues due to susceptible organisms. *N. gonorrhoeae*: as an alternate choice of treatment for gonorrhea in patients allergic to the penicillins. Before treatment of gonorrhea, the possibility of concomitant infection due to *T. pallidum* should be excluded.
Unlabeled/Investigational Use Treatment of *Toxoplasma gondii* to prevent transmission from mother to fetus
Local Anesthetic/Vasoconstrictor Precautions No information available to require special precautions
Effects on Dental Treatment No significant effects or complications reported
Common Adverse Effects Frequency not defined.
Central nervous system: Paresthesia (rare)
Dermatologic: Rash, urticaria, pruritus, angioedema (rare)
Gastrointestinal: Nausea, vomiting, diarrhea, pseudomembranous colitis (rare)
Hepatic: Transaminases increased
Miscellaneous: Anaphylactic shock (rare)
Restrictions Not available in U.S.
Mechanism of Action Inhibits growth of susceptible organisms; mechanism not established.
Drug Interactions
Cytochrome P450 Effect: Substrate of CYP3A4 (major)
Increased Effect/Toxicity: CYP3A4 inhibitors may increase the levels/effects of spiramycin; example inhibitors include azole antifungals, clarithromycin, diclofenac, doxycycline, erythromycin, imatinib, isoniazid, nefazodone, nicardipine, propofol, protease inhibitors, quinidine, telithromycin, and verapamil.

Decreased Effect: Spiramycin has been reported to decrease carbidopa absorption and decrease levodopa concentrations. CYP3A4 inducers may decrease the levels/effects of spiramycin; example inducers include aminoglutethimide, carbamazepine, nafcillin, nevirapine, phenobarbital, phenytoin, and rifamycins.

Pregnancy Risk Factor Not assigned (other macrolides rated B); C per expert analysis

---

Spirapril (SPYE ra pril)

Generic Available No

Pharmacologic Category Angiotensin-Converting Enzyme (ACE) Inhibitor

Use Management of mild to severe hypertension; treatment of left ventricular dysfunction after myocardial infarction

Local Anesthetic/Vasoconstrictor Precautions No information available to require special precautions

Effects on Dental Treatment Key adverse event(s) related to dental treatment: Orthostatic hypotension.

Common Adverse Effects Frequency not defined.

Cardiovascular: Hypotension (orthostatic), angioedema

Central nervous system: Headache, dizziness, migraine headache (exacerbation of), hypoesthesia

Dermatologic: Skin rash

Gastrointestinal: Nausea, diarrhea, vomiting

Neuromuscular & skeletal: Back pain

Ocular: Conjunctivitis

Respiratory: Cough

Restrictions Not available in U.S.

Mechanism of Action ACE inhibitor; inhibits renin-angiotensin system

Drug Interactions

Increased Effect/Toxicity: Potassium supplements, co-trimoxazole (high dose), angiotensin II receptor antagonists (eg, candesartan, losartan, irbesartan), or potassium-sparing diuretics (amiloride, spironolactone, triamterene) may result in elevated serum potassium levels when combined with ramipril. ACE inhibitor effects may be increased by phenothiazines or probenecid (increases levels of captopril). ACE inhibitors may increase serum concentrations/effects of lithium.

Diuretics have additive hypotensive effects with ACE inhibitors, and hypovolemia increases the potential for adverse renal effects of ACE inhibitors. In patients with compromised renal function, coadministration with NSAIDs may result in further deterioration of renal function. Allopurinol and ACE inhibitors may cause a higher risk of hypersensitivity reaction when taken concurrently.

Decreased Effect: Aspirin (high dose) may reduce the therapeutic effects of ACE inhibitors; at low dosages this does not appear to be significant. Rifampin may decrease the effect of ACE inhibitors. Antacids may decrease the bioavailability of ACE inhibitors (may be more likely to occur with captopril); separate administration times by 1-2 hours. NSAIDs, specifically indomethacin, may reduce the hypotensive effects of ACE inhibitors. More likely to occur in low renin or volume dependent hypertensive patients.

Pharmacodynamics/Kinetics

Absorption: 53% to 60%; delayed by high fat meals

Half-life elimination, serum: 1-2 hours

Pregnancy Risk Factor C (1st trimester); D (2nd and 3rd trimesters)

Spiriva® see Tiotropium on page 1494

Spironolactone (speer on oh LAK tone)

Related Information

Cardiovascular Diseases on page 1636

U.S. Brand Names Aldactone®

Canadian Brand Names Aldactone®; Novo-Spiroton

Mexican Brand Names Aldactone®; Aldactone-A®

Generic Available Yes

Pharmacologic Category Diuretic, Potassium-Sparing; Selective Aldosterone Blocker

Use Management of edema associated with excessive aldosterone excretion; hypertension; congestive heart failure; primary hyperaldosteronism; hypokalemia; treatment of hirsutism; cirrhosis of liver accompanied by edema or ascites

(Continued)

Spironolactone *(Continued)*

Unlabeled/Investigational Use Female acne (adjunctive therapy); hirsutism; hypertension (pediatric); diuretic (pediatric)

Local Anesthetic/Vasoconstrictor Precautions No information available to require special precautions

Effects on Dental Treatment No significant effects or complications reported

Common Adverse Effects Incidence of adverse events is not always reported. (Mean daily dose: 26 mg)

Cardiovascular: Edema (2%, placebo 2%)

Central nervous system: Disorders (23%, placebo 21%) which may include drowsiness, lethargy, headache, mental confusion, drug fever, ataxia, fatigue

Dermatologic: Maculopapular, erythematous cutaneous eruptions, urticaria, hirsutism, eosinophilia

Endocrine & metabolic: Gynecomastia (men 9%; placebo 1%), breast pain (men 2%; placebo 0.1%), serious hyperkalemia (2%, placebo 1%), hyponatremia, dehydration, hyperchloremic metabolic acidosis in decompensated hepatic cirrhosis, inability to achieve or maintain an erection, irregular menses, amenorrhea, postmenopausal bleeding

Gastrointestinal: Disorders (29%, placebo 29%) which may include anorexia, nausea, cramping, diarrhea, gastric bleeding, ulceration, gastritis, vomiting

Genitourinary: Disorders (12%, placebo 11%)

Hematologic: Agranulocytosis

Hepatic: Cholestatic/hepatocellular toxicity

Renal: Increased BUN concentration

Respiratory: Disorders (32%, placebo 34%)

Miscellaneous: Deepening of the voice, anaphylactic reaction, breast cancer

Dosage To reduce delay in onset of effect, a loading dose of 2 or 3 times the daily dose may be administered on the first day of therapy. Oral:

Children:

Diuretic, hypertension (unlabeled use): Children 1-17 years: Initial: 1 mg/kg/day divided every 12-24 hours (maximum dose: 3.3 mg/kg/day, up to 100 mg/day)

Diagnosis of primary aldosteronism (unlabeled use): 125-375 mg/m^2/day in divided doses

Adults:

Edema, hypokalemia: 25-200 mg/day in 1-2 divided doses

Hypertension (JNC 7): 25-50 mg/day in 1-2 divided doses

Diagnosis of primary aldosteronism: 100-400 mg/day in 1-2 divided doses

Acne in women (unlabeled use): 25-200 mg once daily

Hirsutism in women (unlabeled use): 50-200 mg/day in 1-2 divided doses

CHF, severe (with ACE inhibitor and a loop diuretic ± digoxin): 12.5-25 mg/day; maximum daily dose: 50 mg (higher doses may occasionally be used). In the RALES trial, 25 mg every other day was the lowest maintenance dose possible.

Note: If potassium >5.4 mEq/L, consider dosage reduction.

Elderly: Initial: 25-50 mg/day in 1-2 divided doses, increasing by 25-50 mg every 5 days as needed.

Dosing interval in renal impairment:

Cl_{cr} 10-50 mL/minute: Administer every 12-24 hours.

Cl_{cr} <10 mL/minute: Avoid use.

Mechanism of Action Competes with aldosterone for receptor sites in the distal renal tubules, increasing sodium chloride and water excretion while conserving potassium and hydrogen ions; may block the effect of aldosterone on arteriolar smooth muscle as well

Contraindications Hypersensitivity to spironolactone or any component of the formulation; anuria; acute renal insufficiency; significant impairment of renal excretory function; hyperkalemia; pregnancy (pregnancy-induced hypertension - per expert analysis)

Warnings/Precautions Avoid potassium supplements, potassium-containing salt substitutes, a diet rich in potassium, or other drugs that can cause hyperkalemia. Monitor for fluid and electrolyte imbalances. Gynecomastia is related to dose and duration of therapy. Diuretic therapy should be carefully used in severe hepatic dysfunction; electrolyte and fluid shifts can cause or exacerbate encephalopathy. Discontinue use prior to adrenal vein catheterization. When evaluating a heart failure patient for spironolactone treatment, creatinine should be ≤2.5 mg/dL in men or ≤2 mg/dL in women and potassium <5 mEq/L.

Drug Interactions

Increased Effect/Toxicity: Concurrent use of spironolactone with other potassium-sparing diuretics, potassium supplements, angiotensin receptor antagonists, co-trimoxazole (high dose), and ACE inhibitors can increase the risk of hyperkalemia, especially in patients with renal impairment. Cholestyramine can cause hyperchloremic acidosis in cirrhotic patients; avoid concurrent use.

Decreased Effect: The effects of digoxin (loss of positive inotropic effect) and mitotane may be reduced by spironolactone. Salicylates and NSAIDs (indomethacin) may decrease the natriuretic effect of spironolactone.

Ethanol/Nutrition/Herb Interactions
Food: Food increases absorption.
Herb/Nutraceutical: Avoid natural licorice (due to mineralocorticoid activity)

Dietary Considerations Should be taken with food to decrease gastrointestinal irritation and to increase absorption. Excessive potassium intake (eg, salt substitutes, low-salt foods, bananas, nuts) should be avoided.

Pharmacodynamics/Kinetics
Duration of action: 2-3 days
Protein binding: 91% to 98%
Metabolism: Hepatic to multiple metabolites, including canrenone (active)
Half-life elimination: 78-84 minutes
Time to peak, serum: 1-3 hours (primarily as the active metabolite)
Excretion: Urine and feces

Pregnancy Risk Factor C/D in pregnancy-induced hypertension (per expert analysis)

Dosage Forms TAB: 25 mg, 50 mg, 100 mg

Spironolactone and Hydrochlorothiazide see Hydrochlorothiazide and Spironolactone on page 778

Sporanox® see Itraconazole on page 873

Sportscreme® [OTC] see Triethanolamine Salicylate on page 1535

Sprintec™ see Ethinyl Estradiol and Norgestimate on page 613

SSD® see Silver Sulfadiazine on page 1393

SSD® AF see Silver Sulfadiazine on page 1393

SSKI® see Potassium Iodide on page 1260

S.T. 37® [OTC] see Hexylresorcinol on page 771

Stadol® see Butorphanol on page 243

Stagesic® see Hydrocodone and Acetaminophen on page 779

Stalevo™ see Levodopa, Carbidopa, and Entacapone on page 912

StanGard® see Fluoride on page 671

StanGard® Perio see Fluoride on page 671

Stannous Fluoride see Fluoride on page 671

Stanozolol (stan OH zoe lole)

U.S. Brand Names Winstrol®
Generic Available No
Pharmacologic Category Anabolic Steroid
Use Prophylactic use against hereditary angioedema
Local Anesthetic/Vasoconstrictor Precautions No information available to require special precautions
Effects on Dental Treatment No significant effects or complications reported
Common Adverse Effects
Male:
Postpubertal:
>10%:
Dermatologic: Acne
Endocrine & metabolic: Gynecomastia
Genitourinary: Bladder irritability, priapism
1% to 10%:
Central nervous system: Insomnia, chills
Endocrine & metabolic: Decreased libido, hepatic dysfunction
Gastrointestinal: Nausea, diarrhea
Genitourinary: Prostatic hyperplasia (elderly)
Hematologic: Iron deficiency anemia, suppression of clotting factors
Prepubertal:
>10%:
Dermatologic: Acne
Endocrine & metabolic: Virilism
1% to 10%:
Central nervous system: Chills, insomnia, factors
Dermatologic: Hyperpigmentation
Gastrointestinal: Diarrhea, nausea
Hematologic: Iron deficiency anemia, suppression of clotting
(Continued)

Stanozolol (Continued)

Female:

>10%: Endocrine & metabolic: Virilism

1% to 10%:

Central nervous system: Chills, insomnia

Endocrine & metabolic: Hypercalcemia

Gastrointestinal: Nausea, diarrhea

Hematologic: Iron deficiency anemia, suppression of clotting factors

Hepatic: Hepatic dysfunction

Restrictions C-III

Mechanism of Action Synthetic testosterone derivative with similar androgenic and anabolic actions

Drug Interactions

Increased Effect/Toxicity: ACTH, adrenal steroids may increase risk of edema and acne. Stanozolol enhances the hypoprothrombinemic effects of oral anticoagulants and enhances the hypoglycemic effects of insulin and sulfonylureas (oral hypoglycemics).

Pharmacodynamics/Kinetics

Metabolism: Hepatic

Excretion: Urine (90%); feces (6%)

Pregnancy Risk Factor X

Starlix® *see* Nateglinide *on page 1094*

Staticin® [DSC] *see* Erythromycin *on page 562*

Stavudine (STAV yoo deen)

Related Information

HIV Infection and AIDS *on page 1662*

U.S. Brand Names Zerit®

Canadian Brand Names Zerit®

Mexican Brand Names Zerit®

Generic Available No

Synonyms d4T

Pharmacologic Category Antiretroviral Agent, Reverse Transcriptase Inhibitor (Nucleoside)

Use Treatment of HIV infection in combination with other antiretroviral agents

Local Anesthetic/Vasoconstrictor Precautions No information available to require special precautions

Effects on Dental Treatment No significant effects or complications reported

Common Adverse Effects All adverse reactions reported below were similar to comparative agent, zidovudine, except for peripheral neuropathy, which was greater for stavudine. Selected adverse events reported as monotherapy or in combination therapy include:

>10%:

Central nervous system: Headache

Dermatologic: Rash

Gastrointestinal: Nausea, vomiting, diarrhea

Hepatic: Hepatic transaminases increased

Neuromuscular & skeletal: Peripheral neuropathy

Miscellaneous: Amylase increased

1% to 10%: Hepatic: Bilirubin increased

Mechanism of Action Stavudine is a thymidine analog which interferes with HIV viral DNA dependent DNA polymerase resulting in inhibition of viral replication; nucleoside reverse transcriptase inhibitor

Drug Interactions

Increased Effect/Toxicity: Risk of pancreatitis may be increased with concurrent didanosine use; cases of fatal lactic acidosis have been reported with this combination when used during pregnancy (use only if clearly needed). Risk of hepatotoxicity or pancreatitis may be increased with concurrent hydroxyurea use. Zalcitabine may increase risk of peripheral neuropathy; concurrent use not recommended.

Decreased Effect: Zidovudine inhibits intracellular phosphorylation of stavudine; concurrent use not recommended. Doxorubicin may inhibit intracellular phosphorylation of stavudine; use with caution. Ribavirin may inhibit intracellular phosphorylation of stavudine; use with caution.

Pharmacodynamics/Kinetics

Distribution: V_d: 0.5 L/kg

Bioavailability: 86.4%

Metabolism: Undergoes intracellular phosphorylation to an active metabolite

Half-life elimination: 1-1.6 hours
Time to peak, serum: 1 hour
Excretion: Urine (40% as unchanged drug)
Pregnancy Risk Factor C

Sterapred® *see* PredniSONE *on page 1271*

Sterapred® DS *see* PredniSONE *on page 1271*

STI571 *see* Imatinib *on page 817*

Stimate™ *see* Desmopressin *on page 437*

Sting-Kill [OTC] *see* Benzocaine *on page 190*

St. Joseph® Adult Aspirin [OTC] *see* Aspirin *on page 145*

Stop® *see* Fluoride *on page 671*

Strattera® *see* Atomoxetine *on page 156*

Streptase® *see* Streptokinase *on page 1417*

Streptokinase (strep toe KYE nase)

Related Information
Cardiovascular Diseases *on page 1636*
U.S. Brand Names Streptase®
Canadian Brand Names Streptase®
Mexican Brand Names Streptase®
Generic Available No
Synonyms SK
Pharmacologic Category Thrombolytic Agent
Use Thrombolytic agent used in treatment of recent severe or massive deep vein thrombosis, pulmonary emboli, myocardial infarction, and occluded arteriovenous cannulas
Local Anesthetic/Vasoconstrictor Precautions No information available to require special precautions
Effects on Dental Treatment No significant effects or complications reported
Common Adverse Effects As with all drugs which may affect hemostasis, bleeding is the major adverse effect associated with streptokinase. Hemorrhage may occur at virtually any site. Risk is dependent on multiple variables, including the dosage administered, concurrent use of multiple agents which alter hemostasis, and patient predisposition (including hypertension). Rapid lysis of coronary artery thrombi by thrombolytic agents may be associated with reperfusion-related atrial and/or ventricular arrhythmia.

>10%:
  Cardiovascular: Hypotension
  Local: Injection site bleeding
1% to 10%:
  Central nervous system: Fever (1% to 4%)
  Dermatologic: Bruising, rash, pruritus
  Gastrointestinal: Gastrointestinal hemorrhage, nausea, vomiting
  Genitourinary: Genitourinary hemorrhage
  Hematologic: Anemia
  Neuromuscular & skeletal: Muscle pain
  Ocular: Eye hemorrhage, periorbital edema
  Respiratory: Bronchospasm, epistaxis
  Miscellaneous: Diaphoresis hemorrhage, gingival hemorrhage

Additional cardiovascular events associated with use in MI: Asystole, AV block, cardiac arrest, cardiac tamponade, cardiogenic shock, electromechanical dissociation, heart failure, mitral regurgitation, myocardial rupture, pericardial effusion, pericarditis, pulmonary edema, recurrent ischemia/infarction, thromboembolism, ventricular tachycardia

Mechanism of Action Activates the conversion of plasminogen to plasmin by forming a complex, exposing plasminogen-activating site, and cleaving a peptide bond that converts plasminogen to plasmin; plasmin degrades fibrin, fibrinogen and other procoagulant proteins into soluble fragments; effective both outside and within the formed thrombus/embolus

Drug Interactions
Increased Effect/Toxicity: The risk of bleeding with streptokinase is increased by oral anticoagulants (warfarin), heparin, low molecular weight heparins, and drugs which affect platelet function (eg, NSAIDs, dipyridamole, ticlopidine, clopidogrel, IIb/IIIa antagonists). Although concurrent use with aspirin and heparin may increase the risk of bleeding. Aspirin and heparin were used concomitantly with streptokinase in the majority of patients in clinical studies of MI.
(Continued)

Streptokinase *(Continued)*

Decreased Effect: Antifibrinolytic agents (aminocaproic acid) may decrease effectiveness to thrombolytic agents.

Pharmacodynamics/Kinetics

Onset of action: Activation of plasminogen occurs almost immediately

Duration: Fibrinolytic effect: Several hours; Anticoagulant effect: 12-24 hours

Half-life elimination: 83 minutes

Excretion: By circulating antibodies and the reticuloendothelial system

Pregnancy Risk Factor C

Streptomycin *(strep toe MYE sin)*

Related Information

Tuberculosis *on page 1673*

Generic Available Yes

Synonyms Streptomycin Sulfate

Pharmacologic Category Antibiotic, Aminoglycoside; Antitubercular Agent

Use Part of combination therapy of active tuberculosis; used in combination with other agents for treatment of streptococcal or enterococcal endocarditis, mycobacterial infections, plague, tularemia, and brucellosis

Local Anesthetic/Vasoconstrictor Precautions No information available to require special precautions

Effects on Dental Treatment No significant effects or complications reported

Common Adverse Effects Frequency not defined.

Cardiovascular: Hypotension

Central nervous system: Neurotoxicity, drowsiness, headache, drug fever, paresthesia

Dermatologic: Skin rash

Gastrointestinal: Nausea, vomiting

Hematologic: Eosinophilia, anemia

Neuromuscular & skeletal: Arthralgia, weakness, tremor

Otic: Ototoxicity (auditory), ototoxicity (vestibular)

Renal: Nephrotoxicity

Respiratory: Difficulty in breathing

Mechanism of Action Inhibits bacterial protein synthesis by binding directly to the 30S ribosomal subunits causing faulty peptide sequence to form in the protein chain

Drug Interactions

Increased Effect/Toxicity: Increased/prolonged effect with depolarizing and nondepolarizing neuromuscular blocking agents. Concurrent use with amphotericin or loop diuretics may increase nephrotoxicity.

Pharmacodynamics/Kinetics

Absorption: I.M.: Well absorbed

Distribution: To extracellular fluid including serum, abscesses, ascitic, pericardial, pleural, synovial, lymphatic, and peritoneal fluids; crosses placenta; small amounts enter breast milk

Protein binding: 34%

Half-life elimination: Newborns: 4-10 hours; Adults: 2-4.7 hours, prolonged with renal impairment

Time to peak: Within 1 hour

Excretion: Urine (90% as unchanged drug); feces, saliva, sweat, and tears (<1%)

Pregnancy Risk Factor D

Streptomycin Sulfate *see Streptomycin on page 1418*

Streptozocin *(strep toe ZOE sin)*

U.S. Brand Names Zanosar®

Canadian Brand Names Zanosar®

Generic Available No

Synonyms NSC-85998

Pharmacologic Category Antineoplastic Agent, Alkylating Agent

Use Treatment of metastatic islet cell carcinoma of the pancreas, carcinoid tumor and syndrome, Hodgkin's disease, palliative treatment of colorectal cancer

Local Anesthetic/Vasoconstrictor Precautions No information available to require special precautions

Effects on Dental Treatment No significant effects or complications reported

Common Adverse Effects

>10%:

Gastrointestinal: Nausea and vomiting (100%)

Hepatic: Increased LFTs

Miscellaneous: Hypoalbuminemia

Renal: BUN increased, Cl_{cr} decreased, hypophosphatemia, nephrotoxicity (25% to 75%), proteinuria, renal dysfunction (65%), renal tubular acidosis

1% to 10%:

Endocrine & metabolic: Hypoglycemia (6%)

Gastrointestinal: Diarrhea (10%)

Local: Pain at injection site

Mechanism of Action Interferes with the normal function of DNA by alkylation and cross-linking the strands of DNA, and by possible protein modification

Drug Interactions

Increased Effect/Toxicity: Doxorubicin toxicity may be increased with concurrent use of streptozocin. Manufacturer recommends doxorubicin dosage adjustment be considered.

Decreased Effect: Phenytoin results in negation of streptozocin cytotoxicity.

Pharmacodynamics/Kinetics

Duration: Disappears from serum in 4 hours

Distribution: Concentrates in liver, intestine, pancreas, and kidney

Metabolism: Rapidly hepatic

Half-life elimination: 35-40 minutes

Excretion: Urine (60% to 70% as metabolites); exhaled gases (5%); feces (1%)

Pregnancy Risk Factor D

Stresstabs® B-Complex [OTC] see Vitamin B Complex Combinations on page 1581

Stresstabs® B-Complex + Iron [OTC] see Vitamin B Complex Combinations on page 1581

Stresstabs® B-Complex + Zinc [OTC] see Vitamin B Complex Combinations on page 1581

Striant® see Testosterone on page 1462

Stri-dex® [OTC] see Salicylic Acid on page 1374

Stri-dex® Body Focus [OTC] see Salicylic Acid on page 1374

Stri-dex® Facewipes To Go™ [OTC] see Salicylic Acid on page 1374

Stri-dex® Maximum Strength [OTC] see Salicylic Acid on page 1374

Stromectol® see Ivermectin on page 877

Strong Iodine Solution see Potassium Iodide and Iodine on page 1260

Strovite® Forte see Vitamins (Multiple/Oral) on page 1582

SU11248 see Sunitinib on page 1434

Sublimaze® see Fentanyl on page 644

Suboxone® see Buprenorphine and Naloxone on page 232

Subutex® see Buprenorphine on page 231

Succinylcholine (suks in il KOE leen)

U.S. Brand Names Quelicin®

Canadian Brand Names Quelicin®

Mexican Brand Names Anectine®

Generic Available No

Synonyms Succinylcholine Chloride; Suxamethonium Chloride

Pharmacologic Category Neuromuscular Blocker Agent, Depolarizing

Use Adjunct to general anesthesia to facilitate both rapid sequence and routine endotracheal intubation and to relax skeletal muscles during surgery; to reduce the intensity of muscle contractions of pharmacologically- or electrically-induced convulsions; does not relieve pain or produce sedation

Local Anesthetic/Vasoconstrictor Precautions No information available to require special precautions

Effects on Dental Treatment No significant effects or complications reported

Common Adverse Effects

>10%:

Ocular: Increased intraocular pressure

Miscellaneous: Postoperative stiffness

1% to 10%:

Cardiovascular: Bradycardia, hypotension, cardiac arrhythmia, tachycardia

Gastrointestinal: Intragastric pressure, salivation

Causes of prolonged neuromuscular blockade: Excessive drug administration; cumulative drug effect, decreased metabolism/excretion (hepatic and/or renal impairment); accumulation of active metabolites; electrolyte imbalance

(Continued)

Succinylcholine (Continued)

(hypokalemia, hypocalcemia, hypermagnesemia, hypernatremia); hypothermia; drug interactions; increased sensitivity to muscle relaxants (eg, neuromuscular disorders such as myasthenia gravis or polymyositis)

Mechanism of Action Acts similar to acetylcholine, produces depolarization of the motor endplate at the myoneural junction which causes sustained flaccid skeletal muscle paralysis produced by state of accommodation that develops in adjacent excitable muscle membranes

Drug Interactions
Increased Effect/Toxicity:

Increased toxicity: Anticholinesterase drugs (neostigmine, physostigmine, or pyridostigmine) in combination with succinylcholine can cause cardiorespiratory collapse; cyclophosphamide, oral contraceptives, lidocaine, thiotepa, pancuronium, lithium, magnesium salts, aprotinin, chloroquine, metoclopramide, terbutaline, and procaine enhance and prolong the effects of succinylcholine

Prolonged neuromuscular blockade: Inhaled anesthetics, local anesthetics, calcium channel blockers, antiarrhythmics (eg, quinidine or procainamide), antibiotics (eg, aminoglycosides, tetracyclines, vancomycin, clindamycin), immunosuppressants (eg, cyclosporine)

Pharmacodynamics/Kinetics

Onset of action: I.M.: 2-3 minutes; I.V.: Complete muscular relaxation: 30-60 seconds

Duration: I.M.: 10-30 minutes; I.V.: 4-6 minutes with single administration

Metabolism: Rapidly hydrolyzed by plasma pseudocholinesterase

Pregnancy Risk Factor C

Succinylcholine Chloride see Succinylcholine on page 1419

Sucraid® see Sacrosidase on page 1373

Sucralfate (soo KRAL fate)

Related Information

Management of Patients Undergoing Cancer Therapy on page 1728

U.S. Brand Names Carafate®

Canadian Brand Names Apo-Sucralate®; Novo-Sucralate; Nu-Sucralate; PMS-Sucralate; Sulcrate®; Sulcrate® Suspension Plus

Generic Available Yes

Synonyms Aluminum Sucrose Sulfate, Basic

Pharmacologic Category Gastrointestinal Agent, Miscellaneous

Use Short-term management of duodenal ulcers; maintenance of duodenal ulcers

Unlabeled/Investigational Use Gastric ulcers; suspension may be used topically for treatment of stomatitis due to cancer chemotherapy and other causes of esophageal and gastric erosions; GERD, esophagitis; treatment of NSAID mucosal damage; prevention of stress ulcers; postsclerotherapy for esophageal variceal bleeding

Local Anesthetic/Vasoconstrictor Precautions No information available to require special precautions

Effects on Dental Treatment No significant effects or complications reported

Common Adverse Effects 1% to 10%: Gastrointestinal: Constipation

Dosage Oral:

Children: Dose not established, doses of 40-80 mg/kg/day divided every 6 hours have been used

Stomatitis (unlabeled use): 2.5-5 mL (1 g/10 mL suspension), swish and spit or swish and swallow 4 times/day

Adults:

Stress ulcer prophylaxis: 1 g 4 times/day

Stress ulcer treatment: 1 g every 4 hours

Duodenal ulcer:

Treatment: 1 g 4 times/day on an empty stomach and at bedtime for 4-8 weeks, or alternatively 2 g twice daily; treatment is recommended for 4-8 weeks in adults, the elderly may require 12 weeks

Maintenance: Prophylaxis: 1 g twice daily

Stomatitis (unlabeled use): 1 g/10 mL suspension, swish and spit or swish and swallow 4 times/day

Dosage comment in renal impairment: Aluminum salt is minimally absorbed (<5%), however, may accumulate in renal failure

Mechanism of Action Forms a complex by binding with positively charged proteins in exudates, forming a viscous paste-like, adhesive substance. This selectively forms a protective coating that protects the lining against peptic acid, pepsin, and bile salts.

Contraindications Hypersensitivity to sucralfate or any component of the formulation

Warnings/Precautions Successful therapy with sucralfate should not be expected to alter the posthealing frequency of recurrence or the severity of duodenal ulceration; use with caution in patients with chronic renal failure who have an impaired excretion of absorbed aluminum. Because of the potential for sucralfate to alter the absorption of some drugs, separate administration (take other medication 2 hours before sucralfate) should be considered when alterations in bioavailability are believed to be critical

Drug Interactions

Decreased Effect: Sucralfate may alter the absorption of digoxin, phenytoin (hydantoins), warfarin, ketoconazole, quinidine, quinolones, tetracycline, theophylline. Because of the potential for sucralfate to alter the absorption of some drugs; separate administration (take other medications at least 2 hours before sucralfate). The potential for decreased absorption should be considered when alterations in bioavailability are believed to be critical.

Ethanol/Nutrition/Herb Interactions Food: Sucralfate may interfere with absorption of vitamin A, vitamin D, vitamin E, and vitamin K.

Dietary Considerations Administer with water on an empty stomach.

Pharmacodynamics/Kinetics

Onset of action: Paste formation and ulcer adhesion: 1-2 hours

Duration: Up to 6 hours

Absorption: Oral: <5%

Distribution: Acts locally at ulcer sites; unbound in GI tract to aluminum and sucrose octasulfate

Metabolism: None

Excretion: Urine (small amounts as unchanged compounds)

Pregnancy Risk Factor B

Dosage Forms SUSP, oral: (Carafate®): 1 g/10 mL (420 mL). **TAB** (Carafate®): 1 g

Sucrets® [OTC] *see* Dyclonine *on page 525*

Sucrets® Original [OTC] *see* Hexylresorcinol *on page 771*

Sudafed® [OTC] *see* Pseudoephedrine *on page 1309*

Sudafed® 12 Hour [OTC] *see* Pseudoephedrine *on page 1309*

Sudafed® 24 Hour [OTC] *see* Pseudoephedrine *on page 1309*

Sudafed® Children's [OTC] *see* Pseudoephedrine *on page 1309*

Sudafed® Children's Cold & Cough [OTC] *see* Pseudoephedrine and Dextromethorphan *on page 1311*

Sudafed® Non-Drying Sinus [OTC] *see* Guaifenesin and Pseudoephedrine *on page 755*

Sudafed PE™ [OTC] *see* Phenylephrine *on page 1226*

Sudafed® Severe Cold [OTC] *see* Acetaminophen, Dextromethorphan, and Pseudoephedrine *on page 44*

Sudafed® Sinus & Allergy [OTC] *see* Chlorpheniramine and Pseudoephedrine *on page 325*

Sudafed® Sinus and Cold [OTC] *see* Acetaminophen and Pseudoephedrine *on page 38*

Sudafed® Sinus Headache [OTC] *see* Acetaminophen and Pseudoephedrine *on page 38*

Sudafed® Sinus Nighttime [OTC] *see* Triprolidine and Pseudoephedrine *on page 1542*

Sudal® 12 *see* Chlorpheniramine and Pseudoephedrine *on page 325*

Sudodrin [OTC] *see* Pseudoephedrine *on page 1309*

SudoGest [OTC] *see* Pseudoephedrine *on page 1309*

SudoGest Children's [OTC] *see* Pseudoephedrine and Dextromethorphan *on page 1311*

SudoGest Sinus [OTC] *see* Acetaminophen and Pseudoephedrine *on page 38*

Sudo-Tab® [OTC] *see* Pseudoephedrine *on page 1309*

Sufenta® *see* Sufentanil *on page 1421*

Sufentanil (soo FEN ta nil)

U.S. Brand Names Sufenta®
Canadian Brand Names Sufenta®
Generic Available Yes
(Continued)

Sufentanil (Continued)

Synonyms Sufentanil Citrate

Pharmacologic Category Analgesic, Narcotic; General Anesthetic

Use Analgesic supplement in maintenance of balanced general anesthesia

Local Anesthetic/Vasoconstrictor Precautions No information available to require special precautions

Effects on Dental Treatment No significant effects or complications reported

Common Adverse Effects

>10%:
Cardiovascular: Bradycardia, hypotension
Central nervous system: Somnolence
Gastrointestinal: Nausea, vomiting
Respiratory: Respiratory depression

1% to 10%:
Cardiovascular: Cardiac arrhythmia, orthostatic hypotension
Central nervous system: CNS depression, confusion
Gastrointestinal: Biliary spasm
Ocular: Blurred vision

Restrictions C-II

Mechanism of Action Binds to opioid receptors throughout the CNS. Once receptor binding occurs, effects are exerted by opening K+ channels and inhibiting Ca++ channels. These mechanisms increase pain threshold, alter pain perception, inhibit ascending pain pathways; short-acting narcotic

Drug Interactions

Cytochrome P450 Effect: Substrate of CYP3A4 (major)

Increased Effect/Toxicity: Additive effect/toxicity with CNS depressants or beta-blockers. May increase response to neuromuscular-blocking agents. CYP3A4 inhibitors may increase the levels/effects of sufentanil; example inhibitors include azole antifungals, clarithromycin, diclofenac, doxycycline, erythromycin, imatinib, isoniazid, nefazodone, nicardipine, propofol, protease inhibitors, quinidine, telithromycin, and verapamil.

Pharmacodynamics/Kinetics

Onset of action: 1-3 minutes
Duration: Dose dependent
Metabolism: Primarily hepatic

Pregnancy Risk Factor C

Sufentanil Citrate see Sufentanil on page 1421
Sular® see Nisoldipine on page 1117
Sulbactam and Ampicillin see Ampicillin and Sulbactam on page 120

Sulconazole (sul KON a zole)

U.S. Brand Names Exelderm®

Canadian Brand Names Exelderm®

Generic Available No

Synonyms Sulconazole Nitrate

Pharmacologic Category Antifungal Agent, Topical

Use Treatment of superficial fungal infections of the skin, including tinea cruris (jock itch), tinea corporis (ringworm), tinea versicolor, and possibly tinea pedis (athlete's foot, cream only)

Local Anesthetic/Vasoconstrictor Precautions No information available to require special precautions

Effects on Dental Treatment No significant effects or complications reported

Common Adverse Effects 1% to 10%:
Dermatologic: Itching
Local: Burning, stinging, redness

Mechanism of Action Substituted imidazole derivative which inhibits metabolic reactions necessary for the synthesis of ergosterol, an essential membrane component. The end result is usually fungistatic; however, sulconazole may act as a fungicide in *Candida albicans* and *Candida parapsilosis* during certain growth phases.

Drug Interactions

Cytochrome P450 Effect: Inhibits CYP1A2 (weak), 2A6 (weak), 2C8/9 (weak), 2C19 (weak), 2D6 (weak), 2E1 (weak), 3A4 (weak)

Pharmacodynamics/Kinetics

Absorption: Topical: ~8.7% percutaneously
Excretion: Primarily urine

Pregnancy Risk Factor C

Sulconazole Nitrate see Sulconazole on page 1422

Sulfabenzamide, Sulfacetamide, and Sulfathiazole
(sul fa BENZ a mide, sul fa SEE ta mide, & sul fa THYE a zole)

Related Information
Sulfacetamide *on page 1423*
U.S. Brand Names V.V.S.®
Generic Available Yes
Synonyms Triple Sulfa
Pharmacologic Category Antibiotic, Vaginal
Use Treatment of *Haemophilus vaginalis* vaginitis
Local Anesthetic/Vasoconstrictor Precautions No information available to require special precautions
Effects on Dental Treatment No significant effects or complications reported
Common Adverse Effects Frequency not defined.
Dermatologic: Pruritus, urticaria, Stevens-Johnson syndrome
Local: Local irritation
Miscellaneous: Allergic reactions
Mechanism of Action Interferes with microbial folic acid synthesis and growth via inhibition of para-aminobenzoic acid metabolism
Pharmacodynamics/Kinetics
Absorption: Absorption from vagina is variable and unreliable
Metabolism: Primarily via acetylation
Excretion: Urine
Pregnancy Risk Factor C (avoid if near term)

Sulfacetamide (sul fa SEE ta mide)

U.S. Brand Names Bleph®-10; Carmol® Scalp; Klaron®; Ovace™
Canadian Brand Names Cetamide™; Diosulf™
Mexican Brand Names Ceta Sulfa®
Generic Available Yes: Ointment, solution
Synonyms Sodium Sulfacetamide; Sulfacetamide Sodium
Pharmacologic Category Antibiotic, Ophthalmic; Antibiotic, Sulfonamide Derivative
Use
Ophthalmic: Treatment and prophylaxis of conjunctivitis due to susceptible organisms; corneal ulcers; adjunctive treatment with systemic sulfonamides for therapy of trachoma
Dermatologic: Scaling dermatosis (seborrheic); bacterial infections of the skin; acne vulgaris
Local Anesthetic/Vasoconstrictor Precautions No information available to require special precautions
Effects on Dental Treatment No significant effects or complications reported
Common Adverse Effects Frequency not defined.
Cardiovascular: Edema
Dermatologic: Burning, erythema, irritation, itching, stinging, Stevens-Johnson syndrome
Ocular (following ophthalmic application): Burning, conjunctivitis, conjunctival hyperemia, corneal ulcers, irritation, stinging
Miscellaneous: Allergic reactions, systemic lupus erythematosus
Mechanism of Action Interferes with bacterial growth by inhibiting bacterial folic acid synthesis through competitive antagonism of PABA
Drug Interactions
Decreased Effect: Silver containing products are incompatible with sulfacetamide solutions.
Pharmacodynamics/Kinetics
Half-life elimination: 7-13 hours
Excretion: When absorbed, primarily urine (as unchanged drug)
Pregnancy Risk Factor C

Sulfacetamide and Fluorometholone
(sul fa SEE ta mide & flure oh METH oh lone)

Related Information
Fluorometholone *on page 674*
Sulfacetamide *on page 1423*
U.S. Brand Names FML-S®
Generic Available No
(Continued)

Sulfacetamide and Fluorometholone *(Continued)*

Synonyms Fluorometholone and Sulfacetamide

Pharmacologic Category Antibiotic/Corticosteroid, Ophthalmic

Use Steroid-responsive inflammatory ocular conditions where infection is present or there is a risk of infection

Local Anesthetic/Vasoconstrictor Precautions No information available to require special precautions

Effects on Dental Treatment No significant effects or complications reported

Mechanism of Action
See individual agents.

Pregnancy Risk Factor C

Sulfacetamide and Prednisolone
(sul fa SEE ta mide & pred NIS oh lone)

Related Information
PrednisoLONE *on page 1268*
Sulfacetamide *on page 1423*

U.S. Brand Names Blephamide®

Canadian Brand Names Blephamide®; Dioptimyd®

Generic Available Yes: Solution

Synonyms Prednisolone and Sulfacetamide

Pharmacologic Category Antibiotic/Corticosteroid, Ophthalmic

Use Steroid-responsive inflammatory ocular conditions where infection is present or there is a risk of infection; ophthalmic suspension may be used as an otic preparation

Local Anesthetic/Vasoconstrictor Precautions No information available to require special precautions

Effects on Dental Treatment No significant effects or complications reported

Mechanism of Action Interferes with bacterial growth by inhibiting bacterial folic acid synthesis through competitive antagonism of PABA; decreases inflammation by suppression of migration of polymorphonuclear leukocytes and reversal of increased capillary permeability; suppresses the immune system by reducing activity and volume of the lymphatic system

Pregnancy Risk Factor C

Sulfacetamide Sodium *see* Sulfacetamide *on page 1423*

SulfaDIAZINE (sul fa DYE a zeen)

Generic Available Yes

Pharmacologic Category Antibiotic, Sulfonamide Derivative

Use Treatment of urinary tract infections and nocardiosis; adjunctive treatment in toxoplasmosis; uncomplicated attack of malaria

Unlabeled/Investigational Use Rheumatic fever prophylaxis

Local Anesthetic/Vasoconstrictor Precautions No information available to require special precautions

Effects on Dental Treatment No significant effects or complications reported

Mechanism of Action Interferes with bacterial growth by inhibiting bacterial folic acid synthesis through competitive antagonism of PABA

Pregnancy Risk Factor B/D (at term)

Sulfadoxine and Pyrimethamine
(sul fa DOKS een & peer i METH a meen)

Related Information
Pyrimethamine *on page 1317*

U.S. Brand Names Fansidar®

Generic Available No

Synonyms Pyrimethamine and Sulfadoxine

Pharmacologic Category Antimalarial Agent

Use Treatment of *Plasmodium falciparum* malaria in patients in whom chloroquine resistance is suspected; malaria prophylaxis for travelers to areas where chloroquine-resistant malaria is endemic

Local Anesthetic/Vasoconstrictor Precautions No information available to require special precautions

Effects on Dental Treatment No significant effects or complications reported

Common Adverse Effects Frequency not defined.
Cardiovascular: Myocarditis (allergic), pericarditis (allergic), periorbital edema

Central nervous system: Ataxia, hallucinations, headache, polyneuritis, seizure

Dermatologic: Photosensitivity, Stevens-Johnson syndrome, erythema multiforme, toxic epidermal necrolysis, rash

Endocrine & metabolic: Thyroid function dysfunction

Gastrointestinal: Anorexia, atrophic glossitis, gastritis, pancreatitis, vomiting

Genitourinary: Crystalluria

Hematologic: Megaloblastic anemia, leukopenia, thrombocytopenia, pancytopenia

Hepatic: Hepatic necrosis, hepatitis

Neuromuscular & skeletal: Tremors

Renal: BUN increased, interstitial nephritis, renal failure, serum creatinine increased

Respiratory: Respiratory failure, alveolitis (resembling eosinophilic or allergic)

Miscellaneous: Anaphylactoid reaction, drug fever, hypersensitivity, Lupus-like syndrome, periarteritis nodosum

Mechanism of Action Sulfadoxine interferes with bacterial folic acid synthesis and growth via competitive inhibition of para-aminiobenzoic acid; pyrimethamine inhibits microbial dihydrofolate reductase, resulting in inhibition of tetrahydrofolic acid synthesis

Drug Interactions

Cytochrome P450 Effect: Pyrimethamine: **Inhibits** CYP2C8/9 (moderate), 2D6 (moderate)

Increased Effect/Toxicity: Effect of oral hypoglycemics (rare, but severe) may occur. Combination with methenamine may result in crystalluria; avoid use. May increase methotrexate-induced bone marrow suppression. NSAIDs and salicylates may increase sulfonamide concentrations. Pyrimethamine may increase the levels/effects of amiodarone, amphetamines, selected beta-blockers, dextromethorphan, fluoxetine, glimepiride, glipizide, lidocaine, mirtazapine, nateglinide, nefazodone, paroxetine, phenytoin, pioglitazone, risperidone, ritonavir, rosiglitazone, sertraline, thioridazine, tricyclic antidepressants, venlafaxine, warfarin, and other CYP2C8/9 and 2D6 substrates.

Decreased Effect: Cyclosporine concentrations may be decreased; monitor levels and renal function. PABA (para-aminobenzoic acid - may be found in some vitamin supplements): interferes with the antibacterial activity of sulfonamides; avoid concurrent use. Pyrimethamine may decrease the levels/effects of CYP2D6 prodrug substrates (eg, codeine, hydrocodone, oxycodone, tramadol).

Pharmacodynamics/Kinetics

Absorption: Well absorbed

Distribution: Sulfadoxine: Well distributed like other sulfonamides; Pyrimethamine: Widely distributed, mainly in blood cells, kidneys, lungs, liver, and spleen

Metabolism: Pyrimethamine: Hepatic; Sulfadoxine: None

Half-life elimination: Pyrimethamine: 80-95 hours; Sulfadoxine: 5-8 days

Time to peak, serum: 2-8 hours

Excretion: Urine (as unchanged drug and several unidentified metabolites)

Pregnancy Risk Factor C/D (at term)

Sulfamethoxazole and Trimethoprim
(sul fa meth OKS a zole & trye METH oh prim)

Related Information
Sexually-Transmitted Diseases *on page 1674*
Trimethoprim *on page 1538*

U.S. Brand Names Bactrim™; Bactrim™ DS; Septra®; Septra® DS

Canadian Brand Names Apo-Sulfatrim®; Novo-Trimel; Novo-Trimel D.S.; Nu-Cotrimox; Septra® Injection

Generic Available Yes

Synonyms Co-Trimoxazole; SMZ-TMP; Sulfatrim; TMP-SMZ; Trimethoprim and Sulfamethoxazole

Pharmacologic Category Antibiotic, Miscellaneous; Antibiotic, Sulfonamide Derivative

Use
Oral treatment of urinary tract infections due to *E. coli*, *Klebsiella* and *Enterobacter* sp, *M. morganii*, *P. mirabilis* and *P. vulgaris*; acute otitis media in children; acute exacerbations of chronic bronchitis in adults due to susceptible strains of *H. influenzae* or *S. pneumoniae*; treatment and prophylaxis of *Pneumocystis carinii* pneumonitis (PCP); traveler's diarrhea due to enterotoxigenic *E. coli*; treatment of enteritis caused by *Shigella flexneri* or *Shigella sonnei*
(Continued)

Sulfamethoxazole and Trimethoprim *(Continued)*

I.V. treatment or severe or complicated infections when oral therapy is not feasible, for documented PCP, empiric treatment of PCP in immune compromised patients; treatment of documented or suspected shigellosis, typhoid fever, *Nocardia asteroides* infection, or other infections caused by susceptible bacteria

Unlabeled/Investigational Use Cholera and *Salmonella*-type infections and nocardiosis; chronic prostatitis; as prophylaxis in neutropenic patients with *P. carinii* infections, in leukemics, and in patients following renal transplantation, to decrease incidence of PCP; treatment of *Cyclospora* infection, typhoid fever, *Nocardia asteroides* infection

Local Anesthetic/Vasoconstrictor Precautions No information available to require special precautions

Effects on Dental Treatment No significant effects or complications reported

Common Adverse Effects The most common adverse reactions include gastrointestinal upset (nausea, vomiting, anorexia) and dermatologic reactions (rash or urticaria). Rare, life-threatening reactions have been associated with co-trimoxazole, including severe dermatologic reactions and hepatotoxic reactions. Most other reactions listed are rare, however, frequency cannot be accurately estimated.

Cardiovascular: Allergic myocarditis

Central nervous system: Confusion, depression, hallucinations, seizure, aseptic meningitis, peripheral neuritis, fever, ataxia, kernicterus in neonates

Dermatologic: Rashes, pruritus, urticaria, photosensitivity; rare reactions include erythema multiforme, Stevens-Johnson syndrome, toxic epidermal necrolysis, exfoliative dermatitis, and Henoch-Schönlein purpura

Endocrine & metabolic: Hyperkalemia (generally at high dosages), hypoglycemia

Gastrointestinal: Nausea, vomiting, anorexia, stomatitis, diarrhea, pseudomembranous colitis, pancreatitis

Hematologic: Thrombocytopenia, megaloblastic anemia, granulocytopenia, eosinophilia, pancytopenia, aplastic anemia, methemoglobinemia, hemolysis (with G6PD deficiency), agranulocytosis

Hepatic: Hepatotoxicity (including hepatitis, cholestasis, and hepatic necrosis), hyperbilirubinemia, transaminases increased

Neuromuscular & skeletal: Arthralgia, myalgia, rhabdomyolysis

Renal: Interstitial nephritis, crystalluria, renal failure, nephrotoxicity (in association with cyclosporine), diuresis

Respiratory: Cough, dyspnea, pulmonary infiltrates

Miscellaneous: Serum sickness, angioedema, periarteritis nodosa (rare), systemic lupus erythematosus (rare)

Dosage Dosage recommendations are based on the trimethoprim component. Double-strength tablets are equivalent to sulfamethoxazole 800 mg and trimethoprim 160 mg.

Children >2 months:

General dosing guidelines:

Mild-to-moderate infections: Oral: 8-12 mg TMP/kg/day in divided doses every 12 hours

Serious infection:

Oral: 20 mg TMP/kg/day in divided doses every 6 hours

I.V.: 8-12 mg TMP/kg/day in divided doses every 6 hours

Acute otitis media: Oral: 8 mg TMP/kg/day in divided doses every 12 hours for 10 days

Urinary tract infection:

Treatment:

Oral: 6-12 mg TMP/kg/day in divided doses every 12 hours

I.V.: 8-10 mg TMP/kg/day in divided doses every 6, 8, or 12 hours for up to 4 days with serious infections

Prophylaxis: Oral: 2 mg TMP/kg/dose daily or 5 mg TMP/kg/dose twice weekly

Pneumocystis:

Treatment: Oral, I.V.: 15-20 mg TMP/kg/day in divided doses every 6-8 hours

Prophylaxis: Oral, 150 mg TMP/m²/day in divided doses every 12 hours for 3 days/week; dose should not exceed trimethoprim 320 mg and sulfamethoxazole 1600 mg daily

Alternative prophylaxis dosing schedules include:

150 mg TMP/m²/day as a single daily dose 3 times/week on consecutive days

or

150 mg TMP/m²/day in divided doses every 12 hours administered 7 days/week

or

150 mg TMP/m²/day in divided doses every 12 hours administered 3 times/week on alternate days

Shigellosis:
  Oral: 8 mg TMP/kg/day in divided doses every 12 hours for 5 days
  I.V.: 8-10 mg TMP/kg/day in divided doses every 6, 8, or 12 hours for up to 5 days

Cyclospora (unlabeled use): Oral, I.V.: 5 mg TMP/kg twice daily for 7-10 days

Adults:
  Urinary tract infection:
    Oral: One double-strength tablet every 12 hours
      Duration of therapy: Uncomplicated: 3-5 days; Complicated: 7-10 days
        Pyelonephritis: 14 days
        Prostatitis: Acute: 2 weeks; Chronic: 2-3 months
    I.V.: 8-10 mg TMP/kg/day in divided doses every 6, 8, or 12 hours for up to 14 days with severe infections

  Chronic bronchitis: Oral: One double-strength tablet every 12 hours for 10-14 days

  Meningitis (bacterial): I.V.: 10-20 mg TMP/kg/day in divided doses every 6-12 hours

  Shigellosis:
    Oral: One double strength tablet every 12 hours for 5 days
    I.V.: 8-10 mg TMP/kg/day in divided doses every 6, 8, or 12 hours for up to 5 days

  Travelers' diarrhea: Oral: One double strength tablet every 12 hours for 5 days

  Sepsis: I.V.: 20 TMP/kg/day divided every 6 hours

  Pneumocystis carinii:
    Prophylaxis: Oral: 1 double strength tablet daily or 3 times/week
    Treatment: Oral, I.V.: 15-20 mg TMP/kg/day in 3-4 divided doses

  Cyclospora (unlabeled use): Oral, I.V.: 160 mg TMP twice daily for 7-10 days

  Nocardia (unlabeled use): Oral, I.V.:
    Cutaneous infections: 5 mg TMP/kg/day in 2 divided doses
    Severe infections (pulmonary/cerebral): 10-15 mg TMP/kg/day in 2-3 divided doses. Treatment duration is controversial; an average of 7 months has been reported.
    Note: Therapy for severe infection may be initiated I.V. and converted to oral therapy (frequently converted to approximate dosages of oral solid dosage forms: 2 DS tablets every 8-12 hours). Although not widely available, sulfonamide levels should be considered in patients with questionable absorption, at risk for dose-related toxicity, or those with poor therapeutic response.

Dosing adjustment in renal impairment: Oral, I.V.:
  Cl$_{cr}$ 15-30 mL/minute: Administer 50% of recommended dose
  Cl$_{cr}$ <15 mL/minute: Use is not recommended

Mechanism of Action Sulfamethoxazole interferes with bacterial folic acid synthesis and growth via inhibition of dihydrofolic acid formation from para-aminobenzoic acid; trimethoprim inhibits dihydrofolic acid reduction to tetrahydrofolate resulting in sequential inhibition of enzymes of the folic acid pathway

Contraindications Hypersensitivity to any sulfa drug, trimethoprim, or any component of the formulation; porphyria; megaloblastic anemia due to folate deficiency; infants <2 months of age; marked hepatic damage; severe renal disease; pregnancy (at term)

Warnings/Precautions Use with caution in patients with G6PD deficiency, impaired renal or hepatic function or potential folate deficiency (malnourished, chronic anticonvulsant therapy, or elderly); maintain adequate hydration to prevent crystalluria; adjust dosage in patients with renal impairment. Injection vehicle contains benzyl alcohol and sodium metabisulfite.

Chemical similarities are present among sulfonamides, sulfonylureas, carbonic anhydrase inhibitors, thiazides, and loop diuretics (except ethacrynic acid). Use in patients with sulfonamide allergy is specifically contraindicated in product labeling, however, a risk of cross-reaction exists in patients with allergy to any of these compounds; avoid use when previous reaction has been severe.

Fatalities associated with severe reactions including Stevens-Johnson syndrome, toxic epidermal necrolysis, hepatic necrosis, agranulocytosis, aplastic anemia and other blood dyscrasias; discontinue use at first sign of rash. Elderly patients appear at greater risk for more severe adverse reactions. May cause hypoglycemia, particularly in malnourished, or patients with renal or (Continued)

Sulfamethoxazole and Trimethoprim *(Continued)*

hepatic impairment. Use with caution in patients with porphyria or thyroid dysfunction. Slow acetylators may be more prone to adverse reactions. Caution in patients with allergies or asthma. May cause hyperkalemia (associated with high doses of trimethoprim). Incidence of adverse effects appears to be increased in patients with AIDS.

Drug Interactions

Cytochrome P450 Effect:

Sulfamethoxazole: **Substrate** of CYP2C8/9 (major), 3A4 (minor); **Inhibits** CYP2C8/9 (moderate)

Trimethoprim: **Substrate** (major) of CYP2C8/9, 3A4; **Inhibits** CYP2C8/9 (moderate)

Increased Effect/Toxicity: Sulfamethoxazole/trimethoprim may increase toxicity of methotrexate. Sulfamethoxazole/trimethoprim may increase the serum levels of procainamide. Concurrent therapy with pyrimethamine (in doses >25 mg/week) may increase the risk of megaloblastic anemia. Sulfamethoxazole/trimethoprim may increase the levels/effects of amiodarone, fluoxetine, glimepiride, glipizide, nateglinide, phenytoin, pioglitazone, rosiglitazone, sertraline, warfarin, and other CYP2C8/9 substrates.

ACE Inhibitors, angiotensin receptor antagonists, or potassium-sparing diuretics may increase the risk of hyperkalemia. Concurrent use with cyclosporine may result in an increased risk of nephrotoxicity when used with sulfamethoxazole/trimethoprim. Trimethoprim may increase the serum concentration of dapsone.

Decreased Effect: The levels/effects of sulfamethoxazole may be decreased by carbamazepine, phenobarbital, phenytoin, rifampin, rifapentine, secobarbital, and other CYP2C8/9 inducers. Although occasionally recommended to limit or reverse hematologic toxicity of high-dose sulfamethoxazole/trimethoprim, concurrent use has been associated with a decreased effectiveness in treating *Pneumocystis carinii*.

Ethanol/Nutrition/Herb Interactions Herb/Nutraceutical: Avoid dong quai, St John's wort (may also cause photosensitization).

Dietary Considerations Should be taken with 8 oz of water on empty stomach.

Pharmacodynamics/Kinetics

Absorption: Oral: Almost completely, 90% to 100%

Protein binding: SMX: 68%, TMP: 45%

Metabolism: SMX: N-acetylated and glucuronidated; TMP: Metabolized to oxide and hydroxylated metabolites

Half-life elimination: SMX: 9 hours, TMP: 6-17 hours; both are prolonged in renal failure

Time to peak, serum: Within 1-4 hours

Excretion: Both are excreted in urine as metabolites and unchanged drug

Effects of aging on the pharmacokinetics of both agents has been variable; increase in half-life and decreases in clearance have been associated with reduced creatinine clearance

Pregnancy Risk Factor C/D (at term - expert analysis)

Dosage Forms Note: The 5:1 ratio (SMX:TMP) remains constant in all dosage forms. **INJ, solution:** Sulfamethoxazole 80 mg and trimethoprim 16 mg per mL (5 mL, 10 mL, 30 mL). **SUSP, oral:** Sulfamethoxazole 200 mg and trimethoprim 40 mg per 5 mL (480 mL); (Septra®): Sulfamethoxazole 200 mg and trimethoprim 40 mg per 5 mL (480 mL). **TAB:** Sulfamethoxazole 400 mg and trimethoprim 80 mg; (Bactrim™, Septra®): Sulfamethoxazole 400 mg and trimethoprim 80 mg. **TAB, double strength:** Sulfamethoxazole 800 mg and trimethoprim 160 mg; (Bactrim™ DS, Septra® DS): Sulfamethoxazole 800 mg and trimethoprim 160 mg

Sulfamylon® *see* Mafenide *on page 959*

Sulfasalazine *(sul fa SAL a zeen)*

U.S. Brand Names Azulfidine®; Azulfidine® EN-tabs®; Sulfazine; Sulfazine EC

Canadian Brand Names Alti-Sulfasalazine; Salazopyrin®; Salazopyrin En-Tabs®

Generic Available Yes

Synonyms Salicylazosulfapyridine

Pharmacologic Category 5-Aminosalicylic Acid Derivative

Use Management of ulcerative colitis; enteric coated tablets are also used for rheumatoid arthritis (including juvenile rheumatoid arthritis) in patients who inadequately respond to analgesics and NSAIDs

Unlabeled/Investigational Use Ankylosing spondylitis, collagenous colitis, Crohn's disease, psoriasis, psoriatic arthritis, juvenile chronic arthritis

Local Anesthetic/Vasoconstrictor Precautions No information available to require special precautions

Effects on Dental Treatment No significant effects or complications reported

Common Adverse Effects

>10%:

Central nervous system: Headache (33%)

Dermatologic: Photosensitivity

Gastrointestinal: Anorexia, nausea, vomiting, diarrhea (33%), gastric distress

Genitourinary: Reversible oligospermia (33%)

<3%:

Dermatologic: Urticaria/pruritus (<3%)

Hematologic: Hemolytic anemia (<3%), Heinz body anemia (<3%)

Additional events reported with sulfonamides and/or 5-ASA derivatives: Cholestatic jaundice, eosinophilia pneumonitis, erythema multiforme, fibrosing alveolitis, hepatic necrosis, Kawasaki-like syndrome, SLE-like syndrome, pericarditis, seizure, transverse myelitis

Mechanism of Action Acts locally in the colon to decrease the inflammatory response and systemically interferes with secretion by inhibiting prostaglandin synthesis

Drug Interactions

Increased Effect/Toxicity: Sulfasalazine may increase hydantoin levels. Effects of thiopental, oral hypoglycemics, and oral anticoagulants may be increased. Sulfasalazine may increase the risk of myelosuppression with azathioprine, mercaptopurine, or thioguanine (due to TPMT inhibition); may also increase the toxicity of methotrexate. Risk of thrombocytopenia may be increased with thiazide diuretics. Concurrent methenamine may increase risk of crystalluria.

Decreased Effect: Decreased effect with iron, digoxin and PABA or PABA metabolites of drugs (eg, procaine, proparacaine, tetracaine).

Pharmacodynamics/Kinetics

Absorption: 10% to 15% as unchanged drug from small intestine

Distribution: Small amounts enter feces and breast milk

Metabolism: Via colonic intestinal flora to sulfapyridine and 5-aminosalicylic acid (5-ASA); following absorption, sulfapyridine undergoes N-acetylation and ring hydroxylation while 5-ASA undergoes N-acetylation

Half-life elimination: 5.7-10 hours

Excretion: Primarily urine (as unchanged drug, components, and acetylated metabolites)

Pregnancy Risk Factor B/D (at term)

Sulfatrim see Sulfamethoxazole and Trimethoprim on page 1425

Sulfazine see Sulfasalazine on page 1428

Sulfazine EC see Sulfasalazine on page 1428

SulfiSOXAZOLE (sul fi SOKS a zole)

U.S. Brand Names Gantrisin®

Canadian Brand Names Novo-Soxazole; Sulfizole®

Generic Available Yes: Tablet

Synonyms Sulfisoxazole Acetyl; Sulphafurazole

Pharmacologic Category Antibiotic, Sulfonamide Derivative

Use Treatment of urinary tract infections, otitis media, *Chlamydia*; nocardiosis

Local Anesthetic/Vasoconstrictor Precautions No information available to require special precautions

Effects on Dental Treatment No significant effects or complications reported

Mechanism of Action Interferes with bacterial growth by inhibiting bacterial folic acid synthesis through competitive antagonism of PABA

Pregnancy Risk Factor B/D (near term)

Sulfisoxazole Acetyl see SulfiSOXAZOLE on page 1429

Sulfisoxazole and Erythromycin see Erythromycin and Sulfisoxazole on page 568

Sulfonated Phenolics in Aqueous Solution
(SUL fo NATE ed fe NOL iks in AYE kwee us so LU shun)

U.S. Brand Names Debacterol®

Generic Available No

Pharmacologic Category Aphthous Ulcer Treatment Agent

Dental Use Therapeutic cauterization in the treatment of oral mucosal lesions (aphthous stomatitis, gingivitis, moderate to severe periodontitis)

(Continued)

Sulfonated Phenolics in Aqueous Solution *(Continued)*

Local Anesthetic/Vasoconstrictor Precautions No information available to require special precautions

Effects on Dental Treatment No significant effects or complications reported

Significant Adverse Effects Frequency not defined: Local: Irritation upon administration

Dental Usual Dosing Apply applicator tip to the lesion as directed (see Dental Comment)

Mechanism of Action Semiviscous, chemical cautery agent which provides controlled, focal debridement and sterilization of necrotic tissues; relieving pain, sealing damaged tissue, and providing local antiseptic action

Contraindications For external use only

Warnings/Precautions For topical use only. Debacterol® is not intended for the treatment of cold sores and fever blisters. Prolonged use of Debacterol® on normal tissue should be avoided. If ingested, do not induce vomiting; immediately dilute with milk or water and get medical help or contact a Poison Control Center. If eye exposure occurs, immediately remove contact lenses, irrigate eyes for at least 15 minutes with lukewarm water, and contact a physician. Safety and efficacy in children <12 years have not been established.

Pregnancy Risk Factor C

Breast-Feeding Considerations Unknown if excreted in breast milk; use with caution

Dosage Forms Debacterol® single-use applicator package: Prefilled cotton swab applicator and drying cotton swab: 0.2 mL (30% sulfuric acid, 22% sulfonated phenolics in aqueous solution) [also supplied as one box of 12 single-use applicator packages]

Dental Comment Prior to application/treatment, the ulcerated mucosal area should be thoroughly dried using the drying swab. After drying lesion, hold applicator "swab" with the colored ring end up. Bend the colored ring tip gently to the side until it snaps to release liquid inside. Liquid flows down into the white tip applicator. Apply the Debacterol® coated applicator tip to the dried ulcer area for at least 5 seconds, but no more than 10 seconds. Use rolling motion to completely cover the entire ulcer bed and ulcer rim. A "stinging" sensation is experienced immediately upon application. Debacterol® will not harm normal mucosa when used as directed. Thoroughly rinse out the mouth with water and spit out the rinse water. If the ulcer pain returns shortly after rinsing with water, it is an indication that some part of the ulcer was not covered. Repeat application one more time following directions above. One application per ulcer is usually sufficient. If excess irritation occurs during use, a rinse with sodium bicarbonate (baking soda) solution will neutralize the reaction (use 0.5 teaspoon in 120 mL water). It is not recommended that more than one Debacterol® treatment session be performed on an individual ulcer.

Selected Readings

Rhodus NL and Bereuter J, "An Evaluation of a Chemical Cautery Agent and an Anti-inflammatory Ointment for the Treatment of Recurrent Aphthous Stomatitis: A Pilot Study," *Quintessence Int,* 1998, 29(12):769-73.

Sulindac *(sul IN dak)*

Related Information

Rheumatoid Arthritis, Osteoarthritis, and Osteoporosis *on page 1668*
Temporomandibular Dysfunction (TMD) *on page 1724*

U.S. Brand Names Clinoril®

Canadian Brand Names Apo-Sulin®; Novo-Sundac; Nu-Sundac

Generic Available Yes

Pharmacologic Category Nonsteroidal Anti-inflammatory Drug (NSAID), Oral

Use Management of inflammatory disease, osteoarthritis, rheumatoid disorders, acute gouty arthritis, ankylosing spondylitis, bursitis/tendonitis of shoulder

Local Anesthetic/Vasoconstrictor Precautions No information available to require special precautions

Effects on Dental Treatment NSAID formulations are known to reversibly decrease platelet aggregation via mechanisms different than observed with aspirin. The dentist should be aware of the potential of abnormal coagulation. Caution should also be exercised in the use of NSAIDs in patients already on anticoagulant therapy with drugs such as warfarin (Coumadin®).

Common Adverse Effects

1% to 10%:

Cardiovascular: Edema (1% to 3%)

Central nervous system: Dizziness (3% to 9%), headache(3% to 9%), nervousness (1% to 3%)

Dermatologic: Rash (3% to 9%), pruritus (1% to 3%)

Gastrointestinal: Gastrointestinal: GI pain (10%), constipation (3% to 9%), diarrhea (3% to 9%), dyspepsia (3% to 9%), nausea (3% to 9%), abdominal cramps (1% to 3%), anorexia (1% to 3%), flatulence (1% to 3%), vomiting (1% to 3%)

Otic: Tinnitus (1% to 3%)

Restrictions A medication guide should be dispensed with each prescription. A template for the required MedGuide can be found on the FDA website at: http://www.fda.gov/medwatch/SAFETY/2005/safety05.htm#NSAID

Dosage Oral:

Children: Dose not established

Adults: **Note:** Maximum daily dose: 400 mg

Osteoarthritis, rheumatoid arthritis, ankylosing spondylitis: 150 mg twice/daily

Bursitis/tendonitis: 200 mg twice daily; usual treatment: 7-14 days

Acute gouty arthritis: 200 mg twice daily; usual treatment: 7 days

Dosing adjustment in renal impairment: Not recommended with advanced renal impairment; if required, decrease dose and monitor closely

Dosing adjustment in hepatic impairment: Dose reduction is necessary; discontinue if abnormal liver function tests occur

Mechanism of Action Inhibits prostaglandin synthesis by decreasing the activity of the enzyme, cyclooxygenase, which results in decreased formation of prostaglandin precursors

Contraindications Hypersensitivity to sulindac, aspirin, other NSAIDs, or any component of the formulation; perioperative pain in the setting of coronary artery bypass surgery (CABG); pregnancy (3rd trimester)

Warnings/Precautions NSAIDs are associated with an increased risk of adverse cardiovascular events, including MI, stroke, and new onset or worsening of pre-existing hypertension. Use caution with fluid retention, CHF or hypertension. Use of NSAIDs can compromise existing renal function. Sulindac is not recommended for patients with advanced renal disease. Use caution in patients with renal lithiasis; sulindac metabolites have been reported as components of renal stones. Use hydration in patients with a history of renal stones. Use with caution in patients with decreased hepatic function. May require dosage adjustment in hepatic dysfunction; sulfide and sulfone metabolites may accumulate.

NSAIDs may increase risk of gastrointestinal irritation, ulceration, bleeding, and perforation. Use the lowest effective dose for the shortest duration of time, consistent with individual patient goals, to reduce risk of cardiovascular or GI adverse events.

NSAIDs may cause serious skin adverse events including exfoliative dermatitis, Stevens-Johnson syndrome (SJS) and toxic epidermal necrolysis (TEN). Anaphylactoid reactions may occur. Do not use in patients who experience bronchospasm, asthma, rhinitis, or urticaria with NSAID or aspirin therapy.

Withhold for at least 4-6 half-lives prior to surgical or dental procedures.

Drug Interactions

Increased Effect/Toxicity: Sulindac may increase effect/toxicity of anticoagulants (bleeding), antiplatelet agents (bleeding), aminoglycosides, bisphosphonates (GI irritation), corticosteroids (GI irritation), cyclosporine (nephrotoxicity), lithium, methotrexate, pemetrexed, treprostinil (bleeding), vancomycin.

Decreased Effect: May reduce effect of some diuretics and antihypertensive effect of beta-blockers, ACE inhibitors, angiotensin II inhibitors, hydralazine. Dimethyl sulfoxide may decrease active metabolite of sulindac; combination may cause peripheral neuropathy. Cholestyramine (and other bile acid sequestrants) may decrease the absorption of NSAIDs; separate by at least 2 hours.

Ethanol/Nutrition/Herb Interactions

Ethanol: Avoid ethanol (may enhance gastric mucosal irritation).

Food: Food may decrease the rate but not the extent of oral absorption. The therapeutic effect of sulindac may be decreased if taken with food.

Herb/Nutraceutical: Avoid alfalfa, anise, bilberry, bladderwrack, bromelain, cat's claw, celery, coleus, cordyceps, dong quai, evening primrose, feverfew, fenugreek, garlic, ginger, ginkgo biloba, red clover, horse chestnut, grapeseed, green tea, ginseng, guggul, horse chestnut seed, horseradish, licorice, prickly ash, red clover, reishi, SAMe, sweet clover, turmeric, white willow (all have additional antiplatelet activity).

Dietary Considerations Drug may cause GI upset, bleeding, ulceration, perforation; take with food or milk to minimize GI upset.

Pharmacodynamics/Kinetics

Onset of action: Analgesic: ~1 hour

Duration: 12-24 hours

Absorption: 90%

(Continued)

Sulindac *(Continued)*

Metabolism: Hepatic; prodrug metabolized to sulfide metabolite (active) for therapeutic effects and to sulfone metabolites (inactive)

Half-life elimination: Parent drug: ~8 hours; Active metabolite: ~16 hours

Excretion: Urine (50%, primarily as inactive metabolites); feces (25%, primarily as metabolites)

Pregnancy Risk Factor C/D (3rd trimester)

Dosage Forms TAB: 150 mg, 200 mg; (Clinoril®): 200 mg

Sulphafurazole *see* SulfiSOXAZOLE *on page 1429*

Sumatriptan *(soo ma TRIP tan SUKS i nate)*

U.S. Brand Names Imitrex®

Canadian Brand Names Apo-Sumatriptan®; Gen-Sumatriptan; Imitrex®; Imitrex® DF; Novo-Sumatriptan; PMS-Sumatriptan; Sandoz-Sumatriptan

Mexican Brand Names Imigran®

Generic Available No

Synonyms Sumatriptan Succinate

Pharmacologic Category Serotonin 5-HT$_{1D}$ Receptor Agonist

Use

Oral, SubQ: Acute treatment of migraine with or without aura

SubQ: Acute treatment of cluster headache episodes

Local Anesthetic/Vasoconstrictor Precautions No information available to require special precautions

Effects on Dental Treatment Key adverse event(s) related to dental treatment: Bad taste, hyposalivation (tablet), mouth/tongue discomfort (injection).

Common Adverse Effects

Injection:

>10%:

Central nervous system: Dizziness (12%), warm/hot sensation (11%)

Local: Pain at injection site (59%)

Neuromuscular & skeletal: Paresthesia (14%)

1% to 10%:

Cardiovascular: Chest pain/tightness/heaviness/pressure (2% to 3%), hyper-/hypotension (1%)

Central nervous system: Burning (7%), feeling of heaviness (7%), flushing (7%), pressure sensation (7%), feeling of tightness (5%), drowsiness (3%), malaise/fatigue (1%), feeling strange (2%), headache (2%), tight feeling in head (2%), cold sensation (1%), anxiety (1%)

Gastrointestinal: Abdominal discomfort (1%), dysphagia (1%)

Neuromuscular & skeletal: Neck, throat, and jaw pain/tightness/pressure (2% to 5%), mouth/tongue discomfort (5%), weakness (5%), myalgia (2%); muscle cramps (1%), numbness (5%)

Ocular: Vision alterations (1%)

Respiratory: Throat discomfort (3%), nasal disorder/discomfort (2%)

Miscellaneous: Diaphoresis (2%)

Nasal spray:

>10%: Gastrointestinal: Bad taste (13% to 24%), nausea (11% to 13%), vomiting (11% to 13%)

1% to 10%:

Central nervous system: Dizziness (1% to 2%)

Respiratory: Nasal disorder/discomfort (2% to 4%), throat discomfort (1% to 2%)

Tablet:

1% to 10%:

Cardiovascular: Chest pain/tightness/heaviness/pressure (1% to 2%), hyper-/hypotension (1%), palpitation (1%), syncope (1%)

Central nervous system: Burning (1%), dizziness (>1%), drowsiness (>1%), malaise/fatigue (2% to 3%), headache (>1%), nonspecified pain (1% to 2%, placebo 1%), vertigo (<1% to 2%), migraine (>1%), sleepiness (>1%)

Gastrointestinal: Diarrhea (1%), nausea (>1%), vomiting (>1%), hyposalivation (>1%)

Genitourinary: Hematuria (1%)

Hematologic: Hemolytic anemia (1%)

Neuromuscular & skeletal: Neck, throat, and jaw pain/tightness/pressure (2% to 3%), paresthesia (3% to 5%), myalgia (1%), numbness (1%)

Otic: Ear hemorrhage (1%), hearing loss (1%), sensitivity to noise (1%), tinnitus (1%)

Respiratory: Allergic rhinitis (1%), dyspnea (1%), nasal inflammation (1%), nose/throat hemorrhage (1%), sinusitis (1%), upper respiratory inflammation (1%)

Miscellaneous: Hypersensitivity reactions (1%), nonspecified pressure/tightness/heaviness (1% to 3%, placebo 2%); warm/cold sensation (2% to 3%, placebo 2%)

Dosage Adults:

Oral: A single dose of 25 mg, 50 mg, or 100 mg (taken with fluids). If a satisfactory response has not been obtained at 2 hours, a second dose may be administered. Results from clinical trials show that initial doses of 50 mg and 100 mg are more effective than doses of 25 mg, and that 100 mg doses do not provide a greater effect than 50 mg and may have increased incidence of side effects. Although doses of up to 300 mg/day have been studied, the total daily dose should not exceed 200 mg. The safety of treating an average of >4 headaches in a 30-day period have not been established.

Intranasal: A single dose of 5 mg, 10 mg, or 20 mg administered in one nostril. A 10 mg dose may be achieved by administering a single 5 mg dose in each nostril. If headache returns, the dose may be repeated once after 2 hours, not to exceed a total daily dose of 40 mg. The safety of treating an average of >4 headaches in a 30-day period has not been established.

SubQ: Up to 6 mg; if side effects are dose-limiting, lower doses may be used. A second injection may be administered at least 1 hour after the initial dose, but not more than 2 injections in a 24-hour period.

Dosage adjustment in renal impairment: Dosage adjustment not necessary

Dosage adjustment in hepatic impairment: Bioavailability of oral sumatriptan is increased with liver disease. If treatment is needed, do not exceed single doses of 50 mg. The nasal spray has not been studied in patients with hepatic impairment, however, because the spray does not undergo first-pass metabolism, levels would not be expected to alter. Use of all dosage forms is contraindicated with severe hepatic impairment.

Mechanism of Action Selective agonist for serotonin (5-HT$_{1D}$ receptor) in cranial arteries to cause vasoconstriction and reduces sterile inflammation associated with antidromic neuronal transmission correlating with relief of migraine

Contraindications Hypersensitivity to sumatriptan or any component of the formulation; patients with ischemic heart disease or signs or symptoms of ischemic heart disease (including Prinzmetal's angina, angina pectoris, myocardial infarction, silent myocardial ischemia); cerebrovascular syndromes (including strokes, transient ischemic attacks); peripheral vascular syndromes (including ischemic bowel disease); uncontrolled hypertension; use within 24 hours of ergotamine derivatives; use within 24 hours of another 5-HT$_1$ agonist; concurrent administration or within 2 weeks of discontinuing an MAO inhibitor, specifically MAO type A inhibitors; management of hemiplegic or basilar migraine; prophylactic treatment of migraine; severe hepatic impairment; not for I.V. administration

Warnings/Precautions

Sumatriptan is indicated only in patients ≥18 years of age with a clear diagnosis of migraine or cluster headache.

Cardiac events (coronary artery vasospasm, transient ischemia, myocardial infarction, ventricular tachycardia/fibrillation, cardiac arrest and death), cerebral/subarachnoid hemorrhage, and stroke have been reported with 5-HT$_1$ agonist administration.

Do not give to patients with risk factors for CAD until a cardiovascular evaluation has been performed; if evaluation is satisfactory, the healthcare provider should administer the first dose and cardiovascular status should be periodically evaluated.

Significant elevation in blood pressure, including hypertensive crisis, has also been reported on rare occasions in patients with and without a history of hypertension. Vasospasm-related reactions have been reported other than coronary artery vasospasm. Peripheral vascular ischemia and colonic ischemia with abdominal pain and bloody diarrhea have occurred.

Use with caution in patients with a history of seizure disorder or in patients with a lowered seizure threshold. Safety and efficacy in pediatric patients have not been established.

Drug Interactions

Increased Effect/Toxicity: Increased toxicity with ergot-containing drugs, avoid use, wait 24 hours from last ergot containing drug (dihydroergotamine, or methysergide) before administering sumatriptan. MAO inhibitors decrease clearance of sumatriptan increasing the risk of systemic sumatriptan toxic

(Continued)

Sumatriptan *(Continued)*

effects. Sumatriptan may enhance CNS toxic effects when taken with selective serotonin reuptake inhibitors (SSRIs) like fluoxetine, fluvoxamine, paroxetine, or sertraline. **Note:** Use cautiously in patients receiving concomitant medications that can lower the seizure threshold.

Pharmacodynamics/Kinetics

Onset of action: ~30 minutes

Distribution: V_d: 2.4 L/kg

Protein binding: 14% to 21%

Metabolism: Hepatic, primarily via MAO-A isoenzyme

Bioavailability: SubQ: 97% ± 16% of that following I.V. injection; Oral: 15%

Half-life elimination: Injection, tablet: 2.5 hours; Nasal spray: 2 hours

Time to peak, serum: 5-20 minutes

Excretion:

Injection: Urine (38% as indole acetic acid metabolite, 22% as unchanged drug)

Nasal spray: Urine (42% as indole acetic acid metabolite, 3% as unchanged drug)

Tablet: Urine (60% as indole acetic acid metabolite, 3% as unchanged drug); feces (40%)

Pregnancy Risk Factor C

Dosage Forms Note: Strength expressed as sumatriptan base. **INJ, solution:** 8 mg/mL (0.5 mL); 12 mg/mL (0.5 mL). **SOLN, intranasal spray:** 5 mg (100 µL unit dose spray device); 20 mg (100 µL unit dose spray device). **TAB:** 25 mg, 50 mg, 100 mg

Sumatriptan Succinate *see* Sumatriptan *on page 1432*

Summer's Eve® Medicated Douche [OTC] *see* Povidone-Iodine *on page 1262*

Summer's Eve® SpecialCare™ Medicated Anti-Itch Cream [OTC] *see* Hydrocortisone *on page 793*

Sumycin® *see* Tetracycline *on page 1467*

Sunitinib (su NIT e nib)

U.S. Brand Names Sutent®

Generic Available No

Synonyms NSC736511; SU11248; Sunitinib Maleate

Pharmacologic Category Antineoplastic Agent, Tyrosine Kinase Inhibitor; Vascular Endothelial Growth Factor (VEGF) Inhibitor

Use Treatment of gastrointestinal stromal tumor (GIST) following failure of or intolerance to imatinib; treatment of advanced renal cell cancer (RCC)

Unlabeled/Investigational Use Treatment of acute myeloid leukemia (AML)

Local Anesthetic/Vasoconstrictor Precautions No information available to require special precautions

Effects on Dental Treatment Key adverse event(s) related to dental treatment: Mucositis/stomatitis (29% to 53%), taste perversion (21% to 43%), oral pain (6%)

Common Adverse Effects

>10%:

Cardiovascular: Hypertension (15% to 28%), edema (peripheral 17%)

Central nervous system: Fatigue (42% to 74%), headache (13% to 25%), fever (15% to 18%), dizziness (16%)

Dermatologic: Rash (14% to 38%), hyperpigmentation (30% to 33%), dry skin (17%), hair color changes (7% to 17%), hand-foot syndrome (12% to 14%), alopecia (5% to 12%)

Endocrine & metabolic: Hyperuricemia (10% to 15%), hypokalemia (12%), dehydration (11%)

Gastrointestinal: Diarrhea (40% to 55%), nausea (31% to 54%), mucositis/stomatitis (29% to 53%), dyspepsia (46%), taste perversion (21% to 43%), vomiting (24% to 37%), constipation (20% to 34%), anorexia (31% to 33%), abdominal pain (20% to 33%), hyperlipasemia (16% to 25%), amylase increased (5% to 17%), glossodynia (15%), flatulence (14%)

Hematologic: Neutropenia (53%; grades 3/4: 10% to 13%), lymphopenia (38%; grades 3/4: 21%), thrombocytopenia (38%; grades 3/4: 3% to 5%), anemia (26%; grades 3/4: 3% to 7%), bleeding (18% to 26%)

Hepatic: AST/ALT increased (39%), alkaline phosphatase increased (24%), hyperbilirubinemia (10% to 16%)

Neuromuscular & skeletal: Arthralgia (12% to 28%), weakness (22%), limb pain (18%), myalgia (14% to 17%), back pain (11% to 17%)

Renal: Creatinine increased (12%)

Respiratory: Dyspnea (10% to 28%), cough (8% to 17%)

1% to 10%:
> Cardiovascular: LVEF decreased (10%; grade 3/4: 1%), DVT (1% to 3%), myocardial ischemia (1%)
> Central nervous system: Neuropathy (peripheral 10%)
> Dermatologic: Skin blistering (7%)
> Endocrine & metabolic: Hypernatremia (10%), hypophosphatemia (9% to 10%), hypothyroidism (4% to 7%), hyperkalemia (6%), hyponatremia (6%)
> Gastrointestinal: Appetite disturbance (9%), oral pain (6%)
> Ocular: Periorbital edema (7%), lacrimation increased (6%)
> Respiratory: Pulmonary embolism (1%)

Restrictions Pharmacies may order sunitinib by contacting McKesson Specialty at 1-800-496-6540 for an Order Authorization Number (OAN). Contact your wholesaler with the OAN; McKesson Specialty will ship the order to the pharmacy and bill through your wholesaler.

Mechanism of Action Exhibits antitumor and antiangiogenic properties by inhibiting multiple receptor tyrosine kinases, including platelet-derived growth factors (PDGFRα and PDGFRβ), vascular endothelial growth factors (VEGFR1, VEGFR2, and VEGFR3), FMS-like tyrosine kinase-3 (FLT3), colony-stimulating factor type 1 (CSF-1R), and glial cell-line-derived neurotrophic factor receptor (RET).

Drug Interactions

Cytochrome P450 Effect: Substrate of CYP3A4 (major)

> **Increased Effect/Toxicity:** CYP3A4 inhibitors may increase the levels/effects of sunitinib (example inhibitors include azole antifungals, clarithromycin, diclofenac, doxycycline, erythromycin, imatinib, isoniazid, nefazodone, nicardipine, propofol, protease inhibitors, quinidine, telithromycin, and verapamil). Ketoconazole may increase the effects of sunitinib.

> **Decreased Effect:** CYP3A4 inducers may decrease the levels/effects of sunitinib (example inducers include aminoglutethimide, carbamazepine, dexamethasone, nafcillin, nevirapine, phenobarbital, and phenytoin. Rifamycins may decrease the effects of sunitinib.

Pharmacodynamics/Kinetics

Distribution: V_d/F: 2230 L
Protein binding: Sunitinib: 95%; SU12662: 90%
Metabolism: Hepatic; primarily metabolized by CYP3A4 to the N-desethyl metabolite SU12662 (active)
Half-life elimination: Sunitinib: 40-60 hours; SU12662: 80-110 hours
Time to peak, plasma: 6-12 hours
Excretion: Feces (61%); urine (16%)

Pregnancy Risk Factor D

Sunitinib Maleate *see* Sunitinib *on page 1434*

Supartz™ *see* Hyaluronate and Derivatives *on page 773*

Superdophilus® [OTC] *see* Lactobacillus *on page 535*

Suprax® *see* Cefixime *on page 287*

Surbex-T® [OTC] *see* Vitamin B Complex Combinations *on page 1581*

Sureprin 81™ [OTC] *see* Aspirin *on page 145*

Surfak® [OTC] *see* Docusate *on page 496*

Surgicel® *see* Cellulose (Oxidized/Regenerated) *on page 300*

Surgicel® Fibrillar *see* Cellulose (Oxidized/Regenerated) *on page 300*

Surgicel® NuKnit *see* Cellulose (Oxidized/Regenerated) *on page 300*

Surmontil® *see* Trimipramine *on page 1540*

Survanta® *see* Beractant *on page 198*

Sustiva® *see* Efavirenz *on page 530*

Sutent® *see* Sunitinib *on page 1434*

Su-Tuss DM *see* Guaifenesin and Dextromethorphan *on page 754*

Su-Tuss®-HD *see* Hydrocodone, Pseudoephedrine, and Guaifenesin *on page 792*

Suxamethonium Chloride *see* Succinylcholine *on page 1419*

Sween Cream® [OTC] *see* Vitamin A and Vitamin D *on page 1580*

Symax SL *see* Hyoscyamine *on page 803*

Symax SR *see* Hyoscyamine *on page 803*

Symbyax™ *see* Olanzapine and Fluoxetine *on page 1141*

Symlin® *see* Pramlintide *on page 1263*

Symmetrel® *see* Amantadine *on page 81*

Sympt-X [OTC] *see* Glutamine *on page 743*

Sympt-X G.I. [OTC] *see* Glutamine *on page 743*

Synacthen *see* Cosyntropin *on page 396*

Synagis® *see* Palivizumab *on page 1179*

Synalar® *see* Fluocinolone *on page 667*

Synalgos®-DC *see* Dihydrocodeine, Aspirin, and Caffeine *on page 475*

Synarel® *see* Nafarelin *on page 1081*

Synera™ *see* Lidocaine and Tetracaine *on page 930*

Synercid® *see* Quinupristin and Dalfopristin *on page 1326*

Syntest D.S. *see* Estrogens (Esterified) and Methyltestosterone *on page 585*

Syntest H.S. *see* Estrogens (Esterified) and Methyltestosterone *on page 585*

Synthroid® *see* Levothyroxine *on page 917*

Synvisc® *see* Hyaluronate and Derivatives *on page 773*

Syrex *see* Sodium Chloride *on page 1400*

SyringeAvitene™ *see* Collagen Hemostat *on page 392*

Syrup of Ipecac *see* Ipecac Syrup *on page 856*

T$_3$ Sodium (error-prone abbreviation) *see* Liothyronine *on page 934*

T$_3$/T$_4$ Liotrix *see* Liotrix *on page 935*

T$_4$ *see* Levothyroxine *on page 917*

T-20 *see* Enfuvirtide *on page 541*

Tabloid® *see* Thioguanine *on page 1476*

Tacrine (TAK reen)

U.S. Brand Names Cognex®

Generic Available No

Synonyms Tacrine Hydrochloride; Tetrahydroaminoacrine; THA

Pharmacologic Category Acetylcholinesterase Inhibitor (Central)

Use Treatment of mild to moderate dementia of the Alzheimer's type

Local Anesthetic/Vasoconstrictor Precautions No information available to require special precautions

Effects on Dental Treatment No significant effects or complications reported

Common Adverse Effects

>10%:

Central nervous system: Headache, dizziness

Gastrointestinal: Nausea, vomiting, diarrhea

Miscellaneous: Transaminases increased

1% to 10%:

Cardiovascular: Flushing

Central nervous system: Confusion, ataxia, insomnia, somnolence, depression, anxiety, fatigue

Dermatologic: Rash

Gastrointestinal: Dyspepsia, anorexia, abdominal pain, flatulence, constipation, weight loss

Neuromuscular & skeletal: Myalgia, tremor

Respiratory: Rhinitis

Mechanism of Action Centrally-acting cholinesterase inhibitor. It elevates acetylcholine in cerebral cortex by slowing the degradation of acetylcholine.

Drug Interactions

Cytochrome P450 Effect: Substrate of CYP1A2 (major); **Inhibits** CYP1A2 (weak)

Increased Effect/Toxicity: CYP1A2 inhibitors may increase the levels/effects of tacrine; example inhibitors include amiodarone, ciprofloxacin, fluvoxamine, ketoconazole, norfloxacin, ofloxacin, and rofecoxib. Tacrine in combination with other cholinergic agents (eg, ambenonium, edrophonium, neostigmine, pyridostigmine, bethanechol), will likely produce additive cholinergic effects. Tacrine in combination with beta-blockers may produce additive bradycardia. Tacrine may increase the levels/effect of succinylcholine and theophylline. in elevated plasma levels. Fluvoxamine, enoxacin, and cimetidine increase tacrine concentrations via enzyme inhibition (CYP1A2). Acetylcholinesterase inhibitors (central) may increase the risk of antipsychotic-related extrapyramidal symptoms.

Decreased Effect: CYP1A2 inducers may decrease the levels/effects of tacrine; example inducers include aminoglutethimide, carbamazepine, phenobarbital, rifampin, and cigarette smoking. Tacrine may worsen Parkinson's disease and inhibit the effects of levodopa. Tacrine may antagonize the therapeutic effect of anticholinergic agents (benztropine, trihexyphenidyl).

Pharmacodynamics/Kinetics

Absorption: Oral: Rapid

Distribution: V$_d$: Mean: 349 L; reduced by food

Protein binding, plasma: 55%

Metabolism: Extensively by CYP450 to multiple metabolites; first pass effect

Bioavailability: Absolute: 17%

Half-life elimination, serum: 2-4 hours; Steady-state: 24-36 hours

Time to peak, plasma: 1-2 hours
Pregnancy Risk Factor C

Tacrine Hydrochloride *see* Tacrine *on page 1436*

Tacrolimus (ta KROE li mus)

U.S. Brand Names Prograf®; Protopic®
Canadian Brand Names Prograf®; Protopic®
Mexican Brand Names Prograf®
Generic Available No
Synonyms FK506
Pharmacologic Category Immunosuppressant Agent; Topical Skin Product
Dental Use Topical: Treatment of severe ulcerative or vesicobullous lesions (usually in consult with patient's physician)
Use
  Oral/injection: Potent immunosuppressive drug used in heart, kidney, or liver transplant recipients
  Topical: Moderate-to-severe atopic dermatitis in patients not responsive to conventional therapy or when conventional therapy is not appropriate
Unlabeled/Investigational Use Potent immunosuppressive drug used in lung, small bowel transplant recipients; immunosuppressive drug for peripheral stem cell/bone marrow transplantation
Local Anesthetic/Vasoconstrictor Precautions No information available to require special precautions
Effects on Dental Treatment No significant effects or complications reported
Significant Adverse Effects
  Oral, I.V.:
    ≥15%:
      Cardiovascular: Chest pain, hypertension, pericardial effusion (heart transplant)
      Central nervous system: Dizziness, headache, insomnia, tremor (headache and tremor are associated with high whole blood concentrations and may respond to decreased dosage)
      Dermatologic: Pruritus, rash
      Endocrine & metabolic: Diabetes mellitus, hyperglycemia, hyper-/hypokalemia, hyperlipemia, hypomagnesemia, hypophosphatemia
      Gastrointestinal: Abdominal pain, constipation, diarrhea, dyspepsia, nausea, vomiting
      Genitourinary: Urinary tract infection
      Hematologic: Anemia, leukocytosis, leukopenia, thrombocytopenia
      Hepatic: Ascites
      Neuromuscular & skeletal: Arthralgia, back pain, paresthesia, tremor, weakness
      Renal: Abnormal kidney function, BUN increased, creatinine increased, oliguria, urinary tract infection
      Respiratory: Atelectasis, bronchitis, dyspnea, increased cough, pleural effusion
      Miscellaneous: CMV infection, infection
    <15%:
      Cardiovascular: Abnormal ECG (QRS or ST segment abnormal), angina pectoris, cardiopulmonary failure, deep thrombophlebitis, heart rate decreased, hemorrhage, hemorrhagic stroke, hypervolemia, hypotension, generalized edema, peripheral vascular disorder, phlebitis, postural hypotension, tachycardia, thrombosis, vasodilation
      Central nervous system: Abnormal dreams, abnormal thinking, agitation, amnesia, anxiety, chills, confusion, depression, dizziness, elevated mood, emotional lability, encephalopathy, hallucinations, nervousness, paralysis, psychosis, quadriparesis, seizure, somnolence
      Dermatologic: Acne, alopecia, cellulitis, exfoliative dermatitis, fungal dermatitis, hirsutism, increased diaphoresis, photosensitivity reaction, skin discoloration, skin disorder, skin ulcer
      Endocrine & metabolic: Acidosis, alkalosis, Cushing's syndrome, decreased bicarbonate, decreased serum iron, diabetes mellitus, hypercalcemia, hypercholesterolemia, hyperphosphatemia, hypoproteinemia, increased alkaline phosphatase
      Gastrointestinal: Anorexia, appetite increased, cramps, duodenitis, dysphagia, enlarged abdomen, esophagitis (including ulcerative), flatulence, gastritis, gastroesophagitis, GI perforation/hemorrhage, ileus, oral moniliasis, pancreatic pseudocyst, rectal disorder, stomatitis, weight gain
      Genitourinary: Bladder spasm, cystitis, dysuria, nocturia, oliguria, urge incontinence, urinary frequency, urinary incontinence, urinary retention, vaginitis
(Continued)

Tacrolimus *(Continued)*

Hematologic: Bruising, coagulation disorder, decreased prothrombin, hypochromic anemia, polycythemia

Hepatic: Abnormal liver function tests, ALT/AST increased, bilirubinemia, cholangitis, cholestatic jaundice, GGT increased, hepatitis (including granulomatous), jaundice, liver damage, increase LDH

Neuromuscular & skeletal: Hypertonia, incoordination, joint disorder, leg cramps, myalgia, myasthenia, myoclonus, nerve compression, neuropathy, osteoporosis

Ocular: Abnormal vision, amblyopia

Otic: Ear pain, otitis media, tinnitus

Renal: Albuminuria, renal tubular necrosis, toxic nephropathy

Respiratory: Asthma, lung disorder, pharyngitis, pneumonia, pneumothorax, pulmonary edema, respiratory disorder, rhinitis, sinusitis, voice alteration

Miscellaneous: Abscess, abnormal healing, allergic reaction, crying, flu-like syndrome, generalized spasm, hernia, herpes simplex, peritonitis, sepsis, writing impaired

Topical:

>10%:

Central nervous system: Headache (5% to 20%), fever (1% to 21%)

Dermatologic: Skin burning (43% to 58%; tends to improve as lesions resolve), pruritus (41% to 46%), erythema (12% to 28%)

Respiratory: Increased cough (18% children)

Miscellaneous: Flu-like syndrome (23% to 28%), allergic reaction (4% to 12%)

Oral, I.V., topical: Postmarketing and/or case reports (limited to important or life-threatening): Acute renal failure, alopecia, anaphylaxis, anaphylactoid reaction, angioedema, ARDS, arrhythmia, atrial fibrillation, atrial flutter, bile duct stenosis, blindness, cardiac arrest, cerebral infarction, cerebrovascular accident, deafness, delirium, depression, DIC, hemiparesis, hemolytic-uremic syndrome, hemorrhagic cystitis, hepatic necrosis, hepatotoxicity, hyperglycemia, leukoencephalopathy, lymphoproliferative disorder (related to EBV), myocardial hypertrophy (associated with ventricular dysfunction; reversible upon discontinuation), MI, neutropenia, pancreatitis (hemorrhagic and necrotizing), pancytopenia, paresthesia, photosensitivity reaction (topical), quadriplegia, QT_c prolongation, respiratory failure, seizure, skin discoloration (topical), Stevens-Johnson syndrome, syncope, toxic epidermal necrolysis, thrombocytopenic purpura, torsade de pointes, TTP, veno-occlusive hepatic disease, venous thrombosis, ventricular fibrillation

Note: Calcineurin inhibitor-induced hemolytic uremic syndrome/thrombotic thrombocytopenic purpura/thrombotic microangiopathy (HUS/TTP/TMA) have been reported (with concurrent sirolimus).

Restrictions An FDA-approved medication guide is available at http://www.fda.gov/cder/Offices/ODS/labeling.htm; distribute to each patient to whom the ointment is dispensed.

Dosage

Oral:

Children: **Notes:** Patients without pre-existing renal or hepatic dysfunction have required (and tolerated) higher doses than adults to achieve similar blood concentrations. It is recommended that therapy be initiated at high end of the recommended adult I.V. and oral dosing ranges; dosage adjustments may be required. If switching from I.V. to oral, the oral dose should be started 8-12 hours after stopping the infusion. Adjunctive therapy with corticosteroids is recommended early post-transplant.

Liver transplant: Initial dose: 0.15-0.20 mg/kg/day in 2 divided doses, given every 12 hours; begin oral dose no sooner than 6 hours post-transplant

Adults: **Notes:** If switching from I.V. to oral, the oral dose should be started 8-12 hours after stopping the infusion. Adjunctive therapy with corticosteroids is recommended early post-transplant.

Heart transplant: Initial dose: 0.075 mg/kg/day in 2 divided doses, given every 12 hours; begin oral dose no sooner than 6 hours post-transplant

Kidney transplant: Initial dose: 0.2 mg/kg/day in 2 divided doses, given every 12 hours; initial dose may be given within 24 hours of transplant, but should be delayed until renal function has recovered; African-American patients may require larger doses to maintain trough concentration

Liver transplant: Initial dose: 0.1-0.15 mg/kg/day in 2 divided doses, given every 12 hours; begin oral dose no sooner than 6 hours post-transplant

I.V.: Children and Adults: **Note:** I.V. route should only be used in patients not able to take oral medications and continued only until oral medication can be tolerated; anaphylaxis has been reported. Begin no sooner than 6 hours post-transplant; adjunctive therapy with corticosteroids is recommended.

Heart transplant: Initial dose: 0.01 mg/kg/day as a continuous infusion

Kidney, liver transplant: Initial dose: 0.03-0.05 mg/kg/day as a continuous infusion

Prevention of graft-vs-host disease: 0.03 mg/kg/day as continuous infusion

Topical: Children ≥2 years and Adults: Atopic dermatitis (moderate to severe): Apply minimum amount of 0.03% or 0.1% ointment to affected area twice daily; rub in gently and completely. Discontinue use when symptoms have cleared. If no improvement within 6 weeks, patients should be re-examined to confirm diagnosis.

Dosing adjustment in renal impairment: Evidence suggests that lower doses should be used; patients should receive doses at the lowest value of the recommended I.V. and oral dosing ranges; further reductions in dose below these ranges may be required.

Tacrolimus therapy should usually be delayed up to 48 hours or longer in patients with postoperative oliguria.

Hemodialysis: Not removed by hemodialysis; supplemental dose is not necessary.

Peritoneal dialysis: Significant drug removal is unlikely based on physiochemical characteristics.

Dosing adjustment in hepatic impairment: Use of tacrolimus in liver transplant recipients experiencing post-transplant hepatic impairment may be associated with increased risk of developing renal insufficiency related to high whole blood levels of tacrolimus. The presence of moderate-to-severe hepatic dysfunction (serum bilirubin >2 mg/dL; Child-Pugh score ≥10) appears to affect the metabolism of tacrolimus. The half-life of the drug was prolonged and the clearance reduced after I.V. administration. The bioavailability of tacrolimus was also increased after oral administration. The higher plasma concentrations as determined by ELISA, in patients with severe hepatic dysfunction are probably due to the accumulation of metabolites of lower activity. These patients should be monitored closely and dosage adjustments should be considered. Some evidence indicates that lower doses could be used in these patients.

Mechanism of Action Suppresses cellular immunity (inhibits T-lymphocyte activation), possibly by binding to an intracellular protein, FKBP-12

Contraindications Hypersensitivity to tacrolimus or any component of the formulation

Warnings/Precautions

Oral/injection: Insulin-dependent post-transplant diabetes mellitus (PTDM) has been reported (1% to 20%); risk increases in African-American and Hispanic kidney transplant patients. Increased susceptibility to infection and the possible development of lymphoma may occur after administration of tacrolimus. Nephrotoxicity and neurotoxicity have been reported, especially with higher doses; to avoid excess nephrotoxicity do not administer simultaneously with cyclosporine; monitoring of serum concentrations (trough for oral therapy) is essential to prevent organ rejection and reduce drug-related toxicity; tonic clonic seizures may have been triggered by tacrolimus. A period of 24 hours should elapse between discontinuation of cyclosporine and the initiation of tacrolimus. Use caution in renal or hepatic dysfunction, dosing adjustments may be required. Delay initiation if postoperative oliguria occurs. Use may be associated with the development of hypertension (common). Myocardial hypertrophy has been reported (rare). Each mL of injection contains polyoxyl 60 hydrogenated castor oil (HCO-60) (200 mg) and dehydrated alcohol USP 80% v/v. Anaphylaxis has been reported with the injection, use should be reserved for those patients not able to take oral medications.

Topical: Topical calcineurin inhibitors have been associated with rare cases of malignancy. Avoid use on malignant or skin conditions (eg cutaneous T-cell lymphoma). Topical calcineurin agents are considered second-line therapies in the treatment of atopic dermatitis/eczema, and should be limited to use in patients who have failed treatment with other therapies. They should be used for short-term and intermittent treatment using the minimum amount necessary for the control of symptoms should be used. Application should be limited to involved areas. Safety of intermittent use for >1 year has not been established.

Should not be used in immunocompromised patients. Do not apply to areas of active viral infection; infections at the treatment site should be cleared prior to therapy. Patients with atopic dermatitis are predisposed to skin infections, and tacrolimus therapy has been associated with risk of developing eczema herpeticum, varicella zoster, and herpes simplex. May be associated with development of lymphadenopathy; possible infectious causes should be investigated. Discontinue use in patients with unknown cause of lymphadenopathy or acute infectious mononucleosis. Not recommended for use in patients with skin disease which may increase systemic absorption (eg, Netherton's syndrome). (Continued)

Tacrolimus (Continued)

Avoid artificial or natural sunlight exposure, even when Protopic® is not on the skin. Safety not established in patients with generalized erythroderma. The use of Protopic® in children <2 years of age is not recommended, particularly since the effect on immune system development is unknown.

Drug Interactions **Substrate** of CYP3A4 (major); **Inhibits** CYP3A4 (weak)

Antacids: Separate administration by at least 2 hours

Anticonvulsants: Carbamazepine, phenobarbital, phenytoin: May decrease tacrolimus blood levels.

Calcium channel blockers: May increase tacrolimus serum concentrations; monitor.

Caspofungin: May decrease tacrolimus serum concentrations.

Cisapride (and metoclopramide): May increase serum concentration of tacrolimus

Cyclosporine: Concomitant use is associated with synergistic immunosuppression and increased nephrotoxicity; give first dose of tacrolimus no sooner than 24 hours after last cyclosporine dose. In the presence of elevated tacrolimus or cyclosporine concentration, dosing of the other usually should be delayed longer.

CYP3A4 inducers: CYP3A4 inducers may decrease the levels/effects of tacrolimus. Example inducers include aminoglutethimide, carbamazepine, nafcillin, nevirapine, phenobarbital, phenytoin, and rifamycins.

CYP3A4 inhibitors: May increase the levels/effects of tacrolimus. Example inhibitors include azole antifungals, clarithromycin, diclofenac, doxycycline, erythromycin, imatinib, isoniazid, nefazodone, nicardipine, propofol, protease inhibitors, quinidine, telithromycin, and verapamil.

Ganciclovir: Nephrotoxicity may be additive with tacrolimus; use caution.

Macrolides: May increase tacrolimus serum concentrations (limited documentation); monitor.

Potassium-sparing diuretics: Tacrolimus use may lead to hyperkalemia; avoid concomitant use

Rifabutin, rifampin: May decrease serum levels of tacrolimus.

Sirolimus: May decrease tacrolimus serum concentrations. Concurrent therapy may increase the risk of HUS/TTP/TMA.

St John's wort: May decrease tacrolimus serum concentrations; avoid concurrent use.

Sucralfate: Separate administration by at least 2 hours

Vaccines (live): Vaccine may be less effective; avoid vaccination during treatment if possible

Voriconazole: Tacrolimus serum concentrations may be increased; monitor serum concentrations and renal function. Decrease tacrolimus dosage by 66% when initiating voriconazole.

Ethanol/Nutrition/Herb Interactions

Ethanol: Localized flushing (redness, warm sensation) may occur at application site of topical tacrolimus following ethanol consumption.

Food: Decreases rate and extent of absorption. High-fat meals have most pronounced effect (35% decrease in AUC, 77% decrease in C_{max}). Grapefruit juice, CYP3A4 inhibitor, may increase serum level and/or toxicity of tacrolimus; avoid concurrent use.

Herb/Nutraceutical: St John's wort: May reduce tacrolimus serum concentrations (avoid concurrent use).

Dietary Considerations Capsule: Take on an empty stomach; be consistent with timing and composition of meals if GI intolerance occurs (per manufacturer).

Pharmacodynamics/Kinetics

Absorption: Better in resected patients with a closed stoma; unlike cyclosporine, clamping of the T-tube in liver transplant patients does not alter trough concentrations or AUC

Oral: Incomplete and variable; food within 15 minutes of administration decreases absorption (27%)

Topical: Serum concentrations range from undetectable to 20 ng/mL (<5 ng/mL in majority of adult patients studied)

Protein binding: 99%

Metabolism: Extensively hepatic via CYP3A4 to eight possible metabolites (major metabolite, 31-demethyl tacrolimus, shows same activity as tacrolimus *in vitro*)

Bioavailability: Oral: Adults: 7% to 28%, Children: 10% to 52%; Topical: <0.5%; Absolute: Unknown

Half-life elimination: Variable, 21-61 hours in healthy volunteers

Time to peak: 0.5-4 hours

Excretion: Feces (~92%); feces/urine (<1% as unchanged drug)

Pregnancy Risk Factor C

Lactation Enters breast milk/contraindicated

Breast-Feeding Considerations Concentrations in breast milk are equivalent to plasma concentrations; breast-feeding is not advised.

Dosage Forms

Capsule (Prograf®): 0.5 mg, 1 mg, 5 mg

Injection, solution (Prograf®): 5 mg/mL (1 mL) [contains dehydrated alcohol 80% and polyoxyl 60 hydrogenated castor oil]

Ointment, topical (Protopic®): 0.03% (30 g, 60 g, 100 g); 0.1% (30 g, 60 g, 100 g)

Tadalafil (tah DA la fil)

U.S. Brand Names Cialis®

Canadian Brand Names Cialis®

Generic Available No

Synonyms GF196960

Pharmacologic Category Phosphodiesterase-5 Enzyme Inhibitor

Use Treatment of erectile dysfunction

Local Anesthetic/Vasoconstrictor Precautions No information available to require special precautions

Effects on Dental Treatment No significant effects or complications reported

Common Adverse Effects

>10%: Central nervous system: Headache (11% to 15%)

2% to 10%:

Cardiovascular: Flushing (2% to 3%)

Gastrointestinal: Dyspepsia (4% to 10%)

Neuromuscular & skeletal: CPK increased (2%), back pain (3% to 6%), myalgia (1% to 4%), limb pain (1% to 3%)

Respiratory: Nasal congestion (2% to 3%)

Dosage Oral: Adults: Erectile dysfunction: 10 mg prior to anticipated sexual activity (dosing range: 5-20 mg); to be given as one single dose and not given more than once daily. **Note:** Erectile function may be improved for up to 36 hours following a single dose; adjust dose.

Elderly: Dosage is based on renal function; refer to "Dosage adjustment in renal impairment"

Dosing adjustment with concomitant medications:

Alpha₁-blockers: If stabilized on either alpha blockers or tadalafil therapy, initiate new therapy with the other agent at the lowest possible dose.

CYP3A4 inhibitors: Dose reduction of tadalafil is recommended with strong CYP3A4 inhibitors. The dose of tadalafil should not exceed 10 mg, and tadalafil should not be taken more frequently than once every 72 hours. Examples of such inhibitors include amprenavir, atazanavir, clarithromycin, conivaptan, delavirdine, diclofenac, fosamprenavir, imatinib, indinavir, isoniazid, itraconazole, ketoconazole, miconazole, nefazodone, nelfinavir, nicardipine, propofol, quinidine, ritonavir, and telithromycin.

Dosage adjustment in renal impairment:

Cl_cr 31-50 mL/minute: Initial dose 5 mg once daily; maximum dose 10 mg not to be given more frequently than every 48 hours.

Cl_cr <30 mL/minute or hemodialysis: Maximum dose 5 mg.

Dosage adjustment in hepatic impairment:

Mild-to-moderate hepatic impairment (Child-Pugh class A or B): Dose should not exceed 10 mg once daily

Severe hepatic impairment: Use is not recommended

Mechanism of Action Does not directly cause penile erections, but affects the response to sexual stimulation. The physiologic mechanism of erection of the penis involves release of nitric oxide (NO) in the corpus cavernosum during sexual stimulation. NO then activates the enzyme guanylate cyclase, which results in increased levels of cyclic guanosine monophosphate (cGMP), producing smooth muscle relaxation and inflow of blood to the corpus cavernosum. Tadalafil enhances the effect of NO by inhibiting phosphodiesterase type 5 (PDE-5), which is responsible for degradation of cGMP in the corpus cavernosum; when sexual stimulation causes local release of NO, inhibition of PDE-5 by tadalafil causes increased levels of cGMP in the corpus cavernosum, resulting in smooth muscle relaxation and inflow of blood to the corpus cavernosum. At recommended doses, it has no effect in the absence of sexual stimulation.

Contraindications Hypersensitivity to tadalafil or any component of the formulation; concurrent use of organic nitrates (nitroglycerin) in any form

Warnings/Precautions There is a degree of cardiac risk associated with sexual activity; therefore, physicians may wish to consider the cardiovascular status of their patients prior to initiating any treatment for erectile dysfunction. (Continued)

Tadalafil *(Continued)*

Use caution in patients with left ventricular outflow obstruction (aortic stenosis or IHSS); may be more sensitive to hypotensive actions. Concurrent use with alpha-adrenergic antagonist therapy may cause symptomatic hypotension; patients should be hemodynamically stable prior to initiating tadalafil therapy at the lowest possible dose. Use caution in patients receiving strong CYP3A4 inhibitors, the elderly, or those with hepatic impairment or renal impairment; dosage adjustment/limitation is needed. Use caution in patients with peptic ulcer disease.

Agents for the treatment of erectile dysfunction should be used with caution in patients with anatomical deformation of the penis (angulation, cavernosal fibrosis, or Peyronie's disease), or in patients who have conditions which may predispose them to priapism (sickle cell anemia, multiple myeloma, leukemia). All patients should be instructed to seek medical attention if erection persists >4 hours. The safety and efficacy of tadalafil with other treatments for erectile dysfunction have not been studied and are, therefore, not recommended as combination therapy.

Rare cases of nonarteritic ischemic optic neuropathy (NAION) have been reported; risk may be increased with history of vision loss. Other risk factors for NAION include heart disease, diabetes, hypertension, smoking, age >50 years, or history of certain eye problems.

Safety and efficacy have not been studied in patients with the following conditions, therefore, use in these patients is not recommended: Arrhythmias, hypotension, uncontrolled hypertension, unstable angina or angina during intercourse, cardiac failure (NYHA Class II or greater), myocardial infarction within the last 3 months, or stroke within the last 6 months. A minority of patients with retinitis pigmentosa have genetic disorders of retinal phosphodiesterases; use is not recommended. Safety and efficacy in children have not been established.

Drug Interactions

Cytochrome P450 Effect: Substrate of CYP3A4 (major)

Increased Effect/Toxicity:

Tadalafil increases the hypotensive effects of alpha1-blockers. Concurrent use with organic nitrates may cause severe hypotension. Antifungals agents (imidazole), macrolide antibiotics (clarithromycin, erythromycin, telithromycin, troleandomycin), protease inhibitors (amprenavir, atazanavir, fosamprenavir, indinavir, lopinavir, nelfinavir, ritonavir, saquinavir), and other CYP3A4 inhibitors may increase tadalafil levels.

Ethanol/Nutrition/Herb Interactions

Ethanol: Substantial consumption of ethanol may increase the risk of hypotension and orthostasis. Lower ethanol consumption has not been associated with significant changes in blood pressure or increase in orthostatic symptoms.

Food: Rate and extent of absorption are not affected by food. Grapefruit juice may increase serum levels/toxicity of tadalafil. Do not give more than a single 10 mg dose of tadalafil more frequently than every 72 hours in patients who regularly consume grapefruit juice.

Dietary Considerations May be taken with or without food.

Pharmacodynamics/Kinetics

Onset: Within 1 hour

Duration: Up to 36 hours

Distribution: V_d: 63 L

Protein binding: 94%

Metabolism: Hepatic, via CYP3A4 to metabolites (inactive)

Half-life elimination: 17.5 hours

Time to peak, plasma: 2 hours

Excretion: Feces (61%, as metabolites); urine (36%, as metabolites)

Pregnancy Risk Factor B

Dosage Forms TAB: 5 mg, 10 mg, 20 mg

Tagamet® *see* Cimetidine *on page 341*

Tagamet® HB 200 [OTC] *see* Cimetidine *on page 341*

TAK-375 *see* Ramelteon *on page 1331*

Talacen® *see* Pentazocine and Acetaminophen *on page 1209*

Talwin® *see* Pentazocine *on page 1208*

Talwin® NX *see* Pentazocine *on page 1208*

TAM *see* Tamoxifen *on page 1443*

Tambocor™ *see* Flecainide *on page 657*

Tamiflu® *see* Oseltamivir *on page 1152*

Tamoxifen (ta MOKS i fen)

U.S. Brand Names Nolvadex® [DSC]; Soltamox™

Canadian Brand Names Apo-Tamox®; Gen-Tamoxifen; Nolvadex®; Nolvadex®-D; Novo-Tamoxifen; Tamofen®

Mexican Brand Names Nolvadex®; Taxus®; Tecnofen®

Generic Available Yes: Tablet

Synonyms ICI-46474; NSC-180973; TAM; Tamoxifen Citrate

Pharmacologic Category Antineoplastic Agent, Estrogen Receptor Antagonist

Use Palliative or adjunctive treatment of advanced breast cancer; reduce the incidence of breast cancer in women at high risk; reduce risk of invasive breast cancer in women with ductal carcinoma *in situ* (DCIS); metastatic female and male breast cancer

Unlabeled/Investigational Use Treatment of mastalgia, gynecomastia, pancreatic carcinoma, melanoma and desmoid tumors; induction of ovulation; treatment of precocious puberty in females, secondary to McCune-Albright syndrome

Local Anesthetic/Vasoconstrictor Precautions No information available to require special precautions

Effects on Dental Treatment No significant effects or complications reported

Common Adverse Effects Note: Differences in the frequency of some adverse events may be related to use for a specific indication.

>10%:

Cardiovascular: Flushing (33% to 41%), hypertension (11%), peripheral edema (11%)

Central nervous system: Pain (3% to 16%), mood changes (12% to 18%), depression (2% to 12%)

Dermatologic: Skin changes (6% to 19%), rash (13%)

Endocrine & metabolic: Hot flashes (3% to 80%), fluid retention (32%), altered menses (13% to 25%), amenorrhea (16%)

Gastrointestinal: Nausea (5% to 26%), weight loss (23%)

Genitourinary: Vaginal bleeding (2% to 23%), vaginal discharge (13% to 55%)

Neuromuscular & skeletal: Weakness (19%), arthritis (14%), arthralgia (11%)

Respiratory: Pharyngitis (14%)

1% to 10%:

Cardiovascular: Chest pain (5%), venous thrombotic events (5%), edema (4%), cardiovascular ischemia (3%), cerebrovascular ischemia (3%), angina (2%), deep venous thrombus (2%), MI (1%)

Central nervous system: Insomnia (9%), dizziness (8%), headache (8%), anxiety (6%), fatigue (4%)

Dermatologic: Alopecia (<1% to 5%)

Endocrine & metabolic: Oligomenorrhea (9%), breast pain (6%), menstrual disorder (6%), breast neoplasm (5%), hypercholesterolemia (4%)

Gastrointestinal: Abdominal pain (9%), weight gain (9%), throat irritation (oral solution 5%), constipation (4% to 8%), diarrhea (7%), dyspepsia (6%), abdominal cramps (1%), anorexia (1%)

Genitourinary: Urinary tract infection (10%), leukorrhea (9%), vaginal hemorrhage (6%), vaginitis (5%), ovarian cyst (3%)

Hematologic: Thrombocytopenia (<1% to 10%), anemia (5%)

Hepatic: SGOT increased (5%), serum bilirubin increased (2%)

Neuromuscular & skeletal: Bone pain (6% to 10%), osteoporosis (7%), fracture (7%), arthrosis (5%), myalgia (5%), paresthesia (5%), musculoskeletal pain (3%)

Ocular: Cataract (7%)

Renal: Serum creatinine increased (up to 2%)

Respiratory: Cough (4% to 9%), dyspnea (8%), bronchitis (5%), sinusitis (5%)

Miscellaneous: Infection/sepsis (up to 9%), diaphoresis (6%), flu-like syndrome (6%), allergic reaction (3%)

Restrictions An FDA-approved medication guide is available at www.AstraZeneca-us.com/pi/Nolvadex.pdf. Distribute to each female patient who is using tamoxifen to decrease risk of developing breast cancer or who has ductal carcinoma *in situ*.

Dosage Oral (refer to individual protocols):

Children: Female: Precocious puberty and McCune-Albright syndrome (unlabeled use): A dose of 20 mg/day has been reported in patients 2-10 years of age; safety and efficacy have not been established for treatment of longer than 1 year duration

(Continued)

Tamoxifen *(Continued)*

Adults:

Breast cancer:

Metastatic (males and females) or adjuvant therapy (females): 20-40 mg/day; daily doses >20 mg should be given in 2 divided doses (morning and evening)

Prevention (high-risk females): 20 mg/day for 5 years

DCIS (females): 20 mg once daily for 5 years

Note: Higher dosages (up to 700 mg/day) have been investigated for use in modulation of multidrug resistance (MDR), but are not routinely used in clinical practice

Induction of ovulation (unlabeled use): 5-40 mg twice daily for 4 days

Mechanism of Action Competitively binds to estrogen receptors on tumors and other tissue targets, producing a nuclear complex that decreases DNA synthesis and inhibits estrogen effects; nonsteroidal agent with potent antiestrogenic properties which compete with estrogen for binding sites in breast and other tissues; cells accumulate in the G_0 and G_1 phases; therefore, tamoxifen is cytostatic rather than cytocidal.

Contraindications Hypersensitivity to tamoxifen or any component of the formulation; concurrent warfarin therapy or history of deep vein thrombosis or pulmonary embolism (when tamoxifen is used for cancer risk reduction); pregnancy

Warnings/Precautions Hazardous agent - use appropriate precautions for handling and disposal. Serious and life-threatening events (including stroke, pulmonary emboli, and uterine malignancy) have occurred at an incidence greater than placebo during use for cancer risk reduction; these events are rare, but require consideration in risk:benefit evaluation. An increased incidence of thromboembolic events has been associated with use for breast cancer; risk may increase with chemotherapy addition; use caution in individuals with a history of thromboembolic events. Use with caution in patients with leukopenia, thrombocytopenia, or hyperlipidemias. Decreased visual acuity, retinopathy, corneal changes, and increased incidence of cataracts have been reported. Hypercalcemia has occurred in patients with bone metastasis. Significant bone loss of the lumbar spine and hip was associated with use in premenopausal women. Liver abnormalities such as cholestasis, fatty liver, hepatitis, and hepatic necrosis have occurred. Hepatocellular carcinomas have been reported in some studies; relationship to treatment is unclear. Endometrial hyperplasia, polyps, endometriosis, uterine fibroids, and ovarian cysts have occurred. Increased risk of uterine or endometrial cancer; monitor. Safety and efficacy in children <2 years of age, or for treatment durations >1 year in children 2-10 years, have not been established.

Drug Interactions

Cytochrome P450 Effect: Substrate of CYP2A6 (minor), 2B6 (minor), 2C9 (major), 2D6 (major), 2E1 (minor), 3A4 (major); **Inhibits** CYP2B6 (weak), 2C8 (moderate), 2C9 (weak), 3A4 (weak)

Increased Effect/Toxicity: Concomitant use of warfarin is contraindicated when used for risk reduction; results in significant enhancement of the anticoagulant effects of warfarin. Tamoxifen may increase the levels/effects of CYP2C8 substrates; example substrates include amiodarone, paclitaxel, pioglitazone, repaglinide, and rosiglitazone. CYP2C9 inhibitors may increase the levels/effects of tamoxifen; example inhibitors include delavirdine, fluconazole, gemfibrozil, ketoconazole, nicardipine, NSAIDs, sulfonamides, and tolbutamide. CYP2D6 inhibitors may increase the levels/effects of tamoxifen; example inhibitors include chlorpromazine, delavirdine, fluoxetine, miconazole, paroxetine, pergolide, quinidine, quinine, ritonavir, and ropinirole. CYP3A4 inhibitors may increase the levels/effects of tamoxifen; example inhibitors include azole antifungals, clarithromycin, diclofenac, doxycycline, erythromycin, imatinib, isoniazid, nefazodone, nicardipine, propofol, protease inhibitors, quinidine, telithromycin, and verapamil. Rifamycin derivatives may increase the metabolism (via CYP isoenzymes) of tamoxifen.

Decreased Effect: CYP2C9 inducers may decrease the levels/effects of tamoxifen; example inducers include carbamazepine, phenobarbital, phenytoin, rifampin, rifapentine, and secobarbital. CYP3A4 inducers may decrease the levels/effects of tamoxifen; example inducers include aminoglutethimide, carbamazepine, nafcillin, nevirapine, phenobarbital, phenytoin, and rifamycins.

Ethanol/Nutrition/Herb Interactions Herb/Nutraceutical: Avoid black cohosh, dong quai in estrogen-dependent tumors. Avoid St John's wort (may decrease levels/effects of tamoxifen).

Pharmacodynamics/Kinetics

Absorption: Well absorbed; tablet and oral solution are bioequivalent

Distribution: High concentrations found in uterus, endometrial and breast tissue

Protein binding: 99%

Metabolism: Hepatic (via CYP3A4) to major metabolites, N-desmethyl tamoxifen (major) and 4-hydroxytamoxifen (minor), and a tamoxifen derivative (minor); undergoes enterohepatic recirculation

Half-life elimination: Distribution: 7-14 hours; Elimination: 5-7 days; Metabolites: 14 days

Time to peak, serum: 5 hours

Excretion: Feces (26% to 51%); urine (9% to 13%)

Pregnancy Risk Factor D

Dosage Forms SOLN, oral: 10 mg/5 mL (150 mL). **TAB:** 10 mg, 20 mg

Tamoxifen Citrate *see* Tamoxifen *on page 1443*

Tamsulosin (tam SOO loe sin)

U.S. Brand Names Flomax®

Canadian Brand Names Flomax®

Mexican Brand Names Secotex®

Generic Available No

Synonyms Tamsulosin Hydrochloride

Pharmacologic Category Alpha$_1$ Blocker

Use Treatment of signs and symptoms of benign prostatic hyperplasia (BPH)

Local Anesthetic/Vasoconstrictor Precautions No information available to require special precautions

Effects on Dental Treatment No significant effects or complications reported

Common Adverse Effects

>10%:

Cardiovascular: Studies specific for orthostatic hypotension: Overall, at least one positive test was observed in 16% of patients receiving 0.4 mg and 19% of patients receiving the 0.8 mg dose. "First-dose" orthostatic hypotension following a 0.4 mg dose was reported as 7% at 4 hours postdose and 6% at 8 hours postdose.

Central nervous system: Headache (19% to 21%), dizziness (15% to 17%)

Genitourinary: Abnormal ejaculation (8% to 18%)

Respiratory: Rhinitis (13% to 18%)

1% to 10%:

Cardiovascular: Chest pain (~4%)

Central nervous system: Somnolence (3% to 4%), insomnia (1% to 2%), vertigo (0.6% to 1%)

Endocrine & metabolic: Libido decreased (1% to 2%)

Gastrointestinal: Diarrhea (4% to 6%), nausea (3% to 4%), stomach discomfort (2% to 3%), bitter taste (2% to 3%)

Neuromuscular & skeletal: Weakness (8% to 9%), back pain (7% to 8%)

Ocular: Amblyopia (0.2% to 2%)

Respiratory: Pharyngitis (5% to 6%), cough (3% to 5%), sinusitis (2% to 4%)

Miscellaneous: Infection (9% to 11%), tooth disorder (1% to 2%)

Dosage Oral: Adults: 0.4 mg once daily ~30 minutes after the same meal each day; dose may be increased after 2-4 weeks to 0.8 mg once daily in patients who fail to respond. If therapy is interrupted for several days, restart with 0.4 mg once daily.

Dosage adjustment in renal impairment:

Cl$_{cr}$ ≥10 mL/minute: No adjustment needed

Cl$_{cr}$ <10 mL/minute: Not studied

Mechanism of Action Tamsulosin is an antagonist of alpha$_{1A}$ adrenoreceptors in the prostate. Smooth muscle tone in the prostate is mediated by alpha$_{1A}$ adrenoreceptors; blocking them leads to relaxation of smooth muscle in the bladder neck and prostate causing an improvement of urine flow and decreased symptoms of BPH. Approximately 75% of the alpha$_1$ receptors in the prostate are of the alpha$_{1A}$ subtype.

Contraindications Hypersensitivity to tamsulosin or any component of the formulation; concurrent use with phosphodiesterase-5 (PDE-5) inhibitors including sildenafil (>25 mg), tadalafil (if tamsulosin dose >0.4 mg/day), or vardenafil

Warnings/Precautions Not intended for use as an antihypertensive drug. May cause orthostasis, syncope or dizziness. Patients should avoid situations where injury may occur as a result of syncope. Rule out prostatic carcinoma before beginning therapy with tamsulosin. Intraoperative Floppy Iris Syndrome occurred most often in patients taking their alpha-1 blocker at the time of cataract surgery, but some cases occurred when the alpha-1 blocker blocker was stopped 2-14 days prior to surgery and as long as 5 weeks to 9 months prior to surgery. The benefit of stopping an alpha-1blocker prior to cataract

(Continued)

Tamsulosin *(Continued)*

surgery has not been established. Rarely, patients with a sulfa allergy have also developed an allergic reaction to tamsulosin; avoid use when previous reaction has been severe.

Drug Interactions

Cytochrome P450 Effect: Substrate (major) of CYP2D6, 3A4

Increased Effect/Toxicity: Alpha-adrenergic blockers and calcium channel blockers may increase risk of hypotension. Risk of first-dose orthostatic hypotension may increase with beta-blockers. Cimetidine may decrease tamsulosin clearance. Blood pressure-lowering effects are additive with sildenafil (use with extreme caution), tadalafil (may be used when tamsulosin dose is ≤0.4 mg/day), and vardenafil (use is contraindicated by the manufacturer).

CYP2D6 inhibitors may increase the levels/effects of tamsulosin; example inhibitors include chlorpromazine, delavirdine, fluoxetine, miconazole, paroxetine, pergolide, quinidine, quinine, ritonavir, and ropinirole. CYP3A4 inhibitors may increase the levels/effects of tamsulosin; example inhibitors include azole antifungals, clarithromycin, diclofenac, doxycycline, erythromycin, imatinib, isoniazid, nefazodone, nicardipine, propofol, protease inhibitors, quinidine, telithromycin, and verapamil.

Decreased Effect: CYP3A4 inducers may decrease the levels/effects of tamsulosin; example inducers include aminoglutethimide, carbamazepine, nafcillin, nevirapine, phenobarbital, phenytoin, and rifamycins.

Ethanol/Nutrition/Herb Interactions

Food: Fasting increases bioavailability by 30% and peak concentration 40% to 70%.

Herb/Nutraceutical: Avoid saw palmetto (due to limited experience with this combination).

Dietary Considerations Take once daily, 30 minutes after the same meal each day.

Pharmacodynamics/Kinetics

Absorption: >90%

Protein binding: 94% to 99%, primarily to alpha$_1$ acid glycoprotein (AAG)

Metabolism: Hepatic via CYP; metabolites undergo extensive conjugation to glucuronide or sulfate

Bioavailability: Fasting: 30% increase

Distribution: V_d: 16 L

Steady-state: By the fifth day of once-daily dosing

Half-life elimination: Healthy volunteers: 9-13 hours; Target population: 14-15 hours

Time to peak: Fasting: 4-5 hours; With food: 6-7 hours

Excretion: Urine (76%, <10% as unchanged drug); feces (21%)

Pregnancy Risk Factor B

Dosage Forms CAP: 0.4 mg

Tamsulosin Hydrochloride *see* Tamsulosin *on page 1445*

Tanac® [OTC] *see* Benzocaine *on page 190*

Tanafed DP™ *see* Dexchlorpheniramine and Pseudoephedrine *on page 443*

Tannate 12 S *see* Carbetapentane and Chlorpheniramine *on page 266*

Tannic-12 *see* Carbetapentane and Chlorpheniramine *on page 266*

Tannic-12 S *see* Carbetapentane and Chlorpheniramine *on page 266*

Tannihist-12 RF *see* Carbetapentane and Chlorpheniramine *on page 266*

TAP-144 *see* Leuprolide *on page 906*

Tapazole® *see* Methimazole *on page 1008*

Tarceva™ *see* Erlotinib *on page 560*

Targretin® *see* Bexarotene *on page 205*

Tarka® *see* Trandolapril and Verapamil *on page 1518*

Tarsum® [OTC] *see* Coal Tar and Salicylic Acid *on page 383*

Tasmar® *see* Tolcapone *on page 1503*

Tavist® Allergy [OTC] *see* Clemastine *on page 359*

Tavist® ND [OTC] *see* Loratadine *on page 946*

Taxol® *see* Paclitaxel *on page 1176*

Taxotere® *see* Docetaxel *on page 494*

Tazarotene *(taz AR oh teen)*

U.S. Brand Names Avage™; Tazorac®
Canadian Brand Names Tazorac®
Generic Available No

Pharmacologic Category Keratolytic Agent

Use Topical treatment of facial acne vulgaris; topical treatment of stable plaque psoriasis of up to 20% body surface area involvement; mitigation (palliation) of facial skin wrinkling, facial mottled hyper/hypopigmentation, and benign facial lentigines

Local Anesthetic/Vasoconstrictor Precautions No information available to require special precautions

Effects on Dental Treatment No significant effects or complications reported

Common Adverse Effects Percentage of incidence varies with formulation and/or strength:

>10%: Dermatologic: Burning/stinging, desquamation, dry skin, erythema, pruritus, skin pain, worsening of psoriasis

1% to 10%: Dermatologic: Contact dermatitis, discoloration, fissuring, hypertriglyceridemia, inflammation, irritation, localized bleeding, rash

Frequency not defined:
Dermatologic: Photosensitization
Neuromuscular & skeletal: Peripheral neuropathy

Mechanism of Action Synthetic, acetylenic retinoid which modulates differentiation and proliferation of epithelial tissue and exerts some degree of anti-inflammatory and immunological activity

Drug Interactions
Increased Effect/Toxicity: Increased toxicity may occur with sulfur, benzoyl peroxide, salicylic acid, resorcinol, or any product with strong drying effects (including alcohol-containing compounds) due to increased drying actions. May augment phototoxicity of sensitizing medications (thiazides, tetracyclines, fluoroquinolones, phenothiazines, sulfonamides).

Pharmacodynamics/Kinetics
Duration: Therapeutic: Psoriasis: Effects have been observed for up to 3 months after a 3-month course of topical treatment

Absorption: Minimal following cutaneous application (≤6% of dose)

Distribution: Retained in skin for prolonged periods after topical application.

Protein binding: >99%

Metabolism: Prodrug, rapidly metabolized via esterases to an active metabolite (tazarotenic acid) following topical application and systemic absorption; tazarotenic acid undergoes further hepatic metabolism

Half-life elimination: 18 hours

Excretion: Urine and feces (as metabolites)

Pregnancy Risk Factor X

Tazicef® see Ceftazidime on page 292

Tazorac® see Tazarotene on page 1446

Taztia XT™ see Diltiazem on page 479

3TC see Lamivudine on page 894

3TC, Abacavir, and Zidovudine see Abacavir, Lamivudine, and Zidovudine on page 23

T-Cell Growth Factor see Aldesleukin on page 61

TCGF see Aldesleukin on page 61

TCN see Tetracycline on page 1467

TDF see Tenofovir on page 1457

Teargen® [OTC] see Artificial Tears on page 143

Teargen® II [OTC] see Artificial Tears on page 143

Tearisol® [OTC] see Artificial Tears on page 143

Tears Again® [OTC] see Artificial Tears on page 143

Tears Again® MC [OTC] see Hydroxypropyl Methylcellulose on page 800

Tears Again® Gel Drops™ [OTC] see Carboxymethylcellulose on page 271

Tears Again® Night and Day™ [OTC] see Carboxymethylcellulose on page 271

Tears Naturale® [OTC] see Artificial Tears on page 143

Tears Naturale® II [OTC] see Artificial Tears on page 143

Tears Naturale® Free [OTC] see Artificial Tears on page 143

Tears Plus® [OTC] see Artificial Tears on page 143

Tears Renewed® [OTC] see Artificial Tears on page 143

TEAS see Triethanolamine Salicylate on page 1535

Tebamide™ see Trimethobenzamide on page 1538

Tegaserod (teg a SER od)

U.S. Brand Names Zelnorm®
Canadian Brand Names Zelnorm®
Mexican Brand Names Zelmac®
Generic Available No
Synonyms HTF919; Tegaserod Maleate
Pharmacologic Category Serotonin 5-HT$_4$ Receptor Agonist
Use Short-term treatment of constipation-predominate irritable bowel syndrome (IBS) in women; treatment of chronic idiopathic constipation
Local Anesthetic/Vasoconstrictor Precautions No information available to require special precautions
Effects on Dental Treatment No significant effects or complications reported
Common Adverse Effects
>10%:
Central nervous system: Headache (15%)
Gastrointestinal: Abdominal pain (12%)
1% to 10%:
Central nervous system: Dizziness (4%), migraine (2%)
Gastrointestinal: Diarrhea (9%; severe <1%), nausea (8%), flatulence (6%)
Neuromuscular & skeletal: Back pain (5%), arthropathy (2%), leg pain (1%)
Mechanism of Action Tegaserod is a partial neuronal 5-HT$_4$ receptor agonist. Its action at the receptor site leads to stimulation of the peristaltic reflex and intestinal secretion, and moderation of visceral sensitivity.
Pharmacodynamics/Kinetics
Distribution: V$_d$: 368 ± 223 L
Protein binding: 98% primarily to α_1-acid glycoprotein
Metabolism: GI: Hydrolysis in the stomach; Hepatic: Oxidation, conjugation, and glucuronidation; metabolite (negligible activity); significant first-pass effect
Bioavailability: Fasting: 10%
Half-life elimination: I.V.: 11 ± 5 hours
Time to peak: 1 hour
Excretion: Feces (~66% as unchanged drug); urine (~33% as metabolites)
Pregnancy Risk Factor B

Tegaserod Maleate *see* Tegaserod *on page 1448*

Tegretol® *see* Carbamazepine *on page 260*

Tegretol®-XR *see* Carbamazepine *on page 260*

Teldrin® HBP [OTC] *see* Chlorpheniramine *on page 323*

Telithromycin (tel ith roe MYE sin)

U.S. Brand Names Ketek®
Canadian Brand Names Ketek®
Generic Available No
Synonyms HMR 3647
Pharmacologic Category Antibiotic, Ketolide
Use Treatment of community-acquired pneumonia (mild-to-moderate) caused by susceptible strains of *Streptococcus pneumoniae* (including multidrug-resistant isolates), *Haemophilus influenzae*, *Chlamydia pneumoniae*, *Moraxella catarrhalis*, and *Mycoplasma pneumoniae*; treatment of bacterial exacerbation of chronic bronchitis caused by susceptible strains of *S. pneumoniae*, *H. influenzae* and *Moraxella catarrhalis*; treatment of acute bacterial sinusitis caused by *Streptococcus pneumoniae*, *Haemophilus influenzae*, *Moraxella catarrhalis*, and *Staphylococcus aureus*
Unlabeled/Investigational Use Approved in Canada for use in the treatment of tonsillitis/pharyngitis due to *S. pyogenes* (as an alternative to beta-lactam antibiotics when necessary/appropriate)
Local Anesthetic/Vasoconstrictor Precautions Telithromycin is associated with prolongation of cardiac repolarization. It produces a block of myocardial potassium currents resulting in prolonged QT$_c$ interval which may give rise to ventricular tachycardia, ventricular fibrillation or torsade de pointes. Vasoconstrictor should be used with caution; if possible, wait until the patients complete their course of antibiotic therapy prior to using vasoconstrictor. The overall risk of ventricular arrhythmias by telithromycin is small and can be further reduced by the cautious use of vasoconstrictor. See Dental Comment.
Effects on Dental Treatment Key adverse event(s) related to dental treatment: Xerostomia (normal salivary flow resumes upon discontinuation), glossitis, stomatitis, and tooth discoloration.

Common Adverse Effects

2% to 10%:

Central nervous system: Headache (2% to 6%), dizziness (3% to 4%)

Gastrointestinal: Diarrhea (10%), nausea (7% to 8%), vomiting (2% to 3%), loose stools (2%), dysgeusia (2%)

≥0.2% to <2%:

Central nervous system: Vertigo, fatigue, somnolence, insomnia

Dermatologic: Rash

Gastrointestinal: Abdominal distension, abdominal pain, anorexia, constipation, dyspepsia, flatulence, gastritis, gastroenteritis, GI upset, glossitis, stomatitis, watery stools, xerostomia

Genitourinary: Vaginal candidiasis

Hematologic: Platelets increased

Hepatic: Transaminases increased, hepatitis

Ocular: Blurred vision, accommodation delayed, diplopia

Miscellaneous: Candidiasis, diaphoresis increased, exacerbation of myasthenia gravis (rare)

Additional effects also reported with telithromycin: Abnormal dreams, anemia, appetite decreased, bundle branch block, cholestasis, coagulation disorder, esophagitis, hyperkalemia, hypersensitivity, hypokalemia, leukopenia, lymphopenia, nervousness, neutropenia, palpitation, pharyngolaryngeal pain, polyuria, pseudomembranous colitis, QT_c prolongation, reflux esophagitis, serum creatinine increased, thrombocytopenia, tooth discoloration, tremor, urine discoloration, vaginal irritation, vasculitis, weakness

Dosage Oral:

Children ≥13 years and Adults: Tonsillitis/pharyngitis (unlabeled U.S. indication): 800 mg once daily for 5 days

Adults:

Acute exacerbation of chronic bronchitis, acute bacterial sinusitis: 800 mg once daily for 5 days

Community-acquired pneumonia: 800 mg once daily for 7-10 days

Dosage adjustment in renal impairment:

U.S. product labeling: Cl_{cr} <30 mL/minute: 600 mg once daily; when renal impairment is accompanied by hepatic impairment, reduce dosage to 400 mg once daily

Canadian product labeling: Cl_{cr} <30 mL/minute: Reduce dose to 400 mg once daily

Hemodialysis: Administer following dialysis

Dosage adjustment in hepatic impairment: No adjustment recommended, unless concurrent severe renal impairment is present

Mechanism of Action Inhibits bacterial protein synthesis by binding to two sites on the 50S ribosomal subunit. Telithromycin has also been demonstrated to alter secretion of IL-1alpha and TNF-alpha; the clinical significance of this immunomodulatory effect has not been evaluated.

Contraindications Hypersensitivity to telithromycin, macrolide antibiotics, or any component of the formulation; concurrent use of cisapride or pimozide

Warnings/Precautions May prolong QT_c interval, leading to a risk of ventricular arrhythmias; closely-related antibiotics have been associated with malignant ventricular arrhythmias and torsade de pointes. Avoid in patients with prolongation of QT_c interval due to congenital causes, history of long QT syndrome, uncorrected electrolyte disturbances (hypokalemia or hypomagnesemia), significant bradycardia (<50 bpm), or concurrent therapy with QT_c-prolonging drugs (eg, class Ia and class III antiarrhythmics). Avoid use in patients with a prior history of confirmed cardiogenic syncope or ventricular arrhythmias while receiving macrolide antibiotics or other QT_c-prolonging drugs. Limited case reports have documented the occurrence of jaundice and serious liver damage; use caution with hepatic impairment or previous history of jaundice, and discontinue with signs/symptoms of liver damage. Use caution in renal impairment. Use caution in patients with myasthenia gravis (use only if suitable alternatives are not available). Inform patients of potential for blurred vision, which may interfere with ability to operate machinery or drive; use caution until effects are known. Safety and efficacy not established in pediatric patients <13 years of age per Canadian approved labeling and <18 years of age per U.S. approved labeling. Pseudomembranous colitis has been reported.

Drug Interactions

Cytochrome P450 Effect: Substrate of CYP1A2 (minor), 3A4 (major); **Inhibits** CYP2D6 (weak), 3A4 (strong)

Increased Effect/Toxicity: Concurrent use of cisapride or pimozide is contraindicated. Concurrent use with antiarrhythmics (eg, class Ia and class

(Continued)

Telithromycin *(Continued)*

III) or other drugs which prolong QT$_c$ (eg, gatifloxacin, mesoridazine, moxiflox-acin, pimozide, sparfloxacin, thioridazine) may be additive; serious arrhythmias may occur. Neuromuscular-blocking agents may be potentiated by telithromycin.

Telithromycin may increase the levels/effects of selected benzodiazepines, calcium channel blockers, cyclosporine, ergot alkaloids, selected HMG-CoA reductase inhibitors, mirtazapine, nateglinide, nefazodone, pimozide, quinidine, sildenafil (and other PDE-5 inhibitors), tacrolimus, venlafaxine, warfarin (monitor), and other CYP3A4 substrates. Selected benzodiazepines (midazolam, triazolam), and selected HMG-CoA reductase inhibitors (atorvastatin, lovastatin and simvastatin) are generally contraindicated with strong CYP3A4 inhibitors. When used with strong CYP3A4 inhibitors, dosage adjustment/limits are recommended for sildenafil and other PDE-5 inhibitors; refer to individual monographs.

The levels/effects of telithromycin may be increased by azole antifungals, clarithromycin, diclofenac, doxycycline, erythromycin, imatinib, isoniazid, nefazodone, nicardipine, propofol, protease inhibitors, quinidine, verapamil, and other CYP3A4 inhibitors.

Decreased Effect: The levels/effects of telithromycin may be decreased by aminoglutethimide, carbamazepine, nafcillin, nevirapine, phenobarbital, phenytoin, rifamycins, and other CYP3A4 inducers; avoid concurrent use.

Dietary Considerations May be taken with or without food.

Pharmacodynamics/Kinetics

Absorption: Rapid
Distribution: 2.9 L/kg
Protein binding: 60% to 70%
Metabolism: Hepatic, via CYP3A4 (50%) and non-CYP-mediated pathways
Bioavailability: 57% (significant first-pass metabolism)
Half-life elimination: 10 hours
Time to peak, plasma: 1 hour
Excretion: Urine (13% unchanged drug, remainder as metabolites); feces (7%)

Pregnancy Risk Factor C

Dosage Forms TAB [film coated]: 300 mg [not available in Canada], 400 mg; (Ketek Pak™) [blister pack]: 400 mg (10s)

Dental Comment

This drug is known to prolong the QT interval. The QT interval is measured as the time and distance between the Q point of the QRS complex and the end of the T wave in the ECG tracing. After adjustment for heart rate, the QT interval is defined as prolonged if it is more than 450 msec in men and 460 msec in women. A long QT syndrome was first described in the 1950s and 60s as a congenital syndrome involving QT interval prolongation and syncope and sudden death. Some of the congenital long QT syndromes were characterized by a peculiar electrocardiographic appearance of the QRS complex involving a premature atria beat followed by a pause, then a subsequent sinus beat showing marked QT prolongation and deformity. This type of cardiac arrhythmia was originally termed "torsade de pointes" (translated from the French as "twisting of the points").

Prolongation of the QT interval is thought to result from delayed ventricular repolarization. The repolarization process within the myocardial cell is due to the efflux of intracellular potassium. The channels associated with this current can be blocked by many drugs and predisposes the electrical propagation cycle to torsade de pointes.

Telithromycin is one of the drugs confirmed to prolong the QT interval and is accepted as having a risk of causing torsade de pointes. The risk of drug-induced torsade de pointes is extremely low when a single QT interval prolonging drug is prescribed. In terms of epinephrine, it is not known what effect vasoconstrictors in the local anesthetic regimen will have in patients with a known history of congenital prolonged QT interval or in patients taking any medication that prolongs the QT interval. Until more information is obtained, it is suggested that the clinician consult with the physician prior to the use of a vasoconstrictor in suspected patients, and that the vasoconstrictor (epinephrine, levonordefrin [Neo-Cobefrin®]) be used with caution.

Selected Readings

Araujo FG, Slifer TL, and Remington JS, "Inhibition of Secretion of Interleukin-1alpha and Tumor Necrosis Factor Alpha by the Ketolide Antibiotic Telithromycin," *Antimicrob Agents Chemother,* 2002, 46(10):3327-30.

Bhargava V, Lenfant B, Perret C, et al, "Lack of Effect of Food on the Bioavailability of a New Ketolide Antibacterial, Telithromycin," *Scand J Infect Dis,* 2002, 34(11):823-6.

Cantalloube C, Bhargava V, Sultan E, et al, "Pharmacokinetics of the Ketolide Telithromycin After Single and Repeated Doses in Patients With Hepatic Impairment," *Int J Antimicrob Agents,* 2003, 22(2):112-21.

Canton R, Morosini M, Enright MC, et al, "Worldwide Incidence, Molecular Epidemiology and Mutations Implicated in Fluoroquinolone-resistant *Streptococcus pneumoniae*: Data From the Global PROTEKT Surveillance Programme," *J Antimicrob Chemother*, 2003, 52(6):944-52.

Carbon C, "A Pooled Analysis of Telithromycin in the Treatment of Community-Acquired Respiratory Tract Infections in Adults," *Infection*, 2003, 31(5):308-17.

Demolis JL, Vacheron F, Cardus S, et al, "Effect of Single and Repeated Oral Doses of Telithromycin on Cardiac QT Interval in Healthy Subjects," *Clin Pharmacol Ther*, 2003, 73(3):242-52.

Perret C, Lenfant B, Weinling E, et al, "Pharmacokinetics and Absolute Oral Bioavailability of an 800-mg Oral Dose of Telithromycin in Healthy Young and Elderly Volunteers," *Chemotherapy*, 2002, 48(5):217-23.

Nieman RB, Sharma K, Edelberg H, et al, "Telithromycin and Myasthenia Gravis," *Clin Infect Dis*, 2003, 37(11):1579.

Quinn J, Ruoff GE, and Ziter PS, "Efficacy and tolerability of 5-day, once-daily telithromycin compared with 10-day, twice-daily clarithromycin for the treatment of group A beta-hemolytic streptococcal tonsillitis/pharyngitis: a multicenter, randomized, double-blind, parallel-group study," *Clin Ther*, 2003, 25(2):422-43.

Ubukata K, Iwata S, and Sunakawa K, "*In vitro* Activities of New Ketolide, Telithromycin, and Eight Other Macrolide Antibiotics Against *Streptococcus pneumoniae* Having mefA and ermB Genes That Mediate Macrolide Resistance," *J Infect Chemother*, 2003, 9(3):221-6.

Zervos MJ, Heyder AM, and Leroy B, "Oral Telithromycin 800 mg Once Daily for 5 Days Versus Cefuroxime Axetil 500 mg Twice Daily for 10 Days in Adults With Acute Exacerbations of Chronic Bronchitis," *J Int Med Res*, 2003, 31(3):157-69.

Telmisartan (tel mi SAR tan)

Related Information
Cardiovascular Diseases *on page 1636*

U.S. Brand Names Micardis®

Canadian Brand Names Micardis®

Generic Available No

Pharmacologic Category Angiotensin II Receptor Blocker

Use Treatment of hypertension; may be used alone or in combination with other antihypertensive agents

Local Anesthetic/Vasoconstrictor Precautions No information available to require special precautions

Effects on Dental Treatment No significant effects or complications reported

Common Adverse Effects May be associated with worsening of renal function in patients dependent on renin-angiotensin-aldosterone system.

1% to 10%:
Cardiovascular: Hypertension (1%), chest pain (1%), peripheral edema (1%)
Central nervous system: Headache (1%), dizziness (1%), pain (1%), fatigue (1%)
Gastrointestinal: Diarrhea (3%), dyspepsia (1%), nausea (1%), abdominal pain (1%)
Genitourinary: Urinary tract infection (1%)
Neuromuscular & skeletal: Back pain (3%), myalgia (1%)
Respiratory: Upper respiratory infection (7%), sinusitis (3%), pharyngitis (1%), cough (2%)
Miscellaneous: Flu-like syndrome (1%)

Dosage Adults: Oral: Initial: 40 mg once daily; usual maintenance dose range: 20-80 mg/day. Patients with volume depletion should be initiated on the lower dosage with close supervision.

Dosage adjustment in hepatic impairment: Supervise patients closely.

Mechanism of Action Angiotensin II acts as a vasoconstrictor. In addition to causing direct vasoconstriction, angiotensin II also stimulates the release of aldosterone. Once aldosterone is released, sodium as well as water are reabsorbed. The end result is an elevation in blood pressure. Telmisartan is a nonpeptide AT1 angiotensin II receptor antagonist. This binding prevents angiotensin II from binding to the receptor thereby blocking the vasoconstriction and the aldosterone secreting effects of angiotensin II.

Contraindications Hypersensitivity to telmisartan or any component of the formulation; hypersensitivity to other A-II receptor antagonists; bilateral renal artery stenosis; pregnancy (2nd and 3rd trimesters)

Warnings/Precautions Avoid use or use a smaller dose in patients who are volume depleted; correct depletion first. Deterioration in renal function can occur with initiation. Use with caution in unilateral renal artery stenosis and pre-existing renal insufficiency; significant aortic/mitral stenosis. Use with caution in patients who have biliary obstructive disorders or hepatic dysfunction.

Drug Interactions
Cytochrome P450 Effect: Inhibits CYP2C19 (weak)

Increased Effect/Toxicity: Telmisartan may increase serum digoxin concentrations. Potassium salts/supplements, co-trimoxazole (high dose), ACE inhibitors, and potassium-sparing diuretics (amiloride, spironolactone, triamterene) may increase the risk of hyperkalemia with telmisartan.

(Continued)

Telmisartan (Continued)

Decreased Effect: Telmisartan decreased the trough concentrations of warfarin during concurrent therapy; however, INR was not changed.

Ethanol/Nutrition/Herb Interactions Herb/Nutraceutical: Avoid dong quai if using for hypertension (has estrogenic activity). Avoid ephedra, yohimbe, ginseng (may worsen hypertension). Avoid garlic (may have increased antihypertensive effect).

Dietary Considerations May be taken without regard to food.

Pharmacodynamics/Kinetics Orally active, not a prodrug

Onset of action: 1-2 hours
  Peak effect: 0.5-1 hours
Duration: Up to 24 hours
Protein binding: >99.5%
Metabolism: Hepatic via conjugation to inactive metabolites; not metabolized via CYP
Bioavailability (dose dependent): 42% to 58%
Half-life elimination: Terminal: 24 hours
Excretion: Feces (97%)
  Clearance: Total body: 800 mL/minute

Pregnancy Risk Factor C (1st trimester); D (2nd and 3rd trimesters)

Dosage Forms TAB: 20 mg, 40 mg, 80 mg

Telmisartan and Hydrochlorothiazide

(tel mi SAR tan & hye droe klor oh THYE a zide)

Related Information

Hydrochlorothiazide *on page 776*
Telmisartan *on page 1451*

U.S. Brand Names Micardis® HCT

Canadian Brand Names Micardis® Plus

Generic Available No

Synonyms Hydrochlorothiazide and Telmisartan

Pharmacologic Category Angiotensin II Receptor Blocker Combination; Antihypertensive Agent, Combination; Diuretic, Thiazide

Use Treatment of hypertension; combination product should not be used for initial therapy

Local Anesthetic/Vasoconstrictor Precautions No information available to require special precautions

Effects on Dental Treatment No significant effects or complications reported

Common Adverse Effects The following reactions have been reported with the combination product; see individual agents for additional adverse reactions that may be expected from each agent.

2% to 10%:
  Central nervous system: Dizziness (5%)
  Gastrointestinal: Diarrhea (3%), nausea (2%)
  Renal: BUN increased (3%)
  Respiratory: Upper respiratory tract infection (8%), sinusitis (4%)
  Miscellaneous: Flu-like syndrome (2%)
<2%: Abdominal pain, back pain, bilirubin increased, bronchitis, dyspepsia, hematocrit decreased, hemoglobin decreased, hypokalemia, liver enzymes increased, pharyngitis, postural hypotension, rash, serum creatinine increased, tachycardia, vomiting; rhabdomyolysis has been reported (rarely) with angiotensin-receptor antagonists

Mechanism of Action

Telmisartan: Telmisartan is an angiotensin receptor antagonist. Angiotensin II acts as a vasoconstrictor. In addition to causing direct vasoconstriction, angiotensin II also stimulates the release of aldosterone. Once aldosterone is released, sodium as well as water are reabsorbed. The end result is an elevation in blood pressure. Telmisartan binds to the AT1 angiotensin II receptor. This binding prevents angiotensin II from binding to the receptor thereby blocking the vasoconstriction and the aldosterone secreting effects of angiotensin II.

Hydrochlorothiazide: Inhibits sodium reabsorption in the distal tubules causing increased excretion of sodium and water as well as potassium and hydrogen ions

Drug Interactions

Cytochrome P450 Effect: Telmisartan: **Inhibits** CYP2C19 (weak)

Increased Effect/Toxicity: See individual agents.

Decreased Effect: See individual agents.

Pharmacodynamics/Kinetics See individual agents.

Pregnancy Risk Factor C (1st trimester); D (2nd and 3rd trimesters)

Temazepam (te MAZ e pam)

U.S. Brand Names Restoril®
Canadian Brand Names Apo-Temazepam®; CO Temazepam; Gen-Temazepam; Novo-Temazepam; Nu-Temazepam; PMS-Temazepam; ratio-Temazepam; Restoril®
Generic Available Yes
Pharmacologic Category Hypnotic, Benzodiazepine
Use Short-term treatment of insomnia
Unlabeled/Investigational Use Treatment of anxiety; adjunct in the treatment of depression; management of panic attacks
Local Anesthetic/Vasoconstrictor Precautions No information available to require special precautions
Effects on Dental Treatment Key adverse event(s) related to dental treatment: Significant xerostomia (normal salivary flow resumes upon discontinuation).
Common Adverse Effects
1% to 10%:
Central nervous system: Confusion, dizziness, drowsiness, fatigue, anxiety, headache, lethargy, hangover, euphoria, vertigo
Dermatologic: Rash
Endocrine & metabolic: Decreased libido
Gastrointestinal: Diarrhea
Neuromuscular & skeletal: Dysarthria, weakness
Ocular: Blurred vision
Miscellaneous: Diaphoresis
Restrictions C-IV
Dosage Oral:
Adults: 15-30 mg at bedtime
Elderly or debilitated patients: 15 mg
Mechanism of Action Binds to stereospecific benzodiazepine receptors on the postsynaptic GABA neuron at several sites within the central nervous system, including the limbic system, reticular formation. Enhancement of the inhibitory effect of GABA on neuronal excitability results by increased neuronal membrane permeability to chloride ions. This shift in chloride ions results in hyperpolarization (a less excitable state) and stabilization.
Contraindications Hypersensitivity to temazepam or any component of the formulation (cross-sensitivity with other benzodiazepines may exist); narrow-angle glaucoma (not in product labeling, however, benzodiazepines are contraindicated); pregnancy
Warnings/Precautions Should be used only after evaluation of potential causes of sleep disturbance. Failure of sleep disturbance to resolve after 7-10 days may indicate psychiatric or medical illness. A worsening of insomnia or the emergence of new abnormalities of thought or behavior may represent unrecognized psychiatric or medical illness and requires immediate and careful evaluation.

Use with caution in elderly or debilitated patients, patients with hepatic disease (including alcoholics), or renal impairment. Use with caution in patients with respiratory disease, or impaired gag reflex. Avoid use inpatients with sleep apnea.

Causes CNS depression (dose-related) resulting in sedation, dizziness, confusion, or ataxia which may impair physical and mental capabilities. Patients must be cautioned about performing tasks which require mental alertness (eg, operating machinery or driving). Use with caution in patients receiving other CNS depressants or psychoactive agents. Effects with other sedative drugs or ethanol may be potentiated. Benzodiazepines have been associated with falls and traumatic injury and should be used with extreme caution in patients who are at risk of these events (especially the elderly).

Use caution in patients with suicidal risk. Use with caution in patients with a history of drug dependence. Benzodiazepines have been associated with dependence and acute withdrawal symptoms on discontinuation or reduction in dose (may occur after as little as 10 days). Acute withdrawal, including seizures, may be precipitated after administration of flumazenil to patients receiving long-term benzodiazepine therapy.

Benzodiazepines have been associated with anterograde amnesia. Paradoxical reactions, including hyperactive or aggressive behavior, have been reported with benzodiazepines, particularly in adolescent/pediatric or psychiatric patients. Does not have analgesic, antidepressant, or antipsychotic properties. (Continued)

Temazepam *(Continued)*

Drug Interactions

Cytochrome P450 Effect: Substrate (minor) of CYP2B6, 2C8/9, 2C19, 3A4

Increased Effect/Toxicity: Temazepam potentiates the CNS depressant effects of narcotic analgesics, barbiturates, phenothiazines, ethanol, antihistamines, MAO inhibitors, sedative-hypnotics, and cyclic antidepressants. Serum levels of temazepam may be increased by inhibitors of CYP3A4, including cimetidine, ciprofloxacin, clarithromycin, clozapine, diltiazem, disulfiram, digoxin, erythromycin, ethanol, fluconazole, fluoxetine, fluvoxamine, grapefruit juice, isoniazid, itraconazole, ketoconazole, labetalol, levodopa, loxapine, metoprolol, metronidazole, miconazole, nefazodone, omeprazole, phenytoin, rifabutin, rifampin, troleandomycin, valproic acid, and verapamil.

Decreased Effect: Oral contraceptives may increase the clearance of temazepam. Temazepam may decrease the antiparkinsonian efficacy of levodopa. Theophylline and other CNS stimulants may antagonize the sedative effects of temazepam. Carbamazepine, rifampin, rifabutin may enhance the metabolism of temazepam and decrease its therapeutic effect.

Ethanol/Nutrition/Herb Interactions

Ethanol: Avoid ethanol (may increase CNS depression).

Food: Serum levels may be increased by grapefruit juice.

Herb/Nutraceutical: St John's wort may decrease temazepam levels. Avoid valerian, St John's wort, kava kava, gotu kola (may increase CNS depression).

Pharmacodynamics/Kinetics

Distribution: V_d: 1.4 L/kg

Protein binding: 96%

Metabolism: Hepatic

Half-life elimination: 9.5-12.4 hours

Time to peak, serum: 2-3 hours

Excretion: Urine (80% to 90% as inactive metabolites)

Pregnancy Risk Factor X

Dosage Forms CAP: 15 mg, 30 mg; (Restoril®): 7.5 mg, 15 mg, 30 mg

Temodar® *see* Temozolomide *on page 1454*

Temovate® *see* Clobetasol *on page 365*

Temovate E® *see* Clobetasol *on page 365*

Temozolomide *(te moe ZOE loe mide)*

U.S. Brand Names Temodar®

Canadian Brand Names Temodal™; Temodar®

Generic Available No

Synonyms NSC-362856; TMZ

Pharmacologic Category Antineoplastic Agent, Alkylating Agent

Use Treatment of adult patients with refractory (first relapse) anaplastic astrocytoma who have experienced disease progression on nitrosourea and procarbazine; newly-diagnosed glioblastoma multiforme

Unlabeled/Investigational Use Glioma, melanoma

Local Anesthetic/Vasoconstrictor Precautions No information available to require special precautions

Effects on Dental Treatment No significant effects or complications reported

Common Adverse Effects Adverse reactions are listed as the combined incidence in studies for treatment of newly-diagnosed glioblastoma multiforme during the maintenance phase (after radiotherapy) and refractory anaplastic astrocytoma in adults.

>10%:

Cardiovascular: Peripheral edema (up to 11%)

Central nervous system: Fatigue (34% to 61%), headache (23% to 41%), fatigue (34% to 61%), convulsions (6% to 23%), hemiparesis (18%), dizziness (5% to 12%), fever (up to 13%), coordination abnormality (up to 11%). In the case of CNS malignancies, it is difficult to distinguish the relative contributions of temozolomide and progressive disease to CNS symptoms.

Dermatologic: Alopecia (55% - maintenance phase after radiotherapy), rash (8% to 13%)

Gastrointestinal: Nausea (49% to 53%), vomiting (29% to 42%), constipation (22% to 33%), anorexia (9% to 27%), diarrhea (10% to 16%)

Hematologic: Lymphopenia (grade 3/4 in 55%), thrombocytopenia (grade 3/4 in 4% to 19%), neutropenia (grade 3/4 in 8% to 14%), leukopenia (grade 3/4 in 11%)

Neuromuscular & skeletal: Weakness (7% to 13%)

Miscellaneous: Viral infection (up to 11%)

1% to 10%:
   Central nervous system: Ataxia (8%), memory impairment (up to 7%), confusion (5%), anxiety (7%), depression (up to 6%), amnesia (up to 10%), paresis (up to 8%), somnolence (up to 9%), insomnia (4% to 10%)
   Dermatologic: Rash (8% to 13%), pruritus (5% to 8%), dry skin (up to 5%), radiation injury (2% - maintenance phase after radiotherapy), erythema (1%)
   Endocrine & metabolic: Hypercorticism (8%), breast pain (up to 6%)
   Gastrointestinal: Dysphagia (up to 7%), abdominal pain (5% to 9%), stomatitis (up to 9%), weight gain (up to 5%)
   Genitourinary: Micturition frequency increased (up to 6%), incontinence (up to 8%), urinary tract infection (up to 8%)
   Hematologic: Anemia (8%; grade 3/4 in up to 4%)
   Neuromuscular & skeletal: Paresthesia (up to 9%), back pain (up to 8%), arthralgia (up to 6%), abnormal gait (up to 6%), myalgia (up to 5%),
   Ocular: Diplopia (5%); vision abnormality (blurred vision, visual deficit, vision changes) (5% to 8%)
   Respiratory: Pharyngitis (up to 8%), sinusitis (up to 6%), cough (5% to 8%), upper respiratory tract infection (up to 8%), dyspnea (5%)
   Miscellaneous: Taste perversion (up to 5%), allergic reaction (up to 3%)

Mechanism of Action Like dacarbazine, temozolomide is converted to the active alkylating metabolite MTIC [(methyl-triazene-1-yl)-imidazole-4-carboxamide]. Unlike dacarbazine, however, this conversion is spontaneous, nonenzymatic, and occurs under physiologic conditions in all tissues to which the drug distributes.

Pharmacodynamics/Kinetics
   Distribution: V_d: Parent drug: 0.4 L/kg
   Protein binding: 15%
   Metabolism: Prodrug, hydrolyzed to the active form, MTIC; MTIC is eventually eliminated as CO_2 and 5-aminoimidazole-4-carboxamide (AIC), a natural constituent in urine
   Bioavailability: 100%
   Half-life elimination: Mean: Parent drug: 1.8 hours
   Time to peak: Empty stomach: 1 hour
   Excretion: Urine (~38%; parent drug 6%); feces 0.8%

Pregnancy Risk Factor D

Tenecteplase (ten EK te plase)

Related Information
   Cardiovascular Diseases *on page 1636*
U.S. Brand Names TNKase™
Canadian Brand Names TNKase™
Generic Available No
Pharmacologic Category Thrombolytic Agent
Use Thrombolytic agent used in the management of acute myocardial infarction for the lysis of thrombi in the coronary vasculature to restore perfusion and reduce mortality.
Unlabeled/Investigational Use Acute MI — combination regimen of tenecteplase (unlabeled dose), abciximab, and heparin (unlabeled dose)
Local Anesthetic/Vasoconstrictor Precautions No information available to require special precautions
Effects on Dental Treatment No significant effects or complications reported
Common Adverse Effects As with all drugs which may affect hemostasis, bleeding is the major adverse effect associated with tenecteplase. Hemorrhage may occur at virtually any site. Risk is dependent on multiple variables, including the dosage administered, concurrent use of multiple agents which alter hemostasis, and patient predisposition. Rapid lysis of coronary artery thrombi by thrombolytic agents may be associated with reperfusion-related arterial and/or ventricular arrhythmia. The incidence of stroke and bleeding increase in patients >65 years.

>10%:
   Hematologic: Bleeding (22% minor: ASSENT-2 trial)
   Local: Hematoma (12% minor)
1% to 10%:
   Central nervous system: Stroke (2%)
   Gastrointestinal: GI hemorrhage (1% major, 2% minor), epistaxis (2% minor)
   Genitourinary: GU bleeding (4% minor)
   Hematologic: Bleeding (5% major: ASSENT-2 trial)
   Local: Bleeding at catheter puncture site (4% minor), hematoma (2% major)
   Respiratory: Pharyngeal bleeding (3% minor)
(Continued)

Tenecteplase *(Continued)*

Additional cardiovascular events associated with use in MI: Cardiogenic shock, arrhythmia, AV block, pulmonary edema, heart failure, cardiac arrest, recurrent myocardial ischemia, myocardial reinfarction, myocardial rupture, cardiac tamponade, pericarditis, pericardial effusion, mitral regurgitation, thrombosis, embolism, electromechanical dissociation, hypotension, fever, nausea, vomiting

Mechanism of Action Initiates fibrinolysis by binding to fibrin and converting plasminogen to plasmin.

Drug Interactions

Increased Effect/Toxicity: Drugs which affect platelet function (eg, NSAIDs, dipyridamole, ticlopidine, clopidogrel, IIb/IIIa antagonists) may potentiate the risk of hemorrhage; use with caution.

Heparin and aspirin: Use with aspirin and heparin may increase bleeding. However, aspirin and heparin were used concomitantly with tenecteplase in the majority of patients in clinical studies.

Warfarin or oral anticoagulants: Risk of bleeding may be increased during concurrent therapy.

Decreased Effect: Aminocaproic acid (antifibrinolytic agent) may decrease effectiveness.

Pharmacodynamics/Kinetics

Distribution: V_d is weight related and approximates plasma volume

Metabolism: Primarily hepatic

Half-life elimination: 90-130 minutes

Excretion: Clearance: Plasma: 99-119 mL/minute

Pregnancy Risk Factor C

Tenex® *see* Guanfacine *on page 758*

Teniposide *(ten i POE side)*

U.S. Brand Names Vumon®
Canadian Brand Names Vumon®
Mexican Brand Names Vumon®
Generic Available No
Synonyms EPT; VM-26
Pharmacologic Category Antineoplastic Agent, Miscellaneous
Use Treatment of acute lymphocytic leukemia, small cell lung cancer
Local Anesthetic/Vasoconstrictor Precautions No information available to require special precautions
Effects on Dental Treatment No significant effects or complications reported
Common Adverse Effects

>10%:

Gastrointestinal: Mucositis (75%); diarrhea, nausea, vomiting (20% to 30%); anorexia

Hematologic: Myelosuppression, leukopenia, neutropenia (95%), thrombocytopenia (65% to 80%), anemia

Onset: 5-7 days

Nadir: 7-10 days

Recovery: 21-28 days

1% to 10%:

Cardiovascular: Hypotension (2%), associated with rapid (<30 minutes) infusions

Dermatologic: Alopecia (9%), rash (3%)

Miscellaneous: Anaphylactoid reactions (5%) (fever, rash, hyper-/hypotension, dyspnea, bronchospasm), usually seen with rapid (<30 minutes) infusions

Mechanism of Action Teniposide does not inhibit microtubular assembly; it has been shown to delay transit of cells through the S phase and arrest cells in late S or early G_2 phase. Teniposide is a topoisomerase II inhibitor, and appears to cause DNA strand breaks by inhibition of strand-passing and DNA ligase action.

Drug Interactions

Cytochrome P450 Effect: Substrate of CYP3A4 (major); **Inhibits** CYP2C8/9 (weak), 3A4 (weak)

Increased Effect/Toxicity: May increase toxicity of methotrexate. Sodium salicylate, sulfamethizole, and tolbutamide displace teniposide from protein-binding sites which could cause substantial increases in free drug levels, resulting in potentiation of toxicity. Concurrent use of vincristine may increase the incidence of peripheral neuropathy. CYP3A4 inhibitors may increase the levels/effects of teniposide; example inhibitors include azole antifungals, clarithromycin, diclofenac, doxycycline, erythromycin, imatinib, isoniazid, nefazodone, nicardipine, propofol, protease inhibitors, quinidine, telithromycin, and verapamil.

Decreased Effect: CYP3A4 inducers may decrease the levels/effects of teniposide; example inducers include aminoglutethimide, carbamazepine, nafcillin, nevirapine, phenobarbital, phenytoin, and rifamycins.

Pharmacodynamics/Kinetics

Distribution: V_d: 0.28 L/kg; Adults: 8-44 L; Children: 3-11 L; mainly into liver, kidneys, small intestine, and adrenals; crosses blood-brain barrier to a limited extent

Protein binding: 99.4%

Metabolism: Extensively hepatic

Half-life elimination: 5 hours

Excretion: Urine (44%, 21% as unchanged drug); feces (≤10%)

Pregnancy Risk Factor D

Tenofovir (te NOE fo veer)

Related Information

HIV Infection and AIDS *on page 1662*

U.S. Brand Names Viread®

Canadian Brand Names Viread®

Generic Available No

Synonyms PMPA; TDF; Tenofovir Disoproxil Fumarate

Pharmacologic Category Antiretroviral Agent, Reverse Transcriptase Inhibitor (Nucleotide)

Use Management of HIV infections in combination with at least two other antiretroviral agents

Local Anesthetic/Vasoconstrictor Precautions No information available to require special precautions

Effects on Dental Treatment No significant effects or complications reported

Common Adverse Effects

>10%:

Central nervous system: Pain (7% to 12%)

Gastrointestinal: Diarrhea (11% to 16%), nausea (8% to 11%),

Neuromuscular & skeletal: Weakness (7% to 11%)

1% to 10%:

Central nervous system: Headache (5% to 8%), depression (4% to 8%; treatment naïve 11%), insomnia (3% to 4%), fever (2% to 4%; treatment naïve 8%), dizziness (1% to 3%)

Dermatologic: Rash event (maculopapular, pustular, or vesiculobullous rash, pruritus or urticaria 5% to 7%; treatment naïve 18%)

Endocrine & metabolic: Amylase increased (9%, treatment naïve)

Gastrointestinal: Vomiting (4% to 7%), abdominal pain (4% to 7%), dyspepsia (3% to 4%), flatulence (3% to 4%), anorexia (3% to 4%), weight loss (2% to 4%)

Hematologic: Neutropenia (1% to 2%)

Hepatic: Transaminases increased (2% to 4%)

Neuromuscular & skeletal: Back pain (3% to 4%; treatment naïve 9%), myalgia (3% to 4%), neuropathy (peripheral 1% to 3%)

Respiratory: Pneumonia (2% to 3%)

Miscellaneous: Diaphoresis (3%)

Mechanism of Action Tenofovir disoproxil fumarate (TDF) is an analog of adenosine 5'-monophosphate; it interferes with the HIV viral RNA dependent DNA polymerase resulting in inhibition of viral replication. TDF is first converted intracellularly by hydrolysis to tenofovir and subsequently phosphorylated to the active tenofovir diphosphate; nucleotide reverse transcriptase inhibitor.

Drug Interactions

Cytochrome P450 Effect: Inhibits CYP1A2 (weak)

Increased Effect/Toxicity: Concurrent use has been noted to increase serum concentrations/exposure to didanosine and its metabolites, potentially increasing the risk of didanosine toxicity (hyperglycemia, pancreatitis, peripheral neuropathy, or lactic acidosis); decreased CD4 cell counts and decreased virologic response have been reported. Use caution and monitor closely; suspend therapy if signs/symptoms of toxicity are present. Drugs which may compete for renal tubule secretion (including acyclovir, cidofovir, ganciclovir, valacyclovir, valganciclovir) may increase the serum concentrations of tenofovir. Drugs causing nephrotoxicity may reduce elimination of tenofovir. Protease inhibitors (especially ritonavir and combinations with ritonavir) may increase serum concentrations of tenofovir.

(Continued)

Tenofovir *(Continued)*

Decreased Effect: Tenofovir may decrease serum concentrations of atazanavir and other protease inhibitors, resulting in a loss of virologic response (specific atazanavir dosing recommendations provided by manufacturer).

Pharmacodynamics/Kinetics

Distribution: 1.2-1.3 L/kg

Protein binding: 7% to serum proteins

Metabolism: Tenofovir disoproxil fumarate (TDF) is converted intracellularly by hydrolysis (by non-CYP enzymes) to tenofovir, then phosphorylated to the active tenofovir diphosphate

Bioavailability: 25% (fasting); increases ~40% with high-fat meal

Half-life elimination: 17 hours

Time to peak, serum: Fasting: 36-84 minutes; With food: 96-144 minutes

Excretion: Urine (70% to 80%) via filtration and active secretion, primarily as unchanged tenofovir

Pregnancy Risk Factor B

Tenofovir and Emtricitabine *see* Emtricitabine and Tenofovir *on page 537*

Tenofovir Disoproxil Fumarate *see* Tenofovir *on page 1457*

Tenoretic® *see* Atenolol and Chlorthalidone *on page 156*

Tenormin® *see* Atenolol *on page 154*

Tenuate® *see* Diethylpropion *on page 467*

Tenuate® Dospan® *see* Diethylpropion *on page 467*

Tequin® [DSC] *see* Gatifloxacin *on page 724*

Tera-Gel™ [OTC] *see* Coal Tar *on page 383*

Terazol® 3 *see* Terconazole *on page 1461*

Terazol® 7 *see* Terconazole *on page 1461*

Terazosin *(ter AY zoe sin)*

Related Information

Cardiovascular Diseases *on page 1636*

U.S. Brand Names Hytrin®

Canadian Brand Names Alti-Terazosin; Apo-Terazosin®; Hytrin®; Novo-Terazosin; Nu-Terazosin; PMS-Terazosin

Mexican Brand Names Adecur®; Hytrin®

Generic Available Yes

Pharmacologic Category Alpha₁ Blocker

Use Management of mild to moderate hypertension; alone or in combination with other agents such as diuretics or beta-blockers; benign prostate hyperplasia (BPH)

Local Anesthetic/Vasoconstrictor Precautions No information available to require special precautions

Effects on Dental Treatment Key adverse event(s) related to dental treatment: Xerostomia (normal salivary flow resumes upon discontinuation).

Common Adverse Effects Asthenia, postural hypotension, dizziness, somnolence, nasal congestion/rhinitis, and impotence were the only events noted in clinical trials to occur at a frequency significantly greater than placebo (p <0.05).

>10%:

Central nervous system: Dizziness, headache

Neuromuscular & skeletal: Muscle weakness

1% to 10%:

Cardiovascular: Edema, palpitation, chest pain, peripheral edema (3%), orthostatic hypotension (3% to 4%), tachycardia

Central nervous system: Fatigue, nervousness, drowsiness

Gastrointestinal: Dry mouth

Genitourinary: Urinary incontinence

Ocular: Blurred vision

Respiratory: Dyspnea, nasal congestion

Dosage Oral: Adults:

Hypertension: Initial: 1 mg at bedtime; slowly increase dose to achieve desired blood pressure, up to 20 mg/day; usual dose range (JNC 7): 1-20 mg once daily

Dosage reduction may be needed when adding a diuretic or other antihypertensive agent; if drug is discontinued for greater than several days, consider beginning with initial dose and retitrate as needed; dosage may be given on a twice daily regimen if response is diminished at 24 hours and hypotensive is observed at 2-4 hours following a dose

Benign prostatic hyperplasia: Initial: 1 mg at bedtime, increasing as needed; most patients require 10 mg day; if no response after 4-6 weeks of 10 mg/day, may increase to 20 mg/day

Mechanism of Action Alpha$_1$-specific blocking agent with minimal alpha$_2$ effects; this allows peripheral postsynaptic blockade, with the resultant decrease in arterial tone, while preserving the negative feedback loop which is mediated by the peripheral presynaptic alpha$_2$-receptors; terazosin relaxes the smooth muscle of the bladder neck, thus reducing bladder outlet obstruction

Contraindications Hypersensitivity to quinazolines (doxazosin, prazosin, terazosin) or any component of the formulation; concurrent use with phosphodiesterase-5 (PDE-5) inhibitors including sildenafil (>25 mg), tadalafil, or vardenafil

Warnings/Precautions Marked orthostatic hypotension, syncope, and loss of consciousness may occur with first dose ("first dose phenomenon"). This reaction is more likely to occur in patients receiving beta-blockers, diuretics, low sodium diets, or first doses >1 mg/dose in adults; avoid rapid increase in dose; use with caution in patients with renal impairment.

Drug Interactions

Increased Effect/Toxicity: Terazosin's hypotensive effect is increased with beta-blockers, diuretics, ACE inhibitors, calcium channel blockers, other antihypertensive medications, sildenafil (use with extreme caution at a dose ≤25 mg), tadalafil (use is contraindicated by the manufacturer), and vardenafil (use is contraindicated by the manufacturer).

Decreased Effect: Decreased antihypertensive response with NSAIDs. Alpha-blockers reduce the response to pressor agents (norepinephrine).

Ethanol/Nutrition/Herb Interactions Herb/Nutraceutical: Avoid dong quai if using for hypertension (has estrogenic activity). Avoid ephedra, yohimbe, ginseng (may worsen hypertension). Avoid saw palmetto. Avoid garlic (may have increased antihypertensive effect).

Dietary Considerations May be taken without regard to meals at the same time each day.

Pharmacodynamics/Kinetics
Onset of action: 1-2 hours
Absorption: Rapid
Protein binding: 90% to 95%
Metabolism: Extensively hepatic
Half-life elimination: 9.2-12 hours
Time to peak, serum: ~1 hour
Excretion: Feces (60%); urine (40%)

Pregnancy Risk Factor C
Dosage Forms CAP: 1 mg, 2 mg, 5 mg, 10 mg

Terbinafine (TER bin a feen)

U.S. Brand Names Lamisil®; Lamisil® AT™ [OTC]
Canadian Brand Names Apo-Terbinafine®; CO Terbinafine; Gen-Terbinafine; Lamisil®; Novo-Terbinafine; PMS-Terbinafine
Mexican Brand Names Lamisil®
Generic Available No
Synonyms Terbinafine Hydrochloride
Pharmacologic Category Antifungal Agent, Oral; Antifungal Agent, Topical
Use Active against most strains of *Trichophyton mentagrophytes*, *Trichophyton rubrum*; may be effective for infections of *Microsporum gypseum* and *M. nanum*, *Trichophyton verrucosum*, *Epidermophyton floccosum*, *Candida albicans*, and *Scopulariopsis brevicaulis*

Oral: Onychomycosis of the toenail or fingernail due to susceptible dermatophytes
Topical: Antifungal for the treatment of tinea pedis (athlete's foot), tinea cruris (jock itch), and tinea corporis (ringworm) [OTC/prescription formulations]; tinea versicolor [prescription formulations]

Local Anesthetic/Vasoconstrictor Precautions No information available to require special precautions

Effects on Dental Treatment No significant effects or complications reported

Common Adverse Effects
Oral: 1% to 10%:
Central nervous system: Headache, dizziness, vertigo
Dermatologic: Rash, pruritus, urticaria
Gastrointestinal: Diarrhea, dyspepsia, abdominal pain, appetite decrease, taste disturbance
Hematologic: Lymphocytopenia
Hepatic: Liver enzymes increased
Ocular: Visual disturbance
(Continued)

Terbinafine (Continued)

Topical: 1% to 10%:
 Dermatologic: Pruritus, contact dermatitis, irritation, burning, dryness
 Local: Irritation, stinging

Mechanism of Action Synthetic allylamine derivative which inhibits squalene epoxidase, a key enzyme in sterol biosynthesis in fungi. This results in a deficiency in ergosterol within the fungal cell wall and results in fungal cell death.

Drug Interactions

Cytochrome P450 Effect: Substrate (minor) of 1A2, 2C8/9, 2C19, 3A4; Inhibits CYP2D6 (strong); Induces CYP3A4 (weak)

Increased Effect/Toxicity: Terbinafine may increase the levels/effects of amphetamines, beta-blockers, dextromethorphan, fluoxetine, lidocaine, mirtazapine, nefazodone, paroxetine, risperidone, ritonavir, thioridazine, tricyclic antidepressants, venlafaxine, and other CYP2D6 substrates. The effects of warfarin may be increased.

Decreased Effect: Terbinafine may decrease the levels/effects of CYP2D6 prodrug substrates (eg, codeine, hydrocodone, oxycodone, tramadol).

Pharmacodynamics/Kinetics

Absorption: Topical: Limited (<5%); Oral: >70%

Distribution: V_d: 2000 L; distributed to sebum and skin predominantly

Protein binding, plasma: >99%

Metabolism: Hepatic; no active metabolites; first-pass effect; little effect on CYP

Bioavailability: Oral: 40%

Half-life elimination:
 Topical: 22-26 hours
 Oral: Terminal half-life: 200-400 hours; very slow release of drug from skin and adipose tissues occurs; effective half-life: ~36 hours

Time to peak, plasma: 1-2 hours

Excretion: Urine (70% to 75%)

Pregnancy Risk Factor B

Terbinafine Hydrochloride *see* Terbinafine *on page 1459*

Terbutaline (ter BYOO ta leen)

Related Information
 Respiratory Diseases *on page 1656*
U.S. Brand Names Brethine®
Canadian Brand Names Bricanyl®
Mexican Brand Names Bricanyl®; Taziken®[tabs]
Generic Available Yes
Synonyms Brethaire [DSC]; Bricanyl [DSC]
Pharmacologic Category Beta$_2$-Adrenergic Agonist
Use Bronchodilator in reversible airway obstruction and bronchial asthma
Unlabeled/Investigational Use Tocolytic agent (management of preterm labor)
Local Anesthetic/Vasoconstrictor Precautions No information available to require special precautions
Effects on Dental Treatment Key adverse event(s) related to dental treatment: Xerostomia (normal salivary flow resumes upon discontinuation).

Common Adverse Effects
>10%:
 Central nervous system: Nervousness, restlessness
 Endocrine & metabolic: Serum glucose increased, serum potassium decreased
 Neuromuscular & skeletal: Trembling

1% to 10%:
 Cardiovascular: Tachycardia, hypertension
 Central nervous system: Dizziness, drowsiness, headache, insomnia
 Gastrointestinal: Xerostomia, nausea, vomiting, bad taste in mouth
 Neuromuscular & skeletal: Muscle cramps, weakness
 Miscellaneous: Diaphoresis

Mechanism of Action Relaxes bronchial smooth muscle by action on beta$_2$-receptors with less effect on heart rate

Drug Interactions
Increased Effect/Toxicity: Increased toxicity with MAO inhibitors, tricyclic antidepressants.
Decreased Effect: Decreased effect with beta-blockers.

Pharmacodynamics/Kinetics
Onset of action: Oral: 30-45 minutes; SubQ: 6-15 minutes

Protein binding: 25%
Metabolism: Hepatic to inactive sulfate conjugates
Bioavailability: SubQ doses are more bioavailable than oral
Half-life elimination: 11-16 hours
Excretion: Urine
Pregnancy Risk Factor B

Terconazole (ter KONE a zole)

Related Information
Sexually-Transmitted Diseases *on page 1674*
U.S. Brand Names Terazol® 3; Terazol® 7
Canadian Brand Names Terazol®
Mexican Brand Names Fungistat®
Generic Available Yes: Cream
Synonyms Triaconazole
Pharmacologic Category Antifungal Agent, Vaginal
Use Local treatment of vulvovaginal candidiasis
Local Anesthetic/Vasoconstrictor Precautions No information available to require special precautions
Effects on Dental Treatment No significant effects or complications reported
Common Adverse Effects 1% to 10%:
Central nervous system; Fever, chills
Gastrointestinal: Abdominal pain
Genitourinary: Vulvar/vaginal burning, dysmenorrhea
Mechanism of Action Triazole ketal antifungal agent; involves inhibition of fungal cytochrome P450. Specifically, terconazole inhibits cytochrome P450-dependent 14-alpha-demethylase which results in accumulation of membrane disturbing 14-alpha-demethylsterols and ergosterol depletion.
Pharmacodynamics/Kinetics Absorption: Extent of systemic absorption after vaginal administration may be dependent on presence of a uterus; 5% to 8% in women who had a hysterectomy versus 12% to 16% in nonhysterectomy women
Pregnancy Risk Factor C

Teriparatide (ter i PAR a tide)

U.S. Brand Names Forteo™
Canadian Brand Names Forteo™
Generic Available No
Synonyms Parathyroid Hormone (1-34); Recombinant Human Parathyroid Hormone (1-34); rhPTH(1-34)
Pharmacologic Category Parathyroid Hormone Analog
Use Treatment of osteoporosis in postmenopausal women at high risk of fracture; treatment of primary or hypogonadal osteoporosis in men at high risk of fracture
Local Anesthetic/Vasoconstrictor Precautions No information available to require special precautions
Effects on Dental Treatment No significant effects or complications reported
Common Adverse Effects 1% to 10%:
Cardiovascular: Chest pain (3%), syncope (3%)
Central nervous system: Dizziness (8%), depression (4%), vertigo (4%)
Dermatologic: Rash (5%)
Endocrine & metabolic: Hypercalcemia (transient increases noted 4-6 hours postdose in 11% of women and 6% of men)
Gastrointestinal: Nausea (9%), dyspepsia (5%), vomiting (3%), tooth disorder (2%)
Genitourinary: Hyperuricemia (3%)
Neuromuscular & skeletal: Arthralgia (10%), weakness (9%), leg cramps (3%)
Respiratory: Rhinitis (10%), pharyngitis (6%), dyspnea (4%), pneumonia (4%)
Miscellaneous: Antibodies to teriparatide (3% of women in long-term treatment; hypersensitivity reactions or decreased efficacy were not associated in preclinical trials)
Restrictions An FDA-approved medication guide is available at http://www.fda.gov/cder/Offices/ODS/labeling.htm; distribute to each patient to whom this medication is dispensed.
Mechanism of Action Teriparatide is a recombinant formulation of endogenous parathyroid hormone (PTH), containing a 34-amino-acid sequence which is identical to the N-terminal portion of this hormone. The pharmacologic activity of teriparatide is similar to the physiologic activity of PTH, stimulating osteoblast function, increasing gastrointestinal calcium absorption, increasing renal tubular
(Continued)

Teriparatide *(Continued)*

reabsorption of calcium. Treatment with teriparatide increases bone mineral density, bone mass, and strength. In postmenopausal women, it has been shown to decrease osteoporosis-related fractures.

Drug Interactions

Increased Effect/Toxicity: Digitalis serum concentrations are not affected, however, transient hypercalcemia may increase risk of digitalis toxicity (case reports).

Pharmacodynamics/Kinetics

Distribution: V_d: 0.12 L/kg

Metabolism: Hepatic (nonspecific proteolysis)

Bioavailability: 95%

Half-life elimination: Serum: I.V.: 5 minutes; SubQ: 1 hour

Excretion: Urine (as metabolites)

Pregnancy Risk Factor C

Terramycin® I.M. [DSC] *see* Oxytetracycline *on page 1174*

Teslac® *see* Testolactone *on page 1462*

TESPA *see* Thiotepa *on page 1479*

Tessalon® *see* Benzonatate *on page 194*

Testim® *see* Testosterone *on page 1462*

Testolactone *(tes toe LAK tone)*

U.S. Brand Names Teslac®

Canadian Brand Names Teslac®

Generic Available No

Pharmacologic Category Androgen

Use Palliative treatment of advanced or disseminated breast carcinoma

Local Anesthetic/Vasoconstrictor Precautions No information available to require special precautions

Effects on Dental Treatment No significant effects or complications reported

Common Adverse Effects Frequency not defined.

Cardiovascular: Edema, blood pressure increased

Central nervous system: Malaise

Dermatologic: Maculopapular rash, alopecia (rare)

Endocrine & metabolic: Hypercalcemia

Gastrointestinal: Anorexia, diarrhea, nausea, edema of the tongue

Neuromuscular & skeletal: Paresthesias, peripheral neuropathies

Miscellaneous: Nail growth disturbance (rare)

Restrictions C-III

Mechanism of Action Testolactone is a synthetic testosterone derivative without significant androgen activity. The drug inhibits steroid aromatase activity, thereby blocking the production of estradiol and estrone from androgen precursors such as testosterone and androstenedione. Unfortunately, the enzymatic block provided by testolactone is transient and is usually limited to a period of 3 months.

Drug Interactions

Increased Effect/Toxicity: Increased effects of oral anticoagulants.

Pharmacodynamics/Kinetics

Absorption: Well absorbed

Metabolism: Hepatic (forms metabolites)

Excretion: Urine

Pregnancy Risk Factor C

Testopel® *see* Testosterone *on page 1462*

Testosterone *(tes TOS ter one)*

U.S. Brand Names Androderm®; AndroGel®; Delatestryl®; Depo®-Testosterone; First® Testosterone; First® Testosterone MC; Striant®; Testim®; Testopel®

Canadian Brand Names Andriol®; Androderm®; AndroGel®; Andropository; Delatestryl®; Depotest® 100; Everone® 200; Virilon® IM

Mexican Brand Names Andriol®; Primoteston Depot®; Sostenon® [Propionate, Phenylpropionate, Isocaproate, Decanoate]

Generic Available Yes: Injection

Synonyms Testosterone Cypionate; Testosterone Enanthate

Pharmacologic Category Androgen

Use

Injection: Androgen replacement therapy in the treatment of delayed male puberty; male hypogonadism (primary or hypogonadotropic); inoperable female breast cancer (enanthate only)

Pellet: Androgen replacement therapy in the treatment of delayed male puberty; male hypogonadism (primary or hypogonadotropic)

Buccal, topical: Male hypogonadism (primary or hypogonadotropic)

Capsule (not available in U.S.): Management of congenital or acquired primary hypogonadism and hypogonadotropic hypogonadism; development and maintenenance of secondary sexual characteristics in males with testosterone deficiency; stimulation of puberty in carefully selected males with clearly delayed puberty not secondary to a pathological disorder; replacement therapy in syndromes with symptoms of deficiency or absence of endogenous testosterone; replacement therapy in impotence or for male climacteric symptoms when the conditions are due to a measured or documented androgen deficiency

Local Anesthetic/Vasoconstrictor Precautions No information available to require special precautions

Effects on Dental Treatment No significant effects or complications reported

Common Adverse Effects Frequency not defined.

Cardiovascular: Flushing, edema

Central nervous system: Excitation, aggressive behavior, sleeplessness, anxiety, mental depression, headache

Dermatologic: Hirsutism (increase in pubic hair growth), acne

Endocrine & metabolic: Menstrual problems (amenorrhea), virilism, breast soreness, gynecomastia, hypercalcemia, hypoglycemia

Gastrointestinal: Nausea, vomiting, GI irritation

Following buccal administration: Bitter taste, gum edema, gum or mouth irritation, gum tenderness, taste perversion

Genitourinary: Bladder irritability, epididymitis, impotence, priapism, prostatic carcinoma, prostatic hyperplasia, PSA increased (up to 18%), testicular atrophy, urination impaired

Hepatic: Hepatic dysfunction, cholestatic hepatitis, hepatic necrosis

Hematologic: Leukopenia, polycythemia, suppression of clotting factors

Miscellaneous: Hypersensitivity reactions

Restrictions C-III

Mechanism of Action Principal endogenous androgen responsible for promoting the growth and development of the male sex organs and maintaining secondary sex characteristics in androgen-deficient males

Drug Interactions

Cytochrome P450 Effect: Substrate (minor) of CYP2B6, 2C8/9, 2C19, 3A4; **Inhibits** CYP3A4 (weak)

Increased Effect/Toxicity: Testosterone may increase the effects warfarin.

Pharmacodynamics/Kinetics

Duration (route and ester dependent): I.M.: Cypionate and enanthate esters have longest duration, ≤2-4 weeks

Absorption: Transdermal gel: ~10% of applied dose

Distribution: Crosses placenta; enters breast milk

Protein binding: 98%; bound to sex hormone-binding globulin (40%) and albumin

Metabolism: Hepatic; forms metabolites, including dihydrotestosterone (DHT) and estradiol (both active)

Half-life elimination: 10-100 minutes

Excretion: Urine (90%); feces (6%)

Pregnancy Risk Factor X

Testosterone Cypionate *see* Testosterone *on page 1462*

Testosterone Enanthate *see* Testosterone *on page 1462*

Testred® *see* MethylTESTOSTERone *on page 1028*

Tetanus Immune Globulin (Human)
(TET a nus i MYUN GLOB yoo lin HYU man)

U.S. Brand Names BayTet™

Canadian Brand Names BayTet™

Generic Available No

Synonyms TIG

Pharmacologic Category Immune Globulin

Use Passive immunization against tetanus; tetanus immune globulin is preferred over tetanus antitoxin for treatment of active tetanus; part of the management of
(Continued)

Tetanus Immune Globulin (Human) *(Continued)*

an unclean, wound in a person whose history of previous receipt of tetanus toxoid is unknown or who has received less than three doses of tetanus toxoid; elderly may require TIG more often than younger patients with tetanus infection due to declining antibody titers with age

Local Anesthetic/Vasoconstrictor Precautions No information available to require special precautions

Effects on Dental Treatment No significant effects or complications reported

Common Adverse Effects
>10%: Local: Pain, tenderness, erythema at injection site
1% to 10%:
  Central nervous system: Fever (mild)
  Dermatologic: Urticaria, angioedema
  Neuromuscular & skeletal: Muscle stiffness
  Miscellaneous: Anaphylaxis reaction

Mechanism of Action Passive immunity toward tetanus
Pharmacodynamics/Kinetics Absorption: Well absorbed
Pregnancy Risk Factor C

Tetanus Toxoid (Adsorbed) (TET a nus TOKS oyd, ad SORBED)

Generic Available No
Pharmacologic Category Toxoid
Use Active immunization against tetanus when combination antigen preparations are not indicated. **Note:** Tetanus and diphtheria toxoids for adult use (Td) is the preferred immunizing agent for most adults and for children after their seventh birthday. Young children should receive trivalent DTaP (diphtheria/tetanus/acellular pertussis), as part of their childhood immunization program, unless pertussis is contraindicated, then TD is warranted.

Local Anesthetic/Vasoconstrictor Precautions No information available to require special precautions

Effects on Dental Treatment No significant effects or complications reported

Common Adverse Effects All serious adverse reactions must be reported to the U.S. Department of Health and Human Services (DHHS) Vaccine Adverse Event Reporting System (VAERS) 1-800-822-7967.
Frequency not defined.
  Cardiovascular: Hypotension
  Central nervous system: Brachial neuritis, fever, malaise, pain
  Gastrointestinal: Nausea
  Local: Edema, induration (with or without tenderness), rash, redness, urticaria, warmth
  Neuromuscular: Arthralgia, Guillain-Barré syndrome
  Miscellaneous: Anaphylactic reaction, Arthus-type hypersensitivity reaction

Mechanism of Action Tetanus toxoid preparations contain the toxin produced by virulent tetanus bacilli (detoxified growth products of *Clostridium tetani*). The toxin has been modified by treatment with formaldehyde so that it has lost toxicity but still retains ability to act as antigen and produce active immunity; the aluminum salt, a mineral adjuvant, delays the rate of absorption and prolongs and enhances its properties; duration ~10 years.

Drug Interactions
Decreased Effect: When used in greater than physiologic doses, corticosteroids lead to decreased effect of vaccine (consider deferring immunization for 1 month after steroid is discontinued). Consider deferring immunization for 1 month after immunosuppressive agent is discontinued (decreased response to vaccine).

Pharmacodynamics/Kinetics Duration: Primary immunization: ~10 years
Pregnancy Risk Factor C

Tetanus Toxoid (Fluid) (TET a nus TOKS oyd FLOO id)

Generic Available No
Synonyms Tetanus Toxoid Plain
Pharmacologic Category Toxoid
Use Indicated as booster dose in the active immunization against tetanus in the rare adult or child who is allergic to the aluminum adjuvant (a product containing adsorbed tetanus toxoid is preferred); not indicated for primary immunization

Unlabeled/Investigational Use Anergy testing (no longer recommended)

Local Anesthetic/Vasoconstrictor Precautions No information available to require special precautions

Effects on Dental Treatment No significant effects or complications reported

Common Adverse Effects All serious adverse reactions must be reported to the U.S. Department of Health and Human Services (DHHS) Vaccine Adverse Event Reporting System (VAERS) 1-800-822-7967.

Frequency not defined.
Cardiovascular: Hypotension
Central nervous system: Brachial neuritis, fever, Guillain-Barré syndrome, malaise
Dermatologic: Rash, urticaria
Gastrointestinal: Nausea
Local: Edema, induration (with or without tenderness), redness, warmth
Neuromuscular & skeletal: Arthralgia
Miscellaneous: Anaphylaxis, Arthus-type hypersensitivity reactions (severe local reaction developing 2-8 hours following injection)

Mechanism of Action Tetanus toxoid preparations contain the toxin produced by virulent tetanus bacilli (detoxified growth products of *Clostridium tetani*). The toxin has been modified by treatment with formaldehyde so that is has lost toxicity but still retains ability to act as antigen and produce active immunity.

Drug Interactions
Increased Effect/Toxicity: Increased bleeding and bruising may occur from I.M. injection in patients on anticoagulants.
Decreased Effect: Decreased effect of vaccine may occur with corticosteroids (greater than physiologic doses) or immunosuppressive agents

Pregnancy Risk Factor C

Tetanus Toxoid Plain *see* Tetanus Toxoid (Fluid) *on page 1464*

Tetrabenazine (tet ra BEN a zeen)

Canadian Brand Names Nitoman™
Pharmacologic Category Central Monoamine-Depleting Agent
Use Treatment of hyperkinetic movement disorders, including Huntington's chorea, hemiballismus, senile chorea, Tourette syndrome, and tardive dyskinesia

Local Anesthetic/Vasoconstrictor Precautions No information available to require special precautions

Effects on Dental Treatment
Key adverse event(s) related to dental treatment: Orthostatic hypotension has been reported; monitor patient during erect posture from dental chair.

Common Adverse Effects Note: Many adverse effects are dose-related and may resolve at lower dosages.
>10%: Central nervous system: Drowsiness (37%), parkinsonism (29%), depression (15%), insomnia (11%)
1% to 10%:
Cardiovascular: Orthostasis (2%)
Central nervous system: Nervousness (10%), anxiety (10%), akathisia (10%), dystonic reaction (3%), confusion (2%), memory impairment (2%), dizziness (1%), headache (1%), hallucination (1%), paresthesia (1%), panic attack (1%), paranoia (1%)
Gastrointestinal: Nausea (5%), vomiting (5%), diarrhea (1%), dysphagia (1%), drooling, epigastric pain
Neuromuscular & skeletal: Tremor (3%), gait disturbance (1%)
Ocular: Blurred vision (1%)
Respiratory: Pharyngeal spasm (1%), pharyngeal pain (1%)
Frequency not defined: Disorientation, fatigue, irritability, neuroleptic malignant syndrome, restlessness, weakness

Restrictions Not available in U.S.

Mechanism of Action Within basal ganglia, interferes with storage of neurotransmitters (including dopamine, serotonin, and norepinephrine) in presynaptic vesicles (likely through actions on vesicle monoamine transporter) resulting in depletion of these neurotransmitters. Tetrabenazine inhibits presynaptic dopamine release and also blocks CNS dopamine receptors. The effects resemble reserpine but with less peripheral activity and a shorter duration of action. Treatment results in symptomatic improvement of hyperkinetic movement disorders, including Huntington's chorea, hemiballismus, senile chorea, Tic and Hille's de la Tourette syndrome, and tardive dyskinesia.

Drug Interactions
Increased Effect/Toxicity: Tetrabenazine may increase the toxicity of cyclic antidepressants; CNS excitation and hypertension may occur during concurrent therapy. Concurrent use of tetrabenazine with antipsychotic agents may result in severe manifestations of dopamine deficiency. Neuroleptic malignant syndrome has been reported. CNS depressants may increase the adverse effects of tetrabenazine.
(Continued)

Tetrabenazine *(Continued)*

Tetrabenazine may increase the toxicity of MAO inhibitors; CNS excitation and hypertension may occur during concurrent therapy. Tetrabenazine should not be administered within 14 days of an MAO inhibitor. Concurrent therapy with reserpine may increase the effect/toxicity of both agents (due to similarities in mechanism of action). In the management of movement disorders, lithium may be additive with tetrabenazine, allowing management at lower dosages of both agents (limited data).

Decreased Effect: Tetrabenazine may reduce the anti-Parkinsonian effect of levodopa; avoid concurrent use.

Pharmacodynamics/Kinetics
Duration of action: 16-24 hours
Metabolism: Hepatic, to hydroxytetrabenazine (primary active moiety)
Bioavailability: Low and erratic (due to extensive first-pass effects)
Excretion: Urine (40% as metabolites); feces (2.5%)

Tetracaine *(TET ra kane)*

Related Information
Mouth Pain, Cold Sore, and Canker Sore Products *on page 1828*
Oral Pain *on page 1692*
Ulcerative and Erosive Disorders *on page 1712*
U.S. Brand Names Pontocaine®; Pontocaine® Niphanoid®
Canadian Brand Names Ametop™; Pontocaine®
Generic Available Yes: Ophthalmic solution, solution for injection
Synonyms Amethocaine Hydrochloride; Tetracaine Hydrochloride
Pharmacologic Category Local Anesthetic
Dental Use Ester-type local anesthetic; applied topically to throat for various diagnostic procedures and on cold sores and fever blisters for pain
Use Spinal anesthesia; local anesthesia in the eye for various diagnostic and examination purposes; topically applied to nose and throat for various diagnostic procedures
Local Anesthetic/Vasoconstrictor Precautions No information available to require special precautions
Effects on Dental Treatment No significant effects or complications reported
Significant Adverse Effects Frequency not defined.
Injection: Note: Adverse effects listed are those characteristics of local anesthetics.
Cardiovascular: Cardiac arrest, hypotension
Central nervous system: Chills, convulsions, dizziness, drowsiness, nervousness, unconsciousness
Gastrointestinal: Nausea, vomiting
Neuromuscular & skeletal: Tremors
Ocular: Blurred vision, pupil constriction
Otic: Tinnitus
Respiratory: Respiratory arrest
Miscellaneous: Allergic reaction
Ophthalmic: Ocular: Chemosis, lacrimation, photophobia, transient stinging
With chronic use: Corneal erosions, corneal healing retardation, corneal opacification (permanent), corneal scarring, keratitis (severe)
Dental Usual Dosing Topical mucous membranes (rhinolaryngology): Adults: Used as a 0.25% or 0.5% solution by direct application or nebulization; total dose should not exceed 20 mg
Dosage Adults:
Ophthalmic: Short-term anesthesia of the eye: 0.5% solution: Instill 1-2 drops; prolonged use (especially for at-home self-medication) is not recommended
Injection: Spinal anesthesia: **Note:** Dosage varies with the anesthetic procedure, the degree of anesthesia required, and the individual patient response; it is administered by subarachnoid injection for spinal anesthesia.
Perineal anesthesia: 5 mg
Perineal and lower extremities: 10 mg
Anesthesia extending up to costal margin: 15 mg; doses up to 20 mg may be given, but are reserved for exceptional cases
Low spinal anesthesia (saddle block): 2-5 mg
Topical mucous membranes (rhinolaryngology): Used as a 0.25% or 0.5% solution by direct application or nebulization; total dose should not exceed 20 mg
Mechanism of Action Ester local anesthetic blocks both the initiation and conduction of nerve impulses by decreasing the neuronal membrane's permeability to sodium ions, which results in inhibition of depolarization with resultant blockade of conduction

Contraindications Hypersensitivity to tetracaine, ester-type anesthetics, aminobenzoic acid, or any component of the formulation; injection should not be used when spinal anesthesia is contraindicated

Warnings/Precautions Use with caution in patients with cardiac disease, hyperthyroidism, abnormal or decreased levels of plasma esterases. Use of the lowest effective dose is recommended. Acutely ill, elderly, debilitated, obstetric patients, or patients with increased intra-abdominal pressure may require decreased doses. Products may contain sodium bisulfite which may cause allergic reactions in some individuals.

Ophthalmic: May delay wound healing. Prolonged use is not recommended. The anesthetized eye should be protected from irritation, foreign bodies, and rubbing to prevent inadvertent damage.

Pharmacodynamics/Kinetics
Onset of action: Anesthetic: Rhinolaryngology: 5-10 minutes
Duration: Rhinolaryngology: ~30 minutes
Metabolism: Hepatic; detoxified by plasma esterases to aminobenzoic acid
Excretion: Urine

Pregnancy Risk Factor C

Lactation Excretion in breast milk unknown/use caution

Dosage Forms [DSC] = Discontinued product
Injection, solution, as hydrochloride [preservative free] (Pontocaine®): 1% [10 mg/mL] (2 mL) [contains sodium bisulfite]
Injection, solution, as hydrochloride [premixed in dextrose 6%] (Pontocaine®): 0.3% [3 mg/mL] (5 mL) [DSC]
Injection, powder for reconstitution, as hydrochloride [preservative free] (Pontocaine® Niphanoid®): 20 mg
Solution, ophthalmic, as hydrochloride: 0.5% [5 mg/mL] (15 mL)
Solution, topical, as hydrochloride (Pontocaine®): 2% [20 mg/mL] (30 mL, 118 mL) [for rhinolaryngology]

Tetracaine and Dextrose (TET ra kane & DEKS trose)

Related Information
Dextrose on page 452
Oral Pain on page 1692
Tetracaine on page 1466
U.S. Brand Names Pontocaine® With Dextrose
Generic Available Yes
Synonyms Dextrose and Tetracaine
Pharmacologic Category Local Anesthetic
Use Spinal anesthesia (saddle block)
Local Anesthetic/Vasoconstrictor Precautions No information available to require special precautions
Effects on Dental Treatment No significant effects or complications reported
Pharmacodynamics/Kinetics See Tetracaine monograph.
Pregnancy Risk Factor C

Tetracaine and Lidocaine see Lidocaine and Tetracaine on page 930

Tetracaine Hydrochloride see Tetracaine on page 1466

Tetracaine Hydrochloride, Benzocaine, Butyl Aminobenzoate, and Benzalkonium Chloride see Benzocaine, Butyl Aminobenzoate, Tetracaine, and Benzalkonium Chloride on page 193

Tetracosactide see Cosyntropin on page 396

Tetracycline (tet ra SYE kleen)

Related Information
Bacterial Infections on page 1697
Gastrointestinal Disorders on page 1654
Periodontal Diseases on page 1705
Sexually-Transmitted Diseases on page 1674
Ulcerative and Erosive Disorders on page 1712
U.S. Brand Names Sumycin®
Canadian Brand Names Apo-Tetra®; Nu-Tetra
Mexican Brand Names Tetra-Atlantis®
Generic Available Yes: Capsule
Synonyms Achromycin; TCN; Tetracycline Hydrochloride
Pharmacologic Category Antibiotic, Tetracycline Derivative
Dental Use Treatment of periodontitis associated with presence of *Actinobacillus actinomycetemcomitans* (AA); as adjunctive therapy in recurrent aphthous ulcers
(Continued)

Tetracycline *(Continued)*

Use Treatment of susceptible bacterial infections of both gram-positive and gram-negative organisms; also infections due to *Mycoplasma*, *Chlamydia*, and *Rickettsia*; indicated for acne, exacerbations of chronic bronchitis, and treatment of gonorrhea and syphilis in patients that are allergic to penicillin; as part of a multidrug regimen for *H. pylori* eradication to reduce the risk of duodenal ulcer recurrence

Local Anesthetic/Vasoconstrictor Precautions No information available to require special precautions

Effects on Dental Treatment Key adverse event(s) related to dental treatment: Esophagitis, superinfections, and candidal superinfection. Opportunistic "superinfection" with *Candida albicans*; tetracyclines are not recommended for use during pregnancy or in children ≤8 years of age since they have been reported to cause enamel hypoplasia and permanent teeth discoloration. The use of tetracyclines should only be used in these patients if other agents are contraindicated or alternative antimicrobials will not eradicate the organism. Long-term use associated with oral candidiasis.

Significant Adverse Effects Frequency not defined.

Cardiovascular: Pericarditis

Central nervous system: Intracranial pressure increased, bulging fontanels in infants, pseudotumor cerebri, paresthesia

Dermatologic: Photosensitivity, pruritus, pigmentation of nails, exfoliative dermatitis

Endocrine & metabolic: Diabetes insipidus syndrome

Gastrointestinal: Discoloration of teeth and enamel hypoplasia (young children), nausea, diarrhea, vomiting, esophagitis, anorexia, abdominal cramps, antibiotic-associated pseudomembranous colitis, staphylococcal enterocolitis, pancreatitis

Hematologic: Thrombophlebitis

Hepatic: Hepatotoxicity

Renal: Acute renal failure, azotemia, renal damage

Miscellaneous: Superinfection, anaphylaxis, hypersensitivity reactions, candidal superinfection

Dental Usual Dosing Periodontitis: Adults: Oral: 250 mg every 6 hours until improvement (usually 10 days)

Dosage Oral:

Children >8 years: 25-50 mg/kg/day in divided doses every 6 hours

Adults: 250-500 mg/dose every 6 hours

Helicobacter pylori eradication: 500 mg 2-4 times/day depending on regimen; requires combination therapy with at least one other antibiotic and an acid-suppressing agent (proton pump inhibitor or H_2 blocker)

Dosing interval in renal impairment:

Cl_{cr} 50-80 mL/minute: Administer every 8-12 hours

Cl_{cr} 10-50 mL/minute: Administer every 12-24 hours

Cl_{cr} <10 mL/minute: Administer every 24 hours

Dialysis: Slightly dialyzable (5% to 20%) via hemo- and peritoneal dialysis or via continuous arteriovenous or venovenous hemofiltration; no supplemental dosage necessary

Dosing adjustment in hepatic impairment: Avoid use or maximum dose is 1 g/day

Mechanism of Action Inhibits bacterial protein synthesis by binding with the 30S and possibly the 50S ribosomal subunit(s) of susceptible bacteria; may also cause alterations in the cytoplasmic membrane

Contraindications Hypersensitivity to tetracycline or any component of the formulation; do not administer to children ≤8 years of age; pregnancy

Warnings/Precautions Use of tetracyclines during tooth development may cause permanent discoloration of the teeth and enamel, hypoplasia and retardation of skeletal development and bone growth with risk being the greatest for children <4 years and those receiving high doses; use with caution in patients with renal or hepatic impairment (eg, elderly); dosage modification required in patients with renal impairment since it may increase BUN as an antianabolic agent; pseudotumor cerebri has been reported with tetracycline use (usually resolves with discontinuation); outdated drug can cause nephropathy; superinfection possible; use protective measure to avoid photosensitivity

Drug Interactions Substrate of CYP3A4 (major); **Inhibits** CYP3A4 (moderate)

Antacids: May decrease tetracycline absorption; separate doses.

Calcium supplements (oral): May decrease tetracycline absorption; separate doses.

CYP3A4 inducers: CYP3A4 inducers may decrease the levels/effects of tetracycline. Example inducers include aminoglutethimide, carbamazepine, nafcillin, nevirapine, phenobarbital, phenytoin, and rifamycins.

CYP3A4 substrates: Tetracycline may increase the levels/effects of CYP3A4 substrates. Example substrates include benzodiazepines, calcium channel blockers, cyclosporine, mirtazapine, nateglinide, nefazodone, sildenafil (and other PDE-5 inhibitors), tacrolimus, and venlafaxine. Selected benzodiazepines (midazolam and triazolam), cisapride, ergot alkaloids, selected HMG-CoA reductase inhibitors (lovastatin and simvastatin), and pimozide are generally contraindicated with strong CYP3A4 inhibitors.

Didanosine: May decrease tetracycline absorption; separate doses.

Digoxin: Tetracyclines may rarely increase digoxin serum levels.

Iron: May decrease tetracycline absorption; separate doses.

Methoxyflurane anesthesia when concurrent with tetracycline may cause fatal nephrotoxicity.

Oral contraceptives: Anecdotal reports suggesting decreased contraceptive efficacy with tetracyclines have been refuted by more rigorous scientific and clinical data.

Quinapril: May decrease tetracycline absorption; separate doses.

Warfarin with tetracyclines may result in increased anticoagulation.

Ethanol/Nutrition/Herb Interactions

Food: Tetracycline serum concentrations may be decreased if taken with dairy products.

Herb/Nutraceutical: Avoid dong quai, St John's wort (may also cause photosensitization)

Pharmacodynamics/Kinetics

Absorption: Oral: 75%

Distribution: Small amount appears in bile
Relative diffusion from blood into CSF: Good only with inflammation (exceeds usual MICs)

CSF:blood level ratio: Inflamed meninges: 25%

Protein binding: ~65%

Half-life elimination: Normal renal function: 8-11 hours; End-stage renal disease: 57-108 hours

Time to peak, serum: Oral: 2-4 hours

Excretion: Urine (60% as unchanged drug); feces (as active form)

Pregnancy Risk Factor D

Lactation Enters breast milk/not recommended (AAP rates "compatible")

Breast-Feeding Considerations Negligible absorption by infant; potential to stain infants' unerupted teeth

Dosage Forms

Capsule, as hydrochloride: 250 mg, 500 mg

Suspension, oral, as hydrochloride (Sumycin®): 125 mg/5 mL (480 mL) [contains sodium benzoate and sodium metabisulfite; fruit flavor]

Tablet, as hydrochloride (Sumycin®): 250 mg, 500 mg

Selected Readings

Gordon JM and Walker CB, "Current Status of Systemic Antibiotic Usage in Destructive Periodontal Disease," *J Periodontol*, 1993, 64(8 Suppl): 760-71.

Rams TE and Slots J, "Antibiotics in Periodontal Therapy: An Update," *Compendium*, 1992, 13(12):1130, 1132, 1134.

Seymour RA and Heasman PA, "Tetracyclines in the Management of Periodontal Diseases. A Review," *J Clin Periodontol*, 1995, 22(1):22-35.

Seymour RA and Heasman PA, "Pharmacological Control of Periodontal Disease. II. Antimicrobial Agents," *J Dent*, 1995, 23(1):5-14

Tetracycline Hydrochloride *see* Tetracycline *on page 1467*

Tetracycline, Metronidazole, and Bismuth Subsalicylate *see* Bismuth Subsalicylate, Metronidazole, and Tetracycline *on page 210*

Tetrafluoroethane and Pentafluoropropane *see* Pentafluoropropane and Tetrafluoroethane *on page 1206*

Tetrahydroaminoacrine *see* Tacrine *on page 1436*

Tetrahydrocannabinol *see* Dronabinol *on page 518*

Tetrahydrocannabinol and Cannabidiol
(TET ra hye droe can NAB e nol & can nab e DYE ol)

Canadian Brand Names Sativex®

Generic Available No

Synonyms Cannabidiol and Tetrahydrocannabinol; Delta-9-Tetrahydrocannabinol and Cannabinol; GW-1000-02; THC and CBD

Pharmacologic Category Analgesic, Miscellaneous

Use
Adjunctive treatment of neuropathic pain in multiple sclerosis

Local Anesthetic/Vasoconstrictor Precautions No information available to require special precautions

(Continued)

Tetrahydrocannabinol and Cannabidiol *(Continued)*

Effects on Dental Treatment Key adverse event(s) related to dental treatment: Xerostomia and changes in salivation (normal salivary flow resumes upon discontinuation), abnormal taste; administered as buccal spray, associated with irritation to the buccal (oral) mucosa.

Common Adverse Effects
>10%:
Central nervous system: Dizziness (41%), fatigue (11%)
Gastrointestinal: Oral application site events (20% to 25%)
1% to 10%:
Cardiovascular: Tachycardia, orthostatic hypotension, syncope
Central nervous system: Headache (9%), somnolence (8%), impaired balance (5%), euphoria (5%), depression (4% to 5%), memory impairment (4%), disorientation (3%), dissociation (3%), vertigo (3%), lethargy (3%)
Endocrine & metabolic: Appetite increased (4%), thirst (3%)
Gastrointestinal: Nausea (10%), xerostomia (8%), application site pain (8%), oral pain (7%), abnormal taste (4%), mucosal irritation/ulceration (3%), vomiting (2%)
Hepatic: ALT increased (2.6%)
Neuromuscular & skeletal: Weakness (4%)
Respiratory: Pharyngitis (4%)
Miscellaneous: Feeling drunk (7%), falls (3%), sensation of heaviness (2%)

Restrictions Not available in U.S.; CDSA-II

Mechanism of Action
Stimulates cannabinoid receptors CB1 and CB2 in the CNS and dorsal root ganglia as well as other sites in the body. Cannabinoid receptors in the pain pathways of the brain and spinal cord mediate cannabinoid-induced analgesia. Peripheral CB2 receptors modulate immune function through cytokine release.

Drug Interactions
Cytochrome P450 Effect:
Substrate (minor) of CYP2C9, 2C19, 2D6, 3A4; Inhibits (weak) CYP1A2, 2C19, 2D6, 3A4
Increased Effect/Toxicity:
CNS depressants: The depressant effects may be additive/synergistic with cannabinoids (includes ethanol, barbiturates, and benzodiazepines).

Pharmacodynamics/Kinetics
Absorption: Rapidly absorbed from the buccal mucosa
Distribution: Widely distributed, particularly to fatty tissues
Protein binding: Extensive
Metabolism: Hepatic, via CYP isoenzymes (2C9, 2C19, 2D6 and 3A4)
Half-life elimination: Initial: 1.3-2.2 hours; terminal half-life may require 24-36 hours (or longer) due to redistribution from fatty tissue
Time to peak, plasma: 2-4 hours
Excretion: As metabolites, urine and feces

Tetrahydrozoline *(tet ra hye DROZ a leen)*

U.S. Brand Names Eye-Sine™ [OTC]; Geneye® [OTC]; Murine® Tears Plus [OTC]; Optigene® 3 [OTC]; Tyzine®; Tyzine® Pediatric; Visine® Advanced Relief [OTC]; Visine® Original [OTC]

Mexican Brand Names Visine®

Generic Available Yes: Ophthalmic solution

Synonyms Tetrahydrozoline Hydrochloride; Tetryzoline

Pharmacologic Category Adrenergic Agonist Agent; Ophthalmic Agent, Vasoconstrictor

Use Symptomatic relief of nasal congestion and conjunctival congestion

Local Anesthetic/Vasoconstrictor Precautions No information available to require special precautions

Effects on Dental Treatment No significant effects or complications reported

Common Adverse Effects
>10%:
Local: Transient stinging
Respiratory: Sneezing
1% to 10%:
Cardiovascular: Tachycardia, palpitation, hypertension, heart rate
Central nervous system: Headache
Neuromuscular & skeletal: Tremor
Ocular: Blurred vision

Mechanism of Action Stimulates alpha-adrenergic receptors in the arterioles of the conjunctiva and the nasal mucosa to produce vasoconstriction

Pharmacodynamics/Kinetics
Onset of action: Decongestant: Intranasal: 4-8 hours
Duration: Ophthalmic vasoconstriction: 2-3 hours
Pregnancy Risk Factor C

Tetrahydrozoline Hydrochloride *see* Tetrahydrozoline *on page 1470*

Tetra Tannate Pediatric *see* Chlorpheniramine, Ephedrine, Phenylephrine, and Carbetapentane *on page 325*

Tetryzoline *see* Tetrahydrozoline *on page 1470*

Teveten® *see* Eprosartan *on page 554*

Teveten® HCT *see* Eprosartan and Hydrochlorothiazide *on page 555*

Tev-Tropin™ *see* Somatropin *on page 1406*

Texacort® *see* Hydrocortisone *on page 793*

TG *see* Thioguanine *on page 1476*

6-TG (error-prone abbreviation) *see* Thioguanine *on page 1476*

THA *see* Tacrine *on page 1436*

Thalidomide (tha LI doe mide)

Related Information
HIV Infection and AIDS *on page 1662*
Ulcerative and Erosive Disorders *on page 1712*
U.S. Brand Names Thalomid®
Canadian Brand Names Thalomid®
Generic Available No
Synonyms NSC-66847
Pharmacologic Category Angiogenesis Inhibitor; Immunosuppressant Agent; Tumor Necrosis Factor (TNF) Blocking Agent
Use Treatment and maintenance of cutaneous manifestations of erythema nodosum leprosum (ENL)
Unlabeled/Investigational Use Treatment of multiple myeloma; Crohn's disease; graft-versus-host reactions after bone marrow transplantation; AIDS-related aphthous stomatitis; Behçet's syndrome; Waldenström's macroglobulinemia; Langerhans cell histiocytosis; may be effective in rheumatoid arthritis, discoid lupus erythematosus, and erythema multiforme
Local Anesthetic/Vasoconstrictor Precautions No information available to require special precautions
Effects on Dental Treatment Key adverse event(s) related to dental treatment: Oral moniliasis (HIV-seropositive patients), toothache, xerostomia (normal salivary flow resumes upon discontinuation), and aphthous stomatitis.
Common Adverse Effects
Controlled clinical trials: ENL:
>10%:
  Central nervous system: Somnolence (38%), headache (13%)
  Dermatologic: Rash (21%)
1% to 10%:
  Cardiovascular: Facial edema (4%), peripheral edema (4%)
  Central nervous system: Malaise (8%), pain (8%), vertigo (8%), dizziness (4%)
  Dermatologic: Pruritus (8%), dermatitis (fungal) (4%), maculopapular rash (4%), nail disorder (4%)
  Gastrointestinal: Constipation (4%), diarrhea, (4%) nausea (4%), oral moniliasis (4%), tooth pain (4%)
  Genitourinary: Impotence (8%)
  Neuromuscular & skeletal: Weakness (8%), back pain (4%), neck pain (4%), neck rigidity (4%), tremor (4%)
  Respiratory: Pharyngitis (4%), rhinitis (4%), sinusitis (4%)

HIV-seropositive:
General: An increased viral load has been noted in patients treated with thalidomide. This is of uncertain clinical significance.
>10%:
  Central nervous system: Somnolence (36% to 38%), dizziness (19%), fever (19% to 22%), headache (17% to 19%)
  Dermatologic: Rash (25%), maculopapular rash (17% to 19%), acne (3% to 11%)
  Gastrointestinal: Diarrhea (11% to 19%), nausea (13%), oral moniliasis (6% to 11%)
  Hematologic: Leukopenia (17% to 25%), anemia (6% to 13%), lymphadenopathy (6% to 13%)
  Hepatic: AST increased (3% to 13%)
(Continued)

Thalidomide *(Continued)*

      Neuromuscular & skeletal: Paresthesia (may be severe and/or irreversible) (6% to 16%), weakness (6% to 22%)

      Renal: Hematuria (11%)

      Miscellaneous: Diaphoresis (13%), lymphadenopathy (6% to 13%)

   1% to 10%:

      Cardiovascular: Peripheral edema (3% to 8%)

      Central nervous system: Nervousness (3% to 9%), insomnia (9%), agitation (9%), pain (3%)

      Dermatologic: Dermatitis (fungal) (6% to 9%), nail disorder (3%), pruritus (3% to 6%)

      Endocrine & metabolic: Hyperlipemia (6% to 9%)

      Gastrointestinal: Anorexia (3% to 9%), constipation (3% to 9%), xerostomia (8% to 9%), flatulence (8%)

      Genitourinary: Impotence (3%)

      Hepatic: LFTs abnormal (9%)

      Neuromuscular & skeletal: Neuropathy (8%), back pain (6%)

      Renal: Albuminuria (3% to 8%)

      Respiratory: Pharyngitis (6% to 8%), sinusitis (3% to 8%)

      Miscellaneous: Accidental injury (6%), infection (6% to 8%)

Restrictions Thalidomide is approved for marketing only under a special distribution program. This program, called the "System for Thalidomide Education and Prescribing Safety" (STEPS® 1-888-423-5436), has been approved by the FDA. Prescribers and pharmacists must be registered with the program. No more than a 4-week supply should be dispensed. Blister packs should be dispensed intact (do not repackage capsules). Prescriptions must be filled within 7 days. Subsequent prescriptions may be filled only if fewer than 7 days of therapy remain on the previous prescription. A new prescription is required for further dispensing (a telephone prescription may not be accepted.)

Dosage Oral:

Cutaneous ENL:

   Initial: 100-300 mg/day taken once daily at bedtime with water (at least 1 hour after evening meal)

      Patients weighing <50 kg: Initiate at lower end of the dosing range

      Severe cutaneous reaction or patients previously requiring high dose may be initiated at 400 mg/day; doses may be divided, but taken 1 hour after meals

   Maintenance: Dosing should continue until active reaction subsides (usually at least 2 weeks), then tapered in 50 mg decrements every 2-4 weeks

      Patients who flare during tapering or with a history or requiring prolonged maintenance should be maintained on the minimum dosage necessary to control the reaction. Efforts to taper should be repeated every 3-6 months, in increments of 50 mg every 2-4 weeks.

Behçet's syndrome (unlabeled use): 100-400 mg/day

Graft-vs-host reactions (unlabeled use): 100-1600 mg/day; usual initial dose: 200 mg 4 times/day for use up to 700 days

AIDS-related aphthous stomatitis (unlabeled use): 200 mg twice daily for 5 days, then 200 mg/day for up to 8 weeks

Discoid lupus erythematosus (unlabeled use): 100-400 mg/day; maintenance dose: 25-50 mg

Mechanism of Action Not fully characterized; has immunomodulatory and antiangiogenic characteristics. Immunologic effects may vary based on conditions; may suppress tumor necrosis factor-alpha production in patients with ENL, yet may increase plasma tumor necrosis factor-alpha levels in HIV-positive patients. Other proposed mechanisms of action include suppression of angiogenesis, prevention of free-radical-mediated DNA damage, increased cell mediated cytotoxic effects, and altered expression of cellular adhesion molecules.

Contraindications Hypersensitivity to thalidomide or any component of the formulation; neuropathy (peripheral); patient unable to comply with STEPS® program; women of childbearing potential unless alternative therapies are inappropriate and adequate precautions are taken to avoid pregnancy; pregnancy

Warnings/Precautions Hazardous agent - use appropriate precautions for handling and disposal. Thalidomide is a known teratogen; effective contraception must be used for at least 4 weeks before initiating therapy, during therapy, and for 4 weeks following discontinuation of thalidomide for women of childbearing potential. Use caution with drugs which may decrease the efficacy of hormonal contraceptives. May cause sedation; patients must be warned to use caution when performing tasks which require alertness. Use caution in patients with renal or hepatic impairment, neurological disorders, or constipation.

Thalidomide has been associated with the development of peripheral neuropathy, which may be irreversible; use caution with other medications which may cause peripheral neuropathy. Consider immediate discontinuation (if clinically appropriate) in patients who develop neuropathy. May cause seizures; use caution in patients with a history of seizures, concurrent therapy with drugs which alter seizure threshold, or conditions which predispose to seizures. May cause neutropenia; discontinue therapy if absolute neutrophil count decreases to <750/mm^3. Use caution in patients with HIV infection; has been associated with increased viral loads.

May cause orthostasis and/or bradycardia; use with caution in patients with cardiovascular disease or in patients who would not tolerate transient hypotensive episodes. Thrombotic events have been reported (generally in patients with other risk factors for thrombosis [neoplastic disease, inflammatory disease, or concurrent therapy with other drugs which may cause thrombosis]). Hypersensitivity, Stevens-Johnson syndrome (SJS) and toxic epidermal necrolyis (TEN) have been reported; withhold therapy and evaluate with skin rashes; permanently discontinued if rash is exfoliative, purpuric, bullous or if SJS or TEN is suspected. Safety and efficacy have not been established in children <12 years of age.

Drug Interactions
  Increased Effect/Toxicity: Thalidomide may enhance the sedative activity of other drugs such as ethanol, barbiturates, reserpine, and chlorpromazine. Thalidomide may be associated with increased risk of serious infection when used in combination with abatacept or anakinra. Thalidomide may increase the risk of vaccinal infection with vaccine (live organism).
  Decreased Effect: Thalidomide may decrease the effect of vaccines (dead organisms).

Ethanol/Nutrition/Herb Interactions
  Ethanol: Avoid ethanol (may increase sedation).
  Herb/Nutraceutical: Avoid cat's claw and echinacea (have immunostimulant properties; consider therapy modifications).

Dietary Considerations Should be taken at least 1 hour after the evening meal.

Pharmacodynamics/Kinetics
  Distribution: V_d: 120 L
  Protein binding: 55% to 66%
  Metabolism: Nonenzymatic hydrolysis in plasma; forms multiple metabolites
  Half-life elimination: 5-7 hours
  Time to peak, plasma: 3-6 hours
  Excretion: Urine (<1% as unchanged drug))

Pregnancy Risk Factor X

Dosage Forms CAP: 50 mg, 100 mg, 200 mg

Selected Readings
  Beckman DA and Brent RL, "Mechanism of Known Environmental Teratogens: Drugs and Chemicals," *Clin Perinatol*, 1986, 13(3):649-87.
  Gunzler V, "Thalidomide in Human Immunodeficiency Virus (HIV) Patients. A Review of Safety Considerations," *Drug Saf*, 1992, 7(2):116-34.
  Hamuryudan V, Mat C, Saip S, et al, "Thalidomide in the Treatment of the Mucocutaneous Lesions of the Behçet Syndrome. A Randomized, Double-Blind, Placebo-Controlled Trial," *Ann Intern Med*, 1998, 128(6):443-50.
  Jacobson JM, Greenspan JS, Spritzler J, et al, "Thalidomide for the Treatment of Oral Aphthous Ulcers in Patients With Human Immunodeficiency Virus Infection. National Institute of Allergy and Infectious Diseases AIDS Clinical Trials Group," *N Engl J Med*, 1997, 336(21):1487-93.
  Levien T, Baker DE, and Ballasiotes AA, "Reviews of Dexrazoxane and Thalidomide," *Hosp Pharm*, 1996, 31(5):487-8, 493-4, 499-500, 504, 508, 510.
  Schuler U and Ehninger G, "Thalidomide: Rationale for Renewed Use in Immunological Disorders," *Drug Saf*, 1995, 12(6):364-9.
  "Thalidomide," *Med Lett Drugs Ther*, 1998, 40(1038):103-4.

Thalitone® *see* Chlorthalidone *on page 332*

Thalomid® *see* Thalidomide *on page 1471*

THAM® *see* Tromethamine *on page 1545*

THC *see* Dronabinol *on page 518*

THC and CBD *see* Tetrahydrocannabinol and Cannabidiol *on page 1469*

Theo-24® *see* Theophylline *on page 1473*

TheoCap™ *see* Theophylline *on page 1473*

Theochron® *see* Theophylline *on page 1473*

Theolate [DSC] *see* Theophylline and Guaifenesin *on page 1475*

Theophylline (thee OFF i lin)

Related Information
  Aminophylline *on page 89*
  Respiratory Diseases *on page 1656*
  (Continued)

Theophylline *(Continued)*

U.S. Brand Names Elixophyllin®; Quibron®-T; Quibron®-T/SR; Theo-24®; TheoCap™; Theochron®; Uniphyl®

Canadian Brand Names Apo-Theo LA®; Novo-Theophyl SR; PMS-Theophylline; Pulmophylline; ratio-Theo-Bronc; Theochron® SR; Theolair™; Uniphyl® SRT

Mexican Brand Names Slo-Bid®; Teolong®; Uni-Dur®

Generic Available Yes: Extended release capsule and tablet, infusion

Synonyms Theophylline Anhydrous

Pharmacologic Category Theophylline Derivative

Use Treatment of symptoms and reversible airway obstruction due to chronic asthma, chronic bronchitis, or COPD

Local Anesthetic/Vasoconstrictor Precautions No information available to require special precautions

Effects on Dental Treatment Prescribe erythromycin products with caution to patients taking theophylline products. Erythromycin will delay the normal metabolic inactivation of theophyllines leading to increased blood levels; this has resulted in nausea, vomiting, and CNS restlessness. Azithromycin does not cause these effects in combination with theophylline products.

Common Adverse Effects

Adverse reactions/theophylline serum level: (Adverse effects do not necessarily occur according to serum levels. Arrhythmia and seizure can occur without seeing the other adverse effects).

　15-25 mcg/mL: GI upset, diarrhea, nausea/vomiting, abdominal pain, nervousness, headache, insomnia, agitation, dizziness, muscle cramp, tremor

　25-35 mcg/mL: Tachycardia, occasional PVC

　>35 mcg/mL: Ventricular tachycardia, frequent PVC, seizure

Uncommon at serum theophylline concentrations ≤20 mcg/mL:

1% to 10%:

　Cardiovascular: Tachycardia

　Central nervous system: Nervousness, restlessness

　Gastrointestinal: Nausea, vomiting

Mechanism of Action Causes bronchodilatation, diuresis, CNS and cardiac stimulation, and gastric acid secretion by blocking phosphodiesterase which increases tissue concentrations of cyclic adenine monophosphate (cAMP) which in turn promotes catecholamine stimulation of lipolysis, glycogenolysis, and gluconeogenesis and induces release of epinephrine from adrenal medulla cells

Drug Interactions

Cytochrome P450 Effect: Substrate of CYP1A2 (major), 2C8/9 (minor), 2D6 (minor), 2E1 (major), 3A4 (major); **Inhibits** CYP1A2 (weak)

Increased Effect/Toxicity: CYP1A2 inhibitors may increase the levels/effects of theophylline; example inhibitors include amiodarone, ciprofloxacin, fluvoxamine, ketoconazole, norfloxacin, ofloxacin, and rofecoxib. CYP2E1 inhibitors may increase the levels/effects of theophylline; example inhibitors include disulfiram, isoniazid, and miconazole. Changes in diet may affect the elimination of theophylline. CYP3A4 inhibitors may increase the levels/effects of theophylline; example inhibitors include azole antifungals, clarithromycin, diclofenac, doxycycline, erythromycin, imatinib, isoniazid, nefazodone, nicardipine, propofol, protease inhibitors, quinidine, telithromycin, and verapamil.

Decreased Effect: CYP1A2 inducers may decrease the levels/effects of theophylline; example inducers include aminoglutethimide, carbamazepine, phenobarbital, and rifampin. CYP3A4 inducers may decrease the levels/effects of theophylline; example inducers include aminoglutethimide, carbamazepine, nafcillin, nevirapine, phenobarbital, phenytoin, and rifamycins.

Pharmacodynamics/Kinetics

Absorption: Oral: Dosage form dependent

Distribution: 0.45 L/kg based on ideal body weight

Metabolism: Children >1 year and Adults: Hepatic; involves CYP1A2, 2E1 and 3A4; forms active metabolites (caffeine and 3-methylxanthine)

Half-life elimination: Highly variable and dependent upon age, liver function, cardiac function, lung disease, and smoking history

Time to peak, serum:

　Oral: Liquid: 1 hour; Tablet, enteric-coated: 5 hours; Tablet, uncoated: 2 hours

　I.V.: Within 30 minutes

Excretion: Urine

　Neonates: 50% unchanged

　Children >3 months and Adults: 10% unchanged

Pregnancy Risk Factor C

Theophylline and Guaifenesin (thee OFF i lin & gwye FEN e sin)

Related Information
  Guaifenesin *on page 752*
  Theophylline *on page 1473*
U.S. Brand Names Elixophyllin-GG®; Quibron®; Theolate [DSC]
Generic Available No
Synonyms Guaifenesin and Theophylline
Pharmacologic Category Theophylline Derivative
Use Symptomatic treatment of bronchospasm associated with bronchial asthma, chronic bronchitis, and pulmonary emphysema
Local Anesthetic/Vasoconstrictor Precautions No information available to require special precautions
Effects on Dental Treatment Prescribe erythromycin products with caution to patients taking theophylline products. Erythromycin will delay the normal metabolic inactivation of theophyllines leading to increased blood levels; this has resulted in nausea, vomiting, and CNS restlessness.
Drug Interactions
  Cytochrome P450 Effect: Theophylline: **Substrate** of CYP1A2 (major), 2C8/9 (minor), 2D6 (minor), 2E1 (major), 3A4 (major); **Inhibits** CYP1A2 (weak)
Pharmacodynamics/Kinetics See individual agents.
Pregnancy Risk Factor C

Theophylline Anhydrous *see* Theophylline *on page 1473*
Theophylline Ethylenediamine *see* Aminophylline *on page 89*
TheraCys® *see* BCG Vaccine *on page 181*
Thera-Flu® Cold and Sore Throat Night Time [OTC] *see* Acetaminophen, Chlorpheniramine, and Pseudoephedrine *on page 43*
Thera-Flur-N® *see* Fluoride *on page 671*
Thera-Flu® Severe Cold Non-Drowsy [OTC] [DSC] *see* Acetaminophen, Dextromethorphan, and Pseudoephedrine *on page 44*
Theragran-M® Advanced Formula [OTC] [DSC] *see* Vitamins (Multiple/Oral) *on page 1582*
Theragran® Heart Right™ [OTC] [DSC] *see* Vitamins (Multiple/Oral) *on page 1582*
Theramycin Z® *see* Erythromycin *on page 562*
Therapeutic Multivitamins *see* Vitamins (Multiple/Oral) *on page 1582*
Theratears® *see* Carboxymethylcellulose *on page 271*
Thermazene® *see* Silver Sulfadiazine *on page 1393*

Thiabendazole (thye a BEN da zole)

U.S. Brand Names Mintezol®
Generic Available No
Synonyms Tiabendazole
Pharmacologic Category Anthelmintic
Use Treatment of strongyloidiasis, cutaneous larva migrans, visceral larva migrans, dracunculiasis, trichinosis, and mixed helminthic infections
Unlabeled/Investigational Use Cutaneous larva migrans (topical application)
Local Anesthetic/Vasoconstrictor Precautions No information available to require special precautions
Effects on Dental Treatment No significant effects or complications reported
Common Adverse Effects Frequency not defined.
  Central nervous system: Seizures, hallucinations, delirium, dizziness, drowsiness, headache, chills
  Dermatologic: Rash, Stevens-Johnson syndrome, pruritus, angioedema
  Endocrine & metabolic: Hyperglycemia
  Gastrointestinal: Anorexia, diarrhea, nausea, vomiting, drying of mucous membranes, abdominal pain
  Genitourinary: Malodor of urine, hematuria, crystalluria, enuresis
  Hematologic: Leukopenia
  Hepatic: Jaundice, cholestasis, hepatic failure, hepatotoxicity
  Neuromuscular & skeletal: Numbness, incoordination
  Ocular: Abnormal sensation in eyes, blurred vision, dry eyes, Sicca syndrome, vision decreased, xanthopsia
  Otic: Tinnitus
  Renal: Nephrotoxicity
  Miscellaneous: Anaphylaxis, hypersensitivity reactions, lymphadenopathy
Mechanism of Action Inhibits helminth-specific mitochondrial fumarate reductase
(Continued)

Thiabendazole (Continued)

Drug Interactions

Cytochrome P450 Effect: Substrate of CYP1A2 (minor); **Inhibits** CYP1A2 (strong)

Increased Effect/Toxicity: Thiabendazole may increase the levels/effects of aminophylline, fluvoxamine, mexiletine, mirtazapine, ropinirole, theophylline, trifluoperazine, and other CYP1A2 substrates.

Pharmacodynamics/Kinetics

Absorption: Rapid and well absorbed

Metabolism: Rapidly hepatic; metabolized to 5-hydroxy form

Half-life elimination: 1.2 hours

Time to peak, plasma: Oral suspension: Within 1-2 hours

Excretion: Urine (90%) and feces (5%) primarily as conjugated metabolites

Pregnancy Risk Factor C

Thiamazole see Methimazole on page 1008

Thiamine (THYE a min)

Canadian Brand Names Betaxin®

Mexican Brand Names Benerva®

Generic Available Yes

Synonyms Aneurine Hydrochloride; Thiamine Hydrochloride; Thiaminium Chloride Hydrochloride; Vitamin B$_1$

Pharmacologic Category Vitamin, Water Soluble

Use Treatment of thiamine deficiency including beriberi, Wernicke's encephalopathy syndrome, and peripheral neuritis associated with pellagra, alcoholic patients with altered sensorium; various genetic metabolic disorders

Local Anesthetic/Vasoconstrictor Precautions No information available to require special precautions

Effects on Dental Treatment No significant effects or complications reported

Mechanism of Action An essential coenzyme in carbohydrate metabolism by combining with adenosine triphosphate to form thiamine pyrophosphate

Pharmacodynamics/Kinetics

Absorption: Oral: Adequate; I.M.: Rapid and complete

Excretion: Urine (as unchanged drug and as pyrimidine after body storage sites become saturated)

Pregnancy Risk Factor A/C (dose exceeding RDA recommendation)

Thiamine Hydrochloride see Thiamine on page 1476

Thiaminium Chloride Hydrochloride see Thiamine on page 1476

Thioguanine (thye oh GWAH neen)

U.S. Brand Names Tabloid®

Canadian Brand Names Lanvis®

Generic Available No

Synonyms 2-Amino-6-Mercaptopurine; NSC-752; TG; 6-TG (error-prone abbreviation); 6-Thioguanine (error-prone abbreviation); Tioguanine

Pharmacologic Category Antineoplastic Agent, Antimetabolite (Purine Antagonist)

Use Treatment of acute myelogenous (nonlymphocytic) leukemia; treatment of chronic myelogenous leukemia and granulocytic leukemia

Local Anesthetic/Vasoconstrictor Precautions No information available to require special precautions

Effects on Dental Treatment Key adverse event(s) related to dental treatment: Stomatitis.

Common Adverse Effects

>10%: Hematologic: Myelosuppressive:

WBC: Moderate

Platelets: Moderate

Onset (days): 7-10

Nadir (days): 14

Recovery (days): 21

1% to 10%:

Dermatologic: Skin rash

Endocrine & metabolic: Hyperuricemia

Gastrointestinal: Mild nausea or vomiting, anorexia, stomatitis, diarrhea

Neuromuscular & skeletal: Unsteady gait

Restrictions The I.V. formulation is not available in U.S./Investigational

Mechanism of Action Purine analog that is incorporated into DNA and RNA resulting in the blockage of synthesis and metabolism of purine nucleotides

Drug Interactions

Increased Effect/Toxicity: Allopurinol can be used in full doses with thioguanine unlike mercaptopurine. Use with busulfan may cause hepatotoxicity and esophageal varices. Aminosalicylates (olsalazine, mesalamine, sulfasalazine) may inhibit TPMT, increasing toxicity/myelosuppression of thioguanine.

Pharmacodynamics/Kinetics

Absorption: 30% (highly variable)

Distribution: Crosses placenta

Metabolism: Hepatic; rapidly and extensively via TPMT to 2-amino-6-methylthioguanine (active) and inactive compounds

Half-life elimination: Terminal: 11 hours

Time to peak, serum: Within 8 hours

Excretion: Urine

Pregnancy Risk Factor D

6-Thioguanine (error-prone abbreviation) *see* Thioguanine *on page 1476*

Thiola® *see* Tiopronin *on page 1494*

Thiopental (thye oh PEN tal)

U.S. Brand Names Pentothal®

Canadian Brand Names Pentothal®

Mexican Brand Names Pentothal Sodico®; Sodipental®

Generic Available No

Synonyms Thiopental Sodium

Pharmacologic Category Anticonvulsant, Barbiturate; Barbiturate; General Anesthetic

Use Induction of anesthesia; adjunct for intubation in head injury patients; control of convulsive states; treatment of elevated intracranial pressure

Local Anesthetic/Vasoconstrictor Precautions No information available to require special precautions

Effects on Dental Treatment No significant effects or complications reported

Mechanism of Action Short-acting barbiturate with sedative, hypnotic, and anticonvulsant properties. Barbiturates depress the sensory cortex, decrease motor activity, alter cerebellar function, and produce drowsiness, sedation, and hypnosis. In high doses, barbiturates exhibit anticonvulsant activity; barbiturates produce dose-dependent respiratory depression.

Pregnancy Risk Factor C

Thiopental Sodium *see* Thiopental *on page 1477*

Thiophosphoramide *see* Thiotepa *on page 1479*

Thioridazine (thye oh RID a zeen)

Canadian Brand Names Apo-Thioridazine®; Mellaril®

Generic Available Yes

Synonyms Thioridazine Hydrochloride

Pharmacologic Category Antipsychotic Agent, Typical, Phenothiazine

Use Management of schizophrenic patients who fail to respond adequately to treatment with other antipsychotic drugs, either because of insufficient effectiveness or the inability to achieve an effective dose due to intolerable adverse effects from those medications

Unlabeled/Investigational Use Psychosis

Local Anesthetic/Vasoconstrictor Precautions Most pharmacology textbooks state that in presence of phenothiazines, systemic doses of epinephrine paradoxically decrease the blood pressure. This is the so called "epinephrine reversal" phenomenon. This has never been observed when epinephrine is given by infiltration as part of the anesthesia procedure. See Dental Comment.

Effects on Dental Treatment Key adverse event(s) related to dental treatment: Xerostomia and changes in salivation (normal salivary flow resumes upon discontinuation). Significant hypotension may occur, especially when the drug is administered parenterally; orthostatic hypotension is due to alpha-receptor blockade, the elderly are at greater risk for orthostatic hypotension.

Tardive dyskinesia; Prevalence rate may be 40% in elderly; development of the syndrome and the irreversible nature are proportional to duration and total cumulative dose over time. Extrapyramidal reactions are more common in elderly with up to 50% developing these reactions after 60 years of age. Drug-induced Parkinson's syndrome occurs often; akathisia is the most common extrapyramidal reaction in elderly.

(Continued)

Thioridazine *(Continued)*

Common Adverse Effects Frequency not defined.

Cardiovascular: Hypotension, orthostatic hypotension, peripheral edema, ECG changes

Central nervous system: EPS (pseudoparkinsonism, akathisia, dystonias, tardive dyskinesia), dizziness, drowsiness, neuroleptic malignant syndrome (NMS), impairment of temperature regulation, lowering of seizure threshold, seizure

Dermatologic: Increased sensitivity to sun, rash, discoloration of skin (blue-gray)

Endocrine & metabolic: Changes in menstrual cycle, libido (changes in), breast pain, galactorrhea, amenorrhea

Gastrointestinal: Constipation, weight gain, nausea, vomiting, stomach pain, xerostomia, nausea, vomiting, diarrhea

Genitourinary: Difficulty in urination, ejaculatory disturbances, urinary retention, priapism

Hematologic: Agranulocytosis, leukopenia

Hepatic: Cholestatic jaundice, hepatotoxicity

Neuromuscular & skeletal: Tremor

Ocular: Pigmentary retinopathy, blurred vision, cornea and lens changes

Respiratory: Nasal congestion

Mechanism of Action Thioridazine is a piperidine phenothiazine which blocks postsynaptic mesolimbic dopaminergic receptors in the brain; exhibits a strong alpha-adrenergic blocking effect and depresses the release of hypothalamic and hypophyseal hormones

Drug Interactions

Cytochrome P450 Effect: Substrate of CYP2C19 (minor), 2D6 (major); Inhibits CYP1A2 (weak), 2C8/9 (weak), 2D6 (moderate), 2E1 (weak)

Increased Effect/Toxicity: Concurrent use fluvoxamine, propranolol, and pindolol. The levels/effects of thioridazine may be increased by chlorpromazine, delavirdine, fluoxetine, miconazole, paroxetine, pergolide, quinidine, quinine, ritonavir, ropinirole, and other CYP2D6 inhibitors. **Thioridazine is contraindicated with strong inhibitors of this enzyme.**

Drugs which alter the QT_c interval may be additive with thioridazine, increasing the risk of malignant arrhythmias; includes type Ia antiarrhythmics, TCAs, and some quinolone antibiotics (sparfloxacin, moxifloxacin and gatifloxacin). **These agents are contraindicated with thioridazine.** Potassium depleting agents may increase the risk of serious arrhythmias with thioridazine (includes many diuretics, aminoglycosides, and amphotericin).

Phenothiazines inhibit the ability of bromocriptine to lower serum prolactin concentrations. The sedative effects of CNS depressants or ethanol may be additive with phenothiazines. Phenothiazines and trazodone may produce additive hypotensive effects. Metoclopramide may increase risk of extrapyramidal symptoms (EPS). Acetylcholinesterase inhibitors (central) may increase the risk of antipsychotic-related EPS. Concurrent use of antihypertensives may result in additive hypotensive effects (particularly orthostasis).

Thioridazine may increase the levels/effects of amphetamines, beta-blockers, dextromethorphan, fluoxetine, lidocaine, mirtazapine, nefazodone, paroxetine, risperidone, ritonavir, tricyclic antidepressants, venlafaxine, and other CYP2D6 substrates. **Concurrent use with fluvoxamine is contraindicated.**

Phenothiazines may produce neurotoxicity with lithium; this is a rare effect. Rare cases of respiratory paralysis have been reported with concurrent use of phenothiazines and polypeptide antibiotics. Naltrexone in combination with thioridazine has been reported to cause lethargy and somnolence. Phenylpropanolamine has been reported to result in cardiac arrhythmias when combined with thioridazine.

Decreased Effect: Aluminum salts may decrease the absorption of phenothiazines. The efficacy of amphetamines may be diminished by antipsychotics; in addition, amphetamines may increase psychotic symptoms; avoid concurrent use. Anticholinergics may inhibit the therapeutic response to phenothiazines and excess anticholinergic effects may occur (includes benztropine, trihexyphenidyl, biperiden, and drugs with significant anticholinergic activity). Chlorpromazine (and possibly other low potency antipsychotics) may diminish the pressor effects of epinephrine. The antihypertensive effects of guanethidine or guanadrel may be inhibited by phenothiazines. Phenothiazines may inhibit the antiparkinsonian effect of levodopa. Enzyme inducers may enhance the hepatic metabolism of phenothiazines; larger doses may be required; includes rifampin, rifabutin, barbiturates, phenytoin, and cigarette smoking.

Thioridazine may decrease the levels/effects of CYP2D6 prodrug substrates (eg, codeine, hydrocodone, oxycodone, tramadol).

Pharmacodynamics/Kinetics
Duration: 4-5 days
Half-life elimination: 21-25 hours
Time to peak, serum: ~1 hour

Pregnancy Risk Factor C

Dental Comment
This drug is known to prolong the QT interval. The QT interval is measured as the time and distance between the Q point of the QRS complex and the end of the T wave in the ECG tracing. After adjustment for heart rate, the QT interval is defined as prolonged if it is more than 450 msec in men and 460 msec in women. A long QT syndrome was first described in the 1950s and 60s as a congenital syndrome involving QT interval prolongation and syncope and sudden death. Some of the congenital long QT syndromes were characterized by a peculiar electrocardiographic appearance of the QRS complex involving a premature atria beat followed by a pause, then a subsequent sinus beat showing marked QT prolongation and deformity. This type of cardiac arrhythmia was originally termed "torsade de pointes" (translated from the French as "twisting of the points").

Prolongation of the QT interval is thought to result from delayed ventricular repolarization. The repolarization process within the myocardial cell is due to the efflux of intracellular potassium. The channels associated with this current can be blocked by many drugs and predisposes the electrical propagation cycle to torsade de pointes.

Thioridazine is one of the drugs confirmed to prolong the QT interval and is accepted as having a risk of causing torsade de pointes. The risk of drug-induced torsade de pointes is extremely low when a single QT interval prolonging drug is prescribed. In terms of epinephrine, it is not known what effect vasoconstrictors in the local anesthetic regimen will have in patients with a known history of congenital prolonged QT interval or in patients taking any medication that prolongs the QT interval. Until more information is obtained, it is suggested that the clinician consult with the physician prior to the use of a vasoconstrictor in suspected patients, and that the vasoconstrictor (epinephrine, levonordefrin [Neo-Cobefrin®]) be used with caution.

Thioridazine Hydrochloride *see* Thioridazine *on page 1477*

Thiosulfuric Acid Disodium Salt *see* Sodium Thiosulfate *on page 1404*

Thiotepa (thye oh TEP a)

Generic Available Yes
Synonyms TESPA; Thiophosphoramide; Triethylenethiophosphoramide; TSPA
Pharmacologic Category Antineoplastic Agent, Alkylating Agent
Use Treatment of superficial tumors of the bladder; palliative treatment of adeno-carcinoma of breast or ovary; lymphomas and sarcomas; controlling intracavi-tary effusions caused by metastatic tumors; I.T. use: CNS leukemia/lymphoma, CNS metastases

Local Anesthetic/Vasoconstrictor Precautions No information available to require special precautions

Effects on Dental Treatment No significant effects or complications reported

Common Adverse Effects
>10%:
Hematopoietic: Dose-limiting toxicity which is dose related and cumulative; moderate to severe leukopenia and severe thrombocytopenia have occurred. Anemia and pancytopenia may become fatal, so careful hemato-logic monitoring is required; intravesical administration may cause bone marrow suppression as well.
Hematologic: Myelosuppressive:
WBC: Moderate
Platelets: Severe
Onset: 7-10 days
Nadir: 14 days
Recovery: 28 days
Local: Pain at injection site
1% to 10%:
Central nervous system: Dizziness, fever, headache
Dermatologic: Alopecia, rash, pruritus, hyperpigmentation with high-dose therapy
Endocrine & metabolic: Hyperuricemia
Gastrointestinal: Anorexia, nausea and vomiting rarely occur
(Continued)

Thiotepa (Continued)

Emetic potential: Low (<10%)
Genitourinary: Hemorrhagic cystitis
Renal: Hematuria
Miscellaneous: Tightness of the throat, allergic reactions

Mechanism of Action Alkylating agent that reacts with DNA phosphate groups to produce cross-linking of DNA strands leading to inhibition of DNA, RNA, and protein synthesis; mechanism of action has not been explored as thoroughly as the other alkylating agents, it is presumed that the aziridine rings open and react as nitrogen mustard; reactivity is enhanced at a lower pH

Drug Interactions

Cytochrome P450 Effect: Inhibits CYP2B6 (weak)

Increased Effect/Toxicity: Other alkylating agents or irradiation used concomitantly with thiotepa intensifies toxicity rather than enhancing therapeutic response. Prolonged muscular paralysis and respiratory depression may occur when neuromuscular blocking agents are administered. Succinylcholine and other neuromuscular blocking agents' action can be prolonged due to thiotepa inhibiting plasma pseudocholinesterase.

Pharmacodynamics/Kinetics

Absorption: Intracavitary instillation: Unreliable (10% to 100%) through bladder mucosa; I.M.: variable
Metabolism: Extensively hepatic
Half-life elimination: Terminal (dose-dependent clearance): 109 minutes
Excretion: Urine (as metabolites and unchanged drug)

Pregnancy Risk Factor D

Thiothixene (thye oh THIKS een)

U.S. Brand Names Navane®
Canadian Brand Names Navane®
Generic Available Yes
Synonyms Tiotixene
Pharmacologic Category Antipsychotic Agent, Typical
Use Management of schizophrenia
Unlabeled/Investigational Use Psychotic disorders
Local Anesthetic/Vasoconstrictor Precautions Most pharmacology textbooks state that in presence of phenothiazines, systemic doses of epinephrine paradoxically decrease the blood pressure. This is the so called "epinephrine reversal" phenomenon. This has never been observed when epinephrine is given by infiltration as part of the anesthesia procedure. See Dental Comment.
Effects on Dental Treatment Key adverse event(s) related to dental treatment: Significant hypotension may occur, especially when the drug is administered parenterally; orthostatic hypotension is due to alpha-receptor blockade, the elderly are at greater risk for orthostatic hypotension.

Tardive dyskinesia: Prevalence rate may be 40% in elderly; development of the syndrome and the irreversible nature are proportional to duration and total cumulative dose over time. Extrapyramidal reactions are more common in elderly with up to 50% developing these reactions after 60 years of age. Drug-induced Parkinson's syndrome occurs often; akathisia is the most common extrapyramidal reaction in elderly.

Common Adverse Effects Frequency not defined.

Cardiovascular: Hypotension, tachycardia, syncope, nonspecific ECG changes
Central nervous system: Extrapyramidal signs (pseudoparkinsonism, akathisia, dystonias, lightheadedness, tardive dyskinesia), dizziness, drowsiness, restlessness, agitation, insomnia
Dermatologic: Discoloration of skin (blue-gray), rash, pruritus, urticaria, photosensitivity
Endocrine & metabolic: Changes in menstrual cycle, libido (changes in), breast pain, galactorrhea, lactation, amenorrhea, gynecomastia, hyperglycemia, hypoglycemia
Gastrointestinal: Weight gain, nausea, vomiting, stomach pain, constipation, xerostomia, increased salivation
Genitourinary: Difficulty in urination, ejaculatory disturbances, impotence
Hematologic: Leukopenia, leukocytes
Neuromuscular & skeletal: Tremors
Ocular: Pigmentary retinopathy, blurred vision
Respiratory: Nasal congestion
Miscellaneous: Diaphoresis

Mechanism of Action Thiothixene is a thioxanthene antipsychotic which elicits antipsychotic activity by postsynaptic blockade of CNS dopamine receptors resulting in inhibition of dopamine-mediated effects; also has alpha-adrenergic blocking activity

Drug Interactions

Cytochrome P450 Effect: Substrate of CYP1A2 (major); **Inhibits** CYP2D6 (weak)

Increased Effect/Toxicity: CYP1A2 inhibitors may increase the levels/ effects of thiothixene; example inhibitors include amiodarone, ciprofloxacin, fluvoxamine, ketoconazole, norfloxacin, ofloxacin, and rofecoxib. Thiothixene and CNS depressants (ethanol, narcotics) may produce additive CNS depressant effects. Thiothixene may increase the effect/toxicity of antihypertensives, benztropine (and other anticholinergic agents), lithium, trazodone, and TCAs. Thiothixene's concentrations may be increased by chloroquine, sulfadoxine-pyrimethamine, and propranolol. Metoclopramide may increase risk of extrapyramidal symptoms (EPS). Acetylcholinesterase inhibitors (central) may increase the risk of antipsychotic-related EPS.

Decreased Effect: CYP1A2 inducers may decrease the levels/effects of thiothixene; example inducers include aminoglutethimide, carbamazepine, phenobarbital, and rifampin. Thiothixene inhibits the activity of guanadrel, guanethidine, levodopa, and bromocriptine. Benztropine (and other anticholinergics) may inhibit the therapeutic response to thiothixene. Thiothixene and low potency antipsychotics may reverse the pressor effects of epinephrine.

Pharmacodynamics/Kinetics

Metabolism: Extensively hepatic

Half-life elimination: >24 hours with chronic use

Pregnancy Risk Factor C

Dental Comment

This drug is known to prolong the QT interval. The QT interval is measured as the time and distance between the Q point of the QRS complex and the end of the T wave in the ECG tracing. After adjustment for heart rate, the QT interval is defined as prolonged if it is more than 450 msec in men and 460 msec in women. A long QT syndrome was first described in the 1950s and 60s as a congenital syndrome involving QT interval prolongation and syncope and sudden death. Some of the congenital long QT syndromes were characterized by a peculiar electrocardiographic appearance of the QRS complex involving a premature atria beat followed by a pause, then a subsequent sinus beat showing marked QT prolongation and deformity. This type of cardiac arrhythmia was originally termed "torsade de pointes" (translated from the French as "twisting of the points").

Prolongation of the QT interval is thought to result from delayed ventricular repolarization. The repolarization process within the myocardial cell is due to the efflux of intracellular potassium. The channels associated with this current can be blocked by many drugs and predisposes the electrical propagation cycle to torsade de pointes.

Thiothixene is one of the drugs confirmed to prolong the QT interval and is accepted as having a risk of causing torsade de pointes. The risk of drug-induced torsade de pointes is extremely low when a single QT interval prolonging drug is prescribed. In terms of epinephrine, it is not known what effect vasoconstrictors in the local anesthetic regimen will have in patients with a known history of congenital prolonged QT interval or in patients taking any medication that prolongs the QT interval. Until more information is obtained, it is suggested that the clinician consult with the physician prior to the use of a vasoconstrictor in suspected patients, and that the vasoconstrictor (epinephrine, levonordefrin [Neo-Cobefrin®]) be used with caution.

Thorets [OTC] *see* Benzocaine *on page 190*

Thrombate III® *see* Antithrombin III *on page 131*

Thrombin-JMI® *see* Thrombin (Topical) *on page 1481*

Thrombin (Topical) (THROM bin, TOP i kal)

U.S. Brand Names Thrombin-JMI®

Generic Available No

Pharmacologic Category Hemostatic Agent

Dental Use Hemostasis whenever minor bleeding from capillaries and small venules is accessible

Use Hemostasis whenever minor bleeding from capillaries and small venules is accessible

Local Anesthetic/Vasoconstrictor Precautions No information available to require special precautions

Effects on Dental Treatment No significant effects or complications reported

(Continued)

Thrombin (Topical) *(Continued)*

Significant Adverse Effects 1% to 10%:
Central nervous system: Fever
Miscellaneous: Allergic type reaction

Dental Usual Dosing Bleeding: Adults: Topical: Use 1000-2000 units/mL of solution where bleeding is profuse; apply powder directly to the site of bleeding or on oozing surfaces; use 100 units/mL for bleeding from skin or mucosal surfaces

Dosage Use 1000-2000 units/mL of solution where bleeding is profuse; apply powder directly to the site of bleeding or on oozing surfaces; use 100 units/mL for bleeding from skin or mucosal surfaces

Mechanism of Action Catalyzes the conversion of fibrinogen to fibrin

Contraindications Hypersensitivity to thrombin or any component of the formulation

Warnings/Precautions Do not inject, for topical use only

Drug Interactions No data reported

Pregnancy Risk Factor C

Dosage Forms Powder for reconstitution, topical:
Thrombin-JMI®: 5000 units, 20,000 units [packaged with diluent]
Thrombin-JMI® Spray Kit: 20,000 units [packaged with diluent and spray pump]
Thrombin-JMI® Syringe Spray Kit: 20,000 units [packaged with diluent, spray tip, and syringe]

Thymocyte Stimulating Factor *see* Aldesleukin *on page 61*

Thyrel® TRH [DSC] *see* Protirelin *on page 1307*

Thyrogen® *see* Thyrotropin Alpha *on page 1483*

Thyroid (THYE roid)

Related Information
Endocrine Disorders and Pregnancy *on page 1659*

U.S. Brand Names Armour® Thyroid; Nature-Throid® NT; Westhroid®

Generic Available Yes

Synonyms Desiccated Thyroid; Thyroid Extract; Thyroid USP

Pharmacologic Category Thyroid Product

Use Replacement or supplemental therapy in hypothyroidism; pituitary TSH suppressants (thyroid nodules, thyroiditis, multinodular goiter, thyroid cancer), thyrotoxicosis, diagnostic suppression tests

Local Anesthetic/Vasoconstrictor Precautions No precautions with vasoconstrictor are necessary if patient is well controlled with thyroid preparations

Effects on Dental Treatment No significant effects or complications reported

Mechanism of Action The primary active compound is T_3 (triiodothyronine), which may be converted from T_4 (thyroxine) and then circulates throughout the body to influence growth and maturation of various tissues; exact mechanism of action is unknown; however, it is believed the thyroid hormone exerts its many metabolic effects through control of DNA transcription and protein synthesis; involved in normal metabolism, growth, and development; promotes gluconeogenesis, increases utilization and mobilization of glycogen stores and stimulates protein synthesis, increases basal metabolic rate

Drug Interactions

Increased Effect/Toxicity: Thyroid may potentiate the hypoprothrombinemic effect of oral anticoagulants. Tricyclic antidepressants (TAD) coadministered with thyroid hormone may increase potential for toxicity of both drugs.

Decreased Effect: Thyroid hormones increase the therapeutic need for oral hypoglycemics or insulin. Cholestyramine can bind thyroid and reduce its absorption. Phenytoin may decrease thyroxine serum levels. Thyroid hormone may decrease effect of oral sulfonylureas.

Pharmacodynamics/Kinetics
Absorption: T_4: 48% to 79%; T_3: 95%; desiccated thyroid contains thyroxine, liothyronine, and iodine (primarily bound)
Metabolism: Thyroxine: Largely converted to liothyronine
Half-life elimination, serum: Liothyronine: 1-2 days; Thyroxine: 6-7 days

Pregnancy Risk Factor A

Thyroid Extract *see* Thyroid *on page 1482*

Thyroid USP *see* Thyroid *on page 1482*

Thyrolar® *see* Liotrix *on page 935*

ThyroSafe™ [OTC] *see* Potassium Iodide *on page 1260*

ThyroShield™ [OTC] *see* Potassium Iodide *on page 1260*

Thyrotropin Alpha (thye roe TROH pin AL fa)

U.S. Brand Names Thyrogen®
Canadian Brand Names Thyrogen®
Generic Available No
Synonyms Human Thyroid Stimulating Hormone; TSH
Pharmacologic Category Diagnostic Agent
Use As an adjunctive diagnostic tool for serum thyroglobulin (Tg) testing with or without radioiodine imaging in the follow-up of patients with well-differentiated thyroid cancer

Potential clinical use:

1. Patients with an undetectable Tg on thyroid hormone suppressive therapy to exclude the diagnosis of residual or recurrent thyroid cancer
2. Patients requiring serum Tg testing and radioiodine imaging who are unwilling to undergo thyroid hormone withdrawal testing and whose treating physician believes that use of a less sensitive test is justified
3. Patients who are either unable to mount an adequate endogenous TSH response to thyroid hormone withdrawal or in whom withdrawal is medically contraindicated

Local Anesthetic/Vasoconstrictor Precautions No information available to require special precautions
Effects on Dental Treatment No significant effects or complications reported
Common Adverse Effects
>10 %: Gastrointestinal: Nausea (11%)
1% to 10%:
Central nervous system: Headache (7%), dizziness (2%), chills (1%), fever (1%)
Gastrointestinal: Vomiting (2%)
Neuromuscular & skeletal: Weakness (3%), paresthesia (2%)
Miscellaneous: Flu-like syndrome (1%)
Adverse reactions which may be related to local edema or hemorrhage at metastatic sites: Acute visual loss, enlargement of locally-recurring papillary carcinoma, laryngeal edema with respiratory distress, stridor
Mechanism of Action A recombinant DNA source of human TSH that serves as an additional diagnostic tool in the follow-up of patients with a history of well-differentiated thyroid cancer. Binding of thyrotropin alpha to TSH receptors on normal thyroid epithelial cells or on well-differentiated thyroid cancer tissue stimulates iodine uptake and organification, and synthesis and secretion of thyroglobulin, triiodothyronine, and thyroxine. In thyroid cancer patients with near total thyroidectomy, thyrotropin is used to stimulate thyroglobulin from residual or remnant thyroid cancer tissue, which prevents the need for thyroid hormone therapy withdrawal.
Pharmacodynamics/Kinetics
Half-life elimination: 25 ± 10 hours
Time to peak: Median: 10 hours (range: 3-24 hours)
Pregnancy Risk Factor C

Thyrotropin Releasing Hormone *see* Protirelin *on page 1307*
L-Thyroxine Sodium *see* Levothyroxine *on page 917*
Tiabendazole *see* Thiabendazole *on page 1475*

Tiagabine (tye AG a been)

U.S. Brand Names Gabitril®
Canadian Brand Names Gabitril®
Generic Available No
Synonyms Tiagabine Hydrochloride
Pharmacologic Category Anticonvulsant, Miscellaneous
Use Adjunctive therapy in adults and children ≥12 years of age in the treatment of partial seizures
Local Anesthetic/Vasoconstrictor Precautions No information available to require special precautions
Effects on Dental Treatment No significant effects or complications reported
Common Adverse Effects
>10%:
Central nervous system: Concentration decreased, dizziness, nervousness, somnolence
Gastrointestinal: Nausea
Neuromuscular & skeletal: Weakness, tremor
(Continued)

Tiagabine *(Continued)*

1% to 10%:

Cardiovascular: Chest pain, edema, hypertension, palpitation, peripheral edema, syncope, tachycardia, vasodilation

Central nervous system: Agitation, ataxia, chills, confusion, difficulty with memory, confusion, depersonalization, depression, euphoria, hallucination, hostility, insomnia, malaise, migraine, paranoid reaction, personality disorder, speech disorder

Dermatologic: Alopecia, bruising, dry skin, pruritus, rash

Gastrointestinal: Abdominal pain, diarrhea, gingivitis, increased appetite, mouth ulceration, stomatitis, vomiting, weight gain/loss

Neuromuscular & skeletal: Abnormal gait, arthralgia, dysarthria, hyper-/hypo-kinesia, hyper-/hypotonia, myasthenia, myalgia, myoclonus, neck pain, paresthesia, reflexes decreased, stupor, twitching, vertigo

Ocular: Abnormal vision, amblyopia, nystagmus

Otic: Ear pain, hearing impairment, otitis media, tinnitus

Respiratory: Bronchitis, cough, dyspnea, epistaxis, pneumonia

Miscellaneous: Allergic reaction, cyst, diaphoresis, flu-like syndrome, lymph-adenopathy

Mechanism of Action The exact mechanism by which tiagabine exerts antiseizure activity is not definitively known; however, *in vitro* experiments demonstrate that it enhances the activity of gamma aminobutyric acid (GABA), the major neuroinhibitory transmitter in the nervous system; it is thought that binding to the GABA uptake carrier inhibits the uptake of GABA into presynaptic neurons, allowing an increased amount of GABA to be available to postsynaptic neurons; based on *in vitro* studies, tiagabine does not inhibit the uptake of dopamine, norepinephrine, serotonin, glutamate, or choline

Drug Interactions

Cytochrome P450 Effect: Substrate of 3A4 (major)

Increased Effect/Toxicity: CYP3A4 inhibitors may increase the levels/effects of tiagabine; example inhibitors include azole antifungals, clarithromycin, diclofenac, doxycycline, erythromycin, imatinib, isoniazid, nefazodone, nicardipine, propofol, protease inhibitors, quinidine, telithromycin, and verapamil. Valproate increased free tiagabine concentrations (*in vitro*) by 40%.

Decreased Effect: CYP3A4 inducers may decrease the levels/effects of tiagabine; example inducers include aminoglutethimide, carbamazepine, nafcillin, nevirapine, phenobarbital, phenytoin, and rifamycins.

Pharmacodynamics/Kinetics

Absorption: Rapid (45 minutes); prolonged with food

Protein binding: 96%, primarily to albumin and α_1-acid glycoprotein

Metabolism: Hepatic via CYP (primarily 3A4)

Bioavailability: Oral: Absolute: 90%

Half-life elimination: 2-5 hours when administered with enzyme inducers; 7-9 hours when administered without enzyme inducers

Time to peak, plasma: 45 minutes

Excretion: Feces (63%); urine (25%); 2% as unchanged drug; primarily as metabolites

Pregnancy Risk Factor C

Tiagabine Hydrochloride *see* Tiagabine *on page 1483*

Tiazac® *see* Diltiazem *on page 479*

Ticar® *see* Ticarcillin *on page 1484*

Ticarcillin *(tye kar SIL in)*

U.S. Brand Names Ticar®

Generic Available No

Synonyms Ticarcillin Disodium

Pharmacologic Category Antibiotic, Penicillin

Use Treatment of susceptible infections such as septicemia, acute and chronic respiratory tract infections, skin and soft tissue infections, and urinary tract infections due to susceptible strains of *Pseudomonas*, and other gram-negative bacteria

Local Anesthetic/Vasoconstrictor Precautions No information available to require special precautions

Effects on Dental Treatment Key adverse event(s) related to dental treatment: Prolonged use of penicillins may lead to development of oral candidiasis.

Common Adverse Effects Frequency not defined.

Central nervous system: Confusion, convulsions, drowsiness, fever, Jarisch-Herxheimer reaction

Dermatologic: Rash

Endocrine & metabolic: Electrolyte imbalance

Gastrointestinal: *Clostridium difficile* colitis

Hematologic: Bleeding, eosinophilia, hemolytic anemia, leukopenia, neutropenia, positive Coombs' reaction, thrombocytopenia

Hepatic: Hepatotoxicity, jaundice

Local: Thrombophlebitis

Neuromuscular & skeletal: Myoclonus

Renal: Interstitial nephritis (acute)

Miscellaneous: Anaphylaxis, hypersensitivity reactions

Mechanism of Action Inhibits bacterial cell wall synthesis by binding to one or more of the penicillin binding proteins (PBPs); which in turn inhibits the final transpeptidation step of peptidoglycan synthesis in bacterial cell walls, thus inhibiting cell wall biosynthesis. Bacteria eventually lyse due to ongoing activity of cell wall autolytic enzymes (autolysins and murein hydrolases) while cell wall assembly is arrested.

Drug Interactions

Increased Effect/Toxicity: Probenecid may increase penicillin levels. Neuromuscular blockers may have an increased duration of action (neuromuscular blockade). Penicillins may increase the exposure to methotrexate during concurrent therapy; monitor.

Decreased Effect: Tetracyclines may decrease penicillin effectiveness. Aminoglycosides may cause physical inactivation of aminoglycosides in the presence of high concentrations of ticarcillin and potential toxicity in patients with mild-moderate renal dysfunction. Although anecdotal reports suggest oral contraceptive efficacy could be reduced by penicillins, this has been refuted by more rigorous scientific and clinical data.

Pharmacodynamics/Kinetics

Absorption: I.M.: 86%

Distribution: Blister fluid, lymph tissue, and gallbladder; low concentrations into CSF increasing with inflamed meninges, otherwise widely distributed; crosses placenta; enters breast milk (low concentrations)

Protein binding: 45% to 65%

Half-life elimination:

Neonates: <1 week old: 3.5-5.6 hours; 1-8 weeks old: 1.3-2.2 hours

Children 5-13 years: 0.9 hour

Adults: 66-72 minutes; prolonged with renal and/or hepatic impairment

Time to peak, serum: I.M.: 30-75 minutes

Excretion: Almost entirely urine (as unchanged drug and metabolites); feces (3.5%)

Pregnancy Risk Factor B

Ticarcillin and Clavulanate Potassium

(tye kar SIL in & klav yoo LAN ate poe TASS ee um)

Related Information

Ticarcillin *on page 1484*

U.S. Brand Names Timentin®

Canadian Brand Names Timentin®

Generic Available No

Synonyms Ticarcillin and Clavulanic Acid

Pharmacologic Category Antibiotic, Penicillin

Use Treatment of infections of lower respiratory tract, urinary tract, skin and skin structures, bone and joint, and septicemia caused by susceptible organisms. Clavulanate expands activity of ticarcillin to include beta-lactamase producing strains of *S. aureus*, *H. influenzae*, *Bacteroides* species, and some other gram-negative bacilli

Local Anesthetic/Vasoconstrictor Precautions No information available to require special precautions

Effects on Dental Treatment Key adverse event(s) related to dental treatment: Prolonged use of penicillins may lead to development of oral candidiasis.

Common Adverse Effects Frequency not defined.

Central nervous system: Confusion, convulsions, drowsiness, fever, Jarisch-Herxheimer reaction

Dermatologic: Rash, erythema multiforme, toxic epidermal necrolysis, Stevens-Johnson syndrome

Endocrine & metabolic: Electrolyte imbalance

Gastrointestinal: *Clostridium difficile* colitis

Hematologic: Bleeding, hemolytic anemia, leukopenia, neutropenia, positive Coombs' reaction, thrombocytopenia

Hepatic: Hepatotoxicity, jaundice

Local: Thrombophlebitis

(Continued)

Ticarcillin and Clavulanate Potassium *(Continued)*

Neuromuscular & skeletal: Myoclonus
Renal: Interstitial nephritis (acute)
Miscellaneous: Anaphylaxis, hypersensitivity reactions

Mechanism of Action Inhibits bacterial cell wall synthesis by binding to one or more of the penicillin binding proteins (PBPs); which in turn inhibits the final transpeptidation step of peptidoglycan synthesis in bacterial cell walls, thus inhibiting cell wall biosynthesis. Bacteria eventually lyse due to ongoing activity of cell wall autolytic enzymes (autolysins and murein hydrolases) while cell wall assembly is arrested.

Drug Interactions

Increased Effect/Toxicity: Probenecid may increase penicillin levels. Neuromuscular blockers may have an increased duration of action (neuromuscular blockade). Penicillins may increase the exposure to methotrexate during concurrent therapy; monitor.

Decreased Effect: Tetracyclines may decrease penicillin effectiveness. Aminoglycosides may cause physical inactivation of aminoglycosides in the presence of high concentrations of ticarcillin and potential toxicity in patients with mild-moderate renal dysfunction. Although anecdotal reports suggest oral contraceptive efficacy could be reduced by penicillins, this has been refuted by more rigorous scientific and clinical data.

Pharmacodynamics/Kinetics

Ticarcillin: See Ticarcillin monograph.

Clavulanic acid:
Protein binding: 9% to 30%
Metabolism: Hepatic
Half-life elimination: 66-90 minutes
Excretion: Urine (45% as unchanged drug)
Clearance: Does not affect clearance of ticarcillin

Pregnancy Risk Factor B

Ticarcillin and Clavulanic Acid *see* Ticarcillin and Clavulanate Potassium *on page 1485*

Ticarcillin Disodium *see* Ticarcillin *on page 1484*

TICE® BCG *see* BCG Vaccine *on page 181*

Ticlid® *see* Ticlopidine *on page 1486*

Ticlopidine *(tye KLOE pi deen)*

Related Information
Cardiovascular Diseases *on page 1636*

U.S. Brand Names Ticlid®

Canadian Brand Names Alti-Ticlopidine; Apo-Ticlopidine®; Gen-Ticlopidine; Novo-Ticlopidine; Nu-Ticlopidine; Rhoxal-ticlopidine; Sandoz-Ticlopidine; Ticlid®

Mexican Brand Names Ticlid®

Generic Available Yes

Synonyms Ticlopidine Hydrochloride

Pharmacologic Category Antiplatelet Agent

Use Platelet aggregation inhibitor that reduces the risk of thrombotic stroke in patients who have had a stroke or stroke precursors. **Note:** Due to its association with life-threatening hematologic disorders, ticlopidine should be reserved for patients who are intolerant to aspirin, or who have failed aspirin therapy. Adjunctive therapy (with aspirin) following successful coronary stent implantation to reduce the incidence of subacute stent thrombosis.

Unlabeled/Investigational Use Protection of aortocoronary bypass grafts, diabetic microangiopathy, ischemic heart disease, prevention of postoperative DVT, reduction of graft loss following renal transplant

Local Anesthetic/Vasoconstrictor Precautions No information available to require special precautions

Effects on Dental Treatment No significant effects or complications reported; if a patient is to undergo elective surgery and an antiplatelet effect is not desired, ticlopidine should be discontinued at least 7 days prior to surgery.

Common Adverse Effects As with all drugs which may affect hemostasis, bleeding is associated with ticlopidine. Hemorrhage may occur at virtually any site. Risk is dependent on multiple variables, including the use of multiple agents which alter hemostasis and patient susceptibility.

>10%:
Endocrine & metabolic: Increased total cholesterol (increases of ~8% to 10% within 1 month of therapy)

Gastrointestinal: Diarrhea (13%)

1% to 10%:

Central nervous system: Dizziness (1%)

Dermatologic: Rash (5%), purpura (2%), pruritus (1%)

Gastrointestinal: Nausea (7%), dyspepsia (7%), gastrointestinal pain (4%), vomiting (2%), flatulence (2%), anorexia (1%)

Hematologic: Neutropenia (2%)

Hepatic: Abnormal liver function test (1%)

Mechanism of Action Ticlopidine is an inhibitor of platelet function with a mechanism which is different from other antiplatelet drugs. The drug significantly increases bleeding time. This effect may not be solely related to ticlopidine's effect on platelets. The prolongation of the bleeding time caused by ticlopidine is further increased by the addition of aspirin in *ex vivo* experiments. Although many metabolites of ticlopidine have been found, none have been shown to account for *in vivo* activity.

Drug Interactions

Cytochrome P450 Effect: Substrate of CYP3A4 (major); **Inhibits** CYP1A2 (weak), 2C8/9 (weak), 2C19 (strong), 2D6 (moderate), 2E1 (weak), 3A4 (weak)

Increased Effect/Toxicity: Ticlopidine may increase effect/toxicity of aspirin, anticoagulants, theophylline, and NSAIDs. Cimetidine may increase ticlopidine blood levels. Ticlopidine may increase the levels/effects of amphetamines, selected beta-blockers, citalopram, dextromethorphan, diazepam, fluoxetine, lidocaine, methsuximide, mirtazapine, nefazodone, paroxetine, phenytoin, sertraline, risperidone, ritonavir, thioridazine, tricyclic antidepressants, venlafaxine, and other CYP2C19 or 2D6 substrates.

Decreased Effect: Decreased effect of ticlopidine with antacids (decreased absorption). Ticlopidine may decrease the effect of digoxin or cyclosporine. The levels/effects of ticlopidine may be decreased by aminoglutethimide, carbamazepine, nafcillin, nevirapine, phenobarbital, phenytoin, rifamycins, and other CYP3A4 inducers. Ticlopidine may decrease the levels/effects of CYP2D6 prodrug substrates (eg, codeine, hydrocodone, oxycodone, tramadol).

Pharmacodynamics/Kinetics

Onset of action: ~6 hours

Peak effect: 3-5 days; serum levels do not correlate with clinical antiplatelet activity

Metabolism: Extensively hepatic; has at least one active metabolite

Half-life elimination: 24 hours

Pregnancy Risk Factor B

Ticlopidine Hydrochloride *see* Ticlopidine *on page 1486*

TIG *see* Tetanus Immune Globulin (Human) *on page 1463*

Tigan® *see* Trimethobenzamide *on page 1538*

Tigecycline (tye ge SYE kleen)

U.S. Brand Names Tygacil™

Generic Available No

Synonyms GAR-936

Pharmacologic Category Antibiotic, Glycylcycline

Use Treatment of complicated skin and skin structure infections caused by susceptible organisms, including methicillin-resistant *Staphylococcus aureus* and vancomycin-sensitive *Enterococcus faecalis*; treatment of complicated intra-abdominal infections

Local Anesthetic/Vasoconstrictor Precautions No information available to require special precautions

Effects on Dental Treatment Key adverse events(s) related to dental treatment: Tigecycline is structurally similar to tetracycline. Therefore, tigecycline is not recommended for use in pregnancy or in children ≤8 years of age. Permanent discoloration of the teeth may occur if used during tooth development.

Common Adverse Effects Note: Frequencies relative to placebo are not available; some frequencies are lower than those experienced with comparator drugs.

>10%: Gastrointestinal: Nausea (25% to 30%; severe in 1%), vomiting (20%; severe in 1%), diarrhea (13%)

2% to 10%:

Cardiovascular: Hypertension (5%), peripheral edema (3%), hypotension (2%), phlebitis (2%)

Central nervous system: Fever (7%), headache (6%), dizziness (4%), pain (4%), insomnia (2%)

Dermatologic: Pruritus (3%), rash (2%)

(Continued)

Tigecycline *(Continued)*

Endocrine & metabolic: Hypoproteinemia (5%), hyperglycemia (2%), hypokalemia (2%)

Gastrointestinal: Abdominal pain (7%), constipation (3%), dyspepsia (3%)

Hematologic: Thrombocythemia (6%), anemia (4%), leukocytosis (4%)

Hepatic: SGPT increased (6%), SGOT increased (4%), alkaline phosphatase increased (4%), amylase increased (3%), bilirubin increased (2%), LDH increased (4%)

Local: Reaction to procedure (9%)

Neuromuscular & skeletal: Weakness (3%)

Renal: BUN increased (2%)

Respiratory: Cough increased (4%), dyspnea (3%), pulmonary physical finding (2%)

Miscellaneous: Abnormal healing (4%), infection (8%), abscess (3%), diaphoresis increased (2%)

Mechanism of Action Binds to the 30S ribosomal subunit of susceptible bacteria, inhibiting protein synthesis.

Drug Interactions

Increased Effect/Toxicity: Retinoic acid derivatives may increase risk of pseudotumor cerebri (reported with tetracyclines). Hypoprothrombinemic response of warfarin may be increased with tigecycline; monitor INR closely during initiation or discontinuation.

Decreased Effect: Anecdotal reports of oral contraceptives suggesting decreased contraceptive efficacy with tetracyclines have been refuted by more rigorous scientific and clinical data.

Pharmacodynamics/Kinetics Note: Systemic clearance is reduced by 55% and half-life increased by 43% in moderate hepatic impairment.

Distribution: V_d: 7-9 L/kg; extensive tissue distribution

Protein binding: 71% to 89%

Metabolism: Hepatic, via glucuronidation, N-acetylation, and epimerization to several metabolites, each <10% of the dose

Half-life elimination: Single dose: 27 hours; following multiple doses: 42 hours

Excretion: Urine (33%; with 22% as unchanged drug); feces (59%; primarily as unchanged drug)

Pregnancy Risk Factor D

Tikosyn™ *see* Dofetilide *on page 497*

Tilade® *see* Nedocromil *on page 1095*

Tiludronate *(tye LOO droe nate)*

U.S. Brand Names Skelid®

Generic Available No

Synonyms Tiludronate Disodium

Pharmacologic Category Bisphosphonate Derivative

Use Treatment of Paget's disease of the bone in patients who have a level of serum alkaline phosphatase (SAP) at least twice the upper limit of normal, or who are symptomatic, or who are at risk for future complications of their disease

Local Anesthetic/Vasoconstrictor Precautions No information available to require special precautions

Effects on Dental Treatment Osteonecrosis of the jaw (ONJ), generally associated with local infection and/or tooth extraction and often with delayed healing, has been reported in patients taking bisphosphonates. Most reported cases of bisphosphonate-associated osteonecrosis have been in cancer patients treated with intravenous bisphosphonates. However, some have occurred in patients with postmenopausal osteoporosis taking oral bisphosphonates. Dental surgery may exacerbate ONJ. For patients requiring dental procedures, there are no data available to suggest whether discontinuation of bisphosphonate treatment reduces the risk of ONJ. See Dental Comment.

Common Adverse Effects The following events occurred >2% and at a frequency greater than placebo:

1% to 10%:

Cardiovascular: Chest pain (3%), edema (3%)

Central nervous system: Dizziness (4%), paresthesia (4%)

Dermatologic: Rash (3%), skin disorder (3%)

Gastrointestinal: Nausea (9%), diarrhea (9%), heartburn (5%), vomiting (4%), flatulence (3%)

Neuromuscular & skeletal: Arthrosis (3%)

Ocular: cataract (3%), conjunctivitis (3%), glaucoma (3%)

Respiratory: Rhinitis (5%), sinusitis (5%), cough (3%), pharyngitis (3%)

Mechanism of Action Inhibition of normal and abnormal bone resorption. Inhibits osteoclasts through at least two mechanisms: disruption of the cytoskeletal ring structure, possibly by inhibition of protein-tyrosine-phosphatase, thus leading to the detachment of osteoclasts from the bone surface area and the inhibition of the osteoclast proton pump.

Drug Interactions

Increased Effect/Toxicity: Aminoglycosides may lower serum calcium levels with prolonged administration; concomitant use may have an additive hypocalcemic effect. NSAIDs may enhance the gastrointestinal adverse/toxic effects (increased incidence of GI ulcers) of bisphosphonate derivatives. Bisphosphonate derivatives may enhance the hypocalcemic effect of phosphate supplements.

Decreased Effect: The following agents may decrease the absorption of oral bisphosphonate derivatives: Antacids (aluminum, calcium, magnesium), oral calcium salts, oral iron salts, and oral magnesium salts.

Pharmacodynamics/Kinetics

Onset of action: Delayed, may require several weeks

Absorption: Rapid

Distribution: Widely to bone and soft tissue

Protein binding: 90%, primarily to albumin

Metabolism: Little, if any

Bioavailability: 6%; reduced by food

Half-life elimination: Healthy volunteers: 50 hours; Pagetic patients: 150 hours

Time to peak, plasma: ~2 hours

Excretion: Urine (60% as unchanged drug) within 13 days

Pregnancy Risk Factor C

Dental Comment

Novartis Pharmaceuticals Corporation has notified dental health professionals of the risk of osteonecrosis of the jaw (ONJ) and the use of the bisphosphonates, pamidronate, and zoledronic acid. This warning has not be issued for tiludronate.

Previously, Novartis and the Food and Drug Administration (FDA) had notified healthcare providers of a serious adverse event related to the use of bisphosphonates. Osteonecrosis of the jaw has been reported in patients with cancer who were receiving chemotherapy, corticosteroids, and chronic bisphosphonate therapy. The bisphosphonates involved were pamidronate and zoledronic acid. To date, there are no reported associations between tiludronate and osteonecrosis of the jaw. Dental exams and preventative dentistry should be performed prior to placing patients with risk factors (chemotherapy, corticosteroids, poor oral hygiene) on chronic bisphosphonate therapy. Invasive dental procedures should be avoided during treatment. Product labelings for pamidronate (Aredia®) and zoledronic acid (Zometa®) have been updated. Recently, 63 cases of osteonecrosis associated with the use of bisphosphonates were published (Ruggiero, 2004). In a retrospective review, 56 of the patients received intravenous bisphosphonates for at least one year and 7 patients were on chronic oral therapy. The presenting symptom was a nonhealing extraction socket or an exposed jawbone. These lesions did not show evidence of metastatic disease and required removal of involved bone in most cases. Bisphosphonates are widely used in the management of metastatic bone disease to treat hypercalcemia associated with malignancies and to treat osteoporosis. In the report by Ruggiero et al, the cluster of patients observed to have necrotic lesions in the jaw shared only one common clinical feature, all received chronic bisphosphonate therapy. The necrosis detected was typical of osteoradionecrosis. It was suggested that because of the trend in the use of chronic bisphosphonate therapy, the observation of an associated risk of osteonecrosis of the jaw should alert practitioners to monitor for this previously unrecognized potential complication.

Selected Readings

Ruggiero SL, Mehrotra B, Rosenberg TJ, et al, "Osteonecrosis of the Jaws Associated With the Use of Bisphosphonates: A Review of 63 Cases," *J Oral Maxillofac Surg*, 2004, 62(5):527-34.

Tiludronate Disodium *see* Tiludronate *on page 1488*

Timentin® *see* Ticarcillin and Clavulanate Potassium *on page 1485*

Timolol (TYE moe lole)

Related Information

Cardiovascular Diseases *on page 1636*

U.S. Brand Names Betimol®; Blocadren®; Istalol™; Timoptic®; Timoptic® OcuDose®; Timoptic-XE®

Canadian Brand Names Alti-Timolol; Apo-Timol®; Apo-Timop®; Gen-Timolol; Nu-Timolol; Phoxal-timolol; PMS-Timolol; Tim-AK; Timoptic®; Timoptic-XE®

Generic Available Yes: Excludes hemihydrate ophthalmic solutions

(Continued)

Timolol *(Continued)*

Synonyms Timolol Hemihydrate; Timolol Maleate

Pharmacologic Category Beta-Adrenergic Blocker, Nonselective; Ophthalmic Agent, Antiglaucoma

Use

Ophthalmic: Treatment of elevated intraocular pressure such as glaucoma or ocular hypertension

Oral: Treatment of hypertension and angina; to reduce mortality following myocardial infarction; prophylaxis of migraine

Local Anesthetic/Vasoconstrictor Precautions Epinephrine has interacted with nonselective beta blockers such as propranolol to result in initial hypertensive episode followed by bradycardia. Timolol is also a nonselective beta blocker. Timolol is available as an eye drop and oral dose form. When administered as an eye drop, the significance of a potential systemic interaction with epinephrine is unknown. However, it is suggested that cautionary procedures be used, particularly if vasoconstrictor is used immediately following an ophthalmic dose of timolol taken by the patient. If patients are taking the oral form of timolol, then the significance of a potential systemic interaction is well known and cautionary use of epinephrine is advised.

Effects on Dental Treatment Timolol is a nonselective beta-blocker and may enhance the pressor response to epinephrine, resulting in hypertension and bradycardia. Many nonsteroidal anti-inflammatory drugs, such as ibuprofen and indomethacin, can reduce the hypotensive effect of beta-blockers after 3 or more weeks of therapy with the NSAID. Short-term NSAID use (ie, 3 days) requires no special precautions in patients taking beta-blockers.

Common Adverse Effects

Ophthalmic:

>10%: Ocular: Burning, stinging

1% to 10%:

Cardiovascular: Hypertension

Central nervous system: Headache

Ocular: Blurred vision, cataract, conjunctival injection, itching, visual acuity decreased

Miscellaneous: Infection

Systemic:

1% to 10%:

Cardiovascular: Bradycardia

Central nervous system: Fatigue, dizziness

Respiratory: Dyspnea

Frequency not defined (reported with any dosage form):

Cardiovascular: Angina pectoris, arrhythmia, bradycardia, cardiac failure, cardiac arrest, cerebral vascular accident, cerebral ischemia, edema, hypotension, heart block, palpitation, Raynaud's phenomenon

Central nervous system: Anxiety, confusion, depression, disorientation, dizziness, hallucinations, insomnia, memory loss, nervousness, nightmares, somnolence

Dermatologic: Alopecia, angioedema, pseudopemphigoid, psoriasiform rash, psoriasis exacerbation, rash, urticaria

Endocrine & metabolic: Hypoglycemia masked, libido decreased

Gastrointestinal: Anorexia, diarrhea, dyspepsia, nausea, xerostomia

Genitourinary: Impotence, retoperitoneal fibrosis

Hematologic: Claudication

Neuromuscular & skeletal: Myasthenia gravis exacerbation, paresthesia

Ocular: Blepharitis, conjunctivitis, corneal sensitivity decreased, cystoid macular edema, diplopia, dry eyes, foreign body sensation, keratitis, ocular discharge, ocular pain, ptosis, refractive changes, tearing, visual disturbances

Otic: Tinnitus

Respiratory: Bronchospasm, cough, dyspnea, nasal congestion, pulmonary edema, respiratory failure

Miscellaneous: Allergic reactions, cold hands/feet, Peyronie's disease, systemic lupus erythematosus

Mechanism of Action Blocks both beta$_1$- and beta$_2$-adrenergic receptors, reduces intraocular pressure by reducing aqueous humor production or possibly outflow; reduces blood pressure by blocking adrenergic receptors and decreasing sympathetic outflow, produces a negative chronotropic and inotropic activity through an unknown mechanism

Drug Interactions

Cytochrome P450 Effect: Substrate of CYP2D6 (major); **Inhibits** CYP2D6 (weak)

Increased Effect/Toxicity: CYP2D6 inhibitors may increase the levels/ effects of timolol; example inhibitors include chlorpromazine, delavirdine, fluoxetine, miconazole, paroxetine, pergolide, quinidine, quinine, ritonavir, and ropinirole. The heart rate-lowering effects of timolol are additive with other drugs which slow AV conduction (digoxin, verapamil, diltiazem). Reserpine increases the effects of timolol. Concurrent use of timolol may increase the effects of alpha-blockers (prazosin, terazosin), alpha-adrenergic stimulants (epinephrine, phenylephrine), and the vasoconstrictive effects of ergot alkaloids. Timolol may mask the tachycardia from hypoglycemia caused by insulin and oral hypoglycemics. In patients receiving concurrent therapy, the risk of hypertensive crisis is increased when either clonidine or the beta-blocker is withdrawn. Beta-blockers may increase the action or levels of ethanol, disopyramide, nondepolarizing muscle relaxants, and theophylline although the effects are difficult to predict.

Decreased Effect: Decreased effect of timolol with aluminum salts, barbiturates, calcium salts, cholestyramine, colestipol, NSAIDs, penicillins (ampicillin), rifampin, salicylates, and sulfinpyrazone due to decreased bioavailability and plasma levels. Beta-blockers may decrease the effect of sulfonylureas. Beta-blockers may affect the action or levels of ethanol, disopyramide, nondepolarizing muscle relaxants, and theophylline, although the effects are difficult to predict.

Pharmacodynamics/Kinetics

Onset of action:
  Hypotensive: Oral: 15-45 minutes
    Peak effect: 0.5-2.5 hours
  Intraocular pressure reduction: Ophthalmic: 30 minutes
    Peak effect: 1-2 hours
Duration: ~4 hours; Ophthalmic: Intraocular: 24 hours
Protein binding: 60%
Metabolism: Extensively hepatic; extensive first-pass effect
Half-life elimination: 2-2.7 hours; prolonged with renal impairment
Excretion: Urine (15% to 20% as unchanged drug)

Pregnancy Risk Factor C (manufacturer); D (2nd and 3rd trimesters - expert analysis)

Timolol and Dorzolamide *see* Dorzolamide and Timolol *on page 501*

Timolol Hemihydrate *see* Timolol *on page 1489*

Timolol Maleate *see* Timolol *on page 1489*

Timoptic® *see* Timolol *on page 1489*

Timoptic® OcuDose® *see* Timolol *on page 1489*

Timoptic-XE® *see* Timolol *on page 1489*

Tinactin® Antifungal [OTC] *see* Tolnaftate *on page 1506*

Tinactin® Antifungal Jock Itch [OTC] *see* Tolnaftate *on page 1506*

Tinaderm [OTC] *see* Tolnaftate *on page 1506*

Tinamed® [OTC] *see* Salicylic Acid *on page 1374*

TinBen® [OTC] [DSC] *see* Benzoin *on page 193*

Tindamax™ *see* Tinidazole *on page 1491*

Tine Test *see* Tuberculin Tests *on page 1548*

Ting® Cream [OTC] *see* Tolnaftate *on page 1506*

Tinidazole (tye NI da zole)

U.S. Brand Names Tindamax™
Mexican Brand Names Fasigyn®
Generic Available No
Pharmacologic Category Amebicide; Antibiotic, Miscellaneous; Antiprotozoal, Nitroimidazole
Use Treatment of trichomoniasis caused by *T. vaginalis*; treatment of giardiasis caused by *G. duodenalis* (*G. lamblia*); treatment of intestinal amebiasis and amebic liver abscess caused by *E. histolytica*
Local Anesthetic/Vasoconstrictor Precautions No information available to require special precautions
Effects on Dental Treatment Key adverse event(s) related to dental treatment: Xerostomia and changes in salivation (normal salivary flow resumes upon discontinuation), metallic/bitter taste, oral candidiasis, tongue discoloration, stomatitis, furry tongue. See Dental Comment.
Common Adverse Effects
1% to 10%:
  Central nervous system: Fatigue/malaise (1% to 2%), dizziness (≤1%), headache (≤1%)
(Continued)

Tinidazole *(Continued)*

Gastrointestinal: Metallic/bitter taste (4% to 6%), nausea (3% to 5%), anorexia (2% to 3%), dyspepsia/cramps/epigastric discomfort (1% to 2%), vomiting (1% to 2%), constipation (≤1%)

Neuromuscular & skeletal: Weakness (1% to 2%)

Frequency not defined.

Cardiovascular: Flushing, palpitation

Central nervous system: Ataxia, coma, confusion, convulsions, depression, drowsiness, fever, giddiness, insomnia, vertigo

Dermatologic: Angioedema, pruritus, rash, urticaria

Gastrointestinal: Diarrhea, furry tongue, oral candidiasis, salivation, stomatitis, thirst, tongue discoloration, xerostomia

Genitourinary: Urine darkened, vaginal discharge increased

Hematologic: Leukopenia (transient), neutropenia (transient), thrombocytopenia (reversible)

Hepatic: Transaminases increased

Neuromuscular & skeletal: Arthralgia, arthritis, myalgia, peripheral neuropathy (transient, includes numbness and paresthesia)

Respiratory: Bronchospasm, dyspnea, pharyngitis

Miscellaneous: Burning sensation, *Candida* overgrowth, diaphoresis

Mechanism of Action After diffusing into the organism, it is proposed that tinidazole causes cytotoxicity by damaging DNA and preventing further DNA synthesis.

Drug Interactions

Cytochrome P450 Effect: Substrate of CYP3A4 (minor)

Increased Effect/Toxicity: Specific interaction studies have not been conducted. Refer to Metronidazole monograph *on page 1033*.

Decreased Effect: Specific interaction studies have not been conducted. Refer to Metronidazole monograph *on page 1033*.

Pharmacodynamics/Kinetics

Absorption: Rapid and complete

Distribution: V_d: 50 L

Protein binding: 12%

Metabolism: Hepatic via CYP3A4 (primarily); undergoes oxidation, hydroxylation and conjugation; forms a metabolite

Half-life elimination: 13 hours

Excretion: Urine (20% to 25%); feces (12%)

Pregnancy Risk Factor C

Dental Comment Although this drug is a member of the metronidazole family, there is no specific dental indication for its use. Just as with metronidazole, alcohol in any form is contraindicated while the patient is on this medication because of the danger of a disulfiram-type reaction.

Tinzaparin *(tin ZA pa rin)*

Related Information

Cardiovascular Diseases *on page 1636*

U.S. Brand Names Innohep®

Canadian Brand Names Innohep®

Generic Available No

Synonyms Tinzaparin Sodium

Pharmacologic Category Low Molecular Weight Heparin

Use Treatment of acute symptomatic deep vein thrombosis, with or without pulmonary embolism, in conjunction with warfarin sodium

Local Anesthetic/Vasoconstrictor Precautions No information available to require special precautions

Effects on Dental Treatment No significant effects or complications reported

Common Adverse Effects As with all anticoagulants, bleeding is the major adverse effect of tinzaparin. Hemorrhage may occur at virtually any site. Risk is dependent on multiple variables.

>10%:

Hepatic: Increased ALT (13%)

Local: Injection site hematoma (16%)

1% to 10%:

Cardiovascular: Angina pectoris, chest pain (2%), hyper-/hypotension, tachycardia

Central nervous system: Confusion, dizziness, fever (2%), headache (2%), insomnia, pain (2%)

Dermatologic: Bullous eruption, pruritus, rash (1%), skin disorder

Gastrointestinal: Constipation (1%), dyspepsia, flatulence, nausea (2%), nonspecified gastrointestinal disorder, vomiting (1%)

Genitourinary: Dysuria, urinary retention, urinary tract infection (4%)

Hematologic: Anemia, hematoma, hemorrhage (2%), thrombocytopenia (1%)

Hepatic: Increased AST (9%)

Local: Deep vein thrombosis, injection site hematoma

Neuromuscular & skeletal: Back pain (2%)

Renal: Hematuria (1%)

Respiratory: Dyspnea (1%), epistaxis (2%), pneumonia, pulmonary embolism (2%), respiratory disorder

Miscellaneous: Impaired healing, infection, unclassified reactions

Mechanism of Action Standard heparin consists of components with molecular weights ranging from 4000-30,000 daltons with a mean of 16,000 daltons. Heparin acts as an anticoagulant by enhancing the inhibition rate of clotting proteases by antithrombin III, impairing normal hemostasis and inhibition of factor Xa. Low molecular weight heparins have a small effect on the activated partial thromboplastin time and strongly inhibit factor Xa. The primary inhibitory activity of tinzaparin is through antithrombin. Tinzaparin is derived from porcine heparin that undergoes controlled enzymatic depolymerization. The average molecular weight of tinzaparin ranges between 5500 and 7500 daltons which is distributed as (<10%) 2000 daltons (60% to 72%) 2000-8000 daltons, and (22% to 36%) >8000 daltons. The antifactor Xa activity is approximately 100 int. units/mg.

Drug Interactions

Increased Effect/Toxicity: Drugs which affect platelet function (eg, aspirin, NSAIDs, dipyridamole, ticlopidine, clopidogrel, sulfinpyrazone, dextran) may potentiate the risk of hemorrhage. Thrombolytic agents increase the risk of hemorrhage.

Warfarin: Risk of bleeding may be increased during concurrent therapy. Tinzaparin is commonly continued during the initiation of warfarin therapy to assure anticoagulation and to protect against possible transient hypercoagulability

Pharmacodynamics/Kinetics

Onset of action: 2-3 hours

Distribution: 3-5 L

Half-life elimination: 3-4 hours

Metabolism: Partially metabolized by desulphation and depolymerization

Bioavailability: 87%

Time to peak: 4-5 hours

Excretion: Urine

Pregnancy Risk Factor B

Tinzaparin Sodium see Tinzaparin on page 1492

Tioconazole (tye oh KONE a zole)

U.S. Brand Names 1-Day™ [OTC]; Vagistat®-1 [OTC]

Generic Available No

Pharmacologic Category Antifungal Agent, Vaginal

Use Local treatment of vulvovaginal candidiasis

Local Anesthetic/Vasoconstrictor Precautions No information available to require special precautions

Effects on Dental Treatment No significant effects or complications reported

Common Adverse Effects Frequency not defined.

Central nervous system: Headache

Gastrointestinal: Abdominal pain

Dermatologic: Burning, desquamation

Genitourinary: Discharge, dyspareunia, dysuria, irritation, itching, nocturia, vaginal pain, vaginitis, vulvar swelling

Mechanism of Action A 1-substituted imidazole derivative with a broad antifungal spectrum against a wide variety of dermatophytes and yeasts, including *Trichophyton mentagrophytes*, *T. rubrum*, *T. erinacei*, *T. tonsurans*, *Microsporum canis*, *Microsporum gypseum*, and *Candida albicans*. Both agents appear to be similarly effective against *Epidermophyton floccosum*.

Drug Interactions

Cytochrome P450 Effect: Inhibits CYP1A2 (weak), 2A6 (weak), 2C8/9 (weak), 2C19 (weak), 2D6 (weak), 2E1 (weak)

Pharmacodynamics/Kinetics

Onset of action: Some improvement: Within 24 hours; Complete relief: Within 7 days

Absorption: Intravaginal: Systemic (small amounts)

Distribution: Vaginal fluid: 24-72 hours

(Continued)

Tioconazole *(Continued)*

Excretion: Urine and feces
Pregnancy Risk Factor C

Tioguanine *see* Thioguanine *on page 1476*

Tiopronin (tye oh PROE nin)

U.S. Brand Names Thiola®
Canadian Brand Names Thiola®
Generic Available No
Pharmacologic Category Urinary Tract Product
Use Prevention of kidney stone (cystine) formation in patients with severe homozygous cystinuric who have urinary cystine >500 mg/day who are resistant to treatment with high fluid intake, alkali, and diet modification, or who have had adverse reactions to penicillamine
Local Anesthetic/Vasoconstrictor Precautions No information available to require special precautions
Effects on Dental Treatment No significant effects or complications reported
Pregnancy Risk Factor C

Tiotixene *see* Thiothixene *on page 1480*

Tiotropium (ty oh TRO pee um)

U.S. Brand Names Spiriva®
Canadian Brand Names Spiriva®
Synonyms Tiotropium Bromide Monohydrate
Pharmacologic Category Anticholinergic Agent
Use Maintenance treatment of bronchospasm associated with COPD (bronchitis and emphysema)
Local Anesthetic/Vasoconstrictor Precautions No information available to require special precautions
Effects on Dental Treatment Key adverse event(s) related to dental treatment: Xerostomia (normal salivary flow resumes upon discontinuation) and ulcerative stomatitis.
Common Adverse Effects
>10%:
    Gastrointestinal: Xerostomia (16%)
    Respiratory: Upper respiratory tract infection (41% vs 37% with placebo), sinusitis (11% vs 9% with placebo), pharyngeal irritation (frequency not specified)
1% to 10%:
    Cardiovascular: Angina, edema (dependent, 5%)
    Central nervous system: Paresthesia, depression
    Dermatologic: Rash (4%)
    Endocrine & metabolic: Hypercholesterolemia, hyperglycemia
    Gastrointestinal: Dyspepsia (6%), abdominal pain (5%), constipation (4%), vomiting (4%), reflux, ulcerative stomatitis
    Genitourinary: Urinary tract infection (7%)
    Neuromuscular & skeletal: Myalgia (4%), leg pain, skeletal pain
    Ocular: Cataract
    Respiratory: Pharyngitis (9%), rhinitis (6%), epistaxis (4%), dysphonia, laryngitis
    Miscellaneous: Infection (4%), moniliasis (4%), allergic reaction, herpes zoster
Mechanism of Action Blocks the action of acetylcholine at parasympathetic sites in bronchial smooth muscle causing bronchodilation
Drug Interactions
Cytochrome P450 Effect: Substrate (minor) of CYP2D6, 3A4
Increased Effect/Toxicity: Increased toxicity with anticholinergics or drugs with anticholinergic properties.
Pharmacodynamics/Kinetics
Absorption: Poorly absorbed from GI tract, systemic absorption may occur from lung
Distribution: V_d: 32 L/kg
Protein binding: 72%
Metabolism: Hepatic (minimal), via CYP2D6 and CYP3A4
Bioavailability: Following inhalation, 19.5%; oral solution: 2% to 3%
Half-life elimination: 5-6 days
Time to peak, plasma: 5 minutes (following inhalation)

Excretion: Urine (74% as unchanged drug)
Pregnancy Risk Factor C

Tiotropium Bromide Monohydrate *see* Tiotropium *on page 1494*

Tipranavir (tip RA na veer)

U.S. Brand Names Aptivus®
Generic Available No
Synonyms PNU-140690E; TPV
Pharmacologic Category Antiretroviral Agent, Protease Inhibitor
Use Treatment of HIV-1 infections in combination with ritonavir and other antiretroviral agents; limited to highly treatment experienced or multi-protease inhibitor resistant patients.
Local Anesthetic/Vasoconstrictor Precautions No information available to require special precautions
Effects on Dental Treatment No significant effects or complications reported
Common Adverse Effects Protease inhibitors cause dyslipidemia which includes elevated cholesterol and triglycerides and a redistribution of body fat centrally to cause increased abdominal girth, buffalo hump, facial atrophy, and breast enlargement. These agents also cause hyperglycemia.
>10%:
  Endocrine & metabolic: Hypercholesterolemia (>300 mg/dL: 11%), hypertriglyceridemia (>400 mg/dL: 26%)
  Gastrointestinal: Diarrhea (11%)
  Hepatic: Transaminase increased (ALT or AST: 24%)
2% to 10%:
  Central nervous system: Fever (5%), fatigue (4%), headache (3%), depression (2%)
  Dermatologic: Rash (2%)
  Endocrine & metabolic: Amylase increased (3%)
  Gastrointestinal: Nausea (7%), vomiting (3%), abdominal pain (3%), amylase increased (3%)
  Hematologic: WBC decreased (grade 3-4: 4%)
  Neuromuscular & skeletal: Weakness (2%)
  Respiratory: Bronchitis (3%)
Mechanism of Action Tipranavir is a nonpeptide inhibitor of HIV-1 protease. It binds to the protease activity site and inhibits the activity of the enzyme. HIV protease is required for the cleavage of viral polyprotein precursors into individual functional proteins found in infectious HIV. Inhibition prevents cleavage of these polyproteins, resulting in the formation of immature, noninfectious viral particles.
Drug Interactions
  Cytochrome P450 Effect:
    Substrate of CYP3A4 (major; minimal metabolism when coadministered with ritonavir)
    Ritonavir: **Inhibits** CYP3A4 (strong) and 2D6
  Increased Effect/Toxicity: Note: Listed interactions include interactions resulting from coadministration with ritonavir. Refer to Ritonavir monograph *on page 1359* for additional interaction concerns. The serum concentrations of tipranavir may be increased by ritonavir. This combination is recommended to enhance the effect ("boost") tipranavir.

  Tipranavir/ritonavir may increase the levels/effects of CYP3A4 substrates. Tipranavir/ritonavir may increase the toxicity of benzodiazepines; concurrent use of midazolam and triazolam is specifically contraindicated. Tipranavir may increase serum concentrations of cisapride, increasing the risk of malignant arrhythmias; use is contraindicated. Toxicity of pimozide is significantly increased by tipranavir/ritonavir; concurrent use is contraindicated. Tipranavir/ritonavir may increase serum concentrations/toxicity of several antiarrhythmic agents; contraindicated with amiodarone, bepridil, flecainide, propafenone, and quinidine (use extreme caution with lidocaine). Tipranavir/ritonavir may also increase serum concentrations/effects of calcium channel blockers and immunosuppressants (cyclosporine, sirolimus, tacrolimus).

  Serum concentrations of HMG-CoA reductase inhibitors (atorvastatin, cerivastatin, lovastatin, simvastatin) may be increased by tipranavir/ritonavir, increasing the risk of myopathy/rhabdomyolysis. Lovastatin and simvastatin are not recommended. Use lowest possible dose of atorvastatin. Fluvastatin and pravastatin may be safer alternatives. Serum concentrations of rifabutin may be increased by tipranavir/ritonavir; dosage adjustment of rifabutin is required.
(Continued)

Tipranavir (Continued)

The toxicity of ergot alkaloids (dihydroergotamine, ergotamine, ergonovine, methylergonovine) is increased by tipranavir; concurrent use is contraindicated. Effects of hypoglycemic agents may be altered by tipranavir/ritonavir. Concurrent therapy with tipranavir may increase serum concentrations of normeperidine, and decrease serum concentrations of meperidine. The serum concentrations of sildenafil, tadalafil, and vardenafil may be increased by tipranavir/ritonavir; dose adjustment and limitations related to ritonavir coadministration must be recognized.

Concurrent use of disulfiram with tipranavir oral solution is contraindicated due to risk of adverse reaction (due to alcohol content of formulation). Clarithromycin may increase serum concentrations of tipranavir. Tipranavir/ritonavir may increase serum concentrations of clarithromycin. Use with caution and adjust dose of clarithromycin during concurrent therapy in renally impaired patients.

Decreased Effect: CYP3A4 inducers may decrease the levels/effects of tipranavir. Example inducers include aminoglutethimide, carbamazepine, nafcillin, nevirapine, phenobarbital, phenytoin, and rifamycins. When coadministered with ritonavir, reduction of tipranavir serum concentrations is unlikely. Rifampin may decrease serum concentrations of tipranavir. Concurrent use of rifampin is not recommended. The effect of methadone may be reduced by tipranavir (dosage increase may be required).

Serum concentrations of protease inhibitors may be decreased by tipranavir. Concurrent therapy with amprenavir, lopinavir, or saquinavir is not recommended. Tipranavir/ritonavir may decrease serum concentrations of nucleoside reverse transcriptase inhibitors (NRTIs, including abacavir, didanosine, and zidovudine); administer tipranavir/ritonavir 2 hours before or after didanosine.

Pharmacodynamics/Kinetics
Absorption: Incomplete (percentage not established)
Protein binding: 99%
Metabolism: Hepatic, via CYP3A4 (minimal when coadministered with ritonavir)
Bioavailability: Not established
Half-life elimination: 6 hours
Excretion: Feces (82%); urine (4%); primarily as unchanged drug (when coadministered with ritonavir)
Pregnancy Risk Factor C

Tirofiban (tye roe FYE ban)

Related Information
Cardiovascular Diseases *on page 1636*
U.S. Brand Names Aggrastat®
Canadian Brand Names Aggrastat®
Mexican Brand Names Agrastat®
Generic Available No
Synonyms MK383; Tirofiban Hydrochloride
Pharmacologic Category Antiplatelet Agent, Glycoprotein IIb/IIIa Inhibitor
Use In combination with heparin, is indicated for the treatment of acute coronary syndrome, including patients who are to be managed medically and those undergoing PTCA or atherectomy. In this setting, it has been shown to decrease the rate of a combined endpoint of death, new myocardial infarction or refractory ischemia/repeat cardiac procedure.
Local Anesthetic/Vasoconstrictor Precautions No information available to require special precautions
Effects on Dental Treatment No significant effects or complications reported
Common Adverse Effects Bleeding is the major drug-related adverse effect. Patients received background treatment with aspirin and heparin. Major bleeding was reported in 1.4% to 2.2%; minor bleeding in 10.5% to 12%; transfusion was required in 4% to 4.3%.
>1% (nonbleeding adverse events):
Cardiovascular: Bradycardia (4%), coronary artery dissection (5%), edema (2%)
Central nervous system: Dizziness (3%), fever (>1%), headache (>1%), vasovagal reaction (2%)
Gastrointestinal: Nausea (>1%)
Genitourinary: Pelvic pain (6%)
Hematologic: Thrombocytopenia: <90,000/mm^3 (1.5%), <50,000/mm^3 (0.3%)
Neuromuscular & skeletal: Leg pain (3%)
Miscellaneous: Diaphoresis (2%)

Mechanism of Action A reversible antagonist of fibrinogen binding to the GP IIb/IIIa receptor, the major platelet surface receptor involved in platelet aggregation. When administered intravenously, it inhibits *ex vivo* platelet aggregation in a dose- and concentration-dependent manner. When given according to the recommended regimen, >90% inhibition is attained by the end of the 30-minute infusion. Platelet aggregation inhibition is reversible following cessation of the infusion.

Drug Interactions

Increased Effect/Toxicity: Use of tirofiban with aspirin and heparin is associated with an increase in bleeding over aspirin and heparin alone; however, efficacy of tirofiban is improved. Risk of bleeding is increased when used with thrombolytics, oral anticoagulants, NSAIDs, dipyridamole, ticlopidine, and clopidogrel. Avoid concomitant use of other IIb/IIIa antagonists. Cephalosporins which contain the MTT side chain may theoretically increase the risk of hemorrhage.

Decreased Effect: Levothyroxine and omeprazole decrease tirofiban levels; however, the clinical significance of this interaction remains to be demonstrated.

Pharmacodynamics/Kinetics
Distribution: 35% unbound
Metabolism: Minimally hepatic
Half-life elimination: 2 hours
Excretion: Urine (65%) and feces (25%) primarily as unchanged drug
Clearance: Elderly: Reduced by 19% to 26%

Pregnancy Risk Factor B

Tirofiban Hydrochloride *see* Tirofiban *on page 1496*

Tiseb® [OTC] *see* Salicylic Acid *on page 1374*

Tisit® [OTC] *see* Pyrethrins and Piperonyl Butoxide *on page 1315*

Tisit® Blue Gel [OTC] *see* Pyrethrins and Piperonyl Butoxide *on page 1315*

Tisseel® VH Kit *see* Fibrin Sealant Kit *on page 653*

Titralac™ [OTC] *see* Calcium Carbonate *on page 248*

Titralac™ Extra Strength [OTC] *see* Calcium Carbonate *on page 248*

Titralac® Plus [OTC] *see* Calcium Carbonate and Simethicone *on page 249*

Tizanidine (tye ZAN i deen)

U.S. Brand Names Zanaflex®
Canadian Brand Names Apo-Tizanidine®; Zanaflex®
Generic Available Yes: Tablet
Synonyms Sirdalud®
Pharmacologic Category Alpha$_2$-Adrenergic Agonist
Use Skeletal muscle relaxant used for treatment of muscle spasticity
Unlabeled/Investigational Use Tension headaches, low back pain, and trigeminal neuralgia
Local Anesthetic/Vasoconstrictor Precautions No information available to require special precautions
Effects on Dental Treatment Key adverse event(s) related to dental treatment: Significant xerostomia (normal salivary flow resumes upon discontinuation).

Common Adverse Effects
>10%:
  Cardiovascular: Hypotension (16% to 33%)
  Central nervous system: Somnolence (48%), dizziness (16%)
  Gastrointestinal: Xerostomia (49%)
  Neuromuscular & skeletal: Weakness (41%)
1% to 10%:
  Cardiovascular: Bradycardia (2% to 10%)
  Central nervous system: Nervousness (3%), speech disorder (3%)
  Gastrointestinal: Constipation (4%), vomiting (3%), pharyngitis (3%)
  Genitourinary: UTI (10%), urinary frequency (3%)
  Hepatic: Liver enzymes increased (3%)
  Neuromuscular & skeletal: Dyskinesia (3%)
  Ocular: Blurred vision (3%)
  Respiratory: Rhinitis (3%)
  Miscellaneous: Infection (6%), flu-like syndrome (3%)

Dosage
Adults: 2-4 mg 3 times/day
  Usual initial dose: 4 mg, may increase by 2-4 mg as needed for satisfactory reduction of muscle tone every 6-8 hours to a maximum of three doses in any 24 hour period
(Continued)

Tizanidine *(Continued)*

Maximum dose: 36 mg/day

Dosing adjustment in renal/hepatic impairment: May require dose reductions or less frequent dosing

Mechanism of Action An alpha$_2$-adrenergic agonist agent which decreases excitatory input to alpha motor neurons; an imidazole derivative chemically-related to clonidine, which acts as a centrally acting muscle relaxant with alpha$_2$-adrenergic agonist properties; acts on the level of the spinal cord

Contraindications Hypersensitivity to tizanidine or any component of the formulation; concomitant therapy with ciprofloxacin or fluvoxamine

Warnings/Precautions

Reduce dose in patients with liver or renal disease. May cause significant orthostatic hypotension or bradycardia; use with caution in patients with hypotension or cardiac disease. Tizanidine clearance is reduced by more than 50% in elderly patients with renal insufficiency (Cl$_{cr}$ <25 mL/minute) compared to healthy elderly subjects; this may lead to a longer duration of effects and, therefore, should be used with caution in renally impaired patients.

Drug Interactions

Increased Effect/Toxicity:

Additive hypotensive effects may be seen with diuretics, other alpha adrenergic agonists, ciprofloxacin, or antihypertensives; CNS depression with baclofen or other CNS depressants. CYP1A2 Inhibitors may increase the levels/effects of tizanidine; example inhibitors include amiodarone, ciprofloxacin (contraindicated), fluvoxamine (contraindicated), ketoconazole, norfloxacin, ofloxacin, and rofecoxib. Oral contraceptives may decrease the clearance of tizanidine.

Ethanol/Nutrition/Herb Interactions

Ethanol: Avoid ethanol (may increase CNS depression).

Food: The tablet and capsule dosage forms are not bioequivalent when administered with food. Food increases both the time to peak concentration and the extent of absorption for both the tablet and capsule. However, maximal concentrations of tizanidine achieved when administered with food were increased by 30% for the tablet, but decreased by 20% for the capsule. Under fed conditions, the capsule is approximately 80% bioavailable relative to the tablet.

Herb/Nutraceutical: Avoid valerian, St John's wort, kava kava, gotu kola (may increase CNS depression). Avoid black cohosh, California poppy, coleus, golden seal, hawthorn, mistletoe, periwinkle, quinine, shepherd's purse (may increase hypotensive effects).

Pharmacodynamics/Kinetics

Duration: 3-6 hours

Bioavailability: 40%

Metabolism: Extensively hepatic

Half-life elimination: 2 hours

Time to peak, serum:

Fasting state: Capsule, tablet: 1 hour

Fed state: Capsule: 3-4 hours, Tablet: 1.5 hours

Excretion: Urine (60%); feces (20%)

Pregnancy Risk Factor C

Dosage Forms CAP: 2 mg, 4 mg, 6 mg **TAB:** 2 mg, 4 mg

TMP *see* Trimethoprim *on page 1538*

TMP-SMZ *see* Sulfamethoxazole and Trimethoprim *on page 1425*

TMZ *see* Temozolomide *on page 1454*

TNKase™ *see* Tenecteplase *on page 1455*

TOBI® *see* Tobramycin *on page 1498*

TobraDex® *see* Tobramycin and Dexamethasone *on page 1499*

Tobramycin *(toe bra MYE sin)*

U.S. Brand Names AKTob®; TOBI®; Tobrex®

Canadian Brand Names Apo-Tobramycin®; PMS-Tobramycin; TOBI®; Tobrex®

Mexican Brand Names Tobrex®; Trazil®

Generic Available Yes: Excludes ophthalmic ointment, solution for nebulization

Synonyms Tobramycin Sulfate

Pharmacologic Category Antibiotic, Aminoglycoside; Antibiotic, Ophthalmic

Use Treatment of documented or suspected infections caused by susceptible gram-negative bacilli including *Pseudomonas aeruginosa*; topically used to treat superficial ophthalmic infections caused by susceptible bacteria. Tobramycin solution for inhalation is indicated for the management of cystic fibrosis patients (>6 years of age) with *Pseudomonas aeruginosa*.

Local Anesthetic/Vasoconstrictor Precautions No information available to require special precautions

Effects on Dental Treatment No significant effects or complications reported

Common Adverse Effects

Injection: Frequency not defined:

Central nervous system: Confusion, disorientation, dizziness, fever, headache, lethargy, vertigo

Dermatologic: Exfoliative dermatitis, itching, rash, urticaria

Endocrine & metabolic: Serum calcium, magnesium, potassium, and/or sodium decreased

Gastrointestinal: Diarrhea, nausea, vomiting

Hematologic: Anemia, eosinophilia, granulocytopenia, leukocytosis, leukopenia, thrombocytopenia

Hepatic: ALT, AST, bilirubin, and/or LDH increased

Local: Pain at the injection site

Otic: Hearing loss, tinnitus, ototoxicity (auditory), ototoxicity (vestibular), roaring in the ears

Renal: BUN increased, cylindruria, serum creatinine increased, oliguria, proteinuria

Inhalation:

>10%:

Gastrointestinal: Sputum discoloration (21%)

Respiratory: Voice alteration (13%)

1% to 10%:

Central nervous system: Malaise (6%)

Otic: Tinnitus (3%)

Mechanism of Action Interferes with bacterial protein synthesis by binding to 30S and 50S ribosomal subunits resulting in a defective bacterial cell membrane

Drug Interactions

Increased Effect/Toxicity: Increased antimicrobial effect of tobramycin with extended spectrum penicillins (synergistic). Neuromuscular blockers may have an increased duration of action (neuromuscular blockade). Amphotericin B, cephalosporins, and loop diuretics may increase the risk of nephrotoxicity.

Pharmacodynamics/Kinetics

Absorption: I.M.: Rapid and complete

Distribution: V_d: 0.2-0.3 L/kg; Pediatrics: 0.2-0.7 L/kg; to extracellular fluid including serum, abscesses, ascitic, pericardial, pleural, synovial, lymphatic, and peritoneal fluids; crosses placenta; poor penetration into CSF, eye, bone, prostate

Protein binding: <30%

Half-life elimination:

Neonates: ≤1200 g: 11 hours; >1200 g: 2-9 hours

Adults: 2-3 hours; directly dependent upon glomerular filtration rate

Adults with impaired renal function: 5-70 hours

Time to peak, serum: I.M.: 30-60 minutes; I.V.: ~30 minutes

Excretion: Normal renal function: Urine (~90% to 95%) within 24 hours

Pregnancy Risk Factor D (injection, inhalation); B (ophthalmic)

Tobramycin and Dexamethasone
(toe bra MYE sin & deks a METH a sone)

Related Information

Dexamethasone *on page 439*
Tobramycin *on page 1498*

U.S. Brand Names TobraDex®

Canadian Brand Names Tobradex®

Generic Available No

Synonyms Dexamethasone and Tobramycin

Pharmacologic Category Antibiotic/Corticosteroid, Ophthalmic

Use Treatment of external ocular infection caused by susceptible gram-negative bacteria and steroid responsive inflammatory conditions of the palpebral and bulbar conjunctiva, lid, cornea, and anterior segment of the globe

Local Anesthetic/Vasoconstrictor Precautions No information available to require special precautions

Effects on Dental Treatment No significant effects or complications reported

Common Adverse Effects Unless otherwise noted, frequency not defined.

Dermatologic: Allergic contact dermatitis, delayed wound healing

(Continued)

Tobramycin and Dexamethasone *(Continued)*

Ocular: Cataract formation, conjunctival erythema (<4%), glaucoma, intraocular pressure increased, keratitis, lacrimation, lid itching (<4%), lid swelling (<4%), optic nerve damage, secondary infection

Mechanism of Action Refer to individual monographs for Dexamethasone and Tobramycin

Drug Interactions

Cytochrome P450 Effect: Dexamethasone: **Substrate** of CYP3A4 (minor); **Induces** CYP2A6 (weak), 2B6 (weak), 2C8 (weak), 2C9 (weak), 3A4 (weak)

Increased Effect/Toxicity: See individual agents.

Decreased Effect: See individual agents.

Pharmacodynamics/Kinetics

Absorption: Into aqueous humor

Time to peak, serum: 1-2 hours in the cornea and aqueous humor

Pregnancy Risk Factor C

Tobramycin and Loteprednol Etabonate *see* Loteprednol and Tobramycin *on page 953*

Tobramycin Sulfate *see* Tobramycin *on page 1498*

Tobrex® *see* Tobramycin *on page 1498*

Tocainide *(toe KAY nide)*

Related Information

Cardiovascular Diseases *on page 1636*

U.S. Brand Names Tonocard® [DSC]

Generic Available No

Synonyms Tocainide Hydrochloride

Pharmacologic Category Antiarrhythmic Agent, Class Ib

Use Suppression and prevention of symptomatic life-threatening ventricular arrhythmias

Unlabeled/Investigational Use Trigeminal neuralgia

Local Anesthetic/Vasoconstrictor Precautions No information available to require special precautions

Effects on Dental Treatment No significant effects or complications reported

Common Adverse Effects

>10%:

Central nervous system: Dizziness (8% to 15%)

Gastrointestinal: Nausea (14% to 15%)

1% to 10%:

Cardiovascular: Tachycardia (3%), bradycardia/angina/palpitation (0.5% to 1.8%), hypotension (3%)

Central nervous system: Nervousness (0.5% to 1.5%), confusion (2% to 3%), headache (4.6%), anxiety, incoordination, giddiness, vertigo

Dermatologic: Rash (0.5% to 8.4%)

Gastrointestinal: Vomiting (4.5%), diarrhea (4% to 5%), anorexia (1% to 2%), loss of taste

Neuromuscular & skeletal: Paresthesia (3.5% to 9%), tremor (dose related: 2.9% to 8.4%), ataxia (dose related: 2.9% to 8.4%), hot and cold sensations

Ocular: Blurred vision (~1.5%), nystagmus (1%)

Note: Rare, potentially severe hematologic reactions, have occurred (generally within the first 12 weeks of therapy). These may include agranulocytosis, bone marrow depression, aplastic anemia, hypoplastic anemia, hemolytic anemia, anemia, leukopenia, neutropenia, thrombocytopenia, and eosinophilia.

Mechanism of Action Class 1B antiarrhythmic agent; suppresses automaticity of conduction tissue, by increasing electrical stimulation threshold of ventricle, His-Purkinje system, and spontaneous depolarization of the ventricles during diastole by a direct action on the tissues; blocks both the initiation and conduction of nerve impulses by decreasing the neuronal membrane's permeability to sodium ions, which results in inhibition of depolarization with resultant blockade of conduction

Drug Interactions

Cytochrome P450 Effect: Inhibits CYP1A2 (weak)

Increased Effect/Toxicity: Tocainide may increase serum levels of caffeine and theophylline.

Decreased Effect: Decreased tocainide plasma levels with cimetidine, phenobarbital, phenytoin, rifampin, and other hepatic enzyme inducers.

Pharmacodynamics/Kinetics

Absorption: Oral: 99% to 100%

Distribution: V_d: 1.62-3.2 L/kg

Protein binding: 10% to 20%
Metabolism: Hepatic to inactive metabolites; negligible first-pass effect
Half-life elimination: 11-14 hours; Renal and hepatic impairment: 23-27 hours
Time to peak, serum: 30-160 minutes
Excretion: Urine (40% to 50% as unchanged drug)
Pregnancy Risk Factor C

Tocainide Hydrochloride *see* Tocainide *on page 1500*

Today® Sponge [OTC] *see* Nonoxynol 9 *on page 1124*

Tofranil® *see* Imipramine *on page 820*

Tofranil-PM® *see* Imipramine *on page 820*

TOLAZamide (tole AZ a mide)

Related Information
Endocrine Disorders and Pregnancy *on page 1659*
U.S. Brand Names Tolinase® [DSC]
Canadian Brand Names Tolinase®
Generic Available Yes
Pharmacologic Category Antidiabetic Agent, Sulfonylurea
Use Adjunct to diet for the management of mild to moderately severe, stable, type 2 diabetes mellitus (noninsulin dependent, NIDDM)
Local Anesthetic/Vasoconstrictor Precautions No information available to require special precautions
Effects on Dental Treatment Use salicylates with caution in patients taking tolazamide due to potential increased hypoglycemia; NSAIDs such as ibuprofen and naproxen may be safely used. Tolazamide-dependent diabetics (noninsulin dependent, type 2) should be appointed for dental treatment in morning in order to minimize chance of stress-induced hypoglycemia.
Common Adverse Effects Frequency not defined.
Central nervous system: Headache, dizziness
Dermatologic: Rash, urticaria, photosensitivity
Endocrine & metabolic: Hypoglycemia, SIADH
Gastrointestinal: Anorexia, nausea, vomiting, diarrhea, constipation, heartburn, epigastric fullness
Hematologic: Aplastic anemia, hemolytic anemia, bone marrow suppression, thrombocytopenia, agranulocytosis
Hepatic: Cholestatic jaundice
Renal: Diuretic effect
Mechanism of Action Stimulates insulin release from the pancreatic beta cells; reduces glucose output from the liver; insulin sensitivity is increased at peripheral target sites
Drug Interactions
Increased Effect/Toxicity: Salicylates, anticoagulants, H_2 antagonists, TCAs, MAO inhibitors, beta-blockers, and thiazides may increase effect of sulfonylureas.
Decreased Effect: Many drugs, including corticosteroids, beta-blockers, and thiazides may alter response to oral hypoglycemics.
Pharmacodynamics/Kinetics
Onset of action: 4-6 hours
Duration: 10-24 hours
Protein binding: >98%
Metabolism: Extensively hepatic to one active and three inactive metabolites
Half-life elimination: 7 hours
Excretion: Urine
Pregnancy Risk Factor D

Tolazoline (tole AZ oh leen)

U.S. Brand Names Priscoline® [DSC]
Generic Available No
Synonyms Benzazoline Hydrochloride; Tolazoline Hydrochloride
Pharmacologic Category Vasodilator
Use Treatment of persistent pulmonary vasoconstriction and hypertension of the newborn (persistent fetal circulation), peripheral vasospastic disorders
Local Anesthetic/Vasoconstrictor Precautions No information available to require special precautions
Effects on Dental Treatment No significant effects or complications reported
Common Adverse Effects Frequency not defined.
Cardiovascular: Hyper-/hypotension, peripheral vasodilation, tachycardia, arrhythmia
(Continued)

Tolazoline *(Continued)*

Endocrine & metabolic: Hypochloremic alkalosis
Gastrointestinal: GI bleeding, abdominal pain, nausea, diarrhea
Hematologic: Thrombocytopenia, increased agranulocytosis, pancytopenia
Local: Burning at injection site
Neuromuscular & skeletal: Increased pilomotor activity
Ocular: Mydriasis
Renal: Acute renal failure, oliguria
Respiratory: Pulmonary hemorrhage
Miscellaneous: Increased secretions

Mechanism of Action Competitively blocks alpha-adrenergic receptors to produce brief antagonism of circulating epinephrine and norepinephrine; reduces hypertension caused by catecholamines and causes vascular smooth muscle relaxation (direct action); results in peripheral vasodilation and decreased peripheral resistance

Drug Interactions

Increased Effect/Toxicity: Disulfiram reaction may possibly be seen with concomitant ethanol use.

Decreased Effect: Decreased effect (vasopressor) of epinephrine followed by a rebound increase in blood pressure.

Pharmacodynamics/Kinetics

Half-life elimination: Neonates: 3-10 hours; prolonged with renal impairment
Time to peak, serum: Within 30 minutes
Excretion: Urine (primarily as unchanged drug)

Pregnancy Risk Factor C

Tolazoline Hydrochloride *see* Tolazoline *on page 1501*

TOLBUTamide *(tole BYOO ta mide)*

Related Information
Endocrine Disorders and Pregnancy *on page 1659*
Canadian Brand Names Apo-Tolbutamide®
Mexican Brand Names Diaval®; Rastinon®
Generic Available Yes
Synonyms Tolbutamide Sodium
Pharmacologic Category Antidiabetic Agent, Sulfonylurea
Use Adjunct to diet for the management of mild to moderately severe, stable, type 2 diabetes mellitus (noninsulin dependent, NIDDM)
Local Anesthetic/Vasoconstrictor Precautions No information available to require special precautions
Effects on Dental Treatment Use salicylates with caution in patients taking tolazamide due to potential increased hypoglycemia; NSAIDs such as ibuprofen and naproxen may be safely used. Tolbutamide-dependent diabetics (noninsulin dependent, type 2) should be appointed for dental treatment in morning in order to minimize chance of stress-induced hypoglycemia.
Common Adverse Effects Frequency not defined.

Cardiovascular: Venospasm
Central nervous system: Headache, dizziness
Dermatologic: Skin rash, urticaria, photosensitivity
Endocrine & metabolic: Hypoglycemia, SIADH
Gastrointestinal: Constipation, diarrhea, heartburn, anorexia, epigastric fullness, taste alteration
Hematologic: Aplastic anemia, hemolytic anemia, bone marrow suppression, thrombocytopenia, leukopenia, agranulocytosis
Hepatic: Cholestatic jaundice
Otic: Tinnitus
Miscellaneous: Hypersensitivity reaction, disulfiram-like reactions

Mechanism of Action Stimulates insulin release from the pancreatic beta cells; reduces glucose output from the liver; insulin sensitivity is increased at peripheral target sites, suppression of glucagon may also contribute

Drug Interactions

Cytochrome P450 Effect: Substrate of CYP2C8/9 (major), 2C19 (minor); **Inhibits** CYP2C8/9 (strong)

Increased Effect/Toxicity: A number of drugs increase the effect of first-generation sulfonylureas (tolbutamide) including salicylates, chloramphenicol, anticoagulants, H_2 antagonists, tricyclic antidepressants, MAO inhibitors, beta-blockers, and thiazide diuretics. CYP2C8/9 inhibitors may increase the levels/effects of tolbutamide; example inhibitors include delavirdine, fluconazole, gemfibrozil, ketoconazole, nicardipine, NSAIDs, and sulfonamides.

Decreased Effect: CYP2C8/9 inducers may decrease the levels/effects of tolbutamide; example inducers include carbamazepine, phenobarbital, phenytoin, rifampin, rifapentine, and secobarbital. Drugs with increase glucose (corticosteroids, thiazides) may decrease the effect of tolbutamide.

Pharmacodynamics/Kinetics

Onset of action: Peak effect: Hypoglycemic action: Oral: 1-3 hours

Duration: Oral: 6-24 hours

Absorption: Oral: Rapid

Distribution: V_d: 6-10 L; increased with decreased albumin concentrations

Protein binding: 95% to 97%, primarily to albumin

Metabolism: Hepatic to hydroxymethyltolbutamide (mildly active) and carboxytolbutamide (inactive); metabolism does not appear to be affected by age

Half-life elimination: Plasma: 4-25 hours; Elimination: 4-9 hours

Time to peak, serum: 3-5 hours

Excretion: Urine (<2% as unchanged drug, primarily as metabolites)

Pregnancy Risk Factor D

Tolbutamide Sodium *see* TOLBUTamide *on page 1502*

Tolcapone (TOLE ka pone)

U.S. Brand Names Tasmar®
Mexican Brand Names Tasmar®
Generic Available No
Pharmacologic Category Anti-Parkinson's Agent, COMT Inhibitor
Use Adjunct to levodopa and carbidopa for the treatment of signs and symptoms of idiopathic Parkinson's disease

Local Anesthetic/Vasoconstrictor Precautions No information available to require special precautions

Effects on Dental Treatment Dopaminergic therapy in Parkinson's disease (ie, treatment with levodopa) is associated with orthostatic hypotension. Tolcapone enhances levodopa bioavailability and may increase the occurrence of hypotension/syncope in the dental patient. The patient should be carefully assisted from the chair and observed for signs of orthostatic hypotension.

Common Adverse Effects

>10%:

Cardiovascular: Orthostatic hypotension (17%)

Central nervous system: Sleep disorder (24% to 25%), excessive dreaming (16% to 21%), somnolence (14% to 18%), dizziness (6% to 13%), headache (10% to 11%), confusion (10% to 11%)

Gastrointestinal: Nausea (30% to 35%), anorexia (19% to 23%), diarrhea (16% to 18%)

Neuromuscular & skeletal: Dyskinesia (42% to 51%), dystonia (19% to 22%), muscle cramps (17% to 18%)

1% to 10%:

Cardiovascular: Syncope (4% to 5%), chest pain (1% to 3%), hypotension (2%), palpitation

Central nervous system: Hallucinations (8% to 10%), fatigue (3% to 7%), loss of balance (2% to 3%), agitation (1%), euphoria (1%), hyperactivity (1%), malaise (1%), panic reaction (1%), irritability (1%), mental deficiency (1%), fever (1%), depression, hypoesthesia, tremor, speech disorder, vertigo, emotional lability, hyperkinesia

Dermatologic: Alopecia (1%), bleeding (1%), tumor (1%), rash

Gastrointestinal: Vomiting (8% to 10%), constipation (6% to 8%), xerostomia (5% to 6%), abdominal pain (5% to 6%), dyspepsia (3% to 4%), flatulence (2% to 4%) tooth disorder

Genitourinary: UTI (5%), hematuria (4% to 5%), urine discoloration (2% to 3%), urination disorder (1% to 2%), uterine tumor (1%), incontinence, impotence

Hepatic: Transaminases increased (1% to 3%; 3 times ULN, usually with first 6 months of therapy)

Neuromuscular & skeletal: Paresthesia (1% to 3%), hyper-/hypokinesia (1% to 3%), arthritis (1% to 2%), neck pain (2%), stiffness (2%), myalgia, rhabdomyolysis

Ocular: Cataract (1%), eye inflammation (1%)

Otic: Tinnitus

Respiratory: Upper respiratory infection (5% to 7%), dyspnea (3%), sinus congestion (1% to 2%), bronchitis, pharyngitis

Miscellaneous: Diaphoresis (4% to 7%), influenza (3% to 4%), burning (1% to 2%), flank pain, injury, infection

Restrictions A patient signed consent form acknowledging the risks of hepatic injury should be obtained by the treating physician.

(Continued)

Tolcapone *(Continued)*

Mechanism of Action Tolcapone is a selective and reversible inhibitor of catechol-o-methyltransferase (COMT). In the presence of a decarboxylase inhibitor (eg, carbidopa), COMT is the major degradation pathway for levodopa. Inhibition of COMT leads to more sustained plasma levels of levodopa and enhanced central dopaminergic activity.

Drug Interactions

Cytochrome P450 Effect: Inhibits CYP2C9 (weak)

Increased Effect/Toxicity: Tolcapone may decrease the metabolism and increase the side effects of COMT substrates (eg, apomorphine, bitolterol, dobutamine, dopamine, epinephrine, norepinephrine, isoproterenol, isoethamine, and methyldopa). Effects on mental status may be additive with other CNS depressants; includes barbiturates, benzodiazepines, TCAs, antipsychotics, ethanol, narcotic analgesics, and other sedative-hypnotics. Concurrent use of nonselective MAO inhibitors with tolcapone may increase the risk of cardiovascular side effects; selective MAO inhibitors (eg, selegiline ≤10 mg/day) appear to pose limited risk.

Pharmacodynamics/Kinetics

Absorption: Rapid

Distribution: 9 L

Protein binding: >99.0%

Metabolism: Glucuronidation to inactive metabolite

Bioavailability: 65%

Half-life elimination: 2-3 hours

Time to peak: ~2 hours

Excretion: Urine (60% as metabolites); feces (40%)

Pregnancy Risk Factor C

Tolectin® see Tolmetin *on page 1504*

Tolinase® [DSC] see TOLAZamide *on page 1501*

Tolmetin *(TOLE met in)*

Related Information

Rheumatoid Arthritis, Osteoarthritis, and Osteoporosis *on page 1668*

Temporomandibular Dysfunction (TMD) *on page 1724*

U.S. Brand Names Tolectin®

Generic Available Yes

Synonyms Tolmetin Sodium

Pharmacologic Category Nonsteroidal Anti-inflammatory Drug (NSAID), Oral

Use Treatment of rheumatoid arthritis and osteoarthritis, juvenile rheumatoid arthritis

Local Anesthetic/Vasoconstrictor Precautions No information available to require special precautions

Effects on Dental Treatment NSAID formulations are known to reversibly decrease platelet aggregation via mechanisms different than observed with aspirin. The dentist should be aware of the potential of abnormal coagulation. Caution should also be exercised in the use of NSAIDs in patients already on anticoagulant therapy with drugs such as warfarin (Coumadin®).

Common Adverse Effects 1% to 10%:

Cardiovascular: Chest pain, hypertension, edema

Central nervous system: Headache, dizziness, drowsiness, depression

Dermatologic: Skin irritation

Endocrine & metabolic: Weight gain/loss

Gastrointestinal: Heartburn, abdominal pain, diarrhea, flatulence, vomiting, constipation, gastritis, peptic ulcer, nausea

Genitourinary: Urinary Tract Infection

Hematologic: Elevated BUN, transient decreases in hemoglobin/hematocrit

Ocular: Visual disturbances

Otic: Tinnitus

Restrictions A medication guide should be dispensed with each prescription. A template for the required MedGuide can be found on the FDA website at: http://www.fda.gov/medwatch/SAFETY/2005/safety05.htm#NSAID

Dosage Oral:

Children ≥2 years:

Anti-inflammatory: Initial: 20 mg/kg/day in 3 divided doses, then 15-30 mg/kg/day in 3 divided doses

Analgesic: 5-7 mg/kg/dose every 6-8 hours

Adults: 400 mg 3 times/day; usual dose: 600 mg to 1.8 g/day; maximum: 2 g/day

Mechanism of Action Inhibits prostaglandin synthesis by decreasing the activity of the enzyme, cyclooxygenase, which results in decreased formation of prostaglandin precursors

Contraindications Hypersensitivity to tolmetin, aspirin, other NSAIDs, or any component of the formulation; perioperative pain in the setting of coronary artery bypass surgery (CABG); pregnancy (3rd trimester or near term)

Warnings/Precautions NSAIDs are associated with an increased risk of adverse cardiovascular events, including MI, stroke, and new onset or worsening of pre-existing hypertension. Risk may be increased with duration of use or pre-existing cardiovascular risk-factors or disease. Carefully evaluate individual cardiovascular risk profiles prior to prescribing. Use caution with fluid retention, CHF or hypertension.

Use of NSAIDs can compromise existing renal function. Renal toxicity can occur in patient with impaired renal function, dehydration, heart failure, liver dysfunction, those taking diuretics and ACEI and the elderly. Rehydrate patient before starting therapy. Monitor renal function closely. Use caution in patients with advanced renal disease.

NSAIDs may increase risk of gastrointestinal irritation, ulceration, bleeding, and perforation. These events may occur at any time during therapy and without warning. Use caution with a history of GI disease (bleeding or ulcers), concurrent therapy with aspirin, anticoagulants and/or corticosteroids, smoking, use of alcohol, the elderly or debilitated patients.

Use the lowest effective dose for the shortest duration of time, consistent with individual patient goals, to reduce risk of cardiovascular or GI adverse events. Alternate therapies should be considered for patients at high risk.

NSAIDs may cause serious skin adverse events including exfoliative dermatitis, Stevens-Johnson syndrome (SJS) and toxic epidermal necrolysis (TEN). Anaphylactoid reactions may occur, even without prior exposure; patients with "aspirin triad" (bronchial asthma, aspirin intolerance, rhinitis) may be at increased risk. Do not use in patients who experience bronchospasm, asthma, rhinitis, or urticaria with NSAID or aspirin therapy.

Use with caution in patients with decreased hepatic function. Closely monitor patients with any abnormal LFT. Severe hepatic reactions (eg, fulminant hepatitis, liver failure) have occurred with NSAID use, rarely; discontinue if signs or symptoms of liver disease develop, or if systemic manifestations occur.

The elderly are at increased risk for adverse effects (especially peptic ulceration, CNS effects, renal toxicity) from NSAIDs even at low doses.

Withhold for at least 4-6 half-lives prior to surgical or dental procedures. Safety and efficacy have not been established in children <2 years of age.

Drug Interactions
Increased Effect/Toxicity: Increased toxicity of digoxin, methotrexate, cyclosporine, lithium, insulin, sulfonylureas, potassium-sparing diuretics, and aspirin.

Decreased Effect: Decreased effect with aspirin. Decreased effect of thiazides and furosemide. NSAIDs may decrease the antihypertensive effect of ACE inhibitors, beta-blockers, hydralazine, and angiotensin antagonists. Cholestyramine (and other bile acid sequestrants) may decrease the absorption of NSAIDs; separate by at least 2 hours.

Ethanol/Nutrition/Herb Interactions
Ethanol: Avoid ethanol (may enhance gastric mucosal irritation).

Food: Tolmetin peak serum concentrations may be decreased if taken with food or milk.

Herb/Nutraceutical: Avoid alfalfa, anise, bilberry, bladderwrack, bromelain, cat's claw, celery, coleus, cordyceps, dong quai, evening primrose, feverfew, fenugreek, garlic, ginger, ginkgo biloboa, red clover, horse chestnut, grapeseed, green tea, ginseng, guggul, horse chestnut seed, horseradish, licorice, prickly ash, red clover, reishi, SAMe, sweet clover, turmeric, white willow (all have additional antiplatelet activity).

Dietary Considerations Should be taken with food, milk, or antacids to decrease GI adverse effects. Sodium content of 200 mg: 0.8 mEq.

Pharmacodynamics/Kinetics
Onset of action: Analgesic: 1-2 hours; Anti-inflammatory: Days to weeks

Absorption: Well absorbed

Bioavailability: Reduced 16% with food or milk

Half-life elimination: Biphasic: Rapid: 1-2 hours; Slow: 5 hours

Time to peak, serum: 30-60 minutes

Excretion: Urine (as inactive metabolites or conjugates) within 24 hours

Pregnancy Risk Factor C/D (3rd trimester)

Dosage Forms CAP: 400 mg. **TAB:** 200 mg, 600 mg; (Tolectin®): 600 mg

Tolmetin Sodium *see* Tolmetin *on page 1504*

Tolnaftate (tole NAF tate)

U.S. Brand Names Aftate® Antifungal [OTC] [DSC]; Blis-To-Sol® [OTC]; Fungi-Guard [OTC]; Gold Bond® Antifungal [OTC]; Podactin Powder [OTC]; Q-Naftate [OTC]; Tinactin® Antifungal [OTC]; Tinactin® Antifungal Jock Itch [OTC]; Tinaderm [OTC]; Ting® Cream [OTC]

Canadian Brand Names Pitrex

Mexican Brand Names Tinaderm®

Generic Available Yes: Cream, powder, solution, swabs

Pharmacologic Category Antifungal Agent, Topical

Use Treatment of tinea pedis, tinea cruris, tinea corporis

Local Anesthetic/Vasoconstrictor Precautions No information available to require special precautions

Effects on Dental Treatment No significant effects or complications reported

Common Adverse Effects Frequency not defined.
Dermatologic: Pruritus, contact dermatitis
Local: Irritation, stinging

Mechanism of Action Distorts the hyphae and stunts mycelial growth in susceptible fungi

Pharmacodynamics/Kinetics Onset of action: 24-72 hours

Pregnancy Risk Factor C

Tolterodine (tole TER oh deen)

U.S. Brand Names Detrol®; Detrol® LA

Canadian Brand Names Detrol®; Detrol® LA; Unidet®

Mexican Brand Names Detrusitol®

Generic Available No

Synonyms Tolterodine Tartrate

Pharmacologic Category Anticholinergic Agent

Use Treatment of patients with an overactive bladder with symptoms of urinary frequency, urgency, or urge incontinence

Local Anesthetic/Vasoconstrictor Precautions No information available to require special precautions

Effects on Dental Treatment The anticholinergic effects of tolterodine are selective for the urinary bladder rather than salivary glands; xerostomia and changes in salivation (normal salivary flow resumes upon discontinuation).

Common Adverse Effects As reported with immediate release tablet, unless otherwise specified
>10%: Gastrointestinal: Dry mouth (35%; extended release capsules 23%)
1% to 10%:
Cardiovascular: Chest pain (2%)
Central nervous system: Headache (7%; extended release capsules 6%), somnolence (3%; extended release capsules 3%), fatigue (4%; extended release capsules 2%), dizziness (5%; extended release capsules 2%), anxiety (extended release capsules 1%)
Dermatologic: Dry skin (1%)
Gastrointestinal: Abdominal pain (5%; extended release capsules 4%), constipation (7%; extended release capsules 6%), dyspepsia (4%; extended release capsules 3%), diarrhea (4%), weight gain (1%)
Genitourinary: Dysuria (2%; extended release capsules 1%)
Neuromuscular & skeletal: Arthralgia (2%)
Ocular: Abnormal vision (2%; extended release capsules 1%), dry eyes (3%; extended release capsules 3%)
Respiratory: Bronchitis (2%), sinusitis (extended release capsules 2%)
Miscellaneous: Flu-like syndrome (3%), infection (1%)

Dosage
Oral: Adults: Treatment of overactive bladder:
Immediate release tablet: 2 mg twice daily; the dose may be lowered to 1 mg twice daily based on individual response and tolerability
Dosing adjustment in patients concurrently taking CYP3A4 inhibitors: 1 mg twice daily
Extended release capsule: 4 mg once a day; dose may be lowered to 2 mg daily based on individual response and tolerability

Dosing adjustment in patients concurrently taking CYP3A4 inhibitors: 2 mg daily

Elderly: Safety and efficacy in patients >64 years was found to be similar to that in younger patients; no dosage adjustment is needed based on age

Dosing adjustment in renal impairment: Use with caution (studies conducted in patients with Cl_{cr} 10-30 mL/minute):
Immediate release tablet: 1 mg twice daily
Extended release capsule: 2 mg daily

Dosing adjustment in hepatic impairment:
Immediate release tablet: 1 mg twice daily
Extended release capsule: 2 mg daily

Mechanism of Action Tolterodine is a competitive antagonist of muscarinic receptors. In animal models, tolterodine demonstrates selectivity for urinary bladder receptors over salivary receptors. Urinary bladder contraction is mediated by muscarinic receptors. Tolterodine increases residual urine volume and decreases detrusor muscle pressure.

Contraindications Hypersensitivity to tolterodine or any component of the formulation; urinary retention; gastric retention; uncontrolled narrow-angle glaucoma; myasthenia gravis

Warnings/Precautions Use with caution in patients with bladder flow obstruction, may increase the risk of urinary retention. Use with caution in patients with gastrointestinal obstructive disorders (ie, pyloric stenosis), may increase the risk of gastric retention. Use with caution in patients with controlled (treated) narrow-angle glaucoma; metabolized in the liver and excreted in the urine and feces, dosage adjustment is required for patients with renal or hepatic impairment. Tolterodine has been associated with QT_c prolongation at high (supratherapeutic) doses. The manufacturer recommends caution in patients with congenital prolonged QT or in patients receiving concurrent therapy with QT_c-prolonging drugs (class Ia or III antiarrhythmics). However, the mean change in QT_c even at supratherapeutic dosages was less than 15 msec. Individuals who are poor metabolizers via CYP2D6 or in the presence of inhibitors of CYP2D6 and CYP3A4 may be more likely to exhibit prolongation. Dosage adjustment is recommended in patients receiving CYP3A4 inhibitors (a lower dose of tolterodine is recommended). Safety and efficacy in pediatric patients have not been established.

Drug Interactions
Cytochrome P450 Effect: Substrate of CYP2C8/9 (minor), 2C19 (minor), 2D6 (major), 3A4 (major)
Increased Effect/Toxicity: CYP2D6 inhibitors may increase the levels/effects of tolterodine, which may include QT_c prolongation; example inhibitors include chlorpromazine, delavirdine, fluoxetine, miconazole, paroxetine, pergolide, quinidine, quinine, ritonavir, and ropinirole. No dosage adjustment was needed in patients coadministered tolterodine and fluoxetine. CYP3A4 inhibitors may increase the levels/effects of tolterodine, which may include QT_c prolongation; example inhibitors include azole antifungals, clarithromycin, diclofenac, doxycycline, erythromycin, imatinib, isoniazid, nefazodone, nicardipine, propofol, protease inhibitors, quinidine, telithromycin, and verapamil. Concomitant use with systemic anticholinergic agents may increase the risk of anticholinergic side effects. Use with pramlintide may result in increased slowing of gut motility. Additive effects on QT_c prolongation may occur with concurrent therapy with QT_c prolonging agents.
Decreased Effect: CYP3A4 inducers may decrease the levels/effects of tolterodine; example inducers include aminoglutethimide, carbamazepine, nafcillin, nevirapine, phenobarbital, phenytoin, and rifamycins. Use with acetylcholinesterase inhibitors may result in reduced therapeutic efficacy.

Ethanol/Nutrition/Herb Interactions
Food: Increases bioavailability (~53% increase) of tolterodine tablets, but does not affect the pharmacokinetics of tolterodine extended release capsules; adjustment of dose is not needed. As a CYP3A4 inhibitor, grapefruit juice may increase the serum level and/or toxicity of tolterodine, but unlikely secondary to high oral bioavailability.
Herb/Nutraceutical: St John's wort (*Hypericum*) appears to induce CYP3A enzymes.

Pharmacodynamics/Kinetics
Absorption: Immediate release tablet: Rapid; ≥77%
Distribution: I.V.: V_d: 113 ± 27 L
Protein binding: >96% (primarily to alpha$_1$-acid glycoprotein)
Metabolism: Extensively hepatic, primarily via CYP2D6 (some metabolites share activity) and 3A4 usually (minor pathway). In patients with a genetic deficiency of CYP2D6, metabolism via 3A4 predominates. Forms three active metabolites.
(Continued)

Tolterodine *(Continued)*

Bioavailability: Immediate release tablet: Increased 53% with food
Half-life elimination:
Immediate release tablet: Extensive metabolizers: ~2 hours; Poor metabolizers: ~10 hours
Extended release capsule: Extensive metabolizers: ~7 hours; Poor metabolizers: ~18 hours

Time to peak: Immediate release tablet: 1-2 hours; Extended release tablet: 2-6 hours

Excretion: Urine (77%); feces (17%); excreted primarily as metabolites (<1% unchanged drug) of which the active 5-hydroxymethyl metabolite accounts for 5% to 14% (<1% in poor metabolizers)

Pregnancy Risk Factor C
Dosage Forms CAP, extended release (Detrol® LA): 2 mg, 4 mg. **TAB** (Detrol®): 1 mg, 2 mg

Tolterodine Tartrate *see* Tolterodine *on page 1506*

Tomocat® *see* Barium *on page 179*

Tomocat® 1000 *see* Barium *on page 179*

Tomoxetine *see* Atomoxetine *on page 156*

Tonocard® [DSC] *see* Tocainide *on page 1500*

Tonopaque *see* Barium *on page 179*

Topamax® *see* Topiramate *on page 1508*

Topicaine® [OTC] *see* Lidocaine *on page 920*

Topicort® *see* Desoximetasone *on page 438*

Topicort®-LP *see* Desoximetasone *on page 438*

Topiramate *(toe PYRE a mate)*

U.S. Brand Names Topamax®
Canadian Brand Names Gen-Topiramate; Novo-Topiramate; PMS-Topiramate; Sandoz-Topiramate; Topamax®
Mexican Brand Names Topamax®
Generic Available No
Pharmacologic Category Anticonvulsant, Miscellaneous
Use Monotherapy or adjunctive therapy for partial onset seizures and primary generalized tonic-clonic seizures; adjunctive treatment of seizures associated with Lennox-Gastaut syndrome; prophylaxis of migraine headache
Unlabeled/Investigational Use Infantile spasms, neuropathic pain, cluster headache
Local Anesthetic/Vasoconstrictor Precautions No information available to require special precautions
Effects on Dental Treatment Key adverse event(s) related to dental treatment: Gingivitis and xerostomia (normal salivary flow resumes upon discontinuation).
Common Adverse Effects Adverse events are reported for placebo-controlled trials of adjunctive therapy in adult and pediatric patients. Unless otherwise noted, the percentages refer to incidence in epilepsy trials. Note: A wide range of dosages were studied; incidence of adverse events was frequently lower in the pediatric population studied.

>10%:
Central nervous system: Dizziness (4% to 32%), ataxia (6% to 16%), somnolence (15% to 29%), psychomotor slowing (3% to 21%), nervousness (9% to 19%), memory difficulties (2% to 14%), speech problems (2% to 13%), fatigue (9% to 30%), difficulty concentrating (5% to 14%), depression (9% to 13%), confusion (4% to 14%)
Endocrine & metabolic: Serum bicarbonate decreased (dose-related: 7% to 67%; marked reductions [to <17 mEq/L] 1% to 11%)
Gastrointestinal: Nausea (6% to 12%; migraine trial: 14%), weight loss (8% to 13%), anorexia (4% to 24%)
Neuromuscular & skeletal: Paresthesia (1% to 19%; migraine trial: 35% to 51%)
Ocular: Nystagmus (10% to 11%), abnormal vision (<1% to 13%)
Respiratory: Upper respiratory infection (migraine trial: 12% to 13%)
Miscellaneous: Injury (6% to 14%)
1% to 10%:
Cardiovascular: Chest pain (2% to 4%), edema (1% to 2%), bradycardia (1%), pallor (up to 1%), hypertension (1% to 2%)
Central nervous system: Abnormal coordination (4%), hypoesthesia (1% to 2%; migraine trial: 8%), convulsions (1%), depersonalization (1% to 2%),

apathy (1% to 3%), cognitive problems (3%), emotional lability (3%), agitation (3%), aggressive reactions (2% to 9%), tremor (3% to 9%), stupor (1% to 2%), mood problems (4% to 9%), anxiety (2% to 10%), insomnia (4% to 8%), appetite increased (1%), neurosis (1%), vertigo (1% to 2%)

Dermatologic: Pruritus (migraine trial: 2% to 4%), skin disorder (1% to 3%), alopecia (2%), dermatitis (up to 2%), hypertrichosis (up to 2%), rash erythematous (up to 2%), eczema (up to 1%), seborrhea (up to 1%), skin discoloration (up to 1%)

Endocrine & metabolic: Hot flashes (1% to 2%); metabolic acidosis (hyperchloremia, nonanion gap), dehydration, breast pain (up to 4%), menstrual irregularities (1% to 2%), hypoglycemia (1%), libido decreased (<1% to 2%)

Gastrointestinal: Dyspepsia (2% to 7%), abdominal pain (5% to 7%), constipation (3% to 5%), xerostomia (2% to 4%), fecal incontinence (1%), gingivitis (1%), diarrhea (2%; migraine trial: 11%), vomiting (1% to 3%), gastroenteritis (1% to 3%), GI disorder (1%), dysgeusia (2% to 4%; migraine trial: 12% to 15%), dysphagia (1%), flatulence (1%), GERD (1%), glossitis (1%), gum hyperplasia (1%), weight increase (1%)

Genitourinary: Impotence, dysuria/incontinence (<1% to 4%), prostatic disorder (2%), UTI (2% to 3%), premature ejaculation (migraine trial: 3%), cystitis (2%)

Hematologic: Leukopenia (1% to 2%), purpura (8%), hematoma (1%), prothrombin time increased (1%), thrombocytopenia (1%)

Neuromuscular & skeletal: Myalgia (2%), weakness (3% to 6%), back pain (1% to 5%), leg pain (2% to 4%), rigors (1%), hypertonia, arthralgia (1% to 7%), gait abnormal (2% to 8%), involuntary muscle contractions (2%; migraine trial: 4%), skeletal pain (1%), hyperkinesia (up to 5%), hyporeflexia (up to 2%)

Ocular: Conjunctivitis (1%), diplopia (2% to 10%), myopia (up to 1%)

Otic: Hearing decreased (1% to 2%), tinnitus (1% to 2%), otitis media (migraine trial: 1% to 2%)

Renal: Nephrolithiasis, renal calculus (migraine trial: 2%), hematuria (<1% to 2%)

Respiratory: Pharyngitis (3% to 6%), sinusitis (4% to 6%; migraine trial: 8% to 10%), epistaxis (1% to 4%), rhinitis (4% to 7%), dyspnea (1% to 2%), pneumonia (5%), coughing (migraine trial: 2% to 3%), bronchitis (migraine trial: 3%)

Miscellaneous: Flu-like symptoms (3% to 7%), allergy (2% to 3%), body odor (up to 1%), fever (migraine trial: 1% to 2%), viral infection (migraine trial: 3% to 4%), infection (<1% to 2%), diaphoresis (≤1%), thirst (2%)

Dosage Oral: **Note:** Do not abruptly discontinue therapy; taper dosage gradually to prevent rebound seizure.

Monotherapy: Children ≥10 years and Adults: Partial onset seizure and primary generalized tonic-clonic seizure: Initial: 25 mg twice daily; may increase weekly by 50 mg/day up to 100 mg twice daily (week 4 dose); thereafter, may further increase weekly by 100 mg/day up to the recommended maximum of 200 mg twice daily.

Adjunctive therapy:

Children 2-16 years:

Partial onset seizure or seizure associated with Lennox-Gastaut syndrome: Initial dose titration should begin at 25 mg (or less, based on a range of 1-3 mg/kg/day) nightly for the first week; dosage may be increased in increments of 1-3 mg/kg/day (administered in 2 divided doses) at 1- or 2-week intervals to a total daily dose of 5-9 mg/kg/day

Primary generalized tonic-clonic seizure: Use initial dose listed above, but use slower initial titration rate; titrate to recommended maintenance dose by the end of 8 weeks

Adolescents ≥17 years and Adults:

Partial onset seizures: Initial: 25-50 mg/day (given in 2 divided doses) for 1 week; increase at weekly intervals by 25-50 mg/day until response; usual maintenance dose: 100-200 mg twice daily. Doses >1600 mg/day have not been studied.

Primary generalized tonic-clonic seizures: Use initial dose as listed above for partial onset seizures, but use slower initial titration rate; titrate upwards to recommended dose by the end of 8 weeks; usual maintenance dose: 200 mg twice daily. Doses >1600 mg/day have not been studied.

Adults:

Migraine prophylaxis: Initial: 25 mg/day (in the evening), titrated at weekly intervals in 25 mg increments, up to the recommended total daily dose of 100 mg/day given in 2 divided doses

Cluster headache (unlabeled use): Initial: 25 mg/day, titrated at weekly intervals in 25 mg increments, up to 200 mg/day

(Continued)

Topiramate *(Continued)*

Neuropathic pain (unlabeled use): Initial: 25 mg/day, titrated at weekly intervals in 25-50 mg increments to target dose of 400 mg daily in 2 divided doses. Reported dosage range studied: 25-800 mg/day

Dosing adjustment in renal impairment: Cl_{cr} <70 mL/minute: Administer 50% dose and titrate more slowly

Hemodialysis: Supplemental dose may be needed during hemodialysis

Dosing adjustment in hepatic impairment: Clearance may be reduced

Mechanism of Action Anticonvulsant activity may be due to a combination of potential mechanisms: Blocks neuronal voltage-dependent sodium channels, enhances GABA(A) activity, antagonizes AMPA/kainate glutamate receptors, and weakly inhibits carbonic anhydrase.

Contraindications Hypersensitivity to topiramate or any component of the formulation

Warnings/Precautions Use with caution in patients with hepatic, respiratory, or renal impairment. Topiramate may decrease serum bicarbonate concentrations (up to 67% of patients); treatment-emergent metabolic acidosis is less common. Risk may be increased in patients with a predisposing condition (organ dysfunction, ketogenic diet, or concurrent treatment with other drugs which may cause acidosis). Metabolic acidosis may occur at dosages as low as 50 mg/day. Monitor serum bicarbonate as well as potential complications of chronic acidosis (nephrolithiasis, osteomalacia, and reduced growth rates in children). The risk of kidney stones is about 2-4 times that of the untreated population, the risk of this event may be reduced by increasing fluid intake.

Cognitive dysfunction, psychiatric disturbances (mood disorders), and sedation (somnolence or fatigue) may occur with topiramate use; incidence may be related to rapid titration and higher doses. Topiramate may also cause paresthesia and ataxia. Topiramate has been associated with secondary angle-closure glaucoma in adults and children, typically within 1 month of initiation; discontinue in patients with acute onset of decreased visual acuity or ocular pain. Hyperammonemia with or without encephalopathy may occur with concomitant valproate administration; use with caution in patients with inborn errors of metabolism or decreased hepatic mitochondrial activity. Topiramate may be associated (rarely) with severe oligohydrosis and hyperthermia, most frequently in children; use caution and monitor closely during strenuous exercise, during exposure to high environmental temperature, or in patients receiving drugs with anticholinergic activity.

Avoid abrupt withdrawal of topiramate therapy, it should be withdrawn/tapered slowly to minimize the potential of increased seizure frequency. Safety and efficacy have not been established in children <2 years of age for adjunctive treatment and <10 years of age for monotherapy. No adequate and well-controlled studies have been conducted in pregnant women; use only if benefit clearly outweighs risk.

Drug Interactions

Cytochrome P450 Effect: Inhibits CYP2C19 (weak); **Induces** CYP3A4 (weak)

Increased Effect/Toxicity: Concomitant administration with other CNS depressants will increase its sedative effects. Coadministration with acetazolamide: may increase the chance of nephrolithiasis and/or hyperthermia. Topiramate may increase phenytoin concentration by 25%. Concurrent administration with anticholinergic drugs may increase the risk of oligohydrosis and/or hyperthermia (includes drugs with high anticholinergic activity such as antihistamines, cyclic antidepressants, and antipsychotics); use caution.

Decreased Effect: Phenytoin can decrease topiramate levels by as much as 48%, carbamazepine reduces it by 40%. Digoxin levels and ethinyl estradiol blood levels are decreased when coadministered with topiramate. Hyperammonemia (with or without encephalopathy) has been reported in patients who tolerated valproic acid or topiramate alone; these drugs may modestly decrease the serum concentrations of the other drug.

Ethanol/Nutrition/Herb Interactions

Ethanol: Avoid ethanol (may increase CNS depression).

Food: Ketogenic diet may increase the possibility of acidosis.

Herb/Nutraceutical: Avoid evening primrose (seizure threshold decreased).

Pharmacodynamics/Kinetics

Absorption: Good, rapid; unaffected by food

Protein binding: 15% to 41% (inversely related to plasma concentrations)

Metabolism: Hepatic via P450 enzymes

Bioavailability: 80%

Half-life elimination: Mean: Adults: Normal renal function: 21 hours; shorter in pediatric patients; clearance is 50% higher in pediatric patients

Time to peak, serum: ~2-4 hours

Excretion: Urine (~70% to 80% as unchanged drug)

Dialyzable: ~30%

Pregnancy Risk Factor C

Dosage Forms CAP, sprinkle: 15 mg, 25 mg. **TAB:** 25 mg, 50 mg, 100 mg, 200 mg

TOPO *see* Topotecan *on page 1511*

Toposar® *see* Etoposide *on page 626*

Topotecan (toe poe TEE kan)

U.S. Brand Names Hycamtin®

Canadian Brand Names Hycamtin™

Generic Available No

Synonyms Hycamptamine; NSC-609699; SK and F 104864; SKF 104864; SKF 104864-A; TOPO; Topotecan Hydrochloride; TPT

Pharmacologic Category Antineoplastic Agent, Natural Source (Plant) Derivative

Use Treatment of ovarian cancer, small cell lung cancer

Unlabeled/Investigational Use Investigational: Treatment of nonsmall cell lung cancer, sarcoma (pediatrics)

Local Anesthetic/Vasoconstrictor Precautions No information available to require special precautions

Effects on Dental Treatment No significant effects or complications reported

Common Adverse Effects

>10%:

Central nervous system: Headache, fatigue, fever, pain

Dermatologic: Alopecia (reversible), rash

Gastrointestinal: Nausea, vomiting, diarrhea, constipation, abdominal pain, stomatitis, anorexia

Hematologic: Myelosuppressive: Principle dose-limiting toxicity; white blood cell count nadir is 8-11 days and is more frequent than thrombocytopenia (at lower doses); recover is usually within 21 days and cumulative toxicity has not been noted.

Neuromuscular & skeletal: Weakness

Respiratory: Dyspnea (22%), cough

1% to 10%:

Hepatic: Transient increases in liver enzymes

Neuromuscular & skeletal: Paresthesia

Mechanism of Action Binds to topoisomerase I and stabilizes the cleavable complex so that religation of the cleaved DNA strand cannot occur. This results in the accumulation of cleavable complexes and single-strand DNA breaks. Topotecan acts in S phase.

Drug Interactions

Increased Effect/Toxicity: Concurrent administration of TPT and G-CSF in clinical trials results in severe myelosuppression. If G-CSF is to be used, manufacturer recommends that it should not be initiated until 24 hours after the completion of treatment with topotecan. Concurrent *in vitro* exposure to TPT and the topoisomerase II inhibitor etoposide results in no altered effect; sequential exposure results in potentiation. Concurrent exposure to TPT and 5-azacytidine results in potentiation both *in vitro* and *in vivo*. Myelosuppression was more severe when given in combination with cisplatin.

Pharmacodynamics/Kinetics

Absorption: Oral: ~30%

Distribution: V_{dss} of the lactone is high (mean: 87.3 L/mm^2; range: 25.6-186 L/mm^2), suggesting wide distribution and/or tissue sequestering

Protein binding: 35%

Metabolism: Undergoes a rapid, pH-dependent opening of the lactone ring to yield a relatively inactive hydroxy acid in plasma

Half-life elimination: 2-3 hours

Excretion: Urine (30%) within 24 hours

Pregnancy Risk Factor D

Topotecan Hydrochloride *see* Topotecan *on page 1511*

Toprol-XL® *see* Metoprolol *on page 1030*

Toradol® *see* Ketorolac *on page 886*

Toremifene (TORE em i feen)

U.S. Brand Names Fareston®
Canadian Brand Names Fareston®
Mexican Brand Names Fareston®
Generic Available No
Synonyms FC1157a; Toremifene Citrate
Pharmacologic Category Antineoplastic Agent, Estrogen Receptor Antagonist
Use Treatment of advanced breast cancer; management of desmoid tumors and endometrial carcinoma
Local Anesthetic/Vasoconstrictor Precautions No information available to require special precautions
Effects on Dental Treatment No significant effects or complications reported
Common Adverse Effects
>10%:
   Endocrine & metabolic: Vaginal discharge, hot flashes
   Gastrointestinal: Nausea, vomiting
   Miscellaneous: Diaphoresis
1% to 10%:
   Cardiovascular: Thromboembolism: Toremifene has been associated with the occurrence of venous thrombosis and pulmonary embolism; arterial thrombosis has also been described in a few case reports; cardiac failure, MI, edema
   Central nervous system: Dizziness
   Endocrine & metabolic: Hypercalcemia may occur in patients with bone metastases; galactorrhea and vitamin deficiency, menstrual irregularities
   Genitourinary: Vaginal bleeding or discharge, endometriosis, priapism, possible endometrial cancer
   Ocular: Ophthalmologic effects (visual acuity changes, cataracts, or retinopathy), corneal opacities, dry eyes
Mechanism of Action Nonsteroidal, triphenylethylene derivative. Competitively binds to estrogen receptors on tumors and other tissue targets, producing a nuclear complex that decreases DNA synthesis and inhibits estrogen effects. Nonsteroidal agent with potent antiestrogenic properties which compete with estrogen for binding sites in breast and other tissues; cells accumulate in the G_0 and G_1 phases; therefore, toremifene is cytostatic rather than cytocidal.
Drug Interactions
   Cytochrome P450 Effect: Substrate of CYP1A2 (minor), 3A4 (major)
   Increased Effect/Toxicity: Concurrent therapy with warfarin results in significant enhancement of anticoagulant effects; has been speculated that a decrease in antitumor effect of tamoxifen may also occur due to alterations in the percentage of active tamoxifen metabolites.
   Decreased Effect: CYP3A4 inducers may decrease the levels/effects of toremifene; example inducers include aminoglutethimide, carbamazepine, nafcillin, nevirapine, phenobarbital, phenytoin, and rifamycins.
Pharmacodynamics/Kinetics
   Absorption: Well absorbed
   Distribution: V_d: 580 L
   Protein binding, plasma: >99.5%, primarily to albumin
   Metabolism: Extensively hepatic, principally by CYP3A4 to N-demethyl-toremifene, which is also antiestrogenic but with weak *in vivo* antitumor potency
   Half-life elimination: ~5 days
   Time to peak, serum: ~3 hours
   Excretion: Primarily feces; urine (10%) during a 1-week period
Pregnancy Risk Factor D

Toremifene Citrate *see* Toremifene *on page 1512*

Torsemide (TORE se mide)

Related Information
   Cardiovascular Diseases *on page 1636*
U.S. Brand Names Demadex®
Generic Available Yes: Tablet
Pharmacologic Category Diuretic, Loop
Use Management of edema associated with congestive heart failure and hepatic or renal disease; used alone or in combination with antihypertensives in treatment of hypertension; I.V. form is indicated when rapid onset is desired

Local Anesthetic/Vasoconstrictor Precautions No information available to require special precautions

Effects on Dental Treatment No significant effects or complications reported

Common Adverse Effects 1% to 10%:

Cardiovascular: Edema (1.1%), ECG abnormality (2%), chest pain (1.2%)

Central nervous system: Headache (7.3%), dizziness (3.2%), insomnia (1.2%), nervousness (1%)

Endocrine & metabolic: Hyperglycemia, hyperuricemia, hypokalemia

Gastrointestinal: Diarrhea (2%), constipation (1.8%), nausea (1.8%), dyspepsia (1.6%), sore throat (1.6%)

Genitourinary: Excessive urination (6.7%)

Neuromuscular & skeletal: Weakness (2%), arthralgia (1.8%), myalgia (1.6%)

Respiratory: Rhinitis (2.8%), cough increase (2%)

Mechanism of Action Inhibits reabsorption of sodium and chloride in the ascending loop of Henle and distal renal tubule, interfering with the chloride-binding cotransport system, thus causing increased excretion of water, sodium, chloride, magnesium, and calcium; does not alter GFR, renal plasma flow, or acid-base balance

Drug Interactions

Cytochrome P450 Effect: Substrate of CYP2C8/9 (major); **Inhibits** CYP2C19 (weak)

Increased Effect/Toxicity: Torsemide-induced hypokalemia may predispose to digoxin toxicity and may increase the risk of arrhythmia with drugs which may prolong QT interval, including type Ia and type III antiarrhythmic agents, cisapride, and some quinolones (sparfloxacin, gatifloxacin, and moxifloxacin). The risk of toxicity from lithium and salicylates (high dose) may be increased by loop diuretics. Hypotensive effects and/or adverse renal effects of ACE inhibitors and NSAIDs are potentiated by bumetanide-induced hypovolemia. The effects of peripheral adrenergic-blocking drugs or ganglionic blockers may be increased by bumetanide.

Torsemide may increase the risk of ototoxicity with other ototoxic agents (aminoglycosides, cis-platinum), especially in patients with renal dysfunction. Synergistic diuretic effects occur with thiazide-type diuretics. Diuretics tend to be synergistic with other antihypertensive agents, and hypotension may occur.

Decreased Effect: Torsemide action may be reduced with probenecid. Diuretic action may be impaired in patients with cirrhosis and ascites if used with salicylates. Glucose tolerance may be decreased when used with sulfonylureas. CYP2C8/9 inducers may decrease the levels/effects of torsemide; example inducers include carbamazepine, phenobarbital, phenytoin, rifampin, rifapentine, and secobarbital. Torsemide efficacy may be decreased with NSAIDs.

Pharmacodynamics/Kinetics

Onset of action: Diuresis: 30-60 minutes

Peak effect: 1-4 hours

Duration: ~6 hours

Absorption: Oral: Rapid

Protein binding, plasma: ~97% to 99%

Metabolism: Hepatic (80%) via CYP

Bioavailability: 80% to 90%

Half-life elimination: 2-4; Cirrhosis: 7-8 hours

Excretion: Urine (20% as unchanged drug)

Pregnancy Risk Factor B

Touro™ CC see Guaifenesin, Pseudoephedrine, and Dextromethorphan on page 757

Touro™ Allergy see Brompheniramine and Pseudoephedrine on page 223

Touro® DM see Guaifenesin and Dextromethorphan on page 754

Touro LA® see Guaifenesin and Pseudoephedrine on page 755

tPA see Alteplase on page 77

TPT see Topotecan on page 1511

TPV see Tipranavir on page 1495

tRA see Tretinoin (Oral) on page 1524

Trace Metals (trase MET als)

Related Information

Chromium on page 1618

Iodine on page 852

Selenium on page 1383

(Continued)

Trace Metals *(Continued)*

U.S. Brand Names Iodopen®; Molypen®; M.T.E.-4®; M.T.E.-5®; M.T.E.-6®; M.T.E.-7®; Multitrace™-4; Multitrace™-4 Neonatal; Multitrace™-4 Pediatric; Multitrace™-5; Neotrace-4®; Pedtrace-4®; P.T.E.-4®; P.T.E.-5®; Selepen®

Generic Available Yes

Synonyms Chromium; Copper; Iodine; Manganese; Molybdenum; Neonatal Trace Metals; Selenium; Zinc

Pharmacologic Category Trace Element, Parenteral

Use Prevention and correction of trace metal deficiencies

Local Anesthetic/Vasoconstrictor Precautions No information available to require special precautions

Effects on Dental Treatment No significant effects or complications reported

Pregnancy Risk Factor C

Tracleer® *see* Bosentan *on page 215*

Tramadol *(TRA ma dole)*

Related Sample Prescriptions
Moderate/Moderately Severe Oral Pain *on page 1734*

U.S. Brand Names Ultram®; Ultram® ER

Canadian Brand Names Ultram®

Mexican Brand Names Nobligan®; Prontofort®; Tradol®

Generic Available Yes: Excludes extended release tablet

Synonyms Tramadol Hydrochloride

Pharmacologic Category Analgesic, Non-narcotic

Dental Use Relief of moderate to moderately-severe dental pain

Use Relief of moderate to moderately-severe pain

Local Anesthetic/Vasoconstrictor Precautions No information available to require special precautions

Effects on Dental Treatment Key adverse event(s) related to dental treatment: Xerostomia and changes in salivation (normal salivary flow resumes upon discontinuation). See Dental Comment.

Significant Adverse Effects

>10%:

Cardiovascular: Flushing (8% to 16%)

Central nervous system: Dizziness (16% to 33%), headache (8% to 32%), insomnia (7% to 11%), somnolence (7% to 25%)

Dermatologic: Pruritus (6% to 12%)

Gastrointestinal: Constipation (12% to 46%), nausea (15% to 40%)

Neuromuscular & skeletal: Weakness (4% to 12%)

1% to 10%:

Cardiovascular: Chest pain (1% to <5%), postural hypotension (2% to 5%), vasodilation (1% to <5%)

Central nervous system: Agitation, anxiety (1% to <5%), confusion (1% to <5%), coordination impaired (1% to <5%), depression (1% to <5%), emotional lability, euphoria, hallucinations, hypoesthesia, lethargy, malaise, nervousness (1% to <5%), pain, pyrexia, restlessness

Dermatologic: Dermatitis, rash

Endocrine & metabolic: Hot flashes (2% to 9%), menopausal symptoms (1% to <5%)

Gastrointestinal: Abdominal pain, anorexia (<6%), diarrhea (5% to 10%), dry mouth (5% to 10%), dyspepsia, flatulence, vomiting (5% to 9%), weight loss

Genitourinary: Urinary frequency (1% to <5%), urinary retention (1% to <5%), urinary tract infection (1% to <5%)

Neuromuscular & skeletal: Arthralgia (1% to <5%), hypertonia (1% to <5%), rigors (<4%), paresthesia (1% to <5%), spasticity (1% to <5%), tremor (1% to <5%), creatinine phosphokinase increased

Ocular: Blurred vision (1% to <5%), miosis (1% to <5%)

Respiratory: Bronchitis (1% to <5%), cough (1% to <5%), dyspnea (1% to <5%), pharyngitis (1% to <5%), rhinorrhea (1% to <5%), sinusitis (1% to <5%)

Miscellaneous: Diaphoresis (2% to 6%), flu-like syndrome (<2%)

<1% (Limited to important or life-threatening): Allergic reaction, amnesia, anaphylactoid reactions, anaphylaxis, angioedema, bronchospasm, cataracts, cholecystitis, cholelithiasis, cognitive dysfunction, concentration difficulty, creatinine increased, deafness, gastrointestinal bleeding, hepatitis, hyper-/hypotension, liver failure, MI, migraine, myocardial ischemia, night sweats, pancreatitis, peripheral ischemia, pulmonary edema, pulmonary embolism,

seizure, serotonin syndrome, Stevens-Johnson syndrome, suicidal tendency, syncope, toxic epidermal necrolysis, vertigo

A withdrawal syndrome may occur with abrupt discontinuation; includes anxiety, diarrhea, hallucinations (rare), nausea, pain, piloerection, rigors, sweating, and tremor. Uncommon discontinuation symptoms may include severe anxiety, panic attacks, or paresthesia.

Dental Usual Dosing Moderate-to-severe dental pain: Oral:

Adults:

Immediate release formulation: 50-100 mg every 4-6 hours (not to exceed 400 mg/day)

For patients not requiring rapid onset of effect, tolerability may be improved by starting dose at 25 mg/day and titrating dose by 25 mg every 3 days, until reaching 25 mg 4 times/day. Dose may then be increased by 50 mg every 3 days as tolerated, to reach dose of 50 mg 4 times/day.

Extended release formulation: 100 mg once daily; titrate every 5 days (maximum: 300 mg/day)

Elderly: >75 years:

Immediate release: 50 mg every 6 hours (not to exceed 300 mg/day); see dosing adjustments for renal and hepatic impairment.

Extended release formulation: See adult dosing.

Dosage Moderate-to-severe chronic pain: Oral:

Adults:

Immediate release formulation: 50-100 mg every 4-6 hours (not to exceed 400 mg/day)

For patients not requiring rapid onset of effect, tolerability may be improved by starting dose at 25 mg/day and titrating dose by 25 mg every 3 days, until reaching 25 mg 4 times/day. Dose may then be increased by 50 mg every 3 days as tolerated, to reach dose of 50 mg 4 times/day.

Extended release formulation: 100 mg once daily; titrate every 5 days (maximum: 300 mg/day)

Elderly: >75 years:

Immediate release: 50 mg every 6 hours (not to exceed 300 mg/day); see dosing adjustments for renal and hepatic impairment.

Extended release formulation: See adult dosing.

Dosing adjustment in renal impairment:

Immediate release: Cl_{cr} <30 mL/minute: Administer 50-100 mg dose every 12 hours (maximum: 200 mg/day)

Extended release: Should not be used in patients with Cl_{cr} < 30 mL/minute

Dosing adjustment in hepatic impairment:

Immediate release: Cirrhosis: Recommended dose: 50 mg every 12 hours

Extended release: Should not be used in patients with severe (Child-Pugh Class C) hepatic dysfunction

Mechanism of Action Binds to μ-opiate receptors in the CNS causing inhibition of ascending pain pathways, altering the perception of and response to pain; also inhibits the reuptake of norepinephrine and serotonin, which also modifies the ascending pain pathway

Contraindications Hypersensitivity to tramadol, opioids, or any component of the formulation; opioid-dependent patients; acute intoxication with alcohol, hypnotics, centrally-acting analgesics, opioids, or psychotropic drugs

Ultram® ER (extended release formulation): Additional contraindications: Severe (Cl_{cr} <30 mL/minute) renal dysfunction, severe (Child-Pugh Class C) hepatic dysfunction

Warnings/Precautions Should be used only with extreme caution in patients receiving MAO inhibitors. May cause CNS depression and/or respiratory depression, particularly when combined with other CNS depressants. Use with caution and reduce dosage when administered to patients receiving other CNS depressants. An increased risk of seizures may occur in patients receiving serotonin reuptake inhibitors (SSRIs or anorectics), tricyclic antidepressants, other cyclic compounds (including cyclobenzaprine, promethazine), neuroleptics, MAO inhibitors, or drugs which may lower seizure threshold. Patients with a history of seizures, or with a risk of seizures (head trauma, metabolic disorders, CNS infection, or malignancy, or during ethanol/drug withdrawal) are also at increased risk.

Elderly patients and patients with chronic respiratory disorders may be at greater risk of adverse events. Use with caution in patients with increased intracranial pressure or head injury. Avoid use in patients who are suicidal or addiction prone. Use caution in heavy alcohol users. Use caution in treatment of acute abdominal conditions; may mask pain. Use tramadol with caution and reduce dosage in patients with liver disease or renal dysfunction. Not recommended during pregnancy or in nursing mothers. Tolerance or drug dependence may result from extended use (withdrawal symptoms have been reported); abrupt discontinuation should be avoided. Tapering of dose at the (Continued)

Tramadol *(Continued)*

time of discontinuation limits the risk of withdrawal symptoms. Safety and efficacy in pediatric patients <18 years of age have not been established; use in this population is not recommended.

Drug Interactions Substrate of CYP2B6 (minor), 2D6 (major), 3A4 (minor)

Carbamazepine: Tramadol metabolism is increased by carbamazepine. Avoid concurrent use; increases risk of seizures.

Cyclobenzaprine: May enhance the neuroexcitatory and/or seizure-potentiating effect of tramadol.

CYP2D6 inhibitors: May decrease the effects of tramadol. Example inhibitors include chlorpromazine, delavirdine, fluoxetine, miconazole, paroxetine, pergolide, quinidine, quinine, ritonavir, and ropinirole.

Ethanol: Tramadol may enhance the CNS depressant effect of ethanol.

MAO inhibitors: May increase the neuroexcitatory effects or risk of seizures. Examples of inhibitors include isocarboxazid, linezolid, phenelzine, selegiline, and tranylcypromine.

Naloxone: May increase the risk of seizures (if administered in tramadol overdose).

Quinidine: May increase the tramadol serum concentrations and decrease serum concentrations of M1

SSRIs: May increase the neuroexcitatory effects or risk of seizures with tramadol. Examples of SSRIs include citalopram, escitalopram, fluoxetine, fluvoxamine, paroxetine, sertraline.

Serotonin modulators: May enhance the adverse/toxic effects of tramadol. The development of serotonin syndrome may occur.

Sibutramine: May enhance the serotonergic effects of tramadol. Avoid concurrent use.

Tricyclic antidepressants: May increase the risk of seizures.

Ethanol/Nutrition/Herb Interactions

Ethanol: Avoid ethanol (may increase CNS depression).

Food:

Immediate release: Does not affect the rate or extent of absorption.

Extended release: Reduced C_{max} and AUC and T_{max} occurred 3 hours earlier when taken with a high-fat meal.

Herb/Nutraceutical: Avoid valerian, St John's wort, kava kava, gotu kola (may increase CNS depression).

Dietary Considerations May be taken with or without food. Extended release formulation: Be consistent; always give with food or always give on an empty stomach.

Pharmacodynamics/Kinetics

Onset of action: ~1 hour

Duration of action: 9 hours

Absorption: Rapid and complete

Distribution: V_d: 2.5-3 L/kg

Protein binding, plasma: 20%

Metabolism: Extensively hepatic via demethylation, glucuronidation, and sulfation; has pharmacologically active metabolite formed by CYP2D6 (M1; O-desmethyl tramadol)

Bioavailability: Immediate release: 75%; Extended release: 85% to 90% as compared to immediate release.

Half-life elimination: Tramadol: ~6-8 hours; Active metabolite: 7-9 hours; prolonged in elderly, hepatic or renal impairment

Time to peak: Immediate release: 2 hours; Extended release: 12 hours

Excretion: Urine (30% as unchanged drug; 60% as metabolites)

Pregnancy Risk Factor C

Lactation Enters breast milk/contraindicated

Breast-Feeding Considerations Not recommended for postdelivery analgesia in nursing mothers.

Dosage Forms

Tablet, as hydrochloride: 50 mg

Ultram®: 50 mg

Tablet, extended release, as hydrochloride:

Ultram® ER: 100 mg, 200 mg, 300 mg

Dental Comment Literature reports suggest that the efficacy of tramadol in oral surgery pain is equivalent to the combination of aspirin and codeine. One study (Olson et al 1990) showed acetaminophen and dextropropoxyphene combination to be superior to tramadol and another study showed tramadol to be superior to acetaminophen and dextropropoxyphene combination. Tramadol appears to be at least equal to if not better than codeine alone. Seizures have been reported with the use of tramadol.

Selected Readings

Collins M, Young I, Sweeney P, et al, "The Effect of Tramadol on Dento-Alveolar Surgical Pain," *Br J Oral Maxillofac Surg,* 1997, 35(1):54-8.

Doroschak AM, Bowles WR, and Hargreaves KM, "Evaluation of the Combination of Flurbiprofen and Tramadol for Management of Endodontic Pain," *J Endod,* 1999, 25(10):660-3.

Kahn LH, Alderfer RJ, and Graham DJ, "Seizures Reported With Tramadol," *JAMA,* 1997, 278(20):1661.

Lewis KS and Han NH, "Tramadol: A New Centrally Acting Analgesic," *Am J Health Syst Pharm,* 1997, 54(6):643-52.

Moore PA, "Pain Management in Dental Practice: Tramadol vs. Codeine Combinations," *J Am Dent Assoc,* 1999, 130(7):1075-9.

Moore PA, Crout RJ, Jackson DL, et al, "Tramadol Hydrochloride: Analgesic Efficacy Compared With Codeine, Aspirin With Codeine, and Placebo After Dental Extraction," *J Clin Pharmacol,* 1998, 38(6):554-60.

Roelofse JA and Payne KA, "Oral Tramadol: Analgesic Efficacy in Children Following Multiple Dental Extractions," *Eur J Anaesthesiol,* 1999, 16(7):441-7.

Sunshine A, "New Clinical Experience With Tramadol," *Drugs,* 1994, 47(Suppl 1):8-18.

Sunshine A, Olson NZ, Zighelboim I, et al, "Analgesic Oral Efficacy of Tramadol Hydrochloride in Postoperative Pain," *Clin Pharmacol Ther,* 1992; 51(6):740-6.

Wynn RL, "Tramadol (Ultram) - A New Kind of Analgesic," *Gen Dent,* 1996, 44(3):216-8,220.

Tramadol Hydrochloride *see* Tramadol *on page 1514*

Tramadol Hydrochloride and Acetaminophen *see* Acetaminophen and Tramadol *on page 39*

Trandate® *see* Labetalol *on page 891*

Trandolapril (tran DOE la pril)

Related Information
Cardiovascular Diseases *on page 1636*

U.S. Brand Names Mavik®

Canadian Brand Names Mavik™

Mexican Brand Names Gopten®

Generic Available No

Pharmacologic Category Angiotensin-Converting Enzyme (ACE) Inhibitor

Use Management of hypertension alone or in combination with other antihypertensive agents; treatment of left ventricular dysfunction after myocardial infarction

Unlabeled/Investigational Use As a class, ACE inhibitors are recommended in the treatment of systolic congestive heart failure

Local Anesthetic/Vasoconstrictor Precautions No information available to require special precautions

Effects on Dental Treatment No significant effects or complications reported

Common Adverse Effects Note: Frequency ranges include data from hypertension and heart failure trials. Higher rates of adverse reactions have generally been noted in patients with CHF. However, the frequency of adverse effects associated with placebo is also increased in this population.

>1%:

Cardiovascular: Hypotension (<1% to 11%), bradycardia (<1% to 4.7%), intermittent claudication (3.8%), stroke (3.3%)

Central nervous system: Dizziness (1.3% to 23%), syncope (5.9%), asthenia (3.3%)

Endocrine & metabolic: Elevated uric acid (15%), hyperkalemia (5.3%), hypocalcemia (4.7%)

Gastrointestinal: Dyspepsia (6.4%), gastritis (4.2%)

Neuromuscular & skeletal: Myalgia (4.7%)

Renal: Elevated BUN (9%), elevated serum creatinine (1.1% to 4.7%) Respiratory: Cough (1.9% to 35%)

Mechanism of Action Trandolapril is an ACE inhibitor which prevents the formation of angiotensin II from angiotensin I. Trandolapril must undergo enzymatic hydrolysis, mainly in liver, to its biologically active metabolite, trandolaprilat. A CNS mechanism may also be involved in the hypotensive effect as angiotensin II increases adrenergic outflow from the CNS. Vasoactive kallikrein's may be decreased in conversion to active hormones by ACE inhibitors, thus, reducing blood pressure.

Drug Interactions
Increased Effect/Toxicity: Potassium supplements, co-trimoxazole (high dose), angiotensin II receptor antagonists (eg, candesartan, losartan, irbesartan), or potassium-sparing diuretics (amiloride, spironolactone, triamterene) may result in elevated serum potassium levels when combined with trandolapril. ACE inhibitor effects may be increased by phenothiazines or probenecid (increases levels of captopril). ACE inhibitors may increase serum concentrations/effects of lithium.

(Continued)

Trandolapril *(Continued)*

Diuretics have additive hypotensive effects with ACE inhibitors, and hypovolemia increases the potential for adverse renal effects of ACE inhibitors. In patients with compromised renal function, coadministration with NSAIDs may result in further deterioration of renal function. Allopurinol and ACE inhibitors may cause a higher risk of hypersensitivity reaction when taken concurrently.

Decreased Effect: Aspirin (high dose) may reduce the therapeutic effects of ACE inhibitors; at low dosages this does not appear to be significant. Rifampin may decrease the effect of ACE inhibitors. Antacids may decrease the bioavailability of ACE inhibitors (may be more likely to occur with captopril); separate administration times by 1-2 hours. NSAIDs, specifically indomethacin, may reduce the hypotensive effects of ACE inhibitors. More likely to occur in low renin or volume dependent hypertensive patients.

Pharmacodynamics/Kinetics
Onset of action: 1-2 hours
Peak effect: Reduction in blood pressure: 6 hours
Duration: Prolonged; 72 hours after single dose
Absorption: Rapid
Distribution: Trandolaprilat (active metabolite) is very lipophilic in comparison to other ACE inhibitors
Protein binding: 80%
Metabolism: Hepatically hydrolyzed to active metabolite, trandolaprilat
Half-life elimination:
Trandolapril: 6 hours; Trandolaprilat: Effective: 10 hours, Terminal: 24 hours
Time to peak: Parent: 1 hour; Active metabolite trandolaprilat: 4-10 hours
Excretion: Urine (as metabolites)
Clearance: Reduce dose in renal failure; creatinine clearances ≤30 mL/minute result in accumulation of active metabolite

Pregnancy Risk Factor C (1st trimester)/D (2nd and 3rd trimesters)

Trandolapril and Verapamil *(tran DOE la pril & ver AP a mil)*

Related Information
Trandolapril *on page 1517*
Verapamil *on page 1571*
U.S. Brand Names Tarka®
Canadian Brand Names Tarka®
Generic Available No
Synonyms Verapamil and Trandolapril
Pharmacologic Category Antihypertensive Agent, Combination
Use Combination drug for the treatment of hypertension, however, not indicated for initial treatment of hypertension; replacement therapy in patients receiving separate dosage forms (for patient convenience); when monotherapy with one component fails to achieve desired antihypertensive effect, or when dose-limiting adverse effects limit upward titration of monotherapy
Local Anesthetic/Vasoconstrictor Precautions No information available to require special precautions
Effects on Dental Treatment No significant effects or complications reported
Common Adverse Effects See individual agents.
Drug Interactions
Cytochrome P450 Effect: Verapamil: **Substrate** of CYP1A2 (major), 2B6 (minor), 2C8/9 (minor), 2C19 (minor), 2E1 (minor), 3A4 (major); **Inhibits** CYP1A2 (weak), 2C8/9 (weak), 2D6 (weak), 3A4 (moderate)
Pharmacodynamics/Kinetics See individual agents.
Pregnancy Risk Factor C/D (2nd and 3rd trimesters)

Tranexamic Acid *(tran eks AM ik AS id)*

U.S. Brand Names Cyklokapron®
Canadian Brand Names Cyklokapron®
Generic Available No
Pharmacologic Category Antihemophilic Agent
Use Short-term use (2-8 days) in hemophilia patients during and following tooth extraction to reduce or prevent hemorrhage
Unlabeled/Investigational Use Has been used as an alternative to aminocaproic acid for subarachnoid hemorrhage
Local Anesthetic/Vasoconstrictor Precautions No information available to require special precautions
Effects on Dental Treatment No significant effects or complications reported (see Dental Comment)

Common Adverse Effects
>10%: Gastrointestinal: Nausea, diarrhea, vomiting
1% to 10%:
  Cardiovascular: Hypotension, thrombosis
  Ocular: Blurred vision
Mechanism of Action Forms a reversible complex that displaces plasminogen from fibrin resulting in inhibition of fibrinolysis; it also inhibits the proteolytic activity of plasmin
Drug Interactions
  Increased Effect/Toxicity: Chlorpromazine may increase cerebral vasospasm and ischemia. Coadministrations of Factor IX complex or anti-inhibitor coagulant concentrates may increase risk of thrombosis.
Pharmacodynamics/Kinetics
  Half-life elimination: 2-10 hours
  Excretion: Urine (>90% as unchanged drug)
Pregnancy Risk Factor B
Dental Comment Antifibrinolytic drugs are useful for the control of bleeding after dental extractions in patients with hemophilia because the oral mucosa and saliva are rich in plasminogen activators. In a clinical trial, tranexamic acid reduced recurrent bleeding and the amount of clotting-factor-replacement therapy needed. In adults, the oral dose was 20-25 mg/kg tranexamic acid every 8 hours until the dental sockets were completely healed. Mouthwashes containing tranexamic acid are effective for preventing oral bleeding in patients with hemophilia and in patients requiring dental extraction while receiving long-term oral anticoagulant therapy.

Immediately before dental extraction in hemophilic patients, administer 10 mg/kg tranexamic acid I.V. together with replacement therapy. Following surgery, a dose of 25 mg/kg may be given orally 3-4 times/day for 2-8 days.

Transamine Sulphate see Tranylcypromine on page 1519
Transderm Scop® see Scopolamine on page 1380
trans-Retinoic Acid see Tretinoin (Oral) on page 1524
Trans-Ver-Sal® [OTC] see Salicylic Acid on page 1374
Tranxene® SD™ see Clorazepate on page 378
Tranxene® SD™-Half Strength see Clorazepate on page 378
Tranxene® T-Tab® see Clorazepate on page 378

Tranylcypromine (tran il SIP roe meen)

U.S. Brand Names Parnate®
Canadian Brand Names Parnate®
Generic Available No
Synonyms Transamine Sulphate; Tranylcypromine Sulfate
Pharmacologic Category Antidepressant, Monoamine Oxidase Inhibitor
Use Treatment of major depressive episode without melancholia
Unlabeled/Investigational Use Post-traumatic stress disorder
Local Anesthetic/Vasoconstrictor Precautions Attempts should be made to avoid use of vasoconstrictor due to possibility of hypertensive episodes with monoamine oxidase inhibitors
Effects on Dental Treatment Key adverse event(s) related to dental treatment: Orthostatic hypotension. Avoid use as an analgesic due to toxic reactions with MAO inhibitors.
Common Adverse Effects Frequency not defined.
  Cardiovascular: Edema, orthostatic hypotension, palpitations, tachycardia
  Central nervous system: Agitation, akinesia, anxiety, ataxia, chills, confusion, disorientation, dizziness, drowsiness, fatigue, headache, hyper-reflexia, insomnia, mania, memory loss, restlessness, sleep disturbances, twitching
  Dermatologic: Alopecia, cystic acne (flare), pruritus, rash, urticaria, scleroderma (localized)
  Endocrine & metabolic: Hypernatremia, hypermetabolic syndrome; sexual dysfunction (anorgasmia, ejaculatory disturbances, impotence); SIADH
  Gastrointestinal: Abdominal pain, anorexia, constipation, diarrhea, nausea, vomiting, weight gain, xerostomia
  Genitourinary: Incontinence, urinary retention
  Hematologic: Agranulocytosis, anemia, leukopenia, thrombocytopenia
  Hepatic: Hepatitis
  Neuromuscular & skeletal: Akinesis, muscle spasm, myoclonus, numbness, paresthesia, tremor, weakness
  Ocular: Blurred vision, glaucoma
  Otic: Tinnitus
  Miscellaneous: Diaphoresis
  (Continued)

Tranylcypromine *(Continued)*

Restrictions A medication guide concerning the use of antidepressants in children and teenagers can be found on the FDA website at http://www.fda.gov/cder/Offices/ODS/labeling.htm. It should be dispensed to parents or guardians of children and teenagers receiving this medication.

Mechanism of Action Tranylcypromine is a nonhydrazine monoamine oxidase inhibitor. It increases endogenous concentrations of epinephrine, norepinephrine, dopamine, and serotonin through inhibition of the enzyme (monoamine oxidase) responsible for the breakdown of these neurotransmitters.

Drug Interactions

Cytochrome P450 Effect: Inhibits CYP1A2 (moderate), 2A6 (strong), 2C8/9 (weak), 2C19 (moderate), 2D6 (moderate), 2E1 (weak), 3A4 (weak)

Increased Effect/Toxicity: Tranylcypromine may enhance the adverse effects of ethanol (CNS depression), amphetamines (hypertension), general anesthetics (hypotension), atomoxetine (CNS toxicity), buspirone (hypertension), CYP1A2 substrates, CYP2A6 substrates, CYP2C19 substrates, CYP2D6 substrates, dexmethylphenidate (hypertension), disulfiram (delirium), levodopa (hypertension), lithium (CNS toxicity), methylphenidate (hypertension), mirtazapine (CNS toxicity), rauwolfia alkaloids, and thioridazine. Tranylcypromine may enhance the vasopressor effects of alpha-/beta-agonists and enhance the hypertensive effects of alpha$_1$-agonists. Altretamine may enhance the orthostatic effects of tranylcypromine. Anticholinergics may enhance the side effects of tranylcypromine. Concurrent use of anorexiants, cyclobenzaprine, dextromethorphan, meperidine, SSRIs/SNRIs, serotonin 5-HT$_{1D}$ receptor agonist, sibutramine, and tricyclic antidepressants may result in a serotonin syndrome. Concurrent use of bupropion may lead to hypertensive crisis. COMT inhibitors may cause adverse/toxic effects. Pramlintide may increase anticholinergic effects of tranylcypromine. Serotonin modulators may enhance the adverse/toxic effects of tranylcypromine. Tramadol may increase the neuroexcitatory and seizure-potentiating effects of tranylcypromine.

Decreased Effect: Acetylcholinesterase inhibitors decrease tranylcypromine's anticholinergic side effects. Tranylcypromine may decrease the effects of CYP2D6 prodrug substrates, and false neurotransmitters (guanadrel, methyldopa).

Pharmacodynamics/Kinetics

Onset of action: Therapeutic: 2 days to 3 weeks continued dosing

Half-life elimination: 90-190 minutes

Time to peak, serum: ~2 hours

Excretion: Urine

Pregnancy Risk Factor C

Tranylcypromine Sulfate *see* Tranylcypromine *on page 1519*

Trastuzumab *(tras TU zoo mab)*

U.S. Brand Names Herceptin®

Canadian Brand Names Herceptin®

Mexican Brand Names Herceptin®

Generic Available No

Pharmacologic Category Antineoplastic Agent, Monoclonal Antibody; Monoclonal Antibody

Use Treatment of metastatic breast cancer whose tumors overexpress the HER-2/*neu* protein

Unlabeled/Investigational Use Treatment of ovarian, gastric, colorectal, endometrial, lung, bladder, prostate, and salivary gland tumors

Local Anesthetic/Vasoconstrictor Precautions No information available to require special precautions

Effects on Dental Treatment No significant effects or complications reported

Common Adverse Effects Note: The most common adverse effects are infusion-related, occurring in up to 40% of patients, consisting of fever and chills (mild to moderate, often with other systemic symptoms). Treatment with acetaminophen, diphenhydramine, and/or meperidine is usually effective.

>10%:

Central nervous system: Pain (47%), fever (36%), chills (32%), headache (26%), insomnia (14%), dizziness (13%)

Dermatologic: Rash (18%)

Gastrointestinal: Nausea (33%), diarrhea (25%), vomiting (23%), abdominal pain (22%), anorexia (14%)

Neuromuscular & skeletal: Weakness (42%), back pain (22%)

Respiratory: Cough (26%), dyspnea (22%), rhinitis (14%), pharyngitis (12%)

Miscellaneous: Infection (20%); infusion reaction (40%, chills and fever most common)

1% to 10%:

Cardiovascular: Peripheral edema (10%), edema (8%), CHF (7%), tachycardia (5%)

Central nervous system: Paresthesia (9%), depression (6%), peripheral neuritis (2%), neuropathy (1%)

Dermatologic: Herpes simplex (2%), acne (2%)

Genitourinary: Urinary tract infection (5%)

Hematologic: Anemia (4%), leukopenia (3%)

Neuromuscular & skeletal: Bone pain (7%), arthralgia (6%)

Respiratory: Sinusitis (9%)

Miscellaneous: Flu syndrome (10%), accidental injury (6%), allergic reaction (3%)

Mechanism of Action Trastuzumab is a monoclonal antibody which binds to the extracellular domain of the human epidermal growth factor receptor 2 protein (HER-2); it mediates antibody-dependent cellular cytotoxicity against cells which overproduce HER-2

Drug Interactions

Increased Effect/Toxicity: Paclitaxel may result in a decrease in clearance of trastuzumab, increasing serum concentrations. Combined use with anthracyclines may increase the incidence/severity of cardiac dysfunction. Monoclonal antibodies may increase the risk for allergic reactions to trastuzumab due to the presence of HACA antibodies. Trastuzumab may increase the incidence of neutropenia and/or febrile neutropenia when used in combination with myelosuppressive chemotherapy.

Pharmacodynamics/Kinetics

Distribution: V_d: 44 mL/kg

Half-life elimination: Mean: 5.8 days (range: 1-32 days)

Pregnancy Risk Factor B

Trasylol® see Aprotinin on page 135

Travatan® see Travoprost on page 1521

Travoprost (TRA voe prost)

U.S. Brand Names Travatan®

Canadian Brand Names Travatan®

Mexican Brand Names Travatan®

Generic Available No

Pharmacologic Category Ophthalmic Agent, Antiglaucoma; Prostaglandin, Ophthalmic

Use Reduction of elevated intraocular pressure in patients with open-angle glaucoma or ocular hypertension who are intolerant of the other IOP-lowering medications or insufficiently responsive (failed to achieve target IOP determined after multiple measurements over time) to another IOP-lowering medication

Local Anesthetic/Vasoconstrictor Precautions No significant effects or complications reported

Effects on Dental Treatment No information available to require special precautions

Mechanism of Action A selective FP prostanoid receptor agonist which lowers intraocular pressure by increasing outflow

Pregnancy Risk Factor C

Trazodone (TRAZ oh done)

U.S. Brand Names Desyrel®

Canadian Brand Names Alti-Trazodone; Apo-Trazodone®; Apo-Trazodone D®; Desyrel®; Gen-Trazodone; Novo-Trazodone; Nu-Trazodone; PMS-Trazodone; ratio-Trazodone

Generic Available Yes

Synonyms Trazodone Hydrochloride

Pharmacologic Category Antidepressant, Serotonin Reuptake Inhibitor/Antagonist

Use Treatment of depression

Unlabeled/Investigational Use Potential augmenting agent for antidepressants, hypnotic

Local Anesthetic/Vasoconstrictor Precautions Trazodone inhibits reuptake of both serotonin and norepinephrine and also blocks some serotonin receptors. No precautions with vasoconstrictors appear to be necessary.

(Continued)

Trazodone *(Continued)*

Effects on Dental Treatment Key adverse event(s) related to dental treatment: Significant xerostomia (normal salivary flow resumes upon discontinuation).

Common Adverse Effects

>10%:

Central nervous system: Dizziness, headache, sedation

Gastrointestinal: Nausea, xerostomia

Ocular: Blurred vision

1% to 10%:

Cardiovascular: Syncope, hyper-/hypotension, edema

Central nervous system: Confusion, decreased concentration, fatigue, incoordination

Gastrointestinal: Diarrhea, constipation, weight gain/loss

Neuromuscular & skeletal: Tremor, myalgia

Respiratory: Nasal congestion

Restrictions A medication guide concerning the use of antidepressants in children and teenagers can be found on the FDA website at http://www.fda.gov/cder/Offices/ODS/labeling.htm. It should be dispensed to parents or guardians of children and teenagers receiving this medication.

Dosage Oral: Therapeutic effects may take up to 6 weeks to occur; therapy is normally maintained for 6-12 months after optimum response is reached to prevent recurrence of depression

Children 6-12 years: Depression (unlabeled use): Initial: 1.5-2 mg/kg/day in divided doses; increase gradually every 3-4 days as needed; maximum: 6 mg/kg/day in 3 divided doses

Adolescents: Depression (unlabeled use): Initial: 25-50 mg/day; increase to 100-150 mg/day in divided doses

Adults:

Depression: Initial: 150 mg/day in 3 divided doses (may increase by 50 mg/day every 3-7 days); maximum: 600 mg/day

Sedation/hypnotic (unlabeled use): 25-50 mg at bedtime (often in combination with daytime SSRIs); may increase up to 200 mg at bedtime

Elderly: 25-50 mg at bedtime with 25-50 mg/day dose increase every 3 days for inpatients and weekly for outpatients, if tolerated; usual dose: 75-150 mg/day

Mechanism of Action Inhibits reuptake of serotonin, causes adrenoreceptor subsensitivity, and induces significant changes in 5-HT presynaptic receptor adrenoreceptors. Trazodone also significantly blocks histamine (H_1) and alpha$_1$-adrenergic receptors.

Contraindications Hypersensitivity to trazodone or any component of the formulation

Warnings/Precautions Antidepressants increase the risk of suicidal thinking and behavior in children and adolescents with major depressive disorder (MDD) and other depressive disorders; consider risk prior to prescribing. All patients must be closely monitored for clinical worsening, suicidality, or unusual changes in behavior, especially during the initiation of therapy or following an increase or decrease in dosage. When used in children, the child's family or caregiver should be instructed to closely observe the patient and communicate condition with healthcare provider. A medication guide should be dispensed with each prescription. **Trazodone is not FDA approved for use in children.**

The possibility of a suicide attempt is inherent in major depression and may persist until remission occurs. Use caution in high-risk patients. Worsening depression and severe abrupt suicidality that are not part of the presenting symptoms may require discontinuation or modification of drug therapy. The patient's family or caregiver should be alerted to monitor patients for the emergence of suicidality and associated behaviors (such as agitation, irritability, hostility, impulsivity, and hypomania) and call healthcare provider.

May worsen psychosis in some patients or precipitate a shift to mania or hypomania in patients with bipolar disorder. Patients presenting with depressive symptoms should be screened for bipolar disorder. Monotherapy in patients with bipolar disorder should be avoided. **Trazodone is not FDA approved for the treatment of bipolar depression.**

Priapism, including cases resulting in permanent dysfunction, has occurred with the use of trazodone. Not recommended for use in a patient during the acute recovery phase of MI. Trazodone should be initiated with caution in patients who are receiving concurrent or recent therapy with a MAO inhibitor.

The risks of sedation and/or postural hypotension are high relative to other antidepressants. Trazodone frequently causes sedation, which may result in impaired performance of tasks requiring alertness (eg, operating machinery or driving). Sedative effects may be additive with other CNS depressants and ethanol. Use with caution in patients with a history of cardiovascular disease (including previous MI, stroke, tachycardia, or conduction abnormalities). The risk of conduction abnormalities with this agent is low relative to other antidepressants.

Consider discontinuing, when possible, prior to elective surgery. Therapy should not be abruptly discontinued in patients receiving high doses for prolonged periods. Use caution in patients with a previous seizure disorder or condition predisposing to seizures such as brain damage, alcoholism, or concurrent therapy with other drugs which lower the seizure threshold. Use with caution in patients with hepatic or renal dysfunction and in elderly patients.

Drug Interactions
  Cytochrome P450 Effect: Substrate of CYP2D6 (minor), 3A4 (major); **Inhibits** CYP2D6 (moderate), 3A4 (weak)
  Increased Effect/Toxicity: Trazodone, in combination with other serotonergic agents (buspirone, MAO inhibitors), may produce additive serotonergic effects, including serotonin syndrome. Trazodone, in combination with other psychotropics (low potency antipsychotics), may result in additional hypotension. Fluoxetine may inhibit the metabolism of trazodone resulting in elevated plasma levels.

  Trazodone may increase the levels/effects of amphetamines, beta-blockers, dextromethorphan, fluoxetine, lidocaine, mirtazapine, nefazodone, paroxetine, risperidone, ritonavir, thioridazine, tricyclic antidepressants, venlafaxine, and other CYP2D6 substrates. The levels/effects of trazodone may be increased by azole antifungals, clarithromycin, diclofenac, doxycycline, erythromycin, imatinib, isoniazid, nefazodone, nicardipine, propofol, protease inhibitors, quinidine, telithromycin, verapamil, and other CYP3A4 inhibitors.
  Decreased Effect: Trazodone inhibits the hypotensive response to clonidine. The levels/effects of trazodone may be decreased by aminoglutethimide, carbamazepine, nafcillin, nevirapine, phenobarbital, phenytoin, rifamycins, and other CYP3A4 inducers. Trazodone may decrease the levels/effects of CYP2D6 prodrug substrates (eg, codeine, hydrocodone, oxycodone, tramadol).

Ethanol/Nutrition/Herb Interactions
  Ethanol: Avoid ethanol (may increase CNS depression).
  Food: Time to peak serum levels may be increased if trazodone is taken with food.
  Herb/Nutraceutical: Avoid valerian, St John's wort, SAMe, kava kava (may increase risk of serotonin syndrome and/or excessive sedation).

Pharmacodynamics/Kinetics
  Onset of action: Therapeutic (antidepressant): 1-3 weeks; sleep aid: 1-3 hours
  Protein binding: 85% to 95%
  Metabolism: Hepatic via CYP3A4 to an active metabolite (mCPP)
  Half-life elimination: 7-8 hours, two compartment kinetics
  Time to peak, serum: 30-100 minutes; delayed with food (up to 2.5 hours)
  Excretion: Primarily urine; secondarily feces

Pregnancy Risk Factor C
Dosage Forms TAB: 50 mg, 100 mg, 150 mg, 300 mg

Trazodone Hydrochloride *see* Trazodone *on page 1521*

Trecator® *see* Ethionamide *on page 618*

Trelstar™ Depot *see* Triptorelin *on page 1544*

Trelstar™ LA *see* Triptorelin *on page 1544*

Trental® *see* Pentoxifylline *on page 1212*

Treprostinil (tre PROST in il)

U.S. Brand Names Remodulin®
Generic Available No
Synonyms Treprostinil Sodium
Pharmacologic Category Vasodilator
Use Treatment of pulmonary arterial hypertension (PAH) in patients with NYHA Class II-IV symptoms to decrease exercise-associated symptoms; to diminish clinical deterioration when transitioning from epoprostenol (I.V.)
Local Anesthetic/Vasoconstrictor Precautions No information available to require special precautions
Effects on Dental Treatment No significant effects or complications reported
Common Adverse Effects
  >10%:
    Cardiovascular: Vasodilation (11%)
    Central nervous system: Headache (27%)
    Dermatologic: Rash (14%)
(Continued)

Treprostinil *(Continued)*

Gastrointestinal: Diarrhea (25%), nausea (22%)
Local: Infusion site pain (SubQ 85%, may improve after several months of therapy); infusion site reaction (SubQ 83%)
Miscellaneous: Jaw pain (13%)
1% to 10%:
Cardiovascular: Edema (9%), hypotension (4%)
Central nervous system: Dizziness (9%)
Dermatologic: Pruritus (8%)

Mechanism of Action Treprostinil is a direct dilator of both pulmonary and systemic arterial vascular beds; also inhibits platelet aggregation.

Drug Interactions
Increased Effect/Toxicity: Concomitant use of treprostinil with other agents that inhibit platelet aggregation (eg, NSAIDs, ASA, antiplatelet agents, salicylates) or promote anticoagulation (eg, warfarin) may increase the risk of bleeding.

Pharmacodynamics/Kinetics
Absorption: SubQ: Rapidly and completely
Distribution: 14 L/70 kg lean body weight
Protein binding: 91%
Metabolism: Hepatic (enzymes unknown); forms metabolites
Bioavailability: 100%
Half-life elimination: Terminal: 2-4 hours
Excretion: Urine (79% - 4% as unchanged drug, 64% as metabolites); feces (13%)

Pregnancy Risk Factor B

Treprostinil Sodium *see* Treprostinil *on page 1523*

Tretinoin and Mequinol *see* Mequinol and Tretinoin *on page 994*

Tretinoin, Fluocinolone Acetonide, and Hydroquinone *see* Fluocinolone, Hydroquinone, and Tretinoin *on page 669*

Tretinoin (Oral) *(TRET i noyn, oral)*

U.S. Brand Names Vesanoid®
Canadian Brand Names Vesanoid®
Generic Available No
Synonyms All-*trans*-Retinoic Acid; ATRA; NSC-122758; Ro 5488; tRA; *trans*-Retinoic Acid
Pharmacologic Category Antineoplastic Agent, Miscellaneous
Use Induction of remission in patients with acute promyelocytic leukemia (APL), French American British (FAB) classification M3 (including the M3 variant)
Local Anesthetic/Vasoconstrictor Precautions No information available to require special precautions
Effects on Dental Treatment Key adverse event(s) related to dental treatment: Xerostomia (normal salivary flow resumes upon discontinuation).
Common Adverse Effects Virtually all patients experience some drug-related toxicity, especially headache, fever, weakness and fatigue. These adverse effects are seldom permanent or irreversible nor do they usually require therapy interruption.
>10%:
Cardiovascular: Peripheral edema (52%), chest discomfort (32%), edema (29%), arrhythmias (23%), flushing (23%), hypotension (14%), hypertension (11%)
Central nervous system: Headache (86%), fever (83%), malaise (66%), pain (37%), dizziness (20%), anxiety (17%), insomnia (14%), depression (14%), confusion (11%)
Dermatologic: Skin/mucous membrane dryness (77%), pruritus (20%), rash (54%), alopecia (14%)
Endocrine & metabolic: Hypercholesterolemia and/or hypertriglyceridemia (60%)
Gastrointestinal: Nausea/vomiting (57%), liver function tests increased (50% to 60%), GI hemorrhage (34%), abdominal pain (31%), mucositis (26%), diarrhea (23%), constipation (17%), dyspepsia (14%), abdominal distention (11%), weight gain (23%), weight loss (17%), xerostomia, anorexia (17%)
Hematologic: Hemorrhage (60%), leukocytosis (40%), disseminated intravascular coagulation (26%)
Local: Phlebitis (11%), injection site reactions (17%)
Neuromuscular & skeletal: Bone pain (77%), myalgia (14%), paresthesia (17%)
Ocular: Visual disturbances (17%)

Otic: Earache/ear fullness (23%)

Renal: Renal insufficiency (11%)

Respiratory: Upper respiratory tract disorders (63%), dyspnea (60%), respiratory insufficiency (26%), pleural effusion (20%), pneumonia (14%), rales (14%), expiratory wheezing (14%), dry nose

Miscellaneous: Infection (58%), shivering (63%), retinoic acid-acute promyelocytic leukemia syndrome (25%), diaphoresis increased (20%)

1% to 10%:

Cardiovascular: Cerebral hemorrhage (9%), pallor (6%), cardiac failure (6%), cardiac arrest (3%), MI (3%), enlarged heart (3%), heart murmur (3%), ischemia, stroke (3%), myocarditis (3%), pericarditis (3%), pulmonary hypertension (3%), secondary cardiomyopathy (3%)

Central nervous system: Intracranial hypertension (9%), agitation (9%), hallucination (6%), agnosia (3%), aphasia (3%), cerebellar edema (3%), cerebral hemorrhage (9%), seizures (3%), coma (3%), CNS depression (3%), dysarthria (3%), encephalopathy (3%), hypotaxia (3%), light reflex absent (3%), spinal cord disorder (3%), unconsciousness (3%), dementia (3%), forgetfulness (3%), somnolence (3%), slow speech (3%), hypothermia (3%)

Dermatologic: Cellulitis (8%), photosensitivity

Endocrine & metabolic: Acidosis

Gastrointestinal: Hepatosplenomegaly (9%), hepatitis (3%), ulcer (3%)

Genitourinary: Dysuria (9%), acute renal failure (3%), micturition frequency (3%), renal tubular necrosis (3%), enlarged prostate (3%)

Hepatic: Ascites (3%), hepatitis

Neuromuscular & skeletal: Tremor (3%), leg weakness (3%), hyporeflexia, dysarthria, facial paralysis, hemiplegia, flank pain, asterixis, abnormal gait (3%), bone inflammation (3%)

Ocular: Dry eyes, visual acuity change (6%), visual field deficit (3%)

Otic: Hearing loss

Renal: Acute renal failure, renal tubular necrosis

Respiratory: Lower respiratory tract disorders (9%), pulmonary infiltration (6%), bronchial asthma (3%), pulmonary/larynx edema

Miscellaneous: Face edema

Mechanism of Action Tretinoin appears to bind one or more nuclear receptors and inhibits clonal proliferation and/or granulocyte differentiation

Drug Interactions

Cytochrome P450 Effect: Substrate (minor) of CYP2A6, 2B6, 2C8/9; **Inhibits** CYP2C8/9 (weak); **Induces** CYP2E1 (weak)

Increased Effect/Toxicity: Ketoconazole increases the mean plasma AUC of tretinoin. Concurrent use with antifibrinolytic agents (eg, aminocaproic acid, aprotinin, tranexamic acid) may increase risk of thrombosis. Concurrent use with tetracyclines may increase risk of pseudotumor cerebri.

Pharmacodynamics/Kinetics

Protein binding: >95%

Metabolism: Hepatic via CYP; primary metabolite: 4-oxo-all-*trans*-retinoic acid

Half-life elimination: Terminal: Parent drug: 0.5-2 hours

Time to peak, serum: 1-2 hours

Excretion: Urine (63%); feces (30%)

Pregnancy Risk Factor D

Tretinoin (Topical) (TRET i noyn, TOP i kal)

U.S. Brand Names Avita®; Renova®; Retin-A®; Retin-A® Micro

Canadian Brand Names Rejuva-A®; Retin-A®; Retin-A® Micro; Retinova®

Generic Available Yes: Cream, gel

Synonyms Retinoic Acid; *trans*-Retinoic Acid; Vitamin A Acid

Pharmacologic Category Retinoic Acid Derivative

Use Treatment of acne vulgaris; photodamaged skin; palliation of fine wrinkles, mottled hyperpigmentation, and tactile roughness of facial skin as part of a comprehensive skin care and sun avoidance program

Unlabeled/Investigational Use Some skin cancers

Local Anesthetic/Vasoconstrictor Precautions No information available to require special precautions

Effects on Dental Treatment No significant effects or complications reported

Common Adverse Effects

>10%: Dermatologic: Excessive dryness, erythema, scaling of the skin, pruritus

1% to 10%:

Dermatologic: Hyperpigmentation or hypopigmentation, photosensitivity, initial acne flare-up

Local: Edema, blistering, stinging

(Continued)

Tretinoin (Topical) *(Continued)*

Mechanism of Action Keratinocytes in the sebaceous follicle become less adherent which allows for easy removal; inhibits microcomedone formation and eliminates lesions already present

Drug Interactions

Cytochrome P450 Effect: Substrate (minor) of CYP2A6, 2B6, 2C8/9; **Inhibits** CYP2C8/9 (weak); **Induces** CYP2E1 (weak)

Increased Effect/Toxicity: Topical application of sulfur, benzoyl peroxide, salicylic acid, resorcinol, or any product with strong drying effects potentiates adverse reactions with tretinoin.

Photosensitizing medications (thiazides, tetracyclines, fluoroquinolones, phenothiazines, sulfonamides) augment phototoxicity and should not be used when treating palliation of fine wrinkles, mottled hyperpigmentation, and tactile roughness of facial skin.

Pharmacodynamics/Kinetics

Absorption: Minimal

Metabolism: Hepatic for the small amount absorbed

Excretion: Urine and feces

Pregnancy Risk Factor C

Trexall™ *see* Methotrexate *on page 1012*

TRH *see* Protirelin *on page 1307*

Triacetin *(trye a SEE tin)*

U.S. Brand Names Myco-Nail [OTC]

Generic Available No

Synonyms Glycerol Triacetate

Pharmacologic Category Antifungal Agent, Topical

Use Fungistat for athlete's foot and other superficial fungal infections

Local Anesthetic/Vasoconstrictor Precautions No information available to require special precautions

Effects on Dental Treatment No significant effects or complications reported

Triacin-C® [DSC] *see* Triprolidine, Pseudoephedrine, and Codeine *on page 1543*

Triaconazole *see* Terconazole *on page 1461*

Triamcinolone *(trye am SIN oh lone)*

Related Information

Respiratory Diseases *on page 1656*

Ulcerative and Erosive Disorders *on page 1712*

Related Sample Prescriptions

Mild Lichen Planus *on page 1745*

Recurrent Aphthous Stomatitis *on page 1744*

U.S. Brand Names Aristocort®; Aristocort® A; Aristospan®; Azmacort®; Kenalog®; Kenalog-10®; Kenalog-40®; Nasacort® AQ; Triderm®; Tri-Nasal®

Canadian Brand Names Aristospan®; Kenalog®; Kenalog® in Orabase; Nasacort® AQ; Oracort; Triaderm; Trinasal®

Mexican Brand Names Triamsicort®

Generic Available Yes: Cream, lotion, ointment, paste

Synonyms Triamcinolone Acetonide, Aerosol; Triamcinolone Acetonide, Parenteral; Triamcinolone Diacetate, Oral; Triamcinolone Diacetate, Parenteral; Triamcinolone Hexacetonide; Triamcinolone, Oral

Pharmacologic Category Corticosteroid, Adrenal; Corticosteroid, Inhalant (Oral); Corticosteroid, Nasal; Corticosteroid, Systemic; Corticosteroid, Topical

Dental Use Oral, topical: Adjunctive treatment and temporary relief of symptoms associated with oral inflammatory lesions and ulcerative lesions resulting from trauma

Use

Nasal inhalation: Management of seasonal and perennial allergic rhinitis in patients ≥6 years of age

Oral inhalation: Control of bronchial asthma and related bronchospastic conditions

Oral topical: Adjunctive treatment and temporary relief of symptoms associated with oral inflammatory lesions and ulcerative lesions resulting from trauma

Systemic: Adrenocortical insufficiency, rheumatic disorders, allergic states, respiratory diseases, systemic lupus erythematosus (SLE), and other diseases requiring anti-inflammatory or immunosuppressive effects

Topical: Inflammatory dermatoses responsive to steroids

Local Anesthetic/Vasoconstrictor Precautions No information available to require special precautions

Effects on Dental Treatment Key adverse event(s) related to dental treatment: Ulcerative esophagitis, perioral dermatitis, atrophy of oral mucosa, burning, and irritation.

Significant Adverse Effects

Systemic: Frequency not defined:

Cardiovascular: Angioedema, bradycardia, CHF, hypertension, myocardial rupture (following recent MI), thrombophlebitis, vasculitis

Central nervous system: Convulsions, depression, emotional instability, fever, headache, intracranial pressure increased, neuropathy, paresthesia, personality changes, vertigo

Dermatologic: Acne, allergic dermatitis, bruising, cutaneous atrophy, dry/scaly skin, ecchymoses, facial erythema, petechiae, photosensitivity, rash, striae, thin/fragile skin, wound healing impaired

Endocrine & metabolic: Adrenocortical/pituitary unresponsiveness (particularly during stress), carbohydrate tolerance decreased, cushingoid state, diabetes mellitus (manifestations of latent disease), fluid retention, growth suppression (children), hirsutism, hypokalemic alkalosis, menstrual irregularities, negative nitrogen balance, potassium loss, sodium retention

Gastrointestinal: Abdominal distention, bowel perforation, diarrhea, dyspepsia, nausea, oral *Monilia* (oral inhaler), pancreatitis, peptic ulcer, ulcerative esophagitis, weight gain

Hepatic: Hepatomegaly

Local: Skin atrophy (at the injection site)

Neuromuscular & skeletal: Calcinosis (following intra-articular or intralesional injection), Charcot-like arthropathy, femoral/humeral head aseptic necrosis, muscle mass decreased, muscle weakness, osteoporosis, pathologic fracture of long bones, steroid myopathy, tendon rupture, vertebral compression fractures

Ocular: Blindness (periocular injections), cataracts, intraocular pressure increased, exophthalmos, glaucoma, subcapsular cataract

Respiratory: Cough increased (nasal spray), epistaxis (nasal inhaler/spray), pharyngitis (nasal spray/oral inhaler), sinusitis (oral inhaler), voice alteration (oral inhaler)

Miscellaneous: Abnormal fat deposition (moon face), anaphylactoid reaction, anaphylaxis, diaphoresis increased, suppression to skin tests

Topical: Frequency not defined:

Dermatologic: Itching, allergic contact dermatitis, dryness, folliculitis, skin infection (secondary), itching, hypertrichosis, acneiform eruptions, hypopigmentation, skin maceration, skin atrophy, striae, miliaria, perioral dermatitis, atrophy of oral mucosa

Local: Burning, irritation

Dental Usual Dosing Oral inflammatory lesions/ulcers: Adults: Oral topical: Press a small dab (about ¼ inch) to the lesion until a thin film develops; a larger quantity may be required for coverage of some lesions. For optimal results, use only enough to coat the lesion with a thin film; do not rub in.

Triamcinolone Dosing

	Acetonide	Hexacetonide
Intrasynovial	5-40 mg	
Intralesional	1-30 mg (usually 1 mg per injection site); 10 mg/mL suspension usually used	Up to 0.5 mg/sq inch affected area
Sublesional	1-30 mg	
Systemic I.M.	2.5-60 mg/dose (usual adult dose: 60 mg; may repeat with 20-100 mg dose when symptoms recur)	
Intra-articular	2.5-40 mg	2-20 mg average
large joints	5-15 mg	10-20 mg
small joints	2.5-5 mg	2-6 mg
Tendon sheaths	2.5-10 mg	
Intradermal	1 mg/site	

(Continued)

Triamcinolone *(Continued)*

Dosage The lowest possible dose should be used to control the condition; when dose reduction is possible, the dose should be reduced gradually. Parenteral dose is usually ⅓ to ½ the oral dose given every 12 hours. In life-threatening situations, parenteral doses larger than the oral dose may be needed.

Injection:

Acetonide:

Intra-articular, intrabursal, tendon sheaths: Adults: Initial: Smaller joints: 2.5-5 mg, larger joints: 5-15 mg

Intradermal: Adults: Initial: 1 mg

I.M.: Range: 2.5-60 mg/day

Children 6-12 years: Initial: 40 mg

Children >12 years and Adults: Initial: 60 mg

Hexacetonide: Adults:

Intralesional, sublesional: Up to 0.5 mg/square inch of affected skin

Intra-articular: Range: 2-20 mg

Intranasal: Perennial allergic rhinitis, seasonal allergic rhinitis:

Nasal spray:

Children 6-11 years: 110 mcg/day as 1 spray in each nostril once daily.

Children ≥12 years and Adults: 220 mcg/day as 2 sprays in each nostril once daily

Nasal inhaler:

Children 6-11 years: Initial: 220 mcg/day as 2 sprays in each nostril once daily

Children ≥12 years and Adults: Initial: 220 mcg/day as 2 sprays in each nostril once daily; may increase dose to 440 mcg/day (given once daily or divided and given 2 or 4 times/day)

Oral: Adults:

Acute rheumatic carditis: Initial: 20-60 mg/day; reduce dose during maintenance therapy

Acute seasonal or perennial allergic rhinitis: 8-12 mg/day

Adrenocortical insufficiency: Range 4-12 mg/day

Bronchial asthma: 8-16 mg/day

Dermatological disorders, contact/atopic dermatitis: Initial: 8-16 mg/day

Ophthalmic disorders: 12-40 mg/day

Rheumatic disorders: Range: 8-16 mg/day

SLE: Initial: 20-32 mg/day, some patients may need initial doses ≥48 mg; reduce dose during maintenance therapy

Oral inhalation: Asthma:

Children 6-12 years: 100-200 mcg 3-4 times/day **or** 200-400 mcg twice daily; maximum dose: 1200 mcg/day

Children >12 years and Adults: 200 mcg 3-4 times/day **or** 400 mcg twice daily; maximum dose: 1600 mcg/day

Oral topical: Oral inflammatory lesions/ulcers: Press a small dab (about ¼ inch) to the lesion until a thin film develops. A larger quantity may be required for coverage of some lesions. For optimal results use only enough to coat the lesion with a thin film; do not rub in.

Topical:

Cream, Ointment: Apply thin film to affected areas 2-4 times/day

Spray: Apply to affected area 3-4 times/day

Mechanism of Action Decreases inflammation by suppression of migration of polymorphonuclear leukocytes and reversal of increased capillary permeability; suppresses the immune system by reducing activity and volume of the lymphatic system; suppresses adrenal function at high doses

Contraindications Hypersensitivity to triamcinolone or any component of the formulation; systemic fungal infections; serious infections (except septic shock or tuberculous meningitis); primary treatment of status asthmaticus; fungal, viral, or bacterial infections of the mouth or throat (oral topical formulation)

Warnings/Precautions May cause suppression of hypothalamic-pituitary-adrenal (HPA) axis, particularly in younger children or in patients receiving high doses for prolonged periods. Particular care is required when patients are transferred from systemic corticosteroids to inhaled products due to possible adrenal insufficiency or withdrawal from steroids, including an increase in allergic symptoms. Patients receiving 20 mg per day of prednisone (or equivalent) may be most susceptible. Fatalities have occurred due to adrenal insufficiency in asthmatic patients during and after transfer from systemic corticosteroids to aerosol steroids; aerosol steroids do **not** provide the systemic steroid needed to treat patients having trauma, surgery, or infections. With-drawal and discontinuation of the corticosteroid should be done slowly and carefully

Use with caution in patients with hypothyroidism, cirrhosis, nonspecific ulcerative colitis and patients at increased risk for peptic ulcer disease. Corticosteroids should be used with caution in patients with diabetes, hypertension, osteoporosis, glaucoma, cataracts, or tuberculosis. Use caution in hepatic impairment. Do not use occlusive dressings on weeping or exudative lesions and general caution with occlusive dressings should be observed; discontinue if skin irritation or contact dermatitis should occur; do not use in patients with decreased skin circulation; avoid the use of high potency steroids on the face.

Because of the risk of adverse effects, systemic corticosteroids should be used cautiously in the elderly, in the smallest possible dose, and for the shortest possible time. Azmacort® (metered dose inhaler) comes with its own spacer device attached and may be easier to use in older patients.

Controlled clinical studies have shown that orally-inhaled and intranasal corticosteroids may cause a reduction in growth velocity in pediatric patients. (In studies of orally-inhaled corticosteroids, the mean reduction in growth velocity was approximately 1 centimeter per year [range 0.3-1.8 cm per year] and appears to be related to dose and duration of exposure.) The growth of pediatric patients receiving inhaled corticosteroids, should be monitored routinely (eg, via stadiometry). To minimize the systemic effects of orally-inhaled and intranasal corticosteroids, each patient should be titrated to the lowest effective dose.

May suppress the immune system, patients may be more susceptible to infection. Use with caution in patients with systemic infections or ocular herpes simplex. Avoid exposure to chickenpox and measles. Injection suspension contains benzyl alcohol; benzyl alcohol has been associated with the "gasping syndrome" in neonates and low-birth-weight infants.

Oral topical: Discontinue if local irritation or sensitization should develop. If significant regeneration or repair of oral tissues has not occurred in seven days, re-evaluation of the etiology of the oral lesion is advised.

Drug Interactions
Decreased effect: Barbiturates, phenytoin, rifampin increase metabolism of triamcinolone; vaccine and toxoid effects may be reduced

Increased effect: Salmeterol: The addition of salmeterol has been demonstrated to improve response to inhaled corticosteroids (as compared to increasing steroid dosage).

Increased toxicity: Salicylates may increase risk of GI ulceration

Ethanol/Nutrition/Herb Interactions
Ethanol: Avoid ethanol (may enhance gastric mucosal irritation).

Food: Triamcinolone interferes with calcium absorption.

Herb/Nutraceutical: Avoid cat's claw, echinacea (have immunostimulant properties).

Dietary Considerations May be taken with food to decrease GI distress.

Pharmacodynamics/Kinetics
Duration: Oral: 8-12 hours

Absorption: Topical: Systemic

Time to peak: I.M.: 8-10 hours

Half-life elimination: Biologic: 18-36 hours

Pregnancy Risk Factor C

Lactation Excretion in breast milk unknown/use caution

Breast-Feeding Considerations It is not known if triamcinolone is excreted in breast milk, however, other corticosteroids are excreted. Prednisone and prednisolone are excreted in breast milk; the AAP considers them to be "usually compatible" with breast-feeding. Hypertension was reported in a nursing infant when a topical corticosteroid was applied to the nipples of the mother.

Dosage Forms
Aerosol for oral inhalation, as acetonide (Azmacort®): 100 mcg per actuation (20 g) [240 actuations]

Aerosol, topical, as acetonide (Kenalog®): 0.2 mg/2-second spray (63 g)

Cream, as acetonide: 0.025% (15 g, 80 g, 454 g); 0.1% (15 g, 80 g, 454 g, 2270 g); 0.5% (15 g)

Aristocort® A: 0.025% (15 g, 60 g); 0.1% (15 g, 60 g); 0.5% (15 g) [contains benzyl alcohol]

Triderm®: 0.1% (30 g, 85 g)

Injection, suspension, as acetonide:

Kenalog-10®: 10 mg/mL (5 mL) [contains benzyl alcohol; not for I.V. or I.M. use]

Kenalog-40®: 40 mg/mL (1 mL, 5 mL, 10 mL) [contains benzyl alcohol; not for I.V. or intradermal use]

(Continued)

Triamcinolone *(Continued)*

Injection, suspension, as hexacetonide (Aristospan®): 5 mg/mL (5 mL); 20 mg/mL (1 mL, 5 mL) [contains benzyl alcohol; not for I.V. use]

Lotion, as acetonide: 0.025% (60 mL); 0.1% (60 mL)

Ointment, topical, as acetonide: 0.025% (15 g, 80 g, 454 g); 0.1% (15 g, 80 g, 454 g); 0.5% (15 g)

Aristocort® A: 0.1% (15 g, 60 g)

Paste, oral, topical, as acetonide: 0.1% (5 g)

Solution, intranasal, as acetonide [spray] (Tri-Nasal®): 50 mcg/inhalation (15 mL) [120 doses]

Suspension, intranasal, as acetonide [spray] (Nasacort® AQ): 55 mcg/inhalation (16.5 g) [120 doses]

Tablet (Aristocort®): 4 mg [contains lactose and sodium benzoate]

Triamcinolone Acetonide, Aerosol *see* Triamcinolone *on page 1526*

Triamcinolone Acetonide (Dental Paste)
(trye am SIN oh lone a SEE toe nide paste)

Related Information
Triamcinolone *on page 1526*

Canadian Brand Names Oracort®

Generic Available Yes

Pharmacologic Category Anti-inflammatory Agent; Corticosteroid, Topical

Dental Use For adjunctive treatment and for the temporary relief of symptoms associated with oral inflammatory lesions and ulcerative lesions resulting from trauma

Local Anesthetic/Vasoconstrictor Precautions No information available to require special precautions

Effects on Dental Treatment No significant effects or complications reported

Significant Adverse Effects No data reported

Dental Usual Dosing Oral inflammatory lesions/ulcers: Adults: Topical: Press a small dab (about ¼ inch) to the lesion until a thin film develops. A larger quantity may be required for coverage of some lesions. For optimal results use only enough to coat the lesion with a thin film.

Dosage Press a small dab (about ¼ inch) to the lesion until a thin film develops. A larger quantity may be required for coverage of some lesions. For optimal results use only enough to coat the lesion with a thin film.

Mechanism of Action Decreases inflammation by suppression of migration of polymorphonuclear leukocytes and reversal of increased capillary permeability; suppresses the immune system by reducing activity and volume of the lymphatic system; suppresses adrenal function at high doses

Contraindications Hypersensitivity to triamcinolone or any component of the formulation; contraindicated in the presence of fungal, viral, or bacterial infections of the mouth or throat

Warnings/Precautions Patients with tuberculosis, peptic ulcer or diabetes mellitus should not be treated with any corticosteroid preparation without the advice of the patient's physician. Normal immune responses of the oral tissues are depressed in patients receiving topical corticosteroid therapy. Virulent strains of oral microorganisms may multiply without producing the usual warning symptoms of oral infections. The small amount of steroid released from the topical preparation makes systemic effects very unlikely. If local irritation or sensitization should develop, the preparation should be discontinued. If significant regeneration or repair of oral tissues has not occurred in seven days, re-evaluation of the etiology of the oral lesion is advised.

Drug Interactions No data reported

Pharmacodynamics/Kinetics
Absorption: Systemic
Half-life elimination, serum: Biological: 18-36 hours

Pregnancy Risk Factor C

Dosage Forms Paste, oral, topical, as acetonide: 0.1% (5 g)

Triamcinolone Acetonide, Parenteral *see* Triamcinolone *on page 1526*

Triamcinolone and Nystatin *see* Nystatin and Triamcinolone *on page 1134*

Triamcinolone Diacetate, Oral *see* Triamcinolone *on page 1526*

Triamcinolone Diacetate, Parenteral *see* Triamcinolone *on page 1526*

Triamcinolone Hexacetonide *see* Triamcinolone *on page 1526*

Triamcinolone, Oral *see* Triamcinolone *on page 1526*

Triaminic® Allerchews™ [OTC] *see* Loratadine *on page 946*

Triaminic® Cold and Allergy [OTC] *see* Chlorpheniramine and Pseudoephedrine *on page 325*

Triaminic® Cough [OTC] *see* Pseudoephedrine and Dextromethorphan *on page 1311*

Triaminic® Cough and Sore Throat Formula [OTC] *see* Acetaminophen, Dextromethorphan, and Pseudoephedrine *on page 44*

Triaminic® Cough & Nasal Congestion [OTC] *see* Pseudoephedrine and Dextromethorphan *on page 1311*

Triaminic® Thin Strips™ Cough and Runny Nose [OTC] *see* DiphenhydrAMINE *on page 483*

Triaminic® Thin Strips™ Long Acting Cough [OTC] *see* Dextromethorphan *on page 451*

Triamterene (trye AM ter een)

Related Information
Cardiovascular Diseases *on page 1636*
U.S. Brand Names Dyrenium®
Generic Available No
Pharmacologic Category Diuretic, Potassium-Sparing
Use Alone or in combination with other diuretics in treatment of edema and hypertension; decreases potassium excretion caused by kaliuretic diuretics
Local Anesthetic/Vasoconstrictor Precautions No information available to require special precautions
Effects on Dental Treatment No significant effects or complications reported
Common Adverse Effects 1% to 10%:
Cardiovascular: Hypotension, edema, CHF, bradycardia
Central nervous system: Dizziness, headache, fatigue
Gastrointestinal: Constipation, nausea
Respiratory: Dyspnea
Mechanism of Action Interferes with potassium/sodium exchange (active transport) in the distal tubule, cortical collecting tubule and collecting duct by inhibiting sodium, potassium-ATPase; decreases calcium excretion; increases magnesium loss
Drug Interactions
Increased Effect/Toxicity: ACE inhibitors or spironolactone can cause hyperkalemia, especially in patients with renal impairment, potassium-rich diets, or on other drugs causing hyperkalemia; avoid concurrent use or monitor closely. Potassium supplements may further increase potassium retention and cause hyperkalemia; avoid concurrent use.
Pharmacodynamics/Kinetics
Onset of action: Diuresis: 2-4 hours
Duration: 7-9 hours
Absorption: Unreliable
Pregnancy Risk Factor B (manufacturer); D (expert analysis)

Triamterene and Hydrochlorothiazide *see* Hydrochlorothiazide and Triamterene *on page 778*

Triaz® *see* Benzoyl Peroxide *on page 194*

Triaz® Cleanser *see* Benzoyl Peroxide *on page 194*

Triazolam (trye AY zoe lam)

Related Information
Sedation *on page 1727*
Related Sample Prescriptions
Sedation (Prior to Dental Treatment) *on page 1746*
U.S. Brand Names Halcion®
Canadian Brand Names Apo-Triazo®; Gen-Triazolam; Halcion®
Mexican Brand Names Halcion®
Generic Available Yes
Pharmacologic Category Hypnotic, Benzodiazepine
Dental Use Oral premedication before dental procedures
Use Short-term treatment of insomnia
Local Anesthetic/Vasoconstrictor Precautions No information available to require special precautions
Effects on Dental Treatment No significant effects or complications reported (see Dental Comment)
Significant Adverse Effects
>10%: Central nervous system: Drowsiness, anteriograde amnesia
1% to 10%:
Central nervous system: Headache, dizziness, nervousness, lightheadedness, ataxia
(Continued)

Triazolam *(Continued)*

Gastrointestinal: Nausea, vomiting

<1% (Limited to important or life-threatening): Confusion, depression, euphoria, memory impairment

Restrictions C-IV

Dental Usual Dosing Note: Onset of action is rapid, patient should be in bed when taking medication

Preprocedure sedation: Adults: Oral: 0.25 mg taken the evening before oral surgery; or 0.25 mg 1 hour before procedure

Dosage Oral (onset of action is rapid, patient should be in bed when taking medication):

Children <18 years: Dosage not established

Adults:

Hypnotic: 0.125-0.25 mg at bedtime (maximum dose: 0.5 mg/day)

Preprocedure sedation (dental): 0.25 mg taken the evening before oral surgery; or 0.25 mg 1 hour before procedure

Elderly: Insomnia (short-term use): 0.0625-0.125 mg at bedtime; maximum dose: 0.25 mg/day

Dosing adjustment/comments in hepatic impairment: Reduce dose or avoid use in cirrhosis

Mechanism of Action Binds to stereospecific benzodiazepine receptors on the postsynaptic GABA neuron at several sites within the central nervous system, including the limbic system, reticular formation. Enhancement of the inhibitory effect of GABA on neuronal excitability results by increased neuronal membrane permeability to chloride ions. This shift in chloride ions results in hyperpolarization (a less excitable state) and stabilization.

Contraindications Hypersensitivity to triazolam or any component of the formulation (cross-sensitivity with other benzodiazepines may exist); concurrent therapy with atazanavir, ketoconazole, itraconazole, nefazodone, and ritonavir; pregnancy

Warnings/Precautions Should be used only after evaluation of potential causes of sleep disturbance. Failure of sleep disturbance to resolve after 7-10 days may indicate psychiatric or medical illness. A worsening of insomnia or the emergence of new abnormalities of thought or behavior may represent unrecognized psychiatric or medical illness and requires immediate and careful evaluation. Prescription should be written for a maximum of 7-10 days and should not be prescribed in quantities exceeding a 1-month supply. Abrupt discontinuation after sustained use (generally >10 days) may cause withdrawal symptoms.

An increase in daytime anxiety may occur after as few as 10 days of continuous use, which may be related to withdrawal reaction in some patients. Anterograde amnesia may occur at a higher rate with triazolam than with other benzodiazepines. Use with caution in elderly or debilitated patients, patients with hepatic disease (including alcoholics), or renal impairment. Use with caution in patients with respiratory disease or impaired gag reflex. Avoid use in patients with sleep apnea.

Causes CNS depression (dose-related) resulting in sedation, dizziness, confusion, or ataxia which may impair physical and mental capabilities. Patients must be cautioned about performing tasks which require mental alertness (eg, operating machinery or driving). Use with caution in patients receiving other CNS depressants or psychoactive agents. Effects with other sedative drugs or ethanol may be potentiated. Benzodiazepines have been associated with falls and traumatic injury and should be used with extreme caution in patients who are at risk of these events (especially the elderly).

Use caution with potent CYP3A4 inhibitors, as they may significantly decreased the clearance of triazolam. Use caution in patients with depression, particularly if suicidal risk may be present. Use with caution in patients with a history of drug dependence. Benzodiazepines have been associated with dependence and acute withdrawal symptoms on discontinuation or reduction in dose. Acute withdrawal, including seizures, may be precipitated after administration of flumazenil to patients receiving long-term benzodiazepine therapy.

Paradoxical reactions, including hyperactive or aggressive behavior have been reported with benzodiazepines, particularly in adolescent/pediatric or psychiatric patients. Does not have analgesic, antidepressant, or antipsychotic properties.

Drug Interactions Substrate of CYP3A4 (major); **Inhibits** CYP2C8/9 (weak)

CNS depressants: Sedative effects and/or respiratory depression may be additive with CNS depressants; includes ethanol, barbiturates, narcotic analgesics, and other sedative agents; monitor for increased effect

CYP3A4 inducers: CYP3A4 inducers may decrease the levels/effects of triazolam. Example inducers include aminoglutethimide, carbamazepine, nafcillin, nevirapine, phenobarbital, phenytoin, and rifamycins.

CYP3A4 inhibitors: May increase the levels/effects of triazolam. Example inhibitors include azole antifungals, clarithromycin, diclofenac, doxycycline, erythromycin, imatinib, isoniazid, nefazodone, nicardipine, propofol, protease inhibitors, quinidine, telithromycin, and verapamil.

Isoniazid: Isoniazid may increase triazolam levels.

Levodopa: Therapeutic effects may be diminished in some patients following the addition of a benzodiazepine; limited/inconsistent data

Oral contraceptives: May decrease the clearance and increase the half-life of triazolam; monitor for increased triazolam effect

Ranitidine: Ranitidine may increase triazolam levels.

Theophylline: May partially antagonize some of the effects of benzodiazepines; monitor for decreased response; may require higher doses for sedation

Ethanol/Nutrition/Herb Interactions

Ethanol: Avoid ethanol (may increase CNS depression).

Food: Food may decrease the rate of absorption. Triazolam serum concentration may be increased by grapefruit juice; avoid concurrent use.

Herb/Nutraceutical: St John's wort may decrease levels. Avoid valerian, St John's wort, kava kava, gotu kola (may increase CNS depression).

Pharmacodynamics/Kinetics

Onset of action: Hypnotic: 15-30 minutes

Duration: 6-7 hours

Distribution: V_d: 0.8-1.8 L/kg

Protein binding: 89%

Metabolism: Extensively hepatic

Half-life elimination: 1.7-5 hours

Excretion: Urine as unchanged drug and metabolites

Pregnancy Risk Factor X

Lactation Excretion in breast milk unknown/not recommended

Breast-Feeding Considerations It is not known if triazolam is excreted in breast milk; however, other benzodiazepines are known to be excreted in breast milk. The AAP rates use of related agents as "of concern" and breast-feeding is not recommended.

Dosage Forms Tablet: 0.125 mg, 0.25 mg [contains sodium benzoate]

Dental Comment Triazolam (0.25 mg) 1 hour prior to dental procedure has been used as an oral preop sedative.

Triazolam is a benzodiazepine and is being used in dentistry as a preprocedural oral sedative. There has been recent interest in its use as an orally titratable sedative to render anxious patients at ease during difficult dental procedures. This technique has been referred to as enteral conscious sedation (ECS) and oral conscious sedation (OCS).

Triazolam has the shortest half-life of all the orally administered benzodiazepines. Although midazolam is shorter, it is used parenterally, not orally. The relatively fast onset of action (15-30 minutes) of triazolam offers an advantage in its use as an oral sedative. The clinician is reminded that no kinetic data has been reported with multiple titration doses of triazolam, a technique often used in the ECS/OCS regimen.

Selected Readings

Berthold CW, Dionne RA, and Corey SE, "Comparison of Sublingually and Orally Administered Triazolam for Premedication Before Oral Surgery," *Oral Surg Oral Med Oral Pathol Oral Radiol Endod*, 1997, 84(2):119-24.

Berthold CW, Schneider A, and Dionne RA, "Using Triazolam to Reduce Dental Anxiety," *J Am Dent Assoc*, 1993, 124(11):58-64.

Dionne R, "Oral Sedation," *Compend Contin Educ Dent*, 1998, 19(9):868-70.

Flanagan D, "Oral Triazolam Sedation in Implant Dentistry," *J Oral Implantol*, 2004, 30(2):93-7.

Goodchild JH, Feck AS, and Silverman MD, "Anxiolysis in General Dental Practice," *Dent Today*, 2003, 22(3):106-11.

Kaufman E, Hargreaves KM, and Dionne RA, "Comparison of Oral Triazolam and Nitrous Oxide With Placebo and Intravenous Diazepam for Outpatient Premedication," *Oral Surg Oral Med Oral Pathol*, 1993, 75(2):156-64.

Kurzrock M, "Triazolam and Dental Anxiety," *J Am Dent Assoc*, 1994, 125(4):358, 360.

Lieblich SE and Horswell B, "Attenuation of Anxiety in Ambulatory Oral Surgery Patients With Oral Triazolam," *J Oral Maxillofac Surg*, 1991, 49(8):792-7.

Matear DW and Clarke D, "Considerations for the Use of Oral Sedation in the Institutionalized Geriatric Patient During Dental Interventions: A Review of the Literature," *Spec Care Dentist*, 1999, 19(2):56-63.

Milgrom P, Quarnstrom FC, Longley A, et al, "The Efficacy and Memory Effects of Oral Triazolam Premedication in Highly Anxious Dental Patients," *Anesth Prog*, 1994, 41(3):70-6.

Quarnstrom F, "Should Dentists Do Oral Sedation?" *Dent Today*, 2004, 23(3):16-8.

Tribavirin *see* Ribavirin *on page 1343*

Tricalcium Phosphate *see* Calcium Phosphate (Tribasic) *on page 251*

Tricardio B *see* Folic Acid, Cyanocobalamin, and Pyridoxine *on page 697*

Tri-Chlor® see Trichloroacetic Acid on page 1534
Trichlor Fresh Pac™ see Trichloroacetic Acid on page 1534
Trichloroacetaldehyde Monohydrate see Chloral Hydrate on page 312

Trichloroacetic Acid (trye klor oh a SEE tik AS id)

U.S. Brand Names Tri-Chlor®; Trichlor Fresh Pac™
Generic Available Yes
Pharmacologic Category Keratolytic Agent
Use Chemical used in compounding agents for the treatment of warts, skin resurfacing (chemical peels)
Local Anesthetic/Vasoconstrictor Precautions No information available to require special precautions
Effects on Dental Treatment No significant effects or complications reported

Trichloromonofluoromethane and Dichlorodifluoromethane see Dichlorodifluoromethane and Trichloromonofluoromethane on page 458

Triclosan and Fluoride (trye KLOE san & FLOR ide)

Related Information
Fluoride on page 671
Periodontal Diseases on page 1705
U.S. Brand Names Colgate Total®
Generic Available No
Synonyms Fluoride and Triclosan (Dental)
Pharmacologic Category Antibacterial, Dental; Mineral, Oral (Topical)
Dental Use Anticavity, antigingivitis, antiplaque toothpaste
Use Used exclusively in dental applications
Local Anesthetic/Vasoconstrictor Precautions No information available to require special precautions
Effects on Dental Treatment No significant effects or complications reported (see Dental Comment)
Significant Adverse Effects No data reported
Dental Usual Dosing Prevention of dental caries and gingivitis: Adults: Oral: Brush teeth thoroughly after each meal or at least twice daily
Dosage Brush teeth thoroughly after each meal or at least twice daily
Mechanism of Action Triclosan is an antibacterial agent which helps to prevent gingivitis with regular use. Fluoride promotes remineralization of decalcified enamel, inhibits the cariogenic microbial process in dental plaque, and increases tooth resistance to acid dissolution
Warnings/Precautions Antigingivitis and antiplaque effects have not been determined in children <6 years of age. If an amount greater than used for brushing is swallowed, seek professional assistance of contact a poison control center immediately
Pregnancy Risk Factor No data reported
Dosage Forms
Gel, oral [toothpaste]: Triclosan 0.30% and sodium fluoride 0.24% (119 g, 170 g, 221 g)
Paste, oral [toothpaste]: Triclosan 0.30% and sodium fluoride 0.24% (119 g, 170 g, 221 g)
Dental Comment It has been shown that stannous fluoride and triclosan when formulated into a toothpaste vehicle provide plaque inhibitory effects. To provide a longer retention time of the triclosan in plaque, a polymer has been added to the toothpaste vehicle. The polymer is known as PVM/MA which stands for polyvinylmethyl ether/maleic acid copolymer, and is listed as an inactive ingredient (PVM/MA Copolymer) on the manufacturer's label. Studies have reported that the retention of triclosan in plaque (exceeding the minimal inhibitory concentration) after polymer application was 14 hours after brushing. Ongoing studies are evaluating the effects of triclosan/copolymer on alveolar bone loss. Rosling et al. have reported that the daily use of Colgate Total® reduced (1) the frequency of deep periodontal pockets and (2) the number of sites that exhibited additional probing attachment and bone loss.

Selected Readings

Binney A, Addy M, Owens J, et al, "A Comparison of Triclosan and Stannous Fluoride Toothpastes for Inhibition of Plaque Regrowth. A Crossover Study Designed to Access Carry Over," J Clin Periodontol, 1997, 24(3):166-70.
Ellwood RP, Worthington HV, Blinkhorn AS, et al, "Effect of a Triclosan/Copolymer Dentifrice on the Incidence of Periodontal Attachment Loss in Adolescents," J Clin Periodontol, 1998, 25(5):363-7.
Mandel ID, "The New Toothpastes," J Calif Dent Assoc, 1998, 26(3):186-90.
Rosling B, Wannfors B, Volpe AR, et al, "The Use of a Triclosan/Copolymer Dentifrice May Retard the Progression of Periodontitis," J Clin Periodontol, 1997, 24(12):873-80.

TriCor® *see* Fenofibrate *on page 639*
Tricosal *see* Choline Magnesium Trisalicylate *on page 335*
Triderm® *see* Triamcinolone *on page 1526*
Tridesilon® *see* Desonide *on page 437*
Tridione® *see* Trimethadione *on page 1538*

Triethanolamine Polypeptide Oleate-Condensate
(trye eth a NOLE a meen pol i PEP tide OH lee ate-KON den sate)

U.S. Brand Names Cerumenex® [DSC]
Canadian Brand Names Cerumenex®
Generic Available No
Pharmacologic Category Otic Agent, Cerumenolytic
Use Removal of ear wax (cerumen)
Local Anesthetic/Vasoconstrictor Precautions No information available to require special precautions
Effects on Dental Treatment No significant effects or complications reported
Mechanism of Action Emulsifies and disperses accumulated cerumen
Pregnancy Risk Factor C

Triethanolamine Salicylate (TROLE a meen)

U.S. Brand Names Aspercreme® [OTC]; Flex-Power [OTC]; Mobisyl® [OTC]; Myoflex® [OTC]; Sportscreme® [OTC]
Canadian Brand Names Antiphlogistine Rub A-535 No Odour; Myoflex®
Generic Available Yes: Cream
Synonyms TEAS; Triethanolamine Salicylate; Trolamine Salicylate
Pharmacologic Category Analgesic, Topical; Salicylate; Topical Skin Product
Use Relief of pain of muscular aches, rheumatism, neuralgia, sprains, arthritis on intact skin
Local Anesthetic/Vasoconstrictor Precautions No information available to require special precautions
Effects on Dental Treatment No significant effects or complications reported
Common Adverse Effects 1% to 10%:
Central nervous system: Confusion, drowsiness
Gastrointestinal: Nausea, vomiting, diarrhea
Respiratory: Hyperventilation

Triethylenethiophosphoramide *see* Thiotepa *on page 1479*

Trifluoperazine (trye floo oh PER a zeen)

Canadian Brand Names Apo-Trifluoperazine®; Novo-Trifluzine; PMS-Trifluoperazine; Terfluzine
Mexican Brand Names Flupazine®[tabs]; Stelazine®
Generic Available Yes
Synonyms Trifluoperazine Hydrochloride
Pharmacologic Category Antipsychotic Agent, Typical, Phenothiazine
Use Treatment of schizophrenia
Unlabeled/Investigational Use Management of psychotic disorders
Local Anesthetic/Vasoconstrictor Precautions Most pharmacology textbooks state that in presence of phenothiazines, systemic doses of epinephrine paradoxically decrease the blood pressure. This is the so called "epinephrine reversal" phenomenon. This has never been observed when epinephrine is given by infiltration as part of the anesthesia procedure.
Effects on Dental Treatment Key adverse event(s) related to dental treatment: Significant hypotension may occur, especially when the drug is administered parenterally; orthostatic hypotension is due to alpha-receptor blockade, the elderly are at greater risk for orthostatic hypotension.

Tardive dyskinesia: Prevalence rate may be 40% in elderly; development of the syndrome and the irreversible nature are proportional to duration and total cumulative dose over time. Extrapyramidal reactions are more common in elderly with up to 50% developing these reactions after 60 years of age. Drug-induced Parkinson's syndrome occurs often; akathisia is the most common extrapyramidal reaction in elderly.
Common Adverse Effects Frequency not defined.
Cardiovascular: Hypotension, orthostatic hypotension, cardiac arrest
(Continued)

Trifluoperazine *(Continued)*

Central nervous system: Extrapyramidal signs (pseudoparkinsonism, akathisia, dystonias, tardive dyskinesia), dizziness, headache, neuroleptic malignant syndrome (NMS), impairment of temperature regulation, lowering of seizure threshold

Dermatologic: Increased sensitivity to sun, rash, discoloration of skin (blue-gray), photosensitivity

Endocrine & metabolic: Changes in menstrual cycle, libido (changes in), breast pain, hyperglycemia, hypoglycemia, gynecomastia, lactation, galactorrhea

Gastrointestinal: Constipation, weight gain, nausea, vomiting, stomach pain, xerostomia

Genitourinary: Difficulty in urination, ejaculatory disturbances, urinary retention, priapism

Hematologic: Agranulocytosis, leukopenia, pancytopenia, thrombocytopenic purpura, eosinophilia, hemolytic anemia, aplastic anemia

Hepatic: Cholestatic jaundice, hepatotoxicity

Neuromuscular & skeletal: Tremor

Ocular: Pigmentary retinopathy, cornea and lens changes

Respiratory: Nasal congestion

Mechanism of Action Trifluoperazine is a piperazine phenothiazine antipsychotic which blocks postsynaptic mesolimbic dopaminergic receptors in the brain; exhibits alpha-adrenergic blocking effect and depresses the release of hypothalamic and hypophyseal hormones

Drug Interactions

Cytochrome P450 Effect: Substrate of CYP1A2 (major)

Increased Effect/Toxicity: CYP1A2 inhibitors may increase the levels/effects of trifluoperazine; example inhibitors include amiodarone, ciprofloxacin, fluvoxamine, ketoconazole, norfloxacin, ofloxacin, and rofecoxib. Trifluoperazine's effects on CNS depression may be additive when trifluoperazine is combined with CNS depressants (narcotic analgesics, ethanol, barbiturates, cyclic antidepressants, antihistamines, or sedative-hypnotics). Trifluoperazine may increase the effects/toxicity of anticholinergics, antihypertensives, lithium (rare neurotoxicity), trazodone, or valproic acid. Concurrent use with TCA may produce increased toxicity or altered therapeutic response. Chloroquine and propranolol may increase trifluoperazine concentrations. Hypotension may occur when trifluoperazine is combined with epinephrine. May increase the risk of arrhythmia when combined with antiarrhythmics, cisapride, pimozide, sparfloxacin, or other drugs which prolong QT interval. Metoclopramide may increase risk of extrapyramidal symptoms (EPS). Acetylcholinesterase inhibitors (central) may increase the risk of antipsychotic-related EPS.

Decreased Effect: CYP1A2 inducers may decrease the levels/effects of trifluoperazine; example inducers include aminoglutethimide, carbamazepine, phenobarbital, and rifampin. Phenothiazines inhibit the effects of levodopa, guanadrel, guanethidine, and bromocriptine. Benztropine (and other anticholinergics) may inhibit the therapeutic response to trifluoperazine and excess anticholinergic effects may occur. Cigarette smoking may enhance the hepatic metabolism of trifluoperazine. Trifluoperazine and possibly other low potency antipsychotics may reverse the pressor effects of epinephrine.

Pharmacodynamics/Kinetics

Metabolism: Extensively hepatic

Half-life elimination: >24 hours with chronic use

Pregnancy Risk Factor C

Trifluoperazine Hydrochloride *see* Trifluoperazine *on page 1535*

Trifluorothymidine *see* Trifluridine *on page 1536*

Trifluridine *(trye FLURE i deen)*

Related Information

Systemic Viral Diseases *on page 1675*

U.S. Brand Names Viroptic®

Canadian Brand Names SAB-Trifluridine; Viroptic®

Generic Available Yes

Synonyms F_3T; Trifluorothymidine

Pharmacologic Category Antiviral Agent, Ophthalmic

Use Treatment of primary keratoconjunctivitis and recurrent epithelial keratitis caused by herpes simplex virus types I and II

Local Anesthetic/Vasoconstrictor Precautions No information available to require special precautions

Effects on Dental Treatment No significant effects or complications reported

Mechanism of Action Interferes with viral replication by incorporating into viral DNA in place of thymidine, inhibiting thymidylate synthetase resulting in the formation of defective proteins

Pregnancy Risk Factor C

Triglide™ see Fenofibrate on page 639

Triglycerides, Medium Chain see Medium Chain Triglycerides on page 972

Trihexyphenidyl (trye heks ee FEN i dil)

Canadian Brand Names Apo-Trihex®
Mexican Brand Names Hipokinon®
Generic Available Yes
Synonyms Artane; Benzhexol Hydrochloride; Trihexyphenidyl Hydrochloride
Pharmacologic Category Anti-Parkinson's Agent, Anticholinergic; Anticholinergic Agent
Use Adjunctive treatment of Parkinson's disease; treatment of drug-induced extrapyramidal symptoms
Local Anesthetic/Vasoconstrictor Precautions No information available to require special precautions
Effects on Dental Treatment Key adverse event(s) related to dental treatment: Xerostomia, dry throat (normal salivary flow resumes upon discontinuation). Prolonged xerostomia may contribute to discomfort and dental disease (ie, caries, periodontal disease, and oral candidiasis).
Common Adverse Effects Frequency not defined.
    Cardiovascular: Tachycardia
    Central nervous system: Confusion, agitation, euphoria, drowsiness, headache, dizziness, nervousness, delusions, hallucinations, paranoia
    Dermatologic: Dry skin, increased sensitivity to light, rash
    Gastrointestinal: Constipation, xerostomia, dry throat, ileus, nausea, vomiting, parotitis
    Genitourinary: Urinary retention
    Neuromuscular & skeletal: Weakness
    Ocular: Blurred vision, mydriasis, increase in intraocular pressure, glaucoma, blindness (long-term use in narrow-angle glaucoma)
    Respiratory: Dry nose
    Miscellaneous: Diaphoresis (decreased)
Mechanism of Action Exerts a direct inhibitory effect on the parasympathetic nervous system. It also has a relaxing effect on smooth musculature; exerted both directly on the muscle itself and indirectly through parasympathetic nervous system (inhibitory effect)
Drug Interactions
    Increased Effect/Toxicity: Central and/or peripheral anticholinergic syndrome can occur when administered with amantadine, rimantadine, narcotic analgesics, phenothiazines and other antipsychotics (especially with high anticholinergic activity), tricyclic antidepressants, MAO inhibitors, quinidine and some other antiarrhythmics, and antihistamines. CNS depressants (cannabinoids, ethanol, barbiturates, and narcotic analgesics) may have additive effects with trihexyphenidyl; an abuse potential exits.

    Decreased Effect: May increase gastric degradation of levodopa and decrease the amount of levodopa absorbed by delaying gastric emptying; the opposite may be true for digoxin. Therapeutic effects of cholinergic agents (tacrine, donepezil, rivastigmine, galantamine) and neuroleptics may be antagonized.

Pharmacodynamics/Kinetics
    Onset of action: Peak effect: ~1 hour
    Half-life elimination: 3.3-4.1 hours
    Time to peak, serum: 1-1.5 hours
    Excretion: Primarily urine
Pregnancy Risk Factor C

Trihexyphenidyl Hydrochloride see Trihexyphenidyl on page 1537

Tri-K® see Potassium Acetate, Potassium Bicarbonate, and Potassium Citrate on page 1257

Trileptal® see Oxcarbazepine on page 1159

Tri-Levlen® see Ethinyl Estradiol and Levonorgestrel on page 602

Trilisate® [DSC] see Choline Magnesium Trisalicylate on page 335

Tri-Luma™ see Fluocinolone, Hydroquinone, and Tretinoin on page 669

TriLyte™ see Polyethylene Glycol-Electrolyte Solution on page 1253

Trimazide [DSC] see Trimethobenzamide on page 1538

Trimethadione (trye meth a DYE one)

U.S. Brand Names Tridione®
Generic Available No
Synonyms Troxidone
Pharmacologic Category Anticonvulsant, Oxazolidinedione
Use Control absence (petit mal) seizures refractory to other drugs
Local Anesthetic/Vasoconstrictor Precautions No information available to require special precautions
Effects on Dental Treatment No significant effects or complications reported
Mechanism of Action An oxazolidinedione with anticonvulsant sedative properties; elevates the cortical and basal seizure thresholds, and reduces the synaptic response to low frequency impulses
Pregnancy Risk Factor D

Trimethobenzamide (trye meth oh BEN za mide)

U.S. Brand Names Tebamide™; Tigan®; Trimazide [DSC]
Canadian Brand Names Tigan®
Generic Available Yes
Synonyms Trimethobenzamide Hydrochloride
Pharmacologic Category Anticholinergic Agent; Antiemetic
Use Treatment of nausea and vomiting
Local Anesthetic/Vasoconstrictor Precautions No information available to require special precautions
Effects on Dental Treatment No significant effects or complications reported
Common Adverse Effects Frequency not defined.
  Cardiovascular: Hypotension
  Central nervous system: Coma, depression, disorientation, dizziness, drowsiness, EPS, headache, opisthotonos, Parkinson-like syndrome, seizure
  Gastrointestinal: Diarrhea
  Hematologic: Blood dyscrasias
  Hepatic: Jaundice
  Neuromuscular & skeletal: Muscle cramps
  Ocular: Blurred vision
  Miscellaneous: Hypersensitivity reactions
Mechanism of Action Acts centrally to inhibit the medullary chemoreceptor trigger zone
Pharmacodynamics/Kinetics
  Onset of action: Antiemetic: Oral: 10-40 minutes; I.M.: 15-35 minutes
  Duration: 3-4 hours
  Absorption: Rectal: ~60%
  Bioavailability: Oral: 60% to 100%
  Half-life elimination: 7-9 hours
  Time to peak: Oral: 45 minutes; I.M.: 30 minutes
  Excretion: Urine (30% to 50%)
Pregnancy Risk Factor C

Trimethobenzamide Hydrochloride *see* Trimethobenzamide *on page 1538*

Trimethoprim (trye METH oh prim)

U.S. Brand Names Primsol®; Proloprim®
Canadian Brand Names Apo-Trimethoprim®
Generic Available Yes: Tablet
Synonyms TMP
Pharmacologic Category Antibiotic, Miscellaneous
Use Treatment of urinary tract infections due to susceptible strains of *E. coli*, *P. mirabilis*, *K. pneumoniae*, *Enterobacter* sp and coagulase-negative *Staphylococcus* including *S. saprophyticus*; acute otitis media in children; acute exacerbations of chronic bronchitis in adults; in combination with other agents for treatment of toxoplasmosis, *Pneumocystis carinii*; treatment of superficial ocular infections involving the conjunctiva and cornea
Local Anesthetic/Vasoconstrictor Precautions No information available to require special precautions
Effects on Dental Treatment No significant effects or complications reported
Common Adverse Effects Frequency not defined.
  Central nervous system: Aseptic meningitis (rare), fever
  Dermatologic: Maculopapular rash (3% to 7% at 200 mg/day; incidence higher with larger daily doses), erythema multiforme (rare), exfoliative dermatitis

(rare), pruritus (common), phototoxic skin eruptions, Stevens-Johnson syndrome (rare), toxic epidermal necrolysis (rare)

Endocrine & metabolic: Hyperkalemia, hyponatremia

Gastrointestinal: Epigastric distress, glossitis, nausea, vomiting

Hematologic: Leukopenia, megaloblastic anemia, methemoglobinemia, neutropenia, thrombocytopenia

Hepatic: Liver enzyme elevation, cholestatic jaundice (rare)

Renal: BUN and creatinine increased

Miscellaneous: Anaphylaxis, hypersensitivity reactions

Mechanism of Action Inhibits folic acid reduction to tetrahydrofolate, and thereby inhibits microbial growth

Drug Interactions

Cytochrome P450 Effect: Substrate (major) of CYP2C8/9, 3A4; **Inhibits** CYP2C8/9 (moderate)

Increased Effect/Toxicity: Increased effect/toxicity/levels of phenytoin. Concurrent use with ACE inhibitors increases risk of hyperkalemia. Increased myelosuppression with methotrexate. May increase levels of digoxin. Concurrent use with dapsone may increase levels of dapsone and trimethoprim. Concurrent use with procainamide may increase levels of procainamide and trimethoprim. Trimethoprim may increase the levels/effects of amiodarone, fluoxetine, glimepiride, glipizide, nateglinide, phenytoin, pioglitazone, rosiglitazone, sertraline, warfarin, and other CYP2C8/9 substrates.

Decreased Effect: The levels/effects of trimethoprim may be decreased by aminoglutethimide, carbamazepine, nafcillin, nevirapine, phenobarbital, phenytoin, rifampin, rifapentine, secobarbital, and other CYP2C8/9 or 3A4 inducers.

Pharmacodynamics/Kinetics

Absorption: Readily and extensive

Distribution: Widely into body tissues and fluids (middle ear, prostate, bile, aqueous humor, CSF); crosses placenta; enters breast milk

Protein binding: 42% to 46%

Metabolism: Partially hepatic

Half-life elimination: 8-14 hours; prolonged with renal impairment

Time to peak, serum: 1-4 hours

Excretion: Urine (60% to 80%) as unchanged drug

Pregnancy Risk Factor C

Trimethoprim and Polymyxin B
(trye METH oh prim & pol i MIKS in bee)

Related Information

Polymyxin B *on page 1253*

Trimethoprim *on page 1538*

U.S. Brand Names Polytrim®

Canadian Brand Names PMS-Polytrimethoprim; Polytrim™

Generic Available Yes

Synonyms Polymyxin B and Trimethoprim

Pharmacologic Category Antibiotic, Ophthalmic

Use Treatment of surface ocular bacterial conjunctivitis and blepharoconjunctivitis

Local Anesthetic/Vasoconstrictor Precautions No information available to require special precautions

Effects on Dental Treatment No significant effects or complications reported

Pregnancy Risk Factor C

Trimethoprim and Sulfamethoxazole *see* Sulfamethoxazole and Trimethoprim *on page 1425*

Trimetrexate (tri me TREKS ate)

U.S. Brand Names NeuTrexin®

Generic Available No

Synonyms NSC-352122; Trimetrexate Glucuronate

Pharmacologic Category Antineoplastic Agent, Miscellaneous

Use Alternative therapy for the treatment of moderate-to-severe *Pneumocystis jiroveci* pneumonia (PCP) in immunocompromised patients, including patients with acquired immunodeficiency syndrome (AIDS), who are intolerant of, or are refractory to, sulfamethoxazole/trimethoprim therapy or for whom sulfamethoxazole/trimethoprim and pentamidine are contraindicated

(Continued)

Trimetrexate *(Continued)*

Unlabeled/Investigational Use Treatment of nonsmall cell lung cancer, metastatic colorectal cancer, metastatic head and neck cancer, pancreatic adenocarcinoma, cutaneous T-cell lymphoma

Local Anesthetic/Vasoconstrictor Precautions No information available to require special precautions

Effects on Dental Treatment Key adverse event(s) related to dental treatment: Stomatitis.

Common Adverse Effects
>10%:
Hematologic: Neutropenia (30%)
Hepatic: AST increased (14%), ALT increased (11%)
1% to 10%:
Central nervous system: Fever (8%), confusion (3%), fatigue (2%)
Dermatologic: Rash/pruritus (6%)
Endocrine & metabolic: Hyponatremia (5%), hypocalcemia (2%)
Gastrointestinal: Nausea/vomiting (5%), stomatitis
Hematologic: Thrombocytopenia (10%), anemia (7%)
Hepatic: Alkaline phosphatase increased (5%), bilirubin increased (2%)
Neuromuscular & skeletal: Peripheral neuropathy
Miscellaneous: Flu-like illness; hypersensitivity/allergic reactions (chills, rigors); anaphylactoid reactions (acute hypotension, loss of consciousness)

Mechanism of Action Trimetrexate is a folate antimetabolite that inhibits DNA synthesis by inhibition of dihydrofolate reductase (DHFR); DHFR inhibition reduces the formation of reduced folates and thymidylate synthetase, resulting in inhibition of purine and thymidylic acid synthesis.

Drug Interactions
Increased Effect/Toxicity: Zidovudine may increase the myelotoxicity of trimetrexate; discontinue zidovudine during trimetrexate treatment. Trimetrexate may increase toxicity (infections) of live virus vaccines.

Pharmacodynamics/Kinetics
Distribution: V_d: 0.62 L/kg
Protein binding: 80% to 90% (concentration dependent)
Metabolism: Extensively hepatic: O-demethylation followed by conjugation to glucuronide or sulfate (major); N-demethylation and oxidation (minor)
Half-life elimination: 9-18 hours (11 hours with leucovorin)
Excretion: Urine (10% to 40% as unchanged drug); feces (<1% to 8%)

Pregnancy Risk Factor D

Trimetrexate Glucuronate *see* Trimetrexate *on page 1539*

Trimipramine *(trye MI pra meen)*

U.S. Brand Names Surmontil®
Canadian Brand Names Apo-Trimip®; Nu-Trimipramine; Rhotrimine®; Surmontil®
Generic Available No
Synonyms Trimipramine Maleate
Pharmacologic Category Antidepressant, Tricyclic (Tertiary Amine)
Use Treatment of depression

Local Anesthetic/Vasoconstrictor Precautions Use with caution; epinephrine and levonordefrin have been shown to have an increased pressor response in combination with TCAs

Effects on Dental Treatment Key adverse event(s) related to dental treatment: Xerostomia (normal salivary flow resumes upon discontinuation). Long-term treatment with TCAs, such as trimipramine, increases the risk of caries by reducing salivation and salivary buffer capacity.

Common Adverse Effects Frequency not defined.
Cardiovascular: Arrhythmias, hyper-/hypotension, tachycardia, palpitation, heart block, stroke, MI
Central nervous system: Headache, exacerbation of psychosis, confusion, delirium, hallucinations, nervousness, restlessness, delusions, agitation, insomnia, nightmares, anxiety, seizure, drowsiness
Dermatologic: Photosensitivity, rash, petechiae, itching
Endocrine & metabolic: Sexual dysfunction, breast enlargement, galactorrhea, SIADH
Gastrointestinal: Xerostomia, constipation, increased appetite, nausea, unpleasant taste, weight gain, diarrhea, heartburn, vomiting, anorexia, trouble with gums, decreased lower esophageal sphincter tone may cause GE reflux
Genitourinary: Difficult urination, urinary retention, testicular edema
Hematologic: Agranulocytosis, eosinophilia, purpura, thrombocytopenia

Hepatic: Cholestatic jaundice, increased liver enzymes

Neuromuscular & skeletal: Tremors, numbness, tingling, paresthesia, incoordination, ataxia, peripheral neuropathy, extrapyramidal symptoms

Ocular: Blurred vision, eye pain, disturbances in accommodation, mydriasis, increased intraocular pressure

Otic: Tinnitus

Miscellaneous: Allergic reactions

Restrictions A medication guide concerning the use of antidepressants in children and teenagers can be found on the FDA website at http://www.fda.gov/cder/Offices/ODS/labeling.htm. It should be dispensed to parents or guardians of children and teenagers receiving this medication.

Mechanism of Action Increases the synaptic concentration of serotonin and/or norepinephrine in the central nervous system by inhibition of their reuptake by the presynaptic neuronal membrane

Drug Interactions

Cytochrome P450 Effect: Substrate (major) of CYP2C19, 2D6, 3A4

Increased Effect/Toxicity: Pressor response to I.V. epinephrine, norepinephrine, and phenylephrine may be enhanced in patients receiving TCAs (**Note:** Effect is unlikely with epinephrine or levonordefrin dosages typically administered as infiltration in combination with local anesthetics). Trimipramine increases the effects of amphetamines, anticholinergics, other CNS depressants (sedatives, hypnotics, or ethanol), chlorpropamide, tolazamide, and warfarin. When used with MAO inhibitors, hyperpyrexia, hypertension, tachycardia, confusion, seizures, and **deaths have been reported** (serotonin syndrome). Serotonin syndrome has also been reported with ritonavir (rare).

CYP2C19 inhibitors may increase the levels/effects of trimipramine; example inhibitors include delavirdine, fluconazole, fluvoxamine, gemfibrozil, isoniazid, omeprazole, and ticlopidine. CYP2D6 inhibitors may increase the levels/effects of trimipramine; example inhibitors include chlorpromazine, delavirdine, fluoxetine, miconazole, paroxetine, pergolide, quinidine, quinine, ritonavir, and ropinirole. CYP3A4 inhibitors may increase the levels/effects of trimipramine; example inhibitors include azole antifungals, clarithromycin, diclofenac, doxycycline, erythromycin, imatinib, isoniazid, nefazodone, nicardipine, propofol, protease inhibitors, quinidine, telithromycin, and verapamil. Use of lithium with a TCA may increase the risk for neurotoxicity. Phenothiazines may increase concentration of some TCAs and TCAs may increase concentration of phenothiazines. Combined use of beta-agonists or drugs which prolong QT$_c$ (including quinidine, procainamide, disopyramide, cisapride, sparfloxacin, gatifloxacin, moxifloxacin) with TCAs may predispose patients to cardiac arrhythmias.

Decreased Effect: CYP2C19 inducers may decrease the levels/effects of trimipramine; example inducers include aminoglutethimide, carbamazepine, phenytoin, and rifampin. Trimipramine inhibits the antihypertensive response to bethanidine, clonidine, debrisoquin, guanadrel, guanethidine, guanabenz, and guanfacine. Cholestyramine and colestipol may bind TCAs and reduce their absorption; monitor for altered response. CYP3A4 inducers may decrease the levels/effects of trimipramine; example inducers include aminoglutethimide, carbamazepine, nafcillin, nevirapine, phenobarbital, phenytoin, and rifamycins.

Pharmacodynamics/Kinetics

Distribution: V$_d$: 17-48 L/kg

Protein binding: 95%; free drug: 3% to 7%

Metabolism: Hepatic; significant first-pass effect

Bioavailability: 18% to 63%

Half-life elimination: 16-40 hours

Excretion: Urine

Pregnancy Risk Factor C

Trimipramine Maleate *see* Trimipramine *on page 1540*

Trimox® *see* Amoxicillin *on page 106*

Tri-Nasal® *see* Triamcinolone *on page 1526*

TriNessa™ *see* Ethinyl Estradiol and Norgestimate *on page 613*

Tri-Norinyl® *see* Ethinyl Estradiol and Norethindrone *on page 608*

Trinsicon® *see* Vitamin B Complex Combinations *on page 1581*

Triostat® *see* Liothyronine *on page 934*

Tripelennamine (tri pel ENN a meen)

U.S. Brand Names PBZ®; PBZ-SR®

Generic Available Yes

(Continued)

Tripelennamine *(Continued)*

Synonyms Tripelennamine Citrate; Tripelennamine Hydrochloride

Pharmacologic Category Antihistamine

Use Perennial and seasonal allergic rhinitis and other allergic symptoms including urticaria

Local Anesthetic/Vasoconstrictor Precautions No information available to require special precautions

Effects on Dental Treatment Key adverse event(s) related to dental treatment: Xerostomia and changes in salivation (normal salivary flow resumes upon discontinuation). Chronic use of antihistamines will inhibit salivary flow, particularly in elderly patients; this may contribute to periodontal disease and oral discomfort.

Common Adverse Effects

>10%:

Central nervous system: Slight to moderate drowsiness

Respiratory: Thickening of bronchial secretions

1% to 10%:

Central nervous system: Headache, fatigue, nervousness, dizziness

Gastrointestinal: Appetite increase, weight gain, nausea, diarrhea, abdominal pain, xerostomia

Neuromuscular & skeletal: Arthralgia

Respiratory: Pharyngitis

Mechanism of Action Competes with histamine for H_1-receptor sites on effector cells in the gastrointestinal tract, blood vessels, and respiratory tract

Drug Interactions

Cytochrome P450 Effect: Inhibits CYP2D6 (moderate)

Increased Effect/Toxicity: Increased effect/toxicity with alcohol, CNS depressants, and MAO inhibitors. Tripelennamine may increase the levels/effects of amphetamines, beta-blockers, dextromethorphan, fluoxetine, lidocaine, mirtazapine, nefazodone, paroxetine, risperidone, ritonavir, thioridazine, tricyclic antidepressants, venlafaxine, and other CYP2D6 substrates.

Decreased Effect: Tripelennamine may decrease the levels/effects of CYP2D6 prodrug substrates (eg, codeine, hydrocodone, oxycodone, tramadol).

Pharmacodynamics/Kinetics

Onset of action: Antihistaminic: 15-30 minutes

Duration: 4-6 hours (up to 8 hours with PBZ-SR®)

Metabolism: Almost completely hepatic

Excretion: Urine

Pregnancy Risk Factor B

Tripelennamine Citrate *see* Tripelennamine *on page 1541*

Tripelennamine Hydrochloride *see* Tripelennamine *on page 1541*

Triphasil® *see* Ethinyl Estradiol and Levonorgestrel *on page 602*

Triple Antibiotic *see* Bacitracin, Neomycin, and Polymyxin B *on page 176*

Triple Sulfa *see* Sulfabenzamide, Sulfacetamide, and Sulfathiazole *on page 1423*

Tri-Previfem™ *see* Ethinyl Estradiol and Norgestimate *on page 613*

Triprolidine and Pseudoephedrine
(trye PROE li deen & soo doe e FED rin)

Related Information

Pseudoephedrine *on page 1309*

U.S. Brand Names Actifed® Cold and Allergy [OTC]; Allerfrim® [OTC]; Aphedrid™ [OTC]; Aprodine® [OTC]; Genac® [OTC]; Silafed® [OTC]; Sudafed® Sinus Nighttime [OTC]; Tri-Sudo® [OTC]

Canadian Brand Names Actifed®

Generic Available Yes

Synonyms Pseudoephedrine and Triprolidine

Pharmacologic Category Alpha/Beta Agonist; Antihistamine

Use Temporary relief of nasal congestion, decongest sinus openings, running nose, sneezing, itching of nose or throat and itchy, watery eyes due to common cold, hay fever, or other upper respiratory allergies

Local Anesthetic/Vasoconstrictor Precautions Use with caution since pseudoephedrine is a sympathomimetic amine which could interact with epinephrine to cause a pressor response

Effects on Dental Treatment Key adverse event(s) related to dental treatment: Pseudoephedrine: Xerostomia (normal salivary flow resumes upon discontinuation). Chronic use of antihistamines will inhibit salivary flow, particularly in elderly patients; this may contribute to periodontal disease and oral discomfort.

Common Adverse Effects Frequency not defined.

Cardiovascular: Tachycardia

Central nervous system: Drowsiness, nervousness, insomnia, transient stimulation, headache, fatigue, dizziness

Respiratory: Thickening of bronchial secretions, pharyngitis

Gastrointestinal: Appetite increase, weight gain, nausea, diarrhea, abdominal pain, xerostomia

Genitourinary: Dysuria

Neuromuscular & skeletal: Arthralgia, weakness

Miscellaneous: Diaphoresis

Mechanism of Action Refer to Pseudoephedrine monograph

Triprolidine is a member of the propylamine (alkylamine) chemical class of H_1-antagonist antihistamines. As such, it is considered to be relatively less sedating than traditional antihistamines of the ethanolamine, phenothiazine, and ethylenediamine classes of antihistamines. Triprolidine has a shorter half-life and duration of action than most of the other alkylamine antihistamines. Like all H_1-antagonist antihistamines, the mechanism of action of triprolidine is believed to involve competitive blockade of H_1-receptor sites resulting in the inability of histamine to combine with its receptor sites and exert its usual effects on target cells. Antihistamines do not interrupt any effects of histamine which have already occurred. Therefore, these agents are used more successfully in the prevention rather than the treatment of histamine-induced reactions.

Drug Interactions

Cytochrome P450 Effect: Triprolidine: **Inhibits** CYP2D6 (weak)

Increased Effect/Toxicity: Increased toxicity with MAO inhibitors or drugs with MAO inhibiting activity such as linezolid or furazolidone (hypertensive crisis). May increase toxicity of sympathomimetics, CNS depressants, and alcohol.

Decreased Effect: Decreased effect of guanethidine, reserpine, methyldopa.

Pharmacodynamics/Kinetics See Pseudoephedrine monograph.

Pregnancy Risk Factor C

Triprolidine, Codeine, and Pseudoephedrine see Triprolidine, Pseudoephedrine, and Codeine on page 1543

Triprolidine, Pseudoephedrine, and Codeine
(trye PROE li deen, soo doe e FED rin, & KOE deen)

Related Information

Codeine on page 385

Pseudoephedrine on page 1309

U.S. Brand Names Triacin-C® [DSC]

Canadian Brand Names CoActifed®; Covan®; ratio-Cotridin

Generic Available No

Synonyms Codeine, Pseudoephedrine, and Triprolidine; Codeine, Triprolidine, and Pseudoephedrine; Pseudoephedrine, Codeine, and Triprolidine; Pseudoephedrine, Triprolidine, and Codeine; Triprolidine, Codeine, and Pseudoephedrine

Pharmacologic Category Antihistamine/Decongestant/Antitussive

Use Symptomatic relief of upper respiratory symptoms and cough

Local Anesthetic/Vasoconstrictor Precautions Use with caution since pseudoephedrine is a sympathomimetic amine which could interact with epinephrine to cause a pressor response

Effects on Dental Treatment Key adverse event(s) related to dental treatment: Pseudoephedrine: Xerostomia (normal salivary flow resumes upon discontinuation).

Common Adverse Effects Frequency not defined.

Cardiovascular: Hypotension

Central nervous system: Sedation, dizziness, drowsiness, increased ICP, lightheadedness, dysphoria, euphoria, headache, agitation, hallucinations, seizure, respiratory depression

Dermatologic: Pruritus, rash

Gastrointestinal: Constipation, nausea, vomiting, anorexia, xerostomia, taste disturbance, biliary tract spasm

Genitourinary: Urinary retention, urinary tract spasm

Neuromuscular & skeletal: Muscle tremor, paresthesia, muscular rigidity (rare)

Ocular: Blurred vision, nystagmus

(Continued)

Triprolidine, Pseudoephedrine, and Codeine
(Continued)

Miscellaneous: Diaphoresis, physical or psychological dependence with continued use, withdrawal syndrome

Restrictions C-V (CDSA-I)

Drug Interactions

Cytochrome P450 Effect:

Triprolidine: **Inhibits** CYP2D6 (weak)

Codeine: **Substrate** of CYP2D6 (major), 3A4 (minor); **Inhibits** CYP2D6 (weak)

Pharmacodynamics/Kinetics See Pseudoephedrine and Codeine monographs.

Pregnancy Risk Factor C

TripTone® [OTC] see DimenhyDRINATE on page 481

Triptoraline see Triptorelin on page 1544

Triptorelin (trip toe REL in)

U.S. Brand Names Trelstar™ Depot; Trelstar™ LA

Canadian Brand Names Trelstar™ Depot

Generic Available No

Synonyms AY-25650; CL-118,532; D-Trp(6)-LHRH; Triptoraline; Triptorelin Pamoate; Tryptoreline

Pharmacologic Category Gonadotropin Releasing Hormone Agonist

Use Palliative treatment of advanced prostate cancer as an alternative to orchiectomy or estrogen administration

Unlabeled/Investigational Use Treatment of endometriosis, growth hormone deficiency, hyperandrogenism, *in vitro* fertilization, ovarian carcinoma, pancreatic carcinoma, precocious puberty, uterine leiomyomata

Local Anesthetic/Vasoconstrictor Precautions No information available to require special precautions

Effects on Dental Treatment No significant effects or complications reported

Common Adverse Effects As reported with Trelstar™ Depot and Trelstar™ LA; frequency of effect may vary by product:

>10%:

Central nervous system: Headache (30% to 60%)

Endocrine & metabolic: Hot flashes (95% to 100%), glucose increased, hemoglobin decreased, RBC count decreased

Hepatic: Alkaline phosphatase increased, ALT increased, AST increased

Neuromuscular & skeletal: Skeletal pain (12% to 13%)

Renal: BUN increased

1% to 10%:

Cardiovascular: Leg edema (6%), hypertension (4%), chest pain (2%), peripheral edema (1%)

Central nervous system: Dizziness (1% to 3%), pain (2% to 3%), emotional lability (1%), fatigue (2%), insomnia (2%)

Dermatologic: Rash (2%), pruritus (1%)

Endocrine & metabolic: Alkaline phosphatase increased (2%), breast pain (2%), gynecomastia (2%), libido decreased (2%), tumor flare (8%)

Gastrointestinal: Nausea (3%), anorexia (2%), constipation (2%), dyspepsia (2%), vomiting (2%), abdominal pain (1%), diarrhea (1%)

Genitourinary: Dysuria (5%), impotence (2% to 7%), urinary retention (1%), urinary tract infection (1%)

Hematologic: Anemia (1%)

Local: Injection site pain (4%)

Neuromuscular & skeletal: Leg pain (2% to 5%), back pain (3%), arthralgia (2%), leg cramps (2%), myalgia (1%), weakness (1%)

Ocular: Conjunctivitis (1%), eye pain (1%)

Respiratory: Cough (2%), dyspnea (1%), pharyngitis (1%)

Postmarketing and/or case reports: Anaphylaxis, angioedema, hypersensitivity reactions, spinal cord compression, renal dysfunction

Mechanism of Action Causes suppression of ovarian and testicular steroidogenesis due to decreased levels of LH and FSH with subsequent decrease in testosterone (male) and estrogen (female) levels. After chronic and continuous administration, usually 2-4 weeks after initiation, a sustained decrease in LH and FSH secretion occurs.

Drug Interactions

Increased Effect/Toxicity: Not studied. Hyperprolactinemic drugs (dopamine antagonists such as antipsychotics, and metoclopramide) are contraindicated.

Decreased Effect: Not studied. Hyperprolactinemic drugs (dopamine antagonists such as antipsychotics, and metoclopramide) are contraindicated.

Pharmacodynamics/Kinetics

Absorption: Oral: Not active

Distribution: V_d: 30-33 L

Protein binding: None

Metabolism: Unknown; unlikely to involve CYP; no known metabolites

Half-life elimination: 2.8 ± 1.2 hours

Moderate to severe renal impairment: 6.5-7.7 hours

Hepatic impairment: 7.6 hours

Time to peak: 1-3 hours

Excretion: Urine (42% as intact peptide); hepatic

Pregnancy Risk Factor X

Triptorelin Pamoate *see* Triptorelin *on page 1544*

Tris Buffer *see* Tromethamine *on page 1545*

Tris(hydroxymethyl)aminomethane *see* Tromethamine *on page 1545*

Trisodium Calcium Diethylenetriaminepentaacetate (Ca-DTPA) *see* Diethylene Triamine Penta-Acetic Acid *on page 466*

Tri-Sprintec™ *see* Ethinyl Estradiol and Norgestimate *on page 613*

Tri-Sudo® [OTC] *see* Triprolidine and Pseudoephedrine *on page 1542*

Trivalent Inactivated Influenza Vaccine (TIV) *see* Influenza Virus Vaccine *on page 833*

Tri-Vent™ DM *see* Guaifenesin, Pseudoephedrine, and Dextromethorphan *on page 757*

Tri-Vent™ DPC *see* Chlorpheniramine, Phenylephrine, and Dextromethorphan *on page 326*

Tri-Vent™ HC *see* Hydrocodone, Carbinoxamine, and Pseudoephedrine *on page 789*

Trivora® *see* Ethinyl Estradiol and Levonorgestrel *on page 602*

Trizivir® *see* Abacavir, Lamivudine, and Zidovudine *on page 23*

Trobicin® [DSC] *see* Spectinomycin *on page 1412*

Trocaine® [OTC] *see* Benzocaine *on page 190*

Trolamine Salicylate *see* Triethanolamine Salicylate *on page 1535*

Tromethamine (troe METH a meen)

U.S. Brand Names THAM®

Generic Available No

Synonyms Tris Buffer; Tris(hydroxymethyl)aminomethane

Pharmacologic Category Alkalinizing Agent, Parenteral

Use Correction of metabolic acidosis associated with cardiac bypass surgery or cardiac arrest; to correct excess acidity of stored blood that is preserved with acid citrate dextrose; to prime the pump-oxygenator during cardiac bypass surgery; indicated in infants needing alkalinization after receiving maximum sodium bicarbonate (8-10 mEq/kg/24 hours); (advantage of THAM® is that it alkalinizes without increasing pCO_2 and sodium)

Local Anesthetic/Vasoconstrictor Precautions No information available to require special precautions

Effects on Dental Treatment No significant effects or complications reported

Common Adverse Effects 1% to 10%:

Cardiovascular: Venospasm

Local: Tissue irritation, necrosis with extravasation

Mechanism of Action Acts as a proton acceptor, which combines with hydrogen ions to form bicarbonate buffer, to correct acidosis

Pharmacodynamics/Kinetics

Absorption: 30% of dose is not ionized

Excretion: Urine (>75%) within 3 hours

Pregnancy Risk Factor C

Tronolane® Cream [OTC] *see* Pramoxine *on page 1264*

Tronolane® Suppository [OTC] *see* Phenylephrine *on page 1226*

Tropicacyl® *see* Tropicamide *on page 1545*

Tropicamide (troe PIK a mide)

U.S. Brand Names Mydral™; Mydriacyl®; Tropicacyl®

Canadian Brand Names Diotrope®; Mydriacyl®

Generic Available Yes

(Continued)

Tropicamide *(Continued)*

Synonyms Bistropamide

Pharmacologic Category Ophthalmic Agent, Mydriatic

Use Short-acting mydriatic used in diagnostic procedures; as well as preoperatively and postoperatively; treatment of some cases of acute iritis, iridocyclitis, and keratitis

Local Anesthetic/Vasoconstrictor Precautions No information available to require special precautions

Effects on Dental Treatment No significant effects or complications reported

Mechanism of Action Prevents the sphincter muscle of the iris and the muscle of the ciliary body from responding to cholinergic stimulation

Pregnancy Risk Factor C

Tropicamide and Hydroxyamphetamine *see* Hydroxyamphetamine and Tropicamide *on page 799*

Trospium (TROSE pee um)

U.S. Brand Names Sanctura™

Canadian Brand Names Trosec

Generic Available No

Synonyms Trospium Chloride

Pharmacologic Category Anticholinergic Agent

Use Treatment of overactive bladder with symptoms of urgency, incontinence, and urinary frequency

Local Anesthetic/Vasoconstrictor Precautions No information available to require special precautions

Effects on Dental Treatment Key adverse event(s) related to dental treatment: Significant xerostomia and changes in salivation (normal salivary flow resumes upon discontinuation).

Common Adverse Effects
>10%: Gastrointestinal: Xerostomia (20%)
1% to 10%:
Cardiovascular: Tachycardia, heart rate increase
Central nervous system: Headache (4%), fatigue (2%)
Dermatologic: Dry skin
Gastrointestinal: Constipation (10%), abdominal pain (2%), dyspepsia (1%), flatulence (1%), abdominal distention, vomiting, dysgeusia
Genitourinary: Urinary retention (1%)
Ocular: Dry eyes (1%), blurred vision

Mechanism of Action Trospium antagonizes the effects of acetylcholine on muscarinic receptors in cholinergically innervated organs. It reduces the smooth muscle tone of the bladder.

Pharmacodynamics/Kinetics
Absorption: <10%
Distribution: V_d: 395 L, primarily in plasma
Protein binding: 50% to 85% *in vitro*
Metabolism: Hypothesized to be via esterase hydrolysis and conjugation; forms metabolites
Bioavailability: ~10%
Half-life elimination: 20 hours; severe renal insufficiency (Cl_{cr} <30 mL/minute): ~33 hours
Time to peak, plasma: 5-6 hours
Excretion: Feces primarily (85%); urine (~6%; mostly as unchanged drug)

Pregnancy Risk Factor C

Trospium Chloride *see* Trospium *on page 1546*

Trovafloxacin (TROE va floks a sin)

U.S. Brand Names Trovan® [DSC]

Mexican Brand Names Trovan®

Generic Available No

Synonyms Alatrofloxacin Mesylate; CP-99,219-27

Pharmacologic Category Antibiotic, Quinolone

Use Should be used only in life- or limb-threatening infections
Treatment of nosocomial pneumonia, community-acquired pneumonia, complicated intra-abdominal infections, gynecologic/pelvic infections, complicated skin and skin structure infections

Local Anesthetic/Vasoconstrictor Precautions No information available to require special precautions

Effects on Dental Treatment No significant effects or complications reported

Common Adverse Effects Note: Fatalities have occurred in patients developing hepatic necrosis.

1% to 10% (range reported in clinical trials):

Central nervous system: Dizziness (2% to 11%), lightheadedness (<1% to 4%), headache (1% to 5%)

Dermatologic: Rash (<1% to 2%), pruritus (<1% to 2%)

Gastrointestinal: Nausea (4% to 8%), abdominal pain (<1% to 1%), vomiting, diarrhea

Genitourinary: Vaginitis (<1% to 1%)

Hepatic: Increased LFTs

Local: Injection site reaction, pain, or inflammation

Mechanism of Action Inhibits DNA-gyrase in susceptible organisms; inhibits relaxation of supercoiled DNA and promotes breakage of double-stranded DNA

Drug Interactions

Increased Effect/Toxicity: Trovafloxacin may increase the effects/toxicity of glyburide and warfarin. Concomitant use with corticosteroids may increase the risk of tendon rupture. Probenecid may increase trovafloxacin levels.

Decreased Effect: Concurrent administration of metal cations, including most antacids, oral electrolyte supplements, quinapril, sucralfate, some didanosine formulations (chewable/buffered tablets and pediatric powder for oral suspension), and other highly-buffered oral drugs, may decrease quinolone levels; separate doses.

Pharmacodynamics/Kinetics

Distribution: Concentration in most tissues greater than plasma or serum

Protein binding: 76%

Metabolism: Hepatic conjugation; glucuronidation 13%, acetylation 9%

Bioavailability: 88%

Half-life elimination: 9-12 hours

Time to peak, serum: Oral: Within 2 hours

Excretion: Feces (43% as unchanged drug); urine (6% as unchanged drug)

Pregnancy Risk Factor C

Trovan® [DSC] *see* Trovafloxacin *on page 1546*

Troxidone *see* Trimethadione *on page 1538*

Trusopt® *see* Dorzolamide *on page 501*

Truvada® *see* Emtricitabine and Tenofovir *on page 537*

Trypsin, Balsam Peru, and Castor Oil
(TRIP sin, BAL sam pe RUE, & KAS tor oyl)

Related Information

Castor Oil *on page 279*

U.S. Brand Names Granulex®; Xenaderm™

Generic Available Yes: Spray

Synonyms Balsam Peru, Trypsin, and Castor Oil; Castor Oil, Trypsin, and Balsam Peru

Pharmacologic Category Protectant, Topical

Use Treatment of decubitus ulcers, varicose ulcers, debridement of eschar, dehiscent wounds and sunburn; promote wound healing; reduce odor from necrotic wounds

Local Anesthetic/Vasoconstrictor Precautions No information available to require special precautions

Effects on Dental Treatment No significant effects or complications reported

Common Adverse Effects Frequency not defined: Local: Temporary stinging at application site

Mechanism of Action Trypsin is used to debride necrotic tissue; balsam peru stimulates circulation at the wound site and may be mildly bactericidal; castor oil improves epithelialization, acts as a protectant covering and helps reduce pain

Tryptoreline *see* Triptorelin *on page 1544*

TSH *see* Thyrotropin Alpha *on page 1483*

TSPA *see* Thiotepa *on page 1479*

TST *see* Tuberculin Tests *on page 1548*

T-Stat® [DSC] *see* Erythromycin *on page 562*

Tuberculin Purified Protein Derivative *see* Tuberculin Tests *on page 1548*

Tuberculin Skin Test *see* Tuberculin Tests *on page 1548*

Tuberculin Tests (too BER kyoo lin tests)

U.S. Brand Names Aplisol®; Tubersol®
Generic Available No
Synonyms Mantoux; PPD; Tine Test; TST; Tuberculin Purified Protein Derivative; Tuberculin Skin Test
Pharmacologic Category Diagnostic Agent
Use Skin test in diagnosis of tuberculosis, cell-mediated immunodeficiencies
Local Anesthetic/Vasoconstrictor Precautions No information available to require special precautions
Effects on Dental Treatment No significant effects or complications reported
Common Adverse Effects Frequency not defined.
 Dermatologic: Ulceration, necrosis, vesiculation
 Local: Pain at injection site
Mechanism of Action Tuberculosis results in individuals becoming sensitized to certain antigenic components of the *M. tuberculosis* organism. Culture extracts called tuberculins are contained in tuberculin skin test preparations. Upon intracutaneous injection of these culture extracts, a classic delayed (cellular) hypersensitivity reaction occurs. This reaction is characteristic of a delayed course (peak occurs >24 hours after injection, induration of the skin secondary to cell infiltration, and occasional vesiculation and necrosis). Delayed hypersensitivity reactions to tuberculin may indicate infection with a variety of nontuberculosis mycobacteria, or vaccination with the live attenuated mycobacterial strain of *M. bovis* vaccine, BCG, in addition to previous natural infection with *M. tuberculosis*.
Pharmacodynamics/Kinetics
 Onset of action: Delayed hypersensitivity reactions: 5-6 hours
  Peak effect: 48-72 hours
 Duration: Reactions subside over a few days
Pregnancy Risk Factor C

Tubersol® *see* Tuberculin Tests *on page 1548*
Tucks® Anti-Itch [OTC] *see* Hydrocortisone *on page 793*
Tucks® Hemorrhoidal [OTC] *see* Pramoxine *on page 1264*
Tuinal® [DSC] *see* Amobarbital and Secobarbital *on page 104*
Tums® [OTC] *see* Calcium Carbonate *on page 248*
Tums® E-X [OTC] *see* Calcium Carbonate *on page 248*
Tums® Extra Strength Sugar Free [OTC] *see* Calcium Carbonate *on page 248*
Tums® Smoothies™ [OTC] *see* Calcium Carbonate *on page 248*
Tums® Ultra [OTC] *see* Calcium Carbonate *on page 248*
Tussafed® *see* Carbinoxamine, Pseudoephedrine, and Dextromethorphan *on page 269*
Tussafed® HC *see* Hydrocodone, Phenylephrine, and Guaifenesin *on page 791*
Tussend® Expectorant *see* Hydrocodone, Pseudoephedrine, and Guaifenesin *on page 792*
Tussi-12® *see* Carbetapentane and Chlorpheniramine *on page 266*
Tussi-12® D *see* Carbetapentane, Phenylephrine, and Pyrilamine *on page 267*
Tussi-12® DS *see* Carbetapentane, Phenylephrine, and Pyrilamine *on page 267*
Tussi-12 S™ *see* Carbetapentane and Chlorpheniramine *on page 266*
Tussigon® *see* Hydrocodone and Homatropine *on page 786*
Tussin [OTC] *see* Guaifenesin *on page 752*
TussiNate™ *see* Hydrocodone, Phenylephrine, and Diphenhydramine *on page 791*
Tussionex® *see* Hydrocodone and Chlorpheniramine *on page 784*
Tussi-Organidin® NR *see* Guaifenesin and Codeine *on page 753*
Tussi-Organidin® S-NR *see* Guaifenesin and Codeine *on page 753*
Tussizone-12 RF™ *see* Carbetapentane and Chlorpheniramine *on page 266*
T-Vites [OTC] *see* Vitamins (Multiple/Oral) *on page 1582*
Twelve Resin-K *see* Cyanocobalamin *on page 399*
Twilite® [OTC] *see* DiphenhydrAMINE *on page 483*
Twinject™ *see* Epinephrine *on page 546*
Twinrix® *see* Hepatitis A Inactivated and Hepatitis B (Recombinant) Vaccine *on page 766*
Tycolene [OTC] *see* Acetaminophen *on page 31*
Tycolene Maximum Strength [OTC] *see* Acetaminophen *on page 31*
Tygacil™ *see* Tigecycline *on page 1487*
Tylenol® [OTC] *see* Acetaminophen *on page 31*

Tylenol® 8 Hour [OTC] *see* Acetaminophen *on page 31*

Tylenol® Allergy Complete [OTC] *see* Acetaminophen, Chlorpheniramine, and Pseudoephedrine *on page 43*

Tylenol® Allergy Sinus [OTC] [DSC] *see* Acetaminophen, Chlorpheniramine, and Pseudoephedrine *on page 43*

Tylenol® Arthritis Pain [OTC] *see* Acetaminophen *on page 31*

Tylenol® Children's [OTC] *see* Acetaminophen *on page 31*

Tylenol® Children's with Flavor Creator [OTC] *see* Acetaminophen *on page 31*

Tylenol® Children's Plus Cold Nighttime [OTC] *see* Acetaminophen, Chlorpheniramine, and Pseudoephedrine *on page 43*

Tylenol® Cold Day Non-Drowsy [OTC] *see* Acetaminophen, Dextromethorphan, and Pseudoephedrine *on page 44*

Tylenol® Cold, Infants [OTC] *see* Acetaminophen and Pseudoephedrine *on page 38*

Tylenol® Extra Strength [OTC] *see* Acetaminophen *on page 31*

Tylenol® Flu Non-Drowsy Maximum Strength [OTC] *see* Acetaminophen, Dextromethorphan, and Pseudoephedrine *on page 44*

Tylenol® Infants [OTC] *see* Acetaminophen *on page 31*

Tylenol® Junior [OTC] *see* Acetaminophen *on page 31*

Tylenol® PM [OTC] *see* Acetaminophen and Diphenhydramine *on page 38*

Tylenol® Severe Allergy [OTC] *see* Acetaminophen and Diphenhydramine *on page 38*

Tylenol® Sinus, Children's [OTC] *see* Acetaminophen and Pseudoephedrine *on page 38*

Tylenol® Sinus Day Non-Drowsy [OTC] *see* Acetaminophen and Pseudoephedrine *on page 38*

Tylenol® With Codeine *see* Acetaminophen and Codeine *on page 35*

Tylox® *see* Oxycodone and Acetaminophen *on page 1165*

Typhim Vi® *see* Typhoid Vaccine *on page 1549*

Typhoid Vaccine (TYE foid vak SEEN)

Related Information
Immunizations (Vaccines) *on page 1786*

U.S. Brand Names Typhim Vi®; Vivotif Berna®

Generic Available No

Synonyms Typhoid Vaccine Live Oral Ty21a

Pharmacologic Category Vaccine

Use Typhoid vaccine: Live, attenuated Ty21a typhoid vaccine should not be administered to immunocompromised persons, including those known to be infected with HIV. Parenteral inactivated vaccine is a theoretically safer alternative for this group.

Parenteral: Promotes active immunity to typhoid fever for patients intimately exposed to a typhoid carrier or foreign travel to a typhoid fever endemic area

Oral: For immunization of children >6 years of age and adults who expect intimate exposure of or household contact with typhoid fever, travelers to areas of world with risk of exposure to typhoid fever, and workers in microbiology laboratories with expected frequent contact with *S. typhi*

Local Anesthetic/Vasoconstrictor Precautions No information available to require special precautions

Effects on Dental Treatment No significant effects or complications reported

Common Adverse Effects All serious adverse reactions must be reported to the U.S. Department of Health and Human Services (DHHS) Vaccine Adverse Event Reporting System (VAERS) 1-800-822-7967.

Oral: 1% to 10%:
Central nervous system: Headache, fever
Dermatologic: Rash
Gastrointestinal: Abdominal discomfort, stomach cramps, diarrhea, nausea, vomiting

Injection:
>10%:
Central nervous system: Headache (13% to 20%), fever (3% to 11%), malaise (4% to 24%)
Dermatologic: Local tenderness (13% to 98%), induration (5% to 15%), pain at injection site (7% to 41%)

1% to 10%:
Central nervous system: Fever ≥100°F (2%)
Gastrointestinal: Nausea (2% to 8%), diarrhea (3% to 4%), vomiting (2%)
Local: Erythema at injection site (4% to 5%)

(Continued)

Typhoid Vaccine (Continued)

Neuromuscular & skeletal: Myalgia (3% to 7%)

Mechanism of Action Virulent strains of *Salmonella typhi* cause disease by penetrating the intestinal mucosa and entering the systemic circulation via the lymphatic vasculature. One possible mechanism of conferring immunity may be the provocation of a local immune response in the intestinal tract induced by oral ingesting of a live strain with subsequent aborted infection. The ability of *Salmonella typhi* to produce clinical disease (and to elicit an immune response) is dependent on the bacteria having a complete lipopolysaccharide. The live attenuate Ty21a strain lacks the enzyme UDP-4-galactose epimerase so that lipopolysaccharide is only synthesized under conditions that induce bacterial autolysis. Thus, the strain remains avirulent despite the production of sufficient lipopolysaccharide to evoke a protective immune response. Despite low levels of lipopolysaccharide synthesis, cells lyse before gaining a virulent phenotype due to the intracellular accumulation of metabolic intermediates.

Drug Interactions

Decreased Effect: Antibiotics (systemic) and mefloquine may decrease the effect of oral live attenuated Ty21a vaccine (Vivotif Berna®); delay vaccine administration for at least 24 hours after administration of these drugs.

Pharmacodynamics/Kinetics

Onset of action: Immunity to *Salmonella typhi*: Oral: ~1 week

Duration: Immunity: Oral: ~5 years; Parenteral: ~3 years

Pregnancy Risk Factor C

Typhoid Vaccine Live Oral Ty21a *see* Typhoid Vaccine *on page 1549*

Tysabri® *see* Natalizumab *on page 1093*

Tyzine® *see* Tetrahydrozoline *on page 1470*

Tyzine® Pediatric *see* Tetrahydrozoline *on page 1470*

506U78 *see* Nelarabine *on page 1097*

U-90152S *see* Delavirdine *on page 429*

UCB-P071 *see* Cetirizine *on page 306*

UK-88,525 *see* Darifenacin *on page 424*

UK92480 *see* Sildenafil *on page 1390*

UK109496 *see* Voriconazole *on page 1582*

Ulcerease® [OTC] *see* Phenol *on page 1223*

Ultiva® *see* Remifentanil *on page 1338*

Ultracet™ *see* Acetaminophen and Tramadol *on page 39*

Ultra Freeda Iron Free [OTC] *see* Vitamins (Multiple/Oral) *on page 1582*

Ultra Freeda with Iron [OTC] *see* Vitamins (Multiple/Oral) *on page 1582*

Ultram® *see* Tramadol *on page 1514*

Ultram® ER *see* Tramadol *on page 1514*

Ultra Mide® [OTC] *see* Urea *on page 1551*

Ultraprin [OTC] *see* Ibuprofen *on page 808*

Ultrase® *see* Pancrelipase *on page 1183*

Ultrase® MT *see* Pancrelipase *on page 1183*

Ultra Tears® [OTC] *see* Artificial Tears *on page 143*

Ultravate® *see* Halobetasol *on page 760*

Ultravist® *see* Iopromide *on page 855*

Umecta® *see* Urea *on page 1551*

Unasyn® *see* Ampicillin and Sulbactam *on page 120*

Undecylenic Acid and Derivatives

(un de sil EN ik AS id & dah RIV ah tivs)

U.S. Brand Names Fungi-Nail® [OTC]

Generic Available No

Synonyms Zinc Undecylenate

Pharmacologic Category Antifungal Agent, Topical

Use Treatment of athlete's foot (tinea pedis); ringworm (except nails and scalp)

Local Anesthetic/Vasoconstrictor Precautions No information available to require special precautions

Effects on Dental Treatment No significant effects or complications reported

Unicap M® [OTC] *see* Vitamins (Multiple/Oral) *on page 1582*

Unicap Sr® [OTC] *see* Vitamins (Multiple/Oral) *on page 1582*

Unicap T™ [OTC] *see* Vitamins (Multiple/Oral) *on page 1582*

Uni-Cof *see* Pseudoephedrine, Dihydrocodeine, and Chlorpheniramine *on page 1312*

Uniphyl® *see* Theophylline *on page 1473*

Uniretic® *see* Moexipril and Hydrochlorothiazide *on page 1059*

Uni-Senna [OTC] *see* Senna *on page 1384*

Unisom® Maximum Strength SleepGels® [OTC] *see* DiphenhydrAMINE *on page 483*

Unisom® SleepTabs® [OTC] *see* Doxylamine *on page 517*

Unithroid® *see* Levothyroxine *on page 917*

Univasc® *see* Moexipril *on page 1058*

Unna's Boot *see* Zinc Gelatin *on page 1597*

Unna's Paste *see* Zinc Gelatin *on page 1597*

Unoprostone (yoo noe PROS tone)

Canadian Brand Names Rescula®

Generic Available No

Synonyms Unoprostone Isopropyl

Pharmacologic Category Ophthalmic Agent, Antiglaucoma; Prostaglandin, Ophthalmic

Use To lower intraocular pressure (IOP) in patients with open-angle glaucoma or ocular hypertension; should be used in patients who are not tolerant of, or failed treatment with other IOP-lowering medications

Local Anesthetic/Vasoconstrictor Precautions No information available to require special precautions

Effects on Dental Treatment No significant effects or complications reported

Mechanism of Action The exact mechanism of action is unknown; however, unoprostone decreases IOP by increasing the outflow of aqueous humor. Cardiovascular and pulmonary function were not affected in clinical studies. IOP was decreased by 3-4 mm Hg in patients with a mean baseline IOP of 23 mm Hg.

Pregnancy Risk Factor C

Unoprostone Isopropyl *see* Unoprostone *on page 1551*

Urea (yoor EE a)

U.S. Brand Names Amino-Cerv™; Aquacare® [OTC]; Aquaphilic® With Carbamide [OTC]; Carmol® 10 [OTC]; Carmol® 20 [OTC]; Carmol® 40; Carmol® Deep Cleaning; Cerovel™; DPM™ [OTC]; Gormel® [OTC]; Keralac™; Keralac™ Nailstik; Lanaphilic® [OTC]; Nutraplus® [OTC]; Rea-Lo® [OTC]; Ultra Mide® [OTC]; Umecta®; Ureacin® [OTC]; Vanamide™

Canadian Brand Names UltraMide 25™; Uremol®; Urisec®

Mexican Brand Names Derma Keri®; Dermoplast®

Generic Available Yes: Excludes ointment, shampoo

Synonyms Carbamide

Pharmacologic Category Diuretic, Osmotic; Keratolytic Agent; Topical Skin Product

Use

Topical: Keratolytic agent to soften nails or skin; OTC: Moisturizer for dry, rough skin

Vaginal: Treatment of cervicitis

Local Anesthetic/Vasoconstrictor Precautions No information available to require special precautions

Effects on Dental Treatment No significant effects or complications reported

Common Adverse Effects Frequency not defined: Topical: Local: Transient stinging, local irritation

Mechanism of Action

Topical: Urea softens hyperkeratotic areas by dissolving the intracellular matrix, resulting in loosening the horny layer of the skin, or softening and debridement of the nail plate

Vaginal: Urea aids in debridement, promotes epithelialization and prevents excessive tissue formation

Pregnancy Risk Factor C

Urea and Hydrocortisone (yoor EE a & hye droe KOR ti sone)

Related Information

Hydrocortisone *on page 793*

Urea *on page 1551*

U.S. Brand Names Carmol-HC®

Canadian Brand Names Ti-U-Lac® H; Uremol® HC

Generic Available No

(Continued)

Urea and Hydrocortisone *(Continued)*

Synonyms Hydrocortisone and Urea

Pharmacologic Category Corticosteroid, Topical

Use Inflammation of corticosteroid-responsive dermatoses

Local Anesthetic/Vasoconstrictor Precautions No information available to require special precautions

Effects on Dental Treatment No significant effects or complications reported

Drug Interactions

Cytochrome P450 Effect: Hydrocortisone: **Substrate** of CYP3A4 (minor); **Induces** CYP3A4 (weak)

Pharmacodynamics/Kinetics See individual agents.

Pregnancy Risk Factor C

Urea, Chlorophyllin, and Papain *see* Chlorophyllin, Papain, and Urea *on page 319*

Ureacin® [OTC] *see* Urea *on page 1551*

Urea Peroxide *see* Carbamide Peroxide *on page 264*

Urecholine® *see* Bethanechol *on page 204*

Urex® *see* Methenamine *on page 1007*

Urimar-T *see* Methenamine, Sodium Biphosphate, Phenyl Salicylate, Methylene Blue, and Hyoscyamine *on page 1008*

Urimax® [DSC] *see* Methenamine, Sodium Biphosphate, Phenyl Salicylate, Methylene Blue, and Hyoscyamine *on page 1008*

Urispas® *see* Flavoxate *on page 656*

Uristat® [OTC] *see* Phenazopyridine *on page 1220*

Urocit®-K *see* Potassium Citrate *on page 1259*

Urofollitropin *see* Follitropins *on page 698*

Uro-KP-Neutral® *see* Potassium Phosphate and Sodium Phosphate *on page 1261*

Uro-Mag® [OTC] *see* Magnesium Oxide *on page 962*

Uroxatral® *see* Alfuzosin *on page 68*

Urso 250™ *see* Ursodiol *on page 1552*

Ursodeoxycholic Acid *see* Ursodiol *on page 1552*

Ursodiol *(ER soe dye ole)*

U.S. Brand Names Actigall®; Urso 250™; Urso Forte™

Canadian Brand Names Urso®

Mexican Brand Names Ursofalk®

Generic Available Yes: Capsule

Synonyms Ursodeoxycholic Acid

Pharmacologic Category Gallstone Dissolution Agent

Use Actigall®: Gallbladder stone dissolution; prevention of gallstones in obese patients experiencing rapid weight loss; Urso®: Primary biliary cirrhosis

Unlabeled/Investigational Use Liver transplantation

Local Anesthetic/Vasoconstrictor Precautions No information available to require special precautions

Effects on Dental Treatment No significant effects or complications reported

Common Adverse Effects

>10%:

Central nervous system: Headache (up to 25%), dizziness (up to 17%)

Gastrointestinal: In treatment of primary biliary cirrhosis: Constipation (up to 26%)

1% to 10%:

Dermatologic: Rash (<1% to 3%), alopecia (<1% to 5%)

Gastrointestinal:

In gallstone dissolution: Most GI events (diarrhea, nausea, vomiting) are similar to placebo and attributable to gallstone disease.

In treatment of primary biliary cirrhosis: Diarrhea (1%)

Hematologic: Leukopenia (3%)

Miscellaneous: Allergy (5%)

Mechanism of Action Decreases the cholesterol content of bile and bile stones by reducing the secretion of cholesterol from the liver and the fractional reabsorption of cholesterol by the intestines. Mechanism of action in primary biliary cirrhosis is not clearly defined.

Drug Interactions

Decreased Effect: Decreased effect with aluminum-containing antacids, cholestyramine, colestipol, clofibrate, and oral contraceptives (estrogens).

Pharmacodynamics/Kinetics

Metabolism: Undergoes extensive enterohepatic recycling; following hepatic conjugation and biliary secretion, the drug is hydrolyzed to active ursodiol, where it is recycled or transformed to lithocholic acid by colonic microbial flora

Half-life elimination: 100 hours

Excretion: Feces

Pregnancy Risk Factor B

Urso Forte™ *see* Ursodiol *on page 1552*

UTI Relief® [OTC] *see* Phenazopyridine *on page 1220*

Uvadex® *see* Methoxsalen *on page 1018*

Vaccinia Immune Globulin (Intravenous)
(vax IN ee a i MYUN GLOB yoo lin IN tra VEE nus)

U.S. Brand Names CNJ-016™

Generic Available No

Synonyms VIGIV

Pharmacologic Category Immune Globulin

Use Treatment of infectious complications of smallpox (vaccinia virus) vaccination, such as eczema vaccinatum, progressive vaccinia, and severe generalized vaccinia; vaccinia infections in individuals with concurrent skin conditions or accidental virus exposure to eyes (except vaccinia keratitis), mouth, or other areas where viral infection would pose significant risk

Local Anesthetic/Vasoconstrictor Precautions No information available to require special precautions

Effects on Dental Treatment No significant effects or complications reported

Common Adverse Effects Note: Actual frequency varies by dose, rate of infusion and specific product used

Cardiovascular: Flushing

Central nervous system: Cold or hot feeling, dizziness, fatigue, headache, pain, pallor, pyrexia

Dermatologic: Erythema, urticaria

Gastrointestinal: Abdominal pain, appetite decreased, nausea, vomiting

Local: Injection site reaction

Neuromuscular & skeletal: Arthralgia, back pain, paraesthesia, muscle cramp, rigors, tremor, weakness

Miscellaneous: Diaphoresis

Mechanism of Action Antibodies obtained from pooled human plasma of individuals immunized with the smallpox vaccine provide passive immunity

Drug Interactions

Decreased Effect: Vaccina immune globulin may interfere with immune response to live virus vaccines (eg, polio, measles, mumps, and rubella); live virus vaccinations should be deferred until 6 months after administration of VIGIV; if given shortly before receiving VIGIV, revaccination with the live virus may be necessary (consult individual products for guidance)

Pharmacodynamics/Kinetics

Distribution: V_d: CNJ-016™ (Cangene product): 6630 L

Half-life elimination:

CNJ-016™ (Cangene product): 30 days (range 13-67 days)

DynPort product: 22 days

Pregnancy Risk Factor C

Vagifem® *see* Estradiol *on page 574*

Vagi-Gard® [OTC] *see* Povidone-Iodine *on page 1262*

Vagistat®-1 [OTC] *see* Tioconazole *on page 1493*

Valacyclovir (val ay SYE kloe veer)

Related Information

Acyclovir *on page 49*

Sexually-Transmitted Diseases *on page 1674*

Systemic Viral Diseases *on page 1675*

Related Sample Prescriptions

Herpes Simplex (Recurrent) *on page 1742*

Shingles (Varicella-Zoster Virus) *on page 1742*

U.S. Brand Names Valtrex®

Canadian Brand Names Valtrex®

Generic Available No

(Continued)

Valacyclovir *(Continued)*

Synonyms Valacyclovir Hydrochloride

Pharmacologic Category Antiviral Agent, Oral

Dental Use Treatment of herpes labialis (cold sores)

Use Treatment of herpes zoster (shingles) in immunocompetent patients; treatment of first-episode genital herpes; episodic treatment of recurrent genital herpes; suppression of recurrent genital herpes and reduction of heterosexual transmission of genital herpes in immunocompetent patients; suppression of genital herpes in HIV-infected individuals; treatment of herpes labialis (cold sores)

Local Anesthetic/Vasoconstrictor Precautions No information available to require special precautions

Effects on Dental Treatment No significant effects or complications reported

Significant Adverse Effects

>10%: Central nervous system: Headache (14% to 35%)

1% to 10%:

Central nervous system: Dizziness (2% to 4%), depression (0% to 7%)

Endocrine: Dysmenorrhea (≤1% to 8%)

Gastrointestinal: Abdominal pain (2% to 11%), vomiting (<1% to 6%), nausea (6% to 15%)

Hematologic: Leukopenia (≤1%), thrombocytopenia (≤1%)

Hepatic: AST increased (1% to 4%)

Neuromuscular & skeletal: Arthralgia (≤1 to 6%)

<1% (Limited to important or life-threatening): Acute hypersensitivity reactions (angioedema, anaphylaxis, dyspnea, pruritus, rash, urticaria); aggression, agitation, alopecia, aplastic anemia, ataxia, coma, confusion, dysarthria, encephalopathy, erythema multiforme, hallucinations (auditory and visual), hemolytic uremic syndrome (HUS), hepatitis, leukocytoclastic vasculitis, mania, photosensitivity reaction, psychosis, rash, renal failure, seizure, thrombotic thrombocytopenic purpura/hemolytic uremic syndrome, tremor

Dental Usual Dosing Herpes labialis (cold sores): Adolescents and Adults: Oral: 2 g twice daily for 1 day (separate doses by ~12 hours)

Dosage Oral:

Adolescents and Adults: Herpes labialis (cold sores): 2 g twice daily for 1 day (separate doses by ~12 hours)

Adults:

Herpes zoster (shingles): 1 g 3 times/day for 7 days

Genital herpes:

Initial episode: 1 g twice daily for 10 days

Recurrent episode: 500 mg twice daily for 3 days

Reduction of transmission: 500 mg once daily (source partner)

Suppressive therapy:

Immunocompetent patients: 1000 mg once daily (500 mg once daily in patients with <9 recurrences per year)

HIV-infected patients (CD4 ≥100 cells/mm^3): 500 mg twice daily

Dosing interval in renal impairment:

Herpes zoster: Adults:

Cl$_{cr}$ 30-49 mL/minute: 1 g every 12 hours

Cl$_{cr}$ 10-29 mL/minute: 1 g every 24 hours

Cl$_{cr}$ <10 mL/minute: 500 mg every 24 hours

Genital herpes: Adults:

Initial episode:

Cl$_{cr}$ 10-29 mL/minute: 1 g every 24 hours

Cl$_{cr}$ <10 mL/minute: 500 mg every 24 hours

Recurrent episode: Cl$_{cr}$ <10-29 mL/minute: 500 mg every 24 hours

Suppressive therapy: Cl$_{cr}$ <10-29 mL/minute:

For usual dose of 1 g every 24 hours, decrease dose to 500 mg every 24 hours

For usual dose of 500 mg every 24 hours, decrease dose to 500 mg every 48 hours

HIV-infected patients: 500 mg every 24 hours

Herpes labialis: Adolescents and Adults:

Cl$_{cr}$ 30-49 mL/minute: 1 g every 12 hours for 2 doses

Cl$_{cr}$ 10-29 mL/minute: 500 mg every 12 hours for 2 doses

Cl$_{cr}$ <10 mL/minute: 500 mg as a single dose

Hemodialysis: Dialyzable (~33% removed during 4-hour session); administer dose postdialysis

Chronic ambulatory peritoneal dialysis/continuous arteriovenous hemofiltration dialysis: Pharmacokinetic parameters are similar to those in patients with ESRD; supplemental dose not needed following dialysis

Mechanism of Action Valacyclovir is rapidly and nearly completely converted to acyclovir by intestinal and hepatic metabolism. Acyclovir is converted to acyclovir monophosphate by virus-specific thymidine kinase then further converted to acyclovir triphosphate by other cellular enzymes. Acyclovir triphosphate inhibits DNA synthesis and viral replication by competing with deoxyguanosine triphosphate for viral DNA polymerase and being incorporated into viral DNA.

Contraindications Hypersensitivity to valacyclovir, acyclovir, or any component of the formulation

Warnings/Precautions Hazardous agent - use appropriate precautions for handling and disposal. Thrombotic thrombocytopenic purpura/hemolytic uremic syndrome has occurred in immunocompromised patients (at doses of 8 g/day); use caution and adjust the dose in elderly patients or those with renal insufficiency and in patients receiving concurrent nephrotoxic agents. For genital herpes, treatment should begin as soon as possible after the first signs and symptoms (within 72 hours of onset of first diagnosis or within 24 hours of onset of recurrent episodes). For herpes zoster, treatment should begin within 72 hours of onset of rash. For cold sores, treatment should begin at with earliest symptom (tingling, itching, burning). Safety and efficacy in prepubertal patients have not been established.

Drug Interactions

Cimetidine: Decreased renal clearance of acyclovir; no dosage adjustment needed in patients with normal renal function

Probenecid: Decreased renal clearance of acyclovir; no dosage adjustment needed in patients with normal renal function

Dietary Considerations May be taken with or without food.

Pharmacodynamics/Kinetics

Absorption: Rapid

Distribution: Acyclovir is widely distributed throughout the body including brain, kidney, lungs, liver, spleen, muscle, uterus, vagina, and CSF

Protein binding: 13.5% to 17.9%

Metabolism: Hepatic; valacyclovir is rapidly and nearly completely converted to acyclovir and L-valine by first-pass effect; acyclovir is hepatically metabolized to a very small extent by aldehyde oxidase and by alcohol and aldehyde dehydrogenase (inactive metabolites)

Bioavailability: ~55% once converted to acyclovir

Half-life elimination: Normal renal function: Adults: Acyclovir: 2.5-3.3 hours, Valacyclovir: ~30 minutes; End-stage renal disease: Acyclovir: 14-20 hours

Excretion: Urine, primarily as acyclovir (88%); **Note:** Following oral administration of radiolabeled valacyclovir, 46% of the label is eliminated in the feces (corresponding to nonabsorbed drug), while 47% of the radiolabel is eliminated in the urine.

Pregnancy Risk Factor B

Lactation Enters breast milk/use caution

Breast-Feeding Considerations Peak concentrations in breast milk range from 0.5-2.3 times the corresponding maternal acyclovir serum concentration. This is expected to provide a nursing infant with a dose of acyclovir equivalent to ~0.6 mg/kg/day following ingestion of valacyclovir 500 mg twice daily by the mother. Use with caution while breast-feeding.

Dosage Forms Caplet: 500 mg, 1000 mg

Valacyclovir Hydrochloride *see* Valacyclovir *on page 1553*

Valcyte™ *see* Valganciclovir *on page 1555*

Valganciclovir (val gan SYE kloh veer)

Related Information
Ganciclovir *on page 722*

U.S. Brand Names Valcyte™

Canadian Brand Names Valcyte™

Generic Available No

Synonyms Valganciclovir Hydrochloride

Pharmacologic Category Antiviral Agent

Use Treatment of cytomegalovirus (CMV) retinitis in patients with acquired immunodeficiency syndrome (AIDS); prevention of CMV disease in high-risk patients (donor CMV positive/recipient CMV negative) undergoing kidney, heart, or kidney/pancreas transplantation

Local Anesthetic/Vasoconstrictor Precautions No information available to require special precautions

Effects on Dental Treatment No significant effects or complications reported

(Continued)

Valganciclovir *(Continued)*

Common Adverse Effects

>10%:

Central nervous system: Fever (31%), headache (9% to 22%), insomnia (16%)

Gastrointestinal: Diarrhea (16% to 41%), nausea (8% to 30%), vomiting (21%), abdominal pain (15%)

Hematologic: Granulocytopenia (11% to 27%), anemia (8% to 26%)

Ocular: Retinal detachment (15%)

1% to 10%:

Central nervous system: Peripheral neuropathy (9%), paresthesia (8%), seizure (<5%), psychosis, hallucinations (<5%), confusion (<5%), agitation (<5%)

Hematologic: Thrombocytopenia (8%), pancytopenia (<5%), bone marrow depression (<5%), aplastic anemia (<5%), bleeding (potentially life-threatening due to thrombocytopenia <5%)

Renal: Decreased renal function (<5%)

Miscellaneous: Local and systemic infection, including sepsis (<5%); allergic reaction (<5%)

Mechanism of Action Valganciclovir is rapidly converted to ganciclovir in the body. The bioavailability of ganciclovir from valganciclovir is increased 10-fold compared to the oral ganciclovir. A dose of 900 mg achieved systemic exposure of ganciclovir comparable to that achieved with the recommended doses of intravenous ganciclovir of 5 mg/kg. Ganciclovir is phosphorylated to a substrate which competitively inhibits the binding of deoxyguanosine triphosphate to DNA polymerase resulting in inhibition of viral DNA synthesis.

Drug Interactions

Increased Effect/Toxicity: Reported for ganciclovir: Immunosuppressive agents may increase hematologic toxicity of ganciclovir. Imipenem/cilastatin may increase seizure potential. Oral ganciclovir increases blood levels of zidovudine, although zidovudine decreases steady-state levels of ganciclovir. Since both drugs have the potential to cause neutropenia and anemia, some patients may not tolerate concomitant therapy with these drugs at full dosage. Didanosine levels are increased with concurrent ganciclovir. Other nephrotoxic drugs (eg, amphotericin and cyclosporine) may have additive nephrotoxicity with ganciclovir.

Decreased Effect: Reported for ganciclovir: A decrease in blood levels of ganciclovir AUC may occur when used with didanosine.

Pharmacodynamics/Kinetics

Absorption: Well absorbed; high-fat meal increases AUC by 30%

Distribution: Ganciclovir: V_d: 15.26 L/1.73 m²; widely to all tissues including CSF and ocular tissue

Protein binding: 1% to 2%

Metabolism: Converted to ganciclovir by intestinal mucosal cells and hepatocytes

Bioavailability: With food: 60%

Half-life elimination: Ganciclovir: 4.08 hours; prolonged with renal impairment; Severe renal impairment: Up to 68 hours

Excretion: Urine (primarily as ganciclovir)

Pregnancy Risk Factor C

Valganciclovir Hydrochloride *see* Valganciclovir *on page 1555*

Valium® *see* Diazepam *on page 454*

Valorin [OTC] *see* Acetaminophen *on page 31*

Valorin Extra [OTC] *see* Acetaminophen *on page 31*

Valproate Semisodium *see* Valproic Acid and Derivatives *on page 1556*

Valproate Sodium *see* Valproic Acid and Derivatives *on page 1556*

Valproic Acid *see* Valproic Acid and Derivatives *on page 1556*

Valproic Acid and Derivatives
(val PROE ik AS id & dah RIV ah tives)

U.S. Brand Names Depacon®; Depakene®; Depakote® Delayed Release; Depakote® ER; Depakote® Sprinkle®

Canadian Brand Names Alti-Divalproex; Apo-Divalproex®; Depakene®; Epival® I.V.; Gen-Divalproex; Novo-Divalproex; Nu-Divalproex; PMS-Valproic Acid; PMS-Valproic Acid E.C.; Rhoxal-valproic; Sandoz-Valproic

Mexican Brand Names Cryoval®; Depakene®; Epival®; Leptilan®; Valprosid®

Generic Available Yes: Capsule (excluding sprinkle), injection, syrup

Synonyms Dipropylacetic Acid; Divalproex Sodium; DPA; 2-Propylpentanoic Acid; 2-Propylvaleric Acid; Valproate Semisodium; Valproate Sodium; Valproic Acid

Pharmacologic Category Anticonvulsant, Miscellaneous

Use Monotherapy and adjunctive therapy in the treatment of patients with complex partial seizures; monotherapy and adjunctive therapy of simple and complex absence seizures; adjunctive therapy patients with multiple seizure types that include absence seizures; treatment of acute or mixed manic episodes associated with bipolar disorder; migraine prophylaxis

Mania associated with bipolar disorder (Depakote®)

Migraine prophylaxis (Depakote®, Depakote® ER)

Unlabeled/Investigational Use Behavior disorders (eg, agitation, aggression) in patients with dementia (based on the results of several randomized, controlled trials, there is little evidence to support this use); status epilepticus

Local Anesthetic/Vasoconstrictor Precautions No information available to require special precautions

Effects on Dental Treatment No significant effects or complications reported

Common Adverse Effects

Adverse reactions reported when used as monotherapy for complex partial seizure:

>10%:

Central nervous system: Headache (up to 31%), somnolence (7% to 30%), dizziness (12% to 25%), insomnia (1% to 15%), nervousness (1% to 11%), pain (up to 11%)

Dermatologic: Alopecia (6% to 24%)

Gastrointestinal: Nausea (15% to 48%), vomiting (7% to 27%), diarrhea (7% to 23%), abdominal pain (7% to 23%), dyspepsia (7% to 23%), anorexia (11% to 12%)

Hematologic: Thrombocytopenia (1% to 24%)

Neuromuscular & skeletal: Tremor (1% to 57%), weakness (6% to 27%)

Ocular: Diplopia (up to 16%), amblyopia/blurred vision (8% to 12%)

Miscellaneous: Infection (1% to 20%), flu-like symptoms (1% to 12%)

1% to 10%:

Cardiovascular: Arrhythmia, chest pain, edema, hyper-/hypotension, palpitation, peripheral edema (1% to 8%), postural hypotension, tachycardia, vasodilatation

Central nervous system: Abnormal dreams, agitation, amnesia (5% to 7%), anxiety, catatonic reaction, chills, confusion, depression, emotional lability, hallucinations, hypokinesia, malaise, personality disorder, psychosis, reflexes increased, sleep disorder, speech disorder, tardive dyskinesia, thinking abnormal (up to 6%), vertigo

Dermatologic: Bruising, discoid lupus erythematosus, dry skin, erythema nodosum, furunculosis, macropapular rash, petechia, pruritus, rash, seborrhea, vesiculobullous rash

Endocrine & metabolic: Amenorrhea, dysmenorrhea, hypoproteinemia, metrorrhagia

Gastrointestinal: Dysphagia, eructation, fecal incontinence, flatulence, gastroenteritis, glossitis, gum hemorrhage, hematemesis, appetite increased, mouth ulceration, pancreatitis, periodontal abscess, taste perversion, weight gain (1% to 9%), stomatitis, constipation, dry mouth, tooth disorder, weight loss (up to 6%)

Genitourinary: Cystitis, urinary frequency, urinary incontinence, UTI, vaginitis

Hematologic: Anemia, bleeding time increased, leukopenia

Hepatic: AST/ALT increased

Neuromuscular & skeletal: Abnormal gait, arthralgia, arthrosis, ataxia (up to 8%), back pain (1% to 8%), hypertonia, leg cramps, myalgia, myasthenia, neck rigidity, paresthesia, twitching

Ocular: Abnormal vision, conjunctivitis, dry eye, eye pain, nystagmus (7% to 8%), photophobia

Otic: Deafness, otitis media, tinnitus (1% to 7%)

Respiratory: Bronchitis, epistaxis, hiccup, increased cough, pneumonia, rhinitis, sinusitis

Additional adverse effects: Frequency not defined:

Cardiovascular: Bradycardia

Central nervous system: Aggression, behavioral deterioration, cerebral atrophy (reversible), dementia, encephalopathy (rare), hostility, hyperactivity, hypoesthesia, parkinsonism

Dermatologic: Cutaneous vasculitis, erythema multiforme, photosensitivity, Stevens-Johnson syndrome, toxic epidermal necrolysis (rare)

Endocrine & metabolic: Breast enlargement, galactorrhea, hyperammonemia, hyponatremia, inappropriate ADH secretion, parotid gland swelling, polycystic ovary disease (rare), abnormal thyroid function tests

(Continued)

Valproic Acid and Derivatives *(Continued)*

Genitourinary: Enuresis

Hematologic: Anemia, aplastic anemia, bone marrow suppression, eosinophilia, hematoma formation, hemorrhage, hypofibrinogenemia, intermittent porphyria, lymphocytosis, macrocytosis, pancytopenia

Hepatic: Bilirubin increased, hyperammonemic encephalopathy (in patients with UCD)

Neuromuscular & skeletal: Asterixis, bone pain, dysarthria

Ocular: Seeing "spots before the eyes"

Renal: Fanconi-like syndrome (rare, in children)

Miscellaneous: Anaphylaxis, carnitine decreased, hyperglycinemia, lupus

Postmarketing and/or case reports: Life-threatening pancreatitis (2 cases out of 2416 patients), occurring at the start of therapy or following years of use, has been reported in adults and children. Some cases have been hemorrhagic with rapid progression of initial symptoms to death. Cases have also been reported upon rechallenge. Severe hypersensitivity reactions with organ dysfunction have been reported; symptoms include fever and rash along with organ dysfunction, eosinophilia, and hematologic depression (thrombocytopenia, neutropenia).

Dosage

Seizures:

Children ≥10 years and Adults:

Oral: Initial: 10-15 mg/kg/day in 1-3 divided doses; increase by 5-10 mg/kg/day at weekly intervals until therapeutic levels are achieved; maintenance: 30-60 mg/kg/day. Adult usual dose: 1000-2500 mg/day. **Note:** Regular release and delayed release formulations are usually given in 2-4 divided doses/day, extended release formulation (Depakote® ER) is usually given once daily. Conversion to Depakote® ER from a stable dose of Depakote® may require an increase in the total daily dose between 8% and 20% to maintain similar serum concentrations.

Children receiving more than one anticonvulsant (ie, polytherapy) may require doses up to 100 mg/kg/day in 3-4 divided doses

I.V.: Administer as a 60-minute infusion (≤20 mg/minute) with the same frequency as oral products; switch patient to oral products as soon as possible. Alternatively, rapid infusions have been given: ≤15 mg/kg over 5-10 minutes (1.5-3 mg/kg/minute).

Rectal (unlabeled): Dilute syrup 1:1 with water for use as a retention enema; loading dose: 17-20 mg/kg one time; maintenance: 10-15 mg/kg/dose every 8 hours

Status epilepticus (unlabeled use): Adults:

Loading dose: I.V.: 15-25 mg/kg administered at 3 mg/kg/minute.

Maintenance dose: I.V. infusion: 1-4 mg/kg/hour; titrate dose as needed based upon patient response and evaluation of drug-drug interactions

Mania: Adults: Oral: 750-1500 mg/day in divided doses; dose should be adjusted as rapidly as possible to desired clinical effect; a loading dose of 20 mg/kg may be used; maximum recommended dosage: 60 mg/kg/day

Extended release tablets: Initial: 25 mg/kg/day given once daily; dose should be adjusted as rapidly as possible to desired clinical effect; maximum recommended dose: 60 mg/kg/day.

Migraine prophylaxis: Adults: Oral:

Extended release tablets: 500 mg once daily for 7 days, then increase to 1000 mg once daily; adjust dose based on patient response; usual dosage range 500-1000 mg/day

Delayed release tablets: 250 mg twice daily; adjust dose based on patient response, up to 1000 mg/day

Elderly: Elimination is decreased in the elderly. Studies of elderly patients with dementia show a high incidence of somnolence. In some patients, this was associated with weight loss. Starting doses should be lower and increases should be slow, with careful monitoring of nutritional intake and dehydration. Safety and efficacy for use in patients >65 years have not been studied for migraine prophylaxis.

Dosing adjustment in renal impairment: A 27% reduction in clearance of unbound valproate is seen in patients with Cl$_{cr}$ <10 mL/minute. Hemodialysis reduces valproate concentrations by 20%, therefore no dose adjustment is needed in patients with renal failure. Protein binding is reduced, monitoring only total valproate concentrations may be misleading.

Dosing adjustment/comments in hepatic impairment: Reduce dose. Clearance is decreased with liver impairment. Hepatic disease is also associated with decreased albumin concentrations and 2- to 2.6-fold increase in the unbound fraction. Free concentrations of valproate may be elevated while total concentrations appear normal.

Mechanism of Action Causes increased availability of gamma-aminobutyric acid (GABA), an inhibitory neurotransmitter, to brain neurons or may enhance the action of GABA or mimic its action at postsynaptic receptor sites

Contraindications Hypersensitivity to valproic acid, derivatives, or any component of the formulation; hepatic dysfunction; urea cycle disorders

Warnings/Precautions

Hepatic failure resulting in fatalities has occurred in patients; children <2 years of age are at considerable risk; other risk factors include organic brain disease, mental retardation with severe seizure disorders, congenital metabolic disorders, and patients on multiple anticonvulsants. Hepatotoxicity has been reported after 3 days to 6 months of therapy. Monitor patients closely for appearance of malaise, weakness, facial edema, anorexia, jaundice, and vomiting.

May cause teratogenic effects such as neural tube defects (eg, spina bifida). Use in women of childbearing potential requires that benefits of use in mother be weighed against the potential risk to fetus, especially when used for conditions not associated with permanent injury or risk of death (eg, migraine).

May cause severe thrombocytopenia, inhibition of platelet aggregation and bleeding; tremors may indicate overdosage; use with caution in patients receiving other anticonvulsants. Cases of life-threatening pancreatitis, occurring at the start of therapy or following years of use, have been reported in adults and children. Some cases have been hemorrhagic with rapid progression of initial symptoms to death. Hypersensitivity reactions affecting multiple organs have been reported in association with valproic acid use; may include dermatologic and/or hematologic changes (eosinophilia, neutropenia, thrombocytopenia) or symptoms of organ dysfunction.

Hyperammonemia and/or encephalopathy, sometimes fatal, have been reported following the initiation of valproate therapy and may be present with normal transaminase levels. Ammonia levels should be measured in patients who develop unexplained lethargy and vomiting, or changes in mental status. Discontinue therapy if ammonia levels are increased and evaluate for possible urea cycle disorder (UCD). Although rare genetic disorders, UCD evaluation should be considered for the following patients, prior to the start of therapy: History of unexplained encephalopathy or coma; encephalopathy associated with protein load; pregnancy or postpartum encephalopathy; unexplained mental retardation; history of elevated plasma ammonia or glutamine; history of cyclical vomiting and lethargy; episodic extreme irritability, ataxia; low BUN or protein avoidance; family history of UCD or unexplained infant deaths (particularly male); signs or symptoms of UCD (hyperammonemia, encephalopathy, respiratory alkalosis).

In vitro studies have suggested valproate stimulates the replication of HIV and CMV viruses under experimental conditions. The clinical consequence of this is unknown, but should be considered when monitoring affected patients.

Anticonvulsants should not be discontinued abruptly because of the possibility of increasing seizure frequency; valproate should be withdrawn gradually to minimize the potential of increased seizure frequency, unless safety concerns require a more rapid withdrawal. Concomitant use with clonazepam may induce absence status.

CNS depression may occur with valproate use. Patients must be cautioned about performing tasks which require mental alertness (operating machinery or driving). Effects with other sedative drugs or ethanol may be potentiated.

Drug Interactions

Cytochrome P450 Effect: For valproic acid: **Substrate** (minor) of CYP2A6, 2B6, 2C8/9, 2C19, 2E1; **Inhibits** CYP2C8/9 (weak), 2C19 (weak), 2D6 (weak), 3A4 (weak); **Induces** CYP2A6 (weak)

Increased Effect/Toxicity: Absence seizures have been reported in patients receiving VPA and clonazepam. Valproic acid may increase, decrease, or have no effect on carbamazepine and phenytoin levels. Valproic acid may increase serum concentrations of carbamazepine - epoxide (active metabolite). Valproic acid may increase serum concentrations of lamotrigine, phenobarbital, tricyclic antidepressants, and zidovudine. Macrolide antibiotics (clarithromycin, erythromycin, troleandomycin), felbamate, and isoniazid may inhibit the metabolism of valproic acid. Aspirin or other salicylates may displace valproic acid from protein-binding sites, leading to acute toxicity. When combined with topiramate, hyperammonemia with or without encephalopathy has been reported in patients who tolerated either drug alone.

(Continued)

Valproic Acid and Derivatives *(Continued)*

Decreased Effect: Carbapenem antibiotics (ertapenem, imipenem, meropenem) may decrease valproic acid concentrations to subtherapeutic levels; monitor.

Ethanol/Nutrition/Herb Interactions

Ethanol: Avoid ethanol (may increase CNS depression).

Food: Food may delay but does not affect the extent of absorption. Valproic acid serum concentrations may be decreased if taken with food. Milk has no effect on absorption.

Herb/Nutraceutical: Avoid evening primrose (seizure threshold decreased)

Dietary Considerations Valproic acid may cause GI upset; take with large amount of water or food to decrease GI upset. May need to split doses to avoid GI upset.

Coated particles of divalproex sodium may be mixed with semisolid food (eg, applesauce or pudding) in patients having difficulty swallowing; particles should be swallowed and not chewed

Valproate sodium oral solution will generate valproic acid in carbonated beverages and may cause mouth and throat irritation; do not mix valproate sodium oral solution with carbonated beverages; sodium content of valproate sodium syrup (5 mL): 23 mg (1 mEq)

Pharmacodynamics/Kinetics

Distribution: Total valproate: 11 L/1.73 m^2; free valproate 92 L/1.73 m^2

Protein binding (dose dependent): 80% to 90%

Metabolism: Extensively hepatic via glucuronide conjugation and mitochondrial beta-oxidation. The relationship between dose and total valproate concentration is nonlinear; concentration does not increase proportionally with the dose, but increases to a lesser extent due to saturable plasma protein binding. The kinetics of unbound drug are linear.

Bioavailability: Extended release: 90% of I.V. dose and 81% to 90% of delayed release dose

Half-life elimination: (increased in neonates and with liver disease): Children: 4-14 hours; Adults: 9-16 hours

Time to peak, serum: 1-4 hours; Divalproex (enteric coated): 3-5 hours

Excretion: Urine (30% to 50% as glucuronide conjugate, 3% as unchanged drug)

Pregnancy Risk Factor D

Dosage Forms CAP, as valproic acid (Depakene®): 250 mg. **CAP, sprinkles, as divalproex sodium (Depakote® Sprinkle®):** 125 mg. **INJ, solution, as valproate sodium (Depacon®):** 100 mg/mL (5 mL). **SYR, as valproic acid:** 250 mg/5 mL (480 mL); (Depakene®): 250 mg/5 mL (480 mL). **TAB, delayed release, as divalproex sodium (Depakote®):** 125 mg, 250 mg, 500 mg. **TAB, extended release, as divalproex sodium (Depakote® ER):** 250 mg, 500 mg

Selected Readings

Redington K, Wells C, and Petito F, "Erythromycin and Valproic Acid Interaction," *Ann Intern Med*, 1992, 116(10):877-8.

Valrubicin *(val ROO bi sin)*

U.S. Brand Names Valstar® [DSC]

Canadian Brand Names Valstar®; Valtaxin®

Generic Available No

Synonyms AD3L; *N*-trifluoroacetyladriamycin-14-valerate

Pharmacologic Category Antineoplastic Agent, Anthracycline

Use Intravesical therapy of BCG-refractory carcinoma *in situ* of the urinary bladder

Local Anesthetic/Vasoconstrictor Precautions No information available to require special precautions

Effects on Dental Treatment No significant effects or complications reported

Common Adverse Effects

>10%: Genitourinary: Frequency (61%), dysuria (56%), urgency (57%), bladder spasm (31%), hematuria (29%), bladder pain (28%), urinary incontinence (22%), cystitis (15%), urinary tract infection (15%)

1% to 10%:

Cardiovascular: Chest pain (2%), vasodilation (2%), peripheral edema (1%)

Central nervous system: Headache (4%), malaise (4%), dizziness (3%), fever (2%)

Dermatologic: Rash (3%)

Endocrine & metabolic: Hyperglycemia (1%)

Gastrointestinal: Abdominal pain (5%), nausea (5%), diarrhea (3%), vomiting (2%), flatulence (1%)

Genitourinary: Nocturia (7%), burning symptoms (5%), urinary retention (4%), urethral pain (3%), pelvic pain (1%), hematuria (microscopic) (3%)

Hematologic: Anemia (2%)

Neuromuscular & skeletal: Weakness (4%), back pain (3%), myalgia (1%)

Respiratory: Pneumonia (1%)

Mechanism of Action Blocks function of DNA topoisomerase II; inhibits DNA synthesis, causes extensive chromosomal damage, and arrests cell development; unlike other anthracyclines, does not appear to intercalate DNA

Drug Interactions

Increased Effect/Toxicity: No specific drug interactions studies have been performed. Systemic exposure to valrubicin is negligible, and interactions are unlikely.

Decreased Effect: No specific drug interactions studies have been performed. Systemic exposure to valrubicin is negligible, and interactions are unlikely.

Pharmacodynamics/Kinetics

Absorption: Well absorbed into bladder tissue, negligible systemic absorption. Trauma to mucosa may increase absorption, and perforation greatly increases absorption with significant systemic myelotoxicity.

Metabolism: Negligible after intravesical instillation and 2 hour retention

Excretion: Urine when expelled from urinary bladder (98.6% as intact drug; 0.4% as *N*-trifluoroacetyladriamycin)

Pregnancy Risk Factor C

Valsartan (val SAR tan)

Related Information

Cardiovascular Diseases *on page 1636*

U.S. Brand Names Diovan®

Canadian Brand Names Diovan®

Generic Available No

Pharmacologic Category Angiotensin II Receptor Blocker

Use Alone or in combination with other antihypertensive agents in the treatment of essential hypertension; treatment of heart failure (NYHA Class II-IV); reduction of cardiovascular mortality in patients with left ventricular dysfunction post-myocardial infarction

Local Anesthetic/Vasoconstrictor Precautions No information available to require special precautions

Effects on Dental Treatment No significant effects or complications reported

Common Adverse Effects

>10%: Central nervous system: Dizziness (2% to 17%)

1% to 10%:

Cardiovascular: Hypotension (6% to 7%), postural hypotension (2%)

Central nervous system: Fatigue (2% to 3%)

Endocrine & metabolic: Serum potassium increased (4% to 10%), hyperkalemia (<1% to 2%)

Gastrointestinal: Diarrhea (5%), abdominal pain (2%)

Hematologic: Neutropenia (2%)

Neuromuscular & skeletal: Arthralgia (3%), back pain (3%)

Renal: Creatinine increased >50% (4%)

Respiratory: Cough (3%)

Miscellaneous: Viral infection (3%)

Dosage Adults: Oral:

Hypertension: Initial: 80 mg or 160 mg once daily (in patients who are not volume depleted); dose may be increased to achieve desired effect; maximum recommended dose: 320 mg/day

Heart failure: Initial: 40 mg twice daily; titrate dose to 80-160 mg twice daily, as tolerated; maximum daily dose: 320 mg

Left ventricular dysfunction after MI: Initial: 20 mg twice daily; titrate dose to target of 160 mg twice daily as tolerated; may initiate ≥12 hours following MI

Dosing adjustment in renal impairment: No dosage adjustment necessary if Cl_{cr} >10 mL/minute.

Dosing adjustment in hepatic impairment (mild - moderate): ≤80 mg/day

Dialysis: Not significantly removed

Mechanism of Action Valsartan produces direct antagonism of the angiotensin II (AT2) receptors, unlike the ACE inhibitors. It displaces angiotensin II from the AT1 receptor and produces its blood pressure lowering effects by antagonizing AT1-induced vasoconstriction, aldosterone release, catecholamine release, arginine vasopressin release, water intake, and hypertrophic responses. This action results in more efficient blockade of the cardiovascular effects of angiotensin II and fewer side effects than the ACE inhibitors.

(Continued)

Valsartan *(Continued)*

Contraindications Hypersensitivity to valsartan or any component of the formulation; hypersensitivity to other A-II receptor antagonists; bilateral renal artery stenosis; pregnancy (2nd and 3rd trimesters)

Warnings/Precautions During the initiation of therapy, hypotension may occur, particularly in patients with heart failure or post-MI patients. Use extreme caution with concurrent administration of potassium-sparing diuretics or potassium supplements, in patients with mild to moderate hepatic dysfunction (adjust dose), in those who may be sodium/water depleted (eg, on high-dose diuretics), and in the elderly; avoid use in patients with CHF, unilateral renal artery stenosis, aortic/mitral valve stenosis, coronary artery disease, or hypertrophic cardiomyopathy, if possible

Drug Interactions

Cytochrome P450 Effect: Inhibits CYP2C8/9 (weak)

Increased Effect/Toxicity: Valsartan blood levels may be increased by cimetidine and monoxidine; clinical effect is unknown. Concurrent use of potassium salts/supplements, co-trimoxazole (high dose), ACE inhibitors, and potassium-sparing diuretics (amiloride, spironolactone, triamterene) may increase the risk of hyperkalemia.

Decreased Effect: Phenobarbital, ketoconazole, troleandomycin, sulfaphenazole

Ethanol/Nutrition/Herb Interactions

Food: Decreases rate and extent of absorption by 50% and 40%, respectively.

Herb/Nutraceutical: Avoid dong quai if using for hypertension (has estrogenic activity). Avoid ephedra, yohimbe, ginseng (may worsen hypertension). Avoid garlic (may have increased antihypertensive effect).

Dietary Considerations Avoid salt substitutes which contain potassium. May be taken with or without food.

Pharmacodynamics/Kinetics

Onset of antihypertensive effect: 2 weeks (maximal: 4 weeks)

Distribution: V_d: 17 L (adults)

Protein binding: 95%, primarily albumin

Metabolism: To inactive metabolite

Bioavailability: 25% (range 10% to 35%)

Half-life elimination: 6 hours

Time to peak, serum: 2-4 hours

Excretion: Feces (83%) and urine (13%) as unchanged drug

Pregnancy Risk Factor C/D (2nd and 3rd trimesters)

Dosage Forms TAB: 40 mg, 80 mg, 160 mg, 320 mg

Valsartan and Hydrochlorothiazide
(val SAR tan & hye droe klor oh THYE a zide)

Related Information

Cardiovascular Diseases *on page 1636*

Hydrochlorothiazide *on page 776*

Valsartan *on page 1561*

U.S. Brand Names Diovan HCT®

Canadian Brand Names Diovan HCT®

Generic Available No

Synonyms Hydrochlorothiazide and Valsartan

Pharmacologic Category Angiotensin II Receptor Blocker Combination; Antihypertensive Agent, Combination; Diuretic, Thiazide

Use Treatment of hypertension (not indicated for initial therapy)

Local Anesthetic/Vasoconstrictor Precautions No information available to require special precautions

Effects on Dental Treatment No significant effects or complications reported

Common Adverse Effects Percentages reported with combination product; other reactions have been reported (see individual agents for additional information)

1% to 10%:

Central nervous system: Dizziness (9%; dose related), fatigue (5%)

Endocrine & metabolic: Hypokalemia (3%)

Gastrointestinal: Diarrhea (3%)

Respiratory: Cough (3%), nasopharyngitis (3%)

Drug Interactions

Cytochrome P450 Effect: Valsartan: Inhibits CYP2C8/9 (weak)

Increased Effect/Toxicity: See individual agents.

Decreased Effect: See individual agents.

Pharmacodynamics/Kinetics See individual agents.

Pregnancy Risk Factor C/D (2nd and 3rd trimester)

Valstar® [DSC] *see* Valrubicin *on page 1560*

Valtrex® *see* Valacyclovir *on page 1553*

Vanamide™ *see* Urea *on page 1551*

Vancocin® *see* Vancomycin *on page 1563*

Vancomycin (van koe MYE sin)

Related Information
Cardiovascular Diseases *on page 1636*

U.S. Brand Names Vancocin®

Canadian Brand Names Vancocin®

Generic Available Yes: Injection

Synonyms Vancomycin Hydrochloride

Pharmacologic Category Antibiotic, Miscellaneous

Use Treatment of patients with infections caused by staphylococcal species and streptococcal species; used orally for staphylococcal enterocolitis or for antibiotic-associated pseudomembranous colitis produced by *C. difficile*

Local Anesthetic/Vasoconstrictor Precautions No information available to require special precautions

Effects on Dental Treatment Key adverse event(s) related to dental treatment: Bitter taste. The "red man syndrome" characterized by skin rash and hypotension is not an allergic reaction but rather is associated with too rapid infusion of the drug. To alleviate or prevent the reaction, infuse vancomycin at a rate of ≥30 minutes for each 500 mg of drug being administered (eg, 1 g over ≥60 minutes); 1.5 g over ≥90 minutes.

Common Adverse Effects
Oral:
>10%: Gastrointestinal: Bitter taste, nausea, vomiting
1% to 10%:
Central nervous system: Chills, drug fever
Hematologic: Eosinophilia
Parenteral:
>10%:
Cardiovascular: Hypotension accompanied by flushing
Dermatologic: Erythematous rash on face and upper body (red neck or red man syndrome - infusion rate related)
1% to 10%:
Central nervous system: Chills, drug fever
Dermatologic: Rash
Hematologic: Eosinophilia, reversible neutropenia

Dosage Initial dosage recommendation:
Neonates: I.V.:
Postnatal age ≤7 days:
<1200 g: 15 mg/kg/dose every 24 hours
1200-2000 g: 10 mg/kg/dose every 12 hours
>2000 g: 15 mg/kg/dose every 12 hours
Postnatal age >7 days:
<1200 g: 15 mg/kg/dose every 24 hours
≥1200 g: 10 mg/kg/dose every 8 hours
Infants >1 month and Children: I.V.:
40 mg/kg/day in divided doses every 6 hours
Prophylaxis for bacterial endocarditis:
Dental, oral, or upper respiratory tract surgery: 20 mg/kg 1 hour prior to the procedure
GI/GU procedure: 20 mg/kg plus gentamicin 2 mg/kg 1 hour prior to surgery
Infants >1 month and Children with staphylococcal central nervous system infection: I.V.: 60 mg/kg/day in divided doses every 6 hours
Adults: I.V.:
With normal renal function: 1 g **or** 10-15 mg/kg/dose every 12 hours
Hospital-acquired pneumonia (HAP): 15 mg/kg/dose every 12 hours (American Thoracic Society/ATS guidelines)
Meningitis *(Pneumococcus* or *Staphylococcus)*: 30-45 mg/kg/day in divided doses every 8-12 hours **or** 500-750 mg every 6 hours (with third-generation cephalosporin for PCN-resistant *Streptococcus pneumoniae*); maximum dose: 2-3 g/day
Prophylaxis for bacterial endocarditis:
Dental, oral, or upper respiratory tract surgery: 1 g 1 hour before surgery
GI/GU procedure: 1 g plus 1.5 mg/kg gentamicin 1 hour prior to surgery
(Continued)

Vancomycin (Continued)

Antibiotic lock technique (for catheter infections): 2 mg/mL in SWI/NS or D₅W; instill 3-5 mL into catheter port as a flush solution instead of heparin lock (**Note:** Do not mix with any other solutions)

Intrathecal: Vancomycin is available as a powder for injection and may be diluted to 1-5 mg/mL concentration in preservative-free 0.9% sodium chloride for administration into the CSF
Neonates: 5-10 mg/day
Children: 5-20 mg/day
Adults: Up to 20 mg/day

Oral: Pseudomembranous colitis produced by *C. difficile*:
Neonates: 10 mg/kg/day in divided doses
Children: 40 mg/kg/day in divided doses, added to fluids
Adults: 125 mg 4 times/day for 10 days

Dosing interval in renal impairment (vancomycin levels should be monitored in patients with any renal impairment):
Cl_{cr} >60 mL/minute: Start with 1 g or 10-15 mg/kg/dose every 12 hours
Cl_{cr} 40-60 mL/minute: Start with 1 g or 10-15 mg/kg/dose every 24 hours
Cl_{cr} <40 mL/minute: Will need longer intervals; determine by serum concentration monitoring
Hemodialysis: Not dialyzable (0% to 5%); generally not removed; exception minimal-moderate removal by some of the newer high-flux filters; dose may need to be administered more frequently; monitor serum concentrations
Continuous ambulatory peritoneal dialysis (CAPD): Not significantly removed; administration via CAPD fluid: 15-30 mg/L (15-30 mcg/mL) of CAPD fluid
Continuous arteriovenous hemofiltration: Dose as for Cl_{cr} 10-40 mL/minute

Mechanism of Action Inhibits bacterial cell wall synthesis by blocking glycopeptide polymerization through binding tightly to D-alanyl-D-alanine portion of cell wall precursor

Contraindications Hypersensitivity to vancomycin or any component of the formulation; avoid in patients with previous severe hearing loss

Warnings/Precautions Use with caution in patients with renal impairment or those receiving other nephrotoxic or ototoxic drugs; dosage modification required in patients with impaired renal function (especially elderly)

Drug Interactions
Increased Effect/Toxicity: Increased toxicity with other ototoxic or nephrotoxic drugs. Increased neuromuscular blockade with most neuromuscular blocking agents.

Dietary Considerations May be taken with food.

Pharmacodynamics/Kinetics
Absorption: Oral: Poor; I.M.: Erratic; Intraperitoneal: ~38%
Distribution: Widely in body tissues and fluids. except for CSF
Relative diffusion from blood into CSF: Good only with inflammation (exceeds usual MICs)
CSF:blood level ratio: Normal meninges: Nil; Inflamed meninges: 20% to 30%
Protein binding: 10% to 50%
Half-life elimination: Biphasic: Terminal:
Newborns: 6-10 hours
Infants and Children 3 months to 4 years: 4 hours
Children >3 years: 2.2-3 hours
Adults: 5-11 hours; significantly prolonged with renal impairment
End-stage renal disease: 200-250 hours
Time to peak, serum: I.V.: 45-65 minutes
Excretion: I.V.: Urine (80% to 90% as unchanged drug); Oral: Primarily feces

Pregnancy Risk Factor C

Dosage Forms CAP (Vancocin®): 125 mg, 250 mg. **INF** [premixed in iso-osmotic dextrose] (Vancocin®): 500 mg (100 mL); 1 g (200 mL). **INJ, powder for reconstitution:** 500 mg, 1 g, 5 g, 10 g

Vancomycin Hydrochloride *see* Vancomycin *on page 1563*

Vandazole™ *see* Metronidazole *on page 1033*

Vaniqa™ *see* Eflornithine *on page 532*

Vanos™ *see* Fluocinonide *on page 670*

Vanoxide-HC® *see* Benzoyl Peroxide and Hydrocortisone *on page 195*

Vanquish® Extra Strength Pain Reliever [OTC] *see* Acetaminophen, Aspirin, and Caffeine *on page 41*

Van R Gingibraid® *see* Epinephrine (Racemic) and Aluminum Potassium Sulfate *on page 550*

Vantas™ *see* Histrelin *on page 772*

Vantin® *see* Cefpodoxime *on page 290*

Vaprisol® *see* Conivaptan *on page 393*

VAQTA® see Hepatitis A Vaccine on page 767

Vardenafil (var DEN a fil)

U.S. Brand Names Levitra®
Canadian Brand Names Levitra®
Mexican Brand Names Levitra®
Generic Available No
Synonyms Vardenafil Hydrochloride
Pharmacologic Category Phosphodiesterase-5 Enzyme Inhibitor
Use Treatment of erectile dysfunction
Local Anesthetic/Vasoconstrictor Precautions No information available to require special precautions
Effects on Dental Treatment No significant effects or complications reported
Common Adverse Effects
>10%:
  Cardiovascular: Flushing (11%)
  Central nervous system: Headache (15%)
2% to 10%:
  Central nervous system: Dizziness (2%)
  Gastrointestinal: Dyspepsia (4%), nausea (2%)
  Neuromuscular & skeletal: CPK increased (2%)
  Respiratory: Rhinitis (9%), sinusitis (3%)
  Miscellaneous: Flu-like syndrome (3%)
Dosage Oral: Adults: Erectile dysfunction: 10 mg 60 minutes prior to sexual activity; dosing range: 5-20 mg; to be given as one single dose and not given more than once daily
Dosing adjustment with concomitant medications:
  Alpha blocker (dose should be stable at time of vardenafil initiation): Initial vardenafil dose: 5 mg/24 hours; if an alpha blocker is added to vardenafil therapy, it should be initiated at the smallest possible dose, and titrated carefully.
  Erythromycin: Maximum vardenafil dose: 5 mg/24 hours
  Indinavir: Maximum vardenafil dose: 2.5 mg/24 hours
  Itraconazole:
    200 mg/day: Maximum vardenafil dose: 5 mg/24 hours
    400 mg/day: Maximum vardenafil dose: 2.5 mg/24 hours
  Ketoconazole:
    200 mg/day: Maximum vardenafil dose: 5 mg/24 hours
    400 mg/day: Maximum vardenafil dose: 2.5 mg/24 hours
  Ritonavir: Maximum vardenafil dose: 2.5 mg/72 hours
Elderly ≥65 years: Initial: 5 mg 60 minutes prior to sexual activity; to be given as one single dose and not given more than once daily
Dosage adjustment in renal impairment: Dose adjustment not needed for mild, moderate, or severe impairment; use has not been studied in patients on renal dialysis
Dosage adjustment in hepatic impairment: Child-Pugh class B: Initial: 5 mg 60 minutes prior to sexual activity (maximum dose: 10 mg); to be given as one single dose and not given more than once daily
Mechanism of Action Does not directly cause penile erections, but affects the response to sexual stimulation. The physiologic mechanism of erection of the penis involves release of nitric oxide (NO) in the corpus cavernosum during sexual stimulation. NO then activates the enzyme guanylate cyclase, which results in increased levels of cyclic guanosine monophosphate (cGMP), producing smooth muscle relaxation and inflow of blood to the corpus cavernosum. Vardenafil enhances the effect of NO by inhibiting phosphodiesterase type 5 (PDE-5), which is responsible for degradation of cGMP in the corpus cavernosum; when sexual stimulation causes local release of NO, inhibition of PDE-5 by vardenafil causes increased levels of cGMP in the corpus cavernosum, resulting in smooth muscle relaxation and inflow of blood to the corpus cavernosum; at recommended doses, it has no effect in the absence of sexual stimulation.
Contraindications Hypersensitivity to vardenafil or any component of the formulation; concurrent use of organic nitrates (nitroglycerin; scheduled dosing or as needed)
Warnings/Precautions There is a degree of cardiac risk associated with sexual activity; therefore, physicians may wish to consider the patient's cardiovascular status prior to initiating any treatment for erectile dysfunction. Use caution in patients with anatomical deformation of the penis (angulation, cavernosal fibrosis, or Peyronie's disease) and in patients who have conditions which may predispose them to priapism (sickle cell anemia, multiple myeloma, (Continued)

Vardenafil *(Continued)*

leukemia). Patients should be instructed to seek medical attention if erection persists >4 hours.

Not recommended for use in patients with congenital QT prolongation or those taking Class Ia or III antiarrhythmics. Concomitant use with alpha blockers may cause hypotension; safety of this combination may be affected by other antihypertensives and intravascular volume depletion. Patients should be hemodynamically stable prior to initiating therapy. Use caution with alpha blockers, effective CYP3A4 inhibitors, the elderly, or those with hepatic impairment (Child-Pugh class B); dosage adjustment is needed.

Rare cases of nonarteritic ischemic optic neuropathy (NAION) have been reported; risk may be increased with history of vision loss. Other risk factors for NAION include heart disease, diabetes, hypertension, smoking, age >50 years, or history of certain eye problems.

Safety and efficacy have not been studied in patients with the following conditions, therefore, use in these patients is not recommended at this time: Hypotension, uncontrolled hypertension, unstable angina, severe cardiac failure; a life-threatening arrhythmia, myocardial infarction, or stroke within the last 6 months; severe hepatic impairment (Child-Pugh class C); end-stage renal disease requiring dialysis; retinitis pigmentosa or other degenerative retinal disorders. The safety and efficacy of vardenafil with other treatments for erectile dysfunction have not been studied and are not recommended as combination therapy.

Drug Interactions

Cytochrome P450 Effect: Substrate of CYP2C (minor), 3A5 (minor), 3A4 (major)

Increased Effect/Toxicity: CYP3A4 inhibitors may increase the levels/effects of vardenafil; example inhibitors include azole antifungals, clarithromycin, diclofenac, doxycycline, erythromycin, imatinib, isoniazid, nefazodone, nicardipine, propofol, protease inhibitors, quinidine, telithromycin, and verapamil. Nitroglycerin may lead to excessive hypotension; concomitant use is contraindicated. Alpha-blockers may also lead to excessive hypotension; initiate vardenafil at lowest possible dose if patient is stabilized on alpha blocker; initiate alpha-blocker at lowest possible dose and titrate cautiously in patients on a stable dose of vardenafil.

Ethanol/Nutrition/Herb Interactions

Food: High-fat meals decrease maximum serum concentration 18% to 50%. Serum concentrations/toxicity may be increased with grapefruit juice; avoid concurrent use.

Dietary Considerations May take with or without food

Pharmacodynamics/Kinetics

Absorption: Rapid

Distribution: V_d: 208 L; <0.01% found in semen 1.5 hours after dose

Metabolism: Hepatic via CYP3A4 (major), CYP2C and 3A5 (minor); forms metabolite (active)

Bioavailability: 15%; Elderly (≥65 years): 52%; Hepatic impairment (Child-Pugh class B): 160%

Half-life elimination: Terminal: Vardenafil and metabolite: 4-5 hours

Time to peak, plasma: 0.5-2 hours

Excretion: Feces (91% to 95% as metabolites); urine (2% to 6%)

Clearance: 56 L/hour

Pregnancy Risk Factor B

Dosage Forms TAB, film-coated: 2.5 mg, 5 mg, 10 mg, 20 mg

Vardenafil Hydrochloride *see* Vardenafil *on page 1565*

Varicella, Measles, Mumps, and Rubella Vaccine *see* Measles, Mumps, Rubella, and Varicella Virus Vaccine *on page 967*

Varicella-Zoster Immune Globulin (Human)
(var i SEL a- ZOS ter i MYUN GLOB yoo lin HYU man)

Related Information
Immunizations (Vaccines) *on page 1786*

Generic Available No

Synonyms VZIG

Pharmacologic Category Immune Globulin

Use Passive immunization of susceptible patients who are at a greater risk of complications following significant exposure to varicella

Restrict administration to those patients meeting the following criteria:
Immunocompromised children including those with neoplastic disease (eg, leukemia or lymphoma); congenital or acquired immunodeficiency; immuno-suppressive therapy with steroids, antimetabolites or other immunosuppressive treatment regimens

Newborn of mother who had onset of varicella (chickenpox) within 5 days before delivery or within 48 hours after delivery (not indicated if the mother has zoster)

Premature infants (≥28 weeks gestation) whose mother has no history of chickenpox

Premature infants (<28 weeks gestation or ≤1000 g) regardless of maternal history

Immunocompromised adults

Significant exposure includes:
Continuous household contact

Playmate contact (>1 hour play indoors)

Hospital contact (in same 2-4 bedroom or adjacent beds in a large ward or prolonged face-to-face contact with an infectious staff member or patient)

Local Anesthetic/Vasoconstrictor Precautions No information available to require special precautions

Effects on Dental Treatment No significant effects or complications reported

Common Adverse Effects 1%: Local: Discomfort at the site of injection (pain, redness, edema)

Mechanism of Action Antibodies obtained from pooled human plasma of individuals with high titers of varicella-zoster provide passive immunity

Drug Interactions
Decreased Effect:
VZIG may interfere with the immune response; do not administer live virus vaccines within 5 months of VZIG administration

Pharmacodynamics/Kinetics Duration: ~3 weeks

Pregnancy Risk Factor C

Vaseretic® *see* Enalapril and Hydrochlorothiazide *on page 541*

Vasocon®-A [OTC] [DSC] *see* Naphazoline and Antazoline *on page 1088*

Vasodilan® [DSC] *see* Isoxsuprine *on page 871*

Vasopressin (vay soe PRES in)

U.S. Brand Names Pitressin®
Canadian Brand Names Pressyn®; Pressyn® AR
Generic Available No
Synonyms ADH; Antidiuretic Hormone; 8-Arginine Vasopressin
Pharmacologic Category Antidiuretic Hormone Analog; Hormone, Posterior Pituitary
Use Treatment of diabetes insipidus; prevention and treatment of postoperative abdominal distention; differential diagnosis of diabetes insipidus
Unlabeled/Investigational Use Adjunct in the treatment of GI hemorrhage and esophageal varices; pulseless arrest (ventricular tachycardia [VT]/ventricular fibrillation [VF], asystole/pulseless electrical activity [PEA]); vasodilatory shock (septic shock)
Local Anesthetic/Vasoconstrictor Precautions No information available to require special precautions
Effects on Dental Treatment No significant effects or complications reported
Common Adverse Effects Frequency not defined.
Cardiovascular: Arrhythmia, asystole (>0.4 units/minute), blood pressure increased, cardiac output decreased (>0.4 units/minute), chest pain, MI, vasoconstriction (with higher doses), venous thrombosis
Central nervous system: Pounding in the head, fever, vertigo
Dermatologic: Ischemic skin lesions, circumoral pallor, urticaria
Gastrointestinal: Abdominal cramps, flatulence, mesenteric ischemia, nausea, vomiting
Genitourinary: Uterine contraction
Neuromuscular & skeletal: Tremor
Respiratory: Bronchial constriction
Miscellaneous: Diaphoresis
Mechanism of Action Increases cyclic adenosine monophosphate (cAMP) which increases water permeability at the renal tubule resulting in decreased urine volume and increased osmolality; causes peristalsis by directly stimulating the smooth muscle in the GI tract; direct vasoconstrictor without inotropic or chronotropic effects
(Continued)

Vasopressin *(Continued)*

Drug Interactions
Increased Effect/Toxicity: Chlorpropamide, urea, clofibrate, carbamazepine, and fludrocortisone potentiate antidiuretic response.

Decreased Effect: Lithium, epinephrine, demeclocycline, heparin, and ethanol block antidiuretic activity to varying degrees.

Pharmacodynamics/Kinetics
Onset of action: Nasal: 1 hour

Duration: Nasal: 3-8 hours; I.M., SubQ: 2-8 hours

Metabolism: Nasal/Parenteral: Hepatic, renal

Half-life elimination: Nasal: 15 minutes; Parenteral: 10-20 minutes

Excretion: Nasal: Urine; SubQ: Urine (5% as unchanged drug) after 4 hours

Pregnancy Risk Factor C

Vasotec® *see* Enalapril *on page 538*

VCF™ [OTC] *see* Nonoxynol 9 *on page 1124*

VCR *see* VinCRIStine *on page 1576*

Veetids® *see* Penicillin V Potassium *on page 1205*

Veg-Pancreatin 4X [OTC] *see* Pancreatin *on page 1183*

Velcade® *see* Bortezomib *on page 215*

Velivet™ *see* Ethinyl Estradiol and Desogestrel *on page 592*

Velosef® *see* Cephradine *on page 304*

Venlafaxine *(VEN la faks een)*

U.S. Brand Names Effexor®; Effexor® XR

Canadian Brand Names Effexor® XR

Mexican Brand Names Efexor®

Generic Available No

Pharmacologic Category Antidepressant, Serotonin/Norepinephrine Reuptake Inhibitor

Use Treatment of major depressive disorder; generalized anxiety disorder (GAD), social anxiety disorder (social phobia); panic disorder

Unlabeled/Investigational Use Obsessive-compulsive disorder (OCD); hot flashes; neuropathic pain; attention-deficit/hyperactivity disorder (ADHD)

Local Anesthetic/Vasoconstrictor Precautions Although venlafaxine is not a tricyclic antidepressant, it does block norepinephrine reuptake within CNS synapses as part of its mechanisms. It has been suggested that vasoconstrictor be administered with caution and to monitor vital signs in dental patients taking antidepressants that affect norepinephrine in this way. This is particularly important in patients taking venlafaxine, which has been noted to produce a sustained increase in diastolic blood pressure and heart rate as a side effect.

Effects on Dental Treatment Key adverse event(s) related to dental treatment: Significant xerostomia (normal salivary flow resumes upon discontinuation); may contribute to oral discomfort, especially in the elderly

Common Adverse Effects
>10%:

Central nervous system: Headache (25% to 34%), insomnia (15% to 23%), somnolence (12% to 23%), dizziness (11% to 20%), nervousness (6% to 13%)

Gastrointestinal: Nausea (21% to 37%), xerostomia (12% to 22%), anorexia (8% to 20%), constipation (8% to 15%)

Genitourinary: Abnormal ejaculation/orgasm (2% to 16%)

Neuromuscular & skeletal: Weakness (8% to 17%)

Miscellaneous: Diaphoresis (10% to 14%)

1% to 10%:

Cardiovascular: Hypertension (dose related; 3% in patients receiving <100 mg/day, up to 13% in patients receiving >300 mg/day); vasodilation (3% to 4%); palpitation (3%), tachycardia (2%), chest pain (2%), postural hypotension (1%), edema

Central nervous system: Abnormal dreams (3% to 7%), anxiety (5% to 6%), yawning (3% to 5%), agitation (2% to 4%), chills (3%), confusion (2%), abnormal thinking (2%), depersonalization (1%), depression (1% to 3%), chills, fever, migraine, amnesia, hypoethesia, trismus, vertigo

Dermatologic: Rash (3%), pruritus (1%), bruising

Endocrine & metabolic: Libido decreased (3% to 9%)

Gastrointestinal: Diarrhea (6% to 8%), vomiting (3% to 6%), dyspepsia (5%), abdominal pain (4%), flatulence (3% to 4%), taste perversion (2%), weight loss (1% to 4%), appetite increased, weight gain

Genitourinary: Impotence (4% to 10%), urinary frequency (3%), impaired urination (2%), urinary retention (1%), prostatic disorder

Neuromuscular & skeletal: Tremor (4% to 5%), hypertonia (3%), paresthesia (2% to 3%), twitching (1% to 2%), neck pain, arthralgia

Ocular: Abnormal or blurred vision (4% to 6%), mydriasis (2%

Otic: Tinnitus (2%)

Respiratory: Pharyngitis (7%), sinusitis (2%), cough increased, dyspnea

Miscellaneous: Infection (6%), flu-like syndrome (6%), trauma (2%)

Restrictions A medication guide concerning the use of antidepressants in children and teenagers can be found on the FDA website at http://www.fda.gov/cder/Offices/ODS/labeling.htm. It should be dispensed to parents or guardians of children and teenagers receiving this medication.

Dosage Oral:

Children and Adolescents:

ADHD (unlabeled use): Initial: 12.5 mg/day

Children <40 kg: Increase by 12.5 mg/week to maximum of 50 mg/day in 2 divided doses

Children ≥40 kg: Increase by 25 mg/week to maximum of 75 mg/day in 3 divided doses.

Mean dose: 60 mg or 1.4 mg/kg administered in 2-3 divided doses

Adults:

Depression:

Immediate-release tablets: 75 mg/day, administered in 2 or 3 divided doses, taken with food; dose may be increased in 75 mg/day increments at intervals of at least 4 days, up to 225-375 mg/day

Extended-release capsules: 75 mg once daily taken with food; for some new patients, it may be desirable to start at 37.5 mg/day for 4-7 days before increasing to 75 mg once daily; dose may be increased by up to 75 mg/day increments every 4 days as tolerated, up to a maximum of 225 mg/day

GAD, social anxiety disorder: Extended-release capsules: 75 mg once daily taken with food; for some new patients, it may be desirable to start at 37.5 mg/day for 4-7 days before increasing to 75 mg once daily; dose may be increased by up to 75 mg/day increments every 4 days as tolerated, up to a maximum of 225 mg/day

Panic disorder: Extended-release capsules: 37.5 mg once daily for 1 week; may increase to 75 mg daily, with subsequent weekly increases of 75 mg/day up to a maximum of 225 mg/day.

Obsessive-compulsive disorder (unlabeled use): Titrate to usual dosage range of 150-300 mg/day; however, doses up to 375 mg daily have been used; response may be seen in 4 weeks

Neuropathic pain (unlabeled use): Dosages evaluated varied considerably based on etiology of chronic pain, but efficacy has been shown for many conditions in the range of 75-225 mg/day; onset of relief may occur in 1-2 weeks, or take up to 6 weeks for full benefit.

Hot flashes (unlabeled use): Doses of 37.5-75 mg/day have demonstrated significant improvement of vasomotor symptoms after 4-8 weeks of treatment; in one study, doses >75 mg/day offered no additional benefit; however, higher doses (225 mg/day) may be beneficial in patients with perimenopausal depression.

Attention-deficit disorder (unlabeled use): Initial: Doses vary between 18.75 to 75 mg/day; may increase after 4 weeks to 150 mg/day; if tolerated, doses up to 225 mg/day have been used

Note: When discontinuing this medication after more than 1 week of treatment, it is generally recommended that the dose be tapered. If venlafaxine is used for 6 weeks or longer, the dose should be tapered over 2 weeks when discontinuing its use.

Dosing adjustment in renal impairment: Cl_{cr} 10-70 mL/minute: Decrease dose by 25%; decrease total daily dose by 50% if dialysis patients; dialysis patients should receive dosing after completion of dialysis

Dosing adjustment in moderate hepatic impairment: Reduce total daily dosage by 50%

Mechanism of Action Venlafaxine and its active metabolite o-desmethylvenlafaxine (ODV) are potent inhibitors of neuronal serotonin and norepinephrine reuptake and weak inhibitors of dopamine reuptake. Venlafaxine and ODV have no significant activity for muscarinic cholinergic, H_1-histaminergic, or alpha$_2$-adrenergic receptors. Venlafaxine and ODV do not possess MAO-inhibitory activity.

Contraindications Hypersensitivity to venlafaxine or any component of the formulation; use of MAO inhibitors within 14 days; should not initiate MAO inhibitor within 7 days of discontinuing venlafaxine

Warnings/Precautions Antidepressants increase the risk of suicidal thinking and behavior in children and adolescents with major depressive disorder (MDD) and other depressive disorders; consider risk prior to prescribing. All patients

(Continued)

Venlafaxine *(Continued)*

must be closely monitored for clinical worsening, suicidality, or unusual changes in behavior, especially during the initiation of therapy or following an increase or decrease in dosage. When used in children, the child's family or caregiver should be instructed to closely observe the patient and communicate condition with healthcare provider. Reduced growth rate has been observed with venlafaxine therapy in children. A medication guide should be dispensed with each prescription. **Venlafaxine is not FDA approved for use in children.**

The possibility of a suicide attempt is inherent in major depression and may persist until remission occurs. Use caution in high-risk patients. Worsening depression and severe abrupt suicidality that are not part of the presenting symptoms may require discontinuation or modification of drug therapy. The patient's family or caregiver should be alerted to monitor patients for the emergence of suicidality and associated behaviors (such as agitation, irritability, hostility, impulsivity, and hypomania) and call healthcare provider.

May worsen psychosis in some patients or precipitate a shift to mania or hypomania in patients with bipolar disorder. Patients presenting with depressive symptoms should be screened for bipolar disorder. Monotherapy in patients with bipolar disorder should be avoided. **Venlafaxine is not FDA approved for the treatment of bipolar depression.**

The potential for severe reactions exists when used with MAO inhibitors (myoclonus, diaphoresis, hyperthermia, NMS features, seizures, and death). May cause sustained increase in blood pressure or tachycardia; dose related and increases are generally modest (12-15 mmHg diastolic). Control pre-existing hypertension perior to initiation of venlafaxine. Use caution in patients with recent history of MI, unstable heart disease, or hyperthyroidism; may cause increase in anxiety, nervousness, insomnia; may cause weight loss (use with caution in patients where weight loss is undesirable); may cause increases in serum cholesterol. Use caution with hepatic or renal impairment. Venlafaxine has been associated with the development of SIADH and hyponatremia.

May increase the risks associated with electroconvulsive therapy. Use cautiously in patients with a history of seizures. The risks of cognitive or motor impairment, as well as the potential for anticholinergic effects are very low. May cause or exacerbate sexual dysfunction. May impair platelet aggregation, resulting in bleeding.

Abrupt discontinuation or dosage reduction after extended (≥6 weeks) therapy may lead to agitation, dysphoria, nervousness, anxiety, and other symptoms. When discontinuing therapy, dosage should be tapered gradually over at least a 2-week period. If intolerable symptoms occur following a decrease in dosage or upon discontinuation of therapy, then resuming the previous dose with a more gradual taper should be considered. Use caution in patients with increased intraocular pressure or at risk of acute narrow-angle glaucoma.

Drug Interactions

Cytochrome P450 Effect: Substrate of CYP2C8/9 (minor), 2C19 (minor), 2D6 (major), 3A4 (major); Inhibits CYP2B6 (weak), 2D6 (weak), 3A4 (weak)

Increased Effect/Toxicity: Concurrent use of MAO inhibitors (phenelzine, isocarboxazid), or drugs with MAO inhibitor activity (linezolid) may result in serotonin syndrome; should not be used within 2 weeks of each other. Selegiline may have a lower risk of this effect, particularly at low dosages, due to selectivity for MAO type B. In addition, concurrent use of buspirone, lithium, meperidine, nefazodone, selegiline, serotonin agonists (sumatriptan, naratriptan), sibutramine, SSRIs, trazodone, or tricyclic antidepressants may increase the risk of serotonin syndrome. Serum levels of haloperidol may be increased by venlafaxine. CYP2D6 inhibitors may increase the levels/effects of venlafaxine; example inhibitors include chlorpromazine, delavirdine, fluoxetine, miconazole, paroxetine, pergolide, quinidine, quinine, ritonavir, and ropinirole. CYP3A4 inhibitors may increase the levels/effects of venlafaxine; example inhibitors include azole antifungals, clarithromycin, diclofenac, doxycycline, erythromycin, imatinib, isoniazid, nefazodone, nicardipine, propofol, protease inhibitors, quinidine, telithromycin, and verapamil.

Decreased Effect: Serum levels of indinavir may be reduced be venlafaxine (AUC reduced by 28%); clinical significance not determined. CYP3A4 inducers may decrease the levels/effects of venlafaxine; example inducers include aminoglutethimide, carbamazepine, nafcillin, nevirapine, phenobarbital, phenytoin, and rifamycins.

Ethanol/Nutrition/Herb Interactions

Ethanol: Avoid ethanol (may increase CNS effects).

Herb/Nutraceutical: Avoid valerian, St John's wort, SAMe, kava kava, tryptophan (may increase risk of serotonin syndrome and/or excessive sedation).

Dietary Considerations Should be taken with food.

Pharmacodynamics/Kinetics

Absorption: Oral: 92% to 100%; food has no significant effect on the absorption of venlafaxine or formation of the active metabolite O-desmethylvenlafaxine (ODV)

Distribution: At steady state: Venlafaxine 7.5 ± 3.7 L/kg, ODV 5.7 ± 1.8 L/Kg

Protein binding: Bound to human plasma protein: Venlafaxine 27%, ODV 30%

Metabolism: Hepatic via CYP2D6 to active metabolite, O-desmethylvenlafaxine (ODV); other metabolites include N-desmethylvenlafaxine and N,O-didesmethylvenlafaxine

Bioavailability: Absolute: ~45%

Half-life elimination: Venlafaxine: 3-7 hours; ODV: 9-13 hours; Steady-state, plasma: Venlafaxine/ODV: Within 3 days of multiple-dose therapy; prolonged with cirrhosis (Adults: Venlafaxine: ~30%, ODV: ~60%) and with dialysis (Adults: Venlafaxine: ~180%, ODV: ~142%)

Time to peak:
Immediate release: Venlafaxine: 2 hours, ODV: 3 hours
Extended release: Venlafaxine: 5.5 hours, ODV: 9 hours

Excretion: Urine (~87%, 5% as unchanged drug, 29% as unconjugated ODV, 26% as conjugated ODV, 27% as minor inactive metabolites) within 48 hours

Clearance at steady state: Venlafaxine: 1.3 ± 0.6 L/hour/kg, ODV: 0.4 ± 0.2 L/hour/kg

Clearance decreased with:
Cirrhosis: Adults: Venlafaxine: ~50%, ODV: ~30%
Severe cirrhosis: Adults: Venlafaxine: ~90%
Renal impairment (Cl_{cr} 10-70 mL/minute): Adults: Venlafaxine: ~24%
Dialysis: Adults: Venlafaxine: ~57%, ODV: ~56%; due to large volume of distribution, a significant amount of drug is not likely to be removed.

Pregnancy Risk Factor C

Dosage Forms CAP, extended release (Effexor® XR): 37.5 mg, 75 mg, 150 mg. TAB (Effexor®): 25 mg, 37.5 mg, 50 mg, 75 mg, 100 mg

Selected Readings

Ganzberg S, "Psychoactive Drugs," *ADA Guide to Dental Therapeutics,* 2nd edition, Chapter 21, Chicago, IL: ADA Publishing, 2000, 381.

Venofer® *see* Iron Sucrose *on page 862*

Ventavis™ *see* Iloprost *on page 816*

Ventolin® HFA *see* Albuterol *on page 58*

VePesid® *see* Etoposide *on page 626*

Veracolate [OTC] *see* Bisacodyl *on page 209*

Verapamil (ver AP a mil)

Related Information

Cardiovascular Diseases *on page 1636*

U.S. Brand Names Calan®; Calan® SR; Covera-HS®; Isoptin® SR; Verelan®; Verelan® PM

Canadian Brand Names Alti-Verapamil; Apo-Verap®; Calan®; Chronovera®; Covera®; Gen-Verapamil; Gen-Verapamil SR; Isoptin® SR; Novo-Veramil SR; Nu-Verap

Mexican Brand Names Cronovera®; Dilacoran®

Generic Available Yes: Excludes controlled onset products

Synonyms Iproveratril Hydrochloride; Verapamil Hydrochloride

Pharmacologic Category Antiarrhythmic Agent, Class IV; Calcium Channel Blocker

Use Orally for treatment of angina pectoris (vasospastic, chronic stable, unstable) and hypertension; I.V. for supraventricular tachyarrhythmias (PSVT, atrial fibrillation, atrial flutter)

Unlabeled/Investigational Use Migraine; hypertrophic cardiomyopathy; bipolar disorder (manic manifestations)

Local Anesthetic/Vasoconstrictor Precautions No information available to require special precautions

Effects on Dental Treatment Key adverse event(s) related to dental treatment: Gingival hyperplasia. Calcium channel blockers (CCB) have been reported to cause gingival hyperplasia (GH). Verapamil induced GH has appeared 11 months or more after subjects took daily doses of 240-360 mg. The severity of hyperplastic syndrome does not seem to be dose-dependent. Gingivectomy is only successful if CCB therapy is discontinued. GH regresses markedly 1 week after CCB discontinuance with all symptoms resolving in 2 months. If a patient must continue CCB therapy, begin a program of professional cleaning and patient plaque control to minimize severity and growth rate of gingival tissue.

(Continued)

Verapamil *(Continued)*

Common Adverse Effects

>10%: Gastrointestinal: Gingival hyperplasia (19%)

1% to 10%:

Cardiovascular: Bradycardia (1.4% oral, 1.2% I.V.); first-, second-, or third-degree AV block (1.2% oral, unknown I.V.); CHF (1.8% oral); hypotension (2.5% oral, 3% I.V.); peripheral edema (1.9% oral), symptomatic hypotension (1.5% I.V.); severe tachycardia (1% I.V.)

Central nervous system: Dizziness (3.3% oral, 1.2% I.V.), fatigue (1.7% oral), headache (2.2% oral, 1.2% I.V.)

Dermatologic: Rash (1.2% oral)

Gastrointestinal: Constipation (12% up to 42% in clinical trials), nausea (2.7% oral, 0.9% I.V.)

Respiratory: Dyspnea (1.4% oral)

Dosage

Children: SVT:

I.V.:

<1 year: 0.1-0.2 mg/kg over 2 minutes; repeat every 30 minutes as needed

1-15 years: 0.1-0.3 mg/kg over 2 minutes; maximum: 5 mg/dose, may repeat dose in 15 minutes if adequate response not achieved; maximum for second dose: 10 mg/dose

Oral (dose not well established):

1-5 years: 4-8 mg/kg/day in 3 divided doses **or** 40-80 mg every 8 hours

>5 years: 80 mg every 6-8 hours

Adults:

SVT: I.V.: 2.5-5 mg (over 2 minutes); second dose of 5-10 mg (~0.15 mg/kg) may be given 15-30 minutes after the initial dose if patient tolerates, but does not respond to initial dose; maximum total dose: 20 mg

Angina: Oral: Initial dose: 80-120 mg 3 times/day (elderly or small stature: 40 mg 3 times/day); range: 240-480 mg/day in 3-4 divided doses

Hypertension: Oral:

Immediate release: 80 mg 3 times/day; usual dose range (JNC 7): 80-320 mg/day in 2 divided doses

Sustained release: 240 mg/day; usual dose range (JNC 7): 120-360 mg/day in 1-2 divided doses; 120 mg/day in the elderly or small patients (no evidence of additional benefit in doses >360 mg/day).

Extended release:

Covera-HS®: Usual dose range (JNC 7): 120-360 mg once daily (once-daily dosing is recommended at bedtime)

Verelan® PM: Usual dose range: 200-400 mg once daily at bedtime

Dosing adjustment in renal impairment: Cl_{cr} <10 mL/minute: Administer at 50% to 75% of normal dose.

Dialysis: Not dializable (0% to 5%) via hemo- or peritoneal dialysis; supplemental dose is not necessary.

Dosing adjustment/comments in hepatic disease: Reduce dose in cirrhosis, reduce dose to 20% to 50% of normal and monitor ECG.

Mechanism of Action
Inhibits calcium ion from entering the "slow channels" or select voltage-sensitive areas of vascular smooth muscle and myocardium during depolarization; produces a relaxation of coronary vascular smooth muscle and coronary vasodilation; increases myocardial oxygen delivery in patients with vasospastic angina; slows automaticity and conduction of AV node.

Contraindications
Hypersensitivity to verapamil or any component of the formulation; severe left ventricular dysfunction; hypotension (systolic pressure <90 mm Hg) or cardiogenic shock; sick sinus syndrome (except in patients with a functioning artificial pacemaker); second- or third-degree AV block (except in patients with a functioning artificial pacemaker); atrial flutter or fibrillation and an accessory bypass tract (WPW, Lown-Ganong-Levine syndrome)

Warnings/Precautions
Use with caution in sick-sinus syndrome, severe left ventricular dysfunction, hepatic or renal impairment, hypertrophic cardiomyopathy (especially obstructive), abrupt withdrawal may cause increased duration and frequency of chest pain; avoid I.V. use in neonates and young infants due to severe apnea, bradycardia, or hypotensive reactions; elderly may experience more constipation and hypotension. Monitor ECG and blood pressure closely in patients receiving I.V. therapy particularly in patients with supraventricular tachycardia. May prolong recovery from nondepolarizing neuromuscular-blocking agents.

Drug Interactions

Cytochrome P450 Effect: **Substrate** of CYP1A2 (minor), 2B6 (minor), 2C8/9 (minor), 2C18 (minor), 2E1 (minor), 3A4 (major); **Inhibits** CYP1A2 (weak), 2C8/9 (weak), 2D6 (weak), 3A4 (moderate)

Increased Effect/Toxicity: Use of verapamil with amiodarone, beta-blockers, or flecainide may lead to bradycardia and decreased cardiac output. Aspirin and concurrent verapamil use may increase bleeding times. Lithium neurotoxicity may result when verapamil is added. Effect of nondepolarizing neuromuscular blocker is prolonged by verapamil. Grapefruit juice may increase verapamil serum concentrations. Blood pressure-lowering effects may be additive with sildenafil, tadalafil, and vardenafil (use caution).

Cisapride levels may be increased by verapamil, potentially resulting in life-threatening arrhythmias; avoid concurrent use. Verapamil may increase the levels/effects of selected benzodiazepines, other calcium channel blockers, cyclosporine, ergot alkaloids, selected HMG-CoA reductase inhibitors, mirtazapine, nateglinide, nefazodone, pimozide, quinidine, risperidone, sildenafil (and other PDE-5 inhibitors), tacrolimus, telithromycin, venlafaxine, and other CYP3A4 substrates. In addition, serum concentrations of the following drugs may be increased by verapamil: Alfentanil, digoxin, doxorubicin, ethanol, prazosin, and theophylline. Verapamil may increase colchicine toxicity (especially nephrotoxicity).

The levels/effects of verapamil may be increased by azole antifungals, clarithromycin, diclofenac, doxycycline, erythromycin, imatinib, isoniazid, nefazodone, nicardipine, propofol, protease inhibitors, quinidine, telithromycin, and other CYP3A4 inhibitors.

Decreased Effect: The levels/effects of verapamil may be decreased by aminoglutethimide, carbamazepine, nafcillin, nevirapine, phenobarbital, phenytoin, rifamycins, and other CYP3A4 inducers. Lithium levels may be decreased by verapamil. Nafcillin decreases plasma concentration of verapamil.

Ethanol/Nutrition/Herb Interactions

Ethanol: Avoid or limit ethanol (may increase ethanol levels).

Food: Grapefruit juice may increase the serum concentration of verapamil; avoid concurrent use.

Herb/Nutraceutical: St John's wort may decrease levels. Avoid dong quai if using for hypertension (has estrogenic activity). Avoid ephedra, yohimbe, ginseng (may worsen arrhythmia or hypertension). Avoid garlic (may have increased antihypertensive effect).

Dietary Considerations Calan® SR and Isoptin® SR products may be taken with food or milk, other formulations may be administered without regard to meals; sprinkling contents of Verelan® or Verelan® PM capsule onto applesauce does not affect oral absorption.

Pharmacodynamics/Kinetics

Onset of action: Peak effect: Oral: Immediate release: 1-2 hours; I.V.: 1-5 minutes

Duration: Oral: Immediate release tablets: 6-8 hours; I.V.: 10-20 minutes

Protein binding: 90%

Metabolism: Hepatic via multiple CYP isoenzymes; extensive first-pass effect

Bioavailability: Oral: 20% to 35%

Half-life elimination: Infants: 4.4-6.9 hours; Adults: Single dose: 2-8 hours, Multiple doses: 4.5-12 hours; prolonged with hepatic cirrhosis

Excretion: Urine (70%, 3% to 4% as unchanged drug); feces (16%)

Pregnancy Risk Factor C

Dosage Forms CAP, extended release, controlled onset (Verelan® PM): 100 mg, 200 mg, 300 mg. **CAPLET, sustained release** (Calan® SR): 120 mg, 180 mg, 240 mg. **CAP, sustained release** (Verelan®): 120 mg, 180 mg, 240 mg, 360 mg. **INJ, solution:** 2.5 mg/mL (2 mL, 4 mL). **TAB:** 80 mg, 120 mg; (Calan®): 40 mg, 80 mg, 120 mg. **TAB, extended release:** 120 mg, 180 mg, 240 mg. **TAB, extended release, controlled onset** (Covera HS®): 180 mg, 240 mg. **TAB, sustained release** (Isoptin® SR): 120 mg, 180 mg, 240 mg

Selected Readings

Wynn RL, "Update on Calcium Channel Blocker Induced Gingival Hyperplasia," *Gen Dent*, 1995, 43(3):218-22.

Verapamil and Trandolapril *see* Trandolapril and Verapamil *on page 1518*

Verapamil Hydrochloride *see* Verapamil *on page 1571*

Verelan® *see* Verapamil *on page 1571*

Verelan® PM *see* Verapamil *on page 1571*

Vermox® [DSC] *see* Mebendazole *on page 968*

Versed *see* Midazolam *on page 1040*

Versiclear™ *see* Sodium Thiosulfate *on page 1404*

Verteporfin (ver te POR fin)

U.S. Brand Names Visudyne®
Canadian Brand Names Visudyne®
Generic Available No
Pharmacologic Category Ophthalmic Agent
Use Treatment of predominantly classic subfoveal choroidal neovascularization due to macular degeneration, presumed ocular histoplasmosis, or pathologic myopia
Unlabeled/Investigational Use Predominantly occult subfoveal choroidal neovascularization
Local Anesthetic/Vasoconstrictor Precautions No information available to require special precautions
Effects on Dental Treatment No significant effects or complications reported
Mechanism of Action Following intravenous administration, verteporfin is transported by lipoproteins to the neovascular endothelium in the affected eye(s), including choroidal neovasculature and the retina. Verteporfin then needs to be activated by nonthermal red light, which results in local damage to the endothelium, leading to temporary choroidal vessel occlusion.
Pregnancy Risk Factor C

Vesanoid® see Tretinoin (Oral) on page 1524
VESIcare® see Solifenacin on page 1405
Vexol® see Rimexolone on page 1351
VFEND® see Voriconazole on page 1582
Viactiv® Multivitamin [OTC] see Vitamins (Multiple/Oral) on page 1582
Viadur® see Leuprolide on page 906
Viagra® see Sildenafil on page 1390
Vibramycin® see Doxycycline (Systemic) on page 514
Vibra-Tabs® see Doxycycline (Systemic) on page 514
Vicks® 44® Cough Relief [OTC] see Dextromethorphan on page 451
Vicks® 44D Cough & Head Congestion [OTC] see Pseudoephedrine and Dextromethorphan on page 1311
Vicks® 44E [OTC] see Guaifenesin and Dextromethorphan on page 754
Vicks® Casero™ [OTC] see Guaifenesin on page 752
Vicks® DayQuil® Multi-Symptom Cold and Flu [OTC] see Acetaminophen, Dextromethorphan, and Pseudoephedrine on page 44
Vicks® Pediatric Formula 44E [OTC] see Guaifenesin and Dextromethorphan on page 754
Vicks Sinex® 12 Hour [OTC] see Oxymetazoline on page 1172
Vicks Sinex® 12 Hour Ultrafine Mist [OTC] see Oxymetazoline on page 1172
Vicks® Sinex® Nasal Spray [OTC] see Phenylephrine on page 1226
Vicks® Sinex® UltraFine Mist [OTC] see Phenylephrine on page 1226
Vicodin® see Hydrocodone and Acetaminophen on page 779
Vicodin® ES see Hydrocodone and Acetaminophen on page 779
Vicodin® HP see Hydrocodone and Acetaminophen on page 779
Vicon Forte® see Vitamins (Multiple/Oral) on page 1582
Vicoprofen® see Hydrocodone and Ibuprofen on page 787
Vi-Daylin® + Iron Liquid [OTC] [DSC] see Vitamins (Multiple/Oral) on page 1582
Vi-Daylin® Liquid [OTC] [DSC] see Vitamins (Multiple/Oral) on page 1582
Vidaza™ see Azacitidine on page 167
Videx® see Didanosine on page 465
Videx® EC see Didanosine on page 465

Vigabatrin (vye GA ba trin)

Canadian Brand Names Sabril®
Mexican Brand Names Sabril®
Generic Available No
Pharmacologic Category Anticonvulsant, Miscellaneous
Use Active management of partial or secondary generalized seizures not controlled by usual treatments; treatment of infantile spasms
Unlabeled/Investigational Use Spasticity, tardive dyskinesias
Local Anesthetic/Vasoconstrictor Precautions No information available to require special precautions
Effects on Dental Treatment No significant effects or complications reported

Common Adverse Effects

>10%:

Central nervous system: Fatigue (27%), headache (26%), drowsiness (22%), dizziness (19%), depression (13%), tremor (11%), agitation (11%). **Note:** In pediatric use, hyperactivity (hyperkinesia, agitation, excitation, or restlessness) was reported in 11% of patients.

Endocrine & metabolic: Weight gain (12%)

Ophthalmic: Visual field defects, abnormal vision (11%)

1% to 10%:

Cardiovascular: Edema (dependent), chest pain

Central nervous system: Amnesia, confusion, paresthesia, impaired concentration, insomnia, anxiety, emotional lability, abnormal thinking, speech disorder, vertigo, aggression, nervousness, personality disorder

Dermatologic: Rash (5%, similar to placebo), skin disorder

Endocrine & metabolic: Increased appetite, dysmenorrhea, menstrual disorder

Gastrointestinal: Nausea, diarrhea, abdominal pain, constipation, vomiting

Genitourinary: Urinary tract infection

Hematologic: Purpura

Neuromuscular & skeletal: Ataxia, arthralgia, back pain, abnormal coordination, abnormal gait, weakness, hyporeflexia, arthrosis

Ophthalmologic: Nystagmus, diplopia, eye pain

Otic: Ear pain

Respiratory: Throat irritation, nasal congestion, upper respiratory tract infection, sinusitis

Restrictions Not available in U.S.

Mechanism of Action Irreversibly inhibits gamma-aminobutyric acid transaminase (GABA-T), increasing the levels of the inhibitory compound gamma amino butyric acid (GABA) within the brain. Duration of effect is dependent upon rate of GABA-T resynthesis.

Drug Interactions

Decreased Effect: Serum concentrations of phenytoin and phenobarbital may be decreased by vigabatrin.

Pharmacodynamics/Kinetics

Duration (rate of GABA-T resynthesis dependent): Variable (not strictly correlated to serum concentrations)

Absorption: Rapid

Metabolism: Minimal

Half-life elimination: 5-8 hours; Elderly: Up to 13 hours

Time to peak: 2 hours

Excretion: Urine (70%, as unchanged drug)

Pregnancy Risk Factor Not assigned; contraindicated per manufacturer

Vigamox™ *see* Moxifloxacin *on page 1069*

VIGIV *see* Vaccinia Immune Globulin (Intravenous) *on page 1553*

VinBLAStine (vin BLAS teen)

Mexican Brand Names Lemblastine®

Generic Available Yes

Synonyms NSC-49842; Vinblastine Sulfate; VLB

Pharmacologic Category Antineoplastic Agent, Natural Source (Plant) Derivative; Antineoplastic Agent, Vinca Alkaloid

Use Treatment of Hodgkin's and non-Hodgkin's lymphoma, testicular, lung, head and neck, breast, and renal carcinomas, Mycosis fungoides, Kaposi's sarcoma, histiocytosis, choriocarcinoma, and idiopathic thrombocytopenic purpura

Local Anesthetic/Vasoconstrictor Precautions No information available to require special precautions

Effects on Dental Treatment Key adverse event(s) related to dental treatment: Stomatitis, metallic taste, and jaw pain.

Common Adverse Effects

>10%:

Dermatologic: Alopecia

Endocrine & metabolic: SIADH

Gastrointestinal: Diarrhea (less common), stomatitis, anorexia, metallic taste

Hematologic: May cause severe bone marrow suppression and is the dose-limiting toxicity of VLB (unlike vincristine); severe granulocytopenia and thrombocytopenia may occur following the administration of VLB and nadir 5-10 days after treatment

Myelosuppression (primarily leukopenia, may be dose limiting)

Onset: 4-7 days

Nadir: 5-10 days

(Continued)

VinBLAStine *(Continued)*

Recovery: 4-21 days

1% to 10%:

Cardiovascular: Hypertension, Raynaud's phenomenon

Central nervous system: Depression, malaise, headache, seizure

Dermatologic: Rash, photosensitivity, dermatitis

Endocrine & metabolic: Hyperuricemia

Gastrointestinal: Constipation, abdominal pain, nausea (mild), vomiting (mild), paralytic ileus, stomatitis

Genitourinary: Urinary retention

Neuromuscular & skeletal: Jaw pain, myalgia, paresthesia

Respiratory: Bronchospasm

Mechanism of Action Vinblastine binds to tubulin and inhibits microtubule formation, therefore, arresting the cell at metaphase by disrupting the formation of the mitotic spindle; it is specific for the M and S phases. Vinblastine may also interfere with nucleic acid and protein synthesis by blocking glutamic acid utilization.

Drug Interactions

Cytochrome P450 Effect: Substrate of CYP2D6 (minor), 3A4 (major); **Inhibits** CYP2D6 (weak), 3A4 (weak)

Increased Effect/Toxicity: CYP3A4 inhibitors may increase the levels/effects of vinblastine; example inhibitors include azole antifungals, clarithromycin, diclofenac, doxycycline, erythromycin, imatinib, isoniazid, nefazodone, nicardipine, propofol, protease inhibitors, quinidine, telithromycin, and verapamil.

Previous or simultaneous use with mitomycin-C has resulted in acute shortness of breath and severe bronchospasm within minutes or several hours after vinca alkaloid injection and may occur up to 2 weeks after the dose of mitomycin. Mitomycin-C in combination with administration of VLB may cause acute shortness of breath and severe bronchospasm, onset may be within minutes or several hours after VLB injection.

Decreased Effect: CYP3A4 inducers may decrease the levels/effects of vinblastine; example inducers include aminoglutethimide, carbamazepine, nafcillin, nevirapine, phenobarbital, phenytoin (may reduce vinblastine serum concentrations), and rifamycins.

Pharmacodynamics/Kinetics

Distribution: V_d: 27.3 L/kg; binds extensively to tissues; does not penetrate CNS or other fatty tissues; distributes to liver

Protein binding: 99%

Metabolism: Hepatic to active metabolite

Half-life elimination: Biphasic: Initial: 0.164 hours; Terminal: 25 hours

Excretion: Feces (95%); urine (<1% as unchanged drug)

Pregnancy Risk Factor D

Vinblastine Sulfate *see* VinBLAStine *on page 1575*

Vincasar PFS® *see* VinCRIStine *on page 1576*

VinCRIStine *(vin KRIS teen)*

U.S. Brand Names Vincasar PFS®

Canadian Brand Names Vincasar® PFS®

Mexican Brand Names Citomid®; Vintec®

Generic Available Yes

Synonyms LCR; Leurocristine Sulfate; NSC-67574; VCR; Vincristine Sulfate

Pharmacologic Category Antineoplastic Agent, Natural Source (Plant) Derivative; Antineoplastic Agent, Vinca Alkaloid

Use Treatment of leukemias, Hodgkin's disease, non-Hodgkin's lymphomas, Wilms' tumor, neuroblastoma, rhabdomyosarcoma

Local Anesthetic/Vasoconstrictor Precautions No information available to require special precautions

Effects on Dental Treatment No significant effects or complications reported

Common Adverse Effects

>10%: Dermatologic: Alopecia (20% to 70%)

1% to 10%:

Cardiovascular: Orthostatic hypotension or hypertension, hyper-/hypotension

Central nervous system: CNS depression, confusion, cranial nerve paralysis, fever, headache, insomnia, motor difficulties, seizure

Intrathecal administration of vincristine has uniformly caused death; vincristine should never be administered by this route. Neurologic effects of vincristine may be additive with those of other neurotoxic agents and spinal cord irradiation.

Dermatologic: Rash

Endocrine & metabolic: Hyperuricemia

Gastrointestinal: Abdominal cramps, anorexia, bloating, constipation (and possible paralytic ileus secondary to neurologic toxicity), diarrhea, metallic taste, nausea (mild), oral ulceration, vomiting, weight loss

Genitourinary: Bladder atony (related to neurotoxicity), dysuria, polyuria, urinary retention

Hematologic: Leukopenia (mild), thrombocytopenia, myelosuppression (onset: 7 days; nadir: 10 days; recovery: 21 days)

Local: Phlebitis, tissue irritation and necrosis if infiltrated

Neuromuscular & skeletal: Cramping, jaw pain, leg pain, myalgia, numbness, weakness

Peripheral neuropathy: Frequently the dose-limiting toxicity of vincristine. Most frequent in patients >40 years of age; occurs usually after an average of 3 weekly doses, but may occur after just one dose. Manifested as loss of the deep tendon reflexes in the lower extremities, numbness, tingling, pain, paresthesia of the fingers and toes (stocking glove sensation), and "foot drop" or "wrist drop."

Ocular: Optic atrophy, photophobia

Mechanism of Action Binds to tubulin and inhibits microtubule formation; therefore arresting the cell at metaphase by disrupting the formation of the mitotic spindle; it is specific for the M and S phases. Vincristine may also interfere with nucleic acid and protein synthesis by blocking glutamic acid utilization.

Drug Interactions

Cytochrome P450 Effect: **Substrate** of CYP3A4 (major); **Inhibits** CYP3A4 (weak)

Increased Effect/Toxicity: Vincristine should be given 12-24 hours before asparaginase to minimize toxicity (may decrease the hepatic clearance of vincristine). Acute pulmonary reactions may occur with mitomycin-C. Previous or simultaneous use with mitomycin-C has resulted in acute shortness of breath and severe bronchospasm within minutes or several hours after vinca alkaloid injection and may occur up to 2 weeks after the dose of mitomycin.

CYP3A4 inhibitors may increase the levels/effects of vincristine. Example inhibitors include azole antifungals, clarithromycin, diclofenac, doxycycline, erythromycin, imatinib, isoniazid, nefazodone, nicardipine, propofol, protease inhibitors, quinidine, telithromycin, and verapamil. Digoxin plasma levels and renal excretion may decrease with combination chemotherapy including vincristine. Nifedipine may increase the levels/effects of vincristine.

Decreased Effect: Digoxin levels may decrease with combination chemotherapy. CYP3A4 inducers may decrease the levels/effects of vincristine; example inducers include aminoglutethimide, carbamazepine, nafcillin, nevirapine, phenobarbital, phenytoin, and rifamycins.

Pharmacodynamics/Kinetics

Absorption: Oral: Poor

Distribution: V_d: 163-165 L/m^2; Poor penetration into CSF; rapidly removed from bloodstream and tightly bound to tissues; penetrates blood-brain barrier poorly

Protein binding: 75%

Metabolism: Extensively hepatic

Half-life elimination: Terminal: 24 hours

Excretion: Feces (~80%); urine (<1% as unchanged drug)

Pregnancy Risk Factor D

Vincristine Sulfate see VinCRIStine on page 1576

Vindesine (VIN de seen)

Generic Available No

Synonyms DAVA; Deacetyl Vinblastine Carboxamide; Desacetyl Vinblastine Amide Sulfate; DVA; Eldisine Lilly 99094; Lilly CT-3231; NSC-245467; Vindesine Sulfate

Pharmacologic Category Antineoplastic Agent, Vinca Alkaloid

Unlabeled/Investigational Use Investigational: Management of acute lymphocytic leukemia, chronic myelogenous leukemia; breast, head, neck, and lung cancers; lymphomas (Hodgkin's and non-Hodgkin's)

Local Anesthetic/Vasoconstrictor Precautions No information available to require special precautions

Effects on Dental Treatment Key adverse event(s) related to dental treatment: Loss of taste and facial paralysis.

(Continued)

Vindesine (Continued)

Common Adverse Effects

>10%:

Central nervous system: Pyrexia, malaise (up to 60%)

Dermatologic: Alopecia (6% to 92%)

Gastrointestinal: Mild nausea and vomiting (7% to 27%), constipation (10% to 17%) - related to the neurotoxicity

Hematologic: Leukopenia (50%) and thrombocytopenia (14% to 26%), may be dose-limiting; thrombocytosis (20% to 28%)

Nadir: 6-12 days

Recovery: Days 14-18

Neuromuscular & skeletal: Paresthesias (40% to 70%); loss of deep tendon reflexes (35% to 60%, may be dose-limiting); myalgia (up to 60%)

1% to 10%:

Dermatologic: Rashes

Gastrointestinal: Loss of taste

Hematologic: Anemia

Local: Phlebitis

Neuromuscular & skeletal: Facial paralysis

Restrictions Not available in U.S./Investigational

Mechanism of Action Vindesine is a semisynthetic vinca alkaloid, having a mechanism of action similar to the other vinca derivatives. It arrests cell division in metaphase through inhibition of microtubular formation of the mitotic spindle. The drug is cell-cycle specific for the S phase.

Pharmacodynamics/Kinetics

Distribution: V_d: 8 L/kg; minimal distribution to adipose tissue or CNS

Metabolism: Hepatic

Half-life elimination:

Triphasic; Alpha: 2 minutes; Beta: 1 hour

Terminal: 24 hours

Excretion: Feces; urine (~3% to 25% of dose as unchanged drug)

Vindesine Sulfate see Vindesine on page 1577

Vinorelbine (vi NOR el been)

U.S. Brand Names Navelbine®

Canadian Brand Names Navelbine®; Vinorelbine Injection, USP

Mexican Brand Names Navelbine®

Generic Available Yes

Synonyms Dihydroxydeoxynorvinkaleukoblastine; NVB; Vinorelbine Tartrate

Pharmacologic Category Antineoplastic Agent, Natural Source (Plant) Derivative; Antineoplastic Agent, Vinca Alkaloid

Use Treatment of nonsmall cell lung cancer

Unlabeled/Investigational Use Treatment of breast cancer, ovarian carcinoma, Hodgkin's disease, non-Hodgkin's lymphoma

Local Anesthetic/Vasoconstrictor Precautions No information available to require special precautions

Effects on Dental Treatment No significant effects or complications reported

Common Adverse Effects

>10%:

Central nervous system: Fatigue (27%)

Dermatologic: Alopecia (12%)

Gastrointestinal: Nausea (44%, severe <2%) and vomiting (20%) are most common and are easily controlled with standard antiemetics; constipation (35%), diarrhea (17%)

Emetic potential: Moderate (30% to 60%)

Hematologic: May cause severe bone marrow suppression and is the dose-limiting toxicity of vinorelbine; severe granulocytopenia (90%) may occur following the administration of vinorelbine; leukopenia (92%), anemia (83%)

Myelosuppressive:

WBC: Moderate - severe

Onset: 4-7 days

Nadir: 7-10 days

Recovery: 14-21 days

Hepatic: Elevated SGOT (67%), elevated total bilirubin (13%)

Local: Injection site reaction (28%), injection site pain (16%)

Neuromuscular & skeletal: Weakness (36%), peripheral neuropathy (20% to 25%)

1% to 10%:
  Cardiovascular: Chest pain (5%)
  Gastrointestinal: Paralytic ileus (1%)
  Hematologic: Thrombocytopenia (5%)
  Local: Phlebitis (7%)
  Neuromuscular & skeletal: Mild to moderate peripheral neuropathy manifested by paresthesia and hyperesthesia, loss of deep tendon reflexes (<5%); myalgia (<5%), arthralgia (<5%), jaw pain (<5%)
  Respiratory: Dyspnea (3% to 7%)

Mechanism of Action Semisynthetic vinca alkaloid which binds to tubulin and inhibits microtubule formation, therefore, arresting the cell at metaphase by disrupting the formation of the mitotic spindle; it is specific for the M and S phases. Vinorelbine may also interfere with nucleic acid and protein synthesis by blocking glutamic acid utilization.

Drug Interactions
  Cytochrome P450 Effect: Substrate of CYP2D6 (minor), 3A4 (major); **Inhibits** CYP2D6 (weak), 3A4 (weak)
  Increased Effect/Toxicity: Previous or simultaneous use with mitomycin-C has resulted in acute shortness of breath and severe bronchospasm within minutes or several hours after vinca alkaloid injection and may occur up to 2 weeks after the dose of mitomycin. CYP3A4 inhibitors may increase the levels/effects of vinorelbine; example inhibitors include azole antifungals, clarithromycin, diclofenac, doxycycline, erythromycin, imatinib, isoniazid, nefazodone, nicardipine, propofol, protease inhibitors, quinidine, telithromycin, and verapamil. Incidence of granulocytopenia is significantly higher in cisplatin/vinorelbine combination therapy than with single-agent vinorelbine.
  Decreased Effect: CYP3A4 inducers may decrease the levels/effects of vinorelbine; example inducers include aminoglutethimide, carbamazepine, nafcillin, nevirapine, phenobarbital, phenytoin, and rifamycins.

Pharmacodynamics/Kinetics
  Absorption: Unreliable; must be given I.V.
  Distribution: V_d: 25.4-40.1 L/kg; binds extensively to human platelets and lymphocytes (79.6% to 91.2%)
  Protein binding: 80% to 90%
  Metabolism: Extensively hepatic to two metabolites, deacetylvinorelbine (active) and vinorelbine N-oxide
  Bioavailability: Oral: 26% to 45%
  Half-life elimination: Triphasic: Terminal: 27.7-43.6 hours
  Excretion: Feces (46%); urine (18%, 10% to 12% as unchanged drug)
  Clearance: Plasma: Mean: 0.97-1.26 L/hour/kg

Pregnancy Risk Factor D

Vinorelbine Tartrate *see* Vinorelbine *on page 1578*

Viokase® *see* Pancrelipase *on page 1183*

Viosterol *see* Ergocalciferol *on page 556*

Viracept® *see* Nelfinavir *on page 1098*

Viramune® *see* Nevirapine *on page 1104*

Virazole® *see* Ribavirin *on page 1343*

Viread® *see* Tenofovir *on page 1457*

Virilon® *see* MethylTESTOSTERone *on page 1028*

Viroptic® *see* Trifluridine *on page 1536*

Viroxyn® [OTC] *see* Benzalkonium Chloride and Isopropyl Alcohol *on page 189*

Viscoat® *see* Chondroitin Sulfate and Sodium Hyaluronate *on page 336*

Visicol® *see* Sodium Phosphates *on page 1403*

Visine-A™ [OTC] *see* Naphazoline and Pheniramine *on page 1088*

Visine® Advanced Relief [OTC] *see* Tetrahydrozoline *on page 1470*

Visine® L.R. [OTC] *see* Oxymetazoline *on page 1172*

Visine® Original [OTC] *see* Tetrahydrozoline *on page 1470*

Visipaque™ *see* Iodixanol *on page 853*

Vistaril® *see* HydrOXYzine *on page 801*

Vistide® *see* Cidofovir *on page 339*

Visudyne® *see* Verteporfin *on page 1574*

Vita-C® [OTC] *see* Ascorbic Acid *on page 143*

Vitacon Forte *see* Vitamins (Multiple/Oral) *on page 1582*

Vitamin C *see* Ascorbic Acid *on page 143*

Vitamin D₂ *see* Ergocalciferol *on page 556*

Vitamin D₃ *see* Alendronate and Cholecalciferol *on page 66*

Vitamin A (VYE ta min aye)

U.S. Brand Names Aquasol A®; Palmitate-A® [OTC]

Generic Available Yes: Capsule

Synonyms Oleovitamin A

Pharmacologic Category Vitamin, Fat Soluble

Use Treatment and prevention of vitamin A deficiency; parenteral (I.M.) route is indicated when oral administration is not feasible or when absorption is insufficient (malabsorption syndrome)

Local Anesthetic/Vasoconstrictor Precautions No information available to require special precautions

Effects on Dental Treatment No significant effects or complications reported

Common Adverse Effects 1% to 10%:

Central nervous system: Irritability, vertigo, lethargy, malaise, fever, headache

Dermatologic: Drying or cracking of skin

Endocrine & metabolic: Hypercalcemia

Gastrointestinal: Weight loss

Ocular: Visual changes

Miscellaneous: Hypervitaminosis A

Mechanism of Action Needed for bone development, growth, visual adaptation to darkness, testicular and ovarian function, and as a cofactor in many biochemical processes

Drug Interactions

Increased Effect/Toxicity: Retinoids may have additive adverse effects.

Decreased Effect: Cholestyramine resin decreases absorption of vitamin A. Neomycin and mineral oil may also interfere with vitamin A absorption.

Pharmacodynamics/Kinetics

Absorption: Vitamin A in dosages **not** exceeding physiologic replacement is well absorbed after oral administration; water miscible preparations are absorbed more rapidly than oil preparations; large oral doses, conditions of fat malabsorption, low protein intake, or hepatic or pancreatic disease reduces oral absorption

Distribution: Large amounts concentrate for storage in the liver; enters breast milk

Metabolism: Conjugated with glucuronide; undergoes enterohepatic recirculation

Excretion: Feces

Pregnancy Risk Factor A/X (dose exceeding RDA recommendation)

Vitamin A Acid see Tretinoin (Topical) on page 1525

Vitamin A and Vitamin D (VYE ta min aye & VYE ta min dee)

Related Information

Vitamin A on page 1580

U.S. Brand Names A and D® Original [OTC]; Baza® Clear [OTC]; Sween Cream® [OTC]

Generic Available Yes: Capsule, ointment

Synonyms Cod Liver Oil

Pharmacologic Category Topical Skin Product

Use Temporary relief of discomfort due to chapped skin, diaper rash, minor burns, abrasions, as well as irritations associated with ostomy skin care

Local Anesthetic/Vasoconstrictor Precautions No information available to require special precautions

Effects on Dental Treatment No significant effects or complications reported

Common Adverse Effects Frequency not defined: Local: Irritation

Pregnancy Risk Factor B

Vitamin B$_1$ see Thiamine on page 1476

Vitamin B$_2$ see Riboflavin on page 1345

Vitamin B$_3$ see Niacin on page 1105

Vitamin B$_5$ see Pantothenic Acid on page 1186

Vitamin B$_6$ see Pyridoxine on page 1316

Vitamin B$_{12}$ see Cyanocobalamin on page 399

Vitamin B Complex Combinations
(VYE ta min bee KOM pleks kom bi NAY shuns)

U.S. Brand Names Allbee® C-800 [OTC]; Allbee® C-800 + Iron [OTC]; Allbee® with C [OTC]; Apatate® [OTC]; Diatx™; DiatxFe™; Gevrabon® [OTC]; Neph-Plex® Rx; Nephrocaps®; Nephron FA®; Nephro-Vite®; Nephro-Vite® Rx; Stress-tabs® B-Complex [OTC]; Stresstabs® B-Complex + Iron [OTC]; Stresstabs® B-Complex + Zinc [OTC]; Surbex-T® [OTC]; Trinsicon®; Z-Bec® [OTC]

Generic Available Yes

Synonyms B Complex Combinations; B Vitamin Combinations

Pharmacologic Category Vitamin

Use Supplement for use in the wasting syndrome in chronic renal failure, uremia, impaired metabolic functions of the kidney, dialysis; labeled for OTC use as a dietary supplement

Local Anesthetic/Vasoconstrictor Precautions No information available to require special precautions

Effects on Dental Treatment No significant effects or complications reported

Common Adverse Effects Frequency not defined.
Central nervous system: Somnolence
Dermatologic: Itching
Gastrointestinal: Bloating, constipation, diarrhea, flatulence, nausea, vomiting
Hematologic: Peripheral vascular thrombosis, polycythemia vera
Neuromuscular & skeletal: Paresthesia
Miscellaneous: Allergic reaction

Pregnancy Risk Factor A (RDA recommended doses)

Vitamin E (VYE ta min ee)

U.S. Brand Names Alph-E [OTC]; Alph-E-Mixed [OTC]; Aquasol E® [OTC]; Aquavit-E [OTC]; d-Alpha-Gems™ [OTC]; E-Gems® [OTC]; E-Gems Elite® [OTC]; E-Gems Plus® [OTC]; Ester-E™ [OTC]; Gamma E-Gems® [OTC]; Gamma-E Plus [OTC]; High Gamma Vitamin E Complete™ [OTC]; Key-E® [OTC]; Key-E® Kaps [OTC]

Generic Available Yes

Synonyms d-Alpha Tocopherol; dl-Alpha Tocopherol

Pharmacologic Category Vitamin, Fat Soluble

Use Dietary supplement

Unlabeled/Investigational Use To reduce the risk of bronchopulmonary dysplasia or retrolental fibroplasia in infants exposed to high concentrations of oxygen; prevention and treatment of tardive dyskinesia and Alzheimer's disease; prevention and treatment of hemolytic anemia secondary to vitamin E deficiency

Local Anesthetic/Vasoconstrictor Precautions No information available to require special precautions

Effects on Dental Treatment No significant effects or complications reported

Common Adverse Effects Frequency not defined.
Central nervous system: Fatigue, headache, weakness
Dermatologic: Contact dermatitis with topical preparation
Endocrine & metabolic: Gonadal dysfunction
Gastrointestinal: Diarrhea, intestinal cramps, nausea
Neuromuscular & skeletal: Weakness
Ocular: Blurred vision

Mechanism of Action Prevents oxidation of vitamin A and C; protects polyunsaturated fatty acids in membranes from attack by free radicals and protects red blood cells against hemolysis

Drug Interactions
Increased Effect/Toxicity: Vitamin E may alter the effect of vitamin K actions on clotting factors resulting in an increase hypoprothrombinemic response to warfarin; monitor.
Decreased Effect: Vitamin E may impair the hematologic response to iron in children with iron-deficiency anemia; monitor.

Pharmacodynamics/Kinetics
Absorption: Oral: Depends on presence of bile; reduced in conditions of malabsorption, in low birth weight premature infants, and as dosage increases; water miscible preparations are better absorbed than oil preparations
Distribution: To all body tissues, especially adipose tissue, where it is stored
Metabolism: Hepatic to glucuronides
Excretion: Feces

Pregnancy Risk Factor A/C (dose exceeding RDA recommendation)

Vitamin G see Riboflavin on page 1345
Vitamin K₁ see Phytonadione on page 1233

Vitamins (Multiple/Oral) (VYE ta mins, MUL ti pul/OR al)

U.S. Brand Names Centrum® [OTC]; Centrum® Performance™ [OTC]; Centrum® Silver® [OTC]; Geriation [OTC]; Geritol Complete® [OTC]; Geritol Extend® [OTC]; Geritol® Tonic [OTC]; Glutofac®-MX; Glutofac®-ZX; Gynovite® Plus [OTC]; Hemocyte Plus®; Hi-Kovite [OTC; Iberet® [OTC]; Iberet®-500 [OTC]; Monocaps [OTC]; Multiret Folic 500; Ocuvite® [OTC]; Ocuvite® Extra® [OTC]; Ocuvite® Lutein [OTC]; Olay® Vitamins Complete Women's [OTC]; Olay® Vitamins Complete Women's 50+[OTC]; Olay® Vitamins Even Complexion [OTC]; One-A-Day® 50 Plus Formula [OTC]; One-A-Day® Active Formula [OTC]; One-A-Day® Carb Smart [OTC]; One-A-Day® Cholesterol Plus™ [OTC]; One-A-Day® Essential Formula [OTC]; One-A-Day® Maximum Formula [OTC]; One-A-Day® Men's Formula [OTC]; One-A-Day® Today [OTC]; One-A-Day® Weight Smart [OTC; One-A-Day® Women's Formula [OTC]; Optivite® P.M.T. [OTC]; PreserVision® AREDS [OTC]; PreserVision® Lutein [OTC]; Quintabs [OTC]; Quintabs-M [OTC]; Replace [OTC]; Replace with Iron [OTC]; Repliva 21/7™; Strovite® Forte; Theragran® Heart Right™ [OTC] [DSC]; Theragran-M® Advanced Formula [OTC] [DSC]; T-Vites [OTC]; Ultra Freeda Iron Free [OTC]; Ultra Freeda with Iron [OTC]; Unicap M® [OTC]; Unicap Sr® [OTC]; Unicap T™ [OTC]; Viactiv® Multivitamin [OTC]; Vicon Forte®; Vi-Daylin® + Iron Liquid [OTC] [DSC]; Vi-Daylin® Liquid [OTC] [DSC]; Vitacon Forte; Xtramins [OTC]

Generic Available Yes

Synonyms Multiple Vitamins; Therapeutic Multivitamins; Vitamins, Multiple (Oral); Vitamins, Multiple (Therapeutic); Vitamins, Multiple With Iron

Pharmacologic Category Vitamin

Use Prevention/treatment of vitamin and mineral deficiencies; labeled for OTC use as a dietary supplement

Local Anesthetic/Vasoconstrictor Precautions No information available to require special precautions

Effects on Dental Treatment No significant effects or complications reported

Pregnancy Risk Factor A (at RDA recommended dose)

Vitamins, Multiple (Therapeutic) see Vitamins (Multiple/Oral) on page 1582
Vitamins, Multiple With Iron see Vitamins (Multiple/Oral) on page 1582
Vitelle™ Irospan® [OTC] [DSC] see Ferrous Sulfate and Ascorbic Acid on page 651
Vitrase® see Hyaluronidase on page 774
Vitrasert® see Ganciclovir on page 722
Vitravene™ [DSC] see Fomivirsen on page 700
Vitrax® see Hyaluronate and Derivatives on page 773
Vitussin see Hydrocodone and Guaifenesin on page 785
Vivactil® see Protriptyline on page 1307
Viva-Drops® [OTC] see Artificial Tears on page 143
Vivaglobin® see Immune Globulin (Subcutaneous) on page 826
Vivarin® [OTC] see Caffeine on page 245
Vivelle® see Estradiol on page 574
Vivelle-Dot® see Estradiol on page 574
Vivitrol™ see Naltrexone on page 1086
Vivotif Berna® see Typhoid Vaccine on page 1549
VLB see VinBLAStine on page 1575
VM-26 see Teniposide on page 1456
Voltaren® see Diclofenac on page 459
Voltaren Ophthalmic® see Diclofenac on page 459
Voltaren®-XR see Diclofenac on page 459

Voriconazole (vor i KOE na zole)

U.S. Brand Names VFEND®
Canadian Brand Names VFEND®
Generic Available No
Synonyms UK109496
Pharmacologic Category Antifungal Agent, Oral; Antifungal Agent, Parenteral
Use Treatment of invasive aspergillosis; treatment of esophageal candidiasis; treatment of candidemia (in non-neutropenic patients); treatment of *Candida*

deep tissue infections; treatment of serious fungal infections caused by *Scedosporium apiospermum* and *Fusarium* spp (including *Fusarium solani*) in patients intolerant of, or refractory to, other therapy

Local Anesthetic/Vasoconstrictor Precautions No information available to require special precautions (see Dental Comment)

Effects on Dental Treatment Key adverse event(s) related to dental treatment: Xerostomia (normal salivary flow resumes upon discontinuation).

Common Adverse Effects
>10%: Ocular: Visual changes (photophobia, color changes, increased or decreased visual acuity, or blurred vision occur in ~21%)

1% to 10%:
Cardiovascular: Tachycardia (2% to 3%), hyper-/hypotension (2%), vasodilation (2%), peripheral edema (1%)

Central nervous system: Fever (6%), chills (4%), headache (3%), hallucinations (3%), dizziness (1%)

Dermatologic: Rash (6%), pruritus (1%)

Endocrine & metabolic: Hypokalemia (2%), hypomagnesemia (1%)

Gastrointestinal: Nausea (5% to 6%), vomiting (4% to 5%), abdominal pain (2%), diarrhea (1%), xerostomia (1%)

Hematologic: Thrombocytopenia (1%)

Hepatic: Alkaline phosphatase increased (4%), transaminases increased (2% to 3%), AST increased (2%), ALT increased (2%), cholestatic jaundice (1%)

Ocular: Chromatopsia (1%), photophobia (2% to 3%)

Dosage
Usual dosage ranges:
Children <12 years: Dosage not established
Children ≥12 years and Adults:
Oral: 100-300 mg every 12 hours
I.V.: 6 mg/kg every 12 hours for 2 doses; followed by maintenance dose of 4 mg/kg every 12 hours

Indication-specific dosing: Children ≥12 years and Adults:
Aspergillosis (invasive) and other serious fungal infections: I.V.: Initial: Loading dose: 6 mg/kg every 12 hours for 2 doses; followed by maintenance dose of 4 mg/kg every 12 hours

Candidemia and other deep tissue *Candida* infections: I.V.: Initial: Loading dose 6 mg/kg every 12 hours for 2 doses; followed by maintenance dose of 3-4 mg/kg every 12 hours

Note: Conversion to oral dosing:
Patients <40 kg: 100 mg every 12 hours; increase to 150 mg every 12 hours in patients who fail to respond adequately
Patients ≥40 kg: 200 mg every 12 hours; increase to 300 mg every 12 hours in patients who fail to respond adequately

Endophthalmitis, fungal: I.V.: 6 mg/kg every 12 hours for 2 doses, then 200 mg orally twice daily

Esophageal candidiasis: Oral:
Patients <40 kg: 100 mg every 12 hours
Patients ≥40 kg: 200 mg every 12 hours
Note: Treatment should continue for a minimum of 14 days, and for at least 7 days following resolution of symptoms.

Dosage adjustment in patients unable to tolerate treatment:
I.V.: Dose may be reduced to 3 mg/kg every 12 hours
Oral: Dose may be reduced in 50 mg increments to a minimum dosage of 200 mg every 12 hours in patients weighing ≥40 kg (100 mg every 12 hours in patients <40 kg)

Dosage adjustment in patients receiving concomitant phenytoin:
I.V.: Increase maintenance dosage to 5 mg/kg every 12 hours
Oral: Increase dose from 200 mg to 400 mg every 12 hours in patients ≥40 kg (100 mg to 200 mg every 12 hours in patients <40 kg)

Dosage adjustment in patients receiving concomitant cyclosporine:
Reduce cyclosporine dose by ½ and monitor closely.

Dosage adjustment in renal impairment: In patients with Cl_{cr} <50 mL/minute, accumulation of the intravenous vehicle (SBECD) occurs. After initial loading dose, oral voriconazole should be administered to these patients, unless an assessment of the benefit:risk to the patient justifies the use of I.V. voriconazole. Monitor serum creatinine and change to oral voriconazole therapy when possible.
Hemodialysis: Oral dosage adjustment not required.

Dosage adjustment in hepatic impairment:
Mild-to-moderate hepatic dysfunction (Child-Pugh Class A and B): Following standard loading dose, reduce maintenance dosage by 50%
Severe hepatic impairment: Should only be used if benefit outweighs risk; monitor closely for toxicity

(Continued)

Voriconazole *(Continued)*

Mechanism of Action Interferes with fungal cytochrome P450 activity, decreasing ergosterol synthesis (principal sterol in fungal cell membrane) and inhibiting fungal cell membrane formation.

Contraindications Hypersensitivity to voriconazole or any component of the formulation (cross-reaction with other azole antifungal agents may occur but has not been established, use caution); coadministration of CYP3A4 substrates which may lead to QT$_c$ prolongation (cisapride, pimozide, or quinidine); coadministration with barbiturates (long acting), carbamazepine, efavirenz, ergot alkaloids, rifampin, rifabutin, ritonavir (≥800 mg/day), and sirolimus; pregnancy (unless risk:benefit justifies use)

Warnings/Precautions Visual changes are commonly associated with treatment. Patients should be warned to avoid tasks which depend on vision, including operating machinery or driving. Changes are reversible on discontinuation following brief exposure/treatment regimens (≤28 days).

Serious hepatic reactions (including hepatitis, cholestasis, and fulminant hepatic failure) have occurred during treatment, primarily in patients with serious concomitant medical conditions. However, hepatotoxicity has occurred in patients with no identifiable risk factors. Use caution in patients with pre-existing hepatic impairment (dose adjustment required).

Voriconazole tablets contain lactose; avoid administration in hereditary galactose intolerance, Lapp lactase deficiency, or glucose-galactose malabsorption. Suspension contains sucrose; use caution with fructose intolerance, sucrose-isomaltase deficiency, or glucose-galactose malabsorption. Avoid/limit use of intravenous formulation in patients with renal impairment; intravenous formulation contains excipient sulfobutyl ether beta-cyclodextrin (SBECD), which may accumulate in renal insufficiency. Infusion-related reactions may occur with intravenous dosing. Consider discontinuation of infusion if reaction is severe.

Use caution in patients with an increased risk of arrhythmia (concurrent QT$_c$-prolonging drugs, hypokalemia, cardiomyopathy, or prior cardiotoxic therapy). Correct electrolyte abnormalities before initiating therapy. Use caution in patients receiving concurrent non-nucleoside reverse transcriptase inhibitors (efavirenz is contraindicated).

Avoid use in pregnancy, unless an evaluation of the potential benefit justifies possible risk to the fetus. Safety and efficacy have not been established in children <12 years of age.

Drug Interactions

Cytochrome P450 Effect: Substrate of CYP2C9 (major), 2C19 (major), 3A4 (minor); **Inhibits** CYP2C9 (weak), 2C19 (weak), 3A4 (moderate)

Increased Effect/Toxicity: Voriconazole increases serum levels/effects of efavirenz, ergot alkaloids, pimozide, quinidine, rifabutin, and sirolimus; concurrent use contraindicated. Voriconazole increases serum levels/effects of benzodiazepines (metabolized by oxidation; eg, alprazolam, diazepam, triazolam, midazolam), buspirone, busulfan, calcium channel blockers (eg, felodipine, nifedipine, verapamil), cisapride, CYP2C9 substrates, CYP3A4 substrates, cyclosporine, HMG-CoA reductase inhibitors (except pravastatin and fluvastatin), methadone, omeprazole, phenytoin, sulfonylureas, tacrolimus, trimetrexate, warfarin, and vinca alkaloids. Use with QT$_c$-prolonging agents may increase risk of malignant arrhythmia

Decreased Effect: Barbiturates (phenobarbital, secobarbital), carbamazepine, efavirenz, rifampin, and ritonavir (≥800 mg/day) decrease serum levels/effects of voriconazole; concurrent use is contraindicated. CYP2C9 inducers, CYP2C19 inducers, and phenytoin decrease serum levels/effects of voriconazole.

Ethanol/Nutrition/Herb Interactions

Food: May decrease voriconazole absorption. Voriconazole should be taken 1 hour before or 1 hour after a meal.

Herb/Nutraceutical: St John's wort may decrease voriconazole levels.

Dietary Considerations Oral: Should be taken 1 hour before or 1 hour after a meal. Voriconazole tablets contain lactose; avoid administration in hereditary galactose intolerance, Lapp lactase deficiency, or glucose-galactose malabsorption. Suspension contains sucrose; use caution with fructose intolerance, sucrose-isomaltase deficiency, or glucose-galactose malabsorption.

Pharmacodynamics/Kinetics

Absorption: Well absorbed after oral administration

Distribution: V$_d$: 4.6 L/kg

Protein binding: 58%

Metabolism: Hepatic, via CYP2C19 (major pathway) and CYP2C9 and CYP3A4 (less significant); saturable (may demonstrate nonlinearity)

Bioavailability: 96%

Half-life elimination: Variable, dose-dependent

Time to peak: 1-2 hours

Excretion: Urine (as inactive metabolites)

Pregnancy Risk Factor D

Dosage Forms INJ, powder for reconstitution: 200 mg. **POWDER, oral suspension:** 200 mg/5 mL (70 mL). **TAB:** 50 mg, 200 mg

Dental Comment

This drug is known to prolong the QT interval. The QT interval is measured as the time and distance between the Q point of the QRS complex and the end of the T wave in the ECG tracing. After adjustment for heart rate, the QT interval is defined as prolonged if it is more than 450 msec in men and 460 msec in women. A long QT syndrome was first described in the 1950s and 60s as a congenital syndrome involving QT interval prolongation and syncope and sudden death. Some of the congenital long QT syndromes were characterized by a peculiar electrocardiographic appearance of the QRS complex involving a premature atria beat followed by a pause, then a subsequent sinus beat showing marked QT prolongation and deformity. This type of cardiac arrhythmia was originally termed "torsade de pointes" (translated from the French as "twisting of the points").

Prolongation of the QT interval is thought to result from delayed ventricular repolarization. The repolarization process within the myocardial cell is due to the efflux of intracellular potassium. The channels associated with this current can be blocked by many drugs and predisposes the electrical propagation cycle to torsade de pointes.

Voriconazole is one of the drugs confirmed to prolong the QT interval and is accepted as having a risk of causing torsade de pointes. The risk of drug-induced torsade de pointes is extremely low when a single QT interval prolonging drug is prescribed. In terms of epinephrine, it is not known what effect vasoconstrictors in the local anesthetic regimen will have in patients with a known history of congenital prolonged QT interval or in patients taking any medication that prolongs the QT interval. Until more information is obtained, it is suggested that the clinician consult with the physician prior to the use of a vasoconstrictor in suspected patients, and that the vasoconstrictor (epinephrine, levonordefrin [Neo-Cobefrin®]) be used with caution.

VoSol® HC *see* Acetic Acid, Propylene Glycol Diacetate, and Hydrocortisone *on page 45*

VoSpire ER® *see* Albuterol *on page 58*

VP-16 *see* Etoposide *on page 626*

VP-16-213 *see* Etoposide *on page 626*

Vumon® *see* Teniposide *on page 1456*

Vusion™ *see* Miconazole and Zinc Oxide *on page 1040*

V.V.S.® *see* Sulfabenzamide, Sulfacetamide, and Sulfathiazole *on page 1423*

Vytone® *see* Iodoquinol and Hydrocortisone *on page 853*

Vytorin™ *see* Ezetimibe and Simvastatin *on page 631*

VZIG *see* Varicella-Zoster Immune Globulin (Human) *on page 1566*

Warfarin (WAR far in)

Related Information

Cardiovascular Diseases *on page 1636*

U.S. Brand Names Coumadin®; Jantoven™

Canadian Brand Names Apo-Warfarin®; Coumadin®; Gen-Warfarin; Taro-Warfarin

Generic Available Yes: Tablet

Synonyms Warfarin Sodium

Pharmacologic Category Anticoagulant, Coumarin Derivative

Use Prophylaxis and treatment of venous thrombosis, pulmonary embolism and thromboembolic disorders; atrial fibrillation with risk of embolism and as an adjunct in the prophylaxis of systemic embolism after myocardial infarction

Unlabeled/Investigational Use Prevention of recurrent transient ischemic attacks and to reduce risk of recurrent myocardial infarction

Local Anesthetic/Vasoconstrictor Precautions No information available to require special precautions

Effects on Dental Treatment Signs of warfarin overdose may first appear as bleeding from gingival tissue; consultation with prescribing physician is advisable prior to surgery to determine temporary dose reduction or withdrawal of medication.

(Continued)

Warfarin *(Continued)*

Common Adverse Effects As with all anticoagulants, bleeding is the major adverse effect of warfarin. Hemorrhage may occur at virtually any site. Risk is dependent on multiple variables, including the intensity of anticoagulation and patient susceptibility.

Additional adverse effects are often related to idiosyncratic reactions, and the frequency cannot be accurately estimated.

Cardiovascular: Vasculitis, edema, hemorrhagic shock

Central nervous system: Fever, lethargy, malaise, asthenia, pain, headache, dizziness, stroke

Dermatologic: Rash, dermatitis, bullous eruptions, urticaria, pruritus, alopecia

Gastrointestinal: Anorexia, nausea, vomiting, stomach cramps, abdominal pain, diarrhea, flatulence, gastrointestinal bleeding, taste disturbance, mouth ulcers

Genitourinary: Priapism, hematuria

Hematologic: Hemorrhage, leukopenia, unrecognized bleeding sites (eg, colon cancer) may be uncovered by anticoagulation, retroperitoneal hematoma, agranulocytosis

Hepatic: Hepatic injury, jaundice, transaminases increased

Neuromuscular & skeletal: Paresthesia, osteoporosis

Respiratory: Hemoptysis, epistaxis, pulmonary hemorrhage, tracheobronchial calcification

Miscellaneous: Hypersensitivity/allergic reactions

Skin necrosis/gangrene, due to paradoxical local thrombosis, is a known but rare risk of warfarin therapy. Its onset is usually within the first few days of therapy and is frequently localized to the limbs, breast or penis. The risk of this effect is increased in patients with protein C or S deficiency.

"Purple toes syndrome," caused by cholesterol microembolization, also occurs rarely. Typically, this occurs after several weeks of therapy, and may present as a dark, purplish, mottled discoloration of the plantar and lateral surfaces. Other manifestations of cholesterol microembolization may include rash; livedo reticularis; gangrene; abrupt and intense pain in lower extremities; abdominal, flank, or back pain; hematuria, renal insufficiency; hypertension; cerebral ischemia; spinal cord infarction; or other symptom of vascular compromise.

Dosage

Oral:

Infants and Children: 0.05-0.34 mg/kg/day; infants <12 months of age may require doses at or near the high end of this range; consistent anticoagulation may be difficult to maintain in children <5 years of age

Adults: Initial dosing must be individualized. Consider the patient (hepatic function, cardiac function, age, nutritional status, concurrent therapy, risk of bleeding) in addition to prior dose response (if available) and the clinical situation. Start 5-10 mg daily for 2 days. Adjust dose according to INR results; usual maintenance dose ranges from 2-10 mg daily (individual patients may require loading and maintenance doses outside these general guidelines).

Note: Lower starting doses may be required for patients with hepatic impairment, poor nutrition, CHF, elderly, high risk of bleeding, or patients that are debilitated. Higher initial doses may be reasonable in selected patients (ie, receiving enzyme-inducing agents and with low risk of bleeding).

I.V. (administer as a slow bolus injection): 2-5 mg/day

Dosing adjustment/comments in hepatic disease: Monitor effect at usual doses; the response to oral anticoagulants may be markedly enhanced in obstructive jaundice (due to reduced vitamin K absorption) and also in hepatitis and cirrhosis (due to decreased production of vitamin K-dependent clotting factors); prothrombin index should be closely monitored

Mechanism of Action Interferes with hepatic synthesis of vitamin K-dependent coagulation factors (II, VII, IX, X)

Contraindications Hypersensitivity to warfarin or any component of the formulation; hemorrhagic tendencies; hemophilia; thrombocytopenia purpura; leukemia; recent or potential surgery of the eye or CNS; major regional lumbar block anesthesia or surgery resulting in large, open surfaces; patients bleeding from the GI, respiratory, or GU tract; threatened abortion; aneurysm; ascorbic acid deficiency; history of bleeding diathesis; prostatectomy; continuous tube drainage of the small intestine; polyarthritis; diverticulitis; emaciation; malnutrition; cerebrovascular hemorrhage; eclampsia/pre-eclampsia; blood dyscrasias; severe uncontrolled or malignant hypertension; severe hepatic disease; pericarditis or pericardial effusion; subacute bacterial endocarditis; visceral carcinoma; following spinal puncture and other diagnostic or therapeutic procedures with potential for significant bleeding; history of warfarin-induced necrosis; an unreliable, noncompliant patient; alcoholism; patient who has a history of falls or is a significant fall risk; pregnancy

Warnings/Precautions Hypersensitivity to warfarin or any component of the formulation; hemorrhagic tendencies; hemophilia; thrombocytopenia purpura; leukemia; recent or potential surgery of the eye or CNS; major regional lumbar block anesthesia or surgery resulting in large, open surfaces; patients bleeding from the GI, respiratory, or GU tract; threatened abortion; aneurysm; ascorbic acid deficiency; history of bleeding diathesis; prostatectomy; continuous tube drainage of the small intestine; polyarthritis; diverticulitis; emaciation; malnutrition; cerebrovascular hemorrhage; eclampsia/pre-eclampsia; blood dyscrasias; severe uncontrolled or malignant hypertension; severe hepatic disease; pericarditis or pericardial effusion; subacute bacterial endocarditis; visceral carcinoma; following spinal puncture and other diagnostic or therapeutic procedures with potential for significant bleeding; history of warfarin-induced necrosis; an unreliable, noncompliant patient; alcoholism; patient who has a history of falls or is a significant fall risk; pregnancy

Drug Interactions

Cytochrome P450 Effect: Substrate of CYP1A2 (minor), 2C8/9 (major), 2C19 (minor), 3A4 (minor); Inhibits CYP2C8/9 (moderate), 2C19 (weak)

Increased Effect/Toxicity: Serum levels/effects of warfarin may be increased by: acetaminophen (>1.3 g for > 1 week), allopurinol, amiodarone, androgens, antifungal agents (imidazole), capecitabine, cephalosporins, cimetidine, COX-2 inhibitors, CYP2C8/9 inhibitors (moderate/strong), disulfiram, drotrecogin alfa, etoposide, fibric acid derivatives, fluconazole, fluorouracil, glucagon, HMG-CoA reductase inhibitors, ifosfamide, leflunomide, macrolide antibiotics, metronidazole, NSAIDs (nonselective), orlistat, phenytoin, propafenone, propoxyphene, proton pump inhibitors (omeprazole), quinidine, quinolone antibiotics, ropinirole, salicylates, SSRIs, sulfinpyrazone, sulfonamide derivatives, tetracycline derivatives, thyroid products, tigecycline, treprostinil, tricyclic antidepressants, vitamin A, vitamin E, voriconazole, zafirlukast, and zileuton.

Decreased Effect: Serum levels/effects of warfarin may be decreased by: aminoglutethimide, antithyroid agents, aprepitant, azathioprine, barbiturates, bile acid sequestrants, bosentan, carbamazepine, CYP2C8/9 inducers (strong), dicloxacillin, glutethimide, griseofulvin, hormonal contraceptives (estrogens and progestins), mercaptopurine, nafcillin, phytonadione, rifamycin derivatives, and sulfasalazine.

Ethanol/Nutrition/Herb Interactions

Ethanol: Avoid ethanol. Acute ethanol ingestion (binge drinking) decreases the metabolism of warfarin and increases PT/INR. Chronic daily ethanol use increases the metabolism of warfarin and decreases PT/INR.

Food: The anticoagulant effects of warfarin may be decreased if taken with foods rich in vitamin K. Vitamin E may increase warfarin effect. Cranberry juice may increase warfarin effect.

Herb/Nutraceutical: Cranberry, fenugreek, ginkgo biloba, glucosamine, may enhance bleeding or increase warfarin's effect. Ginseng (American), coenzyme Q$_{10}$, and St John's wort may decrease warfarin levels and effects. Avoid alfalfa, anise, bilberry, bladderwrack, bromelain, cat's claw, celery, coleus, cordyceps, dong quai, evening primrose oil, fenugreek, feverfew, garlic, ginger, ginkgo biloba, ginseng (American), ginseng (Panax), ginseng (Siberian), grape seed, green tea, guggul, horse chestnut seed, horseradish, licorice, prickly ash, red clover, reishi, same (s-adenosylmethionine), sweet clover, turmeric, and white willow (all have additional antiplatelet activity).

Dietary Considerations Foods high in vitamin K (eg, beef liver, pork liver, green tea and leafy green vegetables) inhibit anticoagulant effect. Do not change dietary habits once stabilized on warfarin therapy; a balanced diet with a consistent intake of vitamin K is essential; avoid large amounts of alfalfa, asparagus, broccoli, Brussels sprouts, cabbage, cauliflower, green teas, kale, lettuce, spinach, turnip greens, watercress decrease efficacy of warfarin. It is recommended that the diet contain a CONSISTENT vitamin K content of 70-140 mcg/day. Check with healthcare provider before changing diet.

Pharmacodynamics/Kinetics

Onset of action: Anticoagulation: Oral: 36-72 hours

Peak effect: Full therapeutic effect: 5-7 days; INR may increase in 36-72 hours

Duration: 2-5 days

Absorption: Oral: Rapid

Metabolism: Hepatic

Half-life elimination: 20-60 hours; Mean: 40 hours; highly variable among individuals

Pregnancy Risk Factor X

(Continued)

Warfarin *(Continued)*

Dosage Forms INJ, powder for reconstitution (Coumadin®): 5 mg. **TAB** (Coumadin®, Jantoven™): 1 mg, 2 mg, 2.5 mg, 3 mg, 4 mg, 5 mg, 6 mg, 7.5 mg, 10 mg

Selected Readings

Jeske AH, Suchko GD, ADA Council on Scientific Affairs and Division of Science, et al, "Lack of a Scientific Basis for Routine Discontinuation of Oral Anticoagulation Therapy Before Dental Treatment," *J Am Dent Assoc*, 2003, 134(11):1492-7.

Little JW, Miller CS, Henry RG, et al, "Antithrombotic Agents: Implications in Dentistry," *Oral Surg Oral Med Oral Pathol Oral Radiol Endod*, 2002, 93(5):544-51.

Scully C and Wolff A, "Oral Surgery in Patients on Anticoagulant Therapy," *Oral Surg Oral Med Oral Pathol Oral Radiol Endod*, 2002, 94(1):57-64.

Warfarin Sodium *see* Warfarin *on page 1585*

Wart-Off® Maximum Strength [OTC] *see* Salicylic Acid *on page 1374*

4-Way® 12 Hour [OTC] *see* Oxymetazoline *on page 1172*

4-Way® Saline Moisturizing Mist [OTC] *see* Sodium Chloride *on page 1400*

WelChol® *see* Colesevelam *on page 389*

Wellbutrin® *see* BuPROPion *on page 233*

Wellbutrin XL™ *see* BuPROPion *on page 233*

Wellbutrin SR® *see* BuPROPion *on page 233*

Westcort® *see* Hydrocortisone *on page 793*

Westhroid® *see* Thyroid *on page 1482*

Wigraine® *see* Ergotamine and Caffeine *on page 559*

WinRho® SDF *see* Rh₀(D) Immune Globulin *on page 1342*

Winstrol® *see* Stanozolol *on page 1415*

Wound Wash Saline™ [OTC] *see* Sodium Chloride *on page 1400*

WR-2721 *see* Amifostine *on page 83*

WR-139007 *see* Dacarbazine *on page 415*

WR-139013 *see* Chlorambucil *on page 313*

WR-139021 *see* Carmustine *on page 273*

Wycillin [DSC] *see* Penicillin G Procaine *on page 1204*

Xalatan® *see* Latanoprost *on page 900*

Xanax® *see* Alprazolam *on page 73*

Xanax XR® *see* Alprazolam *on page 73*

Xeloda® *see* Capecitabine *on page 255*

Xenaderm™ *see* Trypsin, Balsam Peru, and Castor Oil *on page 1547*

Xenical® *see* Orlistat *on page 1150*

Xibrom™ *see* Bromfenac *on page 221*

Xifaxan™ *see* Rifaximin *on page 1350*

Xigris® *see* Drotrecogin Alfa *on page 522*

Xolair® *see* Omalizumab *on page 1144*

Xopenex® *see* Levalbuterol *on page 907*

Xopenex HFA™ *see* Levalbuterol *on page 907*

X-Prep® [OTC] [DSC] *see* Senna *on page 1384*

X-Seb T® Pearl [OTC] *see* Coal Tar and Salicylic Acid *on page 383*

X-Seb T® Plus [OTC] *see* Coal Tar and Salicylic Acid *on page 383*

Xtramins [OTC] *see* Vitamins (Multiple/Oral) *on page 1582*

Xylocaine® *see* Lidocaine *on page 920*

Xylocaine® MPF *see* Lidocaine *on page 920*

Xylocaine® MPF With Epinephrine *see* Lidocaine and Epinephrine *on page 924*

Xylocaine® Viscous *see* Lidocaine *on page 920*

Xylocaine® With Epinephrine *see* Lidocaine and Epinephrine *on page 924*

Xylometazoline *(zye loe met AZ oh leen)*

U.S. Brand Names Otrivin® [OTC] [DSC]; Otrivin® Pediatric [OTC] [DSC]

Canadian Brand Names Balminil

Generic Available No

Synonyms Xylometazoline Hydrochloride

Pharmacologic Category Vasoconstrictor, Nasal

Use Symptomatic relief of nasal and nasopharyngeal mucosal congestion

Local Anesthetic/Vasoconstrictor Precautions No information available to require special precautions

Effects on Dental Treatment No significant effects or complications reported

Common Adverse Effects Frequency not defined.

Cardiovascular: Palpitations

Central nervous system: Drowsiness, dizziness, seizure, headache

Ocular: Blurred vision, ocular irritation, photophobia

Miscellaneous: Diaphoresis

Mechanism of Action Stimulates alpha-adrenergic receptors in the arterioles of the conjunctiva and the nasal mucosa to produce vasoconstriction

Pharmacodynamics/Kinetics

Onset of action: Intranasal: Local vasoconstriction: 5-10 minutes

Duration: 5-6 hours

Pregnancy Risk Factor C

Xylometazoline Hydrochloride *see* Xylometazoline *on page 1588*

Xyrem® *see* Sodium Oxybate *on page 1402*

Y-90 Zevalin *see* Ibritumomab *on page 807*

Yasmin® *see* Ethinyl Estradiol and Drospirenone *on page 595*

Yaz *see* Ethinyl Estradiol and Drospirenone *on page 595*

YM087 *see* Conivaptan *on page 393*

YM-08310 *see* Amifostine *on page 83*

Yocon® *see* Yohimbine *on page 1589*

Yodoxin® *see* Iodoquinol *on page 853*

Yohimbine (yo HIM bine)

Related Information

Yohimbe *on page 1634*

U.S. Brand Names Aphrodyne®; Yocon®

Canadian Brand Names PMS-Yohimbine; Yocon®

Generic Available Yes

Synonyms Yohimbine Hydrochloride

Pharmacologic Category Miscellaneous Product

Unlabeled/Investigational Use Treatment of SSRI-induced sexual dysfunction; weight loss; impotence; sympatholytic and mydriatic; may have activity as an aphrodisiac

Local Anesthetic/Vasoconstrictor Precautions No information available to require special precautions

Effects on Dental Treatment No significant effects or complications reported

Common Adverse Effects Frequency not defined.

Cardiovascular: Tachycardia, hypertension, hypotension (orthostatic), flushing

Central nervous system: Anxiety, mania, hallucinations, irritability, dizziness, psychosis, insomnia, headache, panic attacks

Gastrointestinal: Nausea, vomiting, anorexia, salivation

Neuromuscular & skeletal: Tremors

Miscellaneous: Antidiuretic action, diaphoresis

Mechanism of Action Derived from the bark of the yohimbe tree (*Corynanthe yohimbe*), this indole alkaloid produces a presynaptic alpha$_2$-adrenergic blockade. Peripheral autonomic effect is to increase cholinergic and decrease adrenergic activity; yohimbine exerts a stimulating effect on the mood and a mild antidiuretic effect.

Drug Interactions

Cytochrome P450 Effect: Substrate of CYP2D6 (minor); Inhibits CYP2D6 (weak)

Increased Effect/Toxicity: Caution with other CNS acting drugs. When used in combination with CYP3A4 inhibitors, serum level and/or toxicity of yohimbine may be increased; inhibitors include amiodarone, cimetidine, clarithromycin, erythromycin, delavirdine, diltiazem, dirithromycin, disulfiram, fluoxetine, fluvoxamine, grapefruit juice, indinavir, itraconazole, ketoconazole, metronidazole, nefazodone, nevirapine, propoxyphene, quinupristin-dalfopristin, ritonavir, saquinavir, verapamil, zafirlukast, zileuton; monitor for altered response. MAO inhibitors or drugs with MAO inhibition (linezolid, furazolidone) theoretically may increase toxicity or adverse effects

Pharmacodynamics/Kinetics

Duration of action: Usually 3-4 hours, but may last 36 hours

Absorption: 33%

Distribution: V$_d$: 0.3-3 L/kg

Half-life elimination: 0.6 hour

Yohimbine Hydrochloride *see* Yohimbine *on page 1589*

Z4942 *see* Ifosfamide *on page 815*

Zaditor™ *see* Ketotifen *on page 890*

Zafirlukast (za FIR loo kast)

Related Information
  Respiratory Diseases *on page 1656*
U.S. Brand Names Accolate®
Canadian Brand Names Accolate®
Mexican Brand Names Accolate®
Generic Available No
Synonyms ICI-204,219
Pharmacologic Category Leukotriene-Receptor Antagonist
Use Prophylaxis and chronic treatment of asthma in adults and children ≥5 years of age

Local Anesthetic/Vasoconstrictor Precautions No information available to require special precautions

Effects on Dental Treatment No significant effects or complications reported

Common Adverse Effects
  >10%: Central nervous system: Headache (13%)
  1% to 10%:
    Central nervous system: Dizziness (2%), pain (2%), fever (2%)
    Gastrointestinal: Nausea (3%), diarrhea (3%), abdominal pain (2%), vomiting (2%), dyspepsia (1%)
    Hepatic: SGPT increased (2%)
    Neuromuscular & skeletal: Back pain (2%), myalgia (2%), weakness (2%)
    Miscellaneous: Infection (4%)

Mechanism of Action Zafirlukast is a selectively and competitive leukotriene-receptor antagonist (LTRA) of leukotriene D4 and E4 (LTD4 and LTE4), components of slow-reacting substance of anaphylaxis (SRSA). Cysteinyl leukotriene production and receptor occupation have been correlated with the pathophysiology of asthma, including airway edema, smooth muscle constriction and altered cellular activity associated with the inflammatory process, which contribute to the signs and symptoms of asthma.

Drug Interactions
  Cytochrome P450 Effect: Substrate of CYP2C9 (major); **Inhibits** CYP1A2 (weak), 2C8 (weak), 2C9 (moderate), 2C19 (weak), 2D6 (weak), 3A4 (weak)
  Increased Effect/Toxicity: Zafirlukast concentrations are increased by aspirin. Zafirlukast may increase theophylline levels. Zafirlukast may increase the levels/effects of bosentan, dapsone, fluoxetine, glimepiride, glipizide, losartan, montelukast, nateglinide, paclitaxel, phenytoin, warfarin, zafirlukast, and other CYP2C9 substrates.
  Decreased Effect: The levels/effects of zafirlukast may be decreased by carbamazepine, phenobarbital, phenytoin, rifampin, rifapentine, secobarbital, and other CYP2C9 inducers. Zafirlukast concentrations may be reduced by erythromycin.

Pharmacodynamics/Kinetics
  Protein binding: >99%, primarily to albumin
  Metabolism: Extensively hepatic via CYP2C9
  Bioavailability: Reduced 40% with food
  Half-life elimination: 10 hours
  Time to peak, serum: 3 hours
  Excretion: Urine (10%); feces
Pregnancy Risk Factor B

Zagam® [DSC] *see* Sparfloxacin *on page 1411*

Zalcitabine (zal SITE a been)

Related Information
  HIV Infection and AIDS *on page 1662*
U.S. Brand Names Hivid®
Canadian Brand Names Hivid®
Generic Available No
Synonyms ddC; Dideoxycytidine
Pharmacologic Category Antiretroviral Agent, Reverse Transcriptase Inhibitor (Nucleoside)
Use In combination with at least two other antiretrovirals in the treatment of patients with HIV infection; it is not recommended that zalcitabine be given in combination with didanosine, stavudine, or lamivudine due to overlapping toxicities, virologic interactions, or lack of clinical data

Local Anesthetic/Vasoconstrictor Precautions No information available to require special precautions

Effects on Dental Treatment Key adverse event(s) related to dental treatment: Oral ulcerations.

Common Adverse Effects

>10%:
Central nervous system: Fever (5% to 17%), malaise (2% to 13%)
Neuromuscular & skeletal: Peripheral neuropathy (28%)

1% to 10%:
Central nervous system: Headache (2%), dizziness (1%), fatigue (4%), seizure (1.3%)
Dermatologic: Rash (2% to 11%), pruritus (3% to 5%)
Endocrine & metabolic: Hypoglycemia (2% to 6%), hyponatremia (4%), hyperglycemia (1% to 6%)
Gastrointestinal: Nausea (3%), dysphagia (1% to 4%), anorexia (4%), abdominal pain (3% to 8%), vomiting (1% to 3%), diarrhea (<1% to 10%), weight loss, oral ulcers (3% to 7%), increased amylase (3% to 8%)
Hematologic: Anemia (occurs as early as 2-4 weeks), granulocytopenia (usually after 6-8 weeks)
Hepatic: Abnormal hepatic function (9%), hyperbilirubinemia (2% to 5%)
Neuromuscular & skeletal: Myalgia (1% to 6%), foot pain
Respiratory: Pharyngitis (2%), cough (6%), nasal discharge (4%)

Mechanism of Action Purine nucleoside (cytosine) analog, zalcitabine or 2′,3′-dideoxycytidine (ddC) is converted to active metabolite ddCTP; lack the presence of the 3′-hydroxyl group necessary for phosphodiester linkages during DNA replication. As a result viral replication is prematurely terminated. ddCTP acts as a competitor for binding sites on the HIV-RNA dependent DNA polymerase (reverse transcriptase) to further contribute to inhibition of viral replication.

Drug Interactions

Increased Effect/Toxicity: Amphotericin, foscarnet, and aminoglycosides may potentiate the risk of developing peripheral neuropathy or other toxicities associated with zalcitabine by interfering with the renal elimination of zalcitabine. Other drugs associated with peripheral neuropathy include chloramphenicol, cisplatin, dapsone, disulfiram, ethionamide, glutethimide, gold, hydralazine, iodoquinol, isoniazid, metronidazole, nitrofurantoin, phenytoin, ribavirin, and vincristine. Concomitant use with zalcitabine may increase risk of peripheral neuropathy. Concomitant use of zalcitabine with didanosine is not recommended. Concomitant use of ribavirin and nucleoside analogues may increase the risk of developing lactic acidosis (includes adefovir, didanosine, lamivudine, stavudine, zalcitabine, zidovudine).

Decreased Effect: It is not recommended that zalcitabine be given in combination with didanosine, stavudine, or lamivudine due to overlapping toxicities, virologic interactions, or lack of clinical data. Doxorubicin and lamivudine have been shown *in vitro* to decrease zalcitabine phosphorylation. Magnesium/aluminum-containing antacids and metoclopramide may decrease the absorption of zalcitabine.

Pharmacodynamics/Kinetics
Absorption: Well, but variable; decreased 39% with food
Distribution: Minimal data available; variable CSF penetration
Protein binding: <4%
Metabolism: Intracellularly to active triphosphorylated agent
Bioavailability: >80%
Half-life elimination: 2.9 hours; Renal impairment: ≤8.5 hours
Excretion: Urine (>70% as unchanged drug)

Pregnancy Risk Factor C

Zaleplon (ZAL e plon)

U.S. Brand Names Sonata®
Canadian Brand Names Sonata®; Starnoc®
Generic Available No
Pharmacologic Category Hypnotic, Nonbenzodiazepine
Dental Use Has not be established
Use Short-term (7-10 days) treatment of insomnia (has been demonstrated to be effective for up to 5 weeks in controlled trial)
Local Anesthetic/Vasoconstrictor Precautions No information available to require special precautions
Effects on Dental Treatment Key adverse event(s) related to dental treatment: Xerostomia (normal salivary flow resumes upon discontinuation).
Common Adverse Effects
1% to 10%:
Cardiovascular: Peripheral edema, chest pain
(Continued)

Zaleplon (Continued)

Central nervous system: Amnesia, anxiety, depersonalization, dizziness, hallucinations, hypoesthesia, somnolence, vertigo, malaise, depression, lightheadedness, impaired coordination, fever, migraine

Dermatologic: Photosensitivity reaction, rash, pruritus

Gastrointestinal: Abdominal pain, anorexia, colitis, dyspepsia, nausea, constipation, xerostomia

Genitourinary: Dysmenorrhea

Neuromuscular & skeletal: Paresthesia, tremor, myalgia, weakness, back pain, arthralgia

Ocular: Abnormal vision, eye pain

Otic: Hyperacusis

Miscellaneous: Parosmia

Restrictions C-IV

Mechanism of Action Zaleplon is unrelated to benzodiazepines, barbiturates, or other hypnotics. However, it interacts with the benzodiazepine GABA receptor complex. Nonclinical studies have shown that it binds selectively to the brain omega-1 receptor situated on the alpha subunit of the GABA-A receptor complex.

Drug Interactions

Cytochrome P450 Effect: Substrate of CYP3A4 (minor)

Increased Effect/Toxicity: Zaleplon potentiates the CNS effects of CNS depressants, including ethanol, anticonvulsants, antipsychotics, barbiturates, benzodiazepines, narcotic agonists, and other sedative agents. Cimetidine increases concentrations of zaleplon. Avoid concurrent use or use 5 mg zaleplon as starting dose in patient receiving cimetidine.

Pharmacodynamics/Kinetics

Onset of action: Rapid

Peak effect: ~1 hour

Duration: 6-8 hours

Absorption: Rapid and almost complete

Distribution: V_d: 1.4 L/kg

Protein binding: 60% ± 15%

Metabolism: Extensive, primarily via aldehyde oxidase to form 5-oxo-zaleplon and to a lesser extent by CYP3A4 to desethylzaleplon; all metabolites are pharmacologically inactive

Bioavailability: 30%

Half-life elimination: 1 hour

Time to peak, serum: 1 hour

Excretion: Urine (primarily metabolites, <1% as unchanged drug)

Clearance: Plasma: Oral: 3 L/hour/kg

Pregnancy Risk Factor C

Zanaflex® see Tizanidine on page 1497

Zanamivir (za NA mi veer)

Related Information

Systemic Viral Diseases on page 1675

U.S. Brand Names Relenza®

Canadian Brand Names Relenza®

Generic Available No

Pharmacologic Category Antiviral Agent; Neuraminidase Inhibitor

Use Treatment of uncomplicated acute illness due to influenza virus A and B; treatment should only be initiated in patients who have been symptomatic for no more than 2 days. Prophylaxis against influenza virus A and B

Local Anesthetic/Vasoconstrictor Precautions No information available to require special precautions

Effects on Dental Treatment No significant effects or complications reported

Common Adverse Effects Most adverse reactions occurred at a frequency which was less than or equal to the control (lactose vehicle).

>10%:

Central nervous system: Headache (prophylaxis 13% to 24%; treatment 2%)

Gastrointestinal: Throat/tonsil discomfort/pain (prophylaxis 8% to 19%)

Respiratory: Cough (prophylaxis 7% to 17%; treatment ≤2%), nasal signs and symptoms (prophylaxis 12%; treatment 2%)

Miscellaneous: Viral infection (prophylaxis 3% to 13%)

1% to 10%:

Central nervous system: Fever/chills (prophylaxis 5% to 9%; treatment <1.5%), fatigue (prophylaxis 5% to 8%; treatment <1.5%), malaise (prophylaxis 5% to 8%; treatment <1.5%), dizziness (treatment 1% to 2%)

Dermatologic: Urticaria (treatment <1.5%)

Gastrointestinal: Anorexia/appetite decreased (prophylaxis 2% to 4%), nausea (prophylaxis 1% to 2%; treatment ≤3%), diarrhea (prophylaxis 2%; treatment 2% to 3%), vomiting (prophylaxis 1% to 2%; treatment 1% to 2%) abdominal pain (treatment <1.5%)

Neuromuscular & skeletal: Muscle pain (prophylaxis 3% to 8%), musculoskeletal pain (prophylaxis 6%), arthralgia/articular rheumatism (prophylaxis 2%), arthralgia (treatment <1.5%), myalgia (treatment <1.5%)

Respiratory: Infection (ear/nose/throat; prophylaxis 2%; treatment 2% to 5%), sinusitis (treatment 3%), bronchitis (treatment 2%), nasal inflammation (prophylaxis 1%)

Mechanism of Action Zanamivir inhibits influenza virus neuraminidase enzymes, potentially altering virus particle aggregation and release.

Drug Interactions

Decreased Effect: Zanamivir may diminish the therapeutic effect of live, attentuated influenza virus vaccine (FluMist™). The manufacturer of FluMist™ recommends that the administration of anti-influenza virus medications be avoided during the period beginning 48 hours prior to vaccine administration and ending 2 weeks after vaccine.

Pharmacodynamics/Kinetics

Absorption: Inhalation: 4% to 17%

Protein binding, plasma: <10%

Metabolism: None

Half-life elimination, serum: 2.5-5.1 hours

Excretion: Urine (as unchanged drug); feces (unabsorbed drug)

Pregnancy Risk Factor C

Zanosar® see Streptozocin on page 1418

Zantac® see Ranitidine on page 1334

Zantac 75® [OTC] see Ranitidine on page 1334

Zantac 150™ [OTC] see Ranitidine on page 1334

Zantac® EFFERdose® see Ranitidine on page 1334

Zapzyt® [OTC] see Benzoyl Peroxide on page 194

Zapzyt® Acne Wash [OTC] see Salicylic Acid on page 1374

Zapzyt® Pore Treatment [OTC] see Salicylic Acid on page 1374

Zarontin® see Ethosuximide on page 619

Zaroxolyn® see Metolazone on page 1030

Zavesca® see Miglustat on page 1047

Z-Bec® [OTC] see Vitamin B Complex Combinations on page 1581

Z-Cof DM see Guaifenesin, Pseudoephedrine, and Dextromethorphan on page 757

Z-Cof LA™ see Guaifenesin and Dextromethorphan on page 754

ZD1033 see Anastrozole on page 126

ZD1839 see Gefitinib on page 727

ZDV see Zidovudine on page 1594

ZDV, Abacavir, and Lamivudine see Abacavir, Lamivudine, and Zidovudine on page 23

Zeasorb®-AF [OTC] see Miconazole on page 1039

Zebeta® see Bisoprolol on page 211

Zebutal™ see Butalbital, Acetaminophen, and Caffeine on page 239

Zegerid® see Omeprazole and Sodium Bicarbonate on page 1146

Zeldox see Ziprasidone on page 1598

Zelnorm® see Tegaserod on page 1448

Zemaira® see Alpha₁-Proteinase Inhibitor on page 73

Zemplar® see Paricalcitol on page 1187

Zenapax® see Daclizumab on page 416

Zeneca 182,780 see Fulvestrant on page 713

Zephiran® [OTC] see Benzalkonium Chloride on page 188

Zephrex® see Guaifenesin and Pseudoephedrine on page 755

Zephrex LA® see Guaifenesin and Pseudoephedrine on page 755

Zerit® see Stavudine on page 1416

Zestoretic® see Lisinopril and Hydrochlorothiazide on page 938

Zestril® see Lisinopril on page 936

Zetar® [OTC] see Coal Tar on page 383

Zetia™ see Ezetimibe on page 630

Zevalin® see Ibritumomab on page 807

Ziac® see Bisoprolol and Hydrochlorothiazide on page 212

Ziagen® see Abacavir on page 22

Ziconotide (zi KOE no tide)

U.S. Brand Names Prialt®

Generic Available No

Pharmacologic Category Analgesic, Non-narcotic; Calcium Channel Blocker, N-Type

Use Management of severe chronic pain in patients requiring intrathecal (I.T.) therapy and are intolerant or refractory to other therapies

Local Anesthetic/Vasoconstrictor Precautions No information available to require special precautions

Effects on Dental Treatment No significant effects or complications reported

Common Adverse Effects Percentages reported when using the slow (21-day) titration schedule; frequencies may be higher with faster titration.

>10%:

Central nervous system: Dizziness (47%), somnolence (22%), confusion (18%), ataxia (16%), headache (15%), memory impairment (12%), pain (11%)

Gastrointestinal: Nausea (41%), diarrhea (19%), vomiting (15%)

Neuromuscular & skeletal: Weakness (22%), gait disturbances (15%), hypertonia (11%)

2% to 10%:

Cardiovascular: Chest pain, edema, hyper-/hypotension, postural hypotension, tachycardia, vasodilation

Central nervous system: Anxiety (9%), speech disorder (9%), aphasia (8%), dysesthesia (7%), fever (7%), hallucinations (7%), nervousness (7%), vertigo (7%), agitation, chills, depression, dreams abnormal, emotional lability, hostility, hyperesthesia, insomnia, malaise, meningitis, paranoid reaction, stupor

Dermatologic: Bruising, cellulitis, dry skin, pruritus, rash

Endocrine & metabolic: Hypokalemia

Gastrointestinal: Anorexia (10%), abdominal pain, constipation, dehydration, dyspepsia, taste perversion, weight loss, xerostomia

Genitourinary: Urinary retention (9%), dysuria, urinary incontinence, urinary tract infection, urination impaired

Hematologic: Anemia

Local: Catheter complication, catheter site pain, pump site complication, pump site mass, pump site pain

Neuromuscular & skeletal: Paresthesia (7%), arthralgia, arthritis, back pain, CPK increased (<2%), incoordination, leg cramps, myalgia, myasthenia, neck pain, neck rigidity, neuralgia, reflexes decreased, tremor

Ocular: Vision abnormal (10%), nystagmus (8%), diplopia, photophobia,

Otic: Tinnitus

Respiratory: Bronchitis, cough, dyspnea, pharyngitis, pneumonia, rhinitis, sinusitis

Miscellaneous: CSF abnormalities, diaphoresis, flu-like syndrome, infection

Mechanism of Action Ziconotide selectively binds to N-type voltage sensitive calcium channels located on the afferent nerves of the dorsal horn in the spinal cord. This binding is thought to block N-type calcium channels, leading to a blockade of excitatory neurotransmitter release and reducing sensitivity to painful stimuli.

Drug Interactions

Increased Effect/Toxicity: May enhance the adverse/toxic effects of other CNS depressants

Pharmacodynamics/Kinetics

Distribution: I.T.: V_d: ~140 mL

Protein binding: 50%

Metabolism: Metabolized via endopeptidases and exopeptidases present on multiple organs including kidney, liver, lung; degraded to peptide fragments and free amino acids

Half-life elimination: I.V.: 1-1.6 hours (plasma); I.T.: 2.9-6.5 hours (CSF)

Excretion: I.V.: Urine (<1%)

Pregnancy Risk Factor C

Zidovudine (zye DOE vyoo deen)

Related Information

HIV Infection and AIDS *on page 1662*
Systemic Viral Diseases *on page 1675*

U.S. Brand Names Retrovir®

Canadian Brand Names AZT™; Retrovir®

Mexican Brand Names Isadol®; Retrovir AZT®

Generic Available Yes: Tablet

Synonyms Azidothymidine; AZT (error-prone abbreviation); Compound S; ZDV

Pharmacologic Category Antiretroviral Agent, Reverse Transcriptase Inhibitor (Nucleoside)

Use Management of patients with HIV infections in combination with at least two other antiretroviral agents; for prevention of maternal/fetal HIV transmission as monotherapy

Unlabeled/Investigational Use Postexposure prophylaxis for HIV exposure as part of a multidrug regimen

Local Anesthetic/Vasoconstrictor Precautions No information available to require special precautions

Effects on Dental Treatment No significant effects or complications reported

Common Adverse Effects

>10%:
  Central nervous system: Severe headache (42%), fever (16%)
  Dermatologic: Rash (17%)
  Gastrointestinal: Nausea (46% to 61%), anorexia (11%), diarrhea (17%), pain (20%), vomiting (6% to 25%)
  Hematologic: Anemia (23% in children), leukopenia, granulocytopenia (39% in children)
  Neuromuscular & skeletal: Weakness (19%)

1% to 10%:
  Central nervous system: Malaise (8%), dizziness (6%), insomnia (5%), somnolence (8%)
  Dermatologic: Hyperpigmentation of nails (bluish-brown)
  Gastrointestinal: Dyspepsia (5%)
  Hematologic: Changes in platelet count
  Neuromuscular & skeletal: Paresthesia (6%)

Mechanism of Action Zidovudine is a thymidine analog which interferes with the HIV viral RNA dependent DNA polymerase resulting in inhibition of viral replication; nucleoside reverse transcriptase inhibitor

Drug Interactions

Cytochrome P450 Effect: Substrate (minor) of CYP2A6, 2C8/9, 2C19, 3A4

Increased Effect/Toxicity: Coadministration of zidovudine with drugs that are nephrotoxic (amphotericin B), cytotoxic (flucytosine, vincristine, vinblastine, doxorubicin, interferon), inhibit glucuronidation or excretion (acetaminophen, cimetidine, indomethacin, lorazepam, probenecid, aspirin), or interfere with RBC/WBC number or function (acyclovir, ganciclovir, pentamidine, dapsone). Clarithromycin may increase blood levels of zidovudine (although total body exposure was unaffected, peak plasma concentrations were increased). Valproic acid significantly increases zidovudine's blood levels (believed due to inhibition first pass metabolism). Concomitant use of ribavirin and nucleoside analogues may increase the risk of developing lactic acidosis (includes adefovir, didanosine, lamivudine, stavudine, zalcitabine, zidovudine).

Decreased Effect: *In vitro* evidence suggests zidovudine's antiretroviral activity may be antagonized by doxorubicin and ribavirin; avoid concurrent use. Zidovudine may decrease the antiviral activity of stavudine (based on *in vitro* data); avoid concurrent use.

Pharmacodynamics/Kinetics

Absorption: Oral: 66% to 70%

Distribution: Significant penetration into the CSF; crosses placenta
  Relative diffusion from blood into CSF: Adequate with or without inflammation (exceeds usual MICs)
  CSF:blood level ratio: Normal meninges: ~60%

Protein binding: 25% to 38%

Metabolism: Hepatic via glucuronidation to inactive metabolites; extensive first-pass effect

Half-life elimination: Terminal: 60 minutes

Time to peak, serum: 30-90 minutes

Excretion:
  Oral: Urine (72% to 74% as metabolites, 14% to 18% as unchanged drug)
  I.V.: Urine (45% to 60% as metabolites, 18% to 29% as unchanged drug)

Pregnancy Risk Factor C

Zidovudine, Abacavir, and Lamivudine see Abacavir, Lamivudine, and Zidovudine on page 23

Zidovudine and Lamivudine
(zye DOE vyoo deen & la MI vyoo deen)

Related Information
HIV Infection and AIDS *on page 1662*
Lamivudine *on page 894*
Zidovudine *on page 1594*
U.S. Brand Names Combivir®
Canadian Brand Names Combivir®
Generic Available No
Synonyms AZT + 3TC (error-prone abbreviation); Lamivudine and Zidovudine
Pharmacologic Category Antiretroviral Agent, Reverse Transcriptase Inhibitor (Nucleoside)
Use Treatment of HIV infection when therapy is warranted based on clinical and/or immunological evidence of disease progression. Combivir® given twice daily, provides an alternative regimen to lamivudine 150 mg twice daily plus zidovudine 600 mg/day in divided doses; this drug form reduces capsule/tablet intake for these two drugs to 2 per day instead of up to 8.
Local Anesthetic/Vasoconstrictor Precautions No information available to require special precautions
Effects on Dental Treatment No significant effects or complications reported
Common Adverse Effects See individual agents.
Mechanism of Action The combination of zidovudine and lamivudine are believed to act synergistically to inhibit reverse transcriptase via DNA chain termination after incorporation of the nucleoside analogue as well as to delay the emergence of mutations conferring resistance
Drug Interactions
Cytochrome P450 Effect: Zidovudine: **Substrate** (minor) of CYP2A6, 2C8/9, 2C19, 3A4
Increased Effect/Toxicity: See individual agents.
Decreased Effect: See individual agents.
Pharmacodynamics/Kinetics See individual agents.
Pregnancy Risk Factor C

Zilactin-L® [OTC] *see* Lidocaine *on page 920*
Zilactin®-B [OTC] *see* Benzocaine *on page 190*
Zilactin Toothache and Gum Pain® [OTC] *see* Benzocaine *on page 190*

Zileuton (zye LOO ton)

Related Information
Respiratory Diseases *on page 1656*
U.S. Brand Names Zyflo®
Generic Available No
Pharmacologic Category 5-Lipoxygenase Inhibitor
Use Prophylaxis and chronic treatment of asthma in children ≥12 years of age and adults
Local Anesthetic/Vasoconstrictor Precautions No information available to require special precautions
Effects on Dental Treatment No significant effects or complications reported
Common Adverse Effects
>10%: Central nervous system: Headache (25%)
1% to 10%:
Central nervous system: Pain (8%)
Gastrointestinal: Dyspepsia (8%), nausea (6%), abdominal pain (5%)
Hematologic: Leukopenia (1%)
Hepatic: ALT increased (2%)
Neuromuscular & skeletal: Asthenia (4%), myalgia (3%)
Frequency not defined:
Cardiovascular: Chest pain
Central nervous system: Dizziness, fever, insomnia, malaise, nervousness, somnolence
Dermatologic: Pruritus
Gastrointestinal: Constipation, flatulence, vomiting
Genitourinary: Urinary tract infection, vaginitis
Neuromuscular & skeletal: Arthralgia, hypertonia, neck pain/rigidity
Ocular: Conjunctivitis
Miscellaneous: Lymphadenopathy
Mechanism of Action Specific 5-Lipoxygenase inhibitor which inhibits leukotriene formation. Leukotrienes augment neutrophil and eosinophil migration,

neutrophil and monocyte aggregation, leukocyte adhesion, increased capillary permeability and smooth muscle contraction (which contribute to inflammation, edema, mucous secretion, and bronchoconstriction in the airway of the asthmatic.)

Drug Interactions

Cytochrome P450 Effect: Substrate (minor) of CYP1A2, 2C8/9, 3A4; **Inhibits** CYP1A2 (weak)

Increased Effect/Toxicity: Zileuton may increase the serum concentration/effects of theophylline, propranolol, and warfarin; monitor and reduce doses accordingly.

Pharmacodynamics/Kinetics

Absorption: Rapid

Distribution: 1.2 L/kg

Protein binding: 93%

Metabolism: Several metabolites in plasma and urine; metabolized by CYP1A2, 2C9, and 3A4

Bioavailability: Unknown

Half-life elimination: 2.5 hours

Time to peak, serum: 1.7 hours

Excretion: Urine (~95% primarily as metabolites); feces (~2%)

Pregnancy Risk Factor C

Zinacef® see Cefuroxime on page 295

Zinc see Trace Metals on page 1513

Zincate® see Zinc Sulfate on page 1598

Zinc Chloride (zink KLOR ide)

Generic Available Yes

Pharmacologic Category Trace Element

Use Cofactor for replacement therapy to different enzymes helps maintain normal growth rates, normal skin hydration and senses of taste and smell

Local Anesthetic/Vasoconstrictor Precautions No information available to require special precautions

Effects on Dental Treatment No significant effects or complications reported

Pregnancy Risk Factor C

Zinc Diethylenetriaminepentaacetate (Zn-DTPA) see Diethylene Triamine Penta-Acetic Acid on page 466

Zincfrin® [OTC] see Phenylephrine and Zinc Sulfate on page 1228

Zinc Gelatin (zink JEL ah tin)

U.S. Brand Names Gelucast®

Generic Available Yes

Synonyms Dome Paste Bandage; Unna's Boot; Unna's Paste; Zinc Gelatin Boot

Pharmacologic Category Topical Skin Product

Use As a protectant and to support varicosities and similar lesions of the lower limbs

Local Anesthetic/Vasoconstrictor Precautions No information available to require special precautions

Effects on Dental Treatment No significant effects or complications reported

Common Adverse Effects 1% to 10%: Local: Irritation

Zinc Gelatin Boot see Zinc Gelatin on page 1597

Zincon® [OTC] see Pyrithione Zinc on page 1318

Zinc Oxide (zink OKS ide)

U.S. Brand Names Ammens® Medicated Deodorant [OTC]; Balmex® [OTC]; Boudreaux's® Butt Paste [OTC]; Critic-Aid Skin Care® [OTC]; Desitin® [OTC]; Desitin® Creamy [OTC]

Canadian Brand Names Zincofax®

Generic Available Yes: Ointment

Synonyms Base Ointment; Lassar's Zinc Paste

Pharmacologic Category Topical Skin Product

Use Protective coating for mild skin irritations and abrasions, soothing and protective ointment to promote healing of chapped skin, diaper rash

Local Anesthetic/Vasoconstrictor Precautions No information available to require special precautions

(Continued)

Zinc Oxide (Continued)

Effects on Dental Treatment No significant effects or complications reported
Common Adverse Effects 1% to 10%: Local: Skin sensitivity, irritation
Mechanism of Action Mild astringent with weak antiseptic properties

Zinc Oxide and Miconazole Nitrate *see* Miconazole and Zinc Oxide *on page 1040*

Zinc Sulfate (zink SUL fate)

U.S. Brand Names Orazinc® [OTC]; Zincate®
Canadian Brand Names Anuzinc; Rivasol
Generic Available Yes
Synonyms ZnSO$_4$ (error-prone abbreviation)
Pharmacologic Category Trace Element
Use Zinc supplement (oral and parenteral); may improve wound healing in those who are deficient
Local Anesthetic/Vasoconstrictor Precautions No information available to require special precautions
Effects on Dental Treatment No significant effects or complications reported
Pregnancy Risk Factor C

Zinc Sulfate and Phenylephrine *see* Phenylephrine and Zinc Sulfate *on page 1228*

Zinc Undecylenate *see* Undecylenic Acid and Derivatives *on page 1550*

Zinecard® *see* Dexrazoxane *on page 446*

Ziox™ *see* Chlorophyllin, Papain, and Urea *on page 319*

Ziprasidone (zi PRAY si done)

U.S. Brand Names Geodon®
Generic Available No
Synonyms Zeldox; Ziprasidone Hydrochloride; Ziprasidone Mesylate
Pharmacologic Category Antipsychotic Agent, Atypical
Use Treatment of schizophrenia; treatment of acute manic or mixed episodes associated with bipolar disorder with or without psychosis; acute agitation in patients with schizophrenia
Unlabeled/Investigational Use Tourette's syndrome
Local Anesthetic/Vasoconstrictor Precautions No information available to require special precautions (see Dental Comment)
Effects on Dental Treatment Key adverse event(s) related to dental treatment: Xerostomia (normal salivary flow resumes upon discontinuation).
Common Adverse Effects Note: Although minor QT$_c$ prolongation (mean 10 msec at 160 mg/day) may occur more frequently (incidence not specified), clinically-relevant prolongation (>500 msec) was rare (0.06%) and less than placebo (0.23%).

>10%:
  Central nervous system: Extrapyramidal symptoms (2% to 31%), somnolence (8% to 31%), headache (3% to 18%), dizziness (3% to 16%)
  Gastrointestinal: Nausea (4% to 12%)
1% to 10%:
  Cardiovascular: Chest pain (5%), postural hypotension (5%), hypertension (2% to 3%), bradycardia (2%), tachycardia (2%), vasodilation (1%), facial edema, orthostatic hypotension
  Central nervous system: Akathisia (2% to 10%), anxiety (2% to 5%) insomnia (3%), agitation (2%), speech disorder (2%), personality disorder (2%), psychosis (1%), akinesia, amnesia, ataxia, chills, confusion, coordination abnormal, delirium, dystonia, fever, hostility, hypothermia, oculogyric crisis, vertigo
  Dermatologic: Rash (4%), fungal dermatitis (2%)
  Endocrine & metabolic: Dysmenorrhea (2%)
  Gastrointestinal: Weight gain (10%), constipation (2% to 9%), dyspepsia (1% to 8%), diarrhea (3% to 5%), vomiting (3% to 5%), salivation increased (4%), xerostomia (1% to 5%), tongue edema (3%), abdominal pain (2%), anorexia (2%), dysphagia (2%), rectal hemorrhage (2%), tooth disorder (1%), buccoglossal syndrome
  Genitourinary: Priapism (1%)
  Local: Injection site pain (7% to 9%)
  Neuromuscular & skeletal: Weakness (2% to 6%), hypoesthesia (2%), myalgia (2%), paresthesia (2%), back pain (1%), cogwheel rigidity (1%),

hypertonia (1%), abnormal gait, choreoathetosis, dysarthria, dyskinesia, hyper-/hypokinesia, hypotonia, neuropathy, tremor, twitching

Ocular: Vision abnormal (3% to 6%), diplopia

Respiratory: Infection (8%), rhinitis (1% to 4%), cough (3%), pharyngitis (3%), dyspnea (2%)

Miscellaneous: Diaphoresis (2%), furunculosis (2%), flu-like syndrome (1%), photosensitivity reaction, withdrawal syndrome

Mechanism of Action Ziprasidone is a benzylisothiazolylpiperazine antipsychotic. The exact mechanism of action is unknown. However, *in vitro* radioligand studies show that ziprasidone has high affinity for D_2, D_3, 5-HT$_{2A}$, 5-HT$_{1A}$, 5-HT$_{2C}$, 5-HT$_{1D}$, and alpha$_1$ adrenergic; moderate affinity for histamine H$_1$ receptors; and no appreciable affinity for alpha$_2$ adrenergic receptors, beta adrenergic, 5-HT$_3$, 5-HT$_4$, cholinergic, mu, sigma, or benzodiazepine receptors. Ziprasidone functions as an antagonist at the D_2, 5-HT$_{2A}$, and 5-HT$_{1D}$ receptors and as an agonist at the 5-HT$_{1A}$ receptor. Ziprasidone moderately inhibits the reuptake of serotonin and norepinephrine.

Drug Interactions

Cytochrome P450 Effect: Substrate (minor) of CYP1A2, 3A4; **Inhibits** CYP2D6 (weak), 3A4 (weak)

Increased Effect/Toxicity:

Ketoconazole may increase serum concentrations of ziprasidone. Other CYP3A4 inhibitors may share this potential.

Concurrent use with QT$_c$-prolonging agents may result in additive effects on cardiac conduction, potentially resulting in malignant or lethal arrhythmias. Concurrent use is contraindicated; includes amiodarone, arsenic trioxide, bretylium, chlorpromazine, cisapride; class Ia antiarrhythmics (quinidine, procainamide); dofetilide, dolasetron, droperidol, halofantrine, ibutilide, levomethadyl, mefloquine, mesoridazine, pentamidine, pimozide, probucol; some quinolone antibiotics (moxifloxacin, sparfloxacin, gatifloxacin); sotalol, tacrolimus, and thioridazine. Potassium- or magnesium-depleting agents (diuretics, aminoglycosides, cyclosporine, and amphotericin B) may increase the risk of QT$_c$ prolongation. Antihypertensive agents may increase the risk of orthostatic hypotension. CNS depressants may increase the degree of sedation caused by ziprasidone. Metoclopramide may increase risk of extrapyramidal symptoms (EPS). Acetylcholinesterase inhibitors (central) may increase the risk of antipsychotic-related EPS.

Decreased Effect: Carbamazepine may decrease serum concentrations of ziprasidone. Other enzyme-inducing agents may share this potential. Amphetamines may decrease the efficacy of ziprasidone. Ziprasidone may inhibit the efficacy of levodopa.

Pharmacodynamics/Kinetics

Absorption: Well absorbed

Distribution: V$_d$: 1.5 L/kg

Protein binding: 99%, primarily to albumin and alpha$_1$-acid glycoprotein

Metabolism: Extensively hepatic, primarily via aldehyde oxidase; less than $\frac{1}{3}$ of total metabolism via CYP3A4 and CYP1A2 (minor)

Bioavailability: Oral (with food): 60% (up to twofold increase with food); I.M.: 100%

Half-life elimination: Oral: 7 hours; I.M.: 2-5 hours

Time to peak: Oral: 6-8 hours; I.M.: ≤60 minutes

Excretion: Feces (66%) and urine (20%) as metabolites; little as unchanged drug (1% urine, 4% feces)

Clearance: 7.5 mL/minute/kg

Pregnancy Risk Factor C

Dental Comment

This drug is known to prolong the QT interval. The QT interval is measured as the time and distance between the Q point of the QRS complex and the end of the T wave in the ECG tracing. After adjustment for heart rate, the QT interval is defined as prolonged if it is more than 450 msec in men and 460 msec in women. A long QT syndrome was first described in the 1950s and 60s as a congenital syndrome involving QT interval prolongation and syncope and sudden death. Some of the congenital long QT syndromes were characterized by a peculiar electrocardiographic appearance of the QRS complex involving a premature atria beat followed by a pause, then a subsequent sinus beat showing marked QT prolongation and deformity. This type of cardiac arrhythmia was originally termed "torsade de pointes" (translated from the French as "twisting of the points").

Prolongation of the QT interval is thought to result from delayed ventricular repolarization. The repolarization process within the myocardial cell is due to the efflux of intracellular potassium. The channels associated with this current can be blocked by many drugs and predisposes the electrical propagation cycle to torsade de pointes.

(Continued)

Ziprasidone *(Continued)*

Ziprasidone is one of the drugs confirmed to prolong the QT interval and is accepted as having a risk of causing torsade de pointes. The risk of drug-induced torsade de pointes is extremely low when a single QT interval prolonging drug is prescribed. In terms of epinephrine, it is not known what effect vasoconstrictors in the local anesthetic regimen will have in patients with a known history of congenital prolonged QT interval or in patients taking any medication that prolongs the QT interval. Until more information is obtained, it is suggested that the clinician consult with the physician prior to the use of a vasoconstrictor in suspected patients, and that the vasoconstrictor (epinephrine, levonordefrin [Neo-Cobefrin®]) be used with caution.

Ziprasidone Hydrochloride *see* Ziprasidone *on page 1598*

Ziprasidone Mesylate *see* Ziprasidone *on page 1598*

Zithromax® *see* Azithromycin *on page 171*

Zithromax® TRI-PAK™ *see* Azithromycin *on page 171*

Zithromax® Z-PAK® *see* Azithromycin *on page 171*

ZM-182,780 *see* Fulvestrant *on page 713*

Zmax™ *see* Azithromycin *on page 171*

Zn-DTPA *see* Diethylene Triamine Penta-Acetic Acid *on page 466*

ZNP® Bar [OTC] *see* Pyrithione Zinc *on page 1318*

ZnSO₄ (error-prone abbreviation) *see* Zinc Sulfate *on page 1598*

Zocor® *see* Simvastatin *on page 1394*

Zoderm® *see* Benzoyl Peroxide *on page 194*

Zofran® *see* Ondansetron *on page 1147*

Zofran® ODT *see* Ondansetron *on page 1147*

Zoladex® *see* Goserelin *on page 750*

Zoledronate *see* Zoledronic Acid *on page 1600*

Zoledronic Acid *(ZOE le dron ik AS id)*

U.S. Brand Names Zometa®
Canadian Brand Names Aclasta®; Zometa®
Mexican Brand Names Zometa®
Generic Available No
Synonyms CGP-42446; Zoledronate
Pharmacologic Category Antidote; Bisphosphonate Derivative
Use Treatment of hypercalcemia of malignancy, multiple myeloma, bone metastases of solid tumors
Unlabeled/Investigational Use Investigational: Prevention of bone metastases from breast or prostate cancer; treatment of metabolic bone diseases
Local Anesthetic/Vasoconstrictor Precautions No information available to require special precautions
Effects on Dental Treatment Key adverse event(s) related to dental treatment: Mucositis.

Osteonecrosis of the jaw (ONJ), generally associated with local infection and/or tooth extraction and often with delayed healing, has been reported in patients taking bisphosphonates. Most reported cases of bisphosphonate-associated osteonecrosis have been in cancer patients treated with intravenous bisphosphonates. However, some have occurred in patients with postmenopausal osteoporosis taking oral bisphosphonates. Dental surgery may exacerbate ONJ. For patients requiring dental procedures, there are no data available to suggest whether discontinuation of bisphosphonate treatment reduces the risk of ONJ. See Dental Comment.

Common Adverse Effects
>10%:
Cardiovascular: Leg edema (5% to 21%), hypotension (11%)
Central nervous system: Fatigue (39%), fever (32% to 44%), headache (5% to 19%), dizziness (18%), insomnia (15% to 16%), anxiety (11% to 14%), depression (14%), agitation (13%), confusion (7% to 13%), hypoesthesia (12%)
Dermatologic: Alopecia (12%), dermatitis (11%)
Endocrine & metabolic: Dehydration (14%), hypophosphatemia (12% to 13%), hypokalemia (12%), hypomagnesemia (11%)
Gastrointestinal: Nausea (29% to 46%), constipation (27% to 31%), vomiting (14% to 32%), diarrhea (17% to 24%), anorexia (9% to 22%), abdominal pain (14% to 16%), weight loss (16%), appetite decreased (13%)
Genitourinary: Urinary tract infection (12% to 14%)
Hematologic: Anemia (22% to 33%), neutropenia (12%)

Neuromuscular & skeletal: Bone pain (55%), weakness (24%), myalgia (23%), arthralgia (5% to 21%), back pain (15%), paresthesia (15%), limb pain (14%), skeletal pain (12%), rigors (11%)

Renal: Renal deterioration (8% to 40%)

Respiratory: Dyspnea (22% to 27%), cough (12% to 22%)

Miscellaneous: Cancer progression (16%), moniliasis (12%)

1% to 10%:

Cardiovascular: Chest pain

Central nervous system: Somnolence

Endocrine & metabolic: Hypocalcemia (1%), hypermagnesemia (2%)

Gastrointestinal: Dysphagia (5% to 10%), dyspepsia (10%), mucositis, stomatitis (8%), sore throat (8%)

Hematologic: Thrombocytopenia (10%), pancytopenia, granulocytopenia

Neuromuscular & skeletal: Asthenia

Renal: Serum creatinine increased (2%)

Respiratory: Pleural effusion, upper respiratory tract infection (10%)

Miscellaneous: Metastases, nonspecifc infection

Symptoms of hypercalcemia include polyuria, nephrolithiasis, anorexia, nausea, vomiting, constipation, weakness, fatigue, confusion, stupor, and coma. These may not be drug-related adverse events, but related to the underlying metabolic condition.

Dosage I.V.: Adults:

Hypercalcemia of malignancy (albumin-corrected serum calcium ≥12 mg/dL): 4 mg (maximum) given as a single dose. Wait at least 7 days before considering retreatment. Dosage adjustment may be needed in patients with decreased renal function following treatment.

Multiple myeloma or metastatic bone lesions from solid tumors: 4 mg every 3-4 weeks

Note: Patients should receive a daily calcium supplement and multivitamin containing vitamin D

Paget's disease (Aclasta®, not available in U.S.): 5 mg infused over at least 15 minutes. **Note:** Data concerning retreatment is not available.

Dosage adjustment in renal impairment: Mild-to-moderate renal impairment:

Zometa®:

Cl_{cr} >60 mL/minute: 4 mg

Cl_{cr} 50-60 mL/minute: 3.5 mg

Cl_{cr} 40-49 mL/minute: 3.3 mg

Cl_{cr} 30-39 mL/minute: 3 mg

Cl_{cr} <30 mL/minute: Not recommended

Aclasta® [not available in U.S.]: Cl_{cr} >30 mL/minute: No adjustment recommended.

Dosage adjustment for renal toxicity:

Hypercalcemia of malignancy: Evidence of renal deterioration: Evaluate risk versus benefit.

Bone metastases: Evidence of renal deterioration: Discontinue further dosing until renal function returns to within 10% of baseline: renal deterioration defined as follows:

Normal baseline creatinine: Increase of 0.5 mg/dL

Abnormal baseline creatinine: Increase of 1 mg/dL

Reinitiate dose at the same dose administered prior to treatment interruption.

Dosage adjustment in hepatic impairment: Specific guidelines are not available.

Mechanism of Action A bisphosphonate which inhibits bone resorption via actions on osteoclasts or on osteoclast precursors; inhibits osteoclastic activity and skeletal calcium release induced by tumors. Decreases serum calcium and phosphorus, and increases their elimination.

Contraindications Hypersensitivity to zoledronic acid, other bisphosphonates, or any component of the formulation; pregnancy

Warnings/Precautions Bisphosphonate therapy has been associated with osteonecrosis, primarily of the jaw; this has been observed mostly in cancer patients, but also in patients with postmenopausal osteoporosis and other diagnoses. Dental exams and preventative dentistry should be performed prior to placing patients with risk factors on chronic bisphosphonate therapy. Invasive dental procedures should be avoided during treatment.

Use caution in renal dysfunction; dosage adjustment required. In cancer patients, renal toxicity has been reported with doses >4 mg or infusions administered over 15 minutes. Risk factors for renal deterioration include pre-existing renal insufficiency and repeated doses of zoledronic acid and other bisphosphonates. Dehydration and the use of other nephrotoxic drugs which may contribute to renal deterioration should be identified and managed. Use is not recommended in patients with severe renal impairment (serum creatinine >3 mg/dL) and bone metastases (limited data); use in patients with hypercalcemia (Continued)

Zoledronic Acid (Continued)

of malignancy and severe renal impairment should only be done if the benefits outweigh the risks. Renal function should be assessed prior to treatment; if decreased after treatment, additional treatments should be withheld until renal function returns to within 10% of baseline. Adequate hydration is required during treatment (urine output ~2 L/day); avoid overhydration, especially in patients with heart failure; diuretics should not be used before correcting hypovolemia. Renal deterioration, resulting in renal failure and dialysis has occurred in patients treated with zoledronic acid after single and multiple infusions at recommended doses of 4 mg over 15 minutes. **Note:** When used in the treatment of Paget's disease (Aclasta® — not available in the U.S.), significant renal deterioration has not been observed with the usual 5 mg unit-dose.

Infrequent reports of severe (and occasionally debilitating) bone, joint, and/or muscle pain during bisphosphonate treatment; onset of pain ranged from a single day to several months, with relief in most cases upon discontinuation of the drug. Some patients experienced recurrence when rechallenged with same drug or another bisphosphonate.

Use caution in patients with aspirin-sensitive asthma (may cause bronchoconstriction), hepatic dysfunction, and the elderly. Women of childbearing age should be advised against becoming pregnant. Safety and efficacy in pediatric patients have not been established.

Drug Interactions

Increased Effect/Toxicity: Aminoglycosides may lower serum calcium levels with prolonged administration; concomitant use may have an additive hypocalcemic effect. NSAIDs may enhance the gastrointestinal adverse/toxic effects (increased incidence of GI ulcers) of bisphosphonate derivatives. Bisphosphonate derivatives may enhance the hypocalcemic effect of phosphate supplements.

Decreased Effect: The following agents may decrease the absorption of oral bisphosphonate derivatives: Antacids (aluminum, calcium, magnesium), oral calcium salts, oral iron salts, and oral magnesium salts.

Dietary Considerations Multiple myeloma or metastatic bone lesions from solid tumors: Take daily calcium supplement (500 mg) and daily multivitamin (with 400 int. units vitamin D).

Pharmacodynamics/Kinetics

Onset of action: Maximum effect may not been seen for 7 days

Distribution: Binds to bone

Protein binding: ~22%

Half-life elimination: Triphasic; Terminal: 146 hours

Excretion: Urine (39% ± 16% as unchanged drug) within 24 hours; feces (<3%)

Pregnancy Risk Factor D

Dosage Forms INF, solution [premixed] (Aclasta® [CAN]): 5 mg (100 mL) [not available in U.S.]. **INJ, solution:** 4 mg/5 mL (5 mL)

Dental Comment

"Dear Dental Health Professional" Letter Issued for Intravenous Bisphosphonates, Pamidronate and Zoledronic Acid, Regarding the Risk of Osteonecrosis of the Jaw (ONJ) in Cancer Patients - May 2005

Novartis Pharmaceuticals Corporation has notified dental health professionals of the risk of **osteonecrosis of the jaw (ONJ)** and the use of the bisphosphonates, pamidronate, and zoledronic acid. Often observed in patients receiving chemotherapy and corticosteroids, reports of ONJ (the majority being associated with dental procedures) have been documented in cancer patients. Consequently, the manufacturer recommends that a dental examination precede therapy in cancer patients beginning I.V. bisphosphonate therapy. Additionally, invasive dental procedures should be avoided during therapy; patients developing ONJ while on bisphosphonate therapy should not have invasive dental procedures because the condition may be exacerbated. It has not been determined whether the discontinuation of bisphosphonate therapy in patients requiring dental surgery decreases the risk of ONJ. The treating health-care professional is encouraged to assess the benefits and risks.

Additional information is available at: http://www.fda.gov/medwatch/SAFETY/2005/safety05.htm#zometa2, or by contacting Novartis Oncology Medical Services at 1-888-669-6682.

Previously, Novartis and the Food and Drug Administration (FDA) had notified healthcare providers of a serious adverse event related to the use of bisphosphonates. Osteonecrosis of the jaw has been reported in patients with cancer who were receiving chemotherapy, corticosteroids, and chronic bisphosphonate therapy. Dental exams and preventative dentistry should be performed prior to placing patients with risk factors (chemotherapy, corticosteroids, poor oral hygiene) on chronic bisphosphonate therapy. Invasive dental procedures should be avoided during treatment. Product labeling for pamidronate (Aredia®) and zoledronic acid (Zometa®) have been updated. Recently, 63 cases of osteonecrosis associated with the use of bisphosphonates were published (Ruggiero, 2004). In a retrospective review, 56 of the patients received intravenous bisphosphonates for at least 1 year and 7 patients were on chronic oral therapy. The presenting symptom was a nonhealing extraction socket or an exposed jawbone. These lesions did not show evidence of metastatic disease and required removal of involved bone in most cases.

Bisphosphonates are widely used in the management of metastatic bone disease to treat hypercalcemia associated with malignancies and to treat osteoporosis. In the report by Ruggiero et al, the cluster of patients observed to have necrotic lesions in the jaw shared only one common clinical feature, all received chronic bisphosphonate therapy. The necrosis detected was typical of osteoradionecrosis. It was suggested that because of the trend in the use of chronic bisphosphonate therapy, the observation of an associated risk of osteonecrosis of the jaw should alert practitioners to monitor for this previously unrecognized potential complication.

Selected Readings
Ruggiero SL, Mehrotra B, Rosenberg TJ, et al, "Osteonecrosis of the Jaws Associated With the Use of Bisphosphonates: A Review of 63 Cases," *J Oral Maxillofac Surg*, 2004, 62(5):527-34.

Zolmitriptan (zohl mi TRIP tan)

U.S. Brand Names Zomig®; Zomig-ZMT™
Canadian Brand Names Zomig®; Zomig® Nasal Spray; Zomig® Rapimelt
Mexican Brand Names Zomig®
Generic Available No
Synonyms 311C90
Pharmacologic Category Serotonin 5-HT$_{1D}$ Receptor Agonist
Use Acute treatment of migraine with or without aura
Local Anesthetic/Vasoconstrictor Precautions No information available to require special precautions
Effects on Dental Treatment Key adverse event(s) related to dental treatment: Xerostomia (normal salivary flow resumes upon discontinuation).
Common Adverse Effects Percentages noted from oral preparations.
1% to 10%:
Cardiovascular: Chest pain (2% to 4%), palpitation (up to 2%)
Central nervous system: Dizziness (6% to 10%), somnolence (5% to 8%), pain (2% to 3%), vertigo (≤2%)
Gastrointestinal: Nausea (4% to 9%), xerostomia (3% to 5%), dyspepsia (1% to 3%), dysphagia (≤2%)
Neuromuscular & skeletal: Paresthesia (5% to 9%), weakness (3% to 9%), warm/cold sensation (5% to 7%), hypoesthesia (1% to 2%), myalgia (1% to 2%), myasthenia (up to 2%)
Miscellaneous: Neck/throat/jaw pain (4% to 10%), diaphoresis (up to 3%), allergic reaction (up to 1%)
Mechanism of Action Selective agonist for serotonin (5-HT$_{1B}$ and 5-HT$_{1D}$ receptors) in cranial arteries to cause vasoconstriction and reduce sterile inflammation associated with antidromic neuronal transmission correlating with relief of migraine
Drug Interactions
Cytochrome P450 Effect: Substrate of CYP1A2 (minor)
Increased Effect/Toxicity: Ergot-containing drugs may lead to vasospasm; cimetidine, MAO inhibitors, oral contraceptives, propranolol increase levels of zolmitriptan; concurrent use with SSRIs and sibutramine may lead to serotonin syndrome.
Pharmacodynamics/Kinetics
Onset of action: 0.5-1 hour
Absorption: Well absorbed
Distribution: V$_d$: 7 L/kg
Protein binding: 25%
Metabolism: Converted to an active N-desmethyl metabolite (2-6 times more potent than zolmitriptan)
Half-life elimination: 2.8-3.7 hours
Bioavailability: 40%
Time to peak, serum: Tablet: 1.5 hours; Orally-disintegrating tablet and nasal spray: 3 hours
Excretion: Urine (~60% to 65% total dose); feces (30% to 40%)
Pregnancy Risk Factor C

Zoloft® *see Sertraline on page 1385*

Zolpidem (zole PI dem)

U.S. Brand Names Ambien®; Ambien CR™
Generic Available No
Synonyms Zolpidem Tartrate
Pharmacologic Category Hypnotic, Nonbenzodiazepine
Dental Use Has not been established
Use Short-term treatment of insomnia (sleep onset and/or sleep maintenance)
Local Anesthetic/Vasoconstrictor Precautions No information available to require special precautions
Effects on Dental Treatment Key adverse event(s) related to dental treatment: Xerostomia (normal salivary flow resumes upon discontinuation).
Common Adverse Effects Actual frequency may be dosage form, dose and/or age dependent

>10%: Central nervous system: Dizziness, headache, somnolence

1% to 10%:

Cardiovascular: Blood pressure increased, chest discomfort, palpitation

Central nervous system: Anxiety, apathy, amnesia, ataxia, attention disturbance, body temperature increased, confusion, depersonalization, depression, disinhibition, disorientation, drowsiness, drugged feeling, euphoria, fatigue, fever, hallucinations, hypoesthesia, insomnia, memory disorder, lethargy, lightheadedness, mood swings, stress

Dermatologic: Rash, urticaria, wrinkling

Endocrine & metabolic: Menorrhagia

Gastrointestinal: Abdominal discomfort, abdominal pain, abdominal tenderness, appetite disorder, constipation, diarrhea, dyspepsia, flatulence, gastroenteritis, gastroesophageal reflux, hiccup, nausea, vomiting, xerostomia

Genitourinary: Urinary tract infection

Neuromuscular & skeletal: Arthralgia, back pain, balance disorder, myalgia, neck pain, paresthesia, psychomotor retardation, tremor, weakness

Ocular: Asthenopia, blurred vision, depth perception altered, diplopia, visual disturbance, red eye

Otic: Labyrinthitis, tinnitus, vertigo

Renal: Dysuria

Respiratory: Pharyngitis, sinusitis, upper respiratory tract infection, throat irritation

Miscellaneous: Allergy, binge eating, flu-like symptoms

Restrictions C-IV; not available in Canada

Dosage Oral:

Adults:

Ambien®: 10 mg immediately before bedtime; maximum dose: 10 mg
Ambien CR™: 12.5 mg immediately before bedtime

Elderly:

Ambien®: 5 mg immediately before bedtime
Ambien CR™: 6.25 mg immediately before bedtime

Dosing adjustment in renal impairment: Dose adjustment not required; monitor closely

Hemodialysis: Not dialyzable

Dosing adjustment in hepatic impairment:

Ambien®: 5 mg
Ambien CR™: 6.25 mg

Mechanism of Action Structurally dissimilar to benzodiazepines. Selective hypnotic effects (with minor anxiolytic, myorelaxant and anticovulsant properties) mediated through selective affinity for the alpha-1 subunit of the omega-1 (benzodiazepine) receptor located on the GABA$_A$ receptor complex. Agonism at this site enhances GABA-ergic chloride conductance hyperpolarizing neuronal membranes thereby reducing the responsiveness to excitatory signals.

Contraindications Hypersensitivity to zolpidem or any component of the formulation

Warnings/Precautions Should be used only after evaluation of potential causes of sleep disturbance. Failure of sleep disturbance to resolve after 7-10 days may indicate psychiatric or medical illness. Use with caution in patients with depression. Abnormal thinking and behavioral changes have been associated with sedative-hypnotics. Sedative/hypnotics may produce withdrawal symptoms following abrupt discontinuation. Causes CNS depression, which may impair physical and mental capabilities. Effects with other sedative drugs or ethanol may be potentiated. Use caution in the elderly; dose adjustment recommended. Closely monitor elderly or debilitated patients for impaired cognitive or motor performance. Avoid use in patients with sleep apnea or a history of sedative-hypnotic abuse. Use caution with hepatic impairment; dose adjustment required. Prescriptions should be written for the smallest effective dose (especially in the elderly) and for the smallest quantity consistent with good patient care (especially with depression). Safety and efficacy have not been established in pediatric patients.

Drug Interactions

Cytochrome P450 Effect: Substrate of CYP1A2 (minor), 2C8/9 (minor), 2C19 (minor), 2D6 (minor), 3A4 (major)

Increased Effect/Toxicity: Use of zolpidem in combination with other centrally-acting drugs may produce additive CNS depression. CYP3A4 inhibitors may increase the levels/effects of zolpidem; example inhibitors include azole antifungals, clarithromycin, diclofenac, doxycycline, erythromycin, imatinib, isoniazid, nefazodone, nicardipine, propofol, protease inhibitors, quinidine, telithromycin, troleandomycin, and verapamil.

Decreased Effect: CYP3A4 inducers may decrease the levels/effects of zolpidem; example inducers include aminoglutethimide, carbamazepine, nafcillin, nevirapine, phenobarbital, phenytoin, and rifamycins.

Ethanol/Nutrition/Herb Interactions

Ethanol: Avoid ethanol (may increase CNS depression).

Food: Maximum plasma concentration and bioavailability are decreased with food; time to peak plasma concentration is increased; half-life remains unchanged.

Herb/Nutraceutical: St John's wort may decrease zolpidem levels. Avoid valerian, St John's wort, kava kava, gotu kola (may increase CNS depression).

Dietary Considerations
For faster sleep onset, do not administer with (or immediately after) a meal.

Pharmacodynamics/Kinetics

Onset of action: 30 minutes

Duration: 6-8 hours

Absorption: Rapid

Distribution: Very low amounts enter breast milk

Protein binding: 92%

Metabolism: Hepatic, primarily via CYP3A4 (~60%), to inactive metabolites

Half-life elimination: 2.5-2.8 hours (range 1.4-4.5 hours); Cirrhosis: Up to 9.9 hours

Time to peak, plasma: 2 hours; 4 hours with food

Excretion: As metabolites in urine, bile, feces

Pregnancy Risk Factor C

Dosage Forms TAB: (Ambien®): 5 mg, 10 mg; (Ambien® PAK™) [dose pack]: 5 mg (30s). TAB, extended release (Ambien CR™): 6.25 mg, 12.5 mg

Selected Readings

Garnier R, Guerault E, Muzard D, et al, "Acute Zolpidem Poisoning - Analysis of 344 Cases," *J Toxicol Clin Toxicol*, 1994, 32(4):391-404.

Holm KJ and Goa KL, "Zolpidem: An Update of Its Pharmacology, Therapeutic Efficacy and Tolerability in the Treatment of Insomnia," *Drugs*, 2000, 59(4):865-89.

Lange CL, "Medication-Associated Somnambulism," *J Am Acad Child Adolesc Psychiatry*, 2005, 44(3):211-2.

Langtry HD and Benfield P, "Zolpidem: A Review of Its Pharmacodynamic and Pharmacokinetic Properties and Therapeutic Potential," *Drugs*, 1990, 40(2):291-313.

Lheureux P, Debailleul G, De Witte O, et al, "Zolpidem Intoxication Mimicking Narcotic Overdose: Response to Flumazenil," *Hum Exp Toxicol*, 1990, 9(2):105-7.

Meram D and Descotes J, "Acute Poisoning By Zolpidem," *Rev Med Interne*, 1989, 10(5):466.

Mercurio M, De Roos F, and Hoffman RS, "Zolpidem (Ambien®): Exposure Assessment of a New Nonbenzodiazepine GABA Agonist," *Vet Hum Toxicol*, 1994, 36:371.

Pacifici GM, Viani A, Rizzo G, et al, "Plasma Protein Binding of Zolpidem in Liver and Renal Insufficiency," *Int J Clin Pharmacol Ther Toxicol*, 1988, 26(9):439-43.

Queneau PE, Koch J, Hrusovsky S, et al, "Cytolytic Hepatitis Related to Zolpidem," 1st International Symposium on Hepatology and Clinical Pharmacology Liver and Drugs, Abstract, 1994, 39.

Salva P and Costa J, "Clinical Pharmacokinetics and Pharmacodynamics of Zolpidem. Therapeutic Implications," *Clin Pharmacokinet*, 1995, 29(3):142-53.

Sanger DJ, "The Pharmacology and Mechanisms of Action of New Generation, Non-Benzodiazepine Hypnotic Agents," *CNS Drugs*, 2004, 18 (Suppl 1):9-15.

Simcox DA, "Zolpidem-Associated Falls," *Consult Pharm*, 1995, 10:1378-80.

Zolpidem Tartrate see Zolpidem on page 1604

Zometa® see Zoledronic Acid on page 1600

Zomig® see Zolmitriptan on page 1603

Zomig-ZMT™ see Zolmitriptan on page 1603

Zonalon® see Doxepin on page 505

Zone-A® see Pramoxine and Hydrocortisone on page 1264

Zone-A Forte® see Pramoxine and Hydrocortisone on page 1264

Zonegran® see Zonisamide on page 1606

Zonisamide (zoe NIS a mide)

U.S. Brand Names Zonegran®
Canadian Brand Names Zonegran®
Generic Available Yes
Pharmacologic Category Anticonvulsant, Miscellaneous
Use Adjunct treatment of partial seizures in children >16 years of age and adults with epilepsy

Unlabeled/Investigational Use Bipolar disorder
Local Anesthetic/Vasoconstrictor Precautions No information available to require special precautions
Effects on Dental Treatment Key adverse event(s) related to dental treatment: Xerostomia (normal salivary flow resumes upon discontinuation) and abnormal taste.
Common Adverse Effects Adjunctive Therapy: Frequencies noted in patients receiving other anticonvulsants:

>10%:
  Central nervous system: Somnolence (17%), dizziness (13%)
  Gastrointestinal: Anorexia (13%)
1% to 10%:
  Central nervous system: Headache (10%), agitation/irritability (9%), fatigue (8%), tiredness (7%), ataxia (6%), confusion (6%), decreased concentration (6%), memory impairment (6%), depression (6%), insomnia (6%), speech disorders (5%), mental slowing (4%), anxiety (3%), nervousness (2%), schizophrenic/schizophreniform behavior (2%), difficulty in verbal expression (2%), status epilepticus (1%), tremor (1%), convulsion (1%), hyperesthesia (1%), incoordination (1%)
  Dermatologic: Rash (3%), bruising (2%), pruritus (1%)
  Gastrointestinal: Nausea (9%), abdominal pain (6%), diarrhea (5%), dyspepsia (3%), weight loss (3%), constipation (2%), dry mouth (2%), taste perversion (2%), vomiting (1%)
  Neuromuscular & skeletal: Paresthesia (4%), weakness (1%), abnormal gait (1%)
  Ocular: Diplopia (6%), nystagmus (4%), amblyopia (1%)
  Otic: Tinnitus (1%)
  Respiratory: Rhinitis (2%), pharyngitis (1%), increased cough (1%)
  Miscellaneous: Flu-like syndrome (4%) accidental injury (1%)
Mechanism of Action The exact mechanism of action is not known. May stabilize neuronal membranes and suppress neuronal hypersynchronization through action at sodium and calcium channels. Does not affect GABA activity.

Drug Interactions
  Cytochrome P450 Effect: Substrate of CYP2C19 (minor), 3A4 (major)
  Increased Effect/Toxicity: Sedative effects may be additive with other CNS depressants; monitor for increased effect (includes barbiturates, benzodiazepines, narcotic analgesics, ethanol, and other sedative agents). CYP3A4 inhibitors may increase the levels/effects of zonisamide; example inhibitors include azole antifungals, clarithromycin, diclofenac, doxycycline, erythromycin, imatinib, isoniazid, nefazodone, nicardipine, propofol, protease inhibitors, quinidine, telithromycin, and verapamil.
  Decreased Effect: CYP3A4 inducers may decrease the levels/effects of zonisamide; example inducers include aminoglutethimide, carbamazepine, nafcillin, nevirapine, phenobarbital, phenytoin, and rifamycins.

Pharmacodynamics/Kinetics
Distribution: V_d: 1.45 L/kg
Protein binding: 40%
Metabolism: Hepatic via CYP3A4; forms N-acetyl zonisamide and 2-sulfamoyl-lacetyl phenol (SMAP)
Half-life elimination: 63 hours
Time to peak: 2-6 hours
Excretion: Urine (62%, 35% as unchanged drug, 65% as metabolites); feces (3%)

Pregnancy Risk Factor C

Zopiclone (ZOE pi clone)

Canadian Brand Names Alti-Zopiclone; Apo-Zopiclone®; Gen-Zopiclone; Imovane®; Novo-Zopiclone; Nu-Zopiclone; PMS-Zopiclone; Rhovane®; Rhoxal-zopiclone; Riva-Zopiclone; Sandoz-Zopiclone
Mexican Brand Names Imovane®
Generic Available Yes

Pharmacologic Category Hypnotic, Nonbenzodiazepine

Dental Use Has not been established

Use Symptomatic relief of transient and short-term insomnia

Local Anesthetic/Vasoconstrictor Precautions No information available to require special precautions

Effects on Dental Treatment Key adverse event(s) related to dental treatment: Coated tongue, dry mouth, halitosis, taste alteration (bitter taste, common).

Common Adverse Effects Frequency not defined.

Cardiovascular: Palpitations

Central nervous system: Agitation, anterograde amnesia, anxiety, asthenia, chills, confusion, depression, dizziness, drowsiness, euphoria, headache, hostility, memory impairment, nervousness, nightmares, somnolence, speech abnormalities

Dermatological: Rash, spots on skin

Endocrine & metabolic: Anorexia; libido decreased; alkaline phosphatase, ALT, and AST increased; appetite increased

Gastrointestinal: Constipation, coated tongue, diarrhea, dry mouth, dyspepsia, halitosis, nausea, taste alteration (bitter taste, common), vomiting

Neuromuscular & skeletal: Hypotonia, impaired coordination, limb heaviness, muscle spasms, paresthesia, tremor

Ocular: Amblyopia

Respiratory: Dyspnea

Miscellaneous: Diaphoresis

Restrictions Not available in U.S.

Mechanism of Action Zopiclone is a cyclopyrrolone derivative and has a pharmacological profile similar to benzodiazepines. Zopiclone reduces sleep latency, increases duration of sleep, and decreases the number of nocturnal awakenings.

Drug Interactions

Cytochrome P450 Effect: Substrate (major) of CYP2C8/9, 3A4

Increased Effect/Toxicity: Zopiclone may produce additive CNS depressant effects when coadministered with ethanol, sedatives, antihistamines, anticonvulsants, or psychotropic medications. CYP2C8/9 inhibitors may increase the levels/effects of zopiclone; example inhibitors include delavirdine, fluconazole, gemfibrozil, ketoconazole, nicardipine, NSAIDs, and sulfonamides. CYP3A4 inhibitors may increase the levels/effects of zopiclone; example inhibitors include azole antifungals, clarithromycin, diclofenac, doxycycline, erythromycin, imatinib, isoniazid, nefazodone, nicardipine, propofol, protease inhibitors, quinidine, telithromycin, and verapamil.

Decreased Effect: CYP2C8/9 inducers may decrease the levels/effects of zopiclone; example inducers include carbamazepine, phenobarbital, phenytoin, rifampin, rifapentine, and secobarbital. CYP3A4 inducers may decrease the levels/effects of zopiclone; example inducers include aminoglutethimide, carbamazepine, nafcillin, nevirapine, phenobarbital, phenytoin, and rifamycins.

Pharmacodynamics/Kinetics

Absorption: Elderly: 75% to 94%

Distribution: Rapidly from vascular compartment

Protein binding: ~45%

Metabolism: Extensively hepatic

Half-life elimination: 5 hours; Elderly: 7 hours; Hepatic impairment: 11.9 hours

Time to peak, serum: <2 hours; Hepatic impairment: 3.5 hours

Excretion: Urine (75%); feces (16%)

Pregnancy Risk Factor Not assigned; similar agents rated D

Zorbtive™ see Somatropin on page 1406

Zorcaine™ see Articaine and Epinephrine on page 139

ZORprin® see Aspirin on page 145

Zostrix® [OTC] see Capsaicin on page 256

Zostrix®-HP [OTC] see Capsaicin on page 256

Zosyn® see Piperacillin and Tazobactam Sodium on page 1245

Zovia™ see Ethinyl Estradiol and Ethynodiol Diacetate on page 597

Zovirax® see Acyclovir on page 49

Ztuss™ Tablet see Hydrocodone, Pseudoephedrine, and Guaifenesin on page 792

Zyban® see BuPROPion on page 233

Zydone® see Hydrocodone and Acetaminophen on page 779

Zyflo® see Zileuton on page 1596

Zylet™ see Loteprednol and Tobramycin on page 953

Zyloprim® see Allopurinol on page 70

Zymar™ *see* Gatifloxacin *on page 724*
Zyprexa® *see* Olanzapine *on page 1139*
Zyprexa® Zydis® *see* Olanzapine *on page 1139*
Zyrtec® *see* Cetirizine *on page 306*
Zyrtec-D 12 Hour™ *see* Cetirizine and Pseudoephedrine *on page 307*
Zyvox™ *see* Linezolid *on page 933*

NATURAL PRODUCTS: HERBAL AND DIETARY SUPPLEMENTS

Medical problem: " I have a toothache."
2000 BC response: "Here, eat this root."
1000 AD: "That root is heathen; here, say this prayer."
1850 AD: "That prayer is superstitious; here, drink this potion."
1940 AD: "That potion is snake oil; here, swallow this pill."
1985 AD: "That pill is ineffective; here, take this new antibiotic."
2000 AD: "That antibiotic is artificial; here, eat this root."

Adapted from an anonymous Internet communication.

INTRODUCTION

For centuries, Eastern and Western civilizations have attributed a large number of medical uses to plants and herbs. Over time, modern scientific methodologies have emerged from some of these remedies. Conversely, some of these agents have fallen into less popularity as more medical knowledge has evolved. In spite of this dichotomy, herbal and natural therapies for treatment of common medical ailments have become exceedingly popular. In America, people consistently seek out natural products that may be able to offset some perceived ailment or assist in the prevention of an ailment. One area of particular interest to those individuals using herbal or natural remedies has commonly been weight loss. There are numerous systemic considerations when some of the natural products that have been attributed weight loss powers are utilized. Many of these products are sold under the blanket of dietary supplements and, therefore, have avoided some of the more stringent Food and Drug Administration legislation. However, in 1994, that legislation was modified to include herbs, vitamins, minerals, and amino acids that may be taken as dietary supplements and the federal guidelines were further modified in 1999. This information must be made available to patients taking these types of products.

The real concern lies in the fact that health claims need not be approved by the FDA, but advertisements must include a disclaimer saying that the product has not yet been fully evaluated. Claims of medicinal use/value are often drawn from popular use, not necessarily from scientific studies. Safety is a concern when these agents are taken in combination with other prescription drugs due to the medical risk which might result. Many of these natural products may have real medicinal value but caution on the part of the dental clinician is prudent. It is impossible to cover all of the natural products, therefore, this chapter has been limited to some of the most popular dietary and herbal supplements and natural remedies used by patients you might treat and what we know about the effects of some of these agents on the body's various systems.

EFFECTS ON VARIOUS SYSTEMS

CARDIOVASCULAR SYSTEM

CONGESTIVE HEART FAILURE

(Diuretics, Xanthine derivatives, Licorice, Ginseng, Aconite)

Alisma plantago, bearberry (*Arctostaphylos uva-ursi*), buchu (*Barosma betulina*), couch grass, dandelion, horsetail rush, juniper, licorice, and xanthine derivatives exert varying degrees of diuretic action. Many patients with congestive heart failure (CHF) are already taking a diuretic medication. By taking products containing one or more of these components, patients already on diuretic medications may increase their risk for dehydration.

Ginseng and licorice can potentially worsen congestive heart failure and edema by causing fluid retention. Aconite has varying effects on the heart that itself could lead to heart failure. Patients with CHF should be advised to consult with their healthcare provider before using products containing any of these components.

HYPERTENSION/HYPOTENSION

(Diuretics, Ginkgo biloba, Ginseng, Hawthorn, Ma-huang, Xanthine derivatives)

The stimulant properties of ginseng and ma-huang could worsen pre-existing hypertension. Elevated blood pressure has been reported as a side effect of ginseng. Although ma-huang contains ephedrine, a known vasoconstrictor, ma-huang's effect on blood pressure varies between individuals. Ma-huang can cause hypotension or hypertension. Due to its unpredictable effects, patients with pre-existing hypertension should use caution when using natural products containing ma-huang. Providers should caution patients with labile hypertension against the use of ginseng.

The diuretic effect of xanthine derivatives and other diuretic components could increase the effects of antihypertensive medications, increasing the risk for hypotension. Hawthorn and ginkgo biloba can cause vasodilation increasing the hypotensive effects of antihypertensive medication. Patients susceptible to hypotension or patients taking antihypertensive medication should use caution when taking products containing xanthine derivatives or diuretics. Patients with pre-existing hypertension or hypotension who wish to use products containing these components should be closely monitored by a healthcare professional for changes in blood pressure control.

ARRHYTHMIAS

(Ginseng)

It has been reported that ginseng may increase the risk of arrhythmias, although it is unclear whether this effect is due to the actual ingredient (ginseng) or other possible impurities. Patients at risk for arrhythmias should be cautioned against the use of products containing ginseng without first consulting with their healthcare provider.

CENTRAL NERVOUS SYSTEM

(Aconite, Ginseng, Xanthine derivatives)

Aconite and hawthorn have potentially sedating effects, and aconite also contains various alkaloids and traces of ephedrine. Some documented central nervous system (CNS) effects of aconite include sedation, vertigo, and incoordination. Hawthorn has been reported to exert a depressive effect on the CNS leading to sedation.

Ginseng, ma-huang, and xanthine derivatives can exert a stimulant effect on the central nervous system. Some of the CNS effects of ginseng include nervousness, insomnia, and euphoria. The action of ma-huang is due to the presence of ephedrine and pseudoephedrine. Ma-huang exerts a stimulant action on the CNS similar to decongestant/weight-loss products (Dexatrim®, etc) thus causing nervousness, insomnia, and anxiety. Kola nut, green tea, guarana, and yerba mate contain varying amounts of caffeine, a xanthine derivative. Stimulant properties exerted by these herbs are expected to be comparable to those of caffeine, including insomnia, nervousness, and anxiety.

Products containing aconite and hawthorn should be used with caution in patients with known history of depression, vertigo, or syncope. Ginseng or xanthine derivatives should be avoided in patients with history of insomnia or anxiety. Use of natural products with these components may contribute to a worsening of a patient's pre-existing medical condition. Patients taking CNS-active medications should avoid or use extreme caution when using preparations containing any of the above components. These components may interact directly or indirectly with CNS-active medications causing an increase or decrease in overall effect.

ENDOCRINE SYSTEM

DIABETES MELLITUS

(Chromium, Glucomannan, Ginseng, Hawthorn, Ma-huang, Periploca, Spirulina)

Ma-huang and spirulina both may increase glucose levels. This could cause a decrease in glucose control, thereby, increasing a patient's risk for hyperglycemia. Patients with diabetes or glucose intolerance should avoid using ma-huang and spirulina containing products.

Chromium, ginseng, glucomannan, periploca (*gymneme sylvestre*), and hawthorn should be used with caution in patients being treated for diabetes. These ingredients may reduce glucose levels increasing the risk for hypoglycemia in patients who are already taking a hypoglycemic agent. Patients with diabetes who wish to use products containing these ingredients should be closely monitored for fluctuations in blood glucose levels.

GASTROINTESTINAL SYSTEM

PEPTIC ULCER DISEASE

(Betaine Hydrochloride, White Willow)

Betaine hydrochloride is a source of hydrochloric acid. The acid released from betaine hydrochloride could aggravate an existing ulcer. White willow, like aspirin, contains salicylates.

Aspirin has been known to induce gastric damage by direct irritation on the gastric mucosa and by an indirect systemic effect. As a result, patients with a history of peptic ulcer disease or gastritis are informed to avoid use of aspirin and other salicylate derivatives. These precautions should also apply to white willow. Patients with a history of peptic ulcer disease or gastritis should not use products containing white willow or betaine hydrochloride as either could exacerbate ulcers.

INFLAMMATORY BOWEL DISEASE

(Cascara Sagrada, Senna, Dandelion)

Cascara sagrada and senna are stimulant laxatives. Their laxative effect is exerted by stimulation of peristalsis in the colon and by inhibition of water and electrolyte secretion. The laxative effect produced by these herbs could induce an exacerbation of inflammatory bowel disease. Patients with a history of inflammatory bowel disease should avoid using products containing cascara sagrada or senna, and use caution when taking products containing dandelion which may also have a laxative effect.

OBSTRUCTION/ILEUS

(Glucomannan, Kelp, Psyllium)

Glucomannan, kelp, and psyllium act as bulk laxatives. In the presence of water, bulk laxatives swell or form a viscous solution adding extra bulk in the gastrointestinal tract. The resulting mass is thought to stimulate peristalsis. In the presence of an ileus, these laxatives could cause an obstruction.

If sufficient water is not consumed when taking a bulk laxative, a semisolid mass can form resulting in an obstruction. Any patient who wishes to take a natural product containing kelp, psyllium, or glucomannan should drink sufficient water to decrease the risk of obstruction. This may be of concern in particular disease states such as CHF or other cases where excess fluid intake may influence the existing disease presentation. Patients with a suspected obstruction or ileus should avoid using products containing kelp, psyllium, or glucomannan without consent of their primary healthcare provider.

HEMATOLOGIC SYSTEM

ANTICOAGULATION THERAPY & COAGULATION DISORDERS

(Horsetail Rush, Ginseng, Ginkgo Biloba, Guarana, White Willow)

Horsetail rush, ginseng, ginkgo biloba, guarana, and white willow can potentially affect platelet aggregation and bleeding time. Ginkgo biloba, ginseng, guarana, and white willow inhibit platelet aggregation resulting in an increase in bleeding time. Horsetail rush, on the other hand, may decrease bleeding time. Patients with coagulation disorders or patients on anticoagulation therapy may be sensitive to the effects on coagulation by these components and should, therefore, avoid use of products containing any of these components.

EFFECTS ON VARIOUS SYSTEMS *(Continued)*

OTHER

PHENYLKETONURIA

(Aspartame, Spirulina)

Patients with phenylketonuria should not use products containing aspartame or spirulina. Aspartame, a common artificial sweetener, is metabolized to phenylalanine, while spirulina contains phenylalanine.

GOUT

(Diuretics, White Willow)

Patients with a history of gout should avoid using natural products containing components with diuretic action or white willow. By increasing urine output, ingredients with diuretic action may concentrate uric acid in the blood increasing the risk of gout in these patients. White willow, like aspirin, may inhibit excretion of urate resulting in an increase in uric acid concentration. The increase in urate levels could cause precipitation of uric acid resulting in an exacerbation of gout.

ALPHABETICAL LISTING OF NATURAL PRODUCTS

Aesculus hippocastanum see Horse Chestnut *on page 1626*

ALA see Flaxseed Oil *on page 1622*

Allium savitum see Garlic *on page 1622*

Aloe

Synonyms Aloe Barbadensis; Aloe Capensis; Aloe vera; Cape

Pharmacologic Category Herb; Topical Skin Product

Use Aloe has been used as an analgesic, antibacterial, antifungal, antiviral, anti-inflammatory, emollient/moisturizer, laxative, wound-healing, and hypoglycemic agent. Topical treatment of minor burns, cuts, and skin irritations, including irritant and roentgen dermatitis. Aloe has been used as an oral rinse for gums and soft tissue. Aloe has been used to reduce discomfort following oral and periodontal surgery and in reducing pain from mouth ulcers. Aloe has been shown to reduce bleeding times after dental surgery and to accelerate the healing process after surgeries. When placed over an extraction site immediately after a tooth has been removed, the application of aloe resulted in significant reduction in postoperative pain, swelling, and bleeding. Aloe promotes wound healing and shows tremendous therapeutic value in a wide variety of soft tissue injuries including tissue insults within the oral cavity. Juice may be taken internally for digestive disorders (eg, constipation, peptic ulcers, irritable bowel syndrome) and as a blood purifier; root ingested for colic. Gel used in many cosmetic and pharmaceutical formulations.

Local Anesthetic/Vasoconstrictor Precautions No information available to require special precautions

Effects on Bleeding None reported

Warnings/Precautions Use with caution in diabetics and those taking hypoglycemic agents or insulin; may lower blood sugar. Some juice products may have high sodium content. Some wound healing may be delayed when administered topically. May alter GI absorption of other herbs or drugs. Avoid other herbs with hypoglycemic or laxative properties. Chronic ingestion of juice may lead to electrolyte abnormalities, especially potassium (if not using as laxative, look for juice products that do not contain the chemical anthranoids responsible for laxative properties); should not be used as a laxative for >2 weeks.

Aloe Barbadensis see Aloe *on page 1614*

Aloe Capensis see Aloe *on page 1614*

Aloe vera see Aloe *on page 1614*

Alpha-linolenic Acid see Flaxseed Oil *on page 1622*

Alpha-lipoate see Alpha-Lipoic Acid *on page 1614*

Alpha-Lipoic Acid

Synonyms Alpha-lipoate; Lipoic Acid; Thioctic acid

Pharmacologic Category Nutritional Supplement

Use Antioxidant; treatment of diabetes, diabetic neuropathy, glaucoma; prevention of cataracts and neurologic disorders including stroke

Local Anesthetic/Vasoconstrictor Precautions No information available to require special precautions

Effects on Bleeding None reported

Warnings/Precautions Use with caution in individuals predisposed to hypoglycemia including those receiving antidiabetic agents.

Altamisa see Feverfew *on page 1621*

Amber Touch-and-Feel see St John's Wort *on page 1632*

American Coneflower see Echinacea *on page 1620*

Anas comosus see Bromelain *on page 1616*

Andro see Androstenedione *on page 1614*

Androstenedione

Synonyms Andro

Pharmacologic Category Nutraceutical

Use Androgenic, anabolic; Athletic performance and libido enhancement; believed to facilitate faster recovery from exercise, increase strength, and promote muscle development in response to training (studies inconclusive)

Local Anesthetic/Vasoconstrictor Precautions No information available to require special precautions

Effects on Bleeding None reported

Warnings/Precautions Use with caution in individuals with CHF, prostate conditions, or hormone-sensitive tumors. The FDA requires specific labeling noting that it "contains steroid hormones that may cause breast enlargement, testicular shrinkage, and infertility in males, and increased facial/body hair, voice-deepening, and clitoral enlargement in females." Avoid herbs with hypertensive properties. Increased cancer risk, decrease in HDL cholesterol.

Angelica sinensis see Dong Quai *on page 1620*

Arctostaphylos uva-ursi see Uva Ursi *on page 1633*

Asian Ginseng *see* Ginseng, Panax *on page 1623*

Astragalus

Synonyms *Astragalus membranaceus*; Milk Vetch

Pharmacologic Category Herb

Use Adaptogen, antibacterial, diuretic, immunostimulant/immunosupportive, radioprotective, vasodilator; treatment of cancer (adjunct to chemotherapy/radiation), hepatitis, peripheral vascular diseases, respiratory infections; disease resistance, stamina, tissue oxygenation; promotes adrenal cortical function

Unlabeled/Investigational: Treatment of HIV/AIDS; antiaging

Local Anesthetic/Vasoconstrictor Precautions No information available to require special precautions

Effects on Bleeding None reported

Warnings/Precautions Use with caution in individuals with acute infection, especially when fever is present.

Astragalus membranaceus see Astragalus *on page 1615*

Awa *see* Kava *on page 1627*

Bachelor's Button *see* Feverfew *on page 1621*

Bearberry *see* Uva Ursi *on page 1633*

Bifidobacterium bifidum / Lactobacillus acidophilus

Related Information
Lactobacillus on page 535

Pharmacologic Category Antidiarrheal; Gastrointestinal Agent, Miscellaneous

Use Antidiarrheal, digestive aid; treatment of GI complaints.
B. bifidum: Maintenance of anaerobic microflora in the colon; treatment of Crohn's disease, diarrhea, ulcerative colitis
L. acidophilus: Recolonization of the GI tract with beneficial bacteria during and after antibiotic use; treatment of constipation, infant diarrhea, lactose intolerance

Local Anesthetic/Vasoconstrictor Precautions No information available to require special precautions

Effects on Bleeding None reported

Warnings/Precautions There are no warnings or reports of toxicity.

Bilberry

Synonyms *Vaccinium myrtillus*

Pharmacologic Category Herb

Use Anticoagulant, antioxidant; treatment of ophthalmic disorders (cataracts, diabetic retinopathy, day/night blindness, diminished visual acuity, macular degeneration, myopia) and vascular disorders (phlebitis, varicose veins); helps maintain capillary integrity and reduce hyperpermeability

Local Anesthetic/Vasoconstrictor Precautions No information available to require special precautions

Effects on Bleeding May see increased bleeding due to inhibition of platelet aggregation

Warnings/Precautions Use with caution in diabetics (may lower blood sugar), individuals with a history of bleeding, hemostatic or drug-related hemostatic disorders, those taking anticoagulants (eg, aspirin or aspirin-containing products, NSAIDs, and warfarin) or antiplatelet agents (eg, ticlopidine, clopidogrel, and dipyridamole), hypoglycemic agents or insulin. Avoid other herbs with anticoagulant/antiplatelet and/or hypoglycemic properties. May alter absorption of calcium, copper, magnesium, and zinc due to tannins. Discontinue at least 14 days prior to dental or surgical procedures.

Black Cohosh

Synonyms *Cimicifuga racemosa*

Pharmacologic Category Herb

Use Analgesic, anti-inflammatory, phytoestrogenic; treatment of rheumatoid arthritis, mild depression, vasomotor symptoms of menopause and premenstrual syndrome (PMS)

Local Anesthetic/Vasoconstrictor Precautions No information available to require special precautions

Effects on Bleeding None reported

Warnings/Precautions Use with caution in individuals taking hormonal contraceptives or receiving hormone replacement therapy (HRT), those with endometrial cancer, history of estrogen-dependent tumors, hypotension, thromboembolic disease, stroke, or salicylate allergy (unknown whether amount of salicylic acid may affect platelet aggregation or have other effects associated with salicylates). Monitor serum hormone levels after 6 months of therapy. Avoid other hypotensive or phytoestrogenic herbs.

Black Susans *see* Echinacea *on page 1620*

BN-52063 *see* Ginkgo Biloba *on page 1622*

Bromelain

Synonyms *Anas comosus*

Pharmacologic Category Herb

Use Anticoagulant, anti-inflammatory, digestive aid; treatment of arthritis, dyspepsia, sinusitis

Local Anesthetic/Vasoconstrictor Precautions No information available to require special precautions

Effects on Bleeding May cause increased bleeding due to inhibition of platelet aggregation

Warnings/Precautions Use with caution in individuals with cardiovascular disease (eg, CHF, hypertension), GI ulceration, history of bleeding, hemostatic or drug-related hemostatic disorders, those taking anticoagulants (eg, aspirin or aspirin-containing products, NSAIDs, warfarin), or antiplatelet agents (eg, ticlopidine, clopidogrel, dipyridamole). Avoid other herbs with anticoagulant/antiplatelet properties. Discontinue at least 14 days prior to dental or surgical procedures.

Calendula

Synonyms *Calendula officinalis*

Pharmacologic Category Herb

Use Analgesic, anti-inflammatory, antimicrobial (antibacterial, antifungal, antiviral), antiprotozoal, antiseptic, antispasmodic, immunostimulant, wound-healing agent; treatment of minor burns, cuts, and other skin irritation

Local Anesthetic/Vasoconstrictor Precautions No information available to require special precautions

Effects on Bleeding None reported

Warnings/Precautions Use with caution in individuals with plant allergies.

Calendula officinalis *see* Calendula *on page 1616*

Camellia sinensis *see* Green Tea *on page 1625*

Cape *see* Aloe *on page 1614*

Capsicum annuum *see* Cayenne *on page 1617*

Capsicum frutescens *see* Cayenne *on page 1617*

Carnitine

Synonyms L-Carnitine

Pharmacologic Category Amino Acid

Use Treatment of CHF, hyperlipidemia, male infertility; athletic performance enhancement, weight loss

Local Anesthetic/Vasoconstrictor Precautions No information available to require special precautions

Effects on Bleeding None reported

Warnings/Precautions L-carnitine appears to be safe; there are no reports of toxicity due to overdosing. Avoid D- or D,L-carnitine since this form can interfere with the body's own production of L-carnitine and can produce a relative carnitine deficiency. Carnitine should not be used by people with cardiovascular diseases.

Cascara

Synonyms Cascara Sagrada
Pharmacologic Category Laxative
Use Temporary relief of constipation; sometimes used with milk of magnesia ("black and white" mixture)
Local Anesthetic/Vasoconstrictor Precautions No information available to require special precautions
Effects on Bleeding None reported
Warnings/Precautions Excessive use can lead to electrolyte imbalance, fluid imbalance, vitamin deficiency, steatorrhea, osteomalacia, cathartic colon, and dependence; should be avoided during nursing because it may have a laxative effect on the infant

Cascara Sagrada *see* Cascara *on page 1617*

Cat's Claw

Synonyms *Uncaria tomentosa*
Pharmacologic Category Herb
Use Anticoagulant, anti-inflammatory, antimicrobial (antibacterial, antifungal, antiviral), antiplatelet, antioxidant, immunosupportive; treatment of allergies and minor infections or inflammatory conditions
Local Anesthetic/Vasoconstrictor Precautions No information available to require special precautions
Effects on Bleeding May cause increased bleeding due to inhibition of platelet aggregation
Warnings/Precautions Use with caution in individuals taking anticoagulants (eg, aspirin or aspirin-containing products, NSAIDs, warfarin) or antiplatelet agents (eg, clopidogrel, dipyridamole, ticlopidine), therapeutic immunosuppression or I.V. immunoglobulin therapy (eg, transplant recipients), those with a history of bleeding, and hemostatic or drug-related hemostatic disorders. Avoid other herbs with anticoagulant/antiplatelet properties. Discontinue at least 14 days prior to dental or surgical procedures.

Cayenne

Related Information
  Capsaicin *on page 256*
Synonyms *Capsicum annuum*; *Capsicum frutescens*
Pharmacologic Category Herb
Use Analgesic, anti-inflammatory, digestive stimulant, sympathomimetic; treatment of arthritis (osteo and rheumatoid), diabetic neuropathy, postmastectomy pain syndrome, postherpetic neuralgia, pruritus, psoriasis; appetite suppressant, bronchial relaxation, cardiovascular circulatory support, decongestant
Local Anesthetic/Vasoconstrictor Precautions No information available to require special precautions
Effects on Bleeding None reported
Warnings/Precautions Use with caution in individuals with GI ulceration, hypertension, and those taking MAO inhibitors. May alter GI absorption of other herbs or drugs; avoid other herbs with hypertensive or sympathomimetic properties.

Centella asiatica *see* Gotu Kola *on page 1624*

Chamomile

Synonyms *Matricaria chamomilla*; *Matricaria recutita*
Pharmacologic Category Herb
Use Antibacterial, anti-inflammatory, antispasmodic, antiulcer agent, anxiolytic, appetite stimulant, carminative, digestive aid, sedative (mild); treatment of eczema and psoriasis, hemorrhoids, inflammatory skin conditions, indigestion and irritable bowel syndrome (IBS), insomnia, leg ulcers, mastitis, premenstrual syndrome (PMS)
Local Anesthetic/Vasoconstrictor Precautions No information available to require special precautions
(Continued)

Chamomile *(Continued)*

Effects on Bleeding None reported

Warnings/Precautions Use with caution in individuals with allergies and asthma (cross sensitivity may occur in those with allergies to asters, chrysanthemums, daisies, feverfew, sunflowers, or ragweed), and those taking anticoagulants, antiplatelets, and sedatives. Avoid other herbs with allergenic, anticoagulant, or antiplatelet properties.

Chasteberry

Synonyms Chastetree; *Vitex agnus-castus*

Pharmacologic Category Herb

Use Treatment of acne vulgaris, amenorrhea, corpus luteum insufficiency, endometriosis, hyperprolactinemia, lactation insufficiency, menopausal symptoms, premenstrual syndrome [PMS]

Local Anesthetic/Vasoconstrictor Precautions No information available to require special precautions

Effects on Bleeding None reported

Warnings/Precautions Use with caution in individuals taking hormonal contraceptives or receiving hormone replacement therapy (HRT). Avoid other phytoprogestogenic herbs.

Chastetree *see* Chasteberry *on page 1618*

Chinese angelica *see* Dong Quai *on page 1620*

Chondroitin Sulfate

Pharmacologic Category Nutraceutical

Use Treatment of osteoarthritis

Local Anesthetic/Vasoconstrictor Precautions No information available to require special precautions

Effects on Bleeding None reported

Warnings/Precautions No known toxicity or serious side effects

Chromium

Related Information

Trace Metals *on page 1513*

Pharmacologic Category Nutraceutical

Use Treatment of hyper- and hypoglycemia, hyperlipidemia, hypercholesterolemia, obesity

Local Anesthetic/Vasoconstrictor Precautions No information available to require special precautions

Effects on Bleeding None reported

Warnings/Precautions There are no warnings or reports of toxicity when taken according to manufacturer's labeled instructions.

Cimicifuga racemosa see Black Cohosh *on page 1616*

Citrus paradisi see Grapefruit Seed *on page 1625*

Coenzyme 1 *see* Nicotinamide Adenine Dinucleotide *on page 1629*

Coenzyme Q₁₀

Synonyms CoQ₁₀; Ubiquinone

Pharmacologic Category Nutraceutical

Use Antioxidant; treatment of angina, breast cancer, cardiovascular diseases (eg, CHF), chronic fatigue syndrome, diabetes, hypertension, muscular dystrophy, obesity, periodontal disease

Local Anesthetic/Vasoconstrictor Precautions No information available to require special precautions

Effects on Bleeding None reported

Warnings/Precautions Avoid other agents with hypoglycemic properties.

Comb Flower *see* Echinacea *on page 1620*

Comphor of the Poor *see* Garlic *on page 1622*

CoQ₁₀ *see* Coenzyme Q₁₀ *on page 1618*

Cranberry

Synonyms *Vaccinium macrocarpon*
Pharmacologic Category Herb
Use Treatment of urinary tract infection and prevention of nephrolithiasis
Local Anesthetic/Vasoconstrictor Precautions No information available to require special precautions
Effects on Bleeding None reported
Warnings/Precautions There are no warnings or reports of toxicity.

Crataegus laevigata see Hawthorn *on page 1626*
Crataegus monogyna see Hawthorn *on page 1626*
Crataegus oxyacantha see Hawthorn *on page 1626*
Crataegus pinnatifida see Hawthorn *on page 1626*

Creatine

Pharmacologic Category Nutraceutical
Use Athletic performance enhancement, energy production, and protein synthesis for muscle building
Local Anesthetic/Vasoconstrictor Precautions No information available to require special precautions
Effects on Bleeding None reported
Warnings/Precautions There are no warnings or reports of toxicity when taken according to manufacturer's labeled instructions.

Curcuma longa see Turmeric *on page 1632*

Dehydroepiandrosterone

Synonyms DHEA
Pharmacologic Category Nutraceutical
Use Antiaging; treatment of depression, diabetes, fatigue, lupus
Local Anesthetic/Vasoconstrictor Precautions No information available to require special precautions
Effects on Bleeding None reported
Warnings/Precautions Use with caution in individuals with diabetes, hepatic dysfunction, or those predisposed to hypoglycemia (monitor blood glucose and dosage of antidiabetic agents). Avoid other agents with hypoglycemic properties.

Devil's Claw

Synonyms *Harpagophytum procumbens*
Pharmacologic Category Herb
Use Anti-inflammatory, cardiotonic; treatment of back pain, gout, osteoarthritis, and other inflammatory conditions
Local Anesthetic/Vasoconstrictor Precautions No information available to require special precautions
Effects on Bleeding May see increased bleeding due to inhibition of platelet aggregation
Warnings/Precautions Use with caution in individuals with history of bleeding, hemostatic or drug-related hemostatic disorders, and those taking anticoagulants (eg, aspirin or aspirin-containing products, NSAIDs, warfarin) or antiplatelet agents (eg, clopidogrel, dipyridamole, ticlopidine), antiarrhythmic agents, or cardiac glycosides (eg, digoxin). Avoid herbs with anticoagulant/antiplatelet properties. Discontinue at least 14 days prior to dental or surgical procedures.

DHA *see* Docosahexaenoic Acid *on page 1620*
DHEA *see* Dehydroepiandrosterone *on page 1619*
Dimethyl Sulfone *see* Methyl Sulfonyl Methane *on page 1629*
Dioscorea villosa see Wild Yam *on page 1634*
DMSO$_2$ *see* Methyl Sulfonyl Methane *on page 1629*

Docosahexaenoic Acid

Synonyms DHA

Pharmacologic Category Nutraceutical

Use Treatment of Alzheimer's disease, attention deficit disorder (ADD) and attention deficit hyperactivity disorder (ADHD), Crohn's disease, diabetes, eczema and psoriasis, hypertension, hypertriglyceridemia, and rheumatoid arthritis; coronary heart disease risk reduction

Local Anesthetic/Vasoconstrictor Precautions No information available to require special precautions

Effects on Bleeding None reported

Warnings/Precautions Use caution with individuals taking anticoagulants (eg, aspirin or aspirin-containing products, NSAIDs, warfarin) or antiplatelet agents (eg, clopidogrel, dipyridamole, ticlopidine), insulin or oral hypoglycemics. Avoid herbs with anticoagulant/antiplatelet properties; may intensify the blood-thinning effect

Dong Quai

Synonyms *Angelica sinensis*; Chinese angelica

Pharmacologic Category Herb

Use Anabolic, anticoagulant; treatment of amenorrhea, anemia, dysmenorrhea, hypertension, menopausal symptoms, premenstrual syndrome (PMS); female vitality

Local Anesthetic/Vasoconstrictor Precautions No information available to require special precautions

Effects on Bleeding Has potential for decreasing platelet aggregation and may increase bleeding

Warnings/Precautions May alter hemostasis, potentiate effects of warfarin, and/or cause photosensitization; use with caution in lactation, pregnancy, cardiovascular or cerebrovascular disease, endometrial cancer, estrogen-dependent tumors, hemostatic or drug-related hemostatic disorders, history of bleeding, hypotension, stroke, thromboembolic disease, and individuals taking anticoagulants (eg, aspirin or aspirin-containing products, NSAIDs, warfarin), antiplatelet agents (eg, clopidogrel, dipyridamole, ticlopidine), antihypertensive medications, hormonal contraceptives or hormone replacement therapy (HRT), or steroids. Avoid other herbs with anabolic, anticoagulant, or antiplatelet properties. Discontinue at least 14 days prior to dental or surgical procedures.

Echinacea

Synonyms American Coneflower; Black Susans; Comb Flower; *Echinacea angustifolia*; *Echinacea purpurea*; Indian Head; Purple Coneflower; Scury Root; Snakeroot

Pharmacologic Category Herb

Use Antibacterial, antihyaluronidase, anti-infective, anti-inflammatory, antiviral, immunostimulant, wound-healing agent; treatment of arthritis, chronic skin complaints, cold, flu, sore throat, tonsillitis, minor upper respiratory tract infections, urinary tract infections

Local Anesthetic/Vasoconstrictor Precautions No information available to require special precautions

Effects on Bleeding None reported

Warnings/Precautions Use as a preventative treatment should be discouraged; may alter immunosuppression; long-term use may cause immunosuppression. Individuals allergic to asters, chamomile, chrysanthemums, daisies, feverfew, sunflowers, or ragweed may display cross-allergy potential (rare but severe); avoid other allergenic herbs. Use with caution in individuals with renal impairment.

Echinacea angustifolia see Echinacea on page 1620

Echinacea purpurea see Echinacea on page 1620

EGb see Ginkgo Biloba on page 1622

Eleutherococcus senticosus see Ginseng, Siberian on page 1623

English Hawthorn see Hawthorn on page 1626

Ethyl Esters of Omega-3 Fatty Acids see Omega-3-Acid Ethyl Esters on page 1621

Evening Primrose

Synonyms Evening Primrose Oil; *Oenothera biennis*

Pharmacologic Category Herb

Use Anticoagulant, anti-inflammatory, hormone stimulant; treatment of atopic eczema and psoriasis, attention deficit disorder (ADD) and attention deficit hyperactivity disorder (ADHD), dermatitis, diabetic neuropathy, endometriosis, hyperglycemia, irritable bowel syndrome (IBS), multiple sclerosis (MS), omega-6 fatty acid supplementation, premenstrual syndrome (PMS), menopausal symptoms, rheumatoid arthritis

Local Anesthetic/Vasoconstrictor Precautions No information available to require special precautions

Effects on Bleeding May see increased bleeding due to inhibition of platelet aggregation

Warnings/Precautions Use with caution in individuals with a history of bleeding, hemostatic or drug-related hemostatic disorders, those taking anticoagulants (eg, aspirin or aspirin-containing products, NSAIDs, warfarin) or antiplatelet agents (eg, clopidogrel, dipyridamole, ticlopidine). Avoid other herbs with anticoagulant/antiplatelet properties. Discontinue at least 14 days prior to dental or surgical procedures.

Evening Primrose Oil *see* Evening Primrose *on page 1621*

Eye Balm *see* Golden Seal *on page 1624*

Eye Root *see* Golden Seal *on page 1624*

Featherfew *see* Feverfew *on page 1621*

Featherfoil *see* Feverfew *on page 1621*

Feverfew

Synonyms Altamisa; Bachelor's Button; Featherfew; Featherfoil; Nosebleed; *Tanacetum parthenium*; Wild Quinine

Pharmacologic Category Herb

Use Anticoagulant/anti-inflammatory, antiprostaglandin, antispasmodic, digestive aid, emmenagogue, sedative; prophylaxis and treatment of migraine headaches and rheumatoid arthritis; treatment of fever, hypertension, premenstrual syndrome (PMS), tinnitus

Local Anesthetic/Vasoconstrictor Precautions No information available to require special precautions

Effects on Bleeding May see increased bleeding due to inhibition of platelet aggregation

Warnings/Precautions Use with caution in individuals with a history of bleeding, hemostatic disorders or drug-related hemostatic problems, and those taking anticoagulants (eg, aspirin or aspirin-containing products, NSAIDs, warfarin), antiplatelet agents (eg, clopidogrel, dipyridamole, ticlopidine), or medications with serotonergic properties. Abrupt discontinuation may increase migraine frequency. May alter absorption of calcium, copper, magnesium, and zinc due to tannins. Avoid other herbs with allergenic, anticoagulant, or antiplatelet properties. Discontinue at least 14 days prior to dental or surgical procedures.

Fish Oil *see* Omega-3-Acid Ethyl Esters *on page 1621*

Omega-3-Acid Ethyl Esters

Synonyms Ethyl Esters of Omega-3 Fatty Acids; Fish Oil

Pharmacologic Category Nutraceutical

Use Antiatherogenic, anticoagulant/antiplatelet, anti-inflammatory; prevention and treatment of cardiovascular diseases; treatment of arteriosclerosis, arthritis, Crohn's disease, diabetes, dyslipidemia, dysmenorrhea, eczema and psoriasis, glaucoma, hypercholesterolemia, hypertension, hypertriglyceridemia; memory enhancement

Local Anesthetic/Vasoconstrictor Precautions No information available to require special precautions

Effects on Bleeding None reported

Warnings/Precautions Use caution with individuals taking anticoagulants (eg, aspirin or aspirin-containing products, NSAIDs, warfarin) or antiplatelet agents (eg, clopidogrel, dipyridamole, ticlopidine), insulin or oral hypoglycemics. Avoid herbs with anticoagulant/antiplatelet properties; may intensify the blood-thinning effect.

Flaxseed Oil

Synonyms ALA; Alpha-linolenic Acid

Pharmacologic Category Nutraceutical

Use Antioxidant, antiatherogenic; treatment of eczema and psoriasis, hypertension, hypercholesterolemia, hypertriglyceridemia; contains 3 times more omega-3 than omega-6 and may be used to help reverse the imbalance between omega-3 and omega-6 (estimated optimal ratio between omega-3 and omega-6 fatty acids is about 1:4 and ratio for many in U.S. is 1:20 to 1:30)

Local Anesthetic/Vasoconstrictor Precautions No information available to require special precautions

Effects on Bleeding None reported

Warnings/Precautions Use with caution in individuals with plant allergies, those taking anticoagulants (eg, aspirin or aspirin-containing products, NSAIDs, warfarin) or antiplatelet agents (eg, clopidogrel, dipyridamole, ticlopidine), insulin or oral hypoglycemics. Avoid herbs with allergenic, anticoagulant, or antiplatelet properties; may intensify the blood-thinning effect.

Garlic

Synonyms *Allium savitum*; Comphor of the Poor; Nectar of the Gods; Poor Mans Treacle; Rustic Treacle; Stinking Rose

Pharmacologic Category Herb

Use Antibiotic, anticoagulant/antiplatelet (potent), anti-inflammatory, antioxidant (aged extract improves benefits), antitumor agent, immunosupportive; treatment of hypercholesterolemia, hypertension, hypertriglyceridemia, hypoglycemia; may decrease thrombosis

Local Anesthetic/Vasoconstrictor Precautions No information available to require special precautions

Effects on Bleeding May see increased bleeding due to potent platelet inhibition

Warnings/Precautions Use with caution in diabetics (may lower blood sugar), individuals taking anticoagulants (eg, aspirin or aspirin-containing products, NSAIDs, warfarin), antihypertensives, antiplatelet agents (eg, clopidogrel, dipyridamole, ticlopidine), hypoglycemic agents or insulin, hypolipidemic agents, and those with a history of bleeding, hemostatic or drug-related hemostatic disorders; may cause GI distress in sensitive individuals. Avoid other herbs with allergenic, anticoagulant/antiplatelet, hypoglycemic, or hypolipidemic properties. Discontinue at least 14 days prior to dental or surgical procedures.

GBE *see* Ginkgo Biloba *on page 1622*

Ginger

Synonyms *Zingiber officinale*

Pharmacologic Category Herb

Use Analgesic, anticoagulant, antiemetic (lack of sedative effects is advantageous over other antiemetics), anti-inflammatory (musculoskeletal), digestive aid; treatment of amenorrhea (Chinese remedy), arthritis, colds, culinary herb, dyspepsia, flu, headaches, motion sickness, nausea/vomiting (eg, from chemotherapy/radiation)

Local Anesthetic/Vasoconstrictor Precautions No information available to require special precautions

Effects on Bleeding Very high doses may inhibit platelet aggregation

Warnings/Precautions Use with caution in diabetics, individuals with a history of bleeding, hemostatic or drug-related hemostatic disorders, those taking anticoagulants (eg, aspirin or aspirin-containing products, NSAIDs, warfarin), antiplatelet agents (eg, clopidogrel, dipyridamole, ticlopidine), cardiac glycosides (eg, digoxin), hypolipidemic agents, hypoglycemic agents, or insulin. Has cardioactive constituents; avoid large and/or prolonged doses. Avoid other herbs with anticoagulant/antiplatelet, hypertensive, hyperlipidemic, or hypoglycemic properties. Discontinue at least 14 days prior to dental or surgical procedures.

Ginkgo Biloba

Synonyms BN-52063; EGb; GBE; ginkgold; Ginkgopowder; Ginkogink; Kaveri; Kew Tree; Maidenhair Tree; Oriental Plum Tree; Rökan; Silver Apricot; Superginkgo; Tanakan; Tanakene; Tebonin; Tramisal; Valverde; Vasan; Vital

Pharmacologic Category Herb

Use Anticoagulant/antiplatelet, antioxidant

Per Commission E: Treatment of primary degenerative dementia, vascular dementia, and demential syndromes (eg, memory deficit), depressive emotional conditions, headache, and tinnitus

Treatment of Alzheimer's disease, arterial insufficiency and intermittent claudication (European remedy), cerebral vascular disease (dementia), macular degeneration, resistant depression, traumatic brain injury, tinnitus, visual disorders, vertigo of vascular origin

Local Anesthetic/Vasoconstrictor Precautions No information available to require special precautions

Effects on Bleeding May see increased bleeding due to inhibition of platelet aggregation; antagonizes platelet activating factor (PAF)

Warnings/Precautions Use with caution in individuals with a history of bleeding, hemostatic drug-related hemostatic disorders, those taking anticoagulants (eg, aspirin or aspirin-containing products, NSAIDs, warfarin) or antiplatelet agents (eg, clopidogrel, dipyridamole, ticlopidine), and MAO inhibitors. Cross reactivity for contact dermatitis (due to fruit pulp) exists with poison ivy and poison oak; may last for 10 days (washing skin within 10 minutes may prevent reaction or topical corticosteroids may be helpful). Fruit pulp contains ginkolic acids which are allergens (seeds are not sensitizing). Admit individuals with neurologic abnormalities after ingestion or ingestions >2 pieces of fruit; pyridoxine may be useful after ingestion of ginkgo seeds or kernels. Avoid other herbs with anticoagulant/antiplatelet properties. Discontinue at least 2-3 weeks prior to surgery; use with caution following recent surgery or trauma.

ginkgold *see* Ginkgo Biloba *on page 1622*
Ginkgopowder *see* Ginkgo Biloba *on page 1622*
Ginkogink *see* Ginkgo Biloba *on page 1622*

Ginseng, Panax

Synonyms Asian Ginseng; *Panax ginseng*
Pharmacologic Category Herb
Use Adaptogen, adrenal tonic, anticoagulant, cardiotonic, hormone stimulant, immunostimulant; support in chemotherapy and radiation (decreases weight loss), postsurgical recovery (stabilize white blood cell counts), endurance

Local Anesthetic/Vasoconstrictor Precautions Has potential to interact with epinephrine and levonordefrin to result in increased BP; use vasoconstrictor with caution

Effects on Bleeding May have antiplatelet effects

Warnings/Precautions Use with caution in elderly or individuals with cardiovascular disease (eg, hypertension), history of bleeding, hemostatic or drug-related hemostatic disorders, and those receiving anticoagulants (eg, aspirin or aspirin-containing products, NSAIDs, warfarin) or antiplatelet agents (eg, clopidogrel, dipyridamole, ticlopidine), hormonal contraceptives, MAO inhibitors, stimulants (eg, OTC decongestants, caffeine), and those receiving hormonal replacement therapy (HRT). May cause "Ginseng Abuse Syndrome"; monitor for signs/symptoms. Avoid other herbs with allergenic, anticoagulant/antiplatelet or hypertensive properties. Discontinue at least 14 days prior to dental or surgical procedures.

Ginseng, Siberian

Synonyms *Eleutherococcus senticosus*; Siberian Ginseng
Pharmacologic Category Herb
Use Adaptogen, anticoagulant, antiviral, immunosupportive; treatment of arteriosclerosis, chronic inflammatory disease, diabetes, hypertension; adaptation to stress, athletic performance enhancement, energy production

Local Anesthetic/Vasoconstrictor Precautions Has potential to interact with epinephrine and levonordefrin to result in increased BP; use vasoconstrictor with caution

Effects on Bleeding May have antiplatelet effects

Warnings/Precautions Use with caution in the elderly or individuals with cardiovascular disease (eg, CHF, hypertension), history of bleeding, hemostatic or drug-related hemostatic disorders, those taking anticoagulants (eg, aspirin or aspirin-containing products, NSAIDs, warfarin) or antiplatelet agents (eg, clopidogrel, dipyridamole, ticlopidine), antihypertensive agents, digoxin, hexobarbital, hypoglycemic agents or insulin, and steroids. Extensive or prolonged use may heighten estrogenic activity. Avoid other herbs with allergenic, anabolic, anticoagulant/antiplatelet, or hypertensive properties. Discontinue at least 14 days prior to dental or surgical procedures.

Glucosamine

Synonyms Glucosamine Hydrochloride; Glucosamine Sulfate
Pharmacologic Category Nutraceutical
Use Treatment of bursitis, gout, osteoarthritis, rheumatoid arthritis, tendonitis
Local Anesthetic/Vasoconstrictor Precautions No information available to require special precautions
Effects on Bleeding None reported
Warnings/Precautions Use with caution in diabetics (may cause insulin resistance) and those taking oral anticoagulants (may increase effect). Avoid other herbs with hyperglycemic properties.

Glucosamine Hydrochloride *see* Glucosamine *on page 1624*
Glucosamine Sulfate *see* Glucosamine *on page 1624*

Glutathione

Synonyms L-Glutathione
Pharmacologic Category Nutraceutical
Use Peptic ulcer diseases; support of immune function; hepatoprotection
Local Anesthetic/Vasoconstrictor Precautions No information available to require special precautions
Effects on Bleeding None reported
Warnings/Precautions There are no warnings or reports of toxicity.

Glycocome *see* Licorice *on page 1627*
Glycyrrhiza glabra *see* Licorice *on page 1627*
Goatweed *see* St John's Wort *on page 1632*

Golden Seal

Synonyms Eye Balm; Eye Root; *Hydrastis canadensis*; Indian Eye; Jaundice Root; Orange Root; Turmeric Root; Yellow Indian Paint; Yellow Root
Pharmacologic Category Herb
Use Antibacterial, antifungal, anti-inflammatory, coagulant; treatment of bronchitis, cystitis, gastritis, infectious diarrhea, inflammation of mucosal membranes, hemorrhoids, postpartum hemorrhage
Local Anesthetic/Vasoconstrictor Precautions No information available to require special precautions
Effects on Bleeding None reported
Warnings/Precautions Efficacy not established in clinical studies. High doses (2-3 g) may cause hypotension or GI distress; toxic doses (18 g) reported to induce CNS depression. Overdose associated with myocardial damage and respiratory failure; extended use of high doses associated with delirium, GI disorders, hallucinations, and neuroexcitation. May alter liver enzymes. Use with caution in individuals with history of bleeding, hemostatic or drug-related hemostatic disorders, hypotension, those taking anticoagulants (aspirin or aspirin-containing products, NSAIDs, and warfarin) or antiplatelet agents (ticlopidine, clopidogrel, and dipyridamole). Avoid other herbs with coagulant or hypotensive properties.

Gotu Kola

Synonyms *Centella asiatica*
Pharmacologic Category Herb
Use Diuretic (mild), sedative (high doses), thermogenic, thyroid-stimulant, wound-healing agent; treatment of hemorrhoids, hypertension, poor circulation, psoriasis, tumors, varicose veins, venous insufficiency, and wounds from infection, inflammation, trauma, or surgery (scar reduction); memory enhancement; modulation/support of connective tissue synthesis; Ayurvedic medicine uses for revitalizing nerves and brain cells; Eastern healers use for emotional disorders (eg, depression) thought to be rooted in physical problems; alcoholic extract was used to treat leprosy in Western medicine
Local Anesthetic/Vasoconstrictor Precautions No information available to require special precautions
Effects on Bleeding None reported
Warnings/Precautions Advise caution when driving or operating machinery; large doses may be sedating. Use with caution in individuals taking sedatives (eg, anxiolytics, benzodiazepines); effects may be additive with other CNS depressants. Topical administration may cause contact dermatitis in sensitive

individuals. High or prolonged doses may elevate cholesterol levels. Avoid other allergenic, hyperglycemic, or thyroid-stimulating herbs.

Grapefruit Seed

Synonyms *Citrus paradisi*; GSE
Pharmacologic Category Herb
Use Antibiotic, antimycotic, antiparasitic, antiprotozoan, antimicrobial (antibacterial, antifungal, antiviral), disinfectant, immunostimulant; treatment of GI complaints, herpes, various bacterial and fungal infections (eg, *Candida albicans*, *Salmonella*), inflammatory conditions of the gums, parasites; facial cleanser, water disinfectant; used topically for antifungal and antibiotic effects
Local Anesthetic/Vasoconstrictor Precautions No information available to require special precautions
Effects on Bleeding None reported
Warnings/Precautions GSE is not the equivalent of grapefruit juice but since grapefruit juice/pulp has been associated with the inhibition of drug metabolism via cytochrome P450 isoenzyme 3A4 (CYP3A4), resulting in a number of drug interactions, it is reasonable to avoid the concurrent use of grapefruit seed extract in individuals receiving astemizole, cisapride, terfenadine and other medications metabolized by this pathway.

Grape Seed

Synonyms *Vitis vinifera*
Pharmacologic Category Herb
Use Anticoagulant/antiplatelet, anti-inflammatory, antioxidant (potent), and source of potent free radical scavengers; treatment of allergies and asthma, arterial/venous insufficiency (capillary fragility, intermittent claudication, poor circulation, varicose veins); improves peripheral circulation; treatment of gingivitis
Local Anesthetic/Vasoconstrictor Precautions No information available to require special precautions
Effects on Bleeding May see increase in bleeding due to inhibition of platelet aggregation
Warnings/Precautions Use with caution in individuals with history of bleeding, hemostatic or drug-related hemostatic problems, those taking anticoagulants (eg, aspirin or aspirin-containing products, NSAIDs, warfarin) or antiplatelet agents (eg, clopidogrel, dipyridamole, ticlopidine). Avoid other herbs with anticoagulant/antiplatelet properties. May alter absorption of calcium, copper, magnesium, and zinc due to tannins. Discontinue use at least 14 days before dental or surgical procedures.

Grape Skin

Synonyms Resveratrol
Pharmacologic Category Herb
Use Antioxidant; cardioprotectant; antiplatelet
Local Anesthetic/Vasoconstrictor Precautions No information available to require special precautions
Effects on Bleeding May see increased bleeding due to inhibition of platelet aggregation
Warnings/Precautions None reported

Green Tea

Synonyms *Camellia sinensis*
Pharmacologic Category Herb
Use Antibacterial, anticarcinogen, antioxidant, astringent, anticoagulant/antiplatelet, antifungal, antiviral, diuretic, immunosupportive; prophylaxis and treatment of cancer, cardiovascular disease, hypercholesterolemia
Local Anesthetic/Vasoconstrictor Precautions No information available to require special precautions
Effects on Bleeding May see increased bleeding due to inhibition of platelet aggregation
Warnings/Precautions Use caffeinated products with caution in individuals with cardiovascular disease, peptic ulcer, and those taking other stimulants (eg, decongestants). Use with caution in individuals with a history of bleeding, hemostatic or drug-related hemostatic disorders, those taking anticoagulants (aspirin (Continued)

Green Tea *(Continued)*

or aspirin-containing products, NSAIDs, warfarin) or antiplatelet agents (eg, ticlopidine, clopidogrel, dipyridamole). Addition of milk to any tea may significantly lower antioxidant potential. May alter absorption of calcium, copper, magnesium, and zinc due to tannins. Avoid other herbs with anticoagulant/antiplatelet properties. Discontinue at least 14 days prior to dental or surgical procedures.

GSE *see* Grapefruit Seed *on page 1625*

Harpagophytum procumbens see Devil's Claw *on page 1619*

Haw *see* Hawthorn *on page 1626*

Hawthorn

Synonyms *Crataegus laevigata*; *Crataegus monogyna*; *Crataegus oxyacantha*; *Crataegus pinnatifida*; English Hawthorn; Haw; Maybush; Whitehorn

Pharmacologic Category Herb

Use Cardiotonic, sedative, vasodilator; treatment of cardiovascular abnormalities (eg, arrhythmia, angina, CHF, hyper- or hypotension, peripheral vascular diseases, tachycardia); used synergistically with digoxin (Europe)

Local Anesthetic/Vasoconstrictor Precautions No information available to require special precautions

Effects on Bleeding None reported

Warnings/Precautions Use with caution in individuals taking ACE inhibitors and antihypertensive agents (may lower BP further). Avoid other herbs with hypotensive properties.

Horse Chestnut

Synonyms *Aesculus hippocastanum*

Pharmacologic Category Herb

Use Analgesic, anticoagulant/antiplatelet, anti-inflammatory, cardiotonic, sedative, wound-healing agent; treatment of varicose veins, hemorrhoids, other venous insufficiencies, deep vein thrombosis, lower extremity edema

Local Anesthetic/Vasoconstrictor Precautions No information available to require special precautions

Effects on Bleeding Inhibits platelet aggregation; may see increased bleeding

Warnings/Precautions Use with caution in individuals with a history of bleeding, hemostatic or drug-related hemostatic disorders, hepatic or renal impairment, and those taking anticoagulants (eg, aspirin or aspirin-containing products, NSAIDs, warfarin) or antiplatelets (eg, clopidogrel, dipyridamole, ticlopidine). Avoid other herbs with anticoagulant/antiplatelet or parasympathomimetic properties. May alter GI absorption of other herbs, minerals, or drugs (especially calcium, copper, magnesium, and zinc) due to tannins. Discontinue at least 14 days prior to dental or surgical procedures.

Huperzia serrata see HuperzineA *on page 1626*

HuperzineA

Synonyms *Huperzia serrata*

Pharmacologic Category Herb

Use Acetylcholinesterase inhibitor; treatment of senile dementia and Alzheimer's disease

Local Anesthetic/Vasoconstrictor Precautions No information available to require special precautions

Effects on Bleeding None reported

Warnings/Precautions Use with caution in individuals taking AChE inhibitors (eg, donepezil or tacrine). Avoid cholinergic drugs and other herbs with parasympathomimetic properties.

Hydrastis canadensis see Golden Seal *on page 1624*

Hypercium perforatum see St John's Wort *on page 1632*

Indian Eye *see* Golden Seal *on page 1624*

Indian Head *see* Echinacea *on page 1620*

Isoflavones *see* Soy Isoflavones *on page 1632*

Jaundice Root *see* Golden Seal *on page 1624*

Johimbe *see* Yohimbe *on page 1634*

Kava

Synonyms Awa; Kava Kava; Kew; *Piper methysticum*; Tonga
Pharmacologic Category Herb
Use Anxiolytic, diuretic, sedative; treatment of insomnia, nervous anxiety, postischemic episodes, stress; skeletal muscle relaxation
Local Anesthetic/Vasoconstrictor Precautions No information available to require special precautions
Effects on Bleeding None reported
Warnings/Precautions The FDA Center for Food Safety and Applied Nutrition (CFSAN) notified healthcare professionals and consumers of the potential risk of severe liver associated with the use of kava-containing dietary supplements. Recently, more than 20 cases of hepatitis, cirrhosis, and liver failure have been reported in Europe, with at least one individual requiring a liver transplant. Given these reports, individuals with hepatic impairment or those taking drugs which can affect the liver, should consult a physician before using supplements containing kava. Physicians are urged to closely evaluate these individuals for potential liver complications. Discontinue if yellow discoloration of skin, hair, or nails occurs (temporary; caused by extended continuous use). Accommodative disturbances (eg, enlargement of the pupils and disturbances of the oculomotor equilibrium) have been described.

Use with caution in individuals taking antianxiety or antidepressant agents, diuretics, hypnotic or sedative agents, alprazolam, or alcohol. May cause sedation; advise caution when driving or operating heavy machinery. Long-term use has resulted in rash. Avoid other herbs with diuretic properties. Discontinue if depression occurs (per Commission E, should not be used >3 months without medical supervision).

Kava Kava see Kava on page 1627
Kaveri see Ginkgo Biloba on page 1622
Kew see Kava on page 1627
Kew Tree see Ginkgo Biloba on page 1622
Klamath Weed see St John's Wort on page 1632
Lakriment Neu see Licorice on page 1627
Laurus Sassafras see Sassafras Oil on page 1631
L-Carnitine see Carnitine on page 1616

Lemon Balm/Melissa

Synonyms *Melissa officinalis*
Pharmacologic Category Herb
Use Antiviral (oral herpes virus)
Local Anesthetic/Vasoconstrictor Precautions No information available to require special precautions
Effects on Bleeding None reported
Warnings/Precautions There are no warnings or reports of toxicity.

L-Glutathione see Glutathione on page 1624

Licorice

Synonyms Glycocome; Glycyrrhiza glabra; Lakriment Neu; Liquorice; Sweet Root; Ulgastrin Neo
Pharmacologic Category Herb
Use Adaptogen, adrenocorticotropic, antidote, anti-inflammatory, antimicrobial (antibacterial, antifungal, antiviral), antioxidant, antispasmodic, antitussive, detoxification agent, emollient, emmenagogue (high doses), expectorant, immunostimulant, laxative (mild), phytoestrogenic; treatment of abdominal pain, Addison's disease, adrenal insufficiency, age spots, arthritis, asthma, atherosclerosis, benign prostatic hyperplasia (BPH), bronchitis, burns, cancer, candidiasis, carbuncle, chronic gastritis, circulatory disorders, colic, colitis, cold/flu, constipation, contact dermatitis, cough, debility, diabetes, diphtheria, diverticulosis, dizziness, dropsy, duodenal ulcer, dyspepsia, excessive thirst, fever, gastric ulcer, gastritis, hay fever, heart palpitation, heartburn, hemorrhoids, hypercholesterolemia, hyperglycemia, hypotension, inflammation, irritable bowel syndrome (IBS), laryngitis, liver disorders, malaria, menopausal symptoms, menstrual cramps, nausea, peptic ulcer, poisoning (eg, ethanol, atropine, chloral hydrate, cocaine, snakebite), pharyngitis, polyuria, rheumatism, rash, sore throat, stress, tetanus, vertigo; adjunct in long-term cortisone treatment
(Continued)

Licorice (Continued)

Per Commission E: GI ulceration, upper/lower respiratory tract infections; foodstuff in candy, chewing gum, chewing tobacco, and cough preparations

Local Anesthetic/Vasoconstrictor Precautions No information available to require special precautions

Effects on Bleeding None reported

Warnings/Precautions Use caution in diabetics, individuals with plant allergies, hypertension, and those taking antihypertensive agents, cardiac glycosides, corticosteroids, diuretics, hormonal contraceptives, laxatives, nitrofurantoin, or receiving hormone replacement therapy (HRT). Avoid other herbs that may be aldosterone synergistic (eg, horehound), hypertensive, or phytoestrogenic.

Lipoic Acid see Alpha-Lipoic Acid on page 1614
Liquorice see Licorice on page 1627

Lutein

Pharmacologic Category Nutraceutical
Use Antioxidant; treatment of cataracts and macular degeneration
Local Anesthetic/Vasoconstrictor Precautions No information available to require special precautions
Effects on Bleeding None reported
Warnings/Precautions There are no warnings or reports of toxicity.

Lycopene

Pharmacologic Category Nutraceutical
Use Treatment of atherosclerosis, macular degeneration; prevention of cancer (especially prostate)
Local Anesthetic/Vasoconstrictor Precautions No information available to require special precautions
Effects on Bleeding None reported
Warnings/Precautions There are no warnings or reports of toxicity.

Maidenhair Tree see Ginkgo Biloba on page 1622

Mastic

Synonyms Pistacia lentiscus
Pharmacologic Category Herb
Use Antibacterial; treatment of dyspepsia, gastric and duodenal ulcers, halitosis
Local Anesthetic/Vasoconstrictor Precautions No information available to require special precautions
Effects on Bleeding None reported
Warnings/Precautions Use all herbal supplements with extreme caution in children <2 years of age and in pregnancy or lactation. Some herbs are contraindicated in pregnancy or lactation; make sure to observe warnings. Use with caution in individuals on medication and with pre-existing medical conditions. Always review for potential herb-drug interactions (HDIs) and other warnings. Large and prolonged doses may increase the potential for adverse effects. Herbs may cause transient adverse effects such as nausea, vomiting, and GI distress due to a variety of chemical constituents. Caution should be used in individuals having known allergies to plants.

Matricaria chamomilla see Chamomile on page 1617
Matricaria recutita see Chamomile on page 1617
Maybush see Hawthorn on page 1626
Melaleuca alternifolia see Melaleuca Oil on page 1628

Melaleuca Oil

Synonyms Melaleuca alternifolia; Tea Tree Oil
Pharmacologic Category Herb
Use Analgesic, anti-inflammatory, antibacterial, antifungal, antiseptic, antiviral, disinfectant, immunosupportive, wound-healing agent; treatment of acne, allergy and cold symptoms, minor bruises/burns/cuts, dental plaque, gum inflammation, insect bites, eczema and psoriasis, fungal infections (eg, athlete's foot, oral thrush), hair lice, herpes, muscle pain, respiratory tract infections (eg,

bronchitis), toothache, warts; aromatherapy, facial skin toner, household disinfectant (to remove dust mites and lice from laundry), insect repellent, massage oil

Local Anesthetic/Vasoconstrictor Precautions No information available to require special precautions

Effects on Bleeding None reported

Warnings/Precautions Contains cineole; may cause rash in sensitive individuals if applied directly to skin undiluted. Store in dark glass bottle; may react badly with some polymer plastics.

Melatonin

Synonyms N-Acetyl-5-methoxytryptamine
Pharmacologic Category Nutraceutical
Use Antioxidant; treatment of sleep disorders (eg, jet lag, insomnia, neurologic problems, shift work), aging, cancer; supports immune system
Local Anesthetic/Vasoconstrictor Precautions No information available to require special precautions
Effects on Bleeding None reported
Warnings/Precautions Avoid agents that may cause additional CNS depression.

Melissa officinalis see Lemon Balm/Melissa *on page 1627*

Methyl Sulfonyl Methane

Synonyms Dimethyl Sulfone; $DMSO_2$; MSM
Pharmacologic Category Nutraceutical
Use Analgesic, anti-inflammatory; treatment of interstitial cystitis, lupus, and osteoarthritis
Local Anesthetic/Vasoconstrictor Precautions No information available to require special precautions
Effects on Bleeding None reported
Warnings/Precautions There are no warnings or reports of toxicity when taken according to manufacturer's labeled instructions.

Milk Thistle

Synonyms *Silybum marianum*
Pharmacologic Category Herb
Use Antidote (Death Cap mushroom), antioxidant (hepatoprotective, including drug toxicities); treatment of acute/chronic hepatitis, jaundice, and stimulation of bile secretion/cholagogue
Local Anesthetic/Vasoconstrictor Precautions No information available to require special precautions
Effects on Bleeding None reported
Warnings/Precautions There are no warnings or reports of toxicity when taken according to manufacturer's labeled instructions.

Milk Vetch see Astragalus *on page 1615*
Monascus purpureus see Red Yeast Rice *on page 1630*
MSM see Methyl Sulfonyl Methane *on page 1629*
N-Acetyl-5-methoxytryptamine see Melatonin *on page 1629*
NADH see Nicotinamide Adenine Dinucleotide *on page 1629*
Nectar of the Gods see Garlic *on page 1622*

Nicotinamide Adenine Dinucleotide

Synonyms Coenzyme 1; NADH
Pharmacologic Category Nutraceutical
Use Treatment of chronic fatigue, Parkinson's disease; increases stamina and energy
Local Anesthetic/Vasoconstrictor Precautions No information available to require special precautions
Effects on Bleeding None reported
Warnings/Precautions There are no warnings or reports of toxicity when taken according to manufacturer's labeled instructions.

Nosebleed see Feverfew *on page 1621*
Oenothera biennis see Evening Primrose *on page 1621*

Orange Root *see* Golden Seal *on page 1624*
Oriental Plum Tree *see* Ginkgo Biloba *on page 1622*
Palmetto Scrub *see* Saw Palmetto *on page 1631*
Panax ginseng see Ginseng, Panax *on page 1623*

Parsley

Synonyms *Petroselinum crispum*
Pharmacologic Category Herb
Use Halitosis; antibacterial, antifungal
Local Anesthetic/Vasoconstrictor Precautions No information available to require special precautions
Effects on Bleeding None reported
Warnings/Precautions There are no warnings or reports of toxicity.

Passiflora spp *see* Passion Flower *on page 1630*

Passion Flower

Synonyms *Passiflora* spp
Pharmacologic Category Herb
Use Sedative
Local Anesthetic/Vasoconstrictor Precautions No information available to require special precautions
Effects on Bleeding None reported
Warnings/Precautions Advise caution when driving or operating heavy machinery. Use with caution in individuals taking antianxiety agents or antidepressants and other sedatives; reported in animal studies to increase sleeping time induced by hexobarbital.

Pausinystalia yohimbe see Yohimbe *on page 1634*
Petroselinum crispum see Parsley *on page 1630*
Piper methysticum see Kava *on page 1627*
Pistacia lentiscus see Mastic *on page 1628*
Poor Mans Treacle *see* Garlic *on page 1622*
Purple Coneflower *see* Echinacea *on page 1620*

Quercetin

Pharmacologic Category Nutraceutical
Use Antioxidant
Local Anesthetic/Vasoconstrictor Precautions No information available to require special precautions
Effects on Bleeding None reported
Warnings/Precautions There are no warnings or reports of toxicity.

Radix *see* Valerian *on page 1633*
Red Valerian *see* Valerian *on page 1633*

Red Yeast Rice

Synonyms *Monascus purpureus*
Pharmacologic Category Herb
Use Antibiotic, anti-inflammatory, antioxidant, HMG-CoA reductase inhibitor; treatment of hypercholesterolemia, hypertension, hypertriglyceridemia
Local Anesthetic/Vasoconstrictor Precautions No information available to require special precautions
Effects on Bleeding None reported
Warnings/Precautions Use with caution in individuals with a history of bleeding, hemostatic or drug-related hemostatic disorders, and those taking anticoagulants (eg, aspirin or aspirin-containing products, NSAIDs, warfarin) or antiplatelet agents (eg, clopidogrel, dipyridamole, ticlopidine), cyclosporine, erythromycin, itraconazole, niacin, HMG-CoA reductase inhibitors (associated with rare but serious adverse effects, including hepatic and skeletal muscle disorders), and other hyperlipidemic agents. Avoid other herbs with hyperlipidemic properties. Discontinue at the first sign of hepatic dysfunction; discontinue at least 14 days prior to dental or surgical procedures.

Resveratrol *see* Grape Skin *on page 1625*
Rosin Rose *see* St John's Wort *on page 1632*
Rustic Treacle *see* Garlic *on page 1622*

Rökan see Ginkgo Biloba on page 1622
Sabal serrulata see Saw Palmetto on page 1631
Sabasilis serrulatae see Saw Palmetto on page 1631
S-adenosylmethionine see SAMe on page 1631

SAMe

Synonyms S-adenosylmethionine
Pharmacologic Category Nutritional Supplement
Use Treatment of depression
Local Anesthetic/Vasoconstrictor Precautions No information available to require special precautions
Effects on Bleeding None reported
Warnings/Precautions Use caution when combining with other antidepressants, tryptophan, or 5-HTP; ineffective in the treatment of depressive symptoms associated with bipolar disorder

Sassafras albidum see Sassafras Oil on page 1631

Sassafras Oil

Synonyms Laurus Sassafras; Sassafras albidum; Sassafras radix; Sassafras varifolium; Sassafrax
Pharmacologic Category Herb
Use Demulcent; treatment of inflammation of the eyes, insect bites, rheumatic pain; used in the past as a flavoring for beer, sauces, and tea
Local Anesthetic/Vasoconstrictor Precautions No information available to require special precautions
Effects on Bleeding None reported
Warnings/Precautions Ingestion can result in poisoning or death (dose-dependent). Sassafras tea can contain as much as 200 mg (3 mg/kg) of safrole; emesis (within 30 minutes) can be considered for ingestion >5 mL (considered lethal).

Sassafras radix see Sassafras Oil on page 1631
Sassafras varifolium see Sassafras Oil on page 1631
Sassafrax see Sassafras Oil on page 1631

Saw Palmetto

Synonyms Palmetto Scrub; Sabal serrulata; Sabasilis serrulatae; Serenoa repens
Pharmacologic Category Herb
Use Antiandrogen, anti-inflammatory; treatment of benign prostatic hyperplasia (BPH)
Local Anesthetic/Vasoconstrictor Precautions No information available to require special precautions
Effects on Bleeding None reported
Warnings/Precautions Not FDA approved; use with caution in individuals on alpha-adrenergic blocking agents and finasteride.

Schisandra

Synonyms Schizandra chinensis
Pharmacologic Category Herb
Use Adaptogen, anti-inflammatory, antioxidant, antitussive, hepatoprotective, immunostimulant; treatment of cancer, chronic diarrhea, cough, diabetes, diaphoresis, fatigue, hepatitis; adjunct support for chemotherapy and radiation, detoxification, energy production, health tonic
Local Anesthetic/Vasoconstrictor Precautions No information available to require special precautions
Effects on Bleeding None reported
Warnings/Precautions May alter metabolism of many drugs; use with caution in individuals taking calcium channel blockers.

Schizandra chinensis see Schisandra on page 1631
Scury Root see Echinacea on page 1620
Serenoa repens see Saw Palmetto on page 1631

Shark Cartilage

Pharmacologic Category Nutraceutical
Use Treatment of cancer, osteoarthritis, and rheumatoid arthritis
Local Anesthetic/Vasoconstrictor Precautions No information available to require special precautions
Effects on Bleeding None reported
Warnings/Precautions There are no warnings or reports of toxicity.

Siberian Ginseng *see* Ginseng, Siberian *on page 1623*
Silver Apricot *see* Ginkgo Biloba *on page 1622*
Silybum marianum *see* Milk Thistle *on page 1629*
Snakeroot *see* Echinacea *on page 1620*

Soy Isoflavones

Synonyms Isoflavones
Pharmacologic Category Nutraceutical
Use Estrogenic (weak); treatment of bone loss, hypercholesterolemia, menopausal symptoms
Local Anesthetic/Vasoconstrictor Precautions No information available to require special precautions
Effects on Bleeding None reported
Warnings/Precautions May alter response to hormone replacement therapy; use with caution in individuals with history of thromboembolism or stroke

Stinking Rose *see* Garlic *on page 1622*

St John's Wort

Synonyms Amber Touch-and-Feel; Goatweed; *Hypercium perforatum*; Klamath Weed; Rosin Rose
Pharmacologic Category Herb
Use Antibacterial, anti-inflammatory, antiviral (high doses), anxiolytic, wound-healing agent; treatment of AIDS (popular due to possible antiretroviral activity), anxiety and stress, insomnia; mild to moderate depression; bruises, muscle soreness, and sprains; vitiligo

Per Commission E: Psychovegetative disorders, depressive moods, anxiety and/or nervous unrest; oily preparations for dyspeptic complaints; oily preparations externally for treatment of post-therapy of acute and contused injuries, myalgia, first degree burns
Local Anesthetic/Vasoconstrictor Precautions No information available to require special precautions
Effects on Bleeding None reported
Warnings/Precautions May be photosensitizing; use caution with drugs metabolized by CYP3A3/4 and tyramine-containing foods (eg, cheese, wine). Use with caution in individuals taking antidepressants, cardiac glycosides, MAO inhibitors, narcotics, reserpine, stimulants, and SSRIs. High does may elevate LFTs (reversible). May alter absorption of calcium, copper, magnesium, and zinc due to tannins. Interacts with many drugs.

Superginkgo *see* Ginkgo Biloba *on page 1622*
Sweet Root *see* Licorice *on page 1627*
Tanacetum parthenium *see* Feverfew *on page 1621*
Tanakan *see* Ginkgo Biloba *on page 1622*
Tanakene *see* Ginkgo Biloba *on page 1622*
Tea Tree Oil *see* Melaleuca Oil *on page 1628*
Tebonin *see* Ginkgo Biloba *on page 1622*
Thioctic acid *see* Alpha-Lipoic Acid *on page 1614*
Tonga *see* Kava *on page 1627*
Tramisal *see* Ginkgo Biloba *on page 1622*

Turmeric

Synonyms *Curcuma longa*
Pharmacologic Category Herb
Use Anti-inflammatory, antioxidant, antiplatelet, antirheumatic; treatment of rheumatoid arthritis and other inflammatory conditions, hypercholesterolemia, and hyperlipidemia

Local Anesthetic/Vasoconstrictor Precautions No information available to require special precautions

Effects on Bleeding May see increased bleeding due to inhibition of platelet aggregation

Warnings/Precautions Use with caution in individuals with history of bleeding, hemostatic or drug-related hemostatic disorders, and those taking anticoagulants (eg, aspirin or aspirin-containing products, NSAIDs, warfarin) or antiplatelet agents (eg, clopidogrel, dipyridamole, ticlopidine). Discontinue at least 14 days prior to dental or surgical procedures.

Turmeric Root *see* Golden Seal *on page 1624*

Ubiquinone *see* Coenzyme Q$_{10}$ *on page 1618*

Ulgastrin Neo *see* Licorice *on page 1627*

Uncaria tomentosa *see* Cat's Claw *on page 1617*

Uva Ursi

Synonyms *Arctostaphylos uva-ursi*; Bearberry

Pharmacologic Category Herb

Use Analgesic, antiseptic, astringent, diuretic; treatment and prevention of urinary tract infections; prevention of kidney stones; treatment of bladder infections, urethritis, and a variety of renal disorders (eg, cystitis, nephritis, nephrolithiasis)

Local Anesthetic/Vasoconstrictor Precautions No information available to require special precautions

Effects on Bleeding None reported

Warnings/Precautions May cause green-brown discoloration of urine; may alter GI absorption of other herbs, minerals, or drugs (especially calcium, copper, magnesium, and zinc) due to tannins. Use caution with individuals taking diuretics; avoid other herbs with diuretic properties.

Vaccinium macrocarpon *see* Cranberry *on page 1619*

Vaccinium myrtillus *see* Bilberry *on page 1615*

Valerian

Synonyms Radix; Red Valerian; *Valeriana edulis*; *Valeriana wallichi*

Pharmacologic Category Herb

Use Antispasmotic, anxiolytic, sedative (mild); treatment of anxiety and panic attacks, headache, intestinal cramps, nervous tension during PMS and menopause, restless motor syndrome and muscle spasms, sleep disorders (eg, insomnia, jet lag)

Per Commission E: Treatment of sleep disorders based on nervous conditions, restlessness

Local Anesthetic/Vasoconstrictor Precautions No information available to require special precautions

Effects on Bleeding None reported

Warnings/Precautions Advise caution when driving or operating heavy machinery. Use only valepotriate and baldrinal-free supplements in children <12 years of age due to potential mutagenic properties. Use with caution in individuals taking antianxiety or antidepressant agents, antipsychotics, histamines, and hypnotics/sedatives. Avoid herbs with sedative properties.

Valeriana edulis *see* Valerian *on page 1633*

Valeriana wallichi *see* Valerian *on page 1633*

Valverde *see* Ginkgo Biloba *on page 1622*

Vanadium

Pharmacologic Category Mineral

Use Treatment of type 1 and type 2 diabetes

Local Anesthetic/Vasoconstrictor Precautions No information available to require special precautions

Effects on Bleeding None reported

Warnings/Precautions May alter glucose regulation; use with caution in diabetics, those predisposed to hypoglycemia, or taking hypoglycemic agents (eg, insulin). Monitor blood sugar and dosage of these agents; may require adjustment (should be carefully coordinated among the individual's healthcare providers).

Vasan *see* Ginkgo Biloba *on page 1622*

Vital *see* Ginkgo Biloba *on page 1622*

Vitex agnus-castus see Chasteberry *on page 1618*
Vitis vinifera see Grape Seed *on page 1625*
Whitehorn see Hawthorn *on page 1626*
Wild Quinine see Feverfew *on page 1621*

Wild Yam

Synonyms *Dioscorea villosa*
Pharmacologic Category Herb
Use Anti-inflammatory, antispasmodic, cholagogue, diuretic (high doses), expectorant (high doses); treatment of diverticulitis, dysmenorrhea, intestinal colic, menopausal symptoms, nausea, premenstrual syndrome (PMS), rheumatic and other inflammatory conditions; female vitality
Local Anesthetic/Vasoconstrictor Precautions No information available to require special precautions
Effects on Bleeding None reported
Warnings/Precautions Use with caution in individuals with a history of stroke or thromboembolic disease and those taking steroids, hormonal contraceptives, or receiving hormone replacement therapy (HRT). Use in children, or women during lactation or pregnancy is not recommended. Overdose may result in poisoning. Avoid other anabolic herbs.

Yellow Indian Paint see Golden Seal *on page 1624*
Yellow Root see Golden Seal *on page 1624*

Yohimbe

Related Information
Yohimbine *on page 1589*
Synonyms Johimbe; *Pausinystalia yohimbe*; Yohimbehe cortex
Pharmacologic Category Herb
Use Anesthetic (local), antiatherogenic, antiviral, aphrodesiac, stimulant, sympathomimetic, thermogenic, vasodilator, vasopressomimetic; treatment of angina pectoris, arteriosclerosis, exhaustion, male erectile dysfunction
Local Anesthetic/Vasoconstrictor Precautions Has potential to interact with epinephrine and levonordefrin to result in increased BP; use vasoconstrictor with caution
Effects on Bleeding None reported
Warnings/Precautions Toxic doses may trigger cardiac failure, hypotension, and psychosis. Use with caution in individuals with diabetes, GI ulceration, or osteoporosis. Avoid other herbs with hypertensive, parasympathomimetic, sympathomimetic, thyroid-stimulating, or vasopressomimetic properties.

Yohimbehe cortex see Yohimbe *on page 1634*
Zingiber officinale see Ginger *on page 1622*

ORAL MEDICINE TOPICS

PART I:

DENTAL MANAGEMENT
AND THERAPEUTIC CONSIDERATIONS
IN MEDICALLY-COMPROMISED PATIENTS

This first part of the chapter focuses on common medical conditions and their associated drug therapies with which the dentist must be familiar. Patient profiles with commonly associated drug regimens are described.

TABLE OF CONTENTS

Cardiovascular Diseases 1636

Gastrointestinal Disorders 1654

Respiratory Diseases. 1656

Endocrine Disorders and Pregnancy. 1659

HIV Infection and AIDS 1662

Rheumatoid Arthritis, Osteoarthritis, and Osteoporosis 1668

Tuberculosis 1673

Sexually-Transmitted Diseases 1674

Systemic Viral Diseases 1675

Antibiotic Prophylaxis – Preprocedural Guidelines for Dental
Patients 1680

CARDIOVASCULAR DISEASES

Cardiovascular disease is the most prevalent human disease affecting over 60 million Americans and this group of diseases accounts >50% of all deaths in the United States. Surgical and pharmacological therapy have resulted in many cardiovascular patients living healthy and profitable lives. Consequently, patients presenting to the dental office may require treatment planning modifications related to the medical management of their cardiovascular disease. For the purposes of this text, we will cover coronary artery disease (CAD) including angina pectoris and myocardial infarction, cardiac arrhythmias, heart failure, and hypertension.

CARDIOVASCULAR DRUGS AND DENTAL CONSIDERATIONS

Some of the drug listings are redundant because the drugs are used to treat more than one cardiovascular disorder. As a convenience to the reader, each table has been constructed as a stand alone listing of drugs for the given disorder. The dental implications of these cardiovascular drugs are listed in Tables 8 and 9. Each of these 2 tables is a consolidation of the drugs from Tables 1-7. The more frequent cardiovascular, respiratory, and central nervous system adverse reactions which you may see in the dental patient are described in Table 8. Table 9 describes the effects on dental treatment reported for these drugs. It is suggested that the reader use Tables 8 and 9 to check for potential effects which could occur in the medicated cardiovascular dental patients.

CORONARY ARTERY DISEASE

Any long-term decrease in the delivery of oxygen to the heart muscle can lead to the condition ischemic heart disease. Often arteriosclerosis and atherosclerosis result in a narrowing of the coronary vessels' lumina and are the most common causes of vascular ischemic heart disease. Other causes such as previous infarct, mitral valve regurgitation, and ruptured septa may also lead to ischemia in the heart muscle. The two most common major conditions that result from ischemic heart disease are angina pectoris and myocardial infarction. Sudden death, a third category, can likewise result from ischemia.

To the physician, the most common presenting sign or symptom of ischemic heart disease is chest pain. This chest pain can be of a transient nature as in angina pectoris or the result of a myocardial infarction. It is now believed that sudden death represents a separate occurrence that essentially involves the development of a lethal cardiac arrhythmia or coronary artery spasm leading to an acute shutdown of the heart muscle blood supply. Risk factors in patients for coronary atherosclerosis include cigarette smoking, elevated blood lipids, hypertension, as well as diabetes mellitus, age, and gender (male).

Coronary artery disease (CAD) is the cause of about half of all deaths in the United States. CAD has been shown to be correlated with the levels of plasma cholesterol and/ or triacylglycerol-containing lipoprotein particles. Primary prevention focuses on averting the development of CAD. In contrast, secondary prevention of (CAD) focuses on therapies to reduce morbidity and mortality in patients with clinically documented CAD.

Lipid-lowering and cardioprotective drugs provide significant risk-reducing benefits in the secondary prevention of CAD. By reducing the levels of total and low density cholesterol through the inhibition of hydroxymethylglutaryl coenzyme A (HMG-CoA) reductase, statin drugs significantly improve survival. Cardioprotective drug therapy includes antiplatelet/ anticoagulant agents to inhibit platelet adhesion, aggregation and blood coagulation; beta-blockers to lower heart rate, contractility and blood pressure; and the angiotensin-converting enzyme (ACE) inhibitors to lower peripheral resistance and workload. For a listing of these drugs, see Table 1.

Table 1.
DRUGS USED IN THE TREATMENT OF CAD

Reduction of Total and Low-Density Cholesterol Levels

    Bile Acid Sequestrant

        Colesevelam *on page 389*

    HMG-CoA Reductase Inhibitors

        Fluvastatin *on page 693*

        Lovastatin *on page 953*

        Pravastatin *on page 1265*

        Simvastatin *on page 1394*

        Atorvastatin *on page 158*

    Fibrate Group

        Fenofibrate *on page 639*

        Gemfibrozil *on page 730*

    Bile Acid Resins

        Cholestyramine Resin *on page 334*

        Colestipol *on page 390*

    Nicotinic Acid

Cardioprotective Therapy

    Antiplatelet / Anticoagulant Agents

        Aspirin *on page 145*

        Clopidogrel *on page 376*

        Ticlopidine *on page 1486*

        Warfarin *on page 1585*

    Beta-Adrenergic Receptor Blockers

        Atenolol *on page 154*

        Metoprolol *on page 1030*

        Propranolol *on page 1301*

    Angiotensin-Converting Enzyme (ACE) Inhibitors

        Captopril *on page 257*

        Enalapril *on page 538*

        Fosinopril *on page 707*

        Lisinopril *on page 936*

        Ramipril *on page 1332*

ANGINA PECTORIS

(EMPHASIS ON UNSTABLE ANGINA)

Numerous physiologic triggers can initiate the rupture of plaque in coronary blood vessels. Rupture leads to the activation, adhesion and aggregation of platelets, and the activation of the clotting cascade, resulting in the formation of occlusive thrombus. If this process leads to the complete occlusion of the artery, acute myocardial infarction with ST-segment elevation occurs. Alternatively, if the process leads to severe stenosis and the artery remains patent, unstable angina occurs. Triggers which induce unstable angina include physical exertion, mechanical stress due to an increase in cardiac contractility, pulse rate, blood pressure, and vasoconstriction.

Unstable angina accounts for more than 1 million hospital admissions annually. In 1989, Braunwald devised a classification system according to the severity of the clinical manifestations of angina. These manifestations are defined as acute angina while at rest (within 48 hours before presentation), subacute angina while at rest (within the previous month but not within the 48 hours before presentation), or new onset of accelerated (progressively more severe) angina. The system also classifies angina according to the clinical circumstances in which unstable angina develops, defined as either angina in the presence or absence of other conditions (ie, fever, hypoxia, tachycardia, thyrotoxicosis) and whether or not ECG abnormalities are present. Recently, the term "acute coronary syndrome" has been used to describe the range of conditions that includes unstable angina, non-Q-wave myocardial infarction, and Q-wave myocardial infarction.

Pharmacologic therapy to treat unstable angina includes antiplatelet drugs, antithrombin therapy, and conventional antianginal therapy with beta-blockers, nitrates, and calcium channel blockers. These drug groups and selected agents are listed in Table 3.

CARDIOVASCULAR DISEASES (Continued)

Antiplatelet Drugs

Aspirin reduces platelet aggregation by blocking platelet cyclo-oxygenase through irreversible acetylation. This action prevents the formation of thromboxane A_2. A number of studies have confirmed that aspirin reduces the risk of death from cardiac causes and fatal and nonfatal myocardial infarction by approximately 50% to 70% in patients presenting with unstable angina. Ticlopidine is a second-line alternative to aspirin in the treatment of unstable angina and is also used as adjunctive therapy with aspirin to prevent thrombosis after placement of intracoronary stents. Ticlopidine blocks ADP-mediated platelet aggregation. Clopidogrel inhibits platelet aggregation by affecting the ADP-dependent activation of the glycoprotein IIb/IIIa complex. Clopidogrel is chemically related to ticlopidine, but has fewer side effects.

Platelet Glycoprotein IIb / IIIa Receptor Antagonists

Antagonists of glycoprotein IIb/IIIa, a receptor on the platelet for adhesive proteins, inhibit the final common pathway involved in adhesion, activation and aggregation. Presently, there exist three classes of inhibitors. One class is murine-human chimeric antibodies of which abciximab is the prototype. The other two classes are the synthetic peptide forms (eg, eptifibatide) and the synthetic nonpeptide forms (eg, tirofiban). These agents, in combination with heparin and aspirin, have been used to treat unstable angina, significantly reducing the incidence of death or myocardial infarction.

Antithrombin Drugs

Unfractionated heparin, in combination with aspirin, is used to treat unstable angina. Unfractionated heparin consists of polysaccharide chains which bind to antithrombin III, causing a conformational change that accelerates the inhibition of thrombin and factor Xa. Unfractionated heparin is therefore an indirect thrombin inhibitor. Unfractionated heparin can only be administered intravenously. Low-molecular-weight heparins (LMWH) have a more predictable pharmacokinetic profile than the unfractionated heparin and can be administered subcutaneously. These heparins have a mechanism of action and use similar to unfractionated heparin.

The direct antithrombins decrease thrombin activity in a manner independent of any actions on antithrombin III. Two such direct antithrombins are lepirudin (also known as recombinant hirudin) and argatroban. These agents are highly specific, direct thrombin inhibitor with each molecule capable of binding to one molecule of thrombin and inhibiting its thrombogenic activity. Direct antithrombins are used for the prevention or reduction of ischemic complications associated with unstable angina.

Warfarin (Coumadin®) elicits its anticoagulant effect by interfering with the hepatic synthesis of vitamin K-dependent coagulation factors II, VII, IX, and X. Although warfarin appears to be somewhat effective after myocardial infarction in preventing death or recurrent myocardial infarction, its effectiveness in the treatment of acute coronary syndrome is questionable. Combination therapy with aspirin and heparin followed by warfarin has resulted in reduced incidence of recurrent angina, myocardial infarction, death, or all three at 14 days as compared with aspirin alone. In contrast, another study however failed to show any additional benefit in the treatment of acute coronary syndrome using a combination of aspirin and warfarin compared to aspirin alone.

Conventional Antianginal Therapy: Beta-Blockers, Nitrates, Calcium Channel Blockers

Current thinking is that there is a definite link between unstable angina and acute myocardial infarction. In this regard, beta-blockers are currently recommended as first-line agents in all acute coronary syndromes. A meta-analysis of studies involving 4700 patients with unstable angina demonstrated a 13% reduction in the risk of myocardial infarction among patients treated with beta-blockers. The various preparations of beta-blockers appear to have equal efficacy. The effects of beta-blockers are thought to be due to their ability to decrease myocardial oxygen demand.

Nitrates, such as nitroglycerin, are widely used in the management of unstable angina. Nitrates elicit a number of effects including a reduction in oxygen demand, arteriolar vasodilation, augmentation of collateral coronary blood flow and frequency of coronary vasospasm. Intravenous nitroglycerin is one of the first line therapies for unstable angina because of the ease of dose titration and the rapid resolution of effects. Continuous nitrate therapy with oral and transdermal patch preparations has resulted in tolerance to the beneficial effects of nitrates. A 6- to 8-hour daily nitrate-free interval will minimize the tolerance phenomenon. Also, supplemental use of vitamin C appears to prevent nitrate tolerance.

Calcium channel blockers such as nifedipine, verapamil, and diltiazem cause coronary vasodilation and reduced blood pressure. Because of these actions, the calcium channel blockers were thought to be a drug group which could be effective in the treatment of unstable angina. However, a meta analysis of studies in which patients with unstable angina were treated with calcium channel blockers found no effect of the drugs on the incidence of death or myocardial infarction. More recently, it has been shown that treatment with diltiazem and verapamil may result in increased survival and reduced rates of reinfarction in patients with acute coronary syndrome. Current thinking suggests that calcium channel blockers should be used in patients in whom beta-blockers are contraindicated or in those with refractory symptoms after treatments with aspirin, nitrates, or beta-blockers.

Dental Management

The dental management of the patient with angina pectoris may include sedation techniques for complicated procedures (see "Sedation" on page 1727), to limit the extent of procedures, and to limit the use of local anesthesia containing 1:100,000 epinephrine to two capsules. Anesthesia without a vasoconstrictor might also be selected. The appropriate use of a vasoconstrictor in anesthesia, however, should be weighed against the necessity to maximize anesthesia. Complete history and appropriate referral and consultation with the patient's physician for those patients who are known to be at risk for angina pectoris is recommended.

MYOCARDIAL INFARCTION

Myocardial infarction is the leading cause of death in the United States. It is an acute irreversible ischemic event that produces an area of myocardial necrosis in the heart tissue. If a patient has a previous history of myocardial infarction, he/she may be taking a variety of drugs (ie, antihypertensives, lipid lowering drugs, ACE inhibitors, and antianginal medications) to not only prevent a second infarct, but to treat the long-term associated ischemic heart disease. Postmyocardial infarction patients are often taking anticoagulants such as warfarin and antiplatelet agents such as aspirin. Consultation with the prescribing physician by the dentist is necessary prior to invasive procedures. Temporary dose reduction may allow the dentist to proceed with very invasive procedures. Most procedures, however, can be accomplished without changing the anticoagulant therapy at all, using local hemostasis techniques.

> Aspirin on page 145
> Warfarin on page 1585

Thrombolytic drugs, that might dissolve hemostatic plugs, may also be given on a short-term basis immediately following an infarct and include:

> Alteplase on page 77
> Reteplase on page 1341
> Streptokinase on page 1417
> Tenecteplase on page 1455

Alteplase [tissue plasminogen activator (TPA)] is also currently in use for acute myocardial infarction. Following myocardial infarction and rehabilitation, outpatients may be placed on anticoagulants (such as coumadin), diuretics, beta-adrenergic blockers, ACE inhibitors to reduce blood pressure, and calcium channel blockers. Depending on the presence or absence of continued angina pectoris, patients may also be taking nitrates, beta-blockers, or calcium channel blockers as indicated for treatment of angina.

BETA-ADRENERGIC BLOCKING AGENTS CATEGORIZED ACCORDING TO SPECIFIC PROPERTIES

Alpha-Adrenergic Blocking Activity

> Labetalol on page 891

Intrinsic Sympathomimetic Activity

> Acebutolol on page 28
> Pindolol on page 1240

Long Duration of Action and Fewer CNS Effects

> Acebutolol on page 28
> Atenolol on page 154
> Betaxolol on page 203
> Nadolol on page 1079

Beta₁-Receptor Selectivity

> Acebutolol on page 28
> Atenolol on page 154
> Metoprolol on page 1030

Nonselective (blocks both beta₁- and beta₂-receptors)

> Betaxolol on page 203
> Labetalol on page 891
> Nadolol on page 1079
> Pindolol on page 1240
> Propranolol on page 1301
> Timolol on page 1489

CARDIOVASCULAR DISEASES *(Continued)*

ARRHYTHMIAS

Abnormal cardiac rhythm can develop spontaneously and survivors of a myocardial infarction are often left with an arrhythmia. An arrhythmia is any alteration or disturbance in the normal rate, rhythm, or conduction through the cardiac tissue. This is known as a cardiac arrhythmia. Abnormalities in rhythm can occur in either the atria or the ventricles. Various valvular deformities, drug effects, and chemical derangements can initiate arrhythmias. These arrhythmias can be a slowing of the heart rate (<60 beats/minute) as defined in bradycardia or tachycardia resulting in a rapid heart beat (usually >150 beats/minute). The dentist will encounter a variety of treatments for management of arrhythmias. Usually, underlying causes such as reduced cardiac output, hypertension, and irregular ventricular beats will require treatment. Pacemaker therapy is also sometimes used. Indwelling pacemakers may require supplementation with antibiotics, and consultation with the physician is certainly appropriate. Sinus tachycardia is often treated with drugs such as:

> Propranolol *on page 1301*
>
> Quinidine *on page 1324*

Beta-blockers are often used to slow cardiac rate and diazepam may be helpful when anxiety is a contributing factor in arrhythmia. When atrial flutter and atrial fibrillation are diagnosed, drug therapy is usually required.

> Digitoxin *on page 471*
>
> Digoxin *on page 471*

Atrial fibrillation (AF) is an arrhythmia characterized by multiple electrical activations in the atria resulting in scattered and disorganized depolarization and repolarization of the myocardium. Atrial contraction can lead to an irregular and rapid rate of ventricular contraction. The prevalence of atrial fibrillation within the US population ranges between 1% and 4%, with the incidence increasing with age. It is often associated with rheumatic valvular disease and nonvalvular conditions including coronary artery disease and hypertension. Coronary artery disease is present in about one-half of the patients with atrial fibrillation. Atrial fibrillation is a major risk factor for systemic and cerebral embolism. It is thought that thrombi develop as a result of stasis in the dilated left atrium and is dislodged by sudden changes in cardiac rhythm. About 10% of all strokes in patients >60 years of age are caused by atrial fibrillation.

The cornerstones of drug therapy for atrial fibrillation are the restoration and maintenance of a normal sinus rhythm through the use of antiarrhythmic drugs, ventricular rate control through the use of beta-blockers, digitalis drugs or calcium channel blockers, and stroke prevention through the use of anticoagulants.

Antiarrhythmic Drugs

Cardiac rhythm is conducted through the sinoatrial (SA) and atrioventricular (AV) nodes, bundle branches, and Purkinje fibers. Electrical impulses are transmitted within this system by the opening and closing of sodium and potassium channels. Antiarrhythmic drugs are classified by which channel they act upon, a classification known as Vaughan Williams after the author of the published paper. The Class I agents act primarily on sodium channels, and the Class III agents act on potassium channels. In addition, there are subclassifications within the Class I agents according to effects of the drug on conduction and refractoriness within the Purkinje and ventricular tissues. Class IA agents show moderate depression of conduction and prolongation of repolarization. Class IB agents show modest depression of conduction and shortening of repolarization. Class IC agents show marked depression of conduction and mild or no effect on repolarization. Class IA and IC agents are effective in the treatment of atrial fibrillation. Class IB agents (ie, lidocaine, phenytoin) are not used to treat atrial fibrillation, but are effective in treating ventricular arrhythmias. Class II drugs are the beta-adrenergic blocking drugs and Class IV are the calcium channel blockers. Table 2 lists the drugs and the categories used to treat atrial fibrillation.

Table 2.
DRUGS USED IN THE TREATMENT OF ATRIAL FIBRILLATION

Class I Antiarrhythmic Agents

    Disopyramide *on page 491*
    Flecainide *on page 657*
    Moricizine *on page 1064*
    Procainamide *on page 1283*
    Propafenone *on page 1293*
    Quinidine *on page 1324*

Class II Antiarrhythmic Agents (Beta-Adrenergic Blockers)
    Cardioselective (Beta₁-Receptor Block only)

        Acebutolol *on page 28*
        Atenolol *on page 154*
        Betaxolol *on page 46*
        Metoprolol *on page 1030*

    Noncardioselective (Beta₁- and Beta₂-Receptor Block)

        Nadolol *on page 1079*
        Penbutolol *on page 1199*
        Pindolol *on page 1240*
        Propranolol *on page 1301*
        Timolol *on page 1489*

Class III Antiarrhythmic Agents

    Amiodarone *on page 90*
    Dofetilide *on page 497*
    Ibutilide *on page 813*
    Sotalol *on page 1409*

Class IV Antiarrhythmic Agents (Calcium Channel Blockers)

    Diltiazem *on page 479*
    Verapamil *on page 1571*

Anticoagulant Agents

    Aspirin *on page 145*
    Warfarin *on page 1585*

Source: USP DI, Volumes I and II, Update, April, 1998.

Restoring and Maintaining Normal Sinus Rhythm

Cardioversion induced by drugs can usually restore sinus rhythm in patients with atrial fibrillation. Class I drugs (moricizine), Class IA drugs (disopyramide, procainamide, quinidine), Class IC drugs (flecainide, propafenone), and Class III antiarrhythmics (amiodarone, sotalol) are all effective in restoring normal sinus rhythm. Success rates may vary greatly and are complicated by the high rate of spontaneous conversion. The drugs used for pharmacologic conversion are also used to maintain sinus rhythm.

Ventricular Rate Control

It is accepted practice to treat patients with medication when the resting ventricular rate is >110 beats/minute. Digoxin, calcium channel blockers, and beta-adrenergic blockers are used in the regulation of ventricular rate. Digoxin increases the vagal tone to the AV node, calcium channel blockers slow the AV nodal conduction, and the beta-adrenergic blocking drugs decrease the sympathetic activation of the AV nodal conduction.

ANTICOAGULANT THERAPY

Over the last thirty years, there has been an increasing use of drugs that relate to the clotting mechanisms in patients. These drugs have included the wide spread use of aspirin as well as an increasing use of anticoagulants found in warfarin as well as synthetic drugs that also have anticoagulation effects. Many patients with ischemic heart disease, atherosclerosis, those with atrial fibrillation and in patients at high risk for stroke, we find the increased use of these anticoagulants. Large numbers of these patients are receiving oral anticoagulation therapy as out patients. The dental clinician is often faced with the decision as to how to manage these patients prior to dental procedures. Key factors regarding the patient receiving anticoagulation therapy include:

- What is the thromboembolytic risk for this patient?

- What is the bleeding risk of the dental procedure planned?

- If an invasive procedure is planned in the face of a high thromboembolytic risk, what is the managing physician's opinion on altering the dosage of anticoagulation therapy?

Often times, to access these factors, consultation with a patient's physician is necessary. However, recent reviews have suggested by Jeske, 2003 and others in our suggested readings list have argued that inappropriate adjustments in anticoagulation therapy create far greater risk for the patient than the risk of hemorrhage during most dental

CARDIOVASCULAR DISEASES (Continued)

procedures. Therefore, the scientific evidence does not support changing regimens of anticoagulation therapy in many, perhaps even most instances. However, this decision can only be determined by weighing the factors described above and discussing the situation with the patient's physician.

Table 3.
DRUGS USED TO MANAGE UNSTABLE ANGINA

Antiplatelet Drugs

    Aspirin *on page 145*

    Clopidogrel *on page 376*

    Ticlopidine *on page 1486*

    Glycoprotein IIb / IIIa Receptor Antagonists

        Abciximab *on page 26*

        Eptifibatide *on page 556*

        Tirofiban *on page 1496*

Antithrombin Drugs

    Indirect Thrombin Inhibitors

        Heparin (unfractionated) *on page 765*

        Low molecular weight heparins

            Dalteparin *on page 418*

            Enoxaparin *on page 542*

            Tinzaparin *on page 1492*

    Direct Thrombin Inhibitors

        Lepirudin *on page 904*

        Argatroban *on page 136*

    Dicumarols

        Warfarin *on page 1585*

Conventional Antianginal Drugs

    Beta-Blockers

        Atenolol *on page 154*

        Bisoprolol *on page 211*

        Carteolol *on page 274*

        Nadolol *on page 1079*

        Propranolol *on page 1301*

    Nitrates

        Isosorbide Dinitrate *on page 866*

        Isosorbide Mononitrate *on page 868*

        Nitroglycerin *on page 1120*

    Calcium Channel Blockers

        Diltiazem *on page 479*

        Nifedipine *on page 1112*

        Verapamil *on page 1571*

Evaluating Antiplatelet Response

Partial thromboplastin time and bleeding time (IVY) are appropriate measures for platelet dysfunction. Aspirin, ticlopidine (Ticlid®), and other new drugs, such as Clopidogrel (Plavix®), are actually considered antiplatelet drugs, whereas oral Coumadin® is considered an oral anticoagulant. Aspirin works by inhibiting cyclo-oxygenase which is an enzyme involved in the platelet system associated with clot formation. As little as one aspirin (300 mg dose) can result in an alteration in this enzyme pathway. Although aspirin is cleared from the circulation very quickly (within 15-30 minutes), the effect on the life of the platelet may last up to 7-10 days. Most routine dental procedures can be accomplished with no change in these medications using aggressive local hemostasis efforts and prudent treatment planning.

Evaluating Coumadin® Response

The effects of Coumadin® on the coagulation within patients, occur by way of the vitamin K-dependent clotting mechanism and are generally monitored by measuring the prothrombin time known as the PT. Often to prevent venous thrombosis, a patient will be maintained at approximately 1.5 times their normal prothrombin time. Other anticoagulant goals such as prevention of arterial thromboembolism, as in patients with artificial heart valves, may require 2-2.5 times the normal prothrombin time. It is important for the clinician to obtain not only the accurate PT but also the International Normalized Ratio (INR) for the patient. This ratio is calculated by dividing the patient's PT by the mean normal PT for the laboratory, which is determined by using the International Sensitivity Index (ISI) to adjust for the lab's reagents.

The response to oral anticoagulants varies greatly in patients and should be monitored regularly. The dental clinician planning an invasive procedure should consider not only what the patient can tell them from a historical point-of-view, but also when the last monitoring test was performed. In general, most dental procedures can be performed in patients that are 1.5-2.5 times normal or less. Most researchers further suggest that 2.5-3 times normal pose little risk in most dental patients and procedures, but these values may be misleading unless the INR is also determined. When in doubt, the prudent dental clinician would consult with the patient's physician and obtain current prothrombin time and INR in order to evaluate fully and plan for his patients.

Coumadin®-Like Anticoagulants

Dicumarol
Warfarin *on page 1585*

Platelet Aggregation Inhibitors

Aspirin *on page 145*
Clopidogrel *on page 376*
Eptifibatide *on page 556*
Ticlopidine *on page 1486*
Tirofiban *on page 1496*

Anticoagulant, Other

Lepirudin *on page 904*

Antiplatelet Agent

Aspirin and Dipyridamole *on page 150*

Regarding dental management patients that are already taking warfarin, the use of analgesics is implicated as a potential source of drug interaction. In an article by Hayek in *JAMA*, it was found that patients taking warfarin for anticoagulation identified the use of dangerously elevated INRs and the fact was discovered that they concomitantly had been taking acetaminophen (not necessarily with their physician's recommendation). The study of the international normalized ratio (INR) in these patients has indicated that additional factors independently influence the INR, as well as the potential interaction with acetaminophen. Potential effects on the INR are greatest in patients taking acetaminophen at high doses over a protracted time period. Short term pain management with acetaminophen poses little risk. These factors included advanced malignancy, patients who did not take their warfarin properly (therefore, took more than was necessary), changes in oral intake of liquids or solids, acute diarrhea leading to dehydration, alcohol consumption, and vitamin K intake.

The mechanisms of these augmenting factors for enhancement of the INR are that the cytochrome P450 system, present in the liver, is also affected by changes in metabolism associated with these factors. For instance, the metabolism of alcohol in the liver alters its ability to manage the CYP450 enzyme system necessary for warfarin, therefore, enhancing its presence and potentially increasing the half-life of warfarin. As oral intake of nutrients declines in patients with either diarrhea or reduced intake of liquids and/or solids, absorption of vitamin K is reduced and the vitamin K dependent system of metabolism of warfarin changes, therefore increasing warfarin blood levels. These factors, along with the liver metabolism of acetaminophen, have resulted in the increased concern that patients, who may be taking acetaminophen as an analgesic or for other reasons, may be at risk for enhancing or elevating, inadvertently, their anticoagulation effect of warfarin. The dentist should be aware of this potential interaction in prescribing any drug containing acetaminophen or in recommending that a patient use an analgesic for relief of even mild pain on a prolonged basis. Therefore, the dentist must be concerned with these factors and is referred to the discussion in the Oral Pain section *on page 1692* for more consideration (adapted from *JAMA*, March 4, 1998, Vol 279, No 9).

Acetaminophen *on page 31*

Although not used specifically for this purpose, numerous herbal medicines and natural dietary supplements have been associated with inhibition of platelet aggregation or other anticoagulation effects, and therefore may lead to increased bleeding during invasive dental procedures. Current reports include bilberry, bromelain, cat's claw, devil's claw, dong quai, evening primrose, feverfew, garlic (irreversible inhibition), ginger (only at very high doses), ginkgo biloba, ginseng, grape seed, green tea, horse chestnut, and turmeric.

References

Carter G, Goss AN, Lloyd J, et al, "Current Concepts of the Management of Dental Extractions for Patients Taking Warfarin," *Aust Dent J*, 2003, 48(2):89-96.

Jeske AH, Suchko GD, ADA Council on Scientific Affairs and Division of Science, et al, "Lack of a Scientific Basis for Routine Discontinuation of Oral Anticoagulation Therapy Before Dental Treatment," *J Am Dent Assoc*, 2003, 134(11):1492-7.

Little JW, Miller CS, Henry RG, et al, "Antithrombotic Agents: Implications in Dentistry," *Oral Surg Oral Med Oral Pathol Oral Radiol Endod*, 2002, 93(5):544-51.

Lockhart PB, Gibson J, Pond SH, et al, "Dental Management Considerations for the Patient With an Acquired Coagulopathy. Part 2: Coagulopathies From Drugs," *Br Dent J*, 2003, 195(9):495-501.

CARDIOVASCULAR DISEASES (Continued)

HEART FAILURE

Heart failure is a condition in which the heart is unable to pump sufficient blood to meet the needs of the body. It is caused by impaired ability of the cardiac muscle to contract or by an increased workload imposed on the heart. Most frequently, the underlying cause of heart failure is coronary artery disease. Other contributory causes include hypertension, diabetes, idiopathic dilated cardiomyopathy, and valvular heart disease. It is estimated that heart failure affects approximately 5 million Americans. The New York Heart Association functional classification is regarded as the standard measure to describe the severity of a patient's symptom. Class I is characterized by having no limitation of physical activity. There is no dyspnea, fatigue, palpitations, or angina with ordinary physical activity. There is no objective evidence of cardiovascular dysfunction. Class II includes those patients having slight limitation of physical activity. These patients experience fatigue, palpitations, dyspnea, or angina with ordinary physical activity, but are comfortable at rest. There is evidence of minimal cardiovascular dysfunction. Class III is characterized by marked limitation of activity. Less than ordinary physical activity causes fatigue, palpitations, dyspnea, or angina, but patients are comfortable at rest. There is objective evidence of moderately severe cardiovascular dysfunction. Class IV is characterized by the inability to carry out any physical activity without discomfort. Symptoms of heart failure or anginal syndrome may be present even at rest, and any physical activity undertaken increases discomfort. There is objective evidence of severe cardiovascular dysfunction. Drug classes and the specific agents used to treat heart failure are listed in Table 4.

Table 4.
DRUGS USED IN THE TREATMENT OF HEART FAILURE

Angiotensin-Converting Enzyme Inhibitors (ACE)[1]
> Benazepril *on page 185*
> Captopril *on page 257*
> Enalapril *on page 538*
> Fosinopril *on page 707*
> Lisinopril *on page 936*
> Perindopril Erhumine *on page 1216*
> Quinapril *on page 1322*
> Ramipril *on page 1332*
> Trandolapril *on page 1517*

Diuretics
> **Thiazides**
>> Hydrochlorothiazide *on page 776*
> **Loop Diuretics**
>> Furosemide *on page 715*
> **Potassium-Sparing Agents**
>> Spironolactone *on page 1413*

Digitalis Glycosides
> Digoxin *on page 471*
> Digitoxin *on page 471*

Beta-Adrenergic Receptor Blockers
> Bisoprolol *on page 211*
> Carvedilol *on page 275*
> Metoprolol *on page 1030*

Catecholamines
> Dobutamine *on page 493*
> Dopamine

Supplemental Agents
> **Direct-Acting Vasodilators**
>> Hydralazine *on page 775*
>> Nitroglycerin *on page 1120*
>> Nitroprusside *on page 1122*
> **Phosphodiesterase Inhibitors**
>> Inamrinone *on page 827*
>> Milrinone *on page 1048*

[1]Regarded as the cornerstone of treatment of heart failure and should be used routinely and early in all patients.

From USP DI, Volumes I and II, Update, December 1998.

Drug Classes and Specific Agents Used to Treat Heart Failure

Angiotensin-converting enzyme (ACE) inhibitors reduce left ventricular volume and filling pressure while decreasing total peripheral resistance. They induce cardiac output (modestly) and natriuresis. ACE inhibitors are usually used in all patients with heart failure if no contraindication or intolerance exists. This group of drugs is considered the cornerstone of treatment and are used routinely and early if pharmacologic treatment is indicated.

Diuretics increase sodium chloride and water excretion resulting in reduction of preload, thus relieving the symptoms of pulmonary congestion associated with heart failure. They may also reduce myocardial oxygen demand. The thiazides, loop diuretics, and potassium-sparing agents are all useful in reducing preload by way of their diuretic actions.

Digitalis glycosides have been used in the treatment of heart failure for more than 200 years. Digitalis drugs increase cardiac output by a direct positive inotropic action on the myocardium. This increased cardiac output results in decreased venous pressure, reduced heart size, and diminished compensatory tachycardia.

Beta-adrenergic receptor blocking drugs (beta-blockers) are used in the treatment of heart failure because of their beneficial effect in reducing mortality. A meta-analysis of randomized clinical trials showed that the beta-blockers significantly reduced all causes of cardiac-related deaths, with carvedilol (Coreg®) showing the greatest efficacy. The overall risk of death was reduced by over 30%.

Other drugs used in the treatment of heart failure are referred to as supplemental agents. The direct-acting vasodilators reduce excessive vasoconstriction and reduce workload of the failing heart. The catecholamines and phosphodiesterase inhibitors are alternative agents with positive inotropic effects, are effective for short-term therapy, and have not been demonstrated to prolong life during long-term therapy.

Treatment of arrhythmias often can result in oral manifestations including oral ulcerations with drugs such as procainamide, lupus-like lesions, as well as xerostomia.

HYPERTENSION

In the United States, almost 50 million adults, 25-74 years of age, have hypertension. Hypertension is defined as systolic blood pressure ≥140 mm Hg, and/or diastolic pressure >90 mm Hg. People with blood pressure above normal are considered at increased risk of developing damage to the heart, kidney, brain, and eyes, resulting in premature morbidity and mortality.

Recently, the Joint National Committee on Prevention, Detection, Evaluation, and Treatment of High Blood Pressure, released its 7th Report in the summer of 2003. The highlights of the new report are that several of the categories have been renamed to connote changes in philosophy towards earlier treatment and intervention for patients with elevated blood pressure.

Also, there is an increased importance in the elevation of systolic blood pressure for people >50 years of age. The category of high normal blood pressure has now been replaced with the term prehypertension for those patients with systolic blood pressure of 120-139 mm Hg and for those with diastolic blood pressure of 80-89 mm Hg. The remaining stages of hypertension have been broken into simply two categories: Stage 1 and Stage 2. Stage 1 diastolic pressure is 90-99 mm Hg and systolic pressure is 140-159 mm Hg, whereas in Stage 2, diastolic pressure >100 mm Hg or systolic pressure >160 mm Hg are the respective cut-off for treatment decisions. This greatly simplifies the classification of blood pressure.

In addition, the 7th Joint National Committee Report highlights the importance of life style modifications in controlling blood pressure along with pharmacologic intervention. Thiazide diuretics have again been considered one of the most important treatments in uncomplicated hypertension and their benefits of lowering blood pressure have been greatly emphasized. The role of dentistry in detection as well as assisting in compliance for patients, has been clearly emphasized in this report.

The suggested initial goals of drug therapy are the maintenance of an arterial pressure of ≤140/90 mm Hg with concurrent control of other modifiable cardiovascular risk factors. Further reduction to 130/85 mm Hg should be pursued if cardiovascular and cerebrovascular function is not compromised. The Hypertension Optimal Treatment (HOT) randomized trial using patients 50-80 years of age found that the lowest incidence of major cardiovascular events and the lowest risk of cardiovascular mortality occurred at a mean diastolic blood pressure of 82.6 and 86.5 mm Hg respectively.

CARDIOVASCULAR DISEASES *(Continued)*

Table 5.
CLASSIFICATION OF BLOOD PRESSURE
FOR ADULTS ≥18 YEARS OF AGE

BP Classification	Systolic BP (mm Hg)	Diastolic BP (mm Hg)
Normotensive	<120	<80
Prehypertension[1]	120-139	80-89
Stage 1 hypertension[2]	140-159	90-99
Stage 2 hypertension[3]	≥160	≥100

[1]Not taking antihypertensive drugs and not acutely ill. When systolic and diastolic blood pressures fall into different categories, the higher category should be selected to classify the individual's blood pressure status. In addition to classifying stages of hypertension on the basis of average blood pressure levels, clinicians should specify presence or absence of target organ disease and additional risk factors. The specificity is important for risk classification and treatment.

[2]Optimal blood pressure with respect to cardiovascular risk is below 120/80 mm Hg. However, unusually low readings should be evaluated for clinical significance.

[3]Based on the average of two or more readings taken at each of two or more visits after an initial screening.

Adapted from Chobanian AV, Bakris GL, Black HR, et al, Joint National Committee on Prevention, Detection, Evaluation, and Treatment of High Blood Pressure. National Heart, Lung, and Blood Institute; National High Blood Pressure Education Program Coordinating Committee. Seventh Report of the Joint National Committee on Prevention, Detection, Evaluation, and Treatment of High Blood Pressure, *Hypertension*, 2003, 42(6):1206-52.

Table 6.
LIFESTYLE MODIFICATIONS TO MANAGE HYPERTENSION[1-3]

Modification	Recommendation	Approximate Systolic Reduction (Range)
Weight reduction	Maintain normal body weight (body mass index 18.5-24.9 kg/m²)	5-20 mm of mercury/ 10 kg weight loss[4]
Adopt DASH[5] eating plan	Consume a diet rich in fruits, vegetables, and low fat dairy products with a reduced content of saturated and total fat	8-14 mm Hg[6]
Dietary sodium reduction	Reduce dietary sodium intake to ≤100 mmol/day (2.4 g sodium or 6 g sodium chloride)	2-8 mm Hg[7]
Physical activity	Engage in regular aerobic physical activity such as brisk walking (≥30 minutes/day, most days of the week)	4-9 mm Hg[8]
Moderation of alcohol consumption	Limit consumption to ≤2 drinks (1 oz or 30 mL ethanol); (eg, 24 oz beer, 10 oz wine, or 3 oz 80-proof whiskey) per day in most men and to ≤1 drink/day in women and lighter weight people	2-4 mm Hg[9]

[1]Adapted from U.S. Department of Health and Human Services; National Institutes of Health; National Heart, Lung, and Blood Institute; National High Blood Pressure Education Program

[2]Overall cardiovascular risk education can be achieved by cessation of smoking

[3]The effects of implementing these modifications are dose- and time-dependent and could be greater for some people

[4]The trials of Hypertension Prevention Collaborative Research Group; He and colleagues

[5]DASH: Dietary Approaches to Stop Hypertension

[6]Sacks and colleagues; Vollmer and colleagues

[7]Sacks and colleagues; Vollmer and colleagues; Chobanian and Hill

[8]Kelley and Kelley; Whelton and colleagues

[9]Xin and colleagues

CLASSES OF DRUGS USED IN THE TREATMENT OF HYPERTENSION

> Diuretics
> Beta-adrenergic receptor blocking agents (beta-blockers)
> Alpha₁-adrenergic receptor blocking agents (alpha₁-blockers)
> Agents which have both alpha- and beta-adrenergic blocking properties (alpha-/beta-blockers)
> Angiotensin-converting enzyme (ACE) inhibitors
> Angiotensin II receptor blockers
> Calcium channel blocking agents
> Supplemental agents such as central-acting alpha₂-adrenergic receptor agonists and direct-acting peripheral vasodilators.

Table 7 lists the drug categories and representative agents used to treat hypertension. Combination drugs are now available to supply several classes of these drugs.

Table 7.
DRUG CATEGORIES AND REPRESENTATIVE AGENTS USED IN THE TREATMENT OF HYPERTENSION[1]

Diuretics
Thiazide Types
Chlorothiazide *on page 322*
Chlorthalidone *on page 332*
Hydrochlorothiazide *on page 776*
Indapamide *on page 828*
Methyclothiazide *on page 1020*
Metolazone *on page 1030*
Polythiazide *on page 1255*
Loops
Bumetanide *on page 227*
Ethacrynic Acid *on page 590*
Furosemide *on page 715*
Torsemide *on page 1512*
Potassium-Sparing
Amiloride *on page 85*
Spironolactone *on page 1413*
Triamterene *on page 1531*
Potassium-Sparing Combinations
Hydrochlorothiazide and Spironolactone *on page 778*
Hydrochlorothiazide and Triamterene *on page 778*

Beta-Blockers
Cardioselective
Acebutolol *on page 28*
Atenolol *on page 154*
Betaxolol *on page 203*
Bisoprolol *on page 211*
Metoprolol *on page 1030*
Sotalol *on page 1409*
Noncardioselective
Carteolol *on page 274*
Carvedilol *on page 275*
Nadolol *on page 1079*
Penbutolol *on page 1199*
Pindolol *on page 1240*
Propranolol *on page 1301*
Timolol *on page 1489*

Alpha₁-Blocker
Doxazosin *on page 503*
Prazosin *on page 1267*
Reserpine *on page 1340*
Terazosin *on page 1458*

Alpha- / Beta-Blocker
Carvedilol *on page 275*
Labetalol *on page 891*

Angiotensin-Converting Enzyme (ACE) Inhibitors
Benazepril *on page 185*
Captopril *on page 257*
Enalapril *on page 538*
Fosinopril *on page 707*
Lisinopril *on page 936*
Moexipril *on page 1058*
Quinapril *on page 1322*
Ramipril *on page 1332*
Trandolapril *on page 1517*

Angiotensin-Converting Enzyme (ACE) Inhibitor / Diuretic Combination
Captopril and Hydrochlorothiazide *on page 259*
Enalapril and Hydrochlorothiazide *on page 541*
Lisinopril and Hydrochlorothiazide *on page 938*

Angiotensin II Receptor Blockers
Candesartan *on page 252*
Eprosartan *on page 554*
Irbesartan *on page 858*
Losartan *on page 950*
Telmisartan *on page 1451*
Valsartan *on page 1561*

Angiotensin II Receptor Blocker / Diuretic Combination
Candesartan + Hydrochlorothiazide *on page 254*
Irbesartan + Hydrochlorothiazide *on page 860*
Valsartan + Hydrochlorothiazide *on page 1562*

CARDIOVASCULAR DISEASES *(Continued)*

(continued)

Calcium Channel Blockers
Amlodipine *on page 100*
Diltiazem *on page 479*
Felodipine *on page 638*
Isradipine *on page 871*
Nicardipine *on page 1107*
Nifedipine *on page 1112*
Nisoldipine *on page 1117*
Verapamil *on page 1571*
Supplemental Agents
Central-Acting Alpha₂-Agonist
Clonidine *on page 373*
Guanabenz *on page 758*
Guanfacine *on page 758*
Methyldopa *on page 1021*
Direct-Acting Peripheral Vasodilator
Hydralazine *on page 775*
Minoxidil *on page 1051*

[1]Source: USP DI, Volumes I and II, Update, November 1998.

Current Thinking Regarding Antihypertensive Drug Selection

Medications in the first eight categories in Table 7 were held to be equally effective in two large-scale studies reported in the *New England Journal of Medicine* and the *Journal of the American Medical Association*, and that any of the medications could be used initially for monotherapy. According to the Seventh Report of the Joint National Committee on Prevention, Detection, Evaluation, and Treatment of High Blood Pressure (JNC VI), diuretics or beta-blockers are recommended as initial therapy for uncomplicated hypertension. If a diuretic is selected as initial therapy, a thiazide diuretic is preferred in patients with normal renal function. If necessary, potassium replacement or concurrent treatment with a potassium-sparing agent may prevent hypokalemia. Loop diuretics are used in patients with impaired renal function or who cannot tolerate thiazides. Diuretics are well tolerated and inexpensive. They are considered the drugs of choice for treating isolated systolic hypertension in the elderly.

Beta-blockers are the agents of choice in patients with coronary artery disease or supraventricular arrhythmia, and in young patients with hyperdynamic circulation. Beta-blockers are alternatives for initial therapy and are more effective in Caucasian patients than in African-American patients. Beta-blockers are not considered first choice drugs in elderly patients with uncomplicated hypertension. The beta-blocking drug carvedilol also selectively blocks alpha₁ receptors and has been shown to reduce mortality in hypertensive patients.

Alpha₁-adrenergic blocking agents can be used as initial therapy. The alpha₁-blocking agent prazosin and related drugs have an added advantage in treating hypertensive patients with coexisting hyperlipidemia since these medications seem to have beneficial effects on lipid levels. Selective blockade of the post-synaptic alpha₁-receptors by prazosin and related agents reduces peripheral vascular resistance and systemic blood pressure. In addition, all alpha₁-adrenergic blocking agents relieve symptoms of benign prostatic hyperplasia.

ACE inhibitors are the preferred drugs for patients with coexisting heart failure. They are useful as initial therapy in hypertensive patients with kidney damage or diabetes mellitus with proteinuria, and in Caucasian patients. No clinically relevant differences have been found among the available ACE inhibitors. The ACE inhibitors are well tolerated by young, physically active patients, and the elderly. The most common adverse effect of the ACE inhibitors is dry cough. Angiotensin II receptor blockers produce hemodynamic effects similar to ACE inhibitors while avoiding dry cough. These agents are similar to the ACE inhibitors in potency and are useful for initial therapy.

Calcium channel blocking agents are effective as initial therapy in both African-American and Caucasian patients, and are well tolerated by the elderly. These agents inhibit entry of calcium ion into cardiac cells and smooth muscle cells of the coronary and systemic vasculature. Nifedipine (Procardia®) and amlodipine (Norvasc®) are more potent as peripheral vasodilators than diltiazem (Cardizem®). Long-acting formulations of the calcium channel blockers have been shown to be very safe despite some earlier reports that short-acting calcium channel blockers were associated with a 60% increase in heart attacks among hypertensive patients given a short-acting calcium antagonist.

Supplemental antihypertensive agents include the central-acting alpha₂ agonists and direct-acting vasodilators. These agents are less commonly prescribed for initial therapy because of the impressive effectiveness of the other drug groups. Clonidine (Catapres®) lowers blood pressure by activating inhibitory alpha₂ receptors in the CNS, thus reducing sympathetic outflow. It lowers both supine and standing blood pressure by reducing total peripheral resistance. Hydralazine (Apresoline®) reduces blood pressure by directly relaxing arteriolar smooth muscle. Hydralazine is given orally for the management of chronic hypertension, usually with a diuretic and a beta-blocker.

The most common oral side effects of the management of the hypertensive patient are related to the antihypertensive drug therapy. A dry sore mouth can be caused by diuretics and central-acting adrenergic inhibitors. Occasionally, lichenoid reactions can occur in patients taking quinidine and methyldopa. The thiazides are occasionally also implicated. Lupus-like face rashes can be seen in patients taking calcium channel blockers as well.

Table 8.
CARDIOVASCULAR / RESPIRATORY / NERVOUS SYSTEM EFFECTS
CAUSED BY DRUGS USED FOR CARDIOVASCULAR DISORDERS[1]

Agent	Incidence	Adverse Effect
Alpha₁-Blocker		
Prazosin (Minipress®)	*More frequent*	Orthostatic hypotension, dizziness
	Less frequent	Heart Palpitations
	Rare	Angina
Alpha-/ Beta-Blocker		
Carvedilol (Coreg®)	*More frequent*	Bradycardia, postural hypotension, dizziness
	Rare	A-V block, hypertension, hypotension, palpitations, vertigo, nervousness, asthma
Angiotensin-Converting Enzyme (ACE) Inhibitors		
Benazepril (Lotensin®)	*Less frequent*	Dizziness, insomnia, headache
	Rare	Hypotension, bronchitis
Captopril (Capoten®)	*Less frequent*	Tachycardia, insomnia, transient cough, dizziness, headache
	Rare	Hypotension
Enalapril (Vasotec®)	*Less frequent*	Chest pain, palpitations, tachycardia, syncope, dizziness, dyspnea
	Rare	Angina pectoris, asthma
Fosinopril (Monopril®)	*Less frequent*	Orthostatic hypotension, dizziness, cough, headache Syncope, insomnia
	Rare	
Lisinopril (Prinivil®)	*Less frequent*	Hypotension, dizziness
	Rare	Angina pectoris, orthostatic hypotension, rhythm disturbances, tachycardia
Moexipril (Univasc®)	*Less frequent*	Hypotension, peripheral edema, headache, dizziness, fatigue, cough, pharyngitis, upper respiratory infection, sinusitis
	Rare	Chest pain, myocardial infarction, palpitations, arrhythmias, syncope, CVA, orthostatic hypotension, dyspnea, bronchospasm
Perindopril Erbumine (Aceon®)	*Less frequent*	Headache, dizziness, cough[2]
	Rare	Hypotension
Quinapril (Accupril®)	*Less frequent*	Hypotension, dizziness, headache, cough
	Rare	Orthostatic hypotension, angina, insomnia
Ramipril (Altace®)	*Less frequent*	Tachycardia, dizziness, headache, cough
	Rare	Hypotension
Trandolapril (Mavrik®)	*Less frequent*	Tachycardia, headache, dizziness, cough[3]
	Rare	Hypotension
Angiotensin-Converting Enzyme Inhibitor / Diuretic Combination		
Captopril/HCTZ (Capozide®)	*Less frequent*	Tachycardia, palpitations, chest pain, dizziness
	Rare	Hypotension
Angiotensin II Receptor Blockers		
Candesartan (Atacand®)	*Less frequent*	Chest pain, flushing
	Rare	Myocardial infarction, tachycardia, angina, palpitations, dyspnea
Losartan (Cozaar®)	*Less frequent*	Hypotension without reflex tachycardia, dizziness
	Rare	Orthostatic hypotension, angina, A-V block (second degree), CVA, palpitations, tachycardia, sinus bradycardia, flushing, dyspnea
Angiotensin II Receptor Blocker / Diuretic Combination		
Candesartan (Atacand HCT™) + HCTZ	*Less frequent*	Chest pain, flushing
	Rare	Myocardial infarction, tachycardia, angina, palpitations, dyspnea
Irbesartan/HCTZ (Avalide®)		Effects unavailable
Valsartan/HCTZ (Diovan HCT®)		Effects unavailable

CARDIOVASCULAR DISEASES *(Continued)*

Agent	Incidence	Adverse Effect
Antiplatelet / Anticoagulant Agents		
Abciximab (ReoPro®)	*More frequent*	Hypotension, pain
	Less frequent	Bradycardia
Aspirin	*Less frequent or Rare*	Anaphylactoid reaction, bronchospastic allergic reaction
Clopidogrel (Plavix®)	*Less frequent*	Chest pain, edema, hypertension, headache, dizziness, depression, fatigue, dyspnea, rhinitis, bronchitis, coughing, upper respiratory infection, syncope, palpitations, cardiac failure, paresthesia, vertigo, atrial fibrillation, neuralgia
Eptifibatide (Integrilin®)	*More frequent*	Hypotension, bleeding
Ticlopidine (Ticlid®)	*Less frequent*	Dizziness
	Rare	Peripheral neuropathy, angioedema, vasculitis, allergic pneumonitis
Tirofiban (Aggrastat®)	*More frequent*	Bleeding
	Less frequent	Bradycardia, dizziness, headache
Warfarin (Coumadin®)	*Less frequent*	Hemoptysis
	Rare	Fever, purple toes syndrome
Beta-Blockers		
Acebutolol (Sectral®)	*Less frequent*	Chest pain, bradycardia, hypotension, dizziness, dyspepsia, dyspnea
	Rare	Ventricular arrhythmias
Atenolol (Tenormin®)	*Less frequent*	Bradycardia, hypotension, chest pain, dizziness, dyspepsia, dyspnea
	Rare	Ventricular arrhythmias
Betaxolol (Kerlone®)	*Less frequent*	Bradycardia, palpitations, dizziness
	Rare	Chest pain
Bisoprolol (Zebeta®)	*More frequent*	Lethargy
	Less frequent	Hypotension, chest pain, bradycardia, headache, dizziness, insomnia, cough
Labetalol (Normodyne®, Trandate®)	*Less frequent*	Orthostatic hypotension, dizziness, nasal congestion
	Rare	Bradycardia, chest pain
Metoprolol (Lopressor®)	*More frequent*	Dizziness
	Less frequent	Bradycardia, heartburn, wheezing
	Rare	Chest pain, confusion
Nadolol (Corgard®)	*More frequent*	Bradycardia
	Less frequent	Dizziness, dyspepsia, wheezing
	Rare	Congestive heart failure, orthostatic hypotension, confusion, paresthesia
Penbutolol (Levatol®)	*Less frequent*	Congestive heart failure, dizziness
	Rare	Bradycardia, chest pain, hypotension, confusion
Pindolol (Visken®)	*More frequent*	Dizziness
	Less frequent	Congestive heart failure, dyspnea
Propranolol (Inderal®)	*More frequent*	Bradycardia
	Less frequent	Congestive heart failure, dizziness, wheezing
	Rare	Chest pain, hypotension, bronchospasm
Timolol (Blocadren®)	*Less frequent*	Bradycardia, dizziness, dyspnea
	Rare	Chest pain, congestive heart failure
Calcium Channel Blockers		
Amlodipine (Norvasc®)	*Less frequent*	Palpitations, dizziness, dyspnea
	Rare	Hypotension, bradycardia, arrhythmias
Diltiazem (Cardizem®)	*Less frequent*	Bradycardia, dizziness
	Rare	Dyspepsia, paresthesia, tremor
Nifedipine (Procardia®)	*More frequent*	Flushing, dizziness
	Less frequent	Palpitations, hypotension, dyspnea
	Rare	Tachycardia, syncope
Verapamil (Calan®)	*Less frequent*	Bradycardia, congestive heart failure, hypotension
	Rare	Chest pain, hypotension (excessive)
Class I Antiarrhythmics		
Disopyramide (Norpace®)	*More frequent*	Exacerbation of angina pectoris, dizziness
	Less frequent	Hypotension, hypertension, tachycardia, dyspnea
	Rare	Syncope, flushing, hyperventilation
Flecainide (Tambocor™)	*More frequent*	Dizziness, dyspnea
	Less frequent	Palpitations, chest pain, tachycardia, tremor
	Rare	Bradycardia, nervousness, paresthesia
Procainimide (Pronestyl®)	*Less frequent*	Tachycardia, dizziness, lightheadedness
	Rare	Hypotension, confusion, disorientation
Propafenone (Rythmol®)	*More frequent*	Dizziness
	Less frequent	Palpitations, angina, bradycardia, loss of balance, dyspepsia, dyspnea
	Rare	Paresthesia
Quinidine (Quinaglute®)	*Less frequent*	Hypotension, syncope, lightheadedness, wheezing
	Rare	Confusion, vertigo, angina, edema

Agent	Incidence	Adverse Effect
Class III Antiarrhythmics		
Amiodarone (Cordarone®)	More frequent	Dizziness, tremor, paresthesia, dyspnea
	Less frequent	Congestive heart failure, bradycardia, tachycardia
	Rare	Hypotension
Sotalol (Betapace®)	More frequent	Bradycardia, chest pain, palpitations, fatigue, dizziness, lightheadedness, dyspnea
	Less frequent	CHF, hypotension, proarrhythmia, syncope, reduced peripheral circulation, edema, asthma, upper respiratory problems
	Rare	Diaphoresis, clouded sensorium, fever, lack of coordination
Digitalis Glycosides		
Digoxin (Lanoxicaps®, Lanoxin®) Digitoxin	Rare	Atrial tachycardia, sinus bradycardia, ventricular fibrillation, vertigo
Diuretics		
Thiazide type	Rare	Hypotension
Loops	More frequent	Orthostatic hypotension, dizziness
Potassium-sparing	Less frequent	Hypotension, bradycardia, dizziness
	Rare	Flushing
Potassium-sparing combination	Rare	Dizziness
HMG-CoA Reductase Inhibitors		
Atorvastatin Fluvastatin Lovastatin Pravastatin Simvastatin	Less frequent	Headache, dizziness
Nitrates		
Nitroglycerins	More frequent	Postural hypotension, flushing, headache, dizziness
	Rare	Reflex tachycardia, bradycardia, arrhythmia
Supplemental Drugs for Heart Failure		
Inamrinone	Less frequent	Arrhythmia, chest pain
Dobutamine (Dobutrex®)	Less frequent	Tachycardia, chest pain
	Rare	Headache, dyspnea
Hydralazine	More frequent	Tachycardia, headache
	Less frequent	Hypotension, nasal congestion
	Rare	Edema, dizziness
Milrinone (Primacor®)	More frequent	Arrhythmias
	Less frequent	Chest pain
Nitroprusside sodium (Nitropress®)	Less frequent	Palpitations, headache
Supplemental Drugs for Hypertension		
Central-Acting Alpha₂-Agonists		
Clonidine (Catapres®)	More frequent	Dizziness
	Less frequent	Orthostatic hypotension, nervousness/agitation
	Rare	Palpitations, tachycardia, bradycardia, congestive heart failure
Direct-Acting		
Hydralazine	More frequent	Tachycardia, headache
	Less frequent	Hypotension, nasal congestion
	Rare	Edema, dizziness

Legend: % of incidence: More frequent = >10%, less frequent = 1% to 10%, rare = <1%.

[1]Source: Professional package insert for individual agents or United States Pharmacopeial Dispensing Information. *Drug Information for the Health Care Professional*, Vol I, 19th ed, Rockville, MD: The United States Pharmacopeial Convention, Inc, 1999.

[2]Incidence greater in women 3:1.

[3]More frequent in women.

CARDIOVASCULAR DISEASES *(Continued)*

Table 9.
CARDIOVASCULAR DRUGS
DENTAL DRUG INTERACTIONS
AND EFFECTS ON DENTAL TREATMENT

Alpha₁-Blocker	
Prazosin (Minipress®)	Significant orthostatic hypotension a possibility; monitor patient when getting out of dental chair; significant dry mouth in up to 10% of patients.
Alpha- / Beta-Blocker	
Carvedilol (Coreg®)	See Nonselective Beta-Blockers
ACE Inhibitors	The NSAID indomethacin reduces the hypotensive effects of ACE inhibitors. Effects of other NSAIDs such as ibuprofen not considered significant.
Angiotensin-Converting Enzyme Inhibitor / Diuretic Combination	
Captopril/HCTZ (Capozide®)	No effect or complications on dental treatment reported.
Angiotensin II Receptor Blockers	
Candesartan (Atacand®)	No effect or complications on dental treatment reported.
Losartan (Cozaar®)	
Antiplatelet / Anticoagulant Agents	
Aspirin	May cause a reduction in the serum levels of NSAIDs if they are used to manage post-operative pain.
Clopidogrel (Plavix®)	If a patient is to undergo elective surgery and an antiplatelet effect is not desired, clopidogrel should be discontinued 7 days prior to surgery.
Eptifibatide (Integrilin®)	Bleeding may occur while patient is medicated with eptifibatide; platelet function is restored in about 4 hours following discontinuation.
Warfarin (Coumadin®)	Signs of warfarin overdose may first appear as bleeding from gingival tissue; consultation with prescribing physician is advisable prior to surgery to determine temporary dose reduction or withdrawal of medication.
Beta-Blockers	
Cardioselective	Cardioselective beta-blockers (ie, atenolol) have no effect or complications on dental treatment reported.
Noncardioselective	Any of the noncardioselective beta-blockers (ie, nadolol, penbutolol, pindolol, propranolol, timolol) may enhance the pressor response to vasoconstrictor epinephrine resulting in hypertension and reflex bradycardia. Although not reported, it is assumed that similar effects could be caused with levonordefrin (Neo-Cobefrin®). Use either vasoconstrictor with caution in hypertensive patients medicated with noncardioselective beta-adrenergic blockers.
Calcium Channel Blockers	Cause gingival hyperplasia in approximately 1% of the general population taking these drugs. There have been fewer reports with diltiazem and amlodipine than with other CBs such as nifedipine. The hyperplasia will usually disappear with cessation of drug therapy. Consultation with the physician is suggested
Class I Antiarrhythmics	
Disopyramide (Norpace®)	Increased serum levels and toxicity with erythromycin. High incidence of anticholinergic effect manifested as dry mouth and throat.
Flecainide (Tambocor™)	No effects or complications on dental treatment reported.
Procainimide (Pronestyl®)	Systemic lupus-like syndrome has been reported resulting in joint pain and swelling, pains with breathing, skin rash.
Propafenone (Rythmol®)	Greater than 10 % experience significantly reduced salivary flow; taste disturbance, bitter or metallic taste
Quinidine (Quinaglute®)	Secondary anticholinergic effects may decrease salivary flow, especially in middle-aged and elderly patients; known to contribute to caries, periodontal disease, and oral candidiasis.
Class III Antiarrhythmics	
Amiodarone	Bitter or metallic taste has been reported.
Digitalis Glycosides	Use vasoconstrictor with caution due to risk of cardiac arrhythmias. Sensitive gag reflex induced by digitalis drugs may cause difficulty in taking dental impressions.
Diuretics	
Thiazide type	No effects or complications on dental treatment reported.
Loops	NSAIDs may increase chloride and tubular water reuptake to counter-act loop type diuretics.
Potassium-sparing	No effects or complications on dental treatment reported.
Potassium-sparing combination	No effects or complications on dental treatment reported.

HMG-CoA Reductase Inhibitors	Concurrent use of erythromycin, clarithromycin, and some of the statin drugs may result in rhabdomyolysis.
Nitrates	No effects or complications on dental treatment reported.
Supplemental Drugs for Heart Failure	
Inamrinone Milrinone (Primacor®)	No effects or complications on dental treatment reported
Supplemental Drugs for Hypertension	
Central-Acting Alpha$_2$-Agonists	
Clonidine (Catapres®)	Greater than 10% of patients experience significant dry mouth.
Direct-Acting	
Hydralazine	No effect or complications on dental treatment reported.

References

Chobanian AV, Bakris GL, Black HR, et al, "The Seventh Report of the Joint National Committee on Prevention, Detection, Evaluation, and Treatment of High Blood Pressure: The JNC 7 Report," *JAMA*, 2003, 289(19):2560-72.

Chobanian AV and Hill M, "National Heart, Lung, and Blood Institute Workshop on Sodium and Blood Pressure: A Critical Review of Current Scientific Evidence," *Hypertension*, 2000, 35(4):858-63.

"Effects of Weight Loss and Sodium Reduction Intervention on Blood Pressure and Hypertension Incidence in Overweight People With High-Normal Blood Pressure. The Trials of Hypertension Prevention, Phase II. The Trials of Hypertension Prevention Collaborative Research Group," *Arch Intern Med*, 1997, 157(6):657-67.

He J, Whelton PK, Appel LJ, et al, "Long-Term Effects of Weight Loss and Dietary Sodium Reduction on Incidence of Hypertension," *Hypertension*, 2000, 35(2):544-9.

Kelley GA and Kelley KS, "Progressive Resistance Exercise and Resting Blood Pressure: A Meta-Analysis of Randomized Controlled Trials," *Hypertension*, 2000, 35(3):838-43.

Sacks FM, Svetkey LP, Vollmer WM, et al, "Effects on Blood Pressure of Reduced Dietary Sodium and the Dietary Approaches to Stop Hypertension (DASH) Diet. DASH-Sodium Collaborative Research Group," *N Engl J Med*, 2001, 344(1):3-10.

Vollmer WM, Sacks FM, Ard J, et al, "Effects of Diet and Sodium Intake on Blood Pressure: Subgroup Analysis of the DASH-Sodium Trial," *Ann Intern Med*, 2001, 135(12):1019-28.

Whelton SP, Chin A, Xin X, et al, "Effect of Aerobic Exercise on Blood Pressure: A Meta-Analysis of Randomized, Controlled Trials," *Ann Intern Med*, 2002, 136(7):493-503.

Xin X, He J, Frontini MG, et al, "Effects of Alcohol Reduction on Blood Pressure: A Meta-Analysis of Randomized Controlled Trials," *Hypertension*, 2001, 38(5):1112-7.

GASTROINTESTINAL DISORDERS

The oral cavity and related structures comprise the first part of the gastrointestinal tract. Diseases affecting the oral cavity are often reflected in GI disturbances. In addition, the oral cavity may indeed reflect diseases of the GI tract, including ulcers, polyps, and liver and gallbladder diseases. The first oral condition that may reflect or be reflected in GI disturbances is that of taste. Typically, complaints of taste abnormalities are presented to the dentist. The sweet, saline, sour, and bitter taste sensations all vary in quality and intensity and are affected by the olfactory system. Often, anemic conditions are reflected in changes in the tongue, resulting in taste aberrations.

Gastric and duodenal ulcers represent the primary diseases that can reflect themselves in the oral cavity. Gastric reflux and problems with food metabolism often present as acid erosions to the teeth and occasionally, changes in the mucosal surface as well. Patients may be encountered that may be identified, upon diagnosis, as harboring the organism *Helicobacter pylori*. Treatment with antibiotics can oftentimes aid in correcting the ulcerative disease.

Proton Pump and Gastric Acid Secretion Inhibitors

Lansoprazole *on page 896*

Lansoprazole, Amoxicillin, and Clarithromycin *on page 898*

Lansoprazole and Naproxen *on page 898*

Omeprazole *on page 1145*

Pantoprazole *on page 1184*

Histamine H₂ Antagonist

Cimetidine *on page 341*

Famotidine *on page 635*

Nizatidine *on page 1123*

Ranitidine *on page 1334*

The oral aspects of gastrointestinal disease are often nonspecific and are related to the patient's gastric reflux problems. Intestinal polyps occasionally present as part of the "Peutz-Jeghers Syndrome", resulting in pigmented areas of the peri-oral region that resemble freckles. The astute dentist will need to differentiate these from melanin pigmentation, while at the same time encouraging the patient to perhaps seek evaluation for an intestinal disorder.

Diseases of the liver and gallbladder system are complex. Most of the disorders that the dentist is interested in are covered in the section Systemic Viral Diseases *on page 1675*. All of the new drugs, including interferons, are mentioned in this section.

Multiple Drug Regimens for the Treatment of *H. pylori* Infection

Drug	Dosages	Duration of Therapy
H$_2$-receptor antagonist[1] *plus*	Any one given at appropriate dose	4 weeks
Bismuth *on page 210* *plus*	525 mg 4 times/day	2 weeks
Metronidazole *on page 1033* *plus*	250 mg 4 times/day	2 weeks
Tetracycline *on page 1467*	500 mg 4 times/day	2 weeks
Proton pump inhibitor[1] *plus*	Esomeprazole 40 mg once daily	10 days
Clarithromycin *on page 355* *plus*	500 mg twice daily	10 days
Amoxicillin *on page 106*	1000 mg twice daily	10 days
Proton pump inhibitor[1] *plus*	Lansoprazole 30 mg twice daily or Omeprazole 20 mg twice daily	10-14 days
Clarithromycin *on page 355* *plus*	500 mg twice daily	10-14 days
Amoxicillin *on page 106*	1000 mg twice daily	10-14 days
Proton pump inhibitor[1] *plus*	Rabeprazole 20 mg twice daily	7 days
Clarithromycin *on page 355* *plus*	500 mg twice daily	7 days
Amoxicillin *on page 106*	1000 mg twice daily	7 days
Proton pump inhibitor *plus*	Lansoprazole 30 mg twice daily or Omeprazole 20 mg twice daily	2 weeks
Clarithromycin *on page 355* *plus*	500 mg twice daily	2 weeks
Metronidazole *on page 1033*	500 mg twice daily	2 weeks
Proton pump inhibitor *plus*	Lansoprazole 30 mg once daily or Omeprazole 20 mg once daily	2 weeks
Bismuth *on page 210* *plus*	525 mg 4 times/day	2 weeks
Metronidazole *on page 1033* *plus*	500 mg 3 times/day	2 weeks
Tetracycline *on page 1467*	500 mg 4 times/day	2 weeks

[1]FDA-approved regimen

Modified from Howden CS and Hunt RH, "Guidelines for the Management of *Helicobacter pylori* Infection," *AJG*, 1998, 93:2336.

RESPIRATORY DISEASES

Diseases of the respiratory system put dental patients at increased risk in the dental office because of their decreased pulmonary reserve, the medications they may be taking, drug interactions between these medications, medications the dentist may prescribe, and in some patients with infectious respiratory diseases, a risk of disease transmission.

The respiratory system consists of the nasal cavity, the nasopharynx, the trachea, and the components of the lung including, of course, the bronchi, the bronchioles, and the alveoli. The diseases that affect the lungs and the respiratory system can be separated by location of affected tissue. Diseases that affect the lower respiratory tract are often chronic, although infections can also occur. Three major diseases that affect the lower respiratory tract are often encountered in the medical history for dental patients. These include chronic bronchitis, emphysema, and asthma. Diseases that affect the upper respiratory tract are usually of the infectious nature and include sinusitis and the common cold. The upper respiratory tract infections may also include a wide variety of nonspecific infections, most of which are also caused by viruses. Influenza produces upper respiratory type symptoms and is often caused by orthomyxoviruses. Herpangina is caused by the Coxsackie type viruses and results in upper respiratory infections in addition to pharyngitis or sore throat. One serious condition, known as croup, has been associated with *Haemophilus influenzae* infections. Other more serious infections might include respiratory syncytial virus, adenoviruses, and parainfluenza viruses.

The respiratory symptoms that are often encountered in both upper respiratory and lower respiratory disorders include cough, dyspnea (difficulty in breathing), the production of sputum, hemoptysis (coughing up blood), a wheeze, and occasionally chest pain. One additional symptom, orthopnea (difficulty in breathing when lying down), is often used by the dentist to assist in evaluating the patient with the condition, pulmonary edema. This condition results from either respiratory disease or congestive heart failure.

No effective drug treatments are available for the management of many of the upper respiratory tract viral infections. However, amantadine (sold under the brand name Symmetrel®) is a synthetic drug given orally (200 mg/day) and has been found to be effective against some strains of influenza. Treatment other than for influenza includes supportive care products, available over-the-counter. These might include antihistamines for symptomatic relief of the upper respiratory congestion, antibiotics to combat secondary bacterial infections, and in severe cases, fluids, when patients have become dehydrated during the illness (see Pharmacologic Category Index for selection). The treatment of herpangina may include management of the painful ulcerations of the oropharynx. The dentist may become involved in managing these lesions in a similar way to those seen in other acute viral infections (see Systemic Viral Diseases *on page 1675*).

SINUSITIS

Sinusitis also represents an upper respiratory infection that often comes under the purview of the practicing dentist. Acute sinusitis, characterized by nasal obstruction, fever, chills, and midface head pain, may be encountered by the dentist and discovered as part of a differential workup for other facial or dental pain. Chronic sinusitis may likewise produce similar dental symptoms. Dental drugs of choice may include ephedrine or nasal drops, antihistamines, and analgesics. These drugs sometimes require supplementation with antibiotics. Most commonly, broad spectrum antibiotics such as ampicillin are prescribed. These are often combined with antral lavage to re-establish drainage from the sinus area. Surgical intervention, such as a Caldwell-Luc procedure opening into the sinus, is rarely necessary and many of the second generation antibiotics, such as cephalosporins, are used successfully in treating the acute and chronic sinusitis patient (see Antibiotic Prophylaxis *on page 1680*).

Gatifloxacin *on page 724*

Moxifloxacin *on page 1069*

LOWER RESPIRATORY DISEASES

Lower respiratory tract diseases, including asthma, chronic bronchitis, and emphysema are often identified in dental patients. Asthma is an intermittent respiratory disorder that produces recurrent bronchial smooth muscle spasm, inflammation of the bronchial mucosa, and hypersecretion of mucus. The incidence of childhood asthma appears to be increasing and may be related to the presence of pollutants such as sulfur dioxide and indoor cigarette smoke. The end result is widespread narrowing of the airways and decreased ventilation with increased airway resistance, especially to expiration. Asthmatic patients often suffer from asthmatic attacks when stimulated by respiratory tract infections, exercise, and cold air. Medications such as aspirin and some NSAIDs, as well as cholinergic and beta-adrenergic blocking drugs, can also trigger asthmatic attacks in addition to chemicals, smoke, and emotional anxiety.

The classical chronic obstructive pulmonary diseases (COPD) of chronic bronchitis and emphysema are both characterized by chronic airflow obstructions during normal ventilatory efforts. They often occur in combination in the same patient and their treatment is similar. One common finding is that the patient is often a smoker. The dentist can play a role in reinforcement of smoking cessation in patients with chronic respiratory diseases.

Treatments include a variety of drugs depending on the severity of the symptoms and the respiratory compromise upon full respiratory evaluation. Patients who are having acute and chronic obstructive pulmonary attacks may be susceptible to infection and antibiotics such as penicillin, ampicillin, tetracycline, or sulfamethoxazole-trimethoprim are often used to eradicate susceptible infective organisms. Corticosteroids, as well as a wide variety of respiratory stimulants, are available in inhalant and/or oral forms. In patients using inhalant medication, oral candidiasis is occasionally encountered.

Amantadine *on page 81*
Analgesics
Antibiotics
Antihistamines
Decongestants
Epinephrine *on page 546*
Gatifloxacin *on page 724*
Moxifloxacin *on page 1069*

SPECIFIC DRUGS USED IN THE TREATMENT OF CHRONIC RESPIRATORY CONDITIONS

Beta$_2$-Selective Agonists

Albuterol *on page 58*
Metaproterenol *on page 1000*
Pirbuterol *on page 1248*
Salmeterol *on page 1375*
Terbutaline *on page 1460*

Methylxanthines

Aminophylline *on page 89*
Theophylline *on page 1473*

Mast Cell Stabilizer

Cromolyn *on page 397*
Nedocromil *on page 1095*

Corticosteroids

Beclomethasone *on page 183*
Dexamethasone *on page 439*
Flunisolide *on page 667*
Fluticasone *on page 686*
Mometasone Furoate *on page 1060*
Prednisone *on page 1271*
Triamcinolone *on page 1526*

Anticholinergics

Ipratropium *on page 857*

Leukotriene Receptor Antagonists

Montelukast *on page 1062*
Zafirlukast *on page 1590*

5-Lipoxygenase Inhibitors

Zileuton *on page 1596*

Other respiratory diseases include tuberculosis and sarcoidosis which are considered to be restrictive granulomatous respiratory diseases (see Tuberculosis *on page 1673*). Sarcoidosis is a condition that at one time was thought to be similar to tuberculosis, however, it is a multisystem disorder of unknown origin which has as a characteristic lymphocytic and mononuclear phagocytic accumulation in epithelioid granulomas within the lung. It occurs worldwide but shows a slight increased prevalence in temperate climates. The treatment of sarcoidosis is usually one that corresponds to its usually benign course, however, many patients are placed on corticosteroids at the level of 40-60 mg of prednisone daily. This treatment is continued for a protracted period of time. As in any disease requiring steroid therapy, consideration of adrenal suppression is necessary. Alteration of steroid dosage prior to stressful dental procedures may be necessary, usually increasing the steroid dosage prior to and during the stressful procedures and then gradually returning the patient to the original dosage over several days. Many dentists prefer to use the Medrol® Dosepak®, however, consultation with the patient's physician regarding dose selection is always advised. Even in the absence of evidence of adrenal suppression, consultation with the prescribing physician for appropriate dosing and timing of procedures is advisable.

Prednisone *on page 1271*

RESPIRATORY DISEASES *(Continued)*

RELATIVE POTENCY OF ENDOGENOUS AND SYNTHETIC CORTICOSTEROIDS

Agent	Equivalent Dose (mg)
Short-Acting (8-12 h)	
Cortisol	20
Cortisone acetate	25
Intermediate-Acting (18-36 h)	
Prednisolone	5
Prednisone	5
Methylprednisolone	4
Triamcinolone	4
Long-Acting (36-54 h)	
Betamethasone	0.75
Dexamethasone	0.75

Potential drug interactions for the respiratory disease patient exist. An acute sensitivity to aspirin-containing drugs and some of the nonsteroidal anti-inflammatory drugs is a threat for the asthmatic patient. Barbiturates and narcotics may occasionally precipitate asthmatic attacks as well. Erythromycin, clarithromycin, and ketoconazole are contraindicated in patients who are taking theophylline due to potential enhancement of theophylline toxicity. Patients that are taking steroid preparations as part of their respiratory therapy may require alteration in dosing prior to stressful dental procedures. The physician should be consulted.

> Barbiturates
> Clarithromycin *on page 355*
> Erythromycin *on page 562*
> Ketoconazole *on page 880*

ENDOCRINE DISORDERS AND PREGNANCY

The human endocrine system manages metabolism and homeostasis. Numerous glandular tissues produce hormones that act in broad reactions with tissues throughout the body. Cells in various organ systems may be sensitive to the hormone, or they release, in reaction to the hormone, a second hormone that acts directly on another organ. Diseases of the endocrine system may have importance in dentistry. For the purposes of this section, we will limit our discussion to diseases of the thyroid tissues, diabetes mellitus, and conditions requiring the administration of synthetic hormones, and pregnancy.

THYROID

Thyroid diseases can be classified into conditions that cause the thyroid to be overactive (hyperthyroidism) and those that cause the thyroid to be underactive (hypothyroidism). Clinical signs and symptoms associated with hyperthyroidism may include goiter, heat intolerance, tremor, weight loss, diarrhea, and hyperactivity. Thyroid hormone production can be tested by TSH levels and additional screens may include radioactive iodine uptake or a pre-T_4 (tetraiodothyronine, thyroxine) assay or iodine index or total serum T_3 (triiodothyronine). The results of thyroid function tests may be altered by ingestion of antithyroid drugs such as propylthiouracil, estrogen-containing drugs, and organic and inorganic iodides. When a diagnosis of hyperthyroidism has been made, treatment usually begins with antithyroid drugs which may include propranolol coupled with radioactive iodides as well as surgical procedures to reduce thyroid tissue. Generally, the beta-blockers are used to control cardiovascular effects of excessive T_4. Propylthiouracil or methimazole are the most common antithyroid drugs used. The dentist should be aware that epinephrine is definitely contraindicated in patients with uncontrolled hyperthyroidism.

Diseases and conditions associated with hypothyroidism may include bradycardia, drowsiness, cold intolerance, thick dry skin, and constipation. Generally, hypothyroidism is treated with replacement thyroid hormone until a euthyroid state is achieved. Various preparations are available, the most common is levothyroxine, commonly known as Synthroid® or Levothroid®, and is generally the drug of choice for thyroid replacement therapy.

Drugs to Treat Hypothyroidism

Levothyroxine *on page 917*
Liothyronine *on page 934*
Liotrix *on page 935*
Thyroid *on page 1482*

Drugs to Treat Hyperthyroidism

Methimazole *on page 1008*
Potassium Iodide *on page 1260*
Propranolol *on page 1301*
Propylthiouracil *on page 1305*

DIABETES

Diabetes mellitus refers to a condition of prolonged hyperglycemia associated with either abnormal production or lack of production of insulin. Commonly known as Type 1 diabetes, insulin-dependent diabetes (IDDM) is a condition where there are absent or deficient levels of circulating insulin therefore triggering tissue reactions associated with prolonged hyperglycemia. The kidney's attempt to excrete the excess glucose and the organs that do not receive adequate glucose essentially are damaged. Small vessels and arterial vessels in the eye, kidney, and brain are usually at the greatest risk. Generally, blood sugar levels between 70-120 mg/dL are considered to be normal. Inadequate insulin levels allow glucose to rise to greater than the renal threshold which is 180 mg/dL, and such elevations prolonged lead to organ damage.

The goals of treatment of the diabetic are to maintain metabolic control of the blood glucose levels and to reduce the morbid effects of periodic hyperglycemia. Insulin therapy is the primary mechanism to attain management of consistent insulin levels. Insulin preparations are categorized according to their duration of action. Generally, NPH or intermediate-acting insulin and long-acting insulin can be used in combination with short-acting or regular insulin to maintain levels consistent throughout the day.

In Type 2 or noninsulin-dependent diabetes (NIDDM), the receptor for insulin in the tissues is generally down regulated and the glucose, therefore, is not utilized at an appropriate rate. There is perhaps a stronger genetic basis for noninsulin-dependent diabetes than for Type 1. Treatment of the diabetes Type 2 patient is generally directed toward early nonpharmacologic intervention, mainly weight reduction, moderate exercise, and lower plasma-glucose concentrations. Oral hypoglycemic agents as seen in the list below are often used to maintain blood sugar levels. Thirty percent of Type 2

ENDOCRINE DISORDERS AND PREGNANCY *(Continued)*

diabetics require insulin, as well as, oral hypoglycemics in order to manage their diabetes. Generally, the two classes of oral hypoglycemics are the sulfonylureas and the biguanides. The sulfonylureas are prescribed more frequently and they stimulate beta cell production of insulin, increase glucose utilization, and tend to normalize glucose metabolism in the liver. The uncontrolled diabetic may represent a challenge to the dental practitioner.

Glycosylated hemoglobin or glycol-hemoglobin assays have emerged as a "gold standard" by which glycemic control is measured in diabetic patients. The test does not rely on the patient's ability to monitor their daily blood glucose levels and is not influenced by acute changes in blood glucose or by the interval since the last meal. Glycohemoglobin is formed when glucose reacts with hemoglobin A in the blood and is composed of several fractions. Numerous assay methods have been developed, however, they vary in their precision. Dental clinicians are advised to be aware of the laboratory's particular standardization procedures when requesting glycosylated hemoglobin values. One major advantage of the glycosylated hemoglobin assay is that it provides an overview of the level of glucose in the life span of the red blood cell population in the patient, and therefore is a measure of overall glycemic control for the previous six to twelve weeks. Thus, clinicians use glycosylated hemoglobin values to determine whether their patient is under good control, on average. These assays have less value in medication dosing decisions. Blood glucose monitoring methods are actually better in that respect. The values of glycosylated hemoglobin are expressed as a percentage of the total hemoglobin in the red blood cell population and a normal value is considered to be <6%. The goal is generally for diabetic patients to remain at <7% and values >8% would constitute a worrisome signal. Medical conditions such as anemias or any red blood cell disease, numerous levels of myelosuppression, or pregnancy can artificially lower glycosylated hemoglobin values.

See Insulin Regular *on page 841*

Oral Hypoglycemic Agents

Acarbose *on page 28*

Chlorpropamide *on page 331*

Glimepiride *on page 738*

Glipizide *on page 740*

Glyburide *on page 744*

Glyburide and Metformin *on page 745*

Metformin *on page 1001*

Miglitol *on page 1046*

Nateglinide *on page 1094*

Repaglinide *on page 1339*

Tolazamide *on page 1501*

Tolbutamide *on page 1502*

Adjunct Therapy

Metoclopramide *on page 1029*

Oral manifestations of uncontrolled diabetes might include abnormal neutrophil function resulting in a poor response to periodontal pathogens. Increased risk of gingivitis and periodontitis in these patients is common. Candidiasis is also a frequent occurrence. Denture-sore mouth may be more prominent. Poor wound-healing following extractions may be one of the complications encountered.

HORMONAL THERAPY

Two uses of hormonal supplementation include oral contraceptives and estrogen replacement therapy. Drugs used for contraception interfere with fertility by inhibiting release of follicle stimulating hormone, luteinizing hormone, and by preventing ovulation. There are few oral side effects; however, moderate gingivitis, similar to that seen during pregnancy, has been reported. The dentist should be aware that decreased effect of oral contraceptives has been reported with most antibiotics (see individual monographs for specific details). It is therefore recommended that dental professionals, when prescribing antibiotics to oral contraceptive users, advise them of this interaction and suggest consulting their physician for additional barrier contraception during antibiotic therapy.

The combination estradiol cypionate and medroxyprogesterone acetate has recently been approved. It is a single monthly injection and has similar warnings and guidelines. However, it's use with antibiotics have not been firmly established. Therefore, discussion/consultation with the patient's OB/GYN physician is indicated.

Drugs commonly encountered include:

Estradiol *on page 574*
Levonorgestrel *on page 916*
Medroxyprogesterone *on page 972*
Mestranol and Norethindrone *on page 999*
Norethindrone *on page 1125*
Norgestrel *on page 1127*

Estrogens or derivatives are usually prescribed as replacement therapy following menopause or cyclic irregularities and to inhibit osteoporosis. The following list of drugs may interact with antidepressants and barbiturates. New tissue-specific estrogens like Evista® may help with the problem of osteoporosis.

Estrogens (Conjugated/Equine) *on page 580*
Estrogens (Conjugated A/Synthetic) *on page 578*
Estrogens (Esterified) *on page 584*
Estrogens (Conjugated/Equine) and Medroxyprogesterone *on page 583*
Estrogens (Esterified) and Methyltestosterone *on page 585*
Estropipate *on page 586*
Raloxifene *on page 1329*

PREGNANCY

Normal endocrine and physiologic functions are altered during pregnancy. Endogenous estrogens and progesterone increase and placental hormones are secreted. Thyroid stimulating hormone and growth hormone also increase. Cardiovascular changes can result and increased blood volume can lead to blood pressure elevations and transient heart murmurs. Generally, in a normal pregnancy, oral gingival changes will be limited to gingivitis. Alteration of treatment plans might include limiting administration of all drugs to emergency procedures only during the first and third trimesters and medical consultation regarding the patients' status for all elective procedures. Limiting dental care throughout pregnancy to preventive procedures is not unreasonable. The effects on dental treatment of the "morning after pill" (Plan B® and PREVEN®) and the abortifacient, mifepristone *on page 1045*, have not been documented at this time.

HIV INFECTION AND AIDS

Human immunodeficiency virus (HIV) represents agents HIV-1 and HIV-2 that produce a devastating systemic disease. The virus causes disease by leading to elevated risk of infections in patients and, from our experience over the last 18 years, there clearly are oral manifestations associated with these patients. Also, there has been a revolution in infection control in our dental offices over the last two decades due to our expanding knowledge of this infectious agent. Infection control practices have been elevated to include all of the infectious agents with which dentists often come into contact. These might include, in addition to HIV, hepatitis viruses (of which the serotypes include A, B, C, D, E, F, and G; see Occupational Exposure to Bloodborne Pathogens (Standard/Universal Precautions)*on page 1770*), the herpes viruses (see Systemic Viral Diseases *on page 1675*); STDs such as syphilis, gonorrhea, and papillomavirus (see Sexually-Transmitted Diseases *on page 1674*).

Acquired immunodeficiency syndrome (AIDS) has been recognized since early 1981 as a unique clinical syndrome manifest by opportunistic infections or by neoplasms complicating the underlying defect in the cellular immune system. These defects are now known to be brought on by infection and pathogenesis with human immunodeficiency virus 1 or 2 (HIV-1 is the predominant serotype identified). The major cellular defect brought on by infection with HIV is a depletion of T-cells, primarily the sub-type, T-helper cells, known as CD4+ cells. Over these years, our knowledge regarding HIV infection and the oral manifestations often associated with patients with HIV or AIDS, has increased dramatically. Populations of individuals known to be at high risk of HIV transmission include homosexuals, intravenous drug abuse patients, transfusion recipients, patients with other sexually transmitted diseases, and patients practicing promiscuous sex.

The definitions of AIDS have also evolved over this period of time. The natural history of HIV infection along with some of the oral manifestations can be reviewed in Table 1. The risk of developing these opportunistic infections increases as the patient progresses to AIDS.

Table 1.
NATURAL HISTORY OF HIV INFECTION/ORAL MANIFESTATIONS

Time From Transmission (Average)	Observation	CD4 Cell Count
0	Viral transmissions	Normal: 1000 ($\pm$500/mm³)
2-4 weeks	Self-limited infectious mononucleosis-like illness with fever, rash, leukopenia, mucocutaneous ulcerations (mouth, genitals, etc), thrush	Transient decrease
6-12 weeks	Seroconversion (rarely requires ≥3 months for seroconversion)	Normal
0-8 years	Healthy/asymptomatic HIV infection; peripheral/persistent generalized lymphadenopathy; HPV, thrush, OHL; RAU, periodontal diseases, salivary gland diseases; dermatitis	≥500/mm³ gradual reduction with average decrease of 50-80/mm³/year
4-8 years	Early symptomatic HIV infection previously called (AIDS-related complex): Thrush, vaginal candidiasis (persistent, frequent and/or severe), cervical dysplasia/CA Hodgkin's lymphoma, B-cell lymphoma, oral hairy leukoplakia, salivary gland diseases, ITP, xerostomia, dermatitis, shingles; RAU, herpes simplex, HPV, bacterial infections, periodontal diseases, molluscum contagiosum, other physical symptoms: fever, weight loss, fatigue	≥300-500/mm³
6-10 years	AIDS: Wasting syndrome, *Candida* esophagitis, Kaposi's sarcoma, HIV-associated dementia, disseminated *M. avium*, Hodgkin's or B-cell lymphoma, herpes simplex >30 days; PCP; cryptococcal meningitis, other systemic fungal infections; CMV	<200/mm³

Natural history indicates course of HIV infection in absence of antiretroviral treatment. Adapted from Bartlett JG, "A Guide to HIV Care from the AIDS Care Program of the Johns Hopkins Medical Institutions," 2nd ed.

PCP -*Pneumocystis carinii* pneumonia; ITP -idiopathic thrombocytopenia purpura; HPV - human papilloma virus; OHL - oral hairy leukoplakia; RAU - recurrent aphthous ulcer

Patients with HIV infection and/or AIDS are seen in dental offices throughout the country. In general, it is the dentist's obligation to treat HIV individuals including patients of record and other patients who may seek treatment when the office is accepting new patients. These patients are protected under the Americans with Disabilities Act and the dentist has an obligation as described. Two excellent publications, one by the American Dental Association and the other by the American Academy of Oral Medicine, outline the dentist's responsibility as well as a very detailed explanation of dental management protocols for HIV patients. These protocols, however, are evolving just as our knowledge of HIV has evolved. New drugs and their interactions present the dentist with continuous need for updates regarding the appropriate management of HIV patients. Diagnostic tests, including determining viral load in combination with the CD4 status, now are used to modify a patient's treatment in ways that allow them to remain relatively illness-free for longer periods of time. This places more of a responsibility on the dental practice team to be aware of drug changes, of new drugs, and of the appropriate oral management in such patients.

Our knowledge of AIDS allows us to properly treat these patients while protecting ourselves, our staff, and other patients in the office. All types of infectious disease require consistent practices in our dental offices known as Standard/Universal Precautions (see Occupational Exposure to Bloodborne Pathogens Standard/Universal Precautions *on page 1770*). The office team that utilizes these precautions appropriately is well protected against passage of infectious agents. These agents include sexually transmitted disease agents, the highly virulent hepatitis viruses, and the less virulent but always worrisome HIV. In general, an office that is practicing standard/universal precautions is one that is considered safe for patients and staff. Throughout this spectrum, HIV is placed somewhere in the middle, in terms of infection risk in the dental office. Other sexually transmitted diseases and infectious diseases such as tuberculosis represent a greater threat to the dentist than HIV itself. However, due to the grave danger of HIV infection, many of our precautions have been instituted to assist the dentist in protecting himself, his staff, and other patients in situations where the office may be involved in treating a patient that is HIV positive.

As in the management of all medically compromised patients, the appropriate care of HIV patients begins with a complete and thorough history. This history must allow the dentist to identify risk factors in the development of HIV, as well as, identify those patients known to be HIV positive. Knowledge of all medications prescribed to patients at risk is also important.

The current antiretroviral therapy used to treat patients with HIV infection and/or AIDS includes three primary classifications of drugs. These are the nucleoside analogs, protease inhibitors, and the non-nucleoside/nucleotide analogs (analogs refers to chemicals that can substitute competitively for naturally produced cell components such as found in DNA, RNA, or proteins). The newest drugs include several nucleoside analogs, abacavir (Ziagen®), subprotease inhibitors, amprenavir, and several non-nucleoside analogs, efavirenz (Sustiva®), and adefovir. Finding the perfect "cocktail" of anti-HIV medications still eludes clinicians. This is partly due to the fact that therapies are still too novel and the patient's years too few to study. Numerous recently-published studies have indicated that combinations of drugs are far better than individual drug therapy. Several of these studies have looked at two drug combinations, particularly between nucleoside analogs, in combination with protease inhibitors. The newer drugs (non-nucleoside analogs) have added the possibility of a triple "cocktail". Recently several studies indicated that this three-drug combination may be the best in managing HIV infection.

When HIV was first discovered, the efforts for monitoring HIV infection focused on the CD4 blood levels and the ratios between the helper cells, suppressor cells within the patient's immune system. These markers were used to indicate success or failure of drug therapies as patients moved through HIV pathogenesis toward AIDS. More recently, however, the advent of protease inhibitors has allowed clinicians to monitor the actual presence of viral RNA within the patient and the term viral load has become the focus of therapy monitoring. The availability of better therapies and our rapidly expanding knowledge of molecular biology of the HIV virus have created new opportunities to control the AIDS epidemic. Cases can be monitored quite closely looking at the number of copy units or virions within the patient's bloodstream as an indication in combination with other infections and/or declining or increasing CD4 numbers to establish prognostic values for the patient's success. Long-term survival of patients infected with HIV has been accomplished by monitoring and adjusting therapy to these numbers.

Comprehensive coordinated approaches, that have been advocated by researchers, have sought to establish national standards for HIV reporting, greater access to effective newly approved medications, improved access to individual physicians treating HIV patients, and continued protection of patient's privacy. These goals allow the reporting of studies that suggest that combination therapies, some of which have been tried in less controlled individual patient treatments, may prove useful in larger populations of HIV-infected individuals. As these studies are reported, the dental clinician should be aware that patients' drug therapies change rapidly, various combinations may be tried, and the side effects and interactions as described in the chapter on drug interactions and the CYP system will also emerge. The dentist must be aware of these potential interactions with seemingly innocuous drugs such as clarithromycin, erythromycin, and some of the sedative drugs that a dentist may utilize in their practice as well as some of the analgesics. These drug interactions may be the most important part of monitoring that the dentist provides in helping to manage a situation. Some of the antiviral drugs more commonly used for HIV, AIDS, Asymptomatic, CD4 <500, and the newer drugs (ie, protease inhibitors, nucleoside analogs, and non-nucleoside nucleotide analogs) are listed in Table 2.

HIV INFECTION AND AIDS *(Continued)*

Table 2. EXAMPLES OF DRUGS

Nucleoside Analogs	Protease Inhibitors	Non-nucleoside / Nucleotide Analogs
Zidovudine	Saquinavir	Nevirapine
(Retrovir®, AZT, SDV)	(Invirase®)	(Viramune®)
Didanosine	Ritonavir	Delavirdine
(Videx®, ddi)	(Norvir®)	(Rescriptor®)
Zalcitabine	Indinavir	Efavirenz
(Hivid®, ddc)	(Crixivan®)	(Sustiva®)
Stavudine	Nelfinavir	Adefovir
(Zerit®, d4T)	(Viracept®)	(HepSera™)
Lamivudine	Amprenavir	
(Epivir®)	(Agenerase®)	
Abacavir	Fosamprenavir	
(Ziagen®)	(Lexiva™)	

The presence of other infections is an important part of the health history. Appropriate medical consultation may be mandated after a health history in order to accomplish a complete evaluation of the patients at risk. Uniformity in the taking of a history from a patient is the dentist's best plan for all patients so that no selectivity or discrimination can be implicated.

An appropriate review of symptoms may also identify oral and systemic conditions that may be present in aggressive HIV disease. Medical physical examination may reveal pre-existing or developing intra- or extra-oral signs/symptoms of progressive disease. Aggressive herpes simplex, herpes zoster, papillomavirus, Kaposi's sarcoma or lymphoma are among the disorders that might be identified. In addition to these, intra-oral examination may raise suspicion regarding fungal infections, angular cheilitis, squamous cell carcinoma, and recurrent aphthous ulcers. The dentist should be vigilant in all patients regardless of HIV risk.

It will always be up to the dental practitioner to determine whether testing for HIV should be recommended following the history and physical examination of a new patient. Because of the severe psychological implications of learning of HIV positivity for a patient, the dentist should be aware that there are appropriate referral sites where psychological counseling and appropriate discrete testing for the patient is available. The dentist's office should have these sites available for referral should the patient be interested. Candid discussions, however, with the patient regarding risk factors and/or other signs or symptoms in their history and physical condition that may indicate a higher HIV risk than the normal population, should be an area the dentist feels comfortable in broaching with any new patient. Oftentimes, it is appropriate to recommend testing for other infectious diseases should risk factors be present. For example, testing for hepatitis B may be appropriate for the patient and along with this the dentist could recommend that the patient consider HIV testing. Because of the legal issues involved, anonymity for HIV testing may be appropriate and it is always up to the patient to follow the doctor's recommendations.

When a patient has either given a positive history of knowing that they are HIV positive or it has been determined after referral for consultation, the dentist should be aware of the AIDS-defining illnesses. Of course, current medical status and drug therapy that the patient may be undergoing is of equal importance. The dentist, through medical consultation and regular follow-up with the patient's physician, should be made aware of the CD4 count (Table 3), the viral load, and the drugs that the patient is taking. The presence of other AIDS-defining illnesses as well as complications, such as higher risk of endocarditis and the risk of other systemic infections such as tuberculosis, are extremely important for the dentist. These may make an impact on the dental treatment plan in terms of the selection of preprocedural antibiotics or the use of oral medications to treat opportunistic infections in or around the oral cavity.

Table 3. CD4+ LYMPHOCYTE COUNT AND PERCENTAGE AS RELATED TO THE RISK OF OPPORTUNISTIC INFECTION

CD4+ Cells/mm³	CD4+ Percentage[1]	Risk of Opportunistic Infection
>600	32-60	No increased risk
400-500	<29	Initial immune suppression
200-400	14-28	Appearance of opportunistic infections, some may be major
<200	<14	Severe immune suppression. AIDS diagnosis. Major opportunistic infections. Although variable, prognosis for surviving greater than 3 years is poor
<50	—	Although variable, prognosis for surviving greater than 1 year is poor

[1]Several studies have suggested that the CD4+ percentage demonstrates less variability between measurements, as compared to the absolute CD4+ cell count. CD4+ percentages may therefore give a clearer impression of the course of disease.

Adapted from Glick M and Silverman S, "Dental Management of HIV-Infected Patients," *J Am Dent Assoc* (Supplement to Reviewers), 1995.

AIDS-defining illnesses such as candidiasis, recurrent pneumonia, or lymphoma are clearly important to the dentist. Chemotherapy that might be being given to the patient for treatment for any or all of these disorders can have implications in terms of the patient's response to simple dental procedures.

Drug therapies have become complex in the treatment of HIV/AIDS. Because of the moderate successes with protease inhibitors and the drug combination therapies, more patients are living longer and receiving more dental care throughout their lives. Drug therapies are often tailored to the current CD4 count in combination with the viral load. In general, patients with high CD4 counts are usually at lower risk for complications in the dental office than patients with low CD4 counts. However, the presence of a high viral load with or without a stable CD4 count may be indicative or a more rapid progression of the HIV/AIDS disease process than had previously been thought. Patients with a high viral load and a declining CD4 count are considered to have the greatest risk and the poorest prognosis of all the groups.

Other organ damage, such as liver compromise potentially leading to bleeding disorders, can be found as the disease progresses to AIDS. Liver dysfunction may be related to pre-existing hepatic diseases due to previous infection with a hepatitis virus such as hepatitis B or other drug toxicities associated with the treatment of AIDS. The dentist must have available current prothrombin and partial thromboplastin times (PT and PTT) in order to accurately evaluate any risk of bleeding abnormality. Platelet count and liver function studies are also important. Potential drug interactions include some antibiotics, as well as any anticoagulating drugs, which may be contraindicated in such patients. It may be necessary to avoid NSAIDs, as well as aspirin. (See Pharmacology of Drug Metabolism and Interactions *on page 1754*).

The use of preprocedural antibiotics is another issue in the HIV patient. As the absolute neutrophil count declines during the progression of AIDS, the use of antibiotics as a preprocedural step prior to dental care may be necessary. If protracted treatment plans are necessary, the dentist should receive updated information as the patient receives such from their physician. It is always important that the dentist have current CD4 counts, viral load assay, as well as liver function studies, AST and ALT, and bleeding indicators including platelet count, PT, and PTT. If any other existing conditions such as cardiac involvement or joint prostheses are involved, antibiotic coverage may also be necessary. However, these determinations are no different than in the non-HIV population and this subject is covered in Antibiotic Prophylaxis - Preprocedural Guidelines for Dental Patients *on page 1680*. Use the table of Normal Blood Values *on page 1814* as a general guideline for provision of dental care.

The consideration of current blood values is important in long-term care of any medically compromised patient and in particular the HIV-positive patient. Preventive dental care is likewise valuable in these patients, however, the dentist's approach should be no different than as with all patients. See Table 4 for oral lesions commonly associated with HIV disease and a brief description of their usual treatment (see Part II of this Oral Medicine chapter for more detailed descriptions of these common oral lesions).

The clinician should be aware that several of the protease inhibitors have now been associated with drug interactions. Some of these drug interactions include therapies that the dentist may be utilizing. The basis for these drug interactions with protease inhibitors is the inhibition of cytochrome P450 isoforms, which are important in normal liver function and metabolism of drugs. A detailed description of the mechanisms of inhibition can be found in Pharmacology of Drug Metabolism and Interactions *on page 1754*, as well as a table illustrating some known drug interactions with antiviral therapy and drugs commonly prescribed in the dental office. The metabolism of these drugs could be affected by the patient's antiviral therapy.

The dentist should also review office protocol for Occupational Exposure to Bloodborne Pathogens (Standard/Universal Precautions) *on page 1770* and the answers to "Frequently Asked Questions" at the end of this section.

HIV INFECTION AND AIDS *(Continued)*

Table 4. ORAL LESIONS COMMONLY SEEN IN HIV/AIDS

Condition	Management
Oral candidiasis Angular cheilitis	See "Fungal Infections" *on page 1707*
Oral hairy leukoplakia	See "Systemic Viral Diseases" *on page 1675*
Periodontal diseases Linear gingivitis Ulcerative periodontitis	See "Bacterial Infections" *on page 1697*
Herpes simplex Herpes zoster	Acyclovir - see "Systemic Viral Diseases" *on page 1675*
Chronic aphthous ulceration	Palliation / Thalidomide (Thalomid®)
Salivary gland disease	Referral
Human papillomavirus	Laser / Surgical excision
Kaposi's sarcoma	See "Antibiotic Prophylaxis" *on page 1680* Biopsy / Laser
Non-Hodgkin's lymphoma	Biopsy / Referral
Tuberculosis	Referral

Dapsone *on page 421*
Delavirdine *on page 429*
Didanosine *on page 465*
Indinavir *on page 829*
Lamivudine *on page 894*
Lopinavir and Ritonavir *on page 943*
Nelfinavir *on page 1098*
Ritonavir *on page 1359*
Stavudine *on page 1416*
Thalidomide *on page 1471*
Tenofovir *on page 1457*
Zalcitabine *on page 1590*
Zidovudine *on page 1594*
Zidovudine and Lamivudine *on page 1596*

FREQUENTLY ASKED QUESTIONS

How does one get AIDS, aside from having unprotected sex?

Our current knowledge about the immunodeficiency virus is that it is carried via semen, contaminated needles, blood products, transfusion products not tested, and potentially in other fluids of the body. Patients at highest risk include I.V. drug-abusers, those receiving multiple transfusions with blood that has not been screened for HIV, or patients practicing unprotected sex with multiple partners, where the history of the partner may not be as clear as the patient would like.

Are patients safe from AIDS or HIV infection when they present to the dentist office?

Our current knowledge indicates that the answer is an unequivocal "yes". The patient is protected because dental offices are practicing stanard/universal precautions, using antimicrobial handwashing agents, gloves, face masks, eye protection, special clothing, aerosol control, and instrument soaking and autoclaving. All of these procedures stop potential transmission to a new patient, as well as, allow for easy disposal of contaminated office supplies for elimination of microbes by an antimicrobial technique, should they be contaminated through treatment of another patient. These precautions are mandated by OSHA requirements (see Occupational Exposure to Bloodborne Pathogens Standard/Universal Precautions *on page 1770*).

What is the most common opportunistic infection that HIV-positive patients suffer that may be important in dentistry?

The most common opportunistic infection important to dentistry is oral candidiasis. This disease can present as white plaques, red areas, or angular cheilitis occurring at the corners of the mouth. Management of such lesions is appropriate by the dentist and is described in this handbook (see Fungal Infections *on page 1707*). Other oral complications include HIV-associated periodontal disease, as well as the other conditions outlined in Table 4. Of great concern to the dentist is the risk of tuberculosis. In many HIV-positive patients, tuberculosis has become a serious, life-threatening opportunistic infection. The dentist should be aware that appropriate referral for anyone showing such respiratory signs and symptoms would be prudent.

Can one patient infect another through unprotected sex if the other patient has tested negative for HIV?

Yes, there is always the possibility that a sexual partner may be in the early window of time when plasma viremia is not at a detectable level. The antibody response to plasma viremia may be slightly delayed and diagnostic testing may not indicate HIV positivity. This window of time represents a period when the patient may be infectious but not show up yet on normal diagnostic testing.

Can HIV be passed by oral fluids?

As our knowledge about HIV has evolved, we have thought that HIV is inactivated in saliva by an agent possibly associated with secretory leukocyte protease inhibitors known as SLPI. There is, however, a current resurgence in our interest in oral transmission because some research indicates that in moderate to advanced periodontal lesions or other oral lesions where there is tissue damage, the presence of a serous exudate may increase the risk of transmission. The dentist should be aware of this ongoing research and attempt to renew knowledge regularly so that any future breakthroughs will be noted.

RHEUMATOID ARTHRITIS, OSTEOARTHRITIS, AND OSTEOPOROSIS

RA AND OSTEOARTHRITIS MANAGEMENT

Arthritis and its variations represent the most common chronic musculoskeletal disorders of man. The conditions can essentially be divided into rheumatoid, osteoarthritic, and polyarthritic presentations. Differences in age of onset and joint involvement exist and it is now currently believed that the diagnosis of each may be less clear than previously thought. These autoinflammatory diseases have now been shown to affect young and old alike. Criteria for a diagnosis of rheumatoid arthritis include a positive serologic test for rheumatoid factor, subcutaneous nodules, affected joints on opposite sides of the body, and clear radiographic changes. The hematologic picture includes moderate normocytic hypochromic anemia, mild leukocytosis, and mild thrombocytopenia. During acute inflammatory periods, C-reactive protein is elevated and IgG and IgM (rheumatoid factors) can be detected. Osteoarthritis lacks these diagnostic features.

Other systemic conditions, such as systemic lupus erythematosus and Sjögren's syndrome, are often found simultaneously with some of the arthritic conditions. The treatment of arthritis includes the use of slow-acting and rapid-acting anti-inflammatory agents ranging from the gold salts to aspirin (see following listings). Long-term usage of these drugs can lead to numerous adverse effects including bone marrow suppression, platelet suppression, and oral ulcerations. The dentist should be aware that steroids (usually prednisone) are often prescribed along with the listed drugs and are often used in dosages sufficient to induce adrenal suppression. Adjustment of dosing prior to invasive dental procedures may be indicated along with consultation with the managing physician. Alteration of steroid dosage prior to stressful dental procedures may be necessary, usually increasing the steroid dosage prior to and during the stressful procedures and then gradually returning the patient to the original dosage over several days. Even in the absence of evidence of adrenal suppression, consultation with the prescribing physician for appropriate dosing and timing of procedures is advisable.

Antirheumatic, Disease Modifying

> Adalimumab *on page 52*

Gold Salts

> Auranofin *on page 166*
> Aurothioglucose

Metabolic Inhibitor

> Leflunomide *on page 901*
> Methotrexate *on page 1012*

Immunomodulator

> Etanercept *on page 588*

Nonsteroidal Anti-inflammatory Agents

> Aminosalicylic Acid *on page 89*
> Choline Magnesium Trisalicylate *on page 335*
> Diclofenac *on page 459*
> Diflunisal *on page 468*
> Etodolac *on page 623*
> Fenoprofen *on page 642*
> Flurbiprofen *on page 683*
> Ibuprofen *on page 808*
> Indomethacin *on page 830*
> Ketoprofen *on page 883*
> Ketorolac *on page 886*
> Magnesium Salicylate *on page 962*
> Meclofenamate *on page 970*
> Mefenamic Acid *on page 973*
> Nabumetone *on page 1077*
> Naproxen *on page 1089*
> Oxaprozin *on page 1155*
> Piroxicam *on page 1248*
> Salsalate *on page 1376*
> Sulindac *on page 1430*
> Tolmetin *on page 1504*

COX-2 Inhibitor NSAID

Celecoxib *on page 296*

Combination NSAID Product to Prevent GI Distress

Diclofenac and Misoprostol *on page 462*

Salicylates

Aspirin *on page 145*
Choline Magnesium Trisalicylate *on page 335*
Salsalate *on page 1376*

Other

Hydroxychloroquine *on page 799*
Prednisone *on page 1271*

ANTI-INFLAMMATORY AGENTS USED IN THE TREATMENT OF RA AND OSTEOARTHRITIS

Drug	Adverse Effects
SLOW-ACTING	
Gold Salts	
Aurothioglucose; Auranofin; Gold Sodium Thiomalate	GI intolerance, diarrhea; leukopenia, thrombocytopenia, and/or anemia; skin and oral eruptions; possible nephrotoxicity and hepatotoxicity
Metabolic Inhibitor	
Leflunomide (Arava™)	Diarrhea, respiratory tract infection
Methotrexate	Oral ulcerations, leukopenia
Immunomodulator	
Etanercept (Enbrel®)	Headache, respiratory tract infection, positive ANA
Other	
Hydroxychloroquine (Plaquenil®)	Usually mild and reversible; ophthalmic complications
Prednisone	Insomnia, nervousness, indigestion, increased appetite
RAPID-ACTING	
Salicylates	
Aspirin	Inhibition of platelet aggregation; gastrointestinal (GI) irritation, ulceration, and bleeding; tinnitus; teratogenicity
Choline magnesium trisalicylate (Trilisate®) Salsalate	GI irritation and ulceration, weakness, skin rash, hemolytic anemia, troubled breathing
Other Nonsteroidal Anti-inflammatory Drugs	
Diclofenac (Cataflam®, Voltaren®); Diflunisal (Dolobid®); Etodolac (Lodine®); Fenoprofen calcium (Nalfon®); Flurbiprofen (Ansaid®); Ibuprofen (Motrin®); Indomethacin (Indocin®); Ketoprofen; Ketorolac (Toradol®); Meclofenamate; Nabumetone (Relafen®); Naproxen (Naprosyn®); Oxaprozin (Daypro®); Piroxicam (Feldene®); Salsalate (Mono-Gesic®, Salflex®); Sulindac (Clinoril®); Tolmetin (Tolectin®)	GI irritation, ulceration, and bleeding; inhibition of platelet aggregation; displacement of protein-bound drugs (eg, oral anticoagulants, sulfonamides, and sulfonylureas); headache; vertigo; mucocutaneous rash or ulceration; parotid enlargement
COX-2 Inhibitor NSAID	
Celecoxib (Celebrex®) Rofecoxib (Vioxx®) Valdecoxib (Bextra®)	Headache, dyspepsia, upper respiratory tract infection, sinusitis
COMBINATION NSAID PRODUCT TO PREVENT GI DISTRESS	
Diclofenac and Misoprostol (Arthrotec®)	Inhibition of platelet aggregation; displacement of protein-bound drugs (eg, oral anticoagulants, sulfonamides, and sulfonylureas); headache; vertigo; mucocutaneous rash or ulceration; parotid enlargement; diarrhea

RHEUMATOID ARTHRITIS, OSTEOARTHRITIS, AND OSTEOPOROSIS *(Continued)*

OSTEOPOROSIS MANAGEMENT

PREVALENCE

Osteoporosis effects 25 million Americans of which 80% are women; 27% of American women >80 years of age have osteopenia and 70% of American women >80 years of age have osteoporosis.

CONSEQUENCES

1.3 million bone fractures annually (low impact/nontraumatic) and pain, pulmonary insufficiency, decreased quality of life, and economic costs; >250,000 hip fractures per year with a 20% mortality rate.

RISK FACTORS

Advanced age, female, chronic renal disease, hyperparathyroidism, Cushing's disease, hypogonadism/anorexia, hyperprolactinemia, cancer, large and prolonged dose heparin or glucocorticoids, anticonvulsants, hyperthyroidism (current or history, or excessive thyroid supplements), sedentary, excessive exercise, early menopause, oophorectomy without hormone replacement, excessive aluminum-containing antacid, smoking, methotrexate.

DIAGNOSIS/MONITORING

DXA bone density, history of fracture (low impact or nontraumatic), compressed vertebrae, decreased height, hump-back appearance. Osteomark™ urine assay measures bone breakdown fragments and may help assess therapy response earlier than DXA but diagnostic value is uncertain as Osteomark™ does not reveal extent of bone loss. Bone markers may be tested to evaluate effectiveness of antiresorptive urine therapy.

PREVENTION

1. Adequate dietary calcium (eg, dairy products)

2. Vitamin D (eg, fortified dairy products, cod, fatty fish)

3. Weight-bearing exercise (eg, walking) as tolerated

4. Calcium supplement of 1000-1500 mg <u>elemental</u> calcium daily (divided in 500 mg increments); women >65 years on estrogen replacement therapy supplement 1000 mg <u>elemental</u> calcium; women >65 not receiving estrogens and men >55 years supplement 1500 mg <u>elemental</u> calcium. To minimize constipation add fiber and start with 500 mg/day for several months, then increase to 500 mg twice daily taken at different times than fiber. Chewable and liquid products are available. Calcium carbonate is given with food to enhance bioavailability. Calcium citrate may be given without regards to meals.

   - Contraindications: Hypercalcemia, ventricular fibrillation
   - Side effects: Constipation, anorexia
   - Drug interactions: Fiber, tetracycline, iron supplement, minerals

5. Vitamin D Supplement: 400-800 units daily (often satisfied by 1-2 multivitamins or fortified milk) in addition to calcium or a combined calcium and vitamin D supplement and/or >15 minutes direct sunlight/day. Some elderly, especially with significant renal or liver disease cannot metabolize (activate) vitamin D and require calcitriol 0.25 mcg orally twice daily or adjusted per serum calcium level, the active form of vitamin D; can check 1,25 OH vitamin D level to confirm need for calcitriol.

   - Contraindications: Hypercalcemia (weakness, headache, drowsiness, nausea, diarrhea), hypercalciuria and renal stones
   - Side effects (uncommon): Hypercalcemia (see above)
   - Monitor 24-hour urine and serum calcium if using >1000 units/day

6. Estrogen: Especially useful if bone density <80% of average plus symptoms of estrogen deficiency or cardiac disease. Bone density increases over 1-2 years then plateaus. This is considered 1st line therapy unless contraindicated due to medicinal history (see below) or risk:benefit assessment which leads to decision to avoid HRT (hormone replacement therapy). **Note:** Estrogens should not be used to prevent coronary heart disease.

- Contraindications: Pregnancy, breast or estrogen-dependent cancer, undiagnosed abnormal genital bleeding, active thrombophlebitis, or history of thromboembolism during previous estrogen or oral contraceptive therapy or pregnancy. Pretreatment mammogram, gynecological exam are advised along with routine breast exam because of an increased risk of breast cancer with long-term use.

- Dose: Conjugated estrogen of 0.625 mg/day or its equivalent (continuous therapy preferred).

- Side effects: Vaginal spotting/bleeding, nausea, vomiting, breast tenderness/enlargement, amenorrheic with extended use.
  Initiate therapy slowly (side effects are more common and severe in women without estrogen for many years). Administer with medroxyprogesterone acetate (MPA) 2.5-5 mg daily, or another oral progesterone, in women with uterus (unopposed estrogen can cause endometrial cancer). MPA can increase vaginal bleeding, increase weight, edema, mood changes.

- Drug interactions: May increase corticosteroid effect, monitor for need to decrease corticosteroid dose.

7. Selective estrogen receptor modulators: Selective-estrogen receptor modulators (SERMs) are nonsteroidal modulators of estrogen-receptor mediated reactions. The key difference between these agents and estrogen replacement therapies is the potential to exert tissue specific effects. Due to their chemical differences, these agents retain some of estrogen's beneficial effects on bone metabolism and lipid levels, but differ in their actions on breast and endometrial tissues, potentially limiting adverse effects related to nonspecific hormone stimulation. Among the SERMs, tamoxifen retains stimulatory effects in endometrial tissue, while raloxifene does not stimulate endometrial or breast tissue, limiting the potential for endometrial or breast cancer related to this agent. Raloxifene is the only SERM which has been approved by the FDA for osteoporosis prevention.

   It should be noted that the effects on bone observed with SERMs appear to be less than that observed with estrogen replacement. In one study, the effect of raloxifene on hip bone mineral density was approximately half of that observed with conjugated estrogens. In addition, the effects on lipid profiles are less than with estrogen replacement. Finally, SERMs do not block the vasomotor effects observed with menopause, which may limit compliance with therapy. As with estrogen replacement, raloxifene has been associated with an increased risk of thromboembolism and is contraindicated in patients with a history of thromboembolic disease.

8. Estradiol, as well as various combination therapies, including ethinyl estradiol with norethindrone (Femhrt®) and ethinyl with norgestimate (Ortho-Prefest™), have been approved for the prevention of osteoporosis (see Estradiol *on page 574*).

TREATMENT

1. Calcium, vitamin D, exercise, and estrogen: As above

2. Bisphosphonates:

   Consider if patient is intolerant of, or refuses estrogen or it is contraindicated, especially if severe osteoporosis (ie, ≥2.5 standard deviations below average young adult bone density, T-score, or history of low impact or nontraumatic fracture). Increasing bone density of hip and spine observed for at least 3 years (ie, no plateau as seen with estrogen).

   Contraindications: Hypocalcemia, not advised if existing gastrointestinal disorders (eg, esophageal disorders such as reflux, sensitive stomach).

   - Alendronate (Fosamax®): Dose: 10 mg once daily or 70 mg/week (treatment dose for osteoporosis; not recommended if creatinine clearance <35 mL/minute). Osteopenia: 5 mg per day or 35 mg/week for prevention.

   - Risedronate (Actonel®): Dose: 5 mg daily or 35 mg/week for treatment or prevention

   Take before breakfast on an empty stomach with 6-8 ounces tap water (not mineral water, coffee, or juice) and remain upright or raise head of bed for bedridden patients at least 30 degree angle for at least 30 minutes (otherwise may cause ulcerative esophagitis) before eating or drinking.

   Note: Some bisphosphonates (usually those given to prevent skeletal related events in cancer) have been associated with an uncommon but serious side effect known as osteonecrosis of the jaw (ONJ). The dentist should be aware of the expanding literature and research on this subject.

   Therapy with calcium and vitamin D is advised, but must be given at a different time of day than alendronate.

RHEUMATOID ARTHRITIS, OSTEOARTHRITIS, AND OSTEOPOROSIS *(Continued)*

- Side effects (well tolerated): Difficulty swallowing, heartburn, abdominal discomfort, nausea (GI side effects increase with aspirin products), arthralgia/myalgia, constipation, diarrhea, headache, esophagitis.

- Drug interactions: None known to date.

3. Etidronate Disodium: Not FDA approved for postmenopausal osteoporosis and can decrease the quality of bone formation, therefore, change to alendronate.

4. Calcitonin (nasal; Miacalcin®): Indicated if estrogen refused, intolerant, or contraindicated. Potential analgesic effect.

   - Contraindications: Hypersensitivity to salmon protein or gelatin diluent; 1 spray (200 units) into 1 nostril daily (alternate right and left nostril daily); 5 days on and 2 days off is also effective; alternate day administration not effective. If used only for pain, can decrease dose once pain is controlled.

   - Side effects (few): Nasal dryness and irritation (periodically inspect); adequate dietary or supplemental calcium + vitamin D is essential.

   Subcutaneous route (100 units daily): Many side effects (eg, nausea, flushing, anorexia) and the discomfort/inconvenience of injection.

5. Fall prevention: Minimize psychoactive and cardiovascular drugs (monitor BP for orthostasis), give diuretics early in the day, environmental safety check.

	% Elemental Calcium	Elemental Calcium
Calcium gluconate (various)	9	500 mg = 45 mg
Calcium glubionate (Neo-Calglucon®)	6.5	1.8 g = 115 g/5 mL
Calcium lactate (various)	13	325 mg = 42.25 mg
Calcium citrate (Citrical®)	21	950 mg = 200 mg
Effervescent tabs (Citrical Liquitab®)		2376 mg = 500 mg
Calcium acetate Phos-Ex 250® Phos-Lo®	25	1000 mg = 250 mg 667 mg = 169 mg
Calcium phosphate, tribasic (Posture®)	39	1565.2 mg = 600 mg
Calcium carbonate Tums® Oscal-500® oral suspension Caltrate 600®	40	1.2 g = 500 mg 1.2 g/5 mL = 500 mg 1.5 g = 600 mg

References

Ashworth L, "Focus on Alendronate. A Nonhormonal Option for the Treatment of Osteoporosis in Postmenopausal Women," *Formulary*, 1996, 31:23-30.

Johnson SR, "Should Older Women Use Estrogen Replacement," *J Am Geriatr Soc*, 1996, 44:89-90.

Liberman UA, Weiss SR, and Brool J, "Effect of Oral Alendronate on Bone-Mineral Density and the Incidence of Fracture in Postmenopausal Osteoporosis," *N Engl J Med*, 1995, 333:1437-43.

"New Drugs for Osteoporosis," *Med Lett Drugs Ther*, 1996, 38:1-3.

NIH Consensus Development Panel on Optimal Calcium Intake, *JAMA*, 1994, 272:1942-8.

TUBERCULOSIS

Tuberculosis is caused by the organism *Mycobacterium tuberculosis* as well as a variety of other mycobacteria including *M. bovis*, *M. avium-intracellulare*, and *M. kansasii*. Diagnosis of tuberculosis can be made from a skin test and a positive chest x-ray as well as acid-fast smears of cultures from respiratory secretions. Nucleic acid probes and polymerase chain reaction (PCR) to identify nucleic acid of *M. tuberculosis* have recently become useful.

The treatment of tuberculosis is based on the general principle that multiple drugs should reduce infectivity within 2 weeks and that failures in therapy may be due to noncompliance with the long-term regimens necessary. General treatment regimens last 6-12 months.

Isoniazid-resistant and multidrug-resistant mycobacterial infections have become an increasingly significant problem in recent years. TB as an opportunistic disease in HIV-positive patients has also risen. Combination drug therapy has always been popular in TB management and the advent of new antibiotics has not diminished this need.

ANTITUBERCULOSIS DRUGS

Bactericidal Agents

Capreomycin *on page 256*
*Isoniazid *on page 864*
Kanamycin *on page 878*
*Pyrazinamide *on page 1314*
Rifabutin *on page 1345*
*Rifampin *on page 1346*
*Streptomycin *on page 1418*

Bacteriostatic Agents

Cycloserine *on page 405*
*Ethambutol *on page 591*
Ethionamide *on page 618*
Aminosalicyllic Acid *on page 89*

*Drugs of choice.

SEXUALLY-TRANSMITTED DISEASES

Sexually transmitted diseases (STDs) represent a group of infectious diseases that include bacterial, fungal, and viral etiologies. Several related infections are covered elsewhere. Gonorrhea and syphilis will be covered here.

The management of a patient with a STD begins with identification. Paramount to the correct management of patients with a history of gonorrhea or syphilis is when the condition was diagnosed, how and with what agent it was treated, did the condition recur, and are there any residual signs and symptoms potentially indicating active or recurrent disease. With standard/universal precautions, the patient with *Neisseria gonorrhoea* or *Treponema pallidum* infection poses little threat to the dentist; however, diagnosis of oral lesions may be problematic. Gonococcal pharyngitis, primary syphilitic lesions (chancre), secondary syphilitic lesions (mucous patch), and tertiary lesions (gumma) may be identified by the dentist.

Drugs used in treatment of gonorrhea/syphilis include:

Cefixime *on page 287*

Ceftriaxone *on page 294*

Ciprofloxacin *on page 343*

Doxycycline *on page 514*

Ofloxacin *on page 1137*

Penicillin G Benzathine *on page 1202*

Penicillin G (Parenteral/Aqueous) *on page 1203*

Spectinomycin (alternate) *on page 1412*

The drugs listed above are often used alone or in stepped regimens, particularly when there is concomitant *Chlamydia* infection or when there is evidence of disseminated disease. The proper treatment for syphilis depends on the state of the disease.

SYSTEMIC VIRAL DISEASES

HEPATITIS

The hepatitis viruses are a group of DNA and RNA viruses that produce symptoms associated with inflammation of the liver. Currently, hepatitis A through G have been identified by immunological testing; however, hepatitis A through E have received most attention in terms of disease identification. Recently, however, there has been increased interest in hepatitis viruses F and G, particularly as relate to healthcare professionals. Our knowledge is expanding rapidly in this area and the clinician should be alert to changes in the literature that might update their knowledge. Hepatitis F, for instance, remains a diagnosis of exclusion effectively being non-A, B, C, D, E, or G. Whereas, hepatitis G has serologic testing available, however, not commercially at this time. Research evaluations of various antibody and RT-PCR tests for hepatitis G are under development at this time.

Signs and symptoms of viral hepatitis in general are quite variable. Patients infected may range from asymptomatic to experiencing flu-like symptoms only. In addition, fever, nausea, joint muscle pain, jaundice, and hepatomegaly along with abdominal pain can result from infection with one of the hepatitis viruses. The virus also can create an acute or chronic infection. Usually following these early symptoms or the asymptomatic period, the patient may recover or may go on to develop chronic liver dysfunction. Liver dysfunction may be represented primarily by changes in liver function tests known as LFTs and these primarily include aspartate aminotransferase known as AST and alanine aminotransferase known as ALT. In addition, for A, B, C, D, and E there are serologic tests for either antigen, antibody, or both. Of hepatitis A through G, five forms have both acute and chronic forms whereas A and E appear to only create acute disease. There are differences in the way clinicians may approach a known postexposure to one of the hepatitis viruses. In many instances, gamma globulin may be used, however, the indications for gamma globulin as a drug limit their use to several of the viruses only. The dental clinician should be aware that the gastroenterologist may choose to give gamma globulin off-label.

Hepatitis A

Hepatitis A virus is an enteric virus that is a member of the Picornavirus family along with Coxsackie viruses and poliovirus. Previously known as infectious hepatitis, hepatitis A has been detected in humans for centuries. It causes acute hepatitis, often transmitted by oral-fecal contamination and having an incubation period of approximately 30 days. Typically, constitutional symptoms are present and jaundice may occur. Drug therapy that the dentist may encounter in a patient being treated for hepatitis A would primarily include immunoglobulin. Hepatitis A vaccine (inactivated) is an FDA-approved vaccine indicated in the prevention of contracting hepatitis A in exposed or high-risk individuals. Candidates at high-risk for HAV infection include persons traveling internationally to highly endemic areas, individuals with chronic liver disease, individuals engaging in high-risk sexual behavior, illicit drug-users, persons with high-risk occupational exposure, hemophiliacs or other persons receiving blood products, pediatric populations, and food handlers in high-risk environments. Two formulations of hepatitis A vaccine are available, Havrix® and VAQTA®. Each is administered as an injection in the deltoid region and both are available in pediatric and adult dosages.

Hepatitis B

Hepatitis B virus is previously known as serum hepatitis and has particular trophism for liver cells. Hepatitis B virus causes both acute and chronic disease in susceptible patients. The incubation period is often long and the diagnosis might be made by serologic markers even in the absence of symptoms. No drug therapy for acute hepatitis B is known; however, chronic hepatitis has recently been successfully-treated with Interferon Alfa-2b.

Hepatitis C

Hepatitis C virus was described in 1988 and has been formerly classified as non-A/non-B. It is clear that hepatitis C represents a high percentage of the transfusion-associated hepatitis that is seen. Treatment of acute hepatitis C infection is generally supportive. Interferon Alfa-2a therapy has been used with some success recently and interferon-alfa may be beneficial with hepatitis C-related chronic hepatitis.

SYSTEMIC VIRAL DISEASES (Continued)

Hepatitis D

Hepatitis D, previously known as the delta agent, is a virus that is incomplete in that it requires previous infection with hepatitis B in order to be manifested. In the past, no antiviral therapy has been effective, however, Interferon Alfa-2b is currently being investigated for unlabeled use in hepatitis D.

Hepatitis E

Hepatitis E virus is an RNA virus that represents a proportion of the previously classified non-A/non-B diagnoses. There is currently no antiviral therapy against hepatitis E.

Hepatitis F

Hepatitis F, as was mentioned, remains a diagnosis of exclusion. There are no known immunological tests available for identification of hepatitis F at present and currently the Centers for Disease Control have not come out with specific guidelines or recommendations. It is thought, however, that hepatitis F is a bloodborne virus and it has been used as a diagnosis in several cases of post-transfusion hepatitis.

Hepatitis G

Hepatitis G virus (HGV) is the newest hepatitis and is also assumed to be a bloodborne virus. Similar in family to hepatitis C, it is thought to occur concomitantly with hepatitis C and appears to be even more prevalent in some blood donors than hepatitis C. Occupational transmission of HGV is currently under study (see the references for updated information) and currently there are no specific CDC recommendations for postexposure to an HGV individual as the testing for identification remains experimental.

For further information, refer to the following:

Occupational Exposure to Bloodborne Pathogens on page 1770

Immunizations (Vaccines) on page 1786

Hepatitis A Vaccine on page 767

Hepatitis A (Inactivated) and Hepatitis B (Recombinant) Vaccine on page 766

Hepatitis B Immune Globulin on page 768

Hepatitis B Vaccine on page 769

Immune Globulin, Intramuscular on page 823

Immune Globulin, Intravenous on page 824

Interferon Alfa-2a on page 842

Interferon Alfa-2b on page 844

Interferon Alfa-2b and Ribavirin on page 847

Peginterferon Alfa-2a on page 1195

Peginterferon Alfa-2b on page 1197

TYPES OF HEPATITIS VIRUS

Features	A	B	C	D	E	F	G
Incubation Period	2-6 wks	8-24 wks	2-52 wks	3-13 wks	3-6 wks	Unknown	Unknown
Onset	Abrupt	Insidious	Insidious	Abrupt	Abrupt	Insidious	Insidious
Symptoms							
Jaundice	Adults: 70% to 80%; Children: 10%	25%	25%	Varies	Unknown	Unknown	Unknown
Asymptomatic patients	Adults: 50%; Children: Most	~75%	~75%	Rare	Rare	Common	Common
Routes of Transmission							
Fecal/Oral	Yes	No	No	No	Yes	Unknown	Unknown
Parenteral	Rare	Yes	Yes	Yes	No		
Sexual	No	Yes	Possible	Yes	No		
Perinatal	No	Yes	Possible	Possible	No		
Water/Food	Yes	No	No	No	Yes		
Sequelae (% of patients)							
Chronic state	No	Adults: 6% to 10%; Children: 25% to 50%; Infants: 70% to 90%	>75%	10% to 15%	No	Unknown	Likely
Case-Fatality Rate	0.6%	1.4%	1% to 2%	30%	1% to 2% Pregnant women: 20%	Unknown	Unknown

PRE-EXPOSURE RISK FACTORS FOR HEPATITIS B

Healthcare factors:

Healthcare workers[1]

Special patient groups (eg, adolescents, infants born to HB$_s$Ag–positive mothers, military personnel, etc)

Hemodialysis patients[2]

Recipients of certain blood products[3]

Lifestyle factors:

Homosexual and bisexual men

Intravenous drug-abusers

Heterosexually active persons with multiple sexual partners or recently acquired sexually transmitted diseases

Environmental factors:

Household and sexual contacts of HBV carriers

Prison inmates

Clients and staff of institutions for the mentally handicapped

Residents, immigrants, and refugees from areas with endemic HBV infection

International travelers at increased risk of acquiring HBV infection

[1]The risk of hepatitis B virus (HBV) infection for healthcare workers varies both between hospitals and within hospitals. Hepatitis B vaccination is recommended for all healthcare workers with blood exposure.

[2]Hemodialysis patients often respond poorly to hepatitis B vaccination; higher vaccine doses or increased number of doses are required. A special formulation of one vaccine is now available for such persons (Recombivax HB®, 40 mcg/mL). The anti-HB$_s$ (antibody to hepatitis B surface antigen) response of such persons should be tested after they are vaccinated, and those who have not responded should be revaccinated with 1-3 additional doses.

Patients with chronic renal disease should be vaccinated as early as possible, ideally before they require hemodialysis. In addition, their anti- HB$_s$ levels should be monitored at 6- to 12-month intervals to assess the need for revaccination.

[3]Patients with hemophilia should be immunized subcutaneously, not intramuscularly.

POSTEXPOSURE PROPHYLAXIS FOR HEPATITIS B[1]

Exposure	Hepatitis B Immune Globulin	Hepatitis B Vaccine
Perinatal	0.5 mL I.M. within 12 hours of birth	0.5 mL[2] I.M. within 12 hours of birth (no later than 7 days), and at 1 and 6 months[3]; test for HB$_s$Ag and anti-HB$_s$ at 12-15 months
Sexual	0.06 mL/kg I.M. within 14 days of sexual contact; a second dose should be given if the index patient remains HB$_s$Ag-positive after 3 months and hepatitis B vaccine was not given initially	1 mL I.M. at 0, 1, and 6 months for homosexual and bisexual men and regular sexual contacts of persons with acute and chronic hepatitis B
Percutaneous; exposed person unvaccinated		
Source known HB$_s$Ag-positive	0.06 mL/kg I.M. within 24 hours	1 mL I.M. within 7 days, and at 1 and 6 months[4]
Source known, HB$_s$Ag status unknown	Test source for HB$_s$Ag; if source is positive, give exposed person 0.06 mL/kg I.M. once within 7 days	1 mL I.M. within 7 days, and at 1 and 6 months[4]
Source not tested or unknown	Nothing required	1 mL I.M. within 7 days, and at 1 and 6 months
Percutaneous; exposed person vaccinated		
Source known HB$_s$Ag-positive	Test exposed person for anti-HB$_s$[5]. If titer is protective, nothing is required; if titer is not protective, give 0.06 mL/kg within 24 hours	Review vaccination status[6]
Source known, HB$_s$Ag status unknown	Test source for HB$_s$Ag and exposed person for anti-HB$_s$. If source is HB$_s$Ag-negative, or if source is HB$_s$Ag-positive but anti-HB$_s$ titer is protective, nothing is required. If source is HB$_s$Ag-positive and anti-HB$_s$ titer is not protective or if exposed person is a known nonresponder, give 0.06 mL/kg I.M. within 24 hours. A second dose of hepatitis B immune globulin can be given 1 month later if a booster dose of hepatitis B vaccine is not given.	Review vaccination status[6]

(table continued on next page)

SYSTEMIC VIRAL DISEASES *(Continued)*

POSTEXPOSURE PROPHYLAXIS FOR HEPATITIS B[1] *(continued)*

Exposure	Hepatitis B Immune Globulin	Hepatitis B Vaccine
Source not tested or unknown	Test exposed person for anti-HB$_s$. If anti-HB$_s$ titer is protective, nothing is required. If anti-HB$_s$ titer is not protective, 0.06 mL/kg may be given along with a booster dose of hepatitis B vaccine.	Review vaccination status[6]

[1]HB$_s$Ag = hepatitis B surface antigen; anti-HB$_s$ = antibody to hepatitis B surface antigen; I.M. = intramuscularly; SRU = standard ratio units.

[2]Each 0.5 mL dose of plasma-derived hepatitis B vaccine contains 10 mcg of HB$_s$Ag; each 0.5 mL dose of recombinant hepatitis B vaccine contains 5 mcg or 10 mcg of HB$_s$Ag.

[3]If hepatitis B immune globulin and hepatitis B vaccine are given simultaneously, they should be given at separate sites.

[4]If hepatitis B vaccine is not given, a second dose of hepatitis B immune globulin should be given 1 month later.

[5]Anti-HB$_s$ titers <10 SRU by radioimmunoassay or negative by enzyme immunoassay indicate lack of protection. Testing the exposed person for anti-HB$_s$ is not necessary if a protective level of antibody has been shown within the previous 24 months.

[6]If the exposed person has not completed a three-dose series of hepatitis B vaccine, the series should be completed. Test the exposed person for anti-HB$_s$. If the antibody level is protective, nothing is required. If an adequate antibody response in the past is shown on retesting to have declined to an inadequate level, a booster dose (1 mL) of hepatitis B vaccine should be given. If the exposed person has inadequate antibody or is a known nonresponder to vaccination, a booster dose can be given along with one dose of hepatitis B immune globulin.

HERPES

The herpes viruses not only represent a topic of specific interest to the dentist due to oral manifestations, but are widespread as systemic infections. Herpes simplex virus is also of interest because of its central nervous system infections and its relationship as one of the viral infections commonly found in AIDS patients. Oral herpes infections will be covered elsewhere. Treatment of herpes simplex primary infection includes acyclovir. Ganciclovir is an alternative drug and foscarnet is also occasionally used. Epstein-Barr virus is a member of the herpesvirus family and produces syndromes important in dentistry, including infectious mononucleosis with the commonly found oral pharyngitis and petechial hemorrhages, as well as being the causative agent of Burkitt's lymphoma. The relationship between Epstein-Barr virus to oral hairy leukoplakia in AIDS patients has not been shown to be one of cause and effect; however, the presence of Epstein-Barr in these lesions is consistent. Currently, there is no accepted treatment for Epstein-Barr virus, although acyclovir has been shown in *in vitro* studies to have some efficacy. Varicella-zoster virus is another member of the herpesvirus family and is the causative agent of two clinical entities, chickenpox and shingles, or herpes zoster. Oral manifestations of both chickenpox and herpes zoster include vesicular eruptions often leading to confluent mucosal ulcerations. Acyclovir is the drug of choice for treatment of herpes zoster infections.

There are other herpes viruses that produce disease in man and animals. These viruses have no specific treatment, therefore, incidence is thought to be less common than those mentioned and the specific treatment is not determined at present. The role of some of these viruses in concomitant infection with the HIV and other coinfection viruses is still under study.

ANTIVIRALS

AGENTS OF ESTABLISHED EFFECTIVENESS

Viral Infection	Drug
Cytomegalovirus	
Retinitis	Ganciclovir, Foscarnet
Pneumonia	Ganciclovir
Hepatitis viruses	
Chronic hepatitis A & B	Hepatitis A (Inactivated) and Hepatitis B (Recombinant) Vaccine
Chronic hepatitis C	Interferon Alfa-2a, Interferon Alfa-2b, Interferon Alfa-2b and Ribavirin, Peginterferon Alfa-2a, Peginterferon Alfa-2b
Chronic hepatitis B	Interferon Alfa-2b
Herpes simplex virus	
Orofacial herpes	
First episode	Acyclovir[1], Valacyclovir
Recurrence	Acyclovir[1], Penciclovir[1], Valacyclovir
Genital herpes	
First episode, recurrence, suppression	Acyclovir, Valacyclovir
Encephalitis	Acyclovir
Mucocutaneous disease in immunocompromised	Acyclovir
Neonatal	Acyclovir
Keratoconjunctivitis	Trifluridine Vidarabine
Influenza A virus	Amantadine, Oseltamivir, Rimantadine, Zanamivir
Papillomavirus	
Condyloma acuminatum	Interferon Alfa-2b, Imiquimod (Aldara™): (use for oral lesions is under study)
Respiratory syncytial virus	Ribavirin
Varicella-zoster virus	
Varicella in normal children	Acyclovir
Varicella in immunocompromised	Acyclovir
Herpes zoster in immunocompromised	Acyclovir
Herpes zoster in normal hosts	Acyclovir, Famciclovir, Valacyclovir

[1]Although acyclovir is often used for these infections, penciclovir and valacyclovir are specifically approved for herpes labialis. The clinician is referred to the monographs.

Acyclovir *on page 49*
Amantadine *on page 81*
Atovaquone *on page 160*
Cidofovir *on page 339*
Famciclovir *on page 633*
Fomivirsen *on page 700*
Foscarnet *on page 703*
Ganciclovir *on page 722*
Hepatitis B Immune Globulin *on page 768*
Imiquimod *on page 821*
Immune Globulin, Intramuscular *on page 823*
Interferon Alfa-2a *on page 842*
Interferon Alfa-2b *on page 844*
Interferon Alfa-2b and Ribavirin *on page 847*
Interferon Alfa-n3 *on page 848*
Oseltamivir *on page 1152*
Peginterferon Alfa-2a *on page 1195*
Peginterferon Alfa-2b *on page 1197*
Penciclovir *on page 1200*
Ribavirin *on page 1343*
Rifabutin *on page 1345*
Rimantadine *on page 1351*
Trifluridine *on page 1536*
Valacyclovir *on page 1553*
Zanamivir *on page 1592*

ANTIBIOTIC PROPHYLAXIS

PREPROCEDURAL GUIDELINES FOR DENTAL PATIENTS

INTRODUCTION

In dental practice, the clinician is often confronted with a decision to prescribe antibiotics. The focus of this section is on the use of antibiotics as a preprocedural treatment in the prevention of adverse infectious sequelae in the two most commonly encountered situations: prevention of endocarditis and prosthetic implants.

The criteria for preprocedural decisions begins with patient evaluation. An accurate and complete medical history is always the initial basis for any prescriptive treatments on the part of the dentist. These prescriptive treatments can include ordering appropriate laboratory tests, referral to the patient's physician for consultation, or immediate decision to prescribe preprocedural antibiotics. The dentist should also be aware that antibiotic coverage of the patient might be appropriate due to diseases that are covered elsewhere in this text, such as human immunodeficiency virus, cavernous thrombosis, undiagnosed or uncontrolled diabetes, lupus, renal failure, and periods of neutropenia as are often associated with cancer chemotherapy. In these instances, medical consultation is almost always necessary in making antibiotic decisions in order to tailor the treatment and dosing to the individual patient's needs.

Note: The ADA Council on Scientific Affairs recently restated the dentist's responsibility when prescribing antibiotics to oral contraceptive users (*JADA*, 2002, 133:880). It is recommended that dental professionals advise these patients to consult their physician for additional barrier contraception due to potential reduction in the efficacy of oral contraceptives from antibiotic interaction.

All tables or figures in this chapter were adapted from the ADA Advisory Statement: "Antibiotic Prophylaxis for Dental Patients With Total Joint Replacement," *J Am Dent Assoc*, 1997, 128:1004-8 or from Dajani AS, Taubert KA, Wilson W, et al, "Prevention of Bacterial Endocarditis. Recommendations by the American Heart Association," *JAMA*, 1997, 7(22):1794-801.

PREVENTION OF BACTERIAL ENDOCARDITIS

Guidelines for the prevention of bacterial endocarditis have been updated by the American Heart Association with approval by the Council of Scientific Affairs of the American Dental Association. These guidelines supercede those issued and published in 1990. They were developed to more clearly define the situations of antibiotic use, to reduce costs to the patient, to reduce gastrointestinal adverse effects, and to improve patient compliance. Highlights of the current recommendations are shown in Table 1 and the specific antibiotic regimens are listed in Table 2 and further illustrated in Figure 1.

Amoxicillin is an amino-type penicillin with an extended spectrum of antibacterial action compared to penicillin VK. The pharmacology of amoxicillin as a dental antibiotic has been reviewed previously in *General Dentistry*. The suggested regimen for standard general prophylaxis is a dose of 2 g 1 hour before the procedure. A follow-up dose is no longer necessary. This dose of amoxicillin is lower than the previous dosing regimen of 3 g 1 hour before the procedure and then 1.5 g 6 hours after the initial dose. Dajani, et al, stated that the 2 g dose of amoxicillin resulted in adequate serum levels for several hours making the second dose unnecessary, both because of a prolonged serum level of amoxicillin above the minimal inhibitory concentration for oral streptococci, and an inhibitory activity of 6-14 hours by amoxicillin against streptococci. The new pediatric dose is 50 mg/kg orally 1 hour before the procedure and not to exceed the adult dose. Amoxicillin is available in capsules (250 mg and 500 mg), chewable tablets (125 mg, 200 mg, 250 mg, 400 mg), and liquid suspension (400 mg/5 mL). The retail cost of generic capsules and tablets ranges from 20-30 cents each and suspension is approximately $12 per 100 mL.

For examples of sample prescriptions see Bacterial Endocarditis (Prevention) on page 1732

The dentist should be vigilant in reviewing literature for updates. The guidelines for antibiotic prophylaxis continue to be reviewed and it is likely that additional modifications to the recommendations will be published in the near future.

Table 1.
HIGHLIGHTS OF THE NEWEST GUIDELINES
FOR ENDOCARDITIS PREVENTION

No.	Change From Old Guidelines
1.	Oral initial dosing for amoxicillin has been reduced to 2 g.
2.	Follow-up antibiotic dose is no longer recommended.
3.	Erythromycin is no longer recommended for penicillin-allergic patients.
4.	Clindamycin and other alternatives have been recommended to replace the erythromycin regimens.
5.	Clearer guidelines for prophylaxis decisions for patients with mitral valve prolapse have been developed.

For individuals unable to take oral medications, intramuscular or intravenous ampicillin is recommended for both adults and children (Table 2). It is to be given 30 minutes before the procedure at the same doses used for the oral amoxicillin medication. Ampicillin is also an amino-type penicillin having an antibacterial spectrum similar to amoxicillin. Ampicillin is not absorbed from the GI tract as effectively as amoxicillin and, therefore, is not recommended for oral use.

Table 2.
PROPHYLACTIC REGIMENS FOR BACTERIAL ENDOCARDITIS
FOR DENTAL PROCEDURES

Situation	Agent	Regimen[1]
Standard general prophylaxis	Amoxicillin *on page 106*	Adults: 2 g orally 1 hour before procedure Children: 50 mg/kg orally 1 hour before procedure
Unable to take oral medications	Ampicillin *on page 117*	Adults: 2 g I.M. or I.V. within 30 minutes before procedure Children: 50 mg/kg I.M. or I.V. within 30 minutes before procedure
Allergic to penicillin	Clindamycin *on page 361* or	Adults: 600 mg orally 1 hour before procedure Children: 20 mg/kg orally 1 hour before procedure
	Cephalexin *on page 301* or Cefadroxil *on page 281*	Adults: 2 g orally 1 hour before procedure Children: 50 mg/kg orally 1 hour before procedure
	Azithromycin *on page 171* or Clarithromycin *on page 355*	Adults: 500 mg orally 1 hour before procedure Children: 15 mg/kg orally 1 hour before procedure
Allergic to penicillin and unable to take oral medications	Clindamycin *on page 361* or	Adults: 600 mg I.V. within 30 minutes before procedure Children: 20 mg/kg I.V. within 30 minutes before procedure
	Cefazolin *on page 283*	Adults: 1 g I.M. or I.V. within 30 minutes before procedure Children: 25 mg/kg I.M. or I.V. within 30 minutes before procedure

[1]Total children's dose should not exceed adult dose.

Note: Cephalosporins should not be used in individuals with immediate-type hypersensitivity reaction (urticaria, angioedema, or anaphylaxis) to penicillins.

Individuals who are allergic to the penicillins, such as amoxicillin or ampicillin, should be treated with an alternate antibiotic. The new guidelines have suggested a number of alternate agents including clindamycin, cephalosporins, azithromycin, and clarithromycin. Clindamycin (Cleocin®) occupies an important niche in dentistry as a useful and effective antibiotic and it was a recommended alternative agent for the prevention of bacterial endocarditis in the previous guidelines. In the new guidelines, the oral adult dose is 600 mg 1 hour before the procedure. A follow-up dose is not necessary. Clindamycin is available as 300 mg capsules; thus 2 capsules will provide the recommended dose. The children's oral dose for clindamycin is 20 mg/kg 1 hour before the procedure. Clindamycin is also available as flavored granules for oral solution. When reconstituted with water, each bottle yields a solution containing 75 mg/5 mL. Intravenous clindamycin is recommended in adults and children who are allergic to penicillin and unable to take oral medications. Refer to Table 2 for the intravenous doses of clindamycin.

Clindamycin was developed in the 1960s as a semisynthetic derivative of lincomycin which was found in the soil organism, *Streptomyces lincolnensis*, near Lincoln, Nebraska. It is commercially available as the hydrochloride salt to improve solubility in the GI tract. Clindamycin is antibacterial against most aerobic Gram-positive cocci including staphylococci and streptococci, and against many types of anaerobic Gram-negative and Gram-positive organisms. It has been used over the years in

ANTIBIOTIC PROPHYLAXIS *(Continued)*

dentistry as an alternative to penicillin and erythromycins for the treatment of oral-facial infections. For a review, see Wynn and Bergman.

The mechanism of antibacterial action of clindamycin is the same as erythromycin. It inhibits protein synthesis in susceptible bacteria resulting in the inhibition of bacterial growth and replication. Following oral administration of a single dose of clindamycin (150 mg, 300 mg, or 600 mg) on an empty stomach, 90% of the dose is rapidly absorbed into the bloodstream and peak serum concentrations are attained within 45-80 minutes. Administration with food does not markedly impair absorption into the bloodstream. Clindamycin serum levels exceed the minimum inhibitory concentration (MIC) for bacterial growth for at least 6 hours after the recommended dose of 600 mg. The serum half-life is 2-3 hours.

Adverse effects of clindamycin after a single dose are virtually nonexistent. Although it is estimated that 1% of patients taking clindamycin will develop symptoms of pseudomembranous colitis, these symptoms usually develop after 9-14 days of clindamycin therapy. These symptoms have never been reported in patients taking an acute dose for the prevention of endocarditis.

In lieu of clindamycin, penicillin-allergic individuals may receive cephalexin (Keflex®) or cefadroxil (Duricef®) provided that they have not had an immediate-type sensitivity reaction such as anaphylaxis, urticaria, or angioedema to penicillins. These antibiotics are first-generation cephalosporins having an antibacterial spectrum of action similar to amoxicillin and ampicillin. They elicit a bactericidal action by inhibiting cell wall synthesis in susceptible bacteria. The recommended adult prophylaxis dose for either of these drugs is 2 g 1 hour before the procedure. Again, no follow-up dose is needed. The children's oral dose for cephalexin and cefadroxil is 50 mg/kg 1 hour before the procedure. Cephalexin is supplied as capsules (250 mg and 500 mg) and tablets (250 mg, 500 mg, 1 g). Cefadroxil is supplied as 500 mg capsules and 1 g tablets. Both antibiotics are available in the form of powder for oral suspension at concentrations of 125 mg and 250 mg (cefadroxil also available as 500 mg/5 mL).

For those individuals (adults and children) allergic to penicillin and unable to take oral medicines, parenteral cefazolin (Ancef®) may be used, provided that they do not have the sensitivities described previously and footnoted in Table 2. Cefazolin is also a first-generation cephalosporin. Please note that the parenteral cefazolin can be given I.M. or I.V. (refer to Table 2 for the adult and children's doses of parenteral cefazolin).

Azithromycin (Zithromax®) and clarithromycin (Biaxin®) are members of the erythromycin-class of antibiotics known as the macrolides. The pharmacology of these drugs has been reviewed previously in *General Dentistry*. The erythromycins have been available for use in dentistry and medicine since the mid 1950s. Azithromycin and clarithromycin represent the first additions to this class in >40 years. The adult prophylactic dose for either drug is 500 mg 1 hour before the procedure with no follow-up dose. The pediatric prophylactic dose of azithromycin and clarithromycin is 15 mg/kg orally 1 hour before the procedure. Although the erythromycin family of drugs are known to inhibit the hepatic metabolism of theophylline and carbamazepine to enhance their effects, azithromycin has not been shown to affect the liver metabolism of these drugs.

Azithromycin is well absorbed from the gastrointestinal tract and is extensively taken up from the circulation into tissues with a slow release from those tissues. It reaches peak serum levels in 2-4 hours and serum half-life is 68 hours. Zithromax® is supplied as 250 mg (retail cost ranges from $7-$8 each) and 600 mg tablets (approximately $15 each). It is also available for oral suspension, supplied as single-dose packets containing 1 g each (approximately $60 for 3 packets). Azithromycin is not yet available as a generic drug.

Clarithromycin (Biaxin®) achieves peak plasma concentrations in 3 hours and maintains effective serum concentrations over a 12-hour period. Reports indicate that it probably interacts with theophylline and carbamazepine by elevating the plasma concentrations of the two drugs. Biaxin® is supplied as 250 mg and 500 mg tablets (retail cost approximately $4 each) and 500 mg extended release tablets (approximately $5 each). It is also available as suspension, supplied as 125 mg/100 mL and 125 mg/50 mL (approximately $20 per 50 mL). Clarithromycin is not yet available as a generic drug.

Amoxicillin *on page 106*

Ampicillin *on page 117*

Azithromycin *on page 171*

Cefadroxil *on page 281*

Cefazolin *on page 283*

Cephalexin *on page 301*

Clarithromycin *on page 355*

Clindamycin *on page 361*

Clinical Considerations for Dentistry

See Figure 1 on page 1688.

The clinician should review carefully those detailed dental procedures in Table 3 to determine those treatment conditions where prophylaxis is, or is not, recommended. In general, in patients with cardiac conditions where prophylaxis is recommended (Table 4), invasive dental procedures where bleeding is likely to be induced from hard or soft tissues (Table 3) should be preceded by antibiotic coverage (Table 2). Clearly, the production of significant bacteremia during a dental procedure is the major risk factor. Patients with a suspicious history of a cardiac condition who are in need of an immediate dental procedure should be prophylaxed with an appropriate antibiotic prior to the procedure(s) until medical evaluation has been completed and the risk level determined. If unanticipated bleeding develops during a procedure in an at-risk patient, appropriate antibiotics should be given immediately. The efficacy of this action is based on animal studies and is possibly effective ≤2 hours after the bacteremia.

Table 3.
DENTAL PROCEDURES AND PREPROCEDURAL ANTIBIOTICS

Endocarditis or Prosthesis Prophylaxis Recommended Due to Likely Significant Bacteremia[1]
Dental extractions
Periodontal procedures including surgery, subgingival placement of antibiotic fibers/strips, scaling and root planing, probing, recall maintenance
Dental implant placement and reimplantation of avulsed teeth
Endodontic (root canal) instrumentation or surgery only beyond the apex
Initial placement of orthodontic bands but not brackets
Intraligamentary local anesthetic injections
Prophylactic cleaning of teeth or implants where bleeding is anticipated
Endocarditis Prophylaxis Not Recommended Due to Usually Insignificant Bacteremia
Restorative dentistry[2] (operative and prosthodontic) with or without retraction cord[3]
Local anesthetic injections (nonintraligamentary)
Intracanal endodontic treatment; postplacement and build-up[3]
Placement of rubber dam[3]
Postoperative suture removal
Placement of removable prosthodontic/orthodontic appliances
Oral impressions[3]
Fluoride treatments
Taking of oral radiographs
Orthodontic appliance adjustment
Shedding of primary teeth
[3]In general, the presence of moderate to severe gingival inflammation may elevate these procedures to a higher risk of bacteremia.

[1]Prophylaxis is recommended for patients with high- and moderate-risk cardiac as well as high-risk prosthesis conditions

[2]This includes restoration of decayed teeth and replacement of missing teeth

[3]Clinical judgment may indicate antibiotic use in any circumstances that may create significant bleeding.

Patients with moderate to advanced gingival inflammatory disease and/or periodontitis should be considered at greater risk of bacteremia. However, the ongoing daily risk of self-induced bacteremia in these patients is currently thought to be minimal as compared to the bacteremia during dental procedures. The clinician may wish to consider the use of a preprocedural antimicrobial rinse in addition to antibiotic prophylaxis and, of course, efforts should always focus on improving periodontal health during dental care. If a series of dental procedures is planned, the clinician must judge whether an interval between procedures, requiring prophylaxis, should be scheduled. The literature supports 9- to 14-day intervals as ideal to minimize the risk of emergence of resistant organisms. Since serum levels of the standard amoxicillin dose may be adequate for 6-14 hours depending on the specific organism challenge, the clinician may have to consider the efficacy of a second dose if multiple procedures are planned over the course of a single day.

ANTIBIOTIC PROPHYLAXIS *(Continued)*

Table 4.
CARDIAC CONDITIONS PREDISPOSING TO ENDOCARDITIS

Endocarditis Prophylaxis Recommended
High-Risk Category
Prosthetic cardiac valves, including bioprosthetic and homograft valves
Previous bacterial endocarditis
Complex cyanotic congenital heart disease (eg, single ventricle states, transposition of the great arteries, tetralogy of Fallot)
Surgically constructed systemic pulmonary shunts or conduits
Moderate-Risk Category
Most other congenital cardiac malformations (other than above and below)
Acquired valvar dysfunction (eg, rheumatic heart disease)
Hypertrophic cardiomyopathy
Mitral valve prolapse with valvar regurgitation and/or thickened leaflets[1]
Endocarditis Prophylaxis Not Recommended
Negligible-Risk Category (no greater risk than the general population)
Isolated secundum atrial septal defect
Surgical repair of atrial septal defect, ventricular septal defect, or patent ductus arteriosus (without residual defects beyond 6 mo)
Previous coronary artery bypass graft surgery
Mitral valve prolapse without valvar regurgitation
Physiologic, functional, or innocent heart murmurs
Previous Kawasaki disease without valvar dysfunction
Previous rheumatic fever without valvar dysfunction
Cardiac pacemakers (intravascular and epicardial) and implanted defibrillators

[1]**Specific risk for patients with a history of fenfluramine or dexfenfluramine (fen-phen or Redux®) use, has not been determined. Such patients should have medical evaluation for potential cardiac damage, as currently recommended by the FDA.**

For patients with suspected or confirmed mitral valve prolapse (MVP), the risk of infection as well as other complications such as tachycardia, syncope, congestive heart failure, or progressive regurgitation are variable. The risk depends on age and severity of MVP. The decision to recommend prophylaxis in such patients is oftentimes controversial but it is generally agreed that the determination of regurgitation is the most predictive (see Algorithm Figure 2 at the end of this chapter). Therefore, patients with MVP with mitral regurgitation require prophylaxis. If the regurgitation is undetermined and the patient is in need of an immediate procedure, then prophylaxis should be given in any case and the patient referred for further evaluation. If echocardiographic or Doppler studies demonstrate regurgitation, then prophylaxis would be recommended routinely. If no regurgitation can be demonstrated by these studies, then MVP alone does not require prophylaxis.

PREPROCEDURAL ANTIBIOTICS FOR PROSTHETIC IMPLANTS

A significant number of dental patients have had total joint replacements or other implanted prosthetic devices. Prior to performing dental procedures that might induce bacteremia, the dentist must consider the use of antibiotic prophylaxis in these patients. Until recently, only the American Heart Association had taken a formal stance on implanted devices by suggesting guidelines for the use of antibiotic prophylaxis in patients with prosthetic heart valves. These guidelines and the recent guidelines for prevention of bacterial endocarditis have been published in *General Dentistry*.

The use of antibiotics in patients with other prosthetic devices, including total joint replacements has remained controversial because of several issues. Late infections of implanted prosthetic devices have rarely been associated with microbial organisms of oral origin. Secondly, since late infections in such patients are often not reported, data is lacking to substantiate or refute this potential. Also, there is general acceptance that patients with acute infections at distant sites such as the oral cavity may be at greater risk of infection of an implanted prosthetic device. Periodontal disease has been implicated as a distant site infection. Since antibiotics are associated with allergies and other adverse reactions, and because the frequent use of antibiotics may lead to emergence of resistant organisms, any perceived benefit of antibiotic prophylaxis must always be weighed against known risks of toxicity, allergy, or potential microbial resistance.

Recently, an advisory group made up of representatives from the American Dental Association and the American Academy of Orthopaedic Surgeons published a statement in the *Journal of the American Dental Association* on the use of antibiotics prior to dental procedures in patients with total joint replacements. The statement concluded that antibiotic prophylaxis should not be prescribed routinely for most dental patients with total joint replacements or for any patients with pins, plates, and screws. However, in an attempt to base the guidelines on available scientific evidence, the advisory group stated that certain patients may be potential risks for joint infection thus justifying the use of prophylactic antibiotics. Those conditions considered by the advisory group to be associated with potential elevated risk of joint infections are listed in Table 5. The dentist should carefully review the patient's history to ensure identification of those medical problems leading to potential elevated risks of joint infections as listed in Table 5. Where appropriate, medical consultation with the patient's internist or orthopedist may be prudent to assist in this determination. The orthopedist should be queried specifically, as to the status of the joint prosthesis itself.

Table 5.
PATIENTS WITH POTENTIAL ELEVATED RISK OF JOINT INFECTION

Inflammatory arthropathies: Rheumatoid arthritis, systemic lupus erythematosus
Disease-, drug-, or radiation-induced immunosuppression
Insulin-dependent diabetes
First 2 years following joint replacement
Previous prosthetic joint infections
Patients with acute infections at a distant site
Hemophilia
Malnourishment[1]
Patients with malignancies[1]
Patients with HIV infection[1]

[1]Source: American Dental Association; American Academy of Orthopedic Surgeons, "Antibiotic Prophylaxis for Dental Patients With Total Joint Replacements," *J Am Dent Assoc*, 2003, 134(7):895-9.

Patients who present with elevated risks of joint infections, in which the dentist is going to perform any procedures associated with a high risk of bacteremia, need to receive preprocedural antibiotics. Those dental procedures associated with high risk of bacteremia are listed in Table 3. Patients undergoing dental procedures involving low risk of bacteremia, probably do not require premedication even though the patient may be in the category of elevated risk of joint infections. Patients with an acute oral infection or moderate to severe gingival inflammation and/or periodontitis must be considered at higher risk for bacteremia during dental procedures than those without active dental disease. In these patients, as in all patients, the dental clinician should aggressively treat these oral conditions striving for optimum oral health. The listing of low bacteremia risks in Table 3 may need to be reconsidered, depending on the patient's oral health.

For examples of sample prescriptions see Prosthetic Joint Late Infections (Prevention) *on page 1733.*

ANTIBIOTIC REGIMENS

The antibiotic prophylaxis regimens as suggested by the advisory panel are listed in Table 6. These regimens are not exactly the same as those listed in Table 2 (for prevention of endocarditis) and must be reviewed carefully to avoid confusion. Cephalexin, cephradine, or amoxicillin may be used in patients not allergic to penicillin. The selected antibiotic is given as a single 2 g dose 1 hour before the procedure. A follow-up dose is not recommended. Cephalexin (Keflex®) and amoxicillin were described earlier in this section. Cephradine (Velosef®) is a first-generation cephalosporin-type antibiotic, effective against anaerobic bacteria and aerobic Gram-positive bacteria. It is predominantly used to treat infections of the bones and joints, lower respiratory tract, urinary tract, skin, and soft tissues.

Parenteral cefazolin (Ancef®) or ampicillin are the recommended antibiotics for patients unable to take oral medications (see Table 6 for doses). Cefazolin is a first-generation cephalosporin, effective against anaerobes and aerobic Gram-positive bacteria. Ampicillin is an aminopenicillin (described earlier). For patients allergic to penicillin, clindamycin is the recommended antibiotic of choice. Clindamycin is active against aerobic and anaerobic streptococci, most staphylococci, the *Bacteroides*, and the *Actinomyces* families of bacteria. The recommended oral and parenteral doses of clindamycin in the joint prosthetic patient are listed in Table 6 below.

Table 6.
ANTIBIOTIC REGIMENS FOR PATIENTS WITH PROSTHETIC IMPLANTS

Patients not allergic to penicillin:	Cephalexin, cephradine, or amoxicillin:	2 g orally 1 hour prior to the procedure
Patients not allergic to penicillin and unable to take oral medications:	Cefazolin: or Ampicillin:	1 g I.M. or I.V. 1 hour prior to the procedure 2 g I.M. or I.V. 1 hour prior to the procedure
Patients allergic to penicillin:	Clindamycin:	600 mg orally 1 hour prior to dental procedure
Patients allergic to penicillin and unable to take oral medications:	Clindamycin:	600 mg I.V. 1 hour prior to the procedure

ANTIBIOTIC PROPHYLAXIS *(Continued)*

Amoxicillin *on page 106*
Ampicillin *on page 117*
Cefazolin *on page 283*
Cephalexin *on page 301*
Cephradine *on page 304*
Clindamycin *on page 361*

Clinical Considerations for Dentistry

See Figure 3 on page 1689.

The frequency of postinsertion infections in patients who have undergone total joint replacement or prosthetic device placement is variable. The most common cause of infection with all devices is found to be from contamination at the time of surgical insertions. The presence of an acute distant infection at a site other than the joint, however, appears to be a risk factor for late infection of these devices. The rationale by the American Dental Association and the American Academy of Orthopedic Surgeons in their advisory statement has been to provide guidelines to minimize the use of antibiotics to the first 2 years following total joint replacement. As more data are collected, these recommendations may be revised. However, it is thought to be prudent for the dental clinician to fully evaluate all patients with respect to history and or physical findings prior to determining the risk.

If a procedure considered to be low risk for bacteremia is performed in a patient at risk for joint complications, and inadvertent bleeding occurs, then an appropriate antibiotic should be given immediately. Although this is not ideal, animal studies suggest that it may be useful. Likewise, in patients where concern exists over joint complications and a medical consultation cannot be immediately obtained, the patient should be treated as though antibiotic coverage is necessary until such time that an appropriate consultation can be completed. The presence of an acute oral infection, in addition to any pre-existing dental conditions, may increase the risk of late infection at the prosthetic joint. Even though most late joint infections are caused by *Staphylococcus* sp, the risk of bacteremia involving another organism, predominant in an acute infection, may increase the risk of joint infection.

The dentist may also need to consider the question of multiple procedures over a period of time. Procedures planned over a period of several days would best be rescheduled at intervals of 9-14 days. The risk of emergence of resistant organisms in patients receiving multiple short-term doses of antibiotics has been shown to be greater than those receiving antibiotics over longer intervals of time.

FREQUENTLY ASKED QUESTIONS

If the patient is presently taking antibiotics for some other ailment, is prophylaxis still necessary?

If a patient is already taking antibiotics for another condition, prophylaxis should be accomplished with a drug from another class. For example, in the patient who is not allergic to penicillin who is taking erythromycin for a medical condition such as mycoplasma infection, amoxicillin would be the drug of choice for prophylaxis. Also, in the penicillin-allergic patient taking clindamycin, prophylaxis would best be accomplished with azithromycin or clarithromycin. The new guidelines restated the position that doses of antibiotics for prevention of recurrence of rheumatic fever are thought to be inadequate to prevent bacterial endocarditis and prophylaxis should be accomplished with the full dose of a drug from another class.

Can clindamycin be used safely in patients with gastrointestinal disorders?

If a patient has a history of inflammatory bowel disease and is allergic to penicillin, azithromycin or clarithromycin should be selected over clindamycin. In patients with a negative history of inflammatory bowel disease, clindamycin has not been shown to induce colitis following a single-dose administration.

Why do the suggested drug regimens for patients with joint prostheses resemble so closely the regimens for the prevention of bacterial endocarditis?

Bacteremia is the predisposing risk factor for the development of endocarditis in those patients at risk due to a cardiac condition. Likewise, the potential of bacteremia during dental procedures is considered to be the risk factor in some late joint prostheses infections, even though this risk is presumed to be much lower.

How do we determine those patients who have had joint replacement complications?

Patients who have had complications during the initial placement of a total joint would be those who had infection following placement, those with recurrent pain, or those who have had previous joint replacement failures. If the patient reports even minor complications, a medical consultation with the orthopedist would be the most appropriate action for the dentist.

Is prophylaxis required in patients with pins, screws, or plates often used in orthopedic repairs?

There is currently no evidence supporting use of antibiotics following the placement of pins, plates, or screws. Breast implants, dental implants, and implanted lenses in the eye following cataract surgery are also all thought to be at minimal risk for infection following dental procedures. Therefore, no antibiotic prophylaxis is recommended in these situations. There is, however, some evidence indicating elevated risk of infection following some types of penile implants and some vascular access devices, used during chemotherapy. It is recommended that the dentist discuss such patients with the physician prior to determining the need for antibiotics.

What should I do if medical consultation results in a recommendation that differs from the published guidelines endorsed by the American Dental Association?

The dentist is ultimately responsible for treatment recommendations. Ideally, by communicating with the physician, a consensus can be achieved that is either in agreement with the guidelines or is based on other established medical reasoning.

What is the best antibiotic modality for treating dental infections?

Penicillin is still the drug of choice for treatment of infections in and around the oral cavity. Phenoxy-methyl penicillin (Pen VK®) has long been the most commonly-selected antibiotic. In penicillin-allergic individuals, erythromycin may be an appropriate consideration. If another drug is sought, clindamycin prescribed 300 mg as a loading dose followed by 150 mg 4 times/day would be an appropriate regimen for a dental infection. In general, if there is no response to Pen VK®, then Augmentin® may be a good alternative in the nonpenicillin-allergic patient because of its slightly altered spectrum. Recommendations would include that the patient should take the drug with food.

Is there cross-allergenicity between the cephalosporins and penicillin?

The incidence of cross-allergenicity is 5% to 8% in the overall population. If a patient has demonstrated a Type I hypersensitivity reaction to penicillin, namely urticaria or anaphylaxis, then this incidence would increase to 20%.

Is there definitely an interaction between contraception agents and antibiotics?

There are well founded interactions between contraceptives and antibiotics. The best instructions that a patient could be given by their dentist are that should an antibiotic be necessary and the dentist is aware that the patient is on contraceptives, and if the patient is using chemical contraceptives, the patient should seriously consider additional means of contraception during the antibiotic management.

Are antibiotics necessary in diabetic patients?

In the management of diabetes, control of the diabetic status is the key factor relative to all morbidity issues. If a patient is well controlled, then antibiotics will likely not be necessary. However, in patients where the control is questionable or where they have recently been given a different drug regimen for their diabetes or if they are being titrated to an appropriate level of either insulin or oral hypoglycemic agents during these periods of time, the dentist might consider preprocedural antibiotics to be efficacious.

Do nonsteroidal anti-inflammatory drugs interfere with blood pressure medication?

At the current time there is no clear evidence that NSAIDs interfere with any of the blood pressure medications that are currently in use.

Is a patient who has taken phentermine at risk for cardiac problems just like a patient who took "fen-phen"?

No, there is often confusion with these drug names. "Fen-phen" referred to a combined use of fenfluramine and phentermine and it is this combination that has led to the FDA statement (see Table 4). The single drug phentermine has not been implicated in this current concern over cardiac complications.

ANTIBIOTIC PROPHYLAXIS *(Continued)*

Figure 1
Preprocedural Dental Action Plan for Patients With a History Indicative of Elevated Endocarditis Risk

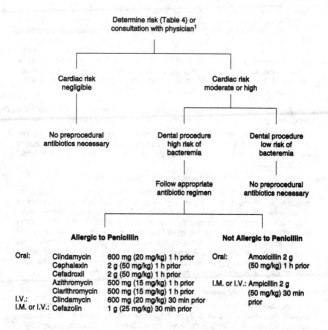

Dosages for children are in parentheses and should never exceed adult dose. Cephalosporins should be avoided in patients with previous Type I hypersensitivity reactions to penicillin due to some evidence of cross-allergenicity.

[1]For Emergency Dental Care, the clinician should attempt phone consultation. If unable to contact patient's physician or determine risk, the patient should be treated as though there is moderate or high risk of cardiac complication and follow the algorithm.

Figure 2
Patient With Suspected Mitral Valve Prolapse

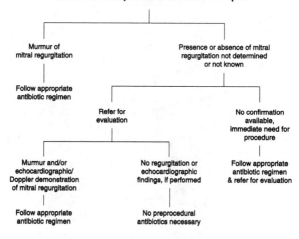

Figure 3
Preprocedural Dental Action Plan for
Patients With Prosthetic Implants

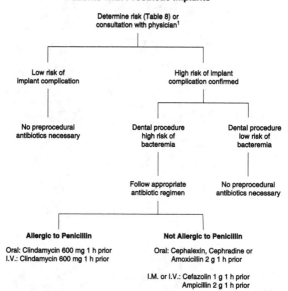

Cephalosporins should be avoided in patients with previous Type I hypersensitivity reactions to penicillin due to some evidence of cross allergenicity.

[1]For Emergency Dental Care the clinician should attempt phone consultation. If unable to contact patient's physician or determine risk, the patient should be treated as though there is high risk of implant complication and follow the algorithm.

ORAL MEDICINE TOPICS

PART II:

DENTAL MANAGEMENT AND THERAPEUTIC CONSIDERATIONS IN PATIENTS WITH SPECIFIC ORAL CONDITIONS AND OTHER MEDICINE TOPICS

This second part of the chapter focuses on therapies the dentist may choose to prescribe for patients suffering from oral disease or who are in need of special care. Some overlap between these sections has resulted from systemic conditions that have oral manifestations and vice-versa. Cross-references to the descriptions and the monographs for individual drugs described elsewhere in this handbook allow for easy retrieval of information. Example prescriptions of selected drug therapies for each condition are presented so that the clinician can evaluate alternate approaches to treatment, since there is seldom a single drug of choice.

Drug prescriptions shown represent prototype drugs and popular prescriptions and are examples only. The pharmacologic category index is available for cross-referencing if alternatives and additional drugs are sought.

TABLE OF CONTENTS

Oral Pain 1692

Bacterial Infections 1697

Periodontal Diseases 1705

Fungal Infections 1707

Viral Infections 1709

Ulcerative and Erosive Disorders 1712

Dentin Hypersensitivity, High Caries Index, and Xerostomia 1714

Temporomandibular Dysfunction (TMD) 1724

Sedation 1727

Management of Patients Undergoing Cancer Therapy 1728

ORAL PAIN

PAIN PREVENTION

For the dental patient, the prevention of pain aids in relieving anxiety and reduces the probability of stress during dental care. For the practitioner, dental procedures can be accomplished more efficiently in a "painless" situation. Appropriate selection and use of local anesthetics is one of the foundations for success in this arena. Local anesthetics listed below include drugs for the most commonly confronted dental procedures. Ester anesthetics are no longer available in dose form for dental injections, and historically had a higher incidence of allergic manifestations due to the formation of the metabolic byproduct, para-aminobenzoic acid. Articaine, which has an ester side chain, is rapidly metabolized to a non-PABA acid and, hence, functions as an amide and has a low allergic potential. The amides, in general, have an almost negligible allergic rate, and only one well-documented case of amide allergy has been reported by Seng, et al. Although injectable diphenhydramine (Benadryl®) has been used in an attempt to provide anesthesia in patients allergic to all the local anesthetics, it is no longer recommended in this context. The vehicle for injectable diphenhydramine can cause tissue necrosis.

The potential interaction between acetaminophen and warfarin has been recently raised in the literature. The cytochrome P450 system of drug metabolism for these vitamin K dependent metabolic pathways has raised the possibility that prolonged use of acetaminophen may inadvertently enhance, to dangerous levels, the anticoagulation effect of warfarin. As monitored by the INR, the effects of these drugs may be one and one-half to two times greater than as expected from the warfarin dosage alone. This potential interaction could be of importance in selecting an analgesic/antipyretic drug for the dental patient.

LOCAL ANESTHETICS

Articaine and Epinephrine [U.S.] *on page 139*

Bupivacaine *on page 228*

Bupivacaine and Epinephrine *on page 228*

Chloroprocaine *on page 320*

Levobupivacaine *on page 909*

Lidocaine *on page 920*

Lidocaine (Transoral) *on page 931*

Lidocaine and Epinephrine *on page 924*

Mepivacaine Dental Anesthetic *on page 989*

Mepivacaine and Levonordefrin *on page 991*

Prilocaine *on page 1277*

Prilocaine and Epinephrine *on page 1278*

Ropivacaine *on page 1366*

Tetracaine *on page 1466*

Tetracaine and Dextrose *on page 1467*

The selection of a vasoconstrictor with the local anesthetic must be based on the length of the procedure to be performed, the patient's medical status (epinephrine is contraindicated in patients with uncontrolled hyperthyroidism), and the need for hemorrhage control. The following table lists some of the common drugs with their duration of action. Transoral patches with lidocaine are now available (DentiPatch®) and the new long-acting amide injectable, Ropivacaine (Naropin®) may be useful for postoperative pain management.

DENTAL ANESTHETICS
(Average Duration by Route)

Product	Infiltration	Inferior Alveolar Block
Articaine HCl 4% and epinephrine 1:100,000	60 minutes	60 minutes
Carbocaine® HCl 2% with Neo-Cobefrin® 1:20,000 (mepivacaine HCl and levonordefrin)	50 minutes	60-75 minutes
Duranest® Injection (etidocaine)	5-10 hours	5-10 hours
Citanest® Plain 4% (prilocaine)	20 minutes	2.5 hours
Citanest Forte® with Epinephrine (prilocaine with epinephrine)	2.25 hours	3 hours
Lidocaine HCl 2% and epinephrine 1:100,000	60 minutes	90 minutes
Marcaine® HCl 0.5% with epinephrine 1:200,000 (bupivacaine and epinephrine)	60 minutes	5-7 hours

The use of articaine 4% with epinephrine 1:100,000 solution for mandibular blocks has been associated occasionally with parasthesia, (*J Am Dent Assoc*, 2001, 132(2):177-85).

The use of preinjection topical anesthetics can assist in pain prevention (see also Viral Infections *on page 1709* and Ulcerative and Erosive Disorders *on page 1712*). Some clinicians are also using EMLA® (eutectic mixture of local anesthetic with lidocaine and prilocaine) as a topical. Skin patch available by Astra not currently approved for oral use.

Benzocaine *on page 190*

Lidocaine *on page 920*

Lidocaine Transoral *on page 931*

Tetracaine *on page 1466*

PAIN MANAGEMENT

The patient with existing acute or chronic oral pain requires appropriate treatment and sensitivity on the part of the dentist, all for the purpose of achieving relief from the oral source of pain. Pain can be divided into mild, moderate, and severe levels and requires a subjective assessment by the dentist based on knowledge of the dental procedures to be performed, the presenting signs and symptoms of the patient, and the realization that most dental procedures are invasive often leading to pain once the patient has left the dental office. The practitioner must be aware that the treatment of the source of the pain is usually the best management. If infection is present, treatment of the infection will directly alleviate the patient's discomfort. However, a patient who is not in pain tends to heal better and it is wise to adequately cover the patient for any residual or recurrent discomfort suffered. Likewise, many of the procedures that the dentist performs have pain associated with them. Much of this pain occurs after leaving the dentist office due to an inflammatory process or a healing process that has been initiated. It is difficult to assign specific pain levels (mild, moderate, or severe) for specific procedures; however, the dentist should use his or her prescribing capacity judiciously so that overmedication is avoided.

The following categories of drugs and appropriate example prescriptions for each follow. These include management of mild pain with aspirin products, acetaminophen, and some of the nonsteroidal noninflammatory agents. Management of moderate pain includes codeine, Vicodin®, Vicodin ES®, Lorcet® 10/650; and Motrin® in the 800 mg dosage. Severe pain may require treatment with Percodan®, Percocet®, or Demerol®. All prescription pain preparations should be closely monitored for efficacy and discontinued if the pain persists or requires a higher level formulation. Combination drugs such as the recently released Combunox™ containing 5 mg of oxycodone and 400 mg of ibuprofen have proven usefulness in acute moderately severe to severe pain management.

The chronic pain patient represents a particular challenge for the practitioner. Some additional drugs that may be useful in managing the patient with chronic pain of neuropathic origin are covered in the temporomandibular dysfunction section *on page 1724*. It is always incumbent on the practitioner to reevaluate the diagnosis, source of pain, and treatment, whenever prolonged use of analgesics (narcotic or non-narcotic) is contemplated. Drugs such as Dilaudid® are not recommended for management of dental pain in most states.

Narcotic analgesics can be used on a short-term basis or intermittently in combination with non-narcotic therapy in the chronic pain patient. Judicious prescribing, monitoring, and maintenance by the practitioner is imperative, particularly whenever considering the use of a narcotic analgesic due to the abuse and addiction liabilities.

ORAL PAIN (Continued)

MILD PAIN

Acetaminophen *on page 31*

Aspirin (various products) *on page 145*

Diflunisal *on page 468*

Ibuprofen *on page 808*

Ketoprofen *on page 883*

Lansoprazole *on page 896*

Lansoprazole and Naproxen *on page 898*

Naproxen *on page 1089*

MODERATE / MODERATELY SEVERE PAIN

Aspirin and Codeine *on page 149*

Dihydrocodeine, Aspirin, and Caffeine *on page 475*

Hydrocodone and Acetaminophen *on page 779*

Hydrocodone and Ibuprofen *on page 787*

Acetaminophen and Tramadol *on page 39*

Ibuprofen (various products) *on page 808*

An additional class of NSAIDs has been approved and indicated in the treatment of arthritis, COX-2 inhibitors. Celecoxib (Celebrex®) has been approved for use in oral pain management.

The following is a guideline to use when prescribing codeine with either aspirin or acetaminophen (Tylenol®):

Codeine No. 2 = codeine 15 mg

Codeine No. 3 = codeine 30 mg

Codeine No. 4 = codeine 60 mg

Example: ASA No. 3 = aspirin 325 mg + codeine 30 mg

HYDROCODONE PRODUCTS

Available hydrocodone oral products are listed in the following table and are scheduled as C-III controlled substances, indicating that prescriptions may either be oral or written. Thus, the prescriber may call–in a prescription to the pharmacy for any of these hydrocodone products. All the formulations are combined with acetaminophen except for Vicoprofen®, which contains ibuprofen, and Lortab® ASA and Damason–P®, which all contain aspirin. Most of these brand name drugs are available generically and the pharmacist will dispense the generic equivalent if available, unless the prescriber indicates otherwise.

HYDROCODONE ANALGESIC COMBINATION ORAL PRODUCTS
(All Products DEA Schedule C-III)

Hydrocodone is available under numerous brand names with varying dosages and in combination with aspirin or ibuprofen.					
Hydrocodone Bitartrate	Acetaminophen (APAP[1])	Other	Brand Name	Generic Available	Form
2.5 mg	500 mg	–	Lortab® 2.5/500	Yes	Tablet
5 mg	400 mg	–	Zydone®	No	Tablet
5 mg	500 mg	–	Vicodin®; Dolagesic®; Hy-Phen®; Hydrocet®; Anexsia® 5/500; Lortab®5/500	Yes	Tablet
5 mg	500 mg	–	Polygesic®; Lorcet-HD®	Yes	Capsule
7.5 mg	400 mg	–	Zydone®	No	Tablet
7.5 mg	500 mg	–	Lortab® 7.5/500	Yes	Tablet
7.5 mg	650 mg	–	Anexsia® 7.5/650; Lorcet Plus®	Yes	Tablet
7.5 mg	750 mg	–	Vicodin ES®	Yes	Tablet
10 mg	400 mg	–	Zydone®	No	Tablet
10 mg	325 mg	–	Norco®	No	Tablet
10 mg	500 mg	–	Lortab® 10/500	Yes	Tablet

HYDROCODONE ANALGESIC COMBINATION ORAL PRODUCTS
(All Products DEA Schedule C-III) (continued)

Hydrocodone is available under numerous brand names with varying dosages and in combination with aspirin or ibuprofen.					
Hydrocodone Bitartrate	Acetaminophen (APAP[1])	Other	Brand Name	Generic Available	Form
10 mg	650 mg	–	Lorcet®	Yes	Tablet
10 mg	660 mg	–	Vicodin HP®; Anexsia® 10/660	Yes	Tablet
10 mg	750 mg	–	Maxidone™	No	Tablet
7.5 mg/15 mL	500 mg/15 mL	–	Lortab® Elixir	Yes	Elixir
5 mg	–	Aspirin 500 mg	Lortab® ASA; Damason–P®	Yes	Tablet
7.5 mg	–	Ibuprofen 200 mg	Vicoprofen®	No	Tablet

[1]APAP is the common acronym for acetaminophen and is the abbreviation of the chemical name N-acetylparaminophenol.

The following are the usual adult doses of the hydrocodone oral products as listed by the most recent edition of the Drug Information for the Health Care Professional (USPDI).

1 or 2 tablets containing 2.5 mg of hydrocodone and 500 mg of acetaminophen every 4-6 hours; or

1 tablet containing 5 mg of hydrocodone and 500 mg acetaminophen every 4-6 hours as needed, with dosage being increased to 2 tablets every 6 hours, if necessary; or

1 capsule containing 5 mg of hydrocodone and 500 mg of acetaminophen every 4-6 hours as needed, with dosage being increased to 2 capsules every 6 hours if necessary; or

1 tablet containing 7.5 mg hydrocodone and 650 mg of acetaminophen every 4-6 hours as needed, with dosage being increased to 2 tablets every 6 hours if necessary; or

1 tablet containing 7.5 mg hydrocodone and 750 mg of acetaminophen every 4-6 hours as needed; or

1 tablet containing 10 mg of hydrocodone and 650 mg acetaminophen every 4-6 hours as needed.

For the elixir (Lortab®), the recommended dose is 1 tablespoonful every 4-6 hours when necessary for pain.

For the aspirin products (Lortab® ASA and Damason-P®), the recommended dose is 1 or 2 tablets every 4-6 hours as needed.

For the ibuprofen product (Vicoprofen®), the recommended dose is 1 or 2 tablets every 4-6 hours as needed. The manufacturer recommends that the maximum dose of Vicoprofen® should not exceed 5 tablets in 24 hours.

The usual adult prescribing limits for the combination hydrocodone-acetaminophen products is up to 40 mg of hydrocodone and up to 4000 mg (4 g) of acetaminophen in a 24-hour period.

SEVERE PAIN

Meperidine on page 983

Oxycodone on page 1163

Oxycodone and Acetaminophen on page 1165

Oxycodone and Aspirin on page 1168

Oxycodone and Ibuprofen on page 1170

Oxycodone is available in a variety of dosages and combinations under numerous brand names. A new combination of Oxycodone hydrochloride with ibuprofen has been used in Phase III clinical trials at Forest Laboratories and is currently awaiting approval.

ORAL PAIN *(Continued)*

SAMPLE PRESCRIPTIONS

Rx:

Ibuprofen 800 mg tablets
Disp: 16 tablets
Sig: Take 1 tablet 3 times/day as needed for pain

Note: Also available as 600 mg tablets

Rx:

Lortab® 5 mg
Disp: 16 tablets
Sig: Take 1 or 2 tablets every 4 hours as needed for pain; not to exceed 8 tablets in 24 hours

Note: Restrictions: C-III; no refills
Ingredients: Hydrocodone 5 mg and acetaminophen 500 mg; available as generic equivalent

For additional sample prescriptions see Oral Pain *on page 1734*

BACTERIAL INFECTIONS

Dental infection can occur for any number of reasons, primarily involving pulpal and periodontal infections. Secondary infections of the soft tissues as well as sinus infections pose special treatment challenges. The drugs of choice in treating most oral infections have been selected because of their efficacy in providing adequate blood levels for delivery to the oral tissues and their proven usefulness in managing dental infections. Penicillin remains the primary drug for treatment of dental infections of pulpal origin. The management of soft tissue infections may require the use of additional drugs.

OROFACIAL INFECTIONS

The basis of all infections is the successful multiplication of a microbial pathogen on or within a host. The pathogen is usually defined as any microorganism that has the capacity to cause disease. If the pathogen is bacterial in nature, antibiotic therapy is often indicated.

DIFFERENTIAL DIAGNOSIS OF ODONTOGENIC INFECTIONS

In choosing the appropriate antibiotic for therapy of a given infection, a number of important factors must be considered. First, the identity of the organism must be known. In odontogenic infections involving dental or periodontal structures, this is seldom the case. Secondly, accurate information regarding antibiotic susceptibility is required. Again, unless the organism has been identified, this is not possible. And thirdly, host factors must be taken into account, in terms of ability to absorb an antibiotic, to achieve appropriate host response. When clinical evidence of cellulitis or odontogenic infection has been found and the cardinal signs of swelling, inflammation, pain, and perhaps fever are present, the selection by the clinician of the appropriate antibiotic agent may lead to eradication.

CAUSES OF ODONTOGENIC INFECTIONS

Most acute orofacial infections are of odontogenic origin. Dental caries, resulting in infection of dental pulp, is the leading cause of odontogenic infection.

The major causative organisms involved in dental caries have been identified as members of the viridans (alpha-hemolytic) streptococci and include *Streptococcus mutans*, *Streptococcus sobrinus*, and *Streptococcus milleri*. Once the bacteria have breached the enamel they invade the dentin and eventually the dental pulp. An inflammatory reaction occurs in the pulp tissue resulting in necrosis and a lower tissue oxidation-reduction potential. At this point, the bacterial flora changes from predominantly aerobic to a more obligate anaerobic flora. The anaerobic gram-positive cocci (*Peptostreptococcus* species), and the anaerobic gram-negative rods, including *Bacteroides, Prevotella, Porphyromonas,* and *Fusobacterium* are most frequently present. An abscess usually forms at the apex of the involved tooth resulting in destruction of bone. Depending on the effectiveness of the host resistance and the virulence of the bacteria, the infection may spread through the marrow spaces, perforate the cortical plate, and enter the surrounding soft tissues.

The other major source of odontogenic infection arises from the anaerobic bacterial flora that inhabits the periodontal and supporting structures of the teeth. The most important potential pathogenic anaerobes within these structures are *Actinobacillus actinomycetemcomitans, Prevotella intermedius, Porphyromonas gingivalis, Fusobacterium nucleatum,* and *Eikenella corrodens*.

Most odontogenic infections (70%) have mixed aerobic and anaerobic flora. Pure aerobic infections are much less common and comprise ~5% incidence. Pure anaerobic infections make up the remaining 25% of odontogenic infections. Clinical correlates suggest that early odontogenic infections are characterized by rapid spreading and cellulitis with the absence of abscess formation. The bacteria are predominantly aerobic with gram-positive, alpha-hemolytic streptococci (*S. viridans*) the predominant pathogen. As the infection matures and becomes more severe, the microbial flora becomes a mix of aerobes and anaerobes. The anaerobes present are determined by the characteristic flora associated with the site of origin, whether it be pulpal or periodontal. Finally, as the infectious process becomes controlled by host defenses, the flora becomes primarily anaerobic. For example, Lewis and MacFarlane found a predominance of facultative oral streptococci in the early infections (<3 days of symptoms) with the later predominance of obligate anaerobes.

In a review of severe odontogenic infections, it was reported that Brook, et al, observed that 50% of odontogenic deep facial space infections yielded anaerobic bacteria only. Also, 44% of these infections yielded a mix of aerobic and anaerobic flora. The results of a study published in 1998 by Sakamoto, et al, were also described in the review. The study confirmed that odontogenic infections usually result from a synergistic interaction among several bacterial species and usually consist of an oral streptococcus and an oral anaerobic gram-negative rod. Sakamoto and his group reported a high level of the

BACTERIAL INFECTIONS *(Continued)*

Streptococcus milleri group of aerobic gram-positive cocci, and high levels of oral anaer-obes, including the *Peptostreptococcus* species and the *Prevotella, Porphyromonas,* and *Fusobacterium* species.

Oral streptococci, especially of the *Streptococcus milleri* group, can invade soft tissues initially, thus preparing an environment conducive to growth of anaerobic bacteria. Obli-gate oral anaerobes are dependent on nutrients synthesized by the aerobes. Thus the anaerobes appear approximately 3 days after onset of symptoms. Early infections are thus caused primarily by the aerobic streptococci (exquisitely sensitive to penicillin) and late infections are caused by the anaerobes (frequently resistant to penicillin).

It appears logical, as Flynn has noted, to separate infections presenting early in their course from those presenting later when selecting empiric antibiotics of choice for odon-togenic infections.

If the patient is not allergic to penicillin, penicillin VK still remains the empiric antibiotic of first choice to treat mild or early odontogenic infections (see Table 1). In penicillin allergy, clindamycin clearly remains the alternative antibiotic for treatment of mild or early infec-tions. Secondary alternative antibiotics still recognized as useful in these conditions are cephalexin (Keflex®), or other first generation cephalosporins available in oral dose forms. The first generation cephalosporins can be used in both penicillin-allergic and nonallergic patients, providing that the penicillin allergy is not the anaphylactoid type.

PENICILLIN VK

The spectrum of antibacterial action of penicillin VK is consistent with most of the organisms identified in odontogenic infections (see Table 2). Penicillin VK is a beta-lactam antibiotic, as are all the penicillins and cephalosporins, and is bactericidal against gram-positive cocci and the major pathogens of mixed anaerobic infections. It elicits virtually no adverse effects in the absence of allergy and is relatively low in cost. Adverse drug reactions occurring in >10% of patients include mild diarrhea, nausea, and oral candidiasis. To treat odontogenic infections and other orofacial infections, the usual dose for adults and children >12 years of age is 500 mg every 6 hours for at least 7 days (see Table 4). The daily dose for children ≤12 years of age is 25-50 mg/kg of body weight in divided doses every 6-8 hours (see Table 4). The patient must be instructed to take the penicillin continuously for the duration of therapy.

After oral dosing, penicillin VK achieves peak serum levels within 1 hour. Penicillin VK may be given with meals, however, blood concentrations may be slightly higher when penicillin is given on an empty stomach. The preferred dosing is 1 hour before meals or 2 hours after meals to ensure maximum serum levels. Penicillin VK diffuses into most body tissues, including oral tissues, soon after dosing. Hepatic metabolism accounts for <30% of the elimination of penicillins. Elimination is primarily renal. The nonmetabolized peni-cillin is excreted largely unchanged in the urine by glomerular filtration and active tubular secretion. Penicillins cross the placenta and are distributed in breast milk. Penicillin VK, like all beta-lactam antibiotics, causes death of bacteria by inhibiting synthesis of the bacterial cell wall during cell division. This action is dependent on the ability of penicillins to reach and bind to penicillin-binding proteins (PBPs) located on the inner membrane of the bacterial cell wall. PBPs (which include transpeptidases, carboxypeptidases, and endopeptidases) are enzymes that are involved in the terminal stages of assembling and reshaping the bacterial cell wall during growth. Penicillins and beta-lactams bind to and inactivate PBPs resulting in lysis of the cell due to weakening of the cell wall.

Penicillin VK is considered a "narrow spectrum" antibiotic. This class of antibiotics produces less alteration of normal microflora thereby reducing the incidence of superin-fection. Also, its bactericidal action will reduce the numbers of microorganisms resulting in less reliance on host-phagocyte mechanisms for eradication of the pathogen.

Among patients, 0.7% to 10% are allergic to penicillins. There is no evidence that any single penicillin derivative differs from others in terms of incidence or severity when administered orally. About 85% of allergic reactions associated with penicillin VK are delayed and take >2 days to develop. This allergic response manifests as skin rashes characterized as erythema and bullous eruptions. This type of allergic reaction is mild, reversible, and usually responds to concurrent antihistamine therapy, such as diphenhy-dramine (Benadryl®). Severe reactions of angioedema have occurred, characterized by marked swelling of the lips, tongue, face, and periorbital tissues. Patients with a history of penicillin allergy must never be given penicillin VK for treatment of infections. The alternative antibiotic is clindamycin. If the allergy is the delayed type and not the anaphy-lactoid type, a first generation cephalosporin may be used as an alternate antibiotic.

CLINDAMYCIN

In the event of penicillin allergy, clindamycin is clearly an alternative of choice in treating mild or early odontogenic infections (see Table 1). It is highly effective against almost all oral pathogens. Clindamycin is active against most aerobic gram-positive cocci, including staphylococci, *S. pneumoniae*, other streptococci, and anaerobic gram-negative and gram-positive organisms, including bacteroides (see Table 3). Clindamycin is not effec-tive against mycoplasma or gram-negative aerobes. It inhibits protein synthesis in bacteria through binding to the 50 S subunit of bacterial ribosomes. Clindamycin has bacteriostatic actions at low concentrations, but is known to elicit bactericidal effects against susceptible bacteria at higher concentrations of drug at the site of infection.

The usual adult oral dose of clindamycin to treat orofacial infections of odontogenic origin is 150-450 mg every 6 hours for 7-10 days. The usual daily oral dose for children is 8-25 mg/kg in 3-4 equally divided doses (see Table 4).

Following oral administration of a 150 mg or a 300 mg dose on an empty stomach, 90% of the dose is rapidly absorbed into the bloodstream and peak serum concentrations are attained in 45-60 minutes. Administration with food does not markedly impair absorption into the bloodstream. Clindamycin serum levels exceed the minimum inhibitory concentration for bacterial growth for at least 6 hours after the recommended doses. The serum half-life is 2-3 hours. Clindamycin is distributed effectively to most body tissues, including saliva and bone. Its small molecular weight enables it to more readily enter bacterial cytoplasm to penetrate bone. It is partially metabolized in the liver to active and inactive metabolites and is excreted in the urine, bile, and feces.

Adverse effects caused by clindamycin can include abdominal pain, nausea, vomiting, and diarrhea. Hypersensitivity reactions are rare, but have resulted in skin rash. Approximately 1% of clindamycin users develop pseudomembranous colitis characterized by severe diarrhea, abdominal cramps, and excretion of blood or mucus in the stools. The mechanism is disruption of normal bacterial flora of the colon, which leads to colonization of the bacterium *Clostridium difficile*. This bacterium releases endotoxins that cause mucosal damage and inflammation. Symptoms usually develop 2-9 days after initiation of therapy, but may not occur until several weeks after taking the drug. If significant diarrhea develops, clindamycin therapy should be discontinued immediately. Theoretically, any antibiotic can cause antibiotic-associated colitis and clindamycin probably has an undeserved reputation associated with this condition.

Sandor, et al, also notes that odontogenic infections are typically polymicrobial and that anaerobes outnumber aerobes by at least four-fold. The penicillins have historically been used as the first-line therapy in these cases, but increasing rates of resistance have lowered their usefulness. Bacterial resistance to penicillins is predominantly achieved through production of beta-lactamases. Clindamycin, because of its relatively broad spectrum of activity and resistance to beta-lactamase degradation, is an attractive first-line therapy in treatment of odontogenic infections.

FIRST GENERATION CEPHALOSPORINS

Antibiotics of this class, which are available in oral dosage forms, include cefadroxil (Duricef®), cephalexin (Keflex®), and cephradine (Velosef®). The first generation cephalosporins are alternates to penicillin VK in the treatment of odontogenic infections based on bactericidal effectiveness against the oral streptococci. These drugs are most active against gram-positive cocci, but are not very active against many anaerobes. First generation cephalosporins are indicated as alternatives in early infections because they are effective in killing the aerobes. First generation cephalosporins are active against gram-positive staphylococci and streptococci, but not enterococci. They are active against many gram-negative aerobic bacilli, including *E. coli, Klebsiella,* and *Proteus mirabilis*. They are inactive against methicillin-resistant *S. aureus* and penicillin-resistant *S. pneumoniae*. The gram-negative aerobic cocci, *Moraxella catarrhalis*, portrays variable sensitivity to first generation cephalosporins.

Cephalexin (Keflex®) is the first generation cephalosporin often used to treat odontogenic infections. The usual adult dose is 250-1000 mg every 6 hours with a maximum of 4 g/day. Children's dose is 25-50 mg/kg/day in divided doses every 6 hours; for severe infections: 50-100 mg/kg/day in divided doses every 6 hours with a maximum dose of 3 g/day (see Table 4).

Cephalexin (Keflex®) causes diarrhea in about 1% to 10% of patients. About 90% of the cephalexin is excreted unchanged in urine.

SECOND GENERATION CEPHALOSPORINS

The second generation cephalosporins such as cefaclor (Ceclor®) have better activity against some of the anaerobes including some *Bacteroides, Peptococcus,* and *Peptostreptococcus* species. Cefaclor (Ceclor®) and cefuroxime (Ceftin®) have been used to treat early stage infections. These antibiotics have the advantage of twice-a-day dosing. The usual oral adult dose of cefaclor is 250-500 mg every 8 hours (or daily dose can be given in 2 divided doses) for at least 7 days. Children's dose is 20-40 mg/kg/day divided every 8-12 hours with a maximum dose of 2 g/day. The usual adult oral dose of cefuroxime is 250-500 mg twice daily. Children's dose is 20 mg/kg/day (maximum 500 mg/day) in 2 divided doses.

The cephalosporins inhibit bacterial cell wall synthesis by binding to one or more of the penicillin-binding proteins (PBPs), which in turn inhibits the final transpeptidation step of peptidoglycan synthesis in bacterial cell walls, thus inhibiting cell wall biosynthesis. Bacteria eventually lyse due to ongoing activity of cell wall autolytic enzymes while cell wall assembly is arrested.

BACTERIAL INFECTIONS *(Continued)*

BACTERIAL RESISTANCE TO ANTIBIOTICS

If a patient with an early stage odontogenic infection does not respond to penicillin VK within 24-36 hours, it is evidence of the presence of resistant bacteria. Bacterial resistance to the penicillins is predominantly achieved through the production of beta-lactamase. A switch to beta-lactamase-stable antibiotics should be made. For example, Kuriyama, et al, reported that past beta-lactam administration increases the emergence of beta-lactamase-producing bacteria and that beta-lactamase-stable antibiotics should be prescribed to patients with unresolved infections who have received beta-lactams. These include either clindamycin or amoxicillin/clavulanic acid (Augmentin®). Doses are listed in Table 4.

In the past, all *S. viridans* species were uniformly susceptible to beta-lactam antibiotics. However, over the years, there has been a significant increase in resistant strains. Resistance may also be due to alteration of penicillin-binding proteins. Consequently, drugs which combine a beta-lactam antibiotic with a beta-lactamase inhibitor, such as amoxicillin/clavulanic acid (Augmentin®), may no longer be more effective than the penicillin VK alone. In these situations, clindamycin is the recommended alternate antibiotic.

Evidence suggests that empirical use of penicillin VK as the first-line drug in treating early odontogenic infections is still the best way to ensure the minimal production of resistant bacteria to other classes of antibiotics, since any overuse of clindamycin or amoxicillin/clavulanic acid (Augmentin®) is minimized in these situations. There is concern that overuse of clindamycin could contribute to development of clindamycin-resistant pathogens.

In late odontogenic infections, it is suggested that clindamycin be considered the first-line antibiotic to treat these infections. The dose of clindamycin would be the same as that used to treat early infections (see Table 4). In these infections, anaerobic bacteria usually predominate. Since penicillin spectrum includes anaerobes, penicillin VK is also useful as an empiric drug of first choice in these infections. It has been reported, however, that the penicillin resistance rate among patients with serious and late infections is in the 35% to 50% range. Therefore, if penicillin is the drug of first choice and the patient does not respond within 24-36 hours, a resistant pathogen should be suspected and a switch to clindamycin be made. Clindamycin, because of its relatively broad spectrum of activity and resistance to beta-lactamase degradation, is an attractive first-line therapy in the treatment of these infections. Another alternative is to add a second drug to the penicillin (eg, metronidazole [Flagyl®]). Consequently, for those infections not responding to treatment with penicillin, the addition of a second drug (eg, metronidazole), not a beta-lactam or macrolide, is likely to be more effective. Bacterial resistance to metronidazole is very rare. The metronidazole dose is listed in Table 4.

Nonionized metronidazole is readily taken up by anaerobic organisms. Its selectivity for anaerobic bacteria is a result of the ability of these organisms to reduce metronidazole to its active form within the bacterial cell. The electron transport proteins necessary for this reaction are found only in anaerobic bacteria. Reduced metronidazole then disrupts DNA's helical structure, thereby inhibiting bacterial nucleic acid synthesis leading to death of the organism. Consequently, metronidazole is not effective against gram-positive aerobic cocci and most *Actinomyces, Lactobacillus,* and *Proprionibacterium* species. Since most odontogenic infections are mixed aerobic and anaerobic, metronidazole should rarely be used as a single agent. Alternatively, one can switch to a beta-lactamase resistant drug (eg, amoxicillin/clavulanic acid [Augmentin®]). The beta-lactamase resistant penicillins including methicillin, oxacillin, cloxacillin, dicloxacillin, and nafcillin, are only effective against gram-positive cocci and have no activity against anaerobes, hence, should not be used to treat the late stage odontogenic infections.

RESISTANCE IN ODONTOGENIC INFECTIONS

Recently, there has been an alarming increase in the incidence of resistant bacterial isolates in odontogenic infections. Many anaerobic bacteria have developed resistance to beta-lactam antibiotics via production of beta-lactamase enzymes. These include several species of *Prevotella, Porphyromonas, Fusobacterium nucleatum,* and *Campylobacter gracilus. Fusobacterium*, especially in combination with *S. viridans* species, has been associated with severe odontogenic infections. Often, they are resistant to macrolides. Clindamycin is the empiric drug of first choice in these patients.

SEVERE INFECTIONS

In patients hospitalized for severe odontogenic infections, I.V. antibiotics are indicated and clindamycin is the clear empiric antibiotic of choice. Alternative antibiotics include an I.V. combination of penicillin and metronidazole or I.V. ampicillin-sulbactam (Unasyn®). Clindamycin, I.V. cephalosporins (if penicillin allergy is not the anaphylactoid type), and ciprofloxacin have been used in patients allergic to penicillins. Flynn notes that *Eikenella corrodens*, an occasional oral pathogen, is resistant to clindamycin. Ciprofloxacin is an excellent antibiotic for this organism.

ERYTHROMYCIN, CLARITHROMYCIN, AND AZITHROMYCIN

In the past, erythromycins were considered highly effective antibiotics for treating odontogenic infections, especially in penicillin allergy. At the present time, however, the current high resistance rates of both oral streptococci and oral anaerobes have rendered the entire macrolide family of antibiotics obsolete for odontogenic infections. Montgomery has noted that resistance develops rapidly to macrolides and there may be cross-resistance between erythromycin and newer macrolides, particularly among streptococci and staphylococci. Hardee has stated that erythromycin is no longer very useful because of resistant pathogens. The antibacterial spectrum of the erythromycin family is similar to penicillin VK. Erythromycins are effective against streptococcus, staphylococcus, and gram-negative aerobes, such as *H. influenzae, M. catarrhalis, N. gonorrhoeae, Bordetella pertussis,* and *Legionella pneumophilia.* Erythromycins are considered narrow spectrum antibiotics.

Both azithromycin and clarithromycin have been used to treat acute odontogenic infections. This is because of the following spectrum of actions: Clarithromycin shows good activity against many gram-positive and gram-negative aerobic and anaerobic organisms. It is active against methicillin-sensitive *S. aureus* and most streptococcus species. *S. aureus* strains resistant to erythromycin are resistant to clarithromycin. Clarithromycin is active against *H. influenzae.* It is similar to erythromycin in effectiveness against anaerobic gram-positive cocci and *Bacteroides sp.* Clarithromycin has been suggested as an alternative antibiotic if the prescriber wants to give an antibiotic from the macrolide family (see Table 3). The recommended oral adult dose is 500 mg twice daily for 7 days.

Azithromycin is active against staphylococci, including *S. aureus* and *S. epidermidis,* as well as streptococci, such as *S. pyogenes* and *S. pneumoniae.* Erythromycin-resistant strains of staphylococcus, enterococcus, and streptococcus, including methicillin-resistant *S. aureus,* are also resistant to azithromycin. It has excellent activity against *H. influenzae.* Inhibition of anaerobes, such as *Clostridium perfringens,* is better with azithromycin than with erythromycin. Inhibition of *Bacteroides fragilis* and other bacteroides species by azithromycin is comparable to erythromycin. Both azithromycin and clarithromycin are presently recommended as alternatives in the prophylactic regimen for prevention of bacterial endocarditis.

AMOXICILLIN

Some clinicians select amoxicillin over penicillin VK as the penicillin of choice to empirically treat odontogenic infections. Except for coverage of *Haemophilus influenzae* in acute sinus and otitis media infections, amoxicillin does not offer any advantage over penicillin VK for treatment of odontogenic infections. It is less effective than penicillin VK for aerobic gram-positive cocci, and similar to penicillin for coverage of anaerobes. Although it does provide coverage against gram-negative enteric bacteria, this is not needed to treat odontogenic infections, except in immunosuppressed patients where these organisms may be present. If one adheres to the principle of using the most effective narrow spectrum antibiotic, amoxicillin should not be favored over penicillin VK.

Note: The ADA Council on Scientific Affairs recently published a review on the subject of antibiotic interaction with oral contraceptives in which a clear statement of the dental professional's responsibility was made. In essence, it was concluded that in any situation where a dentist is planning to prescribe a course of antibiotics, alternative/additional means of contraception should be recommended to the oral contraceptive users. Specifically, patients should be told about the potential for antibiotics to lower the usefulness of oral contraceptives and advised to consult their physician about nonhormonal contraceptive techniques while continuing their oral contraceptive regimen. Even though there is minimal scientific data supporting this position, the risk of possible unwanted pregnancies warrants this simple approach for professionals licensed to prescribe antibiotics (*JADA*, 2002, 133:880).

The following tables have been adapted from Wynn RL, Bergman SA, Meiller TF, et al. "Antibiotics in Treating Orofacial Infections of Odontogenic Origin," *Gen Dent*, 2001, 47(3):238-52.

Amoxicillin and Clavulanate Potassium *on page 108*
Amoxicillin *on page 106*
Ceftibuten *on page 292*
Cefditoren *on page 285*
Cephalexin *on page 301*
Chlorpheniramine *on page 323*
Chlorhexidine Gluconate *on page 316*
Clarithromycin *on page 355*
Clindamycin *on page 361*
Dicloxacillin *on page 463*
Erythromycin *on page 562*
Gatifloxacin *on page 724*
Gemifloxacin *on page 731*
Loratadine and Pseudoephedrine *on page 947*
Metronidazole *on page 1033*
Mouthwash, Antiseptic *on page 1069*
Moxifloxacin *on page 1069*
Oxymetazoline *on page 1172*
Penicillin V Potassium *on page 1205*
Pseudoephedrine *on page 1309*
Tetracycline *on page 1467*

BACTERIAL INFECTIONS *(Continued)*

Table 1.
EMPIRIC ANTIBIOTICS OF CHOICE FOR
ODONTOGENIC INFECTIONS

Type of Infection	Antibiotic of Choice
Early (first 3 days of symptoms)	Penicillin VK, amoxicillin Clindamycin Cephalexin (or other first generation cephalosporin)[1]
No improvement in 24-36 hours	Beta-lactamase-stable antibiotic: Clindamycin or amoxicillin / clavulanic acid
Penicillin allergy	Clindamycin Cephalexin (if penicillin allergy is not anaphylactoid type) Clarithromycin (Biaxin®)[2]
Late (>3 days)	Clindamycin Penicillin VK-metronidazole, amoxicillin-metronidazole
Penicillin allergy	Clindamycin

[1]For better patient compliance, second generation cephalosporins (cefaclor; cefuroxime) at twice daily dosing have been used; see text.

[2]A macrolide useful in patients allergic to penicillin, given as twice daily dosing for better patient compliance; see text.

Table 2.
PENICILLIN VK: ANTIBACTERIAL SPECTRUM

Gram-Positive Cocci	**Oral Anaerobes**
Streptococci	*Bacteroides*
Nonresistant staphylococci[1]	*Porphyromonas*
Pneumococci	*Prevotella*
	Peptococci
Gram-Negative Cocci	*Peptostreptococci*
Neisseria meningitides	*Actinomyces*
Neisseria gonorrhoeae	*Veillonella*
	Eubacterium
Gram-Positive Rods	*Eikenella*
Bacillus	*Capnocytophaga*
Corynebacterium	*Campylobacter*
Clostridium	*Fusobacterium*
	Others

[1]Nonresistant staphylococcus represents a small portion of community-acquired strains of *S. aureus* (5% to 15%). Most strains of *S. aureus* and *S. epidermidis* produce beta-lactamases, which destroy penicillins.

Table 3.
CLINDAMYCIN: ANTIBACTERIAL SPECTRUM[1]

Gram-Positive Cocci	Anaerobes[2]
Streptococci[3]	**Gram-Negative Bacilli**
S. aureus[4]	*Bacteroides* species including *B. fragilis*
Penicillinase and nonpenicillinase-producing staphylococcus	*B. melaninogenicus* *Fusobacterium* species
S. epidermidis	**Gram-Positive Nonsporeforming Bacilli**
Pneumococci	*Propionibacterium*
	Eubacterium
	Actinomyces species
	Gram-Positive Cocci
	Peptococcus
	Peptostreptococcus
	Microaerophilic streptococci

[1]*In vitro* activity against isolates; information from manufacturer's package insert

[2]*Clostridia* are more resistant than most anaerobes to clindamycin. Most *Clostridium perfringens* are susceptible but *C. sporogens* and *C. tertium* are frequently resistant.

[3]Except *S. faecalis*

[4]Some staph strains originally resistant to erythromycin rapidly develop resistance to clindamycin.

Table 4.
ORAL DOSE RANGES OF ANTIBIOTICS USEFUL IN TREATING ODONTOGENIC INFECTIONS[1]

Antibiotic	Dosage	
Clinicians must select specific dose and regimen from ranges available to be prescribed based on clinical judgment		
	Children	Adults
Penicillin VK	≤12 years: 25-50 mg/kg body weight in equally divided doses q6-8h for at least 7 days; maximum dose: 3 g/day	>12 years: 500 mg q6h for at least 7 days
Clindamycin	8-25 mg/kg in 3-4 equally divided doses	150-450 mg q6h for at least 7 days; maximum dose: 1.8 g/day
Cephalexin (Keflex®)	25-50 mg/kg/d in divided doses q6h severe infection: 50-100 mg/kg/d in divided doses q6h; maximum dose: 3 g/24 h	250-1000 mg q6h; maximum dose: 4 g/day
Amoxicillin	<40 kg: 20-40 mg (amoxicillin)/kg/d in divided doses q8h >40 kg: 250-500 mg q8h or 875 mg q12h for at least 7 days; maximum dose 2 g/day	>40 kg: 250-500 mg q8h or 875 mg q12h for at least 7 days; maximum dose: 2 g/day
Amoxicillin/clavulanic acid (Augmentin®)	<40 kg: 20-40 mg (amoxicillin)/kg/d in divided doses q8h >40 kg: 250-500 mg q8h or 875 mg q12h for at least 7 days; maximum dose 2 g/day	>40 kg: 250-500 mg q8h or 875 mg q12h for at least 7 days; maximum dose: 2 g/day
Metronidazole (Flagyl®)		500 mg q6-8h for 7-10 days; maximum dose: 4 g/day

[1]For doses of other antibiotics, see monographs

SAMPLE PRESCRIPTIONS

Rx:

Penicillin V potassium 500 mg

Disp: 40 tablets

Sig: Take 1 tablet 4 times/day for 7-10 days (consider a loading dose of 1 g for acute infection)

Rx:

Clindamycin 300 mg

Disp: 40 capsules

Sig: Take 1 capsule 4 times/day for 7-10 days

Note: Prescription for patients allergic to penicillin

Rx:

Amoxicillin 500 mg

Disp: 30 capsules or tablets

Sig: Take 1 capsule or tablet 3 times/day for 7-10 days

For additional sample prescriptions see Bacterial Infections and Periodontal Diseases *on page 1736*

SINUS INFECTION TREATMENT

Sinus infections represent a common condition which may present with confounding dental complaints. Treatment is sometimes instituted by the dentist, but due to the often chronic and recurrent nature of sinus infections, early involvement of an otolaryngologist is advised. These infections may require antibiotics of varying spectrum as well as requiring the management of sinus congestion. Although amoxicillin is usually adequate, many otolaryngologists go directly to Augmentin®. Second-generation cephalosporins and clarithromycin are sometimes used depending on the chronicity of the problem.

For examples of sample prescriptions see Sinus Infection Treatment *on page 1738*

BACTERIAL INFECTIONS *(Continued)*

FREQUENTLY ASKED QUESTIONS

What is the best antibiotic modality for treating dental infections?

Penicillin is still the drug of choice for treatment of infections in and around the oral cavity. Phenoxy-methyl penicillin (Pen VK) long has been the most commonly selected antibiotic. In penicillin-allergic individuals, erythromycin may be an appropriate consideration. If another drug is sought, clindamycin prescribed 300 mg as a loading dose followed by 150 mg 4 times/day would be an appropriate regimen for a dental infection. In general, if there is no response to Pen VK, then Augmentin® may be a good alternative in the nonpenicillin-allergic patient because of its slightly altered spectrum. Recommendations would include that the patient should take the drug with food.

Is there cross-allergenicity between the cephalosporins and penicillin?

The incidence of cross-allergenicity is 5% to 8% in the overall population. If a patient has demonstrated a Type I hypersensitivity reaction to penicillin, namely urticaria or anaphylaxis, then this incidence would increase to 20%.

Is there definitely an interaction between contraception agents and antibiotics?

There are well founded interactions between contraceptives and antibiotics. The best instructions that a patient could be given by their dentist are that should an antibiotic be necessary and the dentist is aware that the patient is on contraceptives, and if the patient is using chemical contraceptives, the patient should seriously consider additional means of contraception during the antibiotic management.

Are antibiotics necessary in diabetic patients?

In the management of diabetes, control of the diabetic status is the key factor relative to all morbidity issues. If a patient is well controlled, then antibiotics will likely not be necessary. However, in patients where the control is questionable or where they have recently been given a different drug regimen for their diabetes or if they are being titrated to an appropriate level of either insulin or oral hypoglycemic agents during these periods of time, the dentist might consider preprocedural antibiotics to be efficacious.

Do nonsteroidal anti-inflammatory drugs interfere with blood pressure medication?

At the current time there is no clear evidence that NSAIDs interfere with any of the blood pressure medications that are currently in usage.

PERIODONTAL DISEASES

Periodontal diseases are common to mankind affecting, according to some epidemiologic studies, greater than 80% of the worldwide population. The conditions refer primarily to diseases that are caused by accumulations of dental plaque and the subsequent immune response of the host to the bacteria and toxins present in this plaque. Although most of the organisms that have been implicated in advanced periodontal diseases are anaerobic in nature, some aerobes contribute by either coaggregation with the anaerobic species or direct involvement with specific disease types.

Periodontal condition, as a group of diseases, affects the soft tissues supporting the teeth (ie, gingiva) leading to the term gingivitis or inflammation of gingival structures and those conditions that affect the bone and ligament supporting the teeth (ie, periodontitis) resulting from the infection and/or inflammation of these structures. Diseases of the periodontia can be further subdivided into various types including adult periodontitis, early onset periodontitis, prepubertal periodontitis, and rapidly progressing periodontitis. In addition, specific conditions associated with predisposing immunodeficiency disease, such as those found in HIV-infected patients, create further subclassifications of the periodontal diseases, some of which are covered in those chapters associated with those conditions.

It is well accepted that control of most periodontal diseases requires, at the very minimum, appropriate mechanical cleansing of the dentition and the supporting structures by the patient. These efforts include brushing, some type of interdental cleaning, preferably with either floss or other aids, as well as appropriate sulcular cleaning usually with a brush.

Following appropriate dental treatment by the general dental practitioner and/or the periodontist, aids to these efforts by the patient might include the use of chemical agents to assist in the control of the periodontal diseases, or to prevent periodontal diseases. There are many available chemical agents on the market, only some of which are approved by the American Dental Association. Several have been tested utilizing guidelines published in 1986 by the American Dental Association for assessment of agents that claim efficacy in the management of periodontal diseases. These chemical agents include chlorhexidine (Peridex®, PerioGard®), which are bisbiguanides and benzalkonium chloride, which is a quaternary compound. Chlorhexidine, in various concentrations, has shown efficacy in reducing plaque and gingivitis in patients with short-term utilization. Some side effects include staining of the dentition which is reversible by dental prophylaxis. Chlorhexidine demonstrates the concept of substantivity, indicating that after its use, it has a continued effect in reducing the ability of plaque to form. It has been shown to be useful in a variety of periodontal conditions including acute necrotizing ulcerative gingivitis and healing studies. Some disturbances in taste and accumulation of calculus have been reported, however, chlorhexidine is the most applicable chemical agent of the bisbiguanides that has been studied to date.

Other chemical agents available as mouthwashes include the phenol compound Listerine Antiseptic®. These compounds are primarily restricted to prototype agents; the first to be approved by the ADA being Listerine Antiseptic®. Listerine Antiseptic® has been shown to be effective against plaque and gingivitis in long-term studies and comparable to chlorhexidine in these long-term investigations. However, chlorhexidine performs better than Listerine Antiseptic® in short-term investigations. Triclosan, the chemical agent found in the toothpaste Total®, has been recently approved by the FDA and is an aid in the prevention of gingivitis. Antiplaque activity of triclosan is enhanced with the addition of zinc citrate and there are no serious side effects to the use of triclosan. Sanguinarine is a principle herbal extract used for antiplaque activity. It is an alkyloid from the plant *Sanguinaria canadensis* and has some antimicrobial properties perhaps due to its enzyme activity. Zinc citrate and zinc chloride have often been added to toothpastes as well as enzymes such as mucinase, mutanase, and dextrinase which have demonstrated varying results in studies. Some commercial anionic surfactants are available on the market which include aminoalcohols and the agent Plax® which essentially is comprised of sodium thiosulfate as a surfactant. Recent studies have shown Plax® to have some efficacy when it is added to triclosan.

Long-term use of prescription medications, including antibiotics, is seldom recommended and is not in any way a substitute for general dental/periodontal therapies. As adjunctive therapy, however, benefit has been shown and the new formulations of doxycycline (Periostat® and Atridox™), are recommended for long-term or repetitive treatments. It should be noted that the manufacturer's claims indicate that Periostat® functions as a collagenase inhibitor not as an antibiotic at recommended low doses for long-term therapy. Atridox™, however, functions as an antibiotic and is not recommended for constant long-term therapy, but rather in repetitive applications as necessary. Prescription medications used in efforts to treat periodontal diseases have historically included the use of antibiotics such as tetracycline although complications with use with young patients have often precluded their prescription. Doxycycline is often preferred to tetracycline in low doses. This broad-spectrum bacteriostatic agent has shown efficacy against a wide variety of bacterial organisms found in periodontal disease. Minocycline slow-release (Arestin™) has recently been approved.

PERIODONTAL DISEASES *(Continued)*

The drug metronidazole is a nitromidazole. It is an agent that was originally used in treatment of protozoan infections and some anaerobic bacteria. It is bactericidal and has a good absorption and distribution throughout the body. The studies using metronidazole have suggested that it has a variety of uses in periodontal treatment and can be used as adjunct in both acute necrotizing ulcerative gingivitis and has specific efficacy against spirochetes, bacteria, and some *Porphyromonas* species. Clindamycin is a derivative of vancomycin and has been useful in treatment of suppurative periodontal lesions. However, long-term use is precluded by its complicating toxicities associated with colitis and gastrointestinal problems.

Research has also shown that various combination therapies of metronidazole and tetracycline for juvenile periodontitis and metronidazole with amoxicillin for rapidly progressive disease can be useful. The use of other prescription drugs including nonsteroidal anti-inflammatory, as well as other antibacterial agents, have been under study. Effects on prostaglandins of NSAIDs may indirectly slow periodontal disease progression. New research is currently underway in this regard. Perhaps, in combination therapy with some of the antibiotics, these drugs may assist in reducing the patient's immune response or inflammatory response to the presence of disease-causing bacteria.

Of greatest interest has been the improvement in technology for delivery of chemical agents to the periodontally-diseased site. These systems include biodegradable gelatins and biodegradable chips that can be placed under the gingiva and deliver antibacterial agents directly to the site as an adjunct to periodontal treatment. The initial therapy of mechanical debridement by the periodontal therapist is essential prior to using any chemical agent, and the dentist should be aware that the development of newer agents does not substitute for appropriate periodontal therapy and maintenance. The trade names of the gelatin chips and subgingival delivery systems include Periochip®, Atridox®, and Periostat®.

In addition to the periodontal therapy, consideration of the patient's pre-existing or developing medical conditions are important in the management of the periodontal patient. Several diseases illustrate these points most acutely. The reader is referred to the chapters on Diabetes, Cardiovascular Disease, Pregnancy, Respiratory Disease, HIV, and Cancer Chemotherapy. It has long been accepted that uncontrolled diabetes may predispose to periodontal lesions. Now, under current investigation is the hypothesis that pre-existing periodontal diseases may make it more difficult for a diabetic patient to come under control. In addition, the inflammatory response and immune challenge that is ongoing in periodontal disease appears to be implicated in the development of coronary artery disease as well as an increased risk of myocardial infarction and/or stroke. The accumulation of intra-arterial plaques appears enhanced by the presence of the inflammatory response often seen systemically in patients suffering with periodontal disease. The American Heart Association is currently considering recommendations regarding antibiotic prophylaxis in patients with cardiovascular disease. In addition, the clinician is referred to the section on preprocedural antibiotics in the text for a consideration of antibiotic usage in patients that may be at risk for infective endocarditis. Other conditions including pregnancy and respiratory diseases such as COPD, HIV, and cancer therapy must be considered in the overall view of periodontal diseases. The reader is referred to the sections within the text.

Amoxicillin *on page 106*
Minocycline Hydrochloride (Periodontal)*on page 1050*
Benzalkonium Chloride *on page 188*
Chlorhexidine Gluconate *on page 316*
Clindamycin *on page 361*
Doxycycline Hyclate (Periodontal) *on page 512*
Listerine Antiseptic®*on page 1069*
Metronidazole *on page 1033*
NSAIDs see Oral Pain section *on page 1692*
Tetracycline *on page 1467*
Triclosan and Fluoride *on page 1534*

For examples of sample prescriptions see Bacterial Infections and Periodontal Diseases *on page 1736*

FUNGAL INFECTIONS

Oral fungal infections can result from alteration in oral flora, immunosuppression, and underlying systemic diseases that may allow the overgrowth of these opportunistic organisms. These systemic conditions might include diabetes, long-term xerostomia, adrenal suppression, anemia, and chemotherapy-induced myelosuppression for the management of cancer. The use of oral inhalers that include steroids, such as Advair™ Diskus®, have been implicated in the enhancing of the risk of fungal overgrowth. Drugs of choice in treating fungal infections are amphotericin B, ciclopirox olamine, clotrimazole, itraconazole, ketoconazole, fluconazole, naftifine hydrochloride, nystatin, and oxiconazole. Patients being treated for fungal skin infections may also be using topical antifungal preparations coupled with a steroid such as triamcinolone. Clinical presentation might include pseudomembranous, atrophic, and hyperkeratotic forms. Fungus has also been implicated in denture stomatitis and symptomatic geographic tongue.

Nystatin (Mycostatin®) is effective topically in the treatment of candidal infections of the skin and mucous membrane. The drug is extremely well tolerated and appears to be nonsensitizing. In persons with denture stomatitis in which monilial organisms play at least a contributory role, it is important to soak the prosthesis overnight in a nystatin suspension. Nystatin ointment can be placed in the denture during the daytime much like a denture adhesive. Medication should be continued for at least 48 hours after disappearance of clinical signs in order to prevent relapse. Patients must be re-evaluated after 14 days of therapy. Predisposing systemic factors must be reconsidered if the oral fungal infection persists. Topical applications rely on contact of the drug with the lesions. Therefore, 4-5 times daily with a dissolving troche or pastille is appropriate. Concern over the presence of sugar in the troches and pastilles has led practitioners to sometimes prescribe the vaginal suppository formulation for off-labeled oral use. Clotrimazole troches are also useful as a topical therapy.

MANAGEMENT OF FUNGAL INFECTIONS REQUIRING SYSTEMIC MEDICATION

If the patient is refractory to topical treatment, consideration of a systemic route might include Diflucan® or Nizoral®. Also, when the patient cannot tolerate topical therapy, ketoconazole (Nizoral®) is an effective, well tolerated, systematic drug for mucocutaneous candidiasis. Concern over liver function and possible drug interactions must be considered.

Voriconazole (VFEND®) is indicated for treatment of serious fungal infections in patients intolerant of, or refractory to, other therapy.

SAMPLE PRESCRIPTION FOR SYSTEMIC TREATMENT

Rx:

Diflucan® 100 mg tablets

Disp: 22 tablets

Sig: Take 2 tablets day 1, then 1 tablet/day until gone

Note: Sometimes a shorter course is adequate. However, oral infections commonly are more difficult to eradicate and even a second course may be necessary.

Ingredient: Fluconazole

For additional sample prescriptions see Fungal Infections *on page 1740*

MANAGEMENT OF ANGULAR CHEILITIS

Angular cheilitis may represent the clinical manifestation of a multitude of etiologic factors. Cheilitis-like lesions may result from local habits, from a decrease in the intermaxillary space, or from nutritional deficiency. More commonly, angular cheilitis represents a mixed infection coupled with an inflammatory response involving *Candida albicans* and other organisms. The drug of choice is now formulated to contain nystatin

FUNGAL INFECTIONS *(Continued)*

and triamcinolone and the effect is excellent. In addition, an off-label use of iodoquinol and hydrocortisone has also been reported to be effective in the treatment of angular cheilitis.

Amphotericin B (Conventional) *on page 113*
Clotrimazole *on page 379*
Fluconazole *on page 659*
Ketoconazole *on page 880*
Nystatin *on page 1133*
Nystatin and Triamcinolone *on page 1134*
Voriconazole *on page 1582*

Note: Consider Peridex® oral rinse, or Listerine® antiseptic oral rinse for long-term control in immunosuppressed patients.

SAMPLE PRESCRIPTIONS FOR TOPICAL TREATMENT

Rx:

Nystatin 100,000 units/mL oral suspension
Disp: 300 mL
Sig: Rinse with 1 teaspoon (5 mL) for 2 minutes 4-5 times/day and expectorate

Rx:

Mycelex® 10 mg troches
Disp: 70 troches
Sig: Dissolve 1 troche in mouth 5 times/day until gone; leave any prostheses out during treatment

Ingredient: Clotrimazole

For additional sample prescriptions see Fungal Infections *on page 1740*

VIRAL INFECTIONS

Oral viral infections are most commonly caused by herpes simplex viruses and Coxsackie viruses. Oral pharyngeal infections and upper respiratory infections are commonly caused by the Coxsackie group A viruses. Soft tissue viral infections, on the other hand, are most often caused by the herpes simplex viruses. Herpes zoster or varicella-zoster virus, which is one of the herpes family of viruses, can likewise cause similar viral eruptions involving the mucosa.

The diagnosis of an acute viral infection is one that begins by ruling out bacterial etiology and having an awareness of the presenting signs and symptoms associated with viral infection. Acute onset and vesicular eruption on the soft tissues generally favors a diagnosis of viral infection. Unfortunately, vesicles do not remain for a great length of time in the oral cavity; therefore, the short-lived vesicles rupture leaving ulcerated bases as the only indication of their presence. These ulcers, however, are generally small in size and only when left unmanaged, coalesce to form larger, irregular ulcerations. Distinction should be made between the commonly occurring intraoral ulcers (aphthous ulcerations) which do not have a viral etiology and the lesions associated with intraoral herpes. The management of an oral viral infection may be palliative for the most part; however, with the advent of acyclovir we now have a family of drugs that can assist in managing primary and secondary infection. Human *Papillomavirus* is implicated in a number of oral lesions, the most common of which is *Condyloma acuminatum*. Recently, Aldara® has been approved for genital warts; oral use is under study.

It should be noted that herpes can present as a primary infection (gingivostomatitis), recurrent lip lesions (herpes labialis), and intraoral ulcers (recurrent intraoral herpes), involving the oral and perioral tissues. Primary infection is a systemic infection that leads to acute gingivostomatitis involving multiple tissues of the buccal mucosa, lips, tongue, floor of the mouth, and the gingiva. Treatment of primary infections utilizes acyclovir in combination with supportive care. Topical anesthetic used in combination with Benadryl® 0.5% in a saline vehicle was found to be an effective oral rinse in the symptomatic treatment of primary herpetic gingivostomatitis; however, Dyclone® is no longer available. Other agents for symptomatic and supportive treatment include commercially available elixir of Benadryl®, Xylocaine® viscous, Orajel® (OTC), and antibiotics to prevent secondary infections. Systemic supportive therapy should include forced fluids, high concentration protein, vitamin and mineral food supplements, and rest.

Antivirals

Abreva™ (OTC) *on page 495*

Acyclovir *on page 49*

Imiquimod *on page 821*

L-Lysine *on page 959*

Nelfinavir *on page 1098*

Penciclovir *on page 1200*

Valacyclovir *on page 1553*

Viroxyn® *on page 189*

Supportive Therapy

Diphenhydramine *on page 483*

Lidocaine *on page 920*

Prevention of Secondary Bacterial Infection

Penicillin V Potassium *on page 1205*

SUPPORTIVE CARE FOR PAIN AND PREVENTION OF SECONDARY INFECTION

Primary infections often become secondarily infected with bacteria, requiring antibiotics. Dietary supplement may be necessary. Options are presented due to variability in patient compliance and response.

VIRAL INFECTIONS (Continued)

RECURRENT HERPETIC INFECTIONS

Following this primary infection, the herpesvirus remains latent until such time as it has the opportunity to recur. The etiology of this latent period and the degree of viral shedding present during latency is currently under study; however, it is thought that some trigger in the mucosa or the skin causes the virus to begin to replicate. This process may involve Langerhans cells which are immunocompetent antigen-presenting cells resident in all epidermal surfaces. The virus replication then leads to eruptions in tissues surrounding the mouth. The most common form of recurrence is the lip lesion or herpes labialis, however, intraoral recurrent herpes also occurs with some frequency. Prevention of recurrences has been attempted with lysine (OTC) 500-1000 mg/day but response has been variable. Herpes zoster outbreaks can involve the oral and facial tissues although this is uncommon. Valacyclovir is the drug of choice.

Water-soluble bioflavonoid-ascorbic acid complex, now available as Peridin-C®, may be helpful in reducing the signs and symptoms associated with recurrent herpes simplex virus infections. As with all agents used, the therapy is more effective when instituted in the early prodromal stage of the disease process.

PREVENTATIVE SAMPLE PRESCRIPTIONS

Rx:

L-Lysine (OTC) 500 mg

Sig: Take 2 tablets/day as preventive; increase to 4 tablets/day if prodrome or recurrence begins

Rx:

Citrus bioflavonoids and ascorbic acid tablets 400 mg (Peridin-C®)

Disp: 10 tablets

Sig: Take 2 tablets at once, then 1 tablet 3 times/day for 3 days

Where a recurrence is usually precipitated by exposure to sunlight, the lesion may be prevented by the application to the area of a sunscreen, with a high skin protection factor (SPF) in the range of 10-15.

SUPPORTIVE CARE FOR PAIN AND MAINTENANCE OF NUTRITION DURING ORAL VIRAL INFECTIONS

Rx:

Benadryl® liquid 12.5 mg/5mL

Disp: 4 oz bottle

Sig: Rinse with 1-2 teaspoonfuls every 2 hours and expectorate

Note: Benadryl® is available as a generic diphenhydramine liquid.

Rx:

Benadryl® liquid 12.5 mg/5 mL (mix 50/50) with Kaopectate®

Disp: 8 oz total

Sig: Rinse with 1-2 teaspoonfuls every 2 hours and expectorate.

Note: Maalox® can be used in place of Kaopectate® if constipation is a problem. Benadryl® is available as a generic diphenhydramine liquid.

Rx:

Xylocaine® viscous 2%

Disp: 450 mL bottle

Sig: Swish with 1 tablespoon 4 times/day and spit out

Ingredient: Lidocaine

Rx:

Meritene®

Disp: 1 lb can (plain, chocolate, eggnog flavors)

Sig: Take 3 servings daly; prepare as indicated on can

Ingredient: Proteine-vitamin-mineral food supplement

PRESCRIPTIVE TREATMENT

Acyclovir (Zovirax®) possesses antiviral activity against herpes simplex types 1 and 2. Historically, ophthalmic ointments were used topically to treat recurrent mucosal and skin lesions. These do not penetrate well on the skin lesions, thereby providing questionable relief of symptoms. If recommended, use should be closely monitored. Penciclovir, an active metabolite of famciclovir, has been specifically approved in a cream for treatment of recurrent herpes lesions. Valacyclovir has recently been approved for treatment of herpes labialis (see monograph for dosing). The FDA has also approved acyclovir cream for treatment of herpes labialis in adults and adolescents but the product is currently under regulatory review (check www.biovail for status). Biovail Corporation has acquired exclusive marketing and distribution rights for Zovirax® ointment and cream from the manufacturer, GlaxoSmithKline. Recently, in addition to docosanol (Abreva®), another new over-the-counter preparation for treatment of recurrent herpes labialis has been approved. Benzalkonium chloride and isopropyl alcohol (Viroxyn®) is an alcohol/benzalkonium chloride medication in a single dose applicator kit (3 pack) that is marketed to reduce the duration and symptoms of cold sores.

SAMPLE PRESCRIPTIONS

Rx:

    Zovirax 200 mg capsules
    Disp: 50 or 60 capsules
    Sig: Take 1 capsule 5 times/day for 10 days or 2 capsules 3 times/day for 10 days

    Ingredient: Acyclovir

Rx:

    Denavir® topical ointment 5%
    Disp: 1.5 g tube
    Sig: Apply locally as directed to lesion every 2 hours during waking hours (begin when symptoms first occur)

    Ingredient: Penciclovir

For additional sample prescriptions see Viral Infections *on page 1742*

ULCERATIVE AND EROSIVE DISORDERS

RECURRENT APHTHOUS STOMATITIS

Kenalog® in Orabase is indicated for the temporary relief of symptoms associated with infrequent recurrences of minor aphthous lesions and ulcerative lesions resulting from trauma. More severe forms of recurrent aphthous stomatitis may be treated with an oral suspension of tetracycline. The agent appears to reduce the duration of symptoms and decrease the rate of recurrence by reducing secondary bacterial infection. Its use is contraindicated during the last half of pregnancy, infancy, and childhood to the age of 8 years. *Lactobacillus acidophilus* preparations (Bacid®, Lactinex®) are occasionally effective for reducing the frequency and severity of the lesions. Debacterol® has recently been approved. Patients with long-standing history of recurrent aphthous stomatitis should be evaluated for iron, folic acid, and vitamin B_{12} deficiencies. Regular use of Listerine® antiseptic has been shown in clinical trials to reduce the severity, duration, and frequency of aphthous stomatitis. Debacterol® has recently been approved. Chlorhexidine oral rinses 20 mL for 30 seconds 2-3 times/day have also demonstrated efficacy in reducing the duration of aphthae. With both of these products, however, patient intolerance of the burning from the alcohol content is of concern. Viractin® has been approved for symptomatic relief. Immunocompromised patients such as those with AIDS may have severe ulcer recurrences and the drug thalidomide has been approved for these patients.

Amlexanox *on page 99*
Attapulgite *on page 165*
Chlorhexidine Gluconate *on page 316*
Clobetasol *on page 365*
Dexamethasone *on page 439*
Diphenhydramine *on page 483*
Fluocinonide ointment with Orabase *on page 670*
Debacterol® *on page 1429*
Lactobacillus on page 535
Metronidazole *on page 1033*
Mouthwash, Antiseptic *on page 1069*
Prednisone *on page 1271*
Tetracaine *on page 1466*
Tetracycline liquid *on page 1467*
Thalidomide *on page 1471*
Triamcinolone Acetonide Dental Paste *on page 1530*

EROSIVE LICHEN PLANUS AND MAJOR APHTHAE

Elixir of dexamethasone (Decadron®), a potent anti-inflammatory agent, is used topically in the management of acute episodes of erosive lichen planus and major aphthae. Continued supervision of the patient during treatment is essential and the dentist must be aware that treatment of any secondary infections such as fungal overgrowth may be essential in gaining control of the erosive lesions.

For examples of sample prescriptions see Ulcerative and Erosive Disorders *on page 1744*

NECROTIZING ULCERATING PERIODONTITIS
(HIV Periodontal Disease)

Initial Treatment *(In-Office)*
Gentle debridement
Note: Ensure patient has no iodine allergies

Betadine® rinse *on page 1262*

At-Home Treatment
Listerine® antiseptic rinse (20 mL for 30 seconds twice daily)
Peridex® rinse *on page 316*
Metronidazole (Flagyl®) 7-10 days *on page 1033*

Follow-Up Therapy
Proper dental cleaning, including scaling and root planing (repeat as needed)
Continue Peridex® and Listerine® rinse (indefinitely)

BURNING TONGUE SYNDROME, SYMPTOMATIC GEOGRAPHIC TONGUE, MILD-TO-MODERATE FORMS OF ULCERATIONS AND EROSIONS

Burning mouth syndrome is extremely difficult to both diagnose and treat. Initially, systemic factors, including changes in patient's medication, control of diabetes (if the disease is present), concomitant xerostomia, and the presence of fungal infections often complicate the diagnosis and management of burning mouth syndrome. Once these systemic and/or local factors have been eliminated, oftentimes the patient presents with minimal clinically-visible changes and only the subjective complaint of burning mouth. In these instances, a variety of drugs, including clonazepam 0.25-3 mg/day is sometimes used; also the drugs amitriptyline 25-100 mg/day, nortriptyline 10-50 mg/day, gabapentin 900-1500 mg/day, and doxepin as a cream, applied to the lateral borders of the tongue and the areas affected, are sometimes utilized. These drugs should be selected and managed in collaboration with the patient's physician, particularly since many of these patients suffering with burning mouth syndrome have complicated medical histories including the use of additional medications that could be affected.

Elixir of Benadryl®, a potent antihistamine, is used in the oral cavity primarily as a mild topical anesthetic agent for the symptomatic relief of certain allergic deficiencies which should be ruled out as possible etiologies for the oral condition under treatment. It is often used alone as well as in solutions with agents such as Kaopectate® or Maalox® to assist in coating the oral mucosa. Benadryl® can also be used in capsule form.

DENTIN HYPERSENSITIVITY, HIGH CARIES INDEX, AND XEROSTOMIA

DENTIN HYPERSENSITIVITY

Suggested steps in resolving dentin hypersensitivity when a thorough exam has ruled-out any other source for the problem:

Treatment Steps

- Home treatment with a desensitizing toothpaste containing potassium nitrate (used to brush teeth as well as a thin layer applied, each night for 2 weeks)
- If needed, in office potassium oxalate (Protect® by Butler) and/or in office fluoride iontophoresis
- If sensitivity is still not tolerable to the patient, consider pumice then dentin adhesive and unfilled resin or composite restoration overlaying a glass ionomer base

Home Products (all contain nitrate as active ingredient):

Promise®

Denquel®

Sensodyne®

Dentifrice Products *on page 1815*

Other major brand name companies have added ingredients to their dentifrice product lines that also make hypersensitivity claims.

ANTICARIES AGENTS

Fluoride (Gel 0.4%, Rinse 0.05%) *on page 671*

New toothpastes with triclosan such as Colgate Total® show promise for combined treatment/prevention of caries, plaque, and gingivitis. The use of 5% sodium fluoride varnishes (Duraflor® and Duraphat®) have been encouraged by cariologists for the prevention of decay in persons of high-risk populations.

FLUORIDES

Used for the prevention of demineralization of the tooth structure secondary to xerostomia. For patients with long-term or permanent xerostomia, daily application is accomplished using custom applicator trays, such as omnivac. Patients with porcelain crowns should use a neutral pH fluoride (see Fluoride monograph *on page 671*). Final selection of a fluoride product and/or saliva replacement/stimulant product must be based on patient comfort, taste, and ultimately, compliance. Experience has demonstrated that, often times, patients must try various combinations to achieve the greatest effect and their highest comfort levels. The presence of mucositis during cancer management complicates the clinician's selection of products.

See also Oral Rinse Products *on page 1831*

OVER-THE-COUNTER (OTC) PRODUCTS

Form	Brand Name	Strength / Size
Gel, topical (stannous fluoride)	Gel-Kam® (cinnamon, fruit, mint flavors)	0.4% [0.1%] (65 g, 105 g, 122 g)
	Gel-Tin® (lime, grape, cinnamon, raspberry, mint, orange flavors)	0.4% [0.1%] (60 g, 120 g)
	Stop® (grape, cinnamon, bubblegum, piña colada, mint flavors)	0.4% [0.1%] (60 g, 120 g)
Rinse, topical (as sodium)	ACT®, Fluorigard®	0.05% [0.02%] (90 mL, 180 mL, 300 mL, 360 mL, 480 mL)
	Listermint® with Fluoride	0.02% [0.01%] (180 mL, 300 mL, 360 mL, 480 mL, 540 mL, 720 mL, 960 mL, 1740 mL)

PRESCRIPTION ONLY (Rx) PRODUCTS

Form	Brand Name	Strength / Size
Drops, oral (as sodium)		0.275 mg/drop [0.125 mg/drop]
	Fluoritab®, Flura-Drops®	0.55 mg/drop [0.25 mg/drop] (22.8 mL, 24 mL)
	Karidium®, Luride®	0.275 mg/drop [0.125 mg/drop] (30 mL, 60 mL)
	Pediaflor®	1.1 mg/mL [0.5 mg/mL] (50 mL)
Gel-Drops	Thera-Flur® (lime flavor), Thera-Flur-N®	1.1% [0.55%] (24 mL)
Gel, topical		
Acidulated phosphate fluoride	Minute-Gel® (spearmint, strawberry, grape, apple-cinnamon, cherry cola, bubblegum flavors)	1.23% (480 mL)
Sodium fluoride	Karigel® (orange flavor)	1.1% [0.5%]
	Karigel®-N	1.1% [0.5%]
	PreviDent® (mint, berry, cherry, fruit sherbet flavors)	1.1% [0.5%] (24 g, 30 g, 60 g, 120 g, 130 g, 250 g)
Lozenge (as sodium)	Flura-Loz® (raspberry flavor)	2.2 mg [1 mg]
Rinse, topical (as sodium)	Fluorinse®, Point-Two®	0.2% [0.09%] (240 mL, 480 mL, 3780 mL)
Solution, oral (as sodium)	Phos-Flur® (cherry, cinnamon, grape, wintergreen flavors)	0.44 mg/mL [0.2 mg/mL] (250 mL, 500 mL, 3780 mL)
Tablet (as sodium)		1.1 mg [0.5 mg]; 2.2 mg [1 mg]
	Fluor-A-Day®	0.55 mg [0.25 mg]
	Fluor-A-Day®, Fluoritab®, Luride® Lozi-Tab®, Pharmaflur®	1.1 mg [0.5 mg]
Chewable	Fluor-A-Day®, Fluoritab®, Karidium®, Luride® Lozi-Tab®, Luride®-SF Lozi-Tab®, Pharmaflur®	2.2 mg [1 mg]
Oral	Flura®, Karidium®	2.2 mg [1 mg]
Varnish	Duraflor®, Duraphat®	5% [50 mg/mL] (10 mL)

Tables copied from Newland, JR, Meiller, TF, Wynn, RL, et al, *Oral Soft Tissue Diseases*, 2nd ed, Hudson (Cleveland), OH: Lexi-Comp, Inc, 2002.

ANTIMICROBIAL ORAL RINSE

Chlorhexidine Gluconate (Peridex®) *on page 316*

Mouthwash (Antiseptic) (Listerine®) *on page 1069*

For examples of sample prescriptions see Antimicrobial Rinses *on page 1739*

MANAGEMENT OF SIALORRHEA

In patients suffering with medical conditions that result in hypersalivation, the dentist may determine that it is appropriate to use an atropine sulfate medication to achieve a dry field for dental procedures or to reduce excessive drooling. Currently there is one ADA approved medication sold under the name of Sal-Tropine™. See Atropine Sulfate Dental Tablets *on page 164*.

XEROSTOMIA

Xerostomia refers to the subjective sensation of a dry mouth. Numerous factors can play a role in the patient's perception of dry mouth. Changes in salivary function caused by drugs, surgical intervention, or treatment of cancer are among the leading causes of xerostomia. Other factors including aging, smoking, mouth breathing, and the immune complex of disorders, Sjögren's syndrome, can also be implicated in a patient's perception of xerostomia. Human immunodeficiency virus (HIV) may produce xerostomia when viral changes in salivary glands are present. Xerostomia affects women more frequently than men and is also more common in older individuals. Some alteration in salivary function naturally occurs with age, but it is extremely difficult to quantify the effects. Xerostomia and salivary gland hypofunction in the elderly population are contributory to deterioration in the quality of life.

Once a diagnosis of xerostomia or salivary gland hypofunction is made and possible causes confirmed, treatment for the condition usually involves management of the underlying disease and avoidance of unnecessary medications. In addition, good hydration is

DENTIN HYPERSENSITIVITY, HIGH CARIES INDEX, AND XEROSTOMIA *(Continued)*

essential and water is the drink of choice. Also, the use of artificial saliva substitutes, selected chewing gums, and/or toothpastes formulated to treat xerostomia, is often warranted. In more difficult cases, such as patients receiving radiotherapy for cancer of the head and neck regions or patients with Sjögren's syndrome, systemic cholinergic stimulants may be administered if no contraindications exist.

CLINICAL PRODUCT USE

Because of the complex nature of xerostomia, management by the dental clinician is difficult. Treatment success is also difficult to assess and is often unsatisfactory. The salivary stimulants, pilocarpine and cevimeline, may aid in some conditions but are only approved for use as sialogogues in patients receiving radiotherapy and in Sjögren's patients, specifically as described above. Artificial salivas are available as over-the-counter products and represent the potential for continuous application by the patient to achieve comfort for their xerostomic condition.

The role of the clinician in attempting treatment of dry mouth is to first achieve a differential diagnosis and to ensure that other conditions are not simultaneously present. For example, many patients suffer burning mouth syndrome or painful oral tissues with no obvious etiology accompanying dry mouth. Also, higher caries incidence may be associated with changes in salivary flow. As previously mentioned, Sjögren's syndrome represents an immune complex of disorders that can affect the eyes, oral tissues, and other organ systems. The reader is referred to current oral pathology or oral medicine text for review of signs and symptoms of Sjögren's syndrome.

Treatment of cancer often leads to dry mouth. Surgical intervention removing salivary tissue due to the presence of a salivary gland tumor results in loss of salivary function. Also, many of the chemotherapeutic agents produce transitory changes in salivary flow, such that the patient may perceive a dry mouth during chemotherapy. Most notably related to salivary dysfunction is the use of radiation regimens to head and neck tissues. Tumors in or about salivary gland tissue, the oral cavity, and oropharynx are most notably sensitive to radiation therapy and subsequent dry mouth. In the head and neck, therapeutic radiation is commonly used in treatment of squamous cell carcinomas and lymphomas. The radiation level necessary to destroy malignant cells ranges from 40-70 Gy. Salivary tissue is extremely sensitive to radiation changes. Radiation dosages >30 Gy are sufficient to permanently change salivary function. In addition to the mucositis and subsequent secondary infection by fungal colonization or viral exacerbation, oral tissues can become exceptionally dry due to the effects of radiation on salivary glands. In fact, permanent damage to salivary gland tissue within the beam path produces significant levels of xerostomia in most patients. Some recovery may be noted by the patient. Most often, the effects are permanent and even progressive as the radiation dosage increases.

Artificial salivas do not produce any protectant or stimulation of the salivary gland. The use of pilocarpine and cevimeline as salivary stimulants in pre-emptive treatment, as well as postradiation treatment, have been shown to have some efficacy in management of dry mouth. The success rate, however, still is often unsatisfactory and post-treatment management by the dentist usually requires fluoride supplements to prevent radiation-induced caries due to dry mouth. Also, management of dry mouth through patient use of the artificial salivary gel, solutions and sprays, or other over-the-counter products for dry mouth (eg, chewing gum, toothpaste, mouthwash, swab-sticks) is highly recommended. The use of pilocarpine or cevimeline should only be considered by the dentist in consultation with the managing physician. The oftentimes severe and widespread cholinergic side effects of pilocarpine and cevimeline mandate close monitoring of the patient.

The use of artificial salivary substitutes is less problematic for the dentist. The dentist should, in considering selection of a drug, base his or her decision on patient compliance and comfort. Salivary substitutes presently on the market may have some benefit in terms of electrolyte balance and salivary consistency. However, the ultimate decision needs to be based on patients' taste, their willingness to use the medication ad libitum, and improvement in their comfort related to dry mouth. Many of the drugs are pH balanced to reduce additional risk of dental demineralization or caries. Oftentimes, the dentist must try numerous medications, one at a time, prior to finding one which gives the patient some comfort. Another gauge of acceptability is to investigate whether the artificial saliva substitute has the American Dental Association's seal of approval. Most of the currently accepted saliva substitute products have been evaluated by the ADA.

In general, considerations that the clinician might use in a prescribed regimen would be that saliva substitutes are meant to be used regularly throughout the day by the patient to achieve comfort during meals, reduce tissue abrasion, and prevent salivary stagnation on teeth. Other than these, there are no specific recommendations for patients. Recommendations by the dentist need to be tailored to the patient's acceptance. Salivary substitutes may provide an allergic potential in patients who are sensitive to some of the preservatives present in artificial saliva products. In addition to this allergic potential, there is a risk of microbial contamination by placement of the salivary substitute container in close contact with the oral cavity.

Patient education regarding the use of saliva substitutes is also part of the clinical approach. The patient with chronic xerostomia should be educated about regular professional care, high performance in dental hygiene, the need to re-evaluate oral soft tissue pathology, and any changes that might occur long term. In patients with severe xerostomia, artificial salivary medications should be given in combination with topical fluoride treatment programs designed by the dentist to reduce caries.

DENTIN HYPERSENSITIVITY, HIGH CARIES INDEX, AND XEROSTOMIA (Continued)

PRODUCTS AND DRUGS TO TREAT DRY MOUTH

Medication	Manufacturer and Phone Number	Product Type	Manufacturer's Description	Indication	Ingredients	Directions for Use	Form and Availability
				Artificial Salivas (OTC)			
Biotene® OralBalance® Mouth Moisturizing Gel	Laclede Professional Products, Inc (800) 922-5856	Gel	Sugar-free oral lubricant; relieves dry mouth symptoms up to 8 hours; soothes and protects oral tissue to promote healing; helps to inhibit harmful bacteria; improves retention under dentures	Relieves symptoms of dry mouth; burning, itching, cotton palate, sore tissue swallowing difficulties	Contains the "Biotene® protective salivary enzyme system Active: Glucose oxidase (2000 units), lactoperoxidase (3000 units), lysozyme (5 mg), lactoferrin (5 mg) Other: Hydrogenated starch, xylitol, hydroxyethyl cellulose, glycerate polyhydrate, aloe vera	Using a clean fingertip, apply a 1" ribbon of gel on tongue; add additional amount of gel on other dry; use as needed	1.4 oz tube; available at mass merchandise stores, food stores, and drugstores
BreathTech™ Plaque Fighter Mouth Spray	Omnii Oral Pharmaceuticals (800) 445-3386	Pump dispenser	Plaque inhibitor in vanilla-mint flavor for breath malodor or reduced salivary flow	Treats the discomfort of oral dryness	Microdent® patented plaque-inhibitor formula	Spray directly into mouth; spread over teeth and tissue with tongue	18 mL pump dispenser; order directly from manufacturer
Moi-Stir® Moistening Solution	Kingswood Laboratories, Inc (800) 968-7772	Pump spray	Saliva supplement for moistening of mouth and mucosal area	Nontherapeutic treatment of dry mouth; intended for comfort only	Water, sorbitol, sodium carboxymethylcellulose, methylparaben, propylparaben, potassium chloride, sodium chloride, flavoring	Spray directly into mouth as necessary to treat drying conditions	4 oz spray bottle; order directly from manufacturer or various distributors
MouthKote® Oral Moisturizer	Parnell Pharmaceuticals, Inc (800) 457-4276	Aqueous solution	Pleasant lemon-lime flavored oral moisturizer to lubricate and protect oral tissue	Treats the discomfort of oral dryness caused by medications, disease, surgery, irradiation, aging	Water, xylitol, sorbitol, yerba santa, citric acid, ascorbic acid, flavor, sodium benzoate, sodium saccharin	Swirl 1 or 2 teaspoonfuls in mouth for 8-10 seconds; swallow or spit out; shake well before using	2 oz and 8 oz bottles; available at drugstores or order directly from manufacturer

PRODUCTS AND DRUGS TO TREAT DRY MOUTH (continued)

Medication	Manufacturer and Phone Number	Product Type	Manufacturer's Description	Indication	Ingredients	Directions for Use	Form and Availability
Oasis® Moisturizing Mouthwash	GlaxoSmithKline (800) 777-2500	Oral moisturizer, aqueous solution	Moisturizing mouthwash for a dry mouth indication	Moisturizes mouth and helps it from drying out	Active: Glycerin Other: Water, sorbitol, poloxamer 338, PEG-60 hydrogenated castor oil, cellulose gum, cetylpyridinium chloride, copovidone, disodium phosphate, flavor, methylparaben, propylparaben, sodium benzoate, sodium phosphate, sodium saccharin, xanthan gum, FD&C blue #1	Rinse for 30 seconds with 1 ounce of mouthwash first thing in the morning and before going to bed or as needed; do not swallow; use as part of an effective oral hygiene program	16 oz bottle
Optimoist™ Oral Moisturizer	Colgate Oral Pharmaceuticals (800) 225-3756	Oral moisturizer, aqueous solution	Pleasant tasting saliva substitute for instant relief of dry mouth and throat without demineralizing tooth enamel	Treats the discomfort of oral dryness	Deionized water, xylitol, calcium phosphate monobasic, citric acid, sodium hydroxide, sodium benzoate, flavoring, acesulfame potassium, hydroxyethylcellulose, polysorbate 20 and sodium monofluorophosphate (fluoride concentration is 2 parts per million)	Spray directly into mouth to relieve dry mouth discomfort; may be swallowed or expectorated; use as needed	2 oz and 12 oz bottles; available at mass merchandise stores, food stores, and drugstores
Salivart® Synthetic Saliva, Aqueous Solution	Gebauer Co (800) 321-9348	Aerosol aqueous spray	Oral moisturizer for patients with reduced salivary flow	Replacement therapy for patients complaining of xerostomia	Sodium carboxymethylcellulose, sorbitol, sodium chloride, potassium chloride, calcium chloride dihydrate, magnesium chloride hexahydrate, potassium phosphate dibasic, purified water, nitrogen (propellant)	Spray directly into mouth or throat for 1-2 seconds; use as needed	2.48 fl oz (75 g); available at most drugstores or directly from manufacturer
Other Dry Mouth Products (OTC)							
Biotene® Dry Mouth Gum	Laclede Professional Products, Inc (800) 922-9348	Chewing gum	Sugar-free; helps stimulate saliva flow; fights cause/ effect of bad breath; reduces plaque	Treats oral dryness	Active: Lactoperoxidase (0.11 Units), glucose oxidase (0.15 Units) Other: Sorbitol, gum base, xylitol, hydrogenated glucose, potassium thiocyanate	Chew 1 or 2 pieces; use as needed	Each package contains 17 pieces; available at drugstores or directly from manufacturer

DENTIN HYPERSENSITIVITY, HIGH CARIES INDEX, AND XEROSTOMIA *(Continued)*

PRODUCTS AND DRUGS TO TREAT DRY MOUTH *(continued)*

Medication	Manufacturer and Phone Number	Product Type	Manufacturer's Description	Indication	Ingredients	Directions for Use	Form and Availability
Biotene® Dry Mouth Toothpaste	Laclede Professional Products, Inc (800) 922-9348	Toothpaste	Reduces harmful bacteria which cause cavities, periodontal disease, and oral infections	Use in place of regular toothpaste for dry mouth	Active: Lactoperoxidase (15,000 Units), glucose oxidase (10,000 Units), lysozyme (16 mg), sodium monofluorophosphate Other: Sorbitol, glycerin, calcium pyrophosphate, hydrated silica, xylitol, isoceteth-20, cellulose gum, flavoring, sodium benzoate, beta-d-glucose, potassium thiocyanate	Use in place of regular toothpaste; rinse toothbrush before applying; brush for 2 minutes; rinse lightly	4.5 oz tube; available at drugstores or directly from manufacturer
Biotene® Gentle Mouthwash	Laclede Professional Products, Inc (800) 922-9348	Mouthwash	Alcohol-free; strong antibacterial formula neutralizes mouth odors; soothes as it cleans to protect teeth and oral tissue	Treats dry mouth or oral irritations	Lysozyme, lactoferrin, glucose oxidase, lactoperoxidase	Use 15 mL (1 tablespoonful); swish thoroughly for 30 seconds and spit out; for dry throat, sip 1 tablespoonful of mouthwash 2-3 times/ day	Available at drugstores or directly from manufacturer
Moi-Stir® Oral Swabsticks	Kingswood Laboratories, Inc (800) 968-7772	Swabsticks	Lubricates and moistens mouth and mucosal area	Lubricates and moistens mouth and mucosal area	Water, sorbitol, sodium carboxymethylcellulose, methylparaben, propylparaben, potassium chloride, sodium chloride, flavoring	Gently swab all intraoral surfaces of mouth, gums, tongue, palate, buccal mucosa, gingival, teeth, and lips where uncomfortable dryness exists	3 swabsticks/packet; 100 packets/case; order directly from manufacturer or from various distributors.
Oasis® Moisturizing Mouth Spray	GlaxoSmithKline (800) 777-2500	Oral moisturizer	Moisturizing mouth spray for a dry mouth indication	Moisturizes mouth and helps it from drying out	Active: Glycerin 35% (prediluted) Other: Cetylpyridinium chloride, copovidone, flavor, methylparaben, PEG-60 hydrogenated castor oil, propylparaben, sodium benzoate, sodium saccharin, water, xanthan gum, xylitol	Use as required up to a maximum of 30 times or 60 sprays a day; spray 1-2 times into the affected area of mouth; do not rinse out	1 oz bottle

PRODUCTS AND DRUGS TO TREAT DRY MOUTH (continued)

Medication	Manufacturer and Phone Number	Product Type	Manufacturer's Description	Indication	Ingredients	Directions for Use	Form and Availability
Cholinergic Salivary Stimulants (Rx)							
Cevimeline (Evoxac®)	Snow Brand Pharmaceuticals (800) 475-6473			Treats symptoms of dry mouth in patients with Sjögren's syndrome	Active: Cevimeline 30 mg Other: Lactose monohydrate, hydroxypropyl cellulose, magnesium stearate	1 capsule (30 mg) 3 times/day	30 mg capsules
Pilocarpine (Salagen®)	MGI Pharmaceuticals, Inc (800) 562-5580			Treats xerostomia caused by radiation therapy in patients with head/neck cancer, Sjögren's syndrome	Active: Pilocarpine 5 mg Other: Carnauba wax, hydroxypropyl methylcellulose, iron oxide, microcrystalline cellulose, stearic acid, titanium dioxide	1-2 tablets (5 mg) 3-4 times/day, not to exceed 30 mg/day	5 mg tablets

DENTIN HYPERSENSITIVITY, HIGH CARIES INDEX, AND XEROSTOMIA *(Continued)*

CHOLINERGIC SALIVARY STIMULANTS (PRESCRIPTION ONLY)

Pilocarpine (Dental) (Salagen® *on page 1235*), approved in 1994, and cevimeline (Evoxac® *on page 310*), approved in 2000, are cholinergic drugs which stimulate salivary flow. They stimulate muscarinic-type acetylcholine receptors in salivary glands within the parasympathetic division of the autonomic nervous system, causing an increase in serous-type saliva. Thus, they are considered cholinergic, muscarinic-type (parasympathomimetic) drugs. Due to significant side effects caused by these drugs, they are available by prescription only.

Pilocarpine (Salagen®) is indicated for the treatment of xerostomia caused by radiation therapy in patients with head and neck cancer and xerostomia in patients suffering from Sjögren's syndrome. The usual adult dosage is 1-2 tablets (5 mg) 3-4 times/day, not to exceed 30 mg/day. Patients should be treated for a minimum of 90 days for optimum effect. The most frequent adverse side effect is perspiration, which occurs in about 30% of patients who use 5 mg 3 times/day. Other adverse effects (in about 10% of patients) are nausea, rhinitis, chills, frequent urination, dizziness, headache, lacrimation, and pharyngitis. Salagen® is contraindicated for patients with uncontrolled asthma and narrow-angle glaucoma.

The salivary-stimulative effects of oral pilocarpine have been documented since the late 1960s and 1970s. Pilocarpine has been documented to overcome xerostomia from different causes. More recent studies confirm its effectiveness in improving salivary flow in patients undergoing irradiation therapy for head and neck cancer. A capstone study by Johnson, et al, reported the effects of pilocarpine in 208 irradiation patients at 39 different treatment sites. Salagen®, at a dose of 5 mg 3 times/day, improved salivation in 44% of patients, compared with 25% in the placebo group. They concluded that treatment with pilocarpine (Salagen®) produced the best overall outcome with respect to saliva production and relief of symptoms of xerostomia in patients undergoing irradiation therapy.

Additional studies have been published showing the effectiveness of pilocarpine (Salagen®) in stimulating salivary flow in patients suffering from Sjögren's syndrome and the FDA has recently approved the use of Salagen® for this indication.

Recent reports suggest that pre-emptive use of pilocarpine may be effective in protecting salivary glands during therapeutic irradiation; further studies are needed to confirm this. As of this publication date, the use of pilocarpine has not been approved to treat xerostomia induced by chronic medication. Pilocarpine could be used as a sialagogue for individuals with xerostomia induced by antidepressants and other medications. However, the potential for serious drug interactions is a concern and more studies are needed to clarify the safety and effectiveness of pilocarpine when given in the presence of other medications.

Cevimeline (Evoxac®) is indicated for treatment of symptoms of dry mouth in patients with Sjögren's syndrome. The usual dosage in adults is 1 capsule (30 mg) 3 times/day. Cevimeline (Evoxac®) is supplied in 30 mg capsules. Some adverse effects reported for Evoxac® include increased sweating (19%), rhinitis (11%), sinusitis (12%), and upper respiratory infection (11%). Evoxac® is contraindicated for patients with uncontrolled asthma, narrow-angle glaucoma, acute iritis, and other conditions where miosis is undesirable.

OTHER DRUGS IMPLICATED IN XEROSTOMIA

>10%	1% to 10%
Alprazolam	Acrivastine and Pseudoephedrine
Amitriptyline hydrochloride	Albuterol
Amoxapine	Amantadine hydrochloride
Anisotropine methylbromide	Amphetamine sulfate
Atropine sulfate	Astemizole (withdrawn from market)
Belladonna and Opium	Azatadine maleate
Benztropine mesylate	Beclomethasone dipropionate
Bupropion	Bepridil hydrochloride
Chlordiazepoxide	Bitolterol mesylate
Clomipramine hydrochloride	Brompheniramine maleate
Clonazepam	Carbinoxamine and Pseudoephedrine
Clonidine	Chlorpheniramine maleate
Clorazepate dipotassium	Clemastine fumarate
Cyclobenzaprine	Clozapine
Desipramine hydrochloride	Cromolyn sodium
Diazepam	Cyproheptadine hydrochloride
Dicyclomine hydrochloride	Dexchlorpheniramine maleate
Diphenoxylate and Atropine	Dextroamphetamine sulfate
Doxepin hydrochloride	Dimenhydrinate
Ergotamine	Diphenhydramine hydrochloride
Estazolam	Disopyramide phosphate
Flavoxate	Doxazosin
Flurazepam hydrochloride	Dronabinol
Glycopyrrolate	Ephedrine sulfate
Guanabenz acetate	Flumazenil
Guanfacine hydrochloride	Fluvoxamine
Hyoscyamine sulfate	Gabapentin
Interferon alfa-2a	Guaifenesin and Codeine
Interferon alfa-2b	Guanadrel sulfate
Interferon alfa-N3	Guanethidine sulfate
Ipratropium bromide	Hydroxyzine
Isoproterenol	Hyoscyamine, Atropine, Scopolamine, and Phenobarbital
Isotretinoin	Imipramine
Loratadine	Isoetharine
Lorazepam	Levocabastine hydrochloride
Loxapine	Levodopa
Maprotiline hydrochloride	Levodopa and Carbidopa
Methscopolamine bromide	Levorphanol tartrate
Molindone hydrochloride	Meclizine hydrochloride
Nabilone	Meperidine hydrochloride
Nefazodone	Methadone hydrochloride
Oxybutynin chloride	Methamphetamine hydrochloride
Oxazepam	Methyldopa
Paroxetine	Metoclopramide
Phenelzine sulfate	Morphine sulfate
Prochlorperazine	Nortriptyline hydrochloride
Propafenone hydrochloride	Ondansetron
Protriptyline hydrochloride	Oxycodone and Acetaminophen
Quazepam	Oxycodone and Aspirin
Reserpine	Pentazocine
Selegiline hydrochloride	Phenylpropanolamine hydrochloride
Temazepam	Prazosin hydrochloride
Thiethylperazine maleate	Promethazine hydrochloride
Trihexyphenidyl hydrochloride	Propoxyphene
Trimipramine maleate	Pseudoephedrine
Venlafaxine	Risperidone
	Sertraline hydrochloride
	Terazosin
	Terbutaline sulfate

TEMPOROMANDIBULAR DYSFUNCTION (TMD)

Temporomandibular dysfunction comprises a broad spectrum of signs and symptoms. Although TMD presents in patterns, diagnosis is often difficult. Evaluation and treatment is time-intensive and no single therapy or drug regimen has been shown to be universally beneficial.

The thorough diagnostician should perform a screening examination for the temporomandibular joint on all patients. Ideally, a baseline maximum mandibular opening along with lateral and protrusive movement evaluation should be performed. Secondly, the joint area should be palpated and an adequate exam of the muscles of mastication and the muscles of the neck and shoulders should be made. These muscle would include the elevators of the mandible (masseter, internal pterygoid, and temporalis); the depressors of the mandible (including the external pterygoid and digastric); extrusive muscles (including the temporalis and digastric), and protrusive muscles (including the external and internal pterygoids). These muscles also account for lateral movement of the mandible. The clinician should also be alert to indicators of dysfunction, primarily a history of pain with jaw function, chronic history of joint noise (although this can often be misinterpreted), pain in the muscles of the neck, limited jaw movement, pain in the actual muscles of mastication, and headache or even earache. The signs and symptoms are extremely variable and the clinician should be alert for any or all of these areas of interest. Because of the complexity of both evaluation and diagnosis, the general dentist often finds it too time consuming to spend the countless hours evaluating and treating the temporomandibular dysfunction patient. Therefore, oral medicine specialists trained in temporomandibular evaluation and treatment often accept referrals for the management of these complicated patients.

The Oral Medicine specialist in TMD management, the physical therapist interested in head and neck pain, and the Oral and Maxillofacial surgeon will all work together with the referring general dentist to accomplish successful patient treatment. Table 1 lists the wide variety of treatment alternatives available to the team. Depending on the diagnosis, one or more of the therapies might be selected. For organic diseases of the joint not responding to nonsurgical approaches, a wide variety of surgical techniques are available (Table 2).

ACUTE TMD

Acute TMD oftentimes presents alone or as an episode during a chronic pattern of signs and symptoms. Trauma, such as a blow to the chin or the side of the face, can result in acute TMD. Occasionally, similar symptoms will follow a lengthy wide open mouth dental procedure.

The condition usually presents as continuous deep pain in the TMJ. If edema is present in the joint, the condyle sometimes can be displaced which will cause abnormal occlusion of the posterior teeth on the affected side. The diagnosis is usually based on the history and clinical presentation. Management of the patient includes:

1. Restriction of all mandibular movement to function in a pain-free range of motion
2. Soft diet
3. NSAIDs (eg, Anaprox® DS 1 tablet every 12 hours for 7-10 days)
4. Moist heat applications to the affected area for 15-20 minutes, 4-6 times/day
5. Consideration of a muscle relaxant, such as Methocarbamol (Robaxin®) *on page 1009*, adult patient of average height/weight, two (500 mg) tablets at bedtime; daytime dose can be tailored to patient

Additional therapies could include referral to a physical therapist for ultrasound therapy 2-4 times/week and a single injection of steroid in the joint space. A team approach with an oral maxillofacial surgeon for this procedure may be helpful. Spray and stretch with Fluori-methane® is often helpful for rapid relief of trismus.

Dichlorodifluoromethane and Trichloromonofluoromethane *on page 458*

CHRONIC TMD

Following diagnosis which is often problematic, the most common therapeutic modalities include:

- Explaining the problem to the patient
- Recommending a soft diet:

    Diet should consist of soft foods (eg, eggs, yogurt, casseroles, soup, ground meat).

    Avoid chewing gum, salads, large sandwiches, and hard fruit.

- Reducing stress; moist heat application 4-6 times/day for 15-20 minutes coupled with a monitored exercise program will be beneficial. Usually, working with a physical therapist is ideal.

- Medications include analgesics, anti-inflammatories, tranquilizers, and muscle relaxants

MEDICATION OPTIONS

Most commonly used medication (NSAIDs)

Choline Magnesium Trisalicylate *on page 335*

Diclofenac *on page 459*

Diflunisal *on page 468*

Etodolac *on page 623*

Fenoprofen *on page 642*

Flurbiprofen *on page 683*

Ibuprofen *on page 808*

Indomethacin *on page 830*

Ketoprofen *on page 883*

Ketorolac *on page 886*

Magnesium Salicylate *on page 962*

Meclofenamate *on page 970*

Mefenamic Acid *on page 973*

Nabumetone *on page 1077*

Naproxen *on page 1089*

Oxaprozin *on page 1155*

Piroxicam *on page 1248*

Salsalate *on page 1376*

Sulindac *on page 1430*

Tolmetin *on page 1504*

Tranquilizers and muscle relaxants, when used appropriately, can provide excellent adjunctive therapy. These drugs are primarily used for a short period of time to manage acute pain. In low dosages, amitriptyline is often used to treat chronic pain and occasionally migraine headache. Two new drugs similar to the prototype drug, amitriptyline, have recently been approved for use in adults only, for treatment of acute migraine with or without aura: Almotriptan malate (Axert™ [tablets]; Pharmacia Corp) and frovatriptan succinate (Frova™ [tablets]; Elan). Selective serotonin reuptake inhibitors (SSRIs) are sometimes used in the management of chronic neuropathic pain, particularly in patients not responding to amitriptyline. Recently, gabapentin (Neurontin®) has been approved for chronic pain. Problems of inducing bruxism with SSRIs, however, have been reported and may preclude their use. Clinicians attempting to evaluate any patient with bruxism or involuntary muscle movement, who is simultaneously being treated with an SSRI, should be aware of this potential association.

See individual monographs for dosing instructions.

Common minor tranquilizers include:

Alprazolam *on page 73*

Diazepam *on page 454*

Lorazepam *on page 947*

Chronic neuropathic pain management:

Amitriptyline *on page 93*

Carbamazepine *on page 260*

Gabapentin *on page 717*

Acute migraine management:

Almotriptan *on page 71*

Frovatriptan *on page 712*

Rizatriptan *on page 1363*

TEMPOROMANDIBULAR DYSFUNCTION (TMD) *(Continued)*

Common muscle relaxants include:
Chlorzoxazone *on page 333*
Cyclobenzaprine *on page 401*
Methocarbamol *on page 1009*
Orphenadrine *on page 1151*

Note: Muscle relaxants and tranquilizers should generally be prescribed with an analgesic or NSAID to relieve pain as well.

Narcotic analgesics can be used on a short-term basis or intermittently in combination with non-narcotic therapy in the chronic pain patient. Judicious prescribing, monitoring, and maintenance by the practitioner is imperative whenever considering the use of narcotic analgesics due to the abuse and addiction liabilities.

Table 1.
TMD - NONSURGICAL THERAPIES

1. Moist heat and cold spray

2. Injections in muscle trigger areas (procaine)

3. Exercises (passive, active)

4. Medications
   a. Muscle relaxants
   b. Minerals
   c. Multiple vitamins (Ca, B_6, B_{12})

5. Orthopedic craniomandibular repositioning appliance (splints)

6. Biofeedback, acupuncture

7. Physiotherapy: TMJ muscle therapy

8. Myofunctional therapy

9. TENS (transcutaneous electrical neural stimulation), Myo-Monitor

10. Dental therapy
    a. Equilibration (coronoplasty)
    b. Restoring occlusion to proper vertical dimension of maxilla to mandible by orthodontics, dental restorative procedures, orthognathic surgery, permanent splint, or any combination of these

Table 2.
TMD – SURGICAL THERAPIES

1. Cortisone injection into joint (with local anesthetic)

2. Bony and/or fibrous ankylosis: requires surgery (osteoarthrotomy with prosthetic appliance)

3. Chronic subluxation: requires surgery, depending on problem (possibly eminectomy and/or prosthetic implant)

4. Osteoarthritis: requires surgery, depending on problem
   a. Arthroplasty with implant
   b. Meniscectomy with implant
   c. Arthroplasty with repair of disc and/or implant
   d. Implant with Silastic insert

5. Rheumatoid arthritis
   a. Arthroplasty with implant with Silastic insert
   b. "Total" TMJ replacement

6. Tumors: require osteoarthrotomy – removal of tumor and restoring of joint when possible

7. Chronic disc displacement: requires repair of disc and possible removal of bone from condyle

SEDATION

Anxiety constitutes the most frequently found psychiatric problem in the general population. Anxiety can range from simple phobias to severe debilitating anxiety disorders. Functional results of this anxiety can, therefore, range from simple avoidance of dental procedures to panic attacks when confronting stressful situations such as seen in some patients regarding dental visits. Many patients claim to be anxious over dental care when in reality they simply have not been managed with modern techniques of local anesthesia, the availability of sedation, or the caring dental practitioner.

The dentist may detect anxiety in patients during the treatment planning evaluation phase of the care. The anxious person may appear overly alert, may lean forward in the dental chair during conversation or may appear concerned over time, possibly using this as a guise to require that they cut short their dental visit. Anxious persons may also show signs of being nervous by demonstrating sweating, tension in their muscles including their temporomandibular musculature, or they may complain of being tired due to an inability to obtain an adequate night's sleep.

The management of such patients requires a methodical approach to relaxing the patient, discussing their dental needs, and then planning, along with the patient the best way to accomplish dental treatment in the presence of their fears, both real or imagined. Consideration may be given to sedation to assist with managing the patient. This sedation can be oral or parenteral, or inhalation in the case of nitrous oxide. The dentist must be adequately trained in administering the sedative of choice, as well as in monitoring the patient during the sedated procedures. Numerous medications are available to achieve the level of sedation usually necessary in the dental office: Valium®, Ativan®, Xanax®, Vistaril®, Serax®, and BuSpar® represent a few. BuSpar® is soon to be available as a transdermal patch. These oral sedatives can be given prior to dental visits as outlined in the following prescriptions. They have the advantage of allowing the patient a good night's sleep prior to the day of the procedures and providing on-the-spot sedation during the procedures. Nitrous oxide represents an in the office administered sedative that is relatively safe, but requires additional training and carefully planned monitoring protocols of any auxiliary personnel during the inhalation procedures. Both the oral and the inhalation techniques can, however, be applied in a very useful manner to manage the anxious patient in the dental office.

Alprazolam *on page 73*
Buspirone *on page 236*
Diazepam *on page 454*
Hydroxyzine *on page 801*
Lorazepam *on page 947*
Nitrous Oxide *on page 1122*
Oxazepam *on page 1157*
Triazolam *on page 1531*

Note: Although various sedatives have been used for preprocedure sedation, no specific regimens or protocols have been established. Guidelines for use are still under study.

Fluoxetine *on page 675*
Fluvoxamine *on page 694*
Paroxetine *on page 1188*
Sertraline *on page 1385*

For examples of sample prescriptions see Sedation (Prior to Dental Treatment) *on page 1746*

MANAGEMENT OF PATIENTS
UNDERGOING CANCER THERAPY

CANCER PATIENT DENTAL PROTOCOL

The objective in treatment of a patient with cancer is eradication of the disease. Oral complications, such as mucosal ulceration, xerostomia, bleeding, and infections can cause significant morbidity and may compromise systemic treatment of the patient. With proper oral evaluation before systemic treatment, many of the complications can be minimized or prevented.

MUCOSITIS

Normal oral mucosa acts as a barrier against chemical and food irritants and oral microorganisms. Disruption of the mucosal barrier can therefore lead to secondary infection, increased pain, delayed healing, and decreased nutritional intake.

Mucositis is inflammation of the mucous membranes. It is a common reaction to chemotherapy and radiation therapy. It is first seen as an erythematous patch. The mucosal epithelium becomes thin as a result of the killing of the rapidly dividing basal layer mucosal cells. Seven to ten days after cytoreduction chemotherapy and between 1000 cGy and 3000 cGy of radiation to the head and neck, mucosal tissues begin to desquamate and eventually develop into frank ulcerations. The mucosal integrity is broken and is secondarily infected by normal oral flora. The resultant ulcerations can also act as a portal of entry for pathogenic organisms into the patient's bloodstream and may lead to systemic infections. These ulcerations often force interruption of therapy.

Certain chemotherapeutic agents, such as 5-fluorouracil, methotrexate, and doxorubicin, are more commonly associated with the development of oral mucositis. Treatment of oral mucositis is mainly palliative, but steps should be taken to minimize secondary pathogenic infections. Culture and sensitivity data should be obtained to select appropriate therapy for the bacterial, viral, or fungal organisms found.

Prevention of radiation mucositis is difficult. Stents can be constructed to prevent irradiation of uninvolved tissues. The use of multiple ports and fractionation of therapy into smaller doses over a longer period of time can reduce the severity. Fractured restorations, sharp teeth, and ill-fitted prostheses can damage soft tissues and lead to additional interruption of mucosal barriers. Correction of these problems before radiation therapy can diminish these complications.

CHEMOTHERAPY

Chemotherapy for neoplasia also frequently results in oral complications. Infections and mucositis are the most common complications seen in patients receiving chemotherapy. Also occurring frequently are pain, altered nutrition, and xerostomia, which can significantly affect the quality of life.

RADIATION CARIES

Dental caries that sometimes follows radiation therapy is called radiation caries. It usually develops in the cervical region of the teeth adjacent to the gingiva, often affecting many teeth. It is secondary to the damage done to the salivary glands and is initiated by dental plaque, but its rapid progress is due to changes in saliva. In addition to the diminution in the amount of saliva, both the salivary pH and buffering capacity are diminished, which decreases anticaries activity of saliva. Oral bacteria also change with xerostomia leading to the increase in caries activity.

SALIVARY CHANGES

Chemotherapy is not thought to directly alter salivary flow, but alterations in taste and subjective sensations of dry mouth are relatively common complaints. Patients with mucositis and graft-vs-host disease following bone marrow or stem cell transplantation often demonstrate signs and symptoms of xerostomia. Radiation does directly affect salivary production. Radiation to the salivary glands produces fibrosis and alters the production of saliva. If all the major salivary glands are in the field, the decrease in saliva can be dramatic and the serous portion of the glands seems to be most severely affected. The saliva produced is increased in viscosity, which contributes to food retention and increased plaque formation. These xerostomic patients have difficulty in managing a normal diet. Normal saliva also has bacteriostatic properties that are diminished in these patients.

The dental management recommendations for patients undergoing chemotherapy, bone marrow transplantation, and/or radiation therapy for the treatment of cancer are based primarily on clinical observations. The following protocols will provide a conservative, consistent approach to the dental management of patients undergoing chemotherapy or bone marrow transplantation. Many of the cancer chemotherapy drugs produce oral side effects including mucositis, oral ulceration, dry mouth, acute infections, and taste aberrations. Cancer drugs include antibiotics, alkylating agents, antimetabolites, DNA inhibitors, hormones, and cytokines.

All patients undergoing chemotherapy or bone marrow transplantation for malignant disease should have the following baseline:

A. Panoramic radiograph

B. Dental consultation and examination

C. Dental prophylaxis and cleaning (if the neutrophil count is >1500/mm^3 and the platelet count is >50,000/mm^3)

    –   Prophylaxis and cleaning will be deferred if the patient's neutrophil count is <1500 and the platelet count is <50,000. Oral hygiene recommendations will be made. These levels are arbitrary guidelines and the dentist should consider the patient's oral condition and planned procedure relative to hemorrhage and level of bacteremia.

D. Oral Hygiene: Patients should be encouraged to follow normal hygiene procedures. Addition of a chlorhexidine mouth rinse such as Peridex® or PerioGard® *on page 316* is usually helpful. If the patient develops oral mucositis, tolerance of such alcohol-based products may be limited.

E. If the patient develops mucositis, bacterial, viral, and fungal cultures should be obtained. Sucralfate suspension in either a pharmacy-prepared form or Carafate® suspension, as well as Benadryl® *on page 483* or Xylocaine® viscous *on page 920* can assist in helping the patient to tolerate food. Patients may also require systemic analgesics for pain relief depending on the presence of mucositis. Positive fungal cultures may require a nystatin swish-and-swallow prescription or the selection of another antifungal agent (see Fungal Infections *on page 1707*).

F. The determination of performing dental procedures must be based on the goal of preventing infection during periods of neutropenia. Timing of procedures must be coordinated with the patient's hematologic status.

G. If oral surgery is required, at least 7-10 days of healing should be allowed before the anticipated date of bone marrow suppression (eg, ANC <1000/mm^3 and/or platelet count of 50,000/mm^3).

H. Daily use of topical fluorides is recommended for those who have received radiation therapy to the head and neck region involving salivary glands. Any patients with prolonged xerostomia subsequent to graft-vs-host disease and/or chemotherapy can also be considered for fluoride supplement. Use the fluoride-containing mouthwashes (Act®, Fluorigard®, etc) each night before going to sleep; swish, hold 1-2 minutes, spit out or use prescription fluorides (gels or rinses); apply daily for 1-4 minutes as directed; if mouth is sore (mucositis), use flavorless/colorless gels (Thera-Flur®, Gel-Kam®). Improvement in salivary flow following radiation therapy to the head and neck has been noted with Salagen® *on page 1235* or Evoxac™ *on page 310*. Custom trays can be produced by the clinician for the patient's home use using heat-formed materials such as omnivac.

Benzonatate *on page 194*
Cevimeline *on page 310*
Chlorhexidine Gluconate *on page 316*
Diphenhydramine *on page 483*
Lidocaine *on page 920*
Pilocarpine (Oral) *on page 1235*
Povidone-Iodine *on page 1262*
Sucralfate *on page 1420*

ORAL CARE PRODUCTS

BACTERIAL PLAQUE CONTROL

Patients should use an extra soft bristle toothbrush and dental floss for removal of plaque. Sponge/foam sticks and lemon-glycerine swabs do not adequately remove bacterial plaque.

CHOLINERGIC AGENTS

See Products for Xerostomia *on page 1714*

Used for the treatment of xerostomia caused by radiation therapy in patients with head and neck cancer and from Sjögren's syndrome

Cevimeline *on page 310*
Pilocarpine (Oral) *on page 1235*

FLUORIDES

See Fluorides in the Dentin Hypersensitivity, High Caries Index, and Xerostomia section.

Used for the prevention of demineralization of the tooth structure secondary to xerostomia. For patients with long-term or permanent xerostomia, daily application is accomplished using custom gel applicator trays, such as omnivac. Patients with porcelain crowns should use a neutral pH fluoride (see Fluoride monograph *on page 671*). Final

MANAGEMENT OF PATIENTS UNDERGOING CANCER THERAPY *(Continued)*

selection of a fluoride product and/or saliva replacement/stimulant product must be based on patient comfort, taste, and ultimately, compliance. Experience has demonstrated that, often times, patients must try various combinations to achieve the greatest effect and their highest comfort levels. The presence of mucositis during cancer management complicates the clinician's selection of products.

SALIVA SUBSTITUTES

See Products for Xerostomia *on page 1714*

ORAL AND LIP MOISTURIZERS/LUBRICANTS

See Mouth Pain, Cold Sore, and Canker Sore Products *on page 1828*

Note: Water-based gels should first be used to provide moisture to dry oral tissues.

Surgi-Lube®
K-Y Jelly®
Oral Balance®
Mouth Moisturizer®

PALLIATION OF PAIN

See Mouth Pain, Cold Sore, and Canker Sore Products *on page 1828*

Note: Palliative pain preparations should be monitored for efficacy.

- For relief of pain associated with isolated ulcerations, topical anesthetic and protective preparations may be used.

    Orabase-B® with 20% benzocaine *on page 190*

- For generalized oral pain:

    Chloraseptic Spray® (OTC) anesthetic spray without alcohol *on page 1223*
    Ulcer-Ease® anesthetic/analgesic mouthrinse
    Xylocaine® 2% viscous *on page 920*
    Note: May anesthetize swallowing mechanism and cause aspiration of food; caution patient against using too close to eating; lack of sensation may also allow patient to damage intact mucosa
    Tantum Mouthrinse® (benzydamine hydrochloride); may be diluted as required
    Note: Available only in Canada and Europe

PATIENT PREPARED PALLIATIVE MIXTURES

Coating agents:

Maalox® *on page 80*
Mylanta® *on page 81*
Kaopectate® *on page 165*

These products can be mixed with Benadryl® elixir (50:50):

Diphenhydramine (Benadryl®) *on page 483*
Mouth Pain, Cold Sore, and Canker Sore Products *on page 1828*

Topical anesthetics (diphenhydramine chloride):

Benadryl® elixir or Benylin® cough syrup *on page 483*
Note: Choose product with lowest alcohol and sucrose content; ask pharmacist for assistance

PHARMACY PREPARATIONS

A pharmacist may also prepare the following solutions for relief of generalized oral pain:

Benadryl-Lidocaine Solution

Diphenhydramine injectable 1.5 mL (50 mg/mL) *on page 483*
Xylocaine viscous 2% (45 mL) *on page 920*
Magnesium aluminum hydroxide solution (45 mL)
Swish and hold 1 teaspoonful in mouth for 30 seconds; do not use too close to eating

ORAL MEDICINE TOPICS

PART III:

SAMPLE PRESCRIPTIONS

Drug prescriptions shown represent prototype drugs and popular prescriptions and are examples only. The pharmacologic category index is available for cross-referencing if alternatives and additional drugs are sought.

TABLE OF CONTENTS

Bacterial Endocarditis (Prevention) 1732

Prosthetic Joint Late Infections (Prevention) 1733

Oral Pain 1734

Bacterial Infections and Periodontal Diseases 1736

Sinus Infection Treatment 1738

Antimicrobial Rinses 1739

Fungal Infections 1740

Viral Infections 1742

Ulcerative and Erosive Disorders 1744

Sedation (Prior to Dental Treatment) 1746

BACTERIAL ENDOCARDITIS (PREVENTION)

General Prescription Comments

Prescriptions dispense amounts are for 3 visits. These numbers can be adjusted for each patient treatment plan.

Sample Prescriptions

Rx:
Amoxicillin 500 mg
Disp: 12 tablets
Sig: 4 tablets (2 g) 1 hour prior to dental visit and repeat at each appointment

Rx:
Clindamycin 150 mg
Disp: 12 capsules
Sig: 4 capsules (600 mg) 1 hour prior to dental visit and repeat at each appointment

Rx:
Cephalexin 500 mg
Disp: 12 tablets
Sig: 4 tablets (2 g) 1 hour prior to dental visit and repeat at each appointment

Rx:
Azithromycin 500 mg
Disp: 3 tablets
Sig: 1 tablet 1 hour prior to dental visit and repeat at each appointment

PROSTHETIC JOINT LATE INFECTIONS (PREVENTION)

General Prescription Comments

Prescriptions dispense amounts are for 3 visits. These numbers can be adjusted for each patient treatment plan.

Sample Prescriptions

Rx:

Amoxicillin 500 mg
Disp: 12 tablets
Sig: 4 tablets (2 g) 1 hour prior to dental visit and repeat at each appointment

Rx:

Clindamycin 150 mg
Disp: 12 capsules
Sig: 4 capsules (600 mg) 1 hour prior to dental visit and repeat at each appointment

Rx:

Cephalexin 500 mg
Disp: 12 tablets
Sig: 4 tablets (2 g) 1 hour prior to dental visit and repeat at each appointment

ORAL PAIN

Mild / Moderate Oral Pain

General Prescription Comments

Closely monitor and re-evaluate response at least every 2 weeks. If response is inadequate, re-evaluate diagnosis, medication choice, and dosage.

Sample Prescriptions

Rx:

Acetaminophen 325 mg tablets
Disp: To be determined by practitioner
Sig: Take 2-3 tablets every 4 hours

Note: Products include Tylenol® and others.
Note: Acetaminophen can be given if patient has allergies, bleeding problems, or stomach upset secondary to aspirin or NSAIDs.

Rx:

Ibuprofen 200 mg tablets
Disp: To be determined by practitioner
Sig: Take 1-2 tablets every 4 hours

Note: Ibuprofen is an available OTC as Advil®, Motrin® IB, Nuprin®, and many store brand generic names. NSAIDs should not be combined with aspirin. NSAIDs may increase post-treatment bleeding. Use with caution in patients receiving anticoagulants or antiplatelet drugs.

Rx:

Naproxen sodium 220 mg tablets
Disp: To be determined by practitioner
Sig: Take 1-2 tablets every 8 hours

Note: Naproxen sodium is an available OTC as Aleve® and many store brand generic names.

Rx:

Ibuprofen 400 mg tablets
Disp: 20 tablets
Sig: Take 1 tablet every 4-6 hours as needed for pain

Note: Prescription strength ibuprofen is available as the brand name Motrin®.

Rx:

Dolobid® 500 mg tablets
Disp: 16 tablets
Sig: Take 2 tablets initially, then 1 tablet every 8-12 hours as needed for pain
Ingredient: Diflunisal

Moderate / Moderately Severe Oral Pain

General Prescription Comments

Closely monitor and re-evaluate response at least every 2 weeks. If response is inadequate, re-evaluate diagnosis, medication choice, and dosage.

Sample Prescriptions

Rx:

Ibuprofen 800 mg tablets
Disp: 16 tablets
Sig: Take 1 tablet 3 times/day as needed for pain

Note: Also available as 600 mg tablets.

Rx:

Tramadol 50 mg tablets
Disp: 36 tablets
Sig: Take 1-2 tablets every 4-6 hours as needed for pain

Note: Also available as the brand name Ultram®.

Rx:

Ultracet™ tablets
Disp: 36 tablets
Sig: Take 2 tablets every 4-6 hours as needed for pain, not to exceed 8 tablets in 24 hours

Ingredients: Acetaminophen 325 mg and tramadol 37.5 mg

Rx:
    Darvocet-N® 100 tablets
    Disp: 36 tablets
    Sig: Take 1 tablet every 4 hours as needed for pain, not to exceed 6 tablets in 24 hours

    Ingredients: Propoxyphene napsylate 100 mg and acetaminophen 650 mg

Rx:
    Vicoprofen® tablets
    Disp: 16 tablets
    Sig: Take 1-2 tablets every 4-6 hours as needed for pain
    Note: Restrictions: C-III; no refills
    Ingredients: Hydrocodone 7.5 mg and ibuprofen 200 mg; available as generic equivalent

Rx:
    Vicodin® ES tablets
    Disp: 16 tablets
    Sig: Take 1 tablet every 4-6 hours as needed for pain
    Note: Restrictions: C-III; no refills
    Ingredients: Hydrocodone bitartrate 7.5 mg and acetaminophen 750 mg; available as generic equivalent. Also available as Vicodin® tablets: Ingredients: Hydrocodone bitartrate 5 mg and acetaminophen 500 mg; take 1 tablet every 4 hours as needed for pain.

Rx:
    Lortab® 5 mg
    Disp: 16 tablets
    Sig: Take 1 or 2 tablets every 4 hours as needed for pain; not to exceed 8 tablets in 24 hours
    Note: Restrictions: C-III; no refills
    Ingredients: Hydrocodone 5 mg and acetaminophen 500 mg; available as generic equivalent

Rx:
    Tylenol® #3
    Disp: 16 tablets
    Sig: Take 1 tablet every 4 hours as needed for pain
    Note: Restrictions: C-III; no refills
    Ingredients: Codeine 30 mg and acetaminophen 300 mg; available as generic equivalent

Rx:
    Naproxen 275 mg tablets
    Disp: 16 tablets
    Sig: Take 2 tablets initially, then one tablet 3 times/day as needed for pain

Severe Oral Pain

General Prescription Comments

Closely monitor and re-evaluate response at least every 2 weeks. If response is inadequate, re-evaluate diagnosis, medication choice, and dosage.

Liquid volumes are suggested for a typical 2-week course. Check with pharmacist for available sizes.

Cream and ointment tube sizes may vary based on availability. Refer to individual monograph or check with pharmacist for available sizes.

Sample Prescriptions

Rx:
    Percocet® tablets or Tylox® capsules
    Disp: 16 tablets or capsules
    Sig: Take 1 tablet or capsule every 6 hours as needed for pain
    Note: Restrictions: C-II; no refills
    Ingredients: Oxycodone 5 mg and acetaminophen 325 mg (Tylox® contains acetaminophen 500 mg); available as generic equivalent; triplicate prescription required in some states

Rx:
    Combunox™ tablets
    Disp: 16 tablets
    Sig: Take 1 tablet every 6 hours as needed for pain
    Note: Restrictions: C-II; no refills
    Ingredients: Oxycodone 5 mg and ibuprofen 400 mg; not available as generic equivalent; triplicate prescription required in some states

Rx:
    Demerol® 50 mg tablets
    Disp: 16 tablets
    Sig: Take 1 tablet every 4 hours as needed for pain
    Note: Restrictions: C-II; no refills
    Ingredients: Meperidine; triplicate prescription required in some states

BACTERIAL INFECTIONS AND PERIODONTAL DISEASES

General Prescription Comments

Closely monitor and re-evaluate response at least every 2 weeks. If response is inadequate, re-evaluate diagnosis, medication choice, and dosage.

Sample Prescriptions

Rx:

Penicillin V potassium 500 mg
Disp: 40 tablets
Sig: Take 1 tablet 4 times/day for 7-10 days (consider a loading dose of 1 g for acute infection)

Rx:

Clindamycin 150 mg
Disp: 40 capsules
Sig: Take 1 capsule 4 times/day for 7-10 days

Note: Prescription for patients allergic to penicillin

Rx:

Clindamycin 300 mg
Disp: 40 capsules
Sig: Take 1 capsule 4 times/day for 7-10 days

Note: Prescription for patients allergic to penicillin

Rx:

Azithromycin 250 mg
Disp: 1 Z-Pak®
Sig: 2 tablets day 1, then 1 tablet/day until gone

OTHER ANTIBIOTICS:

Rx:

Amoxicillin 250 mg
Disp: 30 capsules
Sig: Take 1 capsule 3 times/day for 7-10 days

Rx:

Amoxicillin 500 mg
Disp: 30 capsules or tablets
Sig: Take 1 capsule or tablet 3 times/day for 7-10 days

Rx:

Amoxicillin 875 mg
Disp: 20 tablets
Sig: Take 1 tablet twice daily

Rx:

Augmentin® 250 mg
Disp: 30 tablets
Sig: Take 1 tablet 3 times/day for 7-10 days

Rx:

Augmentin® 500 mg
Disp: 30 tablets
Sig: Take 1 tablet 3 times/day for 7-10 days

Rx:

Augmentin® 875 mg
Disp: 20 tablets
Sig: Take 1 tablet twice daily for 7-10 days

Rx:

Augmentin XR™ 1000 mg
Disp: 20 tablets
Sig: Take 1 tablet twice daily for 7-10 days

Rx:

Cephalexin 250 mg
Disp: 40 capsules
Sig: Take 1 capsule 4 times/day for 7-10 days

Rx:

Metronidazole 500 mg
Disp: 40 tablets
Sig: Take 1 tablet 4 times/day for 7-10 days

Rx:

Erythromycin 250 mg
Disp: 40 tablets
Sig: Take 1 tablet 4 times/day for 7-10 days

Note: Prescription for patients allergic to penicillin

Rx:

Zithromax® TRI-PAK™ 500 mg
Disp: 1 PAK
Sig: Follow package insert directions until gone

Ingredient: Azithromycin

Rx:

Levaquin® 500 mg
Disp: 10 tablets
Sig: Take 1 tablet/day until gone

SINUS INFECTION TREATMENT

General Prescription Comments

Closely monitor and re-evaluate response at least every 2 weeks. If response is inadequate, re-evaluate diagnosis, medication choice, and dosage.

Sinus infections are not usually true infections. Some clinicians however, couple the medications listed below with antibiotics such as amoxicillin or Augmentin®. when they are uncertain.

Sample Prescriptions

Rx:

Afrin® nasal spray [OTC]
Disp: 15 mg
Sig: Spray once in each nostril every 6-8 hours for no more than 3 days

Ingredient: Oxymetazoline

Rx:

Sudafed® 60 mg tablets [OTC]
Disp: 30 tablets
Sig: Take 1 tablet every 4-6 hours as needed for congestion

Ingredient: Pseudoephedrine

Rx:

Chlor-Trimeton® 4 mg [OTC]
Disp: 14 tablets
Sig: Take 1 tablet twice daily

Ingredient: Chlorpheniramine

ANTIMICROBIAL ORAL RINSE

General Prescription Comments

Closely monitor and re-evaluate response at least every 2 weeks. If response is inadequate, re-evaluate diagnosis, medication choice, and dosage.

Liquid volumes for antimicrobial rinses are suggested for a typical 1 month course. Check with pharmacist for available sizes.

Sample Prescriptions

Rx:

> Chlorhexidine gluconate 0.12% oral rinse
> Disp: 32 oz bottle
> Sig: Rinse with ½ oz twice daily for 30 seconds and expectorate
>
> **Note:** Chlorhexidine gluconate available as the following brands: Peridex®, Perio-Gard®

Rx:

> Listerine® antiseptic mouthwash [OTC]
> Disp: Bottle
> Sig: 20 mL, swish for 30 seconds twice daily

FUNGAL INFECTIONS

Topical Fungal Infections

General Prescription Comments

Closely monitor and re-evaluate response at least every 2 weeks. If response is inadequate, re-evaluate diagnosis, medication choice, and dosage.

Liquid volumes are suggested for a typical 2-week course. Check with pharmacist for available sizes.

Cream and ointment tube sizes may vary based on availability. Refer to individual monograph or check with pharmacist for available sizes.

Sample Prescriptions

Rx:
Nystatin 100,000 units/mL oral suspension
Disp: 300 mL
Sig: Rinse with 1 teaspoon (5 mL) for 2 minutes 4-5 times/day and expectorate

Rx:
Nystatin ointment
Disp: 45 g tube
Sig: Apply locally as directed with a thin coat to inner surface of denture and the
affected area 4-5 times/day

Rx:
Mycelex® 10 mg troches
Disp: 70 troches
Sig: Dissolve 1 troche in mouth 5 times/day until gone; leave any prostheses out
during treatment

Ingredient: Clotrimazole

Rx:
Nizoral® 2% cream
Disp: 45 g tube
Sig: Apply locally as directed with a thin coat to inner surface of denture and
affected areas after meals

Ingredient: Ketoconazole

Systemic Fungal Infections

General Prescription Comments

Note: Decision to use systemic antifungals should be based on diagnostic culture results
or positive smear.

Closely monitor and re-evaluate response at least every 2 weeks. If response is inadequate, re-evaluate diagnosis, medication choice, and dosage.

Sample Prescriptions

Rx:
Nizoral® 200 mg tablets
Disp: 20 tablets
Sig: Take 1 tablet daily

Ingredient: Ketoconazole

Rx:
Diflucan® 100 mg tablets
Disp: 22 tablets
Sig: Take 2 tablets day 1, then 1 tablet/day until gone

Note: Sometimes a shorter course is adequate. However, oral infections commonly
are more difficult to eradicate and even a second course may be necessary.
Ingredient: Fluconazole

Angular Cheilitis

General Prescription Comments

Closely monitor and re-evaluate response at least every 2 weeks. If response is inadequate, re-evaluate diagnosis, medication choice, and dosage.

Cream and ointment tube sizes may vary based on availability. Refer to individual monograph or check with pharmacist for available sizes.

Sample Prescriptions

Rx:

Iodoquinol and hydrocortisone cream
Disp: 45 g tube
Sig: Apply locally as directed 3-4 times/day for 10 days to 2 weeks and then re-evaluate

Note: Available sizes may include 15 g, 30 g, 45 g, and 60 g tubes. Other associated etiologies for angular cheilitis must also be considered such as loss of vertical dimension, trauma, and vitamin deficiencies.

Rx:

Nystatin and triamcinolone acetonide ointment
Disp: 45 g tube
Sig: Apply locally as directed to affected area 4 times/day for 10 days to 2 weeks and then re-evaluate

Note: Available sizes may include 15 g, 30 g, 45 g, and 60 g tubes. Other associated etiologies for angular cheilitis must also be considered such as loss of vertical dimension, trauma, and vitamin deficiencies.

VIRAL INFECTIONS

Herpes Simplex (Primary)

General Prescription Comments

Closely monitor and re-evaluate response at least every 2 weeks. If response is inadequate, re-evaluate diagnosis, medication choice, and dosage.

Sample Prescriptions

Rx:
> Zovirax 200 mg capsules
> Disp: 50 or 60 capsules
> Sig: Take 1 capsule 5 times/day for 10 days or 2 capsules 3 times/day for 10 days
>
> Ingredient: Acyclovir

Herpes Simplex (Recurrent)

General Prescription Comments

Closely monitor and re-evaluate response at least every 2 weeks. If response is inadequate, re-evaluate diagnosis, medication choice, and dosage.

Cream and ointment tube sizes may vary based on availability. Refer to individual monograph or check with pharmacist for available sizes.

Sample Prescriptions

Rx:
> Denavir® topical ointment 5%
> Disp: 1.5 g tube
> Sig: Apply locally as directed to lesion every 2 hours during waking hours (begin
>   when symptoms first occur)
>
> Ingredient: Penciclovir

Rx:
> Famciclovir 125 mg
> Disp: 10 tablets
> Sig: 1 tablet twice daily for 5 days

Rx:
> Valacyclovir 500 mg
> Disp: 8 caplets
> Sig: 4 caplets twice daily for 1 day (separate doses by 12 hours)

Rx:
> Abreva® cream [OTC]
> Disp: 2 g tube
> Sig: Apply to lesion 5 times/day during waking hours for 4 days (begin when
>   symptoms first occur)
>
> Ingredient: Docosanol

Rx:
> Viroxyn® [OTC]
> Disp: 1 pack of 3 individual swab kits
> Sig: Apply locally as directed at first symptoms of recurrence
>
> Ingredient: Benzalkonium 0.13% in isopropyl alcohol

Shingles (Varicella-Zoster Virus)

General Prescription Comments

Closely monitor and re-evaluate response at least every 2 weeks. If response is inadequate, re-evaluate diagnosis, medication choice, and dosage.

Sample Prescriptions

Rx:
> Zovirax® 200 mg capsules
> Disp: 200 capsules
> Sig: Take 4 capsules 5 times/day for 10 days
>
> Ingredient: Acyclovir

Rx:
    Valtrex® HCl 500 mg caplets
    Disp: 42 caplets
    Sig: Take 2 caplets 3 times/day for 7 days

    Note: Use with caution in immunocompromised patients.
    Ingredient: Valacyclovir

Rx:
    Famciclovir 500 mg
    Disp: 21 tablets
    Sig: 1 tablet 3 times/day for 7 days

ULCERATIVE AND EROSIVE DISORDERS

Recurrent Aphthous Stomatitis

General Prescription Comments

Some intraoral uses are off-label. Write directions as "use locally as directed" and closely monitor and re-evaluate response at least every 2 weeks. If response is inadequate, re-evaluate diagnosis, medication choice, and dosage.

Liquid volumes are suggested for a typical 2-week course. Check with pharmacist for available sizes.

Cream and ointment tube sizes may vary based on availability. Refer to individual monograph or check with pharmacist for available sizes.

Sample Prescriptions

Rx:
Amlexanox oral paste 5%
Disp: 5 g tube
Sig: Apply locally as directed, 4 times/day until area heals

Rx:
Orabase® Protective Barrier [OTC]
Disp: 1 package
Sig: Apply locally as directed, every 6 hours as needed

Rx:
Benadryl® liquid 12.5 mg/5 mL (mix 50/50) with Kaopectate®
Disp: 8 oz total
Sig: Rinse with 1-2 teaspoonfuls every 2 hours and expectorate.

Note: Maalox® can be used in place of Kaopectate® if constipation is a problem. Benadryl® is available as a generic diphenhydramine liquid.

Rx:
Benadryl® liquid 12.5 mg/5mL / Kaopectate® / Lidocaine viscous (mix 1/3, 1/3, 1/3)
Disp: 8 oz total
Sig: Rinse with 1-2 teaspoonfuls every 2 hours and expectorate

Note: Maalox® can be used in place of Kaopectate® if constipation is a problem. Benadryl® is available as a generic diphenhydramine liquid. Lidocaine viscous is available as a prescription only.

Rx:
Benadryl® liquid 12.5 mg/5mL
Disp: 4 oz bottle
Sig: Rinse with 1-2 teaspoonfuls every 2 hours and expectorate

Note: Benadryl® is available as a generic diphenhydramine liquid.

Rx:
Kenalog® in Orabase 0.1%
Disp: 5 g tube
Sig: Apply locally as directed to the lesion after each meal and at bedtime

Ingredient: Triamcinolone acetonide

Rx:
Lidex® 0.05% gel
Disp: 45 g tube
Sig: Apply locally as directed to lesion 4 times daily

Ingredient: Fluocinonide 0.05%

Rx:
Temovate® 0.05%
Disp: 45 g tube
Sig: Apply locally as directed a small quantity with a Q-tip to affected area 3-4 times/day

Ingredient: Clobetasol propionate

Rx:
Valisone® 0.1%
Disp: 45 g tube
Sig: Apply locally as directed a small quantity with a Q-tip to affected area 3-4 times/day

Ingredient: Betamethasone valerate

Rx:
Decadron® elixir 0.5 mg/5 mL
Disp: 300 mL
Sig: Rinse with 1 teaspoon for 2 minutes 4 times/day and expectorate

Ingredient: Dexamethasone

Note: Depending on severity of ulceration, instructions can be tailored to include swallowing initial doses and then tapering to every other dose eventually over 4-7 days to no swallowing. See Erosive Lichen Planus and Major Aphthae for more examples.

Mild Lichen Planus

General Prescription Comments

Some intraoral uses are off-label. Write directions as "use locally as directed" and closely monitor and re-evaluate response at least every 2 weeks. If response is inadequate, re-evaluate diagnosis, medication choice, and dosage.

Cream and ointment tube sizes may vary based on availability. Refer to individual monograph or check with pharmacist for available sizes.

Sample Prescriptions

Rx:

Kenalog® in Orabase 0.1%
Disp: 5 g tube
Sig: Apply locally as directed by coating the lesion with a thin film after each meal and at bedtime

Ingredient: Triamcinolone 0.1%

Rx:

Lidex® 0.05% gel
Disp: 45 g tube
Sig: Apply locally as directed to lesion 4 times daily

Ingredient: Fluocinonide 0.05%

Erosive Lichen Planus and Major Aphthae

General Prescription Comments

Some intraoral uses are off-label. Write directions as "use locally as directed" and closely monitor and re-evaluate response at least every 2 weeks. If response is inadequate, re-evaluate diagnosis, medication choice, and dosage.

Liquid volumes are suggested for a typical 2-week course. Check with pharmacist for available sizes.

Cream and ointment tube sizes may vary based on availability. Refer to individual monograph or check with pharmacist for available sizes.

Sample Prescriptions

Rx:

Decadron® 0.5 mg/5 mL elixir
Disp: 400 mL bottle
Sig: For 3 days, rinse with 1 tablespoonful (15 mL) 4 times/day and swallow; then for 3 days, rinse with 1 teaspoonful (5 mL) 4 times/day and swallow; then for 3 days, rinse with 1 teaspoonful (5 mL) 4 times/day and swallow every other time. Then for 3 days rinse with 1 teaspoonful (5 mL) 4 times/day and expectorate. Continue the rinse and expectorate mode for 2 minutes but discontinue medication when mouth becomes completely comfortable.

Ingredient: Dexamethasone; the practitioner can tailor this rinse, hold expectorate and/or swallow prescription to the severity and lesion location for each individual patient.

Rx:

Temovate® 0.05% cream
Disp: 15 g tube
Sig: Apply locally as directed 4-5 times/day

Ingredient: Clobetasol; high potency topical steroid

Rx:

Prednisone 5 mg tablets
Disp: 40 tablets
Sig: Take 5 tablets in the morning for 5 days, then 5 tablets in the morning every other day until gone

Rx:

Prednisone 10 mg tablets
Disp: 50 tablets
Sig: Take 4 tablets in the morning for 5 days, then decrease by 1 tablet on each successive series of 5 days

Rx:

Medrol® Dose Pak
Disp: 1 Pack
Sig: Follow package insert directions until gone

Ingredient: Methylprednisolone

SEDATION
(PRIOR TO DENTAL TREATMENT)

General Prescription Comments

Closely monitor and re-evaluate response at least every 2 weeks. If response is inadequate, re-evaluate diagnosis, medication choice, and dosage.

Sample Prescriptions

Rx:

Valium® 5 mg
Disp: 6 tablets
Sig: Take 1 tablet in evening before going to bed and 1 tablet 1 hour before appointment

Note: Also available as 2 mg and 10 mg.
Ingredient: Diazepam

Rx:

Ativan® 1 mg
Disp: 4 tablets
Sig: Take 2 tablets in evening before going to bed and 2 tablets 1 hour before appointment

Note: Also available as 0.5 mg and 2 mg.
Ingredient: Lorazepam

Rx:

Xanax® 0.5 mg
Disp: 4 tablets
Sig: Take 1 tablet in evening before going to bed and 1 tablet 1 hour before appointment

Ingredient: Alprazolam

Rx:

Vistaril® 25 mg
Disp: 16 capsules
Sig: Take 2 capsules in evening before going to bed and 2 capsules 1 hour before appointment

Ingredient: Hydroxyzine

Rx:

Halcion® 0.25 mg
Disp: 4 tablets
Sig: Take 1 tablet in evening before going to bed and 1 tablet 1 hour before appointment

Ingredient: Triazolam

Rx:

Serax 10 mg
Disp: 2 capsules
Sig: Take 1 capsule before bed and 1 capsule 30 minutes before appointment

Ingredient: Oxazepam

APPENDIX

TABLE OF CONTENTS

Abbreviations and Measurements

Abbreviations, Acronyms, and Symbols 1748
Standard Conversions 1752
    Apothecary / Metric Equivalents 1752
    Pounds / Kilograms Conversion 1753

Pharmacology of Drug Metabolism and Interactions 1754

Infectious Disease Information

Occupational Exposure to Bloodborne Pathogens
    (Standard / Universal Precautions) 1770
Immunizations (Vaccines) 1786
Tuberculosis Treatment..................................... 1800
Treatment of Sexually Transmitted Infections 1811

Laboratory Values

Normal Blood Values.. 1814

Over-the-Counter Dental Products

Dentifrice Products 1815
Mouth Pain, Cold Sore, and Canker Sore Products 1828
Oral Rinse Products 1831

Miscellaneous

Top 200 Most Prescribed Drugs in 2005 1834
Dental Drug Use in Pregnancy and Breast-Feeding.............. 1836
Vasoconstrictor Interactions With Antidepressants 1839

ABBREVIATIONS, ACRONYMS, AND SYMBOLS

Abbreviation	Meaning
<	less than
>	greater than
≤	less than or equal to
≥	greater than or equal to
a̅a̅, aa	of each
AA	Alcoholics Anonymous
ABG	arterial blood gases
ac	before meals or food
ACA	Adult Children of Alcoholics
ACLS	advanced cardiac life support
ad	to, up to
a.d.	right ear
ADHD	attention-deficit/hyperactivity disorder
ADLs	activities of daily living
ad lib	at pleasure
AIDS	acquired immune deficiency syndrome
AIMS	Abnormal Involuntary Movement Scale
a.l.	left ear
ALS	amyotrophic lateral sclerosis
AM	morning
AMA	against medical advice
amp	ampul
amt	amount
aq	water
aq. dest.	distilled water
ARC	AIDS-related complex
ARDS	adult respiratory distress syndrome
ARF	acute renal failure
a.s.	left ear
ASAP	as soon as possible
a.u.	each ear
AUC	area under the curve
BDI	Beck Depression Inventory
bid	twice daily
BLS	basic life support
bm	bowel movement
BMI	body mass index
bp	blood pressure
BPH	benign prostatic hyperplasia
BPRS	Brief Psychiatric Rating Scale
BSA	body surface area
c	a gallon
c̄	with
CA	cancer
CABG	coronary artery bypass graft
CAD	coronary artery disease
cal	calorie
cap	capsule
CBT	cognitive behavioral therapy
cc	cubic centimeter
CCL	creatinine clearance
CF	cystic fibrosis
CGI	Clinical Global Impression
CIE	chemotherapy-induced emesis
cm	centimeter
CIV	continuous I.V. infusion
CNS	central nervous system
comp	compound
cont	continue

Abbreviation	Meaning
COPD	chronic obstructive pulmonary disease
CRF	chronic renal failure
CT	computed tomography
d	day
DBP	diastolic blood pressure
d/c	discontinue
dil	dilute
disp	dispense
div	divide
DOE	dyspnea on exertion
DSC	discontinued
DSM-IV	Diagnostic and Statistical Manual
DTs	delirium tremens
dtd	give of such a dose
DVT	deep vein thrombosis
Dx	diagnosis
ECG	electrocardiogram
ECT	electroconvulsive therapy
EEG	electroencephalogram
elix, el	elixir
emp	as directed
EPS	extrapyramidal side effects
ESRD	end stage renal disease
et	and
EtOH	alcohol
ex aq	in water
f, ft	make, let be made
FDA	Food and Drug Administration
FMS	fibromyalgia syndrome
g	gram
GA	Gamblers Anonymous
GAD	generalized anxiety disorder
GAF	Global Assessment of Functioning Scale
GABA	gamma-aminobutyric acid
GERD	gastroesophageal reflux disease
GFR	glomerular filtration rate
GITS	gastrointestinal therapeutic system
gr	grain
gtt	a drop
GVHD	graft versus host disease
h	hour
HAM-A	Hamilton Anxiety Scale
HAM-D	Hamilton Depression Scale
hs	at bedtime
HSV	herpes simplex virus
HTN	hypertension
IBD	inflammatory bowel disease
IBS	irritable bowel syndrome
ICH	intracranial hemorrhage
IHSS	idiopathic hypertrophic subaortic stenosis
I.M.	intramuscular
IOP	intraocular pressure
IU	international unit
I.V.	intravenous
kcal	kilocalorie
kg	kilogram
KIU	kallikrein inhibitor unit
L	liter
LAMM	L-α-acetyl methadol
liq	a liquor, solution
LVH	left ventricular hypertrophy
M	mix; Molar

ABBREVIATIONS, ACRONYMS, AND SYMBOLS (Continued)

Abbreviation	Meaning
MADRS	Montgomery Asbery Depression Rating Scale
MAOIs	monamine oxidase inhibitors
mcg	microgram
MDEA	3,4-methylene-dioxy amphetamine
m. dict	as directed
MDMA	3,4-methylene-dioxy methamphetamine
mEq	milliequivalent
mg	milligram
mixt	a mixture
mL	milliliter
mm	millimeter
mM	millimolar
MMSE	mini mental status examination
MPPP	l-methyl-4-proprionoxy-4-phenyl pyridine
MR	mental retardation
MRI	magnetic resonance imaging
MS	multiple sclerosis
NF	National Formulary
NKA	no known allergies
NMS	neuroleptic malignant syndrome
no.	number
noc	in the night
non rep	do not repeat, no refills
NPO	nothing by mouth
NSAID	nonsteroidal anti-inflammatory drug
NV	nausea and vomiting
O, Oct	a pint
OA	osteoarthritis
OCD	obsessive-compulsive disorder
o.d.	right eye
o.l.	left eye
o.s.	left eye
o.u.	each eye
PANSS	Positive and Negative Symptom Scale
PAT	paroxysmal artrial tachycardia
pc, post cib	after meals
PCP	phencyclidine
PD	Parkinson's disease
PE	pulmonary embolus
per	through or by
PID	pelvic inflammatory disease
PM	afternoon or evening
P.O.	by mouth
PONV	postoperative nausea and vomiting
P.R.	rectally
prn	as needed
PSVT	paroxysmal superventricular tachycardia
PTA	prior to admission
PTSD	post-traumatic stress disorder
PUD	peptic ulcer disease
pulv	a powder
PVD	peripheral vascular disease
q	every
qad	every other day
qd	every day, daily
qh	every hour
qid	four times a day
qod	every other day
qs	a sufficient quantity
qs ad	a sufficient quantity to make
qty	quantity

Abbreviation	Meaning
qv	as much as you wish
RA	rheumatoid arthritis
REM	rapid eye movement
Rx	take, a recipe
rep	let it be repeated
$\bar{s}$	without
sa	according to art
SAH	subarachnoid hemorrhage
sat	saturated
SBE	subacute bacterial endocarditis
SBP	systolic blood pressure
SIADH	syndrome of inappropriate antidiuretic hormone secretion
sig	label, or let it be printed
SL	sublingual
SLE	systemic lupus erythematosus
SOB	shortness of breath
sol	solution
solv	dissolve
$\overline{ss}$	one-half
sos	if there is need
SSKI	saturated solution of potassium iodide
SSRIs	selective serotonin reuptake inhibitors
stat	at once, immediately
STD	sexually transmitted disease
SubQ	subcutaneous
supp	suppository
SVT	supraventricular tachycardia
Sx	symptom
syr	syrup
tab	tablet
tal	such
TCA	tricyclic antidepressant
TD	tardive dyskinesia
tid	three times a day
TKO	to keep open
TPN	total parenteral nutrition
tr, tinct	tincture
trit	triturate
tsp	teaspoonful
Tx	treatment
ULN	upper limits of normal
ung	ointment
URI	upper respiratory infection
USAN	United States Adopted Names
USP	United States Pharmacopeia
UTI	urinary tract infection
u.d., ut dict	as directed
v.o.	verbal order
VTE	venous thromboembolism
VZV	varicella zoster virus
w.a.	while awake
x3	3 times
x4	4 times
YBOC	Yale Brown Obsessive-Compulsive Scale
YMRS	Young Mania Rating Scale

STANDARD CONVERSIONS

APOTHECARY / METRIC EQUIVALENTS

Approximate Liquid Measures

Basic equivalent: 1 fluid ounce = 30 mL

Examples:

1 gallon	3800 mL	15 minims	1 mL
1 quart	960 mL	10 minims	0.6 mL
1 pint	480 mL	1 gallon	128 fluid ounces
8 fluid ounces	240 mL	1 quart	32 fluid ounces
4 fluid ounces	120 mL	1 pint	16 fluid ounces

Approximate Household Equivalents

1 teaspoonful	5 mL	1 tablespoonful	15 mL

Weights

Basic equivalents:

1 ounce = 30 g   15 grains = 1 g

Examples:

4 ounces	120 g	1/100 grain	600 mcg
2 ounces	60 g	1/150 grain	400 mcg
10 grains	600 mg	1/200 grain	300 mcg
7 1/2 grains	500 mg		
1 grain	60 mg	16 ounces	1 pound

Metric Conversions

Basic equivalents:

1 g	1000 mg	1 mg	1000 mcg

Examples:

5 g	5000 mg	5 mg	5000 mcg
0.5 g	500 mg	0.5 mg	500 mcg
0.05 g	50 mg	0.05 mg	50 mcg

Exact Equivalents

1 g	=	15.43 grains (gr)	0.1 mg =	1/600 gr
1 mL	=	16.23 minims	0.12 mg =	1/500 gr
1 minim	=	0.06 mL	0.15 mg =	1/400 gr
1 gr	=	64.8 mg	0.2 mg =	1/300 gr
1 pint (pt)	=	473.2 mL	0.3 mg =	1/200 gr
1 oz	=	28.35 g	0.4 mg =	1/150 gr
1 lb	=	453.6 g	0.5 mg =	1/120 gr
1 kg	=	2.2 lb	0.6 mg =	1/100 gr
1 qt	=	946.4 mL	0.8 mg =	1/80 gr
			1 mg =	1/65 gr

Solids[1]

1/4 grain	=	15 mg
1/2 grain	=	30 mg
1 grain	=	60 mg
1 1/2 grains	=	90 mg
5 grains	=	300 mg
10 grains	=	600 mg

[1]Use exact equivalents for compounding and calculations requiring a high degree of accuracy.

POUNDS / KILOGRAMS CONVERSION

1 pound = 0.45359 kilograms
1 kilogram = 2.2 pounds

lb	=	kg	lb	=	kg	lb	=	kg
1		0.45	70		31.75	140		63.50
5		2.27	75		34.02	145		65.77
10		4.54	80		36.29	150		68.04
15		6.80	85		38.56	155		70.31
20		9.07	90		40.82	160		72.58
25		11.34	95		43.09	165		74.84
30		13.61	100		45.36	170		77.11
35		15.88	105		47.63	175		79.38
40		18.14	110		49.90	180		81.65
45		20.41	115		52.16	185		83.92
50		22.68	120		54.43	190		86.18
55		24.95	125		56.70	195		88.45
60		27.22	130		58.91	200		90.72
65		29.48	135		61.24			

PHARMACOLOGY OF DRUG METABOLISM AND INTERACTIONS

Most drugs are eliminated from the body, at least in part, by being chemically altered to less lipid-soluble products (ie, metabolized), and thus are more likely to be excreted via the kidneys or the bile. Phase I metabolism includes drug hydrolysis, oxidation, and reduction, and results in drugs that are more polar in their chemical structure, while Phase II metabolism involves the attachment of an additional molecule onto the drug (or partially metabolized drug) in order to create an inactive and/or more water soluble compound. Phase II processes include (primarily) glucuronidation, sulfation, glutathione conjugation, acetylation, and methylation.

Virtually any of the Phase I and II enzymes can be inhibited by some xenobiotic or drug. Some of the Phase I and II enzymes can be induced. Inhibition of the activity of metabolic enzymes will result in increased concentrations of the substrate (drug), whereas induction of the activity of metabolic enzymes will result in decreased concentrations of the substrate. For example, the well-documented enzyme-inducing effects of phenobarbital may include a combination of Phase I and II enzymes. Phase II glucuronidation may be increased via induced UDP-glucuronosyltransferase (UGT) activity, whereas Phase I oxidation may be increased via induced cytochrome P450 (CYP) activity. However, for most drugs, the primary route of metabolism (and the primary focus of drug-drug interaction) is Phase I oxidation, and specifically, metabolism.

CYP enzymes may be responsible for the metabolism (at least partial metabolism) of approximately 75% of all drugs, with the CYP3A subfamily responsible for nearly half of this activity. Found throughout plant, animal, and bacterial species, CYP enzymes represent a superfamily of xenobiotic metabolizing proteins. There have been several hundred CYP enzymes identified in nature, each of which has been assigned to a family (1, 2, 3, etc), subfamily (A, B, C, etc), and given a specific enzyme number (1, 2, 3, etc) according to the similarity in amino acid sequence that it shares with other enzymes. Of these many enzymes, only a few are found in humans, and even fewer appear to be involved in the metabolism of xenobiotics (eg, drugs). The key human enzyme subfamilies include CYP1A, CYP2A, CYP2B, CYP2C, CYP2D, CYP2E, and CYP3A.

CYP enzymes are found in the endoplasmic reticulum of cells in a variety of human tissues (eg, skin, kidneys, brain, lungs), but their predominant sites of concentration and activity are the liver and intestine. Though the abundance of CYP enzymes throughout the body is relatively equally distributed among the various subfamilies, the relative contribution to drug metabolism is (in decreasing order of magnitude) CYP3A4 (nearly 50%), CYP2D6 (nearly 25%), CYP2C8/9 (nearly 15%), then CYP1A2, CYP2C19, CYP2A6, and CYP2E1. Owing to their potential for numerous drug-drug interactions, those drugs that are identified in preclinical studies as substrates of CYP3A enzymes are often given a lower priority for continued research and development in favor of drugs that appear to be less affected by (or less likely to affect) this enzyme subfamily.

Each enzyme subfamily possesses unique selectivity toward potential substrates. For example, CYP1A2 preferentially binds medium-sized, planar, lipophilic molecules, while CYP2D6 preferentially binds molecules that possess a basic nitrogen atom. Some CYP subfamilies exhibit polymorphism (ie, multiple allelic variants that manifest differing catalytic properties). The best described polymorphism involve CYP2C9, CYP2C19, and CYP2D6. Individuals possessing "wild type" gene alleles exhibit normal functioning CYP capacity. Others, however, possess allelic variants that leave the person with a subnormal level of catalytic potential (so called "poor metabolizers"). Poor metabolizers would be more likely to experience toxicity from drugs metabolized by the affected enzymes (or less effects if the enzyme is responsible for converting a prodrug to it's active form as in the case of codeine). The percentage of people classified as poor metabolizers varies by enzyme and population group. As an example, approximately 7% of Caucasians and only about 1% of Orientals appear to be CYP2D6 poor metabolizers.

CYP enzymes can be both inhibited and induced by other drugs, leading to increased or decreased serum concentrations (along with the associated effects), respectively. Induction occurs when a drug causes an increase in the amount of smooth endoplasmic reticulum, secondary to increasing the amount of the affected CYP enzymes in the tissues. This "revving up" of the CYP enzyme system may take several days to reach peak activity, and likewise, may take several days, even months, to return to normal following discontinuation of the inducing agent.

CYP inhibition occurs via several potential mechanisms. Most commonly, a CYP inhibitor competitively (and reversibly) binds to the active site on the enzyme, thus preventing the substrate from binding to the same site, and preventing the substrate from being metabolized. The affinity of an inhibitor for an enzyme may be expressed by an inhibition constant (Ki) or IC50 (defined as the concentration of the inhibitor required to cause 50% inhibition under a given set of conditions). In addition to reversible competition for an enzyme site, drugs may inhibit enzyme activity by binding to sites on the enzyme other than that to which the substrate would bind, and thereby cause a change in the functionality or physical structure of the enzyme. A drug may also bind to the enzyme in an irreversible (ie, "suicide") fashion. In such a case, it is not the concentration of drug at the enzyme site that is important (constantly binding and releasing), but the number of molecules available for binding (once bound, always bound).

Although an inhibitor or inducer may be known to affect a variety of CYP subfamilies, it may only inhibit one or two in a clinically important fashion. Likewise, although a substrate is known to be at least partially metabolized by a variety of CYP enzymes, only one or two enzymes may contribute significantly enough to its overall metabolism to warrant concern when used with potential inducers or inhibitors. Therefore, when attempting to predict the level of risk of using two drugs that may affect each other via altered CYP function, it is important to identify the relative effectiveness of the inhibiting/inducing drug on the CYP subfamilies that significantly contribute to the metabolism of the substrate. The contribution of a specific CYP pathway to substrate metabolism should be considered not only in light of other known CYP pathways, but also other nonoxidative pathways for substrate metabolism (eg, glucuronidation) and transporter proteins (eg, P-glycoprotein) that may affect the presentation of a substrate to a metabolic pathway.

SMOKING AND DRUG METABOLISM

Another area of intense interest involves smoking effects on drug metabolism, as well as, the effects of smoking cessation drugs. A review of the literature suggests that at least a dozen drugs interact with cigarette smoke in a clinically significant manner. Polycyclic aromatic hydrocarbons (PAHs) are largely responsible for enhancing drug metabolism. Cigarette smoke induces an increase in the concentration of CYP1A2, the isoenzyme responsible for metabolism of theophylline. Theophylline is, therefore, eliminated more quickly in smokers than in nonsmokers. As a result of hepatic induction of CYP1A2, serum concentrations of theophylline have been shown to be reduced in smokers. Cigarette smoking may substantially reduce tacrine plasma concentrations. The manufacturer states that mean plasma tacrine concentrations in smokers are about one-third of the concentration in nonsmokers (presumably after multiple doses of tacrine).

Patients with insulin-dependent diabetes who smoke heavily may require a higher dosage of insulin than nonsmokers. Cigarette smoking may also reduce serum concentrations of flecainide. Although the mechanism of this interaction is unknown, enhanced hepatic metabolism is possible. Propoxyphene, a pain reliever, has been found to be less effective in heavy smokers than in nonsmokers. The mechanism for the inefficacy of propoxyphene in smokers compared with nonsmokers may be enhanced biotransformation.

Frankl and Soloff reported in a study of five young, healthy, chronic smokers that propranolol, followed by smoking, significantly decreased cardiac output and significantly increased blood pressure and peripheral resistance compared with smoking alone. Steady-state concentrations of propranolol were found to be lower in smokers than in nonsmokers. Lastly, the incidence of drowsiness associated with the use of diazepam and chlordiazepoxide showed that drowsiness was less likely to occur in smokers than in nonsmokers. Smoking probably acts by producing arousal of the central nervous system rather than by accelerating metabolism and reducing concentrations of these drugs in the brain. Finally, the interaction between smoking and oral contraceptives is complex and may be deadly. Women >35 years of age who smoke >15 cigarettes daily may be at increased risk of myocardial infarction.

The norepinephrine and serotonin reuptake inhibitors, as a new class of smoking cessation drugs, have also received attention relative to metabolic interactions. In vitro studies indicate that bupropion is primarily metabolized to hydroxybupropion by the CYP2B6 isoenzyme. Therefore, the potential exists for a drug interaction between Zyban® and drugs that affect the CYP2B6 isoenzyme metabolism (eg, orphenadrine and cyclophosphamide). The hydroxybupropion metabolite of bupropion does not appear to be metabolized by the cytochrome P450 isoenzymes. No systemic data have been collected on the metabolism of Zyban® following concomitant administration with other drugs, or alternatively, the effect of concomitant administration of Zyban® on the metabolism of other drugs.

Animal data, however, indicated that bupropion may be an inducer of drug-metabolizing enzymes in humans. However, following chronic administration of bupropion, 100 mg 3 times/day, to 8 healthy male volunteers for 14 days, there was no evidence of induction of its own metabolism. Because bupropion is extensively metabolized, coadministration of other drugs may affect its clinical activity. Certain drugs may induce the metabolism of bupropion (eg, carbamazepine, phenobarbital, phenytoin), while other drugs may inhibit its metabolism (eg, cimetidine). Studies in animals demonstrated that the acute toxicity of bupropion is enhanced by the MAO inhibitor, phenelzine.

Limited clinical data suggest a higher incidence of adverse experiences in patients receiving concurrent administration of bupropion and levodopa. Administration of Zyban® to patients receiving levodopa concurrently should be undertaken with caution, using small initial doses and gradual dosage increases. Concurrent administration of Zyban® and agents that lower the seizure threshold should be undertaken only with extreme caution. Physiological changes resulting from smoking cessation itself, with or without treatment with Zyban®, may alter the pharmacokinetics of some concomitant medications, which may require dosage adjustment.

PHARMACOLOGY OF DRUG METABOLISM AND INTERACTIONS (Continued)

INTERACTIONS BETWEEN CIGARETTE SMOKE AND DRUGS

Drug	Mechanism	Effect on Cigarette Smokers
Theophylline	Induction of the CYP1A2 isoenzyme	May lead to reduced theophylline serum concentrations and decreased clinical effect; elimination of theophylline is considerably more rapid
Tacrine	Induction of the CYP1A2 isoenzyme	Effectiveness of tacrine may be decreased
Insulin	Decreased insulin absorption; may be related to peripheral vasoconstriction	Insulin-dependent diabetics who smoke heavily may require a 15% to 30% higher dose of insulin than nonsmokers
Flecainide	Unknown	May reduce flecainide serum concentrations
Propoxyphene	Unknown	May require higher dosage of propoxyphene to achieve analgesic effects
Propranolol	Increased release of catacholamines (eg, epinephrine) in smokers	May have increased blood pressure and heart rate relative to nonsmokers; consider effects on prevention of angina pectoris and stroke
Diazepam	Unclear as to whether pharmacokinetics are altered or end-organ responsiveness is decreased	May require larger doses of diazepam and chlordiazepoxide to achieve sedative effects

Adapted from Schein, JR, "Cigarette Smoking and Clinically Significant Drug Interactions," *Ann Pharmacother*, 1995, 29(11):1139-47.

SUMMARY

Once a drug has been metabolized in the liver, it is eliminated through several different mechanisms. One is directly through bile, into the intestine, and eventually excreted in feces. More commonly, the metabolites and the original drug pass back into the liver from the general circulation and are carried to other organs and tissues. Eventually, these metabolites are excreted through the kidney. In the kidney, the drug and its metabolites may be filtered by the glomerulus or secreted by the renal tubules into the urine. From the kidney, some of the drug may be reabsorbed and pass back into the blood. The drug may also be carried to the lung. If the drug or its metabolite is volatile, it can pass from the blood into the alveolar air and be eliminated in the breath. To a minor extent, drugs and metabolites can be excreted by sweat and saliva. In nursing mothers, drugs are also excreted in mother's milk.

The clinical considerations of drug metabolism may affect which other drugs can and should be administered. Drug tolerance may be a consideration, in that larger doses of a drug may be necessary to obtain effect in patients in which the metabolism is extremely rapid. These interactions, via cytochrome P450 or its isoforms, can occasionally be used beneficially to increase/maintain blood levels of one drug by administering a second drug. Dental clinicians should attempt to stay current on this topic of drug interactions as knowledge evolves.

HOW TO USE THE TABLES

The following CYP SUBSTRATES, INHIBITORS, and INDUCERS tables provide a clinically relevant perspective on drugs that are affected by, or affect, cytochrome P450 (CYP) enzymes. Not all human, drug-metabolizing CYP enzymes are specifically (or separately) included in the tables. Some enzymes have been excluded because they do not appear to significantly contribute to the metabolism of marketed drugs (eg, CYP2C18). Others have been combined in recognition of the difficulty in distinguishing their metabolic activity one from another, or the clinical practicality of doing so (eg, CYP2C8/9, CYP3A4). In the case of CYP3A4, the industry routinely uses this single enzyme designation to represent all enzymes in the CYP3A subfamily. CYP3A7 is present in fetal livers. It is effectively absent from adult livers. CYP3A4 (adult) and CYP3A7 (fetal) appear to share similar properties in their respective hosts. The impact of CYP3A7 in fetal and neonatal drug interactions has not been investigated.

The **CYP Substrates table** contains a list of drugs reported to be metabolized, at least in part, by one or more CYP enzymes. An enzyme that appears to play a clinically significant (major) role in a drug's metabolism is indicated by "●", and an enzyme whose role appears to be clinically insignificant (minor) is indicated by "○". A clinically significant designation is the result of a two-phase review. The first phase considered the contribution of each CYP enzyme to the overall metabolism of the drug. The enzyme pathway was considered potentially clinically relevant if it was responsible for at least 30% of the metabolism of the drug. If so, the drug was subjected to a second phase. The second phase considered the clinical relevance of a substrate's concentration being increased twofold, or decreased by one-half (such as might be observed if combined with an effective CYP inhibitor or inducer, respectively). If either of these changes was considered to present a clinically significant concern, the CYP pathway for the drug was designated "major." If neither change would appear to present a clinically significant concern, or if the CYP enzyme was responsible for a smaller portion of the overall metabolism (ie, <30%), the pathway was designated "minor."

The **CYP Inhibitors table** contains a list of drugs that are reported to inhibit one or more CYP enzymes. Enzymes that are strongly inhibited by a drug are indicated by "●". Enzymes that are moderately inhibited are indicated by "◑". Enzymes that are weakly inhibited are indicated by "○". The designations are the result of a review of published clinical reports, available Ki data, and assessments published by other experts in the field. As it pertains to Ki values set in a ratio with achievable serum drug concentrations ([I]) under normal dosing conditions, the following parameters were employed: [I]/Ki ≥1 = strong; [I]/Ki 0.1-1 = moderate; [I]/Ki <0.1 = weak.

The **CYP Inducers table** contains a list of drugs that are reported to induce one or more CYP enzymes. Enzymes that appear to be effectively induced by a drug are indicated by "●", and enzymes that do not appear to be effectively induced are indicated by "○". The designations are the result of a review of published clinical reports and assessments published by experts in the field.

In general, clinically significant interactions are more likely to occur between substrates and either inhibitors or inducers of the same enzyme(s), all of which have been indicated by "●". However, these assessments possess a degree of subjectivity, at times based on limited indications regarding the significance of CYP effects of particular agents. An attempt has been made to balance a conservative, clinically-sensitive presentation of the data with a desire to avoid the numbing effect of a "beware of everything" approach. Even so, other potential interactions (ie, those involving enzymes indicated by "○") may warrant consideration in some cases. It is important to note that information related to CYP metabolism of drugs is expanding at a rapid pace, and thus, the contents of this table should only be considered to represent a "snapshot" of the information available at the time of publication.

Selected Readings

Bjornsson TD, Callaghan JT, Einolf HJ, et al, "The Conduct of *in vitro* and *in vivo* Drug-Drug Interaction Studies: A PhRMA Perspective," *J Clin Pharmacol*, 2003, 43(5):443-69.

Drug-Drug Interactions, Rodrigues AD, ed, New York, NY: Marcel Dekker, Inc, 2002.

Hersh EV and Moore PA, "Drug Interactions in Dentistry: The Importance of Knowing Your CYP's," *J Am Dent Assoc*, 2004, 135(3):298-311.

Levy RH, Thummel KE, Trager WF, et al, eds, *Metabolic Drug Interactions*, Philadelphia, PA: Lippincott Williams & Wilkins, 2000.

Michalets EL, "Update: Clinically Significant Cytochrome P-450 Drug Interactions," *Pharmacotherapy*, 1998, 18(1):84-112.

Thummel KE and Wilkinson GR, "*In vitro* and *in vivo* Drug Interactions Involving Human CYP3A," *Annu Rev Pharmacol Toxicol*, 1998, 38:389-430.

Wynn RL and Meiller TF, "CYP Enzymes and Adverse Drug Reactions," *Gen Dent*, 1998, 46(5):436-8.

Zhang Y and Benet LZ, "The Gut as a Barrier to Drug Absorption: Combined Role of Cytochrome P450 3A and P-Glycoprotein," *Clin Pharmacokinet*, 2001, 40(3):159-68.

Selected Websites

http://www.gentest.com

http://www.imm.ki.se/CYPalleles

http://medicine.iupui.edu/flockhart

http://www.mhc.com/Cytochromes

PHARMACOLOGY OF DRUG METABOLISM AND INTERACTIONS (Continued)

CYP Substrates

● = major substrate
○ = minor substrate

Drug	1A2	2A6	2B6	2C8	2C9	2C19	2D6	2E1	3A4
Acetaminophen	○	○			○		○	○	○
Albendazole	○								○
Albuterol									●
Alfentanil									●
Almotriptan							○		○
Alosetron	○				●				○
Alprazolam									●
Aminophylline	●							○	○
Amiodarone	○			●		○	○		●
Amitriptyline	○		○		○	○	●		○
Amlodipine									●
Amoxapine							●		
Amphetamine							○		
Amprenavir					○				●
Aprepitant	○					○			●
Argatroban									○
Aripiprazole							●		●
Aspirin					○				
Atazanavir									●
Atomoxetine						○	●		
Atorvastatin									●
Azelastine	○					○	○		○
Azithromycin									○
Benzphetamine			○						●
Benztropine							○		
Betaxolol	●						●		
Bexarotene									○
Bezafibrate									○
Bisoprolol							○		●
Bortezomib	○				○	○	○		●
Bosentan					●				●
Brinzolamide									○
Bromazepam									●
Bromocriptine									●
Budesonide									●
Bupivacaine	○					○	○		○
Buprenorphine									●
BuPROPion	○	○	●			○		○	○
BusPIRone							○		●
Busulfan									●
Caffeine	●				○		○	○	○
Candesartan					○				
Capsaicin								○	
Captopril							●		
Carbamazepine				○					●
Carisoprodol						●			
Carteolol							○		
Carvedilol	○				●		●	○	○
Celecoxib					●				○
Cerivastatin									●
Cetirizine									○
Cevimeline							○		○
Chlordiazepoxide									●
Chloroquine							●		●
Chlorpheniramine							○		●
ChlorproMAZINE	○						●		○
ChlorproPAMIDE					○				
Chlorzoxazone	○	○					○	●	○
Cilostazol	○					●	○		●
Cinacalcet	○						○		○
Cisapride	○	○	○		○	○			●
Citalopram						●	○		●
Clarithromycin									●
Clobazam						●			●

CYP Substrates (continued)

Drug	1A2	2A6	2B6	2C8	2C9	2C19	2D6	2E1	3A4
Clofibrate									○
ClomiPRAMINE	●					●	●		○
Clonazepam									○
Clopidogrel	○								●
Clorazepate									○
Clozapine	●	○			○	○	○		○
Cocaine									●
Codeine[1]							●		○
Colchicine									●
Conivaptan									●
Cyclobenzaprine	●						○		○
Cyclophosphamide[2]		○	●		○	○			●
CycloSPORINE									●
Dacarbazine	●							●	
Dantrolene									●
Dapsone				○	●	○		○	●
Delavirdine							○		●
Desipramine	○						●		
Desogestrel						●			
Dexamethasone									○
Dexmedetomidine		●							
Dextroamphetamine							●		
Dextromethorphan		○			○	○	●	○	○
Diazepam	○		○		○	●			●
Diclofenac	○		○	○	○	○	○		○
Digitoxin									●
Digoxin									○
Dihydrocodeine[1]							●		
Dihydroergotamine									●
Diltiazem					○				●
Dirithromycin									○
Disopyramide									●
Disulfiram	○	○	○				○	○	○
Docetaxel									●
Dofetilide									○
Dolasetron						○			○
Domperidone									○
Donepezil							○		○
Dorzolamide					○				○
Doxepin	●						●		●
DOXOrubicin							●		●
Doxycycline									●
Drospirenone									○
Duloxetine	●						●		
Dutasteride									○
Efavirenz			●						○
Eletriptan									●
Enalapril									●
Enflurane								●	
Eplerenone									●
Ergoloid mesylates									●
Ergonovine									●
Ergotamine									●
Erythromycin			○						●
Escitalopram							●		●
Esomeprazole						●			○
Estazolam									○
Estradiol	●	○	○		○	○	○	○	●
Estrogens, conjugated A/synthetic	●	○	○		○	○	○	○	●
Estrogens, conjugated equine	●	○	○		○	○	○	○	●
Estrogens, conjugated esterified	●		○		○			○	●
Estrone	●		○		○			○	●
Estropipate	●		○		○			○	●
Ethinyl estradiol					○				●
Ethosuximide									●
Etonogestrel									○
Etoposide	○								●
Exemestane								○	●
Felbamate								○	●

PHARMACOLOGY OF DRUG METABOLISM AND INTERACTIONS (Continued)

CYP Substrates (continued)

Drug	1A2	2A6	2B6	2C8	2C9	2C19	2D6	2E1	3A4
Felodipine									●
Fenofibrate									○
Fentanyl									●
Fexofenadine									○
Finasteride									○
Flecainide	○						●		
Fluoxetine	○		○		●	○	●	○	○
Fluphenazine							●		
Flurazepam									●
Flurbiprofen					○				
Flutamide	●								●
Fluticasone									●
Fluvastatin					○		○		○
Fluvoxamine	●						●		
Formoterol		○			○	○	○		
Fosamprenavir (as amprenavir)					○				●
Fosphenytoin (as phenytoin)					●	●			○
Frovatriptan	○								
Fulvestrant									○
Galantamine							○		○
Gefitinib									●
Gemfibrozil									○
Glimepiride					●				
GlipiZIDE					●				
Granisetron									○
Guanabenz	●								
Halazepam									○
Halofantrine					○		○		●
Haloperidol	○						●		●
Halothane		○	○		○		○	●	○
Hydrocodone[1]							●		
Hydrocortisone									○
Ibuprofen					○	○			
Ifosfamide[3]		○	○	○	○	○			●
Imatinib	○				○	○	○		●
Imipramine	○		○			●	●		○
Imiquimod	○								○
Indinavir							○		●
Indomethacin					○	○			
Irbesartan					○				
Irinotecan			●						●
Isoflurane								●	
Isoniazid								●	
Isosorbide									●
Isosorbide dinitrate									●
Isosorbide mononitrate									●
Isradipine									●
Itraconazole									●
Ivermectin									○
Ketamine			●		●				●
Ketoconazole									●
Labetalol							●		
Lansoprazole					○	●			●
Letrozole		○							●
Levobupivacaine	○								○
Levonorgestrel									●
Lidocaine	○	○			○		●		●
Lomustine							●		
Lopinavir									○
Loratadine							○		○
Losartan					●				●
Lovastatin									●
Maprotiline							●		
MedroxyPROGESTERone									●
Mefenamic acid					○				
Mefloquine									●

CYP Substrates *(continued)*

Drug	1A2	2A6	2B6	2C8	2C9	2C19	2D6	2E1	3A4
Meloxicam					○				○
Mephobarbital			○		○	●			
Mestranol⁴					●				●
Methadone					○	○	○		●
Methamphetamine							●		
Methoxsalen		○							
Methsuximide						●			
Methylergonovine									●
Methylphenidate							●		
MethylPREDNISolone									○
Metoclopramide	○						○		
Metoprolol						○	●		
Mexiletine	●						●		
Miconazole									●
Midazolam			○						●
Mifepristone									○
Miglustat									●
Mirtazapine	●				○		●		●
Moclobemide						●	●		
Modafinil									●
Mometasone furoate									○
Montelukast					●				●
Moricizine									●
Morphine sulfate							○		
Naproxen	○				○				
Nateglinide					●				
Nefazodone							●		●
Nelfinavir					○	●	○		●
Nevirapine			○				○		●
NiCARdipine	○				○		○	○	●
Nicotine	○	○	○		○	○	○	○	○
NIFEdipine							○		●
Nilutamide						●			
Nimodipine									●
Nisoldipine									●
Nitrendipine									●
Norelgestromin									○
Norethindrone									●
Norgestrel									●
Nortriptyline	○					○	●		○
Olanzapine	○						○		
Omeprazole		○			○	●	○		○
Ondansetron	○				○		○	○	●
Orphenadrine	○		○				○		○
Oxybutynin									○
Oxycodone¹							●		
Paclitaxel				●	●				●
Palonosetron	○						○		○
Pantoprazole						●			○
Paroxetine							●		
Pentamidine						●			
Pergolide									●
Perphenazine	○				○	○	●		○
Phencyclidine									●
Phenobarbital					○	●		○	
Phenytoin					●	●			○
Pimecrolimus									○
Pimozide	●								●
Pindolol							●		
Pioglitazone				●					●
Pipotiazine							●		●
Piroxicam					○				
Pravastatin									○
Prazepam									○
PrednisoLONE									○
PredniSONE									○
Primaquine									●
Procainamide							●		
Progesterone	○	○			○		●	○	●
Proguanil	○					○			○

PHARMACOLOGY OF DRUG METABOLISM AND INTERACTIONS (Continued)

CYP Substrates (continued)

Drug	1A2	2A6	2B6	2C8	2C9	2C19	2D6	2E1	3A4
Promethazine			●				●		
Propafenone	○						●		○
Propofol	○	○	●		●	○	○	○	○
Propranolol	●					○	●		○
Protriptyline							●		
Quazepam									○
Quetiapine							○		●
Quinidine					○			○	●
Quinine	○					○			●
Rabeprazole						●			●
Ranitidine	○					○	○		
Ranolazine							○		●
Repaglinide				●					●
Rifabutin									●
Riluzole	●								
Risperidone							●		○
Ritonavir	○		○				○		●
Rofecoxib					○				
Ropinirole	●								○
Ropivacaine	○		○				○		○
Rosiglitazone				●	○				
Rosuvastatin					○				○
Salmeterol									●
Saquinavir							○		●
Selegiline	○	○	●		●		○		○
Sertraline			○		○	●	●		○
Sevoflurane		○	○					●	○
Sibutramine									●
Sildenafil					○				●
Simvastatin									●
Sirolimus									●
Sorafenib									○
Spiramycin									●
Sufentanil									●
SulfaDIAZINE					●			○	○
Sulfamethoxazole					●				○
Sulfinpyrazone					●				○
SulfiSOXAZOLE					●				
Sunitinib									●
Tacrine	●								
Tacrolimus									●
Tamoxifen		○	○		●		●	○	●
Tamsulosin							●		●
Telithromycin	○								●
Temazepam			○		○	○			○
Teniposide									●
Terbinafine	○				○	○			○
Testosterone			○		○	○			○
Tetracycline									●
Theophylline	●				○		○	●	●
Thiabendazole	○								
Thioridazine						○	●		
Thiothixene	●								
Tiagabine									●
Ticlopidine									●
Timolol							●		
Tinidazole									○
Tiotropium							○		○
TOLBUTamide					●	○			
Tolcapone		○							○
Tolterodine					○	○	●		●
Toremifene	○								●
Torsemide				○	●				
Tramadol[1]			○				●		○
Trazodone							○		●
Tretinoin		○	○	●	○				
Triazolam									●

CYP Substrates *(continued)*

Drug	1A2	2A6	2B6	2C8	2C9	2C19	2D6	2E1	3A4
Trifluoperazine	●								
Trimethadione					○	○		●	○
Trimethoprim					●				●
Trimipramine						●	●		●
Troleandomycin									●
Valdecoxib					○				○
Valproic acid		○	○		○	○		○	
Vardenafil									●
Venlafaxine					○	○	●		●
Verapamil	○			○	○		○		●
VinBLAStine									●
VinCRIStine									●
Vinorelbine							○		●
Voriconazole					●	●			○
Warfarin	○				●	○			○
Yohimbine							○		
Zafirlukast					●				
Zaleplon									○
Zidovudine		○			○	○			○
Zileuton	○				○				○
Ziprasidone	○								○
Zolmitriptan	○								
Zolpidem	○				○	○	○		●
Zonisamide							○		●
Zopiclone					●				●
Zuclopenthixol							●		

[1]This opioid analgesic is bioactivated *in vivo* via CYP2D6. Inhibiting this enzyme would decrease the effects of the analgesic. The active metabolite might also affect, or be affected by, CYP enzymes.
[2]Cyclophosphamide is bioactivated *in vivo* to acrolein via CYP2B6 and 3A4. Inhibiting these enzymes would decrease the effects of cyclophosphamide.
[3]Ifosfamide is bioactivated *in vivo* to acrolein via CYP3A4. Inhibiting this enzyme would decrease the effects of ifosfamide.
[4]Mestranol is bioactivated *in vivo* to ethinyl estradiol via CYP2C8/9. See Ethinyl Estradiol for additional CYP information.

PHARMACOLOGY OF DRUG METABOLISM AND INTERACTIONS (Continued)

CYP Inhibitors

● = strong inhibitor
◐ = moderate inhibitor
○ = weak inhibitor

Drug	1A2	2A6	2B6	2C8	2C9	2C19	2D6	2E1	3A4
Acebutolol							○		
Acetaminophen									○
AcetaZOLAMIDE									○
Albendazole	○								
Alosetron	○							○	
Amiodarone	●	◐	○		◐	○	◐		◐
Amitriptyline	○				○	○	○	○	
Amlodipine	◐	○	○	○	○		○		○
Amphetamine							○		
Amprenavir						○			●
Anastrozole	○			○	○				○
Aprepitant					○	○			◐
Atazanavir	○			●	○				●
Atorvastatin									○
Azelastine			○		○	○	○		○
Azithromycin									○
Bepridil							○		
Betamethasone									○
Betaxolol							○		
Biperiden							○		
Bortezomib	○				○	◐	○		○
Bromazepam								○	
Bromocriptine	○								○
Buprenorphine	○	○				○	○		
BuPROPion							○		
Caffeine	●								◐
Candesartan				○	○				
Celecoxib			◐				○		
Cerivastatin									○
Chloramphenicol					○				○
Chloroquine							◐		
Chlorpheniramine							○		
ChlorproMAZINE							●	○	
Chlorzoxazone							○	○	
Cholecalciferol					○	○	○		
Cimetidine	◐				○	◐	◐	○	◐
Cinacalcet							○		
Ciprofloxacin	●								○
Cisapride							○		○
Citalopram	○		○			○	○		
Clarithromycin	○								●
Clemastine							○		○
Clofazimine									○
Clofibrate		○							
ClomiPRAMINE							◐		
Clopidogrel					○				
Clotrimazole	○	○	○	○	○	○	○	○	◐
Clozapine	○				○	○	◐	○	○
Cocaine							●		○
Codeine							○		
Conivaptan									●
Cyclophosphamide									○
CycloSPORINE					○				◐
Danazol									○
Delavirdine	○				●	●	●		●
Desipramine		◐	◐				◐	○	◐
Dexmedetomidine	○				○		●		○
Dextromethorphan							○		
Diazepam						○			○
Diclofenac	◐				○			○	●
Dihydroergotamine									○
Diltiazem					○		○		◐

CYP Inhibitors *(continued)*

Drug	1A2	2A6	2B6	2C8	2C9	2C19	2D6	2E1	3A4
Dimethyl sulfoxide					○	○			
DiphenhydrAMINE							◐		
Disulfiram	○	○	○		○		○	●	○
Docetaxel									○
Dolasetron							○		
DOXOrubicin			◐				○		○
Doxycycline									◐
Drospirenone	○				○	○			○
Duloxetine							◐		
Econazole								○	
Efavirenz					○	○			○
Enoxacin	●								●
Entacapone	○	○			○	○	○	○	○
Eprosartan					○				
Ergotamine									○
Erythromycin	○								◐
Escitalopram							○		
Estradiol	○			○					
Estrogens, conjugated A/synthetic	○								
Estrogens, conjugated equine	○								
Ethinyl estradiol	○		○	○		○			○
Ethotoin						○			
Etoposide					○				○
Felbamate						○			
Felodipine				◐	○		○		○
Fenofibrate		○		◐	◐	○			
Fentanyl									○
Fexofenadine							○		
Flecainide							○		
Fluconazole	○				●	●			◐
Fluoxetine	◐		○		○	◐	●		○
Fluphenazine	○				○		○	○	
Flurazepam								○	
Flurbiprofen					●				
Flutamide	○								
Fluvastatin	○			○	◐		○		○
Fluvoxamine	●		○		○	●	○		○
Fosamprenavir (as amprenavir)						○			●
Gefitinib						○	○		
Gemfibrozil	◐			●	●	●			
Glyburide				○					○
Grapefruit juice									◐
Halofantrine							○		
Haloperidol							◐		◐
HydrALAZINE									○
HydrOXYzine							○		
Ibuprofen					●				
Ifosfamide									○
Imatinib					○		○		●
Imipramine	○					○	◐	○	
Indinavir					○	○			●
Indomethacin					●	○			
Interferon alfa-2a	○								
Interferon alfa-2b	○								
Interferon gamma-1b	○							○	
Irbesartan				◐	◐		○		○
Isoflurane			○						
Isoniazid	○	◐			○	●	◐	◐	●
Isradipine									○
Itraconazole									●
Ketoconazole	●	◐	○	●	●	◐	◐		●
Ketoprofen					○				
Labetalol							○		
Lansoprazole					○	◐	○		○
Leflunomide					○				
Letrozole		●				○			
Lidocaine	●						◐		◐
Lomefloxacin	○								
Lomustine							○		○

PHARMACOLOGY OF DRUG METABOLISM AND INTERACTIONS *(Continued)*

CYP Inhibitors *(continued)*

Drug	1A2	2A6	2B6	2C8	2C9	2C19	2D6	2E1	3A4
Loratadine				O		◐	O		
Losartan	O			◐	◐	O			O
Lovastatin					O		O		O
Mefenamic acid					●				
Mefloquine							O		O
Meloxicam					O				
Mephobarbital									
Mestranol	O		O			O			O
Methadone							◐		O
Methimazole	O	O	O		O	O	◐	O	O
Methotrimeprazine							O		
Methoxsalen	●	●			O	O	O	O	O
Methsuximide						O			
Methylphenidate							O		
MethylPREDNISolone				O					O
Metoclopramide							O		
Metoprolol							O		
Metronidazole					O				◐
Metyrapone		O							
Mexiletine	●								
Miconazole	◐	●	O		●	●	●	◐	●
Midazolam				◐	O				O
Mifepristone							O		O
Mirtazapine	O								O
Mitoxantrone									O
Moclobemide	O					O	O		
Modafinil	O	O			O	●		O	O
Montelukast				●	O				
Nalidixic acid	O								
Nateglinide					O				
Nefazodone	O		O	O			O		●
Nelfinavir	O		O		O	O	O		●
Nevirapine	O						O		O
NiCARdipine					●	◐	◐		●
Nicotine		O						O	
NIFEdipine	◐				O		O		O
Nilutamide						O			
Nisoldipine	O								O
Nitrendipine									O
Nizatidine									O
Norfloxacin	●								◐
Nortriptyline							O	O	
Ofloxacin	●								
Olanzapine	O				O	O	O		O
Omeprazole	O				◐	●	O		O
Ondansetron	O				O		O		
Orphenadrine	O	O	O		O	O	O	O	O
Oxcarbazepine						O			
Oxprenolol							O		
Oxybutynin				O			O		O
Pantoprazole						◐			
Paroxetine	O		◐		O	O	●		O
Peginterferon alfa-2a	O								
Peginterferon alfa-2b	O								
Pentamidine					O	O	O		O
Pentoxifylline	O								
Pergolide							●		O
Perphenazine	O						O		
Phencyclidine									O
Pilocarpine		O						O	O
Pimozide						O	O	O	O
Pindolol							O		
Pioglitazone			◐	O	O	O	◐		
Piroxicam					●				
Pravastatin					O		O		O
Praziquantel							O		
PrednisoLONE									O

CYP Inhibitors (continued)

Drug	1A2	2A6	2B6	2C8	2C9	2C19	2D6	2E1	3A4
Primaquine	●						○		○
Probenecid						○			
Progesterone					○	○			○
Promethazine							○		
Propafenone	○						○		
Propofol	◑				○	◑	○	○	●
Propoxyphene					○		○		○
Propranolol	○						○		
Pyrimethamine					◑		◑		
Quinidine					○		●		●
Quinine				◑	◑		●		○
Quinupristin									○
Rabeprazole				◑		◑	○		○
Ranitidine	○						○		
Ranolazine							○		○
Risperidone							○		○
Ritonavir				●	○	○	●	○	●
Rofecoxib	○						●		
Ropinirole	○						●		
Rosiglitazone				◑	○	○	○		
Saquinavir					○	○	○		◑
Selegiline	○	○			○	○	○	○	○
Sertraline	○		◑	○	○	◑	◑	○	◑
Sildenafil	○				○	○	○	○	○
Simvastatin				○	○		○		
Sirolimus									○
Sorafenib			○	○					
Sulconazole	○	○			○	○	○	○	○
SulfaDIAZINE					●				
Sulfamethoxazole					◑				
Sulfinpyrazone					◑				
SulfiSOXAZOLE					●				
Tacrine	○								○
Tacrolimus									○
Tamoxifen			○	◑	○				●
Telithromycin							○		●
Telmisartan						○			
Teniposide					○				○
Tenofovir	○								
Terbinafine							●		
Testosterone									○
Tetracycline									◑
Theophylline	○								
Thiabendazole	●								
Thioridazine	○				○		◑	○	
Thiotepa			○				○		
Thiothixene							○		
Ticlopidine	○				○	●	◑	○	○
Timolol							○		
Tioconazole	○	○			○	○	○	○	
Tocainide	○								
TOLBUTamide				○	●				
Tolcapone					○				
Topiramate						○			
Torsemide						○			
Tranylcypromine	◑	●			○	○	◑	◑	○
Trazodone							◑		○
Tretinoin					○				
Triazolam				○	○				
Trimethoprim					◑	◑			
Tripelennamine							◑		
Triprolidine							○		
Troleandomycin									◑
Valdecoxib				○	○	○			
Valproic acid					○	○	○		○
Valsartan					○				
Venlafaxine			○				○		○
Verapamil		○			○		○		◑
VinBLAStine							○		○
VinCRIStine									○

PHARMACOLOGY OF DRUG METABOLISM AND INTERACTIONS (Continued)

CYP Inhibitors (continued)

Drug	1A2	2A6	2B6	2C8	2C9	2C19	2D6	2E1	3A4
Vinorelbine							○		○
Voriconazole					○	○			◑
Warfarin					◑	○			
Yohimbine							○		
Zafirlukast	○			◑	◑	○	○		○
Zileuton	◑								
Ziprasidone							○		○

CYP Inducers

● = effectively induced
○ = not effectively induced

Drug	1A2	2A6	2B6	2C8	2C9	2C19	2D6	2E1	3A4
Aminoglutethimide	●					●			●
Amobarbital		●							
Aprepritant					○				○
Bexarotene									○
Bosentan					○				○
Calcitriol									○
Carbamazepine	●		●	●	●	●			●
Clofibrate			○						
Colchicine				○	○			○	○
Cyclophosphamide			○	○	○				
Dexamethasone		○	○	○	○				○
Dicloxacillin									○
Efavirenz (in liver only)			○						○
Estradiol									○
Estrogens, conjugated A/synthetic									○
Estrogens, conjugated equine									○
Exemestane									○
Felbamate									○
Fosphenytoin (as phenytoin)			●	●	●	●			●
Griseofulvin	○			○	○				○
Hydrocortisone									○
Ifosfamide				○	○				
Insulin preparations	○								
Isoniazid (after D/C)								○	
Lansoprazole	○								
MedroxyPROGESTERone									○
Mephobarbital		○							
Metyrapone									○
Modafinil	○		○						○
Moricizine	○								●
Nafcillin									●
Nevirapine			●						●
Norethindrone						○			
Omeprazole	○								
Oxcarbazepine									●
Paclitaxel									○
Pantoprazole	○								●
Pentobarbital			●						●
Phenobarbital	●	●	●	●	●				●
Phenytoin			●	●	●	●			●
Pioglitazone									○
PredniSONE						○			○
Primaquine	○								
Primidone[1]	●		●	●	●				●
Rifabutin									●
Rifampin	●	●	●	●	●	●			●
Rifapentine				●	●				●
Ritonavir (long-term)	○			○	○				○
Rofecoxib									○
Secobarbital		●			●	●			
Sulfinpyrazone									○
Terbinafine									○
Topiramate									○
Tretinoin								○	
Troglitazone									○
Valproic acid		○							

[1]Primidone is partially metabolized to phenobarbital. See Phenobarbital for additional CYP information.

OCCUPATIONAL EXPOSURE TO BLOODBORNE PATHOGENS (STANDARD / UNIVERSAL PRECAUTIONS)

OVERVIEW AND REGULATORY CONSIDERATIONS

Every healthcare employee, from nurse to housekeeper, has some (albeit small) risk of exposure to HIV and other viral agents such as hepatitis B and Jakob-Creutzfeldt agent. The incidence of HIV-1 transmission associated with a percutaneous exposure to blood from an HIV-1 infected patient is approximately 0.3% per exposure.[1] In 1989, it was estimated that 12,000 United States healthcare workers acquired hepatitis B annually.[2] An understanding of the appropriate procedures, responsibilities, and risks inherent in the collection and handling of patient specimens is necessary for safe practice and is required by Occupational Safety and Health Administration (OSHA) regulations.

The Occupational Safety and Health Administration published its "Final Rule on Occupational Exposure to Bloodborne Pathogens" in the Federal Register on December 6, 1991. OSHA has chosen to follow the Center for Disease Control (CDC) definition of universal precautions. The Final Rule provides full legal force to universal precautions and requires employers and employees to treat blood and certain body fluids as if they were infectious. The Final Rule mandates that healthcare workers must avoid parenteral contact and must avoid splattering blood or other potentially infectious material on their skin, hair, eyes, mouth, mucous membranes, or on their personal clothing. Hazard abatement strategies must be used to protect the workers. Such plans typically include, but are not limited to, the following:

- safe handling of sharp items ("sharps") and disposal of such into puncture resistant containers
- gloves required for employees handling items soiled with blood or equipment contaminated by blood or other body fluids
- provisions of protective clothing when more extensive contact with blood or body fluids may be anticipated (eg, surgery, autopsy, or deliveries)
- resuscitation equipment to reduce necessity for mouth to mouth resuscitation
- restriction of HIV- or hepatitis B-exposed employees to noninvasive procedures

OSHA has specifically defined the following terms: **Occupational exposure** means reasonably anticipated skin, eye mucous membrane, or parenteral contact with blood or other potentially infectious materials that may result from the performance of an employee's duties. **Other potentially infectious materials** are human body fluids including semen, vaginal secretions, cerebrospinal fluid, synovial fluid, pleural fluid, pericardial fluid, peritoneal fluid, amniotic fluid, saliva in dental procedures, and body fluids that are visibly contaminated with blood, and all body fluids in situations where it is difficult or impossible to differentiate between body fluids; any unfixed tissue or organ (other than intact skin) from a human (living or dead); and HIV-containing cell or tissue cultures, organ cultures, and HIV- or HBV-containing culture medium or other solutions, and blood, organs, or other tissues from experimental animals infected with HIV or HBV. An **exposure incident** involves specific eye, mouth, other mucous membrane, nonintact skin, or parenteral contact with blood or other potentially infectious materials that results from the performance of an employee's duties.[3] It is important to understand that some exposures may go unrecognized despite the strictest precautions.

A written Exposure Control Plan is required. Employers must provide copies of the plan to employees and to OSHA upon request. Compliance with OSHA rules may be accomplished by the following methods.

- **Universal precautions (UPs)** means that all human blood and certain body fluids are treated as if known to be infectious for HIV, HBV, and other bloodborne pathogens. UPs do not apply to feces, nasal secretions, saliva, sputum, sweat, tears, urine, or vomitus unless they contain visible blood.
- **Engineering controls (ECs)** are physical devices which reduce or remove hazards from the workplace by eliminating or minimizing hazards or by isolating the worker from exposure. Engineering control devices include sharps disposal containers, self-resheathing syringes, etc.
- **Work practice controls (WPCs)** are practices and procedures that reduce the likelihood of exposure to hazards by altering the way in which a task is performed. Specific examples are the prohibition of two-handed recapping of needles, prohibition of storing food alongside potentially contaminated material, discouragement of pipetting fluids by mouth, encouraging handwashing after removal of gloves, safe handling of contaminated sharps, and appropriate use of sharps containers.
- **Personal protective equipment (PPE)** is specialized clothing or equipment worn to provide protection from occupational exposure. PPE includes gloves, gowns, laboratory coats (the type and characteristics will depend upon the task and degree of exposure anticipated), face shields or masks, and eye protection. Surgical caps or hoods and/or shoe covers or boots are required in instances in which gross contamination can reasonably be anticipated (eg, autopsies, orthopedic surgery). If PPE is penetrated by blood or any contaminated material, the item must be removed immediately or as soon as feasible. **The employer must provide and launder or dispose of all PPE at no cost to the employee.** Gloves must be worn when there is a reasonable anticipation of hand contact with potentially infectious material, including a patient's mucous membranes or nonintact skin. Disposable

gloves must be changed as soon as possible after they become torn or punctured. Hands must be washed after gloves are removed. OSHA has revised the PPE standards, effective July 5, 1994, to include the requirement that the employer certify in writing that it has conducted a hazard assessment of the workplace to determine whether hazards are present that will necessitate the use of PPE. Also, verification that the employee has received and understood the PPE training is required.[4]

Housekeeping protocols: OSHA requires that all bins, cans, and similar receptacles, intended for reuse which have a reasonable likelihood for becoming contaminated, be inspected and decontaminated immediately or as soon as feasible upon visible contamination and on a regularly scheduled basis. Broken glass that may be contaminated must not be picked up directly with the hands. Mechanical means (eg, brush, dust pan, tongs, or forceps) must be used. Broken glass must be placed in a proper sharps container.

Employers are responsible for teaching appropriate clean-up procedures for the work area and personal protective equipment. A 1:10 dilution of household bleach is a popular and effective disinfectant. It is prudent for employers to maintain signatures or initials of employees who have been properly educated. If one does not have written proof of education of universal precautions teaching, then by OSHA standards, such education never happened.

Pre-exposure and postexposure protocols: OSHA's Final Rule includes the provision that employees, who are exposed to contamination, be offered the hepatitis B vaccine at no cost to the employee. Employees may decline; however, a declination form must be signed. The employee must be offered free vaccine if he/she changes his/her mind. Vaccination to prevent the transmission of hepatitis B in the healthcare setting is widely regarded as sound practice.[5] In the event of exposure, a confidential medical evaluation and follow-up must be offered at no cost to the employee. Follow-up must include collection and testing of blood from the source individual for HBV and HIV if permitted by state law if a blood sample is available. If a postexposure specimen must be specially drawn, the individual's consent is usually required. Some states may not require consent for testing of patient blood after accidental exposure. One must refer to state and/or local guidelines for proper guidance.

The employee follow-up must also include appropriate postexposure prophylaxis, counseling, and evaluation of reported illnesses. The employee has the right to decline baseline blood collection and/or testing. If the employee gives consent for the collection but not the testing, the sample must be preserved for 90 days in the event that the employee changes his/her mind within that time. Confidentiality related to blood testing must be ensured. **The employer does not have the right to know the results** of the testing of either the source individual or the exposed employee.

MANAGEMENT OF HEALTHCARE WORKER EXPOSURES TO HBV, HCV, AND HIV

Adapted from Updated U.S. Public Health Service Guidelines for the Management of Occupational Exposures to HIV and Recommendations for Postexposure Prophylaxis, "Recommended HIV Postexposure Prophylaxis (PEP) for Percutaneous Injuries," *MMWR Recomm Rep*, 2005, 54(RR-9):3-17.

Likelihood of transmission of HIV-1 from occupational exposure is 0.2% per parenteral exposure (eg, needlestick) to blood from HIV infected patients. Factors that increase risk for occupational transmission include advanced stages of HIV in source patient, hollow bore needle puncture, a poor state of health or inexperience of healthcare worker (HCW). After first aid is initiated, the healthcare worker should report exposure to a supervisor and to the institution's occupational medical service for evaluation. All parenteral exposures should be treated equally until they can be evaluated by the occupational medicine service, who will then determine the actual risk of exposure. Counselling regarding risk of exposure, antiviral prophylaxis, plans for follow up, exposure prevention, sexual activity, and providing emotional support and response to concerns are necessary to support the exposed healthcare worker. Additional information should be provided to healthcare workers who are pregnant or planning to become pregnant.

Immediate actions include aggressive first aid at the puncture site (eg, scrubbing site with povidone-iodine solution or soap and water for 10 minutes) or at mucus membrane site (eg, saline irrigation of eye for 15 minutes), followed by immediate reporting to the hospital's occupational medical service where a thorough investigation should be performed, including identification of the source, type of exposure, volume of inoculum, timing of exposure, extent of injury, appropriateness of first aid, as well as psychological status of the healthcare worker. HIV serologies should be performed on the healthcare worker and HIV risk counselling should begin at this point. Although the data are not clear, antiviral prophylaxis may be offered to healthcare workers who are parenterally or mucous membrane exposed. If used, antiretroviral prophylaxis should be initiated within 1-2 hours after exposure.

OCCUPATIONAL EXPOSURE TO BLOODBORNE PATHOGENS (STANDARD / UNIVERSAL PRECAUTIONS) *(Continued)*

Factors to Consider in Assessing the Need for Follow-up of Occupational Exposures

- **Type of exposure**
    - Percutaneous injury
    - Mucous membrane exposure
    - Nonintact skin exposure
    - Bites resulting in blood exposure to either person involved
- **Type and amount of fluid/tissue**
    - Blood
    - Fluids containing blood
    - Potentially infectious fluid or tissue (semen; vaginal secretions; and cerebro-spinal, synovial, pleural, peritoneal, pericardial, and amniotic fluids)
    - Direct contact with concentrated virus
- **Infectious status of source**
    - Presence of HB_sAg
    - Presence of HCV antibody
    - Presence of HIV antibody
- **Susceptibility of exposed person**
    - Hepatitis B vaccine and vaccine response status
    - HBV, HCV, HIV immune status

Evaluation of Occupational Exposure Sources

Known sources

- Test known sources for HB_sAg, anti-HCV, and HIV antibody
    - Direct virus assays for routine screening of source patients are **not** recommended
    - Consider using a rapid HIV-antibody test
    - If the source person is **not** infected with a bloodborne pathogen, baseline testing or further follow-up of the exposed person is **not** necessary
- For sources whose infection status remains unknown (eg, the source person refuses testing), consider medical diagnoses, clinical symptoms, and history of risk behaviors
- Do not test discarded needles for bloodborne pathogens

Unknown sources

- For unknown sources, evaluate the likelihood of exposure to a source at high risk for infection
    - Consider the likelihood of bloodborne pathogen infection among patients in the exposure setting

Recommended Postexposure Prophylaxis for Exposure to Hepatitis B Virus

Vaccination and Antibody Response Status of Exposed Workers[1]	Treatment		
	Source HB$_s$Ag[2]-Positive	Source HB$_s$Ag[2]-Negative	Source Unknown or Not Available for Testing
Unvaccinated	HBIG[3] x 1 and initiate HB vaccine series[4]	Initiate HB vaccine series	Initiate HB vaccine series
Previously vaccinated			
Known responder[5]	No treatment	No treatment	No treatment
Known nonresponder[6]	HBIG x 1 and initiate revaccination or HBIG x 2[7]	No treatment	If known high risk source, treat as if source was HB$_s$Ag-positive
Antibody response unknown	Test exposed person for anti-HB$_s$[8] 1. If adequate,[5] no treatment is necessary 2. If inadequate,[6] administer HBIG x 1 and vaccine booster	No treatment	Test exposed person for anti-HB$_s$ 1. If adequate,[4] no treatment is necessary 2. If inadequate,[4] administer vaccine booster and recheck titer in 1-2 months

[1]Persons who have previously been infected with HBV are immune to reinfection and do not require postexposure prophylaxis.

[2]Hepatitis B surface antigen.

[3]Hepatitis B immune globulin; dose is 0.06 mL/kg intramuscularly.

[4]Hepatitis B vaccine.

[5]A responder is a person with adequate levels of serum antibody to HB$_s$Ag (ie, anti-HB$_s$ ≥10 mIU/mL).

[6]A nonresponder is a person with inadequate response to vaccination (ie, serum anti-HB$_s$ <10 mIU/mL).

[7]The option of giving one dose of HBIG and reinitiating the vaccine series is preferred for nonresponders who have not completed a second 3-dose vaccine series. For persons who previously completed a second vaccine series but failed to respond, two doses of HBIG are preferred.

[8]Antibody to HB$_s$Ag.

OCCUPATIONAL EXPOSURE TO BLOODBORNE PATHOGENS (STANDARD / UNIVERSAL PRECAUTIONS) (Continued)

Recommended HIV Postexposure Prophylaxis (PEP) for Percutaneous Injuries

Exposure Type	HIV-Positive, Class 1[1]	HIV-Positive, Class 2[1]	Infection Status of Source		HIV-Negative
			Source of Unknown HIV Status[2]	Unknown Source[3]	
Less severe[4]	Recommend basic 2-drug PEP	Recommend expanded ≥3-drug PEP	Generally, no PEP warranted; however, consider basic 2-drug PEP[5] for source with HIV risk factors[6]	Generally, no PEP warranted; consider basic 2-drug PEP[5] in settings in which exposure to HIV-infected persons is likely	No PEP warranted
More severe[7]	Recommend expanded 3-drug PEP	Recommend expanded ≥3-drug PEP	Generally, no PEP warranted; however consider basic 2-drug PEP[5] for source with HIV risk factors[6]	Generally, no PEP warranted; consider basic 2-drug PEP[5] in settings in which exposure to HIV-infected persons is likely	No PEP warranted

[1]HIV-positive, class 1 – asymptomatic HIV infection or known low viral load (eg, <1500 ribonucleic acid copies/mL). HIV-positive, class 2 – symptomatic HIV infection, AIDS, acute seroconversion, or known high viral load. If drug resistance is a concern, obtain expert consultation. Initiation of PEP should not be delayed pending expert consultation, and, because expert consultation alone cannot substitute for face-to-face counseling, resources should be available to provide immediate evaluation and follow-up care for all exposures.

[2]For example, deceased source person with no samples available for HIV testing.

[3]For example, a needle from a sharps disposal container.

[4]For example, solid needle or superficial injury.

[5]The recommendation "consider PEP" indicates that PEP is optional; a decision to initiate PEP should be based on a discussion between the exposed person and the treating clinician regarding the risks versus benefits of PEP.

[6]If PEP is offered and administered and the source is later determined to be HIV-negative, PEP should be discontinued.

[7]For example, large-bore hollow needle, deep puncture, visible blood on device, or needle used in patient's artery or vein.

Recommended HIV Postexposure Prophylaxis (PEP) for Mucous Membrane Exposures and Nonintact Skin[1] Exposures

Exposure Type	HIV-Positive, Class 1[2]	HIV-Positive, Class 2[2]	Source of Unknown HIV Status[3]	Unknown Source[4]	HIV-Negative
			Infection Status of Source		
Small volume[5]	Consider basic 2-drug PEP[6]	Recommend basic 2-drug PEP	Generally, no PEP warranted[7]	Generally, no PEP warranted	No PEP warranted
Large volume[8]	Recommend basic 2-drug PEP	Recommend expanded ≥3-drug PEP	Generally, no PEP warranted; however, consider basic 2-drug PEP[6] for source with HIV risk factors[7]	Generally, no PEP warranted; however, consider basic 2-drug PEP[6] in settings in which exposure to HIV-infected persons is likely	No PEP warranted

[1]For skin exposures, follow-up is indicated only if evidence exists of compromised skin integrity (eg, dermatitis, abrasion, or open wound).

[2]HIV-positive, class 1 – asymptomatic HIV infection or known low viral load (eg, <1500 ribonucleic acid copies/mL). HIV-positive, class 2 – symptomatic HIV infection, AIDS, acute seroconversion, or known high viral load. If drug resistance is a concern, obtain expert consultation. Initiation of PEP should not be delayed pending expert consultation, and, because expert consultation alone cannot substitute for face-to-face counseling, resources should be available to provide immediate evaluation and follow-up care for all exposures.

[3]For example, deceased source person with no samples available for HIV testing.

[4]For example, splash from inappropriately disposed blood.

[5]For example, a few drops.

[6]The recommendation "consider PEP" indicates that PEP is optional; a decision to initiate PEP should be based on a discussion between the exposed person and the treating clinician regarding the risks versus benefits of PEP.

[7]If PEP is offered and administered and the source is later determined to be HIV-negative, PEP should be discontinued.

[8]For example, a major blood splash.

OCCUPATIONAL EXPOSURE TO BLOODBORNE PATHOGENS (STANDARD / UNIVERSAL PRECAUTIONS) *(Continued)*

Situations for Which Expert[1] Consultation for HIV Postexposure Prophylaxis Is Advised

- **Delayed (ie, later than 24-36 hours) exposure report**
    - The interval after which there is no benefit from postexposure prophylaxis (PEP) is undefined

- **Unknown source (eg, needle in sharps disposal container or laundry)**
    - Decide use of PEP on a case-by-case basis
    - Consider the severity of the exposure and the epidemiologic likelihood of HIV exposure
    - Do not test needles or sharp instruments for HIV

- **Known or suspected pregnancy in the exposed person**
    - Does not preclude the use of optimal PEP regimens
    - Do not deny PEP solely on the basis of pregnancy

- **Resistance of the source virus to antiretroviral agents**
    - Influence of drug resistance on transmission risk is unknown
    - Selection of drugs to which the source person's virus is unlikely to be resistant is recommended, if the source person's virus is unknown or suspected to be resistant to ≥1 of the drugs considered for the PEP regimen
    - Resistance testing of the source person's virus at the time of the exposure is not recommended

- **Toxicity of the initial PEP regimen**
    - Adverse symptoms, such as nausea and diarrhea, are common with PEP
    - Symptoms can often be managed without changing the PEP regimen by prescribing antimotility and/or antiemetic agents
    - Modification of dose intervals (ie, administering a lower dose of drug more frequently throughout the day, as recommended by the manufacturer), in other situations, might help alleviate symptoms

[1]Local experts and/or the National Clinicians' Postexposure Prophylaxis Hotline (PEPline 1-888-448-4911).

Occupational Exposure Management Resources

National Clinicians' Postexposure Prophylaxis Hotline (PEPline)
Run by University of California-San Francisco/San Francisco General Hospital staff; supported by the Health Resources and Services Administration Ryan White CARE Act, HIV/AIDS Bureau, AIDS Education and Training Centers, and CDC

Phone: (888) 448-4911
Internet: http://www.ucsf.edu/hivcntr

Needlestick!
A website to help clinicians manage and document occupational blood and body fluid exposures. Developed and maintained by the University of California, Los Angeles (UCLA), Emergency Medicine Center, UCLA School of Medicine, and funded in part by CDC and the Agency for Healthcare Research and Quality.

Internet: http://www.needlestick.mednet.ucla.edu

Hepatitis Hotline

Phone: (888) 443-7232
Internet: http://www.cdc.gov/hepatitis

Reporting to CDC:
Occupationally acquired HIV infections and failures of PEP

Phone: (800) 893-0485

HIV Antiretroviral Pregnancy Registry

Phone: (800) 258-4263
Fax: (800) 800-1052
Address: 1410 Commonwealth Drive, Suite 215
Wilmington, NC 28405
Internet: http://www.glaxowellcome.com/preg_reg/antiretroviral

Food and Drug Administration
Report unusual or severe toxicity to antiretroviral agents

Phone: (800) 332-1088
Address: MedWatch
HF-2, FDA
5600 Fishers Lane
Rockville, MD 20857
Internet: http://www.fda.gov/medwatch

HIV/AIDS Treatment Information Service

Internet: http://www.aidsinfo.nih.gov

OCCUPATIONAL EXPOSURE TO BLOODBORNE PATHOGENS (STANDARD / UNIVERSAL PRECAUTIONS) *(Continued)*

Management of Occupational Blood Exposures

Provide immediate care to the exposure site

- Wash wounds and skin with soap and water
- Flush mucous membranes with water

Determine risk associated with exposure by:

- Type of fluid (eg, blood, visibly bloody fluid, other potentially infectious fluid or tissue, and concentrated virus)
- Type of exposure (ie, percutaneous injury, mucous membrane or nonintact skin exposure, and bites resulting in blood exposure)

Evaluate exposure source

- Assess the risk of infection using available information
- Test known sources for HB$_s$Ag, anti-HCV, and HIV antibody (consider using rapid testing)
- For unknown sources, assess risk of exposure to HBV, HCV, or HIV infection
- Do not test discarded needle or syringes for virus contamination

Evaluate the exposed person

- Assess immune status for HBV infection (ie, by history of hepatitis B vaccination and vaccine response)

Give PEP for exposures posing risk of infection transmission

- HBV: See Recommended Postexposure Prophylaxis for Exposure to Hepatitis B Virus Table
- HCV: PEP not recommended
- HIV: See Recommended HIV Postexposure Prophylaxis for Percutaneous Injuries Table and Recommended HIV Postexposure Prophylaxis for Mucous Membrane Exposures and Nonintact Skin Exposures Table

    – Initiate PEP as soon as possible, preferably within hours of exposure
    – Offer pregnancy testing to all women of childbearing age not known to be pregnant
    – Seek expert consultation if viral resistance is suspected
    – Administer PEP for 4 weeks if tolerated

Perform follow-up testing and provide counseling

- Advise exposed persons to seek medical evaluation for any acute illness occurring during follow-up

    HBV exposures

    - Perform follow-up anti-HB$_s$ testing in persons who receive hepatitis B vaccine

        – Test for anti-HB$_s$ 1-2 months after last dose of vaccine
        – Anti-HB$_s$ response to vaccine cannot be ascertained if HBIG was received in the previous 3-4 months

    HCV exposures

    - Perform baseline and follow-up testing for anti-HCV and alanine amino-transferase (ALT) 4-6 months after exposures
    - Perform HCV RNA at 4-6 months if earlier diagnosis of HCV infection is desired
    - Confirm repeatedly reactive anti-HCV enzyme immunoassays (EIAs) with supplemental tests

    HIV exposures

    - Perform HIV antibody testing for at least 6 months postexposure (eg, at baseline, 6 weeks, 3 months, and 6 months)
    - Perform HIV antibody testing if illness compatible with an acute retroviral syndrome occurs
    - Advise exposed persons to use precautions to prevent secondary transmission during the follow-up period
    - Evaluate exposed persons taking PEP within 72 hours after exposure and monitor for drug toxicity for at least 2 weeks

Basic and Expanded HIV Postexposure Prophylaxis Regimens

BASIC REGIMENS

Zidovudine (Retrovir®; ZDV; AZT) + lamivudine (Epivir®; 3TC); available as Combivir®

Preferred dosing
- ZDV: 300 mg twice daily or 200 mg three times daily, with food; total: 600 mg daily
- 3TC: 300 mg once daily or 150 mg twice daily
- Combivir®: One tablet twice daily

Dosage forms
- ZDV: 100 mg capsule, 10 mg/mL injection solution, 50 mg/5 mL oral syrup, 300 mg tablet
- 3TC: 10 mg/mL oral solution, 150 mg or 300 mg tablet
- Combivir®: Tablet, 300 mg ZDV + 150 mg 3TC

Advantages
- ZDV associated with decreased risk for HIV transmission
- ZDV used more often than other drugs for PEP for healthcare personnel (HCP)
- Serious toxicity rare when used for PEP
- Side effects predictable and manageable with antimotility and antiemetic agents
- Can be used by pregnant HCP
- Can be given as a single tablet (Combivir®) twice daily

Disadvantages
- Side effects (especially nausea and fatigue) common and might result in low adherence
- Source-patient virus resistance to this regimen possible
- Potential for delayed toxicity (oncogenic/teratogenic) unknown

Zidovudine (Retrovir®; ZDV; AZT) + emtricitabine (Emtriva®; FTC)

Preferred dosing
- ZDV: 300 mg twice daily or 200 mg three times daily, with food; total: 600 mg/day, in 2-3 divided doses
- FTC: 200 mg (one capsule) once daily

Dosage forms
- ZDV: See above
- FTC: 200 mg capsule, 10 mg/mL oral solution

FTC general comments
- Nucleoside analogue; same structure as 3TC, except fluoride residue at position 5 on pyrimidine ring
- Same resistance and safety profile as 3TC
- No apparent advantage over 3TC; tolerability and virologic response rates appear better than regimens containing ddI + d4T

Advantages
- ZDV: See above
- FTC
  - Convenient (once daily)
  - Well tolerated
  - Long intracellular half-life (~40 hours)

Disadvantages
- ZDV: See above
- FTC
  - Rash perhaps more frequent than with 3TC
  - No long-term experience with this drug
  - Cross resistance to 3TC
  - Hyperpigmentation among non-Caucasians with long-term use: 3%

Tenofovir DF (Viread®; TDF) + lamivudine (Epivir®; 3TC)

Preferred dosing
- TDF: 300 mg once daily
- 3TC: 300 mg once daily or 150 mg twice daily

Dosage forms
- TDF: 300 mg tablet
- 3TC: See above

Advantages
- 3TC: See above
- TDF
  - Convenient dosing (single pill once daily)
  - Resistance profile activity against certain thymidine analogue mutations
  - Well tolerated

OCCUPATIONAL EXPOSURE TO BLOODBORNE PATHOGENS (STANDARD / UNIVERSAL PRECAUTIONS) *(Continued)*

Disadvantages
- TDF
  - Same class warnings as nucleoside reverse transcriptase inhibitors (NRTIs)
  - Drug interactions
  - Increased TDF concentrations among persons taking atazanavir and lopinavir/ritonavir; need to monitor patients for TDF-associated toxicities
- Preferred dosage of atazanavir if used with TDF: 300 mg + ritonavir 100 mg once daily + TDF 300 mg once daily

Tenofovir DF (Viread®; TDF) + emtricitabine (Emtriva®; FTC); available as Truvada®
Preferred dosing
- TDF: 300 mg once daily
- FTC: 200 mg once daily
- As Truvada®: One tablet daily

Dosage forms
- TDF: 300 mg tablet
- FTC: See FTC
- Truvada® (TDF 300 mg plus FTC 200 mg)

Advantages
- FTC: See above
- TDF
  - Convenient dosing (single pill once daily)
  - Resistance profile activity against certain thymidine analogue mutations
  - Well tolerated

Disadvantages
- TDF
  - Same class warnings as NRTIs
  - Drug interactions
  - Increased TDF concentrations among persons taking atazanavir and lopinavir/ritonavir; need to monitor patients for TDF-associated toxicities
  - Preferred dosing of atazanavir if used with TDF: 300 mg + ritonavir 100 mg once daily + TDF 300 mg once daily

ALTERNATE BASIC REGIMENS

Lamivudine (Epivir®; 3TC) + stavudine (Zerit®; d4T)
Preferred dosing
- 3TC: 300 mg once daily or 150 mg twice daily
- d4T: 40 mg twice daily (can use lower doses of 20-30 mg twice daily if toxicity occurs; equally effective but less toxic among HIV-infected patients with peripheral neuropathy); 30 mg twice daily if body weight is <60 kg

Dosage forms
- 3TC: See above
- d4T: 1 mg/mL powder for oral solution, 15 mg, 20 mg, 30 mg, and 40 mg capsule

Advantages
- 3TC: See above
- d4T: Gastrointestinal (GI) side effects rare

Disadvantages
- Possibility that source-patient virus is resistant to this regimen
- Potential for delayed toxicity (oncogenic/teratogenic) unknown

Emtricitabine (Emtriva®; FTC) + stavudine (Zerit®; d4T)
Preferred dosing
- FTC: 200 mg daily
- d4T: 40 mg twice daily (can use lower doses of 20-30 mg twice daily if toxicity occurs; equally effective but less toxic among HIV-infected patients who developed peripheral neuropathy); if body weight is <60 kg, 30 mg twice daily

Dosage forms
- FTC: See above
- d4T: See above

Advantages
- 3TC and FTC: See above; d4T's GI side effects rare

Disadvantages
- Potential that source-patient virus is resistant to this regimen
- Unknown potential for delayed toxicity (oncogenic/teratogenic) unknown

Lamivudine (Epivir®; 3TC) + didanosine (Videx®; ddl)

Preferred dosing
- 3TC: 300 mg once daily or 150 mg twice daily
- ddl: Videx® chewable/dispersible buffered tablets can be administered on an empty stomach as either 200 mg twice daily or 400 mg once daily. Patients must take at least two of the appropriate strength tablets at each dose to provide adequate buffering and prevent gastric acid degradation of ddl. Because of the need for adequate buffering, the 200 mg strength tablet should be used only as a component of a once-daily regimen. The dose is either 200 mg twice daily or 400 mg once daily for patients weighing >60 kg and 125 mg twice daily or 250 mg once daily for patients weighing >60 kg.

Dosage forms
- 3TC: 150 mg or 300 mg tablets
- ddl: 125 mg, 200 mg, 250 mg, 400 mg delayed-release capsule; 25 mg, 50 mg, 100 mg, 150 mg, or 200 mg buffered white tablet

Advantages
- ddl: Once-daily dosing option
- 3TC: See above

Disadvantages
- Tolerability: Diarrhea more common with buffered preparation than with enteric-coated preparation
- Associated with toxicity: Peripheral neuropathy, pancreatitis, and lactic acidosis
- Must be taken on empty stomach except with TDF
- Drug interactions
- 3TC: See above

Emtricitabine (Emtriva®; FTC) + didanosine (Videx®; ddl)

Preferred dosing
- FTC: 200 mg once daily
- ddl: See above

Dosage forms
- ddl: See above
- FTC: See above

Advantages
- ddl: See above
- FTC: See above

Disadvantages
- Tolerability: Diarrhea more common with buffered than with enteric-coated preparation
- Associated with toxicity: Peripheral neuropathy, pancreatitis, and lactic acidosis
- Must be taken on empty stomach except with TDF
- Drug interactions
- FTC: See above

PREFERRED EXPANDED REGIMEN

Basic regimen plus:

Lopinavir / Ritonavir (Kaletra®; LPV/RTV)

Preferred dosing
- LPV/RTV: 400 mg/100 mg = 3 capsules twice daily with food

Dosage forms
- LPV/RTV: 133 mg/33 mg capsules

Advantages
- Potent HIV protease inhibitor
- Generally well-tolerated

Disadvantages
- Potential for serious or life-threatening drug interactions
- Might accelerate clearance of certain drugs, including oral contraceptives (requiring alternative or additional contraceptive measures for women taking these drugs)
- Can cause severe hyperlipidemia, especially hypertriglyceridemia
- GI (eg, diarrhea) events common

OCCUPATIONAL EXPOSURE TO BLOODBORNE PATHOGENS (STANDARD / UNIVERSAL PRECAUTIONS) *(Continued)*

ALTERNATE EXPANDED REGIMEN

Basic regimen plus one of the following:

Atazanavir (Reyataz®; ATV) ± ritonavir (Norvir®; RTV)
Preferred dosing
- ATV: 400 mg once daily, unless used in combination with TDF, in which case ATV should be boosted with RTV, preferred dosing of ATV 300 mg + RTV: 100 mg once daily

Dosage forms
- ATV: 100 mg, 150 mg, and 200 mg capsules
- RTV: 100 mg capsule

Advantages
- Potent HIV protease inhibitor
- Convenient dosing – once daily
- Generally well tolerated

Disadvantages
- Hyperbilirubinemia and jaundice common
- Potential for serious or life-threatening drug interactions
- Avoid coadministration with proton pump inhibitors
- Separate antacids and buffered medications by 2 hours and H_2-receptor antagonists by 12 hours to avoid decreasing ATV levels
- Caution should be used with ATV and products known to induce PR prolongation (eg, diltiazem)

Fosamprenavir (Lexiva™; FOSAPV) ± ritonavir (Norvir®; RTV)
Preferred dosing
- FOSAPV: 1400 mg twice daily (without RTV)
- FOSAPV: 1400 mg once daily + RTV 200 mg once daily
- FOSAPV: 700 mg twice daily + RTV 100 mg twice daily

Dosage forms
- FOSAPV: 700 mg tablets
- RTV: 100 mg capsule

Advantages
- Once daily dosing when given with ritonavir

Disadvantages
- Tolerability: GI side effects common
- Multiple drug interactions. Oral contraceptives decrease fosamprenavir concentrations.
- Incidence of rash in healthy volunteers, especially when used with low doses of ritonavir. Differentiating between early drug-associated rash and acute seroconversion can be difficult and cause extraordinary concern for the exposed person.

Indinavir (Crixivan®; IDV) ± ritonavir (Norvir®; RTV)
Preferred dosing
- IDV 800 mg + RTV 100 mg twice daily without regard to food

Alternative dosing
- IDV: 800 mg every 8 hours, on an empty stomach

Dosage forms
- IDV: 200 mg, 333 mg, and 400 mg capsule
- RTV: 100 mg capsule

Advantages
- Potent HIV inhibitor

Disadvantages
- Potential for serious or life-threatening drug interactions
- Serious toxicity (eg, nephrolithiasis) possible; consumption of 8 glasses of fluid/day required
- Hyperbilirubinemia common; must avoid this drug during late pregnancy
- Requires acid for absorption and cannot be taken simultaneously with ddI, chewable/dispersible buffered tablet formulation (doses must be separated by ≥1 hour)

Saquinavir (Invirase®; SQV) + ritonavir (Norvir®; RTV)
Preferred dosing
- SQV: 1000 mg (given as Invirase®) + RTV 100 mg, twice daily
- SQV: Five capsules twice daily + RTV: One capsule twice daily

Dosage forms
- SQV (Invirase®): 200 mg capsule
- RTV: 100 mg capsule

Advantages
- Generally well-tolerated, although GI events common

Disadvantages
- Potential for serious or life-threatening drug interactions
- Substantial pill burden

Nelfinavir (Viracept®; NFV)

Preferred dosing
- NFV: 1250 mg (2 x 625 mg or 5 x 250 mg tablets), twice daily with a meal

Dosage forms
- NFV: 250 mg or 625 mg tablet

Advantages
- Generally well-tolerated

Disadvantages
- Diarrhea or other GI events common
- Potential for serious and/or life-threatening drug interactions

Efavirenz (Sustiva®; EFV)

Preferred dosing
- EFV: 600 mg daily, at bedtime

Dosage forms
- EFV: 50 mg, 100 mg, 200 mg capsules
- EFV: 600 mg tablet

Advantages
- Does not require phosphorylation before activation and might be active earlier than other antiretroviral agents (a theoretic advantage of no demonstrated clinical benefit)
- Once daily dosing

Disadvantages
- Drug associated with rash (early onset) that can be severe and might rarely progress to Stevens-Johnson syndrome
- Differentiating between early drug-associated rash and acute seroconversion can be difficult and cause extraordinary concern for the exposed person
- Central nervous system side effects (eg, dizziness, somnolence, insomnia, or abnormal dreaming) common; severe psychiatric symptoms possible (dosing before bedtime might minimize these side effects)
- Teratogen; should not be used during pregnancy
- Potential for serious or life-threatening drug interactions

ANTIRETROVIRAL AGENTS GENERALLY NOT RECOMMENDED FOR USE AS PEP

Nevirapine (Viramune®; NVP)

Disadvantages
- Associated with severe hepatotoxicity (including at least one case of liver failure requiring liver transplantation in an exposed person taking PEP)
- Associated with rash (early onset) that can be severe and progress to Stevens-Johnson syndrome
- Differentiating between early drug-associated rash and acute seroconversion can be difficult and cause extraordinary concern for the exposed person
- Drug interactions: Can lower effectiveness of certain antiretroviral agents and other commonly used medicines

Delavirdine (Rescriptor®; DLV)

Disadvantages
- Drug associated with rash (early onset) that can be severe and progress to Stevens-Johnson syndrome
- Multiple drug interactions

Abacavir (Ziagen®; ABC)

Disadvantages
- Severe hypersensitivity reactions can occur, usually within the first 6 weeks
- Differentiating between early drug-associated rash/hypersensitivity and acute seroconversion can be difficult

Zalcitabine (Hivid®; ddC)

Disadvantages
- Three times a day dosing
- Tolerability
- Weakest antiretroviral agent

OCCUPATIONAL EXPOSURE TO BLOODBORNE PATHOGENS (STANDARD / UNIVERSAL PRECAUTIONS) *(Continued)*

ANTIRETROVIRAL AGENT FOR USE AS PEP ONLY WITH EXPERT CONSULTATION

Enfuvirtide (Fuzeon™; T20)

Preferred dosing

- T20: 90 mg (1 mL) twice daily by subcutaneous injection

Dosage forms

- T20: Single-dose vial, reconstituted to 90 mg/mL

Advantages

- New class
- Unique viral target; to block cell entry
- Prevalence of resistance low

Disadvantages

- Twice-daily injection
- Safety profile: Local injection site reactions
- Never studied among antiretroviral-naive or HIV-negative patients
- False-positive EIA HIV antibody tests might result from formation of anti-T20 antibodies that cross-react with anti-gp41 antibodies

HAZARDOUS COMMUNICATION

Communication regarding the dangers of bloodborne infections through the use of labels, signs, information, and education is required. Storage locations (eg, refrigerators and freezers, waste containers) that are used to store, dispose of, transport, or ship blood or other potentially infectious materials require labels. The label background must be red or bright orange with the biohazard design and the word biohazard in a contrasting color. The label must be part of the container or affixed to the container by permanent means.

Education provided by a qualified and knowledgeable instructor is mandated. The sessions for employees must include:

- accessible copies of the regulation
- general epidemiology of bloodborne diseases
- modes of bloodborne pathogen transmission
- an explanation of the exposure control plan and a means to obtain copies of the written plan
- an explanation of the tasks and activities that may involve exposure
- the use of exposure prevention methods and their limitations (eg, engineering controls, work practices, personal protective equipment)
- information on the types, proper use, location, removal, handling, decontamination, and disposal of personal protective equipment)
- an explanation of the basis for selection of personal protective equipment
- information on the HBV vaccine, including information on its efficacy, safety, and method of administration and the benefits of being vaccinated (ie, the employee must understand that the vaccine and vaccination will be offered free of charge)
- information on the appropriate actions to take and persons to contact in an emergency involving exposure to blood or other potentially infectious materials
- an explanation of the procedure to follow if an exposure incident occurs, including the method of reporting the incident
- information on the postexposure evaluation and follow-up that the employer is required to provide for the employee following an exposure incident
- an explanation of the signs, labels, and color coding
- an interactive question-and-answer period

RECORD KEEPING

The OSHA Final Rule requires that the employer maintain both education and medical records. The medical records must be kept confidential and be maintained for the duration of employment plus 30 years. They must contain a copy of the employee's HBV vaccination status and postexposure incident information. Education records must be maintained for 3 years from the date the program was given.

OSHA has the authority to conduct inspections without notice. Penalties for cited violation may be assessed as follows:

Serious violations. In this situation, there is a substantial probability of death or serious physical harm, and the employer knew, or should have known, of the hazard. A violation of this type carries a mandatory penalty of up to $7000 for each violation.

Other-than-serious violations. The violation is unlikely to result in death or serious physical harm. This type of violation carries a discretionary penalty of up to $7000 for each violation.

Willful violations. These are violations committed knowingly or intentionally by the employer and have penalties of up to $70,000 per violation with a minimum of $5000 per violation. If an employee dies as a result of a willful violation, the responsible party, if convicted, may receive a personal fine of up to $250,000 and/or a 6-month jail term. A corporation may be fined $500,000.

Large fines frequently follow visits to laboratories, physicians' offices, and healthcare facilities by OSHA Compliance Safety and Health Offices (CSHOS). Regulations are vigorously enforced. A working knowledge of the final rule and implementation of appropriate policies and practices is imperative for all those involved in the collection and analysis of medical specimens.

Effectiveness of universal precautions in averting exposure to potentially infectious materials has been documented.[7] Compliance with appropriate rules, procedures, and policies, including reporting exposure incidents, is a matter of personal professionalism and prudent self-preservation.

Footnotes

1. Henderson DK, Fahey BJ, Willy M, et al, "Risk for Occupational Transmission of Human Immunodeficiency Virus Type 1 (HIV-1) Associated With Clinical Exposures. A Prospective Evaluation," *Ann Intern Med*, 1990, 113(10):740-6.
2. Niu MT and Margolis HS, "Moving Into a New Era of Government Regulation: Provisions for Hepatitis B Vaccine in the Workplace, *Clin Lab Manage Rev*, 1989, 3:336-40.
3. Bruning LM, "The Bloodborne Pathogens Final Rule — Understanding the Regulation," *AORN Journal*, 1993, 57(2):439-40.
4. "Rules and Regulations," *Federal Register*, 1994, 59(66):16360-3.
5. Schaffner W, Gardner P, and Gross PA, "Hepatitis B Immunization Strategies: Expanding the Target," *Ann Intern Med*, 1993, 118(4):308-9.
6. Fahey BJ, Beekmann SE, Schmitt JM, et al, "Managing Occupational Exposures to HIV-1 in the Healthcare Workplace," *Infect Control Hosp Epidemiol*, 1993, 14(7):405-12.
7. Wong ES, Stotka JL, Chinchilli VM, et al, "Are Universal Precautions Effective in Reducing the Number of Occupational Exposures Among Healthcare Workers?" *JAMA*, 1991, 265(9):1123-8.

References

Buehler JW and Ward JW, "A New Definition for AIDS Surveillance," *Ann Intern Med*, 1993, 118(5):390-2.

Brown JW and Blackwell H, "Complying With the New OSHA Regs, Part 1: Teaching Your Staff About Biosafety," *MLO*, 1992, 24(4)24-8. Part 2: "Safety Protocols No Lab Can Ignore," 1992, 24(5):27-9. Part 3: "Compiling Employee Safety Records That Will Satisfy OSHA," 1992, 24(6):45-8.

Department of Labor, Occupational Safety and Health Administration, "Occupational Exposure to Bloodborne Pathogens; Final Rule (29 CFR Part 1910.1030), "*Federal Register*, December 6, 1991, 64004-182.

Gold JW, "HIV-1 Infection: Diagnosis and Management," *Med Clin North Am*, 1992, 76(1):1-18.

"Hepatitis B Virus: A Comprehensive Strategy for Eliminating Transmission in the United States Through Universal Childhood Vaccination," Recommendations of the Immunization Practices Advisory Committee (ACIP), *MMWR Morb Mortal Wkly Rep*, 1991, 40(RR-13):1-25.

"Mortality Attributable to HIV Infection/AIDS — United States," *MMWR Morb Mortal Wkly Rep*, 1991, 40(3):41-4.

National Committee for Clinical Laboratory Standards, "Protection of Laboratory Workers From Infectious Disease Transmitted by Blood, Body Fluids, and Tissue," NCCLS Document M29-T, Villanova, PA: NCCLS, 1989, 9(1).

"Nosocomial Transmission of Hepatitis B Virus Associated With a Spring-Loaded Fingerstick Device — California," *MMWR Morb Mortal Wkly Rep*, 1990, 39(35):610-3.

Polish LB, Shapiro CN, Bauer F, et al, "Nosocomial Transmission of Hepatitis B Virus Associated With the Use of a Spring-Loaded Fingerstick Device," *N Engl J Med*, 1992, 326(11):721-5.

"Recommendations for Preventing Transmission of Human Immunodeficiency Virus and Hepatitis B Virus to Patients During Exposure-Prone Invasive Procedures," *MMWR Morb Mortal Wkly Rep*, 1991, 40(RR-8):1-9.

"Update: Acquired Immunodeficiency Syndrome — United States," *MMWR Morb Mortal Wkly Rep*, 1992, 41(26):463-8.

"Update: Transmission of HIV Infection During an Invasive Dental Procedure — Florida," *MMWR Morb Mortal Wkly Rep*, 1991, 40(2):21-7, 33.

"Update: Universal Precautions for Prevention of Transmission of Human Immunodeficiency Virus, Hepatitis B Virus, and Other Bloodborne Pathogens in Healthcare Settings," *MMWR Morb Mortal Wkly Rep*, 1988, 37(24):377-82, 387-8.

"U.S. Public Health Service Guidelines for the Management of Occupational Exposures to HBV, HCV, and HIV and Recommendations for Postexposure Prophylaxis," *MMWR Morb Mortal Wkly Rep*, 2001, 50(RR-11).

IMMUNIZATIONS[1] (VACCINES[2])

Drug	Use	Stability	Dosage and Administration
Anthrax vaccine (adsorbed)[2,3] BioThrax™	Immunization against *Bacillus anthracis*, recommended for individuals who may come in contact with animal products which come from anthrax endemic areas and may be contaminated with *Bacillus anthracis* spores; postexposure prophylaxis in combination with antibiotics, recommended for high-risk persons such as veterinarians and others handling potentially infected animals; routine immunization for the general population is not recommended. The Department of Defense is implementing an anthrax vaccination program against the biological warfare agent anthrax, which will be administered to all active duty and reserve personnel. **Note:** Safety and efficacy not established for adults >65 years of age.	Store under refrigeration at 2°C to 8°C (36°F to 46°F). Do not freeze. Do not mix with other injections or use the same site. Shake well before use; do not use if discolored or contains particulate matter.	SubQ: Children ≥18 years and Adults: Three injections of 0.5 mL each given 2 weeks apart, followed by three additional injections given at 6, 12, and 18 months; booster at 1-year intervals Massage site to disperse the vaccine postinjection. It is not necessary to restart the series if a dose is not given on time; resume as soon as practical.
BCG vaccine[6] TheraCys®; TICE® BCG	Immunization against tuberculosis; treatment of bladder cancer; immunotherapy for cancer; treatment of bladder cancer; strongly recommended for infants and children with negative tuberculin skin tests who are at high risk of intimate and prolonged exposure to persistently untreated or ineffectively treated patients with infectious pulmonary tuberculosis; cannot be removed from the source of exposure; cannot be placed on long-term preventive therapy; and are continuously exposed with tuberculosis who have bacilli resistant to isoniazid and rifampin; recommended for tuberculin-negative infants and children in groups in which the rate of new infections exceeds 1% per year and for whom the usual surveillance and treatment programs have been attempted but are not operationally feasible	Refrigerate; protect from light. Use TICE® BCG within 2 hours of mixing.	Children >1 month and Adults: **Immunization against tuberculosis** (TICE® BCG): 0.2-0.3 mL percutaneous; initial lesion usually appears after 10-14 days consisting of small red papule at injection site and reaches maximum diameter of 3 mm in 4-6 weeks. Conduct postvaccinal tuberculin test (ie, 5 TU of PPD) in 2-3 months; if test is negative, repeat vaccination. **Immunotherapy for bladder cancer:** *Intravesical treatment:* Instill into bladder for 2 hours *TheraCys®:* One dose instilled into bladder once weekly for 6 weeks followed by one treatment at 3, 6, 12, 18, and 24 months *TICE® BCG:* One dose instilled into the bladder once weekly for 6 weeks followed by once monthly for 6-12 months (should only be given intravesicularly or percutaneously)
Diphtheria and tetanus toxoid[6,6]	Active immunity against diphtheria and tetanus when pertussis vaccine is contraindicated; tetanus prophylaxis in wound management	Refrigerate.	I.M.: **Children: 6 weeks to 1 year of age:** DT: Three 0.5 mL doses at least 4 weeks apart; administer a reinforcing dose 6-12 months after third injection. **Children >1-6 years:** DT: Two 0.5 mL doses at least 4 weeks apart; reinforcing dose 6-12 months after second injection **Children 4-6 years:** Booster: DT: 0.5 mL; not necessary if all 4 doses were given after fourth birthday; administer doses at 10-year intervals with adult preparation. **Children ≥7 years and Adults:** Td: 2 primary doses of 0.5 mL each, given at an interval of 4-6 weeks; third (reinforcing) dose of 0.5 mL 6-12 months later; booster every 10 years
Diphtheria, tetanus toxoids, and acellular pertussis vaccine[5,6] Daptacel®; Infanrix®; Tripedia®	Active immunization of children from 6 weeks of age through seventh birthday for prevention of diphtheria, tetanus, and pertussis	Refrigerate at 2°C to 8°C (35°F to 46°F); do not freeze.	I.M. (anterolateral aspect of thigh or deltoid muscle of upper arm): **Children 6 weeks through 6 years of age** (use same product for all 3 doses): Three doses of 0.5 mL, usually given at 2-, 4-, and 6 months of age; may be repeated every 4-8 weeks; booster: fourth dose given at ~15-20 months of age, but at least 6 months after third dose. Fifth dose given at 5-6 years of age, prior to starting school or kindergarten (if the fourth dose is given at 4 years of age, the fifth dose may be omitted.) **Children ≥7 years and Adults:** Adult Td preparation is the preferred agent.

Drug	Use	Stability	Dosage and Administration
Diphtheria, tetanus toxoids, acellular pertussis vaccine and *Haemophilus influenzae* b conjugate vaccine (combined)[2,5] TriHIBit®	Active immunization of children 15-18 months of age for prevention of diphtheria, tetanus, pertussis, and invasive disease caused by *H. influenzae* type b	Should be used within 30 minutes of reconstitution.	I.M.: Children >15 months of age: 0.5 mLTriHIBit® is Tripedia® vaccine used to reconstitute ActHIB® (*Haemophilus* b conjugate) vaccine. The combination can be used for the DTaP dose given at 15-18 months when Tripedia® was used for the initial doses and a primary series of HIB vaccine has been given.
Diphtheria, tetanus toxoids, acellular pertussis, hepatitis B (recombinant), and poliovirus (inactivated) vaccine[5,6] Pediarix™	Active immunization against diphtheria, tetanus, pertussis, hepatitis B virus (all known subtypes), and poliomyelitis (caused by poliovirus types 1, 2, and 3)	Store under refrigeration of 2°C to 8°C (36°F to 46°F). Do not freeze; discard if frozen. Do not administer additional vaccines or immunoglobulins at the same site, or use the same syringe. Shake well prior to use; do not use unless a homogeneous, turbid, white suspension forms.	I.M. (anterolateral aspects of the thigh or the deltoid muscle of the upper arm): **Immunization:** Vaccination usually begins at 2 months, but may be started as early as 6 weeks of age: 0.5 mL; repeat in 6-8 week intervals (preferably 8-week) for a total of 3 doses. **Children previously vaccinated with one or more components and who are also scheduled to receive all vaccine components** (safety and efficacy not established): *Hepatitis B vaccine:* Infants born of HBsAg-negative mothers who received 1 dose of hepatitis B vaccine at birth may be given Pediarix™. Infants who received 1 or more doses of hepatitis B vaccine (recombinant) may be given Pediarix™ to complete the hepatitis B series. *Diphtheria and tetanus toxoids, and acellular pertussis vaccine (DTaP):* Infants previously vaccinated with 1 or 2 doses of Infanrix® may use Pediarix™ to complete the first 3 doses of the series; use of Pediarix™ to complete DTaP vaccination started with products other than Infanrix® is not recommended. *Inactivated polio vaccine (IPV):* Infants previously vaccinated with 1 or 2 doses of IPV may use Pediarix™ to complete the first 3 doses of the series.

IMMUNIZATIONS[1] (VACCINES[2]) *(Continued)*

Drug	Use	Stability	Dosage and Administration
Haemophilus b conjugate vaccine[2,6] ActHIB®; HibTITER®; PedvaxHIB®	Routine immunization of children 2 months to 5 years of age against invasive disease caused by *H. influenzae*; unimmunized children 5 years of age with a chronic illness known to be associated with increased risk of *Haemophilus influenzae* type b disease, specifically, persons with anatomic or functional asplenia or sickle cell anemia or those who have undergone splenectomy, should receive Hib vaccine. *Haemophilus* b conjugate vaccines are not indicated for prevention of bronchitis or other infections due to *H. influenzae* in adults; adults with specific dysfunction or certain complement deficiencies who are at especially high risk of *H. influenzae* type b infection (HIV-infected adults); patients with Hodgkin's disease (vaccinated at least 2 weeks before the initiation of chemotherapy or 3 months after the end of chemotherapy)	Keep in refrigerator; may be frozen (not diluent) without affecting potency. Reconstituted Hib-Imune® remains stable for only 8 hours, whereas HibVAX® remain stable for 30 days when refrigerated.	**Note:** The same brand drug should be used throughout the vaccination series. If vaccine previously used is unknown, infants (2-6 months of age) should be given a primary series of three doses. Have epinephrine 1:1000 available. I.M.: Children: 0.5 mL as a single dose administered according to one of the following "brand-specific" schedules (boosters to be given at least 2 months after previous dose): **HibTITER®:** Age at 1st dose: *2-6 months:* 3 doses, 2 months apart; booster in 15 months *7-11 months:* 2 doses, 2 months apart; booster in 15 months *12-14 months:* 1 dose; booster in 15 months *15-60 months:* 1 dose; no booster **PedvaxHIB®:** Age at 1st dose: *2-6 months:* 2 doses, 2 months apart; booster in 12 months *7-11 months:* 2 doses, 2 months apart; booster in 15 months *12-14 months:* 1 dose; booster in 15 months *15-60 months:* 1 dose; no booster **ProHIBIT®:** Age at 1st dose: 15-60 months: 1 dose; no booster
Hepatitis A vaccine[2,5,6] Havrix®; VAQTA®	Protection against hepatitis A or for populations at risk: travelers to developing countries, household and sexual contact with persons infected with hepatitis A, child day care employees, patients with chronic liver disease, illicit drug users, male homosexuals, institutional workers (eg, institutions for the mentally and physically handicapped persons, prisons, etc), and healthcare workers who may be exposed to hepatitis A virus (eg, laboratory employees); protection lasts for ~15 years		**Note:** Use caution in patients with serious active infection, cardiovascular disease, or pulmonary disorders; treatment for anaphylactic reactions should be immediately available. I.M. (deltoid muscle): **Havrix®:** *Children 12 months -18 years:* 720 ELISA units (0.5 mL) with a booster dose of 720 ELISA units 6-12 months following primary immunization *Adults:* 1440 ELISA units (1 mL) with a booster 6-12 months following primary immunization **VAQTA®:** *Children 12 months - 18 years:* 25 units (0.5 mL) with 25 units (0.5 mL); booster in 6-18 months *Adults:* 50 units (1 mL) with 50 units (1 mL); booster in 6-18 months

Drug	Use	Stability	Dosage and Administration
Hepatitis A (inactivated) and hepatitis B (recombinant) vaccine[2,5,6] Twinrix®	Active immunization against disease caused by hepatitis A virus and hepatitis B virus (all known subtypes) in populations desiring protection against or at high risk of exposure to these viruses; travelers to areas of intermediate/high endemicity for **both** HAV and HBV; those at increased risk of HBV infection due to behavioral or occupational factors; patients with chronic liver disease; laboratory workers who handle live HAV and HBV; healthcare workers, police, and other personnel who render first aid or medical assistance; workers who come in contact with sewage; employees of day care centers and correctional facilities; patients/staff of hemodialysis units; male homosexuals; patients frequently receiving blood products; military personnel; users of injectable illicit drugs; close household contacts of patients with hepatitis A and hepatitis B infection	Store in refrigerator at 2°C to 8°C (36°F to 46°F). Do not freeze (discard if frozen). Do not use the same syringe or site as additional vaccines or immunoglobulins. Shake well prior to use; do not dilute.	I.M. (deltoid muscle): Adults: Three doses (1 mL each) given on a 0-, 1-, and 6-month schedule
Hepatitis B immune globulin BayHep B®; HepaGam B™; Nabi-HB®	Provide prophylactic passive immunity to hepatitis B infection to those individuals exposed; newborns of mothers known to be hepatitis B surface antigen positive; not indicated for treatment of active hepatitis B infections; ineffective in the treatment of chronic active hepatitis B infection	Refrigerate at 2°C to 8°C (36°F to 46°F); do not freeze.	HBIG may be administered at the same time (but at a different site) or up to 1 month preceding hepatitis B vaccination without impairing the active immune response. I.M. (gluteal or deltoid region): **Newborns:** Hepatitis B: 0.5 mL as soon after birth as possible (within 12 hours); may repeat at 3 months in order for a higher rate of prevention of the carrier state to be achieved. At this time, an active vaccination program with the vaccine may begin. **Infants <12 months:** Household exposure prophylaxis: 0.5 mL (to be administered if mother or primary caregiver has acute HBV infection) **Adults:** Postexposure prophylaxis: 0.06 mL/kg as soon as possible after exposure (ie, within 24 hours of needlestick, ocular, or mucosal exposure or within 14 days of sexual exposure); usual dose: 3-5 mL; repeat at 28-30 days after exposure

IMMUNIZATIONS[1] (VACCINES[2]) *(Continued)*

Drug	Use	Stability	Dosage and Administration
Hepatitis B vaccine Engerix-B®; Recombivax HB®	Immunization against infection caused by all known subtypes of hepatitis B virus in individuals considered at high risk of potential exposure to hepatitis B virus or HB$_s$Ag-positive materials. Immunity will last ~5-7 years.	Refrigerate at 2°C to 8°C (36°F to 46°F); do not freeze. Shake well prior to withdrawal and use.	It is possible to interchange the vaccines for completion of a series or for booster doses; the antibody produced in response to each type of vaccine is comparable, however, the quantity of the vaccine will vary. Administer with caution in patients receiving anticoagulant therapy. SubQ injection may be administered in patients at risk of hemorrhage which may result in an increased incidence of local reactions and a reduced therapeutic effect. Refer to specific product labeling for dosing. I.M. (deltoid muscle): **Adults:** Immunization regimen consists of 3 doses (0, 1, and 6 months); first dose given on the elected date; second dose given 1 month later; third dose given 6 months after the first dose **Recombivax HB®:** *Children 11-15 years* (10 mcg/mL adult formulation): First dose of 1 mL given on the elected date, second dose given 4-6 months later **Engerix-B®:** *Children ≥10 years:* (10 mcg/0.5 mL formulation): High-risk children: 0.5 mL at 0, 1, 2, and 12 months; lower-risk children ages 5-10 who are candidates for an extended administration schedule may receive an alternative regimen of 0.5 mL at 0, 12, and 24 months.; if booster is needed, revaccinate with 0.5 mL. *Adolescents 11-19 years* (20 mcg/mL formulation): 1 mL at 0, 1, and 6 months. High-risk adolescents: 1 mL at 0, 1, 2, and 12 months; lower-risk adolescents 11-16 years who are candidates for an extended administration schedule may receive an alternative regimen of 0.5 mL (using the 10 mcg/0.5 mL) formulation at 0, 12, and 24 months; if booster is needed, revaccinate with 20 mcg *Adults ≥ 20 years:* High-risk adults (20 mcg/mL formulation): 1 mL at 0, 1, 2, and 12 months; if booster dose is needed, revaccinate with 1 mL

Drug	Use	Stability	Dosage and Administration
Immune globulin (intramuscular) BayGam®	Household and sexual contacts of persons with hepatitis A, measles, varicella, and possibly rubella; travelers to high-risk areas outside tourist routes; staff, attendees, and parents of diapered attendees in daycare center outbreaks For travelers, IG is not an alternative to careful selection of foods and water; frequent travelers should be tested for hepatitis A antibody, and immune hemolytic anemia, and neutropenia (with TTP, I.V. route is usually used).	Refrigerate; do not freeze. Do not mix with other medications.	Skin testing should not be performed as local irritation can occur and be misinterpreted as a positive reaction. Immune globulin can interfere with the antibody response to parenterally administered live virus vaccines. I.M.: **Hepatitis A:** Pre-exposure prophylaxis upon travel into endemic areas (hepatitis A vaccine preferred): 0.02 mL/kg for anticipated risk 1-3 months; 0.06 mL/kg for anticipated risk >3 months; repeat approximate dose every 4-6 months if exposure continues. Postexposure prophylaxis: 0.02 mL/kg given within 2 weeks of exposure **Measles:** Prophylaxis: 0.25 mL/kg/dose (max: 15 mL) given within 6 days of exposure followed by live attenuated measles vaccine in 3 months or at 15 months of age (whichever is later) **Leukemia, lymphoma, immunodeficiency disorders, generalized malignancy, or those receiving immunosuppressive therapy:** 0.5 mL/kg (max: 15 mL). **Poliomyelitis:** Prophylaxis: 0.3 mL/kg/dose as a single dose **Rubella:** Prophylaxis: 0.55 mL/kg/dose within 72 hours of exposure **Varicella:** Prophylaxis: 0.6-1.2 mL/kg (varicella-zoster immune globulin preferred) within 72 hours of exposure **IgG deficiency:** 1.3 mL/kg, then 0.66 mL/kg in 3-4 weeks **Hepatitis B:** Prophylaxis: 0.06 mL/kg/dose (HBIG preferred)
Influenza virus vaccine Fluarix™; fluMist®; Fluvirin®; Fluzone®	Provide active immunity to influenza virus strains contained in the vaccine; for high-risk persons including those ≥65 years of age; residents of nursing homes and other chronic-care facilities that house persons of any age with chronic medical conditions; adults and children with chronic disorders of the pulmonary or cardiovascular systems (asthma); adults and children who have required regular medical follow-up or hospitalization during the preceding year because of chronic metabolic diseases (including diabetes mellitus), renal dysfunction, hemoglobinopathies, or immunosuppression (including immunosuppression caused by medications); children and adolescents (6 months to 18 years of age) who are receiving long-term aspirin therapy and therefore, may be at risk for developing Reye's syndrome after influenza; women who will be in the 2nd or 3rd trimester of pregnancy during the influenza season. Otherwise healthy children aged 6-23 months, healthy persons who may transmit influenza to those at risk, and others who are interested in immunization to influenza virus should receive the vaccine as long as supply is available.	Store between 2°C to 8°C (36°F to 46°F). Potency is destroyed by freezing; do not use if product has been frozen. Suspension should be shaken well prior to use; inspect for particulate matter and discoloration prior to administration. **Note:** Previous year vaccines should not be used to prevent present year influenza.	I.M.: (deltoid muscle in adults and older children; anterolateral aspect of the thigh in infants and young children): *Previously unvaccinated children <9 years:* 2 doses given >1 month apart **Fluarix™:** *Adults:* 0.5 mL/dose (1 dose) **Fluzone®:** *Children 6-35 months:* 0.25 mL/dose (1 or 2 doses) *Children 3-8 years:* 0.5 mL/dose (1 or 2 doses) *Children ≥9 years and Adults:* 0.5 mL/dose (1 dose) **Fluvirin®:** *Children 4-8 years:* 0.5 mL/dose (1 or 2 doses) *Children ≥9 years and Adults:* 0.5 mL/dose (1 dose) **Intranasal: fluMist®:** *Children 5-8 years, previously not vaccinated with influenza vaccine:* Initial season: Two 0.5 mL doses separated by 6-10 weeks *Children 5-8 years, previously vaccinated with influenza vaccine:* 0.5 mL/dose (1 dose) *Children ≥9 years and Adults ≤49 years:* 0.5 mL/dose (1 dose)

Drug	Use	Stability	Dosage and Administration
Japanese encephalitis virus vaccine (inactivated) JE-VAX®	Active immunization against Japanese encephalitis for children ≥ 1 year of age and adults who plan to spend 1 month or more in endemic areas in Asia (especially persons traveling during the transmission season or visiting rural area); older adults >55 years of age should be considered for vaccination (due to increased risk of developing symptomatic illness after infection) Those planning travel to or residence in endemic areas should consult the Travel Advisory Service (Central Campus) for specific advice; consider vaccination for shorter trips to epidemic areas or extensive outdoor activities in Japanese endemic areas. Because of the potential for severe adverse reactions, Japanese encephalitis vaccine is not recommended for all persons travelling to or residing in Asia.	Refrigerate at 2°C to 8°C. Do not freeze. Discard 8 hours after reconstitution.	Severe adverse reactions may occur within minutes following vaccination or up to 17 days later; most reactions occur within 10 days (majority within 48 hours). Observe vaccinees for 30 minutes after vaccination; warn them of the possibility of delayed generalized urticaria and to remain where medical care is readily available for 10 days following any dose of the vaccine. U.S. recommended primary immunization schedule: **SubQ:** **Children 1-3 years:** Three 0.5 mL doses given on days 0, 7, and 30 **Children >3 years and Adults:** Three 1 mL doses given on days 0, 7, and 30; give third dose on day 14 when time does not permit waiting **Booster:** After 2 years, or according to current recommendation **Note:** Abbreviated schedules should be used only when necessary due to time constraints. Two doses a week apart produce immunity in about 80% of recipients; the longest regimen yields highest titers after 6 months. Travel should not commence ≤10 days after the last dose of vaccine, to allow adequate antibody formation and recognition of any delayed adverse reaction. Advise concurrent use of other means to reduce the risk of mosquito exposure when possible, including bed nets, insect repellents, protective clothing, avoidance of travel in endemic areas, and avoidance of outdoor activity during twilight and evening periods.
Measles, mumps, and rubella vaccines (combined) M-M-R® II	Prophylaxis for measles, mumps, and rubella	Prior to reconstitution, store the powder at 2°C to 8°C (36°F to 46°F) or colder (freezing does not affect potency). Protect from light. Diluent may be stored with powder or at room temperature.	SubQ (outer aspect of the upper arm): Infants >12 months: Administer 0.5 mL, then repeat at 4-6 years of age. If the second dose was not received, the schedule should be completed by the 11- to 12-year-old visit. If there is risk of exposure to measles, single-antigen measles vaccine should be administered at 6-11 months of age with a second dose (of MMR) at >12 months of age. **Note:** MMR vaccine should be given within 3 months of immune globulin or whole blood. Have epinephrine available during and after administration. Should not be administered to severely immunocompromised persons with the exception of asymptomatic children with HIV (ACIP and AAP recommendation). Severely immunocompromised patients and symptomatic HIV-infected patients who are exposed to measles should receive immune globulin, regardless of prior vaccination status. Defer immunization during any acute illness. Females should not become pregnant within 3 months of vaccination.
Measles virus vaccine (live) Attenuvax®	Immunization for adults born after 1957 without documentation of live vaccine on or after first birthday, physician-diagnosed measles, or laboratory evidence of immunity should be vaccinated, ideally with two doses of vaccine separated by no less than 1 month; for those previously vaccinated with one dose of measles vaccine, revaccination is recommended for students entering colleges and other institutions of higher education, for healthcare workers at the time of employment, and for international travelers who visit endemic areas.	Refrigerate at 2°C to 8°C. Discard if left at room temperature for over 8 hours. Protect from light.	SubQ (outer aspect of upper arm): Children ≥15 months and Adults: 0.5 mL; no routine booster.

Drug	Use	Stability	Dosage and Administration
Meningococcal polysaccharide vaccine (groups A, C, Y, and W-135) Menomune®-A/C/Y/W-135	Immunization of children≥2 years of age and adults in epidemic or endemic areas as might be determined in a population delineated by neighborhood, school, dormitory, or other reasonable boundary; the prevalent serogroup in such a situation should match a serogroup in the vaccine. Individuals at particular high-risk include persons with terminal component complement deficiencies and those with anatomic or function asplenia. For use with travelers visiting areas of a country that are recognized as having hyperendemic or epidemic meningococcal disease. Vaccinations should be considered for household or institutional contacts of persons with meningococcal disease as an adjunct to appropriate antibiotic chemoprophylaxis as well as medical and laboratory personnel at risk of exposure to meningococcal disease.	Store at 2°C to 8°C (35°F to 46°F).	SubQ: One dose (0.5 mL); individuals who are sensitive to thimerosal should receive single-dose pack (reconstituted with 0.78 mL vial without preservative); the need for booster is unknown; have epinephrine 1:1000 available
Mumps virus vaccine (live/attenuated) Mumpsvax®	Mumps prophylaxis by promoting active immunity **Note:** Trivalent measles-mumps-rubella (M-M-R®) vaccine is the preferred agent for most children and many adults. Persons born prior to 1957 are generally considered immune and need not be vaccinated.	Refrigerate; protect from light. Discard within 8 hours after reconstitution.	SubQ (outer aspect of upper arm): Children ≥15 months and Adults: 0.5 mL; no booster
Plague vaccine	Vaccinate selected travelers to countries where avoidance of rodents and fleas is impossible; laboratory and field personnel working with *Yersinia pestis* organisms possibly resistant to antimicrobials; those engaged in *Yersinia pestis* aerosol experiments or in field operations in areas with enzootic plague where regular exposure to potentially infected wild rodents, rabbits, or their fleas cannot be prevented; prophylactic antibiotics may be indicated following definite exposure, whether or not the exposed persons have been vaccinated.		I.M.: Three doses: First dose 1 mL, second dose (0.2 mL) 1 month later; third dose (0.2 mL) 5 months after the second dose; booster at 1- to 2-year intervals if exposure continues

IMMUNIZATIONS[1] (VACCINES[2]) *(Continued)*

Drug	Use	Stability	Dosage and Administration
Pneumococcal conjugate vaccine (7-valent) Prevnar®	Immunization of infants and toddlers against active disease caused by *Streptococcus pneumoniae* due to serotypes included in the vaccine	Store refrigerated at 2°C to 8°C (36°F to 46°F).	Use of the pneumococcal conjugate vaccine does not replace the use of the 23-valent vaccine in children >24 months of age with sickle cell disease, asplenia, HIV infection, chronic illness, or if immunocompromised. I.M. **Infants: 2-6 months:** 0.5 mL at approximately 2 month-interval for 3 consecutive doses, followed by a fourth dose of 0.5 mL at 12-15 months of age. The first dose may be given as young as 2 months of age, but is typically given at 6 weeks of age. In case of a moderate shortage of vaccine, defer the fourth dose until shortage is resolved; in case of a severe shortage of vaccine, defer third and fourth doses until shortage is resolved. **Infants and Children (previously unvaccinated):** *7-11 months:* 0.5 mL for a total of 3 doses; 2 doses at least 4 weeks apart, followed by a third dose after the 1-year birthday, separated from the second dose by at least 2 months *12-23 months:* 0.5 mL for a total of two doses, separated by at least 2 months *24-59 months:* *Healthy Children:* 0.5 mL as a single dose. *Children with sickle cell disease, asplenia, HIV infection, chronic illness, or immunocompromising conditions (not including bone marrow transplants with results pending):* Use PPV23 (pneumococcal polysaccharide vaccine, polyvalent) at 12- and 24-months until studies are complete): 0.5 mL for a total of 2 doses, separated by 2 months **Children (previously vaccinated with a lapse in vaccination administration):** *7-11 months:* Previously received 1 or 2 doses PCV7: 0.5 mL dose at 7-11 months of age, followed by a second dose ≥2 months later at 12-15 months of age. *12-23 months:* Previously received 1 dose before 12 months: 0.5 mL dose, followed by a second dose ≥2 months later. Previously received 2 doses before 12 months: 0.5 mL dose ≥2 months after the most recent dose. *24-59 months:* Any incomplete schedule: 0.5 mL as a single dose. **Note:** Patients with chronic diseases or immunosuppressing conditions should receive 2 doses ≥2 months apart.

Drug	Use	Stability	Dosage and Administration
Pneumococcal polysaccharide vaccine (polyvalent) Pneumovax® 23	For children >2 years of age and adults who are at increased risk of pneumococcal disease and its complications because of underlying health conditions; older adults, including those ≥65 years of age	Refrigerate.	SubQ, I.M. (deltoid muscle or lateral migthigh): **Children >2 years and Adults:** 0.5 mL; have epinephrine (1:1000) available. **Revaccination** should be considered if: ≥6 years have elapsed since initial vaccination; for patients who received 14-valent pneumococcal vaccine and are at highest risk (asplenic) for fatal infection; at ≥6 years in patients with nephrotic syndrome, renal failure, or transplant recipients; and 3-5 years in children with nephrotic syndrome, asplenia, or sickle cell disease. Use with caution in individuals who have had episodes of pneumococcal infection within the preceeding 3 years; may result in increased reactions to vaccine or cause relapse in patients with stable idiopathic thrombocytopenia purpura. **Previously vaccinated with PCV7 vaccine:** *With sickle cell disease, asplenia, immunocompromised or HIV infection:* 0.5 mL at 2 years of age and 2 months after last dose of PCV7; revaccination with PPV23 should be given 5 years for children >10 years of age and every 3-5 years for children 10 years of age; revaccination should not be administered <3 years after the previous PPV23 dose *With chronic illness:* 0.5 mL at 2 years of age and 2 months after last dose of PCV7; revaccination with PPV23 is not recommended *Following bone marrow transplant (use of PCV7 under study):* Administer one dose PPV23 at 12- and 24-months following BMT.
Poliovirus vaccine (inactivated) IPOL®	All children should receive four doses of IPV (at age 2 months, age 4 months, between ages 6-18 months, and between ages 4-6 years). OPV supplies are expected to be very limited in the United States after inventories are depleted. ACIP reaffirms its support for the global eradication initiative and use of OPV as the vaccine of choice to eradicate polio where it is endemic. Oral poliovirus vaccine (OPV), if available, may be used only for the following special circumstances: Mass vaccination campaigns to control outbreaks of paralytic polio; unvaccinated children who will be traveling within 4 weeks to areas where polio is endemic or epidemic (these children may accept the recommended number of vaccine injections; children of parents who do not accept the recommended number of vaccine injections; children of parents who do not receive OPV only for the third or fourth dose or both; healthcare providers should administer OPV only after discussing the risk for VAPP with parents or caregivers)		**Infants 6-12 weeks of age:** Oral: 0.5 mL; second dose 6-8 weeks after first dose (commonly at 4 months); third dose 8-12 months after second dose (commonly at 18 months) **Older Children and Adults** (adolescents through 18 years of age): SubQ: Two 0.5 mL doses 4-8 weeks apart and a third dose of 0.5 mL 6-12 months after second dose. Enhanced-potency inactivated poliovirus vaccine (E-IPV) is preferred for primary vaccination of adults, two doses 4-8 weeks apart, a third dose 6-12 months after the second. For adults with a completed primary series and for whom a booster is indicated, either OPV or E-IPV can be given (E-IPV preferred). If immediate protection is needed, either OPV or E-IPV is recommended. **Booster:** All children who have received primary immunization series, should receive a single follow-up dose and all children who have not should complete primary series.

IMMUNIZATIONS[1] (VACCINES[2]) *(Continued)*

Drug	Use	Stability	Dosage and Administration
Rabies immune globulin (human) BayRab®; Imogam® Rabies-HT	Part of postexposure prophylaxis of persons with rabies exposure who lack a history of pre-exposure or postexposure prophylaxis with rabies vaccine or a recently documented neutralizing antibody response to previous rabies vaccination; it is preferable to give RIG with the first dose of vaccine, but it can be given up to 8 days after vaccination. **Note:** RIG should always be administered in conjunction with rabies vaccine (HDCV) regimen (as soon as possible after the first dose of vaccine, up to 8 days). Persons with an adequate titer and those who have been completely immunized with rabies vaccine should not receive RIG, only booster doses of HDCV.	Refrigerate.	I.M. (gluteal muscle): 20 units/kg in a single dose Infiltrate half of the dose locally around the wound; administer the remainder I.M.
Rabies virus vaccine Imovax® Rabies; RabAvert®	**Pre-exposure immunization:** Vaccinate persons with greater than usual risk due to occupation or avocation including veterinarians, rangers, animal handlers, certain laboratory workers, and persons living in or visiting countries for >1 month where rabies is a constant threat. Complete pre-exposure prophylaxis does not eliminate the need for additional therapy with rabies vaccine after a rabies exposure. **Postexposure prophylaxis:** If a bite from a carrier animal is unprovoked and it is not captured and rabies is present in that species and area, administer rabies immune globulin (RIG) and the vaccine as indicated.	Refrigerate at 2°–8°C (36°–46°F); do not freeze. Protect from light. Use reconstituted vaccine immediately.	I.M. (deltoid muscle, in adults and older children; outer aspect of the thigh for younger children): **Pre-exposure prophylaxis:** 1 mL on days 0, 7, and 21-28; prolonging the interval between doses does not interfere with immunity achieved after concluding dose of the basic series. **Postexposure prophylaxis** (Cleanse wound with soap and water first;): *Persons not previously immunized:* 20 units/kg body weight, half infiltrated at bite site if possible, remainder I.M. and 5 doses of rabies vaccine, 1 mL on days 0, 3, 7, 14, and 28 *Persons who have have previously received postexposure prophylaxis, pre-exposure series, or have a documented adequate rabies antibody titer:* 1 mL of either vaccine on days 0 and 3; do not administer RIG *Booster* (for occupational or other continuing risk): 1 mL every 2-5 years (or based on antibody titers)
Rubella virus vaccine (live) Meruvax® II	Selective active immunization against rubella; recommended for persons from 12 months of age to puberty; all adults lacking documentation of live vaccine on or after first birthday, or laboratory evidence of immunity should be vaccinated (particularly women of childbearing age; young adults who work in or congregate in hospitals, colleges, and on military bases; susceptible travelers) **Note:** Trivalent measles-mumps-rubella (M-M-R® II) vaccine is the preferred agent for most children and many adults. Persons born prior to 1957 are generally considered immune and need not be vaccinated.	Refrigerate; store at 2°C to 8°C (36°F to 46°F). Discard reconstituted vaccine after 8 hours. Ship vaccine at 10°C; may use dry ice. Protect from light.	Children ≥12 months and Adults: SubQ (outer aspect of upper arm): 0.5 mL; avoid injection into blood vessel.

Drug	Use	Stability	Dosage and Administration
Smallpox vaccine[4] Dryvax®	Active immunization against vaccinia virus, the causative agent of smallpox. ACIP recommends vaccination of laboratory workers at risk of exposure from cultures or contaminated animals which may be a source of vaccinia or related Orthopoxviruses capable of causing infections in humans (monkeypox, cowpox, or variola). Revaccination is recommended every 10 years. In October 2002, the FDA approved the licensing of the current stockpile of smallpox vaccine. This approval allows the vaccine to be distributed and administered in the event of a smallpox attack.	Store at 2°C to 8°C (36°F to 46°F). Do not freeze.	Using a bifurcated needle, 1 drop of vaccine is introduced into the superficial layers of the skin using a multiple-puncture technique. The skin over the insertion of the deltoid muscle or the posterior aspect of the arm over the triceps are the preferred sites for vaccination. A single-use bifurcated needle should be dipped carefully into the reconstituted vaccine (following removal of rubber stopper). Visually confirm that the needle picks up a drop of vaccine solution. Deposit the drop of vaccine onto clean, dry skin at the vaccination site. Holding the bifurcated needle perpendicular to the skin, punctures are to be made rapidly into the superficial skin of the vaccination site. The puncture strokes should be vigorous enough to allow a trace of blood to appear after approximately 15-20 seconds. Wipe off any remaining vaccine with dry sterile gauze. To prevent transmission of the virus, cover vaccination site with gauze and cover gauze with a semipermeable barrier or clothing. Good handwashing prevents inadvertent inoculation. Dispose of all materials in a biohazard waste container. All materials must be burned, boiled, or autoclaved. If no evidence of vaccine take is apparent after 7 days, the individual may be vaccinated again.
Tetanus immune globulin (human) BayTet™	Passive immunization against tetanus (tetanus immune globulin is preferred over tetanus antitoxin for treatment of active tetanus); part of the management of an unclean wound in a person whose history of previous receipt of tetanus toxoid is unknown or who has received less than three doses of tetanus toxoid; elderly may require TIG more often than younger patients with tetanus infection due to declining antibody titers with age.	Refrigerate at 2°C to 8°C (36°F to 46°F). Never administer tetanus toxoid (Td) and TIG in the same syringe (toxoid will be neutralized).	Toxoid may be given at a separate site. Have epinephrine 1:1000 available. Boosters will be necessary. I.M.: **Prophylaxis:** Children: 4 units/kg (some recommend administering 250 units to small children) Adults: 250 units **Treatment:** Children: 500-3000 units (infiltrate some solution locally around the wound) Adults: 3000-6000 units
Tetanus toxoid (adsorbed)	Selective induction of active immunity against tetanus toxoid fluid. Tetanus and diphtheria toxoids for adult use (Td) is the preferred immunizing agent for most adults and/or children after 7 years of age. Young children should receive trivalent DTwP or DTaP (diphtheria/tetanus/pertussis – whole cell or acellular), as part of their childhood immunization program, unless pertussis is contraindicated, then TD is warranted. **Note:** Not equivalent to tetanus toxoid fluid.	Refrigerate; do not freeze.	Have epinephrine 1:1000 available. Avoid injection into a blood vessel. I.M. (midthigh laterally or deltoid): Adults: 0.5 mL; repeat 0.5 mL at 4-8 weeks after the first dose and at 6-12 months after the second dose; booster every 5-10 years
Tetanus toxoid (fluid)	Detection of delayed hypersensitivity and assessment of cell-mediated immunity; active immunization against tetanus in the rare adult or child who is allergic to the aluminum adjuvant (a product containing adsorbed tetanus toxoid is preferred)	Refrigerate.	Have epinephrine 1:1000 available. Anergy testing: Adults: Intradermal: 0.1 mL (Td, TD, DTaP/DTwP recommended): Three doses of 0.5 mL I.M. or SubQ at 4- to 8-week intervals; give fourth dose 6-12 months after third dose; booster: 0.5 mL I.M. SubQ every 10 years

IMMUNIZATIONS[1] (VACCINES[2]) *(Continued)*

Drug	Use	Stability	Dosage and Administration
Typhoid vaccine Typhim Vi®; Vivotif Berna®	**Parenteral:** Promotes active immunity to typhoid fever for patients intimately exposed to a typhoid carrier or foreign travel to a typhoid fever endemic area. **Oral:** Immunization of children >6 years and adults who expect intimate exposure of or household contact with typhoid fever, travelers to areas of the world with a risk of exposure to typhoid fever, and workers in microbiology laboratories with expected frequent contact with *S. typhi*. **Typhoid vaccine:** Live, attenuated typhoid vaccine should not be administered to immunocompromised persons, including those known to be infected with HIV (parenteral inactivated vaccine is a theoretically safer alternative for this group)	Refrigerate, do not freeze; if mistakenly placed in a freezer, remove as soon as possible and place in refrigerator (potency unaffected). Can be used if exposed to temperature ≤60°F.	**I.M. (deltoid muscle): Typhim Vi®: Children ≥2 years and Adults:** 0.5 mL (25 mcg) injection in given at least 2 weeks prior to expected exposure; reimmunization: 0.5 mL single dose every 2 years is currently recommended for repeated or continued exposure **Oral: Children ≥6 years and Adults:** Swallow 1 capsule whole (do not chew) 1 hour before a meal with cold or lukewarm drink on alternate days (day 1, 3, 5, and 7) for a total of 4 doses; booster every 5 years (full course). **Note:** Not all recipients of typhoid vaccine will be fully protected against typhoid fever. Unless a complete immunization schedule is followed, an optimum immune response may not be achieved.
Varicella virus vaccine Varivax®	The American Association of Pediatrics recommends that the chickenpox vaccine should be given to all healthy children between 12 months of age to 18 years. Children 12 months of age to 13 years who have not been immunized or who have not had chickenpox should receive 1 vaccination while children 13-18 years of age require 2 vaccinations 4-8 weeks apart. The vaccine has been added to the childhood immunization schedule for infants 12-28 months of age and children 11-12 years of age who have not been vaccinated previously or who have not had the disease. It is recommended to be given with the measles, mumps, and rubella (MMR) vaccine.	Store powder in freezer at -15°C (5°F); may be stored under refrigeration for up to 72 continuous hours prior to reconstitution. Protect from light. Discard vaccine if not used within 72 hours. Store diluent separately at room temperature or in refrigerator.	SubQ: **Children 12 months to 12 years:** 0.5 mL **Children ≥12 years to Adults:** SubQ: 2 doses of 0.5 mL separated by 4-8 weeks.
Varicella-zoster immune globulin (human)	Passive immunization of susceptible immunodeficient patients after exposure to varicella. Most effective if begun within 96 hours of exposure. There is no evidence that VZIG modifies established varicella-zoster infections. **Restrict administration to:** Patients with neoplastic disease (leukemia, lymphoma); congenital or acquired immunodeficiency; immunosuppressive therapy with steroids, antimetabolites, or other immunosuppressive treatment regimens; newborns or mothers who had onset of chickenpox within 5 days before delivery or within 48 hours after delivery; premature infant (≥28 weeks gestation) whose mother has no history of chickenpox; premature infants (<28 weeks gestation or ≤1000 g VZIG) regardless of maternal history. **One of the following types of exposure to chickenpox or zoster patients may warrant administration:** Continuous household contact; playmate contact (>1 hour play indoors); hospital contact (in same 2-4 bedroom or adjacent beds in a large play ward or prolonged face-to-face contact with an infectious staff member of patient); susceptible to varicella-zoster; age <15 years (administer to immunocompromised adolescents and adults and to other older patients on an individual basis). An acceptable alternative to VZIG prophylaxis is to treat varicella, if it occurs, with high-dose I.V. acyclovir.	Refrigerate at 2°C to 8°C.	I.M. (gluteal muscle or large muscle mass): 125 units/10 kg (22 lb); maximum dose: 625 units (5 vials); minimum dose: 125 units; do not administer fractional doses. High-risk susceptible patients who are exposed again more than 3 weeks after a prior dose of VZIG should receive another full dose; there is no evidence VZIG modifies established varicella-zoster infections.

Drug	Use	Stability	Dosage and Administration
Yellow fever vaccine YF-VAX®	Induction of active immunity against yellow fever virus, primarily among persons traveling or living in areas where yellow fever infection exists. (Some countries require a valid international Certification of Vaccination showing receipt of vaccine; if a pregnant woman is to be vaccinated only to satisfy an international requirement, efforts should be made to obtain a waiver letter.) The WHO requires revaccination every 10 years to maintain traveler's vaccination certificate.	Do not use vaccine unless shipping case contains some dry ice on arrival; must be shipped on dry ice. Maintain vaccine at continuous temperature of -30°C to 5°C (-22°F to 41°F). Use within 1 hour of reconstitution.	SubQ: 0.5 mL single dose 10 days to 10 years before travel; booster every 10 years

¹Contact Poison Control Center.

²Federal law requires that date of administration, name of vaccine manufacturer, lot number of vaccine, and administering person's name, title, and address be entered into the patient's permanent medical record.

³Not commercially available in the U.S.; presently, all anthrax vaccine lots are owned by the U.S. Department of Defense. The Centers for Disease Control (CDC) does not currently recommend routine vaccination of the general public.

⁴The bulk of current supplies have been designated for use by the U.S. military. Bioterrorism experts have proposed immunization of first responders (including police, fire, and emergency workers), but these plans may not be implemented until additional stocks of vaccine are licensed. Recommendations for use in response to bioterrorism are regularly updated by the CDC, and may be found at www.cdc.gov.

⁵For patients at risk of hemorrhage following intramuscular injection, the ACIP recommends "it should be administered intramuscularly if, in the opinion of the physician familiar with the patients bleeding risk, the vaccine can be administered with reasonable safety by this route. If the patient receives antihemophilia or other similar therapy, intramuscular vaccination can be scheduled shortly after such therapy is administered. A fine needle (23 gauge or smaller) can be used for the vaccination and firm pressure applied to the site (without rubbing) for at least 2 minutes. The patient should be instructed concerning the risk of hematoma from the injection."

⁶All serious adverse reactions must be reported to the U.S. Department of Health and Human Services (DHHS) Vaccine Adverse Event Reporting System (VAERS), 1-800-822-7967.

TUBERCULOSIS TREATMENT

Tuberculin Skin Test Recommendations[1]

Children for whom immediate skin testing is indicated:

- Contacts of persons with confirmed or suspected infectious tuberculosis (contact investigation); this includes children identified as contacts of family members or associates in jail or prison in the last 5 years

- Children with radiographic or clinical findings suggesting tuberculosis

- Children immigrating from endemic countries (eg, Asia, Middle East, Africa, Latin America)

- Children with travel histories to endemic countries and/or significant contact with indigenous persons from such countries

Children who should be tested annually for tuberculosis[2]:

- Children infected with HIV or living in household with HIV-infected persons

- Incarcerated adolescents

Children who should be tested every 2-3 years[2]:

- Children exposed to the following individuals: HIV-infected, homeless, residents of nursing homes, institutionalized adolescents or adults, users of illicit drugs, incarcerated adolescents or adults, and migrant farm workers. Foster children with exposure to adults in the preceding high-risk groups are included.

Children who should be considered for tuberculin skin testing at ages 4-6 and 11-16 years:

- Children whose parents immigrated (with unknown tuberculin skin test status) from regions of the world with high prevalence of tuberculosis; continued potential exposure by travel to the endemic areas and/or household contact with persons from the endemic areas (with unknown tuberculin skin test status) should be an indication for repeat tuberculin skin testing

- Children without specific risk factors who reside in high-prevalence areas; in general, a high-risk neighborhood or community does not mean an entire city is at high risk; rates in any area of the city may vary by neighborhood, or even from block to block; physicians should be aware of these patterns in determining the likelihood of exposure; public health officials or local tuberculosis experts should help clinicians identify areas that have appreciable tuberculosis rates

Children at increased risk of progression of infection to disease: Those with other medical risk factors, including diabetes mellitus, chronic renal failure, malnutrition, and congenital or acquired immunodeficiencies deserve special consideration. Without recent exposure, these persons are not at increased risk of acquiring tuberculosis infection. Underlying immune deficiencies associated with these conditions theoretically would enhance the possibility for progression to severe disease. Initial histories of potential exposure to tuberculosis should be included on all of these patients. If these histories or local epidemiologic factors suggest a possibility of exposure, immediate and periodic tuberculin skin testing should be considered. An initial Mantoux tuberculin skin test should be performed before initiation of immunosuppressive therapy in any child with an underlying condition that necessitates immunosuppressive therapy.

---

[1]BCG immunization is not a contraindication to tuberculin skin testing.

[2]Initial tuberculin skin testing is at the time of diagnosis or circumstance, beginning as early as at age 3 months.

Adapted from "Report of the Committee on Infectious Diseases," *2003 Red Book*®, 26th ed, 646.

Table 1. Tuberculosis Prophylaxis
Infection Without Disease (Positive Tuberculin Test)[1]

Specific Circumstances/ Organism	Comments	Regimen
Regardless of age (see INH Preventive Therapy)	Rx indicated	INH (5 mg/kg/d, maximum: 300 mg/d for adults, 10 mg/kg/d not to exceed 300 mg/d for children). Results with 6 months of treatment are nearly as effective as 12 months (65% vs 75% reduction in disease). *Am Thoracic Society* (6 months), *Am Acad Pediatrics*, 1991 (9 months). If CXR is abnormal, treat for 12 months. In HIV-positive patient, treatment for a minimum of 12 months, some suggest longer. Monitor transaminases monthly (*MMWR Morb Mortal Wkly Rep* 1989, 38:247).
Age <35 y	Rx indicated	Reanalysis of earlier studies favors INH prophylaxis for 6 months (if INH-related hepatitis case fatality rate is <1% and TB case fatality is ≥6.7%, which appears to be the case, monitor transaminases monthly (*Arch Int Med*, 1990, 150:2517).
INH-resistant organisms likely	Rx indicated	Data on efficacy of alternative regimens is currently lacking. Regimens include ETB + RIF daily for 6 months. PZA + RIF daily for 2 months, then INH + RIF daily until sensitivities from index case (if available) known, then if INH-CR, discontinue INH and continue RIF for 9 months, otherwise INH + RIF for 9 months (this latter is *Am Acad Pediatrics*, 1991 recommendation).
INH + RIF resistant organisms likely	Rx indicated	Efficacy of alternative regimens is unknown; PZA (25-30 mg/kg/d P.O.) + ETB (15-25 mg/kg/d P.O.) (at 25 mg/kg ETB, monitoring for retrobulbar neuritis required), for 6 months unless HIV-positive, then 12 months; PZA + ciprofloxacin (750 mg P.O. bid) or ofloxacin (400 mg P.O. bid) x 6-12 months (*MMWR Morb Mortal Wkly Rep*, 1992, 41(RR11):68).

INH = isoniazid; RIF = rifampin; KM = kanamycin; ETB = ethambutol
SM = streptomycin; CXR = chest x-ray; Rx = treatment
See also guidelines for interpreting PPD in "Skin Testing for Delayed Hypersensitivity."
[1]Tuberculin test (TBnT). The standard is the Mantoux test, 5 TU PPD in 0.1 mL diluent stabilized with Tween 80. Read at 48-72 hours measuring maximum diameter of induration. A reaction ≥5 mm is defined as positive in the following: positive HIV or risk factors, recent close case contacts, CXR consistent with healed TBc. ≥10 mm is positive in foreign-born in countries of high prevalence, injection drug users, low income populations, nursing home residents, patients with medical conditions which increase risk (see above, preventive treatment). ≥15 mm is positive in all others (*Am Rev Resp Dis*, 1990, 142:725). Two-stage TBnT: Use in individuals to be tested regularly (ie, healthcare workers). TBn reactivity may decrease over time but be boosted by skin testing. If unrecognized, individual may be incorrectly diagnosed as recent converter. If first TBnT is reactive but <10 mm, repeat 5 TU in 1 week, if then ≥10 mm = positive, not recent conversion (*Am Rev Resp Dis*, 1979, 119:587).

TUBERCULOSIS TREATMENT *(Continued)*

Changes From Prior Recommendations on Tuberculin Testing and Treatment of Latent Tuberculosis Infection (LTBI)

Tuberculin Testing

- Emphasis on targeted tuberculin testing among persons at high risk for recent LTBI or with clinical conditions that increase the risk for tuberculosis (TB), regardless of age; testing is discouraged among persons at lower risk

- For patients with organ transplants and other immunosuppressed patients (eg, persons receiving the equivalent of ≥15 mg/day prednisone for 1 month or more), 5 mm of induration rather than 10 mm of induration rather than 10 mm of induration as a cut-off level for tuberculin positivity

- A tuberculin skin test conversion is defined as in increase of ≥10 mm of induration within a 2-year period, regardless of age

Treatment of Latent Tuberculosis Infection

- For human immunodeficiency virus (HIV)-negative persons, isoniazid given for 9 months is preferred over 6-month regimens

- For HIV-positive persons and those with fibrotic lesions on chest x-ray consistent with previous TB, isoniazid should be given for 9 months instead of 12 months

- For HIV-negative and HIV-positive persons, rifampin and pyrazinamide should be given for 2 months

- For HIV-negative and HIV-positive persons, rifampin should be given for 4 months

Clinical and Laboratory Monitoring

- Routine baseline and follow-up laboratory monitoring can be eliminated in most persons with LTBI, except for those with HIV infection, pregnant women (or those in the immediate postpartum period), and persons with chronic liver disease or those who use alcohol regularly

- Emphasis on clinical monitoring for signs and symptoms of possible adverse effects, with prompt evaluation and changes in treatment, as indicated

Adapted from *MMWR*, 2000, 49(RR-6).

Table 2. Recommended Treatment Regimens for Drug-Susceptible Tuberculosis in Infants, Children, and Adolescents

Infection or Disease Category	Regimen	Remarks
Latent tuberculosis infection (positive tuberculin skin test, no disease):		
• Isoniazid-susceptible	9 months of isoniazid once a day	If daily therapy is not possible, directly observed therapy twice a week may be used for 9 months.
• Isoniazid-resistant	6 months of rifampin once a day	
• Isoniazid-rifampin-resistant[1]	Consult a tuberculosis specialist	
Pulmonary and extrapulmonary (except meningitis)	2 months of isoniazid, rifampin, and pyrazinamide daily, followed by 4 months of isoniazid and rifampin[2]	If possible drug resistance is a concern, another drug (ethambutol or aminoglycoside) is added to the initial 3-drug therapy until drug susceptibilities are determined. Directly observed therapy is highly desirable.
		If hilar adenopathy only, a 6-month course of isoniazid and rifampin is sufficient.
		Drugs can be given 2 or 3 times/week under directly observed therapy in the initial phase if nonadherence is likely.
Meningitis	2 months of isoniazid, rifampin, pyrazinamide, and aminoglycoside or ethionamide, once a day, followed by 7-10 months of isoniazid and rifampin once a day or twice a week (9-12 months total)	A fourth drug, usually an aminoglycoside, is given with initial therapy until drug susceptibility is known.
		For patients who may have acquired tuberculosis in geographic areas where resistance to streptomycin is common, capreomycin, kanamycin, or amikacin may be used instead of streptomycin.

[1]Duration of therapy is longer for human immunodeficiency virus (HIV)-infected people, and additional drugs may be indicated.

[2]Medications should be administered daily for the first 2 weeks to 2 months of treatment and then can be administered 2-3 times/week by directly observed therapy.

Adapted from "Report of the Committee on Infectious Diseases," *2003 Red Book®*, 26th ed, 649.

TUBERCULOSIS TREATMENT *(Continued)*

Table 3. Recommended Drug Regimens for Treatment of Latent Tuberculosis Infection in Children

Drug	Interval and Duration	Comments
Isoniazid	Daily for 9 mo	This includes treatment for any child <5 years old who is exposed to household members or other close contacts who are potentially infectious even if skin test is negative
	Twice weekly for 9 mo	
Rifampin	Daily for 4-9 mo	No controlled trials; only to be used in INH intolerant or resistant
Rifampin-pyrazinamide	Daily for 3 mo	No controlled trials; only to be used in INH intolerant or resistant

Modified from *MMWR*, 2000, 14(RR-6).

Table 4. Recommended Drug Regimens for Treatment of Latent Tuberculosis Infection in Adults

Drug	Interval and Duration	Comments	Rating[1] (Evidence)[2] HIV⁻	Rating[1] (Evidence)[2] HIV⁺
Isoniazid	Daily for 9 months[3,4]	In HIV-infected patients, isoniazid may be administered concurrently with nucleoside reverse transcriptase inhibitors (NRTIs), protease inhibitors, or non-nucleoside reverse transcriptase inhibitors (NNRTIs)	A (II)	A (II)
	Twice weekly for 9 months[3,4]	Directly observed therapy (DOT) must be used with twice-weekly dosing	B (II)	B (II)
Isoniazid	Daily for 6 months[4]	Not indicated for HIV-infected persons, those with fibrotic lesions on chest radiographs, or children	B (I)	C (I)
	Twice weekly for 6 months[4]	DOT must be used with twice-weekly dosing	B (II)	C (I)
Rifampin	Daily for 4 months	For persons who cannot tolerate pyrazinamide	B (II)	B (III)
		For persons who are contacts of patients with isoniazid-resistant, rifampin-susceptible TB who cannot tolerate pyrazinamide		
Rifampin plus pyrazinamide	Daily for 2 months	May also be offered to persons who are contacts of pyrazinamide patients with isoniazid-resistant, rifampin-susceptible TB	B (II)	A (I)
		In HIV-infected patients, protease inhibitors or NNRTIs should generally not be administered concurrently with rifampin. Rifabutin can be used as an alternative for patients treated with indinavir, nelfinavir, amprenavir, ritonavir, or efavirenz, and possibly with nevirapine or soft-gel saquinavir[5]		
	Twice weekly for 2-3 months	DOT must be used with twice-weekly dosing	C (II)	C (I)

[1]Strength of recommendation: A = preferred; B = acceptable alternative; C = offer when A and B cannot be given.

[2]Quality of evidence: I = randomized clinical trial data; II = data from clinical trials that are not randomized or were conducted in other populations; III = expert opinion.

[3]Recommended regimen for children <18 years of age.

[4]Recommended regimens for pregnant women. Some experts would use rifampin and pyrazinamide for 2 months as an alternative regimen in HIV-infected pregnant women, although pyrazinamide should be avoided during the first trimester.

[5]Rifabutin should not be used with hard-gel saquinavir or delavirdine. When used with other protease inhibitors or NNRTIs, dose adjustment of rifabutin may be required.

Adapted from *MMWR Recomm Rep*, 2000, 49(RR6).

Table 5. TB Drugs in Special Situations

Drug	Pregnancy[1]	CNS TB Disease	Renal Insufficiency
Isoniazid	Safe	Good penetration	Normal clearance
Rifampin	Safe	Fair penetration Penetrates inflamed meninges (10% to 20%)	Normal clearance
Pyrazinamide	Avoid	Good penetration	Clearance reduced Decrease dose or prolong interval
Ethambutol	Safe	Penetrates inflamed meninges only (4% to 64%)	Clearance reduced Decrease dose or prolong interval
Streptomycin	Avoid	Penetrates inflamed meninges only	Clearance reduced Decrease dose or prolong interval
Capreomycin	Avoid	Penetrates inflamed meninges only	Clearance reduced Decrease dose or prolong interval
Kanamycin	Avoid	Penetrates inflamed meninges only	Clearance reduced Decrease dose or prolong interval
Ethionamide	Do not use	Good penetration	Normal clearance
Para-amino-salicylic acid	Safe	Penetrates inflamed meninges only (10% to 50%)	Incomplete data on clearance
Cycloserine	Avoid	Good penetration	Clearance reduced Decrease dose or prolong interval
Ciprofloxacin	Do not use	Fair penetration (5% to 10%) Penetrates inflamed meninges (50% to 90%)	Clearance reduced Decrease dose or prolong interval
Ofloxacin	Do not use	Fair penetration (5% to 10%) Penetrates inflamed meninges (50% to 90%)	Clearance reduced Decrease dose or prolong interval
Amikacin	Avoid	Penetrates inflamed meninges only	Clearance reduced Decrease dose or prolong interval
Clofazimine	Avoid	Penetration unknown	Clearance probably normal

[1]Safe = the drug has not been demonstrated to have teratogenic effects.

Avoid = data on the drug's safety are limited, or the drug is associated with mild malformations (as in the aminoglycosides).

Do not use = studies show an association between the drug and premature labor, congenital malformations, or teratogenicity.

TUBERCULOSIS TREATMENT *(Continued)*

Table 6. Recommendations for Coadministering Different Antiretroviral
Drugs With the Antimycobacterial Drugs Rifabutin and Rifampin

Antiretroviral	Use in Combination with Rifabutin	Use in Combination with Rifampin	Comments
Saquinavir[1]			
Hard-gel capsules (HGC)	Possibly[2], if antiretroviral regimen also includes ritonavir	Possibly, if antiretroviral regimen also includes ritonavir	Coadministration of saquinavir SGC with usual-dose rifabutin (300 mg/day or 2-3 times/week) is a possibility. However, the pharmacokinetic data and clinical experience for this combination are limited.
Soft-gel capsules (SGC)	Probably[3]	Possibly, if antiretroviral regimen also includes ritonavir	The combination of saquinavir SGC or saquinavir HGC and ritonavir, coadministered with 1) usual-dose rifampin (600 mg/day or 2-3 times/week), or 2) reduced-dose rifabutin (150 mg 2-3 times/week) is a possibility. However, the pharmacokinetic data and clinical experience for these combinations are limited. Coadministration of saquinavir or saquinavir SGC with rifampin is not recommended because rifampin markedly decreases concentrations of saquinavir.
Ritonavir	Probably	Probably	If the combination of ritonavir and rifabutin is used, then a substantially reduced-dose rifabutin regimen (150 mg 2-3 times/week) is recommended. Coadministration of ritonavir with usual-dose rifampin (600 mg/day or 2-3 times/week) is a possibility, though pharmacokinetic data and clinical experience are limited.
Indinavir	Yes	No	There is limited, but favorable, clinical experience with coadministration of indinavir[4] with a reduced daily dose of rifabutin (150 mg) or with the usual dose of rifabutin (300 mg 2-3 times/week). Coadministration of indinavir with rifampin is not recommended because rifampin markedly decreases concentrations of indinavir.
Nelfinavir	Yes	No	There is limited, but favorable, clinical experience with coadministration of nelfinavir[5] with a reduced daily dose of rifabutin (150 mg) or with the usual dose of rifabutin (300 mg 2-3 times/week). Coadministration of nelfinavir with rifampin is not recommended because rifampin markedly decreases concentrations of nelfinavir.
Amprenavir	Yes	No	Coadministration of amprenavir with a reduced daily dose of rifabutin (150 mg) or with the usual dose of rifabutin (300 mg 2-3 times/week) is a possibility, but there is no published clinical experience. Coadministration of amprenavir with rifampin is not recommended because rifampin markedly decreases concentrations of amprenavir.
Nevirapine	Yes	Possibly	Coadministration of nevirapine with usual-dose rifabutin (300 mg/day or 2-3 times/week) is a possibility based on pharmacokinetic study data. However, there is no published clinical experience for this combination. Data are insufficient to assess whether dose adjustments are necessary when rifampin is coadministered with nevirapine. Therefore, rifampin and nevirapine should be used only in combination if clearly indicated and with careful monitoring.
Delavirdine	No	No	Contraindicated because of the marked decrease in concentrations of delavirdine when administered with either rifabutin or rifampin.

Table 6. Recommendations for Coadministering Different Antiretroviral Drugs With the Antimycobacterial Drugs Rifabutin and Rifampin (continued)

Antiretroviral	Use in Combination with Rifabutin	Use in Combination with Rifampin	Comments
Efavirenz	Probably	Probably	Coadministration of efavirenz with increased-dose rifabutin (450 mg/day or 600 mg/day, or 600 mg 2-3 times/week) is a possibility, though there is no published clinical experience. Coadministration of efavirenz[6] with usual-dose rifampin (600 mg/day or 2-3 times/week) is a possibility, though there is no published clinical experience.

[1]Usual recommended doses are 400 mg twice daily for each of these protease inhibitors and 400 mg of ritonavir.

[2]Despite limited data and clinical experience, the use of this combination is potentially successful.

[3]Based on available data and clinical experience, the successful use of this combination is likely.

[4] Usual recommended dose is 800 mg every 8 hours; some experts recommend increasing the indinavir dose to 1000 mg every 8 hours if indinavir is used in combination with rifabutin.

[5]Usual recommended dose is 750 mg 3 times/day or 1250 mg twice daily; some experts recommend increasing the nelfinavir dose to 1000 mg if the 3-times/day dosing is used and nelfinavir is used in combination with rifabutin.

[6]Usual recommended dose is 600 mg/day; some experts recommend increasing the efavirenz dose to 800 mg/day if efavirenz is used in combination with rifampin.

Updated March 2000 from www.aidsinfo.nih.gov -"Updated Guidelines for the Use of Rifabutin or Rifampin for the Treatment and Prevention of Tuberculosis Among HIV-Infected Patients Taking Protease Inhibitors or Non-nucleoside Reverse Transcriptase Inhibitors," *MMWR*, March 10, 2000, 49(09):185-9.

Table 7. Criteria for Tuberculin Positivity, by Risk Group

Reaction ≥5 mm of Induration	Reaction ≥10 mm of Induration	Reaction ≥15 mm of Induration
HIV-positive persons	Recent immigrants (ie, within the last 5 years) from high prevalence countries	Persons with no risk factors for TB
Recent contacts of tuberculosis (TB) case patients	Injection drug users	
Fibrotic changes on chest radiograph consistent with prior TB	Residents and employees[1] of the following high risk congregate settings: prisons and jails, nursing homes and other long-term facilities for the elderly, hospitals and other healthcare facilities, residential facilities for patients with AIDS, and homeless shelters	
Patients with organ transplant and other immunosuppressed patients (receiving the equivalent of ≥15 mg/day of prednisone for 1 month)[2]	Mycobacteriology laboratory personnel	
	Persons with the following clinical conditions that place them at high risk: silicosis, diabetes mellitus, chronic renal failure, some hematologic disorders (eg, leukemias and lymphomas), other specific malignancies (eg, carcinoma of the head or neck and lung), weight loss of ≥10% of ideal body weight, gastrectomy, and jejunoileal bypass	
	Children <4 years of age or infants, children, and adolescents exposed to adults at high-risk	

[1]For persons who are otherwise at low risk and are tested at the start of employment, a reaction of ≥15 mm induration is considered positive.

[2]Risk of TB in patients treated with corticosteroids increases with higher dose and longer duration.

Modified from *MMWR Morb Mortal Wkly Rep*, 2000, 49(RR-6).

TUBERCULOSIS TREATMENT *(Continued)*

Table 8. Recommendations, Rankings, and Performance Indicators for Treatment of Patients With Tuberculosis (TB)

Recommendation	Ranking[1] (Evidence)[2]	Performance Indicator
Obtain bacteriologic confirmation and susceptibility testing for patients with TB or suspected of having TB	A (II)	90% of adults with or suspected of having TB have 3 cultures for mycobacteria obtained before initiation of antituberculosis therapy (50% of children 0-12 y)
Place persons with suspected or confirmed smear-positive pulmonary or laryngeal TB in respiratory isolation until noninfectious	A (II)	90% of persons with sputum smear-positive TB remain in respiratory isolation until smear converts to negative
Begin treatment of patients with confirmed or suspected TB disease with one of the following drug combinations, depending on local resistance patterns: INH + RIF + PZA **or** INH + RIF + PZA + EMB **or** INH + RIF + PZA + SM	A (III)	90% of all patients with TB are started on INH + RIF + PZA + EMB or SM in geographic areas where >4% of TB isolates are resistant to INH
Report each case of TB promptly to the local public health department	A (III)	100% of persons with active TB are reported to the local public health department within 1 week of diagnosis
Perform HIV testing for all patients with TB	A (III)	80% of all patients with TB have HIV status determined within 2 months of a diagnosis of TB
Treat patients with TB caused by a susceptible organism for 6 months, using an ATS/CDC-approved regimen	A (I)	90% of all patients with TB complete 6 months of therapy with 12 months of beginning treatment
Re-evaluate patients with TB who are smear positive at 3 months for possible nonadherence or infection with drug-resistant bacilli	A (III)	90% of all patients with TB who are smear positive at 3 months have sputum culture/susceptibility testing performed within 1 month of the 3-month visit
Add ≥2 new antituberculosis agents when TB treatment failure is suspected	A (II)	100% of patients with TB with suspected treatment failure are prescribed ≥2 new antituberculosis agents
Perform tuberculin skin testing on all patients with a history of ≥1 of the following: HIV infection, I.V. drug use, homelessness, incarceration, or contact with a person with pulmonary TB	A (II)	80% of persons in the indicated population groups receive tuberculin skin test and return for reading
Administer treatment for latent TB infection to all persons with latent TB infection, unless it can be documented that they received such treatment previously	A (I)	75% of patients with positive tuberculin skin tests who are candidates for treatment for latent TB infection complete a course of therapy within 12 months of initiation

Note: ATS/CDC = American Thoracic Society and Centers for Disease Control and Prevention; EMB = ethambutol; INH = isoniazid; PZA = pyrazinamide; RIF = rifampin; SM = streptomycin.

[1]Strength of recommendation: A = preferred; B = acceptable alternative; C = offer when A and B cannot be given.

[2]Quality of evidence: I = randomized clinical trial data; II = data from clinical trials that are not randomized or were conducted in other populations; III = expert opinion.

Adapted from the Infectious Diseases Society of America, *Clinical Infectious Diseases*, 2000, 31:633-9.

Table 9. Drug Regimens for Culture-Positive Pulmonary Tuberculosis Caused by Drug-Susceptible Organisms

Initial Phase			Continuation Phase			Range of Total Doses (minimal duration)	Rating[1] (Evidence)[2]	
Regimen	Drugs	Interval and Doses[3] (minimal duration)	Regimen	Drugs	Interval and Doses[3,4] (minimal duration)		HIV-	HIV+
1	INH RIF PZA EMB	Seven days per week for 56 doses (8 wk) or 5 d/wk for 40 doses (8 wk)[5]	1a	INH/RIF	Seven days per week for 126 doses (18 wk) or 5 d/wk for 90 doses (18 wk)[5]	182-130 (26 wk)	A (I)	A (II)
			1b	INH/RIF	Twice weekly for 36 doses (18 wk)	92-76 (26 wk)	A (I)	A (II)[6]
			1c[7]	INH/RPT	Once weekly for 18 doses (18 wk)	74-58 (26 wk)	B (I)	E (I)
2	INH RIF PZA EMB	Seven days per week for 14 doses (2 wk), then twice weekly for 12 doses (6 wk) or 5 d/wk for 10 doses (2 wk)[5], then twice weekly for 12 doses (6 wk)	2a	INH/RIF	Twice weekly for 36 doses (18 wk)	62-58 (26 wk)	A (II)	B (II)[6]
			2b[7]	INH/RPT	Once weekly for 18 doses (18 wk)	44-40 (26 wk)	B (I)	E (I)
3	INH RIF PZA EMB	Three times weekly for 24 doses (8 wk)	3a	INH/RIF	Three times weekly for 54 doses (18 wk)	78 (26 wk)	B (I)	B (II)
4	INH RIF EMB	Seven days per week for 56 doses (8 wk) or 5 d/wk for 40 doses (8 wk)[5]	4a	INH/RIF	Seven days per week for 217 doses (31 wk) or 5 d/wk for 155 doses (31 wk)[5]	273-195 (39 wk)	C (I)	C (II)
			4b	INH/RIF	Twice weekly for 62 doses (31 wk)	118-102 (39 wk)	C (I)	C (II)

Definition of abbreviations: EMB = ethambutol; INH = isoniazid; PZA = pyrazinamide; RIF = rifampin; RPT = rifapentine.

[1]Definitions of evidence ratings: A = preferred; B = acceptable alternative; C = offer when A and B cannot be given; E = should never be given.

[2]Definitions of evidence ratings: I = randomized clinical trial; II = data from clinical trials that were not randomized or were conducted in other populations; III = expert opinion.

[3]When directly observed therapy (DOT) is used, drugs may be given 5 days/week and the necessary number of doses adjusted accordingly. Although there are no studies that compare five with seven daily doses, extensive experience indicates this would be an effective practice.

[4]Patients with cavitation on initial chest radiograph and positive cultures at completion of 2 months of therapy should receive a 7-month (31-week; either 217 doses daily or 62 doses [twice weekly]) continuation phase.

[5]Five-day/week administration is always given by DOT. Rating for 5 day/week regimens is AIII.

[6]Not recommended for HIV-infected patients with CD4+ cell counts <100 cells/µL.

[7]Options 1c and 2b should be used only in HIV-negative patients who have negative sputum smears at the time of completion of 2 months of therapy and who do not have cavitation on initial chest radiograph. For patients started on this regimen and found to have a positive culture from the 2-month specimen, treatment should be extended an extra 3 months.

Adapted from *MMWR*, 2003, 52(RR11).

TUBERCULOSIS TREATMENT *(Continued)*

Table 10. Suggested Pyrazinamide Doses, Using Whole Tablets, for Adults Weighing 40-90 kg

	Weight (kg)[1]		
	40-55	56-75	76-90
Daily, mg (mg/kg)	1000 (18.2-25)	1500 (20-26.8)	2000[2] (22.2-26.3)
Thrice weekly, mg (mg/kg)	1500 (27.3-37.5)	2500 (33.3-44.6)	3000[2] (33.3-39.5)
Twice weekly, mg (mg/kg)	2000 (36.4-50)	3000 (40-53.6)	4000[2] (44.4-52.6)

[1]Based on estimated lean body weight
[2]Maximum dose regardless of weight.

Table 11. Suggested Ethambutol Doses, Using Whole Tablets, for Adults Weighing 40-90 kg

	Weight (kg)[1]		
	40-55	56-75	76-90
Daily, mg (mg/kg)	800 (14.5-20)	1200 (16-21.4)	1600[2] (17.8-21.1)
Thrice weekly, mg (mg/kg)	1200 (21.8-30)	2000 (26.7-35.7)	2400[2] (26.7-31.6)
Twice weekly, mg (mg/kg)	2000 (36.4-50)	2800 (37.3-50)	4000[2] (44.4-52.6)

[1]Based on estimated lean body weight
[2]Maximum dose regardless of weight.

TREATMENT OF SEXUALLY TRANSMITTED INFECTIONS

Type or Stage	Drugs of Choice / Dosage	Alternatives
CHLAMYDIAL INFECTION AND RELATED CLINICAL SYNDROMES[1]		
Urethritis, cervicitis, conjunctivitis, or proctitis (except lymphogranuloma venereum)		
	Azithromycin 1 g oral once **or** Doxycycline[2,3] 100 mg oral bid x 7 d	Ofloxacin[3] 300 mg oral bid x 7 d **or** Levofloxacin[3] 500 mg oral once/d x 7 d **or** Erythromycin[4] 500 mg oral qid x 7 d
Infection in pregnancy		
	Azithromycin 1 g oral once **or** Amoxicillin 500 mg oral tid x 7 d	Erythromycin[4] 500 mg oral qid x 7 d
Neonatal ophthalmia or pneumonia		
	Azithromycin 20 mg/kg oral once daily x 3 d	Erythromycin 12.5 mg/kg oral qid x 14 d[6]
Lymphogranuloma venereum		
	Doxycycline[2,3] 100 mg oral bid x 21 d	Erythromycin[4] 500 mg oral qid x 21 d
EPIDIDYMITIS		
	Ofloxacin 300 mg bid x 10 d **or** Levofloxacin 500 mg oral once daily x 10 d	Ceftriaxone 250 mg I.M. once **followed by** doxycycline[2] 100 mg oral bid x 10 d
GONORRHEA[6]		
Disseminated gonococcal infection		
	Ceftriaxone 1 g I.M. or I.V. q24h	Cefotaxime 1 g I.V. q8h **or** Ceftizoxime 1 g I.V. q8h **or** For persons allergic to β-lactam drugs: Ciprofloxacin 400 mg I.V. q12h **or** Levofloxacin 250 mg I.V. once daily **or** Ofloxacin 400 mg I.V. q12h **or** Spectinomycin 2 g I.M. q12h All regimens should be continued for 24-48 hours after improvement begins, at which time therapy may be switched to one of the following regimens to complete a full week of antimicrobial therapy: Cefixime 400 mg oral bid **or** Ciprofloxacin 500 mg oral bid **or** Levofloxacin 500 mg oral once daily **or** Ofloxacin 400 mg oral bid
Gonococcal meningitis and endocarditis		
	Ceftriaxone 1-2 g I.V. q12h	
Urethral, cervical, rectal, or pharyngeal		
	Cefixime 400 mg oral once **or** Ceftriaxone 125 mg I.M. once	Cefpodoxime 400 mg oral once **or** Ciprofloxacin[3,7] 500 mg oral once **or** Ofloxacin[3,7] 400 mg oral once **or** Levofloxacin[3,7] 250 mg oral once **or** Spectinomycin 2 g I.M. once[8]
PELVIC INFLAMMATORY DISEASE		
– parenteral	Cefotetan 2 g I.V. q12h **or** cefoxitin 2 g I.V. q6h **plus** doxycycline[3] 100 mg oral or I.V. q12h, until improved **followed by** doxycycline[3] 100 mg oral bid to complete 14 d[10] **or** Clindamycin 900 mg I.V. q8h **plus** gentamicin 2 mg/kg I.V. once, then 1.5 mg/kg I.V. q8h,[11] until improved **followed by** doxycycline[3] 100 mg oral bid to complete 14 d[10]	Ofloxacin[3] 400 mg I.V. q12h **or** levofloxacin[3] 500 mg I.V. once daily **plus** metronidazole 500 mg I.V. q8h[9] **or** Ampicillin/sulbactam 3 g I.V. q6h **plus** doxycycline[3] 100 mg oral or I.V. q12h **All continued until improved, then followed by** doxycycline[3] 100 mg oral bid to complete 14 d[10]
– oral	Ofloxacin[3] 400 mg bid x 14 d **or** Levofloxacin[3] 500 mg once daily x 14 d ± metronidazole[9] 500 mg bid x 14 d **or** Ceftriaxone 250 mg I.M. once **followed by** doxycycline[3,12] 100 mg bid x 14 d	Cefoxitin 2 g once **plus** probenecid 1 g oral once **followed by** doxycycline[3,12] 100 mg bid x 14 d
TRICHOMONIASIS		
	Metronidazole 2 g oral once **or** Tinidazole 2 g oral once	Metronidazole 375 or 500 mg oral bid x 7 d
BACTERIAL VAGINOSIS		
	Metronidazole 500 mg oral bid x 7 d **or** Metronidazole gel 0.75%[14] 5 g intravaginally once or twice daily x 5 d **or** Clindamycin 2% cream[14] 5 g intravaginally qhs x 3-7 d	Metronidazole 2 g oral once[13] or Flagyl ER® 750 mg once daily x 7 d **or** Clindamycin 300 mg oral bid x 7 d **or** Clindamycin ovules[14] 100 mg intravaginally once daily x 3 d

TREATMENT OF SEXUALLY TRANSMITTED INFECTIONS
(Continued)

Type or Stage	Drugs of Choice / Dosage	Alternatives
VULVOVAGINAL CANDIDIASIS		
	Intravaginal butoconazole, clotrimazole, miconazole, terconazole, or tioconazole[15] **or** Fluconazole 150 mg oral once	Nystatin 100,000 unit vaginal tablet once daily x 14 d
SYPHILIS		
Early (primary, secondary, or latent <1 y)		
	Penicillin G benzathine 2.4 million units I.M. once[16]	Doxycycline[3] 100 mg oral bid x 14 d
Late (>1 year's duration, cardiovascular, gumma, late-latent)		
	Penicillin G benzathine 2.4 million units I.M. weekly x 3 wk	Doxycycline[3] 100 mg oral bid x 4 wk
Neurosyphilis[17]		
	Penicillin G 3-4 million units I.V. q4h or 24 million units continuous I.V. infusion x 10-14 d	Penicillin G procaine 2.4 million units I.M. daily **plus** probenecid 500 mg qid oral, both x 10-14 d **or** Ceftriaxone 2 g I.V. once daily x 10-14 d
Congenital		
	Penicillin G 50,000 units/kg I.V. q8-12h for 10-14 d **or** Penicillin G procaine 50,000 units/kg I.M. daily for 10-14 d	
CHANCROID[18]		
	Azithromycin 1 g oral once **or** Ceftriaxone 250 mg I.M. once	Ciprofloxacin[3] 500 mg oral bid x 3 d **or** Erythromycin[4] 500 mg oral qid x 7 d
GENITAL WARTS[19]		
	Trichloroacetic or bichloroacetic acid, or podophyllin[3] or liquid nitrogen 1-2 times/wk until resolved **or** Imiquimod 5% 3 times/wk x 16 wk **or** Podofilox 0.5% bid x 3 d, 4 days rest, then repeated up to 4 times	Surgical removal **or** Laser surgery **or** Intralesional interferon
GENITAL HERPES		
First episode		
	Acyclovir 400 mg oral tid x 7-10 d **or** Famciclovir 250 mg oral tid x 7-10 d **or** Valacyclovir 1 g oral bid x 7-10 d	Acyclovir 200 mg oral 5 times/d x 7-10 d
Severe (hospitalized patients)		
	Acyclovir 5-10 mg/kg I.V. q8h x 5-7 d	
Suppression of recurrences[20]		
	Acyclovir 400 mg oral bid **or** Famciclovir 250 mg oral bid **or** Valacyclovir 500 mg - 1 g once daily[21]	Acyclovir 200 mg oral, 2-5 times/d
Episodic treatment of recurrences[22]		
	Acyclovir 800 mg oral tid x 2 d or 400 mg oral tid x 3-5 d[23] **or** Famciclovir 125 mg oral bid x 3-5 d[23] **or** Valacyclovir 500 mg oral bid x 3 d	
GRANULOMA INGUINALE		
	TMP-SMZ 1 double-strength tablet oral bid for a minimum of 3 wk **or** Doxycycline 100 oral bid for a minimum of 3 wk	Ciprofloxacin 750 mg oral bid for a minimum of 3 wk **or** Erythromycin base 500 mg oral qid for a minimum of 3 wk **or** Azithromycin 1 g oral once per week for a minimum of 3 weeks

[1]Related clinical syndromes include nonchlamydial nongonococcal urethritis and cervicitis.

[2]Or oral tetracycline 500 mg qid.

[3]Not recommended in pregnancy.

[4]Erythromycin ethylsuccinate 800 mg may be substituted for erythromycin base 500 mg; erythromycin estolate is contraindicated in pregnancy.

[5]Pyloric stenosis has been associated with use of erythromycin in newborns.

[6]All patients should also receive a course of treatment effective for *Chlamydia*.

[7]Fluoroquinolones should not be used to treat gonorrhea acquired in Asia, Hawaii, Israel, or other areas where fluoroquinolone-resistant strains of *N. gonorrhoeae* are common.

[8]Recommended only for use during pregnancy in patients allergic to β-lactams. Not effective for pharyngeal infection.

[9]Some clinicians believe the addition of metronidazole is not required.

[10]Or clindamycin 450 mg oral qid to complete 14 days.

[11]A single daily dose of 3 mg/kg is likely to be effective, but has not been studied in pelvic inflammatory disease.

[12]Some experts would add metronidazole 500 mg bid.

[13]Higher relapse rate with single dose, but useful for patients who may not comply with multiple-dose therapy.

[14]In pregnancy, topical preparations have not been effective in preventing premature delivery; oral metronidazole has been effective in some studies.

[15]For preparations and dosage of topical products, see *Med Lett Drugs Ther*, 1994, 36:81; single-dose therapy is not recommended.

[16]Some experts recommend a repeat dose after 7 days, especially in patients with HIV infection or pregnant women.

[17]Patients allergic to penicillin should be desensitized and treated with penicillin.

[18]All regimens, especially single-dose ceftriaxone, are less effective in HIV-infected patients.

[19]Recommendations for external genital warts. Liquid nitrogen can also be used for vaginal, urethral, and oral warts. Podofilox or imiquimod can be used for urethral meatus warts. Trichloroacetic or bichloroacetic acid can be used for anal warts.

[20]Some Medical Letter consultants discontinue preventive treatment for 1-2 months once a year to reassess the frequency of recurrence.

[21]Use 500 mg once daily in patients with <10 recurrences per year and 500 mg bid or 1 g daily in patients with <10 recurrences per year.

[22]Antiviral therapy is variably effective for episodic treatment of recurrences; only effective if started early.

[23]No published data are available to support 3 days' use.

Adapted from "Sexually Transmitted Diseases Treatment Guidelines 2002," *MMWR Morb Mortal Wkly Rep*, 2002, 51(RR-6).

Adapted from "Drugs for Sexually Transmitted Infections," *Treatment Guidelines From The Medical Letter*®, 2004, 2(26):70-2.

NORMAL BLOOD VALUES

Test	Range of Normal Values
Complete Blood Count (CBC)	
White blood cells	4,500-11,000
Red blood cells (male)	4.6-6.2 x 10^6 μL
Red blood cells (female)	4.2-5.4 x 10^6 μL
Platelets	150,000-450,000
Hematocrit (male)	40% to 54%
Hematocrit (female)	38% to 47%
Hemoglobin (male)	13.5-18 g/dL
Hemoglobin (female)	12-16 g/dL
Mean corpuscular volume (MCV)	80-96 $μm^3$
Mean corpuscular hemoglobin (MCH)	27-31 pg
Mean corpuscular hemoglobin concentration (MCHC)	32% to 36%
Differential White Blood Cell Count (%)	
Segmented neutrophils	56
Bands	3.0
Eosinophils	2.7
Basophils	0.3
Lymphocytes	34.0
Monocytes	4.0
Hemostasis	
Bleeding time (BT)	2-8 minutes
Prothrombin time (PT)	10-13 seconds
Activated partial thromboplastin time (aPTT)	25-35 seconds
Serum Chemistry	
Glucose (fasting)	70-110 mg/dL
Blood urea nitrogen (BUN)	8-23 mg/dL
Creatinine (male)	0.1-0.4 mg/dL
Creatinine (female)	0.2-0.7 mg/dL
Bilirubin, indirect (unconjugated)	0.3 mg/dL
Bilirubin, direct (conjugated)	0.1-1 mg/dL
Calcium	9.2-11 mg/dL
Magnesium	1.8-3 mg/dL
Phosphorus	2.3-4.7 mg/dL
Serum Electrolytes	
Sodium (Na^+)	136-142 mEq/L
Potassium (K^+)	3.8-5 mEq/L
Chloride (Cl^-)	95-103 mEq/L
Bicarbonate (HCO_3^-)	21-28 mmol/L
Serum Enzymes	
Alkaline phosphatase	20-130 IU/L
Alanine aminotransferase (ALT) (formerly called SGPT)	4-36 units/L
Aspartate aminotransferase (AST) (formerly called SGOT)	8-33 units/L
Amylase	16-120 Somogyi units/dL
Creatine kinase (CK) (male)	55-170 units/L
Creatine kinase (CK) (female)	30-135 units/L

DENTIFRICE PRODUCTS

Brand Name	Abrasive Ingredient	Therapeutic Ingredient	Foaming Agent
Aim® Baking Soda Gel	Hydrated silica, sodium bicarbonate	Sodium monofluorophosphate 0.7% (fluoride 0.14%)	Sodium lauryl sulfate
	Other Ingredients: Sorbitol and related polyols, water, glycerin, SD alcohol 38B, flavor, cellulose gum, sodium saccharin, blue #1, yellow #10		
Aim® Extra Strength Gel	Hydrated silica	Sodium monofluorophosphate 1.2%	Sodium lauryl sulfate
	Other Ingredients: Sorbitol, water, PEG-32, SD alcohol 38B, flavor, cellulose gum, sodium saccharin, sodium benzoate, blue #1, yellow #10		
Aim® Regular Strength	Hydrated silica	Sodium monofluorophosphate 0.8% (fluoride 0.14%)	Sodium lauryl sulfate
	Other Ingredients: Sorbitol and other related polyols, water, glycerin, SD alcohol 38B, flavor, cellulose gum, sodium saccharin, blue #1, yellow #10		
Aim® Tartar Control Gel	Hydrated silica	Sodium monofluorophosphate 0.8% (fluoride 0.14%)	Sodium lauryl sulfate
	Other Ingredients: Sorbitol and related polyols, water, glycerin, zinc citrate trihydrate, SD alcohol 38B, flavor, cellulose gum, sodium saccharin, blue #1, yellow #10		
Aquafresh® Baking Soda Toothpaste	Calcium carbonate, hydrated silica, sodium bicarbonate	Sodium monofluorophosphate	Sodium lauryl sulfate
	Other Ingredients: Calcium carrageenan, cellulose gum, colors, flavor, glycerin, PEG-8, sodium benzoate, sodium saccharin, sorbitol, titanium dioxide, water		
Aquafresh® Extra Fresh Toothpaste[1]	Hydrated silica, calcium carbonate	Sodium monofluorophosphate	Sodium lauryl sulfate
	Other Ingredients: Sorbitol, water, glycerin, PEG-8, titanium dioxide, cellulose gum, flavor, sodium saccharin, sodium benzoate, calcium carrageenan, colors		
Aquafresh® Extreme Clean® Arctic Cool	Precipitated silica	Sodium fluoride 0.15%	Sodium lauryl sulfate
	Other Ingredients: Cocamidopropyl betaine, D&C red #30, flavor, glycerin, PEG-8, sodium saccharin, sorbitol, synthetic iron oxide, titanium dioxide, water, xanthan gum		
Aquafresh® Extreme Clean® Original Experience	Precipitated silica	Sodium fluoride 0.15%	Sodium lauryl sulfate
	Other Ingredients: Cocamidopropyl betaine, D&C red #30, flavor, PEG-8, sodium saccharin, sorbitol, iron oxide, titanium dioxide, water, xanthan gum		
Aquafresh® Extreme Clean® EMPOWERMINT	Precipitated silica	Sodium fluoride 0.15%	Sodium lauryl sulfate
	Other Ingredients: Cocamidopropyl betaine, D&C red #30, flavor, glycerin, PEG-8, sodium saccharin, sorbitol, synthetic iron oxide, titanium dioxide, water, xanthan gum		
Aquafresh® Extreme Clean® Whitening	Precipitated silica	Sodium fluoride 0.15%	Sodium lauryl sulfate
	Other Ingredients: Cocamidopropyl betaine, D&C red #30, flavor, glycerin, PEG-8, sodium saccharin, sorbitol, synthetic iron oxide, titanium dioxide, water, xanthan gum		
Aquafresh® for Kids Toothpaste[1]	Hydrated silica, calcium carbonate	Sodium monofluorophosphate	Sodium lauryl sulfate
	Other Ingredients: Sorbitol, water, glycerin, PEG-8, titanium dioxide, cellulose gum, flavor, sodium saccharin, calcium carrageenan, sodium benzoate, colors		
Aquafresh® Gum Care Toothpaste	Hydrated silica, calcium carbonate	Sodium monofluorophosphate	Sodium lauryl sulfate
	Other Ingredients: Calcium carrageenan, cellulose gum, colors, flavor, PEG-8, sodium benzoate, sodium saccharin, sorbitol, titanium dioxide, water		
Aquafresh® Multi-Action Whitening	Hydrated silica	Sodium fluoride 0.15%	Sodium lauryl sulfate
	Other Ingredients: D&C red #30 lake, D&C yellow #10 lake, FD&C blue #1 lake, flavor, glycerin, PEG-8, povidone K30, sodium benzoate, sodium hydroxide, sodium saccharin, sodium tripolyphosphate, sorbitol, titanium dioxide, water, xanthan gum		

DENTIFRICE PRODUCTS *(Continued)*

Brand Name	Abrasive Ingredient	Therapeutic Ingredient	Foaming Agent
Aquafresh® Multi-Action Whitening with Triclene® Stain & Tartar Defense™	Hydrated silica	Sodium fluoride 0.15%	Sodium lauryl sulfate
	Other Ingredients: D&C red #30 lake, D&C yellow #10 lake, FD&C blue #1 lake, flavor, glycerin, PEG-8, povidone K30, sodium benzoate, sodium hydroxide, sodium saccharin, sodium tripolyphosphate, sorbitol, titanium dioxide, water, xanthan gum		
Aquafresh® Sensitive Toothpaste	Hydrated silica	Potassium nitrate, sodium fluoride	Sodium lauryl sulfate
	Other Ingredients: Colors, flavor, glycerin, sodium benzoate, sodium saccharin, sorbitol, titanium dioxide, water, xanthan gum		
Aquafresh® Sensitive® Maximum Strength	Hydrated silica	Sodium fluoride 0.15%, potassium nitrate 5%	Sodium lauryl sulfate
	Other Ingredients: D&C red #30 lake, FD&C blue #1 lake, flavor, glycerin, sodium benzoate, sodium hydroxide, sodium saccharin, sorbitol, titanium dioxide, water, xanthan gum		
Aquafresh® Tartar Control Toothpaste[1]	Hydrated silica	Sodium fluoride	Sodium lauryl sulfate
	Other Ingredients: Tetrapotassium pyrophosphate, tetrasodium pyrophosphate, sorbitol, glycerin, PEG-8, flavor, xanthan gum, sodium saccharin, sodium benzoate, colors, titanium dioxide, water		
Aquafresh® Triple Protection Toothpaste[1]	Hydrated silica, calcium carbonate	Sodium monofluorophosphate	Sodium lauryl sulfate
	Other Ingredients: PEG-8, sorbitol, cellulose gum, sodium benzoate, titanium dioxide, calcium carrageenan, flavor, sodium saccharin, colors, water		
Aquafresh® Whitening Gel or Toothpaste	Hydrated silica	Sodium fluoride	Sodium lauryl sulfate
	Other Ingredients: Colors, flavor, glycerin, PEG-8, sodium benzoate, sodium hydroxide, sodium saccharin, sodium tripolyphosphate, sorbitol, titanium dioxide, water, xanthan gum		
Arm & Hammer Advance Breath Care™ Cool Fresh Toothpaste	Calcium carbonate poloxamer 407, sodium bicarbonate	Sodium monofluorophosphate 0.76%	
	Other Ingredients: Water, glycerin, sodium citrate dihydrate, flavor, cellulose gum, cocamidopropyl betaine, zinc, citrate trihydrate, sodium saccharin, titanium dioxide		
Arm & Hammer Advance White™ Toothpaste for Sensitive Teeth	Silica, sodium bicarbonate	Sodium fluoride 0.243%, potassium nitrate 5%	
	Other Ingredients: Cellulose gum, cocamidopropyl betaine, flavor, glycerin, sorbitol, titanium dioxide, water		
Arm & Hammer Advance White™ with Baking Soda & Peroxide	Sodium bicarbonate, silica	Sodium fluoride	Sodium lauryl sulfate
	Other Ingredients: Flavor, PEG-8, poloxapol 1220, sodium carbonate peroxide, sodium lauroyl sarcosinate, sodium saccharin, tetrasodium pyrophosphate, water		
Arm & Hammer Advance White™ with Baking Soda Tartar Control	Sodium bicarbonate, hydrated silica	Sodium fluoride	Sodium lauryl sulfate
	Other Ingredients: Cellulose gum, flavor, glycerin, sodium lauroyl sarcosinate, sodium saccharin, sorbitol, tetrasodium pyrophosphate, titanium dioxide, water		
Arm & Hammer Advance White™ with Gel Micro-Polishers Gel	Sodium bicarbonate, hydrated silica	Sodium fluoride 0.24%	Sodium lauryl sulfate
	Other Ingredients: Cellulose gum, FD&C blue #1, FD&C yellow #5, flavor, glycerin, sodium lauroyl sarcosinate, sodium saccharin, sorbitol, tetrasodium pyrophosphate, water		
Arm & Hammer Complete Care™ Extra Whitening	Silica, sodium bicarbonate	Sodium fluoride 0.24%	Sodium lauryl sulfate
	Other Ingredients: PEG-8, PEG/PPG-116/66 copolymer, sodium carbonate peroxide, sodium lauroyl sarcosinate, sodium saccharin, flavor, zinc citrate trihydrate, water		

Brand Name	Abrasive Ingredient	Therapeutic Ingredient	Foaming Agent
Arm & Hammer Dental Care Tartar Control	Sodium bicarbonate	Sodium fluoride 0.24%	Sodium lauryl sulfate
	Other Ingredients: Water, glycerin, tetrasodium pyrophosphate, PEG-8, sodium saccharin, flavors, cellulose gum, sodium lauroyl sarcosinate		
Arm & Hammer Enamel Care™	Hydrated silica	Sodium fluoride 0.24%	Sodium lauryl sulfate
	Other Ingredients: Glycerin, sodium bicarbonate, water, sorbitol, calcium sulfate, sodium sulfate, flavor, dipotassium phosphate, sodium carbonate, sodium saccharin, cellulose gum, xanthan gum, methylparaben, propylparaben, blue 1, may contain sodium lauroyl sarcosinate		
Arm & Hammer Multi-Benefit PeroxiCare Baking Soda & Peroxide Toothpaste	Sodium bicarbonate, sodium carbonate peroxide, silica	Sodium fluoride 0.24%	Sodium lauryl sulfate
	Other Ingredients: PEG/PPG-38/8 copolymer, PEG/PPG-116/66 copolymer, water, flavor, sodium saccharin, sodium lauroyl sarcosinate, hydrogenated starch hydrolysate, gum Arabic, D&C green #5		
Arm & Hammer PeroxiCare Baking Soda & Peroxide	Sodium bicarbonate, silica	Sodium fluoride 0.24%	Sodium lauryl sulfate
	Other Ingredients: PEG/PPG-38/8 copolymer, PEG/PPG-116/66 copolymer, milled sodium percarbonate, sodium lauroyl sarcosinate, sodium saccharin, flavor, water		
Arm & Hammer P.M.™ Bold Mint	Sodium bicarbonate, silica	Sodium fluoride	Sodium lauryl sulfate
	Other Ingredients: Flavor, PEG-B, poloxapol 1220, sodium percarbonate, sodium lauroyl sarcosinate, sodium saccharin, water, zinc citrate trihydrate		
Arm & Hammer P.M.™ Fresh Mint	Aluminum oxide, hydrated silica	Sodium monofluorophosphate	Sodium lauryl sulfate
	Other Ingredients: Cellulose gum, flavor, glycerin, sodium saccharin, sorbital, water, zinc citrate trihydrate		
Biotene® Antibacterial Dry Mouth Toothpaste	Hydrated silica, calcium pyrophosphate	Lactoperoxidase, glucose oxidase, lysozyme, sodium monofluorophosphate (0.76%)	
	Other Ingredients: Sorbitol, glycerin, xylitol, isoceteth-20, cellulose gum, flavor, sodium benzoate, beta-d-glucose, potassium thiocyanate		
Close-Up® Baking Soda Toothpaste (mint)	Hydrated silica, sodium bicarbonate	Sodium monofluorophosphate 0.79% (fluoride 0.15%)	Sodium lauryl sulfate
	Other Ingredients: Sorbitol and related polyols, water, glycerin, SD alcohol 38B, flavor, cellulose gum, sodium saccharin, sodium benzoate, red #33, red #40, titanium dioxide		
Close-Up® Classic Red Gel	Hydrated silica	Sodium monofluorophosphate 0.8% (fluoride 0.14%)	Sodium lauryl sulfate
	Other Ingredients: Sorbitol and related polyols, water, glycerin, SD alcohol 38B, flavor, cellulose gum, sodium saccharin, sodium chloride, red #33, red #40		
Close-Up® Cool Mint Gel	Hydrated silica	Sodium monofluorophosphate 0.79% (fluoride 0.15%)	Sodium lauryl sulfate
	Other Ingredients: Sorbitol, water, glycerin, SD alcohol 38B, flavor, cellulose gum, sodium saccharin, polysorbate 20, blue #1, mica, red #33, titanium dioxide		
Close-Up® Original Red Whitening Toothpaste	Hydrated silica	Sodium monofluorophosphate 0.8% (fluoride 0.14%)	Sodium lauryl sulfate
	Other Ingredients: Sorbitol and related polyols, water, glycerin, SD alcohol 38B, flavor, cellulose gum, sodium saccharin, sodium chloride, red #30 lake, titanium dioxide, blue #1		
Close-Up® Tartar Control Gel (mint)	Hydrated silica	Sodium monofluorophosphate 0.79% (fluoride 0.15%)	Sodium lauryl sulfate
	Other Ingredients: Sorbitol and related polyols, water, glycerin, zinc citrate trihydrate, SD alcohol 38B, flavor, cellulose gum, sodium saccharin, red #33, red #40, **caffeine free**		

DENTIFRICE PRODUCTS (Continued)

Brand Name	Abrasive Ingredient	Therapeutic Ingredient	Foaming Agent
Close-Up® Tartar Control Whitening Toothpaste	Hydrated silica	Sodium monofluorophosphate 0.8% (fluoride 0.14%)	Sodium lauryl sulfate
	Other Ingredients: Sorbitol and related polypols, water, glycerin, SD alcohol 38B, flavor, zinc citrate trihydrate, cellulose gum, sodium saccharin, titanium dioxide, blue #1, yellow #10		
Colgate® Baking Soda & Peroxide Tartar Control Toothpaste[1]	Hydrated silica, sodium bicarbonate	Sodium monofluorophosphate 0.76%	Sodium lauryl sulfate
	Other Ingredients: Glycerin, propylene glycol, water, pentasodium triphosphate, tetrasodium pyrophosphate, titanium dioxide, flavor, sodium hydroxide, calcium peroxide, sodium saccharin, carrageenan, cellulose gum, FD&C blue #1, D&C yellow #10		
Colgate® Baking Soda & Peroxide Whitening Toothpaste[1]	Hydrated silica, sodium bicarbonate, aluminum oxide	Sodium monofluorophosphate 0.76%	Sodium lauryl sulfate
	Other Ingredients: Glycerin, polypylene glycol, water, pentasodium triphosphate, tetrasodium pyrophosphate, titanium dioxide, flavor, sodium hydroxide, calcium peroxide, sodium saccharin, carrageenan, cellulose gum, **dietetically sucrose free**		
Colgate® Baking Soda Tartar Control Gel or Toothpaste	Hydrated silica, sodium bicarbonate	Sodium fluoride 0.243%	Sodium lauryl sulfate
	Other Ingredients: Glycerin, tetrasodium pyrophosphate, PVM/MA copolymer, cellulose gum, flavor, sodium saccharin, sodium hydroxide, titanium dioxide (paste), FD&C blue #1, D&C yellow #10 (gel), **dietetically sucrose free**		
Colgate® Cavity Protection Toothpaste	Dicalcium phosphate dihydrate	Sodium monofluorophosphate 0.15%	Sodium lauryl sulfate
	Other Ingredients: Water, glycerin, sorbitol, cellulose gum, flavor, tetrapotassium pyrophosphate, sodium saccharin		
Colgate® Herbal White	Hydrated silica	Sodium monofluorophosphate 0.76%	Sodium lauryl sulfate
	Other Ingredients: Calcium carbonate, water, sorbitol, flavor, sodium carbonate, sodium hydroxide, cellulose gum, sodium saccharin, carrageenan, xanthan gum, parabens, balm mint extract, fennel extract, FD&C blue No. 1, D&C yellow No. 10		
Colgate® Luminous™ Paradise Fresh	Hydrated silica	Sodium fluoride 0.24%	Sodium lauryl sulfate
	Other Ingredients: Sorbitol, water, PEG-12, flavor, cellulose gum, tetrasodium pyrophosphate, cocoamidopropyl betaine, sodium saccharin, mica, titanium dioxide, FD&C red #40, FD&C blue #1		
Colgate® Junior Gel[1]	Hydrated silica	Sodium fluoride 0.243%	Sodium lauryl sulfate
	Other Ingredients: Sorbitol, water, PEG-12, flavor, tetrasodium pyrophosphate, cellulose gum, sodium saccharin, mica, titanium dioxide, colorants, **dietetically sucrose free**		
Colgate® MaxFresh™	Hydrated silica	Sodium fluoride 0.24%	Sodium lauryl sulfate
	Other Ingredients: Sorbitol, water, PEG-12, flavor, cellulose gum, tetrasodium pyrophosphate, cocoamidopropyl betaine, sodium saccharin, methylcellulose, FD&C red #40		
Colgate® Platinum™ Whitening Toothpaste[1]	Silica, aluminum oxide	Sodium monofluorophosphate	Sodium lauryl sulfate
	Other Ingredients: Water, hydrated silica, sorbitol, glycerin, PEG-12, tetrapotassium pyrophosphate, PVM/MA copolymer, flavor, sodium hydroxide, sodium saccharin, titanium dioxide		
Colgate® Platinum™ Whitening with Baking Soda Toothpaste[1]	Sodium bicarbonate, aluminum oxide	Sodium monofluorophosphate 0.76%	Sodium lauryl sulfate
	Other Ingredients: Water, glycerin, PEG-12, tetrapotassium pyrophosphate, PVM/MA copolymer, flavor, sodium hydroxide, sodium saccharin, titanium dioxide, cellulose gum		
Colgate® Sensitive Maximum Strength Toothpaste	Hydrated silica, sodium bicarbonate	Potassium nitrate 5%, stannous fluoride 0.45%	Sodium lauryl sulfate
	Other Ingredients: Glycerin and/or sorbitol, water, PEG-40 castor oil, PEG-12, poloxamer 407, sodium citrate, flavor, titanium dioxide, sodium hydroxide, cellulose gum, xanthan gum, sodium saccharin, stannous chloride, citric acid, tetrasodium pyrophosphate, FD&C Blue No. 1		

Brand Name	Abrasive Ingredient	Therapeutic Ingredient	Foaming Agent
Colgate® Sensitive Plus Whitening	Hydrated silica, Sodium bicarbonate	Potassium nitrate 5% antisensitivity (FDA required amount), Stannous Fluoride 0.45% (0.15% w/v fluoride ion)	Sodium lauryl sulfate
	Other Ingredients: Glycerin and/or sorbitol, water, PEG-40 castor oil, PEG-12, poloxamer 405, sodium citrate, flavor, titanium dioxide, sodium hydroxide, cellulose gum, xanthan gum, sodium saccharin, stannous chloride, citric acid, tetrasodium pyrophosphate, mica, FD&C blue No. 1, D&C yellow No. 10		
Colgate® Simply White®	Silica	Sodium fluoride 0.24%	Sodium lauryl sulfate
	Other Ingredients: Water, glycerin, sorbitol, PEG-12, pentasodium triphosphate, flavor, carbomer, hydrogen peroxide, sodium hydroxide, tetrasodium pyrophosphate, PVM/MA copolymer, cellulose gum, sodium saccharin, sodium magnesium silicate, xanthan gum, carrageenan, phosphoric acid, manganese gluconate, butylated hydroxytoluene, titanium dioxide, FD&C blue No. 1		
Colgate® Simply White®	Silica	Sodium fluoride 0.24%	Sodium lauryl sulfate
	Other Ingredients: Water, glycerin, sorbitol, PEG-12, pentasodium triphosphate, flavor, carbomer, hydrogen peroxide, sodium hydroxide, tetrasodium pyrophosphate, PVM/MA copolymer, cellulose gum, sodium saccharin, sodium magnesium silicate, xanthan gum, carrageenan, phosphoric acid, manganese gluconate, butylated hydroxytoluene, titanium dioxide, FD&C blue No. 1		
Colgate® Sparkling White™ Vanilla Mint	Hydrated silica, mica	Sodium fluoride 0.24%	Sodium lauryl sulfate
	Other Ingredients: Sorbitol, water, PEG-12, flavor, cellulose gum, tetrasodium pyrophosphate, cocoamidopropyl betaine, sodium saccharin, FD&C yellow #6		
Colgate® Tartar Control Plus Whitening	Hydrated silica, aluminum oxide	Sodium monofluorophosphate 0.76%	Sodium lauryl sulfate
	Other Ingredients: Water, sorbitol, glycerin, pentasodium triphosphate, tetrasodium pyrophosphate, PVM/MA copolymer, cellulose gum, flavor, sodium hydroxide, titanium dioxide, sodium saccharin, carrageenan		
Colgate® Toothpaste[1]	Dicalcium phosphate dihydrate	Sodium monofluorophosphate 0.76%	Sodium lauryl sulfate
	Other Ingredients: Glycerin, cellulose gum, tetrasodium pyrophosphate, sodium saccharin, flavor, **dietetically sucrose free**		
Colgate® Total® Advanced Fresh Gel	Hydrated silica	Sodium fluoride 0.24%, triclosan 0.3%	Sodium lauryl sulfate
	Other Ingredients: Water, glycerin, sorbitol, PVM/MA copolymer, flavor, cellulose gum, sodium hydroxide, propylene glycol, carrageenan, sodium saccharin, FD&C blue No. 1, D&C yellow No. 10		
Colgate® Total® Toothpaste	Hydrated silica	Sodium fluoride 0.243%, triclosan 0.3%	Sodium lauryl sulfate
	Other Ingredients: Water, glycerin, sorbitol, PVM/MA copolymer, cellulose gum, flavor, sodium hydroxide, propylene glycol, carrageenan, sodium saccharin, titanium dioxide		
Colgate® Total® Clean Mint Paste[1]	Hydrated silica	Triclosan 0.30%, sodium fluoride 0.24%	Sodium lauryl sulfate
	Other Ingredients: Water, glycerin, sorbitol, PVM/MA copolymer, cellulose gum, flavor, sodium hydroxide, propylene glycol, carrageenan, sodium saccharin, titanium dioxide		
Colgate® Total® Mint Stripe™ Gel[1]	Hydrated silica, mica	Triclosan 0.30%, sodium fluoride 0.24%	Sodium lauryl sulfate
	Other Ingredients: Water, glycerin, sorbitol, PVM/MA copolymer, cellulose gum, flavor, sodium saccharin, titanium dioxide, FD&C blue #1, D&C yellow #10		
Colgate® Total® Fresh Stripe Toothpaste	Hydrated silica	Sodium fluoride 0.243%, triclosan 0.3%	Sodium lauryl sulfate
	Other Ingredients: Water, glycerin, sorbitol, PVM/MA copolymer, cellulose gum, flavor, sodium hydroxide, propylene glycol, carrageenan, sodium saccharin, mica, titanium dioxide, FD&C blue #1, D&C yellow #10		
Colgate® Total® Whitening Gel[1]	Hydrated silica, mica	Triclosan 0.30%, sodium fluoride 0.24%	Sodium lauryl sulfate
	Other Ingredients: Water, glycerin, sorbitol, PVM/MA copolymer, cellulose gum, flavor, sodium hydroxide, propylene glycol, carrageenan, sodium saccharin, titanium dioxide, FD&C blue #1		

DENTIFRICE PRODUCTS *(Continued)*

Brand Name	Abrasive Ingredient	Therapeutic Ingredient	Foaming Agent
Colgate® Total® Whitening Paste[1]	Hydrated silica	Triclosan 0.30%, sodium fluoride 0.24%	Sodium lauryl sulfate
	Other Ingredients: Water, glycerin, sorbitol, PVM/MA copolymer, cellulose gum, flavor, sodium hydroxide, propylene glycol, carrageenan, sodium saccharin, titanium dioxide		
Colgate® Winterfresh Gel[1]	Hydrated silica	Sodium fluoride 0.243%	Sodium lauryl sulfate
	Other Ingredients: Sorbitol, water, PEG-12, flavor, tetrasodium pyrophosphate, cellulose gum, sodium saccharin, FD&C blue #1, **dietetically sucrose free**		
Colgate® Whitening Oxygen Bubbles Brisk Mint®	Hydrated silica, sodium bicarbonate	Sodium fluoride 0.24%	Sodium lauryl sulfate
	Other Ingredients: Glycerin, sorbitol, propylene glycol, aluminum oxide, water, pentasodium triphosphate, tetrasodium pyrophosphate, flavor, sodium hydroxide, calcium peroxide, sodium saccharin, carrageenan, cellulose gum, titanium dioxide		
Crest® Baking Soda Tartar Protection Gel or Toothpaste (mint)[1]	Hydrated silica, sodium bicarbonate	Sodium fluoride 0.243%	Sodium lauryl sulfate
	Other Ingredients: Water, glycerin, sorbitol, tetrasodium pyrophosphate, PEG-6, flavor, cellulose gum, sodium saccharin, titanium dioxide (paste), FD&C blue #1 (gel), disodium pyrophosphate, tetrapotassium pyrophosphate, carbomer 956, xanthan gum, FD&C yellow #5 (gel)		
Crest® Baking Soda & Peroxide Whitening with Tarter Protection	Hydrated silica, sodium bicarbonate	Sodium fluoride 0.24%	Sodium lauryl sulfate
	Other Ingredients: Glycerin, water, propylene glycol, sorbitol, . tetrasodium pyrophosphate, sorbitol, PEG-12, flavor, sodium hydroxide, sodium saccharin, poloxamer 407, xanthan gum, calcium peroxide, titanium dioxide, blue #1		
Crest® Cavity Protection with Baking Soda Gel or Toothpaste[1] (mint)	Hydrated silica, sodium bicarbonate	Sodium fluoride 0.243%	Sodium lauryl sulfate
	Other Ingredients: Sorbitol, water, glycerin, sodium carbonate, flavor, cellulose gum; sodium saccharin, titanium dioxide (paste), FD&C blue #1 (gel)		
Crest® Cavity Protection Gel (cool mint)[1]	Hydrated silica	Sodium fluoride 0.243%	Sodium lauryl sulfate
	Other Ingredients: Sorbitol, water, trisodium phosphate, flavor, sodium phosphate, xanthan gum, sodium saccharin, carbomer 956, FD&C blue #1, carbomer 940A		
Crest® Cavity Protection Toothpaste[1] (icy mint or regular)	Hydrated silica	Sodium fluoride 0.243%	Sodium lauryl sulfate
	Other Ingredients: Sorbitol, water, glycerin (mint), trisodium phosphate, flavor, sodium phosphate, cellulose gum (mint), xanthan gum (regular), sodium saccharin, carbomer 956, titanium dioxide, FD&C blue #1. carbomer 940A		
Crest® Extra Whitening Gel or Toothpaste	Hydrated silica	Sodium fluoride 0.15%	Sodium lauryl sulfate, poloxamer 407
	Other Ingredients: Sorbitol, water, glycerin, tetrasodium pyrophosphate, sodium carbonate, carboxymethylcellulose sodium, titanium dioxide, carnauba wax, sodium saccharin, flavor, FD&C blue #1, FD&C yellow #5, PEG-6, sodium bicarbonate[2]		
Crest® for Kids Cavity Protection Gel	Hydrated silica	Sodium fluoride 0.243%	Sodium lauryl sulfate
	Other Ingredients: Sorbitol, water, trisodium phosphate, sodium phosphate, xanthan gum, flavor, sodium saccharin, carbomer 956, mica, titanium dioxide, FD&C blue #1		
Crest® Gum Care Gel or Toothpaste	Hydrated silica	Stannous fluoride 0.454%	Sodium lauryl sulfate
	Other Ingredients: Sorbitol, water, stannous chloride, titanium dioxide (paste), flavor, sodium hydroxide, sodium saccharin, sodium carrageenan, FD&C blue #1 (gel), sodium gluconate, hydroxyethylcellulose		
Crest® Multicare Gel or Toothpaste (cool mint, fresh mint)	Hydrated silica, sodium bicarbonate	Sodium fluoride 0.243%	Sodium lauryl sulfate
	Other Ingredients: Tetrasodium pyrophosphate, xylitol, water, glycerin, PEG-6, poloxamer 407, sodium carbonate, flavor, cellulose gum, xanthan gum, sodium saccharin, titanium dioxide, FD&C blue #1, FD&C yellow #5 (cool mint)		

Brand Name	Abrasive Ingredient	Therapeutic Ingredient	Foaming Agent
Crest® Sensitivity Protection Toothpaste[1] (mild mint)	Hydrated silica	Potassium nitrate 5%, sodium fluoride 0.15%	Sodium lauryl sulfate
	Other Ingredients: Water, glycerin, sorbitol, trisodium phosphate, cellulose gum, flavor, xanthan gum, sodium saccharin, titanium dioxide, **dye free**		
Crest® Sensitivity Whitening Plus Scope	Hydrated silica	Potassium nitrate 5%, sodium fluoride 0.24%	Sodium lauryl sulfate
	Other Ingredients: Water, glycerin, sorbitol, trisodium phosphate, flavor, cellulose guym, alcohol (1.09%), xanthan gum, sodium saccharin, sucralose, polysorbate 80, sodium benzoate, cetylpyridinium chloride, benzoic acid, polyethylene, iron oxides, titanium dioxide, blue #1 aluminum lake, yellow #10 aluminum lake, blue #1, yellow #5		
Crest® Tartar Protection Gel[1] (fresh mint, smooth mint)		Sodium fluoride 0.243%	Sodium lauryl sulfate
	Other Ingredients: Water, sorbitol, glycerin, tetrapotassium pyrophosphate, PEG-6, disodium pyrophosphate, tetrasodium pyrophosphate, flavor, xanthan gum, sodium saccharin, carbomer 956, FD&C blue #1, FD&C yellow #5 (smooth mint)		
Crest® Tartar Protection Toothpaste[1] (original flavor)	Silica	Sodium fluoride 0.243%	Sodium lauryl sulfate
	Other Ingredients: Water, sorbitol, glycerin, tetrapotassium pyrophosphate, PEG-6, disodium pyrophosphate, tetrasodium pyrophosphate, flavor, xanthan gum, sodium saccharin, carbomer 956, titanium dioxide, FD&C blue #1		
Crest® Vivid White™	Hydrated silica	Sodium fluoride 0.243%	Sodium lauryl sulfate
	Other ingredients: Glycerin, water, sorbitol, sodium hexametaphosphate, propylene glycol, flavor, PEG-12, cocamidopropyl betaine, carbomer 956, sodium saccharin, poloxamer 407, polyethylene oxide, xanthan gum, sodium hydroxide, cellulose gum, titanium dioxide		
Crest® Whitening Expressions Extreme Herbal Mint	Hydrated silica	Sodium fluoride 0.243%	Sodium lauryl sulfate
	Other ingredients: Sorbitol, water, glycerin, tetrasodium pyrophosphate, PEG-6, flavor, disodium pyrophosphate, xanthan gum, sodium saccharin, carbomer 956, sucralose, polyethylene, titanium dioxide, blue 1 aluminum lake, yellow 11 aluminum lake		
Crest® Whitening Expressions Fresh Citrus Breeze	Hydrated silica	Sodium fluoride 0.243%	Sodium lauryl sulfate
	Other ingredients: Sorbitol, water, glycerin, tetrasodium pyrophosphate, PEG-6, flavor, disodium pyrophosphate, xanthan gum, sodium saccharin, carnuba wax, carbomer 956, sucralose, titanium dioxide, yellow 6		
Crest® Whitening Plus Scope®	Hydrated silica	Sodium fluoride 0.243% (0.15% w/v fluoride ion)	Sodium lauryl sulfate
	Other ingredients: Water, sorbitol, glycerin, tetrapotassium pyrophosphate, PEG-6, disodium pyrophosphate, tetrasodium pyrophosphate, flavor, alcohol (1.14%), xanthan gum, sodium saccharin, carbomer 956, polysorbate 80, sodium benzoate, cetylpyridinium chloride, benzoic acid, domiphen bromide (.0002 w/v%)		
Dr. Tichenor's Toothpaste	Hydrated silica	Sodium fluoride	Sodium lauryl sulfate
	Other Ingredients: Water, glycerin, sorbitol, insoluble sodium metaphosphate, peppermint oil, cellulose gum, sodium saccharin, sodium phosphate, titanium dioxide, magnesium aluminum silicate, **dye free**		
Enamelon® All-Family Toothpaste	Hydrated silica	Sodium fluoride (fluoride 0.14%)	Sodium lauryl sulfate
	Other Ingredients: Water, glycerin, sorbitol, monoammonium phosphate, calcium sulfate, xanthan gum, flavor, PEG-60 hydrogenated castor oil, sodium saccharin, ammonium chloride, cellulose gum, titanium dioxide, magnesium chloride, methylparaben, propylparaben, FD&C blue #1		
First Teeth™ Baby Gel		Lactoperoxidase 0.7 units/g, lactoferrin, glucose oxidase	Sodium lauryl sulfate
	Other Ingredients: Water, glycerin, sorbitol, pectin, xylitol, flavor, aloe vera, propylene glycol		
Fluoride Foam™[1,3]	**Ingredients:** Fluoride 1.23% (from sodium fluoride and hydrogen fluoride), water, phosphoric acid, poloxamer, sodium saccharin, flavor		
Fluorigard® Anti-Cavity Liquid[1,3]	**Ingredients:** Sodium fluoride 0.05%, ethyl alcohol, pluronic F108 and F127, sweetener, flavor, glycerin, sorbitol, preservatives, **dye free, gluten free**		

DENTIFRICE PRODUCTS (Continued)

Brand Name	Abrasive Ingredient	Therapeutic Ingredient	Foaming Agent
Gleem® Toothpaste	Hydrated silica	Sodium fluoride 0.243%	Sodium lauryl sulfate
	Other Ingredients: Sorbitol, water, trisodium phosphate, flavors, sodium phosphate, xanthan gum, sodium saccharin, carbomer 956, titanium dioxide, **dye free**		
Listerine® Essential Care Gel	Hydrated silica	Anticavity: Sodium monofluorophosphate 0.76% (0.13% W/V fluoride ion Antiplaque/ Antigingivitis: Eucalyptol 0.738%, menthol 0.340%, methyl salicylate 0.480%, thymol 0.511%	Sodium lauryl sulfate
	Other Ingredients: Water, sorbitol, glycerin, flavors, cellulose gum, sodium saccharin, phosphoric acid, FD&C blue #10, sodium phosphate, benzoic acid, PEG-32, and xanthan gum		
Listerine® Gel or Toothpaste (cool mint)	Hydrated silica	Sodium monofluorophosphate	Sodium lauryl sulfate
	Other Ingredients: Water, sorbitol, glycerin, flavors, cellulose gum, sodium saccharin, phosphoric acid, FD&C blue #10, sodium phosphate, benzoic acid, titanium dioxide (paste), xanthan gum		
Listerine® Tartar Control Gel or Toothpaste (cool mint)	Hydrated silica	Sodium fluoride	Sodium lauryl sulfate
	Other Ingredients: Water, sorbitol, glycerin, PEG-32, flavor, cellulose gum, sodium saccharin, tetrapotassium pyrophosphate, FD&C blue #1, D&C yellow #10, titanium dioxide (paste)		
Mentadent® Advanced Whitening Gel or Toothpaste	Hydrated silica, sodium bicarbonate	Sodium fluoride 0.15%	Sodium lauryl sulfate, hydrogen peroxide
	Other Ingredients: Zinc citrate trihydrate, water, sorbitol, glycerin, poloxamer 407, PEG-32, SD alcohol 38B, flavor, cellulose gum, sodium saccharin, phosphoric acid, blue #1, titanium dioxide		
Mentadent® Gum Care Gel or Toothpaste	Hydrated silica, sodium bicarbonate	Sodium fluoride 0.24% (fluoride 0.15%)	Sodium lauryl sulfate, hydrogen peroxide
	Other Ingredients: Zinc citrate trihydrate (1.8%), water, sorbitol, glycerin, poloxamer 407, PEG-32, SD alcohol 38B, flavor, cellulose gum, sodium saccharin, menthol, methyl salicylate, phosphoric acid, green #3, titanium dioxide		
Mentadent® Sensitive Plus™	Hydrated silica, sodium bicarbonate	Potassium nitrate (5%), sodium fluoride	Sodium lauryl sulfate, hydrogen peroxide
	Other Ingredients: Water, glycerin, sorbitol, poloxamer 407, PEG-32, SD alcohol, cellulose gum, sodium saccharin, phosphoric acid, blue #1, titanium dioxide		
Mentadent® Tartar Control Gel or Toothpaste	Hydrated silica, sodium bicarbonate	Sodium fluoride 0.24%	Sodium lauryl sulfate, hydrogen peroxide
	Other Ingredients: Water, sorbitol, glycerin, poloxamer 407, PEG-32, zinc citrate, SD alcohol 38B, flavor, cellulose gum, sodium saccharin, phosphoric acid, blue #1, titanium dioxide, menthol		
Mentadent® with Baking Soda & Peroxide Gel or Toothpaste[1]	Hydrated silica, sodium bicarbonate	Sodium fluoride 0.24% (fluoride 0.15%)	Sodium lauryl sulfate, hydrogen peroxide
	Other Ingredients: Water, sorbitol, glycerin, poloxamer 407, PEG-32, SD alcohol 38B, flavor, cellulose gum, sodium saccharin, phosphoric acid, blue #1, titanium dioxide		
My First Colgate® Gel[1]	Hydrated silica	Sodium fluoride 0.243%	Sodium lauryl sulfate
	Other Ingredients: Water, sorbitol, PEG-12, flavor, tetrasodium pyrophosphate, cellulose gum, sodium saccharin, FD&C red #40, D&C red #33, **dietetically sucrose free**		
Natural Dentist™ Herbal Toothpaste & Gum Therapy, Cinnamon Flavored	Calcium carbonate	Sodium monofluorophosphate	Sodium lauryl sulfate
	Other Ingredients: Vegetable glycerin, aloe vera gel, sodium carrageenan, echinacea, goldenseal, calendula, bloodroot, bee propolis, grapefruit seed extract, sodium bicarbonate[2], cinnamon oil		

Brand Name	Abrasive Ingredient	Therapeutic Ingredient	Foaming Agent
Natural Dentist™ Herbal Toothpaste & Gum Therapy, Mint Flavored	Calcium carbonate	Sodium monofluorophosphate	Sodium lauryl sulfate
	Other Ingredients: Vegetable glycerin, aloe vera gel, sodium carrageenan, echinacea, goldenseal, calendula, bloodroot, bee propolis, grapefruit seed extract, sodium bicarbonate[2], spearmint and peppermint oils		
Natural White® Toothpaste	Hydrated silica	Sodium fluoride	Sodium lauryl sulfate
	Other Ingredients: Sorbitol, water, glycerin, sodium benzoate, titanium dioxide, flavor, cellulose gum, **dietetically sucrose free**		
Natural White® Baking Soda Toothpaste	Calcium carbonate	Sodium monofluorophosphate	Sodium lauryl sulfate
	Other Ingredients: Sorbitol, water, glycerin, sodium bicarbonate[2], carrageenan, natural flavor, **dietetically sucrose free**		
Natural White® Fights Plaque Toothpaste	Hydrated silica	Sodium fluoride	Sodium lauryl sulfate
	Other Ingredients: Sorbitol, water, glycerin, sodium benzoate, titanium dioxide, flavor, cellulose gum, **dietetically sucrose free**		
Natural White® Sensitive Toothpaste	Hydrated silica	Sodium monofluorophosphate, potassium nitrate	Sodium lauryl sulfate
	Other Ingredients: Sorbitol, water, glycerin, flavor, FD&C red #40, sodium benzoate, titanium dioxide, sodium saccharin, **dietetically sucrose free**		
Natural White® Tartar Control Toothpaste	Hydrated silica	Sodium fluoride	Sodium lauryl sulfate
	Other Ingredients: Sorbitol, water, glycerin, xanthan gum, tetrapotassium pyrophosphate, titanium dioxide, cellulose gum, flavor, sodium benzoate, FD&C blue #1, D&C yellow #10, **dietetically sucrose free**		
Natural White® with Peroxide Gel		Hydrogen peroxide	
	Other Ingredients: Water, glycerin, flavor, dipotassium phosphate, sodium saccharin, phosphoric acid, poloxamer, **dietetically sucrose free**		
Oxyfresh Toothpaste	Fine chalk	Oxygene® (stabilized chlorine dioxide)	Sodium lauryl sulfate
	Other Ingredients: Purified deionized water, sorbitol, glycerin, carrageenan, natural flavors, sodium saccharin		
Orajel® Baby Tooth & Gum Cleanser Gel			
	Other Ingredients: Poloxamer 407 (2%), simethicone (0.12%), Microdent, carboxymethylcellulose, sodium, citric acid, flavor, glycerin, methylparaben, potassium sorbate, propylene glycol, propylparaben, water, sodium saccharin, sorbitol, **fluoride free**		
Orajel® Gold Sensitive Teeth Gel for Adults	Hydrated silica	Potassium nitrate 5%, sodium monofluorophosphate 0.2%	Sodium lauryl sulfate
	Other Ingredients: FD&C blue #1, flavor, glycerin, sodium lauroyl sarcosinate, sodium saccharin, sorbitol, xanthan gum		
Pearl Drops® Toothpolish Paste	Hydrated silica, calcium pyrophosphate, dicalcium phosphate, aluminum hydroxide	Sodium monofluorophosphate	Sodium lauryl sulfate
	Other Ingredients: Water, sorbitol, glycerin, PEG-12, flavor, cellulose gum, trisodium phosphate, sodium phosphate, sodium saccharin, **dietetically sucrose free, dye free**		
Pearl Drops® Toothpolish Gel	Hydrated silica	Sodium monofluorophosphate	Sodium lauryl sulfate
	Other Ingredients: Sorbitol, water, glycerin, PEG-12, flavor, cellulose gum, sodium saccharin, FD&C blue #1, FD&C yellow #10, **dietetically sucrose free**		
Pearl Drops® Whitening Extra Strength Paste	Hydrated silica, calcium pyrophosphate, dicalcium phosphate	Sodium monofluorophosphate	Sodium lauryl sulfate
	Other Ingredients: Water, sorbitol, glycerin, PEG-12, flavor, cellulose gum, trisodium phosphate, sodium phosphate, sodium saccharin, titanium dioxide, **dietetically sucrose free, dye free**		
Pearl Drops® Whitening Gel (icy cool mint)	Hydrated silica	Sodium monofluorophosphate	Sodium lauryl sulfate
	Other Ingredients: Sorbitol, water, glycerin, PEG-12, flavor, cellulose gum, sodium saccharin, FD&C blue #1, FD&C yellow #10, **dietetically sucrose free**		

DENTIFRICE PRODUCTS *(Continued)*

Brand Name	Abrasive Ingredient	Therapeutic Ingredient	Foaming Agent
Pepsodent® Baking Soda Toothpaste	Hydrated silica	Sodium monofluorophosphate 0.8% (fluoride (0.14%)	Sodium lauryl sulfate
	Other Ingredients: Sorbitol, water, sodium bicarbonate², PEG-32, SD alcohol 38B, flavor, cellulose gum, sodium saccharin, titanium dioxide		
Pepsodent® Original Toothpaste	Hydrated silica	Sodium monofluorophosphate 0.8% (fluoride (0.14%)	Sodium lauryl sulfate
	Other Ingredients: Sorbitol and related polyols, water, glycerin, SD alcohol 38B, flavor, cellulose gum, sodium saccharin, titanium dioxide		
Pepsodent® Tartar Control Toothpaste	Hydrated silica	Sodium monofluorophosphate 0.8% (fluoride 0.14%)	Sodium lauryl sulfate
	Other Ingredients: Sorbitol and related polyols, water, glycerin, SD alcohol 38B, zinc citrate trihydrate, flavor, cellulose gum, sodium saccharin, titanium dioxide, blue #1, yellow #1		
Pete & Pam™ Gel (premeasured strips)	Hydrated silica	Sodium monofluorophosphate 0.76%	Sodium lauroyl sarcosinate
	Other Ingredients: Sorbitol, water, glycerin, xanthan gum, polysorbate 20, sodium benzoate, pluronic P84, FD&C blue #1, FD&C red #33, FD&C yellow #5, flavor, xylitol		
Promise® Toothpaste	Dicalcium phosphate	Potassium nitrate, sodium monofluorophosphate	Sodium lauryl sulfate
	Other Ingredients: Water, hydroxyethylcellulose, flavor, sodium saccharin, methylparaben, propylparaben, D&C yellow #10, FD&C blue #1, glycerin, sorbitol, silicon dioxide, **dietetically sucrose free**		
Q-Dent – The Antioxidant Toothpaste	Silica	Sodium fluoride 0.15%	Sodium lauryl sulfate
	Other Ingredients: Sorbitol, water, glycerin, tetrasodium pyrophosphate, tetrapotassium pyrophosphate, PEG-300, flavor, coenzyme Q_{10}, cellulose gum, titanium dioxide, sodium saccharin, FD&C blue #1		
Q-Dent – The Coenzyme Q_{10} Toothpaste	Silica	Sodium fluoride 0.15%	Sodium lauryl sulfate
	Other Ingredients: Sorbitol, water, glycerin, tetrasodium pyrophosphate, tetrapotassium pyrophosphate, PEG-300, flavor, coenzyme Q_{10}, cellulose gum, sodium saccharin, FD&C blue #1		
Reach Act Adult Anti-Cavity Treatment Liquid (cinnamon, mint)[3]	**Ingredients:** Sodium fluoride 0.05%, cetylpyridinium chloride, D&C red #33 (cinnamon), EDTA calcium disodium, FD&C yellow #5, flavor, glycerin, monobasic sodium phosphate, dibasic sodium phosphate, poloxamer 407, polysorbate 80 (cinnamon), polysorbate 20 (mint), propylene glycol, sodium benzoate, sodium saccharin, water, FD&C green #3 (mint), menthol (mint), methyl salicylate (mint), potassium sorbate (mint), **alcohol free**		
Reach Act for Kids[1,3]	**Ingredients:** Sodium fluoride 0.05%, cetylpyridinium chloride, D&C red #33, EDTA calcium disodium, flavor, glycerin, monobasic sodium phosphate, dibasic sodium phosphate, poloxamer 407, polysorbate 80, propylene glycol, sodium benzoate, sodium saccharin, water, **alcohol free**		
Rembrandt® Age-Defying Adult Toothpaste (original or mint)	Dicalcium orthophosphate, soft silica	Sodium monofluorophosphate (fluoride 0.15%)	
	Other Ingredients: Trihydroxy propane, perhydrol urea, aluminum oxide, acetylated pectins, sodium citrate, iridium, papain, carboxyl polymethylene, saccharin, propylene glycol, flavor		
Rembrandt® Age-Defying™ Whitening Toothpaste	Silica	Sodium fluoride 0.15%	Sodium lauryl sulfate
	Other Ingredients: Glycerin, dicalcium phosphate, acylated amylopectins, alumina oxide, carbamide peroxide, sodium citrate, flavor, papain, citric acid, EDTA, sodium saccharin		
Rembrandt® Age-Defying Adult Formula Mouthwash[3]	**Ingredients:** Sodium fluoride 0.05%, water, glycerin, hydrogen peroxide solution, sodium citrate, polyoxyl 40 hydrogenated castor oil, flavor, cocamidopropyl betaine, citric acid, sodium benzoate, sodium saccharin, sodium hydroxide, **alcohol free**		
Rembrandt® Daily Whitening Gel	Silica	Sodium monofluorophosphate (fluoride 0.15%)	Carbamide peroxide, sodium lauryl sulfate
	Other Ingredients: Glycerin, sodium citrate, carbopol, triethanolamine, flavor		

Brand Name	Abrasive Ingredient	Therapeutic Ingredient	Foaming Agent
Rembrandt® Extra Whitening Fluoride Toothpaste for Canker Sore Sufferers	Silica	Sodium fluoride 0.15%	
	Other Ingredients: Dicalcium phosphate, glycerin, water, xylitol, alumina, sodium citrate, natural flavors, cocamidopropyl betaine, sodium carrageenan, papain, citric acid, sodium saccharin		
Rembrandt® Intense Stain Removal with Alumasil®	Silica	Sodium fluoride 0.15%	Sodium lauryl sulfate
	Other Ingredients: Dicalcium phosphate, glycerin, sorbitol, water, alumina, sodium citrate, cocamidopropyl betaine, flavor, papain, sodium carrageenan, citric acid, sodium saccharin, methylparaben, vitamin E, FD&C blue No. 1, FD&C yellow No. 5		
Rembrandt® Naturals Toothpaste	Silica	0.15% fluoride ion from sodium monofluorophosphate wt/vol%	None
	Other Ingredients: Water (artesian springs), dicalcium phosphate (from monetite, a mineral), glycerine (by-product of vegetable soap), xylitol (from birch trees), cocamidopropyl betaine (from coconut), flavor (spearmint, peppermint, other natural sources), sodium citrate (from citrus fruit), stevia (from stevia plant), papain (from papaya plant), sodium carrageenan (from seaweed), citric acid and vitamin C (from citrus fruit), ginkgo extract, raspberry leaf extract. Also available containing aloe vera and echinacea or papaya and ginseng.		
Rembrandt® Plus with Active Dental Peroxide Superior Whitening Toothpaste Minty Fresh Flavor	Silica	Sodium fluoride 0.15%	Sodium lauryl sulfate
	Other Ingredients: Glycerin, carbamide peroxide, alumina, acylated amylopectins, flavors, sodium citrate, propylene glycol, cocamidopropyl betaine, papain, carbomer, sodium saccharin, EDTA		
Rembrandt® Whitening Baking Soda Toothpaste	Sodium bicarbonate, silica	Sodium monofluorophosphate (fluoride 0.15%)	Sodium lauryl sulfate
	Other Ingredients: Glycerin, sorbitol, alumina, water, sodium citrate, sodium carrageenan, papain, flavor, sodium hydroxide, FD&C blue #1, sodium saccharin		
Rembrandt® Whitening Canker Sore Prevention Toothpaste	Dicalcium phosphate, silica	Sodium monofluorophosphate (fluoride 0.15%)	
	Other Ingredients: Water, glycerin, xylitol, sodium citrate, natural flavors, sodium carrageenan, papain, citric acid, **dye free**		
Rembrandt® Whitening Natural Toothpaste	Dicalcium phosphate, silica	Sodium monofluorophosphate	
	Other Ingredients: Water, glycerin, xylitol, sodium citrate, natural flavors, sodium carrageenan, papain, citric acid, **dye free**		
Rembrandt® Whitening Sensitive Toothpaste	Dicalcium phosphate dihydrate	Potassium nitrate 5%, sodium monofluorophosphate 0.76%	Sodium lauryl sulfate
	Other Ingredients: Glycerin, sorbitol, water, alumina, papain, sodium citrate, flavor, carboxymethylcellulose sodium, sodium saccharin, methylparaben, FD&C red #40, citric acid		
Rembrandt® Whitening Toothpaste (mint or original)	Dicalcium phosphate dihydrate	Sodium monofluorophosphate 0.76%	Sodium lauryl sulfate
	Other Ingredients: Glycerin, sorbitol, water, alumina, sodium citrate, flavor, sodium carrageenan, papain, sodium saccharin, methylparaben, citric acid, FD&C blue #1, FD&C yellow #5		
Revelation® Toothpowder	Calcium carbonate		Vegetable soap powder
	Other Ingredients: Methyl salicylate, menthol, **dye free**		
Sensodyne® Baking Soda Toothpaste	Sodium bicarbonate, silica	Potassium nitrate, sodium fluoride	Sodium lauryl sulfate
	Other Ingredients: Water, glycerin, flavor, hydroxyethylcellulose, titanium dioxide, sodium saccharin, **dietetically sucrose free, dye free**		
Sensodyne® Cool Gel	Silica	Potassium nitrate, sodium fluoride	Sodium methyl cocoyl taurate
	Other Ingredients: Water, sorbitol, glycerin, sodium carboxymethylcellulose, flavor, sodium saccharin, FD&C blue #1, trisodium phosphate, **dietetically sucrose free**		

DENTIFRICE PRODUCTS *(Continued)*

Brand Name	Abrasive Ingredient	Therapeutic Ingredient	Foaming Agent
Sensodyne® Extra Whitening Toothpaste	Silica	Potassium nitrate, sodium monofluorophosphate	Sodium lauryl sulfate
	Other Ingredients: Water, flavor, glycerin, PEG-12, PEG-75, sodium carbonate, sodium saccharin, titanium dioxide, calcium peroxide, **dietetically sucrose free**		
Sensodyne® Tartar Control Toothpaste	Hydrated silica, silica, sodium bicarbonate	Potassium nitrate, sodium fluoride	Cocamidopropyl betaine
	Other Ingredients: Cellulose gum, flavor, glycerin, sodium saccharin, tetrasodium pyrophosphate, titanium dioxide, water		
Sensodyne® Toothpaste[1] (fresh mint)	Dicalcium phosphate	Potassium nitrate, sodium monofluorophosphate	Sodium lauryl sulfate
	Other Ingredients: Water, glycerin, sorbitol, hydroxymethylcellulose, flavor, sodium saccharin, methylparaben, propylparaben, D&C yellow #10, FD&C blue #1, silicon dioxide, **dietetically sucrose free**		
Sensodyne® Toothpaste (original)	Silica	Potassium nitrate, sodium fluoride	Sodium methyl cocoyl taurate
	Other Ingredients: Water, glycerin, sorbitol, cellulose gum, titanium dioxide, sodium saccharin, flavor, D&C red #28, trisodium phosphate		
Slimer® Gel[1]	Hydrated silica	Sodium fluoride 0.15%	
	Other Ingredients: Sorbitol, water, glycerin, PEG-32, flavor, ethyl alcohol, propylene glycol, glyceryl triacetate, cellulose gum, sodium saccharin, sodium benzoate, FD&C blue #1, FD&C red #33, **dietetically sucrose free**		
Thermodent Toothpaste	Diatomaceous earth, silica	Strontium chloride hexahydrate	Sodium methyl cocoyl taurate
	Other Ingredients: Sorbitol, glycerin, titanium dioxide, guar gum, PEG-40 stearate, hydroxyethylcellulose, flavor, preservative, water		
Tom's® Natural Baking Soda with Propolis & Myrrh Toothpaste	Calcium carbonate, sodium bicarbonate		Sodium lauryl sulfate
	Other Ingredients: Glycerin, water, carrageenan, peppermint oil, myrrh, propolis, **fluoride free**		
Tom's® Natural Baking Soda, Calcium, and Fluoride Toothpaste	Calcium carbonate, sodium bicarbonate	Sodium monofluorophosphate	Sodium lauryl sulfate
	Other Ingredients: Glycerin, water, carrageenan, peppermint oil, xylitol		
Tom's® Natural Calcium and Fluoride Toothpaste[1]	Calcium carbonate	Sodium monofluorophosphate	Sodium lauryl sulfate
	Other Ingredients: Glycerin; water; carrageenan; xylitol (spearmint); cinnamon, fennel oil, or spearmint; peppermint oil (cinnamon, spearmint)		
Tom's® Natural Calcium and Fluoride Toothpaste	Calcium carbonate, hydrated silica	Sodium monofluorophosphate	Sodium lauryl sulfate
	Other Ingredients: Glycerin, water, carrageenan, xylitol, natural wintergreen oil		
Tom's® Natural for Children with Calcium and Fluoride Toothpaste	Calcium carbonate, hydrated silica	Sodium monofluorophosphate	Sodium lauryl sulfate
	Other Ingredients: Glycerin, fruit extracts, carrageenan, water		
Tom's® Natural with Propolis and Myrrh Toothpaste	Calcium carbonate		Sodium lauryl sulfate
	Other Ingredients: Glycerin; water; carrageenan; spearmint, peppermint, cassia, or fennel oil; propolis; myrrh, **fluoride free**		
Topol® Plus Whitening Gel with Calcium Toothpaste	Hydrated silicas	Sodium monofluorophosphate	Sodium lauryl sulfate
	Other Ingredients: Water, sorbitol and glycerin, calcium carbonate, PEG-6, disodium phosphate, flavor, xanthan gum, sodium saccharin, methylparaben and propylparaben, FD&C blue #1		
Topol® Plus Whitening Toothpaste with Baking Soda	Hydrated silicas, sodium bicarbonate	Sodium monofluorophosphate	Sodium lauryl sulfate
	Other Ingredients: Water, glycerin, sorbitol, PEG-6, disodium phosphate, flavor, xanthan gum, sodium saccharin, titanium dioxide, methylparaben, propylparaben		
Topol® Plus Whitening Toothpaste with Natural Papain	Hydrated silicas, calcium carbonate	Sodium monofluorophosphate	Sodium lauryl sulfate
	Other Ingredients: Water, sorbitol, glycerin, PEG-6, disodium phosphate, flavor, xanthan gum, sodium saccharin, methylparaben, propylparaben, FD&C Blue #1		

Brand Name	Abrasive Ingredient	Therapeutic Ingredient	Foaming Agent
Topol® Smoker's Toothpaste	Hydrated silicas	Sodium monofluorophosphate	Sodium lauryl sulfate
	Other Ingredients: Sorbitol, deionized water, glycerin, PEG-6, flavor, xanthan gum, titanium dioxide, sodium saccharin, methylparaben, propylparaben zirconium silicate		
Topol® Smoker's Peppermint Toothpaste		Sodium monofluorophosphate	
Ultra Brite® Baking Soda & Peroxide Toothpaste	Hydrated silica, sodium bicarbonate	Sodium monofluorophosphate 0.76%	Sodium lauryl sulfate
	Other Ingredients: Glycerin, water, propylene glycol, cellulose gum, flavor, sodium saccharin, titanium dioxide, sodium hydroxide, calcium peroxide, carrageenan, **dietetically sucrose free**		
Ultra Brite® Gel	Hydrated silica	Sodium monofluorophosphate 0.76%	Sodium lauryl sulfate
	Other Ingredients: Sorbitol, water, PEG-12, flavor, cellulose gum, sodium saccharin, FD&C blue #1, D&C red #33		
Ultra Brite® Toothpaste	Hydrated silica, alumina	Sodium monofluorophosphate 0.76%	Sodium lauryl sulfate
	Other Ingredients: Glycerin, cellulose gum, sorbitol, carrageenan gum, titanium dioxide, sodium saccharin, flavor, tetrasodium pyrophosphate, **dietetically sucrose free**		
Viadent® Fluoride Gel	Hydrated silica	Sodium monofluorophosphate 0.8%	Sodium lauryl sulfate
	Other Ingredients: Sodium saccharin, zinc chloride, teaberry flavor, sodium carboxymethylcellulose, sorbitol, sanguinaria extract		
Viadent® Fluoride Toothpaste	Hydrated silica	Sodium monofluorophosphate 0.8%	Sodium lauryl sulfate
	Other Ingredients: Sorbitol, titanium dioxide, carboxymethylcellulose, flavor, sodium saccharin, citric acid, zinc chloride, anhydrous sanguinaria extract, citric acid		
Viadent® Original Toothpaste	Dicalcium phosphate		Sodium lauryl sulfate
	Other Ingredients: Glycerin, sorbitol, titanium dioxide, zinc chloride, carrageenan, flavor, sodium saccharin, citric acid, sanguinaria extract, **fluoride free**		
Vince Tooth Powder	Calcium carbonate, sodium carbonate, tricalcium phosphate		
	Other Ingredients: Sodium alum, sodium perborate monohydrate, magnesium trisilicate, sodium saccharin, flavor, D&C red		

[1]Carries American Dental Association (ADA) seal indicating safety and efficacy.

[2]Sodium bicarbonate can also be considered an abrasive.

[3]Topical fluoride product

Adapted with permission from *Nonprescription Products: Formulations & Features, Companion to the Handbook of Nonprescription Drugs*, 11th ed, Washington, DC, American Pharmaceutical Association, 1998, 344-58.

MOUTH PAIN, COLD SORE, AND CANKER SORE PRODUCTS

Brand Name	Anesthetic / Analgesic	Other Ingredients
Abreva™ [OTC]		**Cream:** Docosanol 10%, benzyl alcohol, light mineral oil, propylene glycol, purified water, sucrose distearate, sucrose stearate
Anbesol® Baby Gel (grape, original)	Benzocaine 7.5%	Benzoic acid (grape), carbomer 934P, D&C red #33, EDTA disodium, FD&C blue #1 (grape), flavor (grape), glycerin, methylparaben (grape), PEG, propylparaben (grape), saccharin, purified water, clove oil (original)
Anbesol® Gel or Liquid	Benzocaine 6.3% (gel), 6.4% (liquid); phenol 0.5%	**Gel:** Alcohol 70%, glycerin, carbomer 934P, D&C red #33, D&C yellow #10, FD&C blue #1, FD&C yellow #6, flavor, camphor **Liquid:** Alcohol 70%, potassium iodide, povidone iodine, camphor, menthol, glycerin
Anbesol® Maximum Strength Gel or Liquid	Benzocaine 20%	Alcohol 60%, carbomer 934P (gel), D&C yellow #10, FD&C blue #1, FD&C red #40, flavor, PEG, saccharin
Aveeno® Active Naturals™		White petrolatum, alcohol, lanolin oil, mineral oil, propolis extract, water
Baby® Gumz	Benzocaine 10%	PEG 8 and 32, **alcohol free, dietetically sucrose free**
Banadyne-3	Benzocaine 5%	Dimethicone, methol, propylene glycol, SD alcohol
Benzodent® Denture Analgesic Ointment[1]	Benzocaine 20%	8-hydroxyquinoline sulfate, petrolatum, sodium carboxymethylcellulose, color, eugenol
Blistex® Lip Medex Ointment	Camphor 1%, menthol 1%, phenol 0.5%	Petrolatum, cocoa butter, flavor, lanolin, mixed waxes, oil of cloves
Blistex® Medicated Ointment	Menthol 0.6%, camphor 0.5%, phenol 0.5%	Water, mixed waxes, mineral oil, petrolatum, lanolin
Campho-Phenique® Cold Sore Gel[2]	Camphor 10.8%, phenol 4.7%	Eucalyptus oil, colloidal silicon dioxide, glycerin, light mineral oil, **alcohol free**
Cankaid® Liquid		Carbamide peroxide 10%[3], citric acid monohydrate, sodium citrate, dihydrate, EDTA disodium
Carmex Lip Balm Ointment	Menthol, camphor, salicylic acid, phenol	Alum, fragrance, petrolatum, lanolin, cocoa butter, wax, **alcohol free, dye free, gluten free, dietetically sucrose free**
Cepacol® Viractin®	Tetracaine 2%	Water, ethoxydiglycol, hydroxyethyl cellulose, maleated soybean oil, sodium lauryl sulfate, methylparaben, propylparaben, eucalyptus oil
Chap Stick® Medicated Lip Balm (stick, ointment)	Camphor 1%, menthol 0.6%, phenol 0.5%	**Stick:** Petrolatum 41%, paraffin wax, mineral oil, cocoa butter, 2-octyl dodecanol, arachidyl propionate, polyphenylmethylsiloxane 556, white wax, isopropyl lanolate, carnauba wax, isopropyl myristate, lanolin, fragrance, methylparaben, propylparaben, oleyl alcohol, cetyl alcohol **Ointment:** Petrolatum (jar 60%, tube 67%), microcrystalline wax, mineral oil, cocoa butter, lanolin, paraffin war (jar), fragrance, methylparaben, propylparaben
Dent's® Double-Action Kit (tablets, drops)	Benzocaine 20% (drops), acetaminophen 325 mg (tablet)	**Drops:** Denatured alcohol 74%, chlorobutanol anhydrous 0.09%, propylene glycol, FD&C red #40, eugenol
Dent's® Extra Strength Toothache Gum	Benzocaine 20%	Petrolatum, cotton and wax base, beeswax, FD&C red #40 aluminum lake, eugenol
Dent's® Maxi-Strength Toothache Treatment Drops	Benzocaine 20%	Denatured alcohol 74%, chlorobutanol anhydrous 0.09%, propylene glycol, FD&C red #40, eugenol
Dent-Zel-Ite® Oral Mucosal Analgesic Liquid	Benzocaine 5%, camphor	Alcohol 81%, wintergreen, glycerin, **dye free**
Dent-Zel-Ite® Temporary Dental Filling Liquid	Camphor	Alcohol 56.18%, sandarac gum, methyl salicylate
Dent-Zel-Ite® Toothache Relief Drops	Eugenol 85%, camphor	Alcohol 13.5%, wintergreen
Dentapaine® Gel	Benzocaine 20%	Glycerin, oil of cloves, sodium saccharin, methylparaben, PEG 400 and 4000, water, **alcohol free, dye free, gluten free, dietetically sucrose free**
Dr. Hand's® Teething Gel or Lotion	Menthol	SD alcohol 38B (gel 10%, lotion 11%), sterilized water, carbomer 940, witch hazel, polysorbate 80, sodium hydroxide, simethicone, D&C red #33, FD&C red #3

Brand Name	Anesthetic / Analgesic	Other Ingredients
Gly-Oxide® Liquid		Carbamide peroxide 10%[3], citric acid, flavor, glycerin, propylene glycol, sodium stannate, water
Herpecin-L®		Octinoxate, oxybenzone, meradimate, octisalate, dimethacone, sunflower oil, petrolatum, ozokerite, mineral oil, microcrystalline wax, talc, titanium dioxide, beeswax, mellissa extract, cetyl lactate, glyceryl laurate, flavor, lysine, ascorbyl palmitate, tocopheryl acetate, pyridoxine HCl, panthenol, BHT (244-014)
Herpecin-L® Cold Sore Lip Balm Stick[2]		Padimate O 7%, allantoin 0.5%, titanium dioxide, beeswax, cetyl esters, flavor, octyldodecanol, paraffin, petrolatum, sesame oil, vitamins B6, C and E
Hurricaine® Aerosol[1] (wild cherry)	Benzocaine 20%	PEG, saccharin, flavor, alcohol, **dye free, gluten free, sulfite free**
Hurricaine® Gel[1] (wild cherry, pina colada, watermelon)	Benzocaine 20%	PEG, saccharin, flavor, **alcohol free, dye free, gluten free, sulfite free**
Hurricaine® Liquid[1] (wild cherry, pina colada)	Benzocaine 20%	PEG, saccharin, flavor, **alcohol free, dye free, gluten free, dietetically sucrose free**
Kank-A® Professional Strength Liquid[1]	Benzocaine 20%	Benzoin tincture compound, cetylpyridinium chloride, ethylcellulose, SD alcohol 24%, dimethyl isosorbide, castor oil, flavor, tannic acid, propylene glycol, saccharin, benzyl alcohol
Lipclear™ Lysine Plus™		Zinc oxide, l-lysine, vitamin A, vitamin D, vitamin E, olive oil, yellow beeswax, goldenseal extract, propolis extract, calendula extract, echinacea extract, cajeput oil, tea tree oil, gum benzoin tincture, honey, lithium carbonate (3x)
Lip-Ex® Ointment	Phenol, camphor, salicylic acid, menthol	Petrolatum, cherry flavor
Lipmagik® Liquid	Benzocaine 6.3%, phenol 0.5%	Alcohol 70%, **dye free, sulfite free, gluten free**
Little Teethers® Oral Pain Relief Gel	Benzocaine 7.5%	Carbomer, glycerin, flavor, potassium sorbate, acesulfame K, PEGs, **alcohol free, dye free, dietetically sodium free, dietetically sucrose free**
Medadyne® Liquid	Benzocaine 10%, menthol, camphor, benzyl alcohol	Benzalkonium chloride, tannic acid, flavor, SD alcohol, thymol
Novitra™		Zincum oxydatum (2x), HPUS, alpha tocopherol, benzalkonium chloride, setyl alcohol, cocoa butter, glyceryl monostearate, glycine, modified lanolin, methylparaben, PEG 8000, propylparaben, water, sodium lauryl sulfate
Numzident® Adult Strength Gel	Benzocaine 10%	PEG-8, glycerin, PEG-75, sodium saccharin, purified water, flavor
Numzit® Teething Gel	Benzocaine 7.5%	PEG-8, PEG-75, sodium saccharin, clove oil, peppermint oil, purified water
Orabase® Baby Gel[1]	Benzocaine 7.5%	Glycerin, PEG, carbopol, preservative, sweetener, flavor, **alcohol free**
Orabase® Gel	Benzocaine 15%	Ethanol, propylene glycol, ethylcellulose, tannic acid, salicylic acid, flavor, sodium saccharin
Orabase® Lip Cream	Benzocaine 5%, menthol 0.5%, camphor, phenol	Allantoin 1%, carboxymethylcellulose sodium, veegum, Tween 80, phenonip, PEG, biopure, talc, kaolin, lanolin, petrolatum, oil of clove, hydrated silica, **alcohol free**
Orabase® Plain Paste[1]		Pectin, gelatin, carboxymethylcellulose sodium, polyethylene, mineral oil, flavor, preservative, guar, tragacanth, **alcohol free**
Orabase-B® with Benzocaine Paste[1]	Benzocaine 20%	Plasticized hydrocarbon gel, guar, carboxymethylcellulose, tragacanth, pectin, preservatives, flavor, **alcohol free**
Oragesic Solution	Benzyl alcohol 2%, menthol	Water, sorbitol, polysorbate 20, sodium chloride, yerba santa, saccharin, flavor, **sulfite free**
Orajel® Baby Gel or Liquid	Benzocaine 7.5%	**Gel:** FD&C red #40, flavor, glycerin, PEGs, sodium saccharin, sorbic acid, sorbitol, **alcohol free** **Liquid:** Not applicable
Orajel® Baby Nighttime Gel	Benzocaine 10%	FD&C red #40, flavor, glycerin, PEGs, sodium saccharin, sorbic acid, sorbitol, **alcohol free**
Orajel® CoverMed Cream (tinted light, medium)	Dyclonine HCl 1%	Allantoin 0.5%
Orajel® Denture Gel	Benzocaine 20%	Cellulose gum, gelatin, menthol, methyl salicylate, pectin, plasticized hydrocarbon gel, PEG, sodium saccharin

MOUTH PAIN, COLD SORE, AND CANKER SORE PRODUCTS *(Continued)*

Brand Name	Anesthetic / Analgesic	Other Ingredients
Orajel® Maximum Strength Gel	Benzocaine 20%	Clove oil, flavor, PEGs, sodium saccharin, sorbic acid
Orajel® Mouth-Aid Gel or Liquid	Benzocaine 20%	**Gel:** Zinc chloride 0.1%, benzalkonium chloride 0.02%. allantoin, carbomer, EDTA disodium, peppermint oil, PEG, polysorbate 60, propyl gallate, propylene glycol, purified water, povidone, sodium saccharin, sorbic acid, stearyl alcohol **Liquid:** Ethyl alcohol 44.2%
Orajel® PM Cream	Benzocaine 20%	
Orajel® Periostatic Spot Treatment Oral Cleanser		Carbamide peroxide 15%[3], citric acid, EDTA disodium, flavor, methylparaben, PEG, purified water, sodium chloride, sodium saccharin
Orajel® Periostatic Super Cleaning Oral Rinse		Hydrogen peroxide 1.5%[3], ethyl alcohol 4%
Orajel® Regular Strength Gel	Benzocaine 10%	Clove oil, flavor, PEGs, sodium saccharin, sorbic acid
Peroxyl® Hygienic Dental Rinse		Hydrogen peroxide 1.5%[3], alcohol 5%, pluronic F108, sorbitol, sodium saccharin, dye, polysorbate 20, mint flavor, **gluten free, sulfite free**
Peroxyl® Oral Spot Treatment Gel		Hydrogen peroxide 1.5%[3], ethyl alcohol 5%, pluronic F108, sorbitol, sodium saccharin, dye, polysorbate 20, mint flavor, dye, pluronic F127, **gluten free, dietetically sucrose free**
Proxigel® Gel[2]	Menthol	Carbamide peroxide 10%[3], glycerin, carbomer, phosphoric acid, triethanolamine, flavor, **dye free, gluten free, dietetically sucrose free**
Red Cross® Canker Sore Medication Ointment[2]	Benzocaine 20%, phenol	Carbomer 974P, mineral oil, petrolatum, propylparaben
Red Cross® Toothache Medication Drops	Eugenol 85%	Sesame oil
Retre-Gel®[2]	Benzocaine 5%, menthol 1%	Glycerin 20%
Tanac® Medicated Gel	Dyclonine HCl 1%	Allantoin 0.5%
Tanac® No Sting Liquid	Benzocaine 10%	Benzalkonium chloride 0.125%, saccharin
Zilactin® Gel	Benzyl alcohol 10%	**Gluten free**
Zilactin® Baby Gel	Benzocaine 10%	**Alcohol free, dye free, gluten free**
Zilactin®-B Gel	Benzocaine 10%	**Gluten free**
Zilactin®-L Liquid	Lidocaine 2.5%	Boric acid, propylene glycol, water, salicylic acid, SD alcohol 37, tannic acid

[1] Carries American Dental Association (ADA) seal indicating safety and efficacy

[2] Agent for cold sore treatment only

[3] Agent for debridement or wound cleansing

Adapted with permission from *Nonprescription Products: Formulations & Features, Companion to the Handbook of Nonprescription Drugs*, 11th ed, Washington, DC, American Pharmaceutical Association, 1998, 338-40.

ORAL RINSE PRODUCTS

Brand Name	Active Ingredients	Other Ingredients
ACT® Anticavity Fluoride Rinse, Bubble Gum Blowout™	Cetylpyridinium chloride	Sodium fluoride 0.05%, D&C red #33, calcium EDTA, flavor, glycerin, monobasic and dibasic sodium phosphates, poloxamer 407, polysorbate 80, propylene glycol, sodium benzoate, water, sodium saccharin, **alcohol free**
ACT® Anticavity Fluoride Treatment Rinse, Mint	Cetylpyridinium chloride	Sodium fluoride 0.05%, D&C red #33, calcium EDTA, FD&C yellow #5, flavor, glycerin, monobasic and dibasic sodium phosphates, poloxamer 407, polysorbate 80, propylene glycol, sodium benzoate, sodium saccharin, water, **alcohol free**
Arm & Hammer Advance Breath Care™ Cool Fresh Mint Mouthwash	Alcohol 15%, cetylpyridinium chloride, zinc citrate	Water, glycerin and/or sorbitol, sodium bicarbonate, sodium citrate, poloxamer 407, flavor, sucrose and/or sodium saccharin, D&C green #5, FD&C yellow #5
Arm & Hammer Advance Breath Care™ Icy Fresh Mint Mouthwash	Alcohol 15%, cetylpyridinium chloride, zinc citrate	Water, glycerin and/or sorbitol, sodium bicarbonate, sodium citrate, poloxamer 407, flavor, sucrose and/or sodium saccharin, D&C green #5
Astring-O-Sol® Liquid	SD alcohol 38B 75.6%, methyl salicylate	Water, myrrh extract, zinc chloride, citric acid
Betadine® Mouthwash Gargle	Alcohol 8%	Povidone-iodine 0.5%, glycerin, sodium saccharin, flavor
Biotene® Alcohol-Free Mouthwash	Lysozyme (40 mg), lactoferrin (15 mg), glucose oxidase (2500 units), lactoperoxidase (2500 units)	Water, xylitol, hydrogenated starch, propylene glycol, hydroxyethylcellulose, aloe vera, peppermint, poloxamer 407, sodium benzoate, **alcohol free**
Biotene® Mouthwash	Lysozyme (6 mg), lactoferrin (6 mg), glucose oxidase (4000 units), zinc gluconate	Water, xylitol, hydrogenated starch, propylene glycol, hydroxy ethylcellulose, aloe vera, natural peppermint, poloxamer 407, calcium lactate, sodium benzoate, benzoic acid
Cepacol® Mouthwash/Gargle	Alcohol 14%, cetylpyridinium chloride 0.05%	EDTA disodium, color, flavor, glycerin, polysorbate 80, saccharin, sodium biphosphate, sodium phosphate, water, **gluten free, dietetically sucrose free**
Cepacol® Mouthwash/Gargle (mint)	Alcohol 14.5%, cetylpyridinium chloride 0.5%	Color, flavor, glucono delta-lactone, glycerin, poloxamer 407, sodium saccharin, sodium gluconate, water, **gluten free, dietetically sucrose free**
Crest® Pro-Health™ Rinse	Cetylpyridinium chloride 0.07%	Water, glycerin, flavor, poloxamer 407, sodium saccharin, blue #1
Dr. Tichenor's® Antiseptic Liquid	SDA alcohol 38B 70%	Oil of peppermint, extract of arnica, water, **dye free, gluten free**
Lavoris Crystal Fresh	SD alcohol 38-B, zantrate (citric acid, zinc oxide, sodium hydroxide)	Purified spring water, glycerin, poloxamer 407, saccharin, polysorbate 80, flavors
Lavoris Mint Mouthwash	Zinc chloride and/or zinc oxide, aromatic oils	Glycerin
Lavoris Original Cinnamon Mouthwash	Zinc chloride and/or zinc oxide, aromatic oils	Glycerin
Lavoris Original Mouthwash	SD alcohol 38-B, zinc chloride, zantrate (zinc oxide, sodium hydroxide, citric acid)	Water, glycerin, poloxamer 407, saccharin, clove oil, polysorbate 80, flavor, D&C red #6 and #33
Lavoris Peppermint Mouthwash	SD alcohol 38-B, zantrate (sodium hydroxide, citric acid, zinc oxide)	Water, glycerin, poloxamer 407, polysorbate 80, peppermint oil, saccharin, FD&C blue #4
Listerine®	Eucalyptol 0.092%, menthol 0.042%, methyl salicylate 0.06%, thymol 0.064%	Water, alcohol (21.6%), sorbitol solution, flavoring, poloxamer 407, benzoic acid, zinc chloride, sodium benzoate, sucralose, sodium saccharin, FD&C blue #1

ORAL RINSE PRODUCTS *(Continued)*

Brand Name	Active Ingredients	Other Ingredients
Listerine®[1] Liquid	Alcohol 26.9%, eucalyptol 0.092%, thymol 0.064%, methyl salicylate 0.06%, menthol 0.042%	Benzoic acid, poloxamer 407, caramel, water, sodium benzoate
Listerine®[1] Liquid (freshburst, cool mint)	Alcohol 21.6%, eucalyptol 0.092%, thymol 0.064%, methyl salicylate 0.06%, menthol 0.042%	Water, sorbitol solution, poloxamer 407, benzoic acid, flavor, sodium saccharin, sodium citrate, citric acid, FD&C green #3, D&C yellow #10 (freshburst)
Listerine® Whitening Pre-Brush	Alcohol 8%, hyrdogen peroxide	Water, glycerin, alcohol (8%), flavor, poloxamer 407, sodium lauryl sulfate, sodium citrate, sodium saccharin, sucralose
Mentadent® Mouthwash (cool mint, fresh mint)	Alcohol 10%	Water, sorbitol, sodium bicarbonate, hydrogen peroxide, poloxamer 407, sodium lauryl sulfate, flavor, polysorbate 20, methyl salicylate (cool mint), sodium saccharin, phosphoric acid, blue #1, yellow #5 (cool mint)
Oasis® Moisturizing Mouthwash	Glycerin	Water, sorbitol, poloxamer 338, PEG-60 hydrogenated castor oil, cellulose gum, cetylpyridinium chloride, copovidone, disodium phosphate, flavor, methylparaben, propylparaben, sodium benzoate, sodium phosphate, sodium saccharin, xanthan gum, FD&C blue #1
Oasis® Moisturizing Mouth Spray	Glycerin 35% (prediluted)	Cetylpyridinium chloride, copovidone, flavor, methylparaben, PEG-60 hydrogenated castor oil, propylparaben, sodium benzoate, sodium saccharin, water, xanthan gum, xylitol
Oxyfresh Fresh Mint Mouthrinse	Oxygene® (stabilized chlorine dioxide)	Purified deionized water, xylitol, mint oils, sodium benzoate, **alcohol free**
Oxyfresh Fresh Mint with Fluoride Mouthrinse	Oxygene® (stabilized chlorine dioxide)	Sodium fluoride (0.05%), purified deionized water, xylitol, mint oils, sodium benzoate, **alcohol free**
Oxyfresh Fresh Mint with Zinc Mouthrinse	Oxygene® (stabilized chlorine dioxide), zinc acetate	Purified deionized water, xylitol, sodium citrate, peppermint oil, **alcohol free**
Oxyfresh Original Mint Mouthrinse	Oxygene® (stabilized chlorine dioxide)	Purified deionized water, mint oils, sodium benzoate, **alcohol free**
Oxyfresh Professional Strength Zinc Mouthrinse	Oxygene® (stabilized chlorine dioxide), zinc acetate	Purified deionized water, xylitol, sodium citrate, peppermint oil, **alcohol free**
Oxyfresh Unflavored Mouthrinse	Oxygene® (stabilized chlorine dioxide)	Purified deionized water, sodium benzoate, **alcohol free**
Plax® Advanced Formula (mint sensation)	Alcohol 8.7%	Water, sorbitol solution, tetrasodium pyrophosphate, benzoic acid, flavor, poloxamer 407, sodium benzoate, sodium lauryl sulfate, sodium saccharin, xanthan gum, FD&C blue #1
Plax® Advanced Formula (original, SoftMINT)	Alcohol 8.7%	Sodium lauryl sulfate, water, sorbitol solution, sodium benzoate, tetrasodium pyrophosphate, benzoic acid, poloxamer 407, sodium saccharin, flavor (SoftMINT), xanthan gum (SoftMINT), flavor enhancer (SoftMINT), FD&C blue #1 (SoftMINT), FD&C yellow #5 (SoftMINT)
Rembrandt® Naturals Mouthwash		Spring water, glycerin, xylitol, sodium citrate, vitamin C, stevia, citric acid, dicalcium phosphate, cocamidopropyl betain, flavor, ginkgo extract, raspberry leaf extract, alcohol free. Also available with papaya and ginseng or aloe and echinacea
S.T. 37® Solution	Hexylresorcinol 0.1%	Glycerin, propylene glycol, citric acid, EDTA disodium, sodium bisulfite, sodium citrate

Brand Name	Active Ingredients	Other Ingredients
Scope® Baking Soda	SD alcohol 38F 9.9%, cetylpyridinium chloride, domiphen bromide	Sorbitol, sodium bicarbonate, sodium saccharin, flavor
Scope® (cool peppermint)	SD alcohol 38F 14%, cetylpyridinium chloride, domiphen bromide	Purified water, glycerin, poloxamer 407, sodium saccharin, sodium benzoate, N-ethylmethylcarboxamide, benzoic acid, FD&C blue #1, flavor
Targon® Smokers' Mouthwash (clean taste)	SDA alcohol 38B 15.6%	Water, glycerin, polyoxyl 40 hydrogenated caster oil, sodium lauryl sulfate, dibasic sodium phosphate, benzoic acid, sodium saccharin, caramel powder, **dietetically sucrose free**
Targon® Smokers' Mouthwash (original)	SDA alcohol 38B 16%	Water, sodium saccharin, sodium benzoate, glycerin, sodium lauryl sulfate, FD&C green #3, FD&C yellow #5, polyoxyl 40 hydrogenated castor oil, **dietetically sucrose free**
Tom's of Maine® Natural Mouthwash (cinnamon, original)	Menthol	Water, glycerin, aloe vera juice, witch hazel, poloxamer 335, spearmint oil, ascorbic acid, **alcohol free**
Viadent Advanced Care Oral Rinse	Cetylpyridium chloride 0.05%	Purified water, sorbitol, ethyl alcohol (5.5% w/w), glycerin, propylene glycol, PEG-40 sorbitan diisostearate, flavor, sodium benzoate, sodium saccharin, FD&C yellow No. 6

[1]Carries American Dental Association (ADA) seal indicating safety and efficacy

Note: SD alcohol refers to "specially denatured" alcohol

Adapted with permission from *Nonprescription Products: Formulations & Features, Companion to the Handbook of Nonprescription Drugs*, 11th ed, Washington, DC, American Pharmaceutical Association, 1998, 341-2.

TOP 200 MOST PRESCRIBED DRUGS IN 2005*

1.	Hydrocodone and Acetaminophen	52.	Tramadol
2.	Lipitor®	53.	Ciprofloxacin
3.	Amoxicillin	54.	Lotrel®
4.	Lisinopril	55.	Ranitidine
5.	Hydrochlorothiazide	56.	Allegra®
6.	Atenolol	57.	Levoxyl®
7.	Furosemide (oral)	58.	Diovan®
8.	Alprazolam	59.	Enalapril
9.	Toprol-XL®	60.	Diazepam
10.	Albuterol (aerosol)	61.	Naproxen
11.	Norvasc®	62.	Fluconazole
12.	Levothyroxine	63.	Lisinopril and Hydrochlorothiazide
13.	Synthroid®	64.	Klor-Con®
14.	Metformin	65.	Altace®
15.	Zoloft®	66.	Wellbutrin XL™
16.	Lexapro®	67.	Celebrex®
17.	Ibuprofen	68.	Viagra®
18.	Cephalexin	69.	Doxycycline
19.	Ambien®	70.	Zetia™
20.	Zithromax® Z-Pak®	71.	Avandia®
21.	Prednisone (oral)	72.	Lovastatin
22.	Nexium®	73.	Diovan HCT®
23.	Triamterene and Hydrochlorothiazide	74.	Carisoprodol
24.	Propoxyphene-N and Acetaminophen	75.	Yasmin® 28
		76.	Allopurinol
25.	Zocor®	77.	Clonidine
26.	Singulair®	78.	Methylprednisolone (tablet)
27.	Prevacid®	79.	Actos®
28.	Metoprolol	80.	Pravachol®
29.	Fluoxetine	81.	Actonel®
30.	Lorazepam	82.	Ortho Evra™
31.	Plavix®	83.	Citalopram
32.	Oxycodone and Acetaminophen	84.	Verapamil SR
33.	Amoxicillin and Clavulanate Potassium	85.	Isosorbide Mononitrate
		86.	Penicillin VK
34.	Advair Diskus®	87.	Glyburide
35.	Fosamax®	88.	Zithromax® (suspension)
36.	Effexor® XR	89.	Adderall XR®
37.	Warfarin	90.	Nasonex®
38.	Paroxetine	91.	Folic Acid
39.	Clonazepam	92.	Seroquel®
40.	Zyrtec®	93.	Cozaar®
41.	Protonix®	94.	Tricor®
42.	Potassium Chloride	95.	Coreg®
43.	Acetaminophen and Codeine	96.	Concerta®
44.	Trimethoprim and Sulfamethoxazole	97.	Vytorin™
		98.	Lantus®
45.	Gabapentin	99.	Promethazine (tablet)
46.	Premarin® (tablet)	100.	Mobic®
47.	Flonase®	101.	Flomax®
48.	Trazodone	102.	Crestor®
49.	Cyclobenzaprine	103.	Glipizide (extended release)
50.	Amitriptyline	104.	Ortho Tri-Cyclen® Lo
51.	Levaquin®	105.	Temazepam

106.	Omeprazole	153.	Nabumetone
107.	Omnicef®	154.	Zyprexa®
108.	Albuterol (solution for oral inhalation)	155.	Lamictal®
		156.	Zyrtec® (syrup)
109.	Risperdal®	157.	Glycolax™
110.	Aciphex®	158.	Acyclovir
111.	Digitek®	159.	Propranolol
112.	Spironolactone	160.	Nasacort® AQ
113.	Valtrex®	161.	Aricept®
114.	Xalatan®	162.	Butalbital, Acetaminophen, and Caffeine
115.	Metformin (extended release)		
116.	Hyzaar®	163.	Niaspan®
117.	Zithromax®	164.	Azithromycin
118.	Quinapril	165.	Depakote®
119.	Clindamycin (systemic)	166.	Buspirone
120.	Metronidazole (tablet)	167.	Tri-Sprintec™
121.	Triamcinolone Acetonide Paste (topical)	168.	Methotrexate
		169.	OxyContin®
122.	Topamax®	170.	Rhinocort® Aqua®
123.	Combivent®	171.	Benicar HCT®
124.	Benazepril	172.	Terazosin
125.	Gemfibrozil	173.	Skelaxin®
126.	Avapro®	174.	Betamethasone and Clotrimazole
127.	Amaryl®	175.	Cialis®
128.	TriNessa™	176.	Avalide®
129.	Estradiol (oral)	177.	Fexofenadine
130.	Hydroxyzine	178.	Ortho Tri-Cyclen®
131.	Metoclopramide	179.	Bupropion SR
132.	Allegra-D® 12 Hour	180.	Benzonatate
133.	Doxazosin	181.	Patanol®
134.	Coumadin® (tablet)	182.	Quinine
135.	Glipizide	183.	Cartia XT™
136.	Diclofenac	184.	Humalog®
137.	Evista®	185.	Paxil CR®
138.	Diltiazem CD	186.	Aviane™
139.	Detrol® LA	187.	Lanoxin®
140.	Meclizine	188.	Amphetamine and Dextroamphetamine
141.	Metformin and Glyburide		
142.	Strattera®	189.	Famotidine
143.	Cymbalta®	190.	Digoxin
144.	Nitrofurantoin	191.	Levothroid®
145.	Promethazine and Codeine	192.	Nifedipine ER
146.	Benicar®	193.	Nortriptyline
147.	Mirtazapine	194.	Tussionex®
148.	Bisoprolol and Hydrochlorothiazide	195.	NitroQuick®
		196.	Phenytoin
149.	Clarinex®	197.	Endocet®
150.	Oxycodone	198.	Etodolac
151.	Minocycline	199.	Atenolol and Chlorthalidone
152.	Imitrex® (oral)	200.	Phentermine

*Based on units dispensed in U.S.
Source: Verispan Scott-Levin, SPA

DENTAL DRUG USE IN PREGNANCY AND BREAST-FEEDING[1]

Drug	FDA Pregnancy Category	Use During Pregnancy	Use During Breast-Feeding
Acetaminophen	B	Yes	Yes
Acetaminophen and codeine	C	Low dose for short duration	Yes (with caution)
Acetaminophen and tramadol	C	No information	No information
Acyclovir	B	No information	No information
Alclometasone	C	Yes	No information
Alprazolam	D	Avoid	Avoid
Amitriptyline	C	Yes	Avoid
Amlexanox	B	Yes	Yes
Ammonia spirit (aromatic)	C	No information	No information
Amoxicillin	B	Yes	Yes
Amoxicillin and clavulanate potassium	B	Yes	Yes
Ampicillin	B	Yes	Yes
Ampicillin and sulbactam	B	Yes	Yes
Articaine hydrochloride and epinephrine (U.S.)	C	Yes	Yes
Aspirin	C/D	Not in third trimester	Avoid
Aspirin and codeine	D	Not in third trimester	Avoid
Atropine sulfate (dental tablets)	C	Yes	Avoid
Azithromycin	B	Yes	Yes
Beclomethasone	C	Yes	Avoid
Benzocaine	C	Yes	Yes
Betamethasone and clotrimazole	C	Yes	No information
Bupivacaine	C	Yes	Yes
Bupivacaine and epinephrine	C	Yes	Yes
Butalbital, acetaminophen, caffeine, and codeine	C/D	Not in third trimester	Avoid
Carbamazepine	D	Avoid	Avoid
Carbamide peroxide	C	Yes	Yes
Carisoprodol	C	Yes	Avoid
Carisoprodol and aspirin	C/D	Not in third trimester	Avoid
Carisoprodol, aspirin, and codeine	C/D	Not in third trimester	Avoid
Cefaclor	B	Yes	Yes
Cefadroxil	B	Yes	Yes
Cefazolin	B	Yes	Yes
Cefditoren	B	Yes	Yes
Celecoxib	C/D	No information	No information
Cephalexin	B	Yes	Yes
Cephradine	B	Yes	Yes
Cevimeline	C	No information	No information
Ciprofloxacin	C	Yes	Avoid
Clarithromycin	C	Yes	Yes
Clindamycin	B	Yes	Yes
Clobetasol	C	Yes	Yes
Clonazepam	D	Avoid	Avoid
Clotrimazole	C (troches)	Yes	Yes
Cloxacillin	B	Yes	Yes
Codeine	C	Low dose for short duration	Yes (with caution)
Cyclobenzaprine	B	Yes	No information
Dexamethasone	C	Yes	No information
Diazepam	D	Avoid	Avoid
Dibucaine	C	Yes	Yes
Diclofenac	B/D	Not in third trimester	Yes
Dicloxacillin	B	Yes	Yes
Diflunisal	C/D	Not in third trimester	Yes
Diphenhydramine	B	Yes	Yes
Doxycycline hyclate (periodontal)	D	Avoid	Avoid
Doxycycline (subantimicrobial)	D	Avoid	Avoid

Drug	FDA Pregnancy Category	Use During Pregnancy	Use During Breast-Feeding
Epinephrine	C	Yes	Yes
Erythromycin	B	Yes (avoid estolate)	Yes
Eszopiclone	C	Yes	No information
Etidocaine and epinephrine	B	Yes	Yes
Etodolac	C/D	Not in third trimester	Yes
Famciclovir	B	Yes	No information
Fentanyl	C/D	Yes (with caution)	Yes
Fluocinolone	C	Yes	No information
Fluocinonide	C	Yes	No information
Fluconazole	C	Yes	Yes
Flurbiprofen	C/D	Not in third trimester	Yes
Gabapentin	C	Yes	Avoid
Halobetasol	C	Yes (with caution)	Yes (with caution)
Hydrocodone and acetaminophen	C	Low dose for short duration	Yes (with caution)
Hydrocodone and aspirin	D	Not in third trimester	Avoid
Hydrocodone and ibuprofen	C/D	Not in third trimester	Yes (with caution)
Hydrocortisone	C	Yes	No information
Ibuprofen	B/D	Not in third trimester	Yes
Iodoquinol and hydrocortisone	C	Yes	No information
Ketoconazole	C	Yes	Yes
Ketoprofen	B/D	Not in third trimester	Yes
Ketorolac	C/D	Not in third trimester	Yes
Lidocaine	B	Yes	Yes
Lidocaine and epinephrine	B	Yes	Yes
Lidocaine and prilocaine	B	Yes	Yes
Lorazepam	D	Avoid	Avoid
Meperidine	B/D	Low dose for short duration	Yes (with caution)
Mepivacaine	C	Yes	Yes
Mepivacaine (dental anesthetic)	C	Yes	Yes
Mepivacaine and levonordefrin	C	Yes	Yes
Methocarbamol	C	Yes	No information
Methohexital	C	Yes	Yes
Methylprednisolone	C	Yes	No information
Metronidazole	B	Yes (with caution)	Yes (with caution)
Midazolam	D	Avoid	Avoid
Minocycline	D	Avoid	Avoid
Minocycline hydrochloride (periodontal)	D	Avoid	Avoid
Naloxone	C	Yes	Yes
Naproxen	B/D	Not in third trimester	Yes
Nicotine	D	Avoid	Avoid
Nitrous oxide[2]	None reported	Acute use in patients: Yes (with caution)	Acute use in patients: Yes
Nortriptyline	D	Avoid	Avoid
Nystatin	B/C	Yes	Yes
Nystatin and triamcinolone	C	Yes	No information
Oxycodone	B/D	Low dose for short duration	Yes
Oxycodone and acetaminophen	C/D	Low dose for short duration	Yes
Oxycodone and aspirin	D	Not in third trimester	Avoid
Oxycodone and ibuprofen	C/D	Not in third trimester	Yes (with caution)
Oxygen	None reported	Yes	Yes
Palifermin	C	Yes	No information
Penciclovir	B	Yes	Yes
Penicillin V potassium	B	Yes	Yes

DENTAL DRUG USE IN PREGNANCY AND BREAST-FEEDING[1]
(Continued)

Drug	FDA Pregnancy Category	Use During Pregnancy	Use During Breast-Feeding
Pentazocine and acetaminophen	C	Low dose for short duration	Yes (with caution)
Pilocarpine (dental)	C	Yes	Avoid
Pimecrolimus	C	Yes	No information
Prednisolone	C	Yes	Yes (with caution)
Prednisone	B	Yes	Yes
Prilocaine	B	Yes	Yes
Prilocaine and epinephrine	C	Yes	Yes
Propantheline	C	Yes	Yes
Propoxyphene and acetaminophen	C	Low dose for short duration	Yes (with caution)
Propoxyphene, aspirin, and caffeine	D	Not in third trimester	Avoid
Rofecoxib	C/D	No information	No information
Sulfonated phenolics in aqueous solution	C	Yes	Yes
Telithromycin	C	Yes	Yes (with caution)
Tetracaine	C	Yes	Yes
Tetracycline	D	Avoid	Avoid
Tetracycline (periodontal)	C	Avoid	Avoid
Tramadol	C	No (labor and delivery)	No
Triamcinolone acetonide paste	C	Yes	No information
Triazolam	X	Avoid	Avoid
Valacyclovir	B	Yes	Yes
Valdecoxib	C/D	No information	No information
Zaleplon	C	Yes	Avoid
Zolpidem	B	Yes	Yes (with caution)

[1]Pregnant or breast-feeding women should be encouraged to consult a physician prior to the use of any prescription or nonprescription medication. Additional information concerning other medications may be found in individual drug monographs.

[2]Female dental personnel to avoid chronic exposure to unscavenged nitrous oxide.

References:

Della-Giustina K and Chow G, "Medications in Pregnancy and Lactation," *Emerg Med Clin North Am*, 2003, 21(3):585-613.

Drug Information for the Health Care Professional, 20th ed, Vol 1, Rockville, MD: Medical Economics Company, 2000.

Haas DA, Pynn BR, and Sands TD, "Drug Use for the Pregnant or Lactating Patient," *Gen Dent*, 2000, 48(1):54-60.

Mariotti AJ, "Agents That Affect the Fetus and Nursing Infant," *ADA Guide to Dental Therapeutics*, 2nd ed, Chicago IL: ADA Publishing, 2000, 594-5.

VASOCONSTRICTOR INTERACTIONS WITH ANTIDEPRESSANTS

Antidepressant	Effects with Epinephrine, Levonordefrin	Contraindicated	Recommendation
Tricyclics			
Amitriptyline (Elavil® [DSC])	Epinephrine = increased pressor response; cardiac dysrhythmias	No	Potentially dangerous; use minimal amounts with caution in local anesthetics
Amoxapine			
Clomipramine (Anafranil®)	Levonordefrin = increased pressor response		
Desipramine (Norpramin®)			
Doxepin (Prudoxin™, Sinequan®, Zonalon®)			
Imipramine (Tofranil-PM®, Tofranil®)			
Nortriptyline (Pamelor®)			
Protriptyline (Vivactil®)			
Trimipramine (Surmontil®)			
Serotonin / Norepinephrine Reuptake Inhibitor			
Venlafaxine (Effexor® XR, Effexor®)	No adverse interactions reported	No	Suggest caution since venlafaxine blocks norepinephrine uptake in CNS
Serotonin Only Reuptake Inhibitors			
Citalopram (Celexa™)	No adverse interactions reported	No	No precautions appear to be necessary
Escitalopram (Lexapro™)			
Fluoxetine (Prozac® Weekly™, Prozac®, Sarafem™)			
Fluvoxamine			
Paroxetine (Paxil CR™, Paxil®, Pexeva™)			
Sertraline (Zoloft®)			
Central Alpha-2 Antagonist			
Mirtazapine (Remeron SolTab®, Remeron®)	No adverse interactions reported	No	Suggest caution since mirtazapine increases release of norepinephrine
Dopamine Reuptake Inhibitor			
Bupropion (Wellbutrin SR®, Wellbutrin XL™, Wellbutrin®, Zyban®)	No adverse interactions reported	No	Part of the mechanism of bupropion is to block norepinephrine reuptake within CNS; it has been suggested that vasoconstrictor be administered with caution
Others			
Duloxetine (Cymbalta®)	No adverse interactions reported	No	Part of the mechanism of duloxetine is to block norepinephrine reuptake within CNS; it has been suggested that vasoconstrictor be administered with caution
Maprotiline	Potential for increased pressor response	No	Potentially dangerous; use minimal amounts with caution in local anesthetics
MAO Inhibitors			
Isocarboxazid (Marplan®)	No effects on blood pressure or heart rate reported; however, potential exists for slight increase in pressor response	No	Use vasoconstrictor with caution
Phenelzine (Nardil®)			
Tranylcypromine (Parnate®)			

VASOCONSTRICTOR INTERACTIONS WITH ANTIDEPRESSANTS *(Continued)*

Antidepressant	Effects with Epinephrine, Levonordefrin	Contraindicated	Recommendation
Serotonin Reuptake Inhibitor / Serotonin Antagonist			
Nefazodone (Serzone® [DSC])	No adverse interactions reported	No	No precautions appear to be necessary
Trazodone (Desyrel®)			

Naftalin LW and Yagiela JA, "Vasoconstrictors: Indications and Precautions," *Dent Clin North Am*, 2002, 46(4):733-46.

Wynn RL, "Antidepressant Medications," *Gen Dent*, 1992, 40(3):192-7.

Yagiela JA, "Adverse Drug Interactions in Dental Practice: Interactions Associated With Vasoconstrictors. Part V of a Series," *J Am Dent Assoc*, 1999, 130(5):701-9.

Yagiela JA, "Injectable and Topical Local Anesthetics," *ADA Guide to Dental Therapeutics*, 2nd ed, Chicago, IL: ADA Publishing, 2000, 1-16.

PHARMACOLOGIC CATEGORY INDEX

Abortifacient
Carboprost Tromethamine 270
Dinoprostone 482
Mifepristone 1045

Acetylcholinesterase Inhibitor
Physostigmine 1232
Pyridostigmine 1315

Acetylcholinesterase Inhibitor (Central)
Donepezil 500
Galantamine 720
Rivastigmine 1361
Tacrine 1436

Acne Products
Adapalene 54
Isotretinoin 869

Activated Prothrombin Complex Concentrate (aPCC)
Anti-inhibitor Coagulant Complex 130

Adjuvant, Chemoprotective Agent (Cytoprotective)
Amifostine 83

Adjuvant, Radiosensitizing Agent
Cladribine 354

Adrenergic Agonist Agent
Carbinoxamine and Pseudoephedrine 268
DOBUTamine 493
Epinephrine (Racemic) and Aluminum Potassium Sulfate 550
Oxymetazoline 1172
Phenylephrine and Zinc Sulfate 1228
Propylhexedrine 1305
Tetrahydrozoline 1470

Adrenergic Agonist Agent, Ophthalmic
Hydroxyamphetamine and Tropicamide 799

Aldehyde Dehydrogenase Inhibitor
Disulfiram 492

Alkalinizing Agent
Sodium Bicarbonate 1400

Alkalinizing Agent, Oral
Citric Acid, Sodium Citrate, and Potassium Citrate 354
Potassium Citrate 1259
Potassium Citrate and Citric Acid 1259
Sodium Citrate and Citric Acid 1401

Alkalinizing Agent, Parenteral
Tromethamine 1545

Alpha₁ Agonist
Midodrine 1044
Naphazoline 1087

Alpha₁ Blocker
Alfuzosin 68
Doxazosin 503
Phenoxybenzamine 1224
Phentolamine 1226
Prazosin 1267
Tamsulosin 1445
Terazosin 1458

Alpha₁ Blocker, Ophthalmic
Dapiprazole 421

Alpha₂-Adrenergic Agonist
Clonidine 373
Dexmedetomidine 444
Guanabenz 758
Guanfacine 758
Tizanidine 1497

Alpha₂ Agonist, Ophthalmic
Apraclonidine 133
Brimonidine 220

Alpha-Adrenergic Inhibitor
Methyldopa 1021

Alpha/Beta Agonist
Acetaminophen and Pseudoephedrine 38
Chlorpheniramine and Pseudoephedrine 325
Dexchlorpheniramine and Pseudoephedrine 443
Dipivefrin 489
Ephedrine 545
Epinephrine 546
Epinephrine (Racemic) 549
Epinephrine (Racemic) and Aluminum Potassium Sulfate 550
Guaifenesin and Pseudoephedrine 755
Norepinephrine 1125
Phenylephrine 1226
Pseudoephedrine 1309
Triprolidine and Pseudoephedrine 1542

5 Alpha-Reductase Inhibitor
Dutasteride 524
Finasteride 655

Amebicide
Iodoquinol 853
Metronidazole 1033
Paromomycin 1188
Tinidazole 1491

Amino Acid
Carnitine 1616
Glutamine 743

Aminoquinoline (Antimalarial)
Chloroquine 320
Hydroxychloroquine 799
Primaquine 1281

5-Aminosalicylic Acid Derivative
Balsalazide 179
Mesalamine 996
Olsalazine 1144
Sulfasalazine 1428

Ammonium Detoxicant
Lactulose 893
Neomycin 1100

Amylinomimetic
Pramlintide 1263

Anabolic Steroid
Oxymetholone 1173
Stanozolol 1415

Analgesic Combination (Narcotic)
Acetaminophen, Caffeine, and Dihydrocodeine 42
Belladonna and Opium 184
Butalbital, Acetaminophen, Caffeine, and Codeine 239
Butalbital, Aspirin, Caffeine, and Codeine 241
Hydrocodone and Acetaminophen 779
Hydrocodone and Aspirin 782
Meperidine and Promethazine . . 986
Pentazocine and Acetaminophen 1209
Propoxyphene and Acetaminophen 1298
Propoxyphene, Aspirin, and Caffeine 1300

Analgesic, Miscellaneous
Acetaminophen 31
Acetaminophen and
  Diphenhydramine 38
Acetaminophen and
  Pseudoephedrine 38
Acetaminophen and Tramadol . . . 39
Acetaminophen, Aspirin, and
  Caffeine 41
Acetaminophen,
  Chlorpheniramine, and
  Pseudoephedrine 43
Acetaminophen,
  Isometheptene, and
  Dichloralphenazone 44
Pregabalin 1274
Tetrahydrocannabinol and
  Cannabidiol 1469

Analgesic, Narcotic
Acetaminophen and Codeine 35
Alfentanil 67
Aspirin and Codeine. 149
Buprenorphine 231
Buprenorphine and Naloxone . . . 232
Butorphanol 243
Codeine 385
Dihydrocodeine, Aspirin, and
  Caffeine 475
Fentanyl 644
Hydrocodone and Ibuprofen 787
Hydromorphone 797
Levorphanol 916
Meperidine 983
Methadone 1004
Morphine Sulfate 1065
Nalbuphine 1083
Opium Tincture 1149
Oxycodone 1163
Oxycodone and
  Acetaminophen 1165
Oxycodone and Aspirin 1168
Oxycodone and Ibuprofen 1170
Oxymorphone. 1174
Paregoric 1187
Pentazocine 1208
Propoxyphene 1297
Remifentanil 1338
Sufentanil 1421

Analgesic, Non-narcotic
Acetaminophen and
  Phenyltoloxamine 38
Acetaminophen and Tramadol . . .39
Methotrimeprazine 1016
Tramadol 1514
Ziconotide 1594

Analgesic, Topical
Capsaicin 256
Dichlorodifluoromethane and
  Trichloromonofluoromethane
  458
Lidocaine 920
Lidocaine and Tetracaine 930
Triethanolamine Salicylate 1535

Analgesic, Urinary
Pentosan Polysulfate Sodium
  1211
Phenazopyridine 1220

Androgen
Danazol 419
Fluoxymesterone 679
MethylTESTOSTERone 1028
Nandrolone 1087
Oxandrolone 1155
Testolactone 1462
Testosterone 1462

Anesthetic/Corticosteroid
Lidocaine and Hydrocortisone . . 928

Anesthetic, Topical
Pramoxine and Hydrocortisone
  1264
Pentafluoropropane and
  Tetrafluoroethane 1206
Phenol 1223

Angiogenesis Inhibitor
Lenalidomide 903
Thalidomide 1471

Angiotensin II Receptor Blocker
Candesartan 252
Eprosartan 554
Irbesartan. 858
Losartan. 950
Olmesartan 1142
Telmisartan 1451
Valsartan 1561

Angiotensin II Receptor Blocker Combination
Candesartan and
  Hydrochlorothiazide 254
Eprosartan and
  Hydrochlorothiazide 555
Irbesartan and
  Hydrochlorothiazide 860
Losartan and
  Hydrochlorothiazide 952
Olmesartan and
  Hydrochlorothiazide 1143
Telmisartan and
  Hydrochlorothiazide 1452
Valsartan and
  Hydrochlorothiazide 1562

Angiotensin-Converting Enzyme (ACE) Inhibitor
Benazepril 185
Captopril 257
Cilazapril 340
Enalapril. 538
Fosinopril 707
Lisinopril 936
Moexipril 1058
Perindopril Erbumine 1216
Quinapril 1322
Quinapril and
  Hydrochlorothiazide 1323
Ramipril 1332
Spirapril 1413
Trandolapril 1517

Anorexiant
Benzphetamine 195
Diethylpropion 467
Phendimetrazine 1220
Phentermine. 1224
Sibutramine 1389

Antacid
Aluminum Hydroxide 79
Aluminum Hydroxide and
  Magnesium Carbonate 79
Aluminum Hydroxide and
  Magnesium Hydroxide 80
Aluminum Hydroxide and
  Magnesium Trisilicate 80
Aluminum Hydroxide,
  Magnesium Hydroxide, and
  Simethicone 81
Calcium Carbonate 248
Calcium Carbonate and
  Magnesium Hydroxide 249
Calcium Carbonate and
  Simethicone 249
Famotidine, Calcium
  Carbonate, and
  Magnesium Hydroxide 636
Magaldrate and Simethicone . . . 960
Magnesium Hydroxide 961
Magnesium Sulfate 963

Sodium Bicarbonate 1400

Anthelmintic
Albendazole 57
Ivermectin 877
Mebendazole 968
Piperazine 1246
Praziquantel 1266
Pyrantel Pamoate 1314
Thiabendazole 1475

Antiandrogen
Nilutamide 1115

Antianxiety Agent, Miscellaneous
Aspirin and Meprobamate 151
BusPIRone 236
Meprobamate 993

Antiarrhythmic Agent, Class I
Moricizine 1064

Antiarrhythmic Agent, Class Ia
Disopyramide 491
Procainamide 1283
Quinidine 1324

Antiarrhythmic Agent, Class Ib
Lidocaine 920
Mexiletine 1037
Phenytoin 1228
Tocainide 1500

Antiarrhythmic Agent, Class Ic
Flecainide 657
Propafenone 1293

Antiarrhythmic Agent, Class II
Acebutolol 28
Esmolol 571
Propranolol 1301
Sotalol 1409

Antiarrhythmic Agent, Class III
Amiodarone 90
Bretylium 219
Dofetilide 497
Ibutilide 813
Sotalol 1409

Antiarrhythmic Agent, Class IV
Adenosine 55
Digitoxin 471
Digoxin 471
Verapamil 1571

Antibacterial, Dental
Triclosan and Fluoride 1534

Antibacterial, Oral Rinse
Delmopinol 430

Antibiotic, Aminoglycoside
Amikacin 84
Gentamicin 734
Kanamycin 878
Neomycin 1100
Streptomycin 1418
Tobramycin 1498

Antibiotic, Carbacephem
Loracarbef 945

Antibiotic, Carbapenem
Ertapenem 561
Imipenem and Cilastatin 819
Meropenem 996

Antibiotic, Cephalosporin
Cefditoren 285

Antibiotic, Cephalosporin (First Generation)
Cefadroxil 281
Cefazolin 283
Cephalexin 301
Cephalothin 303
Cephradine 304

Antibiotic, Cephalosporin (Second Generation)
Cefaclor 279
Cefotetan 289
Cefoxitin 290
Cefprozil 291
Cefuroxime 295

Antibiotic, Cephalosporin (Third Generation)
Cefdinir 284
Cefixime 287
Cefotaxime 288
Cefpodoxime 290
Ceftazidime 292
Ceftibuten 292
Ceftizoxime 293
Ceftriaxone 294

Antibiotic, Cephalosporin (Fourth Generation)
Cefepime 287

Antibiotic/Corticosteroid, Ophthalmic
Loteprednol and Tobramycin . . . 953
Neomycin, Polymyxin B, and
  Dexamethasone 1101
Neomycin, Polymyxin B, and
  Hydrocortisone 1101
Neomycin, Polymyxin B, and
  Prednisolone 1102
Prednisolone and Gentamicin
  1271
Sulfacetamide and
  Fluorometholone 1423
Sulfacetamide and
  Prednisolone 1424
Tobramycin and
  Dexamethasone 1499

Antibiotic/Corticosteroid, Otic
Ciprofloxacin and
  Dexamethasone 348
Ciprofloxacin and
  Hydrocortisone 348
Neomycin, Polymyxin B, and
  Hydrocortisone 1101

Antibiotic, Cyclic Lipopeptide
Daptomycin 423

Antibiotic, Glycylcycline
Tigecycline 1487

Antibiotic, Irrigation
Polymyxin B 1253

Antibiotic, Ketolide
Telithromycin 1448

Antibiotic, Lincosamide
Clindamycin 361
Lincomycin 932

Antibiotic, Macrolide
Azithromycin 171
Clarithromycin 355
Dirithromycin 490
Erythromycin 562
Erythromycin and Sulfisoxazole
  568
Spiramycin 1412

Antibiotic, Macrolide Combination
Erythromycin and Sulfisoxazole
  568
Lansoprazole, Amoxicillin, and
  Clarithromycin 898

Antibiotic, Miscellaneous
Aztreonam 175
Bacitracin 175
Capreomycin 256
Chloramphenicol 314

Colistimethate 390
CycloSERINE 405
Dapsone 421
Fosfomycin 706
Methenamine 1007
Methenamine, Sodium
    Biphosphate, Phenyl
    Salicylate, Methylene Blue,
    and Hyoscyamine 1008
Metronidazole 1033
Nitrofurantoin 1119
Pentamidine 1207
Polymyxin B 1253
Rifabutin 1345
Rifampin 1346
Rifampin and Isoniazid 1348
Rifampin, Isoniazid, and
    Pyrazinamide 1348
Rifaximin 1350
Spectinomycin 1412
Sulfamethoxazole and
    Trimethoprim 1425
Tinidazole 1491
Trimethoprim 1538
Vancomycin 1563

Antibiotic, Ophthalmic
Bacitracin 175
Bacitracin and Polymyxin B 176
Bacitracin, Neomycin, and
    Polymyxin B 176
Bacitracin, Neomycin,
    Polymyxin B, and
    Hydrocortisone 177
Ciprofloxacin 343
Erythromycin 562
Gatifloxacin 724
Gentamicin 734
Moxifloxacin 1069
Neomycin, Polymyxin B, and
    Gramicidin 1101
Sulfacetamide 1423
Tobramycin 1498
Trimethoprim and Polymyxin B
    1539

Antibiotic, Oral Rinse
Chlorhexidine Gluconate 316

Antibiotic, Otic
Bacitracin, Neomycin,
    Polymyxin B, and
    Hydrocortisone 177

Antibiotic, Oxazolidinone
Linezolid 933

Antibiotic, Penicillin
Amoxicillin 106
Amoxicillin and Clavulanate
    Potassium 108
Ampicillin 117
Ampicillin and Sulbactam 120
Carbenicillin 265
Cloxacillin 380
Dicloxacillin 463
Lansoprazole, Amoxicillin, and
    Clarithromycin 898
Nafcillin 1082
Oxacillin 1153
Penicillin V Potassium 1205
Penicillin G Benzathine 1202
Penicillin G Benzathine and
    Penicillin G Procaine 1203
Penicillin G (Parenteral/
    Aqueous) 1203
Penicillin G Procaine 1204
Piperacillin 1244
Piperacillin and Tazobactam
    Sodium 1245
Ticarcillin 1484
Ticarcillin and Clavulanate
    Potassium 1485

Antibiotic, Quinolone
Ciprofloxacin 343
Gatifloxacin 724
Gemifloxacin 731
Levofloxacin 913
Lomefloxacin 941
Moxifloxacin 1069
Nalidixic Acid 1083
Norfloxacin 1126
Ofloxacin 1137
Sparfloxacin 1411
Trovafloxacin 1546

Antibiotic, Streptogramin
Quinupristin and Dalfopristin . . 1326

Antibiotic, Sulfonamide
    Derivative
Erythromycin and Sulfisoxazole
    568
Sulfacetamide 1423
SulfaDIAZINE 1424
Sulfamethoxazole and
    Trimethoprim 1425
SulfiSOXAZOLE 1429

Antibiotic, Tetracycline
    Derivative
Bismuth Subsalicylate,
    Metronidazole, and
    Tetracycline 210
Demeclocycline 431
Doxycycline Hyclate
    (Periodontal) 512
Doxycycline (Subantimicrobial) . . 514
Doxycycline (Systemic) 514
Minocycline 1049
Minocycline Hydrochloride
    (Periodontal) 1050
Oxytetracycline 1174
Tetracycline 1467

Antibiotic, Topical
Bacitracin 175
Bacitracin and Polymyxin B 176
Bacitracin, Neomycin, and
    Polymyxin B 176
Bacitracin, Neomycin,
    Polymyxin B, and
    Hydrocortisone 177
Bacitracin, Neomycin,
    Polymyxin B, and
    Pramoxine 177
Benzalkonium Chloride 188
Benzoin 193
Chlorhexidine Gluconate 316
Erythromycin 562
Gentamicin 734
Gentian Violet 735
Hexachlorophene 771
Mafenide 959
Metronidazole 1033
Mupirocin 1073
Neomycin 1100
Neomycin and Polymyxin B . . . 1100
Oxychlorosene 1163
Silver Nitrate 1392
Silver Sulfadiazine 1393

Antibiotic, Vaginal
Sulfabenzamide,
    Sulfacetamide, and
    Sulfathiazole 1423

Anticholinergic/Adrenergic
    Agonist
Phenylephrine and
    Scopolamine 1227

Anticholinergic Agent
Atropine 161
Benztropine 196
Biperiden 208

Chlordiazepoxide and
  Methscopolamine 316
Darifenacin 424
Dicyclomine 464
Edrophonium and Atropine 529
Glycopyrrolate 747
Hyoscyamine 803
Hyoscyamine, Atropine,
  Scopolamine, and
  Phenobarbital 804
Ipratropium 857
Mepenzolate 983
Methscopolamine 1019
Procyclidine 1288
Propantheline 1295
Scopolamine 1380
Solifenacin 1405
Tiotropium 1494
Tolterodine 1506
Trihexyphenidyl 1537
Trimethobenzamide 1538
Trospium 1546

**Anticholinergic Agent,
  Ophthalmic**
Atropine 161
Cyclopentolate 402
Homatropine 772

Anticoagulant
Antithrombin III 131
Danaparoid 418
Heparin 765

**Anticoagulant, Coumarin
  Derivative**
Acenocoumarol 30
Warfarin 1585

**Anticoagulant, Thrombin
  Inhibitor**
Argatroban 136
Bivalirudin 213
Lepirudin 904

Anticonvulsant, Barbiturate
Pentobarbital 1210
Phenobarbital 1221
Thiopental 1477

Anticonvulsant, Hydantoin
Ethotoin 619
Fosphenytoin 710
Phenytoin 1228

Anticonvulsant, Miscellaneous
AcetaZOLAMIDE 45
Carbamazepine 260
Felbamate 637
Gabapentin 717
Lamotrigine 895
Levetiracetam 908
Magnesium Sulfate 963
Oxcarbazepine 1159
Pregabalin 1274
Primidone 1281
Tiagabine 1483
Topiramate 1508
Valproic Acid and Derivatives
  1556
Vigabatrin 1574
Zonisamide 1606

Anticonvulsant, Oxazolidinedione
Trimethadione 1538

Anticonvulsant, Succinimide
Ethosuximide 619
Methsuximide 1019

Anticystine Agent
Cysteamine 412

**Antidepressant, Alpha-2
  Antagonist**
Mirtazapine 1052

**Antidepressant,
  Dopamine-Reuptake
  Inhibitor**
BuPROPion 233

**Antidepressant, Monoamine
  Oxidase Inhibitor**
Isocarboxazid 863
Phenelzine 1221
Selegiline 1382
Tranylcypromine 1519

**Antidepressant, Selective
  Serotonin Reuptake
  Inhibitor**
Citalopram 351
Escitalopram 568
Fluoxetine 675
Fluvoxamine 694
Olanzapine and Fluoxetine 1141
Paroxetine 1188
Sertraline 1385

**Antidepressant, Serotonin/
  Norepinephrine Reuptake
  Inhibitor**
Duloxetine 523
Venlafaxine 1568

**Antidepressant, Serotonin
  Reuptake Inhibitor/
  Antagonist**
Nefazodone 1096
Trazodone 1521

Antidepressant, Tetracyclic
Maprotiline 964

**Antidepressant, Tricyclic
  (Secondary Amine)**
Amoxapine 105
Desipramine 434
Nortriptyline 1128
Protriptyline 1307

**Antidepressant, Tricyclic
  (Tertiary Amine)**
Amitriptyline 93
Amitriptyline and
  Chlordiazepoxide 97
Amitriptyline and Perphenazine
  97
ClomiPRAMINE 370
Doxepin 505
Imipramine 820
Trimipramine 1540

Antidiabetic Agent
Pramlintide 1263

**Antidiabetic Agent,
  Alpha-Glucosidase
  Inhibitor**
Acarbose 28
Miglitol 1046

Antidiabetic Agent, Biguanide
Glipizide and Metformin 741
Glyburide and Metformin 745
Metformin 1001
Pioglitazone and Metformin . . . 1242
Rosiglitazone and Metformin . . 1369

**Antidiabetic Agent, Incretin
  Mimetic**
Exenatide 629

Antidiabetic Agent, Insulin
Insulin Aspart 835
Insulin Aspart Protamine and
  Insulin Aspart 836
Insulin Detemir 836
Insulin Glargine 837
Insulin Glulisine 837
Insulin Inhalation 837

Insulin Lispro 839
Insulin Lispro Protamine and
    Insulin Lispro 839
Insulin NPH 840
Insulin NPH and Insulin
    Regular 840
Insulin Regular 841

Antidiabetic Agent, Meglitinide
    Derivative
Nateglinide 1094
Repaglinide 1339

Antidiabetic Agent, Sulfonylurea
ChlorproPAMIDE 331
Gliclazide 737
Glimepiride 738
GlipiZIDE 740
Glipizide and Metformin 741
GlyBURIDE 744
Glyburide and Metformin 745
Rosiglitazone and Glimepiride
    1369
TOLAZamide 1501
TOLBUTamide 1502

Antidiabetic Agent,
    Thiazolidinedione
Pioglitazone 1241
Pioglitazone and Metformin . . . 1242
Rosiglitazone 1367
Rosiglitazone and Glimepiride
    1369
Rosiglitazone and Metformin . . 1369

Antidiarrheal
Attapulgite 165
Bifidobacterium bifidum /
    Lactobacillus acidophilus . . 1615
Bismuth 210
Bismuth Subsalicylate,
    Metronidazole, and
    Tetracycline 210
Difenoxin and Atropine 467
Diphenoxylate and Atropine 487
Kaolin and Pectin 879
Loperamide 942
Loperamide and Simethicone . . . 943
Octreotide 1135
Opium Tincture 1149
Polycarbophil 1252
Psyllium 1313

Antidiuretic Hormone Analog
Vasopressin 1567

Antidote
Acetylcysteine 46
Aluminum Hydroxide 79
Amifostine 83
Amyl Nitrite 124
Atropine 161
Calcitonin 246
Calcium Acetate 248
Calcium Carbonate 248
Charcoal 311
Deferasirox 427
Deferoxamine 428
Diethylene Triamine
    Penta-Acetic Acid 466
Digoxin Immune Fab 474
Dimercaprol 482
Edrophonium 528
Edrophonium and Atropine 529
Epinephrine 546
Epinephrine and
    Chlorpheniramine 549
Ferric Hexacyanoferrate 650
Flumazenil 665
Fomepizole 699
Glucagon 742
Insulin Regular 841
Ipecac Syrup 856
Leucovorin 905

Nalmefene 1084
Naloxone 1084
Naltrexone 1086
Pamidronate 1181
Protamine Sulfate 1306
Sodium Thiosulfate 1404
Zoledronic Acid 1600

Antidote, Hypoglycemia
Dextrose 452

Antiemetic
Aprepitant 134
Dexamethasone 439
Dolasetron 498
Dronabinol 518
Droperidol 519
Fructose, Dextrose, and
    Phosphoric Acid 713
Granisetron 751
HydrOXYzine 801
Meclizine 969
Metoclopramide 1029
Ondansetron 1147
Palonosetron 1180
Prochlorperazine 1285
Promethazine 1290
Trimethobenzamide 1538

Antiflatulent
Aluminum Hydroxide,
    Magnesium Hydroxide, and
    Simethicone 81
Calcium Carbonate and
    Simethicone 249
Loperamide and Simethicone . . 943
Magaldrate and Simethicone . . 960
Simethicone 1394

Antifungal Agent, Ophthalmic
Natamycin 1093

Antifungal Agent, Oral
Fluconazole 659
Flucytosine 662
Griseofulvin 752
Itraconazole 873
Ketoconazole 880
Terbinafine 1459
Voriconazole 1582

Antifungal Agent, Oral
    Nonabsorbed
Clotrimazole 379
Nystatin 1133

Antifungal Agent, Parenteral
Amphotericin B Cholesteryl
    Sulfate Complex 112
Amphotericin B (Conventional) . . 113
Amphotericin B (Lipid
    Complex) 115
Amphotericin B (Liposomal) 116
Anidulafungin 128
Caspofungin 278
Fluconazole 659
Micafungin 1038
Voriconazole 1582

Antifungal Agent, Topical
Betamethasone and
    Clotrimazole 202
Butenafine 242
Ciclopirox 338
Clotrimazole 379
Econazole 526
Gentian Violet 735
Iodoquinol and Hydrocortisone . . 853
Ketoconazole 880
Miconazole 1039
Miconazole and Zinc Oxide . . . 1040
Naftifine 1082
Nystatin 1133
Nystatin and Triamcinolone . . . 1134
Oxiconazole 1160

Sertaconazole 1385
Sulconazole 1422
Terbinafine 1459
Tolnaftate 1506
Triacetin 1526
Undecylenic Acid and
    Derivatives 1550

Antifungal Agent, Vaginal
Butoconazole 242
Clotrimazole 379
Metronidazole and Nystatin . . . 1036
Miconazole 1039
Nystatin 1133
Terconazole 1461
Tioconazole 1493

Antigout Agent
Colchicine and Probenecid 388

Antihemophilic Agent
Antihemophilic Factor (Human)
    129
Antihemophilic Factor
    (Recombinant) 130
Anti-inhibitor Coagulant
    Complex 130
Desmopressin 437
Factor IX 632
Factor IX Complex (Human) . . 633
Factor VIIa (Recombinant) 632
Tranexamic Acid 1518

Antihistamine
Acetaminophen,
    Chlorpheniramine, and
    Pseudoephedrine 43
Acetaminophen,
    Dextromethorphan, and
    Pseudoephedrine 44
Acrivastine and
    Pseudoephedrine 47
Azelastine 170
Carbetapentane,
    Phenylephrine, and
    Pyrilamine 267
Carbinoxamine 268
Cetirizine 306
Chlorpheniramine 323
Chlorpheniramine and
    Pseudoephedrine 325
Clemastine 359
Cyclizine 400
Cyproheptadine 412
Dexchlorpheniramine 443
Dexchlorpheniramine and
    Pseudoephedrine 443
Dihydrocodeine,
    Chlorpheniramine, and
    Phenylephrine 476
DimenhyDRINATE 481
DiphenhydrAMINE 483
Doxylamine 517
HydrOXYzine 801
Meclizine 969
Olopatadine 1143
Phenindamine 1221
Promethazine 1290
Tripelennamine 1541
Triprolidine and
    Pseudoephedrine 1542

Antihistamine/Analgesic
Chlorpheniramine and
    Acetaminophen 324

Antihistamine/Antitussive
Bromodiphenhydramine and
    Codeine 223
Carbetapentane and
    Chlorpheniramine 266
Hydrocodone and
    Chlorpheniramine 784
Promethazine and Codeine . . . 1291

Promethazine and
    Dextromethorphan 1292

**Antihistamine/Decongestant/
    Anticholinergic**
Chlorpheniramine,
    Phenylephrine, and
    Methscopolamine 327

**Antihistamine/Decongestant/
    Antitussive**
Carbetapentane,
    Phenylephrine, and
    Pyrilamine 267
Carbinoxamine,
    Pseudoephedrine, and
    Dextromethorphan 269
Chlorpheniramine, Ephedrine,
    Phenylephrine, and
    Carbetapentane 325
Chlorpheniramine,
    Phenylephrine, and
    Dextromethorphan 326
Chlorpheniramine,
    Pseudoephedrine, and
    Codeine 329
Dihydrocodeine,
    Chlorpheniramine, and
    Phenylephrine 476
Hydrocodone, Carbinoxamine,
    and Pseudoephedrine 789
Hydrocodone, Phenylephrine,
    and Diphenhydramine 791
Promethazine, Phenylephrine,
    and Codeine 1293
Pseudoephedrine,
    Dihydrocodeine, and
    Chlorpheniramine 1312
Triprolidine, Pseudoephedrine,
    and Codeine 1543

**Antihistamine/Decongestant/
    Antitussive/Expectorant**
Chlorpheniramine,
    Phenylephrine, Codeine,
    and Potassium Iodide 328

**Antihistamine/Decongestant
    Combination**
Brompheniramine and
    Pseudoephedrine 223
Cetirizine and
    Pseudoephedrine 307
Chlorpheniramine and
    Phenylephrine 324
Chlorpheniramine,
    Phenylephrine, and
    Phenyltoloxamine 328
Dexbrompheniramine and
    Pseudoephedrine 442
Diphenhydramine and
    Pseudoephedrine 487
Fexofenadine and
    Pseudoephedrine 653
Loratadine and
    Pseudoephedrine 947
Promethazine and
    Phenylephrine 1292

**Antihistamine/Decongestant
    Combination, Nonsedating**
Desloratadine and
    Pseudoephedrine 436

Antihistamine, H_1 Blocker
Carbinoxamine and
    Pseudoephedrine 268

**Antihistamine, H_1 Blocker,
    Ophthalmic**
Emedastine 534
Epinastine 546
Ketotifen 890
Levocabastine 910

Antihistamine, Nonsedating
Desloratadine 435
Fexofenadine 652
Loratadine 946

Antihypertensive
Diazoxide 457
Oxprenolol 1161
Quinapril and
  Hydrochlorothiazide 1323

Antihypertensive Agent, Combination
Amlodipine and Benazepril 102
Atenolol and Chlorthalidone 156
Benazepril and
  Hydrochlorothiazide 187
Bisoprolol and
  Hydrochlorothiazide 212
Candesartan and
  Hydrochlorothiazide 254
Captopril and
  Hydrochlorothiazide 259
Clonidine and Chlorthalidone . . 376
Enalapril and Felodipine 540
Enalapril and
  Hydrochlorothiazide 541
Eprosartan and
  Hydrochlorothiazide 555
Fosinopril and
  Hydrochlorothiazide 709
Hydralazine and
  Hydrochlorothiazide 775
Hydrochlorothiazide and
  Spironolactone 778
Hydrochlorothiazide and
  Triamterene 778
Irbesartan and
  Hydrochlorothiazide 860
Lisinopril and
  Hydrochlorothiazide 938
Losartan and
  Hydrochlorothiazide 952
Methyldopa and
  Hydrochlorothiazide 1022
Moexipril and
  Hydrochlorothiazide 1059
Nadolol and
  Bendroflumethiazide 1080
Olmesartan and
  Hydrochlorothiazide 1143
Prazosin and Polythiazide 1268
Propranolol and
  Hydrochlorothiazide 1305
Telmisartan and
  Hydrochlorothiazide 1452
Trandolapril and Verapamil . . . 1518
Valsartan and
  Hydrochlorothiazide 1562

Antihypoglycemic Agent
Diazoxide 457

Anti-inflammatory Agent
Balsalazide 179
Colchicine and Probenecid 388
Dexamethasone 439
Flavocoxid 656
Triamcinolone Acetonide
  (Dental Paste) 1530

Anti-inflammatory Agent, Ophthalmic
Dexamethasone 439

Anti-inflammatory, Locally Applied
Amlexanox 99
Carbamide Peroxide 264
Maltodextrin 963

Antilipemic Agent, 2-Azetidinone
Ezetimibe 630
Ezetimibe and Simvastatin 631

Antilipemic Agent, Bile Acid Sequestrant
Cholestyramine Resin 334
Colesevelam 389
Colestipol 390

Antilipemic Agent, Fibric Acid
Fenofibrate 639
Gemfibrozil 730

Antilipemic Agent, HMG-CoA Reductase Inhibitor
Amlodipine and Atorvastatin 101
Aspirin and Pravastatin 151
Atorvastatin 158
Ezetimibe and Simvastatin 631
Fluvastatin 693
Lovastatin 953
Niacin and Lovastatin 1107
Pravastatin 1265
Rosuvastatin 1370
Simvastatin 1394

Antilipemic Agent, Miscellaneous
Niacin 1105
Niacin and Lovastatin 1107

Antimalarial Agent
Atovaquone and Proguanil 160
Halofantrine 761
Mefloquine 975
Pyrimethamine 1317
Quinine 1326
Sulfadoxine and
  Pyrimethamine 1424

Antimicrobial Mouth Rinse
Mouthwash (Antiseptic) 1069

Antimigraine Agent
Frovatriptan 712

Antineoplastic Agent
Amsacrine 123
Bortezomib 215
Carmustine 273

Antineoplastic Agent, Alkylating Agent
Busulfan 237
Carboplatin 270
Chlorambucil 313
Cisplatin 350
Cyclophosphamide 403
Estramustine 578
Ifosfamide 815
Lomustine 941
Melphalan 979
Oxaliplatin 1154
Procarbazine 1284
Streptozocin 1418
Temozolomide 1454
Thiotepa 1479

Antineoplastic Agent, Alkylating Agent (Nitrogen Mustard)
Ifosfamide 815

Antineoplastic Agent, Alkylating Agent (Nitrosourea)
Carmustine 273

Antineoplastic Agent, Alkylating Agent (Triazene)
Dacarbazine 415

Antineoplastic Agent, Anthracenedione
Mitoxantrone 1055

Antineoplastic Agent, Anthracycline
DAUNOrubicin Citrate
  (Liposomal) 425
DAUNOrubicin Hydrochloride . . . 426
DOXOrubicin 509

DOXOrubicin (Liposomal) 511
Epirubicin 550
Idarubicin 814
Valrubicin 1560

Antineoplastic Agent, Antiandrogen
Bicalutamide 207
Flutamide 686
Nilutamide 1115

Antineoplastic Agent, Antibiotic
Bleomycin 214
Dactinomycin 417
Idarubicin 814
Mitomycin 1054
Pentostatin 1211

Antineoplastic Agent, Antimetabolite
Capecitabine 255
Cladribine 354
Cytarabine 413
Cytarabine (Liposomal) 414
Hydroxyurea 800
Mercaptopurine 995
Nelarabine 1097
Pemetrexed 1198

Antineoplastic Agent, Antimetabolite (Antifolate)
Methotrexate 1012
Pemetrexed 1198

Antineoplastic Agent, Antimetabolite (Purine Antagonist)
Cladribine 354
Clofarabine 367
Cytarabine 413
Fludarabine 663
Pentostatin 1211
Thioguanine 1476

Antineoplastic Agent, Antimetabolite (Pyrimidine)
Azacitidine 167

Antineoplastic Agent, Antimetabolite (Pyrimidine Antagonist)
Floxuridine 659
Fluorouracil 674
Gemcitabine 729

Antineoplastic Agent, Antimicrotubular
Paclitaxel 1176
Paclitaxel (Protein Bound) 1177

Antineoplastic Agent, Aromatase Inactivator
Exemestane 628

Antineoplastic Agent, Aromatase Inhibitor
Aminoglutethimide 87
Letrozole 904

Antineoplastic Agent, DNA Adduct-Forming Agent
Carmustine 273

Antineoplastic Agent, DNA Binding Agent
Aminocamptothecin 86
Amonafide 104
Carmustine 273

Antineoplastic Agent, Estrogen Receptor Antagonist
Fulvestrant 713
Tamoxifen 1443
Toremifene 1512

Antineoplastic Agent, Hormone
Estramustine 578
Megestrol 976

Antineoplastic Agent, Hormone Antagonist
Mifepristone 1045

Antineoplastic Agent, Hormone (Estrogen/Nitrogen Mustard)
Estramustine 578

Antineoplastic Agent, Miscellaneous
Alitretinoin 69
Altretamine 78
Asparaginase 144
Bexarotene 205
Denileukin Diftitox 432
Mitotane 1055
Pegaspargase 1194
Porfimer 1256
Teniposide 1456
Tretinoin (Oral) 1524
Trimetrexate 1539

Antineoplastic Agent, Monoclonal Antibody
Alemtuzumab 63
Bevacizumab 204
Cetuximab 308
Gemtuzumab Ozogamicin . . . 732
Ibritumomab 807
Rituximab 1360
Trastuzumab 1520

Antineoplastic Agent, Natural Source (Plant) Derivative
Docetaxel 494
Irinotecan 860
Paclitaxel 1176
Paclitaxel (Protein Bound) 1177
Topotecan 1511
VinBLAStine 1575
VinCRIStine 1576
Vinorelbine 1578

Antineoplastic Agent, Podophyllotoxin Derivative
Etoposide 626
Etoposide Phosphate 627

Antineoplastic Agent, Tyrosine Kinase Inhibitor
Erlotinib 560
Gefitinib 727
Imatinib 817
Sorafenib 1407
Sunitinib 1434

Antineoplastic Agent, Vinca Alkaloid
VinBLAStine 1575
VinCRIStine 1576
Vindesine 1577
Vinorelbine 1578

Antiparasitic Agent, Topical
Lindane 933
Permethrin 1218
Pyrethrins and Piperonyl Butoxide 1315

Anti-Parkinson's Agent, Anticholinergic
Benztropine 196
Biperiden 208
Orphenadrine 1151
Procyclidine 1288
Trihexyphenidyl 1537

Anti-Parkinson's Agent, COMT Inhibitor
Entacapone 543

Levodopa, Carbidopa, and
    Entacapone 912
Tolcapone 1503

**Anti-Parkinson's Agent,
    Dopamine Agonist**
Amantadine 81
Apomorphine 132
Bromocriptine 222
Carbidopa 267
Levodopa and Carbidopa 911
Levodopa, Carbidopa, and
    Entacapone 912
Pergolide 1213
Pramipexole 1262
Ropinirole 1365

**Anti-Parkinson's Agent, MAO
    Type B Inhibitor**
Selegiline 1382

Antiplaque Agent
Mouthwash (Antiseptic) 1069

Antiplatelet Agent
Aspirin and Dipyridamole 150
Cilostazol 340
Clopidogrel 376
Dipyridamole 489
Ticlopidine 1486

**Antiplatelet Agent, Glycoprotein
    IIb/IIIa Inhibitor**
Abciximab 26
Eptifibatide 556
Tirofiban 1496

Antiprogestin
Mifepristone 1045

Antiprotozoal
Atovaquone 160
Eflornithine 532
Furazolidone 714
Nitazoxanide 1117

Antiprotozoal, Nitroimidazole
Metronidazole 1033
Metronidazole and Nystatin . . . 1036
Tinidazole 1491

Antipsoriatic Agent
Anthralin 128

Antipsychotic Agent, Atypical
Aripiprazole 138
Clozapine 382
Olanzapine 1139
Olanzapine and Fluoxetine 1141
Quetiapine 1319
Risperidone 1356
Ziprasidone 1598

Antipsychotic Agent, Typical
Droperidol 519
Haloperidol 762
Loxapine 955
Molindone 1059
Pimozide 1238
Thiothixene 1480

**Antipsychotic Agent, Typical,
    Phenothiazine**
Amitriptyline and Perphenazine
    97
ChlorproMAZINE 329
Fluphenazine 680
Mesoridazine 997
Perphenazine 1218
Prochlorperazine 1285
Thioridazine 1477
Trifluoperazine 1535

**Antipsychotic Agent, Typical,
    Phenothiazine, Piperidine**
Pericyazine 1214
Pipotiazine 1246

**Antiretroviral Agent, Fusion
    Protein Inhibitor**
Enfuvirtide 541

**Antiretroviral Agent, Protease
    Inhibitor**
Amprenavir 122
Atazanavir 152
Fosamprenavir 702
Indinavir 829
Lopinavir and Ritonavir 943
Nelfinavir 1098
Ritonavir 1359
Saquinavir 1377
Tipranavir 1495

**Antiretroviral Agent, Reverse
    Transcriptase Inhibitor
    (Non-nucleoside)**
Delavirdine 429
Efavirenz 530
Nevirapine 1104

**Antiretroviral Agent, Reverse
    Transcriptase Inhibitor
    (Nucleoside)**
Abacavir 22
Abacavir and Lamivudine 23
Abacavir, Lamivudine, and
    Zidovudine 23
Adefovir 54
Didanosine 465
Emtricitabine 536
Emtricitabine and Tenofovir 537
Entecavir 544
Lamivudine 894
Stavudine 1416
Zalcitabine 1590
Zidovudine 1594
Zidovudine and Lamivudine . . . 1596

**Antiretroviral Agent, Reverse
    Transcriptase Inhibitor
    (Nucleotide)**
Emtricitabine and Tenofovir 537
Tenofovir 1457

**Antirheumatic, Disease
    Modifying**
Abatacept 25
Adalimumab 52
Anakinra 125
Etanercept 588
Infliximab 832
Leflunomide 901

Antirheumatic Miscellaneous
Hyaluronate and Derivatives . . . 773

Antiseptic, Ophthalmic
Povidone-Iodine 1262

Antiseptic, Oral Mouthwash
Cetylpyridinium 309

Antiseptic, Topical
Benzalkonium Chloride and
    Isopropyl Alcohol 189
Hexylresorcinol 771
Iodine 852
Povidone-Iodine 1262

Antiseptic, Vaginal
Povidone-Iodine 1262

**Antispasmodic Agent,
    Gastrointestinal**
Atropine 161
Clidinium and
    Chlordiazepoxide 360
Hyoscyamine, Atropine,
    Scopolamine, and
    Phenobarbital 804
Mepenzolate 983

Antispasmodic Agent, Urinary
Belladonna and Opium 184
Flavoxate 656
Oxybutynin 1162

Antithyroid Agent
Methimazole 1008
Potassium Iodide 1260
Potassium Iodide and Iodine . . 1260
Propylthiouracil 1305

Antitrypsin Deficiency Agent
Alpha$_1$-Proteinase Inhibitor 73

Antitubercular Agent
Capreomycin 256
CycloSERINE 405
Ethambutol 591
Ethionamide 618
Isoniazid. 864
Pyrazinamide 1314
Rifabutin 1345
Rifampin. 1346
Rifapentine 1349
Streptomycin 1418

Antitussive
Acetaminophen,
    Dextromethorphan, and
    Pseudoephedrine 44
Benzonatate 194
Carbetapentane,
    Phenylephrine, and
    Pyrilamine 267
Codeine 385
Dextromethorphan 451
Dihydrocodeine,
    Chlorpheniramine, and
    Phenylephrine 476
Guaifenesin and Codeine 753
Guaifenesin and
    Dextromethorphan 754
Guaifenesin,
    Dextromethorphan, and
    Phenylephrine 756
Hydrocodone and Homatropine
    786
Hydrocodone, Phenylephrine,
    and Diphenhydramine 791

Antitussive/Decongestant
Hydrocodone and
    Pseudoephedrine 788
Hydrocodone,
    Chlorpheniramine,
    Phenylephrine,
    Acetaminophen, and
    Caffeine 790
Pseudoephedrine and
    Dextromethorphan 1311

Antitussive/Decongestant/
Expectorant
Dihydrocodeine,
    Pseudoephedrine, and
    Guaifenesin 476
Guaifenesin, Pseudoephedrine,
    and Codeine 756
Guaifenesin, Pseudoephedrine,
    and Dextromethorphan . . . 757
Hydrocodone, Phenylephrine,
    and Guaifenesin 791
Hydrocodone,
    Pseudoephedrine, and
    Guaifenesin 792

Antitussive/Expectorant
Hydrocodone and Guaifenesin . . 785

Antiviral Agent
Acyclovir 49
Cidofovir. 339
Famciclovir 633
Foscarnet 703
Ganciclovir 722

Interferon Alfa-2b and Ribavirin
    847
Oseltamivir 1152
Penciclovir 1200
Ribavirin 1343
Valganciclovir 1555
Zanamivir 1592

Antiviral Agent, Adamantane
Amantadine 81
Rimantadine 1351

Antiviral Agent, Ophthalmic
Fomivirsen 700
Trifluridine 1536

Antiviral Agent, Oral
Valacyclovir 1553

Antiviral Agent, Topical
Docosanol 495

Aphthous Ulcer Treatment Agent
Sulfonated Phenolics in
    Aqueous Solution 1429

Appetite Stimulant
Dronabinol 518
Megestrol 976

Aromatase Inhibitor
Aminoglutethimide 87
Anastrozole 126

Astringent
Aluminum Chloride 78
Epinephrine (Racemic) and
    Aluminum Potassium
    Sulfate 550

Barbiturate
Amobarbital 104
Amobarbital and Secobarbital . . 104
Butabarbital 238
Butalbital, Acetaminophen, and
    Caffeine 239
Butalbital, Acetaminophen,
    Caffeine, and Codeine 239
Butalbital, Aspirin, and Caffeine
    241
Butalbital, Aspirin, Caffeine,
    and Codeine 241
Mephobarbital 986
Methohexital. 1010
Pentobarbital 1210
Phenobarbital 1221
Primidone. 1281
Secobarbital 1381
Thiopental 1477

Benzodiazepine
Alprazolam 73
Amitriptyline and
    Chlordiazepoxide 97
Bromazepam 220
Chlordiazepoxide 315
Chlordiazepoxide and
    Methscopolamine 316
Clidinium and
    Chlordiazepoxide 360
Clobazam. 364
Clonazepam 371
Clorazepate 378
Diazepam 454
Estazolam 573
Lorazepam 947
Midazolam 1040
Oxazepam 1157
Quazepam 1318

Beta$_1$- & Beta$_2$-Adrenergic
Agonist Agent
Isoproterenol 865

Beta$_2$-Adrenergic Agonist
Albuterol 58
Fenoterol Solution 644

Fluticasone and Salmeterol 690
Formoterol 701
Levalbuterol 907
Metaproterenol 1000
Pirbuterol 1248
Salmeterol 1375
Terbutaline 1460

Beta-Adrenergic Blocker
Dorzolamide and Timolol 501

**Beta-Adrenergic Blocker,
Noncardioselective**
Oxprenolol 1161

**Beta-Adrenergic Blocker,
Nonselective**
Levobunolol 909
Metipranolol 1028
Nadolol 1079
Nadolol and
Bendroflumethiazide 1080
Propranolol 1301
Sotalol 1409
Timolol 1489

Beta Blocker, Beta₁ Selective
Atenolol 154
Betaxolol 203
Bisoprolol 211
Esmolol 571
Metoprolol 1030
Metoprolol and
Hydrochlorothiazide 1032

**Beta Blocker With
Alpha-Blocking Activity**
Carvedilol 275
Labetalol 891

**Beta Blocker With Intrinsic
Sympathomimetic Activity**
Acebutolol 28
Carteolol 274
Penbutolol 1199
Pindolol 1240

Biological, Miscellaneous
Glatiramer Acetate 736

Biological Response Modulator
Aldesleukin 61
BCG Vaccine 181
Oprelvekin 1149

Bisphosphonate Derivative
Alendronate 64
Alendronate and
Cholecalciferol 66
Etidronate and Calcium 620
Etidronate Disodium 621
Ibandronate 805
Pamidronate 1181
Risedronate 1352
Risedronate and Calcium 1354
Tiludronate 1488
Zoledronic Acid 1600

Blood Modifiers
Hemin 764
Pentastarch 1208

Blood Product Derivative
Antihemophilic Factor (Human)
. . . . 129
Anti-inhibitor Coagulant
Complex 130
Antithrombin III 131
Aprotinin 135
Factor IX 632
Factor IX Complex (Human) . . 633
Factor VIIa (Recombinant) 632

Blood Viscosity Reducer Agent
Pentoxifylline 1212

Bronchodilator
Ipratropium and Albuterol 857

Calcimimetic
Cinacalcet 342

Calcium Channel Blocker
Amlodipine 100
Amlodipine and Atorvastatin 101
Diltiazem 479
Felodipine 638
Isradipine 871
NiCARdipine 1107
NIFEdipine 1112
Nimodipine 1116
Nisoldipine 1117
Verapamil 1571

**Calcium Channel Blocker,
N-Type**
Ziconotide 1594

Calcium-Lowering Agent
Gallium Nitrate 721

Calcium Salt
Calcium Acetate 248
Calcium Carbonate 248
Calcium Chloride 250
Calcium Citrate 250
Calcium Glubionate 250
Calcium Gluconate 250
Calcium Lactate 251
Calcium Phosphate (Tribasic) . . 251
Etidronate and Calcium 620
Risedronate and Calcium 1354

Caloric Agent
Fat Emulsion 637

Carbonic Anhydrase Inhibitor
AcetaZOLAMIDE 45
Brinzolamide 220
Dichlorphenamide 459
Dorzolamide 501
Dorzolamide and Timolol 501
Methazolamide 1006

Cardiac Glycoside
Digoxin 471

Cardioprotectant
Dexrazoxane 446

**Cardiovascular Agent,
Miscellaneous**
Ranolazine 1336

Cathartic
Sodium Phosphates 1403

Cauterizing Agent, Topical
Silver Nitrate 1392

**Central Monoamine-Depleting
Agent**
Reserpine 1340
Tetrabenazine 1465

**Central Nervous System
Depressant**
Sodium Oxybate 1402

**Central Nervous System
Stimulant**
Dexmethylphenidate 445
Methylphenidate 1023

Chelating Agent
Deferasirox 427
Edetate Calcium Disodium 527
Edetate Disodium 527
Penicillamine 1201

Cholinergic Agonist
Acetylcholine 46
Ambenonium 82
Bethanechol 204
Carbachol 260

Cevimeline 310
Edrophonium 528
Edrophonium and Atropine 529
Guanidine 759
Pilocarpine (Ophthalmic) 1234
Pilocarpine (Oral) 1235

Colchicine
Colchicine 388

Colony Stimulating Factor
Darbepoetin Alfa 423
Epoetin Alfa 552
Filgrastim 654
Pegfilgrastim 1195
Sargramostim 1378

Contraceptive
Ethinyl Estradiol and
Desogestrel 592
Ethinyl Estradiol and
Drospirenone 595
Ethinyl Estradiol and
Ethynodiol Diacetate 597
Ethinyl Estradiol and
Etonogestrel 600
Ethinyl Estradiol and
Levonorgestrel 602
Ethinyl Estradiol and
Norelgestromin 605
Ethinyl Estradiol and
Norethindrone 608
Ethinyl Estradiol and
Norgestimate 613
Ethinyl Estradiol and
Norgestrel 616
Levonorgestrel 916
MedroxyPROGESTERone 972
Mestranol and Norethindrone . . . 999
Nonoxynol 9 1124
Norethindrone 1125
Norgestrel 1127

Corticosteroid, Adrenal
Triamcinolone 1526

Corticosteroid, Inhalant (Oral)
Beclomethasone 183
Budesonide 224
Flunisolide 667
Fluticasone 686
Fluticasone and Salmeterol . . . 690
Mometasone Furoate 1060
Triamcinolone 1526

Corticosteroid, Nasal
Beclomethasone 183
Budesonide 224
Flunisolide 667
Fluticasone 686
Mometasone Furoate 1060
Triamcinolone 1526

Corticosteroid, Ophthalmic
Bacitracin, Neomycin,
Polymyxin B, and
Hydrocortisone 177
Dexamethasone 439
Fluocinolone 667
Fluorometholone 674
Loteprednol 953
Medrysone 973
PrednisoLONE 1268
Rimexolone 1351

Corticosteroid, Otic
Bacitracin, Neomycin,
Polymyxin B, and
Hydrocortisone 177

Corticosteroid, Rectal
Hydrocortisone 793

Corticosteroid, Systemic
Betamethasone 199
Budesonide 224

Corticotropin 395
Cortisone 395
Dexamethasone 439
Fludrocortisone 664
Hydrocortisone 793
MethylPREDNISolone 1025
PrednisoLONE 1268
PredniSONE 1271
Triamcinolone 1526

Corticosteroid, Topical
Alclometasone 60
Amcinonide 83
Bacitracin, Neomycin,
Polymyxin B, and
Hydrocortisone 177
Betamethasone 199
Betamethasone and
Clotrimazole 202
Clobetasol 365
Clocortolone 367
Desonide 437
Desoximetasone 438
Dexamethasone 439
Diflorasone 468
Fluocinolone 667
Fluocinolone, Hydroquinone,
and Tretinoin 669
Fluocinonide 670
Flurandrenolide 681
Fluticasone 686
Halcinonide 760
Halobetasol 760
Hydrocortisone 793
Iodoquinol and Hydrocortisone . . 853
Mometasone Furoate 1060
Nystatin and Triamcinolone . . 1134
Prednicarbate 1268
Triamcinolone 1526
Triamcinolone Acetonide
(Dental Paste) 1530
Urea and Hydrocortisone 1551

Corticosteroid, Topical (Medium Potency)
Fluticasone 686

Cosmetic Agent, Implant
Poly-L-Lactic Acid 1253

Cough Preparation
Guaifenesin and Codeine 753
Guaifenesin and
Dextromethorphan 754

Decongestant
Carbetapentane,
Phenylephrine, and
Pyrilamine 267
Carbinoxamine and
Pseudoephedrine 268
Dihydrocodeine,
Chlorpheniramine, and
Phenylephrine 476
Guaifenesin and Phenylephrine
. . . . 754
Guaifenesin,
Dextromethorphan, and
Phenylephrine 756
Hydrocodone, Phenylephrine,
and Diphenhydramine 791

Decongestant/Analgesic
Pseudoephedrine and
Ibuprofen 1311

Dental Gases
Nitrous Oxide 1122
Oxygen 1172

Depigmenting Agent
Fluocinolone, Hydroquinone,
and Tretinoin 669
Hydroquinone 798

Diagnostic Agent
Adenosine 55
Arginine 137
Benzylpenicilloyl-polylysine 198
Cosyntropin 396
Edrophonium 528
Glucagon 742
Gonadorelin 749
Indocyanine Green 830
Potassium Perchlorate 1261
Proparacaine and Fluorescein
. . . . 1296
Protirelin 1307
Secretin 1381
Sermorelin Acetate 1384
Sincalide 1396
Thyrotropin Alpha 1483
Tuberculin Tests 1548

Diagnostic Agent, Ophthalmic
Hydroxypropyl Methylcellulose . . 800

Dietary Supplement
Lactobacillus 535
Levocarnitine 910

Disinfectant, Antibacterial (Topical)
Sodium Hypochlorite Solution
. . . . 1402

Diuretic, Carbonic Anhydrase Inhibitor
AcetaZOLAMIDE 45
Dichlorphenamide 459
Methazolamide 1006

Diuretic, Combination
Amiloride and
Hydrochlorothiazide 85

Diuretic, Loop
Bumetanide 227
Ethacrynic Acid 590
Furosemide 715
Torsemide 1512

Diuretic, Osmotic
Urea 1551

Diuretic, Potassium-Sparing
Amiloride 85
Eplerenone 551
Hydrochlorothiazide and
Triamterene 778
Spironolactone 1413
Triamterene 1531

Diuretic, Thiazide
Candesartan and
Hydrochlorothiazide 254
Chlorothiazide 322
Chlorthalidone 332
Eprosartan and
Hydrochlorothiazide 555
Hydrochlorothiazide 776
Hydrochlorothiazide and
Triamterene 778
Irbesartan and
Hydrochlorothiazide 860
Losartan and
Hydrochlorothiazide 952
Methyclothiazide 1020
Metoprolol and
Hydrochlorothiazide 1032
Nadolol and
Bendroflumethiazide 1080
Olmesartan and
Hydrochlorothiazide 1143
Polythiazide 1255
Quinapril and
Hydrochlorothiazide 1323
Telmisartan and
Hydrochlorothiazide 1452

Diuretic, Thiazide-Related
Indapamide 828
Metolazone 1030

Dopamine Agonist
Fenoldopam 641

Echinocandin
Anidulafungin 128
Caspofungin 278
Micafungin 1038

Electrolyte Supplement, Oral
Calcium Carbonate 248
Calcium Gluconate 250
Magnesium L-aspartate
Hydrochloride 962
Magnesium Oxide 962
Potassium Acetate, Potassium
Bicarbonate, and
Potassium Citrate 1257
Potassium Bicarbonate 1257
Potassium Bicarbonate and
Potassium Chloride 1258
Potassium Bicarbonate and
Potassium Citrate 1258
Potassium Chloride 1258
Potassium Gluconate 1259
Potassium Phosphate 1261
Potassium Phosphate and
Sodium Phosphate 1261
Sodium Bicarbonate 1400
Sodium Phosphates 1403

Electrolyte Supplement, Parenteral
Ammonium Chloride 103
Calcium Chloride 250
Calcium Gluconate 250
Magnesium Sulfate 963
Potassium Acetate 1257
Potassium Chloride 1258
Potassium Phosphate 1261
Sodium Bicarbonate 1400
Sodium Chloride 1400
Sodium Phosphates 1403

Endothelin Antagonist
Bosentan 215

Enzyme
Agalsidase Beta 55
Alglucerase 68
Dornase Alfa 501
Galsulfase 721
Hyaluronidase 774
Imiglucerase 819
Lactase 892
Laronidase 900
Pancreatin 1183
Pancrelipase 1183
Pegademase Bovine 1193
Rasburicase 1337

Enzyme, Gastrointestinal
Sacrosidase 1373

Enzyme Inhibitor
Aminoglutethimide 87
Miglustat 1047

Enzyme Inhibitor, Topoisomerase I Inhibitor
Aminocamptothecin 86

Enzyme Inhibitor, Topoisomerase II Inhibitor
Amonafide 104

Enzyme, Topical Debridement
Chlorophyllin, Papain, and
Urea 319
Collagenase 391
Papain and Urea 1186

Enzyme, Urate-Oxidase (Recombinant)
Rasburicase 1337

Epidermal Growth Factor Receptor (EGFR) Inhibitor
Cetuximab 308
Erlotinib 560

Ergot Derivative
Belladonna, Phenobarbital, and Ergotamine 185
Bromocriptine 222
Cabergoline 244
Dihydroergotamine 477
Ergoloid Mesylates 557
Ergonovine 558
Ergotamine 558
Ergotamine and Caffeine 559
Methylergonovine 1022
Pergolide 1213

Estrogen and Progestin Combination
Drospirenone and Estradiol . . . 520
Estradiol and Norethindrone . . . 575
Estradiol and Norgestimate . . . 576
Estrogens (Conjugated/Equine) and Medroxyprogesterone . . 583
Estrogens (Esterified) and Methyltestosterone 585
Ethinyl Estradiol and Desogestrel 592
Ethinyl Estradiol and Drospirenone 595
Ethinyl Estradiol and Ethynodiol Diacetate 597
Ethinyl Estradiol and Etonogestrel 600
Ethinyl Estradiol and Levonorgestrel 602
Ethinyl Estradiol and Norelgestromin 605
Ethinyl Estradiol and Norethindrone 608
Ethinyl Estradiol and Norgestimate 613
Ethinyl Estradiol and Norgestrel 616
Mestranol and Norethindrone . . . 999

Estrogen Derivative
Estradiol 574
Estrogens (Conjugated A/Synthetic) 578
Estrogens (Conjugated/Equine) 580
Estrogens (Esterified) 584
Estropipate 586

Expectorant
Guaifenesin 752
Guaifenesin and Codeine 753
Guaifenesin and Dextromethorphan 754
Guaifenesin and Phenylephrine 754
Guaifenesin and Potassium Guaiacolsulfonate 755
Guaifenesin and Pseudoephedrine 755
Potassium Iodide 1260

Factor Xa Inhibitor
Fondaparinux 700

GABA Agonist/Glutamate Antagonist
Acamprosate 27

Gallstone Dissolution Agent
Ursodiol 1552

Ganglionic Blocking Agent
Mecamylamine 968

Gastrointestinal Agent, Miscellaneous
Bifidobacterium bifidum / Lactobacillus acidophilus . . 1615
Chlorophyll 319
Glutamic Acid 743
Infliximab 832
Lansoprazole, Amoxicillin, and Clarithromycin 898
Lubiprostone 957
Saliva Substitute 1374
Sucralfate 1420

Gastrointestinal Agent, Prokinetic
Cisapride 348
Metoclopramide 1029

Gastrointestinal Agent, Stimulant
Dexpanthenol 446

General Anesthetic
Etomidate 625
Fentanyl 644
Ketamine 880
Nitrous Oxide 1122
Propofol 1296
Sufentanil 1421
Thiopental 1477

Genitourinary Irrigant
Sorbitol 1408

Glutamate Inhibitor
Riluzole 1350

Gold Compound
Auranofin 166
Gold Sodium Thiomalate 748

Gonadotropin
Chorionic Gonadotropin (Recombinant) 337
Follitropins 698
Gonadorelin 749
Lutropin Alfa 958
Menotropins 982

Gonadotropin Releasing Hormone Agonist
Goserelin 750
Histrelin 772
Leuprolide 906
Nafarelin 1081
Triptorelin 1544

Gonadotropin Releasing Hormone Antagonist
Abarelix 24
Cetrorelix 307
Ganirelix 723

Growth Factor
Darbepoetin Alfa 423

Growth Factor, Platelet-Derived
Becaplermin 182

Growth Hormone
Mecasermin 968
Sermorelin Acetate 1384
Somatropin 1406

Hemostatic Agent
Aluminum Chloride 78
Aminocaproic Acid 86
Aprotinin 135
Cellulose (Oxidized/Regenerated) 300
Collagen (Absorbable) 391
Collagen Hemostat 392
Desmopressin 437
Fibrin Sealant Kit 653
Gelatin (Absorbable) 728
Thrombin (Topical) 1481

Herb
Aloe 1614

Astragalus 1615
Bilberry. 1615
Black Cohosh 1616
Bromelain 1616
Calendula 1616
Cat's Claw 1617
Cayenne 1617
Chamomile 1617
Chasteberry 1618
Cranberry 1619
Devil's Claw 1619
Dong Quai 1620
Echinacea 1620
Evening Primrose 1621
Feverfew 1621
Garlic 1622
Ginger 1622
Ginkgo Biloba 1622
Ginseng, Panax 1623
Ginseng, Siberian 1623
Golden Seal 1624
Gotu Kola 1624
Grapefruit Seed 1625
Grape Seed 1625
Grape Skin 1625
Green Tea 1625
Hawthorn 1626
Horse Chestnut 1626
HuperzineA 1626
Kava 1627
Lemon Balm/Melissa 1627
Licorice 1627
Mastic 1628
Melaleuca Oil 1628
Milk Thistle 1629
Parsley 1630
Passion Flower 1630
Red Yeast Rice 1630
Sassafras Oil 1631
Saw Palmetto 1631
Schisandra 1631
St John's Wort 1632
Turmeric 1632
Uva Ursi 1633
Valerian 1633
Wild Yam 1634
Yohimbe 1634

Histamine H$_1$ Antagonist
Hydrocodone, Phenylephrine,
  and Diphenhydramine 791

Histamine H$_2$ Antagonist
Cimetidine 341
Famotidine 635
Famotidine, Calcium
  Carbonate, and
  Magnesium Hydroxide 636
Nizatidine 1123
Ranitidine 1334

Homocystinuria, Treatment Agent
Betaine Anhydrous 199

Hormone
Calcitonin 246

Hormone Antagonist, Anti-Adrenal
Aminoglutethimide 87

Hormone, Posterior Pituitary
Vasopressin 1567

Human Growth Factor
Oprelvekin 1149

4-Hydroxyphenylpyruvate Dioxygenase Inhibitor
Nitisinone 1118

Hypnotic, Benzodiazepine
Flurazepam 681
Temazepam 1453
Triazolam 1531

Hypnotic, Nonbenzodiazepine
Chloral Hydrate 312
Eszopiclone 587
Ramelteon 1331
Zaleplon 1591
Zolpidem 1604
Zopiclone 1606

Immune Globulin
Hepatitis B Immune Globulin . . . 768
Immune Globulin
  (Intramuscular) 823
Immune Globulin (Intravenous)
  824
Immune Globulin
  (Subcutaneous) 826
Rabies Immune Globulin
  (Human) 1328
Rh$_o$(D) Immune Globulin . . . 1342
Tetanus Immune Globulin
  (Human) 1463
Vaccinia Immune Globulin
  (Intravenous) 1553
Varicella-Zoster Immune
  Globulin (Human) 1566

Immunosuppressant Agent
Antithymocyte Globulin
  (Equine) 131
Azathioprine 168
CycloSPORINE 406
Daclizumab 416
Efalizumab 529
Lenalidomide 903
Muromonab-CD3 1074
Mycophenolate 1075
Pimecrolimus 1237
Sirolimus 1397
Tacrolimus 1437
Thalidomide 1471

Interferon
Interferon Alfa-2a 842
Interferon Alfa-2b 844
Interferon Alfa-2b and Ribavirin
  847
Interferon Alfa-n3 848
Interferon Beta-1a 849
Interferon Beta-1b 850
Interferon Gamma-1b 851
Peginterferon Alfa-2a 1195
Peginterferon Alfa-2b 1197

Interleukin-1 Receptor Antagonist
Anakinra 125

Intravenous Nutritional Therapy
Dextrose 452

Iodinated Contrast Media
Diatrizoate Meglumine 453
Diatrizoate Meglumine and
  Diatrizoate Sodium 453
Diatrizoate Meglumine and
  Iodipamide Meglumine 453
Diatrizoate Sodium 454
Iodipamide Meglumine 853
Iodixanol 853
Iopamidol 855
Iothalamate Meglumine 855
Iothalamate Sodium 855
Ioversol 856
Ioxaglate Meglumine and
  Ioxaglate Sodium 856

Iron Salt
Ferric Gluconate 649
Ferrous Fumarate 650
Ferrous Gluconate 651
Ferrous Sulfate 651
Ferrous Sulfate and Ascorbic
  Acid 651

Iron Dextran Complex 862
Iron Sucrose 862
Polysaccharide-Iron Complex . . 1254

Keratinocyte Growth Factor
Palifermin 1178

Keratolytic Agent
Anthralin 128
Cantharidin 254
Podofilox 1251
Podophyllum Resin 1251
Salicylic Acid 1374
Tazarotene 1446
Trichloroacetic Acid 1534
Urea 1551

Laxative
Cascara 1617
Magnesium Hydroxide and
  Mineral Oil 961
Methylcellulose 1021

Laxative, Bowel Evacuant
Sodium Phosphates 1403

Laxative, Bulk-Producing
Polycarbophil 1252
Psyllium 1313

Laxative, Miscellaneous
Castor Oil 279

Laxative, Osmotic
Glycerin 747
Lactulose 893
Polyethylene Glycol 3350 1253
Polyethylene Glycol-Electrolyte
  Solution 1253
Sorbitol 1408

Laxative, Saline
Magnesium Citrate 960
Magnesium Sulfate 963

Laxative, Stimulant
Bisacodyl 209
Senna 1384

Laxative/Stool Softener
Docusate and Casanthranol 496

Leprostatic Agent
Clofazimine 369

Leukotriene-Receptor Antagonist
Montelukast 1062
Zafirlukast 1590

Lipase Inhibitor
Orlistat 1150

5-Lipoxygenase Inhibitor
Zileuton 1596

Lithium
Lithium 939

Local Anesthetic
Articaine and Epinephrine 139
Benzocaine 190
Benzocaine, Butyl
  Aminobenzoate,
  Tetracaine, and
  Benzalkonium Chloride 193
Bupivacaine 228
Bupivacaine and Epinephrine . . . 228
Cetylpyridinium and
  Benzocaine 309
Chloroprocaine 320
Cocaine 384
Dibucaine 458
Ethyl Chloride 620
Ethyl Chloride and
  Dichlorotetrafluoroethane . . . 620
Hexylresorcinol 771
Levobupivacaine 909
Lidocaine 920
Lidocaine and Bupivacaine . . . 924

Lidocaine and Epinephrine 924
Lidocaine and Prilocaine 928
Lidocaine and Tetracaine 930
Mepivacaine 987
Mepivacaine and Levonordefrin
  991
Mepivacaine (Dental
  Anesthetic) 989
Pramoxine 1264
Prilocaine 1277
Prilocaine and Epinephrine . . . 1278
Procaine 1284
Proparacaine and Fluorescein
  1296
Ropivacaine 1366
Tetracaine 1466
Tetracaine and Dextrose 1467

Local Anesthetic, Ophthalmic
Proparacaine 1296

Local Anesthetic, Oral
Benzydamine 197
Dyclonine 525

Local Anesthetic, Transoral
Lidocaine (Transoral) 931

Low Molecular Weight Heparin
Dalteparin 418
Enoxaparin 542
Tinzaparin 1492

Lubricant, Ocular
Hydroxypropyl Methylcellulose . . 800
Sodium Chloride 1400

Lung Surfactant
Beractant 198
Calfactant 251
Poractant Alfa 1255

Magnesium Salt
Magnesium Chloride 960
Magnesium Citrate 960
Magnesium Gluconate 961
Magnesium Hydroxide 961
Magnesium Sulfate 963

Mast Cell Stabilizer
Cromolyn 397
Lodoxamide 940
Nedocromil 1095
Pemirolast 1199

Mineral
Vanadium 1633

Mineral, Oral (Topical)
Triclosan and Fluoride 1534

Miscellaneous Product
Yohimbine 1589

Monoclonal Antibody
Adalimumab 52
Alefacept 62
Basiliximab 180
Efalizumab 529
Infliximab 832
Palivizumab 1179
Rituximab 1360
Trastuzumab 1520

**Monoclonal Antibody,
   Anti-Asthmatic**
Omalizumab 1144

**Monoclonal Antibody, Selective
   Adhesion-Molecule
   Inhibitor**
Natalizumab 1093

Mouthwash
Mouthwash (Antiseptic) 1069

Mucolytic Agent
Acetylcysteine 46

Natriuretic Peptide, B-Type, Human
Nesiritide 1103

Neuraminidase Inhibitor
Oseltamivir 1152
Zanamivir 1592

Neuromuscular Blocker Agent, Depolarizing
Succinylcholine 1419

Neuromuscular Blocker Agent, Toxin
Botulinum Toxin Type A 217
Botulinum Toxin Type B 218

N-Methyl-D-Aspartate Receptor Antagonist
Memantine 979

Nonsteroidal Anti-inflammatory Drug (NSAID)
Diclofenac 459

Nonsteroidal Anti-inflammatory Drug (NSAID), COX-2 Selective
Celecoxib 296

Nonsteroidal Anti-inflammatory Drug (NSAID), Ophthalmic
Bromfenac 221
Diclofenac 459
Flurbiprofen 683
Ketorolac 886
Nepafenac 1103

Nonsteroidal Anti-inflammatory Drug (NSAID), Oral
Diclofenac 459
Diclofenac and Misoprostol 462
Diflunisal 468
Etodolac 623
Fenoprofen 642
Flurbiprofen 683
Hydrocodone and Ibuprofen 787
Ibuprofen 808
Indomethacin 830
Ketoprofen 883
Ketorolac 886
Lansoprazole and Naproxen 898
Meclofenamate 970
Mefenamic Acid 973
Meloxicam 977
Nabumetone 1077
Naproxen 1089
Oxaprozin 1155
Oxycodone and Ibuprofen 1170
Piroxicam 1248
Sulindac 1430
Tolmetin 1504

Nonsteroidal Anti-inflammatory Drug (NSAID), Parenteral
Indomethacin 830
Ketorolac 886

Nonsteroidal Aromatase Inhibitor
Aminoglutethimide 87

Norepinephrine Reuptake Inhibitor, Selective
Atomoxetine 156

Nutraceutical
Androstenedione 1614
Chondroitin Sulfate 1618
Chromium 1618
Coenzyme Q$_{10}$ 1618
Creatine 1619
Dehydroepiandrosterone 1619
Docosahexaenoic Acid 1620
Flaxseed Oil 1622
Glucosamine 1624

Glutathione 1624
Lutein 1628
Lycopene 1628
Melatonin 1629
Methyl Sulfonyl Methane 1629
Nicotinamide Adenine Dinucleotide 1629
Omega-3-Acid Ethyl Esters . . . 1621
Quercetin 1630
Shark Cartilage 1632
Soy Isoflavones 1632

Nutritional Supplement
Alpha-Lipoic Acid 1614
Cysteine 412
Fluoride 671
Glucose Polymers 743
L-Lysine 959
Medium Chain Triglycerides 972
SAMe 1631

Ophthalmic Agent
Pegaptanib 1193
Verteporfin 1574

Ophthalmic Agent, Antiglaucoma
AcetaZOLAMIDE 45
Bimatoprost 208
Brimonidine 220
Brinzolamide 220
Carbachol 260
Carteolol 274
Cyclopentolate and Phenylephrine 403
Dichlorphenamide 459
Dipivefrin 489
Dorzolamide 501
Echothiophate Iodide 526
Latanoprost 900
Levobunolol 909
Methazolamide 1006
Metipranolol 1028
Phenylephrine 1226
Pilocarpine (Ophthalmic) 1234
Timolol 1489
Travoprost 1521
Unoprostone 1551

Ophthalmic Agent, Miotic
Acetylcholine 46
Carbachol 260
Echothiophate Iodide 526
Pilocarpine (Ophthalmic) 1234

Ophthalmic Agent, Miscellaneous
Artificial Tears 143
Balanced Salt Solution 178
Carboxymethylcellulose 271
Glycerin 747
Hydroxypropyl Cellulose 800
Olopatadine 1143
Pemirolast 1199

Ophthalmic Agent, Mydriatic
Atropine 161
Homatropine 772
Phenylephrine 1226
Tropicamide 1545

Ophthalmic Agent, Toxin
Botulinum Toxin Type A 217

Ophthalmic Agent, Vasoconstrictor
Dipivefrin 489
Naphazoline 1087
Naphazoline and Antazoline . . . 1088
Naphazoline and Pheniramine 1088
Tetrahydrozoline 1470

Ophthalmic Agent, Viscoelastic
Chondroitin Sulfate and Sodium Hyaluronate 336
Hyaluronate and Derivatives . . . 773

Otic Agent, Analgesic
Antipyrine and Benzocaine 130

Otic Agent, Anti-infective
Acetic Acid, Propylene Glycol
Diacetate, and
Hydrocortisone 45
m-Cresyl Acetate 966

Otic Agent, Cerumenolytic
Antipyrine and Benzocaine 130
Carbamide Peroxide 264
Triethanolamine Polypeptide
Oleate-Condensate 1535

Ovulation Stimulator
Chorionic Gonadotropin
(Human) 336
Chorionic Gonadotropin
(Recombinant) 337
ClomiPHENE 369
Follitropins 698
Lutropin Alfa 958
Menotropins 982

Oxytocic Agent
Oxytocin 1175

Parathyroid Hormone Analog
Teriparatide 1461

Pediculocide
Lindane 933
Pyrethrins and Piperonyl
Butoxide 1315

Peritoneal Dialysate, Osmotic
Icodextrin 814

Phenothiazine Derivative
Promethazine 1290

Phosphate Binder
Calcium Acetate 248
Lanthanum 899
Sevelamer 1388

Phosphodiesterase-5 Enzyme
Inhibitor
Sildenafil 1390
Tadalafil 1441
Vardenafil 1565

Phosphodiesterase Enzyme
Inhibitor
Cilostazol 340
Inamrinone 827
Milrinone 1048

Phospholipase A$_2$ Inhibitor
Anagrelide 124

Photosensitizing Agent, Topical
Aminolevulinic Acid 88

Plasma Volume Expander
Dextran 447
Dextran 1 447

Plasma Volume Expander,
Colloid
Hetastarch 770

Polypeptide Hormone
Iohexol 854

Probiotic
Lactobacillus 535

Progestin
Levonorgestrel 916
MedroxyPROGESTERone 972
Megestrol 976
Norethindrone 1125
Norgestrel 1127
Progesterone 1289

Prostaglandin
Alprostadil 76
Carboprost Tromethamine 270
Diclofenac and Misoprostol 462
Dinoprostone 482
Epoprostenol 553
Iloprost 816
Misoprostol 1053

Prostaglandin, Ophthalmic
Bimatoprost 208
Latanoprost 900
Travoprost 1521
Unoprostone 1551

Proteasome Inhibitor
Bortezomib 215

Protectant, Topical
Aluminum Hydroxide 79
Trypsin, Balsam Peru, and
Castor Oil 1547

Protein C (Activated)
Drotrecogin Alfa 522

Proton Pump Inhibitor
Esomeprazole 572
Lansoprazole 896
Lansoprazole and Naproxen . . . 898
Omeprazole 1145
Omeprazole and Sodium
Bicarbonate 1146
Pantoprazole 1184
Rabeprazole 1327

Psoralen
Methoxsalen 1018

Radiological/Contrast Media,
Ionic
Diatrizoate Meglumine 453
Diatrizoate Meglumine and
Diatrizoate Sodium 453
Diatrizoate Meglumine and
Iodipamide Meglumine 453
Diatrizoate Sodium 454
Iodipamide Meglumine 853
Iothalamate Meglumine 855
Iothalamate Sodium 855
Ioxaglate Meglumine and
Ioxaglate Sodium 856

Radiological/Contrast Media,
Nonionic
Ferumoxides 652
Gadoteridol 719
Iodixanol 853
Iohexol 854
Iopamidol 855
Iopromide 855
Ioversol 856

Radiological/Contrast Media,
Paramagnetic Agent
Gadopentetate Dimeglumine . . . 719

Radiopaque Agents
Barium 179

Radiopharmaceutical
Ibritumomab 807

Rauwolfia Alkaloid
Reserpine 1340

Recombinant Human
Erythropoietin
Darbepoetin Alfa 423

Respiratory Stimulant
Ammonia Spirit (Aromatic) 103
Doxapram 502

Retinoic Acid Derivative
Fluocinolone, Hydroquinone,
and Tretinoin 669
Isotretinoin 869
Mequinol and Tretinoin 994
Tretinoin (Topical) 1525

Salicylate
Aminosalicylic Acid 89

Aspirin 145
Aspirin and Pravastatin 151
Choline Magnesium
    Trisalicylate 335
Magnesium Salicylate 962
Salsalate 1376
Triethanolamine Salicylate 1535

Scabicidal Agent
Crotamiton 398
Lindane 933
Permethrin 1218

Sclerosing Agent
Ethanolamine Oleate 591
Morrhuate Sodium 1068
Sodium Tetradecyl 1404

Sedative
Dexmedetomidine 444
Promethazine 1290

**Selective 5-HT$_3$ Receptor
    Antagonist**
Alosetron 72
Dolasetron 498
Granisetron 751
Ondansetron 1147
Palonosetron 1180

Selective Aldosterone Blocker
Eplerenone 551
Spironolactone 1413

**Selective Estrogen Receptor
    Modulator (SERM)**
Raloxifene 1329

**Serotonin 5-HT$_{1B, 1D}$ Receptor
    Agonist**
Eletriptan 533
Frovatriptan 712

**Serotonin 5-HT$_{1D}$ Receptor
    Agonist**
Almotriptan 71
Naratriptan 1092
Rizatriptan 1363
Sumatriptan 1432
Zolmitriptan 1603

**Serotonin 5-HT$_4$ Receptor
    Agonist**
Tegaserod 1448

Shampoo, Pediculocide
Pyrethrins and Piperonyl
    Butoxide 1315

Skeletal Muscle Relaxant
Baclofen 178
Carisoprodol 271
Carisoprodol and Aspirin 272
Carisoprodol, Aspirin, and
    Codeine 273
Chlorzoxazone 333
Cyclobenzaprine 401
Dantrolene 420
Metaxalone 1001
Methocarbamol 1009
Orphenadrine 1151
Orphenadrine, Aspirin, and
    Caffeine 1152

**Skin and Mucous Membrane
    Agent**
Imiquimod 821

**Skin and Mucous Membrane
    Agent, Miscellaneous**
Hyaluronate and Derivatives . . . 773

Smoking Cessation Aid
BuPROPion 233
Nicotine 1109

Sodium Salt
Sodium Chloride 1400

Somatostatin Analog
Octreotide 1135

Spermicide
Nonoxynol 9 1124

Stimulant
Caffeine 245
Dextroamphetamine 447
Dextroamphetamine and
    Amphetamine 448
Doxapram 502
Ergotamine and Caffeine 559
Methamphetamine 1005
Modafinil 1057
Pemoline 1199

Stool Softener
Docusate 496

**Substance P/Neurokinin 1
    Receptor Antagonist**
Aprepitant 134

Substituted Benzimidazole
Esomeprazole 572
Lansoprazole 896
Omeprazole 1145
Omeprazole and Sodium
    Bicarbonate 1146
Pantoprazole 1184
Rabeprazole 1327

Theophylline Derivative
Aminophylline 89
Dyphylline 526
Theophylline 1473
Theophylline and Guaifenesin
    1475

Thrombolytic Agent
Alteplase 77
Reteplase 1341
Streptokinase 1417
Tenecteplase 1455

Thyroid Product
Levothyroxine 917
Liothyronine 934
Liotrix 935
Thyroid 1482

Topical Skin Product
Aloe 1614
Aluminum Sulfate and Calcium
    Acetate 81
Aminolevulinic Acid 88
Becaplermin 182
Bentoquatam 188
Benzoin 193
Benzoyl Peroxide 194
Benzoyl Peroxide and
    Hydrocortisone 195
Calcipotriene 246
Camphor and Phenol 252
Capsaicin 256
Chloroxine 322
Clindamycin and Benzoyl
    Peroxide 364
Coal Tar 383
Coal Tar and Salicylic Acid . . . 383
Dexpanthenol 446
Doxepin 505
Eflornithine 532
Erythromycin 562
Erythromycin and Benzoyl
    Peroxide 567
Imiquimod 821
Lactic Acid 893
Lactic Acid and Ammonium
    Hydroxide 893
Lanolin, Cetyl Alcohol,
    Glycerin, Petrolatum, and
    Mineral Oil 896
Minoxidil 1051
Monobenzone 1062

Neomycin, Polymyxin B, and
  Hydrocortisone 1101
Pimecrolimus 1237
Podofilox 1251
Povidone-Iodine 1262
Pyrithione Zinc 1318
Tacrolimus 1437
Triethanolamine Salicylate 1535
Urea 1551
Vitamin A and Vitamin D 1580
Zinc Gelatin 1597
Zinc Oxide 1597

Topical Skin Product, Acne
Azelaic Acid 169
Benzoyl Peroxide 194
Benzoyl Peroxide and
  Hydrocortisone 195
Clindamycin and Benzoyl
  Peroxide 364
Erythromycin 562
Erythromycin and Benzoyl
  Peroxide 567

**Topical Skin Product,
  Antibacterial**
Silver Nitrate 1392

Toxoid
Tetanus Toxoid (Adsorbed) . . . 1464
Tetanus Toxoid (Fluid) 1464

Trace Element
Zinc Chloride 1597
Zinc Sulfate 1598

Trace Element, Parenteral
Selenium 1383
Trace Metals 1513

**Tumor Necrosis Factor (TNF)
  Blocking Agent**
Adalimumab 52
Etanercept 588
Infliximab 832
Lenalidomide 903
Thalidomide 1471

Tyrosine Hydroxylase Inhibitor
Metyrosine 1036

**Urea Cycle Disorder (UCD)
  Treatment Agent**
Sodium Phenylbutyrate 1403

Uricosuric Agent
Colchicine and Probenecid 388
Probenecid 1282

Urinary Acidifying Agent
Potassium Acid Phosphate . . . 1257

Urinary Tract Product
Acetohydroxamic Acid 46
Cellulose Sodium Phosphate . . . 301
Citric Acid, Magnesium
  Carbonate, and
  Glucono-Delta-Lactone . . . 353
Cysteamine 412
Tiopronin 1494

Vaccine
Anthrax Vaccine (Adsorbed) . . . 128
BCG Vaccine 181
Diphtheria, Tetanus Toxoids,
  Acellular Pertussis,
  Hepatitis B (Recombinant),
  and Poliovirus (Inactivated)
  Vaccine 488
Haemophilus b Conjugate
  Vaccine 534
Hepatitis A Inactivated and
  Hepatitis B (Recombinant)
  Vaccine 766
Hepatitis A Vaccine 767
Hepatitis B Vaccine 769
Influenza Virus Vaccine 833

Japanese Encephalitis Virus
  Vaccine (Inactivated) 877
Meningococcal Polysaccharide
  (Groups A / C / Y and
  W-135) Diphtheria Toxoid
  Conjugate Vaccine 980
Meningococcal Polysaccharide
  Vaccine (Groups A, C, Y,
  and W-135) 981
Mumps Virus Vaccine (Live/
  Attenuated) 1072
Pneumococcal Conjugate
  Vaccine (7-Valent) 1250
Poliovirus Vaccine (Inactivated)
  1252
Rabies Virus Vaccine 1329
Rotavirus Vaccine 1371
Rubella Virus Vaccine (Live) . . 1372
Typhoid Vaccine 1549

Vaccine, Live Virus
Measles, Mumps, and Rubella
  Vaccines (Combined) . . . 966
Measles, Mumps, Rubella, and
  Varicella Virus Vaccine . . . 967
Measles Virus Vaccine (Live) . . 967

**Vascular Endothelial Growth
  Factor (VEGF) Inhibitor**
Bevacizumab 204
Pegaptanib 1193
Sorafenib 1407
Sunitinib 1434

Vasoconstrictor
Epinephrine (Racemic) 549
Epinephrine (Racemic) and
  Aluminum Potassium
  Sulfate 550
Oxymetazoline 1172

Vasoconstrictor, Nasal
Xylometazoline 1588

Vasodilator
Amyl Nitrite 124
Dipyridamole 489
HydrALAZINE 775
Isosorbide Dinitrate 866
Isosorbide Dinitrate and
  Hydralazine 867
Isosorbide Mononitrate 868
Isoxsuprine 871
Minoxidil 1051
Nesiritide 1103
Nitroglycerin 1120
Nitroprusside 1122
Papaverine 1186
Tolazoline 1501
Treprostinil 1523

Vasodilator, Peripheral
Nylidrin 1133

Vasodilator, Pulmonary
Nitric Oxide 1118

Vasopressin Analog, Synthetic
Desmopressin 437

Vasopressin Antagonist
Conivaptan 393

Vitamin
Ferrous Sulfate and Ascorbic
  Acid 651
Folic Acid, Cyanocobalamin,
  and Pyridoxine 697
Vitamin B Complex
  Combinations 1581
Vitamins (Multiple/Oral) 1582

Vitamin D Analog
Alendronate and
  Cholecalciferol 66
Calcipotriene 246
Calcitriol 247

Cholecalciferol 334
Dihydrotachysterol 478
Doxercalciferol 508
Ergocalciferol 556
Paricalcitol 1187

Vitamin A Derivative
Mequinol and Tretinoin 994

Vitamin, Fat Soluble
Beta-Carotene 198
Phytonadione 1233
Vitamin A 1580
Vitamin E 1581

Vitamin, Topical
Mequinol and Tretinoin 994

Vitamin, Water Soluble
Ascorbic Acid 143
Cyanocobalamin 399
Folic Acid 697
Hydroxocobalamin 798
Leucovorin 905
Niacin 1105
Niacinamide 1106
Pantothenic Acid 1186
Potassium P-Aminobenzoate . . 1261
Pyridoxine 1316
Riboflavin 1345
Thiamine 1476

Xanthine Oxidase Inhibitor
Allopurinol 70

ALPHABETICAL INDEX

1370-999-397 see Anagrelide 124
A₁-PI see Alpha₁-Proteinase
  Inhibitor 73
A200® Lice [OTC] see Permethrin
  1218
A-200® Maximum Strength [OTC]
  see Pyrethrins and Piperonyl
  Butoxide 1315
A and D® Original [OTC] see
  Vitamin A and Vitamin D 1580
Abacavir 22
Abacavir and Lamivudine 23
Abacavir, Lamivudine, and
  Zidovudine 23
Abacavir Sulfate see Abacavir 22
Abacavir Sulfate and Lamivudine
  see Abacavir and Lamivudine . . . 23
Abarelix 24
Abatacept 25
Abbott-43818 see Leuprolide 906
ABC see Abacavir 22
ABCD see Amphotericin B
  Cholesteryl Sulfate Complex . . 112
Abciximab 26
Abelcet® see Amphotericin B (Lipid
  Complex) 115
Abenol® (Can) see Acetaminophen
  31
Abilify® see Aripiprazole 138
ABLC see Amphotericin B (Lipid
  Complex) 115
A/B Otic see Antipyrine and
  Benzocaine 130
Abraxane™ see Paclitaxel (Protein
  Bound) 1177
Abreva® [OTC] see Docosanol 495
Absorbable Cotton see Cellulose
  (Oxidized/Regenerated) 300
Absorbable Gelatin Sponge see
  Gelatin (Absorbable) 728
9-AC see Aminocamptothecin 86
AC 2993 see Exenatide 629
Acamprosate 27
Acamprosate Calcium see
  Acamprosate 27
Acanol® (Mex) see Loperamide . . . 942
Acarbose 28
A-Caro-25® see Beta-Carotene . . . 198
ACC® (Mex) see Acetylcysteine . . . 46
Accolate® see Zafirlukast 1590
AccuNeb™ see Albuterol 58
Accupril® see Quinapril 1322
Accuretic® see Quinapril and
  Hydrochlorothiazide 1323
Accutane® see Isotretinoin 869
Accuzyme® see Papain and Urea
  1186
ACE see Captopril 257
Acebutolol 28
Acebutolol Hydrochloride see
  Acebutolol 28
Acenocoumarin see
  Acenocoumarol 30
Acenocoumarol 30
Aceon® see Perindopril Erbumine
  1216
Acephen™ [OTC] see
  Acetaminophen 31
Acetadiazol® (Mex) see
  AcetaZOLAMIDE 45
Acetadote® see Acetylcysteine 46
Acetafen® (Mex) see
  Acetaminophen 31
Acetaminophen 31
Acetaminophen and
  Chlorpheniramine see
  Chlorpheniramine and
  Acetaminophen 324
Acetaminophen and Codeine 35
Acetaminophen and
  Diphenhydramine 38

Acetaminophen and Hydrocodone
  see Hydrocodone and
  Acetaminophen 779
Acetaminophen and Oxycodone
  see Oxycodone and
  Acetaminophen 1165
Acetaminophen and Pentazocine
  see Pentazocine and
  Acetaminophen 1209
Acetaminophen and
  Phenyltoloxamine 38
Acetaminophen and Propoxyphene
  see Propoxyphene and
  Acetaminophen 1298
Acetaminophen and
  Pseudoephedrine 38
Acetaminophen and Tramadol 39
Acetaminophen, Aspirin, and
  Caffeine 41
Acetaminophen, Butalbital, and
  Caffeine see Butalbital,
  Acetaminophen, and Caffeine . . 239
Acetaminophen, Caffeine, and
  Dihydrocodeine 42
Acetaminophen, Caffeine, Codeine,
  and Butalbital see Butalbital,
  Acetaminophen, Caffeine, and
  Codeine 239
Acetaminophen, Caffeine,
  Hydrocodone,
  Chlorpheniramine, and
  Phenylephrine see
  Hydrocodone,
  Chlorpheniramine,
  Phenylephrine,
  Acetaminophen, and Caffeine . . 790
Acetaminophen, Chlorpheniramine,
  and Pseudoephedrine 43
Acetaminophen,
  Dextromethorphan, and
  Pseudoephedrine 44
Acetaminophen,
  Dichloralphenazone, and
  Isometheptene see
  Acetaminophen,
  Isometheptene, and
  Dichloralphenazone 44
Acetaminophen, Isometheptene,
  and Dichloralphenazone 44
Acetaminophen, Pseudoephedrine,
  and Chlorpheniramine see
  Acetaminophen,
  Chlorpheniramine, and
  Pseudoephedrine 43
Acetasol® HC see Acetic Acid,
  Propylene Glycol Diacetate,
  and Hydrocortisone 45
AcetaZOLAMIDE 45
Acetic Acid, Hydrocortisone, and
  Propylene Glycol Diacetate see
  Acetic Acid, Propylene Glycol
  Diacetate, and Hydrocortisone . . 45
Acetic Acid, Propylene Glycol
  Diacetate, and Hydrocortisone . . 45
Acetohydroxamic Acid 46
Acetoxyl® (Can) see Benzoyl
  Peroxide 194
Acetoxymethylprogesterone see
  MedroxyPROGESTERone 972
Acetylcholine 46
Acetylcholine Chloride see
  Acetylcholine 46
Acetylcysteine 46
Acetylcysteine Sodium see
  Acetylcysteine 46
Acetylcysteine Solution (Can) see
  Acetylcysteine 46
Acetylsalicylic Acid see Aspirin . . . 145
Achromycin® see Tetracycline . . . 1467
Aciclovir see Acyclovir 49

Acidulated Phosphate Fluoride see Fluoride 671
Acifur® (Mex) see Acyclovir 49
Acilac (Can) see Lactulose 893
AcipHex® see Rabeprazole 1327
Aclasta® (Can) see Zoledronic Acid 1600
Acloral® (Mex) see Ranitidine 1334
Aclovate® see Alclometasone 60
4-(9-Acridinylamino) Methanesulfon-m-Anisidide see Amsacrine 123
Acridinyl Anisidide see Amsacrine . . 123
Acrivastine and Pseudoephedrine . . . 47
ACT see Dactinomycin 417
Act-D see Dactinomycin 417
ACTH see Corticotropin 395
ActHIB® see Haemophilus b Conjugate Vaccine 534
Acticin® see Permethrin 1218
Actidose-Aqua® [OTC] see Charcoal 311
Actidose® with Sorbitol [OTC] see Charcoal 311
Actifed® (Can) see Triprolidine and Pseudoephedrine 1542
Actifed® Cold and Allergy [OTC] see Triprolidine and Pseudoephedrine 1542
Actifed® Cold and Sinus [OTC] see Acetaminophen, Chlorpheniramine, and Pseudoephedrine 43
Actigall® see Ursodiol 1552
Actilyse® (Mex) see Alteplase 77
Actimmune® see Interferon Gamma-1b 851
Actinomycin see Dactinomycin 417
Actinomycin D see Dactinomycin . . . 417
Actinomycin Cl see Dactinomycin . . 417
Actiq® see Fentanyl 644
Activase® see Alteplase 77
Activase® rt-PA (Can) see Alteplase 77
Activated Carbon see Charcoal 311
Activated Charcoal see Charcoal . . . 311
Activated Dimethicone see Simethicone 1394
Activated Ergosterol see Ergocalciferol 556
Activated Methylpolysiloxane see Simethicone 1394
Activated Protein C, Human, Recombinant see Drotrecogin Alfa 522
Activella® see Estradiol and Norethindrone 575
Actonel® see Risedronate 1352
Actonel® and Calcium see Risedronate and Calcium 1354
Actoplus Met™ see Pioglitazone and Metformin 1242
Actos® see Pioglitazone 1241
ACT® [OTC] see Fluoride 671
ACT® Plus [OTC] see Fluoride 671
ACT® x2™ [OTC] see Fluoride 671
Acular® see Ketorolac 886
Acular LS™ see Ketorolac 886
Acular® PF see Ketorolac 886
Acupril® (Mex) see Quinapril 1322
ACV see Acyclovir 49
Acycloguanosine see Acyclovir 49
Acyclovir 49
Aczone™ see Dapsone 421
AD3L see Valrubicin 1560
Adagen® see Pegademase Bovine 1193
Adalat® (Mex) see NIFEdipine 1112
Adalat® XL® (Can) see NIFEdipine 1112
Adalat® CC see NIFEdipine 1112

Adalat Oros® (Mex) see NIFEdipine 1112
Adalat Retard® (Mex) see NIFEdipine 1112
Adalimumab 52
Adalken® (Mex) see Penicillamine 1201
Adamantanamine Hydrochloride see Amantadine 81
Adapalene 54
Adderall® see Dextroamphetamine and Amphetamine 448
Adderall XR® see Dextroamphetamine and Amphetamine 448
Adecur® (Mex) see Terazosin 1458
Adefovir 54
Adefovir Dipivoxil see Adefovir 54
Adel® (Mex) see Clarithromycin . . . 355
Adenocard® see Adenosine 55
Adenoscan® see Adenosine 55
Adenosine 55
Adenosine Injection, USP (Can) see Adenosine 55
ADH see Vasopressin 1567
Adipex-P® see Phentermine 1224
Adoxa™ see Doxycycline (Systemic) 514
Adrecort® (Mex) see Dexamethasone 439
Adrenalin® see Epinephrine 546
Adrenaline see Epinephrine 546
Adrenocorticotropic Hormone see Corticotropin 395
ADR (error-prone abbreviation) see DOXOrubicin 509
Adria see DOXOrubicin 509
Adriamycin® (Can) see DOXOrubicin 509
Adriamycin PFS® see DOXOrubicin 509
Adriamycin RDF® see DOXOrubicin 509
Adriblastina® (Mex) see DOXOrubicin 509
Adriblastina RD® (Mex) see DOXOrubicin 509
Adrucil® see Fluorouracil 674
Adsorbent Charcoal see Charcoal . . 311
Advair Diskus® see Fluticasone and Salmeterol 690
Advantage-S™ [OTC] see Nonoxynol 9 1124
Advate see Antihemophilic Factor (Recombinant) 130
Advicor® see Niacin and Lovastatin 1107
Advil® (Can) see Ibuprofen 808
Advil® Children's [OTC] see Ibuprofen 808
Advil® Cold, Children's [OTC] see Pseudoephedrine and Ibuprofen 1311
Advil® Cold & Sinus (Can) see Pseudoephedrine and Ibuprofen 1311
Advil® Cold & Sinus [OTC] see Pseudoephedrine and Ibuprofen 1311
Advil® Infants' [OTC] see Ibuprofen 808
Advil® Junior [OTC] see Ibuprofen . . 808
Advil® Migraine [OTC] see Ibuprofen 808
Advil® [OTC] see Ibuprofen 808
Aerius® (Can) see Desloratadine . . . 435
AeroBid® see Flunisolide 667
AeroBid®-M see Flunisolide 667
Aerosial® (Mex) see Budesonide . . . 224
Aesculus hippocastanum see Horse Chestnut 1626

Afazol Grin® (Mex) see
　　Naphazoline 1087
Afeditab™ CR see NIFEdipine 1112
Afrin® (Mex) see Oxymetazoline . . 1172
Afrin® Extra Moisturizing [OTC] see
　　Oxymetazoline 1172
Afrin® Original [OTC] see
　　Oxymetazoline 1172
Afrin® Severe Congestion [OTC]
　　see Oxymetazoline 1172
Afrin® Sinus [OTC] see
　　Oxymetazoline 1172
Aftate® Antifungal [OTC] [DSC] see
　　Tolnaftate 1506
Afungil® (Mex) see Fluconazole . . . 659
A.f. Valdecasas® (Mex) see Folic
　　Acid 697
AG see Aminoglutethimide 87
Agalsidase Beta 55
Agenerase® see Amprenavir 122
Agglad ofteno® (Mex) see
　　Brimonidine 220
Aggrastat® see Tirofiban 1496
Aggrenox® see Aspirin and
　　Dipyridamole 150
AgNO₃ see Silver Nitrate 1392
Agrastat® (Mex) see Tirofiban 1496
Agrylin® see Anagrelide 124
AGT see Aminoglutethimide 87
AHA see Acetohydroxamic Acid 46
AH-Chew II see Chlorpheniramine,
　　Phenylephrine, and
　　Methscopolamine 327
AH-chew® D [OTC] [DSC] see
　　Phenylephrine 1226
AH-Chew® [DSC] see
　　Chlorpheniramine,
　　Phenylephrine, and
　　Methscopolamine 327
AHF (Human) see Antihemophilic
　　Factor (Human) 129
AHF (Recombinant) see
　　Antihemophilic Factor
　　(Recombinant) 130
A-hydroCort see Hydrocortisone . . . 793
AICC see Anti-inhibitor Coagulant
　　Complex 130
Airomir (Can) see Albuterol 58
Akacin® (Mex) see Amikacin 84
AK-Con™ see Naphazoline 1087
AK-Dilate® see Phenylephrine 1226
Akineton® see Biperiden 208
Akne-Mycin® see Erythromycin 562
Akorazol® (Mex) see Ketoconazole
　　. 880
AK-Pentolate® [DSC] see
　　Cyclopentolate 402
AK-Poly-Bac® see Bacitracin and
　　Polymyxin B 176
AK-Pred® see PrednisoLONE 1268
AKTob® see Tobramycin 1498
AK-Tracin® [DSC] see Bacitracin . . 175
AK-Trol® [DSC] see Neomycin,
　　Polymyxin B, and
　　Dexamethasone 1101
Akwa Tears® [OTC] see Artificial
　　Tears 143
ALA see Flaxseed Oil 1622
Alamag [OTC] see Aluminum
　　Hydroxide and Magnesium
　　Hydroxide 80
Alamag Plus [OTC] see Aluminum
　　Hydroxide, Magnesium
　　Hydroxide, and Simethicone 81
Alamast® see Pemirolast 1199
Alatrofloxacin Mesylate see
　　Trovafloxacin 1546
Alavert™ Allergy and Sinus [OTC]
　　see Loratadine and
　　Pseudoephedrine 947
Alavert® [OTC] see Loratadine 946

Albalon® see Naphazoline 1087
Albalon®-A Liquifilm (Can) see
　　Naphazoline and Antazoline . . . 1088
Albendazole 57
Albenza® see Albendazole 57
Albert® Glyburide (Can) see
　　GlyBURIDE 744
Albert® Pentoxifylline (Can) see
　　Pentoxifylline 1212
Alboral® (Mex) see Diazepam 454
Alboz® (Mex) see Omeprazole 1145
Albuterol 58
Albuterol and Ipratropium see
　　Ipratropium and Albuterol 857
Albuterol Sulfate see Albuterol 58
Alcaine® see Proparacaine 1296
Alcalak [OTC] see Calcium
　　Carbonate 248
Alclometasone 60
Alclometasone Dipropionate see
　　Alclometasone 60
Alcomicin® (Can) see Gentamicin . . 734
Aldactazide® see
　　Hydrochlorothiazide and
　　Spironolactone 778
Aldactazide 25® (Can) see
　　Hydrochlorothiazide and
　　Spironolactone 778
Aldactazide 50® (Can) see
　　Hydrochlorothiazide and
　　Spironolactone 778
Aldactone® see Spironolactone . . . 1413
Aldactone-A® (Mex) see
　　Spironolactone 1413
Aldara™ see Imiquimod 821
Aldesleukin 61
Aldex™ see Guaifenesin and
　　Phenylephrine 754
Aldomet® (Mex) see Methyldopa . . 1021
Aldoril® see Methyldopa and
　　Hydrochlorothiazide 1022
Aldroxicon I [OTC] see Aluminum
　　Hydroxide, Magnesium
　　Hydroxide, and Simethicone 81
Aldroxicon II [OTC] see Aluminum
　　Hydroxide, Magnesium
　　Hydroxide, and Simethicone 81
Aldurazyme® see Laronidase 900
Alefacept 62
Alemtuzumab 63
Alendronate 64
Alendronate and Cholecalciferol 66
Alendronate Sodium see
　　Alendronate 64
Alendronate Sodium and
　　Cholecalciferol see
　　Alendronate and
　　Cholecalciferol 66
Alenic Alka Tablet [OTC] see
　　Aluminum Hydroxide and
　　Magnesium Trisilicate 80
Aleprozil® (Mex) see Omeprazole
　　. 1145
Alepsal® (Mex) see Phenobarbital
　　. 1221
Aler-Cap [OTC] see
　　DiphenhydrAMINE 483
Aler-Dryl [OTC] see
　　DiphenhydrAMINE 483
Aler-Tab [OTC] see
　　DiphenhydrAMINE 483
Alertec® (Can) see Modafinil 1057
Alesse® see Ethinyl Estradiol and
　　Levonorgestrel 602
Aleve® [OTC] see Naproxen 1089
Alfaken® (Mex) see Lisinopril 936
Alfenta® see Alfentanil 67
Alfentanil 67
Alfentanil Hydrochloride see
　　Alfentanil 67

Alfentanil Injection, USP (Can) *see*
  Alfentanil 67
Alferon® N *see* Interferon Alfa-n3 . . . 848
Alfuzosin 68
Alfuzosin Hydrochloride *see*
  Alfuzosin 68
Alglucerase 68
Alimta® *see* Pemetrexed 1198
Alin® (Mex) *see* Dexamethasone . . . 439
Alin Depot® (Mex) *see*
  Dexamethasone 439
Alinia® *see* Nitazoxanide 1117
Alitretinoin 69
Alka-Mints® [OTC] *see* Calcium
  Carbonate 248
Alka-Seltzer Plus® Cold and Cough
  [OTC] *see* Chlorpheniramine,
  Phenylephrine, and
  Dextromethorphan 326
Alka-Seltzer Plus® Cold and Sinus
  Liqui-Gels [OTC] *see*
  Acetaminophen and
  Pseudoephedrine 38
Alka-Seltzer® Plus Cold
  Liqui-Gels® [OTC] *see*
  Acetaminophen,
  Chlorpheniramine, and
  Pseudoephedrine 43
Alka-Seltzer® Plus Flu Liqui-Gels®
  [OTC] *see* Acetaminophen,
  Dextromethorphan, and
  Pseudoephedrine 44
Alkeran® *see* Melphalan 979
Allbee® C-800 + Iron [OTC] *see*
  Vitamin B Complex
  Combinations 1581
Allbee® C-800 [OTC] *see* Vitamin
  B Complex Combinations 1581
Allbee® with C [OTC] *see* Vitamin
  B Complex Combinations 1581
Allegra® *see* Fexofenadine 652
Allegra-D® (Can) *see* Fexofenadine
  and Pseudoephedrine 653
Allegra-D® 12 Hour *see*
  Fexofenadine and
  Pseudoephedrine 653
Allegra-D® 24 Hour *see*
  Fexofenadine and
  Pseudoephedrine 653
Aller-Chlor® [OTC] *see*
  Chlorpheniramine 323
Allerdryl® (Can) *see*
  DiphenhydrAMINE 483
Allerest® Maximum Strength
  Allergy and Hay Fever [OTC]
  see Chlorpheniramine and
  Pseudoephedrine 325
Allerfrim® [OTC] *see* Triprolidine
  and Pseudoephedrine 1542
Allergen® *see* Antipyrine and
  Benzocaine 130
AllerMax® [OTC] *see*
  DiphenhydrAMINE 483
Allernix (Can) *see*
  DiphenhydrAMINE 483
Allersol® *see* Naphazoline 1087
Allerx™ *see* Chlorpheniramine and
  Phenylephrine 324
Allfen-DM *see* Guaifenesin and
  Dextromethorphan 754
Allfen Jr *see* Guaifenesin 752
Allfen (reformulation) *see*
  Guaifenesin and Potassium
  Guaiacolsulfonate 755
Allium sativum see Garlic 1622
Alloprin® (Can) *see* Allopurinol 70
Allopurinol 70
Allopurinol Sodium *see* Allopurinol . . . 70
All-*trans*-Retinoic Acid *see*
  Tretinoin (Oral) 1524

Almacone Double Strength® [OTC]
  see Aluminum Hydroxide,
  Magnesium Hydroxide, and
  Simethicone 81
Almacone® [OTC] *see* Aluminum
  Hydroxide, Magnesium
  Hydroxide, and Simethicone 81
Almora® [OTC] *see* Magnesium
  Gluconate 961
Almotriptan 71
Almotriptan Malate *see* Almotriptan
  71
Alocril® *see* Nedocromil 1095
Aloe 1614
Aloe Barbadensis *see* Aloe 1614
Aloe Capensis *see* Aloe 1614
Aloe vera *see* Aloe 1614
Aloe Vesta® 2-n-1 Antifungal [OTC]
  see Miconazole 1039
Aloid® (Mex) *see* Miconazole 1039
Alomide® *see* Lodoxamide 940
Alophen® [OTC] *see* Bisacodyl 209
Aloprim™ *see* Allopurinol 70
Alora® *see* Estradiol 574
Alosetron 72
Aloxi® *see* Palonosetron 1180
Alpha₁-Antitrypsin *see*
  Alpha₁-Proteinase Inhibitor 73
Alpha₁-PI *see* Alpha₁-Proteinase
  Inhibitor 73
Alpha₁-Proteinase Inhibitor 73
Alpha₁-Proteinase Inhibitor, Human
  see Alpha₁-Proteinase Inhibitor
  73
Alphadinal® (Mex) *see* Naphazoline
  1087
Alpha-Galactosidase-A (Human,
  Recombinant) *see* Agalsidase
  Beta 55
Alphagan® (Can) *see* Brimonidine . . 220
Alphagan® P *see* Brimonidine 220
Alpha-linolenic Acid *see* Flaxseed
  Oil 1622
Alpha-lipoate *see* Alpha-Lipoic Acid
  1614
Alpha-Lipoic Acid 1614
Alphanate® *see* Antihemophilic
  Factor (Human) 129
AlphaNine® SD *see* Factor IX 632
Alphaquin HP® *see* Hydroquinone . . 798
Alph-E-Mixed [OTC] *see* Vitamin E
  1581
Alph-E [OTC] *see* Vitamin E 1581
Alprazolam 73
Alprazolam Intensol® *see*
  Alprazolam 73
Alprostadil 76
Alquimid® (Mex) *see* Ifosfamide . . . 815
Alrex® *see* Loteprednol 953
Altace® *see* Ramipril 1332
Altachlore [OTC] *see* Sodium
  Chloride 1400
Altafrin *see* Phenylephrine 1226
Altamisa *see* Feverfew 1621
Altamist [OTC] *see* Sodium
  Chloride 1400
Altarussin DM [OTC] *see*
  Guaifenesin and
  Dextromethorphan 754
Altaryl [OTC] *see*
  DiphenhydrAMINE 483
Altenal® (Mex) *see* Clotrimazole . . . 379
Alteplase 77
Alteplase, Recombinant *see*
  Alteplase 77
Alteplase, Tissue Plasminogen
  Activator, Recombinant *see*
  Alteplase 77
Alter-H!2® (Mex) *see* Ranitidine . . . 1334
ALternaGEL® [OTC] *see* Aluminum
  Hydroxide 79

Alti-Alprazolam (Can) see
  Alprazolam 73
Alti-Amiodarone (Can) see
  Amiodarone 90
Alti-Amoxi-Clav (Can) see
  Amoxicillin and Clavulanate
  Potassium 108
Alti-Azathioprine (Can) see
  Azathioprine 168
Alti-Captopril (Can) see Captopril . . . 257
Alti-Clindamycin (Can) see
  Clindamycin 361
Alti-Clobazam (Can) see Clobazam
  364
Alti-Clonazepam (Can) see
  Clonazepam 371
Alti-Desipramine (Can) see
  Desipramine 434
Alti-Diltiazem CD (Can) see
  Diltiazem 479
Alti-Divalproex (Can) see Valproic
  Acid and Derivatives 1556
Alti-Doxazosin (Can) see
  Doxazosin 503
Alti-Flunisolide (Can) see
  Flunisolide 667
Alti-Fluoxetine (Can) see
  Fluoxetine 675
Alti-Flurbiprofen (Can) see
  Flurbiprofen 683
Alti-Fluvoxamine (Can) see
  Fluvoxamine 694
Alti-Ipratropium (Can) see
  Ipratropium 857
Alti-Metformin (Can) see Metformin
  1001
Alti-Minocycline (Can) see
  Minocycline 1049
Alti-MPA (Can) see
  MedroxyPROGESTERone 972
Alti-Nadolol (Can) see Nadolol . . . 1079
Alti-Nortriptyline (Can) see
  Nortriptyline 1128
Alti-Ranitidine (Can) see Ranitidine
  1334
Alti-Salbutamol (Can) see Albuterol
  58
Alti-Sotalol (Can) see Sotalol 1409
Alti-Sulfasalazine (Can) see
  Sulfasalazine 1428
Alti-Terazosin (Can) see Terazosin
  1458
Alti-Ticlopidine (Can) see
  Ticlopidine 1486
Alti-Timolol (Can) see Timolol 1489
Alti-Trazodone (Can) see
  Trazodone 1521
Alti-Verapamil (Can) see Verapamil
  1571
Alti-Zopiclone (Can) see Zopiclone
  1606
Altoprev™ see Lovastatin 953
Altretamine 78
Altrical® (Mex) see Calcitriol 247
Aluminum Chloride 78
Aluminum Hydroxide 79
Aluminum Hydroxide and
  Magnesium Carbonate 79
Aluminum Hydroxide and
  Magnesium Hydroxide 80
Aluminum Hydroxide and
  Magnesium Trisilicate 80
Aluminum Hydroxide, Magnesium
  Hydroxide, and Simethicone 81
Aluminum Potassium Sulfate and
  Epinephrine (Racemic) (Dental)
  see Epinephrine (Racemic)
  and Aluminum Potassium
  Sulfate 550
Aluminum Sucrose Sulfate, Basic
  see Sucralfate 1420
Aluminum Sulfate and Calcium
  Acetate 81
Alupent® see Metaproterenol 1000
Alvidina® (Mex) see Ranitidine . . . 1334
Alzam® (Mex) see Alprazolam 73
Amantadine 81
Amantadine Hydrochloride see
  Amantadine 81
Amaryl® see Glimepiride 738
Amatine® (Can) see Midodrine 1044
Ambenonium 82
Ambenonium Chloride see
  Ambenonium 82
Amber Touch-and-Feel see St
  John's Wort 1632
Ambien® see Zolpidem 1604
Ambien CR™ see Zolpidem 1604
Ambifed-G see Guaifenesin and
  Pseudoephedrine 755
Ambifed-G DM see Guaifenesin,
  Pseudoephedrine, and
  Dextromethorphan 757
AmBisome® see Amphotericin B
  (Liposomal) 116
Amcef® (Mex) see Ceftriaxone 294
Amcinonide 83
Amcort® (Can) see Amcinonide 83
Ameblin® (Mex) see Metronidazole
  1033
Amerge® see Naratriptan 1092
Americaine® Hemorrhoidal [OTC]
  see Benzocaine 190
Americaine® [OTC] see
  Benzocaine 190
American Coneflower see
  Echinacea 1620
A-Methapred see
  MethylPREDNISolone 1025
Amethocaine Hydrochloride see
  Tetracaine 1466
Amethopterin see Methotrexate . . . 1012
Ametop™ (Can) see Tetracaine . . . 1466
Amevive® see Alefacept 62
Amfepramone see Diethylpropion . . . 467
AMG 073 see Cinacalcet 342
Amibid DM see Guaifenesin and
  Dextromethorphan 754
Amicar® see Aminocaproic Acid 86
Amidal see Guaifenesin and
  Phenylephrine 754
Amidate® see Etomidate 625
Amidrine see Acetaminophen,
  Isometheptene, and
  Dichloralphenazone 44
Amifostine 83
Amigesic® see Salsalate 1376
Amikacin 84
Amikacin Sulfate see Amikacin 84
Amikacin Sulfate Injection, USP
  (Can) see Amikacin 84
Amikafur® (Mex) see Amikacin 84
Amikalem® (Mex) see Amikacin 84
Amikason's® (Mex) see Amikacin . . . 84
Amikayect® (Mex) see Amikacin 84
Amikin® see Amikacin 84
Amiloride 85
Amiloride and Hydrochlorothiazide . . 85
Amiloride Hydrochloride see
  Amiloride 85
2-Amino-6-Mercaptopurine see
  Thioguanine 1476
2-Amino-6-Methoxypurine
  Arabinoside see Nelarabine . . . 1097
2-Amino-6-Trifluoromethoxy-benzothiazole
  see Riluzole 1350
Aminobenzylpenicillin see
  Ampicillin 117
Aminocamptothecin 86
9-Aminocamptothecin see
  Aminocamptothecin 86
Aminocaproic Acid 86

Amino-Cerv™ see Urea 1551
Aminoglutethimide 87
Aminolevulinic Acid 88
Aminolevulinic Acid Hydrochloride
  see Aminolevulinic Acid 88
Aminophylline 89
Aminosalicylate Sodium see
  Aminosalicylic Acid 89
Aminosalicylic Acid 89
4-Aminosalicylic Acid see
  Aminosalicylic Acid 89
5-Aminosalicylic Acid see
  Mesalamine 996
Aminoxin® [OTC] see Pyridoxine . . 1316
Amiodarone 90
Amiodarone Hydrochloride see
  Amiodarone 90
Amiodarone Hydrochloride for
  Injection® (Can) see
  Amiodarone 90
Ami-Tex LA see Guaifenesin and
  Phenylephrine 754
Ami-Tex PSE see Guaifenesin and
  Pseudoephedrine 755
Amitiza™ see Lubiprostone 957
Amitone® [OTC] [DSC] see
  Calcium Carbonate 248
Amitriptyline 93
Amitriptyline and Chlordiazepoxide . . 97
Amitriptyline and Perphenazine 97
Amitriptyline Hydrochloride see
  Amitriptyline 93
AMJ 9701 see Palifermin 1178
A.M.K.® (Mex) see Amikacin 84
AmLactin® [OTC] see Lactic Acid
  and Ammonium Hydroxide 893
Amlexanox 99
Amlodipine 100
Amlodipine and Atorvastatin 101
Amlodipine and Benazepril 102
Amlodipine Besylate see
  Amlodipine 100
Ammens® Medicated Deodorant
  [OTC] see Zinc Oxide 1597
Ammonapse see Sodium
  Phenylbutyrate 1403
Ammonia Spirit (Aromatic) 103
Ammonium Chloride 103
Ammonium Lactate see Lactic Acid
  and Ammonium Hydroxide 893
Amnesteem™ see Isotretinoin 869
Amobarbital 104
Amobarbital and Secobarbital 104
Amobarbital Sodium see
  Amobarbital 104
Amobarbital Sodium and
  Secobarbital Sodium see
  Amobarbital and Secobarbital . . 104
Amonafide 104
Amonafide Hydrochloride see
  Amonafide 104
Amoxapine 105
Amoxicillin 106
Amoxicillin and Clavulanate
  Potassium 108
Amoxicillin and Clavulanic Acid see
  Amoxicillin and Clavulanate
  Potassium 108
Amoxicillin, Lansoprazole, and
  Clarithromycin see
  Lansoprazole, Amoxicillin, and
  Clarithromycin 898
Amoxicillin Trihydrate see
  Amoxicillin 106
Amoxil® see Amoxicillin 106
Amoxycillin see Amoxicillin 106
Amphadase™ see Hyaluronidase . . 774
Amphetamine and
  Dextroamphetamine see
  Dextroamphetamine and
  Amphetamine 448

Amphocin® see Amphotericin B
  (Conventional) 113
Amphojel® (Can) see Aluminum
  Hydroxide 79
Amphotec® see Amphotericin B
  Cholesteryl Sulfate Complex . . . 112
Amphotericin B Cholesteryl Sulfate
  Complex 112
Amphotericin B Colloidal
  Dispersion see Amphotericin B
  Cholesteryl Sulfate Complex . . . 112
Amphotericin B (Conventional) 113
Amphotericin B Desoxycholate see
  Amphotericin B (Conventional) . . 113
Amphotericin B (Lipid Complex) . . . 115
Amphotericin B (Liposomal) 116
Ampicillin 117
Ampicillin and Sulbactam 120
Ampicillin Sodium see Ampicillin . . 117
Ampicillin Trihydrate see Ampicillin
  117
Amprenavir 122
AMPT see Metyrosine 1036
Amrinone Lactate see Inamrinone . . 827
AMSA see Amsacrine 123
Amsacrine 123
Amsa P-D (Can) see Amsacrine . . . 123
Amyl Nitrite 124
Amylobarbitone see Amobarbital . . 104
Amytal® see Amobarbital 104
AN100226 see Natalizumab 1093
Anadrol® see Oxymetholone 1173
Anafranil® see ClomiPRAMINE . . . 370
Anagrelide 124
Anagrelide Hydrochloride see
  Anagrelide 124
Anakinra 125
Ana-Kit® see Epinephrine and
  Chlorpheniramine 549
Analpram-HC® see Pramoxine and
  Hydrocortisone 1264
AnaMantle® HC see Lidocaine and
  Hydrocortisone 928
Anandron® (Can) see Nilutamide . . 1115
Anaprox® see Naproxen 1089
Anaprox® DS see Naproxen 1089
Anas comosus see Bromelain 1616
Anaspaz® see Hyoscyamine 803
Anastrozole 126
Anatrast see Barium 179
Anbesol® Baby (Can) see
  Benzocaine 190
Anbesol® Baby [OTC] see
  Benzocaine 190
Anbesol® Cold Sore Therapy
  [OTC] see Benzocaine 190
Anbesol® Jr. [OTC] see
  Benzocaine 190
Anbesol® Maximum Strength [OTC]
  see Benzocaine 190
Anbesol® [OTC] see Benzocaine . . 190
Ancef® see Cefazolin 283
Ancobon® see Flucytosine 662
Andehist DM NR Drops see
  Carbinoxamine,
  Pseudoephedrine, and
  Dextromethorphan 269
Andehist NR Drops see
  Carbinoxamine and
  Pseudoephedrine 268
Andehist NR Syrup see
  Brompheniramine and
  Pseudoephedrine 223
Andox® (Mex) see Acetaminophen . . 31
Andriol® (Can) see Testosterone . . 1462
Andro see Androstenedione 1614
Androderm® see Testosterone 1462
AndroGel® see Testosterone 1462
Android® see
  MethylTESTOSTERone 1028

Andropository (Can) see
  Testosterone 1462
Androstenedione 1614
Anectine® (Mex) see
  Succinylcholine 1419
Anestacon® see Lidocaine 920
Aneurine Hydrochloride see
  Thiamine 1476
Anexate® (Can) see Flumazenil 665
Anexsia® see Hydrocodone and
  Acetaminophen 779
Anextuss see Guaifenesin,
  Dextromethorphan, and
  Phenylephrine 756
Angelica sinensis see Dong Quai . . 1620
Angeliq® see Drospirenone and
  Estradiol 520
Angiomax® see Bivalirudin 213
Angiotrofin® (Mex) see Diltiazem . . . 479
Anglix® (Mex) see Nitroglycerin . . . 1120
Anhydrous Glucose see Dextrose . . 452
Anidulafungin 128
Anistal® (Mex) see Ranitidine 1334
Anolor 300 see Butalbital,
  Acetaminophen, and Caffeine . . 239
Ansaid® (Can) see Flurbiprofen 683
Ansaid® [DSC] see Flurbiprofen 683
Ansamycin see Rifabutin 1345
Antabuse® see Disulfiram 492
Antagon® see Ganirelix 723
Antara™ see Fenofibrate 639
Antazoline and Naphazoline see
  Naphazoline and Antazoline . . . 1088
Anthraforte® (Can) see Anthralin . . . 128
Anthralin 128
Anthranol® (Can) see Anthralin 128
Anthrascalp® (Can) see Anthralin . . . 128
Anthrax Vaccine (Adsorbed) 128
Anti-4 Alpha Integrin see
  Natalizumab 1093
Anti-CD11a see Efalizumab 529
Anti-CD20 Monoclonal Antibody
  see Rituximab 1360
Antidigoxin Fab Fragments, Ovine
  see Digoxin Immune Fab 474
Antidiuretic Hormone see
  Vasopressin 1567
Antihemophilic Factor (Human) 129
Antihemophilic Factor
  (Recombinant) 130
Anti-inhibitor Coagulant Complex . . . 130
Antiphlogistine Rub A-535 No
  Odour (Can) see
  Triethanolamine Salicylate 1535
Antipyrine and Benzocaine 130
Antiseptic Mouthwash see
  Mouthwash (Antiseptic) 1069
Antithrombin III 131
Antithymocyte Globulin (Equine) . . . 131
Antithymocyte Immunoglobulin see
  Antithymocyte Globulin
  (Equine) 131
Antitumor Necrosis Factor Apha
  (Human) see Adalimumab 52
Anti-VEGF Monoclonal Antibody
  see Bevacizumab 204
Antivert® see Meclizine 969
Antizol® see Fomepizole 699
Anucort-HC® see Hydrocortisone . . . 793
Anu-Med [OTC] see Phenylephrine
  1226
Anusol-HC® see Hydrocortisone . . . 793
Anusol® HC-1 [OTC] see
  Hydrocortisone 793
Anusol® Ointment [OTC] see
  Pramoxine 1264
Anuzinc (Can) see Zinc Sulfate . . . 1598
Anzemet® see Dolasetron 498
APAP see Acetaminophen 31
APAP and Tramadol see
  Acetaminophen and Tramadol . . . 39

Apatate® [OTC] see Vitamin B
  Complex Combinations 1581
ApexiCon™ see Diflorasone 468
ApexiCon™ E see Diflorasone 468
Aphedrid™ [OTC] see Triprolidine
  and Pseudoephedrine 1542
Aphrodyne® see Yohimbine 1589
Aphthasol® see Amlexanox 99
Apidra® see Insulin Glulisine 837
Aplisol® see Tuberculin Tests 1548
Aplonidine see Apraclonidine 133
Apo-Acebutolol® (Can) see
  Acebutolol 28
Apo-Acetaminophen® (Can) see
  Acetaminophen 31
Apo-Acetazolamide® (Can) see
  AcetaZOLAMIDE 45
Apo-Acyclovir® (Can) see Acyclovir
  49
Apo-Alendronate® (Can) see
  Alendronate 64
Apo-Allopurinol® (Can) see
  Allopurinol 70
Apo-Alpraz® (Can) see Alprazolam
  73
Apo-Amiloride® (Can) see
  Amiloride 85
Apo-Amilzide® (Can) see Amiloride
  and Hydrochlorothiazide 85
Apo-Amiodarone® (Can) see
  Amiodarone 90
Apo-Amitriptyline® (Can) see
  Amitriptyline 93
Apo-Amoxi® (Can) see Amoxicillin . . 106
Apo-Amoxi-Clav® (Can) see
  Amoxicillin and Clavulanate
  Potassium 108
Apo-Ampi® (Can) see Ampicillin . . . 117
Apo-Atenol® (Can) see Atenolol . . . 154
Apo-Azathioprine® (Can) see
  Azathioprine 168
Apo-Azithromycin® (Can) see
  Azithromycin 171
Apo-Baclofen® (Can) see Baclofen
  178
Apo-Beclomethasone® (Can) see
  Beclomethasone 183
Apo-Benazepril® (Can) see
  Benazepril 185
Apo-Benztropine® (Can) see
  Benztropine 196
Apo-Benzydamine® (Can) see
  Benzydamine 197
Apo-Bisacodyl® (Can) see
  Bisacodyl 209
Apo-Bromazepam® (Can) see
  Bromazepam 220
Apo-Bromocriptine® (Can) see
  Bromocriptine 222
Apo-Buspirone® (Can) see
  BusPIRone 236
Apo-Butorphanol® (Can) see
  Butorphanol 243
Apo-Cal® (Can) see Calcium
  Carbonate 248
Apo-Calcitonin® (Can) see
  Calcitonin 246
Apo-Capto® (Can) see Captopril . . . 257
Apo-Carbamazepine® (Can) see
  Carbamazepine 260
Apo-Carvedilol® (Can) see
  Carvedilol 275
Apo-Cefaclor® (Can) see Cefaclor . . 279
Apo-Cefadroxil® (Can) see
  Cefadroxil 281
Apo-Cefuroxime® (Can) see
  Cefuroxime 295
Apo-Cephalex® (Can) see
  Cephalexin 301
Apo-Cetirizine® (Can) see
  Cetirizine 306

Apo-Chlorax® (Can) see Clidinium
  and Chlordiazepoxide 360
Apo-Chlordiazepoxide® (Can) see
  Chlordiazepoxide 315
Apo-Chlorhexadine® (Can) see
  Chlorhexidine Gluconate 316
Apo-Chlorpromazine® (Can) see
  ChlorproMAZINE 329
Apo-Chlorpropamide® (Can) see
  ChlorproPAMIDE 331
Apo-Chlorthalidone® (Can) see
  Chlorthalidone 332
Apo-Cimetidine® (Can) see
  Cimetidine 341
Apo-Ciproflox® (Can) see
  Ciprofloxacin 343
Apo-Citalopram® (Can) see
  Citalopram 351
Apo-Clindamycin® (Can) see
  Clindamycin 361
Apo-Clobazam® (Can) see
  Clobazam 364
Apo-Clomipramine® (Can) see
  ClomiPRAMINE 370
Apo-Clonazepam® (Can) see
  Clonazepam 371
Apo-Clonidine® (Can) see
  Clonidine 373
Apo-Clorazepate® (Can) see
  Clorazepate 378
Apo-Cloxi® (Can) see Cloxacillin . . . 380
Apo-Clozapine® (Can) see
  Clozapine 382
Apo-Cromolyn® (Can) see
  Cromolyn 397
Apo-Cyclobenzaprine® (Can) see
  Cyclobenzaprine 401
Apo-Cyclosporine® (Can) see
  CycloSPORINE 406
Apo-Desipramine® (Can) see
  Desipramine 434
Apo-Desmopressin® (Can) see
  Desmopressin 437
Apo-Dexamethasone® (Can) see
  Dexamethasone 439
Apo-Diazepam® (Can) see
  Diazepam 454
Apo-Diclo® (Can) see Diclofenac . . . 459
Apo-Diclo Rapide® (Can) see
  Diclofenac 459
Apo-Diclo SR® (Can) see
  Diclofenac 459
Apo-Diflunisal® (Can) see Diflunisal
  468
Apo-Diltiaz® (Can) see Diltiazem . . . 479
Apo-Diltiaz CD® (Can) see
  Diltiazem 479
Apo-Diltiaz SR® (Can) see
  Diltiazem 479
Apo-Dimenhydrinate® (Can) see
  DimenhyDRINATE 481
Apo-Dipyridamole FC® (Can) see
  Dipyridamole 489
Apo-Divalproex® (Can) see
  Valproic Acid and Derivatives
  1556
Apo-Docusate-Calcium® (Can) see
  Docusate 496
Apo-Docusate-Sodium® (Can) see
  Docusate 496
Apo-Doxazosin® (Can) see
  Doxazosin 503
Apo-Doxepin® (Can) see Doxepin . . 505
Apo-Doxy® (Can) see Doxycycline
  (Systemic) 514
Apo-Doxy Tabs® (Can) see
  Doxycycline (Systemic) 514
Apo-Erythro Base® (Can) see
  Erythromycin 562
Apo-Erythro E-C® (Can) see
  Erythromycin 562

Apo-Erythro-ES® (Can) see
  Erythromycin 562
Apo-Erythro-S® (Can) see
  Erythromycin 562
Apo-Etidronate® (Can) see
  Etidronate Disodium 621
Apo-Etodolac® (Can) see Etodolac
  623
Apo-Famotidine® (Can) see
  Famotidine 635
Apo-Fenofibrate® (Can) see
  Fenofibrate 639
Apo-Feno-Micro® (Can) see
  Fenofibrate 639
Apo-Ferrous Gluconate® (Can) see
  Ferrous Gluconate 651
Apo-Ferrous Sulfate® (Can) see
  Ferrous Sulfate 651
Apo-Flavoxate® (Can) see
  Flavoxate 656
Apo-Flecainide® (Can) see
  Flecainide 657
Apo-Fluconazole® (Can) see
  Fluconazole 659
Apo-Flunisolide® (Can) see
  Flunisolide 667
Apo-Fluoxetine® (Can) see
  Fluoxetine 675
Apo-Fluphenazine® (Can) see
  Fluphenazine 680
Apo-Fluphenazine Decanoate®
  (Can) see Fluphenazine 680
Apo -Flurazepam® (Can) see
  Flurazepam 681
Apo-Flurbiprofen® (Can) see
  Flurbiprofen 683
Apo-Flutamide® (Can) see
  Flutamide 686
Apo-Fluvoxamine® (Can) see
  Fluvoxamine 694
Apo-Folic® (Can) see Folic Acid 697
Apo-Fosinopril® (Can) see
  Fosinopril 707
Apo-Furosemide® (Can) see
  Furosemide 715
Apo-Gabapentin® (Can) see
  Gabapentin 717
Apo-Gain® (Can) see Minoxidil . . . 1051
Apo-Gemfibrozil® (Can) see
  Gemfibrozil 730
Apo-Gliclazide® (Can) see
  Gliclazide 737
Apo-Glyburide® (Can) see
  GlyBURIDE 744
Apo-Haloperidol® (Can) see
  Haloperidol 762
Apo-Haloperidol LA® (Can) see
  Haloperidol 762
Apo-Hydralazine® (Can) see
  HydrALAZINE 775
Apo-Hydro® (Can) see
  Hydrochlorothiazide 776
Apo-Hydroxyquine® (Can) see
  Hydroxychloroquine 799
Apo-Hydroxyurea® (Can) see
  Hydroxyurea 800
Apo-Hydroxyzine® (Can) see
  HydrOXYzine 801
Apo-Ibuprofen® (Can) see
  Ibuprofen 808
Apo-Imipramine® (Can) see
  Imipramine 820
Apo-Indapamide® (Can) see
  Indapamide 828
Apo-Indomethacin® (Can) see
  Indomethacin 830
Apo-Ipravent® (Can) see
  Ipratropium 857
Apo-ISDN® (Can) see Isosorbide
  Dinitrate 866

Apo-ISMN (Can) *see* Isosorbide
   Mononitrate 868
Apo-K® (Can) *see* Potassium
   Chloride 1258
Apo-Keto® (Can) *see* Ketoprofen . . . 883
Apo-Ketoconazole® (Can) *see*
   Ketoconazole 880
Apo-Keto-E® (Can) *see* Ketoprofen
   883
Apo-Ketorolac® (Can) *see*
   Ketorolac 886
Apo-Ketorolac Injectable® (Can)
   see Ketorolac 886
Apo-Keto SR® (Can) *see*
   Ketoprofen 883
Apo-Ketotifen® (Can) *see* Ketotifen
   890
Apokyn™ *see* Apomorphine . . 132
Apo-Labetalol® (Can) *see* Labetalol
   891
Apo-Lactulose® (Can) *see*
   Lactulose 893
Apo-Lamotrigine® (Can) *see*
   Lamotrigine 895
Apo-Leflunomide® (Can) *see*
   Leflunomide 901
Apo-Levobunolol® (Can) *see*
   Levobunolol 909
Apo-Levocarb® (Can) *see*
   Levodopa and Carbidopa 911
Apo-Levocarb® CR (Can) *see*
   Levodopa and Carbidopa 911
Apo-Lisinopril® (Can) *see* Lisinopril
   936
Apo-Lithium® (Can) *see* Lithium 939
Apo-Lithium® Carbonate SR (Can)
   see Lithium 939
Apo-Loperamide® (Can) *see*
   Loperamide 942
Apo-Loratadine® (Can) *see*
   Loratadine 946
Apo-Lorazepam® (Can) *see*
   Lorazepam 947
Apo-Lovastatin® (Can) *see*
   Lovastatin 953
Apo-Loxapine® (Can) *see* Loxapine
   955
Apo-Medroxy® (Can) *see*
   MedroxyPROGESTERone 972
Apo-Mefenamic® (Can) *see*
   Mefenamic Acid 973
Apo-Mefloquine® (Can) *see*
   Mefloquine 975
Apo-Megestrol® (Can) *see*
   Megestrol 976
Apo-Meloxicam® (Can) *see*
   Meloxicam 977
Apo-Metformin® (Can) *see*
   Metformin 1001
Apo-Methazide® (Can) *see*
   Methyldopa and
   Hydrochlorothiazide 1022
Apo-Methazolamide® (Can) *see*
   Methazolamide 1006
Apo-Methoprazine® (Can) *see*
   Methotrimeprazine 1016
Apo-Methotrexate® (Can) *see*
   Methotrexate 1012
Apo-Methyldopa® (Can) *see*
   Methyldopa 1021
Apo-Methylphenidate® SR (Can)
   see Methylphenidate 1023
Apo-Metoclop® (Can) *see*
   Metoclopramide 1029
Apo-Metoprolol® (Can) *see*
   Metoprolol 1030
Apo-Metronidazole® (Can) *see*
   Metronidazole. 1033
Apo-Midazolam® (Can) *see*
   Midazolam 1040

Apo-Minocycline® (Can) *see*
   Minocycline 1049
Apo-Misoprostol® (Can) *see*
   Misoprostol 1053
Apomorphine 132
Apomorphine Hydrochloride *see*
   Apomorphine 132
Apomorphine Hydrochloride
   Hemihydrate *see* Apomorphine
   132
Apo-Nabumetone® (Can) *see*
   Nabumetone 1077
Apo-Nadol® (Can) *see* Nadolol 1079
Apo-Napro-Na® (Can) *see*
   Naproxen 1089
Apo-Napro-Na DS® (Can) *see*
   Naproxen 1089
Apo-Naproxen® (Can) *see*
   Naproxen 1089
Apo-Naproxen SR® (Can) *see*
   Naproxen 1089
Apo-Nifed® (Can) *see* NIFEdipine
   1112
Apo-Nifed PA® (Can) *see*
   NIFEdipine 1112
Apo-Nitrofurantoin® (Can) *see*
   Nitrofurantoin 1119
Apo-Nizatidine® (Can) *see*
   Nizatidine 1123
Apo-Norflox® (Can) *see* Norfloxacin
   1126
Apo-Nortriptyline® (Can) *see*
   Nortriptyline 1128
Apo-Oflox® (Can) *see* Ofloxacin . . . 1137
Apo-Ofloxacin® (Can) *see*
   Ofloxacin 1137
Apo-Omeprazole® (Can) *see*
   Omeprazole 1145
Apo-Oxaprozin® (Can) *see*
   Oxaprozin 1155
Apo-Oxazepam® (Can) *see*
   Oxazepam 1157
Apo-Paroxetine® (Can) *see*
   Paroxetine 1188
Apo-Pentoxifylline SR® (Can) *see*
   Pentoxifylline 1212
Apo-Pen VK® (Can) *see* Penicillin
   V Potassium 1205
Apo-Pergolide® (Can) *see*
   Pergolide 1213
Apo-Perphenazine® (Can) *see*
   Perphenazine 1218
Apo-Pimozide® (Can) *see*
   Pimozide 1238
Apo-Pindol® (Can) *see* Pindolol . . . 1240
Apo-Piroxicam® (Can) *see*
   Piroxicam 1248
Apo-Pravastatin® (Can) *see*
   Pravastatin 1265
Apo-Prazo® (Can) *see* Prazosin . . . 1267
Apo-Prednisone® (Can) *see*
   PredniSONE 1271
Apo-Primidone® (Can) *see*
   Primidone 1281
Apo-Procainamide® (Can) *see*
   Procainamide 1283
Apo-Prochlorperazine® (Can) *see*
   Prochlorperazine 1285
Apo-Propafenone® (Can) *see*
   Propafenone 1293
Apo-Propranolol® (Can) *see*
   Propranolol 1301
Apo-Quin-G® (Can) *see* Quinidine
   1324
Apo-Quinidine® (Can) *see*
   Quinidine 1324
Apo-Quinine® (Can) *see* Quinine . . 1326
Apo-Ranitidine® (Can) *see*
   Ranitidine 1334
Apo-Salvent® (Can) *see* Albuterol . . . 58

Apo-Selegiline® (Can) see
  Selegiline 1382
Apo-Sertraline® (Can) see
  Sertraline 1385
Apo-Simvastatin® (Can) see
  Simvastatin 1394
Apo-Sotalol® (Can) see Sotalol . . . 1409
Apo-Sucralate® (Can) see
  Sucralfate 1420
Apo-Sulfatrim® (Can) see
  Sulfamethoxazole and
  Trimethoprim 1425
Apo-Sulin® (Can) see Sulindac . . . 1430
Apo-Sumatriptan® (Can) see
  Sumatriptan 1432
Apo-Tamox® (Can) see Tamoxifen
  1443
Apo-Temazepam® (Can) see
  Temazepam 1453
Apo-Terazosin® (Can) see
  Terazosin 1458
Apo-Terbinafine® (Can) see
  Terbinafine 1459
Apo-Tetra® (Can) see Tetracycline
  1467
Apo-Theo LA® (Can) see
  Theophylline 1473
Apo-Thioridazine® (Can) see
  Thioridazine 1477
Apo-Ticlopidine® (Can) see
  Ticlopidine 1486
Apo-Timol® (Can) see Timolol . . . 1489
Apo-Timop® (Can) see Timolol 1489
Apo-Tizanidine® (Can) see
  Tizanidine 1497
Apo-Tobramycin® (Can) see
  Tobramycin 1498
Apo-Tolbutamide® (Can) see
  TOLBUTamide 1502
Apo-Trazodone® (Can) see
  Trazodone 1521
Apo-Trazodone D® (Can) see
  Trazodone 1521
Apo-Triazide® (Can) see
  Hydrochlorothiazide and
  Triamterene 778
Apo-Triazo® (Can) see Triazolam . . 1531
Apo-Trifluoperazine® (Can) see
  Trifluoperazine 1535
Apo-Trihex® (Can) see
  Trihexyphenidyl 1537
Apo-Trimethoprim® (Can) see
  Trimethoprim 1538
Apo-Trimip® (Can) see
  Trimipramine 1540
Apo-Verap® (Can) see Verapamil . . 1571
Apo-Warfarin® (Can) see Warfarin
  1585
Apo-Zopiclone® (Can) see
  Zopiclone 1606
APPG see Penicillin G Procaine . . 1204
Apra Children's [OTC] see
  Acetaminophen 31
Apraclonidine 133
Apraclonidine Hydrochloride see
  Apraclonidine 133
Aprepitant 134
Apresazide [DSC] see Hydralazine
  and Hydrochlorothiazide 775
Apresoline® (Can) see
  HydrALAZINE 775
Apresoline [DSC] see
  HydrALAZINE 775
April® see Ethinyl Estradiol and
  Desogestrel 592
Aprodine® [OTC] see Triprolidine
  and Pseudoephedrine 1542
Aprotinin 135
Aprovel® (Mex) see Irbesartan 858
Aptivus® see Tipranavir 1495
Aquacare® [OTC] see Urea 1551

Aquachloral® Supprettes® see
  Chloral Hydrate 312
Aquacort® (Can) see
  Hydrocortisone 793
AquaLase™ see Balanced Salt
  Solution 178
AquaMEPHYTON® (Can) see
  Phytonadione 1233
Aquanil™ HC (Mex) see
  Hydrocortisone 793
Aquanil™ HC [OTC] see
  Hydrocortisone 793
Aquaphilic® With Carbamide [OTC]
  see Urea 1551
AquaSite® [OTC] see Artificial
  Tears 143
Aquasol A® see Vitamin A 1580
Aquasol E® [OTC] see Vitamin E . . 1581
Aquatensen® (Can) see
  Methyclothiazide 1020
Aquavit-E [OTC] see Vitamin E . . . 1581
Aqueous Procaine Penicillin G see
  Penicillin G Procaine 1204
Ara-C see Cytarabine 413
Arabinosylcytosine see Cytarabine . . 413
Aralast see Alpha₁-Proteinase
  Inhibitor 73
Aralen® see Chloroquine 320
Aranelle™ see Ethinyl Estradiol
  and Norethindrone 608
Aranesp® see Darbepoetin Alfa 423
Arava® see Leflunomide 901
Arctostaphylos uva-ursi see Uva
  Ursi 1633
Aredia® see Pamidronate 1181
Arestin™ see Minocycline
  Hydrochloride (Periodontal) 1050
Argatroban 136
Arginine 137
Arginine Hydrochloride see
  Arginine 137
8-Arginine Vasopressin see
  Vasopressin 1567
Aricept® see Donepezil 500
Aricept® ODT see Donepezil 500
Aricept® RDT (Can) see Donepezil
  500
Arimidex® see Anastrozole 126
Aripiprazole 138
Aristocort® see Triamcinolone 1526
Aristocort® A see Triamcinolone . . . 1526
Aristospan® see Triamcinolone 1526
Arixtra® see Fondaparinux 700
Arlidin® (Can) see Nylidrin 1133
A.R.M® [OTC] see
  Chlorpheniramine and
  Pseudoephedrine 325
Armour® Thyroid see Thyroid 1482
Aromasin® see Exemestane 628
Aropax® (Mex) see Paroxetine 1188
Arranon® see Nelarabine 1097
ArthriCare® for Women Extra
  Moisturizing [OTC] see
  Capsaicin 256
ArthriCare® for Women Multi-Action
  [OTC] see Capsaicin 256
ArthriCare® for Women Silky Dry
  [OTC] see Capsaicin 256
ArthriCare® for Women Ultra
  Strength [OTC] [DSC] see
  Capsaicin 256
Arthrotec® see Diclofenac and
  Misoprostol 462
Articaine and Epinephrine 139
Artificial Tears 143
ASA see Aspirin 145
5-ASA see Mesalamine 996
Asacol® see Mesalamine 996
Asacol® 800 (Can) see
  Mesalamine 996

Asaphen (Can) see Aspirin 145
Asaphen E.C. (Can) see Aspirin . . . 145
Ascorbic Acid 143
Ascorbic Acid and Ferrous Sulfate
    see Ferrous Sulfate and
    Ascorbic Acid 651
Ascriptin® Extra Strength [OTC]
    see Aspirin 145
Ascriptin® [OTC] see Aspirin 145
Asendin [DSC] see Amoxapine 105
Asian Ginseng see Ginseng,
    Panax 1623
Asmanex® Twisthaler® see
    Mometasone Furoate 1060
Asparaginase 144
Aspart Insulin see Insulin Aspart . . . 836
Aspercin Extra [OTC] see Aspirin . . . 145
Aspercin [OTC] see Aspirin 145
Aspercreme® [OTC] see
    Triethanolamine Salicylate 1535
Aspergum® [OTC] see Aspirin 145
Aspirin 145
Aspirin, Acetaminophen, and
    Caffeine see Acetaminophen,
    Aspirin, and Caffeine 41
Aspirin and Carisoprodol see
    Carisoprodol and Aspirin 272
Aspirin and Codeine 149
Aspirin and Dipyridamole 150
Aspirin and Extended-Release
    Dipyridamole see Aspirin and
    Dipyridamole 150
Aspirin and Hydrocodone see
    Hydrocodone and Aspirin 782
Aspirin and Meprobamate 151
Aspirin and Oxycodone see
    Oxycodone and Aspirin 1168
Aspirin and Pravastatin 151
Aspirin, Caffeine and
    Acetaminophen see
    Acetaminophen, Aspirin, and
    Caffeine 41
Aspirin, Caffeine, and Butalbital
    see Butalbital, Aspirin, and
    Caffeine 241
Aspirin, Caffeine, and
    Propoxyphene see
    Propoxyphene, Aspirin, and
    Caffeine 1300
Aspirin, Caffeine, Codeine, and
    Butalbital see Butalbital,
    Aspirin, Caffeine, and Codeine
    241
Aspirin, Carisoprodol, and Codeine
    see Carisoprodol, Aspirin, and
    Codeine 273
Aspirin Free Anacin® Maximum
    Strength [OTC] see
    Acetaminophen 31
Aspirin, Orphenadrine, and
    Caffeine see Orphenadrine,
    Aspirin, and Caffeine 1152
Astelin® see Azelastine 170
AsthmaNefrin® see Epinephrine
    (Racemic) 549
Astracaine® (Can) see Articaine
    and Epinephrine 139
Astracaine® Forte (Can) see
    Articaine and Epinephrine 139
Astragalus 1615
Astragalus membranaceus see
    Astragalus 1615
Astramorph/PF™ see Morphine
    Sulfate 1065
AT-III see Antithrombin III 131
Atacand® see Candesartan 252
Atacand HCT™ see Candesartan
    and Hydrochlorothiazide 254
Atacand® Plus (Can) see
    Candesartan and
    Hydrochlorothiazide 254

Atarax® (Can) see HydrOXYzine . . . 801
Atasol® (Can) see Acetaminophen . . . 31
Atazanavir 152
Atazanavir Sulfate see Atazanavir . . 152
Atenolol 154
Atenolol and Chlorthalidone 156
ATG see Antithymocyte Globulin
    (Equine) 131
Atgam® see Antithymocyte
    Globulin (Equine) 131
Athos® (Mex) see
    Dextromethorphan 451
Atisuril® (Mex) see Allopurinol 70
Ativan® see Lorazepam 947
Atomoxetine 156
Atomoxetine Hydrochloride see
    Atomoxetine 156
Atorvastatin 158
Atorvastatin Calcium and
    Amlodipine Besylate see
    Amlodipine and Atorvastatin 101
Atovaquone 160
Atovaquone and Proguanil 160
ATRA see Tretinoin (Oral) 1524
Atridox™ see Doxycycline Hyclate
    (Periodontal) 512
AtroPen® see Atropine 161
Atropine 161
Atropine and Difenoxin see
    Difenoxin and Atropine 467
Atropine and Diphenoxylate see
    Diphenoxylate and Atropine 487
Atropine-Care® see Atropine 161
Atropine, Hyoscyamine,
    Scopolamine, and
    Phenobarbital see
    Hyoscyamine, Atropine,
    Scopolamine, and
    Phenobarbital 804
Atropine Sulfate see Atropine 161
Atropine Sulfate and Edrophonium
    Chloride see Edrophonium and
    Atropine 529
Atropine Sulfate (Dental Tablets) . . . 164
Atrovent® see Ipratropium 857
Atrovent® HFA see Ipratropium 857
A/T/S® see Erythromycin 562
Attapulgite 165
Attenuvax® see Measles Virus
    Vaccine (Live) 967
Audifluor® (Mex) see Fluoride 671
Augmentin® see Amoxicillin and
    Clavulanate Potassium 108
Augmentin ES-600® see
    Amoxicillin and Clavulanate
    Potassium 108
Augmentin XR™ see Amoxicillin
    and Clavulanate Potassium 108
Auralgan® (Can) see Antipyrine
    and Benzocaine 130
Auranofin 166
Aurodex see Antipyrine and
    Benzocaine 130
Aurolate® see Gold Sodium
    Thiomalate 748
Auroto see Antipyrine and
    Benzocaine 130
Autoplex® T [DSC] see
    Anti-inhibitor Coagulant
    Complex 130
AVA see Anthrax Vaccine
    (Adsorbed) 128
Avagard™ [OTC] see Chlorhexidine
    Gluconate 316
Avage™ see Tazarotene 1446
Avalide® see Irbesartan and
    Hydrochlorothiazide 860
Avandamet™ see Rosiglitazone
    and Metformin 1369
Avandaryl™ see Rosiglitazone and
    Glimepiride 1369

Avandia® see Rosiglitazone 1367
Avapro® see Irbesartan 858
Avapro® HCT see Irbesartan and
  Hydrochlorothiazide 860
Avastin® see Bevacizumab 204
Avaxim® (Can) see Hepatitis A
  Vaccine 767
Avaxim®-Pediatric (Can) see
  Hepatitis A Vaccine 767
Avelox® see Moxifloxacin 1069
Avelox® I.V. see Moxifloxacin 1069
Aventyl® (Can) see Nortriptyline . . . 1128
Aviane™ see Ethinyl Estradiol and
  Levonorgestrel 602
Avinza® see Morphine Sulfate 1065
Avita® see Tretinoin (Topical) 1525
Avitene® see Collagen Hemostat . . . 392
Avitene® Flour see Collagen
  Hemostat 392
Avitene® Ultrafoam see Collagen
  Hemostat 392
Avitene® UltraWrap™ see Collagen
  Hemostat 392
Avodart™ see Dutasteride 524
Avonex® see Interferon Beta-1a . . . 849
Awa see Kava 1627
Axert™ see Almotriptan 71
Axid® see Nizatidine 1123
Axid® AR [OTC] see Nizatidine . . . 1123
Axofor® (Mex)
  Hydroxocobalamin 798
AY-25650 see Triptorelin 1544
Aygestin® see Norethindrone 1125
Ayr® Baby Saline [OTC] see
  Sodium Chloride 1400
Ayr® Saline No-Drip [OTC] see
  Sodium Chloride 1400
Ayr® Saline [OTC] see Sodium
  Chloride 1400
Az® (Mex) see Azelastine 170
Azacitidine 167
AZA-CR see Azacitidine 167
Azactam® see Aztreonam 175
5-Azacytidine see Azacitidine 167
Azanplus® (Mex) see Ranitidine . . . 1334
Azantac® (Mex) see Ranitidine 1334
Azasan® see Azathioprine 168
Azathioprine 168
Azathioprine Sodium see
  Azathioprine 168
Azatrilem® (Mex) see Azathioprine . . 168
5-AZC see Azacitidine 167
Azelaic Acid 169
Azelastine 170
Azelastine Hydrochloride see
  Azelastine 170
Azelex® see Azelaic Acid 169
Azidothymidine see Zidovudine . . . 1594
Azidothymidine, Abacavir, and
  Lamivudine see Abacavir,
  Lamivudine, and Zidovudine 23
Azithromycin 171
Azithromycin Dihydrate see
  Azithromycin 171
Azmacort® see Triamcinolone 1526
AZO-Gesic® [OTC] see
  Phenazopyridine 1220
Azopt® see Brinzolamide 220
AZO-Standard® [OTC] see
  Phenazopyridine 1220
AZT™ (Can) see Zidovudine 1594
AZT + 3TC (error-prone
  abbreviation) see Zidovudine
  and Lamivudine 1596
AZT, Abacavir, and Lamivudine
  see Abacavir, Lamivudine, and
  Zidovudine 23
AZT (error-prone abbreviation) see
  Zidovudine 1594
Azthreonam see Aztreonam 175
Aztreonam 175

Azulfidine® see Sulfasalazine 1428
Azulfidine® EN-tabs® see
  Sulfasalazine 1428
B-D™ Glucose [OTC] see Dextrose
  452
B 9273 see Alefacept 62
BA-16038 see Aminoglutethimide . . . 87
Babee® Cof Syrup [OTC] see
  Dextromethorphan 451
BAC see Benzalkonium Chloride . . . 188
Bachelor's Button see Feverfew . . . 1621
Bacid® (Can) see Lactobacillus 535
Bacid® [OTC] see Lactobacillus 535
Baciguent® (Can) see Bacitracin . . . 175
Baciguent® [OTC] see Bacitracin . . . 175
BaciIM® see Bacitracin 175
Baciject® see Bacitracin 175
Bacillus Calmette-Guérin (BCG)
  Live see BCG Vaccine 181
Bacitracin 175
Bacitracin and Polymyxin B 176
Bacitracin, Neomycin, and
  Polymyxin B 176
Bacitracin, Neomycin, Polymyxin B,
  and Hydrocortisone 177
Bacitracin, Neomycin, Polymyxin B,
  and Pramoxine 177
Baclofen 178
BactoShield® CHG [OTC] see
  Chlorhexidine Gluconate 316
Bactrim™ see Sulfamethoxazole
  and Trimethoprim 1425
Bactrim™ DS see
  Sulfamethoxazole and
  Trimethoprim 1425
Bactroban® see Mupirocin 1073
Bactroban® Nasal see Mupirocin . . 1073
Baking Soda see Sodium
  Bicarbonate 1400
BAL see Dimercaprol 482
Balacet 325™ see Propoxyphene
  and Acetaminophen 1298
Balanced Salt Solution 178
BAL in Oil® see Dimercaprol 482
Balmex® [OTC] see Zinc Oxide . . . 1597
Balminil (Can) see Xylometazoline
  1588
Balminil Decongestant (Can) see
  Pseudoephedrine 1309
Balminil DM D (Can) see
  Pseudoephedrine and
  Dextromethorphan 1311
Balminil DM + Decongestant +
  Expectorant (Can) see
  Guaifenesin, Pseudoephedrine,
  and Dextromethorphan 757
Balminil DM E (Can) see
  Guaifenesin and
  Dextromethorphan 754
Balminil Expectorant (Can) see
  Guaifenesin 752
Balnetar® (Can) see Coal Tar 383
Balnetar® [OTC] see Coal Tar 383
Balsalazide 179
Balsalazide Disodium see
  Balsalazide 179
Balsam Peru, Trypsin, and Castor
  Oil see Trypsin, Balsam Peru,
  and Castor Oil 1547
Baltussin see Dihydrocodeine,
  Chlorpheniramine, and
  Phenylephrine 476
Bancap HC® see Hydrocodone
  and Acetaminophen 779
Band-Aid® Hurt-Free™ Antiseptic
  Wash [OTC] see Lidocaine 920
Banophen® Anti-Itch [OTC] see
  DiphenhydrAMINE 483
Banophen® [OTC] see
  DiphenhydrAMINE 483
Baraclude™ see Entecavir 544

Baricon™ see Barium 179
Baridium® [OTC] see
  Phenazopyridine 1220
Barium 179
Barium Sulfate see Barium 179
Barobag® see Barium 179
Baro-Cat® see Barium 179
Barosperse® see Barium 179
Basaljel® (Can) see Aluminum
  Hydroxide 79
Base Ointment see Zinc Oxide 1597
Basiliximab 180
Bausch & Lomb® Computer Eye
  Drops [OTC] see Glycerin 747
BAY 43-9006 see Sorafenib 1407
Bayer® Aspirin Extra Strength
  [OTC] see Aspirin 145
Bayer® Aspirin [OTC] see Aspirin . . . 145
Bayer® Aspirin Regimen Adult Low
  Strength [OTC] see Aspirin 145
Bayer® Aspirin Regimen Children's
  [OTC] see Aspirin 145
Bayer® Aspirin Regimen Regular
  Strength [OTC] see Aspirin 145
Bayer® Extra Strength Arthritis
  Pain Regimen [OTC] see
  Aspirin 145
Bayer® Plus Extra Strength [OTC]
  see Aspirin 145
Bayer® Women's Aspirin Plus
  Calcium [OTC] see Aspirin 145
BayGam® see Immune Globulin
  (Intramuscular) 823
BayHep B® see Hepatitis B
  Immune Globulin 768
BayRab® see Rabies Immune
  Globulin (Human) 1328
BayRho-D® Full-Dose see Rho(D)
  Immune Globulin 1342
BayRho-D® Mini-Dose see Rho(D)
  Immune Globulin 1342
BayTet™ see Tetanus Immune
  Globulin (Human) 1463
Baza® Antifungal [OTC] see
  Miconazole 1039
Baza® Clear [OTC] see Vitamin A
  and Vitamin D 1580
B-Caro-T™ see Beta-Carotene 198
BCG, Live see BCG Vaccine 181
BCG Vaccine 181
BCG Vaccine U.S.P.
  (percutaneous use product)
  see BCG Vaccine 181
BCI-Fluoxetine (Can) see
  Fluoxetine 675
BCI-Gabapentin (Can) see
  Gabapentin 717
BCI-Metformin (Can) see
  Metformin 1001
BCI-Ranitidine (Can) see
  Ranitidine 1334
BCI-Simvastatin (Can) see
  Simvastatin 1394
BCNU see Carmustine 273
B Complex Combinations see
  Vitamin B Complex
  Combinations 1581
Bearberry see Uva Ursi 1633
Bear-E-Yum® CT see Barium 179
Bear-E-Yum® GI see Barium 179
Bebulin® VH see Factor IX
  Complex (Human) 633
Becaplermin 182
Beclomethasone 183
Beclomethasone Dipropionate see
  Beclomethasone 183
Beconase® AQ see
  Beclomethasone 183
Behenyl Alcohol see Docosanol 495
Bekidiba Dex® (Mex) see
  Dextromethorphan 451

Belladonna Alkaloids With
  Phenobarbital see
  Hyoscyamine, Atropine,
  Scopolamine, and
  Phenobarbital 804
Belladonna and Opium 184
Belladonna, Phenobarbital, and
  Ergotamine 185
Bellamine S see Belladonna,
  Phenobarbital, and Ergotamine
  185
Bellergal® Spacetabs® (Can) see
  Belladonna, Phenobarbital, and
  Ergotamine 185
Bel-Tabs see Belladonna,
  Phenobarbital, and Ergotamine
  185
Benadryl® (Can) see
  DiphenhydrAMINE 483
Benadryl® Allergy and Sinus
  Fastmelt™ [OTC] see
  Diphenhydramine and
  Pseudoephedrine 487
Benadryl® Allergy [OTC] see
  DiphenhydrAMINE 483
Benadryl® Allergy/Sinus [OTC] see
  Diphenhydramine and
  Pseudoephedrine 487
Benadryl® Children's Allergy and
  Cold Fastmelt™ [OTC] see
  Diphenhydramine and
  Pseudoephedrine 487
Benadryl® Children's Allergy and
  Sinus [OTC] see
  Diphenhydramine and
  Pseudoephedrine 487
Benadryl® Children's Allergy
  Fastmelt™ [OTC] see
  DiphenhydrAMINE 483
Benadryl® Children's Allergy [OTC]
  see DiphenhydrAMINE 483
Benadryl® Dye-Free Allergy [OTC]
  see DiphenhydrAMINE 483
Benadryl® Injection see
  DiphenhydrAMINE 483
Benadryl® Itch Stopping Extra
  Strength [OTC] see
  DiphenhydrAMINE 483
Benadryl® Itch Stopping [OTC] see
  DiphenhydrAMINE 483
Benaxima® (Mex) see Cefotaxime . . 288
Benaxona® (Mex) see Ceftriaxone . . 294
Benazepril 185
Benazepril and Hydrochlorothiazide
  187
Benazepril Hydrochloride see
  Benazepril 185
Benazepril Hydrochloride and
  Amlodipine Besylate see
  Amlodipine and Benazepril 102
Bencelin® (Mex) see Penicillin G
  Benzathine 1202
Bendapar® (Mex) see Albendazole
  57
Bendroflumethiazide and Nadolol
  see Nadolol and
  Bendroflumethiazide 1080
Benecid® (Mex) see Probenecid . . . 1282
BeneFix® see Factor IX 632
Beneflur® (Can) see Fludarabine . . . 663
Benemid [DSC] see Probenecid . . . 1282
Benerva® (Mex) see Thiamine 1476
Benicar® see Olmesartan 1142
Benicar HCT® see Olmesartan and
  Hydrochlorothiazide 1143
Benoquin® see Monobenzone 1062
Benoxyl® (Can) see Benzoyl
  Peroxide 194
Bentoquatam 188
Bentyl® see Dicyclomine 464
Bentylol® (Can) see Dicyclomine . . . 464

Benuryl™ (Can) see Probenecid ... 1282
Benylin® 3.3 mg-D-E (Can) see
Guaifenesin, Pseudoephedrine,
and Codeine 756
Benylin® D for Infants (Can) see
Pseudoephedrine 1309
Benylin® Adult [OTC] [DSC] see
Dextromethorphan 451
Benylin® DM-D (Can) see
Pseudoephedrine and
Dextromethorphan 1311
Benylin® DM-D-E (Can) see
Guaifenesin, Pseudoephedrine,
and Dextromethorphan 757
Benylin® DM-E (Can) see
Guaifenesin and
Dextromethorphan 754
Benylin® E Extra Strength (Can)
see Guaifenesin 752
Benylin® Expectorant [OTC] [DSC]
see Guaifenesin and
Dextromethorphan 754
Benylin® Pediatric [OTC] [DSC]
see Dextromethorphan 451
Benzac® see Benzoyl Peroxide 194
Benzac® AC see Benzoyl Peroxide
.... 194
Benzac® AC Wash see Benzoyl
Peroxide 194
BenzaClin® see Clindamycin and
Benzoyl Peroxide 364
Benzac® W see Benzoyl Peroxide . 194
Benzac W® Gel (Can) see Benzoyl
Peroxide 194
Benzac® W Wash see Benzoyl
Peroxide 194
Benzaderm® (Mex) see Benzoyl
Peroxide 194
Benzagel® see Benzoyl Peroxide ... 194
Benzagel® Wash [DSC] see
Benzoyl Peroxide 194
Benzalkonium Chloride........... 188
Benzalkonium Chloride and
Isopropyl Alcohol 189
Benzalkonium Chloride,
Benzocaine, Butyl
Aminobenzoate, and
Tetracaine Hydrochloride see
Benzocaine, Butyl
Aminobenzoate, Tetracaine,
and Benzalkonium Chloride 193
Benzamycin® see Erythromycin
and Benzoyl Peroxide 567
Benzamycin® Pak see
Erythromycin and Benzoyl
Peroxide 567
Benzanil® (Mex) see Penicillin G
Benzathine 1202
Benza® [OTC] see Benzalkonium
Chloride 188
Benzashave® see Benzoyl
Peroxide 194
Benzathine Benzylpenicillin see
Penicillin G Benzathine 1202
Benzathine Penicillin G see
Penicillin G Benzathine 1202
Benzazoline Hydrochloride see
Tolazoline 1501
Benzedrex® [OTC] see
Propylhexedrine 1305
Benzene Hexachloride see
Lindane 933
Benzetacil® (Mex) see Penicillin G
Benzathine 1202
Benzhexol Hydrochloride see
Trihexyphenidyl 1537
Benziq™ see Benzoyl Peroxide 194
Benziq™ LS see Benzoyl Peroxide
.... 194
Benzisoquinolinedione see
Amonafide 104

Benzmethyzin see Procarbazine .. 1284
Benzocaine 190
Benzocaine and Antipyrine see
Antipyrine and Benzocaine..... 130
Benzocaine and Cetylpyridinium
Chloride see Cetylpyridinium
and Benzocaine 309
Benzocaine, Butyl Aminobenzoate,
Tetracaine, and Benzalkonium
Chloride 193
Benzodent® [OTC] see Benzocaine
.... 190
Benzo-Ginestryl® (Mex) see
Estradiol................. 574
Benzoin 193
Benzonatate 194
Benzoyl Peroxide 194
Benzoyl Peroxide and Clindamycin
see Clindamycin and Benzoyl
Peroxide.................. 364
Benzoyl Peroxide and
Erythromycin see Erythromycin
and Benzoyl Peroxide 567
Benzoyl Peroxide and
Hydrocortisone 195
Benzphetamine 195
Benzphetamine Hydrochloride see
Benzphetamine 195
Benztropine 196
Benztropine Mesylate see
Benztropine 196
Benzydamine 197
Benzydamine Hydrochloride see
Benzydamine 197
Benzylpenicillin Benzathine see
Penicillin G Benzathine 1202
Benzylpenicillin Potassium see
Penicillin G (Parenteral/
Aqueous) 1203
Benzylpenicillin Sodium see
Penicillin G (Parenteral/
Aqueous) 1203
Benzylpenicilloyl-polylysine 198
Beractant 198
Berotec® (Can) see Fenoterol 644
9-Beta-D-Ribofuranosyladenine see
Adenosine 55
Betacaine® (Can) see Lidocaine.... 920
Beta-Carotene 198
Betaderm (Can) see
Betamethasone 199
Betadine® (Can) see
Povidone-Iodine 1262
Betadine® First Aid Antibiotics +
Moisturizer [OTC] see
Bacitracin and Polymyxin B 176
Betadine® Ophthalmic see
Povidone-Iodine 1262
Betadine® [OTC] see
Povidone-Iodine 1262
Betagan® see Levobunolol 909
Beta-HC® see Hydrocortisone 793
Betaine Anhydrous 199
Betaject™ (Can) see
Betamethasone 199
Betaloc® (Can) see Metoprolol 1030
Betaloc® Durules® (Can) see
Metoprolol 1030
BetaMed [OTC] see Pyrithione
Zinc 1318
Betamethasone 199
Betamethasone and Clotrimazole ... 202
Betamethasone Dipropionate see
Betamethasone 199
Betamethasone Dipropionate,
Augmented see
Betamethasone 199
Betamethasone Sodium Phosphate
see Betamethasone 199
Betamethasone Valerate see
Betamethasone 199

Betapace® see Sotalol 1409
Betapace AF® see Sotalol 1409
Betasept® [OTC] see Chlorhexidine
    Gluconate 316
Betaseron® see Interferon Beta-1b . . 850
Betatar® Gel [OTC] see Coal Tar . . . 383
Beta-Val® see Betamethasone 199
Betaxin® (Can) see Thiamine 1476
Betaxolol 203
Betaxolol Hydrochloride see
    Betaxolol 203
Bethanechol 204
Bethanechol Chloride see
    Bethanechol 204
Betimol® see Timolol 1489
Betnesol® (Can) see
    Betamethasone 199
Betnovate® (Can) see
    Betamethasone 199
Betoptic® S see Betaxolol 203
Bevacizumab 204
Bexarotene 205
BG 9273 see Alefacept 62
BI-007 see Paclitaxel (Protein
    Bound) 1177
Biaxin® see Clarithromycin 355
Biaxin® XL see Clarithromycin 355
Bicalutamide 207
Bicillin® L-A see Penicillin G
    Benzathine 1202
Bicillin® C-R see Penicillin G
    Benzathine and Penicillin G
    Procaine 1203
Bicillin® C-R 900/300 see Penicillin
    G Benzathine and Penicillin G
    Procaine 1203
Bicitra® see Sodium Citrate and
    Citric Acid 1401
Biclin® (Mex) see Amikacin 84
BiCNu® see Carmustine 273
BIDA see Amonafide 104
BiDil® see Isosorbide Dinitrate and
    Hydralazine 867
Bifidobacterium bifidum /
    Lactobacillus acidophilus 1615
Bilberry 1615
Biltricide® see Praziquantel 1266
Bimatoprost 208
Biocef® see Cephalexin 301
Biofed [OTC] see
    Pseudoephedrine 1309
Biolon™ see Hyaluronate and
    Derivatives 773
Bion® Tears [OTC] see Artificial
    Tears 143
BioQuin® Durules™ (Can) see
    Quinidine 1324
Biosint® (Mex) see Cefotaxime 288
Bio-Statin® see Nystatin 1133
BioThrax™ see Anthrax Vaccine
    (Adsorbed) 128
Biperiden 208
Biperiden Hydrochloride see
    Biperiden 208
Biperiden Lactate see Biperiden 208
Bisac-Evac™ [OTC] see Bisacodyl . . 209
Bisacodyl 209
Bisacodyl Uniserts® [OTC] see
    Bisacodyl 209
bis-chloronitrosourea see
    Carmustine 273
Bismatrol see Bismuth 210
Bismuth 210
Bismuth Subgallate see Bismuth . . . 210
Bismuth Subsalicylate see Bismuth
    210
Bismuth Subsalicylate,
    Metronidazole, and
    Tetracycline 210

Bismuth Subsalicylate,
    Tetracycline, and
    Metronidazole see Bismuth
    Subsalicylate, Metronidazole,
    and Tetracycline 210
Bisoprolol 211
Bisoprolol and Hydrochlorothiazide
    212
Bisoprolol Fumarate see Bisoprolol
    211
Bistropamide see Tropicamide . . . 1545
Bivalirudin 213
BL4162A see Anagrelide 124
Black Cohosh 1616
Black Draught Tablets [OTC] see
    Senna 1384
Black Susans see Echinacea 1620
Bladuril® (Mex) see Flavoxate 656
Blanoxan® (Mex) see Bleomycin . . . 214
Blastocarb® (Mex) see Carboplatin
    270
Blastolem® (Mex) see Cisplatin 350
Blenoxane® see Bleomycin 214
Bleo see Bleomycin 214
Bleolem® (Mex) see Bleomycin 214
Bleomycin 214
Bleomycin Injection, USP (Can)
    see Bleomycin 214
Bleomycin Sulfate see Bleomycin . . 214
Bleph®-10 see Sulfacetamide 1423
Blephamide® see Sulfacetamide
    and Prednisolone 1424
Blis-To-Sol® [OTC] see Tolnaftate
    1506
BLM see Bleomycin 214
Blocadren® see Timolol 1489
Blokium® (Mex) see Atenolol 154
BMS-232632 see Atazanavir 152
BMS 337039 see Aripiprazole 138
BN-52063 see Ginkgo Biloba 1622
Bonamine™ (Can) see Meclizine . . . 969
Bondronat® (Can) see Ibandronate
    805
Bonine® (Can) see Meclizine 969
Bonine® [OTC] see Meclizine 969
Boniva® see Ibandronate 805
Bontril® (Can) see
    Phendimetrazine 1220
Bontril PDM® see Phendimetrazine
    1220
Bontril® Slow-Release see
    Phendimetrazine 1220
Bortezomib 215
Bosentan 215
B&O Supprettes® see Belladonna
    and Opium 184
Botox® see Botulinum Toxin Type
    A 217
Botox® Cosmetic see Botulinum
    Toxin Type A 217
Botulinum Toxin Type A 217
Botulinum Toxin Type B 218
Boudreaux's® Butt Paste [OTC]
    see Zinc Oxide 1597
Bovine Lung Surfactant see
    Beractant 198
Bravelle® see Follitropins 698
Breathe Right® Saline [OTC] see
    Sodium Chloride 1400
Brethaire [DSC] see Terbutaline . . . 1460
Brethine® see Terbutaline 1460
Bretylium 219
Bretylium Tosylate see Bretylium . . . 219
Brevibloc® see Esmolol 571
Brevicon® see Ethinyl Estradiol
    and Norethindrone 608
Brevicon® 0.5/35 (Can) see Ethinyl
    Estradiol and Norethindrone 608
Brevicon® 1/35 (Can) see Ethinyl
    Estradiol and Norethindrone 608
Brevital® (Can) see Methohexital . . 1010

Brevital® Sodium see Methohexital 1010
Brevoxyl® see Benzoyl Peroxide . . 194
Brevoxyl® Cleansing see Benzoyl Peroxide 194
Brevoxyl® Wash see Benzoyl Peroxide 194
Bricanyl® (Can) see Terbutaline . . . 1460
Bricanyl [DSC] see Terbutaline . . . 1460
Brimonidine 220
Brimonidine Tartrate see Brimonidine 220
Brinzolamide 220
Brioschi® [OTC] see Sodium Bicarbonate 1400
British Anti-Lewisite see Dimercaprol 482
BRL 43694 see Granisetron 751
Brofed® see Brompheniramine and Pseudoephedrine 223
Bromaline® [OTC] see Brompheniramine and Pseudoephedrine 223
Bromaxefed RF see Brompheniramine and Pseudoephedrine 223
Bromazepam 220
Bromelain 1616
Bromfenac 221
Bromfenac Sodium see Bromfenac 221
Bromfenex® see Brompheniramine and Pseudoephedrine 223
Bromfenex® PD see Brompheniramine and Pseudoephedrine 223
Bromhist-NR see Brompheniramine and Pseudoephedrine 223
Bromhist Pediatric see Brompheniramine and Pseudoephedrine 223
Bromocriptine 222
Bromocriptine Mesylate see Bromocriptine 222
Bromodiphenhydramine and Codeine 223
Brompheniramine and Pseudoephedrine 223
Brompheniramine Maleate and Pseudoephedrine Hydrochloride see Brompheniramine and Pseudoephedrine 223
Brompheniramine Maleate and Pseudoephedrine Sulfate see Brompheniramine and Pseudoephedrine 223
Broncho Saline® [OTC] see Sodium Chloride 1400
Brontex® see Guaifenesin and Codeine 753
BSS® see Balanced Salt Solution . . 178
BSS Plus® see Balanced Salt Solution 178
BTX-A see Botulinum Toxin Type A 217
B-type Natriuretic Peptide (Human) see Nesiritide 1103
Bubbli-Pred™ [DSC] see PrednisoLONE 1268
Budeprion™ SR see BuPROPion . . . 233
Budesonide 224
Buffered Aspirin and Pravastatin Sodium see Aspirin and Pravastatin 151
Bufferin® Extra Strength [OTC] see Aspirin 145
Bufferin® [OTC] see Aspirin 145
Buffinol Extra [OTC] see Aspirin.... 145
Buffinol [OTC] see Aspirin 145
Bufigen® (Mex) see Nalbuphine . . . 1083

Bumedyl® (Mex) see Bumetanide . . . 227
Bumetanide 227
Bumex® see Bumetanide 227
Buphenyl® see Sodium Phenylbutyrate 1403
Bupivacaine 228
Bupivacaine and Epinephrine 228
Bupivacaine and Lidocaine see Lidocaine and Bupivacaine . . . 924
Bupivacaine Hydrochloride see Bupivacaine 228
Buprenex® see Buprenorphine 231
Buprenorphine 231
Buprenorphine and Naloxone 232
Buprenorphine Hydrochloride see Buprenorphine 231
Buprenorphine Hydrochloride and Naloxone Hydrochloride Dihydrate see Buprenorphine and Naloxone 232
Buproban™ see BuPROPion 233
BuPROPion 233
Burinex® (Can) see Bumetanide ... 227
Burnamycin [OTC] see Lidocaine . . 920
Burn Jel [OTC] see Lidocaine 920
Burn-O-Jel [OTC] see Lidocaine . . 920
Buscapina® (Mex) see Scopolamine 1380
Buscopan® (Can) see Scopolamine 1380
BuSpar® see BusPIRone 236
Buspirex (Can) see BusPIRone . . . 236
BusPIRone 236
Buspirone Hydrochloride see BusPIRone 236
Bustab® (Can) see BusPIRone ... 236
Busulfan 237
Busulfex® see Busulfan 237
Butabarbital 238
Butalbital, Acetaminophen, and Caffeine 239
Butalbital, Acetaminophen, Caffeine, and Codeine 239
Butalbital, Aspirin, and Caffeine . . . 241
Butalbital, Aspirin, Caffeine, and Codeine 241
Butalbital Compound see Butalbital, Aspirin, and Caffeine 241
Butalbital Compound and Codeine see Butalbital, Aspirin, Caffeine, and Codeine 241
Butenafine 242
Butenafine Hydrochloride see Butenafine 242
Butisol Sodium® see Butabarbital . . 238
Butoconazole 242
Butoconazole Nitrate see Butoconazole 242
Butorphanol 243
Butorphanol Tartrate see Butorphanol 243
Butyl Aminobenzoate, Tetracaine Hydrochloride, Benzocaine, and Benzalkonium Chloride see Benzocaine, Butyl Aminobenzoate, Tetracaine, and Benzalkonium Chloride 193
Buvacaina® (Mex) see Bupivacaine 228
B Vitamin Combinations see Vitamin B Complex Combinations 1581
BW-430C see Lamotrigine 895
BW524W91 see Emtricitabine 536
Byetta™ see Exenatide 629
C1H see Alemtuzumab 63
C2B8 see Rituximab 1360
C2B8 Monoclonal Antibody see Rituximab 1360
C7E3 see Abciximab 26

C8-CCK see Sincalide 1396
311C90 see Zolmitriptan 1603
C225 see Cetuximab 308
C-500-GR™ [OTC] see Ascorbic
 Acid 143
Cabergoline 244
Ca-DTPA see Diethylene Triamine
 Penta-Acetic Acid 466
Caduet® see Amlodipine and
 Atorvastatin 101
CaEDTA see Edetate Calcium
 Disodium 527
Caelyx® (Mex) see DOXOrubicin . . 509
Cafcit® see Caffeine 245
Cafergor® (Can) see Ergotamine
 and Caffeine 559
Cafergot® see Ergotamine and
 Caffeine 559
Caffedrine® [OTC] see Caffeine . . . 245
Caffeine 245
Caffeine, Acetaminophen, and
 Aspirin see Acetaminophen,
 Aspirin, and Caffeine 41
Caffeine, Acetaminophen,
 Butalbital, and Codeine see
 Butalbital, Acetaminophen,
 Caffeine, and Codeine 239
Caffeine and Ergotamine see
 Ergotamine and Caffeine 559
Caffeine and Sodium Benzoate
 see Caffeine 245
Caffeine, Aspirin, and
 Acetaminophen see
 Acetaminophen, Aspirin, and
 Caffeine 41
Caffeine Citrate see Caffeine 245
Caffeine, Dihydrocodeine, and
 Acetaminophen see
 Acetaminophen, Caffeine, and
 Dihydrocodeine 42
Caffeine, Hydrocodone,
 Chlorpheniramine,
 Phenylephrine, and
 Acetaminophen see
 Hydrocodone,
 Chlorpheniramine,
 Phenylephrine,
 Acetaminophen, and Caffeine . . 790
Caffeine, Orphenadrine, and
 Aspirin see Orphenadrine,
 Aspirin, and Caffeine 1152
Caffeine, Propoxyphene, and
 Aspirin see Propoxyphene,
 Aspirin, and Caffeine 1300
Caladryl® Clear [OTC] see
 Pramoxine 1264
CalaMycin® Cool and Clear [OTC]
 see Pramoxine 1264
Calan® see Verapamil 1571
Calan® SR see Verapamil 1571
Calcarb 600 [OTC] see Calcium
 Carbonate 248
Calcibind® see Cellulose Sodium
 Phosphate 301
Calci-Chew® [OTC] see Calcium
 Carbonate 248
Calciferol™ see Ergocalciferol 556
Calcijex® see Calcitriol 247
Calcimar® (Can) see Calcitonin . . . 246
Calci-Mix® [OTC] see Calcium
 Carbonate 248
Calcipotriene 246
Calcite-500 (Can) see Calcium
 Carbonate 248
Calcitonin 246
Calcitonin (Salmon) see Calcitonin . . 246
Cal-Citrate® 250 [OTC] see
 Calcium Citrate 250
Calcitriol 247
Calcium Acetate 248

Calcium Acetate and Aluminum
 Sulfate see Aluminum Sulfate
 and Calcium Acetate 81
Calcium Acetylhomotaurinate see
 Acamprosate 27
Calcium and Risedronate see
 Risedronate and Calcium 1354
Calcium Carbonate 248
Calcium Carbonate and Etidronate
 Disodium see Etidronate and
 Calcium 620
Calcium Carbonate and
 Magnesium Hydroxide 249
Calcium Carbonate and
 Simethicone 249
Calcium Carbonate, Magnesium
 Hydroxide, and Famotidine see
 Famotidine, Calcium
 Carbonate, and Magnesium
 Hydroxide 636
Calcium Chloride 250
Calcium Citrate 250
Calcium Disodium Edetate see
 Edetate Calcium Disodium 527
Calcium Disodium Versenate® see
 Edetate Calcium Disodium 527
Calcium EDTA see Edetate
 Calcium Disodium 527
Calcium Glubionate 250
Calcium Gluconate 250
Calcium Lactate 251
Calcium Leucovorin see
 Leucovorin 905
Calcium Pantothenate see
 Pantothenic Acid 1186
Calcium Phosphate (Tribasic) 251
Calcium-Sandoz® (Mex) see
 Calcium Glubionate 250
Caldecort® [OTC] see
 Hydrocortisone 793
Calendula 1616
Calendula officinalis see Calendula
 1616
Calfactant 251
Cal-Gest [OTC] see Calcium
 Carbonate 248
Callergy Clear [OTC] see
 Pramoxine 1264
Cal-Mint [OTC] see Calcium
 Carbonate 248
Calmylin with Codeine (Can) see
 Guaifenesin, Pseudoephedrine,
 and Codeine 756
Calsan® (Mex) see Calcium
 Carbonate 248
Caltine® (Can) see Calcitonin 246
Caltrate® (Can) see Calcium
 Carbonate 248
Caltrate® 600 [OTC] see Calcium
 Carbonate 248
Caltrate® Select (Can) see Calcium
 Carbonate 248
Camellia sinensis see Green Tea
 1625
Camila™ see Norethindrone 1125
Campath® see Alemtuzumab 63
Campath-1H see Alemtuzumab 63
Campho-Phenique® [OTC] see
 Camphor and Phenol 252
Camphor and Phenol 252
Camphorated Tincture of Opium
 (error-prone synonym) see
 Paregoric 1187
Campral® see Acamprosate 27
Camptosar® see Irinotecan 860
Camptothecin-11 see Irinotecan 860
Canasa™ see Mesalamine 996
Cancidas® see Caspofungin 278
Candesartan 252
Candesartan and
 Hydrochlorothiazide 254

Candesartan Cilexetil *see*
  Candesartan 252
Candesartan Cilexetil and
  Hydrochlorothiazide *see*
  Candesartan and
  Hydrochlorothiazide 254
Candimon® (Mex) *see* Clotrimazole
  379
Candistatin® (Can) *see* Nystatin . . . 1133
Canef® (Mex) *see* Fluvastatin 693
Canesten® Topical (Can) *see*
  Clotrimazole 379
Canesten® Vaginal (Can) *see*
  Clotrimazole 379
Cankaid® [OTC] *see* Carbamide
  Peroxide. 264
Cannabidiol and
  Tetrahydrocannabinol *see*
  Tetrahydrocannabinol and
  Cannabidiol 1469
Canthacur® (Can) *see* Cantharidin . . 254
Cantharidin. 254
Cantharone® (Can) *see*
  Cantharidin 254
Cantil® (Can) *see* Mepenzolate 983
Cantil® [DSC] *see* Mepenzolate 983
Capastat® Sulfate *see*
  Capreomycin 256
Cape *see* Aloe 1614
Capecitabine 255
Capex™ *see* Fluocinolone 667
Capital® and Codeine *see*
  Acetaminophen and Codeine 35
Capitrol® (Can) *see* Chloroxine 322
Capitrol® [DSC] *see* Chloroxine 322
Capoten® *see* Captopril 257
Capozide® *see* Captopril and
  Hydrochlorothiazide 259
Capreomycin 256
Capreomycin Sulfate *see*
  Capreomycin 256
Capsagel® [OTC] *see* Capsaicin . . 256
Capsaicin 256
Capsicum annuum see Cayenne . . 1617
Capsicum frutescens see Cayenne
  1617
Captopril 257
Captopril and Hydrochlorothiazide . . 259
Captral® (Mex) *see* Captopril 257
Capzasin-HP® [OTC] *see*
  Capsaicin 256
Capzasin-P® [OTC] *see* Capsaicin . . 256
Carac™ *see* Fluorouracil 674
Carafate® *see* Sucralfate 1420
Carapres® (Can) *see* Clonidine 373
Carbac® (Mex) *see* Loracarbef 945
Carbachol 260
Carbacholine *see* Carbachol 260
Carbamazepine 260
Carbamide *see* Urea 1551
Carbamide Peroxide 264
Carbamylcholine Chloride *see*
  Carbachol 260
Carbastat® [DSC] *see* Carbachol . . . 260
Carbatrol® *see* Carbamazepine 260
Carbaxefed DM RF *see*
  Carbinoxamine,
  Pseudoephedrine, and
  Dextromethorphan 269
Carbaxefed RF *see* Carbinoxamine
  and Pseudoephedrine 268
Carbazep® (Mex) *see*
  Carbamazepine 260
Carbazina® (Mex) *see*
  Carbamazepine 260
Carbenicillin 265
Carbenicillin Indanyl Sodium *see*
  Carbenicillin 265
Carbetapentane and
  Chlorpheniramine 266

Carbetapentane, Ephedrine,
  Phenylephrine, and
  Chlorpheniramine *see*
  Chlorpheniramine, Ephedrine,
  Phenylephrine, and
  Carbetapentane 325
Carbetapentane, Phenylephrine,
  and Pyrilamine 267
Carbetapentane Tannate and
  Chlorpheniramine Tannate *see*
  Carbetapentane and
  Chlorpheniramine 266
Carbidopa 267
Carbidopa and Levodopa *see*
  Levodopa and Carbidopa 911
Carbidopa, Levodopa, and
  Entacapone *see* Levodopa,
  Carbidopa, and Entacapone. . . . 912
Carbihist *see* Carbinoxamine 268
Carbinoxamine 268
Carbinoxamine and
  Pseudoephedrine 268
Carbinoxamine, Dextromethorphan,
  and Pseudoephedrine *see*
  Carbinoxamine,
  Pseudoephedrine, and
  Dextromethorphan 269
Carbinoxamine Maleate *see*
  Carbinoxamine 268
Carbinoxamine PD *see*
  Carbinoxamine 268
Carbinoxamine, Pseudoephedrine,
  and Dextromethorphan 269
Carbinoxamine, Pseudoephedrine,
  and Hydrocodone *see*
  Hydrocodone, Carbinoxamine,
  and Pseudoephedrine 789
Carbinoxamine Tannate *see*
  Carbinoxamine 268
Carbocaine® *see* Mepivacaine 987
Carbocaine® 2% with
  Neo-Cobefrin® *see*
  Mepivacaine and Levonordefrin
  991
Carbolic Acid *see* Phenol 1223
Carbolit® (Mex) *see* Lithium 939
Carbolith™ (Can) *see* Lithium 939
Carboplatin. 270
Carboprost *see* Carboprost
  Tromethamine 270
Carboprost Tromethamine 270
Carbose D *see*
  Carboxymethylcellulose 271
Carbotec® (Mex) *see* Carboplatin . . . 270
Carboxine *see* Carbinoxamine 268
Carboxine-PSE *see* Carbinoxamine
  and Pseudoephedrine 268
Carboxymethylcellulose 271
Carboxymethylcellulose Sodium
  see Carboxymethylcellulose 271
Cardene® *see* NiCARdipine 1107
Cardene® I.V. *see* NiCARdipine . . . 1107
Cardene® SR *see* NiCARdipine 1107
Cardinit® (Mex) *see* Nitroglycerin . . 1120
Cardipril® (Mex) *see* Captopril 257
Cardispan® (Mex) *see*
  Levocarnitine 910
Cardizem® *see* Diltiazem 479
Cardizem® CD *see* Diltiazem 479
Cardizem® LA *see* Diltiazem 479
Cardizem® SR (Can) *see* Diltiazem
  479
Cardizem® SR [DSC] *see*
  Diltiazem 479
Cardura® *see* Doxazosin 503
Cardura-1™ (Can) *see* Doxazosin . . 503
Cardura-2™ (Can) *see* Doxazosin . . 503
Cardura-4™ (Can) *see* Doxazosin . . 503
Cardura® XL *see* Doxazosin. 503
Carexan® (Mex) *see* Itraconazole . . 873

Carimune™ NF see Immune
    Globulin (Intravenous) 824
Carindacillin see Carbenicillin 265
Carisoprodate see Carisoprodol 271
Carisoprodol 271
Carisoprodol and Aspirin 272
Carisoprodol, Aspirin, and Codeine
    273
Carmol® 10 [OTC] see Urea 1551
Carmol® 20 [OTC] see Urea 1551
Carmol® 40 see Urea 1551
Carmol® Deep Cleaning see Urea
    1551
Carmol-HC® see Urea and
    Hydrocortisone 1551
Carmol® Scalp see Sulfacetamide
    1423
Carmustine 273
Carmustinum see Carmustine 273
Carnitine 1616
Carnitor® see Levocarnitine 910
Carnotprim® (Mex) see
    Metoclopramide 1029
Carrington Antifungal [OTC] see
    Miconazole 1039
Carteolol 274
Carteolol Hydrochloride see
    Carteolol 274
Carter's Little Pills® (Can) see
    Bisacodyl 209
Cartia XT™ see Diltiazem 479
Cartrol® see Carteolol 274
Cartrol® Oral (Can) see Carteolol . . . 274
Carvedilol 275
Casanthranol and Docusate see
    Docusate and Casanthranol 496
Cascara 1617
Cascara Sagrada see Cascara 1617
Casodex® see Bicalutamide 207
Caspofungin 278
Caspofungin Acetate see
    Caspofungin 278
Castellani Paint Modified [OTC]
    see Phenol 1223
Castor Oil 279
Castor Oil, Trypsin, and Balsam
    Peru see Trypsin, Balsam
    Peru, and Castor Oil 1547
Cataflam® see Diclofenac 459
Catapres® see Clonidine 373
Catapres-TTS® see Clonidine 373
Cathflo® Activase® see Alteplase . . . 77
Cat's Claw 1617
Caverject® see Alprostadil 76
Caverject Impulse® see Alprostadil
    76
CaviRinse™ (Can) see Fluoride 671
Cayenne 1617
CB-1348 see Chlorambucil 313
CBDCA see Carboplatin 270
CBZ see Carbamazepine 260
CC-5013 see Lenalidomide 903
CCNU see Lomustine 941
2-CdA see Cladribine 354
CDDP see Cisplatin 350
CDX see Bicalutamide 207
Ceclor® (Can) see Cefaclor 279
Cecon® [OTC] see Ascorbic Acid . . . 143
Cedax® see Ceftibuten 292
Cedocard®-SR (Can) see
    Isosorbide Dinitrate 866
CEE see Estrogens (Conjugated/
    Equine) 580
CeeNU® see Lomustine 941
Cefaclor 279
Cefadroxil 281
Cefadroxil Monohydrate see
    Cefadroxil 281
Cefamox® (Mex) see Cefadroxil 281
Cefaxona® (Mex) see Ceftriaxone . . 294
Cefazolin 283

Cefazolin Sodium see Cefazolin 283
Cefdinir 284
Cefditoren 285
Cefditoren Pivoxil see Cefditoren . . . 285
Cefepime 287
Cefepime Hydrochloride see
    Cefepime 287
Cefixime 287
Cefizox® see Ceftizoxime 293
Cefotan® (Can) see Cefotetan 289
Cefotan® [DSC] see Cefotetan 289
Cefotaxime 288
Cefotaxime Sodium see
    Cefotaxime 288
Cefotetan 289
Cefotetan Disodium see Cefotetan . . 289
Cefoxitin 290
Cefoxitin Sodium see Cefoxitin 290
Cefpodoxime 290
Cefpodoxime Proxetil see
    Cefpodoxime 290
Cefprozil 291
Cefradil® (Mex) see Cefotaxime 288
Ceftazidime 292
Ceftibuten 292
Ceftin® see Cefuroxime 295
Ceftizoxime 293
Ceftizoxime Sodium see
    Ceftizoxime 293
Ceftrex® (Mex) see Ceftriaxone 294
Ceftriaxone 294
Ceftriaxone Sodium see
    Ceftriaxone 294
Cefuracet® (Mex) see Cefuroxime . . 295
Cefuroxime 295
Cefuroxime Axetil see Cefuroxime . . 295
Cefuroxime Sodium see
    Cefuroxime 295
Cefzil® see Cefprozil 291
Celebrex® see Celecoxib 296
Celecoxib 296
Celestone® see Betamethasone 199
Celestone® Soluspan® see
    Betamethasone 199
Celexa® see Citalopram 351
CellCept® see Mycophenolate 1075
Cellugel® see Hydroxypropyl
    Methylcellulose 800
Cellulose (Oxidized/Regenerated) . . 300
Cellulose Sodium Phosphate 301
Celluvisc™ (Can) see
    Carboxymethylcellulose 271
Celontin® see Methsuximide 1019
Celulose Grin® (Mex) see
    Hydroxypropyl Methylcellulose . . 800
Cenestin® see Estrogens
    (Conjugated A/Synthetic) 578
Centany™ see Mupirocin 1073
Centella asiatica see Gotu Kola . . . 1624
Centrum® [OTC] see Vitamins
    (Multiple/Oral) 1582
Centrum® Performance™ [OTC]
    see Vitamins (Multiple/Oral) . . . 1582
Centrum® Silver® [OTC] see
    Vitamins (Multiple/Oral) 1582
Cepacol® (Can) see
    Cetylpyridinium and
    Benzocaine 309
Cepacol® Antibacterial Mouthwash
    Gold [OTC] see
    Cetylpyridinium 309
Cepacol® Antibacterial Mouthwash
    [OTC] see Cetylpyridinium 309
Cepacol® Sore Throat [OTC] see
    Benzocaine 190
Cepastat® Extra Strength [OTC]
    see Phenol 1223
Cepastat® [OTC] see Phenol 1223
Cephalexin 301
Cephalexin Monohydrate see
    Cephalexin 301

Cephalothin 303
Cephalothin Sodium see
    Cephalothin 303
Cephradine 304
Ceptaz® [DSC] see Ceftazidime . . . 292
Cerebyx® see Fosphenytoin 710
Ceredase® see Alglucerase 68
Cerezyme® see Imiglucerase 819
Cerovel™ see Urea 1551
Certuss-D® see Guaifenesin,
    Dextromethorphan, and
    Phenylephrine 756
Cerubidine® see DAUNOrubicin
    Hydrochloride 426
Cerumenex® (Can) see
    Triethanolamine Polypeptide
    Oleate-Condensate 1535
Cerumenex® [DSC] see
    Triethanolamine Polypeptide
    Oleate-Condensate 1535
Cervidil® see Dinoprostone 482
C.E.S.® (Can) see Estrogens
    (Conjugated/Equine) 580
Cesia™ see Ethinyl Estradiol and
    Desogestrel 592
Cesol® (Mex) see Praziquantel . . . 1266
Cetacaine® see Benzocaine, Butyl
    Aminobenzoate, Tetracaine,
    and Benzalkonium Chloride 193
Cetacort® see Hydrocortisone 793
Cetafen Cold® [OTC] see
    Acetaminophen and
    Pseudoephedrine 38
Cetafen Extra® [OTC] see
    Acetaminophen 31
Cetafen® [OTC] see
    Acetaminophen 31
Cetamide™ (Can) see
    Sulfacetamide 1423
Ceta-Plus® see Hydrocodone and
    Acetaminophen 779
Ceta Sulfa® (Mex) see
    Sulfacetamide 1423
Cetirizine 306
Cetirizine and Pseudoephedrine . . . 307
Cetirizine Hydrochloride see
    Cetirizine 306
Cetirizine Hydrochloride and
    Pseudoephedrine
    Hydrochloride see Cetirizine
    and Pseudoephedrine 307
Cetoxil® (Mex) see Cefuroxime . . . 295
Cetrorelix 307
Cetrorelix Acetate see Cetrorelix . . . 307
Cetrotide® see Cetrorelix 307
Cetuximab 308
Cetylpyridinium 309
Cetylpyridinium and Benzocaine . . . 309
Cetylpyridinium Chloride see
    Cetylpyridinium 309
Cetylpyridinium Chloride and
    Benzocaine see
    Cetylpyridinium and
    Benzocaine 309
Cevalin® (Mex) see Ascorbic Acid . . 143
Cevi-Bid® [OTC] see Ascorbic Acid
    143
Cevimeline 310
Cevimeline Hydrochloride see
    Cevimeline 310
CFDN see Cefdinir 284
CG see Chorionic Gonadotropin
    (Human) 336
CGP-42446 see Zoledronic Acid . . 1600
CGP-57148B see Imatinib 817
C-Gram [OTC] see Ascorbic Acid . . 143
CGS-20267 see Letrozole 904
Chamomile 1617
Charcadole® (Can) see Charcoal . . 311
Charcadole®, Aqueous (Can) see
    Charcoal 311
Charcadole® TFS (Can) see
    Charcoal 311
Char-Caps [OTC] see Charcoal . . . 311
CharcoAid G® [OTC] [DSC] see
    Charcoal 311
Charcoal 311
Charcoal Plus® DS [OTC] see
    Charcoal 311
Charcocaps® [OTC] see Charcoal . . 311
Chasteberry 1618
Chastetree see Chasteberry 1618
CheeTah® see Barium 179
Cheracol® see Guaifenesin and
    Codeine 753
Cheracol® D [OTC] see
    Guaifenesin and
    Dextromethorphan 754
Cheracol® [OTC] see Phenol 1223
Cheracol® Plus [OTC] see
    Guaifenesin and
    Dextromethorphan 754
Cheratussin AC see Guaifenesin
    and Codeine 753
CHG see Chlorhexidine Gluconate . . 316
Chiggerex [OTC] see Benzocaine
    190
Chiggertox® [OTC] see Benzocaine
    190
Children's Advil® Cold (Can) see
    Pseudoephedrine and
    Ibuprofen 1311
Children's Dimetapp® Elixir Cold &
    Allergy [OTC] see
    Brompheniramine and
    Pseudoephedrine 223
Children's Kaopectate® [OTC]
    [DSC] see Attapulgite 165
Children's Pepto [OTC] see
    Calcium Carbonate 248
Children's Motion Sickness Liquid
    (Can) see DimenhyDRINATE . . . 481
Chinese angelica see Dong Quai . . 1620
Chirocaine® (Can) see
    Levobupivacaine 909
Chirocaine® [DSC] see
    Levobupivacaine 909
Chloral see Chloral Hydrate 312
Chloral Hydrate 312
Chlorambucil 313
Chlorambucilum see Chlorambucil . . 313
Chloraminophene see
    Chlorambucil 313
Chloramphenicol 314
ChloraPrep® [OTC] see
    Chlorhexidine Gluconate 316
Chloraseptic® Gargle [OTC] see
    Phenol 1223
Chloraseptic® Mouth Pain [OTC]
    see Phenol 1223
Chloraseptic® Rinse [OTC] see
    Phenol 1223
Chloraseptic® Spray for Kids [OTC]
    see Phenol 1223
Chloraseptic® Spray [OTC] see
    Phenol 1223
Chlorbutinum see Chlorambucil . . . 313
Chlordiazepoxide 315
Chlordiazepoxide and Amitriptyline
    Hydrochloride see Amitriptyline
    and Chlordiazepoxide 97
Chlordiazepoxide and Clidinium
    see Clidinium and
    Chlordiazepoxide 360
Chlordiazepoxide and
    Methscopolamine 316
Chlorhexidine Gluconate 316
Chlormeprazine see
    Prochlorperazine 1285

Chlor-Mes-D *see*
Chlorpheniramine,
Phenylephrine, and
Methscopolamine 327
2-Chlorodeoxyadenosine *see*
Cladribine 354
Chloroethane *see* Ethyl Chloride . . . 620
Chloromag® *see* Magnesium
Chloride 960
Chloromycetin® (Can) *see*
Chloramphenicol 314
Chloromycetin® Sodium Succinate
see Chloramphenicol 314
Chloromycetin® Succinate (Can)
see Chloramphenicol 314
Chlorophyll 319
Chlorophyllin *see* Chlorophyll 319
Chlorophyllin Copper Complex
Sodium, Papain, and Urea *see*
Chlorophyllin, Papain, and
Urea 319
Chlorophyllin, Papain, and Urea 319
Chloroprocaine 320
Chloroprocaine Hydrochloride *see*
Chloroprocaine 320
Chloroquine 320
Chloroquine Phosphate *see*
Chloroquine 320
Chlorothiazide 322
Chloroxine 322
Chlorpheniramine 323
Chlorpheniramine, Acetaminophen,
and Pseudoephedrine *see*
Acetaminophen,
Chlorpheniramine, and
Pseudoephedrine 43
Chlorpheniramine and
Acetaminophen 324
Chlorpheniramine and
Carbetapentane *see*
Carbetapentane and
Chlorpheniramine 266
Chlorpheniramine and
Phenylephrine 324
Chlorpheniramine and
Pseudoephedrine 325
Chlorpheniramine, Ephedrine,
Phenylephrine, and
Carbetapentane 325
Chlorpheniramine, Hydrocodone,
Phenylephrine,
Acetaminophen, and Caffeine
see Hydrocodone,
Chlorpheniramine,
Phenylephrine,
Acetaminophen, and Caffeine . . 790
Chlorpheniramine Maleate *see*
Chlorpheniramine 323
Chlorpheniramine Maleate and
Hydrocodone Bitartrate *see*
Hydrocodone and
Chlorpheniramine 784
Chlorpheniramine Maleate and
Phenylephrine Hydrochloride
see Chlorpheniramine and
Phenylephrine 324
Chlorpheniramine Maleate and
Pseudoephedrine
Hydrochloride *see*
Chlorpheniramine and
Pseudoephedrine 325
Chlorpheniramine Maleate,
Dihydrocodeine Bitartrate, and
Phenylephrine Hydrochloride
see Dihydrocodeine,
Chlorpheniramine, and
Phenylephrine 476
Chlorpheniramine, Phenylephrine,
and Dextromethorphan 326
Chlorpheniramine, Phenylephrine,
and Methscopolamine 327

Chlorpheniramine, Phenylephrine,
and Phenyltoloxamine 328
Chlorpheniramine, Phenylephrine,
Codeine, and Potassium Iodide
. . . . 328
Chlorpheniramine,
Pseudoephedrine, and
Acetaminophen *see*
Acetaminophen,
Chlorpheniramine, and
Pseudoephedrine 43
Chlorpheniramine,
Pseudoephedrine, and
Codeine 329
Chlorpheniramine,
Pseudoephedrine, and
Dihydrocodeine *see*
Pseudoephedrine,
Dihydrocodeine, and
Chlorpheniramine 1312
Chlorpheniramine Tannate and
Phenylephrine Tannate *see*
Chlorpheniramine and
Phenylephrine 324
Chlorpheniramine Tannate and
Pseudoephedrine Tannate *see*
Chlorpheniramine and
Pseudoephedrine 325
Chlorphen [OTC] *see*
Chlorpheniramine 323
ChlorproMAZINE 329
Chlorpromazine Hydrochloride *see*
ChlorproMAZINE 329
ChlorproPAMIDE 331
Chlorthalidone 332
Chlorthalidone and Atenolol *see*
Atenolol and Chlorthalidone 156
Chlorthalidone and Clonidine *see*
Clonidine and Chlorthalidone . . . 376
Chlor-Trimeton® Allergy D [OTC]
see Chlorpheniramine and
Pseudoephedrine 325
Chlor-Trimeton® [OTC] *see*
Chlorpheniramine 323
Chlor-Tripolon® (Can) *see*
Chlorpheniramine 323
Chlor-Tripolon ND® (Can) *see*
Loratadine and
Pseudoephedrine 947
Chlorzoxazone 333
Cholecalciferol 334
Cholecalciferol and Alendronate
see Alendronate and
Cholecalciferol 66
Cholestyramine Resin 334
Choline Magnesium Trisalicylate . . . 335
Cholografin® Meglumine *see*
Iodipamide Meglumine 853
Chondroitin Sulfate 1618
Chondroitin Sulfate and Sodium
Hyaluronate 336
Chooz® [OTC] *see* Calcium
Carbonate 248
Choriogonadotropin Alfa *see*
Chorionic Gonadotropin
(Recombinant) 337
Chorionic Gonadotropin (Human) . . . 336
Chorionic Gonadotropin
(Recombinant) 337
Chromium *see* Trace Metals 1513
Chronovera® (Can) *see* Verapamil
. . . . 1571
CI-1008 *see* Pregabalin 1274
Cialis® *see* Tadalafil 1441
Cicloferon® (Mex) *see* Acyclovir 49
Ciclopirox 338
Ciclopirox Olamine *see* Ciclopirox . . 338
Cidecin *see* Daptomycin 423
Cidofovir 339
Cilazapril 340

Cilazapril Monohydrate see
    Cilazapril 340
Cilostazol 340
Ciloxan® see Ciprofloxacin 343
Cimetase® (Mex) see Cimetidine . . . 341
Cimetidine 341
Cimicifuga racemosa see Black
    Cohosh 1616
Cimogal® (Mex) see Ciprofloxacin . . 343
Cinacalcet 342
Cinacalcet Hydrochloride see
    Cinacalcet 342
Cipralex® (Can) see Escitalopram . . 568
Cipro® see Ciprofloxacin 343
Cipro® XL (Can) see Ciprofloxacin . . 343
Ciprobiotic® (Mex) see
    Ciprofloxacin 343
Ciprodex® see Ciprofloxacin and
    Dexamethasone 348
Ciproflox® (Mex) see Ciprofloxacin . . 343
Ciprofloxacin 343
Ciprofloxacin and Dexamethasone . . 348
Ciprofloxacin and Hydrocortisone . . . 348
Ciprofloxacin Hydrochloride see
    Ciprofloxacin 343
Ciprofloxacin Hydrochloride and
    Dexamethasone see
    Ciprofloxacin and
    Dexamethasone 348
Ciprofloxacin Hydrochloride and
    Hydrocortisone see
    Ciprofloxacin and
    Hydrocortisone 348
Ciprofur® (Mex) see Ciprofloxacin . . 343
Cipro® HC see Ciprofloxacin and
    Hydrocortisone 348
Ciproxina® (Mex) see Ciprofloxacin
    343
Cipro® XR see Ciprofloxacin 343
Cisapride 348
Cisplatin 350
13-cis-Retinoic Acid see
    Isotretinoin 869
Cisticid® (Mex) see Praziquantel . . 1266
Citalopram 351
Citalopram Hydrobromide see
    Citalopram 351
Citanest® Forte (Can) see
    Prilocaine and Epinephrine . . . 1278
Citanest® Forte Dental see
    Prilocaine and Epinephrine . . . 1278
Citanest® Plain see Prilocaine 1277
Citomid® (Mex) see
    VinCRIStine 1576
Citracal® [OTC] see Calcium
    Citrate 250
Citrate of Magnesia see
    Magnesium Citrate 960
Citric Acid and d-gluconic Acid
    Irrigant see Citric Acid,
    Magnesium Carbonate, and
    Glucono-Delta-Lactone 353
Citric Acid and Potassium Citrate
    see Potassium Citrate and
    Citric Acid 1259
Citric Acid Bladder Mixture see
    Citric Acid, Magnesium
    Carbonate, and
    Glucono-Delta-Lactone 353
Citric Acid, Magnesium Carbonate,
    and Glucono-Delta-Lactone 353
Citric Acid, Magnesium
    Hydroxycarbonate, D-Gluconic
    Acid, Magnesium Acid Citrate,
    and Calcium Carbonate see
    Citric Acid, Magnesium
    Carbonate, and
    Glucono-Delta-Lactone 353
Citric Acid, Sodium Citrate, and
    Potassium Citrate 354

Citro-Mag® (Can) see Magnesium
    Citrate 960
Citrovorum Factor see Leucovorin . . 905
Citrucel® [OTC] see
    Methylcellulose 1021
Citrus paradisi see Grapefruit Seed
    1625
CL-118,532 see Triptorelin 1544
Cl-719 see Gemfibrozil 730
CL-825 see Pentostatin 1211
CL-184116 see Porfimer 1256
Cladribine 354
Claforan® see Cefotaxime 288
Claravis™ see Isotretinoin 869
Clarinex® see Desloratadine 435
Clarinex-D® 12 Hour see
    Desloratadine and
    Pseudoephedrine 436
Clarinex-D® 24 Hour see
    Desloratadine and
    Pseudoephedrine 436
Claripel™ see Hydroquinone 798
Clarithromycin 355
Clarithromycin, Lansoprazole, and
    Amoxicillin see Lansoprazole,
    Amoxicillin, and Clarithromycin . . 898
Claritin® (Can) see Loratadine 946
Claritin® 24 Hour Allergy [OTC]
    see Loratadine 946
Claritin-D® 12-Hour [OTC] see
    Loratadine and
    Pseudoephedrine 947
Claritin-D® 24-Hour [OTC] see
    Loratadine and
    Pseudoephedrine 947
Claritin® Allergic Decongestant
    (Can) see Oxymetazoline 1172
Claritin® Extra (Can) see
    Loratadine and
    Pseudoephedrine 947
Claritin® Hives Relief [OTC] see
    Loratadine 946
Claritin® Kids (Can) see Loratadine
    946
Claritin® Liberator (Can) see
    Loratadine and
    Pseudoephedrine 947
Clarityne® (Mex) see Loratadine 946
Clarus™ (Can) see Isotretinoin 869
Clavulanic Acid and Amoxicillin see
    Amoxicillin and Clavulanate
    Potassium 108
Clavulin® (Can) see Amoxicillin
    and Clavulanate Potassium 108
Clear Eyes® ACR [OTC] see
    Naphazoline 1087
Clear Eyes® Extra Relief [OTC]
    see Naphazoline 1087
Clearplex [OTC] see Benzoyl
    Peroxide 194
Clemastine 359
Clemastine Fumarate see
    Clemastine 359
Cleocin® see Clindamycin 361
Cleocin HCl® see Clindamycin 361
Cleocin Pediatric® see Clindamycin
    361
Cleocin Phosphate® see
    Clindamycin 361
Cleocin T® see Clindamycin 361
Clexane® (Mex) see Enoxaparin . . . 542
Clidinium and Chlordiazepoxide 360
Climaderm® (Mex) see Estradiol . . . 574
Climara® see Estradiol 574
Clinac™ BPO see Benzoyl
    Peroxide 194
Clindagel® see Clindamycin 361
ClindaMax™ see Clindamycin 361
Clindamycin 361
Clindamycin and Benzoyl Peroxide
    364

Clindamycin Hydrochloride see
    Clindamycin 361
Clindamycin Injection, USP (Can)
    see Clindamycin 361
Clindamycin Palmitate see
    Clindamycin 361
Clindamycin Phosphate see
    Clindamycin 361
Clindamycin Phosphate and
    Benzoyl Peroxide see
    Clindamycin and Benzoyl
    Peroxide 364
Clindazyn® (Mex) see Clindamycin
    361
Clindesse™ see Clindamycin 361
Clindets® see Clindamycin 361
Clindoxyl® (Can) see Clindamycin . . 361
Clinoril® see Sulindac 1430
Clobazam 364
Clobazam-10 (Can) see Clobazam
    364
Clobetasol 365
Clobetasol Propionate see
    Clobetasol 365
Clobevate® see Clobetasol 365
Clobex® see Clobetasol 365
Clocortolone 367
Clocortolone Pivalate see
    Clocortolone 367
Cloderm® see Clocortolone 367
Clofarabine 367
Clofarex see Clofarabine 367
Clofazimine 369
Clofazimine Palmitate see
    Clofazimine 369
Clolar™ see Clofarabine 367
Clomid® see ClomiPHENE 369
ClomiPHENE 369
Clomiphene Citrate see
    ClomiPHENE 369
ClomiPRAMINE 370
Clomipramine Hydrochloride see
    ClomiPRAMINE 370
Clonapam (Can) see Clonazepam . . 371
Clonazepam 371
Clonidine 373
Clonidine and Chlorthalidone 376
Clonidine Hydrochloride see
    Clonidine 373
Clopidogrel 376
Clopidogrel Bisulfate see
    Clopidogrel 376
Clorazepate 378
Clorazepate Dipotassium see
    Clorazepate 378
Clorimet® (Mex) see
    Metoclopramide 1029
Clorpactin® WCS-90 [OTC] see
    Oxychlorosene 1163
Clorpres® see Clonidine and
    Chlorthalidone 376
Clostedal® (Mex) see
    Carbamazepine 260
Clotrimaderm (Can) see
    Clotrimazole 379
Clotrimazole 379
Clotrimazole and Betamethasone
    see Betamethasone and
    Clotrimazole 202
Cloxacillin 380
Cloxacillin Sodium see Cloxacillin . . 380
Clozapine 382
Clozaril® see Clozapine 382
CMA-676 see Gemtuzumab
    Ozogamicin 732
CNJ-016™ see Vaccinia Immune
    Globulin (Intravenous) 1553
CoActifed® (Can) see Triprolidine,
    Pseudoephedrine, and
    Codeine 1543

Coagulant Complex Inhibitor see
    Anti-inhibitor Coagulant
    Complex 130
Coagulation Factor VIIa see Factor
    VIIa (Recombinant) 632
CO Alendronate (Can) see
    Alendronate 64
Coal Tar 383
Coal Tar and Salicylic Acid 383
CO Azithromycin (Can) see
    Azithromycin 171
CO Bicalutamide (Can) see
    Bicalutamide 207
Cocaine 384
Cocaine Hydrochloride see
    Cocaine 384
CO Ciprofloxacin (Can) see
    Ciprofloxacin 343
CO Citalopram (Can) see
    Citalopram 351
CO Clomipramine (Can) see
    ClomiPRAMINE 370
CO Clonazepam (Can) see
    Clonazepam 371
Codeine 385
Codeine, Acetaminophen,
    Butalbital, and Caffeine see
    Butalbital, Acetaminophen,
    Caffeine, and Codeine 239
Codeine and Acetaminophen see
    Acetaminophen and Codeine 35
Codeine and
    Bromodiphenhydramine see
    Bromodiphenhydramine and
    Codeine 223
Codeine and Butalbital Compound
    see Butalbital, Aspirin,
    Caffeine, and Codeine 241
Codeine and Guaifenesin see
    Guaifenesin and Codeine 753
Codeine and Promethazine see
    Promethazine and Codeine . . . 1291
Codeine, Aspirin, and Carisoprodol
    see Carisoprodol, Aspirin, and
    Codeine 273
Codeine, Butalbital, Aspirin, and
    Caffeine see Butalbital, Aspirin,
    Caffeine, and Codeine 241
Codeine, Chlorpheniramine, and
    Pseudoephedrine see
    Chlorpheniramine,
    Pseudoephedrine, and
    Codeine 329
Codeine, Chlorpheniramine,
    Phenylephrine, and Potassium
    Iodide see Chlorpheniramine,
    Phenylephrine, Codeine, and
    Potassium Iodide 328
Codeine Contin® (Can) see
    Codeine 385
Codeine, Guaifenesin, and
    Pseudoephedrine see
    Guaifenesin, Pseudoephedrine,
    and Codeine 756
Codeine Phosphate see Codeine . . . 385
Codeine Phosphate and Aspirin
    see Aspirin and Codeine 149
Codeine, Promethazine, and
    Phenylephrine see
    Promethazine, Phenylephrine,
    and Codeine 1293
Codeine, Pseudoephedrine, and
    Triprolidine see Triprolidine,
    Pseudoephedrine, and
    Codeine 1543
Codeine Sulfate see Codeine 385
Codeine, Triprolidine, and
    Pseudoephedrine see
    Triprolidine, Pseudoephedrine,
    and Codeine 1543

Codiclear® DH see Hydrocodone and Guaifenesin 785
Cod Liver Oil see Vitamin A and Vitamin D 1580
Coenzyme 1 see Nicotinamide Adenine Dinucleotide 1629
Coenzyme Q₁₀ 1618
CO Fluoxetine (Can) see Fluoxetine 675
Cogentin® see Benztropine 196
Co-Gesic® see Hydrocodone and Acetaminophen 779
CO Glimepiride (Can) see Glimepiride 738
Cognex® see Tacrine 1436
CO Ipra-Sal (Can) see Ipratropium and Albuterol 857
Colace® (Can) see Docusate 496
Colace® Adult/Children Suppositories [OTC] see Glycerin 747
Colace® Infant/Children Suppositories [OTC] see Glycerin 747
Colace® [OTC] see Docusate 496
Colax-C® (Can) see Docusate 496
Colazal® see Balsalazide 179
ColBenemid see Colchicine and Probenecid 388
Colchicine 388
Colchicine and Probenecid 388
Colchiquim® (Mex) see Colchicine .. 388
Coldcough PD see Dihydrocodeine, Chlorpheniramine, and Phenylephrine 476
Coldtuss DR see Chlorpheniramine, Phenylephrine, and Dextromethorphan 326
Colesevelam 389
Colestid® see Colestipol 390
Colestipol 390
Colestipol Hydrochloride see Colestipol 390
CO Levetiracetam (Can) see Levetiracetam 908
Colgate Total® see Triclosan and Fluoride 1534
Colistimethate 390
Colistimethate Sodium see Colistimethate 390
CollaCote® see Collagen (Absorbable) 391
Collagen see Collagen Hemostat ...392
Collagen (Absorbable) 391
Collagen Absorbable Hemostat see Collagen Hemostat 392
Collagenase 391
Collagen Hemostat 392
CollaPlug® see Collagen (Absorbable) 391
CollaTape® see Collagen (Absorbable) 391
Colocort® see Hydrocortisone 793
CO Lovastatin (Can) see Lovastatin 953
Colufase® (Mex) see Nitazoxanide 1117
Coly-Mycin® M see Colistimethate .. 390
Colyte® see Polyethylene Glycol-Electrolyte Solution 1253
Combantrin™ (Can) see Pyrantel Pamoate 1314
Comb Flower see Echinacea 1620
CombiPatch® see Estradiol and Norethindrone 575
Combipres® [DSC] see Clonidine and Chlorthalidone 376
Combivent® see Ipratropium and Albuterol 857

Combivir® see Zidovudine and Lamivudine 1596
Combunox™ see Oxycodone and Ibuprofen 1170
CO Meloxicam (Can) see Meloxicam 977
Comhist® see Chlorpheniramine, Phenylephrine, and Phenyltoloxamine 328
CO Mirtazapine (Can) see Mirtazapine 1052
Commit™ [OTC] see Nicotine 1109
Compazine® (Can) see Prochlorperazine 1285
Comphor of the Poor see Garlic ..1622
Compound E see Cortisone 395
Compound F see Hydrocortisone ...793
Compound S see Zidovudine 1594
Compound S, Abacavir, and Lamivudine see Abacavir, Lamivudine, and Zidovudine 23
Compound W® One Step Wart Remover [OTC] see Salicylic Acid 1374
Compound W® [OTC] see Salicylic Acid 1374
Compoz® Nighttime Sleep Aid [OTC] see DiphenhydrAMINE ..483
Compro™ see Prochlorperazine ...1285
Comtan® see Entacapone 543
Comtrex® Flu Therapy Day/Night [OTC] see Acetaminophen, Chlorpheniramine, and Pseudoephedrine 43
Comtrex® Flu Th erapy Nighttime [OTC] see Acetaminophen, Chlorpheniramine, and Pseudoephedrine 43
Comtrex® Maximum Strength Sinus and Nasal Decongestant [OTC] [DSC] see Acetaminophen, Chlorpheniramine, and Pseudoephedrine 43
Comtrex® Non-Drowsy Cold and Cough Relief [OTC] see Acetaminophen, Dextromethorphan, and Pseudoephedrine 44
Comtrex® Sore Throat Maximum Strength [OTC] see Acetaminophen 31
Conazol® (Mex) see Ketoconazole .. 880
Conceptrol® [OTC] see Nonoxynol 9 1124
Concerta® see Methylphenidate ...1023
Condyline™ (Can) see Podofilox ..1251
Condylox® see Podofilox 1251
Congestac® [OTC] see Guaifenesin and Pseudoephedrine 755
Conivaptan 393
Conivaptan Hydrochloride see Conivaptan 393
Conjugated Estrogen and Methyltestosterone see Estrogens (Esterified) and Methyltestosterone 585
CO Norfloxacin (Can) see Norfloxacin 1126
Conray® see Iothalamate Meglumine 855
Conray® 30 see Iothalamate Meglumine 855
Conray® 43 see Iothalamate Meglumine 855
Conray® 400 see Iothalamate Sodium 855
Constulose® see Lactulose 893
Contac® Cold 12 Hour Relief Non Drowsy (Can) see Pseudoephedrine 1309

Contac® Cold and Sore Throat,
Non Drowsy, Extra Strength
(Can) see Acetaminophen and
Pseudoephedrine 38
Contac® Cold-Chest Congestion,
Non Drowsy, Regular Strength
(Can) see Guaifenesin and
Pseudoephedrine 755
Contac® Complete (Can) see
Acetaminophen,
Dextromethorphan, and
Pseudoephedrine 44
Contac® Cough, Cold and Flu Day
& Night™ (Can) see
Acetaminophen,
Dextromethorphan, and
Pseudoephedrine 44
Contac® Severe Cold and Flu/
Non-Drowsy [OTC] see
Acetaminophen,
Dextromethorphan, and
Pseudoephedrine 44
Contact® Cold [OTC] see
Pseudoephedrine 1309
Controlip® (Mex) see Fenofibrate . . . 639
ControlRx® see Fluoride 671
CO Paroxetine (Can) see
Paroxetine 1188
Copaxone® see Glatiramer Acetate
. . . . 736
Copegus® see Ribavirin 1343
Copolymer-1 see Glatiramer
Acetate 736
Copper see Trace Metals 1513
CO Pravastatin (Can) see
Pravastatin 1265
CoQ10 see Coenzyme Q10 1618
CO Ranitidine (Can) see Ranitidine
. . . . 1334
Cordarone® see Amiodarone 90
Cordran® see Flurandrenolide 681
Cordran® SP see Flurandrenolide . . 681
Cordron-D NR see Carbinoxamine
and Pseudoephedrine 268
Cordron-DM NR see
Carbinoxamine,
Pseudoephedrine, and
Dextromethorphan 269
Coreg® see Carvedilol 275
Corfen DM see Chlorpheniramine,
Phenylephrine, and
Dextromethorphan 326
Corgard® see Nadolol 1079
Coricidin HBP® Chest Congestion
and Cough [OTC] see
Guaifenesin and
Dextromethorphan 754
Coricidin HBP® Cold and Flu
[OTC] see Chlorpheniramine
and Acetaminophen 324
Corlopam® see Fenoldopam 641
Cormax® see Clobetasol 365
Coronex® (Can) see Isosorbide
Dinitrate 866
Corotrend® (Mex) see NIFEdipine
. . . . 1112
Correctol® Tablets [OTC] see
Bisacodyl 209
Cortaid® Intensive Therapy [OTC]
see Hydrocortisone 793
Cortaid® Maximum Strength [OTC]
see Hydrocortisone 793
Cortaid® Sensitive Skin [OTC] see
Hydrocortisone 793
Cortamed® (Can) see
Hydrocortisone 793
Cortef® see Hydrocortisone 793
Cortenema® (Can) see
Hydrocortisone 793
Corticool® [OTC] see
Hydrocortisone 793

Corticotropin 395
Corticotropin, Repository see
Corticotropin 395
Cortifoam® see Hydrocortisone 793
Cortimyxin® (Can) see Neomycin,
Polymyxin B, and
Hydrocortisone 1101
Cortisol see Hydrocortisone 793
Cortisone 395
Cortisone Acetate see Cortisone . . . 395
Cortisporin® Cream see Neomycin,
Polymyxin B, and
Hydrocortisone 1101
Cortisporin® Ointment see
Bacitracin, Neomycin,
Polymyxin B, and
Hydrocortisone 177
Cortisporin® Ophthalmic see
Neomycin, Polymyxin B, and
Hydrocortisone 1101
Cortisporin® Otic see Neomycin,
Polymyxin B, and
Hydrocortisone 1101
Cortisporin® Topical Ointment
(Can) see Bacitracin,
Neomycin, Polymyxin B, and
Hydrocortisone 177
Cortizone®-10 Maximum Strength
[OTC] see Hydrocortisone 793
Cortizone®-10 Plus Maximum
Strength [OTC] see
Hydrocortisone 793
Cortizone®-10 Quick Shot [OTC]
see Hydrocortisone 793
Cortrosyn® see Cosyntropin 396
Corvert® see Ibutilide 813
Coryphen® Codeine (Can) see
Aspirin and Codeine 149
Corzide® see Nadolol and
Bendroflumethiazide 1080
CO Simvastatin (Can) see
Simvastatin 1394
Cosmegen® see Dactinomycin 417
Cosopt® see Dorzolamide and
Timolol 501
CO Sotalol (Can) see Sotalol 1409
CO Sumatriptan (Can) see
Sumatriptan 1432
Cosyntropin 396
Cotazym® (Can) see Pancrelipase
. . . . 1183
CO Temazepam (Can) see
Temazepam 1453
CO Terbinafine (Can) see
Terbinafine 1459
Co-Trimoxazole see
Sulfamethoxazole and
Trimethoprim 1425
Coumadin® see Warfarin 1585
Covan® (Can) see Triprolidine,
Pseudoephedrine, and
Codeine 1543
Covera® (Can) see Verapamil 1571
Covera-HS® see Verapamil 1571
Coversyl® (Can) see Perindopril
Erbumine 1216
Co-Vidarabine see Pentostatin 1211
Coviracil see Emtricitabine 536
Cozaar® see Losartan 950
CO Zopiclone (Can) see Zopiclone
. . . . 1606
CP-99,219-27 see Trovafloxacin . . 1546
CP358774 see Erlotinib 560
CPC see Cetylpyridinium 309
C-Phed Tannate see
Chlorpheniramine and
Pseudoephedrine 325
CPM see Cyclophosphamide 403
CPT-11 see Irinotecan 860
CPZ see ChlorproMAZINE 329
Cranberry 1619

Crantex ER see Guaifenesin and
    Phenylephrine 754
Crantex HC see Hydrocodone,
    Phenylephrine, and
    Guaifenesin 791
Crantex LA see Guaifenesin and
    Phenylephrine 754
Crataegus laevigata see Hawthorn
    1626
Crataegus monogyna see
    Hawthorn 1626
Crataegus oxyacantha see
    Hawthorn 1626
Crataegus pinnatifida see
    Hawthorn 1626
Creatine 1619
Credaxol® (Mex) see Ranitidine . . . 1334
Crema Blanca® (Mex) see
    Hydroquinone 798
Cremosan® (Mex) see
    Ketoconazole 880
Creomulsion® Cough [OTC] see
    Dextromethorphan 451
Creomulsion® for Children [OTC]
    see Dextromethorphan 451
Creon® (Mex) see Pancreatin 1183
Creon® 5 (Can) see Pancrelipase
    1183
Creon® 10 (Can) see Pancrelipase
    1183
Creon® 20 (Can) see Pancrelipase
    1183
Creon® 25 (Can) see Pancrelipase
    1183
Creo-Terpin® [OTC] see
    Dextromethorphan 451
Crestor® see Rosuvastatin 1370
Cresylate® see m-Cresyl Acetate . . . 966
Crinone® see Progesterone 1289
Critic-Aid Skin Care® [OTC] see
    Zinc Oxide 1597
Crixivan® see Indinavir 829
Crolom® see Cromolyn 397
Cromoglycic Acid see Cromolyn 397
Cromolyn 397
Cromolyn Sodium see Cromolyn . . . 397
Cronovera® (Mex) see Verapamil . . 1571
Crosseal™ see Fibrin Sealant Kit . . . 653
Crotamiton 398
Crude Coal Tar see Coal Tar 383
Cruex® Cream [OTC] see
    Clotrimazole 379
Cryoperacid® (Mex) see
    Loperamide 942
Cryopril® (Mex) see Captopril 257
Cryoval®[caps] (Mex) see Valproic
    Acid and Derivatives 1556
Cryselle™ see Ethinyl Estradiol and
    Norgestrel 616
Crystalline Penicillin see Penicillin
    G (Parenteral/Aqueous) 1203
Crystal Violet see Gentian Violet . . . 735
Crystodigin see Digitoxin 471
CsA see CycloSPORINE 406
CSP see Cellulose Sodium
    Phosphate 301
CTLA-4Ig see Abatacept 25
CTM see Chlorpheniramine 323
CTX see Cyclophosphamide 403
Cubicin® see Daptomycin 423
Culturelle® [OTC] see Lactobacillus
    535
Cuprimine® see Penicillamine 1201
Curasore® [OTC] see Pramoxine . . . 1264
Curcuma longa see Turmeric 1632
Curosurf® see Poractant Alfa 1255
Cutaclin® (Mex) see Clindamycin . . . 361
Cutar® [OTC] see Coal Tar 383
Cutivate® see Fluticasone 686
CyA see CycloSPORINE 406
Cyanocobalamin 399
Cyanocobalamin, Folic Acid, and
    Pyridoxine see Folic Acid,
    Cyanocobalamin, and
    Pyridoxine 697
Cyclen® (Can) see Ethinyl
    Estradiol and Norgestimate 613
Cyclessa® see Ethinyl Estradiol
    and Desogestrel 592
Cyclizine 400
Cyclizine Hydrochloride see
    Cyclizine 400
Cyclizine Lactate see Cyclizine 400
Cyclobenzaprine 401
Cyclobenzaprine Hydrochloride see
    Cyclobenzaprine 401
Cyclocort® see Amcinonide 83
Cyclogyl® see Cyclopentolate 402
Cyclomen® (Can) see Danazol 419
Cyclomydril® see Cyclopentolate
    and Phenylephrine 403
Cyclopentolate 402
Cyclopentolate and Phenylephrine . . 403
Cyclopentolate Hydrochloride see
    Cyclopentolate 402
Cyclophosphamide 403
CycloSERINE 405
Cyclosporin A see CycloSPORINE . . 406
CycloSPORINE 406
Cyklokapron® see Tranexamic Acid
    1518
Cylate® see Cyclopentolate 402
Cylert® [DSC] see Pemoline 1199
Cylex® [OTC] see Benzocaine 190
Cymbalta® see Duloxetine 523
Cymevene® (Mex) see Ganciclovir . . 722
Cyproheptadine 412
Cyproheptadine Hydrochloride see
    Cyproheptadine 412
Cystadane® see Betaine
    Anhydrous 199
Cystagon® see Cysteamine 412
Cysteamine 412
Cysteamine Bitartrate see
    Cysteamine 412
Cysteine 412
Cysteine Hydrochloride see
    Cysteine 412
Cystistat® (Can) see Hyaluronate
    and Derivatives 773
Cysto-Conray® II see Iothalamate
    Meglumine 855
Cystografin® see Diatrizoate
    Meglumine 453
Cystografin® Dilute see Diatrizoate
    Meglumine 453
Cystospaz® see Hyoscyamine 803
Cystospaz-M® [DSC] see
    Hyoscyamine 803
CYT see Cyclophosphamide 403
Cytadren® see Aminoglutethimide . . . 87
Cytarabine 413
Cytarabine Hydrochloride see
    Cytarabine 413
Cytarabine (Liposomal) 414
Cytomel® see Liothyronine 934
Cytosar® (Can) see Cytarabine 413
Cytosar-U® see Cytarabine 413
Cytosine Arabinosine
    Hydrochloride see Cytarabine . . . 413
Cytotec® see Misoprostol 1053
Cytovene® see Ganciclovir 722
Cytoxan® see Cyclophosphamide . . 403
Cytra-2 see Sodium Citrate and
    Citric Acid 1401
Cytra-3 see Citric Acid, Sodium
    Citrate, and Potassium Citrate . . 354
Cytra-K see Potassium Citrate and
    Citric Acid 1259
Cēpacol® Dual Action Maximum
    Strength [OTC] see Dyclonine . . 525
D2E7 see Adalimumab 52

D₃ see Cholecalciferol 334
D-3-Mercaptovaline see
    Penicillamine 1201
d4T see Stavudine 1416
D₅W see Dextrose 452
D₁₀W see Dextrose 452
D₂₅W see Dextrose 452
D₃₀W see Dextrose 452
D₄₀W see Dextrose 452
D₅₀W see Dextrose 452
D₆₀W see Dextrose 452
D₇₀W see Dextrose 452
DAB₃₈₉IL-2 see Denileukin Diftitox . . 432
Dabex® (Mex) see Metformin 1001
Dacarbazine 415
Dacex-DM see Guaifenesin,
    Dextromethorphan, and
    Phenylephrine 756
Daclizumab 416
DACT see Dactinomycin 417
Dactinomycin 417
DAD see Mitoxantrone 1055
Dairyaid® (Can) see Lactase 892
Dakin's Solution see Sodium
    Hypochlorite Solution 1402
Daktarin® (Mex) see Miconazole . . 1039
Dalacin V® (Mex) see Clindamycin . . 361
Dalacin® C (Can) see Clindamycin . . 361
Dalacin® T (Can) see Clindamycin . . 361
Dalacin® Vaginal (Can) see
    Clindamycin 361
Dalisol® (Mex) see Leucovorin 905
Dallergy® see Chlorpheniramine,
    Phenylephrine, and
    Methscopolamine 327
Dallergy-JR® see Chlorpheniramine
    and Phenylephrine 324
Dalmane® see Flurazepam 681
d-Alpha-Gems™ [OTC] see Vitamin
    E 1581
d-Alpha Tocopherol see Vitamin E
    1581
Dalteparin 418
Damason-P® see Hydrocodone
    and Aspirin 782
Danaparoid 418
Danaparoid Sodium see
    Danaparoid 418
Danazol 419
Danocrine® (Can) see Danazol 419
Danocrine® [DSC] see Danazol 419
Dantrium® see Dantrolene 420
Dantrolene 420
Dantrolene Sodium see Dantrolene
    420
Daonil® (Mex) see GlyBURIDE 744
Dapcin see Daptomycin 423
Dapiprazole 421
Dapiprazole Hydrochloride see
    Dapiprazole 421
Dapsone 421
Daptomycin 423
Daranide® see Dichlorphenamide . . 459
Daraprim® see Pyrimethamine 1317
Darbepoetin Alfa 423
Darifenacin 424
Darifenacin Hydrobromide see
    Darifenacin 424
Darvocet A500™ see
    Propoxyphene and
    Acetaminophen 1298
Darvocet-N® 50 see Propoxyphene
    and Acetaminophen 1298
Darvocet-N® 100 see
    Propoxyphene and
    Acetaminophen 1298
Darvon® see Propoxyphene 1297
Darvon® Compound [DSC] see
    Propoxyphene, Aspirin, and
    Caffeine 1300
Darvon-N® see Propoxyphene 1297

Datril® (Mex) see Acetaminophen . . . 31
Daunomycin see DAUNOrubicin
    Hydrochloride 426
DAUNOrubicin Citrate (Liposomal) . . 425
DAUNOrubicin Hydrochloride 426
DaunoXome® see DAUNOrubicin
    Citrate (Liposomal) 425
DAVA see Vindesine 1577
Dayhist® Allergy [OTC] see
    Clemastine 359
1-Day™ [OTC] see Tioconazole . . . 1493
Daypro® see Oxaprozin 1155
Daytrana™ see Methylphenidate . . 1023
dCF see Pentostatin 1211
DDAVP® see Desmopressin 437
ddC see Zalcitabine 1590
ddI see Didanosine 465
Deacetyl Vinblastine Carboxamide
    see Vindesine 1577
1-Deamino-8-D-Arginine
    Vasopressin see
    Desmopressin 437
Debacterol® see Sulfonated
    Phenolics in Aqueous Solution
    1429
Debrox® [OTC] see Carbamide
    Peroxide 264
Decadron® see Dexamethasone . . . 439
Decadronal® (Mex) see
    Dexamethasone 439
Decadron® (Mex) see
    Dexamethasone 439
Decadron® Phosphate [DSC] see
    Dexamethasone 439
Deca-Durabolin® (Can) see
    Nandrolone 1087
Decahist-DM see Carbinoxamine,
    Pseudoephedrine, and
    Dextromethorphan 269
Decapinol® see Delmopinol 430
De-Chlor DM see
    Chlorpheniramine,
    Phenylephrine, and
    Dextromethorphan 326
De-Chlor DR see
    Chlorpheniramine,
    Phenylephrine, and
    Dextromethorphan 326
De-Chlor G see Hydrocodone,
    Phenylephrine, and
    Guaifenesin 791
Declomycin® see Demeclocycline . . 431
Deconamine® see
    Chlorpheniramine and
    Pseudoephedrine 325
Deconamine® SR see
    Chlorpheniramine and
    Pseudoephedrine 325
Deconsal® II see Guaifenesin and
    Phenylephrine 754
Deep Sea [OTC] see Sodium
    Chloride 1400
Deferasirox 427
Deferoxamine 428
Deferoxamine Mesylate see
    Deferoxamine 428
Dehistine see Chlorpheniramine,
    Phenylephrine, and
    Methscopolamine 327
Dehydral® (Can) see Methenamine
    1007
Dehydrobenzperidol® (Mex) see
    Droperidol 519
Dehydroepiandrosterone 1619
Del Aqua® see Benzoyl Peroxide . . . 194
Delatestryl® see Testosterone 1462
Delavirdine 429
Delestrogen® see Estradiol 574
Delfen® [OTC] see Nonoxynol 9 . . . 1124
Delmopinol 430

Delmopinol Hydrochloride see
  Delmopinol 430
Delsym® [OTC] see
  Dextromethorphan 451
Delta-9-tetrahydro-cannabinol see
  Dronabinol 518
Delta-9-Tetrahydrocannabinol and
  Cannabinol see
  Tetrahydrocannabinol and
  Cannabidiol 1469
Delta-9 THC see Dronabinol 518
Delta-D® see Cholecalciferol 334
Deltacortisone see PredniSONE . . 1271
Deltadehydrocortisone see
  PredniSONE 1271
Deltahydrocortisone see
  PrednisoLONE 1268
Demadex® see Torsemide 1512
Demeclocycline 431
Demeclocycline Hydrochloride see
  Demeclocycline 431
Demerol® see Meperidine 983
4-Demethoxydaunorubicin see
  Idarubicin 814
Demethylchlortetracycline see
  Demeclocycline 431
Demser® see Metyrosine 1036
Demulen® see Ethinyl Estradiol
  and Ethynodiol Diacetate 597
Demulen® 30 (Can) see Ethinyl
  Estradiol and Ethynodiol
  Diacetate 597
Denavir® see Penciclovir 1200
Denileukin Diftitox 432
Denorex® Original Therapeutic
  Strength [OTC] see Coal Tar . . 383
Denta 5000 Plus see Fluoride 671
DentaGel see Fluoride 671
Dentapaine [OTC] see Benzocaine
  190
DentiPatch® see Lidocaine
  (Transoral) 931
Dent's Ear Wax [OTC] see
  Carbamide Peroxide 264
Dent's Extra Strength Toothache
  [OTC] see Benzocaine 190
Dent's Maxi-Strength Toothache
  [OTC] see Benzocaine 190
Denvar® (Mex) see Cefixime 287
Deoxycoformycin see Pentostatin . . 1211
2'-Deoxycoformycin see
  Pentostatin 1211
Depacon® see Valproic Acid and
  Derivatives 1556
Depade® see Naltrexone 1086
Depakene® see Valproic Acid and
  Derivatives 1556
Depakote® Delayed Release see
  Valproic Acid and Derivatives . . 1556
Depakote® ER see Valproic Acid
  and Derivatives 1556
Depakote® Sprinkle® see Valproic
  Acid and Derivatives 1556
Depen® see Penicillamine 1201
DepoCyt™ see Cytarabine
  (Liposomal) 414
DepoDur™ see Morphine Sulfate . . 1065
Depo®-Estradiol see Estradiol 574
Depo-Medrol® see
  MethylPREDNISolone 1025
Depo-Prevera® (Can) see
  MedroxyPROGESTERone 972
Depo-Provera® see
  MedroxyPROGESTERone 972
Depo-Provera® Contraceptive see
  MedroxyPROGESTERone 972
depo-subQ provera 104™ see
  MedroxyPROGESTERone 972
Depotest® 100 (Can) see
  Testosterone 1462

Depo®-Testosterone see
  Testosterone 1462
De prenyl see Selegiline 1382
DermaFungal [OTC] see
  Miconazole 1039
Dermagran® AF [OTC] see
  Miconazole 1039
Dermagran® [OTC] see Aluminum
  Hydroxide 79
Derma Keri® (Mex) see Urea 1551
Dermalog® (Mex) see Halcinonide . . 760
Dermamycin® [OTC] see
  DiphenhydrAMINE 483
Dermarest Dricort® [OTC] see
  Hydrocortisone 793
Dermarest® Insect Bite [OTC] see
  DiphenhydrAMINE 483
Dermarest® Plus [OTC] see
  DiphenhydrAMINE 483
Dermarest® Skin Correction Cream
  Plus [OTC] see Hydroquinone . . 798
Derma-Smoothe/FS® see
  Fluocinolone 667
Dermatop® see Prednicarbate 1268
Dermazene® see Iodoquinol and
  Hydrocortisone 853
DermaZinc™ [OTC] see Pyrithione
  Zinc 1318
Dermazole (Can) see Miconazole
  1039
Dermifun® (Mex) see Miconazole . . 1039
Dermoplast® (Mex) see Urea 1551
Dermoplast® Antibacterial [OTC]
  see Benzocaine 190
Dermoplast® Pain Relieving [OTC]
  see Benzocaine 190
Dermovate® (Can) see Clobetasol . . 365
Dermox® (Mex) see Methoxsalen . . 1018
Dermtex® HC [OTC] see
  Hydrocortisone 793
Desacetyl Vinblastine Amide
  Sulfate see Vindesine 1577
Desferal® see Deferoxamine 428
Desiccated Thyroid see Thyroid . . . 1482
Desipramine 434
Desipramine Hydrochloride see
  Desipramine 434
Desitin® Creamy [OTC] see Zinc
  Oxide 1597
Desitin® [OTC] see Zinc Oxide 1597
Desloratadine 435
Desloratadine and
  Pseudoephedrine 436
Desmethylimipramine
  Hydrochloride see Desipramine
  434
Desmopressin 437
Desmopressin Acetate see
  Desmopressin 437
Desocort® (Can) see Desonide . . . 437
Desogen® see Ethinyl Estradiol
  and Desogestrel 592
Desogestrel and Ethinyl Estradiol
  see Ethinyl Estradiol and
  Desogestrel 592
Desonide 437
DesOwen® see Desonide 437
Desoximetasone 438
Desoxyephedrine Hydrochloride
  see Methamphetamine 1005
Desoxyn® see Methamphetamine
  1005
Desoxyphenobarbital see
  Primidone 1281
Desparasil® (Mex) see Piperazine
  1246
Desquam-X® see Benzoyl Peroxide
  194
Desquam-E™ see Benzoyl
  Peroxide 194
Desyrel® see Trazodone 1521

Detane® [OTC] see Benzocaine 190
Detemir Insulin see Insulin Detemir
.... 836
Detrol® see Tolterodine 1506
Detrol® LA see Tolterodine 1506
Detrusitol® (Mex) see Tolterodine .. 1506
Devil's Claw 1619
Dex4® Glucose [OTC] see
  Dextrose 452
Dexagrin® (Mex) see
  Dexamethasone 439
Dexalone® [OTC] see
  Dextromethorphan 451
Dexamethasone 439
Dexamethasone and Ciprofloxacin
  see Ciprofloxacin and
  Dexamethasone 348
Dexamethasone and Tobramycin
  see Tobramycin and
  Dexamethasone 1499
Dexamethasone Intensol® see
  Dexamethasone 439
Dexamethasone, Neomycin, and
  Polymyxin B see Neomycin,
  Polymyxin B, and
  Dexamethasone 1101
Dexamethasone Sodium
  Phosphate see
  Dexamethasone 439
Dexasone® (Can) see
  Dexamethasone 439
Dexbrompheniramine and
  Pseudoephedrine 442
Dexchlorpheniramine 443
Dexchlorpheniramine and
  Pseudoephedrine 443
Dexchlorpheniramine Maleate see
  Dexchlorpheniramine 443
Dexcon-DM see Guaifenesin,
  Dextromethorphan, and
  Phenylephrine 756
Dexcon-PE see Guaifenesin,
  Dextromethorphan, and
  Phenylephrine 756
Dexedrine® see
  Dextroamphetamine 447
Dexferrum® see Iron Dextran
  Complex 862
Dexiron™ (Can) see Iron Dextran
  Complex 862
Dexmedetomidine 444
Dexmedetomidine Hydrochloride
  see Dexmedetomidine 444
Dexmethylphenidate 445
Dexmethylphenidate Hydrochloride
  see Dexmethylphenidate 445
DexPak® TaperPak® see
  Dexamethasone 439
Dexpanthenol 446
Dex PC see Chlorpheniramine,
  Phenylephrine, and
  Dextromethorphan 326
Dexrazoxane 446
Dextran 447
Dextran 1 447
Dextran 40 see Dextran 447
Dextran 70 see Dextran 447
Dextran, High Molecular Weight
  see Dextran 447
Dextran, Low Molecular Weight
  see Dextran 447
Dextroamphetamine 447
Dextroamphetamine and
  Amphetamine 448
Dextroamphetamine Sulfate see
  Dextroamphetamine 447
Dextromethorphan 451

Dextromethorphan,
  Acetaminophen, and
  Pseudoephedrine see
  Acetaminophen,
  Dextromethorphan, and
  Pseudoephedrine 44
Dextromethorphan and
  Guaifenesin see Guaifenesin
  and Dextromethorphan 754
Dextromethorphan and
  Promethazine see
  Promethazine and
  Dextromethorphan 1292
Dextromethorphan and
  Pseudoephedrine see
  Pseudoephedrine and
  Dextromethorphan 1311
Dextromethorphan, Carbinoxamine,
  and Pseudoephedrine see
  Carbinoxamine,
  Pseudoephedrine, and
  Dextromethorphan 269
Dextromethorphan,
  Chlorpheniramine, and
  Phenylephrine see
  Chlorpheniramine,
  Phenylephrine, and
  Dextromethorphan 326
Dextromethorphan, Guaifenesin,
  and Pseudoephedrine see
  Guaifenesin, Pseudoephedrine,
  and Dextromethorphan 757
Dextromethorphan,
  Pseudoephedrine, and
  Carbinoxamine see
  Carbinoxamine,
  Pseudoephedrine, and
  Dextromethorphan 269
Dextropropoxyphene see
  Propoxyphene 1297
Dextrose........................ 452
Dextrose and Tetracaine see
  Tetracaine and Dextrose 1467
Dextrose, Levulose and
  Phosphoric Acid see Fructose,
  Dextrose, and Phosphoric Acid
  713
Dextrose Monohydrate see
  Dextrose 452
Dextrostat® see
  Dextroamphetamine 447
DFMO see Eflornithine 532
DHA see Docosahexaenoic Acid .. 1620
DHAD see Mitoxantrone......... 1055
DHAQ see Mitoxantrone......... 1055
DHE see Dihydroergotamine 477
D.H.E. 45® see Dihydroergotamine
  477
DHEA see
  Dehydroepiandrosterone 1619
DHPG Sodium see Ganciclovir 722
DHS™ Sal [OTC] see Salicylic Acid
  1374
DHS™ Targel [OTC] see Coal Tar .. 383
DHS™ Tar [OTC] see Coal Tar 383
DHS™ Zinc [OTC] see Pyrithione
  Zinc 1318
DHT™ [DSC] see
  Dihydrotachysterol 478
DHT™ Intensol™ [DSC] see
  Dihydrotachysterol 478
Diabeta see GlyBURIDE 744
DiabetAid™ Antifungal Foot Bath
  [OTC] see Miconazole 1039
DiabetAid Gingivitis Mouth Rinse
  [OTC] see Cetylpyridinium 309
Diabetic Tussin C® see
  Guaifenesin and Codeine...... 753
Diabetic Tussin® Allergy Relief
  [OTC] see Chlorpheniramine ... 323

Diabetic Tussin® DM Maximum Strength [OTC] see Guaifenesin and Dextromethorphan 754
Diabetic Tussin® DM [OTC] see Guaifenesin and Dextromethorphan 754
Diabetic Tussin® EX [OTC] see Guaifenesin 752
Diabinese® see ChlorproPAMIDE . . . 331
DiaBeta® see GlyBURIDE 744
Diamicron® (Can) see Gliclazide . . . 737
Diamicron® MR (Can) see Gliclazide 737
Diaminocyclohexane Oxalatoplatinum see Oxaliplatin 1154
Diaminodiphenylsulfone see Dapsone 421
Diamode [OTC] see Loperamide . . . 942
Diamox® (Can) see AcetaZOLAMIDE 45
Diamox® Sequels® see AcetaZOLAMIDE 45
Diarr-Eze (Can) see Loperamide . . . 942
Diasorb® [OTC] see Attapulgite 165
Diastat® see Diazepam 454
Diastat® AcuDial™ see Diazepam . . 454
Diastat® Rectal Delivery System (Can) see Diazepam 454
Diatrizoate Meglumine 453
Diatrizoate Meglumine and Diatrizoate Sodium 453
Diatrizoate Meglumine and Iodipamide Meglumine 453
Diatrizoate Sodium 454
Diatrizoate Sodium and Diatrizoate Meglumine see Diatrizoate Meglumine and Diatrizoate Sodium 453
Diatx™ see Vitamin B Complex Combinations 1581
DiatxFe™ see Vitamin B Complex Combinations 1581
Diaval® (Mex) see TOLBUTamide 1502
Diazemuls® (Can) see Diazepam . . 454
Diazepam 454
Diazepam Intensol® see Diazepam 454
Diazoxide 457
Dibasona® (Mex) see Dexamethasone 439
Dibenzyline® see Phenoxybenzamine 1224
Dibucaine 458
DIC see Dacarbazine 415
Dichloralphenazone, Acetaminophen, and Isometheptene see Acetaminophen, Isometheptene, and Dichloralphenazone 44
Dichloralphenazone, Isometheptene, and Acetaminophen see Acetaminophen, Isometheptene, and Dichloralphenazone 44
6,7-Dichloro-1,5-Dihydroimidazo [2,1b] quinazolin-2(3H)-one Monohydrochloride see Anagrelide 124
Dichlorodifluoromethane and Trichloromonofluoromethane . . . 458
Dichlorotetrafluoroethane and Ethyl Chloride see Ethyl Chloride and Dichlorotetrafluoroethane . . 620
Dichlorphenamide 459
Dichysterol see Dihydrotachysterol . . 478
Diclofenac 459
Diclofenac and Misoprostol 462
Diclofenac Potassium see Diclofenac 459
Diclofenac Sodium see Diclofenac . . 459
Diclofenamide see Dichlorphenamide 459
Diclotride® (Mex) see Hydrochlorothiazide 776
Dicloxacillin 463
Dicloxacillin Sodium see Dicloxacillin 463
Dicyclomine 464
Dicyclomine Hydrochloride see Dicyclomine 464
Dicycloverine Hydrochloride see Dicyclomine 464
Di-Dak-Sol see Sodium Hypochlorite Solution 1402
Didanosine 465
Dideoxycytidine see Zalcitabine . . . 1590
Dideoxyinosine see Didanosine 465
Didrex® see Benzphetamine 195
Didrocal™ (Can) see Etidronate and Calcium 620
Didronel® see Etidronate Disodium 621
Diethylene Triamine Penta-Acetic Acid 466
Diethylpropion 467
Diethylpropion Hydrochloride see Diethylpropion 467
Difenoxin and Atropine 467
Differin® see Adapalene 54
Differin® XP (Can) see Adapalene . . 54
Diflorasone 468
Diflorasone Diacetate see Diflorasone 468
Diflucan® see Fluconazole 659
Diflunisal 468
Difoxacil® (Mex) see Norfloxacin . . 1126
Digezanol® (Mex) see Albendazole 57
Digibind® see Digoxin Immune Fab 474
DigiFab™ see Digoxin Immune Fab 474
Digital HD see Barium 179
Digitek® see Digoxin 471
Digitoxin 471
Digoxin 471
Digoxin CSD (Can) see Digoxin 471
Digoxin Immune Fab 474
Dihematoporphyrin Ether see Porfimer 1256
Dihistine® DH see Chlorpheniramine, Pseudoephedrine, and Codeine 329
Dihydrocodeine, Aspirin, and Caffeine 475
Dihydrocodeine Bitartrate, Acetaminophen, and Caffeine see Acetaminophen, Caffeine, and Dihydrocodeine 42
Dihydrocodeine Bitartrate, Pseudoephedrine Hydrochloride, and Chlorpheniramine Maleate see Pseudoephedrine, Dihydrocodeine, and Chlorpheniramine 1312
Dihydrocodeine, Chlorpheniramine, and Phenylephrine 476
Dihydrocodeine Compound see Dihydrocodeine, Aspirin, and Caffeine 475
Dihydrocodeine, Pseudoephedrine, and Guaifenesin 476
DiHydro-CP see Pseudoephedrine, Dihydrocodeine, and Chlorpheniramine 1312

Dihydroergotamine 477
Dihydroergotamine Mesylate see
    Dihydroergotamine 477
Dihydroergotoxine see Ergoloid
    Mesylates 557
Dihydrogenated Ergot Alkaloids
    see Ergoloid Mesylates 557
DiHydro-GP see Dihydrocodeine,
    Pseudoephedrine, and
    Guaifenesin 476
Dihydrohydroxycodeinone see
    Oxycodone 1163
Dihydromorphinone see
    Hydromorphone 797
Dihydrotachysterol 478
Dihydroxyanthracenedione
    Dihydrochloride see
    Mitoxantrone 1055
1,25 Dihydroxycholecalciferol see
    Calcitriol 247
Dihydroxydeoxynorvinkaleukoblastine
    see Vinorelbine 1578
Dihydroxypropyl Theophylline see
    Dyphylline 526
Diiodohydroxyquin see Iodoquinol . . 853
Dilacoran® (Mex) see Verapamil . . 1571
Dilacor® XR see Diltiazem 479
Dilantin® see Phenytoin 1228
Dilatrate®-SR see Isosorbide
    Dinitrate 866
Dilatrend® (Mex) see Carvedilol . . . 275
Dilaudid® see Hydromorphone 797
Dilaudid-HP® see Hydromorphone . . 797
Dilaudid-HP-Plus® (Can) see
    Hydromorphone 797
Dilaudid® Sterile Powder (Can) see
    Hydromorphone 797
Dilaudid-XP® (Can) see
    Hydromorphone 797
Dilor® see Dyphylline 526
Diltia XT® see Diltiazem 479
Diltiazem 479
Diltiazem HCl ER® (Can) see
    Diltiazem 479
Diltiazem Hydrochloride see
    Diltiazem 479
Diltiazem Hydrochloride Injection
    (Can) see Diltiazem 479
Dimefor® (Mex) see Metformin 1001
DimenhyDRINATE 481
Dimercaprol 482
Dimetapp® 12-Hour Non-Drowsy
    Extentabs® [OTC] see
    Pseudoephedrine 1309
Dimetapp® Cold and Congestion
    [OTC] see Guaifenesin,
    Pseudoephedrine, and
    Dextromethorphan 757
Dimetapp® Decongestant Infant
    [OTC] see Pseudoephedrine . . 1309
Dimetapp® Infant Decongestant
    Plus Cough [OTC] see
    Pseudoephedrine and
    Dextromethorphan 1311
β,β-Dimethylcysteine see
    Penicillamine 1201
Dimethyl Sulfone see Methyl
    Sulfonyl Methane 1629
Dimethyl Triazeno Imidazole
    Carboxamide see Dacarbazine
    415
Dinate® (Can) see
    DimenhyDRINATE 481
Dinoprostone 482
Diocaine® (Can) see Proparacaine
    1296
Diocarpine (Can) see Pilocarpine
    (Ophthalmic) 1234
Diochloram® (Can) see
    Chloramphenicol 314

Diocto C® [DSC] [OTC] see
    Docusate and Casanthranol 496
Diocto® [OTC] see Docusate 496
Dioctyl Calcium Sulfosuccinate see
    Docusate 496
Dioctyl Sodium Sulfosuccinate see
    Docusate 496
Diodex® (Can) see
    Dexamethasone 439
Diodoquin® (Can) see Iodoquinol . . 853
Diogent® (Can) see Gentamicin . . . 734
Diomycin® (Can) see Erythromycin
    562
Dionephrine® (Can) see
    Phenylephrine 1226
Diopentolate® (Can) see
    Cyclopentolate 402
Diopred® (Can) see PrednisoLONE
    1268
Dioptic's Atropine Solution (Can)
    see Atropine 161
Dioptimyd® (Can) see
    Sulfacetamide and
    Prednisolone 1424
Dioptrol® (Can) see Neomycin,
    Polymyxin B, and
    Dexamethasone 1101
Dioscorea villosa see Wild Yam . . 1634
Diosulf™ (Can) see Sulfacetamide
    1423
Diotame® [OTC] see Bismuth 210
Diotrope® (Can) see Tropicamide . . 1545
Diovan® see Valsartan 1561
Diovan HCT® see Valsartan and
    Hydrochlorothiazide 1562
Diovol® (Can) see Aluminum
    Hydroxide and Magnesium
    Hydroxide 80
Diovol® Ex (Can) see Aluminum
    Hydroxide and Magnesium
    Hydroxide 80
Diovol Plus® (Can) see Aluminum
    Hydroxide, Magnesium
    Hydroxide, and Simethicone 81
Dipentum® see Olsalazine 1144
Diphen® AF [OTC] see
    DiphenhydrAMINE 483
Diphenhist [OTC] see
    DiphenhydrAMINE 483
DiphenhydrAMINE 483
Diphenhydramine and
    Acetaminophen see
    Acetaminophen and
    Diphenhydramine 38
Diphenhydramine and
    Pseudoephedrine 487
Diphenhydramine Citrate see
    DiphenhydrAMINE 483
Diphenhydramine Hydrochloride
    see DiphenhydrAMINE 483
Diphenhydramine, Hydrocodone,
    and Phenylephrine see
    Hydrocodone, Phenylephrine,
    and Diphenhydramine 791
Diphenhydramine Tannate see
    DiphenhydrAMINE 483
Diphen® [OTC] see
    DiphenhydrAMINE 483
Diphenoxylate and Atropine 487
Diphenylhydantoin see Phenytoin . . 1228
Diphtheria and Tetanus Toxoids
    and Acellular Pertussis
    Adsorbed, Hepatitis B
    (Recombinant) and Inactivated
    Poliovirus Vaccine Combined
    see Diphtheria, Tetanus
    Toxoids, Acellular Pertussis,
    Hepatitis B (Recombinant), and
    Poliovirus (Inactivated) Vaccine
    488

Diphtheria CRM₁₉₇ Protein see Pneumococcal Conjugate Vaccine (7-Valent) 1250
Diphtheria CRM₁₉₇ Protein Conjugate see Haemophilus b Conjugate Vaccine 534
Diphtheria, Tetanus Toxoids, Acellular Pertussis, Hepatitis B (Recombinant), and Poliovirus (Inactivated) Vaccine 488
Diphtheria Toxoid Conjugate see Haemophilus b Conjugate Vaccine 534
Dipivalyl Epinephrine see Dipivefrin 489
Dipivefrin 489
Dipivefrin Hydrochloride see Dipivefrin 489
Diprivan® see Propofol 1296
Diprolene® see Betamethasone . . 199
Diprolene® AF see Betamethasone 199
Diprolene® Glycol (Can) see Betamethasone 199
Dipropylacetic Acid see Valproic Acid and Derivatives 1556
Diprosone® (Can) see Betamethasone 199
Dipyridamole 489
Dipyridamole and Aspirin see Aspirin and Dipyridamole . . . 150
Dirithromycin 490
Disalicylic Acid see Salsalate . . . 1376
Disodium Cromoglycate see Cromolyn 397
Disodium Thiosulfate Pentahydrate see Sodium Thiosulfate 1404
d-Isoephedrine Hydrochloride see Pseudoephedrine 1309
Disopyramide 491
Disopyramide Phosphate see Disopyramide 491
DisperMox™ [DSC] see Amoxicillin 106
Disulfiram 492
Dithioglycerol see Dimercaprol . . 482
Dithranol see Anthralin 128
Ditropan® see Oxybutynin 1162
Ditropan® XL see Oxybutynin . . . 1162
Diuril® see Chlorothiazide 322
Divalproex Sodium see Valproic Acid and Derivatives 1556
Dixarit® (Can) see Clonidine . . . 373
5071-1DL(6) see Megestrol 976
dl-Alpha Tocopherol see Vitamin E 1581
4-DMDR see Idarubicin 814
DMSO₂ see Methyl Sulfonyl Methane 1629
DNA-Derived Humanized Monoclonal Antibody see Alemtuzumab 63
DNase see Dornase Alfa 501
DNR see DAUNOrubicin Hydrochloride 426
Doak® Tar [OTC] see Coal Tar . . . 383
Doan's® Extra Strength [OTC] see Magnesium Salicylate 962
Doan's® [OTC] see Magnesium Salicylate 962
Dobuject® (Mex) see DOBUTamine 493
DOBUTamine 493
Dobutamine Hydrochloride see DOBUTamine 493
Dobutamine Injection, USP (Can) see DOBUTamine 493
Dobutrex® (Can) see DOBUTamine 493
Docetaxel 494
Docosahexaenoic Acid 1620

Docosanol 495
Docusate 496
Docusate and Casanthranol 496
Docusate Calcium see Docusate . . 496
Docusate Potassium see Docusate 496
Docusate Sodium see Docusate . . 496
Docusoft Plus™ [DSC] [OTC] see Docusate and Casanthranol . . . 496
Docusoft-S™ [OTC] see Docusate . . 496
Dofetilide 497
Dofus [OTC] see Lactobacillus . . . 535
DOK™ [OTC] see Docusate 496
Dolasetron 498
Dolasetron Mesylate see Dolasetron 498
Dolgic® LQ see Butalbital, Acetaminophen, and Caffeine . . 239
Dolgic® Plus see Butalbital, Acetaminophen, and Caffeine . . 239
Dolobid® [DSC] see Diflunisal . . . 468
Dolophine® see Methadone 1004
Dom-Benzydamine (Can) see Benzydamine 197
Dom-Citalopram (Can) see Citalopram 351
Dom-Clobazam (Can) see Clobazam 364
Domeboro® [OTC] see Aluminum Sulfate and Calcium Acetate . . . 81
Dome Paste Bandage see Zinc Gelatin 1597
Dom-Fenofibrate Supra (Can) see Fenofibrate 639
Dom-Mefenamic Acid (Can) see Mefenamic Acid 973
Dom-Methimazole (Can) see Methimazole 1008
Dom-Sumatriptan (Can) see Sumatriptan 1432
Dom-Topiramate (Can) see Topiramate 1508
Donepezil 500
Dong Quai 1620
Donnatal® see Hyoscyamine, Atropine, Scopolamine, and Phenobarbital 804
Donnatal Extentabs® see Hyoscyamine, Atropine, Scopolamine, and Phenobarbital 804
Dopram® see Doxapram 502
Doral® see Quazepam 1318
Dormicum® (Mex) see Midazolam 1040
Dornase Alfa 501
Doryx® see Doxycycline (Systemic) 514
Dorzolamide 501
Dorzolamide and Timolol 501
Dorzolamide Hydrochloride see Dorzolamide 501
DOS® [OTC] see Docusate 496
DOSS see Docusate 496
Dostinex® see Cabergoline 244
Dovonex® see Calcipotriene 246
Doxapram 502
Doxapram Hydrochloride see Doxapram 502
Doxazosin 503
Doxazosin Mesylate see Doxazosin 503
Doxepin 505
Doxepin Hydrochloride see Doxepin 505
Doxercalciferol 508
Doxidan® [DSC] [OTC] see Docusate and Casanthranol . . . 496
Doxidan® (reformulation) [OTC] see Bisacodyl 209

Doxil® see DOXOrubicin
(Liposomal) 511
Doxolem® (Mex) see DOXOrubicin
. . . . 509
DOXOrubicin 509
Doxorubicin Hydrochloride see
DOXOrubicin 509
Doxorubicin Hydrochloride
(Liposomal) see DOXOrubicin
(Liposomal) 511
DOXOrubicin (Liposomal) 511
Doxotec® (Mex) see DOXOrubicin . . 509
Doxy-100® see Doxycycline
(Systemic) 514
Doxycin (Can) see Doxycycline
(Systemic) 514
Doxycycline Calcium see
Doxycycline (Systemic) 514
Doxycycline Hyclate see
Doxycycline (Systemic) 514
Doxycycline Hyclate (Periodontal) . . 512
Doxycycline Monohydrate see
Doxycycline (Systemic) 514
Doxycycline (Subantimicrobial) . . . 514
Doxycycline (Systemic) 514
Doxylamine 517
Doxylamine Succinate see
Doxylamine 517
Doxytec (Can) see Doxycycline
(Systemic) 514
DPA see Valproic Acid and
Derivatives 1556
DPE see Dipivefrin 489
D-Penicillamine see Penicillamine
. . . . 1201
DPH see Phenytoin 1228
DPM™ [OTC] see Urea 1551
Drafilyn® (Mex) see Aminophylline . . 89
Dramamine® (Mex) see
DimenhyDRINATE 481
Dramamine® Less Drowsy Formula
[OTC] see Meclizine 969
Dramamine® [OTC] see
DimenhyDRINATE 481
Drenural® (Mex) see Bumetanide . . 227
Drisdol® see Ergocalciferol 556
Dristan® Long Lasting Nasal (Can)
see Oxymetazoline 1172
Dristan® N.D. (Can) see
Acetaminophen and
Pseudoephedrine 38
Dristan® N.D., Extra Strength
(Can) see Acetaminophen and
Pseudoephedrine 38
Dristan® Sinus [OTC] see
Pseudoephedrine and
Ibuprofen 1311
Dritho-Scalp® see Anthralin 128
Drituss DM see Guaifenesin and
Dextromethorphan 754
Drixoral® (Can) see
Dexbrompheniramine and
Pseudoephedrine 442
Drixoral® Cold & Allergy [OTC] see
Dexbrompheniramine and
Pseudoephedrine 442
Drixoral® Nasal (Can) see
Oxymetazoline 1172
Drixoral® ND (Can) see
Pseudoephedrine 1309
Drize®-R see Chlorpheniramine,
Phenylephrine, and
Methscopolamine 327
Dronabinol 518
Droperidol 519
Droperidol Injection, USP (Can)
see Droperidol 519
Drospirenone and Estradiol 520
Drospirenone and Ethinyl Estradiol
see Ethinyl Estradiol and
Drospirenone 595

Drotrecogin Alfa 522
Drotrecogin Alfa, Activated see
Drotrecogin Alfa 522
Droxia® see Hydroxyurea 800
Dr. Scholl's® Callus Remover
[OTC] see Salicylic Acid 1374
Dr. Scholl's® Clear Away [OTC]
see Salicylic Acid 1374
DSCG see Cromolyn 397
D-Ser(But)6,Azgly10-LHRH see
Goserelin 750
DSS see Docusate 496
D-S-S® [OTC] see Docusate 496
DSS With Casanthranol see
Docusate and Casanthranol 496
DTIC® (Can) see Dacarbazine 415
DTIC-Dome® see Dacarbazine . . . 415
DTO (error-prone abbreviation) see
Opium Tincture 1149
DTPA see Diethylene Triamine
Penta-Acetic Acid 466
D-Trp(6)-LHRH see Triptorelin . . . 1544
Duac™ see Clindamycin and
Benzoyl Peroxide 364
Dulcolan® (Mex) see Bisacodyl . . 209
Dulcolax® (Can) see Bisacodyl . . . 209
Dulcolax® Milk of Magnesia [OTC]
see Magnesium Hydroxide 961
Dulcolax® [OTC] see Bisacodyl . . 209
Dulcolax® Stool Softener [OTC]
see Docusate 496
Dull-C® [OTC] see Ascorbic Acid . . 143
Duloxetine 523
Duloxetine Hydrochloride see
Duloxetine 523
Duocaine™ see Lidocaine and
Bupivacaine 924
Duofilm® (Can) see Salicylic Acid . . 1374
DuoFilm® [OTC] see Salicylic Acid
. . . . 1374
Duoforte® 27 (Can) see Salicylic
Acid 1374
DuoNeb™ see Ipratropium and
Albuterol 857
DuoPlant® (Mex) see Salicylic Acid
. . . . 1374
DuoPlant® [DSC] [OTC] see
Salicylic Acid 1374
Duotan PD see
Dexchlorpheniramine and
Pseudoephedrine 443
DuP 753 see Losartan 950
Durabolin® (Can) see Nandrolone
. . . . 1087
Duracef® (Mex) see Cefadroxil . . . 281
Duraclon™ see Clonidine 373
Duradoce® (Mex) see
Hydroxocobalamin 798
Duradrin® see Acetaminophen,
Isometheptene, and
Dichloralphenazone 44
Duragesic® see Fentanyl 644
Duralith® (Can) see Lithium 939
Duramist® Plus [OTC] see
Oxymetazoline 1172
Duramorph® see Morphine Sulfate
. . . . 1065
Duraphen™ II DM see Guaifenesin,
Dextromethorphan, and
Phenylephrine 756
Duraphen™ DM see Guaifenesin,
Dextromethorphan, and
Phenylephrine 756
Duraphen™ Forte see Guaifenesin,
Dextromethorphan, and
Phenylephrine 756
Durater® (Mex) see Famotidine . . . 635
Duration® [OTC] see
Oxymetazoline 1172
Duratuss® DM see Guaifenesin
and Dextromethorphan 754

Duricef® see Cefadroxil 281
Durolane® (Can) see Hyaluronate
    and Derivatives 773
Dutasteride 524
Duvoid® (Can) see Bethanechol 204
DVA see Vindesine 1577
D-Vi-Sol® (Can) see Cholecalciferol
   334
DW286 see Gemifloxacin 731
Dyazide® see Hydrochlorothiazide
    and Triamterene 778
Dycill® (Can) see Dicloxacillin 463
Dyclonine 525
Dyclonine Hydrochloride see
    Dyclonine 525
Dygase see Pancrelipase 1183
Dynabac® [DSC] see Dirithromycin
   490
Dynacin® see Minocycline 1049
DynaCirc® (Can) see Isradipine ...871
DynaCirc® CR see Isradipine 871
DynaCirc® [DSC] see Isradipine 871
Dyna-Hex® [OTC] see
    Chlorhexidine Gluconate 316
Dynex see Guaifenesin and
    Pseudoephedrine 755
Dyphylline 526
Dyrenium® see Triamterene 1531
Dytan™ see DiphenhydrAMINE 483
E2 and DRSP see Drospirenone
    and Estradiol 520
7E3 see Abciximab 26
E2020 see Donepezil 500
EarSol® HC see Hydrocortisone ...793
Easprin® see Aspirin 145
Ebixa® (Can) see Memantine 979
Ecaten® (Mex) see Captopril 257
Echinacea 1620
Echinacea angustifolia see
    Echinacea 1620
Echinacea purpurea see
    Echinacea 1620
Echothiophate Iodide 526
EC-Naprosyn® see Naproxen 1089
E. coli Asparaginase see
    Asparaginase 144
Econazole 526
Econazole Nitrate see Econazole ..526
Econopred® Plus see
    PrednisoLONE 1268
Ecostatin® (Can) see Econazole ...526
Ecostigmine Iodide see
    Echothiophate Iodide 526
Ecotrin® Low Strength [OTC] see
    Aspirin 145
Ecotrin® Maximum Strength [OTC]
    see Aspirin 145
Ecotrin® [OTC] see Aspirin 145
Ectosone (Can) see
    Betamethasone 199
Ed A-Hist® see Chlorpheniramine
    and Phenylephrine 324
Edathamil Disodium see Edetate
    Disodium 527
Edecrin® see Ethacrynic Acid 590
Edenol® (Mex) see Furosemide 715
Edetate Calcium Disodium 527
Edetate Disodium 527
Edex® see Alprostadil 76
Edrophonium 528
Edrophonium and Atropine 529
Edrophonium Chloride see
    Edrophonium 528
Edrophonium Chloride and
    Atropine Sulfate see
    Edrophonium and Atropine 529
EDTA (Calcium Disodium) see
    Edetate Calcium Disodium 527
EDTA (Disodium) see Edetate
    Disodium 527
E.E.S.® see Erythromycin 562

Efalizumab 529
Efavirenz 530
Efexor® (Mex) see Venlafaxine ...1568
Effer-K™ see Potassium
    Bicarbonate and Potassium
    Citrate 1258
Effexor® see Venlafaxine 1568
Effexor® XR see Venlafaxine 1568
Eflone® [DSC] see
    Fluorometholone 674
Eflornithine 532
Eflornithine Hydrochloride see
    Eflornithine 532
Efudex® see Fluorouracil 674
EGb see Ginkgo Biloba 1622
E-Gems Elite® [OTC] see Vitamin
    E 1581
E-Gems® [OTC] see Vitamin E ...1581
E-Gems Plus® [OTC] see Vitamin
    E 1581
EHDP see Etidronate Disodium 621
Elantan® (Mex) see Isosorbide
    Mononitrate 868
Elavil see Amitriptyline 93
Eldepryl® see Selegiline 1382
Eldisine Lilly 99094 see Vindesine
   1577
Eldopaque® (Can) see
    Hydroquinone 798
Eldopaque Forte® see
    Hydroquinone 798
Eldopaque® [OTC] see
    Hydroquinone 798
Eldoquin® (Can) see Hydroquinone
   798
Eldoquin Forte® see Hydroquinone
   798
Eldoquin® [OTC] see Hydroquinone
   798
Electrolyte Lavage Solution see
    Polyethylene Glycol-Electrolyte
    Solution 1253
Elestat™ see Epinastine 546
Eletriptan 533
Eletriptan Hydrobromide see
    Eletriptan 533
Eleutherococcus senticosus see
    Ginseng, Siberian 1623
Elidel® see Pimecrolimus 1237
Eligard® see Leuprolide 906
Elimite® see Permethrin 1218
Elipten see Aminoglutethimide 87
Elitek™ see Rasburicase 1337
Elixophyllin® see Theophylline ...1473
Elixophyllin-GG® see Theophylline
    and Guaifenesin 1475
ElixSure™ Congestion [OTC] see
    Pseudoephedrine 1309
ElixSure™ Cough [OTC] see
    Dextromethorphan 451
ElixSure™ Fever/Pain [OTC] [DSC]
    see Acetaminophen 31
ElixSure™ IB [OTC] see Ibuprofen ..808
Ellence® see Epirubicin 550
Elmiron® see Pentosan Polysulfate
    Sodium 1211
Elocom® (Can) see Mometasone
    Furoate 1060
Elocon® see Mometasone Furoate
   1060
Eloxatin™ see Oxaliplatin 1154
Elspar® see Asparaginase 144
Eltor® (Can) see Pseudoephedrine
   1309
Eltroxin® (Can) see Levothyroxine ..917
Emadine® see Emedastine 534
Embeline™ see Clobetasol 365
Embeline™ E see Clobetasol 365
Emcyt® see Estramustine 578
Emedastine 534

Emedastine Difumarate *see*
Emedastine 534
Emend® *see* Aprepitant 134
Emetrol® [OTC] *see* Fructose,
Dextrose, and Phosphoric Acid
. . . . 713
Emko® [OTC] [DSC] *see*
Nonoxynol 9. 1124
EMLA® *see* Lidocaine and
Prilocaine. 928
Emo-Cort® (Can) *see*
Hydrocortisone 793
Emsam® *see* Selegiline 1382
Emtricitabine 536
Emtricitabine and Tenofovir 537
Emtriva® *see* Emtricitabine 536
Emulsoil® [OTC] [DSC] *see* Castor
Oil 279
ENA 713 *see* Rivastigmine. 1361
Enablex® *see* Darifenacin. 424
Enaladil® (Mex) *see* Enalapril 538
Enalapril. 538
Enalapril and Felodipine. 540
Enalapril and Hydrochlorothiazide . . . 541
Enalaprilat *see* Enalapril. 538
Enalapril Maleate *see* Enalapril 538
Enbrel® *see* Etanercept 588
Encare® [OTC] *see* Nonoxynol 9 . . . 1124
Encort™ *see* Hydrocortisone 793
Endal® *see* Guaifenesin and
Phenylephrine 754
Endal® HD *see* Hydrocodone,
Phenylephrine, and
Diphenhydramine 791
Endantadine® (Can) *see*
Amantadine 81
EndoAvitene® *see* Collagen
Hemostat 392
Endocet® *see* Oxycodone and
Acetaminophen 1165
Endodan® (Can) *see* Oxycodone
and Aspirin. 1168
Endodan® [DSC] *see* Oxycodone
and Aspirin. 1168
Endo®-Levodopa/Carbidopa (Can)
see Levodopa and Carbidopa . . 911
Endoplus® (Mex) *see* Albendazole . . 57
Endrate® *see* Edetate Disodium 527
Enduron® (Can) *see*
Methyclothiazide 1020
Enduron® [DSC] *see*
Methyclothiazide 1020
Enemeez® [OTC] *see* Docusate 496
Enerjets [OTC] *see* Caffeine 245
Enfamil® Glucose *see* Dextrose 452
Enfuvirtide 541
Engerix-B® *see* Hepatitis B
Vaccine 769
Engerix-B® and Havrix® *see*
Hepatitis A Inactivated and
Hepatitis B (Recombinant)
Vaccine 766
English Hawthorn *see* Hawthorn . . 1626
Enhanced-potency Inactivated
Poliovirus Vaccine *see*
Poliovirus Vaccine (Inactivated)
. . . . 1252
Enhancer *see* Barium. 179
Eni® (Mex) *see* Ciprofloxacin 343
Enlon® *see* Edrophonium 528
Enlon-Plus™ *see* Edrophonium and
Atropine. 529
Enoxaparin. 542
Enoxaparin Injection (Can) *see*
Enoxaparin. 542
Enoxaparin Sodium *see*
Enoxaparin. 542
Enpresse™ *see* Ethinyl Estradiol
and Levonorgestrel 602
Entacapone 543

Entacapone, Carbidopa, and
Levodopa *see* Levodopa,
Carbidopa, and Entacapone. . . . 912
Entacyl® (Can) *see* Piperazine . . . 1246
Entecavir 544
Enterex® Glutapak-10® [OTC] *see*
Glutamine 743
Enteropride® (Mex) *see* Cisapride . . 348
Entertainer's Secret® [OTC] *see*
Saliva Substitute 1374
Entex® *see* Guaifenesin and
Phenylephrine 754
Entex® ER *see* Guaifenesin and
Phenylephrine 754
Entex® LA *see* Guaifenesin and
Phenylephrine 754
Entex® PSE *see* Guaifenesin and
Pseudoephedrine 755
Entocort® (Can) *see* Budesonide . . . 224
Entocort® EC *see* Budesonide . . . 224
Entrobar® *see* Barium 179
EntroEase® *see* Barium 179
Entrophen® (Can) *see* Aspirin 145
Entsol® [OTC] *see* Sodium
Chloride 1400
Enulose® *see* Lactulose 893
Enzone® *see* Pramoxine and
Hydrocortisone 1264
Epamin® (Mex) *see* Phenytoin . . . 1228
Ephedrine. 545
Ephedrine, Chlorpheniramine,
Phenylephrine, and
Carbetapentane *see*
Chlorpheniramine, Ephedrine,
Phenylephrine, and
Carbetapentane 325
Ephedrine Sulfate *see* Ephedrine . . . 545
Epidermal Thymocyte Activating
Factor *see* Aldesleukin. 61
Epifoam® *see* Pramoxine and
Hydrocortisone 1264
Epilem® (Mex) *see* Epirubicin 550
Epinastine 546
Epinastine Hydrochloride *see*
Epinastine 546
Epinephrine 546
Epinephrine and Articaine
Hydrochloride *see* Articaine
and Epinephrine. 139
Epinephrine and Chlorpheniramine
. . . . 549
Epinephrine and Lidocaine *see*
Lidocaine and Epinephrine 924
Epinephrine and Prilocaine
(Dental) *see* Prilocaine and
Epinephrine 1278
Epinephrine Bitartrate *see*
Epinephrine 546
Epinephrine Bitartrate and
Bupivacaine Hydrochloride *see*
Bupivacaine and Epinephrine . . . 228
Epinephrine Hydrochloride *see*
Epinephrine 546
Epinephrine (Racemic) 549
Epinephrine (Racemic) and
Aluminum Potassium Sulfate 550
EpiPen® *see* Epinephrine 546
EpiPen® Jr *see* Epinephrine 546
Epipodophyllotoxin *see* Etoposide . . 626
EpiQuin™ Micro *see* Hydroquinone
. . . . 798
Epirubicin 550
Epitol® *see* Carbamazepine 260
Epival® (Mex) *see* Valproic Acid
and Derivatives 1556
Epival® I.V. (Can) *see* Valproic
Acid and Derivatives 1556
Epivir® *see* Lamivudine 894
Epivir-HBV® *see* Lamivudine 894
Eplerenone 551
EPO *see* Epoetin Alfa 552

Epoetin Alfa 552
Epogen® see Epoetin Alfa 552
Epomax® (Mex) see Epoetin Alfa . . . 552
Epoprostenol 553
Epoprostenol Sodium see
  Epoprostenol 553
Eprex® (Can) see Epoetin Alfa 552
Eprosartan 554
Eprosartan and
  Hydrochlorothiazide 555
Eprosartan Mesylate and
  Hydrochlorothiazide see
  Eprosartan and
  Hydrochlorothiazide 555
Epsilon Aminocaproic Acid see
  Aminocaproic Acid 86
Epsom Salts see Magnesium
  Sulfate 963
EPT see Teniposide 1456
Eptacog Alfa (Activated) see
  Factor VIIa (Recombinant) 632
Eptifibatide 556
Epzicom™ see Abacavir and
  Lamivudine 23
Equagesic® see Aspirin and
  Meprobamate 151
Equalactin® [OTC] see
  Polycarbophil 1252
Equalizer Gas Relief [OTC] see
  Simethicone 1394
Equanil see Meprobamate 993
Equetro™ see Carbamazepine 260
Eranz® (Mex) see Donepezil 500
Eraxis™ see Anidulafungin 128
Erbitux® see Cetuximab 308
Ergocalciferol 556
Ergoloid Mesylates 557
Ergomar® see Ergotamine 558
Ergometrine Maleate see
  Ergonovine 558
Ergonovine 558
Ergonovine Maleate see
  Ergonovine 558
Ergotamine 558
Ergotamine and Caffeine 559
Ergotamine Tartrate see
  Ergotamine 558
Ergotamine Tartrate and Caffeine
  see Ergotamine and Caffeine . . . 559
Ergotamine Tartrate, Belladonna,
  and Phenobarbital see
  Belladonna, Phenobarbital, and
  Ergotamine 185
Ergotrate® see Ergonovine 558
Erlotinib 560
Erlotinib Hydrochloride see
  Erlotinib 560
Errin™ see Norethindrone 1125
Ertaczo™ see Sertaconazole 1385
Ertapenem 561
Ertapenem Sodium see Ertapenem
  561
Erwinase® (Can) see Asparaginase
  144
Erwinia Asparaginase see
  Asparaginase 144
Eryacnen® (Mex) see Erythromycin
  562
Erybid™ (Can) see Erythromycin . . . 562
Eryc® see Erythromycin 562
Eryderm® see Erythromycin 562
Erygel® see Erythromycin 562
EryPed® see Erythromycin 562
Ery-Tab® see Erythromycin 562
Erythrocin® see Erythromycin 562
Erythromycin 562
Erythromycin and Benzoyl
  Peroxide 567
Erythromycin and Sulfisoxazole 568
Erythromycin Base see
  Erythromycin 562

Erythromycin Estolate see
  Erythromycin 562
Erythromycin Ethylsuccinate see
  Erythromycin 562
Erythromycin Gluceptate see
  Erythromycin 562
Erythromycin Lactobionate see
  Erythromycin 562
Erythromycin Stearate see
  Erythromycin 562
Erythropoiesis Stimulating Protein
  see Darbepoetin Alfa 423
Erythropoietin see Epoetin Alfa 552
Escitalopram 568
Escitalopram Oxalate see
  Escitalopram 568
Esclim® see Estradiol 574
Eserine® (Can) see Physostigmine
  1232
Eserine Salicylate see
  Physostigmine 1232
Esgic® see Butalbital,
  Acetaminophen, and Caffeine . . 239
Esgic-Plus™ see Butalbital,
  Acetaminophen, and Caffeine . . 239
Eskalith CR® see Lithium 939
Eskalith [DSC] see Lithium 939
Eskazole® (Mex) see Albendazole . . . 57
Esmolol 571
Esmolol Hydrochloride see Esmolol
  571
Esomeprazole 572
Esomeprazole Magnesium see
  Esomeprazole 572
Esoterica® Regular [OTC] see
  Hydroquinone 798
Espacil® (Mex) see Scopolamine . . 1380
Especol® [OTC] see Fructose,
  Dextrose, and Phosphoric Acid
  713
Estalis® (Can) see Estradiol and
  Norethindrone 575
Estalis-Sequi® (Can) see Estradiol
  and Norethindrone 575
Estar® (Can) see Coal Tar 383
Estazolam 573
Ester-E™ [OTC] see Vitamin E . . . 1581
Esterified Estrogen and
  Methyltestosterone see
  Estrogens (Esterified) and
  Methyltestosterone 585
Esterified Estrogens see Estrogens
  (Esterified) 584
Estrace® see Estradiol 574
Estraderm® see Estradiol 574
Estraderm MTX® (Mex) see
  Estradiol 574
Estraderm TTS® (Mex) see
  Estradiol 574
Estradiol 574
Estradiol Acetate see Estradiol 574
Estradiol and Drospirenone see
  Drospirenone and Estradiol 520
Estradiol and NGM see Estradiol
  and Norgestimate 576
Estradiol and Norethindrone 575
Estradiol and Norgestimate 576
Estradiol Cypionate see Estradiol . . . 574
Estradiol Hemihydrate see
  Estradiol 574
Estradiol Transdermal see
  Estradiol 574
Estradiol Valerate see Estradiol 574
Estradot® (Can) see Estradiol 574
Estramustine 578
Estramustine Phosphate Sodium
  see Estramustine 578
Estrasorb™ see Estradiol 574
Estratab® (Can) see Estrogens
  (Esterified) 584

Estratest® *see* Estrogens (Esterified) and Methyltestosterone 585
Estratest® H.S. *see* Estrogens (Esterified) and Methyltestosterone 585
Estring® *see* Estradiol 574
EstroGel® *see* Estradiol 574
Estrogenic Substances, Conjugated *see* Estrogens (Conjugated/Equine) 580
Estrogens (Conjugated A/ Synthetic).................. 578
Estrogens (Conjugated/Equine) 580
Estrogens (Conjugated/Equine) and Medroxyprogesterone 583
Estrogens (Esterified) 584
Estrogens (Esterified) and Methyltestosterone 585
Estropipate 586
Estrostep® Fe *see* Ethinyl Estradiol and Norethindrone 608
Eszopiclone 587
ETAF *see* Aldesleukin 61
Etanercept 588
Ethacrynate Sodium *see* Ethacrynic Acid 590
Ethacrynic Acid 590
Ethambutol 591
Ethambutol Hydrochloride *see* Ethambutol 591
Ethamolin® *see* Ethanolamine Oleate 591
Ethanolamine Oleate 591
EtheDent™ *see* Fluoride 671
Ethezyme™ *see* Papain and Urea 1186
Ethezyme™ 830 *see* Papain and Urea...................... 1186
Ethinyl Estradiol and Desogestrel ... 592
Ethinyl Estradiol and Drospirenone 595
Ethinyl Estradiol and Ethynodiol Diacetate 597
Ethinyl Estradiol and Etonogestrel .. 600
Ethinyl Estradiol and Levonorgestrel 602
Ethinyl Estradiol and NGM *see* Ethinyl Estradiol and Norgestimate 613
Ethinyl Estradiol and Norelgestromin.............. 605
Ethinyl Estradiol and Norethindrone 608
Ethinyl Estradiol and Norgestimate .. 613
Ethinyl Estradiol and Norgestrel 616
Ethiofos *see* Amifostine 83
Ethionamide 618
Ethmozine® *see* Moricizine 1064
Ethosuximide 619
Ethotoin 619
Ethoxynaphthamido Penicillin Sodium *see* Nafcillin 1082
Ethyl Aminobenzoate *see* Benzocaine 190
Ethyl Chloride 620
Ethyl Chloride and Dichlorotetrafluoroethane 620
Ethyl Esters of Omega-3 Fatty Acids *see* Omega-3-Acid Ethyl Esters 1621
Ethylphenylhydantoin *see* Ethotoin .. 619
Ethynodiol Diacetate and Ethinyl Estradiol *see* Ethinyl Estradiol and Ethynodiol Diacetate 597
Ethyol® *see* Amifostine 83
Etibi® (Can) *see* Ethambutol 591
Etidronate and Calcium 620
Etidronate Disodium 621
Etodolac 623
Etodolic Acid *see* Etodolac 623

Etomidate 625
Etonogestrel and Ethinyl Estradiol *see* Ethinyl Estradiol and Etonogestrel 600
Etopophos® *see* Etoposide Phosphate 627
Etopos® (Mex) *see* Etoposide 626
Etoposide 626
Etoposide Phosphate 627
Etrafon® (Can) *see* Amitriptyline and Perphenazine 97
Eudal®-SR *see* Guaifenesin and Pseudoephedrine 755
Euflex® (Can) *see* Flutamide 686
Euflexxa™ *see* Hyaluronate and Derivatives 773
Euglucon® (Can) *see* GlyBURIDE .. 744
Eulexin® *see* Flutamide 686
Eurax® *see* Crotamiton 398
Eutirox® (Mex) *see* Levothyroxine .. 917
Evac-U-Gen [OTC] *see* Senna 1384
Evening Primrose 1621
Evening Primrose Oil *see* Evening Primrose 1621
Everone® 200 (Can) *see* Testosterone 1462
Evista® *see* Raloxifene 1329
Evoclin™ *see* Clindamycin 361
Evoxac® *see* Cevimeline 310
Evra® (Can) *see* Ethinyl Estradiol and Norelgestromin 605
Exact® Acne Medication [OTC] *see* Benzoyl Peroxide 194
Excedrin® Extra Strength [OTC] *see* Acetaminophen, Aspirin, and Caffeine 41
Excedrin® Migraine [OTC] *see* Acetaminophen, Aspirin, and Caffeine 41
Excedrin® P.M. [OTC] *see* Acetaminophen and Diphenhydramine 38
Exelderm® *see* Sulconazole 1422
Exelon® *see* Rivastigmine 1361
Exemestane 628
Exenatide 629
Exendin-4 *see* Exenatide 629
Exjade® *see* Deferasirox 427
ex-lax® Maximum Strength [OTC] *see* Senna 1384
ex-lax® [OTC] *see* Senna 1384
Exorex® *see* Coal Tar 383
Extendryl *see* Chlorpheniramine, Phenylephrine, and Methscopolamine 327
Extendryl JR *see* Chlorpheniramine, Phenylephrine, and Methscopolamine 327
Extendryl SR *see* Chlorpheniramine, Phenylephrine, and Methscopolamine 327
Extraneal® *see* Icodextrin 814
Exubera® *see* Insulin Inhalation 837
EYE001 *see* Pegaptanib 1193
Eye Balm *see* Golden Seal 1624
Eye Root *see* Golden Seal 1624
Eye-Sine™ [OTC] *see* Tetrahydrozoline 1470
Eyestil (Can) *see* Hyaluronate and Derivatives 773
Eye-Stream® (Can) *see* Balanced Salt Solution................ 178
EZ-Char™ [OTC] *see* Charcoal 311
Ezetimibe 630
Ezetimibe and Simvastatin 631
Ezetrol® (Can) *see* Ezetimibe 630
E•R•O [OTC] *see* Carbamide Peroxide 264
F_3T *see* Trifluridine 1536

Fabrazyme® see Agalsidase Beta . . . 55
Factive® see Gemifloxacin 731
Factor VIII (Human) see
    Antihemophilic Factor (Human)
    129
Factor VIII (Recombinant) see
    Antihemophilic Factor
    (Recombinant) 130
Factor IX 632
Factor IX Complex (Human) 633
Factor VIIa (Recombinant) 632
Factrel® see Gonadorelin 749
Famciclovir 633
Famotidine 635
Famotidine, Calcium Carbonate,
    and Magnesium Hydroxide 636
Famotidine Omega (Can) see
    Famotidine 635
Famoxal® (Mex) see Famotidine . . 635
Famvir® see Famciclovir 633
Fansidar® see Sulfadoxine and
    Pyrimethamine 1424
Fareston® see Toremifene 1512
Farmorubicin® (Mex) see Epirubicin
    550
Farmotex® (Mex) see Famotidine . . . 635
Fasigyn® (Mex) see Tinidazole 1491
Faslodex® see Fulvestrant 713
Fasturtec® (Can) see Rasburicase
    1337
Fat Emulsion 637
FazaClo® see Clozapine 382
5-FC see Flucytosine 662
FC1157a see Toremifene 1512
Featherfew see Feverfew 1621
Featherfoil see Feverfew 1621
Feiba VH see Anti-inhibitor
    Coagulant Complex 130
Feiba VH Immuno (Can) see
    Anti-inhibitor Coagulant
    Complex 130
Felbamate 637
Felbatol® see Felbamate 637
Feldene® see Piroxicam 1248
Feliberal® (Mex) see Enalapril 538
Felodipine 638
Felodipine and Enalapril see
    Enalapril and Felodipine 540
Fem7® (Mex) see Estradiol 574
Femara® see Letrozole 904
femhrt® see Ethinyl Estradiol and
    Norethindrone 608
Femilax™ [OTC] see Bisacodyl . . . 209
Femiron® [OTC] see Ferrous
    Fumarate 650
Fem-Prin® [OTC] see
    Acetaminophen, Aspirin, and
    Caffeine 41
Femring™ see Estradiol 574
Femstat® One (Can) see
    Butoconazole 242
Femtrace® see Estradiol 574
Fenidantoin® (Mex) see
    Phenytoin 1228
Fenitron® (Mex) see
    Phenytoin 1228
Fenofibrate 639
Fenoldopam 641
Fenoldopam Mesylate see
    Fenoldopam 641
Fenoprofen 642
Fenoprofen Calcium see
    Fenoprofen 642
Fenoterol 644
Fenoterol Hydrobromide see
    Fenoterol 644
Fentanyl 644
Fentanyl Citrate see Fentanyl 644
Fentanyl Citrate Injection, USP
    (Can) see Fentanyl 644

Feosol® [OTC] see Ferrous Sulfate
    651
Feostat® [OTC] [DSC] see Ferrous
    Fumarate 650
Feratab® [OTC] see Ferrous
    Sulfate 651
Fer-Gen-Sol [OTC] see Ferrous
    Sulfate 651
Fergon® [OTC] see Ferrous
    Gluconate 651
Feridex I.V.® see Ferumoxides 652
Fer-In-Sol® (Can) see Ferrous
    Sulfate 651
Fer-In-Sol® [OTC] see Ferrous
    Sulfate 651
Fer-Iron® [OTC] see Ferrous
    Sulfate 651
Fermalac (Can) see Lactobacillus . . 535
Ferodan™ (Can) see Ferrous
    Sulfate 651
Fero-Grad 500® [OTC] see Ferrous
    Sulfate and Ascorbic Acid 651
Ferretts [OTC] see Ferrous
    Fumarate 650
Ferrex 150 [OTC] see
    Polysaccharide-Iron Complex . . 1254
Ferric (III) Hexacyanoferrate (II)
    see Ferric Hexacyanoferrate . . . 650
Ferric Gluconate 649
Ferric Hexacyanoferrate 650
Ferrlecit® see Ferric Gluconate 649
Ferro-Sequels® [OTC] see Ferrous
    Fumarate 650
Ferrous Fumarate 650
Ferrous Gluconate 651
Ferrous Sulfate 651
Ferrous Sulfate and Ascorbic Acid . . 651
Ferumoxides 652
Ferval® (Mex) see Ferrous
    Fumarate 650
FeSO₄ see Ferrous Sulfate 651
Fe-Tinic™ 150 [OTC] [DSC] see
    Polysaccharide-Iron Complex . . 1254
FeverALL® [OTC] see
    Acetaminophen 31
Feverfew 1621
Fexofenadine 652
Fexofenadine and
    Pseudoephedrine 653
Fexofenadine Hydrochloride see
    Fexofenadine 652
Fiberall® see Psyllium 1313
Fibercon® (Mex) see Polycarbophil
    1252
FiberCon® [OTC] see Polycarbophil
    1252
FiberEase™ [OTC] see
    Methylcellulose 1021
Fiber-Lax® [OTC] see
    Polycarbophil 1252
Fibrin Sealant Kit 653
Fibro-XL [OTC] see Psyllium 1313
Fibro-Lax [OTC] see Psyllium 1313
Filgrastim 654
Finacea™ see Azelaic Acid 169
Finasteride 655
Fioricet® see Butalbital,
    Acetaminophen, and Caffeine . . 239
Fioricet® with Codeine see
    Butalbital, Acetaminophen,
    Caffeine, and Codeine 239
Fiorinal® see Butalbital, Aspirin,
    and Caffeine 241
Fiorinal®-C 1/2 (Can) see
    Butalbital, Aspirin, Caffeine,
    and Codeine 241
Fiorinal®-C 1/4 (Can) see
    Butalbital, Aspirin, Caffeine,
    and Codeine 241

Fiorinal® With Codeine see
  Butalbital, Aspirin, Caffeine,
  and Codeine 241
First® Testosterone see
  Testosterone 1462
First® Testosterone MC see
  Testosterone 1462
Fisalamine see Mesalamine 996
Fish Oil see Omega-3-Acid Ethyl
  Esters 1621
Fixoten® (Mex) see Pentoxifylline . . 1212
FK506 see Tacrolimus 1437
Flagenase® (Mex) see
  Metronidazole. 1033
Flagyl® see Metronidazole 1033
Flagyl ER® see Metronidazole 1033
Flagyl I.V. RTU™ see
  Metronidazole. 1033
Flagystatin® (Can) see
  Metronidazole and Nystatin . . . 1036
Flamazine® (Can) see Silver
  Sulfadiazine 1393
Flarex® see Fluorometholone 674
Flavan see Flavocoxid 656
Flavocoxid 656
Flavonoid see Flavocoxid 656
Flavoxate 656
Flavoxate Hydrochloride see
  Flavoxate 656
Flaxseed Oil 1622
Flecainide 657
Flecainide Acetate see Flecainide . . 657
Fleet® Accu-Prep [OTC] see
  Sodium Phosphates 1403
Fleet® Babylax® [OTC] see
  Glycerin 747
Fleet® Bisacodyl Enema [OTC] see
  Bisacodyl 209
Fleet Enema® (Can) see Sodium
  Phosphates 1403
Fleet® Enema [OTC] see Sodium
  Phosphates 1403
Fleet® Glycerin Suppositories
  Maximum Strength [OTC] see
  Glycerin 747
Fleet® Glycerin Suppositories
  [OTC] see Glycerin 747
Fleet® Liquid Glycerin
  Suppositories [OTC] see
  Glycerin 747
Fleet® Phospho-Soda® Oral
  Laxative (Can) see Sodium
  Phosphates 1403
Fleet® Phospho-Soda® [OTC] see
  Sodium Phosphates 1403
Fleet® Sof-Lax® [OTC] see
  Docusate 496
Fleet® Sof-Lax® Overnight [DSC]
  [OTC] see Docusate and
  Casanthranol 496
Fleet® Stimulant Laxative [OTC]
  see Bisacodyl 209
Fletcher's® Castoria® [OTC] see
  Senna 1384
Flexeril® see Cyclobenzaprine 401
Flexitec (Can) see
  Cyclobenzaprine 401
Flex-Power [OTC] see
  Triethanolamine Salicylate 1535
Flixonase® (Mex) see Fluticasone . . 686
Flixotide® (Mex) see Fluticasone . . 686
Flo-Coat see Barium 179
Flolan® see Epoprostenol 553
Flomax® see Tamsulosin 1445
Flomax® CR (Can) see Tamsulosin
  1445
Flonase® see Fluticasone 686
Flora-Q™ [OTC] see Lactobacillus . 535
Florazole® ER (Can) see
  Metronidazole. 1033

Fiorical® [OTC] see Calcium
  Carbonate 248
Florinef® see Fludrocortisone 664
Florone® see Diflorasone 468
Flovent® Diskus® (Can) see
  Fluticasone 686
Flovent® HFA see Fluticasone 686
Floxacin® (Mex) see Norfloxacin . . 1126
Floxin® see Ofloxacin 1137
Floxin Otic Singles see Ofloxacin . . 1137
Floxuridine 659
Fluarix™ see Influenza Virus
  Vaccine 833
Flubenisolone see Betamethasone . . 199
Flucaine® see Proparacaine and
  Fluorescein 1296
Fluconazole 659
Fluconazole Injection (Can) see
  Fluconazole 659
Fluconazole Omega (Can) see
  Fluconazole 659
Flucytosine 662
Fludara® see Fludarabine 663
Fludarabine 663
Fludarabine Phosphate see
  Fludarabine 663
Fludrocortisone. 664
Fludrocortisone Acetate see
  Fludrocortisone 664
Fluken® (Mex) see Flutamide 686
Flulem® (Mex) see Flutamide 686
Flumadine® see Rimantadine 1351
Flumazenil 665
Flumazenil Injection (Can) see
  Flumazenil 665
Flumazenil Injection, USP (Can)
  see Flumazenil. 665
fluMist® see Influenza Virus
  Vaccine 833
Flunisolide 667
Fluocinolone 667
Fluocinolone Acetonide see
  Fluocinolone 667
Fluocinolone, Hydroquinone, and
  Tretinoin. 669
Fluocinonide. 670
Fluohydrisone Acetate see
  Fludrocortisone 664
Fluohydrocortisone Acetate see
  Fludrocortisone 664
Fluoracaine® see Proparacaine
  and Fluorescein 1296
Fluor-A-Day see Fluoride 671
Fluorescein and Proparacaine see
  Proparacaine and Fluorescein
  1296
Fluoride 671
Fluoride and Triclosan (Dental) see
  Triclosan and Fluoride 1534
Fluorigard® [OTC] see Fluoride 671
Fluori-Methane® see
  Dichlorodifluoromethane and
  Trichloromonofluoromethane . . . 458
Fluorinse® see Fluoride 671
5-Fluorocytosine see Flucytosine . . 662
Fluorodeoxyuridine see Floxuridine
  659
9α-Fluorohydrocortisone Acetate
  see Fludrocortisone 664
Fluorometholone 674
Fluorometholone and
  Sulfacetamide see
  Sulfacetamide and
  Fluorometholone 1423
Fluor-Op® [DSC] see
  Fluorometholone 674
Fluoroplex® see Fluorouracil 674
Fluorouracil 674
5-Fluorouracil see Fluorouracil 674
Fluotic® (Can) see Fluoride 671

Fluoxac® (Mex) see
    Fluoxetine 675
Fluoxetine 675
Fluoxetine and Olanzapine see
    Olanzapine and Fluoxetine 1141
Fluoxetine Hydrochloride see
    Fluoxetine 675
Fluoxymesterone 679
Flupazine® (Mex) see
    Trifluoperazine 1535
Fluphenazine 680
Fluphenazine Decanoate see
    Fluphenazine 680
Flura-Drops® see Fluoride 671
Flurandrenolide 681
Flurandrenolone see
    Flurandrenolide 681
Flurazepam 681
Flurazepam Hydrochloride see
    Flurazepam 681
Flurbiprofen 683
Flurbiprofen Sodium see
    Flurbiprofen 683
Flurinol® (Mex) see Epinastine 546
5-Flurocytosine see Flucytosine ... 662
Fluro-Ethyl® see Ethyl Chloride
    and Dichlorotetrafluoroethane .. 620
Flutamide 686
Fluticasone 686
Fluticasone and Salmeterol 690
Fluticasone Propionate see
    Fluticasone 686
Fluvastatin 693
Fluviral S/F® (Can) see Influenza
    Virus Vaccine 833
Fluvirin® see Influenza Virus
    Vaccine 833
Fluvoxamine 694
Fluxid™ see Famotidine 635
Fluzone® see Influenza Virus
    Vaccine 833
Flynoken® (Mex) see Leucovorin ... 905
FML® see Fluorometholone 674
FML® Forte see Fluorometholone ... 674
FML-S® see Sulfacetamide and
    Fluorometholone 1423
Focalin™ see Dexmethylphenidate .. 445
Focalin™ XR see
    Dexmethylphenidate 445
Foille® [OTC] see Benzocaine 190
Folacin see Folic Acid 697
Folacin, Vitamin B₁₂, and Vitamin
    B₆ see Folic Acid,
    Cyanocobalamin, and
    Pyridoxine 697
Folate see Folic Acid 697
Folbee see Folic Acid,
    Cyanocobalamin, and
    Pyridoxine 697
Folgard® [OTC] see Folic Acid,
    Cyanocobalamin, and
    Pyridoxine 697
Folgard RX 2.2® [DSC] see Folic
    Acid, Cyanocobalamin, and
    Pyridoxine 697
Folic Acid 697
Folic Acid, Cyanocobalamin, and
    Pyridoxine 697
Folinic Acid see Leucovorin 905
Follistim® AQ see Follitropins 698
Follitrin® (Mex) see Follitropins .. 698
Follitropin Alfa see Follitropins ... 698
Follitropin Alpha see Follitropins ... 698
Follitropin Beta see Follitropins ... 698
Follitropins 698
Foltx® see Folic Acid,
    Cyanocobalamin, and
    Pyridoxine 697
Fomepizole 699
Fomivirsen 700

Fomivirsen Sodium see Fomivirsen
    700
Fondaparinux 700
Fondaparinux Sodium see
    Fondaparinux 700
Foradil® (Can) see Formoterol 701
Foradil® Aerolizer™ see Formoterol
    701
Formoterol 701
Formoterol Fumarate see
    Formoterol 701
Formula EM [OTC] see Fructose,
    Dextrose, and Phosphoric Acid
    713
Formulation R™ [OTC] see
    Phenylephrine 1226
Formulex® (Can) see Dicyclomine .. 464
5-Formyl Tetrahydrofolate see
    Leucovorin 905
Fortamet™ see Metformin 1001
Fortaz® see Ceftazidime 292
Forteo™ see Teriparatide 1461
Fortical® see Calcitonin 246
Fortovase® (Can) see Saquinavir .. 1377
Fortovase® [DSC] see Saquinavir
    1377
Fortum® (Mex) see Ceftazidime 292
Fosamax® see Alendronate 64
Fosamax Plus D™ see Alendronate
    and Cholecalciferol 66
Fosamprenavir 702
Fosamprenavir Calcium see
    Fosamprenavir 702
Fosavance (Can) see Alendronate
    and Cholecalciferol 66
Foscarnet 703
Foscavir® see Foscarnet 703
Fosfocil® (Mex) see Fosfomycin 706
Fosfomycin 706
Fosfomycin Tromethamine see
    Fosfomycin 706
Fosinopril 707
Fosinopril and Hydrochlorothiazide .. 709
Fosinopril Sodium see Fosinopril .. 707
Fosphenytoin 710
Fosphenytoin Sodium see
    Fosphenytoin 710
Fosrenol™ see Lanthanum 899
Fostex® 10% BPO [OTC] see
    Benzoyl Peroxide 194
Fotexina® (Mex) see Cefotaxime ... 288
Fototar® [OTC] see Coal Tar 383
Fragmin® see Dalteparin 418
Freezone® [OTC] see Salicylic
    Acid 1374
Fresenizol® (Mex) see
    Metronidazole 1033
Fresofol® (Mex) see Propofol 1296
Frisium® (Can) see Clobazam 364
Froben® (Can) see Flurbiprofen ... 683
Froben-SR® (Can) see Flurbiprofen
    683
Frova® see Frovatriptan 712
Frovatriptan 712
Frovatriptan Succinate see
    Frovatriptan 712
Froxal® (Mex) see Cefuroxime 295
Fructose, Dextrose, and
    Phosphoric Acid 713
Frusemide see Furosemide 715
FS see Fibrin Sealant Kit 653
FTC see Emtricitabine 536
FU see Fluorouracil 674
5-FU see Fluorouracil 674
FUDR® see Floxuridine 659
5-FUDR see Floxuridine 659
Fulvestrant 713
Fungi-Guard [OTC] see Tolnaftate
    1506
Fungi-Nail® [OTC] see Undecylenic
    Acid and Derivatives 1550

Fungistat® (Mex) see Terconazole
.... 1461
Fungizone® (Can) see
Amphotericin B (Conventional) . . 113
Fungoid® Tincture [OTC] see
Miconazole 1039
Fung-O® [OTC] see Salicylic Acid
.... 1374
Fungoral® (Mex) see Ketoconazole
.... 880
Furadantin® see Nitrofurantoin 1119
Furazolidone 714
Furazosin see Prazosin 1267
Furosemide 715
Furosemide Injection, USP (Can)
see Furosemide 715
Furosemide Special (Can) see
Furosemide 715
Furoxona® (Mex) see Furazolidone
.... 714
Furoxone® (Can) see Furazolidone
.... 714
Fuxol® (Mex) see Furazolidone 714
Fuzeon™ see Enfuvirtide 541
FXT (Can) see Fluoxetine 675
Gabapentin................... 717
Gabitril® see Tiagabine 1483
Gadopentetate Dimeglumine 719
Gadoteridol 719
Galantamine 720
Galantamine Hydrobromide see
Galantamine 720
Galecin® (Mex) see Clindamycin . . . 361
Galidrin® (Mex) see Ranitidine 1334
Gallium Nitrate 721
Galsulfase 721
Gamikal® (Mex) see Amikacin 84
Gamimune® N (Can) see Immune
Globulin (Intravenous) 824
Gamma Benzene Hexachloride
see Lindane 933
Gamma E-Gems® [OTC] see
Vitamin E 1581
Gamma-E Plus [OTC] see Vitamin
E 1581
Gammagard® Liquid see Immune
Globulin (Intravenous) 824
Gammagard® S/D see Immune
Globulin (Intravenous) 824
Gamma Globulin see Immune
Globulin (Intramuscular) 823
Gamma Hydroxybutyric Acid see
Sodium Oxybate 1402
Gammaphos see Amifostine 83
Gammar®-P I.V. see Immune
Globulin (Intravenous) 824
Gamunex® see Immune Globulin
(Intravenous) 824
Ganciclovir 722
Ganidin NR see Guaifenesin 752
Ganirelix 723
Ganirelix Acetate see Ganirelix 723
Ganite™ see Gallium Nitrate 721
Gani-Tuss DM NR see Guaifenesin
and Dextromethorphan........ 754
Gani-Tuss® NR see Guaifenesin
and Codeine 753
Gantrisin® see SulfiSOXAZOLE . . . 1429
GAR-936 see Tigecycline 1487
Garamicina® (Mex) see Gentamicin
.... 734
Garamycin® (Can) see Gentamicin
.... 734
Garlic 1622
Gas-X® Extra Strength [OTC] see
Simethicone 1394
Gas-X® Maximum Strength [OTC]
see Simethicone 1394
Gas-X® [OTC] see Simethicone . . . 1394
GasAid [OTC] see Simethicone . . . 1394

Gas Ban™ [OTC] see Calcium
Carbonate and Simethicone 249
Gascop® (Mex) see Albendazole 57
Gastrocrom® see Cromolyn 397
Gastrografin® see Diatrizoate
Meglumine and Diatrizoate
Sodium................... 453
Gatifloxacin 724
Gaviscon® Extra Strength [OTC]
see Aluminum Hydroxide and
Magnesium Carbonate 79
Gaviscon® Liquid [OTC] see
Aluminum Hydroxide and
Magnesium Carbonate 79
Gaviscon® Tablet [OTC] see
Aluminum Hydroxide and
Magnesium Trisilicate......... 80
GBE see Ginkgo Biloba 1622
G-CSF see Filgrastim 654
G-CSF (PEG Conjugate) see
Pegfilgrastim 1195
GCV Sodium see Ganciclovir 722
Gd-DTPA see Gadopentetate
Dimeglumine 719
Gd-HP-DO3A see Gadoteridol 719
Gebauer's Ethyl Chloride® see
Ethyl Chloride 620
Gebauer's Instant Ice™ [OTC] see
Pentafluoropropane and
Tetrafluoroethane 1206
Gebauer's Pain Ease® see
Pentafluoropropane and
Tetrafluoroethane 1206
Gebauer's Spray and Stretch® see
Pentafluoropropane and
Tetrafluoroethane 1206
Gefitinib 727
Gelatin (Absorbable) 728
Gelclair® see Maltodextrin 963
Gelfilm® see Gelatin (Absorbable) . . 728
Gelfoam® see Gelatin (Absorbable)
.... 728
Gel-Kam® [OTC] see Fluoride ... 671
Gel-Kam® Rinse see Fluoride 671
Gelucast® see Zinc Gelatin 1597
Gelusil® (Can) see Aluminum
Hydroxide, Magnesium
Hydroxide, and Simethicone 81
Gelusil® Extra Strength (Can) see
Aluminum Hydroxide and
Magnesium Hydroxide 80
Gelusil® [OTC] see Aluminum
Hydroxide, Magnesium
Hydroxide, and Simethicone 81
Gemcitabine 729
Gemcitabine Hydrochloride see
Gemcitabine 729
Gemfibrozil 730
Gemifloxacin 731
Gemifloxacin Mesylate see
Gemifloxacin 731
Gemtuzumab Ozogamicin 732
Gemzar® see Gemcitabine 729
Gen-Acebutolol (Can) see
Acebutolol 28
Genaced™ [OTC] see
Acetaminophen, Aspirin, and
Caffeine 41
Genac® [OTC] see Triprolidine and
Pseudoephedrine 1542
Gen-Acyclovir (Can) see Acyclovir . . . 49
Genahist® [OTC] see
DiphenhydrAMINE 483
Gen-Alendronate (Can) see
Alendronate 64
Gen-Alprazolam (Can) see
Alprazolam 73
Gen-Amilazide (Can) see Amiloride
and Hydrochlorothiazide........ 85
Gen-Amiodarone (Can) see
Amiodarone 90

Gen-Amoxicillin (Can) see
   Amoxicillin 106
Gen-Anagrelide (Can) see
   Anagrelide 124
Genapap™ Children [OTC] see
   Acetaminophen 31
Genapap™ Extra Strength [OTC]
   see Acetaminophen 31
Genapap™ Infant [OTC] see
   Acetaminophen 31
Genapap™ [OTC] see
   Acetaminophen 31
Genapap™ Sinus Maximum
   Strength [OTC] see
   Acetaminophen and
   Pseudoephedrine 38
Genaphed® [OTC] see
   Pseudoephedrine 1309
Genasal [OTC] see Oxymetazoline
   1172
Genasoft® [OTC] see Docusate . . 496
Genasoft® Plus [DSC] [OTC] see
   Docusate and Casanthranol 496
Genasyme® [OTC] see
   Simethicone 1394
Gen-Atenolol (Can) see Atenolol . . . 154
Genaton Tablet [OTC] see
   Aluminum Hydroxide and
   Magnesium Trisilicate 80
Genatuss DM® [OTC] see
   Guaifenesin and
   Dextromethorphan 754
Gen-Azathioprine (Can) see
   Azathioprine 168
Gen-Baclofen (Can) see Baclofen . . 178
Gen-Beclo (Can) see
   Beclomethasone 183
Gen-Bromazepam (Can) see
   Bromazepam 220
Gen-Budesonide AQ (Can) see
   Budesonide 224
Gen-Buspirone (Can) see
   BusPIRone 236
Gen-Captopril (Can) see Captopril . . 257
Gen-Carbamazepine CR (Can) see
   Carbamazepine 260
Gen-Cimetidine (Can) see
   Cimetidine 341
Gen-Ciprofloxacin (Can) see
   Ciprofloxacin 343
Gen-Citalopram (Can) see
   Citalopram 351
Gen-Clobetasol (Can) see
   Clobetasol 365
Gen-Clomipramine (Can) see
   ClomiPRAMINE 370
Gen-Clonazepam (Can) see
   Clonazepam 371
Gen-Clozapine (Can) see
   Clozapine 382
Gen-Combo Sterinebs (Can) see
   Ipratropium and Albuterol 857
Gen-Cyclobenzaprine (Can) see
   Cyclobenzaprine 401
Gen-Diltiazem (Can) see Diltiazem
   479
Gen-Diltiazem CD (Can) see
   Diltiazem 479
Gen-Divalproex (Can) see Valproic
   Acid and Derivatives 1556
Gen-Doxazosin (Can) see
   Doxazosin 503
Genebs Extra Strength [OTC] see
   Acetaminophen 31
Genebs [OTC] see Acetaminophen
   31
Genemicin® (Mex) see Gentamicin
   734
Generlac see Lactulose 893

Genesec® [OTC] see
   Acetaminophen and
   Phenyltoloxamine 38
Gen-Etidronate (Can) see
   Etidronate Disodium 621
Geneye® [OTC] see
   Tetrahydrozoline 1470
Gen-Famotidine (Can) see
   Famotidine 635
Gen-Fenofibrate Micro (Can) see
   Fenofibrate 639
Genfiber® [OTC] see Psyllium 1313
Gen-Fluconazole (Can) see
   Fluconazole 659
Gen-Fluoxetine (Can) see
   Fluoxetine 675
Gen-Gabapentin (Can) see
   Gabapentin 717
Gen-Gemfibrozil (Can) see
   Gemfibrozil 730
Gen-Glybe (Can) see GlyBURIDE . . 744
Gengraf® see CycloSPORINE 406
Gen-Hydroxychloroquine (Can) see
   Hydroxychloroquine 799
Gen-Hydroxyurea (Can) see
   Hydroxyurea 800
Gen-Indapamide (Can) see
   Indapamide 828
Gen-Ipratropium (Can) see
   Ipratropium 857
Genkova® (Mex) see Gentamicin . . . 734
Gen-Lamotrigine (Can) see
   Lamotrigine 895
Gen-Levothyroxine (Can) see
   Levothyroxine 917
Gen-Lovastatin (Can) see
   Lovastatin 953
Gen-Medroxy (Can) see
   MedroxyPROGESTERone 972
Gen-Meloxicam (Can) see
   Meloxicam 977
Gen-Metformin (Can) see
   Metformin 1001
Gen-Minocycline (Can) see
   Minocycline 1049
Gen-Mirtazapine (Can) see
   Mirtazapine 1052
Gen-Nabumetone (Can) see
   Nabumetone 1077
Gen-Naproxen EC (Can) see
   Naproxen 1089
Gen-Nitro (Can) see Nitroglycerin
   1120
Gen-Nizatidine (Can) see
   Nizatidine 1123
Gen-Nortriptyline (Can) see
   Nortriptyline 1128
Genoptic® [DSC] see Gentamicin . . . 734
Genotropin® see Somatropin 1406
Genotropin Miniquick® see
   Somatropin 1406
Genoxal® (Mex) see
   Cyclophosphamide 403
Gen-Oxybutynin (Can) see
   Oxybutynin 1162
Gen-Paroxetine (Can) see
   Paroxetine 1188
Gen-Pindolol (Can) see Pindolol . . 1240
Gen-Piroxicam (Can) see
   Piroxicam 1248
Genpril® [OTC] see Ibuprofen 808
Gen-Ranidine (Can) see Ranitidine
   1334
Genrex® (Mex) see Gentamicin 734
Gen-Salbutamol (Can) see
   Albuterol 58
Gen-Selegiline (Can) see
   Selegiline 1382
Gen-Sertraline (Can) see Sertraline
   1385

Gen-Simvastatin (Can) see
   Simvastatin 1394
Gen-Sotalol (Can) see Sotalol 1409
Gen-Sumatriptan (Can) see
   Sumatriptan 1432
Gentabac® (Mex) see Gentamicin . . 734
Gentacin® (Mex) see Gentamicin . . . 734
Genta Grin® (Mex) see Gentamicin
   734
Gentak® see Gentamicin 734
Gentamicin 734
Gentamicin and Prednisolone see
   Prednisolone and Gentamicin
   1271
Gentamicin Injection, USP (Can)
   see Gentamicin 734
Gentamicin Sulfate see Gentamicin
   734
Gen-Tamoxifen (Can) see
   Tamoxifen 1443
Gentarim® (Mex) see Gentamicin . . 734
Gentazaf® (Mex) see Gentamicin . . 734
Genteal® (Can) see Hydroxypropyl
   Methylcellulose 800
GenTeal® Mild [OTC] see
   Hydroxypropyl Methylcellulose . . 800
GenTeal® [OTC] see
   Hydroxypropyl Methylcellulose . . 800
Gen-Temazepam (Can) see
   Temazepam 1453
Gen-Terbinafine (Can) see
   Terbinafine 1459
Gentian Violet 735
Gen-Ticlopidine (Can) see
   Ticlopidine 1486
Gen-Timolol (Can) see Timolol 1489
Gen-Tizanidine (Can) see
   Tizanidine 1497
Gentlax® (Can) see Bisacodyl 209
Gentlax® [OTC] [DSC] see
   Bisacodyl 209
Gen-Topiramate (Can) see
   Topiramate 1508
Gentran® see Dextran 447
Gen-Trazodone (Can) see
   Trazodone 1521
Gen-Triazolam (Can) see
   Triazolam 1531
Gen-Verapamil (Can) see
   Verapamil 1571
Gen-Verapamil SR (Can) see
   Verapamil 1571
Gen-Warfarin (Can) see Warfarin . . 1585
Gen-Zopiclone (Can) see
   Zopiclone 1606
Geocillin® see Carbenicillin 265
Geodon® see Ziprasidone 1598
Geref® (Mex) see Sermorelin
   Acetate 1384
Geref® Diagnostic see Sermorelin
   Acetate 1384
Geriation [OTC] see Vitamins
   (Multiple/Oral) 1582
Geri-Hydrolac™-12 [OTC] see
   Lactic Acid and Ammonium
   Hydroxide 893
Geri-Hydrolac™ [OTC] see Lactic
   Acid and Ammonium
   Hydroxide 893
Geritol Complete® [OTC] see
   Vitamins (Multiple/Oral) 1582
Geritol Extend® [OTC] see
   Vitamins (Multiple/Oral) 1582
Geritol® Tonic [OTC] see Vitamins
   (Multiple/Oral) 1582
German Measles Vaccine see
   Rubella Virus Vaccine (Live) . . 1372
Gevrabon® [OTC] see Vitamin B
   Complex Combinations 1581
GF196960 see Tadalafil 1441
GG see Guaifenesin 752

GHB see Sodium Oxybate 1402
G.I.® (Mex) see Gentamicin 734
GI87084B see Remifentanil 1338
Giltuss® see Guaifenesin,
   Dextromethorphan, and
   Phenylephrine 756
Giltuss HC® see Hydrocodone,
   Phenylephrine, and
   Guaifenesin 791
Giltuss Pediatric® see Guaifenesin,
   Dextromethorphan, and
   Phenylephrine 756
Giltuss TR® see Guaifenesin,
   Dextromethorphan, and
   Phenylephrine 756
Ginedisc® (Mex) see Estradiol 574
Ginger 1622
Ginkgo Biloba 1622
ginkgold see Ginkgo Biloba 1622
Ginkgopowder see Ginkgo Biloba
   1622
Ginkogink see Ginkgo Biloba 1622
Ginseng, Panax 1623
Ginseng, Siberian 1623
Gladase® see Papain and Urea . . . 1186
Glargine Insulin see Insulin
   Glargine 837
Glatiramer Acetate 736
Gleevec® see Imatinib 817
Gliadel® see Carmustine 273
Gliadel Wafer® (Can) see
   Carmustine 273
Glibenclamide see GlyBURIDE 744
Glibenil® (Mex) see GlyBURIDE 744
Gliclazide 737
Glimepiride 738
Glimepiride and Rosiglitazone
   Maleate see Rosiglitazone and
   Glimepiride 1369
Glioten® (Mex) see Enalapril 538
GlipiZIDE 740
Glipizide and Metformin 741
Glipizide and Metformin
   Hydrochloride see Glipizide
   and Metformin 741
Glivec see Imatinib 817
Gln see Glutamine 743
GlucaGen® see Glucagon 742
GlucaGen® Diagnostic Kit see
   Glucagon 742
GlucaGen® HypoKit™ see
   Glucagon 742
Glucagon 742
Glucagon Diagnostic Kit [DSC] see
   Glucagon 742
Glucagon Emergency Kit see
   Glucagon 742
Glucagon Hydrochloride see
   Glucagon 742
Glucal® (Mex) see GlyBURIDE 744
Glucobay® (Mex) see Acarbose 28
Glucocerebrosidase see
   Alglucerase 68
GlucoNorm® (Can) see
   Repaglinide 1339
Glucophage® see Metformin 1001
Glucophage® XR see Metformin . . . 1001
Glucosamine 1624
Glucosamine Hydrochloride see
   Glucosamine 1624
Glucosamine Sulfate see
   Glucosamine 1624
Glucose see Dextrose 452
Glucose Monohydrate see
   Dextrose 452
Glucose Polymers 743
Glucotrol® see GlipiZIDE 740
Glucotrol® XL see GlipiZIDE 740
Glucovance® see Glyburide and
   Metformin 745
Glucoven® (Mex) see GlyBURIDE . . 744

Glu-K® [OTC] see Potassium
  Gluconate 1259
Glulisine Insulin see Insulin
  Glulisine 837
Glumetza® (Can) see Metformin . . 1001
Glupitel® (Mex) see GlipiZIDE 740
Glutamic Acid 743
Glutamic Acid Hydrochloride see
  Glutamic Acid 743
Glutamine 743
Glutathione 1624
Glutofac®-MX see Vitamins
  (Multiple/Oral) 1582
Glutofac®-ZX see Vitamins
  (Multiple/Oral) 1582
Glutol™ [OTC] see Dextrose 452
Glutose™ [OTC] see Dextrose 452
Glybenclamide see GlyBURIDE 744
Glybenzcyclamide see GlyBURIDE
  744
GlyBURIDE 744
Glyburide and Metformin 745
Glyburide and Metformin
  Hydrochloride see Glyburide
  and Metformin 745
Glycerin 747
Glycerol see Glycerin 747
Glycerol Guaiacolate see
  Guaifenesin 752
Glycerol Triacetate see Triacetin . . 1526
Glyceryl Trinitrate see Nitroglycerin
  1120
Glycocome see Licorice 1627
GlycoLax™ see Polyethylene
  Glycol 3350 1253
Glycon (Can) see Metformin 1001
Glycopyrrolate 747
Glycopyrrolate Injection, USP
  (Can) see Glycopyrrolate 747
Glycopyrronium Bromide see
  Glycopyrrolate 747
Glycosum see Dextrose 452
Glycyrrhiza glabra see Licorice . . . 1627
Glydiazinamide see GlipiZIDE 740
Glynase® PresTab® see
  GlyBURIDE 744
Gly-Oxide® [OTC] see Carbamide
  Peroxide. 264
Glyquin® see Hydroquinone 798
Glyquin-XM™ see Hydroquinone . . . 798
Glyset® see Miglitol 1046
GM-CSF see Sargramostim 1378
GMD-Azithromycin (Can) see
  Azithromycin 171
GMD-Fluconazole (Can) see
  Fluconazole 659
GMD-Gemfibrozil (Can) see
  Gemfibrozil. 730
GMD-Sertraline (Can) see
  Sertraline 1385
GnRH see Gonadorelin 749
GnRH Agonist see Histrelin 772
Goatweed see St John's Wort 1632
Gold Bond® Antifungal [OTC] see
  Tolnaftate 1506
Golden Seal 1624
Gold Sodium Thiomalate 748
GoLYTELY® see Polyethylene
  Glycol-Electrolyte Solution 1253
Gonadorelin 749
Gonadorelin Acetate see
  Gonadorelin 749
Gonadorelin Hydrochloride see
  Gonadorelin 749
Gonadotropin Releasing Hormone
  see Gonadorelin 749
Gonak™ [OTC] see Hydroxypropyl
  Methylcellulose. 800
Gonal-f® see Follitropins 698
Gonal-f® RFF see Follitropins 698

Gonioscopic Ophthalmic Solution
  see Hydroxypropyl
  Methylcellulose. 800
Goniosoft™ see Hydroxypropyl
  Methylcellulose. 800
Goniosol® [OTC] [DSC] see
  Hydroxypropyl Methylcellulose . . 800
Good Sense Sleep Aid [OTC] see
  Doxylamine 517
Goody's® Extra Strength Headache
  Powder [OTC] see
  Acetaminophen, Aspirin, and
  Caffeine 41
Goody's® Extra Strength Pain
  Relief [OTC] see
  Acetaminophen, Aspirin, and
  Caffeine 41
Goody's PM® Powder [OTC] see
  Acetaminophen and
  Diphenhydramine 38
Gopten® (Mex) see Trandolapril . . 1517
Gordofilm® [OTC] see Salicylic
  Acid 1374
Gordon Boro-Packs [OTC] see
  Aluminum Sulfate and Calcium
  Acetate. 81
Gormel® [OTC] see Urea 1551
Goserelin 750
Goserelin Acetate see Goserelin . . 750
Gotu Kola 1624
GP 47680 see Oxcarbazepine . . . 1159
Gramicidin, Neomycin, and
  Polymyxin B see Neomycin,
  Polymyxin B, and Gramicidin . . 1101
Granisetron 751
Granulex® see Trypsin, Balsam
  Peru, and Castor Oil 1547
Granulocyte Colony Stimulating
  Factor see Filgrastim 654
Granulocyte Colony Stimulating
  Factor (PEG Conjugate) see
  Pegfilgrastim 1195
Granulocyte-Macrophage Colony
  Stimulating Factor see
  Sargramostim 1378
Grapefruit Seed 1625
Grape Seed 1625
Grape Skin 1625
Gravol® (Can) see
  DimenhyDRINATE 481
Green Tea 1625
Grifulvin® V see Griseofulvin 752
Griseofulvin 752
Griseofulvin Microsize see
  Griseofulvin 752
Griseofulvin Ultramicrosize see
  Griseofulvin 752
Grisovin® (Mex) see Griseofulvin . . 752
Gris-PEG® see Griseofulvin 752
GSE see Grapefruit Seed 1625
Guaicon DM [OTC] see
  Guaifenesin and
  Dextromethorphan 754
Guaicon DMS [OTC] see
  Guaifenesin and
  Dextromethorphan 754
Guaifed® see Guaifenesin and
  Phenylephrine 754
Guaifed-PD® see Guaifenesin and
  Phenylephrine 754
Guaifen-C see Guaifenesin and
  Codeine 753
Guaifenesin 752
Guaifenesin AC see Guaifenesin
  and Codeine 753
Guaifenesin and Codeine 753
Guaifenesin and
  Dextromethorphan 754

Guaifenesin and Hydrocodone see Hydrocodone and Guaifenesin . . 785
Guaifenesin and Phenylephrine 754
Guaifenesin and Phenylephrine Tannate see Guaifenesin and Phenylephrine 754
Guaifenesin and Potassium Guaiacolsulfonate 755
Guaifenesin and Pseudoephedrine . . 755
Guaifenesin and Theophylline see Theophylline and Guaifenesin 1475
Guaifenesin, Dextromethorphan, and Phenylephrine 756
Guaifenesin, Dextromethorphan Hydrobromide, and Phenylephrine Hydrochloride see Guaifenesin, Dextromethorphan, and Phenylephrine 756
Guaifenesin, Dihydrocodeine, and Pseudoephedrine see Dihydrocodeine, Pseudoephedrine, and Guaifenesin 476
Guaifenesin, Hydrocodone, and Pseudoephedrine see Hydrocodone, Pseudoephedrine, and Guaifenesin 792
Guaifenesin, Hydrocodone Bitartrate, and Phenylephrine Hydrochloride see Hydrocodone, Phenylephrine, and Guaifenesin 791
Guaifenesin, Pseudoephedrine, and Codeine 756
Guaifenesin, Pseudoephedrine, and Dextromethorphan 757
Guaifenex® DM see Guaifenesin and Dextromethorphan 754
Guaifenex® GP see Guaifenesin and Pseudoephedrine 755
Guaifenex® PSE see Guaifenesin and Pseudoephedrine 755
Guaimax-D® see Guaifenesin and Pseudoephedrine 755
Guaituss AC see Guaifenesin and Codeine 753
Guanabenz 758
Guanabenz Acetate see Guanabenz 758
Guanfacine 758
Guanfacine Hydrochloride see Guanfacine 758
Guanidine 759
Guanidine Hydrochloride see Guanidine 759
Guia-D see Guaifenesin and Dextromethorphan 754
Guiatuss™ DAC® see Guaifenesin, Pseudoephedrine, and Codeine 756
Guiatuss-DM® [OTC] see Guaifenesin and Dextromethorphan 754
Guiatuss™ [OTC] see Guaifenesin . . 752
Gum Benjamin see Benzoin 193
GW506U78 see Nelarabine 1097
GW-1000-02 see Tetrahydrocannabinol and Cannabidiol 1469
GW433908G see Fosamprenavir . . . 702
Gynazole-1® see Butoconazole 242
Gyne-Lotrimin® 3 [OTC] see Clotrimazole 379
Gynodiol® see Estradiol 574
Gynol II® [OTC] see Nonoxynol 9 1124
Gyno-Myfungar® (Mex) see Oxiconazole 1160

Gynovite® Plus [OTC] see Vitamins (Multiple/Oral) 1582
Habitrol® (Can) see Nicotine 1109
Haemophilus b Conjugate Vaccine . . 534
Haemophilus b Oligosaccharide Conjugate Vaccine see Haemophilus b Conjugate Vaccine 534
Haemophilus b Polysaccharide Vaccine see Haemophilus b Conjugate Vaccine 534
HAES-steril® (Mex) see Hetastarch 770
Halcinonide 760
Halcion® see Triazolam 1531
Haldol® see Haloperidol 762
Haldol decanoas® (Mex) see Haloperidol 762
Haldol® Decanoate see Haloperidol 762
Haley's M-O see Magnesium Hydroxide and Mineral Oil 961
Halfprin® [OTC] see Aspirin 145
Halobetasol 760
Halobetasol Propionate see Halobetasol 760
Halofantrine 761
Halofantrine Hydrochloride see Halofantrine 761
Halog® see Halcinonide 760
Haloperidol 762
Haloperidol Decanoate see Haloperidol 762
Haloperidol Injection, USP (Can) see Haloperidol 762
Haloperidol-LA (Can) see Haloperidol 762
Haloperidol Lactate see Haloperidol 762
Haloperidol-LA Omega (Can) see Haloperidol 762
Haloperidol Long Acting (Can) see Haloperidol 762
Haloperil® (Mex) see Haloperidol . . . 762
Halotestin® see Fluoxymesterone . . . 679
HandClens® [OTC] see Benzalkonium Chloride 188
Harpagophytum procumbens see Devil's Claw 1619
Havrix® see Hepatitis A Vaccine . . . 767
Havrix® and Engerix-B® see Hepatitis A Inactivated and Hepatitis B (Recombinant) Vaccine 766
Haw see Hawthorn 1626
Hawthorn 1626
HbCV see Haemophilus b Conjugate Vaccine 534
HBIG see Hepatitis B Immune Globulin 768
hBNP see Nesiritide 1103
HbOC see Haemophilus b Conjugate Vaccine 534
hCG see Chorionic Gonadotropin (Human) 336
HCTZ (error-prone abbreviation) see Hydrochlorothiazide 776
HD 85® see Barium 179
HD 200® Plus see Barium 179
HDA® Toothache [OTC] see Benzocaine 190
HDCV see Rabies Virus Vaccine . . 1329
Head & Shoulders® Citrus Breeze [OTC] see Pyrithione Zinc 1318
Head & Shoulders® Classic Clean 2-In-1 [OTC] see Pyrithione Zinc 1318
Head & Shoulders® Classic Clean [OTC] see Pyrithione Zinc 1318

Head & Shoulders® Dry Scalp Care [OTC] see Pyrithione Zinc 1318
Head & Shoulders® Extra Volume [OTC] see Pyrithione Zinc ... 1318
Head & Shoulders® Leave-in Treatment [OTC] see Pyrithione Zinc ... 1318
Head & Shoulders® Refresh [OTC] see Pyrithione Zinc 1318
Head & Shoulders® Sensitive Care [OTC] see Pyrithione Zinc ... 1318
Head & Shoulders® Smooth & Silky 2-In-1 [OTC] see Pyrithione Zinc 1318
Healon® see Hyaluronate and Derivatives 773
Healon®5 see Hyaluronate and Derivatives 773
Healon GV® see Hyaluronate and Derivatives 773
Hectorol® see Doxercalciferol 508
Helidac® see Bismuth Subsalicylate, Metronidazole, and Tetracycline 210
Helistat® see Collagen Hemostat . 392
Helitene® see Collagen Hemostat . 392
Helixate® FS see Antihemophilic Factor (Recombinant)......... 130
Hemabate ® see Carboprost Tromethamine 270
Hemiacidrin see Citric Acid, Magnesium Carbonate, and Glucono-Delta-Lactone 353
Hemin 764
Hemobion® (Mex) see Ferrous Sulfate 651
Hemocyte® [OTC] see Ferrous Fumarate 650
Hemocyte Plus® see Vitamins (Multiple/Oral).............. 1582
Hemodent™ see Aluminum Chloride 78
Hemofil® M see Antihemophilic Factor (Human) 129
Hemorrhoidal HC see Hydrocortisone 793
Hemril®-30 see Hydrocortisone ... 793
HepaGam B™ see Hepatitis B Immune Globulin 768
Hepalean® (Can) see Heparin 765
Hepalean® Leo (Can) see Heparin . 765
Hepalean®-LOK (Can) see Heparin 765
Heparin 765
Heparin Calcium see Heparin 765
Heparin Cofactor I see Antithrombin III 131
Heparin Lock Flush see Heparin .. 765
Heparin Sodium see Heparin 765
Hepatitis A Inactivated and Hepatitis B (Recombinant) Vaccine 766
Hepatitis A Vaccine 767
Hepatitis B Immune Globulin 768
Hepatitis B Inactivated Virus Vaccine (plasma derived) see Hepatitis B Vaccine 769
Hepatitis B Inactivated Virus Vaccine (recombinant DNA) see Hepatitis B Vaccine 769
Hepatitis B (Recombinant) and Hepatitis A Inactivated Vaccine see Hepatitis A Inactivated and Hepatitis B (Recombinant) Vaccine 766
Hepatitis B Vaccine 769
HepFlush®-10 see Heparin 765
Hep-Lock® see Heparin 765
Hepsera™ see Adefovir 54

Heptovir® (Can) see Lamivudine ... 894
Herceptin® see Trastuzumab 1520
Herklin Shampoo® (Mex) see Lindane 933
HES see Hetastarch 770
Hespan® see Hetastarch 770
Hetastarch 770
Hexabrix™ see Ioxaglate Meglumine and Ioxaglate Sodium 856
Hexachlorocyclohexane see Lindane 933
Hexachlorophene 771
Hexalen® see Altretamine 78
Hexamethylenetetramine see Methenamine 1007
Hexamethylmelamine see Altretamine 78
Hexit™ (Can) see Lindane 933
HEXM see Altretamine 78
Hextend® see Hetastarch 770
Hexylresorcinol 771
Hibiclens® [OTC] see Chlorhexidine Gluconate 316
Hibidil® 1:2000 (Can) see Chlorhexidine Gluconate 316
Hibistat® [OTC] see Chlorhexidine Gluconate 316
Hib Polysaccharide Conjugate see Haemophilus b Conjugate Vaccine 534
HibTITER® see Haemophilus b Conjugate Vaccine 534
Hidantoina® (Mex) see Phenytoin . . 1228
Hidroquin® (Mex) see Hydroquinone 798
High Gamma Vitamin E Complete™ [OTC] see Vitamin E 1581
Hi-Kovite [OTC see Vitamins (Multiple/Oral)............. 1582
Hipocol® (Mex) see Niacin 1105
Hipokinon® (Mex) see Trihexyphenidyl 1537
Hiprex® see Methenamine 1007
Hirulog see Bivalirudin 213
Histade™ see Chlorpheniramine and Pseudoephedrine 325
Hista-Vent® DA see Chlorpheniramine, Phenylephrine, and Methscopolamine 327
Histex™ see Chlorpheniramine and Pseudoephedrine 325
Histex™ I/E see Carbinoxamine 268
Histex™ CT see Carbinoxamine ... 268
Histex™ HC see Hydrocodone, Carbinoxamine, and Pseudoephedrine 789
Histex™ PD see Carbinoxamine 268
Histex™ PD-12 see Carbinoxamine 268
Histex™ SR see Brompheniramine and Pseudoephedrine 223
Histrelin 772
Histrelin Acetate see Histrelin 772
Histussin D® see Hydrocodone and Pseudoephedrine 788
Hi-Vegi-Lip [OTC] see Pancreatin 1183
Hivid® see Zalcitabine 1590
HMG Massone® (Mex) see Menotropins 982
HMM see Altretamine 78
HMR 3647 see Telithromycin 1448
HMS Liquifilm® [DSC] see Medrysone 973
Hold® DM [OTC] see Dextromethorphan 451
Homatropine.................... 772

Homatropine and Hydrocodone
see Hydrocodone and
Homatropine 786
Homatropine Hydrobromide see
Homatropine 772
Horse Antihuman Thymocyte
Gamma Globulin see
Antithymocyte Globulin
(Equine) 131
Horse Chestnut 1626
H.P. Acthar® Gel see Corticotropin
. . . . 395
Hp-PAC® (Can) see Lansoprazole,
Amoxicillin, and Clarithromycin . . 898
HTF919 see Tegaserod 1448
hu1124 see Efalizumab 529
Humalog® see Insulin Lispro 839
Humalog® Mix 25 (Can) see Insulin
Lispro Protamine and Insulin
Lispro 839
Humalog® Mix 50/50™ (Can) see Insulin
Lispro Protamine and Insulin
Lispro 839
Humalog® Mix 75/25™ see Insulin
Lispro Protamine and Insulin
Lispro 839
Human Antitumor Necrosis Factor
Alpha see Adalimumab 52
Human Diploid Cell Cultures
Rabies Vaccine see Rabies
Virus Vaccine 1329
Human Growth Hormone see
Somatropin 1406
Humanized IgG1 Anti-CD52
Monoclonal Antibody see
Alemtuzumab 63
Human LFA-3/IgG(1) Fusion
Protein see Alefacept 62
Human Thyroid Stimulating
Hormone see Thyrotropin
Alpha 1483
Humate-P® see Antihemophilic
Factor (Human) 129
Humatin® see Paromomycin 1188
Humatrope® see Somatropin 1406
Humegon® (Can) see Chorionic
Gonadotropin (Human) 336
Humibid® CS [OTC] [DSC] see
Guaifenesin and
Dextromethorphan 754
Humibid® e [OTC] see Guaifenesin
. . . . 752
Humibid® LA (reformulation) see
Guaifenesin and Potassium
Guaiacolsulfonate 755
Humira® see Adalimumab 52
Humulin® 20/80 (Can) see Insulin
NPH and Insulin Regular 840
Humulin® 50/50 see Insulin NPH
and Insulin Regular 840
Humulin® 70/30 see Insulin NPH
and Insulin Regular 840
Humulin® N see Insulin NPH 840
Humulin® R see Insulin Regular . . 841
Humulin® R (Concentrated) U-500
see Insulin Regular 841
Huperzia serrata see HuperzineA
. . . . 1626
HuperzineA 1626
Hurricaine® [OTC] see Benzocaine
. . . . 190
HXM see Altretamine 78
Hyalgan® see Hyaluronate and
Derivatives 773
Hyaluronan see Hyaluronate and
Derivatives 773
Hyaluronate and Derivatives 773
Hyaluronic Acid see Hyaluronate
and Derivatives 773
Hyaluronidase 774
Hycamptamine see Topotecan 1511

Hycamtin® see Topotecan 1511
hycet™ see Hydrocodone and
Acetaminophen 779
Hycoclear Tuss see Hydrocodone
and Guaifenesin 785
Hycodan® see Hydrocodone and
Homatropine 786
Hycomine® Compound see
Hydrocodone,
Chlorpheniramine,
Phenylephrine,
Acetaminophen, and Caffeine . . 790
Hycort™ (Can) see Hydrocortisone . . 793
Hycotuss® see Hydrocodone and
Guaifenesin 785
Hydase™ see Hyaluronidase 774
Hydeltra T.B.A.® (Can) see
PrednisoLONE 1268
Hydergine® (Can) see Ergoloid
Mesylates 557
Hydergine [DSC] see Ergoloid
Mesylates 557
Hyderm (Can) see Hydrocortisone . . 793
HydrALAZINE 775
Hydralazine and
Hydrochlorothiazide 775
Hydralazine and Isosorbide
Dinitrate see Isosorbide
Dinitrate and Hydralazine 867
Hydralazine Hydrochloride see
HydrALAZINE 775
Hydramine® [OTC] see
DiphenhydrAMINE 483
Hydrastis canadensis see Golden
Seal 1624
Hydrated Chloral see Chloral
Hydrate 312
Hydrea® see Hydroxyurea 800
Hydrisalic™ [OTC] see Salicylic
Acid 1374
Hydrochlorothiazide 776
Hydrochlorothiazide and Amiloride
see Amiloride and
Hydrochlorothiazide 85
Hydrochlorothiazide and Benazepril
see Benazepril and
Hydrochlorothiazide 187
Hydrochlorothiazide and Bisoprolol
see Bisoprolol and
Hydrochlorothiazide 212
Hydrochlorothiazide and Captopril
see Captopril and
Hydrochlorothiazide 259
Hydrochlorothiazide and Enalapril
see Enalapril and
Hydrochlorothiazide 541
Hydrochlorothiazide and
Eprosartan see Eprosartan and
Hydrochlorothiazide 555
Hydrochlorothiazide and Fosinopril
see Fosinopril and
Hydrochlorothiazide 709
Hydrochlorothiazide and
Hydralazine see Hydralazine
and Hydrochlorothiazide 775
Hydrochlorothiazide and Irbesartan
see Irbesartan and
Hydrochlorothiazide 860
Hydrochlorothiazide and Lisinopril
see Lisinopril and
Hydrochlorothiazide 938
Hydrochlorothiazide and Losartan
see Losartan and
Hydrochlorothiazide 952
Hydrochlorothiazide and
Methyldopa see Methyldopa
and Hydrochlorothiazide 1022
Hydrochlorothiazide and Metoprolol
see Metoprolol and
Hydrochlorothiazide 1032

Hydrochlorothiazide and Metoprolol Tartrate see Metoprolol and Hydrochlorothiazide 1032
Hydrochlorothiazide and Moexipril see Moexipril and Hydrochlorothiazide 1059
Hydrochlorothiazide and Olmesartan Medoxomil see Olmesartan and Hydrochlorothiazide 1143
Hydrochlorothiazide and Propranolol see Propranolol and Hydrochlorothiazide 1305
Hydrochlorothiazide and Quinapril see Quinapril and Hydrochlorothiazide 1323
Hydrochlorothiazide and Spironolactone 778
Hydrochlorothiazide and Telmisartan see Telmisartan and Hydrochlorothiazide 1452
Hydrochlorothiazide and Triamterene 778
Hydrochlorothiazide and Valsartan see Valsartan and Hydrochlorothiazide 1562
Hydrocil® Instant [OTC] see Psyllium 1313
Hydrocodone and Acetaminophen . . 779
Hydrocodone and Aspirin 782
Hydrocodone and Chlorpheniramine 784
Hydrocodone and Guaifenesin 785
Hydrocodone and Homatropine 786
Hydrocodone and Ibuprofen 787
Hydrocodone and Pseudoephedrine 788
Hydrocodone Bitartrate, Carbinoxamine Maleate, and Pseudoephedrine Hydrochloride see Hydrocodone, Carbinoxamine, and Pseudoephedrine 789
Hydrocodone Bitartrate, Phenylephrine Hydrochloride, and Diphenhydramine Hydrochloride see Hydrocodone, Phenylephrine, and Diphenhydramine 791
Hydrocodone, Carbinoxamine, and Pseudoephedrine 789
Hydrocodone, Chlorpheniramine, Phenylephrine, Acetaminophen, and Caffeine . . 790
Hydrocodone, Phenylephrine, and Diphenhydramine 791
Hydrocodone, Phenylephrine, and Guaifenesin 791
Hydrocodone, Pseudoephedrine, and Guaifenesin 792
Hydrocodone Tannate and Chlorpheniramine Tannate see Hydrocodone and Chlorpheniramine 784
Hydrocortisone 793
Hydrocortisone Acetate see Hydrocortisone 793
Hydrocortisone, Acetic Acid, and Propylene Glycol Diacetate see Acetic Acid, Propylene Glycol Diacetate, and Hydrocortisone . . . 45
Hydrocortisone and Benzoyl Peroxide see Benzoyl Peroxide and Hydrocortisone 195
Hydrocortisone and Ciprofloxacin see Ciprofloxacin and Hydrocortisone 348
Hydrocortisone and Iodoquinol see Iodoquinol and Hydrocortisone . . 853
Hydrocortisone and Lidocaine see Lidocaine and Hydrocortisone . . 928

Hydrocortisone and Pramoxine see Pramoxine and Hydrocortisone 1264
Hydrocortisone and Urea see Urea and Hydrocortisone 1551
Hydrocortisone, Bacitracin, Neomycin, and Polymyxin B see Bacitracin, Neomycin, Polymyxin B, and Hydrocortisone 177
Hydrocortisone Butyrate see Hydrocortisone 793
Hydrocortisone, Neomycin, and Polymyxin B see Neomycin, Polymyxin B, and Hydrocortisone 1101
Hydrocortisone Probutate see Hydrocortisone 793
Hydrocortisone Sodium Succinate see Hydrocortisone 793
Hydrocortisone Valerate see Hydrocortisone 793
Hydro DP see Hydrocodone, Phenylephrine, and Diphenhydramine 791
Hydro-GP see Hydrocodone, Phenylephrine, and Guaifenesin 791
Hydromet® see Hydrocodone and Homatropine 786
Hydromorph Contin® (Can) see Hydromorphone 797
Hydromorph-IR® (Can) see Hydromorphone 797
Hydromorphone 797
Hydromorphone HP (Can) see Hydromorphone 797
Hydromorphone HP® 10 (Can) see Hydromorphone 797
Hydromorphone HP® 20 (Can) see Hydromorphone 797
Hydromorphone HP® 50 (Can) see Hydromorphone 797
Hydromorphone HP® Forte (Can) see Hydromorphone 797
Hydromorphone Hydrochloride see Hydromorphone 797
Hydromorphone Hydrochloride Injection, USP (Can) see Hydromorphone 797
Hydropane® see Hydrocodone and Homatropine 786
Hydroquinol see Hydroquinone 798
Hydroquinone 798
Hydroquinone, Fluocinolone Acetonide, and Tretinoin see Fluocinolone, Hydroquinone, and Tretinoin 669
Hydro-Tussin™-CBX see Carbinoxamine and Pseudoephedrine 268
Hydro-Tussin™ DHC see Pseudoephedrine, Dihydrocodeine, and Chlorpheniramine 1312
Hydro-Tussin™ DM see Guaifenesin and Dextromethorphan 754
Hydro-Tussin™ EXP see Dihydrocodeine, Pseudoephedrine, and Guaifenesin 476
Hydro-Tussin™ HD see Hydrocodone, Pseudoephedrine, and Guaifenesin 792
Hydro-Tussin™ XP see Hydrocodone, Pseudoephedrine, and Guaifenesin 792

HydroVal® (Can) see
  Hydrocortisone 793
Hydroxocobalamin 798
Hydroxyamphetamine and
  Tropicamide 799
Hydroxyamphetamine
  Hydrobromide and Tropicamide
  see Hydroxyamphetamine and
  Tropicamide 799
4-Hydroxybutyrate see Sodium
  Oxybate 1402
Hydroxycarbamide see
  Hydroxyurea. 800
Hydroxychloroquine 799
Hydroxychloroquine Sulfate see
  Hydroxychloroquine 799
Hydroxydaunomycin Hydrochloride
  see DOXOrubicin 509
1α-Hydroxyergocalciferol see
  Doxercalciferol 508
Hydroxyethylcellulose see Artificial
  Tears 143
Hydroxyethyl Starch see
  Hetastarch 770
Hydroxyldaunorubicin
  Hydrochloride see
  DOXOrubicin 509
Hydroxypropyl Cellulose 800
Hydroxypropyl Methylcellulose 800
Hydroxyurea. 800
HydrOXYzine 801
Hydroxyzine Hydrochloride see
  HydrOXYzine 801
Hydroxyzine Hydrochloride
  Injection, USP (Can) see
  HydrOXYzine 801
Hydroxyzine Pamoate see
  HydrOXYzine 801
HydroZone Plus [OTC] see
  Hydrocortisone 793
Hygroton see Chlorthalidone 332
Hylaform® see Hyaluronate and
  Derivatives 773
Hylaform® Plus see Hyaluronate
  and Derivatives 773
Hylan Polymers see Hyaluronate
  and Derivatives 773
Hylenex® see Hyaluronidase 774
Hyoscine Butylbromide see
  Scopolamine 1380
Hyoscine Hydrobromide see
  Scopolamine 1380
Hyoscyamine 803
Hyoscyamine, Atropine,
  Scopolamine, and
  Phenobarbital 804
Hyoscyamine, Methenamine,
  Sodium Biphosphate, Phenyl
  Salicylate, and Methylene Blue
  see Methenamine, Sodium
  Biphosphate, Phenyl Salicylate,
  Methylene Blue, and
  Hyoscyamine 1008
Hyoscyamine Sulfate see
  Hyoscyamine 803
Hyosine see Hyoscyamine 803
Hypaque™-76 see Diatrizoate
  Meglumine and Diatrizoate
  Sodium 453
Hypaque-Cysto™ see Diatrizoate
  Meglumine 453
Hypaque™ Meglumine see
  Diatrizoate Meglumine 453
Hypaque™ Sodium see Diatrizoate
  Sodium 454
Hypericum perforatum see St
  John's Wort 1632
HyperHep B® (Can) see Hepatitis
  B Immune Globulin 768
Hyperstat® see Diazoxide 457

HypoTears [OTC] see Artificial
  Tears 143
HypoTears PF [OTC] see Artificial
  Tears 143
Hypromellose see Hydroxypropyl
  Methylcellulose 800
Hytakerol® (Can) see
  Dihydrotachysterol 478
Hytakerol® [DSC] see
  Dihydrotachysterol 478
HyTan™ see Hydrocodone and
  Chlorpheniramine 784
Hytinic® [OTC] see
  Polysaccharide-Iron Complex . . 1254
Hytone® see Hydrocortisone 793
Hytrin® see Terazosin 1458
Hyzaar® see Losartan and
  Hydrochlorothiazide 952
Hyzaar® DS (Can) see Losartan
  and Hydrochlorothiazide 952
Ibandronate 805
Ibandronate Sodium see
  Ibandronate 805
Iberet®-500 [OTC] see Vitamins
  (Multiple/Oral) 1582
Iberet® [OTC] see Vitamins
  (Multiple/Oral) 1582
Ibidomide Hydrochloride see
  Labetalol 891
Ibritumomab 807
Ibritumomab Tiuxetan see
  Ibritumomab 807
Ibu-200 [OTC] see Ibuprofen 808
Ibuprofen 808
Ibuprofen and Hydrocodone see
  Hydrocodone and Ibuprofen 787
Ibuprofen and Oxycodone see
  Oxycodone and Ibuprofen 1170
Ibuprofen and Pseudoephedrine
  see Pseudoephedrine and
  Ibuprofen 1311
Ibutilide 813
Ibutilide Fumarate see Ibutilide . . . 813
IC-Green® see Indocyanine Green . 830
ICI-182,780 see Fulvestrant 713
ICI-204,219 see Zafirlukast 1590
ICI-46474 see Tamoxifen 1443
ICI-118630 see Goserelin 750
ICI-176334 see Bicalutamide 207
ICI-D1033 see Anastrozole 126
ICL670 see Deferasirox 427
Icodextrin 814
ICRF-187 see Dexrazoxane 446
Idamycin® (Can) see Idarubicin . . . 814
Idamycin PFS® see Idarubicin 814
Idarubicin 814
Idarubicin Hydrochloride see
  Idarubicin 814
IDEC-C2B8 see Rituximab 1360
IDR see Idarubicin 814
Ifa Norex® (Mex) see
  Diethylpropion 467
Ifa Reduccing "S"® (Mex) see
  Phentermine 1224
Ifex® see Ifosfamide 815
IFLrA see Interferon Alfa-2a 842
Ifolem® (Mex) see Ifosfamide 815
Ifosfamide 815
Ifoxan® (Mex) see Ifosfamide 815
IG see Immune Globulin
  (Intramuscular) 823
IgG4-Kappa Monoclonal Antibody
  see Natalizumab 1093
IGIM see Immune Globulin
  (Intramuscular) 823
Ikatin® (Mex) see Gentamicin 734
IL-1Ra see Anakinra 125
IL-2 see Aldesleukin 61
IL-11 see Oprelvekin 1149
Iliadin® (Mex) see Oxymetazoline . . 1172
Iloprost 816

Iloprost Tromethamine see Iloprost 816
Ilosone® (Mex) see Erythromycin .. 562
Ilsatec® (Mex) see Lansoprazole .. 896
Imatinib 817
Imatinib Mesylate see Imatinib 817
IMC-C225 see Cetuximab 308
Imdur® see Isosorbide Mononitrate 868
IMI 30 see Idarubicin 814
IMid-3 see Lenalidomide 903
Imidazole Carboxamide see Dacarbazine 415
Imidazole Carboxamide Dimethyltriazene see Dacarbazine 415
Imiglucerase 819
Imigran® (Mex) see Sumatriptan .. 1432
Imipemide see Imipenem and Cilastatin 819
Imipenem and Cilastatin 819
Imipramine 820
Imipramine Hydrochloride see Imipramine 820
Imipramine Pamoate see Imipramine 820
Imiquimod 821
Imitrex® see Sumatriptan 1432
Imitrex® DF (Can) see Sumatriptan 1432
Imitrex® Nasal Spray (Can) see Sumatriptan 1432
ImmuCyst® (Can) see BCG Vaccine 181
Immune Globulin (Intramuscular) ... 823
Immune Globulin (Intravenous) 824
Immune Globulin (Subcutaneous) .. 826
Immune Globulin Subcutaneous (Human) see Immune Globulin (Subcutaneous) 826
Immune Serum Globulin see Immune Globulin (Intramuscular) 823
Immunine® VH (Can) see Factor IX 632
Imodium® (Can) see Loperamide ... 942
Imodium® A-D [OTC] see Loperamide 942
Imodium® Advanced see Loperamide and Simethicone .. 943
Imogam® Rabies-HT see Rabies Immune Globulin (Human) 1328
Imogam® Rabies Pasteurized (Can) see Rabies Immune Globulin (Human) 1328
Imovane® (Can) see Zopiclone ... 1606
Imovax® Rabies see Rabies Virus Vaccine 1329
Imuran® see Azathioprine 168
In-111 Zevalin see Ibritumomab ... 807
Inamrinone 827
Inapsine® see Droperidol 519
Increlex™ see Mecasermin 968
Indapamide 828
Indarzona® (Mex) see Dexamethasone 439
Inderal® see Propranolol 1301
Inderal® LA see Propranolol 1301
Inderide® see Propranolol and Hydrochlorothiazide 1305
Indian Eye see Golden Seal 1624
Indian Head see Echinacea 1620
Indinavir 829
Indinavir Sulfate see Indinavir 829
Indocid® P.D.A. (Can) see Indomethacin 830
Indocin® see Indomethacin 830
Indocin® I.V. see Indomethacin 830
Indocin® SR see Indomethacin 830
Indocyanine Green 830

Indo-Lemmon (Can) see Indomethacin 830
Indometacin see Indomethacin 830
Indomethacin 830
Indomethacin Sodium Trihydrate see Indomethacin 830
Indotec (Can) see Indomethacin ... 830
INF-alpha 2 see Interferon Alfa-2b .. 844
Infantaire Gas Drops [OTC] see Simethicone 1394
Infantaire [OTC] see Acetaminophen 31
Infants' Tylenol® Cold Plus Cough Concentrated Drops [OTC] see Acetaminophen, Dextromethorphan, and Pseudoephedrine 44
Infasurf® see Calfactant 251
INFeD® see Iron Dextran Complex 862
Inflamase® Mild (Can) see PrednisoLONE 1268
Infliximab 832
Infliximab, Recombinant see Infliximab 832
Influenza Virus Vaccine 833
Influenza Virus Vaccine (Purified Surface Antigen) see Influenza Virus Vaccine 833
Influenza Virus Vaccine (Split-Virus) see Influenza Virus Vaccine 833
Influenza Virus Vaccine (Trivalent, Live) see Influenza Virus Vaccine 833
Infufer® (Can) see Iron Dextran Complex 862
Infumorph® see Morphine Sulfate .. 1065
INH see Isoniazid 864
Inhaled Insulin see Insulin Inhalation 837
Inhibace® (Can) see Cilazapril ... 340
Inhibitron® (Mex) see Omeprazole 1145
Inibace® (Mex) see Cilazapril 340
Innohep® see Tinzaparin 1492
InnoPran XL™ see Propranolol ... 1301
INOmax® see Nitric Oxide 1118
Insect Sting Kit see Epinephrine and Chlorpheniramine 549
Insogen® (Mex) see ChlorproPAMIDE 331
Insoluble Prussian Blue see Ferric Hexacyanoferrate 650
Inspra™ see Eplerenone 551
Insta-Glucose® [OTC] see Dextrose 452
Instat™ see Collagen Hemostat ... 392
Instat™ MCH see Collagen Hemostat 392
Insulin Aspart 835
Insulin Aspart and Insulin Aspart Protamine see Insulin Aspart Protamine and Insulin Aspart ... 836
Insulin Aspart Protamine and Insulin Aspart 836
Insulin Detemir 836
Insulin Glargine 837
Insulin Glulisine 837
Insulin Inhalation 837
Insulin Lispro 839
Insulin Lispro and Insulin Lispro Protamine see Insulin Lispro Protamine and Insulin Lispro ... 839
Insulin Lispro Protamine and Insulin Lispro 839
Insulin NPH 840
Insulin NPH and Insulin Regular ... 840
Insulin Regular 841

Insulin Regular and Insulin NPH
  see Insulin NPH and Insulin
  Regular 840
Intal® *see* Cromolyn 397
Integrilin® *see* Eptifibatide 556
α-2-interferon *see* Interferon
  Alfa-2b 844
Interferon Alfa-2a 842
Interferon Alfa-2a (PEG Conjugate)
  see Peginterferon Alfa-2a 1195
Interferon Alfa-2b 844
Interferon Alfa-2b and Ribavirin 847
Interferon Alfa-2b and Ribavirin
  Combination Pack *see*
  Interferon Alfa-2b and Ribavirin
  847
Interferon Alfa-2b (PEG Conjugate)
  see Peginterferon Alfa-2b 1197
Interferon Alfa-n3 848
Interferon Beta-1a 849
Interferon Beta-1b 850
Interferon Gamma-1b 851
Interleukin-1 Receptor Antagonist
  see Anakinra 125
Interleukin-2 *see* Aldesleukin 61
Interleukin-11 *see* Oprelvekin 1149
Intralipid® *see* Fat Emulsion 637
Intravenous Fat Emulsion *see* Fat
  Emulsion 637
Intrifiban *see* Eptifibatide 556
Intron® A *see* Interferon Alfa-2b 844
Intropaste *see* Barium 179
Invanz® *see* Ertapenem 561
Inversine® *see* Mecamylamine 968
Invirase® *see* Saquinavir 1377
Iodex [OTC] *see* Iodine 852
Iodine 852
Iodipamide Meglumine 853
Iodipamide Meglumine and
  Diatrizoate Meglumine *see*
  Diatrizoate Meglumine and
  Iodipamide Meglumine 453
Iodixanol 853
Iodoflex™ *see* Iodine 852
Iodopen® *see* Trace Metals 1513
Iodoquinol 853
Iodoquinol and Hydrocortisone 853
Iodosorb® *see* Iodine 852
Iohexol 854
Ionamin® *see* Phentermine 1224
Ionil® (Mex) *see* Salicylic Acid 1374
Ionil® [OTC] *see* Salicylic Acid 1374
Ionil Plus® (Mex) *see* Salicylic Acid
  1374
Ionil® Plus [OTC] *see* Salicylic Acid
  1374
Ionil T® [OTC] *see* Coal Tar 383
Ionil T® Plus [OTC] *see* Coal Tar . . . 383
Iopamidol 855
Iophen-C NR *see* Guaifenesin and
  Codeine 753
Iophen DM NR *see* Guaifenesin
  and Dextromethorphan 754
Iophen NR *see* Guaifenesin 752
Iopidine® *see* Apraclonidine 133
Iopromide 855
Iosat™ [OTC] *see* Potassium
  Iodide 1260
Iothalamate Meglumine 855
Iothalamate Sodium 855
Ioversol 856
Ioxaglate Meglumine and Ioxaglate
  Sodium 856
Ioxaglate Sodium and Ioxaglate
  Meglumine *see* Ioxaglate
  Meglumine and Ioxaglate
  Sodium 856
Ipecac Syrup 856
Iplex™ *see* Mecasermin 968
IPM Wound Gel™ [OTC] *see*
  Hyaluronate and Derivatives . . . 773

IPOL® *see* Poliovirus Vaccine
  (Inactivated) 1252
Ipratropium 857
Ipratropium and Albuterol 857
Ipratropium Bromide *see*
  Ipratropium 857
I-Prin [OTC] *see* Ibuprofen 808
Iproveratril Hydrochloride *see*
  Verapamil 1571
IPV *see* Poliovirus Vaccine
  (Inactivated) 1252
Iquix® *see* Levofloxacin 913
Irbesartan 858
Irbesartan and Hydrochlorothiazide
  860
Ircon® [OTC] *see* Ferrous
  Fumarate 650
IRESSA® *see* Gefitinib 727
Irinotecan 860
Irinotecan Hydrochloride Trihydrate
  (Can) *see* Irinotecan 860
Iron Dextran Complex 862
Iron Fumarate *see* Ferrous
  Fumarate 650
Iron Gluconate *see* Ferrous
  Gluconate 651
Iron-Polysaccharide Complex *see*
  Polysaccharide-Iron Complex . . 1254
Iron Sucrose 862
Iron Sulfate *see* Ferrous Sulfate 651
Iron Sulfate and Vitamin C *see*
  Ferrous Sulfate and Ascorbic
  Acid 651
Irtan® (Mex) *see* Nedocromil 1095
Isadol® (Mex) *see* Zidovudine 1594
Isavir® (Mex) *see* Acyclovir 49
ISD *see* Isosorbide Dinitrate 866
ISDN *see* Isosorbide Dinitrate 866
ISG *see* Immune Globulin
  (Intramuscular) 823
ISMN *see* Isosorbide Mononitrate . . . 868
Ismo® *see* Isosorbide Mononitrate . . 868
Isoamyl Nitrite *see* Amyl Nitrite 124
Isobamate *see* Carisoprodol 271
Isocarboxazid 863
Isochron™ *see* Isosorbide Dinitrate
  866
Isodine® (Mex) *see*
  Povidone-Iodine 1262
Isoflavones *see* Soy Isoflavones . . 1632
Isoket® (Mex) *see* Isosorbide
  Dinitrate 866
Isometheptene, Acetaminophen,
  and Dichloralphenazone *see*
  Acetaminophen,
  Isometheptene, and
  Dichloralphenazone 44
Isometheptene,
  Dichloralphenazone, and
  Acetaminophen *see*
  Acetaminophen,
  Isometheptene, and
  Dichloralphenazone 44
Isoniazid 864
Isoniazid and Rifampin *see*
  Rifampin and Isoniazid 1348
Isoniazid, Rifampin, and
  Pyrazinamide *see* Rifampin,
  Isoniazid, and Pyrazinamide . . 1348
Isonicotinic Acid Hydrazide *see*
  Isoniazid 864
Isonipecaine Hydrochloride *see*
  Meperidine 983
Isophane Insulin *see* Insulin NPH . . 840
Isophane Insulin and Regular
  Insulin *see* Insulin NPH and
  Insulin Regular 840
Isophosphamide *see* Ifosfamide 815

Isopropyl Alcohol Tincture of
Benzylkonium Chloride *see*
Benzalkonium Chloride and
Isopropyl Alcohol 189
Isoproterenol 865
Isoproterenol Hydrochloride *see*
Isoproterenol 865
Isoptin® SR *see* Verapamil 1571
Isopto® Atropine *see* Atropine 161
Isopto® Carbachol *see* Carbachol . . 260
Isopto® Carpine *see* Pilocarpine
(Ophthalmic) 1234
Isopto® Eserine (Can) *see*
Physostigmine 1232
Isopto® Homatropine *see*
Homatropine 772
Isopto® Hyoscine *see* Scopolamine
. . . . 1380
Isopto® Tears (Can) *see*
Hydroxypropyl Methylcellulose . . 800
Isopto® Tears [OTC] *see* Artificial
Tears 143
Isorbid® (Mex) *see* Isosorbide
Dinitrate 866
Isordil® *see* Isosorbide Dinitrate 866
Isosorbide Dinitrate 866
Isosorbide Dinitrate and
Hydralazine 867
Isosorbide Mononitrate 868
Isotamine® (Can) *see* Isoniazid 864
Isotretinoin 869
Isotrex® (Can) *see* Isotretinoin 869
Isovue® *see* Iopamidol 855
Isovue-M® *see* Iopamidol 855
Isovue Multipack® *see* Iopamidol . . . 855
Isox® (Mex) *see* Itraconazole 873
Isoxsuprine 871
Isoxsuprine Hydrochloride *see*
Isoxsuprine 871
Isradipine 871
Istalol™ *see* Timolol 1489
Isuprel® *see* Isoproterenol 865
Itch-X® [OTC] *see* Pramoxine 1264
Itraconazole 873
Itranax® (Mex) *see* Itraconazole 873
Iveegam EN *see* Immune Globulin
(Intravenous) 824
Iveegam Immuno® (Can) *see*
Immune Globulin (Intravenous)
. . . . 824
Ivermectin 877
IVIG *see* Immune Globulin
(Intravenous) 824
IvyBlock® [OTC] *see* Bentoquatam . . 188
Ivy-Rid® [OTC] *see* Benzocaine 190
IvySoothe® [OTC] *see*
Hydrocortisone 793
Izadima® (Mex) *see* Ceftazidime . . . 292
Jamp® Travel Tablet (Can) *see*
DimenhyDRINATE 481
Jantoven™ *see* Warfarin 1585
Japanese Encephalitis Virus
Vaccine (Inactivated) 877
Jaundice Root *see* Golden Seal . . . 1624
JE-VAX® *see* Japanese
Encephalitis Virus Vaccine
(Inactivated) 877
Johimbe *see* Yohimbe 1634
Jolivette™ *see* Norethindrone 1125
Junel™ *see* Ethinyl Estradiol and
Norethindrone 608
Junel™ Fe *see* Ethinyl Estradiol
and Norethindrone 608
Just for Kids™ [OTC] *see* Fluoride . . 671
K-10® (Can) *see* Potassium
Chloride 1258
Kadian® *see* Morphine Sulfate 1065
Kala® [OTC] *see* *Lactobacillus* 535
Kaletra® *see* Lopinavir and
Ritonavir 943

Kaliolite® (Mex) *see* Potassium
Bicarbonate 1257
Kalmz [OTC] *see* Fructose,
Dextrose, and Phosphoric Acid
. . . . 713
Kanamycin 878
Kanamycin Sulfate *see* Kanamycin
. . . . 878
Kank-A® (Can) *see* Cetylpyridinium
and Benzocaine 309
Kanka® Soft Brush™ [OTC] *see*
Benzocaine 190
Kantrex® *see* Kanamycin 878
Kaodene® NN [OTC] [DSC] *see*
Kaolin and Pectin 879
Kaolin and Pectin 879
Kaon-Cl-10® *see* Potassium
Chloride 1258
Kaon-Cl® 20 *see* Potassium
Chloride 1258
Kao-Paverin® [OTC] *see*
Loperamide 942
Kaopectate® (Can) *see* Attapulgite . . 165
Kaopectate® Advanced Formula
[OTC] [DSC] *see* Attapulgite . . . 165
Kaopectate® Extra Strength [OTC]
see Bismuth 210
Kaopectate® Maximum Strength
Caplets [OTC] [DSC] *see*
Attapulgite 165
Kaopectate® [OTC] *see* Bismuth . . 210
Kaopectolin *(new formulation)*
[OTC] *see* Bismuth 210
Kao-Spen® [OTC] [DSC] *see*
Kaolin and Pectin 879
Kapectolin [OTC] [DSC] *see*
Kaolin and Pectin 879
Kariva™ *see* Ethinyl Estradiol and
Desogestrel 592
Kasmal® (Mex) *see* Ketotifen 890
Kava 1627
Kava Kava *see* Kava 1627
Kaveri *see* Ginkgo Biloba 1622
Kay Ciel® *see* Potassium Chloride
. . . . 1258
K-Citra® (Can) *see* Potassium
Citrate 1259
KCl *see* Potassium Chloride 1258
K-Dur® (Mex) *see* Potassium
Bicarbonate 1257
K-Dur® 10 *see* Potassium Chloride
. . . . 1258
K-Dur® 20 *see* Potassium Chloride
. . . . 1258
Keflex® *see* Cephalexin 301
Keftab® (Can) *see* Cephalexin 301
Kelnor™ *see* Ethinyl Estradiol and
Ethynodiol Diacetate 597
Kemadrin® *see* Procyclidine 1288
Kenalog® *see* Triamcinolone 1526
Kenalog-10® *see* Triamcinolone . . . 1526
Kenalog-40® *see* Triamcinolone . . . 1526
Kenalog® in Orabase (Can) *see*
Triamcinolone 1526
Kenoket® (Mex) *see* Clonazepam . . 371
Kenolan® (Mex) *see* Captopril 257
Kenopril® (Mex) *see* Enalapril 538
Kentadin® (Mex) *see* Pentoxifylline
. . . . 1212
Kenzoflex® (Mex) *see* Ciprofloxacin
. . . . 343
Keoxifene Hydrochloride *see*
Raloxifene 1329
Kepivance™ *see* Palifermin 1178
Keppra® *see* Levetiracetam 908
Keralac™ *see* Urea 1551
Keralac™ Nailstik *see* Urea 1551
Keralyt® [OTC] *see* Salicylic Acid . . 1374
Kerlone® *see* Betaxolol 203
Kerr Insta-Char® [OTC] *see*
Charcoal 311

Ketalar® see Ketamine 880
Ketalin® (Mex) see Ketamine 880
Ketamine 880
Ketamine Hydrochloride see
  Ketamine 880
Ketamine Hydrochloride Injection,
  USP (Can) see Ketamine . . . 880
Ketek® see Telithromycin 1448
Ketoconazole 880
Ketoderm® (Can) see
  Ketoconazole 880
Ketoprofen 883
Ketorolac 886
Ketorolac Tromethamine see
  Ketorolac 886
Ketorolac Tromethamine Injection,
  USP (Can) see Ketorolac 886
Ketotifen 890
Ketotifen Fumarate see Ketotifen . . 890
Kew see Kava 1627
Kew Tree see Ginkgo Biloba 1622
Key-E® Kaps [OTC] see Vitamin E
  1581
Key-E® [OTC] see Vitamin E 1581
Keygesic [OTC] see Magnesium
  Salicylate 962
KI see Potassium Iodide 1260
Kidkare Decongestant [OTC] see
  Pseudoephedrine 1309
Kidrolase® (Can) see Asparaginase
  144
Kineret® see Anakinra 125
Kinestase® (Mex) see Cisapride . . . 348
Kinevac® see Sincalide 1396
Kivexa™ (Can) see Abacavir and
  Lamivudine 23
Klamath Weed see St John's Wort
  1632
Klaricid® (Mex) see Clarithromycin . . 355
Klaron® see Sulfacetamide 1423
Klean-Prep® (Can) see
  Polyethylene Glycol-Electrolyte
  Solution 1253
Klonopin® see Clonazepam 371
K-Lor® see Potassium Chloride 1258
Klor-Con® see Potassium Chloride
  1258
Klor-Con® 8 see Potassium
  Chloride 1258
Klor-Con® 10 see Potassium
  Chloride 1258
Klor-Con®/25 see Potassium
  Chloride 1258
Klor-Con® M see Potassium
  Chloride 1258
Klor-Con®/EF see Potassium
  Bicarbonate and Potassium
  Citrate 1258
Klyndaken® (Mex) see Clindamycin
  361
K-Lyte® see Potassium
  Bicarbonate and Potassium
  Citrate 1258
K-Lyte/Cl® see Potassium
  Bicarbonate and Potassium
  Chloride 1258
K-Lyte/Cl® 50 [DSC] see
  Potassium Bicarbonate and
  Potassium Chloride 1258
K-Lyte® DS see Potassium
  Bicarbonate and Potassium
  Citrate 1258
Kodet SE [OTC] see
  Pseudoephedrine 1309
Koffex DM-D (Can) see
  Pseudoephedrine and
  Dextromethorphan 1311
Koffex DM + Decongestant +
  Expectorant (Can) see
  Guaifenesin, Pseudoephedrine,
  and Dextromethorphan 757

Koffex DM-Expectorant (Can) see
  Guaifenesin and
  Dextromethorphan 754
Koffex Expectorant (Can) see
  Guaifenesin 752
Kogenate® (Can) see
  Antihemophilic Factor
  (Recombinant) 130
Kogenate® FS see Antihemophilic
  Factor (Recombinant) 130
Kolephrin® #1 see Guaifenesin and
  Codeine 753
Kolephrin® GG/DM [OTC] see
  Guaifenesin and
  Dextromethorphan 754
Kolephrin® [OTC] see
  Acetaminophen,
  Chlorpheniramine, and
  Pseudoephedrine 43
Konaderm® (Mex) see
  Ketoconazole 880
Konakion (Can) see Phytonadione
  1233
Konsyl-D® [OTC] see Psyllium . . . 1313
Konsyl® Easy Mix [OTC] see
  Psyllium 1313
Konsyl® Fiber Tablets [OTC] see
  Polycarbophil 1252
Konsyl® Orange [OTC] see
  Psyllium 1313
Konsyl® [OTC] see Psyllium 1313
Koptin® (Mex) see Kanamycin 878
Kovia® see Papain and Urea 1186
Koāte®-DVI see Antihemophilic
  Factor (Human) 129
K-Pek II [OTC] see Loperamide . . . 942
K-Phos® MF see Potassium
  Phosphate and Sodium
  Phosphate 1261
K-Phos® Neutral see Potassium
  Phosphate and Sodium
  Phosphate 1261
K-Phos® No. 2 see Potassium
  Phosphate and Sodium
  Phosphate 1261
K-Phos® Original see Potassium
  Acid Phosphate 1257
K+ Potassium see Potassium
  Chloride 1258
Kristalose™ see Lactulose 893
Kronofed-A® see Chlorpheniramine
  and Pseudoephedrine 325
Kronofed-A®-Jr see
  Chlorpheniramine and
  Pseudoephedrine 325
K-Tab® see Potassium Chloride . . . 1258
kutrase® see Pancreatin 1183
ku-zyme® see Pancreatin 1183
ku-zyme® HP see Pancrelipase . . . 1183
Kwelcof® see Hydrocodone and
  Guaifenesin 785
Kwellada-P™ (Can) see Permethrin
  1218
Kytril® see Granisetron 751
L-749,345 see Ertapenem 561
L-M-X™ 4 [OTC] see Lidocaine . . . 920
L-M-X™ 5 [OTC] see Lidocaine . . . 920
L 754030 see Aprepitant 134
LA 20304a see Gemifloxacin 731
Labetalol 891
Labetalol Hydrochloride see
  Labetalol 891
Labetalol Hydrochloride Injection,
  USP (Can) see Labetalol 891
Lac-Hydrin® see Lactic Acid and
  Ammonium Hydroxide 893
Lac-Hydrin® Five [OTC] see Lactic
  Acid and Ammonium
  Hydroxide 893
Laciken® (Mex) see Acyclovir 49

LAClotion™ see Lactic Acid and Ammonium Hydroxide 893
Lacrisert® see Hydroxypropyl Cellulose 800
Lactaid® Extra Strength [OTC] [DSC] see Lactase 892
Lactaid® Fast Act [OTC] see Lactase 892
Lactaid® Original [OTC] see Lactase 892
Lactaid® Ultra [OTC] [DSC] see Lactase 892
Lactase 892
Lactic Acid 893
Lactic Acid and Ammonium Hydroxide 893
LactiCare-HC® (Mex) see Hydrocortisone 793
LactiCare® [OTC] see Lactic Acid . 893
Lactinex™ [OTC] see Lactobacillus 535
Lactinol® see Lactic Acid 893
Lactinol-E® see Lactic Acid 893
Lactobacillus 535
Lactobacillus acidophilus see Lactobacillus 535
Lactobacillus bifidus see Lactobacillus 535
Lactobacillus bulgaricus see Lactobacillus 535
Lactobacillus casei see Lactobacillus 535
Lactobacillus paracasei see Lactobacillus 535
Lactobacillus reuteri see Lactobacillus 535
Lactobacillus rhamnosus GG see Lactobacillus 535
Lacto-Bifidus [OTC] see Lactobacillus 535
Lactoflavin see Riboflavin 1345
Lacto-Key [OTC] see Lactobacillus 535
Lacto-Pectin [OTC] see Lactobacillus 535
Lacto-TriBlend [OTC] see Lactobacillus 535
Lactrase® [OTC] see Lactase 892
Lactulax® (Mex) see Lactulose . . . 893
Lactulose 893
Ladakamycin see Azacitidine 167
Ladogal® (Mex) see Danazol 419
Lakriment Neu see Licorice 1627
L-AmB see Amphotericin B (Liposomal) 116
Lamictal® see Lamotrigine 895
Lamisil® see Terbinafine 1459
Lamisil® AT™ [OTC] see Terbinafine 1459
Lamivudine 894
Lamivudine, Abacavir, and Zidovudine see Abacavir, Lamivudine, and Zidovudine . . . 23
Lamivudine and Abacavir see Abacavir and Lamivudine 23
Lamivudine and Zidovudine see Zidovudine and Lamivudine . . . 1596
Lamotrigine 895
Lamprene® (Can) see Clofazimine . 369
Lamprene® [DSC] see Clofazimine 369
Lanacane® Maximum Strength [OTC] see Benzocaine 190
Lanacane® [OTC] see Benzocaine . 190
Lanaphilic® [OTC] see Urea 1551
Lanexat® (Mex) see Flumazenil . . . 665
Lanolin, Cetyl Alcohol, Glycerin, Petrolatum, and Mineral Oil 896
Lanoxicaps® see Digoxin 471
Lanoxin® see Digoxin 471
Lansoprazole 896

Lansoprazole, Amoxicillin, and Clarithromycin 898
Lansoprazole and Naproxen 898
Lanthanum 899
Lanthanum Carbonate see Lanthanum 899
Lantus® see Insulin Glargine 837
Lantus® OptiSet® (Can) see Insulin Glargine 837
Lanvis® (Can) see Thioguanine . . . 1476
Lapase see Pancrelipase 1183
Laracit® (Mex) see Cytarabine 413
Largactil® (Can) see ChlorproMAZINE 329
Lariam® see Mefloquine 975
Laronidase 900
Lasix® see Furosemide 715
Lasix® Special (Can) see Furosemide 715
L-asparaginase see Asparaginase . . 144
Lassar's Zinc Paste see Zinc Oxide 1597
Lastet® (Mex) see Etoposide 626
Latanoprost 900
Latotryd® (Mex) see Erythromycin . 562
Lauricin® (Mex) see Erythromycin . 562
Lauritran® (Mex) see Erythromycin . 562
Laurus Sassafras see Sassafras Oil 1631
Laxilose (Can) see Lactulose 893
l-Bunolol Hydrochloride see Levobunolol 909
L-Carnitine see Levocarnitine 910
LCD see Coal Tar 383
LCR see VinCRIStine 1576
L-Deprenyl see Selegiline 1382
LDP-341 see Bortezomib 215
Lectopam® (Can) see Bromazepam 220
Ledertrexate® (Mex) see Methotrexate 1012
Ledoxina® (Mex) see Cyclophosphamide 403
Leena™ see Ethinyl Estradiol and Norethindrone 608
Leflunomide 901
Legatrin PM® [OTC] see Acetaminophen and Diphenhydramine 38
Lemblastine® (Mex) see VinBLAStine 1575
Lemon Balm/Melissa 1627
Lenalidomide 903
Lenpryl® (Mex) see Captopril 257
Lepirudin 904
Lepirudin (rDNA) see Lepirudin . . . 904
Leptilan® (Mex) see Valproic Acid and Derivatives 1556
Leptopsique® (Mex) see Perphenazine 1218
Lertamine® (Mex) see Loratadine . . . 946
Lertamine-D® (Mex) see Pseudoephedrine 1309
Lescol® see Fluvastatin 693
Lescol® XL see Fluvastatin 693
Lessina™ see Ethinyl Estradiol and Levonorgestrel 602
Letrozole 904
Leucovorin 905
Leucovorin Calcium see Leucovorin 905
Leukeran® see Chlorambucil 313
Leukine® see Sargramostim 1378
Leunase® (Mex) see Asparaginase 144
Leuprolide 906
Leuprolide Acetate see Leuprolide . . 906
Leuprorelin Acetate see Leuprolide 906
Leurocristine Sulfate see VinCRIStine 1576

Leustatin® see Cladribine 354
Levalbuterol 907
Levalbuterol Hydrochloride see
   Levalbuterol 907
Levalbuterol Tartrate see
   Levalbuterol 907
Levall 5.0 see Hydrocodone,
   Phenylephrine, and
   Guaifenesin 791
Levall G see Guaifenesin and
   Pseudoephedrine 755
Levaquin® see Levofloxacin 913
Levarterenol Bitartrate see
   Norepinephrine. 1125
Levate® (Can) see Amitriptyline 93
Levatol® see Penbutolol 1199
Levbid® see Hyoscyamine 803
Levemir® see Insulin Detemir 836
Levetiracetam 908
Levitra® see Vardenafil 1565
Levlen® see Ethinyl Estradiol and
   Levonorgestrel 602
Levlite™ see Ethinyl Estradiol and
   Levonorgestrel 602
Levobunolol 909
Levobunolol Hydrochloride see
   Levobunolol 909
Levobupivacaine 909
Levocabastine 910
Levocabastine Hydrochloride see
   Levocabastine 910
Levocarnitine 910
Levocina® (Mex) see
   Methotrimeprazine 1016
Levodopa and Carbidopa 911
Levodopa, Carbidopa, and
   Entacapone 912
Levo-Dromoran® see Levorphanol . . 916
Levofloxacin 913
Levomepromazine see
   Methotrimeprazine 1016
Levonordefrin and Mepivacaine
   Hydrochloride see Mepivacaine
   and Levonordefrin . . . .
   991
Levonorgestrel 916
Levonorgestrel and Ethinyl
   Estradiol see Ethinyl Estradiol
   and Levonorgestrel 602
Levophed® see Norepinephrine 1125
Levora® see Ethinyl Estradiol and
   Levonorgestrel 602
Levorphanol 916
Levorphanol Tartrate see
   Levorphanol 916
Levorphan Tartrate see
   Levorphanol 916
Levothroid® see Levothyroxine 917
Levothyroxine 917
Levothyroxine Sodium (Can) see
   Levothyroxine. 917
Levoxyl® see Levothyroxine 917
Levsin® see Hyoscyamine 803
Levsinex® see Hyoscyamine 803
Levsin/SL® see Hyoscyamine 803
Levulan® (Can) see Aminolevulinic
   Acid 88
Levulan® Kerastick® see
   Aminolevulinic Acid 88
Levulose, Dextrose and
   Phosphoric Acid see Fructose,
   Dextrose, and Phosphoric Acid
   713
Lexapro® see Escitalopram 568
Lexiva™ see Fosamprenavir 702
Lexotan® (Mex) see Bromazepam . . 220
Lexxel® see Enalapril and
   Felodipine 540
LFA-3/IgG(1) Fusion Protein,
   Human see Alefacept 62
L-Glutamine see Glutamine 743
L-Glutathione see Glutathione 1624

LHRH see Gonadorelin 749
LH-RH Agonist see Histrelin 772
l-Hyoscyamine Sulfate see
   Hyoscyamine 803
Librax® (Can) see Clidinium and
   Chlordiazepoxide 360
Librax® [original formulation] see
   Clidinium and
   Chlordiazepoxide 360
Librax® [reformulation] [DSC] see
   Chlordiazepoxide and
   Methscopolamine 316
Librium® see Chlordiazepoxide. 315
Lice-Aid [OTC] see Pyrethrins and
   Piperonyl Butoxide 1315
Licide® [OTC] see Pyrethrins and
   Piperonyl Butoxide 1315
Licorice. 1627
LidaMantle® see Lidocaine 920
Lida-Mantle® HC see Lidocaine
   and Hydrocortisone 928
Lidemol® (Can) see Fluocinonide . . 670
Lidex® see Fluocinonide 670
Lidex-E® see Fluocinonide 670
Lidocaine 920
Lidocaine and Bupivacaine. 924
Lidocaine and Epinephrine 924
Lidocaine and Hydrocortisone 928
Lidocaine and Prilocaine 928
Lidocaine and Tetracaine 930
Lidocaine Hydrochloride see
   Lidocaine 920
Lidocaine Hydrochloride and
   Bupivacaine Hydrochloride see
   Lidocaine and Bupivacaine 924
Lidocaine (Transoral) 931
Lidodan™ (Can) see Lidocaine 920
Lidoderm® see Lidocaine 920
LidoSite™ see Lidocaine and
   Epinephrine 924
LID-Pack® (Can) see Bacitracin
   and Polymyxin B 176
Lignocaine Hydrochloride see
   Lidocaine 920
Lilly CT-3231 see Vindesine 1577
Limbitrol® see Amitriptyline and
   Chlordiazepoxide 97
Limbitrol® DS see Amitriptyline and
   Chlordiazepoxide 97
Limbrel™ see Flavocoxid 656
Lin-Amox (Can) see Amoxicillin . . . 106
Lin-Buspirone (Can) see
   BusPIRone 236
Lincocin® see Lincomycin 932
Lincomycin 932
Lincomycin Hydrochloride see
   Lincomycin 932
Lindane 933
Linessa® (Can) see Ethinyl
   Estradiol and Desogestrel 592
Linezolid. 933
Lin-Sotalol (Can) see Sotalol 1409
Lioresal® see Baclofen 178
Liotec (Can) see Baclofen 178
Liothyronine 934
Liothyronine Sodium see
   Liothyronine 934
Liotrix 935
Lipancreatin see Pancrelipase 1183
Lipidil® (Mex) see Fenofibrate 639
Lipidil EZ® (Can) see Fenofibrate . . 639
Lipidil Micro® (Can) see
   Fenofibrate 639
Lipidil Supra® (Can) see
   Fenofibrate 639
Lipitor® see Atorvastatin 158
Lipofen™ see Fenofibrate 639
Lipoic Acid see Alpha-Lipoic Acid
   1614
Liposyn® II (Can) see Fat Emulsion
   637

Liposyn® III see Fat Emulsion 637
Lipram 4500 see Pancrelipase 1183
Lipram-CR see Pancrelipase 1183
Lipram-PN see Pancrelipase 1183
Lipram-UL see Pancrelipase 1183
Liquibid-D see Guaifenesin and
    Phenylephrine 754
Liquibid-PD see Guaifenesin and
    Phenylephrine 754
Liqui-Coat HD® see Barium 179
Liquid Antidote see Charcoal 311
Liquid Barosperse® see Barium 179
Liquifilm® Tears [OTC] see Artificial
    Tears 143
Liquorice see Licorice 1627
Lisinopril 936
Lisinopril and Hydrochlorothiazide . . 938
Lispro Insulin see Insulin Lispro . . . 839
Lithane™ (Can) see Lithium 939
Litheum® (Mex) see Lithium 939
Lithium 939
Lithium Carbonate see Lithium 939
Lithium Citrate see Lithium 939
Lithobid® see Lithium 939
Lithostat® see Acetohydroxamic
    Acid 46
Live Attenuated Influenza Vaccine
    (LAIV) see Influenza Virus
    Vaccine 833
Livostin® (Can) see Levocabastine . . 910
Livostin® [DSC] see Levocabastine
    910
L-Lysine 959
L-Lysine Hydrochloride see
    L-Lysine 959
LMD® see Dextran 447
LNg 20 see Levonorgestrel 916
Locoid® see Hydrocortisone 793
Locoid Lipocream® see
    Hydrocortisone 793
Lodine® (Can) see Etodolac 623
Lodine® XL [DSC] see Etodolac . . . 623
Lodine® [DSC] see Etodolac 623
Lodosyn® see Carbidopa 267
Lodoxamide 940
Lodoxamide Tromethamine see
    Lodoxamide 940
Lodrane® see Brompheniramine
    and Pseudoephedrine 223
Lodrane® 12D see
    Brompheniramine and
    Pseudoephedrine 223
Lodrane® LD see
    Brompheniramine and
    Pseudoephedrine 223
Loestrin® see Ethinyl Estradiol and
    Norethindrone 608
Loestrin™ 1.5/30 (Can) see Ethinyl
    Estradiol and Norethindrone 608
Loestrin® 24 Fe see Ethinyl
    Estradiol and Norethindrone 608
Loestrin® Fe see Ethinyl Estradiol
    and Norethindrone 608
Lofibra™ see Fenofibrate 639
LoHist-D see Chlorpheniramine
    and Pseudoephedrine 325
L-OHP see Oxaliplatin 1154
LoKara™ see Desonide 437
Lomacin® (Mex) see Lomefloxacin . . 941
Lomefloxacin 941
Lomefloxacin Hydrochloride see
    Lomefloxacin 941
Lomine (Can) see Dicyclomine 464
Lomotil® see Diphenoxylate and
    Atropine 487
Lomustine 941
Loniten® see Minoxidil 1051
Lonol® (Mex) see Benzydamine 197
Lonox® see Diphenoxylate and
    Atropine 487

Lo/Ovral® see Ethinyl Estradiol and
    Norgestrel 616
Loperacap (Can) see Loperamide . . 942
Loperamide 942
Loperamide and Simethicone 943
Loperamide Hydrochloride see
    Loperamide 942
Lopid® see Gemfibrozil 730
Lopinavir and Ritonavir 943
Lopremone see Protirelin 1307
Lopresor® (Mex) see Metoprolol . . . 1030
Lopressor® see Metoprolol 1030
Lopressor HCT® see Metoprolol
    and Hydrochlorothiazide 1032
Loprox® see Ciclopirox 338
Lorabid® see Loracarbef 945
Loracarbef 945
Loratadine 946
Loratadine and Pseudoephedrine . . 947
Lorazepam 947
Lorazepam Injection, USP (Can)
    see Lorazepam 947
Lorazepam Intensol® see
    Lorazepam 947
Lorcet® 10/650 see Hydrocodone
    and Acetaminophen 779
Lorcet®-HD [DSC] see
    Hydrocodone and
    Acetaminophen 779
Lorcet® Plus see Hydrocodone and
    Acetaminophen 779
Loroxide® [OTC] see Benzoyl
    Peroxide 194
Lortab® see Hydrocodone and
    Acetaminophen 779
Losartan 950
Losartan and Hydrochlorothiazide . . 952
Losartan Potassium see Losartan . . 950
Losec® (Can) see Omeprazole 1145
Losec MUPS® (Can) see
    Omeprazole 1145
Lotemax® see Loteprednol 953
Lotensin® see Benazepril 185
Lotensin® HCT see Benazepril and
    Hydrochlorothiazide 187
Loteprednol 953
Loteprednol and Tobramycin 953
Loteprednol Etabonate see
    Loteprednol 953
Loteprednol Etabonate and
    Tobramycin see Loteprednol
    and Tobramycin 953
Lotrel® see Amlodipine and
    Benazepril 102
Lotriderm® (Can) see
    Betamethasone and
    Clotrimazole 202
Lotrimin® (Mex) see Clotrimazole . . . 379
Lotrimin AF® (Mex) see
    Miconazole 1039
Lotrimin® AF Athlete's Foot Cream
    [OTC] see Clotrimazole 379
Lotrimin® AF Athlete's Foot
    Solution [OTC] see
    Clotrimazole 379
Lotrimin® AF Jock Itch Cream
    [OTC] see Clotrimazole 379
Lotrimin® AF Jock Itch Powder
    Spray [OTC] see Miconazole
    1039
Lotrimin® AF Powder/Spray [OTC]
    see Miconazole 1039
Lotrimin® Ultra™ [OTC] see
    Butenafine 242
Lotrisone® see Betamethasone and
    Clotrimazole 202
Lotronex® see Alosetron 72
Lovastatin 953
Lovastatin and Niacin see Niacin
    and Lovastatin 1107
Lovenox® see Enoxaparin 542

Lovenox® HP (Can) see
    Enoxaparin 542
Low-Ogestrel® see Ethinyl
    Estradiol and Norgestrel 616
Loxapac® IM (Can) see Loxapine . . . 955
Loxapine 955
Loxapine Succinate see Loxapine . . 955
Loxitane® see Loxapine 955
Lozide® (Can) see Indapamide . . . 828
Lozi-Flur™ see Fluoride 671
Lozol® see Indapamide 828
L-PAM see Melphalan 979
LRH see Gonadorelin 749
L-Sarcolysin see Melphalan 979
LTA® 360 see Lidocaine 920
LTG see Lamotrigine 895
Lu-26-054 see Escitalopram 568
Lubiprostone 957
Lubriderm® Fragrance Free [OTC]
    see Lanolin, Cetyl Alcohol,
    Glycerin, Petrolatum, and
    Mineral Oil 896
Lubriderm® [OTC] see Lanolin,
    Cetyl Alcohol, Glycerin,
    Petrolatum, and Mineral Oil 896
Lucidex [OTC] see Caffeine 245
Ludiomil® (Mex) see Maprotiline 964
Lufyllin® see Dyphylline 526
Lugol's Solution see Potassium
    Iodide and Iodine 1260
Lumigan® see Bimatoprost 208
Luminal® Sodium see
    Phenobarbital 1221
Lumitene™ see Beta-Carotene 198
Lunesta™ see Eszopiclone 587
LupiCare™ II Psoriasis [OTC] see
    Salicylic Acid 1374
LupiCare™ Dandruff [OTC] see
    Salicylic Acid 1374
LupiCare™ Psoriasis [OTC] see
    Salicylic Acid 1374
Lupron® see Leuprolide 906
Lupron Depot® see Leuprolide 906
Lupron Depot-Ped® see Leuprolide
    906
Lurdex® (Mex) see Albendazole 57
Luride® see Fluoride 671
Luride® Lozi-Tab® see Fluoride . . . 671
Lustra® see Hydroquinone 798
Lustra-AF™ see Hydroquinone 798
Lutein 1628
Luteinizing Hormone Releasing
    Hormone see Gonadorelin 749
Lutera™ see Ethinyl Estradiol and
    Levonorgestrel 602
Lutrepulse™ (Can) see
    Gonadorelin 749
Lutropin Alfa 958
Luveris® see Lutropin Alfa 958
Luvox® (Can) see Fluvoxamine 694
Luxiq® see Betamethasone 199
LY139603 see Atomoxetine 156
LY146032 see Daptomycin 423
LY170053 see Olanzapine 1139
LY231514 see Pemetrexed 1198
LY248686 see Duloxetine 523
LY303366 see Anidulafungin 128
LY2148568 see Exenatide 629
Lycopene 1628
Lyderm® (Can) see Fluocinonide . . . 670
Lymphocyte Immune Globulin see
    Antithymocyte Globulin
    (Equine) 131
Lymphocyte Mitogenic Factor see
    Aldesleukin 61
Lyrica® see Pregabalin 1274
Lysinyl [OTC] see L-Lysine 959
Lysodren® see Mitotane 1055
M-M-R® II see Measles, Mumps,
    and Rubella Vaccines
    (Combined) 966

Maalox® Max [OTC] see Aluminum
    Hydroxide, Magnesium
    Hydroxide, and Simethicone 81
Maalox® [OTC] see Aluminum
    Hydroxide, Magnesium
    Hydroxide, and Simethicone 81
Maalox® Quick Dissolve [OTC] see
    Calcium Carbonate 248
Maalox® Total Stomach Relief®
    [OTC] see Bismuth 210
Mabicrol® (Mex) see Clarithromycin
    355
Mabthera® (Mex) see Rituximab . . . 1360
Macrobid® see Nitrofurantoin 1119
Macrodantin® see Nitrofurantoin . . . 1119
Macrodantina® (Mex) see
    Nitrofurantoin 1119
Macugen® see Pegaptanib 1193
Mafenide 959
Mafenide Acetate see Mafenide 959
Magaldrate and Simethicone 960
Mag Delay® [OTC] see Magnesium
    Chloride 960
Mag G® [OTC] see Magnesium
    Gluconate 961
Maginex™ DS [OTC] see
    Magnesium L-aspartate
    Hydrochloride 962
Maginex™ [OTC] see Magnesium
    L-aspartate Hydrochloride 962
Magnesia Magma see Magnesium
    Hydroxide 961
Magnesium L-aspartate
    Hydrochloride 962
Magnesium Carbonate and
    Aluminum Hydroxide see
    Aluminum Hydroxide and
    Magnesiu m Carbonate 79
Magnesium Chloride 960
Magnesium Citrate 960
Magnesium Gluconate 961
Magnesium Hydroxide 961
Magnesium Hydroxide, Aluminum
    Hydroxide, and Simethicone
    see Aluminum Hydroxide,
    Magnesium Hydroxide, and
    Simethicone 81
Magnesium Hydroxide and
    Aluminum Hydroxide see
    Aluminum Hydroxide and
    Magnesium Hydroxide 80
Magnesium Hydroxide and
    Calcium Carbonate see
    Calcium Carbonate and
    Magnesium Hydroxide 249
Magnesium Hydroxide and Mineral
    Oil 961
Magnesium Hydroxide, Famotidine,
    and Calcium Carbonate see
    Famotidine, Calcium
    Carbonate, and Magnesium
    Hydroxide 636
Magnesium Oxide 962
Magnesium Salicylate 962
Magnesium Sulfate 963
Magnesium Trisilicate and
    Aluminum Hydroxide see
    Aluminum Hydroxide and
    Magnesium Trisilicate 80
Magnevist® see Gadopentetate
    Dimeglumine 719
Magnidol® (Mex) see
    Acetaminophen 31
Magonate® [OTC] see Magnesium
    Gluconate 961
Magonate® Sport [OTC] [DSC] see
    Magnesium Gluconate 961
Mag-Ox® 400 [OTC] see
    Magnesium Oxide 962
Mag-SR® [OTC] see Magnesium
    Chloride 960

Magtrate® [OTC] see Magnesium Gluconate 961
MAH see Magnesium L-aspartate Hydrochloride 962
Maidenhair Tree see Ginkgo Biloba 1622
Malarone® see Atovaquone and Proguanil 160
Malarone® Pediatric (Can) see Atovaquone and Proguanil 160
Maltodextrin 963
m-AMSA see Amsacrine 123
Mandelamine® see Methenamine . . 1007
Mandrake see Podophyllum Resin 1251
Manganese see Trace Metals 1513
Mantoux see Tuberculin Tests 1548
Mapap Children's [OTC] see Acetaminophen 31
Mapap Extra Strength [OTC] see Acetaminophen 31
Mapap Infants [OTC] see Acetaminophen 31
Mapap [OTC] see Acetaminophen . . 31
Mapap Sinus Maximum Strength [OTC] see Acetaminophen and Pseudoephedrine 38
Mapezine® (Can) see Carbamazepine 260
Mapluxin® (Mex) see Digoxin 471
Maprotiline 964
Maprotiline Hydrochloride see Maprotiline 964
Marcaine® see Bupivacaine 228
Marcaine® Spinal see Bupivacaine . . 228
Marcaine® with Epinephrine see Bupivacaine and Epinephrine . . . 228
Marezine® [OTC] see Cyclizine 400
Margesic® H see Hydrocodone and Acetaminophen 779
Marinol® see Dronabinol 518
Marplan® see Isocarboxazid 863
Marvelon® (Can) see Ethinyl Estradiol and Desogestrel 592
Mastic 1628
Matricaria chamomilla see Chamomile 1617
Matricaria recutita see Chamomile 1617
Matulane® see Procarbazine 1284
3M™ Avagard™ [OTC] see Chlorhexidine Gluconate . . . 316
Mavik® see Trandolapril 1517
Maxair™ Autohaler™ see Pirbuterol 1248
Maxalt® see Rizatriptan 1363
Maxalt-MLT® see Rizatriptan 1363
Maxalt RPD™ (Can) see Rizatriptan 1363
Maxaquin® (Mex) see Lomefloxacin 941
Maxaquin® [DSC] see Lomefloxacin 941
Maxidex® see Dexamethasone 439
Maxidone™ see Hydrocodone and Acetaminophen 779
Maxifed® see Guaifenesin and Pseudoephedrine 755
Maxifed DM see Guaifenesin, Pseudoephedrine, and Dextromethorphan 757
Maxifed-G® see Guaifenesin and Pseudoephedrine 755
Maxiphen DM see Guaifenesin, Dextromethorphan, and Phenylephrine 756
Maxipime® see Cefepime 287
Maxitrol® see Neomycin, Polymyxin B, and Dexamethasone 1101
Maxi-Tuss HCG see Hydrocodone and Guaifenesin 785

Maxivate® see Betamethasone 199
Maxzide® see Hydrochlorothiazide and Triamterene 778
Maxzide®-25 see Hydrochlorothiazide and Triamterene 778
May Apple see Podophyllum Resin 1251
Maybush see Hawthorn 1626
3M™ Cavilon™ Skin Cleanser [OTC] see Benzalkonium Chloride 188
MCH see Collagen Hemostat 392
m-Cresyl Acetate 966
MCT see Medium Chain Triglycerides 972
MCT Oil® (Can) see Medium Chain Triglycerides 972
MCT Oil® [OTC] see Medium Chain Triglycerides 972
MCV4 see Meningococcal Polysaccharide (Groups A / C / Y and W-135) Diphtheria Toxoid Conjugate Vaccine 980
MD-76®R see Diatrizoate Meglumine and Diatrizoate Sodium 453
MD-Gastroview® see Diatrizoate Meglumine and Diatrizoate Sodium 453
MDL 73,147EF see Dolasetron 498
Measles, Mumps, and Rubella Vaccines (Combined) 966
Measles, Mumps, Rubella, and Varicella Virus Vaccine 967
Measles Virus Vaccine (Live) 967
Mebaral® see Mephobarbital 986
Mebendazole 968
Mecamylamine 968
Mecamylamine Hydrochloride see Mecamylamine 968
Mecasermin 968
Mecasermin (rDNA Origin) see Mecasermin 968
Mecasermin Rinfabate see Mecasermin 968
Meclizine 969
Meclizine Hydrochloride see Meclizine 969
Meclofenamate 970
Meclofenamate Sodium see Meclofenamate 970
Meclomen® (Can) see Meclofenamate 970
Meclomid® (Mex) see Metoclopramide 1029
Meclozine Hydrochloride see Meclizine 969
Med-Diltiazem (Can) see Diltiazem 479
Medebar® Plus see Barium 179
Medescan® see Barium 179
Medicinal Carbon see Charcoal 311
Medicinal Charcoal see Charcoal . . . 311
Medicone® [OTC] see Phenylephrine 1226
Medigesic® see Butalbital, Acetaminophen, and Caffeine . . 239
Mediplast® [OTC] see Salicylic Acid 1374
Medi-Synal [OTC] see Acetaminophen and Pseudoephedrine 38
Medium Chain Triglycerides 972
Medrol® see MethylPREDNISolone 1025
MedroxyPROGESTERone 972
Medroxyprogesterone Acetate see MedroxyPROGESTERone 972

Medroxyprogesterone and
  Estrogens (Conjugated) see
  Estrogens (Conjugated/Equine)
  and Medroxyprogesterone 583
Medrysone 973
Mefenamic-250 (Can) see
  Mefenamic Acid 973
Mefenamic Acid 973
Mefloquine 975
Mefloquine Hydrochloride see
  Mefloquine 975
Mefoxin® see Cefoxitin 290
Megace® see Megestrol 976
Megace® ES see Megestrol 976
Megace® OS (Can) see Megestrol . . 976
Megadophilus® [OTC] see
  Lactobacillus 535
Megestrol 976
Megestrol Acetate see Megestrol . . . 976
Meladinina® (Mex) see
  Methoxsalen 1018
Melaleuca alternifolia see
  Melaleuca Oil 1628
Melaleuca Oil 1628
Melanex® see Hydroquinone 798
Melatonin 1629
Melfiat® see Phendimetrazine 1220
Melissa officinalis see Lemon
  Balm/Melissa 1627
Mellaril® (Can) see Thioridazine . . . 1477
Meloxicam 977
Melpaque HP® see Hydroquinone . . 798
Melphalan 979
Melquin-3® see Hydroquinone 798
Melquin HP® see Hydroquinone 798
Memantine 979
Memantine Hydrochloride see
  Memantine 979
Menactra® see Meningococcal
  Polysaccharide (Groups A / C /
  Y and W-135) Diphtheria
  Toxoid Conjugate Vaccine 980
Menest® see Estrogens (Esterified)
  584
Meningitec® (Can) see
  Meningococcal Polysaccharide
  (Groups A / C / Y and W-135)
  Diphtheria Toxoid Conjugate
  Vaccine 980
Meningococcal Polysaccharide
  (Groups A / C / Y and W-135)
  Diphtheria Toxoid Conjugate
  Vaccine 980
Meningococcal Polysaccharide
  Vaccine (Groups A, C, Y, and
  W-135) 981
Menomune®-A/C/Y/W-135 see
  Meningococcal Polysaccharide
  Vaccine (Groups A, C, Y, and
  W-135) 981
Menopur® see Menotropins 982
Menostar™ see Estradiol 574
Menotropins 982
Mentax® see Butenafine 242
292 MEP (Can) see Aspirin and
  Meprobamate 151
Mepenzolate 983
Mepenzolate Bromide see
  Mepenzolate 983
Mepergan see Meperidine and
  Promethazine 986
Meperidine 983
Meperidine and Promethazine 986
Meperidine Hydrochloride see
  Meperidine 983
Meperitab® see Meperidine 983
Mephobarbital 986
Mephyton® see Phytonadione 1233
Mepivacaine 987
Mepivacaine and Levonordefrin 991
Mepivacaine (Dental Anesthetic) . . . 989

Mepivacaine Hydrochloride see
  Mepivacaine 987
Meprobamate 993
Meprobamate and Aspirin see
  Aspirin and Meprobamate 151
Mepron® see Atovaquone 160
Mequinol and Tretinoin 994
Mercaptopurine 995
6-Mercaptopurine see
  Mercaptopurine 995
Mercapturic Acid see
  Acetylcysteine 46
Meridia® see Sibutramine 1389
Meropenem 996
Merrem® (Can) see Meropenem . . . 996
Merrem® I.V. see Meropenem 996
Meruvax® II see Rubella Virus
  Vaccine (Live) 1372
Mesalamine 996
Mesalazine see Mesalamine 996
Mesasal® (Can) see Mesalamine . . . 996
M-Eslon® (Can) see Morphine
  Sulfate 1065
Mesoridazine 997
Mesoridazine Besylate see
  Mesoridazine 997
Mestinon® see Pyridostigmine 1315
Mestinon®-SR (Can) see
  Pyridostigmine 1315
Mestinon® Timespan® see
  Pyridostigmine 1315
Mestranol and Norethindrone 999
Metacortandralone see
  PrednisoLONE 1268
Metadate® CD see
  Methylphenidate 1023
Metadate® ER see
  Methylphenidate 1023
Metadol™ see Methadone . . 1004
Metaglip™ see Glipizide and
  Metformin 741
Metamucil® (Can) see Psyllium . . . 1313
Metamucil® [OTC] see Psyllium . . . 1313
Metamucil® Plus Calcium [OTC]
  see Psyllium 1313
Metamucil® Smooth Texture [OTC]
  see Psyllium 1313
Metaproterenol 1000
Metaproterenol Sulfate see
  Metaproterenol 1000
Metaxalone 1001
Metclopramide Hydrochloride
  Injection (Can) see
  Metoclopramide 1029
Metformin 1001
Metformin and Glipizide see
  Glipizide and Metformin 741
Metformin and Glyburide see
  Glyburide and Metformin 745
Metformin and Rosiglitazone see
  Rosiglitazone and Metformin . . 1369
Metformin Hydrochloride see
  Metformin 1001
Metformin Hydrochloride and
  Pioglitazone Hydrochloride see
  Pioglitazone and Metformin . . . 1242
Metformin Hydrochloride and
  Rosiglitazone Maleate see
  Rosiglitazone and Metformin . . 1369
Methadone 1004
Methadone Diskets® see
  Methadone 1004
Methadone Hydrochloride see
  Methadone 1004
Methadone Intensol™ see
  Methadone 1004
Methadose® see Methadone 1004
Methaminodiazepoxide
  Hydrochloride see
  Chlordiazepoxide 315
Methamphetamine 1005

Methamphetamine Hydrochloride
   see Methamphetamine 1005
Methazolamide 1006
Methenamine 1007
Methenamine Hippurate see
   Methenamine 1007
Methenamine Mandelate see
   Methenamine 1007
Methenamine, Sodium
   Biphosphate, Phenyl Salicylate,
   Methylene Blue, and
   Hyoscyamine 1008
Methergine® see Methylergonovine
   1022
Methimazole 1008
Methitest™ see
   MethylTESTOSTERone 1028
Methocarbamol 1009
Methohexital 1010
Methohexital Sodium see
   Methohexital 1010
Methotrexate 1012
Methotrexate Sodium see
   Methotrexate 1012
Methotrimeprazine 1016
Methotrimeprazine Hydrochloride
   see Methotrimeprazine 1016
Methoxsalen 1018
Methoxypsoralen see Methoxsalen
   1018
8-Methoxypsoralen see
   Methoxsalen 1018
Methscopolamine 1019
Methscopolamine Bromide see
   Methscopolamine 1019
Methscopolamine,
   Chlorpheniramine, and
   Phenylephrine see
   Chlorpheniramine,
   Phenylephrine, and
   Methscopolamine 327
Methscopolamine Nitrate and
   Chlordiazepoxide
   Hydrochloride see
   Chlordiazepoxide and
   Methscopolamine 316
Methsuximide 1019
Methyclothiazide 1020
Methylacetoxyprogesterone see
   MedroxyPROGESTERone 972
Methylcellulose 1021
Methyldopa 1021
Methyldopa and
   Hydrochlorothiazide 1022
Methyldopate Hydrochloride see
   Methyldopa 1021
Methylene Blue, Methenamine,
   Sodium Biphosphate, Phenyl
   Salicylate, and Hyoscyamine
   see Methenamine, Sodium
   Biphosphate, Phenyl Salicylate,
   Methylene Blue, and
   Hyoscyamine 1008
Methylergometrine Maleate see
   Methylergonovine 1022
Methylergonovine 1022
Methylergonovine Maleate see
   Methylergonovine 1022
Methylin® see Methylphenidate . . . 1023
Methylin® ER see
   Methylphenidate 1023
Methylmorphine see Codeine 385
Methylphenidate 1023
Methylphenidate Hydrochloride see
   Methylphenidate 1023
Methylphenobarbital see
   Mephobarbital 986
Methylphenoxy-Benzene
   Propanamine see Atomoxetine
   156

Methylphenyl Isoxazolyl Penicillin
   see Oxacillin 1153
Methylphytyl Napthoquinone see
   Phytonadione 1233
MethylPREDNISolone 1025
6-α-Methylprednisolone see
   MethylPREDNISolone 1025
Methylprednisolone Acetate (Can)
   see MethylPREDNISolone 1025
Methylprednisolone Sodium
   Succinate see
   MethylPREDNISolone 1025
4-Methylpyrazole see Fomepizole . . 699
Methylrosaniline Chloride see
   Gentian Violet 735
Methyl Sulfonyl Methane 1629
MethylTESTOSTERone 1028
Meticel Ofteno® (Mex) see
   Hydroxypropyl Methylcellulose . . 800
Meticorten® (Mex) see
   PredniSONE 1271
Metipranolol 1028
Metipranolol Hydrochloride see
   Metipranolol 1028
Metoclopramide 1029
Metolazone 1030
Metoprolol 1030
Metoprolol and Hydrochlorothiazide
   1032
Metoprolol Succinate see
   Metoprolol 1030
Metoprolol Tartrate see Metoprolol
   1030
Metoprolol Tartrate and
   Hydrochlorothiazide see
   Metoprolol and
   Hydrochlorothiazide 1032
Metoprolol Tartrate Injection, USP
   (Can) see Metoprolol 1030
MetroCream® see Metronidazole . . 1033
MetroGel® see Metronidazole 1033
MetroGel-Vaginal® see
   Metronidazole 1033
MetroLotion® see Metronidazole . . . 1033
Metronidazole 1033
Metronidazole and Nystatin 1036
Metronidazole, Bismuth
   Subsalicylate, and Tetracycline
   see Bismuth Subsalicylate,
   Metronidazole, and
   Tetracycline 210
Metronidazole Hydrochloride see
   Metronidazole 1033
Metyrosine 1036
Mevacor® see Lovastatin 953
Mevinolin see Lovastatin 953
Mexiletine 1037
Mexitil® [DSC] see Mexiletine 1037
M-FA-142 see Amonafide 104
MG 217® Medicated Tar [OTC] see
   Coal Tar 383
MG 217® [OTC] see Coal Tar 383
MG217 Sal-Acid® [OTC] see
   Salicylic Acid 1374
MgSO₄ (error-prone abbreviation)
   see Magnesium Sulfate 963
Miacalcic® [salmon] (Mex) see
   Calcitonin 246
Miacalcin® see Calcitonin 246
Miacalcin® NS (Can) see
   Calcitonin 246
Mi-Acid™ Double Strength [OTC]
   see Calcium Carbonate and
   Magnesium Hydroxide 249
Mi-Acid Maximum Strength [OTC]
   see Aluminum Hydroxide,
   Magnesium Hydroxide, and
   Simethicone 81
Mi-Acid [OTC] see Aluminum
   Hydroxide, Magnesium
   Hydroxide, and Simethicone 81

Micaderm® [OTC] see Miconazole ... 1039
Micafungin ... 1038
Micafungin Sodium see Micafungin ... 1038
Micanol® (Can) see Anthralin ... 128
Micardis® see Telmisartan ... 1451
Micardis® HCT see Telmisartan and Hydrochlorothiazide ... 1452
Micardis® Plus (Can) see Telmisartan and Hydrochlorothiazide ... 1452
Micatin® (Can) see Miconazole ... 1039
Micatin® Athlete's Foot [OTC] see Miconazole ... 1039
Micatin® Jock Itch [OTC] see Miconazole ... 1039
Miccil® (Mex) see Bumetanide ... 227
Miconazole ... 1039
Miconazole and Zinc Oxide ... 1040
Miconazole Nitrate see Miconazole ... 1039
Micostatin® (Mex) see Nystatin ... 1133
Micostyl® (Mex) see Econazole ... 526
Micozole (Can) see Miconazole ... 1039
MICRhoGAM® see Rh₀(D) Immune Globulin ... 1342
Microfibrillar Collagen Hemostat see Collagen Hemostat ... 392
Microgestin™ see Ethinyl Estradiol and Norethindrone ... 608
Microgestin™ Fe see Ethinyl Estradiol and Norethindrone ... 608
Micro-Guard® [OTC] see Miconazole ... 1039
microK® see Potassium Chloride ... 1258
microK® 10 see Potassium Chloride ... 1258
Micro-K Extencaps® (Can) see Potassium Chloride ... 1258
Microlut® (Mex) see Levonorgestrel ... 916
Micronase® see GlyBURIDE ... 744
microNefrin® see Epinephrine (Racemic) ... 549
Micronor® see Norethindrone ... 1125
Microrgan® (Mex) see Ciprofloxacin ... 343
Microzide™ see Hydrochlorothiazide ... 776
Midamor® [DSC] see Amiloride ... 85
Midazolam ... 1040
Midazolam Hydrochloride see Midazolam ... 1040
Midazolam Injection (Can) see Midazolam ... 1040
Midodrine ... 1044
Midodrine Hydrochloride see Midodrine ... 1044
Midol® Cramp and Body Aches [OTC] see Ibuprofen ... 808
Midol® Extended Relief see Naproxen ... 1089
Midrin® see Acetaminophen, Isometheptene, and Dichloralphenazone ... 44
Mifeprex® see Mifepristone ... 1045
Mifepristone ... 1045
Miglitol ... 1046
Miglustat ... 1047
Migquin see Acetaminophen, Isometheptene, and Dichloralphenazone ... 44
Migranal® see Dihydroergotamine ... 477
Migratine see Acetaminophen, Isometheptene, and Dichloralphenazone ... 44
Migrazone® see Acetaminophen, Isometheptene, and Dichloralphenazone ... 44

Migrin-A see Acetaminophen, Isometheptene, and Dichloralphenazone ... 44
Mi-Ke-Son's® (Mex) see Ketoconazole ... 880
Milk of Magnesia see Magnesium Hydroxide ... 961
Milk Thistle ... 1629
Milk Vetch see Astragalus ... 1615
Milophene® (Can) see ClomiPHENE ... 369
Milrinone ... 1048
Milrinone Lactate see Milrinone ... 1048
Miltown® [DSC] see Meprobamate ... 993
Mindal DM [DSC] see Guaifenesin and Dextromethorphan ... 754
Mineral Oil, Petrolatum, Lanolin, Cetyl Alcohol, and Glycerin see Lanolin, Cetyl Alcohol, Glycerin, Petrolatum, and Mineral Oil ... 896
Minestrin™ 1/20 (Can) see Ethinyl Estradiol and Norethindrone ... 608
Minidyne® [OTC] see Povidone-Iodine ... 1262
Minipres® (Mex) see Prazosin ... 1267
Minipress® see Prazosin ... 1267
Minirin® (Can) see Desmopressin ... 437
Minitran™ see Nitroglycerin ... 1120
Minizide® see Prazosin and Polythiazide ... 1268
Minocin® see Minocycline ... 1049
Minocycline ... 1049
Minocycline Hydrochloride see Minocycline ... 1049
Minocycline Hydrochloride (Periodontal) ... 1050
Minodiab® (Mex) see GlipiZIDE ... 740
Min-Ovral® (Can) see Ethinyl Estradiol and Levonorgestrel ... 602
Minox (Can) see Minoxidil ... 1051
Minoxidil ... 1051
Mintab DM see Guaifenesin and Dextromethorphan ... 754
Mintezol® see Thiabendazole ... 1475
Mintox Extra Strength [OTC] see Aluminum Hydroxide, Magnesium Hydroxide, and Simethicone ... 81
Mintox Plus [OTC] see Aluminum Hydroxide, Magnesium Hydroxide, and Simethicone ... 81
Miochol-E® see Acetylcholine ... 46
Miostat® see Carbachol ... 260
MiraLax™ see Polyethylene Glycol 3350 ... 1253
Mirapex® see Pramipexole ... 1262
Miraphen PSE see Guaifenesin and Pseudoephedrine ... 755
Mircette® see Ethinyl Estradiol and Desogestrel ... 592
Mirena® see Levonorgestrel ... 916
Mirtazapine ... 1052
Misoprostol ... 1053
Misoprostol and Diclofenac see Diclofenac and Misoprostol ... 462
Mitocin® (Mex) see Mitomycin ... 1054
Mitomycin ... 1054
Mitomycin-X see Mitomycin ... 1054
Mitomycin-C see Mitomycin ... 1054
Mitotane ... 1055
Mitoxantrone ... 1055
Mitoxantrone Hydrochloride CL-232315 see Mitoxantrone ... 1055
Mitoxantrone Injection® (Can) see Mitoxantrone ... 1055
Mitozantrone see Mitoxantrone ... 1055
Mitrazol™ [OTC] see Miconazole ... 1039
Mitroken® (Mex) see Ciprofloxacin ... 343
Mitroxone® (Mex) see Mitoxantrone ... 1055

MK383 see Tirofiban 1496
MK462 see Rizatriptan 1363
MK594 see Losartan 950
MK0826 see Ertapenem 561
MK 869 see Aprepitant 134
MLN341 see Bortezomib 215
MMF see Mycophenolate 1075
MMR see Measles, Mumps, and
   Rubella Vaccines (Combined) . 966
Moban® see Molindone 1059
Mobic® see Meloxicam 977
Mobicox® (Can) see Meloxicam 977
Mobisyl® [OTC] see
   Triethanolamine Salicylate 1535
Modafinil 1057
Modane® Bulk [OTC] see Psyllium
   1313
Modane Tablets® [OTC] see
   Bisacodyl 209
Modecate® (Can) see
   Fluphenazine 680
Modecate® Concentrate (Can) see
   Fluphenazine 680
Modicon® see Ethinyl Estradiol and
   Norethindrone 608
Modified Dakin's Solution see
   Sodium Hypochlorite Solution
   1402
Modified Shohl's Solution see
   Sodium Citrate and Citric Acid
   1401
Modical® [OTC] see Glucose
   Polymers 743
Moduret™ (Can) see Amiloride 85
Moexipril 1058
Moexipril and Hydrochlorothiazide
   1059
Moexipril Hydrochloride see
   Moexipril 1058
Moi-Stir® [OTC] see Saliva
   Substitute 1374
Moisture® Eyes [OTC] see Artificial
   Tears 143
Moisture® Eyes PM [OTC] see
   Artificial Tears 143
Molindone 1059
Molindone Hydrochloride see
   Molindone 1059
Molybdenum see Trace Metals . . . 1513
Molypen® see Trace Metals 1513
MOM see Magnesium Hydroxide . . . 961
Momentum® [OTC] see
   Magnesium Salicylate 962
Mometasone Furoate 1060
MOM/Mineral Oil Emulsion see
   Magnesium Hydroxide and
   Mineral Oil 961
Monacolin K see Lovastatin 953
Monarc® M see Antihemophilic
   Factor (Human) 129
Monascus purpureus see Red
   Yeast Rice 1630
Monistat® (Can) see Miconazole . . 1039
Monistat® 1 Combination Pack
   [OTC] see Miconazole 1039
Monistat® 3 (Can) see Miconazole
   1039
Monistat® 3 [OTC] see Miconazole
   1039
Monistat® 7 [OTC] see Miconazole
   1039
Monistat-Derm® see Miconazole . . 1039
Monitan® (Can) see Acebutolol 28
Monobenzone 1062
Monocaps [OTC] see Vitamins
   (Multiple/Oral) 1582
Monoclate-P® see Antihemophilic
   Factor (Human) 129
Monoclonal Antibody see
   Muromonab-CD3 1074
Monocor® (Can) see Bisoprolol 211

Monodox® see Doxycycline
   (Systemic) 514
Monoethanolamine see
   Ethanolamine Oleate 591
Monoket® see Isosorbide
   Mononitrate 868
Mono Mack® (Mex) see Isosorbide
   Mononitrate 868
MonoNessa™ see Ethinyl Estradiol
   and Norgestimate 613
Mononine® see Factor IX 632
Monopril® see Fosinopril 707
Monopril-HCT® see Fosinopril and
   Hydrochlorothiazide 709
Montelukast 1062
Montelukast Sodium see
   Montelukast 1062
Monurol™ see Fosfomycin 706
8-MOP® see Methoxsalen 1018
More Attenuated Enders Strain see
   Measles Virus Vaccine (Live) . . . 967
MoreDophilus® [OTC] see
   Lactobacillus 535
Moricizine 1064
Moricizine Hydrochloride see
   Moricizine 1064
Morning After Pill see Ethinyl
   Estradiol and Norgestrel 616
Morphine HP® (Can) see Morphine
   Sulfate 1065
Morphine LP® Epidural (Can) see
   Morphine Sulfate 1065
Morphine Sulfate 1065
Morrhuate Sodium 1068
M.O.S.® 10 (Can) see Morphine
   Sulfate 1065
M.O.S.® 20 (Can) see Morphine
   Sulfate 1065
M.O.S.® 30 (Can) see Morphine
   Sulfate 1065
Mosco® Corn and Callus Remover
   [OTC] see Salicylic Acid 1374
M.O.S.-SR® (Can) see Morphine
   Sulfate 1065
M.O.S.-Sulfate® (Can) see
   Morphine Sulfate 1065
Motofen® see Difenoxin and
   Atropine 467
Motrin® see Ibuprofen 808
Motrin® (Children's) (Can) see
   Ibuprofen 808
Motrin® Children's [OTC] see
   Ibuprofen 808
Motrin® Cold and Sinus [OTC] see
   Pseudoephedrine and
   Ibuprofen 1311
Motrin® Cold, Children's [OTC] see
   Pseudoephedrine and
   Ibuprofen 1311
Motrin® IB (Can) see Ibuprofen 808
Motrin® IB [OTC] see Ibuprofen 808
Motrin® Infants' [OTC] see
   Ibuprofen 808
Motrin® Junior Strength [OTC] see
   Ibuprofen 808
Mouthkote® [OTC] see Saliva
   Substitute 1374
Mouthwash (Antiseptic) 1069
Moxifloxacin 1069
Moxifloxacin Hydrochloride see
   Moxifloxacin 1069
Moxilin® see Amoxicillin 106
4-MP see Fomepizole 699
6-MP see Mercaptopurine 995
MPA see
   MedroxyPROGESTERone 972
MPA and Estrogens (Conjugated)
   see Estrogens (Conjugated/
   Equine) and
   Medroxyprogesterone 583

MPSV4 see Meningococcal Polysaccharide Vaccine (Groups A, C, Y, and W-135) . . 981

MS Contin® see Morphine Sulfate 1065

MS-IR® (Can) see Morphine Sulfate 1065

MSM see Methyl Sulfonyl Methane 1629

MSO₄ (error-prone abbreviation) see Morphine Sulfate . . . 1065

MTA see Pemetrexed 1198

MTC see Mitomycin 1054

M.T.E.-4® see Trace Metals 1513

M.T.E.-5® see Trace Metals 1513

M.T.E.-6® see Trace Metals 1513

M.T.E.-7® see Trace Metals 1513

MTX (error-prone abbreviation) see Methotrexate 1012

Mucinex®-D [OTC] see Guaifenesin and Pseudoephedrine . . . 755

Mucinex® DM [OTC] see Guaifenesin and Dextromethorphan 754

Mucinex® [OTC] see Guaifenesin . . 752

Mucomyst® (Can) see Acetylcysteine 46

Multidex® [OTC] see Maltodextrin . 963

Multiple Vitamins see Vitamins (Multiple/Oral) 1582

Multiret Folic 500 see Vitamins (Multiple/Oral) 1582

Multitargeted Antifolate see Pemetrexed 1198

Multitrace™-4 see Trace Metals . . . 1513

Multitrace™-4 Neonatal see Trace Metals 1513

Multitrace™-4 Pediatric see Trace Metals 1513

Multitrace™-5 see Trace Metals . . . 1513

Mumps, Measles and Rubella Vaccines, Combined see Measles, Mumps, and Rubella Vaccines (Combined) 966

Mumps, Rubella, Varicella, and Measles Vaccine see Measles, Mumps, Rubella, and Varicella Virus Vaccine 967

Mumpsvax® see Mumps Virus Vaccine (Live/Attenuated) 1072

Mumps Virus Vaccine (Live/Attenuated) 1072

Munobal® (Mex) see Felodipine . . . 638

Mupirocin 1073

Mupirocin Calcium see Mupirocin . . 1073

Murine® Ear Wax Removal System [OTC] see Carbamide Peroxide 264

Murine® Tears [OTC] see Artificial Tears 143

Murine® Tears Plus [OTC] see Tetrahydrozoline 1470

Muro 128® [OTC] see Sodium Chloride 1400

Murocel® [OTC] see Artificial Tears 143

Murocoll-2® see Phenylephrine and Scopolamine 1227

Muromonab-CD3 1074

Muse® see Alprostadil 76

Muse® Pellet (Can) see Alprostadil 76

Mutamycin® see Mitomycin 1054

Myambutol® see Ethambutol 591

Myamine™ see Micafungin 1038

Mycelex® see Clotrimazole 379

Mycelex®-3 [OTC] see Butoconazole 242

Mycelex®-7 [OTC] see Clotrimazole 379

Mycelex® Twin Pack [OTC] see Clotrimazole 379

Mycinaire™ [OTC] see Sodium Chloride 1400

Mycinettes® [OTC] see Benzocaine 190

Mycobutin® see Rifabutin 1345

Mycodib® (Mex) see Ketoconazole . . 880

Mycolog®-II [DSC] see Nystatin and Triamcinolone 1134

Myco-Nail [OTC] see Triacetin 1526

Mycophenolate 1075

Mycophenolate Mofetil see Mycophenolate 1075

Mycophenolate Sodium see Mycophenolate 1075

Mycophenolic Acid see Mycophenolate 1075

Mycostatin® see Nystatin 1133

Mydfrin® see Phenylephrine 1226

Mydral™ see Tropicamide 1545

Mydriacyl® see Tropicamide 1545

Myfortic® see Mycophenolate 1075

Myfungar® (Mex) see Oxiconazole 1160

Mykrox® (Can) see Metolazone . . . 1030

Mylanta™ (Can) see Aluminum Hydroxide and Magnesium Hydroxide 80

Mylanta® Children's [OTC] see Calcium Carbonate 248

Mylanta® Double Strength (Can) see Aluminum Hydroxide, Magnesium Hydroxide, and Simethicone 81

Mylanta® Extra Strength (Can) see Aluminum Hydroxide, Magnesium Hydroxide, and Simethicone 81

Mylanta® Gas Maximum Strength [OTC] see Simethicone 1394

Mylanta® Gas [OTC] see Simethicone 1394

Mylanta® Gelcaps® [OTC] see Calcium Carbonate and Magnesium Hydroxide 249

Mylanta® Liquid [OTC] see Aluminum Hydroxide, Magnesium Hydroxide, and Simethicone 81

Mylanta® Maximum Strength Liquid [OTC] see Aluminum Hydroxide, Magnesium Hydroxide, and Simethicone 81

Mylanta® Regular Strength (Can) see Aluminum Hydroxide, Magnesium Hydroxide, and Simethicone 81

Mylanta® Supreme [OTC] see Calcium Carbonate and Magnesium Hydroxide 249

Mylanta® Ultra [OTC] see Calcium Carbonate and Magnesium Hydroxide 249

Myleran® see Busulfan 237

Mylicon® Infants [OTC] see Simethicone 1394

Mylocel™ see Hydroxyurea 800

Mylotarg® see Gemtuzumab Ozogamicin 732

Myobloc® see Botulinum Toxin Type B 218

Myochrysine® (Can) see Gold Sodium Thiomalate 748

Myoflex® (Can) see Triethanolamine Salicylate 1535

Myoflex® [OTC] see Triethanolamine Salicylate 1535

Myotonachol® (Can) see Bethanechol 204

myrac™ see Minocycline 1049

Mysoline® see Primidone 1281
Mytelase® see Ambenonium 82
Mytussin® AC see Guaifenesin and
   Codeine 753
Mytussin® DAC see Guaifenesin,
   Pseudoephedrine, and
   Codeine 756
N-9 see Nonoxynol 9 1124
Na2EDTA see Edetate Disodium . . 527
Nabi-HB® see Hepatitis B Immune
   Globulin 768
NAB-Paclitaxel see Paclitaxel
   (Protein Bound) 1177
Nabumetone 1077
NAC see Acetylcysteine 46
N-Acetyl-5-methoxytryptamine see
   Melatonin 1629
N-Acetyl-L-cysteine see
   Acetylcysteine 46
N-Acetylcysteine see
   Acetylcysteine 46
N-Acetyl-P-Aminophenol see
   Acetaminophen 31
NaCl see Sodium Chloride 1400
NADH see Nicotinamide Adenine
   Dinucleotide 1629
Nadib® (Mex) see GlyBURIDE 744
Nadolol 1079
Nadolol and Bendroflumethiazide . . 1080
Nafarelin 1081
Nafarelin Acetate see Nafarelin . . . 1081
Nafcillin 1082
Nafcillin Sodium see Nafcillin 1082
Nafidimide see Amonafide 104
Naftifine 1082
Naftifine Hydrochloride see
   Naftifine 1082
Naftin® see Naftifine 1082
Naglazyme™ see Galsulfase 721
NaHCO₃ see Sodium Bicarbonate
   1400
Nalbuphine 1083
Nalbuphine Hydrochloride see
   Nalbuphine 1083
Nalcrom® (Can) see Cromolyn 397
Nalcryn® (Mex) see Nalbuphine . . . 1083
Naldecon Senior EX® [OTC] [DSC]
   see Guaifenesin 752
Nalex®-A see Chlorpheniramine,
   Phenylephrine, and
   Phenyltoloxamine 328
Nalfon® see Fenoprofen 642
Nalidixic Acid 1083
Nalidixinic Acid see Nalidixic Acid
   1083
Nallpen® (Can) see Nafcillin 1082
N-allylnoroxymorphine
   Hydrochloride see Naloxone . . 1084
Nalmefene 1084
Nalmefene Hydrochloride see
   Nalmefene 1084
Naloxone 1084
Naloxone and Buprenorphine see
   Buprenorphine and Naloxone . . . 232
Naloxone Hydrochloride see
   Naloxone 1084
Naloxone Hydrochloride and
   Pentazocine Hydrochloride see
   Pentazocine 1208
Naloxone Hydrochloride Dihydrate
   and Buprenorphine
   Hydrochloride see
   Buprenorphine and Naloxone . . 232
Naloxone Hydrochloride Injection®
   (Can) see Naloxone 1084
Naltrexone 1086
Naltrexone Hydrochloride see
   Naltrexone 1086
Namenda™ see Memantine 979
Nandrolone 1087

Nandrolone Decanoate see
   Nandrolone 1087
Nandrolone Phenpropionate see
   Nandrolone 1087
Naphazoline 1087
Naphazoline and Antazoline 1088
Naphazoline and Pheniramine . . . 1088
Naphazoline Hydrochloride see
   Naphazoline 1087
Naphcon-A® (Can) see
   Naphazoline and Pheniramine
   1088
Naphcon-A® [OTC] see
   Naphazoline and Pheniramine
   1088
Naphcon Forte® (Can) see
   Naphazoline 1087
Naphcon® [OTC] see Naphazoline
   1087
NapraPAC™ see Lansoprazole and
   Naproxen 898
Naprelan® see Naproxen 1089
Naprosyn® see Naproxen 1089
Naproxen 1089
Naproxen and Lansoprazole see
   Lansoprazole and Naproxen . . . 898
Naproxen Sodium see Naproxen . . 1089
Naramig® (Mex) see Naratriptan . . 1092
Naratriptan 1092
Naratriptan Hydrochloride see
   Naratriptan 1092
Narcan® [DSC] see Naloxone 1084
Narcanti® (Mex) see Naloxone . . . 1084
Nardil® see Phenelzine 1221
Naropin® see Ropivacaine 1366
Nasacort® AQ see Triamcinolone . . 1526
NasalCrom® [OTC] see Cromolyn . . 397
Nasalide® (Can) see Flunisolide . . 667
Nasal Moist® [OTC] see Sodium
   Chloride 1400
NaSal™ [OTC] see Sodium
   Chloride 1400
Nasarel® see Flunisolide 667
Nasatab® LA see Guaifenesin and
   Pseudoephedrine 755
Nascobal® see Cyanocobalamin . . 399
Nasonex® see Mometasone
   Furoate 1060
Natacyn® see Natamycin 1093
Natalizumab 1093
Natamycin 1093
Nateglinide 1094
Natrecor® see Nesiritide 1103
Natriuretic Peptide see Nesiritide . . 1103
Natulan® (Can) see Procarbazine
   1284
Natural Fiber Therapy [OTC] see
   Psyllium 1313
Natural Lung Surfactant see
   Beractant 198
Nature's Tears® [OTC] see
   Artificial Tears 143
Nature-Throid® NT see Thyroid . . . 1482
Nausea Relief [OTC] see Fructose,
   Dextrose, and Phosphoric Acid
   713
Nauseatol (Can) see
   DimenhyDRINATE 481
Nausetrol® [OTC] see Fructose,
   Dextrose, and Phosphoric Acid
   713
Navane® see Thiothixene 1480
Navelbine® see Vinorelbine 1578
Naxen® (Can) see Naproxen 1089
Na-Zone® [OTC] see Sodium
   Chloride 1400
NC-722665 see Bicalutamide 207
n-Docosanol see Docosanol 495
NebuPent® see Pentamidine 1207
Necon® 0.5/35 see Ethinyl
   Estradiol and Norethindrone 608

Necon® 1/35 see Ethinyl Estradiol and Norethindrone 608
Necon® 1/50 see Mestranol and Norethindrone 999
Necon® 7/7/7 see Ethinyl Estradiol and Norethindrone 608
Necon® 10/11 see Ethinyl Estradiol and Norethindrone 608
Nectar of the Gods see Garlic 1622
Nedocromil 1095
Nedocromil Sodium see Nedocromil 1095
Nefazodone 1096
Nefazodone Hydrochloride see Nefazodone 1096
NegGram® (Can) see Nalidixic Acid 1083
NegGram® [DSC] see Nalidixic Acid 1083
Nelarabine 1097
Nelfinavir 1098
Nembutal® see Pentobarbital 1210
Nembutal® Sodium (Can) see Pentobarbital 1210
Neobes® (Mex) see Diethylpropion
. . . . 467
NeoCeuticals™ Acne Spot Treatment [OTC] see Salicylic Acid 1374
Neodol® (Mex) see Acetaminophen
. . . . 31
Neodolito® (Mex) see Acetaminophen 31
Neofomiral® (Mex) see Fluconazole
. . . . 659
Neo-Fradin™ see Neomycin 1100
Neomicol® (Mex) see Miconazole . . 1039
Neomycin 1100
Neomycin and Polymyxin B 1100
Neomycin, Bacitracin, and Polymyxin B see Bacitracin, Neomycin, and Polymyxin B . . . 176
Neomycin, Bacitracin, Polymyxin B, and Hydrocortisone see Bacitracin, Neomycin, Polymyxin B, and Hydrocortisone 177
Neomycin, Bacitracin, Polymyxin B, and Pramoxine see Bacitracin, Neomycin, Polymyxin B, and Pramoxine 177
Neomycin, Polymyxin B, and Dexamethasone 1101
Neomycin, Polymyxin B, and Gramicidin 1101
Neomycin, Polymyxin B, and Hydrocortisone 1101
Neomycin, Polymyxin B, and Prednisolone 1102
Neomycin Sulfate see Neomycin . . . 1100
Neonatal Trace Metals see Trace Metals 1513
Neopulmonier® (Mex) see Dextromethorphan 451
Neoral® see CycloSPORINE 406
Neo-Rx see Neomycin 1100
Neosporin® (Can) see Neomycin, Polymyxin B, and Gramicidin . . 1101
Neosporin® AF [OTC] see Miconazole 1039
Neosporin® G.U. Irrigant see Neomycin and Polymyxin B . . . 1100
Neosporin® Irrigating Solution (Can) see Neomycin and Polymyxin B 1100
Neosporin® Neo To Go® [OTC] see Bacitracin, Neomycin, and Polymyxin B 176
Neosporin® Ophthalmic Ointment (Can) see Bacitracin, Neomycin, and Polymyxin B . . . 176

Neosporin® Ophthalmic Ointment [DSC] see Bacitracin, Neomycin, and Polymyxin B . . . 176
Neosporin® Ophthalmic Solution see Neomycin, Polymyxin B, and Gramicidin 1101
Neosporin® + Pain Ointment [OTC] see Bacitracin, Neomycin, Polymyxin B, and Pramoxine . . . 177
Neosporin® Topical [OTC] see Bacitracin, Neomycin, and Polymyxin B 176
NeoStrata® AHA [OTC] see Hydroquinone 798
NeoStrata® HQ (Can) see Hydroquinone 798
Neo-Synephrine® (Can) see Phenylephrine 1226
Neo-Synephrine® 12 Hour Extra Moisturizing [OTC] see Oxymetazoline 1172
Neo-Synephrine® 12 Hour [OTC] see Oxymetazoline 1172
Neo-Synephrine® Extra Strength [OTC] see Phenylephrine 1226
Neo-Synephrine® Mild [OTC] see Phenylephrine 1226
Neo-Synephrine® Ophthalmic [DSC] see Phenylephrine 1226
Neo-Synephrine® Regular Strength [OTC] see Phenylephrine 1226
Neotrace-4® see Trace Metals 1513
Nepafenac 1103
NephPlex® Rx see Vitamin B Complex Combinations 1581
Nephro-Calci® [OTC] see Calcium Carbonate 248
Nephrocaps® see Vitamin B Complex Combinations 1581
Nephro-Fer® [OTC] see Ferrous Fumarate 650
Nephron FA® see Vitamin B Complex Combinations 1581
Nephro-Vite® see Vitamin B Complex C ombinations 1581
Nephro-Vite® Rx see Vitamin B Complex Combinations 1581
Nesacaine® see Chloroprocaine . . . 320
Nesacaine®-CE (Can) see Chloroprocaine 320
Nesacaine®-MPF see Chloroprocaine 320
Nesiritide 1103
Neugal® (Mex) see Ranitidine 1334
Neugeron® (Mex) see Carbamazepine 260
Neulasta® see Pegfilgrastim 1195
Neuleptil® (Can) see Pericyazine . 1214
Neumega® see Oprelvekin 1149
Neupogen® see Filgrastim 654
Neurontin® see Gabapentin 717
Neurosine® (Mex) see BusPIRone . . 236
Neut® see Sodium Bicarbonate . . . 1400
NeutraCare® see Fluoride 671
NeutraGard® Advanced see Fluoride 671
NeutraGard® [OTC] see Fluoride . . . 671
NeutraGard® Plus see Fluoride 671
Neutra-Phos®-K [OTC] see Potassium Phosphate 1261
Neutra-Phos® [OTC] see Potassium Phosphate and Sodium Phosphate 1261
NeuTrexin® see Trimetrexate 1539
Neutrogena® Acne Mask [OTC] see Benzoyl Peroxide 194
Neutrogena® Acne Wash [OTC] see Salicylic Acid 1374
Neutrogena® Body Clear™ [OTC] see Salicylic Acid 1374

Neutrogena® Clear Pore [OTC] see
    Salicylic Acid 1374
Neutrogena® Clear Pore Shine
    Control [OTC] see Salicylic
    Acid 1374
Neutrogena® Healthy Scalp [OTC]
    see Salicylic Acid 1374
Neutrogena® Maximum Strength T/
    Sal® [OTC] see Salicylic Acid
    1374
Neutrogena® On The Spot® Acne
    Patch [OTC] see Salicylic Acid
    1374
Neutrogena® On The Spot® Acne
    Treatment [OTC] see Benzoyl
    Peroxide. 194
Neutrogena® T/Gel Extra Strength
    [OTC] see Coal Tar 383
Neutrogena® T/Gel [OTC] see Coal
    Tar 383
Neutrogena® T/Gel Stubborn Itch
    Control [OTC] see Coal Tar 383
Nevanac™ see Nepafenac 1103
Nevirapine 1104
New-Fill® see Poly-L-Lactic Acid . . 1253
Nexavar® see Sorafenib 1407
Nexium® see Esomeprazole 572
NFV see Nelfinavir 1098
Niacin 1105
Niacinamide 1106
Niacin and Lovastatin 1107
Niacor® see Niacin 1105
Niar® (Mex) see Selegiline 1382
Niaspan® see Niacin 1105
Niastase® (Can) see Factor VIIa
    (Recombinant) 632
NiCARdipine 1107
Nicardipine Hydrochloride see
    NiCARdipine 1107
Nicoderm® (Can) see Nicotine 1109
NicoDerm® CQ® [OTC] see
    Nicotine 1109
Nicomide-T™ see Niacinamide 1106
Nicorette® (Can) see Nicotine 1109
Nicorette® [OTC] see Nicotine 1109
Nicorette® Plus (Can) see Nicotine
    1109
Nicotinamide see Niacinamide 1106
Nicotinamide Adenine Dinucleotide
    1629
Nicotine 1109
Nicotinell TTS® (Mex) see Nicotine
    1109
Nicotinic Acid see Niacin 1105
Nicotinic Acid Amide see
    Niacinamide 1106
Nicotrol® (Can) see Nicotine. 1109
Nicotrol® Inhaler see Nicotine 1109
Nicotrol® NS see Nicotine 1109
Nicotrol® Patch [OTC] see Nicotine
    1109
Nicoumalone see Acenocoumarol . . 30
Nidagel™ (Can) see Metronidazole
    1033
Nidrozol® (Mex) see Metronidazole
    1033
Nifediac™ CC see NIFEdipine 1112
Nifedical™ XL see NIFEdipine 1112
NIFEdipine 1112
Nifedipres® (Mex) see NIFEdipine
    1112
Niferex® 150 [OTC] see
    Polysaccharide-Iron Complex . . 1254
Niferex® [OTC] see
    Polysaccharide-Iron Complex . . 1254
Niftolid see Flutamide 686
Nilandron® see Nilutamide 1115
Nilstat (Can) see Nystatin 1133
Nilutamide 1115
Nimodipine 1116
Nimotop® see Nimodipine 1116

Nipent® see Pentostatin 1211
Niravam™ see Alprazolam 73
Nisoldipine 1117
Nistaken® (Mex) see
    Propafenone 1293
Nitalapram see Citalopram 351
Nitazoxanide 1117
Nitisinone 1118
Nitoman™ (Can) see
    Tetrabenazine 1465
Nitradisc® (Mex) see Nitroglycerin
    1120
Nitrek® see Nitroglycerin 1120
Nitric Oxide 1118
4'-Nitro-3'-Trifluoromethylisobutyrantide
    see Flutamide 686
Nitro-Bid® see Nitroglycerin 1120
Nitroderm TTS® (Mex) see
    Nitroglycerin 1120
Nitro-Dur® see Nitroglycerin 1120
Nitrofurantoin 1119
Nitroglycerin 1120
Nitroglycerin Injection, USP (Can)
    see Nitroglycerin 1120
Nitroglycerol see Nitroglycerin 1120
Nitrol® (Can) see Nitroglycerin 1120
Nitrolingual® see Nitroglycerin 1120
Nitropress® see Nitroprusside 1122
Nitroprusside 1122
Nitroprusside Sodium see
    Nitroprusside 1122
NitroQuick® see Nitroglycerin 1120
Nitrostat® see Nitroglycerin 1120
Nitro-Tab® see Nitroglycerin 1120
NitroTime® see Nitroglycerin 1120
Nitrous Oxide 1122
Nivoflox® (Mex) see Ciprofloxacin . . 343
Nix® (Can) see Permethrin 1218
Nix® [OTC] see Permethrin 1218
Nizatidine 1123
Nizoral® see Ketoconazole 880
Nizoral® A-D [OTC] see
    Ketoconazole 880
N-Methylhydrazine see
    Procarbazine 1284
Nobligan® (Mex) see Tramadol . . . 1514
No Doz® Maximum Strength [OTC]
    see Caffeine. 245
Nolahist® (Can) see Phenindamine
    1221
Nolahist® [OTC] [DSC] see
    Phenindamine 1221
Nolvadex® (Can) see Tamoxifen . . 1443
Nolvadex®-D (Can) see Tamoxifen
    1443
Nolvadex® [DSC] see Tamoxifen . . 1443
Nonoxynol 9 1124
Nora-BE™ see Norethindrone 1125
Noradrenaline see Norepinephrine
    1125
Noradrenaline Acid Tartrate see
    Norepinephrine 1125
Norboral® (Mex) see GlyBURIDE . . 744
Norciden® (Mex) see Danazol 419
Norco® see Hydrocodone and
    Acetaminophen 779
Nordeoxyguanosine see
    Ganciclovir 722
Nordette® see Ethinyl Estradiol and
    Levonorgestrel 602
Norditropin® see Somatropin 1406
Norditropin® NordiFlex® see
    Somatropin 1406
Norelgestromin and Ethinyl
    Estradiol see Ethinyl Estradiol
    and Norelgestromin 605
Norepinephrine 1125
Norepinephrine Bitartrate see
    Norepinephrine 1125
Norethindrone 1125

Norethindrone Acetate see
Norethindrone 1125
Norethindrone Acetate and Ethinyl
Estradiol see Ethinyl Estradiol
and Norethindrone 608
Norethindrone and Estradiol see
Estradiol and Norethindrone. . . . 575
Norethindrone and Mestranol see
Mestranol and Norethindrone . . . 999
Norethisterone see Norethindrone
. . . . 1125
Norfenon® (Mex) see Propafenone
. . . . 1293
Norflex™ see Orphenadrine 1151
Norfloxacin 1126
Norfloxacine® (Can) see
Norfloxacin 1126
Norgesic™ see
Orphenadrine, Aspirin, and
Caffeine 1152
Norgesic™ [DSC] see
Orphenadrine, Aspirin, and
Caffeine 1152
Norgesic™ Forte (Can) see
Orphenadrine, Aspirin, and
Caffeine 1152
Norgesic™ Forte [DSC] see
Orphenadrine, Aspirin, and
Caffeine 1152
Norgestimate and Estradiol see
Estradiol and Norgestimate 576
Norgestimate and Ethinyl Estradiol
see Ethinyl Estradiol and
Norgestimate 613
Norgestrel 1127
Norgestrel and Ethinyl Estradiol
see Ethinyl Estradiol and
Norgestrel 616
Norinyl® 1+35 see Ethinyl Estradiol
and Norethindrone 608
Norinyl® 1+50 see Mestranol and
Norethindrone 999
Noritate® see Metronidazole 1033
Norlutate® (Can) see
Norethindrone 1125
Normal Saline see Sodium
Chloride 1400
Normodyne® (Can) see Labetalol . . . 891
Noroxin® see Norfloxacin 1126
Norpace® see Disopyramide 491
Norpace® CR see Disopyramide . . . 491
Norplant® Implant (Can) see
Levonorgestrel 916
Norpramin® see Desipramine 434
Norpril® (Mex) see Enalapril . . . 538
Nor-QD® see Norethindrone 1125
Nortemp Children's [OTC] see
Acetaminophen 31
Nortrel™ see Ethinyl Estradiol and
Norethindrone 608
Nortrel™ 7/7/7 see Ethinyl Estradiol
and Norethindrone 608
Nortriptyline 1128
Nortriptyline Hydrochloride see
Nortriptyline 1128
Norvas® (Mex) see Amlodipine . . . 100
Norvasc® see Amlodipine 100
Norventyl (Can) see Nortriptyline . . 1128
Norvir® see Ritonavir 1359
Norvir® SEC (Can) see Ritonavir . . 1359
Nosebleed see Feverfew 1621
Novahistex® DM Decongestant
(Can) see Pseudoephedrine
and Dextromethorphan. 1311
Novahistex® DM Decongestant
Expectorant (Can) see
Guaifenesin, Pseudoephedrine,
and Dextromethorphan. 757

Novahistex® Expectorant with
Decongestant (Can) see
Guaifenesin and
Pseudoephedrine 755
Novahistine® DM Decongestant
(Can) see Pseudoephedrine
and Dextromethorphan. 1311
Novahistine® DM Decongestant
Expectorant (Can) see
Guaifenesin, Pseudoephedrine,
and Dextromethorphan. 757
Novamilor (Can) see Amiloride and
Hydrochlorothiazide 85
Novamoxin® (Can) see Amoxicillin . . 106
Novantrone® see Mitoxantrone 1055
Novarel™ see Chorionic
Gonadotropin (Human). 336
Novasen (Can) see Aspirin 145
Novo-5 ASA (Can) see
Mesalamine 996
Novo-Acebutolol (Can) see
Acebutolol 28
Novo-Alendronate (Can) see
Alendronate 64
Novo-Alprazol (Can) see
Alprazolam 73
Novo-Amiodarone (Can) see
Amiodarone 90
Novo-Ampicillin (Can) see
Ampicillin 117
Novo-Atenol (Can) see Atenolol . . . 154
Novo-Azathioprine (Can) see
Azathioprine 168
Novo-Azithromycin (Can) see
Azithromycin 171
Novo-Benzydamine (Can) see
Benzydamine 197
Novo-Bicalutamide (Can) see
Bicalutamide 207
Novo-Bisoprolol (Can) see
Bisoprolol 211
Novo-Bromazepam (Can) see
Bromazepam 220
Novo-Bupropion SR (Can) see
BuPROPion 233
Novo-Buspirone (Can) see
BusPIRone 236
Novocain® see Procaine. 1284
Novo-Captopril (Can) see Captopril
. . . . 257
Novo-Carbamaz (Can) see
Carbamazepine 260
Novo-Carvedilol (Can) see
Carvedilol 275
Novo-Cefaclor (Can) see Cefaclor . . 279
Novo-Cefadroxil (Can) see
Cefadroxil. 281
Novo-Chloroquine (Can) see
Chloroquine 320
Novo-Chlorpromazine (Can) see
ChlorproMAZINE 329
Novo-Cholamine (Can) see
Cholestyramine Resin 334
Novo-Cholamine Light (Can) see
Cholestyramine Resin 334
Novo-Cilazapril (Can) see
Cilazapril 340
Novo-Cimetidine (Can) see
Cimetidine 341
Novo-Ciprofloxacin (Can) see
Ciprofloxacin 343
Novo-Citalopram (Can) see
Citalopram 351
Novo-Clavamoxin (Can) see
Amoxicillin and Clavulanate
Potassium 108
Novo-Clindamycin (Can) see
Clindamycin 361
Novo-Clobazam (Can) see
Clobazam 364

Novo-Clobetasol (Can) see
  Clobetasol 365
Novo-Clonazepam (Can) see
  Clonazepam 371
Novo-Clonidine (Can) see
  Clonidine 373
Novo-Clopate (Can) see
  Clorazepate 378
Novo-Cloxin (Can) see Cloxacillin . . 380
Novo-Cycloprine (Can) see
  Cyclobenzaprine 401
Novo-Difenac (Can) see Diclofenac
  459
Novo-Difenac K (Can) see
  Diclofenac 459
Novo-Difenac-SR (Can) see
  Diclofenac 459
Novo-Diflunisal (Can) see Diflunisal
  468
Novo-Digoxin (Can) see Digoxin . . . 471
Novo-Diltiazem (Can) see Diltiazem
  479
Novo-Diltiazem-CD (Can) see
  Diltiazem 479
Novo-Diltiazem HCl ER (Can) see
  Diltiazem 479
Novo-Dimenate (Can) see
  DimenhyDRINATE 481
Novo-Dipam (Can) see Diazepam . . 454
Novo-Divalproex (Can) see
  Valproic Acid and Derivatives
  1556
Novo-Docusate Calcium (Can) see
  Docusate 496
Novo-Docusate Sodium (Can) see
  Docusate 496
Novo-Doxazosin (Can) see
  Doxazosin 503
Novo-Doxepin (Can) see Doxepin . . 505
Novo-Doxylin (Can) see
  Doxycycline (Systemic) 514
Novo-Famotidine (Can) see
  Famotidine 635
Novo-Fenofibrate (Can) see
  Fenofibrate 639
Novo-Ferrogluc (Can) see Ferrous
  Gluconate 651
Novo-Fluconazole (Can) see
  Fluconazole 659
Novo-Fluoxetine (Can) see
  Fluoxetine 675
Novo-Flurprofen (Can) see
  Flurbiprofen 683
Novo-Flutamide (Can) see
  Flutamide 686
Novo-Fluvoxamine (Can) see
  Fluvoxamine 694
Novo-Fosinopril (Can) see
  Fosinopril 707
Novo-Furantoin (Can) see
  Nitrofurantoin 1119
Novo-Gabapentin (Can) see
  Gabapentin 717
Novo-Gemfibrozil (Can) see
  Gemfibrozil 730
Novo-Gesic (Can) see
  Acetaminophen 31
Novo-Gliclazide (Can) see
  Gliclazide 737
Novo-Glimepiride (Can) see
  Glimepiride 738
Novo-Glyburide (Can) see
  GlyBURIDE 744
Novo-Herklin 2000® (Mex) see
  Permethrin 1218
Novo-Hydrazide (Can) see
  Hydrochlorothiazide 776
Novo-Hydroxyzin (Can) see
  HydrOXYzine 801
Novo-Hylazin (Can) see
  HydrALAZINE 775

Novo-Indapamide (Can) see
  Indapamide 828
Novo-Ipramide (Can) see
  Ipratropium 857
Novo-Keto (Can) see Ketoprofen . . . 883
Novo-Ketoconazole (Can) see
  Ketoconazole 880
Novo-Keto-EC (Can) see
  Ketoprofen 883
Novo-Ketorolac (Can) see
  Ketorolac 886
Novo-Ketotifen (Can) see Ketotifen
  890
Novo-Lamotrigine (Can) see
  Lamotrigine 895
Novo-Leflunomide (Can) see
  Leflunomide 901
Novo-Levobunolol (Can) see
  Levobunolol 909
Novo-Levocarbidopa (Can) see
  Levodopa and Carbidopa 911
Novo-Levofloxacin (Can) see
  Levofloxacin 913
Novo-Lexin (Can) see Cephalexin . . 301
Novolin® 70/30 see Insulin NPH
  and Insulin Regular 840
Novolin® ge 10/90 (Can) see
  Insulin NPH and Insulin
  Regular 840
Novolin® ge 20/80 (Can) see
  Insulin NPH and Insulin
  Regular 840
Novolin® ge 30/70 (Can) see
  Insulin NPH and Insulin
  Regular 840
Novolin® ge 40/60 (Can) see
  Insulin NPH and Insulin
  Regular 840
Novolin® ge 50/50 (Can) see
  Insulin NPH and Insulin
  Regular 840
Novolin® ge NPH (Can) see Insulin
  NPH 840
Novolin® ge Toronto (Can) see
  Insulin Regular 841
Novolin® N see Insulin NPH 840
Novolin® R see Insulin Regular 841
NovoLog® see Insulin Aspart 835
NovoLog® Mix 70/30 see Insulin
  Aspart Protamine and Insulin
  Aspart 836
Novo-Loperamide (Can) see
  Loperamide 942
Novo-Lorazepam (Can) see
  Lorazepam 947
Novo-Lovastatin (Can) see
  Lovastatin 953
Novo-Maprotiline (Can) see
  Maprotiline 964
Novo-Medrone (Can) see
  MedroxyPROGESTERone 972
Novo-Meloxicam (Can) see
  Meloxicam 977
Novo-Mepro (Can) see
  Meprobamate 993
Novo-Metformin (Can) see
  Metformin 1001
Novo-Methacin (Can) see
  Indomethacin 830
Novo-Metoprolol (Can) see
  Metoprolol 1030
Novo-Mexiletine (Can) see
  Mexiletine 1037
Novo-Minocycline (Can) see
  Minocycline 1049
Novo-Mirtazapine (Can) see
  Mirtazapine 1052
Novo-Misoprostol (Can) see
  Misoprostol 1053
Novo-Nabumetone (Can) see
  Nabumetone 1077

Novo-Nadolol (Can) see Nadolol . . 1079
Novo-Naproc EC (Can) see
Naproxen 1089
Novo-Naprox (Can) see Naproxen
. . . . 1089
Novo-Naprox Sodium (Can) see
Naproxen 1089
Novo-Naprox Sodium DS (Can)
see Naproxen 1089
Novo-Naprox SR (Can) see
Naproxen 1089
Novo-Nifedin (Can) see NIFEdipine
. . . . 1112
Novo-Nizatidine (Can) see
Nizatidine 1123
Novo-Norfloxacin (Can) see
Norfloxacin 1126
Novo-Nortriptyline (Can) see
Nortriptyline 1128
Novo-Ofloxacin (Can) see
Ofloxacin 1137
Novo-Oxybutynin (Can) see
Oxybutynin 1162
Novo-Paroxetine (Can) see
Paroxetine 1188
Novo-Pen-VK (Can) see Penicillin
V Potassium 1205
Novo-Peridol (Can) see
Haloperidol 762
Novo-Pheniram (Can) see
Chlorpheniramine 323
Novo-Pindol (Can) see Pindolol . . . 1240
Novo-Pirocam (Can) see Piroxicam
. . . . 1248
Novo-Pramine (Can) see
Imipramine 820
Novo-Pranol (Can) see Propranolol
. . . . 1301
Novo-Pravastatin (Can) see
Pravastatin 1265
Novo-Prazin (Can) see Prazosin . . 1267
Novo-Prednisolone (Can) see
PrednisoLONE 1268
Novo-Prednisone (Can) see
PredniSONE 1271
Novo-Profen (Can) see Ibuprofen . . 808
Novo-Propamide (Can) see
ChlorproPAMIDE 331
Novo-Purol (Can) see Allopurinol . . . 70
Novoquin® (Mex) see Ciprofloxacin
. . . . 343
Novo-Quinidin (Can) see Quinidine
. . . . 1324
Novo-Quinine (Can) see Quinine . . 1326
Novo-Ranidine (Can) see
Ranitidine 1334
NovoRapid® (Can) see Insulin
Aspart 836
Novo-Rythro Estolate (Can) see
Erythromycin 562
Novo-Rythro Ethylsuccinate (Can)
see Erythromycin 562
Novo-Selegiline (Can) see
Selegiline 1382
Novo-Semide (Can) see
Furosemide 715
Novo-Sertraline (Can) see
Sertraline 1385
NovoSeven® see Factor VIIa
(Recombinant) 632
Novo-Simvastatin (Can) see
Simvastatin 1394
Novo-Sorbide (Can) see Isosorbide
Dinitrate 866
Novo-Sotalol (Can) see Sotalol . . . 1409
Novo-Soxazole (Can) see
SulfiSOXAZOLE 1429
Novo-Spiroton (Can) see
Spironolactone 1413

Novo-Spirozine (Can) see
Hydrochlorothiazide and
Spironolactone 778
Novo-Sucralate (Can) see
Sucralfate 1420
Novo-Sumatriptan (Can) see
Sumatriptan 1432
Novo-Sundac (Can) see Sulindac
. . . . 1430
Novo-Tamoxifen (Can) see
Tamoxifen 1443
Novo-Temazepam (Can) see
Temazepam 1453
Novo-Terazosin (Can) see
Terazosin 1458
Novo-Terbinafine (Can) see
Terbinafine 1459
Novo-Theophyl SR (Can) see
Theophylline 1473
Novo-Ticlopidine (Can) see
Ticlopidine 1486
Novo-Topiramate (Can) see
Topiramate 1508
Novo-Trazodone (Can) see
Trazodone 1521
Novo-Triamzide (Can) see
Hydrochlorothiazide and
Triamterene 778
Novo-Trifluzine (Can) see
Trifluoperazine 1535
Novo-Trimel (Can) see
Sulfamethoxazole and
Trimethoprim 1425
Novo-Trimel D.S. (Can) see
Sulfamethoxazole and
Trimethoprim 1425
Novo-Triptyn (Can) see
Amitriptyline 93
Novo-Veramil SR (Can) see
Verapamil 1571
Novo-Warfarin (Can) see Warfarin
. . . . 1585
Novoxapram® (Can) see
Oxazepam 1157
Novo-Zopiclone (Can) see
Zopiclone 1606
Nozinan® (Can) see
Methotrimeprazine 1016
NPH Insulin see Insulin NPH 840
NPH Insulin and Regular Insulin
see Insulin NPH and Insulin
Regular 840
NRS® [OTC] see Oxymetazoline . . . 1172
NSC-740 see Methotrexate 1012
NSC-752 see Thioguanine 1476
NSC-755 see Mercaptopurine 995
NSC-3053 see Dactinomycin 417
NSC-3088 see Chlorambucil 313
NSC-10363 see Megestrol 976
NSC-13875 see Altretamine 78
NSC-15200 see Gallium Nitrate . . . 721
NSC-26271 see
Cyclophosphamide 403
NSC-26980 see Mitomycin 1054
NSC-27640 see Floxuridine 659
NSC-38721 see Mitotane 1055
NSC-49842 see VinBLAStine 1575
NSC-63878 see Cytarabine 413
NSC-66847 see Thalidomide 1471
NSC-67574 see VinCRIStine 1576
NSC-77213 see Procarbazine 1284
NSC-82151 see DAUNOrubicin
Hydrochloride 426
NSC-85998 see Streptozocin 1418
NSC-89199 see Estramustine 578
NSC-102816 see Azacitidine 167
NSC-106977 (Erwinia) see
Asparaginase 144
NSC-109229 (E. coli) see
Asparaginase 144
NSC-109724 see Ifosfamide 815

NSC-122758 see Tretinoin (Oral) . . 1524
NSC-123127 see DOXOrubicin 509
NSC-125066 see Bleomycin 214
NSC-125973 see Paclitaxel 1176
NSC-147834 see Flutamide 686
NSC-180973 see Tamoxifen 1443
NSC-218321 see Pentostatin 1211
NSC-245467 see Vindesine 1577
NSC-249992 see Amsacrine 123
NSC-256439 see Idarubicin 814
NSC-266046 see Oxaliplatin 1154
NSC-301739 see Mitoxantrone . . . 1055
NSC-308847 see Amonafide 104
NSC-352122 see Trimetrexate 1539
NSC-362856 see Temozolomide . . . 1454
NSC-373364 see Aldesleukin 61
NSC-377526 see Leuprolide 906
NSC-409962 see Carmustine 273
NSC-603071 see
    Aminocamptothecin 86
NSC-606864 see Goserelin 750
NSC606869 see Clofarabine 367
NSC-609699 see Topotecan 1511
NSC-616348 see Irinotecan 860
NSC-628503 see Docetaxel 494
NSC-644954 see Pegaspargase . . . 1194
NSC-673089 see Paclitaxel 1176
NSC-687451 see Rituximab 1360
NSC-698037 see Pemetrexed 1198
NSC-704865 see Bevacizumab . . . 204
NSC-706725 see Raloxifene 1329
NSC-712807 see Capecitabine 255
NSC-714692 see Cetuximab 308
NSC-714744 see Denileukin
    Diftitox 432
NSC-715055 see Gefitinib 727
NSC-718781 see Erlotinib 560
NSC-719345 see Letrozole 904
NSC-720568 see Gemtuzumab
    Ozogamicin 732
NSC-728729 see Infliximab 832
NSC736511 see Sunitinib 1434
NTG see Nitroglycerin 1120
N-trifluoroacetyladriamycin-14-valerate
    see Valrubicin 1560
NTZ® (Mex) see Nitazoxanide 1117
Nu-Acebutolol (Can) see
    Acebutolol 28
Nu-Acyclovir (Can) see Acyclovir 49
Nu-Alprax (Can) see Alprazolam . . . 73
Nu-Amilzide (Can) see Amiloride
    and Hydrochlorothiazide 85
Nu-Amoxi (Can) see Amoxicillin . . . 106
Nu-Ampi (Can) see Ampicillin 117
Nu-Atenol (Can) see Atenolol 154
Nu-Baclo (Can) see Baclofen 178
Nubain® see Nalbuphine 1083
Nu-Beclomethasone (Can) see
    Beclomethasone 183
Nu-Bromazepam (Can) see
    Bromazepam 220
Nu-Buspirone (Can) see
    BusPIRone 236
Nu-Capto (Can) see Captopril 257
Nu-Carbamazepine (Can) see
    Carbamazepine 260
Nu-Cefaclor (Can) see Cefaclor . . . 279
Nu-Cephalex (Can) see
    Cephalexin 301
Nu-Cimet (Can) see Cimetidine . . . 341
Nu-Clonazepam (Can) see
    Clonazepam 371
Nu-Clonidine (Can) see Clonidine . . 373
Nu-Cloxi (Can) see Cloxacillin 380
Nucofed® Expectorant see
    Guaifenesin, Pseudoephedrine,
    and Codeine 756
Nucofed® Pediatric Expectorant
    see Guaifenesin,
    Pseudoephedrine, and
    Codeine 756

Nu-Cotrimox (Can) see
    Sulfamethoxazole and
    Trimethoprim 1425
Nu-Cromolyn (Can) see Cromolyn . . 397
Nu-Cyclobenzaprine (Can) see
    Cyclobenzaprine 401
Nu-Desipramine (Can) see
    Desipramine 434
Nu-Diclo (Can) see Diclofenac 459
Nu-Diclo-SR (Can) see Diclofenac . . 459
Nu-Diflunisal (Can) see Diflunisal . . . 468
Nu-Diltiaz (Can) see Diltiazem 479
Nu-Diltiaz-CD (Can) see Diltiazem . . 479
Nu-Divalproex (Can) see Valproic
    Acid and Derivatives 1556
Nu-Doxycycline (Can) see
    Doxycycline (Systemic) 514
Nu-Erythromycin-S (Can) see
    Erythromycin 562
Nu-Famotidine (Can) see
    Famotidine 635
Nu-Fenofibrate (Can) see
    Fenofibrate 639
Nu-Fluoxetine (Can) see
    Fluoxetine 675
Nu-Flurprofen (Can) see
    Flurbiprofen 683
Nu-Fluvoxamine (Can) see
    Fluvoxamine 694
Nu-Gabapentin (Can) see
    Gabapentin 717
Nu-Gemfibrozil (Can) see
    Gemfibrozil 730
Nu-Glyburide (Can) see
    GlyBURIDE 744
Nu-Hydral (Can) see HydrALAZINE
    775
Nu-Ibuprofen (Can) see Ibuprofen . . 808
Nu-Indapamide (Can) see
    Indapamide 828
Nu-Indo (Can) see Indomethacin . . . 830
Nu-Ipratropium (Can) see
    Ipratropium 857
Nu-Iron® 150 [OTC] see
    Polysaccharide-Iron Complex . . 1254
Nu-Ketoprofen (Can) see
    Ketoprofen 883
Nu-Ketoprofen-E (Can) see
    Ketoprofen 883
NuLev™ see Hyoscyamine 803
Nu-Levocarb (Can) see Levodopa
    and Carbidopa 911
Nullo® [OTC] see Chlorophyll 319
Nu-Loraz (Can) see Lorazepam . . . 947
Nu-Lovastatin (Can) see Lovastatin
    953
Nu-Loxapine (Can) see Loxapine . . . 955
NuLYTELY® see Polyethylene
    Glycol-Electrolyte Solution 1253
Nu-Medopa (Can) see Methyldopa
    1021
Nu-Mefenamic (Can) see
    Mefenamic Acid 973
Nu-Megestrol (Can) see Megestrol . . 976
Nu-Metformin (Can) see Metformin
    1001
Nu-Metoclopramide (Can) see
    Metoclopramide 1029
Nu-Metop (Can) see Metoprolol . . . 1030
Numorphan® see Oxymorphone . . . 1174
Nu-Naprox (Can) see Naproxen . . . 1089
Nu-Nifed (Can) see NIFEdipine . . . 1112
Nu-Nizatidine (Can) see Nizatidine
    1123
Nu-Nortriptyline (Can) see
    Nortriptyline 1128
Nu-Oxybutyn (Can) see
    Oxybutynin 1162
Nu-Pentoxifylline SR (Can) see
    Pentoxifylline 1212

Nu-Pen-VK (Can) see Penicillin V
Potassium 1205
Nupercainal® Hydrocortisone
Cream [OTC] see
Hydrocortisone 793
Nupercainal® [OTC] see Dibucaine
. . . . 458
Nu-Pindol (Can) see Pindolol 1240
Nu-Pirox (Can) see Piroxicam . . . 1248
Nu-Prazo (Can) see Prazosin 1267
Nu-Prochlor (Can) see
Prochlorperazine 1285
Nu-Propranolol (Can) see
Propranolol. 1301
Nuquin HP® see Hydroquinone . . . 798
Nu-Ranit (Can) see Ranitidine . . . 1334
Nu-Selegiline (Can) see Selegiline
. . . . 1382
Nu-Sertraline (Can) see Sertraline
. . . . 1385
Nu-Sotalol (Can) see Sotalol 1409
Nu-Sucralate (Can) see Sucralfate
. . . . 1420
Nu-Sundac (Can) see Sulindac . . . 1430
Nu-Tears® II [OTC] see Artificial
Tears 143
Nu-Tears® [OTC] see Artificial
Tears 143
Nu-Temazepam (Can) see
Temazepam 1453
Nu-Terazosin (Can) see Terazosin
. . . . 1458
Nu-Tetra (Can) see Tetracycline . . 1467
Nu-Ticlopidine (Can) see
Ticlopidine 1486
Nu-Timolol (Can) see Timolol 1489
Nutracort® see Hydrocortisone 793
Nutralox® [OTC] see Calcium
Carbonate 248
Nutraplus® [OTC] see Urea 1551
Nu-Trazodone (Can) see
Trazodone 1521
NutreStore™ see Glutamine 743
Nu-Triazide (Can) see
Hydrochlorothiazide and
Triamterene 778
Nu-Trimipramine (Can) see
Trimipramine 1540
Nutropin® see Somatropin 1406
Nutropin AQ® see Somatropin 1406
Nutropine® (Can) see Somatropin
. . . . 1406
NuvaRing® see Ethinyl Estradiol
and Etonogestrel 600
Nu-Verap (Can) see Verapamil . . . 1571
Nu-Zopiclone (Can) see Zopiclone
. . . . 1606
NVB see Vinorelbine 1578
NVP see Nevirapine 1104
Nyaderm (Can) see Nystatin 1133
Nyamyc™ see Nystatin 1133
Nydrazid® [DSC] see Isoniazid 864
Nylidrin 1133
Nystatin 1133
Nystatin and Triamcinolone 1134
Nystat-Rx® see Nystatin 1133
Nystop® see Nystatin 1133
Nytol® (Can) see
DiphenhydrAMINE 483
Nytol® Extra Strength (Can) see
DiphenhydrAMINE 483
Nytol® Quick Caps [OTC] see
DiphenhydrAMINE 483
Nytol® Quick Gels [OTC] see
DiphenhydrAMINE 483
NäSop™ see Phenylephrine 1226
Nõstrilla® [OTC] see
Oxymetazoline 1172
Obezine® [DSC] see
Phendimetrazine 1220
OCBZ see Oxcarbazepine 1159

Occlusal™-HP (Can) see Salicylic
Acid 1374
Occlusal®-HP [OTC] see Salicylic
Acid 1374
Ocean® [OTC] see Sodium
Chloride 1400
Ocean® for Kids [OTC] see
Sodium Chloride 1400
Octagam® see Immune Globulin
(Intravenous) 824
Octostim® (Can) see
Desmopressin 437
Octreotide 1135
Octreotide Acetate see Octreotide
. . . . 1135
Octreotide Acetate Injection (Can)
see Octreotide 1135
Octreotide Acetate Omega (Can)
see Octreotide 1135
Ocuclear® (Mex) see
Oxymetazoline 1172
OcuCoat® [OTC] see Artificial
Tears 143
OcuCoat® PF [OTC] see Artificial
Tears 143
Ocufen® see Flurbiprofen 683
Ocuflox® see Ofloxacin 1137
Ocupress® [DSC] see Carteolol . . . 274
Ocupress® Ophthalmic (Can) see
Carteolol 274
Ocuvite® Extra® [OTC] see
Vitamins (Multiple/Oral) 1582
Ocuvite® Lutein [OTC] see
Vitamins (Multiple/Oral) 1582
Ocuvite® [OTC] see Vitamins
(Multiple/Oral). 1582
Oenothera biennis see Evening
Primrose 1621
Oesclim® (Can) see Estradiol 574
Ofloxacin 1137
Ogastro® (Mex) see Lansoprazole . 896
Ogen® see Estropipate 586
Ogestrel® see Ethinyl Estradiol and
Norgestrel 616
OGMT see Metyrosine 1036
OGT-918 see Miglustat 1047
OKT3 see Muromonab-CD3 1074
Olanzapine 1139
Olanzapine and Fluoxetine 1141
Olanzapine and Fluoxetine
Hydrochloride see Olanzapine
and Fluoxetine 1141
Olay® Vitamins Complete Women's
50+[OTC] see Vitamins
(Multiple/Oral). 1582
Olay® Vitamins Complete Women's
[OTC] see Vitamins (Multiple/
Oral) 1582
Olay® Vitamins Even Complexion
[OTC] see Vitamins (Multiple/
Oral) 1582
Oleovitamin A see Vitamin A 1580
Oleum Ricini see Castor Oil 279
Olexin® (Mex) see Omeprazole . . . 1145
Olmesartan. 1142
Olmesartan and
Hydrochlorothiazide 1143
Olmesartan Medoxomil see
Olmesartan 1142
Olmesartan Medoxomil and
Hydrochlorothiazide see
Olmesartan and
Hydrochlorothiazide 1143
Olopatadine 1143
Olsalazine 1144
Olsalazine Sodium see Olsalazine
. . . . 1144
Olux® see Clobetasol 365
Omalizumab 1144
Omega-3-Acid Ethyl Esters 1621
Omeprazole 1145

Omeprazole and Sodium
  Bicarbonate 1146
Omnicef® see Cefdinir 284
Omnii Gel™ [OTC] see Fluoride 671
Omnipaque™ see Iohexol 854
Oncaspar® see Pegaspargase 1194
Oncotice™ (Can) see BCG Vaccine
   181
Ondansetron 1147
Ondansetron Hydrochloride see
  Ondansetron 1147
One-A-Day® 50 Plus Formula
  [OTC] see Vitamins (Multiple/
  Oral) 1582
One-A-Day® Active Formula [OTC]
  see Vitamins (Multiple/Oral) . . . 1582
One-A-Day® Carb Smart [OTC]
  see Vitamins (Multiple/Oral) . . . 1582
One-A-Day® Cholesterol Plus™
  [OTC] see Vitamins (Multiple/
  Oral) 1582
One-A-Day® Essential Formula
  [OTC] see Vitamins (Multiple/
  Oral) 1582
One-A-Day® Maximum Formula
  [OTC] see Vitamins (Multiple/
  Oral) 1582
One-A-Day® Men's Formula [OTC]
  see Vitamins (Multiple/Oral) . . . 1582
One-A-Day® Today [OTC] see
  Vitamins (Multiple/Oral) 1582
One-A-Day® Weight Smart [OTC
  see Vitamins (Multiple/Oral) . . . 1582
One-A-Day® Women's Formula
  [OTC] see Vitamins (Multiple/
  Oral) 1582
Onofin-K® (Mex) see Ketoconazole
   880
ONTAK® see Denileukin Diftitox 432
Onxol™ see Paclitaxel 1176
Ony-Clear [OTC] [DSC] see
  Benzalkonium Chloride 188
OPC-13013 see Cilostazol 340
OPC-14597 see Aripiprazole 138
OP-CCK see Sincalide 1396
Opcon-A® [OTC] see Naphazoline
  and Pheniramine 1088
Operand® Chlorhexidine Gluconate
  [OTC] see Chlorhexidine
  Gluconate 316
Operand® [OTC] see
  Povidone-Iodine 1262
Ophthetic® see Proparacaine 1296
Ophtho-Dipivefrin® (Can) see
  Dipivefrin 489
Ophtho-Tate® (Can) see
  PrednisoLONE 1268
Opium and Belladonna see
  Belladonna and Opium 184
Opium Tincture 1149
Opium Tincture, Deodorized see
  Opium Tincture 1149
Oprad® (Mex) see Amikacin 84
Oprelvekin 1149
Opthaflox® (Mex) see Ciprofloxacin
   343
Opthavir® (Mex) see Acyclovir 49
Optho-Bunolol® (Can) see
  Levobunolol 909
Opticrom® see Cromolyn 397
Optifree® (Mex) see Pancreatin 1183
Optigene® 3 [OTC] see
  Tetrahydrozoline 1470
Optimyxin® (Can) see Bacitracin
  and Polymyxin B 176
Optimyxin Plus® (Can) see
  Neomycin, Polymyxin B, and
  Gramicidin 1101
OptiPranolol® see Metipranolol 1028
Optiray® see Ioversol 856
Optivar® see Azelastine 170

Optivite® P.M.T. [OTC] see
  Vitamins (Multiple/Oral) 1582
Optomicin® (Mex) see
  Erythromycin 562
o,p'-DDD see Mitotane 1055
Orabase® with Benzocaine [OTC]
  see Benzocaine 190
Oracit® see Sodium Citrate and
  Citric Acid 1401
Oracort (Can) see Triamcinolone . . 1526
Orajel® Baby Daytime and
  Nighttime [OTC] see
  Benzocaine 190
Orajel® Baby Teething Nighttime
  [OTC] see Benzocaine 190
Orajel® Baby Teething [OTC] see
  Benzocaine 190
Orajel® Denture Plus [OTC] see
  Benzocaine 190
Orajel® Maximum Strength [OTC]
  see Benzocaine 190
Orajel® Medicated Toothache
  [OTC] see Benzocaine 190
Orajel® Mouth Sore [OTC] see
  Benzocaine 190
Orajel® Multi-Action Cold Sore
  [OTC] see Benzocaine 190
Orajel® Perioseptic® Spot
  Treatment [OTC] see
  Carbamide Peroxide 264
Orajel PM® [OTC] see Benzocaine
   190
Orajel® Ultra Mouth Sore [OTC]
  see Benzocaine 190
Oramorph SR® see Morphine
  Sulfate 1065
Orange Root see Golden Seal 1624
Oranor® (Mex) see Norfloxacin . . . 1126
Oranyl [OTC] see
  Pseudoephedrine 1309
Orap® see Pimozide 1238
Orapred® see PrednisoLONE 1268
Oraquix® see Lidocaine and
  Prilocaine 928
OraRinse™ [OTC] see Maltodextrin
   963
Orazinc® [OTC] see Zinc Sulfate . . 1598
Orciprenaline Sulfate see
  Metaproterenol 1000
Orelox® (Mex) see Cefpodoxime . . . 290
Orencia® see Abatacept 25
Orfadin® see Nitisinone 1118
Orgalutran® (Can) see Ganirelix . . . 723
Organ-1 NR see Guaifenesin 752
Organidin® NR see Guaifenesin . . . 752
Orgaran® (Can) see Danaparoid . . . 418
Oriental Plum Tree see Ginkgo
  Biloba 1622
Orlistat 1150
Ornex® Maximum Strength [OTC]
  see Acetaminophen and
  Pseudoephedrine 38
Ornex® [OTC] see Acetaminophen
  and Pseudoephedrine 38
ORO-Clense (Can) see
  Chlorhexidine Gluconate 316
Orphenace® (Can) see
  Orphenadrine 1151
Orphenadrine 1151
Orphenadrine, Aspirin, and
  Caffeine 1152
Orphenadrine Citrate see
  Orphenadrine 1151
Orphengesic [DSC] see
  Orphenadrine, Aspirin, and
  Caffeine 1152
Orphengesic Forte [DSC] see
  Orphenadrine, Aspirin, and
  Caffeine 1152
Ortho® 0.5/35 (Can) see Ethinyl
  Estradiol and Norethindrone 608

Ortho® 1/35 (Can) see Ethinyl
  Estradiol and Norethindrone 608
Ortho® 7/7/7 (Can) see Ethinyl
  Estradiol and Norethindrone 608
Ortho-Cept® see Ethinyl Estradiol
  and Desogestrel 592
Orthoclone® (Mex) see
  Muromonab-CD3 1074
Orthoclone OKT® 3 see
  Muromonab-CD3 1074
Ortho-Cyclen® see Ethinyl Estradiol
  and Norgestimate 613
Ortho-Est® see Estropipate 586
Ortho Evra® see Ethinyl Estradiol
  and Norelgestromin 605
Ortho-Novum® see Ethinyl
  Estradiol and Norethindrone . . . 608
Ortho-Novum® 1/50 see Mestranol
  and Norethindrone 999
Ortho Prefest see Estradiol and
  Norgestimate 576
Ortho Tri-Cyclen® see Ethinyl
  Estradiol and Norgestimate 613
Ortho Tri-Cyclen® Lo see Ethinyl
  Estradiol and Norgestimate 613
Orthovisc® see Hyaluronate and
  Derivatives 773
Ortopsique® (Mex) see Diazepam . . 454
Orudis® KT [OTC] [DSC] see
  Ketoprofen 883
Oruvail® (Can) see Ketoprofen 883
Orvaten™ see Midodrine 1044
Os-Cal® (Can) see Calcium
  Carbonate 248
Os-Cal® 500 [OTC] see Calcium
  Carbonate 248
Oseltamivir 1152
Oseum® [salmon] (Mex) see
  Calcitonin 246
OSI-774 see Erlotinib 560
Osiren® (Mex) see Omeprazole . . . 1145
Osmoglyn® [DSC] see Glycerin . . . 747
OsmoPrep™ see Sodium
  Phosphates 1403
Osteocit® (Can) see Calcium
  Citrate 250
Osteomin® (Mex) see Calcium
  Carbonate 248
Ostoforte® (Can) see Ergocalciferol
  556
Oticaine see Benzocaine 190
Otocaine™ see Benzocaine 190
Otrivin® [OTC] [DSC] see
  Xylometazoline 1588
Otrivin® Pediatric [OTC] [DSC] see
  Xylometazoline 1588
Outgro® [OTC] see Benzocaine 190
Ovace™ see Sulfacetamide 1423
Ovcon® see Ethinyl Estradiol and
  Norethindrone 608
Ovidrel® see Chorionic
  Gonadotropin (Recombinant) . . 337
Ovol® (Can) see Simethicone 1394
Ovral® (Can) see Ethinyl Estradiol
  and Norgestrel 616
Ovrette® (Can) see Norgestrel 1127
Ovrette® [DSC] see Norgestrel 1127
Oxacillin 1153
Oxacillin Sodium see Oxacillin . . . 1153
Oxaliplatin 1154
Oxandrin® see Oxandrolone 1155
Oxandrolone 1155
Oxaprozin 1155
Oxazepam 1157
Oxcarbazepine 1159
Oxeze® Turbuhaler® (Can) see
  Formoterol 701
Oxiconazole 1160
Oxiconazole Nitrate see
  Oxiconazole 1160

Oxidized Regenerated Cellulose
  see Cellulose (Oxidized/
  Regenerated) 300
Oxifungol® (Mex) see Fluconazole . . 659
Oxiken® (Mex) see DOBUTamine . . 493
Oxilapine Succinate see Loxapine . 955
Oxipor® VHC [OTC] see Coal Tar . . 383
Oxistat® see Oxiconazole 1160
Oxitraklin® (Mex) see
  Oxytetracycline 1174
Oxpam® (Can) see Oxazepam 1157
Oxpentifylline see Pentoxifylline . . 1212
Oxpram® (Can) see Oxazepam . . . 1157
Oxprenolol 1161
Oxprenolol Hydrochloride see
  Oxprenolol 1161
Oxsoralen® see Methoxsalen 1018
Oxsoralen-Ultra® see Methoxsalen
  1018
Oxy 10® Balanced Medicated Face
  Wash [OTC] see Benzoyl
  Peroxide 194
Oxy 10® Balance Spot Treatment
  [OTC] see Benzoyl Peroxide . . . 194
Oxy Balance® Deep Pore [OTC]
  see Salicylic Acid 1374
Oxy Balance® [OTC] see Salicylic
  Acid 1374
Oxybutynin 1162
Oxybutynin Chloride see
  Oxybutynin 1162
Oxychlorosene 1163
Oxychlorosene Sodium see
  Oxychlorosene 1163
Oxycocet® (Can) see Oxycodone
  and Acetaminophen 1165
Oxycodan® (Can) see Oxycodone
  and Aspirin 1168
Oxycodone 1163
Oxycodone and Acetaminophen . . . 1165
Oxycodone and Aspirin 1168
Oxycodone and Ibuprofen 1170
Oxycodone Hydrochloride see
  Oxycodone 1163
OxyContin® see Oxycodone 1163
Oxyderm™ (Can) see Benzoyl
  Peroxide 194
Oxydose™ see Oxycodone 1163
OxyFast® see Oxycodone 1163
Oxygen 1172
OxyIR® see Oxycodone 1163
Oxylin® (Mex) see Oxymetazoline
  1172
Oxymetazoline 1172
Oxymetazoline Hydrochloride see
  Oxymetazoline 1172
Oxymetholone 1173
Oxymorphone 1174
Oxymorphone Hydrochloride see
  Oxymorphone 1174
Oxytetracycline 1174
Oxytetracycline Hydrochloride see
  Oxytetracycline 1174
Oxytocin 1175
Oxytrol® see Oxybutynin 1162
Oysco 500 [OTC] see Calcium
  Carbonate 248
Oyst-Cal 500 [OTC] see Calcium
  Carbonate 248
P-V Tussin Tablet see
  Hydrocodone and
  Pseudoephedrine 788
P-071 see Cetirizine 306
Pacerone® see Amiodarone 90
Pacis™ (Can) see BCG Vaccine . . . 181
Pacitran® (Mex) see Diazepam 454
Paclitaxel 1176
Paclitaxel (Protein Bound) 1177
Pain-A-Lay® [OTC] see Phenol . . . 1223
Pain Eze [OTC] see
  Acetaminophen 31

Pain-Off [OTC] see
Acetaminophen, Aspirin, and
Caffeine 41
Palafer® (Can) see Ferrous
Fumarate 650
Palane® (Mex) see Enalapril . . . 538
Palgic see Carbinoxamine 268
Palgic®-D see Carbinoxamine and
Pseudoephedrine 268
Palgic®-DS see Carbinoxamine
and Pseudoephedrine 268
Palifermin 1178
Palivizumab 1179
Palladone™ [Withdrawn] see
Hydromorphone 797
Palmer's® Skin Success Acne
Cleanser [OTC] see Salicylic
Acid 1374
Palmer's® Skin Success Acne
[OTC] see Benzoyl Peroxide . . . 194
Palmer's® Skin Success Eventone®
Fade Cream [OTC] see
Hydroquinone 798
Palmetto Scrub see Saw Palmetto
. . . . 1631
Palmitate-A® [OTC] see Vitamin A
. . . . 1580
Palonosetron 1180
Palonosetron Hydrochloride see
Palonosetron 1180
Pamelor® see Nortriptyline 1128
Pamidronate 1181
Pamidronate Disodium® (Can) see
Pamidronate 1181
Pamine® see Methscopolamine . . . 1019
Pamine® Forte see
Methscopolamine 1019
p-Aminoclonidine see
Apraclonidine 133
Pamix™ [OTC] see Pyrantel
Pamoate 1314
Pamprin® Maximum Strength All
Day Relief [OTC] see
Naproxen 1089
Pan-2400™ [OTC] see Pancreatin
. . . . 1183
Panafil® see Chlorophyllin, Papain,
and Urea 319
Panax ginseng see Ginseng,
Panax 1623
Pan-B Antibody see Rituximab 1360
Pancof® see Pseudoephedrine,
Dihydrocodeine, and
Chlorpheniramine 1312
Pancof®-EXP see Dihydrocodeine,
Pseudoephedrine, and
Guaifenesin 476
Pancof®-PD see Dihydrocodeine,
Chlorpheniramine, and
Phenylephrine 476
Pancrease® (Mex) see Pancreatin
. . . . 1183
Pancrease® [DSC] see
Pancrelipase 1183
Pancrease® MT see Pancrelipase
. . . . 1183
Pancreatin 1183
Pancreatin 4X [OTC] see
Pancreatin 1183
Pancreatin 8X [OTC] see
Pancreatin 1183
Pancrecarb MS® see Pancrelipase
. . . . 1183
Pancrelipase 1183
Pandel® see Hydrocortisone 793
Pangestyme™ CN see
Pancrelipase 1183
Pangestyme™ EC see
Pancrelipase 1183
Pangestyme™ MT see
Pancrelipase 1183

Pangestyme™ UL see
Pancrelipase 1183
Panglobulin® NF see Immune
Globulin (Intravenous) 824
Panhematin® see Hemin 764
Panixine DisperDose™ [DSC] see
Cephalexin 301
Panlor® DC see Acetaminophen,
Caffeine, and Dihydrocodeine . . . 42
Panlor® SS see Acetaminophen,
Caffeine, and Dihydrocodeine . . . 42
PanMist®-DM [DSC] see
Guaifenesin, Pseudoephedrine,
and Dextromethorphan 757
PanMist®-JR see Guaifenesin and
Pseudoephedrine 755
PanMist®-LA see Guaifenesin and
Pseudoephedrine 755
PanMist®-S see Guaifenesin and
Pseudoephedrine 755
Panokase® see Pancrelipase 1183
Panokase® 16 see Pancrelipase . . 1183
PanOxyl® see Benzoyl Peroxide . . 194
PanOxyl®-AQ see Benzoyl
Peroxide 194
PanOxyl® Aqua Gel see Benzoyl
Peroxide 194
PanOxyl® Bar [OTC] see Benzoyl
Peroxide 194
Panretin® see Alitretinoin 69
Panthoderm® [OTC] see
Dexpanthenol 446
Panto™ IV (Can) see Pantoprazole
. . . . 1184
Pantoloc® (Can) see Pantoprazole
. . . . 1184
Pantomicina® (Mex) see
Erythromycin 562
Pantoprazole 1184
Pantothenic Acid 1186
Pantothenyl Alcohol see
Dexpanthenol 446
Pantozol® (Mex) see Pantoprazole
. . . . 1184
Papain and Urea 1186
Papain, Urea, and Chlorophyllin
see Chlorophyllin, Papain, and
Urea 319
Papaverine 1186
Papaverine Hydrochloride see
Papaverine 1186
Para-Aminosalicylate Sodium see
Aminosalicylic Acid 89
Paracetamol see Acetaminophen . . . 31
Parafon Forte® (Can) see
Chlorzoxazone 333
Parafon Forte® DSC see
Chlorzoxazone 333
Paraplatin® see Carboplatin 270
Paraplatin-AQ (Can) see
Carboplatin 270
Parathyroid Hormone (1-34) see
Teriparatide 1461
Para-Time SR® see Papaverine . . . 1186
Parcopa™ see Levodopa and
Carbidopa 911
Paregoric 1187
Paremyd® see
Hydroxyamphetamine and
Tropicamide 799
Paricalcitol 1187
Pariet® (Can) see Rabeprazole . . . 1327
Pariprazole see Rabeprazole 1327
Parlodel® see Bromocriptine 222
Parnate® see Tranylcypromine 1519
Paromomycin 1188
Paromomycin Sulfate see
Paromomycin 1188
Paroxetine 1188
Paroxetine Hydrochloride see
Paroxetine 1188

Paroxetine Mesylate see
  Paroxetine 1188
Parsley 1630
Partusisten® (Mex) see Fenoterol . . . 644
Parvolex® (Can) see Acetylcysteine
  46
PAS see Aminosalicylic Acid 89
Paser® see Aminosalicylic Acid 89
Passiflora spp see Passion Flower
  1630
Passion Flower 1630
Patanol® see Olopatadine 1143
Pathocil® (Can) see Dicloxacillin . . . 463
Pausinystalia yohimbe see
  Yohimbe 1634
Pavabid [DSC] see Papaverine . . . 1186
Paxil® see Paroxetine 1188
Paxil CR® see Paroxetine 1188
PBZ® see Tripelennamine 1541
PBZ-SR® see Tripelennamine 1541
PCA (error-prone abbreviation) see
  Procainamide 1283
PCE® see Erythromycin 562
PCEC see Rabies Virus Vaccine . . 1329
PCM see Chlorpheniramine,
  Phenylephrine, and
  Methscopolamine 327
PCM Allergy see
  Chlorpheniramine,
  Phenylephrine, and
  Methscopolamine 327
PCV7 see Pneumococcal
  Conjugate Vaccine (7-Valent)
  1250
Pectin and Kaolin see Kaolin and
  Pectin 879
PediaCare® Children's Long Acting
  Cough Plus Cold [OTC] see
  Pseudoephedrine and
  Dextromethorphan 1311
PediaCare® Children's Medicated
  Freezer Pops Long Acting
  Cough [OTC] see
  Dextromethorphan 451
PediaCare® Cold and Allergy
  [OTC] see Chlorpheniramine
  and Pseudoephedrine 325
PediaCare® Decongestant Infants
  [OTC] see Pseudoephedrine . . 1309
PediaCare® Infants' Decongestant
  & Cough [OTC] see
  Pseudoephedrine and
  Dextromethorphan 1311
PediaCare® Infants' Long-Acting
  Cough [OTC] see
  Dextromethorphan 451
Pediacof® [DSC] see
  Chlorpheniramine,
  Phenylephrine, Codeine, and
  Potassium Iodide 328
Pediaflor® [DSC] see Fluoride 671
Pediapred® see PrednisoLONE . . . 1268
Pedia Relief Cough and Cold
  [OTC] see Pseudoephedrine
  and Dextromethorphan 1311
Pedia Relief Infants [OTC] see
  Pseudoephedrine and
  Dextromethorphan 1311
Pediarix™ see Diphtheria, Tetanus
  Toxoids, Acellular Pertussis,
  Hepatitis B (Recombinant), and
  Poliovirus (Inactivated) Vaccine
  488
Pediatex™ see Carbinoxamine 268
Pediatex™ 12 see Carbinoxamine . . 268
Pediatex™-D see Carbinoxamine
  and Pseudoephedrine 268
Pediatex™ DM [DSC] see
  Carbinoxamine,
  Pseudoephedrine, and
  Dextromethorphan 269

Pediatric Digoxin CSD (Can) see
  Digoxin 471
Pediatrix (Can) see
  Acetaminophen 31
Pediazole® see Erythromycin and
  Sulfisoxazole 568
Pedi-Boro® [OTC] see Aluminum
  Sulfate and Calcium Acetate 81
Pedi-Dri® see Nystatin 1133
PediOtic® see Neomycin,
  Polymyxin B, and
  Hydrocortisone 1101
Pedisilk® [OTC] see Salicylic Acid
  1374
Pedtrace-4® see Trace Metals 1513
PedvaxHIB® see Haemophilus b
  Conjugate Vaccine 534
PEG see Polyethylene Glycol 3350
  1253
PEG-L-asparaginase see
  Pegaspargase 1194
Pegademase Bovine 1193
Peganone® see Ethotoin 619
Pegaptanib 1193
Pegaptanib Sodium see
  Pegaptanib 1193
Pegaspargase 1194
Pegasys® see Peginterferon
  Alfa-2a 1195
Pegfilgrastim 1195
Peginterferon Alfa-2a 1195
Peginterferon Alfa-2b 1197
PEG-Intron® see Peginterferon
  Alfa-2b 1197
PegLyte® (Can) see Polyethylene
  Glycol-Electrolyte Solution 1253
Pegylated Interferon Alfa-2a see
  Peginterferon Alfa-2a 1195
Pegylated Interferon Alfa-2b see
  Peginterferon Alfa-2b 1197
PemADD® CT [DSC] see Pemoline
  1199
PemADD® [DSC] see Pemoline . . . 1199
Pemetrexed 1198
Pemetrexed Disodium see
  Pemetrexed 1198
Pemirolast 1199
Pemoline 1199
Penbutolol 1199
Penbutolol Sulfate see Penbutolol
  1199
Penciclovir 1200
Penicillamine 1201
Penicillin V Potassium 1205
Penicillin G Benzathine 1202
Penicillin G Benzathine and
  Penicillin G Procaine 1203
Penicillin G (Parenteral/Aqueous) . . 1203
Penicillin G Potassium see
  Penicillin G (Parenteral/
  Aqueous) 1203
Penicillin G Procaine 1204
Penicillin G Procaine and
  Benzathine Combined see
  Penicillin G Benzathine and
  Penicillin G Procaine 1203
Penicillin G Sodium see Penicillin
  G (Parenteral/Aqueous) 1203
Penicilloyl-polylysine see
  Benzylpenicilloyl-polylysine 198
Penlac® see Ciclopirox 338
Pennsaid® (Can) see Diclofenac . . 459
Pentafluoropropane and
  Tetrafluoroethane 1206
Pentahydrate see Sodium
  Thiosulfate 1404
Pentam-300® see Pentamidine 1207
Pentamidine 1207
Pentamidine Isethionate see
  Pentamidine 1207

Pentamycetin® (Can) see
  Chloramphenicol 314
Pentasa® see Mesalamine 996
Pentaspan® see Pentastarch 1208
Pentastarch 1208
Penta-Triamterene HCTZ (Can)
  see Hydrochlorothiazide and
  Triamterene 778
Pentavalent Human-Bovine
  Reassortant Rotavirus Vaccine
  see Rotavirus Vaccine 1371
Pentazocine 1208
Pentazocine and Acetaminophen . . 1209
Pentazocine Hydrochloride see
  Pentazocine 1208
Pentazocine Hydrochloride and
  Acetaminophen see
  Pentazocine and
  Acetaminophen 1209
Pentazocine Hydrochloride and
  Naloxone Hydrochloride see
  Pentazocine 1208
Pentazocine Lactate see
  Pentazocine 1208
Pentetate Calcium Trisodium see
  Diethylene Triamine
  Penta-Acetic Acid 466
Pentetate Zinc Trisodium see
  Diethylene Triamine
  Penta-Acetic Acid 466
Pentobarbital 1210
Pentobarbital Sodium see
  Pentobarbital 1210
Pentosan Polysulfate Sodium 1211
Pentostatin 1211
Penthotal® see Thiopental 1477
Pentothal Sodico® (Mex) see
  Thiopental 1477
Pentoxifylline 1212
Pentoxil® see Pentoxifylline 1212
Pen VK see Penicillin V Potassium
  1205
Pepcid® see Famotidine 635
Pepcid® AC (Can) see Famotidine . . 635
Pepcid® AC [OTC] see Famotidine
  635
Pepcid® Complete [OTC] see
  Famotidine, Calcium
  Carbonate, and Magnesium
  Hydroxide 636
Pepcidine® (Mex) see Famotidine . . 635
Pepcid® I.V. (Can) see Famotidine . . 635
Pepevit® (Mex) see Niacin 1105
Pepto-Bismol® Maximum Strength
  [OTC] see Bismuth 210
Pepto-Bismol® [OTC] see Bismuth . . 210
Perchloracap® [DSC] see
  Potassium Perchlorate 1261
Percocet® see Oxycodone and
  Acetaminophen 1165
Percocet®-Demi (Can) see
  Oxycodone and
  Acetaminophen 1165
Percodan® see Oxycodone and
  Aspirin 1168
Percogesic® Extra Strength [OTC]
  see Acetaminophen and
  Diphenhydramine 38
Percogesic® [OTC] see
  Acetaminophen and
  Phenyltoloxamine 38
Perdiem® Overnight Relief [OTC]
  see Senna 1384
Pergolide 1213
Pergolide Mesylate see Pergolide
  1213
Pergonal® [DSC] see Menotropins . . 982
Periactin® see Cyproheptadine 412
Peri-Colace® [DSC] [OTC] see
  Docusate and Casanthranol 496
Pericyazine 1214

Peridane® (Mex) see Pentoxifylline
  1212
Peridex® see Chlorhexidine
  Gluconate 316
Peridol (Can) see Haloperidol . . 762
Perindopril Erbumine 1216
PerioChip® see Chlorhexidine
  Gluconate 316
PerioGard® see Chlorhexidine
  Gluconate 316
PerioMed™ see Fluoride 671
Periostat® see Doxycycline
  (Subantimicrobial) 514
Permax® see Pergolide 1213
Permethrin 1218
Perphenazine 1218
Perphenazine and Amitriptyline
  Hydrochloride see Amitriptyline
  and Perphenazine 97
Persantine® see Dipyridamole 489
Pestarin® (Mex) see Rifampin 1346
Pethidine Hydrochloride see
  Meperidine 983
Petroselinum crispum see Parsley
  1630
Pevaryl Lipogel® (Mex) see
  Econazole 526
Pexeva® see Paroxetine 1188
Pexicam® (Can) see Piroxicam . . 1248
PFA see Foscarnet 703
Pfizerpen® see Penicillin G
  (Parenteral/Aqueous) 1203
Pfizerpen-AS® (Can) see Penicillin
  G Procaine 1204
PGE₁ see Alprostadil 76
PGE₂ see Dinoprostone 482
PGI₂ see Epoprostenol 553
PGX see Epoprostenol 553
Phanasin® Diabetic Choice [OTC]
  see Guaifenesin 752
Phanasin® [OTC] see Guaifenesin . . 752
Phanatuss® DM [OTC] see
  Guaifenesin and
  Dextromethorphan 754
Pharmaflur® see Fluoride 671
Pharmaflur® 1.1 see Fluoride 671
Pharmorubicin® (Can) see
  Epirubicin 550
Phazyme™ (Can) see Simethicone
  1394
Phazyme® Quick Dissolve [OTC]
  see Simethicone 1394
Phazyme® Ultra Strength [OTC]
  see Simethicone 1394
Phenabid DM® see
  Chlorpheniramine,
  Phenylephrine, and
  Dextromethorphan 326
Phenadoz™ see Promethazine 1290
Phenaseptic [OTC] see Phenol 1223
PhenaVent™ see Guaifenesin and
  Phenylephrine 754
PhenaVent™ D see Guaifenesin
  and Phenylephrine 754
PhenaVent™ Ped see Guaifenesin
  and Phenylephrine 754
Phenazo™ (Can) see
  Phenazopyridine 1220
Phenazopyridine 1220
Phenazopyridine Hydrochloride see
  Phenazopyridine 1220
Phendimetrazine 1220
Phendimetrazine Tartrate see
  Phendimetrazine 1220
Phenelzine 1221
Phenelzine Sulfate see Phenelzine
  1221
Phenergan® see Promethazine . . . 1290
Phenindamine 1221
Phenindamine Tartrate see
  Phenindamine 1221

Pheniramine and Naphazoline see
Naphazoline and Pheniramine
.... 1088
Phenobarbital 1221
Phenobarbital, Belladonna, and
Ergotamine Tartrate see
Belladonna, Phenobarbital, and
Ergotamine 185
Phenobarbital, Hyoscyamine,
Atropine, and Scopolamine see
Hyoscyamine, Atropine,
Scopolamine, and
Phenobarbital 804
Phenobarbital Sodium see
Phenobarbital 1221
Phenobarbitone see Phenobarbital
.... 1221
Phenol 1223
Phenol and Camphor see
Camphor and Phenol 252
Phenol EZ® [OTC] see Phenol 1223
Phenoxybenzamine 1224
Phenoxybenzamine Hydrochloride
see Phenoxybenzamine 1224
Phenoxymethyl Penicillin see
Penicillin V Potassium 1205
Phentermine 1224
Phentermine Hydrochloride see
Phentermine 1224
Phentolamine 1226
Phentolamine Mesylate see
Phentolamine 1226
Phenylalanine Mustard see
Melphalan 979
Phenylazo Diamino Pyridine
Hydrochloride see
Phenazopyridine 1220
Phenylephrine 1226
Phenylephrine and
Chlorpheniramine see
Chlorpheniramine and
Phenylephrine 324
Phenylephrine and Cyclopentolate
see Cyclopentolate and
Phenylephrine 403
Phenylephrine and Promethazine
see Promethazine and
Phenylephrine 1292
Phenylephrine and Scopolamine .. 1227
Phenylephrine and Zinc Sulfate ... 1228
Phenylephrine, Chlorpheniramine,
and Dextromethorphan see
Chlorpheniramine,
Phenylephrine, and
Dextromethorphan 326
Phenylephrine, Chlorpheniramine,
and Dihydrocodeine see
Dihydrocodeine,
Chlorpheniramine, and
Phenylephrine 476
Phenylephrine, Chlorpheniramine,
and Methscopolamine see
Chlorpheniramine,
Phenylephrine, and
Methscopolamine 327
Phenylephrine, Chlorpheniramine,
and Phenyltoloxamine see
Chlorpheniramine,
Phenylephrine, and
Phenyltoloxamine 328
Phenylephrine, Chlorpheniramine,
Codeine, and Potassium Iodide
see Chlorpheniramine,
Phenylephrine, Codeine, and
Potassium Iodide 328
Phenylephrine, Diphenhydramine,
and Hydrocodone see
Hydrocodone, Phenylephrine,
and Diphenhydramine 791

Phenylephrine, Ephedrine,
Chlorpheniramine, and
Carbetapentane see
Chlorpheniramine, Ephedrine,
Phenylephrine, and
Carbetapentane 325
Phenylephrine, Guaifenesin, and
Hydrocodone see
Hydrocodone, Phenylephrine,
and Guaifenesin 791
Phenylephrine Hydrochloride see
Phenylephrine 1226
Phenylephrine Hydrochloride and
Guaifenesin see Guaifenesin
and Phenylephrine 754
Phenylephrine Hydrochloride,
Guaifenesin, and
Dextromethorphan
Hydrobromide see
Guaifenesin,
Dextromethorphan, and
Phenylephrine 756
Phenylephrine, Hydrocodone,
Chlorpheniramine,
Acetaminophen, and Caffeine
see Hydrocodone,
Chlorpheniramine,
Phenylephrine,
Acetaminophen, and Caffeine .. 790
Phenylephrine, Promethazine, and
Codeine see Promethazine,
Phenylephrine, and Codeine .. 1293
Phenylephrine Tannate see
Phenylephrine 1226
Phenylephrine Tannate,
Carbetapentane Tannate, and
Pyrilamine Tannate see
Carbetapentane,
Phenylephrine, and Pyrilamine .. 267
Phenylethylmalonylurea see
Phenobarbital 1221
Phenylgesic® [OTC] see
Acetaminophen and
Phenyltoloxamine 38
Phenylisohydantoin see Pemoline
.... 1199
Phenyl Salicylate, Methenamine,
Methylene Blue, Sodium
Biphosphate, and
Hyoscyamine see
Methenamine, Sodium
Biphosphate, Phenyl Salicylate,
Methylene Blue, and
Hyoscyamine 1008
Phenyltoloxamine and
Acetaminophen see
Acetaminophen and
Phenyltoloxamine 38
Phenyltoloxamine,
Chlorpheniramine, and
Phenylephrine see
Chlorpheniramine,
Phenylephrine, and
Phenyltoloxamine 328
Phenytek™ see Phenytoin 1228
Phenytoin 1228
Phenytoin Sodium see Phenytoin .. 1228
Phenytoin Sodium, Extended see
Phenytoin 1228
Phenytoin Sodium, Prompt see
Phenytoin 1228
Phillips'® M-O [OTC] see
Magnesium Hydroxide and
Mineral Oil 961
Phillips'® Fibercaps [OTC] see
Polycarbophil 1252
Phillips'® Milk of Magnesia [OTC]
see Magnesium Hydroxide 961
Phillips'® Stool Softener Laxative
[OTC] see Docusate 496
pHisoHex® see Hexachlorophene .. 771

PHL-Citalopram (Can) see
   Citalopram 351
Phos-Flur® see Fluoride 671
Phos-Flur® Rinse [OTC] see
   Fluoride 671
PhosLo® see Calcium Acetate 248
Phos-NaK see Potassium
   Phosphate and Sodium
   Phosphate 1261
Phospha 250™ Neutral see
   Potassium Phosphate and
   Sodium Phosphate 1261
Phosphate, Potassium see
   Potassium Phosphate 1261
Phospholine Iodide® see
   Echothiophate Iodide 526
Phosphonoformate see Foscarnet . . 703
Phosphonoformic Acid see
   Foscarnet 703
Phosphorated Carbohydrate
   Solution see Fructose,
   Dextrose, and Phosphoric Acid
   713
Phosphoric Acid, Levulose and
   Dextrose see Fructose,
   Dextrose, and Phosphoric Acid
   713
Photofrin® see Porfimer 1256
Phoxal-timolol (Can) see Timolol . . 1489
Phrenilin® With Caffeine and
   Codeine see Butalbital, Aspirin,
   Caffeine, and Codeine 241
p-Hydroxyampicillin see Amoxicillin
   106
Phyllocontin® (Can) see
   Aminophylline 89
Phyllocontin®-350 (Can) see
   Aminophylline 89
Phylloquinone see Phytonadione . . 1233
Physostigmine 1232
Physostigmine Salicylate see
   Physostigmine 1232
Physostigmine Sulfate see
   Physostigmine 1232
Phytomenadione see Phytonadione
   1233
Phytonadione 1233
α₁-PI see Alpha₁-Proteinase
   Inhibitor 73
Pidorubicin see Epirubicin 550
Pidorubicin Hydrochloride see
   Epirubicin 550
Pilocar® see Pilocarpine
   (Ophthalmic) 1234
Pilocarpine Hydrochloride see
   Pilocarpine (Ophthalmic) 1234
Pilocarpine Nitrate see Pilocarpine
   (Ophthalmic) 1234
Pilocarpine (Ophthalmic) 1234
Pilocarpine (Oral) 1235
Pilopine HS® see Pilocarpine
   (Ophthalmic) 1234
Piloptic® see Pilocarpine
   (Ophthalmic) 1234
Pima® see Potassium Iodide 1260
Pimaricin see Natamycin 1093
Pimecrolimus 1237
Pimozide 1238
Pin-X® [OTC] see Pyrantel
   Pamoate 1314
Pindolol 1240
Pink Bismuth see Bismuth 210
PIO see Pemoline 1199
Pioglitazone 1241
Pioglitazone and Metformin 1242
Piperacillin 1244
Piperacillin and Tazobactam
   Sodium 1245
Piperacillin Sodium see Piperacillin
   1244

Piperacillin Sodium and
   Tazobactam Sodium see
   Piperacillin and Tazobactam
   Sodium 1245
Piperazine 1246
Piperazine Citrate see Piperazine
   1246
Piperazine Estrone Sulfate see
   Estropipate 586
Piper methysticum see Kava 1627
Piperonyl Butoxide and Pyrethrins
   see Pyrethrins and Piperonyl
   Butoxide 1315
Piportil® L₄ (Can) see Pipotiazine . . 1246
Piportil L4® (Mex) see
   Pipotiazine 1246
Pipotiazine 1246
Pipotiazine Palmitate see
   Pipotiazine 1246
Pirbuterol 1248
Pirbuterol Acetate see Pirbuterol . . 1248
Piroxicam 1248
p-Isobutylhydratropic Acid see
   Ibuprofen 808
Pistacia lentiscus see Mastic 1628
Pit see Oxytocin 1175
Pitocin® see Oxytocin 1175
Pitressin® see Vasopressin 1567
Pitrex (Can) see Tolnaftate 1506
Pix Carbonis see Coal Tar 383
PLA see Poly-L-Lactic Acid 1253
Plan B® see Levonorgestrel 916
Plantago Seed see Psyllium 1313
Plantain Seed see Psyllium 1313
Plaquenil® see Hydroxychloroquine
   799
Plaretase® 8000 see Pancrelipase
   1183
Plasil® (Mex) see Metoclopramide
   1029
Platinol® (Mex) see Cisplatin 350
Platinol®-AQ [DSC] see Cisplatin . . 350
Plavix® see Clopidogrel 376
Plegine® (Can) see
   Phendimetrazine 1220
Plenaxis™ [DSC] see Abarelix 24
Plendil® see Felodipine 638
Pletal® see Cilostazol 340
PMPA see Tenofovir 1457
PMS-Amantadine (Can) see
   Amantadine 81
PMS-Amitriptyline (Can) see
   Amitriptyline 93
PMS-Amoxicillin (Can) see
   Amoxicillin 106
PMS-Anagrelide (Can) see
   Anagrelide 124
PMS-Atenolol (Can) see Atenolol . . 154
PMS-Azithromycin (Can) see
   Azithromycin 171
PMS-Baclofen (Can) see Baclofen . . 178
PMS-Benzydamine (Can) see
   Benzydamine 197
PMS-Bethanechol (Can) see
   Bethanechol 204
PMS-Bicalutamide (Can) see
   Bicalutamide 207
PMS-Brimonidine Tartrate (Can)
   see Brimonidine 220
PMS-Bromocriptine (Can) see
   Bromocriptine 222
PMS-Buspirone (Can) see
   BusPIRone 236
PMS-Butorphanol (Can) see
   Butorphanol 243
PMS-Captopril (Can) see Captopril
   257
PMS-Carbamazepine (Can) see
   Carbamazepine 260
PMS-Carvedilol (Can) see
   Carvedilol 275

PMS-Cefaclor (Can) *see* Cefaclor . . 279
PMS-Chloral Hydrate (Can) *see*
 Chloral Hydrate 312
PMS-Cholestyramine (Can) *see*
 Cholestyramine Resin 334
PMS-Cimetidine (Can) *see*
 Cimetidine 341
PMS-Ciprofloxacin (Can) *see*
 Ciprofloxacin 343
PMS-Citalopram (Can) *see*
 Citalopram 351
PMS-Clobazam (Can) *see*
 Clobazam 364
PMS-Clonazepam (Can) *see*
 Clonazepam 371
PMS-Deferoxamine (Can) *see*
 Deferoxamine 428
PMS-Desipramine (Can) *see*
 Desipramine 434
PMS-Desonide (Can) *see*
 Desonide 437
PMS-Dexamethasone (Can) *see*
 Dexamethasone 439
PMS-Dicitrate (Can) *see* Sodium
 Citrate and Citric Acid 1401
PMS-Diclofenac (Can) *see*
 Diclofenac 459
PMS-Diclofenac SR (Can) *see*
 Diclofenac 459
PMS-Diphenhydramine (Can) *see*
 DiphenhydrAMINE 483
PMS-Dipivefrin (Can) *see*
 Dipivefrin 489
PMS-Docusate Calcium (Can) *see*
 Docusate 496
PMS-Docusate Sodium (Can) *see*
 Docusate 496
PMS-Erythromycin (Can) *see*
 Erythromycin 562
PMS-Fenofibrate Micro (Can) *see*
 Fenofibrate 639
PMS-Fluorometholone (Can) *see*
 Fluorometholone 674
PMS-Fluoxetine (Can) *see*
 Fluoxetine 675
PMS-Fluphenazine Decanoate
 (Can) *see* Fluphenazine 680
PMS-Fluvoxamine (Can) *see*
 Fluvoxamine 694
PMS-Gabapentin (Can) *see*
 Gabapentin 717
PMS-Gemfibrozil (Can) *see*
 Gemfibrozil 730
PMS-Glyburide (Can) *see*
 GlyBURIDE 744
PMS-Haloperidol LA (Can) *see*
 Haloperidol 762
PMS-Hydrochlorothiazide (Can)
 see Hydrochlorothiazide 776
PMS-Hydromorphone (Can) *see*
 Hydromorphone 797
PMS-Hydroxyzine (Can) *see*
 HydrOXYzine 801
PMS-Indapamide (Can) *see*
 Indapamide 828
PMS-Ipratropium (Can) *see*
 Ipratropium 857
PMS-Isoniazid (Can) *see* Isoniazid . . 864
PMS-Isosorbide (Can) *see*
 Isosorbide Dinitrate 866
PMS-Lactulose (Can) *see*
 Lactulose 893
PMS-Lamotrigine (Can) *see*
 Lamotrigine 895
PMS-Levobunolol (Can) *see*
 Levobunolol 909
PMS-Lindane (Can) *see* Lindane . . . 933
PMS-Lithium Carbonate (Can) *see*
 Lithium 939
PMS-Lithium Citrate (Can) *see*
 Lithium 939

PMS-Loperamide (Can) *see*
 Loperamide 942
PMS-Lorazepam (Can) *see*
 Lorazepam 947
PMS-Lovastatin (Can) *see*
 Lovastatin 953
PMS-Loxapine (Can) *see* Loxapine
 955
PMS-Mefenamic Acid (Can) *see*
 Mefenamic Acid 973
PMS-Meloxicam (Can) *see*
 Meloxicam 977
PMS-Metformin (Can) *see*
 Metformin 1001
PMS-Methylphenidate (Can) *see*
 Methylphenidate 1023
PMS-Metoprolol (Can) *see*
 Metoprolol 1030
PMS-Minocycline (Can) *see*
 Minocycline 1049
PMS-Mirtazapine (Can) *see*
 Mirtazapine 1052
PMS-Morphine Sulfate SR (Can)
 see Morphine Sulfate 1065
PMS-Nizatidine (Can) *see*
 Nizatidine 1123
PMS-Norfloxacin (Can) *see*
 Norfloxacin 1126
PMS-Nortriptyline (Can) *see*
 Nortriptyline 1128
PMS-Nystatin (Can) *see* Nystatin . . 1133
PMS-Ofloxacin (Can) *see*
 Ofloxacin 1137
PMS-Oxazepam (Can) *see*
 Oxazepam 1157
PMS-Oxybutynin (Can) *see*
 Oxybutynin 1162
PMS-Oxycodone-Acetaminophen
 (Can) *see* Oxycodone and
 Acetaminophen 1165
PMS-Paroxetine (Can) *see*
 Paroxetine 1188
PMS-Phenobarbital (Can) *see*
 Phenobarbital 1221
PMS-Pindolol (Can) *see* Pindolol . . 1240
PMS-Polytrimethoprim (Can) *see*
 Trimethoprim and Polymyxin B
 1539
PMS-Pravastatin (Can) *see*
 Pravastatin 1265
PMS-Procyclidine (Can) *see*
 Procyclidine 1288
PMS-Pseudoephedrine (Can) *see*
 Pseudoephedrine 1309
PMS-Ranitidine (Can) *see*
 Ranitidine 1334
PMS-Salbutamol (Can) *see*
 Albuterol 58
PMS-Sertraline (Can) *see*
 Sertraline 1385
PMS-Simvastatin (Can) *see*
 Simvastatin 1394
PMS-Sotalol (Can) *see* Sotalol 1409
PMS-Sucralate (Can) *see*
 Sucralfate 1420
PMS-Sumatriptan (Can) *see*
 Sumatriptan 1432
PMS-Temazepam (Can) *see*
 Temazepam 1453
PMS-Terazosin (Can) *see*
 Terazosin 1458
PMS-Terbinafine (Can) *see*
 Terbinafine 1459
PMS-Theophylline (Can) *see*
 Theophylline 1473
PMS-Timolol (Can) *see* Timolol . . . 1489
PMS-Tobramycin (Can) *see*
 Tobramycin 1498
PMS-Topiramate (Can) *see*
 Topiramate 1508

PMS-Trazodone (Can) see
Trazodone 1521
PMS-Trifluoperazine (Can) see
Trifluoperazine 1535
PMS-Valproic Acid (Can) see
Valproic Acid and Derivatives
. . . . 1556
PMS-Valproic Acid E.C. (Can) see
Valproic Acid and Derivatives
. . . . 1556
PMS-Yohimbine (Can) see
Yohimbine 1589
PMS-Zopiclone (Can) see
Zopiclone 1606
Pneumococcal 7-Valent Conjugate
Vaccine see Pneumococcal
Conjugate Vaccine (7-Valent)
. . . . 1250
Pneumococcal Conjugate Vaccine
(7-Valent) 1250
Pneumotussin® see Hydrocodone
and Guaifenesin 785
PNU-140690E see Tipranavir 1495
Podactin Cream [OTC] see
Miconazole 1039
Podactin Powder [OTC] see
Tolnaftate 1506
Podocon-25® see Podophyllum
Resin 1251
Podofilm® (Can) see Podophyllum
Resin 1251
Podofilox 1251
Podophyllin see Podophyllum
Resin 1251
Podophyllum Resin 1251
Poliovirus Vaccine (Inactivated) . . . 1252
Polocaine® see Mepivacaine 987
Polocaine® 2% and Levonordefrin
1:20,000 (Can) see
Mepivacaine and Levonordefrin
. . . . 991
Polocaine® Dental see
Mepivacaine 987
Polocaine® MPF see Mepivacaine . . 987
Poly-L-Lactic Acid 1253
Polycarbophil 1252
Polycitra® see Citric Acid, Sodium
Citrate, and Potassium Citrate . . 354
Polycitra®-K see Potassium Citrate
and Citric Acid 1259
Polycitra®-LC see Citric Acid,
Sodium Citrate, and Potassium
Citrate 354
Polycose® [OTC] see Glucose
Polymers 743
Poly-Dex™ see Neomycin,
Polymyxin B, and
Dexamethasone 1101
Polyethylene Glycol 3350 1253
Polyethylene Glycol-Electrolyte
Solution 1253
Polygam® S/D see Immune
Globulin (Intravenous) 824
Polymyxin B 1253
Polymyxin B and Bacitracin see
Bacitracin and Polymyxin B 176
Polymyxin B and Neomycin see
Neomycin and Polymyxin B . . . 1100
Polymyxin B and Trimethoprim see
Trimethoprim and Polymyxin B
. . . . 1539
Polymyxin B, Bacitracin, and
Neomycin see Bacitracin,
Neomycin, and Polymyxin B . . . 176
Polymyxin B, Bacitracin, Neomycin,
and Hydrocortisone see
Bacitracin, Neomycin,
Polymyxin B, and
Hydrocortisone 177

Polymyxin B, Neomycin, and
Dexamethasone see
Neomycin, Polymyxin B, and
Dexamethasone 1101
Polymyxin B, Neomycin, and
Gramicidin see Neomycin,
Polymyxin B, and Gramicidin . . 1101
Polymyxin B, Neomycin, and
Hydrocortisone see Neomycin,
Polymyxin B, and
Hydrocortisone 1101
Polymyxin B, Neomycin, and
Prednisolone see Neomycin,
Polymyxin B, and Prednisolone
. . . . 1102
Polymyxin B, Neomycin, Bacitracin,
and Pramoxine see Bacitracin,
Neomycin, Polymyxin B, and
Pramoxine 177
Polymyxin B Sulfate see Polymyxin
B 1253
Poly-Pred® see Neomycin,
Polymyxin B, and Prednisolone
. . . . 1102
Poly-Rx see Polymyxin B 1253
Polysaccharide-Iron Complex 1254
Polysporin® Ophthalmic see
Bacitracin and Polymyxin B 176
Polysporin® Topical [OTC] see
Bacitracin and Polymyxin B 176
Polytar® [OTC] see Coal Tar 383
Polythiazide 1255
Polythiazide and Prazosin see
Prazosin and Polythiazide . . . 1268
Polytrim® see Trimethoprim and
Polymyxin B 1539
Polyvinyl Alcohol see Artificial
Tears 143
Polyvinylpyrrolidone with Iodine
see Povidone-Iodine 1262
Ponstel® see Mefenamic Acid . . . 973
Pontocaine® see Tetracaine 1466
Pontocaine® Niphanoid® see
Tetracaine 1466
Pontocaine® With Dextrose see
Tetracaine and Dextrose 1467
Poor Mans Treacle see Garlic 1622
Poractant Alfa 1255
Porfimer 1256
Porfimer Sodium see Porfimer 1256
Portia™ see Ethinyl Estradiol and
Levonorgestrel 602
Post Peel Healing Balm [OTC] see
Hydrocortisone 793
Posture® [OTC] see Calcium
Phosphate (Tribasic) 251
Potaba® see Potassium
P-Aminobenzoate 1261
Potassium Acetate 1257
Potassium Acetate, Potassium
Bicarbonate, and Potassium
Citrate 1257
Potassium Acetate, Potassium
Citrate, and Potassium
Bicarbonate see Potassium
Acetate, Potassium
Bicarbonate, and Potassium
Citrate 1257
Potassium Acid Phosphate 1257
Potassium Bicarbonate 1257
Potassium Bicarbonate and
Potassium Chloride 1258
Potassium Bicarbonate and
Potassium Chloride
(Effervescent) see Potassium
Bicarbonate and Potassium
Chloride 1258
Potassium Bicarbonate and
Potassium Citrate 1258

Potassium Bicarbonate and Potassium Citrate (Effervescent) see Potassium Bicarbonate and Potassium Citrate 1258

Potassium Bicarbonate, Potassium Acetate, and Potassium Citrate see Potassium Acetate, Potassium Bicarbonate, and Potassium Citrate 1257

Potassium Bicarbonate, Potassium Citrate, and Potassium Acetate see Potassium Acetate, Potassium Bicarbonate, and Potassium Citrate 1257

Potassium Chloride 1258
Potassium Citrate 1259
Potassium Citrate and Citric Acid . . 1259
Potassium Citrate, Citric Acid, and Sodium Citrate see Citric Acid, Sodium Citrate, and Potassium Citrate 354

Potassium Citrate, Potassium Acetate, and Potassium Bicarbonate see Potassium Acetate, Potassium Bicarbonate, and Potassium Citrate 1257

Potassium Citrate, Potassium Bicarbonate, and Potassium Acetate see Potassium Acetate, Potassium Bicarbonate, and Potassium Citrate 1257

Potassium Gluconate 1259
Potassium Guaiacolsulfonate and Guaifenesin see Guaifenesin and Potassium Guaiacolsulfonate 755

Potassium Iodide 1260
Potassium Iodide and Iodine 1260
Potassium Iodide, Chlorpheniramine, Phenylephrine, and Codeine see Chlorpheniramine, Phenylephrine, Codeine, and Potassium Iodide 328

Potassium P-Aminobenzoate 1261
Potassium Perchlorate 1261
Potassium Phosphate 1261
Potassium Phosphate and Sodium Phosphate 1261

Povidine™ [OTC] see Povidone-Iodine 1262

Povidone-Iodine 1262
PPD see Tuberculin Tests 1548
PPI-149 see Abarelix 24
PPL see Benzylpenicilloyl-polylysine . . . 198

PPS see Pentosan Polysulfate Sodium 1211

Pramidal® (Mex) see Loperamide . . . 942
Pramipexole 1262
Pramlintide 1263
Pramlintide Acetate see Pramlintide 1263

Pramosone® see Pramoxine and Hydrocortisone 1264

Pramox® HC (Can) see Pramoxine and Hydrocortisone 1264

Pramoxine 1264
Pramoxine and Hydrocortisone . . . 1264
Pramoxine Hydrochloride see Pramoxine 1264

Pramoxine, Neomycin, Bacitracin, and Polymyxin B see Bacitracin, Neomycin, Polymyxin B, and Pramoxine . . . 177

Prandase® (Can) see Acarbose 28
Prandin® see Repaglinide 1339
Pravachol® see Pravastatin 1265

Pravacol® (Mex) see Pravastatin . . 1265
Pravastatin 1265
Pravastatin and Aspirin see Aspirin and Pravastatin 151

Pravastatin Sodium see Pravastatin 1265

Pravigard™ PAC [DSC] see Aspirin and Pravastatin 151

Prax® [OTC] see Pramoxine 1264
Prazidec® (Mex) see Omeprazole 1145

Praziquantel 1266
Prazolit® (Mex) see Omeprazole . . . 1145
Prazosin 1267
Prazosin and Polythiazide 1268
Prazosin Hydrochloride see Prazosin 1267

Precedex™ see Dexmedetomidine . . 444
Precose® see Acarbose 28
Pred Forte® see PrednisoLONE . . . 1268
Pred-G® see Prednisolone and Gentamicin 1271

Pred Mild® see PrednisoLONE 1268
Prednicarbate 1268
Prednidib® (Mex) see PredniSONE 1271

PrednisoLONE 1268
Prednisolone Acetate see PrednisoLONE 1268

Prednisolone Acetate, Ophthalmic see PrednisoLONE 1268

Prednisolone and Gentamicin 1271
Prednisolone and Sulfacetamide see Sulfacetamide and Prednisolone 1424

Prednisolone, Neomycin, and Polymyxin B see Neomycin, Polymyxin B, and Prednisolone 1102

Prednisolone Sodium Phosphate see PrednisoLONE 1268

Prednisolone Sodium Phosphate, Ophthalmic see PrednisoLONE 1268

PredniSONE 1271
Prednisone Intensol™ see PredniSONE 1271

Prefest™ see Estradiol and Norgestimate 576

Pregabalin 1274
Pregnenedione see Progesterone 1289

Pregnyl® see Chorionic Gonadotropin (Human) 336

Prelone® see PrednisoLONE 1268
Prelu-2® [DSC] see Phendimetrazine 1220

Premarin® see Estrogens (Conjugated/Equine) 580

Premjact® [OTC] see Lidocaine 920
Premphase® see Estrogens (Conjugated/Equine) and Medroxyprogesterone 583

Premplus® (Can) see Estrogens (Conjugated/Equine) and Medroxyprogesterone 583

Prempro™ see Estrogens (Conjugated/Equine) and Medroxyprogesterone 583

Preparation H® Hydrocortisone [OTC] see Hydrocortisone 793

Prepcat see Barium 179
Pre-Pen® [DSC] see Benzylpenicilloyl-polylysine . . . 198

Prepidil® see Dinoprostone 482
Prepulsid® (Mex) see Cisapride 348
Preservative-Free Cosopt® (Can) see Dorzolamide and Timolol . . . 501

PreserVision® AREDS [OTC] see Vitamins (Multiple/Oral) 1582

PreserVision® Lutein [OTC] see
  Vitamins (Multiple/Oral) 1582
Pressyn® (Can) see Vasopressin . . 1567
Pressyn® AR (Can) see
  Vasopressin 1567
Pretz-D® [OTC] see Ephedrine 545
Pretz® [OTC] see Sodium Chloride
  1400
Prevacid® see Lansoprazole 896
Prevacid® NapraPAC™ see
  Lansoprazole and Naproxen . . . 898
Prevacid® SoluTab™ see
  Lansoprazole 896
Prevalite® see Cholestyramine
  Resin 334
PREVEN® see Ethinyl Estradiol
  and Levonorgestrel 602
Prevex® B (Can) see
  Betamethasone 199
Prevex® HC (Can) see
  Hydrocortisone 793
PreviDent® see Fluoride 671
PreviDent® 5000 Plus™ see
  Fluoride 671
Previfem™ see Ethinyl Estradiol
  and Norgestimate 613
Prevnar® see Pneumococcal
  Conjugate Vaccine (7-Valent)
  1250
Prevpac® see Lansoprazole,
  Amoxicillin, and Clarithromycin . . 898
Prialt® see Ziconotide 1594
Priftin® see Rifapentine 1349
Prilocaine 1277
Prilocaine and Epinephrine 1278
Prilocaine and Lidocaine see
  Lidocaine and Prilocaine 928
Prilosec® see Omeprazole 1145
Prilosec OTC™ [OTC] see
  Omeprazole 1145
Primaclone see Primidone 1281
Primacor® see Milrinone 1048
Primaquine 1281
Primaquine Phosphate see
  Primaquine 1281
Primatene® Mist [OTC] see
  Epinephrine 546
Primaxin® see Imipenem and
  Cilastatin 819
Primidone 1281
Primogyn® (Mex) see Estradiol 574
Primoteston Depot® (Mex) see
  Testosterone 1462
Primsol® see Trimethoprim 1538
Principen® see Ampicillin 117
Princol® (Mex) see Lincomycin 932
Prinivil® see Lisinopril 936
Prinzide® see Lisinopril and
  Hydrochlorothiazide 938
Priorix™ (Can) see Measles,
  Mumps, and Rubella Vaccines
  (Combined) 966
Priscoline® [DSC] see Tolazoline . . 1501
Pristinamycin see Quinupristin and
  Dalfopristin 1326
Privine® [OTC] see Naphazoline . . . 1087
ProAmatine® see Midodrine 1044
Probenecid 1282
Probenecid and Colchicine see
  Colchicine and Probenecid 388
Procainamide 1283
Procainamide Hydrochloride see
  Procainamide 1283
Procaine 1284
Procaine Amide Hydrochloride see
  Procainamide 1283
Procaine Benzylpenicillin see
  Penicillin G Procaine 1204
Procaine Hydrochloride see
  Procaine 1284

Procaine Penicillin G see Penicillin
  G Procaine 1204
Procanbid® see Procainamide 1283
Procan® SR (Can) see
  Procainamide 1283
Procarbazine 1284
Procarbazine Hydrochloride see
  Procarbazine 1284
Procardia® see NIFEdipine 1112
Procardia XL® see NIFEdipine 1112
Procef® (Mex) see Cefprozil 291
Procephal® (Mex) see
  Erythromycin 562
Procetofene see Fenofibrate 639
Prochieve™ see Progesterone 1289
Prochlorperazine 1285
Prochlorperazine Edisylate see
  Prochlorperazine 1285
Prochlorperazine Maleate see
  Prochlorperazine 1285
Procrit® see Epoetin Alfa 552
Proctocort® see Hydrocortisone . . . 793
ProctoCream® HC see
  Hydrocortisone 793
Proctofene see Fenofibrate 639
ProctoFoam®-HC see Pramoxine
  and Hydrocortisone 1264
ProctoFoam® NS [OTC] see
  Pramoxine 1264
Procto-Kit™ see Hydrocortisone . . . 793
Procto-Pak™ see Hydrocortisone . . 793
Proctosert see Hydrocortisone 793
Proctosol-HC® see Hydrocortisone . 793
Proctozone-HC™ see
  Hydrocortisone 793
Procyclidine 1288
Procyclidine Hydrochloride see
  Procyclidine 1288
Procytox® (Can) see
  Cyclophosphamide 403
Profasi® HP (Can) see Chorionic
  Gonadotropin (Human) 336
Profen II® see Guaifenesin and
  Pseudoephedrine 755
Profen II DM® see Guaifenesin,
  Pseudoephedrine, and
  Dextromethorphan 757
Profen Forte® see Guaifenesin and
  Pseudoephedrine 755
Profen Forte™ DM see
  Guaifenesin, Pseudoephedrine,
  and Dextromethorphan 757
Profilnine® SD see Factor IX
  Complex (Human) 633
Proflavanol C™ (Can) see Ascorbic
  Acid 143
Progesterone 1289
Progestin see Progesterone 1289
Proglycem® see Diazoxide 457
Prograf® see Tacrolimus 1437
Proguanil and Atovaquone see
  Atovaquone and Proguanil 160
ProHance® see Gadoteridol 719
Proken M® (Mex) see Metoprolol . . 1030
Prolaken® (Mex) see Metoprolol . . . 1030
Prolastin® see Alpha₁-Proteinase
  Inhibitor 73
Proleukin® see Aldesleukin 61
Prolex™-D see Guaifenesin and
  Phenylephrine 754
Prolixin Decanoate® see
  Fluphenazine 680
Prolixin® [DSC] see Fluphenazine . . 680
Proloprim® see Trimethoprim 1538
Promethazine 1290
Promethazine and Codeine 1291
Promethazine and
  Dextromethorphan 1292
Promethazine and Meperidine see
  Meperidine and Promethazine . . 986
Promethazine and Phenylephrine . . 1292

Promethazine Hydrochloride *see*
Promethazine 1290
Promethazine, Phenylephrine, and
Codeine 1293
Promethegan™ *see* Promethazine
. . . . 1290
Prometrium® *see* Progesterone . . . 1289
Promit® *see* Dextran 1 447
Pronap-100® *see* Propoxyphene
and Acetaminophen 1298
Pronestyl®-SR (Can) *see*
Procainamide 1283
Pronto® Complete Lice Killing Kit
[OTC] *see* Pyrethrins and
Piperonyl Butoxide 1315
Prontofort® (Mex) *see* Tramadol . . . 1514
Pronto® Lice Control (Can) *see*
Pyrethrins and Piperonyl
Butoxide 1315
Pronto® Plus Hair and Scalp
Masque [OTC] *see* Pyrethrins
and Piperonyl Butoxide 1315
Pronto® Plus Mousse [OTC] *see*
Pyrethrins and Piperonyl
Butoxide 1315
Pronto® Plus Warm Oil Treatment
and Conditioner [OTC] *see*
Pyrethrins and Piperonyl
Butoxide 1315
Pronto® Plus with Natural Extracts
and Oils [OTC] *see* Pyrethrins
and Piperonyl Butoxide 1315
Propaderm® (Can) *see*
Beclomethasone 183
Propafenone 1293
Propafenone Hydrochloride *see*
Propafenone 1293
Propantheline 1295
Propantheline Bromide *see*
Propantheline 1295
Propa pH [OTC] *see* Salicylic Acid
. . . . 1374
Proparacaine 1296
Proparacaine and Fluorescein 1296
Proparacaine Hydrochloride *see*
Proparacaine 1296
Propecia® *see* Finasteride 655
Propeshia® (Mex) *see* Finasteride . . 655
Propess® (Mex) *see* Dinoprostone . . 482
Propine® *see* Dipivefrin 489
Proplex® T *see* Factor IX Complex
(Human) 633
Propofol 1296
Propoxyphene 1297
Propoxyphene and Acetaminophen
. . . . 1298
Propoxyphene, Aspirin, and
Caffeine 1300
Propoxyphene Hydrochloride *see*
Propoxyphene 1297
Propoxyphene Hydrochloride and
Acetaminophen *see*
Propoxyphene and
Acetaminophen 1298
Propoxyphene Hydrochloride,
Aspirin, and Caffeine *see*
Propoxyphene, Aspirin, and
Caffeine 1300
Propoxyphene Napsylate *see*
Propoxyphene 1297
Propoxyphene Napsylate and
Acetaminophen *see*
Propoxyphene and
Acetaminophen 1298
Propranolol 1301
Propranolol and
Hydrochlorothiazide 1305
Propranolol Hydrochloride *see*
Propranolol 1301

Proprinal® Cold and Sinus [OTC]
see Pseudoephedrine and
Ibuprofen 1311
Proprinal [OTC] *see* Ibuprofen 808
Propulsid® *see* Cisapride 348
Propylene Glycol Diacetate, Acetic
Acid, and Hydrocortisone *see*
Acetic Acid, Propylene Glycol
Diacetate, and Hydrocortisone . . . 45
Propylhexedrine 1305
2-Propylpentanoic Acid *see*
Valproic Acid and Derivatives
. . . . 1556
Propylthiouracil 1305
Propyl-Thyracil® (Can) *see*
Propylthiouracil 1305
2-Propylvaleric Acid *see* Valproic
Acid and Derivatives 1556
ProQuad® *see* Measles, Mumps,
Rubella, and Varicella Virus
Vaccine 967
Proquin® XR *see* Ciprofloxacin 343
Proscar® *see* Finasteride 655
ProSom® *see* Estazolam 573
Prostacyclin *see* Epoprostenol 553
Prostacyclin PGI₂ *see* Iloprost 816
Prostaglandin E₁ *see* Alprostadil 76
Prostaglandin E₂ *see* Dinoprostone
. . . . 482
Prostin E₂® *see* Dinoprostone 482
Prostin® VR (Can) *see* Alprostadil . . . 76
Prostin VR Pediatric® *see*
Alprostadil 76
Protamine Sulfate 1306
Protein C (Activated), Human,
Recombinant *see* Drotrecogin
Alfa 522
Protein-Bound Paclitaxel *see*
Paclitaxel (Protein Bound) 1177
Prothrombin Complex Concentrate
see Factor IX Complex
(Human) 633
Protirelin 1307
Protonix® *see* Pantoprazole 1184
Protopic® *see* Tacrolimus 1437
Protriptyline 1307
Protriptyline Hydrochloride *see*
Protriptyline 1307
Proventil® *see* Albuterol 58
Proventil® HFA *see* Albuterol 58
Provera® *see*
MedroxyPROGESTERone 972
Provigil® *see* Modafinil 1057
Proviodine (Can) *see*
Povidone-Iodine 1262
Provisc® *see* Hyaluronate and
Derivatives 773
Proxymetacaine *see* Proparacaine
. . . . 1296
Prozac® *see* Fluoxetine 675
Prozac® Weekly™ *see* Fluoxetine . . . 675
PRP-OMP *see* Haemophilus b
Conjugate Vaccine 534
PRP-T *see* Haemophilus b
Conjugate Vaccine 534
Prudoxin™ *see* Doxepin 505
Prussian Blue *see* Ferric
Hexacyanoferrate 650
Prymaccone *see* Primaquine 1281
PS-341 *see* Bortezomib 215
Pseudoephedrine 1309
Pseudoephedrine, Acetaminophen,
and Chlorpheniramine *see*
Acetaminophen,
Chlorpheniramine, and
Pseudoephedrine 43
Pseudoephedrine, Acetaminophen,
and Dextromethorphan *see*
Acetaminophen,
Dextromethorphan, and
Pseudoephedrine 44

Pseudoephedrine and Acetaminophen see Acetaminophen and Pseudoephedrine 38

Pseudoephedrine and Brompheniramine see Brompheniramine and Pseudoephedrine 223

Pseudoephedrine and Carbinoxamine see Carbinoxamine and Pseudoephedrine 268

Pseudoephedrine and Chlorpheniramine see Chlorpheniramine and Pseudoephedrine 325

Pseudoephedrine and Desloratadine see Desloratadine and Pseudoephedrine 436

Pseudoephedrine and Dexbrompheniramine see Dexbrompheniramine and Pseudoephedrine 442

Pseudoephedrine and Dextromethorphan 1311

Pseudoephedrine and Diphenhydramine see Diphenhydramine and Pseudoephedrine 487

Pseudoephedrine and Fexofenadine see Fexofenadine and Pseudoephedrine 653

Pseudoephedrine and Guaifenesin see Guaifenesin and Pseudoephedrine 755

Pseudoephedrine and Hydrocodone see Hydrocodone and Pseudoephedrine 788

Pseudoephedrine and Ibuprofen . . 1311

Pseudoephedrine and Loratadine see Loratadine and Pseudoephedrine 947

Pseudoephedrine and Triprolidine see Triprolidine and Pseudoephedrine 1542

Pseudoephedrine, Carbinoxamine, and Dextromethorphan see Carbinoxamine, Pseudoephedrine, and Dextromethorphan 269

Pseudoephedrine, Chlorpheniramine, and Acetaminophen see Acetaminophen, Chlorpheniramine, and Pseudoephedrine 43

Pseudoephedrine, Chlorpheniramine, and Codeine see Chlorpheniramine, Pseudoephedrine, and Codeine 329

Pseudoephedrine, Chlorpheniramine, and Dihydrocodeine see Pseudoephedrine, Dihydrocodeine, and Chlorpheniramine 1312

Pseudoephedrine, Codeine, and Triprolidine see Triprolidine, Pseudoephedrine, and Codeine 1543

Pseudoephedrine, Dextromethorphan, and Acetaminophen see Acetaminophen, Dextromethorphan, and Pseudoephedrine 44

Pseudoephedrine, Dextromethorphan, and Carbinoxamine see Carbinoxamine, Pseudoephedrine, and Dextromethorphan 269

Pseudoephedrine, Dextromethorphan, and Guaifenesin see Guaifenesin, Pseudoephedrine, and Dextromethorphan 757

Pseudoephedrine, Dihydrocodeine, and Chlorpheniramine 1312

Pseudoephedrine, Guaifenesin, and Codeine see Guaifenesin, Pseudoephedrine, and Codeine 756

Pseudoephedrine Hydrochloride see Pseudoephedrine 1309

Pseudoephedrine Hydrochloride and Acrivastine see Acrivastine and Pseudoephedrine 47

Pseudoephedrine Hydrochloride and Cetirizine Hydrochloride see Cetirizine and Pseudoephedrine 307

Pseudoephedrine Hydrochloride, Guaifenesin, and Dihydrocodeine Bitartrate see Dihydrocodeine, Pseudoephedrine, and Guaifenesin 476

Pseudoephedrine, Hydrocodone, and Carbinoxamine see Hydrocodone, Carbinoxamine, and Pseudoephedrine 789

Pseudoephedrine, Hydrocodone, and Guaifenesin see Hydrocodone, Pseudoephedrine, and Guaifenesin 792

Pseudoephedrine Sulfate see Pseudoephedrine 1309

Pseudoephedrine Tannate and Dexchlorpheniramine Tannate see Dexchlorpheniramine and Pseudoephedrine 443

Pseudoephedrine, Triprolidine, and Codeine see Triprolidine, Pseudoephedrine, and Codeine 1543

Pseudofrin (Can) see Pseudoephedrine 1309

Pseudo GG TR see Guaifenesin and Pseudoephedrine 755

Pseudomonic Acid A see Mupirocin 1073

Pseudovent™ see Guaifenesin and Pseudoephedrine 755

Pseudovent™ 400 see Guaifenesin and Pseudoephedrine 755

Pseudovent™ DM see Guaifenesin, Pseudoephedrine, and Dextromethorphan 757

Pseudovent™-Ped see Guaifenesin and Pseudoephedrine 755

P & S™ Liquid Phenol (Can) see Phenol 1223

Psorcon® (Can) see Diflorasone 468

Psorcon® e™ see Diflorasone 468

Psoriatec™ see Anthralin 128

PsoriGel® [OTC] [DSC] see Coal Tar 383

Psyllium 1313

Psyllium Hydrophilic Mucilloid see Psyllium 1313

P.T.E.-4® see Trace Metals 1513

P.T.E.-5® see Trace Metals 1513

Pteroylglutamic Acid see Folic Acid 697

PTU (error-prone abbreviation) see
  Propylthiouracil. 1305
Pulmicort® (Can) see Budesonide . . 224
Pulmicort Respules® see
  Budesonide 224
Pulmicort Turbuhaler® see
  Budesonide. 224
Pulmophylline (Can) see
  Theophylline. 1473
Pulmozyme® see Dornase Alfa . . . 501
Pulsol® (Mex) see Enalapril 538
Puralube® Tears [OTC] see
  Artificial Tears 143
Puregon® (Can) see Follitropins . . . 698
Puregon® (Mex) see
  Follitropins. 698
Purge® [OTC] see Castor Oil 279
Purified Chick Embryo Cell see
  Rabies Virus Vaccine 1329
Purinethol® see Mercaptopurine . . . 995
Purple Coneflower see Echinacea
  1620
PVP-I see Povidone-Iodine 1262
Pyrantel Pamoate. 1314
Pyrazinamide 1314
Pyrazinamide, Rifampin, and
  Isoniazid see Rifampin,
  Isoniazid, and Pyrazinamide . . 1348
Pyrazinoic Acid Amide see
  Pyrazinamide. 1314
Pyrethrins and Piperonyl Butoxide
  1315
Pyridium® see Phenazopyridine . . . 1220
Pyridostigmine 1315
Pyridostigmine Bromide see
  Pyridostigmine 1315
Pyridoxine 1316
Pyridoxine, Folic Acid, and
  Cyanocobalamin see Folic
  Acid, Cyanocobalamin, and
  Pyridoxine 697
Pyridoxine Hydrochloride see
  Pyridoxine. 1316
Pyrilamine, Phenylephrine, and
  Carbetapentane see
  Carbetapentane,
  Phenylephrine, and Pyrilamine . . 267
Pyrimethamine 1317
Pyrimethamine and Sulfadoxine
  see Sulfadoxine and
  Pyrimethamine 1424
Pyrinyl Plus® [OTC] see Pyrethrins
  and Piperonyl Butoxide 1315
Pyrithione Zinc 1318
Q-Bid DM see Guaifenesin and
  Dextromethorphan 754
Q-Dryl [OTC] see
  DiphenhydrAMINE 483
Q-Naftate [OTC] see Tolnaftate . . . 1506
Q-Tussin DM [OTC] see
  Guaifenesin and
  Dextromethorphan 754
Q-Tussin [OTC] see Guaifenesin . . . 752
Quaternium-18 Bentonite see
  Bentoquatam 188
Quazepam 1318
Quelicin® see Succinylcholine 1419
Quenalin [OTC] see
  DiphenhydrAMINE 483
Quercetin 1630
Questran® see Cholestyramine
  Resin 334
Questran® Light see
  Cholestyramine Resin 334
Questran® Light Sugar Free (Can)
  see Cholestyramine Resin 334
Quetiapine 1319
Quetiapine Fumarate see
  Quetiapine. 1319
Quibron® see Theophylline and
  Guaifenesin 1475

Quibron®-T see Theophylline 1473
Quibron®-T/SR see Theophylline . . 1473
Quinalbarbitone Sodium see
  Secobarbital 1381
Quinapril 1322
Quinapril and Hydrochlorothiazide
  1323
Quinapril Hydrochloride see
  Quinapril 1322
Quinaretic see Quinapril and
  Hydrochlorothiazide 1323
Quinate® (Can) see Quinidine 1324
Quinidine 1324
Quinidine Gluconate see Quinidine
  1324
Quinidine Polygalacturonate see
  Quinidine 1324
Quinidine Sulfate see Quinidine . . . 1324
Quinine. 1326
Quinine-Odan™ (Can) see Quinine
  1326
Quinine Sulfate see Quinine. 1326
Quinoflox® (Mex) see Ciprofloxacin
  343
Quinol see Hydroquinone 798
Quintabs-M [OTC] see Vitamins
  (Multiple/Oral) 1582
Quintabs [OTC] see Vitamins
  (Multiple/Oral) 1582
Quintasa® (Can) see Mesalamine . . 996
Quintex HC see Hydrocodone,
  Phenylephrine, and
  Guaifenesin 791
Quinupristin and Dalfopristin 1326
Quixin™ see Levofloxacin 913
QVAR® see Beclomethasone 183
R 14-15 see Erlotinib 560
R & C™ II (Can) see Pyrethrins
  and Piperonyl Butoxide 1315
R & C™ Shampoo/Conditioner
  (Can) see Pyrethrins and
  Piperonyl Butoxide 1315
R-3827 see Abarelix. 24
RabAvert® see Rabies Virus
  Vaccine 1329
Rabeprazole 1327
Rabies Immune Globulin (Human)
  1328
Rabies Virus Vaccine 1329
Racepinephrine see Epinephrine . . . 546
Radiogardase™ see Ferric
  Hexacyanoferrate 650
Radix see Valerian 1633
Raductil® (Mex) see Sibutramine . . 1389
rAHF see Antihemophilic Factor
  (Recombinant) 130
R-albuterol see Levalbuterol 907
Raloxifene 1329
Raloxifene Hydrochloride see
  Raloxifene 1329
Ramace® (Mex) see Ramipril 1332
Ramelteon 1331
Ramipril 1332
Ranexa™ see Ranolazine 1336
Raniclor™ see Cefaclor 279
Ranifur® (Mex) see Ranitidine
  1334
Ranifur® (Mex) see Ranitidine
  1334
Ranisen® (Mex) see Ranitidine . . . 1334
Ranitidine 1334
Ranitidine Hydrochloride see
  Ranitidine 1334
Ranolazine 1336
Rapamune® see Sirolimus 1397
Raphon [OTC] see Epinephrine . . . 546
Raptiva® see Efalizumab 529
Rasburicase 1337
Rastinon® (Mex) see
  TOLBUTamide 1502

ratio-Aclavulanate (Can) see
  Amoxicillin and Clavulanate
  Potassium 108
ratio-Acyclovir (Can) see Acyclovir ... 49
ratio-Alendronate (Can) see
  Alendronate 64
ratio-Amcinonide (Can) see
  Amcinonide 83
ratio-Azithromycin (Can) see
  Azithromycin 171
ratio-Benzydamine (Can) see
  Benzydamine 197
ratio-Bicalutamide (Can) see
  Bicalutamide 207
ratio-Brimonidine (Can) see
  Brimonidine 220
ratio-Carvedilol (Can) see
  Carvedilol 275
ratio-Cefuroxime (Can) see
  Cefuroxime 295
ratio-Ciprofloxacin (Can) see
  Ciprofloxacin 343
ratio-Citalopram (Can) see
  Citalopram 351
ratio-Clarithromycin (Can) see
  Clarithromycin 355
ratio-Clobazam (Can) see
  Clobazam 364
ratio-Cotridin (Can) see
  Triprolidine, Pseudoephedrine,
  and Codeine 1543
ratio-Diltiazem CD (Can) see
  Diltiazem 479
ratio-Emtec (Can) see
  Acetaminophen and Codeine 35
ratio-Famotidine (Can) see
  Famotidine 635
ratio-Fenofibrate MC (Can) see
  Fenofibrate 639
ratio-Fosinopril (Can) see
  Fosinopril 707
ratio-Glimepiride (Can) see
  Glimepiride 738
ratio-Glyburide (Can) see
  GlyBURIDE 744
ratio-Inspra-Sal (Can) see Albuterol
  58
ratio-Ketorolac (Can) see Ketorolac
  886
ratio-Lamotrigine (Can) see
  Lamotrigine 895
ratio-Lenoltec (Can) see
  Acetaminophen and Codeine ... 35
ratio-Lovastatin (Can) see
  Lovastatin 953
ratio-Methotrexate (Can) see
  Methotrexate 1012
ratio-Mometasone (Can) see
  Mometasone Furoate 1060
ratio-Morphine SR (Can) see
  Morphine Sulfate 1065
ratio-Paroxetine (Can) see
  Paroxetine 1188
ratio-Pentoxifylline (Can) see
  Pentoxifylline 1212
ratio-Pravastatin (Can) see
  Pravastatin 1265
ratio-Salbutamol (Can) see
  Albuterol 58
ratio-Sertraline (Can) see
  Sertraline 1385
ratio-Simvastatin (Can) see
  Simvastatin 1394
ratio-Temazepam (Can) see
  Temazepam 1453
ratio-Theo-Bronc (Can) see
  Theophylline 1473
ratio-Trazodone (Can) see
  Trazodone 1521
Raudil® (Mex) see Ranitidine 1334
Razadyne™ see Galantamine 720

Razadyne™ ER see Galantamine .. 720
Reactine™ (Can) see Cetirizine 306
Reactine® Allergy and Sinus (Can)
  see Cetirizine and
  Pseudoephedrine 307
Rea-Lo® [OTC] see Urea 1551
ReAzo [OTC] see Phenazopyridine
  1220
Rebetol® see Ribavirin 1343
Rebetron® see Interferon Alfa-2b
  and Ribavirin 847
Rebif® see Interferon Beta-1a 849
Reclipsen® see Ethinyl Estradiol
  and Desogestrel 592
Recofol® (Mex) see Propofol 1296
Recombinant α-L-Iduronidase
  (Glycosaminoglycan
  α-L-Iduronohydrolase) see
  Laronidase 900
Recombinant Hirudin see Lepirudin
  904
Recombinant Human
  Deoxyribonuclease see
  Dornase Alfa 501
Recombinant Human Follicle
  Stimulating Hormone see
  Follitropins 698
Recombinant Human Insulin-Like
  Growth Factor-1 see
  Mecasermin 968
Recombinant Human Interleukin-11
  see Oprelvekin 1149
Recombinant Human Luteinizing
  Hormone see Lutropin Alfa 958
Recombinant Human Parathyroid
  Hormone (1-34) see
  Teriparatide 1461
Recombinant Human
  Platelet-Derived Growth Factor
  B see Becaplermin 182
Recombinant Interleukin-11 see
  Oprelvekin 1149
Recombinant
  N-Acetylgalactosamine
  4-Sulfatase see Galsulfase 721
Recombinant Plasminogen
  Activator see Reteplase 1341
Recombinate™ see Antihemophilic
  Factor (Recombinant) 130
Recombivax HB® see Hepatitis B
  Vaccine 769
Rectacaine [OTC] see
  Phenylephrine 1226
Redactiv® (Mex) see Rifaximin 1350
Red Cross™ Canker Sore [OTC]
  see Benzocaine 190
Redoxon® (Mex) see Ascorbic Acid
  143
Reductil® (Mex) see Sibutramine . 1389
Red Valerian see Valerian 1633
Red Yeast Rice 1630
Reese's® Pinworm Medicine [OTC]
  see Pyrantel Pamoate 1314
ReFacto® see Antihemophilic
  Factor (Recombinant) 130
Refenesen Plus [OTC] see
  Guaifenesin and
  Pseudoephedrine 755
Refludan® see Lepirudin 904
Refresh Liquigel™ [OTC] see
  Carboxymethylcellulose 271
Refresh® [OTC] see Artificial Tears
  143
Refresh Plus® (Can) see
  Carboxymethylcellulose 271
Refresh Plus® [OTC] see Artificial
  Tears 143
Refresh Tears® (Can) see
  Carboxymethylcellulose 271
Refresh Tears® [OTC] see Artificial
  Tears 143

Regaine® (Mex) see Minoxidil 1051
Regitine® (Can) see Phentolamine
.... 1226
Regitine [DSC] see Phentolamine
.... 1226
Reglan® see Metoclopramide 1029
Regonol® see Pyridostigmine 1315
Regranex® see Becaplermin 182
Regulact® (Mex) see Lactulose 893
Regular Insulin see Insulin Regular
.... 841
Regulex® (Can) see Docusate 496
Reguloid® [OTC] see Psyllium 1313
Rejuva-A® (Can) see Tretinoin
    (Topical) 1525
Relacon-DM see Guaifenesin,
    Pseudoephedrine, and
    Dextromethorphan 757
Relafen® see Nabumetone 1077
Relefact® TRH (Can) see Protirelin
.... 1307
Relenza® see Zanamivir 1592
Relief® [OTC] see Phenylephrine .. 1226
Relisorm L® (Mex) see
    Gonadorelin 749
Relpax® see Eletriptan 533
Remeron® see Mirtazapine 1052
Remeron® RD (Can) see
    Mirtazapine 1052
Remeron SolTab® see Mirtazapine
.... 1052
Reme-T™ [OTC] see Coal Tar 383
Remicade® see Infliximab 832
Remifentanil 1338
Reminyl® (Can) see Galantamine .. 720
Reminyl® [DSC] see Galantamine .. 720
Remodulin® see Treprostinil 1523
Renacidin® see Citric Acid,
    Magnesium Carbonate, and
    Glucono-Delta-Lactone 353
Renagel® see Sevelamer 1388
Renedil® (Can) see Felodipine 638
Renese® see Polythiazide 1255
Renitec® (Mex) see Enalapril 538
Reno-30® see Diatrizoate
    Meglumine 453
Reno-60® see Diatrizoate
    Meglumine 453
RenoCal-76® see Diatrizoate
    Meglumine and Diatrizoate
    Sodium...................... 453
Reno-Dip® see Diatrizoate
    Meglumine 453
Renografin®-60 see Diatrizoate
    Meglumine and Diatrizoate
    Sodium...................... 453
Renova® see Tretinoin (Topical)... 1525
ReoPro® see Abciximab 26
Repaglinide 1339
Repan® see Butalbital,
    Acetaminophen, and Caffeine .. 239
Replace [OTC] see Vitamins
    (Multiple/Oral) 1582
Replace with Iron [OTC] see
    Vitamins (Multiple/Oral) 1582
Repliva 21/7™ see Vitamins
    (Multiple/Oral) 1582
Reprexain™ see Hydrocodone and
    Ibuprofen 787
Repronex® see Menotropins....... 982
Requip® see Ropinirole 1365
Rescon GG see Guaifenesin and
    Phenylephrine 754
Rescon-Jr see Chlorpheniramine
    and Phenylephrine 324
Rescriptor® see Delavirdine 429
Rescula® (Can) see Unoprostone
.... 1551
Reserpine 1340
Resource® GlutaSolve® [OTC] see
    Glutamine 743

Respa-DM® see Guaifenesin and
    Dextromethorphan 754
Respaire®-60 SR see Guaifenesin
    and Pseudoephedrine 755
Respaire®-120 SR see Guaifenesin
    and Pseudoephedrine 755
Restasis® see CycloSPORINE 406
Restoril® see Temazepam 1453
Restylane® see Hyaluronate and
    Derivatives 773
Resveratrol see Grape Skin 1625
Retavase® see Reteplase 1341
Reteplase 1341
Retin-A® see Tretinoin (Topical) .. 1525
Retin-A® Micro see Tretinoin
    (Topical) 1525
Retinoic Acid see Tretinoin
    (Topical) 1525
Retinova® (Can) see Tretinoin
    (Topical) 1525
Retisert™ see Fluocinolone 667
Retrovir® see Zidovudine 1594
Retrovir AZT® (Mex) see
    Zidovudine 1594
Revapol® (Mex) see Mebendazole .. 968
Revatio™ see Sildenafil 1390
Reversol® see Edrophonium 528
Revex® see Nalmefene 1084
ReVia® see Naltrexone 1086
Revitalose C-1000® (Can) see
    Ascorbic Acid 143
Revlimid® see Lenalidomide...... 903
Reyataz® see Atazanavir 152
rFSH-alpha see Follitropins 698
rFSH-beta see Follitropins 698
rFVIIa see Factor VIIa
    (Recombinant) 632
R-Gene® see Arginine 137
rGM-CSF see Sargramostim 1378
rhASB see Galsulfase 721
r-hCG see Chorionic Gonadotropin
    (Recombinant) 337
Rheomacrodex® (Mex) see
    Dextran 447
Rheumatrex® see Methotrexate ... 1012
rhFSH-alpha see Follitropins 698
rhFSH-beta see Follitropins 698
r-h α-GAL see Agalsidase Beta 55
RhIG see Rho(D) Immune Globulin
.... 1342
rhIGF-1 see Mecasermin 968
rhIGF-1/rhIGFBP-3 see
    Mecasermin 968
rhIL-11 see Oprelvekin 1149
Rhinalar® (Can) see Flunisolide .. 667
Rhinall [OTC] see Phenylephrine .. 1226
Rhinocort® (Mex) see Budesonide .. 224
Rhinocort® Aqua® see Budesonide
.... 224
Rhinocort® Turbuhaler® (Can) see
    Budesonide 224
r-hLH see Lutropin Alfa 958
Rho(D) Immune Globulin 1342
Rho(D) Immune Globulin (Human)
    see Rho(D) Immune Globulin .. 1342
Rho®-Clonazepam (Can) see
    Clonazepam 371
Rhodacine® (Can) see
    Indomethacin 830
Rhodis™ (Can) see Ketoprofen 883
Rhodis-EC™ (Can) see Ketoprofen
.... 883
Rhodis SR™ (Can) see Ketoprofen
.... 883
RhoGAM® see Rho(D) Immune
    Globulin 1342
RholGIV see Rho(D) Immune
    Globulin 1342
RholVIM see Rho(D) Immune
    Globulin 1342

Rho®-Loperamine (Can) see
    Loperamide 942
Rho®-Metformin (Can) see
    Metformin 1001
Rho®-Nitro (Can) see Nitroglycerin
    1120
Rhophylac® see Rh₀(D) Immune
    Globulin 1342
Rho®-Sotalol (Can) see Sotalol . . 1409
Rhotral (Can) see Acebutolol 28
Rhotrimine® (Can) see
    Trimipramine 1540
Rhovane® (Can) see Zopiclone . . 1606
Rhoxal-acebutolol (Can) see
    Acebutolol 28
Rhoxal-amiodarone (Can) see
    Amiodarone 90
Rhoxal-anagrelide (Can) see
    Anagrelide 124
Rhoxal-atenolol (Can) see Atenolol
    154
Rhoxal-ciprofloxacin (Can) see
    Ciprofloxacin 343
Rhoxal-citalopram (Can) see
    Citalopram 351
Rhoxal-cyclosporine (Can) see
    CycloSPORINE 406
Rhoxal-diltiazem CD (Can) see
    Diltiazem 479
Rhoxal-diltiazem SR (Can) see
    Diltiazem 479
Rhoxal-fluoxetine (Can) see
    Fluoxetine 675
Rhoxal-fluvoxamine (Can) see
    Fluvoxamine 694
Rhoxal-gliclazide (Can) see
    Gliclazide 737
Rhoxal-minocycline (Can) see
    Minocycline 1049
Rhoxal-mirtazapine (Can) see
    Mirtazapine 1052
Rhoxal-nabumetone (Can) see
    Nabumetone 1077
Rhoxal-orphendrine (Can) see
    Orphenadrine 1151
Rhoxal-paroxetine (Can) see
    Paroxetine 1188
Rhoxal-ranitidine (Can) see
    Ranitidine 1334
Rhoxal-salbutamol (Can) see
    Albuterol 58
Rhoxal-sertraline (Can) see
    Sertraline 1385
Rhoxal-ticlopidine (Can) see
    Ticlopidine 1486
Rhoxal-valproic (Can) see Valproic
    Acid and Derivatives 1556
Rhoxal-zopiclone (Can) see
    Zopiclone 1606
rhPTH(1-34) see Teriparatide 1461
rHuEPO-α see Epoetin Alfa 552
rHu-KGF see Palifermin 1178
rhuMAb-E25 see Omalizumab 1144
rhuMAb-VEGF see Bevacizumab . . 204
Ribasphere™ see Ribavirin 1343
Ribavirin 1343
Ribavirin and Interferon Alfa-2b
    Combination Pack see
    Interferon Alfa-2b and Ribavirin
    847
Ribo-100 see Riboflavin 1345
Riboflavin 1345
Rid-A-Pain Dental Drops [OTC]
    see Benzocaine 190
Ridaura® see Auranofin 166
Ridene® (Mex) see NiCARdipine . . 1107
RID® Maximum Strength [OTC]
    see Pyrethrins and Piperonyl
    Butoxide 1315
RID® Mousse (Can) see Pyrethrins
    and Piperonyl Butoxide 1315

Rid® Spray [OTC] see Permethrin
    1218
Rifabutin 1345
Rifadin® see Rifampin 1346
Rifamate® see Rifampin and
    Isoniazid 1348
Rifampicin see Rifampin 1346
Rifampin 1346
Rifampin and Isoniazid 1348
Rifampin, Isoniazid, and
    Pyrazinamide 1348
Rifapentine 1349
Rifater® see Rifampin, Isoniazid,
    and Pyrazinamide 1348
Rifaximin 1350
rIFN-A see Interferon Alfa-2a 842
rIFN beta-1a see Interferon
    Beta-1a 849
rIFN beta-1b see Interferon
    Beta-1b 850
RIG see Rabies Immune Globulin
    (Human) 1328
rIL-11 see Oprelvekin 1149
Rilutek® see Riluzole 1350
Riluzole 1350
Rimactan® (Mex) see Rifampin . . . 1346
Rimantadine 1351
Rimantadine Hydrochloride see
    Rimantadine 1351
Rimexolone 1351
Rimsalin® (Mex) see Lincomycin . . . 932
Riomet™ see Metformin 1001
Riopan Plus® Double Strength
    [OTC] [DSC] see Magaldrate
    and Simethicone 960
Riopan Plus® [OTC] [DSC] see
    Magaldrate and Simethicone . . 960
Riphenidate (Can) see
    Methylphenidate 1023
Risedronate 1352
Risedronate and Calcium 1354
Risedronate Sodium see
    Risedronate 1352
Risedronate Sodium and Calcium
    Carbonate see Risedronate
    and Calcium 1354
Risperdal® see Risperidone 1356
Risperdal® M-Tab® see
    Risperidone 1356
Risperdal® Consta™ see
    Risperidone 1356
Risperidone 1356
Ritalin® see Methylphenidate 1023
Ritalin® LA see Methylphenidate . . 1023
Ritalin-SR® see Methylphenidate . . 1023
Ritmolol® (Mex) see Metoprolol . . 1030
Ritonavir 1359
Ritonavir and Lopinavir see
    Lopinavir and Ritonavir 943
Rituxan® see Rituximab 1360
Rituximab 1360
Riva-Atenolol (Can) see Atenolol . . 154
Riva-Cloxacillin (Can) see
    Cloxacillin 380
Riva-Diclofenac (Can) see
    Diclofenac 459
Riva-Diclofenac-K (Can) see
    Diclofenac 459
Riva-Dicyclomine (Can) see
    Dicyclomine 464
Riva-Famotidine (Can) see
    Famotidine 635
Riva-Loperamine (Can) see
    Loperamide 942
Riva-Lorazepam (Can) see
    Lorazepam 947
Riva-Naproxen (Can) see
    Naproxen 1089
Rivanase AQ (Can) see
    Beclomethasone 183

Riva-Norfloxacin (Can) see
  Norfloxacin 1126
Riva-Oxazepam (Can) see
  Oxazepam 1157
Riva-Simvastatin (Can) see
  Simvastatin 1394
Rivasol (Can) see Zinc Sulfate 1598
Rivastigmine 1361
Rivastigmine Tartrate see
  Rivastigmine 1361
Riva-Zide (Can) see
  Hydrochlorothiazide and
  Triamterene 778
Riva-Zopiclone (Can) see
  Zopiclone 1606
Rivotril® (Can) see Clonazepam . . . 371
Rizatriptan 1363
rLFN-α2 see Interferon Alfa-2b 844
RMS® see Morphine Sulfate 1065
Ro 5488 see Tretinoin (Oral) 1524
Roaccutan® (Mex) see Isotretinoin . . 869
Robafen® AC see Guaifenesin and
  Codeine 753
Robafen DM [OTC] see
  Guaifenesin and
  Dextromethorphan 754
Robaxin® see Methocarbamol 1009
Robidrine® (Can) see
  Pseudoephedrine 1309
Robinul® see Glycopyrrolate 747
Robinul® Forte see Glycopyrrolate . . 747
Robitussin® (Can) see Guaifenesin
  752
Robitussin® CF [OTC] see
  Guaifenesin, Pseudoephedrine,
  and Dextromethorphan 757
Robitussin® Childrens Cough &
  Cold (Can) see
  Pseudoephedrine and
  Dextromethorphan 1311
Robitussin® Cold and Congestion
  [OTC] see Guaifenesin,
  Pseudoephedrine, and
  Dextromethorphan 757
Robitussin® Cough and Cold Infant
  [OTC] see Guaifenesin,
  Pseudoephedrine, and
  Dextromethorphan 757
Robitussin® Cough and Congestion
  [OTC] see Guaifenesin and
  Dextromethorphan 754
Robitussin® Cough & Cold® (Can)
  see Guaifenesin,
  Pseudoephedrine, and
  Dextromethorphan 757
Robitussin® CoughGels™ [OTC]
  see Dextromethorphan 451
Robitussin® DM (Can) see
  Guaifenesin and
  Dextromethorphan 754
Robitussin® DM Infant [OTC] see
  Guaifenesin and
  Dextromethorphan 754
Robitussin® DM [OTC] see
  Guaifenesin and
  Dextromethorphan 754
Robitussin® Honey Cough [OTC]
  see Dextromethorphan 451
Robitussin® Maximum Strength
  Cough & Cold [OTC] see
  Pseudoephedrine and
  Dextromethorphan 1311
Robitussin® Maximum Strength
  Cough [OTC] see
  Dextromethorphan 451
Robitussin® [OTC] see Guaifenesin
  . . . . α2 752
Robitussin® Pediatric Cough &
  Cold [OTC] see
  Pseudoephedrine and
  Dextromethorphan 1311

Robitussin® Pediatric Cough [OTC]
  see Dextromethorphan 451
Robitussin-PE® [OTC] see
  Guaifenesin and
  Pseudoephedrine 755
Robitussin® Severe Congestion
  [OTC] see Guaifenesin and
  Pseudoephedrine 755
Robitussin® Sugar Free Cough
  [OTC] see Guaifenesin and
  Dextromethorphan 754
Rocaltrol® see Calcitriol 247
Rocephin® see Ceftriaxone 294
Rofact™ (Can) see Rifampin 1346
Roferon-A® see Interferon Alfa-2a . . 842
Rogaine® (Can) see Minoxidil 1051
Rogaine® Extra Strength for Men
  [OTC] see Minoxidil 1051
Rogaine® for Men [OTC] see
  Minoxidil 1051
Rogaine® for Women [OTC] see
  Minoxidil 1051
Rogitine® (Can) see Phentolamine
  1226
Rolaids® Extra Strength [OTC] see
  Calcium Carbonate and
  Magnesium Hydroxide 249
Rolaids® [OTC] see Calcium
  Carbonate and Magnesium
  Hydroxide 249
Rolaids® Softchews [OTC] see
  Calcium Carbonate 248
Romazicon® see Flumazenil 665
Romilar® (Mex) see
  Dextromethorphan 451
Romilar® AC see Guaifenesin and
  Codeine 753
Romir® (Mex) see Captopril 257
Romycin® see Erythromycin 562
Rondec®-DM Drops [DSC] see
  Carbinoxamine,
  Pseudoephedrine, and
  Dextromethorphan 269
Rondec®-DM [reformulation] see
  Chlorpheniramine,
  Phenylephrine, and
  Dextromethorphan 326
Rondec® Drops [DSC] see
  Carbinoxamine and
  Pseudoephedrine 268
Rondec® [reformulation] see
  Chlorpheniramine and
  Phenylephrine 324
Rondec® Syrup [DSC] see
  Brompheniramine and
  Pseudoephedrine 223
Rondec® Tablets see
  Carbinoxamine and
  Pseudoephedrine 268
Rondec-TR® see Carbinoxamine
  and Pseudoephedrine 268
Ropinirole 1365
Ropinirole Hydrochloride see
  Ropinirole 1365
Ropivacaine 1366
Ropivacaine Hydrochloride see
  Ropivacaine 1366
Rosiglitazone 1367
Rosiglitazone and Glimepiride 1369
Rosiglitazone and Metformin 1369
Rosiglitazone Maleate and
  Metformin Hydrochloride see
  Rosiglitazone and Metformin . . . 1369
Rosin Rose see St John's Wort . . . 1632
Rosuvastatin 1370
Rosuvastatin Calcium see
  Rosuvastatin 1370
RotaTeq® see Rotavirus Vaccine . . 1371
Rotavirus Vaccine 1371
Rotavirus Vaccine, Pentavalent
  see Rotavirus Vaccine 1371

Rowasa® see Mesalamine 996
Roxanol™ see Morphine Sulfate. . . 1065
Roxanol 100™ see Morphine
    Sulfate. 1065
Roxanol™-T [DSC] see Morphine
    Sulfate. 1065
Roxicet™ see Oxycodone and
    Acetaminophen 1165
Roxicet™ 5/500 see Oxycodone
    and Acetaminophen 1165
Roxicodone™ see Oxycodone 1163
Roxicodone™ Intensol™ see
    Oxycodone. 1163
Roychlor® (Can) see Potassium
    Chloride. 1258
Rozerem™ see Ramelteon 1331
RP-6976 see Docetaxel 494
RP-54274 see Riluzole 1350
RP-59500 see Quinupristin and
    Dalfopristin 1326
r-PA see Reteplase 1341
rPDGF-BB see Becaplermin 182
RS-25259 see Palonosetron 1180
RS-25259-197 see Palonosetron . . 1180
R-Tanna see Chlorpheniramine
    and Phenylephrine 324
RTCA see Ribavirin 1343
RU 0211 see Lubiprostone 957
RU-486 see Mifepristone 1045
RU-23908 see Nilutamide 1115
RU-38486 see Mifepristone 1045
Rubella, Measles and Mumps
    Vaccines, Combined see
    Measles, Mumps, and Rubella
    Vaccines (Combined) 966
Rubella, Varicella, Measles, and
    Mumps Vaccine see Measles,
    Mumps, Rubella, and Varicella
    Virus Vaccine 967
Rubella Virus Vaccine (Live) 1372
Rubeola Vaccine see Measles
    Virus Vaccine (Live) 967
Rubex® see DOXOrubicin 509
Rubidomycin Hydrochloride see
    DAUNOrubicin Hydrochloride . . . 426
Rubilem® (Mex) see DAUNOrubicin
    Hydrochloride. 426
Rulox No. 1 [DSC] see Aluminum
    Hydroxide and Magnesium
    Hydroxide. 80
Rulox [OTC] see Aluminum
    Hydroxide and Magnesium
    Hydroxide. 80
Rum-K® see Potassium Chloride . . 1258
Rustic Treacle see Garlic 1622
Rynatan® see Chlorpheniramine
    and Phenylephrine 324
Rynatan® Pediatric Suspension
    see Chlorpheniramine and
    Phenylephrine 324
Rynatuss® see Chlorpheniramine,
    Ephedrine, Phenylephrine, and
    Carbetapentane 325
Rynatuss® Pediatric [DSC] see
    Chlorpheniramine, Ephedrine,
    Phenylephrine, and
    Carbetapentane 325
Rythmodan® (Can) see
    Disopyramide 491
Rythmodan®-LA (Can) see
    Disopyramide 491
Rythmol® see Propafenone 1293
Rythmol® Gen-Propafenone (Can)
    see Propafenone 1293
Rythmol® SR see Propafenone . . . 1293
Rökan see Ginkgo Biloba 1622
Rēv-Eyes™ see Dapiprazole 421
S-2® see Epinephrine (Racemic) . . 549
S2® [OTC] see Epinephrine 546
S-(+)-3-isobutylgaba see
    Pregabalin 1274

Sabal serrulata see Saw Palmetto
    1631
Sabasilis serrulatae see Saw
    Palmetto 1631
SAB-Dimenhydrinate (Can) see
    DimenhyDRINATE 481
SAB-Gentamicin (Can) see
    Gentamicin. 734
Sab-Prenase (Can) see
    PrednisoLONE 1268
Sabril® (Can) see Vigabatrin 1574
SAB-Trifluridine (Can) see
    Trifluridine 1536
Sacrosidase 1373
S-adenosylmethionine see SAMe . . 1631
Safe Tussin® [OTC] see
    Guaifenesin and
    Dextromethorphan 754
Saizen® see Somatropin 1406
Sal-Acid [OTC] see Salicylic Acid
    1374
SalAc® [OTC] see Salicylic Acid . . . 1374
Salactic® [OTC] see Salicylic Acid
    1374
Salagen® see Pilocarpine (Oral) . . . 1235
Salazopyrin® (Can) see
    Sulfasalazine 1428
Salazopyrin En-Tabs® (Can) see
    Sulfasalazine 1428
Salbu-2 (Can) see Albuterol 58
Salbu-4 (Can) see Albuterol 58
Salbulin Autohaler® (Mex) see
    Albuterol. 58
Salbutamol see Albuterol 58
Salbutamol and Ipratropium see
    Ipratropium and Albuterol 857
Salflex® (Can) see Salsalate 1376
Salicylazosulfapyridine see
    Sulfasalazine 1428
Salicylic Acid 1374
Salicylic Acid and Coal Tar see
    Coal Tar and Salicylic Acid 383
Salicylsalicylic Acid see Salsalate
    1376
SalineX® [OTC] see Sodium
    Chloride 1400
Salivart® [OTC] see Saliva
    Substitute 1374
Saliva Substitute 1374
Saliva Substitute™ [OTC] see
    Saliva Substitute 1374
Salix® [OTC] see Saliva Substitute
    1374
Salk Vaccine see Poliovirus
    Vaccine (Inactivated) 1252
Salmeterol 1375
Salmeterol and Fluticasone see
    Fluticasone and Salmeterol 690
Salmeterol Xinafoate see
    Salmeterol 1375
Salmocide® (Mex) see
    Furazolidone 714
Salofalk® (Can) see Mesalamine . . 996
Sal-Plant® [OTC] see Salicylic Acid
    1374
Salsalate 1376
Salt see Sodium Chloride 1400
Sal-Tropine™ see Atropine 161
SAMe 1631
Sanctura™ see Trospium 1546
Sandimmune® see CycloSPORINE
    406
Sandimmune® I.V. (Can) see
    CycloSPORINE 406
Sandostatin® see Octreotide 1135
Sandostatin LAR® see Octreotide
    1135
Sandoz-Acebutolol (Can) see
    Acebutolol 28
Sandoz Amiodarone (Can) see
    Amiodarone 90

Sandoz-Anagrelide (Can) *see*
  Anagrelide 124
Sandoz-Atenolol (Can) *see*
  Atenolol 154
Sandoz-Azithromycin (Can) *see*
  Azithromycin 171
Sandoz-Bicalutamide (Can) *see*
  Bicalutamide 207
Sandoz-Clonazepam (Can) *see*
  Clonazepam 371
Sandoz-Cyclosporine (Can) *see*
  CycloSPORINE 406
Sandoz-Diltiazem CD (Can) *see*
  Diltiazem 479
Sandoz-Diltiazem T (Can) *see*
  Diltiazem 479
Sandoz-Estradiol Derm 50 (Can)
  see Estradiol 574
Sandoz-Estradiol Derm 75 (Can)
  see Estradiol 574
Sandoz-Estradiol Derm 100 (Can)
  see Estradiol 574
Sandoz-Fluoxetine (Can) *see*
  Fluoxetine 675
Sandoz-Gliclazide (Can) *see*
  Gliclazide 737
Sandoz-Glimepiride (Can) *see*
  Glimepiride 738
Sandoz-Glyburide (Can) *see*
  GlyBURIDE 744
Sandoz-Lovastatin (Can) *see*
  Lovastatin 953
Sandoz-Metformin FC (Can) *see*
  Metformin 1001
Sandoz-Metoprolol (Can) *see*
  Metoprolol 1030
Sandoz-Mirtazapine (Can) *see*
  Mirtazapine 1052
Sandoz-Mirtazapine FC (Can) *see*
  Mirtazapine 1052
Sandoz-Nabumetone (Can) *see*
  Nabumetone 1077
Sandoz-Paroxetine (Can) *see*
  Paroxetine 1188
Sandoz-Pravastatin (Can) *see*
  Pravastatin 1265
Sandoz-Simvastatin (Can) *see*
  Simvastatin 1394
Sandoz-Sumatriptan (Can) *see*
  Sumatriptan 1432
Sandoz-Ticlopidine (Can) *see*
  Ticlopidine 1486
Sandoz-Topiramate (Can) *see*
  Topiramate 1508
Sandoz-Valproic (Can) *see*
  Valproic Acid and Derivatives
  1556
Sandoz-Zopiclone (Can) *see*
  Zopiclone 1606
Sani-Supp® [OTC] *see* Glycerin 747
Sans Acne® (Can) *see*
  Erythromycin 562
Santyl® *see* Collagenase 391
Saquinavir 1377
Saquinavir Mesylate *see*
  Saquinavir 1377
Sarafem® *see* Fluoxetine 675
Sargramostim 1378
Sarna® HC (Can) *see*
  Hydrocortisone 793
Sarna® Sensitive *see* Pramoxine . . 1264
Sarnol®-HC [OTC] *see*
  Hydrocortisone 793
Sassafras albidum see Sassafras
  Oil 1631
Sassafras Oil 1631
Sassafras radix see Sassafras Oil
  1631
Sassafras varifolium see Sassafras
  Oil 1631
Sassafrax see Sassafras Oil 1631

Sativex® (Can) *see*
  Tetrahydrocannabinol and
  Cannabidiol 1469
Saw Palmetto 1631
SB-265805 *see* Gemifloxacin 731
SC 33428 *see* Idarubicin 814
Scabisan® (Mex) *see* Lindane 933
SCH 13521 *see* Flutamide 686
Schisandra 1631
Schizandra chinensis see
  Schisandra 1631
SCIG *see* Immune Globulin
  (Subcutaneous) 826
S-Citalopram *see* Escitalopram 568
Scleromate® *see* Morrhuate
  Sodium 1068
Scopace™ *see* Scopolamine 1380
Scopolamine 1380
Scopolamine and Phenylephrine
  see Phenylephrine and
  Scopolamine 1227
Scopolamine Butylbromide *see*
  Scopolamine 1380
Scopolamine Hydrobromide *see*
  Scopolamine 1380
Scopolamine, Hyoscyamine,
  Atropine, and Phenobarbital
  see Hyoscyamine, Atropine,
  Scopolamine, and
  Phenobarbital 804
Scot-Tussin DM® Cough Chasers
  [OTC] *see* Dextromethorphan . . 451
Scot-Tussin® Expectorant [OTC]
  see Guaifenesin 752
Scot-Tussin® Senior [OTC] *see*
  Guaifenesin and
  Dextromethorphan 754
Sculptra™ *see* Poly-L-Lactic Acid . . 1253
Scury Root *see* Echinacea 1620
SDZ ENA 713 *see* Rivastigmine . 1361
Seasonale® *see* Ethinyl Estradiol
  and Levonorgestrel 602
Seba-Gel™ *see* Benzoyl Peroxide . . 194
Sebcur® (Can) *see* Salicylic Acid . 1374
Sebcur/T® (Can) *see* Coal Tar and
  Salicylic Acid 383
Secobarbital 1381
Secobarbital and Amobarbital *see*
  Amobarbital and Secobarbital . . 104
Secobarbital Sodium *see*
  Secobarbital 1381
Seconal® *see* Secobarbital 1381
Secotex® (Mex) *see* Tamsulosin . 1445
SecreFlo™ *see* Secretin 1381
Secretin 1381
Secretin, Human *see* Secretin 1381
Secretin, Porcine *see* Secretin 1381
Sectral® *see* Acebutolol 28
Secura® Antifungal [OTC] *see*
  Miconazole 1039
Sedalito® (Mex) *see*
  Acetaminophen 31
Sefulken® (Mex) *see* Diazoxide 457
Selax® (Can) *see* Docusate 496
Select™ 1/35 (Can) *see* Ethinyl
  Estradiol and Norethindrone 608
Selectadril® (Mex) *see* Metoprolol
  1030
Selecto® (Mex) *see* Pancreatin . . . 1183
Selectofur® (Mex) *see*
  Furosemide 715
Selegil® (Mex) *see* Metronidazole
  1033
Selegiline 1382
Selegiline Hydrochloride *see*
  Selegiline 1382
Selenicaps [OTC] *see* Selenium . . 1383
Selenimin [OTC] *see* Selenium . . . 1383
Selenium 1383
Selepen® *see* Selenium 1383
Seloken® (Mex) *see* Metoprolol . . . 1030

Selpiran-S® (Mex) see
  Scopolamine 1380
Semprex®-D see Acrivastine and
  Pseudoephedrine 47
Senexon [OTC] see Senna 1384
Senna 1384
Senna-Gen® [OTC] see Senna . . . 1384
Sennatural™ [OTC] see Senna . . . 1384
Senokot® [OTC] see Senna 1384
Sensibit® (Mex) see Loratadine . . 946
Sensipar® see Cinacalcet 342
Sensorcaine® see Bupivacaine . . . 228
Sensorcaine®-MPF see
  Bupivacaine 228
Sensorcaine®-MPF with
  Epinephrine see Bupivacaine
  and Epinephrine 228
Sensorcaine® with Epinephrine see
  Bupivacaine and Epinephrine . . 228
Septanest® N (Can) see Articaine
  and Epinephrine 139
Septanest® SP (Can) see Articaine
  and Epinephrine 139
Septocaine™ see Articaine and
  Epinephrine 139
Septra® see Sulfamethoxazole and
  Trimethoprim 1425
Septra® DS see Sulfamethoxazole
  and Trimethoprim 1425
Septra® Injection (Can) see
  Sulfamethoxazole and
  Trimethoprim 1425
Serax® see Oxazepam 1157
Serenoa repens see Saw Palmetto
  1631
Serentil® (Can) see Mesoridazine . . 997
Serentil® [DSC] see Mesoridazine . . 997
Serevent® (Can) see Salmeterol . . 1375
Serevent® Diskus® see Salmeterol
  1375
Sermorelin Acetate 1384
Serocryptin® (Mex) see
  Bromocriptine 222
Seromycin® see CycloSERINE 405
Serophene® see ClomiPHENE . . . 369
Seropram® (Mex) see Citalopram . . 351
Seroquel® see Quetiapine 1319
Serostim® see Somatropin 1406
Sertaconazole 1385
Sertaconazole Nitrate see
  Sertaconazole 1385
Sertraline 1385
Sertraline Hydrochloride see
  Sertraline 1385
Serutan® [OTC] see Psyllium 1313
Servigenta® (Mex) see Gentamicin
  734
Serviradine® (Mex) see Ranitidine
  1334
Servizol® (Mex) see Metronidazole
  1033
Serzone see Nefazodone 1096
Sevelamer 1388
Sevelamer Hydrochloride see
  Sevelamer 1388
Shark Cartilage 1632
Shur-Seal® [OTC] [DSC] see
  Nonoxynol 9 1124
Siberian Ginseng see Ginseng,
  Siberian 1623
Sibutramine 1389
Sibutramine Hydrochloride
  Monohydrate see Sibutramine
  1389
Sigafam® (Mex) see Famotidine . . . 635
Silace [OTC] see Docusate 496
Siladryl® Allergy [OTC] see
  DiphenhydrAMINE 483
Siladryl® DAS [OTC] see
  DiphenhydrAMINE 483

Silafed® [OTC] see Triprolidine and
  Pseudoephedrine 1542
Silapap® Children's [OTC] see
  Acetaminophen 31
Silapap® Infants [OTC] see
  Acetaminophen 31
Sildec see Carbinoxamine and
  Pseudoephedrine 268
Sildec-DM see Carbinoxamine,
  Pseudoephedrine, and
  Dextromethorphan 269
Sildenafil 1390
Silexin [OTC] see Guaifenesin and
  Dextromethorphan 754
Silfedrine Children's [OTC] see
  Pseudoephedrine 1309
Silphen DM [OTC] see
  Dextromethorphan 451
Silphen® [OTC] see
  DiphenhydrAMINE 483
Sil-Tex see Guaifenesin and
  Phenylephrine 754
Siltussin DAS [OTC] see
  Guaifenesin 752
Siltussin DM DAS [OTC] see
  Guaifenesin and
  Dextromethorphan 754
Siltussin DM [OTC] see
  Guaifenesin and
  Dextromethorphan 754
Siltussin SA [OTC] see
  Guaifenesin 752
Silvadene® see Silver Sulfadiazine
  1393
Silver Apricot see Ginkgo Biloba . . 1622
Silver Nitrate 1392
Silver Sulfadiazine 1393
Silybum marianum see Milk Thistle
  1629
Simethicone 1394
Simethicone, Aluminum Hydroxide,
  and Magnesium Hydroxide see
  Aluminum Hydroxide,
  Magnesium Hydroxide, and
  Simethicone 81
Simethicone and Calcium
  Carbonate see Calcium
  Carbonate and Simethicone 249
Simethicone and Loperamide
  Hydrochloride see Loperamide
  and Simethicone 943
Simethicone and Magaldrate see
  Magaldrate and Simethicone . . 960
Similac® Glucose see Dextrose . . . 452
Simply Cough® [OTC] see
  Dextromethorphan 451
Simply Saline® Baby [OTC] see
  Sodium Chloride 1400
Simply Saline® Nasal Moist® [OTC]
  see Sodium Chloride 1400
Simply Saline® [OTC] see Sodium
  Chloride 1400
Simply Sleep® (Can) see
  DiphenhydrAMINE 483
Simply Sleep® [OTC] see
  DiphenhydrAMINE 483
Simply Stuffy™ [OTC] see
  Pseudoephedrine 1309
Simulect® see Basiliximab 180
Simvastatin 1394
Sina-12X see Guaifenesin and
  Phenylephrine 754
Sincalide 1396
Sinedol® (Mex) see
  Acetaminophen 31
Sinemet® see Levodopa and
  Carbidopa 911
Sinemet® CR see Levodopa and
  Carbidopa 911
Sinequan® (Can) see Doxepin 505
Sinequan® [DSC] see Doxepin 505

Sinestron® (Mex) see Lorazepam ... 947
Singulair® see Montelukast 1062
Sinogan® (Mex) see
  Methotrimeprazine 1016
Sinografin® see Diatrizoate
  Meglumine and Iodipamide
  Meglumine 453
Sinozzard® (Mex) see Prazosin .. 1267
Sintrom® (Can) see
  Acenocoumarol 30
Sinus-Relief [OTC] see
  Acetaminophen and
  Pseudoephedrine 38
Sinutab® Non Drowsy (Can) see
  Acetaminophen and
  Pseudoephedrine 38
Sinutab® Sinus & Allergy (Can)
  see Acetaminophen,
  Chlorpheniramine, and
  Pseudoephedrine 43
Sinutab® Sinus Allergy Maximum
  Strength [OTC] see
  Acetaminophen,
  Chlorpheniramine, and
  Pseudoephedrine 43
Sinutab® Sinus [OTC] see
  Acetaminophen and
  Pseudoephedrine 38
SINUvent® PE see Guaifenesin
  and Phenylephrine 754
Siqual®[caps] (Mex) see
  Fluoxetine 675
Sirdalud® see Tizanidine 1497
Sirolimus 1397
SK see Streptokinase 1417
SK and F 104864 see Topotecan
  1511
Skeeter Stik [OTC] see
  Benzocaine 190
Skelaxin® see Metaxalone 1001
Skelid® see Tiludronate 1488
SKF 104864 see Topotecan 1511
SKF 104864-A see Topotecan 1511
Skin Care™ [OTC] see Pyrithione
  Zinc 1318
Sleep-ettes D [OTC] see
  DiphenhydrAMINE 483
Sleepinal® [OTC] see
  DiphenhydrAMINE 483
Slo-Bid® (Mex) see Theophylline .. 1473
Slo-Niacin® [OTC] see Niacin 1105
Slow FE® [OTC] see Ferrous
  Sulfate 651
Slow-K® (Can) see Potassium
  Chloride 1258
Slow-Mag® [OTC] see Magnesium
  Chloride 960
Slow-Trasicor® (Can) see
  Oxprenolol 1161
Smelling Salts see Ammonia Spirit
  (Aromatic) 103
SMZ-TMP see Sulfamethoxazole
  and Trimethoprim 1425
Snakeroot see Echinacea 1620
(+)-(S)-N-Methyl-γ-(1-naphthyloxy)-
  2-thiophenepropylamine
  Hydrochloride see Duloxetine .. 523
Sodipental® (Mex) see
  Thiopental 1477
Sodium 4-Hydroxybutyrate see
  Sodium Oxybate 1402
Sodium L-Triiodothyronine see
  Liothyronine 934
Sodium Acid Carbonate see
  Sodium Bicarbonate 1400
Sodium Benzoate and Caffeine
  see Caffeine 245

Sodium Bicarbonate 1400
Sodium Biphosphate,
  Methenamine, Methylene Blue,
  Phenyl Salicylate, and
  Hyoscyamine see
  Methenamine, Sodium
  Biphosphate, Phenyl Salicylate,
  Methylene Blue, and
  Hyoscyamine 1008
Sodium Cellulose Phosphate see
  Cellulose Sodium Phosphate .. 301
Sodium Chloride............... 1400
Sodium Citrate and Citric Acid ... 1401
Sodium Citrate, Citric Acid, and
  Potassium Citrate see Citric
  Acid, Sodium Citrate, and
  Potassium Citrate 354
Sodium Edetate see Edetate
  Disodium 527
Sodium Etidronate see Etidronate
  Disodium 621
Sodium Ferric Gluconate see
  Ferric Gluconate 649
Sodium Fluoride see Fluoride 671
Sodium Hyaluronate see
  Hyaluronate and Derivatives ... 773
Sodium Hyaluronate and
  Chondroitin Sulfate see
  Chondroitin Sulfate and
  Sodium Hyaluronate 336
Sodium Hydrogen Carbonate see
  Sodium Bicarbonate 1400
Sodium Hypochlorite Solution..... 1402
Sodium Hyposulfate see Sodium
  Thiosulfate 1404
Sodium Nafcillin see Nafcillin 1082
Sodium Nitroferricyanide see
  Nitroprusside 1122
Sodium Nitroprusside see
  Nitroprusside 1122
Sodium Oxybate 1402
Sodium PAS see Aminosalicylic
  Acid 89
Sodium-PCA and Lactic Acid see
  Lactic Acid 893
Sodium Phenylbutyrate 1403
Sodium Phosphate and Potassium
  Phosphate see Potassium
  Phosphate and Sodium
  Phosphate 1261
Sodium Phosphates 1403
Sodium Sulfacetamide see
  Sulfacetamide 1423
Sodium Tetradecyl 1404
Sodium Tetradecyl Sulfate see
  Sodium Tetradecyl 1404
Sodium Thiosulfate 1404
Sodium Thiosulphate see Sodium
  Thiosulfate 1404
Soflax™ (Can) see Docusate 496
Solagé™ see Mequinol and
  Tretinoin 994
Solaquin® (Can) see Hydroquinone
  798
Solaquin Forte® see Hydroquinone
  798
Solaquin® [OTC] see Hydroquinone
  798
Solaraze® see Diclofenac 459
Solarcaine® Aloe Extra Burn Relief
  [OTC] see Lidocaine 920
Solia™ see Ethinyl Estradiol and
  Desogestrel 592
Solifenacin 1405
Solifenacin Succinate see
  Solifenacin 1405
Solodyn™ see Minocycline 1049
Soltamox™ see Tamoxifen 1443
Solu-Cortef® see Hydrocortisone ... 793
Solugel® (Can) see Benzoyl
  Peroxide................... 194

Solu-Medrol® see
   MethylPREDNISolone 1025
Soluver® (Can) see Salicylic Acid . . 1374
Soluver® Plus (Can) see Salicylic
   Acid 1374
Soma® see Carisoprodol 271
Soma® Compound see
   Carisoprodol and Aspirin 272
Soma® Compound w/Codeine see
   Carisoprodol, Aspirin, and
   Codeine 273
Somatrem see Somatropin 1406
Somatropin 1406
Sominex® Maximum Strength
   [OTC] see DiphenhydrAMINE . . 483
Sominex® [OTC] see
   DiphenhydrAMINE 483
Somnote® see Chloral Hydrate . . . 312
Sonata® see Zaleplon 1591
Sophixin® (Mex) see Ciprofloxacin . 343
Sorafenib 1407
Sorafenib Tosylate see Sorafenib
   1407
Sorbitol 1408
Sorine® see Sotalol 1409
Sostenon® [Propionate,
   Phenylpropionate, Isocaproate,
   Decanoate] (Mex) see
   Testosterone 1462
Sotacor® (Can) see Sotalol 1409
Sotalol 1409
Sotalol Hydrochloride see Sotalol . . 1409
Sotradecol® see Sodium
   Tetradecyl 1404
Sotret® see Isotretinoin 869
Soy Isoflavones 1632
Spacol [DSC] see Hyoscyamine . . . 803
Spacol T/S [DSC] see
   Hyoscyamine 803
Sparfloxacin 1411
SPD417 see Carbamazepine 260
Spectazole® see Econazole 526
Spectinomycin 1412
Spectinomycin Hydrochloride see
   Spectinomycin 1412
Spectracef™ see Cefditoren 285
Spectrocin Plus™ [OTC] see
   Bacitracin, Neomycin,
   Polymyxin B, and Pramoxine . . . 177
SPI 0211 see Lubiprostone 957
Spiramycin 1412
Spirapril 1413
Spiriva® see Tiotropium 1494
Spironolactone 1413
Spironolactone and
   Hydrochlorothiazide see
   Hydrochlorothiazide and
   Spironolactone 778
Sporanox® see Itraconazole 873
Sportscreme® [OTC] see
   Triethanolamine Salicylate 1535
Sprintec™ see Ethinyl Estradiol
   and Norgestimate 613
SSD® see Silver Sulfadiazine 1393
SSD® AF see Silver Sulfadiazine . . 1393
SSKI® see Potassium Iodide 1260
S.T. 37® [OTC] see
   Hexylresorcinol. 771
Stadol® see Butorphanol 243
Stagesic® see Hydrocodone and
   Acetaminophen 779
Stalevo™ see Levodopa,
   Carbidopa, and Entacapone . . . 912
StanGard® see Fluoride 671
StanGard® Perio see Fluoride 671
Stannous Fluoride see Fluoride . . . 671
Stanozolol 1415
Starlix® see Nateglinide 1094
Starnoc® (Can) see Zaleplon 1591
Statex® (Can) see Morphine
   Sulfate 1065

Staticin® [DSC] see Erythromycin . . . 562
Statobex® (Can) see
   Phendimetrazine 1220
Stavudine 1416
Stelazine® (Mex) see
   Trifluoperazine 1535
Stemetil® (Can) see
   Prochlorperazine 1285
Stenox® (Mex) see
   Fluoxymesterone 679
Sterapred® see PredniSONE 1271
Sterapred® DS see PredniSONE . . 1271
STI571 see Imatinib 817
Stiemycin® (Mex) see Erythromycin
   562
Stieprox® (Can) see Ciclopirox 338
Stimate™ see Desmopressin 437
Sting-Kill [OTC] see Benzocaine . . . 190
Stinking Rose see Garlic 1622
St John's Wort 1632
St. Joseph® Adult Aspirin [OTC]
   see Aspirin 145
Stop® see Fluoride 671
Strattera® see Atomoxetine 156
Streptase® see Streptokinase 1417
Streptokinase 1417
Streptomycin 1418
Streptomycin Sulfate see
   Streptomycin 1418
Streptozocin 1418
Stresstabs® B-Complex + Iron
   [OTC] see Vitamin B Complex
   Combinations 1581
Stresstabs® B-Complex [OTC] see
   Vitamin B Complex
   Combinations 1581
Stresstabs® B-Complex + Zinc
   [OTC] see Vitamin B Complex
   Combinations 1581
Striant® see Testosterone 1462
Stri-dex® Body Focus [OTC] see
   Salicylic Acid 1374
Stri-dex® Facewipes To Go™
   [OTC] see Salicylic Acid 1374
Stri-dex® Maximum Strength [OTC]
   see Salicylic Acid 1374
Stri-dex® [OTC] see Salicylic Acid
   1374
Strifon Forte® (Can) see
   Chlorzoxazone 333
Stromectol® see Ivermectin 877
Strong Iodine Solution see
   Potassium Iodide and Iodine . . 1260
Strovite® Forte see Vitamins
   (Multiple/Oral) 1582
SU11248 see Sunitinib 1434
Sublimaze® see Fentanyl 644
Suboxone® see Buprenorphine and
   Naloxone 232
Subutex® see Buprenorphine 231
Succinylcholine 1419
Succinylcholine Chloride see
   Succinylcholine 1419
Sucraid® see Sacrosidase 1373
Sucralfate 1420
Sucrets® Original [OTC] see
   Hexylresorcinol. 771
Sucrets® [OTC] see Dyclonine . . . 525
Sudafed® (Mex) see
   Pseudoephedrine 1309
Sudafed® 12 Hour [OTC] see
   Pseudoephedrine 1309
Sudafed® 24 Hour [OTC] see
   Pseudoephedrine 1309
Sudafed® Children's Cold & Cough
   [OTC] see Pseudoephedrine
   and Dextromethorphan 1311
Sudafed® Children's [OTC] see
   Pseudoephedrine 1309

Sudafed® Cold & Cough Extra Strength (Can) see Acetaminophen, Dextromethorphan, and Pseudoephedrine 44
Sudafed® Decongestant (Can) see Pseudoephedrine 1309
Sudafed® Head Cold and Sinus Extra Strength (Can) see Acetaminophen and Pseudoephedrine 38
Sudafed® Non-Drying Sinus [OTC] see Guaifenesin and Pseudoephedrine 755
Sudafed® [OTC] see Pseudoephedrine 1309
Sudafed PE™ [OTC] see Phenylephrine 1226
Sudafed® Severe Cold [OTC] see Acetaminophen, Dextromethorphan, and Pseudoephedrine 44
Sudafed® Sinus Advance (Can) see Pseudoephedrine and Ibuprofen 1311
Sudafed® Sinus & Allergy [OTC] see Chlorpheniramine and Pseudoephedrine 325
Sudafed® Sinus and Cold [OTC] see Acetaminophen and Pseudoephedrine 38
Sudafed® Sinus Headache [OTC] see Acetaminophen and Pseudoephedrine 38
Sudafed® Sinus Nighttime [OTC] see Triprolidine and Pseudoephedrine 1542
Sudal® 12 see Chlorpheniramine and Pseudoephedrine 325
Sudodrin [OTC] see Pseudoephedrine 1309
SudoGest Children's [OTC] see Pseudoephedrine and Dextromethorphan 1311
SudoGest [OTC] see Pseudoephedrine 1309
SudoGest Sinus [OTC] see Acetaminophen and Pseudoephedrine 38
Sudo-Tab® [OTC] see Pseudoephedrine 1309
Sufenta® see Sufentanil 1421
Sufentanil 1421
Sufentanil Citrate see Sufentanil .. 1421
Sufisal® (Mex) see Pentoxifylline .. 1212
Sufortan® (Mex) see Penicillamine 1201
Sufortanon® (Mex) see Penicillamine 1201
Suiflox® (Mex) see Ciprofloxacin ... 343
Sular® see Nisoldipine 1117
Sulbactam and Ampicillin see Ampicillin and Sulbactam 120
Sulconazole 1422
Sulconazole Nitrate see Sulconazole 1422
Sulcrate® (Can) see Sucralfate ... 1420
Sulcrate® Suspension Plus (Can) see Sucralfate 1420
Sulfabenzamide, Sulfacetamide, and Sulfathiazole 1423
Sulfacetamide 1423
Sulfacetamide and Fluorometholone 1423
Sulfacetamide and Prednisolone .. 1424
Sulfacetamide Sodium see Sulfacetamide 1423
SulfaDIAZINE 1424
Sulfadoxine and Pyrimethamine ... 1424
Sulfamethoxazole and Trimethoprim 1425

Sulfamylon® see Mafenide 959
Sulfasalazine 1428
Sulfatrim see Sulfamethoxazole and Trimethoprim 1425
Sulfazine see Sulfasalazine 1428
Sulfazine EC see Sulfasalazine ... 1428
SulfiSOXAZOLE 1429
Sulfisoxazole Acetyl see SulfiSOXAZOLE 1429
Sulfisoxazole and Erythromycin see Erythromycin and Sulfisoxazole 568
Sulfizole® (Can) see SulfiSOXAZOLE 1429
Sulfonated Phenolics in Aqueous Solution 1429
Sulindac 1430
Sulphafurazole see SulfiSOXAZOLE 1429
Sumatriptan 1432
Sumatriptan Succinate see Sumatriptan 1432
Summer's Eve® Medicated Douche [OTC] see Povidone-Iodine .. 1262
Summer's Eve® SpecialCare™ Medicated Anti-Itch Cream [OTC] see Hydrocortisone 793
Sumycin® see Tetracycline 1467
Sun-Benz® (Can) see Benzydamine 197
Sunitinib 1434
Sunitinib Maleate see Sunitinib ... 1434
Supartz™ see Hyaluronate and Derivatives 773
Superdophilus® [OTC] see Lactobacillus 535
Superginkgo see Ginkgo Biloba .. 1622
Supeudol® (Can) see Oxycodone .. 1163
Suplasyn® (Can) see Hyaluronate and Derivatives 773
Supositorios Senosiain® (Mex) see Glycerin 747
Suprax® see Cefixime 287
Surbex-T® [OTC] see Vitamin B Complex Combinations 1581
Surepin 81™ [OTC] see Aspirin ... 145
Surfak® [OTC] see Docusate 496
Surgicel® see Cellulose (Oxidized/ Regenerated) 300
Surgicel® Fibrillar see Cellulose (Oxidized/Regenerated) 300
Surgicel® NuKnit see Cellulose (Oxidized/Regenerated) 300
Surmontil® see Trimipramine 1540
Survanta® see Beractant 198
Sustiva® see Efavirenz 530
Sutent® see Sunitinib 1434
Su-Tuss DM see Guaifenesin and Dextromethorphan 754
Su-Tuss®-HD see Hydrocodone, Pseudoephedrine, and Guaifenesin 792
Suxamethonium Chloride see Succinylcholine 1419
Sween Cream® [OTC] see Vitamin A and Vitamin D 1580
Sweet Root see Licorice 1627
Symax SL see Hyoscyamine 803
Symax SR see Hyoscyamine 803
Symbyax™ see Olanzapine and Fluoxetine 1141
Symlin® see Pramlintide 1263
Symmetrel® see Amantadine 81
Sympt-X G.I. [OTC] see Glutamine 743
Sympt-X [OTC] see Glutamine 743
Synacthen see Cosyntropin 396
Synagis® see Palivizumab 1179
Synalar® see Fluocinolone 667
Synalgos®-DC see Dihydrocodeine, Aspirin, and Caffeine 475

Synarel® see Nafarelin 1081

Syn-Diltiazem® (Can) see Diltiazem 479

Synera™ see Lidocaine and Tetracaine 930

Synercid® see Quinupristin and Dalfopristin 1326

Synphasic® (Can) see Ethinyl Estradiol and Norethindrone 608

Syntest D.S. see Estrogens (Esterified) and Methyltestosterone 585

Syntest H.S. see Estrogens (Esterified) and Methyltestosterone 585

Synthroid® see Levothyroxine 917

Syntocinon® (Can) see Oxytocin . . 1175

Synvisc® see Hyaluronate and Derivatives 773

Syrex see Sodium Chloride 1400

SyringeAvitene™ see Collagen Hemostat 392

Syrup of Ipecac see Ipecac Syrup . . 856

Syscor® (Mex) see Nisoldipine 1117

Systen® (Mex) see Estradiol 574

T₃ Sodium (error-prone abbreviation) see Liothyronine . . 934

T₃/T₄ Liotrix see Liotrix 935

T₄ see Levothyroxine 917

T-20 see Enfuvirtide 541

642® Tablet see Propoxyphene 1297

Tabloid® see Thioguanine 1476

Tacex® (Mex) see Ceftriaxone 294

Tacrine 1436

Tacrine Hydrochloride see Tacrine 1436

Tacrolimus 1437

Tadalafil 1441

Tafil® (Mex) see Alprazolam 73

Tagal® (Mex) see Ceftazidime 292

Tagamet® see Cimetidine 341

Tagamet® HB (Can) see Cimetidine 341

Tagamet® HB 200 [OTC] see Cimetidine 341

TAK-375 see Ramelteon 1331

Talacen® see Pentazocine and Acetaminophen 1209

Talpramin® (Mex) see Imipramine . . 820

Talwin® see Pentazocine 1208

Talwin® NX see Pentazocine 1208

TAM see Tamoxifen 1443

Tambocor™ see Flecainide 657

Tamiflu® see Oseltamivir 1152

Tamofen® (Can) see Tamoxifen 1443

Tamoxifen 1443

Tamoxifen Citrate see Tamoxifen . . 1443

Tamsulosin 1445

Tamsulosin Hydrochloride see Tamsulosin 1445

Tanacetum parthenium see Feverfew 1621

Tanac® [OTC] see Benzocaine 190

Tanafed DP™ see Dexchlorpheniramine and Pseudoephedrine 443

Tanakan see Ginkgo Biloba 1622

Tanakene see Ginkgo Biloba 1622

Tannate 12 S see Carbetapentane and Chlorpheniramine 266

Tannic-12 see Carbetapentane and Chlorpheniramine 266

Tannic-12 S see Carbetapentane and Chlorpheniramine 266

Tannihist-12 RF see Carbetapentane and Chlorpheniramine 266

Tantum® (Can) see Benzydamine . . 197

TAP-144 see Leuprolide 906

Tapazole® see Methimazole 1008

Taporin® (Mex) see Cefotaxime 288

Tarceva™ see Erlotinib 560

Targel® (Can) see Coal Tar 383

Targretin® see Bexarotene 205

Tarka® see Trandolapril and Verapamil 1518

Taro-Carbamazepine Chewable (Can) see Carbamazepine 260

Taro-Desoximetasone (Can) see Desoximetasone 438

Taro-Sone® (Can) see Betamethasone 199

Taro-Warfarin (Can) see Warfarin 1585

Tarsum® [OTC] see Coal Tar and Salicylic Acid 383

Tasedan® (Mex) see Estazolam 573

Tasmar® see Tolcapone 1503

Tavist® (Mex) see Clemastine 359

Tavist® Allergy [OTC] see Clemastine 359

Tavist® ND [OTC] see Loratadine . . 946

Tavor® (Mex) see Oxybutynin 1162

Taxifur® (Mex) see Ceftazidime 292

Taxol® see Paclitaxel 1176

Taxotere® see Docetaxel 494

Taxus® (Mex) see Tamoxifen 1443

Tazarotene 1446

Tazicef® see Ceftazidime 292

Taziken® (Mex) see Terbutaline 1460

Tazocin® (Can) see Piperacillin and Tazobactam Sodium 1245

Tazorac® see Tazarotene 1446

Taztia XT™ see Diltiazem 479

3TC® (Can) see Lamivudine 894

3TC, Abacavir, and Zidovudine see Abacavir, Lamivudine, and Zidovudine 23

T-Cell Growth Factor see Aldesleukin 61

TCGF see Aldesleukin 61

TCN see Tetracycline 1467

TDF see Tenofovir 1457

Teardrops® (Can) see Artificial Tears 143

Teargen® II [OTC] see Artificial Tears 143

Teargen® [OTC] see Artificial Tears 143

Tearisol® [OTC] see Artificial Tears 143

Tears Again® MC [OTC] see Hydroxypropyl Methylcellulose . . 800

Tears Again® Gel Drops™ [OTC] see Carboxymethylcellulose 271

Tears Again® Night and Day™ [OTC] see Carboxymethylcellulose 271

Tears Again® [OTC] see Artificial Tears 143

Tears Naturale® II [OTC] see Artificial Tears 143

Tears Naturale® Free [OTC] see Artificial Tears 143

Tears Naturale® [OTC] see Artificial Tears 143

Tears Plus® [OTC] see Artificial Tears 143

Tears Renewed® [OTC] see Artificial Tears 143

TEAS see Triethanolamine Salicylate 1535

Tea Tree Oil see Melaleuca Oil . . . 1628

Tebamide™ see Trimethobenzamide 1538

Tebonin see Ginkgo Biloba 1622

Tebrazid™ (Can) see Pyrazinamide 1314

Tecnal C 1/2 (Can) see Butalbital,
Aspirin, Caffeine, and Codeine
................................241
Tecnal C 1/4 (Can) see Butalbital,
Aspirin, Caffeine, and Codeine
................................241
Tecnofen® (Mex) see
Tamoxifen 1443
Tecnoplatin® (Mex) see Cisplatin ...350
Tegaserod 1448
Tegaserod Maleate see Tegaserod
................................1448
Tegretol® see Carbamazepine 260
Tegretol®-XR see Carbamazepine ..260
Teldrin® HBP [OTC] see
Chlorpheniramine 323
Telithromycin 1448
Telmisartan 1451
Telmisartan and
Hydrochlorothiazide 1452
Telzir® (Can) see Fosamprenavir ...702
Temazepam 1453
Temgesic® (Mex) see
Buprenorphine 231
Temodal™ (Can) see
Temozolomide 1454
Temodar® see Temozolomide 1454
Temovate® see Clobetasol 365
Temovate E® see Clobetasol 365
Temozolomide 1454
Temperal® (Mex) see
Acetaminophen 31
Tempra® (Can) see
Acetaminophen 31
Tenecteplase 1455
Tenex® see Guanfacine 758
Teniposide 1456
Tenofovir 1457
Tenofovir and Emtricitabine see
Emtricitabine and Tenofovir 537
Tenofovir Disoproxil Fumarate see
Tenofovir 1457
Tenolin (Can) see Atenolol 154
Tenoretic® see Atenolol and
Chlorthalidone 156
Tenormin® see Atenolol 154
Tenuate® see Diethylpropion 467
Tenuate® Dospan® see
Diethylpropion 467
Teolong® (Mex) see Theophylline
................................1473
Tequin® (Can) see Gatifloxacin 724
Tequin® [DSC] see Gatifloxacin 724
Tera-Gel™ [OTC] see Coal Tar 383
Terazol® (Can) see Terconazole ..1461
Terazol® 3 see Terconazole 1461
Terazol® 7 see Terconazole 1461
Terazosin 1458
Terbac® (Mex) see Ceftriaxone 294
Terbinafine 1459
Terbinafine Hydrochloride see
Terbinafine 1459
Terbutaline 1460
Terconazole 1461
Terfluzine (Can) see
Trifluoperazine 1535
Teriparatide 1461
Termizol® (Mex) see Ketoconazole
................................880
Terramicina® (Mex) see
Oxytetracycline 1174
Terramycin® (Can) see
Oxytetracycline 1174
Terramycin® I.M. [DSC] see
Oxytetracycline 1174
Tesalon® (Mex) see Benzonatate ..194
Teslac® see Testolactone 1462
TESPA see Thiotepa 1479
Tessalon® see Benzonatate 194
Testim® see Testosterone 1462
Testolactone 1462

Testopel® see Testosterone 1462
Testosterone 1462
Testosterone Cypionate see
Testosterone 1462
Testosterone Enanthate see
Testosterone 1462
Testred® see
MethylTESTOSTERone 1028
Tetanus Immune Globulin (Human)
................................1463
Tetanus Toxoid (Adsorbed) 1464
Tetanus Toxoid (Fluid) 1464
Tetanus Toxoid Plain see Tetanus
Toxoid (Fluid) 1464
Tetra-Atlantis® (Mex) see
Tetracycline 1467
Tetrabenazine 1465
Tetracaine 1466
Tetracaine and Dextrose 1467
Tetracaine and Lidocaine see
Lidocaine and Tetracaine 930
Tetracaine Hydrochloride see
Tetracaine 1466
Tetracaine Hydrochloride,
Benzocaine, Butyl
Aminobenzoate, and
Benzalkonium Chloride see
Benzocaine, Butyl
Aminobenzoate, Tetracaine,
and Benzalkonium Chloride 193
Tetracosactide see Cosyntropin ...396
Tetracycline 1467
Tetracycline Hydrochloride see
Tetracycline 1467
Tetracycline, Metronidazole, and
Bismuth Subsalicylate see
Bismuth Subsalicylate,
Metronidazole, and
Tetracycline 210
Tetrafluoroethane and
Pentafluoropropane see
Pentafluoropropane and
Tetrafluoroethane 1206
Tetrahydroaminoacrine see Tacrine
................................1436
Tetrahydrocannabinol see
Dronabinol 518
Tetrahydrocannabinol and
Cannabidiol 1469
Tetrahydrozoline 1470
Tetrahydrozoline Hydrochloride see
Tetrahydrozoline 1470
Tetra Tannate Pediatric see
Chlorpheniramine, Ephedrine,
Phenylephrine, and
Carbetapentane 325
Tetryzoline see Tetrahydrozoline ..1470
Teveten® see Eprosartan 554
Teveten® HCT see Eprosartan and
Hydrochlorothiazide 555
Teveten® Plus (Can) see
Eprosartan and
Hydrochlorothiazide 555
Tev-Tropin™ see Somatropin 1406
Texacort® see Hydrocortisone 793
Texate® (Mex) see Methotrexate ..1012
TG see Thioguanine 1476
6-TG (error-prone abbreviation)
see Thioguanine 1476
THA see Tacrine 1436
Thalidomide 1471
Thalitone® see Chlorthalidone 332
Thalomid® see Thalidomide 1471
THAM® see Tromethamine 1545
THC see Dronabinol 518
THC and CBD see
Tetrahydrocannabinol and
Cannabidiol 1469
Theo-24® see Theophylline 1473
TheoCap™ see Theophylline 1473
Theochron® see Theophylline 1473

Theochron® SR (Can) see
    Theophylline 1473
Theolair™ (Can) see Theophylline
    1473
Theolate [DSC] see Theophylline
    and Guaifenesin 1475
Theophylline 1473
Theophylline and Guaifenesin 1475
Theophylline Anhydrous see
    Theophylline 1473
Theophylline Ethylenediamine see
    Aminophylline 89
TheraCys® see BCG Vaccine 181
Thera-Flu® Cold and Sore Throat
    Night Time [OTC] see
    Acetaminophen,
    Chlorpheniramine, and
    Pseudoephedrine 43
Thera-Flur-N® see Fluoride 671
Thera-Flu® Severe Cold
    Non-Drowsy [OTC] [DSC] see
    Acetaminophen,
    Dextromethorphan, and
    Pseudoephedrine 44
Theragran-M® Advanced Formula
    [OTC] [DSC] see Vitamins
    (Multiple/Oral) 1582
Theragran® Heart Right™ [OTC]
    [DSC] see Vitamins (Multiple/
    Oral) 1582
Theramycin Z® see Erythromycin . . . 562
Therapeutic Multivitamins see
    Vitamins (Multiple/Oral) 1582
Theratears® see
    Carboxymethylcellulose 271
Thermazene® see Silver
    Sulfadiazine 1393
Thiabendazole 1475
Thiamazole see Methimazole . . . 1008
Thiamine 1476
Thiamine Hydrochloride see
    Thiamine 1476
Thiaminium Chloride Hydrochloride
    see Thiamine 1476
Thioctic acid see Alpha-Lipoic Acid
    1614
Thioguanine 1476
6-Thioguanine (error-prone
    abbreviation) see Thioguanine
    1476
Thiola® see Tiopronin 1494
Thiopental 1477
Thiopental Sodium see Thiopental
    1477
Thiophosphoramide see Thiotepa
    1479
Thioridazine 1477
Thioridazine Hydrochloride see
    Thioridazine 1477
Thiosulfuric Acid Disodium Salt see
    Sodium Thiosulfate 1404
Thiotepa 1479
Thiothixene 1480
Thorets [OTC] see Benzocaine . . . 190
Thrombate III® see Antithrombin III
    131
Thrombin-JMI® see Thrombin
    (Topical) 1481
Thrombin (Topical) 1481
Thymocyte Stimulating Factor see
    Aldesleukin 61
Thyrel® TRH [DSC] see Protirelin . . 1307
Thyrogen® see Thyrotropin Alpha
    1483
Thyroid 1482
Thyroid Extract see Thyroid 1482
Thyroid USP see Thyroid 1482
Thyrolar® see Liotrix 935
ThyroSafe™ [OTC] see Potassium
    Iodide 1260

ThyroShield™ [OTC] see
    Potassium Iodide 1260
Thyrotropin Alpha 1483
Thyrotropin Releasing Hormone
    see Protirelin 1307
L-Thyroxine Sodium see
    Levothyroxine 917
Tiabendazole see Thiabendazole . . 1475
Tiagabine 1483
Tiagabine Hydrochloride see
    Tiagabine 1483
Tiamol® (Can) see Fluocinonide . . . 670
Tiazac® see Diltiazem 479
Tiazac® XC (Can) see Diltiazem . . . 479
Ticar® see Ticarcillin 1484
Ticarcillin 1484
Ticarcillin and Clavulanate
    Potassium 1485
Ticarcillin and Clavulanic Acid see
    Ticarcillin and Clavulanate
    Potassium 1485
Ticarcillin Disodium see Ticarcillin
    1484
TICE® BCG see BCG Vaccine 181
Ticlid® see Ticlopidine 1486
Ticlopidine 1486
Ticlopidine Hydrochloride see
    Ticlopidine 1486
TIG see Tetanus Immune Globulin
    (Human) 1463
Tigan® see Trimethobenzamide . . . 1538
Tigecycline 1487
Tikosyn™ see Dofetilide 497
Tilade® see Nedocromil 1095
Tilaire® (Mex) see Nedocromil 1095
Tilazem® (Mex) see Diltiazem 479
Tiludronate 1488
Tiludronate Disodium see
    Tiludronate 1488
Tim-AK (Can) see Timolol 1489
Timentin® see Ticarcillin and
    Clavulanate Potassium 1485
Timolol 1489
Timolol and Dorzolamide see
    Dorzolamide and Timolol 501
Timolol Hemihydrate see Timolol . . 1489
Timolol Maleate see Timolol 1489
Timoptic® see Timolol 1489
Timoptic® OcuDose® see Timolol . . 1489
Timoptic-XE® see Timolol 1489
Tinactin® Antifungal Jock Itch
    [OTC] see Tolnaftate 1506
Tinactin® Antifungal [OTC] see
    Tolnaftate 1506
Tinaderm® (Mex) see Tolnaftate . . . 1506
Tinaderm [OTC] see Tolnaftate . . . 1506
Tinamed® [OTC] see Salicylic Acid
    1374
TinBen® [OTC] [DSC] see Benzoin
    193
Tindamax™ see Tinidazole 1491
Tine Test see Tuberculin Tests . . . 1548
Ting® Cream [OTC] see Tolnaftate
    1506
Tiniazol® (Mex) see Ketoconazole . . 880
Tinidazole 1491
Tinzaparin 1492
Tinzaparin Sodium see Tinzaparin
    1492
Tioconazole 1493
Tioguanine see Thioguanine 1476
Tiopronin 1494
Tiotixene see Thiothixene 1480
Tiotropium 1494
Tiotropium Bromide Monohydrate
    see Tiotropium 1494
Tipranavir 1495
Tirocal® (Mex) see Calcitriol 247
Tirofiban 1496
Tirofiban Hydrochloride see
    Tirofiban 1496

Tiroidine® (Mex) see
Levothyroxine 917
Tiseb® [OTC] see Salicylic Acid . . . 1374
Tisit® Blue Gel [OTC] see
Pyrethrins and Piperonyl
Butoxide 1315
Tisit® [OTC] see Pyrethrins and
Piperonyl Butoxide 1315
Tisseel® VH see Fibrin Sealant Kit . . 653
Titralac® Extra Strength [OTC] see
Calcium Carbonate 248
Titralac™ [OTC] see Calcium
Carbonate 248
Titralac® Plus [OTC] see Calcium
Carbonate and Simethicone 249
Ti-U-Lac® H (Can) see Urea and
Hydrocortisone 1551
Tizanidine 1497
TMP see Trimethoprim 1538
TMP-SMZ see Sulfamethoxazole
and Trimethoprim 1425
TMZ see Temozolomide 1454
TNKase™ see Tenecteplase 1455
TOBI® see Tobramycin 1498
TobraDex® see Tobramycin and
Dexamethasone 1499
Tobramycin 1498
Tobramycin and Dexamethasone . . 1499
Tobramycin and Loteprednol
Etabonate see Loteprednol and
Tobramycin 953
Tobramycin Sulfate see
Tobramycin 1498
Tobrex® see Tobramycin 1498
Tocainide 1500
Tocainide Hydrochloride see
Tocainide 1500
Today® Sponge [OTC] see
Nonoxynol 9 1124
Tofranil® see Imipramine 820
Tofranil-PM® see Imipramine 820
TOLAZamide 1501
Tolazoline 1501
Tolazoline Hydrochloride see
Tolazoline 1501
TOLBUTamide 1502
Tolbutamide Sodium see
TOLBUTamide 1502
Tolcapone 1503
Tolectin® see Tolmetin 1504
Tolinase® (Can) see TOLAZamide
. . . . 1501
Tolinase® [DSC] see TOLAZamide
. . . . 1501
Tolmetin 1504
Tolmetin Sodium see Tolmetin 1504
Tolnaftate 1506
Tolterodine 1506
Tolterodine Tartrate see
Tolterodine 1506
Tomocat® see Barium 179
Tomocat® 1000 see Barium 179
Tomoxetine see Atomoxetine 156
Tondex® (Mex) see Gentamicin 734
Tonga see Kava 1627
Tonocalcin® [salmon] (Mex) see
Calcitonin 246
Tonocard® [DSC] see Tocainide . . . 1500
Tonopaque see Barium 179
Topamax® see Topiramate 1508
Top-Dal® (Mex) see
Loperamide 942
Topicaine® [OTC] see Lidocaine . . . 920
Topicort® see Desoximetasone 438
Topicort®-LP see Desoximetasone . . 438
Topilene® (Can) see
Betamethasone 199
Topiramate 1508
Topisone® (Can) see
Betamethasone 199
TOPO see Topotecan 1511

Toposar® see Etoposide 626
Topotecan 1511
Topotecan Hydrochloride see
Topotecan 1511
Toprol-XL® see Metoprolol 1030
Topsyn® (Can) see Fluocinonide . . 670
Toradol® see Ketorolac 886
Toradol® IM (Can) see Ketorolac . . . 886
Toremifene 1512
Toremifene Citrate see Toremifene
. . . . 1512
Torsemide 1512
Touro™ CC see Guaifenesin,
Pseudoephedrine, and
Dextromethorphan 757
Touro™ Allergy see
Brompheniramine and
Pseudoephedrine 223
Touro® DM see Guaifenesin and
Dextromethorphan 754
Touro LA® see Guaifenesin and
Pseudoephedrine 755
tPA see Alteplase 77
TPT see Topotecan 1511
TPV see Tipranavir 1495
tRA see Tretinoin (Oral) 1524
Trace Metals 1513
Tracleer® see Bosentan 215
Tradol® (Mex) see Tramadol 1514
Tramacet (Can) see
Acetaminophen and Tramadol . . 39
Tramadol 1514
Tramadol Hydrochloride see
Tramadol 1514
Tramadol Hydrochloride and
Acetaminophen see
Acetaminophen and Tramadol . . 39
Tramisal see Ginkgo Biloba 1622
Trandate® see Labetalol 891
Trandolapril 1517
Trandolapril and Verapamil 1518
Tranexamic Acid 1518
Transamine Sulphate see
Tranylcypromine 1519
Transderm-V® (Can) see
Scopolamine 1380
Transderm-Nitro® (Can) see
Nitroglycerin 1120
Transderm Scōp® see
Scopolamine 1380
Trans-Plantar® (Can) see Salicylic
Acid 1374
trans-Retinoic Acid see Tretinoin
(Oral) 1524
Trans-Ver-Sal® (Can) see Salicylic
Acid 1374
Trans-Ver-Sal® [OTC] see Salicylic
Acid 1374
Tranxene® (Mex) see Clorazepate . . 378
Tranxene® SD™ see Clorazepate . . . 378
Tranxene® SD™-Half Strength see
Clorazepate 378
Tranxene® T-Tab® see
Clorazepate 378
Tranylcypromine 1519
Tranylcypromine Sulfate see
Tranylcypromine 1519
Trasicor® (Can) see Oxprenolol . . . 1161
Trastuzumab 1520
Trasylol® see Aprotinin 135
Travatan® see Travoprost 1521
Travoprost 1521
Trazil® (Mex) see Tobramycin 1498
Trazodone 1521
Trazodone Hydrochloride see
Trazodone 1521
Trecator® see Ethionamide 618
Trelstar™ Depot see Triptorelin . . . 1544
Trelstar® LA see Triptorelin 1544
Trental® see Pentoxifylline 1212
Treprostinil 1523

Treprostinil Sodium see Treprostinil
. . . . 1523
Tretinoin and Mequinol see
    Mequinol and Tretinoin. 994
Tretinoin, Fluocinolone Acetonide,
    and Hydroquinone see
    Fluocinolone, Hydroquinone,
    and Tretinoin 669
Tretinoin (Oral) 1524
Tretinoin (Topical) 1525
Trexall™ see Methotrexate 1012
TRH see Protirelin 1307
Triacetin 1526
Triacin-C® [DSC] see Triprolidine,
    Pseudoephedrine, and
    Codeine 1543
Triaconazole see Terconazole 1461
Triaderm (Can) see Triamcinolone
. . . . 1526
Triaken® (Mex) see Ceftriaxone 294
Triamcinolone 1526
Triamcinolone Acetonide, Aerosol
    see Triamcinolone 1526
Triamcinolone Acetonide (Dental
    Paste) 1530
Triamcinolone Acetonide,
    Parenteral see Triamcinolone
. . . . 1526
Triamcinolone and Nystatin see
    Nystatin and Triamcinolone . . . 1134
Triamcinolone Diacetate, Oral see
    Triamcinolone. 1526
Triamcinolone Diacetate,
    Parenteral see Triamcinolone
. . . . 1526
Triamcinolone Hexacetonide see
    Triamcinolone. 1526
Triamcinolone, Oral see
    Triamcinolone. 1526
Triaminic® Allerchews™ [OTC] see
    Loratadine 946
Triaminic® Cold & Allergy (Can)
    see Chlorpheniramine and
    Pseudoephedrine 325
Triaminic® Cold and Allergy [OTC]
    see Chlorpheniramine and
    Pseudoephedrine 325
Triaminic® Cough and Sore Throat
    Formula [OTC] see
    Acetaminophen,
    Dextromethorphan, and
    Pseudoephedrine 44
Triaminic® Cough & Nasal
    Congestion [OTC] see
    Pseudoephedrine and
    Dextromethorphan 1311
Triaminic® Cough [OTC] see
    Pseudoephedrine and
    Dextromethorphan 1311
Triaminic® Thin Strips™ Cough and
    Runny Nose [OTC] see
    DiphenhydrAMINE 483
Triaminic® Thin Strips™ Long
    Acting Cough [OTC] see
    Dextromethorphan 451
Triamsicort® (Mex) see
    Triamcinolone. 1526
Triamterene 1531
Triamterene and
    Hydrochlorothiazide see
    Hydrochlorothiazide and
    Triamterene 778
Triatec-8 (Can) see
    Acetaminophen and Codeine 35
Triatec-8 Strong (Can) see
    Acetaminophen and Codeine 35
Triatec-30 (Can) see
    Acetaminophen and Codeine 35
Triaz® see Benzoyl Peroxide 194
Triaz® Cleanser see Benzoyl
    Peroxide. 194

Triazolam 1531
Tribavirin see Ribavirin 1343
Tricalcium Phosphate see Calcium
    Phosphate (Tribasic) 251
Tricardio B see Folic Acid,
    Cyanocobalamin, and
    Pyridoxine 697
Tri-Chlor® see Trichloroacetic Acid
. . . . 1534
Trichlor Fresh Pac™ see
    Trichloroacetic Acid 1534
Trichloroacetaldehyde
    Monohydrate see Chloral
    Hydrate 312
Trichloroacetic Acid 1534
Trichloromonofluoromethane and
    Dichlorodifluoromethane see
    Dichlorodifluoromethane and
    Trichloromonofluoromethane . . . 458
Triclosan and Fluoride 1534
TriCor® see Fenofibrate 639
Tricosal see Choline Magnesium
    Trisalicylate 335
Tri-Cyclen® (Can) see Ethinyl
    Estradiol and Norgestimate 613
Tri-Cyclen® Lo (Can) see Ethinyl
    Estradiol and Norgestimate 613
Triderm® see Triamcinolone 1526
Tridesilon® see Desonide 437
Tridione® see Trimethadione 1538
Triethanolamine Polypeptide
    Oleate-Condensate 1535
Triethanolamine Salicylate 1535
Triethylenethiophosphoramide see
    Thiotepa 1479
Trifluoperazine 1535
Trifluoperazine Hydrochloride see
    Trifluoperazine 1535
Trifluorothymidine see Trifluridine . . 1536
Trifluridine 1536
Triglide™ see Fenofibrate 639
Triglycerides, Medium Chain see
    Medium Chain Triglycerides 972
Trihexyphenidyl 1537
Trihexyphenidyl Hydrochloride see
    Trihexyphenidyl 1537
Tri-K® see Potassium Acetate,
    Potassium Bicarbonate, and
    Potassium Citrate 1257
Trikacide (Can) see Metronidazole
. . . . 1033
Trileptal® see Oxcarbazepine 1159
Tri-Levlen® see Ethinyl Estradiol
    and Levonorgestrel 602
Trilisate® [DSC] see Choline
    Magnesium Trisalicylate 335
Tri-Luma™ see Fluocinolone,
    Hydroquinone, and Tretinoin . . . 669
TriLyte™ see Polyethylene
    Glycol-Electrolyte Solution 1253
Trimazide [DSC] see
    Trimethobenzamide 1538
Trimethadione 1538
Trimethobenzamide 1538
Trimethobenzamide Hydrochloride
    see Trimethobenzamide 1538
Trimethoprim 1538
Trimethoprim and Polymyxin B 1539
Trimethoprim and
    Sulfamethoxazole see
    Sulfamethoxazole and
    Trimethoprim 1425
Trimetrexate 1539
Trimetrexate Glucuronate see
    Trimetrexate 1539
Trimipramine 1540
Trimipramine Maleate see
    Trimipramine 1540
Trimox® see Amoxicillin 106
Tri-Nasal® see Triamcinolone 1526

TriNessa™ *see* Ethinyl Estradiol and Norgestimate 613
Trinipatch® 0.2 (Can) *see* Nitroglycerin 1120
Trinipatch® 0.4 (Can) *see* Nitroglycerin 1120
Trinipatch® 0.6 (Can) *see* Nitroglycerin 1120
Tri-Norinyl® *see* Ethinyl Estradiol and Norethindrone 608
Trinsicon® *see* Vitamin B Complex Combinations 1581
Triostat® *see* Liothyronine 934
Tripelennamine 1541
Tripelennamine Citrate *see* Tripelennamine 1541
Tripelennamine Hydrochloride *see* Tripelennamine 1541
Triphasil® *see* Ethinyl Estradiol and Levonorgestrel 602
Triple Antibiotic *see* Bacitracin, Neomycin, and Polymyxin B . . 176
Triple Sulfa *see* Sulfabenzamide, Sulfacetamide, and Sulfathiazole 1423
Tri-Previfem™ *see* Ethinyl Estradiol and Norgestimate 613
Triprolidine and Pseudoephedrine 1542
Triprolidine, Codeine, and Pseudoephedrine *see* Triprolidine, Pseudoephedrine, and Codeine 1543
Triprolidine, Pseudoephedrine, and Codeine 1543
TripTone® [OTC] *see* DimenhyDRINATE 481
Triptoraline *see* Triptorelin 1544
Triptorelin 1544
Triptorelin Pamoate *see* Triptorelin 1544
Triquilar® (Can) *see* Ethinyl Estradiol and Levonorgestrel . . . 602
Tris Buffer *see* Tromethamine 1545
Tris(hydroxymethyl)aminomethane *see* Tromethamine 1545
Trisodium Calcium Diethylenetriaminepentaacetate (Ca-DTPA) *see* Diethylene Triamine Penta-Acetic Acid 466
Tri-Sprintec™ *see* Ethinyl Estradiol and Norgestimate 613
Tri-Sudo® [OTC] *see* Triprolidine and Pseudoephedrine 1542
Tritace® (Mex) *see* Ramipril 1332
Trivagizole-3® (Can) *see* Clotrimazole 379
Trivalent Inactivated Influenza Vaccine (TIV) *see* Influenza Virus Vaccine 833
Tri-Vent™ DM *see* Guaifenesin, Pseudoephedrine, and Dextromethorphan 757
Tri-Vent™ DPC *see* Chlorpheniramine, Phenylephrine, and Dextromethorphan 326
Tri-Vent™ HC *see* Hydrocodone, Carbinoxamine, and Pseudoephedrine 789
Trivora® *see* Ethinyl Estradiol and Levonorgestrel 602
Trixilem® (Mex) *see* Methotrexate 1012
Triyotex® (Mex) *see* Liothyronine . . . 934
Trizivir® *see* Abacavir, Lamivudine, and Zidovudine 23
Trobicin® (Mex) *see* Spectinomycin 1412
Trobicin® [DSC] *see* Spectinomycin 1412
Trocaine® [OTC] *see* Benzocaine . . . 190
Trolamine Salicylate *see* Triethanolamine Salicylate 1535
Trombovar® (Can) *see* Sodium Tetradecyl 1404
Tromethamine 1545
Tronolane® Cream [OTC] *see* Pramoxine 1264
Tronolane® Suppository [OTC] *see* Phenylephrine 1226
Tropicacyl® *see* Tropicamide 1545
Tropicamide 1545
Tropicamide and Hydroxyamphetamine *see* Hydroxyamphetamine and Tropicamide 799
Tropyn Z® (Mex) *see* Atropine 161
Trosec (Can) *see* Trospium 1546
Trospium 1546
Trospium Chloride *see* Trospium . . 1546
Trovafloxacin 1546
Trovan® (Mex) *see* Trovafloxacin . . 1546
Trovan® [DSC] *see* Trovafloxacin . . 1546
Troxidone *see* Trimethadione 1538
Trusopt® *see* Dorzolamide 501
Truvada® *see* Emtricitabine and Tenofovir 537
Trypsin, Balsam Peru, and Castor Oil 1547
Tryptoreline *see* Triptorelin 1544
TSH *see* Thyrotropin Alpha 1483
TSPA *see* Thiotepa 1479
TST *see* Tuberculin Tests 1548
T-Stat® [DSC] *see* Erythromycin 562
Tuberculin Purified Protein Derivative *see* Tuberculin Tests 1548
Tuberculin Skin Test *see* Tuberculin Tests 1548
Tuberculin Tests 1548
Tubersol® *see* Tuberculin Tests . . . 1548
Tucks® Anti-Itch [OTC] *see* Hydrocortisone 793
Tucks® Hemorrhoidal [OTC] *see* Pramoxine 1264
Tuinal® [DSC] *see* Amobarbital and Secobarbital 104
Tukol® (Mex) *see* Guaifenesin 752
Tums® E-X [OTC] *see* Calcium Carbonate 248
Tums® Extra Strength Sugar Free [OTC] *see* Calcium Carbonate . . 248
Tums® [OTC] *see* Calcium Carbonate 248
Tums® Smoothies™ [OTC] *see* Calcium Carbonate 248
Tums® Ultra [OTC] *see* Calcium Carbonate 248
Turmeric 1632
Turmeric Root *see* Golden Seal . . . 1624
Tusical® (Mex) *see* Benzonatate . . . 194
Tusitato® (Mex) *see* Benzonatate . . 194
Tussafed® *see* Carbinoxamine, Pseudoephedrine, and Dextromethorphan 269
Tussafed® HC *see* Hydrocodone, Phenylephrine, and Guaifenesin 791
Tussend® Expectorant *see* Hydrocodone, Pseudoephedrine, and Guaifenesin 792
Tussi-12® *see* Carbetapentane and Chlorpheniramine 266
Tussi-12® D *see* Carbetapentane, Phenylephrine, and Pyrilamine . . 267
Tussi-12® DS *see* Carbetapentane, Phenylephrine, and Pyrilamine . . 267
Tussi-12 S™ *see* Carbetapentane and Chlorpheniramine 266

Tussigon® see Hydrocodone and
   Homatropine 786
TussiNate™ see Hydrocodone,
   Phenylephrine, and
   Diphenhydramine 791
Tussin [OTC] see Guaifenesin 752
Tussionex® see Hydrocodone and
   Chlorpheniramine 784
Tussi-Organidin® NR see
   Guaifenesin and Codeine 753
Tussi-Organidin® S-NR see
   Guaifenesin and Codeine 753
Tussizone-12 RF™ see
   Carbetapentane and
   Chlorpheniramine 266
T-Vites [OTC] see Vitamins
   (Multiple/Oral) 1582
Twelve Resin-K see
   Cyanocobalamin 399
Twilite® [OTC] see
   DiphenhydrAMINE 483
Twinject™ see Epinephrine 546
Twinrix® see Hepatitis A
   Inactivated and Hepatitis B
   (Recombinant) Vaccine 766
Tycolene Maximum Strength [OTC]
   see Acetaminophen 31
Tycolene [OTC] see
   Acetaminophen 31
Tygacil™ see Tigecycline 1487
Tylenol® (Can) see Acetaminophen
   31
Tylenol® 8 Hour [OTC] see
   Acetaminophen 31
Tylenol® Allergy Complete [OTC]
   see Acetaminophen,
   Chlorpheniramine, and
   Pseudoephedrine 43
Tylenol® Allergy Sinus (Can) see
   Acetaminophen,
   Chlorpheniramine, and
   Pseudoephedrine 43
Tylenol® Allergy Sinus [OTC]
   [DSC] see Acetaminophen,
   Chlorpheniramine, and
   Pseudoephedrine 43
Tylenol® Arthritis Pain [OTC] see
   Acetaminophen 31
Tylenol® Children's [OTC] see
   Acetaminophen 31
Tylenol® Children's with Flavor
   Creator [OTC] see
   Acetaminophen 31
Tylenol® Children's Plus Cold
   Nighttime [OTC] see
   Acetaminophen,
   Chlorpheniramine, and
   Pseudoephedrine 43
Tylenol® Cold Day Non-Drowsy
   [OTC] see Acetaminophen,
   Dextromethorphan, and
   Pseudoephedrine 44
Tylenol® Cold Daytime (Can) see
   Acetaminophen,
   Dextromethorphan, and
   Pseudoephedrine 44
Tylenol® Cold, Infants [OTC] see
   Acetaminophen and
   Pseudoephedrine 38
Tylenol® Decongestant (Can) see
   Acetaminophen and
   Pseudoephedrine 38
Tylenol® Elixir with Codeine (Can)
   see Acetaminophen and
   Codeine 35
Tylenol® Extra Strength [OTC] see
   Acetaminophen 31

Tylenol® Flu Non-Drowsy
   Maximum Strength [OTC] see
   Acetaminophen,
   Dextromethorphan, and
   Pseudoephedrine 44
Tylenol® Infants [OTC] see
   Acetaminophen 31
Tylenol® Junior [OTC] see
   Acetaminophen 31
Tylenol No. 1 (Can) see
   Acetaminophen and Codeine 35
Tylenol No. 1 Forte (Can) see
   Acetaminophen and Codeine 35
Tylenol No. 2 with Codeine (Can)
   see Acetaminophen and
   Codeine 35
Tylenol No. 3 with Codeine (Can)
   see Acetaminophen and
   Codeine 35
Tylenol No. 4 with Codeine (Can)
   see Acetaminophen and
   Codeine 35
Tylenol® [OTC] see
   Acetaminophen 31
Tylenol® PM [OTC] see
   Acetaminophen and
   Diphenhydramine 38
Tylenol® Severe Allergy [OTC] see
   Acetaminophen and
   Diphenhydramine 38
Tylenol® Sinus (Can) see
   Acetaminophen and
   Pseudoephedrine 38
Tylenol® Sinus, Children's [OTC]
   see Acetaminophen and
   Pseudoephedrine 38
Tylenol® Sinus Day Non-Drowsy
   [OTC] see Acetaminophen and
   Pseudoephedrine 38
Tylenol® With Codeine (Can) see
   Acetaminophen and Codeine 35
Tylex® (Mex) see Acetaminophen . . . 31
Tylox® see Oxycodone and
   Acetaminophen 1165
Typhim Vi® see Typhoid Vaccine . 1549
Typhoid Vaccine 1549
Typhoid Vaccine Live Oral Ty21a
   see Typhoid Vaccine 1549
Tysabri® see Natalizumab 1093
Tyzine® see Tetrahydrozoline 1470
Tyzine® Pediatric see
   Tetrahydrozoline 1470
Tzoali® (Mex) see
   DiphenhydrAMINE 483
506U78 see Nelarabine 1097
U-90152S see Delavirdine 429
Ubiquinone see Coenzyme Q₁₀ . . . 1618
UCB-P071 see Cetirizine 306
UK-88,525 see Darifenacin 424
UK92480 see Sildenafil 1390
UK109496 see Voriconazole 1582
Ulcedin® (Mex) see Ranitidine 1334
Ulcerease® [OTC] see Phenol 1223
Ulgastrin Neo see Licorice 1627
Ulpax® (Mex) see Lansoprazole . . . 896
Ulsaven® (Mex) see Ranitidine 1334
Ulsen® (Mex) see Omeprazole 1145
Ultiva® see Remifentanil 1338
Ultracaine® D-S (Can) see
   Articaine and Epinephrine 139
Ultracaine® D-S Forte (Can) see
   Articaine and Epinephrine 139
Ultracet™ see Acetaminophen and
   Tramadol 39
Ultra Freeda Iron Free [OTC] see
   Vitamins (Multiple/Oral) 1582
Ultra Freeda with Iron [OTC] see
   Vitamins (Multiple/Oral) 1582
Ultram® see Tramadol 1514
Ultram® ER see Tramadol 1514
UltraMide 25™ (Can) see Urea . . . 1551

Ultra Mide® [OTC] see Urea 1551
Ultramop™ (Can) see Methoxsalen 1018
Ultran® (Mex) see Ranitidine 1334
Ultraprin [OTC] see Ibuprofen 808
Ultraquin™ (Can) see Hydroquinone 798
Ultrase® see Pancrelipase 1183
Ultrase® MT see Pancrelipase 1183
Ultra Tears® [OTC] see Artificial Tears 143
Ultravate® see Halobetasol 760
Ultravist® see Iopromide 855
Umecta® see Urea 1551
Unamol® (Mex) see Cisapride 348
Unasyn® see Ampicillin and Sulbactam 120
Uncaria tomentosa see Cat's Claw 1617
Undecylenic Acid and Derivatives 1550
Unicap M® [OTC] see Vitamins (Multiple/Oral) 1582
Unicap Sr® [OTC] see Vitamins (Multiple/Oral) 1582
Unicap T™ [OTC] see Vitamins (Multiple/Oral) 1582
Uni-Cof see Pseudoephedrine, Dihydrocodeine, and Chlorpheniramine 1312
Unidet® (Can) see Tolterodine 1506
Uni-Dur® (Mex) see Theophylline . . 1473
Unipen® (Can) see Nafcillin 1082
Uniphyl® see Theophylline 1473
Uniphyl® SRT (Can) see Theophylline 1473
Uniretic® see Moexipril and Hydrochlorothiazide 1059
Uni-Senna [OTC] see Senna 1384
Unisom®-2 (Can) see Doxylamine . . 517
Unisom® Maximum Strength SleepGels® [OTC] see DiphenhydrAMINE 483
Unisom® SleepTabs® [OTC] see Doxylamine 517
Unithroid® see Levothyroxine 917
Univasc® see Moexipril 1058
Unna's Boot see Zinc Gelatin 1597
Unna's Paste see Zinc Gelatin 1597
Unoprostone 1551
Unoprostone Isopropyl see Unoprostone 1551
Urasal® (Can) see Methenamine . . 1007
Urea 1551
Urea and Hydrocortisone 1551
Urea, Chlorophyllin, and Papain see Chlorophyllin, Papain, and Urea 319
Ureacin® [OTC] see Urea 1551
Urea Peroxide see Carbamide Peroxide 264
Urecholine® see Bethanechol 204
Uremol® (Can) see Urea 1551
Uremol® HC (Can) see Urea and Hydrocortisone 1551
Urex® see Methenamine 1007
Urimar-T see Methenamine, Sodium Biphosphate, Phenyl Salicylate, Methylene Blue, and Hyoscyamine 1008
Urimax® [DSC] see Methenamine, Sodium Biphosphate, Phenyl Salicylate, Methylene Blue, and Hyoscyamine 1008
Urisec® (Can) see Urea 1551
Urispas® see Flavoxate 656
Uristat® [OTC] see Phenazopyridine 1220
Urocit®-K see Potassium Citrate . . . 1259
Urofollitropin see Follitropins 698

Uro-KP-Neutral® see Potassium Phosphate and Sodium Phosphate 1261
Uro-Mag® [OTC] see Magnesium Oxide 962
Uroxatral® see Alfuzosin 68
Urso® (Can) see Ursodiol 1552
Urso 250™ see Ursodiol 1552
Ursodeoxycholic Acid see Ursodiol 1552
Ursodiol 1552
Ursofalk® (Mex) see Ursodiol 1552
Urso Forte™ see Ursodiol 1552
UTI Relief® [OTC] see Phenazopyridine 1220
Utradol™ (Can) see Etodolac 623
Uvadex® see Methoxsalen 1018
Uva Ursi 1633
Vaccinia Immune Globulin (Intravenous) 1553
Vaccinium macrocarpon see Cranberry 1619
Vaccinium myrtillus see Bilberry . . . 1615
Vagifem® see Estradiol 574
Vagi-Gard® [OTC] see Povidone-Iodine 1262
Vagistat®-1 [OTC] see Tioconazole 1493
Valacyclovir 1553
Valacyclovir Hydrochloride see Valacyclovir 1553
Valcyte™ see Valganciclovir 1555
Valerian 1633
Valeriana edulis see Valerian 1633
Valeriana wallichi see Valerian 1633
Valganciclovir 1555
Valganciclovir Hydrochloride see Valganciclovir 1555
Valisone® Scalp Lotion (Can) see Betamethasone 199
Valium® see Diazepam 454
Valorin Extra [OTC] see Acetaminophen 31
Valorin [OTC] see Acetaminophen . . . 31
Valproate Semisodium see Valproic Acid and Derivatives 1556
Valproate Sodium see Valproic Acid and Derivatives 1556
Valproic Acid see Valproic Acid and Derivatives 1556
Valproic Acid and Derivatives 1556
Valprosid® (Mex) see Valproic Acid and Derivatives 1556
Valrubicin 1560
Valsartan 1561
Valsartan and Hydrochlorothiazide 1562
Valstar® (Can) see Valrubicin 1560
Valstar® [DSC] see Valrubicin 1560
Valtaxin® (Can) see Valrubicin 1560
Valtrex® see Valacyclovir 1553
Valverde see Ginkgo Biloba 1622
Vanadium 1633
Vanamide™ see Urea 1551
Vanceril® AEM (Can) see Beclomethasone 183
Vancocin® see Vancomycin 1563
Vancomycin 1563
Vancomycin Hydrochloride see Vancomycin 1563
Vandazole® see Metronidazole . . . 1033
Vaniqa™ see Eflornithine 532
Vanos™ see Fluocinonide 670
Vanoxide-HC® see Benzoyl Peroxide and Hydrocortisone . . . 195
Vanquish® Extra Strength Pain Reliever [OTC] see Acetaminophen, Aspirin, and Caffeine 41

Van R Gingibraid® see Epinephrine (Racemic) and Aluminum Potassium Sulfate 550
Vantal® (Mex) see Benzydamine . . . 197
Vantas™ see Histrelin 772
Vantin® see Cefpodoxime 290
Vaprisol® see Conivaptan 393
VAQTA® see Hepatitis A Vaccine . . 767
Vardenafil 1565
Vardenafil Hydrochloride see Vardenafil 1565
Varicella, Measles, Mumps, and Rubella Vaccine see Measles, Mumps, Rubella, and Varicella Virus Vaccine 967
Varicella-Zoster Immune Globulin (Human) 1566
Vasan see Ginkgo Biloba 1622
Vaseretic® see Enalapril and Hydrochlorothiazide 541
Vasocon® (Can) see Naphazoline 1087
Vasocon®-A (Can) see Naphazoline and Antazoline . . . 1088
Vasocon®-A [OTC] [DSC] see Naphazoline and Antazoline . . . 1088
Vasodilan® [DSC] see Isoxsuprine . . 871
Vasofyl® (Mex) see Pentoxifylline . . 1212
Vasopressin 1567
Vasotec® see Enalapril 538
Vaxigrip® (Can) see Influenza Virus Vaccine 833
VCF™ [OTC] see Nonoxynol 9 1124
VCR see VinCRIStine 1576
Veetids® see Penicillin V Potassium 1205
Veg-Pancreatin 4X [OTC] see Pancreatin 1183
Velcade® see Bortezomib 215
Velivet™ see Ethinyl Estradiol and Desogestrel 592
Velosef® see Cephradine 304
Venlafaxine 1568
Venofer® see Iron Sucrose 862
Ventavis™ see Iloprost 816
Ventisol® (Mex) see Ketotifen 890
Ventolin® (Can) see Albuterol 58
Ventolin® Diskus (Can) see Albuterol 58
Ventolin® HFA see Albuterol 58
Ventrodisk (Can) see Albuterol 58
VePesid® see Etoposide 626
Veracolate [OTC] see Bisacodyl . . . 209
Verapamil 1571
Verapamil and Trandolapril see Trandolapril and Verapamil . . . 1518
Verapamil Hydrochloride see Verapamil 1571
Verelan® see Verapamil 1571
Verelan® PM see Verapamil 1571
Vermicol® (Mex) see Mebendazole 968
Vermidil® (Mex) see Mebendazole . . 968
Vermin® (Mex) see Mebendazole . . . 968
Vermox® (Can) see Mebendazole . . 968
Vermox® [DSC] see Mebendazole . . 968
Versed see Midazolam 1040
Versiclear™ see Sodium Thiosulfate 1404
Verteporfin 1574
Vertisal® (Mex) see Metronidazole 1033
Vesanoid® see Tretinoin (Oral) 1524
VESIcare® see Solifenacin 1405
Vexol® see Rimexolone 1351
VFEND® see Voriconazole 1582
Viactiv® Multivitamin [OTC] see Vitamins (Multiple/Oral) 1582
Viadur® see Leuprolide 906
Viagra® see Sildenafil 1390

Vibramicina® (Mex) see Doxycycline (Systemic) 514
Vibramycin® see Doxycycline (Systemic) 514
Vibra-Tabs® see Doxycycline (Systemic) 514
Vicks® 44® Cough Relief [OTC] see Dextromethorphan 451
Vicks® 44D Cough & Head Congestion [OTC] see Pseudoephedrine and Dextromethorphan 1311
Vicks® 44E [OTC] see Guaifenesin and Dextromethorphan 754
Vicks® Casero™ [OTC] see Guaifenesin 752
Vicks® DayQuil® Multi-Symptom Cold and Flu [OTC] see Acetaminophen, Dextromethorphan, and Pseudoephedrine 44
Vicks® Pediatric Formula 44E [OTC] see Guaifenesin and Dextromethorphan 754
Vicks Sinex® 12 Hour [OTC] see Oxymetazoline 1172
Vicks Sinex® 12 Hour Ultrafine Mist [OTC] see Oxymetazoline 1172
Vicks® Sinex® Nasal Spray [OTC] see Phenylephrine 1226
Vicks® Sinex® UltraFine Mist [OTC] see Phenylephrine 1226
Vicodin® see Hydrocodone and Acetaminophen 779
Vicodin® ES see Hydrocodone and Acetaminophen 779
Vicodin® HP see Hydrocodone and Acetaminophen 779
Vicon Forte® see Vitamins (Multiple/Oral) 1582
Vicoprofen® see Hydrocodone and Ibuprofen 787
Vi-Daylin® + Iron Liquid [OTC] [DSC] see Vitamins (Multiple/ Oral) 1582
Vi-Daylin® Liquid [OTC] [DSC] see Vitamins (Multiple/Oral) 1582
Vidaza™ see Azacitidine 167
Videx® see Didanosine 465
Videx® EC see Didanosine 465
Vigabatrin 1574
Vigamox™ see Moxifloxacin 1069
VIGIV see Vaccinia Immune Globulin (Intravenous) 1553
Viken® (Mex) see Cefotaxime 288
VinBLAStine 1575
Vinblastine Sulfate see VinBLAStine 1575
Vincasar PFS® see VinCRIStine . . 1576
VinCRIStine 1576
Vincristine Sulfate see VinCRIStine 1576
Vindesine 1577
Vindesine Sulfate see Vindesine . . 1577
Vinorelbine 1578
Vinorelbine Injection, USP (Can) see Vinorelbine 1578
Vinorelbine Tartrate see Vinorelbine 1578
Vintec® (Mex) see VinCRIStine . . . 1576
Viokase® see Pancrelipase 1183
Viosterol see Ergocalciferol 556
Viracept® see Nelfinavir 1098
Viramune® see Nevirapine 1104
Virazole® see Ribavirin 1343
Viread® see Tenofovir 1457
Virilon® see MethylTESTOSTERone 1028
Virilon® IM (Can) see Testosterone 1462

Virlix® (Mex) see Cetirizine 306
Viroptic® see Trifluridine 1536
Viroxyn® [OTC] see Benzalkonium
   Chloride and Isopropyl Alcohol
   189
Viscoat® see Chondroitin Sulfate
   and Sodium Hyaluronate 336
Visicol® see Sodium Phosphates . . 1403
Visine® (Mex) see Tetrahydrozoline
   1470
Visine A.D.® (Mex) see
   Oxymetazoline 1172
Visine® Advanced Allergy (Can)
   see Naphazoline and
   Pheniramine 1088
Visine® Advanced Relief [OTC] see
   Tetrahydrozoline 1470
Visine-A™ [OTC] see Naphazoline
   and Pheniramine 1088
Visine® L.R. [OTC] see
   Oxymetazoline 1172
Visine® Original [OTC] see
   Tetrahydrozoline 1470
Visipaque™ see Iodixanol 853
Visken® (Can) see Pindolol 1240
Vistaril® see HydrOXYzine 801
Vistide® see Cidofovir 339
Visudyne® see Verteporfin 1574
Vita-C® [OTC] see Ascorbic Acid . . . 143
Vitacon Forte see Vitamins
   (Multiple/Oral) 1582
Vital see Ginkgo Biloba 1622
Vitamin C see Ascorbic Acid 143
Vitamin D₂ see Ergocalciferol 556
Vitamin D₃ see Alendronate and
   Cholecalciferol 66
Vitamin A 1580
Vitamin A Acid see Tretinoin
   (Topical) 1525
Vitamin A and Vitamin D 1580
Vitamin B₁ see Thiamine 1476
Vitamin B₂ see Riboflavin 1345
Vitamin B₃ see Niacin 1105
Vitamin B₅ see Pantothenic Acid . . 1186
Vitamin B₆ see Pyridoxine 1316
Vitamin B₁₂ see Cyanocobalamin . . . 399
Vitamin B Complex Combinations
   1581
Vitamin E 1581
Vitamin G see Riboflavin 1345
Vitamin K₁ see Phytonadione 1233
Vitamins (Multiple/Oral) 1582
Vitamins, Multiple (Therapeutic)
   see Vitamins (Multiple/Oral) . . . 1582
Vitamins, Multiple With Iron see
   Vitamins (Multiple/Oral) 1582
Vitelle™ Irospan® [OTC] [DSC] see
   Ferrous Sulfate and Ascorbic
   Acid 651
Viternum® (Mex) see
   Cyproheptadine 412
Vitex agnus-castus see
   Chasteberry 1618
Vitis vinifera see Grape Seed 1625
Vitrase® see Hyaluronidase 774
Vitrasert® see Ganciclovir 722
Vitravene™ (Can) see Fomivirsen . . 700
Vitravene™ [DSC] see Fomivirsen . . 700
Vitrax® see Hyaluronate and
   Derivatives 773
Vitussin see Hydrocodone and
   Guaifenesin 785
Vivactil® see Protriptyline 1307
Viva-Drops® [OTC] see Artificial
   Tears 143
Vivaglobin® see Immune Globulin
   (Subcutaneous) 826
Vivarin® [OTC] see Caffeine 245
Vivelle® see Estradiol 574
Vivelle-Dot® see Estradiol 574
Vivitrol™ see Naltrexone 1086

Vivotif Berna® see Typhoid
   Vaccine 1549
VLB see VinBLAStine 1575
VM-26 see Teniposide 1456
Volmax® (Mex) see Albuterol 58
Voltaren® see Diclofenac 459
Voltaren Ophtha® (Can) see
   Diclofenac 459
Voltaren Ophthalmic® see
   Diclofenac 459
Voltaren Rapide® (Can) see
   Diclofenac 459
Voltaren®-XR see Diclofenac 459
Voluven® (Can) see Hetastarch . . . 770
Vomisin® (Mex) see
   DimenhyDRINATE 481
Voriconazole 1582
VoSol® HC see Acetic Acid,
   Propylene Glycol Diacetate,
   and Hydrocortisone 45
VoSpire ER® see Albuterol 58
VP-16 see Etoposide 626
VP-16-213 see Etoposide 626
Vp-Tec® (Mex) see Etoposide 626
Vumon® see Teniposide 1456
Vusion™ see Miconazole and Zinc
   Oxide 1040
V.V.S.® see Sulfabenzamide,
   Sulfacetamide, and
   Sulfathiazole 1423
Vytone® see Iodoquinol and
   Hydrocortisone 853
Vytorin™ see Ezetimibe and
   Simvastatin 631
VZIG see Varicella-Zoster Immune
   Globulin (Human) 1566
Warfarin 1585
Warfarin Sodium see Warfarin 1585
Wartec® (Can) see Podofilox 1251
Wart-Off® Maximum Strength
   [OTC] see Salicylic Acid 1374
4-Way® 12 Hour [OTC] see
   Oxymetazoline 1172
4-Way® Saline Moisturizing Mist
   [OTC] see Sodium Chloride 1400
WelChol® see Colesevelam 389
Wellbutrin® see BuPROPion 233
Wellbutrin XL™ see BuPROPion . . . 233
Wellbutrin SR® see BuPROPion 233
Westcort® see Hydrocortisone 793
Westhroid™ see Thyroid 1482
Whitehorn see Hawthorn 1626
Wigraine® see Ergotamine and
   Caffeine 559
Wild Quinine see Feverfew 1621
Wild Yam 1634
Winpred™ (Can) see PredniSONE
   1271
WinRho® SDF see Rhₒ(D) Immune
   Globulin 1342
Winstrol® see Stanozolol 1415
Wound Wash Saline™ [OTC] see
   Sodium Chloride 1400
WR-2721 see Amifostine 83
WR-139007 see Dacarbazine 415
WR-139013 see Chlorambucil 313
WR-139021 see Carmustine 273
Wycillin® (Can) see Penicillin G
   Procaine 1204
Wycillin [DSC] see Penicillin G
   Procaine 1204
Wytensin® (Can) see Guanabenz . . . 758
Xalatan® see Latanoprost 900
Xanax® see Alprazolam 73
Xanax TS™ (Can) see Alprazolam . . . 73
Xanax XR® see Alprazolam 73
Xatral (Can) see Alfuzosin 68
Xeloda® see Capecitabine 255
Xenaderm™ see Trypsin, Balsam
   Peru, and Castor Oil 1547
Xenical® see Orlistat 1150

Xibrom™ see Bromfenac 221
Xifaxan™ see Rifaximin 1350
Xigris® see Drotrecogin Alfa 522
Xitocin® (Mex) see Oxytocin 1175
Xolair® see Omalizumab 1144
Xopenex® see Levalbuterol 907
Xopenex HFA™ see Levalbuterol . . . 907
X-Prep® [OTC] [DSC] see Senna . . 1384
X-Seb T® Pearl [OTC] see Coal
    Tar and Salicylic Acid 383
X-Seb T® Plus [OTC] see Coal Tar
    and Salicylic Acid 383
Xtramins [OTC] see Vitamins
    (Multiple/Oral) 1582
Xylocaine® (Mex) see Lidocaine 920
Xylocaine® see Lidocaine 920
Xylocaine® MPF see Lidocaine 920
Xylocaine® MPF With Epinephrine
    see Lidocaine and Epinephrine
    924
Xylocaine® Viscous see Lidocaine . . 920
Xylocaine® With Epinephrine see
    Lidocaine and Epinephrine 924
Xylocard® (Can) see Lidocaine 920
Xylometazoline 1588
Xylometazoline Hydrochloride see
    Xylometazoline 1588
Xyrem® see Sodium Oxybate 1402
Y-90 Zevalin see Ibritumomab 807
Yasmin® see Ethinyl Estradiol and
    Drospirenone 595
Yaz see Ethinyl Estradiol and
    Drospirenone 595
Yectamicina® (Mex) see
    Gentamicin 734
Yectamid® (Mex) see Amikacin 84
Yellow Indian Paint see Golden
    Seal 1624
Yellow Root see Golden Seal 1624
YM087 see Conivaptan 393
YM-08310 see Amifostine 83
Yocon® see Yohimbine 1589
Yodine® (Mex) see
    Povidone-Iodine 1262
Yodoxin® see Iodoquinol 853
Yohimbe 1634
Yohimbehe cortex see Yohimbe . . . 1634
Yohimbine 1589
Yohimbine Hydrochloride see
    Yohimbine 1589
Z4942 see Ifosfamide 815
Zaditen® (Can) see Ketotifen 890
Zaditor™ see Ketotifen 890
Zafimida® (Mex) see Furosemide . . . 715
Zafirlukast 1590
Zagam® [DSC] see Sparfloxacin . . 1411
Zalcitabine 1590
Zaleplon 1591
Zanaflex® see Tizanidine 1497
Zanamivir 1592
Zanosar® see Streptozocin 1418
Zantac® see Ranitidine 1334
Zantac 75® (Can) see Ranitidine . . . 1334
Zantac 75® [OTC] see Ranitidine . . 1334
Zantac 150™ [OTC] see Ranitidine
    1334
Zantac® EFFERdose® see
    Ranitidine 1334
Zapzyt® Acne Wash [OTC] see
    Salicylic Acid 1374
Zapzyt® [OTC] see Benzoyl
    Peroxide 194
Zapzyt® Pore Treatment [OTC] see
    Salicylic Acid 1374
Zarontin® see Ethosuximide 619
Zaroxolyn® see Metolazone 1030
Zavesca® see Miglustat 1047
Z-Bec® [OTC] see Vitamin B
    Complex Combinations 1581

Z-Cof DM see Guaifenesin,
    Pseudoephedrine, and
    Dextromethorphan 757
Z-Cof LA™ see Guaifenesin and
    Dextromethorphan 754
ZD1033 see Anastrozole 126
ZD1839 see Gefitinib 727
ZDV see Zidovudine 1594
ZDV, Abacavir, and Lamivudine
    see Abacavir, Lamivudine, and
    Zidovudine 23
Zeasorb®-AF [OTC] see
    Miconazole 1039
Zebeta® see Bisoprolol 211
Zebutal™ see Butalbital,
    Acetaminophen, and Caffeine . . 239
Zegerid® see Omeprazole and
    Sodium Bicarbonate 1146
Zeldox see Ziprasidone 1598
Zelmac® (Mex) see Tegaserod 1448
Zelnorm® see Tegaserod 1448
Zemaira® see Alpha₁-Proteinase
    Inhibitor 73
Zemplar® see Paricalcitol 1187
Zenapax® see Daclizumab 416
Zeneca 182,780 see Fulvestrant . . 713
Zentel® (Mex) see Albendazole . . . 57
Zephiran® [OTC] see
    Benzalkonium Chloride 188
Zephrex® see Guaifenesin and
    Pseudoephedrine 755
Zephrex LA® see Guaifenesin and
    Pseudoephedrine 755
Zerit® see Stavudine 1416
Zestoretic® see Lisinopril and
    Hydrochlorothiazide 938
Zestril® see Lisinopril 936
Zetar® [OTC] see Coal Tar 383
Zetia™ see Ezetimibe 630
Zevalin® see Ibritumomab 807
Ziac® see Bisoprolol and
    Hydrochlorothiazide 212
Ziagen® see Abacavir 22
Ziconotide 1594
Zidovudine 1594
Zidovudine, Abacavir, and
    Lamivudine see Abacavir,
    Lamivudine, and Zidovudine 23
Zidovudine and Lamivudine 1596
Zilactin® (Can) see Lidocaine 920
Zilactin-L® [OTC] see Lidocaine . . . 920
Zilactin-B® (Can) see Benzocaine . . 190
Zilactin Baby® (Can) see
    Benzocaine 190
Zilactin®-B [OTC] see Benzocaine . . 190
Zilactin Toothache and Gum Pain®
    [OTC] see Benzocaine 190
Zileuton 1596
Zinacef® see Cefuroxime 295
Zinc see Trace Metals 1513
Zincate® see Zinc Sulfate 1598
Zinc Chloride 1597
Zinc Diethylenetriaminepentaacetate
    (Zn-DTPA) see Diethylene
    Triamine Penta-Acetic Acid 466
Zincfrin® (Can) see Phenylephrine
    and Zinc Sulfate 1228
Zincfrin® [OTC] see Phenylephrine
    and Zinc Sulfate 1228
Zinc Gelatin 1597
Zinc Gelatin Boot see Zinc Gelatin
    1597
Zincofax® (Can) see Zinc Oxide . . . 1597
Zincon® [OTC] see Pyrithione Zinc
    1318
Zinc Oxide 1597
Zinc Oxide and Miconazole Nitrate
    see Miconazole and Zinc
    Oxide 1040
Zinc Sulfate 1598

Zinc Sulfate and Phenylephrine
see Phenylephrine and Zinc
Sulfate 1228
Zinc Undecylenate see
Undecylenic Acid and
Derivatives 1550
Zinecard® see Dexrazoxane 446
Zingiber officinale see Ginger 1622
Zinnat® (Mex) see Cefuroxime 295
Ziox™ see Chlorophyllin, Papain,
and Urea 319
Zipra® (Mex) see Ciprofloxacin 343
Ziprasidone 1598
Ziprasidone Hydrochloride see
Ziprasidone 1598
Ziprasidone Mesylate see
Ziprasidone 1598
Zithromax® see Azithromycin 171
Zithromax® TRI-PAK™ see
Azithromycin 171
Zithromax® Z-PAK® see
Azithromycin 171
ZM-182,780 see Fulvestrant 713
Zmax™ see Azithromycin 171
Zn-DTPA see Diethylene Triamine
Penta-Acetic Acid 466
ZNP® (Mex) see Pyrithione Zinc . . 1318
ZNP® Bar [OTC] see Pyrithione
Zinc 1318
ZnSO₄ (error-prone abbreviation)
see Zinc Sulfate 1598
Zocor® see Simvastatin 1394
Zoderm® see Benzoyl Peroxide 194
Zofran® see Ondansetron 1147
Zofran® ODT see Ondansetron . . . 1147
Zoladex® see Goserelin 750
Zoladex® LA (Can) see Goserelin . . 750
Zoledronate see Zoledronic Acid . . 1600
Zoledronic Acid 1600
Zolmitriptan 1603
Zoloft® see Sertraline 1385
Zolpidem 1604
Zolpidem Tartrate see Zolpidem . . . 1604
Zometa® see Zoledronic Acid 1600
Zomig® see Zolmitriptan 1603
Zomig® Nasal Spray (Can) see
Zolmitriptan 1603

Zomig® Rapimelt (Can) see
Zolmitriptan 1603
Zomig-ZMT™ see Zolmitriptan 1603
Zonal® (Mex) see Fluconazole 659
Zonalon® see Doxepin 505
Zone-A® see Pramoxine and
Hydrocortisone 1264
Zone-A Forte® see Pramoxine and
Hydrocortisone 1264
Zonegran® see Zonisamide 1606
Zonisamide 1606
Zopiclone 1606
Zorbtive™ see Somatropin 1406
Zorcaine™ see Articaine and
Epinephrine 139
ZORprin® see Aspirin 145
Zostrix® (Can) see Capsaicin 256
Zostrix® H.P. (Can) see Capsaicin . . 256
Zostrix®-HP [OTC] see Capsaicin . . . 256
Zostrix® [OTC] see Capsaicin 256
Zosyn® see Piperacillin and
Tazobactam Sodium 1245
Zovia™ see Ethinyl Estradiol and
Ethynodiol Diacetate 597
Zovirax® see Acyclovir 49
Ztuss™ Tablet see Hydrocodone,
Pseudoephedrine, and
Guaifenesin 792
Zurcal® (Mex) see Pantoprazole . . . 1184
Zyban® see BuPROPion 233
Zydone® see Hydrocodone and
Acetaminophen 779
Zyflo® see Zileuton 1596
Zylet™ see Loteprednol and
Tobramycin 953
Zyloprim® see Allopurinol 70
Zymar™ see Gatifloxacin 724
Zyprexa® see Olanzapine 1139
Zyprexa® Zydis® see Olanzapine . . 1139
Zyrtec® see Cetirizine 306
Zyrtec-D 12 Hour™ see Cetirizine
and Pseudoephedrine 307
Zyvox™ see Linezolid 933
Zyvoxam® (Can) see Linezolid 933

NOTES

Other Products Offered by Lexi-Comp®

Oral Soft Tissue Diseases
by J. Robert Newland, DDS, MS; Timothy F. Meiller, DDS, PhD; Richard L. Wynn, BSPharm, PhD; and Harold L. Crossley, DDS, PhD

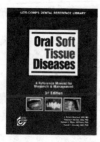

Designed for all dental professionals, a pictorial reference to assist in the diagnosis and management of oral soft tissue diseases (over 160 photos). Easy-to-use, sections include: Diagnosis process: obtaining a history, examining the patient, establishing a differential diagnosis, selecting appropriate diagnostic tests, interpreting the results, etc.; white lesions; red lesions; blistering-sloughing lesions; ulcerated lesions; pigmented lesions; papillary lesions; soft tissue swelling (each lesion is illustrated with a color representative photograph); specific medications to treat oral soft tissue diseases; sample prescriptions; and special topics.

Oral Hard Tissue Diseases
by J. Robert Newland, Dds, Ms

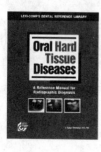

A reference manual for radiographic diagnosis, visually-cued with over 130 high quality radiographs is designed to require little more than visual recognition to make an accurate diagnosis. Each lesion is illustrated by one or more photographs depicting the typical radiographic features and common variations. There are 12 chapters tabbed for easy access: 1) Periapical Radiolucent Lesions; 2) Pericoronal Radiolucent Lesions; 3) Inter-Radicular Radiolucent Lesions; 4) Periodontal Radiolucent Lesions; 5) Radiolucent Lesions Not Associated With Teeth; 6) Radiolucent Lesions With Irregular Margins; 7) Periapical Radiopaque Lesions; 8) Periocoronal Radiopaque Lesions; 9) Inter-Radicular Radiopaque Lesions; 10) Radiopaque Lesions Not Associated With Teeth; 11) Radiopaque Lesions With Irregular Margins; 12) Selected Readings / Alphabetical Index

Dental Office Medical Emergencies
by Timothy F. Meiller, DDS, PhD; Richard L. Wynn, BSPharm, PhD; Ann Marie McMullin, MD; Cynthia Biron, RDH, EMT, MA; and Harold L. Crossley, DDS, PhD

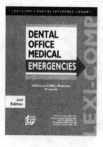

Designed specifically for general dentists during times of emergency. A tabbed paging system allows for quick access to specific crisis events. Created with urgency in mind, it is spiral bound and drilled with a hole for hanging purposes. Contains the following: Basic Action Plan for Stabilization; Allergic / Drug Reactions; Loss of Consciousness / Respiratory Distress / Chest Pain; Altered Sensation / Changes in Affect; Management of Acute Bleeding; Office Preparedness / Procedures and Protocols; Automated External Defibrillator (AED); Oxygen Delivery

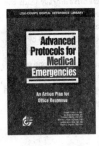
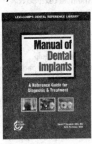
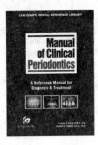

Other Products Offered by Lexi-Comp®

Oral Surgery for the General Dentist
by Lawrence I. Gaum, DDS, FADSA, FICD

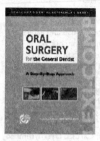

Oral Surgery for the General Dentist literally leads the practitioner through numerous surgical procedures in a well organized fashion. Utilizing a step-by-step approach for a variety of surgical techniques accompanied by detailed color photographs, this manual is filled with fantastic tips and suggestions that have been kept secret from the general dentist for many years. This manual will show how to achieve success, avoid failures, and perform surgery with confidence and expertise.

Clinician's Endodontic Handbook
by Thom C. Dumsha, MS, DDS, MS and James L. Gutmann, DDS, FACD, FICD

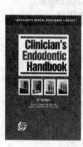

The *Clinician's Endodontic Handbook*, 2nd Edition, was developed as a quick reference to address current issues in clinical endodontics. The easy-to-use format presents the latest techniques, procedures, and materials to the busy practitioner eliminating the need for multiple textbooks.

Features

- Clinical Note sections outline the authors' combined 50 years of endodontic experience
- Frequently Asked Questions are provided to help practitioners communicate more effectively with patients
- Defines root canal therapy: Whys and Why-Nots
- Includes a guide to the diagnosis and treatment of endodontic emergencies
- Facts and rationale behind treating endodontically-involved teeth
- Straight-forward dental trauma management information
- Contains 21 chapters presented in a practical format

Illustrated Handbook of Clinical Dentistry
by Richard A. Lehman, DMD, MPH

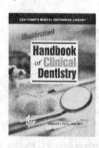

The *Illustrated Handbook of Clinical Dentistry* is an invaluable manual for dentists and dental students that concisely summarizes the major disciplines of clinical dentistry. This handbook is written as an aid for transition into clinical practice, or as a refresher for a seasoned dental professional. It offers a quick reference for basic clinical principles and procedures encountered on a daily basis.

Other Products Offered by Lexi-Comp®

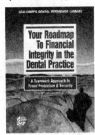
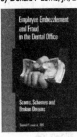
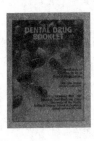

Other Products Offered by Lexi-Comp®

A Patient Guide to Dental Implants

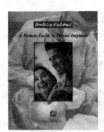

A highly illustrative description of the options available for various types of implants, including a frequently asked question-and-answer section. The flip-chart format allows for display on a desk, if required.

Tabbed sections include:
- Single Tooth Replacement
- Replacement of Several Teeth
- Four-Implant Retained Overdenture
- Two-Implant Retained Overdenture
- Screw-Retained Denture

Additional Features:
- Over 1600 bulleted points of interest
- Over 180 checklist options
- 13 real-life stories
- Over 80 boxed topics of special interest

A Patient Guide to Dental Implants Booklet

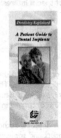

This simplified guide to dental implants will help your patients understand the different options for this procedure. Easy to read and illustrated in a non-frightening way, the diagrams show how single or multiple implants can be achieved.

Useful for reception areas, these leaflets can be supplied in bulk quantities.

Patient Guide to Root Canal Therapy

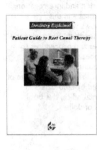

An illustrated, detailed explanation of Root Canal Therapy including a frequently asked question-and-answer section. The flip-chart format allows for display on a desk, if required.

Tabbed sections include:
- What is Root Canal Therapy?
- Access Opening
- Cleaning & Shaping the Root Canal System
- Filling the Root Canal System
- Temporary Restoration
- Permanent Restoration
- Crown Restoration

A Patient Guide to Periodontal Disease

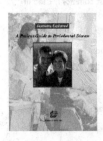

This informative patient guide provides a colorful visual overview of the procedures involved with the treatment of Periodontal Disease. The flip-chart format allows for display on a desk, if required.

Tabbed sections include:
- Healthy Gums
- Gingivitis
- Mild to Moderate Periodontitis
- Advanced Periodontitis
- Treatment Options
- If Left Untreated
- Oral Hygiene Instruction
- Prevention